Harrison's

Principles of Internal Medicine

EDITORS OF PREVIOUS EDITIONS

T. R. Harrison, Editor-in-Chief, Editions 1, 2, 3, 4, 5

W. R. Resnik, Editor, Editions 1, 2, 3, 4, 5

M. M. Wintrobe, Editor, Editions 1, 2, 3, 4, 5
Editor-in-Chief, Editions 6, 7

G. W. Thorn, Editor, Editions 1, 2, 3, 4, 5, 6, 7

R. D. Adams, Editor, Editions 2, 3, 4, 5, 6, 7

P. B. Beeson, Editor, Editions 1, 2

I. L. Bennett, Jr., Editor, Editions 3, 4, 5, 6

E. Braunwald, Editor, Editions 6, 7

K. J. Isselbacher, Editor, Editions 6, 7

R. G. Petersdorf, Editor, Editions 6, 7

Harrison's

Principles of Internal Medicine

Eighth Edition

EDITORS

GEORGE W. THORN *M.D., M.A. (Hon.), LL.D. (Hon.), D.SC. (Hon.), M.D. (Hon.), F.R.C.P. Hersey Professor of the Theory and Practice of Physic, Emeritus, Harvard Medical School; Samuel A. Levine Professor of Medicine, Emeritus, Harvard Medical School; Physician-in-Chief, Emeritus, Peter Bent Brigham Hospital, Boston.*

RAYMOND D. ADAMS *B.A., M.A., M.D., M.A. (Hon.), D.SC. (Hon.), M.D. (Hon.) Bullard Professor of Neuropathology, Harvard Medical School; Chief of Neurology Service and Neuropathologist, Massachusetts General Hospital, Boston.*

EUGENE BRAUNWALD *A.B., M.D., M.A. (Hon.) Hersey Professor of the Theory and Practice of Physic (Medicine), Harvard Medical School; Physician-in-Chief, Peter Bent Brigham Hospital, Boston.*

KURT J. ISSELBACHER *A.B., M.D. Mallinckrodt Professor of Medicine, Harvard Medical School; Physician and Chief, Gastrointestinal Unit, Massachusetts General Hospital, Boston.*

ROBERT G. PETERSDORF *A.B., M.D. Professor and Chairman, Department of Medicine, University of Washington School of Medicine; Physician-in-Chief, University of Washington Hospital, Seattle.*

McGRAW-HILL BOOK COMPANY *New York St. Louis San Francisco Auckland Bogotá Düsseldorf Johannesburg London Madrid Mexico Montreal New Delhi Panama Paris São Paulo Singapore Sydney Tokyo Toronto*

A BLAKISTON PUBLICATION

Library of Congress Cataloging in Publication Data (1 vol. ed.)

Harrison, Tinsley Randolph, date ed.
Harrison's Principles of internal medicine.
"A Blakiston publication."
Includes bibliographies and index.
1. Internal medicine. I. Thorn, George Widmer, date II. Title. III. Title: Principles of internal medicine. [DNLM: 1. Internal medicine. WB100 H322]
RC46.H32 1977 616'.026 76-41901
ISBN 0-07-064518-3

LC CIP DATA (2 vol. ed.)
[RC46.H32 1977b] 616'.026 76-43442
ISBN 0-07-064519-1 (set)

Harrison's
Principles of Internal Medicine

2 3 4 5 6 7 8 9 0 DODO 7 8 3 2 1 0 9 8 7

Foreign Editions

FRENCH (Seventh Edition)—Flammarion, © 1975
ITALIAN (Seventh Edition)—Casa Editrice Dr. Francesco Vallardi, © 1976
POLISH (Fifth Edition)—Panstwowy Zakland Wydawnictw Lekarskich, © 1971
PORTUGUESE (Seventh Edition)—Editora Guanabara Koogan, S.A., © 1977 (est.)
SPANISH (Sixth Edition)—La Prensa Medica Mexicana, © 1973
TURKISH (Sixth Edition)—Mentes, © 1976 (est.)
JAPANESE (Seventh Edition)—Hirokawa, © 1975
GREEK (Sixth Edition)—G. Parissianos © 1974

This book was set in Times Roman by National ShareGraphics, Inc., and Textbook Services, Inc.
The editors were Joseph J. Brehm, Stuart D. Boynton, and Richard S. Laufer.
The indexer was Philip James;
the designer, Barbara Ellwood;
and the production supervisor, Thomas J. LoPinto.
R. R. Donnelley & Sons Company was printer and binder.

*To all those who have taught us,
and especially to our younger colleagues
who continue to teach and inspire us*

contents

An Atlas of Common Lesions Encountered During the Physical Examination of the Skin (Plates 1 to 4):

1-1 Dermatofibroma *1-2* Acrochordon *1-3* Angiokeratoma *1-4* Cafe au lait macules *1-5* Acne

2-1 Dermatophytosis *2-2* Eczematous dermatitis *2-3* Localized lichenification *2-4* Melasma *2-5* Milia *2-6* Psoriasis

3-1 Perleche *3-2* Rosacea *3-3* Seborrheic dermatitis *3-4* Seborrheic keratosis *3-5* Senile angioma *3-6* Senile lentigo

list of contributors

AMERICO ABBRUZZESE, M.D.
Assistant Professor of Medicine, Harvard Medical School; Associate in Medicine, Peter Bent Brigham Hospital, Boston.

RAYMOND D. ADAMS, B.S., M.A., M.D., M.A. (Hon), D.Sc. (Hon), M.D. (Hon)
Bullard Professor of Neuropathology, Harvard Medical School; Chief of Neurology Service and Neuropathologist, Massachusetts General Hospital, Boston.

JOHN W. ADAMSON, M.D.
Associate Professor of Medicine, University of Washington School of Medicine; Head, Division of Hematology, Veterans Administration Hospital, Seattle.

DAVID H. ALPERS, M.D.
Professor of Medicine and Chief, Division of Gastroenterology, Washington University School of Medicine, St. Louis.

ELLIOT ALPERT, M.D.
Associate Professor of Medicine, Harvard Medical School; Assistant Physician, Massachusetts General Hospital, Boston.

ARTHUR K. ASBURY, M.D.
Professor of Neurology, University of Pennsylvania; Chairman, Department of Neurology, University Hospital of Pennsylvania, Philadelphia.

KARL-ERIK ÅSTRÖM, M.D.
Associate Professor of Neuropathology, Harvard Medical School; Associate Neuropathologist, Massachusetts General Hospital, Boston.

K. FRANK AUSTEN, M.D.
Theodore Bevier Bayles Professor of Medicine, Harvard Medical School; Physician-in-Chief, Robert B. Brigham Hospital, Boston.

ROBERT AUSTRIAN, M.D.
John Herr Musser Professor of Research Medicine, University of Pennsylvania Medical Center, The School of Medicine, Philadelphia.

ROSS J. BALDESSARINI, M.D.
Associate Professor of Psychiatry, Harvard Medical School; Chief, Neuropharmacology Laboratories, Psychiatric Research, Massachusetts General Hospital, Boston.

JOSEPH H. BATES, M.D.
Professor of Medicine, University of Arkansas School of Medicine; Chief, Medical Service, Veterans Hospital, Little Rock.

HARRY N. BEATY, M.D.
Professor of Medicine, Department of Medicine, University of Washington School of Medicine; Medical Director, Providence Hospital, Seattle.

JOSEPH R. BERTINO, M.D.
Professor of Medicine and Pharmacology, Department of Pharmacology, Yale University School of Medicine, New Haven.

STUART BONDURANT, M.D.
President and Dean, Albany Medical College, New York; Attending Physician, Albany Medical Center Hospital, Albany.

AREND BOUHUYS, M.D.
Professor of Medicine and Epidemiology; Director, Yale University Lung Research Center, Yale University School of Medicine, New Haven.

ABRAHAM I. BRAUDE, M.D.
Professor of Medicine and Pathology, University of California at San Diego School of Medicine, San Diego.

EUGENE BRAUNWALD, A.B., M.D., M.A. (Hon)
Hersey Professor of the Theory and Practice of Physic (Medicine), Harvard Medical School; Physician-in-Chief, Peter Bent Brigham Hospital, Boston.

MICHAEL S. BROWN, M.D.
Professor of Internal Medicine, Department of Internal Medicine, The University of Texas Health Science Center at Dallas.

ROGER BULGER, M.D.
Chancellor of Health Sciences, Dean, School of Medicine, University of Massachusetts School of Medicine, Worcester.

H. FRANKLIN BUNN, M.D.
Associate Professor of Medicine, Harvard Medical School; Director, Hematology Division, and Physician, Peter Bent Brigham Hospital, Boston.

GEORGE F. CAHILL, JR., M.D.
Professor of Medicine, Harvard Medical School; Director of Research, Joslin Diabetes Foundation, Inc.; Physician, Peter Bent Brigham Hospital, Boston.

JACQUES R. CALDWELL, M.D.
Associate Professor of Medicine, Division of Infectious Diseases, Department of Medicine, University of Florida, Gainesville.

EVAN CALKINS, A.B., M.D.
Professor and Chairman, Department of Medicine, State University of New York at Buffalo School of Medicine; Director, Department of Medicine, Edward J. Meyer Memorial Hospital, Buffalo.

GEORGE P. CANELLOS, M.D.
Associate Professor of Medicine, Harvard Medical School; Chief, Division of Medical Oncology, Sidney Farber Cancer Center; Senior Associate in Medicine, Peter Bent Brigham Hospital, Boston.

CHARLES B. CARPENTER, M.D.
Associate Professor of Medicine, Harvard Medical School; Senior Associate in Medicine, Peter Bent Brigham Hospital, Boston.

CHARLES C.J. CARPENTER, M.D.
Professor and Chairman, Department of Medicine, Case Western Reserve University School of Medicine; Physician-in-Chief, University Hospitals, Cleveland.

GEORGE E. CARTWRIGHT, B.A., M.D.
Professor and Chairman, Department of Medicine, University of Utah College of Medicine; Chief, Medical Service, University Hospital, Salt Lake City.

BAYARD D. CLARKSON, M.D.
Professor of Medicine, Cornell University Medical Center; Attending Physician and Chief Hematology Service, Memorial Hospital, New York.

LEIGHTON E. CLUFF, M.D.
Vice President, The Robert Wood Johnson Foundation, Princeton.

MAX D. COOPER, M.D.
Professor of Pediatrics and Microbiology, Department of Pediatrics, University of Alabama in Birmingham, The Medical Center, Birmingham.

RICHARD A. COOPER, M.D.
Professor of Medicine and Chief, Hematology-Oncology Section, Hospital of the University of Pennsylvania School of Medicine, Philadelphia.

JOHN F. CRIGLER, JR., M.D.
Associate Professor of Pediatrics at Children's Hospital Medical Center, Department of Pediatrics, Harvard Medical School; Chief, Division of Endocrinology, Department of Medicine, Children's Hospital Medical Center, Boston.

EUGENE P. CRONKITE, M.D.
Professor of Medicine, Department of Medicine, State University of New York at Stony Brook; Dean of the Clinical Campus at Brookhaven National Laboratory; Attending Physician, Hospital of the Medical Research Center, Brookhaven National Laboratory, Upton.

DAVID C. DALE, M.D.
Associate Professor, Department of Medicine, University of Washington School of Medicine, Seattle.

JAMES E. DALEN, M.D.
Professor and Chairman, Department of Cardiovascular Medicine, University of Massachusetts Medical School, Worcester.

CHANDLER R. DAWSON, M.D.
Associate Professor in Residence, F.I. Proctor Foundation, University of California Medical Center; Director, WHO International Reference Center for Trachoma, San Francisco.

ROBERT DELONG, M.D.
Assistant Professor of Neurology, Harvard Medical School; Associate Neurologist, Associate Pediatrician, Massachusetts General Hospital, Boston.

VINCENT T. DE VITA, JR., M.D.
Director, Division of Cancer Treatment, National Cancer Institute, National Institutes of Health, Bethesda.

JAMES J. DINEEN, M.D.
Assistant Professor of Medicine; Harvard Medical School; Assistant Physician, Massachusetts General Hospital, Boston.

ROBERT H. DLUHY, M.D.
Associate Professor of Medicine, Harvard Medical School; Associate Director, Endocrine-Hypertension Division, Peter Bent Brigham Hospital, Boston.

HENRI VANDER EECKEN, H.M., M.D.
Professor of Neurology, Faculty of Medicine, University of Ghent; Head of the Department of Neurology, Akademisch Zeikenhuis, Ghent.

KENDALL EMERSON, JR., M.D.
Clinical Professor of Medicine at the Peter Bent Brigham Hospital, Emeritus, Harvard Medical School; Physician, Emeritus, Peter Bent Brigham Hospital, Boston.

KARL ENGELMAN, B.S., M.A. (Hon), M.D.
Associate Professor of Medicine and Pharmacology; Chief, Hypertension and Clinical Pharmacology Section; Director, Clinical Research Center, University of Pennsylvania, School of Medicine, Philadelphia.

FRANKLIN H. EPSTEIN, B.A., M.A. (Hon), M.D.
Herrman L. Blumgart Professor of Medicine, Harvard Medical School; Physician-in-Chief, Beth Israel Hospital, Boston.

STEFAN S. FAJANS, B.S., M.D.
Professor of Internal Medicine, University of Michigan Medical School; Head, Division of Endocrinology and Metabolism and Director, Metabolic Research Unit, University Hospital, Ann Arbor.

ALEXANDER FEFER, M.D.
Professor of Medicine, University of Washington School of Medicine; Attending Physician, University of Washington Hospital, Seattle.

HARRY A. FELDMAN, M.D.
Professor and Chairman, Department of Preventive Medicine, State University of New York Upstate Medical Center, Syracuse.

RICHARD A. FIELD, A.B., M.D.
Associate Clinical Professor of Medicine, Harvard Medical School; Associate Physician, Beth Israel Hospital; Senior Scientist, Retina Foundation, Boston.

C. MILLER FISHER, M.D.
Professor of Neurology, Harvard Medical School; Neurologist and Neuropathologist, Massachusetts General Hospital, Boston.

RUSSELL S. FISHER, B.S., M.D.
Clinical Professor of Forensic Pathology, University of

Maryland School of Medicine; Consultant in Pathology, Greater Baltimore Medical Center, Towson.

ALFRED P. FISHMAN, M.D.
William Maul Measey Professor of Medicine and Director, Cardiovascular-Pulmonary Division, Department of Medicine, University of Pennsylvania; Attending Physician, Hospital of the University of Pennsylvania, Philadelphia.

THOMAS B. FITZPATRICK, M.D., PH.D.
Edward Wigglesworth Professor of Dermatology and Head, Department of Dermatology, Harvard Medical School; Chief, Dermatology Service, Massachusetts General Hospital; Physician, Peter Bent Brigham Hospital; Consultant in Dermatology, Children's Hospital Medical Center, Boston.

EDWARD C. FRANKLIN, M.D.
Professor of Medicine and Head, Division of Rheumatology, Department of Medicine, New York University Medical Center, New York.

DONALD S. FREDRICKSON, M.D.
Director, National Institutes of Health, Bethesda.

LAWRENCE R. FREEDMAN, M.D.
Professor and Chairman, Department of Internal Medicine, University of Lausanne; Chief of Medicine, Centre Hospitalier Universitaire Vaudois, Lausanne.

WILLIAM F. FRIEDMAN, M.D.
Professor of Pediatrics, University of California, San Diego; Chief, Pediatric Cardiology, University Hospital, San Diego.

ALVIN E. FRIEDMAN-KIEN, M.D.
Associate Professor of Dermatology and Microbiology, New York University Medical Center, School of Medicine, New York.

J. BERNARD L. GEE, M.D.
Associate Professor of Medicine, Yale University School of Medicine; Attending Physician, Yale-New Haven Hospital, New Haven.

ELOISE R. GIBLETT, M.D.
Research Professor of Medicine, University of Washington School of Medicine; Head of Immunogenetics, Puget Sound Blood Center, Seattle.

BRUCE C. GILLILAND, M.D.
Associate Professor of Laboratory Medicine and Medicine and Head, Division of Immunology, Department of Laboratory Medicine, University of Washington School of Medicine, Seattle.

GERALD GLICK, A.B., M.D.
Director, Cardiovascular Institute, Department of Medicine, Michael Reese Hospital and Medical Center; Professor of Medicine, University of Chicago Pritzker School of Medicine, Chicago.

ROBERT M. GLICKMAN, M.D.
Assistant Professor of Medicine, Harvard Medical School; Chief of Gastroenterology, Beth Israel Hospital, Boston.

STEPHEN E. GOLDFINGER, M.D.
Associate Professor of Medicine and Associate Dean of Continuing Education, Harvard Medical School; Associate Physician, Massachusetts General Hospital, Boston.

PAUL GOLDHABER, D.D.S.
Dean and Professor of Periodontology, Harvard School of Dental Medicine, Boston.

JOSEPH L. GOLDSTEIN, M.D.
Professor of Internal Medicine and Head, Division of Medical Genetics, Department of Internal Medicine, The University of Texas Health Science Center at Dallas.

HARVEY M. GOLOMB, M.D.
Assistant Professor, Department of Medicine, Section of Hematology/Oncology, University of Chicago, Chicago.

ROBERT W. GRAEBNER, M.D.
Assistant Clinical Professor, Department of Neurology, University of Wisconsin Hospitals, Center for Health Sciences, Madison.

J. THOMAS GRAYSTON, M.D.
Vice President for Health Affairs, Health Sciences Center; Professor, Department of Epidemiology and International Health, University of Washington School of Public Health and Community Medicine, Seattle.

NORTON J. GREENBERGER, M.D.
Professor and Chairman, Department of Medicine, University of Kansas Medical Center, College of Health Sciences, Kansas City.

RICHARD L. GUERRANT, M.D.
Associate Professor of Medicine, Department of Medicine, University of Virginia Medical Center, Charlottesville.

STEPHEN J. GUGGENHEIM, M.D.
Assistant Professor of Pathology and Medicine, University of Colorado Medical Center, Denver.

THOMAS P. HACKETT, M.D.
Professor of Psychiatry, Harvard Medical School; Chief, Psychiatric Service, Massachusetts General Hospital, Boston.

JAMES P. HARNISCH, M.D.
Acting Instructor, Department of Medicine, University of Washington School of Medicine, Seattle.

TINSLEY R. HARRISON, A.B., M.D.
Professor of Medicine, The Medical College of the University of Alabama, Birmingham and Distinguished Professor of the University of Alabama.

DONALD H. HARTER, M.D.
Chairman, Department of Neurology, Northwestern University Medical School, Chicago.

HARLEY A. HAYNES, M.D.
Associate Professor of Dermatology, Harvard Medical School; Director, Dermatology Division, Peter Bent Brigham Hospital, Boston.

THOMAS R. HENDRIX, M.D.
Professor of Medicine and Chief, Gastroenterology Division, Johns Hopkins University School of Medicine, Baltimore.

ROGER B. HICKLER, M.D.
Professor and Chairman, Department of Medicine, University of Massachusetts Medical School; Chief of Medicine, University Hospital, University of Massachusetts Medical Center, Worcester.

PAUL D. HOEPRICH, M.D.
Professor of Medicine and Pathology and Chief, Section of Infectious and Immunologic Diseases, Department of Internal Medicine, University of California, Davis.

KING K. HOLMES, M.D., Ph.D.
Associate Professor of Medicine, University of Washington School of Medicine; Chief, Division of Infectious Diseases, U.S. Public Health Service Hospital, Seattle.

EDWARD W. HOOK, M.D.
Professor and Chairman, Department of Medicine, University of Virginia Medical Center; Physician-in-Chief, University of Virginia Hospital, Charlottesville.

SIDNEY H. INGBAR, M.D.
Professor of Medicine, Harvard Medical School; Director, Thorndike Laboratory of Harvard Medical School, Beth Israel Hospital, Boston.

ROLAND H. INGRAM, JR., M.D.
Associate Professor of Medicine, Harvard Medical School; Director, Respiratory Division, Peter Bent Brigham Hospital, Boston.

KURT J. ISSELBACHER, M.D.
Mallinckrodt Professor of Medicine, Harvard Medical School; Physician and Chief, Gastrointestinal Unit, Massachusetts General Hospital, Boston.

PAUL I. JAGGER, M.D.
Adjunct Professor of Medicine, University of California, School of Medicine, San Diego; Director, Clinical Research Center, University Hospital, San Diego.

CAROL J. JOHNS, M.D.
Associate Professor of Medicine and Director, Medical Clinics, The Johns Hopkins University School of Medicine, Baltimore.

JOSEPH E. JOHNSON, III, M.D.
Professor and Chairman, Department of Medicine, Bowman-Gray School of Medicine, Winston-Salem.

RICHARD L. KAHLER, M.D.
Head, Cardiovascular Division, Scripps Clinic Medical Institutions, La Jolla; Adjunct Associate Professor of Medicine, University of California School of Medicine, San Diego.

BYRON A. KAKULAS, M.D., F.R.A.C.P., M.R.C., Path., F.R.C.P.A.
Professor of Neuropathology, University of Western Australia, Perth; Senior Neuropathologist, Royal Perth Hospital, Perth.

MARTIN J. KELLY, M.D.
Assistant Professor of Psychiatry, Harvard Medical School; Associate Director of Psychiatric Service, Peter Bent Brigham Hospital, Boston.

WILLIAM M. M. KIRBY, M.D.
Professor of Medicine and Head, Division of Infectious Diseases, Department of Medicine, University of Washington School of Medicine, Seattle.

VERNON KNIGHT, M.D.
Professor and Chairman, Department of Microbiology and Immunology, Baylor College of Medicine, Texas Medical Center; Senior Attending Physician, The Methodist Hospital, Houston.

JAN KOCH-WESER, M.D. (on Sabbatical)
Centre de Recherche Merrell International, Strasbourg.

RAYMOND S. KOFF, M.D.
Associate Professor of Medicine, Boston University School of Medicine; Chief, Hepatology Section, Veterans Administration Hospital, Boston.

STEPHEN M. KRANE, M.D., A.M. (Hon), A.B.
Professor of Medicine, Harvard Medical School; Physician and Chief, Arthritis Unit, Massachusetts General Hospital, Boston.

J. THOMAS LAMONT, M. D.
Assistant Professor of Medicine, Harvard Medical School; Associate in Medicine, Division of Gastroenterology, Peter Bent Brigham Hospital, Boston.

ALEXANDER R. LAWTON, M.D.
Associate Professor of Pediatrics and Microbiology, Department of Pediatrics, The University of Alabama in Birmingham, The Medical Center, Birmingham.

G. RICHARD LEE, M.D.
Professor, Department of Internal Medicine, University of Utah College of Medicine, Salt Lake City.

A. MARTIN LERNER, M.D.
Professor of Medicine and Head, Division of Infectious Diseases, Department of Medicine, Wayne State University School of Medicine; Chief, Hutzel Hospital Medical Unit, Detroit.

MICHAEL LESCH, M.D.
Magerstadt Professor of Medicine, Northwestern University School of Medicine; Director, Section of Cardiology, Northwestern Memorial Hospital, Chicago.

NORMAN G. LEVINSKY, M.D.
Wade Professor and Chairman, Division of Medicine, Boston University School of Medicine; Physician-in-Chief and Director, Evans Memorial Department of Clinical Research, University Hospital, Boston.

JOSEPH F. LIPINSKI, M.D.
Assistant Professor of Psychiatry, Harvard Medical School; Assistant in Psychiatry, Massachusetts General Hospital, Boston; Assistant Psychiatrist, McLean Hospital, Belmont.

BERNARD LOWN, M.D.
Professor of Cardiology, Department of Nutrition, Harvard School of Public Health; Physician, Peter Bent Brigham Hospital, Boston.

BERNARD LYTTON, M.B., F.R.C.S.
Professor and Chief, Section of Urology, Yale University School of Medicine; Chief of Urology, Yale-New Haven Medical Center, New Haven.

WALTER C. MacDONALD, M.D.
Associate Professor of Medicine, University of British Columbia, Vancouver.

GERALD L. MANDELL, M.D.
Professor of Medicine, Department of Medicine, University of Virginia Medical Center, Charlottesville.

HENRY J. MANKIN, M.D.
Edith M. Ashley Professor of Orthopedic Surgery, Harvard Medical School; Chief, Orthopedic Service, Massachusetts General Hospital, Boston.

GEORGE V. MANN, ScD., M.D.
Associate Professor of Biochemistry and Medicine, Vanderbilt University School of Medicine, Nashville.

MART MANNIK, M.D.
Professor of Medicine and Adjunct Professor of Microbiology; Head, Division of Rheumatology, Department of Medicine, University of Washington School of Medicine, Seattle.

JOSEPH B. MARTIN, M.D., Ph.D., F.R.C.P.(C)
Professor of Neurology, McGill University; Neurologist-in-Chief, Montreal Neurological Hospital, Montreal.

JANET W. McARTHUR, M.S., M.D.
Professor of Obstetrics and Gynecology, Harvard Medical School; Associate Physician, Massachusetts General Hospital, Boston.

E. REGIS McFADDEN, M.D.
Assistant Professor of Medicine, Harvard Medical School; Associate Physician, Peter Bent Brigham Hospital, Boston.

VICTOR A. McKUSICK, M.D.
Professor and Chairman, Department of Medicine, Johns Hopkins University School of Medicine; Physician-in-Chief, Johns Hopkins Hospital, Baltimore.

JOHN P. MERRILL, M.D.
Professor of Medicine, Harvard Medical School; Chief, Renal Division, Peter Bent Brigham Hospital, Boston.

MARTIN C. MIHM, JR., M.D.
Associate Professor of Pathology, Harvard Medical School; Associate Pathologist and Assistant Dermatologist, Massachusetts General Hospital, Boston.

MYRON MILLER, M.D., F.A.C.P.
Professor of Medicine, State University of New York, Upstate Medical Center; Chief, Medical Service, Veterans Administration Hospital; Attending Physician in Medicine, State University Hospital, Syracuse.

JAY P. MOHR, M.D.
Assistant Professor of Neurology, Harvard Medical School; Associate Neurologist, Massachusetts General Hospital, Boston.

HUGO MOSER, M.D.
Professor of Pediatrics and Neurology, Johns Hopkins Medical School; Director of Kennedy Institute, Baltimore.

KENNETH M. MOSER, M.D.
Professor of Medicine and Director, Pulmonary Division, University of California, San Diego, School of Medicine, San Diego.

ARNOLD M. MOSES, M.D., F.A.C.P.
Professor of Medicine, State University of New York Upstate Medical Center; Chief, Endocrinology Section, Veterans Administration Hospital; Attending Physician in Medicine, State University Hospital, Syracuse.

JOHN MURRAY, M.D.
Professor of Medicine, School of Medicine, University of California, San Francisco; Chief, Chest Service, San Francisco General Hospital, San Francisco.

ROBERT J. MYERBURG, M.D.
Professor of Medicine and Physiology and Director, Division of Cardiology, University of Miami School of Medicine, Miami.

DON H. NELSON, M.D.
Professor of Medicine, Department of Medicine, University of Utah College of Medicine, Salt Lake City.

JAMES C. NIEDERMAN, M.D.
Associate Clinical Professor of Epidemiology and Medicine, Department of Epidemiology and Public Health, Yale University School of Medicine, New Haven.

HYMIE L. NOSSEL, M.D.
Professor of Medicine, College of Physicians and Surgeons, Columbia University; Attending Physician, Presbyterian Hospital, New York.

JOHN A. OATES, M.D.
The Joe and Morris Werthan Professor of Investigative Medicine, Departments of Medicine and Pharmacology, Vanderbilt University School of Medicine; Attending Physician, Vanderbilt University Hospital, Nashville.

ROBERT A. O'ROURKE, M.D.
Professor of Medicine and Director, Division of Cardiovascular Diseases, University of Texas Health Science Center, San Antonio.

MADHUKAR A. PATHAK, M.B., Ph.D.
Principal Associate in Dermatology, Harvard Medical School; Associate Biochemist in Dermatology, Massachusetts General Hospital, Boston.

LAWRENCE L. PELLETIER, JR., M.D.
Assistant Professor of Medicine and Chief, Division of Infectious Diseases, University of North Dakota School of Medicine, Fargo.

PETER PERINE, M.D.
Emergency Medicine, The Mason Clinic, Seattle, Washington.

ROBERT G. PETERSDORF, M.D.
Professor and Chairman, Department of Medicine, University of Washington School of Medicine; Physician-in-Chief, University of Washington Hospital, Seattle.

KIRK L. PETERSON, M.D.
Associate Professor of Medicine, University of California, San Diego, School of Medicine; Director, Cardiac Catheterization Laboratory, University of California Medical Center, San Diego.

JAMES J. PLORDE, M.D.
Associate Professor of Medicine and Laboratory Medicine, Department of Medicine, University of Washington School of Medicine, Seattle.

PETER E. POOL, M.D.
Associate Clinical Professor of Medicine, Cardiovascular Division, University of California, San Diego, School of Medicine, La Jolla.

DAVID C. POSKANZER, M.D., M.P.H.
Associate Professor in Neurology, Harvard Medical School; Associate Neurologist, Epidemiologist, Massachusetts General Hospital, Boston.

JOHN T. POTTS, JR., M.D.
Professor of Medicine, Harvard Medical School; Chief, Endocrine Unit, Massachusetts General Hospital, Boston.

CHARLES H. RAMMELKAMP, JR., M.D., D.Sc. (Hon)
Professor of Medicine and Preventive Medicine, Case Western Reserve University School of Medicine; Director, Department of Medicine, Cleveland Metropolitan General Hospital, Cleveland.

JOEL M. RAPPEPORT, M.D.
Assistant Professor of Medicine, Department of Medicine, Harvard Medical School; Associate in Medicine, Peter Bent Brigham Hospital and Children's Hospital Medical Center, Boston.

C. GEORGE RAY, M.D.
Professor, Laboratory Medicine, Microbiology and Immunology, and Pediatrics, University of Washington School of Medicine, Seattle.

JEAN J. REBEIZ, M.D.
Assistant Professor of Neurology and Neuropathology, American University of Beirut; Neurologist and Neuropathologist, American University Hospital, Beirut, Lebanon.

PETER REICH, M.D.
Associate Professor of Psychiatry and Director, Division of Psychiatry, Peter Bent Brigham Hospital; Director of Psychiatry, Boston Hospital for Women.

E. P. RICHARDSON, JR., M.D.
Professor of Neuropathology, Harvard Medical School; Neurologist and Neuropathologist, Massachusetts General Hospital, Boston.

LESLIE I. ROSE, M.D.
Associate Professor of Medicine, Hahnemann Medical College and Hospital; Director, Section of Endocrinology and Metabolism, Hahnemann Hospital, Philadelphia.

EUGENIA ROSEMBERG, M.D.
Research Professor, University of Massachusetts Medical School; Research Director, Medical Research Institute of Worcester, Inc.; Director of Medical Research, Worcester City Hospital, Worcester.

SAUL A. ROSENBERG, M.D.
Professor of Medicine and Radiology, Stanford University School of Medicine, Stanford.

JOHN ROSS, JR., M.D.
Professor of Medicine and Chief, Cardiovascular Division, Department of Medicine, University of California, San Diego, School of Medicine, La Jolla.

RICHARD S. ROSS, M.D.
Professor of Medicine, Susan and William Clayton Professor of Cardiovascular Disease, Dean of the Medical Faculty, Vice President for the Health Divisions, The Johns Hopkins University School of Medicine, Baltimore.

CYRUS E. RUBIN, M.D.
Professor of Medicine, Division of Gastroenterology, University of Washington School of Medicine, Seattle.

ROBERT H. RUBIN, M.D.
Infectious Disease Unit, Massachusetts General Hospital, Boston.

DAVID C. SABISTON, JR., M.D.
James B. Duke Professor and Chairman, Department of Surgery, Duke University Medical Center, Durham.

FUAD SABRA, M.D., F.A.C.P.
Professor of Neurology and Head of Division of Neurology, Medical School, American University of Beirut; Neurologist, American University Hospital, Beirut.

MARIA Z. SALAM, M.D.
Assistant Professor of Neurology, Harvard Medical School; Clinical and Research Fellow in Children's Neurology, Massachusetts General Hospital, Boston.

HERBERT A. SALTZMAN, M.D.
Professor of Medicine, Duke University School of Medicine; Director, F. G. Hall Laboratory for Environmental Research, Durham.

MERLE A. SANDE, M.D.
Associate Professor, Department of Medicine, University of Virginia Medical Center, Charlottesville.

JAY P. SANFORD, M.D.
Dean, The Uniformed Services, University of the Health Sciences, Office of the Secretary of Defense, Bethesda.

ROBERT W. SCHRIER, M.D.
Professor of Medicine, University of Colorado Department of Medicine; Head, Division of Renal Disease, Colorado General Hospital, University of Colorado Medical Center, Denver.

CHARLES C. SHEPARD, M.D.
Chief, Leprosy and Rickettsial Branch, Virology Division, Bureau of Laboratories, Center for Disease Control, Department of Health, Education and Welfare, Public Health Service, Atlanta.

WILLIAM SILEN, M.D.
Johnson and Johnson Professor of Surgery, Harvard Medical School; Surgeon-in-Chief, Beth Israel Hospital, Boston.

FRED E. SILVERSTEIN, M.D.
Assistant Professor of Medicine, University of Washington School of Medicine; Director, Gastrointestinal Endoscopy Service, University of Washington Hospital, Seattle.

LLOYD H. SMITH, JR., M.D., D.Sc. (Hon)
Professor and Chairman, Department of Medicine, University of California, San Francisco; Chief of the Medical Service, Moffitt Hospital, San Francisco.

PHILIP J. SNODGRASS, M.D.
Professor of Medicine, Indiana University School of Medicine; Chief, Medical Service, Veterans Administration Hospital, Indianapolis.

BURTON E. SOBEL, M.D.
Professor of Medicine, Washington University; Director, Cardiovascular Division, Barnes Hospital, St. Louis.

ARTHUR J. SOBER, M.D.
Instructor in Dermatology, Harvard Medical School; Assistant Dermatologist, Massachusetts General Hospital, Boston.

J. STUART SOELDNER, B.S., M.D.
Associate Professor of Medicine at Peter Bent Brigham Hospital, Harvard Medical School; Senior Associate in Medicine, Peter Bent Brigham Hospital, Boston.

EDMUND H. SONNENBLICK, M.D.
Professor of Medicine and Chief, Division of Cardiology, Department of Medicine, Albert Einstein College of Medicine of Yeshiva University, New York.

WESLEY W. SPINK, M.D., D.Sc. (Hon)
Emeritus Regents' Professor of Medicine and Comparative Medicine, University of Minnesota Health Sciences Center, Minneapolis.

WILLIAM W. STEAD, M.D.
Director, Tuberculosis Program, Arkansas Department of Health; Professor of Medicine, University of Arkansas School of Medicine, Little Rock.

DANIEL J. STECHSCHULTE, M.D.
Associate Professor of Medicine and Director, Division of Allergy, Clinical Immunology and Rheumatology, University of Kansas Medical Center, College of Health Sciences and Hospital, Kansas City.

JURGEN STEINKE, M.D. (Deceased)
Formerly Chief of Endocrinology and Metabolism, Rancho Los Amigos Hospital; Formerly Associate Professor of Medicine, School of Medicine, University of Southern California, Los Angeles.

GENE H. STOLLERMAN, M.D.
Professor and Chairman, Department of Medicine, University of Tennessee College of Medicine; Physician-in-Chief, City of Memphis Hospital, Memphis.

D. EUGENE STRANDNESS, JR., M.D.
Professor of Surgery, Department of Surgery, University of Washington School of Medicine, Seattle.

DAVID H.P. STREETEN, M.B., D.Phil., F.R.C.P., F.A.C.P.
Professor of Medicine and Chief, Section of Endocrinology, State University of New York Upstate Medical Center; Attending Physician in Medicine, State University Hospital, Syracuse.

MELVIN L. TAYMOR, M.D.
Associate Clinical Professor of Obstetrics and Gynecology, Harvard Medical School; Senior Obstetrician and Gynecologist, Boston Hospital for Women, Boston.

GEORGE W. THORN, M.D., M.A. (Hon), LL.D. (Hon), D.Sc. (Hon), M.D. (Hon), F.R.C.P.
Hersey Professor of the Theory and Practice of Physic, Emeritus, Harvard Medical School; Samuel A. Levine Professor of Medicine, Emeritus, Harvard Medical School; Physician-in-Chief, Emeritus, Peter Bent Brigham Hospital, Boston.

GENNARO M. TISI, M.D.
Associate Professor of Medicine, University of California, San Diego, School of Medicine; Chief, Pulmonary Section, Veterans Administration Hospital, San Diego.

MARVIN TURCK, M.D.
Physician-in-Chief, Harborview Medical Center; Professor of Medicine, University of Washington School of Medicine, Seattle.

DAVID D. ULMER, M.D.
Professor and Chairman, Department of Medicine, Charles R. Drew Postgraduate Medical School; Professor of Medicine, University of Southern California School of Medicine; Chief, Department of Internal Medicine, Los Angeles County-Martin Luther King, Jr., General Hospital, Los Angeles.

JOHN E. ULTMAN, M.D.
Professor of Medicine, Section of Hematology/Oncology and Director, University of Chicago Cancer Research Center, University of Chicago, Chicago.

THEODORE B. VAN ITALLIE, M.D.
Professor of Medicine, College of Physicians and Surgeons, Columbia University; Attending Physician, St. Luke's Hospital Center, New York.

MAURICE VICTOR, M.D.
Professor of Neurology, Case-Western Reserve University, School of Medicine; Director, Neurology Service, Cleveland Metropolitan General Hospital, Cleveland.

JAMES FINDLAY WALLACE, M.D.
Associate Professor of Medicine, University of Washington School of Medicine; Head, Division of Ambulatory Medicine and Assistant Physician-in-Chief, University Hospital, Seattle.

JACK R. WANDS, M.D.
Assistant Professor of Medicine, Harvard Medical School; Assistant in Medicine, Massachusetts General Hospital, Boston.

HENRY deF. WEBSTER, M.D.
Head, Section Cellular Neuropathology, National Institute of Neurological Disease and Stroke, National Institutes of Health, Bethesda.

LOUIS WEINSTEIN, B.S., M.S., PH.D., M.D., Sc.D. (Hon)
Visiting Professor of Medicine, Harvard Medical School; Physician, Peter Bent Brigham Hospital, Boston.

LOUIS G. WELT, A.B., M.D. (Deceased)
Formerly Professor of Medicine and Chairman, Department of Internal Medicine, Yale University School of Medicine; Formerly Chief, Medical Service, Yale-New Haven Hospital, New Haven.

JOHN B. WEST, M.D., PH.D.
Professor of Medicine, University of California, San Diego School of Medicine; Physician, University Hospital, University of California, San Diego, Medical Center, San Diego.

GRANT R. WILKINSON, M.D.
Associate Professor of Pharmacology, Vanderbilt University School of Medicine, Nashville.

GORDON H. WILLIAMS, M.D.
Associate Professor of Medicine, Harvard Medical School; Director, Endocrinology-Hypertension Division, Peter Bent Brigham Hospital, Boston.

MAXWELL M. WINTROBE, B.A., M.D., B.Sc. (Med.), PH.D., D.Sc. (Hon. Manit.), D.Sc. (Hon. Utah), M.A.C.P.
Distinguished Professor of Internal Medicine, University of Utah College of Medicine, Salt Lake City.

KENNETH A. WOEBER, M.D.
Professor of Medicine, University of California, San Francisco; Chief, Department of Medicine, Mount Zion Hospital and Medical Center, San Francisco.

SHELDON M. WOLFF, M.D.
Clinical Director, National Institute of Allergy and Infectious Diseases and Chief, Laboratory of Clinical Investigation, National Institute of Allergy and Infectious Diseases, National Institutes of Health, Bethesda.

THEODORE E. WOODWARD, M.D.
Professor of Medicine and Head, Department of Medicine, University of Maryland School of Medicine, Baltimore.

RICHARD J. WURTMAN, M.D.
Professor of Endocrinology and Metabolism, Massachusetts Institute of Technology, Cambridge; Clinical Assistant in Medicine, Massachusetts General Hospital, Boston.

JAMES B. WYNGAARDEN, M.D.
Frederic M. Hanes Professor and Chairman, Department of Medicine, Duke University Medical Center; Chief of Medical Service, Duke Hospital, Durham.

ROBERT R. YOUNG, M.D.
Associate Professor of Neurology, Harvard Medical School; Associate Neurologist and Chief, Clinical Neurophysiology, Massachusetts General Hospital, Boston.

preface

It often is asked why prefaces are written and whether they are ever read. In his famous preface to *Cromwell,* Victor Hugo pointed out that one seldom inspects the cellar of a house after visiting its salons nor examines the roots of a tree after eating its fruit. Admittedly, the readers of this book will judge it by the substance of its contents and its style, not by the pretexts offered by its editors. It could be added that if the guest has returned several times, then surely he knows that the cellar is well stocked. Why then a preface to an eighth edition?

This preface is intended to indicate the ways in which the present edition maintains or diverges from, as the case may be, the original objectives of this book. By doing this, it will be possible to present the objectives of this textbook of medicine to readers unfamiliar with earlier editions.

When the first group of editors met together almost thirty years ago, they decided to write a textbook of medicine which would conform to the *clinical method* which they had found most useful both as students and as teachers. It was thought that such a book should recapitulate the steps in the process of thinking by which a physician reaches a diagnosis, these being the recording of the patient's symptoms and signs, the consideration of the various disorders that can give rise to them, and the effective utilization of measures which will support and confirm or alter the first impressions and lead ultimately to a firm diagosis.

The logical first step consistent with this clinical approach is the consideration of the cardinal manifestations of disease. Patients present themselves with symptoms, not diagnoses. Consequently it is basic to good clinical medicine to appreciate the different causes of various manifestations of disease and to understand how they may be produced. This requires an understanding of physiology and of the ways in which deviations from the normal lead to disorders of one kind or another. For this reason material of fundamental biologic importance was incorporated in the first edition of this book and has been regarded as an essential component ever since.

The revolutionary changes in the curricula of many American medical schools, particularly the abbreviation of the standard courses in the science basic to clinical medicine and the substitution of shorter "core" courses, has imposed, we believe, additional responsibilities on the modern teacher of clinical medicine and on the modern textbook of medicine. The students who embark on their clinical training now, although far more sophisticated in many ways than their predecessors of even one generation ago, may not possess as much understanding of the mechanisms of symptoms and disease processes as is required to deal intelligently with clinical problems. This book recognizes the challenge to education posed by such curricula. Clinical biochemistry and pathophysiology form an integral part of this book but, insofar as possible, are considered within the clinical setting.

The interpretation of symptoms usually is most effectively achieved by proceeding from the general to the particular. Symptoms often can be grouped as syndromes. Syndromes are the consequence of a variety of etiologic factors or disease mechanisms and, if these can be recognized and understood, measures to restore the normal physiologic state can be designed and carried out in a logical, systematic fashion. Furthermore, the method of approaching a diagnosis which is based on an analysis of the symptoms, recognition of the syndrome, and consideration of the various disease mechanisms which may have produced it, ensures consideration of the many possible interpretations of the clinical picture which the patient presents. By pursuing such an approach, it is less likely that a disorder which should be considered will be overlooked. The problem-oriented record, which is discussed in a special chapter in this edition (Chap. 4) facilitates such a logical approach to the consideration of the patient's complaints.

The plan of this book is consistent with this approach. Following a discussion of the editors' general philosophy regarding the approach to the patient (Part One), the Cardinal Manifestations of Disease are considered (Part Two). The mechanisms whereby various symptoms are produced are discussed and an approach to the recognition of the diseases of which they may be manifestations is outlined. Laboratory findings are discussed in relation of the clinical manifestations. Part Three summarizes important Biological Considerations in the Approach to Clinical Medicine and includes sections on Genetics and Human Disease with a discussion of cytogenetics, prenatal diagnosis, and genetic counselling; Clinical Pharmacology with chapters on principles of drug action and reactions to drugs; a section Metabolic Considerations which includes chapters on intermediary metabolism of carbohydrate, fat, and protein, fluid and electrolytes, acidosis and alkalosis; and a section on Immunologic Considerations.

The remainder of the book is concerned with specific disorders and disease entities. In all these sections, the syndromic approach is emphasized insofar as possible. The reader will find at the beginning of most of the sections, either in the introduction and/or in the first chapter, a discussion of the approach to the patient whose clinical manifestations suggest the type of disease considered in that section.

Treatment is discussed in relation to specific disorders or categories of disease (e.g., Chapter 130, Chemotherapy of Infection; Chapter 239, Pharmacologic Treatment of Cardiovascular Disorders) and is described in terms which are as specific as practical.

A deliberate attempt has been made to avoid long bibliographies. The references at the end of the chapters are limited, for the most part, to reviews and monographs which contain comprehensive bibliographies, as well as to a few of the most significant recent articles.

Major sections of the book have been revised for the eighth edition and a number of new chapters and discussions have been included, viz: The Adult Respiratory Distress Syndrome, which is assuming more and more importance in internal medicine; new physiological concepts concerning the mechanism of fluid retention; a discussion of angina pectoris with an evaluation of coronary bypass operations; echocardiography; fiber optic bronchoscopy and hypersensitivity diseases of the lung; a completely rewritten section on hematological diseases including a discussion of bone marrow transplantation; new chapters on host defense mechanisms, emergencies in medicine, oncology, and gastroenterology, the latter containing a discussion of endoscopic techniques, current status of gallstone formation, and inflammatory bowel disease; a reorganized chapter on cerebrovascular disease to make the material more useful to the practicing physician (the common problems are outlined along with clinical approaches to each); the value of computerized axial tomography as a noninvasive technique of examination of the brain and illustrations of its use in the diagnosis of hypertensive hemorrhages, subdural and extradural hematomas, brain tumors, abscesses, hemorrhagic infarcts, hydrocephalus, and cerebral atrophy (this new method has led to the modification of the standard clinical approaches to each of these pathologic states); in the section on endocrinology new chapters on hypothalamic releasing hormones, inappropriate antidiuretic hormone secretion, glucagon and calcitonin secretion and the importance of trace elements in clinical disease, also chapters on fertility control, sexual counseling for the internist, and a discussion of ageing, involution, and senescence.

With the publication of the seventh edition of the Textbook one of its original editors and Editor-in-Chief for that edition, Dr. Maxwell M. Wintrobe, retired. Dr. Wintrobe made major contributions to the Textbook over a period of nearly thirty years, encompassing seven successive editions. It was Dr. Wintrobe and his associates in Salt Lake City who sponsored the unique system of critical review of each new chapter by *medical students* and *house staff* as well as *faculty members,* thus giving the editors very helpful insight as to the needs and ideas of the "consumer." Dr. Wintrobe's advice and counsel will be missed, but his influence undoubtedly will continue to be felt in succeeding editions of the Textbook.

Once again the editors take pleasure in expressing appreciation to our many colleagues who have so generously responded to editorial suggestions. We continue to be indebted to numerous friends and colleagues for valuable criticisms. Among these are: Doctors George Brengelmann, Wayne R. Crill, Ralph E. Cutler, Harvey Featherstone, Alexander Fefer, Philip Fialkow, Clement A. Finch, Robert O. Friedel, Charles J. Goodner, Ted Hansen, Laurence A. Harker, Walter Herrmann, Eugene A. Hessel, Robert S. Hillman, John A. Holcenberg, Robert Jones, Sambasiva Lakshminarayan, Victor Lavis, Leonard Quadracci, John C. Sherris, George Stamatoyannopoulos, Douglas K. Stewart, Paul E. Strandjord, Gary E. Striker, S. Mark Sumi, Phillip D. Swanson, E. Donnall Thomas, and Paul P. Van Arsdel of Seattle, Washington; Sam Masouredis of San Diego; Richard K. Root of New Haven, and Robert S. Gutman of Durham. In addition to the above individuals a large number of the authors listed on pages xxi through xxviii also reviewed and criticized individual chapters.

Of immeasurable help have been our secretarial coworkers. We are especially indebted to Mrs. Freda Foster, Mrs. Hilda Gardner, Mrs. Trudy Geissler, Mrs. Mary Jackson, Miss Patricia Kadlick, Miss Rita Kopps, Mrs. Cynthia Reid, and Mrs. Jana Spellman.

GEORGE W. THORN

RAYMOND D. ADAMS

EUGENE BRAUNWALD

KURT J. ISSELBACHER

ROBERT G. PETERSDORF

PART ONE | THE PHYSICIAN AND THE PATIENT

1 APPROACH TO THE PATIENT

THE EDITORS

No greater opportunity, responsibility, or obligation is given to an individual than that of serving as a physician. In treating the suffering, there is need for technical skill, scientific knowledge, and human understanding. The person who uses these with courage, with humility, and with wisdom will provide a unique service and will build an enduring edifice of character. The physician should ask of destiny no more than this and be content with no less.

THE ART OF MEDICINE In the practice of medicine the physician employs a discipline which seeks to utilize scientific methods and principles in the solution of its problems, but it is one in which, in the end, both science and art are wedded. The crucial importance of understanding the scientific base of modern medicine is well known; the significance of the art of medicine is not as well appreciated. Thus, to extract the telltale clue from a mass of conflicting physical signs and laboratory data the ones that are of crucial significance, to know in a borderline case when to initiate and when to refrain from a line of investigation or treatment involves judgments based on "assimilated" experience. Skill in accomplishing these necessities of medical art is not usually the outcome of laboratory study alone.

Intuition and maturing wisdom are called upon in developing the more personal relations with the patient and the understanding and capacity to peer beneath surface motivations into his behavior. Astute physicians will recognize when the casual mention of an apparently trivial complaint is a device for seeking reassurance regarding a feared disorder such as cancer or heart disease. They will at once know when to probe the more intimate aspects of the patient's life, and when to leave them undiscussed; when to express a bright and reassuring prognosis, and when and how to utter doubt and caution.

Medicine is an art also in the sense that physicians can never be content with the sole aim of endeavoring to clarify the laws of nature; they cannot proceed in their labors with the cool detachment of the scientist whose aim is the winning of the truth, and who, in doing so, conducts a "controlled experiment." Yet it is essential that they maintain objectivity in the study and care of their patients, for this is in the patients' interests; nevertheless, they must use wise judgment and must never forget that their primary and traditional objectives are utilitarian—the prevention and cure of disease and the relief of suffering, whether of body or of mind.

THE PATIENT AS A PERSON The same type of illness presents in a variety of ways depending on the age, personality, and social situation of the patient. Relevant here is the progressive change in social relationships, from a state of complete dependence on parent, family, and teacher, who must supply much of the historical details of an illness, to one of relative independence. At the same time, there are variable degrees of maturation which involve the partial suppression of egocentric drives. These trends and their modification during life experience are the basis of personality; and deviations in these natural developments prevent satisfactory social adjustment. This alone may be the sole reason for seeking medical help, but more often it complicates other illness.

Another aspect of illness that influences the physician-patient relationship is the real or implied significance of disease in the mind of the patient. Any departure from good health involves a potential threat of physical disintegration or crippling disability, and even the most intelligent and best-informed patient should not be considered immune to forebodings just because he refrains from mentioning them. In fact, most patients are more concerned with the possibility of being rendered dependent by illness than with the disease itself. It is especially important that these fears be borne in mind when dealing with the elderly patient, who is rarely unmindful that "the trap is laid" and death is always near.

The attitude of the patient approaching the doctor must always be tinged, for the most part unconsciously, with distaste and dread; his deepest desire will tend to be comfort and relief rather than cure, and his faith and expectation will be directed towards some magical exhibition of these boons. Do not let yourselves believe that however smoothly concealed by education, by reason, and by confidential frankness these strong elements may be, they are ever in any circumstances altogether absent. (Wilfred Trotter)

Illness also constitutes a threat to the individual's status in his social group. Prolonged invalidism during childhood tends inevitably to leave behind an excessive egocentricity, which may become the basis of a lifelong neurosis. In the adult, illness often enforces a return to a posture of dependency, a change usually accompanied by feelings of apprehension and discouragement, sometimes leading to frank anxiety and depression. This explains a number of common psychologic defenses which the patient exercises against illness. He may refuse medical aid; or, if he summons the courage to consult a physician, he may minimize or even fail to mention the very symptom about which he is most deeply concerned. Then, too, there are persons whose emotional stability has been tenuous and uncertain, so that the position of dependency imposed by illness comes as a welcome relief from adult responsibility. They appear to enjoy illness and to resent anything that menaces their state of invalidism. Lesser degrees of this tendency are seen among those who consult the physician at the appearance of every new symptom and who are continuously preoccupied with their past illnesses and operations.

During examination in the relatively neutral domain of the hospital ward a patient's emotional life may seem relatively unimportant. Organic lesions have a way of compelling attention to themselves, and further, it may be less exhausting to limit one's focus to the sphere of physical disease. More time, energy, and experience frequently are necessary to view the patient as an active participant in an enormous moving pageant which includes the personal eccentricities of his forebears, his own fears and patterns of reaction, the roles of poverty, insecurity, and perhaps poor vocational and domestic relations. Yet every experienced physician knows that to explain many of the manifestations of illness, it is necessary to view the patient comprehensively as an organism with a vast repository of past experiences, many of which are vaguely remembered, yet have become the foundation of his current system of meeting daily problems.

THE PHYSICIAN'S RESPONSIBILITIES The physician seeks to respond to and alleviate the patient's complaints, to search out signs of ill health not yet apparent to the patient or of abnormalities which may lead to ill health, and to maintain the patient in a state of well-being. To achieve these goals requires a broad orientation. Illness is never limited to one system, nor necessarily to a single disease, and whether the physician is a family practitioner, an internist who provides "primary care," or a specialist, the patient must be viewed not as an organ system but as a person.

EXAMINATION OF THE WELL PERSON The intelligent practice of preventive medicine is often considered undramatic; yet few areas of medicine are of greater importance to a single individual or to an entire population. In this aspect of medical practice, the physician deals with individuals or groups who are not overtly ill or whose complaints may be unrelated to the disease process which is to be prevented. The use of the periodic physical examination and the ready availability of multiphasic screening tests allow the physician to detect and to intervene in disease processes early in their course, often before the first symptom becomes manifest.

Physicians who examine well individuals are not "wasting their training." More skill is required to recognize the early signs of ill health than to deal with what is obvious to the patient or his family. The discovery and cure of potentially serious disease represent a far greater service to one's patient than ministrations in the course of an incurable condition.

The finding of an elevated arterial blood pressure or an elevated blood sugar, serum uric acid, or cholesterol level in an asymptomatic person or the discussion of milder degrees of nervousness or depression provides an unparalleled opportunity to prevent or retard events of serious consequence. It is not always easy to persuade an asymptomatic person to face a situation he has hoped to avoid or to alter his habits or diet in order to follow a therapeutic program throughout the rest of his life. Nevertheless the value of these efforts is so great that it fully justifies the effort and attention of every physician.

CHANGING PATIENT-PHYSICIAN RELATIONSHIPS The one-to-one patient-physician relationship which traditionally has been the goal of all physicians is changing, primarily because of the changing setting in which medicine is being practiced. In many cases the management of the individual patient requires the active participation of a variety of trained professional personnel—not only physicians, but also nurses, physicians' assistants, dietitians, biochemists, psychologists, and other paramedical personnel. The patient can benefit greatly from such collaboration, but it is the duty of the physician to guide the patient through an illness. In order to carry out this increasingly difficult task, the physician must have some familiarity with the techniques, skills, and objectives of colleagues in the fields allied to medicine. Their findings must be interpreted not as isolated phenomena but rather in terms of the total clinical picture. In giving the patient an opportunity to receive all the benefits of the important advances of science, the physician must retain responsibility for the crucial decisions concerning diagnosis and treatment.

An increasing number of patients is being cared for by groups of physicians, clinics, hospitals, and health-maintenance organizations (HMOs) rather than by a single, independent practitioner. There are many potential advantages in the use of such organized medical groups, but there also are hazards, both to the patient and the physician. The identity of the physician who is primarily and continuously responsible for each particular patient must be clearly defined. It is this physician who must have an overview of a patient's problems and who must maintain familiarity with the patient's reaction to illness, to drugs, and to the challenges of daily living. In addition, since a number of physicians may, at any one time, contribute to the care of a particular patient, and since patients as well as physicians are becoming increasingly mobile, accurate and detailed record keeping assumes progressively greater importance. It is imperative that the physician promptly commit all pertinent data obtained from the clinical and laboratory examinations to the patient's permanent medical record. Only in this way can continuity and high quality in the care of the patient be provided.

THE PHYSICIAN AS A PERSON The examining physician is first a human instrument, subject to reactions arising from events in his or her own biography. This background will strongly influence the physician's responses to and understanding of the patient. The student receives much expert coaching in the methods of physical and laboratory diagnosis, and in these areas will most easily develop the skills that permit a comfortable relationship with the patient. The young physician may feel inadequate in dealing with the patient, for not only is a sense of insecurity inevitable with respect to the patient's problems but also with respect to the newly acquired role of authority and responsibility. Moreover, some reactions may be difficult to control: lack of interest in a patient who presents no fascinating problems of organic disease, irritation at the patient's verbosity or lack of clarity and consistency in reciting his history, or even disappointment because the patient's illness fails to respond to treatment in the expected manner.

To perceive and understand the problems of the patient, the physician requires not simply instruction but emotional maturity and an interest in and concern for other human beings. The physician must learn to be at ease and to establish rapport with persons of every walk of life, realizing that everyone is born with manifold potentialities determined by his genes and has a personality and character shaped by the emotional climate in which he grows and develops. The physician must relate as much to the person who is ill as to the illness for which he seeks relief.

The physician has a special function in society and should be skilled as a psychologist in human behavior as well as a biologist in human disease. With the highly technical knowledge and skills the physician brings to bear upon the patient's physiologic functioning there should also be a feeling of humaneness, a sense of confidence and security based upon the conviction that all will be done that can be done. Such an atmosphere will develop a wholesome personal relationship. The patient must be made to realize that his unique individuality is recognized and that his life's problems are appreciated. This is as important to patients with well-defined organic disease as to those suffering primarily from psychologic and emotional problems.

2 APPROACH TO DISEASE

THE EDITORS

HISTORY The written history of an illness should embody all the facts of medical significance in the life of the patient up to the time that he consults the physician; but, of course, his most recent diseases attract the most attention, for these, obviously, are the reason that he seeks medical advice. Ideally the narration of symptoms should be in the patient's own words, the principal events being presented in the temporal order in which they occurred. However, few patients possess the necessary powers of observation and talent for lucid, coherent description and require guiding questions from the physician, who must at the same time avoid suggesting answers.

Often a symptom which has concerned a patient has little significance, whereas a seemingly minor complaint may be of importance. Therefore the mind of the physician must be constantly alert to the possibility that any event related by the patient, any symptom however trivial or apparently remote, may be the key to the solution of the medical problem. As data are gained from the physical and laboratory examinations, the problems which are presented should be clearly identified.

An informative history is more than an orderly listing of symptoms. Something always is gained by listening to the patient and noting the way in which he talks about his symptoms. Inflection of voice, facial expression, and attitude may betray important clues as to the meaning of the symptoms to the patient. Thus in listening to this recitation, one discovers not only something about the disease but also something about the patient.

With experience one learns the pitfalls of history taking. What patients relate for the most part consists of subjective phenomena filtered through minds that vary in their background of past experience. Patients obviously differ widely in their responses to the same stimuli. Their remarks are variably colored by fear of disease, disability, and death, and by concern over the consequences of illness to their families. Additional difficulties are created by language barriers, by failing intellectual powers which deprive the patient of accurate recall, or by a disorder of consciousness that makes him unaware of his illness. It is not surprising, then, that even the most careful physician may at times despair of collecting factual data and be forced to proceed with evidence that represents little more than an approximation of the truth.

Viewed in another way, the symptom marks, in the patient's mind, a departure from normal health; in the physician's mind, it initiates a process of inductive and deductive reasoning that culminates in diagnosis. In pondering the various possible explanations of a given symptom or clinical state, the physician begins a search for other data, elicited by further questioning of the patient and his family, by physical examination, or by laboratory tests. The symptoms alone sometimes will provide the most certain clue, as in angina pectoris or epilepsy, where physical findings and laboratory data collected between attacks may give no evidence of the existence of disease even when it is manifestly present. In most illnesses, however, the history will not be so decisive, though it may narrow the number of diagnostic possibilities and guide the subsequent investigation.

It is in the taking of the history that the physician's skill, knowledge, and experience are most clearly in evidence. Each symptom is evaluated according to its nature and context; there are times for questioning its credibility and turning to more reliable sources of information, but skepticism must not cause an unusual symptom, or manifestation of some new condition, to be overlooked. Moreover, there are times when an interrogation must be pressed more deeply in search for further details and times when the questions must be broader, because "disease often tells its secrets in a casual parenthesis." And finally, the physician knows how to take advantage of the interview in which the history is gathered to obtain the confidence of the patient and allay apprehension and fear, the first steps in therapy.

The family history, all too often obtained in a routine, cursory fashion, is a leading tool of clinical genetics and can provide important evidence regarding the nature of the patient's complaints. Information regarding symptoms like those of the patient which have occurred in blood relatives, or "run in the family," and knowledge of the ethnic origin of the parents and of consanguinity may be exceedingly helpful. The information must be obtained with tact, however, for patients may be embarrassed by such inquiries. Finally it should be emphasized that the best family history is one which is supported by actual examination of other members of the family. Frequently it is found that some physical deviation from the normal, too subtle to be recognized by a lay person, is quite apparent to the trained observer and that a minor deviation in laboratory data assumes significance when evaluated within a family constellation.

PHYSICAL EXAMINATION Little need be said about the importance of the physical examination, for early in their training physicians learn that physical signs are the objective and verifiable marks of disease. The physical sign represents a solid, indisputable fact. However, its significance is enhanced when it confirms a functional or structural change already evidenced by the patient's history. At other times, the physical sign may stand as the only evidence of disease, especially in those instances in which the history has been inconsistent, confused, or is completely lacking.

If full advantage is to be derived from the physical examination, it must be performed methodically and thoroughly. Although attention has usually been directed by the history to the offending organ or part of the body, the examination must extend to all parts of the body. The patient must be scrutinized literally from head to toe in an objective search for abnormalities that may yield information concerning present and possible future illnesses. Unless the examination procedure is systematic, important parts of it may be forgotten, an error against which even the most skilled clinician must guard. The results of the examination, like the details of the history, should be recorded at the time they are elicited, not hours later when they are subject to the distortions of memory. Many inaccuracies stem from the careless practice of writing or dictating notes long after the examination has terminated.

Skill in physical diagnosis is acquired with experience, but it is not merely technique that determines success in eliciting signs. The detection of a few scattered petechiae or a faint diastolic murmur or a small mass in the abdomen is not a question of keener eyes and ears or more sensitive fingers, but of a mind directed to be alert to these findings. Skill in physical diagnosis reflects a way of thinking more than a way of doing.

All investigations of the body should be regarded as part of the physical examination. The use of various instruments, such as the ophthalmoscope, sphygmomanometer, galvanometer, microscope, or roentgen tube, are mere extensions of the examination to less accessible structures. Proficiency in their use is part of internal medicine.

LABORATORY EXAMINATIONS The marked increase in the number and availability of laboratory diagnostic procedures has inevitably augmented reliance on the knowledge gained from these studies in the solution of clinical problems. It is essential that one bear in mind the limitations of such procedures, which by virtue of their impersonal quality and the complexity of the techniques involved often gain an aura of authority regardless of the fallibility of the individuals or the instruments responsible for carrying out the technical procedures or interpreting the data. One must not be misled by the "magic of numbers!"

Accumulation of laboratory data cannot release the physician from the necessity of careful observation and study of the patient. The wise physician understands the merits and limitations of each source of information, whether it be history, physical examination, or laboratory investigation. The physician also must weigh carefully the hazards and the expense involved in every laboratory procedure.

Laboratory tests rarely are ordered and reported singly. Rather they are produced as "batteries." A common combination is the M-6 which consists of determinations of serum sodium, potassium, carbon dioxide–combining power, chloride, blood urea nitrogen, and blood glucose. More elaborate combinations, one of which is the M-12, are available and report simultaneously serum calcium, phosphate, proteins, albumin, uric acid, cholesterol, and several enzymes. The various combinations of laboratory tests are often useful. For example, they may provide the clue to such nonspecific symptoms as generalized weakness and increased fatigability by revealing an elevated serum calcium which, in turn, would suggest the diagnosis of hyperparathyroidism.

The thoughtful use of screening tests is not to be confused with indiscriminate laboratory testing; it is based on the fact that a group of laboratory determinations which are known to be frequent harbingers of disease can now be carried out on a single specimen of blood at relatively low cost. Biochemical measurements, together with simple laboratory examinations such as blood count, urinalysis, and sedimentation rate, often provide the major clue to the presence of a pathologic process. This is particularly helpful in identifying organic disease in a patient with evident psychologic or emotional problems. At the same time the physician must learn to evaluate occasional abnormalities among the screening tests which may not necessarily connote significant disease. There is nothing more costly and unproductive than the subsequent in-depth work-up following the reporting of an isolated laboratory abnormality in an otherwise well patient.

Discrimination in the ordering of laboratory procedures and judgment in appraising their risk and expense as against the value of the information to be derived from them are important indicators of the effectiveness with which the art and science of medicine have been fused by the individual physician.

THE CLINICAL METHOD AND THE SYNDROMIC APPROACH TO DISEASE The clinical method has as its object the collection of accurate data concerning all the diseases to which human beings are subject, namely, all conditions that "limit life in its powers, enjoyment, and duration." But much more is required in making a diagnosis. Each datum must be interpreted in the light of the known facts of anatomy, physiology, and chemistry. The synthesis of these interpretations yields information concerning the affected organ or body system. Further, from the vantage point afforded by such an anatomic diagnosis the physician may then turn to other data, such as the mode of onset and clinical course of the illness, and to the results of laboratory tests, in order to ascertain the cause of the disease and degree of physiologic impairment.

The clinical method always proceeds in a series of logical steps. The perceptive student will note certain similarities between the clinical method and the scientific method. Each begins with observational data which suggest a series of hypotheses. The latter are tested in the light of further observations, some of which are made in the clinic and others in the laboratory. Finally, a conclusion is reached, which in science is called a *theory* and in medicine a *working diagnosis.* The modus operandi of the clinical method, like that of the scientific method, cannot be reduced to a single principle or a type of inductive or deductive reasoning. It involves both analysis and synthesis, the essential parts of cartesian logic. As a physician, one does not start with an open mind any more than does the scientist, but with one prejudiced from knowledge of recent cases; and the patient's first statement directs one's thinking to certain channels. There is a constant struggle to avoid the bias occasioned by one's own attitude, mood, and interest.

It is particularly in the study of more difficult patients that the logical order of the clinical method becomes most important. Here in particular the physician must carefully list each problem indicated by the patient's complaints and physical and laboratory findings and seek answers to each. Anatomic diagnosis regularly precedes etiological diagnosis. One seldom succeeds in determining the cause and mechanism of a disease before ascertaining which organ has been involved. An intermediate step is syndromic diagnosis. Most physicians attempt consciously or unconsciously to fit a given problem into one of a series of syndromes. The syndrome, in essence, is a group of symptoms and signs of disordered function, related to one another by means of some anatomic, physiologic, or biochemical peculiarity of the organism. It embodies a hypothesis concerning the deranged function of an organ, organ system, or tissue. Congestive heart failure, Cushing's disease, and dementia are examples. In congestive heart failure dyspnea, orthopnea, cyanosis, dependent edema, engorged neck veins, pleural fluid, pulmonary rales, and enlarged liver are known to be connected by a single pathophysiologic mechanism—failure of the heart, leading to salt and water retention and high venous pressure. In Cushing's disease the moon facies, hypertension, diabetes, and osteoporosis are the recognized effects of excess corticosteroids acting on many target organs. In dementia deterioration of memory, incoherent thinking, faulty judgment, etc., are related through a neuroanatomic and a neurophysiologic principle; i.e., all these disordered intellectual functions are related to slow impairment of the function and destruction of the association areas of the cerebrum.

A syndromic diagnosis usually does not necessarily identify the precise cause of an illness, but it greatly narrows the number of possibilities and, thus, suggests whatever further clinical and laboratory studies are required. The derangements of each organ system in human beings are reducible to a relatively small number of syndromes. Diagnosis is greatly simplified if a given clinical problem conforms neatly to a well-defined syndrome. Then one need only turn to a book for a list of the various diseases that may cause it. The search for the cause of an illness that does not conform to a syndrome is much more difficult, for a seemingly infinite number of diseases may then have to be considered. Nevertheless, the principle remains: the clinical method is a orderly intellectual activity which proceeds almost invariably from symptom to sign, to syndrome, to disease.

THE COMPUTER IN MEDICINE The uses of the computer in managing the economic aspects of medical practice are already well established. However, the role of the computer in clinical medicine is still in an evolutionary stage. It has been used successfully in the clinical laboratory for processing data from automated chemical and microbiological determinations. Several centers have successfully developed computerized medical records for hospital and outpatient use. Pharmacy automated information systems are becoming sophisticated and are able to assist in prevention of drug-drug interactions and improved monitoring of therapy. Although these newer developments are noteworthy, computer management of medical data is still in its infancy.

The role of the computer in medical decision making remains elusive but challenging. Several applications have been successful and have made a contribution to patient care and physician education. The educational aspects should not be underestimated because, in this stage of development, the attempt to program medical decisions has already led to a better scientific understanding of the "art" of medical judgment.

The advantages to the physician who can use computer technology are obvious. Much time and effort can be saved with appropriate applications, and more accurate and reliable clinical information can be brought quickly into the hands of the physician.

ACCOUNTABILITY Traditionally, physicians, once licensed to practice medicine, have not had to account for their actions except to their peers. In the past decade, however, there have been increasing demands for physicians to account for the way in which they practice medicine by meeting certain standards prescribed by the federal government. Hospitalized patients whose health care is sponsored by the government (Medicare and Medicaid) have been subjected to utilization review. This means that the physician must defend the duration of a patient's hospitalization if it exceeds preset criteria. This concept has been extended in the form of Professional Standard Review Organizations (PSRO) under whose direction norms and standards for the care of patients are developed. The purpose of these regulations is ostensibly to improve the quality of patient care, and, in some instances, this will undoubtedly happen. An equally important reason for implementing these regulations, however, is to contain spiraling health care costs. There is no question but that the insertion of this type of review will be extended to all phases of medical practice and will inevitably alter not only the practice of medicine but the traditional patient-physician relationship.

Physicians also will be expected to give account of their continuing competence by mandatory continuing education, patient record audit, recertification by examination, and possible relicensure. The American Board of Internal Medicine administered its first voluntary recertification examination in 1974 to nearly 3,400 physicians; a second examination is planned for 1977. The American Board of Family Practice will also administer a recertification examination to its recent diplomates.

COST-EFFECTIVENESS IN MEDICAL CARE As society undertakes greater responsibility for health care, and as the cost of medical care continues to skyrocket, it will become necessary to establish priorities as to where and how the health dollars will be spent. Preventive measures often offer the greatest return per dollar; outstanding examples include vaccination, immunization, reduction in accidents and occupational hazards, and improved environmental control. In a relatively new area the cost of "newborn screening" for metabolic disorders is being evaluated. In 1972 and 1973 the Commonwealth of Massachusetts noted that the cost of collecting and analyzing 200,000 specimens was $355,000 and that the additional costs of evaluating and treating individuals with phenylketonuria and other disorders detected in the survey added $103,000, for a total cost of $458,000. The cost of hospitalization and institutionalization for all affected individuals, it was estimated, would have amounted to more than $800,000 per year, if early detection had not been available. The saving of over $300,000 in one year provides an example of what can be accomplished as economical diagnostic screening procedures become available. In the study just cited, the savings which were reported do not include the potential contribution to society which will be made by successfully treated individuals.

As experience is gained, it will become necessary to evaluate the justifiability of performing prohibitively costly operations which provide only a limited life expectancy as against the pressing need for more primary care centers for those large segments of the population who suffer from inadequate medical services. At the level of the individual patient, it has become extremely important to minimize as far as possible hospital admissions with their very high costs, if total health care is to be provided at a figure which most can afford. This, of course, implies and depends upon a close cooperative effort between patients, their physicians, third-party carriers, and government, and a constant surveillance of those types of procedures which can be conducted safely and effectively on an ambulatory basis. Equally important in reducing total health care expenditures is the need for each physician to monitor carefully the medications prescribed with particular reference to their effectiveness as well as to their relative costs. In the last analysis the public must depend upon the medical profession for leadership and guidance in the manner and method with which the provision of health services is legislated. It is important, however, that consideration of these important socioeconomic aspects of the health delivery system not be permitted to attenuate a physician's primary humane concern for the welfare of the individual patient.

REFERENCE

EDITORIAL: Cost-benefit analysis for newborn screening for metabolic disorders. N Engl J Med 291:1414, 1974

PAUKER SJ, KASSIRER, JP: Therapeutic decision making: a cost-benefit analysis. N Engl J Med 293:229–234, 1975

3 CARE OF THE PATIENT

THE EDITORS

The care of the patient begins with the development of an interpersonal relationship between the patient and his physician, as discussed in Chap. 1. In the absence of a sense of trust and confidence on the part of the patient, the effectiveness of therapeutic measures is diminished. In many instances, when there is confidence in the physician, reassurance alone suffices and is all that is needed. In those cases which for the time being are insusceptible of solution or for which no effective remedy is available, a feeling on the part of the patient that his physician is doing all that is possible is one of the most important therapeutic measures that his physician can provide.

The discovery during the past several decades of therapeutic agents capable of exerting decisive influence on the course of disease has made it essential that the physician have some understanding not only of the disturbed functions induced by disease, but also of the manner of treatment most likely to exert a beneficial effect, and of the risks involved in the proposed therapeutic plan.

Ideally, treatment should strive for the complete restoration of the patient's physical and mental health. When this goal is not attainable, remedies may still be available which will postpone the progress of incurable disease and delay its evil consequences; or, when they can no longer be postponed, they can be rendered tolerable.

IATROGENIC DISORDERS It is the responsibility of the physician to use the new and powerful therapeutic measures wisely, with due regard for their action, cost, and potential dangers. Every medical procedure, whether diagnostic or therapeutic, contains within it the potentiality of harm, but it would be impossible to afford the patient all the benefits of modern scientific medicine if reasonable steps in diagnosis and therapy were withheld because of possible risks. "Reasonable" here implies that the physician has weighed the pros and cons of a procedure and has concluded on rational grounds that the step is advisable or essential for the relief of discomfort or the cure or amelioration of disease. When the deleterious effects of the physician's action exceed the advantages that could have been anticipated, one is justified in designating these undesirable effects as iatrogenic. It is necessary only to recall the dangerous or fatal reactions that occasionally follow the use of antibiotics given for trivial respiratory infections, the gastric hemorrhage or perforation caused by cortisone administered for a mild arthritis, the fatal homologous serum hepatitis that may follow needless transfusions of blood or plasma, or the arterial thrombosis or arrhythmia that may complicate coronary angiography.

But the harm that a physician can do to a patient is not limited to the imprudent use of medication. Equally important are ill-considered or unjustified remarks. Since the patient, no matter how apparently placid, approaches the physician with apprehension, his anxiety may be enhanced by a too-serious demeanor, a flippant remark, or an unexplained conference concerning his illness. Many persons have been led to a cardiac neurosis because the physician expressed a grave prognosis on the basis of a misinterpreted electrocardiogram. Not only the treatment itself but the physician's words and behavior are always capable of causing injury.

The physician must never become so much absorbed in the disease as to forget the patient who is its victim. This exhortation cannot be repeated too often. As the science of medicine advances, it is all too easy to become so fascinated by the manifestations of a malady that one disregards the ailing person, his fears, his concerns about his job and the future of his family, the cost of medical care, and the specter of economic insecurity. Treatment of a patient consists of more than the dispassionate confrontation of a disease. It embodies also the exercise of warmth, compassion, and understanding. In the now famous words of Peabody, "One of the essential qualities of the clinician is interest in humanity, for the secret of the care of the patient is in caring for the patient."

INFORMED CONSENT In an era of rapidly advancing technology, patients progressively will require diagnostic and therapeutic procedures that are painful and that pose some risk. These include all surgical procedures, e.g., biopsies of tissues, radiographic maneuvers involving the insertion of catheters, endoscopy, and many others. In most hospitals and clinics, patients undergoing such procedures are required to sign a form consenting to them. More important, however, is the notion that the patient must understand clearly the risk entailed in these procedures; this is the definition of *informed consent*. It is incumbent upon the physician to explain to the patient clearly, in language that he understands, the procedures he faces. By doing this conscientiously, much of the dread of the unknown that is inherent in hospitalization will be mitigated.

INCURABILITY AND DEATH No problem is more distressing than that presented by the patient with incurable disease, particularly when death is imminent and inevitable. What should the patient and his family be told, what measures should be taken to maintain the patient's life, and how is death to be defined?

There is no ironclad rule that the patient must be told "everything," even if he is an adult and the head of his family. How much the patient is told will depend upon his own desires and character, the wishes of his family, the state of his affairs, and perhaps his religious convictions. First of all, the patient must be given an opportunity to speak to his physician and to ask questions. Patients may find it easier to share their feelings about death with their physician who they realize is likely to be more objective and less emotional than their own family members.

One thing is certain: it is not for you to don the black cap and, assuming the judicial function, take hope away from any patient . . . hope that comes to us all. (William Osler)

Even when the patient directly inquires, "Doctor, am I dying?" the physician must be circumspect and must attempt to determine whether this is a request for information, a demand for reassurance, or even an expression of hostility. Only further exchanges between the patient and his physician can resolve these questions and guide the physician in what to say and how to say it.

The physician should provide or arrange for emotional, physical, and spiritual support, and must be compassionate, unhurried, and open. Pain should be adequately controlled, human dignity maintained, and isolation from family avoided. The last two, in particular, tend to be overlooked in hospitals, where the intrusion of life-sustaining apparatus can so easily detract from attention to the whole person and instead concentrate on the life-threatening disorder.

The physician must also be prepared to deal with the expiatory attitude of the family when a member becomes gravely or hopelessly ill. The meager resources that may represent the savings of a lifetime may be dissipated in weeks of payment for needlessly expensive rooms, nursing services, and futile therapeutic measures. It is difficult for the physician to oppose these gestures too strenuously, for they serve more to bring consolation to the family than to assuage the distress of the patient, but they need not be encouraged.

Physicians also must be prepared to deal with the feelings of guilt that almost invariably afflict the members of a family when parent or child or spouse has died. They must tender what assurance is possible that no fault or stigma of neglect need be attached to the living.

Apart from the anguish of facing the terminal phases of disease, to which patient and family react in highly individualistic ways according to temperament, personal philosophy, and religion, important biologic and medical problems arise as death approaches. One must at each stage in an illness ascertain whether a fatal outcome is inevitable and also whether the patient, should he survive, will suffer a degree of disability that would make life unbearable for him and his family. New concepts of death must also be considered.

Traditionally, in every society, arrest of heart action has been taken as the only valid medical criterion of death. Law books cite this as the only certain proof that human life has ended. But, as every modern physician knows, the heart may sometimes be restored to action, seemingly miraculously, minutes after it has stopped. On the other hand, other vital organs such as the brain may be destroyed, leaving the individual essentially dead as far as his psychic life and personality are concerned, while heart action and circulation are maintained.

Biologically speaking, life, when viewed at a cellular level, is an intricate process of growth and decay in varying proportions at different ages. When decay exceeds growth in organs composed of postmitotic cells such as the musculature and nervous system, where each cell must endure for the lifetime of the individual, death proceeds gradually. This might be termed *cellular death*, and in its most advanced forms organ function may be impaired to a point incompatible with useful life. Of all the organs of man it is the central nervous system, more specifically the brain, that imparts meaningful qualities to life. Without a functioning cerebrum man has none of the attributes that distinguish him from another individual of his own species or from beasts. All awareness of self is permanently effaced; no longer can he think, respond to his physical or social environment, speak, or move. Most thoughtful physicians and many lay people concede that such a state is equivalent to death even though the heart still beats.

Clinical and electrographic criteria are at hand which

permit the reliable diagnosis of cerebral death. According to the report of the staff of the Massachusetts General Hospital and the Harvard Committee on Brain Death, one may assume that death has occurred when, as a consequence usually of hypoxia and hypotension, all signs of receptivity and responsivity are in abeyance, including all brainstem and spinal reflexes (pupillary reactions, ocular movement, blinking, swallowing, breathing, tendon and other spinal reflexes), and the electroencephalogram is isoelectric. Occasionally, intoxications and metabolic disorders may simulate this state; hence the diagnosis requires expert medical evaluation. Under the aforementioned circumstances, to continue with heroic, highly costly, supportive measures merely for the purpose of preserving cardiac function is in actuality against the best interests of patient, family, and society.

Here physicians, on contemplating the broad implications of their actions, must either involve themselves in fruitless supportive care or may have to make the difficult decision to abandon their traditional roles of making every effort to preserve life at any cost. If the medical profession, in accord with social sanction, can be brought to redefine life as a state in which cerebral action subserves awareness of environment and the possibility of expressing intellect, emotion, personality, and character, and can equate the opposite of this with death, the dilemma can be avoided.

A practice which has been adopted and which has proved most acceptable is as follows:

1 The diagnosis of brain death, based on the above criteria, should be corroborated by another physician, and the clinical examination and EEG should be repeated one or more times over a period of 24 hours.
2 The family and nurses should be informed of the irreversibility of brain function but should not be asked or permitted to make the decision as to the continuation of medical treatment.
3 The physician may withdraw supportive medical measures, assuming that nothing more can be offered and that extraordinary measures to maintain heart function need not be employed (in agreement with recommendations of Pope Pius XII and others of the clergy).
4 The possibility that such patients may become sources of organs for grafting should not enter into such decisions, although prior to the cessation of heart action the family may be approached by surgeons and asked whether this would be their wish, or the family may suggest that organs be used for this purpose.

AGING, INVOLUTION, AND SENESCENCE The clinical phenomena with which physicians are customarily concerned depend on pathological derangements of biological processes. These acquire full significance in medicine only when their time sequence is considered with reference to a time scale in the human life cycle called aging. Biologically, age confers on any category of development a quantitative dimension, and from a medical viewpoint a given age represents a specific position on the growth scale. One of the clearest manifestations of disease is a displacement of an individual from the expected position in the chronology of his life cycle.

Certain categories of disease are known to predominate in particular periods of life. Anomalies of development, genetically determined metabolic disease, and certain of the more serious infections tend to declare themselves in infancy and childhood, while neoplasms, vascular diseases, atrophy, and degeneration are peculiar to late adult life. Whereas the accomplished pediatrician is expected to know the time of appearance and disappearance of a large range of reflex and automatic activities, perceptual abilities, and language skills, there has been an unwillingness by physicians to accept involution and aging as a natural and inevitable phase of life. Many physicians are inclined to attribute all changes which occur late in life as reflecting only the cumulative effect of injury and disease.

With advancing age there is a steady, inexorable susceptibility to fatal disease. This susceptibility parallels the decline in rate of body growth, and the diseases to which human beings ultimately succumb do not alter very greatly their predetermined life span. Indeed, if it were possible to avoid them all, the average life span would not be lengthened much beyond 10 years!

The composite of overt bodily changes due to senescence such as cessation of skeletal growth, wrinkling of the skin, graying of the hair, loss of teeth, involution of the sex organs, loss of sensory acuity, bent posture, weakening of muscular power, loss of coordination, rigidity of mind, and forgetfulness are known to all. When considered one by one, it is evident that waning vitality or senescence has a different time of onset and rate of progress in different organ systems. Visual and auditory acuity probably reach their maximum at age 10, whereas intellectual power reaches its peak at about 21 years, and muscular power and coordination at age 25. Senescence appears then to be a diverse, complex process manifesting itself in all structures and functions of the body. The *clinical problem* is to distinguish the declining function of vital organs from the effects superimposed by injury and disease.

Of all the age-related changes in organ systems of the human body, those in the *nervous system* are of paramount importance. The most consistent neurological abnormalities of octogenarians include presbyopia, presbycusis, slowed reaction time, diminution of vibratory sensation, loss of fine coordination, weakening of muscle power, thinness of musculature, and reduced or absent Achilles reflex. Deterioration of the capacity to memorize along with retention of material learned at an earlier age and the relative preservation of verbal skill characterize mental performance in the aged. High intelligence, well-organized habit patterns, and sound judgment compensate for many of the deficiencies. Nerve and muscle cells which cease to divide early and must last the lifetime of the organisms are known to have a variable life span. If accidentally destroyed by disease, they are never replaced. But in the absence of disease there is a steady falloff which begins at about the end of the growth period and continues at an accelerated pace into the senium. Functional deficits in an organ such as the brain are in large measure related to cell loss. From early adult life to the senium the average male brain will decrease approximately 150 g in weight. However, there is a safety factor, i.e., a protective surfeit of cells that must be lost before symptoms appear. Whether cells begin to falter functionally before their final disintegration is not known.

The *skeletal muscles* also lose cells (fibers), and the reduction in their weight parallels that of the brain. After the age of 40 to 50, skeletal *bone* mass begins to decline, at a faster rate in women than in men and at a different rate in different parts of the skeleton. For example, the rate of loss is greater in the metacarpals, in the femoral neck, and in the vertebral bodies than in the midshaft of the femur, the tibia, or the skull. Over the next three or four decades the total loss in skeletal mass may be as much as 30 to 50 percent from a base line at age 30 to 40! Aging effects in the skin, connective, and elastic tissues are well known and induce the expenditures of vast sums on cosmetics and beauty treatments in a desperate effort to counteract them. Fine wrinkling and looseness of the skin, the prominence of temporal vessels, the graying and loss of scalp hair, the tendency to facial hirsutism in women, the formation of senile keratoses, and increased incidence of skin cancers on exposed surfaces represent the more frequent changes.

Since collagen constitutes 40 percent of all proteins in the body and undergoes certain consistent alterations in skin, muscles, bones, joints, and blood vessels, naturally biologists should look at this substance for clues to the aging process. Once the fibers of collagen are laid down, they are not renewed. Although a number of chemical changes occur in collagen and elastin which have been identified with aging, to date there is no information on why these changes occur.

Aging is also associated with changes in respiratory function. Maximum oxygen uptake, ventilation volume, and vital capacity progressively diminish with age. Lung volumes increase owing to diminution in elastic recoil. A special form of senile emphysema seems to parallel aging. It is more difficult to differentiate the cardiovascular effects of aging from those of disease, particularly atherosclerosis and hypertension. Under conditions of maximal exertion the aged person cannot achieve as great an increase in cardiac output. In individuals who have escaped atherosclerosis and hypertension, the heart gradually diminishes in weight with advancing years, and the cardiac muscle cells undergo slight atrophy and accumulate wear-and-tear pigment (see below), the so-called "brown atrophy." The aortic valves thicken, and the mitral ring calcifies. The vessel walls of arteries thicken slightly, the internal elastic lamina becomes reduplicated, and collagenous tissue may become hyalinized. Between the third and eighth decades of life the blood flow through the kidneys diminishes by more than 50 percent. The number of functional units (nephrons) is reduced with age, and there is loss of both glomeruli and collecting tubules.

Among endocrine changes, gonadal deterioration is one of the most constant and inevitable marks of aging. In women the onset of menopause marks the end of the reproductive period; this happens long before aging effects are evident in other organs or tissues. In the male, while sexual vigor diminishes, it has been shown to persist much longer than was formerly believed. The basal metabolic rate falls slowly with age, and this, combined with the reduced activity of elderly individuals, predisposes to weight gain unless dietary intake is reduced appropriately.

The cytological events leading to death of nondividing cells are poorly understood. Accumulation of lipofuscin in the cytoplasm of these cells is a constant phenomenon of sufficient predictability that it can be used as a reliable index of cytological age. Called wear-and-tear pigment, lipochrome, or lipofuscin, these yellow granules form in the cytoplasm of nerve and muscle cells, being derived in all probability from lysosomes or possibly mitochondria. Simultaneously with their formation the cell diminishes in volume, the nucleus becomes smaller, and histological stains reveal a depletion of oxidative as well as phosphorylative enzymes.

It also has been shown in tissue culture that fibroblasts from a human infant divide about 50 times; those from a 20-year-old person, about 30 times; and those from an 80-year-old person, about 20 times. Toward the end of the life cycle chromosomal aberration and peculiarities of cell division begin to appear. What underlies the diminishing capacity of cells to divide? Studies imply that the secret of aging in dividing cells probably relates to an obscure degeneration of inherited information-containing molecules in the cell nucleus which provide the final control of cell division.

The seemingly endless list of diseases found in the elderly at autopsy reflects the effects of both disease and age. But the latter effects, being relatively inapparent, are often overlooked, which is the reason one is so often prompted to ask during the autopsy of an elderly person, "What was the cause of death?" At this point one can also ask, "Is aging as inevitable as it appears? Can the immutable running down of cells and their increasing disposition to neoplastic change be altered?" These are some of the basic biological considerations that await solution. Until answers are obtained, physicians responsible for the care of elderly patients must be satisfied with the attainment of lesser objectives. They must reach an understanding of the common diseases of the senium with an idea of modifying the rate of progress through the application of appropriate physical, psychological, and pharmacological intervention.

4 PROBLEM-ORIENTED MEDICAL RECORD

STEPHEN E. GOLDFINGER
JAMES J. DINEEN

Whatever can be said, can be said clearly.
Whereof one cannot speak, thereof one ought remain silent.
Ludwig Wittgenstein

Medical records, as kept for years, have often failed the purposes of lucid communication, education, and rapid retrieval of stored information. Poorly supported diagnoses, incomplete progress notes, chaotically entered laboratory results, and inadequately expressed plans of management are embarrassingly common findings in records existing at some of the most sophisticated medical institutions. In response to this, the Problem-Oriented Medical Record (POMR) has been devised to provide a method whereby the medical record will better reflect the health problems of patients and the professional responses to them on the part of physicians, nurses, and other major participants in care.

Central to its formulation is the view that the patient's record must be designed so that it expresses specifically what physicians deal with most frequently—the *problems* of patients. While the ultimate goal of clinical taxonomy is directed toward identification of etiology, pathology, and pathologic physiology, in view of their importance as guides to therapy, it would be both unrealistic and dangerous to require a specific diagnosis for a severely dyspneic patient in the absence of reasonably convincing information concerning the reason for his dyspnea. Until the cause can be established, all diagnostic modalities and therapeutic interventions are oriented to the real and immediate problem—*dyspnea.* The same is true of a great variety of symptoms, signs, and laboratory findings which are derived in the process of patient care. A high serum calcium reported in an SMA screening study, a suspicious pigmented skin lesion, or a sudden unexplained deterioration of intellect are examples of worrisome findings that are most appropriately expressed, initially, as *problems.* In each instance, a more refined diagnosis in the absence of further data can only represent guesswork; hence, it may be wrong. As data pertaining to each problem become available, the problem may then be expressed at a higher level of understanding, i.e., hyperparathyroidism, malignant melanoma, or subdural hematoma. By offering the physician a system of record keeping compatible with the most frequent focus of attention in the practice of medicine—the problem—an opportunity is provided to reduce distortion and error.

The second and more fundamental aspect of problem orientation is the systematized display of patient care embodied in records. This is best described by considering the elements of medical care and their dynamic interrelationship, as proposed by Weed (Fig. 4-1).

THE DATA BASE All clinical care must start with a data base. A careful and complete history and a physical examination are of fundamental value to the physician. The POMR stresses the importance of this traditional approach to data collection. However, there may be instances when full information is unobtainable as, for example, in the case of an unidentified unconscious patient brought into the emergency room. His management is nevertheless contingent on data, even though incomplete—primarily the initial physical examination, lumbar puncture, and laboratory results. At the other extreme, one might safely argue that no data base can be absolutely complete on any patient, for a lifetime of psychic and biological events can never be fully recalled, much less transcribed. The POMR brings into focus a defined data base, highlights its deficiencies, and serves as the nucleus for its expansion when desirable. Elements of the data base include:

1 Identifying information (i.e., name, age, sex, race, religion, insurance information, etc.)
2 Patient profile (i.e., occupation, education, marital status, children, hobbies, worries, moods, sleep patterns, habits, etc.)
3 Medical history
  a Chief complaints
  b History of present illnesses
  c Past medical history
  d Review of systems
  e Family history
  f Medications
4 Physical examination
5 Laboratory data and physiologic tests (i.e., complete blood count, electrocardiogram, chest x-ray, creatinine, urinalysis, vital capacity, tonometry, etc.)

It is evident that these components do not constitute anything new to conscientious physicians. In using the POMR, they are asked to *define* the data base and to highlight the abnormalities revealed by it as *problems* with which they must deal. Admittedly, an *ideal* data base has not yet been conceived. Such a construct would depend in part on the population served, the resources at hand, and, most importantly, on the relative cost-benefit of various screening studies in regard to prevention of morbidity. Studies of the value of such tests in these terms may lead to the development of a series of risk-related data bases, each applicable to different groups of individuals. Material obtained for each part of the data base is often organized in the record by standardized formats for display. Although some rather sophisticated examples of such data sheets have been designed, it must be emphasized that the ultimate value of a data base depends on the validity of the information that is entered. An inaccurate history, careless examination of the heart, or a faulty piece of laboratory equipment will yield inaccurate data no matter how clearly the results are recorded. Moreover, it should be recognized that the data base must constantly be supplemented by later entries into the record.

FIGURE 4-1

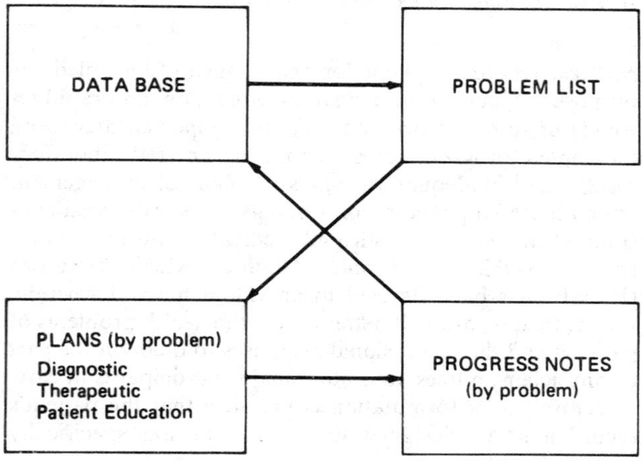

THE PROBLEM LIST From the data at hand, a Master Problem List is formulated. It should include those features in the patient's psychobiological makeup that require continuing attention by the physician and other members of the health team. Thus, the Problem List may contain entries relating to social history (e.g., marital discord), risk factors (e.g., familial polyposis of the colon), symptoms (e.g., hemoptysis), physical findings (e.g., splenomegaly), laboratory tests (e.g., anemia), etc. All problems are expressed at a level of highest understanding. For example, if the cause of gastrointestinal bleeding is known to be a duodenal ulcer, the latter becomes the appropriate entry, unless severe bleeding in itself constitutes a major health hazard.

The Problem List is a *dynamic* entity which is altered as

PROBLEM LIST

No.	Active	Date	Inactive	Date
1	Hypertension	1953		
2	Recurrent bronchitis	1958		
3	Penicillin allergy	1958		
4			S/P pyelonephritis	1960
5	Gallstones	Oct 1975	resolved → Cholecystectomy	Mar 1976
6	Arthralgias	Mar 1976	resolved → #9	June 1976
7	Pleurisy	Mar 1976	resolved → #9	June 1976
8	Proteinuria	Apr 1976	resolved → #9	June 1976
9	SLE	Jun 1976		
10	Unemployment	Nov 1976		

FIGURE 4-2

new information and events dictate. All entries are dated, and a separate column permits the recording of resolved and inactive problems (Fig. 4-2).

When kept in this manner, a Problem List featured at the beginning of a patient record provides a succinct summary of all important health matters and, moreover, serves as a table of contents for entries within the record which are properly labeled according to problem (see below). Satisfactory problem listing clearly requires periodic revision of this inventory. Also necessary is a sense of proportion, so that a variety of minor, self-limited problems (e.g., colds, sprains, minor gastrointestinal upsets) are excluded from the Master Problem List, which might otherwise be unduly cluttered with trivial illnesses. When a number of clearly psychosomatic complaints predominate, they may be grouped together as a single entry, e.g., "Functional Symptoms."

PROBLEM-RELATED PLANS Problems regarded as "active" generally require planning for their proper management. The display of these plans, separately listed for each problem, is of critical importance as a reflection of the physician's response to the problems that have been identified. Plans are recorded under three categories:

1 *Diagnostic:* i.e., laboratory tests, radiological studies, consultations, continued observation, etc.
2 *Therapeutic:* i.e., medications, diet, physiotherapy, corrective surgery, etc.
3 *Patient Education:* i.e., instruction of the patient in various aspects of self-care, education regarding the goal of therapy, the prognosis that has been given to him, etc.

It is not necessary that all three sections be completed for each problem, inasmuch as planning may at times be concerned with only one or two of them. For example:

1 Diarrhea
Dx Stool for occult blood, culture, ova, and parasites, microscopic fat, and muscle fibers
Sigmoidoscopy
Barium enema if persistent
Rx Avoid foods that exacerbate
Propantheline 30 mg 3 i.d.
Pt.Ed. Informed that more information is needed to make a diagnosis, will aim for symptomatic therapy for now

2 Pyuria
Dx BUN
Repeat urinalysis
Urine culture

3 Obesity
Rx 1500 kcal diet
Weight Watchers
Pt.Ed. Dangers of obesity cited. *Goal:* 170 lb

PROGRESS NOTES Progress notes are structured on the basis of those problems which have received attention during the office or hospital visit. (Thus, all problems on the list need not be entered.) In a sense, these notes update the course and management of the problem, following the same general schema already described. They are structured in the following manner:

#Problem
Subjective(S): Interval history
Adherence to program
Objective(O): Physical findings
Reports of laboratory, x-ray, other tests
Assessment(A): Appraisal of progress, interpretation of new findings, etc.
Plan(P):
Diagnostic:
Therapeutic:
Patient Education:

Example:
#3 RHD with mitral stenosis
S: 2 flight dyspnea, mild fatigue. No orthopnea, hemoptysis, ankle edema. Child has strep throat.
Meds: chlorothiazide 500 mg q.d.
O: B. P. 120/70 P. 78 regular.
Neck veins normal, lungs clear.
Grade iii diastolic rumble, wide opening snap. P_2 slightly ↑.
EKG: Early P mitrale, otherwise normal.
A: Stable. Catheterization still not indicated. Risk of strep throat present.
P:
Dx: Cardiac fluoroscopy
Rx: Continue chlorothiazide and penicillin V 250 mg b.i.d.—2 weeks
Pt.Ed: Reinstructed about antibiotic coverage for tooth extractions, scheduled for next month. (Will contact oral surgeon.)

DATA FLOW SHEETS At times, the course and management of a particular problem may be succinctly recorded by using data flow sheets. Many physicians are familiar with this method of making brief-interval record entries on patients with diabetic ketoacidosis or acute gastrointestinal hemorrhage. A number of other conditions—both acute and chronic—lend themselves to this manner of sequential description. Data flow sheets for such problems as hypertension, renal failure, and respiratory insufficiency serve as excellent adjuncts to effective patient care within the POMR.

CLINICAL JUDGMENT This intangible element of patient care is so crucial that it is cited to emphasize that the style of recording in itself is no guarantee of excellence. The *content* of the record—the problems selected from the data base, the nature of the plans evolved, the choice of therapeutic programs—reflects the true quality of the care provided. In this respect, the initials "C. J." might appropriately be placed alongside every arrow in Fig. 4-1 to represent the absolute need for clinical judgment to effectively catalyze the process of sound medical care.

POTENTIAL BENEFITS OF THE PROBLEM-ORIENTED MEDICAL RECORD **Allied health personnel** Several aspects of the POMR facilitate the team approach to patient care. First, the requirement that all members of the health team systematically display their thoughts and actions improves communications and potentiates supervision. Second, the existence of a list of the patient's problems that the health team must manage reduces errors of omission and treatment out of context. Furthermore, the establishment of a plan for each problem leads to clearer assignment of specific tasks to each of its members. Most importantly, the dissection of the health care process into gathering a data base, formulating problems, and designing a plan for the management of each problem provides a useful road map for the intelligent expansion of the role of various allied health personnel. This breakdown helps physicians as team leaders to rethink their role in the health care process and concentrate on the more difficult aspects such as identifying problems from the data base and organizing approaches to these problems, while assigning more routine tasks to other members of the team. Practical experiences in clinical settings as varied as large hospital clinics and rural offices have suggested the value of the POMR in the team approach to patient care.

Education and audit In addition to facilitating patient care, a good medical record should educate its readers and also be subject to audit in its own right. By clearly outlining the physician's logic, the POMR reveals the process of patient care in a manner which can be evaluated. This, in itself, is an educational process. It deemphasizes rote memory and substitutes a record of the logical steps which are being taken to recognize the patient's problems and the physician's capacity to act as a guide in attempting to solve them. Such an endeavor, if begun early, can set the stage for a lifelong educational process of self and peer evaluation through effective record audit.

Clinical research Any record system that clarifies the details of patient-physician interaction can be a powerful tool in clinical research. A clear data base, an organized system for record entries, and the use of data flow sheets serve to facilitate rapid extraction and analysis of clinical information. Efforts to computerize the POMR, if successful, will amass a spectrum of clinical and epidemiologic data that may prove extremely valuable in our understanding of illness and the process of health care.

THE ROLE OF THE POMR IN PATIENT CARE The POMR is a system of record keeping which greatly facilitates data retrieval and at the same time highlights the decision-making role of physicians as they respond to the problems of patients. It should be evident, nevertheless, that it can only serve the goal of improved health care when it is used with a sound intellectual appreciation of disease, based on a full understanding of pathophysiology and a scientific approach to therapy. The tendency for the POMR to compartmentalize problems must not preclude creative, synthetic thinking. At some institutions an Initial Assessment entry is placed before the Problem List to provide an opportunity for the physician to express an overall perspective and to distinguish the major problems from others which are less important. Finally, as emphasized in the preceding chapters, compassion is an element of medical care that can never be adequately displayed by any record system. A possible danger of the POMR is that the emotional needs of patients may receive even less attention by the busy physician who is intent on writing excellent notes. The patient and not the record must remain the primary focus of physician care.

REFERENCES

BJORN JC, CROSS HD: *Problem Oriented Practice,* Chicago: Modern Hospital Press, McGraw-Hill Publications Company, 1970

FEINSTEIN AR: The problems of the "problem-oriented medical record." Ann Int Med 78:751, 1973

GOLDFINGER SE: The problem-oriented record: A critique from a believer. N Engl J Med 288:606, 1973

HURST W, WALKER HK: *The Problem Oriented System.* New York: Medcom Press, 1972

WEED LL: *Medical Records, Medical Education and Patient Care.* Cleveland: Case University Press, 1969

PART TWO | CARDINAL MANIFESTATIONS AND APPROACH TO DISEASE

section 1 | Pain

5
GENERAL CONSIDERATIONS

RAYMOND D. ADAMS

Pain, it has been said, is one of "Nature's earliest signs of morbidity." Few will deny that it stands preeminent among all the sensory experiences by which man judges the existence of disease within himself. There are relatively few maladies that do not have their painful phases, and in many of them pain is a characteristic without which diagnosis must always be in doubt. It seems appropriate, therefore, to begin a section on the cardinal manifestations of disease with a discussion of the more general aspects of pain.

The painful experiences of the sick pose manifold problems for practitioners of medicine, and students should know something of these problems in order to prepare themselves for the task ahead. They must be ready to diagnose disease in patients who have felt only the first rumblings of discomfort, before other symptoms and signs of disease have appeared. To cope effectively with problems of this type requires a sound knowledge of the sensory supply of the viscera and a familiarity with the typical symptoms of many diseases. They will be consulted by some patients who seek treatment for pains that appear to have no obvious structural basis, and further inquiry will disclose that worry, fear, and other troubled emotional states may have aggrandized relatively minor aches and pains. To understand problems of this type requires insight into the psychologic factors which influence behavior and a knowledge of psychiatric disease. Next, they must manage the "difficult pain cases," in which no amount of investigation will bring to light either medical disease or psychiatric illness, and it is here that they will sense the need of a sound and assured clinical approach to the pain problem. Finally, they must care for the patients with intractable pain, often from an established and incurable disease, who demand relief either by drug or by the "less moderate means of surgery." Assessing the possibilities of the latter requires a comprehension of the anatomic pathways of pain.

END ORGANS, AFFERENT TRACTS, AND NUCLEI OF TERMINATION OF PAIN PATHWAYS Pain is a sensation which has its own sensory apparatus. The receptors in the skin and deep structures are fine, freely branching nerve endings which form an intricate network throughout the body. A single primary pain neuron with its cell body in the posterior root ganglion subdivides into many small peripheral branches to supply an area of skin of several square millimeters. The cutaneous area of each neuron overlaps with those of other neurons, so that every spot of skin lies within the domain of two to four neurons. These freely branching nerve endings are also found in many of the other specialized sensory receptors in the skin, such as the Krause end bulbs, the Ruffinian plumes, the Pacinian corpuscles, which may explain why the extremes of hot, cold, and pressure sensation become painful. Free nerve endings may also serve as receptors for other types of sensation. They are the only end organ in the cornea, where touch and temperature as well as pain are felt.

The sensory nerve fibers for pain, as they course through somatic and visceral nerves, are mixed with other sensory and motor fibers. All sensory fibers enter the spinal cord through the posterior roots and enter the brainstem through certain of the cranial nerves. The pain fibers are of two sizes, one very small (2 to 4 μm in diameter), called *C fibers* with a slow conducting velocity, the other somewhat larger (6 to 8 μm), called *A-delta fibers,* with more rapid transmission rates. As the posterior root enters the spinal cord, it separates into two divisions, medial and lateral. The medial division, heavily myelinated, synapses either with large secondary sensory neurons in the posterior horn or with anterior horn cells (serving segmental reflexes), or it passes upward in the posterior columns to the medulla. The lateral division, of thinly myelinated and nonmyelinated fibers, enters the substantia gelatinosa, where it synapses with (1) many small neurons whose axons pass into the posterior and anterior horns of the same and adjacent segments of the spinal cord, also effecting reflex connections, and (2) large secondary sensory neurons some of which will form the lateral spinothalamic tract and others ascend near the gray matter. The neurons on which the afferent root fibers terminate lie in the first and fifth laminae of the posterior horn, and it is postulated that their reactivity is influenced by large afferent touch fibers or by other inhibitory neurons within the spinal gray matter. Through a mechanism still rather obscure two secondary ascending pathways for pain are activated. One is the lateral spinothalamic tract, the cell bodies of which lie in the posterior horns, with axons crossing through the anterior commissure of the spinal cord within one to two segments of the level of entry. The other is a less well-defined, multineuronal chain which extends upward along the reticular part of the gray matter. The lateral spinothalamic tract, joined in the brainstem by the trigeminothalamic tract, courses through the lateral part of the medulla, pons, and midbrain, giving off many collaterals before terminating in the nucleus ventralis posterolateralis and probably in other thalamic nuclei as well (Fig. 5-1). The reticular chain of neurons extends cephalad and finally makes connections through the interlaminar nuclei of the thalamus with the limbic portions of the cerebrum.

The secondary spinothalamic and trigeminothalamic tracts synapse with the tertiary sensory neurons of the thalamus, whose axons extend to the cortex of the parietal lobe. Physiologists are not agreed as to the cortical terminus for the pain fibers, for electrical stimulation of the cortex in the conscious human being seldom produces a painful sensation, and parietal lobe lesions seldom cause central pain. Most of the pain fibers from the periphery cross to the opposite side of the brain; only a small contingent remains ipsilateral.

Segmental innervation As a means of quick orientation to the anatomy of the peripheral pain pathways, it should be remembered that the facial structures and anterior cranium lie in the field of the trigeminal nerves; the back of the head, second cervical; the neck, third cervical; epaulet area, fourth cervical; deltoid area, fifth cervical, radial forearm and thumb, sixth cervical; index finger, seventh cervical; middle finger, eighth cervical; little finger and inner forearm, first thoracic; nipple segment, fifth thoracic; umbilical, tenth thoracic; groin, first lumbar; medial side of knee, third lumbar; great toe, fifth lumbar; little toe, first sacral; back of thigh, second sacral; genitosacral areas, third, fourth, and fifth sacral. The first to fourth thoracic nerve roots are the important sensory pathways for the intrathoracic viscera; the sixth to eighth thoracic, for the upper abdominal organs (Fig. 21-1).

PHYSIOLOGY AND PSYCHOLOGY OF PAIN The stimuli that arouse pain vary for each tissue. Generally the adequate stimuli for skin are those which injure tissue, i.e., pricking, cutting, crushing, burning, and freezing. Interestingly, these same forms of stimulation have little effect when applied to the stomach and intestine. Pain in the gastrointestinal tract is produced instead by local trauma of an engorged or inflamed mucosa, distention or spasm of smooth muscle, and traction on the mesenteric attachment. Pain is induced in skeletal muscles by ischemia (the basis for the condition known as intermittent claudication), as well as by tears of connective tissue sheaths, necrosis, hemorrhage, or the injection of irritating solutions. Prolonged contraction of muscles evokes an aching type of pain. Ischemia, the only proved source of pain in the heart muscle, is responsible for angina pectoris and for the pain of myocardial infarction. Joints are insensitive to pricking, cutting, and cautery, but pain is induced in the synovial membrane by hypertonic saline solution and inflammation. Arteries give rise to pain when pierced with a needle, when induced to pulsate excessively (as in migraine), and in certain diseases of their walls such as exemplified by atherosclerotic thrombosis and arteritis of cranial arteries. Traction and displacement of intracranial vessels and the meningeal structures by which they are supported may cause headache.

In these painful lesions which damage tissues, irritating substances are believed to be liberated and to stimulate nerve endings. Acetylcholine, 5-hydroxytryptamine, histamine, bradykinin, and other similar polypeptides or acid metabolites released by tissue injury have been found to elicit pain when injected intraarterially or applied to the base of a blister. Such substances are viewed as the "mediators" for pain.

The sensory experiences resulting from these several modes of stimulation in the skin and in deep skeletomuscular and visceral structures differ in quality. Integumentary stimuli, at the lowest levels of intensity, evoke sensations of touch, pressure, warmth, cold, or tickle. When increased to the point approaching tissue destruction, pain is added, and the resulting experience is thereafter a mixed one. The painful experience itself is one of pricking or burning. The threshold for burning pain from a thermal stimulus is approximately 2,000 times the threshold for warmth. This relationship of pain to tissue destruction is the basis of a biologic principle—that pain has a protective, or self-preserving, value to the organism.

The threshold for the perception of pain, i.e., the lowest intensity of stimulus recognized as pain, is approximately the same in all persons. It is lowered by inflammation and raised by local anesthetics (e.g., procaine), lesions of the nervous system, and centrally acting analgesic drugs. Distraction and suggestion, by turning attention away from the painful part, reduce the awareness of and the response to pain. Strong emotion (fear or rage) suppresses pain. Neurotic patients in general have the same pain threshold as normal subjects, but their reaction may be excessive or abnormal. The pain threshold of a frontal lobotomized subject is also unchanged, but he reacts little if at all to his pain. The degree of emotional reaction and the verbalization (complaint) also vary with the personality and character of the patient.

Superficial pain Sensory impulses subserving pricking pain, being transmitted by larger pain fibers, have a more rapid rate of conductivity to the nervous system than burning pain. A hot needle applied to the toe, for example, produces a quick, pricking pain and, only 1 to 2 s later, a burning pain. Together they constitute the "double response" of Lewis. Ischemia of nerve, by the application of a tourniquet to a limb, abolishes pricking pain before burning pain. Both types of dermal pain are localized with precision ("local sign"), made possible by the overlap of sensory neurons. Analgesia means the interruption of all pain neurons to an area, and hypalgesia, the interruption of only part of them.

Visceral pain Deep pain (including that of visceral and skeletal structures) has basically the quality of aching, but if intense may be sharp and penetrating ("knifelike"). Occasionally there is a burning type of pain, as in the heartburn of esophageal irritation and rarely in angina pectoris. The pain is felt as being deep to the body surface. The double response is absent, localization is poor, and the margins of the pain are not well delineated, presumably because of the paucity of nerve endings in viscera.

Actually, the pain originating in deep skeletomuscular and visceral structures cannot be localized closer than two to three sensory segments. For example, pain from myocardial disease is felt to arise within the first to fourth or possibly fifth thoracic segments (see Fig. 5-1, showing theoretic distribution of heart pain). Unfortunately, from the standpoint of diagnosis, these spinal segments also receive sensory fibers from other structures—the esophagus, mediastinal contents, bones, muscles, etc.—and diseases of these structures may cause pain that is difficult to distinguish from cardiac pain.

Deep musculoskeletal pain Since deep skeletal pain and visceral pain are mediated through a common deep sensory system, it is not surprising that their characteristics (type, localization, and referral) should be similar. Kellgren has mapped the topography of muscle and tendinous pain by injecting a few milliliters of normal saline solution into the various muscles and noting the location of induced pain. The ache is usually segmental and may spread one to two segments above (less often below) the site injected. A tear or injury in a lumbar muscle may give rise to a pain which, in quality and localization, including radiation into the groin and scrotum, is indistinguishable from the pain of renal colic. A hemorrhage into the right upper rectus muscle mimics the pain of gallbladder colic; and a lesion in a muscle or ligament deep in the chest wall causes pain referred to the left arm, like that of angina. The differentiation of these pains must be made on grounds other than location and reference.

Referred pain Deep visceral and somatic pains tend always to be referred superficially to those structures within a given spinal segment that have the most extensive nerve ramifications and therefore the widest cerebral representation (e.g., there are more sensory nerves in the integument than in the viscera, hence the pain in the latter is projected to the body surface). In the case of myocardial pain, sensory impulses entering the first to fourth thoracic nerves activate a pool of sensory neurons, the largest number of which also receive afferents from the skin of the inner side of the arm ($T_{1\text{-}2}$) and the anterior precordium ($T_{3\text{-}4}$). More of the sensory neurons from the heart enter the left side of the spinal cord than the right. These anatomic and physiologic data explain why cardiac pain is referred predominantly to the substernal, left precordial, and inner brachial zones.

Aberrant reference of pain occurs not infrequently and is explained in terms of the physiologic status of the spinal pool of sensory neurons. As was stated, a single sensory neuron entering one spinal root presynaptically depolarizes to a varying degree a pool of spinal neurons over four or five spinal segments. Pain then should spread to segments adjacent to the painful lesion, where it also causes cutaneous hyperesthesia and, by activating motor neurons, involuntary muscle contraction. If some preexistent disease in *adjacent* somatic segments has already partially depolarized the spinal pool of sensory neurons, a new painful disease which will further depolarize them causes the pain to spread to them. For example, if gallbladder disease, which activates sensory fibers entering at the sixth to eighth thoracic nerve, or cervical arthritis (at the second to eighth cervical nerve) was present before a myocardial infarct, the cardiac pain may then be referred to the upper part of the abdomen or neck. Generally these aberrant referrals occur in segments that are cephalad to the normal segmental distribution of pain because their inhibitory connections are more abundant than those of caudal ones.

Hyperesthesia, hyperalgesia, hyperpathia, involuntary spasms, and other responses It has been customary to use the first two of these terms to designate a lowering of the threshold to touch and pain stimuli and the third for a state of pain with a normal or raised threshold but overreaction. The latter may even occur with anesthesia, as in

FIGURE 5-1
Radiation and sites of reference of cardiac pain (upper), *gallbladder pain* (lower).

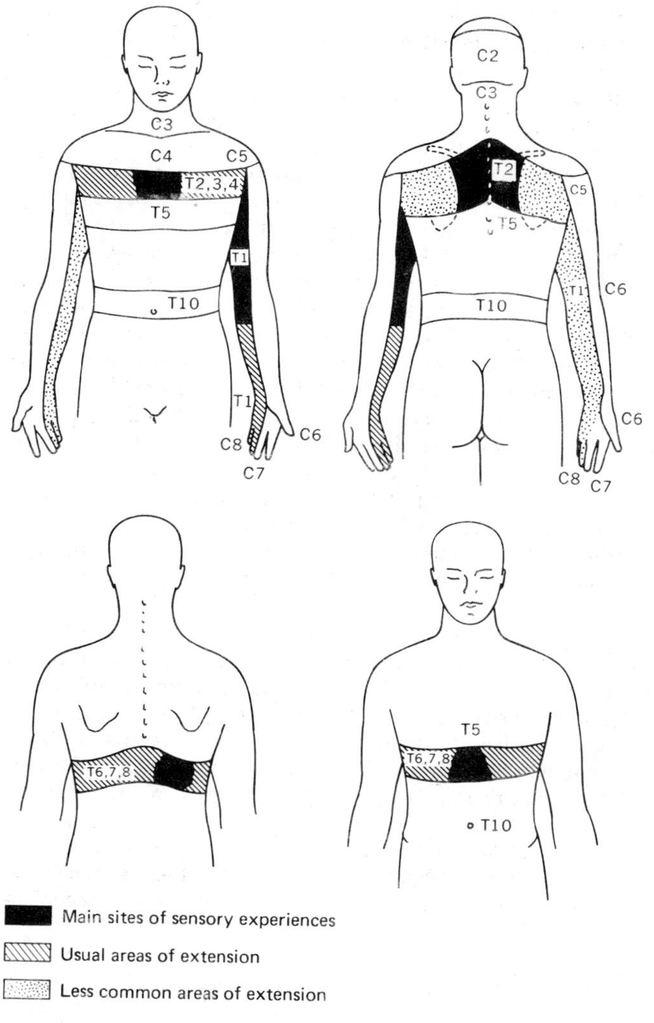

anesthesia dolorosa. Any real distinction between these states is ephemeral. Probably only with inflammation of the skin is the pain threshold consistently lowered. What is most characteristic of all chronically painful states, and these frequently implicate nerves or central nervous structures, is that the part is unusually sensitive to all stimuli, even those which normally do not evoke pain; and the elicited pain is unnatural, radiant, outlasts the initiating stimulus, and is unusually modifiable by fatigue, emotion, etc. One sees listed here many of the characteristics of causalgia, spinal cord pain, phantom pain, zoster neuralgia, thalamic pain, etc. The explanation currently offered for these states is that at the peripheral as well as the central level the system of pain fibers is no longer in equilibrium with other sensory fibers. A kind of inhibition is exerted on the pain system at all times by the small neurons in the substantia gelatinosa, under the control of other afferent as well as descending pathways. Since the largest afferent peripheral nerve fibers suppress the secondary spinal neurons receiving pain impulses, nerve injury, which tends often to destroy some of the larger fibers, then permits their over-response. According to Melzack and Wall, the small neurons of the substantia gelatinosa constitute a kind of "gate control system," which modulates input. The activation of large afferent fibers in a peripheral nerve is said to inhibit the gateway cells. While much of the recent physiological evidence has failed to confirm this gateway hypothesis, it has called attention to some type of mechanism that controls the pain threshold and painful states. Some such segmental mechanism must also be under the influence of descending pathways from the cerebrum and from other spinal segments. One might suppose that the activation of some of the sensory fibers controlling "gateway neurons" could be the basis of the effectiveness of *acupuncture,* though the psychological mechanism of suggestion is more likely. There is a wide range of responses to pain to which attention is drawn. Strong, acute pain causes a startle reaction. Intense, persistent pain is usually accompanied by segment-flexion reflexes (e.g., spasm of a segment of the abdominal wall with visceral disease, flexion of knees and hips with peritoneal irritation, extension of neck with meningitis), autonomic responses, postural adjustments, avoidance movements, and vocalization. The obvious biologic function of segmental spasms is to splint the diseased part and to facilitate healing. The altered state of receptivity of the spinal gray matter accounts for stimuli of nonreceptive-type evoking pain, e.g., for subcutaneous pressure being painful.

As pain sensation may be induced by stimulation of the receptors or by irritation of peripheral nerves or roots, it may be abolished by diseases which affect the peripheral or central nervous system, or by a surgical procedure which accomplishes the same result. Pain in a circumscribed region may be terminated by section of the nerve which supplies that region (neurotomy) or by section of the spinal roots (posterior rhizotomy); pain in a limb or one side of the trunk may be abolished by section of the anterolateral spinothalamic tracts (lateral spinal tractotomy in the spinal cord or tractotomy in the lateral medulla or mesencephalon).

Perception of pain Only upon the arrival of pain impulses at the thalamocortical level of the nervous system is there conscious awareness of the pain stimulus. Clinical study has not informed us of the exact localization of the nervous apparatus for this mental process. It is not entirely abolished by a total hemispherectomy, including the thalamus on one side. It is often said that impulses reaching the thalamus create awareness of the attributes of sensation and that the parietal cortex is necessary for the appreciation of the intensity and localization of the sensation. This seems to be an oversimplification. Probably a close and harmonious relationship between thalamus and cortex must exist in order for a sensory experience to be complete. The traditional separation of sensation (in this instance awareness of pain) and perception (awareness of the nature of the painful stimulus) has been abandoned in favor of the view that sensation, perception, and the various conscious and unconscious responses to a pain stimulus comprise an indivisible process.

Although similar to other sensory or perceptive phenomena in certain respects, such as predictable response to given intensity of stimulus, pain differs in other ways. One of its most remarkable characteristics is the strong feeling tone, or affect, with which it is endowed, nearly always one of unpleasantness. Furthermore, pain does not appear to be subject to negative adaptation. Most stimuli, if applied continuously, soon cease to be effective, whereas pain may persist as long as the stimulus is operative; and, by establishing a central excitatory state, may even outlast the stimulus.

Stereotaxic surgery on the thalamus in cases of intractable pain permits dissection of the anatomy of the pain experience. Lesions in the terminus of the lateral spinothalamic tract in the posterolateral nucleus are said to abolish pain and temperature sensation in the contralateral side of the body while leaving the patient with all his misery or affect of pain. Lesions in the centrum medianum relieve the painful state without altering pain and temperature sensation. Thus, at this level there must also be a balance of inhibitory and facilitatory sensory systems, for one cannot explain intractable pain simply in terms of continuous stimulation of chains of pain neurons.

Psychologic aspects of pain A discussion of this problem could hardly be complete without some reference to the influence of emotional states or to the importance of racial, cultural, and religious factors on the pain response, especially its overt expressions. It is common knowledge that some individuals, by virtue of training, habit, or phlegmatic character, are relatively stoical and that others are excessively responsive to pain. And there are rare individuals who are totally incapable of experiencing pain throughout their lifetime, either from a lack of sensory endings or peripheral sensory apparatus, or from some peculiarity of central reception.

Lastly, it is important to keep in mind the devastating effects of chronic pain. As Ambroise Paré remarked, "There is nothing that abateth so much the strength as paine." Continuous pain can be observed to have an adverse effect on the entire nervous system. There are increased irritability, fatigue, troubled sleep, poor appetite, and loss of emotional stability. Courageous men are reduced to a whimpering, pitiable state that may arouse only the scorn of a healthy person. They are irrational about illness and may make unreasonable demands on family and physician. This condition, which may be termed *pain shock,* once established, requires delicate but firm management. Depression (reactive?) is common. Of course, demand for and dependency on narcotic drugs often complicates the picture.

CLINICAL APPROACH TO THE PATIENT WITH PAIN AS THE PREDOMINANT SYMPTOM One of the first points to keep in mind is that not all pain is the consequence of serious disease. Otherwise healthy individuals have thousands of pains which are part of their daily sensory experience. To mention but a few, there is the momentary, hard pain over an eye, in the temporal region, or in the ear or jaw, which strikes with alarming suddenness; the more persistent ache which arises in some fleshy part, such as the shoulder, neck, thigh, or calf, the darting pain in an arm or leg, the fleeting precordial discomfort that arouses momentarily the thought of heart disease, the breathtaking catch in the side, the cluster of abdominal pains with their associated intestinal rumblings, and the brief discomfort upon movement of a joint. These *normal pains,* as they should be called, occur at all ages, tend to be brief, and depart as obscurely as they come. They acquire medical significance only when elicited by an inquiring physician, or when presented as a complaint by a worried patient; and, of course, they must always be distinguished from the *abnormal pains* of disease.

When pain, by its intensity, duration, and the circumstance of its occurrence, appears to be abnormal or constitutes one of the principal symptoms of disease, an attempt should be made to reach a tentative decision as to its cause and the mechanism of its production. This can usually be accomplished by a thorough interrogation of the patient, in which he is encouraged to relate as accurately as possible the main characteristics of the pain and the circumstances under which it occurs. The physical examination is directed toward a search for evidences of suspected disease and the reproduction of the pain.

Location of pain When the pain is caused by a superficial lesion, the cause and effect are usually so obvious that no problem is posed. It is the deep lesion, whether involving somatic or visceral structures, that causes trouble, and here exact localization becomes especially important. We have already seen that the pain originating from such tissues is no longer sensed as coming from them, but is instead only roughly segmental, i.e., within the territory of the cord segments innervating the structure. The identification of the segments involved is of value, for it sets the limit on the diagnostic possibilities that must be considered, i.e., they are limited to those structures having a corresponding innervation. Thus an epigastric or subxiphoid pain, or one in the opposite region in the back, obliges one to search for its cause in all those structures innervated by the sixth through eighth thoracic cord segments, i.e., the esophagus, stomach, duodenum, pancreas, biliary tract, the upper retroperitoneal structures, as well as the deep somatic tissues in this region. Also, one must consider the possibility that a lesion in a viscus innervated by spinal segments above or below the sixth through eighth thoracic cord segments may at times be the source of pain that has spread outside its normal boundaries and involved the epigastrium (Fig. 5-1).

Provoking and relieving factors These factors are of greater value than quality of pain in providing important data concerning its mechanism. Pain related to breathing, swallowing, and defecation focuses attention on the respiratory apparatus, the esophagus, and the lower part of the intestinal tract, respectively. A pain coming on a few minutes after the beginning of general bodily movement and relieved almost at once by rest indicates ischemia or a neural mechanism as the probable cause (see Chaps. 9 and 10). Pain occurring several hours after meals and relieved by food or alkali suggests the irritative effect of acid on the raw lining of the stomach or duodenum. Pain that is brought on or relieved by certain movements or postures of parts of the body is usually due to diseased skeletal structures (bones, muscles, ligaments). Pain that is enhanced by cough, sneeze, and strain is usually radicular in origin or arises in ligamentous structures. Pain that is increased or altered by cutaneous stimuli is due to disease in sensory tracts in the peripheral or central nervous system.

Quality and time-intensity characteristics of pain Much reliance is put on the patient's choice of words and his account of the intensity of pain. Unfortunately this will depend, in part at least, on his intelligence, his vocabulary, and on what he imagines is taking place. "Crushing" and "squeezing" are commonly employed to describe an anginal pain, and this implication of pressure has some significance, since the pain may depend on an associated involuntary contraction of the pectoral muscles. Another patient with the same disease, however, may describe the pain as "exploding" or "burning." Far more important than the adjective used for pain is the information that it is steady and does not fluctuate. Similarly, the pain of peptic ulcer is frequently designated as "gnawing," but again, the deep, steady quality is more important than the word used to denote it. Gallbladder colic and renal colic are misnomers, if by colic is meant a "paroxysmal abdominal pain due to spasm, obstruction, or distention of any of the hollow viscera." *In both these disorders, the pain tends to be steady.* The aching quality of all deep pains is usually characteristic, but there are also several other informative attributes. A true colicky pain, one that is rhythmic and cramping, suggests an obstructive lesion in a hollow viscus. If the patient is a woman and has had children, it is a good idea to ask whether her "cramp" resembles the pains she had during childbirth. A pain that is steady and varies little or not at all from moment to moment means that the stimulus to pain is steady and unwavering, as in angina pectoris and peptic ulcer. Thus, a pain in the anterior midsternal region whose intensity fluctuates appreciably within the space of a minute or two is not due to angina, even though the history may appear to suggest a relation to exertion. Similarly, a high epigastric pain appearing several hours after a meal and even apparently relieved by food is not caused by an ulcer if the pain fluctuates perceptibly within seconds or a few minutes. The stimulus to ulcer pain does not quickly vary in intensity. A throbbing pain indicates that an arterial pulsation is giving rise to painful stimuli. Sharp, recurrent stabs of pain are caused by disease of nerve roots or sensory ganglions, as exemplified by tic douloureux or tabes, or a single episode may be due to a tear of a muscle or ligament. Once started, in each instance there may be a background of dull, aching pain. Particularly noteworthy here is the abrupt intensification of the dull ache of root pain by cough, sneeze, or strain which momentarily stretches or alters the position of the root.

Mode of onset of pain This factor is also important. A pain reaching its full intensity almost immediately after its appearance suggests a rupture of tissue. The pain of a dissecting aortic aneurysm often develops in this manner. In fact, the suddenness and the severity of the pain, reaching a peak of intensity within seconds or minutes, sometimes provides the first clue in differentiating this type of chest pain from that caused by myocardial infarction. A similarly rapid accession of pain may occur with the rupture of a peptic ulcer.

Duration of pain This is another useful diagnostic attribute. Anginal pain, for example, rarely lasts less than 2 or 3 min or more than 10 to 15 min. Ulcer pain may continue for an hour or more, unless terminated by the ingestion of food or alkali or a tumbler of water.

Severity of pain In any given disease, the severity of pain is subject to wide variation, and also patients differ in their tolerance to it. Therefore, one cannot judge the gravity of an illness solely by the patient's report of the intensity of pain. As a rule, pains that completely interrupt work or pleasurable activity, require opiates for relief, enforce bed rest, or awaken the patient from sound sleep are to be taken more seriously than those which have the opposite characteristics.

Time of occurrence An accurate determination must be made of the temporal aspects of the pain. The relationship of ulcer pain to the preceding meal has already been mentioned. Postural aches come after prolonged activity and disappear with rest; arthritic pains are usually most severe during the first movements after prolonged inactivity. The mechanisms for this latter phenomenon are not known, nor do we understand why painful lesions of the bone, such as those caused by metastatic cancer, are likely to be most disturbing during the night. It is possible that the occurrence or aggravation of the latter types of pain is due to enhanced awareness of painful stimuli at a time when the mind is not distracted by other stimuli; or it may be that the pains are now more easily evoked by unconscious movements made during sleep when protective reflexes are in abeyance.

It should be obvious from these remarks that the full significance of a pain is usually not revealed by any one single characteristic. It is only by combining all these data that one can determine its anatomic site and its mechanism. In general, *the most important and revealing clues are obtained from the answers to the questions: What brings on the pain? What relieves it?* Pain is a subjective manifestation, not a state to be observed or measured. The accuracy of our data depends on the skill with which we frame our questions and on the powers of observation and memory of the person answering them.

Finally, the diagnostic value of measures which *reproduce* and *relieve the pain* should be stressed. Not only are they important for diagnosis, but they convince the patient that the physician understands and can control his pain and the illness behind it. Climbing several flights of stairs under the physician's supervision may settle the question of the presence or absence of angina pectoris. An injection of procaine into the tender area in the chest wall or some other skeletal structure, with complete disappearance of the pain, may establish its skeletal origin and exclude the possibility of visceral disease. Reproducing the distress sometimes caused by aerophagia merely by distending the esophagus or stomach with air, or reproducing the vague but sometimes alarming sensation of pressure in the chest caused by unconscious hyperventilation by having the patient deliberately hyperventilate are other examples of how the principle of the reproduction of pain may be usefully employed.

A systematic interrogation of the patient will not lead to accurate diagnosis in every instance, but the habit of searching for the identifying characteristics of pain will enable the physician to increase his skill in this difficult field. Furthermore, after becoming familiar with the customary responses to these questions, he becomes more alert to the anxious, the hysterical, or the depressed patient who, while complaining of pain, seems incapable of describing any of its details, or is unwilling to do so. Instead, there is preoccupation with theories of what is wrong or with the treatments or mistreatments already given.

Obscure and intractable pains Finally, there will always be cases that defy solution, and the physician must develop a systematic clinical approach to them. There are four discernible groups of such pains: (1) the pain of medical and surgical diseases yet undiagnosable; (2) "psychiatric" pains; (3) "neurologic" pains; (4) pains of indeterminate types.

With respect to group 1, neoplasms in retropharyngeal, posterior mediastinal, and retroperitoneal regions and the spine are among the more frequent causes of pain lasting months before being revealed by the usual methods of diagnosis. In group 2, four psychiatric conditions are associated with pain which may dominate the clinical picture: psychotic depression, hysteria, compensation "neurosis," and the constitutional psychopathy; any one of them may be complicated by drug addiction. Since psychiatric illnesses do not preclude another painful disease, the clinical analysis must of necessity rule out the latter while establishing on the basis of history and physical findings the existence and nature of the former (see Chaps. 344 and 345). In group 3, neurologic diseases of painful type (causalgia, spinal cord injury, discogenic root disease, and thalamic pain syndrome) are usually diagnosable on the basis of the clinical findings (see Chaps. 9 and 21), but the difficult problems are those in which the neurologic disease is accompanied by depression, malingering, compensation "neurosis," or opiate or other drug addiction. The fourth group includes the cases that are left when the first three are excluded. They defy solution. The physician can proceed only by repeatedly reexamining the patient, explaining the need for continued observation, and enlisting the patient's aid and forbearance during this trying period. Asking him to tolerate a certain amount of pain without the use of powerful analgesics is usually effective, particularly when the possibility of drug addiction is explained to him.

In the relatively rare circumstances when all manner of investigation has failed to throw light on the cause and mechanism of the pain, demands for pain-relieving surgery may become increasingly insistent. The physician may, in desperation, turn to measures which are more dangerous than the disease. Here the commonest source of error is to operate unnecessarily on the hysterical patient (see Chap. 344), only to discover too late that each operative procedure is followed by a new pain, often at a higher level than the first. Or depressive psychosis may have masqueraded as a painful state and is operated upon when electric shock therapy would have dramatically terminated the illness. Sometimes a half dozen or more operations are unsuccessfully performed on a single patient. The safest rule to follow in these cases is not to use opiates continuously or to recommend operation for the relief of pain unless a reasonable diagnosis has been made. For the pains of metastatic cancer, the thalamic pain of vascular disease of the brain, and other incurable diseases, the relative advantages of the controlled use of opiates versus lateral spinothalamic tractotomy or frontal lobotomy must be carefully weighed in each patient. The age of the patient, other diseases, life expectancy, and mental state are all of importance in selecting the treatment procedure. Too often an operation on the spinal cord or brain is chosen in preference to narcotics and the controlled use of drugs. Forgotten is the fact that many patients with cancer were formerly kept relatively comfortable and active by the judicious use of morphine and its analogues and were never subjected to costly operations or deprived of any of those qualities of mind and character which are so treasured by their families.

TREATMENT Superficial pain arising in integumentary structures rarely presents a problem in therapy. Acetylsalicylic acid, 0.30 to 0.60 g, or acetaminophen (Tylenol), 0.30 to 0.60 g, orally every 4 h usually suffices. Acetophenetidin may be added. These two drugs are a particularly effective combination when one element of pain is integumentary. Commercial proprietary preparations of these drugs containing caffeine or amphetamines such as ASA compound, Empirin compound, aspirin, or Edrisal are available in most pharmacies. The caffeine or amphetamine is particularly useful if there is central nervous system depression, and often there is advantage to adding a sedative drug. When this type of pain is not effectively controlled by nonnarcotic analgesics, codeine should be given. Usually the addition of small amounts (8 to 30 mg) of codeine phosphate to the standard dose of acetylsalicylic acid and acetophenetidin is effective. A preparation containing codeine phosphate 8 to 30 mg, acetylsalicylic acid 0.23 g, acetophenetidin 0.16 g, and caffeine 0.032 g is commercially available (Empirin compound with codeine phosphate). Codeine, 20 to 45 mg every 3 h, gives fairly effective analgesia with minimal side effects. Adequate rest and relief of muscle tension should also be encouraged. The application of moist heat is usually beneficial. Occasionally cold applications are preferred, but with the exception of cooling packs applied to an inflamed, burning skin or to a causalgia, cold is more likely to aggravate than to soothe the painful condition.

Occasionally integumental and deep pains of skeletal structures are of such severity as to require more powerful narcotic analgesics, such as meperidine hydrochloride (Demerol) in doses of 50 to 100 mg orally or intramuscularly, methadone hydrochloride, 5 to 10 mg orally or subcutaneously, or dihydromorphine hydrochloride (Dilaudid), 1 to 2 mg orally and subcutaneously. These drugs are most useful when sedation is not required. When pain is unusually severe and some degree of euphoria is desired, one of the new drugs such as pentazocine hydrochloride (Talwin) should be given in doses of 50 mg orally or subcutaneously every 3 to 4 h. Morphine, although still a valuable drug in doses of 8 to 15 mg, is not used much because of its habit-forming tendency and the frequently associated nausea and vomiting. Since all these narcotic analgesics are, for the most part, detoxified by the liver, they either should not be used or should be given in only half the usual dosage in cases of liver disease, myxedema, adrenal insufficiency, and other states in which the metabolic rate is reduced. Morphine and related narcotic analgesics tend to cause pruritus and, therefore, should be used with care in patients with skin irritability. The possibility of initiating addiction in susceptible persons must be carefully evaluated in every instance (cf. Chap. 119).

If the patient exhibits mental tension, insomnia, and restlessness, a sedative drug such as phenobarbital or Amytal Sodium may be given with the analgesic agents. Sedative medication, especially the quick-acting barbiturates, should not be used alone for the control of pain, because they sometimes cause excitement and confusion under these circumstances. If psychotic depression is the underlying illness, it should be managed as outlined in Chap. 345.

Visceral pain originating in the stomach, gallbladder, intestines, or heart is usually very poorly controlled by the nonnarcotic analgesics. The narcotic analgesics are the agents of choice, but of course, they should never be given until the physician is certain that the relief of the pain will not mask the state of his patient. If sedation is not desirable and if constipation is a troublesome problem, the newer synthetic analgesics, meperidine in doses of 50 to 100 mg orally or intramuscularly or methadone 5 to 10 mg by mouth or subcutaneously every 4 to 6 h, are recommended. Like morphine, these drugs are habit-forming but less so because they induce milder analgesia, sedation, and euphoria. Patients with severe visceral pain who are also anxious or fearful and unable to relax or sleep should be given morphine sulfate in doses of 8 to 15 mg subcutaneously. The well-known spasmogenic effects of morphine are partially counteracted by atropine sulfate, 0.3 to 0.4 mg. Aminophylline, 0.5 g intravenously, also overcomes much of this undesirable spastic action; a rectal suppository of 0.5 g, although less effective, may be substituted. When pain is due to benign, chronic diseases, every effort should be made to avoid opiate addiction. Here the judicious use of propoxyphene (Darvon), 65 mg q 4 to 6 h; oxycodone hydrochloride (Percodan), 4.5 mg q 6 h, or pentazocine hydrochloride, 50 mg q 3 to 4 h, may prove to be adequate.

Intractable pain due to incurable diseases, such as metastatic carcinoma, is one of the most difficult therapeutic problems. As a rule, one resorts to narcotic drugs because of their strong analgesic action, and habituation is accepted as the lesser of two evils. An alternative is pain-relieving surgery. Section of peripheral nerves, the lateral spinothalamic tracts in the spinal cord (cordotomy) or the lateral part of the medulla, stereotaxic thalamotomy, and lobotomy are relatively safe procedures which have advantages over the continuous use of opiates in selected cases.

REFERENCES

BONICA JJ (ed): *Advances in Neurology,* vol. 4. New York: Raven Press, 1974

FEINDEL WH et al: Pain sensibility in deep somatic structures. J Neurol Neurosurg Psychiatry 11:113, 1948

HARDY JD et al: *Pain Sensations and Reactions,* Baltimore: Williams & Wilkins, 1952

LEWIS T: *Pain,* New York: Macmillan, 1942

MELZACK R, WALL PD: Interaction of fast and slow conducting fiber systems involved in pain and analgesia, in *Pharmacology of Pain,* eds RKS Lim et al, London: Pergamon, 1968

WHITE JC, SWEET WH: *Pain and the Neurosurgeon—A Forty Years Experience,* Springfield, Ill.: Charles C Thomas, 1969

6 HEADACHE

RAYMOND D. ADAMS

The term *headache* should encompass all aches and pains located in the head, but in common language its application is restricted to unpleasant sensations in the region of the cranial vault. Facial, pharyngeal, and cervical pain are put aside as something different and are discussed in Chaps. 9 and 332.

Headache, along with fatigue, hunger, and thirst, represent man's most frequent discomforts. Medically speaking, its significance is often abstruse, for it may stand as a symptomatic expression of disease or of some minor tension or fatigue, incident to the affairs of the day. Fortunately, in most instances it reflects the latter, and only exceptionally does it warn of serious disease seated in intracranial structures. But it is this dual significance, benign and potentially malignant, that keeps the physician on the alert. Systematic approach to the headache problem necessitates a broad knowledge of the medical and surgical diseases of which it is a symptom and a clinical methodology which leaves none of the common and treatable causes unexplored.

GENERAL CONSIDERATIONS In the introductory chapter on pain, reference was made to the necessity, when dealing with any painful state, of determining its quality, location, duration and time course, and conditions which produce, exacerbate, or relieve it. When headache is considered in these terms, a certain amount of useful information is obtained by careful history, but perhaps less than one might expect. Unfortunately, physical examination of the head itself is seldom useful.

As to quality of cephalic pain, the patient is rarely helpful in his description. In fact persistent questioning on that point occasions surprise, for the patient usually assumes that the word *headache* should have conveyed enough information to the examiner about the nature of the discomfort. Most headaches are dull, deeply located, and of aching character, a pain recognizable as of the type that usually arises from structures deep to the skin. Seldom is there reported the superficial burning, smarting, or stinging type of pain localized to the skin. When asked to analogize the sensation to another sensory experience, the patient may make some allusion to tightness, pressure, or bursting feeling, terms which then give clue to a muscular tension or psychologic state.

Queries about the intensity of the pain are seldom of much value since they reflect more the patient's attitude toward the condition and his customary way of reporting things that happen to him than the true severity. As usual, the bluff, hearty person tends to minimize his discomfort, whereas the neurotic dramatizes it. Degree of incapacity is a better index. A severe migraine attack seldom allows performance of the day's work. The pain which awakens the patient from sleep at night, or prevents sleep, is also more likely to have a demonstrable organic basis. As a rule, the most intense cranial pains are those which accompany subarachnoid hemorrhage and meningitis, which have grave implications, or migraine and paroxysmal nocturnal orbitotemporal ("cluster") headaches, which are benign.

Data regarding *location* of the headache are apt to be more informative. If the source is in deep structures (extracranial, subdermal, or intracranial), as is usually the case, the correspondence with the site of the pain is fairly precise. Inflammation of an extracranial artery causes pain well localized to the site of the vessel. Lesions of paranasal sinuses, teeth, eyes, and upper cervical vertebras induce less sharply localized pain but one that is still referred in a regional distribution that is fairly constant. Intracranial lesions in the posterior fossa cause pain in the occipital-nuchal region, homolateral if the lesion is one-sided. Supratentorial lesions induce frontotemporal pains, again homolateral to the lesion if it is on one side. But localization can also be very uninformative or misleading. Ear pain, for example, although it may mean disease in the ear, more often is referred from other regions, and eye pain may be referred from parts as remote as the occiput or cervical spine.

Duration and *time-intensity curve* of headaches in both the attack itself and their life profile are most useful. Of course, the headache of bacterial meningitis or subarachnoid hemorrhage occurs usually in single attacks over a period of days. Single, brief, momentary (1 to 2 s) pains in the cranium are presently uninterpretable and are significant only because they indicate no serious underlying disease. Migraine of the classic type has its onset in the early morning hours or daytime, reaches its peak of severity in a half hour or so, and lasts, unless treated, for several hours up to 1 to 2 days, but often terminated by sleep. In the life history a frequency of more than a single attack every few weeks is exceptional. A migraine patient having several attacks per week usually proves to have a combination of migraine and tension headaches. In contrast to this is the nightly occurrence (2 to 3 h after onset of sleep) over a period of several weeks to months of the rapidly peaking, nonthrobbing orbital or supraorbital pain of cluster headache, which tends to dissipate within an hour. The headache of intracranial tumor characteristically can occur at any time of day or night, interrupt sleep, vary in intensity, and last a few minutes to hours. The life profile is one of increasing frequency and intensity over a period of months. Tension headache, once commenced, may persist continuously for weeks or months, though waxing and waning from hour to hour.

Headache that bears a more or less constant relationship to certain biologic events and also to physical environmental changes may prove to be informative. Premenstrual headaches most typically relate to premenstrual tension during the period of oliguria and edema formation; they usually vanish after the first day of vaginal bleeding. The headaches of cervical arthritis are most typically intense after a period of inactivity, and the first movements in the morning are both difficult and painful. Hypertensive headaches, like those of cerebral tumor, tend to occur on waking in the morning, but, as with all vascular headaches, excitement and tension may provoke them. Headache from infection of nasal sinuses may appear, with clocklike regularity, upon awakening and in midmorning, and is characteristically worsened by stooping. Eyestrain headaches naturally follow prolonged use of the eyes, as in reading, peering for a long time against glaring headlights in traffic, or watching the cinema. Atmospheric cold may evoke pain in the so-called "fibrositic" or "nodular" headache or when the underlying condition is arthritic or neuralgic. Anger, excitement, or irritation may initiate common migraine in certain disposed persons; this is more typical of common migraine than of the classic type.

PAIN-SENSITIVE STRUCTURES AND MECHANISMS OF HEADACHE Understanding of headache has been greatly augmented by the observations of surgeons during operations on man. They inform us that the following cranial structures are sensitive to mechanical stimulation: (1) skin, subcutaneous tissue, muscles, arteries, and periosteum of skull; (2) delicate structures of eye, ear, and nasal cavity; (3) intracranial venous sinuses and their tributary veins; (4) parts of the dura at the base of the brain and the arteries within the dura mater and piarachnoid; (5) the trigeminal, glossopharyngeal, vagus, and first three cervical nerves. The bony skull, much of the piarachnoid and dura, and the parenchyma of the brain lack sensitivity. Interestingly, pain is practically the only sensation produced by stimulation of the listed structures.

The pathways whereby sensory stimuli, whatever their source, are conveyed to the central nervous system are the trigeminal nerves for structures above the tentorium in the anterior and middle fossae of the skull, and the first three cervical nerves for those in the posterior fossa and infradural structures. The ninth and tenth cranial nerves supply part of the posterior fossa and refer the pain to the ear and throat. The tentorium is the border zone between the trigeminal and cervical innervation. The central connections through spinal cord and brainstem to thalamus have already been described and depicted in Chap. 5.

The pain of intracranial disease is referred, by a mechanism already discussed, to some part of the cranium lying within the areas supplied by the aforementioned nerves (the fifth, ninth, and tenth cranial nerves and the first three cervicals). There may be an associated local tenderness of the scalp at the site of reference. Dental or jaw pain may also have cranial reference. The pain of disease in other parts of the body is not referred to the head, although it may initiate headache by other means.

By analysis of several types of headache, Wolff and his colleagues have demonstrated that most "spontaneous" cranial pains can be traced to the operation of one or more of the following mechanisms:

1. Distention, traction, and dilatation of the intracranial or extracranial arteries
2. Traction or displacement of large intracranial veins or the dural envelope in which they lie
3. Compression, traction, or inflammation of sensory cranial and spinal nerves.
4. Voluntary or involuntary spasm and possibly interstitial inflammation and trauma of cranial and cervical muscles
5. Raised intracranial pressure

More specifically, intracranial mass lesions cause headache only if in a position to deform, displace, or exert traction on vessels and dural structures at the base of the brain, and this may happen long before intracranial pressure rises. In fact the artificial induction of high intraspinal and intracranial pressure by the subarachnoid or intraventricular injection of sterile saline solution does not result in headache. Some have interpreted this to mean raised intracranial pressure does not cause headache, a conclusion which is called into question by the demonstrable relief of headache by lumbar puncture and lowering the cerebrospinal fluid (CSF) pressure in some patients. Actually, most patients with high intracranial pressure complain of recurrent bioccipital and bifrontal headache, probably due to traction on vessels or dura. As to localization, the pains follow the patterns mentioned above; those lesions deflecting the falx or pressing on superior longitudinal or straight sinuses induce pain behind or above the eye; if the lateral part of the lateral sinus is involved, the pain is felt in the ear. Displacement of tentorium elicits pain felt in the supraorbital region.

Dilatation of the temporal arteries with stretching of surrounding sensitive structures is believed to be the mechanism of most of the pain of migraine. Extracranial, temporal, and occipital arteries, when involved in giant cell arteritis (cranial or "temporal" arteritis), a disease which usually afflicts individuals over fifty years of age, give rise to headache of dull aching and throbbing type, at first localized and then more diffuse. Characteristically it is severe and persistent over a period of weeks or months. The offending artery, strangely, is not always tender to pressure, yet section of it, as in biopsy, may relieve the pain (Chap. 334). Evolving atherosclerotic thrombosis of internal carotid, anterior, and middle cerebral arteries is sometimes accompanied by pain in the forehead or temple; with vertebral artery thrombosis, the pain is postauricular, and basilar artery thrombosis causes pain to be projected to the occiput and sometimes the forehead.

In *infection* or *blockage* of *paranasal sinuses,* accompanied usually by pain over the antrum or in the forehead (from the ethmoid and sphenoid sinuses the pain localizes around the eyes on one or both sides or in the vertex or other part of the cranium, especially in disease of the sphenoid sinuses), the mechanism involves changes in pressure and irritation of pain-sensitive sinus walls. Usually it is associated with tenderness of the skin in the same distribution. The pain may have two remarkable properties: (1)

When throbbing, it may be abolished by compressing the carotid artery on the same side. (2) It tends to recur and subside at the same hours, i.e., on awakening, with gradual disappearance when the person is upright, and coming again in the late morning hours. The time relations are believed to yield information concerning the mechanism; morning pain is ascribed to the sinuses filling at night, and its relief on arising, from emptying after the erect posture has been assumed. Stooping intensifies the pain by pressure change, as does blowing the nose, sometimes; and inhalant sympathomimetic drugs such as Neo-Synephrine, which reduce swelling and congestion, tend to relieve the pain. Some believe that the highly sensitive orifice of the sinus is the source, but more probably, the pain arises in the sensitive mucous membrane of the sinus. However, it may persist after all purulent secretions have disappeared, probably because of mechanism of blockage of the orifice by boggy membranes and a vacuum or suction effect on the sinus wall *(vacuum sinus headaches).* The condition is relieved when aeration is restored. During air flights both earache and sinus headache tend to occur on descent, when the relative pressure in the blocked viscus falls.

Headache of ocular origin, located as a rule in the orbit, forehead, or temple, is of steady, aching type and tends to follow prolonged use of the eyes in close work. Ocular muscle imbalance is believed to be the mechanism. The main faults are hypermetropia and astigmatism (not myopia), which result in sustained contraction of extraocular as well as frontal, temporal, and even occipital muscles. Correction of the refractive error abolishes the headache. Traction on the extraocular muscles during eye surgery, particularly on the iris, will evoke pain. Another mechanism is involved in the raised intraocular pressure seen in acute glaucoma or iridocyclitis, which causes steady, aching pain in the region of the eye. When intense, it may radiate throughout the distribution of the ophthalmic division of the trigeminal nerve. As for ocular pain in general, it is important that the eyes should always be refracted, but eyestrain is probably not as frequent as one would expect from the wholesale dispensing of spectacles.

The mechanism of *headaches accompanying disease of ligaments, muscles, and apophyseal joints* in the upper part of the spine, which are referred to occiput and nape of neck on the same side, can be in part reproduced by the injection of hypertonic saline solution into these structures. Such pains are especially frequent in late life in rheumatoid and hypertrophic arthritis and tend also to occur after whiplash injuries to the neck. If the pain is arthritic in origin, the first movements after being still for some hours are both stiff and painful. In fact, evocation of pain by active and passive motion of the spine should indicate traumatic or other disease of movable parts. The pain of myofibrositis, evidenced by tender nodules near the cranial insertion of cervical and other muscles, is more obscure. There are no pathologic data as to the nature of these vaguely palpable lesions, and it is uncertain whether the pain actually arises in them. They may represent only the deep tenderness felt in the region of referred pain or the involuntary secondary protective spasm of muscles. Characteristically, the pain is steady (nonthrobbing) and spreads from one to both sides of the head. Exposure to cold or draft may precipitate it. Though severe at times, it seldom prevents sleep. Massage of muscles and heat have unpredictable effects but relieve the pain in some cases.

The *headache of meningeal irritation* (infection or hemorrhage), which is of acute onset, severe, generalized, deep-seated, constant, and especially intense at the base of the skull and associated with stiffness of neck on bending forward, has been ascribed by some authorities to increased intracranial pressure. Indeed the withdrawal of cerebrospinal fluid may afford some relief. But dilatation and congestion of inflamed meningeal vessels must also be a factor. It seems more probable, therefore, that the pain is due to the chemical irritation of nerve endings in the meninges.

Lumbar puncture headache, which is characterized by a steady occipital-nuchal pain but also by frontal pain coming on a few minutes after arising from a recumbent position and relieved within a few minutes by lying down, has as its cause a persistent leakage of CSF into the lumbar tissues through the needle site. The CSF pressure is low (often 0 in the lateral decubitus position), and the injection of sterile isotonic saline solution intrathecally relieves it. The headache is usually increased by compression of the jugular veins and is unaffected by digital obliteration of one carotid artery. It seems probable that in the upright position a low intraspinal and negative intracranial pressure exerts traction on dural attachments and dural sinuses by caudal displacement of the brain. Understandably, then, headache following cisternal puncture is rare. As soon as the leakage of CSF stops and CSF pressure is gradually restored (usually from a few days up to a week or so), the headache disappears. "Spontaneous" low-pressure headache may follow a sneeze or strain, presumably because of rupture of the spinal arachnoid along a nerve root.

The mechanism of the throbbing or steady headache which accompanies febrile illnesses, located in frontal or occipital regions or generalized, is probably vascular. It is much like histamine headache in being relieved on one side by carotid artery compression and on both sides by jugular vein compression or the subarachnoid injection of saline solution. It is increased by shaking the head. It seems probable that the meningeal vessels pulsate unduly and stretch pain-sensitive structures around the base of the brain. In certain cases, however, the pain may be lessened by compression of temporal arteries, and in these cases a component of the headache seems to be derived from the walls of extracranial arteries, as in migraine.

PRINCIPAL CLINICAL VARIETIES OF HEADACHE Usually there is no difficulty in diagnosing the headache of glaucoma, purulent sinusitis, bacterial meningitis, and brain tumor, and a fuller account of these special headaches will be found where these diseases are described in later sections of the book. It is when headache is chronic, recurrent, and unattended by other important signs of disease that the physician faces one of the most difficult medical problems.

The following types of headache should then be considered:

Migraine The term *migraine* refers to periodic, hemicranial, throbbing headaches which usually begin in childhood, adolescence, or early adult life and recur with diminishing frequency during advancing years.

Two closely related clinical syndromes have been identified. The first is called "classic" migraine, the second "common." The classic syndrome is ushered in by a disturbance of neurologic function (hemianopsia or central blindness, hemiparesthetic disturbance, slight speech abnormality or aphasia, or hemiparesis) followed in a few minutes by hemicranial headache, nausea, and vomiting, all of which last for hours or as long as a day or two. The other syndrome is characterized by an unheralded onset of hemicranial or generalized headache with or without nausea and vomiting but following the same temporal pattern. Both headache syndromes respond to ergot preparations, if administered early in the attack. Their genetic nature is evidenced by concurrence in several members of the family of the same and successive generations in 60 to 80 percent of cases; but inheritance is somewhat less clear in the common than the classic variety, perhaps because diagnosis is less accurate.

Classic migraine presents such a dramatic and at times confusing sequence of events that it merits further description. On awakening in the morning, or at any time of day, the patient may have a kind of vague premonition of an attack. Then abruptly there is a disturbance of vision consisting usually of bright spots or dazzling zigzag lines which give way within minutes to scotomatous defects; usually they are bilateral and often of homonymous and congruent pattern (corresponding parts of the field of vision of each eye). Soon thereafter, numbness and tingling of lips, face, hand (on one or both sides), slight confusion of thinking, weakness of an arm or leg, mild aphasia, dizziness and uncertainty of gait, drowsiness, or confusion (rarely coma) are added to the clinical picture. Only one or a few of these neurologic phenomena are present in any given patient, and they tend to occur in the same combination in each attack. They last 5 to 15 min or more, and if the weakness or numbness spreads from one part of the body to another or one symptom follows another, it does so slowly in a period of minutes (not in seconds as in a convulsion). Just as inexplicably as they come, they soon begin to recede, and within minutes they are followed by a unilateral throbbing headache, usually on the side of the cerebral disturbance, which slowly increases in intensity. At its peak, in an hour or so, nausea and vomiting may occur. The headache lasts hours or a day or two and is always the most unpleasant feature of the illness.

Much variation occurs. When this "sick headache," as it is called, is most severe, the patient is forced to lie down and to shun light and noise. Milder forms, especially if partially controlled by medication, do not force withdrawal from accustomed activities. Any one of the three principal components—neurologic derangement, headache, or vomiting—may be absent or occur in different sequence than is described above. Particularly with advancing age there is a tendency for the headache and vomiting to become less severe, finally leaving only the neurologic abnormality. The neurologic symptomatology is also subject to variation. Although visual disturbances are far and away the most common manifestation, they differ in detail from patient to patient; numbness and tingling of the lips and fingers of one hand are probably next in frequency, with transient aphasia or a thickness of speech following in that order. A relatively rare syndrome of vertigo, staggering, drowsiness, and stupor has been delineated by Bickerstaff and called *basilar artery migraine.* Also, he has reported the loss of consciousness at the onset, especially in migrainous young women. Recurrent unilateral headaches associated with extraocular muscle palsies have been called *ophthalmoplegic migraine.* A transient third nerve palsy with associated ptosis of one eyelid is the usual picture; rarely, the abducens nerve is affected and lateral movement is impaired. Hemifacial paralysis is another rare variant. Disturbances of the mind may appear—a strange excitement, an unaccountable irritability or depression, or a slight mental confusion, which is the more common. The headache, though typically hemicranial (the word *migraine* is said to be derived from *megrim,* meaning hemicrania), may be frontal, temporal, or generalized. In children abdominal pain and vomiting may accompany the headache (abdominal migraine). The attacks, instead of beginning in childhood and recurring in the usual fashion every few weeks or months with diminishing frequency in middle and late adult years, may begin in adult life or even middle age or suddenly increase in frequency during menopause or when hypertension and vascular disease develop. The neurologic symptoms, instead of being transitory, may leave a permanent deficit (e.g., a homonymous visual field defect) reminiscent of an ischemic stroke. The use of hormones to prevent pregnancy has increased the frequency and severity of migraine and in several reported instances has resulted in a permanent neurologic deficit.

Between attacks the migrainous patient is essentially normal. For a time, when psychosomatic medicine was much in vogue, there was insistence on a migrainous personality characterized by tenseness, rigidity in thinking, meticulousness, and perfectionism. The migrainous attack was said to occur often during the let-down period, after many days of hard work or stress. But further personality analyses have not borne out these ideas, and the temporal relations between headache and the day's activities have not been consistent. Moreover, the fact that the headaches may begin in early childhood, when the personality is relatively amorphous, would argue against this idea.

During an attack, the electroencephalogram reveals a nonspecific slowing of wave frequencies in one-third to one-half of all patients. Carotid arteriograms show arterial constriction at the onset of the headache, and the cerebral circulation is found by blood flow studies to be slowed early in the attack and speeded up once headache begins. Migraine is frequent, found in an estimated 5 percent of general population; females are slightly more susceptible than males, and there is a tendency for the headaches to occur during the period of premenstrual tension and fluid retention. The migrainous attacks usually cease during pregnancy. Reserpine treatment and estrogens and progesterone may increase their frequency. A few patients have linked their attacks to certain articles of diet, such as chocolate. There is no clear relationship, despite many statements to the contrary, between migraine and vascular malformations of the brain and psychoneurosis. The relationship to epilepsy is less clear; convulsions are slightly increased in frequency in the migrainous patient and his relatives.

Vasodilatation and excessive pulsation of branches of the external carotid artery have been observed during the headache. Further, as the pulsation decreases, either spontaneously or after the administration of ergotamine, the headache disappears. Vasoconstriction was early postulated as the basis of the neurologic symptoms; it has been confirmed in at least one chance carotid arteriogram and has been inferred from prompt abolition of the visual or neurologic disorder upon administration of nitrites. Thus the vascular theory of migraine has come to be accepted, supported further by surgical observations, that the extracranial arteries can be a source of pain. However, it is quite apparent that the theory does not explain why the intracranial and extracranial arteries should periodically undergo spasm and dilatation in the migrainous individual, nor does it account for the nausea and vomiting (infrequent in all other headaches except those due to tumor) or the tenderness and swelling of the temporal vessels and surrounding tissues.

A new hypothesis has been put forth—that the observed vasospasm and later hyperemic pulsations are induced by a release of amines such as norepinephrine and epinephrine and serotonin in individuals whose vessels are peculiarly sensitive. These substances are known to be powerful vasoconstrictors. It was found that some migraine patients during their attack excrete increased amounts of the terminal metabolites of the catecholamines, particularly 5-hydroxyindoleacetic acid (5-HIAA) derived from serotonin, and of vanillylmandelic acid (VMA), a product of norepinephrine and epinephrine. A corresponding reduction in serotonin levels in the blood has also been detected. Other observations in line with this are that (1) reserpine, which reduces the level of serotonin in platelets, brain, and other tissues, may provoke migraine; (2) the injection of serotonin gives partial or complete relief of headache, and (3) a serotonin antagonist, methysergide, wholly prevents attacks. However, it is still difficult to reconcile these data with the finding that a heat-stable polypeptide with some of the properties of bradykinin (one of the plasma kinins) not only can be aspirated from the edematous subcutaneous tissue on the side of the headache but, if reinjected at another site, will cause increased capillary permeability, pain, and lowered skin threshold in the overlying skin. Its algogenic action is potentiated by serotonin. Whether this substance, called *neurokinin,* escapes secondarily during the phase of vasodilatation or initiates the vasodilatation is not known. While this humoral amine theory is incomplete and several of the findings need verification, nonetheless it does promise clarification of the migraine syndrome and possibly other forms of vascular headache.

DIAGNOSIS Classic migraine should occasion no difficulty in diagnosis if the above facts are kept in mind and if a good history is obtained. That is possible, as a rule, for migraine patients tend to be intelligent.

The real difficulties come from three sources: (1) ignorance of the fact that a progressively unfolding neurologic syndrome may be migrainous in origin; (2) lack of appreciation that the neurologic disorder may occur without headache; (3) lack of awareness that recurrent headaches, which may be an isolated phenomenon, may take many forms, some of which may prove difficult to distinguish from the other common types of headache described in this chapter.

Some of these problems merit further elaboration because of their practical importance, as follows:

The neurologic part of the migraine syndrome may resemble focal epilepsy, the clinical picture of a vascular malformation such as an angioma or aneurysm, or some other vascular disease such as a thrombotic or embolic stroke. Here it is the pace of the neurologic symptoms of migraine more than their character that reliably distinguishes the condition from epilepsy. The clinical profile of the aura of epilepsy is measured in seconds, for it depends on spreading neural excitation, in contrast to the slow progression of migraine, which is based on spreading vascular spasm.

Ophthalmoplegic migraine will always suggest a carotid aneurysm, but in relatively few cases has carotid arteriography revealed such an abnormality. Despite many claims that hemicranial painful attacks invariably on the same side of the head (unlike migraine) should raise the question of a vascular malformation, in a large series of cases this has not been confirmed by arteriography. Of course, focal epilepsy, protracted headache, stiff neck and bloody cerebrospinal fluid, a persistent neurologic deficit, and cranial bruit would be indicative of a vascular type of headache associated with angioma or aneurysm. Only in the earlier stages, when periodic throbbing headache is the sole symptom, might it be confused with true migraine.

Attacks indistinguishable from epilepsy may also appear in association with the hypertensive and cerebral arteriosclerotic vascular diseases of late life. Here one is aided by late age of onset, more persistent and frequent headaches, and the evidence of vascular disease of heart, lower extremities, and brain.

A special problem relates to paroxysms of throbbing headache, not hemicranial in distribution, not preceded by a neurologic aura, and not accounted for by other known cause. Are they examples of common migraine? Unfortunately, since diagnosis depends on the interpretation of the patient's description of symptoms and since there is as yet no biologically valid confirmatory laboratory test, the controversy as to where migraine begins and ends is of the armchair type. Favoring the diagnosis of migraine are lifelong history, childhood onset, positive family history, and response of the headache to ergot derivatives.

A variety of episodic attacks have been described as migraine equivalents: attacks of abdominal pain with nausea, vomiting, and diarrhea; pain localized in the thorax, pelvis, and extremities; bouts of fever; transient disturbances in mood (psychic equivalents); recurrent nocturnal orbital (cluster) headache, or migrainous neuralgia. The only advantage of considering such attacks as migrainous is that this view protects some patients from unnecessary diagnostic procedures and surgical intervention—but it may also prevent necessary surgery.

From all this discussion the reader should be left with the idea that the migraine syndromes are rather larger and more protean than the rigid stereotyped descriptions we have given would suggest. In these days of complicated diagnostic procedures it is tempting to take x-rays of the skull and perform arteriography and electroencephalography on every patient. A conservative approach would lead to temporization, reserving a single lateral skull film or EEG for the exceptional case.

Cluster headache This headache is also called *paroxysmal nocturnal cephalalgia, migrainous neuralgia,* and *histamine headache* (Horton's syndrome). It is characterized by male predominance, constant, unilateral orbital localization, and onset within 2 or 3 h after falling asleep (it is infrequent during the waking hours). The pain is usually intense, with lacrimation, blocked nostril, then rhinorrhea, and sometimes flush, miosis, ptosis, and edema of cheek, all lasting approximately an hour or two. It tends to recur nightly for several weeks or a few months (hence the term *cluster*), followed by complete freedom for years. The pain of a given attack may leave as rapidly as it began. Clusters may recur over the years, being possibly more likely in times of stress, prolonged strain, overwork, and with upsetting emotional experiences. Rarely, the condition may occur in daytime and may not cluster but continue for 6, 7, or 8 years. The picture is so characteristic that it cannot be confused with any other disease, though to those unfamiliar with it the possibility of a carotid aneurysm, hemangioma, brain tumor, or sinusitis may be suggested. Appropriate roentgenograms and carotid arteriography will always exclude such conditions but usually are unnecessary. In the differential diagnosis orbital (nasociliary, supraorbital, Sluder's sphenopalatine) neuralgias must also be considered (see Chap. 332).

In the life history profile the clusters of headache may last for weeks. The clusters may be single or recur two, three or more times, with years of freedom in between, during which such precipitating factors as alcohol are no longer effective. Often the pain involves the same orbit in each cluster. Examples are seen in which a cluster may last a year or more.

The relationship of the cluster headache to migraine remains conjectural. A portion of the cases have a background of migraine, which led to the earlier postulation of migrainous neuralgia, but the majority do not.

Tension headache and various other cranial pains with psychiatric disease The headache is usually bilateral, often with diffuse extension over the top of the cranium. Occipital-nuchal localization is also common. Although the sensation may be described as pain, close questioning may uncover other sensations, viz., fullness, tightness, pressure (as if the head is surrounded by a band or in a vise), on which waves of aching pain are engrafted. The onset of a given attack is more gradual than in migraine and not infrequently is added intermittently to a pressure ache which lasts unremittingly for weeks or months. In fact, this is the only type of headache that exhibits the peculiarity of being absolutely continuous day and night for long periods of time. Although sleep may be possible, whenever the patient awakens, the headache is present; the common analgesic remedies have no beneficial effect unless the pain is intense and of aching type.

As to mechanism, the ascription of it to sustained muscle activity, shown by the electromyogram, is only a partial explanation. The continuous pressing quality of milder cephalic sensations at times when the patient is relaxed hardly seems to be attributable to physiologic stimulation and suggests instead that the condition is maintained by focused attention on the head (occasioned sometimes by worry and fear of intracranial disease). Moreover, it must be remembered that all types of headache in their late stages may give rise to muscle tension and that this is of an aching rather than a pressure type. In contrast to migraine, in which pain is periodic and lifelong, with tendency to lessen in late adult years, tension headache occurs more often in middle age and usually coincides with anxiety and depression in the trying times of life. Many premenstrual headaches are of this type, and there is an increased incidence of this type of tension headache at menopause.

Psychologic studies of groups of patients with tension headaches have revealed prominent symptoms of anxiety, hypochondriasis, and, to a lesser extent, depression. When psychiatric syndromes are searched for in headache patients, it is evident that the majority of those with anxiety neurosis, hysteria, obsessive-compulsive neurosis, and schizophrenia, in which anxiety is a prominent symptom, exhibit this type of headache. With endogenous and reactive depressions it is less frequent, though the incidence is increased in the late-life involutional and hypochondriacal states (see Chap. 345). Migraine and traumatic headaches may be complicated by tension headache.

Other odd cephalic pains, e.g., boring pains, "clavus hystericus," may occur in hysteria and raise perplexing problems in diagnosis. Their bizarre character, persistence in the face of every known therapy, absence of other signs of disease, and the presence of the stigmata of the hysterical personality provide the basis for correct diagnosis (see Chap. 344).

Headache of angioma and aneurysm The temporal profile of any given attack shows the onset to be sudden or very acute, with the pain reaching a peak within minutes. Neurologic disturbances such as unilateral numbness, weakness, or aphasia tend to occur after the onset of headache and to outlast it. Should hemorrhage occur, the headache is often extremely severe and localizes more toward the occiput and neck, lasting many days in association with stiff neck. A cranial or cervical bruit and, of course, blood in the cerebrospinal fluid establish the diagnosis, but it may require verification by arteriography. The claim that vascular malformations may give rise to migraine is probably untenable. Statistical data show migraine to be no more frequent in this group of patients than in the general population. Of course, vascular lesions may exist for long periods of time without headache, or the latter may develop many years after other manifestations, such as epilepsy and hemiplegia (see Chap. 334).

TRAUMATIC HEADACHE Severe, chronic, continuous or intermittent headaches appear as the cardinal symptom of two posttraumatic syndromes, separable in each instance from the headache that immediately follows head injury (i.e., that of scalp laceration and contusion with sanguineous cerebrospinal fluid and increased intracranial pressure). The latter lasts several days or a week or two.

Headache of chronic subdural hematoma Headache and dizziness of fluctuating severity, followed by drowsiness, stupor, coma, and hemiparesis, are the usual manifestations of chronic subdural hematoma. The head injury may have been minor and forgotten by patient and family. The headaches are deep-seated, steady, unilateral or generalized, and respond to the usual analgesic drugs. The typical attack profile of the headache and other symptoms is one of increasing frequency and severity over several weeks or months. Diagnosis is now established by arteriography and CAT scan (see Chap. 335).

Headache of posttraumatic nervous instability Here, headache is a prominent feature of a complex syndrome composed of giddiness, fatigability, insomnia, nervousness, trembling, irritability, inability to concentrate, and tearfulness. The pain undergoes many variations from one day to another and also a highly individualized pattern of localization. Often it centers on the site of injury, where there is also tenderness. Reference to throbbing pain as well as pressure is obtained. Particular importance is attached to its persistence, intensification by mental and physical effort, stooping, noise, bright light, and confusion. The patient looks and acts much like a person in an agitated depression, and indeed, many neurologists believe such a state to be a posttraumatic neurosis or depression. The severity and duration of the headache bear no relation to the magnitude of the injury; some of the worst cases have had minor injuries without loss of consciousness, and major injuries may leave no headache in their wake. Unsettled litigation surely prolongs the discomfort and disability. The observation that histamine may reproduce some of the more severe headaches has suggested to some a vascular origin. Cephalic tenderness and aching pain sharply localized to the scar of the scalp laceration represent in all probability a different problem, raising the question of a traumatic neuralgia. With whiplash injuries to the neck, unilateral retroauricular or occipital pain suggests trauma of the corresponding nerves (see Chaps. 9 and 335).

Headaches of brain tumor Headache is the outstanding symptom of cerebral tumor. Unfortunately, the quality of the pain has no specific feature. It tends to be deep-seated, nonthrobbing (or throbbing), and aching or bursting. Attacks last a few minutes to an hour or more and occur once or many times during the day. Activity and frequently change in the position of the head may provoke pain, while rest in bed diminishes its frequency. Nocturnal awakening because of pain, although typical, is by no means diagnostic. Unexpected forceful (projectile) vomiting may punctuate the illness in its later stages. As the tumor grows the pain becomes more frequent and severe; it sometimes is nearly continuous terminally. But there are exceptions, some headaches being mild and tolerable, others as agonizing as that of the headache of bacterial meningitis and subarachnoid hemorrhage. If unilateral, the headache is homolateral to the tumor in 9 out of 10 patients. Supratentorial tumors are felt anterior to the interauricular circumference of the skull; posterior fossa tumors behind this line. Bifrontal and bioccipital headache, coming on after unilateral headaches, signifies the development of increased intracranial pressure.

APPROACH TO THE PATIENT WITH HEADACHE Obviously very different possibilities are raised by a patient who presents himself for the first time in his life with severe headache and another one who has had recurrent headache over a period of years. The chances of uncovering the cause in the first instance are much greater than in the latter, and some of the underlying conditions (meningitis, subarachnoid hemorrhage, epidural hematoma, glaucoma, and purulent sinusitis) are more serious.

In searching for the cause of recurrent headache one should investigate the status of cardiovascular and renal systems by blood pressure and urine examination, eyes (fundoscopic, intraocular pressure, and refraction), the sinuses by transillumination and x-rays, the cranial arteries by palpation (and biopsy?), the cervical spine by effect of passive movement and x-rays, the nervous system by neurologic examination, and psychic function by mental status.

Hypertension is, of course, frequent in the general population and is always difficult to prove as a cause of recurrent headaches. Minor elevations of blood pressure may be a result rather than the cause of nervous tension. No doubt severe hypertension with diastolic blood pressures of over 110 mmHg is regularly associated with headache, and measures which reduce blood pressure can be shown to relieve the headache. But it is the moderate hypertensive when subject to numerous and severe headaches who gives concern. If headache is severe and frequent, there is usually an underlying anxiety or tension state or a common migraine syndrome that is exacerbated by blood vessel disease. The mechanism of the puzzling hypertensive phenomenon of occipital pain, present on awakening in the morning and wearing off during the day, is uncertain.

The adolescent with daily frontal headaches represents a special type of problem. Often their relationship to eyestrain is unclear, and refraction of the eyes and new eyeglasses do not relieve the condition. Anxiety or tension is probably a factor in such cases, but it is difficult to be certain of a causal relationship. Some of the most persistent and inexplicable headaches, which have led to a survey by a battery of diagnostic procedures for tumor, have proved in the end to be caused by depression.

Equally puzzling is the somber, tense adult whose primary complaint is headache, or the migrainous person who in late life or at menopause begins to have daily headaches. Here it becomes important to assess mental status along the lines suggested in Chaps. 14, 26, and 343, looking for evidences of anxiety, depression, and hypochondriasis. The quality and persistence of the headache are suggestive of the possibility of psychiatric illness. Sometimes, a direct question as to the patient's idea of what is the matter may elicit suspicion and fear of brain tumor. Antidepressant drugs, given as an empirical test, may relieve the headache, thus clarifying the diagnosis.

The most worrisome type of patient is the one who has headache of increasing frequency and severity over a period of months or a year or so. Usually it becomes necessary to resort to a complete neurologic survey, including careful inspection of optic disk and roentgenograms of skull, electroencephalogram, lumbar puncture, and radioactive-isotope and CT scanning to rule out brain tumor, abscess, or subdural hematoma.

Every elderly person with severe headache of some few days, or weeks, duration should be considered as possibly having cranial arteritis. Increased sedimentation rate, fever, and anemia may be conjoined, but only in a minority of cases, unfortunately. The finding of a thickened temporal artery is important, and arterial biopsy and response to corticosteroids establish the diagnosis; treatment with corticosteroids often relieves the pain.

TREATMENT The most important steps in the treatment of headache are those measures which uncover and remove the underlying disease or functional disturbance.

For the common everyday headache due to fatigue,

stuffy atmosphere, or excessive use of alcohol and tobacco, it is simple enough to advise avoidance of the offending activity or agent, and symptomatic therapy in the form of acetylsalicylic acid, 0.6 g (some brand of aspirin such as Anacin) will suffice. Some patients who invariably have headache when constipated and hypochondriacs who not infrequently suffer incapacitating headache, fatigue, and depression whenever bowel elimination does not meet their expectation, are not easily helped. Certainly, simple explanation, an anticonstipation regimen, and drugs which counteract depression (see Chap. 345) are preferable to the continuous use of analgesics. Premenstrual headache, if troublesome, can usually be helped by the use of a diuretic compound for the week preceding the menstrual period and a mixture of mild analgesic and tranquilizing medications (acetylsalicylic acid, 0.6 g, and phenobarbital, 30 mg). If the headaches are severe and incapacitating, they should be treated as common migraine.

Migraine may require no treatment at all, other than an explanation of its nature to the patient and a reassurance that it will do him no harm. Some patients know, or allege to know, that certain acts induce attacks, and it is obvious enough that they should be urged to avoid these acts, if possible. In certain persons it has been claimed that the correction of a refractive error, an elimination diet, or psychotherapy for some personality disorder has relieved their migraine. However, this is so exceptional that a cause and effect relationship must be doubted, in view of the variability of the disease itself.

Treatment of the neurologic aura is rarely required because of its brevity. If the deficit is lasting, inhalation of an ampul of amyl nitrate should be tried; used at the first premonition of the attack, the drug may prevent it. The time to initiate treatment of the oncoming headache is during the neurologic disorder. If many of the headaches are mild, the patient may already have learned that 0.6 g acetylsalicylic acid and possibly 5 mg Dexedrine will suffice to control the pain so that he can carry on. More severe attacks respond only to ergot preparations (ergotamine and dihydroergotamine). In such patients the attack can be cut short by the intravenous injection of 1 mg dihydroergotamine methane sulfate or 0.5 mg ergotamine tartrate, the former being less likely to induce vomiting. The injection should be repeated in 30 min, if necessary. When these drugs are administered early (within 30 to 60 min of onset), some 90 percent of patients will be relieved of the headache. Oral medication in the form of three 1-mg tablets, to be held under the tongue until dissolved, and repeated in 2-mg doses every half hour until the headache is relieved or until a total of 9 mg is taken, is almost as effective. Caffeine, 100 mg with 1 mg ergotamine (Cafergot), is a useful combination when taken in the form of a tablet (two at onset of headache and a third in half an hour) or as a rectal suppository (2 mg ergotamine and 100 mg caffeine) if vomiting prevents oral administration.

Because of the danger of prolonged vascular spasm in patients who have vascular disease or are pregnant, ergot preparations must be used cautiously, if at all. Even in healthy individuals more than 10 to 15 mg ergotamine per week is risky. For the frequent atypical migraine headaches, some of which respond poorly to ergot, one should prescribe a preparation containing 150 mg acetylsalicylic acid, 160 mg acetophenetidin, and Dexedrine, 5 mg, with phenobarbital, 30 mg. This can be repeated once or twice in a severe attack. Once the headache has become intense, ergot is of little help, and one must resort to codeine sulfate, 30 mg, or meperidine (Demerol), 50 mg, as the only means of terminating the pain.

In individuals with frequent migrainous attacks (one to three times a week) efforts at prevention are worthwhile. Some success has been obtained with preparations of ergot, 0.5 mg, atropine, 0.3 mg, and phenobarbital, 15 mg (Bellergol) twice or three times a day for a few weeks. Adrenocorticotropic hormone (ACTH) (40 units per day) or prednisone (45 mg per day for 3 to 4 weeks) has also been helpful in some difficult refractory patients. In addition, methysergide (Sansert) in a dose of 6 to 8 mg per day given for several weeks or months has proved to be most promising in reducing the frequency of or abolishing attacks. The main contraindication has been retroperitoneal fibrosis; this complication has been reported in several dozen cases, when the patient has been treated continuously for more than 6 months. Discontinuing treatment for 1 month out of every 6 has greatly reduced the incidence of this complication.

All experienced physicians appreciate the importance of helping the patient rearrange his schedule so as to control his tensions and hard-driving ways of living, so often a feature of many migrainous patients. There is no one way of accomplishing this, but in general, long and costly psychotherapy has not been helpful, or at least one can say there are no substantial data as to its value.

Hypertensive headaches respond to agents which lower blood pressure and relieve muscle tension. Chlorothiazide (Diuril), 250 to 500 mg twice a day, and methyldopa (Aldomet), 250 to 500 mg per day, when combined with a small amount of phenobarbital, 15 mg t.i.d., have given the best results. Meprobamate, 200 mg t.i.d., or chlordiazepoxide HCl (Librium), 5 mg t.i.d., may be administered in place of phenobarbital. For the morning occipital ache a capsule containing sodium nitrite, 30 mg, caffeine sodium benzoate, 0.5 g, and acetophenetidin, 0.6 g, has been useful. A simplified method of treating this kind of headache is to supply the caffeine in a cup of strong black coffee and to give with it acetylsalicylic acid. Blocks under the head of the bed may be helpful.

The muscle tension headaches respond best to massage, relaxation, and a combination of drugs which relieve anxiety (phenobarbital, amobarbital, meprobamate, and chlordiazepoxide HCl) and pain [acetylsalicylic acid, propoxyphene HCl (Darvon), or oxycodone (Percodan)]. Stronger analgesic medication (codeine or meperidine HCl) should be avoided. Psychotherapy may be beneficial in this group of patients.

The headache of the syndrome of posttraumatic nervous instability requires supportive psychotherapy in the form of reassurance and frequent explanation of its benign and transient nature, a program of increasing physical activity, and drugs which allay anxiety and depression. Tender scars from scalp laceration may be novocainized repeatedly (subcutaneous injection of 5 ml of 1% procaine) with some degree of success. Settlement of litigation as soon as possible works to the patient's advantage.

Heat, massage, salicylates, and indomethacin (Indocin)

or phenylbutazone (Butazolidin) usually effect some improvement in those arthritic diseases of the cervical spine which are associated with cervicocranial pain (see Chap. 9).

Corticosteroid therapy is indicated in cranial arteritis to prevent disastrous blindness by occlusion of the ophthalmic arteries. The headaches of cranial tumor often respond surprisingly well to large doses of methylprednisolone acetate and like compounds.

In conclusion, it is well to mention the importance of general hygienic measures. Young physicians in particular are apt to seek a specific therapy for each headache syndrome and give little thought to the general health of the patient. We have observed that most of the recurrent and chronic headaches are likely to be more severe and disabling whenever the patient becomes nervous, sick, and tired. A well-rounded diet, adequate rest, a reasonable amount of physical exercise, and a balanced view of the sources of daily anxieties and how to cope with them should be the goal of all therapeutic programs.

REFERENCES

CHAPMAN LF: A humoral agent implicated in vascular headache of the migraine type. Arch Neurol 3:223, 1960

FRIEDMAN AP: *Research and Clinical Studies in Headache,* Baltimore: Williams & Wilkins, 1967

GRAHAM JR, WOLFF HG: The mechanism of the migraine headache and the action of ergotamine tartrate. Arch Neurol Psychiat 39:737, 1938

LANCE JW: *The Mechanism and Management of Headache,* London: Butterworth, 1969

LANCE JW, HINTZENBERGER H: The control of cranial arteries by humoral mechanisms and its relation to the migraine syndrome. Headache 7:93, 1967

PARRY CH: *Collections from the Unpublished Medical Writing of the Late Caleb Hillier Parry,* vol. 1, London: Underwood, 1825

SICUTERI F: Vasoneuroactive substances and their implication in vascular pain, chap. 2 in *Research and Clinical Studies of Headache,* ed A Friedman, Baltimore: Williams & Wilkins, 1967

SMITH R: *Background of Migraine,* New York: Springer, 1967

VINKEN PJ, BRUYN GW: *Handbook of Clinical Neurology,* vol. 5, *Headache and Cranial Neuralgias,* Amsterdam: North-Holland Publishing Company, 1968

WOLFF HG: *Headache and Other Pain,* Fair Lawn, N. J.: Oxford University Press, 1947

7
PAIN IN THE CHEST

EUGENE BRAUNWALD
T. R. HARRISON

There is little parallelism between the severity of chest pain and the gravity of its cause. Therefore, a frequent problem in patients who complain of chest pain is distinguishing trivial disorders from coronary artery disease and other serious disorders. An incorrect positive diagnosis of a hazardous condition such as angina pectoris is likely to have harmful psychologic and economic consequences, while failure to recognize a serious disorder, such as coronary artery disease or mediastinal tumor, may result in the dangerous delay of much-needed treatment.

The apparently bizarre radiation of pain arising in the thoracic viscera can usually be explained in terms of the known facts concerning nerve supply (Chap. 5). One occasionally sees a patient with extension of pain to a location which cannot be logically explained. In most instances, such a person will be found to have more than one disorder capable of causing pain in the chest. The presence of one condition may affect the radiation of the pain produced by the other disorder. For example, when the pain of angina pectoris extends to the back or abdomen, the patient may be found to have also a significant degree of spinal arthritis or an upper abdominal disorder, such as hiatus hernia, disease of the gallbladder, pancreatitis, or peptic ulcer. The common tendency to assume that the presence of an objective abnormality, such as a hiatus hernia or an electrocardiographic abnormality, necessarily means that an atypical chest pain arises in the stomach or the heart is to be strongly condemned. Such an assumption is justified only if a careful history indicates that the behavior of the pain is entirely compatible with the site of origin suggested by the objective finding.

THE LEFT-ARM MYTH There is a long tradition, widely accepted by physicians and laymen, that pain in the left arm, especially when appearing in conjunction with chest pain, has a unique and ominous significance as being almost certain evidence of the presence of ischemic heart disease. This is a myth that has neither theoretic nor clinical foundation. From a theoretic standpoint, any disorder involving the deep afferent fibers of the left upper thoracic region should be capable of causing pain in the chest, the left arm, or both areas. Hence a pain of trivial significance arising in skeletal tissues innervated by upper (first to fourth) thoracic nerves may produce left-arm-area pain; almost any condition capable of causing pain in the chest may induce radiation to the left arm. Such localization is common not only in patients with coronary disease but also in those with numerous other types of chest pain. Although pain due to myocardial ischemia most frequently is substernal, radiates down the ulnar aspect of the left arm (Chap. 244), and is pressing and constricting in nature, the location, radiation, and quality of pain are of less diagnostic significance than the behavior of the pain, in terms of the conditions which induce it and relieve it.

Most persons also believe that cardiac pain is situated in the region of the left breast, and therefore left inframammary pain is one of the common symptoms that bring the patient to seek medical advice. It differs radically from the pain due to myocardial hypoxia, i.e., angina pectoris, in that it is either momentary, sharp and lancinating, or a long-lasting, dull ache, occasionally accentuated by sharp stabs. Such pain is frequently observed in patients who are tense, easily fatigued, unusually anxious, or psychoneurotic, or who have neurocirculatory asthenia. In contrast to angina pectoris, such precordial pain has no relationship to exertion and may be accompanied by tenderness over the precordium.

Only the more important or common conditions causing chest pain will be considered in this chapter.

PAIN DUE TO OXYGEN DEFICIENCY OF THE MYOCARDIUM

PHYSIOLOGIC CONSIDERATIONS OF THE CORONARY CIRCULATION Pain due to myocardial ischemia occurs when the oxygen supply to the heart is deficient in relation to the oxygen need. The oxygen consumption of this organ is closely related to the physiologic effort made during contraction. It is dependent primarily on three factors: (1) the tension developed by the myocardium, (2) the contractile (inotropic) state of the myocardium, and (3) the heart rate. When these three factors remain constant, or almost so, an elevation of stroke volume produces an efficient type of response because it leads to an increase in the external work of the heart (i.e., in the product of cardiac output and arterial pressure) with little accompanying augmentation of myocardial oxygen requirements. Thus, a rise in flow load causes less increment in myocardial oxygen consumption than does a comparable increase in cardiac work per minute brought about by elevation either of pressure or of heart rate. However, the net effects of these hemodynamic variables depend not on oxygen need alone, but rather on the balance between the demand and the supply of oxygen. The heart is always active, and the coronary venous blood is normally much more desaturated than that from other areas of the body. Thus the removal of more oxygen from each unit of blood, which is one of the adjustments commonly utilized by exercising skeletal muscle, is already employed in the heart in the basal state. Therefore, the heart must rely on an increase in the coronary blood flow for obtaining additional oxygen.

It follows, from hydrodynamic considerations, that the flow of blood through the coronary arteries is directly proportional to the pressure gradient between the aorta and the ventricular myocardium during systole and the ventricular cavity during diastole, but is proportional to the fourth power of the radius of the coronary arteries. Thus a relatively slight alteration in coronary diameter will produce a large change in coronary flow, provided that other factors remain constant. In the normal heart, coronary blood flow occurs primarily during diastole, when it is unopposed by myocardial constriction of the coronary vessels. Coronary flow is regulated primarily by myocardial oxygen needs, probably through the release of vasodilator metabolites, such as adenosine, and through variations in myocardial P_{O_2}. Although changes in coronary blood flow occur with activation of autonomic nerves to the coronary vessels, these alterations result primarily from the effects of these nervous stimuli on myocardial contraction and therefore on the heart's oxygen consumption. The role of direct neural regulation of the coronary vascular bed is controversial.

The coronary dilatation which normally occurs during exercise and emotion results from the increased myocardial metabolism during these conditions and is impaired in patients with fixed coronary narrowing due to coronary arteriosclerosis. Thus, any condition in which increased heart rate, arterial pressure, or myocardial contractility occurs tends, particularly, in the presence of coronary obstruction, to precipitate anginal attacks by increasing myocardial oxygen needs. Bradycardia, when not severe, usually has the opposite effects, and this apparently explains the rarity of angina in patients with complete heart block, even when this disorder is associated with coronary disease.

CAUSES OF MYOCARDIAL HYPOXIA By far the most frequently underlying cause is organic narrowing of the coronary arteries secondary to coronary atherosclerosis. Less frequently, narrowing of the coronary orifices due to syphilitic aortitis or to distortion by a dissecting aneurysm may be responsible. There is no evidence that systemic arterial constriction or increased cardiac contractile activity (rise in heart rate or blood pressure, or increase in contractility due to liberation of catecholamines or adrenergic activity) due to emotion can precipitate angina unless there is also structural narrowing of the coronary vessels.

Aside from conditions which narrow the lumen of the coronary arteries, the only other frequent causes of myocardial hypoxia are disorders, such as aortic stenosis and/or regurgitation (Chap. 243), which cause a marked disproportion between the perfusion pressure and the ventricular work. Under such conditions the rise in left ventricular systolic pressure is not, as in hypertensive states, balanced by a corresponding elevation of aortic perfusion pressure. Therefore, an increase in heart rate is especially harmful in patients with aortic stenosis, because it shortens diastole more than systole and thereby decreases the total available perfusion time per minute.

Patients with marked *right ventricular hypertension* may have exertional pain which is, in most respects identical with that of the common type of angina. It is likely that this discomfort results from relative ischemia of the right ventricle brought about by the increased oxygen needs and by the elevated intramural resistance, with sharp reduction of the normally large systolic pressure gradient which perfuses this chamber. Angina is common in patients with *syphilitic aortitis,* and the relative roles of aortic regurgitation and of coronary ostial narrowing are difficult to assess. The importance of tachycardia, decline in arterial pressure, thyrotoxicosis, or diminution in arterial oxygen content (such as occurs in anemia or arterial hypoxemia) in the production of myocardial hypoxia will be apparent from the above discussion. However, these are precipitating and aggravating factors rather than the underlying cause of angina; as already noted, the latter is, in almost all instances, coronary atherosclerosis.

EFFECTS OF MYOCARDIAL HYPOXIA The most common of these is anginal pain, which is considered in some detail in Chap. 244. It is usually described as a heavy pressure or squeezing, a sensation of strangling or constriction in the chest, a "burning" or "heavy feeling," or difficulty in breathing, and it occurs particularly on walking, especially after meals, on cold days against a wind or uphill. It is not a stabbing pain. It occurs during exertion, following heavy meals, and with anger, excitement, and other emotional states; it is not precipitated by coughing or respiratory movements. When anginal pain is induced by walking, it forces the patient to stop or to reduce his speed; it is characteristically relieved by rest and nitroglycerin. The exact mechanism of the pain stimulus is still unknown, but it is probably related to an accumulation of metabolites within the heart muscle. Anginal pain occurs most typically in the substernal region, anteriorly across the midthorax; it may radiate to or rarely occur alone in the interscapular region, in the arms, shoulders, and teeth. The more severe the attack, the greater the radiation from the substernal areas to the left arm, especially its ulnar aspect. There is considerable variability in the amount of effort required to bring on anginal pain.

As a rule, myocardial infarction is associated with a pain similar in quality and distribution to that of angina but of greater intensity and longer duration. The pain of myocardial infarction is not relieved by rest or by coronary dilator drugs and may require large doses of narcotics. It may be accompanied by diaphoresis, nausea, and hypotension (Chap. 245).

In addition to chest pain, a second effect of myocardial ischemia consists of electrocardiographic changes (Chaps. 233, 244, and 245). Many patients with angina have normal tracings between attacks, and the record may even remain normal during the episode of pain. However, often depression of the S-T segments appears in leads I, II, AVL, or in those from the left precordium during exertion. The finding of S-T segment depressions of a deep, ischemic type during an attack of pain, with a return to normal after the pain subsides, strongly suggests that the pain is anginal in origin. There is strong experimental evidence that such depressions, as well as the elevations which are usually seen in patients with infarction and are observed in a few patients during anginal attacks, are related to alterations in cellular ionic balance (Chap. 233). The value and limitation of electrocardiographic changes occurring after exercise in the diagnosis of angina pectoris are discussed in Chap. 244.

A third effect of myocardial hypoxia is an alteration in myocardial contraction. It has been shown that the left ventricular end-diastolic and pulmonary vascular pressures may rise during anginal attacks, particularly if they are prolonged. This indicates transient depression of left ventricular function, which is presumably induced by the decreased contractility of the ischemic areas. On auscultation a fourth heart sound is also frequently heard during the anginal episode; paradoxic pulsations may be evident on palpation of the precordium and can be recorded by apex cardiography.

Another characteristic effect of myocardial hypoxia is liability to sudden death (Chap. 36). This may never occur, despite thousands of anginal episodes. However, it may supervene early in the disease and even in the first attack. The usual mechanism is probably ventricular fibrillation, but occasionally in patients with impaired atrioventricular conduction sudden death may be due to ventricular standstill.

PAIN DUE TO IRRITATION OF SEROUS MEMBRANES OR JOINTS

PERICARDITIS The visceral surface of the pericardium is ordinarily insensitive to pain, as is the parietal surface, except in its lower portion, which has a relatively small number of pain fibers carried in the phrenic nerves. The pain associated with pericarditis is believed to be due to inflammation of the adjacent parietal pleura. These observations explain why noninfectious pericarditis (that associated with uremia and with myocardial infarction) and cardiac tamponade with relatively mild inflammation are usually painless or accompanied by mild pain, whereas infectious pericarditis, being nearly always more intense and spreading to the neighboring pleura, is usually associated with pain having some pleuritic features, i.e., it is aggravated by breathing, coughing, etc. Since the central part of the diaphragm receives its sensory supply from the phrenic nerve (which arises from the third to fifth cervical segments of the spinal cord), pain arising from the lower parietal pericardium and central tendon of the diaphragm is felt characteristically at the tip of the shoulder, the adjoining trapezius ridge, and the neck. Involvement of the more lateral part of the diaphragmatic pleura, supplied by branches from the sixth to ninth intercostal nerves, causes pain not only in the anterior part of the chest but also in the upper part of the abdomen or corresponding region of the back, thus sometimes simulating the pain of acute cholecystitis or pancreatitis.

Pericarditis causes three distinct types of pain (Chap. 246). (1) By far the commonest is the pleuritic pain, related to respiratory movements and aggravated by cough or deep inspiration, sometimes brought on by swallowing, because the esophagus lies just beyond the posterior portion of the heart, sometimes by change of bodily position. It is sharper, more left-sided, is frequently referred to the neck or flank, and lasts longer than the pain of angina pectoris. This type of pain is due to the pleuritic component of the pleuropericarditis so commonly present in the infectious forms. (2) The next commonest pericardial pain is the steady, crushing substernal pain which mimics that of acute myocardial infarction. The mechanism of this steady substernal pain is not certain, but the pain may arise from marked inflammation of the relatively insensitive inner parietal surface of the pericardium, or from irritated afferent cardiac nerve fibers lying in the periadventitial layers of the superficial coronary arteries. (3) The third type of pain, which is quite uncommon, is synchronous with the heartbeat and is felt at the left border of the heart and left shoulder. Occasionally two and rarely all three types of pain may be present simultaneously.

The painful syndromes which may follow trauma to or operations on the heart (i.e., the postcardiotomy syndrome) or myocardial infarction are discussed in later chapters (Chaps. 245 and 246). Such pains often but not always arise in the pericardium.

Pleural pain is very common; it generally results from stretching of inflamed parietal pleura and may be identical with that of pericarditis. It occurs in fibrinous pleurisy, as well as when pneumonic processes reach the periphery of the lung. Pneumothorax and tumors involving the pleural space may also irritate the parietal pleura and cause pleural pain; the latter is sharp, knifelike, superficial in quality, and its aggravation by each breath and by coughing readily distinguishes it from the deep, dull, steady unwavering pain of myocardial ischemia.

The pain resulting from pulmonary embolism may resemble that of acute myocardial infarction, and in massive embolism it is located substernally. In patients with smaller emboli the pain is located more laterally, is pleuritic in nature, and may be associated with hemoptysis (Chap.

266). Massive pulmonary emboli and other causes of acute pulmonary hypertension may cause severe, persistent substernal pain, presumably due to distention of the pulmonary artery. The pain of mediastinal emphysema (Chap. 264) may be intense and sharp and may radiate from the substernal region to the shoulders; often a distinct crepitus is heard. The pain associated with mediastinitis and mediastinal tumors usually resembles that of pleuritis but is more likely to be maximal in the substernal region, and the associated feeling of constriction or oppression may cause confusion with myocardial infarction. The pain due to *acute dissection of the aorta* or to an expanding aortic aneurysm results from stimulation of the adventitia; it is usually extremely severe, is localized to the center of the chest, lasts for hours, and requires unusually large amounts of analgesics for relief. It often radiates into the back but is not aggravated by changes in position or respiration (Chap. 251).

The *costochondral and chondrosternal articulations* are the commonest sites of anterior chest pain. Objective signs in the form of swelling (Tietze's syndrome), redness, and heat are rare, but sharply localized tenderness is common. The pain may be "neuritic," i.e., darting and lasting for only a few seconds, or a dull ache enduring for hours or days. An associated feeling of tightness due to muscle spasm (see below) is frequent. When the discomfort persists for a few days only, a story of minor trauma or of some unaccustomed physical effort can often be obtained. The variety of this discomfort is common in persons with arthritis of the spine and also in patients with ischemic heart disease, but in many instances no associated disorder is found. It should be emphasized that *pressure on the chondrosternal and costochondral junctions is an essential part of the examination of every patient with chest pain.* A large percentage of patients with costochondral pain, especially those who also have minor and innocent T-wave alterations (Chap. 233), are erroneously labeled as having coronary disease. The dire consequences of such a mistake have already been emphasized.

Pain secondary to *subacromial bursitis* and *arthritis of the shoulder and spine* may be precipitated by exercise of the local area but not by general exertion. It may be brought about by passive movement of the involved area as well as by coughing.

PAIN DUE TO TISSUE DISRUPTION

Rupture or tear of a structure may give rise to pain that sets in abruptly and reaches its peak of intensity almost instantly. Such a story should arouse the suspicion of dissecting aortic aneurysm, pneumothorax, mediastinal emphysema, a cervical disk syndrome, or rupture of the esophagus. However, the patient may be too ill to recall the precise circumstances, or the pain may be atypical and increase gradually in severity. Likewise, other and more benign conditions, such as a slipped costal cartilage or an intercostal muscle cramp, may also produce pain with an abrupt onset.

Dissecting aortic aneurysm usually causes very severe persistent pain located in the anterior chest. It often radiates into the back, and is not intensified by breathing or motion.

CLINICAL ASPECTS OF THE COMMONER CAUSES OF CHEST PAIN

Some of the features of pericarditis have already been described, and those of the more serious causes of chest pain such as myocardial ischemia (angina pectoris and infarction), dissecting aneurysm, and disorders of the pleura, esophagus, stomach, duodenum, and pancreas are considered in the appropriate chapters dealing with these problems. Here, we are concerned with the discussion of those causes which are not considered in more detail elsewhere.

PAIN ARISING IN THE CHEST WALL OR UPPER EXTREMITY This may develop as a result of muscle or ligament strains brought on by unaccustomed exercise and felt in the costochondral or chondrosternal junctions or in the chest wall muscles. We mention the upper extremities and especially the left because of the deeply ingrained legend that pain in the left arm has a specific significance in indicting the heart. Other causes are *osteoarthritis* of the dorsal or thoracic spine and *ruptured cervical disks.* Pain in the left upper extremity and precordium may be due to compression of portions of the brachial plexus by a cervical rib or by spasm and shortening of the scalenus anticus muscle secondary to high fixation of the ribs and sternum. Finally, pains in the upper extremity (shoulder-hand syndrome) and in the pectoral muscles may, through unknown mechanisms, occur in patients with ischemic heart disease.

Skeletal pains in the chest wall or shoulder girdles or arms are usually recognized quite easily. Localized tenderness of the affected area is usually present, and the pain is sometimes clearly related to movements involving the painful locus. Thus deep breathing, turning or twisting of the chest, and movements of the shoulder girdle and arm will elicit and duplicate the pain of which the patient complains. The pain may be very brief, lasting only a few seconds, or full and aching and enduring for hours. The duration is, therefore, likely to be either longer or shorter than untreated anginal pain, which usually lasts for only a few minutes.

These skeletal pains often have a sharp or sticking quality. In addition, there is frequently a feeling of tightness, which is probably due to associated spasm of intercostal or pectoral muscles. This may produce the "morning stiffness" seen in so many skeletal disorders. The discomfort is unaffected by nitroglycerin but often is abolished by infiltration of the painful areas with procaine. When chest wall pain is of recent origin and follows trauma, strain, or some unusual activity involving the pectoral muscles, it presents no problem in diagnosis. However, *long-standing skeletal pain is frequent in persons who also have angina pectoris.* Since both disorders are very common, this association may be coincidental. In other instances, the coronary disease appears to be responsible for the chest wall pain; the exact mechanism is uncertain but probably is similar to that responsible for the well-known shoulder-hand syndrome. This coexistence of the two different types of chest pain in the same patient is a frequent cause of a confusing history, because in the patient's mind the anginal needle may be hidden in the skeletal haystack. Thus every middle-aged or elderly patient who has long-standing anterior chest wall pain merits careful study for the presence of ischemic heart disease.

Detailed questioning may reveal that what was originally thought by the patient to be a single type of discomfort actually comprises two different pains, which, though similar in quality and area, differ in duration and initiating factors. When the history is inconclusive, the exercise electrocardiogram may furnish useful information concerning the existence of myocardial ischemia. In rare instances coronary arteriography may be required. It may be necessary also to learn by direct observation whether exercise alone or postprandial exertion is capable of producing it. Repeated tests may be required, the effects of preceding placebos, as compared with nitroglycerin, on the amount of exertion required to induce the pain being compared. *The confusion created by the presence of innocent skeletal pain impairs the reliability of the history and is probably the commonest cause of errors—both positive and negative—in the diagnosis of angina pectoris.*

ESOPHAGEAL PAIN This usually presents as deep thoracic pain; it results from chemical (acid) irritation of the esophageal mucosa or from spasm of the esophageal muscle in the presence of an intraluminal obstruction, and characteristically follows deglutition. Accompanying dysphagia, regurgitation of undigested food, and weight loss direct attention to the esophagus (see Chaps. 38 and 286).

EMOTIONAL DISORDERS These are also common causes of chest wall pain. Usually, the discomfort is experienced as a sense of "tightness," sometimes called "aching," and occasionally it may be sufficiently severe as to be designated a pain of considerable magnitude. Since the discomfort has almost always the additional quality of tightness or constriction, and, furthermore, since it is often localized beneath the sternum, although it may be felt in other areas of the anterior part of the chest, it is not surprising that this type of pain is frequently confused with that of myocardial ischemia. Ordinarily, it lasts for a half hour or more and may persist for a day or less with slow fluctuation of intensity. The association with fatigue or emotional strain is usually clear, although this may not be recognized by the patient until called to his attention. The pain probably develops through unconscious and prolonged increase of muscle tone (as in frowning in the face, or as can be quickly produced in the hand by rigidly clenching the fist), often enhanced by an accompanying hyperventilation (by causing a contraction of the chest wall muscles similar to the painful tetany of the extremities). When the hyperventilation and/or the associated andrenergic effect due to anxiety also causes innocent changes in the T waves and S-T segments, the confusion with coronary disease is strengthened. However, the long duration of the pain, the lack of any relation to exertion but association rather with fatigue or tension, and the usually periodic occurrence on successive days without any limitation of capacity for exercise usually make the differentiation from ischemic pain quite clear.

As compared with these two causes (the chest wall muscle and ligament strains and the contraction of the pectoral muscles due to reflex influences, fatigue, or tension), the various other conditions that may cause skeletal discomfort are uncommon and readily recognized after appropriate observation: spinal arthritis, herpes zoster, anterior scalene and hyperabduction syndromes, malignant disease of the ribs, etc.

OTHER CAUSES OF CHEST PAIN The several *abdominal disorders* which may at times mimic anginal pain may usually be suspected from the history, which, as in esophageal pain, ordinarily indicates some relationship to swallowing, eating, belching, etc. Pain resulting from gastric or duodenal ulcer (Chap. 287) is epigastric or substernal, commences about 1 to 1 ½ h after meals, and is usually promptly relieved by antacids or milk. The gastrointestinal roentgenogram will be of crucial significance, and roentgenographic examination is also often helpful in differentiating biliary, gastrointestinal, aortic, pulmonary, and skeletal disease pain from angina pectoris. It should be emphasized again that the demonstration of the presence of a coexistent abdominal disorder such as a hiatus hernia does not constitute proof that the chest pain of which the patient complains is due to this. Such disorders are frequently asymptomatic and are not at all uncommon in patients who also have angina pectoris.

Substernal discomfort also frequently occurs in the presence of *tracheobronchitis;* it is described as a burning sensation accentuated by coughing. A variety of *disorders involving the breast,* including inflammatory breast disease, benign and malignant tumors, as well as mastodynia, are common causes of thoracic pain. The localization and superficial swelling and tenderness are of diagnostic importance.

APPROACH TO THE PATIENT WITH PAIN IN THE CHEST

Most persons with this complaint will fall into one of two general groups. The first consists of persons with prolonged and often severe pain without obvious initiating factors. Such persons will frequently be gravely ill. The problem is that of differentiating such serious conditions as myocardial infarction, dissecting aneurysm, and pulmonary embolism from each other and from less grave causes. In some such instances, the careful history will provide significant clues, while objective evidence of crucial importance will appear within the subsequent 2 or 3 days. Thus, when the initial examinations are not decisive, a watch-and-wait policy, with repeated electrocardiograms coupled with measurements of serum enzymes, lung scans, and chest roentgenograms, will commonly provide the correct answer.

The second group of patients comprises those who have brief episodes of pain and are otherwise in apparently excellent health. Here, the resting electrocardiogram will rarely supply decisive information, but records taken during or immediately after exercise will often reveal characteristic changes (Chap. 244). However, in many instances it is the study of the subjective phenomenon, i.e., of the pain itself, that will lead to the diagnosis. Of the several methods of investigation which are available for such patients, three are of cardinal importance.

A detailed and *meticulous history* of the behavior of the pain is the most important method. The location, radiation, quality, intensity, and, especially, duration of the episodes are important. Even more so is the story of the aggravating and alleviating factors. Thus a history of sharp aggravation by breathing, coughing, or other respiratory movements will usually point toward the pericardium (because of the associated pleuropericarditis) or mediastinum as the site, although chest wall pain is likewise affected by respiratory motions. Similarly, a pain which regularly appears on rapid walking and vanishes within a few minutes upon standing still suggests the diagnosis of angina pectoris, although here, once again, a similar story will rarely be obtained from patients with skeletal disorders.

When the history is inconclusive, the *study of the patient at the time of the spontaneous episode* will often supply crucial information. Thus the electrocardiogram, which may be normal both at rest and even during or after exercise in the absence of pain, will occasionally demonstrate striking changes when recorded during an anginal episode. Similarly, radiographic study of the esophagus or of the stomach may show no evidence of cardiospasm or of hiatal hernia except when the observation is made during the pain.

The third method of study represents the *attempt to produce and alleviate the pain at will.* This procedure is necessary only when doubt exists following the history or when needed for psychotherapeutic purposes. Thus the demonstration that a localized pain, which can be reproduced by pressure on the chest, is completely relieved by local infiltration with procaine will often be of conclusive importance in convincing the patient that the heart is not the site.

When, as is not rarely the case, the history is atypical, the correct diagnosis of angina pectoris will often depend in large measure on the response to nitroglycerin. Here, a number of pitfalls should be avoided. If the patient has previously had the drug, careful questioning may be necessary to avoid errors. Thus, relief of pain after its sublingual administration does not necessarily prove that there is a cause-and-effect relationship. It is necessary to be certain that the pain vanishes more rapidly (usually within 5 min) and more completely when the drug is used than when it is not employed. A false negative impression concerning the effect of nitroglycerin may be the result of the use of a deteriorated preparation which has been exposed to light. In doubtful instances, repeated exercise tests, with and without preceding administration of nitroglycerin, are necessary. The demonstration that the time required for a given exercise to produce pain is consistently and considerably longer when it is undertaken within a few minutes after a sublingual nitroglycerin pill than after a placebo may, in some instances, represent the sole method for accurate recognition of angina pectoris. A completely negative response to such repeated tests constitutes almost conclusive evidence against angina.

In patients in whom the question of whether there is coronary disease cannot be resolved despite the aforementioned clinical and laboratory tests, including exercise electrocardiography (Chap. 244), cardiac catheterization and coronary arteriography may be required. A useful stress test that can be carried out at the time of catheterization is to elevate cardiac frequency in stepwise fashion by electrical pacing; the development of S-T segment depressions on the electrocardiogram and the reproduction of the pain support the diagnosis of myocardial ischemia. Coronary arteriography will show severe (more than 60 percent) reduction of the lumen in patients with obstructive coronary artery disease (see Chaps. 235 and 244).

REFERENCES

BRAUNWALD E: Control of myocardial oxygen consumption: Physiologic and clinical considerations. Am J Cardiol 27:416, 1971

—— et al: *Mechanisms of Contraction of the Normal and Failing Heart,* 2d ed., Boston: Little, Brown, 1976

BURCH GE et al: Cardiac causalgia. Am Heart J 76:725, 1968

DRESSLER W: Angina pectoris, in *Clinical Aids in Cardiac Diagnosis,* New York: Grune & Stratton, 1970

HURST JW: Symptoms due to heart disease, in *The Heart,* 3d ed., New York: McGraw-Hill, 1974, p. 140

SELZER A: *Principles of Clinical Cardiology,* p. 21, Philadelphia: Saunders, 1975

PAINE R: Thoracic pain, in *Signs and Symptoms,* 6th ed., ed RS Blacklow, Philadelphia: Lippincott, 1976

WOOD P: The chief symptoms of heart disease, in *Diseases of the Heart and Circulation,* 3d ed., Philadelphia: Lippincott, 1968

8
ABDOMINAL PAIN

WILLIAM SILEN

The correct interpretation of acute abdominal pain is one of the most challenging demands made of any physician. Since proper therapy often requires urgent action, the luxury of the leisurely approach suitable for the study of other conditions is frequently denied. Few other clinical situations demand greater experience and judgment, because the most catastrophic of events may be forecast by the subtlest of symptoms and signs. Nowhere in medicine is a meticulously executed detailed history and physical examination of greater importance. The etiologic classification in Table 8-1, although not complete, forms a useful frame of reference for the evaluation of patients with abdominal pain.

The diagnosis of "acute or surgical abdomen" so often heard in emergency wards is not an acceptable one because of its often misleading and erroneous connotation. The most obvious of "acute abdomens" may not require operative intervention, and the mildest of abdominal pains may herald the onset of an urgently correctible lesion. Any patient with abdominal pain of recent onset requires early and thorough evaluation with specific attempts at accurate diagnosis.

SOME MECHANISMS OF PAIN ORIGINATING IN THE ABDOMEN Inflammation of the parietal peritoneum The pain of parietal peritoneal inflammation is steady and aching in character and is located directly over the inflamed area, its exact reference being possible because it is transmitted by overlapping somatic nerves supplying the parietal peritoneum. The intensity of the pain is dependent upon the type and amount of foreign substance to which the peritoneal surfaces are exposed in a given period of time. For example, the sudden release into the peritoneal cavity of a small quantity of *sterile* acid gastric juice causes much more pain than the same amount of grossly contaminated neutral fecal material. Enzymatically active pancreatic juice incites more pain and inflammation than does the same amount of sterile bile containing no potent enzymes. Blood and urine are often so bland as to go undetected if exposure of the peritoneum has not been sudden and massive. In the case of bacterial contamination, such as in pelvic inflammatory disease, the pain is frequently of low intensity early in the illness until bacterial multiplication has caused the elaboration of irritating substances.

So important is the rate at which the irritating material is applied to the peritoneum that cases of perforated peptic ulcer may be associated with entirely different clinical pictures dependent only upon the rapidity with which the gastric juice enters the peritoneal cavity.

The pain of peritoneal inflammation is invariably accentuated by pressure or changes in tension of the peritoneum, whether produced by palpation or by movement, as in coughing or sneezing. Consequently, the patient with peritonitis lies quietly in bed, preferring to avoid motion, in contrast to the patient with colic, who may writhe incessantly.

TABLE 8-1
Some important causes of abdominal pain

- *I* Pain originating in the abdomen
  - *A* Parietal peritoneal inflammation
    - *1* Bacterial contamination, e.g., perforated appendix, pelvic inflammatory disease
    - *2* Chemical irritation, e.g., perforated ulcer, pancreatitis, mittelschmerz
  - *B* Mechanical obstruction of hollow viscera
    - *1* Obstruction of the small or large intestine
    - *2* Obstruction of the biliary tree
    - *3* Obstruction of the ureter
  - *C* Vascular disturbances
    - *1* Embolism or thrombosis
    - *2* Vascular rupture
    - *3* Pressure or torsional occlusion
    - *4* Sickle-cell anemia
  - *D* Abdominal wall
    - *1* Distortion or traction of mesentery
    - *2* Trauma or infection of muscles
    - *3* Distention of visceral surfaces, e.g., hepatic or renal capsules
- *II* Pain referred from extraabdominal sources
  - *A* Thorax—e.g., pneumonia, referred pain from coronary occlusion
  - *B* Spine—e.g., radiculitis from arthritis
  - *C* Genitalia—e.g., torsion of the testicle
- *III* Metabolic causes
  - *A* Exogenous
    - *1* Black widow spider bite
    - *2* Lead poisoning and others
  - *B* Endogenous
    - *1* Uremia
    - *2* Diabetic coma
    - *3* Porphyria
    - *4* Allergic factors (C′ 1-esterase deficiency)
- *IV* Neurogenic causes
  - *A* Organic
    - *1* Tabes dorsalis
    - *2* Herpes zoster
    - *3* Causalgia and others
  - *B* Functional

Another of the characteristic features of peritoneal irritation is tonic reflex spasm of the abdominal musculature, localized to the involved body segment. The intensity of the tonic muscle spasm accompanying peritoneal inflammation is dependent upon the location of the inflammatory process, the rate at which it develops, and the integrity of the nervous system. Spasm over a perforated retrocecal appendix or perforated ulcer into the lesser peritoneal sac may be minimal or absent because of the protective effect of overlying viscera. As in pain of peritoneal inflammation, a slowly developing process often greatly attenuates the degree of muscle spasm. Catastrophic abdominal emergencies such as a perforated ulcer have been repeatedly associated with minimal or occasionally no detectable pain or muscle spasm in obtunded, seriously ill, debilitated elderly patients or in psychotic patients.

Obstruction of hollow viscera The pain of obstruction of hollow abdominal viscera is classically described as intermittent, or colicky. Yet the lack of a truly cramping character should not be misleading, because distention of a hollow viscus may produce steady pain with only very occasional exacerbations. Although not nearly as well localized as the pain of parietal peritoneal inflammation, some useful generalities can be made concerning its distribution.

The colicky pain of obstruction of small intestine is usually periumbilical or supraumbilical and is poorly localized. As the intestine becomes progressively dilated with loss of muscular tone, the colicky nature of the pain may become less apparent. With superimposed strangulating obstruction, pain may spread in the lower lumbar region if there is traction on the root of the mesentery. Pain arising in the colon is usually perceived in the region involved by the pathologic process.

Sudden distention of the biliary tree produces a steady rather than colicky type of pain; hence the term "biliary colic" is misleading. Acute distention of the gallbladder usually causes pain in the right upper quadrant with radiation to the right posterior region of the thorax or to the tip of the right scapula, and distention of the common bile duct is often associated with pain in the epigastrium radiating to the upper part of the lumbar region. Considerable variation is common, however, so that differentiation between these may be impossible. The typical subscapular pain or lumbar radiation is frequently absent. Gradual dilatation of the biliary tree as in carcinoma of the head of the pancreas may cause no pain or only a mild aching sensation in the epigastrium or right upper quadrant. The pain of distention of the pancreatic ducts is similar to that described for distention of the common bile duct but in addition is very frequently accentuated by recumbency and relieved by the upright position.

Obstruction of the urinary bladder results in dull suprapubic pain, usually low in intensity. Restlessness without specific complaint of pain may be the only sign of a distended bladder in an obtunded patient. In contrast, acute obstruction of the intravesicular portion of the ureter is characterized by severe suprapubic and flank pain which radiates to the penis, scrotum, or inner aspect of the upper region of the thigh. Obstruction of the ureteropelvic junction is felt as pain in the costovertebral angle, whereas obstruction of the remainder of the ureter is associated with flank pain, which often extends into the corresponding side of the abdomen.

Vascular disturbances A frequent misconception, despite abundant experience to the contrary, is that pain associated with intraabdominal vascular disturbances is sudden and catastrophic in nature. The pain of embolism or thrombosis of the superior mesenteric artery or that of impending rupture of an abdominal aortic aneurysm certainly may be severe and diffuse. Yet just as frequently, the patient with occlusion of the superior mesenteric artery has only mild continuous diffuse pain for 2 or 3 days before vascular collapse or findings of peritoneal inflammation appear. The early, seemingly insignificant discomfort is caused by hyperperistalsis rather than peritoneal inflammation. Indeed, absence of tenderness and rigidity in the presence of continuous diffuse pain in a patient likely to have vascular disease is quite characteristic of occlusion of the superior mesenteric artery. Abdominal pain with radiation to the sacral region, flank, or genitalia should always signal the possible presence of a rupturing abdominal aortic aneurysm. This pain may persist over a period of several days before rupture and collapse occur.

Abdominal wall Pain arising from the abdominal wall is usually constant and aching. Movement and pressure accentuate the discomfort and muscle spasm. In the case of hematoma of the rectus sheath, now most frequently encountered in association with anticoagulant therapy, a mass may be present in the lower quadrants of the abdomen. Simultaneous involvement of muscles in other parts of the body usually serves to differentiate myositis of the abdominal wall from an intraabdominal process which might cause pain in the same region.

REFERRED PAIN IN ABDOMINAL DISEASES Pain referred to the abdomen from the thorax, spine, or genitalia may prove a vexing problem in differential diagnosis, because diseases of the upper part of the abdominal cavity such as acute cholecystitis, perforated ulcer, or subphrenic abscesses are frequently associated with intrathoracic complications. A most important, yet often forgotten, dictum is that the possibility of intrathoracic disease must be considered in every patient with abdominal pain, especially if the pain is in the upper part of the abdomen. Systematic questioning and examination directed toward detecting the presence or absence of myocardial or pulmonary infarction, pneumonia, pericarditis, or esophageal disease (the intrathoracic diseases which most often masquerade as abdominal emergencies) will often provide sufficient clues to establish the proper diagnosis. Diaphragmatic pleuritis resulting from pneumonia or pulmonary infarction may cause pain in the right upper quadrant and pain in the supraclavicular area, the latter radiation to be sharply distinguished from the referred subscapular pain caused by acute distention of the extrahepatic biliary tree. The ultimate decision as to the origin of abdominal pain may require deliberate and planned observation over a period of several hours, during which time repeated questioning and examination will provide the proper explanation.

Referred pain of thoracic origin is often accompanied by splinting of the involved hemithorax with respiratory lag and decrease in excursion more marked than that seen in the presence of intraabdominal disease. In addition, apparent abdominal muscle spasm caused by referred pain will diminish during the inspiratory phase of respiration, whereas it is persistent throughout both respiratory phases if it is of abdominal origin. Palpation over the area of referred pain in the abdomen also does not usually accentuate the pain and in many instances actually seems to relieve it. The frequent coexistence of thoracic and abdominal disease may be misleading and confusing, so that differentiation might be difficult or impossible. For example, the patient with known biliary tract disease often has epigastric pain during myocardial infarction, or biliary colic may be referred to the precordium or left shoulder in a patient who has suffered previously from angina pectoris. For the explanation of the radiation of pain to a previously diseased area, see Chap. 5.

Referred pain from the spine, which usually involves compression or irritation of nerve roots, is characteristically intensified by certain motions such as cough, sneeze, or strain and is associated with hyperesthesia over the involved dermatomes. Pain referred to the abdomen from the testicles or seminal vesicles is generally accentuated by the slightest pressure on either of these organs. The abdominal discomfort is of dull aching character and is poorly localized.

METABOLIC ABDOMINAL CRISES Pain of metabolic origin may simulate almost any other type of intraabdominal disease. Here several mechanisms may be at work. In certain instances, such as hyperparathyroidism, the metabolic disease itself may produce an intraabdominal process such as pancreatitis. Primary hyperlipemia may also be accompanied by severe pancreatitis, which can lead to unnecessary laparotomy unless recognized. C′1-esterase deficiency associated with angioneurotic edema is also often associated with episodes of severe abdominal pain. Whenever the cause of abdominal pain is obscure, a metabolic origin must always be considered. Abdominal pain is also the hallmark of familial Mediterranean fever (Chap. 229).

The problem of differential diagnosis is often not readily resolved. The pain of porphyria and of lead colic usually is difficult to distinguish from that of intestinal obstruction, because severe hyperperistalsis is a prominent feature of both. The pain of uremia or diabetes is nonspecific, and the pain and tenderness frequently shift in location and intensity. Diabetic acidosis may be precipitated by acute appendicitis or intestinal obstruction, so that if prompt resolution of the abdominal pain does not result from correction of the metabolic abnormalities, an underlying organic problem should be suspected. Black widow spider bites produce intense pain and rigidity of the abdominal muscles and of the back, an area infrequently involved in disease of intraabdominal origin.

NEUROGENIC CAUSES Causalgic pain may occur in diseases which injure nerves of sensory type. It has a burning character and is usually limited to the distribution of a given peripheral nerve. Normal stimuli such as touch or change in temperature may be transformed into this type of pain, which is also frequently present in a patient at rest. A helpful finding is the demonstration that cutaneous pain spots are now irregularly spaced, and this may be the only indication of an old nerve lesion underlying causalgic pain. Even though the pain may be precipitated by gentle palpation, rigidity of the abdominal muscles is absent, and the respirations are not disturbed. Distention of the abdomen is uncommon, and the pain has no relationship to the intake of food.

Pain arising from spinal nerves or roots comes and goes suddenly and is of a lancinating type (see Chap. 9). It may be caused by herpes zoster, impingement by arthritis, tumors, herniated nucleus pulposus, diabetes, or syphilis. Again it is not associated with food intake, abdominal distention, or changes in respiration. Severe muscle spasm, as in the gastric crises of tabes dorsalis, is common but is either relieved or is not accentuated by abdominal palpation. The pain is made worse by movement of the spine and is usually confined to a few dermatome segments. Hyperesthesia is very common.

Psychogenic pain conforms to none of the aforementioned patterns of disease. Here the mechanism is hard to define. The most common problem is the hysterical adolescent or young women who develops abdominal pain; she frequently loses an appendix and other organs because of it. Ovulation or some other natural event that causes brief mild abdominal discomfort may be maximized as an abdominal catastrophe.

Psychogenic pain varies enormously in type and location but usually has no relation to meals. It is often at its onset markedly accentuated during the night. Nausea and vomiting are rarely observed, although occasionally the patient reports these symptoms. Spasm is seldom induced in the abdominal musculature and if present does not persist, especially if the attention of the patient can be distracted. Persistent localized tenderness is rare, and, if found, the muscle spasm in the area is inconsistent and often absent. Restriction of the depth of respiration is the most common respiratory abnormality, but this is in the nature of a smothering or choking sensation and is part of an anxiety state (see Chap. 14). It occurs in the absence of thoracic splinting or change in the respiratory rate.

APPROACH TO THE PATIENT WITH ABDOMINAL PAIN

There are few abdominal conditions which require such urgent operative intervention that an orderly approach need be abandoned, no matter how ill the patient. Only those patients with exsanguinating hemorrhage must be rushed to the operating room immediately, but in such instances only a few minutes are required to assess the critical nature of the problem. Under these circumstances, all obstacles must be swept aside, adequate access for intravenous fluid replacement obtained, and the operation begun. Many patients of this type have died in the radiology department or the emergency room while awaiting such unnecessary examinations as electrocardiograms or films of the abdomen. *There are no contraindications to operation when massive hemorrhage is present.* Although exceedingly important, this situation fortunately is relatively rare.

Nothing will supplant an orderly painstakingly *detailed history,* which is far more valuable than any laboratory or roentgenologic examination. This kind of history is laborious and time-consuming, making it not especially popular even though a reasonably accurate diagnosis can be made on the basis of the history alone in the majority of cases. The *chronological sequence of events* in the patient's history is often more important than emphasis on the location of pain. If the examiner is sufficiently open-minded and unhurried, asks the proper questions, and listens, the patient will often himself provide the diagnosis. Careful attention should be paid to the extraabdominal regions which may be responsible for abdominal pain. An accurate menstrual history in a female patient is essential. Narcotics or analgesics should be withheld until a definitive diagnosis or a definitive plan has been formulated, because these agents often make it more difficult to secure and to interpret the history and physical findings.

In the examination, simple critical inspection of the patient, e.g., of his facies, position in bed, and respiratory activity, may provide valuable clues. The amount of information to be gleaned is directly proportional to the *gentleness* and thoroughness of the examiner. Once a patient with peritoneal inflammation has been examined in a brusque manner, accurate assessment by the next examiner becomes almost impossible. For example, eliciting rebound tenderness by sudden release of a deeply palpating hand in a patient with suspected peritonitis is cruel and unnecessary. The same information can be obtained by gentle percussion of the abdomen (rebound tenderness on a miniature scale), a maneuver which can be far more precise and localizing. Asking the patient to cough will elicit true rebound tenderness without the need for placing a hand on the abdomen. Furthermore, the brusque demonstration of rebound tenderness will startle and induce protective spasm in a nervous or worried patient in whom true rebound tenderness is not present. A palpable gallbladder will be missed if palpation is so brusque that voluntary muscle spasm becomes superimposed upon involuntary muscular rigidity.

As in history taking, there is no substitute for sufficient time spent in the examination. It is important to remember that abdominal signs may be minimal but nevertheless, if accompanied by consistent symptoms, may be exceptionally meaningful when carefully assessed. Signs may be virtually or actually totally absent in cases of pelvic peritonitis, so that careful *pelvic and rectal examinations are mandatory in every patient with abdominal pain.* The presence of tenderness on pelvic or rectal examination in the absence of other abdominal signs must not lead the examiner to exclude such important operative indications as perforated appendicitis, diverticulitis, twisted ovarian cyst, and many others.

Much attention has been paid to the presence or absence of peristaltic sounds, their quality, and their frequency. Auscultation of the abdomen is probably one of the least rewarding aspects of the physical examination of a patient with abdominal pain. Severe catastrophes, such as strangulating small-intestinal obstruction or perforated appendicitis, may occur in the presence of normal peristalsis. Conversely, when the proximal part of the intestine above an obstruction becomes markedly distended and edematous, peristaltic sounds may lose the characteristics of borborygmi and become weak or absent even when peritonitis is not present. It is usually the severe chemical peritonitis of sudden onset which is associated with the truly silent abdomen. Assessment of the patient's state of hydration is important. The hematocrit and urinalysis permit an accurate estimate of the severity of dehydration, so that adequate replacement can be carried out.

Laboratory examinations may be of enormous value in the assessment of the patient with abdominal pain, yet with but a few exceptions they rarely establish a diagnosis. Leukocytosis should never be the single deciding factor as to whether or not operation is indicated. A white blood cell count greater than 20,000 per mm^3 may be observed with perforation of a viscus, but pancreatitis, acute cholecystitis, pelvic inflammatory disease, and intestinal infarction may be associated with marked leukocytosis. A normal white blood cell count is by no means rare in cases of perforation of abdominal viscera. The diagnosis of anemia may be more helpful than the white blood cell count, especially when combined with the history.

The urinalysis is also of great value in indicating to some degree the state of hydration or to rule out severe renal disease, diabetes, or porphyria. Determination of the blood urea nitrogen, blood sugar, and serum bilirubin levels may also be helpful. The serum amylase determination is overrated, since in carefully controlled series of patients with proved pancreatitis where the determination has been done within the first 72 h, amylase was less than 200 Somogyi units in one-third of the cases, between 200 and 500 in another one-third of the cases, and greater than 500 in one-third. Since many diseases other than pancreatitis, e.g., perforated ulcer, strangulating intestinal obstruction, and acute cholecystitis, may be associated with very marked increase in the serum amylase, great care must be exercised in denying an operation to a patient solely on the basis of an elevated serum amylase level. The determination of the output of urinary amylase and the clearance of amylase are probably more accurate than the estimation of the serum amylase in the diagnosis of pancreatitis.

Abdominal paracentesis has proved to be a safe and effective diagnostic maneuver in patients with acute abdominal pain. It is of special value in patients with blunt trauma to the abdomen where evaluation of the abdomen may be difficult because of other multiple injuries to the spine, pelvis, or ribs and where blood in the peritoneal cavity produces only a very mild peritoneal reaction. The gallbladder is the only organ which may continue to seep fluid following accidental perforation, so that the region of this organ must be assiduously avoided. Determination of the pH of the aspirated fluid to ascertain the site of a perforation is misleading, because even highly acid gastric juice is rapidly buffered by peritoneal exudate.

Plain and upright or lateral decubitus roentgenograms of the abdomen may be of the greatest value. They are usually unnecessary in patients with acute appendicitis or strangulated external hernias. However, in cases of intestinal obstruction, perforated ulcer, and a variety of other conditions, films may be diagnostic. During a search for free air, the patient should be kept in the decubitus or upright position for at least 10 min before the appropriate film is taken lest a small pneumoperitoneum be missed. In rare instances, barium or water-soluble medium examination of the upper part of the gastrointestinal tract may demonstrate partial intestinal obstruction which may elude diagnosis by other means. If there is any question of obstruction of the colon, oral administration of barium sulfate should be avoided. On the other hand, barium enema is of inestimable value in cases of colonic obstruction and should be used with greater frequency where the possibility of perforation does not exist.

Sometimes, even under the best of circumstances with all available auxiliary aids and with the greatest of clinical skill, a definitive diagnosis cannot be established at the time of the initial examination. Nevertheless, despite lack of a clear anatomic diagnosis it may be abundantly clear to an experienced and thoughtful physician and surgeon on clinical grounds alone that operation is indicated. Should that decision be questionable, watchful waiting with repeated questioning and examination will often elucidate the true nature of the illness and indicate the proper course of action.

REFERENCES

COPE Z: *The Early Diagnosis of the Acute Abdomen,* 13th ed., Fair Lawn, N. J.: Oxford University Press, 1968

FITZ RH: Perforating inflammation of the vermiform appendix: With special reference to its early diagnosis and treatment. Trans Assoc Am Physicians 1:107, 1886

LASSER, RB et al: The role of intestinal gas in functional abdominal pain. N Eng J Med 293:524, 1975

SILEN W et al: Strangulation obstruction of the small intestine. Arch Surg 85:121, 1962

STANILAND JR et al: Clinical presentation of acute abdomen: Study of 600 patients. Br Med J 2:393, 1972

9

PAIN IN THE BACK AND NECK

HENRY J. MANKIN
RAYMOND D. ADAMS

The following remarks concern mainly the lower part of the back, since it is most frequently the site of disabling pain. The lower portions of the spine and pelvis, with their many muscular and tendinous attachments, are relatively inaccessible to palpation and inspection. Although certain physical signs and radiographs are helpful, it is often necessary to depend on the patient's description of his pain (which may not be altogether accurate) and his behavior during the execution of certain maneuvers to fully assess the nature of his problem. Seasoned clinicians, for these reasons, come to appreciate the need of a systematic clinical approach, the description of which is one of the main purposes of this chapter.

ANATOMY AND PHYSIOLOGY OF THE LOWER PART OF THE BACK

The bony spine is a complex structure, roughly divisible into two parts. The anterior part consists of a series of cylindrical vertebral bodies, articulated by the intervertebral disks and held together by the anterior and posterior longitudinal ligaments. The posterior part consists of more delicate elements that extend from the vertebral body as pedicles and laminae fused by ligaments to form the vertebral canal. Stout transverse and spinous ligaments project laterally and posteriorly and serve as the attachments of muscles which support and protect the vertebral column. The stability of the spine depends on two types of supporting structures, the ligamentous (passive) and muscular (active). The ligamentous structures are quite strong, but because neither they nor the vertebral body–disk complexes have sufficient integral strength to resist the enormous forces acting on the column during even simple movements, most of the stability is provided by the voluntary and reflex contractions of the sacrospinalis, abdominal, glutei maximi, psoas, and hamstring muscles.

The vertebral and paravertebral structures derive their innervation from the recurrent branches of the spinal nerves. Pain endings and fibers have been demonstrated in the ligaments, muscles, periosteum of bone, outer layers of annulus fibrosus, and synovium of the articular facets. The sensory fibers from these structures and the sacroiliac and lumbosacral joints join to form the sinovertebral nerves which pass via the recurrent branches of the spinal nerves of the first sacral and the fifth to first lumbar vertebrae into the gray matter of the corresponding segments of the spinal cord. Efferent fibers emerge from these segments and extend to the muscles through the same nerves. The sympathetic nerves contribute only to the innervation of blood vessels and appear to play no part in voluntary and reflex movement, though they do contain sensory fibers.

The parts of the back that possess the greatest freedom of movement, and hence are most frequently subject to injury, are the lumbar and cervical. In addition to the voluntary motions required for bending, twisting, and other movements, many actions of the spine are reflex in nature and are the basis of posture.

GENERAL CLINICAL CONSIDERATIONS

TYPES OF LOW BACK PAIN Of the several symptoms of disease of the spine (pain, stiffness or limitation of movement, and deformity), pain is of foremost importance by virtue of its frequency and its disabling effects. Four types of pain may be differentiated: local, referred, radicular, and that arising from secondary (protective) muscular spasm. One must identify these several types of pain by the patient's description, and here reliance is placed mainly on the character, location, and the conditions which modify them. The mechanism of the several types of pain has already been described in Chap. 5.

Local pain is caused by any pathologic process which impinges upon or irritates sensory endings. Involvement of structures which contain no sensory endings is painless. The substance of the vertebral body may be destroyed by tumor, for example, without evocation of pain, whereas lesions of periosteum, synovial membranes, muscles, annulus fibrosus, and ligaments are often exquisitely painful. Although painful states are often accompanied by swelling of the affected tissues, this is not apparent if a deep structure of the back is the site of disease. Local pain is often described as steady but may be intermittent and varies with position or activity. The pain may be sharp or dull and although often diffuse is always felt in or near the affected part of the spine. Often it is associated with reflex splinting of the spine segments by paravertebral muscles. Certain movements or postures which alter the position of the injured tissues aggravate or relieve the pain. Firm pressure or percussion upon superficial structures in the region involved usually evokes tenderness which is of aid in identifying the site of the abnormality.

Referred pain is of two types, that projected from the spine into regions lying within the area of the lumbar and upper sacral dermatomes and that projected from the pelvic and abdominal viscera to the spine. Pain due to diseases of the upper part of the lumbar spine is usually referred to the anterior aspects of the thighs and legs; that from the lower part of the lumbar spine is referred to the gluteal regions, posterior thighs, and calves. Pain of this type, although of deep, aching quality and rather diffuse, tends at times to be superficially projected. In general the referred pain parallels in intensity the local pain in the back. In other words, maneuvers which alter local pain have a similar effect on referred pain, though not with such precision and immediacy as in radicular, or "root," pain. Referred pain may be confused with pain from visceral disease, but the latter is usually described as "deep" and tends to radiate from the abdomen through to the back. Also, the pain is usually unaffected by movement of the spine, does not improve with recumbency, and may be modified by the activity of the involved viscus.

Radicular, or "root," *pain* has some of the characteristics of referred pain but differs in its greater intensity, distal radiation, circumscription to the territory of a root, and the factors which excite it. The mechanism is distortion, stretching, irritation, or compression of a spinal root, most often central to the intervertebral foramen. Although the pain itself is often dull or aching, various maneuvers which increase the irritation of the root may greatly intensify the pain. Nearly always the radiation of pain is from a central position near the spine to some part of the lower extremity. Cough, sneeze, and strain are characteristically evocative maneuvers; but since they may also jar or move the spine, they may aggravate local pain as well. Any motion which stretches the nerve, e.g., forward bending with the knees extended or "straight-leg raising" in disease of the lower part of the lumbar spine, excites radicular pain; jugular vein compression, which raises intraspinal pressure and may cause a shift in the position of the root, may have a similar effect. The fourth and fifth lumbar and first sacral roots, which form the sciatic nerve, cause pain which extends mainly down the posterior aspects of thigh, the postero- and anterolateral aspects of the leg, and into the foot, in the distribution of this nerve—so-called "sciatica." Tingling, paresthesias, and numbness or sensory impairment of the skin, soreness of the skin, and tenderness along the nerve usually accompany radicular pain. Also reflex loss, weakness, atrophy, fascicular twitching, and often stasis edema may occur if motor fibers of the anterior root are involved.

Pain resulting from muscular spasm is usually mentioned in relation to local pain. Muscle spasm may be associated with many disorders of the spine and can produce significant distortions of the normal posture. Chronic tension in muscles may give rise to a dull and sometimes cramping ache. One can in this instance feel the tautness of the sacrospinalis and gluteal muscles and demonstrate by palpation that the pain is localized to them.

Other pains often of undetermined origin are sometimes described by patients with chronic disease of the lower part of the back. In the legs, drawing, pulling, cramping sensations (without involuntary muscle spasm), tearing, throbbing, or jabbing pains, feelings of burning or coldness are difficult to interpret and, like paresthesias and numbness, should always suggest the possibility of nerve or root disease.

Since it is often difficult to obtain physical or laboratory confirmation of painful disease of the lower region of the spine, it is extremely important to obtain an accurate history. In addition to assessing the character and location of the pain, one should determine the factors which aggravate and relieve it, its constancy, and its relationship to recumbancy and such stereotyped movements and maneuvers as forward bending, cough, sneeze, and strain. Frequently the most important lead comes from the knowledge of the mode of onset and circumstances which initiated the pain. Inasmuch as many painful affections of the back are the result of injury incurred during work or in an accident, the possibility of exaggeration or prolongation of pain for purposes of compensation or other personal reasons, or because of hysteria or malingering, must always be kept in mind.

EXAMINATION OF THE LOWER PART OF THE BACK

Much information may be gained by "inspection" of the back, buttocks, and lower extremities in various positions and movements. The normal spine shows a dorsal kyphosis and lumbar lordosis in the saggital plane, which in some individuals may be somewhat exaggerated (swayback). Normally the spine, in the coronal plane, is relatively straight, although slight curvature is frequent, particularly in females. In spinal disorders, one should observe the spine closely for excessive curvature, list, flattening of the normal lumbar arch, presence of a gibbus (a short, sharp, kyphotic angulation usually indicative of a fracture), pelvic tilt or obliquity, or asymmetry of the paravertebral or gluteal musculature. In severe sciatica, one may observe abnormalities of posture of the affected leg, presumably to reduce tension on the irritated part.

The next step in the examination is observation of the spine, hips, and legs during certain motions. During the procedure it is well to remember that no advantage accrues from trying to find out how much the patient can be hurt. Instead, it is much more important to determine when and under what conditions the pain commences. One looks for limitation of the natural motions of the patient as he disrobes and while he is standing, sitting, and reclining. When standing, the motion of forward bending normally produces flattening and reversal of the lumbar lordotic curve and exaggeration of the dorsal curve. With lesions of the lumbosacral region which involve the posterior ligaments, articular facets, or sacrospinalis muscle and with ruptured lumbar disks, protective reflexes prevent stretching of these structures. As a consequence, the sacrospinalis muscles remain taut and limit motion in the lumbar part of the spine. Forward bending then occurs at the hips and at the lumbar-thoracic junction. With disease of the lumbosacral joints and spinal roots, the patient bends in such a way as to avoid tensing the hamstring muscles and putting undue leverage upon the pelvis. In unilateral "sciatica," with its increased curvature toward the side of the lesion, lumbar and lumbosacral motions are splinted, and bending is mainly at the hips; at a certain point the knee on the affected side is flexed to relieve hamstring spasm and tilting of the pelvis, and to slacken the lumbosacral roots and sciatic nerve.

It is sometimes of value to record the degree of flexion achieved by measuring either distance between the fingertips and the floor or by estimating the degree of bending of the spine. Lateral bending is usually less instructive than forward bending. However, in unilateral ligamentous or muscular strain, bending to the opposite side aggravates the pain by stretching the damaged tissues. Moreover, in lateral disk lesions, bending of the spine toward the side from which the trunk lists is restricted. In diseases of the lower part of the spine, flexion while sitting with the hips and knees flexed can normally be performed easily, even to the point of bringing the knees in contact with the chest. The reason is that knee flexion relaxes the tightened hamstring muscles and also relieves stretch of the sciatic nerve.

The study of motions in the reclining position yields the same information as study of motions in the standing and sitting positions, with the difference that there is less intradiskal pressure. With lumbosacral lesions and sciatica, passive lumbar flexion causes little pain and is not limited as long as the hamstrings are relaxed and there is no stretching of the sciatic nerve. With lumbosacral and lumbar spine disease (e.g., arthritis), passive flexion of the hips is free, whereas flexion of the lumbar spine may be impeded and painful. Passive straight-leg raising (possible in most normal individuals up to 90° except in those who have unusually tight hamstrings), like forward bending in the standing posture with the legs straight, places the sciatic nerve and its roots under tension, thereby producing pain. It may also cause an anterior rotation of the pelvis around a transverse axis, increasing stress on the lumbosacral joint, and thus causing pain if this segment is arthritic or otherwise impaired. Consequently, in diseases of the lumbosacral joints and lumbosacral roots, this movement is limited on the affected side and, to a lesser extent, the opposite side. Lasègue's sign (pain and limitation of movement during elevation of the leg when the knee is extended) is a useful test of this condition. Straight-leg raising of the opposite leg may also cause contralateral pain but of lesser degree, believed by some to be a sign of a more extensive lesion, such as an extruded disk fragment, rather than a simple prolapse or protrusion. It is important to remember, however, that the evoked pain is always referred to the diseased side, no matter which leg is flexed.

The motion of hyperextension is best performed with the patient standing or lying prone. If the condition causing back pain is acute, it may be difficult to extend the spine in the standing position. A patient with lumbosacral strain or disk disease can usually extend or hyperextend the spine without aggravation of pain. If there is an active inflammatory process or fracture of the vertebral body or posterior elements, hyperextension may be markedly limited.

Palpation and percussion of the spine are the last steps in the examination. The approach must always be gentle since rough percussion of the designated area of pain may antagonize the patient and only serve to confuse the physician. It is preferable to palpate first those regions which are the least likely to evoke pain. At all times the examiner should know what structures are being palpated (see Fig. 9-1). Localized tenderness is seldom pronounced in disease of the spine because the involved structures are so deep that they rarely give rise to surface tenderness. Mild superficial and poorly localized tenderness signifies only a disease process within the affected segment of the body, i.e., dermatome.

Tenderness over the costovertebral angle often indicates genitourinary disease, adrenal disease (Rogoff's sign), or an injury to the transverse processes of the first or second lumbar vertebra [Fig. 9-1 (1)]. Hypersensitivity on palpation of the transverse processes of the other lumbar vertebrae as well as the overlying sacrospinalis muscles may signify fracture of the transverse process or a strain of muscle attachments. Tenderness of a spinous process or aggravation of pain by the jarring of gentle percussion may be nonspecific but frequently indicates the presence of a disk lesion at the site deep to it, inflammation (as in disk space infection), or pathologic fracture.

FIGURE 9-1

(1) Costovertebral angle. (2) Spinous process and interspinous ligament. (3) Region of articular fifth lumbar to first sacral facet. (4) Dorsum of sacrum. (5) Region of iliac crest. (6) Iliolumbar angle. (7) Spinous processes of fifth lumbar to first sacral vertebrae (tenderness = faulty posture or occasionally spina bifida occulta). (8) Region between posterior superior and posterior inferior spines. Sacroiliac ligaments (tenderness = sacroiliac sprain, often tender with fifth lumbar to first sacral disk). (9) Sacrococcygeal junction (tenderness = sacrococcygeal injury, i.e., sprain or fracture). (10) Region of sacrosciatic notch (tenderness = fourth to fifth lumbar disk rupture and sacroiliac sprain). (11) Sciatic nerve trunk (tenderness = ruptured lumbar disk or sciatic nerve lesion).

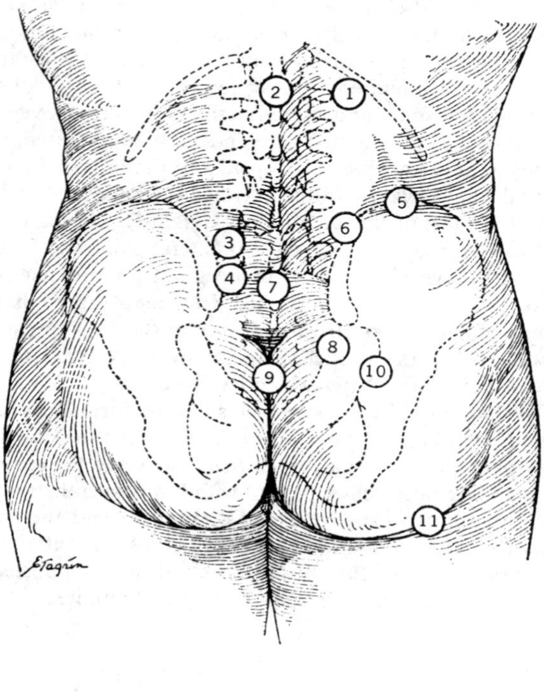

In palpation of the spinous processes, it is important to note any deviation in the lateral plane (this may be indicative of fracture or arthritis) or in the anteroposterior plane. A "step-off" forward displacement of the spinous process may be an important clue to a spondylolisthesis, one segment below the displaced level.

Tenderness in the region of the articular facets between the fifth lumbar and first sacral vertebrae is consistent with disease of a lumbosacral disk [Fig. 9-1 (3)]. It is also frequent in rheumatoid arthritis.

Abdominal, rectal, and pelvic examination and assessment of the status of the peripheral vascular system are additional parts of the examination of the patient with complaints in the lower back which should not be omitted, especially in difficult cases. They may provide evidence of neoplastic disease, inflammation, or other disorders which have caused a pain referred to the lower spine.

Finally, there should be a search for motor, reflex, and sensory changes (see Protrusion of Lumbar Intervertebral Disks, below), particularly in the lower extremities.

SPECIAL LABORATORY PROCEDURES Useful laboratory tests, depending on the nature of the problem and the circumstances, include a complete blood count, erythrocyte sedimentation rate (especially helpful in screening for infection or myeloma), measurement of serum calcium, phosphorus, alkaline phosphatase, acid phosphatase (if one suspects metastatic carcinoma of the prostate), protein electrophoresis, and immunoglobulin electrophoresis, tuberculin test, and tests for febrile agglutinins and rheumatoid factor. Roentgenograms of the lumbar part of the spine should be taken in every case of low back pain and sciatica (preferably with the patient standing) in the anteroposterior, lateral, and oblique planes. Special spot views or stereoscopic or laminographic films may provide further information in certain cases. Examination of the spinal canal with a contrast medium (air or other contrast myelogram) is often of great value, especially if a spinal cord tumor is suspected or if a patient thought to have a disk herniation fails to improve on a conservative regimen. Myelography can be combined with tests of dynamics of the cerebrospinal fluid, and a sample of the fluid should always be removed for cytologic and chemical examination prior to the instillation of the contrast medium (Pantopaque, Myodil, air, or some of the newer contrast media which are resorbed). Injection and removal of Pantopaque require special skill and should not be attempted without previous experience with the procedure. If done properly, the procedure has a very low incidence of significant complications. Recently a new absorbable substance, Dimer X, has been introduced. It is nonirritating to spinal roots, gives excellent visualization, and makes the entire procedure easier. Injection of contrast medium directly into the intervertebral disk (diskograms) has recently become popular but is still controversial. The technique of this procedure is more complicated than that of myelographic examination, and the risk of damage to the disk or nerve roots and the possibility of introduction of infection is not inconsiderable. In the authors' opinion, such a procedure is indicated only under very special circumstances.

PRINCIPAL CONDITIONS WHICH GIVE RISE TO DISABLING PAIN IN THE LOWER PART OF THE BACK

CONGENITAL ANOMALIES OF THE LUMBAR SPINE Anatomic variations of the spine are not at all infrequent, and although rarely of themselves the source of pain and functional derangement, they may predispose an individual to excessive stress because of the altered mechanics or alignment of the spine.

There may be a lack of fusion of the laminae of the neural arch (a spina bifida) of one or several of the lumbar vertebrae or of the sacrum. Hypertrichosis or hyperpigmentation in the sacral area may betray the condition, but in most patients the spine defect remains entirely occult until disclosed by x-ray. The anomaly has greater potentiality for pain if accompanied by malformation of vertebral joints. Usually the pain is induced by injury. There are many other congenital anomalies which affect the lower lumbar vertebrae such as asymmetrical facetal joints, abnormalities of the transverse processes, sacralization of the fifth lumbar vertebra (in which L_5 appears to be firmly fixed to the sacrum), or lumbarization of the first sacral (in which the first sacral looks like a sixth lumbar vertebra). Any one of these is occasionally observed in patients with symptoms referable to the low back, but they occur with equal frequency in individuals with no evidence of low back problem. Their role in the genesis of low back derangement is unclear, but in the authors' opinion, they are rarely the cause of specific symptomatology.

Spondylolysis consists of a bony defect, probably congenital, in the pars interarticularis (a segment near the junction of the pedicle with the lamina) of the lower lumbar area. The defect is best visualized on oblique projections. In some individuals the defect is bilateral. Under the circumstance of single or multiple injuries, the vertebral body, pedicle, and superior articular facet move anteriorly, leaving the posterior elements behind. This latter abnormality, known as *spondylolisthesis,* usually results in symptoms. The patient complains of pain in the low back radiating into the thighs, and there is limitation of motion. Often tenderness is elicited near the segment which has "slipped" forward (most often L_5 or occasionally L_4), and one can feel a "step" on deep palpation of the posterior elements. The pelvis is sometimes rotated and hip flexion limited by hamstring spasm; a variety of neurologic deficits indicative of radiculopathy complete the clinical syndrome. In exceptionally severe cases, the trunk may be shortened and the abdomen protrude, both the result of the forward shift of L_5 on S_1.

TRAUMATIC AFFLICTIONS OF THE LOWER PART OF THE BACK Trauma constitutes the most frequent cause of low back pain.

In severe acute injuries, the examining physician must be careful to avoid further damage. In tests of mobility, all movements must be kept to a minimum until an approximate diagnosis has been made and adequate measures have been instituted for the proper care of the patient. If the patient complains of pain in his back and cannot move his legs, his spine may have been fractured. His neck should not be flexed, nor should he be allowed to sit up. (See Chap. 333 for further discussion of spinal cord injury.)

Sprains, strains, and derangements The terms lumbosacral *sprain* and *strain* are used loosely by most physicians, and it is probably impossible to distinguish between them. The authors prefer the term *low back derangement* or *strain* for minor, self-limited injuries usually associated with lifting a heavy object, a fall, or a sudden deceleration as may occur in an automobile accident. Occasionally these syndromes are more chronic in nature, suggesting that postural, muscular, or arthritic factors may play a role. The patients with low back derangement or strain are often acutely discomfited and may assume unusual postures related to spasm of the sacrospinalis muscles. The pain is usually confined to the lower back and is almost invariably relieved by rest. What formerly was regarded as sacroiliac strain or sprain is now known to be due to disk disease in most instances. This is caused by lifting heavy objects with the spine in a position of imperfect mechanical balance, as when lifting and turning at the same time. Sudden unexpected motion is particularly likely to cause this injury.

The diagnosis of lumbosacral and sacroiliac strains with injury of the various structures of the lower part of the back depends upon the description of the injury, the localization of the pain by the patient, the finding of localized tenderness, and the augmentation of pain when tension is exerted on the involved structures by the appropriate maneuvers. The prompt alleviation of the pain by rest and relaxation indicates the existence of a strain. The rate of recovery depends on the degree of damage, preexisting disk disease, etc. Pain may be immediately relieved by local infiltration of an anesthetic agent, a finding which is also helpful in diagnosis.

Vertebral fractures Fractures of the lumbar vertebral body are usually the result of flexion injuries. Such traumas may occur in a fall from a height (in which case the calcanei may also be fractured) or as a result of an automobile accident or other violence. When fractures occur with minimal trauma (or spontaneously), the bone is presumed to have been previously weakened by some pathologic process. Most of the time, particularly in older individuals, osteoporosis is the cause of such an event, but there are many other underlying systemic disorders such as osteomalacia, hyperparathyroidism, hyperthyroidism, multiple myeloma, metastatic carcinoma, and a large number of local conditions in which the initial symptoms and signs are related to a vertebral fracture. Spasms of the lower lumbar muscles, limitation of motion of the lumbar section of the spine, and the roentgenographic appearance of the damaged lumbar portion (with or without neurologic abnormalities) are the basis of clinical diagnosis. The pain is usually immediate, though occasionally it may be delayed for a few days.

Fractured transverse processes, which are almost always associated with tearing of the paravertebral muscles, are diagnosed by the finding of deep tenderness at the site of the injury, local muscle spasm on one side, and limitation of all movements which stretch the lumbar muscles. Radiologic evidence provides the final confirmation. In some circumstances, extensive tears of the paravertebral musculature may be associated with a hemorrhage into the retroperitoneal space and profound shock. Fractures of multiple transverse processes, although seemingly trivial, should be the object of considerable concern, and the patient carefully watched over the initial period for internal hemorrhage.

Protrusion of lumbar intervertebral disks This condition is now recognized as the major cause of severe and chronic or recurrent low back and leg pain. It is most likely to occur between the fifth lumbar and first sacral vertebrae and, with lessening frequency, between the fourth and fifth lumbar, the third and fourth lumbar, the second and third lumbar, and the first and second lumbar vertebrae. Rare in the thoracic portion of the spine, it is next most frequent between the sixth and seventh and fifth and sixth cervical vertebrae. The cause is usually a flexion injury, but in a considerable proportion of cases no trauma is recalled. Degeneration of the posterior longitudinal ligaments and the annulus fibrosus, which occurs in most adults of middle and advanced years, may have taken place silently or have been manifested by mild, recurrent lumbar ache. A sneeze, lurch, or other trivial movement may then cause the nucleus pulposus to prolapse, pushing the frayed and weakened annulus posteriorly. In more severe cases of disk disease, the nucleus may protrude through the annulus or become extruded to lie as a free fragment in the vertebral canal.

The fully developed syndrome of ruptured intervertebral disk consists of backache, abnormal posture, and limitation of motion of the spine (particularly flexion). Nerve root involvement is indicated by radicular pain, sensory disturbances (paresthesias, hyper- and hyposensitivity in dermatome pattern), coarse twitching and fasciculation, muscle spasms, and impairment of a tendon reflex. Motor abnormalities (weakness and muscle atrophy) may also occur but are usually less prominent than the pain and sensory disorder. Since herniation of the intervertebral lumbar disks most often occurs between the fourth and fifth lumbar vertebrae and the fifth lumbar and first sacral vertebrae with irritation and compression of the fifth lumbar and first sacral roots, respectively, it is important to recognize the clinical characteristics of lesions of these two roots. *Lesions of the fifth lumbar root* produce pain in the region of the hip, groin, posterolateral thigh, lateral calf to the external malleolus, dorsal surface of the foot, and the first or second and third toes. Paresthesias may be in the entire territory or only in the distal parts of these territories. The tenderness is in the lateral gluteal region and near the head of the fibula. Weakness, if present, involves the extensors of the big toe and of the foot. The knee and ankle reflex seldom are definitely diminished; they are usually unchanged. Walking on the heels may be more difficult, because of weakness of dorsiflexion of the foot, and more uncomfortable than walking on the toes. In *lesions of the first sacral root* the pain is felt in the midgluteal region, posterior part of the thigh, posterior region of the calf to the heel, and the plantar surface of the foot and fourth and fifth toes. Tenderness is most pronounced over the midgluteal region (sacroiliac joint), posterior thigh area, and calf. Paresthesias and sensory loss are mainly in the lower leg and outer toes, and weakness, if present, involves the flexor muscles of the foot and toes, abductors of the toes, and hamstring muscles. The ankle reflex is diminished to absent in the majority of cases. Walking on the toes is more difficult, because of weakness of plantar flexors, and more uncomfortable than walking on the heel. With lesions of either root there may be limitation of straight-leg raising during the acute, painful stages.

Low back pain may also be caused by degeneration of the intervertebral disk, without frank extrusion of a fragment of disk tissue. Or the herniation may occur into the adjacent vertebral body, giving rise to a Schmorl's nodule. In such cases there are no signs of nerve root involvement though the back pain may be referred to the thigh and leg.

The rarer *lesions of the fourth and third lumbar roots* give rise to pain in the anterior part of the thigh and knee, with corresponding sensory loss. The knee-jerk is diminished or abolished. An inverted Lasègue sign is positive when the third lumbar root is affected.

The lumbar disk syndromes are usually unilateral. Only with massive derangements of the disk or the extrusion of a large, free fragment into the canal do bilateral symptoms and signs occur, and these may then be associated with paralysis of the sphincters. The pain may be mild or severe. All or part of the above syndrome may be present. There may be back pain with little or no leg pain; rarely only leg pain may be experienced. The rupture of multiple lumbar or lumbar and cervical disks is not infrequent, attesting to a basic disorder of the entire disk including the annulus fibrosus.

When all components of the syndrome are present, the diagnosis is easy; when only one part is present, particularly backache, it may be difficult, especially if there has been no accident. Since similar symptoms may occur without demonstrable disk rupture, other diagnostic procedures are required. Plain roentgenograms usually show no abnormality or at most a narrowing of the intervertebral space, sometimes more on the side of the rupture, or traction spurs, which are indicative of disk degeneration; hence one must resort to Pantopaque or air myelography. This will reveal in most cases an indentation of the lumbar subarachnoid space or deformity of the root sleeve. Occasionally with large lesions there is a complete interruption of the flow of contrast material. Or, conversely, a small ruptured disk may not show, especially at the fifth lumbar to first sacral level where there is a large space between the spinal canal and dura. Some clinics use diskograms (opaque material is injected into the disk) to reveal any evidence of extrusion, but the procedure is risky, and the results are difficult to interpret. The electromyogram is helpful in showing denervation of leg muscles (see Chap. 356). The protein level of the cerebrospinal fluid is elevated in some instances.

Tumor of the spinal canal, epidural or intradural, may produce a syndrome similar to that of ruptured disk (see Chap. 333).

ARTHRITIS Arthritis of the spine is a major cause of backache, cervical pain, and occipital headache.

Osteoarthritis This more frequent type occurs usually in later life and may involve any part of the spine. It is most prevalent in the cervical and lumbar regions, however, and the exact location determines the localization of the symptoms. Patients often complain of pain, centered in the spine, which is increased by motion and is almost invariably associated with complaints of stiffness and limitation of motion. There is a notable absence of systemic symptoms such as fatigue, malaise, and fever, and the pain usually can be relieved by rest. The severity of the symptoms often bears little relation to the radiologic findings; pain may be present when there are minimal findings on an x-ray, and, conversely, marked osteophytic overgrowth with spur formation, ridging, and bridging of vertebrae can be seen in asymptomatic patients in middle and later life. Osteoarthropathic changes in the cervical spine and to a lesser extent in the lumbar spine may by their location compress roots or even the cauda equina or spinal cord, giving rise to the spondylitic form of myelopathy (See Chaps. 333 and 335).

Spondylitic caudal radiculopathy (SCR) is another variant of hypertrophic arthritis. A congenital smallness of the lumbar canal, especially at the L_4 to L_5 level, renders the individual susceptible to either a rupture of an intervertebral disk or arthrosis. The latter condition further narrows the anteroposterior diameter of the canal and leads to compression of lumbosacral roots and even to a block of the spinal canal. The roots are actually caught between the posterior surface of the vertebral body and the ligamentum flavum posterolaterally. Lumbosacral pains are followed by weakening of the lower legs, impairment of ankle and knee reflexes, and numbness and paresthesia in the feet and legs. Extension of the lumbar spine during walking and standing produces or aggravates the neurologic symptoms, and flexion relieves them. The clinical picture and its intermittency correspond to the so-called *intermittent claudication* of the *spinal cord.* Decompression of the spinal canal relieves the symptoms in a considerable proportion of the cases. SCR is the lumbar equivalent of spondylitic cervical myelopathy (SCM), described below. SCR is a cauda equina syndrome, and its differential diagnosis is discussed in Chap. 333, Diseases of the Spinal Cord.

Rheumatoid arthritis and ankylosing spondylitis Arthritic disease of the spine takes two distinct forms—ankylosing spondylitis (the more common) and rheumatoid arthritis.

Patients with *ankylosing spondylitis* (also called Marie-Strümpell arthritis) are usually young men who complain of mild to moderate pain, which early in the course of the disease is centered in the back, and on occasion radiates to the back of the thighs. The symptoms may be vague at first (tired back, "catches" up and down the back, sore back) and intermittent, and the diagnosis may be overlooked for years. Although the pain is recurrent, the complaint and the finding of limitation of movement are constant and progressive and over a period of time tend to dominate the picture. Early in the course, this finding is described as "morning stiffness" or increasing stiffness after periods of inactivity, and may be present long before radiologic changes are manifest. Limitation of chest expansion, tenderness over the sternum, and decreased motion and flexion contractures of the hips may also be present early in the course. The radiologic hallmark of the disease is at first destruction and subsequently obliteration of the sacroiliac joints, followed by bridging between the vertebral bodies by bone to produce the characteristic "bamboo spine." The entire spine becomes immobilized, and usually the pain then subsides. Patterns of restricted movement, indistinguishable from those of ankylosing spondylitis, may accompany Reiter's syndrome, psoriatic arthritis, and inflammatory diseases of the intestine.

Occasionally ankylosing spondylitis is complicated by progressively destructive vertebral lesions. This complication should be suspected whenever the pain returns, after a period of quiescence, or becomes localized. The etiology of these lesions is not known, but they may represent an exaggerated healing response to fracture or excessive production of fibrous inflammatory tissues. Rarely they may result in collapse of a segment of the spine and compression of the spinal cord. Another complication of severe ankylosing spondylitis is bilateral chest involvement which may greatly accentuate the back deformity and increase the disability.

Spinal rheumatoid arthritis tends to be localized to the cervical apophyseal joints and atlantoaxial articulation; the pain, stiffness, and limitation of motion are then in the neck and back of the head. In contrast to ankylosing spondylitis, rheumatoid arthritis is rarely confined to the spine, nor does it lead to significant degrees of intervertebral bridging. Because of major affection of other joints, the diagnosis is relatively easy to make, but significant involvement of the neck may be overlooked. In the advanced stages of the disease, one or several of the vertebrae may be displaced anteriorly, or a synovitis of the atlantoaxial joint may damage the transverse ligament of the atlas, resulting in forward displacement of the atlas on the axis, i.e., atlantoaxial subluxation. In either instance, serious and even life-threatening compression of the spinal cord may occur gradually or suddenly (see Chaps. 333 and 335). Lateral roentgenograms in flexion and extension, performed cautiously, are necessary to visualize dislocation or subluxation.

OTHER DESTRUCTIVE DISEASES Neoplastic, infectious, and metabolic diseases Metastatic carcinoma (breast, lung, prostate, thyroid, kidney, gastrointestinal tract), multiple myeloma, Hodgkin's disease, and reticulum cell sarcoma are the malignant tumors which most frequently involve the spine. Since the primary site may be small, the presenting complaint of such tumors may be pain in the back. The pain tends to be constant and dull, and is often unrelieved by rest. Indeed, it may be worse at night. Radiographic changes may be absent early in the disease, but when they appear, usually are manifest as destructive lesions in one or several vertebral bodies with little or limited involvement of the disk space, even in the face of a compression fracture. A bone scan is often extremely helpful in lighting up "hot spots" indicating areas of bone destruction and reactive bone formation associated with the infiltration by neoplastic tissue and arthritis.

Infection of the vertebral column is usually the result of pyogenic organisms (staphylococci or coliform bacilli) or tubercule bacilli and is often difficult to distinguish on the basis of clinical findings. Patients complain of pain in the back of subacute or chronic nature that is exacerbated by motion but not materially relieved by rest. There is limitation of motion, tenderness over the spine of the involved segments, and pain with jarring of the spine, such as occurs with walking on the heels. Usually, these patients are afebrile and often do not have a leukocytosis although the erythrocyte sedimentation rate is elevated. Radiographs may demonstrate narrowing of a disk space with erosion and destruction of the two adjacent vertebrae. A paravertebral soft tissue mass may be present, indicating an abscess, which may in the case of tuberculosis drain spontaneously, at sites quite remote from the vertebral column.

Special mention should be made of the spinal *epidural abscess* (usually staphylococcal), which necessitates urgent surgical treatment. The symptoms are a localized pain, occurring spontaneously and with percussion and palpation, often with radicular radiation, and a rapidly developing flaccid paraplegia appearing in a febrile patient (see Chap. 337).

In so-called "metabolic bone diseases" (osteoporosis or osteomalacia) a considerable degree of loss of bone substance may occur without any symptoms whatsoever. Many patients with such conditions do, however, complain of aching in the lumbar or thoracic area. This is most likely to occur following an injury, sometimes of trivial degree, which leads to collapse or wedging of a vertebra. Certain movements greatly enhance the pain, and certain positions relieve it. One or more spinal roots may be involved. Paget's disease of the spine is nearly always painless. It may lead to compression of the spinal cord. The recognition of these bone disorders is discussed in some detail elsewhere (Chaps. 355 and 356).

In general, patients thought to have neoplastic, infectious, or metabolic disease of the spine should be thoroughly evaluated by means of radiographs, bone scans, myelography, and appropriate laboratory studies (see above).

REFERRED PAIN FROM VISCERAL DISEASE The pain of disease of the pelvic, abdominal, or thoracic viscera is often felt in the region of the spine; i.e., it is referred to the more posterior parts of the spinal segment which innervates the diseased organ. Occasionally back pain may be the first and only sign. The general rule is that pelvic diseases are referred to the sacral region, lower abdominal diseases to the lumbar region (centering around the second to fourth lumbar vertebrae), and upper abdominal diseases to the lower thoracic spine (eighth thoracic to the first and second lumbar vertebrae). Characteristically there are no local signs or stiffness of the back, and motion is of full range without augmentation of the pain. However, some positions, e.g., flexion of the lumbar area of the spine in the lateral recumbent position, may be more comfortable than others.

Low thoracic and upper lumbar pain in abdominal disease Peptic ulceration or tumor of the wall of the stomach and of the duodenum most typically induces pain in the epigastrium (see Chaps. 7, 8, and 287); but if the posterior wall is involved, and particularly if there is retroperitoneal extension, the pain may be felt in the region of the spine. The pain may be central in location or more intense on one side, or it may be felt in both locations. If very intense, it may seem to encircle the body. It tends to retain the characteristics of pain from the affected organ; e.g., if due to peptic ulceration, it appears about 2 h after a meal and is relieved by food and antacids.

Diseases of the pancreas (peptic ulceration with extension to the pancreas, cholecystitis with pancreatitis, tumor) are apt to cause pain in the back, being more to the right of the spine if the head of the pancreas is involved and to the left if the body and tail are implicated.

Diseases of retroperitoneal structures, e.g., lymphomas, sarcomas, and carcinomas, may evoke pain in this part of the spine with some tendency toward radiation to the lower part of the abdomen, groins, and anterior thighs. A secondary tumor of the iliopsoas region on one side often produces a unilateral lumbar ache with radiation toward the groin and labia or testicle; there may also be signs of involvement of the upper lumbar spinal roots. An aneurysm of the abdominal aorta may induce pain which is localized to this region of the spine but may be felt higher or lower, depending on the location of the lesion.

The sudden appearance of obscure lumbar pain in a patient receiving anticoagulants should arouse the suspicion of retroperitoneal bleeding.

Lumbar pain with lower abdominal diseases Inflammatory diseases of segments of the colon (colitis, diverticulitis) or tumor of the colon cause pain which may be felt in the lower part of the abdomen between the umbilicus and pubis, in the midlumbar region, or in both places. If very intense, the pain may have a beltlike distribution around the body. A lesion in the transverse colon or first part of the descending colon may be central or left-sided, and its level of reference to the back is to the second to third lumbar vertebrae. If the sigmoid colon is implicated, the pain is lower, in the upper sacral region and anteriorly in the midline suprapubic region or left lower quadrant of the abdomen.

Sacral pain in pelvic (urologic and gynecologic) diseases Although gynecologic disorders may manifest themselves by back pain, the pelvis is seldom the site of a disease which causes obscure low back pain. For the most part the diagnosis of painful pelvic lesions is not difficult, for a thorough palpation of structures by abdominal, vaginal, and rectal examination may be supplemented by methods (sigmoidoscopy, barium enema, pyelography, and culdoscopy) which permit adequate visualization of all these parts.

Menstrual pain itself may be felt in the sacral region. It is rather poorly localized, tends to radiate down the legs, and is of a crampy nature. The most important source of chronic back pain from the pelvic organs, however, is the uterosacral ligaments. Endometriosis or carcinoma of the uterus (body or cervix) may invade these structures, while malposition of the uterus may pull on them. The pain is localized centrally in the sacrum below the lumbosacral joint but may be more on one side. In endometriosis the pain begins during the premenstrual phase and often continues until it merges with menstrual pain. Malposition of the uterus (retroversion, descensus, and prolapse) characteristically leads to sacral pain, especially after the patient has been standing for several hours. One may observe the effect of postural influences here as when a fibroma of the uterus pulls on the uterosacral ligaments. Carcinomatous pain due to implication of nerve plexuses is continuous and becomes progressively more severe; it tends to be more intense at night. The primary lesion may be inconspicuous, being overlooked upon pelvic examination. Papanicolaou smears and a pyelogram are the most useful diagnostic procedures. X-ray therapy of these tumors may produce sacral pain consequent to swelling and necrosis of tissue, the so-called "radiation phlegmon of the pelvis." Low back pain with radiation into one or both thighs is a common phenomenon during the last weeks of pregnancy.

Chronic prostatitis, evidenced by prostatic discharge, burning and frequency of urination, and slight reduction in sexual potency, may be attended by a nagging sacral ache; it may be mainly on one side, with radiation into one leg if the seminal vesicle is involved on that side. Carcinoma of the prostate with metastases to the lower part of the spine is another more common cause of sacral or lumbar pain. It may be present without urinary frequency or burning. Spinal nerves may be infiltrated by tumor cells, or the spinal cord itself may be compressed if the epidural space is invaded. The diagnosis is established by rectal examination, roentgenograms of the spine, and measurement of acid phosphatase (particularly the prostatic phosphatase fraction). Lesions of the bladder and testes are usually not accompanied by back pain. When the kidney is the site of disease, the pain is ipsilateral, being felt in the flank or lumbar region.

Visceral derangements of whatever type may intensify the pain of arthritis, and the presence of arthritis may alter the distribution of visceral pain. With disease of the spine in the lumbosacral region, for example, distention of the ampulla of the sigmoid by feces or a bout of colitis may aggravate the arthritic pain. In patients with arthritis of the cervical or thoracic spine, the pain of myocardial ischemia may radiate to the back.

OBSCURE TYPES OF LOW BACK PAIN AND THE QUESTION OF PSYCHIATRIC DISEASE. The practitioner is frequently consulted by persons who complain of low back pain of obscure origin. Usually the disorder is benign in nature and results from some minor derangement, muscular strain, or diskal prolapse. This is particularly true for those lesions which are of acute onset and aggravated by motion, and relieved by rest. Considerably more difficult are patients with chronic pain, especially those who have had prior back surgery or chronic visceral disease, or those who have severe and progressive pain in which neoplasia or infection is considered.

Even when exhaustive studies have been performed, there remains a group of patients in whom no anatomic or pathologic lesion can be found. These patients generally fall into two categories: those with postural back pain and those with psychiatric illness.

Postural back pain Many slender asthenic individuals and some obese middle-aged individuals have discomfort in the back. Their backs ache much of the time, and the pain interferes with effective work. The physical examination is negative except for slack musculature and poor posture. The pain is diffuse in the mid or low region of the back and characteristically is relieved by bed rest and induced by the maintenance of a particular posture over a period of time. Pain in the neck and between the shoulder blades is a common complaint among thin, tense, active women and seems to be related to taut trapezius muscles.

Psychiatric illness Low back pain may be encountered in compensation hysteria and malingering, in anxiety or neurocirculatory asthenia (formerly called neurasthenia), in depression and hypochondriasis, and in many nervous persons whose symptoms and complaints do not fall within any category of psychiatric illness. It is probably correct to assume that pain in the back in such patients usually signifies disease of the spine and adjacent structures, and one should always search for a specific cause. However, even when organic factors are found, the pain may be exaggerated, prolonged, or woven into a pattern of invalidism or disability because of coexistent psychologic factors. This is especially true when there is the possibility of secondary gain (notably compensation). Patients seeking compensation for protracted low back pain without obvious structural disease tend, after a time, to become suspicious, uncooperative, and hostile toward the medical profession or anyone who might question the authenticity of their illness. One notes in them a tendency to describe their pain poorly and to prefer, instead, to discuss the degree of their disability and their mistreatment in the hands of the medical profession. These features and a negative examination of the back should lead one to suspect a psychologic factor. A few patients, usually frank malingerers, adopt the most bizarre attitudes, such as being unable to straighten up or walking with the trunk flexed at almost a right angle (camptocormia) (see Chap. 344).

The depressed and hypochondriac patient represents a troublesome problem, and a common error is to minimize the importance of anxiety and depression or to ascribe them to worry over the illness and its social effects. The more common and minor back ailments, e.g., those due to osteoarthritis and postural ache, are enhanced and rendered intolerable by irritable moodiness and self-concern. Such patients are often subjected to surgical procedures, which prove ineffective. The disability seems excessive for the degree of spinal malfunction, and misery and despair are the prevailing features of the syndrome. One of the more reliable diagnostic measures is the favorable response to drugs that alleviate the depression (see Chap. 345).

PAIN IN THE NECK AND SHOULDER

This topic is discussed to some extent in Chap. 7, Pain in the Chest, and further references are found in Chap. 10, Pain in the Extremities.

It is useful to distinguish here three major categories of painful disease—of the spine, brachial plexus (thoracic outlet), and shoulder. Although pain in these three regions of the body may overlap, the patient himself usually can indicate the site of origin. Pain arising from the cervical spine is felt in the neck and back of the head (though it may be projected to the shoulder and arm), is evoked or enhanced by certain movements or positions of the neck, and is accompanied by tenderness and limitation of motions of the neck. Similarly, pain resulting from abnormalities of the thoracic outlet is experienced in and around the shoulder in the supraclavicular region, or between the shoulders; is induced by the performance of certain tasks with the arm and by certain positions; and is associated with tenderness of structures above the clavicle. There may be a palpable abnormality above the clavicle (aneurysms of the subclavian artery, tumor, cervical rib). The combination of circulatory symptoms and signs referable to the lower part of the brachial plexus, manifested in the hand by obliteration of pulse when the patient holds a full breath with the head tilted back or turned (Adson's test), unilateral Raynaud's phenomenon, trophic changes in the fingers, and sensory loss over the ulnar side of the hand with or without interosseous atrophy, complete the clinical picture. Roentgenograms showing a cervical rib, deformed thoracic outlet, or superior sulcus tumor of the lung (Pancoast's syndrome) corroborate disease in this location. Electromyography and conduction studies of the ulnar nerve are especially helpful in evaluating this problem. Pain, localized to the shoulder region, influenced by motion, and associated with tenderness and limitation of motions (extension, abduction, external and especially internal rotation), points to a tear of the rotator cuff of tendons of the muscles surrounding the shoulder joint or to a calcific tendonitis. Often the term *bursitis* has been loosely used to designate this tendonitis, capsulitis, or muscular tear. Shoulder pain may radiate into the arm or hand, but the sensory, motor, and reflex changes which indicate disease of nerve roots, plexus, or peripheral nerves are absent.

Osteoarthritis of the cervical part of the spine may cause pains which radiate into the back of the head, shoulders, and arms on one or both sides of the thorax. Coincident involvement of nerve roots is manifested by paresthesias, sensory loss, weakness, or deep tendon reflex change. Should bony ridges form in the spinal canal (spondylosis), the spinal cord may be compressed (see Chap. 333). A Pantopaque or air cervical myelogram reveals the degree of encroachment on the spinal canal (narrowing of the canal to less than 11 mm in the anteroposterior diameter) at the level at which the spinal cord is affected. The authors have experienced difficulty in distinguishing spondylosis with or without disk rupture and spinal cord compression from primary neurologic diseases (syringomyelia, amyotrophic lateral sclerosis, or tumor) with an unrelated osteoarthritis of the cervical portion of the spine, particularly at the fifth to sixth and sixth to seventh cervical vertebrae, where the disk spaces are often narrowed in the adult. A combination of nervous tension with osteoarthritis of the cervical part of the spine or a painful injury to ligaments and muscles after an accident in which the neck is forcibly extended and flexed (e.g., whiplash injury to spine) raises extremely vexatious clinical syndromes. If the pain is persistent and limited to the neck, the problem will sometimes prove to have been due to disruption of a disk, but it is often complicated by psychologic factors.

RUPTURED CERVICAL DISKS One of the commonest causes of neck, shoulder, and arm pain is disk herniation in the lower cervical region. As with rupture of the lumbar disks, the complete syndrome includes the disorder of spinal function and evidence of neural involvement. It may develop after trauma either major or minor (sudden hyperextension of the neck, diving, forceful manipulations, etc.). Virtually every patient exhibits an abnormality in range of motion of the neck (limitation and pain). Hyperextension is the movement that most consistently aggravates the pain, although one occasionally sees patients whose principal limitation is in flexion. With laterally situated disk lesions between the fifth and sixth cervical vertebrae, the symptoms and signs are referred to the sixth cervical roots. The full syndrome is characterized by pain felt at the trapezius ridge, tip of the shoulder, anterior upper part of the arm, radial forearm, and often in the thumb; paresthesias and sensory impairment or hypersensitivity in the same regions; tenderness in the area above the spine of the scapula and in the supraclavicular and biceps regions; weakness in flexion of the forearm; diminished to absent biceps and supinator reflexes (triceps retained or exaggerated). When the protruded disk lies between the sixth and seventh cervical vertebrae, the seventh cervical root is involved. Under these circumstances, in the patient with the complete syndrome, the pain is in the region of the shoulder blade, pectoral region and medial axilla, posterolateral upper arm, elbow and dorsal forearm, index and middle fingers, or all the fingers; tenderness is most pronounced over the medial aspect of the shoulder blade opposite the third to fourth thoracic spinous processes, in the supraclavicular area and triceps region; paresthesias and sensory loss are most pronounced in the second and third fingers or tips of all the fingers; weakness is seen in extension of the forearm, in the extension of the wrist, and in the hand grip; the triceps reflex is diminished to absent, and the biceps and supinator reflexes are preserved. Either of these syndromes may be incomplete in that only one of several of the typical findings (e.g., pain) is present. Usually the patient states that cough, sneeze, and downward pressure on the head in the hyperextension position exacerbate pain and traction (even manual) tends to relieve it.

Unlike lumbar disks, the cervical ones, if large and centrally situated, may result in compression of the spinal cord (central disk, all the cord; paracentral disk, part of the cord). The central disk is often nearly painless, and the cord syndrome may simulate a degenerative disease (amyotrophic lateral sclerosis, combined system disease). A common error is to fail to think of a ruptured disk in the cervical region in patients with obscure symptoms in the legs. The diagnosis of ruptured cervical disk should be confirmed by the same laboratory procedures that were mentioned under Spondylosis, above.

OTHER CONDITIONS Metastases to the cervical spine are fortunately less common than to other parts of the vertebral column. They are frequently painful and the cause of disordered root function. Compression fractures or extension of the tumor posteriorly may lead to rapid development of quadriplegia.

Shoulder injuries (rotator cuff), subacromial or subdeltoid bursitis, the frozen shoulder (periarthritis or capsulitis), tendonitis, and arthritis may develop in patients who are otherwise well, but these conditions are also frequent in hemiplegics or in individuals suffering from coronary heart disease. The pain is often severe and extends toward the neck and down the arm into the hand. The dorsum of the latter may tingle without other signs of nerve involvement. Vasomotor changes also may occur in the hand (shoulder-hand syndrome), and after a time, osteoporosis and atrophy of cutaneous and subcutaneous structures occur (Sudeck's atrophy or Sudeck-Leriche syndrome). These conditions fall more within the province of orthopedics than of medicine and are not discussed here in detail. The physician, however, must know that they can often be prevented by proper exercises (Chap. 10).

The *carpal tunnel syndrome,* with paresthesias and numbness in palmar distribution of the median nerve and aching pain which extends up into the forearm, may be mistaken for disease of the shoulder or neck. Similarly, other less common forms of nerve entrapment may involve the ulnar, radial, or median nerves and lead to a mistaken diagnosis of brachial plexus lesion or cervical syndrome. Electromyography and conduction studies are especially helpful in such conditions (Chap. 331).

MANAGEMENT OF BACK PAIN

Without doubt the preventive aspects of back pain are important. There would be many fewer back problems if adults kept their trunk muscles in optimal condition by regular exercise such as swimming, walking briskly, running, and calisthenic programs such as that of the Canadian Air Force. Morning is the ideal time since the back of the older adult tends to stiffen during the night because of inactivity. This happens regardless of whether a bed board or a stiff mattress is used. Sleeping with back hyperextended and sitting for long times in an overstuffed chair or a badly designed auto seat are particularly risky. It is estimated that intradiskal pressures are increased 200 percent by changing from a recumbent to a standing position and by 400 percent by sitting slumped in an easy chair. Correct sitting posture lessens this. Long trips in a car or plane without change in position put maximal strain on disk and ligamentous structures in the spine. Lifting from a position of flexed trunk, as in removing a suitcase from the trunk of a car, is dangerous (always lift with the object close to the body). Sudden strenuous activity without conditioning and warm-up also is likely to cause trouble to disks and their ligamentous envelopes (the commonest sources of back pain); certain families seem disposed.

The following diagrams are useful guides in strengthening trunk muscles (Figs. 9-2 to 9-6).

Muscular and ligamentous strains and minor disk prolapses are usually self-limited, responding to simple measures in a relatively short period of time. The basic principle of therapy is rest in a recumbent position for several days to weeks. When weight bearing is resumed, a light lumbosacral support is usually helpful in continuing the immobilization until the patient is restored to full health. Physical measures such as heat, cold, diathermy, or massage are of limited value; of considerably greater importance are active exercises to both reduce the spasm and improve muscle tone. Analgesic medication should be given liberally during the first few days: codeine, 30 mg, and aspirin, 0.6 g, or pentazocine (Talwin), 50 mg, propoxyphene (Darvon), 65 mg, or meperidine (Demerol), 50 mg.

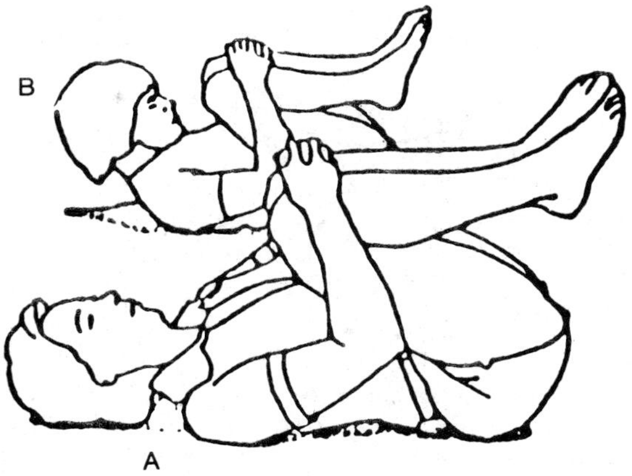

FIGURE 9-3
A *Keeping shoulders flat on floor, draw knees toward chest, clasp hands around knees, and pull knees tightly against chest.* B *Next bring forehead up to knees. (From* U. S. News & World Report. *Copyright 1975* U. S. News & World Report.)

FIGURE 9-2
A *With knees bent, feet flat on floor, and hands clasped behind head, pinch buttocks together, pull in abdomen, and flatten back against floor. At first, hold position for a count of 5, relax for 5, then gradually increase to counts of 20.* B *Next do this same exercise with legs extended and arms raised straight overhead. (From* U. S. News & World Report. *Copyright 1975* U. S. News & World Report.)

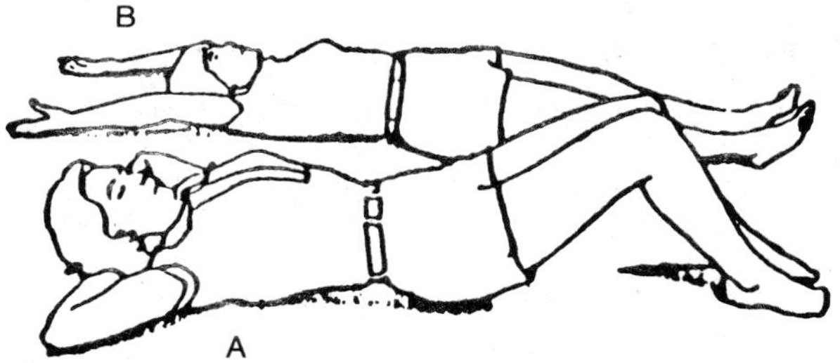

FIGURE 9-4
A *With knees bent, keep feet flat on floor and held or hooked under a heavy piece of furniture to provide leverage.* B *Cross arms on chest, raise head and shoulders, and curl up to a sitting position. Keep back round and pull with abdominal muscles. Lower self slowly. (From* U. S. News & World Report. *Copyright 1975* U. S. News & World Report.)

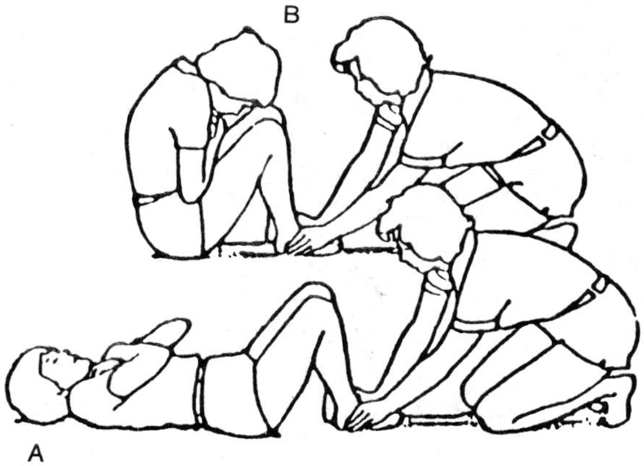

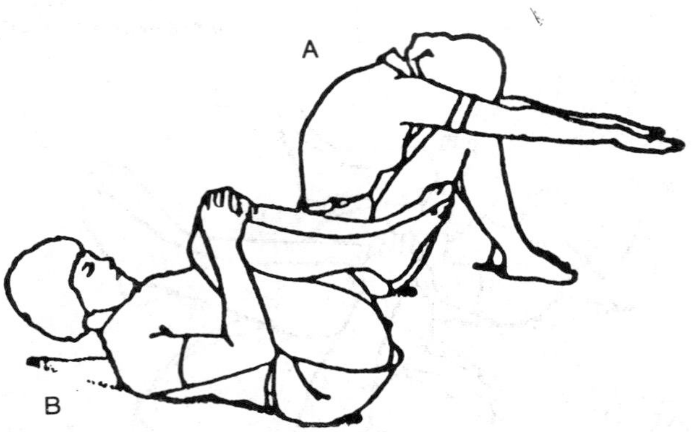

FIGURE 9-5
A *Bend knees, keeping feet flat on floor and arms straight forward. Raise up and touch head to knees.* B *Lower self, then pull knees up tightly against chest and bring forehead up to knees. (From* U. S. News & World Report. *Copyright 1975* U. S. News & World Report.)

Muscle relaxants are often a valuable adjunct, particularly in that such drugs as Valium, 8 to 40 mg in divided doses, and carisoprodol (Soma), 350 mg, twice daily, make bed rest more tolerable. If an inflammatory component is suspected, indomethacin, 75 mg per day (in divided doses), or ibuprofen (Motrin), 400 mg three or four times daily, may be helpful.

In the treatment of an acute or chronic rupture of a lumbar or cervical disk, complete bed rest is essential, and strong analgesic medication may be required. Traction is of little value in lumbar disk disease, and it is best to permit the patient to find the most comfortable position. Cervical traction with a halter may be of considerable benefit to patients with cervical disk syndrome. It can be administered with the patient in recumbency, or after sufficient improvement to allow ambulation, can be performed intermittently in the erect position using special equipment. During the recumbent phase of treatment of lumbar disk disease, exercises to reduce spasm, muscle relaxants, and anti-inflammatory agents as described above may be of considerable value. After 2 to 3 weeks in bed, the patient can be allowed to slowly resume activities, usually with the protection of a brace or light spinal support. Exercise programs designed to increase the strength of the abdominal and gluteal muscles are helpful at this point. The patient may suffer some minor recurrence of the pain but be able to carry on his usual activities, and eventually he will recover. If the pain and neurologic findings do not disappear on prolonged conservative management, or if the patient suffers frequently recurring acute episodes, surgical management may be indicated. This should always be preceded by a myelogram to localize the lesion (and rule out the presence of intra- or extradural tumors). The surgical procedure most often indicated is a hemilaminectomy with excision of the disk involved. Arthrodesis of the involved segments is indicated only in cases in which there is extraordinary instability usually related to an anatomic abnormality (such as spondylolysis) or in the cervical region when an extensive laminectomy has rendered the spine unstable.

FIGURE 9-6
A *Place hands at edge of chair.* B *Bend forward to bring head to knees, pulling in abdomen as you curl forward. Keep weight well back on hips. Release abdominal muscles slowly as you come up. (From* U. S. News & World Report. *Copyright 1975* U. S. News & World Report.)

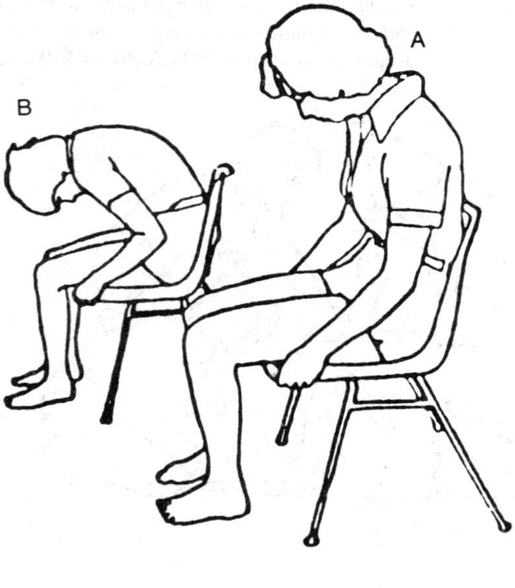

Recently, a new technique, *chemonucleolysis,* has been introduced for the management of moderately severe lumbar disk lesions which do not respond to conservative measures. Chymopapain, a polysaccharide-splitting enzyme of plant origin, is introduced into the damaged nucleus pulposus through a laterally placed fine needle under x-ray control. The enzyme, by its lytic action, causes a decrease in intradiskal pressure and in over half the cases is said to cause a cessation of symptoms. The choice and performance of such procedures as laminectomy, chemonucleolysis, and spinal arthrodesis are subject to many considerations and should be weighed carefully in the light of the patient's occupation, emotional response, compensation status, etc.

Spondylosis of the cervical part of the spine, if painful, is helped by bed rest and traction; if signs of spinal cord involvement are present, a collar to limit movement may halt the progression and even lead to improvement. Decompressive laminectomy or anterior fusion is reserved for severe instances of the disease with advancing neurologic symptoms. The shoulder-hand syndrome may benefit from stellate ganglion blocks or ganglionectomy, but the basic treatment is physiotherapy, with or without prednisone, and surgical procedures are used only as measures of last resort.

REFERENCES

ARMSTRONG JR: *Lumbar Disc Lesions,* 3d ed., Williams & Wilkins, Baltimore, 1965

BRADY LP et al: An evaluation of the electromyogram in the diagnosis of lumbar disk lesion. J Bone & Joint Surg 51A:539–47, 1969

CONVENTRY MB: Anatomy of the intervertebral disk. Clin Orthop 67:9–15, 1969

EDEIKEN J, PITT MJ: The radiologic diagnoses of disk disease. Orthop Clin N Amer 2:405–418, 1971

FRIEDENBERG AB, MILLER WT: Degenerative disk disease of the cervical spine. J Bone & Joint Surg 45A:1171–1183, 1963

GOLUB B, ROVIT R, MANKIN HJ: Cervical and lumbar disk disease: a review. Bull Rheum Dis 21:635, 1971

NAYLOR A: The changes in the human intervertebral disk in degeneration and nuclear prolapse. Orthop Clin N Amer 2:343–358, 1971

WATTS C, KNIGHTON R, ROULHAC G: Chymopapain treatment of intervertebral disk disease. J Neurosurg 42:374–383, 1975

10 PAIN IN THE EXTREMITIES

D. EUGENE STRANDNESS, JR.

INTRODUCTION Pain in the extremities occurs from a wide variety of diseases of the skin and of the musculoskeletal, vascular, and nervous systems. The commoner ones seen in clinical practice are the subject of this chapter.

In the diagnosis of pain of the limbs it is important to classify the pain and localize the site of involvement. Pain may be classified as superficial, deep, and referred. *Superficial pain* arising from either the skin or spreading from adjacent structures such as joints is well localized and is associated with tenderness and hyperalgesia. *Deep pain* arising from fascia, vessels, periosteum, joints, and supporting structures is often poorly localized and dull, and may be associated with muscular rigidity and deep tenderness. *Referred pain* is usually well localized and similar to pain arising from deep structures (Chap. 5). In persons with acute ischemia of the limbs, with threatened loss of viability, both superficial and deep pain are present.

A thorough examination of the limbs must include inspection for evidence of cutaneous manifestations, palpation for masses and tenderness, and auscultation for arterial bruits. Examination of the peripheral pulses at their accessible sites must always be done. A careful neurologic examination looking for changes in reflexes and sensation is also essential.

In most instances an accurate diagnosis can be made or strongly suspected by history and physical examination. Special tests such as arteriography, myelography, and nerve conduction studies are often helpful but are primarily reserved for accurate localization of the disease and determination of the extent of involvement.

PAINFUL SKIN DISEASE The common bacterial and fungous infections may occasionally produce pain, and it can occur in or remote to the involved areas. This is especially true when bacteria have entered the dermis and subcutaneous tissues via the base of the nails or interdigital areas. Depending upon the infecting agent, cellulitis with or without lymphangitis may rapidly ensue and produce local swelling, pain, erythema, and systemic signs of toxicity. If the infection develops in areas such as the pulp of the digits or in plantar or palmar spaces, the pain is severe, throbbing, and may secondarily extend to tendons and joints.

Fungous infections, particularly those of the interdigital areas of the feet, may also become secondarily infected by bacteria, resulting in a spreading cellulitis and lymphangitis. There are also nonbacterial forms of cellulitis. The lymphangitis is diagnosed by the presence of the "red lines" in the involved areas. Pain may also occur in the region of the lymph nodes which drain the infected area and may be the first sign of secondary infection.

Cellulitis, particularly of the lower extremities, may be confused with thrombophlebitis. Differentiating features supporting the diagnosis of cellulitis include: (1) rapidity of onset, (2) prominent cutaneous hyperemia and tenderness, (3) presence of a portal of entry for the infective agent, and (4) the nature of the systemic response (fever, leukocytosis), which is usually much more severe than with thrombophlebitis.

Erythema nodosum (Chap. 55) should be suspected when tender erythematous nodules appear in or under the skin and are associated with fever and joint pains. The articular manifestations often precede the appearance of the nodules. These lesions can be associated with a wide variety of diseases, some of which include tuberculosis, sarcoidosis, coccidioidomycosis, streptococcal infections, and ulcerative colitis. However, in the majority of cases, no underlying disease is found.

MUSCULOSKELETAL PAIN **Bursitis and tendonitis** *Inflammation* of one or more of the bursae may occur as a result of trauma, rheumatoid arthritis, gout, connective tissue disorders, and bacterial infection. The commonly involved bursae are the subdeltoid, olecranon, trochanteric, calcaneal, and prepatellar. When the process is acute, it is characterized by severe local pain and tenderness with marked limitation of activity and mobility. In long-standing cases the symptoms and physical findings are less pronounced. Calcific deposits within the involved bursa develop in some patients and may be seen in an x-ray.

Tenosynovitis of the tendon sheaths of hands or wrists produces pain in restricted regions. Tenosynovitis may arise in association with infection, rheumatoid arthritis, osteoarthritis, or trauma, or occur without explanation. When the sheath of the thumb's abductor longus and extensor brevis tendons at the radial styloid are affected, the condition is called *de Quervain's disease.* The flexor tendons in the palm and finger and the extensor sheaths on the dorsum of the wrist may also be the site of the inflammation. Typically, the pain and tenderness occur in the region of the tendon, and the pain is aggravated by stretching the involved tendons as their muscles contract.

An important variant of tenosynovitis is the *carpal tunnel syndrome,* the symptoms of which may be confused with the thoracic outlet syndrome, cervical disk disease, and local vascular insufficiency. Thickening or swelling of the tendons as they pass through the flexor compartment at the wrist, amyloid deposit with multiple myeloma, or bone enlargement (acromegaly) can exert pressure on the median nerve, causing nocturnal paresthesias and pain in the fingers, wrist, and forearm. As the condition worsens, atrophy of the thenar eminence develops, as well as weakness and sensory loss in the territory of the median nerve. There may be tenderness on pressure over the carpal ligament and electrical tingling in the fingers when the wrist is tapped (Tinel's sign). Nerve conduction may be delayed at the wrist, confirming the diagnosis.

Calcific and *noncalcific tendonitis* is common in the bicipital and supraspinatus tendons, and in the common tendon of origin for the forearm extensors and flexors at the lateral and medial epicondyle of the humerus, respectively (tennis elbow). The diagnosis is suspected by the location of the pain and the painful limitation of motion involved by movement of these tendons.

Painful synovial cysts Cysts of the popliteal space (Baker's cysts) can be an obscure source of pain in the leg. The lesion consists of a cyst in the popliteal fossa, which frequently communicates with the knee joint. While the cause is unknown, such cysts are frequently associated with rheumatoid or osteoarthritis. Trauma may be an inciting factor. Unruptured cysts produce only mild aching in the popliteal space with associated stiffness of the joint. If the cyst ruptures, there is an acute, extensive inflammation of the lower leg with swelling and pain which may be severe. The clinical picture is commonly confused with thrombophlebitis. The diagnosis can easily be made by instilling radiopaque material into the knee joint.

Painful arthritis of extremities Most causes of arthritis can be classified into one of five major groups: (1) infectious, (2) degenerative, (3) posttraumatic, (4) metabolic, and (5) unknown etiology. The synovial membranes and periarticular structures are primarily involved in rheumatoid disease, infectious arthritis, and gout, whereas the cartilage and bone are mainly affected in osteoarthritis and rarer varieties. With acute pyogenic arthritis, gout, and rheumatic fever, the pain is severe even at rest and greatly intensified by even the slightest motion. The local findings of swelling, redness, and heat may be pronounced.

The principal symptom of *osteoarthritis* is pain which is brought on by use and is relieved by rest. Stiffness after sitting and immediately upon rising in the morning is common but seldom persists for more than a few minutes. Some of the more common locations are the terminal phalanges, knees, hips, and spine.

Rheumatoid arthritis most commonly involves the proximal interphalangeal and metacarpophalangeal joints, toes, wrists, ankle, knee, elbow, hip, and shoulder. The onset is often insidious with general fatigue, paresthesias in the extremities, joint pain, and stiffness. The most common symptoms include joint pain at rest which is aggravated by motion. Thickening of the periarticular structures may be marked and accompanied by atrophy of adjacent muscles. Subcutaneous nodules are often found over pressure points. Many of the patients are also subject to cold sensitivity of Raynaud's type. (See Chaps. 359 and 363.)

Gout, a disease usually of men over thirty years of age, manifests itself often in acute episodes. Most frequently the metatarsophalangeal joint is involved; the affected joint is extremely painful and swells markedly within a few hours, becoming hot and dusky red. The process particularly in the acute form may be difficult to distinguish from acute rheumatic fever, gonococcal arthritis, atypical rheumatoid arthritis, traumatic arthritis, cellulitis, suppurative arthritis, and Reiter's syndrome. The presence of tophi and an elevated uric acid clarify the diagnosis. Finding the rod-like crystals of sodium urate in a tophus or synovial fluid establishes the diagnosis with certainty. (See Chap. 107.)

Pyogenic arthritis localizes usually in large joints (hip, knee, and shoulder). Such infections are usually metastatic in origin and remain monoarticular. The cardinal signs of infection, pain, and swelling, and a local increase in temperature with cutaneous hyperemia and fever, usually leave little doubt as to the nature of the condition. In suspected cases the joint must be aspirated to identify the organism by Gram's stain and culture.

Hypertrophic osteoarthropathy, with its characteristic clubbing, periostitis at the ends of long bones, arthritis, and autonomic disorder, causes pain which varies from mild to severe. It is deep and aching pain and along with tenderness is localized to the involved joints and adjacent long bones. This syndrome usually appears in relation to malignancies or suppurative conditions of the lungs, mediastinum, or pleura.

Osteomyelitis Osteomyelitis may occur following open fractures, open surgical reduction of fractures, or from a distant infective focus. Usually the symptoms commence abruptly with severe pain (aggravated by motion), local swelling, exquisite tenderness, chills, and fever. There is nearly always a neutrophilic leukocytosis and elevated sedimentation rate, and blood cultures may be positive. X-ray changes may not be evident until the second week or later. The differential diagnosis includes acute pyogenic arthritis, hemarthrosis (particularly in children), cellulitis, and erysipelas.

Painful disorders of muscle Disorders of muscles are common causes of severe pain in the limbs. Localized tenderness and pain with motion is most commonly seen after trauma or severe exercise. An acute suppurative myositis is nearly always associated with injury and direct inoculation with bacteria. Clostridial myositis (Chap. 158) must be considered in every case of a deep infection occurring secondary to a puncture wound.

A condition frequently confused with ischemic rest pain is the *nocturnal muscle cramp.* This process of unknown cause occurs in both sexes at all ages but is most often a source of complaints in pregnant women, the middle aged, and the elderly. Unusually strenuous activity in the daytime increases the liability to cramp at night especially when the feet are cold. The onset is sudden, usually in one of the muscles of the foot or leg, and it may awaken the patient. The pain subsides with vigorous massage and stretching (Chap. 351) of the part. If frequent and troublesome, 50 mg benadryl taken at bedtime will usually prevent the cramps.

When there is generalized muscle tenderness, weakness, increasing fatigability, and other systemic symptoms, the possibility of polymyositis and dermatomyositis must be considered.

ACUTE ARTERIAL OCCLUSION The clinical picture that results from acute arterial occlusion regardless of its cause is dependent upon the location and extent of the obstruction. If critical areas of the vasculature are involved, a sequence of events unfolds, the first part of which is pain in the most distal portion of the limb. Coldness, paresthesias, numbness, and finally paralysis follow in rapid succession. Irreversible tissue damage, leading to gangrene, will result within 4 to 6 h if the occlusion is complete. Examination of the limb reveals loss of pulses distal to the obstruction, decreased skin temperature, and pallor. It is not possible on clinical grounds alone to distinguish arterial thrombosis from embolism, although a cardiac source of emboli, mitral stenosis, atrial fibrillation, and myocardial infarction tend to favor the latter.

If the collateral circulation is adequate to maintain viability of the tissues, the symptoms are often mild. Under these circumstances there may be no more than a subjective sensation of numbness and coldness of the limb.

Cholesterol emboli arising from ulcerating plaques in the aorta can result in a confusing clinical picture. The emboli are small and may pass to the kidney, gut, and lower extremities, giving rise to hematuria and abdominal pain. In the legs they occlude the digital arteries, manifested as ischemic rest pain which is often bilateral and symmetrical. The skin of the foot may exhibit a curious mottling (livedo reticularis). Cutaneous infarction (gangrene) of the toes may result. Similar changes in the digits may be caused by intravascular clotting (cold agglutinins, platelet thrombosis, etc.).

Certain parts of the leg are especially vulnerable to circulatory insufficiency. For example the pretibial compartment containing the extensor muscles of toes and foot are enveloped by tight sheaths. If overexerted to the point of injury with attendant pain and swelling, the muscles become infarcted and permanently weakened, and even fatal myoglobinuria has been known to occur.

CHRONIC ARTERIAL OCCLUSION **Arteriosclerosis obliterans** Atherosclerosis of large- and medium-sized arteries, the most common vascular disease of man, often leads to symptoms which are induced by exercise (intermittent claudication) but may occur also at rest (ischemic rest pain). The diabetic patient is especially susceptible. The muscle pain which is brought on by exercise and promptly relieved by rest most frequently involves the calf and thigh muscles. If the atherosclerotic narrowing or occlusion involves the aortic and iliac arteries, it may also cause hip and buttock claudication and impotence in the male (Leriche syndrome). Ischemic rest pain, and sometimes attendant ulceration and gangrene, is usually localized to the foot and toes and is usually the consequence of multiple sites of vascular occlusion. Pain at rest is characteristically worse at night and totally or partially relieved by dependency.

The examination of such patients will reveal a loss of one or more peripheral pulses, trophic changes in skin and nails (in advanced cases), and the presence of bruits or thrills over or distal to sites of narrowing. A search should always be made in such patients for an abdominal aortic aneurysm since it is prone to rupture and can be corrected by operation. Arteriography is necessary only for confirmation of the location and extent of the occlusive involvement in planning surgical therapy. The upper extremities distal to the origin of the subclavian artery are rarely involved. Aneurysms of the peripheral arteries do not usually produce pain unless they compress adjacent nerves. Aneurysms of peripheral arteries are of importance primarily because they become the source of distal arterial embolization or undergo thrombosis.

Thromboangiitis obliterans This is a disease of young and middle-aged male cigarette smokers which involves the more distal small and medium arteries of the arms and

legs. A spectrum of symptoms occur which is useful in establishing the diagnosis. These symptoms include (1) instep claudication, (2) migratory thrombophlebitis, (3) cold sensitivity, and (4) hand and forearm claudication. The disease is usually bilateral and should be suspected on physical examination by the location of the pulse deficit. The pedal and wrist pulses are often absent. There is marked rubor of the feet even in the supine position. Ischemic rest pain and ulcers when present are usually very severe, leading to early amputation of the involved part. Some clinicians doubt the existence of this entity, pointing out that most such patients on investigation prove to have an unusually severe form of atherosclerosis (Chap. 334).

PAINFUL VASOSPASTIC DISORDERS In an evaluation of patients with cold sensitivity, it is important to distinguish *Raynaud's disease* from *Raynaud's phenomenon. Raynaud's disease* is a benign, symmetrical disorder of unknown cause which usually has its onset in the late teens or early twenties. Females are most commonly afflicted, and cold and emotional stimuli are the factors which trigger the response in the digits. The fingers become white, then blue, and finally red (the triphasic color response). Pain and paresthesias are common during the ischemic phase. Ulcerations are rarely observed.

Raynaud's phenomenon is always secondary to some underlying problem. The onset may occur at any period of life and may be asymmetrical. Excessive use of hands (e.g., sculling, working with a pneumatic drill) may give rise to it, and often it is associated with one of the connective tissue diseases. When severe it is accompanied by tender, painful fingertip ulcers. It may be the first symptom of the underlying disease. The common disorders associated with this problem are collagen vascular disease, rheumatoid arthritis, thromboangiitis obliterans, dysproteinemias, occupational trauma, and the thoracic outlet syndromes.

ERYTHROMELALGIA This rare disorder of the microvasculature produces a burning pain usually in the toes and forefoot associated with changes in ambient temperature. Each patient has a temperature threshold above which symptoms appear and the feet become bright red and warm. Those afflicted rarely wear stockings or regular shoes since these tend to bring out the symptoms. Patients characteristically relieve the pain by walking on a cold surface or soaking their feet in ice water. On physical examination, the peripheral pulses are intact. The foot and toes have a bright red appearance during the attacks. The disease is usually of unknown cause but has been associated in rare cases with myeloproliferative disorders. In some instances it is the manifestation of a painful neuropathy (Chap. 331).

VENOUS THROMBOSIS The common varieties of inflammation and thrombosis (thrombophlebitis) of the superficial and deep veins during severe illness, prolonged bed rest, trauma, and malignancy may produce pain in the extremities. When the superficial veins are involved, the afflicted areas are tender and firm, with associated edema and erythema of the overlying skin. Leg swelling is not then prominent.

Deep venous thrombosis is often more subtle and difficult to diagnose. Classically there is a dull, diffuse pain associated with muscle tenderness and leg edema. Calf pain with dorsiflexion of the foot may be present. The first symptom of this disorder is often pulmonary embolism, which can be life-threatening or fatal. The physical findings are nonspecific and the only certain way of establishing the diagnosis is venography. Ultrasonic and plethysmographic methods have been found useful in establishing the presence of thrombosis of the major deep veins of the leg. The radioactive fibrinogen (^{125}I) test is the only bedside method capable of detecting early calf vein thrombosis.

Venous thrombosis destroys the valves of veins. This is the principal cause of the *postphlebitic syndrome.* In the upright position the contraction of leg muscles forces blood not only toward the heart but also in the direction of the foot and through the perforating veins. The consequence of the latter is edema, subcutaneous hemorrhage (usually in the region of the medial malleolus), deposition of hemosiderin pigment, cutaneous fibrosis, and ulceration. Dull, diffuse pain that is prolonged by dependency and relieved by elevation of the legs is the usual manifestation. Congenital arteriovenous fistulas can also produce venous hypertension, incompetence of the venous valves, and a clinical picture indistinguishable from the postphlebitic syndrome.

LYMPHEDEMA Obstruction of the lymphatics, either congenital or acquired, leads to the development of brawny edema which may also be associated with a dull, mild, deep pain. The clinical picture is often confused with the postphlebitis syndrome. The edema is firm and does not pit readily. The pattern and location of the swelling provide clues as to its nature. In the legs, involvement of the dorsum of the foot is diagnostic. The swelling does not rapidly disappear with bed rest.

THORACIC OUTLET SYNDROMES Compression of the neurovascular bundle as it leaves the thorax can produce symptoms of numbness, tingling, and pain in the hand or portions of it. The pain and tingling occur only in certain positions, depending upon the anatomic defect present. They immediately disappear when the compression is removed. The diagnosis is suspected by reproducing the symptoms and confirming disappearance of the radial pulse with the arm in the position associated with the problem. It is important to x-ray the neck and shoulder girdle looking for cervical ribs. Nerve conduction studies may also be useful in establishing the diagnosis. Exact classification of the anatomic defect depends upon establishing the site of compression and the position in which symptoms appear. The common causes include not only cervical ribs but also scalenus anterior, costoclavicular, and Wright's syndromes (Chap. 9).

NEUROGENIC LIMB PAIN Many diseases may affect the peripheral nerves and cause pain in the limbs. These include beriberi, rheumatoid arthritis, collagen vascular diseases, and diabetes mellitus. Clues to diagnosis are areflexia, which is usually most prominent in the lower limbs, and distal or other sensory impairment. The pain tends to be of a persistent, burning, and tearing nature and is often associated with tenderness of deep tissues.

Diabetic neuritis may be difficult to diagnose. The diabetic patient often exhibits a loss of deep pain sensation and develops painless, nonhealing ulcers over weight-bearing or pressure-supporting areas. Motor involvement is less common. The ankle and knee jerks are usually absent. There is often a loss of sympathetic tone, and as a result the feet are warm and dry. The problem in such patients is to determine whether the pain is neuropathic, vascular, arthritic, or diskogenic (see Chaps. 9, 331, and 358 for differential diagnosis).

Nerve root compression syndromes A herniated nucleus pulposus is a common disorder which results in nerve root compression with pain radiating into the limbs. The pain is deep and poorly localized to the level of the spine where the disk rupture has occurred and is accompanied by involuntary spasm of paravertebral muscles. If the adjacent nerve roots are compressed, the pain radiates along the corresponding nerve distribution, and there are also numbness and paresthesias. The neurologic findings are discussed in Chap. 9. Degenerative disk disease and osteoarthritis can also produce symptoms similar to those observed with a herniated disk. Plain films of the vertebral column and in some cases myelography may be required to establish the diagnosis.

It has been recognized that degenerative joint disease of the spine or hip, spinal cord neoplasm, and a herniated disk can all cause symptoms in the limbs which gradually develop with activity and are relieved by rest. Since it mimics intermittent claudication, this sequence has been called the *pseudoclaudication syndrome.* Findings which help distinguish this entity from true claudication include the following: (1) Extreme variation in the walk-pain-rest cycle; with ischemic claudication the walking distance is usually constant, with prompt pain relief upon cessation of exercise. (2) The pain most often occurs in the thigh and buttock without calf pain; this variation is not usually seen in chronic arterial occlusion. (3) There is an attendant low back pain or discomfort. (4) Sensory, motor, and reflex changes are present. (5) There are no pulse deficits or associated bruits.

Reflex sympathetic dystrophies *Causalgia* is a syndrome characterized by a constant, spontaneous, severe burning pain which follows partial or more rarely, complete, injury to a peripheral nerve trunk. It is frequently associated with hyperalgesia, hyperesthesia, and vasomotor and sudomotor disturbances. In far advanced cases, there may be associated trophic changes. The diagnosis is not difficult if the clinical picture can be related to evidence of previous injury.

While causalgia is considered a reflex sympathetic dystrophy, it is often classified separately because of its numerous entities which can lead to similar complaints, and it is better to classify them more broadly as minor reflex sympathetic dystrophies. The causes include trauma, surgery, occupational use, myocardial infarction, neurologic disorders (central and peripheral), infections, and vascular disorders. The shoulder-hand syndrome which may follow myocardial infarction is considered to be a reflex dystrophy.

A useful diagnostic test for patients suspected of having

a reflex sympathetic dystrophy is to carry out a sympathetic block. The pain is usually completely relieved, with concomitant modification of the physical findings.

Glomus tumor This neoplasm is a benign tumor which develops at the level of the neuromyoarterial glomus. The lesion is small (a few millimeters in diameter) and most frequently located beneath the nails. These small tumors are exquisitely tender to palpation, which distinguishes them from fibromas, neurofibromas, nevi, angiomas, and subungual melanomas.

Interdigital neuroma When pain occurs in the plantar aspect of the foot and is related to walking or local pressure, an interdigital neuroma should be suspected. Essentially this is a compression neuropathy of a plantar nerve, sometimes called "Morton's toe." The lesion usually develops near the ball of the foot, and during weight bearing there is a numbness of two or three toes (usually 3–4). Applied pressure will reproduce the symptoms described by the patient. Occasionally the small nodule is palpable. Excision of the affected nerve relieves the pain (Chap. 331).

REFERENCES

BRAIN L, WALTON JN: *Brain's Diseases of the Nervous System,* 7th ed., London: Oxford University Press, 1969

FAIRBAIRN JF II et al: *Peripheral Vascular Diseases,* 4th ed., Philadelphia: Saunders, 1972

HOLLANDER JL (ed): *Arthritis and Allied Conditions,* 7th ed., Philadelphia: Lea & Febiger, 1966

section 2 | Alterations in body temperature

11 DISTURBANCES OF HEAT REGULATION

ROBERT G. PETERSDORF

CONTROL OF BODY TEMPERATURE

INTRODUCTION In health, the body temperature of human beings is maintained within a narrow range despite extremes in environmental conditions and physical activity. This is also true for most birds and mammals, and such animals are termed *homeothermic,* or warm-blooded. An almost invariable accompaniment of systemic illness is a disturbance in temperature regulation, usually an abnormal elevation, or *fever.* In fact, fever is such a sensitive and reliable indicator of the presence of disease that thermometry is probably the commonest clinical procedure in use. Even in the absence of a frank febrile response, interference with heat regulation by disease is evident. This may take the form of flushing, pallor, sweating, shivering, and abnormal sensations of cold or warmth, or it may consist of erratic fluctuations of body temperature within normal limits when a patient is at bed rest.

HEAT PRODUCTION The major source of basal heat production is through thyroid thermogenesis and the action of adenosine triphosphatase (ATPase) on the sodium pump of all membranes. The muscles are most important in promoting increased heat production with exercise through increased shivering. Heat production by muscle is of particular importance because the quantity can be varied according to the need. In most circumstances this variation consists of small increases and decreases in the number of nerve impulses to the muscles, causing inapparent tensing or relaxing. When, however, there is a strong stimulus for heat production, muscle activity may increase to the point of shivering, or even to a generalized rigor.

HEAT LOSS Heat is lost from the body in several ways. Small amounts are used in warming food or drink and in the evaporation of moisture from the respiratory tract. Most heat is lost from the surface of the body, by *convection,* i.e., the transfer of heat to a fluid medium. Heat loss by convection depends on the existence of a temperature gradient between the body surface and the ambient air. A second mechanism for heat loss is *radiation,* which may be defined as an exchange of electromagnetic energy between the body and the radiant environment. *Evaporation* is the third major mechanism for dissipating heat and is particularly important when the ambient temperature exceeds that of the body.

The principal method of regulating heat loss is by varying the volume of blood flowing to the surface of the body. A rich circulation in the skin and subcutaneous tissues carries heat to the surface, where it can escape. In addition, sweating increases heat loss by providing water to be vaporized. The sweat, or eccrine, glands are under the control of the sympathetic nerves which, in this instance, mediate cholinergic stimuli. Heat loss by sweating may be tremendous and as much as 1 liter per h of sweat may be elaborated. The amount of heat loss through sweating is also dependent upon the humidity in the air. The greater the humidity, the less the ability to lose heat through sweat.

When there is need for conservation of heat, adrenergic

autonomic stimuli cause a sharp reduction in the blood flow to the surface. This causes vasoconstriction and transforms the skin and subcutaneous tissue into layers of insulation.

HEAT TRANSFER WITHIN THE BODY This depends upon *conduction,* i.e., the transfer of heat between adjacent organs; and by *circulatory convection,* which is governed by bulk movement of body fluids and which is responsible for the transfer of heat between the cells and the bloodstream. It is useful, although oversimplified, to visualize the body as a central core at uniform temperatures surrounded by an insulating shell. The role of the shell as a mediator for heat conservation and heat loss is determined in part by its blood supply and by vasoconstriction or vasodilatation. Although insulation is relatively uniform throughout the body, some parts, such as the digits, are particularly susceptible to cold because of the increased surface-to-volume ratio. Moreover, blood that reaches the digits has already been cooled on the way. Insulation may be enhanced by the addition of clothing.

NEURAL CONTROL OF TEMPERATURE The control of body temperature, integrating the various physical and chemical processes for heat production or loss, is a function of cerebral centers located in the hypothalamus. A high-decerebrate animal displays a normal temperature if the hypothalamus is left intact. On the other hand, an animal whose brainstem has been sectioned loses ability to control body temperature, which consequently tends to vary with the environment, a condition referred to as *poikilothermia.* Animal experiments suggest that the preoptic anterior hypothalamus and some centers in the spinal cord have neurons which respond directly to local temperature and act as a sensor for internal temperature. This function is distinct from the integrative function which responds to temperature-sensitive structures all over the body.

Factors affecting neural control of temperature The temperature-regulating system is a negative feedback control system, and possesses three elements essential to such a system: (1) receptors which sense the existing central temperatures; (2) effector mechanisms, consisting of the vasomotor, sudomotor, and metabolic effectors, and (3) integrative structures which determine whether the existing temperature is too high or too low and which activate the appropriate motor response. It is a negative feedback system because a rise in central temperature initiates mechanisms for losing heat while a fall in central temperature activates mechanisms for heat production and heat conservation. The activation of these effector responses is governed by a central integrative mechanism which may be compared with a thermostat and which responds to a variety of stimuli, such as the sensory impulses engendered in flushing or sweating, behavioral impulses, exercise, endocrine influences, and probably the temperature of the blood circulating through the hypothalamic centers. In a sense all these stimuli reset the thermostat.

A classic example of the endocrine influence on temperature is the effect of menstruation. The mean body temperature of women is higher during the second half of the menstrual cycle than it is between the onset of menstruation and the time of ovulation. The sensations of intense heat followed by diaphoresis that characterize the vasomotor instability experienced by some women at the menopause are undoubtedly the result of endocrine imbalance. The activation of the adrenal medulla in response to cold is another example of the relationship between the endocrine system and the thermoregulatory apparatus.

NORMAL BODY TEMPERATURE It is not practical to designate an exact upper level of normal body temperature because there are small differences among normal persons. There are rare individuals whose temperatures are always elevated slightly above accepted "normal" levels, and there is considerable variation in temperature in a given individual. In general, however, it is safe to regard an oral temperature above 99°F (37.2°C) in a person at bed rest as an indication of disease. The temperature may be as low as 96.5°F (35.8°C) in healthy persons. Rectal temperature is usually 0.5 to 1.0°F higher than oral temperature. In very hot weather the body temperature may be elevated by 0.5 or even 1.0°F.

There is a distinct diurnal variation in body temperature in healthy human beings. Oral readings of 97°F (36.1°C) are relatively common on arising in the morning. Body temperature rises steadily through the day, reaches a peak of 99°F (37.2°C) or greater between 6 P.M. and 10 P.M., and then drops slowly to reach a minimum at 2 A.M. to 4 A.M. Although it has been postulated that this diurnal variation is dependent upon increasing activity during the day and rest at night, the pattern is not reversed in individuals who work at night and sleep during the day for long periods of time. The febrile patterns of most human diseases also tend to follow this normal diurnal pattern. Fevers tend to be higher, to "spike," in the evening, and many patients with febrile disease have relatively normal temperatures in the early morning hours.

Severe or prolonged exercise or very hot baths can produce a transient elevation in body temperature, which is quickly compensated for by increased dissipation of heat from the skin and lungs. Such elevations are not properly classified as fevers. Body temperature is more labile in young children, and transient elevations after relatively slight exertion in warm weather are frequently observed in them.

DISORDERED THERMOREGULATION In exercise, there is a temporary imbalance between heat production and heat loss with prompt reestablishment of normal temperatures at rest due to continuing activation of heat loss mechanisms. In contrast, in fever once a stable body temperature is reached, heat production equals heat loss, but both are greater than in the basal state. Cutaneous blood flow plays a greater role in controlling heat production and heat loss in fever than does sweating. At the beginning of fever, the body temperature as sensed by the thermoreceptors is low and the individual responds physiologically as if he were cold. *Heat production* is increased by shivering, and *heat loss* is decreased by vasoconstriction. These events explain the sensation of cold or the chills that characterize the beginning of fever. Conversely, when the cause of fever is removed, the temperature returns to normal, and the individual responds as if he were warm. Cutaneous vasodilatation, sweating, and inhibition of shivering are the compensatory responses.

Deviations of 5°F (approx. 3.5°C) from the normal body temperature do not interfere appreciably with most bodily functions. Convulsions are common at temperatures higher than 106°F (41.1°C), and irreversible brain damage, presumably due to protein denaturation (impairment of normal enzymic functions), is common when temperatures of 108°F (42.2°C) are reached. Fortunately, when hyperthermia reaches dangerous levels, the mechanisms for heat loss are suddenly activated; consequently, oral temperatures above 106°F (41.1°C) are rare in man. Conversely, when temperatures are lowered to 91°F (32.8°C), loss of consciousness occurs; at 86°F (30°C) poikilothermia sets in, and between 83 and 84°F (28.5°C) slow atrial fibrillation supervenes. Ventricular fibrillation during hypothermia is comparatively rare.

The systemic symptoms accompanying deviations in temperature are poorly understood. For example at temperatures of 102°F (39°C) many patients have malaise, drowsiness, weakness, and generalized aches and pains. Many others, however, feel entirely well. Why some individuals are able to tolerate fever so well while others become markedly ill remains an enigma. Perhaps the inciting stimulus rather than fever per se is the major determinant of systemic complaints.

Diseases of the nervous system Disease of the regulatory centers in the hypothalamus may affect body temperature. Cases have been observed in which there was destruction of the centers controlling heat-conserving mechanisms, with resulting hypothermia. More commonly, cerebral lesions are manifested by hyperthermia; this may occur with tumors, infections, degenerative diseases, or vascular accidents. It is not uncommon in cerebral apoplexy for the temperature to rise to 105 to 107°F (42 to 43°C) during the last few hours before death. Central fever is accompanied by lack of a diurnal variation, absence of sweating, resistance to antipyretic drugs, excessive response to external cooling and loss of consciousness.

Heat stroke ("sunstroke") (see below) is an interesting example of fever due to interference with the controlling mechanism. Here the central mechanisms for cooling seem suddenly to fail and the patient ceases to sweat, despite the fact that his temperature is rising. Some of the highest temperatures ever observed in human beings (112 to 113°F) (44.4°C) have been in cases of heat stroke. A temperature higher than 114°F is not compatible with life.

Increased heat production Patients with thyrotoxicosis have exaggerated heat production mechanisms, and their temperature is often 1 to 2°F above the normal range. Dinitrophenol, a drug once used for weight reduction in obese persons, causes elevation of temperature; this too seems to be caused by increased metabolic activity.

Patients with severe burns tend to be hyperthermic despite the fact that a great deal of heat is lost through denuded skin. Presumably, the pyrexia is the result of a hypermetabolic state. The reason for the increased metabolism remains unknown.

Impairment of heat loss Patients with *congestive heart failure* often have an elevation of body temperature between 0.5 and 1.5°F. Perhaps this elevation is caused by impairment of heat dissipation as a result of diminished cardiac output, decline in cutaneous blood flow (with increasing insulation of the central temperature core), the insulating effect of edema, and the increased heat production incident to the muscular activity of dyspnea. On the other hand, patients with congestive heart failure are likely to have other causes of fever, such as venous thrombosis, pulmonary embolism and infarction, myocardial infarction, rheumatic fever, and urinary tract infection. However, since slight fever is so regularly present even in the absence of such complications, the circulatory disturbance may be responsible.

Patients with skin disorders such as *ichthyosis* or *congenital absence of sweat glands* may have fever in a warm environment because of inability to lose heat from the surface of the body. Similarly, individuals taking *drugs which impair sweating,* such as atropine or propantheline (Pro-Banthine), may have fever in warm weather.

DISEASES ASSOCIATED WITH HIGH TEMPERATURES (HEAT SYNDROMES)

Three clinical syndromes are associated with high environmental temperature: *heat cramps, heat exhaustion,* and *heat pyrexia.* Although each entity may be identified clinically, there is considerable overlap in the changes produced by a high environmental temperature. These alterations are especially prevalent during the first days of a heat wave before effective acclimatization can occur. Prophylaxis by augmenting sodium chloride intake prior to exposure, or by restoring a physiologic balance prior to the onset of overt morbidity, can help prevent the full-blown syndrome, especially heat pyrexia. Children and elderly individuals are particularly susceptible to heat stress. Strenuous physical activity or the presence of an acute or chronic disease may hasten the development of one of the heat syndromes.

ACCLIMATIZATION The basic mechanism by which man accommodates to excessive temperatures is unknown. Acclimatization does not increase the threshold for sweating. However, sweating is the most effective natural means of combating heat stress, and can occur with little or no change in the core temperature of the body. As long as sweating continues, man can withstand remarkably high temperatures, provided water and sodium chloride, the most important physiologic constituents of sweat, are replaced. The concentration of sodium chloride varies between that of interstitial fluid and very low concentrations, and the ability to secrete sweat of low NaCl content is a major mechanism for the conservation of salt in hot weather. Dilatation of the peripheral blood vessels in an attempt to dissipate heat is another well-known phenomenon in hot temperatures. Other alterations include a decrease in total circulating blood volume, a decrease in renal blood flow, an increase of the antidiuretic hormones (ADH) as well as aldosterone. Hyperaldosteronism may result in severe potassium loss, which may be aggravated by replacement of sodium without concomitant repletion of potassium. Initially there is an increase in cardiac output but as heat stress persists, venous return diminishes and heart failure may occur. If environmental temperatures in excess of the body's temperature persist, heat is retained and hyperpyrexia develops.

HEAT CRAMPS Heat cramps, called "miner's cramps" and "stoker's cramps," are the most benign heat syndrome. Cramps are characterized by painful spasms of the voluntary muscles and usually follow strenuous exercise. In general, only individuals in good physical condition develop this syndrome. External temperatures need not exceed the body temperature, and direct exposure to the sun is not necessary. The body temperature is usually not elevated. Muscle cramps usually occur after excessive sweating and may even be precipitated by strenuous exercise in cold environments in untrained persons heavily clothed. Muscles of the extremities bear the brunt of physical activity and hence show the highest incidence of cramps. Physical examination of the patient is normal between the paroxysms. Examination of the blood reveals a concentration of the formed elements and a decreased sodium and chloride concentration. Excretion of these ions in the urine is characteristically low. Treatment consists of sodium chloride; cessation of cramps with replacement of sodium chloride and water is striking and supports the hypothesis that the cause of heat cramps is depletion of these essential electrolytes. Occasionally cramps involve the abdominal musculature, mimicking an intraabdominal emergency. Such patients have had mistaken exploratory surgery performed, often with disatrous results. Replacement of saline prior to surgery would have obviated such operations.

HEAT EXHAUSTION Heat prostration, or heat collapse, is probably the most common heat syndrome. Weakness, vertigo, headache, nausea, anorexia, and faintness may precede collapse. Heat collapse occurs in both physically active and sedentary individuals. The onset is usually sudden and the duration of collapse brief. During the acute stage, the patient looks ashen-gray. The skin is cold and clammy. The pupils are dilated. The blood pressure may be low and the pulse pressure elevated. Since prostration develops before exposure to heat is prolonged, body temperature is subnormal or normal. The duration of exposure and the extent to which sweat is lost determine the degree of hemoconcentration. Treatment consists of removal of the patient to a cool area, and spontaneous recovery then usually takes place. Intravenous administration of saline solution or whole blood is necessary only rarely. The pathogenetic mechanism of heat prostration is not primarily a depletion of water and salt, but it is likely that maintenance of these electrolytes will prevent heat prostration in individuals exposed to high temperatures.

HEAT PYREXIA Heat hyperpyrexia, heat stroke, or sunstroke is most common in individuals with preexisting chronic disease. Among these are arteriosclerosis, diabetes mellitus, alcoholism and disorders in which it may be difficult to lose heat such as ectodermal dysplasia, congenital absence of the sweat glands, or severe scleroderma. Direct exposure to the sun is not a necessary prerequisite. Heat pyrexia may develop during any period of hot weather, but the incidence in temperate climates increases during prolonged heat waves. High humidity is a prerequisite to heat stroke, and patients usually stop sweating before onset of acute symptoms. The cessation of sweating is due to an intrinsic breakdown of the heat regulatory mechanism for reasons not known. There may be few premonitory symptoms of heat stroke, and loss of consciousness may be the first sign. Other patients may complain of headache, vertigo, faintness, abdominal distress, or confusion. Delirium may develop in more severe cases.

Pyrexia and prostration are the significant findings on physical examination. A rectal temperature greater than 106°F (41.1°C) is common and is a grave prognostic sign. Internal body temperatures as high as 112 to 113°F (44.4°C) have been recorded. The skin is hot and dry, and sweating is absent. The pulse rate is increased, and respirations are rapid and weak. The systolic blood pressure may be elevated. The muscles are flaccid, and tendon reflexes may be diminished. Shock is common in fatal cases. Examination of the blood and urine may show few abnormalities. Leukocytosis is characteristic as are proteinuria, cylinduria, and an elevation in BUN. At the onset electrolytes are normal, although the potassium may be diminished. The electrocardiogram may show, in addition to tachycardia and sinus arrhythmia, flattening and subsequent inversion of the T wave and depression of the S-T segment. Diffuse myocardial necrosis with ECG evidence of myocardial infarction has been reported. Other major laboratory abnormalities include thrombocytopenia; prolonged bleeding, clotting, and prothrombin times; afibrinogenemia and fibrinolysis; and consumptive coagulopathy. All these may be responsible for diffuse bleeding. Liver damage is common; it appears 24 to 36 h after admission and is characterized by clinically apparent jaundice and, often, by abnormalities in hepatocellular enzymes. Renal failure is a common complication of heat stroke.

Patients with heat stroke may die within a few hours after being discovered, or may die of complications such as acute renal failure. However, a number of patients will die several weeks after the acute episode, usually of myocardial infarction, heart failure, renal failure, bronchopneumonia or complicating bacteremia. In them autopsy may show extensive parenchymal damage to various organs, either from hyperpyrexia per se or from petechial hemorrhages in the brain, heart, kidneys, or liver.

TREATMENT Heat stroke requires heroic emergency measures. Time is most important. The patient should be placed in a cool place with adequate circulation of fresh air and with most of the clothing removed. Because the pathogenesis of heat stroke involves failure of the heat-regulating mechanism with cessation of sweating, external means of heat dissipation must be employed. The most effective measure is to immerse the patient in an ice-water bath, and there is no effective substitute for this seemingly drastic treatment. An ice-water bath does not induce shock or stimulate significant cutaneous vasoconstriction. The bath should be given with a minimum of delay. The patient should be watched constantly by a nurse or physician and the rectal temperature monitored. The bath may be discontinued when the rectal temperature falls below 101°F (38.3°C), but treatment should be resumed if there is a febrile rebound. Compared with immersion in ice water, other forms of therapy are ineffective. After the bath the patient should be placed in a cool, well-ventilated room. Massage of the skin aids the acceleration of heat loss and stimulates return of the cool peripheral blood to the overheated brain and viscera. Phenothiazine may be given to reduce shivering. Stimulants such as epinephrine and narcotics are contraindicated. Intravenous fluids should be given with monitoring of the central venous pressure and urinary output. Both dehydration and heart failure must be avoided. Fresh blood should be given in case of bleeding, and clear-cut evidence of disseminated intravascular coagulation calls for heparin (7,500 U per hour). Persistent oliguria is an indication for early dialysis.

Malignant hyperthermia Persons with malignant hyperthermia, an autosomally inherited disease of skeletal and cardiac muscle, react to potent inhalational anesthetics such as halothane or skeletal muscle relaxants (succinylcholine) with high fever, muscle rigidity, tachycardia, arrhythmias, hypotension, and mottled cyanosis. Early laboratory abnormalities include respiratory and metabolic acidosis, hyperkalemia and hypermagnesemia, and elevation in blood lactate and pyruvate. The mechanism of the hyperthermic reaction apppears to be related to hypermetabolism in muscle that is induced by a sudden increase in myoplasmic calcium. This, in turn, leads to stimulation of ATPase, increased ATP utilization in the face of falling ATP production, and marked increase in heat production. Sarcolemmal disruption, characterized by severe intracellular biochemical abnormalities, occurs. Late complications include massive skeletal muscle swelling, pulmonary edema, disseminated intravascular coagulation, and acute renal failure. Treatment consists of infusion of procainamide (0.5 to 1.0 mg per kg per min), correction of acidosis, diuretics to induce a myoglobin diuresis, and correction of hyperkalemia.

Between attacks, persons susceptible to malignant hyperthermia may be entirely normal. Some have increased muscle bulk, some have localized areas of muscle weakness, some spontaneous muscle cramps, and a few have generalized muscle weakness. In some of these patients, the creatine phosphokinase (CPK) is elevated, but in many this test is entirely normal. Microscopy of muscle shows marked variation in fiber diameter.

DISEASES ASSOCIATED WITH LOW TEMPERATURES

COLD ACCLIMATIZATION Cold acclimatization represents a state of increased resistance to cold injury and is the result of exposure to a cold but tolerable environment. Adaptive responses consist of circulatory adjustments protecting the temperatures of exposed portions of the body; metabolic adaptation results in greater heat production to compensate for increased heat loss; and behavioral and neural adaptations minimize either the actual cold stress or the discomfort resulting from physiologically tolerable hypothermia. In contrast with heat acclimatization, it is not possible to delineate adaptive physiologic changes to cold. Nevertheless, primitive people live at zero temperatures wearing little or no clothing; pain perception is less in persons, such as fishermen, who work periodically with their hands in ice water; and military personnel shiver less during cold exposure after training in the Arctic. Adaptation may take place either by shivering, with production of excess heat, or, as is the case in Australian aborigines, by a drop of internal temperature with only minimal shivering.

HYPOTHERMIA Hypothermia is far less common than is elevation in temperature but is of considerable importance because it represents a medical emergency which lends itself to treatment.

Accidental hypothermia This is a well-known complication of exposure, and has often been reported during the winter months. It usually occurs in elderly individuals after prolonged exposure, not necessarily to excessively low external temperatures. It is attributed not only to exogenous factors such as a low external environment but also to unknown endogenous factors. The diagnosis of hypothermia has proved elusive largely because *clinical thermometers do not record temperatures below 95°F (35°C). Whenever a patient presents with a temperature in this range the true temperature should be determined with an incubator thermometer or a thermocouple.* Accidental hypothermia has been found in association with myxedema, pituitary insufficiency, Addison's disease, hypoglycemia, cerebrovascular disease, myocardial infarction, terminal cirrhosis, pancreatitis, and ingestion of drugs or alcohol. For example, it is not uncommon to find a derelict in a railroad yard or under a bridge following an alcoholic debauche with a temperature between 85 and 90°F (28.5 to 32.3°C) or lower. These patients usually appear cold and pale and, when their temperatures are very low, give the appearance of having rigor mortis, so stiff is their musculature. Patients with temperatures less than 80°F (26.7°C) are usually unconscious. The pupils are usually miotic, respirations tend to be shallow and slow, there is bradycardia, and most patients are hypotensive. There is often generalized edema. Laboratory data tend to show hemoconcentration, mild azotemia, and metabolic acidosis. Some patients have hypoglycemia while others show evidence of diabetes mellitus. Thyroid function tests give results typical of myxedema in a number of these patients. Some patients have elevations in serum amylase and a few show pancreatitis at autopsy. The electrocardiogram is distorted by muscular tremors, and may show bradycardia or slow atrial fibrillation, and a characteristic J wave (occurring at the junction of the QRS complex and S-T segment).

TREATMENT Therapy should be instituted at once and consists of maintenance of the airway and intravenous administration of glucose and saline and low molecular weight dextran, both to expand blood volume and to prevent the infarctions which have been a hallmark in fatal cases. *External rewarming is contraindicated* because, while it tends to dilate the constricted peripheral blood vessels, it diverts blood from the visceral organs; most patients who have been rewarmed externally have died. On the other hand, restoration of the core temperature by hemodialysis during which the blood is warmed externally or by peritoneal dialysis during which the dialysate is warmed to 98.6°F is helpful. Corticosteroids, vasopressors, and prophylactic antibiotics have not proved valuable. Large volumes of fluid, supplemented by dialysis, is the treatment of choice. The prognosis in accidental hypothermia remains poor, primarily because many of these patients are old and have associated debilitating disease. One young patient was saved even after her temperature dropped to 69°F (20.6°C).

Immersion hypothermia Responses to cold water immersion may be classified as (1) stimulatory, with deep body temperature normal to 95°F (35°C); (2) depressant, with deep body temperature 95 to 86°F (35 to 30°C); and critical, with deep body temperature 86 to 77°F (30 to 25°C).

The long-distance swimmer is able to maintain a normal body temperature for periods of 15 to 25 h or more in water that may plunge skin temperature to 59°F (15°C) or lower, which is some 28°F below deep body temperature, lending support to the concept of a body core insulated by a body shell. The vasoconstriction operative in cold water greatly reduces heat loss. However, there is great individual variability in heat loss in cold water. The relatively obese swimmer may maintain a normal rectal temperature for 2 h without shivering in 61°F (16°C) water. A lean man under the same conditions, despite violent shivering, may experience a fall in rectal temperature of several degrees and become incapacitated from the rigor. In hypersensitive persons, immersion in cold water may be followed by vascular spasm, vomiting, and syncope.

Other compensatory responses include bradycardia, a slight rise in blood pressure, and an early rise in rectal temperature followed by a fall. At 86°F (30°C), atrial fibrillation is common.

TREATMENT Although rewarming in hot water has been recommended in the treatment of immersion hypothermia, the same objections to sudden diversion of cardiac output to peripheral tissues described above apply. Individuals with this problem should be covered with a light blanket and placed in a room with a moderate ambient temperature. Hemodialysis or peritoneal dialysis should be considered.

LOCAL COLD INJURIES Mechanisms of freezing injury These can be divided into phenomena which affect cells and extracellular fluids (direct effects) and those which disrupt the function of organized tissues and the integrity of the circulation (indirect effects).

DIRECT EFFECTS When tissue freezes, ice crystals form and, concomitantly, solutes in the residual liquid become concentrated. The physical dislocation during slow freezing is extreme. Ice crystals many times the size of individual cells form but only in the extracellular spaces. Large ice crystals can develop between cells in soft tissue without producing irreversible injury as long as the percentage of water frozen does not exceed a critical amount. A major source of damage to living cells during freezing and thawing appears to be the strong salt solutions which develop during formation and dissolution of ice; changes in the proportions of lipids and phospholipids in the cell membrane are also of great importance. The discovery of the protective value of such substances as glycerol and dimethylsulfoxide, which enter cells and prevent freezing injury during comparatively slow cooling to low temperatures and rewarming from them, represents a significant advance. This method has been used extensively in banking spermatozoa for subsequent artificial insemination. It has not been possible, however, to protect organs in this manner since the protective substance must be delivered to all cells.

INDIRECT EFFECTS The fulminating vascular reaction and stasis which supervene are associated with production of histamine-like substances which increase the permeability of the capillary bed. Within blood vessels, cellular elements aggregate. Irreversible occlusion of small blood vessels by cell masses has been demonstrated in thawed tissue following freezing injury. The damaged frozen tissue simulates tissue damage produced by burns.

Manifestations Local cold injury may be divided into freezing (frostbite) and nonfreezing (immersion-foot) injuries. The two types may be observed in the same extremity or in different extremities in the same individual, e.g., trench foot and freezing of the hands but not the feet of shipwreck survivors. The diagnosis of freezing versus nonfreezing injury generally can be made on the basis of history and clinical manifestations.

IMMERSION FOOT This entity is observed in shipwreck survivors or in soldiers (trench foot) whose feet have been wet but not freezing cold for prolonged periods. There is primarily injury to nerve and muscle tissue, but no gross or irreparable pathologic changes occur in blood vessels and skin. The clinical picture reflects primary hypoxic trauma giving rise to three clearly recognizable conditions: (1) *ischemia,* denoted by a pale, pulseless extremity; (2) *hyperemia,* characterized by a bounding pulsatile circulation in red, swollen, painful feet; and (3) the *posthyperemic* or recovery period. The initial cold-induced vasoconstriction, increased blood viscosity, and impaired oxygen transport in the ischemic state are aggravated by such factors as malnutrition, general hypothermia, dehydration, and trauma from relatively fixed, pendant extremities. The problem of rewarming is critical in these patients during the stage of ischemia, when overheating of tissue may lead to gangrene. In the state of hyperemia, the red, swollen feet require judicious cooling. Severe cases may show muscular weakness, atrophy, ulceration, and gangrene of superficial areas. Sensitivity to cold and pain on weight bearing, which may cause discomfort for many years, are sequelae even of milder injuries.

FROSTBITE In contrast with immersion foot, in frostbite the blood vessels may be severely and irreparably injured, the circulation of blood ceases, and the vascular bed of the frozen tissue is occluded by agglutinated cell aggregates and thrombi. The cutaneous injury consists in part of separation of the epidermal-dermal interface. Early, the intravascular clumping is reversible. However, with the passage of time, clumped red cells within vessels in injured tissue lose their morphologic identity and take on the appearance of a homogenous, hyalinaceous plug. It has been shown in some, but not all, experimental studies that much of the intravascular aggregation following freezing injury can be reversed and microcirculatory perfusion improved if low molecular weight dextran is given intravenously shortly after injury. Frostbitten tissues unfortunately are often neglected and with thawing become macerated; if this is the situation the method of rewarming is not important. The method of rewarming has been a matter of controversy. It seems most rational to warm the core of the body before treating the local area of frostbite. Following restoration of the core temperature to normal, warming of a frostbitten limb should begin in water at 50 to 59°F (10 to 15°C), which is then increased 9°F (5°C) every 5 min to a maximum of 104°F (40°C).

Most cold injuries do not require warming, and treatment should be conservative and consists of bed rest, elevation of the injured part, tetanus antitoxin, and antibiotics, when indicated; early drainage of blebs and bullae; daily washes with pHisoHex; and early institution of physiotherapy. Surgical amputation and reconstruction is usually not necessary. Regional sympathectomy performed 24 to 48 h after thawing is followed by rapid resolution of edema, earlier demarcation of destroyed tissue, and faster healing. The effect of regional sympathectomy is probably due to ablation of persistent vasospasm and to restoration of cold perception.

Some patients with frostbite have residua consisting of excessive sweating, pain, cold feet, numbness, abnormal color, and pain in the joints. The symptoms are generally worse in the winter and following exposure to cold. These patients also often show abnormal nails, discoloration and pigmentation, hyperhydrosis, and, by x-ray, osteoporosis and cystic defects near the joints. These abnormalities tend to be milder in patients who have had sympathectomies. Most cold injuries are preventable by graded exposure to cold, as well as appropriate clothing in freezing temperatures.

CLINICAL USES OF LOW TEMPERATURES

Localized application Low temperature has been used extensively in recent years. Two outstanding examples are selective destruction by freezing in cryosurgery and preservation of biologic material. Practical advantages of cryogenic surgery are safety and hemostasis; the results in therapeutic management of tumors have been encouraging. The preservation of red blood cells, spermatozoa, and other viable material by low temperature has become possible through use of glycerol to protect cells against freezing. Hypothermia combined with hyperbaric oxygenation has been employed with notable success in preserving organs, chiefly kidneys, for transplantation.

In surgery Periods of ischemia sufficient to permit surgical intervention can be tolerated by organs such as the brain and heart, provided that tissue temperature has been lowered to reduce metabolism before blood supply is interrupted. Hypothermia can be induced with light anesthesia and surface cooling or, more effectively, by means of a pump-oxygenator to provide extracorporeal circulation. Prior to the introduction of this technique, surgical hypothermia was limited to temperatures of about 82.4°F (28°C) and temperatures below 77°F (25°C) were dangerous. At present, extracorporeal circulation has extended the application of hypothermia to temperatures of 10°C or lower. The principal medical problem arises from disturbances in acid-base balance, including large fluctuations in dissolved CO_2 in relation to temperature change, the oxygen debt incurred by some tissues, and an excess in lactic acid production. The oxygen debt is present not only during induction of hypothermia but also during the period of recovery when cardiac function is less than optimal. The body's buffer mechanisms are often inadequate to cope with the shifts in pH and to regulate pH. Therefore intravenous amine type buffers (TRIS or THAM) may need to be used. The addition of hyperbaric oxygen has also improved pH control and has enhanced the period during which ischemia may be maintained safely.

REFERENCES

Brengelman G: Temperature regulation, in *Physiology and Biophysics,* eds TC Ruch and HD Patton, Philadelphia: Saunders, 1973

Britt BA: Malignant hyperthermia: A pharmacogenetic disease of skeletal and cardiac muscle. N Engl J Med 290:1140, 1974

Clinicopathologic Conference: A sixty-five-year-old woman with heat stroke. Am J Med 43:113, 1967

Clowes GHA, Jr, O'Donnel TF, Jr: Current concepts: Heat stroke. N Engl J Med 291:564, 1974

David DM et al: Accidental hypothermia treated by extracorporeal blood-warming. Lancet 1:1036, 1967

Duguid H, Simpson RG: Accidental hypothermia. Lancet 2:1213, 1961

Edelman IS: Thyroid thermogenesis. N Engl J Med 290:1303, 1974

Golding MR et al: The role of sympathectomy in frostbite, with a review of 68 cases. Surgery 57:774, 1965

Knochel JP et al: The renal, cardiovascular, hematologic and serum electrolyte abnormalities of heat stroke. Am J Med 30:299, 1961

Lash RF et al: Accidental profound hypothermia and barbiturate intoxication: A report of rapid "core" rewarming by peritoneal dialysis. JAMA 201:123, 1966

O'Donnel TF, Jr, Clowes GHA, Jr: The circulatory abnormalities of heat stroke. New Engl J Med 287:734, 1972

Penn I, Schwartz SI: Evaluation of low molecular weight dextran in the treatment of frostbite. J Trauma 4:784, 1964

Tolman KG, Cohen A: Accidental hypothermia. Can Med Assoc J 103:1357, 1970

12

CHILLS AND FEVER

ROBERT G. PETERSDORF

In view of the extensive knowledge of physiologic mechanisms controlling body temperature mentioned in Chap. 11, it is surprising that so little is known about the ways in which disease upsets thermoregulation.

Some bacteria, particularly gram-negative species, produce endotoxins which are pyrogenic, and a few viruses also cause fever when injected into man or animals. Many microorganisms, however, possess no demonstrable pyrogenic toxin and, of course, fever accompanies diseases which do not involve invasion of the body by any known parasite. Omitting disorders which may involve cerebral thermoregulatory centers directly, such as brain tumors, intracranial hemorrhage or thrombosis, or heat stroke, the following disease states may be accompanied by fever: (1) All *infections,* whether caused by bacteria, rickettsias, viruses, or more complex parasites, cause fever. (2) *Mechanical trauma,* e.g., a crushing injury, frequently gives rise to fever lasting 1 or 2 days. Not infrequently, however, complicating infection sets in. (3) Many *neoplastic diseases* are associated with fever. In most patients, fever in patients with cancer is related to obstruction or infection produced by the tumor. In some solid tumors, however, fever may be due to the tumor per se, particularly following metastasis to the liver. Tumors which are associated with fever include hypernephroma, carcinoma of the pancreas, lung, or bone, and hepatoma. In tumors of the reticuloendothelial system, including Hodgkin's disease, lymphosarcoma, reticulum cell sarcoma, and acute leukemias, fever may be one of the prominent early manifestations. (4) *Hematopoietic disorders,* e.g., acute hemolytic episodes, may be characterized by pyrexia. (5) *Vascular accidents* of any magnitude e.g., myocardial, pulmonary, and cerebral infarctions, nearly always cause fever. (6) *Diseases due to immune mechanisms* are almost always febrile. These include the collagen diseases, drug fevers, and serum sickness. (7) Certain *acute metabolic disorders,* such as gout, porphyria, hypertriglyceridemia, Fabry's disease, and Addisonian or thyroid crises, sometimes are associated with fever.

PATHOGENESIS OF FEVER Several hypotheses have been offered to explain disturbed temperature regulation in disease. One attributes fever to shifts in body water which interfere with heat production and heat loss. It is true that newborn infants may become febrile when fluid intake is inadequate and that the temperature elevation subsides promptly when fluid is administered. In adults, there are occasional instances of fever associated with extracellular fluid deficit when the ambient temperature is above 90°F. On the other hand, "dehydration" is not ordinarily associated with fever in adults, and the clinical practice of attributing fever to this cause has little basis in fact.

There is little evidence to implicate abnormal thyroid and adrenal function in the pathogenesis of fever. Temperature regulation is normal in Addison's disease and in Cushing's syndrome. Body temperature is slightly above normal in thyrotoxicosis and a little low in myxedema, but these differences are entirely in keeping with the metabolic rate and there is no real evidence of impaired thermoregulation in either disease.

There was a renewal of interest in a role of the endocrines in the pathogenesis of fever with the finding that abnormalities of etiocholanolone metabolism exist in some patients with "periodic fever" (Chap. 229). Although administration of progesterone and some of its congeners, and of etiocholanolone, results in fever in man, there is no evidence that specific steroid fevers (notably etiocholanolone fever) exist.

Tissue injury Because fever is associated with so many diverse disease processes, it seems reasonable that it is determined by some common mechanism, and the common factor in febrile diseases, whether or not they are infectious in origin, is *tissue injury.* The hypothesis which best fits clinical and experimental observations is that fever results from disturbance of cerebral thermoregulation brought about by a product or products of tissue injury. It has been shown experimentally that inflammatory exudates cause fever when injected intravenously into normal animals, and similar results have been obtained in human subjects. The major sources of pyrogenic material are polymorphonuclear and mononuclear leukocytes.

The elements of the febrile response can be illustrated by the sequence of events that follow intravenous injection of killed bacteria or of purified bacterial endotoxin. Following administration of a small amount of typhoid vaccine intravenously in man, the body temperature does not begin to rise until about an hour after the injection. During this interval, the patient notes no discomfort and his appearance is unchanged. Then, rather suddenly, there is malaise, he complains of cold, and within minutes he is burrowing down into the bedclothes, asking for more blankets. He begins to shiver and is soon having a shaking chill which lasts 10 to 20 min. During this time, the skin is pale and cold but the rectal temperature rises steeply. After subsidence of the rigor, the patient gradually feels warmer, the skin circulation increases, and within 2 h he is flushed and complains of feeling feverish. After another hour, profuse sweating begins and the body temperature begins to return toward normal.

Endogenous pyrogen The pathophysiologic counterpart of these clinical events has been worked out to a large extent in experimental animals. Following its injection, endotoxin is removed rapidly from the bloodstream by the fixed phagocytes of the reticuloendothelial system. At the same time there is, in most species, a profound leukopenia, and the leukocytes are marginated along blood vessel walls. During this period the marginated polymorphonuclear leukocytes as well as the fixed reticuloendothelial cells are activated by the endotoxin to release fever-producing substances into the circulation. These humoral factors, which have been called *endogenous pyrogens,* are presumably the substances which act on the thermoregulatory centers to produce fever. They have been found in the bloodstream of animals given endotoxin, antigens (in previously sensitized animals), and antigen-antibody complexes, and those with experimental pneumococcal, streptococcal, staphylococcal, and viral infections. In these situations the cells are activated during phagocytosis and then release their pyrogen. Biologically, endogenous pyrogen found in serum is similar to leukocytic pyrogen derived from sterile inflammatory exudates. Two separate pyrogens have been partially purified, one from polymorphonuclear and the other from mononuclear phagocytes. The pyrogens are somewhat different from one another, but both are basic proteins of low molecular weight. Endogenous pyrogen exists in cells in an inactive precursor form. Activation of the cells is associated with *de novo* protein synthesis, following which the pyrogen is released into the surrounding medium (usually blood) over a relatively long period. Whether endogenous pyrogen is the sole mediator of fever or whether some of the agents which incite its release—such as endotoxin—can activate the thermoregulatory centers directly is unknown.

ACCOMPANIMENTS OF FEVER **Systemic symptoms** The perception of fever by patients varies enormously. Some persons can tell with considerable accuracy whether their body temperatures are elevated; others, notably patients with tuberculosis, may be wholly unaware of body temperature as high as 103°F. Often, also, patients may pay no attention to fever because of other unpleasant symptoms such as headache and pleuritic pain. Pain in the back, generalized myalgias, and arthralgia without arthritis are common in fever. Whether these symptoms reflect the presence of an infectious agent or are merely a nonspecific accompaniment of pyrexia is not clear.

Chills Abrupt onset of fever with a *chill* or *rigor* is characteristic of some diseases and, in the absence of antipyretic drugs, rare in others. Although repeated rigors are typical of pyogenic infection with bacteremia, a similar pattern of fever may occur in noninfectious diseases such as lymphoma. It is important to differentiate a true chill, which is accompanied by teeth chattering and bed shaking, from the chilly sensation which occurs in almost all fevers, particularly those in viral infections. In some instances, however, a true rigor occurs in viremia. Chills may be evoked or perpetuated by the intermittent administration of aspirin or other antipyretics. These agents may cause a sharp depression in temperature, which is followed by compensatory involuntary muscular contractions, i.e., a chill. This unpleasant side effect of antipyretic drugs can be averted by administering these agents frequently and in low doses.

Herpes labialis, so-called fever blister, results from activation of the herpes simplex virus by elevation in temperature and occurs frequently in patients undergoing artificial fever therapy. For reasons which are obscure, fever blisters are common in pneumococcal infections, streptococcosis, malaria, meningococcemia, and rickettsioses but are rare in mycoplasma pneumonia, tuberculosis, brucellosis, smallpox, and typhoid.

Delirium may result from elevation of body temperature and is particularly common in patients with alcoholism, cerebral arteriosclerosis, or senility.

Convulsions are not infrequent in febrile children, especially those with a family history of epilepsy, although febrile convulsions do not, in general, reflect serious cerebral disease.

CLINICAL IMPORTANCE OF FEVER The temperature is a simple, objective, and accurate indicator of a physiologic state and is much less subject to external and psychogenic stimuli than the other vital signs, i.e., the pulse, respiratory rate, and blood pressure. For these reasons, determination of the body temperature assists in estimating the severity of an illness, its course and duration, and the effect of therapy, or even in deciding whether a person has an organic illness.

Benefit of fever There are few infections of man in which pyrexia appears definitely to be beneficial to the host, examples being neurosyphilis and perhaps chronic brucellosis. Certain other diseases, such as uveitis and rheumatoid arthritis, sometimes improve after fever therapy. In experimental animals some pneumococcal and cryptococcal infections have been influenced in favor of the host animal by raising the body temperature. Aged and debilitated patients with infection may have little or no fever, and this is generally interpreted as a bad prognostic sign. In the great majority of infectious diseases, however, there is no reason to believe that pyrexia accelerates phagocytosis, antibody formation, or other defense mechanisms.

Detrimental aspects of fever Fever accelerates all metabolic processes and accentuates weight loss and nitrogen wastage. The work and the rate of the heart are increased. Sweating aggravates loss of salt and water. There may be discomfort due to headache, photophobia, general malaise, or unpleasant sensation of warmth. The rigors and profuse sweats of hectic fevers are particularly unpleasant for the patient. In elderly individuals with overt or potential cardiac or cerebral vascular disease, fever may be particularly deleterious.

MANAGEMENT OF FEVER Since fever ordinarily does little harm and imposes no great discomfort, antipyretic drugs are rarely necessary and may obfuscate the effect of a specific therapeutic agent or of the natural course of the disease. There are situations, however, in which lowering of the body temperature is of vital importance; e.g., heat stroke, postoperative hyperthermia, delirium due to hyperpyrexia, or shock associated with fever and heart failure. Under these circumstances lowering the temperature is indicated. Cooling blankets which can be set at hypothermic temperatures are a highly effective means for external cooling. Alternatively, sponging the body surface with cool saline solution or the application of cool compresses to the skin and forehead may be employed. There is no advantage in sponging with alcohol, which, because of its pungent odor, makes some patients ill. When high internal temperature is combined with cutaneous vasoconstriction, as in heat stroke or postoperative hyperthermia, the cooling measures should be combined with massage of the skin in order to bring blood to the surface, where it may be cooled. Immediate immersion in a tub of ice water should be considered a lifesaving emergency procedure in patients with heat stroke if the internal body temperature is in excess of 108°F (42.2°C). If cooling blankets are available, they are preferable to immersion in ice in most instances.

If antipyretic drugs, such as aspirin (0.3 to 0.6 g), are employed to bring about a fall in temperature, ill effects such as unpleasant diaphoresis, sometimes associated with an alarming fall in blood pressure and the subsequent return of fever and occasionally accompanied by a chill, may occur. These can be mitigated by enforcing a liberal fluid intake and by administering the drug regularly and frequently at 2- to 3-h intervals. Although adrenal steroids are also potent antipyretics, they must be used with caution because of their tendency to precipitate abrupt falls in temperature accompanied by hypotension. The capacity of these drugs to mask other manifestations of infection also constitutes a relative contraindication to their use.

The discomfort of a rigor can be alleviated in many patients by the intravenous injection of calcium gluconate. This procedure will stop the shivering and chilliness but has no influence on the ultimate height of the fever. Severe disruptive rigors sometimes need to be abolished with morphine sulfate (10 to 15 mg subcutaneously).

DIAGNOSTIC CONSIDERATIONS IN FEVER

In many illnesses fever is the most prominent and often the only manifestation of disease. It is not an indication of any particular type of disease; rather it should be considered a reaction to injury comparable to an elevated leukocyte count or a rapid erythrocyte sedimentation rate.

TYPES OF FEVER Fever is classically described as intermittent, remittent, sustained, and relapsing.

An intermittent fever is one in which the temperature falls to normal each day. When the variation between the peak and the nadir is very large, the fever is called *hectic* or *septic.* Intermittent fevers are characteristic in pyogenic infections, particularly abscesses, lymphomas, and miliary tuberculosis.

In remittent fever the temperature falls each day but does not return to normal. Most fevers are remittent, and this type of febrile response is in no way characteristic.

A sustained fever is characterized by persistent elevation without significant diurnal variation. It is exemplified by the fever of untreated typhoid or typhus.

A relapsing fever is one in which short febrile periods occur between one or several days of normal temperature. Examples of relapsing fever are seen in the following conditions:

Malaria (Chap. 215) had vanished from the United States almost completely, but for several years Vietnam war veterans constituted an important and sizable reservoir of this infection, as do other persons recently arrived from foreign countries. It is most unusual, however, for malaria to recur after a symptom-free interval of 1 year or more. Seizures recur at 2- or 3-day intervals, or more irregularly in falciparum infections, depending on the maturation cycle of the parasite. The diagnosis depends on demonstration of the parasites in the blood.

Relapsing fever (Chap. 167) occurs in the southwest part of the United States, as far east as Texas, and in many other parts of the world. The recurrences are related to the cyclic development of parasites. Diagnosis is by demonstration of the spirochetal organisms in stained films of the blood.

Rat-bite fever is brought about by two agents—*Spirillum minus* (Chap. 168) and *Streptobacillus moniliformis* (Chap. 149), both transmitted by the bite of a rat. Both may cause an illness characterized by periodic exacerbations of fever. The clue to the diagnosis depends on obtaining a history of rat bite 1 to 10 weeks previous to the onset of symptoms. The cause can be established by appropriate laboratory procedures.

Localized *pyogenic infections* in rare instances give rise to periodic bouts of fever separated by afebrile and relatively symptom-free intervals. The so-called "Charcot's intermittent biliary fever," i.e., cholangitis with biliary obstruction due to stones, is an example. *Urinary tract infection,* with episodes of ureteral obstruction due to small stones or inspissated pus, can also cause recurrent fever.

Approximately 5 percent of patients with Hodgkin's disease at some time have so-called "Pel-Ebstein fever"—bouts of fever lasting 3 to 10 days, separated by afebrile and asymptomatic periods of 3 to 10 days. These cycles may be repeated regularly over a period of several months. In rare instances this periodicity of the fever has been sufficiently striking to suggest the correct diagnosis before lymphadenopathy or splenomegaly became evident. However, Pel-Ebstein fever may be caused by other diseases, not related to Hodgkin's disease.

EPIDEMIOLOGY OF FEVER The diagnosis of febrile illnesses must take into consideration the context of the epidemiologic setting. For example, an acute 6-day febrile illness in Southeast Asia is probably due to dengue or Chikungunya fevers (Chap. 213), malaria (Chap. 215), scrub typhus (Chap. 185), or leptospirosis (Chap. 166); in a college student in the United States it may represent infectious mononucleosis or some other viral infection; and in an octogenarian following prostatectomy it is probably an indication of urinary tract infection, wound infection, pulmonary infarction, or aspiration pneumonia. Likewise, travelers returning from short trips to foreign countries are much more likely to have febrile illnesses indigenous to their home than to the foreign country they have visited.

RARE VERSUS COMMON DISEASES Most of the time fever is a manifestation of a common disease, and fever associated with a pulmonary infiltrate is much more likely to be due to pneumococcal than to pneumocystis pneumonia. Failure to appreciate this cardinal principle has led to many prolonged and futile diagnostic workups.

FEBRILE ILLNESSES OF SHORT DURATION Acute febrile illnesses of less than 2 weeks' duration are a common occurrence in medical practice. In many instances they run their course, progressing to complete recovery, and a precise diagnosis is not made. In most instances, however, it is safe to assume that the illness is of infectious origin. Although short febrile illnesses may be noninfectious (e.g., allergic fevers due to drugs or serums, thromboembolic disease, hemolytic crises, or gout), they are decidedly in the minority.

Most undiagnosed acute febrile infectious diseases are probably viral and remain undiagnosed because diagnostic methods are unavailable or cumbersome. It is not practical to carry out tests needed to identify all the known viruses, and, furthermore, there must be a considerable number of still unidentified viruses pathogenic for man. In bacterial infections, on the other hand, laboratory diagnosis is simpler, and these infections are often rapidly controlled with chemotherapy.

The following characteristics, though not restricted solely to acute infections, are highly suggestive that infection is present:

1 Abrupt onset
2 High fever, i.e., 102 to 105°F, with or without chills
3 Respiratory symptoms—sore throat, coryza, cough
4 Severe malaise, with muscle or joint pain, photophobia, pain on movement of the eyes, headache
5 Nausea, vomiting, or diarrhea
6 Acute enlargement of lymph nodes or spleen
7 Meningeal signs, with or without spinal fluid pleocytosis
8 Leukocyte count above 12,000 or below 5,000 per mm^3
9 Dysuria, frequency, and flank pain

None of the symptoms or signs listed is encountered only in infection. Many of these features could be seen in acute leukemia or disseminated lupus erythematosus. Nevertheless, in a given instance of acute febrile illness with some or all of the manifestations listed, the probabilities strongly favor infection, and the patient may be given reasonable reassurance that he will probably recover in a week or two, regardless of a precise diagnosis.

It is desirable, of course, to establish an accurate diagnosis, and whatever steps are practicable in the circumstances to establish the cause should be taken. Cultures of the throat, blood, urine, or feces should be obtained before institution of antibacterial chemotherapy. Skin and/or serologic tests should be carried out when indicated.

PROLONGED FEBRILE ILLNESSES Some of the knottiest problems in the field of internal medicine are found in cases of prolonged fever in which the diagnosis remains obscure for weeks or even months. Eventually, however, the true nature of the illness usually reveals itself, since a disease which causes injury sufficient to evoke temperature elevations to 101°F or higher for several weeks does not often subside without leaving some clue as to its nature. The elucidation of problems of this sort calls for skillful application of all diagnostic methods—careful history, thorough physical examination, and the carefully considered use of laboratory examinations and roentgenograms.

Fever of unknown origin (FUO) In some patients fever becomes the dominant sign or symptom in a patient's illness, and when its cause escapes detection it is defined as fever of unknown origin (FUO). It is appropriate to use this term only in patients who have elevations in temperature (>101°F) for a prolonged period (at least 2 to 3 weeks) and in whom the diagnosis cannot be made during at least 1 week of intensive studies. These rigid criteria eliminate from this diagnostic category patients with common bacterial or viral infections, those in whom the diagnosis is obvious, and those whose fever is due to a sequential occurrence of etiologically unrelated diseases, e.g., one who is febrile following a myocardial infarction, who then develops thrombophlebitis that is associated with fever, and in whom this is followed by multiple pulmonary emboli, also a febrile disease. Much of the confusion in the literature concerning causes of FUO is due to failure to define the criteria employed in classifying patients who have had fever of unknown origin.

DISEASES CAUSING PROLONGED FEVERS

Table 12-1 lists some of the diseases which are responsible for prolonged fever. Some of these disorders must initially be considered to be FUO; in others the diagnosis comes to mind readily.

Infection

Infections occupy a less prominent position among causes of prolonged fever now than formerly because of the common practice of administering antibiotics to any patient in whom fever persists for more than a few days. Consequently, many infections are at present being eradicated by more or less "blind" therapy without accurate determination of their nature or location. Nevertheless, patients with infections comprise the greatest percentage of any group with FUO. Many times these infections enjoy protection from host defenses and take the form of localized abscesses, osteomyelitis, or bacterial endocarditis; or the organisms are located intracellularly.

TUBERCULOSIS (Chap. 161) Tuberculosis remains the most prominent cause of FUO. The diagnosis should be considered strongly in dark-skinned persons. Most of these patients do not have pulmonary tuberculosis but extrapulmonary or miliary disease involving the bones, lymph nodes, genital or urinary organs, peritoneum, or liver. Extrapulmonary or miliary tuberculosis may not be detectable by x-ray until late in the course of the disease. Skin test is an important diagnostic tool because, except in severely debilitated patients with overwhelming disease, a negative result, if the test has been properly executed, rules out the possibility of tuberculosis. A positive skin reaction, on the other hand, does not prove that tuberculosis is causing the illness but requires that the diagnosis be kept in mind until another cause for the fever is found.

PYOGENIC INFECTIONS **Upper abdominal infections** These commonly occur in the right upper quadrant and are related to the gallbladder or liver. Patients with such conditions tend to have mild jaundice, abnormality of liver function, high spiking fevers, and leukocytosis. Bacteremia, often due to enteric pathogens or *Salmonella,* is common. Liver scan is a most useful diagnostic tool, although exploratory laparotomy is often necessary for diagnosis and may achieve cure as well.

Lower abdominal infections Appendicitis with perforation and abscess formation is a remarkably common cause of prolonged fever, particularly in elderly patients. Persistent right lower quadrant physical signs along with x-ray abnormalities require surgical exploration.

Renal infections Ordinary pyelonephritis is rarely accompanied by prolonged fever; if pyrexia occurs in these patients, intrarenal or perinephric abscess should be considered. Ureteral obstruction by either a mass of leukocytes or renal epithelium, as in papillary necrosis, may be accompanied by prolonged fever.

Retroperitoneal infection Aneurysms that have become filled with organizing clot and debris may become infected. Enteric pathogens (including *Escherichia coli,* bacteroides, and *Salmonella*), have been isolated frequently from patients with such infections. Surgery is mandatory for both diagnosis and therapy.

BACTERIAL ENDOCARDITIS In the classical subacute form of the disease, a heart murmur is nearly always present; therefore, absence of murmur largely eliminates this disease from consideration. The correct diagnosis is likely to be missed in middle-aged or elderly patients, in whom a heart murmur may not be given much weight. For example, an elderly patient with subacute bacterial endocarditis may first come to the physician's attention following the occurrence of a cerebral embolus and may be regarded as having had a hemorrhage or thrombosis because of arteriosclerosis. The best clinical practice is to culture the blood of *every* patient who has fever and a heart murmur. Bacterial endocarditis without cardiac murmurs is seen most frequently in intravenous drug users who develop infection on the tricuspid valve; every such person with fever should be assumed to have endocarditis until proved otherwise. In addition, antibiotics mask subacute bacterial endocarditis (SBE) because they often render the blood culture negative until they have been excreted or metabolized. For this reason, patients suspected of having SBE who have received antimicrobials should have blood cultures taken for several days after administration of the drugs is discontinued.

BACTEREMIA Neisseria Although rare, chronic meningococcemia (Chap. 136) is a well-known cause of prolonged fever. The arthralgia and rash of this disease are sufficiently evanescent to be missed. When this syndrome appears in a young woman, gonococcemia is much more likely (Chap. 137).

Salmonella (Chap. 140) Typhoid fever is not often a cause of prolonged fever of obscure origin because cultures of feces and blood will be positive and specific antibodies

TABLE 12-1
Common disease entities in the United States causing prolonged fever

- *I* Infections
  - *A* Granulomatous infections
    - *1* Tuberculosis
    - *2* Deep-seated fungus infections
  - *B* Pyogenic infections
    - *1* Upper abdominal infections
      - *a* Cholecystitis (stone), empyema of gallbladder
      - *b* Cholangitis
      - *c* Liver abcess
      - *d* Subhepatic abscess
      - *e* Subphrenic abscess
      - *f* Lesser sac abscess
    - *2* Lower abdominal infections
      - *a* Diverticulitis
      - *b* Appendicitis
    - *3* Pelvic inflammatory disease
    - *4* Renal infections
      - *a* Pyelonephritis (rare)
      - *b* Intrarenal abscess
      - *c* Perinephric abscess
      - *d* Ureteral obstruction
    - *5* Retroperitoneal infections: Infected aortic aneurysm
  - *C* Bacterial endocarditis (acute and subacute)
  - *D* Bacteremias with overt primary focus
    - *1* Meningococcemia
    - *2* Gonococcemia
    - *3* Vibriosis
    - *4* Listeriosis
    - *5* Brucellosis
  - *E* Viral, rickettsial, and chlamydial infections
    - *1* Infectious mononucleosis
    - *2* Cytomegalovirus
    - *3* Coxsackie B virus diseases
    - *4* Q fever (including endocarditis)
    - *5* Psittacosis
  - *F* Parasitic diseases
    - *1* Amebiasis
    - *2* Malaria
    - *3* Trichinosis
  - *G* Spirochetal infections
    - *1* Leptospirosis
    - *2* Relapsing fever
- *II* Neoplasms
  - *A* Solid (localized)
    - *1* Kidney
    - *2* Lung
    - *3* Pancreas
    - *4* Liver
    - *5* Atrial myxoma
  - *B* Metastatic
    - *1* From gastrointestinal tract
    - *2* From lung, kidneys, bone
    - *3* Melanoma
  - *C* Tumors of the reticuloendothelial system
    - *1* Lymphoma, Hodgkin's disease
    - *2* Leukemias
    - *3* Reticulum cell sarcoma, multiple myeloma (rare)
  - *D* Unclassified: Diffuse sarcoma of bone
- *III* Connective tissue disease
  - *A* Rheumatic fever
  - *B* Systemic lupus erythematosus
  - *C* Rheumatoid arthritis (including Still's disease)
  - *D* Temporal arteritis (polymyalgia rheumatica)
  - *E* Hypersensitivity vasculitis
- *IV* Miscellaneous
  - *A* Drug fever
  - *B* Multiple pulmonary emboli
  - *C* Sarcoidosis
  - *D* Thyroiditis
  - *E* Hemolytic states
  - *F* Cryptic trauma with bleeding into enclosed space
  - *G* Regional enteritis and Whipple's disease
  - *H* Granulomatous hepatitis
- *V* Metabolic and inherited diseases
  - *A* Familial Mediterranean fever
  - *B* Hypertriglyceridemia
  - *C* Fabry's disease
- *VI* Pseudogenic fevers
  - *A* Habitual hyperthermia
  - *B* Factitious fever
- *VII* Periodic fevers
  - *A* Cyclic neutropenia
- *VIII* Undiagnosed

will be found in the serum. Other *Salmonella* organisms may, however, cause prolonged febrile illness and may present greater diagnostic difficulties. Repeated culture of the blood or bone marrow may yield the cause of this organism. Eventually, the infection may localize in a joint, pleural cavity, or another metastatic focus. Serologic confirmation of a salmonella infection is sometimes helpful.

BRUCELLOSIS (Chap. 144) This infection should be considered primarily in farmers, veterinarians, or slaughterhouse workers. Arthralgia and myalgia are common, but arthritis is rare. These patients tend to have normal or depressed leukocyte counts, and their sedimentation rate is often normal. In active febrile disease the blood and bone marrow cultures are frequently positive and specific agglutinins are nearly always present in the serum.

VIRAL, RICKETTSIAL, AND CHLAMYDIAL INFECTIONS These are rarely the cause of prolonged fevers, but occasionally patients with Epstein-Barr or cytomegalovirus infections may have febrile illnesses, which are often characterized by spontaneous remissions and exacerbations. Psittacosis may look much like typhoid fever, and Q-fever endocarditis has been a particularly puzzling illness.

PARASITIC DISEASES Amebiasis presents as an FUO, primarily in the form of liver abscess. The diagnosis of malaria demands a history of recent exposure.

Neoplasms

CARCINOMAS AND SARCOMAS Certain malignant processes are especially likely to cause fever. Notable are sarcomas involving bone or lymphoid tissue, hypernephroma, carcinoma of the pancreas or stomach, and primary or metastatic cancer of the liver. Occasionally, the clinical picture is strongly suggestive of pyogenic infection, with hectic fever, chills, sweats, and marked leukocytosis; and patients have been subjected to laparotomy with preoperative diagnoses such as empyema of the gallbladder, localized peritonitis, or liver abscess. An elevated alkaline phosphatase level and abnormal retention of Bromsulphalein (BSP) accompanied by filling defects on a liver scan are important clues to intrahepatic malignancy or other infiltrative hepatic disease.

HODGKIN'S DISEASE AND LYMPHOMAS Fever may be the principal symptom and only objective finding early in the course of Hodgkin's disease, especially when the principal involvement is in the abdominal viscera or retroperitoneal regions. Pel-Ebstein fever is seen in a minority of cases of Hodgkin's disease. The diagnosis of this disorder is usually made by biopsy or occasionally at staging laparotomy.

LEUKEMIAS It is not uncommon for acute leukemia to be mistaken for acute infection at the onset. The acute leukemias are nearly always accompanied by fever, sometimes as high as 105°F (40.6°C). The correct diagnosis is suggested by rapid development of anemia and characteristic changes in peripheral blood and bone marrow. Chronic lymphatic or granulocytic leukemia may be characterized by fever, but such fever is usually due to concomitant infection. Because of the typical changes in circulating leukocytes, fever does not often cause a diagnostic problem. Before it is assumed that fever in a patient with leukemia is due to the blood dyscrasia, infection must be ruled out by appropriate tests and cultures, and sometimes attempts to treat the "most likely" pathogen must be made.

ATRIAL MYXOMA Patients with changing heart murmurs, peripheral embolic phenomena, and joint pains are usually suspected of having bacterial endocarditis, rheumatic fever, or occasionally some other connective tissue disease such as lupus erythematosus. In the face of persistence of these symptoms and signs without a positive diagnosis, echocardiography and angiography should be performed with the possibility that an atrial myxoma may be responsible.

Connective tissue disease

RHEUMATIC FEVER Though rheumatic fever is generally easy to detect in children, the diagnosis in adults may be difficult. Attention to unexplained heart murmurs, arrhythmias, pleural and pericardial rubs, arthralgias, and skin rashes should call the diagnosis to mind. These findings, along with an elevated antistreptolysin titer, C-reactive protein, and other acute phase reactants, contribute to the diagnosis. A prompt response to large doses of aspirin is characteristic of rheumatic fever and provides another diagnostic clue.

SYSTEMIC LUPUS ERYTHEMATOSUS Fever is a common accompaniment of this disease. Of course, in the presence of arthritis, pleuritis, pericarditis, the classical malar rash, and renal failure, the diagnosis is easy. However, often these findings are absent and fever is the major manifestation. Biopsy of many organs, including the kidney, is generally not helpful; the diagnosis must be made by finding LE cells in the blood or bone marrow or by detecting a high titer of antinuclear antibody.

RHEUMATOID ARTHRITIS In its classic form, this disease is not difficult to recognize, but in certain patients who initially have FUO arthritis is absent early in the course of the illness; these patients have primarily fever, hepatosplenomegaly, lymphadenopathy, anemia, and leukocytosis. Joint changes do not appear until late in the disease. This disease often occurs in young adults, and may be considered the adult counterpart of juvenile rheumatoid disease. The diagnosis is made usually only after prolonged observation, in part because serologic tests for rheumatoid disease are characteristically negative.

TEMPORAL ARTERITIS (POLYMYALGIA RHEUMATICA) This is a disease of elderly persons who complain of fever, headache, and pain in the muscles and joints. Overt arthritis is unusual. The sedimentation rate tends to be very rapid, and there may be anemia, leukocytosis, or eosinophilia. Occasionally, the temporal or occipital arteries are inflamed and tender; when this is the case, the diagnosis is easily made by temporal artery biopsy. There may be accompanying visual defects or blindness because of involvement of the retinal artery. This disease responds extremely well to steroids, which may be used as a therapeutic trial.

Miscellaneous causes of fever

SARCOIDOSIS Ordinarily fever is not characteristic of sarcoidosis, but it is prominent in a minority of cases, especially those characterized by arthralgia, hilar lymphadenopathy, and cutaneous lesions resembling erythema nodosum, or in those with extensive hepatic lesions. Diagnosis is suggested by lymphoid enlargement, ocular lesions, and hyperglobulinemia and is clinched by biopsy of skin, lymph nodes, muscle, and liver.

REGIONAL ENTERITIS Inflammatory lesions of the large and small intestine rarely present as FUO, but an occasional patient who has only fever, abdominal pain, and subtle changes in bowel habits will be found to have regional enteritis. Likewise, Whipple's disease may make itself known by fever, without arthritis or malabsorption.

DRUG FEVER This is an important cause of cryptic fever; a careful history of drug intake should be taken in every patient with unexplained fever. Fever due to allergy to one of the antibiotics may become superimposed on the fever of the infection for which the drug was given, resulting in a very confused picture. Often fever is due to common drugs, including sulfonamides, arsenicals, iodides, thiouracils, barbiturates, and laxatives, especially those containing phenolphthalein. Any questions of drug fever can be resolved rapidly by discontinuing all medications. The diagnosis can be further substantiated by giving a test dose of the drug after fever has subsided, but this may result in a very unpleasant or even dangerous reaction.

MULTIPLE PULMONARY EMBOLI Symptomless thrombosis of deep calf or pelvic veins may cause prolonged febrile illness as a result of repeated small pulmonary emboli. These emboli may not be manifested by pleuritic pain or hemoptysis, but cough, dyspnea, or vague thoracic discomfort is likely to be present. Careful examination of the legs and repeated examination of the lungs should reveal the diagnosis. Sometimes these patients come to the physician's attention with a nephrotic syndrome due to renal vein thrombosis. Pelvic thrombophlebitis with or without pulmonary emboli is an important cause of FUO in postpartum patients.

HEMOLYTIC EPISODES Most hemolytic diseases are characterized by bouts of fever, and acute hemolytic crises may give rise to shaking chills and marked elevations of temperature. The difficulty sometimes encountered in differentiating sickle-cell disease from acute rheumatic fever is well known. The presence of these hemolytic disorders is suggested by the more rapid development of anemia than occurs in other febrile illnesses and by the usual accompaniment of reticulocytosis and jaundice. Fever is not characteristic of severe anemia due to external blood loss or of the anemia of uremia.

CRYPTIC TRAUMA Perisplenic and perivesical hematomas, with or without superimposed infection, are among the sites in which accumulated old blood and pus have resulted in prolonged fever.

GRANULOMATOUS HEPATITIS This disease of unknown etiology is not an uncommon cause of FUO. It is probably a manifestation of hypersensitivity. Liver biopsy shows only nonspecific granulomas. The fever generally subsides spontaneously over a period of weeks or months. Sometimes defervescence can be achieved with steroids, but because the diagnosis of tuberculosis can never be ruled out completely, patients in whom steroid therapy is given should also be given antituberculous medication.

HABITUAL HYPERTHERMIA Not infrequently, a patient while not appearing acutely ill has been subject to elevation of body temperature above the "normal" range level, i.e., his temperature has been in the range of 99.0 to 100.5°F (37.2 to 38°C). Prolonged low-grade fever may be a manifestation of serious illness, or it may be a matter of no real consequence. Possibly there are some persons whose "normal" temperatures are in this range. However, there is no certain way of identifying such individuals. The possibilities to be considered in such cases vary considerably according to the age groups concerned. A special problem termed *habitual hyperthermia* is encountered in young females. The patient may have temperatures ranging from 99.0 to 100.5°F regularly or intermittently for years and also usually has a variety of complaints characteristic of psychoneurosis, such as fatigability, insomnia, bowel distress, vague aches, and headache. Prolonged careful study and observation fail to reveal evidence of organic disease. Unfortunately, many of these people go from doctor to doctor and are subjected to a variety of unpleasant, expensive, and even harmful tests, treatments, and operations. The diagnosis of this syndrome can be made with reasonable certainty after a suitable period of observation and study, and if the patient can be convinced of its validity, a real service will have been rendered.

In a patient past middle age, even low-grade fever should always be regarded as a probable indication of organic disease. The possibilities to be considered in this age group are the same as those discussed earlier under Prolonged Febrile Illness.

FACTITIOUS FEVER Rarely, a patient will produce purposeful elevations in temperature. Many methods have been employed to cause the thermometer to register higher than the true temperature. If malingering is suspected, all that is necessary to prove it is to repeat the temperature determination immediately after a high reading has been obtained, with someone remaining at the bedside while the thermometer is in place. Other clues to false elevations in the temperature are a dissociation between pulse and temperature, absence of the normal diurnal variation in temperature, and excessively high fevers [greater than 106°F (41.1°C) in adults] in the absence of chills, sweats, or tachycardia. Some of these malingerers have severe character disorders and are notoriously refractory to psychotherapy, while others, mostly young girls, use this device to ask for psychiatric help, and do well with psychotherapy.

Familial Mediterranean fever (See Chap. 229)

Cyclic neutropenia (See Chap. 63)

DIAGNOSTIC PROCEDURES IN FEVER

With so large a number of possibilities, it is obvious that no single plan can be outlined for the systematic study of every problem in unexplained fever. In any given patient, the history, physical examination, and, most importantly, the epidemiologic setting must determine the diagnostic approach. If the features suggest infectious disease, the main dependence will be upon bacteriologic and immunologic methods, whereas when a person in the "cancer age group" has an obscure febrile disorder the best chance of early diagnosis may lie in x-ray studies and biopsy.

HISTORY Careful elicitation of the patient's past history and the chronologic development of his symptoms may provide important leads. Places of recent residence, contact with domestic or wild animals and birds, preceding acute infectious diseases such as diarrheal illness or boils, or contact with persons with tuberculosis may provide clues to infection. Localizing symptoms may provide a lead to an organ system affected by neoplasm or infection.

PHYSICAL EXAMINATION Careful search is made for skin lesions and for petechial hemorrhages in the ocular fundi, conjunctivas, nail beds, and skin. The lymph nodes are carefully palpated, with special attention to the supraclavicular, axillary, and epitrochlear areas. The finding of a heart murmur may be important. Detection of an abdominal mass may be the first lead to the diagnosis of neoplastic disease. Palpable enlargement of the spleen suggests infection, leukemia, or lymphoma and points away from a diagnosis of solid tumors. Enlargement of the liver and spleen suggests lymphoma, leukemia, chronic infection, or cirrhosis. A large liver without palpable spleen points to liver abscess or metastatic cancer. The rectum and the female pelvic organs may reveal masses or abscesses; the testicles may reveal teratoma or tuberculosis.

LABORATORY TESTS Useful examinations include:

1 Cultures of blood, bone marrow (*Brucella* or *Salmonella*), or other body fluids.
2 Serum enzymes, particularly *alkaline phosphatase* and enzymes that measure hepatocellular function, and serum and urinary amylase.
3 Blood smears for abnormal morphology, parasites, LE cells.
4 Bone marrow examinations for tumor cells, granulomas, LE cells, and abnormal red or white cells. Bone marrow biopsy is superior to aspiration for detection of granulomas and tumor cells.
5 Immunologic tests, i.e., ASLO titers and other acute-phase reactants, antinuclear antibodies, latex fixation tests, and a variety of febrile agglutinins.

ROENTGENOGRAMS The following should be considered:

1 Chest films, which need to be repeated at intervals.
2 Bone x-rays are useful for detecting foci of osteomyelitis or primary or metastatic bone tumors.
3 Intravenous urograms are helpful in finding tumors of the kidney or perinephric or intrarenal abscesses. However, if a renal tumor is suspect on clinical grounds a negative IVP does not rule out the diagnosis, and an aortogram should be performed.
4 Abdominal aortography is useful for diagnosing tumors of the kidney, retroperitoneal mass lesions, and, if selective arterial catheterization is performed, tumors of the liver, pancreas, and gut.
5 Intravenous cholangiograms may be helpful in delineating right upper quadrant pathologic change if the patient is not jaundiced.
6 Visualization of the gallbladder, common bile duct, hepatic ducts, and pancreas may be best accomplished by instilling contrast medium through a flexible endoscope following cannulation of the ampulla of Vater [endoscopic, retrograde choledochopancreatography (ERCP)].
7 Cardiac angiograms and echocardiograms should reveal atrial myxoma.
8 Lymphangiograms are helpful in the diagnosis of abdominal or retroperitoneal lymphomas but may be misleading.
9 Upper gastrointestinal x-rays are rarely useful; films of the small intestine may provide clues to Whipple's disease or regional enteritis, and a barium enema may show diverticulitis or tumor.

RADIOACTIVE SCANS *The liver scan is the single most useful test in the diagnosis of disease in the right upper quadrant.* Lung scans may reveal pulmonary emboli, and simultaneous liver and lung scans are useful in delineating subphrenic abscess. Bone scans may detect osseous metastases more readily than x-rays. Gallium scan may be useful in identifying a cryptic focus of infection or infiltration, but is rarely the only means for doing so.

BIOPSIES Biopsy often is the best means of definitive diagnosis.

1 Bone marrow biopsy may be helpful not only in clarifying the histologic nature of the marrow but also for occasional demonstration of other disease processes such as metastatic carcinoma or granulomas, and for culture.
2 Needle biopsy of the liver is a very useful procedure and can be done with reasonable safety. It may be helpful not only in primary or metastatic disease of the liver, but also because the liver may reveal existence of other diseases such as histoplasmosis, schistosomiasis, brucellosis, tuberculosis, sarcoidosis, or lymphoma.
3 Lymph node biopsy is helpful in diagnosis of many diseases, including the lymphomas, metastatic cancer, tu-

berculosis, and mycotic infections. However, inguinal nodes are notoriously unsatisfactory for biopsy and are too frequently chosen because of their easy accessibility. Axillary, cervical, and supraclavicular nodes are much more likely to yield helpful information, and the node excised need not necessarily be large.

4 Skin and muscle biopsy may be of assistance in the recognition of dermatomyositis, periarteritis nodosa, sarcoidosis, and trichinosis.
5 Lung biopsy may be performed with a needle under direct fluoroscopy. It is of value primarily in solitary mass lesions; diffuse pulmonary disease is rarely diagnosed by needle biopsy; instead, open lung biopsy should be performed. Transbronchial biopsy through a fiberoptic bronchoscope may improve on these results.
6 Renal biopsy is rarely helpful, even in connective tissue disease.
7 Pleural and pericardial biopsy with the hook needle technique should be attempted in the presence of effusion.
8 Biopsy of the temporal artery (see above).
9 Biopsy of other accessible masses should not be neglected.

EXPLORATORY LAPAROTOMY Exploratory laparotomy has been advocated as the most definitive diagnostic maneuver in connection with FUO, but is valuable only when other investigations including history, physical examination, x-rays, and laboratory data point to the abdomen as a likely source of disease. Blind exploration of the abdomen simply because the diagnosis is obscure is to be deprecated. Moreover, often the tissue that is obtained at laparotomy could just as easily have been sampled by external biopsy techniques.

THERAPEUTIC TRIALS It is common practice to give a trial of antibiotic therapy to patients with unidentified febrile disorders. Occasionally, this kind of marksmanship is effective, but in general, "blind" therapy does more harm than good. Undesirable features include drug toxicity, superinfection due to resistant pathogenic bacteria, and interference with accurate diagnosis by cultural methods. Furthermore, a coincidental fall in temperature not due to therapy is likely to be interpreted as response to treatment, with the conclusion that an infectious disease is present. If therapeutic trials are instituted, they should be as specific as possible. Examples are *isoniazid* or *ethambutol* for tuberculosis; *aspirin* for rheumatic fever; *Flagyl* for hepatic amebiasis; *penicillin* and *streptomycin* for enterococcal endocarditis; and *chloramphenicol* for *Salmonella* bacteremia. Shotgun broad-spectrum therapy is contraindicated, because it is unlikely to yield useful information and is more likely to be toxic. Similarly, cortisone or ACTH is nonspecific. These drugs do have an antipyretic effect and produce euphoria in many persons, but the apparent improvement induced by them tells little about the nature of the underlying disease. Temporal arteritis is an exception to this statement.

PROGNOSIS IN FUO The intelligent application of appropriate diagnostic maneuvers should provide the answer in approximately 90 to 95 percent of patients with prolonged obscure febrile illness. Fortunately, the remainder recover spontaneously. Because many of the procedures involved in the diagnosis of FUO are painful, time-consuming, and expensive, it is essential that they be chosen with thoughtfulness and care.

REFERENCES

Atkins E: Fever, in *Signs and Symptoms,* 5th ed., eds McBryde and Blacklow, Philadelphia: Lippincott, 1972

Baker RR, Tumulty PA et al: The value of exploratory laparotomy in fever of undetermined etiology. Johns Hopkins Med J 125:159, 1969

Bodel P: Studies on the mechanism of endogenous pyrogen production: III. Human blood monocytes. J Exp Med 140:954, 1974

Bujak JS et al: Juvenile rheumatoid arthritis presenting in the adult as fever of unknown origin. Medicine 52:431, 1973

Dinarello CA et al: Demonstration and characterization of two distinct human leukocytic pyrogens. J Med 139:1369, 1974

Guerty D et al: Periodic hematopoiesis in human cyclic neutropenia. J Clin Invest 52:3220, 1973

Petersdorf RG, Beeson PB: Fever of unexplained origin: Report of 100 cases. Medicine 40:1, 1961

——, Bennett IL, Jr: Factitious fever. Ann Intern Med 46:1039, 1957

——, Wallace JF: Fever of unknown origin, in *Diagnostic Approaches to Presenting Syndromes,* ed JA Barondess, Baltimore: Williams & Wilkins, 1971, pp. 301–332

Simon HB, Wolff SM: Granulomatous hepatitis and prolonged fever of unknown origin: A study of 13 patients. Medicine 52:1, 1973

Wolff SM et al: Unusual etiologies of fever and their evaluation. Annu Rev Med 26:277, 1975

section 3 | Alterations of nervous function

13
GENERAL CONSIDERATIONS

RAYMOND D. ADAMS

The symptoms and signs of nervous disease are probably the most frequent and complex in all of medicine. To present a lucid exposition of all the many diverse neurological manifestations is difficult in part because the more complex phenomena may be viewed from either a neurologic or psychologic standpoint. The neurologic physician is inclined to assume that all are manifestations of diseases of the nervous system. The psychiatrically minded physician thinks of many of them in terms of abnormal psychologic reactions. Naturally, our bias is more toward the neurologic for it draws on all the accepted principles of medicine and biologic science. But each extreme can be criticized. The aim, therefore, throughout this section is to avoid entanglement in such theoretical problems, to describe as accurately as possible all the more common expressions of disordered nervous function, and to offer the most generally accepted explanations in terms of anatomy, physiology, biochemistry, and psychology. However, in discussing some of the more abstruse, complex cerebral derangements, a particular effort will be made to present both the neurologic and psychologic conceptions, for the latter have received much attention in recent years.

To provide an initial orientation toward the broad field of neuropsychiatry, it is helpful to think of the subject matter as divisible into two main categories: diseases of the nervous system and disorders based on abnormal psychologic reactions. By *disease* we mean any condition which produces a visible lesion in the nervous system or in which there is actual or presumptive evidence of such. By *abnormal psychological reaction* we mean a disorder in psychic life and behavior occasioned by abnormal life experiences and maladjustments in social relations. A brain tumor, delirium tremens, and a confusional psychosis would be considered examples of disease; unusually protracted grief, unexplained anxiety, and a character disorder would fall in the category of psychologic abnormality due to the formation of unusual personality traits after repeated psychic traumas and environmental stresses. All diseases of the neuromuscular apparatus, spinal cord, brainstem, and cerebellum and many of those of the cerebrum, fall within the province of neurology, whereas other of the cerebral diseases (especially if they disturb intellect, emotions, and behavior) are of concern to neurology and psychiatry, and all abnormal psychologic reactions are within the province of psychiatry.

Many nervous disorders are not so easily classified. A psychopathic personality, an anxiety neurosis, or a depressive reaction could be a manifestation of either a disease of the brain or an abnormal psychologic reaction. Schizophrenia and manic-depressive psychosis would presently be classified as genetically determined diseases by neurologists and many psychiatrists even though a lesion has never been demonstrated by the conventional techniques of pathology. Other psychiatrists believe psychogenetic factors to be important.

Our objective in the early part of this book is to single out all the common symptoms and signs of diseases of the nervous system as well as the manifestations of certain abnormal psychologic states. In the section on diseases of organ systems, we subdivide the material, presenting in one section all the common diseases of the nervous system, and in another the major psychiatric disorders.

There are two areas of neuropsychiatry which in a way are even more controversial—the psychosomatic diseases and the sociopathic states. Included under psychosomatic disorders are such conditions as Raynaud's disease, peptic ulcer, ulcerative colitis, bronchial asthma, dysmenorrhea, hypertension, hyperthyroidism, neurodermatitis, rheumatoid arthritis, migraine, and paroxysmal tachycardia. These diseases have been set apart on the basis of three lines of evidence: (1) A large series of observations which have revealed that the malfunctioning organ is excited and possibly deranged by strong emotion and restored to relative normality by tranquility and feelings of security; (2) the discovery in the biographies of such patients of an inordinately high incidence of resentment, hostility, suppressed emotionality, etc.; (3) a demonstrable relationship between onset and exacerbation of the disease and disturbing and frustrating incidents in the patient's life. These psychosomatic diseases differ from the psychoneuroses in that they exhibit different symptoms, are of longer duration, have a known pathologic basis and often a known cause (e.g., allergy in asthma, atopic dermatitis, and hay fever). Finally, the incidence of frank neuroses in this group of diseases is no greater than in the population at large, and neurotics are not more liable to them than normal individuals. For many reasons, not the least of which is that a psychogenic basis has never been proved in any of these diseases, we have chosen to present the relevant facts in the organ systems involved. They are not discussed further in the sections on neurology and psychiatry.

The sociopathies involve so many sociologic, educational, economic, and political factors that they fall almost beyond the orbit of medicine. While a medical position is often of value, particularly if there are questions of nervous disease or major psychiatric disorder, there is no clear evidence that medical opinion contributes significantly to the understanding and management of these problems. For these and other reasons such sociopathic states as amoral conduct, aggression, criminality, and sexual deviation are also eliminated from this section of the book.

14
NERVOUSNESS, ANXIETY, AND DEPRESSION

RAYMOND D. ADAMS

The majority of patients who enter a physician's office or hospital will admit to being nervous, anxious, or depressed. The stress of contemporary society or the prospect of real or imaginary illness is thought to induce these reactions. If they stand in clear relationship to a stressful event or situation, such as worry over economic reverses or grief over the death of a loved one, such states can be accepted as normal. Only when excessively intense and uncontrollable or when accompanied by derangements of visceral function do they become the basis for medical consultation.

Such problems become more abstruse when similar symptoms occur in persons who are not being subjected to immediately stressful or unhappy experiences, and knowledge of such threatening situations, if it exists at all, lies buried in the subconscious mind of the patient. One may assume that it either has been suppressed from consciousness or is part of an elaborate subjective interpretation of which the patient is unaware. The relationship between social stimulus and prevailing anxiety or nervousness can then be discovered only by gentle probings by the psychologically sophisticated physician. But once the connection is established and the problem dealt with realistically, the symptoms become understandable and disappear. One recognizes here all the elements of a *psychoneurotic reaction.* The line of separation between the latter and normal emotional reactions is admittedly ambiguous.

There is still another category of nervousness, anxiety, and depression wherein the emotional states are intense and prolonged but without obvious explanation. Such states may overwhelm the individual and derange him in all his activities. Delving into his unconscious mind or studying his lifelong reaction pattern fails to reveal a plausible psychogenesis. One recognizes here all the elements of a more complete, pervasive *psychotic reaction.* In many such instances a genetic factor appears to operate, and the features of the illness are so stereotyped as to indicate a disease of the parts of the nervous system which control the affective, emotional life. Yet consistent biochemical change in the blood or brain tissue has not been found, and no lesion has been discerned. Therefore treatment must proceed along nonpsychologic lines.

The problem confronting every physician is to recognize all these nuances of reaction and disease which obviously shade into one another, and to determine to what extent they dominate the medical condition of the patient. Some type of therapeutic maneuver must then be initiated, varying from simple reassurance and realistic management of existing personal difficulties, to suppression of symptoms by drugs. Often referral to a psychiatrist is necessary for more expert management, including electrotherapy.

In this chapter the cardinal features of these states are described, together with currently accepted views of their origins. The major diseases of which they may be a part are discussed in Chaps. 344 and 345.

NERVOUSNESS By this vague term the lay person usually refers to a state of restlessness, tension, uneasy apprehension, irritability, or hyperexcitability. But it may connote other states, such as thoughts of suicide, fear of killing one's child or spouse, a distressing hallucination, a paranoid idea, or a frankly hysterical outburst. Careful inquiry as to what the patient means when he complains of nervousness is always a necessary first step.

In its most common signification, a period of nervousness may represent no more than a psychic and behavioral state in which an organism is maximally challenged by difficult personal problems, and there are periods in normal life when this is more likely to happen. For example, adolescence rarely passes without its period of turmoil as the person attempts to emancipate himself from parental dominance or to adjust to scholastic demands or to the opposite sex. The menses are regularly accompanied by increased tension and moodiness, and, of course, the menopause is another critical period. Some persons, because of early patterning or character formation, claim to have been nervous in all their social relationships throughout life; one should then suspect a psychoneurosis or depressive character formation even though performance within the family unit, at school, and at work were adequate. Others complain of a recent development of nervousness, and one must consider such conditions as an upheaval in personal affairs, the first attack or exacerbation of a psychoneurosis, an endogenous depression, an endocrine disease (hyperthyroidism, adrenal corticism, or corticosteroid therapy), or withdrawal from a sedative drug (alcohol, barbiturate). Some patients complain of a nervousness that attends the onset of a medical or neurologic disease; it would then appear to be secondary, occasioned by fear of disability, dependency, or death.

Nervousness, even in its simplest form, is reflected in many important activities of the human organism. There are often a mild somberness of mood, an increased tendency to tears and anger (irritability). Fatigue that bears no proper relationship to activity and rest is frequent, and sleep is often disturbed, as are eating and drinking habits. Headaches may increase in number and intensity. There is a tendency to sweat, tremble, be aware of heart action, feel a bit "queer in the head" or giddy, have an upset stomach, and urinate more often, though these recognized autonomic accompaniments of anxiety are seldom as conspicuous as in anxiety neurosis. Thus, it would appear that nervousness and anxiety constitute a graded series of reactions, the latter in many instances being only a more intense and protracted form of nervousness (see Chap. 344).

THE ANXIETY STATE Anxiety is "the fundamental phenomenon and central problem of the neurosis . . . a nodal point, linking up all kinds of most important questions, a riddle of which the solution must cast a flood of light upon our whole mental life" (Freud). From the viewpoint of the social historian, anxiety is said to be "the most prominent mental characteristic of Occidental civilization" (Willoughby). These comments should inform the reader of the broad implications of this reaction.

The more strictly medical meaning of the term *anxiety,* and the one used in this chapter, is a state characterized by a subjective feeling of fear and uneasy anticipation (apprehension), usually with a definite topical content and associated with the physiologic accompaniments of strong emotion, i.e., breathlessness, choking sensation, palpitation, restlessness, increased muscular tension, tightness in the chest, giddiness, trembling, sweating, and flushing. By *topical content* is meant the idea, person, or object about which the person is anxious. The several vasomotor and visceral alterations that underlie the symptoms are mediated through the autonomic nervous system, particularly the sympathetic part of it, and involve also the thyroid and adrenal glands.

Forms of anxiety Anxiety is manifested in acute episodes, each lasting a few minutes, or as a protracted state that may last for weeks, months, or years. In the acute *attacks,* or *panics* as they are called, the patient is plunged into an inexplicable mental state in which he fears he will die, lose his reason or self-control, become insane, or commit some horrible crime. He is breathless, has a racing heart, chokes, sweats, trembles, and feels gastric distress and anorexia. As a persistent protracted state he experiences fluctuating degrees of nervousness, restlessness, irritability, fatigue, insomnia, intolerance of physical exertion, and pressure or tension headaches. Discrete anxiety attacks and chronic states of anxiety merge into one another.

Episodic anxiety without disorder of mood (i.e., depression) is usually classified as *anxiety neurosis.* The chronic form with prominent exercise intolerance is called *neurocirculatory asthenia.* Anxiety may, however, be combined with other somatic symptoms in hysteria and may be the restraining factor in *phobic neurosis.* Persistent anxiety with insomnia, lassitude, and fatigue, regardless of mood, should always raise suspicion of a *depressive psychosis,* especially if it begins late in life. Panic attacks may also occur at the beginning of a schizophrenic illness. Both anxiety and depression are prominent features of the syndrome of posttraumatic nervous instability (see Chaps. 335, 345, and 346).

Thus, the differential diagnosis of an anxiety state requires that the physician consider all the major syndromes in psychiatry. Often it is but one component of a far more serious condition, one which may result in suicide or some other antisocial act. Also, without the psychic counterparts of fear and apprehension, the visceral symptoms alone should arouse suspicion of thyrotoxicosis, epilepsy, corticosteroid overdosage, pheochromocytoma, hypoglycemia, and menopause.

Physiologic and psychologic basis The cause, mechanism, and biologic meaning of anxiety have been the subjects of much speculation, and completely satisfactory explanations are not possible. The psychologist regards anxiety as anticipatory behavior, i.e., a state of uneasiness about something which may happen in the future. William McDougall spoke of it as "an emotional state arising when a continuing strong desire seems likely to miss its goal." The primary emotion, somewhat muted perhaps, is that of fear, and its arousal under conditions not overtly threatening may be explained by conditioning to some recondite component of a formerly threatening stimulus.

The only well-systematized theory is that put forth by the school of psychoanalysis, which looks upon anxiety as a response to a situation that in some manner undermines the security of the individual. The topical content or cause of potential danger lies in the unconscious mind. The postulated danger is internal rather than external; a primitive drive has been aroused that is not compatible with current social practices, and it can be satisfied only at risk of harm to the person.

Physicians have searched for evidence of impairments of visceral function without success. The neurocirculatory asthenic is in poor physical condition, has an elevated blood lactate level after exercise, and will not tolerate the work or exercise needed to build up his stamina. And even in the resting state lactic acid levels in the blood may be elevated, and infusions containing lactic acid are said to make the symptoms worse. The urinary excretion of epinephrine has been found elevated in some patients; in others, there is an increased urinary excretion of norepinephrine. Aldosterone excretion is raised to two or three times the normal level during intense anxiety. Medical students experiencing fear and anxiety while preparing for an examination also excrete increased amounts of aldosterone. The interpretation of these data (whether primary or secondary) is not certain, but it is becoming increasingly evident that prolonged and diffuse anxiety is a pattern of behavior related to certain biochemical abnormalities of blood, and probably of the brain.

DEPRESSION There are few persons who do not experience periods of discouragement and despair, and these periods become manifestly more frequent in modern society where individual freedom is constrained and one's impulses must be inhibited. As with nervousness and anxiety, depression of mood that is appropriate to a given situation in life is a natural, healthy reaction and seldom is the basis of medical complaint. The patient tends to seek help only when he cannot control his grief or unhappiness. But there are numerous instances in which the patient is miserable, unhappy, and hopeless for reasons which are not apparent. Many of his symptoms are interpreted as ill health, being so similar to those of many disease states as to bring him first to the internist. Sometimes another disease is found (such as chronic hepatitis, brucellosis, postinfluenzal asthenia infections), in which a chronic fatigue is confused with depression; but often an endogenous depression is itself the essential problem. Since the risk of suicide is not inconsiderable if the illness is mistaken for another or overlooked as a complication, an error in diagnosis may be life-threatening.

Information about depression, like that about all psychiatric syndromes, is gained from three sources: the history obtained from the patient, the history obtained from the family or close friend, and the findings on examination.

From the patient and his family it is learned that he has

been "feeling unwell," "low in spirits," "blue," "glum," "unhappy," or "morbid." There has been a change in emotional reactions of which the patient may not be fully aware. Activities that were formerly pleasurable are no longer so. Often, however, change in mood is less conspicuous than reduction in psychic and physical energy. Fatigue is almost invariable; not uncommonly, it is worse in the morning after a night of restless sleep. The words "loss of pep," "weak," "tired," "no energy to work," "my job seems more trying and difficult" appear in the language of the patient. The outlook is pessimistic. The patient is preoccupied with uncontrollable worry over trivialities. With excessive worry the ability to think with accustomed efficiency is reduced; there is complaint that the mind does not function properly, of being forgetful and unable to concentrate. If the patient is naturally of suspicious nature, paranoid tendencies may assert themselves.

Particularly troublesome in medical diagnosis is the patient's tendency to become hypochondriacal about associated diseases. Indeed, most cases formerly diagnosed as hypochondriasis are now regarded as depression. Pain from whatever cause—a stiff joint, a toothache, fleeting abdominal pains, or other troubles such as constipation, frequency of urination, insomnia, pruritus, burning tongue, weight loss—may become an obsessive focus of complaint. The patient passes from doctor to doctor seeking relief from symptoms that would not trouble the average person, and no amount of reassurance relieves his state of mind. The nervousness and anxiety felt by many of these persons may be obscured by their preoccupation with visceral functions.

When examined, the patient's facial expression is often plaintive, troubled, pained, or anguished. His attitude and manner betray his prevailing mood of depression, discouragement, and despondency. In other words, the affective response, which is the outward expression of feeling, is consistent with the depressed mood. During the interview the patient's eyes may be tearful, or he may cry openly. In some there is a kind of immobility of the face that mimics parkinsonism, though others are restless and agitated (pacing, wringing their hands, etc). Occasionally the patient will smile, but the smile impresses one as more of a social gesture than an expression of feeling.

The stream of speech, from which the ideational content is determined, is slow. At times the patient is mute and speaks neither spontaneously nor in response to questions. Again there may be a long pause between questions and answers. The latter are brief and may be monosyllabic. There is a paucity of ideas. The retardation extends to all topics of conversation and affects movement of limbs as well. The most extreme forms of decreased motor activity, rarely seen in the medical clinic, border on stupor.

Content of speech is found to be abnormal if examined carefully. Conversation is replete with pessimistic thoughts, fears, expressions of unworthiness, inadequacy, inferiority, and sometimes guilt. In severe depressions bizarre ideas, delusions about the body ("blood drying up," "bowels are blocked with cement," "I am half dead") may be expressed.

Etiology and mechanism Three theories have emerged concerning the cause of the pathologic depressive state: (1) the endogenous form is hereditary; (2) a biochemical abnormality results in a periodic depletion in the brain of serotonin and norepinephrine; (3) a basic fault in character development exists. These theories, which are not mutually exclusive, are elaborated upon in Chap. 344.

It is the writer's belief that depression is one of the most commonly overlooked diagnoses in clinical medicine. Part of the trouble is with the word itself, which implies being unhappy about something. The persistent or recurrent endogenous depression or involutional depression should be suspected in all chronic states of ill health, hypochondriasis, disability that exceeds manifest signs of a medical disease, neurasthenia, and suicide attempts. Inasmuch as recovery is the rule, the suicide is a tragedy for which the medical profession must often share responsibility.

REFERENCE

FREEDMAN AM, KAPLAN HI: *Comprehensive Textbook of Psychiatry,* chaps. 17, 23, Baltimore: Williams & Wilkins, 1967

15 LASSITUDE AND ASTHENIA

RAYMOND D. ADAMS

The terms *weakness* and *fatigue* are used by patients to describe a variety of subjective complaints which vary in their import and prognostic significance. The different meanings can usually be fitted into the following classification:

1 Lassitude, fatigue, lack of energy, listlessness, and languor. (These terms, though not synonymous, shade into one another; all refer to a weariness and a loss of that sense of well-being typically found in persons healthy of body and mind.)

2 Weakness, loss of strength, paresis, paralysis. These may be persistent or episodic.
   - *a* Persistent weakness: This may be (1) restricted to certain muscles or groups of muscles (see Chap. 17) or (2) more or less generalized, i.e., involving the entire musculature (see Chaps. 17 and 347).
   - *b* Episodic, often recurrent: Attacks of weakness may occur in the periodic paralyses. [Many patients confuse "attacks of weakness" with a diminshed sense of alertness, lightheadedness, feeling of faintness. These usually turn out to be episodes of partial or threatening syncope, attacks of anxiety or vertigo, or seizures (see Chaps. 16, 19, and 24).]

LASSITUDE AND FATIGUE Of all the symptoms in this group these are among the most frequent and abstruse. More than half of all patients entering a general hospital register direct complaint of fatigability or admit to it when questioned. During the Second World War fatigue was so prominent as to be given a separate place in medical nosology, viz., "combat fatigue," which referred to all acute psychiatric illnesses that happened on the battlefield. The common clinical antecedents and accompaniments of fatigue, its significance, and its physiologic and pyschologic bases should, therefore, be matters of common medical knowledge.

Patients who complain of weariness and tiredness have a more or less characteristic way of describing their condition. They say that they "are all in," "have lost pep," "have no ambition" or "no interest," are "turned off" or "fed up." They manifest their condition by showing an indifference to the tasks at hand, by talking much about how hard they are working; they are inclined to sit around or lie down, occupying themselves with trivial tasks. On closer analysis one observes that they have a difficulty in initiating activity and also in sustaining it.

This condition is the familiar aftermath of prolonged labor or great physical exertion, and under such circumstances it is accepted as a normal, physiologic reaction. When, however, the same symptoms or similar ones appear in no relation to such antecedents, they are suspected as being the manifestations of disease.

The physician's task begins, then, with an attempt to determine whether the patient is merely suffering from the physical and mental effects of overwork without realizing it. Overworked, overwrought people are everywhere observable in our society. Their actions are both instructive and pathetic. They seem to be impelled by notions of duty and refuse to think of themselves. Or, as is often the case, some personal inadequacy seems to prevent them from deriving pleasure from any activity except their work, in which they indulge themselves as a kind of defense mechanism. Such persons show their fatigue by other symptoms, such as irritability, restlessness, and sleeplessness. Their symptoms and behavior are best understood by referring to psychologic studies of the effect of fatigue on the normal individual.

Effects of fatigue on the normal person According to several authoritative sources, fatigue has both explicit and implicit effects, grouped under: (1) a series of biochemical and physiologic changes in many organs of the body, (2) an overt disorder in behavior, a reduced output of work, known as *work decrement,* and (3) an expressed dissatisfaction and a subjective feeling of tiredness.

As to the biochemical and physiologic changes, continuous muscular work leads to depletion of muscle glycogen and an accumulation of lactic acid and other metabolites, which in themselves reduce the power of contraction and delay recovery. Extreme degrees of muscle work, in which activity exceeds provision of substrate, results in necrosis of fibers and rise in serum levels of creatine phosphokinase and aldolase even in normal persons. The muscles are slightly swollen and sore for several days. It is said that the injection of blood from a fatigued animal into a rested one will produce overt manifestations of fatigue in the latter. During repeated contractions of muscle, its action is observed to become tremulous, movements are less adept, and the coordination of agonist, antagonist, and synergic muscles is less perfect. The rate of breathing increases, the pulse quickens, the blood pressure rises and pulse pressure widens, and the white blood cell count and metabolic rate are increased. These alterations bear out the hypothesis that fatigue is in part a manifestation of altered metabolism.

The decreased capacity for work or productivity which is a direct consequence of fatigue has been investigated by

industrial psychologists. Their findings show clearly the importance of the motivational factor on work output, whether it be in manual or clerical tasks. Individual differences in energy potential appear to be important, as are differences in physique, intelligence, and temperament.

The subjective feelings of fatigue have been carefully recorded. Aside from feeling weary the tired person is unable to deal effectively with complex problems and tends to be unreasonable, often about trivialities. The number and quality of his associations in psychologic tests are reduced. The ability to deliberate and to reach judgments is impaired; decisions made late at night may appear unsound the next day. The worker after a long, hard day is unable to perform adequately his duties as head of a household; the example of the tired businessman who becomes the proverbial tyrant of the family circle is well known. A disinclination to try and the appearance of ideas of inferiority are other characteristics of the fatigued mind.

Instances of fatigue and lassitude resulting from overwork are not difficult to recognize. A description of the patient's daily routine and a talk with his associates and family will usually suffice. Moreover if he can be persuaded to live at a more reasonable pace and allow time for outside pleasurable activities, his symptoms will promptly subside. A common error in diagnosis, however, is the ascription of fatigue to overwork when actually it is a manifestation of a psychoneurosis or depression.

Fatigue as a manifestation of psychiatric disorder

The great majority of patients who enter a hospital because of unexplained chronic fatigue and lassitude have been found to have some type of psychiatric illness. Formerly this state was called *neurasthenia;* but since fatigue rarely exists as an isolated phenomenon, the current practice is to label such cases according to the total clinical picture. The usual associated symptoms are nervousness, irritability, anxiety, depression, insomnia, headaches, difficulty in concentrating, sexual disorders, and loss of bodily appetites. In one series in a general hospital 75 percent of persons admitted because of chronic fatigue and nervousness were diagnosed, finally, as having *anxiety neurosis* and *tension states.* Depression accounted for another 10 percent, and the remainder of the patients had a miscellany of medical and psychiatric illnesses.

Several features are common to the psychiatric group. The fatigue may be worse in the morning. There is an inclination to lie down and rest, but sleep does not come. The fatigue relates more to some activities than to others. Inquiry as to what was happening when the fatigue was first experienced may reveal an unpleasant event, a grief reaction, a surgical operation, or a medical illness. The feeling of fatigue interferes with mental as well as physical activities. As to the psychic aspects, it is difficult to concentrate during the solution of a problem, or in carrying on an involved conversation.

Depressing emotion, as was already remarked in the previous chapter, has its characteristic effect on impulse life and energy. Also, sleep is poor, with a tendency to early-morning waking, so that such persons are at their worst in the morning, both in spirit and in energy output. Their tendency is to improve as the day wears on, and they even feel fairly normal by evening. It is difficult to decide whether the fatigue is a primary manifestation of disease or is secondary to a lack of interest.

Many physicians question whether all chronically fatigued individuals deviate enough from normal to justify the diagnosis psychoneurosis or depression. Many people in society, because of circumstances beyond their control, have no purpose in life and much idle time. They are bored with the monotony of their routine. Such circumstances are conducive to fatigue, just as the opposite is also true—that a new enterprise that excites optimism and enthusiasm will dispel fatigue. Other individuals seem normal until some adversity is encountered, arousing worry or fear, and then it becomes apparent that their adjustment is unstable. Such reactions are understandable to anyone who has ever had stage fright or "buck fever" and who remembers the sense of physical weakness, the utter incapacity to act, the intellectual chaos that overwhelms the previously well-ordered mind, and the exhaustion which follows.

Psychologic theories The enervating effect of a strong emotion such as anxiety is well known, and it might be supposed that the simple prolongation of the emotional experience would provide a rational explanation for a chronic fatigue of anxiety. But even if true, however, this explanation does not account for the occurrence of emotion at a time when there is no reason for it.

The dynamic schools of psychiatry, particularly the psychoanalytic, have postulated that chronic fatigue, in the broadest sense, is like the anxiety from which it derives; it is a danger signal that something is wrong—that some attitude or activity has been too intense or too persistent. The fatigue is self-preservative, serving not merely as a protection against physical injury but also as a protection of the individual's self-esteem and his confidence in himself. As to mechanism, it is claimed that the fatigue is the result of exhaustion of the store of pyschic energy required to maintain repression of unacceptable ideas. Others, however, claim to have evidence that fatigue is not a negative symptom, a lack or depletion of energy, but an unconscious desire for inactivity. A reciprocal relationship is said to exist between fatigue and anxiety. Both are protective, but anxiety is the more imperative. It calls for the individual to take some positive action to extricate himself from a predicament, whereas fatigue calls for inactivity. Both operate blindly, however, for the person cannot perceive what it is that must be done or stopped. All this happens at the unconscious level.

Some persons are low in impulse and energy throughout life, being more so at times of stress; some psychiatrists believe that they have a constitutional inadequacy. Kahn classifies such individuals as "psychopaths weak in impulse," and points out in his description their inability throughout life to play games vigorously, to compete successfully, to work hard without exhaustion, to withstand or recover quickly from illness, or to assume a dominant role in a social group.

It is obvious that these several psychologic hypotheses could not all be correct, nor could they be applicable to all situations in which chronic fatigue is the complaint. Undoubtedly there are persons who are underactive and weak because of genetic factors or early life experiences. It is equally clear that psychic and physical energy are closely linked to mood. The more chronic varieties of acquired fatigue, without a basis in medical disease, have in nearly all instances a psychologic basis.

Lassitude and fatigue in chronic infection and in endocrine and other medical diseases Infection is another cause of chronic fatigue, though a much less frequent one. Everyone has at some time or other sensed the abrupt onset of extreme exhaustion, the tired ache in the muscles, an inexplicable listlessness, only to discover later that he is "coming down with the flu." In chronic infections such as hepatitis, tuberculosis, brucellosis, infectious mononucleosis, the infection may not be at once evident. But it should always be suspected when the fatigue is out of proportion to other symptoms such as mood change, nervousness, and anxiety. Often this syndrome will begin with an obvious infection but will persist for several weeks after it should have terminated, and it may then be difficult to decide whether there is still a lingering infection or the infection has been complicated by psychiatric illness during convalescence. In many diseases such as infectious hepatitis and brucellosis, infectious mononucleosis, and a host of other systemic viral infections, long-standing neurotic symptoms appear to have been uncovered. Nevertheless it is difficult to dismiss an obscure secondary metabolic disorder consequent to the infection. (See Chap. 345.)

Metabolic and endocrine diseases (see Chaps. 90 and 92) of various types may cause inordinate degrees of lassitude and fatigue. Sometimes there is in addition a true muscular weakness (see Chaps. 16 and 360). In Addison's disease and Simmonds' disease fatigue may dominate the clinical picture. Aldosterone deficiency is another established cause of fatigue (see Chap. 93). In persons with hypothyroidism, with or without frank myxedema, lassitude and sluggishness are frequent complaints. These same symptoms may also be present in patients with hyperthyroidism but are usually less troublesome than nervousness. Uncontrolled diabetes mellitus may be accompanied by excessive fatigability, as are hyperparathyroidism, hypogonadism, and Cushing's disease.

Anemia, when moderate or severe, should be considered as a possible cause of unexplained lassitude. Mild grades of anemia are usually asymptomatic; lassitude is far too often ascribed to it.

Any type of nutritional deficiency may, when severe, cause lassitude, and in its earlier stages this may be the chief complaint. Weight loss and the history of dietary inadequacy may provide the only other clues to the nature of the illness. Many patients feel weak and tired after a myocardial infarct, but usually there is an accompanying depression.

Among neurologic diseases in which fatigability is a prominent symptom should be mentioned the posttraumatic nervous instability syndrome, Parkinson's disease, and multiple sclerosis. The fatigue of Parkinson's disease may precede the recognition of neurologic signs by months or even years. It is probably a reaction to the increasing disability occasioned by subjective awareness of the akinesia. The majority of patients who recover from a stroke complain of being weak and tired. Hot temperatures worsen the fatigue and other symptoms of the multiple sclerotic patient.

Differential diagnosis If one looks critically at the patients who enter a hospital because of lassitude and fatigability (sometimes incorrectly called weakness), it is clear that the most common overlooked diagnoses are psychoneurosis and depression. The correct conclusion can usually be reached by keeping these illnesses in mind as one elicits the principal symptoms of these psychiatric illnesses from patient and family. Difficulty arises when such symptoms are so inconspicuous as not to be appreciated; one comes then to suspect the psychiatric diagnosis only by having eliminated the common medical causes. Observations in the hospital may bear out the existence of a tension state or gloomy mood, as the patient resists attempts to be mobilized. Strong reassurance in combination with a therapeutic trial of 2.5 to 5.0 mg dextroamphetamine morning and noon and 100 to 200 mg sodium amobarbital three times a day may suppress symptoms of which the patient was barely aware and may clarify diagnosis. The danger of mistaking a depression for a neurosis has already been mentioned. Of course the asthenic psychopath is recognized by his actions as revealed in his biography.

Obscure infections such as pulmonary tuberculosis, brucellosis, subclinical hepatitis, subacute bacterial endocarditis, malaria, hookworm, and parasitic infections should be sought by the characteristic symptoms and signs described elsewhere in the book. An endocrine survey is in order in all obscure cases. There should also be a search for occult tumors. The use of a simple "water excretion test" may prove very helpful in identifying an organic component in a patient's fatigue syndrome, since a wide variety of systemic disorders is associated with a delayed diuresis following the ingestion of water. It is thought that the "sick cell" with impaired permeability of cell membrane "traps" water and then releases it slowly. The test consists in the administration of 500 ml water at 8:15, and 8:30 A. M. for a total intake of 1,500 ml with the patient fasting and lying in a horizontal position. Smoking is not permitted. The water should be room temperature, *not cold.* Urine volume is measured hourly for 3 to 4 h. A normal response will usually include a diuresis of 400 to 600 ml in the first, second, and third hours, with a total volume of at least 80 percent in 3 to 4 h (1,200 ml). An impaired response in the horizontal position suggests *organic disease.* The test is inexpensive and simple to administer! It should be remembered that chronic intoxications with barbiturates, alcohol, or bromides, some of which are given to suppress nervousness, may contribute to fatigability.

Finally, when onset of fatigue is rapid and recent, the cause is likely to be an infection, a disturbance in fluid balance, or rapidly developing circulatory failure of either peripheral or cardiac origin.

GENERALIZED WEAKNESS AND ASTHENIA As can be judged from the foregoing remarks, weakness must be distinguished from lassitude and fatigue. The demonstration of reduced muscular power sets the case analysis along rather different lines, for it raises consideration more particularly of diseases of the nervous system or of the musculature.

True neural or myopathic weakness is probably never due to psychologic factors, though the hysteric or malingering patient may claim weakness. Usually this can be detected by the criteria outlined in Chap. 347. In anemia, chronic infection, malignancy, and nutritional depletion (except when polyneuropathy is present), the thin muscles are always stronger during tests of peak contraction than one would expect, though of course strength falls short of that of a healthy individual (see Chap. 347 for description of tests of peak, power, and endurance of muscles).

The proper ascertainment of muscular weakness depends on two lines of inquiry: (1) a history of reduced efficiency; and (2) demonstrable failure in ability to contract the muscles forcefully one or more times. If one proceeds to test each of the major groups of muscles from head to foot, comparing the patient's performance with one's idea of normalcy for man and woman, one may ascertain whether all or certain groups fall below standard. Quantitative and qualitative changes (myasthenia, inverse myasthenia, myotonia, paramyotonia, pathologic cramping) may also be detected by the methods outlined in Chap. 347. The topography of weakness and associated neurologic findings permit distinction between the various types of spinal, peripheral nerve, and myopathic pareses. Rare diseases, difficult to diagnose, that cause inexplicable muscle weakness are masked hyperthyroidism, hyperparathyroidism, ossifying hemangiomas with hypophosphatemia, some of the kalemic periodic paralyses, and hyperinsulinism.

REFERENCES

ADAMS RD: *Principles of Clinical Myology,* Thayer Lectures, Johns Hopkins Medical Journal, 131:24, 1972

MAYER-GROSS W et al: *Clinical Psychiatry,* 3d ed., Baltimore: Williams & Wilkins, 1969

WALTON JN (ed): *Disease of Voluntary Muscle,* 3d ed., London: Churchill, 1975

16
FAINTNESS, SYNCOPE, AND EPISODIC WEAKNESS

RAYMOND D. ADAMS
EUGENE BRAUNWALD

Episodic faintness, lightheadedness or giddiness, and reduced alertness are frequently difficult to distinguish, tending to shade into one another. And the difference between faintness and frank syncope is only quantitative. Types of episodic weakness, such as myasthenia gravis and familial periodic paralysis, which cause striking reduction of muscular strength but no impairment of consciousness, should be set apart (see Chaps. 15 and 350); epilepsy, which is also associated with episodic unconsciousness, differs from syncope in most other respects and is discussed in Chap. 24.

CARDINAL FEATURES

Syncope comprises a generalized weakness of muscles, with inability to stand upright, and a loss of consciousness. The term *faintness,* in contrast, refers to lack of strength, with sensation of impending loss of consciousness. At the beginning of the attack the patient is nearly always in the upright position, either sitting or standing [the Stokes-Adams attack (see Chap. 238) is exceptional in this respect]. Usually the patient is warned of the impending faint by a sense of "feeling badly." He is assailed by giddiness, the floor seems to move, and surrounding objects begin to sway. His senses become confused, he yawns or gapes, there are spots before his eyes, his vision may dim, and his ears may ring. Nausea and sometimes vomiting accompany these symptoms. There is a striking pallor or ashen-gray color of the face, and very often the face and body are bathed in cold perspiration. The deliberate onset may enable the patient to protect himself as he slumps; a hurtful fall is exceptional. If the patient can lie down promptly, the attack may be averted without complete loss of consciousness.

The depth and duration of unconsciousness vary. Sometimes the patient is not completely oblivious of his surroundings, or there may be complete lack of awareness and of capacity to respond. The patient may remain in this state for seconds to minutes or even as long as half an hour. Usually he lies motionless with skeletal muscles relaxed, but a few clonic jerks of the limbs and face may occur in exceptional cases, shortly after the beginning of the unconsciousness. Generalized tonic-clonic convulsions are never a part of syncope. Sphincter control is usually maintained. The pulse is feeble or cannot be felt; the blood pressure may be low, and breathing almost imperceptible. Once the patient is in a horizontal position, perhaps from having fallen, gravitation no longer hinders the flow of blood to the brain. The strength of the pulse then improves, color begins to return to the face, breathing becomes quicker and deeper, and consciousness is regained. There is from this moment onward a correct perception of the environment. The patient is, nevertheless, keenly aware of physical weakness, and if he rises too soon, another faint may be precipitated. Headache and drowsiness, which, with mental confusion, are the usual sequelae of a convulsion, do not follow a syncopal attack.

ETIOLOGY

The list of causes in Table 16-1 is based on established or assumed physiologic mechanisms. The commoner types of faint are reducible to a few simple mechanisms. Syncope results essentially from a sudden impairment of brain metabolism usually brought about by a hypotensive reduction of cerebral blood flow.

Nature has provided man with several mechanisms by which his circulation adjusts to the upright posture. Approximately three-fourths of the systemic blood volume is contained in the venous bed, and any interference with venous return may lead to a reduction in cardiac output. Cerebral blood flow may still be maintained, as long as systemic arterial vasoconstriction occurs; but when this adjustment fails, serious hypotension with resultant cerebral underperfusion to less than half of normal results in syncope. Normally, the pooling of blood in the lower parts of the body is prevented by (1) pressor reflexes which induce constriction of peripheral arteries and arterioles; (2) reflex acceleration of the heart by means of aortic and carotid reflexes; (3) improvement of venous return to the heart by activity of the muscles of the limbs and by increased rate of respiration. Placing a normal person on a tilt table to relax his muscles and tilting him upright slightly diminishes cardiac output, and blood accumulates in the legs to a slight degree. This may then be followed by a slight transitory fall in systolic arterial pressure, and thus may be a means of reproducing faints in patients with defective vasomotor reflexes.

TYPES OF SYNCOPE

VASOVAGAL (VASODEPRESSOR) SYNCOPE This is the common faint that may be experienced by normal persons; it is frequently recurrent, and tends to take place during

TABLE 16-1
Causes of recurrent weakness, faintness, and disturbances of consciousness

- *I* Circulatory (deficient quantity of blood to the brain)
  - *A* Inadequate vasoconstrictor mechanisms
    - *1* Vasovagal (vasodepressor)
    - *2* Postural hypotension
    - *3* Primary autonomic insufficiency
    - *4* Sympathectomy (pharmacologic or surgical)
    - *5* Diseases of central and peripheral nervous systems (Chap. 331)
    - *6* Carotid sinus syncope (see also Bradyarrhythmias, below)
  - *B* Hypovolemia
  - *C* Mechanical reduction of venous return
    - *1* Valsalva's maneuver
    - *2* Cough
    - *3* Micturition
    - *4* Atrial myxoma, ball valve thrombus
  - *D* Reduced cardiac output
    - *1* Obstruction to left ventricular outflow: aortic stenosis, hypertrophic subaortic stenosis
    - *2* Obstruction to pulmonary flow: pulmonic stenosis, primary pulmonary hypertension, pulmonary embolism
    - *3* Myocardial: massive myocardial infarction with pump failure
    - *4* Pericardial: cardiac tamponade
  - *E* Arrhythmias (Chap. 238)
    - *1* Bradyarrhythmias
      - *a* Atrioventricular (AV) block (II° and III°), with Stokes-Adams attacks
      - *b* Ventricular asystole
      - *c* Sinus bradycardia, sinoatrial block, sinus arrest
      - *d* Carotid sinus syncope (see also Inadequate Vasoconstrictor Mechanisms, above)
      - *e* Glossopharyngeal neuralgia (and other painful states)
    - *2* Tachyarrhythmias
      - *a* Episodic ventricular fibrillation with or without associated bradyarrhythmias
      - *b* Ventricular tachycardia
      - *c* Supraventricular tachycardia without AV block
- *II* Other causes of weakness and episodic disturbances of consciousness
  - *A* Altered state of blood to the brain
    - *1* Hypoxia
    - *2* Anemia
    - *3* Diminished CO_2 due to hyperventilation (faintness common, syncope seldom occurs)
    - *4* Hypoglycemia (episodic weakness common, faintness occasional, syncope rare)
  - *B* Cerebral
    - *1* Cerebrovascular disturbances (cerebral ischemic attacks, see Chap. 334)
      - *a* Extracranial vascular insufficiency (basilar-vertebral, carotid)
      - *b* Diffuse spasm of cerebral arterioles (hypertensive encephalopathy)
    - *2* Emotional disturbances, anxiety attacks, and hysterical seizures (see Chaps. 14 and 344)

emotional stress (especially in a warm, crowded room), after an injurious, shocking accident, and during pain. Mild blood loss, poor physical condition, prolonged bed rest, anemia, fever, organic heart disease, and fasting are other factors which increase the possibility of fainting in susceptible individuals. A short premonitory phase is characterized by nausea, perspiration, yawning, epigastric distress, hyperpnea, tachypnea, weakness, confusion, tachycardia, and pupillary dilatation. Physiologically, there is first a marked fall in arterial pressure and systemic resistance which is most notable in the skeletal muscular beds. Cardiac output may be within normal limits, but it fails to exhibit the expected increase which normally occurs with hypotension. It declines when vagal activity leads to marked bradycardia, replacing tachycardia, resulting in further lowering of arterial pressure and reduction of cerebral perfusion. Assumption of the supine posture with elevation of the legs and removal of the offending stimulus will rapidly restore consciousness.

POSTURAL HYPOTENSION WITH SYNCOPE This type of syncope affects persons who have a chronic defect in or variable instability of vasomotor reflexes. Though the character of the syncopal attack differs little from that of the vasovagal or vasodepressor type, the effect of posture is its cardinal feature; sudden arising from a recumbent position or standing still are the circumstances under which it is most likely to happen.

Postural syncope tends to occur under the following conditions: (1) in otherwise normal persons who for some unknown reason have defective postural reflexes; (2) rarely, as part of a syndrome named *primary autonomic insufficiency,* which includes chronic orthostatic hypotension, as well as symptoms of peripheral preganglionic autonomic and extrapyramidal disorder; (3) after physical deconditioning, e.g., after prolonged illness with recumbency, especially in elderly individuals with flabby muscles; (4) after a sympathectomy that has abolished vasopressor reflexes; (5) in diabetic, alcoholic, and other neuropathies, tabes dorsalis, syringomyelia, subacute combined sclerosis, and diseases of the nervous system which cause muscular atrophy and paralysis of vasopressor reflexes; (6) in persons with varicose veins, because of pooling of blood in the abnormally enlarged venous channels; (7) in patients receiving antihypertensive, vasodilator, and tranquilizing or sedative drugs as well as those who may be hypovolemic because of diuretics or excessive sweating.

In the otherwise normal individuals who faint if tilted on a table, it has been found that at first the blood pressure diminishes slightly and then stabilizes at a lower level. Shortly thereafter the compensatory reflexes suddenly fail, and the arterial pressure falls precipitously. This reaction also may be observed in some of the conditions listed above. In others, e.g., after pharmacologic sympathectomy, in diseases of the sympathetic nervous system, and in the unusual condition known as chronic orthostatic hypotension, the arterial pressure never stabilizes after tilting but falls steadily to a level at which cerebral circulation cannot be maintained.

CHRONIC ORTHOSTATIC HYPOTENSION In this condition, occurring as a consequence of *primary autonomic insufficiency,* there is a degeneration of preganglionic and probably postganglionic autonomic neurons, with anhydrosis and other symptoms of sympathetic and parasympathetic paralysis (sphincteric disturbances, impotence, lack of tears, lack of saliva, pupillary paralysis). Extrapyramidal disorders (tremor, ataxia, rigidity) appear in the more advanced stages of the disease. As arterial pressure falls, there are no compensatory tachycardia, pallor, sweating, nausea, or other symptoms. The orthostatic pooling of blood in the abdomen and legs fails to excite a normal degree of vasoconstriction of systemic arterioles, presumably because of the abnormality in the autonomic nervous system and perhaps because of diminished release of catecholamines from the adrenal medulla as well. There is also evidence that patients with this type of postural hypotension are deficient in release of norepinephrine and epinephrine. Repeated attacks may result in mental confusion, slurred speech, and other neurologic signs, though the extrapyramidal disorder appears to be due to the same degenerative process that affects autonomic motor neurons. The combination is called the *Shy-Drager* syndrome. It occurs also in striatonigral degeneration.

Micturition syncope, a condition usually seen in the elderly during or after urination, particularly after arising from the recumbent position, is probably a special type of postural syncope. It has been suggested that vasomotor reflexes from the bladder itself play a contributory part and that vagally medicated bradycardia forms a significant component.

SYNCOPE OF CARDIAC ORIGIN (CARDIAC SYNCOPE) Cardiac syncope results from a sudden reduction in cardiac output, caused most commonly by a cardiac arrhythmia. In normal individuals slow ventricular rates, but above 35 to 40 beats per min, and fast ones not exceeding 150 beats per min do not reduce cerebral blood flow, especially if the person is in the supine position, but changes in pulse rate outside these limits impair cerebral circulation and functions. The upright posture, cerebrovascular disease, anemia, and coronary, myocardial, or valvular disease all reduce the tolerance to alterations in rate.

Complete atrioventricular block is the commonest arrhythmia that leads to fainting, and syncopal episodes associated with this arrhythmia are known as the Stokes-Adams-Morgagni syndrome. The etiology of disturbances in atrioventricular conduction is considered elsewhere (Chap. 238), but in patients with these attacks the block may be persistent or intermittent; it is often preceded or followed by disturbed conduction in one or two of the three fascicles through which the ventricles are normally activated, by second degree atrioventricular block (Mobitz type II), or bifascicular or trifascicular block. When the block is complete and the pacemaker below the block fails to function, syncope occurs. Less commonly a brief bout of ventricular tachycardia or fibrillation is responsible for the syncopal episode. Familial instances of recurrent syncope due to ventricular fibrillation, characterized by a prolonged Q-T interval (sometimes associated with congenital deafness), have been reported.

Stokes-Adams attacks occur usually without more than a momentary sense of weakness, the patient suddenly losing consciousness. After cardiac standstill of more than several seconds, the patient turns pale, falls unconscious, and, as in other types of fainting, may exhibit a few clonic jerks. With longer periods of asystole, the ashen-gray pallor gives way to cyanosis, stertorous breathing, fixed pupils, incontinence, and bilateral Babinski signs. Prolonged confusion and neurologic signs due to cerebral ischemia may persist in some patients, and permanent impairment of mental function may also occur, although focal neurologic signs are rare. Cardiac faints of this type may recur several times a day. Occasionally the heart block is transitory, and the electrocardiogram taken later may not show any arrhythmia.

Less commonly, a decreased rate of discharge of the sinoatrial node leads to syncope. Recurrent attacks of tachyarrhythmias—including atrial flutter and paroxysmal atrial and ventricular tachycardia with normal AV conduction—may also suddenly reduce cardiac output, to a degree sufficient to cause syncope.

In another form of cardiac syncope the heart block is reflexive and is due to irritation of the vagus nerves. Examples of this phenomenon have been observed in patients with esophageal diverticula, mediastinal tumors, gallbladder disease, carotid sinus disease, glossopharyngeal neuralgia, and pleural and pulmonary irritation. However, in these conditions reflex bradycardia is more commonly of the sinoatrial than the atrioventricular type.

Cardiac syncope may also result from *acute massive myocardial infarction,* particularly when associated with cardiogenic shock. *Aortic stenosis* often sets the stage for exertional syncope, most commonly by limiting cardiac output in the face of peripheral vasodilatation, but sometimes during exertion, with resultant myocardial and cerebral ischemia and occasionally arrhythmias. *Idiopathic hypertrophic subaortic stenosis* may also lead to exertional syncope, because of intensified obstruction and/or ventricular arrhythmias (Chap. 247). In *primary pulmonary hypertension* a relatively fixed cardiac output and bouts of acute right ventricular failure may be associated with syncope (Chap. 265). However, vagal reflexes may be involved in this condition as well as in the syncope that occurs with *pulmonary embolism.* Ball valve thrombus in the left atrium, left atrial myxoma, or thrombosis or malfunction of a prosthetic valve may produce sudden mechanical obstruction of the circulation and syncope. *Tetralogy of Fallot* is the congenital cardiac malformation most commonly responsible for syncope. In this condition systemic vasodilatation, perhaps associated with infundibular spasm, greatly increases the right-to-left shunt and produces arterial hypoxia, which leads to syncope.

CAROTID SINUS SYNCOPE The carotid sinus is normally sensitive to stretch and gives rise to sensory impulses carried via the nerve of Hering, a branch of the glossopharyngeal nerve, to the medulla oblongata. Massage of one or both of the carotid sinuses, particularly in elderly persons, causes (1) a reflex cardiac slowing (sinus bradycardia, sinus arrest, or even atrioventricular block), the so-called vagal type of response, (2) a fall of arterial pressure without cardiac slowing, the so-called depressor type of response, and (3) an interference with the circulation of the ipsilateral cerebral hemisphere, the so-called central type. Two or three types of carotid sinus response may coexist.

Syncope due to carotid sinus sensitivity may be initiated by turning of the heart to one side, by a tight collar, or, as in a few reported cases, by shaving over the region of the sinus. But the absence of such stimuli is of no aid in diagnosis, since spontaneous attacks may occur. The attack nearly always begins when the patient is in an upright position, usually when he is standing. The period of unconsciousness seldom lasts longer than a few minutes. The sensorium is immediately clear when consciousness is regained. The majority of the reported cases have been in men. In a patient displaying faintness on compression of one carotid sinus, it is important to distinguish between the benign disorder (hypersensitivity of one carotid sinus) and a much more serious condition—atheromatous narrowing of the opposite carotid or of the basilar artery (see Chap. 334).

Other forms of vasovagal syncope have been described. Exceptionally intense pain of the visceral origin may inhibit cardiac action through vagal stimulation, e.g., cardiac standstill during an attack of gallbladder colic, a lesion of the esophagus or mediastinum, bronchoscopy, pleural or peritoneal taps, intense vertigo from labyrinthine or vestibular disease, and needling of body cavities.

VAGAL AND GLOSSOPHARYNGEAL NEURALGIA This is known occasionally to induce a reflex type of fainting. Again the sequence is always pain, then syncope; in this instance the pain is localized to the base of the tongue, pharynx or larynx, tonsillar area, and ear. It may be triggered by pressure at these sites. Section of the appropriate branches of the ninth or tenth cranial nerve relieves the condition. The cardiovascular effects are attributable to excitation of the dorsal motor nucleus of the vagus via collateral fibers from the nucleus of the tractus solitarius.

TUSSIVE SYNCOPE ("LARYNGEAL VERTIGO") This is a rare condition that results from a paroxysm of coughing, usually in men with chronic bronchitis. After hard coughing the patient suddenly becomes weak and loses consciousness momentarily. The intrathoracic pressure becomes elevated and interferes with the venous return to the heart, as does the Valsalva maneuver (exhaling against a closed glottis). Episodes of faintness and lightheadedness are not infrequent in pertussis and chronic laryngitis.

SYNCOPE ASSOCIATED WITH CEREBROVASCULAR DISEASE This is usually caused by partial or complete occlusion of the large arteries in the neck. Physical activity may then critically reduce blood flow to the upper part of the brainstem, causing abrupt loss of consciousness (see Chap. 334).

PATHOPHYSIOLOGY OF SYNCOPE

In the final analysis the loss of consciousness in these different types of syncope is caused by a change in the nervous elements in those parts of the brain which subserve consciousness. Syncope resembles epilepsy in this respect; yet there is an important difference. In epilepsy, whether major or minor, the arrest in mental function is almost instantaneous, and, as revealed by the electroencephalogram, it is accompanied by a paroxysm of activity in certain groups of cerebral neurons. Syncope, on the other hand, is not so sudden. The difference relates to the essential pathophysiology—a sudden spread of an electric discharge in epilepsy, and the more gradual failure of the cerebral circulation in syncope.

During syncopal attacks, there are demonstrable reductions in cerebral blood flow, cerebral oxygen utilization, and cerebral vascular resistance. The electroencephalogram reveals high-voltage slow waves, two to five per second, coincident with the loss of consciousness. If the ischemia lasts only a few minutes, there are no lasting effects on the brain. If it persists for a longer time, it may result in necrosis of the border zones between the major cerebral and cerebellar arteries.

DIFFERENTIAL DIAGNOSIS OF CONDITIONS INVOLVING EPISODIC WEAKNESS AND FAINTNESS BUT NOT SYNCOPE

ANXIETY ATTACKS AND THE HYPERVENTILATION SYNDROME These are discussed in detail in Chaps. 14, 19, and 344. The giddiness of anxiety is frequently interpreted as a feeling of faintness without actual loss of consciousness. Such symptoms are not accompanied by facial pallor and are not relieved by recumbency. The diagnosis is made on the basis of the associated symptom, and part of the attack can be reproduced by hyperventilation. Two of the mechanisms known to be involved in the attacks are reduction in carbon dioxide as the result of hyperventilation and the release of epinephrine. Hyperventilation results in hypocapnia, alkalosis, increased cerebrovascular resistance, and decreased cerebral blood flow.

HYPOGLYCEMIA When severe, hypoglycemia is usually traceable to a serious disease, such as a tumor of the islets of Langerhans or advanced adrenal, pituitary, or hepatic disease. The clinical picture is one of confusion or even a loss of consciousness. When mild, as is usually the case, hypoglycemia is the reactive type (Chap. 97), occurring 2 to 5 h after eating, and is not usually associated with a disturbance of consciousness. The diagnosis depends on the history, the documentation of reduced blood sugar during an attack, and the reproduction by an injection of insulin of a symptom complex exactly similar to that occurring in the spontaneous attacks.

ACUTE HEMORRHAGE Acute blood loss, usually within the gastrointestinal tract, is an occasional cause of syncope. In the absence of pain and hematemesis the cause of the weakness, faintness, or even unconsciousness may remain obscure until the passage of a black stool.

CEREBRAL ISCHEMIC ATTACKS These occur in some patients with arteriosclerotic narrowings or occlusion of the major arteries of the brain. The main symptoms vary from patient to patient and include dim vision, hemiparesis, numbness of one side of the body, dizziness, and thick speech, and to these may be added an impairment of consciousness. In any one patient all attacks are of identical type and indicate a temporary deficit of the function in a certain region of the brain due to inadequate circulation.

HYSTERICAL FAINTING Hysterical fainting is rather frequent and usually occurs under dramatic circumstances (Chap. 344). The attack is unattended by any outward display of anxiety. The evident lack of change in pulse and blood pressure or color of the skin and mucous membranes distinguishes it from the vasodepressor faint. The diagnosis is based on the bizarre nature of the attack in a person who exhibits the general personality and behavioral characteristics of hysteria.

DIFFERENTIAL DIAGNOSIS OF SEIZURE AND SYNCOPE

More typical varieties of syncope must be distinguished from other disturbances of cerebral function, the most frequent of which is akinetic or some other form of epilepsy (see Chap. 24). The epileptic attack may occur day or night, regardless of the position of the patient; syncope rarely appears when the patient is recumbent, the only common exception being the Stokes-Adams attack. The patient's color does not usually change in epilepsy; pallor is an early and invariable finding in all types of syncope, except chronic orthostatic hypotension and hysteria, and it precedes unconsciousness. Epilepsy is more sudden in onset, and if an aura is present, it rarely lasts longer than a few seconds before consciousness is abolished. The onset of syncope is usually more deliberate and without aura. Injury from falling is frequent in epilepsy and rare in syncope, for the reason that only in epilepsy are protective reflexes instantaneously abolished. Tonic-convulsive movements with upturning eyes are a feature of epilepsy and not of syncope. The period of unconsciouness tends to be longer in epilepsy than in syncope. Urinary incontinence is frequent in epilepsy and rare in syncope, but since it may be observed occasionally in syncope, it cannot be used as a means of excluding epilepsy. The return of consciousness is prompt in syncope, slow in epilepsy. Mental confusion, headache, and drowsiness are common sequelae in epilepsy; physical weakness with clear sensorium characterizes the postsyncopal state. Repeated spells of unconsciousness in a young person at a rate of several per day or month are much more suggestive of epilepsy than of syncope. No one of these points will absolutely differentiate epilepsy from syncope, but taken as a group and supplemented by electroencephalograms, they provide a means of distinguishing the two conditions.

DIFFERENT TYPES OF SYNCOPE Differentiation of the several conditions that diminish cerebral blood flow is discussed in greater detail in Chap. 34.

When faintness is related to reduced cerebral blood flow resulting directly from a disorder of cardiac function, there is likely to be a combination of pallor and cyanosis, with pronounced dyspnea, and often the jugular veins are distended. When, on the other hand, the peripheral circulation is at fault, pallor is usually striking but is not accompanied by cyanosis or respiratory disturbances, and the veins are collapsed. When the primary disturbance lies in the cerebral circulation, the face is likely to be florid and the breathing slow and stertorous. During the attack a heart rate faster than 150 beats per min indicates an ectopic cardiac rhythm, while a striking bradycardia (rate of less than 40) suggests complete heart block. In a patient with faintness or syncope attended by bradycardia, one has to distinguish between the neurogenic reflex and the cardiogenic (Stokes-Adams) types. The electrocardiogram is decisive, but even without it, the Stokes-Adams seizures can be recognized clinically by their longer duration, by the greater constancy of the slow heart rate, by the presence of audible sounds synchronous with atrial contraction, by atrial contraction (A) waves in the jugular venous pulse, and by marked variation in intensity of the first sound, despite the regular rhythm (Chap. 238).

It is of primary importance to know the circumstances and the precipitating and alleviating factors in a given episode of weakness or fainting.

TYPE OF ONSET When the attack begins over the period of a few seconds, carotid sinus syncope, postural hypotension, sudden atrioventricular block, ventricular standstill, or fibrillation is likely. When the symptoms develop gradually during a period of several minutes, hyperventilation or hypoglycemia should be considered. Onset of syncope during or immediately after exertion suggests aortic stenosis and, in elderly subjects, postural hypotension. Exertional syncope is seen occasionally in persons with aortic insufficiency and with severe occlusive disease of cerebral arteries. In patients with ventricular standstill, loss of consciousness occurs several seconds later, followed rapidly by cessation of electroencephalographic activity and then often by brief clonic contractions.

POSITION AT ONSET OF ATTACK Attacks due to hypoglycemia, hyperventilation, or heart block are likely to be independent of posture. Faintness associated with a decline in blood pressure (including carotid sinus attacks) and with ectopic tachycardia usually occurs only in the sitting or standing position, whereas faintness resulting from orthostatic hypotension is apt to set in shortly after change from the recumbent to the standing position.

ASSOCIATED SYMPTOMS Palpitation is likely to be present when the attack is due to anxiety or hyperventilation, to ectopic tachycardia, or to hypoglycemia. Numbness and tingling in the hands and face are frequent accompaniments of hyperventilation. Genuine convulsions during the attack, although characteristic of epilepsy, may occasionally occur with heart block, ventricular standstill, or fibrillation.

DURATION OF ATTACK When the duration is very brief, i.e., a few seconds to a few minutes, carotid sinus syncope or one of the several forms of postural hypotension is most likely. A duration of more than a few minutes but less than an hour suggests hypoglycemia or hyperventilation.

SPECIAL METHODS OF EXAMINATION

In many patients who complain of recurrent weakness or syncope but do not have a spontaneous attack while under observation of the physician, an attempt to reproduce attacks is of great assistance in diagnosis.

When hyperventilation is accompanied by faintness, the pattern of symptoms can be reproduced readily by having the subject breathe rapidly and deeply for 2 to 3 min. This test is often of therapeutic value also, because the underlying anxiety tends to be lessened when the patient learns that he can produce and alleviate the symptoms at will simply by controlling his breathing.

Among other conditions in which the diagnosis is commonly clarified by reproducing the attacks are carotid sinus hypersensitivity (massage of one or the other carotid sinus), orthostatic hypotension and orthostatic tachycardia (observations of pulse rate, blood pressure, and symptoms in the recumbent and standing positions), and tussive syncope (by inducing the Valsalva maneuver). In all these instances the crucial point is not whether symptoms are produced (the procedures mentioned frequently induce symptoms in healthy persons) but whether the exact pattern of symptoms that occurs in the spontaneous attacks is reproduced in all the artificial ones. Careful, continuous monitoring of the electrocardiogram in the hospital or the recording of the electrocardiogram over several hours using a portable lightweight tape recorder in an ambulatory patient may be extremely useful in identifying an arrhythmia responsible for the syncopal episode. Monitoring is most helpful if it shows that the syncopal episode is characterized by a bout of cardiac standstill, extreme bradycardia, or tachyarrhythmia.

The electroencephalogram may be helpful in differentiating syncope from epilepsy. In the interval between epileptic seizures it may show some degree of abnormality in 40 to 80 percent of cases. In the interval between syncopal attacks it should be normal.

TREATMENT

Fainting in most instances is relatively benign. In dealing with patients who have fainted, the physician should think first of those causes of fainting that constitute a therapeutic emergency. Among them are massive internal hemorrhage and myocardial infarction, which may be painless, and cardiac arrhythmias. In an elderly person a sudden faint, without obvious cause, should arouse the suspicion of complete heart block, even though all findings are negative when the physician sees the patient.

If the patient is seen during the preliminary stages of fainting or after he has lost consciousness, he should be placed in a position which permits maximal cerebral blood flow, i.e., with head lowered between the knees, if sitting, or in the supine position. All tight clothing and other constrictions should be loosened and the head turned so that the tongue does not fall back into the throat, blocking the airway. Peripheral irritation, such as sprinkling or dashing cold water on the face and neck or the application of cold moist towels, is helpful. If the temperature is subnormal, the body should be covered with a warm blanket. If available, aromatic spirit of ammonia may be given cautiously by inhalation. Since emesis is frequent, one should be prepared for a possible aspiration. Nothing should be given by mouth until the patient has regained consciousness. Then one-half a teaspoon of aromatic spirit of ammonia in one-half a glass of cold water, or a sip of brandy or whiskey, may be given. The patient should not be permitted to rise until his sense of physical weakness has passed, and he should be watched carefully for a few minutes after rising.

The *prevention* of fainting depends on the mechanisms involved. In the usual vasovagal faint of adolescents, which tends to occur in periods of emotional excitement, fatigue, hunger, etc., it is enough to advise the patient to avoid such circumstances. In postural hypotension the patient should be cautioned against arising suddenly from bed. Instead, he should first exercise his legs for a few seconds, then sit on the edge of the bed and make sure he is not lightheaded or dizzy before he starts to walk. He should sleep with the headposts of the bed elevated on wooden blocks 8 to 12 in. high. A snug elastic abdominal binder and elastic stockings are often helpful. Drugs of the ephedrine group may be useful if they do not cause insomnia. If there are no contraindications, a high intake of sodium chloride, which expands the extracellular fluid volume, may be beneficial.

In the syndrome of chronic orthostatic hypotension, special corticosteroid preparations (Florinef Acetate tablets, 1 to 2 mg per day in divided doses) have given relief in some cases. Binding of the legs (G suit) and sleeping with head and shoulders elevated are helpful.

The treatment of carotid sinus syncope involves first of all instructing the patient in measures that minimize the hazards of a fall (see below). Loose collars should be worn, and the patient should learn to turn the whole body, rather than the head alone, when looking to one side. Atropine or the ephedrine group of drugs should be used, respectively, in patients with pronounced bradycardia or hypotension during attacks. If atropine is not successful, a demand pacemaker should be inserted into the right ventricle. Radiation or surgical denervation of the carotid sinus has apparently yielded favorable results in some patients, but it is rarely necessary. Once it has been concluded that the attacks are due to a narrowing of major cerebral arteries, some of the surgical measures discussed in Chap. 334 must be considered.

The treatment of the various cardiac arrhythmias which may induce syncope is discussed in Chap. 238. The treatment of hypoglycemia will be found in Chap. 97 and of the hyperventilation syndrome and hysterical fainting in Chaps. 14 and 344, respectively.

The chief hazard of a faint in most elderly persons is not the underlying disease but rather fracture or other trauma due to the fall. Therefore, patients subject to recurrent syncope should cover the bathroom floor and bathtub with rubber mats and should have as much of their home carpeted as is feasible. Especially important is the floor space between the bed and the bathroom, because faints are common in elderly persons when walking from bed to toilet. Outdoor walking should be on soft ground rather than hard surfaces, and the patient should avoid standing still, which is more likely to induce an attack than walking.

REFERENCES

HICKLER R: Fainting, chap 33 in *Signs and Symptoms,* 6th ed., ed RS Blacklow, Philadelphia: Lippincott, 1977

LEE JE et al: Episodic unconsciousness, in *Diagnostic Approaches to Presenting Syndromes,* ed JA Barondess, Baltimore: Williams & Wilkins, 1971, pp. 133–167

SELZER A: *Principles of Clinical Cardiology,* Philadelphia: Saunders, 1975, pp. 27, 233, 300, 486

WEISSLER AM, WARREN JV: Syncope and shock, in *The Heart,* 3d ed., ed JW Hurst, New York: McGraw-Hill, 1974, p. 570

WRIGHT KE JR, MCINTOSH MD: Syncope: review of pathophysiological mechanisms. Prog Cardiovasc Dis 13:580–594, 1971

17 MOTOR PARALYSIS

RAYMOND D. ADAMS

Impairments of motor function may be subdivided into (1) paralysis due to affection of lower motor neurons, (2) paralysis due to disorder of upper motor (corticospinal and cortico-brainstem) neurons, (3) abnormalities of coordination (ataxia) due to lesions in the cerebellum, (4) abnormalities of movement and posture due to disease of the extrapyramidal motor system, (5) apraxic or nonparalytic disturbances of purposive movement due to involvement of the cerebrum. The first two types of motor disorder and the cerebral disorders of movement are discussed briefly in the following pages; cerebellar ataxia and extrapyramidal motor abnormalities are considered in Chap. 18.

DEFINITIONS When applied to voluntary muscles, *paralysis* means loss of contraction due to interruption of one of the motor pathways from the cerebrum to the muscle fiber. Lesser degrees of paralysis are sometimes spoken of as *paresis,* but in everyday medical parlance motor paralysis usually stands for either partial or complete loss of function. The word *plegia* comes from the Greek word meaning stroke; and the word *palsy,* from an old French word, has the same meaning as paralysis. It is preferable to use paresis for slight and paralysis or plegia for severe loss of motor function.

PARALYSIS DUE TO DISEASE OF THE LOWER MOTOR NEURONS Each motor nerve cell, through the extensive arborization of the terminal part of its fiber, comes into contact with 100 to 200 or more muscle fibers; altogether they constitute "the motor unit." All the variations in force, range, and type of movement are determined by differences in the number and size of motor units called into activity and the frequency of their action. Feeble movements recruit few units, stronger ones many more units of increasing size. Histochemical methods show that motor units involved in slow, tonic contractions (type I) have muscle fibers rich in oxidative enzymes and mitochondria, and those involved in fast, phasic contractions (type II), more phosphorylase. When a motor neuron becomes diseased, as in progressive muscular atrophy, it may manifest increased irritability, and all the muscle fibers that it controls may discharge sporadically, in isolation from other units. The result of the contraction of one or several such units is a visible twitch, or *fasciculation,* which can be seen and recorded in the electromyogram as a large diphasic or multiphasic action potential. If the motor neuron is destroyed, all the muscle fibers to which it is attached undergo a profound atrophy, namely, denervation atrophy. For some unknown reason the individual denervated muscle fibers now begin to be hypersensitive and to contract spontaneously, though they can no longer do so in response to a nerve impulse as a part of a motor unit. This isolated activity of individual muscle fibers is called *fibrillation* and is so fine that it cannot be seen through the intact skin but can be recorded only as a repetitive short-duration spike potential in the electromyogram. The motor nerve fibers of each anterior root intermingle as the roots join to form plexuses, and although the innervation of the muscles is roughly according to segments of the spinal cord, each large muscle comes to be supplied by two or more roots. In contrast, a single peripheral nerve usually provides the complete motor innervation of a muscle or group of muscles. For this reason the distribution of paralysis due to disease of the anterior horn cells or anterior roots differs from that which follows a lesion of a peripheral nerve.

All motor activity, even the most elementary reflex type, requires the cooperation of several muscles. The analysis of a relatively simple movement, such as clenching the fist, affords some idea of the complexity of the underlying neural arrangements. In this act the primary movement is a contraction of the flexor muscles of the fingers, the flexor digitorum sublimis and profundus, the flexor pollicis longus and brevis, and the abductor pollicis brevis. These muscles act as *agonists,* or *prime movers,* in this act. In order for flexion to be smooth and forceful, the extensor muscles (antagonists) must relax at the same rate at which the flexors contract. The muscles which flex the fingers also flex the wrist; and since it is desired that only the fingers flex, the muscles which extend the wrist must be brought into play to prevent its flexion. The action of the wrist extensors is *synergic,* and these muscles are called synergists in this particular act. Lastly the wrist, elbow, and shoulder must be stabilized by appropriate flexor and extensor muscles, which serve as *fixators.* The coordination of agonists, antagonists, synergists, and fixators involves reciprocal innervation and is managed entirely by segmental spinal reflexes under the guidance of proprioceptive sensory stimuli. Only the agonist movement in a voluntary act is believed to be initiated at a cortical level.

In addition there are many basic motor activities, such as the maintenance of certain postures, stepping movements and others, which do not involve reciprocal innervation. Agonists and antagonists contract simultaneously. The alternating movements of spinal stepping represent an even more basic type of coordination. In the support of the body in an upright posture, when the limb must be as rigid as a pillar, and in shivering the agonists and antagonists must act together. In general, the more delicate the movement, the more precise the coordination between agonist and antagonist muscles.

If all or practically all peripheral motor nerves supplying a muscle are destroyed, all voluntary, postural, and reflex movements are abolished. The muscle becomes soft and yields excessively to passive stretching, a condition known as *flaccidity.* Muscle tone—the slight resistance that normal relaxed muscle offers to passive movement—is reduced (hypotonia or atonia). The denervated muscles undergo extreme atrophy, usually being reduced to 20 to 30 percent of their original bulk within 3 months. The reaction of the muscle to sudden stretch, as by tapping its tendon, is lost. And, finally, it may be demonstrated that the muscle will no longer respond to electric stimuli of short duration, i.e., faradic stimuli, but still responds to currents of long duration, i.e., to galvanic stimuli. This alteration of electric response is known as *Erb's reaction of degeneration.* If only a part of the motor units in the muscles is affected, partial paralysis will ensue. Quantitative testing by determination of strength-duration curves is a means of showing partial denervation, and electromyographic evidence of fibrillations may also be obtained.

The tonus of muscle and the tendon reflexes are known to depend on the muscle spindles and the afferent fibers to which they give origin and on the small anterior horn cells whose axons terminate on the small muscle fibers within the spindles. These small spinal motor neurons are called *gamma neurons,* in contrast to the large *alpha neurons.* Two different gamma neurons are now recognized, one, connected with nuclear bag spindle muscle fibers for phasic actions; the other, with nuclear chain spindle fibers for tonic actions. A tap on a tendon, by stretching the spindle muscle fibers, activates afferent neurons which transmit impulses to alpha motor neurons. The result is the familiar brief muscle contraction or tendon reflex. The spindle muscle fibers are then relaxed (unloaded), which terminates the reflex. Thus the setting of the spindle fibers and the state of excitability of the gamma neurons (normally inhibited by the corticospinal fibers and other supranuclear neurons) determine the level of activity of the tendon reflexes and the responsiveness of muscle to stretch. Other mechanisms of an inhibitory nature, involving Golgi tendon organs, are brought into play in more powerful stretching of muscle.

Lower motor neuron paralysis is the direct result of physiologic arrest or destruction of anterior horn cells or their axons in anterior roots and nerves. The signs and symptoms vary according to the location of the lesion. Probably the most important question for clinical purposes is whether sensory changes coexist. The combination of flaccid, areflexic paralysis and sensory changes usually indicates involvement of mixed motor and sensory nerves or affection of both anterior and posterior roots. If sensory changes are absent, the lesion must be situated in the gray matter of the spinal cord, in the anterior roots, in a purely motor branch of a peripheral nerve, or in motor axons alone. The distinction between nuclear (spinal) and anterior root (radicular) lesions may at times be impossible to make. Spasticity in muscles weakened by a spinal lesion points to the integrity of the segments below the level of the lesion.

PARALYSIS DUE TO DISEASE OF THE CORTICOSPINAL AND CORTICO-BRAINSTEM NEURONS It was formerly believed that the corticospinal tract originated from the large motor cell of Betz in the fifth layer of the precentral convolution. However, there are only about 25,000 to 30,000 Betz cells, whereas the corticospinal tract at the level of the medulla contains approximately 1 million axons. This tract must, therefore, contain many fibers that arise not from the giant Betz cells of the motor cortex (area 4 of Brodmann) but rather from the smaller Betz cells of area 4, the cells of the adjacent precentral cortex (area 6), as well as those of the secondary motor cortex in the superior frontal convolution and postcentral cortex (areas 1, 2, 3, 5, 7). The most critical degeneration studies of van Crevel have shown that when areas 4, 6, 1, 2, 3, 5, and 7 are removed in the cat, if one waits several months, all will be found degenerated and none can be traced to other parts of the cerebral cortex. The corticospinal tract is the only long-fiber connection between the cerebrum and the spinal cord. At the level of the internal capsule these corticospinal fibers are intermingled with many others destined to end in the globus pallidus, substantia nigra, red nucleus, and reticular substance and with others ascending from the thalamus. The fibers to the cranial nerve nuclei become separated at about the level of the midbrain and cross the midline to the contralateral cranial nerve nuclei (Fig. 17-1). These fibers form the corticomesencephalic, corticopontine, and corticobulbar tracts and, since they have functions similar to those of the corticospinal tract, may be included in the pyramidal system of motor neurons. The decussation of the corticospinal tract at the lower end of the medulla is variable in different persons. Most of the crossing fibers come to occupy a position in the posterolateral part of the lateral funiculus; a few cross to form an anterior fasciculus. A small number of fibers, 10 to 20 percent, do not cross but descend ipsilaterally as the uncrossed corticospinal tract. Exceptionally, all of them cross; rarely, none. The termination of the corticospinal tract is in relation to nerve cells in the intermediate zone of gray matter, but not more than 10 to 15 percent establish direct synaptic connection with anterior horn cells. These facts, derived from degeneration studies, must of necessity modify current views of the anatomy of the corticospinal tract and suggest new interpretations.

The motor area of the cerebral cortex is difficult to define. It includes that part of the precentral convolution which contains Betz cells (area 4), but, as already mentioned, it probably extends anteriorly into area 6 and the secondary motor area of the superior frontal convolution and posteriorly into the anterior parietal lobe, where it overlaps the sensory areas. Physiologically it is defined as the region of electrically excitable cortex from which isolated movements can be evoked by stimuli of minimal intensity. The muscle groups of the contralateral face, arm, trunk, and leg are represented in the motor cortex, those of the face being at the lower end of the precentral convolution and those of the leg in the paracentral lobule on the medial surface of the cerebral hemisphere. The parts of the body capable of the most delicate movements have, in general, the largest cortical representation. Very strong stimuli elicit movements from a wide area of premotor frontal and parietal cortex, and the same movements may be obtained from several points. From this it may be assumed that one of the functions of the motor cortex is to synthesize simple movements into an infinite variety of finely graded, highly differentiated patterns.

Corticospinal motor neuron paralysis may be due to lesions in the cerebral cortex, subcortical white matter, internal capsule, brainstem, or spinal cord. Usually much more is involved than the corticospinal, or pyramidal, tract; hence the term pyramidal paralysis is a misnomer. The distribution of the paralysis varies with the locale of the lesion, but there are certain common features. Paralysis due to a lesion of these supranuclear motor neurons always involves a group of muscles, never individual muscles, and if any movement is possible, the proper relationships between antagonists, synergists, and fixators are always preserved. The paralysis never involves all the muscles on one side of the body, even in the hemiplegia resulting from a complete lesion of the internal capsule. Movements that are invariably bilateral, such as those of the eyes, jaw, pharynx, larynx, neck, thorax, and abdomen, are little if at all affected. The hand and arm muscles suffer most severely, the leg muscles next, and of the cranial musculature only the muscles of the lower part of the face and tongue are involved to any significant degree. Corticospinal motor paralysis is rarely complete for any long period of time; in this respect it differs from the total and absolute paralysis due to a complete destruction or interruption of anterior horn cells and their axons. The paralyzed arm may suddenly move during yawning and stretching, and various spinal reflexes can be elicited at all times.

Acute disorders of the corticospinal motor system, at lower levels such as the cervical cord, may not only cause a paralysis of voluntary movement but may also abolish temporarily the spinal reflexes subserved by segments below the lesion. This condition is known as *spinal shock.* After a few days to weeks it disappears and gives way to a phenomenon known as *spasticity.* The latter is a feature of all acute and chronic lesions of the pyramidal system at cerebral, capsular, midbrain, and pontine levels. In cerebral and brainstem lesions it does not usually appear immediately, and in exceptional cases the paralyzed limbs remain flaccid but with reflexes. Spasticity is related to the excessive activity of the released or disinhibited spinal motor neurons. The tendon reflexes are hyperactive, and clonus may appear. The posture of the arm and leg inform us that certain spinal neurons are more active than others. The arm, for example, is maintained in a pronated, flexed position and the leg in an adducted, extended position. Any attempts to extend the arm or flex the leg passively will encounter, after a brief free interval, a resistance which quickly yields (clasp-knife phenomenon). When the limb is

FIGURE 17-1
Diagram of the corticospinal and corticobulbar tracts. Lesion at A *produces ipsilateral oculomotor palsy and contralateral paralysis involving face, arm, and leg. Lesion at* B *causes ipsilateral facial paralysis of peripheral type and contralateral paralysis of arm and leg. Lesion at* b *results in ipsilateral facial weakness of upper motor neuron of central type and contralateral paralysis of arm and leg. (Courtesy of Bergmann and Staehln:* Krankheiten des Nervensystems. *Berlin: Springer-Verlag, 1939.)*

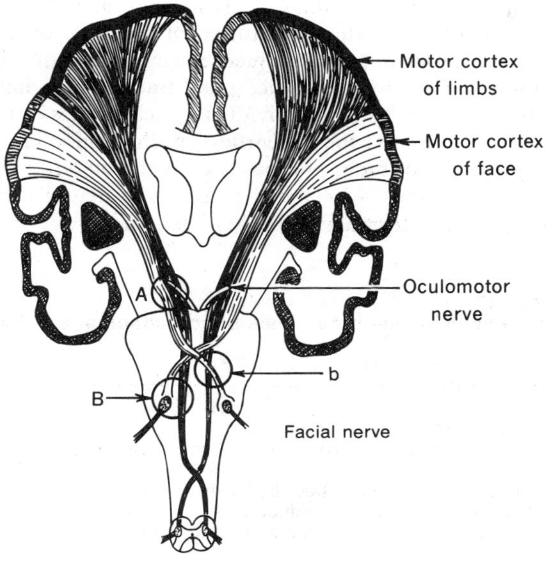

left in the new position, the resistance reappears (lengthening and shortening reactions). The nocifensive spinal flexion reflexes, of which Babinski's sign is a part, are also released, and the cutaneomuscular abdominal and cremasteric reflexes abolished. The flexion reflexes are not an essential component of spasticity. In the hemiplegic patient they are less prominent than in the spinal paraplegic or quadriplegic patient. With cerebral lesions exaggerated stretch and cutaneous cranial reflexes can also be elicited in cranial as well as limb and trunk muscles, and when the corticospinal disorder is bilateral, there is pseudobulbar paralysis (dysarthria, dysphonia, and dysphagia with bifacial paralysis). Flexor and extensor spasms may occur with lesions of the spinal cord but not the cerebrum.

Spasticity may be present when the limbs are not paralyzed but only paretic, and it then produces interesting effects on voluntary movements. Attempts by the patient to move the hemiplegic limbs voluntarily may result in a variety of associated movements. Flexion of the arms results in involuntary pronation; flexion of the leg causes the foot to dorsiflex and evert automatically (Strumpell's tibialis sign). When asked to rotate one arm, the quadriparetic patient makes the same movement in the other (mirror movement). Flexion of one leg is associated with involuntary extension of the other.

Table 17-1 shows the main differences between corticospinal and lower motor neuron syndrome.

APRAXIC OR NONPARALYTIC DISORDERS OF MOTOR FUNCTION Aside from upper and lower motor neuron paralysis with cerebral lesions, there may be loss of purposive movement without paralysis. This is called *apraxia* and may be explained as follows. Many simple actions are acquired by learning or practice. These depend on the formation of movement patterns, particularly those which involve the use of tools and instruments as well as gestures. Once established, they are remembered and may be reproduced under the proper circumstances. Any purposive act may be conceived as occurring in several stages. First, the idea of an act must be aroused in the mind of the subject by an appropriate stimulus situation, perhaps by a spoken command to do something. This idea is then translated into action by excitation of patterns of premotor or motor cortical neurons in proper sequence, which are transmitted to lower centers by the corticospinal tracts. These initiate particular movements of individual muscle groups but also modify or suppress the subcortical mechanisms that control the basic attitudes and postures of the body. In right-handed and most left-handed persons the neural mechanisms for the formulation of an idea of an act (motor schema or image) in response to a spoken command or a verbal stimulus and its reproduction are believed to be centered in the posterior and inferior parts of the left parietal lobe; these areas, near the language mechanism, are connected with the left premotor regions for the control of the right hand and thence with the motor areas of the right cerebral hemisphere through the corpus callosum for the control of the left side.

A failure to execute certain acts in the correct context while retaining the ability to carry out the individual movements upon which such acts depend is the main feature of *apraxia.* The most adequate clinical test of motor deficits of this type is to observe a series of self-initiated actions such as using a comb, a razor, a toothbrush, or a common tool, or gesturing, e.g., waving goodbye, saluting, shaking the fist as though angry, or blowing a kiss. These actions may be called forth by a command or a request to imitate the examiner. Of course, failure to follow a spoken or written request may be due to an aphasia that prevents understanding of what is asked, or an agnosia may prevent recognition of the tool or object to be used. But when these difficulties are excluded, there remains a peculiar motor deficit in which the patient appears to understand but has lost his memory of how to perform a given act, especially if it is called for in an unnatural setting. He may have the idea of what he wants to do or what others command him to do, but he cannot translate the idea of the sequence of movements into a precise, well-executed act. This is sometimes called *ideomotor apraxia.* The failure may be evident both after a spoken command and in requests to imitate the gestures of the examiner. Sometimes these two conditions may be dissociated; the patient, while not aphasic, cannot execute a spoken command but can still imitate the act if it is called forth by gesture. Also if merely given the tool he may use it properly in an automatic fashion.

Apraxia may be limited to one group of muscles, such as tongue or lips, as in Broca's aphasia (Chap. 25), or the loss of commanded actions of the left arm and leg in right-sided hemiplegics (sympathetic apraxia).

If this motor disorder can be singled out, it reflects a specific loss of certain learned patterns of movement (a "specific amnesia," so to speak, analogous to the amnesia of words in aphasia). The added element of mental confusion tends often to obscure the disorder.

DIFFERENTIAL DIAGNOSIS OF PARALYSIS The diagnostic consideration of paralysis may be simplified by the following subdivisions, which relate to the location and distribution of weakness.

Monoplegia The physical examination of patients who complain of weakness of one extremity often discloses an

TABLE 17-1
Differences between paralysis of corticospinal and lower motor neurons

Upper, corticospinal motor paralysis	*Lower, spinomuscular, or nuclear-infranuclear paralysis*
Muscle groups affected diffusely, never individual muscles	Individual muscles may be affected
Atrophy slight and due to disuse	Atrophy pronounced, 70 to 80 percent of total bulk
Spasticity with hyperactivity of the tendon reflexes	Flaccidity and hypotonia of affected muscles with loss of tendon reflexes
Extensor plantar reflex, Babinski's sign	Plantar reflex, if present, is of normal flexor type
Fascicular twitches not produced	Fascicular twitches may be present
Normal reactions to galvanic and faradic current	Loss of faradic reaction, retention of galvanic action (reaction of degeneration)

unnoticed weakness in another limb, and the condition is actually hemiplegia or paraplegia. Or instead of weakness of all the muscles in a limb, only isolated groups are found to be affected. Ataxia, sensory disturbances, or pain in an extremity will often be interpreted by the patient as weakness, as will the mechanical limitation resulting from arthritis or the rigidity of parkinsonism.

In general, the presence or absence of atrophy of muscles in a monoplegic limb can be of diagnostic help.

PARALYSIS WITHOUT MUSCULAR ATROPHY Long-continued disuse of a limb may lead to atrophy, but this is usually not so marked as in diseases that denervate muscles; the tendon reflexes are normal, and the response of the muscles to electric stimulation and the electromyogram are unaltered.

The most frequent cause of monoplegia without muscular wasting is a lesion of the cerebral cortex. Only occasionally does it occur in diseases which interrupt the cortiocospinal tract at the level of the internal capsule, brainstem, or spinal cord. A vascular lesion (thrombosis or embolus) is the commonest cause, and, of course, a tumor or abscess may have the same effect. Multiple sclerosis and spinal cord tumor, early in their course, may cause weakness of one extremity, usually the leg. Weakness due to damage to the corticospinal system is usually accompanied by spasticity, increased reflexes, and an extensor plantar reflex (Babinski's sign), and the electric reactions and electromyogram are normal. However, acute diseases that destroy the motor tracts in the spinal cord may at first (for several days) reduce the tendon reflexes and cause hypotonia *(spinal shock)*. This does not occur in partial or slowly evolving lesions and occurs only to minimal degree in lesions of brainstem and cerebrum. In acute diseases affecting the lower motor neurons the tendon reflexes are always reduced or abolished, but atrophy may not appear for several weeks. Hence one must take into account the mode of onset and the duration of the disease in evaluating the tendon reflexes, muscle tone, and degree of atrophy before reaching an anatomic diagnosis.

PARALYSIS WITH MUSCULAR ATROPHY This is more frequent than paralysis without muscular atrophy. In addition to the paralysis and reduced or abolished tendon reflexes, there may be visible fasciculations. If completely paralyzed, the muscles exhibit an electric reaction of degeneration, and the electromyogram shows reduced numbers of motor units (often of large size), fasciculations at rest, and fibrillations. The lesion may be in the spinal cord, spinal roots, or peripheral nerves. Its location can usually be decided by the distribution of the palsied muscles (whether the pattern is one of nerve, spinal root, or spinal cord involvement), by the associated neurologic symptoms and signs, and by special tests (cerebrospinal fluid examination, roentgenogram of spine, and myelogram).

Brachial atrophic monoplegia is relatively rare, and when present, it should suggest in an infant a brachial plexus trauma, in a child poliomyelitis, in an adult poliomyelitis, syringomyelia, amyotrophic lateral sclerosis, or other brachial plexus lesions. Crural monoplegia is more frequent and may be caused by any lesion of thoracic or lumbar cord, i.e., trauma, tumor, myelitis, multiple sclerosis, etc. Multiple sclerosis almost never causes atrophy, and ruptured intervertebral disk and the many varieties of neuritis rarely paralyze all or most of the muscles of a limb. Muscle dystrophy may begin in one limb, but by the time the patient is seen the typical more or less symmetric pattern of proximal limb and trunk involvement is evident. A unilateral retroperitioneal tumor may paralyze the leg by implicating the entire lumbosacral plexus.

Hemiplegia Loss of strength in arm, leg, and sometimes face on one side of the body is the most frequent distribution of paralysis in man. With rare exceptions (a few unusual cases of poliomyelitis or motor system disease) this pattern of paralysis is due to involvement of the corticospinal tract.

LOCATION OF LESION-PRODUCING HEMIPLEGIA The site or level of the lesion can usually be deduced from the associated neurologic findings. Diseases localized in the cerebral cortex, cerebral white matter (corona radiata), and internal capsule usually evoke weakness or paralysis of the face, arm, and leg on the opposite side. The occurrence of convulsive seizures or the presence of a defect in speech (aphasia), a cortical type of sensory loss (astereognosis, loss of two-point discrimination, etc.), anosognosia, or defects in the visual fields suggest a cortical or subcortical location.

Damage to the corticospinal and cortico-brainstem tracts in the upper portion of the brainstem (see Fig. 17-1) may cause paralysis of the face, arm, and leg on the opposite side. The lesion in such cases is localized by the presence of a paralysis of the muscles supplied by the oculomotor nerve on the same side as the lesion (Weber's syndrome) or other neurologic findings. With low pontine lesions a unilateral abducens or facial palsy is combined with a contralateral weakness or paralysis of the arm and leg (Millard-Gubler syndrome). Lesions of the lowermost part of the brainstem, i.e., in the medulla, affect the tongue and sometimes the pharynx and larynx on one side and arm and leg on the other side. These "crossed paralyses," so common in brainstem diseases, are described in Chap. 332.

Rarely, a homolateral hemiplegia may be caused by a lesion in the lateral column of the cervical spinal cord. At this level, however, the pathologic process often induces bilateral signs, with resulting quadriparesis or quadriplegia. Homolateral paralysis if combined with a loss of vibratory and position sense on the same side and a contralateral loss of pain and temperature (Brown-Séquard syndrome) signifies disease of the spinal cord on one side (Chaps. 21 and 333).

Muscle atrophy of minor degree often follows lesions of the corticospinal system but never reaches the proportions seen in diseases of the lower motor neurons. The atrophy is due to disuse. When the motor cortex and adjacent parts of the parietal lobe are damaged in infancy or childhood, the normal development of the muscles and the skeletal system in the affected limbs is retarded. The palsied limbs and even the trunk on one side are small. This does not occur if the paralysis begins after the greater part of skeletal growth is attained (after puberty). In the hemiplegia due to spinal cord injury muscles at the level of the lesion undergo atrophy as a result of damage to anterior horn cells or ventral roots.

CAUSES OF HEMIPLEGIA In this condition vascular diseases of the cerebrum and brainstem exceed all others in frequency. Trauma (brain contusion, epidural and subdural hemorrhage) ranks second, and other diseases such as brain tumor, brain abscess and encephalitis, demyelinative diseases, complications of meningitis, tuberculosis, and syphilis are of decreasing order of importance.

Paraplegia Paralysis of both lower extremities may occur in diseases of the spinal cord and the spinal roots or of the peripheral nerves. If onset is acute, it may be difficult to distinguish spinal from neural paralysis, for in any acute myelopathy spinal shock may result in abolition of reflexes and flaccidity. As a rule in acute spinal cord diseases with involvement of corticospinal tracts, the paralysis affects all muscles below a given level; and often, if the white matter is extensively damaged, sensory loss below a particular level (loss of pain and temperature sense with lateral spinothalamic tracts and loss of vibratory and position sense with posterior columns) is conjoined. Also, in bilateral disease of the spinal cord, the bladder and bowel sphincters are paralyzed. Alterations of cerebrospinal fluid (dynamic block, increase in protein or cells) are frequent. In peripheral nerve diseases both sensory loss and motor loss tend to involve the distal muscles of the legs more than the proximal ones (an exception is acute idiopathic polyneuritis), and the sphincters are often spared or only briefly deranged in function. Sensory loss, if present, is more likely to consist of distal impairment of touch, vibration, and position sense, with pain and temperature sense spared in many instances. The cerebrospinal fluid protein level may be normal or elevated.

Acute paraplegia beginning at any age is relatively infrequent. Fracture dislocation of the spine with traumatic necrosis of the spinal cord, spontaneous hematomyelia with bleeding from a vascular malformation (angioma, telangiectasis), thrombosis of a spinal artery with infarction (myelomalacia), and dissecting aortic aneurysm or atherosclerotic occlusion of nutrient spinal arteries arising from the aorta with resulting infarction (myelomalacia) are the commonest varieties of sudden paraplegia (or quadriplegia, if the cervical cord is involved). Postinfectious or postvaccinal myelitis, acute demyelinative myelitis (Devic's disease if the optic nerves are affected), necrotizing myelitis, and epidural abscess or tumor with spinal cord compression tend to develop somewhat more slowly, over a period of hours or days, or they may have a acute onset. Poliomyelitis, a purely motor disorder with meningitis, must be distinguished from the other acute myelopathies.

In adult life multiple sclerosis, subacute combined degeneration, spinal cord tumor, ruptured cervical disk and cervical spondylosis, syphilitic meningomyelitis, chronic epidural infections (fungous and other granulomatous diseases), Erb's spastic paraplegia and motor system disease, and syringomyelia represent the most frequently encountered forms of spinal paraplegia. (See Chap. 333 for discussion of these spinal cord diseases.) The several varieties of polyneuritis and polymyositis must be considered in their differential diagnosis, for they, too, may cause paraparesis. Friedreich's ataxia and familial paraplegia, progressive muscular dystrophy, and the chronic varieties of polyneuritis tend to appear during late childhood and adolescence and are slowly progressive.

Quadriplegia All that has been written about the common causes of paraplegia applies to quadriplegia. The lesion is usually in the cervical rather than the thoracic or lumbar segments of the spinal cord. If it is situated in the low cervical segments and involves the anterior half of the spinal cord, as in occlusion of the anterior spinal artery, the arm paralysis may be flaccid and areflexic and the leg paralysis spastic (anterior spinal syndrome). There are only a few points of difference between the common paraplegic and quadriplegic syndromes. Repeated cerebral vascular accidents may lead to bilateral hemiplegia, usually accompanied by pseudobulbar palsy.

Isolated paralysis Paralysis of isolated muscle groups usually indicates a lesion of one or more peripheral nerves. The diagnosis of a lesion of an individual peripheral nerve is made on the presence of weakness or paralysis of the muscle or group of muscles and impairment or loss of sensation in the distribution of the nerve in question (Chap. 331). Complete transection or severe injury to a peripheral nerve is usually followed by atrophy of the muscles it innervates and by loss of their tendon reflexes. Trophic changes in the skin, nails, and subcutaneous tissue may also occur. It is of considerable importance to decide whether the lesion is a temporary one of conduction only (neuropraxia) or whether there has been a pathologic dissolution of continuity, requiring nerve regeneration for recovery. Electromyography may be of value here.

EXAMINATION SCHEME FOR MOTOR PARALYSIS AND APRAXIA The first step is to inspect the paralyzed limb, taking note first of its posture and of the presence or absence of muscle atrophy, hypertrophy, and fascicular twitchings. The patient is then called upon to move each muscle group, and the power and facility of movement are graded and recorded. The range of passive movement is then determined by moving all the joints. This provides information concerning alterations of muscle tone, i.e., hypotonia, spasticity, and rigidity. Dislocations, diseased joints, and ankyloses may also be revealed by these same maneuvers. Muscle bulk is then inspected. Slight atrophy may be due to disuse from any cause, i.e., pain, fixation as the result of a cast, or any type of paralysis. Pronounced atrophy usually occurs only with denervation of several weeks' or months' standing (see Chap. 350).

The tendon reflexes are then tested. The usual routine is to try to elicit the jaw jerk (increased in pseudobulbar palsy) and the supinator, biceps, triceps, quadriceps, and Achilles tendon reflexes. Two cutaneous reflexes are then tested, the abdominal and plantar reflexes.

If there is no evidence of upper or lower motor neuron disease, but certain acts are nonetheless imperfectly performed, one should look for a disorder of postural sensibility or of cerebellar coordination or rigidity with abnormality of posture and movement due to disease of the basal ganglions (Chap. 18). In the absence of these disorders, the possibility of an apraxic disorder may be investigated by watching the patient's own movements and those called forth by specific command and gesture.

Hysterical paralysis may pose problems. Usually it is easily distinguished from chronic lower motor neuron disease by absence of areflexia and severe atrophy. Diagnostic difficulty arises only in certain acute cases of upper motor neuron disease that lack all the usual changes in reflexes and muscle tone. In hysterical paralysis one arm or one leg or all one side of the body may be affected. The hysterical gait is sometimes diagnostic (Chap. 19). Often there is loss of sensation in the paralyzed side, a group of sensory changes that is never seen in organic brain disease. The patient should be asked to move the affected limbs; as he does so, the movement is seen to be slow and jerky, often with contraction of both agonist and antagonist muscles simultaneously or intermittently. Hoover's sign and Babinski's combined leg flexion test are helpful in distinguishing hysterical from organic hemiplegia. To elicit Hoover's sign, the patient, lying on his back, is asked to rise one leg from the bed against resistance; in a normal individual the back of the heel of the contralateral leg is pressed firmly down, and the same is true when the patient with organic hemiplegia attempts to lift the paralyzed leg. The hysteric exerts little force with the good leg or will contract it more strongly under these circumstances than as a primary willed action. To carry out Babinski's combined leg flexion test, a patient with an organic hemiplegia is asked to sit up without using his arms; when he does so, the paralyzed or weak leg flexes at the hip, and the heel is lifted from the bed while the heel of the sound leg is pressed into the bed. This sign is absent in hysterical hemiplegia.

MUSCULAR PARALYSIS AND SPASM UNATTENDED BY VISIBLE CHANGE IN NERVE OR MUSCLE A group of diseases appears to have no basis in visible structural change in motor nerve cells, nerve fibers, motor end plates, and muscular fibers. This group is composed of myasthenia gravis, myotonia congenita (Thomsen's disease), familial periodic paralysis, disorders of potassium, sodium, calcium, and magnesium metabolism, tetany, tetanus, botulinus poisoning, black widow spider bite, and the thyroid myopathies. In these diseases, each of which possesses a fairly distinctive clinical picture, the abnormality is purely biochemical, and even if the patient survives for a long time, no visible microscopic changes develop. An understanding of these diseases requires knowledge of the processes involved in nerve and muscle excitation and the contraction of muscle. They are discussed in Chaps. 350 and 351.

REFERENCE

BRODAL A: *Neurological Anatomy in Relation to Clinical Medicine,* New York: Oxford, 1969

18
TREMOR, CHOREA, ATHETOSIS, ATAXIA, AND OTHER ABNORMALITIES OF MOVEMENT AND POSTURE

RAYMOND D. ADAMS

In this chapter are discussed the automatic, static, and less modifiable postural activities of the human nervous system. These are believed, on good evidence, to be an expression of the function of the *older motor system,* meaning the motor structures in the basal ganglia and brainstem.

In health, the activities of the motor systems of basal ganglia and cerebellum are blended and modulate the corticospinal and cortico-brainstem-spinal systems. The static postural activities of the former are indispensable to the voluntary or willed movements of the latter.

This close association of the corticospinal (formerly pyramidal) and extrapyramidal systems is shown by human disease. Lesions of the corticospinal tracts result not only in paralysis of volitional movements of the contralateral half of the body but in the appearance of a fixed posture or attitude in which the arm is maintained in flexion and the leg in extension (predilection type of Wernicke-Mann or hemiplegic dystonia of Denny-Brown). Similarly, decerebration from a lesion in the upper pons or midbrain releases another posture in which all four extremities are extended and the cervical and thoracolumbar spine dorsiflexed. In these released action patterns one has evidence of extrapyramidal postural and righting reflexes which are mediated through bulbospinal and other brainstem-spinal systems.

The student may be dismayed to read in current articles trenchant criticism of the validity of the concept of the corticospinal tract and the division of the motor system into corticospinal and extrapyramidal. Extremists claim the corticospinal tract may be severed in animals and even in man without lasting motor deficits. But it must be remembered that this tract is so puny in most mammals, even in small monkeys, that it can hardly be compared with that of man, and there has yet to be a pathologically proved example in man of complete interruption of this tract with preserved voluntary motor function.

If an oversimplification may be permitted for clarity of exposition, the extrapyramidal motor system may be subdivided into two parts: (1) the striatopallidonigral and (2) the cerebellar. Disease in either of these parts will result in disturbances of movement and posture without significant paralysis. These two major systems and the symptoms that result when they are diseased are reviewed on the following pages.

BASAL GANGLIA: PHARMACOLOGY AND PATHOLOGIC ANATOMY

As an anatomic entity the basal ganglia have no precise definition. The list of basal structures originally thought to have some part in motor function, such as the caudate and lenticular nuclei, has been greatly expanded by physiologists to include the field of Forel and zona incerta, subthalamic nucleus of Luys, substantia nigra, red nucleus, dentate nucleus of cerebellum, and the reticular formation of the brainstem. The anatomic connections between these structures and other parts of the brain, such as the cerebral cortex and afferent sensory systems, are too intricate to present in a textbook of medicine (cf. Brodal's monograph on neurologic anatomy).

The principal new anatomic datum to emerge in recent years is the central physiologic role of the ventrolateral (and anterior) nucleus of the thalamus. It is a vital link in an ascending fiber system from the lenticular nucleus and cerebellum to the motor cortex. Indeed it would seem that most of the basal ganglionic and cerebellar influence on the motor system is funneled through the ventral plane of thalamic nuclei, thus effecting a number of corticocortical circuits. Descending pathways to the spinal cord are disputed; probably there are polysynaptic descending fibers through the reticular formation of the pons and medulla to the motor neurons of the spinal cord. It is noteworthy that these ascending thalamocortical fibers pass through the internal capsule and cerebral white matter; hence lesions in these parts may simultaneously affect both corticospinal and extrapyramidal systems.

Another exciting development has been the discovery that certain drugs such as the phenothiazines produce extrapyramidal syndromes (Parkinson's disease, athetosis, dystonia, etc.); this has led to a major advance in the chemistry of central neurotransmitters. In man it has been found that the substantia nigra, putamen, and caudatum are rich in dopamine, serotonin, and norepinephrine. Of these substances dopamine has excited the greatest attention; the metabolic pathways involved are depicted in Fig. 94-1. Dopa is seen to be a step in the metabolism not only of norepinephrine but also of melanin. Norepinephrine is an important intercellular transmitter substance in the hypothalamus and peripheral autonomic system; melanin is contained in certain of the neurons of the substantia nigra and other pigmented nuclei of the brainstem. Dopamine has physiologic properties of its own; probably it, too, is a transmitter substance in the parts of the brain where it is concentrated.

The metabolic pathway of serotonin, or 5-hydroxytryptamine, the other postulated neurotransmitter, is shown in Fig. 103-1.

In Parkinson's disease the lenticular nuclei and substantia nigra have a reduced content of dopamine, serotonin, and acetylcholine, and the content of the major metabolite, homovanillic acid, is decreased in these parts and in the cerebrospinal fluid (CSF). A number of the tranquilizing medications, such as reserpine and chlorpromazine, deplete the basal ganglia of these substances. The quantity of dopamine in the striatum and substantia nigra is also decreased, and the administration of L-dopa orally or intravenously replenishes the stores in the basal ganglia, with concomitant improvement in extrapyramidal symptoms. Further information concerning the biochemistry of the catecholamines, serotonin, and norepinephrine may be found in Chaps. 94 and 103.

Some of the most significant facts about clinicopathologic relationships in man are to be found in the writings of a number of famous neurologists. In 1912 S. A. K. Wilson delineated the syndrome of familial lenticular degeneration, and at about the same time Van Woerkem observed a disturbance of basal ganglionic and cerebral function in acquired forms of liver disease. The putamen and globus pallidus were thought to be the main anatomic sites of both types of hepatocerebral degeneration. In 1920 Oskar and Cecile Vogt described a number of other motor disturbances associated with lesions limited to the striatum (putamen and caudatum). Lewy was one of the first to describe the pathology of paralysis agitans, and with the work of Tretiakoff (in postencephalitic forms) and Hassler (in paralysis agitans) at least some of the lesions were localized in the substantia nigra. The thorough studies of Huntington's chorea by Bielschowsky in 1919 related the choreoathetosis to lesions in the caudate nucleus and putamen. A long series of observations, the most recent ones being those of J. Purdon Martin, have related hemiballismus to lesions in the subthalamic nucleus of Luys.

Table 18-1 presents clinicopathologic correlations accepted by many neurologists; however, there is still much uncertainty as to finer details.

The symptoms that lend themselves best to clinical analysis are akinesia, rigidity, chorea, athetosis, dystonia, myoclonus, and tremor.

TABLE 18-1
Clinicopathologic correlations

Symptoms	*Principal location of morbid anatomy*
Unilateral plastic rigidity with static tremor (Parkinson's syndrome)	Contralateral substantia nigra plus (?) other structures
Unilateral hemiballismus and hemichorea	Contralateral subthalamic nucleus of Luys, prerubral area, and Forel's fields
Chronic chorea of Huntington's type	Caudate nucleus, putamen
Athetosis and dystonia	Contralateral putamen or thalamus
Cerebellar ataxia, i.e., intention tremor; slowness in starting and stopping alternating voluntary movements; hypotonia; rebound phenomenon	Homolateral cerebellar hemisphere or middle and inferior cerebellar peduncles, superior brachium conjunctivum (ipsilateral if below the decussation, contralateral if above)
Decerebrate rigidity, i.e., opisthotonos, extension of arms and legs	Lesion usually bilateral in tegmentum, involving upper brainstem, particularly red nucleus or structures between red nucleus and vestibular nuclei
Palatal and facial myoclonus (rhythmic)	Lesion in the central tegmental tract, inferior olivary nucleus, and olivodentate connections
Diffuse myoclonus	Cerebellar cortex (?), thalami (?)

AKINESIA

When extrapyramidal disease is analyzed along classic neurologic lines into primary functional deficits and secondary release effects, akinesia stands as the principal negative or deficit symptom. By the term *akinesia* one refers to the disinclination of the patient to use an affected part of the body, to engage it freely in all the natural actions of the body. In contrast to paralysis, the negative symptom of corticospinal lesions, strength is undiminished in the part, and it can be used effectively in the desired movement. In this respect, too, it is unlike apraxia, where movements are lost because of a lesion which erases the memory of the motor schema that forms a sequence of movements for intended action. The parkinsonian patient exhibits the phenomenon of akinesia most clearly in his extreme underactivity. He sits motionless for long times. In looking to the side he moves his eyes, not his head. In arising from a chair he fails to make all the little adjustments needed (putting feet back, putting hands on arms of chair, etc.). He neglects his affected arm. Yet he is not weak (paretic) or apraxic. Formerly, akinesia was attributed to rigidity, which could reasonably hamper all movements, but now that stereotaxic surgery has been shown to abolish both tremor and rigidity, it becomes clear that the motor deficit, or akinesia, is still there. Strictly interpreted it would appear that, apart from their contribution to the maintenance of postures, the basal ganglia must provide something essential to the performance of the large variety of semiautomatic actions that make up the full repertoire of natural human motility.

ALTERATIONS OF MUSCLE TONE (SPASTICITY, RIGIDITY, HYPOTONIA)

It has been pointed out that muscle tone (the small resistance to muscle stretch offered by healthy muscle) is enhanced in the many conditions that cause a paralysis of voluntary movement by interrupting the corticospinal tract. The special distribution of the increased tone (i.e., greater in antigravity muscles—leg extensors and arm flexors in man), the sudden augmentation of tone with gradual yielding upon quick movement (the lengthening reaction or clasp-knife phenomenon), the absence of resistance upon slow movement and its disappearance in relaxed muscle with "electromyographic silence when relaxed," and exaggerated tendon reflexes are the identifying characteristics of spasticity. This type of hypertonus is believed to be due in some instances to hyperactivity of the small gamma motor neurons, resulting in increase in the sensitivity of the spindle muscle fibers to stretch; in other instances it seems clearly related to excessive activity (or disinhibition) of the larger alpha motor neurons. The "gamma spasticity" is abolished by procaine injection of the motor nerve, which paralyzes the small gamma motor and sensory fibers, leaving the larger ones intact, without weakening the willed contractions of the muscle; the "alpha spasticity" is not affected by procaine.

In the state known as *rigidity* the muscles are continuously or intermittently firm, tense, and prominent; and the resistance to passive movement is intense and even, like that noted in bending a lead pipe or in stretching a strand of toffee. Although rigidity is present in all muscle groups, both flexor and extensor, on the whole it tends to be more prominent in those which maintain a flexed posture, i.e., the flexor muscles of trunk and limbs. It appears to be somewhat greater in the large muscle groups, but this may be merely a question of muscle mass. Certainly the smaller muscles of the face and tongue and even those of the larynx are often affected. Nevertheless, like "gamma spasticity," this rigidity is said to be abolished by procaine, and Foerster earlier demonstrated that it is eradicated by posterior root section. In the electromyographic tracing, motor unit activity is more continuous than in spasticity, persisting even after relaxation.

A special type of rigidity is the *cogwheel phenomenon.* When the hypertonic muscle is passively stretched, the resistance may be rhythmically jerky, as though the resistance of the limb were controlled by a ratchet. A number of different explanations of this phenomenon have been suggested. Wilson postulated that it might be due to a minor form of the lengthening-shortening reaction, but a more likely explanation is an associated static tremor that is masked by rigidity during an attitude of repose but emerges faintly during manipulation.

Rigidity is prominent in extrapyramidal diseases such as paralysis agitans, postencephalitic Parkinson's syndrome, and dystonia musculorum deformans.

The *tension hypertonus of athetosis* differs from both spasticity and rigidity. Strictly speaking, it takes two forms, one which occurs during the involuntary athetotic movement, and another which appears in the absence of any involuntary motion. Clinically these forms of hypertonus are variable from one moment to the next and are paradoxic in that they sometimes disappear during a rapid passive movement or when the limb is passively shaken. The tendon reflexes may be normal or brisk. The lengthening and shortening reactions are absent. This form of variable hypertonus is found in double athetosis and choreoathetosis and in some cases of dystonia musculorum deformans. Usually in Sydenham's and Huntington's chorea a state of hypotonia prevails, sometimes as strikingly as in sensory polyneuropathies and lower motor neuron paralyses.

INVOLUNTARY MOVEMENTS

CHOREA Derived from the Greek word meaning "dance," *chorea* refers to widespread arrhythmic movements of a forcible, rapid, jerky type. These movements are involuntary and are noted for their irregularity, variability, relative speed, and brief duration. They may be simple or quite elaborate and of variable distribution. In some respects they resemble a voluntary movement in their complexity, yet they are never combined into a coordinated act. The patient may, however, incorporate them into a deliberate movement, as if to make them less noticeable. When superimposed on voluntary movements, they may take on a grotesque and exaggerated character. Grimacing and peculiar respiratory sounds may be other expressions of the movement disorder. Usually the movements are discrete, but if very numerous, they may flow into one another; the resultant picture then resembles athetosis. They may be limited to a limb or an arm and leg on one side (hemichorea), or they may involve all parts of the body. Normal volitional movements are, of course, possible, for there is no paralysis, but they too may be excessively quick and poorly sustained. The limbs are often unusually slack, or hypotonic. A choreic movement may be superimposed on a tendon reflex, giving rise to the "hung-up reflex." The tendon reflexes tend to be pendular because of the associated hypotonia; when the knee jerk is elicited with the patient sitting, the leg swings back and forth four or five times, like a pendulum, rather than one or two times as in a normal person.

Chorea appears in typical form in Sydenham's chorea and was noted also in the acute stages of epidemic encephalitis lethargica. It is a feature also of Huntington's chorea (chronic chorea), where the movements tend more typically to be choreoathetotic. Vascular lesions in the subthalamus, particularly those in and near the subthalamic nucleus of Luys, may result in wild flinging movements of the opposite arm and leg (hemiballismus). As these subside, they become almost indistinguishable from chorea. Phenothiazine drugs and, rarely, hyperthyroidism may cause chorea.

ATHETOSIS This term is from a Greek word meaning "unfixed" or "changeable." The condition is characterized by an inability to sustain the fingers and toes, tongue, or any other group of muscles in one position. The maintained posture is interrupted by continuous, slow, sinuous, purposeless movements. These are most pronounced in the digits and the hands but often involve the tongue, throat, and face. One can detect as basic patterns of movement an extension and pronation and flexion and supination of the arm, and alternating flexion and extension of the fingers. They may be unilateral, especially in children who have suffered a hemiplegia at some previous date (posthemiplegic athetosis). The movements are slower than those of chorea, but in many cases gradations between the two (choreoathetosis) are seen. Most athetotic patients exhibit variable degrees of motor deficit due in some instances to associated corticospinal tract disease. Discrete individual movements of the tongue, lips, and hand are often impossible, and attempts to perform such voluntary movements result in a contraction of all the muscles in the limb (an *intention spasm*). Variable degrees of rigidity are generally associated, and these may account for the slower quality of athetosis, in contrast to chorea. It must be admitted, however, that in some cases it is almost impossible to distinguish between chorea and athetosis.

Athetosis or choreoathetosis of all four limbs is a cardinal feature of a curious state known as *double athetosis,* which begins in childhood. Athetosis appearing in the first months of life usually represents a congenital or postnatal condition such as hypoxia, kernicterus, or birth injury. Postmortem examination in some of the cases has disclosed a peculiar pathologic change of probable hypoxic etiology, a status marmoratus in the striatum and thalamus; in others there has been a loss of medullated fibers, a status dysmyelinisatus, in the same regions. In adults athetosis may occur as an episodic illness or persistently in acquired hepatocerebral degeneration, in postphenothiazine dyskinesias, and in certain degenerative diseases.

TORSION SPASM OR DYSTONIA Torsion spasm is closely allied to athetosis, differing only in that the larger axial muscles (those of the trunk and limb girdles) rather than appendicular muscles are involved. It results in bizarre, grotesque movements and positions of the body. The word *dystonia* has been given to these movements but, unfortunately, is also applied to any fixed posture which may be the end result of a disease of the motor system. Thus Denny-Brown speaks of hemiplegic dystonia, the flexion dystonia of parkinsonism, and extensor dystonia with retraction of the head and arching or twisting of the back. If the latter meaning is given, it would be better to speak of athetosis of the trunk as torsion spasms or phasic dystonia, in contrast to fixed dystonia. The former, like athetosis, may show remarkable fluctuations; sometimes the whole musculature of the body may be thrown into spasm by an effort to move an arm or to speak. If mild, the torsion spasm may be limited to the lumbar or cervical muscles or those of one limb and may cease when the body is at rest.

Torsion spasm may be seen in the condition of double athetosis after hypoxic damage to the brain, in kernicterus, and, rarely, in Wilson's hepatolenticular degeneration. It is most characteristic of the syndrome designated *dystonia musculorum deformans* but also occurs in other conditions such as the postphenothiazine dyskinesias and Hallevorden-Spatz disease (Chap. 341).

Chorea, athetosis, and torsion spasm are all closely related. The movements are elaborate and depend for their expression on cortical mechanisms. Paralytic lesions involving the corticospinal tract abolish the involuntary movements. The hypotonia in chorea and some cases of athetosis, the pendular reflexes, and some degree of interference with natural movements are also reminiscent of the syndrome that follows disease of the cerebellum. Lacking, however, are intention tremor and true incoordination or ataxia.

MYOCLONUS This term refers to several different motor disorders, some localized, others diffuse. As in chorea, the myoclonic movement is involuntary and arrhythmic, but it is much faster than chorea, being concluded in a few hundred milliseconds or less. Variations in degree are noteworthy; it may consist of no more than a flick of a single muscle or part of a muscle, but the larger movements always betray its nature, involving as they do a group of muscles. Thus myoclonus may be distinguished from fasciculation. Sensory relationships are another prominent attribute. Flickering light, a series of loud sounds, or abrupt contact with some part of the body may regularly initiate a jerk, sometimes as a direct sensorimotor effect, again through the mechanism of startle. One special variety is evoked by willed movement, presumably through a proprioceptive mechanism. Hence, one may speak of action or intention myoclonus, auditory or visual myoclonus. A series of intense stimuli may recruit a series of myoclonic jerks into a full-blown seizure, as happens often in the familial myoclonic epilepsy syndrome of Unverricht-Lundborg. The pathologic disturbance in the latter is usually a lipid storage disease or an amyloid Lafora body inclusion disease (Chap. 341).

Familial types of myoclonus may persist in almost pure form or in association with mild ataxia over a period of many years. In the child and adult, herpes simplex encephalitis may present as a confusional state and dementia with myoclonus. In the elderly adult diffuse myoclonus and a rapidly evolving dementia are prominent symptoms in Creutzfeldt-Jakob disease. Intention myoclonus is often a sequela to anoxic encephalopathy. Postsomnolescent myoclonic jerks of arms for 20 to 30 min after a night's sleep are reported by some patients with idiopathic epilepsy. In all these diseases the pathologic changes are so widespread that anatomic localization is impossible. The least degrees of lesion causing myoclonus are seemingly located in the thalamus and cerebellum. Indeed cerebellar incoordination and intention tremor are combined with diffuse myoclonus of the action or intention type in several of the aforementioned diseases, i.e., lipidoses and the Lafora body type of myoclonus.

The term *myoclonus* unfortunately has also been assigned to a rather different motor phenomenon—that of repetitious, rhythmic clonus of some part of the "branchial cleft" or craniocervical musculature. An example is "nystagmus of the palate" (rhythmic contractions at the rate of 10 to 50 or more per min of the soft palate, pharyngeal muscles, vocal cords, facial muscles, and diaphragm). The lesions producing this state, which we would prefer to designate as a form of continuous *bulbar, facial,* or *diaphragmatic clonus,* have been situated in all instances in the central tegmental tract, inferior olivary nucleus, or olivocerebellar tract. The causative lesions have been infarcts, tumors, and encephalitic processes.

The main fault with our concept of myoclonus is that it covers too many motor disorders. When movements are grouped according to their brevity or involuntary nature, one must include the normal dormescent start or jerk of a limb as one falls asleep, and the motor components of a natural startle reaction. The obligatory Moro response also falls within the group, as well as the form of epilepsy known as infantile or salaam spasms and the falling spells of the petit mal triad. Metrazol injections cause myoclonus of the limbs, which has been shown to depend on a lower brainstem (medullary reticular) mechanism. Another problem arises on the clinical side in distinguishing diffuse myoclonus from other abrupt involuntary movements such as tremors, chorea, and restricted forms of epilepsy (epilepsia partialis continua). Speed of movement, lack of rhythmicity, and relationships to sensory stimulation prove to be the most reliable identifying features of the larger group of myoclonic disorders. There is an advantage in trying to separate the arrhythmic diffuse form from the rhythmic restricted form in that each stands as a diagnostic attribute of a separate category of nervous diseases.

TREMOR This consists of a more or less regular rhythmic oscillation of a part of the body around a fixed point. The rate varies from three to eight oscillations per second; in a particular person the rate is fairly constant in all affected parts, regardless of the size of the muscle or of the part of the body. Tremors usually involve the distal part of the limbs, the head, tongue, or jaw, and rarely the trunk.

There are many different types of tremor, and only a few are recognized as bearing any meaningful relationship to disease of the extrapyramidal motor system; but since tremors have not been discussed elsewhere, all the different types will be considered here.

Tremors may be subdivided according to their distribution, amplitude, regularity, and relationship to volitional movement. The tremors described in the following paragraphs should be familiar to every physician.

Static (parkinsonian) tremor This is a coarse, rhythmic tremor, with an average rate of four to five beats per second, most often localized in one or both hands, and, occasionally, in the jaw or tongue. Its most characteristic feature is that it occurs when the limb is in an attitude of repose, and willed movement at least temporarily suppresses it. If the tremulous limb is completely relaxed, the tremor usually disappears, but the average patient rarely achieves this state. In some cases the tremor is constant; in others it varies from time to time and with the progress of the disease extends from one group of muscles to another. In paralysis agitans the tremor tends to be rather gentle and more or less limited to the distal muscles, whereas in postencephalitic parkinsonism and hepatolenticular degeneration it often has a wider range and involves proximal muscles. In many cases there is a variable degree of rigidity of a plastic type. The tremor interferes with voluntary movements surprisingly little; it is not uncommon to see a patient who has been trembling violently raise a full glass of water to his lips and drain the contents without spilling a drop. The handwriting of these patients is often small and cramped (micrographia). The gait may be of festinating type. It is the combination of static tremor, slowness of movement, rigidity, and flexed postures without true paralysis that constitutes Parkinson's syndrome (also called *amyostatic* syndrome).

The exact pathologic anatomy of static tremor is unknown. In paralysis agitans and postencephalitic Parkinson's syndrome, the visible lesions are predominantly in the substantia nigra. In hepatocerebral degeneration, where this syndrome is mixed with cerebellar ataxia, the lesions are more diffuse. A similar tremor, without rigidity, slowness of movement, flexed postures, or masked facies, is seen in senile persons. Unlike Parkinson's disease, it does not progress.

Action tremor This term refers to a tremor present when the limbs are actively maintained in a certain position, as when outstretched, and throughout voluntary movement. It may increase slightly as the action of the limbs becomes more precise, but it never approaches the degree of augmentation in fine movement seen in intention tremor. It is easily made to disappear when the limbs are relaxed. Probably some of the *action tremors* are but an exaggeration of normal or physiologic tremor, which ranges from six to eight per second, being slower in childhood and old age. In adults the tremor is of small excursion, has a frequency of seven to eight per second, and is somewhat irregular. The tremor involves the outstretched hand, head, and, less often, the lips and tongue, and it interferes little with voluntary movements such as handwriting and speech. This type of tremor is seen in numerous medical, neurologic, and psychiatric diseases and is therefore more difficult to interpret than static tremor. There are somewhat slower frequencies of action tremor, and instead of rather irregular potentials in both agonist and antagonist muscles, their activity alternates. Either form, when occurring as the only neurologic abnormality in several members of a family, is known as *familial* or *hereditary tremor.* Familial tremor may begin in childhood, but usually comes on later and persists throughout adult life. Being worse when the patient is under observation, it becomes a source of embarrassment because it suggests to the onlooker that the patient is nervous. A curious fact about familial tremors is that one or two drinks of an alcoholic beverage may abolish them, and they may become worse after the effects of the alcohol have worn off. Similar tremors are seen in delirious states, such as delirium tremens, in chronic alcoholism as an isolated symptom ("the morning shakes"), and in general paresis. An action tremor, usually more rapid than the above, is also characteristic of hyperthyroidism and other toxic states, and a similar tremor is frequently observed in patients suffering intense anxiety. In fact it can be reproduced by injections of epinephrine. Severe action tremor may also accompany certain diseases of the basal ganglia, including parkinsonism. Some of the fast-frequency action tremors are suppressed by beta-adrenergic blocking agents (propranolol, 40 mg t.i.d.).

Intention tremor The word *intention* is ambiguous in this context because the tremor itself is not intentional. The term means, instead, that the tremor requires for its full expression the performance of an exacting, precise, willed movement. The term *ataxic tremor* has been suggested because it is always combined with and adds to cerebellar ataxia. The tremor is absent when the limbs are inactive and during the first part of a voluntary movement, but as the action continues and greater precision of movement is demanded (e.g., in touching a target such as the patient's nose or the examiner's finger), a jerky, more or less rhythmic interruption of forward progression, with side-to-side oscillation, appears. It continues for a fraction of a second or so after the act is completed. The tremor may seriously interfere with the patient's performance of skilled acts. Sometimes the head is involved (titubation). This type of tremor invariably indicates disease of the cerebellum and of its connections. When the disease is very severe, every movement, even the lifting of a limb, results in a wide-ranging tremor of such violence as to throw the patient off balance. This latter state is occasionally seen in multiple sclerosis, Wilson's disease, and vascular and other lesions of the midbrain and subthalamus but not of the cerebellum.

Hysterical tremor Hysterical tremors may simulate any of the aforementioned varieties and are difficult to diagnose. One notable feature is that they usually do not correspond to any of the better-known types of organic tremor. Most often they are restricted to a limb, and they are seldom as regular as the static tremors of paralysis agitans. If the affected limb is restrained by the examiner, the tremor may move to another part of the body. It persists during movement and at rest and is less subject to the modifying influences of posture and willed movement than organic tremors are. This manifestation of hysteria is exceedingly rare.

OTHER INVOLUNTARY MOVEMENTS There are other abnormalities of movement, about which only a few words can be said. They vary from simple irritative phenomena to complex psychologically related disorders, such as compulsions, mannerisms, etc.

Spasmodic torticollis This is an intermittent or continuous spasm of sternomastoid, trapezius, and other neck muscles, usually more pronounced on one side, with turning or tipping of the head. It is involuntary and cannot be inhibited and thereby differs from habit spasm or tic. This condition should be considered a form of dystonia. It is worse when the patient sits, stands, or walks, and usually contactual stimulation of the chin or of the back of the head partially alleviates the muscle imbalance. Psychiatric treatment is ineffectual. In severe cases muscle sectioning, neurectomy, or section of the anterior cervical roots has given favorable results.

Other craniocervical spasms Blepharoclonus (inability to keep the eyes open), lingual spasms, "spastic" dysphonia, facial spasms, and cervicothoracic spasms are all special varieties of involuntary movement, appearing usually in late middle life and the senium. Facial, cervical, and thoracic spasms have occurred with striking frequency during phenothiazine medication. Transiency, or nonprogressivity, unresponsiveness to psychotherapy, and uncertain amelioration by all pharmacologic agents characterize most of them. Exceptionally, these disorders are induced by drugs of the phenothiazine class and persist after their discontinuance (tardive or postphenothiazine dyskinesias).

Tics and habit spasms Many persons throughout life are given to habitual movements, such as sniffing, clearing the throat, protruding the chin, or blinking, whenever they become tense. The patient admits that the movements are voluntary and that he feels compelled to make them in order to relieve tension; they can be inhibited for a time by an effort of will but reappear when attention is diverted. In certain cases they become so ingrained that the person is unaware of them and unable to control them. Children between five and ten years of age are especially likely to have habit spasms. The movements are often purposive coordinated acts which normally serve the organism; it is only their incessant repetition when uncalled for that constitutes a habit. Stereotypy is their main identifying feature. Multiple convulsive tics *(Gilles de la Tourette's disease)* constitute a more severe form of the same condition. In children it is best to ignore the habit spasm and at the same time to arrange for more rest and calmer environment. In adults relief of nervous tension by tranquilizing drugs and psychotherapy is helpful, but the disposition to tic formation persists. Mentally backward children and adults often display, when idle, a wide variety of rhythmic body-rocking, head-bobbing, arm-and-finger movements. These are of the nature of mannerisms and have no known basal ganglion pathology.

EXTRAPYRAMIDAL MOTOR DISTURBANCES DUE PRIMARILY TO DISEASES OF THE CEREBELLUM

Isolated lesions in the midline flocculonodular lobe result in grave disturbances of equilibrium. Often the symptoms are exhibited only when the patient attempts to stand and walk. He sways, staggers, titubates, and reels (see below under Disturbance of Movement and Posture). There may be no disturbance in coordination and no intention tremor of the limbs. A midline tumor of the cerebellum such as medulloblastoma, hemorrhage, or other lesion usually produces this syndrome.

Extensive lesions of one cerebellar hemisphere, especially the anterior lobe, cause disturbances in coordination of volitional movements of the ipsilateral arm and leg. This is known as *ataxia.* The movements are characterized by an inappropriate range, rate, and strength of each of the various components of the motor act and by an improper combination of those components. Electromyographic analysis has shown that ataxia is manifested as a decomposition of movement consisting of abnormal duration and timing of bursts of contraction and relaxation of agonists and antagonists of a joint, usually a large one (Carrera and Mettler). This incoordination is also called *asynergia.* The defects are particularly noticeable in acts that require rapid alternation of movements. Slowness in acceleration and deceleration, which is almost invariably present, impedes the performance (dysdiadochokinesis). The direction of projected (purposive) movement is frequently inaccurate. Owing to delay in arresting a movement, the patient may overshoot his mark. The antagonist muscles do not come into play at the proper time, possibly because of the hypotonia that is almost always present. This may be demonstrated by having the patient flex his arm against a resistance that is suddenly released. The patient with cerebellar disease will sometimes strike his face because he fails to check the flexion movement (Holmes rebound phenomenon). In movements requiring accurate direction, as the limb approaches its destination it may stop short and then advance by a more or less rhythmic series of jerks and oscillations (intention tremor). In addition to hypotonia, there may be, in acute cerebellar lesions, some slight weakness.

A similar ataxia, asynergia, and dysmetria, usually with hypotonia and only a little intention tremor, may accompany lesions of the lateral and inferior parts of the cerebellar hemisphere. Bilateral lesions of the cerebellar hemispheres and midline flocculonodular lobe lead to such a severe disturbance in all movements that the patient may be unable to stand or walk or use his limbs effectively. In addition, there are ocular and speech disturbances, namely, nystagmus, dysmetria, and skew deviation of the eyes, and dysarthria. Lesions of the cerebellar peduncles have the same effect as extensive hemispheral lesions. This syndrome, due to involvement of one cerebellar hemisphere, may be observed in a tumor or abscess or in vascular lesions of the brainstem and cerebellar peduncles. The ataxia tends to be bilateral and symmetric in primary atrophy or degeneration of the cerebellum. There have been numerous attempts to explain in physiologic terms the hypotonia, mild degrees of weakness and fatigability, and abnormalities in the rate and regularity of projected movement that accompany cerebellar lesions in man. It has been found that depression of fusimotor (spindle) efferent activity in the spinal cord leads to decreased spindle afferent discharge and lessened tonic facilitation of alpha motor neuron activity. The cerebellar facilitation that is lost with acute lesions is normally mediated through two systems of fibers—the fastigioreticulospinal and the dentatorubrothalamocortical. The latter, acting specifically on cortical areas 4 and 6, is the more important in man. Although the corticospinal tract is probably essential for expression of cerebellar deficits in man, in the primate any pathway subserving specifically projected movements into environment may support tremor and other parts of the syndrome. Tremor, ataxia, and hypotonia seem to be separable, independent entities, but all are believed related to the disturbed fusimotor activity.

A kind of pseudoataxia, especially of gait, may be caused by the improper timing of the components of complex actions, e.g., with defects in postural sense (sensory ataxia) and with slow relaxation of muscles in hypothyroidism (myxedema with ataxia).

SOME GENERAL FEATURES OF ALL EXTRAPYRAMIDAL MOTOR DISTURBANCES

From the above discussion of many special types of motor disorder the reader must not think that they always appear in pure form. Various combinations occur in diseases. For example, Wilson's disease usually presents with a Parkinson-like picture of tremor, rigidity, slowness of movement, and flexion dystonia of trunk, but exceptionally there is athetosis, tonic innervation (inability to relax a voluntary movement), phasic dystonia, and intention tremor. Hallevorden-Spatz disease may take the form of universal rigidity and flexion dystonia or choreoathetosis. Occasionally the degeneration of Huntington's chorea leads to rigidity rather than choreoathetosis. Corticospinal and various of these extrapyramidal disorders may be associated in patients with cerebral diplegia. Nonetheless certain combinations tend to occur with greater or lesser frequency in certain diseases, as discussed in Chaps. 338, 340, and 341.

In broad terms all the extrapyramidal disorders should be viewed in terms of the primary deficit (negative symptom) and of the new phenomena (movements, abnormal postures, tremors, etc.) which have appeared. These latter positive symptoms are presently ascribed to release from or disequilibrium of undamaged motor parts of the nervous system. The clearest negative effect is usually evidenced as an akinesia, or disinclination to use the affected muscles. The difficulty in rapid alternating sequences of movement stands as another negative effect in diseases of both the basal ganglia and the cerebellum. In fact this latter symptom, presenting as a clumsiness, may be the only fault manifest in certain maladroit children. Stress and nervous tension characteristically worsen both the motor deficiency and the abnormal movements in all these extrapyramidal syndromes, just as relaxation helps the motor performance. All the movement disorders are abolished in sleep.

One of the most remarkable discoveries of recent years, to be credited largely to the pioneering efforts of neurosurgeons (Meyer, Cooper), has been the abolition of tremors, rigidity, and involuntary movements of the limbs by a surgical lesion in the medial segment of the globus pallidus or the ventrolateral nucleus of the thalamus. The effects are contralateral. Usually the lesion has been made first by the injection of procaine (Novocain) and then by use of alcohol, cooling and freezing (Cooper), or electrocoagulation (White and Sweet and Leksell). The operation has been successful in temporarily alleviating tremor or rigidity (or both) on one side. The procedure is successful in approximately 80 percent of cases of paralysis agitans, and the postural abnormality in dystonia musculorum deformans and double athetosis has responded somewhat less consistently. The operations have been perfected to the point at which the mortality rate is less than 1 percent, and the risk of hemiplegia or some other sequel is less than 10 percent. Of course, as the disease progresses, the beneficial effects are lost. The therapeutic procedure indicates that the pallidum and ventrolateral nucleus, probably through their connections with the cerebral cortex (motor cortex and its corticospinal pathway), are essential for the expression of these extrapyramidal syndromes. The indications for these surgical procedures are discussed in Chap. 341.

DISTURBANCE OF MOVEMENT AND POSTURE: EXAMINATION AND DIFFERENTIAL DIAGNOSIS

In Chap. 17 the methods of examining the motor system are described at some length, so only a few additional remarks concerning extrapyramidal disorders need be made here. These abnormalities are best demonstrated by seeing the patient in action. If he complains of a limp after walking a distance or of difficulty in climbing stairs, he should be observed under these conditions. Tests of rate, regularity, and coordination of voluntary movement must be sufficiently varied and demanding of the patient's motor coordination to bring out the defect. The physician must cultivate the habit of accurately observing and describing abnormalities of movement and must not be content merely to give the condition a name or to force it into some category such as chorea, tic, or myoclonus. The main postures of the body in all common acts should be noted. Aside from the assessment of muscle power and of gait, the usual test applied to the upper limb is to ask the patient to touch the examiner's fingertip and then the tip of his own nose repeatedly *(finger-to-nose test).* To test the leg, the patient is asked to place his heel on one knee and then to run it down his shin and back to the knee *(heel-to-knee-to-shin test).* Finer movements of the hand may be tested by having the patient successively touch each finger to his thumb, pat his thigh rapidly, or use tools or handle objects. Rapidly alternating movements such as repeatedly touching the index finger with the thumb, pronation and supination of wrist, or opening and closing the hands are valuable tests.

The fully developed extrapyramidal motor syndromes can be recognized without difficulty once the physician has become familiar with the typical pictures. The mental picture of Parkinson's syndrome, with its slowness of movement, poverty of facial expression, and static tremor and rigidity, should be fixed in mind. Similarly, the gross distortions and postural abnormalities of dystonia, whether widespread in trunk muscles or involving only neck muscles, as in spasmodic torticollis, once seen should thereafter be familiar. Athetosis, with its instability of postures and ceaseless movements of fingers and hands; intention spasm, chorea, with its more rapid and complicated movements; and the abrupt movements of myoclonus that flit over the body are other standard syndromes. Characteristic of all is a mild defect in the voluntary use of the affected parts.

The clinical differences between corticospinal and extrapyramidal disorders are summarized in Table 18-2.

Early or mild forms of these conditions, like all medical diseases, may offer special difficulties in diagnosis. Cases of paralysis agitans, seen before the appearance of tremor, are often overlooked. The patient may complain of being nervous and restless or may have experienced an indescribable stiffness and aching in certain parts of the body. Because of the absence of weakness or of reflex changes, the case may be considered psychogenic or rheumatic. It is well to remember that Parkinson's syndrome often begins in a hemiplegic distribution, and for this reason the illness may be misdiagnosed as cerebral thrombosis. A slight masking of the face, a suggestion of a limp, blepharoclonus (uninhibited blinking of eyes when the bridge of the nose is tapped), a mild rigidity, failure of an arm to swing naturally in walking, or loss of certain movements of cooperation will help in diagnosis at this time. Every case presenting the syndrome of Parkinson or other abnormality of movement and posture in adolescence or early adult life should be surveyed for hepatolenticular degeneration by tests of liver function and slit-lamp examination for corneal pigmentation (Kayser-Fleischer ring); if facilities are available, urinary amino-nitrogen excretion and copper excretion should be determined.

Mild or early chorea is often mistaken for simple nervousness. If one sits for a time and watches the patient, the diagnosis will often become evident. There are cases, nonetheless, in which it is impossible to distinguish simple nervousness from early Sydenham's chorea, especially in children, and there is no laboratory test upon which one can depend. The first postural manifestation of dystonia may suggest hysteria, and it is only later, when the fixity of the postural abnormality, the lack of the usual psychologic picture of hysteria, and the relentlessly progressive character of the illness become evident, that accurate diagnosis is reached. Another common error is to assume that a bedfast patient who has complained of dizziness, staggering, and headaches and exhibits no other neurologic abnormality is suffering from hysteria. The flocculonodular cerebellar syndrome is demonstrable only when the patient attempts to stand and walk.

The uncertainty of balance and short-stepped gait (marche à petit pas) in the elderly is often incorrectly attributed to loss of confidence and fear of falling.

TABLE 18-2
Clinical differences between corticospinal and extrapyramidal syndromes

	Corticospinal	*Extrapyramidal*
Character of rigidity	Clasp-knife effect	Plastic, equal throughout (massive movement or intermittent cogwheel rigidity)
Distribution of rigidity	Flexors of arms, extensors of legs	Flexors of all four limbs and trunk
Shortening and lengthening reaction	Present	Absent
Involuntary movements	Absent	Presence of tremors, chorea, athetosis, dystonia
Tendon reflexes	Increased	Normal or slightly increased
Babinski's sign	Present	Absent
Paralysis of voluntary movement	Present	Absent or slight

REFERENCES

BRODAL A: *Neurological Anatomy in Relation to Clinical Medicine,* New York: Oxford, 1969

COOPER IS: *Involuntary Movement Disorders,* New York: Hoeber, 1969

CUMINGS JN: Biochemistry of the basal ganglia, chap. 4 in *Handbook of Clinical Neurology,* vol. 6, eds PJ Vinken and GW

Bruyn, Amsterdam: North Holland Publishing Company, 1968, p. 116

DENNY-BROWN, D: Clinical symptomatology of disease of the basal ganglia, in *Handbook of Clinical Neurology,* vol. 6, eds PJ Vinken and GW Bruyn, Amsterdam: North Holland Publishing Company, 1968, p. 133

19 DIZZINESS, VERTIGO, AND DISORDERS OF GAIT

MAURICE VICTOR
RAYMOND D. ADAMS

Dizziness and other sensations of unbalance occur in a wide variety of diseases. In many instances the clue to an important medical disorder is afforded by the correct analysis of the complaint.

The term *dizziness* covers a number of different sensory experiences—true vertigo, which refers to a feeling of whirling or rotation, as well as nonrotatory swaying, weakness, faintness, and lightheadedness. Blurring of vision, feelings of unreality, syncope, and even petit mal may be incorrectly called dizzy spells; hence a close questioning as to how the patient is using the term becomes a necessary first step in clinical study. A distinction is sometimes drawn between subjective vertigo, meaning a sense of turning one's body, and objective vertigo, an illusion of movement of objects in the environment, but its validity is doubtful.

In this chapter the term *vertigo* is used to refer to all subjective and objective illusions of rotation. *Giddiness* refers to a swaying type of dizziness. *Equilibrium,* the state of equipoise whereby the posture of the body is maintained against the forces of gravity, is deranged in vertigo but is also affected by other disorders as well, e.g., loss of joint or muscle sense (sensory ataxia), cerebellar disease (cerebellar ataxia), and motor abnormalities (spasticity and rigidity, myotonia, and the pseudomyotonia of hypothyroidism). Although these latter conditions are described in Chaps. 17, 18, and 351, their effects on stance and gait are appropriately reviewed in this context.

ANATOMIC, PHYSIOLOGIC, AND PSYCHOLOGIC CONSIDERATIONS Several mechanisms maintain balanced posture and awareness of the body's positions in relation to its surroundings. The most important of these are:

1. Impulses from the retinas of the eyes which are coordinated by ocular motor mechanisms to supply information about the position and movement of the body and its surroundings.
2. Impulses from the labyrinths of the inner ears—specialized spatial proprioceptors whose primary function is to register changes in the direction of motion (either acceleration or deceleration) and position of the body. [N. B. The semicircular canals respond to movement and angular momentum, whereas the otoliths (sense organs of the utricle and saccule) are mainly concerned with orienting the organism with reference to gravitational force.]
3. Impulses from the proprioceptors of joints and muscles—essential to all reflex, postural, and volitional movements. Those of the neck are of special importance in relating the position of the head to that of the rest of the body.

The cerebellum and certain ganglionic centers in the brainstem (particularly the vestibular nuclei, oculomotor nucleus, and red nucleus) and in the basal ganglia are the important coordinators of these sensory data and provide for postural adjustment, upright stance, and locomotion.

Important psychophysiologic mechanisms are also involved in the maintenance of equilibrium and the proper relationship of our bodies to the external world. Early in life we come to coordinate the parts of our body in relation to one another and to perceive that portion of space occupied by our bodies. The construct of these integrated sensory data has been designated by Russell Brain as the *body schema.* The space around our body is said to be represented by another set of data, the *environmental schema.* These two schemata are dynamic and interdependent, since both are simultaneously changed in every activity. For example, we learn to see objects as being stationary when we are moving. Thus, the motion of ourselves and of objects in space is always relative. At times, when sensory information is incomplete, we mistake movement of our surroundings for those of our own body, as in the illusion caused by motion of a neighboring train. A disturbance in the awareness of one's own body schema is postulated by some psychiatrists as the basis of neurotic disorientation and feelings of unreality.

CLINICAL CHARACTERISTICS OF VERTIGO AND GIDDINESS The clinical recognition of *vertigo* proves to be relatively easy when the patient states that objects in the environment turned or moved in one direction or that his head and body whirled. Often, however, he is not so explicit. The feeling may be described as oscillation, or of veering, of being pulled to one side or to the ground, as though drawn by a magnet. Again, the floor or walls may seem to tilt, sink, or rise up. The feeling of impulsion is particularly characteristic.

All but the mildest forms of vertigo are accompanied by perspiration, pallor, nausea, and vomiting. The nystagmus which is invariably present causes objects in the field of vision to move rhythmically in one direction. As a rule the patient can walk only with difficulty, or not at all should the vertigo be intense. A sudden attack may even catapult him to the ground, and only when down does he experience vertigo. Forced to lie down he realizes that one position, usually on one side with eyes closed, reduces the vertigo and nausea, and that the slightest motion of the head aggravates them. One form of vertigo, the benign positional vertigo of Bárány, occurs only for a few seconds after lying down and sitting up. If the vertigo is less severe, the patient can walk unsteadily but may veer to one side. The ataxia of gait with vertigo (vertiginous ataxia) is recognized always as being a "dizziness in the head," not a trouble in the control of the legs and trunk. It is noteworthy that in these circumstances the coordination of the individual movements of the limbs is not impaired—a point of difference from cerebellar disease. There may be headache, especially in the region of the offending ear. Loss of consciousness as part of a vertiginous attack nearly always signifies another type of disorder (seizure or faint).

Giddiness and other types of pseudovertigo are usually described as feelings of swaying, lightheadedness, a swimming sensation, and, more rarely, as though walking on air, "queer in the head," uncertain, about to fall or "pass out." These sensory experiences are particularly common in psychoneurotic and other psychiatric illnesses featured by anxiety attacks. They may be reproduced by hyperventilation, and then it is appreciated that panic and apprehensiveness, palpitation, breathlessness, trembling, and sweating are concurrent.

Other pseudovertiginous symptoms are less definite. In severe anemic states weakness and languor may be attended by a lightheadedness related to postural change and exertion. In the emphysematous patient physical effort may be associated with weakness and peculiar cephalic sensations, and coughing may lead to giddiness and even fainting (tussive syncope) because of impaired return of venous blood to the heart. The dizziness that so often accompanies hypertension is more difficult to evaluate. Sometimes it is an expression of anxiety, or it may be due to an unstable adjustment of cerebral blood flow. *Postural dizziness* is another example of unstable vasomotor reflexes preventing a constancy of cerebral circulation and is notably frequent in persons recently bedfast, in the weak and ill, and the elderly. Abrupt arising from a recumbent or sitting position is followed immediately by a swaying type of dizziness, dimming of vision, and spots before the eyes which last a few seconds. The patient is forced to stand still and steady himself by holding onto a nearby object. A syncopal attack may occur at this time (see Chap. 16).

In practice it is not difficult to separate these types of pseudovertigo from true vertigo for there is none of the feeling of rotation or impulsion so characteristic of the latter. Lacking also are the other ancillary symptoms of true vertigo, namely, nausea, vomiting, tinnitus and deafness, and staggering.

NEUROLOGIC AND OTOLOGIC CAUSES OF VERTIGO Vertigo may constitute the aura of an epileptic seizure, but this event is rare. The lesion is then on the posterolateral aspects of the temporal lobe near the sylvian fissure. A sensation of movement, either of the body away from the side of the lesion or of the environment in the opposite direction, lasts for a few seconds before being submerged in other seizure activity. Vertiginous sensations may rarely serve as a stimulus for *reflex epilepsy* (see Chap. 24), and the test for this form of vertigo provokes the seizure.

Oculomotor disorders are a source of a spatial disorientation simulating dizziness. This is maximal when the patient looks in the direction of action of the paralyzed muscle; it is attributable to the receipt of two conflicting visual images. In fact some normal individuals even experience dizziness for a time when adjusting to bifocal glasses or when looking down from a height.

Whether lesions of the cerebellum can produce vertigo seems to depend on the part of it involved. Large destructive processes in the cerebellar hemispheres and vermis cause no vertigo, unless they extend to central vestibulocerebellar connections.

Labyrinthine (aural) lesions are the usual causes of paroxysmal vertigo. In the classic variety, that of Ménière's disease, the onset is abrupt, the vertigo is clearly of the rotary type, and it lasts a few minutes to hours. Concomitant tinnitus, fullness in the ear, high-tone deafness with auditory recruitment (see Chap. 20), nystagmus, nausea, vomiting, and staggering constitute the full syndrome. The patient preferentially lies with the faulty ear uppermost and is disinclined to look toward the normal side because of exaggeration of the nystagmus and dizziness. The nystagmus is fine, rotatory, and most pronounced when the eyes are turned away from the offending ear. Vertiginous attacks of this type may recur and give rise to mild, chronic states of disequilibrium which may persist for days. Seldom does it last, however, for central mechanisms compensate for permanent deficits of one labyrinth. Chronic vertigo may be complicated by the giddiness of a secondary anxiety state. *Vestibular neuronitis* is a term that refers to severe vertigo, often of several days' duration, without tinnitus or deafness. Its pathologic basis is uncertain. Episodic vertigo occurs in Bárány's benign positional vertigo and the more malignant positional vertigo of posterior fossa tumors and other lesions, and lasts only a few seconds.

Vertigo of acoustic nerve origin, the commonest cause of which is an acoustic neuroma, tends usually to be mild and intermittent (lasting weeks or months). Seldom does it come in discrete attacks separated by free intervals. Vertigo has rarely been observed as the initial symptom with eighth nerve tumors, but the usual sequence is deafness of high-frequency type (without recruitment), followed some years later by chronic vertigo and impaired caloric responses, then cranial nerve palsies (involving the eighth, fifth, and tenth nerves), ipsilateral ataxia of limbs, and headache, the other common signs of a cerebellopontine angle tumor.

Vertigo of brainstem origin implicates vestibular nuclei and their connections. In these cases auditory function is nearly always spared, since the vestibular and cochlear fibers separate upon entering the medulla and pons. The nystagmus which accompanies such central lesions tends to be coarse and protracted; it is more marked on lateral gaze to one side than the other. There may also be a nonrotatory vertical component. The central localization is evidenced further by the attendant signs of involvement of other structures within the brainstem (cranial nerves, sensory and motor tracts, etc.). Mode of onset, duration, and other features of the clinical picture depend upon the nature of the causative disease, usually vascular, neoplastic, or demyelinative.

DIFFERENTIAL DIAGNOSIS As already stated, a careful history and physical examination of the dizzy patient usually afford a basis for separating true vertigo from the swaying dizziness of the hyperventilating, anxious patient and from the other types of pseudovertigo. If the patient is unobservant or imprecise in his descriptions, a helpful tactic is to provoke a number of dissimilar sensations by rotating the patient, irrigating his ears with warm or cold water, by asking him to stoop for a minute and straighten up, and to hyperventilate for 3 min. Should the patient be unable to distinguish among these several types of induced dizziness or to ascertain the similarity of one of the types to his own condition, his history is probably too inaccurate for purposes of diagnosis.

When vertigo is mild or poorly described, small items of the patient's history, such as disinclination to walk during an attack, tendency to list to one side, aggravation by riding in a vehicle, preference for one position, are helpful.

In some patients an attack of vertigo is so abrupt and violent that they are virtually flung to the ground, sometimes with a serious injury. These attacks have been called by the quaint term "otolithic crises of Tumarken," but without proof of involvement of the utricle or saccule. The diagnosis is usually substantiated by the presence of vertigo, nausea, and vomiting while on the ground, distinguishing it from a seizure or faint. Probably it differs from other forms of labyrinthine vertigo only in its severity.

In the differentiation of types of labyrinthine and vestibular nerve disease, inspection of eardrums, x-rays of mastoids, middle ears, and inner ears, and auditory and caloric tests are useful, especially in excluding labyrinthitis. In caloric testing, the patient's head is tilted forward 30° from the horizontal (bringing the horizontal semicircular canal into a vertical plane), which is the position of maximal sensitivity to thermal stimuli. The external auditory meati are irrigated in turn for 40 s with water at 30°C and 44°C (7° below and above body temperature). Cold water induces nystagmus to the opposite side (direction of the fast phase), and warm water to the same side. The nystagmus begins in 20 s and should persist 90 to 120°. Comparison of the two ears reveals which one is paretic or hypersensitive. Special rotational chairs and electronystagmography are other more refined means of assessing disordered labyrinthine function. The diagnosis of benign positional vertigo is settled at the bedside by reproducing a brief vertigo and nystagmus (lasting up to a minute) by moving the patient from the sitting position to recumbency with head to one side in one trial and to the other in the second. Going from a recumbent to a sitting position reverses the direction of vertigo and nystagmus. This specific pattern and its reversibility are not observed in the more malignant positional vertigo of posterior fossa tumors and other lesions.

The association of vertigo with auditory signs and symptoms always signifies a disease process of end organ or eighth nerve. Labyrinthine and auditory tests and neurologic signs of structures adjacent to the eighth cranial nerve separate these two groups of diseases.

Pure vertigo as a manifestation of disease of the brainstem is rare, and the rule we have found trustworthy is that unless other symptoms and signs appear within 1 to 2 weeks, one can nearly always postulate an aural origin and exclude vascular disease of the brainstem. This is true of multiple sclerosis, which may be the explanation of a persistent vertigo in some adolescents or young adults.

DISTURBANCES OF EQUILIBRIUM AND OF GAIT All that has been said above refers in large measure to the patient's awareness of a disorientation in space; however, there are forms of neurologic abnormality with a prominent disequilibrium of the body but no dizziness whatsoever. Since these are manifested most clearly as an impairment of upright stance and locomotion, their evaluation depends on a knowledge of the nervous mechanisms underlying these peculiarly human functions.

Since normal body posture and locomotion require visual information, labyrinthine function, and proprioception, it is of interest to note the effect of deficits in these senses on normal function. A blind man or a normal one who is blindfolded may walk very well. He moves cautiously, to avoid collision with objects, and on smooth pavement shortens his step slightly; with the shortening there is less rocking of the body, and he seems unnaturally stiff. A man without labyrinthine function shows a slight unsteadiness in walking and an inability to descend stairs without holding onto a banister. Running is also difficult. Characteristically, he has great difficulty in focusing on a stationary object when he is moving, so that he cannot drive a car. Proof that he is dependent on visual cues comes from his performance blindfolded, when his unsteadiness and staggering increase to some extent, but usually not to the point of falling. A loss of proprioception, as in a complete lesion in the posterior columns of the spinal cord in the high cervical region, abolishes for a long time the capacity for independent locomotion. After years of training, the patient will still have difficulty in starting to walk and in propelling himself forward. As Purdon Martin has illustrated, he holds his hands in front of his body, bends body and head forward, walks with a wide base with irregular uneven steps but does rock his body. If he loses his balance, he shows no reactions to his posture. If he falls, he cannot arise without help, and he cannot get up from a chair. He is unable to crawl or to get into an "all-fours" posture. When standing, if blindfolded, he immediately falls. Thus the postural reactions are demonstrably more dependent on proprioceptive than on visual or labyrinthine information.

When confronted with a disorder of gait, the examiner must observe the patient's natural stance and the attitude and dominant positions of the legs, trunk, and arms. It is good practice to watch the patient as he walks into the examining room, because he is apt to walk more naturally then than during special tests. He should be asked to stand with his feet together, head erect, with eyes first open and then closed. Swaying due to nervousness may be overcome by asking him to touch the tip of his nose with the finger of first one hand and then the other. Next the patient should be asked to walk forward and backward, with his eyes first open and then closed. Any tendency to reel to one side, as in cerebellar disease, can be checked by having him walk around a chair. When the affected side is toward the chair, the patient tends to walk into it; when it is away from the chair, he veers outward in ever-widening circles. More delicate tests of gait are walking a straight line heel to toe or having the patient arise quickly from a chair, walk briskly, and then stop or turn suddenly. If all these tests are successfully executed, it may be assumed that any difficulty in locomotion is not due to disease of the proprioceptive mechanisms or cerebellum. Detailed neurologic examination is then necessary in order to determine which of the many other possible diseases is responsible for the patient's disorder of gait.

The following abnormal gaits are so distinctive that with a little practice they can be recognized at a glance.

Cerebellar gait The main features of this gait are *wide base* (separation of legs), *unsteadiness, irregularity,* and *lateral reeling.* Steps are uncertain, some are shorter and others longer than intended, and the patient may lurch to one side or the other. The unsteadiness is more prominent on quickly arising from a chair and walking, on stopping suddenly while walking, or on turning abruptly. If the ataxia is severe, the patient cannot stand without assistance. If it is lesser in degree, standing with feet together and head erect, with eyes either open or closed, may be difficult. In its mildest form the ataxia is best demonstrated by having the patient walk a line heel to toe. After two or three steps he loses his balance and must place one foot to the side to avoid falling. Romberg's sign, i.e., marked swaying or falling with the eyes closed but not with the eyes open, is not a feature of cerebellar disease. Compensation may be effected by shortening the step and shuffling, i.e., keeping both feet simultaneously on the ground. The defect in the cerebellar gait is not in antigravity support, steppage, or propulsion but in the coordination of proprioceptive, labyrinthine, and visual information in reflex coordination of movements. The abnormality of gait may or may not be accompanied by other signs of cerebellar incoordination and intention tremor of the arms and legs. The presence of the latter signs depends on involvement of the superior midline structures as distinct from cerebellar hemispheres; if the lesion is unilateral, the signs are always on the same side.

Cerebellar gait is in some instances a predominant symptom in multiple sclerosis, cerebellar tumors, particularly medulloblastoma of the cerebellar vermis, and the cerebellar degenerations. In certain forms of cerebellar degeneration (e.g., the type associated with chronic alcoholism) the disease process reaches a plateau and then remains stable for many years, and the gait disorder, in these circumstances, becomes altered to some extent. The base is wide and the steps are still short, but more regular; the trunk is inclined slightly forward, the arms are held away from the sides, and the gait assumes a somewhat rhythmic quality. In this way the patient can walk for long distances, but he lacks the capacity to make the necessary postural adjustments in response to sudden changes in his position.

A slowness in muscle relaxation as in myxedema may also lead to a kind of gait disorder that simulates a cerebellar defect.

Gait of sensory ataxia This gait is due to an impairment of proprioception resulting from interruption of afferent nerve fibers in the peripheral nerves, posterior roots, posterior columns of the spinal cords, or medial lemnisci; it may also be produced occasionally by a lesion of both parietal lobes. Whatever the location of the lesion, the patient is deprived of knowledge of the position of his limbs. The principal features of the resulting gait disorder are *uncertainty, irregularity,* and the *stamp* of the feet. Hunt characterized this type of gait very well when he said that the ataxic patient is recognized by "his stamp and stick." This form of ataxia is characterized by varying degrees of difficulty in standing and walking, and in advanced cases there is a complete failure of locomotion, although muscular power is retained. The legs are kept far apart to correct the instability, and the patient carefully watches the ground and his legs. As he steps out, the legs are flung abruptly forward and outward, often lifted higher than necessary. The steps are of variable length, and many are attended by an audible stamp as the foot is banged down on the floor. The body is held in a slightly flexed position, and the weight may be supported on the cane that the severely ataxic patient often carries. The incoordination is greatly exaggerated when the patient is deprived of visual cues, as in walking in the dark. Most patients, when asked to stand with feet together and eyes closed, show greatly increased swaying or actual falling (Romberg's sign). It has been said that a lame man whose shoes are not worn in any one place is probably suffering from sensory ataxia. There is invariably a loss of vibratory and position sense in the feet and legs. A disordered gait of this type is observed in tabes dorsalis, Friedreich's ataxia, subacute combined degeneration, syphilitic meningomyelitis, chronic polyneuritis, and those cases of multiple sclerosis in which posterior column disease predominates.

Hemiplegic and paraplegic (spastic) gait In hemiplegia the leg is held stiffly and does not flex freely and gracefully at the knee and hip. It tends to rotate outward and describes a semicircle, first away from and then toward the trunk (circumduction). The foot scrapes along the floor, and the toe and outer side of the sole of the shoe are worn. One can diagnose the hemiplegic gait by hearing the slow rhythmic scuff of the foot along the floor. The other muscles of the body on the affected side are weak and stiff to a variable degree, particularly the arm, which is carried in a flexed position and does not swing naturally. This type of gait disorder is most frequently associated with vascular disease of the brain.

The spastic paraplegic gait is entirely different from the gait of sensory ataxia, though the two may be combined. Each leg is advanced slowly and stiffly with restricted motion at the knee and hip. The patient looks as though he were wading in water. The legs are extended or slightly bent at the knees and may be strongly adducted at the hips, tending almost to cross ("scissors" gait). The steps are regular and short. Movements of the legs are slow, and the patient may be able to advance only with great effort. An easy way to remember the main features of the hemiplegic and paraplegic gait is by the letter S, which begins each of its descriptive adjectives—spastic, slow, scuffing. The defect is in the stepping mechanism and in propulsion, not in support or equilibrium. Cerebral spastic diplegia, multiple sclerosis, syringomyelia, spinal syphilis, combined system disease, spinal cord compression, and familial spinal spastic ataxia are the common causes of spastic paraparesis.

Festinating gait The term *festinating* comes from the Latin *festinare,* to hasten, and appropriately describes the involuntary increase or hastening of the gait that characterizes both paralysis agitans and postencephalitic Parkinson's syndrome. *Rigidity* and *shuffling,* in addition to *festination,* are the cardinal features of this gait. When they are joined to the typical tremors, rigidity, and slowness of movement, there can be little doubt as to the diagnosis.

The general attitude of the patient is one of flexion; rigidity and immobility of the body are other conspicuous features. There is a paucity of the automatic movements made in sitting, standing, and walking; the head does not turn in looking to one side, the arms are seldom folded, and the legs are rarely crossed. The arms are held stiffly as though in preparation for writing, and the facial expression is unblinking and masklike.

In walking, the trunk is bent forward and the arms are carried ahead of the body and do not swing. The legs are stiff and bent at the knees and hips. The steps are short, and the feet barely clear the ground as the patient shuffles along. Once forward or backward locomotion is started, the upper part of the body advances ahead of the lower part, as though the patient were chasing his center of gravity. His steps become more and more rapid, and he may fall if not assisted. This is the festination, and it may occur when the patient is walking forward or backward, taking the form of either propulsion or retropulsion. The defect is in rocking the body from side to side so as to clear the floor and in moving the legs quickly enough to catch the center of gravity in forward propulsion. Other unusual gaits are sometimes observed in the postencephalitic patient. For example, he may be unable to take his first step forward because he cannot lift one foot, or he may be unable to step forward until he hops or takes one step backward; walking may be initiated by a series of short steps that give way to a more normal gait; occasionally such a patient may run better than he walks or walk backwards better than forward.

Athetotic, dystonic, and choreic gaits Diseases that are characterized by involuntary movements and abnormal postures seriously affect gait. In fact, a disturbance of gait may be the initial and dominant manifestation of these diseases, and the testing of gait often serves to provoke abnormalities of movement and posture that are otherwise not conspicuous. The *athetotic* patient often assumes the most grotesque postures. One arm may be held aloft and the other one behind the body with wrist and fingers alternately undergoing slow flexion, extension, and rotation. The head may be inclined in one direction, the lips alternately retract and then purse, and the tongue intermittently protrudes from the mouth. The legs advance slowly and awkwardly, the result of superimposed involuntary movements and postures. Sometimes the foot is plantar-flexed at the ankle, and the weight is carried on the toes; or it may be dorsiflexed or inverted. This type of gait is typical of congenital athetosis and Huntington's chorea.

In *dystonia musculorum deformans* the first symptom may be a limp due to inversion or plantar flexion of the foot or a distortion of the pelvis. The patient stands with one leg rigidly extended or one shoulder elevated. The trunk may be in a position of exaggerated lordosis, and the hips are partly flexed, with a tilting forward of the pelvis. Because of the muscle spasms that deform the body in this manner, the patient may have to walk with knees flexed. The gait may seem normal as the first steps are taken, but as the patient walks, one or both legs become flexed, giving rise to the "dromedary gait." In the more advanced stages walking becomes impossible, owing to torsion of the trunk or the continuous flexion of one leg.

In *Sydenham's chorea* the gait is often bizarre (see Chap. 341). As the patient stands or walks, there is a continuous play of irregular "choreic" movements affecting the face, neck, hands, and, in the advanced stages, the large proximal joints and trunk. The positions of the trunk and upper parts of the body vary with each step. There are jerks of the head, grimacing, squirming, twisting movements of the trunk and limbs, and peculiar respiratory noises.

Drop-foot, steppage, or equine gait This is caused by paralysis of the pretibial and peroneal muscles. The legs must be lifted abnormally high in order for the feet to clear the ground. There is a slapping noise as the foot strokes the floor. The anterior and lateral borders of the sole of the shoe become worn. The steps are regular and even; otherwise, walking is not remarkable. Foot drop may be unilateral or bilateral and occurs in diseases that affect the peripheral nerves of the legs or motor neurons in the spinal cord, such as poliomyelitis, progressive muscular atrophy, and Charcot-Marie-Tooth disease (peroneal muscular atrophy). It may also be observed in patients with peripheral types of muscular dystrophy. The most common cause of unilateral foot drop is compression of the anterior tibial nerve, where it crosses the head of the fibula (see Chap. 331).

Waddling gait This gait is characteristic of progressive muscular dystrophy. The attitude of the body may be straight, but more often the lumbar lordosis is accentuated. The steps are regular but a little uncertain. With each step there is an exaggerated elevation of one hip and depression of the other; once the weight is on the hip it yields to an abnormal degree, so that the upper trunk then inclines to that side. This alternation of lateral trunk movements results in the rolling gait, or *waddle,* a term suggested by Oppenheim. The gluteal musculature is weak and inefficient, although leg muscles may appear well developed. Muscular contractures leading to an equinovarus position of the foot may complicate childhood cases, so that the waddle is combined with circumduction of the legs and "walking on the toes."

Staggering or drunken gait This is characteristic of alcoholic and barbiturate intoxication. The drunken patient totters, reels, tips forward and then backward, threatening each moment to lose his balance and fall. Control over trunk and legs is greatly impaired. The steps are irregular and uncertain. The patient appears stupefied and indifferent to the quality of his performance, but under certain circumstances he can momentarily correct his defect.

The frequently used adjectives *drunken* and *reeling* do not describe aptly the gait of cerebellar disease, except, perhaps, the most acute and severe cases. The intoxicated patient reels in many different directions, unlike the patient with cerebellar disease, and no effort is made to correct the staggering by watching the legs or the ground, as in cerebellar or sensory ataxia. In the drunken patient, despite a wide diversity of excursions of all parts of the body, balance may be exquisitely maintained. In contrast, the patient with cerebellar disease has great difficulty in maintaining his balance if he sways or lurches too far to one side.

Hysterical gait This may take any one of several forms—monoplegic, paraplegic, or hemiplegic. The monoplegic or hemiplegic patient does not lift the foot from the floor while walking; instead, he drags it as a useless member or pushes it ahead of him as though it were a skate. The characteristic circumduction is absent in hysterical hemiplegia, and the typical hemiplegic posture, hyperactive tendon reflexes, and Babinski sign are missing. The hysterical paraplegic cannot very well drag both legs, and usually he depends on a crutch or remains helpless in bed; the muscles may be rigid with pseudocontractures or flaccid. The gait may be quite dramatic. Some patients look as though they were walking on stilts, and others lurch wildly in all directions, actually demonstrating by their gyrations a remarkable ability to make rapid postural adjustments.

Astasia-abasia, in which the patient, though unable to either stand or walk, retains normal use of his legs while in bed, is nearly always hysterical. When such a patient is placed on his feet, he takes a few normal steps and then becomes unable to advance his feet; he lurches wildly and crumples to the floor if not assisted.

Frontal lobe ataxia Equilibrium and the capacity to stand and walk may be severely disturbed by diseases that affect the frontal lobes, particularly their medial parts. Although this disorder of gait is sometimes spoken of as an ataxia or as an *apraxia,* since the difficulty in walking cannot be accounted for by weakness or loss of sensation, it is probably neither. It most likely represents a loss of integration at the cortical and basal ganglionic level of the essential elements of stance and locomotion which were acquired in infancy and are often lost in senility.

The patient assumes a posture of slight flexion, with the feet placed farther apart then normal. He advances slowly, with small, shuffling, hesitant steps. At times the patient halts, unable to advance without great effort, although he does much better with a little assistance. Turning is accomplished by a series of tiny, uncertain steps which are made with one foot, the other being planted on the floor as a pivot. The initiation of walking becomes progressively more difficult, and in advanced cases the patient may be unable to take a step, as though his feet were glued to the floor. Finally he becomes unable to stand or even to sit, and without support he falls backward or to one side.

Some patients are able to make complex movements with their legs, such as drawing imaginary figures, at a time when their gait is seriously impaired. Eventually, however, all movements of the legs become slow and awkward, and the limbs, when passively moved, offer variable resistance (gegenhalten). An inability to turn in bed is highly characteristic, and may eventually become complete. These motor disabilities are usually associated with dementia, but there need be no parallelism in their evolution. Grasping, groping, hyperactive tendon reflexes, and Babinski signs may or may not be present. The end result in many cases is a "cerebral paraplegia in flexion" (Yakovlev), in which the patient lies curled up in bed, immobile and mute, his limbs fixed by contractures in an attitude of flexion.

Senile gait Elderly persons often complain of difficulty in walking, and examination may disclose no abnormality other than the slightly flexed posture of the senile and short uncertain steps, *marche à petit pas.* Speed, balance, and all the graceful, adaptive movements are lost. The exact nature of this gait disorder is not understood. Probably it is the frontal lobe gait disorder. It should be noted, however, that a short-stepped, cautious gait lacks specificity, being a general defensive reaction to all forms of defective locomotion.

REFERENCES

Adams RD, Victor M: *Principles of Neurology,* New York: McGraw-Hill, 1977

Altmann F: Diagnostic significance of vertigo, in *The Vestibular System and Its Diseases,* ed RJ Wolfson, Philadelphia: University of Pennsylvania Press, 1966, p. 353

Dix MR: Modern tests of vestibular function, with special reference to their value in clinical practice. Br Med J 3:317, 1969

Fisher CM: Vertigo in cerebrovascular disease. Arch Otolaryngol 85:529, 1967

Spector M: *Dizziness and Vertigo,* New York: Grune & Stratton, 1967

20 COMMON DISTURBANCES OF VISION, OCULAR MOVEMENT, AND HEARING

MAURICE VICTOR
RAYMOND D. ADAMS

Diseases of the eyes and ears, by virtue of their frequency, unusual nature, and serious consequences, make up separate medical specialties and, therefore, fall outside the field of internal medicine. Yet disturbances of visual and auditory function may be the initial or leading manifestations of many systemic diseases. Of more general interest is the fact that these two senses represent the most finely developed parts of the entire afferent apparatus of the nervous system; hence the study of their disorders may yield important information about neurologic diseases.

THE EYE AND DISORDERS OF VISION The diverse composition of the eye, with its epithelial, vascular, collagenous, neural, and pigmentary tissue, explains why it is a medical microcosm susceptible to manifold diseases. Moreover its transparency makes it accessible to direct inspection by means of an instrument found in the consulting room of every physician and affords an opportunity to inspect directly during life many of the specific lesions of medical diseases.

Since the eye is the organ of vision, it is obvious that degrees of impairment of visual acuity to the point of blindness should stand as the most frequent symptom of eye disease. Strabismus and diplopia, ocular pain, irritation, redness and photophobia, inability to read or recognize objects and people, and drooping or closure of the eyelids are of lesser importance. The impairment of eyesight may be unilateral or bilateral, sudden or gradual, episodic or enduring. The common causes vary with age. In late childhood and adolescence increasing difficulty in focusing the eyes and in seeing clearly usually can be traced to *myopia,* though an optic nerve or suprasellar tumor must be excluded. In middle age *presbyopia* is almost invariable and requires eye refraction and spectacles. Still later in life *cataracts, glaucoma, retinal hemorrhages,* and *detachments* are the most frequent causes of visual disturbance. Episodic blindness in early life is usually due to migraine; later, amaurosis fugax is caused by stenosis of the carotid artery or cranial arteritis. Cerebrovascular disease deranges vision with increasing frequency in late life.

Thus failing eyesight may be due to an abnormality of the refractive media of the eye or to a lesion of the retina or optic nerve or the parts of the brain with which they are connected. In approaching this problem one begins always by inquiring as to precisely what the patient means when he says he cannot see properly, for he may be referring to symptoms as varied as excessive tearing, diplopia, partial syncope, or even giddiness or dizziness. Fortunately his statements can be checked by the measurement of visual activity, a technique which is the single most important part of the ocular examination. If visual acuity is less than 20/20 and cannot be improved by refraction and if the media of the eye are transparent, there is some sensory defect, the nature of which must be ascertained.

In the measurement of visual acuity the *Snellen Chart,* which contains rows of letters of diminishing size (those of each row subtending 5 min of an arc when held at various distances from the eye), is utilized. The letters at the top of the chart subtend 5 min of an arc at a distance of 200 ft; those at the bottom subtend an arc of 5 min at 20 ft. Thus if the patient can see only the top letters at 20 ft, rather than 200 ft, his vision is 20/200; if he sees those at the bottom at this distance, the acuity is 20/20. The patient with a corrected refractive error should wear his eyeglasses for the test; if the visual acuity is then less than 20/20, either his refractive error has not been properly corrected or there is some other reason for it. The former possibility can be ruled out if the patient sees clearly while looking through a pinhole of 2 to 3 mm in a cardboard with his glasses still on. The pinhole permits a narrow shaft of light to fall on the fovea without being refracted.

Light entering the eye is focused on the outer layer of the retina (the rods and cones). Consequently the media (tissues and fluids) through which the light passes must be transparent. These media are the cornea, the aqueous humor of the anterior chamber, the lens, the vitreous humor of the vitreous cavity, and the retina itself. The clarity of these media can be determined ophthalmoscopically, but this examination requires that the pupil be dilated to at least 6 mm in diameter. This is best accomplished by instilling a few drops of 10% phenylephrine (Neo-Synephrine) in each eye after the visual acuity is measured, the pupillary response recorded, and the intraocular pressure estimated. *An attack of angle-closure glaucoma may be precipitated by pupillary dilatation, but this happens rarely and can be controlled by 4% pilocarpine.* The cycloplegic action of phenylephrine lasts only an hour or two. Looking through a +6 ophthalmoscopic lens from a distance of 15 to 20 cm permits the visualization of any opacity in refractive media against the diffuse bright red of reflexed light from the retina. By adjusting the lens of the ophthalmoscope from high + to 0 or − one can "depth-focus" from the cornea to the retina. Clarity of all media means that reduced vision uncorrected by glasses must be due to a lesion in the macula, optic nerve, or structures further back in the visual system.

More specifically the alterations in the refractile media that affect vision have certain medical implications, as follows.

Corneas In hypercalcemia [secondary to sarcoid (Chap. 228)], hyperparathyroidism (Chap. 353), and vitamin D intoxication (Chap. 352), calcium phosphates and carbonates precipitate in the cornea, primarily beneath the epithelium—so-called *band keratopathy* (see Color Plate 7-8); cystine crystals are deposited in cystinosis (Chap. 104), cholesterol esters in hypercholesterolemia (*arcus senilis*) (Chap. 113), chloroquine crystals in treatment of discoid lupus by this drug, and copper in hepatolenticular degeneration [Kayser-Fleischer ring (Chap. 110)]. Opacification (keratitis) of the cornea may also occur after herpes simplex and herpes zoster infections (Chaps. 206 and 189); or it may be combined with uveitis and iritis in Behçet's disease (Chap. 189), Reiter's disease (Chap. 207), Stevens-Johnson disease (Chap. 78), and idiopathic infections. Keratitis may be a manifestation also of congenital syphilis (Chap. 164) and of more innocent states such as drying and injury of eyes during coma.

Aqueous humor The common problem is one of high pressure due to impediment of the outflow of the aqueous fluid. This is termed *glaucoma.* In 90 percent of cases (of the wide-angle type) the cause is unknown; in 5 percent the angle between pupil and lateral cornea is narrow and blocked when the pupil is dilated; and in the remaining 5 percent the condition is secondary to some disease process that blocks outflow channels (inflammatory debris of uveitis, or red blood cells from hemorrhage in the anterior chamber, i.e., hyphema). Glaucoma occurs in 2 percent of all patients over the age of forty; it may be asymptomatic and go unrecognized for years before it progresses to rapid loss of vision. Therefore, the intraocular pressure should be measured routinely, using a Schiotz tonometer. This is a simple procedure which should be practiced by every physician. With the patient supine, a drop of local anesthetic is put into each eye and the tonometer is then placed on the cornea so that the instrument is perfectly vertical. When the tonometer is pressed against the eye, the scale is read and the units are converted into millimeters of mercury from the chart in the tonometer case. The normal pressure is about 15 mmHg. Pressures of 20 to 30 may damage the optic nerve, leading first to a nasal quadrant defect and finally to blindness. With the ophthalmoscope one can see also that the optic disk is excavated.

The lens Opacities form in diabetes mellitus (Chap. 95) and galactosemia ("sugar cataracts," from sustained high levels of blood glucose and galactose, which are changed to sorbitol or dulcitol, the accumulation of which leads to a high osmotic gradient within the lens fibers); in hypoparathyroidism (Chap. 353), which by lowering the concentration of Ca in the aqueous opacifies newly forming lens fibers; after prolonged high doses of chlorpromazine, triparanol, and corticosteroid therapy, which are believed to result in lenticular opacities; and in myotonic dystrophy (Chap. 349), which is associated with a special type of cataract. Weakening of zonular ligaments of lens allows a dislocation (iridodenesis) in both Marfan's syndrome (Chap. 367) and homocystinuria (Color Plate 7-7 and Chap. 103).

Vitreous humor Hemorrhage may occur from rupture of a retinal vessel, causing a shower of black or red dots. It is also seen in diabetes mellitus, where it may occur following rupture of newly formed retinal vessels, in *retinitis proliferans,* or after a retinal tear which may progress to retinal detachment. The vitreous humor may also be affected by deposition of calcium soaps (seen as glistening objects with the ophthalmoscope)—so-called *asteroid hyalosis* of diabetes mellitus.

Retina and optic nerve The search for neurologic explanations of reduced vision begins with an examination of the retina with an ophthalmoscope. This thin (0.4 mm) sheet of transparent tissue and the optic nerve head into which the visual information is channeled are the only parts of the central nervous system that can be inspected during life.

Light entering the eye passes through the full thickness of the retina to reach the receptor layer of rods and cones and underlying pigment epithelium, which contains the visual pigment (rhodopsin). Impulses arising in these photoreceptors are transmitted via secondary neurons, the bipolar cells, to the innermost ganglion cell layer, the axons of which in turn travel through the optic nerve head, optic nerve, chiasm, and optic tracts to the lateral geniculate bodies. These retinal neurons normally acquire a myelin sheath only after piercing the lamina cribrosa. The macular region (two disk diameters or 3 mm lateral to the optic disk) is the most sensitive part of the retina. The vascular supply comes from the ophthalmic branch of the internal carotid artery, which in turn gives origin to the central retinal artery. The latter, upon issuing from the optic disk, divides into four arterioles, which supply the four quadrants of the retina. The ganglion cells and bipolar cells receive their blood supply from these arterioles and their capillaries, whereas photoreceptor elements receive nourishment from the underlying choroidal vascular bed.

These small vessels react in disease like those of corresponding size in the brain. Since the walls of the retinal arterioles are transparent with the ophthalmoscope, what is seen is a column of blood. In arteriosclerosis (usually coexistent with hypertension), the lumens of the vessels are narrowed because of fibrous tissue replacement of the media and thickening of the basement membrane. The light reflection from the vessel then has a different refractive index than the adjacent retinal tissue. Tortuosity of vessels, arteriole-venous compressions, and narrowed segments are other signs of hypertension and arteriolosclerosis. In malignant hypertension there are, in addition, cotton-wool exudates, splinter hemorrhages, and papilledema, and they correlate with similar changes in the intracranial arterioles (Color Plate 8-5). Atheromatous deposits, which form in larger arteries, are seldom observed in the retina because of the small size of the vessels, although occasionally atheromatous and other emboli from the carotid and aorta may reach them. Capillary-venular aneurysms may develop, most often in diabetes mellitus (Color Plates 8-6, 8-7, and 8-8). Since the central retinal vein and artery share a common adventitial sheath, atheromatous plaques in the artery may result in thrombosis of the vein. Round, punctate hemorrhages always lie in the bipolar layer, and flame-shaped ones in the outer ganglion cell layer. Rupture of arterioles on the inner surface of the retina, as occurs with ruptured intracranial saccular aneurysms, hemangiomas, and other conditions causing sudden high elevations of intracranial pressure, permits blood to cover the retina and extend beneath the vitreous humor (subhyaloid hemorrhage).

Aside from visible vascular lesions, other more specific alterations of the retina may impair vision. The most important of these are tears and separations and detachments and degenerations.

1 *Degeneration of the outer receptor layer and subjacent pigment epithelium* occurs as a hereditary trait in retinitis pigmentosa (Color Plate 7-5), and also in Laurence-Moon-Biedl syndrome, progressive ophthalmoplegia, Bassen-Kornzweig disease (Chap. 113), Refsum's disease (Chap. 331), Batten-Mayou juvenile lipid storage disease, and idiopathic senile macular degeneration (Chaps. 113 and 341).
2 *Degeneration in Bruch's membrane* (which supports the layer of pigment epithelium next to the rods and cones) and its repair by fibrosis give rise to angioid streaks typical of pseudoxanthoma elasticum (Chap. 367), Paget's disease (Chap. 356), hyperphosphatemia, and acromegaly (Color Plate 7-6).
3 *Deposits of phenothiazine conjugate with the melanin* of the pigment layer with resulting degeneration of the outer retinal layers. When these drugs are used, the doses should be kept low and the central visual fields tested with small colored test objects.

Sarcoidosis, toxoplasmosis, and *histoplasmosis* involve both the retina and the choroid (Color Plates 8-2 and 8-3). The latter is the site of noninfective inflammatory reactions, often in association with iridocyclitis.

The optic nerves, chiasm, and tracts which constitute the third visual neuron can be inspected only in part, from the foveal or macular region to the optic disk. The latter reflects raised intracranial pressure (papilledema or choked disk), papillitis (a demyelinative disease of the optic nerve), optic nerve atrophy, and glaucoma (Color Plate 7-3).

Central visual disturbances (caused by defects in the retina, optic nerves and tracts, lateral geniculate bodies, geniculocalcarine path, and striate cortex of occipital lobes) are evidenced by changes in the visual fields. In good light, if a cotton pledget on a stick is used to cover first one eye, then the other, the periphery of the patient's visual field can be compared with that of the examiner. The types of visual field defect resulting from lesions in different parts of the visual pathways are shown in Fig. 20-1. A prechiasmal lesion causes either a scotoma (an island of impaired vision within the visual field) or a cut in the peripheral part of the visual field. A small scotoma in the macular part of the visual field may seriously impair visual acuity. Demyelinative, toxic (methyl alcohol, quinine, and certain of the phenothiazine tranquilizing drugs), nutritional (so-called "tobacco-alcohol" amblyopia), and vascular diseases are the usual causes of scotomas. The toxic states are characterized by symmetric bilateral scotomas, and the nutritional disorders by more or less symmetric central scotomas (involving the fixation point) or centrocecal ones (involving both the fixation point and the blind spot). These latter scotomas are predominantly in the distribution of the papillomacular bundle, but their presence does not establish whether the primary effect is on the nerve fibers or the ganglion cells. Demyelinative diseases are characterized by unilateral or asymmetric bilateral scotomas. If the lesion is near the optic disk, there may be swelling of the optic nerve head, i.e., *papillitis,* which can usually be distinguished from papilledema by the marked impairment of vision it produces. Vascular lesions as a rule give rise to unilateral scotomas. The lesions take the form of retinal hemorrhages, hard exudates, or occluded vessels which cause infarction of the retina or, rarely, of the optic nerve. The common cotton-wool patches are in reality small retinal infarcts. Large zones of retinal infarction may follow occlusion of a branch of the central retinal artery (Color Plates 8-4 and 8-5).

Another common defect encountered on visual field examination is concentric constriction. This may be due to papilledema, in which case it is usually accompanied by an enlargement of the blind spot. A concentric constriction of the visual field, at first unilateral and later bilateral, and pallor of the optic disks (optic atrophy) should suggest chronic syphilitic meningo-optic neuritis. Glaucoma is another cause of this type of field defect. Tubular vision, i.e., constriction of the visual field to the same degree regardless of the distance of the visual test stimulus from the eye, is a sign of hysteria. In organic disease, for example, chorioretinitis, the area of the constricted visual field naturally enlarges as the distance between the patient and the stimulus increases.

With most diseases of the optic nerve, the optic nerve will eventually become pale (optic atrophy). This may require several weeks or months to occur, as illustrated by the delay between the sudden blindness of a traumatic severance of one optic nerve and the pallor. If the optic nerve degenerates [e.g., in multiple sclerosis, Leber's hereditary optic atrophy (Chap. 341), or syphilitic optic atrophy], the disk becomes chalk-white, with sharp, clean margins. If the atrophy is secondary to papillitis or papilledema, the margins are obscure and irregular, with pigment deposits in the adjacent retina (Color Plates 7-2 and 7-4).

Hemianopsia means blindness in one-half of the visual field. *Bitemporal hemianopsia* indicates a lesion of the decussating fibers of the optic chiasm and is due usually to tumor of the pituitary gland or of the infundibulum or third ventricle, to meningioma of the diaphragm of the sella, or occasionally to a large suprasellar aneurysm of the circle of Willis. *Homonymous hemianopsia* (a loss of vision in corresponding halves of the visual fields) signifies a lesion of the visual pathway behind the chiasm and, if *complete,* gives no more information than that. *Incomplete homonymous hemianopsia* has more localizing value: if the field defects in the two eyes are identical (*congruous*), the lesion is likely to be in the calcarine cortex; if *incongruous,* the visual fibers in the parietal or temporal lobe are more likely to be implicated. Since the fibers from the peripheral lower quadrants of the retina extend for a variable distance into the temporal lobe, lesions of this lobe may be accompanied by a homonymous upper quadrantic field defect. Parietal lobe lesions may affect the lower quadrants more than the upper.

If the entire optic tract or calcarine cortex on one side is destroyed, there is complete homonymous hemianopsia, including that part of the field supplied by the macula. Incomplete lesions of the optic tract and radiation usually spare central (macular) vision. Apparent macular sparing is frequently due to imperfect fixation of gaze. A lesion of the tip of one occipital lobe produces central homonymous hemianopsia because half the macular fibers of both eyes terminate there. Lesions of both occipital poles (as in embolization of the posterior cerebral arteries) result in bilateral central scotomas; if all the calcarine cortex on both sides is completely destroyed, there is "cortical" blindness. Altitudinal or horizontal hemianopsias are more often due to lesions of the occipital lobes below or above the calcarine sulcus than to lesions of the optic chiasm.

In addition to blindness, i.e., "visual anesthesia," there is another category of visual impairment, which consists of a defect of visual perception, i.e., *visual agnosia.* The patient can see but cannot recognize objects unless he hears, smells, tastes, or palpates them. The failure of visual recognition of words alone is called *alexia.* The ability to recognize visually presented objects and words depends upon the integrity not only of the visual pathways and primary

FIGURE 20-1
Diagram showing the effects on the fields of vision produced by lesions at various points along the optic pathway. A *Complete blindness in left eye;* B *bitemporal hemianopsia;* C *nasal hemianopsia of left eye;* D *right homonymous hemianopsia;* E *and* F *right upper and lower quadrant hemianopsias;* G *right homonymous hemianopsia with preservation of central vision. (From Homans,* A Textbook of Surgery, *Springfield, Ill.: Charles C Thomas, 1945)*

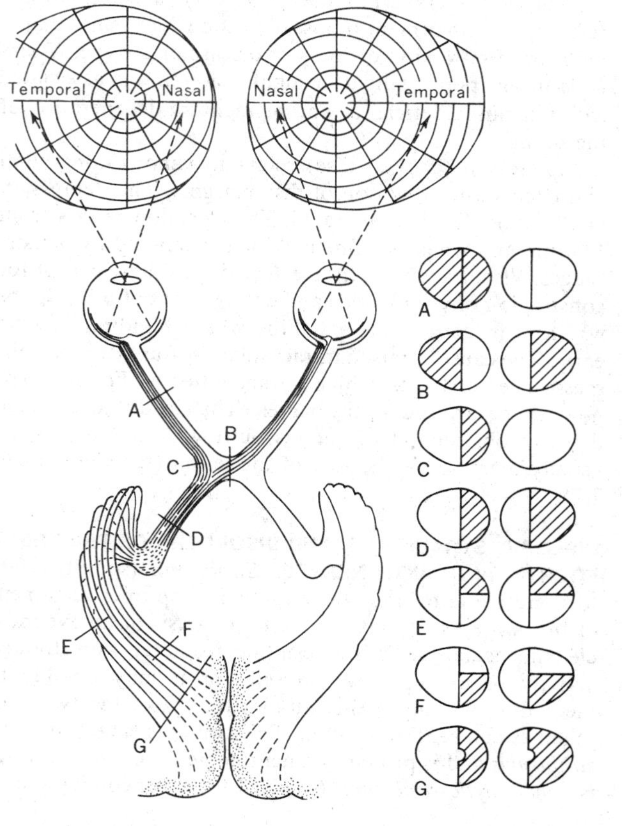

areas of the cerebral cortex but also of those secondary and tertiary visual cortical areas which lie just anterior to them and the angular gyrus of the dominant hemisphere. Visual-object agnosia and alexia result from lesions of these latter areas or from a lesion of the left calcarine cortex combined with one which interrupts the fibers crossing from the right occipital lobe. These subjects are discussed further in Chaps. 21 and 27.

Other disturbances of vision include various types of distortion in which the perceived objects appear too small (micropsia), too large (macropsia), or askew. If this disturbance is in only one eye, a local retinal lesion should be suspected. When bilateral, such phenomena suggest disease of the temporal lobes; the latter may be accompanied by attacks with complex visual hallucinations which actually represent a sensory seizure (Chap. 24).

The optic nerves also contain the afferent fibers for the pupillary reflexes. These fibers leave the optic tract and terminate in the superior colliculi. A lesion of the optic nerve or tracts may abolish the pupillary light reflex; the pupil is dilated and unreactive. Cerebral lesions, on the other hand, leave the pupillary light reflex unaltered. The lack of direct reflex in the blind eye and of consensual reflex in the sound one means that the afferent limb of the reflex arc (optic nerve) is the site of the lesion. A lack of direct light reflex with retention of the consensual reflex places the lesion in the efferent limb of the reflex (the homolateral oculomotor nucleus or nerve). Loss of light reflex without visual impairment or ocular palsy (Argyll Robertson pupillary phenomenon) is thought to be due to a lesion in the superior colliculi or periaqueductal region (see Alterations of Pupils below).

Amaurosis refers to blindness from any cause. *Amblyopia* refers to an impairment or loss of vision which is not due to an error of refraction or to other disease of the eye. *Nyctalopia* means poor twilight or night vision and is associated with vitamin A deficiency and pigmentary degeneration of the retina.

Papilledema (choked disc) refers to venous congestion and edema and elevation of disc margins. The depression of the optic disc is obliterated. The elevation ranges from 1–4 mm and when extreme may be surrounded by hemorrhages. Visual acuity is little affected until late, except for constriction of visual fields and enlargement of blind spots, which is in contrast to papillitis where blindness occurs early. The cause is raised intracranial pressure (tumors, abscesses, hemorrhages) which is transmitted to the subarachnoid space around optic nerves. This leads, after some days, to obstruction of venous outflow from the retinas, usually more so on the side of the lesion (see Color Plate 7-3).

DIPLOPIA, STRABISMUS, AND DISORDERS OF THE THIRD, FOURTH, AND SIXTH NERVES *Strabismus* (squint) refers to a muscle imbalance that results in improper alignment of the two eyes. It may be due to paralysis of an eye muscle, the ocular deviation resulting from the unrestrained activity of the opposing muscle; or it may be due to inequality of tone in the muscles that yoke the two eyes together in a central position. The former is called *paralytic strabismus* and is primarily a neurologic problem; the latter is *nonparalytic strabismus* (referred to as concomitant strabismus if the squinting eye has a full range of movement) and is an ophthalmologic problem. Once binocular fusion is established, any type of ocular imbalance causes diplopia, for the reason that images then fall on disparate or noncorresponding parts of the two retinas. After a time, however, the patient learns to suppress the image of one eye. This almost invariably happens early in concomitant strabismus of congenital nature, and the person grows up with a diminished visual acuity in that eye (*amblyopia ex anopsia*). The vision may remain normal in both eyes when the eyes are used alternately for fixation; this is *alternating strabismus.*

The oculomotor, trochlear, and abducens nerves innervate the extrinsic musculature of the eye. A knowledge of their origin and anatomic relationships is essential to an understanding of the various paralytic ocular syndromes. The oculomotor nucleus consists of several groups of nerve cells ventral to the aqueduct of Sylvius, at the level of the superior colliculi. The nerve cells that innervate the iris and ciliary body are situated anteriorly in the so-called "Edinger-Westphal nucleus." Below this nucleus are the cells for the superior rectus, inferior oblique, internal rectus, and inferior rectus muscles, in that order from above downward. Convergence is under the control of the medial groups of cells, the nucleus of Perlia. The cells of origin of the trochlear nerves are just inferior to those of the oculomotor nerves. The sixth nerve arises at a considerably lower level, from a paired group of cells in the floor of the fourth ventricle at the level of the lower pons. The intrapontine portion of the facial nerve loops around the sixth nerve nucleus before it turns anterolaterally to make its exit; a lesion in this locality usually causes a homolateral paralysis of both lateral rectus and facial muscles.

All three nerves, after leaving the brainstem, course anteriorly and pass through the cavernous sinus, where they come into close proximity with the ophthalmic division of the fifth nerve, and together they enter the orbit through the superior orbital fissure. The oculomotor nerve supplies all the extrinsic ocular muscles except two—the superior oblique and the external rectus—which are innervated by the trochlear and the abducens nerves, respectively. The voluntary part of the levator palpebrae muscle is also supplied by the oculomotor nerve, the involuntary part being under the control of autonomic fibers. Parasympathetic fibers of the oculomotor nerve supply the sphincter pupillae and the ciliary muscles (muscles of accommodation).

Although all the extraocular muscles probably participate in every movement of the eyes, particular muscles move the eyes in certain fields. The lateral rectus rotates the eye outward; the medial rectus, inward. The function of the vertical recti and the oblique muscles varies according to the position of the eye. When the eye is turned outward, the elevators and depressors of the eye are the superior and inferior recti; when the eye is turned inward, they are the inferior and superior oblique muscles, respectively. In contrast, torsion of the eyeball is effected by the oblique muscles when the eye is turned outward, and by the recti when it is turned inward.

Accurate binocular vision is achieved by the associated action of the ocular muscles, which allows a visual stimulus to fall on exactly corresponding parts of the two retinas. Conjugate movement of the eyes is controlled by centers in the cerebral cortex and brainstem. Area 8 in the frontal lobe is the center for voluntary conjugate movements of the eyes to the opposite side. In addition, there is a center in the occipital lobe concerned with contralateral following movements. Fibers from these centers pass to the opposite sides of the brainstem, where they connect with lower centers for conjugate movements: those for the right lateral gaze are thought to be in the proximity of the right abducens nucleus; those for the left lateral gaze are near the left abducens. Simultaneous innervation of one internal rectus and the other external rectus during lateral gaze is mediated through the medial longitudinal fasciculus which connects one abducens nucleus with the opposite oculomotor. The arrangements of nerve cells and fibers for vertical gaze and convergence are situated in the pretectal areas and paramedian zones of the midbrain tegmentum.

OCULAR MUSCLE AND GAZE PALSIES There are three types of paralysis of extraocular muscles: (1) paralysis of isolated ocular muscles, (2) paralysis of conjugate movements (gaze), and (3) syndromes of mixed gaze and ocular muscle paralysis.

Characteristic clinical disturbances result from single lesions of the third, fourth, or sixth cranial nerves. A complete third nerve lesion causes ptosis (since the levator palpebrae is supplied mainly by the third nerve), an inability to rotate the eye upward, downward, or inward; a divergent strabismus due to unopposed action of the lateral rectus muscle; a dilated nonreactive pupil (iridoplegia); and paralysis of accommodation (cycloplegia). When only the muscles of the iris and ciliary body are paralyzed, the condition is termed *internal ophthalmoplegia.* Fourth nerve lesions result in an extorsion of the eye and a weakness of downward gaze most marked when the eye is turned inward, so that patients commonly complain of special difficulty in going downstairs. Head tilting, to the opposite shoulder, is especially characteristic of fourth nerve lesions. This maneuver causes a compensatory intorsion of the lower part of the eye, enabling the patient to obtain binocular vision. Lesions of the sixth nerve result in paralysis of abduction and a convergent strabismus, owing to the unopposed action of the internal rectus muscles. With incomplete sixth nerve palsies, turning the head toward the side of the paretic muscle may overcome diplopia. (The foregoing signs may occur with various degrees of completeness, depending on the severity and site of the lesion or lesions.)

TABLE 20-1
Comparison of lesions within and outside the brainstem

Effect	*Lesions within the brainstem*	*Lesions external to the brainstem*
Involvement of multiple contiguous nerves	±	+
Involvement of sensorimotor tracts	+, often "alternating" or crossed sensory motor palsies	±
Disturbance of consciousness	+	0(+ late)
Evidence of other segmental disturbances of the brainstem such as decerebrate rigidity, tonic neck reflexes, pseudobulbar palsy	+	0(+ late)
X-ray evidence of erosion of cranial bones or enlargement of foramens	0	+

Ocular palsies may be central, i.e., due to a lesion of the nucleus or the intramedullary portion of the cranial nerve, or peripheral. Ophthalmoplegia due to a lesion in the brainstem is usually accompanied by involvement of other cranial nerves or long tracts. Peripheral lesions, which may or may not be solitary, have a great variety of causes; the most common are *aneurysm of the circle of Willis,* tumors of the base of the brain, carcinomatosis of the meninges, herpes zoster, *syphilitic* and other chronic forms of *meningitis.* The third nerve palsy that occurs with diabetes is most often due to infarction of the third nerve, and the prognosis for recovery in such cases, as with other nonprogressive diseases of the peripheral nerve, is usually excellent. The points of difference between lesions within and outside the brainstem are tabulated in Table 20-1, and the various intramedullary and extramedullary cranial nerve syndromes are described in Table 332-1 and 332-2. See also the diagrams in Chap. 334.

Paralysis of conjugate movement (gaze) The term *conjugate gaze,* or *conjugate movement,* refers to the simultaneous movement of the two eyes in the same direction. An acute lesion, such as an infarct, in one frontal lobe may cause paralysis of contralateral gaze, and the eyes will turn toward the side of the lesion. The ocular disorder in this circumstance is temporary (several days' duration). In bilateral frontal lesions the patient may be unable to turn his eyes voluntarily in any direction—up, down, or to the side—but retains fixation and following movements, which are believed to be occipital lobe functions. Gaze paralysis of cerebral origin is not attended by strabismus or diplopia. The usual causes are vascular occlusion with infarction, hemorrhage, and abscess or tumor of the frontal lobe. With certain extrapyramidal disorders, e.g., postencephalitic parkinsonism, Huntington's chorea, and Steele-Richardson disease, ocular movements may be limited in all directions, especially upward. Lesions of the superior colliculi and tegmentum, near the posterior commissure, interfere with voluntary upward gaze, and often movements of convergence as well as the pupillary light reflexes are abolished (Parinaud's syndrome). There also exists a pontine center for conjugate lateral gaze, probably in the vicinity of the abducens nuclei. A lesion here causes ipsilateral gaze palsy, with the eyes turning to the opposite side. Vertical and lateral gaze palsies are combined in the supranuclear ophthalmoplegia syndrome of Steele-Richardson. The palsy is persistent unlike that with cerebral lesions and is frequently accompanied by other signs of midbrain disease. Fully developed forms of gaze paralysis are readily discerned, but lesser degrees may be overlooked unless one pays special attention to the predominant position of the eyes and tests the ability to sustain conjugate movement.

Ocular apraxia on looking to the side is another special gaze disorder. Normally on looking to the side the eyes and head turn together but in this condition the head turns and the eyes actually go in the opposite direction. The head is flung too far, then the eyes "catch up." This may be a solitary congenital abnormality (Cogan), the anatomy of which is unknown, or it may be acquired as in ataxia telangiectasia (see Chap. 342).

In skew deviation, a poorly understood disorder of gaze, the eyes diverge, one looking down, the other up. The deviation is constant in all fields of gaze. It may occur with any lesion of the posterior fossa but particularly with one in the brainstem. The lesion is on the side of the lower eye.

Mixed gaze and ocular paralyses These are always a sign of intrapontine or mesencephalic disease. A lesion of the lower pons in or near the sixth nerve nucleus causes a homolateral paralysis of the lateral rectus muscle and a failure of adduction of the opposite eye, i.e., a combined paralysis of the sixth nerve and of conjugate lateral gaze. Lesions of the medial longitudinal fasciculi interfere with lateral conjugate gaze in another way. When the patient looks to the right, the left eye fails to adduct; when he looks to the left, the right eye fails to adduct. The abducting eye may show nystagmus. This condition is referrred to as *internuclear ophthalmoplegia* and should always be suspected when only adduction of the eyes is affected. If the lesion is in the higher (midbrain) part of the medial longitudinal fasciculus, convergence may be lost, along with paralysis of the medial recti on attempted lateral gaze (anterior internuclear ophthalmoplegia); if the lesion is in the lower (pontine) part, convergence is normal but there may be some degree of associated limitation of conjugate lateral gaze or sixth nerve palsy (posterior internuclear ophthalmoplegia).

NYSTAGMUS This refers to involuntary rhythmic movements of the eyes; it is of two types, oscillating (pendular) and rhythmic (jerk). In jerk nystagmus, the movements are distinctly faster in one direction than the other; in pendular nystagmus, the oscillations are roughly equal in rate for the two directions, although on conjugate lateral gaze, the pendular type may resemble the jerk type, with the fast component to the side of the gaze.

In testing for nystagmus, the eyes should first be examined in the central position and then during upward, downward, and lateral movements. If nystagmus is monocular, each eye should be tested separately, with the other one covered. Labyrinthine nystagmus is most obvious when visual fixation is prevented by shielding the eyes; and brainstem nystagmus and cerebellar nystagmus are brought out best by having the patient fixate on a finger. Labyrinthine nystagmus may vary with the position of the head; hence, these various tests should be performed with the head in several different positions. In particular, the postural nystagmus of Bárány is evoked by hyperextension of the neck, with the patient supine. Optokinetic nystagmus should be tested by asking the patient to look at a rotating cylinder on which several stripes have been painted or at a striped cloth moved across the field of vision.

A few irregular jerks are observed in many normal individuals when the eyes are turned far to the side. These so-called "nystagmoid movements" are probably similar to the tremulousness of a muscle that is contracted maximally. Occasionally a fine rhythmic nystagmus may be found in extreme lateral gaze, but if it is bilateral and disappears as the eyes move a few degrees toward the midline, it usually has no clinical significance.

Pendular nystagmus is found in a variety of conditions in which central vision is lost early in life, such as albinism and in various other diseases of the retina and refractive media. Occasionally it is observed in patients with multiple sclerosis and as a congenital abnormality, even without poor vision. The syndrome of miners' nystagmus, formerly a common cause of industrial disability, occurs after many years of work in comparative darkness. The oscillations of the eyes are very rapid, increase on upward gaze, and are often associated with vertigo, head tremor, and intolerance of light.

Jerk nystagmus is the commoner type. It may be lateral or vertical, particularly on ocular movement in these planes, or it may be rotary. By custom, the direction of the nystagmus is named according to the direction of the fast component. There are several varieties of jerk nystagmus. When one is watching a moving object—e.g., the passing landscape from a train window or a rotating drum with vertical stripes—a rhythmic jerk nystagmus, *optokinetic nystagmus,* normally appears. The slow phase is a result of visual fixation; the quick phase is compensatory. With unilateral cerebral lesions, particularly in the parietooccipital region, optokinetic nystagmus is lost when the moving stimulus, e.g., the drum, moves toward the side of the lesion.

Aside from optokinetic nystagmus, lateral and vertical nystagmus are most frequently due to barbiturate intoxication. Jerk nystagmus may signify disease of the labyrinthine-vestibular apparatus. Labyrinthine stimulation or irritation produces a nystagmus with the fast phase to the opposite side. The slow component reflects the effect of impulses derived from the semicircular canals, and the fast component is a corrective movement. Vestibular-labyrinthine nystagmus may be horizontal, vertical, or, most characteristically, rotary. Vertigo, nausea, vomiting, and staggering are the usual accompaniments (Chap. 19). Brainstem lesions often cause a coarse unidirectional nystagmus, which may be horizontal or vertical; the latter is brought out usually on upward gaze and rarely on downward gaze. The presence of vertical nystagmus is pathognomonic of disease in the tegmentum of the brainstem. Vertigo is inconstant, and signs of disease of other nuclear structures and tracts in the brainstem are frequent. Upward jerk nystagmus of this type is frequent in demyelinative or vascular disease, in tumors, and in Wernicke's disease and syringobulbia. Vertical downward nystagmus is most often associated with the Arnold-Chiari malformation. Cerebellopontine angle tumors cause a coarse bilateral horizontal nystagmus, coarser to the side of the lesion. Nystagmus probably does not occur with cerebellar disease unless the fastigial nuclei and their connections with the vestibular nuclei are involved. The nystagmus that occurs only in the abducting eye and is said to be a pathognomonic sign of multiple sclerosis probably represents an incompletely developed form of internuclear ophthalmoplegia.

Convergence nystagmus is a rhythmic oscillation in which a slow abduction of the eyes in respect to each other is followed by a quick movement of adduction. It is usually accompanied by other types of nystagmus and by one or more features of Parinaud's syndrome. Occasionally there is also a rhythmic retraction movement of the eyes (*nystagmus retractorius*) or eyelids, or a maintained spasm of convergence, best brought out on attempted elevation of the eyes to command. These unusual phenomena all point to a lesion of the upper midbrain tegmentum and are usually manifestations of vascular disease or of pinealoma. *Seesaw nystagmus*—one eye moving up, the other down—is occasionally observed in conjunction with bitemporal hemianopia. Its mechanism is unknown.

Oscillopsia refers to illusory movement of the environment, in which objects seem to move back and forth, to jerk, or to wiggle. It may or may not occur with turning of the eyes and consequent displacement of the image on the retina. *Opsoclonus* is the term applied to either sustained, irregular, conjugate "dancing" movements of the eyes in a horizontal, rotary, and vertical direction or a fast-frequency flutter. The neurologic basis for these movements is not clear, but in most cases they are associated with signs of cerebellar disease.

Ocular dysmetria consists of an overshoot of the eyes on attempted fixation, followed by several cycles of oscillations of diminishing amplitude until precise fixation is attained. The overshoot may occur on eccentric fixation or on refixation in the primary position of gaze. This sign occurs in disease of the cerebellum or its pathways and is analogous to cerebellar dysmetria of the limbs.

ALTERATIONS OF PUPILS Pupil size is determined by the balance of innervation between the dilator and constrictor fibers. The pupillodilator fibers arise in the posterior part of the hypothalamus and descend in the lateral tegmentum of the midbrain, pons, medulla, and cervical spinal cord to the eighth cervical and first thoracic segments, where they synapse with the lateral horn cells. These give rise to preganglionic fibers that synapse in the superior cervical ganglion; the postganglionic fibers course along the internal carotid artery and traverse the cavernous sinus to join the first division of the trigeminal nerve, finally reaching the eyes as the long ciliary nerves. The pupilloconstrictor fibers arise in the nucleus of Edinger-Westphal, join the oculomotor nerve, and synapse in the ciliary ganglion with the postganglionic neurons that innervate the iris and ciliary body.

The pupils are usually equal in size, though if the eyes are turned to one side, the pupil of the abducting eye dilates slightly. Pupil size varies with light intensity; as one pupil constricts under a bright light (direct reflex), the other unexposed pupil does likewise (consensual reflex). Pupillary constriction is also part of the act of convergence and accommodation for near objects.

Interruption of the sympathetic fibers either centrally, between the hypothalamus and their point of exit from the spinal cord (first thoracic segment), or peripherally (superior cervical ganglion in the neck or along the carotid artery) results in miosis and ptosis (because of paralysis of the levator palpebrae), with loss of sweating of the face, and occasionally enophthalmos (Bernard-Horner syndrome). Stimulation or irritation of the pupillodilator fibers has the opposite effect, i.e., lid retraction, slight proptosis, and dilatation of the pupil. The ciliospinal pupillary reflex, evoked by pinching the neck, is effected through these efferent sympathetic fibers. Abnormal dilatation of the pupils (mydriasis), often with loss of pupillary light reflexes, may result from midbrain lesions and is a frequent finding in cases of deep coma. Extreme constriction of the pupils (miosis) is commonly observed with pontine lesions, presumably because of bilateral interruption of the pupillodilator fibers.

The functional integrity of the sympathetic and parasympathetic nerve endings in the iris may be determined by the use of certain drugs. Atropine and homatropine dilate the pupils by paralyzing the parasympathetic nerve endings; physostigmine and pilocarpine constrict them, the former by inhibiting cholinesterase activity at the neuromuscular junction, and the latter by direct stimulation of the sphincter muscle of the iris. Cocaine dilates the pupils by stimulating the sympathetic nerve endings. Morphine acts centrally to constrict the pupils.

In chronic syphilitic meningitis and other forms of late syphilis, particularly tabes dorsalis, the pupils are usually small, irregular, and unequal; they do not dilate properly in response to mydriatic drugs and fail to react to light, although they do constrict on accommodation. In some cases there is an associated atrophy of the iris. This is known as the *Argyll Robertson pupil.* The exact locality of the lesion is not certain; it is generally believed to be in the tectum of the midbrain proximal to the oculomotor nuclei, where the descending pupillodilator fibers are in close proximity to the light-reflex fibers. A dissociation of the light reflex from the accommodation-convergence reaction is sometimes observed with other midbrain lesions, e.g., pinealoma, multiple sclerosis, and diabetes mellitus; in these diseases miosis, irregularity of pupils, and failure to respond to a mydriatic are not constantly present. However, in the usual Argyll Robertson pupillary abnormality of tabes and of diabetic and amyloid polyneuropathy the lesion is probably peripheral, in the oculomotor nerve or ciliary ganglion. Another interesting pupillary abnormality is the myotonic reaction, sometimes referred to as *Adie's pupil.* The patient may complain of blurring of vision or may have suddenly noticed that one pupil is larger than the other. The reaction to light and convergence are absent if tested in the customary manner, although the size of the pupil will change slowly on prolonged stimulation. Once contracted or dilated, the pupils remain in that state for some minutes. The affected pupil reacts promptly to the usual mydriatic and miotic drugs but is usually sensitive to a 2.5% solution of Mecholyl, a strength that will not affect a normal pupil. The myotonic pupil usually appears during the third or fourth decade of life; it may be associated with absence of knee or ankle jerks and hence be mistaken for tabes dorsalis.

Ocular movement, pupillary contraction, and visual acuity may be affected by diseases which alter the contents of the orbit. Usually this is accompanied by bilateral exophthalmos, as in thyroid or pituitary disease (Chap. 92), unilateral exophthalmos with orbital tumors (dermoids, adenoma of lacrimal gland, optic nerve glioma, neurofibroma, metastatic carcinoma, meningioma) or granuloma, or cavernous sinus thrombosis (Chap. 337). Progressive paralysis of the eyelids, which may obstruct vision, occurs separately or as part of an external paralysis, as in ocular dystrophy or in oculopharyngeal dystrophy.

DISTURBANCES OF HEARING *Tinnitus* and *deafness* are frequent symptoms and always indicate disease of the ear or of the auditory nerve and its central connections.

Tinnitus, or ringing in the ears, is a purely subjective phenomenon and may also be reported as a buzzing, whistling, hissing, or roaring sound. It is a very common symptom in adults (present in more than 90 percent). Low-frequency vibratory clicks, pops, roarings, etc., are invariably due to diseases of the middle ear and eustachian tube. High-pitched tonal, nonvibratory tinnitus means disease of the cochlea and eighth nerve. Severe and prolonged tinnitus in the presence of normal hearing is very rare. If tinnitus is localized to one ear and is described as having a low-pitched tonal character, such as ringing or a bell-like tone, and particularly if there is reduced hearing with the recruitment phenomenon (see below), it is probably cochlear in origin. Clicking sounds are caused by intermittent contraction of the tensor tympani. A pulsating tinnitus synchronous with the pulse may be related to an intracranial vascular malformation; however, this symptom must be carefully judged, since introspective persons often report hearing their pulse when lying with one ear on a pillow. Certain drugs such as salicylates and quinine produce tinnitus and transient deafness. Nervous persons are less tolerant of tinnitus than more stable ones; depressed or anxious patients may demand relief from tinnitus that has existed for years.

Examination of hearing should always begin with inspection of the external auditory canal and the tympanic membrane. A ticking watch or whispered words are suitable means of testing hearing at the bedside, the opposite ear being closed by the finger. If there is any suspicion of deafness or a complaint of tinnitus or vertigo, or if the patient is a child with a speech defect, then hearing must be tested further. This can be done with the use of tuning forks of different frequencies, but the most accurate results are obtained by the use of an electric audiometer and the construction of an audiogram which reveals the entire range of hearing at a glance.

Deafness is frequent. In the United States it is estimated that there are more than 6 million persons with hearing loss; in one-third to one-half these persons the loss is hereditary. The deafness is of two types: (1) nerve deafness (also called sensorineural), due to cochlear disease or interruption of nerve fibers, and (2) conduction deafness, due to disease of the middle ear, such as otosclerosis or chronic otitis, or to occlusion of the external auditory canal or eustachian tube. In differentiating these two types, the tuning fork tests are of value. When a vibrating fork of 256-d.v. frequency is held several inches from the ear (the test for air conduction), sound waves can be appreciated only as they are transmitted through the middle ear and are reduced with disease in this location. When the fork is applied to the skull (test for bone conduction), the sound waves are conveyed directly to the cochlea, without the intervention of the middle ear apparatus, and are therefore not reduced or lost. Normally air conduction is better than bone conduction. These principles form the basis for several tests of auditory function.

In *Weber's test,* the vibrating fork is applied to the forehead in the midline. In middle ear deafness the sound is localized in the affected ear; in nerve deafness, in the normal ear. In *Rinné's test,* the vibrating fork is applied to the mastoid process, the other ear being closed by the observer's finger. At the moment the sound ceases, the fork is held at the auditory meatus. In middle ear deafness the sound cannot be heard by air conduction after bone conduction has ceased (abnormal or negative Rinné's test). In nerve deafness the reverse is true (normal or positive Rinné's test), although both air and bone conduction may be quantitatively decreased. In *Schwabach's test,* the patient's bone conduction is compared with that of a normal observer. In general, high-pitched tones are lost in nerve deafness and low-pitched ones in middle ear deafness, but there are frequent exceptions to this rule.

The following audiologic tests, taken together, help distinguish between cochlear and retrocochlear (nerve) lesions. (1) *Auditory recruitment:* the difference in hearing between the two ears is estimated, and the loudness of the stimulus delivered to each ear is then increased by regular increments. In nonrecruiting deafness (characteristic of nerve trunk lesion) the original difference in hearing persists in all comparisons of loudness above threshold. In recruiting deafness (as occurs in Ménière's disease) the more defective ear gains in loudness and finally is equal to the better one. (2) *Speech discrimination:* retrocochlear lesions are indicated by scores indicating less than 25 percent of words recognized. (3) *Short-increment sensitivity index* (SISI), in which the patient responds to a series of twenty 1-decibel (dB) increments in amplitude superimposed on a steady tone of the same frequency presented at a sensation level of 20 dB. The patient's score is the percentage of these 20-dB increments which he is able to detect at a given frequency. Low SISI scores, below 60 percent, point to an end-organ lesion. (4) *Threshold sensitivity* recorded via *Békésy audiometry* for both continuous and interrupted tonal stimuli: four types of tracing may be obtained; the type II tracing is obtained in patients with end-organ lesions, and type III or IV, usually the former, characterizes retrocochlear lesions. (5) *Threshold tone decay:* this test quantifies auditory adaptation and requires only a conventional pure tone audiometer. Retrocochlear lesions yield greater amounts of decay than cochlear ones.

The common causes of middle ear deafness are otitis media, otosclerosis, and rupture of the eardrum. Nerve deafness has many causes. The internal ear may be aplastic from birth (hereditary deaf-mutism), or it may be damaged by rubella in the pregnant mother. Acute purulent meningitis or chronic infection spreading from the middle ear may cause nerve deafness in childhood. The auditory nerve may be involved by tumors of the cerebellopontine angle or by syphilis. Deafness may also result from a demyelinative plaque in the brainstem. A large series of genetically determined syndromes which feature a neural type of deafness, some congenital, others progressive, has recently come to light (see article by Konigsmark). The most interesting of these are dominant progressive nerve deafness, dominant unilateral deafness, dominant low-frequency hearing loss, recessive congenital deafness, sex-linked congenital neural deafness, several types of deafness (neural and conductive) with malformations of external ears, face, and neck (Treacher-Collins disease and Engelmann's diaphyseal dysplasia); hereditary deafness with goiter (Pendred's disease); hereditary heart disease with deafness; hereditary deafness with various combinations of mental retardation, retinitis pigmentosa, and polyneuropathy (as in Hallgren's disease, Alstrom's disease, Refsum's disease); hereditary deafness with skin abnormalities such as albinism, lentigines, piebaldness, white forelock (Waardenburg's disease), onchydystrophy and pegged teeth, atopic dermatitis, anhydrosis.

Of the types of progressive conduction deafness, hereditary otosclerosis is the most frequent (cause of 50 percent of deafness in adulthood). Hysterical deafness may be difficult to distinguish from organic disease. In the case of bilateral deafness, the distinction can be made by observing a blink (cochleoorbicular reflex) or an alteration in skin sweating (psychogalvanic skin reflex) in response to a loud sound. Unilateral hysterical deafness may be detected by an audiometer, with both ears connected, or by whispering into the bell of a stethoscope attached to the patient's ears, closing first one tube and then the other without the patient's knowledge.

In otosclerosis and hereditary sensorineural deafness, vestibular function is usually retained (caloric responses are normal).

REFERENCES

Bender MB: Neurophthalmology, in *Clinical Neurology,* vol. 1, chap. 4, ed AB Baker, New York: Hoeber-Harper, 1962

Cogan DG: *Neurology of the Ocular Muscles,* 2d ed., Springfield, Ill.: Charles C Thomas, 1956

Konigsmark BW: Medical progress. Hereditary deafness in man. N Engl J Med 281:713–720; 774–778; 827–832, 1969

Tillman TW: Special hearing tests in otoneurologic diagnosis. Arch Otolaryngol 89:25–30, 1969

21
DISORDERS OF SENSATION

MAURICE VICTOR
RAYMOND D. ADAMS

Loss or perversion of somatic sensation not infrequently is the principal manifestation of disease of the nervous system. The reason for this is clear enough, since the major anatomic pathways of the sensory system are distinct from those of the motor system and may be selectively disturbed by disease. An understanding of these sensory disorders may provide important leads to neurologic diagnosis.

GENERAL CONSIDERATIONS Unfortunately, space does not permit here a more detailed review of the anatomy of the sensory system or of its physiology. The interested reader may turn to the references at the end of the chapter. The cutaneous distribution of sensory spinal roots may be observed in Fig. 21-1 (see also Chap. 5).

Disorders of the somatic sensory apparatus pose special problems for the patient. He is confronted with derangements of sensation which may be unlike anything he has previously experienced, and he has few words in his vocabulary to describe what he feels. He may say that a limb feels "numb" and "dead" when in fact he means it is weak. Observant individuals may occasionally discover a loss of sensation, for example, inability to feel discomfort on touching an object hot enough to blister the skin or unawareness of articles of clothing and other objects in contact with the skin. But more often disease has induced a new and unnatural series of sensory experiences. If nerves, spinal roots, or spinal tracts are only partially interrupted, a touch may arouse tingling or pricking, meaning presumably that at least some of the remaining touch and pain fibers are functional but are acting abnormally. Tightness and drawing and pulling sensations, a feeling of a band or girdle around the limb or trunk, are common with partial involvement of pressure fibers. Similarly, burning and pain (causalgia) may represent overactivity of surviving thermal and pain fibers. The responsible lesion may be in the peripheral nerve, the lateral spinothalamic tract in the spinal cord or brainstem, or the thalamus. Also, hyperesthesia and hyperpathia are frequent. These abnormal sensations are called *paresthesias,* or *dysesthesias,* if they are unpleasant; and their character and distribution inform us of the anatomy of the lesion involving the sensory system.

EXAMINATION OF SENSATION The examination of sensation is the most difficult part of the neurologic examination. For one thing, test procedures are relatively crude and inadequate. And, embarrassingly often, no objective sensory loss can be demonstrated despite symptoms that clearly indicate the presence of such a deficit. Also, a response to a sensory stimulus is difficult to evaluate objectively, since the examiner's conclusions depend on the patient's inter-

FIGURE 21-1
Distribution of the sensory spinal roots on the surface of the body. (From G Holmes, Introduction to Clinical Neurology, *2d ed., Baltimore: Williams & Wilkins, 1952)*

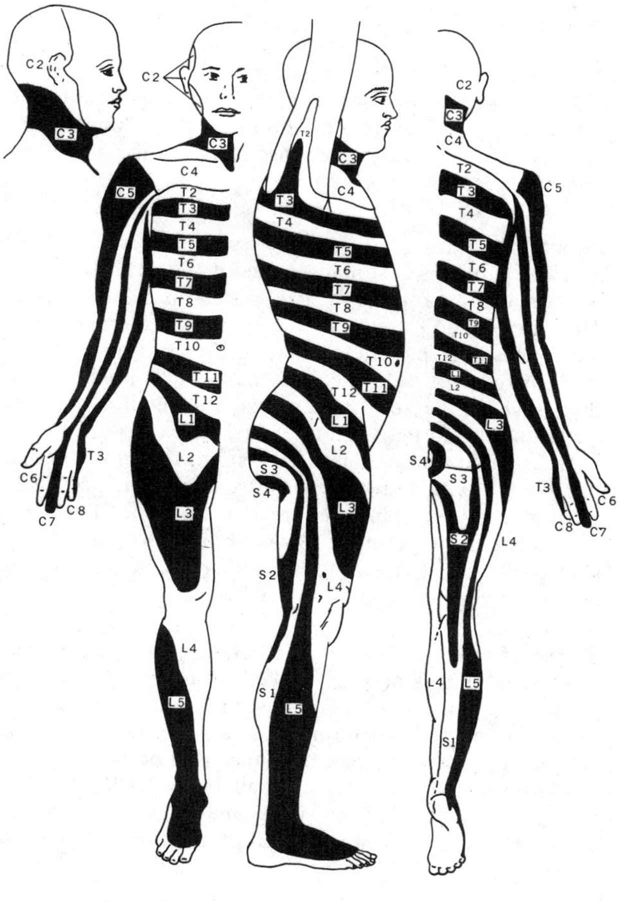

pretations of sensory experiences. This presupposes a general responsiveness, alertness, and a desire to cooperate, as well as intelligence and a certain level of education. Hypersuggestibility and fatigue may interfere with the obtaining of accurate test data.

The detail in which sensation is tested will be determined by the clinical situation. If the patient has no sensory complaints, it is sufficient to examine vibration and position sense in the fingers and toes, to test the appreciation of pain over the face, trunk, and extremities, and to determine whether the sensory findings are the same in symmetric parts of the body. A rough survey of this sort may detect sensory defects of which the patient is unaware. On the other hand, more thorough testing is in order if the patient has complaints referable to the sensory system, or if there is localized atrophy or weakness, ataxia, trophic changes of joints, or painless ulcers.

A few other general principles should be mentioned. One should not press the sensory examination in the presence of fatigue, for an inattentive patient is a poor witness. The examiner must also avoid suggesting symptoms to the patient. After having explained in the simplest terms what is required, he should interpose as few questions and remarks as possible. Consequently, the patient must not be asked, "Do you feel that?" each time he is touched; he should simply be told to say "yes" or "sharp" every time he has been touched or feels pain. The patient should not be permitted to see the part under examination. For short tests it is sufficient that he close his eyes; during more detailed testing it is preferable to screen his eyes from the part being examined. Finally, the findings of the sensory examination should be accurately recorded on a chart.

Sensation is frequently classified as *superficial* (cutaneous, exteroceptive) and *deep* (proprioceptive); the former comprises the modalities of light touch, pain, and temperature; the latter includes the sense of position, passive motion, vibration, and deep pain.

Sense of touch This is usually tested with a wisp of cotton. The patient is first made acquainted with the nature of the stimulus by applying it to a normal part of the body. Then he is asked to say "yes" each time various other parts are touched. A patient simulating sensory loss may say "no" in response to a tactile stimulus. Cornified areas of skin, such as the soles and palms, will require a heavier stimulus than normal, and the hair-clad parts a lighter one because of the numerous nerve endings around the hair follicle. The patient is more sensitive to a moving contactual stimulus of any kind than a stationary one. The gentle movement of the examiner's or preferably the patient's finger tip over his skin is a useful method of mapping out an area of tactile loss.

Sense of pain This is most efficiently estimated by pinprick, although it may be evoked by a great diversity of noxious stimuli. The patient must understand that he is to report the degree of sharpness of the pin, not simply the feeling of contact or pressure of the point or even a special sensation due to penetration of the skin. If the pinpricks are applied rapidly, their effects may be summated and excessive pain may result; therefore, they should be delivered not too rapidly, about one per second, and not over the same spot.

If an area of diminished or absent touch or pain sensation is encountered, its boundaries should be demarcated to determine whether it has a segmental or peripheral nerve distribution or whether sensation is lost below a certain level. Such areas are best delineated by proceeding from the region of impaired sensation toward the normal, and the changes may be confirmed by dragging a pin lightly over the skin.

Deep pressure sense One can estimate this sense simply by pinching or pressing deeply on the tendons and muscles. Pain can often be elicited by heavy pressure even when superficial sensation is diminished; conversely, in some diseases, such as tabetic neurosyphilis, the loss of deep pressure sense may be more prominent.

The following procedure for testing thermal sensation is suggested. The areas of skin to be tested should be exposed for some time before the examination. The test objects should be large, preferably Erlenmeyer flasks containing hot and cold water. Thermometers, which extend into the water through the flask stoppers, indicate the temperature of the water at the moment of testing. At first, extreme degrees of heat and cold (e.g., 10 and 45°C) may be employed to delineate roughly an area of thermal sensory disturbance; the patient will report that the flask feels "less hot" or "less cold" over such an area than over a normal part. If areas of impaired sensation are found, the borders may be accurately determined by moving the flask along the skin from the insensitive to the normal region. The qualitative change should then be quantitated as far as possible by estimating the *differences in temperature* which the patient is able to recognize. The patient is asked to report whether one stimulus is *warmer or colder* than another not whether a given stimulus is warm or cold, since the cooler of the two may be interpreted as warm. The range of temperature difference between the two flasks is gradually narrowed by mixing their contents. A normal person is capable of detecting a difference of 1° when the temperature of the flasks is in the range of 28 to 32°C. In the warm range he should readily recognize differences between 35 and 40°C, and in the cold range, between 10 and 20°C. In many normal older persons and in others with poor peripheral circulation (especially in cold weather), the responses may be modified.

The sensation of heat or cold depends not only on the temperature of the stimulus but also on the duration of the stimulus and the area over which it is applied. This principle may be employed to detect slight degrees of sensory impairment; the patient may be able to distinguish small differences in temperature when the bottom of the flask is applied for 3 s but unable to do so if only the side of the flask is applied for 1 s. Throughout the test procedure, especially when small temperature differences are involved, the area of sensory disturbance should be continually checked against perception in normal parts.

Postural sense and the appreciation of passive movement These modalities are usually lost together, although in any particular case one may be disproportionately affected.

Abnormalities of postural sensation may be revealed in

several ways. When the patient extends his arms in front of him and closes his eyes, the affected arm will wander from its original position; if the fingers are spread apart, they may undergo a series of slow-changing postures ("piano-playing" movements, or *pseudoathetosis*). In attempting to touch the tip of the nose with his index finger, the patient may miss the target repeatedly.

The lack of position sense in the legs may be demonstrated by displacing the limb from its original position and asking the patient to point to his large toe. If postural sensation is defective in both legs, the patient will be unable to maintain his balance with feet together and eyes closed (Romberg's sign). This sign should be interpreted with caution. Even a normal person in the Romberg position will sway slightly more with his eyes closed than open. A patient with lack of balance due to motor disorders or cerebellar disease will also sway more if his visual cues are removed. Only if there is a marked discrepancy between the state of balance with eyes open and closed can one confidently state that the patient shows Romberg's sign, i.e., loss of joint-position sense. Mild degrees of unsteadiness in nervous or suggestible patients may be overcome by diverting their attention, e.g., by having them alternately touch the index finger of each hand to their nose while standing with their eyes closed.

The appreciation of passive movement is first tested in the fingers and toes, and the defect, when present, is reflected maximally in these parts. It is important to grasp the digit firmly at the sides opposite the plane of movement; otherwise the pressure applied by the examiner in displacing the digit may allow the patient to identify the direction of movement. This applies to the testing of the more proximal segments of the limb as well. The patient should be instructed to report each movement as "up" or "down" in relation to the previous stationary position. It is useful to demonstrate the test with a large and easily identified movement, but once the idea is clear to the patient, the smallest detectable changes in position should be tested. The range of movement normally appreciated in the digits is said to be as little as 1°. Clinically, however, defective appreciation of passive movement is judged by comparison with a normal limb or, if bilaterally defective, on the basis of what the examiner has through experience learned to regard as normal. Slight impairment may be disclosed by a slow response or, if the digit is displaced very slowly, by a relative unawareness that movements have occurred; or after the digit has been displaced in the same direction several times, the patient may misjudge the first movement in the opposite direction; or after the examiner has moved the toe, the patient may make a number of small voluntary movements of the toe, in an apparent attempt to determine its position or the direction of the movement.

The sense of vibration This is a composite sensation comprising touch and rapid alterations of deep pressure sense. Its conduction depends on both cutaneous and deep afferent fibers which ascend in the dorsal columns of the cord. It is therefore rarely affected by lesions of single nerves but will be disturbed in cases of polyneuritis and disease of the dorsal columns, medial lemniscus, and thalamus. For this reason, vibration and position sense are usually lost together, although one of them (usually vibration sense) may be affected disproportionately. With advancing age, vibration sense may be diminished at the toes and ankles.

Vibration sense is tested by placing a tuning fork with a low rate (and long duration) of vibration (128 d.v.) over the bony prominences. The examiner must make sure that the patient responds to the vibration, not simply to the pressure of the fork. Although there are mechanical devices to quantitate vibration sense, it is sufficient for clinical purposes to compare the point tested with a normal part of the patient or the examiner. Thus, if the fork is allowed to run down until vibration is no longer appreciated but is still felt at an analogous point on the opposite limb, and if this finding is consistent, one can be certain of a significant impairment of vibration sense. In a similar way, the appreciation of vibration at the tibial tuberosity after it has disappeared in the ankle, or at the iliac portion of the spine after it has disappeared at the tibial tuberosity, is an indication of a peripheral nerve lesion. The level of vibration-sense loss due to spinal cord lesions may be estimated by placing the fork over successive vertebral spines.

DISCRIMINATIVE SENSORY FUNCTIONS Damage to the sensory cortex or to the sensory projections from thalamus to cortex results in a special type of disturbance that affects mainly the patient's ability to make sensory discriminations. Lesions in these structures may disturb postural sense but leave the so-called "primary modalities" (touch, pain, temperature, and vibration sense) relatively little affected. In such a situation, or if a cerebral lesion is suspected on other grounds, discriminative function should be tested further by the following tests:

Two-point discrimination The ability to distinguish two points from one is tested by using a compass, the points of which should be blunt and applied simultaneously and painlessly. The distance at which such a stimulus can be recognized as double varies greatly; 1 mm at the tip of the tongue, 2 to 3 mm on the lips, 3 to 5 mm on the dorsa of the hands and feet, and 4 to 7 cm on the body surface. It is characteristic of the patient with a lesion of the sensory cortex to mistake two points for one, although occasionally the opposite occurs.

Cutaneous localization and number writing The ability to localize cutaneous stimuli is tested by touching various parts of the patient's body and asking him to point to the part touched or the corresponding part on the examiner's limb. Recognition of numbers or letters (these should be larger than 4 cm) or of the direction of lines drawn on the skin also depends on localization of tactile stimuli.

Appreciation of texture, size, and shape Appreciation of texture depends mainly on cutaneous impressions, but the recognition of shape and size of objects is based on impressions from deeper receptors as well. The lack of recognition of shape and form, therefore, though frequently found with cortical lesions, may also be present with lesions of the spinal cord and brainstem because of interruption of tracts transmitting postural and tactile sensation. The latter type of sensory defect, called stereoanesthesia, should be distinguished from astereognosis, which connotes an inability to identify an object by palpation, the primary sense data (touch, pain, temperature, and vibration) being intact. In practice, a pure astereognosis is rarely encountered, and the term is employed where the impairment of superficial and vibratory sensation in the hands is of insufficient severity to account for the defect. Defined in this way, astereognosis may be the product of a lesion in *either* hemisphere, in the postcentral gyrus or the thalamoparietal projections. Astereognosis may be confused with *tactile agnosia.* The latter disorder is due to a lesion lying posterior to the postcentral gyrus of the *dominant* parietal lobe, and causes an inability to recognize an object by touch or handling in *both* hands. In contrast to tactile agnosia the patient with astereognosis may appreciate the size, form, consistency, and weight of an object placed in his hand, and therefore cannot identify it.

Extinction of sensory stimuli and sensory inattention In response to bilateral simultaneous testing of symmetric parts, the patient may acknowledge only the stimulus on the sound side, or he may improperly localize the stimulus on the affected side, whereas stimuli applied to each side separately are properly appreciated. This phenomenon of extinction, or cortical inattention, is characteristic of parietal lobe lesions, the symptoms of which are considered in Chap. 27.

A few other terms require definition, since they may be encountered in descriptions of sensation. *Anesthesia* refers to a loss of all forms of sensation, and *hypesthesia* to a diminution of all sensation. Loss or impairment of specific cutaneous sensations is indicated by an appropriate prefix or suffix, e.g., thermoanesthesia or thermohypesthesia, analgesia (loss of pain) or hypalgesia, tactile anesthesia (loss of sense of touch), and pallanesthesia (loss of vibratory sense). The term *hyperesthesia* requires special mention; although it implies a heightened receptiveness of the nervous system, careful testing will usually demonstrate an underlying sensory defect, i.e., an elevated threshold to tactile, painful, or thermal stimuli; once the stimulus is perceived, however, it may have a severely painful or unpleasant quality (hyperpathia).

SENSORY SYNDROMES Sensory changes may be due to interruption of a single peripheral nerve. These changes will vary with the composition of the nerve involved, depending on whether it is predominantly muscular, cutaneous, or mixed. In lesions of cutaneous nerves, the area of tactile anesthesia is more extensive than the one for pain, because of greater overlapping of pain fibers. Also, because of overlap from adjacent nerves, the area of sensory loss following division of a cutaneous nerve is always less than its anatomic distribution. If a large area of skin is involved, the sensory defect characteristically consists of a central portion, in which all forms of cutaneous sensation are lost, surrounded by a zone of partial loss, which becomes less marked as one proceeds from the center to the periphery. The sense of deep pressure and passive movement is intact because it is carried by special nerve fibers from subcutaneous structures and joints. Along the margin of the hypesthetic zone the skin becomes excessively sensitive. According to Weddell, this is because of collateral regeneration from surrounding healthy nerves into the denervated region (see Chap. 5).

Particular types of lesions differentially affect the fibers in a sensory nerve. Compression paralyzes large touch and pressure fibers more than the small pain, thermal, and autonomic motor fibers; procaine and cocaine have opposite effects.

In lesions involving the brachial and lumbosacral plexuses, the sensory disturbance is no longer confined to the territory of a single nerve and is accompanied by muscle weakness and reflex change.

Sensory changes due to multiple nerve involvement (polyneuropathy) In most instances of polyneuropathy the sensory changes are accompanied by varying degrees of motor and reflex loss. Usually the sensory impairment is symmetric, with notable exceptions in some instances of diabetic and periarteritic neuropathy. Since the longest and largest fibers tend to be the most affected, the sensory loss is most severe over the feet and legs and less severe over the hands. The abdomen, thorax, and face are spared except in the most severe cases. The sensory loss usually involves all the modalities, and although it is manifestly difficult to equate the impairment of pain, touch, temperature, vibration, and position sense, one of these may seemingly be impaired out of proportion to the others. One cannot accurately predict, from the patient's symptoms, which mode of sensation will be disproportionately affected. The term glove-and-stocking anesthesia is frequently employed to describe the sensory loss of polyneuropathy and draws attention to the predominantly distal pattern of involvement. It is an inaccurate term insofar as the border between normal and impaired sensation is not so sharp; the sensory loss shades off gradually. In hysteria, by contrast, the border between normal and absent sensation is usually sharp.

Sensory changes due to involvement of multiple spinal nerve roots Because of considerable overlap from adjacent roots, division of a single sensory root does not produce complete loss of sensation in any area of skin. Compression of a single sensory cervical or lumbar root (e.g., in herniated intervertebral disks) causes varying degrees of impairment of cutaneous sensation in a segmental pattern, however. When two or more roots have been completely divided, a zone of sensory loss can be found in which reduction of pain perception is greater in extent than touch. Surrounding the area of complete loss is a narrow zone of partial loss, in which a raised threshold accompanied by overreaction *(hyperpathia)* may or may not be demonstrated. The presence of muscle paralysis atrophy and reflex loss indicates involvement of ventral roots as well.

Tabetic syndrome This results from damage to the large proprioceptive and other fibers of the posterior lumbosacral roots. It is usually caused by neurosyphilis, less often by meningeal tumors, diabetes mellitus, etc. Numbness or paresthesias and lightning pains are frequent complaints, and areflexia, atonicity of the bladder, abnormalities of gait (Chap. 19), and hypotonia without muscle weakness are found on examination. The sensory loss may consist only of loss of vibration and position sense in the lower extremities, but in severe cases, loss or impairment of superficial or deep pain sense or of touch may be added. The feet and legs are most affected, much less often the arms and trunk.

Complete spinal sensory syndromes In a complete transverse lesion of the spinal cord, all forms of sensation are abolished below a level that corresponds to the lesion. There may be a narrow zone of "hyperesthesia" at the upper margin of the anesthetic zone. During the evolution of such a lesion there may be a discrepancy between the level of the lesion and that of the sensory loss, the latter ascending as the lesion progresses. This can be understood if one conceives of a lesion evolving from the periphery to the center of the cord, affecting first the outermost fibers carrying pain and temperature sensation from the legs. Conversely, a lesion advancing from the center of the cord may affect these modalities in the reverse order.

Partial spinal sensory syndromes (hemisection of the spinal cord—Brown-Séquard syndrome) In rare instances disease is confined to one side of the spinal cord; pain and heat sensation are affected on the opposite side, and proprioceptive sensation is affected on the same side as the lesion. The loss of pain and temperature sensation begins two or three segments below the lesion. An associated motor paralysis on the side of the lesion completes the syndrome. Tactile sensation is not involved, since the fibers from one side of the body are distributed in tracts on both sides of the cord.

Lesions of the central gray matter (syringomyelic syndrome) Since fibers conducting pain and temperature cross the cord in the anterior commissure, a lesion in this location will characteristically abolish these modalities on one or both sides but will spare tactile sensation. The commonest cause of such a lesion is syringomyelia, less often, tumor and hemorrhage. This type of dissociated sensory loss usually occurs in a segmental distribution, and since the lesion frequently involves other parts of the gray matter, varying degrees of segmental amyotrophy and reflex loss may be added. If the lesion has spread to the white matter, corticospinal, spinothalamic, and posterior column signs will be present as well.

Posterior column syndrome There is loss of vibratory and position sense below the lesion, but the senses of pain, temperature, and touch are affected relatively little or not at all. This condition may be difficult to distinguish from an affection of large fibers in sensory roots (tabetic syndrome). In some diseases vibratory sensation may be involved predominantly, whereas in others position sense is more affected. An interruption of proprioceptive fibers may interfere with discriminative sensory function, such as two-point discrimination and recognition of size, shape, and weight; and impairment of these functions may occur with posterior column disease alone. Paresthesias in the form of tingling and "pins-and-needles" sensations or girdle sensations are a common complaint with posterior column disease, and pain stimuli may also produce unpleasant sensations.

The anterior spinal artery syndrome With occlusion of the anterior spinal artery or other destructive lesions that predominantly affect the ventral portion of the cord, there is a relative or absolute sparing of proprioceptive sensation and only a loss of pain and temperature sensation below the level of the lesion. Since the corticospinal tracts and the ventral gray matter also fall within the area of distribution of the anterior spinal artery, paralysis of motor function forms a prominent part of this syndrome.

Disturbances of sensation due to lesions of the brainstem A characteristic feature of lesions of the medulla and lower pons is that in many instances the sensory disturbance is crossed, i.e., there is loss of pain and temperature sensation of one side of the face and of the opposite side of the body. This is accounted for by involvement of the trigeminal tract or nucleus and the lateral spinothalamic tract on one side of the brainstem. This is nearly always due to a lateral medullary infarction (Wallenburg's syndrome). In the upper pons and midbrain, where the spinothalamic tracts and the medical lemniscus become confluent, an appropriately placed lesion may cause a loss of all superficial and deep sensation over the contralateral side of the body. Cranial nerve palsies, cerebellar ataxia, or motor paralysis are often associated (see Chap. 332).

Sensory loss due to a lesion of the thalamus (syndrome of Dejerine-Roussy) Involvement of the nucleus ventralis posterolateralis of the thalamus, usually due to a vascular lesion or tumor, causes loss or diminution of all forms of sensation on the opposite side of the body. Position sense is affected more frequently than any other sensory function, and deep sensory loss is usually, but not always, more profound than cutaneous loss. There may be spontaneous pain or discomfort ("thalamic pain"), sometimes of the most torturing and disabling type, on the affected side of the body; and any form of stimulus may have a diffuse, unpleasant, lingering quality. Emotional disturbance also aggravates the painful state. The thalamic pain syndrome may occasionally accompany lesions of the white matter of the parietal lobe (Chap. 27).

Sensory loss due to lesions in the parietal lobe There is a disturbance mainly of discriminative sensory functions on the opposite side of the body, particularly the face, arm, and leg. Loss of position sense, impaired ability to localize touch and pain stimuli, elevation of two-point threshold, a general inattentiveness to sensory stimuli on one side of the body, and astereognosis (if the lesions is in the dominant hemisphere) are the most prominent findings. With cortical lesions, the patient's reports are variable; one examination may disclose no sensory abnormalities, whereas another does. This type of response is often attributed to hysteria. Other features of parietal lobe symptomatology and the differences between dominant and nondominant parietal lobe syndromes are considered in Chap. 27.

Sensory loss due to suggestion and hysteria Hysterical patients almost never complain spontaneously of cutaneous sensory loss, although they may use the term *numbness* to indicate a paralysis of a limb. Complete hemianesthesia, often with reduced hearing, sight, smell, and taste, as well as impaired vibration sense over only half the skull, is a common finding in hysteria. Anesthesia of one entire limb or a sharply defined sensory loss over part of a limb, not conforming to the distribution of root or cutaneous nerve, is also frequently observed. Postural sensation is rarely affected. The diagnosis of hysterical hemianesthesia is best made by eliciting the other relevant symptoms of hysteria or, if this is not possible, by noting the discrepancies between this type of sensory loss and that which occurs as part of the usual sensory syndromes.

REFERENCES

BRODAL A: The somatic afferent pathways, chap. 2 in *Neurological Anatomy,* New York: Oxford, 1969

MAYO CLINIC: *Clinical Examinations in Neurology,* 3d ed., Philadelphia: Saunders, 1972

MOUNTCASTLE VB: Central nervous mechanisms in sensation, chaps. 61, 62, and 63 in *Medical Physiology,* 12th ed., ed VB Mountcastle, vol. 2, St. Louis: Mosby, 1968

22 COMA AND RELATED DISTURBANCES OF CONSCIOUSNESS

RAYMOND D. ADAMS

The practitioner of medicine is frequently called upon to treat patients whose principal abnormality is an impairment of consciousness, which varies from inattentiveness and simple confusion to coma. In large municipal hospitals it is estimated that as many as 3 percent of total admissions to the emergency ward are due to diseases that have caused coma; although this figure seems high, it serves to emphasize the importance of this class of neurologic diseases and the necessity for every student of medicine to acquire a theoretic as well as a practical knowledge of them.

The terms *consciousness, confusion, stupor, unconsciousness,* and *coma* have been endowed with so many meanings that it is almost impossible to avoid ambiguity in their usage. They are not strictly medical terms, but literary, philosophic, and psychologic ones as well. The word *consciousness* is the most difficult of all. William James once remarked that everyone knew what consciousness was until he attempted to define it. To the psychologist consciousness denotes a state of awareness of one's self and one's environment. Knowledge of one's self, of course, includes all "feelings, attitudes and emotions, impulses, volitions, and the active or striving aspects of conduct" (English)—in short, an awareness of all one's own mental functioning, particularly of the cognitive processes. These can be judged only by the patient's verbal account of his introspections and, indirectly, by his actions. Physicians, being practical persons for the most part, have learned to place greater confidence in their observations of the patient's general behavior and reactions to overt stimuli than in what the patient says. For this reason when they employ the term *consciousness,* they usually do so in its commonest and simplest signification, namely, a state of awareness of the environment. This narrow definition has another advantage in that the word *unconsciousness* is its exact opposite—a state of unawareness of environment or a suspension of those mental activities by which man is made aware of his environment. To add to the ambiguity, psychoanalysts have given the word *unconscious* a still different meaning; for them it stands for the repository of impulses and memories of previous experiences that cannot immediately be recalled to the conscious mind.

DESCRIPTION OF STATES OF NORMAL AND IMPAIRED CONSCIOUSNESS The following definitions, though admittedly unacceptable to most psychologists, are of service to medicine, and they will provide the students with a convenient terminology for describing the mental states of their patients.

Normal consciousness This is the condition of the normal person when fully awake, in which he is responsive to psychologic stimuli and "indicates by his behavior and speech that he has the same awareness of himself and his environment as ourselves." This normal state may fluctuate during the course of the day from keen alertness or deep concentration with a marked constriction of the field of attention to general inattentiveness and drowsiness.

Sleep Sleep is a state of physical and mental inactivity from which the patient may be aroused to normal consciousness. A person in sleep gives little evidence of being aware of himself or his environment, and in this respect he is unconscious. Yet he differs from a comatose patient in that he may still respond to unaccustomed stimuli and at times is capable of some mental activity in the form of dreams, which leave their traces in memory. And, of course, he can be recalled to a state of normal consciousness when stimulated.

Inattention, confusional, and cloudy states of consciousness In these conditions the patient does not take into account all elements of his immediate environment. As in delirium, there is always an element of sensorial clouding or imperceptiveness and distractibility of attention. The term *confusion* lacks precision, for often it is meant to denote an inability to think with customary speed and coherence. Here the difficulty is in defining *thinking,* a term which invariably refers to problem solving and coherence of ideas about a subject.

An inattentive, severely confused person is usually unable to do more than carry out a few simple commands. Few if any thought processes are in operation. His capacity for speech may be limited to a few words or phrases, or he may be voluble. He is unaware of much that goes on around him and does not grasp his immediate situation. A moderately confused person can carry on a simple conversation for short periods of time, but his thinking is slow and incoherent, and he is unable to stay on one topic. He is distractible and at the mercy of every stimulus. Usually he is disoriented in time and place. In mild degrees of confusion the disorder may be so slight that it is overlooked unless the examiner is searching in his analysis of the patient's behavior and conversation. The patient may even be roughly oriented as to time and place and able to speak freely on almost any subject. Only occasional irrelevant remarks betray an incoherence of thinking. Patients with mild or moderately severe confusion may be subjected to psychologic testing. The degree of confusion often varies from one time of day to another and tends to be least pronounced in the early morning. Severe confusion or stupor may resemble semicoma during periods when the patient is drowsy or asleep. Many events that happen to the confused patient leave no trace in his memory; in fact, capacity to recall later the events that transpired in any given period is one of the most delicate tests of mental clarity. However, careful analysis will show the defect to be one of inadequate registration and fixation of items rather than a fault in retentive memory.

Some neurologists regard *delirium* as a state of confusion with excitement and hyperactivity, and in some medical writings the terms *delirium* and *confused-cloudy states* are used interchangeably. It is undoubtedly true that the delirious patient is nearly always confused. However, the inability to sleep, the vivid hallucinations which characterize delirious states, the relative inaccessibility of the patient to other events than those to which he is reacting at any one moment, his extreme agitation and tremulousness, and the tendency to convulse suggest a cerebral disorder of a somewhat different type. The clearest evidence of the relationship of inattention, confusion, stupor, and coma is that the patient may pass through all these states as he becomes comatose or emerges from coma. The author has not observed any such relationship between coma and delirium. These distinctions are drawn with greater clarity in Chap. 26.

At times a patient with certain types of aphasia, especially jargon aphasia, may create the impression of confusion, but close observation will reveal that the disorder is confined to the sphere of language and that behavior is otherwise natural.

Stupor In stupor mental and physical activity are reduced to a minimum. Although inaccessible to many stimuli, the patient opens his eyes, looks at the examiner, and does not appear to be unconscious. Response to spoken commands is either absent or slow and inadequate. As a rule tendon or plantar reflexes are not altered. On the other hand, tremulousness of movement, coarse twitching of muscles, restless or stereotyped motor activity, and grasping and sucking reflexes are not infrequent, depending on the way in which disease affects the nervous system. In psychiatry the term *stupor* means a state in which impressions of the external world are normally received but activity is suspended or marked by negativism, e.g., catatonic stupor of schizophrenia.

Coma The patient who appears to be asleep and is at the same time incapable of sensing or responding adequately to either external stimuli or inner needs is in a state of coma. Coma may vary in degree, and in its deepest stages no reaction of any kind is obtainable. Corneal, pupillary, pharyngeal, tendon, and plantar reflexes are all absent. With lesser degrees of coma pupillary reflexes and ocular movements and other brainstem reflexes are preserved, and there may or may not be extensor rigidity of the limbs and opisthotonos, signs which, as Sherrington showed, indicate decerebration. Respirations are often slow or rapid and may be periodic, i.e., Cheyne-Stokes breathing. In still lighter stages, referred to as *semicoma,* most of the above reflexes can be elicited, and the plantar reflexes may be either flexor or extensor (Babinski's sign). Moreover, pricking or pinching the skin, shaking and shouting at the patient, or an uncomfortable distention of the bladder may cause the patient to stir or moan and his respirations to quicken. Coma differs from sleep in that the patient is unarousable, and from akinetic mutism and the "locked-in" syndromes in which the patient is still receptive but unresponsive.

ELECTROENCEPHALOGRAM AND DISTURBANCES OF CONSCIOUSNESS One of the most delicate confirmations of the fact that these states of altered consciousness are expressions of neurophysiologic changes is the electroencephalogram. In the normal waking state the electrical potentials of the cortical neurons are integrated into regular waves of two frequency ranges, from 8 to 15 per second (alpha rhythm) and from 16 to 25 per second (beta rhythm). These wave forms are established by adolescence, but certain individual differences in general pattern and dominance of alpha waves are maintained throughout adult life. With sleep these cortical potentials slow down, and amplitude (voltage) of the individual waves increases. At one stage in light sleep characteristic bursts of 14 to 16 waves per second appear, the so-called "sleep spindles," and in deep [nonrapid eye movement (NREM)] sleep all the waves of normal frequency and amplitude are replaced by slow ones of high voltage (1¼ to 3 per second). In rapid eye movement (REM) sleep the brain waves return to normal (see Chap. 23). Similarly, some alteration in brain waves occurs in all disturbances of consciousness except the milder degrees of confusion. This alteration usually consists of a disorganization of the electroencephalographic pattern, which shows random, slow waves of high voltage in stages of confusion; more regular, slow, two-to-three-per-second waves of high voltage in stupor and semicoma; and slow waves or even suppression of all organized electrical activity (isoelectric state) in the deep coma of hypoxia and ischemia, the so-called "brain-death syndrome." The electroencephalograms of deep sleep and of light coma resemble each other. However, not all diseases that cause confusion and coma have the same effect on the electroencephalogram. Some, such as barbiturate intoxication, may cause an increase in frequency and amplitude of the brain waves. In epilepsy the disturbance of consciousness is usually attended by paroxysms of "spikes" (fast waves of high amplitude) or by the characteristic alternating slow waves and spikes of petit mal. Other diseases, such as hepatic coma, characteristically cause a slowing in frequency and an increasing amplitude of "brain waves" and special triphasic waves. Whether all metabolic diseases of the brain induce similar changes in the electroencephalogram has not been determined. Probably there are differences among them, some of which may be significant (see Chap. 330).

MORBID ANATOMY AND PHYSIOLOGY OF COMA In recent times there has been some clarification and amplification of earlier neuropathologic observations that the smallest lesions associated with protracted coma are always to be found in the midbrain and thalamus. The essence of more recent neurophysiologic studies, to be found in the writings of Bremer, of Morison and Dempsey, and of Moruzzi and Magoun, is that a systematic series of destructive lesions of spinal cord, medulla, pons, and cerebellum has no effect on the state of consciousness until the level of midbrain and diencephalon (thalamus) is reached. High brainstem transections invariably induce states of prolonged unresponsiveness, whereas stimulation of the upper brainstem reticular formation causes a drowsy or sleeping animal to become suddenly alert and its EEG to change correspondingly. As anesthetic agents abolish consciousness, they are found to suppress the activity of the upper reticular activating system, without interfering, at least at certain levels, with the transmission of specific sensory impulses en route to parietal lobe cortex.

Anatomic studies show the reticular activating system of the upper brainstem to receive collaterals from the specific sensory pathways and to project, not just to the sensory cortex of the parietal lobe, as do the thalamic relay nuclei for somatic sensation, but to the whole of the cerebral cortex. The latter has corticofugal connections which feed back nerve impulses to the reticular formation. Sensory stimulation, it would seem, then, has the double effect of conveying to the brain information about the outside world but also of providing some of the energy for activating those parts of the nervous system on which consciousness depends.

These new data are in line with the older ideas of Herbert Spencer and Hughlings Jackson—that the diencephalon and cerebral cortex always function together as a unit and represent the highest levels of integrative nervous activity, called by Penfield *centrencephalic.* Though anatomic details have yet to be worked out and the precise physiology of the reticular activating system leaves much to be desired, being more complicated than this simple formulation would suggest, nevertheless, as a working idea it will make some of the following neuropathologic observations more comprehensible.

The study of a large series of human cases in which coma has preceded death by several days will bring to light two major types of lesion. In the first group a macroscopically visible lesion such as a tumor, abscess, intracerebral, subarachnoid, subdural, or epidural hemorrhage, massive infarct, or meningitis is demonstrable; usually the lesion involves a portion only of the cortex and white matter, leaving much of the cerebrum intact. Rarely, it is located in the thalamus or midbrain, which would make the coma understandable. But in the other instances the coma will always be related to a temporal lobe-tentorial herniation with compression, ischemia, and secondary hemorrhage in the midbrain and lower thalamus or with downward displacement of the brainstem. A detailed clinical record will show the coma to have coincided with these secondary displacements and herniations. Exceptionally, widespread bilateral damage to the cortex and subcortical white matter will be found—the result of bilateral infarcts or hemorrhages, viral encephalitis, hypoxia, or ischemia—without thalamic or midbrain lesions. In the second group (and this is larger than the first) no visible lesion is seen by the naked eye, and often no abnormality is divulged by any technique of pathology. The lesion, here caused by a metabolic or toxic state, is subcellular or molecular. In some instances the grossly normal brain will reveal a demonstrable cellular change under the light microscope which may be characteristic, e.g., hepatic coma. Usually the microscopic lesions are too diffuse for clinicoanatomic correlation. Thus, pathologic changes are compatible with physiologic deductions—that the state of prolonged coma correlates with lesions of all parts of the cortical-diencephalic systems of neurons, but it is only in the upper brainstem that they may be small and discrete.

MECHANISMS WHEREBY CONSCIOUSNESS IS DISTURBED IN DISEASE Knowledge of diseases of the nervous system is so limited that it is not possible to identify all the different mechanisms by means of which consciousness is disturbed. Already several different ways in which the mesencephalic-diencephalic-cortical systems are deranged have been identified; there are probably many others.

In a number of disease processes there is evidence of direct interference with the metabolic activities of the nerve cells in the cerebral cortex and central thalamic nuclei of the brain. Hypoxia, hypoglycemia, hyper- and hypoosmolar states, acidosis, alkalosis, hyper- and hypokalemia, hyperammonemia, and deficiencies of thiamine, nicotinic acid, vitamin B_{12}, pantothenic acid, and pyridoxine are well-known examples (see Chap. 340). The relevant points for our discussion are that cerebral metabolism or blood flow is reduced in all the metabolic disorders leading to coma. Oxygen values below 2 ml per 100 g brain tissue per min are incompatible with an alert state. In hypoglycemia the cerebral blood flow is normal or above normal, whereas the cerebral metabolic rate is diminished, owing to deficiency of substrate. In thiamine and vitamin B_{12} deficiency the cerebral blood flow is normal or slightly diminished, and the cerebral metabolic rate is diminished, presumably because of insufficiency of coenzymes. Extremes of body temperature, either hyperthermia (temperature over 41°C) or hypothermia (temperature below 35°C), probably induce coma by exerting a nonspecific effect on the metabolic activity of neurons.

Diabetic acidosis, uremia, hepatic coma, and the coma of systemic infections are examples of endogenous intoxications. The identity of the toxic agents is not entirely known. In diabetes acetone bodies (acetoacetic acid, β-hydroxybutyric acid, and acetone) are present in high concentration, and in uremia there is probably accumulation of dialyzable toxins, perhaps phenolic derivatives of the aromatic amino acids. In both conditions "dehydration" and serum acidosis may also play an important role. In many cases of hepatic coma, elevation of blood NH_3 to levels five to six times normal has been found. Lactic acidemia and other organic acids may affect the brain by lowering its pH to less than 7.3. The mode of action of bacterial toxins is unknown. In all these conditions the cerebral metabolic rate tends to be reduced, whereas cerebral blood flow remains normal. In water intoxication the membrane excitability of nerve cells is altered by hyponatremia and changes in intracellular K levels.

Drugs such as barbiturates, bromides, Dilantin, alcohol, glutethimide, and phenothiazines induce coma by their direct suppressive effect on the neurons of the cerebrum and diencephalon. Others such as methyl alcohol and ethylene glycol result in metabolic acidosis. Many additional pharmacologic agents have no direct action on the nervous system but may lead to coma through the mechanism of circulatory collapse and inadequate cerebral blood flow. In toxic and metabolic diseases, although the patient usually approaches coma through stages of drowsiness, confusion, and stupor, and the reverse sequence occurs as he emerges from it, each disease has its special effects, manifesting itself by a characteristic clinical picture. This means that the mechanism and topography of the lesion will be different.

A critical fall in blood pressure, usually to a systolic level below 70 mmHg, affects neural structures by causing a decrease in cerebral blood flow and, secondarily, a diminution in cerebral metabolic rate. If decline in blood pressure is episodic, the corresponding clinical picture is one of physical weakness usually preceding and following the loss of consciousness, the whole process being acute and promptly reversible.

The sudden, violent, and excessive discharge of *epilepsy* is another mechanism. Usually a Jacksonian convulsion has little effect on consciousness until it spreads from one side of the body to the other. Coma immediately ensues, presumably because the spreading of the seizure discharge to central neuronal structures paralyzes their function. Other types of seizure in which consciousness is interrupted from the very beginning are believed to originate in the diencephalon.

Concussion exemplifies still another special pathophysiologic mechanism. In "blunt" head injury it has been shown that there is an enormous increase in intracranial pressure of the order of 200 to 700 lb per in.^{2}, lasting a few thousandths of a second. Either the vibration set up in the skull and transmitted to the brain or this sudden high intracranial pressure is believed to be the basis of the abrupt paralysis of the nervous system that follows head injury. Separate rotatory motion of the brain within the skull is another more likely possibility. Raising the intraventricular pressure to a level approaching diastolic blood pressure has abolished all vital functions in the experimental animal.

As was pointed out above, large, destructive, and space-consuming lesions of the brain, such as hemorrhage, tumor, or abscess, interfere with consciousness in two ways. One is by direct destruction of the midbrain and diencephalon; the other, far more frequent, is by producing herniation of the medial part of the temporal lobe through the opening of the tentorium and crushing the upper brain against the opposite free edge of the tentorium or lateral and downward displacement of brainstem. Here the mechanism is again mechanical, and probably circulatory as well.

CLINICAL APPROACH TO THE COMATOSE PATIENT

Coma is not an independent disease entity but is always a symptomatic expression of disease. Sometimes the underlying disease is perfectly obvious, as when a healthy individual is struck on the head and rendered unconscious. All too often, however, the patient is brought to the hospital in a state of coma, and little or no information about him is immediately available. The physician must then subject the clinical problem to careful scrutiny from many directions. To do this efficiently requires a broad knowledge of disease and a methodical approach that leaves none of the common and treatable causes of coma unexplored.

It should be pointed out that when the comatose patient is seen for the first time, simple therapeutic measures take precedence over diagnostic procedures. In a quick survey one makes sure that the comatose patient has a clear airway and is not in shock (circulatory collapse) or, if trauma has occurred, that he is not bleeding from a wound. In patients who have suffered a head injury there may be a fracture of the cervical vertebrae, and therefore one must be cautious about moving the head and neck lest the spinal cord be inadvertently crushed. There must be an immediate inquiry as to the previous health of the patient: whether he had suffered a head injury or had been seen in a convulsion, and the circumstances in which he was found. The persons who accompany the comatose patient to the hospital should not be permitted to leave until they have been questioned.

Diagnosis The temperature, pulse, respiratory rate, and blood pressure are of aid in diagnosis. Fever suggests a severe systemic infection such as pneumonia, bacterial meningitis, or a brain lesion that has disturbed the temperature-regulating centers. An excessively high body temperature, 41 to 44°C, associated with dry skin should arouse the suspicion of heat stroke. Hypothermia is frequently observed in alcoholic or barbiturate intoxication, extracellular fluid deficit, peripheral circulatory failure, or myxedema. Slow breathing points to morphine, barbiturate intoxication, or hypothyroidism, whereas deep, rapid breathing suggests pneumonia but may occur in diabetic or uremic acidosis (Kussmaul's respiration) or with intracranial diseases, as in central neurogenic hyperpnea. The rapid breathing of pneumonia is often accompanied by an expiratory grunt, cyanosis, and fever. Diseases that elevate the intracranial pressure or damage the brain, especially the brainstem or cerebrum, often cause slow, irregular, or periodic (Cheyne-Stokes) breathing. The pulse rate is less helpful, but if exceptionally slow, it should suggest heart block, or if combined with periodic breathing and hypertension, an increase in intracranial pressure. A tachycardia of 140 heartbeats per min or above calls attention to the possibility of an ectopic cardiac rhythm with insufficiency of cerebral circulation. Marked hypertension occurs in patients with cerebral hemorrhage and hypertensive encephalopathy and, at times, those with increased intracranial pressure, whereas hypotension is the usual finding in the coma of alcohol or barbiturate intoxication, or internal hemorrhage, myocardial infarction, gram-negative bacillary septicemia, and Addison's disease.

Inspection of the skin may also yield valuable information. Cyanosis of the lips and nail beds means inadequate oxygenation. Cherry-red coloration indicates carbon monoxide poisoning. Multiple bruises, and in particular a bruise or boggy area in the scalp, favor cranial trauma. Bleeding from an ear or nose or orbital hemorrhage also raises the possibility of trauma. Puffiness and hyperemia of face and conjunctivas and telangiectasia are the usual stigmas of alcoholism; marked pallor suggests internal hemorrhage. The presence of a maculohemorrhagic rash indicates the possibility of meningococcal infection, staphylococcus endocarditis, typhus, or Rocky Mountain spotted fever. Pellagra may be diagnosed from the typical skin lesions on face and hands. The face may be myxedematous. In pituitary hypoadrenalism the skin is sallow. Excessive sweating suggests hypoglycemia or shock, and dry skin, diabetic acidosis and uremia. Skin turgor is reduced in dehydration. Hemorrhagic blisters will have formed over pressure points if the patient has been motionless for a time.

The odor of the breath may provide clues to the nature of a disease causing coma. The odor of alcohol is easily recognized (except for vodka, which is odorless). The spoiled-fruit odor of diabetic coma, the uriniferous odor of uremia, and the musty fetor of hepatic coma are distinctive enough to be identified by physicians who possess a keen sense of smell.

The next step in the physical examination should give special attention to the status of the nervous system. Although the examination is limited in many ways, careful observation of the stuporous or comatose patient may yield considerable information concerning the function of different parts of the nervous system. One of the most helpful procedures is to sit at the patient's bedside for 5 to 10 min and observe what he does. The predominant postures of the body, the position of the head and eyes, the rate, depth, and rhythm of respiration, and the pulse should be noted. The state of responsiveness should then be estimated by noting the patient's reaction when his name is called and his capacity to execute a simple command or to respond to painful stimuli. The most effective painful stimuli are supraorbital pressure, sternal pressure, or pinching the side of the neck or inner parts of the upper arms or thighs. By grading these stimuli, one may titrate the response, so to speak, and evaluate both the degree of coma and changes from hour to hour in the course of the disease. Vocalization may persist in stupor and light coma and is the first response to be lost. Deft avoidance movements of parts stimulated, and grimacing are preserved in light coma and substantiate the integrity of corticomedullary and corticospinal tracts.

Usually it is possible to determine whether the coma is accompanied by meningeal irritation or focal disease in the cerebrum or brainstem. With meningeal irritation from either bacterial meningitis or subarachnoid hemorrhage, there is resistance to active and passive flexion of the neck but not to extension, turning, or tipping the head. Resistance to movement of the neck in all directions indicates disease of the cervical spine or is part of generalized rigidity. In infants, bulging of the anterior fontanel is at times a more reliable sign of meningeal irritation than stiff neck. A temporal lobe or cerebellar pressure cone or decerebrate rigidity may also limit passive flexion of the neck and may be confused with meningeal irritation.

Evidence of disease of a cerebral hemisphere, diencephalon, midbrain, pons, or medulla can be obtained even though the patient is comatose by noting the residual movement, prevailing postures of the body, respiratory rhythm and frequency, and status of cranial nerves. This is of more than passing importance, because severe and persistent derangements of these functions are frequent with mass lesions of the brain and rare in metabolic disorders (except in terminal stages). A hemiplegia, in most instances, reflects a contralateral hemispheral lesion and is revealed by lack of restless movements, grasp reflex, and avoidance movements. The paralyzed limbs are slack and remain in uncomfortable positions. If lifted from the bed, they "fall flail." The cheek puffs out in expiration on the paralyzed side, and the eyes are often turned away from the paralysis (toward the lesion). Painful stimuli may provoke a moan or grimace on one side and not the other, reflecting a hemianesthesia. A homonymous hemianopsia in a stuporous patient is revealed by attraction of eyes to visual stimuli presented on one side and not the other or lack of blink in reaction to threat on one side.

Of the various tests of brainstem function those which have been most useful are pattern of breathing, pupillary size and reactivity, and ocular movement and oculovestibular reflexes. As to patterns of abnormal breathing in progressive lesions which reduce the state of consciousness from confusion and inattention to stupor and coma, the earliest abnormality with cerebral lesions is the appearance of posthyperventilation apnea (period of apnea after 5 to 10 deep breaths). Its presence indicates bifrontal disease, wherein lies the mechanism, according to Plum, for activating rhythmic breathing when CO_2 is reduced. In coma due to massive cerebral lesions the rate of respiration increases slightly, and as it progresses an irregularity appears which gives way to the waxing-waning Cheyne-Stokes respiration (CSR). This means that the centers in the midbrain now isolated from the cerebrum are rendered more sensitive than usual to CO_2 (hyperventilation drive), and by intermittently reducing plasma CO_2 to low levels a temporary apnea follows. With midbrain–upper pontine lesions a state of *central neurogenic hyperpnea* (CNH), rather like Kussmaul breathing, supervenes. Here respirations are increased in rate (up to 100 per min) and in depth, to the extent that respiratory alkalosis may result. The reflex mechanisms for respiratory control in the lower brainstem have in this instance been released, and the threshold of respiratory activation is low. This respiratory drive continues despite low arterial CO_2 tensions and elevated pH. Oxygen therapy (unlike the hyperventilation of pneumonia, pulmonary congestion, etc.) does not modify the pattern. Low pontine-level lesions sometimes cause *apneustic breathing* (where there is a pause of 2 to 3 s after full inspiration) or other abnormal patterns, such as short cycle clusters [three to four respirations without a waxing or waning followed by a pause (Biot respirations)]; or respiration alternans, in which a few breaths are omitted from time to time. With lesions of the medulla the rhythm of breathing is chaotic, being irregularly interrupted, the breath varying in rate and depth. This has been called "ataxic breathing," not a very appropriate term. The latter progresses to apnea, as may also CSR or CNH; in fact, respiratory arrest is the mode of death of most patients with serious central nervous system disease. As Plum and Fisher both point out, when certain supratentorial brain lesions progress to the point where the temporal lobe and cerebellum herniates, one may observe a succession of respiratory patterns (CSR–CNH–Biot breathing to ataxic breathing), indicating extension of the functional disorder from upper to lower brainstem.

With midbrain lesions the pupils dilate to 4 or 5 mm and become unreactive to light; with severe destruction of the tissue at this level (anoxic pannecrosis), they will finally dilate widely and not respond. Pontine tegmental lesions cause miotic pupils with only slight reaction to strong light. Thus, the preservation of pupillary light reflexes indicates integrity of the pupillary dilatation and constrictive mechanisms in the midbrain. Ciliospinal pupillary dilatation is also lost in brainstem lesions (see Chap. 20). Unilateral

Horner's syndrome (miosis, ptosis, exophthalmos, and reduced sweating) may be observed homolateral to a predominantly one-sided lower brainstem lesion, usually medullary. The pupillary reactions are of great importance, because drug intoxications and metabolic disorders which cause coma leave the pupils unaffected. Exceptions are glutethimide (Doriden) and deep ether anesthesia, which cause the pupils to be of medium size or slightly enlarged and unreactive for several hours; opiates (heroin and morphine), which cause pinpoint pupils with light reflex so small that it can be seen only with a magnifying glass, and atropine poisoning, in which the pupils are widely dilated and fixed.

Ocular movements are altered in a variety of ways. In light coma from metabolic abnormalities the eyes rove from side to side in random fashion like the slow eye movements of light sleep. They disappear as brainstem function becomes depressed. Oculocephalic reflexes (doll's eye movements), elicited by briskly turning or tilting the head, with eyes moving conjugately in the opposite direction, are exaggerated. They are not present in the normal person, and if they are elicitable, evidence is obtained of the integrity of the tegmental structures of the midbrain and pons, which integrate ocular movements, and of the third, fourth, and sixth cranial nerves. Irrigation of each ear with 30 to 100 ml ice water (or just cold water if the patient is not completely comatose) will normally cause nystagmus away from the stimulated side (see Chap. 20). In comatose patients in whom the fast corrective "cortical" phase of nystagmus is lost, the eyes are deflected to the side irrigated with cold water or away from the side irrigated with hot water. The position is held for 2 to 3 min. These oculovestibular reflexes are also lost in brainstem lesions. If only one eye abducts and the other fails to adduct in the lateral conjugate movement, there is indication of interruption of the medial longitudinal fasciculus (on the side of adductor paralysis). Irrigating both ears with ice water with the head extended to 60° will sometimes induce vertical conjugate movements. An abducens palsy (sixth nerve) is reflected by a turning in of the eye because of unopposed action of the abducens muscle. The eyes may be held conjugately to one side at all times in a coma—away from the side of the paralysis with large cerebral lesions (looking at the lesion) and toward the side of the paralysis with unilateral pontine lesions (looking away from the lesion). And during a one-sided seizure, the eyes jerk toward the convulsing side of the face, arm, and leg (opposite the irritative focus). The eyes may be turned down and inward (looking at the nose) in thalamic and upper midbrain lesion (Parinaud's syndrome, see Chap. 20). Retraction and convergence nystagmus and ocular bobbing [brisk downward movements of both eyes with slow elevation to the original position (two or three times a minute)] occur with lesions in the midbrain tegmentum and lower pons, respectively. The major brainstem structural lesions, including temporal lobe herniation, abolish most, if not all, conjugate ocular movements when producing coma, whereas metabolic disorders do not. Barbiturates and diphenylhydantoin (Dilantin) are the only common intoxicating drugs which affect ocular movements, but they leave pupillary reactions intact.

As to the meaning of the forced postures and movements in the comatose patient, it may be said that restless, grasping, picking movements of one arm or arm and leg or all four extremities signify that the corticospinal tract(s) is intact; variable resistance to passive movement (paratonic rigidity) and strong grasping or complex avoidance movements have the same signification, and if they are bilateral, the coma usually is not deep. Focal seizures require an intact corticospinal motor system and are seldom seen in the paralyzed side with massive destruction of a cerebral hemisphere. Often these elaborate forms of semivoluntary movement are present on the "good side" in patients with extensive disease in one hemisphere and probably represent some type of disequilibrium of cortical and subcortical movement patterns. Definite choreic, athetotic, or even hemiballismic movements indicate disorder of the subthalamic and basal ganglionic structures, just as they do in the alert patient. *Decerebrate rigidity,* with jaw clenched, neck retracted, arms and legs stiffly extended and internally rotated, appears in the condition of diencephalic-midbrain compression by temporal lobe pressure cone, with hemorrhages and infarction of the upper pons and midbrain and with certain metabolic disorders such as hypoglycemia and hypoxia. Occasionally the mechanism of the decerebrate posture is unclear, as with certain bilateral subacute encephalitic, demyelinative, and infarctive cerebral lesions. In some instances the lesions are clearly in the cerebral white matter or basal ganglia. *Decorticate rigidity,* with arm or arms in flexion and adduction and leg(s) extended, signifies higher lesions in cerebral white matter, internal capsules, and thalamus. *Diagonal postures,* opposite arms and legs flexed and extended, probably mean supratentorial lesions; extended arms and flexed legs are probably fragments of decerebrate postures and point to midpontine lesions. *Abolition of all postures and movements* indicates acute bilateral corticospinal interruption and low pontine-medullary lesions involving reticular facilitatory (extrapyramidal) mechanisms. The coma is usually profound.

Lower brainstem reflexes are seldom helpful in the analysis of coma. Only in the most profound metabolic comas and intoxications and in the hypoxemic panecrosis of the entire brain (brain-death syndromes) are coughing, swallowing, and spontaneous respirations all abolished. Further, the tendon and plantar reflexes give little indication of what is happening. Tendon reflexes may be preserved until late and may be normal or slightly reduced on the hemiplegic side. The plantar reflexes may be absent or extensor. Only in deep coma or in states of decerebrate rigidity will a cerebral hemiplegia not be detected by flaccidity and motionless arm and leg.

A history of headache before or at the onset of coma, recurrent vomiting, and papilledema afford the best clues to increased intracranial pressure. This can be confirmed by lumbar puncture, which is usually safe unless there is a herniation of the temporal lobe through the tentorium or of the cerebellum through the foramen magnum. In the latter instance the cerebrospinal fluid pressure may not reflect intracranial pressure. Papilledema may develop within 12 to 24 h in brain trauma and brain hemorrhage but, if pronounced, usually signifies brain tumor or abscess, a lesion of longer duration. Multiple retinal or large subhyaloid hemorrhages are usually associated with ruptured saccular aneurysm or hemorrhage from an angioma. Papilledema, with widespread retinal exudates, hemorrhages, and arteriolar changes, is an almost invariable accompaniment of hypertensive encephalopathy. In patients with evidence of increased intracranial pressure, lumbar puncture, although admittedly dangerous because it may promote further herniation, is nevertheless necessary in some instances. See Chap. 20 for further discussion of retinal changes.

Laboratory procedures Unless the diagnosis is established at once by history and physical examination, it is necessary to carry out a number of laboratory procedures. If poisoning is suspected, the gastric contents must be aspirated and saved for later chemical analysis. A catheter is passed into the urinary bladder, and a specimen of urine is obtained for determination of specific gravity, sugar, acetone, and albumin content. Urine of low specific gravity and high protein content is nearly always found in uremia, but proteinuria may also occur for 2 or 3 days after a subarachnoid hemorrhage or with fever. Urine of high specific gravity, glycosuria, and acetonuria are almost invariable in diabetic coma; but glycosuria and hyperglycemia may result from a massive cerebral lesion. If diphenylhydantoin, bromide, or barbiturate intoxication is suspected, it can be verified by special tests for these substances. A blood count is made, and in malarial districts a blood smear is examined for malarial parasites. Neutrophilic leukocytosis occurs in bacterial infections and also with brain hemorrhage and softening. Venous blood should be examined for glucose, nonprotein nitrogen, CO_2, sodium bicarbonate, pH, NH_3, sodium potassium, chlorides, and Ca. The cerebrospinal fluid must be drawn, and the pressure, presence of blood, white cell count, and results of Pandy's test should be recorded. Bloody cerebrospinal fluid occurs in cerebral contusion, subarachnoid hemorrhage, brain hemorrhage, and occasionally with hemorrhagic infarcts due to thrombophlebitis or arterial embolism. If there is pleocytosis, a stained smear of the sediment should be searched for bacteria, and a rough quantitative sugar determination should be done. The standard cerebrospinal fluid formula in bacterial meningitis is elevated pressure, high white cell count (5,000 to 20,000 per mm^3), elevated protein level, and subnormal sugar values. The fluid should be saved for quantitative tests for sugar and protein, and a bacterial culture and Wassermann reaction should be performed. If it is suspected that the pressure is elevated, a No. 22 needle should be used. A very high pressure must be slowly reduced by removal of 10 to 15 ml over a period of 15 to 20 min, and urea, mannitol, or other hypertonic solutions should be given to reduce brain swelling over a longer period of time. Jugular compression tests are obviously contraindicated. X-rays of the skull and CT scan should be obtained as soon as possible after these procedures, preferably between the emergency ward and the hospital room.

CLASSIFICATION OF COMA AND DIFFERENTIAL DIAGNOSIS The demonstration of focal brain disease or meningeal irritation, with cerebrospinal fluid abnormality, helps in differential diagnosis. The diseases that frequently cause coma may be conveniently divided into three classes, as follows:

I Diseases that cause no focal or lateralizing neurologic signs or alteration of the cellular content of the cerebrospinal fluid
- *A* Intoxications (alcohol, barbiturates, opiates, etc.) (Chaps. 118 to 120)
- *B* Metabolic disturbances (diabetic acidosis, uremia, Addisonian crises, hepatic coma, hypoglycemia, hypoxia) (Chap. 340)
- *C* Severe systemic infections (pneumonia, typhoid fever, malaria, Waterhouse-Friderichsen syndrome) (Chap. 136)
- *D* Circulatory collapse (shock) from any cause, and cardiac decompensation in the aged (Chaps. 34 and 129)
- *E* Epilepsy (Chap. 24)
- *F* Hypertensive encephalopathy and eclampsia (Chap. 334)
- *G* Hyperthermia or hypothermia (Chap. 11)
- *H* Concussion (Chap. 335)

II Diseases that cause meningeal irritation, with either blood or an excess of white cells in the cerebrospinal fluid, usually without focal or lateralizing signs
- *A* Subarachnoid hemorrhage from ruptured aneurysm, occasionally trauma (Chap. 334)
- *B* Acute bacterial meningitis (Chap. 337)
- *C* Some forms of virus encephalitis (Chap. 338)
- *D* Acute hemorrhagic leukoencephalitis (Chap. 339)

III Diseases causing focal or lateralizing neurologic signs, with or without changes in cerebrospinal fluid
- *A* Brain hemorrhage (Chap. 334)
- *B* Brain softening due to thrombosis or embolism (Chap. 334)
- *C* Brain abscess (Chap. 337)
- *D* Epidural and subdural hemorrhage and brain contusion (Chap. 335)
- *E* Brain tumor (Chap. 336)
- *F* Miscellaneous, i.e., thrombophlebitis, some forms of virus encephalomyelitis (Chap. 338)

With the clinical tests outlined above clearly in mind, one can usually ascertain whether a patient with coma falls in one of the above categories. Concerning the group of comas without focal, lateralizing, or meningeal signs, which includes most of the secondary metabolic diseases of the brain, intoxications (both exogenous and endogenous), concussion, and postseizure states, it should be pointed out that a previous neurologic disease may have left residues which confuse the clinical picture. An earlier hemiparesis from vascular disease or trauma may reveal itself in an alcoholic or hepatic coma, uremia, or hyperglycemic encephalopathy. Also, in hypertensive encephalopathy, transitory focal signs may sometimes be present. And occasionally, for no understandable reason one leg may seem to move less or one plantar reflex be extensor in a metabolic coma. In actuality, the diagnosis of postepileptic coma or concussion depends on observation of the precipitating event or indirect evidence thereof; usually the diagnosis is not too long obscure, for another fit may occur and recovery of consciousness, once the seizures cease, is usually prompt. The final determination of the exact toxic or metabolic disorder requires the synthesis of a variety of clinical and laboratory data, which are described in other parts of the book.

With respect to the comas of group II, the signs of meningeal irritation (head retraction, stiffness of neck on forward bending, Kernig and Brudzinski leg flexion signs) can usually be elicited in both bacterial meningitis and subarachnoid hemorrhage. However, if the coma becomes deep, stiff neck may disappear or be absent from the beginning. In such cases diagnosis is established by CSF examination. In the coma of bacterial meningitis, unless it is associated with brain swelling and cerebellar herniation, the CSF pressure is not exceptionally high (usually less than 400 mm); if the pressure is high, as death approaches there are signs of compression of the medulla, with fixed, dilated pupils, arrest of respiration, and fall in arterial blood pressure. Patients in coma from ruptured aneurysms also have high CSF pressure and often a massive hemispheral and ventricular extension of the hemorrhage.

In patients with group III type of coma it is the inequality of sensory-motor disturbances in the two arms and legs and the aforementioned changes in respiratory pattern, pupillary and ocular reflexes, and the remaining postural states that provide clues to serious structural lesions in the segmental brainstem apparatus. As the latter become prominent, they may obscure earlier signs of cerebral disease. It is noteworthy that bilateral cerebral infarction or hemorrhage or traumatic necrosis and hemorrhage may resemble the comatose state of metabolic and toxic disease, since brainstem mechanisms may be preserved; contrariwise, hepatic, hypoglycemic, and hypoxic coma will sometimes look like the coma of brainstem lesion by causing decerebrate postures. Usually, however, the CSF pressure is elevated and the fluid sanguineous in massive cerebral hemorrhage. Unilateral infarction due to anterior, middle, or posterior cerebral artery occlusion seldom produces more than a stupor or light coma; if infarction is bilateral, however, coma may be profound. Evidence of brainstem displacement and temporal lobe herniation is manifested by increased or altered ventilation (CSR, CNH), bilateral Babinski signs, dilated pupil and drooped eyelid on the side of the lesion, decerebrate postures, later dilated pupils, and loss of full ocular movements. The coma itself gives no clue as to the nature of the original mass lesion. The terminal pattern of a descending gradient of diencephalic, mesencephalic, pontomedullary paralysis of nervous system is identical in all. Differential diagnosis must depend on the other data.

An error which must be cautioned against is the diagnosis of irreversible coma (brain-death syndrome) on the basis of complete abolition of all brainstem and cerebral activity and isoelectric (flat) EEG if there is hypothermia or evidence of intoxication. Only with hypoxia and cerebral ischemia can this diagnosis be made securely.

Diagnosis has as its prime purpose the direction of therapy, and it matters little to the patient if we diagnose a disease for which we have no treatment. The treatable forms of coma are drug intoxications, toxemia from systemic infections, epidural and subdural hematoma, brain abscess, bacterial and tuberculous meningitis, diabetic acidosis, and hypoglycemia.

RELATIVE INCIDENCE OF DISEASES THAT CAUSE COMA

There have been only a few attempts to determine the relative incidence of diseases that lead to coma. A report from the Boston City Hospital (Solomon and Aring) included the largest series of clinical cases but was heavily skewed by the large local problem of chronic alcoholics, which made up 60 percent of all admissions in coma. Trauma (13 percent), cerebral vascular disease (10 percent), poisonings (3 percent), epilepsy (2.4 percent), diabetes, bacterial meningitis, pneumonia, uremia, and eclampsia followed in that order. In a series of 386 cases of coma of uncertain cause Plum and Posner observed that approximately 40 percent turned out to be metabolic; 25 percent, drug intoxications; and the remainder, neurologic disease of supra- or infratentorial structures.

Of course, figures like these do not provide information concerning coma caused by multiple factors. For example, a patient with a cerebral vascular lesion, old or recent, and diabetes mellitus may lapse into coma during an insulin reaction at a time when there is still sugar in the urine. Only by appreciating the interplay of these several common factors is one likely to reach the correct diagnosis.

The differential diagnosis of diseases that cause focal or lateralizing signs and meningitis is taken up under the discussions of traumatic, neoplastic, vascular, and infective diseases of the brain.

CARE OF THE COMATOSE PATIENT Impaired states of consciousness, regardless of their cause, are often fatal because they not only represent an advanced stage of many diseases but also add their own characteristic burden to the primary disease. The main objective of therapy is, of course, to find the cause of the coma, by utilization of procedures already outlined, and to remove it. Often, however, the disease process is one for which there is no specific therapy; or, as in hypoxia or hypoglycemia, the disease process may already have expended itself before the patient comes to the attention of the physician. Again, the problem may be infinitely complex, for the disturbance may be attributable not to a single cause but rather to several possible factors acting in unison, no one of which could account for the total clinical picture. In lieu of direct therapy, supportive measures must be used, and, indeed, it may be said that the patient's chances of surviving the original disease often depend in large measure on their effectiveness.

The physician must give attention to every vital function in the insensate patient. The following is a brief outline of the more important procedures. In order for them to be carried out successfully, a well-coordinated team of nurses under constant guidance of a physician is needed.

1. If the patient is in shock, this takes precedence over all other abnormalities. The treatment of shock is discussed in Chap. 34.
2. Shallow and irregular respirations and cyanosis require the establishment of a clear airway and oxygen. The patient should be placed in a lateral position so that secretions and vomitus do not enter the tracheobronchial tree. Pharyngeal reflexes are usually suppressed, and therefore an endotracheal tube can be inserted without difficulty. Stagnant secretions should be removed with a suction apparatus as soon as they accumulate, since they will lead to atelectasis and bronchopneumonia. Oxygen can be administered by mask in a 100 percent concentration for 6 to 12 h, alternating with 50 percent concen-

tration for 4 h. The depth of respiration can be increased by the use of 5 to 10 percent carbon dioxide for periods of 3 to 5 min every hour. Atropine should not be given; edema of the lungs and fluid in the tracheobronchial passages are not glandular secretions. Furthermore, atropine thickens this fluid and also may disturb temperature regulation of the body. Aminophylline is helpful in controlling Cheyne-Stokes breathing. Respiratory paralysis dictates the use of endotracheal intubation and a positive pressure respirator, but in the author's experience neither has been effective in comatose states in which there is disorganization of respiratory centers.

3 The temperature-regulating mechanisms may be disturbed, and extreme hypothermia, hyperthermia, or an unrecognized poikilothermia may occur. In hyperthermia, removal of blankets and use of alcohol sponges and cooling solutions are indicated.

4 The bladder should not be permitted to become distended. If the patient does not void, a retention catheter should be inserted. If more than 500 ml urine is found in the bladder, decompression must be carried out slowly over a period of hours. Urine excretion should be kept between 500 and 1,000 ml per day. The patient should not be permitted to lie in a wet or soiled bed.

5 Diseases of the central nervous system may upset the control of water, glucose, and salt. The unconscious patient can no longer adjust his intake of food and fluids by hunger and thirst. Salt-losing and salt-retaining syndromes have both been described with brain disease. Water intoxication and severe hyponatremia may of themselves prove fatal. The maintenance of water and electrolytes is discussed in Chap. 69. If coma is prolonged, the insertion of a stomach tube will ease the problem of feeding the patient and maintaining fluid and electrolyte balance.

6 Aspiration pneumonitis should be avoided by prevention of vomiting (stomach tube), position, and restriction of oral fluids. Should it occur, corticosteroid therapy is beneficial. The legs should be examined each day for signs of phlebothrombosis.

7 If the patient is capable of moving, suitable restraints should be used to prevent a possible fall out of bed.

8 Convulsions should be controlled by measures outlined in Chap. 24.

REFERENCES

FISHER CM: Neurological examination of the comatose patient. Acta Neurol Scand, Suppl 36, 45:5, 1969

PLUM F, POSNER J: *Diagnosis of Stupor and Coma,* 2d ed, Philadelphia: Davis, 1975

23 SLEEP AND ITS ABNORMALITIES

RAYMOND D. ADAMS

NORMAL SLEEP The pattern of sleeping varies in the different epochs of life. A nocturnal predominance begins to appear after the first few weeks of postnatal life, resulting in the biphasic pattern of sleeping and waking which persists throughout adolescence and adult years, unless altered by disease. Not until old age does it break down progressively. Night awakenings then increase in frequency, and the daytime waking period becomes interrupted frequently by paroxysmal bursts of sleep lasting 1 to 10 s (microsleep) and by longer naps. Throughout most of life females need about an hour more sleep than males.

Physiologic mechanisms By means of electroencephalographic analysis five stages of sleep, associated with two alternating physiologic mechanisms, have been defined. Relaxed wakefulness is found to be accompanied by sinusoidal alpha waves of 8 to 12 cycles per second (cps) and low-voltage fast activity of mixed frequency in the EEG; there are the usual associated blinks, eye and limb movements, and moderate tone in all the skeletal muscles. As a person falls asleep and the muscles relax, the eyelids droop, the eyes begin to roll from side to side, and the EEG pattern changes to one of progressively lower voltage and mixed frequency. This is called stage I sleep. As sleep deepens into stage II, bursts of 12- to 14-cps waves (sleep spindles) and high-amplitude, sharp, slow-wave (*k*) complexes appear. By now eye movements have ceased, but muscle tone is maintained. The deep sleep of stages III and IV is featured by an increasing proportion of high-voltage, slow-wave activity in the EEG. In stage V, rapid eye movements return and muscle tension increases in the jaw, whereas the neck, trunk, and limb muscles, after a few quivering, tremulous, or myoclonic movements, become completely slack. The first four stages are called *nonrapid eye movement sleep* (NREMS); the last stage is variously designated as *rapid eye movement sleep* (REMS), *paradoxic sleep* (PS), or *activated sleep* (AS).

In a typical night the normal drowsy adult passes successively through stages I, II, III, and IV of NREMS. After about 70 min, mostly spent in stages III and IV, the first REMS period occurs, usually heralded by an increase in body movements and a shift in the EEG pattern from stage IV to II. This NREMS-REMS cycle (activity-rest cycle of Kleitman) is repeated at about the same interval four to six times during the night, depending on the length of sleep. The first REMS cycle may be brief, and the later cycles include less stage IV NREMS.

There is some evidence that the two alternating physiologic sleep mechanisms for NREMS and REMS lie in the brainstem and are influenced by biogenic amines, particularly 5-hydroxytryptamine (serotonin) and norepinephrine. The serotoninergic neurons are known to be located in the medial tegmentum of the medulla, pons, and lower midbrain and to project upward to the hypothalamus and thalamus and to the orbital frontal and medial temporal (limbic) cortex. Activation of serotoninergic neurons, presumably by factor S (see below), suppresses the higher reticular formation subserving consciousness and causes hypersomnia with increase in NREMS and REMS; their destruction or pharmacologic suppression by serotonin antagonists results in insomnia, with disappearance of both NREMS and REMS. Another group of neurons, presumably responsive to dopamine and norepinephrine, lies in the lateral tegmentum of the pons, the locus ceruleus, substantia nigra, and hypothalamus and are necessary for REMS. Their activation increases REMS and their destruction or suppression by norepinephrine antagonists reduces or abolishes it. However, REMS is primed by NREMS serotoninergic neurons, and the two types of sleep are always closely related. Only under conditions of narcolepsy, cataplexy, and sleep paralysis (see below) is REMS separated from NREMS. Monoamine oxidase inhibitors selectively diminish or abolish REMS. Thus, normal sleep involves both a serotoninergic mechanism and a catecholaminergic or adrenergic mechanism.

The details of the neuropharmacology of sleep have not yet been fully ascertained. In some mysterious way, a product(s) of fatigue or some obscure hypnotoxin activates the serotoninergic neurons subserving NREMS and at the same time suppresses the effects of afferent stimulation of the upper reticular formation. It is not known how neuronal systems of REMS are suppressed for a time during NREMS and periodically become active and interrupt it. The plasma of drowsy or sleeping animals has been shown by Monnier to contain factor delta, a substance with properties that induce somnolence and increase NREMS in alert animals. More recently Pappenheimer and his associates have isolated a factor S from the cerebrospinal fluid and brain of animals deprived of sleep. When injected into rats and rabbits, it induces slow-wave sleep lasting 4 to 6 h. Its molecular weight is about 350, and it is destroyed by pronase, indicating the presence of peptides. Probably it is similar if not identical to the sleep-promoting factor isolated by Nagasaki.

EFFECTS OF SLEEP LOSS Of all the conditions that make for human efficiency and sense of well-being, sleep is one of the most important. Deprived of sleep, experimental animals will die within a few days, no matter how well they are fed, watered, and housed; under similar circumstances human beings suffer a variety of unpleasant symptoms that must be separated from the diseases that cause insomnia.

Human beings deprived of sleep (NREM and REM) for periods of 60 to 200 h experience increasing fatigue and irritability and find it difficult to concentrate, to perceive accurately, and to maintain their orientation. Illusions and hallucinations intrude into consciousness, primarily in the visual and tactile sensory fields, becoming more intense as the period of sleeplessness is prolonged. Performance of motor tasks deteriorates. If the tests are of short duration and of slow pace, the subject can keep up; if speed and perseverance are demanded, he cannot. Incentive to work weakens, and sustained action is interrupted by lapses of attention. Neurologic signs include mild and fleeting nystagmus, a slight tremor of the hands, ptosis of eyelids, expressionless face, and thickness of speech, with mispronunciation and incorrect choice of words. A decrement of alpha waves appears in the EEG, and closing of the eyes no longer generates alpha activity. The concentration of 17-hydroxycorticosteroids increases in the blood, and catecholamine output rises.

Recovery after prolonged sleep deprivation shows that the amount of sleep required is never equal to the amount lost. At first, the subject rapidly falls into stage IV of NREMS, often with "supernormal" slow waves in the EEG and remains there, at the expense of stage II sleep; stage IV is interrupted from time to time by REMS which remains in the usual proportion. But by the second night, REMS rebounds and exceeds that of the predeprivation period. Stage IV NREMS seems, then, to be the most valuable stage in restoring the flagging functions of the nervous system.

The effects of partial and differential deprivation are somewhat different. If prevented night after night from having REMS, subjects show a greater tendency to become hyperactive and emotionally labile, and less able to control their impulses, a state which corresponds to the heightened activity, excessive appetite, and oversexuality of REMS-deprived animals. Differential deprivation of NREMS (stages III and IV) leads, instead, to hyporesponsiveness.

Of course, since the need for sleep is known to vary from person to person in everyday life, it is difficult to decide what is partial sleep deprivation. Some individuals function perfectly on as little as 3 to 4 h per night, and others, who sleep long hours, claim not to obtain the maximum benefit from it.

DERANGEMENTS OF SLEEP **Insomnia** This word signifies want of sleep, and is used popularly to indicate any impairment in its duration, depth, or restorative properties. Quantitative precision as to what constitutes insomnia is impossible because of the uncertainty as to the natural requirement of sleep and also its role in the economy of the human body.

Two classes of insomniacs may be defined: one in which there appears to be a primary disturbance of the normal sleep mechanism, the other in which sleep impairment is secondary to another disease or condition. The latter is encountered frequently in medical practice and may usually be ascribed to pain or some other annoying sensation, or to nervousness, anxiety, and worry.

The term *primary insomnia* should be reserved for those persons who throughout their lives have never enjoyed restful slumber, and in whom none of the usual symptoms of neurosis, depression, or other psychiatric or medical diseases can be elicited. Unlike the rare individuals who seem to thrive on 3 to 4 h sleep a night, they suffer the effects of partial sleep deprivation and resort to drugs and various techniques to induce or maintain sleep. Their life comes so obviously to revolve around sleep that they have been called "sleep pedants" or "sleep hypochondriacs." They sleep for shorter periods than normal persons, awaken more often, spend less time in REMS and more in stage II NREMS, move more often, have more rapid pulse, peripheral vasoconstriction, and higher body temperature, and show a heightened physiologic arousal. Thus their sleep is both quantitatively and qualitatively different from that of "good sleepers."

While there is no doubt that the victims of insomnia, regardless of the cause of their wakefulness, are likely to exaggerate the amount of sleep lost, *primary insomnia* should be recognized as an entity and not passed off as a neurotic quirk.

Of the sensory disorders conducive to abnormal wakefulness, pain in the spine with or without nerve root involvement stands out, as does abdominal discomfort from peptic ulcer and carcinoma. Tired, aching, restless legs, an obscure benign state known as the "restless leg syndrome" (anxietas tibialis), may regularly delay the onset of sleep. Excessive fatigue may give rise to many abnormal muscular sensations of similar nature. Acroparesthesias, peculiar nocturnal tingling and numbness of palms and fingers due to tight carpal ligaments (carpal tunnel syndrome), may awaken the patient at night, as does cluster or histamine headache, which nearly always occurs 2 to 3 h after falling asleep.

Severe insomnia is a more frequent complaint of patients suffering from psychiatric disease (more than 85 percent in one series). Its simplest form occurs in a reactive nervous state in which domestic and business worries keep the patient's mind in a turmoil. Also, vigorous mental activity late at night or excitement which leaves the muscles tense counteracts drowsiness and sleep. Under these circumstances there is difficulty in falling asleep and a tendency to sleep late in the morning. Sleeplessness is also commonly recorded in the histories of patients suffering from psychoneuroses and psychoses.

Illnesses in which anxiety and fear are prominent symptoms usually result in difficulty in falling asleep and light, fitful, or intermittent sleep. Also, disturbing dreams are frequent and may awaken the patient; exceptionally, he may even try to stay awake in order to avoid them. The diurnal-nocturnal timing of sleep is altered, but quality and quantity are little if at all changed. In contrast, the depressive illnesses, particularly the manic-depressive or involutional type, cause either light sleep in the early part of the night or early morning waking and inability to return to sleep. Quantity of sleep is reduced, and nocturnal mobility is increased. The REMS, although not reduced, comes earlier in the night; this is termed the *increased pressure of REMS*. If anxiety is combined with depression, both the above patterns are observed. In states of mania, sleep diminishes and REMS may be abolished. The sleep rhythm may be totally deranged in acute confusional states and delirium, and REMS increases. In the latter the patient may only doze for short periods, both day and night. The total amount and depth of sleep in a 24-h period are reduced. Frightening hallucinations may prevent sleep. The senile and arteriosclerotic patient tends to catnap during the day and then refuses to go to bed at night. His nocturnal sleep is intermittent; its total amount may be either increased or decreased.

Disturbances in the transitional period of sleep As sleep comes on, certain nervous centers may be excited to a burst of insubordinate activity. The result is a sudden start that arouses the incipient sleeper. It may involve one or both legs or the trunk, less often the arms. If the start occurs repeatedly during the process of falling asleep and is a nightly event, it may become a matter of great concern to the patient.

Sensory centers may be disturbed in a similar way, either as an isolated phenomenon or in association with phenomena that induce motion. As the patient drops off to sleep, he may be roused by a sensation that darts through his body. Or a sudden clang or crashing sound disturbs commencing sleep. Sometimes there is a sudden flash of light or a sensation of being lifted and dashed to earth or of being turned. These symptoms are probably similar sensory paroxysms involving the labyrinthine mechanism.

Sleep palsies and acroparesthesias Curious and at times distressing paresthetic disturbances develop during sleep. Everyone is familiar with the phenomenon of an arm or leg "falling asleep." The immobility of the limbs and the maintenance of uncomfortable postures without being aware of them permit pressure to be applied to exposed nerves. The ulnar, radial, and peroneal nerves are quite superficial in places; pressure of the nerve against an underlying bone may interfere with intraneural circulation of the compressed segment. If such pressure is continued for half an hour or longer, a sensory and motor paralysis sometimes referred to as *sleep palsy* may develop. This condition usually lasts only a few minutes or hours, but if the compression is prolonged, the nerve may be severely damaged so that functional recovery awaits regeneration. Unusually deep sleep, as in alcoholic intoxication, renders the patient especially liable to sleep palsies merely because he does not heed the discomfort of an unnatural posture.

Acroparesthesias are frequent in adult women and are not unknown to men. The patient will say that after being asleep for a few hours she is awakened by an intense numbness, tingling, prickling, a feeling of "pins and needles" in her fingers and hands. There are also aching, burning pains or tightness and other unpleasant sensations. At first there is a suspicion of having slept on the arm, but the usual bilaterality and the occurrence regardless of the position of the arms dispel this notion. Usually the paresthesias are in the distribution of the median nerves. Vigorous rubbing of the hands restores normal sensation, and the paresthesias subside within a few minutes, only to return later upon first awakening in the morning. The condition seldom occurs during the daytime unless the patient is lying down or sitting with the arms and hands in one position. When acroparesthesias are frequent, the hands may at all times feel swollen, stiff, clumsy, slightly numb, and sometimes distressingly painful. More severe degrees of this condition merge with the compression syndrome of the median nerve (carpal tunnel syndrome) described in Chaps. 331 and 366.

Nightmares and night terrors (pavor nocturnus) Awakening in a state of terror has happened to nearly everyone. Children are especially susceptible. Fever disposes to it, as may many other conditions, such as indigestion. Bad dreams, stimulated directly by the reading of blood-curdling stories or seeing exciting television programs before bedtime, may be followed by a nightmare. Nightmares differ from night terrors only in the greater intensity of the anxiety and extreme degree of autonomic discharges. In addition there is more vocalization and motor activity, even to the point of running as if pursued.

Then night terror and somnambulism are combined. Gastaut and his associates, who have compared nightmares and night terrors, found the latter to occur in stage IV NREMS often within a half hour of falling asleep. The patient suddenly develops an arousal response (imperfect) with return of alpha rhythm in the EEG and a pattern of extreme motility. Vocalizations, walking, screams, tachycardia (130 to 170 beats per min) and increase in respiratory rate, all lasting a few minutes, may occur.

Such phenomena are of little significance as isolated events in childhood. Indeed, few children have escaped the more frequent experience of nightmare. Only if persistent and frequent do they become matters of pressing medical complaint. Of greater importance is the differentiation of both the nightmare and night terror from nocturnal epilepsy, which also may have a tendency to occur only during a specific stage of sleep. Pharmacologic agents which interfere with the metabolism of either serotonin or norepinephrine offer a possible therapeutic approach to both nightmares and night terrors.

Somnambulism and sleep automatism Examples of sleepwalking occasionally come to the attention of the practicing physician. This condition likewise occurs more often in children than in adults. After being asleep for a time, the patient arises from his bed and walks about the house. He may turn on a light or perform some other familiar act. There is no outward sign of emotion; the eyes are open, and the sleeper is guided by vision, thus avoiding familiar objects. The sight of an unfamiliar object may awaken him. If spoken to, he makes no response; if told to return to bed, he may do so but more often must be led back to it. Sometimes he will mutter strange phrases or sentences over and over. The following morning he usually has no memory of the episode. Talking in one's sleep is probably a minor variant.

Nocturnal epilepsy Paroxysmal abnormalities of the brain waves of the type seen in epilepsy tend to occur in epileptic patients during or shortly after the onset of sleep.

Nocturnal jerks of the legs, also called *nocturnal myoclonus,* are another troublesome symptom because they interfere with sleep night after night. This condition differs from the restless leg syndrome in that involuntary movements occur. Only recently has it been classified as a myoclonic form of epilepsy. It is unaccompanied by all other epileptic manifestations. Anticonvulsant drugs are said to control it, though in two cases the author has had better success with an occasional dose of Pantopon. Obviously an opiate cannot be prescribed for its control.

THE HYPERSOMNIAS *Prolonged states of sleep* are characteristic of patients suffering from encephalitis lethargica (Chap. 338), trypanosomiasis (Chap. 217), and a variety of other diseases localized to the floor and walls of the third ventricle. Small tumors in the posterior hypothalamus and midbrain have been associated with arterial hypotension, diabetes insipidus, and somnolence lasting many weeks. Such patients can be aroused, but if left alone, immediately fall asleep. Tumors of the brain, in general, show a tendency to cause drowsiness and increase in time spent in sleep, but those of the diencephalon more so than any others (e.g., more so than those of the posterior fossa). Traumatic brain lesions and other diseases have been found to produce similar clinical pictures. Myxedema, if severe, may cause hypersomnia.

There are two special varieties of hypersomnia, the Kleine-Levin and Pickwickian syndromes. The Kleine-Levin syndrome consists of periodic hypersomnolence lasting for periods of 2 to 3 weeks and hyperphagia (bulimia). The attacks occur two or three times a year. Onset is usually during adolescence with a striking male predominance. The pathogenesis is obscure. The Pickwickian syndrome of obesity, dyspnea, hypercapnea, and drowsiness are discussed in Chap. 261. This condition may be accompanied by a distressing *sleep apnea.*

NARCOLEPSY AND CATAPLEXY **Narcolepsy** The essential disorder is one of uncontrollable sleepiness. Many times a day the individual is assailed by an uncontrollable desire to sleep. His eyes close, his muscles relax, his breathing slows, and he has all the appearances of a person who is dozing. A noise or a touch is enough to awaken him, and he may feel refreshed momentarily. As a rule the condition begins in adolescence or early adult life. The periods of sleep may occur at any time of day, especially when the patient is physically inactive. The impulse to sleep is so insistent that the victim may be unable to sit through a single class in school or a meeting without at once falling asleep. A given period of sleep usually lasts up to 15 min, seldom as long as an hour unless lying down. At the onset there may be blurring of vision, diplopia, and ptosis which may raise the question of an ophthalmologic disorder. The condition is often associated with cataplexy (70 percent of cases), sleep paralysis (50 percent), and hypnagogic hallucination (25 percent).

Cataplexy This consists of the sudden loss of muscle tone provoked by exaggerated emotion such as excessive laughter or anger. Approximately 70 percent of patients with narcolepsy, if questioned carefully, will admit to having cataplexy. Reference here is made to the curious circumstance that hearty laughter, sadness, or anger will cause the patient's head to fall forward, his jaw to drop open, his knees to buckle, even with falling to the ground, and all with preservation of consciousness. The attack lasts only a minute or two.

The other components of the narcoleptic tetrad are sleep paralysis and hypnagogic hallucinations. In sleep paralysis the individual, as he falls asleep or awakens, becomes conscious of an inability to move or speak. He has the helpless feeling that a word from someone or a touch would break the spell. He recovers in a minute or two. Vivid hallucinations may also occur in this period or separately in a brief nap.

Narcolepsy and cataplexy usually begin in adolescence or early adult life and, once started, continue throughout the adult period, possibly being less frequent in old age. Males are affected more than females, and there is suggestion of a genetic factor. The attack of narcolepsy resembles REMS, as is also true of cataplexy, sleep paralysis, and the hallucinations. The night sleep pattern may also begin with REMS. The EEG is usually normal. No complete pathologic studies are available. There are no other neurologic abnormalities. The condition must be distinguished from the somnolence of obesity, hypothyroidism, heart failure, and excessive use of drugs and alcohol. In these latter cataplexy is always absent.

SLEEP IN RELATION TO MEDICAL DISEASES Patients with a variety of nocturnal medical complaints have been found to undergo other important physiologic changes in relation to certain phases of sleep. Anginal attacks at night appear usually with REMS and peptic ulcer pain increases during REMS when production of hydrochloric acid increases. On the other hand, attacks of bronchial asthma during the night may appear in any phase of sleep.

TREATMENT OF SLEEP DISORDERS **Insomnia** In general, there are three varieties of wakefulness. For best management, treatment should be based on the type exhibited by the patient. One type, infrequently observed in younger patients, is the inability to fall asleep. Individuals affected by this type have become more and more tense during the day and are unable to relax. This type of insomnia usually lasts from 1 to 3 h, and then the individual sinks into an exhausted, deep sleep which continues through the night. For these patients any fairly quick-acting, rapidly destroyed hypnotic such as secobarbital (Seconal), 0.1 g, flurazepam (Dalmane), 30 to 60 mg, chloral hydrate (Noctec), 500 to 1,000 mg, glutethimide (Doriden), 500 mg, or methaqualone (Sopor), 150 to 300 mg, given 15 to 30 min before going to bed is useful in inducing and maintaining sleep. After a week or two, however, their effect wanes. Kales and Kales found only flurazepam to retain its power of reducing sleep latency and awake time after sleep onset.

The second type of insomnia is exhibited by patients who are able to go to sleep but who awaken in 2 or 3 h and lose sleep in the middle of the night. They awaken during the period when sleep normally lightens, and some are alternately awake and asleep all the rest of the night. Often these are sick persons with a debilitating or painful illness which generates more pain and restlessness as muscles relax and leave painful areas unsplinted. In others, fever, sweats, dyspnea, or other distressful symptoms develop and demand attention. Frequently, these patients secure relief from pentobarbital (Nembutal), 0.1 g, or flurazepam (Dalmane), 30 to 60 mg, given at bedtime. For cardiac patients who have Cheyne-Stokes respiration or moderate orthopnea, a rectal suppository of aminophylline, 0.5 g given at bedtime, will frequently relieve the respiratory distress and promote sleep. When pain is a factor in insomnia, acetylsalicylic acid, 0.3 to 0.6 g, should be given with the sedative. Occasionally, codeine phosphate, 30 mg, meperidine (Demerol), 50 mg, or morphine sulfate, 10 to 15 mg, may be required when pain is severe.

The third type of insomnia is seen in patients who go to sleep promptly and sleep well most of the night, only to awaken too early in the morning. Most of these individuals are older persons who turn night into day. They go to bed and get up earlier and earlier so that soon they are sleeping during the day and are alert during the night. Into this category also fall those individuals who are under great tension, worry, or anxiety or are overworked and exhausted. These people sink into bed and sleep through sheer exhaustion, but around 4 or 5 A.M. they awaken with their worries and are unable to get back to sleep. Most of these patients are benefited by barbital, 0.3 g, given with fruit juice or milk at bedtime. For debilitated patients the compressed tablets of insoluble material should be crushed to ensure proper absorption, or sodium barbital should be substituted. Chloral hydrate, 500 mg given with fruit juice at bedtime, is also effective and may be substituted for barbital.

Patients with serious mental agitation, delirium, or excitement who require prompt, easily controlled, relatively safe sedation should receive whiskey, 30 to 60 ml by mouth, or paraldehyde, 15 to 30 ml by mouth in iced fruit juice, or the same dose of the latter by rectum but diluted with 200 ml physiologic saline or 120 ml olive oil. For frankly delirious patients 25 to 50 mg chlorpromazine (t. i. d.) or a similar psychotropic drug has been a most helpful medication. Generally, it is wise to avoid barbiturates with highly agitated patients, since occasionally they may precipitate serious mental confusion, excitement, or even manic tendencies. Chloral hydrate, 1 to 2 g by mouth, is also useful in the management of these individuals and frequently proves more satisfactory than the barbiturates.

A word of caution about oversedation is wise in any discussion of sedative drugs. All too frequently they are abused in that they are given when not needed, the dosage is too great, or the wrong preparation is chosen. These drugs are a common source of constipation, lead to fatigue and lack of energy and strength, and interfere with the patient's recovery from his illness.

When large dosages of quicker-acting barbiturates, 0.4 to 0.6 g daily, or other of the soporific drugs are given for more than a few weeks, there is real danger of habituation, which, once developed, is pernicious in character. Withdrawal, unless accomplished skillfully and in graded steps, may cause serious mental disturbance or precipitate convulsions. The chronic insomniac who has no other symptoms should not be permitted to use sedative drugs as a crutch on which to limp through life. The solution of his problem is rarely to be found in medication. One should search out and correct the underlying difficulty, using medication only as a temporary helpful tool. A good book, pleasure in staying awake, and belief that the human organism will always get as much sleep as needed are helpful.

Since psychologic factors have not been demonstrated in such cases, a conservative program of medical management and pharmacologic treatment is indicated. Diazepam (Valium), which suppresses stage IV NREMS, is helpful in controlling night terrors, and if their differentiation from nocturnal epilepsy is impossible, a trial on diphenylhydantoin sodium (Dilantin sodium) and phenobarbital is indicated. (See Chap. 24 for further information concerning anticonvulsant medication.)

NARCOLEPSY AND CATAPLEXY For narcolepsy and cataplexy there is no therapy which will control all the symptoms. The narcolepsy responds best to (1) strategically placed naps (during lunch hour, before or after dinner, etc.) and (2) the use of analeptic drugs, such as amphetamine sulfate (Benzedrine), methylphenidate (Ritalin), or pipradrol (Meratran). The time of medication should be adjusted to the study or work habits of the patient. The usual dose of amphetamine varies from 5 to 10 mg given three to five times a day. This is ordinarily well tolerated and does not cause wakefulness at night. The dose of Ritalin is 10 to 20 mg thrice daily, and of Meratran, 2.5 to 5.0 mg twice or thrice daily. These have rather little effect on cataplexy but are partially effective in the Kleine-Levin syndrome. Fortunately the latter is less frequent, and some psychiatrists have claimed that it can be controlled by avoidance of emotionally charged situations. The newest addition to the pharmacology of narcolepsy and cataplexy is imipramine (Tofranil), which, in doses of 25 mg three to four times a day, markedly reduces attacks, presumably by abolishing REMS.

REFERENCES

Adams RD, Victor M: *Principles of Neurology,* New York: McGraw-Hill, 1977

Jacobs et al: Eye movements during sleep. I. The pattern in the normal human. Arch Neurol 25:151, 1971

Kales A, Kales JD: Recent findings in the diagnosis and treatment of disturbed sleep. New Engl J Med 290:487, 1974

Pappenheimer JR, Setchell BP: The measurement of cerebral blood flow in the rabbit and sheep. J Physiol (Lond) 226:48P, 1972

24
THE CONVULSIVE STATE AND IDIOPATHIC EPILEPSY

RAYMOND D. ADAMS

The magnitude of the problem of convulsion as a leading manifestation of a medical or neurologic disease can hardly be overstated. The statistics of Hauser and Kurland show that at least 1 million persons in the United States are subject to recurrent seizures and that at least ten times that number consult a physician or go to a hospital at some time in their lives because of a seizure.

A solitary or brief outburst of convulsions may occur during the course of many medical illnesses; its significance derives from the fact that it indicates involvement of the nervous system and by its very nature, if repeated every few minutes, as in status epilepticus, may threaten life. Recurrent convulsions over long periods of life, most of the episodes being more or less identical in type, represent a different sort of problem. On the one hand they may be a manifestation of an ongoing primary neurologic disease that demands diagnosis and therapy, as in brain tumor. On the other, they may call attention to an old burnt-out lesion that began some time in the distant past and remains as a fibroglial scar. Not infrequently the original disease was unnoticed; perhaps it occurred *in utero,* at birth, or during childhood in parts of the brain that were too immature to test; or it may have affected a silent area of the mature brain. Patients with such old lesions, who make up the majority of those with recurrent seizures, are necessarily classified as having "idiopathic epilepsy," because it is impossible to obtain data regarding the original disease. The seizure may be the only sign of the brain abnormality.

The convulsive disorder is the expression of a sudden, excessive, disorderly discharge of neurons in either a structurally normal or diseased cortex. The discharge results in an almost instantaneous disturbance of sensation, loss of consciousness, convulsive movement, or some combination thereof. A terminologic embarrassment arises from the diversity of the clinical manifestations. It seems improper to call a condition a "convulsion" when only an alteration of sensation or of consciousness takes place. The word "seizure" is preferable, as a generic term, and also lends itself to qualification. Motor or convulsive seizure is not, therefore, tautologic, and one may also speak of sensory seizure.

COMMON TYPES OF CONVULSIVE DISORDER The generalized convulsion ranks as the most frequent type, being both a common expression of a number of ongoing diseases and the lasting mark of some obscure disease in the past. As in petit mal, another special type of brief spell, the location of the causative lesion and its cause are unknown. Presumably the generalized seizure involves the entire cerebral cortex and diencephalon. Various other patterns of seizure, such as the psychomotor, which is associated with disease of the temporal lobe, usually have a demonstrable cortical focus, either actively progressing or stationary.

When the idiopathic recurrent types of convulsive disorder are analyzed as a group, as in the survey of nearly 2,000 patients by Lennox, it was found that 51 percent had generalized convulsions; 8 percent, petit mal; and the remaining 41 percent, focal and mixed types, of which psychomotor was the most frequent.

Generalized convulsion (other than grand mal) Certain intercurrent medical diseases manifest themselves at one stage by a seizure or a series of seizures beginning as immediate loss of consciousness, with stiffening, then clonic rhythmic jerking of the limbs or only with the latter. The focality of the initiating lesion may be indicated by tonic or clonic spasm of the muscles of only one part of the body or a turning of eyes and head to one side. Consciousness tends to be reinstated soon after the cessation of the generalized motor activity. A single myoclonic jerk or multiple ones may be a prelude to the major seizure or may follow it or be interspersed between seizures. In some instances, especially in metabolic disorders of the brain, the focal motor seizures may appear first on one side of the body, then on the other, progressing to a generalized seizure.

Generalized convulsion (grand mal) The recurrent generalized seizure of grand mal type is more elaborate and demonstrates more clearly the effect of the epileptic discharge on the physiology of the nervous system. It begins with a sudden loss of consciousness, a cry, a fall to the ground, tonic then clonic movements of muscles of cranium and limbs, sometimes sphincteric incontinence, and other autonomic disorders. The motor activity soon terminates, leaving the patient in a state of coma, which lasts for many minutes or even as long as a half-hour. As the coma recedes, mental confusion, drowsiness, and headache supervene.

Petit mal (minor epilepsy, l'absence) This type of seizure, from the age of four years to adolescence, comes without warning and is notable for its brevity and minimal motor accompaniment. It consists essentially of a brief loss of consciousness, lasting a few seconds. A few three-per-second blinks or jerks of eyelids and sometimes arms may be conjoined. Petit mal may be more variable (atypical) with two-per-second motor and EEG pattern and then is more likely to be combined with sudden falling episodes or single, brief, generalized myoclonic contractions of limbs.

COMMON FOCAL SEIZURE PATTERNS **Psychomotor epilepsy** Certainly this is the most frequent and interesting type of focal seizure pattern. The aura, if it occurs, often takes the form of a complex hallucination or perceptual illusion. There may be an unpleasant smell or taste, or the revival of a complicated visual scene involving people, dwellings, etc., usually taken from past experiences and resembling a dream. Furthermore, the patient's perception of what is seen and heard and his relationship to the outside world are altered. Objects appear to be far away or unreal *(jamais vu);* or strange objects or persons may seem familiar *(déjà vu phenomenon).* Hughlings Jackson applied the term *dreamy state* to these psychic disturbances. In the seizure the patient behaves as though he were partially conscious. He may get up and walk about, unbutton or remove his clothes, attempt to speak, or even continue such habitual acts as driving a car. If he is asked a specific question or given a command, it is evident that he is out of contact with the examiner and does not understand. When restrained, he may resist with great energy and at times may be violent. This type of behavior is said to be *automatic,* presumably because the patient behaves like an automaton. Convulsive movements, when present, are likely to consist of chewing, smacking and licking of the lips, and, less often, tonic spasms of the limbs or turning of the head and eyes to one side.

In any given case one or several of these phenomena may be observed. In the series studied by Lennox and Lennox, which numbered 414 cases, 43 percent of patients displayed some of these motor or psychomotor phenomena; 32 percent, the automatic state; and 25 percent, the psychic changes. Some psychomotor seizures are very brief, lasting only for seconds, and others continue for hours. This calls to mind that the duration of the seizure is an unsatisfactory criterion for classification.

LOCALIZED MOTOR SEIZURES A lesion in one or the other frontal lobe may give rise to a generalized or major convulsive seizure of the type described above, without an introductory aura. In some cases there is a turning movement of the head and eyes to one side, simultaneously with loss of consciousness. It has been postulated that in both types of seizure, the one with and the one without contraversive movements, the discharge from the frontal lobe spreads rapidly into an integrating center such as the thalamus, with immediate loss of consciousness.

The *Jacksonian motor seizure* begins usually with a tonic contraction or a clonic rhythmic twitching of the fingers of one hand, the face on one side, or one foot. The twitching may occur in bursts, or paroxysms. The disorder then spreads, or marches, from the part first affected to other muscles on the same side of the body—from the face to the neck, hand, forearm, arm, trunk, and leg; if the first movement is in the foot, the order is reversed. A high incidence of onset in the lips, fingers, and toes probably is related to the greater cortical representation of these parts of the body. The disease process or focus of excitation is usually the rolandic cortex, area 4 (Fig. 27-1) on the opposite side; in a few cases it has been found in the post-rolandic convolution. Lesions confined to the premotor cortex (area 6) are said to induce tonic contractions of an arm, face, neck, or all of one side of the body. Perspiration and piloerection, sometimes only of the parts of the body involved in a focal motor seizure, suggest that these autonomic functions have cortical representation in the rolandic area.

Another type of focal motor epilepsy consists of rhythmic clonic movements of one group of muscles, usually in the face, arm, or leg. These may continue for a variable period of time, from minutes to weeks or months. The seizure does not occur in bursts or paroxysms and usually does not "march" to other parts of the body. Its localizing value has not been settled. Some patients have a lesion in the opposite sensorimotor areas of the cerebral cortex.

SOMATIC, VISUAL, AND OTHER SENSORY SEIZURES Somatic sensory seizures, either focal or marching to other parts of the body on one side, nearly always indicate a parietal lobe lesion. The usual *sensory disorder* is described as a numbness, a tingling, or a "pins-and-needles" feeling. Other variations are sensations of crawling (formication), buzzing, electricity, or vibration. Pain and thermal sensations are infrequent. The onset is in the lips, fingers, and toes in the majority of cases, and the spread to adjacent parts of the body follows a pattern determined by sensory arrangements in the postcentral (post-rolandic) convolution of the parietal lobe. In the series of Kristiansen and Penfield the seizure focus was found in the postcentral convolution in 24 of 55 cases; it was central, either pre- or post-rolandic, in 18, and precentral in 7 cases. If localized in the cranial muscles, the focus is in the lowest part of the convolution, near the sylvian fissure; if in the foot or leg, the upper part near the superior sagittal sinus is involved.

Lesions in or near the striate cortex of the occipital lobe usually produce a sensation of lights, of darkness, or of color. The patient may tell of seeing stars or moving lights in the visual field on the side opposite the lesion. Sometimes they appear to be straight ahead of the patient. Often, if they occur on only one side of the visual field, he believes only one eye to be affected, the one opposite the lesion, probably because the average person is unaware that he has two corresponding visual fields. It is curious that a seizure arising in one occipital lobe may cause momentary blindness in both eyes. It has been noted that seizures arising in the lateral surface of the occipital lobes (Brodmann's areas 18 and 19) are more likely to cause twinkling or pulsating lights. Complex visual hallucinations are usually due to a focus in the posterior part of the temporal lobe, near its junction with the parietal, and they may be associated with auditory hallucinations. Often the visual images, either those of the hallucination or of objects seen, are distorted or seem too small *(micropsia)* or unnaturally arranged.

Auditory hallucinations are rather infrequent as an initial manifestation of a seizure. Occasionally a patient with a focus in the superior temporal convolution on one side will report a buzzing or a roaring in his ears. A human voice sometimes repeating recognizable words has been noted a few times in patients with lesions in the more posterior part of the dominant temporal lobe.

Vertiginous sensations of a type suggesting vestibular stimulation may be the first symptom of a seizure. The lesion is usually localized in the superior posterior temporal region or at the junction between the parietal and temporal lobes. Occasionally, with a temporal focus, vertigo is followed by an auditory sensation.

Olfactory hallucinations are often associated with disease of the inferior and medial parts of the temporal lobe, usually in the region of the hippocampal convolution or the uncus (hence the term *uncinate seizures,* after Jackson). Usually the smell is exteriorized, i.e., projected to someplace in the environment, and is of a disagreeable nature. Gustatory hallucinations have also been recorded in proved cases of temporal lobe disease. Sensations of thirst and salivation may be associated. Seizures arising in and stimulation of the upper surface of the temporal lobe in the depths of the sylvian fissure during neurosurgical operations have produced peculiar sensations of taste.

Visceral sensations arising in the thorax, epigastrium, and abdomen are among the most frequent of the auras. They are described as a vague, indefinable feeling, a sinking sensation in the pit of the stomach, and a weakness in the epigastrium or substernal area that rises to the throat and head. The seizure discharge may be localized to the upper bank of the sylvian fissure or in the upper intermediate or medial frontal areas near the cingulate gyrus. Palpitation and acceleration of pulse at the beginning of the attack have also been related to a temporal lobe focus.

PSYCHIC PHENOMENA A close relationship between psychic changes and temporal lobe foci has been established. Disease of either temporal lobe may be accompanied by seizures that have many of the characteristics of psychomotor epilepsy. In addition, complex visual and auditory hallucinations with feelings of unreality, and partial or complete interruption of consciousness, may be observed. Compulsive thought or action may recur in a fixed pattern during each seizure. Automatic behavior or even frank psychoses resembling confusional states or schizophrenia, and lasting for hours or days, may be induced by seizure discharges or electrical stimulation of the temporal lobe.

The various motor, sensory, or psychic phenomena may be combined in many different sequences. These presumably indicate the spread of a seizure discharge from one cortical area to another. A flash of light followed by tingling of one side of the body suggests that the epileptic discharge began in the occipital lobe and extended to the somatic sensory areas in the parietal lobe. A smell of something burning, followed by chewing and smacking movements, and then loss of speech would be interpreted as a spread of the seizure discharge from the region of the uncus to the upper parts of the temporal and the inferior frontal lobes. A focal motor seizure followed by a tonic contraction of one side of the body and then by turning of the head and eyes contralaterally would indicate a successive involvement of the motor, premotor, and contraversive cortical field for head and eyes. Little is known about the factors that facilitate or inhibit the spread of seizure discharges from one part of the brain to another.

EVOCATION OF SEIZURES (REFLEX EPILEPSY) Seizures can sometimes be evoked in susceptible persons by a physiologic or psychologic stimulus. Approximately 1 in every 15 patients will have remarked that their seizures occur under special circumstances, such as being exposed to flickering light, passing from darkness to light or the reverse, being startled by a loud noise, hearing a series of monotonous sounds or music, touching, rubbing, or hurting a particular part of the body, making certain movements (e.g., eating, reading, carrying out some complex mental task), or being subjected to fright or other strong emotion. The evoked seizure may be focal (beginning often in the part of the body that has been stimulated) or generalized. In a few instances this reflex epilepsy, as it is called, has been due to a focal cerebral disease, such as a tumor, but more often its cause cannot be ascertained. A special type of reflex myoclonic epilepsy with a strong tendency to familial incidence can be elicited by photic stimulation (photic epilepsy). Another point of interest in these cases of evoked seizure has been the phenomenon of willfully averting the seizure by undertaking some mental task, e.g., thinking about some distracting subject or counting, or by initiating some physical activity.

PATHOPHYSIOLOGY OF THE CONVULSION Reflex epilepsy suggests that epilepsy is a natural state, a physiologic event resulting from excitation and subsequent inhibition of a damaged part of the cerebrum. Eventually the physiologic event that initiates the seizure is a high-voltage discharge of an assemblage of cortical neurons. There need not be a visible lesion for, under the proper circumstances, it can be initiated in entirely normal cerebral cortex, as when the cortex is activated by a drug or injured by hypoxia. But it is the visible focal lesion that has been the most thoroughly investigated. Some of the electrical properties of the cortical focus suggest that its neurons have been deafferented. Deafferented neurons are known to be hypersensitive; they remain chronically in a state of partial depolarization, and the cytoplasmic membranes have an increased permeability which renders them susceptible to activation by hyperthermia, hypoxia, hypoglycemia, and hyponatremia, as well as by repeated sensory (e.g., photic) stimulation and during certain phases of sleep (when hypersynchrony of neurons is known to occur). Another hypothesis is that the lesion of the cortex has resulted in the removal of a normal diencephalic inhibitory effect.

The biochemical studies of the involved clone of neurons of a seizure focus have not clarified the problem. Epileptic foci are known to be sensitive to the facilitatory transmitter substance acetylcholine and to be slower in binding and removing it than normal cerebral cortex; a deficiency of gamma-aminobutyric acid (GABA), the inhibitory transmitter, a disturbance of cytochrome oxidase with decrease in ATP production, a reduction in the Krebs cycle function with a shift to GABA-succinate shunt, a disturbance in local regulation of extracellular K, Na, Ca, Mg are other hypotheses equally lacking of confirmation.

Once the intensity of the seizure discharge exceeds a certain point, it spreads to adjacent cortical and to thalamic and brainstem nuclei. Then it is that the first clinical manifestation of the convulsion begins. Presumably the excitatory activity is fed back from the thalamus to the original focus and to other parts of the forebrain, giving rise to the characteristic high-frequency discharge in the EEG, and there is propagation downward to spinal neurons via corticospinal and reticulospinal pathways. Shortly thereafter a diencephalocortical inhibition begins and intermittently interrupts the focal and generalized seizure discharge, changing it from the persistent discharge of the tonic phase to the intermittent bursts of the clonic phase. These become less and less frequent and finally cease altogether, leaving in their wake strong inhibition or paralysis of the neurons of the epileptic focus. This latter is the basis of *Todd's postepileptic paralysis* which is accompanied by diffuse slow waves in the EEG in all parts of the cerebrum. In petit mal it is thought that the high-voltage spike-slow-wave discharge originates in the thalamus, and this may also be true of some cases of grand mal, in both of which consciousness is at once abolished. On the other hand, atypical petit mal and possibly the typical type as well can be induced by a mesial frontal lesion. Temporal lobe seizures are known to arise in foci in the medial temporal lobe amygdaloid nuclei and hippocampus. Electrical stimulation in these areas reproduces a partial loss of conscious contact with environment, feelings of depersonalization, and automatic behavior.

A discovery of no little importance is that a seizure focus, if active for a time, may establish via commissural connections a secondary focus in the corresponding area of cortex in the opposite hemisphere (mirror focus). The nature of this development is not fully understood. This becomes a source of confusion in trying to identify electrographically the side of the primary lesion.

Severe seizures may disturb the chemistry of the brain by causing hypoxia, acidosis with rise in P_{CO_2}, and an accumulation of lactic acid. Some of these effects are secondary to respiratory spasm, blockage of airway, and excessive muscular activity. These biochemical changes give rise to secondary cerebral lesions. The latter are especially frequent in the temporal lobes and cerebellum and may themselves later become epileptic foci. A violent epileptic discharge of the brain may cause respiratory arrest or cardiac standstill, with death ensuing immediately.

The electroencephalogram provides a delicate proof of Hughlings Jackson's theory of epilepsy—that it is an excessive, disorderly discharge of cortical neurons. At the onset of the focal seizure this is registered in or near the focus as a series of spikes or sharp waves interrupting the normal alpha and beta waves. The clinical spread of the seizure has its electroencephalographic equivalent in the extension of the abnormal electrical waves; with generalization of the seizure (grand mal), the entire electroencephalographic recording surface of the brain exhibits spikes of high voltage. Petit mal is accompanied by a characteristic three-per-second wave-spike complex occurring simultaneously in all cortical leads and presumably taking origin from a diencephalic focus. At first there was thought to be a characteristic electroencephalographic picture for psychomotor epilepsy, but further studies have not confirmed this. The postseizure state, sometimes called *postconvulsive paralysis of cerebral function,* also has its electroencephalographic correlate in random generalized slow waves. With recovery of normal mentation the electroencephalogram returns to normal. If the electroencephalographic tracing is obtained during the interval between seizures, it is abnormal to some degree in approximately 40 percent of fully conscious and 75 percent of sleeping patients.

The epileptic lesion Of the innumerable diseases that are epileptogenic it has not been possible to distinguish the component of lesion that is responsible for the seizures from one that is not. In other words one cannot say from microscopic examination whether any given lesion was epileptic. Gliosis, fibrosis, vascularization, meningocerebral cicatrix have all been incriminated, but they occur as well in nonepileptic foci. Partial disconnection of groups of cortical neurons from those of neighboring cortex, of the other cerebral hemisphere, and of the thalamus seems likely to have occurred. Or certain systems of inhibiting neurons may have been destroyed. Once a gliotic focus of whatever cause, bordered by groups of discharging neurons, becomes epileptogenic, it may remain so throughout the lifetime of the patient.

DISEASES CAUSING SYMPTOMATIC SEIZURES Among the medical diseases which may be complicated by a burst of seizures, the following are the most frequent.

Generalized convulsions mixed in some instances with unilateral muscular contractions of clonic type appear prominently during an abstinence or withdrawal period in patients addicted to *alcohol* or *barbiturates.* Suspicion of this mechanism is raised by the telltale marks of alcoholic excesses or the history of a prolonged nervousness requiring sedation. Also disturbances of sleep, disorientation, illusions, and visual hallucinations often precede and follow the convulsive phase of the illness. The convulsive period lasts several days and is accompanied and followed for several more by a confusional state.

Bacterial meningitis is another type of illness with a strong convulsive tendency, more pronounced in children than in adults. Fever and stiff neck usually provide the clue, and lumbar puncture yields the salient laboratory data.

Uremia is another condition with a prominent convulsive aspect. Of interest is the sequence of events in complete anuria. This condition is tolerated for 2 to 3 days without neurologic signs, and then there is a rapid onset of twitching, trembling, myoclonic jerks, and generalized motor seizures. Tetany may be added (see Chap. 272). The motor display, one of the most dramatic in medicine, lasts several days until the patient sinks into terminal coma or recovers. When this syndrome accompanies lupus erythematosus, delirium tremens, idiopathic epilepsy, or generalized neoplasia, one can nearly always be sure that it has a basis in renal failure.

Cardiac arrest, suffocation or respiratory failure, NO_2 anesthesia, CO poisoning—the common causes of hypoxic encephalopathy—induce a diffuse myoclonic jerking of all the musculature and generalized seizures as soon as cardiac function is resumed. The convulsive phase of this condition may last only a few days, in association with coma, stupor, or confusion; or it may persist indefinitely as an intensive myoclonic-convulsive state.

Other acute illnesses complicated by generalized and multifocal motor seizures are hyponatremia and water intoxication, thyrotoxic storm, hypertensive encephalopathy, porphyria, hypoglycemia, pyridoxine deficiency, argininosuccinic aciduria, and phenylketonuria. Picrotoxin and

Metrazol are two of the most highly convulsant drugs in use, and lead and arsenic the most frequent convulsive metallic intoxicants.

Generalized seizures with or without twitching may occur in the terminal phases of many other illnesses, such as gram-negative septicemias with shock, liver coma, and intractable congestive heart failure.

There are several primary diseases of the brain which are announced by an acute convulsive state. Myoclonic jerking and seizures appear early in acute inclusion-body encephalitis and other forms of viral, treponemal, and parasitic encephalitis, subacute sclerosing encephalitis, as well as in lipid storage diseases, Jakob-Creutzfeldt disease, and diffuse gliomatosis of the brain.

It seems strange that difficult problems of a convulsive nature seldom occur in patients suffering from cerebrovascular disease. Only exceptionally will a cerebral embolus cause a focal fit, though old cortical infarcts arising therefrom become epileptogenic in 20 percent of cases. The rupture of an aneurysm is occasionally marked by one or two generalized convulsions. Thrombotic occlusions of cerebral arteries are almost never convulsive in the opening phases of the stroke. Subcortical hemorrhages in malignant hypertension occasionally become sources of recurrent focal epilepsy. The rare thrombophlebitis with cortical ischemia and infarction is probably the most highly convulsive vascular lesion. Tumor, on the other hand, is a frequent cause of focal or generalized seizures, the latter present in more than 30 percent of cases if located in the central parts of the cerebrum. Nearly 40 percent of cerebral abscesses leave in their wake recurrent convulsions. Cerebral traumatism is the other common convulsive disease. Thirty to forty percent of all penetrating and contusing cerebral injuries will be followed by focal epilepsy. (See Chaps. 335 to 337.)

IDIOPATHIC EPILEPSY Idiopathic epilepsy tends to express itself with maximal frequency at two periods in life, between the ages of two and five years and around puberty. More often than not the first seizure is generalized, though a series of petit mal, "staring spells," may precede its appearance. Up to this moment development may have been normal, and a neurologic examination is likely to disclose no other abnormality. In a smaller proportion other types of seizures (neonatal, infantile spasms, etc.) have occurred earlier in life. Although the seizures may be either of generalized motor type (51 percent of cases) or petit mal (8 percent) in the beginning, as the years pass and the seizures continue, approximately 40 percent of patients will have both these types or psychomotor seizures.

The severity of the convulsive state varies from a single attack every several years to many per day. If the generalized seizures are at all frequent, they pose a constant threat of injury or social embarrassment, often preventing the further education of the child or the gainful occupation of the adult. Of the milder form of disorder, however, sufficient medical control may be achieved so that there is no interference with the normal life activities. In enlightened communities no longer is an intelligent epileptic ostracized by teachers or employers, and virtually all patients without other neurologic abnormalities can find their place in society. If there is evidence of mental retardation, character changes, hemiparesis, etc., as not infrequently happens, the other problems may be more important than the idiopathic epilepsy.

The common diagnostic procedures performed in the interval between seizures are usually uninformative, i.e., the cerebrospinal fluid is normal, x-rays of skull are normal, pneumoencephalogram and arteriograms, where they have been done, are negative. Only the electroencephalogram will demonstrate an abnormality in 40 to 75 percent of cases, either a generalized paroxysmal 3-per-s spike-slow-wave complex (dart-dome), sharp waves, or some other alterations.

Without doubt the appearance of a convulsion poses a serious problem for the patient, his family, and his physician. There is first of all the possibility of its being the initial manifestation of a neurologic disease which will take the life of the patient (e.g., infiltrating glioma). But even if the convulsion is due to a stationary, healed lesion, life expectancy is slightly reduced owing to the danger of injury or, rarely, unexplained death. If seizures are frequent or difficult to control, mentation may be altered: the patient is dull, vague, querulous, and illogically argumentative. If seizures are infrequent and the EEG relatively normal between attacks, prognoses for successful schooling, occupational adjustment, and marriage are excellent. Mental deterioration, fortunately, occurs rarely, contrary to lay opinion, and when it becomes evident over a few weeks, one must suspect (1) wrong initial diagnosis (not idiopathic epilepsy but seizures due to some definable cerebral disease), (2) drug intoxication from anticonvulsant medication, (3) recurrent subclinical seizures, (4) hypoxic–hypotensive crisis during a bout of prolonged seizures, (5) subdural hematoma resulting from head injury.

APPROACH TO THE CLINICAL PROBLEM OF RECURRENT SEIZURES A history of recurrent attacks of loss of consciousness or awareness associated with abnormal movements or confusion is usually sufficient to establish a diagnosis of epilepsy. With such patients a thorough history, a complete physical and neurologic examination, testing of the visual fields, and laboratory studies, including x-ray examination of the skull and an electroencephalogram, should be done. The results of these essential procedures will determine to which of the categories in the above classification the case belongs or whether one must resort to the label of idiopathic epilepsy.

If a patient not known to have been epileptic has an acute illness with frequent generalized or one-sided seizures, a search must be conducted for clinical and laboratory signs of infection, metabolic and endocrine diseases, and intoxications.

If convulsions have occurred in the past, an inquiry as to epilepsy in the family history and occurrence of head trauma or cerebral infections in the past must be made; careful description of the seizure itself, including prodromata, aura, manifestations during the seizure and the postictal period, must be obtained. Seizures in other members of the family favor slightly the diagnosis of *idiopathic epilepsy*. Signs of pulmonary or ear infection or of congenital heart disease with a right-to-left shunt should suggest, in a patient with recently acquired seizures, the possibility of a *brain abscess*. The presence of a heart murmur and fever or of atrial fibrillation favors embolism. Head trauma of a serious nature, followed by seizures after an interval of several weeks to 2 years, indicates that an injury may have given rise to convulsions. A regularly recurring aura, especially of a focal nature, may indicate a localized lesion in the brain. Similarly, a focal convulsive movement at the onset of the seizure probably indicates a localized cerebral lesion. A transient monoplegia or hemiplegia (Todd's paralysis) in the postictal period also has considerable significance in localizing a lesion. In fact, its presence may provide the best clue to a focal brain lesion. A history of other neurologic symptoms such as headache, localized paralysis, or mental changes often indicates the need for special diagnostic studies.

A general physical examination may provide clues to the legion of conditions associated with epilepsy. Protuberances over the skull may suggest an underlying pathologic condition. Vascular nevi over the body, especially over the face and in the retina, may be associated with vascular abnormalities within the skull. Small tumors, often pedunculated, distributed over the body surface bring to mind the diagnosis of von Recklinghausen's disease and, when associated with seizures, may indicate an intracranial glioma or neurofibroma. White spots over the trunk and limbs and sebaceous adenomas of the face point to the diagnosis of tuberous sclerosis. Smallness of an arm or leg indicates a lesion acquired at an early age. Cranial nerve disturbances are also helpful in diagnosis; thus, a sixth-nerve paralysis is often associated with increased intracranial pressure. Localized weakness, differences in reflexes, or the presence of abnormal reflexes, such as Babinski's response, all have localizing value.

The question of what laboratory procedures should be done in cases of epilepsy can be answered only on the basis of the clinical findings. With recent onset of generalized convulsions simple blood chemistry tests are among the first measures to be carried out. The determination of blood glucose helps orient the examiner in instances of hypoglycemia and hyperglycemia; the calcium level provides the main clue to hypocalcemia, the blood urea nitrogen (BUN) to kidney disease, and sodium and potassium levels to multiple metabolic disturbances, including dilutional hyponatremia. X-rays of the skull should be taken in all cases. Significant findings related to increased intracranial pressure include erosion of the clinoid processes and, in infants and children, separation of the sutures. Hyperostoses, erosions of the skull, abnormal vascular markings, and intracranial calcifications are other findings of importance that may appear in skull x-rays. Because of the frequency of cerebral metastases from primary carcinoma of the lung, chest x-rays should be made in all patients suspected of having intracranial neoplasm.

Lumbar puncture can be of considerable value in elucidating the causes of epilepsy. If the history, neurologic examination, or skull x-rays show any abnormality, especially if a focal lesion in the brain is suggested, then a lumbar puncture is mandatory (unless there are signs of high intracranial pressure). Of special importance are determination of the pressure, cell count, total protein, and serologic tests. Increased pressure points to an expanding intracranial lesion. An abnormal cell count usually indicates an infectious process. An elevation only of total protein (greater than 100 mg per 100 ml) favors the diagnosis of a tumor. If the pressure is normal but other symptoms or signs point to a recently acquired, localized brain lesion, an arteriogram or pneumoencephalogram may be needed. If, in addition to localizing signs, the patient shows signs of increased intracranial pressure, whether by papilledema or high cerebrospinal fluid pressure, then a ventriculogram may be preferred to a pneumoencephalogram. However arteriography is now used more frequently than air visualization because of its greater safety, and both are now being superseded by radioactive isotopic scanning and computerized axial tomography. The visualization of the cerebral hemisphere by these procedures may be of particular help to the neurosurgeon in localizing the lesion and in planning a surgical approach to it.

The electroencephalogram, although now routinely employed in the definitive diagnosis of cases with epilepsy, is not absolutely conclusive, since it may be normal in some patients, particularly if the seizures are relatively infrequent, or abnormal in diseases that do not cause epilepsy. The test is of particular value in diagnosing petit mal, for here clinical or subclinical attacks are apt to be frequent enough to register during the electroencephalographic test. Abnormal electrical waves may manifest themselves in other types of epilepsy as well, and the electroencephalogram may be abnormal during the interseizure period, demonstrating either focal or generalized abnormalities of cortical activity. Activation of the electroencephalogram by photic stimulation, drug-induced sleep, or Metazol injection is now standard procedure in many laboratories (see Chap. 330).

The type of clinical study in any given case is dictated to some extent by the age of the patient. Up until early adulthood most patients turn out to have idiopathic epilepsy. With increasing age, the incidence of idiopathic epilepsy becomes less and that of symptomatic epilepsy increases. Thus the appearance of convulsions for the first time in early or middle adult life should be presumptive evidence of brain tumor until every effort has been made to rule it out (see Table 24-1).

TABLE 24-1
Causes of recurrent convulsion in different age groups

Age of onset, yr	*Probable cause*
Infancy, 0–2	Congenital maldevelopment, birth injury; metabolic (hypocalcemia, hypoglycemia), vitamin B_6 deficiency, phenylketonuria
Childhood, 2–10	Birth injury, trauma, infections, thrombosis of cerebral arteries or veins, beginning of idiopathic epilepsy
Adolescence, 10–18	Idiopathic epilepsy, trauma, congenital defects
Early adulthood, 18–35	Trauma, neoplasm, idiopathic epilepsy, alcoholism, drug addiction
Middle age, 35–60	Neoplasm, trauma, vascular disease, alcoholism, drug addiction
Late life, over 60	Vascular disease, degeneration, tumor

DIFFERENTIAL DIAGNOSIS The clinical differences between a seizure and a syncopal attack are presented in Chap. 16 and need not be repeated here. It must be emphasized once again that there is no single criterion for distinguishing between them. The author has erred in calling akinetic seizures simple faints and in mistaking cardiac or carotid sinus faints for seizures. Petit mal may be difficult to identify because of the brevity of attacks. One helpful maneuver is to have the patient count for 5 to 10 min. If he is having petit mal, he will blink or stare, pause in counting, or skip one or two numbers. Hyperventilation is a useful way of evoking this type of seizure. Psychomotor seizures are the most difficult of all to diagnose. These attacks are so variable in character and so likely to induce minor disturbances in conduct rather than obvious interruptions of consciousness that they may be misdiagnosed as temper tantrums, hysteria, psychopathic behavior, or acute psychosis.

A special problem in diagnosis is offered by states of mental dullness and confusion. Epileptic patients as seen in hospital and office practice usually show no mental deterioration, regardless of the type of seizure. Therefore, the appearance of dementia, confusion, or some other derangement of mental function should suggest the possibility of recurrent subclinical seizures not controlled by medication, drug intoxication, postseizure psychosis, or a brain disease that has caused both dementia and seizures. To distinguish these clinical states may require careful observation, along the lines suggested in Chap. 26, and electroencephalography (Chap. 330).

TREATMENT AND MANAGEMENT OF THE CONVULSING AND EPILEPTIC PATIENT **Status epilepticus** Rarely does a single seizure terminate life, although instances do occur presumably from a cardiac arrhythmia, suffocation, or aspiration. Recovery from a single seizure is usually prompt and requires no special treatment.

While the patient is convulsing, it is necessary to protect him from injury and to make sure that there is a clear airway. A soft object that cannot be swallowed may be placed between the teeth to protect the tongue, but once the jaws are set in a tonic spasm, one should not try to force them open because of the risk of breaking teeth.

Once the seizures are under control, further anticonvulsant therapy depends on the nature of the disease. If a causative lesion is eliminated by medication, e.g., meningitis, no further therapy is needed. When seizures are associated with a surgically removable lesion of the brain, such as a tumor or abscess, its excision may eradicate the discharging focus. This is unpredictable, however, for convulsive seizures are relieved in only about 50 percent of cases of meningioma and an even smaller percentage of cases of glioma or abscess of the cerebrum.

A series of seizures without restoration of consciousness between (status epilepticus) is more dangerous and demands admission to a hospital and prompt pharmacotherapy. Often the patient is already receiving a maintenance dose of anticonvulsant medication, but if not, diphenylhydantoin, 400 mg per day, and phenobarbital, 200 mg per day, should be administered. For control of the status epilepticus diazepam (Valium), 5 to 10 mg, or sodium phenobarbital may be given intravenously or intramuscularly. Intravenous injection of Valium should be made slowly over the period of a minute into a large vein and repeated every 2 to 4 h if necessary. Rapid injection may cause apnea or cardiac arrest. The alternative, sodium phenobarbital, may also be given intravenously, in a dose of 200 mg, to be repeated if necessary every 4 h. For *focal* status epilepticus paraldehyde, 1 to 3 ml given slowly by intravenous route or 5 to 10 ml intramuscularly (avoiding nerves), is sometimes useful. Once the cycle of status epilepticus is broken, one may rely on the standard oral or parenteral anticonvulsant medications. If the seizures are not responsive to the above doses of Valium or sodium phenobarbital, it is better for the patient to have a few seizures than to be rendered comatose by increasing doses of medication.

The type of disease causing the seizures and its treatment is another important consideration. Antibiotic medication usually arrests the seizure tendency in bacterial meningitis. NaCl in a 3% solution usually terminates the seizures in hyponatremia, and 5% glucose solution has a similar effect in hypoglycemic seizures. $MgSO_4$ and calcium gluconate often help in uremic seizures. Abstinence seizures cease usually within a few days and are rarely severe and frequent. In all these conditions or in idiopathic epilepsy if status epilepticus occurs, occasional seizures are of less serious consequence than a deepening drug-induced coma from excessive doses of anticonvulsant medication.

Recurrent seizures including idiopathic epilepsy Of course success in the management of patients with epilepsy depends in large measure on the deployment of drugs for the prevention of seizures. If managed well with anticonvulsants, fully 75 percent of patients may have their seizures controlled or reduced in frequency.

The drugs in common use for this purpose are the barbiturates, hydantoins, and oxazoladinediones, and to a lesser extent acetylureas and benzodiazepams. The available products which have received a thorough clinical trial and their daily dosages are listed in Table 24-2.

Certain drugs are more effective in one type of seizure than in another, and it is necessary to use the proper drugs in the optimum dosages for the different types of seizures. If satisfactory results are not obtained with one of the drugs, the others should be tried, but frequent shifting of drugs is not advisable, and each should be given in adequate trial before another is substituted. In some patients a combination of two or more drugs will produce better results than one alone.

Intelligent administration of drugs depends on having the patients chart daily their medication and the number, time, and circumstances of their seizures. Ideally such a base line should be established before medication is begun, since each patient tends to have his own pattern of seizures, but often this is impractical. Changes in medication should be made only when a given program is shown to be inadequate. Frequent measurements of blood levels of diphenylhydantoin, barbiturate and other drugs are useful. For Dilantin, the therapeutic level is 10 to 15 μg per ml, and one-half of patients have side effects at 30 or more μg per ml. These consist of ataxia, slurred speech, staggering, nystagmus, diplopia, mental dullness, forgetfulness, and confusion. Coma occurs when the level exceeds 50 μg. Clinical and electroencephalographic improvement are not obtained if the level is below 10 μg per ml. The therapeutic level for phenobarbital is probably about 10 to 15 μg per ml, though the range varies with the type of barbiturate used. Side effects appear in patients on long-term treatment with phenobarbital above 30 μg per ml.

When changing medication, the dosage of the new drug should be gradually increased to an optimum level at the same time as the dosage of the old drug is gradually decreased. The sudden withdrawal of a drug may lead to status epilepticus, even though a new drug is substituted. Once an anticonvulsant or a combination of anticonvulsants is found to be effective, its use should be maintained for a period of years.

The therapeutic dose for any patient must be determined to some extent by trial and error. Not uncommonly a drug is discarded as being ineffective, whereas a slightly increased dosage would have led to a complete disappearance of all the attacks. It is, however, inadvisable to administer a drug to the point where the patient is so dull and stupid that he is more incapacitated by the toxic effects than by the seizures. There is no evidence to prove that the prolonged administration of anticonvulsant medication is a factor in the development of the mental deterioration that occurs in a small percentage of the patients with convulsive seizures. It is not uncommon to note an improvement in the mental faculties of some patients following control of the seizures by the use of anticonvulsant drugs. The recent claim of pulmonary fibrosis and cerebellar degeneration after prolonged Dilantin therapy seems to be unfounded. An antifolate effect on blood serum and a reduction of protein-bound iodine (without lowering of the BMR) have been reported. Occasionally one of the anticonvulsant drugs (Mysoline or Dilantin) causes a mild polyneuropathy (abolition of reflexes in legs and numb feet). When this happens, the drug should be changed.

Indications for use of specific drugs GRAND MAL SEIZURES For those patients with infrequent grand mal seizures (from one to four per year), phenobarbital can be tried first because of its high therapeutic index and its relatively low toxicity. When the seizures are more frequent, Dilantin is the drug of choice. A combination of Dilantin (0.3 to 0.4 g) and phenobarbital (0.1 to 0.2 g) is more often effective than either of the drugs used alone. When these drugs are used in combination, a full therapeutic dose of each drug must be given. Occasionally, Mesantoin or a combination of this drug with the Dilantin or Mysoline will succeed where Dilantin alone has failed. Only rarely will bromides or a combination of bromides and phenobarbital or Dilantin prove to be more effective.

The toxic effects of phenobarbital, which are drowsiness and mental dullness, nystagmus, and staggering, should be used as indications of excess dosage. Only skin eruption is a contraindication to its further use; otherwise these symptoms can be controlled by reducing the dose. Dilantin almost always leads to hirsutism, hypertrophy of gums, and, as was stated above, ataxia, stupor, or coma if given in excess dosages. If skin rashes and other hypersensitivity phenomena (polyarteritis) occur, discontinuation of the medication is necessary. Reduction of dose controls the other symptoms.

PSYCHOMOTOR ATTACKS Drugs effective in the treatment of grand mal seizures are effective in the treatment of patients with psychomotor attacks. Dilantin, 300 to 400 mg per day, and Mysoline, 750 to 1,000 mg per day, have given the best results. The results on the whole are not as good as in grand mal epilepsy.

PETIT MAL ATTACKS As a rule, drugs effective in the treatment of grand mal and psychomotor seizures are relatively ineffective in the treatment of patients with petit mal attacks. Zarontin, 750 to 1,500 mg per day, has been most

TABLE 24-2
Anticonvulsant medications*,†

Generic name	*Trade name*	*Total daily dose per kg body wt and usual adult dose*	*Principal therapeutic purposes*	*Serum half-life, hr*	*Effective blood level, μg %*	*Toxic level, μg*
Phenobarbital	Luminal	1–5 mg; 60–200 mg	Major seizures; partial seizures; psychomotor seizures; and petit mal	96 ± 12	15	40
Diphenylhydantoin	Dilantin	4–7 mg; 200–500 mg	Major seizures; psychomotor seizures; partial epilepsy	24 ± 12	10	20
Primidone	Mysoline	10–25 mg; 750–1,500 mg	Major seizures; psychomotor seizures; partial epilepsy	12 ± 6	5	12
Ethosuximide	Zarontin	20–30 mg; 1,000–1,500 mg	Petit mal	30 ± 6	40	100
Trimethadione	Tridione	10–25 mg; 500–1,250 mg	Petit mal			
Paramethadione	Paradione	10–25 mg; 500–1,250 mg	Petit mal			
Mephenytoin	Mesantoin	7–12 mg; 300–600 mg	Major seizures; psychomotor seizures; focal epilepsy			
Mephobarbital	Mebaral	2.5–10 mg; 200–500 mg	Same as phenobarbital; myoclonic epilepsy			
Methsuximide	Celontin	10–20 mg; 500–1,000 mg	Petit mal			
Phensuximide	Milontin	10–20 mg; 500–1,250 mg	Petit mal			
Acetazolamide	Diamox	5–15 mg; 250–750 mg	Petit mal; infantile spasms; major seizures			
Diazepam	Valium	0.15–2 mg; 15–30 mg	Petit mal; major seizures; status epilepticus			
Nitrazepam	Mogadon	0.15–2 mg; 10–100 mg	Infantile spasms; myoclonic epilepsy			
Ethotoin	Peganone	10–20 mg; 500–1,000 mg	Major seizures; focal seizures			
ACTH		40–60 units per day	Infantile spasms			
Carbamazepine	Tegretol	10–20 mg; 1,000–1,200 mg	Tonic-clonic seizures; complex partial seizures	12 ± 3	4	8
Benzodiazepine	Clonazepam	1–12 mg/day	Atypical petit mal			

* *Children usually need larger doses than adults, if dose is calculated according to body weight. Excessive drowsiness can often be diminished by dextroamphetamine (Dexedrine), methamphetamine (Desoxyn), or methylphenidate (Ritalin).*
† *This table lists only drugs in common use; for a complete list and discussion consult Penry and Schmidt (see references).*

successful and has the advantage over trimethadione (Tridione), paramethadione (Paradione), and phensuximide (Milontin) in producing less side effects. It is wise to begin with a single dose of 250 mg per day and increase it every week until therapeutic effect is achieved. Toxic symptoms to Tridione and Paradione are skin eruptions and photophobia. Aplastic anemia has been reported; hence monthly blood counts during the first year are indicated. Methsuximide (Celontin), (adult dose 0.3 g three or four times a day) and acetazolamide (Diamox) (adult dose 0.25 to 0.75 g per day) have been useful in controlling difficult cases of petit mal and massive myoclonus in children. Atypical varieties of petit mal (2-per-s wave and spike EEG paroxysms) in association with myoclonus and akinetic falling spells or brief focal tonic or clonic seizures may be exceedingly resistant to medication. Methsuximide (Celontin) and acetazolamide (Diamox) or carbamazepine (Tegretol) (adult dose 1.0 to 1.2 gm per day) have had some success. Clonazepam, recently introduced (1.0 to 4.0 mg t.i.d.), is reported to have controlled atypical petit mal better than Zarontin.

MINOR SEIZURES AND FOCAL ATTACKS The same drugs effective in the treatment of grand mal and psychomotor seizures are effective against minor seizures and focal attacks. Minor seizures, which appear in patients whose grand mal attacks have been controlled, can occasionally be checked by simply increasing the dose of the drug or drugs that the patient is already taking. If the minor attacks are very infrequent and nonincapacitating, no great effort need be made to treat them.

PETIT MAL PLUS OTHER TYPES When patients are subject to petit mal seizures as well as grand mal or psychomotor seizures, they should receive Zarontin plus diphenylhydantoin sodium, phenobarbital, or Mesantoin.

MYOCLONIC EPILEPSY Mebaral (0.2 to 0.5 g) and phenobarbital (0.1 to 0.2 g) have been the most effective agents in this type of seizure. In the treatment of massive myoclonus in infants, ACTH or a combination of Mogadon and Diamox have been most effective.

Surgery has been advocated for the removal of cortical scars secondary to cerebral trauma, of vascular lesions, and birth injuries on the assumption that such scars are surrounded by irritable foci which act as a trigger mechanism for the seizures. Reduction in the frequency of seizures has been reported as a sequel to these operations by a number of neurosurgeons. This treatment should be limited to the group of patients with focal attacks which do not respond to medical therapy. In addition, such lesions should be excised only by neurosurgeons who have facilities for the adequate localization of the lesion. Further medical treatment will still be required for most of these patients after operation.

The anterior tip of the temporal lobe and the amygdaloid nuclei have been removed or destroyed by stereotaxis in patients with psychomotor seizures who have failed to respond to medical therapy and in whom it was possible to demonstrate a temporal lobe focus by electroencephalography. Favorable results have been reported with this procedure by some neurosurgeons, but experience is too limited to evaluate its efficacy. The same may be said of implantation of cerebellar stimulators and section of the corpus callosum to prevent spread of seizure.

Since epilepsy is a long-term medical problem, general hygienic measures are important for they tend to stabilize the neurophysiologic state of the cerebrum. They should include regular hours of sleep, balanced diet, daily exercise, avoidance of constipation, and abstinence from alcohol. With proper safeguards even the more dangerous sports such as swimming and football may be permitted. The uncontrolled epileptic obviously should not be allowed to drive a car, operate unguarded machines, climb to heights, and so forth.

Psychotherapy will help prevent or overcome feelings of inferiority and self-consciousness or shame. Both the patient and his family will benefit from such therapy, and proper attitudes may be established. Oversolicitude and overprotection are to be discouraged. It is important for the patient to live as normal a life as possible.

Every effort should be made to keep children in school, and adults should stay at work. Many communities have a branch of the American Committee against Epilepsy or a vocational rehabilitation center, and advantage should be taken of such facilities. Patients should participate in available recreational activities such as movies, dancing, and parties.

Not infrequently the convulsive disorder is but one manifestation of a widespread static cerebral disease that in itself interferes with education and work. Then realistic planning for activities that lie within the patient's scope is desirable.

REFERENCES

ADAMS RD, VICTOR M: *Principles of Neurology,* New York: McGraw-Hill, 1977

HAUSER WA, KURLAND LT: The epidemiology of epilepsy in Rochester, Minnesota. Epilepsia 16:1, 1975

LENNOX W, LENNOX M: *Epilepsy and Related Disorders,* Boston: Little, Brown, 1960

PENRY JK, DALY DD (eds): *Complex Partial Seizures and Their Treatment,* New York: Raven Press, 1975

SCHMIDT RP, WILDER BJ: Epilepsy, in *Contemporary Neurology Series,* vol. 5, eds F Plum, FH McDowell, Philadelphia: Davis, 1968

25 AFFECTIONS OF SPEECH

JAY P. MOHR
RAYMOND D. ADAMS

Language and speech are of fundamental significance to man both in his social intercourse and his private intellectual life. When disordered as a consequence of disease of the brain, the loss exceeds in gravity even blindness, deafness, and paralysis.

GENERAL CONSIDERATIONS

The terms *speech* and *language* refer to some of the most complex and poorly understood integrating activities of the cerebrum. The terms are not synonymous.

Speech involves the execution of acquired skills by which vocal, manual, auditory, and visual systems are utilized to permit the conveyance of communicative efforts. These skills include: pronunciation of words, variations in stress, intonation, and melody; the production of graphic marks in the accepted spatial orientation; the discrimination of spoken speech and its classification as to speaker; the discrimination of handwritten or printed speech, the visual search patterns involved in scanning a text; and the use of other, less specifiable behaviors. Deficiencies in these skills impede interpersonal communication apart from any separate impairment in language usage; when intact, these skills do not suffice for any but elemental communication, such as that between two individuals who speak languages unfamiliar to each other.

Language has a wider connotation and refers to the selection and serial ordering of individual words according to accepted rules that permit a person using the speech modalities to modify the behavior of another and to externalize that poorly understood cerebral activity referred to as *thinking.* A disturbance of language usage, usually accompanied by a disturbance in speech from cerebral dysfunction, is referred to as *aphasia,* or more properly as *dysphasia* (see below).

CEREBRAL DOMINANCE AND ITS RELATIONSHIP TO SPEECH AND HANDEDNESS

The functional supremacy of one cerebral hemisphere is crucial to language function. There are three ways of determining that the left side of the brain is dominant: (1) the loss of speech when disease occurs in certain parts of the left hemisphere and its preservation in diseases involving corresponding parts of the right hemisphere; (2) the greater facility in the use of the right hand, foot, and eye; (3) the arrest of speech immediately after the injection of amobarbital (Amytal Sodium) or some other drug in the left internal carotid artery. Only (2) and (3) are of use in deciding the cerebral dominance of a living, healthy patient. Unfortunately the Amytal Sodium, or Wada test does not reproduce the syndrome of major hemisphere inactivation. There is only mutism, followed by a brief period of groping for names. Presumably it gives information about the localization of motor output areas rather than of sensory ones.

Of the general population approximately 90 to 95 percent are right-handed; the remainder prefer the left hand. A person is said to be right-handed if he chooses the right hand for intricate, complex acts and is more skillful with it. The preference is more complete in some persons than in others. Most individuals are neither right-handed nor completely left-handed but favor one hand for more complicated tasks.

The reason for hand preference is still controversial. There is strong evidence of a hereditary factor, but the mode of inheritance is uncertain. Learning is also a factor; many children are shifted at an early age from left to right (shifted sinistrals) because it is a handicap to be left-handed in a right-handed world. Many right-handed persons sight with the right eye, and it has been said that eye preference determines hand preference.

Anatomic differences between the dominant and the minor cerebral hemispheres have recently attracted attention. The left plenum temporale, part of Wernicke's language zone, in the left hemisphere, is larger, and other evidence of asymmetries elsewhere are being uncovered; it is suggested that they are related to functional hemispheral differences.

Left-handedness may result from disease of the left cerebral hemisphere in early life; this fact probably accounts for its higher incidence among the feebleminded and brain-injured. Presumably the neural mechanisms for language then become centered in the right cerebral hemisphere. Handedness and cerebral dominance may fail to develop in some individuals; this is particularly true in certain families.

In studies of groups of left-handed individuals who suffer cerebral derangements of speech, it has been noted that approximately 75 percent have had lesions in the left cerebral hemisphere. Further, in those extremely rare cases of aphasia due to right cerebral lesions, the patient is nearly always left-handed, and the speech disorder tends to be less severe and enduring. The latter may take the form of an expressive disturbance, with prominent faults in calculation, implicit unawareness of the neurologic deficits (anosognosia), and visuoconstructive troubles.

The functional capacities of the minor hemisphere in speech are not fully understood despite careful anatomic studies. An additional problem in assessment is the uncertainty as to whether any residual function after lesions of the major hemisphere is due to recovery of parts of its language zones or to the activity solely of the minor hemisphere. The following functions are not disturbed in lesions of the left hemisphere: motor responses of mimicry, social anticipation (smiling, handshaking, modesty reactions) and self-care (washing and feeding), avoidance behavior to noxious stimuli, and capability of training in performances of cross-matching visually presented simple words with pictures.

TYPES OF LANGUAGE DISORDERS ENCOUNTERED IN MEDICAL PRACTICE

These may be divided into four categories:

1 Cerebral disturbances in which there is a loss more or less exclusively of the production and/or comprehension of spoken and/or written speech and language. Such a condition is called *aphasia,* or, in milder degrees, *dysphasia.*

2 Defects in articulation with intact mental functions and normal comprehension and memory of words. These are pure motor disorders of the muscles of articulation and may be due to flaccid or spastic paralysis, rigidity, repetitive spasms (stuttering), or ataxia. The terms *anarthria* and *dysarthria* have been applied to some of these conditions.

3 Loss of voice due to a disease of the larynx or its innervation, with resultant *aphonia* or *dysphonia.*

4 Disturbances of speech that occur with diseases affecting the higher nervous integrations, namely delirium and dementia (see Chaps. 26 and 27). Speech is seldom lost in these conditions but is instead merely deranged as part of a general impairment of all elements of language.

APHASIA OR DYSPHASIA In the scientific study of aphasia one faces formidable problems since there are no experimental models; this prevents the easy testing of hypotheses of speech and language function. The only reliable source materials are humans with cerebral disease, and the study of such cases is hampered by a number of uncontrollable variables such as the difficulty in delineating the basic functional deficit and the changes in symptomatology at different periods in the time-course of the disease. The anatomic site of the lesion is often imprecisely characterized which makes for difficulty in clinicoanatomic and clinicopathologic correlation. And, finally, of theoretical importance is the problem of ascribing normal function to a part of the cerebrum by a study of the abnormal diseased brain.

As a general orientation, most of the lesions that lead to aphasia are known to be located in the perisylvian or *opercular* regions (frontal, temporal, and parietal) that cover the insula of the dominant cerebral hemisphere, i.e., the left in right-handed individuals.

The clinical deficit is most easily demonstrated in the acute phase. The changes that occur with time make estimation of lesion site and size more difficult later on, especially with the smaller lesions. Lesions one or more centimeters in diameter are often found at autopsy in cases whose clinical deficit was evanescent and had faded to functional insignificance within weeks or months. Diseases affecting the cerebral surface gray matter produce a more significant deficit than those more confined to the white matter; tumors, for example, confined as they are largely to the white matter, may reach discouragingly large size before speech or language deficit is evident. The site is more significant than the size of the lesion, for the former determines the qualitative features of the deficit, but the size determines the quantitative features and, in the larger lesions, appears to produce additional qualitative features not present in the smaller lesions. In particular, deficits in speech function are more evident in smaller lesions, while deficits in language and speech functions occur in the larger lesions.

The speech disturbances in sylvian lesions vary with the site of the lesion. Those that lie anteriorly produce deficits in the acts of speaking. These disorders include mutism, impaired articulation, disordered transitions from syllable to syllable, and defective stress, intonation, and melody. Those located more posteriorly produce malpositioning of the oral cavity and some anticipatory errors out of sequence that result in gross mispronunciations of the intended syllables and words, more evident when the expected utterance is lengthy. Lesions grouped around the posterior sylvian fissure including the superior temporal lobe and its auditory gyri are always manifested by disordered discrimination of spoken speech, resulting in poor repetition of speech sounds and understanding of spoken language.

Language deficits are less well understood and less well correlated with anatomic pathology. Many formulations of aphasia envision only one "true" language deficit, the detection of which by any method of testing suffices to label the patient as aphasic. But those formulations based more on pathoanatomic correlations are leaning more toward separation of two large categories of disorder. That disorder reflecting large lesions involving the bulk of the frontal operculum and insula shows *agrammatism,* which features sharply contracted sentence structures, lacking most small grammatical words, often with faulty use of grammar in the words remaining, the surviving words serving mainly predicative or substantive function. Large posterior sylvian lesions show almost the opposite, with substantive elements missing or substituted by approximations (paraphasias) which are related in the means of vocal production (literal paraphasias) or in meaning (verbal paraphasias). Disturbances in understanding language through auditory and visual speech forms affect both types of major lesions, more particularly the cases with posterior lesions.

Lesions in other parts of the cerebrum either cause no disturbance of human communicative skills or alter them only secondarily. An example of the latter is the lesion of the frontal lobes, especially the medial and orbital parts which impair all motor activities, inducing an abulia verging on akinetic mutism. If partial, speech is laconic with long pauses between utterances and an inability to sustain monologue and narrative. Extensive occipital lesions impair reading and reduce the utilization of all visual, lexical stimuli. Thalamic and deep cerebral lesions impair alertness and cause fluctuant states of inattention and disorientation, thereby inducing fragmentation of words (neologisms) and phrases, and protracted uncontrollable talking (logorrhea). Strong stimulation which momentarily stabilizes behavior and speech proves the essential integrity of language mechanisms.

In the initial formulations of cerebral function in the last century, it was easily concluded that lesions of the frontal (motor) regions produced syndromes independent from those of the posterior (sensory) regions and that the dysphasias could be classified as motor (Broca's) or sensory (Wernicke's), and could be further specified as subcortical, cortical, or transcortical in type. Subcortical lesions were envisioned to cut off the main efferent or afferent projections of the cortical "center." Cortical lesions involved the "centers" themselves. Transcortical lesions isolated the "centers" from one another ("conduction" aphasia) or from other regions of the brain. In modern times, the difficulties in attempting to understand the disorders of language usually accompanying the disorders of speech in focal brain disease, the improvements in techniques to document the extent of the lesion, and data available in longitudinal studies have led to a more complex, less pristine evolution of these views.

TYPES OF APHASIA The examination of patients with disturbances of speech and language discloses a number of different abnormalities. Attempts have been made to classify them in terms of their predominant form, their presumed physiologic or psychologic bases, or the anatomy of the underlying diseases. No one of the many schemes has been accepted, and all the great students of language have railed against the premature acceptance of incomplete simplistic theories of language.

The most readily recognized type of aphasia is a complete or global form in which all modes of expression (spoken word, written word, and gesture) as well as the capacity for reading and understanding of spoken words are abolished. If more or less permanent, large perisylvian lesions of the left cerebral hemisphere are demonstrable. A second major type involves the motor, verbal, and executive side of the language and is named *Broca's aphasia.* The lesion is large, involving the bulk of the anterosuperior sylvian operculum and insula, in the territory of supply of the upper division of the left middle cerebral artery. A third major type involves the receptive, sensory, and central aspects of language and is named Wernicke's aphasia, after the German neurologist who differentiated it from Broca's aphasia. The syndrome is ascribed to a large lesion involving the left posterior temporal and parietal regions, in the territory of supply of the lower, posterior division of the left middle cerebral artery. There are in addition a number of so-called *dissociative aphasias* such as "conduction" aphasia, "pure" word deafness, "pure" word blindness, "amnestic" aphasia, and "pure" agraphia, each attributed to smaller lesions within the speech areas or in their afferent and efferent connections. Scrutiny of these syndromes has shown that their anatomy is poorly established, and ideas about them are more in tune with theory of language than observed fact.

The practical student might question the purpose of these classifications. There are several. Many of these syndromes have fairly specific anatomic localizing value and are of clinical assistance to the physician in cases having surgical implications. In addition, the different prognoses attached to several syndromes are helpful in management and in the use of different corrective measures in therapy. And, finally, such data might become the basis of a unified theory of language.

Complete (total) aphasia This syndrome is due to a lesion that destroys a large part of the speech areas of the major cerebral hemisphere. As such, it represents the maximal aphasic deficit possible and shows the least improvement of all aphasic syndromes. Since the middle cerebral artery nourishes all the speech areas, nearly all aphasic syndromes due to vascular occlusion are caused by involvement of this artery or its branches. In complete aphasia, occlusion of the left internal carotid or the middle cerebral artery at its origin is usually responsible. Less often, the syndrome may be caused by a large hemorrhage, tumor, other lesions, or even temporarily as a postictal effect of grand mal epilepsy.

Most patients with total aphasia can say at most a few words; they cannot read or write, and they understand only a few words and phrases of the speech of others. Related signs include right hemiplegia, hemianesthesia, and homonymous hemianopia. The state of consciousness may vary from full alertness to semicoma; in the latter condition the lack of verbal response is obviously difficult to interpret, for the very diagnosis of aphasia presupposes a reasonably alert mind and the relative integrity of other cerebral functions. The alert patient may participate in common gestures of greeting, may show modesty and avoidance reactions, and is able to engage in self-help activities. With the passage of time some degree of understanding of spoken speech may be evident, and a few words of speech may emerge. Early appearance of clearly vocalized stereotyped words, such as "hi," are often falsely encouraging signs and may reflect the uninhibited function of the right hemisphere. Rapid improvement frequently occurs when the main cause is edema, postconvulsive paralysis, or transient metabolic derangements such as infection, or hyponatremia, which worsen old aphasic lesions. Although speech loss from a disintegrating embolus of the left middle artery may be transient, some part of the deficit may persist, being easily demonstrated by presenting the patient with complex words or double negatives in sentences.

Broca's aphasia (frontosuperior sylvian syndromes) This term is used to designate a complex syndrome, predominantly a failure of motor aspects of speaking and writing, with an accompanying *agrammatism* and a variable impairment in language comprehension. Although commonly thought due to a circumscribed lesion in the inferior frontal convolution (Broca's area), this major syndrome is usually the result of a large lesion, involving cortical and subcortical structures along the frontal and superior sylvian fissure including the insula, in the territory of supply of the upper division of the left middle cerebral artery.

The large extent of the lesion, and involvement of the sensorimotor rolandic region, account for the more or less dense right hemiparetic and hemisensory syndrome that almost invariably accompanies the aphasia and usually persists. Initially, a transient right hemianopia and contralateral ocular deviation are observed.

In the acute phase of the syndrome, the entire language mechanism appears inactivated, and the helplessly mute, noncommunicative, and uncomprehending patient presents the syndrome *total aphasia,* indistinguishable by present methods from the form of total aphasia coming from complete middle cerebral artery territory infarction. Within weeks to years, the disorder of comprehension abates somewhat, but remains forever easily detected by formal testing. This improvement in comprehension exceeds that in speaking and writing, where deficits are sufficient to stamp the syndrome traditionally as *motor aphasia.*

In the chronic state of the syndrome, the patient will have severe difficulties in speaking aloud. No longer can he utter a word on command, in conversation, in reading aloud, or in trying to repeat what he hears. Occasionally expletives, or "yes" and "no," can be spoken, usually in the correct context; the few words spoken are uttered in a dysmelodic, jerky fashion (dysprosody). One might suspect the lingual and phonatory apparatus of being paralyzed, but often the patient uses it to lick his lips, chew, swallow, audibly clear his throat, and even to vocalize without the emission of words. The lower part of the face on the right side is weak and sags, and the tongue also deviates to the weak side, usually accompanied by weakness of the right arm and leg. For a time, despite satisfactory comprehension of spoken words and ability to read simple commands, an apraxia of the linguooropharyngeal apparatus is observed in his faulty efforts when asked to smack and make other purposeful movements. In these circumstances imitation of the examiner's actions are better performed than execution of acts on command. Self-initiated actions, by contrast, are often normal. The patient, if he speaks at all, may repeat his few remaining words over and over, as if compelled to do so. Certain stereotyped phrases such as "hi," "good morning," "how are you" seem to be more easily emitted, as are the words of popular songs when sung. When angered or excited, the patient may curse. Thus, it is evident that although "speechless" he is not "wordless." The patient's efforts and facial expressions suggest an awareness of his own ineptitudes and mistakes. Repeated failures cause exasperation and despair.

As the patient improves and in the milder forms of motor aphasia, the patient is able to speak aloud to some degree. Words are enunciated slowly and laboriously. Articulation and the melody of speech (prosody) are impaired. This dysfluency takes the form of improper accent or stress on certain syllables and incorrect phrasing of words in a series and pacing of the speed of word sequences. Speech is sparse and consists mainly of nouns, transitive verbs, and important adjectives; many of the small words (articles, prepositions, conjunctions) are omitted, giving the speech an agrammatic and telegraphic character. The substantive content allows the patient to communicate to some extent despite the gross mechanical and language difficulties. Once fully established, these speech impediments persist and improve only slightly despite years of speech therapy.

Most patients with Broca's aphasia have a correspondingly severe impairment in writing. Should their right hand be paralyzed, they cannot print with their left one; if manual mobility is spared, they fail as completely in writing out their commands or replies to questions as in speaking them. Writing from dictation is impossible, though letters and words can still be copied. On careful testing, communication by writing can be shown superior to that of speaking, suggesting a certain independence between these two acts as vehicles of language.

The lesion of Broca's aphasia is most often an infarction of frontal, anterior parietal, and anterior insular parts of the cerebrum due to embolic occlusion of the upper division of the left middle cerebral artery (MCA). Major putaminal hypertensive hemorrhage is also a common cause. A huge frontal lobe tumor or abscess is occasionally responsible; metastatic lesions, subdural hematoma, and encephalitis are rare causes of the syndrome.

Minor motor aphasia Sharp focal lesions along the anterior and superior sylvian operculum and insula produce remarkably circumscribed effects on the mechanical elaboration of speech which can be observed alone or in combinations, depending on the site and extent of the lesion. However, *none of these focal lesions produces significant or lasting deficits in language usage;* the experienced listener can easily detect the error patterns in speech and, through them, discern the communicative efforts of the sufferer, who is acutely aware of and discouraged by the deficit. The effects on speech of focal opercular lesions take several forms. *Broca's area infarction* involves the lower premotor cortex adjacent to the motor cortex for the oropharynx, larynx, and respiratory apparatus; the infarct interrupts skilled movements of these muscle groups, and the resultant dyspraxia in speech takes the form of impaired transitions between syllables and words, and disruption of the melodic intonation of phrases (dysprosody). Involvement of this region appears insufficient to produce the major syndrome referred to as Broca's aphasia. *Rolandic infarction* involves the sensorimotor cortex itself; poor articulation, lowered volume and pitch of speech, and a nasal quality to the voice reveal the pareses of the involved musculature. *Postcentral, anterior parietal infarction* appears to be associated with errors in the positioning of the oral cavity for individual sounds, syllables, and whole words; the acoustic features of the utterance are often distorted by these malpositions of the oral cavity and strike the listener's ear as literal paraphasias. Since they are easily produced in tests of repeating and reading aloud and occur in conversation, the patient could be labeled as having "conduction" aphasia. The important point with all these minor motor aphasias is that at first they may resemble major motor aphasia except for the excellent understanding of spoken and written words, and the prognosis for nearly full recovery is excellent.

Most lesions sufficiently focal as to produce such circumscribed deficits are embolic in nature. The unusual sequential branching of the upper division of the middle cerebral artery provides a series of separate sites for emboli to lodge. Deeper, larger lesions, or larger emboli involving the stem of the upper division, encompass several deficit types in a single patient, making these individual distinctions less clear, and blend with the major syndromes of Broca's aphasia. Facial, lingual, and sometimes brachial paresis and ideomotor dyspraxia of the face and *left,* nondominant limbs commonly accompany the speech disorder. Most of these syndromes fade in clinical significance within months or years.

Wernicke's aphasia (posterior perisylvian syndrome) This syndrome is said to have two components: (1) an impairment in the hearing of word elements (phonemic hearing), which reflects involvement of auditory association areas or their separation from the angular gyrus, and the proximity of the lesion to the primary auditory cortex of Heschl's transverse gyri; (2) a general impairment of language-dependent behavior, which reveals the major role the auditory region plays in the regulation of language.

The defect in auditory functions is manifested by impaired ability to repeat spoken words. The only words that can be repeated are short ones and those of which the component syllables are widely separated in phonemic composition. A few simple commands may still be executed, but there is failure to carry out complex ones.

The patient gestures freely, talks volubly, and appears strangely unaware of his deficit. The words that he utters are often inappropriate, in the nature of paraphasia, which means substitution of words similar in sound (literal paraphasia) or similar in meaning to the correct one (verbal paraphasia). Speech elements may appear that are not part of the language (neologisms or jargon speech). Hesitancy and lack of fluency, which are constant features of motor speech disorders, may also occur in Wernicke's aphasia. Characteristically, however, they tend to occur chiefly in that part of a spoken phrase that contains the central communicative (predicative) item, such as a key noun, verb, or descriptive phrase. The impression is often conveyed that the patient is constantly "searching" for the correct word and that he has difficulty in finding it. When severely disorganized, the speech may be reduced to an incomprehensible gibberish or jargon.

The general impairment of language-dependent behavior may be more or less dissociated from the deficit in the hearing of words. Although all the sensory and motor apparatus required in the activation and expression of language behavior appears to be intact, the patient is unable to function as a social organism because he is deprived of all means of communication. As already stated, he cannot understand what is said to him, read aloud or silently with comprehension, tell others what he wants or thinks, or write to them. When trying to refer to an object that he sees or feels, he cannot find the name, even though he may be able to repeat it from dictation; nor can he write from dictation the very words that he can copy from sight or touch. His copying performance is notably slow and laborious and conforms to the exact contours of the model (including the examiner's handwriting style) in a servile fashion. When tested in detail he cannot match words that he hears with those that he sees. Yet he can repeat aloud single words that he hears and can match a single word shown to him with that same word when it is mixed with other words. Performance is also impaired on those tasks which require the recognition, on the basis of past experience, of a relationship between two stimuli which are physically dissimilar but verbally equivalent (e.g., the sound of the word "cat"). But the patient can still produce a response that is physically identical to that given (e.g., copying from sight the word "cat").

In time there is nearly always improvement, often to the point that the deficits can be detected only by asking the patient to repeat unfamiliar words from dictation, to name unusual objects, to spell difficult words, or to write complex self-generated sentences.

As a rule, the lesion lies in the posterior sylvian region (temporal and parietal) and is due to an embolic occlusion of the lower division of the left middle cerebral artery. A "slit hemorrhage" in the subcortex of the temporoparietal region or involvement of the temporal isthmus and adjacent white matter by tumor, abscess, or extension of a small putaminal or thalamic hemorrhage may have similar effects. The posterior sylvian region, comprising posterosuperior temporal, opercular supramarginal, and posterior insular gyri, appears to encompass a variety of language functions, since seemingly minor changes in size and locale of the lesion are associated with important variations in the elements of Wernicke's aphasia or lead to *conduction aphasia* or to *pure word deafness.*

Minor posterior sylvian syndromes In time the patient with Wernicke's aphasia always improves, and as he does so a number of lesser syndromes appear. These latter, however, may be present in comparatively pure form from the beginning, when only small restricted lesions involve some part of the aforementioned posterior sylvian territory. Depending on the exact locale of lesion, language behavior dependent on auditory function (hearing spoken words, echoing sounds and speech, relating the spoken to the written word, and finally repeating and writing it) may be deranged partially or in its entirety. The same is true of language behavior dependent upon visual function, when the left posterior parietal lobe is involved.

These partial syndromes include a central type of conduction disorder, pure word deafness, and pure word blindness. Since their effects approximate those predicted by the isolation of certain speech centers from their afferent and/or efferent connections or from one another, we have described them below as dissociation syndromes.

Attempts to correlate complete and partial posterior sylvian syndromes with arteriographic findings during life frequently fail. Since most partial vascular aphasias are due to cerebral embolism, the latter may have lodged in the artery long enough to cause infarction and then disintegrate. The arteriogram done after this happens is normal. Or a fragment of the disintegrating embolus may drift distally but permanently, blocking only a more distal branch, sometimes permitting part of the ischemic tissue to recover. Clinically undiscovered variations in collateral blood flow from adjacent branches of the posterior cerebral artery may alter the extent of the infarct. Thus cases with similar arteriographic appearance or brain scan abnormality may be accompanied by rather different clinical pictures.

Dissociative speech syndromes These disorders are characterized by an interruption of afferent nervous impulses to the language mechanism or efferent ones from these centers to other motor structures. This concept is an interesting one and has had the heuristic value of indicating certain lines of anatomicophysiologic separation of language functions. However, the anatomy of several of the following conditions is far from proved, and the theories that derive from such data as are available lead one to a naïve conception of the language mechanisms in terms of a kind of telephonic circuitry. With these reservations we present the following syndromes.

CENTRAL-TYPE CONDUCTION DISORDER: SEPARATION OF WERNICKE'S AND BROCA'S LANGUAGE AREAS Here the principal abnormality resembles Wernicke's aphasia in certain respects. There is the same paraphasia in self-initiated speech, in repeating what is heard, and in reading aloud. In contrast, no difficulty is shown in comprehending words that are heard or seen. Nor is any element of dysarthria or dysprosody detected. The patient is alert and aware of his deficit. One of the best ways of eliciting the defect is to have the patient repeat nonsense syllables. His mistakes are then manifestly of a type observed in literal paraphasia, i.e., close similarity but detectably different sounds occasioned by improper positioning of the oropharyngeal apparatus. The disorder in repeating from dictation becomes more apparent when the rate of presentation of auditory material is increased and as the uttered words become more polysyllabic. Since nouns are the longest words in the sentence, one may gain an impression that they are specifically affected.

The lesion in autopsied cases is located in the cortex and subcortical white matter in the upper bank of the sylvian fissure, involving the supramarginal gyrus of the inferior parietal lobule and occasionally the posterior part of the superior temporal region. Presumably fiber systems in the insula are interrupted. The usual cause is an embolus in the ascending parietal or posterior temporal branch of the middle cerebral artery. Deeper, larger lesions in position to interrupt the arcuate fasciculus connecting the temporal and frontal lobes usually involve other pathways as well, giving rise to a more extensive speech deficit (central Wernicke's aphasia, or amnestic aphasia). However, these latter types of aphasia, as they regress, may resolve into conduction aphasia. More anterior insular lesions usually include some degree of Broca's aphasia.

"PURE" WORD DEAFNESS This syndrome is characterized by impaired auditory comprehension and inability to repeat what is said or to write to dictation, being similar in this respect to Wernicke's aphasia. Language, by contrast, is intact, as manifested by correctly phrased self-initiated utterances, correct writing, and reading. The patient may declare that he cannot hear, but shouting does not help him, sometimes to his surprise. By audiometric testing no hearing defect is found, or minor abnormalities appear which may well reveal the underlying deficit in individual cases. Ordinary sounds can be distinguished. The patient is forced to depend heavily on visual cues in understanding the remarks of others, and frequently he uses these cues well enough to obviate much of his difficulty. But tests which prevent the use of visual cues readily uncover his deficit. If able to describe his auditory experience, the patient says that words sound like a jumble of noises. Often the syndrome is not pure and elements of paraphasia enter, or other findings indicating a state of mild Wernicke's aphasia exist.

In most recorded autopsy studies the lesion has been bilateral in the superior temporal gyrus, in position to damage the primary auditory cortex in the transverse gyrus of Heschl and its relations to the association areas of the superior, posterior part of the temporal lobe. The few unilateral lesions are localized in this part of the major (dominant) temporal lobe. Requirements of small size and superficiality of the lesion in the cortex and subcortical white matter are best fulfilled by a small embolic occlusion of a branch of the lower division of the middle cerebral artery.

"PURE" WORD BLINDNESS In this state a literate person loses the ability to read and often to name colors. He can no longer name or point on dictated command to visual letter stimuli or the words of which they are composed. However, understanding spoken language, repetition of what is heard, writing to dictation, and conversation are all intact. Often the patient is unaware of the difficulty and registers no complaint; it is discovered almost by accident. In lesser degrees of the affection, reading aloud is possible, but the patient manages only a single letter at a time (this may be seen in otherwise normal patients who have bilateral hemianopia with only central vision remaining); commonly letter or name responses that seem to have little connection with the presented ones are expressed. The response may be corrected and the defect obscured if other visual cues are available, such as the bottle on which the words Coca-Cola appear. The naming of common colors presented singly and of objects is also impaired. When the dominant hemisphere is involved, as it usually is in such cases, there may be a right homonymous hemianopia, an amnestic defect (see Chap. 26), and a hemisensory defect on the right due to involvement of the left occipital lobe, the left fornix and its decussation, and the left thalamus, respectively, a combination which nearly always signifies thrombosis or embolism of the left posterior cerebral artery.

The autopsy of such lesions has usually demonstrated a lesion that destroys the left visual striate cortex (area 17) and visual association areas (18 and 19), as well as the connections of the right visual cortex and association areas with the left angular gyrus. This latter "disconnection" usually is due to interruption of the fibers passing through the posterior part (splenium) of the corpus callosum, which connect the visual association areas of the two hemispheres. A lesion deep in the left parieto-occipital region may also prevent visual information from both occipital lobes reaching the left angular gyrus. In this case the right homonymous hemianopia may be absent. With purely left cerebral lesions, aside from vascular lesions there may be a primary or secondary tumor, or, rarely, multifocal leukoencephalopathy may be the underlying disease.

ISOLATION OF SPEECH AREAS Following prolonged hypotension or carbon monoxide poisoning, widespread cerebral ischemia affects the vascular anatomic border zones linking the major cerebral arteries and their distal branches on the cerebral surfaces, and spreads centripetally into their adjacent territories. The central fields of supply of these arteries are spared. In the middle cerebral artery territory, this sparing leaves largely intact the sylvian region and its speech areas. With much of the rest of the brain out of action in patients who have survived such hypoxic-hypotensive accidents, the speech mechanism is preserved and can be activated by spoken words. There is parrot-like repetition of words and sounds (echolalia) and similar findings which indicate that the auditory-vocal loop remains functional. Scant evidence of comprehension or self-initiated conversation has been observed, findings that are thought to reflect the widespread injury outside the speech regions. The syndrome is of great theoretic interest, and may prove common in cases surviving cardiac arrest.

"PURE" WORD MUTENESS (SUBCORTICAL MOTOR APHASIA) The patient will have lost all capacity to write, to understand spoken words, and to read silently with comprehension. Although usually paretic, the lips, tongue, pharynx, and larynx show none of the apraxic disturbance of Broca's aphasia. With recovery or in milder degrees of the disorder, vocal utterances are dysarthric because of paresis and are extremely slow, with inadequate volume and intonation.

The causative lesion, usually vascular, is located in the premotor cortex, separating it from the motor cortex for face, tongue, and laryngeal movements; or it is located beneath both Broca's convolution and the motor cortex, or in the internal capsule, separating the cerebrum from subcortical motor centers.

AMNESTIC-DYSNOMIC APHASIA This may be a relatively early or an isolated manifestation of disease of the nervous system. The patient loses only the ability to name objects. There are typical pauses in speech, groping for words, and substitution of another word or phrase that conveys the meaning (circumlocution). When shown a series of common objects, the patient may tell of their use instead of giving their names. The difficulty applies not only to objects seen but to the names of things heard or felt. By contrast, other verbal tasks, including recall of the names for letters, digits, and other printed verbal material is almost invariably preserved. That the deficit is principally one of naming is shown by the patient's correct use of the object and, usually, by an ability to point to the correct object on hearing or seeing the name. There is a tendency among patients to attribute their failure to forgetfulness, or to give some other lame excuse for the disability, suggesting that they are not completely aware of the nature of their difficulty.

The causative lesion is usually deep in the temporal lobe, in position, probably, to interrupt connections of sensory speech areas with the hippocampal-parahippocampal regions concerned with learning and memory. Mass lesions, such as a tumor or an otogenic abscess, are the most frequent, and as they enlarge, an upper contralateral quadrantic visual field defect, or Wernicke's aphasia, is added. Occasionally, dysnomia appears with diseases which occlude the temporal branches of the posterior cerebral artery. Alzheimer's disease and senile dementia may begin with a dysnomic or amnestic type of aphasia. By the time the patient's difficulty is fully recognized, other disorders of speech and indifference, apathy, and abulia are conjoined. This deficit may also be discovered in testing patients with a confusional state caused by metabolic, infectious, intoxicative, or other acute medical illnesses, but then it has no certain localizing value.

DISORDERS OF ARTICULATION AND PHONATION In simple dysarthria there is no abnormality of the cortical centers. The dysarthric patient is able to understand perfectly what he hears, and if literate, he reads and has no difficulty in writing, even though he is unable to utter a single intelligible word. This is the strict meaning of being inarticulate.

The act of speaking is a highly coordinated sequence of contractions of the larynx, pharynx, palate, tongue, lips, and respiratory musculature. These are innervated by the hypoglossal, vagal, facial, and phrenic nerves. The nuclei of these nerves are controlled through the corticobulbar tracts by both motor cortices. As with all movements, there are also extrapyramidal influences from the cerebellum and basal ganglia. A current of air is produced by expiration, and the force of it is finely regulated by the activity of the various muscles engaged in speech. *Phonation,* or the production of vocal sounds, is a function of the larynx. Changes in the size and shape of the glottis and in the length and tension of the vocal cords are controlled by the action of the laryngeal muscles. Vibrations are set up and transmitted to the column of air passing over the vocal cords. Sounds thus formed are modified as they pass through the nasopharynx and mouth, which act as resonators. Articulation consists of contractions of the tongue, lips, pharynx, and palate, which interrupt or alter the vocal sounds. Vowels are of laryngeal origin, as are some consonants; but the latter are formed for the most part during articulation. For instance, the consonants *m, b,* and *p* are labial, *l* and *t* are lingual, and *nk* and *ng* are nasoguttural.

Defective articulation and phonation are recognized at once by listening to the patient during ordinary conversation or while he is reading aloud from a newspaper or a book. Test phrases or attempts at rapid repetition of lingual, labial, and guttural consonants (e.g., la-la-la-la or me-me-me-me) bring out the particular abnormality. Disorders of phonation call for a precise analysis of the voice and its apparatus. The movements of the vocal cords should be inspected with the aid of a hand mirror, or, even better, a laryngoscope, and those of the tongue, palate, and pharynx by direct observation.

Defects in articulation may be subdivided into several types: paretic dysarthria, spastic and rigid dysarthria, choreic, myoclonic, and ataxic dysarthria.

Paretic dysarthria This is due to a neural or bulbar (medullary) weakness or paralysis of the articulatory muscles (lower motor neuron paralysis). In the latter condition the shriveled tongue lies inert on the floor of the mouth, and the lips are relaxed and tremulous. Saliva constantly collects in the mouth because of dysphagia, and spills over the lips causing drooling. Speech becomes less and less distinct. There is a special difficulty in the correct utterance of vibratives, such as *r;* as the paralysis becomes more complete, lingual and labial consonants are finally not pronounced at all. Degrees of this abnormality are observed in myasthenia gravis. Bilateral paralysis of the palate may occur with diphtheria, poliomyelitis, and progressive bulbar palsy. Bilateral paralysis of the lips, as in the facial diplegia of idiopathic polyneuritis, interferes with enunciation of labial consonants; *p* and *b* are slurred and sound more like *f* and *v.*

Spastic and rigid dysarthria These are more frequent than the paralytic variety. Diseases that involve the corticobulbar tracts, usually vascular disease or motor system disease, result in the syndrome of pseudobulbar palsy. The patient may have had a minor stroke some time in the past affecting the corticobulbar fibers on one side; but since the bulbar muscles are probably represented in both motor cortices, there is no impairment in speech or swallowing from a unilateral lesion. Should another stroke then occur, involving the other corticobulbar tract and possibly the corticospinal tract at the pontine, midbrain, or capsular level, the patient immediately becomes anarthric or dysarthric and dysphagic. Often the muscles of facial expression on both sides are weakened as well. Unlike bulbar paralysis due to lower motor neuron involvement, this condition entails no atrophy or fasciculation of the paralyzed muscles; the jaw jerk and other facial reflexes soon become exaggerated; the palatal reflexes are retained; emotional control is poor (pathologic laughter and crying); and sometimes breathing becomes periodic (Cheyne-Stokes). When the frontal operculum alone is involved, the speech deficit may be a pure dysarthria but usually without the impairment in emotional control. In the beginning, the patient may be totally anarthric and aphonic, but as he improves, or in mild degrees of the same condition, speech is notably slow, thick, and indistinct, much like that of partial bulbar paralysis.

In paralysis agitans, or postencephalitic Parkinson's syndrome, one observes an extrapyramidal disturbance of articulation. The patient speaks hastily and articulates poorly, slurring over many syllables and trailing off the end of sentences. The words are pronounced hastily. The voice is low-pitched, monotonous, and lacks inflection; voice volume diminishes. In advanced cases speech is almost unintelligible; only whispering is possible. It may happen that the patient finds it impossible to talk while walking but can speak if he sits or lies down.

Pyramidal and extrapyramidal disturbances of speech

may be combined in generalized cerebral diseases such as general paresis, in which slurred speech is one of the cardinal signs.

In many cases of capsular hemiplegia or partially recovered Broca's aphasia the patient is left with a dysarthria that may be difficult to distinguish from a pure articulatory defect. Careful testing of other language functions, especially writing, will reveal the aphasic quality.

Choreic and myoclonic dysarthria In chorea and myoclonus, speech may also be affected in a highly characteristic way. Unlike the defect of pseudobulbar palsy or paralysis agitans, chorea and myoclonus abruptly interrupt the pronunciation of words by the abnormal movements. The idea is best conveyed by the phrase "hiccup speech," in that the breaks are as unexpected as in singultus. Grimacing and other characteristic motor signs must be depended upon for diagnosis.

Ataxic dysarthria This is characteristic of acute and chronic cerebellar lesions. It may be observed in multiple sclerosis, Friedreich's ataxia, cerebellar atrophy, and heat stroke. The principal speech abnormality is slowness; imprecise enunciation, monotony, and unnatural separation of the syllables of words (scanning) are other features. Coordination of speech and respiration are poor. There may not be enough breath to utter certain words, and others may be ejaculated explosively. *Scanning dysarthria* is distinctive, but in some cases, especially if there is a possibility of spastic weakness of the tongue from corticobulbar tract involvement, it is impossible to predict the anatomy of disease from analysis of speech alone. Myoclonic jerks involving the speech musculature may be superimposed on cerebellar ataxia in a number of diseases.

APHONIA AND DYSPHONIA Finally, a few points should be made concerning the group of speech disorders involving disturbances of voice.

Paresis of the respiratory movements, as in poliomyelitis and acute infectious polyneuritis, may affect voice because insufficient air is provided for phonation and speech. Also, disturbances in the rhythm of respiration may interfere with the fluency of speech. This is particularly noticeable in so-called "extrapyramidal diseases," where one may observe that the patient does not allow sufficient air during expiration to complete a phrase. In the latter conditions reduced volume of speech due to limited excursion of the breathing muscles is another common feature; the patient is unable to speak above a whisper or to shout. Whispering speech is also a feature of stupor, but strong stimulation may make the voice audible.

Paresis of both vocal cords causes complete aphonia. There is no voice, and the patient can speak only in whispers. Since the vocal cords normally separate during inspiration, their failure to do so when paralyzed may result in an inspiratory stridor. If one vocal cord is paralyzed, the voice becomes hoarse, low-pitched, and rasping. Involvement of one of the tenth cranial nerves by tumor, for example, may also cause a certain nasality of voice because the posterior nares do not close during phonation. Certain consonants such as *b, p, n,* and *k* are followed by escape of air into the nasal passages. The abnormality is sometimes less pronounced in recumbency and increases when the head is thrown forward. Hoarseness may also be due to structural changes in the vocal cords caused by cigarette smoking, chronic inflammation, polyps, etc.

Another curious condition about which little is known is *spastic dysphonia.* The authors have seen many patients, middle-aged or elderly men and women, otherwise healthy, who gradually lose the ability to speak quietly and fluently. Any effort to speak results in contraction of all the speech musculature so the patient's voice is strained and phonation is labored. This is apparently a neurologic disorder similar to writer's cramp. The patients are not neurotic, and psychotherapy and speech therapy have been ineffective. This condition differs from the stridor caused by spasm of the laryngeal muscles in tetany. It is nonprogressive but in some instances is combined with other of the restricted extrapyramidal disorders such as blepharospasm and spasmodic torticollis.

CLINICAL APPROACH TO LANGUAGE DISORDERS Aphasia In investigating a case of aphasia, it is first necessary to inquire into the patient's native language, his handedness, and his previous education. Many naturally left-handed children are trained to use their right hand for writing; therefore, in determining this point we must ask which hand is used for throwing a ball, threading a needle, or using a spoon and common tools such as a hammer, saw, or bread knife. It is important before the beginning of the examination to determine whether the patient is alert and can be made to participate reliably in testing, as accurate assessment of language depends on these factors. One should quickly ascertain whether the patient has other signs of a gross cerebral lesion such as hemiplegia, facial weakness, homonymous hemianopia, or cortical sensory loss. When hemiplegia, hemianesthesia, and homonymous hemianopia coexist, the aphasic disorder is usually complete or global. Such a constellation of major neurologic signs is seldom associated with the less complete forms of language disorder, the posterior sylvian syndromes, or one of the dissociative syndromes. Dyspraxia of limbs and speech musculature, in response to spoken commands or to visual mimicry, is generally associated with Broca's aphasia and sometimes with Wernicke's aphasia. Bilateral or unilateral homonymous hemianopia without motor weakness tends often to be linked to "pure" word blindness (alexia or dyslexia) or to amnestic-dysnomic aphasia. Bilateral hemiplegias due to extensive frontal lesions are accompanied not infrequently by "pure" word muteness. The special types of aphasia—alexia, "pure" word deafness, etc.—are often associated with evidences of embolism to other parts of the brain or other organs.

Conversational testing permits quick assessment of the motor aspects of speech (praxis and prosody) and apparent language formulation and auditory comprehension.

Disabilities in the purely motor aspects of speech suggest a motor aphasia, and this possibility can be pursued further by tests of repeating from dictation and by special tests of praxis of the oropharyngeal and respiratory apparatus. Disabilities in language formulation in the form of literal paraphasias with impaired comprehension are indicative of Wernicke's aphasia. Impaired comprehension but perfectly normal formulated speech suggest the rare syndrome of pure word deafness. Disorders confined to naming, generally without paraphasias, when other language functions (reading, writing, spelling, etc.) are found adequate, are diagnostic of amnestic dysnomia.

When conversation shows virtually no disabilities, other tests may still be revealing. Reading aloud single letters, words, and text may reveal the dissociative syndrome of pure word blindness, while tests of writing in this syndrome will show little abnormality. Literal and verbal paraphasic errors may appear in milder cases of Wernicke's aphasia as the patient reads aloud from text or from words in the examiner's handwriting. Similar errors appear even more frequently when the patient is asked to explain the text, read aloud, or give his explanation in writing. Should such tests still be unrevealing of deficits, the examiner may find it useful to increase the complexity of the tests. If the patient then succeeds, one may be sure that there is no disorder of adequacy of reception. Adequacy of response channels is next determined by presenting the patient with tasks that permit a response physically identical with the test stimulus. Copying visual stimuli and repeating aloud from auditory stimuli are examples of this kind of testing. Inadequacy of receptive or response channels will then preclude further analysis of the deficit involving that channel in more complex types of tests, except in the unlikely instance that the more complex test is better performed. If reception and response channels are found adequate in these initial tests, they may then be used in tests requiring all types of language function, such as writing from dictation, vocal naming of visual stimuli, matching physically dissimilar stimuli having a name in common (i.e., the word "cow" and a picture of a cow). By utilizing the same test material used in the earlier tests, direct comparison of performances in spoken naming, written naming, and matching can be compared from visual, auditory, and palpated stimuli. A performance profile can be constructed separately for each type of stimulus material tested (i.e., objects, pictures, words, letters, numbers, colors, etc.). The resultant profile can then be used to determine whether the main deficits fall across one or more input or response channels. These data then provide a base line against which later changes may be compared.

Articulatory-phonation disorders Disturbances of articulation point to involvement of a different set of neural structures, such as the motor cortices, the corticobulbar pathways, the seventh, ninth, and tenth nuclei, the brainstem, and extrapyramidal nuclei and tracts. Often it is necessary to use other neurologic findings to decide which of these are implicated in any given case. The important distinction between the pseudobulbar or supranuclear palsies and the bulbar palsies is grasped only with difficulty by the average student. The information obtained by localizing these two major types of dysarthria is extremely helpful in differential diagnosis.

Dysphonia should lead to an investigation of laryngeal disease, either primary or secondary to an abnormality of innervation. Inspection of vocal cords is a necessary step in the clinical study.

TREATMENT The sudden loss of speech would be expected to cause great apprehension, but except for almost pure motor defects, most patients show remarkably little concern. It appears that the very lesion that deprives them of speech also causes a partial loss of insight into their own disability. This reaches almost a ludicrous extreme in some cases of Wernicke's aphasia, in which the patient becomes indignant when others cannot understand his jargon. Nonetheless, as improvement occurs, many patients do become discouraged. Reassurance and a positive program of speech rehabilitation are the best ways of helping the patient at this stage.

The contemporary methods of training and reeducation in overcoming an aphasic defect have never been critically evaluated. Most aphasic difficulties are due to vascular disease of the brain, and nearly always this is accompanied by some degree of spontaneous improvement in the days, weeks, and months that follow the stroke. Sometimes recovery is complete within hours or days; at times not more than a few words are regained after a year or two of assiduous speech training. Nevertheless, it is the opinion of many experts in the field that speech training is worthwhile.

One must decide for each patient whether speech training is needed and when it should be started. As a rule, therapy is not advisable in the first few days of an aphasic illness, because one does not know how lasting it will be. Also, if the patient suffers a severe global aphasia and can neither speak nor understand spoken and written words, the speech therapist is helpless. Under such circumstances, one does well to wait a few weeks until some one of the language functions has begun to return. Then the physician may begin to encourage and help the patient to use the function to a maximal degree. In milder aphasic disorders the patient may be sent to the speech therapist as soon as the illness has stabilized.

The methods of speech training are specialized, and it is advisable to call in a person who has been trained in this field. However, inasmuch as the benefit is largely psychologic, an interested member of the family or a schoolteacher can be of help if a speech therapist is not available.

There is no special treatment for the dysarthric disturbance of speech.

PROGNOSIS The outcome of aphasia depends on the nature of the underlying disease and the magnitude of the lesion within the speech areas. Global aphasias lasting more than a week or two usually have a bad outcome. Seldom is there enough recovery of communicative speech to permit resumption of occupation or profession. Partial aphasias frequently improve, sometimes to a gratifying degree, if of vascular or encephalitic origin. Aphasias due to embolism, whether global or restricted, may disappear in hours to days, like all cerebral embolic deficits, or persist.

REFERENCES

BRAIN R: Aphasia, apraxia, agnosia, chap. 83 in *Neurology,* 2d ed., eds SAK Wilson, N Bruce, vol. 3, Baltimore: William & Wilkins, 1955

GESCHWIND N: Disconnection syndromes in animals and man. Brain 88:237, 585, 1965

MOHR JP: Broca's area and Broca's aphasia, chap. 6, in *Studies in Neurolinguistics,* ed H Whitaker, New York: Academic, 1975

—— and SIDMAN M: Aphasia: Behavioral aspects, chap. 11, pp. 279–298, in *American Handbook of Psychiatry,* vol. 4, ed M Reiser, New York: Basic Books, 1975

NIELSEN JM: *Agnosia, Apraxia, Aphasia: Their Value in Cerebral Localization,* 2d ed., New York: Hafner, 1962

26 DELIRIUM AND OTHER ACUTE CONFUSIONAL STATES

RAYMOND D. ADAMS
MAURICE VICTOR

Every physician sooner or later discovers through clinical experience the need for special competence in assessing the mental faculties of his patients. He must be able to observe with detachment and complete objectivity their character, intelligence, mood, memory, judgment, and other attributes of personality, in much the same fashion as he observes the nutritional state and the color of the mucous membranes. The systematic examination of these affective and cognitive functions permits him to reach certain conclusions regarding mental status, and these are also of value in understanding the patient and his illness. Without the data obtained from the study of the mental status, errors will be made in evaluating the reliability of the patient's history, in diagnosing the neurologic or psychiatric disease from which he suffers, and in conducting any proposed therapeutic program.

DEFINITION OF TERMS

The definition of normal and abnormal states of mind is difficult because the terms used to describe these states have been given so many different meanings in both medical and nonmedical writings. Compounding the difficulty is the fact that the pathophysiology of the confusional states, delirium and dementia, is not fully understood, and the definitions depend on their clinical relationships, with all the lack of precision which this entails. The following nomenclature, though tentative, is useful, and is employed throughout this textbook.

Confusion is a general term denoting an incapacity of the patient to think with customary speed and clarity. This abnormality may depend on any one of several factors. In delirium, for example, inattention and the intrusion of illusory and hallucinatory experiences are mainly responsible. At certain stages in the evolution or devolution of stupor and coma, as indicated in Chap. 22, confusion is aligned with a disorder of consciousness, awareness, and perception. In patients with dementia, confusion is related to a derangement of intellectual function, i.e., an inability to learn, remember, calculate, make appropriate deductions from given premises, reason abstractly, etc.

The term *delirium* is used here to denote a special type of confusional state, acute in onset and transient in nature, and characterized by gross disorientation in the presence of alertness and vigilance, disorders of perception in which illusions and vivid hallucinations are prominent, and overactivity of psychomotor and autonomic nervous system functions. Implicit in the definition are certain nonmedical connotations of the term—intense agitation, frenzied excitement, and creations of the imagination. Most stuporous or demented patients, in contrast to those with delirium, show a *reduced* state of alertness and attentiveness, *decreased* psychomotor activity, and a *relatively slight* tendency to hallucinate. For these reasons, and also because of the particular clinical settings in which they occur, it seems worthwhile to set the delirious states apart from those of depressed consciousness on the one hand and of dementia and amnesia on the other. Such a concept is far from new. To a greater or lesser extent, the terms exogenous reaction type, symptomatic psychosis, toxic psychosis, infective-exhaustive psychosis, and drug, traumatic, or fever delirium all have reference to the syndrome of delirium. All these terms convey the idea of an acute and transient confusional state, occurring in a particular clinical setting and carrying a serious prognosis, by virtue of adding its burden to an already serious medical illness.

The term *amnesia* means loss of the ability to form memories despite an alert state of mind. It presupposes an ability to grasp the problem, to use language normally, and to maintain adequate motivation. The failure is mainly one of retention, recall, and reproduction, and it should be distinguished from states of drowsiness and acute confusion, in which the learned material seems never to have been adequately assimilated.

Dementia means loss of reason or, more particularly, a deterioration of all intellectual or cognitive functions, without clouding or disturbances of perception. Implied in the word is the idea of a gradual enfeeblement of mental powers in a person who formerly possessed a normal mind. *Amentia,* by contrast, indicates a congenital feeblemindedness.

OBSERVABLE BEHAVIOR AND ITS RELATION TO CONFUSION, DELIRIUM, AMNESIA, AND DEMENTIA

The components of mentation and behavior that lend themselves to bedside examination are (1) the processes of sensation and perception; (2) the capacity for memorizing; (3) the ability to think, reason, and form logical conclusions; (4) temperament, mood, and emotion; (5) initiative, impulse, and drive; (6) insight. Of these (1) is sensorial, (2) and (3) may be considered cognitive, (4) affective, and (5) conative or volitional. Insight includes all introspective observations made by the patient concerning his own normal or disordered functioning. Each component of behavior and intellection has its objective side, expressed in the manifest effects of certain stimulus conditions on the patient and his behavioral responses, and its subjective side, expressed in what the patient says he thinks and feels in relation to the stimuli.

DISTURBANCES OF PERCEPTION Perception, i.e., the processes involved in acquiring through the senses a knowledge of the "world about" or of one's own body, involves many things aside from the simple sensory process of being aware of the attributes of a stimulus. It includes the selective focusing and maintaining of attention, elimination of all extraneous stimuli, and recognition of the stimulus by knowing its relationship to personal remembered experience. One must appreciate that the perception of an object undergoes predictable types of derangement in disease. Most often one finds a reduction in the number of perceptions in a given unit of time and failure to synthesize them properly and relate them to the ongoing activities of the mind. Or there may be apparent inattentiveness or fluctuations of attention, distractibility (pertinent and irrelevant stimuli now having equal value), and inability to persist in an assigned task. Qualitative changes also appear, mainly in the form of sensory distortions and misinterpretation and misidentification of objects and persons (illusions); these changes, at least in part, form the basis of hallucinatory experience in which the patient reports and reacts to stimuli not present in his environment. There is an inability to perceive simultaneously all elements of a large complex of stimuli, which is sometimes explained as a "failure of subjective reorganization." These major disturbances in the perceptual sphere, sometimes called "clouding of the sensorium," occur most often in acute confusional states and deliria, but quantitative deficiency may also become evident in the advanced stages of amentia and dementia.

DISTURBANCES OF MEMORY Memory, i.e., the retention of learned experiences, is involved in all mental activities. It may be arbitrarily subdivided into several parts, namely, (1) registration, which includes all that was mentioned under perception; (2) mnemonic integration and retention; (3) recall; and (4) reproduction. In disturbances of perception and attention there may be a complete failure of learning and memory for the reason that the material to be learned was never registered and assimilated. In Korsakoff's amnestic syndrome newly presented material appears to be temporarily registered but cannot be retained for more than a few minutes, and there is nearly always an associated defect in the recall and reproduction of memories formed some days, weeks, or months before the onset of the illness (retrograde amnesia). Dislocation of events in time and the fabrication of stories, *confabulation,* constitutes a third, but not invariable feature of the syndrome. Sound retention with failure of recall is at times a normal state; when it is severe and extends to all events of past life, it is usually due to hysteria or malingering. Proof that the processes of registration and retention are intact under these circumstances comes from hypnosis and suggestion, whereby the lost items are fully recalled and reproduced. In Korsakoff's amnesic state the patient fails on all tests of learning and recent memory, and his behavior accords with his deficiencies of information. Since some aspect of memory is involved to some extent in all mental processes, it becomes the most testable component of mentation and behavior.

DISTURBANCES OF THINKING Thinking, which is central to so many important intellectual activities, remains one of the most elusive of all mental operations. If by thinking we mean selective ordering of symbols for problem solving and capacity to reason and form sound judgments (the usual definition), obviously the working units of most complex experiences of this type are words and numbers. The activity of substituting word and number symbols for the objects for which they stand (symbolization) is a fundamental part of the process. These symbols are formed into ideas or concepts, and the arrangement of new and remembered ideas into certain orders or relationships, according to the rules of logic, constitutes another intricate part of thought. In a general way one may examine thinking for speed and efficiency, ideational content, coherence and logical relationships of ideas, quantity and quality of associations to a given idea, and the propriety of the feeling and behavior engendered by an idea.

Information concerning the thought processes and associative functions is best obtained by analyzing the patient's spontaneous verbal productions and by engaging him in conversation. If he is taciturn or mute, one may then have to depend on his responses to direct questions or upon written material, i.e., letters, etc. One notes the prevailing trends of the patient's thoughts; whether his ideas are reasonable, precise, and coherent or vague, circumstantial, tangential, and irrelevant; and whether his thought processes are shallow and completely fragmented. Disorders of thought are frequent in confusional states and in degenerative and other types of cerebral disease. The organization of thought may be disrupted with fragmentation, repetition, and perseveration. This is spoken of as *incoherence* and marks many acute confusional and delirious states. The patient may be excessively critical, rationalizing, and hairsplitting; this is a type of thinking often manifest in depressive psychoses. Derangements of thinking may also take the form of a flight of ideas. The patient moves nimbly from one idea to another, and his associations are numerous and loosely linked. This is a common feature in hypomanic or manic states. The opposite condition, poverty of ideas, is characteristic both of depression, where it is combined with gloomy thoughts, and of dementing diseases, where it is part of a general reduction in all intellectual activity. Thinking may be distorted in such a way that the patient fails to check his ideas against reality. When a false belief is maintained in spite of normally convincing contradictory evidence, the patient is said to have a *delusion.* Delusion is common to many illnesses, particularly manic-depressive and schizophrenic states. Ideas may seem to the patient to have been implanted in his mind by some outside agency such as radio, television, or atomic energy. These reflect the passivity feelings characteristic of schizophrenic psychoses. Other distortions of logical thought, such as gaps or condensations of logical associations, are also typical of schizophrenia, of which they constitute a diagnostic feature.

DISTURBANCES OF EMOTION, MOOD, AND AFFECT The emotional life of the patient is expressed in a variety of ways. In the first place, rather marked individual differences in basic temperament are to be observed in the normal population; some persons are throughout their life cheerful, gregarious, optimistic, and free from worry, whereas others are just the opposite. The unusually volatile, cyclothymic person is believed to be liable to manic-depressive psychosis, and the suspicious, withdrawn, introverted person to schizophrenia and paranoia. Strong, persistent emotional states such as fear and anxiety may occur as reactions to life situations and may be accompanied by derangements of visceral function. If excessive and disproportionate to the stimulus, they are usually manifestations of an anxiety neurosis or depression. Variations in the degree of responsiveness to emotional stimuli are also frequent and, when excessive and persistent, assume importance. In depression all stimuli tend to enhance the somber mood of unhappiness. Emotional response that is excessively labile, variable from moment to moment, and poorly controlled or uninhibited is a condition common to many diseases of the cerebrum, particularly those involving the corticopontine and corticobulbar pathways. It constitutes a part of the syndrome of pseudobulbar palsy. All emotional expression may be lacking, as in apathetic states or severe depressions, or the patient may be a victim of every trivial problem in daily life; i.e., he cannot control his worries. Finally, the emotional response may be inappropriate to the stimulus, e.g., a depressing or morbid thought may seem amusing and be attended by a smile or arouse no emotional reaction, as in schizophrenia.

Since there are relatively few overt manifestations of temperament, mood, and other emotional experiences described above, the physician must evaluate these states by the appearance of the patient and by verbalized accounts of his feelings. For these purposes it is convenient to divide emotionality into mood and feeling or affect. By *mood* is meant the prevailing emotional state of the individual without reference to the stimuli immediately impinging upon him. It may be pleasant and cheerful or melancholic. The language, e.g., the adjectives used, and the facial expressions, attitudes, postures, and speed of movement most reliably betray the patient's mood. By contrast, *feelings* (or *affect*) are said to be emotional experiences evoked by environmental stimuli.

DISTURBANCES IN IMPULSE Impulse, that basic biologic urge, driving force, or purpose, by which every organism is directed to reach its full potentialities, appears to be another extremely important and observable, though somewhat neglected, dimension of behavior. Again, one notes wide normal variations from one person to another in strength of impulse to action and thought, and these individual differences are present throughout life. One of the most conspicuous pathologic deviations is an apparent constitutional weakness in impulse in certain neurotic persons. Moreover, with many types of cerebral disease (particularly those which involve the posterior orbital parts of the frontal lobes) a reduction in impulse is coupled with an indifference or lack of concern about the consequences of actions. In such cases all other measurable aspects of psychic function may be normal. Extreme degrees of lack of impulse, or *abulia,* sometimes take the form of mutism and immobility called *akinetic mutism.* Psychomotor retardation is a lesser degree of the same state and is a feature of cerebral disease or of depression. In the latter instance mood alteration and extreme fatigability are conjoined.

LOSS OF INSIGHT Insight, the state of being fully aware of the nature and degree of one's deficits, becomes manifestly impaired or abolished in relation to all types of cerebral disease that cause complex disorders of behavior. Rarely does the patient with any of the aforementioned states seek advice or help for his illness. Instead, his family usually brings him to the physician. Thus, it appears that the diseases which produce all these abnormalities not only evoke observable changes in behavior but also alter or reduce the patient's insight.

COMMON SYNDROMES

Delirium

CLINICAL FEATURES These are most perfectly depicted in the alcoholic patient. The symptoms usually develop over a period of 2 or 3 days. The first indications of the approaching attack are difficulty in concentrating, restless irritability, tremulousness, insommia, and poor appetite. One or several generalized convulsions are the initial major symptom in 30 percent of the cases. The patient's rest becomes troubled by unpleasant and terrifying dreams. There may be momentary disorientation or an occasional inappropriate remark.

These initial symptoms rapidly give way to a clinical picture that, in severe cases, is one of the most colorful and dramatic in medicine. The state of consciousness becomes altered; it is clouded in that the patient is inattentive and unable to perceive all elements of his situation. He may talk incessantly and incoherently and looks distressed and perplexed; his expression is in keeping with his vague notions of being annoyed or pursued by someone who seeks to injure him. From his manner and from the content of his speech it is evident that he misinterprets the meaning of ordinary objects and sounds around him and has vivid visual, auditory, and tactile hallucinations, often of a most unpleasant type. At first he can be brought momentarily into touch with reality and may in fact answer questions correctly; but almost at once he relapses into his preoccupied, confused state, gives wrong answers, and is unable to think coherently. The clouding of sensorium is revealed by his inability to repeat or reverse series of digits or to do serial additions or subtractions. As a rule he is oriented. Before long he is unable to shake off his hallucinations even for a second and does not recognize his family or his physician. Tremor and restless movements are usually present and may be violent. Sleep is impossible or occurs only in brief naps. The countenance is flushed, the pupils are dilated, and the conjunctivas are injected; the pulse is rapid, and the temperature may be raised. There is much sweating, and the urine is scanty and of high specific gravity. The signs of overactivity of the autonomic nervous system, more than any other, distinguish delirium from all other confusional states.

The symptoms abate, either suddenly or gradually, after 2 or 3 days, although in exceptional cases they may persist for several weeks. The most certain indication of the end of the attack is the occurrence of sound sleep and of lucid intervals of increasing length. Recovery is usually complete.

Delirium is subject to all degrees of variability, not only from patient to patient but in the same patient from day to day and hour to hour. The entire syndrome may be observed in one patient, and only one or two symptoms in another. In its mildest form, as so often occurs in febrile diseases, it consists of an occasional wandering of the mind and incoherence of verbal expression, interrupted by periods of lucidity. This form, lacking motor and autonomic overactivity, is sometimes referred to as a *quiet delirium* (or *hypokinetic delirium*) and is difficult to distinguish from other confusional states. The more severe form of active delirium and tremulousness, best exemplified by delirium tremens, may progress to a "muttering stupor" and in about 10 percent of patients ends fatally.

MORBID ANATOMY AND PATHOPHYSIOLOGY The brains of patients who have died in delirium tremens usually show no pathologic changes of significance. A number of diseases, however, may cause delirium and also give rise to focal lesions in the brain, such as focal embolic encephalitis, viral encephalitis, Wernicke's disease, or trauma. The topography of these lesions is of particular interest. They tend to be localized in the midbrain and subthalamus and in the temporal lobes, where they involve the reticular activating and limbic systems.

Penfield's studies of the human cortex during surgical exploration clearly indicate the importance of the temporal lobe in producing visual, auditory, and olfactory hallucinations. With subthalamic and midbrain lesions, visual hallucinations may occur that are not unpleasant and may be accompanied by good insight (the peduncular hallucinosis of Lhermitte).

The electroencephalogram in delirium shows nonfocal slow activity in the 5- to 7-per-s range, a state that rapidly returns to normal as the delirium clears. However, in other cases only activity in the fast beta frequency range is seen, and in milder degrees of delirium there is usually no abnormality at all.

An analysis of the several conditions conducive to delirium suggests at least three different physiologic mechanisms. The withdrawal of alcohol, barbiturates, or other sedation drugs, following a period of chronic intoxication is the most common cause of delirium (Chaps. 118 and 120). These drugs are known to have a strong depressant effect on certain areas of the central nervous system; presumably the release and overactivity of these parts, after withdrawal of the drug, are the basis of delirium. In the case of bacterial infections and poisoning by certain drugs, such as atropine and scopolamine, the delirious state probably results from the direct action of the toxin or chemical on these same parts of the brain. Thirdly, destructive lesions, such as acute inclusion body encephalitis of the temporal lobes, may cause delirium by disturbing the function of certain areas.

Acute confusional states associated with reduced mental alertness and responsiveness

In the most typical examples, all mental functions are reduced to some degree, but alertness, attentiveness, and the ability to grasp all elements of the immediate situation suffer most. In the mildest form the patient may pass for normal, and only failure to recollect and reproduce happenings of the past few hours or days reveals the inadequacy of mental function. The more obviously confused patient spends much of his time in idleness, but what he does do may be inappropriate and annoying to others. Only the more automatic acts and verbal responses are properly performed, but these may permit the examiner to obtain from the patient a number of relevant and accurate replies to questions about age, occupation, and residence. Reactions are slow and indecisive, and it is difficult for the patient to sustain a conversation. He may doze during the interview and is observed to sleep more hours each day than is natural or the same number at more irregular intervals. Responses tend to be rather abrupt, brief, and mechanical. Perceptual difficulties are frequent, and voices, common objects, and the actions of other persons are frequently misinterpreted. Often one cannot discern whether the patient hears voices and sees things that do not exist, i.e., whether he is hallucinating, or is merely misinterpreting stimuli in the environment. Inadequate perception and forgetfulness result in a constant state of bewilderment. Failing to recognize his surroundings and having lost all sense of time, he repeats the same question and makes the same remarks over and over again. Irritability may or may not be present. Some patients are extremely suspicious; in fact, a paranoid trend may be the most pronounced and troublesome feature of the illness.

As the confusion deepens, conversation becomes more difficult, and at a certain state the patient no longer notices or responds to much of what is going on around him. Replies to questions may be a single word or a short phrase spoken in a soft tremulous voice or whisper. The patient may be mute. In its most advanced stages confusion gives way to stupor and finally to coma. As the patient improves, he may pass again through the stage of stupor and confusion in the reverse order. All this informs us that at least one category of confusion is but a manifestation of the same disease processes that in their severest form cause coma.

In the most typical cases, this type of confusional state is readily distinguished from delirium; in others with more than the usual degree of irritability and restlessness, one cannot fail to notice the resemblance to delirium. Similarly, certain cases of delirium, in which tremor, vivid hallucinations, vigilant excited attitude, insomnia, and the low convulsive threshold are inconspicuous, are difficult to distinguish from other acute confusional states. The same diagnostic difficulty arises when a delirium is complicated by an illness that superimposes stupor (e.g., delirium tremens with pneumonia or meningitis).

Senile and other dementing brain diseases complicated by medical diseases (beclouded dementia)

Many elderly patients who enter the hospital with medical or surgical illness are mentally confused. Presumably the liability to this state is determined by preexisting brain disease, in this instance senile dementia, which may or may not have been obvious to the family before the onset of the complicating illness. Other cerebral diseases (vascular, neoplastic, demyelinative) may have the same effect of increasing the patient's liability to confusion.

All the clinical features of hypokinetic delirium or of acute confusion may be present. The severity may vary greatly. The confusion may be reflected only in the patient's inability to relate sequentially the history of his illness, or it may be so severe that he is virtually *non compos mentis*.

Although almost any complicating illness may bring out his confusion, it is particularly frequent with infectious disease; with posttraumatic and postoperative states, notably after concussive brain injuries; with the removal of cataracts (in which case the confusion is probably related to being temporarily deprived of vision); and with congestive heart failure, chronic respiratory disease, and severe anemia, especially pernicious anemia. Often it is difficult to determine which of several possible factors is responsible for the confusion in this heterogeneous group of illnesses, and there may be more than one. A cardiac patient with a confusional psychosis may be febrile, have marginally reduced cerebral blood flow, be intoxicated by one or more drugs, or be in electrolyte imbalance.

When the patient recovers from the medical or surgical illness, he usually returns to his premorbid state, though his shortcomings, now drawn to the attention of the family and physician, may be more obvious than before.

Development of acute schizophrenic or manic-depressive psychosis during illness

A certain proportion of psychoses of the schizophrenic or manic-depressive type first become manifest during an acute medical illness or following an operation or parturition. A causal relationship between the two is usually sought but cannot be established. Usually the psychosis began long before but was not recognized. The diagnostic studies of the psychiatric illness must proceed along the lines suggested in Chaps. 345 and 346. Close observation will usually reveal a clear sensorium and relatively intact memory, which permits differentiation from the acute confusional states.

CLASSIFICATION AND DIAGNOSIS (See Table 26-1)

The first step in *diagnosis* is to recognize that the patient is confused. This is obvious in most cases, but, as pointed out above, the mildest form of confusion, particularly when some other acute alteration of personality is prominent, may be overlooked. In these mild forms a careful analysis of the patient's thinking as he gives the history of his illness and the details of his personal life will usually reveal an incoherence. Digit span and serial subtraction of 3s and 7s from 100 are useful bedside tests of the patient's capacity for sustained mental activity. Memory of recent events is one of the most delicate tests of adequate mental function and may be accomplished by having the patient relate all the details of his entry to the hospital, laboratory tests, etc.

Once it is established that the patient is confused, the differential diagnosis must be made among delirium, acute confusional states associated with psychomotor underactivity, and a beclouded dementia. This can be done usually by careful attention to the patient's degree of alertness and wakefulness, his capacity to solve new problems, his memory, accuracy of perception, and hallucinations. The distinction between confusional states and dementia may be difficult at times.

CARE OF THE DELIRIOUS AND CONFUSED PATIENT

The physician must be secure in his ability to manage the delirious and confused patient because such illnesses are observed almost daily on the medical and surgical wards of

TABLE 26-1
Classification of delirium and acute confusional states

I Delirium
- *A* In a medical or surgical illness (no focal or lateralizing neurologic signs; cerebrospinal fluid usually clear)
  - *1* Typhoid fever
  - *2* Pneumonia
  - *3* Septicemia, particularly erysipelas and other streptococcal infections
  - *4* Rheumatic fever
  - *5* Thyrotoxicosis and ACTH intoxication (rare)
  - *6* Postoperative and posttraumatic states
- *B* In neurologic disease that causes focal or lateralizing signs or changes in the cerebrospinal fluid
  - *1* Vascular, neoplastic, or other diseases, particularly those involving the temporal lobes and upper part of the brainstem
  - *2* Cerebral contusion and laceration (traumatic delirium)
  - *3* Acute bacterial and tuberculous meningitis
  - *4* Subarachnoid hemorrhage
  - *5* Encephalitis due to viral causes
- *C* The abstinence states, exogenous intoxications, and postconvulsive states; signs of other medical, surgical, and neurologic illnesses absent or coincidental
  - *1* Withdrawal of alcohol (delirium tremens), barbiturates, and nonbarbiturate sedative drugs, following chronic intoxication (Chaps. 118 and 120)
  - *2* Drug intoxications: camphor, caffeine, ergot, bromides, scopolamine, atropine, amphetamine
  - *3* Postconvulsive delirium

II Acute confusional states associated with psychomotor underactivity
- *A* Associated with a medical or surgical disease (no focal lateralizing neurologic signs; cerebrospinal fluid clear)
  - *1* Metabolic disorders: hepatic stupor, uremia, hypoxia, hypercapnea, hypoglycemia, porphyria
  - *2* Infective fevers
  - *3* Congestive heart failure
  - *4* Postoperative, posttraumatic, and puerperal psychoses
- *B* Associated with drug intoxication (no focal or lateralizing signs; cerebrospinal fluid clear): opiates, barbiturates, bromides, Artane, etc.
- *C* Associated with diseases of the nervous system (the focal or lateralizing neurologic signs and cerebrospinal fluid changes of these conditions are commoner than in delirium)
  - *1* Cerebral vascular disease, tumor, abcess
  - *2* Subdural hematoma
  - *3* Meningitis
  - *4* Encephalitis
- *D* Beclouded dementia, i.e., senile or other brain disease in combination with infective fevers, drug reactions, heart failure, or other medical or surgical disease

a general hospital. Occurring as they do during an infective fever, in the course of another illness such as cardiac failure, or following an injury, operation, or the excessive use of alcohol, they never fail to create grave problems. The physician's program of treatment may constantly be threatened by the patient's agitation, sleeplessness, and uncooperative attitude. The nursing personnel are often sorely taxed by the necessity of providing a satisfactory environment for the convalescence of the patient and, at the same time, maintaining a tranquil atmosphere for the other patients. And the family is appalled by the sudden specter of insanity and all that it entails.

The primary therapeutic effort is directed to the control of the underlying medical disease. Other important objectives are to quiet the patient and protect him against injury. A private nurse, an attendant, or a member of the family should be with the patient at all times if this can be arranged. Depending on how active and vigorous he is, a locked room, screened windows that cannot be opened by the patient, and a low bed or mattress on the floor should be arranged. It is often better to let the patient walk about the room than to tie him into bed, which may excite or frighten him so that he struggles to the point of complete exhaustion and collapse. If he is less active, the patient can usually be kept in bed by leather wrist restraints, a restraining sheet, or a net thrown over the bed. Unless it is contraindicated by the primary disease, the patient should be permitted to sit up or walk about the room part of the day.

All drugs that could possibly be responsible for delirium—particularly opiates, barbiturates, bromides, atropine, hyoscine, cortisone, adrenocorticotropic hormone (ACTH), and salicylates in large doses—should be discontinued (unless withdrawal effects are believed to underlie the illness). Paraldehyde and choral hydrate are trustworthy sedatives under these circumstances. Paraldehyde, which is preferred, may be given orally or rectally in doses of 10 to 12 ml. For oral administration, mixing it with fruit juices makes it more palatable. Chlorpromazine, chlordiazepoxide, and diazepam are often extremely effective if given in full doses, and should be continued until natural sleep is restored. One must be cautious in attempting to suppress agitation completely. To accomplish this may require very large doses of drugs, and vital functions may then be dangerously impaired. The purpose of sedation is to ensure rest and sleep so that the patient does not exhaust himself.

A fluid intake and output chart should be kept, and any fluid and electrolyte deficit should be corrected. The pulse and blood pressure should be recorded at intervals of 2 h in anticipation of circulatory collapse. Transfusions of whole blood and vasopressor drugs may be lifesaving.

Finally, the physician should be aware of many small therapeutic measures that may allay fear and suspicion and reduce the tendency to hallucinations. The room should be kept dimly lighted at night, and if possible the patient should not be moved from one room to another. Every procedure should be explained in detail, even such simple ones as the taking of blood pressure or temperature. The presence of a member of the family may enable the patient to maintain contact with reality.

Most delirious patients tend to recover if they are placed in good hygienic surroundings and competently nursed. The family should be reassured on this point and must also understand that the abnormal behavior and irrational actions of the patient are not willful but rather are symptomatic of a brain disease.

REFERENCES

ADAMS RD, VICTOR M: *Principles of Neurology,* New York: McGraw-Hill, 1977

LIPOWSKI ZJ: Delirium, clouding of consciousness and confusion. J Nerv Ment Dis 145:227, 1967

27
DERANGEMENTS OF INTELLECT AND BEHAVIOR DUE TO DIFFUSE AND FOCAL CEREBRAL DISEASE

RAYMOND D. ADAMS
MAURICE VICTOR

Increasingly, as the number of elderly adults in our population rises, the internist is consulted because an otherwise healthy person begins to lose his capacity to function effectively as head of a family or as a worker. This may have several significations—indicating the beginning of a brain tumor, the formation of a chronic subdural hematoma, or the development of a chronic drug intoxication, a chronic meningoencephalitis (syphilis), degenerative cerebral disease, a chronic, low-pressure hydrocephalus, or a depressive psychosis. In former times when there was little that could be done about any of these clinical states, no great premium was attached to diagnosis. But modern medicine now offers the means of treating several of these conditions and in some instances of restoring the patient to normal health and effectiveness. Early recognition of the underlying pathologic process improves chances of recovery.

THE CLINICAL SYNDROME OF DEMENTIA The term *dementia* usually denotes a clinical state composed of failing memory and loss of other intellectual functions due to chronic progressive degenerative disease of the brain. It may or may not be associated with signs of disease in one or more of the motor, sensory, or speech areas of the cerebrum. The chronicity of the process is ordinarily emphasized, but the illogic of setting apart any one constellation of cerebral symptoms on the basis of their speed of onset, evolution, or duration is obvious. We would like to emphasize that the state of dementia is a generic syndrome of multiple causation and mechanism, and that a diffuse degeneration of neurons is only one of the causes.

The earliest signs of dementia may be so subtle as to escape the notice of even the most discerning physician. Often an observant relative of the patient or an employer is the first to become aware of a certain lack of initiative, irritability, loss of interest, and inability to perform up to the usual standard. Later there is distractibility, inability to think with accustomed clarity, reduced general comprehension, perseveration in speech, action, and thought, and defective memory, especially for recent events. Frequently a change in mood becomes apparent, deviating more often toward depression than elation. The direction of this deviation is said to depend on the previous personality of the patient rather than upon the character of the disease. Excessive lability of mood may also be observed, i.e., easy fluctuation from laughter to tears on slight provocation. Lapses in social graces and conduct occur, and judgment becomes impaired, early in some cases and late in others. Paranoid ideas and delusions may develop. As a rule, the patient has little or no realization of these changes in himself; he lacks insight. As the condition progresses, there is loss of almost all intellectual faculties. Mutism, unresponsiveness, dysarthria, aphasia, and sphincteric incontinence may be added to the clinical picture. In a late stage a secondary physical deterioration also takes place. Food intake, which may be increased in the beginning of the illness, is in the end usually limited, with resulting emaciation. Any febrile illness or metabolic upset induces a marked increase in confusion and even stupor or coma, indicating the precarious state of cerebral compensation. Finally the patient remains in bed most of the time and dies of pneumonia or some other intercurrent infection. This whole process may evolve over a period of months or years, usually the latter.

Many of the alterations of behavior are the direct result of disease of the nervous system; expressed in another way, the symptoms are the primary manifestations of neurologic disease. Others are secondary; i.e., they are reactions to the catastrophe of losing one's mind. For example, the dement is said to seek solitude to hide his affliction and may thus appear asocial or apathetic. Again, excessive orderliness may be an attempt to compensate for failing memory; apprehension, gloom, or irritability may reflect general dissatisfaction with a necessarily restricted life. It would appear that even in a state of fairly advanced deterioration, the patient is still capable of reacting to his illness and to the persons who care for him.

Degenerative diseases may terminate in virtually complete decortication. The patient is unaware of what is happening but lies with eyes open. He no longer responds to spoken commands or speaks. There is no interest in food or drink though they are swallowed if placed in mouth. The facial and limb muscles are stiff with increased tendon reflexes and Babinski signs. Grasping and sucking are prominent. The sphincters are incontinent.

Morbid anatomy and pathologic physiology of dementia Dementia is related usually to obvious structural disease of the cerebrum and the diencephalon. In some, such as Alzheimer's disease, senile dementia, and Pick's disease, the main process appears to be a degeneration and loss of nerve cells in the association areas, with secondary changes in the cerebral white matter. In others, such as Huntington's chorea and other cerebro-basal ganglionic degenerations, loss of neurons in the cerebral cortex is accompanied by a similar degeneration of neurons in the putamen and caudate nuclei and cerebellum. Arteriosclerotic vascular disease results in multiple foci of infarction all through the thalami, basal ganglia, brainstem, and cerebrum and, in the latter, in the motor, sensory, or visual projection areas as well as in the association areas. Severe trauma may cause contusions of cerebral convolutions and white matter as well as necroses and hemorrhages in the midbrain, which underlie protracted stupor, coma, or dementia. Most diseases that produce dementia are quite extensive, and the frontal lobes are affected more often than other parts of the cerebrum.

Mechanisms other than the destruction of brain tissue may operate in some cases. Chronic increased intracranial pressure or chronic hydrocephalus (with large ventricles the pressure may not exceed 180 mm), regardless of cause, is often associated with a general impairment of mental function. Compression of cerebral white matter is the main factor. The compression of one or both of the cerebral hemispheres by chronic subdural hematomas may cause a widespread disturbance of cortical function. A diffuse inflammatory process is at least in part the basis for dementia in syphilis and in neurotropic virus infections such as "inclusion body encephalitis"; presumably there are loss of some neurons and also inflammatory derangement of the function of other neurons. Lastly, several of the toxic and metabolic diseases discussed in Chap. 340 may interfere with nervous function over a period of time and create a clinical picture similar to, if not identical with, that of dementia. One must suppose that the altered biochemical environment has affected the excitability of the neurons.

(Details of all the diseases which cause dementia are found in Chap. 341.)

Bedside classification of dementia

I Diseases in which dementia is usually associated with clinical and laboratory signs of other medical disease
- *A* Hypothyroidism
- *B* Cushing's disease
- *C* Nutritional deficiency states such as pellagra, the Wernicke-Korsakoff syndrome, and subacute combined degeneration of spinal cord and brain (vitamin B_{12} deficiency)
- *D* Neurosyphilis: general paresis and meningovascular syphilis
- *E* Hepatolenticular degeneration, familial and acquired
- *F* Bromidism, chronic barbiturate intoxication

II Diseases in which dementia is associated with other neurologic signs but not with other obvious medical disease
- *A* Invariably associated with other neurologic signs
  - *1* Huntington's chorea (choreoathetosis)
  - *2* Schilder's disease, metachromatic leukodystrophy, and related demyelinative diseases (spastic weakness, pseudobulbar palsy, blindness, deafness)
  - *3* Lipofuscinosis and other lipid-storage diseases (myoclonic seizures, blindness, spasticity, cerebellar ataxia)
  - *4* Myoclonic epilepsy (diffuse myoclonus, generalized seizures, cerebellar ataxia)
  - *5* Jakob-Creutzfeldt disease (diffuse myoclonus)
  - *6* Cerebrocerebellar degeneration (cerebellar ataxia)

   7 Cerebral-basal ganglion degenerations (apraxia-rigidity)
   8 Dementia with spastic paraplegia
   9 Basal ganglia calcification (Fahr's disease and hypoparathyroidism)
   10 Hallevorden-Spatz disease
   11 Dementia with Parkinson's disease
  B Often associated with other neurologic signs
   1 Cerebral arteriosclerosis
   2 Brain tumor
   3 Brain trauma, such as cerebral contusion, midbrain hemorrhage, chronic subdural hematoma
   4 Marchiafava-Bignami disease (often with apraxia and other frontal lobe signs)
   5 Low-pressure hydrocephalus (nearly always with ataxia of gait)
III Diseases in which dementia is usually the only evidence of neurologic or medical disease
  A Alzheimer's disease and senile dementia
  B Pick's disease

Many of these diseases are discussed more fully in other sections of this book. The special features of the dementia that accompanies arteriosclerotic, senile, syphilitic, traumatic, nutritional, and degenerative diseases are discussed in the appropriate chapters.

Differential diagnosis The first task in dealing with this class of patients is to make sure of deterioration of intellect and personality change. It may be necessary to examine the patient several times before one is confident of the clinical findings.

There is always a tendency to assume that mental function is normal if there is complaint only of nervousness, fatigue, insomnia, or vague somatic symptoms, and to label the patients psychoneurotic. *This will be avoided if one keeps in mind that psychoneuroses rarely begin in middle or late adult life.* A practical rule is to assume that all mental illnesses beginning during this period are due either to structural disease of the brain or to a depressive psychosis.

A mild dysphasia must not be mistaken for dementia. The aphasic patient appears uncertain of himself, and his speech may be incoherent. Furthermore, he may be anxious and depressed over his ineptitude. Careful attention to the patient's language performance will lead to the correct diagnosis in most instances. Further observation will disclose that the patient's behavior, except that which is related to the language disorder, is within normal limits.

The depressed patient presents another type of problem. He may remark that his mental function is poor or that he is forgetful and cannot concentrate. Scrutiny of his remarks will show, however, that he actually remembers all the details of his illness and that no qualitative change in mental ability has taken place. His difficulty is either a lack of energy and interest or an anxiety that prevents the focusing of attention on anything except his own problems. Even during mental tests his performance may be impaired by his emotions, in much the same way as that of the worried student during examinations. This condition of emotional blocking is called *experiential confusion.* When the patient is calmed by reassurance and given more time in the performance of tests, his mental function improves, indicating that intellectual deterioration has not occurred. The hypomanic patient fails in tests of intellectual function because of his restlessness and distractibility. It is helpful to remember that the demented patient rarely has sufficient insight to complain of mental deterioration and if he admits to poor memory, he seldom realizes the degree of his disability. The physician must never rely on the patient's statements as to the efficiency of mental function and must always evaluate a poor performance on tests in the light of the emotional state and motivation at the time the test is given.

The neurologic syndromes associated with metabolic or endocrine disorders, i.e., ACTH therapy, hyperthyroidism, Cushing's disease, Addison's disease, or the post-partum state may be difficult to diagnose because of the wide variety of clinical pictures by which they manifest themselves. Some patients appear to be suffering from a dementia, others from an acute confusional psychosis; or if mood change or negativism predominates, a manic-depressive psychosis or schizophrenia is suggested. In these conditions some degree of clouding of sensorium and impairment of intellectual function can usually be recognized, and these findings alone should be enough to exclude schizophrenia and manic-depressive psychosis. It is well to remember that acute onset of mental symptoms always suggests confusional psychosis or delirium. Inasmuch as many of these conditions are completely reversible, they must be distinguished from dementia (see Chap. 26).

Once it is decided that the patient suffers from a dementing disease, the next step is to determine by careful physical examination whether there are other neurologic signs or indications of a particular medical disease. This enables the physician to place the case in one of the three categories in the bedside classification (see list above). X-rays of the skull, electroencephalogram, lumbar puncture, and pneumoencephalogram or preferably computerized axial tomography (CAT) scan should be carried out in most cases. Usually these procedures necessitate admission to a hospital. The final step is to determine by the total clinical picture which disease within any one category the patient has.

KORSAKOFF'S PSYCHOSIS [AMNESIC- (OR AMNESTIC-) CONFABULATORY PSYCHOSIS] These terms are used interchangeably to designate a unique but common disorder of cognitive function, in which memory is deranged out of all proportion to all other components of mentation and behavior. It possesses two salient features which may vary in severity but are always conjoined: (1) an impaired ability to recall events and other information that had been recorded in mind before the onset of the illness (retrograde amnesia); and (2) an impaired ability to acquire new information, i.e., to learn or to form new memories (anterograde amnesia). Other cognitive functions (particularly the capacity for concentration, spatial organization, visual and verbal abstraction), which depend little or not at all on memory, may also be impaired but to a relatively minor degree. The patient tends to be lacking in initiative and spontaneity. Confabulation, meaning false or fabricated accounts of recent events, is present in most cases, especially in the acute phase of the illness.

The definition of Korsakoff's psychosis demands also that certain aspects of behavior and mental function be intact. The patient should be alert, attentive, responsive, and capable of understanding the written and spoken word, of making appropriate deductions from given premises and solving such problems as can be concluded within his forward memory span. These "negative" features are of particular importance because they help to distinguish Korsakoff's psychosis from a number of other disorders in which the basic defect is not necessarily in retentive memory, but in some other psychologic mechanism, e.g., in attention and perception (as in the delirious, confused, or stuporous patient), in recall (as in the hysterical patient), or in volition (as in the patient with frontal lobe disease).

The anatomic structures of particular importance in memory function are the diencephalon (specifically the medial portions of the medial dorsal nuclei of the thalamus) and the hippocampal formations (gyrus dentatus, hippocampus, and parahippocampal gyri). Bilaterally placed lesions in either of these regions derange memory and learning out of all proportion to other cognitive functions, and even unilateral lesions of the dominant hemispheres produce a lesser degree of the same effect. It would appear that the aforementioned anatomic structures are involved in all forms of learning and integration of newly formed memories and that they form a tenuous but vital link between the high-brainstem reticular formation (the integrity of which is necessary to maintain an alert state of mind, a prerequisite for any learning) and the cerebral cortex, which is the locus for special memories such as words, geometric figures, and numbers.

Classification of diseases characterized by an amnesic syndrome

I Amnesic syndrome of sudden onset—usually with gradual but incomplete recovery
- *A* Bilateral hippocampal infarction due to atherosclerotic-thrombotic or embolic occlusion of the posterior cerebral arteries or their inferior temporal branches
- *B* Trauma to the diencephalic or inferomedial temporal regions
- *C* Spontaneous subarachnoid hemorrhage
- *D* Carbon monoxide poisoning and other hypoxic states (rare)

II Amnesia of sudden onset and brief duration with full recovery
- *A* Temporal lobe seizures
- *B* Postconcussive states
- *C* "Transient global amnesia"

III Amnesic syndrome of subacute onset with varying degrees of recovery, usually leaving permanent residue
- *A* Wernicke-Korsakoff disease
- *B* Inclusion body (herpes simplex) encephalitis
- *C* Tuberculous and other forms of meningitis characterized by a granulomatous exudate at the base of the brain

IV Slowly progressive amnesic states
- *A* Tumors involving the walls of the third ventricle and temporal lobes
- *B* Alzheimer's disease and other degenerative disorders

SYNDROMES CAUSED BY DISEASES OF SPECIAL PARTS OF THE CEREBRUM Frontal lobes In Fig. 27-1, it may be seen that the frontal lobes lie anterior to the central, or rolandic, sulcus and superior to the sylvian fissure. They consist of several functionally different parts, which are conventionally designated in the neurologic literature by numbers (according to a scheme devised by Brodmann) and by letters (the scheme of von Economo and Koskinas).

The posterior parts, areas 4 and 6 of Brodmann, are specifically related to motor function. Voluntary movement in man depends on the integrity of these areas, and lesions in them produce spastic paralysis of the contralateral face, arm, and leg. This is discussed in Chap. 17. Lesions limited more or less to the premotor areas (area 6) are accompanied by prominent grasp and sucking reflexes. Lesions in areas 8 and 24 of Brodmann interfere with the mechanism concerned with turning the head and eyes contralaterally. Lesions in areas 44 and 45 of the major hemisphere abolish or reduce verbalization, deglutition, and chewing. Lesions in area 44 of the dominant cerebral hemisphere, usually the left one, have often resulted in loss of verbal expression, the aphasia of Broca. Lesions in the medial limbic or piriform cortex (areas 23 and 24), wherein are bilaterally orga-

FIGURE 27-1
Diagram to show cortical areas, numbered according to the scheme of Brodmann. The speech areas are in black, the three main ones being 39, 41, and 45. The zone marked by vertical stripes in the superior frontal convolution is the secondary motor area which, like Broca's area 45, if stimulated, causes vocal arrest. (Redrawn from Handbuch der Inneren Medizin, *Berlin: Springer-Verlag, 1939)*

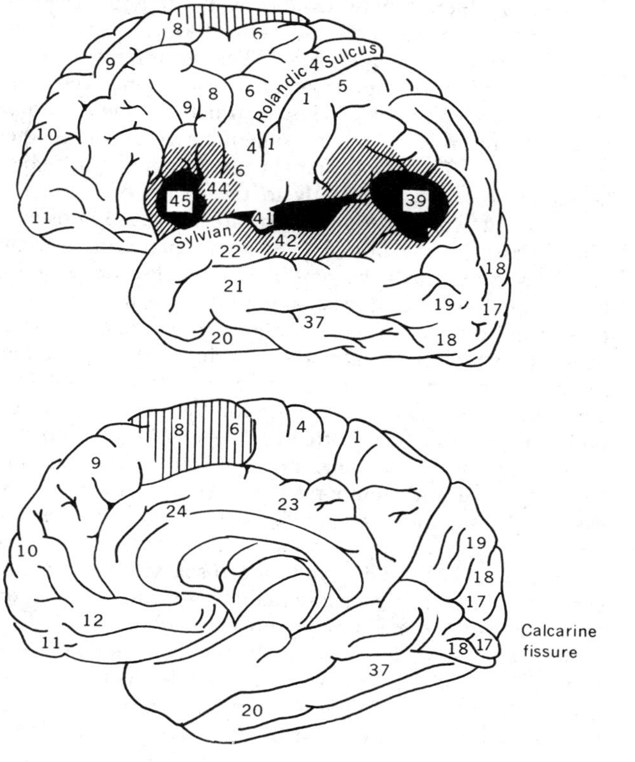

nized the mechanisms controlling respiration, circulation, and micturition, have relatively unclear clinical effects.

The remaining parts of the frontal lobes (areas 9 to 13 of Brodmann), sometimes called the *prefrontal areas,* have less specific and measurable functions. In contrast to the motor areas of the frontal lobes and other areas of the brain, stimulation of the prefrontal areas in man has yielded a paucity of findings. Many patients with gunshot wounds of these areas have shown only mild and inconsistent abnormalities of behavior. Nevertheless, the following groups of symptoms have been observed in patients with large lesions of one or both of the frontal lobes or of the central white matter and the anterior part of the corpus callosum by which they are joined:

1 Change of personality, usually expressed as lack of concern over the consequences of any action, which may take the form of a childish excitement, an inappropriate joking and punning, or an instability and superficiality of emotion, or irritability
2 Slight impairment of intelligence, usually described as lack of concentration, vacillation of attention, inability to carry out planned activity, difficulty in changing from one activity to another, slight loss of recent memory, or lack of initiative and spontaneity
3 Motor abnormalities such as decomposition of gait and upright stance, trunk ataxia of Bruns, abnormal postures, reflex grasping or sucking, incontinence of sphincters, and an apathetic-akinetic-abulic state

Temporal lobes The boundaries of the temporal lobes may be seen in Fig. 27-1. The sylvian fissure separates the superior surface of each temporal lobe from the frontal and anterior parts of the parietal lobes. There is no definite anatomic boundary between the temporal and occipital lobes or between temporal and parietal lobes. The temporal lobe includes the superior, middle, and inferior temporal, fusiform, and hippocampal convolutions and the transverse convolutions of Heschl, which are the auditory receptive area present on the superior surface within the sylvian fissure. The hippocampal convolution was once believed to be related indirectly to the olfactory bulb, but now it is known that lesions here do not cause anosmia. The fibers from the homolateral lower quadrant of each retina course through the central white matter en route to the occipital lobes, and lesions that interrupt them characteristically produce a contralateral homonymous upper quadrant defect of visual fields. Hearing and labyrinthine function, also localized in the temporal lobes, are bilaterally represented, which accounts for the fact that unless both temporal lobes are affected, there is little or no demonstrable loss of hearing. Loss of equilibrium has not been observed with temporal lobe lesions. Extensive disease in the superior and middle convolutions of the left temporal lobe in right-handed individuals results in Wernicke's aphasia. This syndrome, discussed in Chap. 25, consists of jargon aphasia and inability to read, to write, or to understand the meaning of spoken words.

Between the auditory and olfactory projection areas there is a large expanse of temporal lobe which has no assignable function. This is the temporal association area. Dysnomia has been the most frequent symptom in dominant hemisphere lesions. The most careful psychologic studies have shown a difference between cases involving loss of the dominant and the nondominant temporal lobe. With lesions of the dominant side there is impairment in learning auditorially presented material; with nondominant lesions there is a similar failure in tests with visually presented material. In addition, about 20 percent of both right and left lobectomy patients have shown a syndrome similar to that described for the prefrontal parts of the brain; but more significant is the fact that in the other cases little or no defect in personality was exhibited. The study of cases of uncinate epilepsy, with the characteristic dreamy state, olfactory or gustatory hallucinations, and masticatory movements, suggests that all these functions are organized through the temporal lobes. Similarly, stimulation of the posterior parts of the temporal lobes of fully conscious epileptic patients during surgical procedures has brought to light the interesting fact that complex memories and visual and auditory images, some with strong emotional content, can be aroused. Studies of the effect of stimulation of the amygdaloid nucleus, which is in the anterior and medial part of the temporal lobe, have shed additional light on this subject. Symptoms may be evoked not unlike some of those of schizophrenic patients. Complex emotional experiences that have occurred previously may be revived. There are remarkable autonomic effects. Blood pressure rises, pulse increases, respirations are increased in frequency and depth, and the patient looks frightened. Ablation of these nuclei has eliminated uncontrollable rage reactions in psychotic patients. Hippocampal and adjacent convolutions have been excised bilaterally, with a disastrous loss of ability to learn or to establish new memories (Korsakoff's psychosis). All this indicates an important role of the temporal lobes in auditory and visual perception and imagery, in learning and memory, and in the emotional life of the individual.

In summary:

I Effects of unilateral disease of the dominant temporal lobe
- *A* Quadrantic homonymous anopia
- *B* Wernicke's aphasia
- *C* Impairment in verbal tests of material presented through the auditory sense
- *D* Dysnomia or amnesic aphasia

II Effects of unilateral disease of nondominant temporal lobe
- *A* Quadrantic homonymous anopia
- *B* Impairment of mental function with inability to judge spatial relationships in some cases
- *C* Impairment in nonverbal tests of visually presented material

III Effects of bilateral disease
- *A* Korsakoff's amnesic defect
- *B* Apathy and placidity
- *C* Loss of sexual capacity
- *D* Loss of other of the unilateral functions

Parietal lobes It has been known that the postcentral convolution is the terminus of somatic sensory pathways from the opposite half of the body. It has also been learned that destructive lesions here do not abolish cutaneous sensation but instead cause mainly a defect in sensory discrimination with variable impairment of sensation. In other words, pain, touch, and thermal and vibratory sensation are largely retained, whereas stereognosis, sense of position, distinction between single and double contacts (two-point threshold), and the localization of sensory stimuli are lost. There is also the phenomenon of extinction, i.e., if both sides of the body are touched simultaneously, only the stimulus on the normal side is perceived. This type of sensory disturbance, sometimes called *cortical sensory defect,* is discussed in Chap. 21. Later it was noted that extensive lesions deep in the white matter of the parietal lobes produce a contralateral homonymous hemianopia, often incongruous and greater in inferior quadrants, and lesions in the angular gyrus of the dominant hemisphere result in an inability to read.

More recent investigations have centered about the function of the parietal lobes in perception of position in space and of the relationship of the various parts of the body to one another. Since the time of Babinski it has been known that patients with a large lesion of the minor parietal lobe are often unaware of their hemiplegia and hemianesthesia. Babinski called this condition *anosognosia.* Related psychologic disorders are lack of recognition of the left arm and leg, neglect of the left side of the body (as in dressing) and of external space on the left side, and constructional apraxia (an inability to perform the movements of constructing simple figures). All these disorders of parietal lobe function may occur with left-sided lesions as well, but are observed only rarely, being obscured by the commonly associated *aphasia* and *agnosia.*

Another frequent constellation of symptoms, usually referred to as *Gerstmann's syndrome,* occurs only with lesions of the dominant parietal lobe. This consists of inability to write (agraphia), inability to calculate (acalculia), failure to distinguish right from left, and loss of recognition of various fingers and toes. This is a true *agnosia,* since it represents a defect in the formulation and use of symbolic concepts, including the significance of numbers and letters and the names of parts of the body. An ideomotor apraxia may or may not be associated. *Agnosia* and *apraxia* are discussed in Chaps. 17 and 21.

The effects of disease of the parietal lobes may be summarized as follows:

I Effects of unilateral disease of the parietal lobe, right or left
- *A* Cortical sensory syndrome and sensory extinction (or total hemianesthesia with large acute lesions of white matter)
- *B* Mild hemiparesis, unilateral muscular atrophy in children
- *C* Homonymous hemianopia or visual inattention, and sometimes anosognosia, neglect of one-half of the body and of extrapersonal space
- *D* Abolition of opticokinetic nystagmus to one side

II Effects of unilateral disease of the dominant parietal lobe (left hemisphere in right-handed patients), additional phenomena
- *A* Disorders of language (especially alexia)
- *B* Gerstmann's syndrome
- *C* Bimanual astereognosis (tactile agnosia)
- *D* Bilateral apraxia of the ideomotor type

III Effects of nondominant parietal lobe (additional phenomena)
- *A* Dressing apraxia
- *B* Constructional apraxia
- *C* Misidentification of left arm and leg
- *D* Bland mood, indifference to illness, or neurologic defects

In all these lesions, if the disease is sufficiently extensive, there may be a reduction in the capacity to think clearly, inattentiveness, and impaired memory.

Occipital lobes The occipital lobes are the terminus of the geniculocalcarine pathways and are essential for visual sensation and perception. Lesions in one occipital lobe result in homonymous defects in the contralateral visual fields. Most often the defect takes the form of loss of vision in part of or all the homonymous fields. Occasionally patients complain of changes in the form and contour of visually perceived objects (metamorphopsia), as well as illusory displacement of images from one side of the visual field to another (optic alloesthesia), or of abnormal persistence of the visual image after the object has been removed (palinopsia). Bilateral lesions cause "cortical" blindness, a state of blindness without change in optic fundi or pupillary reflexes.

Lesions in Brodmann's areas 18 and 19 of the dominant hemisphere (Fig. 27-1) cause a loss of visual recognition with retention of some degree of visual acuity, a state termed *visual agnosia.* In the classic form of this blindness an individual with intact mental powers is unable to recognize objects, even though by tests of visual acuity and perimetry he appears to see sufficiently well to do so; he is able to recognize objects by tactile or other extravisual sense. In these terms, *alexia,* or inability to read, represents a visual verbal agnosia or "word blindness." The patient can see letters and words but cannot recognize their meaning, although he can still recognize them through tactile or auditory senses.

CORPUS CALLOSUM AND THE DISCONNECTION SYNDROMES A number of clinical syndromes result from interruption of the connections between the two cerebral hemispheres in the corpus callosum or adjacent white matter (commissural syndromes) or between the several parts of one hemisphere (intrahemispheric dissociation syndromes).

When the entire corpus callosum is missing because of a congenital defect or destroyed by a surgical procedure or anterior cerebral artery occlusion (anterior four-fifths), the speech and perceptual areas of the left hemisphere are isolated from those of the right hemisphere. The patient, if blindfolded, is unable to match a stimulus object held in one hand with that in the other hand. Further he cannot match an object seen in the right half of his visual field with one in the left half. If given verbal commands to execute, he performs correctly with the right hand but not with the left. Without vision, objects placed in the right hand are named correctly, but not those in the left. In lesions confined to the posterior fifth of the corpus callosum (splenium), only the visual part of the disconnection syndrome occurs. The occlusion of the left posterior cerebral artery provides the best examples of the latter. Since infarction of the left occipital lobe causes a right homonymous hemianopia, thereafter all visual information needed for activating the speech areas of the left hemisphere must come from the right occipital lobe across the splenium of the corpus callosum. If there is a lesion in the latter the patient cannot read or name colors because the visual information cannot reach the left angular gyrus. There is no difficulty in copying words (though he cannot read what he has written); the visual information for activating the left motor area crosses the corpus callosum more anteriorly. Matching of colors without naming them is done without error.

A disconnection in the anterior third of the corpus callosum, where fiber systems between right and left motor areas pass, results only in failure of the left hand to obey commands, the right one performing perfectly (left-sided motor apraxia). The left one can still imitate the examiner's movements.

Of intrahemispheric disconnections, the following are the most important:

1 Conduction (also called "central") aphasia: the patient has fluent but paraphasic speech and writing with nearly perfect comprehension of spoken or written language.
2 Sympathetic apraxia in Broca's aphasia: a lesion in the subcortical region causes an apraxia of command movements of the left hand.
3 Pure word deafness: although the patient is able to hear and to identify nonverbal sounds, there is loss of ability to comprehend spoken language. The patient's speech remains normal.
4 Alexia and inability to name colors without agraphia: a lesion in the left occipital lobe and splenium of corpus callosum.

OTHER BEHAVIORAL DISORDERS ASSOCIATED WITH CEREBRAL DISEASE When one attempts to categorize all the patients with relatively acute or subacute disorders of mentation and behavior under the section headings above, there are still a considerable number that remain difficult to classify. They present themselves as an almost infinite variety of syndromes in which the following abnormalities of function may occur: reduced or increased levels of speech, thought, and action; disorientation as to time and place; idleness and lack of interest; loss of spontaneity and sense of humor; muteness and hypokinesia, resistiveness and negativism; hostility, lack of observance of social custom, use of abusive and vulgar language; inexplicable fright, euphoria, and lack of proper concern; complaint of visual distortion, of excess sensitivity to sounds; distortions of smell and taste; inability to find the names of objects, to follow a conversation, to think coherently; sexual indiscretion, lack of modesty, and other signs of disinhibition; seizures; disturbances of sleep. Obviously these many symptoms do not all have the same basic significance and the majority possess only relative localizing value. They may be associated with definite hemiparesis, hemihypesthesia, frank aphasia, or homonymous hemianopia, but even without these lateralizing signs they point to the existence of cerebral disease.

Syndromes comprising these elements may be observed in subacute inclusion body encephalitis, Behçet's meningoencephalitis, adult toxoplasmosis, infectious mononucleosis, acute or subacute demyelinative diseases (acute or subacute recurrent multiple sclerosis), granulomatous and other forms of angiitis, gliomatosis cerebri, carcinomatosis with encephalopathy of multifocal type, multiple tumor metastases, acute and subacute bacterial endocarditis, and thrombopenia with multiple-platelet thromboses in small vessels (Moschocowitz's disease). A fuller account of some of these cerebral symptoms is found in descriptions of these diseases.

APPROACH TO THE PATIENT The physician presented with a patient suffering from dementia caused by local cerebral disease must adopt an examination technique designed to expose fully the intellectual defect. Abnormalities of posture, movement, sensation, and reflexes cannot be relied upon for the full demonstration of the neurologic deficit, for it must be remembered that the association areas of the brain may be severely damaged without demonstrable neurologic signs of this type.

Three sources of data are required for the recognition and differential diagnosis of dementing brain disease:

1 A reliable history of the illness
2 Findings on mental examination, i.e., so-called "mental status," as well as on the rest of the neurologic examination
3 Special laboratory procedures, lumbar puncture, x-rays of the skull, electroencephalogram, CAT, and radioactive scanning of the brain, and sometimes pneumoencephalogram

The history should always be supplemented by information obtained from a person other than the patient, because, through lack of insight, the patient is often unaware of his illness; indeed, he may be ignorant even of his chief complaint. Special inquiry should be made about the patient's general behavior, capacity for work, personal habits, and such faculties as memory and judgment.

This performance of an examination of the mental status must be systematic. At a minimum it should include the following:

I Insight (patient's replies to questions about his chief symptoms): What is your difficulty? Are you ill? When did your illness begin?

II Orientation (knowledge of personal identity and present situation): What is your name? What is your occupation? Where do you live? Are you married?
Place: What is the name of the place where you are now? How did you get here? What floor is it on? Where is the bathroom? What are you doing now?
Time: What is the date today? What time of day is it? What meals have you had? When was the last holiday?

III Memory:
Remote: Tell me the names of your children and their birth dates. When were you married? What was your mother's maiden name? What was the name of your first school teacher? What jobs have you held?
Recent past: Tell me about your recent illness (compare with previous statements). What did you have for breakfast today? What is my name or the nurse's name? When did you see me for the first time? What tests were done yesterday? What were the headlines in the newspaper today? Give the patient a simple

story, oral or written, and ask him to recall it after 3 to 5 min.

Immediate recall ("short-term memory"): Repeat these numbers after me (give a series of 3,4,5,6,7,8 digits at speed of one per second). Now when I give a series of numbers, repeat them in reverse order.

Visual span: Show the patient a picture of several objects, ask him to name what he has seen, and note any inaccuracies.

IV General information: Ask about names of presidents, well-known historic dates, the names of large rivers or cities, etc.

V Capacity for sustained mental activity:

Calculation: Test ability to add, substract, multiply, and divide. Subtraction of serial 7s or 3s from 100 is a good test of calculation as well as of concentration.

Abstract thinking: See if the patient can detect similarities and differences between classes of objects, or explain a proverb or a fable.

VI General behavior: Attitudes, general bearing, stream of thought, attentiveness, mood, manner of dress, etc.

VII Special tests of localized cerebral functions: grasping, sucking, aphasia battery, praxis with both hands, cortical sensory function, drawing of clock face, map of United States or Europe, floor plan of house, etc.

In order to enlist the patient's full cooperation, the physician must prepare him for questions of this type. Otherwise, the first reaction will be one of embarrassment or anger because of the implication that his mind is not sound. It should be pointed out to the patient that some individuals are rather forgetful and that it is necessary to ask specific questions in order to form some impression about their degree of nervousness when being examined. Reassurance that these are not tests of intelligence or of sanity is helpful. A more formal and reliable method of examining the mental capacity of adults is the Wechsler-Bellevue test.

The correct diagnosis of treatable forms of senile (over sixty years of age) or presenile (forty to sixty years) dementias, such as general paresis, subdural hematoma, brain tumor, bromide or other chronic drug intoxication, normal-pressure hydrocephalus, pellagra and other deficiency states, and hypothyroidism, is of greater practical importance than the diagnosis of the untreatable ones.

Management of the patient Dementia is a clinical state of the most serious nature, and usually it is worthwhile to admit the patient to the hospital for a period of observation. The physician then has an opportunity to see him several times in a new and fairly constant hospital environment, and certain special procedures such as x-rays of the skull, lumbar puncture, analysis of blood for drugs, basal metabolic rate, an electroencephalogram, and often a pneumonencephalogram can be carried out at this time. The management of the demented patient in the hospital may be relatively simple if he is quiet and cooperative. If the disorder of mental function is severe, a nurse, attendant, or member of the family must stay with him at all times. Provision must be made for adequate food and fluid intake and control of infection, using the same measures outlined for the delirious patient (see Chap. 26).

Once it is established that the patient has an untreatable dementing brain disease, a responsible member of the family should be apprised of the medical facts. The patient should be told that he has a nervous condition for which he is to be given rest and treatment. Nothing is accomplished by telling him more. The family should be given the prognosis, if the diagnosis is sufficiently certain for this to be done. If the dementia is slight and circumstances are suitable, the patient should remain at home, continuing activities of which he is capable. He should be spared responsibility and guarded against injury that might result from imprudent action. If he is still at work, plans for occupational retirement should be carried out. In more advanced stages of the disease mental and physical enfeeblement become pronounced and institutional care should be advised. Seizures should be treated symptomatically. Nerve tonics, vitamins, and hormones are of no value in checking the course of the illness or in regenerating decayed tissue. They may, however, offer some support to the patient and family. Sometimes stimulants in the form of dextroamphetamine, caffeine, and nicotinic acid cause transitory improvement in mental function. Undesirable restlessness, nocturnal wandering, belligerency, or anxiety may be reduced by some of the tranquilizing drugs (see Chap. 121).

REFERENCE

Adams RD, Victor M: *Principles of Neurology,* New York: McGraw-Hill, 1977

section 4 | Alterations in circulatory and respiratory function

28
DISEASES OF THE UPPER RESPIRATORY TRACT

LOUIS WEINSTEIN

Disorders of the upper respiratory tract (nose, nasopharynx, paranasal sinuses, and larynx) are among the commonest forms of human illness. In most instances, they result in discomfort which is more annoying and distracting than disabling, and while they may interfere with the individual's function sufficiently to prevent participation in normal activities, they are not life-threatening nor do they usually lead to serious chronic disability. Less commonly, more serious disorders may present with symptoms referable to the upper respiratory tract.

NOSE

ANOSMIA Total loss of olfactory sense is most common as a transient manifestation of acute infections of the upper respiratory tract. It may be present with chronic nasal obstruction due to edema of the mucosa or marked swelling of the turbinates, with congenital defects, ozena, tumors, (see below), trauma involving the olfactory nerves and nasal polyps.

RHINOPHYMA This is a progressive, deforming, nodular enlargement of the alae nasi due to hypertrophy of sebaceous follicles in association with chronic, severe acne rosacea. There is no specific treatment. Plastic surgery may produce a dramatic degree of improvement.

RHINITIS AND NASAL OBSTRUCTION Intermittent or persistent nasal discharge may be caused by a variety of disorders including hay fever, vasomotor rhinitis and complicating nasal polyposis, acute coryza and other forms of viral rhinitis, the upper respiratory manifestations of measles, syphilis (the "snuffles" of the congenital disease), nasal diphtheria, intranasal foreign bodies, and chronic use of vasoconstrictor drugs.

Acute and self-limited nasal obstruction is usually associated with acute upper respiratory tract infections, most commonly viral. Hypertrophy and inflammation of the turbinates leading to nasal obstruction, with or without persistent nasal discharge, may be caused by allergic reactions. A common reason for difficulty in breathing through the nose is a deviated septum. Menstruation is associated, in some instances, with bogginess of the turbinates to a degree sufficient to produce retardation of airflow through the nose; pregnancy may produce the same phenomenon.

RHINORRHEA Although unilateral nasal discharge may be caused by intranasal foreign bodies, when it is intermittent or persistent, the possibility that it is due to *cerebrospinal fluid (CSF) rhinorrhea* must be considered. This condition may be diagnosed by injecting a marker such as a dye (fluorescein) or a radioactive tracer into the CSF and following its appearance in nasal secretions. A positive reaction for glucose indicates that the nasal discharge is cerebrospinal fluid.

OZENA This is a severe chronic rhinitis of unknown cause, characterized by thick, greenish discharge, mucosal crusts, atrophy of the turbinates, and an offensive odor. Patients eventually become anosmic. Even when the nasal passages are widened and resistance to airflow is decreased, obstruction is a constant complaint. Cultures grow gram-negative bacilli (*Klebsiella, Pseudomonas,* etc.). Treatment, aimed at reducing the odor, includes use of local or systemic antibiotics and large doses of vasodilators (Priscoline, nicotinic acid). Local cleansing by means of repeated saline irrigation is extremely important to eliminate foul-smelling crusts.

PERFORATION OF THE NASAL SEPTUM A variety of conditions may cause perforation of the nasal septum, including chronic nose "picking," prolonged use of potent vasoconstrictors, chronic sniffing of cocaine, cautery of the nasal septum for repeated episodes of epistaxis, tumors of the nose invading the septum, nasal septal surgery, rheumatoid arthritis, syphilis, the espundia type of American leishmaniasis, South American blastomycosis, midline granuloma, Wegener's granulomatosis, and phycomycosis.

EPISTAXIS Probably the commonest cause is nose picking, leading to tearing of the rich network of veins in the anterior nares (Kiesselbach's plexus). Among the infections in which acute nosebleed may develop are typhoid fever, unilateral nasal diphtheria, pertussis, and malaria. Minor epistaxis may also appear in the course of viral infections of the upper respiratory tract. Other causes of intermittent or repeated episodes of epistaxis are atheromas of the nasal vessels, hypertension, vicarious menstruation, bleeding diatheses including thrombocytopenia of different etiologies and deficiencies of clotting factors, polycythemia vera, rhinoliths, acute sinusitis especially involving the ethmoid sinus, tumors of the nose and paranasal sinuses, and nasal angiomas. Episodes of bleeding or the severity of attacks are frequently increased in patients receiving aspirin. Vitamin C and prothrombin deficiency are *not* associated with isolated epistaxis, although this may occur with bleeding from other sites. In hereditary hemorrhagic telangiectasia (Osler-Rendu-Weber syndrome) the only site of bleeding may be the nose; a family history of repeated hemorrhages from this and other sites should suggest this diagnosis.

NASAL FURUNCULOSIS Furuncules involving the internal or external surfaces of the nose pose potential threats to life because of the possibility of spread to the cavernous sinus via the draining veins. When seen in their early stage, they respond rapidly to antimicrobial therapy which should be directed primarily against *Staphylococcus aureus* and given in large doses (Chap. 134). Oral treatment may be adequate in the early stages of the disease, but parenteral therapy is necessary when the constitutional reaction is severe and there is marked edema of the intra- or extranasal tissues. *Under no circumstances should these lesions be squeezed* because of the danger of spread of organisms to intracranial venous sinuses. Also, incision for drainage should not be carried out unless pain becomes severe or the lesion has become large.

NASAL TUMORS Basal cell carcinoma of the skin covering the nose is the commonest malignant tumor of this organ. Rodent ulcer resulting from local spread of a basal-cell lesion may involve not only the skin over the external nasal surface and adjacent areas of the face, but may also invade intranasally and produce marked destruction of the internal structures.

PHARYNX

ACUTE PHARYNGITIS The outstanding symptom of acute pharyngitis, regardless of cause, is a sore throat. About two-thirds of all acute illnesses in families are viral infections of the upper respiratory tract, with varying degrees of pharyngeal discomfort present. The acute pharyngitides can be classified into three groups: (1) Treatable infections, (2) untreatable infections, and (3) noninfectious disorders (Table 28-1).

Physical examination of the pharyngeal mucosa may reveal changes varying in intensity from mild redness and congestion of blood vessels (many viral infections) to intense red-purple color, patchy yellow exudate, hypertrophy of all the lymphoid tissue, and marked vascular injection (e.g., severe disease due to group A *Streptococcus pyogenes*). Symptoms may be variable and may range from a complaint of "scratchy throat" to pain so severe that swallowing of saliva is difficult. The presence of exudate does not establish a specific etiology and may be noted in infections due to *Strep. pyogenes, Hemophilus influenzae, H. parainfluenzae* (children), *Corynebacterium diphtheriae, Strep. pneumoniae* (rare) as well as in some viral diseases, such as those caused by adenovirus. Ulcerations involving the posterior pharyngeal wall and/or tonsils are characteristically present in fusobacterial infections (Plaut-Vincent's angina), pharyngeal tularemia, syphilis (primary chancre), tuberculosis, following local trauma to the pharynx, and in immunosuppressed and agranulocytic patients in whom invasion by fusobacteria or other members of the indigenous pharyngeal microflora takes place. The presence of limited or extensive pseudomembrane does not always indicate a specific microbial cause. While most characteristic of faucial diphtheria, such lesions may be present in infectious mononucleosis, agranulocytosis, staphylococcal pharyngitis, and diffuse injury to the pharyngeal mucosa following direct trauma or chemical or thermal burns.

The tonsils are often involved in the course of viral and bacterial pharyngitis; they may be markedly reddened and swollen and contain exudate in the crypts.

The etiologic diagnosis of acute pharyngitis is difficult to establish on the basis of visual examination of the throat. However, in some instances in which characteristic findings are present, such as the typical pseudomembrane and suggestive odor of diphtheria, severe group A streptococcal infection, the ulceration and anaerobic odor of fusobacterial disease, or the white irregular patches overlying shallow ulcers produced by *Candida,* a specific cause may be suspected.

Cultures of the pharyngeal mucosa, tonsils, or exudate will usually reveal the bacteria responsible for the disease and determine the choice of antimicrobial agent. It should

TABLE 28-1
Etiology of pharyngitis

I Infections
- *A* Treatable
  - *1* Group A *Streptococcus pyogenes*
  - *2* *Hemophilus influenzae*
  - *3* *H. parainfluenzae*
  - *4* *Neisseria gonorrhoeae*
  - *5* *N. meningitidis*
  - *6* *Corynebacterium diphtheriae*
  - *7* *Spirochaeta pallida*
  - *8* *Fusobacterium*
  - *9* *F. tularensis*
  - *10* *Candida*
  - *11* *Cryptococcus*
  - *12* *Histoplasma*
  - *13* *Mycoplasma pneumoniae* (?)
  - *14* *Streptococcus pneumoniae* (?)
  - *15* *Staphylococcus aureus* or gram-negative bacilli are rare and are usually found in neutropenic patients or those treated with antibiotics
- *B* Untreatable
  - *1* Primary
    - *a* Influenza virus
    - *b* Rhinovirus
    - *c* Coxsackie virus A
    - *d* Epstein-Barr virus
    - *e* Echo virus
    - *f* Herpes simplex
    - *g* Reovirus
  - *2* Manifestation of systemic disease
    - *a* Poliomyelitis
    - *b* Measles
    - *c* Chickenpox
    - *d* Smallpox
    - *e* Viral hepatitis
    - *f* Rubella
    - *g* Pertussis

II Noninfectious
- *A* Trauma by heat, sharp objects, etc.
- *B* Inhalation of irritants
- *C* Dehydration—mouth breathing
- *D* Glossopharyngeal neuralgia
- *E* Subacute thyroiditis (tends to be prolonged or frequently recurrent, often associated with low-grade fever)
- *F* Psychogenic (see comment above)
- *G* Monomyelocytic leukemia
- *H* Immunosuppressed state

be stressed, however, that these are not always rewarding. For example, only 70 percent of single throat cultures yield group A *Strep. pyogenes* even when pharyngitis due to this organism is severe. The sore throat of subacute thyroiditis may be relieved occasionally by the administration of thyroid hormone or prednisone. None of the viral pharyngitides is treatable.

PERITONSILLAR CELLULITIS AND ABSCESS (QUINSY) This condition is most often a complication of acute pharyngitis. The organisms commonly involved are group A *Strep. pyogenes* and *Staph. aureus.* The first sign of this disease is marked enlargement of the tonsils which are surrounded by red, edematous pillars. The tonsillar and peritonsillar hypertrophy may progress to a degree threatening occlusion of the upper airway. High-grade fever and leukocytosis are present, and severe rigors may occur. In its early stages, the process is a cellulitis, but, in the absence of therapy, abscess develops, as infection progresses and involves one or both tonsils; at this time, soft grayish-white exudate may cover the tonsillar surfaces. The diagnosis is made purely on the basis of the physical findings. If detected early when only peritonsillar cellulitis is present, administration of a properly selected antimicrobial agent may clear the infection and abort the development of abscess. Antimicrobial therapy alone is inadequate after abscess has developed. The optimal treatment at this stage is incision and drainage of the involved tonsil(s).

PARAPHARYNGEAL SPACE ABSCESS This syndrome is always a complication of acute pharyngitis. Primary or secondary bacterial invasion of one of the tonsils results in the development of an intratonsillar abscess accompanied by considerable edema and inflammatory reaction in the parapharyngeal space. The lesion is usually unilateral; there is frequently very little pharyngeal discomfort, but there is marked tenderness at the angle of the jaw on the same side as the tonsillar abscess. The remainder of the throat frequently has a benign appearance. There is usually considerable fever and leukocytosis. If unrecognized and not treated early in its course, the infection spreads through the tonsillar veins to the jugular vein where it produces thrombophlebitis. Septic emboli from this source may be widely disseminated and cause widespread metastatic thrombosis and infection, a highly fatal syndrome termed *postanginal sepsis.* Early recognition and institution of therapy before spread to the jugular vein results in rapid clearing of the infection.

RETROPHARYNGEAL ABSCESS Infection of the retropharyngeal lymph nodes occurs most often as a complication of acute bacterial pharyngitis in children 3 years of age or younger; these nodes disappear rapidly after this age. Adults usually acquire the disease as a result of injury to the posterior pharyngeal wall by a sharp object, as a complication of neglected acute infections of the middle ear, during the course of tuberculosis, or secondary to suppurative parotitis. A universal symptom is the sensation of a "lump in the throat that cannot be swallowed." Dyspnea that is present in the sitting position and absent when the patient lies on his back and pain on swallowing are common. The voice has a characteristic quality that has been likened to the cry of a duck *(cri du canard).* Cough, snoring, choking, and stertorous breathing are often present. As the abscess enlarges, progressive airway obstruction develops, marked edema and redness of the entire posterior pharynx and cervical lymphadenopathy are common, and there is usually high fever. When recognized early, most retropharyngeal abscesses respond promptly to antimicrobial therapy. Because most of the organisms involved are gram-positive cocci, parenteral administration of a penicillinase-resistant penicillin or a cephalosporin compound is usually effective; in young children, therapy must include agents effective against *H. influenzae.* If the abscess comes to attention late in its course, or if obstruction of the airway is progressing rapidly, the lesion must be drained surgically and chemotherapy must be given before, during, and after the procedure. Tracheostomy may be necessary in far-advanced cases.

TUMORS OF THE TONSILS Carcinoma of the tonsil is the second commonest tumor of the upper airway (osteoma being the commonest; see below). Other neoplastic tonsillar lesions include lymphoma and Hodgkin's disease. Persistence of pain in one enlarged firm tonsil, in the absence of an infectious process, is an indication for biopsy. The presence of fever does not rule out a neoplastic lesion because considerable elevation of the temperature may be present when lymphoma is the cause.

LINGUAL TONSILS These are situated on the posterior borders of the tongue and extend from the circumvallate papillae to the epiglottis. Infection produces lingual pain that may be severe and markedly increased by movement of the tongue. Sore throat is often absent or mild; when the responsible organism is *Strep. pyogenes,* fever is present. Examination of the posterior tongue reveals swelling and redness of the lymphoid masses; yellow exudate is present in the crypts when group A streptococci are the cause of the disease. The pharynx may appear normal or only slightly reddened.

SINUSES

ACUTE SINUSITIS The organisms most often responsible for acute sinusitis are *Strep. pneumoniae,* group A *Strep. pyogenes, Staph. aureus,* and *H. influenzae.* Other bacteria may be involved in patients receiving immunosuppressive therapy, in those who have received antibiotics, or in whom penetrating trauma, local tumors, or vasculitis is a predisposing factor. The etiology of chronic sinusitis may be the same as that of the acute form, but more than one pathogen may be present. In many instances, however, cultures yield only members of the indigenous microflora of the upper respiratory tract.

The commonest predisposing factor of acute purulent sinusitis is viral infection of the upper respiratory tract, which may lead to obstruction of drainage of the paranasal sinuses and the development of localized pain, tenderness, and low-grade fever. These manifestations usually clear as the viral disease subsides. In a number of instances, however, invasion by pyogenic bacteria supervenes and is responsible for the development of purulent sinusitis. Obstruction of meatal drainage of any type or direct introduction of bacteria into the sinuses may lead to the development of acute infection of the paranasal sinuses. Abscesses of the roots of the upper bicuspid or molar teeth that rupture into the maxillary sinuses, swimming and diving, and direct local injury may be inciting mechanisms. Fractures of the bones encompassing the sinuses, especially the frontals and ethmoids, may be followed by infection. Wegener's granulomatosis and tumors of the meatuses of the turbinates may produce the clinical picture of acute or chronic sinusitis. In some of these patients, bacterial infection is superimposed, and these patients are studied only after infection develops, the underlying lesion often being overlooked. This underscores the fact that recurrent or prolonged episodes of sinusitis that are refractory to antimicrobial therapy, or that relapse soon after treatment is discontinued, must be investigated thoroughly for the presence of a noninfectious obstructing lesion.

The diagnosis of acute purulent sinusitis is usually made when constitutional manifestations are present such as fever, chills, pain and tenderness of the involved sinuses, nasal obstruction and recurrent headaches that change in intensity with position and disappear shortly after getting out of bed. Isolation of a pathogenic organism from the nasal secretions or from material draining into the meatuses of the nasal turbinates may help to solidify the diagnosis. When there is marked swelling of the turbinates, they can be shrunk by the local application of cocaine or other potent vasoconstrictors. This exposes the meatuses and permits the collection of exudate draining directly from the involved sinus. Transillumination of the sinuses is also helpful, while radiologic study is of value in identifying the specific sinus involved.

Frontal sinusitis is characterized by pain over the forehead approximately in the area of the underlying sinus. Although the overlying site is usually normal, it may be swollen and reddened over an area outlining the sinuses. Pressure applied over the sinuses and on the lateral edge of the orbital ridges produces pain. Examination of the nasal turbinates shows purulent exudate in the middle meatus if drainage is not prevented by swelling of these structures. Pain, swelling, and tenderness in the anterior portions of the maxillae are the outstanding features of *maxillary sinusitis.* When the infection is severe, pain may be referred to the upper teeth which may become loosened, and hemorrhage may be present in the surrounding tissues. Pus is visible in the middle meatus of the turbinates. The symptoms and signs of *ethmoid sinusitis* are pain in the upper lateral areas of the nose, frontal headache, and redness of the skin and tenderness to pressure over the upper lateral areas of the nasal bones adjacent to the inner canthi of the eyes. Pus is visible in the middle meatus when the anterior cells of the sinus are involved, and in the superior meatus if the posterior cells are infected; in most instances, both areas of the sinus are involved and exudate is present in both meatuses. The manifestations of infection of the *sphenoid sinus* are tenderness and pain over the vertex of the skull, the mastoid bones (in the presence of normal tympanic membranes), and the occipital portion of the head. Rarely, streaks of redness may be detectable over both zygomas as a result of irritation of a branch of the trigeminal nerve that lies in close proximity to the sinus.

Osteomyelitis of the frontal bone is a rare complication of frontal sinusitis. This is characterized by fever, chills, leukocytosis, frontal headache, and the presence of cool, pale edema over the forehead (Pott's puffy tumor). Despite absence of signs of inflammation in the overlying skin, aspiration of the subgaleal area frequently yields purulent exudate. Involvement of the bone in which the ethmoid sinus lies may be manifest by unilateral or bilateral exophthalmos when one or both sinuses are involved. This is usually due to a sterile or pyogenic orbital cellulitis secondary to a "sympathetic" inflammation or perforation of the lamina papyralla, the lateral wall of the sinus, and the medial wall of the orbit. Complications of venous return from the orbits may supervene because of intracranial spread of infection from the sinuses through the diploic veins. Among these are meningitis, infection, and thrombosis of the superficial cerebral veins or cavernous and sagittal venous sinuses, cranial nerve palsies, and extradural abscess.

Bacterial meningitis is also a rare complication of purulent sinusitis, usually involving the frontal sinuses, and associated with cranial osteomyelitis and subdural and brain abscess. Sudden onset of convulsions, hemiplegia, and aphasia in a patient with acute frontal sinusitis should suggest the possibility of subdural abscess with thrombophlebitis of the sagittal sinus or superficial cerebral veins. Infections of the ethmoid sinus may be complicated by paralysis of the third cranial nerve due to invasion of the dural sinuses, or profuse epistaxis as a result of thrombosis of the ethmoidal veins that drain into the cavernous sinus, which may become thrombosed. Chronic or recurrent purulent sinusitis may eventually be responsible for the development of bronchiectasis. An unusual form of chronic sinusitis in association with bronchiectasis and situs inversus is *Kartagener's syndrome.*

CHRONIC SINUSITIS It is difficult to establish the diagnosis of chronic sinusitis in the absence of documented recurrences of acute purulent infection. Many patients complaining of headaches, often frontal in nature, and troubled by obstruction of the nasal airway, may have some degree of tenderness over any of the paranasal sinuses. X-ray examinations of the sinuses often reveal thickening of the mucous membranes. Cultures of the nose or nasal discharge frequently yield no pathogenic organisms. In many instances, an allergic background is present in individuals with this syndrome; in these cases, relief of symptoms is often produced by the judicious use of nasal vasoconstrictors, and treatment is directed to the specific allergy. Occasionally, chronic sinusitis is due to persistent infection, as demonstrated by repeated isolation of a pathogenic organism. However, there is considerable experience to suggest that the manifestations presented by many patients are not related to chronic infection, but are due to other factors such as irritating dusts or gases or excessive exposure to tobacco smoke.

Effective management of acute sinusitis rests on demonstration of a specific pathogenic organism in the secretion present in the nose or drained from the sinuses, testing of the organism for sensitivity to a variety of antimicrobial agents, and administration of the most active agent in adequate dose. The antibiotics most effective for the bacteria most frequently involved in this disease are discussed in Chap. 130. Vasoconstrictors are of help in producing transient relief of symptoms, but must not be used excessively. Surgical drainage may be indicated when infection becomes prolonged or local or intracranial complications develop.

TUMORS OF THE SINUSES The commonest benign tumor of the paranasal sinuses is osteoma. Fifty percent of cases involve the frontal, 40 percent the ethmoid, and 10 percent the maxillary and sphenoid sinuses. The malignant tumors include carcinoma of the maxilla, sarcoma, Burkitt's lymphoma, myeloma, and adenocarcinoma. Melanoma of the nasal cavity may extend into the paranasal sinuses. Other malignant diseases originating in the sinuses may invade the nasal cavity and, because they produce obstruction, lead to consideration of the nose as the primary site of the lesion. A neoplastic lesion should be ruled out in patients who experience repeated episodes of acute sinusitis or who have chronic symptoms, particularly repeated epistaxis in the absence of an identifiable pathogenic organism.

LARYNX

SYMPTOMS AND SIGNS OF LARYNGEAL DISEASE There are three main causes of laryngeal disease: (1) Intralaryngeal lesions, (2) extralaryngeal processes that produce other manifestations by direct pressure on either the larynx or the nerves that supply the vocal cords, and (3) disorders in which either local or diffuse disease of the nervous system leads to dysfunction of the vocal cords. A differential diagnosis of the various disorders of the larynx is presented in Table 28-2.

Hoarseness is the commonest symptom of disorders of the larynx, regardless of etiology. The common denominator of the numerous causes of this symptom is interference with normal phonatory function of the larynx. Both inflammatory and noninflammatory diseases of this organ as well as functional disturbances (hysterical aphonia) may be causative factors. Although hoarseness is usually of short duration with acute self-limited processes such as infections, it may persist for long periods.

Cough is common with any type of laryngeal disease. *Pain* occurs occasionally, while *stridor* and *dyspnea* are uncommon manifestations of laryngeal involvement. However, when present, the latter are ominous because they indicate the development of airway obstruction which may rapidly become complete. Obstruction to breathing is not only associated with intralaryngeal lesions or those which exert pressure directly on this organ, but may occur as a result of neurologic disorders in which paralysis of both vocal cords develops.

The exact cause of laryngeal obstruction can be detected only by direct or indirect examination of the larynx. *This is usually necessary when manifestations have persisted for longer than 2 or 3 weeks.* However, if serious obstruction of the airway develops rapidly in acute disorders of the larynx, laryngoscopic examination should be carried out promptly and tracheostomy performed if necessary.

The three disorders of the larynx described below require specific and early diagnosis because of their life-threatening potential.

ACUTE EPIGLOTTITIS Acute infections of the epiglottis are most commonly caused by *H. influenzae* in children; this organism, as well as the pneumococcus and group A streptococci, may be responsible for the disease in all age groups. The onset of symptoms is often very rapid and is

TABLE 28-2
Differential diagnosis of hoarseness and other manifestations of laryngeal dysfunction

- *I* Intralaryngeal disease
  - *A* Infectious
    - *1* Common cold
    - *2* Viral laryngitis
    - *3* *Hemophilus influenzae*
    - *4* *Membranous laryngitis (Streptococcus pyogenes, Pseudomonas, Fusobacterium)*
    - *5* Diphtheria (laryngeal membrane)
    - *6* Herpes simplex
    - *7* Actinomycosis
    - *8* Candidiasis
    - *9* Blastomycosis
    - *10* Tuberculosis (ulcers)
    - *11* Syphilis (secondary stage, chondritis, gumma)
  - *B* Noninfectious
    - *1* Trauma (edema or hematoma)
    - *2* Vocal cord nodules (singer's nodes)
    - *3* Papillomas of vocal cords
    - *4* Pachyderma of vocal cords
    - *5* Inhalation of smoke, fire, irritating gases, tobacco smoke
    - *6* Leukoplakia of vocal cords
    - *7* Rheumatoid arthritis (involvement of cricoarytenoid joint)
    - *8* Chronic alcoholism
    - *9* Benign tumors
    - *10* Cancer
    - *11* Foreign bodies
- *II* Extralaryngeal disease
  - *A* Lesions in neck [produce hoarseness because of (1) pressure on larynx that interferes with movement of vocal cords, (2) edema secondary to decreased venous and lymphatic drainage, and (3) impingement on laryngeal nerves with paresis or paralysis of cords]
    - *1* Hemorrhages and/or edema due to trauma, severe traction of neck, thyroidectomy, tracheostomy, and biopsy of scalene node
    - *2* Tumors of hypopharynx
    - *3* Tumors of carotid body
    - *4* Thrombophlebitis of jugular bulb
  - *B* Local and systemic disorders outside neck (produce hoarseness by pressure on laryngeal nerves anywhere along the course outside the neck, or paresis or paralysis of the vocal cords as a manifestation of generalized neurologic dysfunction)
    - *1* Local lesions
      - *a* Bacterial meningitis
      - *b* Meningovascular syphilis
      - *c* Infectious mononucleosis (enlarged mediastinal nodes)
      - *d* Angioneurotic edema
      - *e* Mitral stenosis (enlarged pulmonary artery)
      - *f* Aneurysms of arch of aorta, carotid or innominate arteries
      - *g* Ligation or patent ductus arteriosus
      - *h* Tumors of mediastinal structures
      - *i* Tumors of parotid gland
      - *j* Relapsing polychondritis
      - *k* Neoplastic disease of meninges
      - *l* Fracture of base of skull
      - *m* Cancer or nodules of thyroid
      - *n* Goiter
    - *2* Systemic disorders
      - *a* Diphtheria (peripheral neuritis)
      - *b* Poliomyelitis (bulbar)
      - *c* Infectious mononucleosis (nervous system involvement)
      - *d* Herpes zoster
      - *e* Mucoviscidosis
      - *f* Myxedema
      - *g* Acromegaly
      - *h* Wegener's granulomatosis
      - *i* Lupus erythematosus
      - *j* Diabetic neuropathy
      - *k* Poisoning by lead, mercury, arsenic, botulinus toxin

characterized by varying degrees of fever, severe sore throat, pooling of pharyngeal secretions, drooling, and dysphagia. Stridor is rapidly followed by increasing difficulty in breathing as airway obstruction develops. If untreated, there is increasing use of the accessory muscles of respiration followed by cyanosis, prostration, and finally shock.

Examination of the hypopharynx reveals a markedly swollen, cherry-red epiglottis, which may be necrotic when *Strep. pyogenes* is involved. Treatment must be undertaken early, preferably before there is evidence of severe respiratory distress. In such instances, the administration of ampicillin or any other antimicrobial agent effective against the organisms most often involved, together with inhalation of moist air and oxygen, will often prevent progression of the disease. When it is clear that the airway is seriously threatened, tracheostomy, in addition to chemotherapy, is urgently indicated.

FOREIGN BODY Inhalation of a foreign body rapidly produces symptoms. *Pain* is "sticking" in quality and localized to the larynx. *Laryngeal spasm* is usually present. *Dyspnea* may develop as a result of edema and lead to a degree of obstruction sufficient to compromise the airway. There is often a *change in the quality of the voice;* complete *aphonia* may occur. If the inhaled object is sharp, as a chicken bone, there is rapid development of local swelling and progressive obstruction to breathing. Perforation of the larynx may occur and lead to infection that extends from the local site to other areas in the neck and mediastinum. If the inhaled object is lying loosely in the larynx, three diagnostical signs are helpful. These are the *wheeze, palpatory thud* (palpating fingers detect a thud over the larynx during respirations), and *auscultatory slap* (a slapping noise is heard over the larynx as its walls are hit by the foreign body when it moves while breathing). Suspicion of a foreign body makes mirror or laryngoscopic examination an emergency procedure.

CANCER OF THE LARYNX This lesion develops at an average age of 60 years and is ten times more common in men than in women. Cancers of the larynx are of two types: *intrinsic,* arising on the vocal cords (70 percent of the cases), and *extrinsic,* extending beyond the vocal cords. Although hoarseness develops early in the course of intrinsic lesions, it is frequently late in onset with extrinsic ones. The treatment of choice for this disease is surgery.

Small lesions of the middle third of the cord often respond to radiation alone. Total or partial laryngectomy is required in the majority of cases. When the cancer involves the epiglottis and/or the false cords, partial supraglottic laryngectomy is the preferred operative procedure because it does not result in loss of normal speech and has a high chance of cure. In some instances, preoperative irradiation of the larynx and surrounding lymph nodes may help in the eradication of the tumor. About 90 percent of cancers of the larynx are cured if detected and treated early.

REFERENCES

BALLENGER JJ: *Diseases of the Nose, Throat and Ear,* 11th ed., Philadelphia: Lea & Febiger, 1969

DEWEESE DD, SAUNDERS WH: *Textbook of Otolaryngology,* 4th ed., St. Louis: Mosby, 1973

SCOTT-BROWN WG: *Diseases of the Ear, Nose and Throat,* vol. 3. *The Nose,* 3d ed., eds V Ballantine, J Groves, Philadelphia: Lippincott, 1971

——: *Diseases of the Ear, Nose and Throat,* vol. 4. *The Throat,* 3d ed., eds V Ballantine, J Groves, Philadelphia: Lippincott, 1971

29 COUGH AND HEMOPTYSIS

GENNARO M. TISI
EUGENE BRAUNWALD

COUGH

Cough, one of the most frequent cardiorespiratory symptoms, is an explosive expiration which provides a means of clearing the tracheobronchial tree of secretions and foreign bodies.

MECHANISM Coughing may be initiated either voluntarily or reflexly. As a defensive reflex it has both afferent and efferent pathways. The *afferent limb* includes cough receptors within the sensory distribution of the trigeminal, glossopharyngeal, superior laryngeal, and vagus nerves. The *efferent limb* includes the recurrent laryngeal nerve (which causes glottic closure) and the spinal nerves (which cause contraction of the thoracic and abdominal musculature). The *sequence of a cough* includes an appropriate stimulus which initiates a deep inspiration. This is followed by glottic closure, relaxation of the diaphragm, and muscle contraction against a closed glottis so as to produce maximally positive intrathoracic and intraairway pressures. These positive intrathoracic pressures result in a narrowing of the trachea, produced by an infolding of its more compliant posterior membrane. Once the glottis opens, the combination of a large pressure differential between the airways and the atmosphere coupled with this tracheal narrowing produces flow rates through the trachea close to the speed of sound. The shearing forces which are developed aid in the elimination of mucus and foreign materials. A tracheostomy short-circuits glottic closure and therefore decreases the effectiveness of the cough mechanism.

ETIOLOGY Cough is produced by inflammatory, mechanical, chemical, and thermal stimulation of the cough receptors. *Inflammatory* stimuli are initiated by edema and hyperemia of the respiratory mucous membranes, and by irritation from exudative processes. Such stimuli may arise either in the airways (as in laryngitis, tracheitis, bronchitis, and bronchiolitis) or in the alveoli (as in pneumonitis and lung abscess). *Mechanical* stimuli are produced by inhalation of particulate matter, such as dust particles, and by compression of the air passages and pressure or tension upon these structures. Lesions associated with airway compression may be either extramural or intramural in type. The former include aortic aneurysms, granulomas, pulmonary neoplasms, and mediastinal tumors; intramural lesions include bronchogenic carcinoma, bronchial adenoma, foreign bodies, granulomatous endobronchial involvement, and contraction of airway smooth muscle (bronchial asthma). Pressure or tension upon the air passages is usually produced by lesions associated with a decrease in pulmonary compliance. Examples of specific causes include acute and chronic interstitial fibrosis (Chap. 260), pulmonary edema, and atelectasis. *Chemical* stimuli may result from inhalation of irritant gases, including cigarette smoke, and of chemical fumes. Finally, *thermal* stimuli may be produced by inhalation of either very hot or cold air.

DIAGNOSTIC EVALUATION When one is considering the above list of causes, answers to the following general questions will significantly narrow the diagnostic possibilities: Is the cough acute or chronic? Is it productive of sputum or nonproductive? A chronic productive cough may be caused by diseases such as chronic bronchitis, pulmonary tuberculosis, and pulmonary neoplasms. Are the findings on physical examination of the chest normal or abnormal? Is the chest roentgenogram normal or abnormal?

Features of the history, physical examination, chest roentgenogram, screening pulmonary function studies (static lung volumes and dynamic flow rates), and sputum examination may indicate a specific cause. The *history* may indicate specific diagnoses. Acute episodes of cough may be associated with such viral infections as acute tracheobronchitis or pneumonitis or with bacterial bronchopneumonia. Cough associated with an acute febrile episode and associated with hoarseness is usually produced by viral laryngotracheobronchitis. The character of the cough may suggest the anatomic site of involvement: the patient with a "barking" type of cough may have epiglottal involvement, while the cough associated with tracheal or major airway involvement is often loud and "brassy." Cough associated with generalized wheezing may be produced by acute bronchospasm. The time of occurrence of a cough may indicate a specific cause: a cough which occurs selectively at night suggests congestive heart failure; one related to meals suggests a tracheoesophageal fistula, a hiatal hernia, or an esophageal diverticulum; a cough precipitated by a change in position suggests a lung abscess or a localized area of bronchiectasis. The description of sputum or secretions produced in conjunction with the cough may also be helpful: putrid sputum suggests a lung abscess; bloody sputum, bleeding (see Hemoptysis below); frothy and pink-tinged sputum, pulmonary edema; mucoid and massive sputum, alveolar cell carcinoma; purulent and/or large amounts of sputum, lung abscess and bronchiectasis. On *physical examination* the character of the auscultatory findings may suggest the site of disease: inspiratory stridor and wheezing may be present in laryngeal disease; inspiratory and expiratory rhonchi favor tracheal and major airway involvement; coarse subcrepitant inspiratory rales may indicate interstitial fibrosis and/or edema; fine crepitant rales may indicate a process such as pneumonitis or pulmonary edema, which fills the alveoli with fluid. The *chest roentgenogram* may reveal the cause of the cough; it may show an intrapulmonary mass lesion which may be either central or peripheral (Chap. 263), an alveolar filling process which may be pneumonic or nonpneumonic, an area of honeycombing and cyst formation which may indicate an area of localized bronchiectasis, or bilateral hilar adenopathy which may indicate sarcoidosis or a lymphoma. *Screening pulmonary function* studies may also indicate specific diagnoses. Significant expiratory obstruction to airflow (as determined from a forced expiratory flow maneuver), coupled with a history of cough and significant sputum production, suggests that irrespective of other lesions the patient has significant bronchitis. Decreased lung volume (as determined from the static lung volumes) indicates that a restrictive type of lung disease is present—reduction of lung volumes produced by thoracic, pleural, alveolar, or interstitial disease. Finally, a careful *sputum examination* may be more enlightening than a patient's description of the character of his sputum. Examination shows whether the sputum is thin or viscid, purulent or not, foul-smelling or not, blood tinged or not, scant or copious. Gram stain and culture of the deep-cough specimen may reveal a specific bacterial, fungal, or mycoplasmal causation, while sputum cytology may result in a positive diagnosis of a pulmonary neoplasm.

Two features of cough should be highlighted. (1) A cough is often so common in the cigarette smoker as to be ignored or minimized. *Any changes in the nature and character of a chronic cigarette cough should initiate immediate diagnostic evaluation, with particular attention directed to detection of bronchogenic carcinoma.* (2) Female patients are inclined to swallow sputum and not to expectorate as male patients do. This tendency may lead to the incorrect conclusion that a cough in a female patient is irritative and nonproductive.

COMPLICATIONS Three complications may be produced by the coughing mechanism: paroxysms of coughing may precipitate syncope (cough syncope, Chap. 16), and strenuous coughing may produce rupture of an emphysematous bleb and rib fractures. A potential mechanism for cough syncope includes the development of markedly positive intrathoracic and alveolar pressures which decrease venous return, producing a decrease in cardiac output and resultant syncope. Although cough fractures of the ribs may occur in otherwise normal patients, their occurrence should at least raise the possibility of pathologic fractures, which are seen in multiple myeloma, osteoporosis, and osteolytic metastases.

THERAPY Specific treatment of cough depends upon the underlying cause. An irritative, nonproductive cough may be suppressed by an antitussive agent, such as codeine or dextromethorphan, 15 mg q.i.d. These drugs are particularly useful in interrupting prolonged, self-perpetuating paroxysms. However, a cough productive of significant quantities of sputum should not be suppressed, since retention of sputum in the tracheobronchial tree may interfere with alveolar aeration and impair the ability of the lung to resist infection. When secretions are tenacious and thick, adequate hydration, expectorants (such as potassium iodide), and humidification of the air with an ultrasonic nebulizer may be helpful.

HEMOPTYSIS

For purposes of definition hemoptysis includes both blood-streaked sputum and gross hemoptysis. It is apparent that any patient with gross hemoptysis should be given appropriate diagnostic tests so that a specific cause may be found. The patient with blood-streaked sputum should also be studied unless one can be certain that this type of hemoptysis is due to a benign condition. A major pitfall in dealing with hemoptysis is to ascribe recurrent episodes of hemoptysis to a previously established diagnosis, such as chronic bronchiectasis or bronchitis. Such an approach may result in missing a serious but potentially treatable lesion. The safest approach to a recurrent episode of hemoptysis is to treat it as if it were the initial episode and proceed with a complete diagnostic evaluation.

ETIOLOGY AND INCIDENCE Prior to embarking upon an extensive diagnostic workup of hemoptysis, it is essential to determine that the blood is in fact coming from the respiratory tract, not from the nasopharynx or gastrointestinal tract. Once this point is established, the diagnostic tests for hemoptysis may proceed. Although there are numerous single case reports of diseases which have been associated with hemoptysis, Table 29-1 presents the more common disorders.

The incidence of the diagnoses listed in Table 29-1 depends upon the nature of the series reported and whether one includes both gross bleeding and blood streaking of the sputum. If both types of bleeding are included, then the major causes (approximately 60 to 70 percent) are chronic bronchitis and bronchiectasis. If the definition is restricted to gross bleeding (greater than several tablespoons) then the incidence depends upon the type of series reported. Surgical series favor the incidence of mass lesions and operable lesions (carcinoma, 20 percent; localized, segmental, or lobar bronchiectasis, 30 percent). Those from centers with a large tuberculosis population favor this condition (incidence varying between 2 and 40 percent). Combined medical-surgical series include a wider representation of those lesions which present with hemoptysis (carcinoma, 20 percent; bronchiectasis, 30 percent; bronchitis, 15 percent; other inflammatory lesions including tuberculosis, 10 to 20 percent; other lesions including the vascular, traumatic, and hemorrhagic etiologies listed in Table 29-1, 10 percent). Despite the most extensive of evaluations, 5 to 15 percent of cases entailing gross hemoptysis remain undiagnosed.

Two points should be highlighted with reference to diseases associated with hemoptysis: (1) *hemoptysis is rare in metastatic carcinoma to the lung;* (2) *although hemoptysis may occur at some time during the course of a viral or bacterial pneumonia, it is usually scanty and its occurrence should always raise the question of a more serious underlying process.*

DIAGNOSIS The *history* may suggest specific diagnoses: recurrent, chronic hemoptysis in a young, otherwise asymptomatic female favors the diagnosis of a bronchial adenoma; recurrent hemoptysis with chronic, marked sputum production associated with ring shadows, tram lines (abnormal air bronchograms), and cyst formation on the roentgenogram suggests a diagnosis of bronchiectasis; putrid sputum production suggests a lung abscess; weight loss and anorexia in a male smoker over the age of forty years raises the possibility of a bronchogenic carcinoma; a recent history of blunt trauma to the chest suggests a lung contusion; and acute pleuritic chest pain raises the possibility of pulmonary embolism with infarction or some other pleurally based lesion (lung abscess, coccidiomycosis cavity, and vasculitis). Several findings on the *physical examination* may also suggest a specific diagnosis: a pleural friction rub suggests those diagnoses just mentioned in connection with pleuritic pain; the findings of pulmonary hypertension raise the diagnostic possibilities of primary pulmonary hypertension, mitral stenosis, recurrent or chronic thromboembolism, and Eisenmenger's syndrome; a localized wheeze over a major lobar airway suggests an intramural lesion such as a bronchogenic carcinoma or a foreign body; systemic arteriovenous communications or the presence of a murmur over the lung fields suggest the diagnosis of Osler-Weber-Rendu disease with pulmonary AV malformation; evidence of significant expiratory obstruction to airflow coupled with sputum production suggests that whatever other lesion may be present, the patient has significant bronchitis. Finally, the *chest roentgenogram* is critical to diagnosis. The presence of ring shadows favors a diagnosis of bronchiectasis; an air-fluid level, the diagnosis of a lung abscess; and a mass lesion, the diagnosis of a central or peripheral pulmonary neoplasm. A mass lesion which may cause hemoptysis should be distinguished from an area of blood pneumonitis caused by aspiration of blood into contiguous areas.

One of the most demanding diagnostic problems is the identification of the side of bleeding in a patient with normal findings on physical examination and a normal roentgenogram of the chest. A patient with hemoptysis tends to keep the bleeding side dependent. If he did not do this, gravitational drainage would cause aspiration into the noninvolved dependent lung. The patient may also be able to give a history of a burning or deep pain which may localize the side of bleeding; bronchoscopy may then be useful. This procedure generally is most helpful when the bleeding is scant, and of least help when the bleeding is massive, since blood may be aspirated into contiguous airways.

Following the history and physical examination, the

TABLE 29-1
Causes of hemoptysis

1 Inflammatory
- *a* Tuberculosis
- *b* Bronchiectasis
- *c* Lung abcess
- *d* Pneumonia, particularly *Klebsiella*
- *e* Bronchitis

2 Neoplastic
- *a* Bronchogenic carcinoma
- *b* Bronchial adenoma

3 Vascular
- *a* Left ventricular failure
- *b* Mitral stenosis
- *c* Pulmonary thromboembolism
- *d* Primary pulmonary hypertension
- *e* Arteriovenous malformations
- *f* Eisenmenger's syndrome
- *g* Pulmonary vasculitis: Wegener's granulomatosis and Goodpasture's syndrome
- *h* Idiopathic pulmonary hemosiderosis
- *i* Amyloidosis of the respiratory tract

4 Traumatic
- *a* Foreign body
- *b* Lung contusion

5 Hemorrhagic
- *a* Hemorrhagic diathesis
- *b* Anticoagulant therapy

diagnostic approach to a patient with hemoptysis includes whatever specialized studies and procedures are required to make a specific diagnosis. The first step is to obtain a roentgenogram. Usually bronchoscopy is the procedure employed next. The recent introduction of fiberoptic bronchoscopy (Chap. 255) has improved visualization of the upper lobes and included within the range of visualization airways as small as several millimeters in diameter. This endoscopic technique may provide definitive visual, biopsy, or cytologic information. Since direct visualization of more peripheral portions of the airway system is now possible, the indications for bronchography in the evaluation of hemoptysis are being modified. The principal indications for bronchography in such patients are: (1) to establish the presence of localized bronchiectasis (including a sequestered lobe); and (2) to rule out the presence of more generalized bronchiectasis in a patient with localized disease who is regarded as a surgical candidate because of either repetitive hemoptysis or recurrent infections. The recognition of the significance of ring shadows and tram lines on chest x-rays has also reduced the need for bronchography in establishing the diagnosis of bronchiectasis.

THERAPY Since hemoptysis is such an alarming symptom, there is a tendency to overtreat the patient. Usually hemoptysis is scant and will stop spontaneously without specific therapy. If the hemoptysis is substantial, the mainstays of therapy include keeping the patient calm, instituting complete bed rest, excluding unnecessary diagnostic procedures until the hemoptysis has begun to subside, and suppressing cough if it is present and an aggravating feature of the hemoptysis. The emergency care of such a patient demands that intubation and suctioning equipment be at the bedside.

The management of potentially lethal massive hemoptysis remains controversial. The choice between a medical approach and surgical intervention hinges on the words *potentially lethal.* If one could predict in a patient of a given age and clinical status with a particular disease that a particular volume of hemoptysis was a harbinger of exsanguination or massive aspiration, then surgical intervention could be recommended. To date, these variables which affect the natural history of massive hemoptysis have not been analyzed so as to allow such a prediction. However, potentially exsanguinating hemorrhage, exceeding 1,000 ml per 24 h, or serious aspiration despite medical treatment, is ordinarily the indication for surgical treatment which usually consists of lobectomy and requires the prior identification of the site of bleeding.

REFERENCES

BATES DV et al: *Respiratory Function in Disease,* p. 584 ff, Philadelphia: Saunders, 1971

COMMITTEE ON ETIOLOGY OF CHRONIC BRONCHITIS, MEDICAL RESEARCH COUNCIL: Definition and classification of chronic bronchitis. Lancet 1:775, 1965

COMMITTEE ON THERAPY, AMERICAN THORACIC SOCIETY: The management of hemoptysis. Am Rev Resp Dis 93:471, 1966

KARY RC, SMITH JR: Medical history and physical examination in the assessment of pulmonary disease, in *Textbook of Pulmonary Diseases,* 2d ed., ed GL Baum, Boston: Little, Brown, 1974, p. 3

LOUDON RG, SHAW GB: Mechanics of cough in normal subjects and in patients with obstructive respiratory disease. Am Rev Resp Dis 96:666, 1967

PIERCE J: Cough and hemoptysis, chaps. 17, 18, in *Signs and Symptoms,* 6th ed., ed RS Blacklow, Philadelphia: Lippincott, 1977

30 DYSPNEA AND PULMONARY EDEMA

ROLAND H. INGRAM, JR.
EUGENE BRAUNWALD

DYSPNEA

INTRODUCTION For an average 70-kg adult at rest the normal breathing pattern consists of an average frequency of 14 breaths per minute and has a mean tidal volume of 600 ml. It is not surprising that a normal, resting person is unaware of the act of breathing since it originates in the more vegetative portions of the central nervous system and is modulated by both lower central and peripheral vagal pathways. The breathing pattern is changed by a series of higher central and peripheral control mechanisms which can increase ventilation in excess of metabolic demands in conditions such as anxiety and fear, and can increase ventilation appropriate to increased metabolic demands during physical activity. Although a person may become conscious of breathing during mild to moderate exertion, no discomfort is experienced. However, during and following exhausting exertion an individual may become unpleasantly aware of breathing, yet feel reasonably assured that the sensation will be transitory and is appropriate to the level of exercise. Therefore, as a cardinal symptom of diseases affecting the cardiorespiratory system, dyspnea is defined as an *abnormally uncomfortable awareness of breathing.*

Although dyspnea is not painful in the usual sense of the word, it is, like pain, involved with both the perception of a sensation and the reaction to that perception. Thus, since it is a symptom, dyspnea is present whenever a patient complains of it. Patients experience a number of uncomfortable sensations related to breathing and use an even larger number of verbal expressions to describe these sensations, such as "cannot get enough air," "air does not go all the way down," "smothering feeling in the chest," "tightness in the chest," "fatigue in the chest," and a "choking sensation." It may be necessary, therefore, to review meticulously the patient's history in order to ascertain whether the more abstruse descriptions do, in fact, represent dyspnea. Once it is established that a patient does have dyspnea, it is of paramount importance to define the circumstances in which it occurs and to assess associated symptoms. There are situations in which breathing appears labored but in which dyspnea does not occur. For example, the hyperventilation in association with metabolic acidemia is rarely accompanied by dyspnea. On the other hand, patients with apparently normal breathing patterns may complain of shortness of breath.

QUANTITATION OF DYSPNEA The gradation of dyspnea may usefully be based upon the amount of physical exertion required to produce the sensation. In actual practice the major functional classifications of patients with heart or lung disease are based largely on dyspnea in relation to degree of exertion. However, in assessing the severity of dyspnea, it is important to obtain a clear understanding of the patient's general physical condition, work history, and recreational habits. For example, the development of dyspnea in a trained runner upon running 2 mi may signify a more serious disturbance than a similar degree of breathlessness on running a fraction of this distance in a sedentary person. It is also important to note that some patients with lung or heart disease may have such reduced capabilities due to other disease that exertional dyspnea is precluded despite serious impairment of pulmonary or cardiac function; in contrast, others who decrease their physical activities gradually may avoid dyspnea because they do not stress themselves.

Some patterns of dyspnea are not directly related to physical exertion. Sudden and unexpected dyspneic episodes at rest can be associated with pulmonary emboli, spontaneous pneumothorax, or anxiety. Nocturnal episodes of severe paroxysmal dyspnea and diaphoresis are characteristic of congestive heart failure in association with hypertensive cardiovascular disease. Dyspnea upon assuming the supine posture, *orthopnea* (see below), thought to be mainly characteristic of congestive heart failure, may also occur in some patients with asthma and chronic obstruction of the airways and is a regular finding in the rare occurrence of bilateral diaphragmatic paralysis. The term *trepopnea* is used to describe the unusual circumstance in which dyspnea occurs only in the left or right lateral decubitus positions, most often in patients with heart disease, while *platypnea* is dyspnea which occurs only in the upright position. Both of these patterns remain to be fully explained but may be related to positional alterations in ventilation-perfusion relations.

MECHANISMS OF DYSPNEA Physicians usually relate the symptom of dyspnea to a process such as obstruction of the airways or congestive heart failure and generally proceed with further diagnostic and/or therapeutic attempts, having satisfied themselves that they understand the mechanism of the dyspnea. In fact, elucidation of the *actual* mechanism(s) of dyspnea has eluded clinical investigators.

It is well known that dyspnea occurs whenever the work of breathing is excessive. Increased force generation is required of the respiratory muscles to produce a given volume change if the chest wall or lungs are less compliant or if resistance to airflow is increased. Although it is true that an individual is more apt to become dyspneic when the work of breathing is increased, the work theory does not account for the perceptual difference between a deep breath with a normal mechanical load and a normal-sized breath with an increased mechanical load. The work might be the same with both breaths, but the normal one with the increased load will be associated with discomfort. A more appealing theory involves the inappropriateness of length to tension in the respiratory muscles. Campbell has proposed that a sense of discomfort arises when there is misalignment of the nerve spindles, which are sensing tension, in relation to muscle length. This misalignment would lead to the sensation that a person is getting an insufficient breath for the tension generated by the respiratory muscles. Such a theory is difficult to test and, if tested and proved in some circumstances, would still not explain why patients

who are completely paralyzed, either by cord transections or neuromuscular blockade, experience dyspnea although aided by a mechanical ventilator.

In all likelihood a number of different mechanisms operate to different degrees in the various clinical situations in which dyspnea occurs. Perhaps, in some circumstances, dyspnea is evoked by stimulation of receptors in the upper respiratory tract; in others it may originate from receptors in the lungs, airways, respiratory muscles, or some combination of those structures. In general, there is a reasonably good correlation between the severity of dyspnea and the disturbances of pulmonary or cardiac function which are responsible.

DIFFERENTIAL DIAGNOSIS **Obstructive disease of airways** (See also Chaps. 257 and 258.) Obstruction to airflow can be present anywhere from the extrathoracic airways out to the small airways in the periphery of the lung. Large extrathoracic airway obstruction can occur acutely, as with aspiration of food or a foreign body or with angioneurotic edema of the glottis. Circumstantial evidence or testimony from witnesses should cause the physician to suspect aspiration, and an allergic history together with a few scattered hives should raise the possibility of glottic edema. The acute form of upper airway obstruction is a medical emergency. More chronic forms can occur with tumors or with fibrotic stenosis following tracheostomy or prolonged endotracheal intubation. Whether acute or chronic, the cardinal symptom is dyspnea, and the characteristic signs are stridor and retraction of the supraclavicular fossae with inspiration.

Obstruction of intrathoracic airways can occur acutely and intermittently or can be present chronically with worsening during respiratory infections. Acute intermittent obstruction with wheezing is typical of *asthma.* Chronic cough with expectoration is typical of *chronic bronchitis* and *bronchiectasis.* Most often there is a prolongation of expiration and coarse rhonchi which are generalized in chronic bronchitis and may be localized in the case of bronchiectasis. Intercurrent infection results in worsening of the cough, increased expectoration of purulent sputum, and more severe dyspnea. During such episodes the patient may complain of nocturnal paroxysms of dyspnea with wheezing relieved by cough and expectoration of sputum.

Many years of exertional dyspnea progressing to dyspnea at rest characterize the patient with predominant *emphysema,* a condition which is defined as dilatation of the terminal air sacs with disruption of alveolar septa. Although a parenchymal disease by definition, emphysema is invariably accompanied by obstruction of airways. The signs are prominent usage of accessory muscles which lift the anterior thorax, retraction of the lower intercostal spaces with inspiration, distant breath sounds with a hyperresonant percussion note, and end-expiratory wheezes.

With severe chronic bronchitis and/or emphysema, the signs of cor pulmonale may either appear or increase during a respiratory infection. Spirometry and measurements of lung volumes and arterial blood gases (Chap. 254) are not only helpful in establishing a diagnosis but also serve to assess the severity of the process in guiding therapy.

Diffuse parenchymal lung diseases (See also Chap. 260.) This category includes a large number of diseases ranging from acute pneumonia to chronic disorders such as sarcoidosis and the various forms of *pneumoconiosis.* History, physical findings, and radiographic abnormalities often provide clues to the diagnosis. The patients are often tachypneic with arterial P_{CO_2} and P_{O_2} values below normal. Exertion often further reduces the arterial P_{O_2}. Lung volumes are decreased and the lungs are stiffer, i.e., less compliant.

Pulmonary vascular occlusive diseases (See also Chap. 266.) Whether due to repeated emboli or intrinsic vascular disease, right ventricular hypertrophy or signs of right ventricular failure in the absence of obvious parenchymal lung disease should suggest the possibility of pulmonary vascular occlusive disease. Repeated episodes of dyspnea at rest often occur with repeated emboli. A source for emboli, such as phlebitis of a lower extremity or the pelvis, is quite helpful in leading the physician to suspect the diagnosis. Arterial blood gases are almost invariably abnormal, but lung volumes are frequently normal or only minimally abnormal.

Diseases of the chest wall or respiratory muscles (See also Chap. 261.) The physical examination establishes the presence of a chest wall disease such as severe kyphoscoliosis, pectus excavatum, or spondylitis. Although all three of these deformities may be associated with dyspnea, only severe kyphoscoliosis regularly interferes with ventilation sufficiently to produce chronic cor pulmonale and respiratory failure.

Both weakness and paralysis of respiratory muscles can lead to respiratory failure, but most often the signs and symptoms of the neurologic or muscular disorder are more prominently manifested in other systems. A reduced total lung capacity and vital capacity along with an increased residual volume in the absence of apparent heart or lung disease suggests the diagnosis. Such a pattern can be explained by muscle weakness, which can be confirmed by measuring maximal voluntary static pressures.

Anxiety neurosis Dyspnea experienced by someone with an anxiety neurosis is a difficult symptom to evaluate. The signs and symptoms of acute and chronic hyperventilation do not serve to distinguish between anxiety neurosis and other processes, such as recurrent pulmonary emboli. A rather extensive series of pulmonary and cardiac function tests, carried out both at rest and during exercise, may be needed to be certain that anxiety is, in fact, the cause of the dyspnea. Certain clues are helpful in leading one to suspect a psychogenic origin. Frequent sighing respirations and a bizarre, irregular breathing pattern are helpful. Often the breathing pattern returns to normal during sleep.

Heart disease In patients with cardiac disease exertional dyspnea occurs most commonly as a consequence of an elevated pulmonary capillary pressure; aside from uncommon causes such as obstructive disease of the pulmonary veins (Chap. 241), pulmonary capillary hypertension is a consequence of left atrial hypertension, which in turn may be due to left ventricular dysfunction (Chaps. 236 and 237), reduced left ventricular compliance, and mitral stenosis. The elevation of hydrostatic pressure in the pulmonary vascular bed tends to upset the Starling equilibrium (see Pulmonary Edema below) with resulting transudation of fluid into the interstitial space, reducing the compliance of the lungs. A diminution in compliance increases the work of breathing which, to some degree, is minimized by both an increase in frequency of respirations and a reduction in tidal volume. In severe heart disease, usually involving elevation of both pulmonary and systemic venous pressures, hydrothorax develops, further interfering with pulmonary function and intensifying dyspnea. Less commonly, in patients with heart disease, dyspnea is due to a severely diminished cardiac output, resulting in inadequate perfusion of the respiratory muscles and hence their fatigue; dyspnea may also be associated with severe systemic and cerebral anoxia, as occurs during exertion in patients with congenital heart disease and right-to-left shunts (Chap. 241).

Cardiac dyspnea usually begins as breathlessness on strenuous exertion which, over the course of months or years, progresses until the patient is dyspneic at rest. Occasionally, as in patients with massive acute myocardial infarction, the course may be associated with a nonproductive cough developing in the recumbent position, particularly at night.

ORTHOPNEA Orthopnea, i.e., dyspnea in the recumbent position, is characteristic of those forms of heart failure associated with elevations of pulmonary venous and capillary pressures. While orthopnea is usually a symptom of more advanced heart failure than exertional dyspnea, in patients who are physically inactive its onset may actually precede that of exertional dyspnea. Orthopnea is associated with the redistribution of blood from the lower extremities and splanchnic bed to the lungs as the result of the alteration of gravitational forces when the recumbent position is assumed. This augmentation of intrathoracic blood volumes elevates pulmonary venous and capillary pressures which increases the pulmonary closing volume and reduces the vital capacity. An additional factor associated with recumbency is the elevation of the diaphragm, which results in a lower end-expiratory lung volume. This combination of lower end-expiratory lung volume and increase in closing volume results in a significant alteration of alveolar-capillary gas exchange.

PAROXYSMAL (NOCTURNAL) DYSPNEA Also known as *cardiac asthma,* this condition is characterized by attacks of severe shortness of breath which generally occur at night and usually awaken the patient from sleep. The attack is precipitated by stimuli which aggravate the previously existing pulmonary congestion; frequently the total blood volume is augmented at night because of the reabsorption of edema from dependent portions of the body during recumbency; the redistribution of blood volume which takes place results in an increase in intrathoracic blood volume and therefore produces pulmonary congestion. A sleeping patient can tolerate relatively severe pulmonary engorgement and may awaken only when actual pulmonary edema and bronchospasm have developed, with the feeling of suffocation and with wheezing respirations.

CHEYNE-STOKES RESPIRATION See Chap. 237.

DIAGNOSIS The diagnosis of cardiac dyspnea depends on

the recognition of heart disease on the basis of the history and physical examination. There may be a history of antecedent myocardial infarction, third and fourth sound gallops may be audible, and/or there may be evidence of left ventricular enlargement, jugular neck vein distention, and/or peripheral edema. Often there are radiographic signs of heart failure, with evidence of interstitial edema, pulmonary vascular redistribution, and accumulation of fluid in the septal planes and pleural cavity (Chap. 234). Cardiomegaly is often present, but the overall heart size may be normal, particularly in patients with dyspnea due to acute myocardial infarction or mitral stenosis, although an enlarged left atrium is usually evident in the latter condition. The electrocardiogram (Chap. 233) is rarely specific for heart disease and cannot specifically indicate whether a patient's dyspnea is caused by heart disease; however, it is rarely normal in patients with cardiac dyspnea.

Differentiation between cardiac and pulmonary dyspnea In most patients with dyspnea there is obvious clinical evidence of disease of either heart or lungs. The dyspnea of chronic obstructive lung disease tends to develop more gradually than that of heart diseases; exceptions, of course, occur in patients with obstructive lung disease who develop an episode of infectious bronchitis, pneumonia, or pneumothorax, or an exacerbation of asthma. Like patients with cardiac dyspnea, patients with chronic obstructive lung disease may also waken at night with dyspnea, but this is usually associated with sputum production; the dyspnea is relieved after the patient rids himself of secretions.

The difficulty in the distinction between cardiac and pulmonary dyspnea may be compounded by the coexistence of diseases involving both organ systems. Patients with a history of chronic bronchitis or asthma who develop left ventricular failure tend to develop recurrences of bronchoconstriction and wheezing in association with bouts of paroxysmal nocturnal dyspnea and pulmonary edema. This condition, i.e., cardiac asthma, usually occurs in patients with overt clinical evidence of heart disease. Acute cardiac asthma is further differentiated from acute attacks of bronchial asthma by the presence of diaphoresis, more bubbly airways sounds, and the more common occurrence of cyanosis.

It is desirable to carry out pulmonary function testing in patients in whom the etiology of dyspnea is not clear, and these should be helpful in determining whether dyspnea is produced by heart disease, lung disease, abnormalities of the chest wall, or anxiety. In addition to the usual means of assessing patients for heart disease (Chap. 231), the arm-to-tongue circulation time may be useful, since in patients with dyspnea on a cardiac basis it usually exceeds the upper normal limit of 16 s by 4 s or more. Careful observation during the performance of an exercise treadmill test will often help in the identification of the patient who is malingering or whose dyspnea is secondary to anxiety. Under these circumstances the patient usually complains of severe shortness of breath but appears to be breathing either effortlessly or totally irregularly.

PULMONARY EDEMA

An increase in pulmonary venous pressure, which results initially in the engorgement of the pulmonary vasculature, is common in most instances of dyspnea in association with congestive heart failure. The lungs become less compliant, the resistance of small airways increases, and there is an increase in lymphatic flow which apparently serves to maintain a constant pulmonary extravascular fluid volume. At this early stage there is usually mild tachypnea, and, if arterial blood gases are measured, the arterial P_{O_2} and P_{CO_2} are both lowered with an increase in the alveolar to arterial oxygen difference. Tachypnea itself, which might result from stimulation of receptors in the pulmonary interstitium, apparently increases lymphatic flow by augmenting ventilatory pumping of lymphatic vessels. The changes described are seen well in advance of auscultatory findings or radiographic signs pointing to congestive heart failure. If sufficient both in magnitude and duration, the increase in intravascular pressure results in a net gain of fluid in the extravascular space despite further increases in lymphatic flow. It is at this point that symptoms worsen, tachypnea increases, gas exchange deteriorates further, and radiographic changes, such as Kerley B lines and an antigravity redistribution of blood flow, are seen. Even at this intermediate stage, the capillary endothelial intercellular junctions have been shown to widen and allow passage of macromolecules into the interstices. Up to and including this stage, the edema is purely *interstitial.* Sufficient further elevations in intravascular pressure result in disruption of the tighter junctions between alveolar lining cells, and alveolar edema ensues with outpouring of fluid, which contains both red blood cells and macromolecules and floods the airways. At this point *alveolar edema* is present. Full-blown clinical pulmonary edema with bilateral wet rales and rhonchi is now seen, and the chest radiographic changes may show diffuse haziness of the lung fields. Typically, the patient is anxious and perspires freely, and the sputum is frothy and blood-tinged. Gas exchange is more severely compromised with worsening hypoxemia and possibly hypercapnia. Without effective treatment (Chap. 237) progressive acidemia, hypoxemia, and respiratory arrest ensue.

The earlier sequence of fluid accumulation described above follows the Starling law of capillary-interstitial fluid exchange:

$$\text{Fluid accumulation} = K[(Pc + \pi if) - (Pif + \pi pl)] - \text{lymph } Q$$

where K = permeability coefficient
Pc = mean intracapillary pressure
πif = oncotic pressure of interstitial fluid
Pif = mean interstitial fluid pressure
πpl = oncotic pressure of the plasma
lymph Q = lymphatic flow

The pressures tending to move fluid out of the vessel are Pc and πif, which are normally more than offset by pressures tending to move fluid back into the vasculature, i.e., the algebraic sum of Pif and πpl. Implicit in the above equation is that lymphatic flow can increase in the case of imbalance of forces and result in no net accumulation of interstitial fluid. However, in later sequences, with opening of first the endothelial and then the alveolar intercellular junctions, the permeability coefficient changes strikingly. Thus, the initial process of hemodynamic pulmonary edema is one of fluid filtration and clearance. With further increasing pressures, disruption of both structure and function of the alveolar-capillary membrane occurs.

There are several clinical conditions which are associated with pulmonary edema based upon an imbalance of Starling forces other than through primary elevations of pulmonary capillary pressure. Although diminished plasma oncotic pressure in hypoalbuminemic states (e.g., severe liver disease, nephrotic syndrome, protein-losing enteropathy) might be expected to lead to pulmonary edema, the balance of forces normally so strongly favors resorption that even under these conditions some elevation of capillary pressure is necessary before interstitial edema develops. Increased negativity of interstitial pressure has been implicated in the genesis of unilateral pulmonary edema following rapid evacuation of a large pneumothorax. In this situation the findings are apparent only by radiography. Lymphatic blockade secondary to fibrotic and inflammatory diseases or lymphangitic carcinomatosis may lead to interstitial edema. In such instances both clinical and radiographic manifestations are dominated by the underlying disease process.

There are other conditions characterized by increases in the interstitial fluid content of the lungs which begin neither with an imbalance between intravascular and interstitial forces nor with alterations in lymphatics, but rather appear to be associated primarily with disruption of the alveolar-capillary membranes. Experimentally the prototype for such conditions is the pulmonary edema following alloxan administration. Any number of spontaneously occurring or environmental toxic insults are associated with diffuse pulmonary edema which clearly does not have a hemodynamic origin. These conditions are discussed in Chap. 268.

There are three forms of pulmonary edema which have not been clearly related to increased permeability, inadequate lymphatic flow, or an imbalance of Starling forces; hence their precise mechanism remains unexplained. *Narcotic overdose* is a well-recognized antecedent to pulmonary edema. Although illicit use of parenteral heroin has been the most frequent cause, parenteral and oral overdoses of legitimate preparations of morphine, methadone, and dextropropoxyphene have been associated with pulmonary edema. Thus the earlier idea that injected impurities lead to the disorder is untenable. Available evidence suggests that there are alterations in the permeability of alveolar and capillary membranes rather than elevation of pulmonary capillary pressure. *Exposure to high altitude* in association with severe physical exertion is a well-recognized setting for pulmonary edema in unacclimatized, yet otherwise healthy, persons. The mechanism remains obscure, and studies have been conflicting, some suggesting pulmonary venous constriction and others indicating pulmonary arteriolar constriction as the prime mechanisms. *Neurogenic* pulmonary edema has been suspected in patients with central nervous system disorders and without apparent left ventricular dysfunction. Although most experimental equivalents have implicated increased sympathetic nervous system activity, the mechanism whereby sympathetic efferent activity leads to pulmonary edema is not clear.

Treatment of pulmonary edema See Chap. 237.

REFERENCES

CAMPBELL EJM et al: *Breathlessness,* Oxford: Blackwell, 1966

——et al: *The Respiratory Muscles: Mechanisms and Neural Control,* Philadelphia: Saunders, 1970

GOLD W: Dyspnea, chap. 19 in *Signs and Symptoms,* 6th ed., ed RS Blacklow, Philadelphia: Lippincott, 1977

STAUB NC: State of the art review: Pathogenesis of pulmonary edema. Am Rev Resp Dis 109:358, 1974

SZIDON JP et al: The alveolar-capillary membrane and pulmonary edema. N Engl J Med 286:1200, 1972

31 CYANOSIS, HYPOXIA, AND POLYCYTHEMIA

EUGENE BRAUNWALD
RICHARD L. KAHLER
M. M. WINTROBE

CYANOSIS

Cyanosis refers to a bluish color of the skin and mucous membranes resulting from an increased amount of reduced hemoglobin, or of hemoglobin derivatives, in the small blood vessels of those areas. It is usually most marked in the lips, nail beds, ears, and malar eminences. The "red cyanosis" of polycythemia vera (Chap. 315) must be distinguished from the true cyanosis discussed here. A cherry-colored flush, rather than cyanosis, is caused by carboxyhemoglobin (Chap. 116). In *argyria,* the skin is bluish because of the deposition of silver salts, and the discoloration persists despite pressure, unlike cyanotic skin which blanches. The degree of cyanosis is modified by the quality of cutaneous pigment, the color of the blood plasma, and the thickness of the skin, as well as by the state of the cutaneous capillaries. The accurate clinical detection of the presence and degree of cyanosis is difficult, as proved by oximetric studies. Some observers can reliably detect central cyanosis when the arterial saturation has fallen to 85 percent; others may not detect it until the saturation has reached 75 percent.

The increase in the amount of reduced hemoglobin in the cutaneous vessels, which produces cyanosis, may be brought about either by an increase in the quantity of venous blood in the skin as the result of dilatation of the venules and venous ends of the capillaries, or by a decrease in the oxygen saturation in the capillary blood. In general, cyanosis becomes apparent when the mean capillary concentration of reduced hemoglobin exceeds 5 g per 100 ml. It is the *absolute* rather than the *relative* amount of reduced hemoglobin which is important in producing cyanosis. Thus, in a patient with severe anemia the relative amount of reduced hemoglobin in the venous blood may be very large when considered in relation to the total amount of hemoglobin. However, since the latter is markedly lowered, the absolute amount of reduced hemoglobin may still be small, and therefore patients with severe anemia and marked arterial desaturation do not display cyanosis. Conversely, the higher the total hemoglobin content, the greater the tendency toward cyanosis; thus, patients with marked polycythemia tend to be cyanotic at higher levels of arterial oxygen saturation than patients with normal hematocrit values. Likewise, local passive congestion, which causes an increase in the total amount of reduced hemoglobin in the vessels in a given area, may cause cyanosis. Cyanosis also is observed when nonfunctional hemoglobin is present in the blood; as little as 1.5 g per 100 ml methemoglobin or 0.5 g sulfhemoglobin is sufficient to produce cyanosis (Chap. 316).

True cyanosis may be subdivided into *central* and *peripheral* categories. In the *central* type, there is arterial blood unsaturation or an abnormal hemoglobin derivative, and the mucous membranes and skin are both affected. *Peripheral* cyanosis is due to a slowing of blood flow to an area and abnormally great extraction of oxygen from normally saturated arterial blood. It results from vasoconstriction and diminished peripheral blood flow, such as occurs in cold exposure, shock, congestive failure, and peripheral vascular disease. Often, in these conditions, the mucous membranes of the oral cavity or those beneath the tongue may be spared. Clinical differentiation between central and peripheral cyanosis may not always be simple, and in conditions such as cardiogenic shock with pulmonary edema there may be a mixture of both types.

Differential diagnosis

CENTRAL CYANOSIS Decreased arterial oxygen saturation results from a marked reduction in the oxygen tension in the arterial blood. This may be brought about by a decline in the tension of oxygen in the inspired air without sufficient compensatory alveolar hyperventilation to maintain alveolar oxygen tension. Cyanosis does not occur in a significant degree in an ascent to an altitude of 8,000 ft but is marked in a further ascent to 16,000 ft. The reason for this becomes clear on studying the S shape of the oxygen dissociation curve (Fig. 31-1). At 8,000 ft the tension of oxygen in the inspired air is about 120 mmHg, the alveolar tension is approximately 80 mmHg, and the hemoglobin is nearly completely saturated. However, at 16,000 ft the oxygen tensions in atmospheric air and alveolar air are about 85 and 50 mmHg, respectively, and the oxygen dissociation curve shows that the arterial blood is only about 75 percent saturated. This leaves 25 percent of the hemoglobin in the reduced form, an amount likely to be associated with cyanosis in the absence of anemia. Similarly, a mutant hemoglobin with a low affinity for oxygen (Hb Kansas) causes lowered arterial oxygen saturation and resultant central cyanosis.

Seriously *impaired pulmonary function,* through alveolar hypoventilation, perfusion of unventilated or poorly ventilated areas of the lung, or impaired oxygen diffusion, is a common cause of central cyanosis. This may occur acutely, as in extensive pneumonia or in pulmonary edema, or with chronic pulmonary diseases (e.g., emphysema). In the last situation clubbing of the fingers and polycythemia are generally present. However, in many types of chronic pulmonary disease with fibrosis and obliteration of the capillary vascular bed, cyanosis does not occur because there is relatively little perfusion of underventilated areas.

Another cause of decreased arterial oxygen saturation is shunting of systemic venous blood into the arterial circuit. Certain types of congenital heart disease are associated with cyanosis (Chap. 241). Since blood normally flows from a high-pressure to a low-pressure region, in order for a cardiac defect to result in a right-to-left shunt, it must ordinarily be combined with an obstructive lesion distal to the defect or with elevated pulmonary vascular resistance. The commonest congenital cardiac lesion associated with cyanosis is the combination of ventricular septal defect and pulmonary outflow tract obstruction (tetralogy of Fallot). The more severe the obstruction, the greater the degree of right-to-left shunting and resultant cyanosis. The mechanisms for the elevated pulmonary vascular resistance which

FIGURE 31-1

The oxyhemoglobin dissociation curve and factors which affect it. The percentage saturation of hemoglobin is shown on the ordinate, and the P_{O_2} *in millimeters of mercury is shown on the abscissa. Decreases of 2,3-diphosphoglyceric acid (2,3-DPG) concentration,* P_{CO_2}*, or temperature, or increased pH cause a leftward shift in the curve. Conversely, a rightward shift of the curve results from increased 2,3-DPG concentration, temperature, or* P_{CO_2}*, or a decreased pH. Adjustments in blood pH or body temperature have an immediate effect on the affinity of hemoglobin for oxygen, while shifts mediated through 2,3-DPG changes take several hours to occur. A rightward shift in the curve (decreased affinity of hemoglobin for oxygen) results in the release of a greater percentage of oxygen to the tissues.*

During vigorous muscular effort the blood acidity and temperature increase, and an increase in 2,3-DPG concentration has been demonstrated. This causes the dissociation curve to shift rightward and raises the tissue oxygen tension for any given degree of saturation of the hemoglobin, thus making oxygen more available to the exercising muscles. On the other hand, acute exposure to high altitude, with its respiratory alkalosis and rise in pH (opposing the effects of increased 2,3-DPG synthesis), results in a leftward shift of the dissociation curve. (From DR Harkness; by permission of Year Book Medical Publishers)

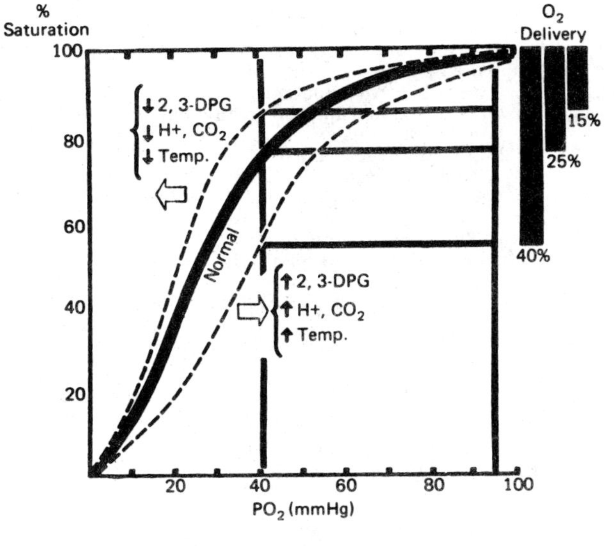

may produce cyanosis in the presence of intra- and extracardiac communications without pulmonic stenosis are discussed elsewhere (Chap. 241). In patients with patent ductus arteriosus, pulmonary hypertension, and right-to-left shunt, differential cyanosis results; i.e., cyanosis occurs in the lower extremities but not in the upper extremities.

Pulmonary arteriovenous fistulas may be congenital or acquired, solitary or multiple, microscopic or massive. The degree of cyanosis produced by these fistulas depends upon their size and number. They occur with some frequency in hereditary hemorrhagic telangiectasia (Chap. 318). Arterial oxygen unsaturation also occurs in some patients with cirrhosis, presumably as a consequence of pulmonary arteriovenous fistulas or portal vein-pulmonary vein anastomoses.

In patients with cardiac or pulmonary right-to-left shunts, the presence and severity of cyanosis depend on the size of the shunt relative to the systemic flow as well as on the oxyhemoglobin saturation of the venous blood. In patients with central cyanosis due to arterial oxygen unsaturation, the severity of cyanosis increases with exercise. With increased extraction of oxygen from the blood by the exercising muscles, the venous blood returning to the right side of the heart is more unsaturated than at rest, and shunting of this blood or its passage through lungs incapable of normal oxygenation intensifies the cyanosis. Also, since the systemic vascular resistance normally decreases with exercise, the right-to-left shunt is augmented by exercise in patients with congenital heart disease and communications between the two sides of the heart. Secondary polycythemia occurs frequently in patients with arterial unsaturation and contributes to the cyanosis.

Cyanosis is produced by small amounts of circulating methemoglobin and by even smaller amounts of sulfhemoglobin (Chap. 316). Although they are uncommon causes of cyanosis, these abnormal hemoglobin pigments should be sought by spectroscopy when cyanosis is not readily explained by malfunction of the circulatory or respiratory systems. Generally, clubbing does not occur with them.

TABLE 31-1
Causes of cyanosis

- *I* Central cyanosis
  - *A* Decreased arterial oxygen saturation
    - *1* Decreased atmospheric pressure—high altitude
    - *2* Impaired pulmonary function
      - *a* Alveolar hypoventilation
      - *b* Uneven relationships between pulmonary ventilation and perfusion
      - *c* Impaired oxygen diffusion
    - *3* Anatomic shunts
      - *a* Certain types of congenital heart disease
      - *b* Pulmonary arteriovenous fistulas
      - *c* Multiple small intrapulmonary shunts
    - *4* Hemoglobin with low affinity for oxygen
  - *B* Hemoglobin abnormalities
    - *1* Methemoglobinemia—hereditary, acquired
    - *2* Sulfhemoglobinemia—acquired
    - *3* Carboxyhemoglobinemia (not true cyanosis)
- *II* Peripheral cyanosis
  - *A* Reduced cardiac output
  - *B* Cold exposure
  - *C* Redistribution of blood flow from extremities
  - *D* Arterial obstruction
  - *E* Venous obstruction

PERIPHERAL CYANOSIS Probably the most common cause of peripheral cyanosis is generalized vasoconstriction resulting from exposure to cold air or water. This is clearly a normal response to the stimulus and is transient. When cardiac output is low, as in severe congestive heart failure or shock, cutaneous vasoconstriction occurs as a compensatory mechanism, so that blood is diverted to more vital areas [central nervous system, heart (Chap. 237)], and intense cyanosis associated with cool extremities may result. Even though the arterial blood is normally saturated, the reduced volume flow through the skin and the reduced oxygen tension at the venous end of the capillary result in cyanosis.

Arterial obstruction to an extremity generally results in pallor and coldness, but there may be associated slight cyanosis. If there is venous obstruction, the extremity is usually congested and markedly cyanotic, and there is true stagnation of blood flow. Venous hypertension, which may be local (as in thrombophlebitis) or generalized (as in tricuspid valve disease or constrictive pericarditis), dilates the subpapillary venous plexuses and intensifies cyanosis.

Certain features are important in arriving at the proper cause of cyanosis.

1 The history, particularly the duration (cyanosis present since birth is usually due to congenital heart disease); possible exposure to drugs or chemicals which may produce abnormal types of hemoglobin.

2 Clinical differentiation of central as opposed to peripheral cyanosis. Objective evidence by physical or radiographic examination of disorders of the respiratory or cardiovascular systems. Massage or gentle warming of a cyanotic extremity will increase peripheral blood flow and abolish peripheral but not central cyanosis.

3 The presence or absence of clubbing of the fingers. Clubbing without cyanosis is frequent in patients with subacute bacterial endocarditis and in association with ulcerative colitis, it may occasionally occur in healthy persons, and in some instances it may be occupational, e.g., in jackhammer operators. Slight cyanosis of the lips and cheeks, without clubbing of the fingers, is common in patients with well-compensated mitral stenosis and is probably due to minimal arterial hypoxia resulting from fibrotic changes in the lungs secondary to long-standing congestion combined with reduction of cardiac output. The combination of cyanosis and clubbing is frequent in many patients with certain types of congenital cardiac disease and is seen occasionally in persons with pulmonary disease such as lung abscess or pulmonary arteriovenous shunts. On the other hand, peripheral cyanosis or acutely developing central cyanosis is not associated with clubbed fingers.

4 Determination of arterial blood oxygen tension or oxygen saturation. Spectroscopic and other examinations of the blood for abnormal types of hemoglobin.

HYPOXIA

The fundamental purpose of the cardiorespiratory system is to deliver oxygen (and substrates) to the cells and to remove carbon dioxide (and other metabolic products) from them. Proper maintenance of this function depends on intact cardiovascular and respiratory systems and a supply of inspired gas containing adequate oxygen. Changes in oxygen and in carbon dioxide tension as well as changes in the intraerythrocytic concentration of certain *organic phosphate compounds,* especially 2,3-diphosphoglyceric acid (2,3-DPG), cause shifts in the oxygen dissociation curve. Increased concentrations of 2,3-DPG shift the oxyhemoglobin dissociation curve to the right, thus decreasing the affinity of hemoglobin for oxygen and releasing a greater percentage of oxygen to the tissues. On the other hand, this advantage may be offset by a decreasing oxygen loading of blood in the lung when the alveolar oxygen tension is very low. Decreased concentrations of 2,3-DPG lead to a diminished delivery of oxygen because of the greater affinity of hemoglobin for oxygen (Fig. 31-1). Intraerythrocytic concentration of 2,3-DPG increases in a variety of conditions characterized by chronic tissue hypoxia; these conditions include chronic anemia, exposure to high altitude, low-output cardiac failure, cyanotic congenital heart disease, and chronic obstructive pulmonary disease. It is one of the important adaptive mechanisms for avoiding tissue hypoxia in these conditions.

When hypoxia occurs as the result of a decline in oxygen tension in the inspired air, respiration is stimulated, alveolar ventilation increases, and the carbon dioxide tension in the alveoli and in the arterial blood falls. This respiratory alkalosis causes a leftward shift in the oxygen dissociation curve, i.e., an increased affinity of hemoglobin for oxygen (Fig. 31-1), and enables a given alveolar oxygen tension to cause a greater degree of oxygen uptake by the hemoglobin (Bohr's effect). Thus, at an alveolar oxygen tension of 55 mmHg, a rise in pH from 7.44 to 7.64 will cause the arterial saturation to increase from 80 to nearly 90 percent.

However, when hypoxia results from interference with the passage of air into the lungs or from the perfusion of poorly ventilated alveoli, carbon dioxide tension usually remains normal or even rises; and the oxygen dissociation curve tends to remain unchanged or move to the right. Under these conditions the percentage saturation of the hemoglobin in the arterial blood at a given level of alveolar oxygen tension does not rise and may even fall. Thus arterial hypoxia and cyanosis are likely to be more marked in proportion to the degree of depression of alveolar oxygen tension when such depression results from pulmonary disease than when the depression occurs as the result of a decline in the partial pressure of oxygen in the inspired air.

ANEMIC HYPOXIA Any decrease in hemoglobin concentration is attended by a corresponding decline in the oxygen-carrying power. The P_{O_2} in the arterial blood remains normal, but the absolute amount of oxygen transported per unit volume of blood is diminished. As the anemic blood passes through the capillaries, and the usual amount of oxygen is removed from it, the P_{O_2} in the venous blood declines to a greater degree than would normally be the case.

CARBON MONOXIDE INTOXICATION (Chap. 116) This condition is accompanied by the equivalent of anemic hypoxia in that the hemoglobin which is combined with the carbon monoxide (carboxyhemoglobin) is unavailable for oxygen transport. In addition, the presence of carboxyhemoglobin increases the affinity of normal hemoglobin for oxygen at low levels of P_{O_2} (i.e., shifts the lower portion

of the dissociation curve of hemoglobin to the left), so that the oxygen can be unloaded only at lower tensions. By such formation of carboxyhemoglobin a given degree of reduction in oxygen-carrying power produces a far greater degree of tissue hypoxia than the equivalent reduction in hemoglobin due to simple anemia.

CIRCULATORY HYPOXIA As in anemic hypoxia, arterial P_{O_2} is normal but venous and tissue P_{O_2} are reduced as a consequence of reduced tissue perfusion in the face of normal tissue oxygen consumption. For this reason the term *stagnant hypoxia* may be used for this condition. Generalized circulatory hypoxia occurs in heart failure, as discussed in Chap. 237.

SPECIFIC ORGAN HYPOXIA Decreased circulation to a specific organ resulting in localized stagnant hypoxia may be due to organic arterial or venous obstruction or may occur as a reflex phenomenon. The latter may occur when vasoconstriction of, for instance, the limbs results from an attempt to maintain adequate perfusion to more vital organs, as in severe congestive heart failure. When organic arterial obliterative disease develops, ischemic hypoxia results, with accompanying pallor. Localized hypoxia may also result from venous obstruction which results in congestion. Edema, which increases the distance through which oxygen diffuses before it reaches the cells, can also cause localized hypoxia.

INCREASED OXYGEN REQUIREMENTS Even if oxygen diffusion into blood perfusing the pulmonary capillary bed is unhampered and the hemoglobin is qualitatively and quantitatively normal, the P_{O_2} in venous blood (hence, capillary and tissue P_{O_2}) may be reduced if the oxygen consumption of the tissues is elevated without a corresponding increase in volume flow per unit of time. Such a situation may be encountered in febrile states and in thyrotoxicosis. Under such conditions the circulation may be considered deficient relative to the metabolic requirements. Thus, this type of metabolic hypoxia is comparable to circulatory hypoxia, in that in both conditions the volume flow of blood is decreased relative to the needs of the tissues; the difference is that in one case the primary defect is the volume flow of blood and in the other the primary defect is an increased oxygen need by the tissues.

Ordinarily, the clinical picture of patients with hypoxia due to an elevated basal metabolic rate is quite different from that in other types of hypoxia; the skin is warm and flushed, owing to increased cutaneous blood flow which dissipates the excessive heat produced, and cyanosis is absent in these patients.

Exercise is a classic example of increased tissue oxygen requirements. The increased demands are normally met by several mechanisms: (1) increasing the cardiac output and thus oxygen delivery to the tissues; (2) preferentially directing the blood to the exercising muscles and away from resting muscles (by changing vascular resistances in various circulatory beds, in some areas by direct effects, in others reflexly); (3) increasing oxygen extraction from the delivered blood and widening the arteriovenous oxygen differences. If the capacity of these mechanisms is exceeded, then hypoxia, especially of the exercising muscles, will result.

IMPROPER OXYGEN UTILIZATION The administration of cyanide (Chap. 116) and several other similarly acting poisons leads to a paradoxic state in which the tissues are unable to utilize oxygen and as a consequence the venous blood tends to have a high oxygen tension. This condition has been termed *histotoxic hypoxia.* Cyanide produces cellular hypoxia by paralyzing the electron-transfer function of cytochrome oxidase so that it cannot pass electrons to oxygen, whereas diphtheria toxin is believed to inhibit the synthesis of one of the cytochromes and thus interfere with oxygen consumption and energy production by the cells involved.

Effects of hypoxia

When hypoxia is general, all parts of the body may suffer some impairment of function, but those parts which are most sensitive to the effects of hypoxia give rise to symptoms which dominate the clinical picture. The *changes in the central nervous system,* particularly the higher centers, are especially important. Acute hypoxia produces impaired judgment, motor incoordination, and a clinical picture closely resembling that of acute alcoholism. When hypoxia is long-standing, the symptoms consist of fatigue, drowsiness, apathy, inattentiveness, delayed reaction time, severe fatigue, and reduced work capacity. As hypoxia becomes more severe, the centers of the brainstem are affected, and death usually results from respiratory failure. With reduction of arterial oxygen tension, cerebrovascular resistance decreases and cerebral blood flow increases, which tends to minimize the cerebral hypoxia. On the other hand when the reduction of arterial P_{O_2} is accompanied by hyperventilation and diminution of P_{CO_2}, cerebrovascular resistance rises, blood flow falls, and hypoxia is enhanced. Compared with the brain, the phylogenetically older spinal cord and peripheral nerves are relatively insensitive to hypoxia. Hypoxia also causes pulmonary arterial constriction, which serves the useful function of shunting blood away from poorly ventilated areas toward better-ventilated portions of the lung. However, it has the disadvantage of causing increased pulmonary vascular resistance and an increased burden on the right ventricle.

A complex disturbance of cellular functions results from the metabolic effects of severe acute hypoxia. In liver and muscles the breakdown of the primary foodstuff, carbohydrate, normally proceeds anaerobically (i.e., without oxidation) to the stage of formation of pyruvic acid. The breakdown of pyruvate requires oxygen, and when this is deficient, increasing proportions of pyruvate are reduced to lactic acid, which cannot be further broken down (Chap. 68). Hence, there is an increase in the blood lactate, with decrease in bicarbonate and a corresponding acidosis. Under these circumstances the total energy obtained from foodstuff breakdown is greatly reduced, and the amount of energy available for continuing resynthesis of energy-rich phosphate compounds becomes inadequate. Impairment of the myriad anabolic reactions which take place in tissues follows. The deficiency of energy-rich phosphate compounds produces a complex disturbance of cellular function.

Most of the useful respiratory response to hypoxia originates in special chemosensitive cells in the carotid and aortic bodies, although the respiratory center is also stimulated directly by oxygen lack. The peripheral chemoreceptors are extremely rugged and continue to function after other tissues have been damaged by hypoxemia. The chemoreceptors are stimulated by a reduction in their oxygen supply below their needs either by lowered arterial P_{O_2} or by lowered blood flow to them. If respiration is stimulated by hypoxia, the resulting increase in ventilation, with loss of carbon dioxide, tends to make the blood more alkaline. On the other hand, the diffusion of additional quantities of lactic acid from the tissues into the blood tends to make the blood more acid. In either case the total amount of bicarbonate, and hence the carbon dioxide-combining power, tends to be diminished. With mild hypoxia there is likely to be respiratory alkalosis; severe hypoxia is attended by metabolic acidosis.

The heart, although relatively sensitive to hypoxia as compared with most of the structures of the body, is less sensitive than the nervous system. Consequently, in the absence of severe coronary artery disease, serious manifestations arising in the nervous system dominate the picture. Diminished oxygen tension in any tissue results in local vasodilatation, and in generalized hypoxia diffuse vasodilatation results in an elevation of total cardiac output. In patients with preexisting heart disease, particularly coronary artery disease, the combination of hypoxia and the requirements of the peripheral tissues for an increase of cardiac output may precipitate congestive heart failure. Prolonged or severe hypoxia may also impair hepatic and renal function.

One of the important mechanisms of compensation for prolonged hypoxia is an increase in the amount of hemoglobin in the blood. This is due not to direct stimulation of the bone marrow but to the effect of an erythropoiesis-stimulating factor (erythropoietin) which originates primarily in the kidneys. Assayable levels of erythropoietin are increased by hypoxia, and its production has been found to be regulated by the balance between tissue oxygen supply and demand.

POLYCYTHEMIA

The term *polycythemia* signifies an increase above the normal in the number of red corpuscles in the circulating blood. This increase is usually, though not always, accompanied by a corresponding increase in the quantity of hemoglobin and in the volume of packed red corpuscles. The increase may or may not be associated with an increase in the total quantity of red blood cells in the body. It is important to distinguish between *absolute* polycythemia (an increase in the total red corpuscle mass) and *relative* polycythemia, which occurs when, through loss of blood plasma, the concentration of the red corpuscles becomes greater than normal in the circulating blood. This may be the consequence of abnormally lowered fluid intake, of the loss of plasma into the interstitial fluid, and of the marked loss of body fluids, such as occurs in persistent vomiting, severe diarrhea, copious sweating, or acidosis (Chap. 70).

Because the term polycythemia is used loosely to refer to

all varieties of increase in the number of red corpuscles, the terms *erythrocytosis* and *erythremia* are preferred in referring to two forms of absolute polycythemia. Erythrocytosis denotes absolute polycythemia which occurs in response to some known stimulus (secondary polycythemia); erythremia (polycythemia rubra vera) refers to the disease of unknown etiology, which is discussed elsewhere (Chap. 315).

Erythrocytosis develops as a consequence of a variety of factors and represents a physiologic response to conditions of hypoxia. Sojourn at high altitudes leads to defective saturation of arterial blood with oxygen and stimulates the production of more red corpuscles. The oxygen saturation, rather than oxygen tension, appears to be the more important determinant of the erythropoietic response to chronic hypoxia (Fig. 31-2). A disorder may set in insidiously after several years of continued residence at high altitudes, leading to the development of a condition known as *chronic mountain sickness* or *seroche* (Monge's disease). Two forms have been described: an *emphysematous type,* in which dyspnea is prominent and bronchitis is common, and an *erythremic type,* in which prominent manifestations are a florid color which turns to cyanosis on mild exertion, mental torpor, fatigue, and headache. Those affected are usually in the fourth to sixth decades. Return to sea level promptly relieves the symptoms. *Brisket disease of cattle,* a disorder of calves grazing at high altitudes in Utah and Colorado, which is characterized by pulmonary hypertension and subsequent failure of the right side of the heart, is not a true counterpart of Monge's disease, since it is not associated with sustained oxygen unsaturation or polycythemia. Living at high altitudes also evokes a number of compensatory reactions which act to increase oxygen delivery to the tissues. These include hyperventilation, which reduces the oxygen gradient between ambient and alveolar air, an augmentation of pulmonary capillary blood volume, a reduction of diffusing capacity, and an increase in cardiac output.

Any chronic pulmonary disease which alters ventilation-perfusion relationships or seriously impairs gas diffusion may produce chronic hypoxemia and lead to erythrocytosis. *Pulmonary arteriovenous fistulas* or *cavernous hemangioma of the lung* may lead to impaired saturation of arterial blood with oxygen, with the consequent development of erythrocytosis and of a clinical picture resembling closely that of certain types of congenital heart disease. The increased blood viscosity secondary to the polycythemia (Fig. 31-3) elevates pulmonary arterial pressure and, combined with the elevation of pulmonary vascular resistance resulting from hypoxia, further elevates right ventricular pressure, contributing to the development or intensification of cor pulmonale (Chap. 267).

The *abnormal ventilatory conditions* present in very obese individuals may cause alveolar hypoventilation and result in arterial unsaturation, erythrocytosis, hypercapnea, and somnolence (the Pickwickian syndrome, Chap. 261). This syndrome is observed less commonly in nonobese persons, in whom decreased sensitivity of the respiratory center to CO_2 may play a role.

The partial shunting of blood from the pulmonary circuit, such as occurs in *congenital heart disease,* causes the most striking erythrocytosis resulting from abnormalities in the heart or lungs. Erythrocyte counts as high as 13 million per mm^3, which are possible only when the red corpuscles are smaller than normal, have been observed in such cases, with volumes of packed red blood cells even as high as 86 ml per 100 ml of blood. As the polycythemia develops, there is a progressive rise in blood viscosity (Fig. 31-3), with the sharpest increase beginning when the volume of packed red blood cells reaches 65 to 70 percent. The commonest defect producing such polycythemia is pulmonary

FIGURE 31-2

Relationship between mean arterial oxygen saturation (percent) and the mean hemoglobin content (g per 100 ml) in healthy male residents at various altitudes. (From Hurtado et al; by permission of Annals of Internal Medicine*)*

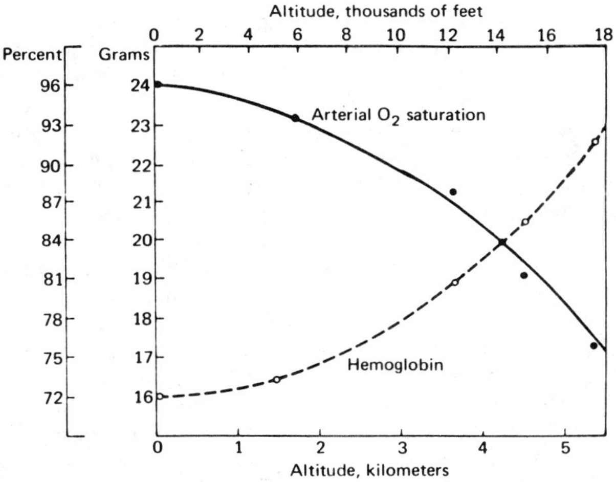

FIGURE 31-3

Correlation of hematocrit value with specific viscosity of the blood. (From Rudolph et al; by permission of Pediatrics*)*

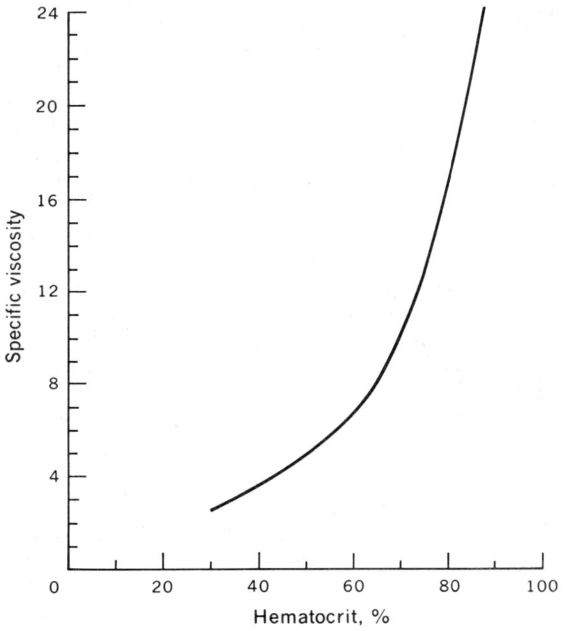

stenosis associated with a right-to-left shunt that allows venous blood to enter the systemic arterial tree without traversing the lungs. Other conditions include transposition of the great arteries, tricuspid atresia, persistent truncus arteriosus, and other less common anomalies, discussed in Chap. 241.

Reduction in red blood cell volume (phlebotomy with reinfusion of the plasma) is sometimes performed in severely symptomatic patients with extremely high hematocrit levels, but it must be carried out slowly and with great caution. It results in a reduction of the elevated blood viscosity which decreases the impedance to flow. When pulmonary blood flow is derived largely from the systemic circuit, as in patients with tetralogy of Fallot and severe pulmonary outflow obstruction, this maneuver reduces systemic O_2 saturation. On the other hand, if pulmonary blood flow is independent of the systemic circuit, as in D-transposition of the great arteries, an increase in pulmonary blood flow occurs.

The polycythemia of cyanotic congenital heart disease may lead to spontaneous thrombosis at any site, including the central nervous system. It may also be accompanied by a variety of blood coagulation defects, including reduced fibrinogen and prothrombin concentrations, as well as thrombocytopenia.

The excessive use of coal-tar derivatives and other forms of chronic poisoning, by producing abnormal hemoglobin pigments such as methemoglobin and sulfhemoglobin (Chap. 316), also may cause erythrocytosis. Carriers of certain abnormal hemoglobins which displace the oxygen dissociation curve to the left and interfere with oxygen unloading in the tissues stimulates the production of erythropoietin and a secondary erythrocytosis unassociated with leukocytosis or thrombocytosis (Chap. 313).

Erythrocytosis is found in *Cushing's syndrome* (Chap. 93) and can be produced by the administration of large amounts of adrenocortical steroids. Especially intriguing are the instances of polycythemia observed in association with various *tumors.* These have been chiefly of two varieties, *infratentorial* and *renal.* The tumors in the posterior fossa of the skull have usually been vascular (hemangioblastomas). The renal tumors have included hypernephroma, adenoma, and sarcoma. Other tumors that have been associated with polycythemia include uterine myoma and hepatic carcinoma. Polycythemia also has been reported in association with polycystic disease of the kidneys and hydronephrosis. However, only a small proportion (0.3 to 2.6 percent) of the various renal disorders mentioned above have been associated with polycythemia. Plasma erythropoietin levels have been found elevated in a number of these patients. Erythropoiesis-stimulating activity has been demonstrated in tumor extracts and in renal cyst fluid, and polycythemia has disappeared after the associated tumor was removed.

The term *stress erythrocytosis* has been applied to the polycythemia seen occasionally in very active, hard-working persons in a state of anxiety, who appear florid but who have none of the characteristic signs of erythremia—no splenomegaly or leukocytosis with immature cells in the blood. In such persons the total red blood cell mass is normal, and the plasma volume is below normal.

The differential diagnosis of polycythemia is discussed in Chap. 315. However, it should be pointed out that in secondary polycythemia with hypoxia, arterial Po_2 is reduced, erythropoietin levels are elevated, while levels of leukocyte alkaline phosphatase and serum vitamin B_{12} are normal. In polycythemia vera, erythropoietin levels are normal or decreased and leukocyte alkaline phosphatase and vitamin B_{12} levels are elevated.

REFERENCES

BATES DV et al: *Respiratory Function in Disease,* Philadelphia: Saunders, 1971, p. 584

DENNIS RC, VITO L, WEISEL RD, VALERI CR, BERGER RL, HECHTMAN HB: Improved myocardial performance following high 2,3 diphosphoglycerate red cells. Transfusions: Surgery 77:741–747, 1975

ERSLEV AJ, GABUZDA TG: *Pathophysiology of Blood,* Philadelphia: Saunders, 1975

GOLD W: Cyanosis, chap. 20 in *Signs and Symptoms,* ed RS Blacklow, 6th ed, Philadelphia: Lippincott, 1977

HARKNESS DR: The regulation of hemoglobin oxygenation, in *Advances in Internal Medicine,* ed GH Stollerman, Chicago: Year Book, 1971, p. 189

HURTADO A: Some clinical aspects of life at high altitudes. Ann Intern Med 53:247, 1960

JEPSON JH, FRANKL W: *Haematological complications in Cardiac Practice,* Philadelphia: Saunders, 1975

ROSENTHAL A, TYLER DC: Effect of red cell volume reduction or pulmonary blood flow in polycythemia of cyanotic congenital heart disease. Am J Cardiol 33:410, 1974

32 EDEMA

EUGENE BRAUNWALD

Edema is defined as an increase in the extravascular (interstitial) component of the extracellular fluid volume, which may increase by several liters before the abnormality is recognized. Therefore, a weight gain of several kilograms usually precedes overt manifestations of edema, and a similar weight loss resulting from diuresis can be induced in a slightly edematous patient before "dry weight" is achieved. *Ascites* (Chap. 44) and *hydrothorax* refer to accumulation of excess fluid in the peritoneal and pleural cavities, respectively, and are considered to be special forms of edema. *Anasarca,* or "dropsy," refers to gross, generalized edema. Depending on its etiology and mechanism, edema may be localized or have a generalized distribution; it is recognized in its generalized form by puffiness of the face, which is most readily apparent in the periorbital areas, and by the persistence of an indentation of the skin following pressure; this is known as "pitting" edema. In its more subtle form, it may be detected by the fact that the rim of the bell of the stethoscope leaves an indentation on the skin of the chest that lasts a few minutes. One of the early symptoms a patient may note is the ring on a finger fitting more snugly than in the past, or difficulty getting into his shoes, particularly in the evening.

PATHOGENESIS A more detailed discussion of the volume and distribution of body fluids is presented in Chap. 69. About one-third of the total body water is confined to the extracellular space. This compartment, in turn, is composed of the plasma volume and the interstitial space. Under ordinary circumstances the plasma volume represents about 25 percent of the extracellular space, and the remainder is interstitial fluid. The forces that regulate the disposition of fluid between these two components of the extracellular compartment are frequently referred to as the Starling forces (see Pulmonary Edema in Chap. 30). In general terms, two forces, the hydrostatic pressure within the vascular system and the colloid oncotic pressure in the interstitial fluid, tend to promote a movement of fluid from the vascular to the extravascular space. In contrast, the colloid oncotic pressure contributed by the plasma proteins, and the hydrostatic pressure within the interstitial fluid, referred to as the *tissue tension,* promote a movement of fluid into the vascular compartment. As a consequence of these forces there is a large movement of water and diffusible solutes from the vascular space at the arteriolar end of the microcirculation and back into the vascular compartment at the venous end. In addition, fluid is returned from the interstitial space into the vascular system by way of the lymphatics, and unless these channels are obstructed, lymph flow tends to increase if there is a tendency toward a net movement of fluid from the vascular compartment to the interstitium. All these forces are usually balanced so that a steady state exists in the size of the intravascular and interstitial compartments, and yet a large exchange between them is permitted. However, should any one of these factors be altered significantly, a net movement of fluid from one component of the extracellular space to the other will occur.

An increase in capillary pressure may readily result from an increase in venous pressure due to local obstruction in venous drainage, to congestive heart failure, or rarely to the simple expansion of the vascular volume by the administration of large volumes of fluid at a rate in excess of the ability of the kidneys to excrete these excesses. The colloid oncotic pressure of the plasma may be reduced owing to any of the factors that may induce hypoalbuminemia, such as malnutrition, liver disease, and loss of protein into the urine or into the gastrointestinal tract, or to a severe catabolic state.

Edema may also result from damage to the capillary endothelium, which increases the permeability of these vessels, permitting the transfer to the interstitial compartment of a fluid containing more protein than usual. Injury to the capillary walls may be the result of chemical, bacterial, thermal, or mechanical agents. Increased capillary permeability may also be a consequence of a hypersensitivity reaction and is characteristic of immune injury. Damage to the capillary endothelium is presumably responsible for inflammatory edema, which is nonpitting, usually localized, and readily recognized by the presence of other signs of inflammation—redness, heat, and tenderness.

In an attempt to formulate a hypothesis concerning the pathophysiology involved in edematous states, it is important to discriminate between the *primary* events, such as venous or lymphatic obstruction, reduction of cardiac output, hypoalbuminemia, or trapping of fluid in spaces such as the peritoneal cavity, and the predictable *secondary* consequences, which include the renal retention of salt and water. There are instances in which an abnormal positive balance of salt and water may, in fact, be the primary disturbance. In these circumstances the edema is a secondary manifestation of the generalized increase in extracellular fluid volume. These special instances are usually related to conditions characterized by an acute reduction in renal function, such as acute tubular necrosis or acute glomerulonephritis (Figs. 32-1 and 34-1).

These circumstances aside, a hypothesis can be advanced which, although admittedly incomplete, leads to improved understanding of the events in a variety of edematous states and enhances the perception of their pathophysiology. The basic premise is that the primary disorder concerns one or more alterations in the Starling forces so that there is a net movement of fluid from the vascular system into the interstitium or into a "third space," or from the arterial compartment of the vascular space into the chambers of the heart or into the venous circulation itself. The *effective arterial blood volume,* an as yet poorly defined parameter of the filling of the arterial tree, is reduced, and a series of physiologic responses which are designed to restore it to normal are set into motion. A key element of these responses is the retention of an increment of salt and water, and in many instances this repairs the deficit of the effective arterial blood volume; often this occurs without the development of overt edema. If, however, the retention of salt and water is insufficient to restore and maintain the effective arterial blood volume, the stimuli are not dissipated, the retention of salt and water continues, and edema develops. The sequence of events described above is operative in a variety of circumstances, including dehydration and hemorrhage. Although there is a reduction of effective arterial blood volume and activation of the entire sequence shown on the right side of Fig. 32-1, including the retention of salt and water, edema does not occur because the total extravascular fluid volume is reduced.

Certain data suggest that the increase in volume of some component(s) of the extracellular space normally promotes the secretion of a natriuretic hormone, also referred to as "third factor." The unambiguous demonstration of such a hormone, its site(s) of secretion, and its characterization is yet to be presented. The retention of sodium is accompanied by an increased reabsorption of water. This is attested to by (1) the usual failure to accumulate edema if sodium is not available in the diet, and (2) the successful use of pharmacologic agents and other measures that promote the excretion of sodium chloride in the urine. In most circumstances the mechanisms responsible for maintaining a normal effective osmolality in the body fluids continue to operate efficiently so that sodium retention promotes thirst and secretion of the antidiuretic hormone, which, in turn, lead to the ingestion and retention of approximately 1 liter water for each 140 mmol sodium retained. Similarly, measures which promote the loss of sodium into the urine are accompanied by the net loss of an equivalent volume of water from the body.

Obstruction of venous and lymphatic drainage of a limb In this condition the hydrostatic pressure in the capillary bed increases so that more fluid is transferred from the vascular to the interstitial space than can be reabsorbed at the venous end of the capillaries; since the alternate route (i.e., the lymphatic channels) is obstructed as well, this event must of necessity cause an increased volume of interstitial fluid in the limb, i.e., a trapping of fluid in the extremity, at the expense of the blood volume in the remainder of the body, thereby reducing effective arterial blood volume and leading to the consequences shown in Fig. 32-1.

As fluid accumulates in the interstitium of the limb, in which venous and lymphatic drainage are obstructed, tissue tension rises until it is great enough to counterbalance the primary alterations in the Starling forces, at which time no further fluid will accumulate in that limb. At this point the additional accumulation of fluid will repair the deficit in plasma volume, and the stimuli to retain more salt and water are dissipated. The net effect is an increase in the volume of interstitial fluid in a local area, and the secondary responses repair the plasma volume deficit incurred by the primary event. This same sequence may be translated to many other edematous states.

Congestive heart failure (See also Chap. 237.) In this disorder it is postulated that the defective systolic emptying of the chambers of the heart promotes an accumulation of blood in the heart and venous circulation at the expense of the arterial volume, and the aforementioned sequence of events (Fig. 32-1) is initiated. In many instances of mild heart failure a small increment of volume may be achieved, which repairs the volume deficit and establishes a new steady state because through the operation of Starling's law of the heart, up to a point an increase in the volume of blood within the chambers of the heart promotes a more forceful contraction and may thereby increase the volume ejected in systole (Fig. 236-7). However, if the cardiac disorder is more severe, retention of fluid cannot repair the deficit in effective arterial blood volume. The increment accumulates in the venous circulation, and the increase in hydrostatic pressure therein promotes the formation of edema. The formation of edema in the lungs (Chap. 30) impairs gas exchange and may induce hypoxia, which embarrasses cardiac function still further.

In addition to the sequence shown on the right-hand side of Fig. 32-1, incomplete ventricular emptying leads to an elevation of ventricular end-diastolic pressure. If the impairment of cardiac function involves the right ventricle primarily, then incomplete ventricular emptying leads to an elevation of right ventricular end-diastolic volume and pressure; as a consequence pressures in the systemic veins and capillaries also rise, thereby augmenting transudation of fluid into the interstitial space and enhancing the likeli-

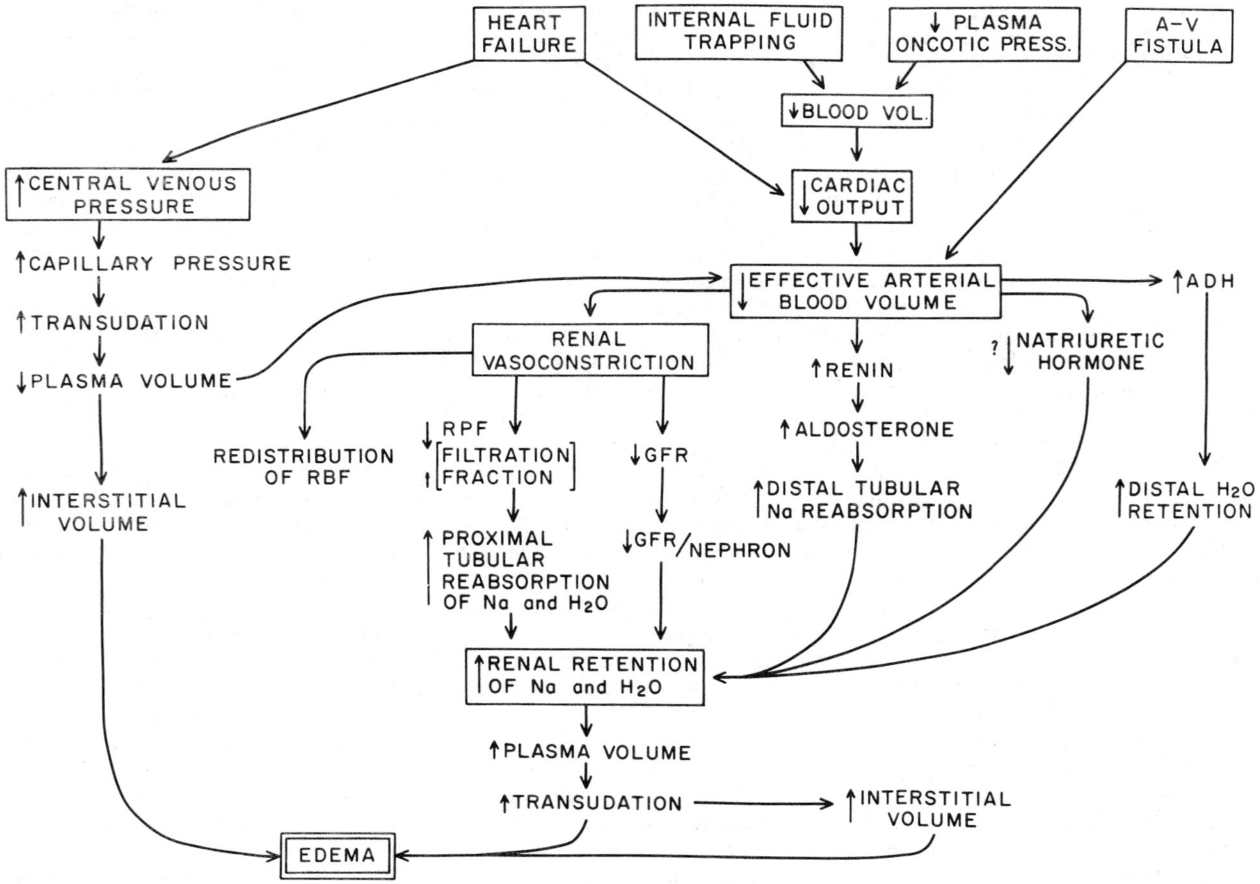

FIGURE 32-1

Sequence of events leading to the formation and retention of salt and water and the development of edema.

hood of peripheral edema. If the impairment of cardiac function involves the left ventricle, then pulmonary venous and capillary pressures rise [leading in some instances to pulmonary edema (Chap. 30)], as does pulmonary artery pressure; this in turn interferes with the systolic emptying of the right ventricle, leading to an elevation of right ventricular end-diastolic and central and systemic venous pressures, enhancing the likelihood of edema formation.

A reduction of cardiac output is associated with a reduction of the effective arterial blood volume as well as of renal blood flow and an elevation of the filtration fraction, i.e., the ratio of glomerular filtration rate to renal plasma flow. In severe heart failure the blood flow to the outer renal cortex, in particular, is significantly reduced with less depression in the more central regions of the kidney, and there is a reduction in the glomerular filtration rate. This constriction of renal cortical vessels appears to play an important role in the retention of salt and water and the formation of edema in heart failure. Indirect evidence suggests that at different stages of heart failure, activation of the sympathetic nervous system and of the renin-angiotensin systems is responsible for renal vasoconstriction. Activation of the former can be counteracted by the administration of alpha-adrenergic blocking agents, a finding which indicates that the elevated renal vascular resistance in heart failure is mediated, at least in part, by sympathetic stimuli.

It is generally agreed that an increase in the tubular reabsorption of glomerular filtrate plays a principal role in the salt and water retention of heart failure. However, the precise site(s) in the system composed of the renal tubules, loops of Henle, and collective ducts which is involved is not clear, nor have the responsible mechanism(s) been identified. Alterations in intrarenal hemodynamics appear to play a significant role. Heart failure, by augmenting renal arteriolar constriction, reduces the hydrostatic pressure and raises the colloid osmotic pressure in the peritubular capillaries, thus enhancing salt and water reabsorption in the proximal tubule. The aforementioned distribution of intrarenal blood flow characteristic of heart failure may be responsible for augmentation of sodium reabsorption in the ascending limb of the loop of Henle.

In addition, the diminished renal blood flow characteristic of all states in which the effective arterial blood volume is reduced is translated by the renal juxtaglomerular cells into a signal for increased renin release (Chap. 93). The specific nature of the signal is complex. One factor involves a baroreceptor mechanism, in which reduced renal perfusion results in incomplete filling of the renal arterioles and diminished stretch of the juxtaglomerular cells, a signal that provides for the elaboration or release, or both, of renin. A second mechanism involves the macula densa; as a result of reduced glomerular filtration the sodium load reaching the distal renal tubules is reduced. This is sensed by the macula densa, which in an as yet undefined manner signals the neighboring juxtaglomerular cells to secrete renin. A third mechanism involves the sympathetic nervous system and circulating catecholamines. Activation of the beta-adrenergic receptors in the juxtaglomerular cells stimulates them to release renin. These three mechanisms generally act in concert.

Renin, an enzyme that has a molecular weight of about 40,000, acts on its substrate, angiotensinogen, an α2-globulin synthesized by the liver, resulting in the elaboration of angiotensin-II, an octapeptide with vasoconstrictor properties. The intrarenal production of angiotensin-II may also contribute to renal vasoconstriction in heart failure and to the salt and water retention in this state. Angiotensin-II also passes through the circulation and stimulates the production of aldosterone by the zona glomerulosa region of the adrenal cortex. In patients with heart failure, not only is aldosterone secretion elevated, but the biologic half-life of aldosterone is prolonged, indicating a reduced catabolic rate and further increasing the plasma level of the hormone. A depression of hepatic blood flow, particularly during exercise, secondary to a reduction in cardiac output, is responsible for the reduced hepatic catabolism of aldosterone.

Although increased quantities of aldosterone have been demonstrated to be secreted in heart failure and other edematous states, augmented levels of aldosterone (or other mineralocorticoids) do not always promote the accumulation of edema, as witnessed by the lack of striking fluid retention in most instances of primary aldosteronism. Furthermore, although normal subjects will retain some salt and water under the influence of a potent mineralocorticoid, such as deoxycorticosterone acetate or 9α-fluorohydrocortisone, the accumulation appears to be self-terminative, despite continued exposure to the steroid and to salt and water. It is probable that the failure of normal subjects to accumulate large quantities of fluid is a consequence of an increase in glomerular filtration rate, other hemodynamic influences, and most importantly the increase in volume which promotes an increased excretion of salt independent of the filtered load of sodium, i.e., through the action of natriuretic substance(s). The role of aldosterone in the accumulation of fluid in edematous states may be more important because these patients are unable to repair the crucial deficit in volume.

Nephrotic syndrome and other hypoalbuminic states (See also Chap. 275.) The primary alteration in this disorder is a diminished colloid oncotic pressure due to massive losses of protein into the urine. This should promote a net movement of fluid into the interstitium and hypovolemia, and initiate the sequence of events described above. As long as the hypoalbuminemia is severe, the salt and water retained cannot be restrained within the vascular compartment, and hence the stimuli to retain salt and water are not abated. A similar sequence of events occurs in other conditions which lead to severe hypoalbuminemia, including severe nutritional deficiency states, protein-losing enteropathy, congenital hypoalbuminemia, and severe, chronic liver disease.

Cirrhosis (See also Chaps. 44 and 301.) The total blood volume in cirrhosis of the liver is commonly increased when the disorder is accompanied by a system of dilated venous radicles and multiple small arteriovenous fistulas. Effective systemic perfusion and the effective arterial blood volume appear to be diminished, probably as a consequence of the passage of blood through these fistulas. The enlarged abdominal venous system resulting from obstruction of the lymphatic drainage of the liver, as well as from portal vein obstruction, also promotes a deficit in the arterial component. These alterations are frequently complicated by the reduced serum albumin characteristic of cirrhosis, which tends to reduce the effective arterial blood volume even further. Initially, the excess interstitial fluid is localized preferentially behind the congested portal venous system and obstructed hepatic lymphatics, i.e., in the peritoneal cavity. In late stages of the disease, particularly when there is hypoalbuminemia, peripheral edema may also be noted.

Idiopathic cyclic edema This syndrome, which occurs predominantly in women, particularly those with psychosocial difficulties, is characterized by periodic episodes of edema, frequently accompanied by abdominal distention. Fairly large, diurnal alterations in weight occur, so that the patient may well weigh several pounds more in the evening than in the morning after having been in the upright posture most of the day. Such large diurnal weight changes suggest an increase in capillary permeability which appears to fluctuate in severity. The fact that it occurs most commonly in women and appears to have some temporal relation to the menstrual cycle suggests that there may be some hormonal influence in the permeability of the vessels which permits the loss of plasma volume into the interstitial space and the sequence of events secondary to a contraction in plasma volume.

The treatment of idiopathic cyclic edema includes a reduction in salt intake, the use of appropriate diuretic agents in anticipation of the edematous episode, beta-adrenergic blocking agents, education in the use of rest in the supine position for several hours each day, the wearing of elastic stockings which are put on prior to arising in the morning, and an attempt to understand the underlying emotional problems. It has been reported that the plasma concentration of cyclic adenosine monophosphate (AMP) is high in patients with idiopathic edema in both the recumbent and upright positions, and its renal clearance, unlike that of creatinine, is low. If a relationship between extracellular cyclic AMP and the action of hormones on beta-adrenergic receptors could be established, the favorable therapeutic effect of propranolol in cases where diuretics alone did not satisfactorily control the disease could be explained.

DIFFERENTIAL DIAGNOSIS As a rule, localized edema can be readily differentiated from generalized edema. The great majority of patients with noninflammatory generalized edema of significant degree suffer from advanced cardiac, renal, hepatic, or nutritional disorders. Consequently, the differential diagnosis of generalized edema should be directed toward implicating or excluding these several conditions.

Localized edema Edema originating from inflammation or hypersensitivity is usually readily identified. Localized edema due to venous or lymphatic obstruction may be caused by thrombophlebitis, chronic lymphangitis, resection of regional lymph nodes, filariasis, etc. Lymph edema is particularly intractable because restriction of lymphatic flow results in increased protein concentration in the interstitial fluid, a circumstance which severely impedes removal of retained fluid.

Edema of heart failure Evidence of heart disease, as manifested by cardiac enlargement and gallop rhythm together with evidence of cardiac failure, such as dyspnea, basilar rales, diminished vital capacity, prolonged circulation time, venous distention, increased venous pressure, and hepatomegaly, usually provides an indication of the pathogenesis of edema resulting from heart failure (see also Chap. 237).

Edema of the nephrotic syndrome Massive proteinuria, severe hypoproteinemia, and in some instances hypercholesterolemia are present. This syndrome may occur during the course of a variety of kidney diseases, which include glomerulonephritis, diabetic glomerulosclerosis, and hypersensitivity reactions. A history of previous renal disease may or may not be elicited (see also Chap. 275).

Edema of acute glomerulonephritis The edema occurring during the acute phases of glomerulonephritis is characteristically associated with hematuria, proteinuria, and hypertension. Although some evidence supports the view that the fluid retention is due to increased capillary permeability, in most instances the edema in this disease results from primary retention of sodium and water by the kidneys owing to renal insufficiency. This state differs from congestive heart failure in that it is characterized by a normal or increased cardiac output, normal or diminished circulation time, a reduction in the packed cell volume, a normal arteriovenous oxygen difference, and failure to respond to a digitalis preparation. Patients commonly have evidence of pulmonary congestion on chest roentgenograms before cardiac enlargement is significant and do not develop orthopnea. If one cannot discriminate between the congested state and congestive heart failure, use of a cardiac glycoside is appropriate, but special care should be taken to avoid digitalis intoxication in a patient with impaired renal function (see also Chap. 274).

Edema of cirrhosis Ascites and evidence of hepatic disease (collateral venous channels, jaundice, and spider angiomas) characterize edema of hepatic origin. The ascites is frequently refractory to treatment because it collects as a result of a combination of obstruction of hepatic lymphatic drainage, portal hypertension, hypoalbuminemia, and relatively high protein content of the ascitic fluid. The latter may be due to escape of a protein-containing fluid through the lymphatic vessels of the liver capsule or through the portal vessels, with their lymphatic drainage impeded. Edema may also occur in other parts of the body in these patients as a result of hypoalbuminemia. Furthermore, the sizable accumulation of ascitic fluid may be expected to increase intraabdominal pressure and impede venous return from the lower extremities; hence, it tends to promote accumulation of edema in this region as well (see also Chap. 301).

Edema of nutritional origin An inadequate diet over a prolonged period may produce hypoproteinemia and edema which may be intensified by beriberi heart disease, in which multiple peripheral arteriovenous fistulas result in reduced effective systemic perfusion and effective arterial blood volume, thereby enhancing edema formation. More striking edema is commonly observed when these famished subjects are provided with an adequate diet. The mechanism responsible for this latter phenomenon is not clear, but the ingestion of more food may increase the quantity of salt taken, which is retained along with water. Edema of nutritional origin may be more apparent than under other circumstances, because the subcutaneous tissue is so depleted of fat that modest collections of edema may be more obvious than they would be in a well-nourished subject.

Distribution The distribution of edema is an important guide to the cause. Thus, edema of one leg or of one or both arms is usually the result of venous and/or lymphatic obstruction. Edema resulting from hypoproteinemia characteristically is generalized, but it is especially evident in the eyelids and face and tends to be most pronounced in the morning because of the recumbent posture assumed during the night. Edema associated with heart failure, on the other hand, tends to be more extensive in the legs and to be accentuated in the evening, a feature also determined largely by posture. In the rare types of cardiac disease, such as tricuspid stenosis and constrictive pericarditis, in which orthopnea may be absent and the patient actually prefers the recumbent posture, the factor of gravity may be equalized and facial edema observed. Less common causes of facial edema include trichinosis, allergic reactions, and myxedema. Unilateral edema occasionally results from lesions in the central nervous system affecting the vasomotor fibers on one side of the body; paralysis also reduces lymphatic and venous drainage on the affected side.

Additional factors in diagnosis The color, thickness, and sensitivity of the skin are significant. Local tenderness and increase in temperature suggest inflammation. Local cyanosis may signify a venous obstruction. In individuals who have had repeated episodes of prolonged edema, the skin over the involved areas may be thickened, hard, and often red.

Measurement of the venous pressure is also of great importance in evaluating edema. Elevation in an isolated part of the body usually reflects localized venous obstruction. Generalized elevation of systemic venous pressure suggests the presence of congestive heart failure, although it may be present in the congested state that accompanies acute renal insufficiency. Ordinarily, significant increase in venous pressure can be recognized by the level at which cervical veins collapse; in doubtful cases and for accurate recording, the central venous pressure should be measured. In patients with obstruction of the superior vena cava, edema is confined to the face, neck, and upper extremities, where the venous pressure is elevated compared with that in the lower extremities. Measurement of venous pressure in the upper extremities is also useful in patients with massive edema of the lower extremities and ascites; it is elevated when the edema is on a cardiac basis (e.g., constrictive pericarditis or tricuspid stenosis), but is normal when it is secondary to cirrhosis.

Determination of the concentration of serum proteins, and especially of serum albumin, clearly differentiates those patients in whom edema is due entirely or in part to diminished intravascular colloid osmotic pressure. The presence of proteinuria affords useful clues. The complete absence of protein in the urine is evidence against, but does not exclude, either cardiac or renal disease as a cause of edema. Slight to moderate proteinuria is the rule in patients with heart failure, whereas persistent massive proteinuria usually reflects the presence of the nephrotic syndrome. Valuable information can also be obtained from other features of the examination. Some of these are the presence or absence of heart disease, the character of the urinary sediment, the dietary history, and a history of alcoholism.

SIGNIFICANT QUESTIONS AND ANSWERS REGARDING A PATIENT WITH EDEMA

1 Is the edema localized or general?

2 If localized, concentrate on those phenomena alluded to above that may be responsible. In this context, localized edema may include hydrothorax, ascites, or both in the absence of congestive heart failure or hypoalbuminemia. Either of these collections may be a consequence of local venous or lymphatic obstruction, as in inflammatory disease or carcinoma. It is a frequent accompaniment of an inflammatory process which involves the pleura or peritoneum, and the cause of the inflammatory process may vary from bacterial invasion to infarction or underlying parenchyma to a diffuse connective tissue disease with vasculitis, etc. In instances of either hydrothorax or ascites, an examination of the characteristics of the fluid is extremely important. This should include bacterial culture, smear with stains for ordinary and less common infectious agents, determination of protein concentration, cell count, and the presence or absence of blood; the cells should be concentrated by centrifugation and preparation for histologic examination for evidences of malignancy and other characteristics.

3 If the edema is generalized: (a) Is there hypoalbuminemia of significant degree, e.g., serum albumin concentration less than 2.5 g per 100 ml? If there is, a history, physical examination, and other laboratory data will help evaluate the question of cirrhosis, severe malnutrition, protein-losing gastroenteropathy, or the nephrotic syndrome as the underlying disorder. (b) Is there evidence of congestive heart failure of a severity to promote generalized edema even in the absence of hypoalbuminemia, or is there evidence of both congestive heart failure and some degree of hypoalbuminemia? (c) Does the patient have an adequate urine output, or is there significant oliguria or even anuria? These abnormalities are discussed in Chaps. 272, 273, and 278. The major differential diagnosis in these instances is frequently the discrimination between overload with fluid and a congested state as opposed to congestive heart failure.

REFERENCES

BRAUNWALD E et al: *Mechanisms of Contraction of the Normal and Failing Heart,* 2d ed., Boston: Little, Brown, 1976

COGGINS CP: Edema, chap. 36 in *Signs and Symptoms,* ed RS Blacklow, Philadelphia: Lippincott, 1977

DE WARDENER HE: The control of sodium excretion, chap. 21 in *Handbook of Physiology, Renal Physiology* 8, eds J. Orloff et al, Washington: The American Physiological Society, 1973, p. 677

DIRKS J et al: Control of extracellular fluid volume and the pathophysiology of edema formation, chap. 14 in *The Kidney,* eds BM Brenner, FC Rector Jr, Philadelphia: Saunders, 1976

EARLEY LE, SCHRIER RW: Intrarenal control of sodium excretion by hemodynamic and physical factors, chap. 22 in *Handbook of Physiology, Renal Physiology* 8, eds J Orloff et al, Washington: The American Physiological Society, 1973, p. 721

GUYTON AC et al: *Circulatory Physiology II: Dynamics and Control of the Body Fluids,* Philadelphia: Saunders, 1975

GUYTON AC: Edema, in *Textbook of Medical Physiology,* 5th ed, Philadelphia: Saunders, 1976, p. 403

LARAGH JH, SEALEY JE: The renin-angiotensin-aldosterone hormonal system and regulation of sodium, potassium and blood pressure homeostasis, chap. 26 in *Handbook of Physiology, Renal Physiology* 8, eds J Orloff et al, Washington: The American Physiological Society, 1973, p. 831

SELDIN DW: Sodium balance and fluid volume. *The Sea Within Us,* ed NS Bricker, New York: Science & Medical Publishing Co, 1975, pp. 4–13

33 PALPITATION

EUGENE BRAUNWALD

Palpitation is a common, disagreeable subjective phenomenon which may be defined as an awareness of the beating of the heart, an awareness most commonly brought about by a change in the heart's rhythm or rate or by an augmentation of its contractility. Palpitation is not pathognomonic of any particular group of disorders; indeed, often it signifies not a primary physical disorder but rather a psychic disturbance. Even when it occurs as a more or less prominent complaint, the diagnosis of the underlying disease is made largely on the basis of other associated symptoms and data. Nevertheless, palpitation is frequently of considerable importance in the minds of patients, who fear that it may indicate heart disease. Concern is all the more pronounced in patients who know or who have been told that they may have heart disease; to them palpitation may seem to be an omen of impending disaster. Since the resulting anxiety may be associated with increased activity of the autonomic nervous system, with consequent increases of the cardiac rate and rhythm and the vigor of contraction, the patient's awareness of these changes may then lead to a vicious cycle, which may ultimately be responsible for his incapacitation.

Palpitation may be described by the patient in various terms, such as "pounding," "fluttering," "flopping," and "skipping," and in most cases it will be obvious that the complaint is of a sensation of disturbed heartbeat. The wide variability in the sensitivity to alterations in cardiac activity among different individuals must be appreciated. Some patients seem to be unaware of the most serious and chaotic dysrhythmias; others are seriously troubled by an occasional extrasystole. Patients with anxiety states often exhibit a lowered threshold at which disorders of rate and rhythm result in palpitation. Indeed, it is not unusual for palpitation to be the major manifestation of the emotional disorder. The awareness of the heartbeat also tends to be more common at night and during introspective moments, but is less marked during activity. Patients with organic heart disease and chronic disorders of cardiac rate, rhythm, or stroke volume tend to accommodate to these abnormalities and are often less sensitive than normal persons to such events. Persistent tachycardia and/or atrial fibrillation may not be accompanied by continual palpitation, in contrast to a sudden, brief alteration in cardiac rate or rhythm which often causes considerable subjective discomfort. Thus, palpitation is particularly prominent when the precipitating cause for increased heart rate or contractility or arrhythmia is recent, transient, and episodic. Conversely, in emotionally well-adjusted individuals palpitation becomes progressively less disconcerting as the cause (e.g., anemia, frequent extrasystoles, complete atrioventricular block) persists.

PATHOGENESIS OF PALPITATION

Under ordinary circumstances the rhythmic heartbeat is imperceptible to the healthy individual of average or placid temperament. Palpitation may be experienced by normal persons who have engaged in strenuous physical effort or have been aroused emotionally or sexually. This type of palpitation is physiologic and represents the normal awareness of an overactive heart—i.e., a heart that is beating at a rapid rate and with an increased contractility. Since palpitation due to overactivity of the heart may occur also in certain pathologic states, e.g., high fever, severe anemia, or thyrotoxicosis, it is commonly assumed that it is the overactivity per se that is responsible for the symptom. However, overactivity of the heart is generally associated with several other alterations in cardiac function, including acceleration of heart rate, more rapid development of intraventricular pressure during isometric contraction, increased intensity of the heart sounds, especially of the first sound, a shorter duration of systole, and a greater ejection velocity.

When palpitation is heavy and regular, it is usually caused by an augmented stroke volume, and it should raise the question of aortic or mitral regurgitation, ventricular septal defect, or of a variety of hyperkinetic circulatory states (anemia, arteriovenous fistula, thyrotoxicosis, and the so-called idiopathic hyperkinetic heart syndrome). It may also occur immediately after the onset of cardiac slowing, as with the sudden development of heart block, or upon the conversion of sinus rhythm from atrial fibrillation. But unusual movements of the heart within the thorax are also frequently the mechanism of palpitation. Thus, the ectopic beat and/or the compensatory pause may be appreciated, since both are associated with alterations in cardiac motion.

IMPORTANT CAUSES OF PALPITATION

Palpitation due to disorders of the mechanism of the heartbeat

(See also Chap. 238)

EXTRASYSTOLES In most cases the diagnosis will be suggested by the patient's story. The premature contraction and postpremature beat are often described as a "flopping," or the patient may say that he feels as if "the heart turns over." The pause following the premature contraction may be felt as an actual cessation of the heartbeat, in contrast with the complete unawareness of pauses of similar duration when atrial fibrillation with a slow ventricular rate occurs. The patient's apprehensions seem to magnify the duration of the interval and sometimes may make him wonder if the heart will ever resume its beat. The first ventricular contraction succeeding the pause may be felt as an unusually vigorous beat and will be described as "pounding" or "thudding."

Usually the identification of the extrasystole as the cause of palpitation is a simple matter. When extrasystoles are numerous, clinical differentiation from atrial fibrillation can be made by any procedure that will bring about a definite increase in the ventricular rate; at increasingly rapid heart rates, the extrasystoles usually diminish in frequency and then disappear, whereas the irregularity of atrial fibrillation increases. Atrioventricular block, with dropped beats, is the only other common arrhythmia with which the premature contraction is likely to be confused; but simple auscultation will reveal the difference.

ECTOPIC TACHYCARDIAS These conditions, which are considered in some detail in Chap. 238, are common and medically important causes of palpitation. Ventricular tachycardia, one of the most serious arrhythmias, rarely is manifested as palpitation; this may be related to the abnormal sequence, and hence impaired coordination and vigor, of ventricular contraction. If the patient is seen between attacks, the diagnosis of ectopic tachycardia and its type will have to depend on the history, but of course the precise diagnosis can be made only when an electrocardiogram and observations on the effect of carotid sinus pressure are made during the episode. Monitoring of the electrocardiogram with a portable tape recording system and asking the patient to record the time of onset and cessation of the palpitations are extremely helpful in determining their cause. The mode of onset and offset gives the most important lead in distinguishing sinus from one of the various forms of ectopic tachycardias; sinus tachycardia commences and ceases over the course of minutes or seconds, but not instantaneously as is characteristic of ectopic rhythms.

Palpitation dependent on organic or functional disturbance originating outside the circulatory system

THYROTOXICOSIS In its fully developed form, thyrotoxicosis will usually be evident and offers little difficulty in the way of diagnosis except in the elderly, in whom so-called apathetic hyperthyroidism may be present. Thyrotoxicosis is particularly likely to be overlooked in the presence of myocardial failure (Chap. 92).

ANEMIA When mild, anemia may cause palpitation during exertion; when severe, palpitation may be present at rest. Appropriate studies of the blood will clarify the situation.

FEVER Palpitation may be present in acute infections, particularly in the early stages, but here the symptom is merely an insignificant phenomenon in the midst of other obviously more important ones. Palpitation may be a prominent symptom in an individual suffering from one of the chronic and sometimes more obscure febrile illnesses, such as tuberculosis, chronic brucellosis, subacute bacterial endocarditis, or acute rheumatic fever with carditis and relatively few or no joint manifestations. The problem is to determine that the underlying cause of the palpitation is an infectious illness or inflammatory process and to carry out the usual procedures to reveal the cause.

HYPOGLYCEMIA Palpitation is often a prominent feature of this condition and appears to be related to release of catecholamines. The diagnosis is confirmed by appropriate blood sugar estimations, by reproduction of the symptom when insulin is administered, and by prompt relief of all symptoms on the administration of glucose (Chap. 97).

TUMORS OF THE ADRENAL MEDULLA (PHEOCHROMOCYTOMAS) Such tumors may give rise to recurrent attacks, including paroxysms of hypertension and palpitation which are identical to those seen following the injection of epinephrine or norepinephrine. This type of tumor is a rather uncommon cause of palpitation and is mentioned chiefly because cure may be effected by surgical removal (Chap. 94). A similar syndrome may be produced when monoamine oxidase (MAO) inhibitor drugs are taken concurrently with sympathomimetic drugs, such as ephedrine or amphetamine.

DRUGS The relationship between the development of palpitation and the use of tobacco, coffee, tea, alcohol, epinephrine, ephedrine, aminophylline, atropine, or thyroid extract is obvious.

Palpitation as a manifestation of the anxiety state

Persons who are healthy physically and well adjusted emotionally may have palpitation under certain circumstances. Thus, during or immediately after vigorous physical exertion or during sudden emotional tension, palpitation is common and is usually associated with sinus tachycardia. In poorly conditioned persons without organic heart disease, the sinus tachycardia of exercise may be excessive and associated with palpitation.

In some patients, palpitation may be one of the outstanding manifestations of an episode of acute anxiety which may never recur. In other persons the palpitation may, with other symptoms, represent prolonged anxiety neurosis or a lifelong disorder characterized by volatile autonomic function. The latter condition has been called *neurocirculatory asthenia* (see Chap. 344). Whether these illnesses are simply an expression of a chronic, deep-seated anxiety state superimposed on a normal autonomic nervous system or whether they depend on instability of the autonomic nervous system is not clear. At any rate, the clinical significance of this differentiation between the transitory and the enduring forms is that the former is often dissipated by firm reassurance from the physician, whereas the latter is usually resistant even to the most thorough and expert psychiatric care. In the latter case, the patient must be treated with most carefully planned psychologic support and tranquilizing medications. This chronic form of palpitation is known by various names such as *Da Costa's syndrome, soldier's heart, effort syndrome, irritable heart, neurocirculatory asthenia,* and *functional cardiovascular disease.* Aside from palpitation, the chief symptoms are those of an anxiety state.

Physical examination usually reveals the typical findings of the hyperkinetic syndrome. These include a left parasternal lift, a precordial or apical systolic murmur, a wide pulse pressure, rapidly rising pulse, and excessive perspiration. The electrocardiogram may display minor depressions of the S-T junction and inversion of T waves and so occasionally lead to a mistaken diagnosis of coronary disease; this is particularly likely to occur when these findings are associated with complaints by the patients of an aching feeling of substernal tightness, commonly present in emotional stress. The presence of any kind of organic disease is one of the commonest causes of the underlying anxiety which frequently precipitates this functional syndrome.

Even when a patient presents undoubted objective evidence of structural cardiac disease, a superimposed anxiety state should be considered responsible for the symptoms when the clinical picture is that which has been described. Normal values for vital capacity and for circulation time make it extremely improbable that the dyspnea that accompanies this type of palpitation is due to organic cardiac disease. It is noteworthy that an anxiety state, in contrast to heart disease, causes a sighing type of dyspnea. Also pain localized to the region of the apex, either brief and lancinating in character or lasting for hours or days and accompanied by hyperesthesia, is due usually to an anxiety state, not to structural cardiac disease. Palpitation associated with organic cardiac disease is nearly always accompanied by arrhythmia or by marked tachycardia, whereas the symptom may exist with regular rhythm and with a heart rate of 80 beats per min or less in patients with the anxiety state. Giddiness due to this syndrome can usually be reproduced by hyperventilation (Chap. 16) or by change from the recumbent to the erect posture.

The *treatment* of the anxiety state with palpitation is difficult and depends on removal of the cause. In many instances a thorough examination of the heart and a statement that it is normal will suffice. Instructions to take more rather than less physical exercise will reinforce these statements. Frequently, the demonstration that the physician can reproduce not only the palpitation but many other symptoms of the anxiety state merely by the subcutaneous injection of 0.5 to 1.0 ml 1:1,000 epinephrine serves to convince the patient that his symptoms are not the result of some mysterious disorder but are rather the effect of a well-understood physiologic mechanism. This is especially true when the initial anxiety has been mainly the result of fear of heart disease. When the anxiety state is a manifestation of chronic anxiety neurosis or depressive psychosis, the symptoms are more likely to persist.

Management of patients with palpitation and the anxiety cardiac syndrome is facilitated by a clear understanding on the physician's part of the mechanisms of the symptoms. The palpitation is probably related to adrenergic stimulation of the heart and to the lower perception threshold. The pain may arise in the intercostal tissues as a result of the pounding of the heart. The hyperventilation with its ensuing train of symptoms (Chap. 16) is analogous to sighing. Explanation of these physiologic mechanisms to the patient and reassurance that they are not indicative of serious disease is one of the most important therapeutic steps.

Table 33-1 summarizes the main points of information to be ascertained in the history in elucidating the significance of palpitation. The recording of the electrocardiogram using a portable tape recorder in an ambulatory subject, and the precise temporal correlation of the cardiac rate and rhythm with the presence of palpitation are extremely useful in the identification or exclusion of a rhythmic disturbance. The effectiveness of antiarrhythmia treatment can also be assessed objectively in this manner, without the necessity of relying only on the patient's subjective symptoms. Beta-adrenergic blockade with propranolol, beginning with 40 mg per day in divided doses, and ranging as high as 240 mg per day, can be extremely effective in patients with palpitation and sinus rhythm or sinus tachycardia. The indications and contraindications for this drug are presented in Chap. 239.

One point merits special emphasis. *As a rule palpitation produces anxiety and fear out of all proportion to its seriousness.* When the cause has been accurately determined and its significance explained to the patient, his concern is often ameliorated and may disappear entirely.

TABLE 33-1
Items to be covered in history

Does the palpitation occur:	*If so, suspect:*
As isolated "jumps" or "skips"?	Extrasystoles
In attacks, known to be of abrupt beginning, with a heart rate of 120 beats/min or over, or regular or irregular rhythm?	Paroxysmal rapid heart action
Independent of exercise or excitement adequate to account for the symptom?	Atrial fibrillation, atrial flutter, thyrotoxicosis, anemia, febrile states, hypoglycemia, anxiety state
In attacks developing rapidly though not absolutely abruptly, unrelated to exertion or excitement?	Hemorrhage, hypoglycemia, tumor of the adrenal medulla
In conjunction with the taking of drugs?	Tobacco, coffee, tea, alcohol, epinephrine, ephedrine, aminophylline, atropine, thyroid extract, monoamine oxidase inhibitors
On standing?	Postural hypotension
In middle-aged women, in conjunction with flushes and sweats?	Menopausal syndrome
When the rate is known to be normal and the rhythm regular?	Anxiety state

REFERENCES

DRESSLER W: *Clinical Aids in Cardiac Diagnosis,* New York: Grune & Stratton, 1970, p. 4

HURST JW et al: *The Heart,* 3d ed., p. 143, New York: McGraw-Hill, 1974

MASSIE E: Palpitation and tachycardia, chap. 16 in *Signs and Symptoms,* 6th ed., ed RS Blacklow, Philadelphia: Lippincott, 1977

SELZER A: *Principles of Clinical Cardiology,* p. 25, Philadelphia: Saunders, 1975

WOOD P: *Diseases of the Heart and Circulation,* 3d ed., Philadelphia: Lippincott, 1968, p. 17

34 HYPOTENSION AND THE SHOCK SYNDROME

KARL ENGELMAN
EUGENE BRAUNWALD

The differential diagnosis of hypotensive states and the development of a rational plan of therapy require understanding of the normal regulation of arterial pressure.

CONTROL OF ARTERIAL PRESSURE Arterial pressure must be maintained at levels sufficient to permit adequate perfusion of the extensive capillary networks in the systemic vascular bed. The level of pressure in the central arterial bed is in a large measure dependent on two factors—the volume of blood ejected by the left ventricle per unit of time, i.e., the cardiac output, and the resistance to blood flow offered by the vessels in the peripheral vascular bed. The resistance of a blood vessel, in turn, varies inversely as the fourth power of its radius, and at any given level of cardiac output arterial pressure is therefore largely dependent upon the degree of constriction of the smooth muscle in the walls of the arterioles. Though resistance to flow also varies with the viscosity of the fluid and the length of the vessels, alterations in these factors are ordinarily of only secondary importance.

Cardiac output is controlled largely by factors which regulate ventricular end-diastolic volume, the level of myocardial contractility, and heart rate (Chap. 236). The autonomic nervous system plays a major role in the maintenance of arterial pressure by its influences on the cardiac output and on the degree of constriction of the resistance (arterioles) and capacitance (venules and veins) vessels. The afferent limbs of the autonomic reflex arcs regulating arterial pressure acutely arise in stretch receptors in the aortic arch and the carotid sinuses. Impulses are transmitted along afferent fibers in the glossopharyngeal and vagus nerves to extensive central autonomic connections in the medulla. Synapses connect not only the sympathetic and parasympathetic nuclei and efferent arcs, but also the cerebral cortex and hypothalamic nuclei which control hormonal secretion via the pituitary gland.

A rapid reduction of arterial pressure diminishes the stimulation of pressoreceptors, which in turn activates sympathetic outflow and inhibits parasympathetic activity. As a result, the vascular smooth muscle in arterioles and veins constricts, while heart rate and myocardial contractility are augmented. In addition, as arterial pressure falls, adrenal medullary secretion increases, along with the output of antidiuretic hormone (ADH), adrenocorticotropic hormone (ACTH), renin, and aldosterone; all these effects act to restore the arterial pressure to control levels. Opposite changes occur if arterial pressure is raised acutely. Thus, the operation of the pressoreceptor and a number of humoral systems normally serve to buffer the body from a variety of influences which would otherwise produce marked alterations in arterial pressure.

MEASUREMENT OF ARTERIAL PRESSURE Arterial pressure is determined clinically with a pneumatic cuff; ordinarily, this indirect method provides slight underestimation of the true arterial pressure. Considerable error may be introduced if proper precautions are not taken in determining blood pressure by this method. The arterial pressure may be significantly underestimated if the air in the cuff is released too rapidly, especially in the presence of bradycardia or an irregular rhythm, or if inadequate inflation of the cuff does not result in complete vascular occlusion. This indirect method is most accurate when, in normal-sized adults, cuffs 12 to 14 cm in width are employed. However, when a cuff of this size is used on children or adults with unusually thin arms, blood pressure may be seriously underestimated, or conversely, it may be overestimated when employed on an arm or thigh greater than 20 cm in girth. Marked vasoconstriction resulting in severely attenuated limb blood flow and/or marked reductions in pulse pressure may also result in serious underestimation of arterial pressure by the auscultatory method. Direct intraarterial recordings may reveal a normal or even an elevated pressure, while the absence of Korotkov sounds makes the pressure unobtainable by the indirect methods.

THE "NORMAL" BLOOD PRESSURE The "normal" blood pressure is difficult to define. Traditional statistical approaches define normality on the basis of values included within two standard deviations of the mean of pressures obtained in a large population of presumably healthy individuals. On this basis 95 percent of the population are defined as being normotensive, with the remaining 5 percent evenly divided between the hypertensive and hypotensive groups. A better definition of abnormality would be based on demonstrated deleterious effects of blood pressure levels exceeding certain limits. If such criteria are used, chronic hypotension would seem to occur very rarely. However, the incidence of hypertension based on casual blood pressure levels exceeding 160/95 mmHg (widely accepted as hazardous) is estimated to be approximately 15 percent in the adult population of the United States, with the incidence in the black population exceeding that in the nonblacks by 50 to 100 percent. Even these statistics may understate the prevalence of hypertension if one accepts the validity of actuarial data indicating that longevity is shortened progressively in adults whose blood pressures exceed 100/60 mmHg. The hazard of hypertension and its major complication, widespread vascular disease, appears to be a function of the level of blood pressure; the hazard rises more steeply with higher levels, especially as they exceed diastolic values of 90 to 95 mmHg (Chap. 250).

ACUTE HYPOTENSION AND SHOCK

Not uncommonly, physicians are called upon to treat patients who acutely develop severe hypotension or shock. These two terms are not synonymous; although shock is usually associated with hypotension, a previously hypertensive patient may be in shock despite an arterial pressure within normal limits, and hypotension may occur in the absence of shock. *Shock* may be defined as a state in which there is widespread, serious reduction of tissue perfusion which, if prolonged, leads to generalized impairment of cellular function.

CAUSES The most common clinical causes of shock are listed in Table 34-1. Since arterial pressure is dependent on cardiac output and peripheral vasomotor tone, marked reductions in either of these variables without a compensatory elevation of the other results in systemic hypotension. Reduction of cardiac output due to hypovolemia or acute myocardial infarction is among the most frequently encountered and easily categorized causes of shock. Failure of neurogenic mechanisms resulting in decreased vasoconstrictor impulses is another well-defined category; in many patients, particularly in the late stages of shock, multiple factors figure in the development of circulatory failure.

Hypovolemia has been studied much more extensively than any other cause of shock; the mechanism of development is usually readily evident and well understood, and therapy, i.e., restoration of blood volume, is both simple and effective if applied before irreversible tissue damage occurs. Whether the primary insult is the external loss of blood, plasma, or water and salt or the internal sequestration of these fluids in a hollow viscus or body cavity, the general effect is similar, i.e., reduced venous return and decreased cardiac output. For purposes of a general discussion of shock, hemorrhagic hypovolemia will be used as the model, but the general reduced tissue perfusion are similar.

TABLE 34-1
Etiologic factors in shock

I Hypovolemia
- *A* External fluid losses
  - *1* Hemorrhage
  - *2* Gastrointestinal
    - *a* Vomiting (pyloric stenosis, intestinal obstruction)
    - *b* Diarrhea
  - *3* Renal
    - *a* Diabetes mellitus
    - *b* Diabetes insipidus
    - *c* Excessive use of diuretics
  - *4* Cutaneous
    - *a* Burns
    - *b* Exudative lesions
    - *c* Perspiration and insensible water loss without replacement
- *B* Internal sequestration
  - *1* Fractures
  - *2* Ascites (peritonitis, pancreatitis, cirrhosis)
  - *3* Intestinal obstruction
  - *4* Hemothorax
  - *5* Hemoperitoneum

II Cardiogenic
- *A* Myocardial infarction
- *B* Arrhythmia (paroxysmal tachycardia or fibrillation, severe bradycardia)
- *C* Severe congestive heart failure with low cardiac output

III Obstruction to blood flow
- *A* Pulmonary embolus
- *B* Tension pneumothorax
- *C* Cardiac tamponade
- *D* Dissecting aortic aneurysm
- *E* Intracardiac (ball valve thrombus, atrial myxoma)

IV Neuropathic
- *A* Drug induced
  - *1* Anesthesia
  - *2* Ganglion-blocking or other antihypertensive drugs
  - *3* "Ingestion" (barbiturates, glutethimide, phenothiazines)
- *B* Spinal cord injury
- *C* Orthostatic hypotension (primary autonomic insufficiency, peripheral neuropathies)

V Other
- *A* Infection
  - *1* Gram-negative septicemia (endotoxin)
  - *2* Other septicemias
- *B* Anaphylaxis
- *C* Endocrine failure (Addison's disease, myxedema)
- *D* Anoxia

Stages of hypovolemic shock Depending upon the severity and rate of development of hypovolemia, the shock syndrome may develop abruptly or evolve gradually. If the precipitating factors progress unabated, the endogenous defense mechanisms, while initially competent to maintain adequate circulation, eventually are extended beyond their capacity for compensation. The development of the shock syndrome may be thought to evolve through several stages which merge with one another:

1 The period in which the blood volume deficit is relatively minor and in which the patient may be asymptomatic. In a previously healthy individual compensation for an acute blood loss of as much as 10 percent of the normal blood volume (as with venesection of 500 ml blood from a donor) is achieved acutely by constriction of the arteriolar bed and an augmentation of heart rate, effects mediated by reflex increases in sympathetic neural discharge of norepinephrine from sympathetic nerve endings and of both norepinephrine and epinephrine from the adrenal medulla. Other responses with more gradual effects include the increased secretion of antidiuretic hormone and the activation of the reninangiotensinaldosterone axis (Chap. 93). Arterial pressure is maintained and cardiac output is normal, or only slightly reduced, primarily as a consequence of selective reductions of blood flow to the skin and muscle beds.

2 With a reduction of blood volume of 15 to 25 percent, cardiac output falls markedly, and despite intense arteriolar constriction in most vascular beds, arterial pressure declines, although proportionately less than cardiac output. Generalized venoconstriction occurs, increasing the fraction of the total blood volume in the central circulation and tending to sustain venous return. With this massive reflex adrenergic discharge there are tachycardia, tachypnea, intense cutaneous vasoconstriction, pallor, diaphoresis, piloerection, oliguria, apprehension, and restlessness. The latter mental signs relate to primary reduction in cerebral circulation due to decreased perfusion pressure rather than to local vasoconstriction. Angina may occur in patients who have intrinsic coronary vascular disease.

3 Once the patient has achieved this state of maximal mobilization of compensatory mechanisms, small additional losses of blood result in rapid deterioration of the circulation, with life-threatening reductions of cardiac output, blood pressure, and tissue perfusion. The duration of this shock state, the severity of tissue anoxia, and the age and underlying physical state of the patient are of primary importance in determining the ultimate outcome. If tissue perfusion is restored rapidly, recovery may be expected. However, if shock persists, the severe vasoconstriction may itself become a complicating factor and by reducing tissue perfusion even further may initiate a vicious cycle leading to an irreversible state due to widespread cellular injury. Blood flow to the brain, heart, and kidneys is further reduced, and severe ischemia of these vital organs leads to irreversible tissue damage which may result in impaired function of the organ and, eventually, death. Impaired coronary perfusion depresses cardiac function, particularly in patients with some coronary vascular obstruction, and this may lead to further lowering of cardiac output, thus perpetuating a vicious cycle. Cardiac function is also depressed by the release of myocardial *depressant factor(s)* from other hypoperfused organs. Reduced flow to the medullary vasomotor center, late in the stage of shock, depresses the activity of compensatory reflexes. Anoxia, hypercapnia, and lactic acidosis result from hypoperfusion of tissues and anaerobic metabolism. These metabolic derangements ultimately result in failure of the energy-requiring active transport systems of cell membranes. The cellular high-energy phosphate reserves are depleted. The integrity of the cells is compromised, and potassium ions, intracellular lysosomal enzymes, peptides, and other vasoactive compounds are released into the circulation. The integrity of capillary membranes is disrupted, and fluid, proteins, and cellular constituents of the blood seep into the extravascular space of tissues.

In profound shock from any cause an additional important factor which may exacerbate status of the microcirculation is widespread disseminated intravascular coagulation (DIC) in the bowel, kidney, and other organs. The resultant ischemia produced in the bowel may further complicate the circulatory compensation as a result of breakdown of the mucosal barrier, leading to entry of bacteria and toxic bacterial products into the circulation. Similar changes in the capillary network of the lungs result in interstitial and alveolar edema and impaired respiratory gas transfer. Because many bacterial substances are potent vasodilators, vasoconstrictor mechanisms may be inhibited, with a further decrease in blood pressure despite intense sympathetic activity.

Just as tissue perfusion may fall to dangerous or even fatal levels because of actual fluid losses or sequestration with diminished venous return, cardiac failure or intrathoracic obstruction to blood flow may have a similar effect. Furthermore, even in the presence of a normal blood volume and cardiac function, "vasomotor collapse" due to drug-induced or neuropathic failure of sympathetic vasomotor activity can result in shock because of reduction of peripheral resistance and the pooling of blood in the venous bed.

Other forms of shock A complex form of shock may result from infection, especially gram-negative bacteremia with endotoxin release. This form of shock is associated with vascular pooling, diminished venous return, and reduced cardiac output. Sometimes there is inadequate vasoconstriction with a decline in perfusion pressures. At other stages there is intense vasoconstriction with tissue damage secondary to reduced perfusion. In anaphylactic shock, release of histamine or a histaminelike substance causes venous dilatation and an attendant increase in vascular capacity and reduction in cardiac output. Also, it results in arteriolar dilatation and a reduction of perfusion pressure, as well as increased capillary permeability with loss of intravascular volume.

TREATMENT This should be directed toward the rapid restoration of cardiac output and tissue perfusion. General supportive measures must be undertaken immediately, sometimes even before the cause of the shock state has been identified. Whether shock results from decreased cardiac output due to a primary reduction in intravascular volume or a reduction of "effective blood volume" with pooling of blood in certain vascular beds, the most effective means of restoring adequate circulation is by the rapid infusion of volume-expanding fluids (whole blood, plasma, plasma substitutes, or isotonic electrolyte solutions). However, when shock is secondary to, or is accompanied by, cardiac failure with increased pulmonary vascular and central venous pressures, the infusion of volume-expanding fluids may result in pulmonary edema. Here attention must be directed toward restoring cardiac function with cardiotonic drugs such as digitalis glycosides and isoproterenol, and an attempt should be made to support arterial pressure at levels sufficient to maintain the coronary perfusion pressure (Chap. 244). Arrhythmias, which may also contribute to the low cardiac output, should be corrected (Chap. 238).

The appearance of the external jugular veins may be helpful in differentiating between shock with high or low central venous pressure. However, catheters inserted into the superior vena cava and, if possible, into the pulmonary artery (a Swan-Ganz balloon-tipped catheter) are the best means for continuously monitoring venous pressure and of considerable value in guiding therapy; such catheters should be inserted in patients with shock whenever possible. Serial measurements of central venous pressure, urine flow rate, heart rate, and the clinical and mental state of the patient often provide more important indexes of the efficacy of therapy than arterial pressure changes. In patients with shock and impaired left ventricular function, e.g., cardiogenic shock due to massive acute myocardial infarction, the balloon-tipped catheter "floated" into the pulmonary artery at the bedside without the aid of fluoroscopy is essential in guiding treatment (Chap. 245).

There is considerable debate concerning the efficacy of vasoconstrictor drugs in shock. In patients with severe peripheral constriction these agents are often ineffective and may actually reduce the already lowered tissue perfusion. However, these drugs are usually helpful in patients with inadequate vasoconstrictor responses. The use of alpha-adrenergic blocking agents or massive doses of adrenal glucocorticoids in shock secondary to gram-negative septicemia with endotoxin release is also a matter of considerable controversy and cannot yet be considered a routine procedure. Following immediate attention to improvement of perfusion, attention should be directed to treating the underlying etiologic factor, such as diabetic acidosis, pneumothorax, or septicemia (Table 34-1).

CHRONIC HYPOTENSION

Although many patients have been treated for chronic "low blood pressure," most of them, with systolic pressures in the range of 90 to 110 mmHg, are normal and may actually have a greater life expectancy than those with higher pressures. Patients with true chronic hypotension may complain of lethargy, weakness, easy fatigability, and dizziness or faintness, especially if arterial pressure is lowered further when the erect position is assumed. These symptoms are presumably due to a decrease in perfusion of the brain, heart, skeletal muscle, and other organs.

Chronic hypotension occasionally results from severe reductions of the cardiac output. The major endocrine causes of chronic hypotension are associated with deficient gluco- and mineralocorticoid secretion and resultant reductions of the intravascular and interstitial fluid volume. Hypotension is usually more pronounced in patients with primary adrenocortical insufficiency than in those with hypopituitarism because secretion of the salt-retaining adrenocortical hormone, aldosterone, is partially preserved in pituitary insufficiency (Chap. 90).

Malnutrition, cachexia, chronic bed rest, and a variety of neurologic disorders may result in chronic hypotension, especially in the standing position. Interference with the neural pathways anywhere between the vasomotor center and the efferent sympathetic nerve endings on the blood vessels or heart may prevent the vasoconstriction and increase in cardiac output which occur as a normal response to a reduction in arterial pressure. Multiple sclerosis, amyotrophic lateral sclerosis, syringomyelia, syphilitic or diabetic tabes dorsalis, peripheral neuropathies, spinal cord section, diabetic neuropathy, extensive lumbodorsal sympathectomy, and the administration of drugs interfering with nerve transmission in the sympathetic nervous system are all associated with orthostatic hypotension. In addition, *idiopathic orthostatic hypotension* (primary autonomic insufficiency), a rare condition in which there is degeneration of central and/or peripheral autonomic nervous structures, may result in such severe orthostatic hypotension that syncope or seizures occur when the patient arises from recumbency. This condition is progressive and characterized by ascending anhydrosis and loss of hair, decreased basal metabolic rate (BMR), reduced norepinephrine production, deficient secretion of lacrimal and salivary glands, ileus, bladder atony, and absence of tachycardia on standing despite the marked reduction of blood pressure.

Specific therapy is not available for most of the neurologic causes of orthostatic hypotension, and treatment with sympathomimetic drugs has not proved effective over prolonged periods. However, the expansion of extracellular volume, which may be achieved with a high-salt diet (10 to 20 g per day), and/or the potent synthetic salt-retaining steroid, 9α-fluorhydrocortisone (0.1 to 0.5 mg per day) may be helpful. Tight, full-length elastic supportive hose to reduce orthostatic pooling of blood in the legs may also be helpful in sustaining arterial pressure, and in the most severe cases pressurized aviator suits may be necessary to permit ambulation.

REFERENCES

ANDERSON RW: Shock and circulatory collapse, chap. 5 in *Gibbon's Surgery of the Chest,* 3d ed., eds DC Sabiston, FC Spencer, Philadelphia: Saunders, 1976, pp. 107–145

CHRISTY JH: Pathophysiology of gram-negative shock. Am Heart J 81:694, 1971

GUYTON AC: Circulatory shock and physiology of its treatment, chap. 28 in *Textbook of Medical Physiology,* 5th ed., Philadelphia: Saunders, 1976, pp. 357–369

NICKERSON M: Vascular adjustments during the development of shock. Can Med Assoc J 103:853, 1971

SCHUMER W, NYHUS, L: *Treatment of Shock: Principles and Practice,* Philadelphia: Lea & Febiger, 1974

TARAZI RC: Sympathomimetic agents in the treatment of shock. Annals Int Med 81:364–371, 1974

WEIL MH et al: Treatment of circulatory shock. JAMA 231:1280–1286, 1975

35
ELEVATION OF ARTERIAL PRESSURE

KARL ENGELMAN
EUGENE BRAUNWALD

Patients with elevations of arterial pressure are usually asymptomatic, and the blood pressure abnormality often arouses attention only incidentally during military, life insurance, or other periodic physical examinations. Because hypertension results in secondary organ damage and a reduced life span, it should be evaluated fully and, when appropriate, treated.

DIAGNOSIS OF HYPERTENSION Often, however, the first question is whether patients with a moderately elevated routine blood pressure recording are truly hypertensive. It is well established that anxiety, discomfort, physical activity, or other stress can acutely and transiently raise arterial pressure. Most persons have a higher pressure when initially examined than after several measurements made in the course of a single visit; in order to establish the diagnosis of hypertension, it is necessary to document in the course of several examinations that arterial pressure remains elevated (Chap. 250). This precaution need not be taken in patients with markedly elevated blood pressure and/or in those in whom significant target organ damage is already manifest. Patients with transient or "labile" hypertension may not require immediate treatment but should be reexamined periodically, since over the course of time they often develop sustained hypertension.

Systolic hypertension in the presence of a normal or reduced diastolic pressure is less likely to be responsible for organ damage, but usually reflects other pathologic processes. It is most commonly seen in elderly patients with decreased compliance of the aortic wall. In patients with severe bradycardia, thyrotoxicosis, severe anemia, fever, aortic valvular insufficiency, arteriovenous shunts or fistulas, and the hyperkinetic heart syndrome, systolic hypertension is due to an elevated stroke volume, often accompanied by a rapid diastolic runoff.

Patients with true systemic hypertension have an increased mean arterial pressure, with elevations of both systolic and diastolic pressures. Regardless of the primary cause, the hemodynamic abnormality in most of these patients is increased vascular resistance, especially at the level of the smaller muscular arteries and arterioles, though a small number of patients may have an increased cardiac output, particularly in the early stages of the illness. In a small fraction of patients, hypertension is associated with hypervolemia, or increased blood viscosity secondary to polycythemia.

ETIOLOGY OF HYPERTENSION A specific cause for the increase in peripheral resistance which is responsible for the elevated arterial pressure cannot be defined for approximately 90 percent of patients with hypertensive disease. Numerous experimental studies have sought to define the role of a variety of components ultimately responsible for idiopathic, or so-called "essential," hypertension. Evidence for the role played by abnormal psychologic stimuli comes from the finding that chronically stressed animals may become hypertensive, and that sedatives and tranquilizers are helpful in the treatment of many hypertensive patients. Another neurogenic mechanism, the resetting of the sensitivity of the pressoreceptors, occurs in hypertensive dogs so that they appear to recognize elevated arterial pressures as normal. The importance of salt intake is suggested by studies showing that rats can be made hypertensive when given excessive dietary salt, and epidemiologic studies have also suggested this as a factor of possible etiologic significance in man; other studies have indicated that increased water and sodium in the walls of arterioles may result in increased peripheral resistance. In addition, hereditary and racial factors seem to play significant roles in the development of hypertension, since this disease is often found in families and is especially prevalent and virulent among certain ethnic groups, such as the American black population.

Using a "systems analysis" approach, Guyton has presented an elegantly reasoned and documented hypothesis that most hypertension results from altered fluid and volume control due to renal or prerenal factors. The essence of this theory is that blood pressure is automatically adjusted to ensure an adequate urine output of salt and water in an attempt to maintain normal fluid volume and balance. This unified explanation can be used to account for hypertension due to salt load, renal artery stenosis, and renal glomerular and parenchymal disease, as well as an excess of aldosterone and sympathetic tone.

A schema for the control of blood pressure is shown in Fig. 35-1. A critical role is played by the blood volume, which in turn is a principal determinant of the venous return to the heart, itself a principal regulator of cardiac output. Autoregulation is an intrinsic vascular phenomenon by which local vessels regulate tissue perfusion; through its operation an increase in cardiac output augments vascular resistance. Arterial pressure is determined by the product of output and resistance. Both the cardiac output and the arterial pressure influence the so-called "effective arterial blood volume," an as yet poorly defined parameter of the filling of the arterial tree, perhaps that portion in which the elusive volume receptors are located. It is the effective arterial blood volume, in turn, which is a principal regulator of

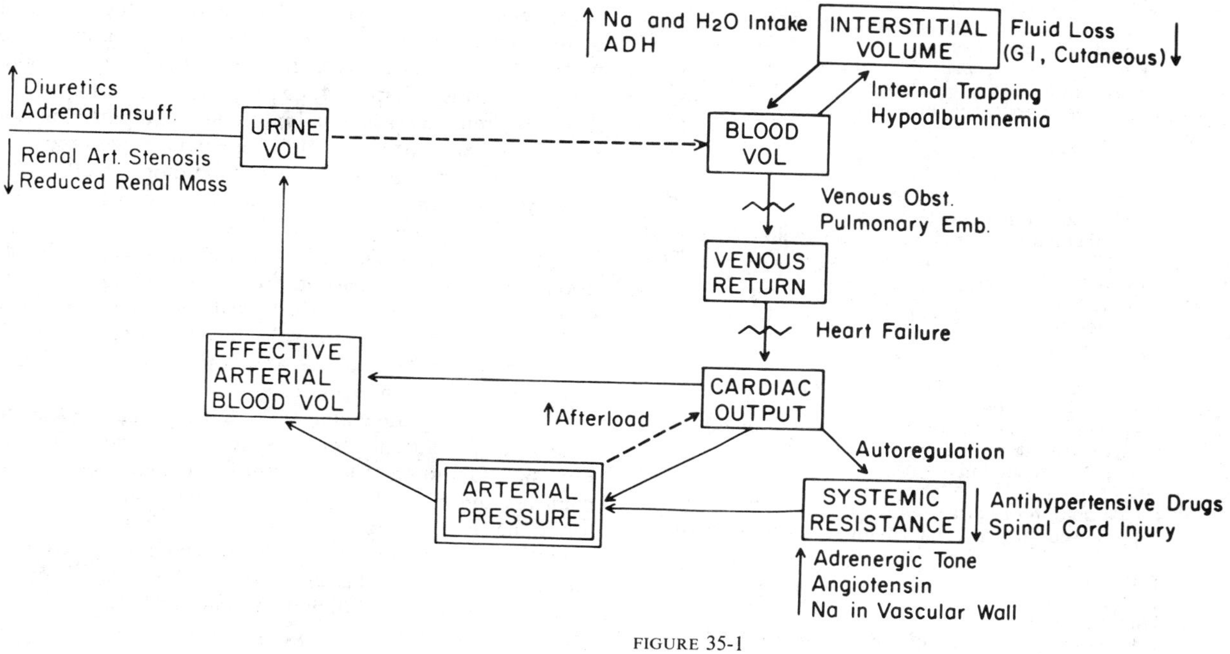

FIGURE 35-1

Schema interrelating arterial pressure, urine formation, blood volume, and cardiac output. ADH = antidiuretic hormone; GI = gastrointestinal. Solid arrows represent stimulatory effects; arrows with broken lines represent inhibitory effects.

the renal handling of salt and water excretion and therefore of urine volume. There are two negative feedbacks in this system: (1) Urine volume will exert an inverse effect on blood volume, and (2) the elevation of arterial pressure, by augmenting cardiac afterload, depresses stroke volume and thereby cardiac output (Fig. 236-6).

A wide variety of physiologic and pathologic influences act on this system. For example, blood volume may be reduced by hemorrhage, by fluid losses from the interstitial space (e.g., gastrointestinal and cutaneous losses), by the redistribution of fluid from the intravascular to the interstitial space (nephrotic syndrome), or by the pathologic sequestration of extracellular fluid (e.g., ascites). Excessive intake or administration of salt and water, administration of mineralocorticoids or their excessive secretion (Chap. 93), or overtransfusion can expand blood volume. Obstruction of systemic venous return and pulmonary embolism can impair venous return to the left ventricle, despite a normal or even augmented blood volume, and the various forms of cardiac failure depress cardiac output despite the capacity of the peripheral vascular bed to return blood to the heart (Chap. 237). Systemic vascular resistance can be augmented by a number of influences such as adrenergic stimuli, circulating angiotensin and catecholamines, and stiffness of the arteriolar walls as a consequence of an increased sodium content, while directly acting vasodilator drugs such as hydralazine and antiadrenergic agents such as guanethidine can exert the opposite effects. Of great potential interest in the etiology of hypertension is the observation that a reduction of the renal parenchymal mass, renal artery stenosis, and renal vasoconstriction, and augmented mineralocorticoid action all tend to reduce urine salt and water loss and thereby inhibit the principal negative feedback, thus tending to elevate arterial pressure, while the administration of diuretics or adrenal insufficiency (Chap. 93) exerts the opposite effect. Thus, a block in the system anywhere upstream of or including the heart will result in edema formation without hypertension, while a block in the system downstream of the heart and including the kidney will result in hypertension usually without edema.

It appears that all the above-mentioned factors play some role in the development of essential hypertension, which might be best regarded as a multifactorial disease related to abnormalities of the regulatory mechanisms normally concerned with the homeostatic control of arterial pressure.

More specific etiologic relationships have been established for a smaller group of patients with systemic hypertension (Table 35-1). Primary renal diseases associated with the development of serious hypertension (as distinguished from renal damage secondary to hypertension) have been recognized for years, although in many cases the exact mechanism of blood pressure elevation is unknown. Hypertension may develop suddenly during the course of acute glomerulonephritis, and it is usually a prominent feature in the late stages of renal damage due to chronic glomerulonephritis (Chap. 274) or pyelonephritis (Chap. 277). Polycystic renal disease, renal infarction, and partial occlusion of the renal artery due to congenital or acquired vascular defects are also implicated as etiologic factors, the latter having been clearly related to activation of the renin-angiotensin-aldosterone pressor system.

The most clearly defined etiologic relationships in the development of hypertension are found among the endocrine disorders. Adrenocortical hormones have also been implicated in the hypertensive syndromes associated with tumors or hyperplasia of the anterior pituitary (Cushing's syndrome, primary hyperaldosteronism, Chap. 93), as well as with various congenital or hereditary enzyme defects (hypertensive adrenogenital syndromes). Secretion of excessive quantities of the pressor catecholamines, norepinephrine and epinephrine, associated with pheochromocytomas, i.e., chromaffin cell tumors arising from the adrenal medulla or sympathetic ganglia, is also commonly associated with hypertension (Chap. 94). Up to 50 percent of patients with acromegaly (Chap. 90) may have hypertension, but the mechanism of their blood pressure elevation is less clear. The presence of these endocrinopathies is usually readily recognizable and distinguishable from essential hypertension by their distinctive clinical and biochemical fea-

TABLE 35-1
Classification of arterial hypertension

- *I* Systolic hypertension with wide pulse pressure
  - *A* Decreased compliance of aorta (arteriosclerosis)
  - *B* Increased stroke volume or cardiac output
    - *1* Arteriovenous fistula
    - *2* Thyrotoxicosis
    - *3* Hyperkinetic heart disease
    - *4* Fever
    - *5* Psychogenic factors
    - *6* Aortic valvular insufficiency
    - *7* Patent ductus arteriosus
- *II* Systolic and diastolic hypertension (increased peripheral vascular resistance)
  - *A* Renal
    - *1* Chronic pyelonephritis
    - *2* Acute and chronic glomerulonephritis
    - *3* Polycystic renal disease
    - *4* Renovascular stenosis or renal infarction
    - *5* Most other severe renal disease (arteriolar nephrosclerosis, diabetic nephropathy, etc.)
  - *B* Endocrine
    - *1* Acromegaly
    - *2* Adrenocortical hyperfunction
      - *a* Cushing's disease and syndrome
      - *b* Primary hyperaldosteronism
      - *c* Congenital or hereditary adrenogenital syndromes (17α-hydroxylase and 11β-hydroxylase defects)
    - *3* Pheochromocytoma
    - *4* Myxedema
  - *C* Neurogenic
    - *1* Psychogenic
    - *2* "Diencephalic syndrome"
    - *3* Familial dysautonomia (Riley-Day)
    - *4* Poliomyelitis (bulbar)
    - *5* Polyneuritis (acute porphyria, lead poisoning)
    - *6* Increased intracranial pressure (acute)
    - *7* Spinal cord section
  - *D* Miscellaneous
    - *1* Coarctation of aorta
    - *2* Increased intravascular volume (excessive transfusion)
    - *3* Polyarteritis nodosa
    - *4* Hypercalcemia
  - *E* Unknown etiology
    - *1* Essential hypertension (>90% of all cases of hypertension)
    - *2* Toxemia of pregnancy
    - *3* Acute intermittent porphyria
    - *4* Oral contraceptives

tures. The clinical differentiations between primary and the various forms of secondary hypertension are detailed in Chap. 250.

EFFECTS OF HYPERTENSION Following an asymptomatic latent period, clinical manifestations which reflect the underlying pathologic sequelae of the hypertensive state usually become apparent. Cardiac, renal, and central nervous system effects due to accelerated vascular damage are most prominent, and if unaltered by therapy, they often ultimately result in symptomatic illness and death.

Effects on heart Cardiac compensation for the excessive workload imposed by increased systemic pressure is at first sustained by left ventricular hypertrophy. Ultimately, the function of this chamber deteriorates, it dilates, and the symptoms and signs of heart failure appear (Chap. 237). Angina pectoris may also occur because of accelerated coronary arterial disease and/or increased myocardial oxygen requirements as a consequence of the increased myocardial mass, which exceeds the capacity of the coronary circulation. On physical examination the heart is enlarged and has a prominent left ventricular impulse. The sound of aortic closure is accentuated, and there may be a faint murmur of aortic insufficiency. Presystolic (atrial) gallop sounds appear frequently in hypertensive heart disease, and a protodiastolic (ventricular), or summation, gallop rhythm may be present. Electrocardiographic changes of left ventricular hypertrophy are common; evidence of ischemia or infarction may be observed late in the disease. The majority of deaths due to hypertension result from myocardial infarction or congestive heart failure.

Neurologic effects The neurologic effects of long-standing hypertension may be divided into retinal and central nervous system changes. Because the retina is the only tissue in which the arteries and arterioles can be examined directly, repeated ophthalmoscopic examination provides the opportunity to observe the progress of the vascular effects of hypertension. The Keith-Wagener-Barker classification of the retinal changes in hypertension (Table 35-2) has provided a simple and excellent means for serial evaluation of the hypertensive patient. Table 35-2 includes both the criteria for grouping the retinal findings of hypertension and the secondary arteriolosclerotic changes. Increasing severity of hypertension is associated with focal spasm and progressive general narrowing of the arterioles, as well as the appearance of hemorrhages, exudates, and papilledema. These retinal lesions often produce scotomas, blurred vision, and even blindness, especially in the presence of papilledema or hemorrhages of the macular area. Hypertensive lesions may develop acutely, and if therapy results in significant reduction of blood pressure, may show rapid resolution. Rarely, these lesions resolve without therapy. In contrast, retinal arteriolosclerosis results from endothelial and muscular proliferation, and it accurately reflects similar changes in other organs. Sclerotic changes do not develop as rapidly as hypertensive lesions, nor do they regress appreciably with therapy. As a consequence of increased wall thickness and rigidity, sclerotic arterioles distort and compress the veins as they cross within their common fibrous sheath, and the reflected light streak from the arterioles is changed by the increased opacity of the vessel wall.

Central nervous system dysfunction also occurs frequently in patients with hypertension. Occipital headaches, most often in the morning, are among the most prominent early symptoms of hypertension. Dizziness, lightheadedness, vertigo, tinnitus, and dimmed vision or syncope may also be observed, but the more serious manifestations are due to vascular occlusion or hemorrhage. With severe long-standing hypertension, patients develop multiple focal or large vascular infarcts or hemorrhages which result in destruction of brain tissue. The focal changes may be manifested as personality or memory deficits, but the larger

TABLE 35-2
Classification of hypertensive and arteriolosclerotic retinopathy

	Hypertension					*Arteriolosclerosis*	
	Arterioles						
Degree	*General narrowing AV ratio**	*Focal spasm†*	*Hemorrhages*	*Exudates*	*Papilledema*	*Arteriolar light reflex*	*AV crossing‡ defects*
Normal	3/4	1/1	0	0	0	Fine yellow line, red blood column	0
Grade I	1/2	1/1	0	0	0	Broadened yellow line, red blood column	Mild depression of vein
Grade II	1/3	2/3	0	0	0	Broad yellow line, "copper wire," blood column not visible	Depression or humping of vein
Grade III	1/4	1/3	+	+	0	Broad white line, "silver wire," blood column not visible	(*a*) Right-angle deviation, tapering, and disappearance of vein under arteriole (*b*) Distal dilatation of vein
Grade IV	Fine, fibrous cords	Obliteration of distal flow	+	+	+	Fibrous cords, blood column not visible	Same as grade III

* *This is the ratio of arteriolar/venous diameters.*
† *This is the ratio of diameters of region of spasm to proximal arteriole.*
‡ *Arteriolar length and tortuosity increase with severity.*

lesions which produce major strokes are responsible for up to 10 to 15 percent of deaths occurring secondary to hypertension.

Renal effects Arteriolosclerotic lesions of the afferent and efferent arterioles and the glomerular capillary tufts are the most common renal vascular lesions in hypertension and result in decreased glomerular filtration rate and tubular dysfunction. Proteinuria and microscopic hematuria occur because of glomerular lesions, and approximately 10 percent of the deaths secondary to hypertension result from renal failure. Blood loss in hypertension occurs not only from renal lesions; epistaxis, hemoptysis, and metrorrhagia also occur more frequently in these patients.

TREATMENT As a consequence of the pathologic changes secondary to the elevated arterial pressure, treatment of patients with systemic hypertension is directed toward lowering pressure in an attempt to halt or reverse the progressive organ damage. In certain instances specific therapy or cure of the primary etiologic factor can be achieved by repair of a stenotic renal artery lesion or coarctation of the aorta, or by removal of a tumor which secretes pressor substances. However, because of the unknown cause of the hypertension in the majority of patients, therapy is directed primarily toward the major physiologic abnormality, i.e., it is designed to lower systemic vascular resistance. Because the sympathetic nervous system plays such an important role in the maintenance of peripheral resistance, many effective antihypertensive drugs act by interfering with the vasoconstrictor impulses mediated by this system (Chap. 250). Other effective means of treating hypertension include reduction of intravascular volume and cardiac output with diuretics and peripheral vasodilatation with drugs which directly relax the vascular smooth muscle (Chap. 250). Although arterial pressure can be reduced in the majority of patients, hypertension is a chronic disease, and a therapeutic program must usually be maintained for the duration of the patient's life.

REFERENCES

GUYTON AC et al: Hypertension: A disease of abnormal circulatory control. Chest 65:328, 1974

——: Regulation of arterial pressure, in *Textbook of Medical Physiology,* 5th ed., Philadelphia: Saunders, 1976, pp. 265–294

HOLLENBERG NK et al: Renal vascular tone in essential and secondary hypertension. Medicine 54:29, 1975

LARAGH JH et al: The renin axis and vasoconstriction volume analysis for understanding and treating renovascular and renal hypertension. Amer J Med 58:4, 1975

PICKERING G: *Hypertension,* 2d ed., New York: Churchill, Livingston, 1974

SCHEIE HG: Evaluation of ophthalmoscopic changes of hypertension and arteriolar sclerosis. AMA Arch Ophthalmol 49:117, 1953

36 SUDDEN CARDIOVASCULAR COLLAPSE AND DEATH

BURTON E. SOBEL
EUGENE BRAUNWALD

Sudden death claims more than 400,000 lives annually in the United States alone. It is a major health problem in the Western world. Despite the liberality of the definition of sudden death of the Joint American Heart Association—International Society of Cardiology Committee (death occurring instantaneously or within an estimated 24 h of the onset of acute symptoms or signs), about half of sudden deaths are virtually instantaneous. A brief period of time, usually only several minutes, elapses between sudden cardiovascular collapse (without effective cardiac output) and irreversible ischemic changes in the central nervous system. Prolonged survival without functional impairment may be the reward for prompt treatment of certain forms of cardiovascular collapse.

MECHANISMS Sudden cardiovascular collapse may be due to (1) dysrhythmia (Chap. 238); (*a*) most commonly, ventricular tachycardia or fibrillation, sometimes occurring following a bradyarrhythmia, or (*b*) less frequently, ventricular asystole or severe bradycardia; (2) a marked, abrupt reduction in cardiac output, such as occurs with mechanical blockade of the circulation; massive pulmonary thromboembolism (Chap. 266) and cardiac tamponade are two examples of this form; (3) sudden ventricular (pump) failure, which may occur in the presence of an acute myocardial infarction (Chap. 244) or critical aortic stenosis (Chap. 243); (4) activation of vasodepressor reflexes, which may contribute to sudden reductions in arterial pressure and heart rate, and which are activated in diverse conditions, including primary pulmonary hypertension (Chap. 265), pulmonary thromboembolism, and the hypersensitive carotid sinus syndrome (Chap. 16).

Sudden death and coronary atherosclerosis Sudden death is primarily a complication of coronary atherosclerosis. More than two-thirds of the cases result from this disorder. In the vast majority of such patients sudden death results from precipitous ventricular fibrillation. However, evidence of coronary occlusion and, indeed, of acute myocardial infarction may not be found at autopsy; nonetheless, acute myocardial ischemia appears to be the precipitating event. Only approximately 40 percent of patients dying from coronary artery disease survive long enough to be hospitalized. The remainder (approximately 300,000 patients per year in the United States) die suddenly before they reach the hospital. In fact, in 25 percent of patients with coronary artery disease, death is the first indication of the presence of the disorder (Chap. 244). By extrapolation from experience in coronary care units, in which control of electrical activity of the heart has affected mortality favorably, it would appear that the incidence of sudden death in the community might be reduced substantially by prophylactic therapy in populations at particularly high risk, if such therapy could be demonstrated to be effective, of low toxicity, and convenient to the patient. However, sudden death may be but one mode of expression of coronary artery disease, and effective prevention of sudden death will almost certainly require reduction in the incidence and severity of this disease.

Factors associated with increased risk of sudden death in nonhospitalized persons When electrocardiograms are recorded for 24 h during the course of normal activities, supraventricular premature contractions are found to occur in most American men over fifty years of age, ventricular premature contractions and complex ventricular dysrhythmias in almost two-thirds, and persistent or transient conduction defects in less than 10 percent. Supraventricular dysrhythmias do not appear to be associated with increased risk of sudden death except when they are a manifestation of the severity of anterior myocardial infarction and presage increased early mortality. On the other hand, conduction abnormalities and certain types of ventricular premature beats, such as those originating from the left ventricle (recognizable by their terminal anterior and rightward vectors), those occurring during the vulnerable period, and those occurring in pairs or salvos do appear to be associated with an increased risk. In general, ventricular dysrhythmias are of greater significance and more ominous in the presence of acute ischemia than its absence. In the asymptomatic patient, ventricular premature contractions should alert the physician to look for more definitive evidence of heart disease, such as other electrocardiographic abnormalities, hypertension, or a history of angina.

Overt coronary artery disease, hypertension, or diabetes mellitus is present in more than 75 percent of persons dying suddenly, and, perhaps more significantly, the incidence of sudden death in persons with at least one of the three abnormalities is substantially increased. Severe coronary artery disease, not necessarily accompanied by morphologic evidence of an acute event, is consistently present in victims of sudden, unexpected death. More than 75 percent of men without known prior coronary artery disease who die suddenly exhibit at least two of the following four risk factors: hypercholesterolemia, hypertension, hyperglycemia, and cigarette smoking. Obesity and electrocardiographic criteria of left ventricular hypertrophy are also associated with an increased incidence. The incidence of sudden death is higher in cigarette smokers than in nonsmokers, perhaps because of the elevation of circulating catecholamines and fatty acids and the production of increased circulating carboxyhemoglobin with consequently diminished oxygen-carrying capacity by the blood. The proclivity of cigarette smoking to cause sudden death is not cumulative and appears to be entirely reversible when smoking is discontinued.

Ventricular premature contractions may be increased or made overt by exercise, and sudden death appears sometimes to follow unusual exertion. On the other hand, the incidence appears to be diminished in subjects engaged in regular, intermittent, strenuous physical activity in comparison with controls in the same socioeconomic group with a more sedentary existence. Cardiovascular collapse on exertion occurs very rarely in patients with ischemic heart disease undergoing exercise testing, and with appropriate personnel and facilities these episodes respond promptly to electrical defibrillation. Rarely also, acute emotional stress may precipitate acute myocardial infarction and sudden death, findings which are in keeping with recent experimental observations of increased susceptibility to ventricular tachycardia and ventricular fibrillation after coronary occlusion in emotionally stressed animals or those with augmented sympathetic activity.

Two major clinical syndromes may be recognized in patients who die suddenly and unexpectedly; both are generally associated with ischemic heart disease. In the larger group, the dysrhythmia, which may be termed *primary ventricular fibrillation,* occurs totally unexpectedly and without preceding symptoms or prodromata. This form is *not* associated with acute myocardial infarction; following resuscitation, there is a propensity for early recurrence, probably reflecting the myocardial electrical instability responsible for the initial episode, and a relatively high 2-year mortality (approximately 50 percent). Clearly, these patients can be salvaged only by a rapidly responsive system, and pharmacologic prophylaxis is required to enhance survival. The second, smaller group consists of patients who, following resuscitation, give evidence of acute myocardial infarction. These patients often exhibit prodromal symptoms—chest pain, dyspnea, and syncope—and show a much lower recurrence and 2-year mortality (15 percent). Survival in this subgroup is similar to that following resuscitation from ventricular fibrillation complicating acute myocardial infarction in the coronary care unit. Thus, it would appear that the propensity for developing ventricular fibrillation at the time of acute infarction is of short duration, while ventricular fibrillation in the absence of acute infarction may be related to a chronic process and is likely to recur.

Other causes of sudden death Sudden cardiovascular collapse may result from a number of disorders other than coronary atherosclerosis (Table 36-1). Severe aortic stenosis (congenital or acquired) with sudden dysrhythmias or pump failure, idiopathic hypertrophic subaortic stenosis, and myocarditis or cardiomyopathy associated with dysrhythmia may be responsible. Massive pulmonary embolism leads to circulatory collapse and death within minutes in approximately 10 percent of patients; some of the remainder succumb gradually with progressive right ventric-

TABLE 36-1
Conditions associated with cardiovascular collapse and sudden death in adults

Ischemic heart disease secondary to coronary atherosclerosis
Valvular heart disease, especially aortic stenosis
Bacterial endocarditis
Myocarditis
Cardiomyopathies (primary myocardial disease and particularly idiopathic hypertrophic subaortic stenosis)
Ruptured or dissecting aortic aneurysm
Coronary embolism
Congenital coronary artery disease
Hereditary Q-T interval prolongation
Sinoatrial node disease
Primary degeneration of the conduction system, sometimes familial
Secondary disease of the conduction system (e.g., amyloid, sarcoid, hemochromatosis, thrombotic thrombocytopenic purpura, myotonia dystrophica)
Cerebrovascular accident, particularly hemorrhage
Pulmonary thromboembolism
Chronic obstructive pulmonary disease
Drug toxicity or idiosyncrasy (e.g., digitalis, quinidine)

ular failure. Acute circulatory collapse may be presaged by smaller emboli occurring at variable intervals before the lethal attack. Accordingly, implementation of therapy during the premonitory sublethal phase, including anticoagulant administration, may be lifesaving (Chap. 266). Sublethal emboli are common in hospitalized patients and can be recognized in at least 40 percent of postmortem examinations when specialized pulmonary arterial injection techniques are utilized. Their clinical manifestations include unexplained or disproportionate dyspnea or tachypnea, hypoxemia, respiratory alkalosis, and hypocapnia. Sinus tachycardia is common. Atrial flutter, chaotic atrial rhythms, and multiple premature atrial beats are compatible with the diagnosis; thrombophlebitis or conditions predisposing to this are also helpful, suggestive signs.

Sudden death with cardiovascular collapse is a rare but always potential complication of bacterial endocarditis (Chap. 132). In this condition it is usually due to relentless progression of congestive heart failure, but it may also result from ventricular fibrillation, complete atrioventricular block, rupture of a sinus of Valsalva, or a septic embolus to the cerebral or coronary vessels. Sudden, unexpected death in infants, so-called "crib death," is responsible for approximately 10,000 deaths per year in the United States. Respiratory infections, abnormalities of the small vessels supplying the sinus and atrioventricular nodes, and abnormally exaggerated cardioinhibitory reflexes may be responsible.

A number of less common causes of sudden death have been recognized increasingly in recent years. Primary degeneration of the atrioventricular conduction system, with or without deposition of calcium or cartilage, may lead to sudden death in the absence of severe coronary atherosclerosis. Trifascicular atrioventricular (AV) block is often seen in these conditions, which account for more than two-thirds of the cases of chronic AV block in adults (Chap. 238). Patients in whom the degree of block is unstable are particularly susceptible to more serious brady- or tachyarrhythmias. Electrocardiographic Q-T interval prolongation, nerve deafness, and autosomal recessive inheritance seem to be associated with a high proportion of cases of ventricular fibrillation. The same electrocardiographic abnormality and electrophysiologic instability without nerve deafness appear to be inherited in an autosomal dominant mode. Electrocardiographic changes in these disorders may be manifest only after exercise, and so they may be more important causes of sudden death than has been generally recognized. Other conditions with Q-T prolongation and increased temporal dispersion of repolarization, such as mitral valve prolapse (the click-murmur syndrome), hypothermia, and phenothiazine, emetine, or quinidine toxicity are rarely associated with sudden death. Sinoatrial arrest or block with depression of lower pacemakers may also lead to asystole. Sudden rupture of a papillary muscle, the ventricular septum, or free wall, usually occurring within the first few days following acute myocardial infarction, occasionally causes sudden death (Chap. 244). Sudden cardiovascular collapse is also a major, frequently the terminal, event in patients with major cerebrovascular accidents (Chap. 334), sudden alterations of intracranial pressure, or lesions affecting the brainstem. It may also occur with asphyxia, and the toxicity of cardioactive drugs such as digitalis and quinidine may result in life-threatening arrhythmias, leading to sudden cardiovascular collapse and, if treatment is not immediate, to death (Chap. 239).

Electrophysiologic mechanisms underlying ventricular fibrillation Available data suggest that potentially lethal ventricular dysrhythmias in patients with acute myocardial infarction result from (1) enhanced automaticity of His-Purkinje fibers, (2) reentry due to locally impaired conduction facilitated by dispersion of the refractory periods in adjacent regions of myocardium and depression of conduction velocity; (3) possible focal reexcitation from current flow between adjacent cells repolarized at disparate times; and (4) conversion of fast (sodium-mediated) to slow (calcium-mediated) depolarizations, favored by reduced transmembrane resting potentials. Local myocardial ischemia, electrolyte and pH changes, exaggerated catecholamine release, elevated circulating free fatty acid levels, and digitalis or quinidine toxicity may prolong the refractory period, depress conduction velocity, and set the stage for reentry rhythms. Enhanced automaticity, repetitive spontaneous after-potentials, and delayed conduction appear to result from slow current, calcium-mediated responses in ischemic zones with low amplitude, slow rising, and prolonged action potentials. These phenomena may be amenable to favorable modification with antiarrhythmic agents such as verapamil, which selectively block the slow (calcium-mediated) responses.

The so-called vulnerable period, corresponding to the ascending limb of the T wave (Chap. 240), represents that portion of the cardiac cycle when temporal dispersion of ventricular refractoriness is normally maximum and, accordingly, when reentrant rhythms leading to sustained, repetitive activity can be initiated most readily. In patients with acute myocardial infarction, the vulnerable period is prolonged and the intensity of stimulus required to evoke repetitive tachycardia or ventricular fibrillation is reduced, so that a single ventricular premature contraction may initiate the rhythm. Electrical shocks of low energy or even a blow struck over the precordium ("thump version") may terminate ventricular tachycardia, presumably by interrupting a reentrant pathway. Since paroxysms of ventricular ectopic beats progressively increase asynchrony of recovery, such paroxysms frequently augur ventricular fibrillation. In addition, since temporal dispersion of refractoriness may be increased in the presence of a slow heart rate, profound bradycardia due to decreased automaticity of the sinus node or AV block may also be particularly dangerous in patients with acute myocardial infarction. Increased automaticity of subsidiary ectopic pacemakers, driven by myocardial catecholamine release, may contribute further to the development of chaotic ventricular rhythms. Electrophysiologic derangements tend to occur with greatest frequency early following the onset of myocardial ischemia or infarction. They may be accentuated by ventricular enlargement (favoring reentry), concomitant metabolic derangements, and deleterious effects of cardioactive drugs. These derangements cause the majority of instantaneous deaths, but they may also occur suddenly and unexpectedly later in the course of an otherwise uncomplicated hospitalization or subsequent convalescence.

Asystole is a less common electrophysiologic mechanism

underlying sudden death due to coronary atherosclerosis. It may occur when impulse formation in the sinus node is impaired or AV block impedes transmission and subsidiary pacemakers fail to function effectively.

PREVENTION OF SUDDEN DEATH The difficulties entailed in ambulatory electrocardiographic monitoring or other procedures for mass screening to detect candidates at risk of sudden death are formidable, since the population at risk comprises more than one-third of all men in the 35- to 74-year age groups. Some patients have prodromata, usually the new development of angina pectoris or an increase in the severity of previously existing angina (Chap. 244) in the weeks or months preceding acute myocardial infarction, and therefore these symptoms also often precede sudden cardiovascular collapse. As already stated, the presence of certain forms of ventricular premature contractions may characterize patients particularly susceptible to sudden death. Unsupervised physical stress, such as jogging, by patients with known ischemic heart disease should be discouraged. Although identification of patients at high risk is particularly important, selection of an effective prophylactic regimen remains difficult, and none has clearly demonstrated effectiveness in reducing the risk. For example, although procainamide is effective in suppressing ventricular dysrhythmias in patients in the coronary care unit, drug toxicity militates against its routine prolonged use in a general ambulatory population. One subset of patients at particularly high risk comprises those successfully resuscitated after prehospital ventricular fibrillation, even when fibrillation occurs without evolution of acute myocardial infarction manifested electrocardiographically or by elevated serum enzymes. Another group comprises all patients surviving acute myocardial infarction. It is reasonable to propose a trial of prophylactic treatment, on an individual basis, of patients with known or suspected coronary artery disease with hazardous or recurrent dysrhythmias or the electrocardiographic characteristics described above. Quinidine gluconate, 330 mg by mouth every 6 h, may be effective in suppressing these dysrhythmias. The dosage may be increased up to 3 g per day if found necessary, unless gastrointestinal disturbances or electrocardiographic evidence of toxicity occurs. The long-acting preparation has the obvious advantage of requiring relatively infrequent dose schedules (b.i.d. or t.i.d.). Patients who tolerate quinidine poorly may do well with procainamide, 500 mg by mouth every 4 h. Ambulatory electrocardiographic monitoring may be particularly helpful in documenting the efficacy of treatment, since the incomplete knowledge regarding the pathogenesis of sudden death makes rational prophylactic drug selection and dosage difficult and a stereotyped regimen for all patients impractical.

Decreased incidence of sudden death in randomized patients surviving acute myocardial infarction has been documented in prospective double-blind studies utilizing alprenolol, a cardioselective beta-adrenergic blocking agent, although the effect of treatment on dysrhythmia was not quantified and the mechanism of apparent protection has not yet been identified.

Delays by the patient, physician, transportation system and in the emergency room after the occurrence of acute myocardial infarction are significant impediments to prevention of sudden death. The median elapsed time between onset of symptoms and hospitalization averages 5 to 8 h in most areas of the United States. Denial by the patient of the seriousness of his condition and indecision by both the patient and physician contribute most to total delay.

Experience gained in Seattle, Wash., has shown that in order to deal effectively on a community-wide basis with the problem of sudden cardiovascular collapse and deaths, it is necessary to develop a system which provides rapid and effective response for these emergencies. Important elements of the system include a city-wide emergency call number through which the system can be activated, a well-trained group of paramedical personnel such as firemen to respond, a short average time of response (under 4 min), and a large number of lay people trained in techniques of resuscitation. Clearly, the success in immediate resuscitation and for long-term survival is directly related to how soon following collapse resuscitation efforts are initiated. The availability of special ambulances (mobile coronary care units) equipped and staffed to handle acute cardiac emergencies appears to reduce delay by increasing community and physician awareness of the urgency of prompt medical attention. Such a system can be effective in resuscitating more than 40 percent of patients who have undergone cardiovascular collapse, and more than 25 percent of such patients are discharged from the hospital.

Therefore, providing instructions to susceptible persons on how to seek medical care on an emergency basis upon the development of symptoms of myocardial infarction is of great importance in the prevention of sudden cardiac death. This strategy includes instructing the patient that prompt entry into an effective emergency care system is not only correct but also what the physician expects of the patient, regardless of whether symptoms suggestive of myocardial infarction occur during the day or night (Chap. 244); this concept means also instructing the patient to bypass the physician and to contact the emergency care system directly.

APPROACH TO THE PATIENT WITH SUDDEN CARDIOVASCULAR COLLAPSE Sudden death can often be averted even when cardiovascular collapse has occurred. In patients experiencing sudden onset of ventricular fibrillation without prior ventricular failure (primary ventricular fibrillation) while they are under observation in the operating room, the cardiac catheterization laboratory, or the coronary care unit, correction of the dysrhythmia is the rule, and the outcome is usually favorable. However, prompt application of definitive therapy for sudden cardiovascular collapse in the community entails formidable practical obstacles, as outlined above.

The development of transvenous and transthoracic cardiac pacemakers (Chap. 238) and the improvement of cardiopulmonary resuscitative maneuvers, including external cardiac massage coupled with artificial respiration, have contributed to effective therapy.

When a patient under close medical observation develops sudden collapse from a dysrhythmia, the immediate goal must be restoration of effective cardiac rhythm. Circulatory collapse must be recognized and confirmed immediately. Its cardinal features are (1) impaired cerebration, syncope, and seizures, (2) absent peripheral arterial pulses, and (3) absent heart sounds. When ventilation immediately preceding the collapse has been adequate, cyanosis may be absent or minimal. Since external cardiac massage can provide only limited cardiac output, definitive restoration of effective rhythm should be the immediate goal, and in the absence of evidence to the contrary, abrupt circulatory collapse should be assumed to be due to ventricular fibrillation. If the physician sees the patient within 50 s of the collapse, time should not be wasted by attempting to achieve oxygenation. An immediate blow to the precordium ("thump version") may be attempted, since this is occasionally effective and takes only seconds. Electrical defibrillation (Chap. 240) should be attempted immediately thereafter, without necessarily even pausing first to record an electrocardiogram on separate equipment, although use of portable defibrillators capable of electrocardiographic recording from the defibrillating electrodes themselves may be helpful. Maximum electrical output, usually 400 W-s, should be used. If these immediate attempts are unsuccessful, external cardiac massage and complete cardiopulmonary resuscitation should be brought into play.

If collapse is due to unequivocal asystole, transthoracic or transvenous electrical pacing should be implemented immediately. Intracardiac epinephrine, 1 ml of 1:1,000 solution diluted 1:10 with intracavitary blood may facilitate the heart's response to artificial pacing or be helpful when a slow ventricular focus is present but ineffective. If these initial definitive measures fail despite adequate technical performance, prompt restitution of a favorable metabolic milieu and monitoring are necessary. This is best accomplished by these three procedures: (1) External cardiac massage. (2) Correction of acid-base balance, often requiring intravenous sodium bicarbonate administration in an initial dose of 1 mg per kg repeated once within 5 to 10 min. Administration of subsequent doses of bicarbonate should be guided by frequent determinations of arterial pH, particularly since intracellular pH may paradoxically increase because permeability to carbon dioxide is so much greater than to bicarbonate. (3) Assessment and correction of electrolyte imbalance. Definitive efforts to restore an effective cardiac rhythm should be attempted again as soon as possible, certainly within minutes. When effective cardiac rhythm is restored but rapidly degenerates again into ventricular tachycardia or fibrillation, lidocaine should be administered as a bolus, 1 mg per kg intravenously, then continued by intravenous infusion at a rate up to 1 to 5 mg/kg/h, and countershock repeated.

Cardiac massage External cardiac massage is designed to lead to the ejection of blood from the heart by manual compression of the ventricles between the sternum and the spine, and cyclic passive ventricular filling. Adherence to several aspects of technique is essential (Fig. 36-1). (1) The patient should be placed supine on a firm surface (a wooden board beneath his back serves well). (2) Compression of the chest should be performed with the heel of one hand on the lower third of the sternum cephalad to the xiphoid process (to avoid lacerations of the liver) and the other hand applied on top of the first. (3) The frequency of external massage should approximate one per second to permit adequate time for ventricular filling. (4) The resuscitator's waist must be higher than the patient's chest in order to permit him to administer the approximately 100-lb force required to depress the anterior chest wall of an adult male the necessary 5 cm per beat. (5) Depression and release of the chest wall should be smooth, with each occupying 50 percent of the cycle, since sudden compression may elicit a pressure wave palpable at the femoral or carotid artery but able to eject little blood. (6) Massage should not be interrupted, even momentarily, since cardiac output increases cumulatively during the first 8 to 10 compressions and even brief interruptions are detrimental. (7) Effective ventilation must be carried out. To accomplish this, the chin must be retracted and the neck fully extended. Mouth-to-mouth or mouth-to-nose technique must be continued throughout the resuscitative effort at a frequency of about 12 per min and monitored by arterial blood gas analyses. If the latter are clearly abnormal, endotracheal intubation should be carried out expeditiously.

Each external cardiac compression limits venous return, and the optimal anticipated cardiac index during external

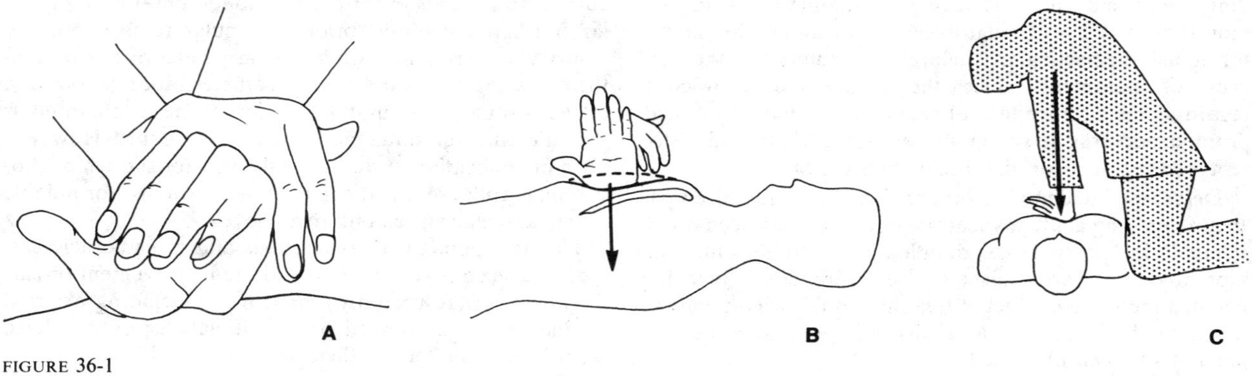

FIGURE 36-1

External cardiac massage. A Position of hands during application of external cardiac massage. B When pressure is applied, the lower portion of the sternum is displaced posteriorly with the palm of the hand. C In order to apply maximal downward pressure, the resuscitator leans far forward, so that his arms are at right angles to the sternum.

massage approximates only 40 percent of the lower limit of normal, well below that seen in most patients after spontaneous ventricular contractions have returned or have been induced by ventricular pacing. Therefore, prompt restoration of effective cardiac rhythm is essential. Rarely, organized electrocardiographic activity unaccompanied by effective cardiac contraction (electromechanical dissociation) may occur and respond to intracardiac epinephrine (1 ml of 1:1,000 solution diluted 1:10 with blood) or calcium gluconate (1 g). Cardiac massage should be terminated as soon as effective cardiac contractions, initiated spontaneously or by ventricular pacing, serve to produce a detectable pulse and systemic arterial blood pressure. Subsequent treatment of dysrhythmias and hypotension and adjustment of intravascular volume should be guided by the same general principles underlying their management in circulatory collapse due to cardiogenic shock (Chap. 244).

The therapeutic approach outlined above is based on several considerations: (1) Irreversible brain damage often occurs after a few (approximately four) minutes of circulatory collapse; (2) the likelihood of restoring effective cardiac rhythm and successfully resuscitating the patient diminishes rapidly with time; (3) 80 to 90 percent survival can be anticipated in patients developing primary ventricular fibrillation, as when undergoing cardiac catheterization or exercise testing, in whom definitive treatment is prompt; (4) survival rates in the general hospital setting are much lower, approximately 20 percent, depending in part on the coexisting or underlying disease process; (5) survival rates in the community approach zero, unless special emergency care systems have been perfected, probably because of unavoidable delays in initiating definitive therapy and limitations of equipment and available personnel; and (6) external cardiac massage can provide only a limited cardiac output. When ventricular fibrillation occurs, the earliest application of electrical countershock is the one most likely to succeed. Thus, when circulatory collapse is a primary event, therapy must be directed toward prompt restoration of effective cardiac rhythm.

Complications External cardiac massage is not free from significant complications, including rib fracture, hemopericardium and tamponade, hemothorax, pneumothorax, liver laceration, fat embolus, and ruptured spleen with late, occult blood loss. However, these complications can be minimized by proper technique and, if appropriately considered, can be readily recognized and often managed effectively. The decision to terminate unsuccessful cardiopulmonary resuscitation is always difficult. In general, if effective cardiac rhythm has not been restored and if the patient's pupils are fixed and dilated despite 30 min or more of cardiac massage, a successful resuscitation cannot be expected.

An important challenge to the medical system is to provide trained medical or paramedical personnel immediately for patients who develop sudden cardiovascular collapse. The development of appropriately staffed "rescue stations" in large factories, office buildings, and sports arenas is one approach that has been proposed since aggressive precoronary care can reduce mortality. However, it is likely that the identification of individuals at high risk and the application of effective preventive measures to this segment of the population will be more satisfactory.

REFERENCES

HINKLE LE JR et al: The frequency of asymptomatic disturbances of cardiac rhythm and conduction in middle-aged man. Am J Cardiol 24:629, 1969

KANNEL WB et al: Precursors of sudden coronary death: Factors related to the incidence of sudden death. Circulation 51:606, 1975

KOTLER MN et al: Prognostic significance of ventricular ectopic beats with respect to sudden death in the late postinfarction period. Circulation 47:959, 1973

KULLER LH, PERPER JA, COOPER MD: Sudden and unexpected death due to arteriosclerotic heart disease, chap. 11, in *Modern Trends in Cardiology*–3, ed MF Oliver, London and Boston: Butterworth, 1975, pp. 292–332

LOWN B, WOLF M: Approaches to sudden death from coronary heart disease. Circulation 44:130, 1971

OLDHAM HN JR: Cardiopulmonary arrest and resuscitation, chap. 10 in *Gibbon's Surgery of the Chest,* 3d ed., eds DC Sabiston, FC Spencer, Philadelphia: Saunders, 1976, pp. 239–255

PANTRIDGE JF et al: *The Acute Coronary Attack.* New York: Grune & Stratton, 1975, 141 pp.

PRINEAS RJ, BLACKBURN H: Sudden coronary death outside hospital. Circulation 52:(Suppl III)287, 1975

SCHAFFER WA, COBB LA: Recurrent ventricular fibrillation and modes of death in survivors of out-of-hospital ventricular fibrillation. N Engl J Med 293:259, 1975

STANDARDS FOR CARDIOPULMONARY RESUSCITATION: Part II—Basic Life Support. JAMA 227:841–851, 1974

WILHELMSSON C et al: Reduction of sudden deaths after myocardial infarction by treatment with alprenolol: Preliminary results. Lancet 7:1157, 1974

section 5 | Alterations in gastrointestinal function

37
ORAL MANIFESTATIONS OF DISEASE

PAUL GOLDHABER

DISTURBANCES OF THE TEETH AND DENTAL TISSUES

DENTAL CARIES, PULPAL AND PERIAPICAL INFECTION, AND SEQUELAE Dental caries, the principal cause of tooth loss up to the fourth decade of life, is characterized by a bacteria-induced progressive destruction of the mineral and organic components of the outer enamel and underlying dentin. Numerous long-term studies have clearly shown that the artificial fluoridation of drinking water supplies to a level of 1 part per million leads to a 50 to 75 percent reduction in the occurrence of dental caries in permanent teeth of children, presumably because of an alteration of the developing enamel crystals during tooth formation which makes them more resistant to acid dissolution.

If the carious lesion progresses unchecked, there is eventual infection of the dental pulp, giving rise to an *acute pulpitis.* During the early stages of pulpitis moderately severe pain may result from thermal changes, particularly cold drinks. As more of the pulp becomes involved because of advanced caries, heat or reclining may stimulate the onset of even more severe and continuous pain. At this stage, damage to the pulp is irreversible, and treatment consists either of extraction or thorough removal of the remaining contents of the pulp chamber and root canals followed by sterilization and filling with an inert material (root canal therapy).

If the pulpitis is not treated, infection may spread beyond the apex of the tooth into the periodontal ligament, giving rise to pain on chewing or percussion. The most common manifestation of periapical disease is the *periapical granuloma,* a localized mass of chronic granulation tissue which slowly expands at the expense of the surrounding alveolar bone. The *chronic periapical granuloma* may present the above symptoms or may be asymptomatic. If allowed to persist untreated the periapical granuloma may give rise to a *periapical cyst* or a *periapical abscess*—all three lesions appearing as radiolucent areas on roentgenograms. The acute periapical abscess may extend into the surrounding bone marrow, resulting in an *osteomyelitis.* More frequently, the abscess perforates the cortical plate and, following the path of least resistance, spreads through various tissue spaces, giving rise to cellulitis and bacteremia, or discharges into the oral cavity, into the maxillary sinus, or through the skin.

The symptoms produced by cellulitis depend on which tissue space is affected. For example, *Ludwig's angina* originates from an infected mandibular molar, involves the submaxillary space, and subsequently extends into the sublingual and submental spaces. Clinically, this is manifested by swelling of the floor of the mouth, elevation of the tongue, and difficulty in swallowing and breathing. With continued swelling, there may be edema of the glottis, necessitating an emergency tracheotomy. Spread of the infection to the parapharyngeal spaces may lead to cavernous sinus thrombosis.

PERIODONTAL DISEASE

After the third decade chronic destructive periodontal disease *(periodontitis)* is responsible for the loss of more teeth than dental caries. It begins as a marginal inflammation of the gingivae (gingivitis), which slowly spreads to involve the underlying alveolar bone and periodontal ligament. As the disease progresses, the alveolar bone is resorbed, resulting in loss of periodontal ligament fiber attachment from the tooth to the bone. The separation of the soft tissue from the tooth surface results in "pocket" formation, the inner aspect of which bleeds readily on probing or spontaneously during chewing. Frank pus sometimes exudes from under the gingival margin, accounting for the use of the now outmoded term "pyorrhea." With continued loss of alveolar bone the involved teeth become mobile. As the periodontal pockets deepen, the pocket orifice may become occluded, leading to the formation of a *periodontal abscess.* The prognosis for teeth with advanced bone loss, extreme mobility, and recurrent abscess formation is usually poor or hopeless, and the usual treatment is extraction.

The most important local etiologic factors associated with this disease are thought to be *poor oral hygiene,* resulting in the accumulation of grossly visible adherent masses of bacteria *(bacterial plaque),* calculus (mineralized bacterial plaque), and food impaction. The margins of overextended fillings also play a role as local irritating factors. Occlusal trauma, particularly due to grinding and clenching habits, may be involved. Therapy is aimed at elimination of these factors and the development of a local environment which can be maintained in health by good oral hygiene.

Systemic factors are thought to modify the response of the host to the local factors, but their nature is more obscure. In some instances, however, there are characteristic alterations in the gingiva in response to a number of specific systemic conditions. For example, during *pregnancy* the gingiva may become edematous and friable, with a raspberry-like appearance of the interdental papillae. Occasionally, a tumorlike mass may develop in an interdental area; this usually regresses following parturition. The use of the anticonvulsant drug *diphenylhydantoin sodium* (Dilantin) frequently results in fibrous hyperplasia of the gingiva, which may actually cover the teeth, interfere with mastication, and cause a serious esthetic problem. A similar clinical picture, although usually more generalized and extensive, occurs in *idiopathic familial fibromatosis.* The latter condition appears to be hereditary.

A relatively common gingival disease, found predominantly in young adults, is *acute necrotizing ulcerative gingivitis* (Vincent's infection; trench mouth). This disease is characterized by tender or painful gingivae, bleeding on pressure, and the pathognomonic sign of papillary or marginal gingival necrosis and ulceration. Clinical evidence suggests that the cause of this disease has a psychosomatic component. Vincent's infection differs from *acute herpetic gingivostomatitis,* with which it is most frequently confused, in that fever or malaise rarely develops, and patients respond rapidly to penicillin or broad-spectrum antibiotics.

It should be noted that both infected periapical lesions and periodontal disease provide potential sources of infection which may spread to other sites. Transient bacteremias have been demonstrated after simple massage of inflamed gingivae, as well as during tooth extraction. The frequent association of tooth extraction with the subsequent occurrence of subacute bacterial endocarditis has led to the prophylactic use of antibiotics in dental patients with a history of rheumatic fever or other evidence of valvular disease.

DISEASES OF THE ORAL MUCOSA AND TONGUE

HEMATOLOGIC DISTURBANCES Oral manifestations are common in both the acute and chronic forms of all types of leukemia, particularly *monocytic leukemia.* They consist of local gingival bleeding, enlargement, and necrosis. Petechiae and ulceration of the oral mucosa may also be evident. Extensive ulcerations of the gingivae, buccal mucosa, lips, soft palate, pharynx, and tonsils may also occur in *agranulocytosis.* In thrombocytopenic states multiple petechiae, ecchymoses, and bleeding gingivae may be observed. The mucous membranes of the oral cavity, including the papillae of the tongue, are atrophic in the *Plummer-Vinson syndrome* (see Chaps. 38, 286). As a result, the tongue is red, smooth, and sore, and there is difficulty in swallowing. Of interest is the finding that the atrophic mucous membranes have a predisposition toward the development of oral carcinoma. The oral symptoms in *pernicious anemia* are similar (see Chap. 310).

VITAMIN DEFICIENCIES *The oral effects of deficiency of the B group of vitamins* involve the soft tissues primarily, giving rise to reddening and ulceration of the oral mucosa and tongue, swelling and burning of the tongue, and fissuring at the corners of the lips *(angular cheilosis).* Severe vitamin C deficiency *(scurvy)* is manifested by petechiae in the oral mucosa; swollen, ulcerated, bleeding gingivae; and loosening of teeth.

PIGMENTATIONS (see Table 37-1) The spread of irregular spots or blotches or brown pigment throughout the oral mucosa, primarily the buccal mucosa, may be the first sign of *Addison's disease.* The pigmentation associated with the *Peutz-Jeghers syndrome* is readily differentiated because of its characteristic distribution around the lips, eyes, and nostrils, as well as its intraoral distribution. Both *lead poisoning* and *bismuth poisoning* may be manifested by a dark line along the gingival margin, particularly in individuals who have poor oral hygiene. Bismuth poisoning may also

TABLE 37-1
Pigmented lesions of the oral mucosa

Condition	*Usual location*	*Clinical features*	*Course*
Black, hairy tongue	Dorsum of tongue	Elongation of filiform papillae of tongue, which take on a brown to black coloration	Long-lasting but may disappear spontaneously
Heavy-metal pigmentation (bismuth, mercury, lead)	Gingival margin	Thin blue-black pigmented line along gingival margin due to prior treatment for syphilis with bismuth or mercury or from accidental absorption of lead	Long-lasting
Amalgam tattoo	Gingiva and mucobuccal fold	Small blue-black pigmented areas associated with embedded amalgam particles in soft tissues; these will show up on radiographs as radiopaque particles	Remains indefinitely
Fordyce's disease	Buccal and labial mucosa	Aggregation of numerous, small yellowish spots just beneath mucosal surface; no subjective symptoms	Remains without apparent change indefinitely
Addison's disease	Any area in mouth but mostly on buccal mucosa	Blotches or spots of bluish-black to dark-brown pigmentation occurring early in the disease accompanied by diffuse pigmentation of skin; other symptoms of adrenal insufficiency	Condition controlled by steroid therapy
Peutz-Jeghers syndrome	Any area in mouth	Dark-brown spots on lips, buccal mucosa, and palate with characteristic distribution of pigment around lips, nose, eyes, and on hands; concomitant intestinal polyposis	Lesions remaining indefinitely
Malignant melanoma	Any area in mouth	May appear as a raised, painless, brown-black lesion or may be amelanotic; may be ulcerated and infected	Early metastasis leading to death

demonstrate pigmented patches elsewhere in the oral mucosa.

INFECTIONS See Tables 37-2 and 37-3.

DERMATOLOGIC DISEASES See Tables 37-2 and 37-3 and Chaps. 54 to 59.

TONGUE ALTERATIONS See Table 37-4.

MALODOROUS BREATH A distinctly unpleasant odor of the breath (halitosis) may emanate from any patient with *infections of the upper part of the respiratory tract,* especially in bronchiectasis and lung abscess. Halitosis may occur with oral sepsis as in *stomatitis, gingivitis,* or extensive *caries.* Some persons who smoke excessively may have halitosis. Occasionally otherwise normal persons will have halitosis without obvious cause. A *fishy odor* of the breath is found in patients with hepatic failure, an *ammoniacal or urinary odor* is found in azotemia, and a *sweet, fruity odor* is typical of diabetic acidosis.

DISEASES OF THE SALIVARY GLANDS

Conditions affecting the salivary glands include mumps parotitis (Chap. 210), Mikulicz's disease, and Sjögren's syndrome (Chap. 359). Inflammation of the salivary glands *(sialadenitis)* is usually associated with the presence of a salivary stone *(sialolithiasis)* in the duct of one of the major salivary glands. The classic history of pain and swelling of the gland at mealtimes is due to the partial blockage of salivary flow by the stone. Localization of the stone may be accomplished by palpation or by roentgenograms with or without the use of an intraductal injection of radiopaque material *(sialography).* Acute or recurrent parotitis, with or without a defined microorganism, may occur in children and is marked by sudden onset of swelling of the whole gland or side of the face, accompanied by suppuration from Stenson's duct.

Xerostomia, or dryness of the mouth, is due to salivary gland dysfunction and may be temporary or permanent. Among the factors which cause temporary dryness are emotional factors (such as fear), infection of the glands, and administration of drugs, such as atropine or antihistamines. Radiation to the area may produce a more permanent xerostomia because of atrophy of the glands. A similar dryness may occur in Sjögren's syndrome.

ORAL CANCER

Oral cancer constitutes more than 5 percent of all human cancers. *Squamous cell carcinoma* is the most common malignant oral tumor, accounting for approximately 90 to 95 percent of all oral malignant tumors. Most of these tumors occur on the lips, primarily the lower lip, rather than intraorally. About half the intraoral tumors involve the tongue, primarily the posterior two-thirds and the lateral borders. The major etiologic factor in lip cancer appears to be exposure to intense sunlight. Predisposing factors for intraoral carcinoma include tobacco (usually in the form of

TABLE 37-2
Vesicular, bullous, or ulcerative lesions of the oral mucosa

Condition	*Usual location*	*Clinical features*	*Course*
VIRAL DISEASES			
Acute herpetic gingivostomatitis (herpes simplex)	Lip and oral mucosa	Labial vesicles which rupture and crust, and intraoral vesicles which quickly ulcerate; extremely painful to pressure; acute gingivitis, fever, malaise, foul odor, and cervical lymphadenopathy; occurs primarily in infants and children	Heals spontaneously in 10–14 days, unless secondarily infected
Recurrent herpes labialis	Mucocutaneous junction of lip	Eruption of groups of vesicles which may coalesce, then rupture and crust; painful to pressure or spicy foods	Lasts about 1 week, but condition may be prolonged if secondary infection occurs
Herpangina (Coxsackie A; also possibly Coxsackie B and echo viruses)	Oral mucosa, pharynx, tongue	Sudden onset of fever, sore throat, and oropharyngeal vesicles usually in children under 4 years, summer months; diffuse pharyngeal injection and vesicles (1–2 mm), grayish white surrounded by red areola; vesicles enlarge and ulcerate	Incubation period 2–9 days; fever for 1–4 days; recovery uneventful
Foot, hand, and mouth disease (Coxsackie A-16)	Oral mucosa, pharynx, palms, and soles	Fever, malaise, headache with oropharyngeal vesicles which become painful, shallow ulcers	Incubation period 2–18 days; lesions heal spontaneously in 2–4 weeks
BACTERIAL OR FUNGOUS DISEASES			
Acute necrotizing ulcerative gingivitis ("trench mouth," Vincent's infection)	Gingiva	Painful, bleeding gingiva characterized by necrosis and ulceration of gingival papillae and margins plus lymphadenopathy and foul odor	Continued destruction of tissue followed by remission, but may recur
Primary syphilis (chancre)	Lesion appears where organism enters body; may occur on lips, tongue, or tonsillar area	Small papule developing rapidly into a large, painless ulcer with indurated border; unilateral lymphadenopathy; chancre and lymph nodes containing spirochetes; serologic tests positive by 3d to 4th weeks	Healing of chancre in 1–2 months, followed by secondary syphilis in 6–8 weeks

TABLE 37-2 *(continued)*

Condition	*Usual location*	*Clinical features*	*Course*
DERMATOLOGIC DISEASES			
Secondary syphilis	Oral mucosa frequently involved with mucous patches, primarily on palate but also at commissures of mouth	Maculopapular lesions of oral mucosa, about 5–10 mm in diameter with central ulceration covered by grayish membrane; eruptions occurring on various mucosal surfaces and skin accompanied by fever, malaise, and sore throat	Lesions may persist from several weeks to a year
Tertiary syphilis	Palate and tongue	Gummatous infiltration of palate or tongue followed by ulceration and fibrosis; atrophy of tongue papillae may produce characteristic bald tongue and glossitis	Gumma may destroy palate, causing complete perforation
Tuberculosis	Tongue, tonsillar area, soft palate	A solitary, irregular ulcer covered by a persistent exudate; ulcer has an undermined, indurated border	Lesion may persist
Cervicofacial actinomycosis	Swellings in region of face, neck, and floor of mouth	Infection may be associated with an extraction, jaw fracture, or eruption of molar tooth; in acute form resembles an acute pyogenic abscess, but contains yellow "sulfur granules" (gram-positive mycelia and their hyphae)	Acute form may last a few weeks; chronic form lasts months or years. Prognosis excellent. Actinomycetes respond to antibiotics (tetracyclines or penicillin) but not to antifungal drugs
Histoplasmosis	Any area in mouth, particularly tongue, gingiva, or palate	Numerous small nodules which may ulcerate; hoarseness and dysphagia may occur because of lesions in larynx, usually associated with fever and malaise	May be fatal
Mucous membrane pemphigoid	Primarily mucous membranes of the oral cavity, but may also involve the eyes, urethra, vagina, and rectum	Painful, grayish-white collapsed vesicles or bullae with peripheral erythematous zone; gingival lesions desquamate, leaving ulcerated area	Protracted course with remissions and exacerbations; involvement of different sites occurs slowly; corticosteroids may control severe cases
Erythema multiforme	Primarily the oral mucosa and skin of hands and feet	Intraoral ruptured bullae surrounded by an inflammatory area; lips may show hemorrhagic crusts; the "iris" or "target" lesion on the skin is pathognomonic; patient may have severe signs of toxicity	Onset very rapid; condition may last 1–2 weeks; may be fatal
Pemphigus vulgaris	Oral mucosa and skin	Ruptured bullae and ulcerated oral areas; mostly in older adults	With repeated recurrence of bullae, toxicity may lead to cachexia, infection, and death within 2 years
NEOPLASTIC DISEASES			
Squamous cell carcinoma	Any area in mouth, most commonly on lower lip, tongue, and floor of mouth	Ulcer with elevated, indurated border; failure to heal, pain not prominent; lesions tend to arise in areas of leukoplakia or in smooth or atrophic tongue	Invades and destroys underlying tissues or may metastasize to regional lymph nodes
Acute leukemia	Gingiva	Gingival swelling and superficial ulcerations followed by hyperplasia of gingiva with extensive necrosis and hemorrhage; deep ulcers may occur elsewhere on the mucosa complicated by secondary infection	Fatal
Lymphosarcoma	Gingiva, palate, tongue, and tonsillar area	Elevated, ulcerated area which may proliferate rapidly, giving the appearance of a traumatic inflammatory lesion; swelling of regional lymph nodes	Fatal
OTHER CONDITIONS			
Recurrent aphthous stomatitis	Any place on oral mucosa	Single or clusters of painful ulcers with surrounding erythematous border, found anywhere on mucosa; lesions may be 1-15 mm in diameter	Lesions heal in 1–2 weeks but may recur monthly or several times a year
Traumatic ulcers	Any place on oral mucosa; dentures frequently responsible for ulcers in vestibule	Localized, discrete ulcerated lesion with red border; produced by accidental biting of mucosa, penetration by a foreign object, or chronic irritation by a denture	Lesion usually heals in 7–10 days when irritant is removed, unless secondarily infected

TABLE 37-3
White lesions of oral mucosa

Condition	*Usual location*	*Clinical features*	*Course*
Pachyderma oris	Any area in mouth	Elevated white lesion due to hyperkeratosis and thickening of the oral epithelium secondary to chronic irritation	Removal of irritant leads to healing in 2–3 weeks
Leukoplakia	Any area in mouth	White patch or raised plaque with sharply defined borders; in more severe cases the lesion is indurated and rough, and may be fissured and eroded; pain not present in early lesions	Carcinoma frequently arises in the more severe type of lesion
Lichen planus	Any area in mouth but most often on buccal mucosa	Varied appearance of lesion due to arrangement of grayish-white papules which coalesce to make up the pattern; a reticular network is most common; oral lesions may precede skin lesions	May disappear spontaneously
Moniliasis (thrush)	Any area in mouth	Creamy white curdlike patches which reveal a raw, bleeding surface when scraped; found in sick infants, debilitated elderly patients, or patients receiving high doses of corticosteroids or broad-spectrum antibiotics	Responds favorably to antifungal therapy after correction of predisposing causes
Chemical burns	Any area in mouth	White slough due to necrosis of epithelium and underlying connective tissue caused by contact with agents (e.g., aspirin) applied locally or the use of undiluted sodium perborate or hydrogen peroxide as a mouthwash; removal of slough leaves a raw, painful surface	Lesion heals in several weeks if not secondarily infected

TABLE 37-4
Alterations of the tongue

Type of change	*Clinical features*
SIZE OR MORPHOLOGY CHANGES	
Macroglossia	Enlarged tongue which may be part of a syndrome found in developmental conditions such as Down's syndrome; may be due to tumor (hemangioma or lymphangioma), metabolic disease (such as primary amyloidosis), or endocrine disturbance (such as acromegaly or cretinism)
Fissured ("scrotal") tongue	Dorsal surface and sides of tongue covered by painless shallow or deep fissures which may collect debris and become irritated
Median rhomboid glossitis	Congenital abnormality of tongue with ovoid, denuded area in the median posterior portion of the tongue
COLOR CHANGES	
"Geographic" tongue ("wandering rash")	Asymptomatic inflammatory condition of the tongue, with rapid loss and regrowth of filiform papillae, leading to appearance of denuded red patches "wandering" across the surface of the tongue
Hairy tongue	Elongation of filiform papillae of the medial dorsal surface area due to failure of keratin layer of the papillae to desquamate normally; brownish-black coloration may be due to staining by tobacco, food, or chromogenic organisms
"Strawberry" and "raspberry" tongue	Appearance of tongue during scarlet fever due to the hypertrophy of fungiform papillae plus changes in the filiform papillae
"Bald" tongue	Complete atrophy of papillae which may occur in pernicious anemia, severe iron-deficiency anemia, pellagra, or syphilis; may be accompanied by painful, burning sensations

cigar or pipe smoking, or snuff placed in the mucobuccal fold), excessive consumption of alcohol, syphilitic glossitis, and the atrophic mucosa of the Plummer-Vinson syndrome. Although numerous instances of carcinoma of the tongue adjacent to a sharp tooth or dental appliance have been reported, animal studies with chronic irritation per se, as well as epidemiologic studies, cast doubt on this apparent relationship. The most common *precancerous lesion* in the oral cavity is *leukoplakia,* a whitish patch on the mucosa that histologically shows hyperkeratosis, acanthosis, and dyskeratosis. *All chronic ulcerative lesions which fail to heal within 1 to 2 weeks should be considered potentially malignant* and must be biopsied in order to make the definitive diagnosis. It is noteworthy that in their early stages intraoral epidermoid carcinomas are rarely painful, in contrast to similar-appearing inflammatory lesions.

The prognosis for patients with carcinoma of the lip is usually good, since these malignant tumors are noted sooner and apparently metastasize later. Patients with carcinoma of the tongue have a poorer prognosis, particularly as the tumor occurs more posteriorly on the tongue. Intraoral carcinomas may spread by direct invasion to the underlying bone. Depending on the site of origin of the intraoral carcinoma, metastases usually spread to the submaxillary or cervical lymph nodes. Death may result from recurrent or uncontrollable disease above the clavicles; metastatic disease beyond the neck; treatment complications; or a second primary cancer, usually in the oral cavity or the upper parts of the gastrointestinal or respiratory tracts.

NEUROLOGIC DISTURBANCES

A number of neurologic disturbances have a direct effect on oral and paraoral structures. *Trigeminal neuralgia* (tic douloureux), is an example of a syndrome involving the trigeminal nerve. It is characterized by extremely severe, unilateral, lancinating pain of the face occurring spontaneously or set off by pressure on a "trigger zone" on the face (see Chap. 332). Facial palsy is a unilateral disturbance of the motor branch of the facial nerve due to either trauma, surgical sectioning, or tumor involvement. When it is of acute onset and unknown cause, possibly a localized infection in the nerve, it is called *Bell's palsy.* It may be due to cranial herpes zoster in some instances. The condition is manifested by drooping of the corner of the mouth, inability to close the eye on the same side, and difficulty in speech and eating. In mild cases the symptoms may disappear spontaneously within a month. Alteration in taste sensation in the anterior two-thirds of the tongue due to disturbance of the sensory component of the facial nerve occurs in some cases and indicates a more central location of the lesion in the nerve (see Chap. 332).

The pain associated with the *glossopharyngeal neuralgia syndrome* is similar in type and intensity to that found in trigeminal neuralgia, being set off by a trigger zone in the pharynx and affecting the posterior region of the tongue, pharynx, soft palate, and ear. Disturbance of the hypoglossal nerve leads to dysfunction of the tongue musculature and atrophy. Bilateral nerve involvement prevents protrusion of the tongue; unilateral involvement leads to deviation of the protruded tongue toward the affected side.

DISTURBANCES OF THE TEMPOROMANDIBULAR JOINT

Pain in the area of the temporomandibular joint frequently causes the patient to seek therapy. It may be due to posterior displacement of the condyle in the fossa leading to displacement of the meniscus and chronic trauma. *Dislocation of the condyle anteriorly* beyond the articular eminence due to sudden stretching or tearing of the capsular ligament may result in a locking of the mandible in an open position. In *osteoarthritis* the clinical signs and symptoms may be minimal despite extensive changes in the condyle. Temporomandibular joint involvement occurs less frequently in *rheumatoid arthritis.* When affected, the joints are swollen and painful, leading to limitation of movement, particularly on arising in the morning. In children the disease may lead to malocclusion. *Ankylosis* on the joint may occur eventually, necessitating a condylectomy (see Chap. 359).

The myofascial pain syndrome, the most common disorder of the temporomandibular joint, is characterized by facial pain and mandibular dysfunction. The pain is often localized in the ear or jaw and may extend to the neck and shoulder. The mandibular dysfunction is manifested by limitation of movement, particularly an inability to open the jaw to the fullest extent. It is thought that such patients have increased musculature tension and hyperexcitable reflexes related to emotional tension. The precipitating factor appears to be the stretching of an abnormal focus of pain which initiates a self-sustaining pain-spasm-pain cycle. Treatment of the pain-dysfunction syndrome involves the use of drugs to relieve the pain, lessen cortical excitability, and relax the muscles. Local anesthetics are used intramuscularly in the region of the trigger zone or as superficial sprays in an attempt to break the pain-spasm-pain cycle.

REFERENCES

BHASKAR SN: *Synopsis of Oral Pathology,* St. Louis: Mosby, 1969

GLICKMAN I: *Clinical Periodontology,* Philadelphia: Saunders, 1972

GOLDMAN HM, COHEN DW (eds): *Periodontal Therapy,* St. Louis: Mosby, 1973

MCCARTHY P, SHKLAR G: *Diseases of the Oral Mucosa,* New York: McGraw-Hill, 1964

MERGENHAGEN SE, SCHERP HW (eds): *Comparative Immunology of the Oral Cavity,* Bethesda, Md.: Dept. Health, Education and Welfare Publication No. (NIH)73–438, 1973

SHAFER WG et al: *A Textbook of Oral Pathology,* Philadelphia: Saunders, 1974

38

DYSPHAGIA

THOMAS R. HENDRIX

Dysphagia, or difficulty in swallowing, is a most reliable symptom and indicates the presence of disease or dysfunction. Dysphagia should never be dismissed as an emotional disturbance or be confused with globus hystericus, a term used to indicate the sensation of a lump or tightness in the throat independent of swallowing.

The most characteristic manifestation of dysphagia is the sensation of food "sticking" somewhere in its passage to the stomach, usually at the level of the obstruction but sometimes referred to the suprasternal notch, even though the obstruction may be at the lower end of the esophagus. Pain may accompany dysphagia, especially if esophageal spasm is induced by the peristaltic waves attempting to force the bolus through the obstruction. If the pain is mild, it tends to be localized to the site of obstruction; if more severe, it radiates more widely, into the base of the neck, angles of the jaw, arms, epigastrium, or back. Sometimes pain, in a sense, may even cause dysphagia, as when the throat is so sore that swallowing is difficult. For further details regarding these symptoms, see Chap. 286.

Normal swallowing is a complex function dependent upon coordination of voluntary muscular structures of the oropharynx, striated muscles protecting the larynx and respiratory passages, as well as relaxation of the esophageal sphincters and the peristaltic wave itself; hence dysphagia may occur as a consequence of derangement or incoordination of any of the elements of the swallowing act as well as narrowing of the lumen by inflammatory stricture or tumor.

For clinical purposes it is useful to consider dysphagia as having either an oropharyngeal or an esophageal origin, because symptoms, etiology, and treatment are usually different for the two types.

OROPHARYNGEAL DYSPHAGIA Symptoms associated with dysphagia caused by disorders of oropharyngeal structures include aspiration with swallowing, regurgitation of fluid into the nose, pharyngeal pain with swallowing, and inability of the tongue to move the bolus into the pharynx. Dilatation and atony of piriform sinuses and pharynx and retention of contrast media in the valleculae are characteristic radiographic findings in patients with pharyngeal dysfunction. In addition, aspiration of contrast medium into the trachea or regurgitation into the nasopharynx and apparent obstruction at the upper esophageal sphincter (cricopharyngeus) may be found.

Neuromuscular disorders are the most common causes

of oropharyngeal dysphagia, which, however, is usually only part of the symptom complex. Examples of these disorders are cerebral vascular accidents which cause pseudobulbar palsy (see Chap. 17) or bulbar palsy, poliomyelitis, motor system disease, diphtheritic polyneuritis, myasthenia gravis, myotonic dystrophies and restricted muscular dystrophies (oculopharyngeal and laryngoesophageal), and dermatomyositis. Ulcerative lesions such as pharyngitis, Vincent's angina, monilia stomatitis, viral infections with herpetic lesions, and retropharyngeal abscess interfere by causing pain and thereby inhibiting the initiation of deglutition. Plummer-Vinson syndrome (Paterson-Kelly syndrome, or sideropenic dysphagia) may also be listed here, since the difficulty in swallowing in this disorder resembles that due to a neuromuscular disorder, although pain may be an additional disturbing feature. Limited pathologic studies have shown both epithelial and muscle atrophy. It is clear that the dysphagia is not due to the characteristic web, or mucosal fold, of the anterior aspect of the cricopharyngeal area, because the web often persists long after the symptoms have been relieved by iron replacement.

Oropharyngeal dysphagia may be caused by narrowing of the lumen of the pharynx or upper esophagus by tumor, granulomatous disease, Zenker's diverticulum, or an enlarged thyroid.

ESOPHAGEAL DYSPHAGIA Symptoms indicating that the cause of dysphagia is to be found in the esophagus range from retrosternal fullness with swallowing to failure of the bolus to pass through the esophagus associated with pain relieved only by regurgitation of the offending bolus. Barium swallows in patients with dysphagia of esophageal origin show segmental narrowing of the esophageal lumen, failure of peristalsis, or both. Abnormalities of peristalsis may be characterized more precisely by intraluminal manometric studies.

Mechanical narrowing of the esophageal lumen is most frequently caused either by carcinoma of the squamous type, arising from the esophagus itself, or by adenocarcinoma of the cardia extending up into the esophagus. Rarely, benign tumors may reach sufficient size to cause dysphagia. Inflammatory strictures most commonly result from reflux esophagitis but are also caused by ingestion of corrosive substances, such as lye, or by trauma from foreign bodies or instrumentation. In addition, a lower esophageal ring may produce dysphagia by obstructing the esophageal lumen. Extrinsic pressure from aneurysms, vascular anomalies, mediastinal tumors, or paraesophageal diaphragmatic hernias may compress the esophageal lumen sufficiently to cause dysphagia. Finally, the motility disturbances associated with diffuse esophageal spasm, cardiospasm, and esophageal reflux may be the basis of dysphagia. Although esophageal peristalsis is absent in the majority of patients with scleroderma, dysphagia does not become a prominent symptom until reflux esophagitis has led to an inflammatory stricture.

DIFFERENTIAL DIAGNOSIS Determination of the basic mechanism responsible for dysphagia is usually a simple matter, but identification of the exact disorder responsible for it may be quite difficult. For example, cancer of the esophagus sometimes presents suddenly rather than gradually, and the roentgenogram may have a smooth, symmetric appearance such as is more commonly seen with benign stricture or cardiospasm; even esophagoscopy may be inconclusive, and biopsy may yield deceptive results if the tissue shows only inflammatory reaction and does not include neoplastic cells. Similarly, neuromuscular disorders and disturbances of esophageal motility interfering with swallowing may be difficult to classify.

Certain symptoms associated with dysphagia, however, have diagnostic value. Hiccups, together with difficulty in swallowing, suggest a lesion at the terminal portion of the esophagus, such as carcinoma, achalasia, or hiatal hernia. Dysphagia followed after an interval of some duration by hoarseness usually means extension of a malignant growth beyond the walls of the esophagus and the involvement of a recurrent laryngeal nerve. When the hoarseness comes first and the dysphagia later, the primary lesion is almost always in the larynx. This combination of laryngeal and pharyngeal symptoms may also occur in polymyositis or dermatomyositis or with any disease causing bilateral involvement of vagus nerves or nuclei (poliomyelitis and polyneuritis). In motor system disease, the most common cause of a mixture of bulbar and pseudobulbar palsy, dysphagia is usually combined with dysphonia and dysarthria; the jaw jerk is hyperactive and the tongue atrophic. Dysphagia and unilateral wheezing virtually always indicate a mediastinal mass involving the esophagus and a main or large bronchus. Coughing with each swallow of food or drink means a fistulous communication between the esophagus and the trachea or a motor disorder in which the larynx is not effectively closed. Coughing occurring some time after swallowing may be due to regurgitation of food, most common in achalasia and Zenker's diverticulum.

DIAGNOSTIC PROCEDURES Examination of the mouth and pharynx should disclose those lesions which impede the transfer of food from the mouth to the esophagus, because of pain or mechanical interference. When lesions of the hypopharynx (e.g., *chronic abscess secondary to tuberculosis of the spine*) or of the larynx (e.g., *tuberculosis* or *carcinoma*) are suspected, examination with a mirror is necessary.

The most important diagnostic technique in the evaluation of dysphagia is a *barium swallow,* which makes it possible to determine whether dysphagia is caused by mechanical obstruction or by esophageal motor abnormality. Absence of esophageal peristalsis can best be demonstrated by barium swallows with the patient in Trendelenburg's position. If there is no peristalsis, barium will remain in the esophagus until the patient is tilted upright. Since the muscular action of the pharynx is so rapid, swallows must be recorded by *cineradiography.* Projection of the film at slow speed permits detection and analysis of abnormalities of pharyngeal function.

If barium swallow shows a lesion within the esophagus or a narrowing of the lumen, *esophagoscopy* is the most direct method for establishing the nature of the lesion. In addition to inspecting the lesion, one should perform biopsies and brushings of the lesion for cytologic examination to differentiate inflammatory from neoplastic lesions. A malignant stricture is not ruled out with certainty, however, if the biopsy shows only normal tissue or chronic inflammation, because tumors of the esophagus often spread beneath the mucosa and may be missed by a superficial biopsy. In such circumstances repeated biopsy or exfoliative cytology is necessary. Cytologic studies by experienced personnel are very accurate in the diagnosis of esophageal cancer.

Motor abnormalities of the pharynx and esophagus may be suspected by viewing the movement of a swallowed radiopaque bolus by fluoroscopy, but to characterize these abnormalities definitely, the motor response of pharynx and esophagus to swallowing must be studied by recording intraluminal pressure from several points simultaneously. Records are best obtained by use of a train of water-filled, perfused catheters connected to external pressure transducers or strain gages. Examination of manometric records of swallows will demonstrate whether the wave is normally propagated over the length of the esophagus, whether the pressure generated by the peristaltic wave is normal and sufficient to propel the bolus, and, finally, whether sphincter relaxation is complete, of adequate duration, and properly coordinated with the peristaltic wave. Combining manometric with cineradiographic techniques has added greatly to understanding pharyngoesophageal function.

REFERENCES

CASTELL DO: The lower esophageal sphincter: Physiologic and clinical aspects. Ann Int Med 83:390, 1975

COHEN BR, WOLF BS: Cineradiographic and intraluminal pressure correlations in the pharynx and esophagus, in *Handbook of Physiology,* sec. 6, vol. IV, ed CF Code, Washington: American Physiology Society, 1968, p. 1841

DONNER MW, SILBIGER DL: Cinefluorographic analysis of pharyngeal swallowing in neuromuscular disorders. Am J Med Sci 251:600, 1966

HARRIS LD: The present status of esophageal manometry. Gastroenterology 50:708, 1966

MACDONALD WC et al: Esophageal exfoliative cytology, a neglected procedure. Ann Intern Med 59:332, 1963

PHILLIPS MM, HENDRIX TR: Dysphagia. Postgrad Med 50:81, 1971

RATTAN S et al: Neural control of the lower esophageal sphincter: influence of the vagus nerves. J Clin Invest 54:899, 1974

39 INDIGESTION

KURT J. ISSELBACHER

"Indigestion" is a term frequently used by patients to describe a multitude of symptoms generally appreciated as distress associated with the intake of food. The term is thus nonspecific and may have a different meaning for the patient and the physician. In approaching the patient with indigestion, it is important for the physician first to elicit a good description of this complaint. To some patients indigestion refers to a feeling that digestion has not proceeded naturally. They may describe a sense of abdominal fullness, pressure, or actual pain. Others may use the term to describe heartburn, belching, distention, or flatulence. These complaints are considered in this chapter. Discussed elsewhere are the closely related symptoms of dysphagia, nausea and vomiting, and anorexia (Chaps. 38 and 40).

Indigestion may occur as a result of disease of the gastrointestinal tract or in association with pathologic states in other organ systems. As a result of systematic clinical and laboratory tests, a definable pathophysiologic process often can be shown to be responsible for the symptoms in a given case of indigestion. Frequently, however, clear etiologic explanation for the patient's complaints of indigestion are not established. Such cases are often designated as "functional indigestion," with a strong implication that psychosomatic factors underlie the complaints. Although it is clear that psychic factors may lead to symptoms of indigestion, the designation of "functional indigestion" is rarely if ever a satisfactory explanation, serving only to rephrase the patient's description of his symptoms. A psychogenic cause should not be assumed until organic causes of indigestion have been thoroughly excluded.

After having ascertained the patient's definition of indigestion, it is also important to determine (1) the location and duration of the discomfort, (2) the temporal relation of the symptoms to the ingestion of food, and (3) the possible relation of the symptoms to the ingestion of specific types of food (e.g., fatty foods, milk, and drugs).

PAIN PATTERNS True visceral abdominal pain as seen in indigestion is mediated over visceral afferent nerves which accompany the abdominal sympathetic pathways (see Chap. 8). Visceral pain is generally described as dull and aching in nature (with a diffuse midline localization) or as fullness or pressure. The location of the discomfort corresponds generally to the segmental level of the affected organ. Abdominal visceral pain can be produced experimentally by artificially increasing pressure in a hollow viscus. Usually this pain is the result of distention or exaggerated muscular contraction of a viscus. Inflammation generally lowers the threshold to such stimuli.

The visceral pain of indigestion should be distinguished from the sharp, lateralized, and localized pain patterns seen in many acute abdominal processes involving the peritoneum. In contrast to true visceral pain, this pain is mediated over cerebrospinal afferent nerves. Again it is of a dull, aching type, whether from inflammation of the viscera or of peritoneal surfaces.

In view of the diffuse nature of true visceral abdominal pain, the main clue comes from the segmental level of the viscus; in any given segmental region there is no way of determining which of several viscera are the source of it (Table 39-1). The following rules, already given in Chap. 5, are useful: *Substernal pain* of gastrointestinal origin usually arises from disorders in the esophagus or cardia of the stomach. Because pain in this area is frequently of cardiac origin, heart disease must be considered carefully and excluded. *Epigastric pain* is generally of gastric, duodenal, biliary, or pancreatic origin. As the pathologic process in the biliary tract and pancreas becomes more intense, it tends to lateralize and localize, e.g., biliary pain to the right upper quadrant and tip of the right scapula and pancreatic pain to the epigastrium, left upper quadrant, and back. *Periumbilical pain* is generally associated with small-intestinal disease. *Pain below the umbilicus* is often of appendiceal, large-intestinal, or pelvic origin.

TEMPORAL RELATIONSHIPS OF PAIN AND INDIGESTION The unraveling of the temporal relationships of the patient's symptoms often provides the most significant diagnostic information. It is important to ascertain whether the symptoms are *constant* (continually present over extended periods of time), as may occur, for example, with an infiltrating gastric carcinoma, or *intermittent,* as in acute gastritis following an alcoholic binge or in association with the use of certain drugs. The symptoms may have a *diurnal* pattern; e.g., pain occurring *nocturnally* and with *recumbency* is seen in esophagitis and hiatus hernia. Symptoms are occasionally *seasonal;* this may occur in peptic ulcer disease, in which some patients experience more discomfort in the spring and autumn.

Another important and often diagnostic feature is the relation of pain or indigestion to ingestion of food. This relationship is especially significant or helpful if symptoms occur either during or minutes after the meal or if they occur several hours (four or more) after eating. *Early postprandial symptoms* may reflect esophageal disease, because they may be associated with disordered swallowing function. In such instances, the distress or other symptoms of indigestion often are experienced substernally. Early postprandial complaints occur also in gastric disorders such as acute gastritis or carcinoma. *Late postprandial indigestion,* i.e., that occurring several hours after eating, may reflect failure of the stomach to empty adequately, as in pyloric stenosis or gastric atony. It may also be a symptom of duodenal ulcer, in which case it classically occurs several hours after the meal, when the ulcerated mucosa is exposed to acid secretions of the stomach unbuffered by food. Conversely, the relief of pain following food ingestion is also seen in patients with peptic ulcer and is presumably due to the neutralization of the acid by the ingested food. Such pain also is typically alleviated quickly by oral antacids. Late postprandial indigestion also may result from impaired digestive and absorptive processes, as in pancreatic insufficiency.

TABLE 39-1
Distribution of visceral pain and examples of disorders frequently involving the specific organ

Organ	*Location of referred pain*	*Frequent disorders*
Esophagus	Substernum, epigastrium	Peptic esophagitis, hiatus hernia, stricture, carcinoma
Stomach	Epigastrium	Gastritis, peptic ulcer, carcinoma
Duodenum (first and second portions)	Epigastrium	Peptic ulcer
Duodenum (third portion, jejunum, and ileum)	Periumbilical	Regional enteritis, lymphoma, gastroenteritis (infectious), intestinal obstruction
Gallbladder	Epigastrium, right upper quadrant, right side of back	Cholelithiasis, cholecystitis
Pancreas	Epigastrium, left side of back	Pancreatitis, pancreatic carcinoma
Liver	Right upper quadrant	Passive congestion of liver, hepatitis, cirrhosis
Colon	Below umbilicus	Ulcerative colitis, carcinoma, partial obstruction

FOOD INTOLERANCE In a number of situations specific foods or types of foods appear to be related to indigestion. Careful documentation of this relationship is sometimes of great help in arriving at an etiologic diagnosis.

Some foods may be poorly tolerated because of their consistency. Patients with esophageal stricture or carcinoma may tolerate liquids well, but the ingestion of solids may be associated with discomfort, especially substernal distress (see Chap. 286). Certain foods may be tolerated poorly because the intestinal tract cannot assimilate them adequately. This may occur following the ingestion of fatty foods in patients with pancreatic or biliary tract disease. Citrus fruits, with their relatively low pH, often provoke symptoms in patients with peptic ulcer disease.

Individuals may lack a specific enzyme required for assimilation of a certain nutrient. Patients may have a deficiency of the mucosal enzyme lactase, which catalyzes the hydrolysis of lactose. When lactase deficiency exists on a congenital or acquired basis (e.g., in sprue, ulcerative colitis) (Chap. 289), the ingestion of milk (which contains lactose) results in abdominal cramps, distention, flatulence, and diarrhea.

There are a number of other conditions or disorders in which specific foods are poorly tolerated. Foods may be poorly tolerated because they initiate *allergic reactions* or exert a deleterious or *toxic effect* on the intestinal tract of susceptible persons (e.g., gluten in patients with nontropical sprue). Finally certain substances may lead to systemic effects because of biochemical defects in the patient which render the substances particularly hazardous. An example of the latter is galactose intolerance in galactosemia (Chap. 112).

The above mechanisms do not explain the majority of clinical situations in which indigestion is associated with the eating of specific foods. For example, a history of fatty-food intolerance or an inability to eat cabbage, cucumbers, or spicy foods is commonly obtained from patients with indigestion. However, the mechanisms underlying the production of symptoms in these circumstances is still unclear.

ADDITIONAL SYNDROMES COMMONLY DESCRIBED AS INDIGESTION Gaseousness, flatulence, aerophagia A number of common clinical syndromes which may be described by the patient as "indigestion" appear to be related to increased quantities of gas in the intestinal tract. About 20 to 60 percent of intraluminal gas represents swallowed air. A degree of air swallowing, or *aerophagia,* occurs in normal persons, and the swallowed air can be observed by the radiologist at fluoroscopy. Under certain circumstances, such as chronic anxiety, poor eating habits, or actual intestinal disease itself, aerophagia may increase in magnitude and lead to symptoms in its own right.

The combination of early postprandial fullness and pressure, relieved by eructation and accompanied by a large amount of air seen in the gastric fundus on roentgenogram, is often referred to as the *magenblase* (i.e., gastric bubble) *syndrome.* Acute gastric distention by swallowed air can occasionally produce sharp pains which may mimic angina pectoris. This sequence of events may be especially perplexing in older patients with coronary artery disease, because it is well recognized that true angina pectoris may itself be precipitated by the ingestion of a large meal. Fatty meals delay gastric emptying and hence the passage of swallowed air down the intestine. This relationship may explain, in part, the prolonged sense of fullness and eructations experienced by many individuals after a fatty meal.

Swallowed air that is not eructated passes on in the intestinal tract and may either produce diffuse abdominal distention or become trapped in the splenic flexure of the colon. Distention of this segment of the colon produces a sensation of left upper quadrant fullness and pressure with radiation to the left side of the chest. This is known as the *splenic flexure syndrome.* Patients will often describe relief of pain with defecation or with the expulsion of flatus. Diagnosis may be made by demonstrating, on physical examination, a note of increased tympany in the extreme left lateral portion of the upper part of the abdomen or by the visualization of large amounts of air in the splenic flexure of the colon by radiography.

A second major source of intestinal gas is the fermentative action of bacteria on carbohydrates and proteins within the lumen. Increased amounts of intraluminal gas production due to this mechanism have been demonstrated in conditions associated with abnormal bacterial colonization of the small intestine and in patients with carbohydrate malabsorption.

Increased gas production may occur following the ingestion of certain foods (e.g., the legumes) which contain significant quantities of nonabsorbable sugars. As in the case of swallowed air, increased amounts of intraluminally produced gas can produce symptoms by causing distention, pain, increased motility (with diarrhea), or flatulence.

Heartburn Heartburn, or pyrosis, is a sensation of warmth or burning located substernally or high in the epigastrium. Experimental studies in human beings have shown that esophageal distention or increased motor activity is associated in most subjects with a feeling of fullness and burning in this area.

Heartburn may occur with organic disease of the intestinal tract and is usually associated with gastroesophageal reflux. This is frequently the case in hiatus hernia. In this setting, heartburn occurs after a large meal or with stooping or bending. Esophageal reflux of acid contents at these times leads to symptoms by either the production of abnormal motor activity or direct mucosal irritation (i.e., esophagitis). Heartburn may arise following the ingestion of certain foods or drugs (e.g., alcohol and aspirin). It may also be seen in the absence of a demonstrable anatomic or motor pathologic condition, in which case it is frequently accompanied by aerophagia and for lack of other explanation is often attributed to psychologic factors.

INDIGESTION DUE TO DISEASE OUTSIDE THE INTESTINAL TRACT A multitude of extraintestinal disease processes may result in indigestion by mechanisms which are poorly understood. Indigestion may be the presenting complaint, for example, in congestive heart failure, uremia, pulmonary tuberculosis, and neoplastic disease. Under these circumstances the symptoms of indigestion may present with no unique features to suggest that they are in fact due to some other systemic disease process. Drugs such as aspirin, corticosteroids, indomethacin, and phenylbutazone affect gastric secretion and are ulcerogenic; thus they may lead to symptoms of indigestion.

DIAGNOSTIC APPROACH TO THE PATIENT WITH INDIGESTION Indigestion represents a challenging and difficult diagnostic problem because of the nonspecific nature of its manifestations. The evaluation of indigestion must include initially a thorough medical workup, with ultimate confirmation or exclusion of pathophysiologic derangements by the appropriate diagnostic procedures.

A careful history should include an assessment of the patient's general medical health, including the possibility of diseases in extraintestinal organ systems which may produce indigestion. Careful evaluation of psychologic factors is crucial, because they often play an etiologic or contributory role in the patient's problem. Of particular importance are anxiety, depressive reactions, and hysteria (Chaps. 344 and 345). Evaluation of the patient's intestinal problem must include an assessment of his nutritional status, changes in weight, and appetite.

A clear and detailed description of the specific symptoms should be obtained, particularly the patient's definition of the term "indigestion." The nature of the pain, its frequency and time of occurrence, its relationship to meals, and the special circumstances which lead to its exacerbation or relief should be elicited. Associated intestinal symptoms such as nausea and vomiting, abnormal bowel habits, steatorrhea, diarrhea, and melena should also be sought. Physical examination rarely establishes the specific diagnosis, but it may be useful in detecting disease in other organ systems (e.g., congestive heart failure) which can affect intestinal physiology.

X-ray examination of the alimentary tract is crucial to the evaluation of indigestion. This may involve examination of the esophagus, stomach, small intestine, colon, and biliary tract. Esophagoscopy, gastroscopy, colonoscopy, or sigmoidoscopy also may be helpful or necessary. Stools should be examined for appearance, occult blood, fat, and muscle fibers. As stated above, careful attempts must be made to exclude nonintestinal disease, especially cardiac disease.

Unfortunately, even after completion of careful diagnostic studies, many cases of indigestion will turn out to have no clear explanation. Some of these are psychogenic and may respond to appropriate psychiatric measures. Others represent physiologic derangements which are undetectable by currently available diagnostic methods. Still others represent actual disease processes in early stages which may be diagnosable by conventional methods at a later date. The ultimate evaluation of indigestion requires, therefore, the utmost in sensitivity, diligence, and patience on the part of the examining physician.

REFERENCES

Calloway DH: Respiratory hydrogen and methane as affected by consumption of gas forming foods. Gastroenterology 51:383, 1966

Coghill NF: Dyspepsia. Br Med J 4:97, 1967

Lasser RB et al: The role of intestinal gas in functional abdominal pain. N Engl J Med 293:524, 1975

Levitt MD: Methane production in the gut. N Engl J Med 291: 528, 1974

40
ANOREXIA, NAUSEA, AND VOMITING

KURT J. ISSELBACHER

ANOREXIA Anorexia, or loss of the desire to eat, is a prominent symptom in a wide variety of intestinal and extraintestinal disorders. It must be clearly differentiated from satiety and from specific food intolerance. Anorexia occurs in many disorders and as a result *by itself is of little specific diagnostic value.* The mechanisms whereby hunger and appetite are modified in various disease states are poorly understood. Normally food intake is regulated by two hypothalamic centers—a lateral "feeding center" and a ventral-medial "satiety center." The latter inhibits the feeding center following a meal leading to the sensation of satiety.

Anorexia is commonly seen in diseases of the gastrointestinal tract and liver. For example, it may precede the appearance of jaundice in hepatitis, or it may be a prominent symptom in gastric carcinoma. In the setting of intestinal disease, anorexia should be clearly differentiated from *sitophobia,* or fear of eating because of subsequent or associated discomfort. In such circumstances, appetite may persist, but the ingestion of food is curtailed nonetheless. Sitophobia may be seen, for example, in regional enteritis (especially with partial obstruction) or in patients with gastric ulcer following partial or total gastrectomy.

Anorexia may also be a prominent feature of severe extraintestinal diseases. For example, anorexia may be profound in severe congestive heart failure and is often associated with cardiac glycoside intoxication. It may be a major symptom in patients with uremia, pulmonary failure, and various endocrinopathies (e.g., hyperparathyroidism, Addison's disease, and panhypopituitarism). Anorexia also often accompanies psychogenic disturbances, such as anxiety or depression.

ANOREXIA NERVOSA Anorexia nervosa is a self-imposed state of cachexia and malnutrition and may at times become life-threatening. It is primarily a disorder of young women which is accompanied by severe psychologic disturbances leading to an abnormal desire to lose weight. The major clinical feature of anorexia nervosa consists of profound weight loss in the absence of other signs of demonstrable organic illness. Although the name implies loss of appetite, these patients also have abnormal eating patterns, with episodes of anorexia and periods of excessive eating. The severe restriction of dietary intake is often in response to an uncontrollable urge to eat. Once anorexia becomes severe, other peculiar habits may develop which are aimed at limiting weight gain. Patients may surreptitiously dispose of food, induce vomiting, or employ laxatives to produce diarrhea. One of the striking findings in these patients is that in spite of their depleted nutritional state they may show hyperactivity and increased alertness.

Anorexia nervosa is accompanied by other psychologic behavior disorders, including withdrawal, obsessions, depression, and occasionally psychotic delusions. Most often anorexia nervosa is associated with excessive concern about obesity and physical appearance. Commonly patients with anorexia nervosa demonstrate a distorted perception of their physical state, denying the presence of any abnormality, and tend to view their emaciated, wasted appearance as normal. When these manifestations represent the major psychologic disturbance, the disorder is referred to as *true* or *primary anorexia nervosa.* However, profound anorexia may also be a major manifestation of psychiatric disorders. Thus in hysterical patients anorexia may be the prominent symptom. Obsessive-compulsive patients may adhere to ritualistic diets, with resulting malnutrition. With severe depression there may be a loss of interest in eating, while the psychotic patient may avoid eating because of a delusional fear of food. These types of anorexia or malnutrition have been referred to as *secondary anorexia nervosa.*

Physical examination of the patient with anorexia nervosa reveals emaciation, often of extreme degree. There may be multiple vitamin deficiencies. The blood pressure, basal metabolism, and body temperature may be subnormal. The skin is often dry and scaly. Sexual maturity is markedly delayed. In female patients amenorrhea is quite common, and the appearance of axillary and pubic hair may be delayed. In general these patients are alert, outwardly cooperative, and of normal intelligence.

Laboratory tests are of value primarily to exclude systemic diseases such as carcinomatosis, miliary tuberculosis, panhypopituitarism, malabsorption states, regional enteritis, or diabetes mellitus. However, some conditions may be falsely diagnosed as anorexia nervosa either when the underlying organic disease is subtle or when it is in its early stages and the history, physical examination, and laboratory tests are not yet diagnostic. This is especially true in regional enteritis.

The hormone patterns of patients with anorexia nervosa are typical of prepubertal or pubertal children; their 24-h luteinizing hormone pattern shows low levels during wakefulness and higher plasma levels during sleep. These changes are reversed with restoration of weight. In differentiating anorexia nervosa from panhypopituitarism, the most significant findings are the preservation of axillary and pubic hair and breast tissue, as well as thyroid and adrenal function.

Treatment of this condition is difficult. In extreme cases it may be necessary to nourish the patient with parenteral or nasogastric feedings. Since patients with anorexia nervosa invariably exhibit severe psychologic disturbances, optimal management necessitates resolution of the patient's distorted ideas about eating. In some patients a period of anorexia will terminate spontaneously. Improvement has also been obtained by the use of *operant reinforcement techniques.* With this approach, access to physical activity, recreation, and personal attention is made contingent on weight gain by the patient. More intensive psychotherapeutic measures are frequently employed; yet often the basic conflicts in patients with anorexia nervosa remain unresolved or are likely to recur.

NAUSEA AND VOMITING Nausea and vomiting may occur independently of each other, but generally they are so closely allied that they may conveniently be considered together. *Nausea* denotes the feeling of the imminent desire to vomit, usually referred to the throat or epigastrium. *Vomiting* refers to the forceful oral expulsion of gastric contents; *retching* denotes the labored rhythmic respiratory activity that frequently precedes emesis. Extremely forceful *projectile vomiting* is a special form of vomiting which has significance because it connotes the presence of increased intracranial pressure.

Nausea often precedes or accompanies vomiting. It is usually associated with diminished functional activity of the stomach and alterations of the motility of the duodenum and small intestine. Accompanying severe nausea there is often evidence of altered autonomic (especially parasympathetic) activity: pallor of the skin, increased perspiration, salivation, and the occasional association of hypotension and bradycardia (vasovagal syndrome). Anorexia is also often present.

Following a period of nausea and a brief interval of retching, a sequence of involuntary visceral and somatic motor events occurs, resulting in emesis. The stomach plays a relatively passive role in the vomiting process, the major ejection force being provided by the abdominal musculature. With relaxation of the gastric fundus and gastroesophageal sphincter, a sharp increase in intraabdominal pressure is brought about by forceful contraction of the diaphragm and abdominal wall. This, together with concomitant annular contraction of the gastric pylorus, results in the expulsion of gastric contents into the esophagus. Increased intrathoracic pressure results in the further movement of esophageal contents into the mouth. Reversal of the normal direction of esophageal peristalsis may play a role in this process. Reflex elevation of the soft palate during the vomiting act prevents the entry of the material into the nasopharynx, whereas reflex closure of the glottis and inhibition of respiration help to prevent pulmonary aspiration.

Repeated emesis may have deleterious effects in a number of different ways. The process of vomiting itself may lead to traumatic rupture or tearing in the region of the cardioesophageal junction, resulting in massive hematemesis, the Mallory-Weiss syndrome. Prolonged vomiting may lead to dehydration and the loss of gastric secretions (especially hydrochloric acid) to metabolic alkalosis with hypokalemia. Finally, in states of central nervous system depression (coma, etc.), gastric contents may be aspirated into the lungs, with a resulting aspiration pneumonitis.

Vomiting mechanism The act of vomiting is under the control of two functionally distinct medullary centers: the *vomiting center* and the *chemoreceptor trigger zone*. The vomiting center controls and integrates the actual act of emesis. It receives afferent stimuli from the intestinal tract and other parts of the body, from higher cortical centers, especially the labyrinthine apparatus, and from the chemoreceptor trigger zone. The important efferent pathways in vomiting are the phrenic nerves (to the diaphragm), the spinal nerves (to the abdominal musculature), and visceral efferent nerves (to the stomach and esophagus).

The chemoreceptor trigger zone is also located in the medulla but by itself is incapable of mediating the act of vomiting. Activation of this zone results in efferent impulses to the medullary vomiting center, which in turn initiates the act of emesis. The chemoreceptor trigger zone can be activated by many stimuli, including drugs such as apomorphine, cardiac glycosides, and ergot alkaloids. Certain of the phenothiazine derivatives appear to antagonize the effects of the above-mentioned drugs on the chemoreceptor trigger zone.

Clinical classification Nausea and vomiting are common manifestations of organic and functional disorders. The precise mechanisms triggering vomiting in the various clinical states are poorly understood, making classification of mechanisms difficult. The categories mentioned below serve to illustrate some of the many disorders which may be accompanied by nausea and vomiting.

Many *acute abdominal emergencies* which lead to the "surgical abdomen" are associated with nausea and vomiting. Notably, vomiting may be seen with inflammation of a viscus as in acute appendicitis or acute cholecystitis, obstruction of the intestine, or acute peritonitis (see Chap. 8).

In many of the disorders involving *chronic indigestion* (see Chap. 39) nausea and vomiting may be prominent. Emesis may be either spontaneous or self-induced and may lead to relief of symptoms, as, for example, in uncomplicated peptic ulcer. Nausea and vomiting may accompany the distention and pain seen in the aerophagic syndromes. Often in patients with chronic indigestion, nausea and vomiting may be provoked by specific foods (e.g., fatty foods), for reasons that are poorly understood.

Acute systemic infections with fever, especially in young children, are frequently accompanied by vomiting and often by severe diarrhea. The mechanism whereby infections remote from the gastrointestinal tract produce these manifestations is unclear. Viral, bacterial, and parasitic infections of the intestinal tract may be associated with severe nausea and vomiting, often with diarrhea. Severe nausea and vomiting may be prominent in viral hepatitis, even before the appearance of jaundice.

Central nervous system disorders which lead to increased intracranial pressure may be accompanied by vomiting, often projectile. Brain swelling due to inflammation, anoxemia, acute hydrocephalus, neoplasms, etc., may thus be complicated by vomiting. Disorders of the labyrinthine apparatus and its central connections which underlie vertigo may be accompanied by vomiting with nausea and retching. Acute labyrinthitis and Ménière's disease are examples of such disturbances. Migraine headaches, tabetic crises, and acute meningitis are additional examples of disorders of the nervous system which may lead to vomiting. In the reactive phase of hypotension with syncope, there may be nausea and vomiting.

Severe nausea and vomiting may be present in *acute myocardial infarction*, especially of the posterior wall of the heart. Nausea and vomiting may also be seen in *congestive heart failure*, perhaps in relation to congestion of the liver. The possibility that these symptoms may be due to drugs (e.g., opiates or digitalis) should always be borne in mind in patients with cardiac disease.

Nausea and vomiting commonly accompany several *endocrinologic disorders*, including diabetic acidosis and adrenal insufficiency, especially adrenal crises. The morning sickness of early pregnancy is another instance of nausea and vomiting possibly related to hormonal changes.

The *side effects of many drugs and chemicals* include nausea and vomiting. In some instances this is because of gastric irritation which stimulates the medullary vomiting center.

Psychogenic vomiting means vomiting which may occur as part of any emotional upset on a transitory basis or more persistently as part of a psychic disturbance. Close observation will usually disclose the condition to be one of regurgitation rather than of vomiting, and weight loss may not correspond at all to the patient's description of the frequency and severity of vomiting. As discussed earlier in this chapter, anorexia nervosa is an emotional disturbance which may be associated not only with anorexia but also with vomiting. Often patients with emotional disorders and vomiting maintain a relatively normal state of nutrition, because a relatively small amount of the ingested food is vomited.

Differential diagnosis Vomiting should be distinguished from *regurgitation,* which refers to the expulsion of food in the absence of nausea and without abdominal diaphragmatic muscular contraction which is part of vomiting. Regurgitation of esophageal contents may occur with esophageal stricture or diverticula. Regurgitation of gastric contents is generally seen with gastroesophageal sphincter incompetence, especially with hiatus hernia or in association with peptic ulcer, usually when pylorospasm supervenes.

The temporal relationships of vomiting to eating may be of help diagnostically. Vomiting which occurs predominantly in the morning is often seen early in pregnancy and uremia. Alcoholic gastritis is commonly accompanied by early-morning emesis, the so-called "dry heaves." Vomiting which occurs shortly after eating may suggest pylorospasm or gastritis. On the other hand, vomiting which occurs 4 to 6 h or longer after eating and involves the elimination of large quantities of undigested food often indicates gastric retention (e.g., diabetic gastric atony or pyloric obstruction).

The character of the vomitus offers clues to the diagnosis. If the vomitus contains free hydrochloric acid, the obstruction may be due to an ulcer; absence of free hydrochloric acid is more compatible with gastric malignancy. A feculent or putrid odor reflects the results of bacterial action on the intestinal contents. Such vomiting may be seen with low-intestinal obstruction, peritonitis, or gastrocolic fistula. Bile is commonly present in gastric contents whenever vomiting is prolonged. It has no significance unless constantly present in large quantities, when it may signify an obstructive lesion below the ampulla of Vater. The presence of blood in the gastric contents usually denotes bleeding from the esophagus, stomach, or duodenum.

REFERENCES

BLINDER BJ et al: Behavior therapy of anorexia nervosa: Effectiveness of activity as a reinforcer of weight gain. Am J Psychiatry 126:8, 1970

BOYAR RM et al: Anorexia nervosa. Immaturity of the 24-hour luteinizing hormone secretory pattern. N Engl J Med 291:861, 1974

HALL, RJC: Normal and abnormal food intake. Gut 16:744, 1975

KANIS JA et al: Anorexia nervosa: A clinical psychiatric and laboratory study. Quart J Med (new series) 43:321, 1974

LUMSDEN K, HOLDEN SW: The act of vomiting in man. Gut 10: 173, 1969

41 CONSTIPATION, DIARRHEA, AND DISTURBANCES OF ANORECTAL FUNCTION

STEPHEN E. GOLDFINGER

NORMAL COLONIC FUNCTION Each day approximately 800 ml of a slurry of dietary residue plus unabsorbed intestinal secretions and cellular debris moves from the small intestine across the ileocecal valve, usually in response to postprandial reflex stimulation. Little of nutritional value remains after the extensive digestive processing and absorption that has occurred in the normal small intestine. The colon converts this liquid ileal effluent to solid fecal material which is advanced to the rectum and evacuated. Thus, normal colonic function involves primarily three physiologic processes: *absorption* of fluid and electrolytes, *contractions* whereby luminal contents are churned, exposed to the mucosa, and eventually transported to the rectum, and finally *defecation.*

Absorption of fluid and electrolytes (See also Chap. 289.) Dehydration of intestinal chyme occurs primarily in the ascending and transverse colon. In the normal adult, daily fecal water excretion averages only 100 ml. Colonic absorption of water is a passive process accompanying the net absorption of sodium and chloride which occurs by active transport against concentration gradients. In addition, bicarbonate is secreted in exchange for chloride, and normally there is a net efflux of potassium across the colonic mucosa into the lumen. The secreted bicarbonate is converted, in part, to carbon dioxide by reacting with acids produced by colonic bacteria. Analysis of fecal electrolyte concentrations in normal subjects reveals considerable variation, but average values for sodium, potassium, chloride, and bicarbonate are 32, 75, 16, and 40 meq per liter, respectively. The hyperosmolality of normal stool, which averages 375 milliosmoles, is largely due to osmotically active organic compounds produced by bacteria.

Factors which tend to cause diarrhea include:

1 Excessive outpouring of fluid from the small intestine into the colon, exceeding the latter's reabsorptive capacity of 2 liters per day. This may occur in association with viral and bacterial enteritis, various malabsorptive diseases of the small intestine, pancreatic tumors secreting gastrin or vasoactive intestinal peptide, and resection of the terminal ileum.

2 Reduced amount or deficient function of colonic mucosa (e.g., subtotal colectomy, diffuse ulcerative colitis).

3 Neural and hormonal stimuli which decrease to-and-fro peristalsis or promote massive propulsive activity (see below) and thus reduce mucosal surface contact time (e.g., exaggerated postprandial motility).

4 Impaired colonic reabsorption of water and electrolytes due to the presence of excessive bile salts and fatty acids. Ineffective ileal reabsorption of bile salts may occur due to ileal resection or disease (regional enteritis). Dihydroxy bile salts inhibit colonic sodium reabsorption and enhance efflux of sodium ions across the mucosa into the lumen leading to watery diarrhea. Fatty acids and hydroxylated long-chain fatty acids produced by bacteria retard colonic electrolyte and water absorption. Increased luminal concentrations of fatty acids may occur in malabsorptive disorders such as sprue.
5 Excessive colonic secretion distal to sites of water reabsorption (e.g., villous adenoma of the rectum).
6 Increased luminal concentrations of nonabsorbed molecules exerting significant osmotic effect (e.g., magnesium-containing cathartics, lactose when individuals with lactase deficiency eat milk products).

Excessively hard stools are usually due to increased absorption of fluid as a result of prolonged contact of the luminal contents with the colonic mucosa consequent to delayed transit. In some instances ingested material such as calcium carbonate can explain "rocklike" feces.

Motility (contraction) patterns of the colon The colon and rectum are extensively innervated by both the sympathetic and parasympathetic systems. Impulses received via these nerve fibers, local neural reflex arcs, and intrinsic contactile responses of smooth muscle all play roles in the coordination of colonic motility. Parasympathetic innervation is generally equated with excitatory stimulation and is believed to dominate the regulation of colonic motor activity; sympathetic tone tends to inhibit cholinergic stimulation. More complex integration of both visceral systems may well occur in a manner that is poorly appreciated.

Basal colonic motor activity consists mainly of haustral shuttling, serving to move luminal contents to and fro by seemingly random segmental contractions of circular smooth muscle. Since no net aboral advance is achieved, it would seem that the principal purpose of these movements is to maximize mucosal surface contact for absorption. With increased parasympathetic tone, such as occurs postprandially, more propulsive activity occurs. This may take the form of aboral contractions across short segments of colon or involve massive peristalsis, which begins in the right or transverse colon and rapidly transports luminal contents to the sigmoid colon and rectum. Massive peristalsis may occur only several times a day. Resultant distention of the rectum initiates the defecatory urge.

It is evident that colonic motility plays an important role in both absorption and movement of contents to the rectum. Aberrations in adrenergic and cholinergic tone, either occurring physiologically or induced by various drugs, tend to have a significant influence on bowel activity. In view of the number of pharmacologic agents that may influence smooth muscle contractility, it is important to take a careful drug history when evaluating patients with constipation or diarrhea of recent onset.

Defecation The defecatory reflex is initiated by acute distention of the rectum. When it is allowed to progress by supraspinal centers, sigmoidal and rectal contractions heighten the pressure within the rectum and also obliterate the rectosigmoidal angle. Concomitant relaxation of the internal and external anal sphincters then permits the evacuation of feces. This can be augmented by an increase in intraabdominal pressure created by the Valsava maneuver (i.e., voluntary closure of the glottis, diaphragmatic fixation, and abdominal-wall contraction). Conversely, defecation may be consciously prevented by the forceful contraction of the striated muscles of the pelvic diaphragm and external anal sphincter. The functional value of voluntary control of defecation requires little elaboration, but the opportunity for individuals to resist the defecatory urge, when abused, may lead to chronic rectal distention, reduced afferent signals, loss of motor tone, and chronic constipation.

DIARRHEA AND CONSTIPATION The bowel habits of apparently healthy persons vary widely. For this reason, the terms *diarrhea* and *constipation* have little meaning except when viewed as a change from the individual's customary pattern. Reasonably detailed information is important in evaluating either abnormality. When patients complain of diarrhea, it is important to obtain an estimate of the volume as well as frequency of fecal output and, in addition, to directly examine a stool sample for consistency, blood, oiliness, and malodor. For example, the repeated elimination of small quantities of solid material admixed with gas has a far different connotation than the same number of movements of voluminous blood-tinged feces. The term *constipation* may be used by the patient to refer to a variety of changes including reduction in frequency of defecation, a constant sensation of rectal fullness with incomplete evacuation of feces, and sometimes painful defecation due to hard stools or perianal pathology. In an assessment of complaints of diarrhea or constipation, it is important to focus on the patient's emotional status since in many instances the recent onset of psychologic stress is the major reason for altered bowel habits. However, it can be hazardous to assume this to be the case, even when the relationship seems convincing. For this reason, the judicious use of laboratory, proctoscopic, and radiologic procedures is recommended to make certain that organic disease will not be overlooked.

Acute diarrhea Diarrhea of abrupt onset occurring in otherwise healthy persons is most often related to an infectious process. A variety of accompanying symptoms are often observed, including fever, headache, anorexia, vomiting, malaise, and myalgia, but they cannot be used to distinguish with certainty between viral, bacterial, and protozoal causes. In most instances, identifiable pathogens are not recovered from the feces. For this reason so-called "nonspecific" diarrhea is usually considered to be of viral etiology. However, the recent demonstration of enterotoxin-producing strains of *Escherichia coli* (see below), which are not distinguishable from "normal flora" on routine culture, suggests that this assumption may often be incorrect and that these organisms may account for a substantial number of cases that were in the past ascribed to viral infection.

Acute diarrhea presumed to be of viral etiology typically

persists for a period of 1 to 3 days; death is extremely rare except in previously debilitated individuals who become severely dehydrated. Abnormal small-intestinal morphology including villous shortening, increase in the number of crypt cells, and increased cellularity of the lamina propria has been described in experimentally infected human volunteers. Unfortunately the techniques of tissue culture and immune electron microscopy used for viral identification are generally not available clinically. The diagnosis of viral diarrhea is supported (but not confirmed) by the absence of polymorphonuclear leukocytes and erythrocytes in stool samples after preparation with Loeffler's methylene blue. Bacterial diarrhea may be suspected if there is a history of a similar and simultaneous illness in individuals who shared contaminated food with the patient. Diarrhea developing within 12 h of the meal is most likely due to ingestion of a preformed toxin (e.g., staphylococcal exotoxin). A lag period of up to 3 days after consumption of contaminated food can occur with salmonellosis.

The pathogenesis of bacterial diarrhea appears to be due to two principal mechanisms, *mucosal invasion* and *enterotoxin-induced hypersecretion.* Bacterial invasion of the colon leads to mucosal hyperemia, edema, leukocytic infiltration, and frank ulceration. Lower abdominal cramps and tenderness are prominent, as are tenesmus and rectal urgency. In severe cases the stool is grossly bloody. At other times, microscopic examination of the stool will reveal erythrocytes along with pus cells. In *shigellosis* defective colonic absorption due to mucosal damage is believed to be the principal cause of diarrhea, but small-intestinal hypersecretion may also occur with some enterotoxin-producing strains of *Shigella.* The prototype of hypersecretory bacterial diarrhea is *cholera,* in which the organism *Vibrio cholerae* remains within the bowel lumen and releases an enterotoxin which stimulates massive secretion of fluid and electrolytes by the small intestine. This may be produced experimentally in animals by placing the enterotoxin, free of the organism itself, into isolated intestinal loops. Hypersecretion reaches a peak at 4 to 6 h and is due to the stimulation of mucosal adenylate cyclase by the toxin. It should be emphasized that in cholera there is no tissue invasion. Mucosal morphology is essentially normal, and intestinal absorptive capacity is preserved. This provides the basis for oral rehydration therapy with solutions containing glucose and sodium chloride, the former stimulating absorption of the latter. Because other species of bacteria, such as *E. coli,* clostridia, and *Salmonella,* have been shown to produce enterotoxins, the finding of an exudate-free stool does not preclude bacterial infection as the cause of diarrhea.

Protozoal infections may also be responsible for acute diarrhea. *Entamoeba histolytica,* prevalent in some areas of the United States, produces an inflammatory colitis which can closely mimic idiopathic ulcerative colitis. Cystic *Giardia lamblia* may be excreted in the stools of asymptomatic individuals, but giardiasis is also a cause of prolonged, watery diarrhea especially in travelers returning from endemic areas where the water supply has been contaminated. In some patients giardiasis is associated with an underlying immunoglobulin deficiency of the IgA type. Careful examination of fresh stools by experienced technicians is required for the diagnosis of protozoal infection. In approximately 50 percent of cases, only examination of duodenal aspirates will reveal the presence of *Giardia.*

Travelers' diarrhea may result from any one or several of the pathogens described above. However, often no known agent is identified, and the etiology is assumed to be viral or due to enterotoxin-producing coliform organisms. Not infrequently prolonged bowel irregularity will occur following the acute illness.

Ulcerative colitis and *regional enteritis* (Crohn's disease) may present with acute diarrhea (Chaps. 290 and 291). Bloody stools and generalized abdominal cramping and tenderness are more apt to occur in the patients with ulcerative colitis; in regional enteritis, the diarrhea tends to be milder, is usually nonbloody, and is associated with right lower quadrant pain and tenderness. Diarrhea may be induced directly or indirectly by *drugs* including parasympathomimetic agents, magnesium-containing antacids, cardiac glycosides, and broad-spectrum antibiotics. In the latter category clindamycin appears to have a particular propensity to cause pseudomembranous colitis. Diarrhea due to *diverticulitis* is usually accompanied by fever, tenesmus, and rectal urgency, together with cramps and tenderness in the left lower quadrant (Chap. 291). When there is no evidence of acute inflammation, diarrhea in the presence of colonic diverticuli is more apt to be due to spastic (irritable) colon which should be regarded as the cause rather than the result of diverticular disease. In elderly and debilitated individuals with *fecal impaction* the presenting symptom may be the frequent expulsion of small amounts of liquid stool due to colonic distention behind the impaction. Acute *psychologic stress* can cause diarrhea at any age.

DIAGNOSTIC APPROACH The appropriate tempo and approach in the evaluation of acute diarrhea depend so heavily on the clinical setting in which it occurs that only very general guidelines can be offered. It is entirely reasonable to withhold studies in mild, self-limited cases such as are seen as part of an epidemic viral illness. When dealing with sporadic severe diarrhea or when a suggestive epidemiologic history is obtained, bacterial cultures and microscopic examination of the stool for parasites and inflammatory cells are appropriate. Proctoscopy is generally reserved for patients with bloody diarrhea, or those who do not show improvement within 5 days. Likewise, radiologic studies should usually be deferred until the initial course of the illness has been observed. In cases of massive fluid loss, measurement of serum electrolytes is useful to aid in determining replacement therapy.

TREATMENT General and nonspecific treatment of acute diarrhea includes rest, encouragement of fluid intake, and prescription of opiate-containing agents by mouth. Intravenous fluid and electrolyte replacement may be desirable and necessary in infants and the elderly. As a result of success achieved with cholera patients, the use of oral glucose-electrolyte solutions is being extended to the treatment of patients with acute diarrhea considered to be due to other enterotoxin-producing bacteria.

Chronic diarrhea Diarrhea persisting for weeks or months, whether constant or intermittent, may be a functional symptom or a manifestation of serious illness. For this reason, it is incumbent upon the physician to search carefully for evidence of organic disease, such as fever, weight loss, malnutrition, anemia, or an increased erythrocyte sedimentation rate. Abdominal tenderness and fever suggest the presence of inflammation. When there is involvement of the large bowel, the major diseases to be considered include ulcerative colitis, Crohn's disease of the colon, amebiasis, and diverticulitis. Crohn's disease of the small intestine (regional enteritis) may involve one or more of its segments. The ileum is most frequently affected. Other diarrheal conditions which may resemble Crohn's disease radiographically include tuberculous and fungal enteritis, lymphosarcoma, amyloidosis, and argentaffin (carcinoid) tumors of the small bowel.

Prolonged diarrhea without evidence of inflammation may reflect impairments of absorption, secretion, or digestion. Selective derangements, such as those due to *bile salt enteropathy* and *lactase deficiency,* are usually not accompanied by weight loss or malnutrition. *Mucosal disorders,* best exemplified by sprue, are frequently associated with weight loss, malodorous stools, abdominal distention, and anemia, and, when more severe, with osteomalacia, hypoprothrombinemia, avitaminotic neuropathies, and tetany. *Pancreatic insufficiency* resulting from chronic pancreatitis, carcinoma, or resection produces steatorrhea and weight loss of varying severity. A number of mechanisms may be responsible for *postgastrectomy diarrhea* (see Chap. 287). These include the dumping syndrome, postvagotomy motility derangements, inadequate stimulation of pancreatic digestive enzymes, and incomplete mixing of these enzymes with food. On rare occasions severe postgastrectomy diarrhea and malnutrition are due to the inadvertent creation by the surgeon of a gastroileostomy instead of a gastrojejunostomy. *Bacterial overgrowth* in the small intestine, as may occur with multiple intestinal diverticulosis and prolonged bowel stasis secondary to disorders of peristalsis (e.g., scleroderma, diabetic visceral neuropathy), can also lead to chronic diarrhea and weight loss. This has been attributed to bacterial deconjugation of bile salts, to consumption of nutrients by the organisms, and to mucosal abnormalities believed to be caused by bacteria or their metabolites (see Chap. 289). At times, diarrhea may accompany stasis in the absence of bacterial overgrowth.

Endocrine disorders that may be accompanied by chronic diarrhea include thyrotoxicosis, adrenal insufficiency, and hypoparathyroidism. The release of potent bioactive humoral agents from neoplastic tissue in the Zollinger-Ellison syndrome (gastrin), medullary carcinoma of the thyroid (calcitonin, prostaglandins), pancreatic cholera syndrome (vasoactive intestinal peptide), and metastatic carcinoid tumors (serotonin, prostaglandins) make diarrhea a prominent feature of these disorders. The passage of excessive amounts of clear liquid, at times sufficient to cause dehydration, occurs in some patients with large villous adenomas of the rectum.

Habitual *cathartic abuse* must be suspected when the cause of prolonged diarrhea remains perplexing. Even if this is denied by the patient, a stool sample should be alkalinized with sodium hydroxide; this will produce a burgundy color if phenolphthalein-containing laxatives have been surreptitiously ingested. The observation of melanosis coli by sigmoidoscopy indicates chronic usage of anthraquinone laxatives.

Constipation Constipation is a common complaint often resulting from the inordinate expectation of "regularity" in bowel-conscious individuals. Stools may be described as infrequent, incomplete, or unduly hard; unusual straining may be required to achieve defecation. A review of the patient's habits may reveal contributory and correctable causes, such as insufficient dietary roughage, lack of exercise, suppression of defecatory urges arising at inconvenient moments, inadequate allotment of time for full defecation, and prolonged travel. Appropriate adjustments of these patterns and reassurance are preferable to the prescription of laxatives and may be all that is required for improvement. When the patient also has symptoms such as fatigue, malaise, headaches, or anorexia, the possibility should be considered that such symptoms reflect an underlying depression of which constipation is but one component. Deranged colonic motility is responsible for the constipation associated with the use of parasympatholytic drugs, the irritable colon syndrome, scleroderma, and Hirschprung's disease.

Hemorrhoids, anal fissures, perineal abscesses, and rectal strictures often prevent easy and adequate stool evacuation; fear of resultant pain may account for delayed or inadequate defecation. When constipation and tenesmus of recent onset are reported, the possibility of carcinoma of the rectum or descending colon must be seriously considered. In such instances sigmoidoscopic and barium enema examinations should be obtained early and are virtually obligatory if fecal blood has been observed or if occult blood is detected on any of three successive stool specimens. Stools of abnormally thin caliber occur in patients with rectal or sigmoid colon carcinoma but are even more commonly due to an irritable colon. Other mechanical causes of constipation include volvulus of the sigmoid colon, diverticulitis, intussusception, and hernias. A variety of metabolic abnormalities, such as hypothyroidism, hypercalcemia, hypokalemia, porphyria, lead poisoning, and dehydration are often associated with constipation. Tremendous retention and impaction of feces may occur in certain neurologic disorders (e.g., spinal cord injury, multiple sclerosis, cerebral palsy, senility), and in these instances, when autonomous regulation of evacuation is unachievable, vigorous and sustained enema programs are often necessary.

IRRITABLE COLON The irritable colon syndrome (also referred to as *spastic colon* and *mucous colitis*) is one of the most frequent gastrointestinal disorders (see Chap. 291). This condition is characterized by periodic or chronic symptoms of alternating diarrhea and constipation with associated cramping and tenesmus. These symptoms are generally associated with psychologic stresses, but the anxiety produced by the bowel disturbance is frequently regarded by the patient as the fundamental cause of the emotional upset. Stools tend to be thin, fragmented, or pelletlike, and accompanied by excessive mucus and gas. Efforts to ameliorate symptoms with mild cathartics or antispasmodic drugs often yield adverse and exaggerated responses. An increased sigmoidal contractility has been demonstrated in this syndrome, but it is not clear whether this is primary or due to psychically generated disturbances of visceral tone. A variety of therapeutic approaches, including the avoidance of foods which tend to upset the patient, addition of bulk-forming agents, judicious use of antispasmodics and tranquilizers, and gentle psychotherapy may provide some relief. If the patient's life goals can be shifted away from the quixotic search for the perfect stool, much can be accomplished. At the same time, it must be remembered that such individuals are not exempt from developing bowel cancer, and any worrisome deviation from their general pattern of derangement must be seriously evaluated.

FLATULENCE A significant amount of flatus is passed each day by normal persons, and the complaint of flatulence may merely reflect a heightened and embarrassing awareness of this natural occurrence. Excessive passage of intestinal gas may be the result of aerophagia or the formation of increased amounts of gas by intestinal bacteria. The latter process can be associated with malabsorption syndromes or significant constipation but is more frequently a consequence of eating foods such as beans, broccoli, and cabbage which have a high content of nondigestible polysaccharides. The oligosaccharides stachyose and raffinose, isolated from beans, are particularly effective substrates for fermentation to carbon dioxide, hydrogen, and methane by colonic flora. The treatment of flatulence is generally undertaken to reduce embarrassment and consists of measures to decrease aerophagia along with avoidance of foods that cause excessive gas.

REFERENCES

DAVENPORT HW: *Physiology of the Digestive Tract,* 3d ed., Chicago: Year Book, 1971

GORBACH SL et al: Travellers' diarrhea and toxigenic *Escherichia coli.* N Engl J Med 292:933, 1975

HARRIS JC et al: Fecal leukocytes in diarrheal illness. Ann Intern Med 76:697, 1972

PHILLIPS SF: Diarrhea: A current view of the pathophysiology. Gastroenterology 63:495, 1972

42
HEMATEMESIS AND MELENA

KURT J. ISSELBACHER
RAYMOND S. KOFF

Hematemesis is defined as the vomiting of blood, and *melena* as the passage of black, tarry stools. These symptoms of gastrointestinal hemorrhage should not only bring the patient to prompt medical attention but, within certain limits, help define the anatomic site of bleeding. Only rarely will exsanguinating gastrointestinal hemorrhage occur without the appearance of altered or gross blood passed by mouth or rectum. The color of vomited blood will vary from red to black depending upon the concentration of hydrochloric acid in the stomach and its admixture with the blood. Thus if vomiting occurs shortly after the onset of bleeding, the vomitus is likely to be red; if there is delay in vomiting, the appearance will be dark-red, black, or of "coffee grounds" appearance. Since blood entering the gastrointestinal tract below the duodenum rarely reenters the stomach, hematemesis usually indicates that the bleeding is proximal to the jejunum.

Melena may occur independently of, or be associated with, hematemesis. Bleeding of sufficient volume to produce hematemesis usually results in melena. The altered color of the blood results from contact with hydrochloric acid in gastric juice to produce hematin. In contrast to hematemesis, melena may result from hemorrhage into the jejunum or ileum provided that transit through the intestine is slow. At least 50 to 100 ml blood must rapidly enter the upper part of the gastrointestinal tract to produce a single black, tarry stool. Following a single-liter episode of hemorrhage, tarry stools will persist for 1 to 3 days. Subsequently the stools return to normal color, but tests for occult blood may be positive for 3 to 8 days.

The passage of red blood per rectum usually denotes lower intestinal bleeding, i.e., bleeding originating below the duodenum. However, if bleeding is massive and rapid enough, red blood may appear per rectum from an upper intestinal or gastric lesion.

Not all black or red stools are due to blood. Black stools may result from the ingestion of iron, charcoal, or bismuth. Red or purple stools are occasionally seen after ingestion of beets or after intravenous administration of sulfobromophthalein. Gastrointestinal bleeding, even if detected only by positive tests for occult blood in the stool, indicates potentially serious disease and must be investigated.

The clinical manifestations of gastrointestinal bleeding are dependent upon the extent of hemorrhage, the rate of bleeding, and associated or coincidental diseases. Unless anemia is present prior to the onset of bleeding, loss of less than 500 ml blood is usually not associated with systemic symptoms. Rapid hemorrhage of greater volume will result in decreased venous return to the heart, decreased cardiac output, reflex vasoconstriction, and increased peripheral resistance. The presence of orthostatic hypotension (i.e., a decrease in blood pressure of more than 10 mmHg on sitting), is a more accurate indicator of blood loss than is tachycardia, and suggests that a volume depletion of 20 percent or more has occurred. The patient may experience syncope, lightheadedness, nausea, sweating, and thirst. He may appear anxious and restless. When blood loss approaches 40 percent of the blood volume, shock with tachycardia and a thready peripheral pulse are usually present. The skin is cold and clammy, and pallor is prominent. Hematocrits will not reflect the blood loss accurately until several hours after the start of the hemorrhage, when hemodilution has occurred. Leukocytosis is found 2 to 5 h after onset of bleeding, and the platelet count rises. Occasionally blood in the intestinal tract is associated with mild fever (100 to 102°F), and the blood urea nitrogen level becomes variably elevated 24 to 48 h after bleeding, because of the breakdown of blood proteins to urea by intestinal bacteria and a decrease in glomerular filtration rate.

ETIOLOGY OF UPPER GASTROINTESTINAL BLEEDING
Swallowed blood resulting from epistaxis, hemoptysis, dental extractions, and tonsillectomy may be vomited or result in melena. A careful history and physical examination will exclude these sources.

The three most common causes of upper gastrointestinal hemorrhage are (1) peptic ulceration, (2) erosive gastritis, and (3) variceal bleeding. These three entities encompass

90 to 95 percent of all cases of upper gastrointestinal bleeding in which a definite lesion can be found.

Peptic ulcer Peptic ulcer disease is probably the most common cause of upper gastrointestinal bleeding. The majority of these ulcers are situated in the duodenum. About 20 to 30 percent of patients with peptic ulcer will have at least one episode of significant gastrointestinal bleeding. When a patient with known peptic ulcer has gastrointestinal hemorrhage, the ulcer is the most probable site of bleeding.

Gastritis Gastritis may be associated with recent heavy alcohol ingestion or with a history of ingestion of salicylates or other drugs. Similarly gastric erosions and superficial ulcerations may occur in "stressful" situations and are often found in patients with intracranial disease, burns, or recent trauma. Erosive gastritis does not produce a clinical syndrome by either history or physical examination. Furthermore it can rarely be diagnosed by radiologic techniques, and gastroscopy is necessary to confirm this diagnosis.

Variceal bleeding Bleeding from esophageal or gastric varices is most frequently associated with portal hypertension due to cirrhosis of the liver. Although in the United States alcoholic cirrhosis is by far the most prevalent form of this disease, variceal hemorrhage may occur in other forms of cirrhosis associated with portal hypertension, especially postnecrotic cirrhosis. Portal vein thrombosis may also lead to variceal hemorrhage in the absence of cirrhosis. Bleeding from varices tends to be abrupt and often massive; however, minor bleeding may occur for days from esophageal varices before it is discovered. Upper gastrointestinal bleeding in a patient with cirrhosis suggests a variceal source, but because as many as 40 percent of patients with cirrhosis may be bleeding from other lesions, e.g., peptic ulceration, bleeding from nonvariceal sites must be excluded.

Other lesions Less common sources of upper gastrointestinal bleeding originating in the esophagus include esophagitis (with or without hiatus hernia), carcinoma, and peptic ulcer of the esophagus. Lacerations of the mucosa of the distal end of the esophagus associated with severe vomiting (the Mallory-Weiss syndrome) are suggested by a history of nonbloody vomiting followed by hematemesis. Though sudden severe hemorrhage is seen in a small number of patients with carcinoma of the stomach, particularly in association with mucosal ulceration, chronic blood loss is a more frequent complication of gastric carcinoma.

Lymphoma, polyps, and other tumors of the stomach and proximal small intestine are relatively uncommon lesions and are therefore unusual sources of hemorrhage. Leiomyoma and leiomyosarcoma of the stomach are notorious as sources of massive bleeding. The Peutz-Jeghers syndrome of small-intestinal polyposis and melanin pigmentation of the lips, mucosa, fingers, and toes may be associated with recurrent melena. Vascular insufficiency of the intestine, including nonocclusive and occlusive disease, may lead to bloody diarrhea or red blood in the stools.

Saccular arteriosclerotic aortic aneurysms may rupture into the upper part of the intestine and are almost invariably fatal. Most commonly rupture occurs into the third portion of the duodenum. Rupture into the intestine may also occur following aortic or renal artery reconstructive surgery. Sudden intestinal bleeding may occur following abdominal trauma and hepatic laceration. Such bleeding should suggest the entry of blood from a damaged liver into the bile ducts, i.e., hemobilia. The latter condition may also result from rupture of a hepatic artery aneurysm, and may be episodic and associated with jaundice.

Primary blood dyscrasias, including leukemia, thrombocytopenic states, the hemophilias, and disseminated intravascular coagulation, may result in significant gastrointestinal bleeding. Polycythemia vera, although associated with an increased incidence of peptic ulceration, may also result in gastrointestinal bleeding because of mesenteric or portal vein thrombosis. Periarteritis nodosa, Henoch-Schönlein purpura, and other vasculitides may lead to gastrointestinal blood loss.

Gastrointestinal bleeding, usually mild although occasionally persistent, may accompany amyloidosis, Osler-Rendu-Weber disease, pseudoxanthoma elasticum, Turner's syndrome, single or multiple intestinal hemangiomas, neurofibromatosis, and Kaposi's sarcoma. Hematemesis and melena occur in uremia, with occult intestinal bleeding being the most common cause. In central nervous system disorders, especially after trauma or surgery, superficial gastric erosions may develop (Cushing's ulcers) and be a cause of upper intestinal bleeding.

ETIOLOGY OF LOWER GASTROINTESTINAL BLEEDING

Anal lesions Small amounts of bright-red blood on the surface of the stool and on toilet tissue are most commonly caused by hemorrhoids. Bleeding from internal or external hemorrhoids is frequently precipitated by straining or passage of hard stools. Anal fissures or fistulas likewise first may come to the attention of the patient as a result of rectal bleeding. Nonspecific proctitis or cryptitis at the anorectal margin is a common source of bleeding. An anal pathologic condition does not preclude other causes and sources of bleeding, such as carcinoma, and these must be sought and excluded.

Rectal and colonic disease Carcinoma of the rectum, rectal polyps, and ulcerative proctitis are the most common bleeding lesions of the rectum. Bleeding from carcinoma in any area of the colon may result in the appearance of gross blood, whether on the stool or mixed with the fecal contents. Bloody diarrhea is often the presenting feature of ulcerative colitis but is less common in granulomatous ileocolitis, although occult blood may be present in the stool. Bleeding may also accompany diarrhea due to infections such as shigellosis, amebiasis, and rarely salmonellosis. In elderly patients chronic blood loss may result from submucosal vascular ectasia (angiodysplasia), often on the right side of the colon. Segmental bowel ischemia (ischemic colitis) may produce bloody diarrhea.

Diverticula Intestinal diverticula may occur in every part of the intestinal tract but are most commonly found in the sigmoid colon. Diverticulosis per se may be the most common cause of massive lower gastrointestinal bleeding. Diverticula to the right of the splenic flexure are more likely to cause important hemorrhage than those in the sigmoid and descending colon. Mild blood loss is more common when inflammation is present, i.e., in diverticulitis. Meckel's diverticulum, a congenital anomaly occurring in about 2 percent of the population and located in the ileum usually 20 to 100 cm proximal to the ileocecal valve, is often associated with bleeding. Ectopic gastric mucosa may be present in about 15 percent of these diverticula and may ulcerate, with profuse or recurrent rectal hemorrhage, particularly in children and young adults.

APPROACH TO THE PATIENT WITH GASTROINTESTINAL BLEEDING The approach to the problem presented by the patient with gross bleeding from the gastrointestinal tract is dependent upon the site, extent, and rate of bleeding. In general the patient with hematemesis is more likely to have bled greater amounts and is more likely to exsanguinate than the patient with melena. There is usually a sense of urgency in the immediate diagnosis and treatment of patients with upper gastrointestinal bleeding. When first seen, the patient may be in shock. Before a complete history and physical examination are undertaken, blood must be obtained for typing and cross matching, and an intravenous infusion of saline solution or other plasma expanders must be started at once.

History A history of epigastric pain relieved by food, milk, or antacids strongly suggests peptic ulcer disease. A history of jaundice and alcoholism suggests chronic liver disease. One must carefully inquire about a recent alcoholic binge or the ingestion of drugs such as aspirin, which may be associated with gastritis or precipitate bleeding from peptic ulcer. Attention must be directed to possible previous episodes of bleeding, vomiting, symptoms of gastrointestinal distress, diarrhea, cramps, weight loss, fever, bleeding from other sites such as the skin and mucous membranes, and a family history of intestinal disease or hemorrhagic diathesis.

Physical examination Initially the examiner must determine whether volume depletion is present on the basis of vital signs and the response to postural alterations. In that event, volume repletion is the immediate priority. Attention may then be directed to excluding a nonintestinal source of blood (i.e., ruling out epistaxis, hemoptysis, pharyngeal lesions). Careful assessment of the skin may reveal the characteristic telangiectasia of Osler-Rendu-Weber disease, the diffuse melanin pigmentation of hemochromatosis, the localized pigmentation of Peutz-Jeghers syndrome, the soft-tissue tumors and multiple sebaceous cysts which occur with colonic polyposis in Gardner's syndrome, or the dermal neurofibromas of neurofibromatosis. The peripheral stigmata of chronic liver disease with hepatosplenomegaly, ascites, and edema suggest the likelihood of portal hypertension and the possibility of bleeding from varices, gastritis, or peptic ulceration. One must look for abdominal tenderness or masses, determine the frequency and character of the bowel sounds, and look for evidence of malignancy such as a Virchow's node or rectal shelf.

Laboratory studies Initial studies include the hematocrit, hemoglobin, careful assessment of red blood cell morphologic features (hypochromic, microcytic red blood cells suggest that blood loss is chronic), white blood cell count, and differential blood cell count. There should be a platelet count, or the adequacy of platelets should be estimated from the blood smear. Prothrombin time, partial thromboplastin time, and other coagulation studies may be in order to exclude primary or secondary clotting defects. Though the initial studies are valuable and essential, repeated evaluation of the laboratory data is important as one follows the clinical course of the bleeding.

DIAGNOSTIC APPROACH The diagnostic approach (see also Chaps. 287 and 301 for additional and detailed discussions) to the patient with gastrointestinal hemorrhage must necessarily be individualized. The initial management of gastrointestinal bleeding may be under the direction of the internist, but it is prudent to consult a surgeon early in the course of the illness in the event that the bleeding cannot be controlled by medical means. It must be emphasized that demonstration of a lesion in a patient with gastrointestinal bleeding should also be accompanied by evidence that this lesion is the site of bleeding. In recent years the availability of experienced endoscopists as well as radiologists with facilities for selective arteriography has increased to the extent that in many medical centers it is possible to have emergency endoscopy, angiographic, and barium studies performed within hours of the patient's admission to the hospital. It is to be hoped that this "vigorous diagnostic approach" will serve to decrease the morbidity and mortality associated with upper gastrointestinal bleeding.

When there is a history of melena or hematemesis or the suspicion of bleeding from the upper part of the gastrointestinal tract, the patient should have a tube passed to empty the stomach and to determine whether the bleeding is in the upper part of the gastrointestinal tract and is still active. Provided that blood volume is maintained, the next diagnostic step will depend on whether the bleeding continues. This is generally determined by vital signs, gastric aspiration, the number, frequency, and consistency of stools, and requirements for blood.

If gastric aspiration suggests that bleeding has stopped, medical treatment may be initiated. Upper gastrointestinal barium studies may then be obtained when the patient's general condition has stabilized. If the conventional barium study is nondiagnostic, esophagogastroscopy may be performed 8 to 12 h later. Some consultants recommend, however, that endoscopy be performed first, with barium studies carried out secondarily.

If upper gastrointestinal bleeding persists, ice water or iced saline lavage may be attempted to slow the bleeding. If bleeding persists, and gastroesophagoscopy and barium studies have not revealed the site of bleeding, the patient should be considered for emergency selective angiography. Angiography may demonstrate the site of active bleeding and, if variceal hemorrhage is suspected, may confirm the presence of varices as well as portal hypertension. Occasionally one may be able to observe the leaking of contrast material from esophageal vessels. Angiography is also valuable in providing information on the patency of the portal, splenic, and left renal veins should surgical decompression of the portal system be contemplated.

When bleeding continues and gastric aspiration fails to reveal fresh bleeding into the stomach, blood loss may be occurring from a lesion beyond the pylorus or ligament of Treitz. In that situation, selective celiac axis and mesenteric artery angiography may be useful to localize the origin of the cryptogenic bleeding. However, extravasation of contrast material into the intestinal lumen can be shown only when bleeding is active and at a rate estimated to be greater than 0.5 ml per min. Arteriography is helpful to reveal the *site of bleeding;* however, the *cause of bleeding* often cannot be determined unless an aneurysm, varix, or vascular malformation is present. A promising approach to the control of persistent bleeding is the continuous administration of vasoconstrictors, such as vasopressin, either by selective superior mesenteric artery infusion (in the case of esophageal varices) or in the case of arterial bleeding by direct infusion of the agent into the vessel leading to the bleeding site (Fig. 42-1). This should be considered a temporary, rather than a definitive, method for the control of bleeding. In some instances in which infusion therapy fails to halt bleeding, transcatheter embolization or thrombus formation with autologous blood clot or other hemostatic material has been attempted. The efficacy and risks of this procedure remain to be determined.

If *variceal hemorrhage* is suspected, massive bleeding persists, and angiography is *not* available, the administration of vasopressin into a peripheral vein (10 to 20 units over a 20- to 30-min period and repeated once or twice every 2 to 4 h) may permit hemostasis by reduction of portal venous pressure. However repeated systemic injections of vasopressin may lead to loss of effectiveness because of tachyphylaxis, and occasionally adverse cardiovascular reactions may occur because of vasoconstrictor effects. It may then be necessary to resort to esophageal tamponade, with a Sengstaken-Blakemore tube. Although tamponade is hazardous because of the occasional occurrence of esophageal erosions or rupture, variceal hemorrhage can frequently be controlled temporarily with the use of this technique. Nevertheless, esophageal tamponade is probably most useful to reduce bleeding and stabilize the patient's condition as a preoperative maneuver.

In the evaluation of *rectal bleeding* (see also Chap. 291) the most important diagnostic procedures are digital examination of the rectum, anoscopy, and proctosigmoidoscopy. Occasionally retrograde bleeding from a distal lesion may be a source of confusion in establishing the site of bleeding on sigmoidoscopic examination. Biopsy of suggestive lesions may be performed through the sigmoidoscope under direct vision. Barium enema examination and air-contrast studies will aid in localizing lesions above the reach of the sigmoidoscope. Superior and inferior mesenteric angiography is very useful for demonstrating the site of active colonic bleeding, and the local infusion of vasoconstrictors through the angiographic catheter has been successful in controlling hemorrhage. Colonoscopy, by means of a flexible fiber optic instrument capable of permitting visualization of the entire large intestine, is currently being evaluated and may prove useful in determining the site and nature of bleeding lesions proximal to the rectosigmoid area. It would appear to be most helpful in the identification of slowly bleeding small lesions not detectable by either barium enema or angiography. Bleeding should not be attributed to hemorrhoids or anal fissures unless other lesions have been excluded. When appropriate, stool culture and examination for ova and parasites should be performed.

The primary consideration in the management of gastrointestinal bleeding, regardless of the source and site of hemorrhage, is the necessity to maintain adequate blood volume and perfusion by blood transfusion during the diagnostic evaluation.

FIGURE 42-1
Angiographic findings on a patient with massive upper gastrointestinal bleeding. Angiographic studies revealed the bleeding to be secondary to hemorrhagic gastritis; it was controlled by the selective left gastric arterial infusion of vasopressin. A *Selective left gastric arteriography demonstrates massive extravasation of contrast material (arrow) from a branch of the left gastric artery.* B *Selective left gastric arteriography during the infusion of 0.1 unit vasopressin per min demonstrates a marked decrease in the caliber of the left gastric artery and cessation of hemorrhage.*

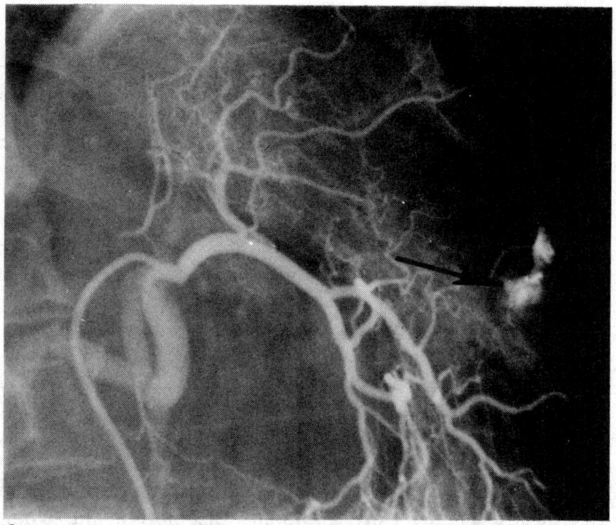

A

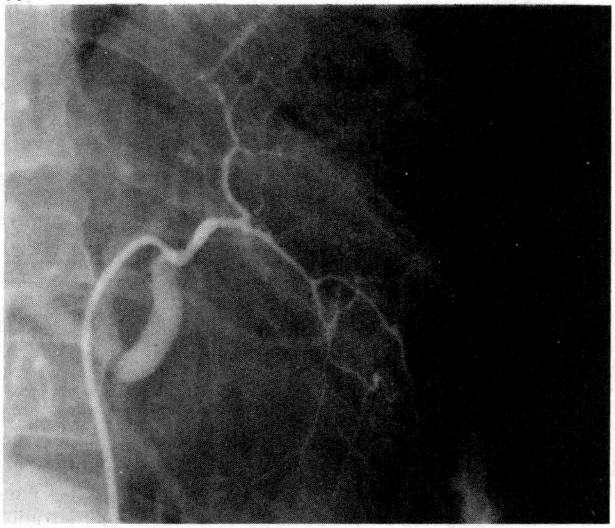

B

REFERENCES

BAUM S et al: Selective mesenteric arterial infusions in the management of massive diverticular hemorrhage. N Engl J Med 288:1269, 1973

CASARELLA WJ et al: "Lower" gastrointestinal tract hemorrhage: New concepts based on arteriography. Am J Roentgenol Radium Ther Nucl Med 121:357, 1974

CONN HO et al: Intraarterial vasopressin in the treatment of upper gastrointestinal hemorrhage; a prospective, controlled clinical trial. Gastroenterology 68:211, 1975

HEDBERG SE: Endoscopy in gastrointestinal bleeding. A systematic approach to diagnosis. Surg Clin North Am 54:549, 1974

MOODY FG: Current concepts: Rectal bleeding. N Engl J Med 290:839, 1974

PALMER ED: Upper gastrointestinal hemorrhage. JAMA 231:853, 1975

43 JAUNDICE AND HEPATOMEGALY

KURT J. ISSELBACHER

JAUNDICE

Jaundice, or *icterus,* refers to the yellow pigmentation of the skin or scleras by bilirubin. This in turn is a result of elevated levels of bilirubin in the bloodstream. Jaundice may be brought to clinical attention by a darkening of the urine or a yellow discoloration of the skin or sclera; the latter often is the site where clinical icterus may first be detected. Scleral pigmentation is attributed to richness of this tissue in elastin, which has a special affinity for bilirubin. Jaundice must be distinguished from other causes of yellow pigmentation such as carotenemia (see Chaps. 57, 86, and 92), which is due to carotenoid pigments in the bloodstream and is associated with a yellowish discoloration of the skin but not of the sclera. Atabrine treatment (see Chap. 215) may produce a yellow color of the skin and urine, but the sclerae are usually only minimally discolored, and when pigment is present, it is seen only in the regions of the sclerae exposed to light.

Normal serum bilirubin concentrations range from 0.5 to 1.0 mg per 100 ml, and normally most of this is unconjugated (see Fig. 43-1). The precise level at which jaundice becomes clinically evident varies, but usually it can be recognized when the total serum bilirubin exceeds 2 to 2.5 mg per 100 ml. Not infrequently in deep jaundice the skin may take on a greenish hue because of the conversion of bilirubin to biliverdin, an oxidation product of bilirubin. Oxidation occurs more readily with conjugated bilirubin, and hence a greenish hue is seen more frequently in conditions with pronounced conjugated hyperbilirubinemia.

Production and metabolism of bilirubin

NORMAL SOURCES OF BILIRUBIN (Fig. 43-2) The greater part of the bilirubin is derived from the catabolism of hemoglobin present in senescent red blood cells. This normally accounts for about 80 to 85 percent of the daily bilirubin production. When a circulating red blood cell reaches the end of its normal life span of approximately 120 days, it is destroyed in the reticuloendothelial system. In the catabolism of hemoglobin, globin is first dissociated from heme, after which the heme moiety is oxidatively cleaved and converted to biliverdin by a microsomal heme oxygenase. This enzyme system requires oxygen and a cofactor, reduced nicotinamide-adenine dinucleotide phosphate (NADPH). Bilirubin is then formed from biliverdin by another enzyme, biliverdin reductase.

About 15 to 20 percent of the bilirubin is derived from sources other than senescent erythrocytes. One source is the *destruction of maturing erythroid cells in the bone marrow,* or so-called "ineffective erythropoiesis" (see Chap. 311). The other is *nonerythroid components,* especially in the liver, and involves the turnover of heme and heme proteins (such as cytochrome, myoglobin, and heme-containing enzymes). These two sources of bilirubin are collectively referred to as the *early labeled fraction,* a term derived from experiments with labeled glycine and delta-aminolevulinic acid (ALA). Thus when labeled glycine is administered to a

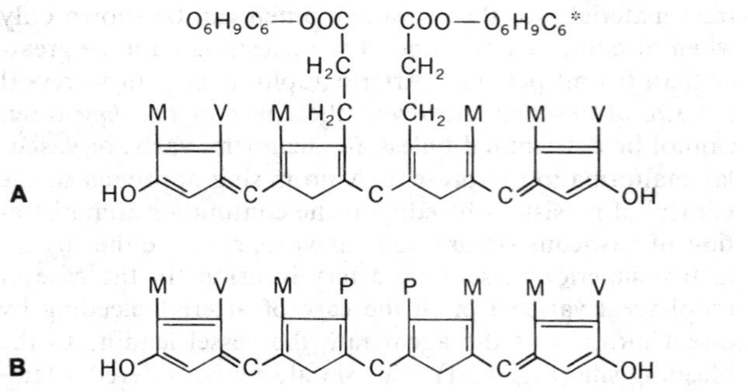

FIGURE 43-1
The chemical structures of conjugated (A) and unconjugated (B) bilirubin. Abbreviations: M = methyl, V = vinyl, P = propionic acid. The asterisk (*) refers to glucuronic acid.

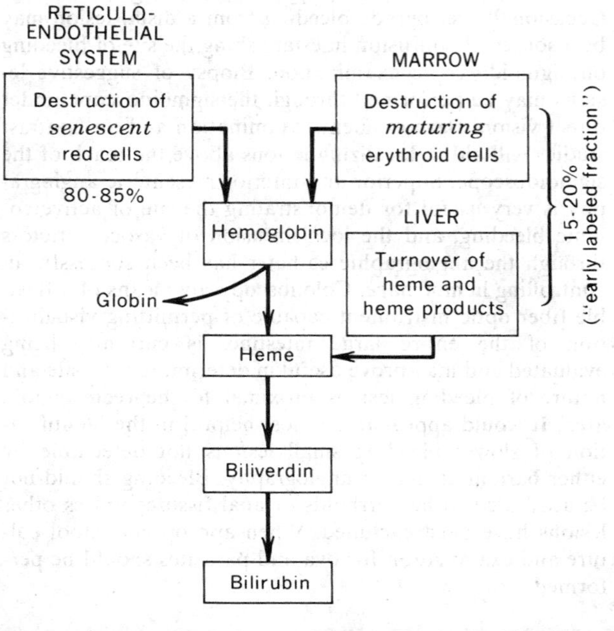

FIGURE 43-2
The sources and precursors of plasma bilirubin.

normal subject, approximately 15 percent of the label appears in stool stercobilinogen in the first 3 to 5 days; 85 percent of the label appears at about 120 days and reflects the bilirubin produced from the normal destruction of senescent red blood cells.

TRANSPORT OF BILIRUBIN Following liberation of bilirubin into the plasma, virtually all the pigment is tightly *bound to albumin.* The maximum binding capacity is 2 moles of bilirubin per mole of albumin. Because in a normal adult this corresponds to plasma unconjugated bilirubin concentrations of 60 to 80 mg per ml, saturation of the binding capacity of the plasma almost never occurs. It is clinically relevant that certain organic anions, such as sulfonamides and salicylates, compete with bilirubin for common binding sites on albumin and may displace bilirubin from albumin, permitting it to enter tissues such as the central nervous system. Most of the evidence for albumin binding has been obtained from studies using unconjugated bilirubin. The conjugated pigment also appears to be bound primarily to albumin, although the binding forces may be different. Some conjugated bilirubin in the plasma is ultrafiltrable.

Bilirubin is found in body fluids (cerebrospinal fluid, joint effusions, cysts, etc.) in proportion to the albumin content of the fluids and is absent from true secretions such as tears, saliva, and pancreatic juice. Scar tissue is rarely bilirubin-stained. The appearance of jaundice is also influenced by blood flow and edema. Paralyzed extremities and edematous areas tend to remain uncolored, and "unilateral" jaundice in patients with hemiplegia and edema may be seen if jaundice develops.

HEPATIC METABOLISM OF BILIRUBIN The liver occupies a central role in the metabolism of the bile pigments. Three distinct phases are recognized: (1) *hepatic uptake,* (2) *conjugation,* and (3) *excretion* into bile. Of these three steps, excretion appears to be the rate-limiting step and the one most susceptible to impairment when the liver cell is damaged.

Uptake Unconjugated bilirubin bound to albumin is presented to the liver cell, and upon entry the pigment and albumin become dissociated. Little is known concerning the uptake phase, but the mechanism is believed to involve the binding of bilirubin to certain cytoplasmic anionic binding proteins referred to as Y and Z proteins or ligandins. Hepatic uptake appears to be reversible.

Conjugation Unconjugated bilirubin is water-insoluble and must be converted to a *water-soluble derivative* in order to be excreted by the liver cell into bile. This is accomplished by the process of conjugation whereby bilirubin is predominantly converted to bilirubin glucuronide (mostly diglucuronide). This reaction occurs in the microsomes or endoplasmic reticulum of the hepatocytes by action of the glucuronyl transferases. The action catalyzed by bilirubin glucuronyl transferase is as follows:

Bilirubin + uridine diphosphate glucuronic acid → bilirubin diglucuronide + uridine diphosphate

As a result of this enzymatic reaction glucuronic acid is attached to the two carboxyl groups of bilirubin (Fig. 43-1). Glucuronyl transferases are also found in kidney and intestine, but the liver is the principal site of conjugated bilirubin formation. The hepatic microsomal glucuronyl transferases are also involved in the formation of glucuronides of other endogenous and exogenous substances (e.g., conjugates of steroids, antibiotics, and salicylates) (see Chap. 296).

The *major* product of conjugation is *bilirubin diglucuronide.* However, bile also contains various amounts of other derivatives, especially glycosidic conjugates with monosaccharides (e.g., glucose, xylose) and disaccharides (e.g., aldobiuronic acid, hexuronosylhexuronic acid). The role of these other conjugates normally and in disease states is unclear.

Excretion or secretion into bile In order for bilirubin to be excreted into bile, *the pigment must be in the conjugated form.* Although the overall process is not well understood, the excretion of conjugated bilirubin into bile appears to be an energy-dependent process and the *rate-limiting* step in the hepatic metabolism of bilirubin. When this step is compromised, two consequences occur: (1) decreased excretion of bilirubin into the bile, and (2) "regurgitation," or reentry of conjugated bilirubin from the liver cells into the bloodstream.

INTESTINAL PHASE OF BILIRUBIN METABOLISM After its appearance in the intestinal lumen, bilirubin glucuronide may be excreted in the stool or metabolized to urobilinogen and related products. Because of its polarity, *conjugated bilirubin is not reabsorbed* by the intestinal mucosa, a mechanism which may serve to rid the body of this pigment.

The formation of urobilinogen from conjugated bilirubin requires the action of bacteria and occurs in the lower part of the small intestine and colon. The bacteria, by stepwise enzymatic reductions, induce the formation of a series of colorless urobilinogens (Fig. 43-3), which react with Ehrlich's aldehyde reagent to produce red aldehyde complexes. Oxidation of the urobilinogens (i.e., *d*-urobilinogen, mesobilirubinogen, and stercobilinogen) leads to colored products, the urobilins. When urobilin is mixed with Schlesinger's solution (zinc acetate in alcohol), zinc complexes are produced which have an intense green fluorescence. Because these compounds are measured together in most quantitative analyses, they usually are referred to collectively as "urobilinogens."

In contrast to conjugated bilirubin, *urobilinogen is reabsorbed* from the small intestine into the portal blood and is thus subject to an enterohepatic circulation. Some urobilinogen is reexcreted by the liver into the bile; the rest is excreted in the urine in an amount usually not exceeding 4 mg daily. When the hepatic excretory mechanism is impaired (e.g., in hepatocellular disease) or the production of bilirubin is greatly increased (e.g., in hemolytic anemia), the urinary urobilinogen may increase significantly.

The normal output of fecal urobilinogen ranges from 50 to 280 mg per day. Under conditions of decreased excretion of conjugated bilirubin into the intestine (e.g., liver disease, bile duct obstruction) or suppression of intestinal flora by antibiotics, fecal output will be diminished. In hemolytic anemia, urinary and fecal urobilinogen excretion is greatly increased.

In a normal person with a blood volume of 5 liters and a hemoglobin concentration of 15 g per 100 ml, the total circulating hemoglobin is 750 g. Because approximately 0.8 percent of the red blood cells are destroyed daily, 6.3 g hemoglobin is released for catabolism. Assuming a quantitative degradation of heme to bilirubin and to urobilinogen, the expected daily output of urobilinogen would be approximately 250 mg plus the additional 15 to 30 mg which would be derived from the other sources described above (i.e., ineffective erythropoiesis, nonhemoglobin heme precursors). Often, however, the amount excreted is considerably less, and it appears likely that there are alternative pathways for hemoglobin degradation not involving bilirubin formation.

RENAL EXCRETION OF BILIRUBIN Normally the urine contains no bilirubin that is detected by the methods usually employed, although traces may be detectable by sensitive spectrophotometric procedures. Unconjugated bilirubin, being tightly bound to albumin, is not filtered by the renal glomeruli, and because there is no tubular secretory process for bilirubin, *unconjugated bilirubin is not excreted in urine.* On the other hand, conjugated bilirubin is less tightly bound to albumin, and a small fraction (about 5 percent) is unbound or associated with low molecular weight proteins or peptides. The non-albumin-bound fraction is dialyzable and is filtered by the renal glomeruli. Thus, in contrast to the unconjugated pigment, a fraction of plasma *conjugated bilirubin appears in the urine.* Bile salts enhance the dialyzability of conjugated bilirubin, and in obstructive jaundice, the elevated level of plasma bile acids may account for an increased renal excretion of conjugated bilirubin. This may also explain why in biliary tract obstruction, serum conjugated bilirubin levels tend to plateau and not to exceed 30 to 40 mg per 100 ml, while with severe hepatocellular injury bilirubin levels higher than this may occur.

Chemical tests for bile pigments

The most widely employed chemical test for the bile pigments in serum is the van den Bergh reaction. In this reaction the bilirubin pigments are diazotized with sulfanilic acid, and the chromogenic products are measured colorimetrically. The van den Bergh reaction can be used to distinguish between unconjugated and conjugated bilirubin because of the different solubility properties of the pigments. When the reaction is carried out in an *aqueous* medium, the water-soluble conjugated bilirubin reacts to give the so-called *direct* van den Bergh reaction. When the reaction is carried out in *methanol,* both conjugated and unconjugated pigments react, giving a measure of the *total* bilirubin level. The total minus the direct-reacting bilirubin give the *indirect* value, which is a measure of the unconjugated bilirubin level.

In the direct van den Bergh reaction, the most accurate measurements are those carried out at 1 min. If the reaction is allowed to proceed longer, a small amount of the unconjugated pigment may begin to react in the aqueous medium. As a result, if the reaction is carried out at 30 min in a patient with unconjugated hyperbilirubinemia, falsely low values for the indirect-reacting bilirubin may be obtained. This serves to emphasize that the direct and indirect van den Bergh reactions represent *approximations* (not absolute measurements) of the conjugated and unconjugated pigments. A summary of the key differences in the properties and reactions of the bilirubin pigments is presented in Table 43-1.

The measurement of bilirubin in the urine may be carried out by the Harrison spot test or with Ictotest[1] tablets. The foam test is also a simple and qualitatively valid procedure. When normal urine is vigorously shaken in a test tube, the foam is absolutely white. In a urine containing bilirubin, the foam will be yellow. This difference may be subtle and may become evident only by comparing a normal urine specimen and one containing bilirubin side by side. Urine urobilinogen may be estimated by the semiquantitative Watson-Schwartz test or the qualitative Diamond test. Fecal measurement must be quantitative to be of value.

Except for concentrated urine, the most common cause of a deep yellow-brown or dark urine is bilirubinuria. However, other mechanisms and diseases associated with a dark urine need to be considered. These include yellow urine due to drugs (e.g., azosulfapyridine); red urine due to porphyria, hemoglobinuria, myoglobinuria, or drugs (e.g., pyridium); and dark-brown or black urine due to homogentisic acid (in ochronosis) or melanin (with melanoma).

APPROACH TO THE PATIENT WITH JAUNDICE

Once jaundice is recognized clinically or chemically, it is important to determine whether it is predominantly due to unconjugated or conjugated hyperbilirubinemia. *A simple clue in this regard is to determine whether bilirubin is present in the urine.* Its absence in the urine suggests unconjugated

[1] *Trademark of Ames Company, Ames, Iowa.*

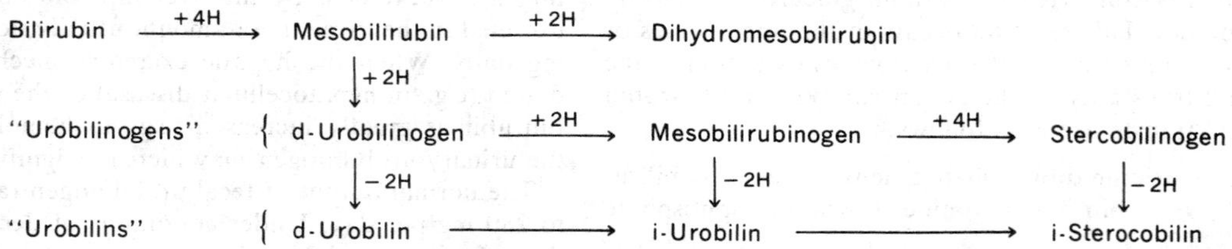

FIGURE 43-3
Chemical steps in the reduction of bilirubin to the urobilinogens and urobilins.

TABLE 43-1
Comparison of the major differences between conjugated and unconjugated bilirubin

Properties and reactions	*Unconjugated*	*Conjugated*
Water solubility	0	+
Affinity for lipids	+	0
Bound to serum albumin	+++	+
Renal excretion	0	+
Van den Bergh reaction	Indirect (total minus direct)	Direct
Lipid membrane permeability	+	0

hyperbilirubinemia (since this pigment is not filtered by the glomerulus); its presence indicates conjugated hyperbilirubinemia. One can then proceed to the direct chemical measurement of the bilirubin pigments in the serum. In predominantly unconjugated hyperbilirubinemia, 80 to 85 percent of the total serum bilirubin is unconjugated (i. e., less than 15 to 20 percent is conjugated). The patient is considered to have predominantly conjugated hyperbilirubinemia when more than 50 percent of the serum bilirubin is of the conjugated type.

An approach to the classification of jaundice based on this important distinction is presented in Table 43-2. Derangements of bilirubin metabolism may occur through any of four mechanisms: (1) overproduction, (2) decreased hepatic uptake, (3) decreased hepatic conjugation, and (4) decreased excretion of bilirubin into bile (due to both intrahepatic and extrahepatic factors). Jaundice may also be described on the basis of the pathogenetic mechanisms or disease processes leading to increased bilirubin levels. Thus, the terms *hemolytic jaundice, hepatocellular jaundice,* and *obstructive* (or cholestatic) *jaundice* are often used.

Though these classifications and terms are helpful, in any one patient more than a single derangement or more than one "type" of jaundice may be present. For example, a patient with cirrhosis may have not only impaired liver cell function (and hence hepatocellular jaundice) but also hemolysis. Furthermore, obstructive jaundice may be due to either *mechanical* obstruction of the biliary radicles or *functional* factors causing impaired hepatic excretion of bilirubin into bile.

In the present chapter a brief description of the major types of jaundice is given. A more detailed discussion of the individual disease entities is found in Chap. 298.

JAUNDICE WITH PREDOMINANTLY UNCONJUGATED BILIRUBIN IN THE SERUM

Overproduction of bilirubin When an increased amount of hemoglobin is released from red blood cells into either the bloodstream or tissues, increased bilirubin production occurs. Hyperbilirubinemia develops when the capacity of the liver to remove the pigment from the circulation is exceeded. In most cases of hemolysis, the total serum bilirubin concentration ranges from 3 to 5 mg per 100 ml. A slight increase in direct-reacting pigment may also be found, but this usually constitutes less than 15 percent of the total serum bilirubin. This finding is probably analogous to the slight elevations of direct-reacting bilirubin which occur when normal subjects are infused with unconjugated bilirubin. Both instances appear to be a reflection of the fact that the rate-limiting step in hepatic bilirubin metabolism is excretion and that when the excretory capacity of the liver is exceeded, some reentry of conjugated bilirubin into the bloodstream occurs. For a detailed description of the causes of increased bilirubin production, see Chap. 298.

Impaired hepatic uptake of bilirubin As indicated previously, the uptake of bilirubin by the liver cell involves dissociation of the pigment from albumin, and presumably binding to certain cytoplasmic proteins (i.e., ligandins). In Gilbert's syndrome and some cases of drug-induced jaundice there may be a derangement in this phase of bilirubin metabolism (see Chap. 298).

Impaired glucuronide conjugation Both acquired and genetic derangements in hepatic glucuronyl transferase occur. In the fetus and at birth, glucuronyl transferase activity is low and appears to account in part for the *neonatal jaundice* normally found between the second and the fifth days of life. There is also a rare hereditary disorder, the Crigler-Najjar syndrome, with either an absence (type I) or a deficiency (type II) of bilirubin glucuronyl transferase leading to pronounced unconjugated hyperbilirubinemia.

Acquired defects in bilirubin glucuronyl transferase activity may be produced by drugs (i.e., enzyme inhibition) or intrinsic liver disease. However, with liver cell damage, the excretory capacity of the liver is impaired to a greater

TABLE 43-2
Classification of jaundice based on underlying derangement of bilirubin metabolism

I Predominantly *unconjugated* hyperbilirubinemia
- *A* Overproduction
  - *1* Hemolysis (intra- and extravascular)
  - *2* Ineffective erythropoiesis
- *B* Impaired hepatic uptake
  - *1* Gilbert's syndrome
  - *2* Drugs (e.g., flavaspidic acid)
  - *3* Prolonged fasting
- *C* Impaired bilirubin conjugation (decreased glucuronyl transferase activity)
  - *1* Hereditary absence or deficiency of transferase (type I and type II Crigler-Najjar syndrome)
  - *2* Gilbert's syndrome
  - *3* "Immaturity" of transferase (neonatal jaundice)
  - *4* Acquired transferase deficiency
    - *a* Drug inhibition (e.g., pregnanediol, chloramphenicol)
    - *b* Hepatocellular disease (hepatitis, cirrhosis)*

II Predominantly *conjugated* hyperbilirubinemia
- *A* Impaired hepatic excretion (intrahepatic defects)
  - *1* Familial or hereditary disorders
    - *a* Dubin-Johnson syndrome; Rotor syndrome
    - *b* Recurrent (benign) intrahepatic cholestasis
    - *c* Cholestatic jaundice of pregnancy
  - *2* Acquired disorders
    - *a* Hepatocellular disease* (e.g., viral or drug-induced hepatitis)
    - *b* Drug-induced cholestasis (e.g., oral contraceptives, methyltestosterone)
- *B* Extrahepatic biliary obstruction (mechanical obstruction, e.g., stones, stricture, tumor of bile duct)

**In hepatocellular disease (hepatitis and cirrhosis) there is usually interference in the three major steps of bilirubin metabolism—uptake, conjugation, and excretion. However, excretion is the rate-limiting step and is usually impaired to the greatest extent. As a result, conjugated hyperbilirubinemia predominates.*

extent than is the conjugating capacity. Therefore in most hepatocellular diseases, the hyperbilirubinemia is predominantly of the conjugated type (see Chap 298).

JAUNDICE WITH PREDOMINANTLY CONJUGATED BILIRUBIN IN THE SERUM Impaired excretion of bilirubin by the liver The impaired excretion of bilirubin into the biliary canaliculi, whether due to functional or mechanical factors, results in predominantly conjugated hyperbilirubinemia and bilirubinuria. The presence of *bilirubin in the urine is evidence of conjugated hyperbilirubinemia* and is a most important point in the differential diagnosis of jaundice. Such findings are identical to those occurring in complete obstruction of the bile duct, emphasizing that *jaundice due to hepatocellular disease can seldom be differentiated from that due to extrahepatic obstruction solely on the basis of changes in bile pigment metabolism.* Indeed there are often instances when the two conditions are not distinguishable by any biochemical criteria, and liver biopsy or other diagnostic procedures are needed for the definitive diagnosis.

When there is interference in the excretion of conjugated bilirubin into bile, by what mechanism does this pigment enter the systemic circulation? Several postulates have been proposed for this "reentry": (1) rupture of the bile canaliculi secondary to the necrosis of the hepatic cells that constitute their walls; (2) occlusion of the canaliculi by inspissated bile or their compression by swollen hepatic cells; (3) obstruction of the terminal intrahepatic bile ducts (cholangioles) by inflammatory cells; (4) altered hepatic cell permeability; and (5) as a result of impaired excretion, accumulation of conjugated bilirubin in the hepatocytes and secondary diffusion into the plasma. Although some of these postulates are speculative, it is likely that several of these mechanisms occur. For example, occasionally in histologic sections, escape of bile through rents in the walls of canaliculi in areas of necrosis is apparent. Also microscopic studies of the liver of rats injected with fluorescent dyes have shown reflux of bile from canaliculi into sinusoids. However, no anatomic damage needs to be invoked, because when unconjugated bilirubin is infused into normal subjects at high rates, conjugated hyperbilirubinemia occurs; this is explained most logically by passive diffusion.

Extrahepatic biliary obstruction Complete obstruction of the extrahepatic bile ducts leads to jaundice with predominantly conjugated hyperbilirubinemia, bilirubinuria, and clay-colored stools. Failure of bile to reach the intestine results in virtual disappearance of urobilinogen from the stool and urine. The concentration of bilirubin rises progressively but then usually plateaus at a level of 30 to 40 mg per 100 ml. To some extent this plateau may be explained by a balance between renal excretion and diversion of bilirubin to other metabolites. In hepatocellular jaundice, such a plateau tends not to occur, and bilirubin levels in excess of 50 mg per 100 ml may be found.

Partial obstruction of the extrahepatic bile ducts can also give rise to jaundice but only if the intrabiliary pressure is increased, because the excretion of bilirubin does not diminish until the intraductile pressure approaches the maximal secretory pressure of approximately 250 mm bile. Jaundice may occur at much lower pressures if the obstruction is complicated by infection of the ducts or hepatocellular injury. Therefore, jaundice, bilirubinuria, and clay-colored stools are inconstant findings in partial biliary obstruction, and the amount of urobilinogen in urine and stool varies with the degree of occlusion.

The functional reserve of the liver is so great that *occlusion of the intrahepatic bile ducts* does not give rise to jaundice unless the drainage of bile from a large segment of the parenchyma is interrupted. Either of the two major hepatic ducts or a large number of secondary radicles may be occluded without production of jaundice. In experimental animals the ducts draining at least 75 percent of the parenchyma must be occluded before jaundice appears.

ADDITIONAL POINTS OF TERMINOLOGY In clinical practice, a patient may be described as having *obstructive,* or *cholestatic,* jaundice. By this is meant that clinically, and especially biochemically, there is little to suggest hepatocellular damage and that the main features point to interference with, or obstruction in, the flow of bile. Typically one would expect such a patient to show (1) predominantly conjugated hyperbilirubinemia, (2) minimal biochemical changes of parenchymal liver damage, and (3) a moderate to a marked increase in the serum alkaline phosphatase level (usually greater than 15 Bodansky units). As emphasized in Chaps. 296 and 297, an *elevated alkaline phosphatase level* in a patient with jaundice or liver disease, in the absence of other disorders such as bone disease, is most suggestive of interference with bile secretion or an infiltrative process in the liver. However, *laboratory tests alone may not permit differentiation of intrahepatic from extrahepatic cholestasis.*

Some clinicians reserve the term obstructive jaundice for those situations in which anatomic obstruction can be demonstrated and use the term cholestatic jaundice for cases of parenchymal liver disease in which the obstructive phase is on a junctional basis. Nevertheless, because these two entities frequently are indistinguishable by clinical and biochemical criteria, the terms obstructive jaundice and cholestatic jaundice are often used interchangeably.

Hepatocellular disorders in which jaundice associated with an obstructive, or cholestatic, phase occurs include (1) occasional cases of viral hepatitis, (2) drug reactions, especially those due to chlorpromazine and methyltestosterone, (3) some cases of alcoholic hepatitis or alcohol-induced fatty liver, (4) jaundice in the last trimester of pregnancy, (5) most cases of Dubin-Johnson or Rotor syndrome, (6) benign recurrent intrahepatic cholestasis, and (7) certain types of postoperative jaundice. These and other conditions are discussed in Chaps. 298 and 299.

In summary, all forms of conjugated hyperbilirubinemia have by definition an impairment in the excretion of bilirubin into bile. In most cases of parenchymal liver disease, a broad derangement is shown by the biochemical tests of liver function. However, when the major detectable alterations of liver function tests include (1) conjugated hyperbilirubinemia and (2) moderate to marked elevation of the serum alkaline phosphatase level, the terms obstructive or cholestatic jaundice may be appropriate. Additional procedures, including operation, are often needed to determine the cause of the cholestasis (see Chaps. 295 and 297).

HEPATOMEGALY

In the supine position, the major part of the liver lies beneath the right rib cage. In some normal persons the liver edge may be palpable 1 to 2 cm below the right costal margin, and a palpable liver edge by itself does not necessarily indicate hepatomegaly. In evaluating liver size by physical examination, two factors other than ability to palpate the liver edge need to be considered, namely, (1) the location of the upper border of liver dullness by percussion, and (2) the body habitus.

Normally, the upper edge of liver dullness on the right side in the midclavicular line is at the level of the fifth rib, but in those of asthenic habitus it may be lower. The liver edge normally descends 1 to 3 cm with deep inspiration. In hypersthenic subjects, the liver may extend over to the left side of the abdominal wall, with the lower edge high and not palpable; in hyposthenic subjects with a very acute costal angle, the liver may lie in the right half of the abdomen, the edge being palpable by as much as 6 to 8 cm below the right costal margin lateral to the right rectus abdominis muscle. Thus, palpability does not necessarily imply hepatomegaly.

In determining liver enlargement by palpation, one should be certain that the liver is being palpated rather than other right upper quadrant masses such as gallbladder, colonic neoplasm, or fecal material in the colon. Liver enlargement is often confirmed by radiologic studies, including hepatic scintiscans, celiac axis angiography, and splenic venography.

In many cases of generalized liver enlargement, the left lobe will be felt in the epigastrium between the xiphoid and umbilicus. The liver should be carefully palpated during deep inspiration to determine whether the edge is tender, regular or irregular, firm or soft, rounded and thickened or sharp. The edge is tender and often rounded with hepatic inflammation, as in hepatitis, or when the liver is acutely congested, as in cardiac decompensation. Pulsation of the liver may be found with tricuspid valvular incompetence. A carcinomatous liver may be rocklike in hardness; the cirrhotic liver is very firm in consistency. The largest livers are often found with carcinoma (primary or metastatic), marked fatty infiltration, congestive cardiac decompensation, Hodgkin's disease, and amyloidosis. Rapid decrease in liver size may occur with improvement of congestive failure, mobilization of fat from the liver, or massive hepatic necrosis.

In a patient with hepatomegaly, auscultation is sometimes helpful. A friction rub may be audible (and palpable) in the right upper quadrant; it is usually due to a recent biopsy, tumor, or perihepatitis. In portal hypertension a venous hum may be audible between the umbilicus and the xiphoid. An arterial murmur or bruit over the liver may indicate tumor, usually hepatoma.

Some of the causes of a palpable liver and hepatomegaly are given in Table 43-3.

TABLE 43-3
Causes of a palpable liver and hepatomegaly

I Palpable liver without hepatomegaly
- *A* Right diaphragm displaced downward (e.g., emphysema, asthma)
- *B* Subdiaphragmatic lesion (e.g., abscess)
- *C* Aberrant lobe of liver (Riedel's lobe)
- *D* Extremely thin or relaxed abdominal muscles
- *E* Occasionally present in normal persons

II Hepatomegaly
- *A* Vascular congestion (e.g., congestive heart failure, hepatic vein thrombosis)
- *B* Bile duct obstruction (e.g., lesion in common duct leading to hepatomegaly and subsequently biliary cirrhosis)
- *C* Infiltrative disorders
  - *1* Bone marrow and reticuloendothelial cells
    - *a* Extramedullary hematopoiesis
    - *b* Leukemia
    - *c* Lymphoma
  - *2* Fat
    - *a* Fatty liver (e.g., secondary to alcohol, diabetes, or toxins)
    - *b* Gaucher's disease and some other lipidoses
  - *3* Glycogen (e.g., diabetes, especially after insulin excess)
  - *4* Amyloid
  - *5* Iron (hemochromatosis and hemosiderosis)
  - *6* Granuloma (tuberculosis, sarcoid)
- *D* Inflammatory disorders
  - *1* Hepatitis—due to drugs or infectious agents
  - *2* Cirrhosis—except in late stages when prolonged scarring may lead to a *small*, shrunken liver
- *E* Tumors—primary or metastatic
- *F* Cysts—polycystic disease, congenital hepatic fibrosis

REFERENCES

ARIAS IM: Inheritable and congenital hyperbilirubinemia. N Engl J Med 285:1416, 1971

BERK PD et al: Unconjugated hyperbilirubinemia: Physiologic evaluation and experimental approaches to therapy. Ann Intern Med 82:552, 1975

BILLING BH, JANSEN FH: Enigma of bilirubin conjugation. Gastroenterology 61:258, 1971

BISSELL DM: Formation and elimination of bilirubin. Gastroenterology 69:519, 1975

CASTELL DO et al: Estimation of liver size by percussion in normal individuals. Ann Intern Med 70:1183, 1969

SCHMID R: Bilirubin metabolism in man. N Engl J Med 287:703, 1972

SHERLOCK S: Jaundice, chap. 10 in *Diseases of the Liver,* 5th ed., Philadelphia: Davis, 1975

THOMPSON RPH, HOFMANN AF: Free and conjugated bile pigments of body fluids: Qualitative analysis by thin layer chromatography. J Lab Clin Med 82:483, 1973

44
ABDOMINAL SWELLING AND ASCITES

ROBERT M. GLICKMAN
KURT J. ISSELBACHER

ABDOMINAL SWELLING Abdominal swelling or distention is a common problem in clinical medicine and may be the initial manifestation of a systemic disease or of otherwise unsuspected abdominal disease. *Subjective* abdominal enlargement, often described as a sensation of fullness or bloating, is usually transient and is often related to a functional gastrointestinal disorder when it is not accompanied by objective physical findings of increased abdominal girth or local swelling. *Obesity* and lumbar lordosis, which may be associated with prominence of the abdomen, may usually be distinguished from true increases in the volume of the peritoneal cavity by history and careful physical examination.

Clinical history Abdominal swelling may first be noticed by the patient because of a progressive increase in belt or clothing size, the appearance of abdominal or inguinal hernias, or the development of a localized swelling. Often, considerable abdominal enlargement has gone unnoticed for weeks or months, either because of coexistent obesity or because the ascites formation has been insidious, without pain or localizing symptoms. Progressive abdominal distention may be associated with a sensation of "pulling" or "stretching" of the flanks or groins and vague low back pain. Localized *pain* usually results from involvement of an abdominal organ (e.g., a passively congested liver, large spleen, or colonic tumor). Pain is uncommon in cirrhosis with ascites and when it is present pancreatitis, hepatoma or peritonitis should be considered. Tense ascites or abdominal tumors may produce increased intraabdominal pressure, resulting in *indigestion* and *heartburn* due to gastroesophageal reflux or *dyspnea, orthopnea,* and *tachypnea* from elevation of the diaphragm. A coexistent pleural effusion, more commonly on the right, presumably due to leakage of ascitic fluid through lymphatic channels in the diaphragm, may also contribute to respiratory embarrassment. The patient with diffuse abdominal swelling should be questioned about increased alcoholic intake, a prior episode of jaundice or hematuria, a change in bowel habits, or a past history of rheumatic heart disease. Such historic information may provide the clues that will lead one to suspect an occult cirrhosis, a colonic tumor with peritoneal seeding, congestive heart failure, or nephrosis.

Physical examination A carefully executed *general physical examination* can yield valuable clues concerning the etiology of abdominal swelling. Thus palmar erythema and spider angiomas suggest an underlying cirrhosis, while supraclavicular adenopathy (Virchow's node) should raise the question of an underlying gastrointestinal malignancy. *Inspection* of the abdomen is an important but often cursorily performed aspect of the abdominal examination. By noting the abdominal contour, one may be able to distinguish localized from generalized swelling. The tensely distended abdomen with tightly stretched skin, bulging flanks, and everted umbilicus is characteristic of ascites. A prominent abdominal venous pattern with the direction of flow away from the umbilicus often is a reflection of portal hypertension; venous collaterals with flow from the lower part of the abdomen toward the umbilicus suggests obstruction of the inferior vena cava; flow downward toward the umbilicus suggests superior vena cava obstruction. "Doming" of the abdomen with visible ridges from underlying intestinal loops is usually due to intestinal obstruction or distention. An epigastric mass, with evident peristalsis proceeding from left to right, usually indicates underlying pyloric obstruction. A liver with metastatic deposits may be visible as a nodular right upper quadrant mass moving with respiration.

Auscultation may reveal the high-pitched, rushing sounds of early intestinal obstruction or a succussion sound due to increased fluid and gas in a dilated hollow viscus. Careful auscultation over an enlarged liver occasionally reveals the harsh bruit of a vascular tumor, especially a hepatoma, or the leathery friction rub of a surface nodule. A venous hum at the umbilicus may signify portal hypertension and an increased collateral blood flow around the liver. A fluid wave and flank dullness which shifts with change in position of the patient are important signs that indicate the presence of peritoneal fluid. In the obese patient, small amounts of fluid may be difficult to demonstrate; on occasion the fluid may be detected by abdominal percussion with the patient on his hands and knees. Doubt about the presence of peritoneal fluid may be resolved by careful paracentesis with a small-gage (No. 19 or 20) needle. Careful percussion should serve to distinguish generalized abdominal enlargement from localized swelling due to an enlarged uterus, ovarian cyst, or distended bladder. Percussion can also outline an abnormally small or large liver. Loss of normal liver dullness may result from massive hepatic necrosis; it may also be a clue to free gas in the peritoneal cavity, as from perforation of a hollow viscus.

Palpation is often difficult with massive ascites, and ballottement of overlying fluid may be the only method of palpating the liver or spleen. A slightly enlarged spleen in association with ascites may be the only evidence of an occult cirrhosis. When there is evidence of portal hypertension, a soft liver suggests that obstruction to portal flow is extrahepatic; a firm liver suggests cirrhosis as the likely cause of the portal hypertension. A very hard or nodular liver is a clue that the liver is infiltrated with tumor, and when accompanied by ascites, it suggests that the latter is due to peritoneal seeding. A pulsatile liver and ascites may be found in tricuspid insufficiency.

An attempt should be made to determine whether a mass is solid or cystic, smooth or irregular, and whether it moves with respiration. The liver, spleen, and gallbladder should descend with respiration unless they are fixed by adhesions or extension of tumor beyond the organ. A fixed mass not descending with respiration may indicate that it is retroperitoneal. Tenderness, especially if localized, may indicate an inflammatory process such as an abscess; it may also be due to stretching of the visceral peritoneum or tumor necrosis. Rectal and pelvic examinations are mandatory; they may reveal otherwise undetected masses due to tumor or infection.

Radiographic and laboratory examinations are essential for confirming or extending the impressions gained on physical examination. Upright and recumbent films of the abdomen may demonstrate the dilated loops of intestine with fluid levels characteristic of intestinal obstruction or the diffuse abdominal haziness and loss of psoas margins suggestive of ascites. A plain film of the abdomen may reveal the distended colon of otherwise unsuspected ulcerative colitis and give valuable information as to the size of the liver and spleen. An irregular and elevated right side of the diaphragm may be a clue to a liver abscess or hepatoma. Studies of the gastrointestinal tract with barium or other contrast media are usually necessary in the search for a primary tumor.

ASCITES In most cases the clinical and laboratory evaluation of the patient with ascites is sufficient to reveal the cause of the fluid accumulation. Often the ascites is a component or complication of cirrhosis, congestive heart failure, nephrosis, or disseminated carcinomatosis. However, even when the cause of ascites seems obvious, it is often important to determine whether another separate or related disease process has supervened. For example, when the patient with compensated cirrhosis and minimal ascites develops progressive ascites that is increasingly difficult to control with sodium restriction or diuretics, the obvious temptation is to attribute the worsening of the clinical picture to progressive liver disease. However, an occult hepatoma, portal vein thrombosis, or even tuberculosis may be responsible for the decompensation. The disappointingly low success of diagnosing tuberculous peritonitis or hepatoma in the patient with cirrhosis and ascites reflects the too-low index of suspicion for the development of such superimposed conditions. Similarly, the patient with congestive heart failure may develop ascites from a disseminated carcinoma with peritoneal seeding. The thorough evaluation of each patient with ascites, even in the presence of an "obvious" cause, will help avoid these errors.

Diagnostic paracentesis (50 to 100 ml) should be part of the routine evaluation of the patient with ascites. The fluid should be examined for its gross appearance, protein content, cell count, and differential cell count, as well as Gram's and acid-fast stains and culture. Cytologic and cell-block examination may disclose an otherwise unsuspected carcinoma. Table 44-1 presents some of the features of ascitic fluid typically found in various disease states. In some disorders, such as cirrhosis, the fluid has the characteristics of a transudate (less than 2.5 g protein per 100 ml and a specific gravity less than 1.016); in others, such as peritonitis, the features are those of an exudate. Although there is variability of the ascitic fluid in any given disease state, some features are sufficiently characteristic to suggest certain diagnostic possibilities. For example, blood-stained fluid with more than 2.5 g protein per 100 ml is unusual in uncomplicated cirrhosis but is consistent with tuberculous peritonitis or neoplasm. Cloudy fluid with a predominance of polymorphonuclear cells, and positive Gram's stain is characteristic of bacterial peritonitis; if the cells are mostly lymphocytes, tuberculosis should be suspected. The complete examination of each fluid is most important, for occasionally only *one* finding may be abnormal. For example, if the fluid is a typical transudate but contains more than 250 white blood cells per mm³, the finding should be recognized as atypical for cirrhosis, nephrosis, or congestive heart failure and should warrant a search for tumor or infection.

Chylous ascites refers to a turbid, milky, or creamy peritoneal fluid due to the presence of thoracic or intestinal lymph. Such a fluid shows Sudan-staining fat globules microscopically, and an increased triglyceride content by chemical examination. A turbid fluid due to leukocytes or tumor cells may be confused with chylous fluid, and it is often helpful to carry out alkalinization and ether extraction of the specimen. Alkali will tend to dissolve cellular proteins and thereby reduce turbidity; ether extraction will lead to clearing if the turbidity of the fluid is due to lipid. Chylous ascites is most often the result of lymphatic ob-

TABLE 44-1
Ascitic fluid characteristics in various disease states

Condition	Gross appearance	Specific gravity	Protein, g/100 ml	Cell count: Red blood cells, >10,000/mm³	Cell count: White blood cells, mm³	Other tests
Cirrhosis	Straw-colored or bile-stained	<1.016 (95%)*	<2.5 (95%)*	1%	<250 (90%)*; predominantly endothelial	
Neoplasm	Straw-colored, hemorrhagic, mucinous, or chylous	Variable, >1.016 (45%)	>2.5 (75%)	20%	>1,000 (50%); variable cell types	Cytology, cell block, peritoneal biopsy
Tuberculous peritonitis	Clear, turbid, hemorrhagic, chylous	Variable, >1.016 (50%)	>2.5 (50%)	7%	>1,000 (70%); usually >70% lymphocytes	Peritoneal biopsy, stain and culture for acid-fast bacilli
Pyogenic peritonitis	Turbid or purulent	If purulent, >1.016	If purulent, >2.5	Unusual	Predominantly polymorphonuclear leukocytes	+Gram's stain, culture
Congestive heart failure	Straw-colored	Variable, <1.016 (60%)	Variable 1.5–5.3	10%	<1,000 (90%); usually mesothelial, mononuclear	
Nephrosis	Straw-colored or chylous	<1.016	<2.5(100%)	Unusual	<250; mesothelial, mononuclear	If chylous, ether extraction, Sudan staining
Pancreatitis, pseudocyst	Turbid, hemorrhagic, or chylous	Variable, often >1.016	Variable, often >2.5	Variable, may be blood stained	Variable	Increased amylase in ascitic fluid and serum

* *Since the conditions of examining fluid and selecting patients were not identical in each series, the percentage figures (in the parentheses) should be taken as an indication of the order of magnitude rather than as the precise incidence of any abnormal finding.*

SOURCE: *The data in this table are a composite of those from several large series (see the first five references at the end of the chapter).*

struction from trauma, tumor, tuberculosis, filariasis (see Chap. 224), or congenital abnormalities. It may also be seen in the nephrotic syndrome.

Rarely, ascitic fluid may be *mucinous* in character, suggesting either pseudomyxoma peritonei (Chap. 294) or rarely a colloid carcinoma of the stomach or colon with peritoneal implants.

On rare occasions a syndrome may be seen of fever and ascites, without infection, occurring several weeks after abdominal surgery. This seems to result from starch (from surgical gloves) introduced into the peritoneum at the time of surgery, with a subsequent foreign-body reaction and ascites formation. Given the proper index of suspicion, diagnosis can be made by paracentesis and finding double refractile particles (i.e., starch) when polarized light is used (Fig. 44-1).

The etiology of ascites may remain uncertain even after the usual diagnostic procedures have been carried out. Under those circumstances a high proportion of the cases will be due to (1) cirrhosis of the liver, (2) carcinomatosis with peritoneal involvement, (3) tuberculous peritonitis, or (4) hepatoma. In all these conditions pronounced weight loss, wasting, anorexia, and fever may be found, and hepatomegaly, splenomegaly, and deranged liver function tests may be present. Procedures such as peritoneal biopsy (Fig. 44-2), peritoneoscopy, liver biopsy, splenoportography, or laparotomy may be necessary to provide the diagnosis. Other less common causes of ascites include constrictive pericarditis, hepatic vein obstruction, myxedema and benign tumors of the ovary, particularly fibroma (Meigs' syndrome, with ascites and hydrothorax). The physiologic and metabolic factors involved in the production of ascites are described in Chap. 301.

FIGURE 44-1
Starch peritonitis. Examination of ascitic fluid under polarized light reveals doubly refractile starch granules.

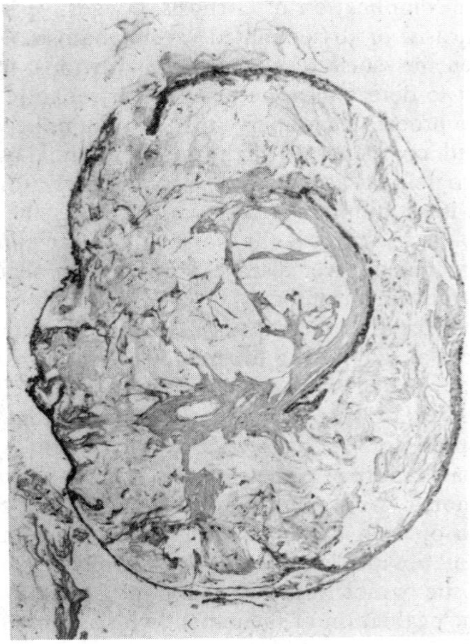

FIGURE 44-2
Peritoneal biopsy of mucinous metastatic ovarian carcinoma. Small nests of tumor cells are visible beneath the peritoneal surface in a mucinous matrix.

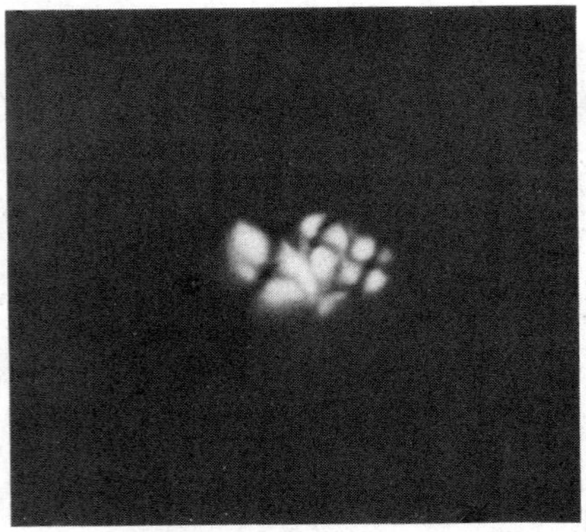

REFERENCES

BERNER C et al: Diagnostic probabilities in patients with conspicuous ascites. Arch Intern Med 113:687, 1964

BORHANMANESH F et al: Tuberculous peritonitis: Prospective study of 32 cases in Iran. Ann Intern Med 76:567, 1972

CODER DM, OLANDER GA: Granulomatous peritonitis caused by starch glove powder. Arch Surg 105:83, 1972

LEVINE H: Needle biopsy of the peritoneum in exudative ascites. Arch Intern Med 120:542, 1967

MALAGELADA JR et al: Origin of fat in chylous ascites of patients with liver cirrhosis. Gastroenterology 67:878, 1974

WARSHAW AL: Diagnosis of starch peritonitis by paracentesis. Lancet 2:1054, 1972

section 6 | Alterations in body weight

45
LOSS OF WEIGHT

(See also Chap. 40)

GEORGE W. THORN

Weight loss, as revealed by history or detected by physical examination, constitutes a cardinal manifestation of disease or disordered bodily function, unless an otherwise normal individual has imposed on himself caloric restriction in an effort to reduce.

Under normal circumstances decreased food intake or total starvation initiates a constellation of metabolic changes designed to reduce energy expenditure and heat loss. Chief among these are reduced basal metabolic rate, lowered body temperature, restricted physical activity, and reduced peripheral blood flow (vasoconstriction). By these means the body attempts to maintain the function of vital organs such as the heart, brain, kidneys, liver, and lungs. These mechanisms are seriously impaired when complications such as fever, vomiting, diarrhea, or dehydration supervene.

Anorexia is a frequent accompaniment of chronic as well as acute disease processes. In the absence of specific abnormalities of gastrointestinal function, loss of appetite may be due to toxic products liberated by microorganisms, by breakdown products of tumor tissue, or by retention of metabolic end products as occurs in late-stage renal and hepatic disease. Hypoosmolality of the body fluid compartment and increased cell water content may give rise to centrally mediated nausea and vomiting through its effect on specific hypothalamic centers. Thus, a patient with malignant hypertension may experience nausea as a consequence of hypertensive cerebrovascular changes in the absence of uremia or, later, as a result of retention of nitrogenous products with progressive renal failure.

In an evaluation of the implication of weight loss, several considerations deserve special attention.

1 Is the patient's history concerning the magnitude and duration of weight loss reliable? Can it be documented by comparison with prior measurements or confirmed by physical examination?
2 Has there been a notable change in appetite or food intake?
3 Has there been evidence of disordered gastrointestinal function with a change in bowel habits?
4 Has there been evidence of polyuria, particularly nocturia?

The determination of the *magnitude of weight loss* is not always easy. Some patients follow changes in weight regularly on bathroom scales or weighing machines, or they have serial physical examinations. Other patients may be vague or uninformed regarding actual changes in weight. Questions regarding a change in waist measurement or collar, suit, dress, or shoe size may provide helpful clues. Physical examination should then confirm this, with its opportunity to detect adipose tissue loss and the presence or absence of edema or dehydration. Special consideration should be given to the valuation of overall weight loss in the presence of edema, as the actual tissue loss in such patients will, of course, greatly exceed the apparent decrease in total body weight.

Weight loss with anorexia and decreased food intake occurs in such a diversified range of acute and chronic diseases as not to be particularly helpful in differential diagnosis. The magnitude of weight loss may reflect either the *seriousness* or the *duration* of the underlying disorder. Thought should be given to the diagnosis of psychologic difficulties such as depression and anorexia nervosa, to generalized endocrine and metabolic disorders such as pituitary-adrenal insufficiency and hyperparathyroidism,

TABLE 45-1
Approach to the patient with weight loss

Appetite normal or increased	*Appetite decreased*
1 Increased caloric utilization *a* Hyperthyroidism *b* Anxiety *c* Drugs—thyroid, amphetamines	*1* Predominantly psychologic *a* Depression* *b* Anorexia nervosa
2 Decreased intestinal absorption *a* Hypermotility, carcinoid *b* Sprue, pancreatic deficiency, and enteropathy	*2* Primarily gastrointestinal *a* Decreased absorption *b* Sprue, enteropathy, etc. *c* Obstruction: neoplasm, adhesions *d* Hepatobiliary disease
3 Abnormal loss *a* Diabetes mellitus (glucosuria) *b* Fistulas *c* Intestinal parasites	*3* Systemic disturbances *a* Malignancy *b* Infection *c* Uremia *d* Cardiovascular disease *e* Endocrine-metabolic *(1)* Adrenal insufficiency *(2)* Hypercalcemia *(3)* Hypokalemia *f* Intoxications: lead, alcohol *g* Hematologic disorders *(1)* Myelofibrosis *(2)* Leukemia

* *Depression with reduced food intake occurs frequently in the elderly, with or without concomitant serious organic diseases. Depression is manifested by one or more of the following changes: (1) Sadness, tendency to cry; (2) loss of interest in work; (3) giving up friends; (4) loss of libido; (5) hypochondriasis.*

and to hepatic and renal disease, as well as to chronic infection, neoplasm, and drug intoxication. Weight loss without a significant change in food consumption would suggest hypermetabolic states, such as thyrotoxicosis and anxiety or gastrointestinal hypermotility.

Of course, particular attention will be given in the history to any abnormality in gastrointestinal function as a cause of weight loss. Here again, one is concerned with *decreased food intake* such as might occur in partial intestinal obstruction; *decreased absorption,* which suggests pancreatic or hepatic disease, spruelike syndromes, regional enteritis, or severe food allergies; or *increased loss of food and fluids* through vomiting, diarrhea, or draining fistulas. Disorders of gastrointestinal function accompany systemic disorders so frequently that the physician must always maintain a high index of suspicion that what appears to be primarily a disorder of gastrointestinal function may actually reflect deep-seated infection, tumor, or renal, hepatic, cardiac, or pulmonary disease. On the other hand, *specific gastrointestinal disorders* may complicate systemic disease; thus, the patient with nausea, vomiting, and renal azotemia may have an associated peptic ulcer.

The presence of polyuria, particularly nocturia, in association with anorexia and weight loss suggests diabetes mellitus, diabetes insipidus, chronic renal disease, and disorders giving rise to *hypercalcemia* or *hypokalemia.*

Physicians should encourage patients to weigh regularly and to maintain a lifelong record of changes in body weight, since alterations in weight so frequently mirror abnormalities in bodily function. Loss of weight may be the first indication of serious organic disease or psychologic disorder, the detection and understanding of which may be measurably enhanced by carefully recorded changes in body weight.

46
GAIN IN WEIGHT. OBESITY

GEORGE W. THORN
GEORGE F. CAHILL, JR.

GENERAL CONSIDERATIONS In the adult an increase in body weight may reflect an increase in adipose tissue, an accumulation of fluid (edema), or both. Weight gain in excess of 1 kg per day almost invariably implies excess fluid retention. A useful indication of excessive fluid retention can be derived from differences in body weight measured in the morning and again in the evening. Normally the evening weight rarely exceeds the morning weight by more than 1 kg unless the patient is retaining excessive fluid. With a weight gain of 1 kg or less during the day the patient will return to his usual weight the following morning. With a gain of more than 1.5 kg he is likely to demonstrate a gain in weight and, ultimately, edema if the condition persists. The increased fluid retention may reflect increased salt and fluid intake (diet), decreased sodium and water excretion (cardiovascular, renal, or hepatic disease), or both. Excess gain in body weight, as measured by differences in morning and evening weight, often provides subtle or early evidence of organic disease. Dietary indiscretions, licorice, and medications, including steroid hormones, may also be responsible. Obese patients can sequester substantial quantities of excessive fluid without necessarily exhibiting edema. This fact can be readily demonstrated by noting the striking response to a diuretic agent, a method of exploitation often utilized by "lose-weight-fast" schemes.

CYCLIC EDEMA

Idiopathic edema, or *"cyclic edema,"* is a syndrome which occurs predominantly in females and is characterized by periodic swelling in the absence of demonstrable organic disease. For a discussion of this syndrome, see Chap. 32.

OBESITY

Obesity constitutes the single most prevalent metabolic disorder in countries or cultures where food supply is abundant. It occurs when the caloric intake exceeds the energy requirement of the body for physical activity and growth. As a result there is an accumulation of fat, which is stored as adipose tissue (see Chap. 68). The excessive adipose tissue may be distributed generally over the body, or it may be localized. The factors controlling the location of adipose tissue are not all known, but pituitary, thyroid, adrenal, and sex hormones play an important role. In the female, excessive adipose tissue is distributed predominantly in the lower part of the trunk and extremities; in the male it is frequently more pronounced in the upper part of the trunk, often sparing the extremities.

For the most part, obesity is preventable. Unfortunately, although the prescription for its cure is uniquely simple, the successful application of the treatment for prolonged periods or a lifetime is most difficult. Hence, relapse with return to the obese status is the rule rather than the exception.

For the elderly, a combination of factors, such as a progressive fall in basal metabolic rate, which accompanies the aging process, and a lessened degree of physical activity with sustained enjoyment of food, sets the stage for increased body weight unless caloric intake is appropriately reduced. The association of obesity with serious disorders such as hypertension, diabetes mellitus, cardiovascular disease, and pulmonary insufficiency should stimulate physicians to do everything in their power to acquaint patients with these facts and to be willing to encourage and *supervise* a long-term, rational approach to the problem.

The amount of body fat can be estimated from whole-body specific gravimetric determinations or from measurement of the thickness of subcutaneous fat folds with skinfold calipers (Montoye et al, 1965). Body fat content can also be determined indirectly from a calculation of lean body mass (radioactive potassium technique). The most practical method, however, uses standard weight-height tables (Table 46-1). The weights recorded in these tables are those associated with the lowest mortality rates as derived from life insurance company data. These data, in which the ideal weight approximates that at age twenty-five, indicate quite clearly that increasing weight during adult life is associated with increased mortality rate. A person is considered overweight if he exceeds the upper range of ideal weight for his body frame. He is considered obese if his weight exceeds by 9 to 10 kg his ideal weight.

ETIOLOGY Hypothalamic relationships It has been shown for years that lesions involving the hypothalamus may lead to obesity. Lesions in the ventromedial nucleus of the hypothalamus induce hyperphagia and obesity, whereas lesions in the lateral hypothalamic area lead to a cessation of eating. On the basis of these findings, a dual mechanism has been postulated for the regulation of food intake: a "satiety" center in the ventromedial nucleus and a "feeding" center in the lateral hypothalamic area. Studies on gold thioglucose-treated mice have demonstrated fiber connections between these two centers. Additional experimental studies suggest that the control of food intake may be mediated by a "glucostat," "lipostat," or "aminostat." It appears that the basic cause of obesity is a derangement of the appetite-controlling mechanisms, permitting the assimilation of more food than is needed.

It has been claimed that certain persons are more efficient than others in their ability to digest, absorb, and utilize food and that they therefore become obese at lower caloric intakes than might be expected. Extensive balance studies on such patients have never substantiated this explanation; at equivalent levels of physical activity and basal metabolism, there seems to be little variation in the required caloric intake. Another consideration concerns the possibility that those patients predisposed to obesity may have been born with more fat cells than the less obese person. Direct determination of adipose cell size by biopsy and subsequent measurement of the isolated cells by techniques developed by Hirsch have permitted calculation of the total fat cell number in the body. The average nonobese adult has approximately 4×10^{10} adipose cells. Individuals who develop obesity in midlife ("middle-aged spread") develop larger fat cells, whereas those who develop obesity through the formative years increase fat cell numbers as well as fat cell size, and their obesity is therefore both hyperplastic and hypertrophic. This potential of forming new fat cells during growth in the presence of overnutrition places emphasis on prevention in childhood. Most studies have shown weight loss in both types of obesity to be associated with a reduction in cell size and no loss of fat cells. The prognosis for successful weight loss and maintenance of the loss in individuals who had been grossly obese through childhood is even poorer than for those developing obesity in midlife, perhaps because of a physiologic hunger drive mediated by the relative paucity of fat per fat cell.

TABLE 46-1
Desirable weight, in pounds, for adults age twenty-five and over (indoor clothing)

Height (in shoes)		*Small frame*	*Medium frame*	*Large frame*
MEN				
5 ft.	2 in.	112–120	118–129	126–141
5	3	115–123	121–133	129–144
5	4	118–126	124–136	132–148
5	5	121–129	127–139	135–152
5	6	124–133	130–143	138–156
5	7	128–137	134–147	142–161
5	8	132–141	138–152	147–166
5	9	136–145	142–156	151–170
5	10	140–150	146–160	155–174
5	11	144–154	150–165	159–179
6		148–158	154–170	164–184
6	1	152–162	158–175	168–189
6	2	156–167	162–180	173–194
6	3	160–171	167–185	178–199
6	4	164–175	172–190	182–204
WOMEN				
4 ft.	10 in.	92–98	96–107	104–119
4	11	94–101	98–110	106–122
5		96–104	101–113	109–125
5	1	99–107	104–116	112–128
5	2	102–110	107–119	115–131
5	3	105–113	110–122	118–134
5	4	108–116	113–126	121–138
5	5	111–119	116–130	125–142
5	6	114–123	120–135	129–146
5	7	118–127	124–139	133–150
5	8	122–131	128–143	137–154
5	9	126–135	132–147	141–158
5	10	130–140	136–151	145–163
5	11	134–144	140–155	149–168
6		138–148	144–159	153–173

HORMONAL ALTERATIONS Anterior pituitary deficiency Anterior pituitary deficiency of a mild degree (Sheehan's syndrome, see Chap. 90) may be accompanied by weight gain. This syndrome, most frequently observed in women after childbirth, is characterized by oligomenorrhea, loss of axillary and pubic hair, secondary hypothyroidism, and adrenal cortical deficiency *without increased pigmentation.*

Hypothyroidism Obesity due to inadequate thyroid hormone may be suspected in a patient who has developed intolerance to cold, whose skin has become dry and coarse, and whose reflexes are prolonged (see Chap. 92). Weight gain associated with a more severe degree of hypothyroidism or myxedema may be due to edema, ascites, and pleural effusion. Gordon and his colleagues believe that some obese patients have a specific block in the utilization of fatty acids by peripheral tissues that can be modified by administration of triiodothyronine, but this observation has not been sustained by other investigators.

Cushing's syndrome Patients exhibit the characteristic "buffalo hump," rounded facies, and truncal obesity with sparing of the extremities (see Chap. 93).

Diabetes mellitus Obesity is both a common accompaniment of and a predisposing factor to the development of diabetes mellitus. As the disease progresses in severity, with glucosuria and ketonuria, weight loss occurs despite an increased appetite. Hypoglycemic manifestations developing 4 to 5 h after meals are characteristic of the so-called "paradoxic" response (see Chap. 95).

Hyperinsulinism Obesity results from excessive food intake secondary to the hypoglycemia induced by primary excessive insulin secretion. The hypoglycemia occurs under fasting conditions, in contrast to "reactive hyperglycemia," which characteristically develops 1 to 2 h after a high carbohydrate intake. The latter also may lead to obesity as the symptoms lead to further excessive food intake (see Chap. 97).

Gonadal deficiency Primary gonadal deficiency appears to predispose to obesity in both males and females. The frequent association of obesity with the menopause and with the eunuchoid state is well documented and suggests a relationship to gonadal deficiency, although psychologic factors may well be an additional factor. It is also well known that the obesity of adolescent children disappears with puberty and that at this time the adult adipose tissue distribution takes place.

FAMILIAL AND CULTURAL EATING HABITS These habits are firmly implanted at an early age. In groups which place great emphasis on food, there is a tendency to overeat. Sometimes the cultural pattern equates success with obesity (witness the common caricature of the obese banker) and encourages the ambitious person to achieve a comfortable corpulence. Moreover, when activity patterns change, eating habits may remain constant, so that the man who has previously been physically active may fail to reduce his caloric intake when he suddenly changes to a sedentary occupation. This tendency may be reinforced by the gradual decline of metabolic rate and of muscular activity which ordinarily accompanies aging.

PSYCHOLOGIC FACTORS Certain persons may have increased appetite for psychologic reasons. Under these circumstances food is used as a substitute for the satisfaction that ordinarily would be derived from other sources. In this respect, these persons resemble the alcoholic, who uses alcohol as a substitute for normal sources of satisfaction, such as friends, family, or success in work. Increased food intake may also be a manifestation of depression or anxiety, and the resulting obesity may aggravate the tendency toward isolation or the ineffectiveness of performance. Reduction of food intake under these circumstances, without recognition and treatment of the underlying emotional disturbance, is usually unsuccessful if not hazardous. Psychologic studies have shown that obese persons eat more as a response to external cues, such as the taste of the food or the environment in which it is served, whereas nonobese individuals eat as a response to as-yet-unidentified "hunger" cues arising from within. Also, obese subjects, once they start eating, continue to do so until either the food is gone or their stomachs are uncomfortably distended. Nonobese subjects more frequently leave food on their plate and stop eating because they have lost their hunger. Again, the analogy with the alcoholic is striking.

THERAPEUTIC CONSIDERATIONS

It is axiomatic that weight reduction, other than that resulting from fluid loss, requires that the caloric intake be less than that utilized. Rapid weight-losing schemes exploit the use of diuretics and dehydration programs which may prove unhealthy as well as illusory. It is essential for patients to appreciate that any program which results in weight loss of more than 0.3 kg per day undoubtedly represents to a considerable extent loss of fluid rather than of tissue. It is also important for a patient to realize that from time to time during the diet program he might gain 0.5 to 1.0 kg as a consequence of cyclic retention of salt and water. This phenomenon may be exaggerated in women at or about the time of ovulation or menstruation. It is also obvious that increased physical activity will assist overall weight loss and that specially designed exercise programs may facilitate the redistribution of adipose tissue.

DIET There is little evidence to support the contention that diets of equivalent caloric value but with differing ratios of carbohydrate, fat, or protein exhibit markedly different weight-reducing potential. Diets relatively high in protein do increase satiety, increase specific dynamic action, and minimize fluctuation in blood glucose level. For long-term weight reduction and maintenance of ideal weight *a diet of modest caloric reduction* has been found more acceptable for most patients. There are patients, however, whose social obligations or temperament require more drastic measures—at least for short periods of time. For such individuals, a "fast" day may be prescribed on a weekly basis. On this day the patient rigidly restricts his diet to 100 to 200 kcal (e.g., clear liquids, tea or coffee without cream or sugar, bouillon, low-calorie carbonated beverages, or skim milk if needed). Or a diet of 800 kcal may be prescribed until sufficient weight reduction has been accomplished, and then the patient may be tested on a diet of 1200, 1500, or 1800 kcal for maintenance (Table 46-2). Prolonged periods of almost total starvation, though providing a very effective means of weight reduction, should be carried out only under strict medical supervi-

TABLE 46-2
Three suggested diets for weight reduction

600 kcal	*1200 kcal*	*2400 kcal*
BREAKFAST		
150 kcal	275 kcal	675 kcal
1/2 grapefruit	1/2 grapefruit	1/2 grapefruit
1 slice bread	1 slice bread	2 slices bread
1/2 cup skim milk	1/2 cup skim milk	1/2 cup milk
	1 egg	1 egg
	1 tsp butter	2 tsps butter
		1 1/2 cups dry cereal
		2 tsps sugar
		jelly
LUNCH		
215 kcal	350 kcal	800 kcal
1/4 cup cottage cheese	2 oz lean meat	4-in. chicken pie
1 slice bread	2 slices bread	1 slice bread
1 apple	1 apple	1/2 cup salad
	1 tsp mayonnaise	2 tsps butter
		3 oz ice cream
DINNER		
235 kcal	575 kcal	925 kcal
2 oz lean meat	4 oz lean meat	3-in. hamburger
1/2 tomato	1/2 cup peas	1/2 cup beans
1/2 cup spinach	1/2 cup potato	1/2 cup potato
1 orange	1 tsp butter	2 tsps butter
	1 cup skim milk	1 roll
	1 cup salad with diet dressing	1 cup coleslaw
		1 slice pie

sion; almost without exception they have proved *ineffective* in the long run in terms of maintaining ideal weight.

Significant reduction in dietary fat will, in many patients, lead to constipation. This will be minimized to some extent by the increased intake of fruit and bulky vegetables, but patients may require supplementary medication such as dioctyl sodium sulfosuccinate (Colace), 100 mg once or twice daily, or liquid petrolatum.

The identification of "chemical diabetes" by means of a glucose tolerance test provides a tremendous incentive for patients to attain their ideal weight. This is also true for patients with cardiovascular disease or those with skeletal disorders which involve the spine, hip, knees, ankles, and feet. Also the value of weight reduction as a means of reducing the level of blood lipids should be emphasized.

Group therapy offers a realistic opportunity for long-term reinforcement of a dietary program. Of the various types of approaches, "behavior modification" appears to have been the most successful. Certainly this approach, which has been publicized by R. B. Stuart in 1967 and by Penick et al in 1971, yielded results far superior to those in a comparably selected group who received classical supportive psychotherapy. The behavioral type of program involves four general principles:

1 Description of the behavior to be controlled. This is essentially a carefully notated record of when, where, and how food is ingested.
2 Modification and control of the discriminatory stimuli governing eating.
3 Development of techniques which control eating.
4 Prompt reinforcement of behavior which delays or controls eating.

It appears that the organization and effective supervision of a program such as this can be carried out by a team with modest psychiatric training.

Patients should understand thoroughly when they undertake a reduction diet that, in all probability, some degree of dietary restriction or discretion will be necessary permanently after ideal weight (Table 46-1) *has been attained.* The desirability of determining body weight each morning should be strongly emphasized and the diet for the day adjusted accordingly. It will be helpful if from time to time the physician or the dietitian reviews the comparative caloric content of foods and alcoholic beverages. Once ideal weight has been attained, a patient should be encouraged to visit his physician every 3 to 6 months. At this time, levels of blood sugar, cholesterol, fatty acids, uric acid, etc., can be checked. Continued interest on the part of the physician is essential for success in this important area of preventive medicine.

TABLE 46-3
Some 200 kcal "snacks" and types of exercise required to "burn" 200 kcal

Snacks (200 kcal)	*Exercise equivalent (200 kcal)*
2 apples	Running 12 min
2 tbsp butter	Swimming 30 min
2 slices bread	Walking 1 h
53 peanuts	Singing 3 h
18 marshmallows	Dishwashing 4 h
24 oz beer	Sitting in front of television 14 h
1 martini	
3 eggs	

EXERCISE (See Chap. 68) Exercise has been endorsed as a method to increase caloric loss. Since body fat has no other way to be eliminated than by oxidation to CO_2, exercise should expedite weight reduction during any hypocaloric regimen. Unfortunately, it is very difficult to induce obese subjects to exercise, particularly for any length of time. Table 46-3 lists the exercise needed to eliminate an extra 200 kcal. It is obvious, therefore, that exercise, although excellent for the circulation and for the psyche, is very minimal in its overall caloric effect when compared to a reduction in caloric intake.

THYROID MEDICATION Obese patients should be examined carefully to rule out endocrine abnormalities. One of the commonest and most treatable of these is hypothyroidism resulting from primary thyroid gland insufficiency. Although obesity may accompany hypothyroidism as a complicating disorder, hypothyroidism itself does not cause true adiposity. Thus, correction of hypothyroidism by thyroid therapy does not usually alter the natural course of the associated exogenous obesity. Primary hypothyroidism complicating obesity can be easily corrected by full replacement doses of thyroid. A useful and reliable form of thyroid medication is liotrix (Euthroid), which contains a physiologic ratio of the two synthetic thyroid hormones, L-thyroxine (levothyroxine, T_4) and L-triiodothyronine (liothyronine, T_3).

A much more controversial situation arises when thyroid replacement therapy is considered as the primary treatment of obesity in the absence of any measurable thyroid abnormality. The rationale for using thyroid in the treatment of obesity may have arisen from a misinterpretation of the basal metabolic rate (BMR) in obese subjects. The BMR may be low normal or slightly reduced in obese patients because of the poor correlation of surface area measurements with true metabolic status. Thus, a low BMR in obesity usually does not represent true hypothyroidism; the diagnosis of thyroid disorder must depend upon more specific thyroid hormone measurements (see Chap. 92).

Supplemental thyroid therapy does not raise the low BMR of obese patients unless pharmacologic doses are prescribed (viz., greater than liotrix-3 or desiccated thyroid, 180 mg daily). Large doses of thyroid hormone are not recommended in obesity, since they eventually cause thyrotoxicity and may precipitate cardiac arrhythmias or congestive heart failure. This is especially likely to occur from the synergistic actions of thyroid in the presence of hypokalemia which may have been induced by the concomitant use of thiazide diuretics. Even more hazardous to the obese patient is the use of amphetamines in combination with thyroid hormone and thiazide diuretic therapy.

APPETITE DEPRESSANTS Unfortunately, no pharmacologic agent is avail[illegible]t this time which acts primarily by depressing the "a[illegible]ter." This type of depression is seen regularly in disease states such as hepatitis and uremia and as a toxic manifestation of drugs such as digitalis.

SUBSTANCES WHICH DEPRESS APPETITE BY INDUCING A SENSE OF WELL-BEING Amphetamine and its derivatives are the prototype of this group of substances. These agents are commonly referred to as "anorexigenic" or "anorectic." There is no evidence to show, however, that their effectiveness results from a depression of the appetite center. Probably as a result of stimulation, or a "lift," the patient's drive toward overeating may be significantly modified, so that as far as he is concerned, the overall effect of the drug is "appetite-depressing." Obviously, drugs which create such a state of euphoria may lead to habituation.

At present a large number of derivatives of amphetamine sulfate (Benzedrine) and closely related compounds is available for clinical use; e.g., dextroamphetamine sulfate (Dexedrine), levoamphetamine sulfate and phosphate, levoamphetamine alginate (Levonor), methamphetamine hydrochloride (Amphedroxyn, Desoxyephedrine, Desoxyn, Desyphed, Dexoval, Desoxyfed, Drinalfa, Efroxine, Methedrine, Norodin, Semoxydrine, Syndrox), phenylpropanolimine (Propadrine), phenmetrazine (Preludin), phenyl-*tert*-butylamine resin (Ionamin), and diethylpropion (Tenuate and Tepanil). The usual dosage of amphetamine sulfate or dextroamphetamine sulfate is 5 mg given 30 to 60 min before meals. It may be necessary in some patients to omit the evening dose because of increased nervousness or sleeplessness. A carefully controlled double-blind study has shown fenfluramine 20 mg 3 times daily or dexamphetamine 5 mg 3 times daily 1 h before meals, the last dose being taken before 5 P.M., to be equivalent in facilitating weight loss and both to have greater effectiveness than a placebo (Stunkard et al, 1973). When drugs related to amphetamine are continued for a prolonged period, weight loss usually ceases after 6 to 8 weeks (minimum), and the patient resumes his usual eating habits unless other forms of treatment have been successful. All the controlled studies utilize a fixed dosage throughout the period of study, since a progressive increase in dosage to overcome whatever process is leading to tolerance would presumably add to the risk of drug misuse or habituation. Periods of treatment with amphetamines for 2 weeks alternating with equal periods without treatment are as effective as continuous treatment. Although serious reactions are rarely encountered with amphetamine and its congeners, the physician must be alert to the sympathomimetic effect of the agents in causing a rise in blood pressure, increased cardiac rate and work, and possible development of cardiac arrhythmias.

METABOLIC STIMULANTS, INCLUDING HORMONES Repeated efforts have been made to discover a nontoxic agent which would maintain a normal metabolic level in the face of weight loss. Dinitrophenol has had the widest use. The consensus today is that its undesirable toxic side reactions make its use unjustified.

In most instances, substances of this type are being employed by physicians or patients in an attempt to induce *weight loss without caloric restricti*[illegible] do this, it is obviously necessary to raise basa[illegible] level *above normal.* There is no known subst[illegible]e used to increase metabolic level above normal for prolonged periods of time without danger of toxicity.

Many laymen think "hormones" the most important cause of obesity and hopefully consider them to be its cure. The well-informed physician recognizes to what a small extent disturbances in hormone secretion are primarily responsible for obesity and how futile most types of hormone therapy are as cures of obesity. One must not underestimate the psychologic reinforcement given to a patient on a reducing program when he reports regularly to his physician for "an injection"!

Male and female gonadal hormones and adrenal cortical hormones have no place in therapy unless specific deficiency of these hormones exists. Claims have been made for the usefulness of injected human chorionic gonadotropin in treatment of obesity (Asher et al, 1973). These conclusions have been challenged by Hirsch and Van Itallie (1973). It seems fair to conclude that the efficacy of human chorionic gonadotropin in the treatment of obesity is at best doubtful and that this agent is unlikely to be of dramatic benefit in the usual case.

A number of features of human growth hormone suggest that it should be potentially useful in the treatment of obesity. This hormone will mobilize fatty acids and deplete body fat without producing a noteworthy degree of nitrogen loss. In addition, it appears to have a calorigenic effect. Long-term administration to obese patients has not been carried out. Exacerbation of glucose intolerance might represent a potential hazard, and ultimate resistance to growth hormone action might be anticipated with available preparations when injected over prolonged periods. Unfortunately the present supply of human growth hormone is far too limited to permit adequate trial.

A specific application of hormones to the treatment of complications of obesity has been reported for progesterone. Many obese patients exhibit the Pickwickian syndrome characterized by alveolar hypoventilation. It has been reported that 100 mg progesterone administered daily intramuscularly increased tidal volume, improved respiratory acidosis, and restored the depressed oxygen saturation of peripheral blood to normal. Narcolepsy disappeared completely. The therapeutic effects of progesterone did not appear to be necessarily associated with weight loss. One month after discontinuance of progesterone therapy, pulmonary function had deteriorated appreciably.

SURGICAL PROCEDURES

In extreme situations in which the patient's life is threatened by obesity, such as respiratory or cardiac failure, severe hypertension, or marked peripheral edema with ulceration, surgical bypass procedures can be done. A current procedure is anastomosis of the jejunum, about a foot below the ligament of Treitz, to the terminal ileum by an end-to-side procedure. More radical procedures have resulted in iron and vitamin deficiencies, and less radical procedures in little or no weight loss. Nevertheless, a small number of patients still either fail to lose weight or else develop some degree of symptomatic malabsorption necessitating restoration of the original anatomic arrangement.

REFERENCES

Asher WL et al: Effect of human chorionic gonadotrophin on

weight loss, hunger, and feeling of well-being. Am J Clin Nutr 26:211–218, 1973

Fogarty Task Force on Obesity: Obesity, U. S. Government Printing Office, 1975

HIRSCH J et al: The treatment of obesity. Am J Clin Nutr 26:1039, 1973

MANN GV: The influence of obesity on health. NEJM 291:178; ibid 226, 1974

MEYERS FH et al: CNS stimulants and antidepressants, in *Review of Medical Pharmacology,* 4th ed., Los Altos, Calif.: Lange, 1974, p. 288

MONTOYE HJ et al: The measurement of body fatness: a study in a total community. Am J Clin Nutr 16:417–427, 1965

PENICK SB et al: Behavior modification in the treatment of obesity. Psychosom Med 33:49, 1971

SALANS LB et al: Adipose cell size and number in nonobese and obese patients. J Clin Invest 52:929, 1973

STUART RB: Behavioral control of overeating. Behav Res Ther 5:357–365, 1967

STUNKARD A et al: Fenfluramine in the treatment of obesity. Lancet 1:503, 1973

section 7 | Alterations in urinary function

47 DYSURIA, INCONTINENCE, AND ENURESIS

BERNARD LYTTON
FRANKLIN H. EPSTEIN

NORMAL MICTURITION An appreciation of the anatomic and physiologic mechanisms involved in micturition is necessary for a rational approach to the difficult problems of urinary incontinence, enuresis, and other disorders of bladder function.

The bladder muscle, or detrusor, consists of interlacing bundles of muscle that arch around the internal vesical orifice and continue down into the urethra, where they are interspersed with elastic fibers. The normal tone of these fibers constitutes the internal vesical sphincter. The bladder receives a dual nerve supply from the autonomic system. The sacral parasympathetic nerves, via the pelvic nerves (second, third, and fourth sacral segments), provide the preganglionic fibers to ganglia of the pelvic plexus and bladder wall, and these give off postganglionic fibers to the detrusor, and posterior urethra. The sympathetic preganglionic fibers (last two dorsal and first two lumbar segments) pass via the lumbar splanchnic nerves to synapse in the paraaortic and pelvic plexuses. The postganglionic fibers supply mainly the blood vessels in the bladder wall and the muscles around the bladder neck and posterior urethra. The sympathetic innervation has little influence on bladder function but is concerned with maintenance of smooth muscle tone around the bladder neck and proximal urethra for continence. Administration of sympathomimetic agents can inhibit satisfactory voiding, and sympathetic blocking, as may occur after treatment with certain psychotropic drugs, can cause stress urinary incontinence. Sympathetic activity is also involved in closure of the bladder neck at the time of ejaculation; removal of the first lumbar sympathetic ganglion bilaterally in men is usually followed by infertility because of retrograde ejaculation and in women may result in stress incontinence.

Afferent fibers subserving the sensations of distention and pain pass mainly via the pelvic nerves to the sacral segments of the spinal cord. Some of these fibers are said to pass via the sympathetic nerves, but it is probable that any residual sensation of bladder filling after section of the sacral nerves results from stretching of the peritoneum overlying the bladder. The internal pudendal nerve supplies motor and sensory fibers from the first, second, and third sacral segments to the external sphincter muscle, urethra, and perineal muscles. The action of the detrusor and sphincter muscles is, therefore, both reflex and voluntary.

Micturition is normally a voluntary act. As the bladder fills, a fairly constant low pressure is maintained by the detrusor muscle as it accommodates itself to the increasing volume. When it reaches its capacity, 400 to 500 ml in the normal adult, the stretch receptors transmit impulses via the pelvic afferent nerves, the sacral reflex center, and the fasciculus gracilis to the brain. This initiates the desire to void. Impulses from the brain, which arise in the paracentral lobules, are transmitted via descending fibers, just anterior to the corticospinal tracts, to the micturition center in the sacral part of the cord and to the pelvic and pudendal nerves to initiate the act of micturition. An initial relaxation of the proximal urethra and perineal muscles precedes detrusor contraction. At this point there is usually tensing of the abdominal muscles and diaphragm, although the resultant rise in abdominal pressure alone cannot initiate voiding normally and is not essential for evacuation. The intravesical pressure rises rapidly to 20 to 60 cm water, the external sphincter and posterior urethra relax, the bladder neck opens, and voiding occurs. Voiding pressure does not usually exceed the normal resting urethral pressure. The opening of the bladder neck is the result of a simultaneous detrusor contraction and relaxation of the smooth muscle of the posterior urethra and skeletal muscle of the external sphincter. Closure of the bladder neck occurs after relaxation of the detrusor because of a return of skeletal and smooth muscle activity. It is apparent that any interference with detrusor activity or the anatomy of the bladder neck will interfere with the opening mechanism and lead to incomplete emptying or some loss of continence.

DYSURIA Dysuria denotes difficulty or pain associated with voiding. It may result from a wide variety of pathologic conditions. Frequency, hesitancy, burning, urgency, and strangury (slow, painful emission of urine) are often referred to under the more general term *dysuria*.

Urgency occurs as a result of trigonal or posterior urethral irritation by inflammation, stones, or tumor. The urge may be so great and so sudden that a patient voids involuntarily.

Frequency of urination in connection with bladder lesions occurs when there is either a decreased capacity or pain on distention. In acute inflammatory lesions, edema and loss of elasticity of the bladder wall cause pain or an urge to void when only a small quantity of urine is present in the bladder. Chronic inflammatory lesions such as tuberculosis produce a similar effect and may proceed to permanently diminished capacity from scarring. Frequency may be an early presenting symptom of primary malignant disease of the bladder, because of induration of the bladder wall as a result of tumor invasion and reactionary inflammatory changes.

The majority of conditions producing these symptoms arise in the bladder and urethra. Diseases of other organs and systems may, by invading, compressing, or distorting the lower part of the urinary tract, produce dysuria. Diseases of the nervous system, which involve the nerve supply of the bladder either centrally, as in tabes and multiple sclerosis, or peripherally, as in diabetic neuropathy, produce difficulty in voiding and sometimes pain when secondary infection occurs as a result of residual urine.

The *evaluation of the condition of a patient with dysuria* must include a complete history and physical examination as well as a complete urologic examination, together with relevant radiologic or laboratory investigations suggested by abnormalities detected during the clinical examination.

Inflammatory lesions in the bladder, prostate, or urethra are the commonest causes of dysuria and frequency. These include bacterial infections, chronic prostatitis in men, and chronic posterior urethrotrigonitis in women. The latter conditions are characterized by chronic inflammatory changes involving the posterior urethra, the prostatic glands in the male, or their anlage in the female—the paraurethral glands. The cause is obscure, and treatment is directed principally toward drainage by prostatic massage and by urethral sounding with instillation of mild astringents in the female. Meatal revision, internal urethrotomy, and posterior urethral fulguration are also advocated in the more persistent cases of posterior urethritis in women. A great deal may be learned from examination of the external urinary meatus. About 20 percent of children with urinary complaints have a degree of meatal stenosis, which may interfere sufficiently with bladder function to result in recurrent infection. Meatal stenosis may be an important cause in the development and persistence of chronic prostatitis in men and chronic posterior urethritis and trigonitis in women. Unsuspected meatal stenosis of long standing may cause trabeculation of the bladder and other manifestations of obstructive uropathy. Meatotomy results in relief or considerable improvement.

A urethral caruncle may produce symptoms of severe discomfort on voiding. This tumor appears as a small cherry-red polyp which may or may not protrude from the posterior lip of the external meatus and is generally exquisitely tender on palpation. The latter feature helps to distinguish it from the commoner condition of urethral prolapse. Excision and fulguration constitute the treatment of choice.

Benign overgrowth of the *prostate* commonly causes frequency, hesitancy, straining, slowing of the stream, and dribbling in older men. Pain is uncommon unless the condition is complicated by infection or vesical calculi.

Frequency and urgency may follow *radiation injury* to the bladder; this is most frequently seen after treatment for carcinoma of the cervix. In the acute phase this condition may be amenable to treatment with "bladder sedatives" containing antispasmodics and with small doses of steroids to combat the inflammatory reaction. The persistence of symptoms or bleeding may necessitate surgical intervention. Symptoms may not appear until several months or years after radiation treatment. Malignant tumors of the intestine, diverticulitis, regional ileitis, or ulcerative colitis may involve the bladder and cause frequency. Fistula formation may result in severe dysuria and pneumaturia and should be suspected in any patient with a prolonged and persistent urinary infection.

Chronic interstitial cystitis, a nonspecific chronic inflammatory disease of the bladder wall which may be manifested by small, shallow, stellate hemorrhagic mucosal ulcers (Hunner's ulcers), gives rise to a fairly characteristic pattern of dysuria. This condition may be the result of an autoimmune reaction. The patients, generally middle-aged women, complain of persistent frequency and often have severe suprapubic pain, relieved by voiding. There may be associated terminal hematuria. The urine contains a few white and red blood cells but no bacteria. Interstitial cystitis may ultimately lead to fibrosis with permanent contraction of the bladder, which may require cystoplasty or urinary diversion.

Frequency without discomfort on voiding may be associated with a normal bladder capacity and may be due to the polyuria of diabetes, to conditions causing hypercalcemia or hypokalemia, to the nocturia of early congestive heart failure, to upper urinary tract obstruction with loss of concentrating ability, or to loss of renal parenchyma resulting in the passage of a large volume of poorly concentrated urine. The absence of nocturia in a patient with frequency suggests that it may be of psychogenic origin or may be due to a polyp or irritative lesion in the posterior urethra that is relieved by recumbency. A patient who complains of recent onset of nocturia should be carefully questioned about diuretic medication.

It should always be remembered that frequency may be due to paradoxic incontinence (see below).

Expanding masses in the pelvis that reduce bladder capacity by external compression are exemplified by pregnancy, large ovarian cysts, and uterine fibroids. A retroverted gravid uterus or pelvic tumor which becomes impacted may result in stretching and elongation of the urethra and produce difficulty in voiding and finally complete retention.

INCONTINENCE **Paradoxic incontinence** True incontinence must be distinguished from paradoxic incontinence, which accompanies bladder distention caused by mechanical or functional obstruction and is characterized by small, frequent, involuntary "overflow" voidings. Response of the bladder muscle to obstruction may be compared with that seen in striated and heart muscle. With chronic obstruction the detrusor hypertrophies, the bladder becomes trabeculated, and this suffices to increase the force of contraction to overcome the block. As soon as a small quantity of urine is voided, the intravesical pressure drops, leaving a residual urine which gradually increases in amount. Ultimately, the detrusor becomes paralyzed by overdistention and complete retention ensues. Overflow incontinence is seen in flaccid neurogenic bladders, when small involuntary voidings occur, as the pressure of accumulating urine overcomes the resistance at the bladder outlet. With loss of a small amount of urine, pressure falls and a large residual is left. Timed voiding using suprapubic pressure, together with the oral administration of large doses of bethanechol chloride, may be helpful in controlling this type of incontinence. Often both neurologic and obstructive elements contribute, as in elderly arteriosclerotic men with prostatic enlargement or in cases of diabetic neuropathy with secondary bladder neck obstruction. The bladder in these patients is flaccid and painless, which may make it difficult to palpate, and the residual urine predisposes to infection.

Congenital incontinence Congenital incontinence may be due to malformations such as vesical exstrophy, epispadias, patent urachus, and ectopic ureteral openings in the female, which are frequently associated with duplications of the renal collecting system. Congenital defects in the spinal cord and chorda equina, which occur in association with spina bifida, sacral anomalies, and meningomyelocele, may result in neurogenic vesical dysfunction.

The results of primary reconstructive surgery in cases of exstrophy are cosmetically satisfactory, but sphincter control is rarely achieved. Furthermore, most of these children have persistent vesicoureteral reflux and infection, which may lead to progressive renal damage. The majority, therefore, are still best treated by some form of urinary diversion with excision of the bladder. The results of urethral and bladder neck reconstruction in simple epispadias are better. The management of neurogenic bladder disturbance is principally directed toward establishing timed reflex voiding, decreasing outlet resistance with diminution of residual urine, and controlling infection. The use of electrical stimulators to promote bladder emptying is still in the experimental phase. When there is progressive renal impairment, due to persistent infection and vesicoureteral reflux, urinary diversion is necessary.

Acquired incontinence This may occur as a result of disease or injury to the spinal cord, as in tabes, multiple sclerosis, and tumor, or following fractures of the spine. The disruption of the neural mechanism in lower motor neuron lesions results in complete relaxation of the detrusor and perineal muscles, but sympathetic tone in the posterior urethra remains unimpaired. Upper motor neuron lesions cause uncontrolled hyperactivity of the detrusor with spasticity of the muscles of the urethra and perineum. This results in uncontrollable, frequent voiding. These contractions are usually associated with a further reflex contraction of the bladder outlet rather than reflex relaxation which normally occurs to decrease outlet resistance. The detrusor contractions are therefore ineffective, and there is residual urine. Mixed or incomplete neural lesions and superadded urinary infection result in marked variations in the clinical manifestations of neurogenic vesical dysfunction. Wetting can be controlled by intermittent self-catheterization in patients with both flaccid and spastic neurogenic bladder dysfunction. Anticholinergic drugs should be given to control detrusor hyperreactivity. Sympatholytic agents (phenoxybenzamine) may be used to decrease posterior urethral resistance in patients with an automatic bladder, but endoscopic external sphincterotomy is required in the more severe cases. Phenoxybenzamine can also be used to control autonomic dysreflexia. Cerebral vascular accidents or senility may produce loss of voluntary control of bladder and bowel function.

Parturition can stretch and disrupt the structures of the pelvic floor and perineum to the point that urethral resistance, though sufficient to maintain continence at rest, gives way under stress of straining or coughing, and incontinence ensues. Such incontinence is probably due to descent of the proximal urethra below the pelvic diaphragm, so that an increase in intraabdominal pressure, which is normally transmitted equally to both bladder and the proximal urethra, is no longer exerted on the proximal urethra. The resultant pressure differential thus exceeds the posterior urethral resistance, and urinary leakage occurs. The descensus is associated with loss of the urethrovesical angle and shortening of the urethra, which may be visualized on cystourethrography. Treatment is directed toward repair of the pelvic floor, with return of the bladder neck above the pelvic diaphragm, restoration of urethral length, and correction of the urethrovesical angle.

Stress incontinence may be aggravated by urgency because of an associated urethrotrigonitis. Relief of the trigonitis will sometimes result in satisfactory control. Uncontrolled spontaneous detrusor contractions may aggravate or simulate stress incontinence. These can generally be controlled with imipramine. Urographic and urodynamic study is helpful in defining the mechanism of the incontinence.

Surgical or *radiation injuries* can produce vesicovaginal and ureterovaginal fistulas. Incontinence in ureterovaginal fistula occurs with normal voiding, but in vesicovaginal fistula there is generally no normal evacuation of the bladder. The treatment of these fistulas is always surgical. Temporary urinary diversion will enable spontaneous closure to occur in some instances. Reconstruction of a damaged ureter is the treatment of choice, but mobilization of the bladder to the pelvic brim, anastomosis to the intact ureter, implantation of the ureter into the intestine, or substitution with an ileal segment may be necessary. Nephrectomy is the simplest procedure in the elderly or debilitated patient or when there are serious technical difficulties, provided there is adequate function in the other kidney.

Injury to the sphincter mechanism may occur with pelvic fractures or after prostatic or bladder neck surgery, especially in elderly patients. Gradual improvement may occur for up to a year after injury. Postsurgical incontinence may be controlled with a penile clamp, but this has the disadvantage of producing edema and occasionally ulceration of the penis or a urethral diverticulum. A condom catheter may lead to maceration of the penile skin and is often difficult to apply. An indwelling catheter often leads to problems of chronic infection. A variety of surgical procedures have been devised to improve control by using some mechanical means to increase urethral resistance; they are only partially successful. Urinary diversion may become necessary in certain cases.

ENURESIS Enuresis implies the unintentional voiding of urine, usually at night, when it is synonymously referred to as bedwetting. The term *enuresis* should be restricted to those in whom there is no gross urologic abnormality.

Micturition in infancy is governed by a simple spinal reflex. Maturation of the nervous system and development of control over the simple reflexes by the higher centers occur during the second year of life. By the age of thirty months, most children have voluntary control over rectal and urinary sphincters. The child who persistently wets the bed after the age of three or who, after a period of control, begins to wet the bed again presents a clinical problem. Enuresis then may be a delay in the development or a loss of bladder control. It may be affected by physical and psychologic factors. There appears to be no constant single cause.

It is estimated that 15 percent of boys and 10 percent of girls at the age of five are enuretic, but by the age of nine only 5 percent of all children remain bedwetters. The majority of children with simple enuresis remain dry at night by the time they reach puberty. Bedwetting is more common among children of parents in the lower income groups. This could be because of the later institution of toilet training.

It is important, early in the management of these patients, to distinguish incontinence due to organic urologic disease from enuresis. Diabetes mellitus or insipidus may occasionally present with enuresis. Renal disease due to glomerulo- or pyelonephritis or sickle-cell disease producing papillary necrosis may cause bedwetting as a result of the increased volumes of urine passed by these patients. A careful evaluation at the outset should exclude chronic retention with dribbling incontinence due to either bladder neck obstruction or neurologic disease. Patients with organic disease of the bladder are usually incontinent during the day as well as at night, although enuretics may also be incontinent during the day. Those with organic disease often have constant dribbling of urine. Occasionally, however, one finds serious degrees of bladder neck obstruction with nocturnal enuresis as the only symptom. Lack of proximal urethral smooth-muscle tone due to sympathetic insufficiency, sometimes associated with spina bifida occulta, may be responsible for wetting, particularly during sleep when the voluntary sphincter is relaxed. A congenital decrease in bladder capacity may be responsible for enuresis; this condition is sometimes familial. The enuresis generally ceases as the child gets older and spends less time asleep. Occasionally a patient with petit mal epilepsy may present the problem of bedwetting. Urinalysis will reveal an unsuspected infection. Enuresis occurring in retarded children or in those with serious psychiatric disturbances requires treatment directed to the management of their primary problem.

Contributory factors such as the child's general health, physical environment, and emotional state should be evaluated, and the parents should be encouraged to adopt an understanding rather than a punitive attitude. Correction of minor urologic abnormalities such as meatal stenosis, balanitis, vulvovaginitis, posterior urethritis, and urethral valves will sometimes lead to relief, but this is perhaps attributable only to dysuria following instrumentation or to the understanding interest shown by the physician. The administration of antiparasympathetic agents to reduce bladder activity, or of amphetamines to lighten sleep, has been advocated, but the results are equivocal. Sympathomimetic drugs are helpful in increasing smooth-muscle tone in the posterior urethra. Imipramine (Tofranil), a mood-elevating drug whose effect is reinforced by its anticholinergic and stimulant properties, given at bedtime, has produced a favorable response in over half the children treated, but may require continuation of treatment for some time. The results of psychotherapy are unconvincing. Considerable success has been claimed for alarm systems which attempt to establish a conditioned reflex. The child is awakened when an electrical circuit is completed by wetting; this method seems to be worth a trial in older children who prove resistant to simpler therapy.

REFERENCES

GRIFFITHS DS: The mechanics of the urethra and of micturition. Br J Urol 45:497, 1974

HODGKINSON CP: Stress urinary incontinence. Am J Obstet Gynecol 108:1141, 1970

POUSSAINT AF, DITMAN KS: A controlled study of imipramine (Tofranil) in the treatment of enuresis. J Pediat 67:283, 1965

WHITESIDE CG, ARNOLD EP: Persistent primary enuresis: A urodynamic assessment. Br Med J 1:364, 1975

48
OLIGURIA, POLYURIA, AND NOCTURIA

GEORGE W. THORN
LOUIS G. WELT

INTRODUCTION

The kidneys provide the main channel for the excretion of water and solutes, and the urine flow and composition are adjusted so as to maintain the internal environment of the body in a remarkably constant steady state. The volume and solute content of the urine in health may vary widely. They are largely dependent on the magnitude and characteristics of the fluid and food ingested and on the quantity of water lost from other routes such as perspiration and insensible water loss. There are many ways in which urine flow can be varied in both health and disease, and it appears essential to review briefly, and in a general fashion, the manner in which urine is formed so that the vicissitudes of life and the impact of disease on urine volume and osmolality may be better understood.

The final bladder urine represents the net effect of a host of reactions that begin with the formation of an almost protein-free ultrafiltrate of plasma in the glomeruli. The quantity of fluid filtered at the glomeruli per unit of time is the net effect of the difference in the chemical potential of the water of plasma and that of the ultrafiltrate as well as the surface area available for filtration. These factors apply to the filtrable solutes as well. The volume of water excreted per unit of time is, then, the difference between the volume filtered and the volume reabsorbed. The quantity of solutes excreted per unit of time is the difference between that which is filtered and that which is reabsorbed or secreted by the renal tubules. Many aspects of these mechanisms remain obscure, but there is a general concept around which a description may be presented and from which implications may be drawn with respect to the influence of a variety of circumstances and disease processes.

The water filtered by the glomeruli is reabsorbed at several areas along the nephron by passive diffusion along osmotic gradients, which, in turn, are established by the active transport of solutes. The osmotic gradient is maximized in the medulla and papilla, owing to the anatomic arrangement of the loops of Henle and their accompanying blood vessels, which permit the establishment of an ever-increasing osmolality as the papilla is approached. This latter mechanism is referred to as the *countercurrent multiplication system.*

The *initial* step in the reabsorption of water, and the step that represents the largest volume, occurs in the proximal convolution of the nephron. The active transport of solutes, which are primarily sodium, chloride, bicarbonate, and glucose, creates an osmotic gradient so that water follows immediately. In this fashion, approximately two-thirds to three-fourths of the filtered solutes and water are reabsorbed by the end of the proximal tubule. The characteristics of this fluid are altered considerably, not only in volume but also in composition. However, it is still iso-osmotic with the parent filtrate.

Another phase in the reabsorption of water occurs in the more distal portions of the nephron, which include the loop of Henle, the distal convolution, and lastly, the collecting ducts. Although the reabsorption at these levels is smaller in volume than that which occurs in the more proximal segment of the nephron, these latter mechanisms are responsible in one circumstance for the formation of a maximally concentrated urine, and in the other circumstances for the formation of a dilute urine. There are, obviously, circumstances wherein the urine osmolality occupies positions intermediate between these polar extremes.

The formation of a *maximally concentrated* urine depends on the presence of antidiuretic hormone, which permits the distal convolution and collecting duct membranes to be completely permeable to water. Micropuncture data reveal that the fluid in the early part of the distal convolution is always hypotonic (whether or not there is maximal antidiuretic hormone activity) to plasma. Furthermore, water is lost between the end of the proximal convolution and the early distal convolution. These two data clearly imply that solutes have been transported in excess of water, and hence some part of the ascending limb is presumably impermeable to water in the presence or absence of the antidiuretic hormone.

In the presence of antidiuretic hormone activity, the fluid within the distal convolution becomes more concentrated. Where one distal convolution meets with another to form a collecting tubule, the fluid is invariably iso-osmotic (in the rodent) with the parent filtrate. As the fluid courses through the collecting duct (in the presence of antidiuretic hormone activity) and is exposed to a fluid with an ever-increasing osmolality, a passive movement of water causes the fluid within the collecting ducts to remain in osmotic equilibrium with the fluid in the interstitium; thus, the intraductal fluid increases in concentration until it exits into the pelvis of the kidney and moves into the bladder.

Allusion has been made to the mechanism whereby the fluid in the interstitium is rendered continuously more hyperosmotic from outer medulla to papillary tip. It is dependent upon the anatomic arrangement of the loops of Henle and their blood vessels and is achieved by the transport of sodium salts (in excess of water) from the ascending limb of the loop. This renders the fluid in the interstitium hyperosmotic to the fluid entering the descending limb of the loop of Henle. This difference in osmolality promotes a movement of water from the descending limb fluid; and, in addition, there is entry of solutes into this portion of the limb. The net result is an increase in the osmolality of the fluid in the descending limb. This same process is repeated over and over again, and the fluid in the limb and interstitium becomes more concentrated along its course. When the fluid reaches the ascending portion of the limb and solutes are transported out of the luminal fluid, this fluid and the interstitium become ever less concentrated; the fluid becomes hypotonic by the time it reaches the early distal convolution.[1]

In this setting the fluid coursing through the collecting ducts is made more hyperosmotic. Since urea can presumably permeate the collecting ducts largely by passive diffusion, urea moves from the collecting system into the interstitium as water moves along the osmotic gradient. In this fashion, urea contributes significantly to the total solute concentration in the medullary and papillary interstitium and serves to counterbalance the concentration of urea within the collecting ducts.

In man, the maximal concentration of the final urine may be as high as 1,200 to 1,400 mOsm per kg water. This may be much higher in rodents, the experimental animals from which the data for this formulation have been obtained.

In contrast, in the "complete" absence of antidiuretic hormone, the fluid in the distal convolution is not only hypotonic to plasma in the earliest portions but remains so and is excreted as bladder urine with the same or even lower osmolality. Data reveal that salt is transported from the distal convolutions and from the collecting ducts themselves. In the absence of antidiuretic hormone, this aids and abets formation of minimally concentrated urine.

In this fashion, one can visualize the manner in which a highly concentrated or a minimally concentrated urine can be formed. Varying amounts of antidiuretic hormone between none and maximal provide a graded response.

[1] *The antidiuretic hormone possibly serves to increase the rate of transport of solutes from the ascending limb in addition to its influence on the permeability of the distal tubular and collecting duct permeability.*

Furthermore, it must be pointed out that even in the two polar situations of maximal antidiuretic hormone activity, or none, the rate of excretion of solutes determines the volume and osmolality of urine. This is to state that a urine may have an osmolality approaching that of the plasma with no antidiuretic hormone activity in the face of a solute diuresis; in contrast, the urine volume may be large and the osmolality may approach that of plasma despite maximal antidiuretic hormone activity in the presence of a solute diuresis. The manner in which a solute diuresis influences urine concentration and volume is not completely clear.

However, within the context of the discussion presented above, it is apparent that a good deal of the water removed from the initial volume of filtrate depends on the active transport of salt and other solutes from the luminal fluid. Even if a constant *percentage* of filtered salt were reabsorbed in the proximal tubule, an increased filtration *rate* would provide a larger volume of fluid to the descending limb of the loop of Henle. Furthermore, to the extent that limitations are placed on the transport of salt from the proximal tubule (owing to the presence in filtrate of a larger concentration of a poorly reabsorbable solute), less water will be reabsorbed. If less salt is transported out of the loop of Henle, or if the flow of fluid through the loop is hastened, the countercurrent multiplier system will operate less efficiently; hence, the maximal osmolality will not be achieved in the interstitium of the medulla and the papilla. By the same token, if the reabsorption of solutes is diminished in the distal convolution (e.g., glucose is not reabsorbable at this site), less water will be reabsorbed and a greater volume will reach the collecting duct system. Hence, a large solute excretion will increase the volume and diminish the osmolality of the final urine despite maximal antidiuretic hormone activity.

In contrast, it will be recalled that the efficient transport of solutes prior to, in, and beyond the distal convoluted tubule, coupled with the relative impermeability to water of these latter structures in the absence of antidiuretic hormone, are responsible for the formation of minimally dilute urine. If reabsorption of solutes is less efficient, owing to the filtered load or to the presence of less readily reabsorbable solutes, it is clear that urine osmolality cannot reach minimally dilute levels. As the solute diuresis becomes more intense, urine osmolality will approach that of the plasma.

In summary, a small solute excretion in the absence of antidiuretic hormone would be anticipated to be accompanied by the most dilute urine, and in the presence of antidiuretic hormone, with the most maximally concentrated urine. Varying quantities of antidiuretic hormone will have obvious influences; the character of the urine anticipated in the presence of maximal antidiuretic hormone activity or none will be modified by the quantity and character of the solute load destined for excretion.

APPROACH TO THE PATIENT WITH OLIGURIA, POLYURIA, OR NOCTURIA

OLIGURIA In patients with oliguria it is necessary to differentiate four major etiologic factors: (1) frank dehydration; (2) reduced effective plasma volume; (3) acute and chronic renal disease; (4) obstruction of the urinary tract.

Dehydration In the face of a diminished volume of body fluids glomerular filtration is diminished and the excretion of solutes is reduced owing to the influence of plasma volume deficit on renal hemodynamics. Frank dehydration can be suspected in a patient with a recent history of reduced fluid and food intake, fever and sweating, vomiting or diarrhea, and excessive diuretic medication. It can be readily confirmed by the presence of dry skin and mucous membranes, sunken eyeballs, flat neck veins, a urine of high specific gravity, and hemoconcentration.

Reduced effective plasma volume Oliguria may also result from congestive heart failure or cirrhosis of the liver. These two conditions are characterized by a diminished effective plasma volume in the presence of edema or ascites. The reduced cardiac output which is characteristic of heart failure leads to reduced renal blood flow and reduced glomerular filtration rate. Cirrhosis of the liver is also frequently associated with diminished renal blood flow, reduced glomerular filtration, and strikingly low urine flow. In both of these disorders the renal tubular reabsorption of sodium is efficient, and this further contributes to a diminished urine volume. The distinguishing features of oliguria due to dehydration, heart failure, or cirrhosis are diminished glomerular filtration rate, a large fractional tubular reabsorption of water (i.e., high urine/plasma creatinine ratio), and an avid and efficient tubular transport of salt as evidenced by a low urinary concentration of sodium. The outstanding difference between patients with oliguria due to frank dehydration and those with cardiac or hepatic disease is "dryness" of the former and the presence of ascites or edema in the latter (see Chap. 32).

Renal insufficiency Oliguria is also characteristic of acute renal disease such as glomerulonephritis, acute tubular necrosis, and renal cortical necrosis. In the case of the glomerulopathies, the low volume is due almost entirely to a drastic reduction in filtration rate. While this also occurs in acute tubular necrosis, other factors as well may contribute to the striking oliguria. In renal cortical necrosis where all elements of the nephron are damaged, total anuria is common. In the patient with chronic or end-stage renal insufficiency, striking reductions in urine flow are also observed frequently. This is primarily a consequence of the magnitude of renal cell mass that is destroyed. In contrast to the oliguria which accompanies dehydration and reduced effective plasma volume, the oliguria of renal parenchymal disease is likely to be accompanied by both diminished glomerular filtration rate and impaired tubular reabsorption of water and salt. These combined deficiencies will be reflected by a low urine/plasma concentration ratio of urea or creatinine; frequently this will be less than 20. The urinary concentration of sodium is in excess of 20 m*M*. (See Chap. 270, Approach to the Patient with Renal Disease, and Chap. 271, Renal Function Tests.)

Obstruction of the urinary tract Obstruction of the lower part of the urinary tract, i.e., from the bladder to the urethral meatus, is common and is due most frequently to stricture, to compression of the prostatic urethra by an enlarged prostate gland, and, less commonly, to congenital malformations. The distended bladder is often felt as a cystic swelling arising from the pelvis. Palpation of the prostate may reveal enlargement. Although it is less common to see oliguria as a consequence of obstruction of the upper part of the urinary tract, it does occur. If an obstruction is suspected, delineation of the upper part of the urinary tract is necessary to establish the diagnosis. (See Chap. 278, Obstructive Uropathy.)

POLYURIA For practical purposes there are four important disorders in which polyuria may present:

1 Diabetes mellitus (solute diuresis)
2 Diabetes insipidus: deficiency of vasopressin
3 Nephrogenic diabetes insipidus and acquired renal lesions
4 Psychogenic polydipsia

Solute diuresis A solute diuresis, as is noted in patients with uncontrolled diabetes mellitus, is almost always accompanied by a large urine flow and complaint of polyuria. A history of weight loss, polyphagia, pruritus, or visual difficulties should suggest a urine examination for glucose and, if positive, for blood sugar determinations (see Chap. 95, Diabetes Mellitus). A solute diuresis may also occur in patients suffering a "reaction to injury" who are unable to utilize protein but are given large quantities of this foodstuff. In such instances protein or amino acids are converted to a very large extent to urea which in turn promotes a large urine flow.

Diabetes insipidus Polyuria associated with polydipsia results from an inability of the patient to synthesize and secrete adequate quantities of vasopressin. As a consequence very large volumes of dilute urine are passed during the day *and night.* Intracranial tumors account for approximately 40 percent of cases. An increasingly frequent cause is surgical procedures in the region of the hypothalamoneurohypophyseal system including implantation of radio isotopes and heavy-particle irradiation. Severe head injuries are a third important cause. In approximately one-third of cases diagnostic procedures are unsuccessful in revealing the cause. Patients with true diabetes insipidus respond dramatically to vasopressin (see Chap. 91).

Nephrogenic diabetes insipidus There are a number of disorders in which the renal tubule is unable to respond appropriately to endogenous or exogenous vasopressin. True *nephrogenic diabetes insipidus* is a hereditary disorder with full expression in males and partial expression in females, which manifests itself early in life. These patients are frequently referred to as "water babies." Management of this condition is difficult since the infants do not respond adequately to any of the available vasopressin preparations (see Chap. 91, Diseases of the Neurohypophysis, and Chap. 281, Other Congenital and Hereditary Disorders of the Kidney and Urinary Tract).

Potassium depletion This condition is commonly associated with inability to concentrate the urine appropriately. The nature of the renal tubular defect is not clear. One of the most striking examples occurs in patients with primary hyperaldosteronism. From a practical point of view if potassium deficiency is suspected and polyuria has not occurred, it can be inferred that potassium depletion is neither severe nor long-standing. The defect is readily reversible with potassium repletion and in the case of excessive mineralocorticoid by the concomitant reduction in sodium intake (see Chap. 69, Fluids and Electrolytes).

Hypercalcemia Excess calcium in the blood is well known to be accompanied by diminished ability to concentrate the urine maximally. Polyuria from this cause may be exhibited by patients with primary hyperparathyroidism, vitamin D intoxication, and hypercalcemia associated with malignant disease and sarcoid (see Chaps. 352 and 353).

Miscellaneous conditions Other examples of acquired renal lesions characterized by inability to concentrate the urine are seen frequently in patients with *chronic renal insufficiency,* particularly the "salt-losing" type. In addition, some rather striking examples of extreme polyuria have been seen in patients with multiple myeloma or amyloidosis as well as after relief of obstructive uropathy. A marked diuresis also characterizes the recovery phase of acute tubular necrosis. In all the above acquired disorders, including hypokalemia and hypercalcemia, vasopressin administration will elicit little or no antidiuretic effect.

NOCTURIA Nocturia may have any of several origins so that the details of the *history* are critically important. It is necessary to know if urination is uncomfortable or painful, whether there is difficulty in starting the stream, whether the urine volumes are small or large, and over what period excessive nighttime passage of urine has been present.

The diurnal rhythm as it relates to urine flow is such that a much larger volume is normally excreted in the waking period. This rhythm is frequently reversed in patients with *edema,* because extracellular fluid accumulates during the day as a consequence of activity and the influence of the upright position. At night, when the patient is supine, the edema is slowly mobilized, and the increased plasma volume leads to increased urinary excretion.

In patients with *renal insufficiency* nocturia is common because urine is excreted at a fairly uniform rate, and hence the normal diurnal rhythm is lost. This may be explained as a consequence of a constant osmotic diuresis per nephron.

Partial obstruction of the bladder (prostatic hypertrophy) is often accompanied by nocturia because the stimulus to void is so frequently present. Lastly, any disorder which results in dysuria is almost certain to promote nocturia. In this instance, as in the case with obstruction of the bladder, nocturia is characterized by frequent but small volumes of urine.

REFERENCES

Black, DAK: *Renal Disease,* 3d ed., Philadelphia: Davis, 1972

Campbell MF, Harrison JH: *Urology,* 3d ed., Philadelphia: Saunders, 1970

McDougal WS, Wright FS: Defect in proximal and distal sodium transport in post-obstructive diuresis. Kidney Int 2:304, 1972

Orloff J, Burg MB: *Metabolic Basis of Inherited Disease,* 3d ed., p. 1567, New York: McGraw-Hill, 1972

Strauss MB, Welt LG: *Diseases of the Kidney,* 2d ed., Boston: Little, Brown, 1972

49 HEMATURIA

BERNARD LYTTON
FRANKLIN H. EPSTEIN

Bleeding from the urinary tract, whether microscopic or gross, is a serious sign. Although a common cause is acute cystitis, it should be regarded with the same gravity as abnormal bleeding from any other body orifice. Women sometimes have difficulty in determining whether bleeding is from the urinary tract, vagina, or rectum. Hematuria is usually classified as initial, terminal, or total. *Total hematuria* indicates that the bleeding occurs throughout the urinary stream and suggests that the bleeding originates from either the kidney or the ureter. *Initial bleeding* is generally associated with lesions in the urethra distal to the bladder neck; *terminal bleeding,* with lesions in the bladder, usually in the area of the trigone. Severe hemorrhage from the bladder, however, will present as total hematuria. These distinctions as to the type of bleeding are, therefore, only rough indications as to the origin of the bleeding; too much reliance should not be placed on them. About 20 percent of the patients who come to the physician with hematuria have it as the only symptom of their urinary tract disease; it is often difficult to persuade these patients to undergo a complete urologic investigation to establish the origin of the bleeding. Ureteral colic is often associated with renal bleeding and is due to the passage of clots.

The finding of an occasional red blood cell in a centrifuged specimen of urine is probably of no significance, since Addis showed that up to 500,000 red cells may normally be excreted in the urine in 12 h. *Vigorous exercise* or even intense excitement may increase the number of red cells, epithelial cells, and casts in the urinary sediment of normal subjects. Microscopic hematuria may also be increased during certain *febrile diseases* without implying serious disease of the kidneys. The presence of red blood cell casts is pathologic and further indicates that the source of the bleeding is in the kidneys rather than in the lower part of the urinary tract. The finding of red cell casts, therefore, may spare the patient unnecessary urological instrumentation, while raising the question of percutaneous renal biopsy to clarify the nature of the nephritis (see Chap. 274).

Certain *dyes* and *pigments,* such as phenolsulfonphthalein, azo dyes, and the indole alkaloids found in beet roots (betanin), may produce red discoloration of the urine, which must be distinguished from bleeding. The appearance of the red dye from beet roots occurs only in certain individuals; it is thought to be related to the degree of absorption of the dye from the gastrointestinal tract. Pink or brown discoloration of the urine may occur as a result of hemoor myoglobinuria or in acute porphyria (see Chap. 109). These may be precipitated by cold, exercise, or drug toxicity, especially in susceptible individuals (see Chap. 313).

Diseases of the renal parenchyma, such as glomerulonephritis, malignant hypertension, polycystic kidneys, renal infarction, renal vein thrombosis, or periarteritis, lupus erythematosus, or poisoning with a nephrotoxic agent, will in most instances be detected by a careful history, physical examination, and the usual laboratory tests. Gross hematuria may occasionally occur in patients with end-stage kidney disease as a result of vascular sclerosis. Bloody urine with little or no proteinuria recurring after respiratory infections and exercise suggests focal nephritis (Berger's disease, idiopathic hematuria; see Chap. 274). Hematuria may result from a disorder of blood clotting, produced by blood dyscrasias, scurvy, or anticoagulant drugs. The increased tendency to bleed in patients on long-term anticoagulant therapy may bring to light another, previously unsuspected, pathologic condition in the urinary tract. Sickle-cell anemia or sickle-cell trait may cause bleeding into the urine from disrupted capillaries and microinfarcts in the renal medulla. The aforementioned conditions account for only a small proportion of all patients with hematuria.

Tumors, urinary tract obstructions, calculi, and *infections* account for the bleeding in about 75 percent of patients with hematuria. Tumors alone account for some 20 percent of all cases. It is therefore mandatory in those patients in whom no other cause is found for the bleeding, to visualize the upper part of the urinary tract by intravenous pyelography supplemented by retrograde pyelography as indicated, and to visualize the bladder and urethra by instrumental examination. Retrograde pyelography may be supplemented by injections of air, rather than opaque dye, when one is trying to delineate suspected small calculi or small tumors in the renal collecting system. Doubtful lesions in the kidney may be further investigated by ultrasound renal scanning, nephrotomography, or aortography (see Chap. 270).

Cystoscopy will readily reveal presence of acute and chronic cystitis, interstitial cystitis, bladder tumors, and vesical calculi. Bleeding from engorged veins in the prostatic urethra due to benign prostatic hypertrophy and prostatitis in men and chronic nonspecific urethritis in women commonly causes hematuria. They should be accepted as the origin of the bleeding only after more serious conditions have been excluded.

Acute cystitis may result in gross hematuria, initially overshadowing all other symptoms. Chronic infections such as tuberculosis of the urinary tract or infection with *Schistosoma haematobium* may also have hematuria as their only presenting symptom. Schistosomiasis causes ulceration of the bladder mucosa at the site of deposition of the ova by the adult flukes which inhabit the venules of the bladder and pelvis. It is probably the commonest cause of hematuria in areas in the Middle East and Africa where it is endemic.

Bleeding associated with the menses should suggest the possibility of endometriosis of the urinary tract, provided contamination from the vagina has been excluded.

Trauma to the kidney nearly always manifests itself as hematuria, which is often painless and may persist for several days. The incidence of renal injury is increasing because of the increased number of serious automobile accidents. The majority of these cases may be treated conservatively with bed rest and careful observation. Follow-up intravenous pyelography should be carried out, because occasionally the renal injury may produce an anatomic deformity leading to obstruction, stone formation, or hypertension. A blow on the lower part of the abdomen when the bladder is distended, particularly in children, in whom the bladder is an abdominal organ, may produce a contusion or rupture of the bladder, giving rise to hematuria.

A small group of about 6 to 8 percent of all cases seen have hematuria for which no obvious source can be detected. Further urologic and hematologic investigation 3 to 4 months after the first episode of bleeding will determine the cause in just under half of these. Patients in whom episodes of hematuria persist should have a renal biopsy at a time when they are bleeding. A focal glomerulitis has been found to be responsible for the bleeding in many of these cases. The condition appears to have a good prognosis for normal renal function. A small number of cases, however, still remain undiagnosed and may have persistent hematuria for which no cause is found over a period of many years.

Arteriovenous malformations responsible for intermittent unexplained bleeding may sometimes be detected by renal angiography. These may in some instances be satisfactorily treated by partial nephrectomy. Intraoperative nephroscopy has been helpful in localizing some of these unusual lesions.

An outline for the investigation of hematuria is summarized in Table 49-1.

REFERENCE

LEADER AJ, CARLTON, CE JR.: Hematuria, in *Urology,* 3d ed., eds MF Campbell, JH Harrison, Philadelphia: Saunders, p. 202

TABLE 49-1
Investigation of hematuria

1 Microscopy of urinary sediment
- *a* RBCs, WBCs + bacteria (Suggest hemorrhagic cystitis)
- *b* RBCs, WBCs (Present in calculi, tumors, interstitial cystitis)
- *c* RBC casts (Indicate parenchymal renal disease)
- *d* Cytology (May reveal urothelial tumor cells)

2 Hematologic evaluation
- *a* Complete blood count, platelet count (To rule out leukemias, thrombocytopenia)
- *b* Bleeding time, prothrombin time, partial thromboplastin time (To exclude clotting disorders, coagulopathy)
- *c* Hemoglobin electrophoresis (If sickle-cell disease is suspected)
- *d* Antinuclear factor (Disseminated lupus erythematosus)

3 Radiologic examination
- *a* Intravenous pyelography (Calculi, tumors, obstruction, renal tumors, polycystic disease, retroperitoneal fibrosis)
- *b* Retrograde pyelography (Only if inadequate visualization on intravenous pyelography or systemic reactions to contrast)
- *c* Arteriography and ultrasonography (To differentiate tumor from cyst and define vascular lesions)

4 Cystoscopy (Urethral lesions, prostatic bladder disease, stones, tumors, diverticula, ureteral orifices, site of bleeding)

5 Renal biopsy (To distinguish specific forms of parenchymal disease, especially vascular disease and glomerulonephritis)

section 8 | Alterations in reproductive and sexual functions

50
DISTURBANCES OF MENSTRUATION

GEORGE W. THORN

Since the normal menstrual cycles depend upon the integrated action of the endocrine and nervous system, it is to be expected that abnormalities in the menstrual cycle may occur in association with a wide variety of systemic disorders as well as with specific pathologic changes in the reproductive organs. (See Chap. 99, Diseases of the Ovary.)

MENARCHE Menarche is an integrated function of the maturation process of the young female. It is preceded by functional and anatomical development of all the required organ systems and begins under normal circumstances very logically following a signal most likely related to body mass. The event occurs during the end of the pubertal process which lasts approximately two years. As such it is in general preceded by a growth spurt and early signs of the appearance and development of secondary sex characteristics. These are important considerations for the physician since a disorder in these sequences, i.e., premature growth spurt, no growth spurt at all, or bleeding without secondary sex characteristics, often points at underlying pathology.

In temperate climates the menstrual cycle usually begins between the ages of twelve and fifteen years. In tropical climates it may appear as early as nine to ten years. During the first year or two the cycles are likely to be irregular, since many are anovulatory. Menarche may be delayed beyond the age of sixteen years on a constitutional basis and often as a familial trait. In such individuals there is no demonstrable organic lesion, and with time normal periods appear. In general, however, delayed menarche, when accompanied by any of the following signs, should be investigated thoroughly:

1 Absence of other secondary sex characteristics
2 Symptoms or signs of absence, malformation, or obstructive pathology of uterus and/or vagina
3 Systemic disorders such as obesity, undernutrition, and those with neurologic and endocrine causes (thyroid, adrenal, diabetes mellitus)
4 Psychiatric disorders
5 Signs of chromosomal disorders

When menarche is delayed beyond the age of eighteen, primary amenorrhea is said to exist.

THE MENSTRUAL CYCLE Physiology The two key events which characterize the normal menstrual cycle are ovulation and menstruation. While cycle *lengths* may vary considerably among individuals from 3 weeks to 6 weeks or longer, ovulation normally occurs 2 weeks before the onset of menstrual flow. These 2 weeks represent the life span of the normal corpus luteum in the absence of fertilization. The variation in cycle length is thus introduced by changes in the duration of the follicular phase preceding ovulation. During this time interval follicular growth and maturation take place, requiring the activity of follicle-stimulating hormone (FSH) and luteinizing hormone (LH). Several follicles show early signs of growth during the first few days of the cycle. However, only one will reach full maturity. The mechanism responsible for the selection of only one follicle is unknown.

During the period of follicular maturation, estrogen secretion is the result of biochemical activity of the follicular apparatus. It is the resulting estrogen level in plasma which appears to give the signal for the sudden release of LH (associated with a smaller increment in FSH secretion) responsible for ovulation or ovum release. Another principal function of estrogen during this part of the cycle consists of the stimulation of the endometrium which exhibits active proliferative changes of its vascular system, glandular tissue, and stroma.

Luteal phase and *secretory phase* are the terms used to describe the time interval from ovulation to the onset of menstruation. At the level of the ovary, a corpus luteum is formed at the follicular site. There is still some question whether in the human further pituitary control is required for its formation and function, the latter consisting primarily of synthesis and secretion of estrogen and progesterone. Peak secretory activity occurs around the ninth day of the life of the corpus luteum (or approximately 3 days before menstruation).

The secretion of progesterone during the latter part of the menstrual cycle induces a variety of physiologic changes throughout the body. Examples are elevation of the basal body temperature, negative nitrogen metabolism, and a natriuretic effect. At the level of the reproductive organs, of foremost importance are a decrease in spontaneous uterine activity of the myometrium and initiation and maintenance of secretion by the glands of the endometrium, manifested by the appearance of glycogen in the cells and glandular lumen. During this process the endometrial glands become increasingly convoluted, while the surrounding stroma is characterized by cellular hypertrophy and edema. There are also characteristic changes of the cervical mucus which undergoes dehydration and consequently loses its viscosity.

Vaginal changes consist mostly of clumping of the superficial cornified cells and the appearance of leukocytes. These changes permit the diagnosis of the presence of the corpus luteum by examination of a vaginal smear.

Menstruation appears to be the direct result of the decrease of hormonal levels. The actual "breakdown" of the endometrium is preceded by a collapse of the spiral arteries of the endometrium with hemorrhage into the lower layers and sloughing of the epithelium except for the basal layer.

Three to seven days of menstrual flow are considered normal for most women. The duration of the menstrual cycle is calculated as the interval between the first day of menstruation up to and including the day prior to the onset of the next period. Despite the varying composition of the many groups of women who have been studied, the duration of the cycle exhibits only minor discrepancies among most individuals.

In adult women, a significant number of all cycles comprise the class "28 days," whereas in adolescence variations in cycle length are more common. A similar pattern occurs toward the end of the reproductive years. Anovulatory bleeding rather than cyclic ovarian activity is a frequent cause for an irregular menstrual bleeding pattern.

The amount of blood loss during menstruation may be of clinical significance, yet it is often difficult to assess. Subjective evaluation by the patient may not be accurate, nor is the commonly practiced method of counting vaginal tampons or perineal pads. There is much variation among women in terms of their habits of changing tampons at various stages of saturation. Methods based on total iron or hemoglobin loss suggest that the total blood loss during menstruation may approximate 60 to 200 ml. Women wearing intrauterine devices often experience a greater blood loss, to the point of depletion of their iron stores.

In the presence of malnutrition, poor dietary habits (common among middle-class American teen-agers), anemias of different etiology, etc., the significance of menstrual blood loss should not be overlooked.

Dysmenorrhea The term *dysmenorrhea* is used to describe painful menstruation. It is generally accepted that strong or abnormal uterine contractions (antiperistalsis) are major etiologic factors in the discomfort experienced by the patient. Peritoneal irritation, resulting from either traction on postinflammatory adhesions or retrograde spillage of menstrual blood, may also play a role. As in all instances involving pain, several factors need to be taken into account: individual attitude toward pain, attitude and interrelation with peers and family, anxiety, etc. The symptomatology covers a wide spectrum ranging from minor abdominal cramps (the most common manifestation) to a picture of intense suffering, with severe cramps, and symptoms suggesting vagal irritation such as diarrhea, bladder tenesmus, vomiting, and fainting spells. In extreme situations, hysterical reactions may occur, particularly when fostered by overanxious, possessive, or protective parents.

The following guidelines are useful when evaluating a patient complaining of painful menstruation:

1 Menstruation following a cycle during which ovulation has taken place is more commonly associated with uterine cramps than bleeding from a proliferative endometrium—so-called anovulatory bleeding.

2 Dysmenorrhea occurring in teen-agers essentially from the onset of menstruation is usually not attributable to identifiable pathology of the pelvic organs. Abnormal uterine contractions have been demonstrated in these patients, and the assumption is usually made by a number of investigators that the etiology is psychosomatic. This assumption is based on the common association with hysterical behavior, difficulties in child-parent interaction, and the frequent finding of other symptoms generally attributed to psychosomatic disorders (headaches, constipation, poor eating habits, etc.). The terms *primary dysmenorrhea, spastic primary dysmenorrhea,* and *essential dysmenorrhea* have been used to describe this situation.

It has been claimed repeatedly that childbirth will afford relief. There are, however, no controlled studies to document this. Furthermore, it remains questionable whether it is the process of childbirth or a general adaptation to the life situation which is responsible for the change. From a practical point of view, it is difficult to consider the promise of a spontaneous cure following childbirth to an unmarried teen-ager as a valid procedure. A more practical approach consists in reassurance involving both father and mother, judicious use of certain analgesics, and the suppression of ovulation with adequate doses of estrogen administered throughout the cycle.

The sudden or gradual onset of painful menstruation following several years of menstrual bleeding with no or minimal discomfort must be interpreted differently. It is usually referred to as *secondary dysmenorrhea.* Diseases of the uterus and the surrounding pelvic structures are commonly found to be responsible for the patient's problem. Thus, a polyp or fibroid may obstruct the cervical canal, requiring more intense uterine contractions to overcome the impediment of menstrual flow. Periuterine adhesions due to infection or endometriosis may lead to a picture resembling peritoneal irritation.

A careful history establishing the time of onset and the possibility of coexisting or preceding illness is of utmost importance. Evidence for pelvic pathology must be sought by inquiring of such symptoms as excessive bleeding, changes in bleeding pattern, vaginal discharge, pain during coitus, etc. A careful pelvic examination often provides the necessary clues. Sometimes, however, it is necessary to complete the examination with an intrauterine exploration such as dilation and curettage or a hysterogram in order to rule out all pathology in the uterine cavity. In contrast to the treatment of primary dysmenorrhea which is mostly symptomatic, patients with secondary dysmenorrhea should be treated with the intent of removing the etiologic factor, i.e., infection, endometriosis.

Premenstrual tension This term is applied to a constellation of symptoms which increase in intensity for 5 to 10 days before menstruation. The most frequent complaints are a sense of abdominal bloating, breast tenderness, headache, irritability, mental depression, and an increase in weight which may be associated with edema of the legs (see Chap. 32, Edema). The abdominal distention and tight feeling may be present without any great increase in weight and often without gaseous distention of the intestines. The wide fluctuations in sex hormone levels which occur during the menstrual cycle with their important effect on electrolyte and water metabolism have been implied as providing critical "triggering" mechanisms for pathophysiologic changes in peripheral tissues as well as in the central nervous system. The exact mechanism, however, remains uncertain.

MENOPAUSE The menopause is characterized by the cessation of ovarian function and menstruation. It is a physiologic phenomenon considered by most authors as a manifestation of the aging process. From an endocrinologic point of view, the most important events are the disappearance of periodic progesterone secretion, the gradual decline of estrogen secretion by the ovary, and the increase of gonadotropins as the result of a lack of negative feedback.

Much clinical symptomatology has been attributed to the loss of ovarian function and, more specifically, the decrease of estrogen levels. The clinician should remain alert to the fact, however, that the aging process involves a considerable number of biological systems in both men and women which are not under the control of estrogens. Furthermore, adaptation of an individual in this age group to a different life style may place demands which in themselves can be anxiety-provoking or otherwise bring about reactions that may account for some of the symptoms observed in these patients.

Menopause occurs usually between the ages of 45 and 55 years. Classic symptoms are menstrual irregularity, increased spacing and cessation of menses, and gradual atrophy of estrogen-dependent anatomic structures (breasts, vulva, vagina, uterus). A precise etiology for hot flashes and palpitation, symptoms frequently experienced by patients in the menopause, has not been established.

Cultural and environmental factors seem to play an important contributory role in the etiology of such symptoms as depression, nervousness, and loss of libido. The physician must remain alert to the fact that cardiovascular disease, hyperthyroidism, and a number of other illnesses may present with symptoms superficially similar to those attributed to the menopause. Similarly, irregular uterine bleeding, although most commonly the result of decreasing ovarian function, must always be suspected to be due to uterine cancer, particularly since it is the only symptom which occurs early enough to permit cure of this disease in many instances.

AMENORRHEA Amenorrhea, or the absence of menstruation, occurs under physiologic conditions preceding menarche, in association with pregnancy and lactation, and following the menopause. A classification of patients suffering from amenorrhea into patients with primary amenorrhea (i.e., having never menstruated) and patients with secondary amenorrhea (cessation of menses for a period of time greater than 3 months) is useful because of the difference in etiologic factors found in the two groups. For example, there is a relatively high incidence of chromosomal disorders in patients with primary amenorrhea. On the other hand, "functional disorders," or the absence of clearly identifiable pathology, characterizes many patients in the group suffering from secondary amenorrhea.

The following guidelines are helpful when evaluating a patient complaining of amenorrhea. The basic requirements for normal menstruation are an intact end organ (uterus and vagina), ovarian function (the secretion of estrogen and progesterone), and an intact, functioning central nervous control system.

1 The pelvic organs can be evaluated by direct examination.
2 An assessment of ovarian function (estrogen and progesterone) can be made by evaluation of a number of endocrine-dependent end organs, i.e., vagina, cervix, uterus, breast. Abnormal ovarian function involving the

secretion of androgens is usually expressed by an increase in sebum secretion, abnormal hair growth, and in extreme cases, masculinizing features.

3 With the exception of galactorrhea, there are no clinical features which permit a ready evaluation of the function of the neuroendocrine system controlling gonadal activity. In an evaluation of the hypothalamic-pituitary ovarian axis, it becomes necessary to consider the following:
   a Lack of proper stimulation of the ovary leads to a clinically demonstrable alteration in steroid secretion (evaluation of the end organ).
   b In the presence of normal hypothalamic-pituitary function, the absence of estrogen secretion will lead to an increase of gonadotropin levels.
   c All other endocrine dysfunctions (i.e., thyroid, adrenal) and metabolic disorders which might affect transmission of the central-nervous-system signal to the ovary and/or ovarian function must be of such magnitude as to be clinically detectable. Specific laboratory tests should be used if the clinical impression suggests the possibility of endocrine or metabolic malfunction which might interfere with the control systems of the ovary and ovarian function itself.

Once adequate general health has been established by physical examination and possibly by a number of specific tests, a determination of gonadotropins will pinpoint primary ovarian failure (elevated gonadotropins) or hypothalamic-pituitary failure (low or normal gonadotropins). The latter is particularly significant when there is proof by clinical observation or laboratory testing for inadequate steroid secretion from the ovary.

Recent studies have shown that disorders of the cyclic function of the hypothalamus may be responsible for a variety of entities associated with amenorrhea. Furthermore, the use of releasing factors for luteinizing hormone is providing some hope for differentiation between hypothalamic and pituitary failure (see Chap. 89). However, diagnostic attempts to identify disorders in these latter two categories require multiple determinations of gonadotropins and are usually not within reach of most clinicians.

Among the most common disorders associated with primary amenorrhea are gonadal dysgenesis (absence of gonadal development, sometimes associated with Turner's syndrome) and agenesis of the uterus and the vagina. The first entity is characterized by absence of ovarian function and high gonadotropins, while patients with faulty development of the Müllerian system are correctly diagnosed following pelvic examination and observation of normal development of secondary sex characteristics.

Patients with hypogonadotropic hypogonadism form a third relatively common group. These individuals are characterized by a lack of secondary sexual characteristics and low gonadotropins.

Patients with secondary amenorrhea should be evaluated from the point of view of onset of their symptoms. If menstrual malfunction can be traced back to within 1 or 2 years of puberty, polycystic ovaries (Stein-Leventhal syndrome) are often present. A sudden cessation of menses at a later date should be correlated with concurring events, i.e., psychologic trauma, iatrogenic intervention, and/or clinical signs or symptoms, suggesting a major illness or malfunction responsible for secondary failure of the ovary. Patients suffering from psychogenic amenorrhea are frequently found in this group. Patients with failure to menstruate following administration of birth control pills for a long period of time (approximately 1 percent of women using oral contraception) have been described in increasing numbers, as have patients with Asherman's syndrome (intrauterine synechiae following curettage).

Individuals in whom amenorrhea is associated with a functioning tumor are in general clinically identifiable by the strong evidence for secretion of specific hormones by the neoplasm (feminizing or virilizing changes, evidence for excess excretion of corticoids, etc.).

Tumors of the central nervous system are rarely identified as cause for amenorrhea. They are more common in the prepubertal age group. In adult women, neurologic symptoms will predominate if the tumor involves structures outside the sella turcica. *Basophile* and *eosinophile* adenomas of the pituitary are associated with excess secretion of ACTH or growth hormone, respectively, and they should be suspected when evidence suggesting disturbed functions dependent on these two hormones appears. The most common pituitary tumor in patients with amenorrhea is the chromophobe adenoma, which is often associated with elevated prolactin levels and results in the symptoms of glactorrhea and amenorrhea.

ABNORMAL UTERINE BLEEDING Abnormal uterine bleeding may be associated with disorders of the endocrine system, anatomic abnormalities, neoplastic changes of the genital tract, complications of pregnancy, pelvic infections, and disorders of the clotting mechanism.

1 *Endocrine dysfunction.* Normal ovarian function is dependent upon a variety of endocrine and nonendocrine factors (see Amenorrhea above). Irregular bleeding as the result of anovulation often precedes the onset of amenorrhea. If an endocrine anomaly is suspected, a useful approach is to search for evidence indicating that ovulation is not occurring.

   In patients with ovulatory cycles, other causes than endocrine malfunction must be considered.

2 *Anatomic abnormalities* such as polyps, fibroids, or carcinoma of the cervix or uterus become causes of abnormal uterine bleeding as age increases. Simple endometrial polyps may be found in women with regular cycles as a cause of pre- and postmenstrual spotting. Fibroids tend to increase the amount of blood lost during menstruation in patients with regular cycles. Intermenstrual spotting and postcoital spotting are commonly found in patients with carcinoma of the cervix. Anovulatory periods and erratic bleeding from spotting to severe hemorrhage are seen in association with carcinoma of the endometrium.

3 Occasionally increased menstrual flow is the first symptom of leukemia or other diseases associated with *clotting disorders.* Some screening tests are therefore indicated in women where diagnostic efforts have failed to establish endocrine or anatomic anomalies.

4 *Pregnancy.* Threatened or incomplete abortions, ectopic pregnancy, and tumors of the placenta are all associated with irregular bleeding. It must be borne in mind that patients with ectopic pregnancy as well as patients about to abort may no longer have a positive result with routine laboratory tests for pregnancy. Pregnancy as a contributing factor to bleeding must thus be ruled out by careful history and physical examination.

5 *Pelvic infections.* The presence of acute or subacute pelvic inflammatory disease often leads to increased menstrual flow as well as prolonged bleeding. Ovarian function may be intact or disturbed according to the degree to which ovarian tissue is involved in the inflammatory process. Endometritis of varying etiology is frequently associated with continuous spotting. Certain forms of endometritis (tuberculosis) may, however, lead to amenorrhea as the result of the destruction of a large part of the endometrial surface and/or interference with the shedding mechanism.

There are a number of other causes of bleeding which should be kept in mind. These are midcycle bleeding (ovulation bleeding), trauma (sometimes associated with foreign bodies in the vagina), bleeding from atrophic vaginitis (postmenopausal patients) and acute vaginitis (*Trichomonas*), and finally bleeding from other sources (urethra, rectum) misinterpreted by the patient as representing vaginal bleeding.

In summary, all complaints of abnormal uterine or vaginal bleeding require utmost attention by the physician. A careful diagnostic workup to arrive at the diagnosis and to rule out a life-threatening pathology is always indicated.

REFERENCES

CHARLES D (ed): Symposium on menstrual disorders. Clin Obstet Gynecol 12:691, 1969

MARSHALL WA, TANNER JM: Variations in pattern of pubertal changes in girls. Arch Dis Child 44:291, 1969

RAKOFF AE: Endocrine mechanisms in psychogenic amenorrhea, chap. 8 in *Endocrinology and Human Behavior,* ed RP Michael, Fair Lawn, N.J.: Oxford University Press, 1968

SCHRIENER WE: The ovary, in *Clinical Endocrinology,* ed A Labhart, Berlin: Springer-Verlag, 1974

SHEARMAN RP: A physiological approach to the differential diagnosis and treatment of primary amenorrhea. J Obstet Gynaecol Br Commonw 75:1101, 1968

——, MAYES B: The investigation and treatment of amenorrhea developing after treatment with oral contraceptives. Int J Fertil 13:321, 1968

TETER J: Diagnosis and classification of the syndromes of ovarian deficiency. Med Gynaecol Sociol 4:3, 1969

51
DISTURBANCES OF SEXUAL FUNCTION

GEORGE W. THORN

GENERAL CONSIDERATIONS More and more frequently patients are consulting their family physicians with regard to problems relating to disturbances of sexual function. There are no available epidemiologic studies that would provide accurate incidence rates for the various types of sexual dysfunctions. Clinics which treat sexual problems find that women request help for sexual problems about eight times as frequently as do men, the chief complaint being failure to achieve orgasm during intercourse, followed by lack of arousal during lovemaking. Men most frequently request treatment for premature ejaculation; impotence is second. The types of sexual problems to be encountered in an individual practice are determined by the age, social class, sex, and race of one's patients and further by one's own ease and readiness to discuss sexual matters. (See also Chap. 52, Sexual Counseling.)

ALTERATIONS IN LIBIDO While the four phases of sexual response as described by Masters and Johnson appear to be similar in men and women, there is one major point of difference—the capacity of some women to experience multiple orgasms in close succession. It has been estimated that between 10 and 30 percent of mature women have never experienced an orgasm, in contrast to the fact that it is extremely rare to find an adult male who has never had an orgasm. The extreme diversity in sexual responsiveness in women has not yet been satisfactorily explained. It seems to reflect at least in part the normal distribution of physiologic patterns of female sexual response. However, as female responsiveness has been seen to change rapidly during treatment, this diversity must also be due to the strong inhibitions placed upon female responsiveness in our culture. In the absence of such restrictions, it is unknown what the typical pattern of responsiveness would be.

Loss of libido Loss of libido may occur as a result of either psychologic or somatic factors. It may be complete in the presence of serious organic disease or with advanced age. On the other hand, lost or diminished libido may occur only under particular circumstances or in relation to a particular person, indicating the predominance of psychologic factors. In instances such as these, it is not unusual for a patient to experience nocturnal penile erection and emission of semen. Although loss of libido may accompany serious endocrine disorders such as anterior pituitary deficiency, Addison's disease, or diabetic acidosis or ketosis, it is not likely to be a primary complaint of the patient under these circumstances since the impairment in general health and activity is so overwhelming. Under these circumstances, it is more likely that the patient's spouse will have noted or called attention to the difficulty. Many of the more potent tranquilizing agents appear to depress libido and interfere with penile erection. On the other hand, patients who manifest depression may show improved sexual performance as a response to antidepressive medication. Alcohol, opiates, and marijuana also appear to depress libido and potency, although by the removal of social inhibitions, they may encourage sexual activity.

For practical purposes it is important to bear in mind that the primary complaint of lost or decreased libido in male patients, in the absence of severe organic disease or advanced age, is almost certainly dependent upon emotional or psychologic disturbances.

General sexual dysfunction (frigidity) Inability on the part of women to participate in or derive a pleasurable experience from the sexual act is a distressing complaint of relatively frequent occurrence. In the past such matters were not brought to the attention of the physician, but fortunately with the changing mores of our society many women now seek medical advice.

The sexual drive of the normal woman is primarily conditioned by psychologic factors, with endocrine functions in a supporting role. The changes in sexual drive produced by alterations in hormonal level are of relatively little importance in contrast to the role of emotional and psychologic factors. In evaluation of patients with sexual complaints a detailed sexual and social history is a necessity. Many experiences in childhood can, later in life, result in incapacity for sexual pleasure. Such experiences develop a climate of fear, insecurity, and dread concerning the whole subject of sex. Couples with sexual problems frequently lack knowledge concerning the basic anatomy and physiology of the male and female genital systems. It is the duty of the physician to teach, by use of detailed diagrams of the genital system, the basic physiology of the sex act. Both partners should be present for the instruction, for there is no such thing as an uninvolved partner in a sexually dysfunctional marriage. It is important for both of the patients to discuss any problems concerning sex with the physician, either separately or together, in order to achieve any measure of success. Learning to permit sexual arousal to occur is a slow process; but by careful attention to the particular problems of each case, a good result can frequently be achieved.

Excessive libido A sudden increase in libido should suggest the possibility of temporal lobe disorders or psychosis. Physicians should also be alert to the possibility that the patient might be using stimulants, such as the amphetamines or cocaine, or that paranoia may exist.

ALTERATIONS IN POTENTIA **Impotence** Impotence implies the presence of sexual desires in a patient who cannot obtain or sustain penile erection. Impotence is rarely of endocrine origin. More frequently it accompanies a neurologic or emotional disorder. An important differentiating point is the history of the occurrence of nocturnal or early-morning erections. This implies that the neurologic and circulatory pathways involved in attaining an erection are intact and indicates that emphasis should be placed on finding a psychologic cause.

In neurologic disorders absence or impairment of parasympathetic nerve activity prevents the development of tumescence of the corpora cavernosa. Impotence is common among patients who suffer disease of the sacral cord segments and their afferent and efferent connections, e.g., cord tumor, tabes, and multiple sclerosis. Approximately one-fourth of male diabetics in the younger age group and about one-half in the fifth decade develop impotence as a consequence of diabetic polyneuritis. Loss of both sexual desire and erection may occur in hypopituitarism, hypothyroidism, and severe eunuchoidism, as well as in association with general debilitating diseases. Patients with trauma to the prostatic urethra and those who have had perineal operations frequently have reduced potentia. Malformation of the genitals such as extreme degrees of epispadias, pseudohermaphroditism, growths and edema of the penis, as well as large hernias, hydroceles, and elephantiasis may interfere with sexual function. In the majority of patients, however, impotence is of psychologic origin. Fears and phobias which arise about the sexual act, as well as feelings of guilt, may be responsible.

Priapism True priapism is a state of sustained erection of the penis not accompanied by sexual desire. It is most frequent in the third or fourth decades and is usually accompanied by pain. Two types are recognized: the sustained and the recurrent nocturnal types. Priapism may result from urethral inflammation, from new growth involving the corpora, or from systemic disease such as leukemia or sickle-cell anemia. Diseases of the spinal cord may be accompanied by penile erections, reflexly induced and sustained for long periods of time. The neural apparatus for the control of sexual function is organized through the lower spinal segments, and hence may function effectively even when completely removed from voluntary control by spinal cord lesions. Recurrent nonsustained, painful priapism is of unknown cause, although it is often associated with prostatitis. Since it frequently subsides spontaneously, the efficacy of therapy is difficult to document.

Premature ejaculation Premature ejaculation has been variously defined by: (1) length of intravaginal containment, (2) percentage of partner's orgasmic response prior to ejaculation, and (3) ejaculation which occurs before either or both partners want it to. Masters and Johnson's study and treatment of 186 men laid to rest the psychoanalytic formulation of latent hostility toward women as the etiologic agent in this condition, showing instead premature ejaculation to be a learned reaction to early coital exposures characterized as time-pressured, guilt-ridden, or with fear of apprehension. There appear to be no personality disorders characteristic of this dysfunction. Masters and Johnson report success rates of 98.8 using the "squeeze technique" to increase the period of arousal before reaching orgasm. In this instance the full cooperation of both partners is required.

Dyspareunia This term refers to pain on intercourse in women. It is complicated diagnostically by the fact that dyspareunia has a variety of subjective and objective origins that create combinations of psychophysiologic distress. Dyspareunia can be separated into those types involving superficial pain and discomfort and those complaints of severe or deep pain during intercourse. In the former case the symptoms would most likely be aching, irritation, itching, or burning in the vagina. Dyspareunia occurring at entry most frequently results from lack of lubrication; it also occurs from decrease in the elasticity and size of the vaginal canal as a result of atrophy or senile or radiation vaginitis or vulvitis, or secondary to mycotic or bacterial infections. Sensitivity reactions to chemicals found in contraceptive creams, foams, and jellies, to rubber in certain diaphragms and condoms, and to frequent douching with commercial preparations can be sufficiently irritating to produce chronic dyspareunia.

Deeper pain or pain after entry may be due to scars secondary to vaginal repair, senile vaginitis, vaginal atresia, or pelvic inflammatory disease, endometriosis, retrodisplacement of the uterus, urethritis, cystitis, or proctitis.

Vaginismus refers to the involuntary spastic contraction

of the muscle group in the outer third of the vaginal barrel in response to perceived attempts at vaginal penetration. Multiple etiologic factors include prior sexual trauma, excessive fears (e.g., pregnancy, cancer), strict religious orthodoxy, and severe dyspareunia. Treatment consists of clinical demonstration of the existence of vaginismus to both partners, an explanation of the involuntary nature of the constriction, and the use of Hegar dilators in graduated sizes by the couple. Masters and Johnson reported successful treatment of all 27 women referred to them for vaginismus.

REFERENCES

BURNS E, THOMPSON I: Priapism, in *Urology,* 3d ed., eds MF Campbell, JH Harrison, Philadelphia: Saunders, 1970, p. 531

ENGLISH OS: The psychosomatic approach in urology, chap. 52 in *Urology,* 3d ed., eds MF Campbell, JH Harrison, Philadelphia: Saunders, 1970

GRACE DA, WINTER CC: Priapism: An appraisal of management of twenty-three patients. J Urol 99:301, 1968

KAPLAN HS: *The New Sex Therapy,* New York: Quadrangle, 1974

MASTERS WH, JOHNSON VE: *Human Sexual Inadequacy,* Boston: Little, Brown, 1970

SCHÖFFLING K et al: Disorders of sexual function in male diabetics. Diabetes 12:519, 1963

52
SEXUAL COUNSELING

PETER REICH

ROLE OF THE FAMILY PHYSICIAN AND INTERNIST

The present-day openness about sexuality does not necessarily mean that persons are better educated on sexual matters. In fact, openness may have led to an increase in misconceptions, such as unreal expectations of sexual performance, and may also have led to an increased awareness of complaints and dissatisfactions. However, this openness does allow patients to discuss problems that they might previously have concealed, thus challenging the physician to provide expertise in this area.

Patients will naturally turn to their personal physician when distressing sexual problems emerge or when they need help with long-term difficulties. For them the physician is recognized as a diagnostician and source of health information, as well as a guide to more specialized care, be it from urologist, gynecologist, psychiatrist, sex counselor, or even attorney, if indicated. In addition to a basic knowledge of sexual anatomy, physiology, and behavior, including recent advances in research on the human sexual response, the physician needs to know the effects of illnesses, operative procedures, and medications upon sexual function. Fortunately, most medical schools now include courses on sexuality in their undergraduate curricula. Postgraduate courses are also widely available, and articles on the medical aspects of sexuality are appearing more frequently in medical journals.

Regardless of his expertise, the physician's attitudes may undermine his usefulness as a sexual counselor. Patients

can sense subtle indications of personal bias in the physician, and whether sexual complaints are reported has been shown to depend to a large extent upon the physician's receptivity. Studies indicate that many practicing physicians feel that they are not competent to deal with sexual problems. Others fear that sexual counseling will be too time-consuming or will lead to an excessive involvement with emotional issues. The physician's own moral and ethical positions or his personal discomfort with areas of sexuality, such as homosexuality or sexual deviance, may inhibit communication. In addition, the potentially seductive aspects of an open discussion of sexuality can be disturbing to both patient and physician. Problems of communication across ethnic, racial, economic, or educational lines also take on special significance.

The objective medical approach to sexual symptoms will reduce tensions and will enable both the patient and the physician to deal with sensitive material. The physician does not need to be a psychotherapist or an expert on sexual behavior to be helpful. Patients who seek sexual advice from physicians are likely to be concerned about medical issues. Often sexual problems reflect fears and misconceptions, and the objective evaluation of the symptoms leads to relief without further treatment. Thus the responsibility of the physician is to establish an accurate and complete diagnosis, including both physiologic and psychologic factors, and in the context of the patient's own background and life style to evaluate the significance of the problem and to know the range of treatments that are available.

Approach to the Patient

Physicians may be called upon to provide sexual counseling in a wide variety of medical and human situations. For example, they may encounter adolescent fears of homosexuality or of sexual inadequacy, marital problems that present with sexual incompatibility, sexual inhibitions after surgery or after myocardial infarction, post-partum frigidity, impotency associated with diabetes, ejaculatory disturbances after prostatectomy, and loss of libido in psychologic depression. Although tensions, anxieties, preconceptions and attitudes, and interpersonal factors must be taken into account, the assessment of a sexual problem is similar to the assessment of a problem involving any other system. A complete history, careful attention to multiple determinants, and thorough evaluation of the patient as a person and of the context of the symptoms will yield a working diagnosis that will enable the physician either to treat the patient or to make an appropriate referral. A detailed guide to the assessment of sexual function has been published by the Group for the Advancement of Psychiatry. Similar guides can be found in standard texts of psychiatry and of obstetrics and gynecology. It is useful to have such a framework in mind when obtaining a sexual history.

More often than in other areas of medicine, the physician needs to take an active role in initiating the discussion of sexual matters. In one survey it was found that the incidence of sexual problems reported by patients increased from 7.9 to 14 percent when the physician routinely asked about the sexual symptoms in the review of systems. In those conditions where sexual problems occur frequently, such as in gynecologic and urogenital surgery, cord injury, ileostomies and colostomies, myocardial infarction, diabetes, and various neurologic conditions, the physician has the responsibility to assess sexual function. Even when the patient initiates the discussion, an active inquiry by the physician will enable the patient to discuss specific and intimate details.

Reassurances about confidentiality may be necessary during the discussion of sexual matters even though such confidentiality is already assumed in the doctor-patient relationship. Confidentiality may be especially important when the physician is also treating other members of the family or when the patient needs to discuss extramarital, deviant, or extralegal behavior.

It is well to keep the dignity of the patient in mind as the history is being taken by observing such simple practices as using scientific words for sexual parts and sexual activities instead of using vernacular or slang expressions in a mistaken effort to put the patient at ease, and by refraining from jokes or other informal remarks even though the patient may try to engage in them himself. Comments that may seem casual to the physician tend to live on in the patient's mind.

While the initial inquiry into sexual matters requires tact and timing, the need to protect the patient from embarrassment should not be overemphasized. Physicians' anticipation of discomfort may lead them to choose an evasive route of inquiry while patients might appreciate a direct question. Some patients may allude to sexual problems with idiomatic phrases, such as "changing nature" or "problems in relationships," and, unless the physician is sensitive to the patient's feelings and language, the reference may be missed and the patient may assume that the physician is not interested in further information. Sometimes sexual problems appear indirectly through other complaints relating to the urogenital system. Much of the tension and uncertainty in obtaining a sexual history can be avoided by including questions about sexual physiology, practices, and satisfaction in the systems review.

The sexual problems of elderly patients are not well understood by most physicians. Physicians may refrain from asking questions because they have incorrectly assumed that sexual satisfactions can no longer be achieved as a result of the aging process. At times the patient will silently accept a loss of sexual function because of misconceptions about the effects of illness or of aging. Depression may be a factor in such instances. Here the questions of the physician, coupled with some reassuring statements about the tendencies of many persons to assume mistakenly they will never be able to enjoy sexual relations again, will bring the issue into the open and awaken new hopes in the patient.

Once a sexual complaint has been elicited, it is important to obtain a detailed history of specific behavior. Terms for sexual disorders may be misused by patients or may be exaggerated or misunderstood. Many sexual complaints reflect misconceptions, ignorance, or fears, and the problems prove to be nonexistent when the behavior is explored in detail. Patients tend to overestimate or to underestimate the extent of a problem, depending upon their psychologic orientation. For example, one woman believed herself to be frigid because her sexual partner, for neurotic reasons of his own, was comparing her in a disparaging way to his previous partners. Much can be learned from the first instance of a sexual problem, from the pattern of behavior since the onset of symptoms, and from inquiring whether the problem is present consistently or varies with the circumstances or nature of the sexual practice.

In every disorder there is always a complex interaction between the physical and the emotional; and every sexual symptom needs to be evaluated in the context of the relationships between the patient and the sexual partners, or in the context of the sexual practices and attitudes of the patient. A past history, including early experiences, attitudes of parents, and attitudes toward childhood sexuality, development, marriage, and pregnancy may be relevant. The relationship of sexual function to general health is always a consideration.

A general physical examination with special attention to an examination of the genitalia is a part of the evaluation of all sexual complaints. At times the patient will conceal or be unaware of abnormalities of the genitalia. On the other hand, even sophisticated patients may harbor irrational misconceptions or feelings of shame about their bodies, and they may need concrete reassurance about the adequacy of their genital apparatus. Unless the physician has pursued the process of evaluating the medical aspects of the complaint, the patient may disregard reassurances that there is no medical basis, if indeed the physician has decided that the problem is psychogenic.

Appropriate laboratory tests to screen for systemic illnesses are indicated along with the specific tests for various endocrinopathies, neurologic conditions, and other systemic disorders that may present with sexual problems (see Chap. 51). Attention to the mental status, including assessment of mood, affect, thought content, judgment, and reality testing, will enable the physician to determine whether the sexual symptom is an aspect of a mental disorder (see Chap. 343). Rarely sexual problems, especially loss of libido, may be the presenting sign of a disorder of the central nervous system; an examination of mental status can pick up early signs of dementia or other manifestations of organic brain conditions.

An understanding of the daily habits of a patient may provide important clues to diagnosis. Fatigue, anxiety, and stress, as well as use of alcohol, drugs, and medications, can influence sexual function. In addition, traumatic events, such as automobile accidents, surgical procedures, or the illness or death of another person, may exert acute or chronic effects on sexual behavior.

DIAGNOSTIC CONSIDERATIONS

The specific disorders of sexual function are discussed in Chap. 51. All of them can vary in severity, from complete loss of function under all circumstances to relatively minor disturbances in specific circumstances or with specific partners. Patients also may vary in their reactions to sexual symptoms, some ignoring or concealing severe disability, others reacting with panic to minor disturbances.

The first consideration is whether the condition is primarily organic or psychogenic. In clinics devoted to sexual counseling, the complaints of 10 to 20 percent of the patients are manifestations of organic problems, while the complaints of the remaining 80 to 90 percent are psychogenic. When significant organic factors are present, a useful distinction can be made between sexual symptoms that arise *directly* from organic disorders, such as structural disorders of the urogenital system, neurologic disorders affecting the innervation of the sexual organs, and endocrinopathies that influence sexual physiology, and those that are *secondary* to changes in general health, such as sexual disturbances associated with rheumatoid arthritis, malignancies, renal failure, and other chronic diseases, and also those that occur with acute debilitating conditions, such as myocardial infarction, major surgery, and hepatitis. With primary organic disorders, patients may need counseling to help them adjust to permanent losses of sexual function if medical measures cannot reverse the process. When sexual disturbances are secondary to changes in health, the effects of organic factors are often overemphasized by both the patient and the physician. Although libido may be affected by general loss of vitality and by toxic and metabolic factors, the sexual disturbances associated with physical illnesses are often the expression of hopelessness, depression, or anxiety and may be perpetuated by the psychologic factors long after the organic problems have disappeared.

The physician can also make significant diagnostic distinctions among psychogenic sexual disturbances. *Primary* psychogenic disturbances, those that have been present since puberty, can be distinguished from *secondary* disturbances, those that represent decompensations from previous adequate levels of function. The former often reflect chronic and deep-seated sexual conflicts. When a patient seeks help for a chronic disturbance, the key diagnostic issue may be why he has come for help at this particular time. A secondary decompensation may be the presenting symptom of a psychologic defeat, loss, or a disturbance in a relationship. Some sexual problems occur in connection with life stresses or transitions, such as retirement, pregnancy, work crises, or bereavement. The prognosis is good providing that the underlying issues are recognized and acknowledged. A disproportionate focus on sexual symptoms can actually perpetuate the problem by reinforcing anxiety about sexual performance.

Some sexual disorders are manifestations of major mental disorders and will respond only to treatment directed at the mental disorders themselves. Diminished sexual responsiveness, impotence, or ejaculatory disturbances may be indications of depression. Bizarre sexual complaints with increased or diminished sexual activity can indicate incipient psychosis. The strange qualities of the symptoms or the intensity of the associated feelings may be the best diagnostic clue. Hypersexuality can occur with the onset of mania. It also may appear as a depressive equivalent, especially in postmenopausal women. Neuroses are often associated with sexual inhibitions.

Alcohol may play a significant role in potency disturbances. Often the first episode of secondary impotence is associated with the use of alcohol, and the midlife depressive syndrome that is often related to secondary impotence may be further complicated by alcohol abuse. Barbiturates and opiates also can cause reduced libido and impotence. Antihypertensive agents, tranquilizers, hypnotics, analgesics, and sedatives all may influence sexual function in the male.

Sexual disturbances may develop after traumatic incidents. For example, impotence can develop after cystoscopic examination or after vasectomy, even though neither procedure has any direct physiologic effect upon potency. An automobile accident can have a similar effect. Pregnancy, contraceptive difficulties, casual but disturbing sexual encounters, and a host of other emotionally significant episodes may cause sudden changes in sexual functioning. The patient may not be aware of the importance of such episodes or may be reluctant to discuss them.

The diligent physician may inadvertently overdiagnose sexual disturbances. Most patients have self-doubts and sexual dissatisfactions even though they are functioning adequately. It is well to have in mind the concept of a threshold of disturbance to separate the normal vicissitudes from the problems that require treatment.

TREATMENT APPROACHES

Some sexual problems will resolve themselves during the evaluation process, especially if it extends over several visits. With those that persist, the physician must decide whether to treat the patients or to refer them elsewhere. Often a brief attempt at office counseling will enable the physician to make this decision. Generally the secondary or reactive psychogenic disorders are more amenable to brief counseling, especially when they occur in response to stress. Sexual problems related to physical illnesses are also appropriately handled by the general physician who also treated the physical disorder.

The technique for counseling cannot be mapped in a formal way. Sufficient time, a relaxed atmosphere, and genuine interest by the physician are necessary. The patient should be encouraged to tell the full story with careful attention to the circumstances surrounding the onset of symptoms, to the attitudes of the patient and partner, to the nature of the patient's relationships, and to factors that might be leading to anxiety or depression. Although it may be necessary to review the physical details of the patient's sexual practices, resolution of symptoms may occur with only indirect reference to sexual techniques. Sexual inadequacies often produce anxiety that in turn leads to further defeats and to inhibition of libido. Without reduction of anxiety and lifting of depression, the process cannot be reversed.

Some physicians will choose not to attempt sexual counseling, while others find it to be a satisfying aspect of medical practice. In either case, it is important for physicians to be familiar with the resources in their communities and to understand the capabilities and limitations of various treatment approaches. Physicians usually have referral relationships with gynecologists, urologists, and psychiatrists. In addition, many communities now have family services and counseling services. Referral should be tailored to the nature of the problem and to the life style and personality of the patient. Some patients would consider discussing the intimate details of a sexual problem only with a gynecologist or urologist. Others would appreciate being directed to a reputable clinic where the new direct behavioral approaches to the treatment of sexual dysfunctions are available.

Referral is often a difficult transition for a patient because it implies turning to a stranger after having confided in a physician who has understood the problem. The patient who comes eagerly to a consultant may lose his motivation when the consultant refers him to a colleague. Some physicians advocate having counselors associated with them in their offices. This system has the advantage of maintaining the personal relationship between counselors and physicians but has the disadvantage of encouraging physicians to rely on counselors for the evaluation of emotional problems rather than carrying through the diagnostic phase themselves. If physicians keep in touch with patients through the process of therapy, it will enable them to learn about the efficacy of the treatment program and to provide support and reassurance.

A few examples will illustrate some of the principles involved in the treatment of patients with sexual disorders.

Patient A. R., a 56-year-old attorney who had recently suffered a myocardial infarct, complained to his physician of loss of libido. He was an energetic, competitive, aggressive, self-made man, who enjoyed athletics and was "top" man in his firm. The physician asked him about the details of his daily life and found that the loss of libido was only one of many inhibitions. He avoided arguments, stopped playing handball, cut his workload, and was losing weight. He also reported insomnia and anorexia. Further questioning revealed fears of sudden death and the fatalistic belief that his days were numbered. He assumed that strict reduction of activity was mandatory. His wife shared his fears and urged him to avoid stress. Together they had decided not to have sexual relations during the period immediately after his heart attack, and now he had no desire to resume. In the course of several sessions of counseling the physician reassured him that his fears were exaggerated, that many patients with heart trouble experienced similar feelings, clarified the extent of his disability, and helped him and his wife to plan realistic resumption of many of his previous activities, including sexual relations.

Patient L. D., a 26-year-old woman, consulted a physician because of frigidity. She had left her husband after 6 years of an unfulfilling marriage, and had sought satisfaction in a series of brief affairs. The interview revealed her to be a restless, competitive, chronically dissatisfied person who was unhappy in her career and who experienced disappointment in her close relationships. After careful evaluation of the physical aspects of her sexual difficulties and experiences, the physician decided that her problem reflected long-standing psychologic conflicts and referred her to a psychiatrist.

Patient M. B., a 34-year-old salesman, complained to his physician of impotence. He was a nervous, insecure, ineffectual man who worked for his older brother. His wife, an active real estate broker, had become withdrawn and bitter. His two adolescent children were involved in minor delinquency. The impotence was confined to his relationship with his wife; in a recent extramarital affair he had performed adequately. He said he was unable to satisfy his wife in any way; she was either withdrawn or overly demanding. The physician determined that the impotency had no organic basis and because of the involved nature of the family conflicts referred the patient to a family service agency where the family could be worked with as a unit. Here the wife was found to be depressed and received psychiatric treatment. Later the patient reported that when her depression improved, his potency returned.

In another instance, patient C. W., a woman with breast cancer, was asked about her marriage. She told her physician that her husband had stopped having sexual relations with her when it was discovered that she had metastatic disease. The physician then asked to see the husband. He confessed to an extramarital affair and the wish to leave his wife. He also was experiencing irrational anger at his wife and feelings of shame and worthlessness. It emerged that the marriage had been an unusually close one and that he could not bear the anticipation of his wife's death. Sexual contact with her reminded him of his impending loss. His anger and the affair were responses to grief. The physician met with him for several sessions. By avoiding a moralistic position and by indicating that many spouses of patients with serious diseases have similar feelings and may even find solace in extramarital relationships, the physician helped him to overcome his shame and to share his grief. The process brought dramatic relief, and with occasional contact with the physician he was able to remain with his wife and be helpful to her throughout her terminal illness.

MARITAL COUNSELING BY THE PHYSICIAN

Almost invariably the evaluation of sexual problems leads to some attention to marital or other sexual relationships. Counseling that focuses primarily on these relationships has been designated *marital counseling.* Instead of the usual medical relationship, which emphasizes the individual patient, the treatment in marital counseling involves both partners visiting the physician together, although each may be seen separately at times.

The specific nature of the marital counseling will depend upon the complaints or upon the time of life of the couple. The main requisite for physicians is a willingness to set aside time for this kind of responsibility and to develop an interest in the functional health of their patients beyond the specific issues raised by disease. The stresses and transitions in the early years of a marriage should be appreciated as well as the pressures children exert. In later years, job problems and conflicts over roles may emerge, as well as the "empty nest" syndrome, then menopausal and midlife issues and the male-depressive syndrome as horizons close in and the realities of aging appear.

It is well to know that most marital problems are not due to sexual difficulties, although sexual problems may be the leading edge, especially in our modern climate where sexual adjustment is so widely publicized. Sexual satisfaction is dependent on the broader aspects of the relationship between partners and on mental and physical health. It is to these deeper levels that the alert physician should probe during marriage counseling. In this sense, the more specific counseling about sexual problems is really dependent upon the successful outcome of marriage counseling. Early in the approach the physician should assess the state of motivation of both partners. If one partner is determined to break up the marriage, the counseling may consist of communicating this to the other partner and perhaps advising legal assistance. On the other hand, apparent determination to seek divorce by either partner needs to be evaluated because it may mask depression, a paranoid reaction, or a hidden problem that is being avoided by flight, such as shame over an affair, fear, illness, or personal failure.

In marital counseling, as with other medical counseling, it is well to avoid giving direct advice about interpersonal relationships. By defining the problem, the physician may enable the patient to arrive at a decision on a course of action. By taking sides in family conflicts or by espousing an ethical position, physicians can inadvertently introduce their own bias or can allow themselves to be manipulated by one of the marital partners.

The internist or family physician is in a strategic position to provide effective marital counseling. As preventive medicine gains importance, marital counseling can provide physicians with great professional satisfaction.

REFERENCES

ABSE DW et al (eds): *Marital and Sexual Counseling in Medical Practice,* 2d ed., Hagerstown, Md.: Harper & Row, 1974

FREEDMAN AM et al (eds): Normal and abnormal sexuality, chap. 24 in *Comprehensive Textbook of Psychiatry,* vol. 2, 2d ed., Baltimore: Williams & Wilkins, 1975, p. 1349

LEVINE SB: Marital sexual dysfunction: Ejaculation disturbances. Ann Intern Med 84:575, 1976

MASTERS WH, JOHNSON VE: *Human Sexual Inadequacy,* Boston: Little, Brown, 1970

TAYLOR RW: Aspects of sexual medicine. Some of the commoner sexual disorders. II. Problems mainly affecting the woman. Br Med J 3:31, 1975

VINCENT C (ed): *Human Sexuality in Medical Education and Practice,* Springfield, Ill.: Charles C Thomas, 1968

53
INFERTILITY AND FERTILITY CONTROL

MELVIN L. TAYMOR

INFERTILITY

DEFINITION Infertility may be defined as the inability to conceive during the course of normal sexual activity. It is generally held that a marriage should not be considered infertile until a year of unprotected coitus has been allowed to pass. However, each couple's problems should be judged individually, and diagnosis and treatment instituted at an earlier or later date as indicated.

ETIOLOGY The two fundamental concepts to be kept in mind are (1) the multiplicity of etiologic factors and (2) the equal responsibility of male and female partners. To delineate these possible factors working either singly or in concert, one need only review the pathways of conception in male and female and the disorders of these pathways that may ensue.

Deficiency of sperm production in quantity and quality accounts for the majority of the *male's* contribution to the problem of infertility. Sperm production may be adversely affected by congenital influences such as germinal aplasia or cryptorchidism, by hormonal deficiencies of the pituitary or thyroid glands, by infection such as mumps orchitis, and by environmental factors such as nutritional deficiencies, noxious chemicals and drugs, radiation, excess local heat, and altitude. There is evidence from animal studies that hereditary factors may play a role in disturbances of the male gamete. Often the cause is not ascertainable by diagnostic methods available at present. Sperm transport is affected by congenital malformations, surgical trauma, and infections. Impotency, an important factor in many cases, commonly has a psychologic basis, although local infection or general systemic disorders may play a contributory role.

Defects in the *female* are related to production of ova and interference with their union with spermatozoa. Vaginal causes are organic or functional. Very often these causes are a combination of organic and psychologic factors. The obstruction may be due to an unruptured hymen, or it may be functional and due to hypertrophy and contraction of the levator ani muscles. Vaginitis itself is not a serious cause of infertility except in its role as a temporary deterrent to coitus. The cervix is one of the most important areas of obstruction to the passage of sperm. During the few days prior to ovulation the endocervical glands secrete a thin, watery mucus that is beneficial to sperm survival and migration. Infection or estrogen deficiency may decrease the quality of the mucus. Too often the offender is an overzealous physician who cauterizes the cervix too deeply and destroys the endocervical glands. Uterine abnormalities are not a common cause of infertility. Infertility can be associated with an anomaly such as bicornate, or double, uterus. Uterine fibroids are more likely to result in repeated abortions rather than the failure to conceive. Tubal occlusion is usually secondary to gonorrheal salpingitis. Bacterial salpingitis, secondary to pelvic peritonitis, appendicitis, abortion, or instrumentation, is more likely to result in partial blockage of the fibrated end of the tube. Nongonorrheal infection is also more likely to result in what is called the *peritoneal factor.* In this condition adhesions may develop between the tube and ovary, or fixation of the ovary may occur. Under these circumstances the chances of union between the sperm and egg are significantly reduced. In addition to infection, the peritoneal factor may be due to endometriosis. Hormonal or endocrine factors are all-important; these may result in deficient corpus luteum function and absence of ovulation.

Immunologic factors may play a significant role in some cases of unexplained infertility.

Finally, emotional factors may play a vital role by interfering with ovulation or by initiating tubal spasm or dyspareunia. However, the fact should be stressed that more often than not, the state of infertility with its accompanying diagnostic and therapeutic maneuvers is more likely to produce serious emotional reactions than are primary emotional factors likely to produce infertility.

TREATMENT The treatment of any defects, minor or major, in either the husband or the wife should be carried out concomitantly so that the total infertility potential of the couple will be raised to an optimum level.

In the *male* with azoospermia, in whom spermatogenesis is normal as shown by testicular biopsy, and in whom a block has been demonstrated, epididymovasostomy can result in return of fertility in 10 to 20 percent of cases. When hormonal studies reveal a deficiency of pituitary gonadotropin, an attempt should be made to rule out various causes of pituitary insufficiency, e.g. pituitary tumors. If no tumor is found, then treatment with human chorionic gonadotropin [5,000 units anterior pituitary-like (APL) extract intramuscularly twice weekly for 2 to 6 months] is indicated. Injections of human menopausal gonadotropins, and more recently of luteinizing-hormone-releasing hormone, have been helpful where there is pituitary or hypothalamic dysfunction. However, sperm deficiencies not associated with a specific pituitary or hypothalamic defect will not respond to pituitary or hypothalamic hormones. Azoospermia or severe oligospermia will not respond in any significant degree to the administration of hormones, vitamins, thyroid preparations, or diet unless a specific deficiency can be demonstrated. In the present state of knowledge, little can be offered in the vast majority of cases of azoospermia or severe oligospermia.

This degree of pessimism should not be carried over to the infertile male with moderate degree of oligospermia (10 to 30 million sperms per ml) or to the male partner of an infertile couple with only a moderately lowered sperm count (30 to 60 million sperms per ml), particularly if one considers the "couple-as-a-unit" concept of infertility. A modest improvement in the sperm count or motility combined with attention to the factors in the female partner may raise the fertility of the couple above a critical level. Avoidance of excess alcohol and tobacco, sufficient sleep and exercise, an optimum diet, adjustment of local excesses of heat, administration of thyroid preparations in minor degrees of hypofunction—all these singly or together may prove of definite benefit. A varicocele has been shown to be a contributing factor in oligospermia, and high ligation of the varicocele has been shown to improve sperm count and quality in a significant number of cases.

In the *female* specific attention should be directed to the cervical factor by correction of unfavorable coital habits, correction of retroversion of the uterus by a pessary, improvement in quality and quantity of preovulatory mucus by the daily administration of small dosages of estrogen (0.1 mg diethylstilbestrol daily for three or four cycles), by the use of a plastic cervical cap, and by the correction of cervicitis by systemic and local antibiotics or by cervical cauterization. Cauterization must be conservative lest more harm than good be produced by cervical stenosis or obliteration of mucus-secreting glands. When cervical stenosis is found, dilation under anesthesia is of definite value. A positive culture of *Mycoplasma* from the cervix should be treated with an appropriate antibiotic, usually tetracycline, 500 mg four times a day for 10 days. Because mycoplasma organisms may reside in the male prostate without symptoms, the male partner should be treated similarly and simultaneously.

Attempts to overcome tubal occlusion by repeated insufflations, diathermy, and high dosage of estrogen occasionally meet with success. Plastic repair of tubes or cornual implantation is followed by success in only 10 to 20 percent of cases. Surgery for tube-ovarian blockade, due to ovaries fixed by endometriosis, peritubal or periovarian adhesions, but associated with essentially normal tubes, results in a higher percentage of success. Infrequent ovulation accompanied by gross irregularity will respond to thyroid preparations when specifically indicated and to the correction of a specific dietary or vitamin deficiency. However, thyroid deficiency occurs very infrequently in a series of infertility problems, and thyroid should not be used empirically. Ovulation accompanied by an inadequate luteal phase should be treated with progesterone preparations (medroxyprogesterone, 2.5 mg daily for 10 days) or injections of human chorionic gonadotropin (HCG, 1,000 units intramuscularly every other day for five doses). Treatment should begin on the fifth or sixth day after the midcycle rise in the basal body temperature. Because luteal-phase deficiencies have been found to be associated with lowered FSH levels in the first half of the cycle, clomiphene citrate, 50 to 100 mg from days 5 to 9 of the cycle, can be utilized.

When absence of ovulation is caused by a specific defect in thyroid function, nutrition, adrenal function, or the psyche, correction of these defects often improves the condition. When amenorrhea or anovulation is caused by gonadotropin deficiency, efforts should first be made to diagnose and treat the cause. The amenorrhea itself and associated infertility can be treated effectively by the administration of gonadotropins, high in FSH and LH activity, prepared from the urine of postmenopausal females (HMG). The usual dosage is 150 to 200 FSH units administered intramuscularly daily for 5 to 12 days. When there is evidence of follicular activity, as indicated by increased levels of estrogen in the urine or increasing fern formation in cervical mucus, 8,000 IU of HCG is administered. Each patient responds differently. Overstimulation can result in enlarged cystic ovaries and multiple pregnancies, so the condition of each patient should be followed carefully. Polycystic ovaries are most susceptible to massive enlargement and possible rupture. Daily measurement of urinary estrogen excretion or estrogen levels in the blood probably provides the safest control of therapy.

Clomiphene citrate, a chemical closely related to stilbestrol, also can stimulate ovulation, and usually should be utilized before gonadotropin therapy is attempted. Clomiphene works by replacing estrogen at the level of the hypothalamus where the estrogen is inhibiting FSH and LH release. Therefore, following the administration of clomiphene, FSH and LH rise, follicular development occurs, and estrogen secretion increases. This in turn triggers the midcycle surge of LH that brings about ovulation. Since patients vary in their degree of hypothalamic pituitary hypofunction, the safest approach is to begin with 50 mg daily for 5 days, gradually increasing the dosage by 50-mg increments. Once a dose level is reached that produces an ovulatory response as noted by the basal body temperature chart, this dose is maintained monthly until pregnancy occurs. Doses as high as 200 mg per day for 5 days have been recommended in resistant cases. Clomiphene should be used with caution in patients suspected of having polycystic ovaries.

Initial reports with luteinizing-hormone-releasing hormone in ovulation induction have been disappointing, but on an experimental basis, it now appears probable that higher doses than those previously used, that is, 500 mIU SC b.i.d. for 10 days, can result in sufficient follicular maturation to bring about normal ovulation.

Psychotherapy is of value in improving the coital habits of the couple, in reducing tubal spasm, and in correcting some deficiencies of hormonal nature. Finally, the manner and attitude of the physician play a role in the outcome by preventing undue feelings of guilt and depression from gaining the upper hand, and by instilling sufficient hope and fortitude to allow the couple to carry through with the tedious and sometimes painful diagnostic testing and therapeutic maneuvers.

FERTILITY CONTROL

INDICATIONS The control of fertility is required when there is a medical contraindication to pregnancy or when a couple desires to avoid conception.

REVIEW OF PHYSIOLOGY A review of the anatomic and physiologic factors involved in reproduction in both the male and female will reveal the many areas that are vulnerable to an attack on normal reproduction.

In the female the ovulatory cycle results from dynamic and integrated shifts in neural impulses, hormonal flow, and tissue growth. Hormones from the hypothalamus (gonadotropin-releasing hormone) stimulate the release of gonadotropins, follicle-stimulating hormone and luteinizing hormone, which in turn causes ovulation and the secretion of the ovarian steroid hormones, estrogen and progesterone.

From the viewpoint of control of conception, these ovarian steroid hormones have a negative feedback effect on the flow of releasing hormones and gonadotropins from the hypothalamus and pituitary. Thus, exogenously administered estrogen or progesterone in adequate dosage, singly or in combination, can inhibit ovulation. Exogenous progesterone has other antifertility effects in that it may affect the normal fallopian tube contractility, alter the endometrial histology, or cause cervical secretions to be unreceptive to sperm penetration.

Another approach concerns the ability of the endometrium to nourish the fertilized gamete, i.e., implantation. Intrauterine devices are believed to work by altering endometrial histology so that implantation does not occur.

In the male the vulnerable areas are spermatogenesis and the transport system.

PHYSIOLOGIC REGULATION The attempt to avoid coitus around the fertile period (rhythm method) has been utilized for years. Lack of success is due to variability of ovulation and longevity of sperm once in the female genital tract. Recent attempts to instruct individuals in the assessment of the characteristic of preovulatory cervical mucus suggest that some improvement in this method may be possible.

TABLE 53-1
Tests for infertility

I In the male.
- *A* Routine.
  - *1* Semen analysis. The semen is delivered into a clean glass container by withdrawal or masturbation. The following characteristics are considered normal:
    - *a* Volume—3 to 5 ml.
    - *b* Sperm count—above 60 million per ml is unquestionably normal, below 30 million per ml unquestionably indicates reduced fertility. The significance of counts between 30 million and 60 million depends upon the quality of motility and the degree of fertility in the female partner. A highly fertile female would be more susceptible to a count of borderline fertility.
    - *c* Motility—40 percent or more still actively motile 4 to 5 h after collection.
    - *d* Morphology—at least 60 percent of the spermatozoa should be of normal size and shape.
  - *2* Examination of prostatic smear—excess leukocytes indicate that infection may play a contributory role.
- *B* Special tests—for the male with reduced fertility as indicated by semen analysis.
  - *1* Evaluation of thyroid function.
  - *2* Testicular biopsy—in most cases this will result in a definitive diagnosis. In only a few cases, however, will it demonstrate a remediable defect.
  - *3* Urinary gonadotropins—these may be low in pituitary deficiency. Excretion is high in primary gonadal failure.
  - *4* Sex chromatin determination.

II In the female.
- *A* Routine.
  - *1* Postcoital test—examination of the cervical mucus for its preovulatory qualities of clarity, spinnbarkeit (ability of the mucus to form a thread 5 to 10 cm in length when stretched between slide and cover slip), ferning (ability of the mucus to form fernlike pattern when dried and examined under low power of microscope), and for the number of viable spermatozoa 8 to 12 h after coitus.
    - *a* Good test—more than 20 active spermatozoa per high-power field.
    - *b* Fair test—5 to 20 spermatozoa per high-power field.
    - *c* Poor test—less than 5 spermatozoa per high-power field. A poor postcoital test in the presence of good preovulatory mucus suggests a semen deficiency, a deficiency of the coital method, or malposition of the cervix. A poor postcoital test combined with poor mucus in the preovulatory phase and a normal semen analysis indicates a hostile cervix either on an inflammatory or an endocrine basis.
  - *2* The evaluation of tubal patency—initially by insufflation with carbon dioxide (Rubin test) and followed at a later date by hysterosalpingography in those cases which show failure of carbon dioxide to pass or who fail to conceive after an interval of time despite a normal Rubin test.
  - *3* Evaluation of ovulation and hormonal factors by:
    - *a* Measurement of basal body temperature, which characteristically shows a sustained rise after ovulation. Studies have shown that actual ovulation may occur as long as 2 days before or 2 days after the beginning of the temperature rise. The value of the temperature chart as an exact indicator of ovulation timing for purposes of timing coitus or insemination treatments can be overestimated.
    - *b* Endometrial biopsy with the demonstration of secretory changes in the endometrium is valid evidence that ovulation has occurred. The presence of endometrium out of phase with the time of biopsy is evidence of a progestational deficiency.
- *B* Special tests should be carried out when indicated.
  - *1* Evaluation of thyroid function.
  - *2* Endocrine assays, such as urinary gonadotropin and 17-ketosteroid determination, in cases of anovulation or inadequate luteal function.
  - *3* Further studies of ovulation timing utilizing vaginal or urinary smears and studies of cervical mucus.
  - *4* Endoscopy, either laparoscopy or culdoscopy, to detect early endometriosis, pelvic adhesions interfering with tubal ovarian functions, or polycystic ovaries.
  - *5* Immune test when semen quality is good and postcoital test is poor.
  - *6* Cervical culture for *Mycoplasma*—when available.

MECHANICAL METHODS Foam, condoms, and diaphragms, which prevent the sperm from reaching the female genital tract, have the advantage of not interfering with normal physiology and thus are accompanied by negligible side effects and complications. However, the relatively high failure rates make these methods less than ideal.

HORMONAL CONTRACEPTIVES The concept of hormonal control of ovulation was formulated in the 1920s, but it was not until 1960 that the availability of cheap orally effective steroids made this approach practical.

Ovulation inhibition Since 1960, a host of preparations have been made available for this purpose. Most are combinations of synthetic estrogen and progestins, but some are sequential pills consisting of estrogen followed by a combination of estrogen and progestin. Through the years, the dose of steroids has been gradually diminished, so that at the present most oral contraceptives contain 1 mg progestin and 50 μg of estrogen. In view of the possible role that estrogen may play in some of the complications, new formulations containing 30 and even 20 μg estrogen are now being marketed. These appear to have less undesirable side effects, but there is a relatively high incidence of irregular and breakthrough bleeding.

With estrogens alone, in a sequential formulation, a daily dose of 80 μg is required (to inhibit ovulation). Therefore, those who are concerned about the possible side effects of estrogen will avoid this approach.

Complications, such as thromboembolism, cerebrovascular accidents, liver disease, hypertension, and "post-pill" amenorrhea, are exceedingly rare, and in many cases it is difficult to establish a causal relationship with certainty. Side effects, such as nausea, headaches, weight gain, are more common and seem to be lessened with the lower dosage of estrogen.

Continuous microdose progesterone therapy In an attempt to avoid the side effects and possible complications of estrogen, continuous low doses of progestins have been utilized (norethindrone 0.035 mg; norgestrel 0.075 mg). These have a lessened contraceptive effect, about 98 percent effective, and although there appears to be lessening of the estrogenic side effects, there is considerable irregular or breakthrough bleeding. The continuous dose of progestins probably exerts its contraceptive effect by a combination of effects on the cervical mucus, endometrium, and hypothalamic-pituitary pathways.

INTERFERENCE WITH IMPLANTATION The intrauterine device (IUD) has returned to popularity since the early 1960s. Although numerous modes of action have been described in animals, it is believed that the site of action in the human is at the level of the endometrium where the foreign-body action of the IUD causes fundamental biochemical changes which prevent implantation of the fertilized gamete. A number of shapes and sizes have been introduced through the years, and the clinician must strive for effectiveness with a minimum of side effects and contraceptive failures. Large IUDs cause irritation, bleeding, and possible infection. Smaller ones may be less effective and may be passed out through the cervix. Two commonly used are the Lippes loop and Dalkon shield, each of which comes in various sizes. Recently IUDs impregnated with copper have become increasingly popular. Because the local release of copper adds to the contraceptive effect, the IUD does not have to be as large. Consequently, it is more comfortable and can be utilized in a nulliparous female, and therefore theoretically it should cause fewer complications without decreased effectiveness. Experiments are also being conducted in which progesterone is slowly released from the IUD, adding to the contraceptive effect.

POSTCOITAL CONTRACEPTION High dosages of estrogen have been utilized as a "morning-after pill." These also appear to work by disrupting the endometrium prior to nidation. Single doses of progestin, such as norgestrel, 400 μg after each coital experience, have also been utilized. This seems to work chiefly by inhibiting ovulation itself.

STERILIZATION

Female Improved methods of ligation of the female fallopian tubes have resulted in a marked increase in the popularity of this approach to contraception. It should be emphasized that this must be considered a permanent approach, despite the occasional successful reanastomosis operation. Improved fiber-optic systems and instrumentation have made laparoscopic division of the tubes, either by cautery or by the use of clips or silastic bands, a relatively simple procedure. With local anesthesia, it can be performed in an ambulatory surgical setting, although for comfort of the patient, general anesthesia is preferable.

Male Because there is as yet no method of effective inhibition of spermatogenesis in a reversible manner without affecting testosterone production, a satisfactory hormonal contraceptive for the male is not available. As a result, ligation of the vas deferens is the common approach to contraception through the male. This is done on an outpatient basis, under local anesthesia, and causes little if any disability. There is a small incidence of psychologic impotence after the procedure. Because of the difficulty of reanastomosis of the vas and the development of sperm antibody, it should be considered a permanent procedure.

REFERENCES

AMELAR RD: *Infertility in Men.* Philadelphia: Davis, 1966

GEMZELL CA: Induction of ovulation with human pituitary gonadotropins. Fertil Steril 13:153, 1962

GOLDZIEHER JW: Current status of female hormonal contraception, in *Progress in Gynecology,* vol. 6, eds ML Taymor, TH Green, New York: Grune & Stratton, 1975, p. 353

PINCUS G: Progestational agents and the control of fertility. Vitam Horm 17:307, 1959

STONE A, WARD ME: Factors responsible for pregnancy in 500 infertility cases. Fertil Steril 7:1, 1956

TAYMOR ML: The induction of ovulation, in *Davis' Gynecology and Obstetrics,* ed JJ Sciarra, Hagerstown, Md.: Harper & Row, in press

——: *Management of Infertility,* Springfield, Ill.: Charles C Thomas, 1969

54
INTERPRETATION OF ALTERATIONS IN THE SKIN

T. B. FITZPATRICK
H. A. HAYNES

CLINICAL EXAMINATION OF THE SKIN

The identification of skin lesions, or alterations, is a problem similar to the recognition of cells in a blood smear; the minute details are of the greatest importance. The individual type of skin lesion (e.g., papule, nodule) can be considered as a letter in the alphabet, forming the basic element for the identification of the pathologic change and often leading to the clinical diagnosis. Lesions may be the presenting complaint of the patient or may be incidental findings during the routine physical examination; or they may be incidental to some major presenting complaint such as fever, cough, arthralgia, and the like. The recognition of the important and nonimportant skin lesions commonly encountered during the routine physical examination of the skin is an important part of the physician's task (Color Plates 1 to 4).

Inasmuch as the identification of skin lesions is the *sine qua non* of dermatologic diagnosis, the examiner's eye is undoubtedly the most important instrument at his disposal. Adequate illumination, preferably with natural light, is necessary. The observation of the skin should begin with an overall, "low-power" general assessment of the completely disrobed patient. The systematic approach to the examination of skin should be as follows: first the fingernails and then the anterior and posterior aspects of the arm; then, in sequence, the scalp, the face, the trunk, the lower extremities, and the skin between the toes; and then the mucous membranes, including the mouth and anogenital areas. The examiner of dermatologic lesions should consider the following points: (1) the specific *type* of lesion, (2) the *configuration,* or *shape* of the lesion, and (3) the *arrangement* of the groups of lesions, such as linear, arciform, annular, polycyclic, herpetiform, zosteriform, and serpiginous.

Types of skin lesions can be classified by determining the topographic level of the lesions in relation to the normal skin (Table 54-1). For example, it is possible to distinguish lesions that are in or that protrude or are superimposed above or below the level of the normal skin. The lesions that are encompassed with the scope of dermatology are listed in Fig. 54-1 and Table 54-1, and the histologic aspects are illustrated in Figs. 54-2 through 54-13.

The shape of the individual lesion and the arrangement of two or more lesions in relation to each other sometimes constitute important diagnostic clues. A *linear arrangement* of lesions often is indicative of an exogenous cause; also, linear lesions may occur because the pathologic process involves a vein, a lymphatic component, or an arteriole. Linearity can often be seen in various types of cutaneous hamartoma involving epidermal cells or melanocytes or even dermal connective tissue. In contrast, *annular and arciform* lesions and *annular and arciform arrangements* are relatively common and therefore only rarely lead to a specific diagnosis. The *iris* lesion, however, a special and important type of annular lesion, may be an erythematous annular macule or papule, with either a purplish papule or vesicle in the center. Iris lesions are characteristic of the erythema-multiforme syndrome. Annular macules may be observed in drug eruptions, secondary syphilis, and lupus erythematosus. Annular lesions with scale often suggest dermatophytosis or pityriasis rosea or psoriasis. The wheals that occur in creeping eruptions and the nodules in late syphilis are arranged in a *serpiginous* (snakelike) pattern.

Lesions that are close to each other are described as *grouped,* and are of relatively little diagnostic value except in the special pattern, *herpetiform,* which is pathognomonic for herpes simplex or herpes zoster. Similarly, the special arrangement, *zosteriform,* follows a dermatome in a bandlike pattern and is characteristically seen in herpes zoster; a zosteriform arrangement of skin nodules is occasionally seen in metastatic carcinoma of the breast. A *reticular* arrangement often results from vascular dilatation and is observed in cutis marmorata and livedo reticularis.

The sites of localization of skin eruptions have been greatly overemphasized, however, in dermatologic diagnosis; of far more importance are the type, shape, and arrangement of the lesions. Eruptions can be classified as *localized* or *generalized;* the term *"total"* (universal) denotes an involvement of all the skin, including the hair and the nails. When the eruption occurs in bilateral and symmetrical distribution, the pathologic stimulus is usually endogenous or is hematogenously disseminated. Bilateral

TABLE 54-1
Types of skin lesion

Flat lesions (in plane of skin)	*Elevated lesions (above plane of skin)*	*Depressed lesions (below plane of skin)*
Macule	Vesicle and bulla	Atrophy§
Infarct*	Pustule	Sclerosis§†
Sclerosis*†	Abscess‡	Erosion
Telangiectasia†	Cyst‡	Excoriation
	Papule	Scar†
	Wheal	Ulcer
	Plaque	Sinus‡
	Nodule‡	Gangrene§
	Vegetation	
	Keratosis	
	Desquamation (scales)	
	Exudate* (crusts)	
	Lichenification	

* *May also be below the plane of the skin.*
† *May also be above the plane of the skin.*
‡ *May also be in or below the plane of the skin.*
§ *May also be in the plane of the skin.*
SOURCE: *TB Fitzpatrick, DP Johnson, Fundamentals of dermatologic diagnosis, in* Dermatology in General Medicine, *eds TB Fitzpatrick et al, New York: McGraw-Hill, 1971*

symmetry is characteristic of hypersensitivity and is a common response to a drug. In photosensitivity eruptions, lesions are localized to the parts of the body that are exposed to sunlight. The exposed areas of the face that are usually spared include the fold of skin in the upper eyelids, the skin of the hair-covered scalp, and the skin below the chin.

LABORATORY AND OTHER AIDS IN EXAMINATION OF THE SKIN

There are certain technical, clinical, and laboratory aids and procedures that are indispensable in the clinical examination and interpretation of skin conditions.

Visual aids

MAGNIFICATION Certain diagnostic signs can be revealed only by magnification of the skin lesions; e.g., the follicular plugging indicative of lupus erythematosus, the fine telangiectasia and raised border indicative of basal-cell carcinoma, and, if present, the bluish color indicative of early primary malignant melanoma. A pocket magnifier (2 to 7X) and a binocular microscope (5 to 40X) are useful.

TRANSILLUMINATION Transillumination, or sidelighting, of skin lesions, which is done in a darkened room, is often required to detect slight degrees of elevation or depression, and is also sometimes useful in estimating the extent of the eruption.

DIASCOPY Diascopy is an indispensable technique for the examination of the skin because it permits the differentiation of purpura from erythematous macules. Diascopy consists of firmly pressing a microscope slide or a piece of clear plastic over the skin lesion; if the lesion is erythematous, the pressure will reveal capillary dilatation rather than an extravasation of blood. Sarcoidosis, lymphoma, and tuberculosis of the skin are suggested if diascopy of the nodules reveals either a characteristic hyaline, yellowish brown, or an "apple-jelly" appearance.

LONG-WAVE ULTRAVIOLET LIGHT, OR WOOD'S LAMP Long-wave ultraviolet light (360 nm), or Wood's lamp, is an essential source of illumination for examination of the skin. Wood's lamp consists of a high-pressure mercury arc lamp with a specially compounded glass filter made of nickel oxide and silica (Wood's filter). This filter permits a band of radiation of 360 nm, which, upon impingement, will reveal fluorescence.

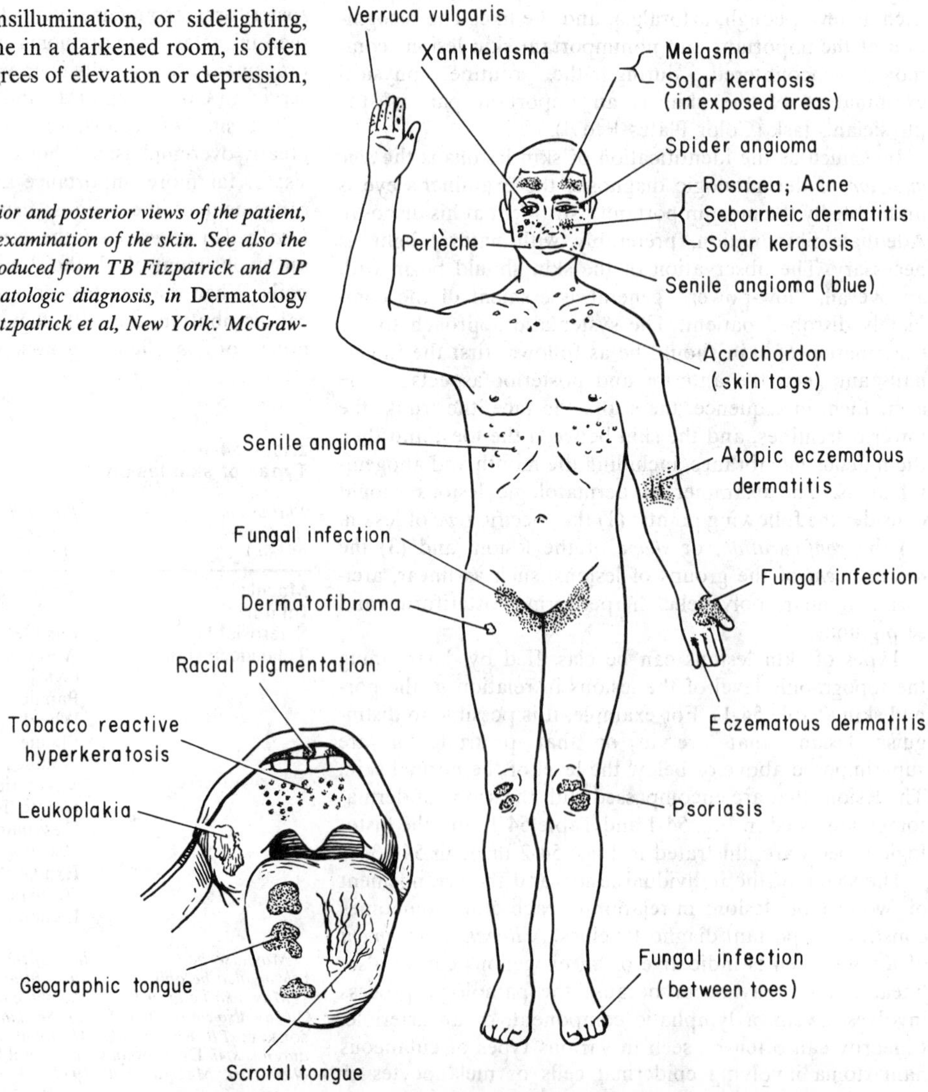

FIGURE 54-1
Common lesions, shown on anterior and posterior views of the patient, encountered during the physical examination of the skin. See also the Color Atlas, Plates 1 to 4. (Reproduced from TB Fitzpatrick and DP Johnson, Fundamentals of dermatologic diagnosis, in Dermatology in General Medicine, *eds TB Fitzpatrick et al, New York: McGraw-Hill, 1971, p. 10)*

An Atlas of common lesions encountered during the physical examination of the skin

The skin and mucous membrane may frequently contain a variety of lesions that are rarely a major complaint (Fig. 52-1). They are, therefore, incidental findings in the general physical examination. The recognition of the "bumps and blemishes" is a necessary first step for the physician, inasmuch as he will be required to distinguish the trivial from the serious and important skin changes. For example, such a serious lesion as a malignant melanoma may be incidentally discovered during a routine physical examination (see color Figs. 6-1, 6-2, 6-3 and the discussion in Chap. 366).

The common disorders of the skin that every physician should be able to recognize are presented in this series of color photographs (Plates 1 to 4).

A

B

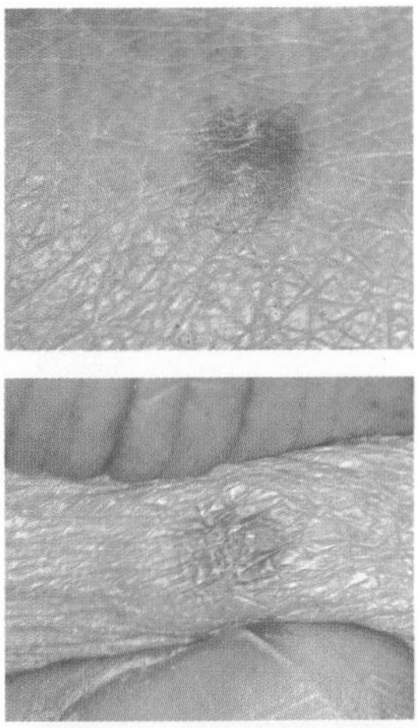

1-1 **Dermatofibroma** is especially common in middle life and in females. The lesions, when pigmented, are occasionally confused with malignant melanoma. They appear as isolated, slightly elevated, hard, button-like nodules *(A)*. In fair-skinned persons, the lesions are not usually skin color, but are pink or dark red, yellowish brown, or gray-black. They are usually less than 1 cm in diameter. A diagnostic sign is that a dermatofibroma dimples or becomes depressed *(B)* when it is laterally compressed; melanocytic nevus and melanoma, however, with which dermatofibroma may be easily confused, become elevated with lateral compression.

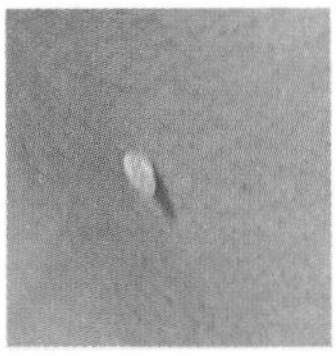

1-2 **Acrochordon** (skin tag) is very common after middle life and appears on the neck, especially in females, in the axillae, and on the upper part of the trunk. The lesions are small (1 to 5 mm), soft, pedunculated papules, usually of normal skin color.

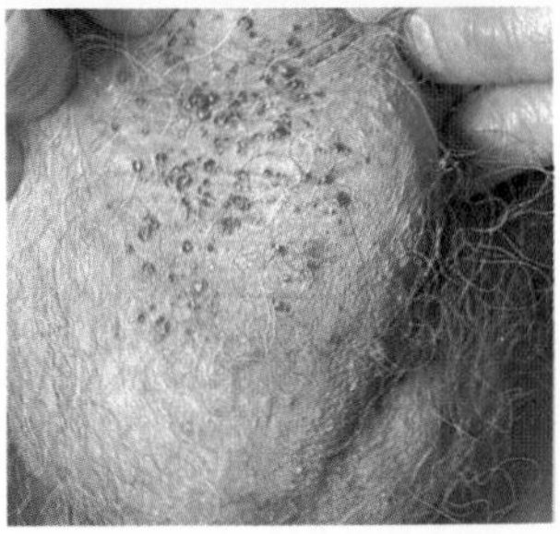

1-3 **Angiokeratomas** are bizarre vascular dilatations that occur under the tongue and on the scrotum and consist of myriads of 2- to 3-mm purplish red papules. They are of no known significance. When they occur on the trunk and extremities, a biopsy is indicated to rule out glycolipid lipidosis, or Fabry's disease.

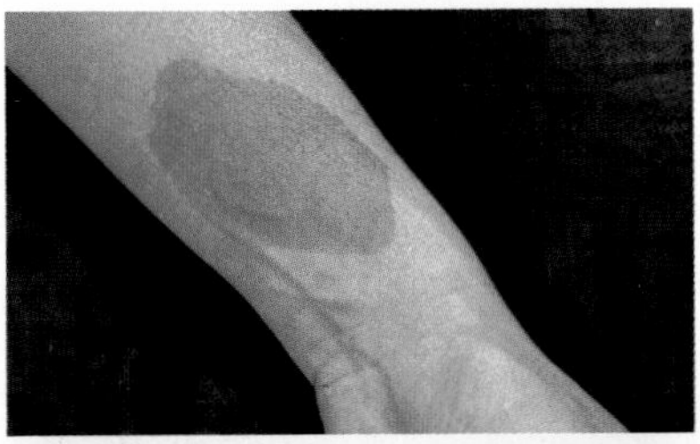

1-4 **Café au lait macules** are found in about 10 percent of the normal population and, in fair-skinned persons, are light-yellowish brown macules, which may also be markers of neurofibromatosis and polyostotic fibrous dysplasia (Albright's syndrome). The presence of six or more café au lait macules with a diameter of 1.5 cm or greater is diagnostic of neurofibromatosis.

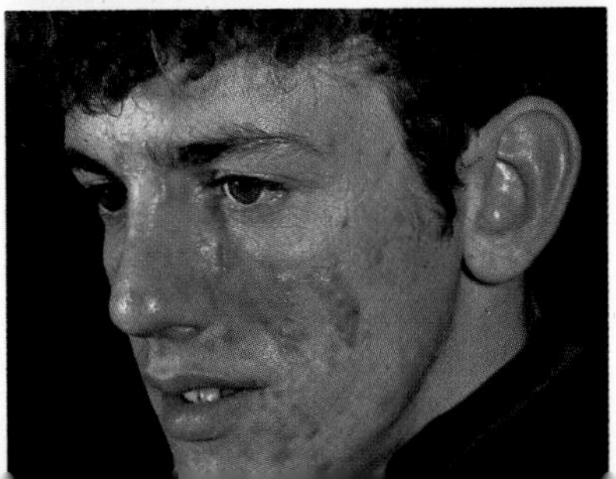

1-5 **Acne** is a condition in which the most characteristic lesion is the comedo, or "blackhead," that later becomes a conical erythematous papule or pustule. A third type of lesion is the "blind boil," which is a dermal cyst without an orifice. This lesion is often associated with atrophic or hypertrophic scarring. Cystic acne may appear with only a very few comedones; also, comedo-like acne may occur with few cysts, or erythematous papules.

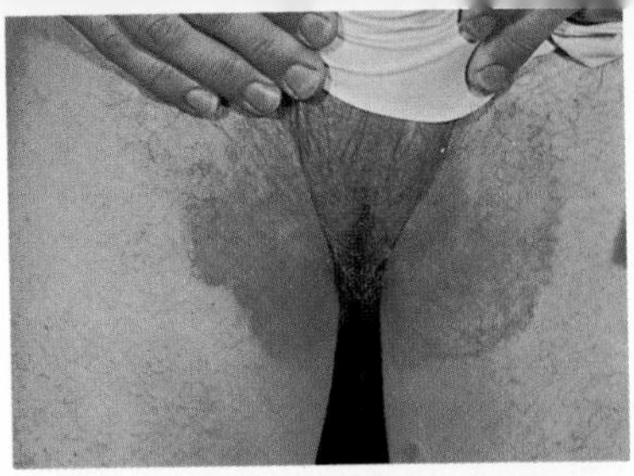

2-1 **Dermatophytosis** is identified by the striking polycyclic, annular shape of the scaling, especially on the feet and hands, where there is often a scalloped pattern. A positive diagnosis of dermatophytosis is quickly established by direct examination of scales from the advancing border; the mycelia are revealed when the scales are immersed in 10% potassium hydroxide or the Swartz stain.

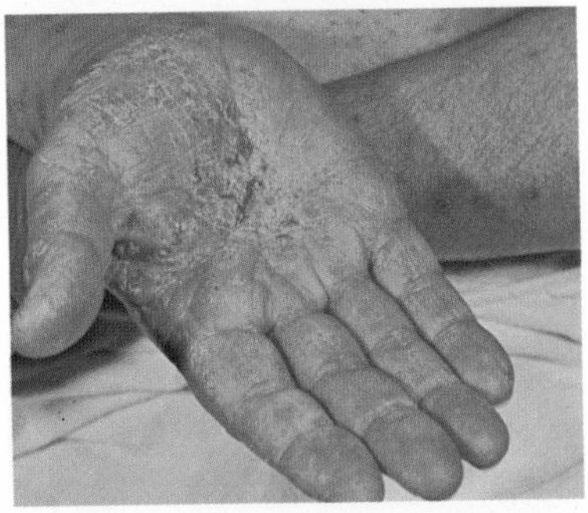

2-2 **Eczematous dermatitis** is a very common cutaneous reaction that is localized to the hands of housewives, to the legs in patients with chronic venous insufficiency, and behind the ears in patients with seborrheic dermatitis. In subacute eczematous dermatitis, there are mild erythema, dry scales, and often small red papules, many of which are excoriated. In chronic eczematous dermatitis, lichenification is the most prominent feature.

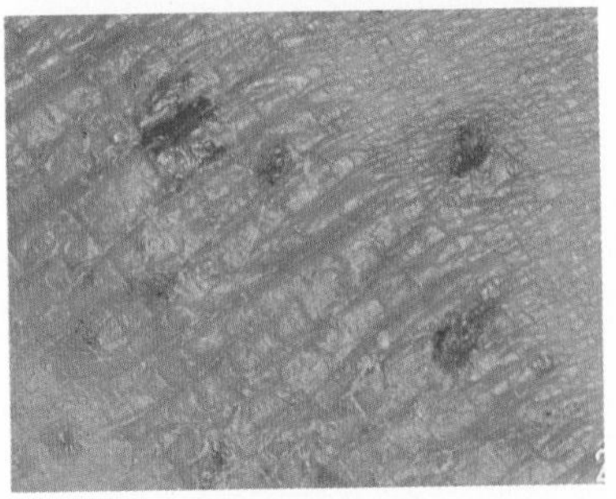

2-3 **Localized lichenification** results from repeated rubbing of the skin and consists of isolated, circumscribed plaques. These single lesions vary in size from 2 to 10 cm and occur most often on the extensor aspect of the forearm and in the scrotal, nuchal, inguinal, and anogenital areas. The perianal and vulvar areas may become diffusely lichenified. Lichenification is thought to be more frequent in persons with an atopic background.

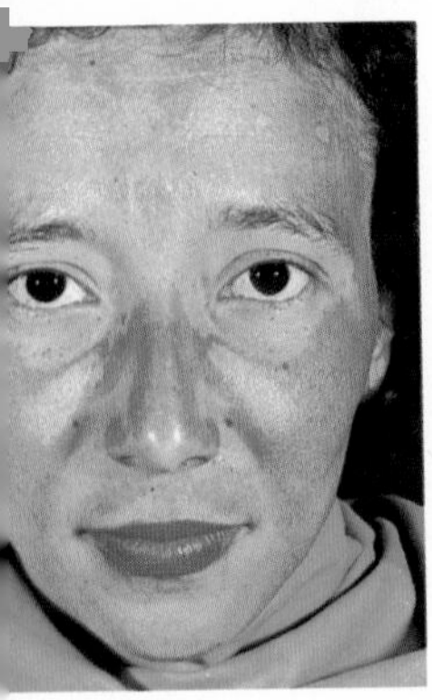

2-4 **Melasma (chloasma)** is the so-called "mask" of pregnancy, but it also occurs in men and in women taking progestational agents. The pigmentation is uniform and is limited to the exposed areas of the face. There is no scaling or epidermal change. In fair-skinned persons, the pigment may be any shade from light tan to a very dark brown. It is most often seen on the cheeks and upper lip, as here, and on the forehead.

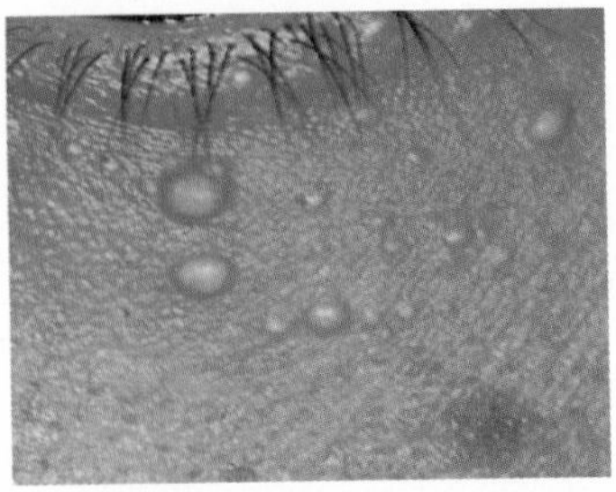

2-5 **Milia** are a collection of lesions occurring most commonly on the face, and consist of tiny (1- to 2-mm) white, hard, rounded, superficial papules. There is no orifice, and the keratinous contents are easily expressed by lateral compression after the making of a tiny incision in the dome of the lesion.

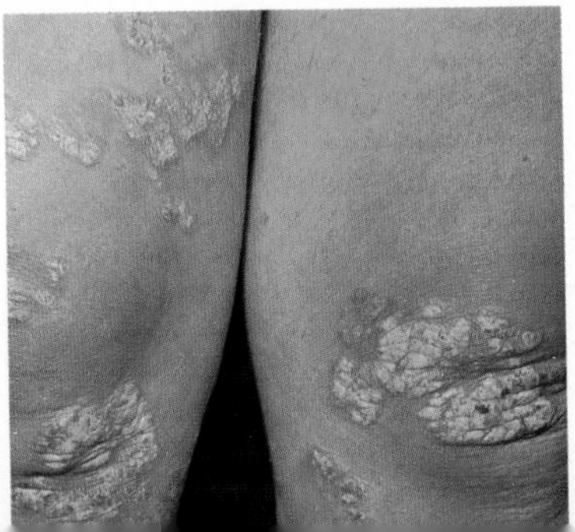

2-6 **Psoriasis,** affecting more than 2 percent of the population, consist of isolating scaling papules or plaques and is quite commonly observed in the routine physical examination. The lesions occur most frequently on the scalp, elbows, and knees. The color and type of scales are the identifying features of the lesions. The scales are either dense and lamellated with peripherally detached edges or loose and branny. The plaques are pink to deep red, and the borders are distinct.

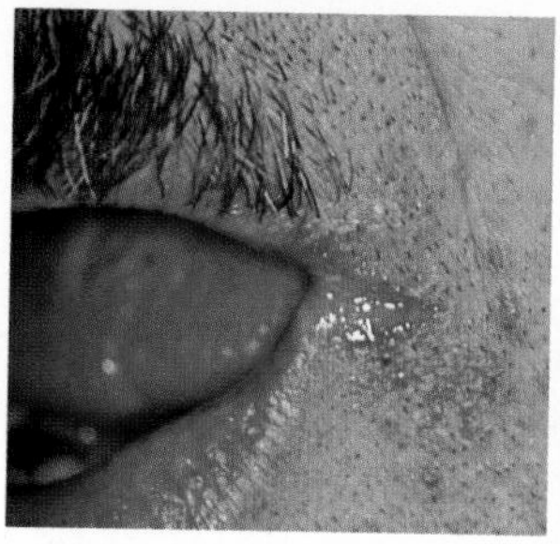

3-1 **Perlèche** consists of painful small fissures at the angles of the mouth, often covered with yellow crusts. Perlèche most often occurs with poorly fitting dentures and in moniliasis and secondary syphilis.

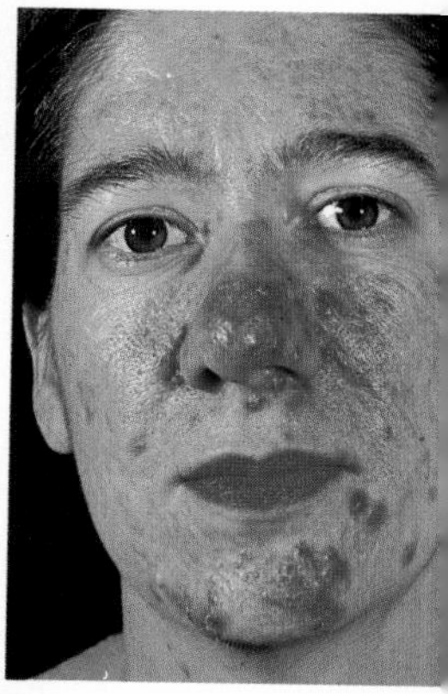

3-2 **Rosacea,** usually limited to the face, consists of tiny, erythematous papules and pustules 1 to 5 mm in size. The pustules, often tiny and sometimes hardly visible, sit on the dome of the papules. The diffuse redness of the face is due to a vasodilatation, as well as to myriads of telangiectases. In males, rhinophyma, a disfiguring enlargement of the nose, may occur.

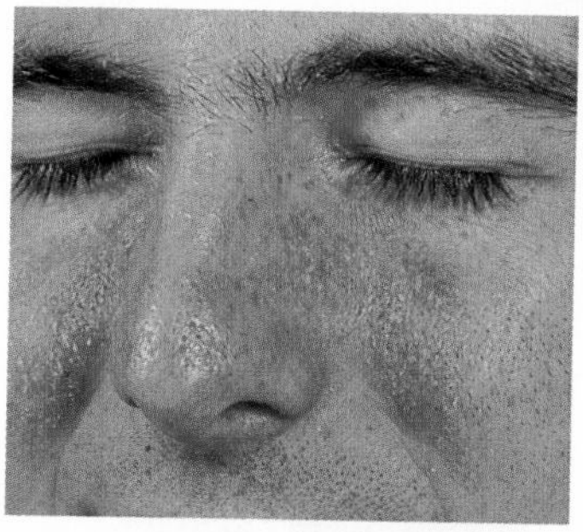

3-3 **Seborrheic dermatitis,** a common disorder found in all age groups, occurs most frequently on the scalp, eyebrows, and nasolabial folds, and behind the ears. Scaling is the prominent feature and is loose and branny; it may be yellow and oily or dry and white. The lesion may become exudative and crusted or eczematous.

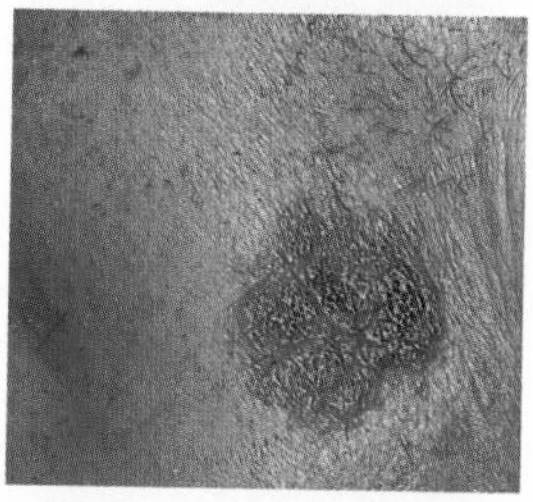

3-4 **Seborrheic keratosis** appears in middle life and may be on the exposed or unexposed areas but is especially common on the trunk. The lesions are irregularly round or oval flat-topped papules or plaques that seem "stuck" on the skin. The margins are distinct, and the surface is often warty or consists of multiple tiny projections (vegetation). In fair-skinned persons, the lesions are light brown at first but, enlarging, become more heavily pigmented and may be confused with malignant melanoma.

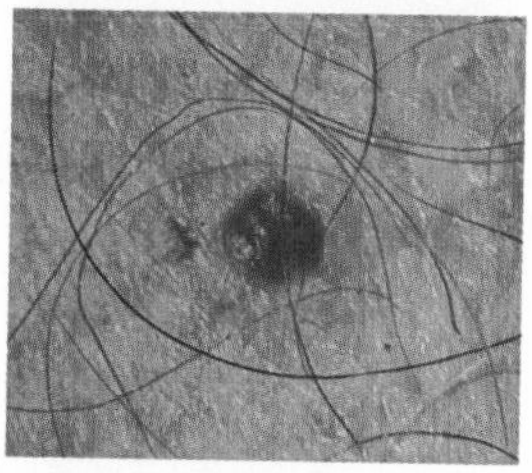

3-5 **Senile angioma ("cherry-red spot")** appears in the third decade. On the lip, the lesion is usually singular and consists of a bluish-red round nodule. On the trunk, the lesions are small (2- to 3-mm), bright red, globular papules.

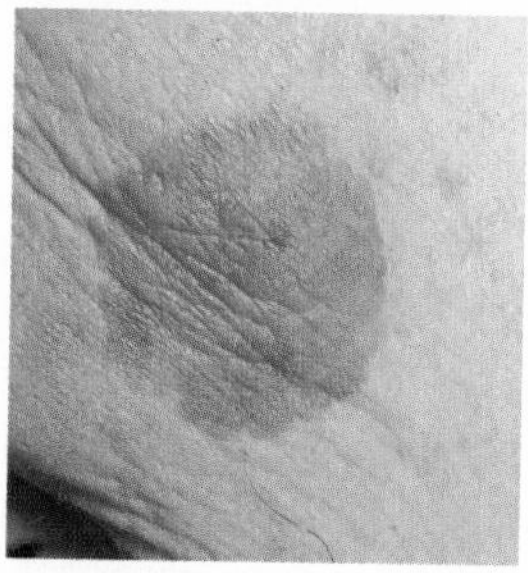

3-6 **Senile lentigo** occurs as a single macule or as a group of isolated, sharply circumscribed macules on the exposed areas, especially on the dorsal surfaces of the hands and arms and on the forehead and cheeks. The macules are usually light yellowish brown, but may be dark brown; the color is somewhat variegated, rather than uniform as it is in a café au lait macule. Rarely, dark brown *papules* develop in these lesions, and then the condition is called *lentigo maligna,* which may slowly develop, over a period of years, into a melanoma (lentigo maligna melanoma).

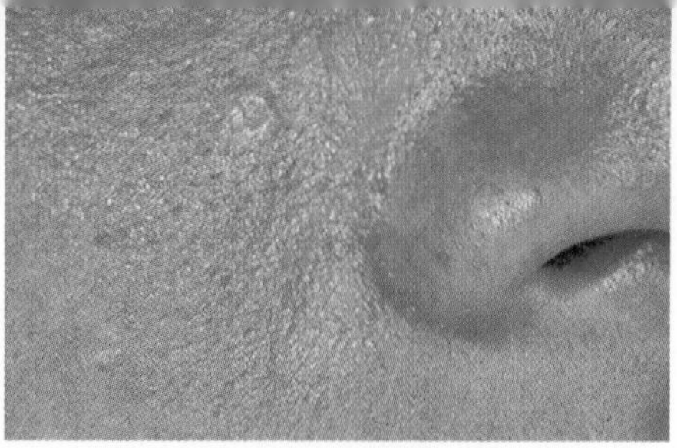

4-1 **Senile sebaceous adenoma** occurs on the face in patients over forty and is often diagnosed as basal-cell carcinoma. The lesions are soft, small, flat-topped papules, varying in size from 1 to 8 mm, and are characterized by a minute central depression from which sebaceous material can be exuded by lateral compression.

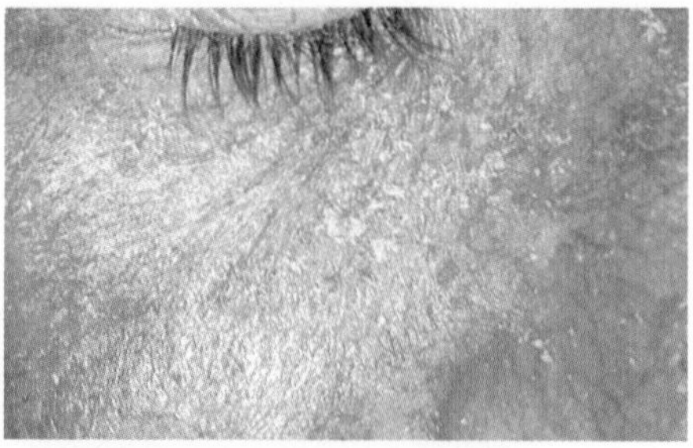

4-2 **Solar keratosis** (1) occurs usually in persons with light skin prone to sunburn or with darker skin after chronic excessive exposure; (2) is strictly limited to exposed skin, especially on the face and dorsal surfaces of the hands; (3) is more easily felt than seen (gritty and sandpaperish); (4) in fair-skinned persons, consists of skin-colored or light brown macules or slightly raised papules with superficial adherent scales not easily removed; (5) is associated with marked wrinkling, telangiectasia, and often diffuse, tiny pale yellow papules indicating solar degeneration of connective tissue ("turkey skin").

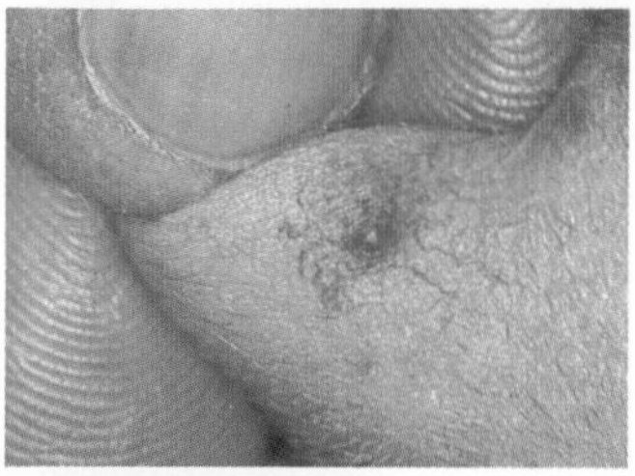

4-3 **Spider nevus** consists of a central, punctate, bright red macule or papule (the body) from which fine red lines radiate like spider legs. There is often a red flare between the radiating vessels. On diascopy, the central body pulsates.

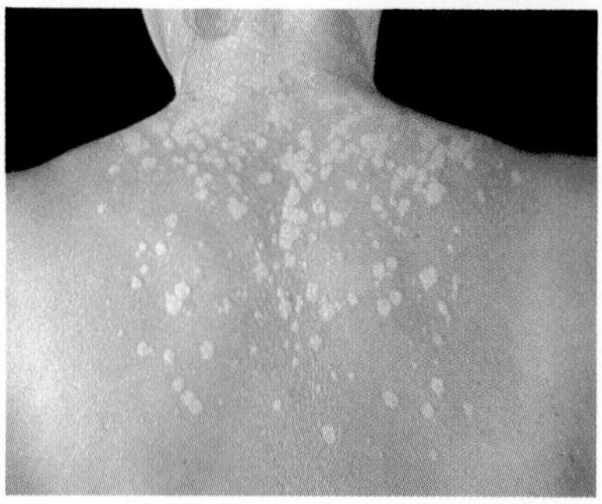

4-4 **Tinea versicolor** is a relatively common disorder occurring primarily on the trunk and appearing in two forms: as scattered, 3- to 5-mm, very slightly scaling brown macules; or as whitish macules that may be confused with vitiligo. The fungal spores and hyphae can be easily demonstrated on direct examination of the scales using the Swartz stain.

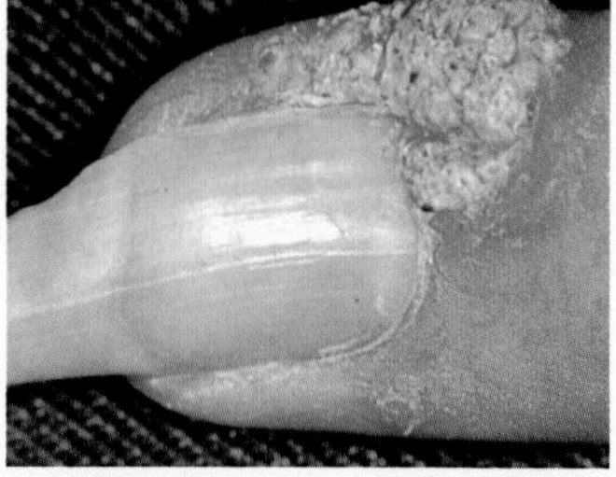

4-5 **Verruca vulgaris** may occur at any age, but it is most common in children. The lesions may be from 0.5 to 2.0 cm, and they are round or oval, firm, skin-colored papules with multiple tiny keratotic, rounded or filiform, projections covering the surface (vegetation). They occur most frequently on the hands and soles.

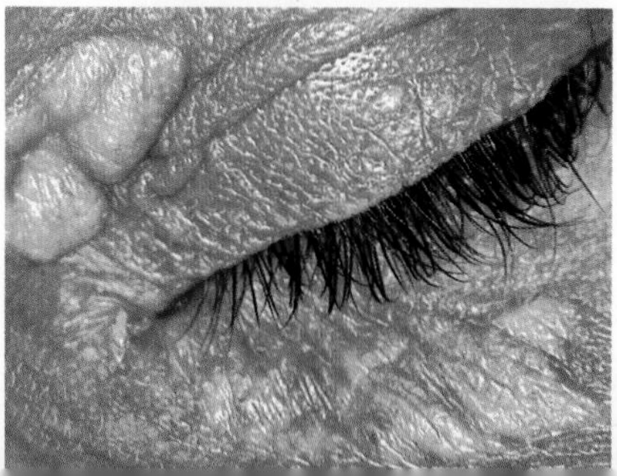

4-6 **Xanthelasma** consists of one or more bright yellow, sharply marginated plaques with no epidermal change, usually occurring on the eyelids. All patients with xanthelasma should be investigated for evidence of plasma lipid abnormalities.

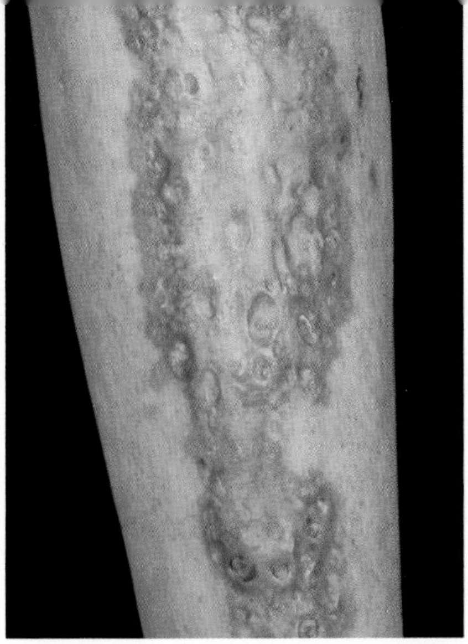

5-1 Necrobiosis lipoidica diabeticorum. Note vivid colors (brown and yellow) and fine, arborizing blood vessels traversing atrophic skin.

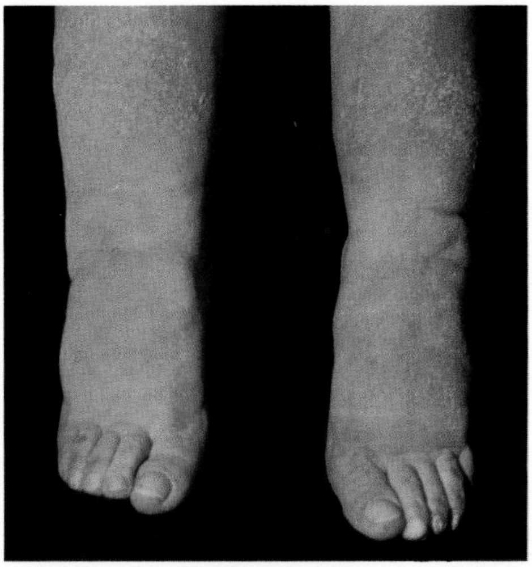

5-2 Pretibial myxedema.

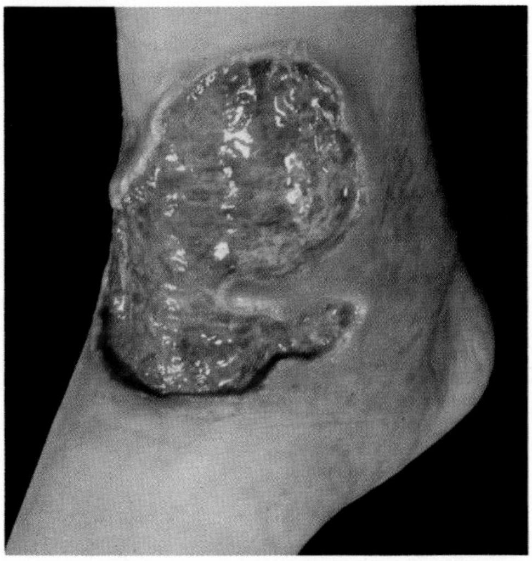

5-3 Pyoderma gangrenosum in a patient with ulcerative colitis.

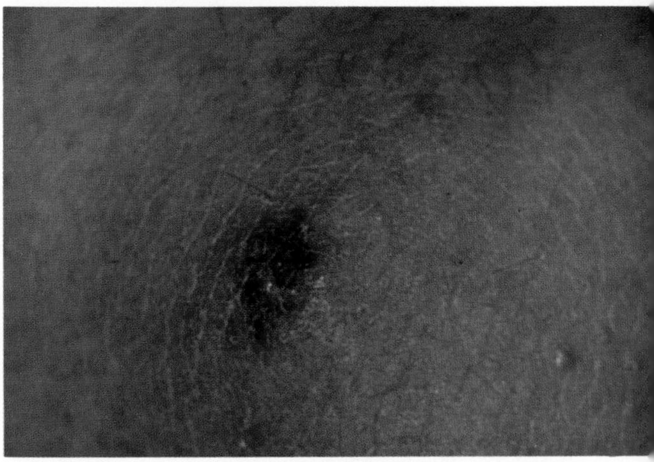

5-4 "Palpable" purpura with inflammation occurring in gonococcemia. An identical lesion may be seen in meningococcemia. staphylococcemia, and systemic vasculitis.

5-5 Tzanck test shows giant epithelial cells on direct smear of vesicle base in varicella.

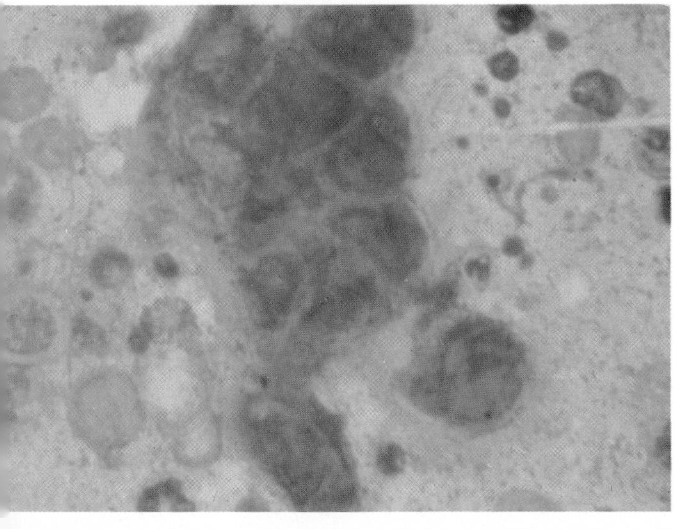

5-6 Hypopigmented ash-leaf-shaped macules in tuberous sclerosis.

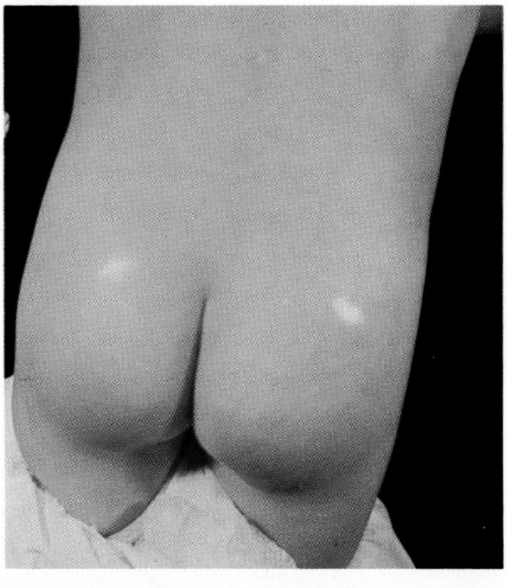

PLATE 6

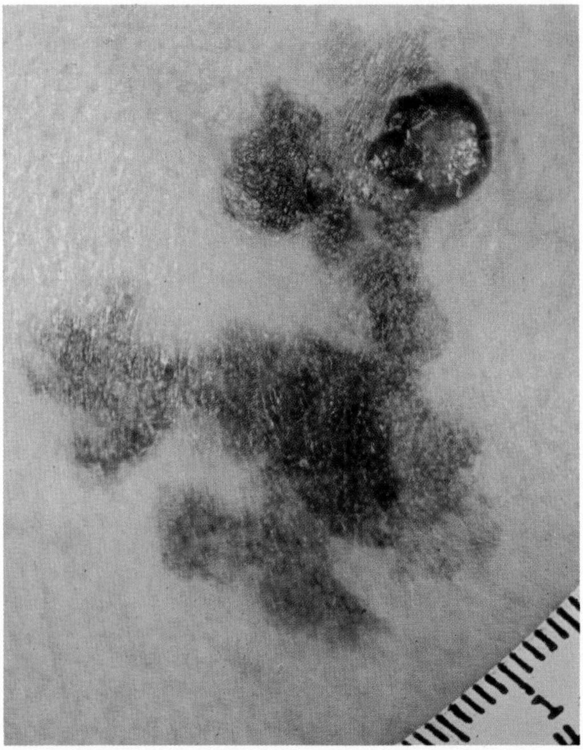

6-1 In Type I malignant melanoma, the lesion is predominantly flat, but there may be a few nodules or papules. The color consists mainly of shades of brown and black, admixed with whitish gray and, occasionally, with reddish brown, bluish gray, and bluish black.

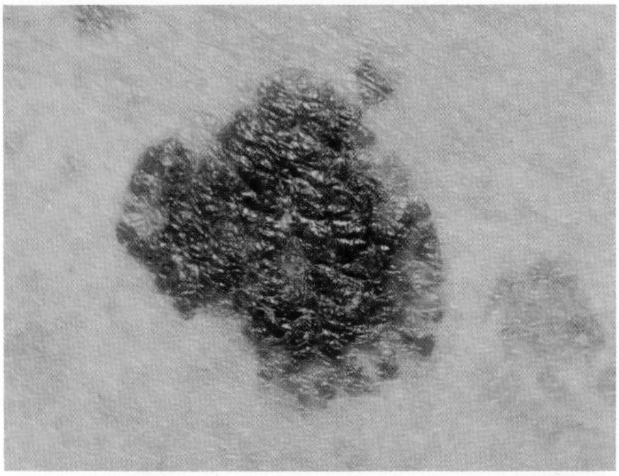

6-2 In Type II malignant melanoma, the lesion is usually just slightly raised in its entirety and is punctuated with papules and, sometimes, nodules. The color consists mainly of brown and black, admixed with bluish red (violaceous), bluish gray, bluish black, reddish brown, and often whitish pink.

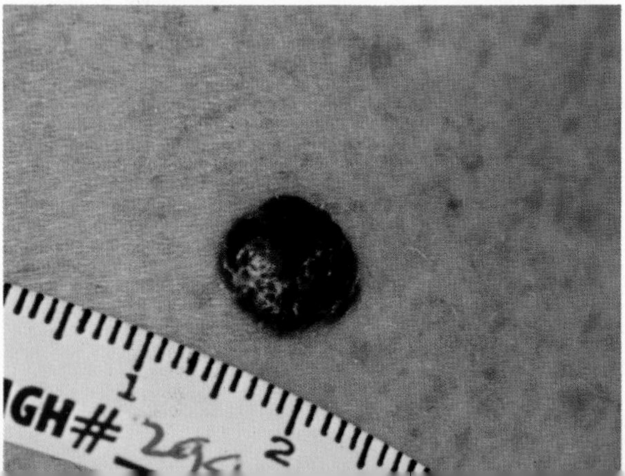

6-3 In Type III malignant melanoma, the lesion is always raised and may be dome-shaped or polypoid. The color is usually uniform bluish black, but there may rarely be shades of reddish blue (purple) or an admixture of bluish black with brown or black.

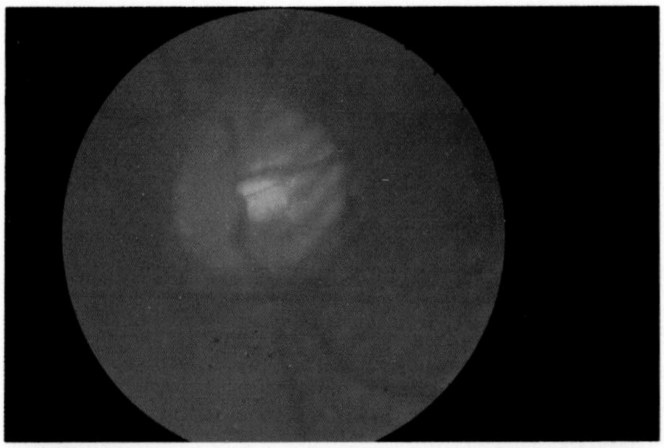

7-1

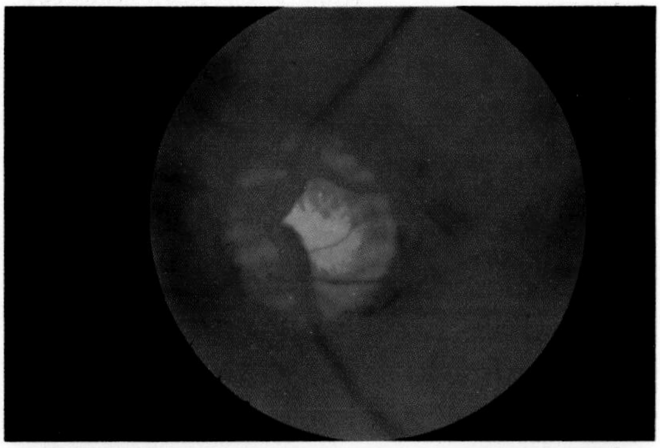

7-2

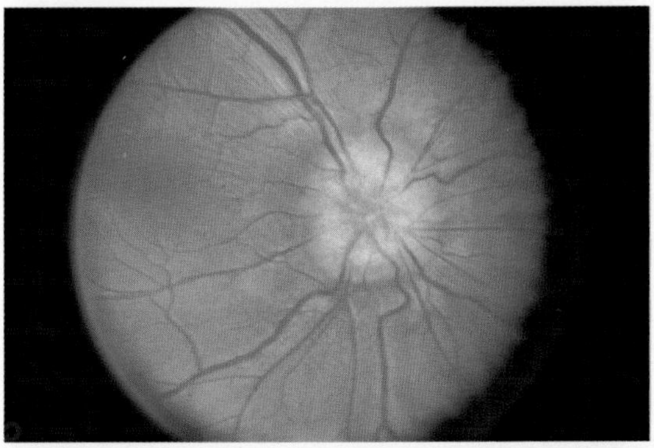

7-3

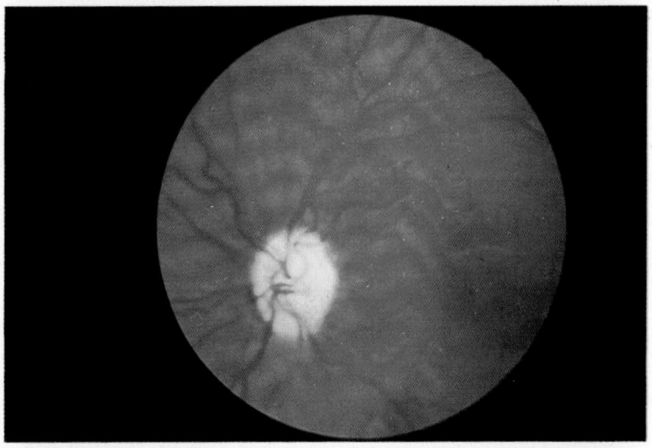

7-4

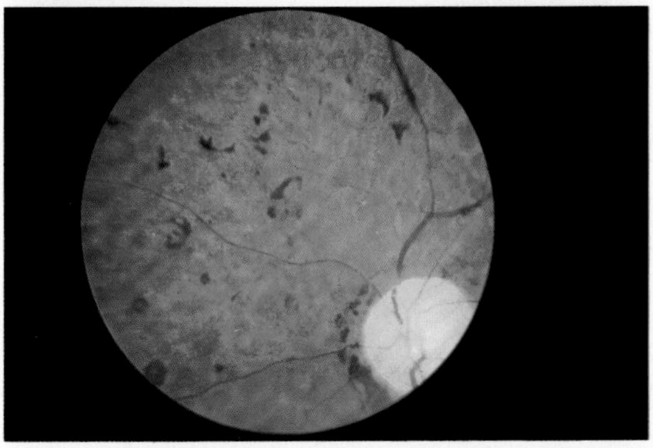

7-5

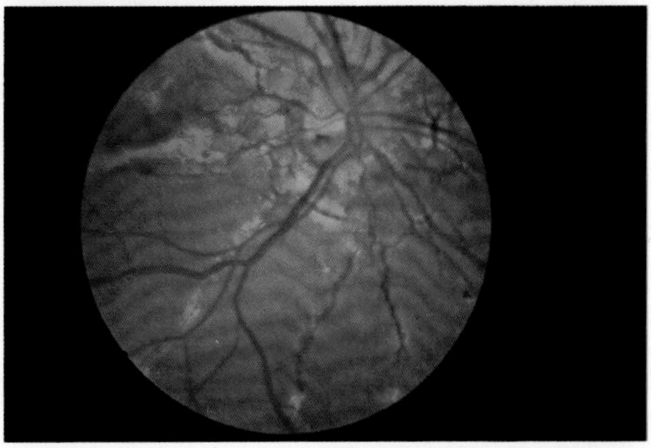

7-6

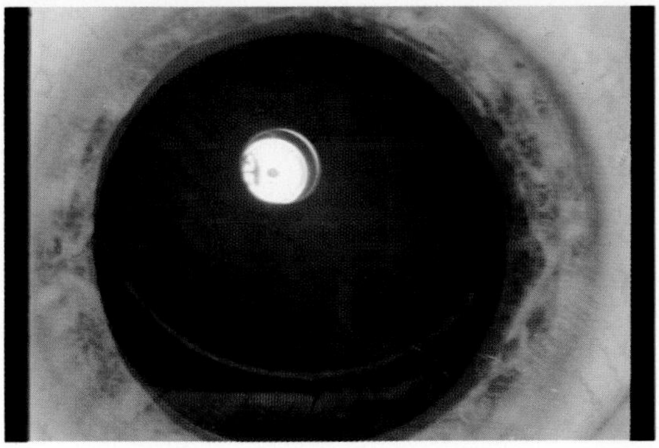

7-7

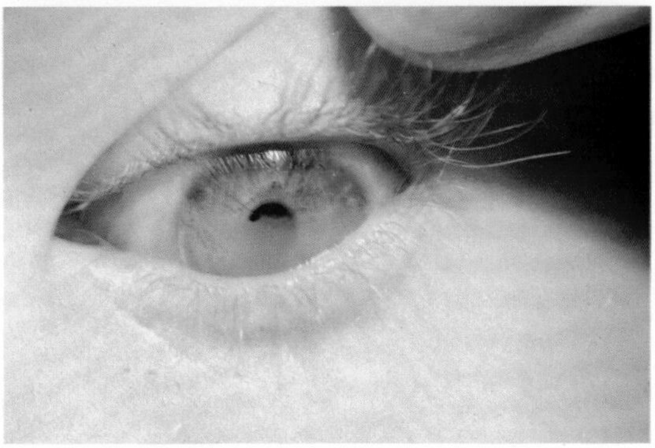

7-8

7-1 Normal optic nervehead, right eye *7-2* Temporal pallor, optic nervehead, left eye. Compare with normal right optic nerve figure 1.
7-3 Papilledema *7-4* Optic atrophy
7-5 Retinitis pigmentosa *7-6* Angioid streaks
7-7 Dislocation of crystalline lens *7-8* Band keratopathy

PLATE 8

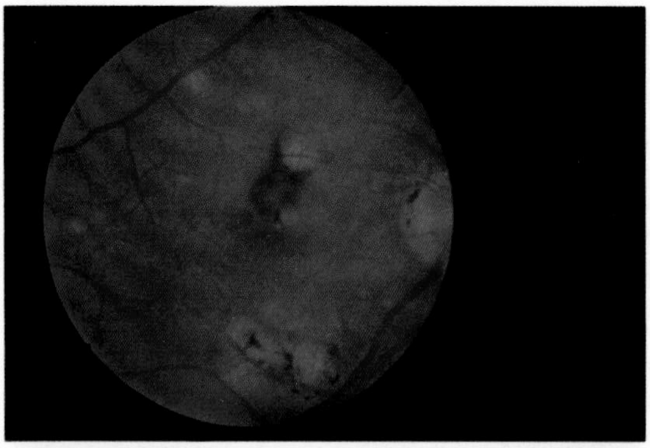

8-1

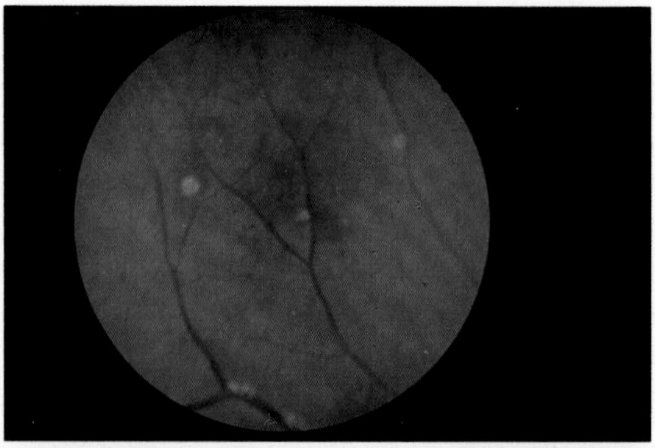

8-2

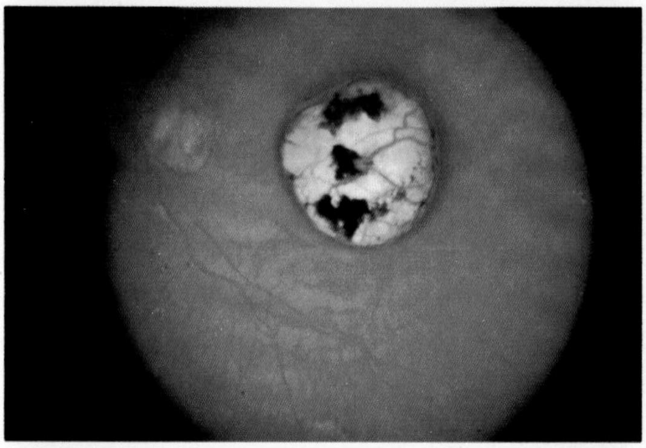

8-3

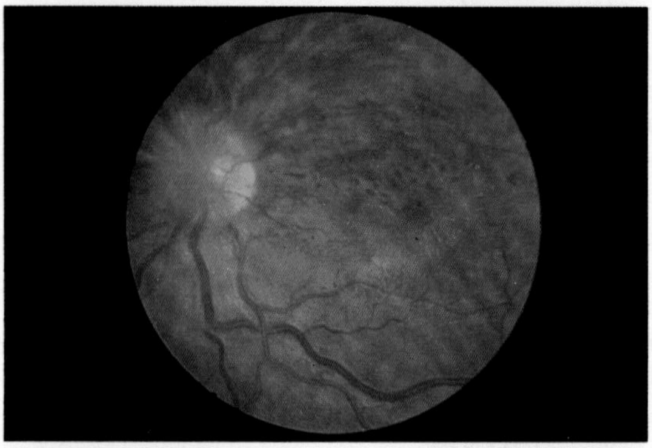

8-4

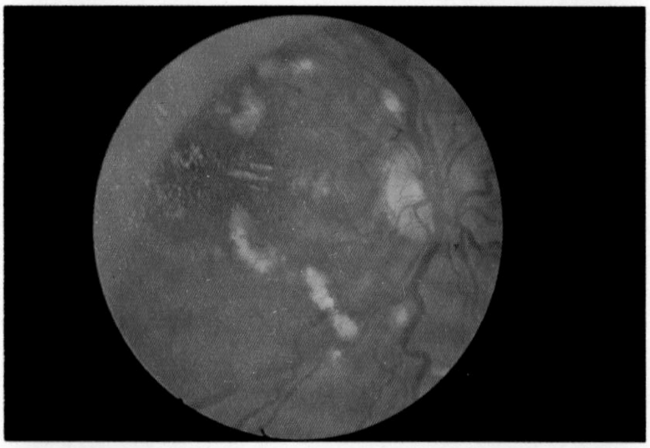

8-5

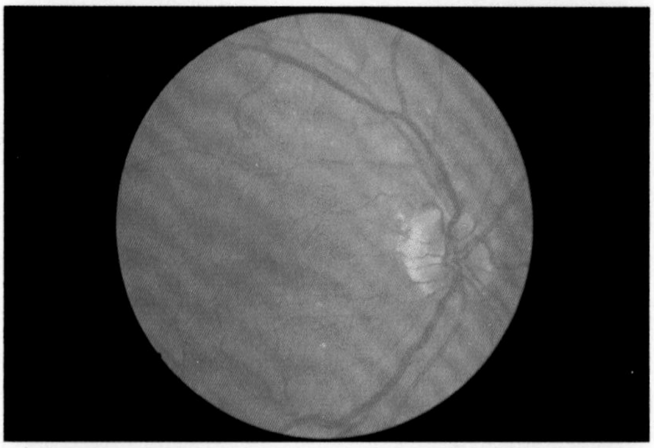

8-6

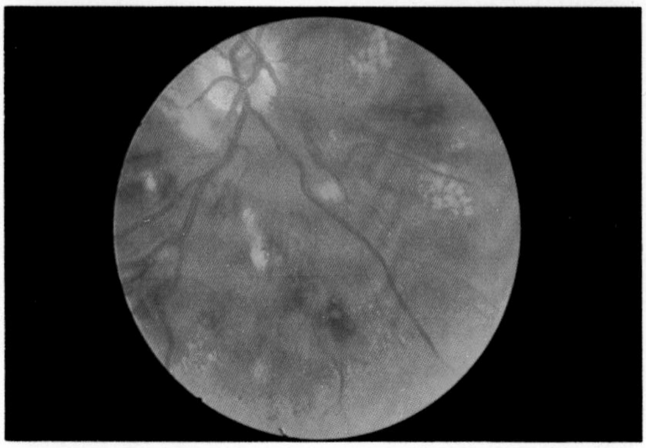

8-7

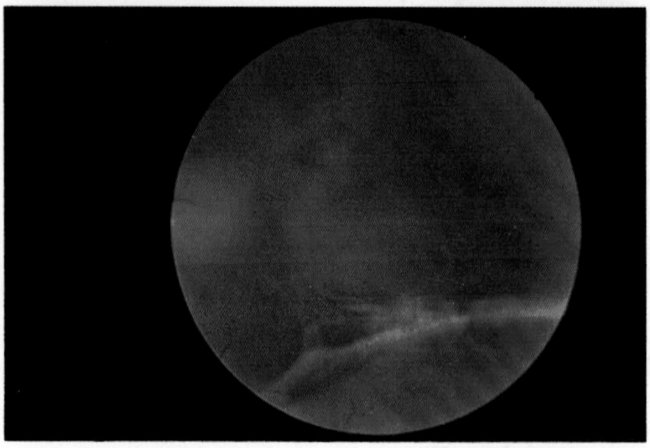

8-8

8-1 Histoplasmosis *8-2* Sarcoid *8-3* Toxoplasmosis
8-4 Occlusion of superior temporal vein with edema of macula
8-5 Hypertensive retinopathy *8-6* Early intraretinal diabetic retinopathy
8-7 Advanced intraretinal diabetic retinopathy
8-8 Advanced extraretinal (proliferative) diabetic retinopathy

This valuable technique can be used for mass screening for the detection of the fluorescence of dermatophytosis *in the hair shaft* in ringworm of the scalp. In internal medicine, however, Wood's lamp is especially important for the detection of the pinkish red fluorescence of the urine of patients with porphyria cutanea tarda; the addition of hydrochloric acid greatly intensifies the fluorescence, owing to the oxidation of porphyrin precursors to porphyrins.

Wood's lamp is also a great help in the estimation of variation in the pigmentation of the skin; it reveals both increased and decreased pigmentation. Inasmuch as melanin is a universal absorber of ultraviolet light, areas of increased melanin will show an increased intensity under Wood's lamp; conversely, areas of decreased melanin will show a decrease in intensity (or an increased reflection) because the ultraviolet light is not absorbed. In this respect, Wood's lamp is the only means of recognizing the sometimes indistinguishable hypomelanotic macules in tuberous sclerosis, a serious, dominantly inherited trait associated with mental retardation. The white spots are present at birth and remain throughout life, and therefore represent important markers of this genetic disorder.

Clinical tests

PATCH-TESTING Patch-testing is primarily used by dermatologists to detect contact sensitivity. The contactants are listed in Fisher's 1973 monograph on the subject.

DARIER'S SIGN One very useful clinical response of the skin, Darier's sign, is used as a test for urticaria pigmentosa, and is evoked by the vigorous rubbing of a pigmented macule with the blunt end of an instrument such as a pen. In urticaria pigmentosa (mastocytosis), a palpable wheal occurs in a few minutes after the physical trauma, owing to the release of histamine by the mast cells in the skin.

Laboratory procedures

EXAMINATION FOR BACTERIA IN CRUSTS AND BIOPSY SPECIMENS Gram's stains and bacterial cultures of exudates should be performed on all lesions consisting of crusts and purulent exudates. Ulcers and nodules should be biopsied by removal of a wedge of tissue which extends from the surface down to the subcutaneous fat. The biopsy specimen should be minced in a sterile mortar and cultured for bacteria (including typical and atypical mycobacteria) and fungi.

EXAMINATION FOR MYCELIA The presence of mycelia may be ascertained by the application of 10% potassium hydroxide to a single tiny portion of scale, which is then gently heated. For fungi, scales and hair should be cultured on Sabouraud's medium.

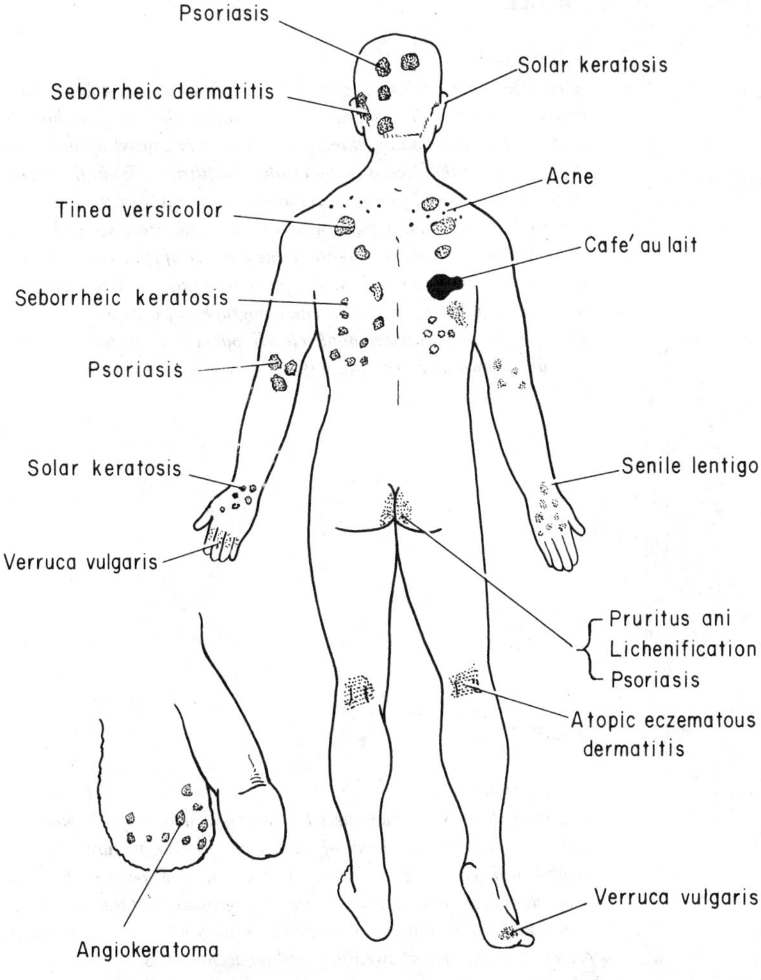

Types of skin lesion

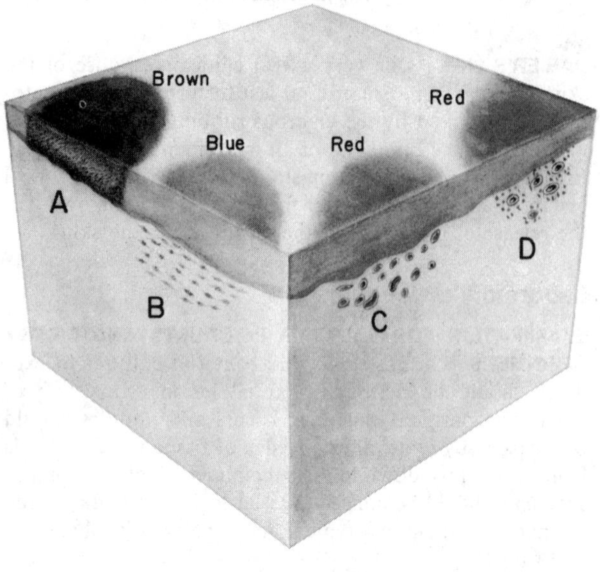

MACULE

FIGURE 54-2
A macule *is a circumscribed area of change in normal skin color without elevation or depression of the surface relative to the surrounding skin. The macules may be of any size and are the result of hypopigmentation (e.g., vitiligo) or hyperpigmentation—melanin* (A) *or hemosiderin* (D)*—such as* café au lait *spots and Mongolian spots* (B), *or permanent vascular abnormalities of the skin, as in a capillary hemangioma or transient capillary dilation (erythema)* (C). *Pressure of a glass slide (diascopy) on the border of a red lesion is a simple and reliable method for detecting the extravasation of red blood cells. If the redness remains under the pressure of the slide, the lesion may be purpuric* (D); *if the redness disappears, the lesion is erythematous and is due to vascular dilation* (C).

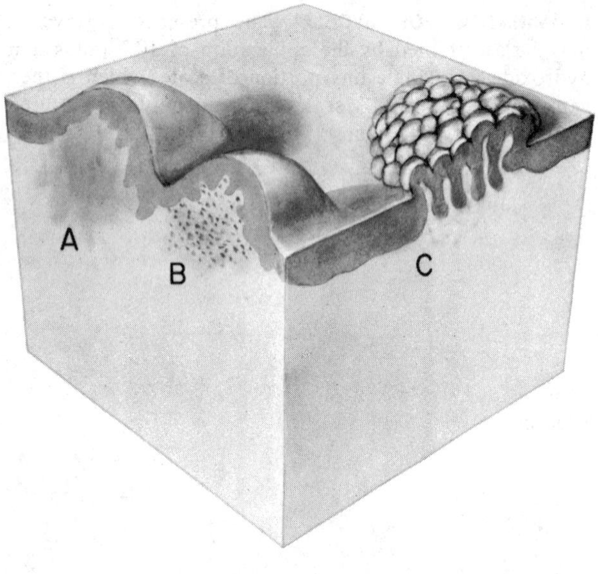

PAPULE

FIGURE 54-3
A papule *is a solid lesion, generally considered as less than 1 cm in diameter. Most of it is elevated above, rather than deep within, the plane of the surrounding skin. The elevation is caused by metabolic deposits* (A) *in the dermis or by localized infiltrates* (B) *in the dermis or by localized hyperplasia of cellular elements* (C) *in the dermis or epidermis. Superficial papules with distinct borders are seen when the lesion is the result of an increase in the number of epidermal cells* (C) *or melanocytes. Deeper dermal papules resulting from cellular infiltrates have indistinct borders. The topography of a papule or plaque may consist of multiple, small, closely packed, projected elevations that are known as a vegetation* (C).

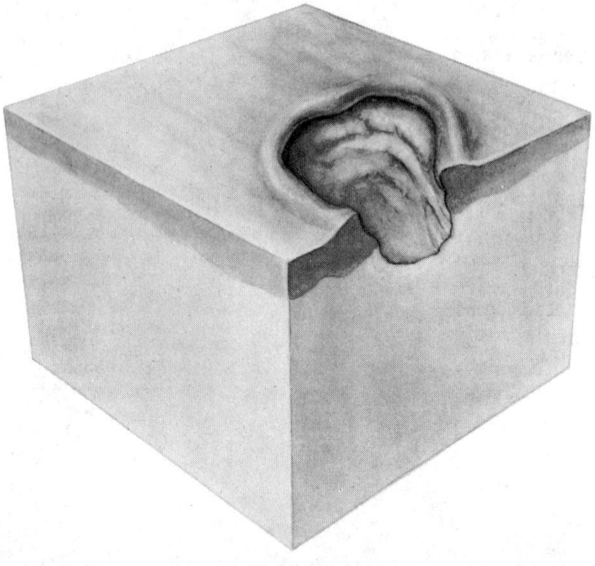

ULCERS

FIGURE 54-4
Ulcers *are lesions in which there has been destruction of the epidermis and the upper papillary layer of the dermis. Certain features that are helpful in determining the cause of ulcers include location, borders, base, discharge, and any associated topographic features of the lesions, such as nodules, excoriations, varicosities, hair distribution, presence or absence of sweating, and adjacent pulses.*

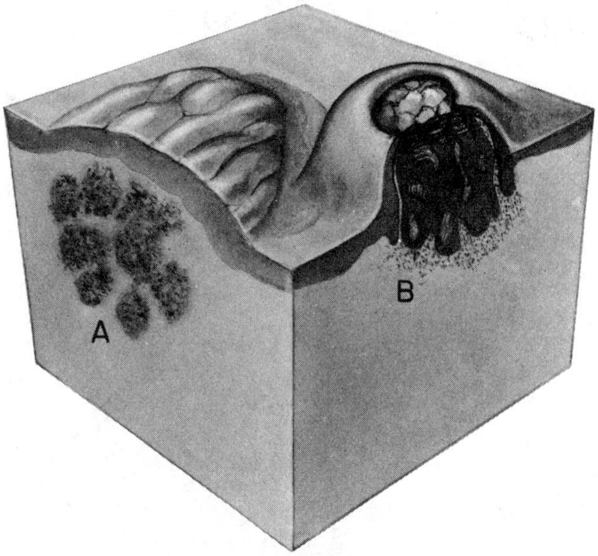

NODULE

FIGURE 54-5
A nodule *is a palpable solid, round, or ellipsoidal lesion deeper than a papule and is in the dermis or subcutaneous tissue* (A) *or in the epidermis* (B). *The depth of involvement rather than the diameter primarily differentiates a nodule from a papule. Nodules result for infiltrates* (A), *neoplasms* (B), *or metabolic deposits in the dermis or subcutaneous tissue and often indicate systemic disease. Late syphilis, tuberculosis, the deep mycoses, lymphoma, and metastatic neoplasms, e.g., can present as cutaneous nodules. Therefore, biopsy should be performed on unidentified persistent nodules, and a portion of excised tissue should be ground in a sterile mortar and cultured for fungi. Nodules can develop as a result of a benign or malignant proliferation of keratinocytes, as in keratoacanthoma* (B), *verruca vulgaris, and squamous-cell and basal-cell carcinoma.*

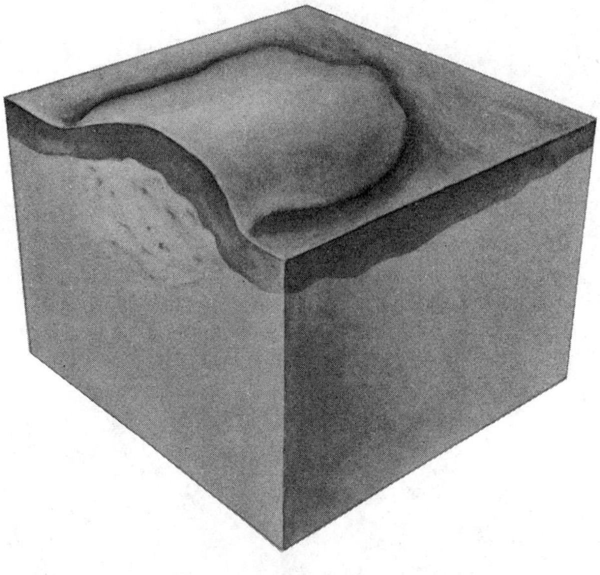

WHEAL

FIGURE 54-6
A wheal *is a rounded or flat-topped, pale-red elevation in the skin that is characteristically evanescent, disappearing within hours. Observation of the borders of wheals that have been traced with a skin-marking pencil reveals that the wheals shift relatively rapidly from the involved to the uninvolved adjacent areas. Wheals are the result of edema in the upper layer of the dermis.*

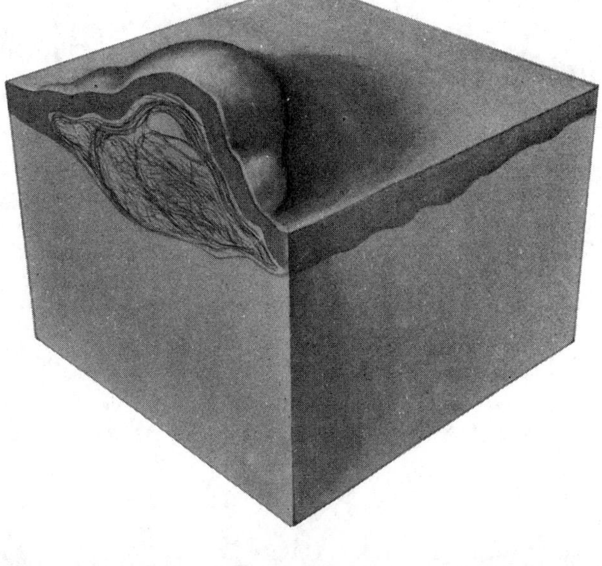

VESICLE

FIGURE 54-7
A vesicle *(less than 0.5 cm) or a* bulla *(more than 0.5 cm) is a circumscribed elevated lesion containing fluid. Often the walls are so thin that they are translucent, and the serum, lymph fluid, blood, or extracellular fluid can be seen. Vesicles and bullae arise from a cleavage at various levels of the skin; the cleavage may be within the epidermis (i.e., intraepidermal vesication), or at the epidermodermal interface (i.e., subepidermal).*

Types of skin lesion (cont.)

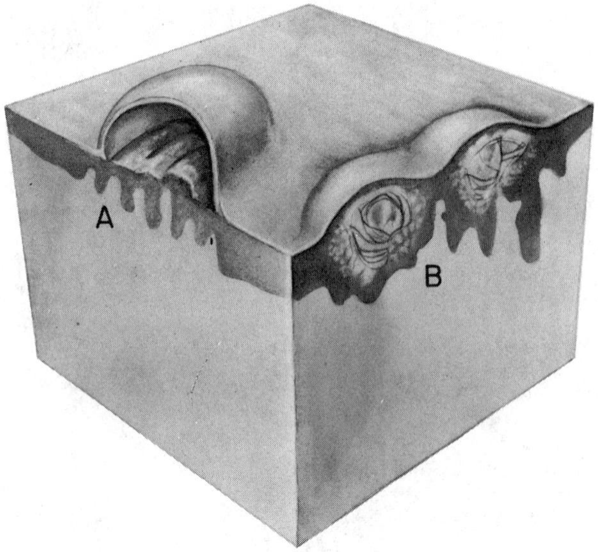

BULLA (A: subcorneal; B: spongiotic)

FIGURE 54-8
When the cleavage is just beneath the stratum corneum, a subcorneal vesicle *or* bulla *results* (A), *as seen in impetigo and subcorneal pustular dermatosis. Intraepidermal vesication may result from intercellular edema, or spongiosis* (B), *as characteristically seen in delayed hypersensitivity reactions of the epidermis (e.g., in contact eczematous dermatitis), and in dyshidrotic eczema* (B). Spongiotic vesicles *may or may not be seen clinically as vesicles.*

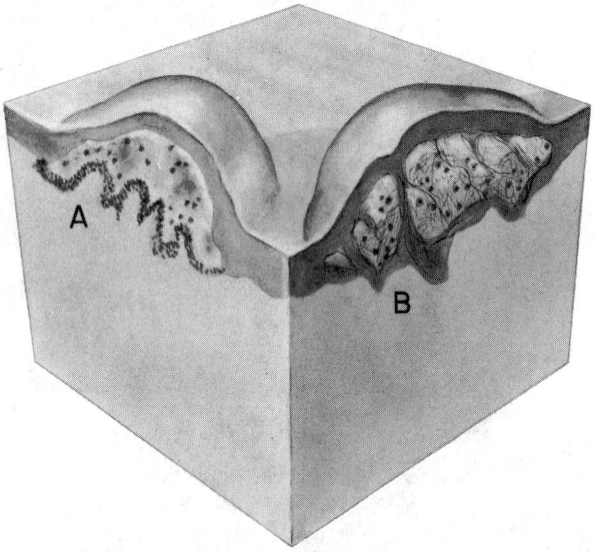

VESICLE (A: acantholytic; B: viral)

FIGURE 54-9
Loss of intercellular bridges, or desmosomes, is known as acantholysis (A), *and this type of intraepidermal vesication is seen in the vesicles or bullae of pemphigus vulgaris; the cleavage is usually just above the basal layer, as in pemphigus vulgaris, but may occur just below the subcorneal layer, as in pemphigus foliaceus. Viruses cause a curious "ballooning degeneration" of epidermal cells* (B), *as in herpes zoster, herpes simplex, variola, and varicella. Vital bullae often have a depressed ("umbilicated") center.*

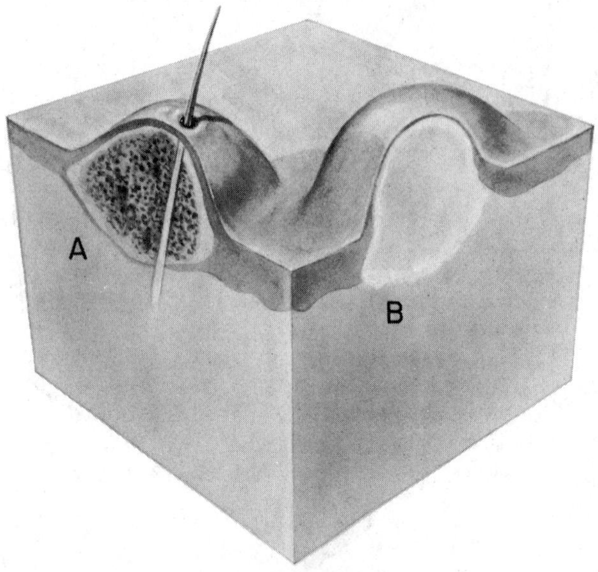

PUSTULE

FIGURE 54-10
A pustule *is a circumscribed elevation of the skin that contains a purulent exudate that may be white, yellow, or greenish yellow. This process may arise in a hair follicle* (A) *or independently* (B). *Pustules may vary in size and shape; follicular pustules, however, are always conical and usually contain a hair in the center. The vesicular lesions of the viral diseases (varicella, variola, vaccinia, herpes simplex, and herpes zoster) may secondarily become pustular. A Gram's stain and culture should be done on all pustules.*

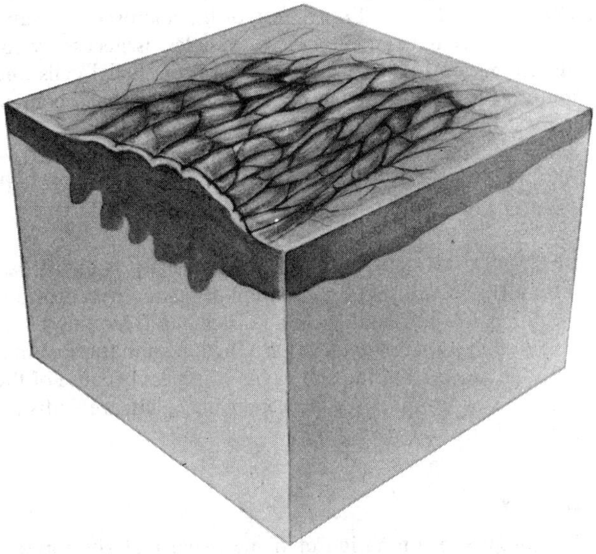

PLAQUE

FIGURE 54-11
A plaque *is an elevation above the skin surface that occupies a relatively large surface area in comparison with its height above the skin. Frequently, it is formed by a confluence of papules, as in psoriasis and mycosis fungoides. Lichenification is a proliferation of keratinocytes and stratum corneum forming a plaquelike structure. The skin appears thickened, and the skin markings are accentuated. The process results from repeated rubbing, and frequently develops in persons with atopy. Lichenification occurs in eczematous dermatitis.*

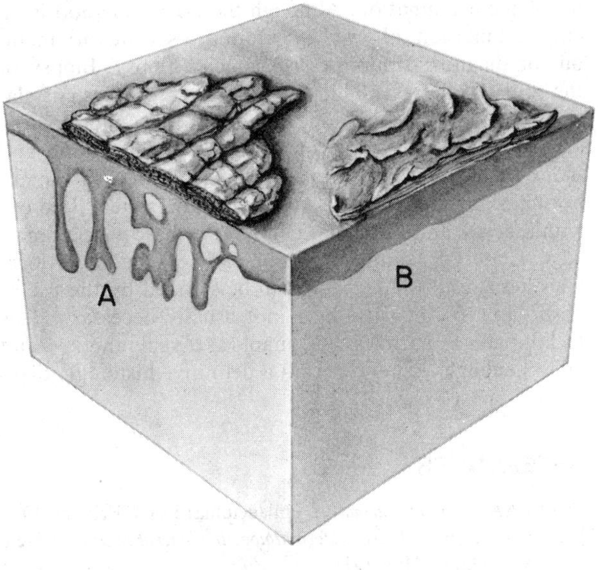

SCALES

FIGURE 54-12
Epidermal cells are completely replaced every 27 days. The end product of this holocrine process is the stratum corneum. This outermost layer of skin, the stratum corneum, normally does not contain nuclei and is imperceptibly lost. With an increased rate of proliferation of epidermal cells, as in psoriasis, the stratum corneum is not formed normally, and the outermost layers of the skin retain their nuclei. These desquamating layers of skin are seen clinically as scales. *Densely adherent scales that have a gritty feel (like sandpaper) result from a localized increase in the stratum corneum and are typically seen in solar keratosis* (B).

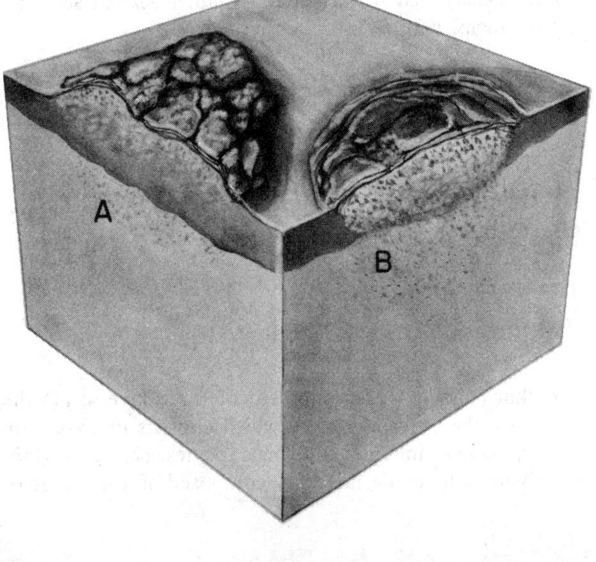

CRUSTS

FIGURE 54-13
Crusts, *resulting when serum, blood, or purulent exudate dries on the skin surface, are the hallmark of pyogenic infection. Crusts may be thin, delicate, and friable* (A) *or thick and adherent* (B). *Crusts are yellow when formed from dried serum, green or yellow-green when formed from purulent exudate, or brown or dark red when formed from blood. Superficial crusts occur as honey-colored, delicate, glistening particulates on the surface* (A) *and are typically seen in impetigo. When the exudate involves the entire epidermis, the crusts may be thick and adherent, and this condition is known as ecthyma* (B).

TZANCK TEST The Tzanck test, or the microscopic examination of cells from the base of vesicles, is necessary for determination of the presence of giant epithelial cells and multinucleated giant cells (Color Plate 5-5) that occur in herpes simplex, herpes zoster, and varicella. Material taken from the base of a vesicle by gentle curettage with a scalpel is spread gently on a glass slide and prepared with Giemsa's or Wright's stain for the examination.

DARKFIELD EXAMINATION OF SERUM FOR TREPONEMA PALLIDUM Darkfield examination of serum from erosions on the male and female genitalia is essential for the detection of *Treponema pallidum.* Darkfield examination of material obtained from the oral cavity is useless because of the presence of nonpathogenic treponemas that are indistinguishable from *T. pallidum.*

Biopsy

Microscopic examination of tissue is particularly applicable in dermatology because the lesions can be subjected to histologic examination. Although the classic method is an elliptical incision followed by suturing, a satisfactory method for diagnostic purposes is "punch" biopsy. Biopsy of the skin, in contrast to biopsy of the liver, enables correlation of gross and microscope pathology. For punch biopsy, a small tubular blade is rotated between the thumb and index finger to cut through the entire thickness of the abnormal skin; the resulting cylinder of skin is then lifted out with forceps, and the skin is cut off at its base with a pointed scissors. This simple operation can be done under local anesthesia, and the bleeding can be stopped by the use of absorbable foam; suturing is not usually necessary. This technique is as harmless and simple as a venipuncture, and allows enough tissue to permit a definitive histologic diagnosis in most cases.

REFERENCES

FISHER AA: *Contact Dermatitis,* Philadelphia: Lea & Febiger, 1973

FITZPATRICK TB et al (eds): *Dermatology in General Medicine,* New York: McGraw-Hill, 1971

ROOK A, WILKINSON DS: The principles of diagnosis, in *Textbook of Dermatology,* ed A Rook et al, Oxford: Blackwell Scientific Publications, 1972, p. 37

55
SKIN LESIONS OF GENERAL MEDICAL SIGNIFICANCE

T. B. FITZPATRICK
H. A. HAYNES

The skin (Fig. 55-1) is composed of three layers: (1) the *epidermis,* the outermost part, which consists of two main cell types, keratinocytes and melanocytes, (2) the *dermis,* upon which the epidermis rests, composed of a mélange of connective-tissue elements, nerves, blood and lymph vessels, glands, appendages, and a few cells (mast cells, histiocytes); and (3) the *panniculus adiposus* (subcutaneous tissue), which acts as a cushion between the epidermis and dermis and the underlying bone. The specialized cells of the epidermis, the keratinocytes, produce and retain in their cytoplasm the scleroprotein keratin. They are constantly turning over, about 27 days being required to complete differentiation and maturation. Maturation of keratinocytes consists of loss of the nucleus, leaving only the cytoplasm. The latter is made up of a highly ordered, two-phase system of keratin filaments embedded in an amorphous matrix, much like the cellulose-lignin system of wood fiber, which is known to be well adapted to withstand shearing and compression forces. The anucleate outermost portion of the epidermis is the *stratum corneum,* which acts as a tough, keratinous membrane. The stratum corneum functions structurally as a "waterproof" wall between the internal fluid milieu and the environment, and is the major barrier of the skin, protecting the body against loss of fluids and entrance of toxic agents. It also serves as a passive membrane—substances move across the skin by passive diffusion in the direction of the concentration gradient.

The skin has a relatively limited number of pathologic responses. If the letters of the alphabet are taken to represent individual skin lesions (see Table 54-1), then words or phrases can be said to represent groups of lesions. The lesions in the majority of patients seen by the general physician can be placed in one of the groups of clinical reactions (Table 55-1) or types of skin lesions listed in Table

FIGURE 55-1
Anatomy of the skin. (Copyright 1967 CIBA Pharmaceutial Company, division of CIBA-Geigy Corporation. Reproduced, with permission from the Clinical Symposia, illustrated by Frank H. Netter, M.D. All rights reserved.)

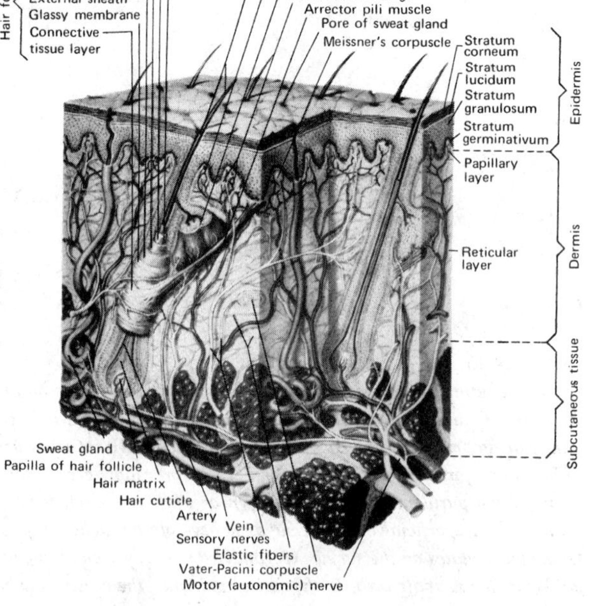

54-1. These skin lesions or clinical reactions may consist of one type of lesion, such as either a vesicle or a nodule, or may consist of aggregates of various types of lesions, such as papules or vesicles, as in erythema multiforme. Just one lesion or several solitary lesions or one or more groups of lesions may be distributed any place on the body. A pathologic process may involve the skin in the form of isolated lesions, as just mentioned, or the pathologic process may involve all the skin so that the borders of the lesions may not be defined; this latter type of diffuse involvement occurs in systemic sclerosis and in pigmentation disorders.

In the physician's attempts to identify the specific types of lesions, it is therefore essential to try to estimate the component of the skin that is *primarily* affected, as the epidermis, the dermis, the blood vessels, or the panniculus adiposus. Inasmuch as there is a finite number of disorders that produce pathologic changes in the various individual components, this method of approach will improve the physician's diagnostic acumen. For example, even though erythema multiforme involves the dermis and the epidermis, the *primary component affected* is the blood vessel, and it is this involvement that explains the erythematous macules; the inflammatory process leads subsequently to the development of the cellular infiltrates seen clinically as papules and to destruction of the basement membrane and the development of bullae.

CLASSIFICATION OF LESIONS ACCORDING TO THE COMPONENT OF THE SKIN PRIMARILY AFFECTED

Epidermis

SCALING MACULES, PAPULES, OR PLAQUES Generalized scaling macules, papules, or plaques are frequent and important diagnostic problems and are usually a presenting complaint of the patient (Figs. 54-2, 54-3, and 54-11).

Sudden onset of symmetrical scaling erythematous macules or papules should suggest that drugs are the etiologic agents. Scaling erythematous papules on the scalp and extensor aspects of the arms and legs are suggestive of *psoriasis;* psoriatic lesions often are accentuated on the sites of repeated trauma, such as the elbows and knees. The papules or plaques of psoriasis often contain a silvery white micaceous scale that is relatively easily removed in layers (see Color Plate 2-6). In psoriasis, there is a severalfold increase in the normal number of the basal cells of the epidermis. This increase in the basal-cell population reduces the turnover time of the epidermis from the normal 27 days to 3 to 4 days. With this shortened interval of epidermal-cell migration from the basal layer to the skin surface, the normal events of cell maturation and keratinization do not occur (see *A* in Fig. 54-12); this failure of maturation is reflected by an array of abnormal morphologic and biochemical changes. In association with the basal-cell hyperplasia, there is enhanced metabolism and accelerated synthesis and degradation of nucleoproteins, resulting in an elevated urinary excretion of nucleic acid metabolites such as uric acid. In addition, there is a proliferation of the subepidermal vasculature that is necessary to support the increased rate of cell division. The large number of cytologic, histologic, histochemical, and biochemical alterations are now known to be the result, rather than the cause, of the disease process. The only main fact known at this time about the fundamental cause of psoriasis is that the predisposition to its development is genetically transmitted. An erosive joint disease, *psoriatic arthritis,* is discussed in Chap. 361.

The treatment of psoriasis still remains in the province of the dermatologist. The most effective treatment in the control of psoriasis, for most patients, is the use of topical corticosteroids with plastic wrap, topical coal-tar preparations, and ultraviolet light or sunlight exposures. Corticosteroids can also be injected directly into small, resistant plaques. Systemic corticosteroids are not only ineffective in psoriasis but may cause generalization of the process and are absolutely contraindicated. With certain patients who are resistant to topical therapy, it has been necessary to use a variety of systemic chemotherapeutic agents, especially methotrexate; the latter has the capacity to inhibit cell replication without a proportionate inhibition of cell function, i.e., keratinization. In 1974, a new form of photochemotherapy was introduced which uses oral methoxsalen and a high-intensity, long-wave ultraviolet light source. This approach may replace many of the other forms of therapy.

TABLE 55-1
Clinical classification of lesions according to the component of the skin primarily affected*

- *I* Affecting the epidermis
  - *A* Keratinocytes and/or stratum corneum
    - *1* Scaling macules, papules, or plaques
    - *2* Vesicles and bullae (erosions follow rupture)
    - *3* Pustules
    - *4* Exudative (impetiginized) lesions
    - *5* Eczematous dermatitis
    - *6* Erythroderma syndrome (exfoliative dermatitis)†
    - *7* Atrophy, diffuse† or circumscribed
  - *B* Melanocytes
    - *1* Hypomelanotic macules
    - *2* Diffuse hypomelanosis†
    - *3* Hypermelanotic (brown) macules
    - *4* Diffuse brown hypermelanosis syndrome†
- *II* Affecting the dermis
  - *A* Connective tissue
    - *1* Papules and nodules (with and without inflammation)
    - *2* Ulcers
    - *3* Sclerosis, diffuse† or circumscribed
    - *4* Edema†
    - *5* Atrophy, diffuse† or circumscribed
  - *B* Blood vessels
    - *1* Morbilliform and scarlatiniform eruptions
    - *2* Urticaria
    - *3* Erythema multiforme syndrome
    - *4* Purpura (with and without inflammation)
    - *5* Infarcts
    - *6* Telangiectasia
- *III* Affecting the panniculus adiposus
  - *A* Nodules
    - *1* Inflammatory, usually tender, red nodules
    - *2* Noninflammatory, usually nontender, nonerythematous nodules
  - *B* Atrophy

* *Not including benign and malignant primary neoplasms of the skin or benign hyperplasias.*
† *Pathologic changes affect large areas of skin; there are no discrete lesions.*

The general physician does not always appreciate the importance of psoriasis as a major cause of disability and of disfigurement. Psoriasis affects between 2 and 8 million persons in the United States.

Symmetrical scaling macules or papules localized on the palms and soles often are presenting signs of *secondary syphilis;* there is very often generalized lymphadenopathy and there may be mouth lesions occurring as erosions.

A relatively common and often baffling generalized scaling eruption is seen in *pityriasis rosea.* In this condition, the scale at the periphery of the lesion is very thin and forms a collarette; the center of the lesion may or may not be scaly. Pityriasis rosea typically has a "fir-tree" type of distribution, especially evident on the back. Very often, but not always, a preceding, single, isolated scaling lesion is present for several days before generalization of the lesions.

Rarely, generalized scaling macules and papules are seen in *dermatophytosis* (Color Plate 2-1) and *candidosis,* and it is therefore necessary that some of the scales be examined for the presence of mycelia.

From the clinician's point of view, *mycotic infections of the skin* may be separated into two major categories, each of which has a different etiology, associated systemic disease, and response to treatment, with only one category responding to the oral antifungal, griseofulvin. The various types of *dermatophytosis* (so-called "ringworm" infections) constitute one category, and all (except tinea versicolor) respond to oral griseofulvin and are confined to the epidermis, hair, toenails, and fingernails. Dermatophytosis is due to three types of fungus: Microsporum, Epidermophyton, and Trichophyton. *Microsporum audouini,* a parasite of humans, is the principal pathogen causing epidemic urban fungous infection of the scalp. *Microsporum canis,* which affects the scalp and also the face, where it causes boggy nodules, is a parasite of animals and originates largely from young (usually) farm animals and pets (kittens, puppies, and calves). *Trichophyton rubrum, Trichophyton mentagrophytes,* and *Epidermophyton floccosum,* which also are parasites of humans, are the agents most usually causing dermatophytosis of the feet, the commonest site of mycotic infection. The type of fungus infecting upper extremities, face, and trunk can be Trichophyton or Microsporum or Epidermophyton.

Inasmuch as Trichophyton, Microsporum, and Epidermophyton are parasites in humans, factors other than just contact might be implicated. Other considerations, such as variation in the host response, based on hereditary factors and mediated, possibly, through increased susceptibility or related to immune factors that have yet to be clearly defined, must be investigated.

The response of these three types of fungus to oral griseofulvin varies. Griseofulvin is highly effective, even in short courses, in fungous infection of the scalp, trunk, and groin, but even prolonged therapy rarely controls infection of the hands, fingernails, or toenails. Topical treatment with any of the antifungals is quite effective in infection of the feet, trunk, and groin, but is without any effect on infection of the fingernails or toenails.

The other major category of mycotic infections is represented by candidiasis (monilial infections). These infections do not respond at all to oral griseofulvin and are caused largely by *Candida albicans,* although occasionally by *C. tropicalis, C. krusei,* and *C. stellatoidea. C. albicans* can exist as a harmless saprophyte in the gastrointestinal tract and in the vagina. It is more common in females, and is most often present in those who are pregnant or who are taking oral contraceptives or broad-spectrum antibiotics. The association with diabetes mellitus, however, is so common that all patients (regardless of sex) with candidiasis should be screened for this disease.

Despite the fact that *C. albicans* is a normal saprophytic fungus in the vagina and gastrointestinal tract, it is rarely isolated from the exposed surface of the normal skin. *C. albicans* can invade the epidermis when the skin is exposed to high humidity and when the skin becomes macerated, and therefore, candidiasis is of common occurrence in the intertriginous areas (under the breasts and in the umbilicus, groin, and axillae), and in the oral, as well as the vaginal, mucous membranes. Chronic paronychia is usually caused by *C. albicans.* Candidiasis also may involve the lungs, urinary tract, and heart (see Chap. 175).

The treatment of candidiasis of the skin and mucous membranes depends on the site of the infection and the type of lesion. Maceration of the skin should be treated by air-drying of the area. Lotions and dusting powders containing nystatin are also very useful for intertriginous areas. Oral administration of nystatin is not of value in cutaneous moniliasis. Unless the male, as well as the female, sexual partner is treated when candidiasis is present, there will be constant retransfer of the infection.

Differentiation between dermatophytosis caused by any of the three types of fungus already mentioned and candidiasis may be difficult, if not impossible, without cultures of the fungus (see Laboratory Procedures in Chap. 54). Direct examination of the scales from a scaling eruption in the intertriginous area is not diagnostic because it may reveal mycelia in both dermatophytosis and candidiasis; spores, however, are seen only in candidiasis. Too often, the general physician starts treatment with topical antifungal agents or with griseofulvin without establishing whether the eruption is a type of dermatophytosis or candidiasis. Inasmuch as candidiasis does not respond to systemic griseofulvin or to most of the topical antifungal agents, prescribing these agents for an eruption that is actually candidiasis results in prolonged disability for the patient. Newer agents such as haloprogin and miconazole are effective against both dermatophytosis and candidiasis.

In the past few years, fungous diseases have assumed a new importance in medicine because of the increased number of patients under treatment with chemotherapeutic agents for leukemia and other neoplasms. Almost all of the saprophytic fungi are now known to invade the tissues of patients who are being treated with chemotherapeutic agents or who have had kidney transplants.

VESICLES AND BULLAE Some diseases may occasionally be associated with vesicles or bullae, such as erythema multiforme or porphyria cutanea tarda, but blisters (vesicles and bullae) are the major feature of a number of disorders: certain bacterial and viral infections; allergic contact dermatitis (such as poison ivy); trauma from mechanical, thermal, or chemical agents; and the bullous diseases of unknown cause (such as pemphigus and pemphigoid).

Grouped vesicles occur in herpes zoster and herpes simplex, whereas scattered discrete vesicles occur in varicella. A helpful sign in determining the nature of the vesicles is the Tzanck test (Color Plate 5-5; see also Laboratory Procedures in Chap. 54). In herpes simplex, herpes zoster, and varicella, there will be clusters of epithelial giant cells, which are absent in vaccinia and variola. Skin biopsy will also establish the nature of the vesicle or bulla, that is, whether it is an intraepidermal (as seen in virus infections and pemphigus) or a subepidermal bulla (as seen in bullous pemphigoid) (Figs. 54-7 to 54-9).

Vesicles arranged in linear streaks are characteristic of poison ivy dermatitis. The most reliable clue to the diagnosis of both allergic and primary-irritant contact dermatitis is the localization of vesicles to the skin areas likely to have been exposed to the agent in question.

Scattered, isolated bullae in adults represent a special and serious problem in diagnosis and treatment. *Bullous pemphigoid* and *pemphigus* are chronic, occurring primarily in adults, and one of them, pemphigus, has serious consequences for the patient. These two disorders need to be distinguished by biopsy of the skin and by the newly available immunofluorescence techniques. It is impossible on the basis of clinical diagnosis alone to distinguish between bullous pemphigoid, which is a chronic and relatively benign disorder and often of limited duration, and *pemphigus vulgaris,* which is a serious disease leading in a relentless course to death, unless treatment with immunosuppressive agents or steroids is instituted. Pemphigus has been divided into four separate entities, but pemphigus vulgaris is the most important for the general physician to recognize. Pemphigus vulgaris may begin in the nasal or oral mucous membrane, and the patient may consult the dentist or otolaryngologist first. The lesions tend to spread in an unpredictable fashion to other parts of the body, but especially seem to localize around the umbilicus and on the scalp and trunk, although there is no specific distribution pattern. Pemphigus vulgaris affects primarily the middle-aged, particularly between the ages of forty and sixty. It rarely occurs before the age of seventeen or after the age of seventy-five years. The clinical lesions appear as flaccid bullae from the beginning; they break easily and rarely become very large. The denuded areas that form at the site of the ruptured bullae increase in size as the epidermis detaches itself. Occasionally, almost the entire surface may be involved by large, denuded areas; this involvement represents a serious problem in the management of secondary infection and in maintenance of fluid balance—more or less the same problems that occur in a severely burned patient. Oral or nasal mucosal lesions occur in nearly all the patients, and more than half have lesions in the mucous membrane of the mouth as the first manifestation of the disease. The disease often starts with only a few lesions in the mouth and may remain limited in extent for several weeks; it then gradually spreads to other parts of the body.

The diagnosis of pemphigus is made on the basis of the light-microscope examination of the biopsy of an early vesicle. The earliest change in pemphigus vulgaris consists of intercellular edema followed by disappearance of intercellular bridges in the lower epidermis (see *A* in Fig. 54-9). This results in loss of cohesion between the epidermal cells (acantholysis) and leads to the formation of clefts and then bullae that are predominantly in the suprabasal locations; in other words, the basal cells, although separated from one another, remain attached to the dermis much like a "row of tombstones."

Immunofluorescence allows detection of antibodies in the serum of patients with pemphigus and bullous pemphigoid and differentiation of these two bullous disorders by the localization of the antibody. The antibodies, which are in the IgG fraction of serum, react with a specific intercellular antigen. The fluorescence is localized to the site of acantholysis in pemphigus; in bullous pemphigoid, however, the antibodies react with the basement membrane, and the fluorescence is localized there.

Treatment of pemphigus with systemic and intradermal corticosteroids, sometimes in combination with methotrexate or azathioprine, is quite successful.

PUSTULES This skin reaction (Fig. 54-10) may result from infections or from sterile inflammation. Pustules may arise from preexisting vesicles of any cause. Infection by pyogenic bacteria, especially staphylococci, as well as by certain fungi and mycobacteria, can produce pustules without a preceding vesicular stage. Noninfectious causes of pustules include acne, pustular psoriasis, and hypersensitivity to drugs, particularly sulfonamides, iodides, or bromides.

EXUDATIVE (IMPETIGINIZED) LESIONS Acute infection with gram-positive cocci can occur as a primary process or may be superimposed on eczematous dermatitis or occasionally on any of the vesicular bullous diseases, and is characterized by the presence of crusts (Fig. 54-13). Such infection on the skin has the same importance as a streptococcal pharyngitis, inasmuch as acute glomerular nephritis develops in a significant percentage of patients with impetiginized dermatitis. Patients with impetiginized dermatitis must therefore be treated with full courses of systemic antibiotics.

ECZEMATOUS DERMATITIS Eczematous dermatitis (Color Plates 2-2 and 2-3) is not a specific disease entity but a characteristic inflammatory response of the skin due to both endogenous and exogenous agents that cause a delayed hypersensitivity reaction. Eczematous dermatitis therefore requires a qualifying etiologic term, e.g., *atopic eczematous dermatitis.* Eczematous dermatitis is sufficiently serious to account for the highest incidence of skin morbidity, responsible for incalculable losses of time and productivity in industry, with approximately one-third of all patients in the United States seen by dermatologists having one or the other of its forms. In Tables 55-2 and 55-3 some of the types of eczematous dermatitis are summarized (*B* in Figs. 54-8 and 54-11).

ERYTHRODERMA SYNDROME (EXFOLIATIVE DERMATITIS) The erythroderma syndrome is an important dermatologic complication that may occur as the result of an extension of a drug reaction, as a generalized spreading of a preexisting dermatosis, such as psoriasis or atopic dermatitis, or in association with lymphoma and leukemia. This syndrome consists of a generalized erythematous scaling eruption involving all of the skin surface, and has important implications in general medicine because of the systemic effects occasioned by the massive and continuous exfoliation of the skin. The severity of the metabolic response to exfoliation depends on the duration and severity of the process itself. Patients with extensive exfoliative dermatitis may have negative nitrogen balance, edema, hypoalbuminemia, and loss of muscle mass. An important feature also in these patients is the large extrarenal water loss, due to the defective cutaneous barrier that leads to markedly increased transepidermal water loss. Serious metabolic effects of chronic exfoliative dermatitis occur when the rate of scaling reaches 17 g per m^2 per 24 h. The etiology of exfoliative dermatitis determines its course: the disease eventually clears in patients with psoriasis or atopic dermatitis, whereas the prognosis is relatively poor in patients with lymphoma and leukemia. Approximately 60 percent of patients with exfoliative dermatitis recover within eight to ten months, 30 percent die, and 10 percent have a persistent problem unresponsive to therapy.

ATROPHY, DIFFUSE OR CIRCUMSCRIBED Epidermal atrophy is manifested by an almost transparent epidermis and is associated with a decrease in the number of epidermal cells. An atrophic epidermis may or may not retain the normal skin markings. Circumscribed epidermal atrophy occurs in discoid lupus erythematosus, in necrobiosis lipoidica diabeticorum, and in striae cutis distensae; diffuse epidermal atrophy occurs with aging and in scleroderma.

The most important atrophic-type disorder is *necrobiosis lipoidica diabeticorum* (NLD) (Color Plate 5-1). These lesions, which are usually asymptomatic, occur more frequently in women and on the areas subject to trauma such as the anterior and lateral surfaces of the lower legs. The lesion begins as a small, reddish, elevated nodule with a sharply circumscribed border, gradually enlarges, and becomes flattened and depressed as the skin becomes atrophic. The brownish-yellow color is prominent, and blood vessels are readily seen because of the atrophic epidermis that is smooth and loses its skin markings entirely. The lesions of NLD are extremely indolent, and shallow ulcerations that are very slow to heal may develop. NLD may occur when diabetes mellitus cannot be detected even by use of most stringent and provocative tests, such as the cortisone-glucose tolerance test. It is characterized by focal changes in the dermis that present as acellular and intense eosinophilic areas of necrosis bordered by inflammation. The inflammatory cells are granulomatous and include epithelioid cells, histiocytes, and multinucleated giant cells. The blood vessels are always involved with endothelial proliferation and sometimes even occlusion of the arterioles and arteries deep within the dermis; the capillary walls are thickened with focal deposits of PAS-positive material.

HYPOMELANOTIC MACULES See Chap. 57.

TABLE 55-2
Various types of eczematous dermatitis* of uncertain etiology

Clinical type	*Suspected pathogenesis*	*Diagnostic considerations*
Atopic eczematous dermatitis	Hereditary predisposition plus precipitating factors	Eczematous dermatitis, especially localized to the antecubital and popliteal fossae and to the face
Lichen simplex chronicus	Hereditary predisposition plus repeated local trauma	One or more lichenified plaques (see Fig. 54-11), especially on neck
Prurigo nodularis	Repeated local trauma	One or more nodules, especially on extremities
"Neurodermatitis"	Hereditary predisposition plus repeated scratching	Generalized or localized eczematous eruption at sites of repeated trauma
Stasis dermatitis	Chronic venous insufficiency	Signs of venous insufficiency
Nummular eczematous dermatitis	Various precipitating factors (contact irritants, xerosis, emotional stress, etc.)	Discrete coin-shaped patches, usually on extremities and trunk
"Dyshidrotic" eczematous dermatitis	Emotional stress plus other factors‡	Vesicles and bullae on palms and soles
Seborrheic dermatitis	Constitutional diathesis	Greasy scaling patches on scalp, eyebrows, and nasolabial area
Various patterns of eczematous dermatitis	Association with gastrointestinal malabsorption	Eczematous eruption in patient with steatorrhea and abnormal biopsy specimens of the jejunal mucosa
"Eczematous-like eruptions"† with systemic disease: Wiskott-Aldrich syndrome; X-linked agammaglobulinemia; Phenylketonuria; Ahistidinemia; Hurler's syndrome; Hartnup disease; Acrodermatitis enteropathica	Metabolic and immunologic disorders	Related features of clinical syndrome plus immunologic deficiency or biochemical abnormality

* *This term is used by many clinicians for at least four types of eczematous dermatitis that may be exclusively localized to the hands (atopic eczematous dermatitis, allergic contact eczematous dermatitis, nummular eczematous dermatitis, and "dyshidrotic" eczematous dermatitis). Possibly, contact irritants to which the hands are frequently exposed may precipitate or aggravate one of the above-mentioned basic types of eczematous dermatitis.*
† *These eruptions are reported in the literature as eczematous dermatitis, but clear, careful clinical descriptions with cutaneous biopsy specimens are frequently lacking.*
‡ *Such as constitutional diathesis and contact dermatitis.*

DIFFUSE HYPOMELANOSIS See Chap. 57.

HYPERMELANOTIC MACULES See Chap. 57.

DIFFUSE BROWN HYPERMELANOSIS SYNDROME See Chap. 57.

Dermis

PAPULES AND NODULES (WITH AND WITHOUT INFLAMMATION) Papules and nodules without epidermal change (i.e., scaling) may be either skin color, erythematous, or even slightly pigmented (yellow or brown). Dermal papules and all nodules require a biopsy for definitive diagnosis because they often represent either processes that have general medical significance, such as sarcoidosis or histiocytosis X, or tuberculosis or lymphoma. Inasmuch as dermal nodules may be present in deep mycotic infections such as coccidioidomycosis, it is necessary to obtain a biopsy, not only to rule out malignancy but to culture a portion of the excised tissue for fungi. Cultures of nodules must be made from minced tissue. The histologic specimen should be carefully studied for the presence of acid-fast bacilli, inasmuch as nodules are the presenting feature of leprosy or tuberculosis; nodules removed from the common areas of localization for leishmaniasis (face and arms) should be carefully examined for the presence of parasites.

Papules and nodules with and without inflammation can occur in disorders of the sebaceous glands. Sebaceous glands are distributed largely on the face and scalp, although they can also occur in the labia minora and on the scrotal skin, trunk, nipples, and eyelids. The sebaceous gland is a holocrine gland in which the entire cell is cast off into the excretory stream. Sebum is a complex lipid mixture of squalene (a major product of the steroid pathway), triglycerides, and wax ester. Sebaceous glands are mostly controlled by direct hormonal stimulation with androgens, derived largely from the gonads in both sexes; in the female, but not in the male, adrenal androgens may be important factors in maintaining sebum production. The major disease of the sebaceous gland in humans is *acne vulgaris* (Color Plate 1-5), which occurs predominantly on the face and, to a lesser degree, on the back, chest, and shoulders. It is characterized by a variety of clinical lesions. These lesions may be either noninflammatory or inflammatory papules and nodules. The noninflammatory papules are called comedones, and these may be either open (blackheads) or closed (whiteheads). The closed comedones are the precursors of large inflammatory nodules and of papules and pustules. In addition, cysts and scars of various sizes may occur, the typical acne scar being a sharply punched-out pit. In the pustular and cystic lesions, despite a large amount of purulent exudate that may be recovered following incision, the lesions are usually sterile but may contain *Corynebacterium acnes.* It is believed that acne develops as a result of a primary inflammation in the follicle wall, and that the follicle partly ruptures, leading to a spilling-out of its components and the development of a perifollicular inflammatory process. The inflammatory infiltrate is lymphocytic but later, as a result of the presence of keratinous material, gram-positive diphtheroids, and sebum, the infiltrate consists essentially of a foreign-body giant-cell reaction.

The initial stimulus to the formation of comedones (both the closed and open type), is not precisely known at this time, but the initial histologic event in comedone formation is excessive keratinization within the follicular canal. It is currently believed that *Corynebacterium acnes* is responsible for lipolysis with a release of fatty acids; it is thought that these fatty acids are capable of producing an inflammatory process in the follicle wall. Acne vulgaris is a serious and important problem, especially common in the adolescent female, and its therapy is complex and prolonged. Moderate to severe acne vulgaris is best treated by a dermatologist utilizing topical agents, incision and drainage of the cystic lesions, ultraviolet-light therapy, and judicious use of systemic antibiotics; x-ray therapy has no place in the treatment of acne vulgaris.

The mechanism of action of antibiotics such as tetracycline is not completely known, but these drugs are known to suppress the number of Corynebacteria and cause a reduction of free fatty acids recoverable from the skin. Inasmuch as the organisms have been shown to have lipolytic activity in vitro, it is presumed that the antibiotic causes this reduction of free fatty acids.

TABLE 55-3
Various types of eczematous dermatitis* of known etiology

Clinical type	*Pathogenesis*	*Diagnostic considerations*
Allergic contact eczematous dermatitis	Chemical allergens (plants, medicaments, cosmetics, metals, fabrics, etc.)	Site and configuration are clues to causal agent; patch tests may confirm diagnosis; avoidance of cause cures eruption
Photoallergic contact eczematous dermatitis	Ultraviolet radiation plus topical chemicals (in soaps, perfumes, citrus fruits, etc.), which then become allergens	Occurs on exposed skin; photopatch tests confirm diagnosis
Polymorphous light-induced eruption—eczematous type	Ultraviolet radiation; sometimes visible light	Occurs on exposed skin; diagnosis implies that all known causes of light-induced eruptions have been eliminated
"Infectious eczematoid dermatitis"	Bacterial products from draining focus (e.g., ear infection)	Occurs near site of infection; responds to treatment of primary infection
Eczematous dermatophytosis	Fungus	Fungi demonstrated in scales or exudate

* *This term is used by many clinicians for at least four types of eczematous dermatitis that may be exclusively localized to the hands (atopic eczematous dermatitis, allergic contact eczematous dermatitis, nummular eczematous dermatitis, and "dyshidrotic" eczematous dermatitis). Possibly, contact irritants to which the hands are frequently exposed may precipitate or aggravate one of the above-mentioned basic types of eczematous dermatitis.*

Estrogens combined with progestins (oral contraceptives) were initially considered effective in controlling acne; however, they have been of only limited value in the treatment of acne in females and cannot be given to males. There is no evidence suggesting that diet has any effect on the course or severity of acne vulgaris. Acne vulgaris may begin as early as the eighth year or may not appear until the twentieth. It lasts for several years and then subsides spontaneously, usually when the patients are in their early twenties. In some patients, however, acne vulgaris may continue into the third and fourth decades.

Pretibial myxedema (PM) also may cause nodules on the legs and dorsa of the feet (Color Plate 5-2). The lesions are usually bilateral and consist of elevated, firm, dermal nodules and plaques that are not easily movable. They may be skin color, pink, or, rarely, brown, and, when diascoped, appear yellow and waxy. The epidermis over the nodules may appear normal or may have a marked verrucous (warty) surface. The pathogenesis of pretibial myxedema is not clear. Pretibial myxedema may occur with hyperthyroidism (Graves' disease) or before or after treatment of hyperthyroidism, and its development does not parallel the ocular changes (if present). The nodules in pretibial myxedema are accumulations of mucopolysaccharides, which can be demonstrated by special staining of the histopathologic material. Long-acting thyroid stimulator (LATS), which is associated in the plasma with immunoglobulin G (7S gamma-globulin), has been implicated in the pathogenesis of pretibial myxedema, exophthalmos, and acropachy; the role of LATS in the pathogenesis of pretibial myxedema has not been established.

ULCERS Ulcers occur as a result of destruction of the epidermis and, at least, the papillary layer of the dermis (Fig. 54-4). All ulcers of the skin that do not heal within a period of a month must be considered to be carcinoma until proved otherwise, and it is essential that a biopsy be obtained to rule out malignancy. Ulcers can be divided into two categories: lesions that occur on the legs and feet, and lesions that occur elsewhere on the body. Ulcers not occurring on the legs are rather uncommon except in primary cancer of the skin or in malignant metastases to the skin. Ulcers arising in nodules with inflammation should be approached in the manner suggested previously for nodules—that is, a biopsy should be obtained, and the tissue examined for bacterial, mycotic, and parasitic diseases. Chancre-like ulcerations and noduloulcerative lesions with regional lymphadenopathy may occur in primary syphilis and primary tuberculosis and in tularemia, anthrax, glanders, and bubonic plague. Isolated noduloulcerative lesions may be seen in sporotrichosis, coccidioidomycosis, leishmaniasis, cryptococcosis, and tertiary syphilis. Serologic studies are necessary in the diagnosis of syphilis.

The most prominent etiologic factors in ulceration on the legs and feet are disturbances of circulation. Chronic venous insufficiency leads to ulceration, especially on the medial aspect of the ankle or lower leg, and the ulcers develop in areas of skin with brownish hemosiderin pigmentation and occasionally where there is edema or sclerosis of the area. Hypertensive or ischemic ulcerations tend to start on the lateral aspect of the ankle. Ulceration can also occur as a result of tissue infarction in areas supplied by either large or small blood vessels (arteries, arterioles); this infarction may occur as the result of occlusion or constriction due to a variety of etiologic factors, in addition to those already mentioned: emboli, thrombosis, cryoagglutinins, macroglobulinemia, cryoglobulinemia, thrombotic thrombocytopenic purpura, polycythemia, systemic lupus erythematosus, Raynaud's phenomenon, arteriosclerosis obliterans, and thromboangiitis obliterans. Ulceration of the lower extremities also occurs in hemolytic anemia, including sickle-cell anemia, thalassemia, and hereditary spherocytosis.

Some ulcers show extensive necrosis of the edges, such as those in *pyoderma gangrenosum* (Color Plate 5-3), an indolent ulcer usually on the lower extremities and often associated with ulcerative colitis or regional ileitis. The ulcers in pyoderma gangrenosum have ragged bluish red overhanging edges and a necrotic base. These lesions often start as pustules or tender red nodules at the site of trauma, and then gradually increase in size until liquefaction necrosis occurs and an irregular ulcer develops. The ulcers are often multiple and may cover large areas of the leg. The histopathologic findings are not specific. The healing of the ulcers usually parallels the activity of the ulcerative colitis, and, inasmuch as the ulceration extends into and involves the reticular layer of the dermis and the subcutis, scarring occurs.

The term *"tropical" ulcer,* in addition to cutaneous leishmaniasis, now also includes ulceration due to cutaneous diphtheria, treponemal disorders (syphilis, yaws, and bejel), and phagedenic ulcer, a chronic ulcer of the feet and legs caused by mixed bacteria that occurs in persons suffering from starvation and neglect.

Ulcers can be associated with peripheral neuropathy ("neuropathic" ulcer, or malum perforans) seen in diabetes mellitus, tabes dorsalis, polyneuritis, leprosy, congenital anesthesia, or hereditary sensory radicular neuropathy.

Anal and perianal ulcers are seen in histiocytosis X and in amebiasis. A hanging-drop preparation is necessary to detect *Entamoeba histolytica.*

Ulcers with artificial and bizarre shapes must be suspected of being self-induced by means of destructive agents such as acid and lighted cigarettes. Factitial ulcers are overstudied and, unfortunately, underdiagnosed by most physicians.

Stony-hard, noduloulcerative lesions, especially around joints (elbows, knees, and fingers) are suggestive of calcinosis cutis or gout; roentgenographic examination enables the detection of calcinosis cutis but shows no opaque bodies in gout.

SCLEROSIS, DIFFUSE OR CIRCUMSCRIBED Diffuse sclerosis of the skin is most often seen on the upper extremities, chest, and face in systemic scleroderma (sometimes called progressive systemic sclerosis). Initially, the skin appears yellowish, and shows slight nonpitting edema; later, however, it becomes indurated, bound down, and may be markedly hyperpigmented. Calcinosis cutis and Raynaud's phenomenon occur commonly.

Circumscribed sclerosis occurs in *morphea,* which consists of one or more round or oval, firm, reddish plaques up to several centimeters in diameter that become white or yellow centrally, often with a lilac-colored, telangiectatic border. This disorder is not associated with any other organ involvement and is a localized cutaneous form of scleroderma. Another type of localized scleroderma is *linear scleroderma,* in which the morphologic change is the same type that is seen in morphea except that the process occurs in bands extending parallel to the long axis of the extremity or along the paramedian line of the forehead and scalp. This form of scleroderma has no relationship to progressive systemic sclerosis.

EDEMA In addition to the various causes of localized edema and generalized edema there is a type of edema of the lower extremities that is not often recognized by the physician. This is a bilateral pedal edema commonly seen in patients with subacute or chronic dermatitis of the lower extremities. This type of edema is most often seen with chronic eczematous dermatitis but is unrelated to cardiac failure or lympathatic obstruction. It is most probably due to an increased permeability as a result of local capillary damage, which is part of the inflammatory process in the skin. The increased capillary permeability leads to an increased transfer of fluid from the intravascular to the extravascular component of the extracellular-fluid space. This type of edema pits and disappears completely when the dermatitis has resolved.

ATROPHY, DIFFUSE OR CIRCUMSCRIBED Dermal atrophy results from a decrease of the papillary or reticular connective tissue and is manifested in the skin as a depression. Circumscribed dermal atrophy may follow trauma, or may occur in association with epidermal atrophy, as in the striae of pregnancy or in Cushing's disease.

Panniculus adiposus (subcutis)

NODULES (INFLAMMATORY, USUALLY TENDER, RED) Nodules in the subcutis may be recognized by the fact that the skin is usually movable over the nodule; occasionally, however, in inflammatory processes, the nodule may involve both the dermis and panniculus adiposus, and the skin will then not be movable over the nodule. Acute, tender, red nodules on the leg are characteristically found in two disorders: *erythema nodosum syndrome* and *nodular subcutaneous fat necrosis* associated with pancreatitis.

The erythema nodosum syndrome refers to the occurrence of multiple bilateral tender nodules appearing principally on the anterior aspect of the lower extremities and occasionally on the upper extremities and face. The erythema nodosum syndrome is associated with a number of disorders that are unrelated to each other.

The nodules in erythema nodosum are only slightly elevated, edematous, and sometimes exquisitely tender. Bruising is a characteristic feature of the disease and is due to hemorrhage, leading to the formation of contusions. The lesions never ulcerate or become indurated and very seldom leave any scarring or atrophy. Erythema nodosum is associated with primary tuberculosis and primary coccidioidomycosis, histoplasmosis, beta-hemolytic streptococcal infections, lymphogranuloma venereum, sarcoidosis, ulcerative colitis, regional enteritis, drugs (penicillin, sulfonamides, bromides, iodides), and oral contraceptives containing ethynylestradiol and norethynodrel.

Tender, red subcutaneous nodules may also appear on

the legs in association with acute pancreatitis and with pancreatic neoplasms and are often erroneously called erythema nodosum. This disorder has been termed *nodular liquefying panniculitis* (NLP). These lesions are distinctive. Their morphologic features are different from those of classic erythema nodosum. The lesions in NLP vary in size from a few millimeters to several centimeters, and, in contrast to the lesions of erythema nodosum, are movable. The lesions of NLP involute in two to three weeks and may leave a hyperpigmented scar that is slightly depressed. The nodules are often associated with abdominal pain and may also be accompanied by fever and arthralgia. Rarely, lesions may be present on other parts of the body besides the legs. Some of the larger nodules may undergo an abscess-like change, becoming fluctuant, and may rupture, exuding a whitish, creamy, or oily viscous material; abscess formation with drainage rarely, if ever, occurs in erythema nodosum. The most common pancreatic neoplasm associated with nodular liquefying panniculitis is an acinous adenocarcinoma of the pancreas. In *Weber-Christian panniculitis,* the subcutaneous nodules, which at first are slightly mobile, become adherent to the overlying skin; then, as the edema subsides in the area of induration, a central depression occurs.

In addition to the above-mentioned entities, various types of vasculitis may also produce tender subcutaneous nodules. Therefore, diagnosis of these lesions often requires an excisional or incisional biopsy.

NODULES (NONINFLAMMATORY, USUALLY NONTENDER, NONERYTHEMATOUS) Movable, painless, noninflammatory-appearing nodules occur around joints in rheumatic fever, rheumatoid arthritis, and in certain metabolic diseases such as xanthoma, gout, and calcinosis. Metastatic carcinoma or metastatic malignant melanoma may appear as movable, nontender subcutaneous nodules. Sarcoidosis may be manifested in the skin solely as subcutaneous nodules on the lower extremities. Subcutaneous nodules also occur in onchocerciasis and loiasis. *Lipomas,* relatively common causes of subcutaneous nodules, are benign tumors composed of adipose tissue and may be single or multiple and are frequently lobulated; they are often rubbery or compressible and occur most often on the trunk and back of the neck and forearms. Occasionally, subcutaneous lipoma may be painful and associated with marked obesity; this condition, known as *Dercum's disease,* occurs especially in middle-aged females.

ATROPHY, DIFFUSE OR CIRCUMSCRIBED Atrophy of the panniculus adiposus produces depressions in the skin; these depressions are seen in progressive lipodystrophy, in liquefying panniculitis, and in the localized fat atrophy that occurs at the site of injections of insulin. About 25 percent of diabetics who receive insulin have this type of atrophy, and, among them, it is more common in females under the age of twenty. The depressed areas of localized fat atrophy show a complete absence of the panniculus, and there is no inflammation. In lipodystrophy, diffuse atrophy of the skin may involve large portions of the body.

Blood vessels

MORBILLIFORM AND SCARLATINIFORM ERUPTIONS Morbilliform (measles-like) and scarlatiniform eruptions are macular and papular exanthems and can be due to drug hypersensitivities, measles, German measles, erythema infectiosum, viral exanthems, rickettsial diseases including endemic murine typhus and Rocky Mountain spotted fever, scarlet fever, and secondary syphilis. Many of the diseases manifested by macules or papules and occurring in acutely ill patients with a fever are listed in Table 55-4.

URTICARIA Urticaria is characterized by wheals, of which the outstanding feature is their persistence for only a few hours (Fig. 54-6). This short duration differentiates urticarial wheals from the otherwise almost identical papules of erythema multiforme, which persist for more than one or two days rather than for a few hours. An acute onset of urticaria is usually related to ingestion of drugs or certain types of foods (shellfish, fresh berries).

Chronic recurrent urticaria is a special problem, and its causes are not easily established. Most patients with chronic recurrent urticaria require a careful search for cryptic diseases such as lymphoma, systemic lupus erythematosus, primary or metastatic carcinoma, intestinal parasites, systemic vasculitis, or dermatomyostis. It is especially important, even in chronic urticarias, to carry out a painstaking interrogation of the patient in search of a history of drugs. Aspirin is one of the commonest drugs causing chronic urticaria and can often be missed even in a careful drug history because many patients do not consider aspirin a drug. It is probably true that some patients with chronic urticaria can relate their problem to emotional stress, but this cause should be considered only after excluding all possible organic causes.

TABLE 55-4
Rash and fever in the acutely ill patient: diagnosis according to type of lesion

DISEASES MANIFESTED BY MACULES OR PAPULES

Drug hypersensitivities	Secondary syphilis
Scarlet fever	Typhus, murine (endemic)
Erythema infectiosum (fifth disease)	Rocky Mountain spotted fever (early lesions)
Measles (rubeola)	Pityriasis rosea
German measles (rubella)	Erythema multiforme
Enterovirus infections (echo and Coxsackie)	Erythema marginatum
	Systemic lupus erythematosus
Adenovirus infections	Dermatomyositis
Viral hepatitis	"Serum sickness" (manifested only as wheals)
Typhoid fever	

DISEASES MANIFESTED BY VESICLES, BULLAE, OR PUSTULES

Drug hypersensitivities	Eczema vaccinatum*
Dermatitis from plants	Variola*
Rickettsial pox	Enterovirus infections (echo and Coxsackie), including hand-foot-mouth disease
Varicella (chickenpox)*	
Generalized herpes zoster*	
Disseminated herpes simplex*	Toxic epidermal necrolysis
Eczema herpeticum*	Erythema multiforme bullosum
Disseminated vaccinia*	

DISEASES MANIFESTED BY PURPURIC MACULES, PURPURIC PAPULES, OR PURPURIC VESICLES

Drug hypersensitivities	Enterovirus infections (echo and Coxsackie)
Bacteremia†	
Meningococcemia (acute or chronic)	Rickettsial diseases:
	Rocky Mountain spotted fever
Gonococcemia	Typhus, louse-borne (epidemic)
Staphylococcemia	"Allergic" vasculitis
Pseudomonas bacteremia	
Subacute bacterial endocarditis	

* *The characteristic lesion of these exanthems is an* umbilicated *papule or vesicle on an erythematous base.*
† *Often presents as infarcts.*
SOURCE: *TB Fitzpatrick, M. Fisher, A color atlas of rashes occurring in the acutely ill febrile patient, in* Dermatology in General Medicine, *eds TB Fitzpatrick et al, New York: McGraw-Hill, 1971*

ERYTHEMA MULTIFORME SYNDROME Erythema multiforme syndrome is a characteristic response of the skin and mucous membranes that is related to a number of different possible etiologies, including infectious agents *(Herpesvirus hominis, Mycoplasma pneumoniae),* and drugs (especially penicillin, antipyretics, barbiturates, hydantoins, and sulfonamides). The major pathology is an acute inflammatory infiltrate around blood vessels and may include degenerative changes in the endothelial cells of the capillaries.

The lesions occur in a characteristic symmetrical distribution and favor the extensor areas of the distal parts of the limbs, the backs of the hands, and the dorsa of the feet; the palms and soles are often involved, even to the exclusion of the dorsal surfaces. Oral lesions, first as blisters and then erosions, occur on the buccal mucous membrane, gums, and tongue, and there is often swelling and crusting of the lips. The syndrome may also include severe toxemia and prostration, high fever, cough, and "patchy" inflammation of the lungs. The skin lesions are often characterized by a vivid redness that gradually becomes duller, and they become more indurated, with the development of centers that are pale or may have bullae; these "target" or "iris" lesions, which are characteristic of erythema multiforme but do not invariably occur, are identified by the clear red area at the periphery that surrounds a pale pink zone and a central livid area, which may contain a bulla.

PURPURA (WITH AND WITHOUT INFLAMMATION) A purpuric eruption demands immediate exploration for its etiology. Purpura arises in the skin of the vascularized dermis and is almost always confined to the dermis. The purpuric macules gradually disappear after days or weeks, depending on their size. Punctate or tiny purpuric spots are termed *petechiae,* larger ($>$2.0 cm) macules are spoken of as *suggillations,* and extensive purpuric macules are called *ecchymoses* (*D* in Fig. 54-2).

Purpura with inflammation is usually "palpable," i.e., papular, and is seen in systemic vasculitis and in bacteremias such as staphylococcemia, gonococcemia (Color Plate 5-4), and meningococcemia. In these bacteremias and in vasculitis, the examination of biopsied skin may establish a diagnosis within 8 h (which is the time required for processing the tissue). Gentle scraping of the purpuric lesions will produce enough material for a Gram's stain; intracellular gram-negative diplococci are occasionally found in the lesions in acute, but not in chronic, meningococcemia, and are rarely found in acute gonococcemia. The differential diagnosis of papable purpuric lesions and infarcts occurring in *systemic vasculitis* as compared with those in chronic meningococcemia is not easy. The skin lesions in systemic vasculitis are usually bilateral, and almost symmetrical, in their distribution. They tend to be concentrated on the lower extremities, especially on the lower portion and around the ankles and the dorsa of the feet. The lesions in chronic meningococcemia are more randomly distributed, with occurrence on the trunk, lower and upper extremities, and face. Nevertheless, in meningococcemia, lesions can occur in a bilateral distribution, which makes the distinction between chronic meningococcemia and systemic vasculitis difficult, if not impossible, at times. The individual lesions in both chronic meningococcemia and systemic vasculitis may be identical, consisting of a mixture of palpable purpura and urticarial-type papules without purpura. Unfortunately, the histologic findings in biopsy specimens of the lesions in both diseases do not permit a distinction. Therefore, a patient with bilaterally distributed palpable purpuric lesions and fever is best treated with antibiotics before the results of blood cultures are available.

Purpura without inflammation is completely macular, and examination of a blood smear can quickly establish the presence of platelets; if platelets are seen in the smear, thrombocytopenic purpura can be safely ruled out as a possibility.

On the lower legs of older people, a great variety of inflammatory skin diseases, including various types of contact dermatitis, may be associated with purpura; under these circumstances, the purpura does not have the same importance as it does when present on the trunk or upper extremities. Perifollicular purpura, however, on the lower extremities (usually accompanied by a follicular hyperkeratosis) is almost pathognomonic of scurvy.

Purpura frequently develops in amyloidosis when the lesions (waxy macules and papules) are pinched. This "pinch" purpura, however, may also occur in the normal skin of patients with thrombocytopenic purpura or in the skin of apparently normal elderly persons. (For a full discussion of the classification and differential diagnosis of purpura, see Chaps. 61 and 317.

INFARCTS Infarcts in the skin are usually not pale like those that occur in the kidney but have a variegated dusky red, grayish hue. They are irregularly shaped macules, sometimes slightly depressed below the plane of the skin, and often surrounded by a pink zone of hyperemia. Infarcts are usually slightly tender.

Cutaneous infarctions are important and often diagnostic signs of serious multisystem disease, including both acute and chronic meningococcemia, streptococcal and staphylococcal septicemia, gonococcemia, pseudomonas septicemia, systemic vasculitis, purpura fulminans, systemic lupus erythematosus and, rarely, dermatomyositis.

TELANGIECTASIA Redness of the skin is most frequently caused by transient dilatation of blood vessels (erythema). In contrast to the color produced by fixed blood pigments, as in purpura, the erythema will disappear under the pressure of a glass or plastic slide (see Diascopy in Chap. 54). Telangiectasia is the condition in which the redness of the skin is the result of a permanent enlargement in the caliber of the blood vessels (which will be revealed by examination with a hand lens) and an increase in the number of the vessels. Telangiectasia may be composed of fine linear branches of blood vessels appearing distinctly red (i.e., not blue), which are often seen on the nose and face, or of confluent macular areas that appear as a permanent erythema. Telangiectasia is the cause of the erythema in discoid and systemic lupus erythematosus, dermatomyositis, and psoriasis.

Telangiectasia may also occur in a scattered, discrete fashion on the upper trunk or on the extremities and is seen characteristically in progressive systemic sclerosis (systemic scleroderma). Telangiectasia occurring around the nail beds, i.e., periungual telangiectasia, is an important diagnostic sign in lupus erythematosus (both discoid and systemic) and in dermatomyositis; these lesions are seen rarely, if at all, in systemic scleroderma.

Sharply outlined, red macules or papules 1 to 2 mm in diameter, with an area of radiating telangiectasia, are seen in *hereditary hemorrhagic telangiectasia* (Chap. 319). These occur on the lips, nasal mucosa, face, and hands.

Generalized telangiectasia occurring in the form of red macules over most of the body surface may be the presenting sign of mastocytosis or urticaria pigmentosa.

Telangiectasia is a prominent and diagnostic feature of *ataxia telangiectasia,* or Louis-Bar's syndrome. Telangiectasia may be present as early as the second year of life but usually develops by the fifth year; it appears first on the bulbar conjunctiva and subsequently involves the ears, the eyelids, the butterfly area of the face, the upper aspect of the chest, and the extremities.

Telangiectasia may occur in a characteristic form known as the *arterial spider,* or spider nevus, spider angioma, or naevus araneus. The main vessel of the spider is an arteriole, and it is usually faintly pulsating, which will show under the diascope. A less common skin lesion usually found with vascular spiders in liver disorders is the telangiectatic *mat* or net, a small red patch composed of intermeshed fine vessels that blanch on pressure. Spider angiomas, usually three or fewer, occur not infrequently in normal children and adults. Numerous spider angiomas often develop during pregnancy or after the ingestion of progestational agents or in rheumatoid arthritis or thyrotoxicosis. Most patients with numerous and prominent vascular spiders, however, have some form of underlying diffuse liver disease, e.g., in alcoholic cirrhosis. The progression of subacute hepatitis is often paralleled by the appearance of crops of spiders, and, in Laënnec's and postnecrotic cirrhosis, almost half the patients have multiple vascular spiders. The mechanism responsible for the development of spider angiomas in liver disease is not known, nor has it been firmly established that the lesions result from disordered metabolism of estrogens by the liver.

REFERENCES

FARBER EM, COX AJ (eds): Psoriasis, in *Proceedings of the International Symposium, Stanford University, 1971,* Stanford, Calif.: Stanford University Press, 1971

FITZPATRICK TB, FISHER M: A color atlas of rashes occurring in the acutely ill febrile patient, in *Dermatology in General Medicine,* eds TB Fitzpatrick et al, New York: McGraw-Hill, 1971

——, JOHNSON DP: Fundamentals of dermatologic diagnosis, in *Dermatology in General Medicine,* eds TB Fitzpatrick et al, New York: McGraw-Hill, 1971

PARRISH JA et al: Photochemotherapy of psoriasis with oral methoxsalen and longwave ultraviolet light. N Engl J Med 291:1207, 1974

56 GENERALIZED PRURITUS

T. B. FITZPATRICK
H. A. HAYNES

Generalized pruritus is a frequent and important problem in differential diagnosis for the general physician. In many patients, intense generalized pruritus is the only symptom. Unfortunately, there are no good studies that have described in detail the special qualities of pruritus that permit a specific diagnosis; in other words, it is not really known what type of pruritus is seen, for example, in obstructive biliary disease as opposed to lymphoma. In the absence of these data, the clinician must rely on the history, physical examination, and laboratory studies to establish the nature of the pruritus.

The most important cause of pruritus is psychogenic, that is, a reaction to stress and strain. This type of pruritus often affects the skin of the scalp, and may be associated with other sensory complaints such as a bitter taste in the mouth or burning of the tongue. Some patients with psychogenic pruritus are convinced that the itching is caused by some sort of parasite in their skin that cannot be seen by themselves or the physician. The patient scratches his skin until the lesions become excoriated, and then asserts that the itching has disappeared, owing, he believes, to removal of the parasite or "germ" by the appearance of bleeding.

Older persons in whom dry skin is a common occurrence may have generalized pruritus unrelated to multisystem disease. Some other older persons, however, usually more than 60 years of age, who do not have obvious dry skin may also have generalized ("senile") pruritus that is intense and does not seem to be caused by emotional stress. This pruritus is usually most severe when the patients disrobe to go to bed, and usually begins in one area, particularly the back, and spreads to involve the entire body. Neither psychogenic nor senile pruritus leads to a loss of sleep.

A subtle and important cause of pruritus without a visible rash may be a reaction to drugs, such as aspirin and, especially, opiates and their derivatives, and quinidine.

The itching that is associated with pediculosis corporis may be so intense that it will interfere with the patient's sleep. This type of eruption is usually relatively easy to diagnose by the linear excoriations that occur along the back, and often the insect can be found in the clothing, particularly along the seams.

For a list of conditions in which generalized pruritus occurs without any evidence of primary skin disease, see Table 56-1.

The pruritus in hepatic disease has no special qualities. Generalized pruritus may frequently be the first sign of biliary cirrhosis and may occur many months before the onset of jaundice. It may be the first sign also of lymphoma, and, rarely, of carcinoma. The pruritus may be of sudden onset and may be very severe from the beginning.

Patients with pruritus associated with obvious skin lesions, such as bullae and papules, should be referred to a dermatologist. Some of the dermatologic disorders in which pruritus is a common symptom include scabies, dermatitis herpetiformis, lichen planus, urticaria, mycosis fungoides, insect bites, and eczematous dermatitis including atopic dermatitis. Many of these disorders require specialized dermatologic approaches, particularly biopsy of the skin, in order to establish the diagnosis.

The treatment of generalized pruritus is unsatisfactory. Not one of the systemic medications has been shown to be effective in generalized pruritus. A topical preparation containing 0.5% menthol and 1% phenol in Nivea oil is somewhat helpful in relieving pruritus temporarily. The topical anesthetics containing benzocaine should be avoided because of the high risk of allergic sensitization. When the patient with pruritus also has insomnia, a hypnotic or a sedative should be prescribed. Antihistamines are of little value except in pruritus due to urticaria. It is a general clinical impression that aspirin is helpful in pruritus of any origin, but this has not been proved. The development of drugs that control pruritus remains one of the great challenges of medical research, and it is paradoxical that, at this juncture, severe pain can be immediately controlled with a variety of agents but there is not one single agent that is so effective for generalized pruritus. The receptors

TABLE 56-1
Conditions associated with generalized pruritus without primary skin lesions

Psychogenic states	*Metabolic and endocrine disorders*	*Malignant neoplasms*	*Drug reactions*	*Infestations*	*Hematologic disease*	*Miscellaneous conditions*
Periods of emotional stress	Obstructive biliary disease	Lymphoma and leukemia	Sensitivity to opium derivatives	Ancylostomiasis (hookworm)	Polycythemia vera†	Dry skin; pregnancy
Delusions of parasitosis	Primary biliary cirrhosis	Abdominal cancer	Sensitivity (subclinical) to miscellaneous drugs	Onchocerciasis		
	Uremia			Pediculosis corporis		
	Hyperthyroidism					
	Hypothyroidism*					
	Diabetes mellitus*					

* *Not definitely proved as causes.*
† *Especially after a bath.*

for the itch stimuli reside in the papillary layer of the dermis, but there are no specific end organs for itching. Itching is a sensation carried principally by unmyelinated slowly conducting fibers of the C group to central neuronal pools in the spinal cord. The stimuli are then carried by the posterior roots of the spinal nerves, and, from the anterolateral spinothalamic tracts, enter the thalamus and then proceed to the sensory area of the gyrus postcentralis of the cortex.

REFERENCE

CAIRNS RJ: The skin and the nervous system, in *Textbook of Dermatology,* eds A Rook et al, Oxford: Blackwell Scientific Publications, 1972, p. 1791

57
PIGMENTATION OF THE SKIN AND DISORDERS OF MELANIN METABOLISM

T. B. FITZPATRICK
H. A. HAYNES

THE MELANOCYTE SYSTEM

DEFINITION OF MELANIN Melanin is the principal pigment in the coloration of human skin, hair, and eyes. In humans, it functions primarily as a screen that shields the dermis from the deleterious effects of solar radiation. Inasmuch as the amount and distribution of melanin in skin and hair are changed in a number of diseases, a detailed study of irregularities of pigmentation may provide important diagnostic clues to diseases in other organs.

Melanin, derived from the Greek word *melas* (black), is the name given to a biochrome of high molecular weight formed when tyrosinase oxidizes the phenol, tyrosine, to dopa. The biochrome is therefore often referred to as tyrosine melanin. Tyrosine melanin is the product of unicellular glands, melanocytes, that secrete melanin particles into epidermal cells. The exact chemical nature of melanin has not been determined because tyrosine melanin (both natural and synthetic) is so extremely insoluble that all attempts to degrade it into identifiable fragments have failed. It is known, however, that all animal melanins contain indoles and are composed basically of indole-5,6-quinone units, in contrast with melanins of plant origin, which contain catechols. From studies with radioactive dopa (dihydroxyphenylalanine) it appears that melanin is a copolymer of dopa-quinone, indole-5,6-quinone, and indole-5,6-quinone-2-carboxylic acid in the ratio of 3:2:1.

BIOSYNTHESIS OF MELANIN Melanocytes are situated at the dermoepidermal interface, in the hair bulb, uveal tract, retinal pigment epithelium, inner ear, and leptomeninges. These scattered groups of cells are known as the melanocyte system, which constitutes a cytologic and biochemical unit, inasmuch as the melanocytes in all these locations (except in the retinal pigment epithelium) are derived from the neural crest (Fig. 57-1) and can hydroxylate tyrosine to dopa and, ultimately, to the pigment tyrosine melanin. The melanocyte system is analogous, but not known to be related, to the chromaffin system. The cells of the chromaffin system also are derived from the neural crest and possess biochemical mechanisms for the hydroxylation of tyrosine to dopa, although by the action of tyrosine hydroxylase, instead of by tyrosinase; unlike melanocytes, they convert dopa to adrenochrome and not to tyrosine melanin. Benign and malignant neoplasms arise in all parts of the melanocyte system except in the retinal pigment epithelium and the hair bulbs.

The melanocytes present at the dermoepidermal interface form a horizontal network that is closely connected to the epidermal cells by means of numerous cytoplasmic processes, or dendrites. This intimate relationship permitting cytocrine transfer of melanin particles (melanosomes) from melanocytes to malpighian cells has been clearly demonstrated by electron microscopy in a study of the fine structure of cortical cells and hair melanocytes and by tissue culture of human epidermis.

FIGURE 57-1
Diagram showing the embryonic origin, dispersal, and developmental fate of melanocytes in man. (By permission from JB Stanbury et al, eds: The Metabolic Basis of Inherited Disease, *2d ed., McGraw-Hill, 1966)*

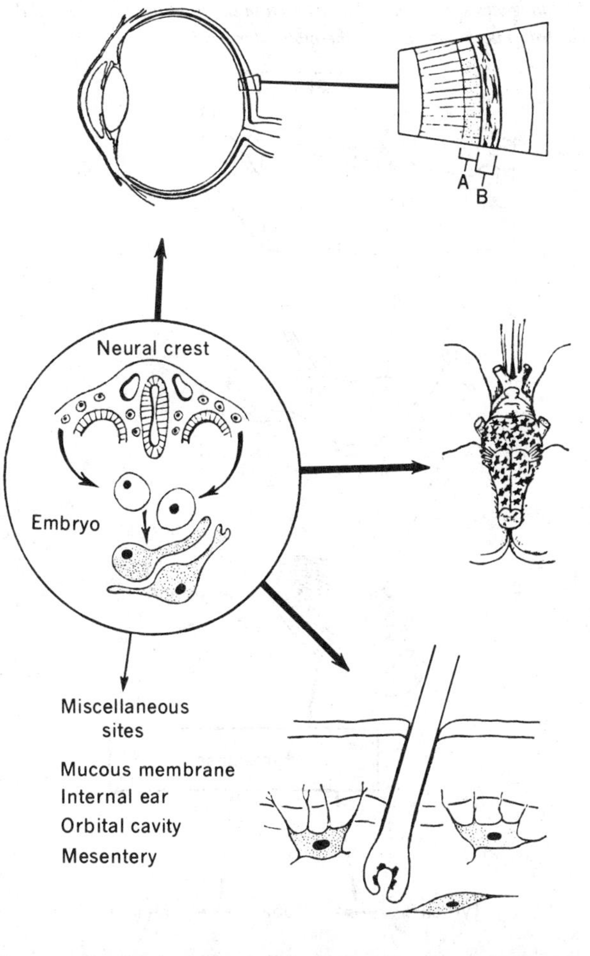

It has been possible to demonstrate by electron microscopy that melanocytes contain specialized organelles with a distinctive internal structure. These organelles, known as *melanosomes,* contain tyrosinase, the melanin synthesizing enzyme. Under normal conditions, melanin is progressively formed and deposited on the surface of melanosomes until they become amorphous particles without detectable tyrosinase activity (Fig. 57-2). Melanosomes are believed to originate in the Golgi area, appearing first as unmelanized vesicles that gradually become dark and increasingly dense.

Tyrosinase is one of a large group of copper-containing aerobic oxidases that catalyze the oxidation of both monohydroxy and *o*-dihydroxy phenols to orthoquinones. In man and other mammals, this oxidase catalyzes the hydroxylation of the melanin precursor, tyrosine, to dopa and dopa-quinone (Fig. 57-3). Tyrosinase is required only for the first step in the biosynthesis of tyrosine melanin, i.e., the orthohydroxylation of tyrosine. It is noteworthy that zinc ions catalyze the conversion of dopa-chrome to 5,6-dihydroxyindole and that melanosomes have been shown to contain zinc in high concentration.

BIOLOGIC PROCESSES UNDERLYING MELANIN PIGMENTATION Melanin pigmentation, as viewed clinically, results from the melanin present in the keratinocytes and also in the melanocytes. Inasmuch as the ratio of keratinocytes to melanocytes in the epidermis is 36:1, it is apparent that the amount of melanin present in the keratinocytes must be the predominant factor in the determination of skin color. The relation of skin color to the location of melanin in the epidermis was studied with the light microscope in Negro Americans of various hues of brown coloration. In lightly pigmented skin, there was a great variation in both the number and location of melanin particles within the epidermis; only scanty melanin deposits were in the malpighian layer, and no deposits were in the stratum corneum. In fact, in the most lightly pigmented skin, the only melanin particles were in the keratinocytes of the basal layer. In the most heavily pigmented skin, there were melanin particles in the keratinocytes of the basal layer, throughout the malpighian cells, and in the stratum corneum.

It is apparent, therefore, from studies of normal skin and of pigmentary disorders, that the intensity of pigmentation, as viewed clinically, depends not only on the rate of melanosome production but also on the number of melanosomes that are transferred to the keratinocytes. Another factor that determines normal and abnormal melanin pigmentation is the degree of melanization of the individual melanosomes. Until recently, three factors—melanosome formation, melanosome melanization, and melanosome secretion—were considered to be the major variables in normal and abnormal melanin pigmentation. In the past few years, however, a fourth variable has been implicated in

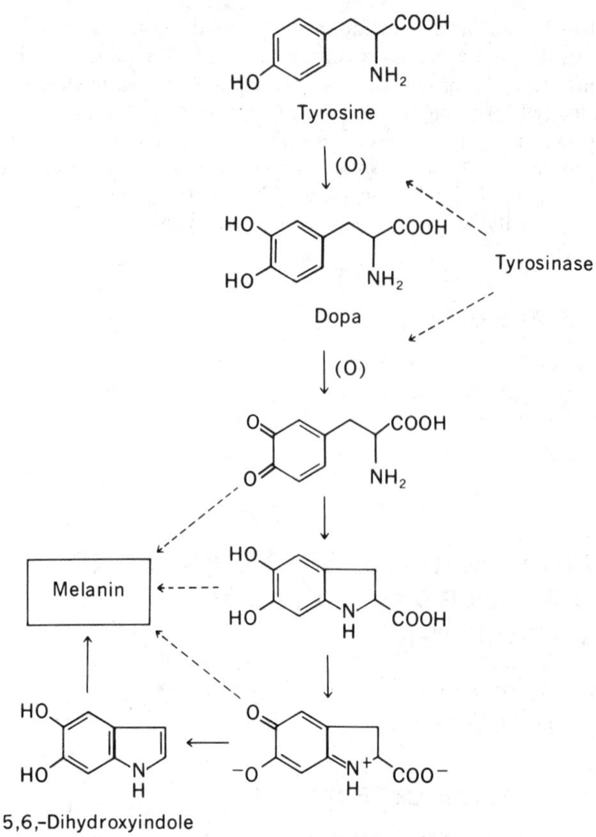

FIGURE 57-3
Biosynthesis of tyrosine melanin.

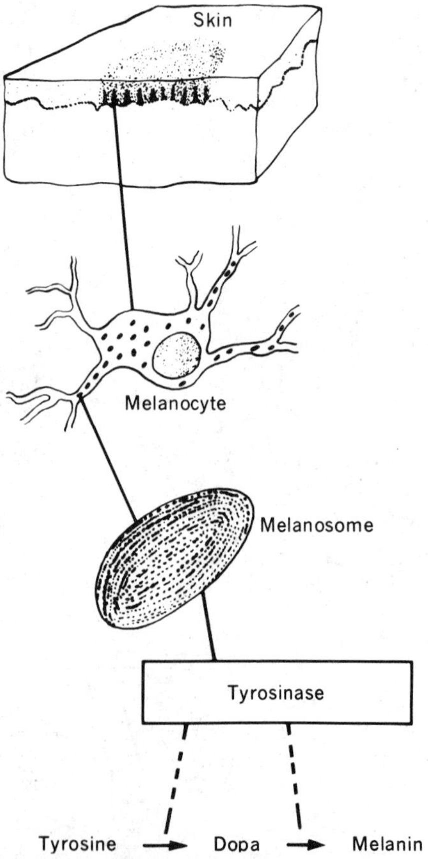

FIGURE 57-2
Melanogenesis in human skin, as seen in the light microscope and the electron microscope and at the molecular level.

melanin pigmentation—i.e., the phenomenon of aggregation and degradation of melanosomes that occurs during their transport in the keratinocytes.

Melanosomes are present in melanocytes mainly as nonaggregated (single), membrane-delimited, discrete organelles. In keratinocytes, however, melanosomes occur either as single, or nonaggregated, particles or as aggregates of three or more within a membrane-delimited organelle. These melanosome-containing organelles resemble the melanosome-containing organelles within macrophages that have been identified as lysosomes. In the epidermal keratinocyte, melanosomes appear to undergo a gradual degradation. In heavily pigmented skin, however, intact melanosomes remain in the stratum corneum, indicating that some melanosomes are apparently not degraded with the lysosomes in the epidermis. Numerous studies in recent years have shown that there appears to be a considerable variation in the arrangement of melanosomes in the nonfollicular keratinocytes in different racial groups. In the keratinocytes of the hair follicle in all racial groups, there are, in the growing phase of the hair growth cycle, single, or nonaggregated, melanosomes. In Negroids and Australian aborigines, however, melanosomes are found, in the epidermal keratinocytes, to be nonaggregated (single), whereas in Caucasoids, Mongoloids, and American Indians, melanosomes are found, in the keratinocytes, to be mostly aggregated, and there is often a suggestion of fragmentation of the melanosomes within these lysosome-like organelles. Some recent observations have shown that the size of the melanosome determines whether or not a melanosome becomes aggregated in the keratinocytes. Melanosomes that are smaller than 1 μm can aggregate in the form of a phagosome and undergo degradation—a process that could gradually decrease the intensity of the coloration.

The pigmentation of the skin is related to four biological processes (Fig. 57-4):

1 Formation of melanosomes in melanocytes
2 Melanization of melanosomes in melanocytes
3 Secretion of melanosomes into keratinocytes
4 Transport of melanosomes by keratinocytes with and without degradation in lysosome-like organelles

Aggregation[1] and dispersion of melanosomes probably play no part in the pigmentary anomalies of humans. Such movement has thus far been observed only in specialized effector cells, melanophores, present only in vertebrates below mammals in the phylogenetic scale; this movement of melanosomes is under neural and hormonal control in these animals.

MELANOCYTE-SYSTEM DISTURBANCES AND ETIOLOGIC FACTORS

Disorders of melanin pigmentation are frequent and important signs of disease in other organ systems (Table 57-1). These disorders of the melanocyte system (Table 57-2) may be classed as hypomelanoses or hypermelanoses and can be divided into three main categories: (1) hypomelano-

FIGURE 57-4
Four biologic processes underlying melanin pigmentation. (1) Formation of melanosomes in melanocytes; (2) melanization of melanosomes in melanocytes; (3) secretion of melanocytes by keratinocytes; and (4) transport of melanocytes by keratinocytes, either with degradation of melanosomes within lysosome-like organelles (in Caucasoids) or without apparent degradation of melanosomes (in Negroids).

Note the difference between the melanosomes in the Negroid and Caucasoid keratinocytes. In the Negroid keratinocytes, the melanosomes are nonaggregated. In the Caucasoid keratinocytes, groups of several melanosomes are aggregated within membrane-limited lysosome-like organelles, and the melanosomes often appear fragmented. (G, Golgi apparatus; N, nucleus; I-IV, the four stages in the development of the melanosome.)

The epidermal melanin unit is shown at the top. The melanocyte supplies melanosomes to a group of keratinocytes.

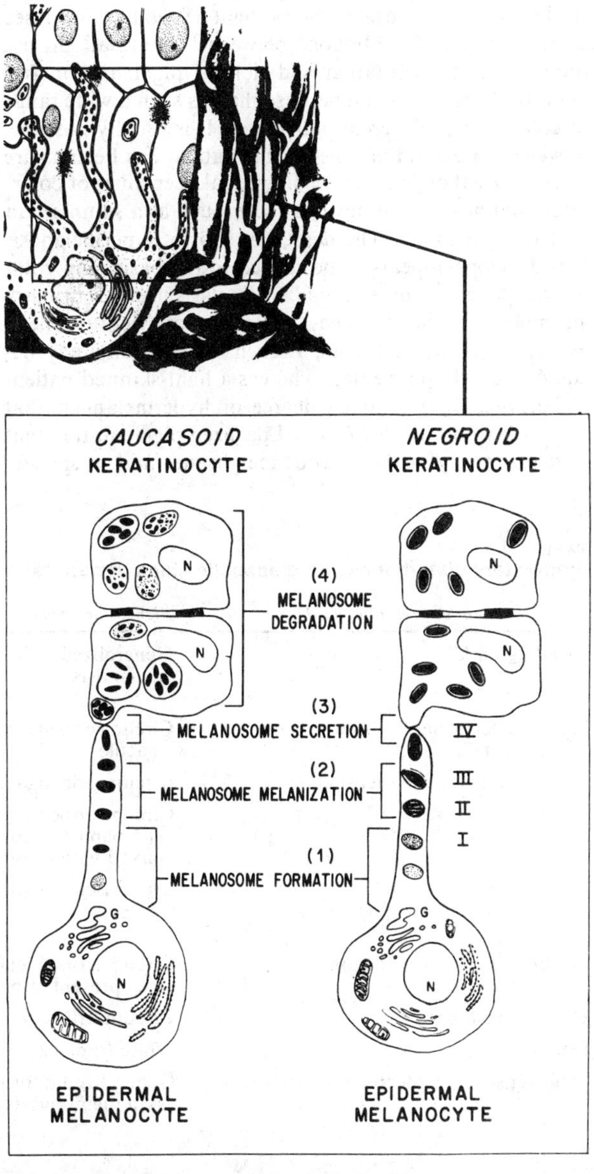

[1] *Aggregation in this sense refers to the clustering of melanosomes around the nucleus of the melanocyte, i.e., the phenomenon that occurs when a frog is placed on a white background; when the frog is placed on a dark background, however, there is movement, or dispersion, of the melanosomes into the dendrites.*

sis, in which paucity or absence of pigment renders the skin white or lighter than normal; (2) hypermelanosis (brown), in which excess pigment produces a brown-to-black color; and (3) hypermelanosis (blue), in which excess pigment produces a blue or slate or gray color. Within the three categories, the pigmentary disorders with similar etiology may be grouped together (Table 57-2). Hypomelanosis (decreased pigmentation) may result from loss of melanocytes, as in thermal burns, or from absence or paucity of melanin. Brown hypermelanosis (see Table 57-2) results, in most instances, from an increase in the activity of epidermal melanocytes, i.e., an increase in the number of melanosomes produced, and not from an increase in the number of these cells. Gray or slate or blue hypermelanosis results from the presence of melanin within dermal phagocytes or ectopic dermal melanocytes, and this clinical color change from brown is related to the Tyndall light-scattering phenomenon.

Recognition of hypomelanosis and of gray or slate or blue hypermelanosis is usually not difficult. When the degree of hypomelanosis is very slight, diagnosis may be facilitated by the use of black light (Wood's lamp; see Chap. 54). Differentiation between abnormal diffuse brown hyperpigmentation and normal pigmentation frequently poses a problem because there is such a wide range of coloration in different individuals. It is usually possible, however, to determine whether the patient has been aware of an unusual or progressive or gradual deepening of coloration that has had no obvious cause, such as a summer tan that has not faded. The degree of brown hypermelanosis that develops appears to be related to the basic skin color of the patient. For example, with the onset of primary adrenocortical insufficiency, a patient of Mediterranean extraction (such as Italian, French, or Spanish) may become intensely pigmented, whereas a light-skinned patient will have only a minimal degree of hypermelanosis that may or may not be detectable. Localized pigmentation that develops newly in the mucous membranes and in specific areas, such as the axillas and palmar creases, is usually easier to identify as a pathologic change than is generalized brown hyperpigmentation.

GENETIC FACTORS *Oculocutaneous albinism* is a mendelian autosomal recessive trait and is characterized by paucity or absence of melanin in the eyes and an unpatterned hypomelanosis of the skin and hair; albinism involving the skin only has not been reported. In this disorder, melanocytes and melanosomes are present, but whatever tyrosinase may be synthesized by the melanocytes must be functionally defective and unable to catalyze the oxidation of tyrosine to melanin. The formation of melanosomes is interrupted in the early stages; few or no mature melanosomes are present in albinotic skin or hair. Oculocutaneous albinism is diagnosed and classified on the basis of ocular and cutaneous findings, and is further classified according to the presence or absence of tyrosinase in the plucked hair follicles of the scalp. In some persons with oculocutaneous albinism, the hair follicles darken when incubated in tyrosine, i.e., *"tyrosinase-positive,"* whereas in others no such darkening occurs, i.e., *"tyrosinase-negative."* These two types are now known to have separate gene loci. The ocular abnormalities in oculocutaneous albinism include hypopigmentation of the fundus oculi, translucence of the irides, and nystagmus. The deficiency of melanin in oculocutaneous albinism has two disturbing consequences for humans: decreased visual acuity and an abnormal degree of intolerance to sunlight. The sensitivity of human albinos to ultraviolet light leads to the development of carcinoma in exposed areas of the skin, especially in albinos living in the tropics.

In *phenylketonuria,* there is a single metabolic block in the conversion of phenylalanine to tyrosine. The condition is associated with subnormal pigmentation of the hair and the iris. The hair of patients with phenylketonuria ranges in color from light blond to dark brown, and it is only by comparison with the hair of siblings that the characteristic dilution of color becomes evident. The diminution of melanin formation results from the fact that the large amounts

TABLE 57-1
Pigmentary disturbances as diagnostic signs in general medicine

Chief complaint or presenting problem	*Pigmentary change*	*Diseases*
"Getting dark"	Generalized diffuse brown hypermelanosis	Addison's disease; hemochromatosis; ACTH-producing tumors; systemic scleroderma
"Abdominal pain"; "brown spots on lips, fingers"	Circumscribed small dark-brown macules	Peutz-Jeghers syndrome
"Brown spots"; hypertension	Circumscribed uniformly brown macules	Neurofibromatosis; Albright's syndrome
"Mole"	Circumscribed polychromic macules and papules (red, white, and blue admixed with brown)	Early primary malignant melanoma
"White spots"	Circumscribed white macules	Leukoderma associated with "vitiligo," Addison's disease, pernicious anemia, thyrotoxicosis
Seizures; mental retardation	Circumscribed leaf-shaped white macules present at birth; poliosis	Tuberous sclerosis
Uveitis; deafness	Circumscribed white macules; poliosis	Vogt-Koyanagi-Harada disease
Deafness	White forelock	Waardenburg's syndrome
"Sun sensitivity"; decreased vision	Generalized diffuse hypomelanosis of skin, hair, and uveal tract	Oculocutaneous albinism

of phenylalanine and its metabolites present in serum and extracellular fluid act as competitive inhibitors of tyrosinase activity, thus blocking melanin synthesis.

Piebaldism, an autosomal dominant trait, involves the skin and the hair but not the eyes. In piebaldism, in addition to the absence of eye involvement, the hypomelanosis occurs in circumscribed areas on the extremities and anterior surface of the thorax, and there is commonly a white forelock. *Waardenburg's syndrome* comprises piebaldism associated with congenital deafness. Electron microscopic studies have revealed that the white areas of the skin lack melanocytes, as in vitiligo (q.v.).

Vitiligo may be localized or generalized. When localized, the hypomelanosis of the skin and hair may be restricted to one region, such as the anogenital area or scalp. When generalized, the pattern of hypomelanosis is quite typical, with lesions particularly on the face, axillae, neck, and extremities, and with loss of pigment in the hair. Idiopathic vitiligo is fairly common, affecting 1 percent of the population. The lesions are completely lacking in pigment, and this snow-whiteness is distinctive and often serves to differentiate vitiligo from other hypomelanoses. Vitiligo is believed to be inherited as an autosomal dominant trait with irregular penetrance. In the majority of cases, vitiligo is idiopathic, but typical vitiligo, as just described, is known to occur with a variety of diseases, such as Addison's disease, hyperthyroidism, hypoparathyroidism, pernicious anemia, and alopecia areata; all of these disorders are believed by some investigators to be caused by autoimmunity. In the differential diagnosis of circumscribed hypomelanosis, there are many disorders with vitiligo-type hypomelanosis of the skin and hair that must be considered (see Table 57-3). Electron microscopic studies of idiopathic vitiligo of the skin reveal a marked reduction or, more commonly, a total absence of detectable melanocytes; this phenomenon suggests, presumably, that the hypomelanosis is the result of a structural defect, rather than a metabolic change, in the existing melanocytes.

In about a third of the patients with vitiligo, it is possible to bring about a permanent repigmentation of vitiligo areas by the use of systemically administered psoralens (furocoumarins), which are available in all countries of the world in various forms. The duration of treatment varies from patient to patient and is determined to a considerable extent by the site of the lesions. Hypomelanotic macules on the face show the most rapid response. Usually, repigmentation is not complete in less than a year.

Tuberous sclerosis is an autosomal dominant trait usually causing mental retardation, seizures, and, more rarely, retinal plaques. The most constant visible clinical features of the disease are white macules on the skin, which are present at birth, thus preceding adenoma sebaceum (the typical facial lesion), which does not occur until the second or even the sixth year after birth. Such immediate diagnosis in an infant enables one to advise the parents about a possible genetic defect in any children born to them. The white macules are isolated and irregularly distributed all over the body but are most frequent on the posterior aspect of the trunk, especially on the buttocks. There may be any number from four to more than a hundred. They are not easily detected in fairskinned infants without the aid of Wood's (ultraviolet) light. The macules occur in two characteristic shapes: (1) lance-ovate lesions in the shape of a leaflet of the mountain-ash tree, usually 3 cm in their longest dimensions (Color Plate 5-6); and (2) polygonal lesions, like a "thumb print" and approximately 1 cm in diameter. The macules are not pure white as in vitiligo or albino skin but are grayish or "off-white." The macules in tuberous sclerosis are hypomelanotic because the melanosomes in the melanocytes synthesize almost no melanin, in contrast to vitiligo, in which the total absence of melanocytes results in the total lack of pigment.

Neurofibromatosis (Recklinghausen's disease) is inherited as a dominant trait. It is characterized by the appearance, usually by the age of three years and primarily on the trunk but also on the extremities, of numerous pale yellowish brown macules (Color Plate 1-4), or *café au lait* spots, that vary in diameter from less than 1 to more than 15 cm. Spotty generalized pigmentation may also be present, especially in the axillae. Often, but not always, a few or myriads of soft, rounded, cone-shaped, or pendulous cutaneous tumors covered by normal skin are seen; these appear in the second or third decade.

The presence of *six or more café au lait spots* with a diameter greater than 1.5 cm is diagnostic of *neurofibromatosis* even when there is no familial history of the condition. In *polyostotic fibrous dysplasia,* however, there are rarely more than *three or four macules,* unilaterally distributed, usually on the buttocks or cervical area. A single, large, isolated *café au lait* spot of neurofibromatosis resembles the pigmented macule of polyostotic fibrous dysplasia *(Albright's disease).* It is possible, however, to detect large pigmented globules in whole mounts of epidermis prepared from the *café au lait* macules of neurofibromatosis; these pigmented globules, macromelanosomes, are not found in the macular pigmented areas present in polyostotic fibrous dysplasia or in the *café au lait* macules that are observed in 10 percent of the normal population.

METABOLIC FACTORS Generalized brown hypermelanosis of the skin is a characteristic manifestation of *hemochromatosis* and *cutaneous porphyria (porphyria cutanea tarda).* The hyperpigmentation observed in hemochromatosis may be grayish brown or brown and be indistinguishable from the hypermelanosis of Addison's disease (see Endocrine Factors below). The diagnosis of hemochromatosis is established by the presence of hemosiderin in the sweat glands of the skin. Porphyria may be recognized by the abnormally large amounts of *uroporphyrin* in the urine, stools, and plasma, and by other characteristic clinical features, such as the presence of bullae, atrophic scars, and milia on the exposed surfaces of the face and hands.

NUTRITIONAL FACTORS In *chronic nutritional deficiency* in general, splotches of dirty-brown hyperpigmentation appear, especially on the trunk. In selective deficiencies, such as when the *deficiency* is *of protein,* as in *kwashiorkor,* or when there is *protein loss* as in *chronic nephrosis, ulcerative colitis,* and *malabsorption syndrome,* there is sometimes an associated change in hair color (which is the only pigmentation change), first to reddish brown and eventually to gray. In other selective deficiencies, such as *sprue,* the brown hypermelanosis may be distributed over any area of the body, whereas, in *pellagra,* it is limited to areas of skin that are exposed to light or to irritation, as in the perineum. In *deficiency of vitamin B_{12},* the hair loses its original color and becomes gray, and there is a general distribution of Addisonian diffuse brown hypermelanosis, which is more prominent around the small joints.

ENDOCRINE FACTORS Diffuse brown hypermelanosis is a striking feature of primary adrenocortical insufficiency (Addison's disease). There is marked accentuation of pigmentation in certain areas, namely, on the pressure points (vertebrae, knuckles, elbows, knees), and in the body folds, palmar creases, and gingival mucous membrane. An identical type of diffuse hyperpigmentation has also been reported to follow adrenalectomy in patients with Cushing's disease. In these patients, there usually are signs and symptoms of pituitary tumors; all the tumors recorded have been chromophobe adenomas. A third example of the Addisonian type of melanosis has been reported in patients with tumors of organs (pancreas, lung) other than the adrenal or pituitary glands. The generalized brown hypermelanosis found in all these conditions results from overproduction of melanocyte-stimulating hormone (MSH) and ACTH. Both MSH and ACTH share common amino acid sequences. It appears that an excess of alpha-melanocyte-stimulating hormone plays the dominant role in the pigmentation that occurs in adrenocortical insufficiency.

TABLE 57-2
Disturbances of human melanin pigmentation

	Classification		
	Hypomelanosis:[1]	*Hypermelanosis*[1]	
Causative factors	*White*	*Brown*	*Gray, slate, or blue*[14]
Genetic factors	Piebaldism[2] Waardenburg's syndrome[2] Canities, premature[2] Vitiligo[2,3] Albinism, oculocutaneous:[4] tyrosinase-positive tyrosinase-negative Albinism, ocular Cross-McKusick-Breen syndrome[4] Hypomelanotic macules in tuberous sclerosis[2,5] Nevus depigmentosus[2,5] Phenylketonuria[6,7] Fanconi's syndrome[6] Neurofibromatosis[2] Ataxia telangiectasia[2]	*Café au lait* and frecklelike macules in neurofibromatosis[2] Melanotic macules in polyostotic fibrous dysplasia (Albright's syndrome)[2] Ephelides (freckles)[2] Lentigines[2] Lentigines with cardiac arrhythmias[2] Neurocutaneous melanosis[2] Xeroderma pigmentosum[2] Acanthosis nigricans, juvenile type[2] Peutz-Jeghers syndrome[2]	Oculodermal melanocytosis (nevus of Ota)[2,14] Dermal melanocytosis (Mongolian spot)[2,14] Blue melanocytic nevus[2,14] Incontinentia pigmenti[2,15]
Metabolic factors		Hemochromatosis[4] Hepatolenticular disease (Wilson's disease)[4] Porphyria (congenital erythropoietic and porphyria variegata and cutanea tarda)[4] Gaucher's disease[11] Niemann-Pick disease[11]	Hemochromatosis[4]
Endocrine factors	Hypopituitarism[4] Addison's disease[2] Hyperthyroidism[2]	ACTH-producing and MSH-producing pituitary and other tumors[4] ACTH therapy[4] Pregnancy[11] Addison's disease[4] Estrogen therapy[12] Melasma[2,13]	
Nutritional factors	Chronic protein deficiency or loss:[6,8] Kwashiorkor Nephrosis Ulcerative colitis Malabsorption syndrome Vitamin B_{12} deficiency[6]	Kwashiorkor[2] Pellagra[11] Sprue[11] Vitamin B_{12} deficiency[11]	Chronic nutritional insufficiency[2]
Chemical and pharmacologic agents	Monobenzyl ether of hydroquinone[2] Chloroquine and hydroxychloroquine[6] Arsenical intoxication[2]	Arsenical intoxication[4] Busulfan administration[4] Photochemical agents (topical or systemic drugs, tar)[2] Berlock dermatosis[2]	Fixed (drug) eruption[2,14] Quinacrine toxicity[4] Chlorpromazine administration[11,16]

Both MSH and ACTH are increased as a result of the decreased output of cortisol by the adrenals. Hypermelanosis of the Addisonian type can be produced in adrenalectomized human subjects by the administration of large amounts of homogeneous ACTH and alpha-MSH.

CHEMICAL FACTORS Chemicals can induce both hypomelanosis and hypermelanosis. Hydroquinone prevents the formation of melanin and is of therapeutic value in treating hypermelanosis. Striking generalized Addisonian hypermelanosis of the skin follows busulfan therapy; the mechanism of action of this drug is not known. Inorganic trivalent arsenicals produce both generalized Addisonian hypermelanosis and scattered macular hypomelanosis, as well as punctate keratoses on the palms and soles. Some phenolic germicides have been shown to cause a vitiligo-like hypomelanosis that may or may not be reversible.

PHYSICAL FACTORS Mechanical trauma, as well as burns caused by heat, ultraviolet light, or alpha, beta, and gamma radiation, can lead to hypomelanosis or hypermelanosis. The effect of these physical agents on pigmentation is determined by the intensity and duration of exposure and is limited to the site of injury. The hypomelanosis results from destruction of melanocytes.

Chronic pruritus (because the skin is constantly scratched

TABLE 57-2 *(continued)*
Disturbances of human melanin pigmentation

	Classification		
	Hypomelanosis[1]	*Hypermelanosis*[1]	
Causative factors	*White*	*Brown*	*Gray, slate, or blue*[14]
Physical agents	Burns: thermal, ultraviolet, and ionizing radiation[2,9] Traumatic injury[2,9]	Ultraviolet light (suntanning)[2] Thermal radiation Alpha, beta, and gamma ionizing radiation[2] Chronic rubbing and scratching[2]	
Inflammation and infection	Pinta[2,9] Leprosy[2,5] Fungal infections (tinea versicolor)[2,5] Pityriasis alba[2,5] Eczematous dermatitis[2,5] Psoriasis[2] Lupus erythematosus, discoid[2]	Lichen planus[2] Lupus erythematosus, discoid[2] Lichen simplex chronicus[2] Atopic dermatitis[11] Psoriasis[2]	Pinta in exposed areas[2] Erythema dyschromicum perstans[2,15]
Neoplasms	In sites of malignant melanoma after disappearance (therapeutic or spontaneous) of tumor[2] Nevus, "halo"[2]	Malignant melanoma[2] Mastocytosis (urticaria pigmentosa)[2] Adenocarcinoma with acanthosis nigricans[2]	Slate-gray dermal pigmentation with metastatic melanoma and melanogenuria[4]
Miscellaneous factors	Vogt-Koyanagi-Harada syndrome[2] Scleroderma, circumscribed or systemic[2] Canities[6] Alopecia areata[10] Horner's syndrome, congenital and acquired[7] Hypomelanosis, guttate, idiopathic[2]	Scleroderma, systemic[4] Chronic hepatic insufficiency[4] Whipple's syndrome[4] Encephalitis, chronic[2] Lentigo, senile ("liver spots")[2]	

[1] *The listing includes the pigmentation disorder itself or the condition with which it is associated.*
[2] *Pigment change is circumscribed.*
[3] *Total loss of pigment in the skin and hair may occur.*
[4] *Pigment change is diffuse, not circumscribed, and there are no identifiable borders.*
[5] *Loss of pigmentation is usually partial (hypomelanosis); viewed with Wood's lamp, the lesions are not completely devoid of pigment (amelanosis), as in vitiligo.*
[6] *Pigment is decreased in the hair.*
[7] *Pigment is decreased in the iris.*
[8] *Hair is gray or reddish.*
[9] *There is a loss of melanocytes.*
[10] *Regrown hair is white.*
[11] *Pigment change may be diffuse or circumscribed.*
[12] *Nipples are affected.*
[13] *Idiopathic or due to progestational agents.*
[14] *Gray, slate, or blue color results from the presence of* dermal *melanocytes or phagocytized melanin in the dermis.*
[15] *Areas of brown may be admixed with the slate-gray and blue discoloration.*
[16] *Pigment has not been definitely identified as melanin.*

SOURCE: *TB Fitzpatrick, MC Mihm Jr, Abnormalities of the melanin pigmentary system, in* Dermatology in General Medicine, *eds TB Fitzpatrick et al, New York: McGraw-Hill, 1971*

and rubbed) such as that associated with chronic biliary tract disease and lymphoma, may lead to generalized brown hypermelanosis.

INFLAMMATORY AND INFECTIOUS FACTORS Circumscribed hypomelanosis is a characteristic feature of *tuberculoid leprosy*. It occurs often in areas of anesthesia, and the degree of pigment loss is only partial; the lesions are lighter in color than the areas of surrounding skin but are not snow-white as in vitiligo. Generalized spotty hyperpigmentation not uncommonly follows *exanthems* and *eruptions due to drugs;* it usually disappears spontaneously within 2 or 3 months.

NEOPLASTIC FACTORS Hypomelanosis is seen in rare instances at the site of a primary or a metastatic *malignant melanoma* that has undergone remission spontaneously or as the result of chemotherapy. During the terminal stages of malignant melanoma, striking generalized blue hypermelanosis of the skin sometimes develops, and large amounts of a conjugated derivative of 5,6-dihydroxyindole are excreted in the urine ("melanogenuria"). This intermediate in the metabolic pathway from tyrosine to melanin can be oxidized to melanin in the absence of tyrosinase, and therefore melanin can be synthesized at almost any site in which oxidation can take place. Consequently, diffuse black pigmentation may develop in the peritoneum, liver, heart, muscle, and dermis of patients during the late stages of malignant melanoma. The brown melanin in the dermal phagocytes appears clinically as blue in the skin because of the Tyndall light-scattering phenomenon.

The multiple, irregular, round or oval, yellowish brown to reddish brown macules and papules characteristic of *urticaria pigmentosa* are related to the presence of melanin in the epidermis that overlies the clusters of mast cells. Urticarial wheals develop when the lesions are stroked vigorously. In rare instances *(systemic mastocytosis),* mast cells infiltrate diffusely into the liver, spleen, gastrointestinal system, and bones, as well as into the skin. Mast-cell leukemia occasionally develops. In children, the skin lesions usually appear in infancy and often clear spontaneously in several years. The usual course is quite benign apart from symptoms of flushing, itching, and urticaria in about 30 percent of patients. Less than 15 percent have vomiting, syncope, or shock. The symptoms are presumed to be due to histamine release from the mast cells and often coincide with increased urinary excretion of free histamines and metabolites. Urinary levels of 5-HIAA are normal. Antihistamines are usually of little benefit.

UNKNOWN FACTORS Generalized brown hypermelanosis of the type seen in Addison's disease is not infrequently associated with *systemic scleroderma* and may appear very early in the course of the disorder. Generalized hyperpigmentation occasionally develops in patients with *chronic hepatic insufficiency*, especially that due to portal cirrhosis. The pathogenesis of the pigmentation in both these conditions is unknown.

Melasma (chloasma) (Color Plate 2-4) occurs in pregnant women and sometimes in women taking oral progestational agents, but it also occurs in nonpregnant women and in men. The lesions consist of large macules with irregular borders on the exposed areas of the face and vary in color from yellow-brown to red-brown and very dark brown.

TABLE 57-3
Circumscribed vitiligo-type hypomelanosis of skin

ASSOCIATED WITH GENETIC DISORDERS	
Present at birth	*Delayed onset*
Piebaldism	Vitiligo
Waardenburg's syndrome	
Nevus depigmentosus	
Tuberous sclerosis	
Neurofibromatosis	
Ataxia telangiectasia	
ASSOCIATED WITH CHEMICALS (OCCUPATIONAL OR THERAPEUTIC)	
Phenolic germicides ("O-Syl," "Phenocide," etc.)	
Hydroquinone	
Hydroquinone, monobenzyl ether of	
Hydroquinone, monomethyl ether of	
ASSOCIATED WITH METABOLIC OR ENDOCRINE DISORDERS	
Addison's disease	
Hyperthyroidism	
Pernicious anemia	
Hypoparathyroidism-Addison's disease-candidiasis syndrome	
ASSOCIATED WITH NEOPLASMS	
Malignant melanoma (in sites of regression)	
Melanocytic nevi ("halo nevi")	
ASSOCIATED WITH INFECTIONS	
Leprosy	
Pinta	
Tinea versicolor	
ASSOCIATED WITH IDIOPATHIC CONDITIONS	
Vogt-Koyangi-Harada syndrome	
Postinflammation: atopic dermatitis, pityriasis alba, psoriasis	

REFERENCES

DEMIS DJ: Mast cell disease (urticaria pigmentosa), in *Clinical Dermatology,* eds DJ Demis et al, New York: Harper & Row, 1974, vol. 1, unit 4–11, p. 1

FITZPATRICK TB et al: The melanocyte system, in *Dermatology in General Medicine,* eds TB Fitzpatrick et al, New York: McGraw-Hill, 1971, p. 117

——, MIHM MC JR: Abnormalities of the melanin pigmentary system, in *Dermatology in General Medicine,* eds TB Fitzpatrick et al, New York: McGraw-Hill, 1971, p. 1591

——, QUEVEDO WC JR: Biologic processes underlying melanin pigmentation and pigmentary disorders, in *Modern Trends in Dermatology,* ed P Borrie, series 4, London: Butterworth, 1971

TODA K et al: Alteration of racial differences in melanosome distribution in human epidermis after exposure to ultraviolet light. Nature [New Biol] 236:143, 1972

58

PHOTOSENSITIVITY AND OTHER REACTIONS TO LIGHT

T. B. FITZPATRICK
M. A. PATHAK

INTRODUCTION

During the last decade, interest in the reaction of human skin to light has been renewed as a result of (1) the widespread use of certain drugs that produce photosensitivity, such as phenothiazines (tranquilizers) and tetracycline and demethychlortetracycline, which alter the cutaneous responses to sunlight, and a steadily growing awareness among investigators and clinicians that many compounds (e.g., sulfonamides and oral hypoglycemic agents) synthesized for various therapeutic purposes can cause cutaneous photosensitivity as a side effect; (2) the incorporation of certain topical antimicrobial agents (e.g., halogenated salicylanilides) into soaps that produce photosensitivity; (3) the increased recognition of, and better diagnostic and therapeutic approaches to, various skin eruptions (papules, plaques, and eczematous and urticarial reactions) of unknown cause and differing morphologic features (i.e., polymorphic photodermatitis) that follow exposure to ultraviolet and visible light; (4) the general public's obsession with sunbathing, resulting in premature aging of the skin (solar elastosis); (5) the establishment of new demographic data indicating that exposure to sunlight is an important cause of basal-cell and squamous-cell carcinoma of the sun-exposed parts of the body; and (6) increased recognition of the fact that sunlight is a major cause of discomfort and photosensitivity reactions in patients with certain types of porphyria, especially for those with erythropoietic protoporphyria.

There are more than 25 human disorders that are either caused by or aggravated by exposure of the skin to sunlight. These range from degenerative and neoplastic changes to disability and discomfort associated with chemically induced photosensitivity reactions.

This discussion will be concerned with: the degenerative and neoplastic conditions associated with solar radiation, such as basal-cell carcinoma, squamous-cell carcinoma, malignant melanoma, solar keratoses (Color Plate 4-2), and chronic sun-induced degeneration; photosensitivity related to drugs; and photosensitivity related to increased plasma levels of photosensitizing porphyrins in patients with all types of porphyria except acute intermittent porphyria.

To understand the photobiology of man's responses to light, it is essential to know about the solar radiation that passes through the atmosphere to the earth's surface.

Electromagnetic emanations from the sun comprise a wide range of radiation and include electric waves, radio waves, infrared rays, visible light, ultraviolet light, roentgen rays, gamma rays, and secondary cosmic rays. The unit of wavelength commonly used to measure ultraviolet and visible light radiation is the nanometer (nm; 10^{-9} m). The shortest wavelengths that reach the surface of the earth through the atmosphere are about 286 to 290 nm. Wavelengths shorter than 290 nm are principally absorbed by ozone in the stratosphere. The solar spectrum that can affect human skin includes wavelengths of 290 to 720 nm.

The amount and type of solar radiation that reach a given part of the earth at any given time are determined by a great variety of factors, such as latitude, time of day, season, altitude, local atmospheric conditions (smog, cloudiness, haze, smoke, dust, fog, humidity, aerosol particles), variations in the thickness of the ozone layer, and height of the sun above the horizon.

Approximately 50 percent of the radiant energy emitted by the sun is present in the visible portion of the spectrum (380 to 720 nm), about 40 percent in the infrared region, and about 10 percent in the ultraviolet region. The damage to skin (sunburn, skin cancer) is evoked by 3 percent of the ultraviolet radiation of wavelengths of from 290 to 320 nm.

Protection against this damage to the "normal" skin has long been the subject of much investigation, and there are many commercially available sunscreens that are satisfactory under certain conditions (Table 58-1). Patients should apply, 45 min *before exposure*, 5% *para*-aminobenzoic acid (PABA) in 50 to 70% ethanol (Table 58-1); PABA-esters in ethanol are less effective. The solution should be reapplied after swimming or after profuse sweating.

SUNBURN AND TANNING

Clinical changes

ERYTHEMA, OR SUNBURN REACTION Erythema is caused principally by radiation of from 290 to 320 nm, with maximum effectiveness at 300 to 307 nm. Light of wavelengths greater than 320 nm (320 to 700 nm) is generally considered to be nonerythemogenic, although prolonged exposure to radiation of 320 to 400 nm (2 h of midday summer sun in northern latitudes) can produce mild sunburn in normal subjects. Wavelengths of 290 to 320 nm are thought to accelerate aging (wrinkling) in the skin and to lead to the development of solar keratoses, carcinoma, and, possibly, some types of malignant melanoma. Wavelengths of the long-wave ultraviolet and visible spectrums are innocuous unless the skin contains either topically applied or ingested photosensitizing agents.

The sunburn reaction is a complex process in which a number of changes occur simultaneously. At present, the nature of the chromophore that absorbs the light energy which initiates the primary photochemical responses is not well established, although the bulk of evidence suggests that nucleic acids (in DNA) are the primary sites for the absorption of radiation of from 290 to 320 nm. Vasodilatation accompanying the sunburn reaction appears to result from the activation and release of one or several chemical mediators (e.g., kinin, serotonin, and also histamine). Ultraviolet radiation appears to have a direct effect on the blood vessels of the upper layer of the dermis (capillaries, venules, and arterioles). The formation of peroxides or peroxy radicals may play an important role in the damage to lysosomal membranes associated with lipid peroxidation.

MELANIN PIGMENTATION, OR TANNING The familiar tanning (increase in melanin pigment) that follows exposure of the skin to solar radiation is known to involve two distinct photobiologic processes. The first, *immediate pigment darkening* (IPD), or darkening of preformed pigment in the epidermis, is elicited by wavelengths of 320 to 720 nm. The second, or *melanogenesis,* is an intricate process that consists of the *erythema response (sunburn)* followed in a few days (4 days usually) by formation of new pigment. Immediate pigment darkening probably represents oxidation of melanin through the production of semiquinone-like free radicals in the melanin polymer; transfer of melanosomes from melanocytes and redistribution of already existing melanosomes within the keratinocytes also may occur.

Melanogenesis involves: (1) increase in the number of functional melanocytes, resulting from increased proliferation of melanocytes, and activation of dormant melanocytes; (2) increased arborization of melanocytic dendrites; (3) increase in the number of melanosomes in melanocytes; (4) increase in tyrosinase activity; and (5) increase in the transfer of melanosomes.

Cellular and molecular changes

HYPERPLASIA Within 72 h after exposure, an increase in the number of epidermal cells is visible in the light microscope and is characterized by a high rate of cell proliferation accompanied by a high rate of mitotic activity. The rate of proliferation of cells decreases after 7 to 10 days, and the thickness of the epidermis gradually returns to normal within the next 30 to 60 days.

DNA AND RNA CHANGES Damage to DNA by sunburn-producing ultraviolet light (230 to 320 nm) results in cell death. The principal photoproducts formed in the DNA of epidermal cells are pyrimidine dimers, which are of the C_4-cyclobutane type and are formed between adjacent pyrimidine bases. DNA and RNA synthesis in the epidermis is inhibited within 1 h after irradiation. By 24 h, new synthesis is evident and, by 60 to 70 h, is maximum.

MITOSIS Inhibition of epidermal mitosis and retardation of basal-cell turnover occurs within 1 h after irradiation. Inhibition of mitosis can persist for 7 to 24 h; it is followed by an acceleration of mitotic rate and basal-cell turnover that reaches a peak by 48 to 72 h and is associated with epidermal hyperplasia. The mitotic cycle appears to be interrupted in the G_2 or in the prophase stage, or in both.

SUN-INDUCED CARCINOMA

The reported epidemiologic evidence clearly implicates solar radiation as a factor in the induction of human skin cancer.

Some studies have established that carcinoma of the skin occurs more frequently on the parts of the body habitually exposed to sunlight; the lesions of the head and hands are concentrated on the nose, central portions of the cheeks, eyelids, and dorsa of the hands. In fair-skinned Caucasoids who easily sunburn, these cancers are limited almost exclusively to the exposed portions of the face, head, neck, arms, and hands. Negroid skin, on the other hand, is remarkably resistant to the development of skin cancer on the exposed surfaces, and a similar resistance is seen among the pigmented Caucasoids (e.g., East Indians), American Indians, and Asiatics. Approximately 80 to 90 percent of basal-cell carcinomas occur on the head and neck, approximately 4 to 8 percent on the trunk, and about 10 to 12 percent on the extremities.

Carcinoma of the exposed skin is more prevalent among persons who are outdoors a great deal (e.g., golfers, farmers, sailors), and is the common cause of cancer in Caucasoids in Australia, South Africa, and the southern parts of the United States.

The reported evidence for a causal relation between sunburn-evoking ultraviolet radiation and the prevalence of human squamous-cell carcinoma and basal-cell carcinoma is overwhelming. The wavelength limit for carcinogenesis

TABLE 58-1
Topical formulations suitable for protection against ultraviolet and visible light and for prevention of sunburn, sun-induced degeneration of the skin and sun-induced carcinoma*

Formulations	*Wavelength range of protection, nm*	*Commercial products*
5% *para*-aminobenzoic acid in 50–70% ethyl alcohol[a]	290–320 (sunburn spectrum or UV-B)	Pabanol (Elder, U.S.A.), Presun (Westwood, U.S.A.)
4% ethylhexyl, *para*-methoxycinnamate, 3% 2-hydroxy-4-methoxybenzophenone 2-phenyl Benzmidazole sulfonic acid in a cream base[a]	290–360	Piz-Buin, Exclusiv Extrem Cream #6[a] and #4[b] (Greiter A.G., Switzerland, Germany, U.S.A.)
2.5% ester of *para*-aminobenzoic acid (isoamyl-*p*-*N*,*N*-dimethyl aminobenzoate) in 50–70% ethyl alcohol[b]	290–320	Block Out (Sea and Ski, U.S.A.), Paba film (Owens, U.S.A.), Spectraban (Stiefel, Germany and United Kingdom)
10% 2-hydroxy-4-methoxybenzophenone 5-sulfonic acid (Sulisobenzone) lotion[b]	290–360	Uval (Dome Laboratories, U.S.A.)
5–10% opaque and light-reflecting pigments like zinc oxide, titanium dioxide, calamine[c]	290–720 (ultraviolet and visible spectrum)	Afil (Texas Pharmaceuticals, U.S.A.), RVPaque (Elder, U.S.A.), Reflecta (Texas Pharmaceuticals, U.S.A.), Covermark (Lydia O'Leary, U.S.A.)
60–180 mg, synthetic beta-carotene[d]	380–600	Solatene (Roche, U.S.A.)

* *Sunscreen should be applied once a day in the morning on the face, neck, and hands; in periods of prolonged sun exposure of over two hours, and after swimming, reapply the sunscreen to the whole body.*
[a] *For sun-sensitive persons who burn easily and tan poorly.*
[b] *For average persons who burn and then tan.*
[c] *Only for patients exhibiting severe hypersensitivity reactions to light who cannot be protected with invisible, cosmetically acceptable sunscreens.*
[d] *An oral preparation for patients with erythropoietic protoporphyria.*

by ultraviolet light has been established at about 290 to 320 nm, which is the same as that for sunburn.

It should be emphasized that, of all the radiation emitted by the sun, ranging from x-rays at the short-wave end of the spectrum to radio waves at the long-wave end, only a portion penetrates the earth's atmosphere; the shortest wavelength of solar radiation recorded at sea level is about 290 nm. This sharp cutoff between the sea level and extraterrestrial distribution in the ultraviolet spectrum is largely, if not exclusively, due to the absorption of harmful radiation by ozone.

Several studies based on the distribution of local populations in the United States, Australia, and Ireland have emphasized that skin cancer develops earlier and more frequently in people who have light skin and freckles, who burn easily and do not tan on exposure to the sun, and who are of mostly Celtic ancestry. Australia, with the highest reported incidence of skin cancer in the world, has a population largely descended from British stock, with about 25 percent claiming Celtic (i.e., Irish, Scottish, and Welsh) extraction. In all three countries surveyed, the persons of Celtic ancestry were found to have a disproportionately high incidence of skin cancer.

All varieties of skin cancer develop in patients with xeroderma pigmentosum, an autosomal recessive trait. This rare defect is representative, in the extreme, of the basic problem of solar radiation and skin cancer. Patients with this disease have a greatly increased susceptibility to malignant tumors of the skin in the light-exposed areas. The characteristic skin manifestations are atrophy, telangiectasia, hyperpigmented macules, keratoses, and ulcerations, all occurring in sun-exposed areas. Within the first few years of life, basal-cell or squamous-cell carcinomas or sarcomas or malignant melanomas develop. An inherited enzyme defect may be responsible, at least in part, for the cancer-forming potential in patients with xeroderma pigmentosum. Cultured fibroblasts from patients with xeroderma pigmentosum are incapable of releasing thymine dimers from DNA and, in consequence, are deficient in their ability to repair their ultraviolet-damaged DNA. It is possible that this enzymatic deficiency results in a high somatic mutation rate of skin cells after sun exposure and, eventually, in cancer formation.

DEGENERATIVE CHANGES OF THE SKIN

Degenerative changes of the skin (wrinkling, telangiectasia, keratoses) are significantly more frequent in white-skinned people living in areas where the intensity of ultraviolet radiation is great (e.g., southwestern U.S.A., Australia, South Africa). The term "solar degeneration" implies a group of changes in the exposed areas of the skin, including wrinkling, atrophy, hypermelanotic and hypomelanotic macules, telangiectasia, yellow papules and plaques, and keratoses. The furrowed and leathery condition of the skin is seen particularly in persons who have fair skin and poor tanning ability and are constantly exposed to the sun. The most conspicuous and characteristic structural change involves biochemical alterations of connective tissues (elastin, as well as collagen). The sunburn-producing radiation (290 to 320 nm) and, possibly also, long-wave ultraviolet radiation (320 to 400 nm) that can penetrate deeply in the dermis are involved in evoking the degenerative changes.

Chronically light-damaged human epidermis shows shortening or flattening of the rete ridges, thinning of the epidermis (decrease in malpighian cells), and many abnormal cells in disorderly arrangement. There is a progressive degeneration in the papillary and subpapillary zones of the dermis. Other changes include: (1) the development of vascular ectasia; (2) accumulation of acid mucopolysaccharides; (3) appearance of abnormal fibrocytes; (4) loss of collagen; (5) degeneration of elastic tissue (referred to as "actinic elastosis"), and disorganization of the connective tissue into amorphous masses.

PHOTOTOXICITY AND PHOTOALLERGY

Sensitivity to sunlight is now regarded as a very common clinical problem. Continuous daily exposure to sun alone may be a major factor responsible for irreversible changes in the human skin, e.g., freckles, telangiectasia, wrinkling, keratosis, atrophy, hypermelanotic and hypomelanotic macules, and carcinomas in the sun-exposed regions.

Apart from these chronic changes, human skin can also become hypersensitive to ultraviolet and visible light. The interface between man and his environment is the skin, and the physical (light) and chemical agents acting directly on it are paramount etiologic or precipitating factors in photosensitivity disorders. Aggravating this situation is the fact that the general public is subjected to an ever-increasing quantity of newer chemicals and is also obsessed with sunbathing.

EFFECT OF DRUGS AND OTHER CHEMICALS PLUS LIGHT

There is now a growing awareness of the relation between certain chemical agents and light in the causation of certain types of dermatitis. These agents include chemicals and drugs that may not act as contact irritants and are generally innocuous to skin in the absence of exposure to light; when the skin is challenged with proper concentrations of the agent and the appropriate wavelengths of light, however, these agents can induce undesirable reactions in the skin.

Many substances occur in nature that have photosensitizing potential and have for a long time been recognized as potentially "toxic." Large numbers of other substances have been synthesized within the past two decades and are used for clinical and commercial purposes without understanding of their incidental "side-effects" that are usually manifested in skin when it is inadvertently exposed to light. The widespread use of certain chemical agents (e.g., tranquilizers and antibiotics) and the development of antimicrobial agents (e.g., halogenated salicylanilides) that are incorporated into soaps and other topical agents have caused many persons to have adverse reactions to light. Several thousand cases of disabling photosensitivity reactions are recognized each year in the United States and elsewhere in industrial workers, agricultural workers, pharmaceutical and cosmetic manufacturing plants, and users of cosmetic preparations, who, in many instances, cannot avoid contact with the causative agent and exposure to either natural or artificial light.

Cutaneous photosensitivity is a general term used in referring to the abnormal reaction of the human skin to the stimulus of light. Drug photosensitivity reactions may be defined clinically as adverse responses manifested by the skin as a result of combined exposure to certain therapeutic or chemical agents and sunlight. The adverse cutaneous reactions can occur in some individuals who have either ingested certain drugs or have been in contact with certain chemicals (Table 58-2). These reactions may include an abnormal sunburn response: edema, papules, macules, vesicles, bullae, or acute eczematous or urticarial reactions. There may be desquamation and hyperpigmentation or hypopigmentation. These adverse photosensitivity reactions are classified into two broad categories: (1) phototoxic reactions, which are common, and (2) photoallergic reactions, which are uncommon.

Phototoxic reactions are those that can be elicited in almost everyone challenged if enough light energy of the appropriate wavelengths and appropriate concentration of the agent are either applied topically or given orally. The reaction produced by light and the offending agent is characterized clinically by an exaggerated sunburn reaction with or without painful edema. The reaction occurs within a few hours (5 to 18 h) after exposure to the sun.

Hyperpigmentation and desquamation also occur. The reaction is usually confined to the site of exposure. If the applied concentration of the implicated agent is high, there may be bullae or small vesicles.

The phototoxic reactions in general should be regarded as the result of abnormal augmentation, due to an association with drugs and other chemicals, of the sunburn response of the skin. It is believed that a deleterious amount of radiant energy is absorbed by the skin and the photosensitizing agents. The photosensitizers are either in the extracellular fluid of the skin after oral ingestion or in the epidermal cells as a result of passive penetration after topical application. The photosensitizing agent absorbs additional quanta of light not only from the sunburn spectrum (290 to 320 nm) but also from the long-wave ultraviolet spectrum (320 to 400 nm) as a result of the formation of a complex between the cellular components (e.g., DNA, RNA, proteins, and lipids) and the sensitizing agent, and thus increases the total amount of absorbed energy. This absorbed energy can directly cause cell damage by creating a covalent linking of the sensitizing molecule to the pyrimidines (e.g., thymine) in the cellular DNA. This linkage, recognized as the formation of cyclobutane photoadducts of the sensitizer and the pyrimidines, can be lethal to the cell. It has been established that photosensitizers like 8-methoxypsoralen and 4,5′,8-trimethylpsoralen selectively undergo a photoaddition reaction with epidermal DNA. In addition, the photosensitizing molecule can transfer the absorbed energy and promote formation of free radicals (molecules with unpaired electrons that are highly reactive) and cause damage to the cell membranes and lysosomes. Drug-induced cutaneous phototoxic reactions may, therefore, reasonably be regarded as the undesirable sequelae of augmentation of the primary photochemical reactions that underlie the sunburn response of skin.

Photoallergy to drugs can be considered to represent an acquired and altered capacity of the skin to respond to light energy in the presence of a photosensitizer, and, presumably, is dependent on an antigen-antibody reaction or a delayed hypersensitivity response mediated by mononuclear cells. The absorbed energy of light seems to promote a photochemical reaction between the drug and the proteins of the skin; the drug acting as a haptenic group either combines directly with the protein to form a photoantigen

TABLE 58-2
Systemic chemicals that induce photosensitivity reactions in humans

Chemical	*Use*	*Clinical findings*	*Action spectrum, nm*
Chlortetracycline; demethylchlortetracycline (Declomycin); oxytetracycline; doxycycline	Antibiotic	Exaggerated sunburn; phototoxicity	290–400
Sulfanilamide; sulfathiazole; sulfapyridine; sulfamethazine; sulfaguanidine; sulfisoxazole; monochlorphenamide	Chemotherapeutic; antibacterial	Phototoxicity; photoallergy	290–320
Carbutamide; tolbutamide (Orinase); chlorpropamide (Diabinease)	Hypoglycemic	Phototoxicity	290–320
Chlorothiazide (Diuril); quinethazone (Hydromox)	Diuretic; antihypertensive	Papules, edema; plaques	290–320
Griseofulvin	Antimycotic	Exaggerated sunburn; phototoxicity; photoallergy	290–400
Nalidixic acid	Antibacterial	Erythema; bullae	290–400
Chlorpromazine (Thorazine); promethazine (Phenergan); mepazine (Stelazine); trimeprazine (Compazine); promazine (Sparine)	Tranquilizer; antihistamine	Exaggerated sunburn; macules, papules, urticaria; gray-blue hyperpigmentation	320–400
Psoralen; 4,5′,8-trimethylpsoralen (Trisoralen); 8-methoxypsoralen (Oxsoralen)	Stimulator of melanin synthesis	Erythema; bullae; hyperpigmentation	320–400
Mestranol and norethynodrel; diethylstilbestrol	Oral contraceptive	Melasma; phototoxicity	?
Chlordiazepoxide (Librium)	Tranquilizer	Eczematous dermatitis	290–320
Triacetyldiphenolisatin	Laxative	Eczematous dermatitis	290–320
Calcium cyclamate; sodium cyclohexylsulfamate	Sweetener	Phototoxicity; photoallergy	290–360

or is altered by the absorbed energy, and this altered haptenic group then reacts with the proteins to form an antigen.

The clinical manifestations in drug-induced photoallergic reactions may range from eczematous or papular lesions, appearing 24 h or more after an exposure, to acute urticarial lesions developing within a few minutes after exposure. The eruption frequently extends beyond the areas that were exposed. In recurrent cases, flare-ups of distant previously uninvolved sites frequently may also occur. The action spectrum (wavelengths that induce cutaneous reactions) is generally in the long-wave range (320 to 400 nm), and less energy is required than is necessary for the production of phototoxic reactions. Histologically, the epidermal changes also are characteristic, although not diagnostic of these various responses. A dense perivascular round-cell infiltrate in the dermis is often seen in both the eczematous and papular responses. Spongiosis and vesiculation are prominent in the eczematous lesions, whereas the urticarial or papular lesions show no remarkable epidermal changes. Some edema and vasodilatation are common in most of these eruptions.

The various clinically important therapeutic agents given systemically and their effects on the skin in the presence of light (whether phototoxic or photoallergic reactions) are listed in Table 58-2. The biologic action spectrums are also given, indicating the range of wavelengths that effectively induces either the phototoxic or photoallergic reactions.

EFFECT OF PLANTS PLUS LIGHT Phytophotodermatitis (phototoxic reactions) can develop as the result of contact with many plants (belonging principally to the families Rutaceae and Umbelliferae) and subsequent exposure of the skin to sunlight. The photodermatitis involves a mild-to-severe erythematous reaction with or without vesicles or bullae. Dense postinflammatory hyperpigmentation is visible within 3 to 5 days. Phytophotodermatitis has also been seen in individuals in contact with carrots, celery, and the oil of Persian limes. Perfumes and colognes containing particular oils are also known to induce hyperpigmentation with or without erythema. The pigmentation in berlock dermatitis occurs in configurations that seem bizarre but actually represent the areas to which the scent was applied; sometimes the hyperpigmentation may be drop-like or pendant-like, and was therefore named accordingly (*bréloque* or *berlocke,* meaning trinket or pendant). This phytophotodermatitis, as well as that which follows contact with various other plants, is thought to be caused by furocoumarins, particularly 5-methoxypsoralen, 8-methoxypsoralen, and other psoralens that are characteristically present in these plants. The combination of exposure to long-wave ultraviolet radiation (320 to 400 nm) and furocoumarins greatly enhances the erythema and the pigmentation response.

Treatment Therapy of acute phototoxic reactions induced by topical or systemic agents is best achieved by removal of the offending agent and avoidance of exposure to the sun, or both. If necessary, the usual dermatologic procedures for minimizing the discomforts of the inflammatory response should be undertaken. However, in instances in which continued systemic use of antibiotic, diuretic, antidiabetic, or tranquilizing drugs is vital, cutaneous photoreactions can be prevented by instructing the patient to remain indoors or by avoiding exposure to sunlight between 10 A.M. and 4 P.M. Generally the problem subsides within a week after discontinuation of the stress (sun and the drug). Sunscreens listed in Table 58-1 also should be prescribed.

EFFECT OF LIGHT ALONE In this category are included several photosensitivity reactions in patients with various types of porphyria. The photosensitivity reactions are related to the overproduction in vivo of proto-, uro- and coproporphyrins and their precursors. In the porphyrias, endogenously synthesized photosensitizing molecules, when exposed to light, cause burning, itching, urticaria, edema, crusting and scarring, vesiculation, atrophy, and many other disabling cutaneous changes. The light-absorbing molecules that are implicated in evoking the cutaneous reactions are undoubtedly the irreversibly oxidized porphyrins that are present in abnormal amounts in red blood cells, plasma, skin, liver, stool, and urine. The photodermatitis is produced by a narrow band of light in the region of 400 to 410 nm, which corresponds to one of the absorption peaks of porphyrins. The most disabling type of photosensitivity reactions are encountered in erythropoietic (congenital) porphyria (Günther's disease) and in erythropoietic protoporphyria (Chap. 109). Symptoms and signs of sensitivity to sunlight occur in early childhood.

The adverse cutaneous responses to sunlight in patients with erythropoietic protoporphyria (EPP) have been found to be ameliorated by oral ingestion of beta-carotene (Chap. 109). Patients who take beta-carotene are able to withstand prolonged exposures to sunlight and experience relief from their usual photosensitivity reactions. In laboratory experiments, beta-carotene was found to be an effective quencher for the "singlet" oxygen which is generated in certain photosensitivity reactions, and therefore presumably acts in the same manner in vivo. During porphyrin-mediated photosensitivity reactions, peroxides are generated; the peroxy radicals apparently are very damaging to the lipid membranes. It is presumed that beta-carotene is preferentially oxidized and, by quenching the "singlet oxygen," inhibits the lipid peroxide formation.

REFERENCES

FITZPATRICK TB et al (eds): *Sunlight and Man,* Tokyo: University of Tokyo Press, 1974

PATHAK MA, EPSTEIN JH: Normal and abnormal reactions of man to light, in *Dermatology in General Medicine,* eds TB Fitzpatrick et al, New York: McGraw-Hill, 1971

—— et al: Evaluation of topical agents that prevent sunburn. New Engl J Med 280:1459, 1969

URBACH F (ed): *The Biologic Effects of Ultraviolet Radiation,* Oxford: Pergamon, 1969

59 HIRSUTISM AND ALOPECIA

T. B. FITZPATRICK
H. A. HAYNES

HIRSUTISM IN WOMEN Forbes described hirsutism as "more hair than is cosmetically acceptable to a woman living in a certain culture." In other words, whether an increased amount of hair is abnormal or normal depends on the ethnic origin of the individual. To determine whether a given degree of hypertrichosis represents hirsutism or a normal quantity of hair for the ethnic group is the major problem for the physician. When hypertrichosis is inherited, it appears at puberty and increases until the early twenties. Forbes suggests that if the menses are regular and the physical examination, including examination of the pelvic organs, does not reveal evidence of a virilizing disorder, then a single assay of urinary 17-ketosteroids and 17-hydroxysteroids should be sufficient to establish whether there is a hormonal disorder.

Hirsutism without any evidence of virilism may appear in acromegaly or in disorders with an excess of glucocorticoid hormone, such as Cushing's syndrome. Also, malignant adrenal tumors may cause atypical syndromes, i.e., a combination of Cushing's syndrome and virilism. Hirsutism can occur in the absence of virilism in porphyria cutanea tarda, in patients receiving androgens or glucocorticoids or diphenylhydantoin sodium (Dilantin).

Hirsutism with virilism is an indication for an assay of plasma testosterone. This assay is particularly indicated in patients with hirsutism and virilism who have urinary 17-ketosteroids that are within the normal range, inasmuch as small amounts of testosterone are capable of causing virilization. Signs of virilism include a low-pitched voice, acne, increased muscularity, and clitoral hypertrophy. Development of male-type recession of the hairline or of general alopecia is a manifestation of virilism and is not a feature of constitutional hirsutism. Hirsutism with virilism may occur as a result of three sources of endogenous adrogen: (1) aberrant *testicular* tissue; (2) *ovarian* tumors, such as arrhenoblastoma and hilus-cell tumors; and (3) *adrenal* tumors, especially malignant tumors of the adrenal cortex, as well as congenital adrenal hyperplasia (adrenogenital syndrome).

Constitutional hirsutism with endocrine dysfunction is the commonest type of hirsutism and is often associated with irregular menses and obesity. The hair appears at puberty and increases until the early twenties, making the distinction from ethnic hirsutism difficult. This syndrome of constitutional hirsutism with endocrine dysfunction may or may not be associated with large polycystic ovaries. Virilism is rarely present, and, if present, is very slight and is represented only by increased sebum secretion or acne with no clitoral hypertrophy or male-pattern baldness. The actual etiology of the endocrine dysfunction in constitutional hirsutism is not known at this time. There have been reports of increased urinary pregnanetriolone in constitutional hirsutism. Suppression of adrenal function by exogenously administered corticosteroids has possibly brought about some improvement in the menstrual irregularities and in the infertility. That the ovaries may be the source of excess androgen production in constitutional hirsutism is suggested by the effects of ovarian wedge resection, which can be beneficial for the sterility that occurs in such hirsute women. Elevated plasma and urinary testosterone levels have been found in some patients with constitutional hirsutism, but, for the most part, these levels appear to be normal in the majority of patients. There have been some reports of qualitative differences of gonadotropin excretion in constitutional hirsutism, including a relative increase in the luteinizing hormone. The use of estrogens to suppress

FIGURE 59-1
Stages in hair cycle. Progressive changes from a growing (anagen) hair to a resting club hair (telogen)—second from right. In the normal human scalp, some 10 percent of the hairs are in the resting phase. In various types of alopecia, this percentage rises sharply and may be readily determined by the number of hairs which are easily removed with gentle traction. (DM Pillsbury and WB Shelley)

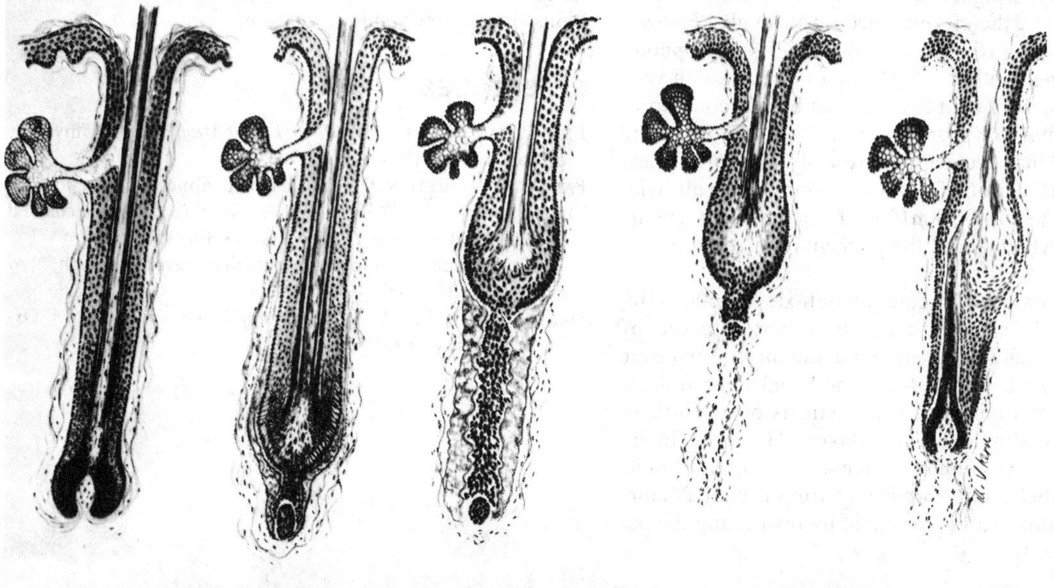

the production of pituitary gonadotropin is a safe, rational, and effective procedure for the treatment of hirsutism.

The cosmetic approach to the treatment of most types of hypertrichosis is quite unsatisfactory except for the permanent removal of the hair follicles by a competent person using electrolysis.

ALOPECIA Hairs plucked from the scalp can be classified as anagen or telogen by the appearance of the hair bulbs (Fig. 59-1). The anagen, or growing, hair roots usually have a sheath surrounding the hair. If the hair is brown or black, the tips will be dark with melanin; the latter can be more easily seen with transmitted light. Telogen hairs, or resting hairs, are club-shaped, the root sheath is absent, and there is a thin epithelial sac surrounding the club.

The scalp has approximately 100,000 hairs; the hair growth cycle is about 2 to 6 years, and the resting period is 3 months. Approximately 70 hairs are normally lost each day from the scalp; the cycle for beard hair is the same. Eyebrows and eyelashes, however, appear to grow for almost 3 months (10 weeks) and then rest for 9 months. The anagen hairs constitute about 85 percent of the population of scalp hairs. In pregnancy, anagen hairs constitute approximately 90 percent during the second and third trimesters, and, therefore, women in the post-partum period note an abnormal loss of hair about 3 months after delivery. This loss is due to the reestablishment of a normal ratio of telogen to anagen hairs.

Alopecia of the scalp, eyebrows, and eyelashes can occur without any visible associated change in the skin (Table 59-1) or secondary to severe local inflammation or scarring, as in discoid lupus erythematosus. Alopecia with scarring or other visible change in the skin usually requires a skin biopsy for diagnosis.

TABLE 59-1
Alopecia and associated conditions*

Condition	*Cause*
ASSOCIATED WITH CIRCUMSCRIBED ALOPECIA (INCLUDING MALE-PATTERN BALDNESS)	
Alopecia areata	Idiopathic
Syphilis, secondary (patchy)	Infection
Trichotillomania	Psychogenic factors
ASSOCIATED WITH DIFFUSE ALOPECIA	
Hypopituitarism,† hypothyroidism,† hyperthyroidism, hypoparathyroidism, pregnancy, postpartum effects	Endocrine factors
Postpyrexia, leprosy†	Infection
Thallium reactions,† anticoagulant administration (prolonged), hypervitaminosis A, therapy with cytotoxic agents	Drug effect
Iron deficiency (with and without anemia), homocystinuria, orotic aciduria (hereditary)	Nutritional and metabolic factors
Lupus erythematosus (systemic); alopecia areata	Idiopathic

**Refers to alopecia primarily involving the scalp, without skin changes.*
†May be limited to lateral one-third of eyebrow.

REFERENCES

BARDIN CE, LIPSETT MB: Testosterone and androstenedione blood production rates in normal women and women with idiopathic hirsutism or polycystic ovaries. J Clin Invest 46:891, 1967

FORBES AP: Hirsutism, in *Dermatology in General Medicine,* eds TB Fitzpatrick et al, New York: McGraw-Hill, 1971

KIRSCHNER MA et al: Effect of estrogen administration on androgen production and plasma luteinizing hormone in hirsute women. J Clin Endocrinol Metab 30:727, 1970

section 10 Hematologic alterations

60
PALLOR AND ANEMIA

MAXWELL W. WINTROBE
G. RICHARD LEE
H. FRANKLIN BUNN

PALLOR

The color of the skin depends on many factors, including the thickness of the epidermis, the quantity and type of pigment contained therein, and the status of the blood vessels, as well as the quantity and nature of the hemoglobin carried within them. Even the nature and fluid content of the subcutaneous tissue are significant factors. It is obvious, therefore, that pallor does not necessarily indicate that anemia is present.
was in their forebears, and may exist in the absence of any true anemia; the flush of excitement, on the other hand, or constant exposure to the sun and wind may produce a ruddy appearance which masks an underlying anemia. The number and pattern of distribution of the finer blood vessels vary among individuals, and, in the same person, vasoconstriction may produce the appearance of pallor, whereas other factors, such as exercise, may lead to the appearance of a "healthier" color. Certain disorders may produce a pallid appearance even though anemia is absent. These disorders include scleroderma, the various nephrotic states, and myxedema. The last two, however, may be accompanied by actual anemia.

Thus, it is evident that the skin itself is an unreliable index of anemia. The mucous membranes, if not inflamed, and the nail beds and palms of the hands, if the hand has not been held in an awkward position and has not been exposed to cold or excessive warmth, are much better. In the palms, the color of the creases is especially significant for they retain their red color even after the intervening skin of the palms has become definitely pale. When the color of the creases is lost, the hemoglobin may be judged as being below 7 g/dl. The color of the conjunctivae may be helpful, but one should not be misled by a coexistent conjunctivitis.

Two factors contribute to the development of pallor in patients with anemia. There is, of course, a decrease in the hemoglobin concentration of blood perfusing the skin and mucous membranes. Also, blood is shunted away from the skin and other peripheral tissues, permitting enhanced blood flow to vital organs. Redistribution of blood flow is an important mode of compensation in anemia (Fig. 60-4).

ANEMIA

Definition and detection Anemia might be most accurately defined as a reduction in the circulating red blood cell mass. However, since the size of the red blood cell mass is not easily measured, such a definition is of limited usefulness. Furthermore, from the standpoint of oxygen transport, concentration is probably more important than total amount of red blood cells or hemoglobin. Certainly, it is more practical to define anemia in terms of concentration per unit volume of blood. In these terms, anemia is a reduction below normal in the volume of packed red blood cells (VPRC), the blood hemoglobin (Hb) concentration per dl, and/or the red blood cell (RBC) count per femtoliter. Under most clinical circumstances, these measurements accurately reflect changes in the red blood cell mass because the total blood volume tends to be kept within relatively narrow limits by a variety of physiologic mechanisms. Nevertheless, in conditions in which blood volume deviates from normal, such as overhydration, dehydration, fluid retention, or significant blood loss, the usual measures of concentration may be misleading. An increase in the plasma volume may give a false impression of anemia. Of greater importance is the fact that an extracellular fluid deficit may mask an underlying anemia.

The hematocrit or packed red blood cell volume is simple, reproducible, and well-suited for routine use in detecting anemia. "Normal" values obtained with the micro method are 1 to 3 percent lower than with the macro method. Also, when anemia is moderately severe, the hematocrit measured by the micro method is less reproducible than by the macro method, making it less suitable for use in calculating erythrocyte indices. The hematocrit also may be calculated from the size and number of cells as determined by electronic counters, but such calculated values do not always agree with results of standard centrifugal methods.

Blood hemoglobin concentration, measured by the cyanmethemoglobin method, also provides accurate information, if properly calibrated. The red blood cell count performed by the hemocytometer method lacks accuracy; when it is performed by an electronic counter, reasonable accuracy is possible if the instrument is calibrated and properly maintained.

Normal values for red blood corpuscles for persons at various ages are presented in the Appendix. In women in the childbearing age group the normal blood values are 10 percent lower than men. These data are for persons living at sea level. At higher altitudes, higher values are found, roughly in proportion to the elevation above sea level. Provided the measurements are accurate, anemia may be defined as a reduction of more than 10 percent below the mean values for the sex. However, since there are variations in normal hemoglobin values of $\pm 10\%$, the line between normal and true anemia is poorly defined.

Physiologic considerations In normal subjects, erythrocytes are produced by the bone marrow and released to the circulation, where they survive approximately 120 days. They are then removed by the "reticuloendothelial," or mononuclear-phagocyte, system in which the hemoglobin is catabolized. It is useful to think of the tissues involved in these processes as if they were one organ, the *erythron,* a concept which is illustrated diagrammatically in Fig. 60-1.

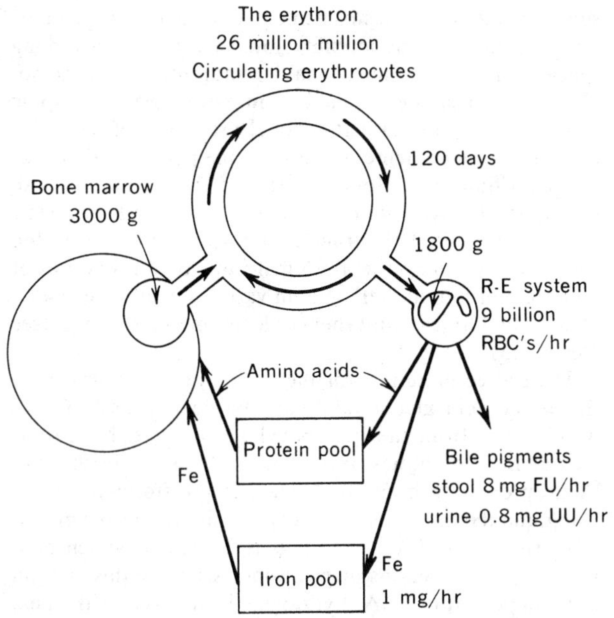

FIGURE 60-1
The amount of blood in circulation represents the balance between production and destruction. In a 70-kg man the circulating red blood corpuscles carry approximately 770 g hemoglobin. Since the average life span of the red blood corpuscles normally is 120 days, the turnover rate per day is the total in the circulation divided by 120. In the average man this comes to approximately 2.16 × 10^{11} red blood corpuscles per day, or 9 billion per h, and 6.4 g hemoglobin per day. From this are derived approximately 21 mg iron per day, 250 mg protoporphyrin, and 6.2 g globin. The iron and globin are reutilized. Of the protoporphyrin derived from the destroyed red blood corpuscles, somewhat less than 250 mg appears as fecal urobilinogen, since there are great variations in completeness of evacuation and also because of variations in the extent to which pigments giving this reaction are produced. Under normal conditions, through increased production and transformation of yellow marrow to red, the bone marrow is capable of approximately a seven- or eightfold increase in production capacity. Consequently, other things being equal, anemia will not develop as the result of increased blood destruction until the life span of the red blood corpuscles has been reduced to less than about 15 to 17 days.

It is apparent that the size of the circulating red blood cell mass is related to the rates of production and destruction. In a normal subject, the two rates are equal; therefore, the red blood cell mass remains constant in size, and the subject can be considered to be in equilibrium. When destruction exceeds production, the red blood cell mass decreases in size, and anemia develops. When production exceeds destruction, the red blood cell mass increases.

Red blood cell production The erythron is maintained within "normal" limits by a well-balanced hormonal mechanism which mediates the response to various normal and abnormal situations. The hormone erythropoietin is a glycoprotein which is thought to be formed by the action of an enzyme produced in the kidney [renal erythropoietic factor (REF) or erythrogenin] on a plasma substance ("erythropoietinogen") of hepatic origin. The kidney, however, in most species (including man) is not the sole source of erythropoietin; removal of the kidneys does not abolish erythropoiesis or cause the complete disappearance of erythropoietin activity in the plasma.

Erythropoietin induces committed stem cells in the marrow to differentiate into pronormoblasts, the earliest recognizable red blood cell precursor. These cells divide three or four times over a 4-day period. During this time, the nucleus becomes smaller, and an increasing amount of hemoglobin is produced in the cytoplasm. Following the last division, the pyknotic nucleus is removed from the normoblast, leaving the reticulocyte which stays in the bone marrow for about two days. The reticulocyte is then released into the general circulation, where it remains for another 24 h before it loses its mitochondria and ribosomes and assumes the morphologic appearance of a mature red blood cell.

Under maximal stimulation, the marrow is capable of increasing its red blood cell production about six- to eightfold. As the erythroid marrow expands, fat is replaced by erythroid cells, and formerly inactive or "yellow" marrow becomes active or "red."

The ultimate stimulus for erythropoietin production is tissue hypoxia, detected by a sensor in the renal parenchyma. Tissue oxygen tension depends on the relative rates of oxygen supply and demand which, in turn, depend on blood flow, blood hemoglobin concentration, hemoglobin oxygen saturation, and hemoglobin oxygen affinity, as discussed in Chap. 31.

In addition to inducing hyperplasia of the erythrocyte precursors, erythropoietin secretion causes red blood cell generation time to be shortened, premature denucleation to occur, and reticulocytes to be released to the blood at an earlier stage of maturity than normally ("shift reticulocytes"). These prematurely released erythrocytes are macrocytic, hypochromic, and polychromatophilic and may undergo reduction in cytoplasmic mass.

Hemoglobin structure and biosynthesis The primary function of the red blood cell is to transport oxygen bound to hemoglobin. Since hemoglobin constitutes about 95 percent of the dry weight of the red blood cell, much of red blood cell production is concerned with hemoglobin synthesis. This molecule has a molecular weight of 64,400 and is made up of a colorless protein, globin, and a prosthetic group, heme. The globin of human adult hemoglobin (hemoglobin A) consists of two pairs of unlike polypeptide chains, α and β chains, which differ from one another in amino acid composition and sequence. One heme group is attached to each of the four chains. Heme, which imparts the red color to the hemoglobin molecule, is a complex of iron and protoporphyrin 9, type III (Fig. 60-2). Like other porphyrin rings, it consists of four pyrrole nuclei connected to one another by methene (=C−) bridges. It is inserted into a nonpolar crevice of each of the four globin chains between two histidine molecules known, respectively, as the proximal (F8, α87, β92) and the distal (E7, α58, β63) histidines. The iron forms a covalent bond with the proximal histidine, and oxygen, when bound, is positioned between iron and the distal histidine.

The structure of heme is identical in all mammals. Because of differences in the amino acid sequences of globin

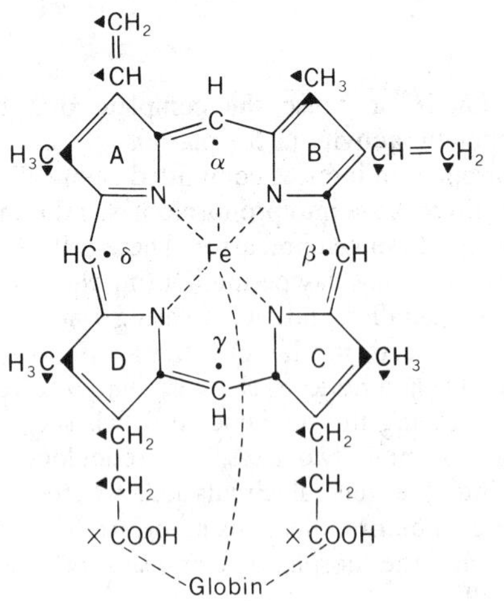

FIGURE 60-2
Chemical structure of heme and its manner of union with globin to form hemoglobin. The carbon atoms derived from the alpha carbon of glycine are represented by ●, those supplied from the methyl carbon of acetate by▲, and those derived from the carboxyl group of acetate by ×. The unmarked carbons are those derived from either the methyl carbon atom of acetate or the carboxyl atom.

subunits, the properties of hemoglobin, such as oxygen affinity, electrophoretic mobility, and solubility, vary among species. The three-dimensional structure of human hemoglobin has been determined from x-ray crystallographic analysis. The important functional properties of hemoglobin such as heme-heme interaction, the pH dependency of oxygen affinity (the Bohr effect), and the interaction with 2,3-diphosphoglycerate can now be understood on a stereochemical basis. This structural information has also been useful in explaining the abnormal functional properties of a number of human hemoglobin variants which are associated with clinical and hematologic manifestations (see Chap. 313).

The source materials for the formation of *porphyrin* are the amino acid glycine and succinyl coenzyme A (CoA), which arises from the tricarboxylic acid cycle. In vitro as well as in vivo studies have clarified the steps in the synthetic process (Fig. 60-3). Acetate is transformed into α-ketoglutarate and this, in the presence of coenzyme A, gives rise to succinyl CoA. This is the site at which pantothenic acid functions in erythropoiesis, since this vitamin is a component of CoA. Pyridoxine is involved in the next step in which the activated form of succinate condenses with a pyridoxal phosphate-glycine-enzyme complex to form delta-aminolevulinic acid (δ-ALA). Two molecules of δ-ALA then condense to form a monopyrrole, porphobilinogen. The subsequent steps leading to the formation of protoporphyrin are shown in the diagram. As discussed in Chap. 109, certain of the porphyrias are due to defects in specific enzymes of porphyrin synthesis. Ultimately proto-

FIGURE 60-3
The biosynthesis of heme. The following abbreviations are used: CoA, coenzyme A; GTP, guanosine triphosphate; GDP, guanosine diphosphate; Pi, inorganic phosphorus; GSH, glutathione; Δ-ALA, delta-aminolevulinic acid; Δ-ALA-DH, delta-aminolevulinate dehydrase; UIS, uroporphyrinogen I synthetase; UIII CoS, uroporphyrinogen III cosynthetase; UD, uroporphyrinogen decarboxylase; CO, coproporphyrinogen oxidase; HS, heme synthetase. Enzymatic steps that occur in mitochondria are shown.

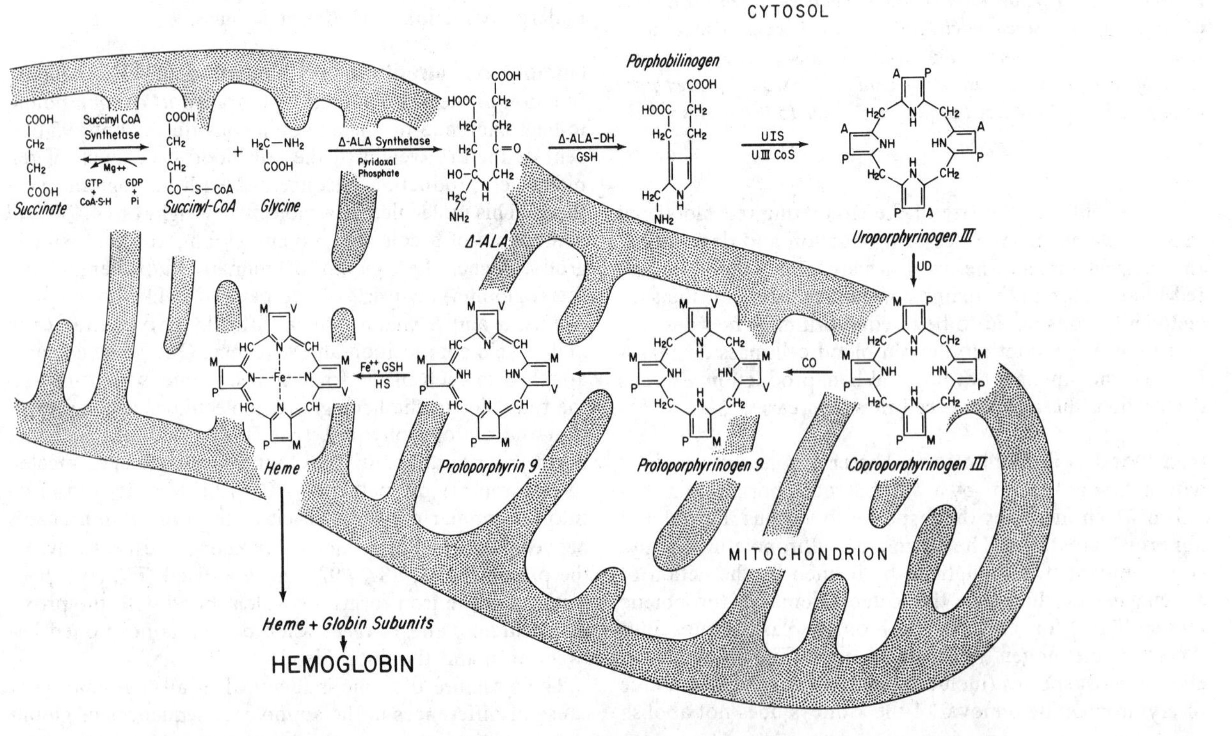

porphyrin is converted to hemoglobin in the presence of iron, globin, and an enzyme, heme synthetase (ferrochelatase). The first and last steps in the heme biosynthetic chain occur in mitochondria. These reactions may be inhibited in the sideroblastic anemias in which mitochondria become laden with iron.

Globin polypeptide chains are produced in the cytoplasm of the red blood cell precursors. The synthesis of each type of globin subunit is directed by a corresponding gene inherited from each parent. In the red blood cells of normal adults, hemoglobin A ($\alpha_2\beta_2$) comprises about 97 percent of the total hemoglobin. The remaining 3 percent is primarily hemoglobin A_2 ($\alpha_2\delta_2$). As discussed in Chap. 313, this minor component is increased in patients with β thalassemia. Hemoglobin F or fetal hemoglobin ($\alpha_2\gamma_2$) is found in trace amounts in adult red blood cells. It is the main hemoglobin component of fetal red cells. During the last 3 months of gestation, γ-chain synthesis switches to β-chain synthesis. However, in certain types of congenital hemolytic anemias such as the β-thalassemias and sickle-cell anemia, the production of γ chains (and therefore of hemoglobin F) persists. In addition, increased levels of hemoglobin F may also be encountered in certain acquired anemias in which there is disordered red cell proliferation.

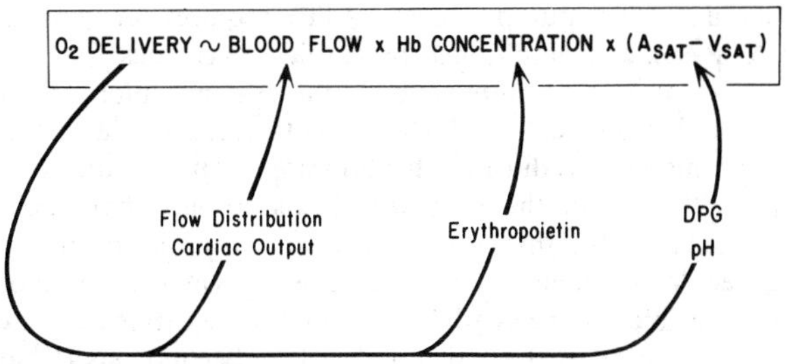

FIGURE 60-4
Oxygen delivered to an organ or tissue is directly proportional to: (1) blood flow; (2) hemoglobin concentration, and (3) the difference in oxygen saturation of the arterial and venous blood. Patients with various types of hypoxia may compensate in the following ways: (1) the distribution of blood flow is altered to maintain oxygenation of vital organs; total cardiac output increases when hypoxia is severe; (2) increased erythropoietin production stimulates erythropoiesis; (3) oxygen unloading is enhanced by a shift to the right in the oxygen dissociation curve, mediated by red blood cell pH and 2,3-DPG.

Hemoglobin function The hemoglobin molecule has been well engineered to perform its primary function, the uptake and unloading of oxygen. In addition, hemoglobin facilitates the transport of carbon dioxide from the tissues to the lungs. During the circulation through the lungs, hemoglobin becomes almost fully saturated with oxygen (1.34 ml O_2 per g hemoglobin). As red blood cells perfuse the capillary beds, oxygen is extracted. Efficient unloading of oxygen at relatively high oxygen tensions is possible because of the sigmoid shape of the oxygen dissociation curve (see Chap. 31 and Fig. 31-1). The affinity of hemoglobin for oxygen is modified by three intracellular cofactors: hydrogen ion, carbon dioxide, and 2,3-diphosphoglycerate (2,3-DPG). Increasing concentrations of each of these three effectors results in a "shift to the right" in the oxygen dissociation curve. In human red blood cells, 2,3-DPG appears to be an important regulator of hemoglobin function. Elevated levels of 2,3-DPG have been noted in various states of hypoxia. The resulting decrease in oxygen affinity permits enhanced oxygen release. The oxygenation of a particular organ or tissue depends on three main factors (depicted in Fig. 60-4): blood flow, oxygen-carrying capacity of the blood (hemoglobin concentration), and the difference between arterial and venous oxygen saturation. The last factor is dependent on the shape and position of the oxygen dissociation curve. Patients with a primary abnormality of one of these three factors depend on adjustments in one or both of the other two in order to maintain optimal tissue oxygenation. For example, patients with anemia have two available modes of compensation: enhanced blood flow and decreased oxygen affinity, mediated by increased levels of 2,3-DPG. Conversely, an individual with a hemoglobin variant having increased oxygen affinity has a primary defect in oxygen unloading. As discussed in Chap. 313, this patient compensates by developing secondary erythrocytosis.

Red blood cell metabolism Since the mature red blood cell contains no nucleus or ribosomes, all the enzymes necessary to maintain the 120-day life span must be in the cell when it enters the circulation. The principal factor essential to normal red cell survival is a regulated source of energy which maintains a flexible membrane and a stable fluid and electrolyte content and protects the cell from endogenous and exogenous oxidants.

About 85 to 90 percent of the energy used by red blood cells is derived from the conversion of glucose to lactate by anaerobic glycolysis. The high energy compound synthesized in this pathway is adenosinetriphosphate (ATP), two molecules of which are produced for each molecule of glucose metabolized. The remaining 10 to 15 percent of erythrocyte energy is derived from the hexosemonophosphate shunt. This pathway helps to protect the red blood cell against oxidant stress. Since no mitochondria are found in mature red blood cells, there is no tricarboxylic acid (Krebs) cycle, and energy from this pathway is not available.

The maintenance of the fluid and electrolyte content of the red blood cell is chiefly a function of its membrane. This is made up of structural proteins (40 to 50 percent) and lipids (35 to 45 percent), as well as carbohydrates (7 to 15 percent). The lipids, consisting of free cholesterol and phospholipids, exchange freely with plasma lipids. The equilibrium between membrane and plasma is affected by plasma bile salt concentration. Alterations in membrane lipids lead to characteristic distortions of erythrocyte shape; e.g., loss of cholesterol leads to spherocytes, cholesterol gain produces target cells. Thorny cells (acanthocytes), found in spur-cell anemia and abetalipoproteinemia, contain excess cholesterol and phospholipid. The structural proteins of the membrane have been only partially characterized. A genetic defect in one of these proteins may lead to the excessive membrane permeability found in hereditary spherocytosis (Chap. 313).

The membrane has the property of selective permeability and is able to facilitate the passage of cations against an ionic gradient. This function is accomplished by a "pump" which exchanges intracellular sodium for extracellular potassium. The pump utilizes ATP, requires an enzyme (ATPase), and is inhibited by cardiac glycosides.

The principal components of the system which protect the red blood cell and its contents from oxidation are glutathione, reduced triphosphopyridine nucleotide (NADPH), and the enzymes glucose 6-phosphate dehydrogenase, glutathione reductase, and glutathione peroxidase. A deficiency in one of these enzymes or in those responsible for the synthesis of glutathione can lead to oxidant damage to the red blood cell and hemolysis (Chap. 313).

Red blood cell destruction At the end of its life span, the red blood cell is removed by components of the mononuclear-phagocyte system, principally the spleen. The factors responsible for the recognition and sequestration of the senescent red blood cell are poorly understood. As it ages in vivo, the erythrocyte may become increasingly rigid and, as a result, have difficulty in traversing the microcirculation including the sinusoids of the spleen. A decrease in the negative surface charge of the older red blood cells may also contribute to their uptake by the reticuloendothelial system.

Hemoglobin catabolism takes place within the reticuloendothelial cell. Iron and amino acids are extracted and subsequently reutilized. Most of the liberated iron is transported as "plasma iron" via the transport protein, transferrin, to the bone marrow where it is used in the synthesis of new hemoglobin. Part of the iron may be retained within the reticuloendothelial cell as ferritin, a ferric iron-protein complex, or as hemosiderin, a more stable and less available form of storage iron. The liberated globin is degraded and is returned to the body pool of amino acids. The porphyrin ring is converted to bile pigments which are excreted. The breakdown of heme is considered in detail in Chap. 43. One mole of carbon monoxide is formed per mole of catabolized heme. Measurement of this compound can serve as an index of the rate of erythrocyte destruction.

Not all the bile pigment is derived from senescent erythrocytes. Studies of stercobilin excretion following the administration of ^{15}N-labeled glycine indicate that normally at least 10 percent (and in diseases such as pernicious anemia, thalassemia, and congenital erythropoietic porphyria, the greater proportion) is probably derived from *ineffective erythropoiesis*, i.e., the destruction of newly formed red blood cells within the marrow or very shortly after their release. In addition, a small amount of "early labeled" bile pigment is derived from a hepatic source.

Bilirubin is converted to urobilinogen in the intestine (see Chap. 43). Urobilinogen consists of a series of colorless compounds, all of which are characterized by a positive Ehrlich's aldehyde reaction, as well as by instability and ease of oxidation to colored pigments, the urobilin group. The transition to urobilins can be hastened by mild oxidizing agents, such as iodine, and this is the basis of Schlesinger's qualitative test (alcoholic zinc acetate) for urobilin.

The amount of urobilinogen extracted in the urine in 24 h (UU) by the normal adult is 0 to 3.5 mg, most frequently 0.5 to 1.5 mg. The normal range for fecal urobilinogen (FU), as calculated from a 4-day period of collection, is 40 to 280 mg per day, usually 100 to 200 mg. The expected values are related to the size of the circulating red blood cell mass; thus, lower values are found in young children. Mean values have been found to increase with age. An important qualification should be added. The administration of certain oral antibiotics causes a marked decrease in the concentration of fecal urobilinogen. The usefulness and limitations of urine and fecal urobilinogen determinations are discussed in Chap. 43.

Pathogenesis of anemia Anemia may develop as the result of blood loss, excessive destruction or inadequate production of red blood cells, or from the various combinations of these processes. The clinical evaluation of an anemic patient is discussed in Chap. 308 and specific anemias are covered in detail in subsequent chapters (Chaps. 309 to 313). Here, certain generalizations may be made.

When *blood loss* is *acute,* the cause of the anemia usually is obvious, although sometimes a large hemorrhage may have occurred under conditions which do not reveal themselves readily (Chap. 308). Chronic loss of blood occurs most commonly from the pelvic organs in women and from the gastrointestinal tract in men. The ultimate result of chronic blood loss is iron deficiency. Iron-deficiency anemia is a very prevalent form of anemia, perhaps the most common, and is discussed in Chap. 309.

Impairment of red blood cell production may be due to either a decrease in the number of functioning erythroid stem cells or an abnormality in the maturation of erythroid precursors. In patients with aplastic anemia there is a marked decrease in the population of erythroid as well as myeloid and thrombopoietic stem cells, resulting in pancytopenia. In rare cases of pure red blood cell anemia, there is a selective diminution of erythroid precursors in the bone marrow. If impairment of red blood cell production is due to marrow fibrosis or invasion by tumor or granulomata, the diseased stroma may cause distortions in red blood cell shape. Normoblasts, teardrop-shaped red blood cells, and immature myeloid cells will be encountered in the peripheral blood. The anemia of uremia is due in part to an inappropriately low level of erythropoietin. In addition, the buildup in the plasma of waste products in the uremic patient may also suppress erythropoiesis independent of erythropoietin. Finally, uremic patients often have a significant reduction in red blood cell survival.

Abnormal maturation of erythroid cells may be due to a defect in hemoglobin synthesis or DNA replication. Iron deficiency, the sideroblastic anemias, and thalassemia involve decreased availability of iron, porphyrin, and globin, the prime constituents required to make hemoglobin. As a result of impaired hemoglobin synthesis, the red blood cells are hypochromic and microcytic. Defective replication of DNA will result in megaloblastic maturation of red blood cell precursors (Chap. 310). This type of abnormal morphology usually reflects a deficiency of folic acid or vitamin B_{12}. In some types of anemias, there is no adequate explanation for defective red blood cell maturation. These include various types of refractory anemias as well as myeloid metaplasia. In this group of anemias ineffective erythropoiesis is often present.

A moderate decrease in red blood cell production is encountered as a consequence of various underlying systemic disorders (Chap. 312). In the anemias of chronic infection and inflammation, a block in the release of iron from the mononuclear-phagocyte system prevents adequate access to red blood cell precursors. As a result, the mature red blood cells are often somewhat hypochromic and microcytic. The anemia secondary to hypothyroidism may represent a physiologic adjustment to decreased oxygen requirement. The pathogenesis of the anemia of liver disease is multifactorial and not well understood. In all these cases, the erythron is functionally intact and morphologically normal. The suppression of erythropoiesis is reversed if the underlying disease regresses or responds to appropriate treatment.

In *hemolytic anemia* (Chap. 313), shortening of red blood cell survival is due to a variety of environmental, membrane, or cytoplasmic factors. In rare cases, mechanical or immunologic damage to the membrane may actually result in the rapid leakage of hemoglobin into the plasma. Such patients with intravascular hemolysis generally have high levels of circulating hemoglobin and hemoglobinuria. More commonly, however, the patient's abnormal red blood cells are recognized and sequestered by phagocytic cells, primarily in the spleen and liver. A common feature of these cells is that they have lost their normal pliability because of some structural or functional defect. As a result, they are trapped in the narrow fenestrations of the mononuclear-phagocyte system. Red blood cells coated with IgG autoantibody bind to specific receptors on the surface of splenic and hepatic macrophages. Because of their spherical shape, the red blood cells of individuals with hereditary spherocytosis are unduly rigid. This abnormality is aggravated by the inimical environment of the spleen. The integrity of the red blood cell membrane may be compromised by other structural abnormalities of the lipoprotein matrix of the membrane or by a defect in intermediary metabolism which affects membrane function such as the maintenance of the sodium-potassium pump. Hemolysis in patients with hemoglobinopathies may be due to the polymerization of hemoglobin (the sickle syndromes) or to the precipitation of hemoglobin within the red blood cell (thalassemias and congenital Heinz body hemolytic anemia). In all cases, abnormalities in shape and decreased deformability of these red blood cells lead to their premature destruction.

All hemolytic anemias are characterized by a compensatory increase in red blood cell production, mediated by erythropoietin. This phenomenon is reflected by erythroid hyperplasia in the bone marrow and an increase in circulating reticulocytes. In addition, other laboratory values such as serum bilirubin, fecal urobilinogen, and haptoglobin can be utilized to document the presence and extent of hemolysis. These are discussed in detail in Chap. 308; the specific hemolytic anemias are covered in Chap. 313.

It must be recognized that, in patients with ailments of long standing, more than one factor may play a role in the development of anemia. Thus, nutritional deficiency because of reduced intake of food or faulty absorption from the gastrointestinal tract, blood loss, the negative nitrogen balance associated with long confinement to bed, and impaired iron metabolism such as that associated with chronic inflammatory conditions, all may play a role.

Signs and symptoms of anemia Anemia should never be thought of as a diagnosis in itself, but rather as a manifestation of an underlying disease process. Thus, the signs and symptoms found in the anemic patient are a mixture of those due to anemia and those due to the underlying disease. Only those symptoms common to all anemias are discussed below; symptoms more specifically related to the underlying disease are dealt with in the chapters dealing with those entities.

CARDIORESPIRATORY SYSTEM Hemoglobin is the vehicle and the cardiovascular system the means of delivery of oxygen to the tissues. When anemia is present, the oxygen-carrying capacity of the blood is reduced. If an equivalent amount of oxygen is to be delivered, blood flow must be increased by means of cardiovascular adjustments. Many of the signs and symptoms of anemia reflect these changes in cardiovascular function.

When anemia is severe (Hb $<$7.5 g/dl), cardiac output increases, owing to an enhancement of both stroke volume and heart rate. The patient may be aware of this increased cardiac activity and complain of palpitation. On examination, tachycardia and an increased pulse pressure may be found, along with increased pulsations over the precordium and major arteries; even capillary pulsation in the fingertips may be detected. The circulation time may be shortened, and there may be a slight rise in atrial pressure.

The adequacy of the cardiovascular adjustments to anemia depends on the degree of the anemia, the rapidity with which it has developed, and the preexisting status of the cardiovascular system. Symptoms are usually present when the blood hemoglobin concentration is less than 7.5 g/dl. If anemia has developed so rapidly that there has been little or no time for physiologic adjustment, symptoms are likely to be prominent and to appear comparatively early; on the other hand, if the anemia has been insidious in onset, the adjustment may be so good that the hemoglobin may be as low as 6 g/dl, without sufficient functional embarrassment occurring for the patient to be seriously handicapped.

The decrease in hemoglobin prevents maximum oxygen flow to tissues; consequently, exercise tolerance is decreased. There may be no symptoms at rest, but signs of oxygen want, such as easy fatigability and dyspnea, develop on exertion. When compensatory adjustments become imperfect or fail, either because of an extreme degree of anemia or because of a previously damaged heart, the clinical picture of cardiac failure ensues (Chap. 237).

Severe anemia may produce a systolic murmur, which is usually most marked at the pulmonic area, but may be heard elsewhere over the precordium, especially at the apex. Very rarely, diastolic murmurs are heard at the base. Over the vessels of the neck, a humming sound, the venous hum, may be heard.

NEUROMUSCULAR SYSTEM Headache, vertigo, faintness, increased sensitivity to cold, tinnitus or roaring in the ears, black spots before the eyes, muscular weakness and easy fatigability, and irritability are common symptoms associated with anemia. Drowsiness develops in severe anemia. Headache due to anemia may be very severe. Delirium is seldom seen.

ALIMENTARY SYSTEM Loss of appetite is not unusual as an accompaniment of anemia. Nausea, flatulence, abdominal discomfort, constipation, diarrhea, vomiting, or abnormal appetite may also be found.

GENITOURINARY SYSTEM Menstrual disturbances (most often amenorrhea) in the female, and loss of libido in the male, are frequently encountered in severe anemia. In other instances, excessive menstrual bleeding accompanies anemia. Slight proteinuria and evidence of distinct renal function impairment may be seen in association with anemia.

EPITHELIAL TISSUES The pallor which accompanies anemia has been discussed. In addition to pallor, loss of normal skin elasticity and tone, thinning of the hair, and purpura and ecchymoses may develop in the chronic forms of anemia.

REFERENCES

BUNN HF et al: *Human Hemoglobins,* Philadelphia: Saunders, 1977

ERSLEV AJ, GABUZDA TG: *Pathophysiology of Blood,* Philadelphia: Saunders, 1975

HARRIS JW, KELLERMEYER RW: *The Red Cell,* Cambridge: Harvard, 1970

HILLMAN RS, FINCH CA: *Red Cell Manual,* Philadelphia: Davis, 1974

SCHMID R (ed): Physiology and disorders of hemoglobin degradation. Semin Hematol 9:1, 1972

WINTROBE MM et al: *Clinical Hematology,* 7th ed., Philadelphia: Lea and Febiger, 1974

61 BLEEDING

HYMIE L. NOSSEL

Bleeding is one of the most serious and significant of the cardinal manifestations of disease. It may occur from a local site or may be generalized. Bleeding associated with a local lesion may be superimposed on either a normal or a defective hemostatic mechanism; in contrast, general bleeding is usually associated with a hemorrhagic diathesis.

LOCAL BLEEDING

In the evaluation of local bleeding, the site, appearance of the blood, signs of blood loss, and evidence for disordered hemostasis should be considered. The sites and common causes of bleeding are listed in Table 61-1. The appearance of the blood may provide a clue as to the cause of the bleeding. Bleeding from the lungs and bronchi is influenced by the degree of aeration and the presence of mucus and pus. In pneumococcal pneumonia the sputum is characteristically rusty. In tuberculosis it is usually bright red. Pus is usually mixed with the blood when infection is present. Massive hemorrhage occasionally occurs in mitral stenosis when a bronchial varicosity ruptures or in tuberculosis when a vessel is eroded. In pulmonary infarction the blood is usually dark red. Blood derived from the gastrointestinal tract may be darkened because of conversion of hemoglobin to brown hematin by gastric acid. Blood vomited from the stomach may be dark ("coffee ground") or bright red if the vomiting is sufficiently rapid. When it appears in the stool, it may be pitch black (melena). Blood derived from the colon is red or brown, and, if inflammation is the cause, mucus or pus is mixed with it (see Chap. 42). If bleeding from the urinary tract is profuse, clots or bright blood may be present in the urine. Small amounts of blood impart a smoky appearance to urine, whereas lesser degrees of hematuria may be detected only by microscopy.

The signs and symptoms of blood loss depend on the amount and rate of bleeding. If very acute, syncope occurs rapidly; with a slower rate of loss, signs and symptoms of peripheral circulatory collapse occur. Shock may occur without external blood loss if a large amount of blood is lost into a serous cavity. Slow and prolonged blood loss will gradually result in symptoms of iron-deficiency anemia.

Local bleeding which is out of proportion to the injury suggests a hemostatic defect. For example, when a patient suffers bleeding following dental extraction sufficient to require blood transfusion, a defect of the coagulation or platelet systems can almost always be defined.

HEMOSTASIS AND ITS DISORDERS

The successful management of patients with a disorder of the hemostatic mechanism depends on accurate diagnosis. Correct diagnosis and rational therapy depend on an understanding of the normal mechanisms for preserving hemostasis.

TABLE 61-1
Locations and causes of localized bleeding

Locations	*Commonest causes*
Skin (petechiae, purpura, ecchymoses)	Thrombocytopenia
Limbs	
Joints	Hemophilia
Intramuscular and subcutaneous hematomas	Hemophilia
Central nervous system	Trauma, hypertension, congenital vascular malformations
Head and neck	
Nose and sinuses	Trauma, inflammation, hypertension, polyps and tumors, hereditary telangiectasia
Ears	Trauma
Optic fundi	Hypertension, nephritis, diabetes, thrombocytopenia, trauma
Chest	
Respiratory tract	Tumors, infections, bronchiectasis, pulmonary embolism, mitral stenosis
Serous cavity	Tumors, tuberculosis, pulmonary infarction
Nipples	Fissure, tumor
Gastrointestinal tract	Esophageal varices, hiatal hernia, peptic ulcer, gastritis, tumors, colitis, hemorrhoids, hereditary telangiectasia
Abdominal cavity	Trauma, splenic rupture, ectopic gestation
Urinary tract	Calculi, infections, glomerulonephritis, tumors, cystitis, prostatic hypertrophy
Vagina	Obstetric and endocrine disorders, tumors

Normal hemostasis comprises mechanisms operative immediately following an injury and those acting over a longer period to maintain hemostasis. The immediate mechanism consists principally of two components: *vasoconstriction* due to active contraction of the smooth muscle cells of the vessel wall, and *plug formation* by masses of aggregated platelets. The maintenance mechanism consists of the *fibrin* (and fibrin clot) produced by the coagulation system.

Platelet plug formation is especially important in capillary hemostasis, while vasoconstriction and fibrin formation seem to be more important in larger vessel hemostasis. These several mechanisms involved in achieving normal hemostasis are interconnected at several points, but for the sake of clarity they will be described as separate entities.

Platelets

The normal platelet count is 150,000 to 400,000 per mm^3. The most accurate method of counting platelets is by electronic particle counting or by phase-contrast microscopy. An estimate of platelet number may be made by examination of the stained peripheral blood smear. With a normal platelet count, several (3 to 10) platelets (individually or in small clumps) should be visible in each oil-immersion field.

STRUCTURE Normal platelets are anucleate bodies 2 to 3 μm in diameter which appear light blue and contain small purple-red granules when stained with Giemsa's solution. With the electron microscope, three distinct structural zones may be identified in the platelet, each related to specific platelet functions. The unique quality of the platelet is its ability to adhere to foreign surfaces and form aggregates in response to a variety of stimuli including thrombin, ADP, and catecholamines. The *peripheral* zone is involved in adhesion, the *cytoplasm* (sol-gel zone) in contraction, and the *organelle* zone in secretion.

The peripheral zone comprises a surface coat of acid mucopolysaccharides (the glycocalyx), the trilaminar plasma unit membrane, and a submembranous area. The surface coat is involved in adhesion, and the membrane provides a trigger mechanism whereby stimuli are transmitted from the exterior into the interior. Specific receptors for thrombin and ADP are present.

The submembranous area and cytoplasmic zone contain the contractile protein *actomyosin* (also termed *thrombosthenin*) in the form of a number of fibrous elements. In the submembranous area, bundles of microtubules encircle the platelet forming a cytoskeleton that stabilizes the cell, permitting it to circulate as a flattened disk. The microtubules are composed of subfilaments which are indistinguishable from microfilaments present in the cytoplasm. The microfilaments are responsible for the centripetal movement and fusion of granules occurring during platelet aggregation, the contraction of pseudopods, and clot retraction.

Distinct components present in the organelle zone include granules, dense bodies, mitochondria, glycogen, and, in an occasional platelet, stacks of flattened saccules resembling a Golgi apparatus. The granules are enclosed by a unit membrane and contain lysosomal enzymes such as acid phosphatase, β-glucuronidase, and cathepsin as well as fibrinogen, actomyosin, ATPase, and adenine nucleotides. The dense bodies are the primary secretory organelles of the platelet and contain serotonin, ADP, catecholamines, and heparin-neutralizing activity termed *platelet factor 4.* Active intermediary metabolism occurs in the mitochondria; ATP is generated from both glycolysis and the tricarboxylic acid cycle, and glycogen and lipid are synthesized. Ribosomes have been detected, consistent with evidence that the platelet has a limited protein synthetic capacity.

DISTRIBUTION AND FATE Platelets are formed in the marrow and released into the circulation. At any moment, about 80 percent of the platelets are in the circulation and 20 percent are in the spleen; free movement occurs between these two pools. If the spleen enlarges markedly, the distribution shifts and up to 80 percent of the platelets may be pooled in the spleen. Survival curves of ^{51}Cr-labeled platelets are linear and suggest that most platelets become senescent and die after a lifespan of about 10 days.

Some platelets appear to be consumed in repairing the minor vascular injuries of daily life. There is evidence that younger platelets are physiologically more active and have higher enzyme concentrations than old platelets. This distinction is most apparent when thrombopoiesis is accelerated in response to increased platelet destruction. Senescent platelets are probably removed by the reticuloendothelial system. In thrombocytopenia due to increased platelet destruction, the destruction is random. Damaged platelets may be removed primarily in the spleen or in both the spleen and the liver. The bone marrow does not contain a reserve of platelets, and if circulating platelets are rapidly destroyed or lost, thrombocytopenia persists for several days until enough new platelets are formed. Governing normal platelet production are one or more humoral factors including *thrombopoietin,* a plasma factor that appears to regulate platelet production.

FUNCTION IN HEMOSTASIS The platelet contributes to hemostasis by forming platelet plugs and by promoting thrombin production. Platelet plug formation may be divided into a number of stages (Fig. 61-1).

Adhesion Platelets adhere to subendothelial structures exposed by trauma. Such structures including collagen fibers and basement membranes. Regularly spaced free amino groups on the collagen molecule are required for platelet adhesion. In addition, a number of plasma proteins, including fibrinogen and von Willebrand factor, are required for normal platelet adherence.

Release reaction Following adherence to collagen, platelets extrude the contents of their granules—a process termed the *release reaction.* This reaction may also be induced by thrombin, and in physiologic hemostasis it is likely that both collagen and thrombin initiate release. The release reaction is inhibited by substances that increase the cyclic adenosine-3′,5′-monophosphate (cyclic AMP) level of the platelet. These agents include a prostaglandin (PGE_1), which increases the activity of adenylate cyclase, an enzyme that converts ATP (adenosine triphosphate) to cyclic AMP, and theophylline, which inhibits phosphodi-

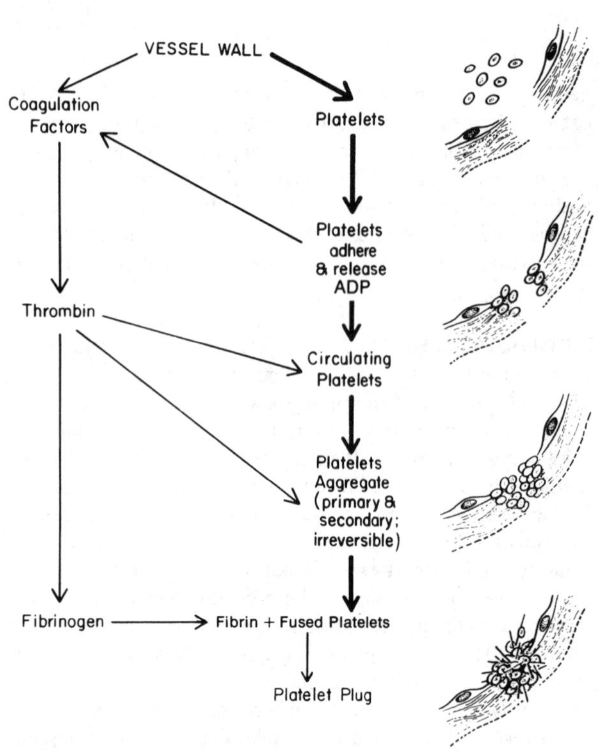

FIGURE 61-1
Platelet plug formation.

esterase, the enzyme that breaks down cyclic AMP. Epinephrine, on the other hand, lowers platelet cyclic AMP levels and facilitates platelet aggregation.

Recent studies indicate that intermediates of prostaglandin synthesis play a major role in mediating the release reaction and consequently second-phase aggregation. When platelets are stimulated by a release-inducer, the enzyme *cyclooxygenase* converts arachidonic acid to a labile endoperoxide intermediate in prostaglandin synthesis. This endoperoxide, termed thromboxane A_2, directly induces the release reaction. Prostaglandin E_2 potentiates the effect of thromboxane A_2, prostaglandin $F_{2}\alpha$ being inactive with regard to platelets (Fig. 61-2). The release reaction involves the extrusion from platelets of a specific group of substances including ADP, serotonin, and heparin-neutralizing activity.

Aggregation The released adenosine diphosphate (ADP) causes additional platelets to aggregate at the site of a vascular injury. How ADP produces aggregation is as yet unclear. Low concentrations of ADP cause only primary platelet aggregation, which is reversible, whereas high concentrations of ADP produce irreversible aggregation. Low concentrations of thrombin or collagen, in addition to causing primary aggregation, stimulate the release of ADP, which promotes secondary irreversible aggregation.

Fusion The action of thrombin produced by the coagulation mechanism leads to fusion. Fibrin (also a product of thrombin action) and fused platelets form a stable hemostatic plug. Platelets themselves participate in clotting reactions which lead to thrombin formation by providing so-called "platelet factor 3." This coagulation factor is actually the platelet membrane itself in a suitable configuration on which the coagulation enzymes and substrates interact and promote clot formation. The platelet membrane surface promotes the coagulation reactions only after the platelets have aggregated. Hence a defect in platelet aggregation will be detected as a defect in activity of platelet factor 3.

Clot retraction Following the in vitro coagulation of blood or platelet-rich plasma, platelets pull the fibrin threads of the clot into a contracted volume and express the fluid trapped in the thrombus. It is uncertain to what extent clot retraction is a necessary component of hemostasis, but the test is simple to do and provides useful information. Clot retraction is readily tested in whole blood or by adding thrombin to platelet-rich plasma and noting the extent of clot retraction 1 h later. Clot retraction is defective in a severe congenital defect of platelet function termed *thrombasthenia,* or when either the platelet count or the fibrinogen concentration is very low.

TESTS OF PLATELET FUNCTION Platelet plugs rapidly stop bleeding from ruptured capillaries and small vessels. The integrity of the platelet plug-forming mechanism is tested by measuring the *bleeding time.* This is most commonly determined by the Ivy bleeding time technique, in which the time is measured for bleeding to cease from three incisions 1 cm long and 1 mm deep in an avascular area of the forearm. Venous return is obstructed by a blood pressure cuff set at 40 mmHg pressure over the upper forearm. The bleeding time is normal in disorders of the coagulation system but is abnormal in the presence of severe thrombocytopenia, defects of platelet function, deficiency of the von Willebrand plasma protein, or total absence of blood fibrinogen. Generally, clinically significant defects in platelet function are found only if the bleeding time is prolonged. Platelet aggregation, a measure of platelet function, may be studied by recording the increase in light transmitted through a cuvette containing continuously stirred platelet-rich plasma when aggregating agents are added to the plasma. The aggregating agents usually tested are collagen, epinephrine, adenosine diphosphate, thrombin, and ristocetin.

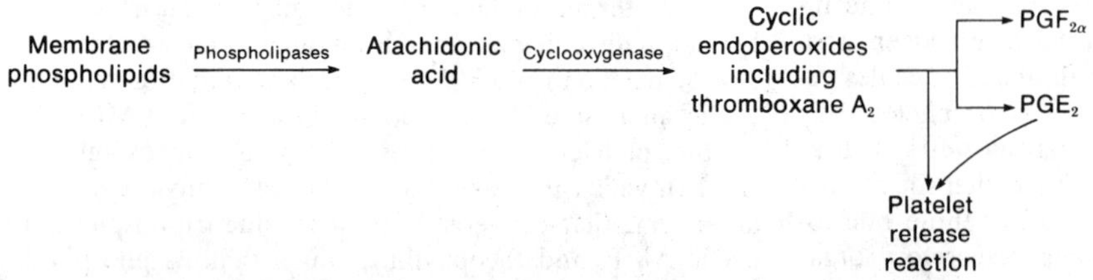

FIGURE 61-2
Role of prostaglandins in platelet release.

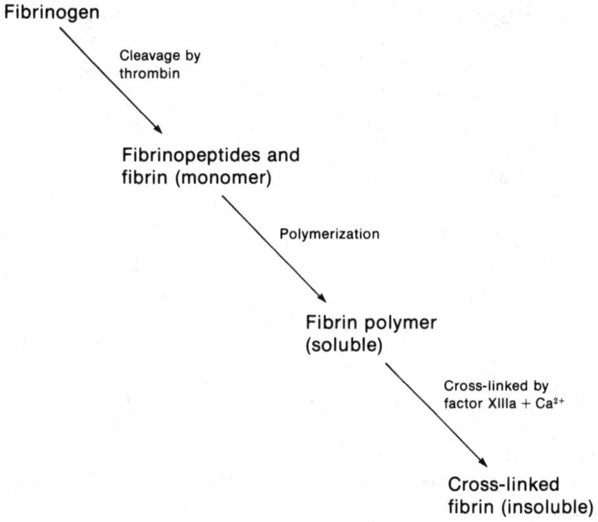

FIGURE 61-3
Steps in cross-linked fibrin formation.

Blood coagulation—mechanism and function

The two main functions of the blood coagulation mechanism are as follows:

1 Production of thrombin which stabilizes the platelet plug
2 Formation of fibrin which mechanically blocks the flow of blood through ruptured vessels.

A number of discrete proenzymes and proteins (termed *coagulation factors*), platelets, and calcium participate in the coagulation process. The process consists of several stages and ends with fibrin formation.

FIBRIN FORMATION The first step is cleavage by thrombin of fibrinopeptides A and B from the fibrinogen molecule, to produce fibrin monomer (Fig. 61-3). When the ratio of fibrin monomer to fibrinogen exceeds 1:5, the fibrin polymerizes and precipitates out of solution to form a visible clot. Polymerized fibrin is soluble in acid and concentrated urea solutions and is hemostatically ineffective. Fibrin polymer is cross-linked by the action of activated factor XIII, which, in the presence of calcium, forms covalent peptide bonds between glutamic and lysine amino acids on adjacent molecules. The resulting product is highly insoluble and is hemostatically very effective.

PROTHROMBIN ACTIVATION Thrombin is formed by the proteolytic cleavage of a proenzyme, prothrombin. The

FIGURE 61-4
Activation of factor X by steps in the extrinsic coagulation pathway.

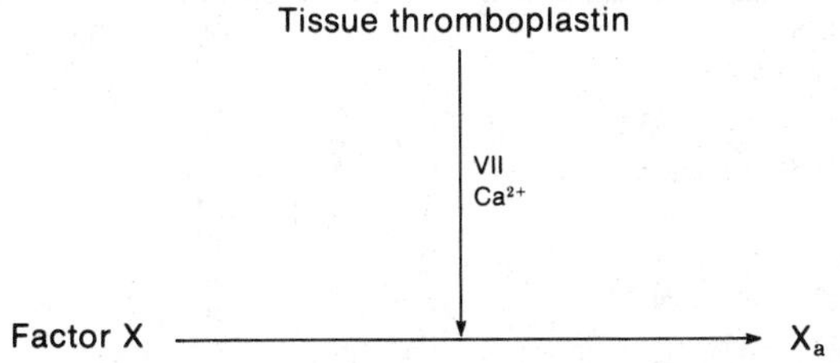

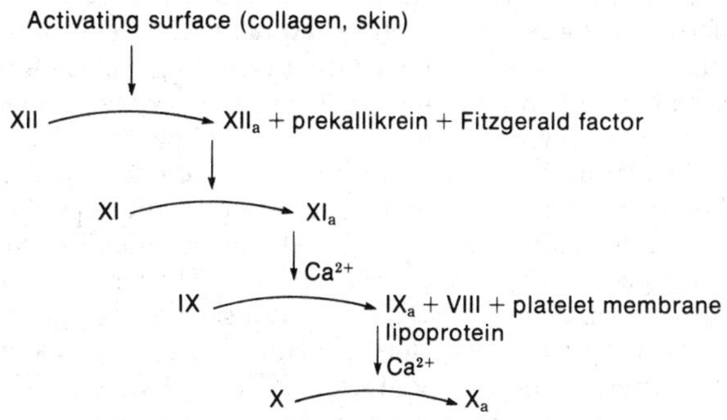

FIGURE 61-5
Activation of factor X by the steps in the intrinsic coagulation pathway.

process is brought about by activated factor X (X_a) in the presence of calcium, platelet membrane lipoprotein, and factor V. Activation of factor X may occur by either of two separate pathways, the extrinsic and the intrinsic. Clinical experience suggests that effective hemostasis requires the participation of both. In the *extrinsic pathway,* a tissue factor (tissue thromboplastin), released from damaged cells, activates factor X in the presence of factor VII and calcium (Fig. 61-4). In the *intrinsic* or *cascade pathway* (Fig. 61-5), the contact of blood with a "foreign" surface, such as collagen or skin, activates factor XII. Activated factor XII, in the presence of prekallikrein and Fitzgerald factor, activates factor XI which, in the presence of calcium, cleaves a peptide from factor IX producing activated factor IX. Activated factor IX proteolytically converts factor X into the activated form (X_a) in the presence of platelet membrane lipoprotein, factor VIII, and calcium.

TESTS OF THE COAGULATION MECHANISM The intrinsic pathway of blood coagulation including fibrin polymerization is tested by measuring the *whole-blood clotting time* and *partial thromboplastin time* (Fig. 61-6).The whole-blood

FIGURE 61-6
Coagulation tests.

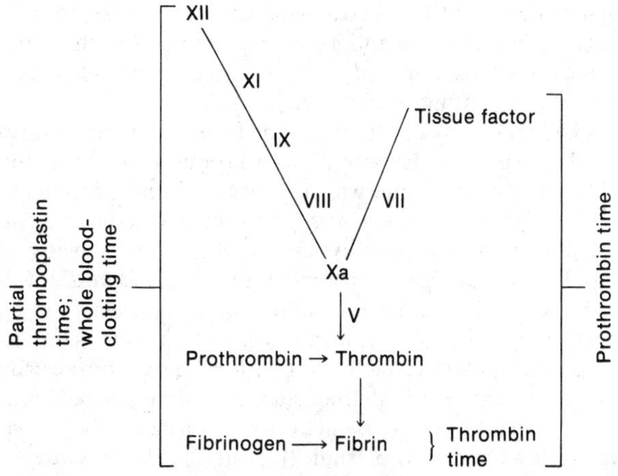

clotting time is the time taken for 1 ml whole blood to clot with controlled temperature (37°C) and exposure of the blood to the glass surface of the test tube. The test is influenced by gross defects in the intrinsic clotting system. The partial thromboplastin time (celite or kaolin cephalin time) is the time required for recalcified citrated plasma to clot. A standardized platelet substitute (cephalin or "partial thromboplastin") and standard surface activation (provided by celite or kaolin) are used to eliminate variability due to the platelet count and surface factors. The test is influenced by moderate defects in the intrinsic clotting system.

The activity of any of the coagulation factors involved in the intrinsic pathway (i.e., factors XII, XI, IX, and VIII) may be measured by comparing the ability of control and test plasma samples to shorten the partial thromboplastin time of a plasma sample known to be deficient in the specific factor.

The extrinsic clotting system is tested by the *one-stage prothrombin time.* In this test, the time taken for recalcified citrated plasma to clot in the presence of tissue thromboplastin is measured. The test is sensitive to defects in the extrinsic clotting system (Figs. 61-4 and 61-6). The activity of factor VII and the common pathway coagulation factors (factors II, V, and X) may be measured by comparing the ability of control and test plasma samples to shorten the prothrombin time of plasma deficient in the specific factor.

The polymerization of fibrinogen is tested by measuring the *thrombin clotting time.* This test measures the time for citrated plasma to clot in the presence of added thrombin. The test is abnormal in the presence of heparin or of acquired or congenital abnormalities of the fibrinogen molecule.

BLOOD FLUIDITY SYSTEM (REGULATOR MECHANISMS) In addition to the coagulation factors, a set of mechanisms exists in the circulation for maintaining the blood in a fluid state. In the absence of this system, sufficient thrombin would be generated by the clotting of only 1 ml blood to coagulate all the fibrinogen in 3 liters blood. The fluidity-maintaining system consists of both cellular and humoral components.

The cellular component comprises the reticuloendothelial system and the liver, both of which specifically remove activated clotting factors and fibrin without affecting precursor (unactivated) coagulation factors. The humoral component consists of several proteins which specifically inactivate the activated coagulation factors. These proteins include antithrombin and α_2-macroglobulin. Antithrombin inactivates thrombin and each of the activated intermediates of the clotting mechanism.

The humoral system includes the fibrinolytic mechanism for dissolving fibrin. Fibrinolysis is produced by the action of an enzyme, plasmin, which is formed from a precursor, plasminogen. Plasminogen is proteolytically converted to plasmin by an extrinsic system in which the activator is supplied by damaged cells present in the blood vessel wall or by an intrinsic system in which the components are all present in the blood. The intrinsic plasmin system is initiated by the contact of factor XII with a foreign surface; by way of a number of intermediates, including prekallikrein and Fitzgerald factor, an activator is formed which converts plasminogen to plasmin (Fig. 61-7). Plasmin attacks

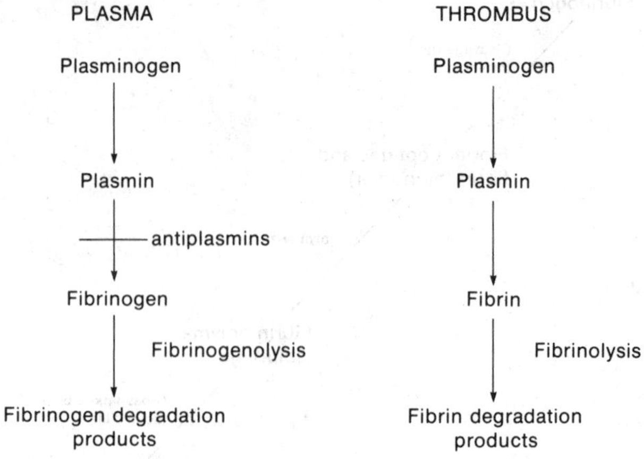

FIGURE 61-7
Plasminogen activation in plasma and in a thrombus and digestion of fibrinogen and fibrin.

peptide bonds involving lysine and digests not only fibrin but also other coagulation factors, including fibrinogen. The products of fibrinogen and fibrin proteolysis are called *fibrinogen degradation products.* These degradation products are of various sizes, and some of the larger molecular fragments prolong the thrombin time. Fibrin polymerization is disrupted by interposition of molecular fragments into the ordered fibrin polymer. Degradation products also inhibit platelet aggregation.

As fibrin is deposited, plasminogen becomes incorporated in the growing thrombus, and is thereby separated from the circulating inhibitors of plasminogen activation so that the plasmin formed is localized at the site of fibrin formation. In this way, discrete local lysis of fibrin can occur without proteolysis of circulating fibrinogen. Clot lysis following fibrin deposition results in release of *fibrin degradation products* into the blood. In those pathologic conditions with extensive intravascular clotting, fibrin degradation products may accumulate in the blood without detectable plasmin levels in the blood sampled from a distant site such as an arm vein.

PRODUCTION, DISTRIBUTION, AND LIFE SPAN OF COAGULATION FACTORS Because the concentrations of all plasma clotting factors, except factor VIII, are depressed in patients with massive liver necrosis, it is thought that hepatic parenchymal cells synthesize all factors except factor VIII. There is evidence that factor VIII is synthes-

TABLE 61-2
Properties of coagulation factors

Factor	*Plasma concentration, μg/ml*	$T^{1}/_{2}$, *h*	*Turnover, μg/ml/24 h*
Fibrinogen	3000	100	600
Prothrombin	150	72	50
V	10	16	15
VII	0.5	5	2
VIII (antihemophilic)	10	12	20
IX	3	24	3
X	15	48	7.5
XI	?	60	?
XII	29	60	12
XIII	20	120	4

ized by endothelial cells but no certainty as to how the coagulant activity of factor VIII comes about. Levels of factor VIII rise sharply after a burst of muscular exercise or an infusion of epinephrine. The rise apparently reflects the release of stores of factor VIII into the circulation. Stress, fever, and infection elevate fibrinogen and factor VIII levels by an unknown mechanism. Gram-negative bacterial endotoxin also stimulates fibrinogen production. Levels of factors VII, VIII, and X and fibrinogen are elevated in pregnancy and in patients using oral contraceptives.

The plasma clotting factors have short intravascular-half-lives compared with other plasma proteins. These can be grouped (in order of decreasing intravascular half-life) as follows (see also Table 61-2):

1 Fibrinogen, factor XIII: 4 to 5 days
2 Prothrombin, factors V, IX, X, XI, and XII: 1 to 3 days
3 Factor VIII: 12 h
4 Factor VII: 5 h

Because of these relatively short half-lives, postoperative prophylaxis or control of bleeding following trauma in a patient with a severe clotting-factor deficiency usually requires repeated replacement therapy during the period of healing.

DIAGNOSTIC APPROACH TO DISORDERS OF HEMOSTASIS

The diagnosis of coagulation disorders is based on both clinical and laboratory evidence. A careful and knowledgeably collected history is essential if the results of laboratory studies are to be properly interpreted.

CLINICAL HISTORY (Table 61-3) A history taken to evaluate hemostasis should answer these questions. (1) Has *abnormal bleeding* or *bruising* occurred either spontaneously or after injury, dental extraction, or surgery? Was there *delayed* or *prolonged* bleeding, suggesting a coagulation disorder, or immediate and transient bleeding, suggesting a platelet disorder? (2) Was there bleeding from the umbilical stump or after circumcision? (3) Is there a history of *prolonged nose bleeds*? Brief epistaxis, stopping within minutes, even if frequent, is usually associated with normal tests of hemostasis.

TABLE 61-3
Clinical distinction between blood coagulation defects and capillary and platelet defects

	Coagulation defects	*Capillary and platelet defects*
Family history	Usually positive	Usually negative
Sex predominance	Males	Females
Type of bleeding	Visceral and intramuscular deep hematomas; usually after trauma	Skin and mucosal surfaces; petechiae and ecchymoses; spontaneous
Duration	Delayed after trauma and persistent	Immediate after trauma; short-lived
Local pressure	Not effective	May stop bleeding

One should try to determine the degree and frequency of the following: (1) *Bruising.* Spontaneous bruises larger than the palm of the hand are generally significant; a history of hematomas and bruises at the sites of injections or immunizations may likewise be suggestive of a hemostatic disorder. (2) *Excessive bleeding from small cuts.* Specific details as to the size of laceration and duration of bleeding should be elicited.

One should question the patient for: (1) evidence of an underlying *systemic disorder* that may be accompanied by defective hemostasis, such as liver disease, systemic lupus erythematosus, uremia, or a hematologic malignancy; (2) a *family history* of bleeding and, if present, the hereditary pattern of transmission; and (3) *drug ingestion.* Drugs that interfere with hemostasis fall into two categories: (1) Drugs that impair formation of the hemostatic plug and (2) drugs that interfere with blood coagulation.

Drugs that impair plug formation include aspirin in ordinary doses, but such prolongation in bleeding time usually remains within the normal range unless platelet function is already abnormal; aspirin should be discontinued several days before surgery. Other drugs which interfere with platelet function are dipyridamole, clofibrate, phenylbutazone, antihistamines, and tranquilizers. The clinical significance of these drugs with respect to hemostasis has yet to be clearly documented.

Drugs that interfere with blood coagulation include heparin and the oral coumarin drugs. Although preoperative patients are rarely receiving parenteral heparin, patients on long-term oral anticoagulant therapy are frequently encountered.

PHYSICAL FINDINGS The patient should be examined for the following.

1 *Abnormal bleeding in the skin.* Ecchymoses suggest abnormal bleeding from relatively large vessels due to a defect in blood clotting. Petechiae, which may be small, require a careful search, particularly around the ankles. Petechiae suggest increased vascular fragility secondary to thrombocytopenia.
2 *Mucosal bleeding.* Look for purpura of the buccal mucosa and the conjunctival surfaces of the eyelids. Hemorrhagic bullae in the mouth are found only in the presence of thrombocytopenia. Hemorrhages in the optic fundi, however, may reflect local eye disease, hypertension, diabetes, severe anemia, or thrombocytopenia.
3 *Hemarthrosis and ankylosis.* These suggest a deficiency of factor VIII or IX.
4 *Hereditary connective tissue disorder.* Abnormal elasticity of the skin and hyperextensibility of the joints (Ehlers-Danlos syndrome) may be associated with vascular bleeding.
5 *Chronic liver disease,* including spider angiomas, palmar erythema, dilated abdominal veins, hepatomegaly, or splenomegaly.

LABORATORY STUDIES **Screening tests** A careful history is the best screening test. Nevertheless, laboratory tests for the integrity of the coagulation and platelet com-

TABLE 61-4
Diagnosis of bleeding disorders involving coagulation

Disorders	*Tests*					
	Prothrombin time	*Partial thromboplastin time*	*Thrombin time*	*Fibrinogen concentration*	*Fibrinogen proteolysis*	*Factor assays*
Congenital deficiency of factor VII	Abnormal	Normal	Normal	Normal	Normal	Specific factor abnormal
Congenital deficiency of factors VIII, IX, XI, XII, Fitzgerald or prekallikrein	Normal	Abnormal	Normal	Normal	Normal	Specific factor abnormal
Deficiency of prothrombin, factor V, factor X, or vitamin K; or coumarin or warfarin effect	Abnormal	Abnormal	Normal	Normal	Normal	Specific factors abnormal
Dysfibrinogenemia, heparin effect	Abnormal	Abnormal	Abnormal	Normal	Normal	Normal
Disseminated intravascular coagulation, liver failure, congenital hypofibrinogenemia	Abnormal	Abnormal	Abnormal	Decreased	Abnormal	Abnormal

ponents of the hemostatic mechanism are indicated under a number of circumstances, including: historical or physical evidence of abnormal hemostasis; family history of abnormal hemostasis; presence of a disorder which may be associated with abnormal hemostasis—e.g., liver disease, systemic lupus erythematosus; and prior to surgical procedures known to be associated with a high incidence of hemorrhage.

Coagulation system tests (Table 61-4) A commonly used set of screening tests for coagulation defects includes: (1) *prothrombin time*; (2) *partial thromboplastin time*; (3) *thrombin clotting time*; and (4) *fibrinogen concentration* (most tests of fibrinogen depend on measuring the concentration of thrombin-clottable protein in the plasma). If one or more of these tests are abnormal, an assessment is made, based on the history as well as the test results, as to the most likely defect. The factor(s) most likely to be abnormal should be specifically assayed, including factor XIII. If all the coagulation system screening tests are normal, no further tests are necessary unless the history strongly suggests abnormal hemostasis.

Platelet system tests (Table 61-5) Basic screening tests include: (1) *the bleeding time* and (2) the *platelet count.*

Tests which screen for defects of platelet function include: (1) clot retraction; (2) activity of platelet factor 3; and (3) platelet aggregation.

If the bleeding time is prolonged and thrombocytopenia is detected, the etiology of the thrombocytopenia should be pursued by a careful history of drug or toxin exposure, physical examination for splenomegaly and systemic disease, a complete blood count, examination of the bone marrow, and tests for systemic lupus erythematosus and platelet antibodies. If the bleeding time is prolonged and the platelet count is normal, tests for von Willebrand's disease and for platelet function should be undertaken (see Chaps. 317 to 319).

REFERENCES

BIGGS R (ed): *Human Blood Coagulation, Haemostasis and Thrombosis,* Oxford: Blackwell, 1972

WEISS HJ: Platelet physiology and abnormalities of platelet function. N Engl J Med 293:531, 1975

TABLE 61-5
Diagnosis of bleeding disorders involving platelets

Platelet disorder	*Tests*		*Platelet function*		
	Bleeding time	*Platelet count*	*Clot retraction*	*Platelet factor 3*	*Platelet aggregation*
Thrombocytopenia	Prolonged	Decreased	Abnormal		
Thrombasthenia	Prolonged	Normal	Abnormal	Abnormal	Abnormal with ADP
Release defects	Prolonged	Normal	Normal	Abnormal	Primary normal; secondary abnormal
Von Willebrand's disease (also has low factor VIII coagulant and antigenic activity)	Prolonged	Normal	Normal	Normal	Abnormal only with ristocetin; normal with ADP, epinephrine, thrombin

WILLIAMS WJ et al (eds): *Hematology,* 2d ed., chaps. 128 to 162, New York: McGraw-Hill (in press)
WINTROBE MM et al: *Clinical Hematology,* 7th ed., Philadelphia: Lea & Febiger, 1974

62
ENLARGEMENT OF LYMPH NODES AND SPLEEN

ALEXANDER FEFER

LYMPH NODES

STRUCTURE AND FUNCTION The principal cells in lymph nodes are the lymphocytes in the lymphoid follicles and the reticuloendothelial cells which line nodal sinuses. Each follicle, located in the cortex of the node, has a germinal center which contains rapidly dividing large lymphocytes (B cells) and macrophages. Surrounding the germinal center is a cuff of densely packed small lymphocytes (T cells) which proliferate at a slower rate and which ultimately leave the node. The chief function of lymphocytes is to respond to antigens presented to the node from the structures being drained. The cells either differentiate into plasma cells and produce antibody (B cells) or enlarge, proliferate, and generate a T-cell-mediated response. The reticuloendothelial cells (histiocytes or macrophages), which can also proliferate, participate in immunity but function chiefly in the phagocytosis of cellular debris and foreign material, e.g., microorganisms which may have gained access to the node from the area being drained by it.

MECHANISMS OF LYMPH NODE ENLARGEMENT Lymphadenopathy may be due to an increase in the number and size of lymphoid follicles with proliferation of lymphocytes or reticuloendothelial cells or to infiltration of the node by cells normally not present in it. Nodal cells proliferate in response to antigens, to other stimuli which evoke greater phagocytic activity, and to unknown stimuli which cause nodal cells to become transformed to lymphoma cells and to proliferate autonomously. Nodes can be infiltrated by leukemia or metastatic carcinoma cells, by polymorphonuclear cells in lymphadenitis, or by metabolite-laden macrophages in the lipid storage diseases.

SIGNIFICANCE OF LYMPHADENOPATHY In normal persons nodes are not palpable or barely palpable. Whether a palpable node is clinically significant depends partly on its location and on the age and occupation of the patient. The number and size of nodes is maximal at puberty. Children are far more likely than adults to respond with lymphoid hyperplasia and generalized adenopathy even to relatively minor stimuli such as mild infection of the upper respiratory tract or skin, and develop appendicitis, mesenteric adenitis, and tonsillitis far more often than do adults.

Lymphadenopathy reflects significant disease more often in the adult than in the child. However, palpable nodes do not always connote serious disease. They may reflect merely the minor trauma to and infections of the structures being drained, such as the hands of a manual laborer (epitrochlear nodes), the upper extremities (axillary), upper respiratory tract and teeth (cervical), and, most frequently, the lower extremities (inguinal). However, enlargement even of those nodes may reflect significant disease. Enlargement of nodes in certain areas must *always* be considered pathologic. These include the posterior auricular, supraclavicular, epitrochlear (not in a manual laborer), popliteal, mediastinal, and abdominal nodes.

DISEASES ASSOCIATED WITH LYMPHADENOPATHY Enlarged nodes may reflect no significant disease, a self-limited benign disease, or a severe or even fatal one. Table 62-1 presents a partial list of the conditions associated with enlarged nodes. The likelihood of each diagnosis varies with age, sex, and geography. Although most patients with significant adenopathy will have either a malignancy, an infection, or a connective tissue disease, the likelihood of each of those conditions is greatest, respectively, in the old, the young, and the female.

PHYSICAL CHARACTERISTICS OF ENLARGED NODES Some nodal characteristics provide clues to diagnosis. Nodes involved by lymphomas or by chronic lymphatic leukemia tend to be large, symmetric, rubbery, firm, movable, discrete, and nontender, whereas nodes in acute leukemia are often tender because of rapid enlargement and concurrent infection. Nodes containing metastatic carcinoma are stony-hard, nontender, well-localized, and bound to surrounding tissues and, therefore, nonmovable. In acute infections, nodes are firm, tender, asymmetric and matted, and the overlying skin may be red and edematous, whereas in chronic infections the nodes are nontender and there is no edema. However, the nodal characteristics are only modestly helpful clues, not pathognomonic signs.

LOCATION OF ENLARGED NODES The extent and location of enlarged nodes also provide diagnostic clues. Generalized adenopathy, i.e., involving more than two separate node groups, is common in non-Hodgkin's lymphomas, chronic lymphocytic leukemia, and the histiocytoses, but

TABLE 62-1
Conditions associated with lymph node enlargement

I Neoplastic
- *A* Hematologic: lymphomas, acute leukemia, chronic lymphocytic leukemia, myeloproliferative syndromes, histiocytoses
- *B* Nonhematologic: carcinomas of head and neck, lung, breast, kidney

II Immunologic or inflammatory
- *A* Infections: pyogenic streptococcal, staphylococcal, and salmonella infections, brucellosis, tuberculosis, syphilis, infectious mononucleosis, cytomegalovirus, infectious hepatitis, rubella, lymphogranuloma venereum, toxoplasmosis, histoplasmosis, coccidioidomycosis, malaria
- *B* Connective tissue diseases: rheumatoid arthritis, systemic lupus erythematosus, dermatomyositis
- *C* Serum sickness
- *D* Reaction to hydantoins
- *E* Sarcoidosis
- *F* Miscellaneous: giant (angiofollicular) lymph node hyperplasia, sinus histiocytosis, dermatopathic lymphadenitis, immunoblastic lymphadenopathy

III Endocrine: hyperthyroidism, Addison's disease

IV Lipid storage diseases: Gaucher's and Niemann-Pick's diseases

not with nonhematologic malignancies. Generalized adenopathy is uncommon in adults with infections except in infectious mononucleosis, brucellosis, cytomegalovirus, tuberculosis, infectious hepatitis, secondary syphilis, toxoplasmosis, and histoplasmosis.

In the absence of generalized adenopathy, enlargement of specific lymph node groups can be helpful diagnostically. Posterior auricular adenopathy suggests rubella. Unilateral anterior auricular adenopathy is associated with lesions of the conjunctiva and eyelids with a resultant oculoglandular syndrome such as is seen with trachoma, tularemia, cat-scratch fever, tuberculosis, syphilis, epidemic keratoconjunctivitis, and swimming pool outbreaks of adenovirus type III pharyngoconjunctival fever. Oropharyngeal or dental infections can occasionally cause cervical adenopathy. Bilateral cervical adenopathy is prominent in tuberculosis, coccidioidomycosis, infectious mononucleosis, toxoplasmosis, sarcoid, lymphomas, and leukemias. However, a unilateral cervical mass often represents a metastasis from an undetected asymptomatic nasopharyngeal tumor. In one study of 1600 patients admitted to surgery with a nonthyroid neck mass, 88 percent of the patients had a malignancy, most often a metastatic tumor or a lymphoma. Therefore, a nonthyroid neck mass in adults, but not children, should be considered neoplastic until proved otherwise and is a strong indication for examination of the mouth, pharynx, nasopharynx, and larynx in search of a malignancy.

Palpable supraclavicular nodes are always abnormal and, in the absence of generalized adenopathy, reflect neoplastic disease in the abdomen or chest. The right node drains parts of the lungs and mediastinum and is involved by intrathoracic lesions especially of the lung and esophagus, whereas the left (Virchow's) node is close to the thoracic duct and is involved by intraabdominal tumor, especially from the stomach, ovary, testis, and kidney. Axillary nodes drain part of the breast and are favorite sites for metastatic breast carcinoma. Epitrochlear nodes often are chronically enlarged bilaterally in secondary lues. Inguinal adenopathy is especially common in lymphogranuloma venereum, chancroid, and syphilis.

Enlarged nodes in certain areas cannot be palpated, but are suspected in the presence of clinical problems which they produce. Enlarged mediastinal or hilar nodes detectable on routine chest x-ray may be asymptomatic or may cause tracheobronchial compression with cough and wheezing, recurrent laryngeal nerve compression with hoarseness and stridor, paralysis of the left leaf of the diaphragm, esophageal compression with dysphagia, superior vena caval compression with swelling of the neck and face, and subclavian vein compression with swelling of the arm. Hilar nodes are often asymmetrically involved by metastatic carcinoma from the lungs and, rarely, from testis and kidney. Bilateral asymmetric mediastinal adenopathy is common with non-Hodgkin's lymphomas and is characteristic of nodular sclerosing Hodgkin's lymphoma. Hilar adenopathy is rarely associated with bacterial or viral pneumonias. It is seen, however, in tuberculosis (usually unilateral) and in coccidioidomycosis (usually bilateral). Bilateral hilar adenopathy is characteristic of sarcoidosis, although tuberculous involvement must be excluded. One study of 100 patients with bilateral hilar adenopathy documented its very frequent association with sarcoidosis and revealed that such adenopathy in patients without symptoms or only with erythema nodosum or uveitis was nearly diagnostic for sarcoidosis. Unlike lymphomatous nodes, hilar nodes in sarcoidosis, coccidioidomycosis, and tuberculosis often show roentgenographically detectable calcification.

Abdominal nodes can enlarge in any disorder which causes generalized adenopathy. However, the cause of intraabdominal or retroperitoneal adenopathy in adults is most often neoplastic, especially lymphomatous. The nodes may cause abdominal pain, nausea, constipation, intestinal obstruction, urinary complaints, backache, fever, ascites, or peripheral edema. If sufficiently large, they can be detected by abdominal, pelvic, or rectal examination, but they are most often detected only by lymphangiography. Lymphatic channels in the feet are injected with a radiopaque dye which then drains into and visualizes the iliac and paraaortic retroperitoneal nodes.

APPROACH TO THE PATIENT WITH ENLARGED LYMPH NODES In most patients, a diagnosis can be made by a careful history and physical examination, hematologic and other laboratory tests, skin tests, and routine x-rays. The association of some diagnoses with age and sex is helpful, e.g., systemic lupus erythematosus in the young female, breast carcinoma in the older female, infectious mononucleosis in the young adult, and chronic lymphocytic leukemia in the old. A history of exposure to potential sources of infection, and of constitutional complaints such as fever, malaise, fatigue, and weight loss, which accompany hematologic malignancies and systemic infections, is important. The duration of symptoms and signs is suggestive. Patients whose nodes are neoplastic tend to present with a longer history—often months—of adenopathy, whereas patients with painful infectious or inflammatory adenopathy often present within days after the nodes appear.

Physical examination should include a search for associated findings of special significance, e.g., splenomegaly for its myriad implications (see below), hepatomegaly for hepatitis and malignancies, skin rashes for viral infections, heart murmurs as in subacute bacterial endocarditis, and evidence of local infection such as chancre. An oral and nasopharyngeal examination for tumor is essential in any patient with a neck mass.

Routine hematologic studies may be diagnostic. The immature cells of leukemia or the atypical lymphocytes of infectious mononucleosis and other viral infections may be detected. A chest x-ray might reveal mediastinal nodes with or without pulmonary nodules or infiltrates. A liver and spleen scan using radioactive material might reveal increased size and defects associated with neoplasia. Cultures of blood, throat, sputum, urine, bone marrow, and other possible infectious sites should be obtained when appropriate, as should special serologic tests such as a test for syphilis and antibody titers for toxoplasmosis and cytomegalovirus. A marrow aspiration is indicated for anemia, thrombocytopenia, or leukopenia and may reveal leukemia or metastatic carcinoma or, when cultured, tuberculosis or other infections. A marrow biopsy is more likely than an aspirate to reveal a lymphoma.

If the above work-up is not diagnostic and a neoplasm or infection for which treatment should not be delayed is suspected, then a lymph node should be biopsied, examined, and cultured. It is best to biopsy cervical or supraclavicular nodes and to avoid axillary or inguinal nodes which are subject to local trauma and infections. Excision biopsy of an entire node provides a look at the nodal architecture. A node biopsy can be diagnostic in lymphoma, carcinoma, infections such as tuberculosis or histoplasmosis, or a granuloma without caseation suggestive of sarcoidosis.

However, in 40 to 60 percent of patients the node biopsy will reveal only reactive hyperplasia and will not yield a specific diagnosis. This failure has been attributed to inability to histologically differentiate conditions such as hydantoin-induced hyperplasia from a true lymphoma, to noninvolvement of the node obtained, or to distortion of the involved node by other processes. If another node is palpable or detectable on chest x-ray, an open biopsy or biopsy via mediastinoscopy should be obtained. If no nodes are evident and lung carcinoma, sarcoidosis, or tuberculosis is considered likely, a biopsy of the scalene node and fat pad in the supraclavicular area should be obtained. However, if despite a nondiagnostic biopsy lymphoma remains a strong possibility, no other nodes are accessible, and progressive disease is apparent, a lymphangiogram is indicated. If abnormal abdominal or retroperitoneal nodes are detected, abdominal laparotomy may be necessary for diagnostic biopsies. However, if the patient with the nondiagnostic biopsy is otherwise well or improving and has no other accessible nodes, watchful waiting is acceptable. Adenopathy secondary to infections will almost always regress within 2 to 3 weeks. However, in several long-term follow-up studies, 25 to 60 percent of patients with nondiagnostic lymph node biopsies were found within a very few months to have lymphomas or carcinomas and, less often, connective tissue disease or infection. The need for careful and frequent follow-up evaluations of such patients and for a node biopsy as nodes become available is obvious.

ENLARGEMENT OF THE SPLEEN

STRUCTURE OF THE SPLEEN Splenic function reflects the specialized cells and unique circulation of this organ. The spleen has a capsule and trabeculae which enclose the white and red pulp. The white pulp consists of periarterial sheaths of lymphocytes with follicles containing germinal centers in which there are plasma cells and macrophages. The red pulp consists of cords of reticulum containing phagocytic macrophages separated from sinuses by a basement membrane. The narrow, tortuous splenic circulation sequesters blood within the pulp and exposes the traversing blood cells to phagocytic cells and to metabolic and immunologic hazards, as well as to barriers which make it necessary for the cells to change their size and shape in order to squeeze through the cords and sinuses and return into the circulation.

FUNCTION OF THE SPLEEN The spleen functions as the largest lymph node. It responds to antigens with proliferation of T lymphocytes in the lymphatic sheath and of the antibody-forming B cells in the germinal centers, as well as with proliferation of phagocytic cells. The phagocytic function of the spleen includes "culling" and "pitting" which occur mostly in the tortuous red pulp. Culling refers to phagocytosis of abnormal whole red blood cells which have been damaged physically or immunologically and of

cells containing nuclei or Howell-Jolly bodies, reticulocytes, siderocytes, target cells, and spherocytes. Pitting refers to the removal of inclusions, e.g., red blood cell nuclei, Heinz bodies, and malarial parasites from red blood cells without destroying the cells. The spleen serves as a reservoir of platelets but not of red blood cells or leukocytes. It normally sequesters 30 to 40 percent of the blood platelets. The spleen is normally the site of blood formation through the fifth fetal month, but not after birth—except in some abnormal conditions.

MECHANISMS OF SPLENIC ENLARGEMENT Like other lymph nodes, the spleen enlarges with reactive proliferation of lymphoma cells, with infiltration by other neoplastic cells, mostly in chronic leukemias, or by lipid-laden macrophages. The spleen also enlarges with extramedullary hemopoiesis, with proliferation of phagocytic cells in response to increased destruction of blood cells, and, uniquely, by vascular congestion in the presence of portal hypertension.

DISEASES ASSOCIATED WITH SPLENOMEGALY Table 62-2 lists the principal conditions associated with splenomegaly, some of which require a brief comment. Any condition which causes generalized lymphadenopathy can cause splenomegaly. Splenomegaly is frequent in infectious mononucleosis, subacute bacterial endocarditis, brucellosis, histoplasmosis, malaria, kala azar, and other parasitic infections. It occurs in 10 to 20 percent of patients with systemic lupus erythematosus and in rheumatoid arthritis which, when associated with splenomegaly and anemia, thrombocytopenia, or, most often, leukopenia, is designated *Felty's syndrome.* The cytopenia often responds to splenectomy.

Lymphomas often involve the spleen even when it is not palpable, and laparotomy to determine the extent of a lymphoma—especially in Hodgkin's disease—always includes splenectomy. The spleen is massively enlarged in myelo-

TABLE 62-2
Conditions associated with splenomegaly

I Immunologic-inflammatory
- *A* Infections: subacute bacterial endocarditis, brucellosis, tuberculosis, infectious mononucleosis, cytomegalovirus, syphilis, histoplasmosis, malaria, kala azar, schistosomiasis
- *B* Connective tissue diseases: rheumatoid arthritis, Felty's syndrome, systemic lupus erythematosus
- *C* Sarcoidosis

II Hematologic disorders
- *A* Neoplastic: lymphomas, histiocytoses, myeloproliferative syndromes (chronic myelocytic leukemia, polycythemia vera, myelofibrosis, and myeloid metaplasia), chronic lymphocytic leukemia, acute leukemia
- *B* Nonneoplastic: hemolytic anemias, e.g., hereditary spherocytosis, autoimmune hemolytic anemia, hemoglobinopathies

III Congestive splenomegaly due to portal hypertension: hepatic cirrhosis, portal or splenic vein thrombosis or stenosis, myeloid metaplasia, vinyl chloride

IV Metabolic-infiltrative: Gaucher's and Niemann-Pick's disease, amyloidosis

V Miscellaneous: cyst, splenic abscess, aneurysm of splenic artery, cavernous hemangioma

proliferative syndromes, especially chronic myelogenous leukemia and myelofibrosis. Splenomegaly may also be prominent in chronic lymphocytic leukemia and may be associated with autoimmune hemolytic anemia. Splenomegaly associated with increased destruction of red blood cells occurs with many hemolytic anemias some of which like hereditary spherocytosis and, sometimes, autoimmune hemolytic anemia, respond dramatically to splenectomy.

Chronic congestive splenomegaly due to portal hypertension (Banti's syndrome, Chap. 320) is associated with gastrointestinal bleeding and pancytopenia. It is usually secondary to cirrhosis of the liver or, less commonly, to portal vein thrombosis. Splenomegaly is often accompanied by the syndrome of hypersplenism (Chap. 320), consisting of a large spleen, anemia, leukopenia or thrombocytopenia, and hyperactivity of the bone marrow. It is often reversed by splenectomy. Hypersplenism may occur in most splenomegalic states (Table 62-2). Its severity does not correlate with the degree of splenic enlargement. However, splenomegaly does not always cause hypersplenism.

APPROACH TO THE PATIENT WITH AN ENLARGED SPLEEN Splenomegaly is common, yet a palpable spleen in an adult is almost always clinically significant. In one study, the spleen was palpable in only 3 percent of students entering an American college and persisted in only a third of them. The spleen is even less likely to be palpable in normal persons beyond college age. Therefore, patients with a palpable spleen but without other signs or symptoms should have at least a spleen scan and complete blood count. Colloid tagged with technetium 99 injected intravenously is taken up by reticuloendothelial cells and visualizes splenic size, shape, and defects suggestive of tumor or abscess. The scan is the best method for detecting an enlarged spleen and for ruling out a nonsplenic mass, e.g., cyst or metastatic tumor, which might cause splenic displacement rather than enlargement. A complete blood count and smear are often helpful or even diagnostic in asymptomatic splenomegalic patients with chronic myelogenous or lymphocytic leukemia.

Since most conditions which cause splenomegaly also cause lymphadenopathy, the approach to diagnosis is that presented in the section on adenopathy (above). The cause of splenomegaly should be determined not by tests on the spleen itself but by tests—possibly including a lymph node biopsy—for diseases known to cause splenomegaly and lymphadenopathy. Splenomegaly in acute leukemia is usually a minor clinical feature—the diagnosis is made by blood count and marrow examinations. Splenomegaly in lymphomas is almost always associated with adenopathy, and the diagnosis made by node biopsy or at laparotomy.

Most conditions which cause splenomegaly without adenopathy can also be suspected and diagnosed by history and physical and laboratory examination. For example, a hemolytic anemia is detectable by routine laboratory tests for anemia and for hemolysis, including reticulocyte counts and serum bilirubin. Specific causes for hemolysis can then be determined by other procedures such as Coombs test, osmotic fragility, and hemoglobin electrophoresis. Similarly, splenomegaly and hypersplenism secondary to portal hypertension caused by cirrhosis of the liver are readily diagnosed by a history of alcoholism or previous liver disease, physical signs of liver dysfunction and portal hypertension, laboratory abnormalities consistent with liver dysfunction and hypersplenism, and radiologic evidence of esophageal varices. The diagnosis of the rare vascular causes of portal hypertension requires angiography.

Some patients with splenomegaly may have systemic symptoms but no nodes available for biopsy. If an underlying lymphoma or serious infection is considered likely but is not detected by the usual examinations, including lymphangiograms, a laparotomy with biopsy of the liver and abdominal nodes, and splenectomy, may be necessary. Appropriate cultures and pathologic examinations are essential. Such laparotomies on patients with splenomegaly of unknown cause have revealed lymphoma in one-third, congestive splenomegaly in one-fourth, and inflammatory disease in one-fifth of patients.

REFERENCES

CHRISTENSEN BE: Pathophysiology of "hypersplenism syndrome." Scand J Haematol 11:5, 1973

MCINTYRE OR, EBAUGH FG JR: Palpable spleens in college freshmen. Ann Intern Med 66:310, 1967

SINCLAIR S et al: Biopsy of enlarged, superficial lymph nodes. JAMA 228:602, 1974

SKANDALAKIS JE et al: Tumors of the neck. Surgery 48:375, 1960

SOLNITZKY OC, JEGHERS H: Lymphadenopathy and disorders of the lymphatic system, in *Signs and Symptoms,* eds CM MacBryde, RS Blacklow, 5th ed., Philadelphia: Lippincott, chap. 26, p. 476, 1970

WEINSTEIN IM: Lymphadenopathy and splenomegaly, in *Hematology,* ed WJ Williams et al, New York: McGraw-Hill, chap. 98, p. 834, 1972

WEISS L, TAVASSOLI M: Anatomical hazards to the passage of erythrocytes through the spleen. Semin Hematol 7:372, 1970

WINTERBAUER RH et al: A clinical interpretation of bilateral hilar adenopathy. Ann Intern Med 78:65, 1973

WINTROBE MM et al: *Clinical Hematology,* 7th ed., Philadelphia: Lea & Febiger, 1974

ZUELZER WW, KAPLAN J: The child with lymphadenopathy. Semin Hematol 12:323, 1975

63 ABNORMALITIES OF LEUKOCYTES

DAVID C. DALE

INTRODUCTION

Alterations of leukocyte counts and functions occur in a wide variety of hematologic, infectious, inflammatory, metabolic, and neoplastic diseases. Because leukocytes are affected by so many diseases, the routine laboratory evaluation of many patients begins with determination of the leukocyte count and the examination of a stained blood smear. From the clinical examination and these blood studies, certain diagnoses can be made or strongly suspected, e.g., leukemia, agranulocytosis, infectious mononucleosis, systemic mastocytosis, and the Chédiak-Higashi syndrome. In patients with infectious and inflammatory diseases, the leukocyte count usually serves as a useful guide to the severity of the disease process. The leukocyte count and blood smear examination plus special studies of leukocyte function also will identify certain patients with heightened susceptibility to infections.

Five types of circulating leukocytes can be identified by their morphology on blood smears: neutrophils, lymphocytes, monocytes, eosinophils, and basophils. It is generally accepted that all these leukocyte types, along with erythrocytes and platelets, derive from a common pluripotent stem cell. However, beyond this common origin, independent regulatory mechanisms govern the production, distribution, and function of each type of leukocyte. For simplicity, inferences are often made about the presence or severity of illness from the total leukocyte count and the differential leukocyte count expressed as a percentage. It is more precise to express the counts of each type of leukocyte in terms of the concentration or absolute count per cubic millimeter of blood. This is usually determined simply by multiplying the total leukocyte count by the percent value. Normal values for blood leukocyte counts are shown in Table 63-1.

NEUTROPHILS

NORMAL PHYSIOLOGY The primary function of neutrophils is phagocytosis, killing and digestion of microorganisms. The cells develop the capacity to perform these special functions in the bone marrow. Early neutrophil precursors, myeloblasts and promyelocytes, differentiate from hematopoietic stem cells by developing an active Golgi apparatus and endoplasmic reticulum and beginning the formation of cytoplasmic granules. The initial or *primary granules* stain reddish-purple with azure dyes; hence they are also called *azurophilic granules.* They contain myeloperoxidase, acid hydrolases, lysozyme, and cationic antibacterial proteins. With further development the cells become myelocytes. At this stage the cytoplasm becomes packed with characteristic secondary or *specific granules* which stain faintly pink with the usual blood stains. These granules contain alkaline phosphatase, collagenase, lactoferrin, lysozyme, and aminopeptidase. Beyond the myelocyte stage, neutrophilic cells do not divide; instead their nuclear chromatin becomes condensed, the cell diminishes modestly in size, and cytoplasmic glycogen accumulates. Normally neutrophils are not released to the blood until the nucleus is segmented, that is, the cells have matured beyond the metamyelocyte and "band" stages.

Approximately 8 to 14 days are required for a cell to move through the sequence of four to six cell divisions and complete maturation, that is, from the myeloblast stage to a mature blood neutrophil. Measurement of the time required for the early developmental stages is difficult, but it

TABLE 63-1
Normal values for concentration of blood leukocytes*

Cell type	*Mean, cells/mm³*	*95% Confidence limits, cells/mm³*
Neutrophil	3,650	1,830–7,250
Lymphocyte	2,500	1,500–4,000
Monocyte	430	200–950
Eosinophil	150	0–700
Basophil	30	0–150

* *Total leukocyte counts from venous blood samples were done in a Coulter counter, and 200 leukocytes were differentiated on Wright's-stained blood smears made on cover glass.*

is clear that there are normally three to four days of neutrophil maturation after cell division is finished. During this time the maturing cells can be released from the bone marrow to the blood under sufficient stress, and therefore they are described as being in the marrow neutrophil reserves. Morphologic and radioisotopic studies on bone marrow indicate that there are normally about 10 times as many nearly mature neutrophils in the marrow as in the blood. The size of the marrow neutrophil reserves can be estimated by administration of endotoxin, etiocholanolone, or glucocorticosteroids and measuring the increase in the neutrophil counts. In normal individuals, these agents roughly double the count or increase blood neutrophils by a minimum of 2,000 cells per mm^3.

The regulation of neutrophil production and release remains poorly understood. Normal individuals maintain their own characteristic neutrophil count, but this is subject to substantial day-to-day variation and is greatly affected by activity and many other factors. A humoral substance has been identified which will stimulate neutrophil release from the bone marrow (neutrophilia-inducing factor). Colony-stimulating factor, a substance present in serum and urine which will stimulate neutrophilic bone marrow cells to grow in tissue culture systems, is another possible neutrophil regulator. The precise physiologic role of these substances is not clear.

The blood serves to transport neutrophils to areas of acute inflammation as well as to the mucosal surfaces of the body where these cells serve to maintain the normal defensive barrier to microbial invasion. Normally only about half of the neutrophils in the vascular system are circulating freely and are described as being in the circulating neutrophil pool. Only these cells are counted in routine blood samples. The other half of the blood neutrophils are loosely adherent to the walls of blood vessels throughout the body in the marginal neutrophil pool. In response to inflammation, neutrophils are shifted to the marginal pool. Certain drugs, i.e., epinephrine, glucocorticosteroids, and other anti-inflammatory agents, may reduce margination.

The neutrophil blood half-disappearance time (blood half-life) is only about 6 to 7 h. Neutrophils leave the vascular compartment by passing between endothelial cells presumably because they are attracted to sites of inflammation by chemotactic factors. Bacteria can release low molecular weight chemotactic substances. Chemotactic factors, specifically C3a, C5a, and C567, are generated from the complement system when plasma reacts with endotoxin, antigen-antibody complexes, and other foreign substances. Kallikrein, plasminogen activator, transfer factor, and other substances will also attract neutrophils.

At the inflammatory site, phagocytosis is facilitated by humoral substances, opsonins, which have coated the surface of the foreign material to be ingested. Immunoglobulins (IgG) and complement (C3) are the best-characterized opsonins. Phagocytosis stimulates numerous intracellular events including increased oxygen consumption, glycogenolysis, glucose oxidation via the hexosemonophosphate shunt, and hydrogen peroxide production. Within the cell, the phagocytized particle is held in a vacuole, and the contents of the secondary and then the primary granules are sequentially emptied into this vacuole. The vacuolar pH is dramatically lowered, and the granule enzymes are activated. The neutrophil possesses a variety of bactericidal mechanisms giving it an "overkill" capacity. The best characterized bactericidal mechanism involves myeloperoxidase combining with hydrogen peroxide and a halide such as iodide or chloride. The system is also effective against viruses, fungi, and *Mycoplasma.* The neutrophil usually degenerates after it digests the phagocytized material. Neutrophils, cellular debris, and digested foreign matter become the pus which characterizes acute inflammation, and to which the residual myeloperoxidase imparts the slightly greenish color.

NEUTROPHILIA An absolute neutrophil count of greater than 10,000 per mm^3 should be regarded as elevated in most patients, although for a few individuals neutrophil counts of 10,000 to 15,000 per mm^3 are normal. The causes of neutrophilia are listed in Table 63-2. Exercise, excitement, epinephrine administration, or stress of any sort will increase the count up to twice the resting level within a few minutes. The duration of this neutrophilia is brief. It is largely due to a shift of cells from the marginal to circulating pool and is not accompanied by an increase in the number of nonsegmented blood neutrophils. Most acute bacterial infections are associated with neutrophilia, especially those that are accompanied by bacteremia, involve substantial amounts of tissue, and are localized in a closed space. This neutrophilia initially occurs because of accelerated release of cells from the bone marrow reserves and is often accompanied by an increase in the number of nonsegmented neutrophils in the blood, i.e., a "shift to the left." With prolonged inflammation from any cause, neutrophil production is stimulated and the bone marrow shows granulocytic hyperplasia. Toxic granulation, due to increased staining of the primary granules, and cytoplasmic vacuolization also occur under these circumstances. In all the usual conditions causing neutrophilia, the counts are generally between 10,000 and 25,000 per mm^3. Persisting neutrophilia with counts greater than 30,000 to 50,000 per mm^3 is called a *leukemoid reaction.* This term is sometimes used to describe any persisting high leukocyte count because this degree of leukocytosis suggests leukemia. Characteristically in a leukemoid reaction the raised count is due predominantly to an increase in mature neutrophils with some increase of band neutrophils and metamyelocytes. Blood myelocytes are rare. The leukocyte alkaline phosphatase is generally high, and the cells do not contain Auer rods. The erythrocyte and platelet counts also are usually not strikingly abnormal. The differentiation between leukemoid reactions, leukemia, and myeloproliferative diseases is discussed further in Chaps. 315 and 325.

NEUTROPENIA Neutrophil counts of less than 2,000 per mm^3 are relatively uncommon in normal individuals although some healthy resting adults, particularly black persons and Yemenite Jews, may have counts as low as 1,000 per mm^3 with no apparent disease. Neutropenia occurs in a wide variety of clinical circumstances (Table 63-3). In general, as the count declines below about 1,000 per mm^3, the risk of infection increases. However, the risk of infection is related to both the nature of the primary disease process and the cell count. For instance, many patients with chronic idiopathic neutropenia have counts of less than 500 per mm^3 for years without infections, whereas few patients with leukemia or aplastic anemia will survive for even a few weeks at these levels without developing an infection.

It is not possible to describe the neutropenias on the basis of kinetic mechanisms analogous to the mechanisms of anemia and thrombocytopenia. Most patients encountered will fit into the following general clinical categories.

Chronic neutropenia without splenomegaly (Chronic idiopathic neutropenia or granulocytopenia, familial benign neutropenia, chronic hypoplastic neutropenia, and chronic benign neutropenia of childhood) Isolated individuals and families are occasionally observed with neutropenia as their sole hematologic abnormality. Characteristically, the spleen is not enlarged. Onset may occur at any age; frequently, the syndrome is recognized on an incidental blood count. In adults, there is a striking female predominance, whereas in children both males and females are affected. Neutrophil counts may be as low as 50 to 200 per mm^3 with only infrequent infections, usually involving the upper respiratory tract. Bacteremia is rare. The blood usually contains normal-appearing mature neutrophils in reduced numbers; blood monocytes are often increased, and hypergammaglobulinemia may be present. The marrow is normocellular and shows few or no mature neutrophils. In a few cases, not readily distinguished from the rest of these patients on clinical grounds, leukoagglutinating antibodies to normal neutrophils have been detected and may be of etiologic significance (chronic idiopathic immunoneutropenia). The disease mechanisms otherwise remain largely unknown. In periods of observation up to 25 years, evolution to leukemia has been reported only extremely rarely. A few children with this disorder have had spontaneous remissions. In a few patients with frequent infections and extremely low counts, alternate-day glucocorticoster-

TABLE 63-2
Causes of neutrophilia

Physiologic: Exercise, excitement, stress, epinephrine
Infections: Chiefly bacterial, also fungal, parasitic, and some viral diseases
Inflammation: Burns, tissue necrosis as in myocardial and pulmonary infarction, collagen vascular diseases, hypersensitivity states, other inflammatory diseases
Metabolic disorders: Ketoacidosis, acute renal failure, eclampsia, acute poisoning
Myeloproliferative diseases: Myelocytic leukemia, myeloid metaplasia, polycythemia vera
Other: Metastatic carcinoma, acute hemorrhage or hemolysis, glucocorticosteroids, lithium therapy, idiopathic

TABLE 63-3
Clinical conditions characterized by neutropenia

Hematologic diseases: Chronic idiopathic neutropenias; cyclic neutropenia; lazy-leukocyte syndrome; Chédiak-Higashi syndrome; leukemia; aplastic anemia
Drug-induced conditions: Agranulocytosis; myelotoxic drugs
Nutritional deficiencies: Vitamin B_{12}; folate, especially in alcoholics; copper
Secondary to other diseases: Infections including typhoid, infectious mononucleosis, malaria, overwhelming sepsis; diseases with splenomegaly, Felty's syndrome, congestive splenomegaly, Gaucher's disease, sarcoidosis; malignancies with marrow infiltration

oids have elevated the neutrophil counts and reduced infections.

Several other groups of patients with chronic neutropenia without splenomegaly can be recognized which have distinctly different clinical characteristics. *Infantile genetic agranulocytosis* is usually a rapidly fatal disorder associated with anemia and atypical, vacuolated marrow precursor cells. *Neutropenia associated with hypogammaglobulinemia* leads to fatal infections at an early age. In *cyclic neutropenia, lazy-leukocyte syndrome,* and *Chédiak-Higashi syndrome,* chronic neutropenia is present but additional neutrophil abnormalities have been observed. Other patients are occasionally encountered with episodic severe neutropenia associated with febrile illnesses. Many other unusual neutropenic disorders have been observed; undoubtedly these neutropenias will be categorized further as their etiologies are better understood.

Cyclic neutropenia This disorder is characterized by the periodic absence of neutrophils from the blood and bone marrow associated with fever, malaise, mouth ulcers, and cervical adenopathy. These findings recur regularly at approximately 21-day intervals. Between episodes the patients are usually well. Symptoms characteristically begin in early childhood, although adult onset has been described. Cyclic fluctuations of other blood leukocytes, platelets, and reticulocytes occur, and bone marrow investigations indicate that the disease is due to a defect in the regulation of hematopoietic cell proliferation. Treatment with glucocorticosteroids, androgens, or splenectomy is not of established benefit; however, early recognition and prompt treatment of infectious complications may be lifesaving.

Neutropenia in the leukemias and aplastic anemia In leukemia, particularly the acute leukemias, neutropenia is frequently present at the time the disease is recognized. The predisposition to infection is severe, in part because the neutrophils which are present may not be functionally normal. The number of neutrophils and other host defenses are further suppressed by chemotherapy. When the neutrophil count is less than 500 per mm^3, especially in patients in relapse, fever and infection should be expected (Chap. 128).

In aplastic anemia, the infection risk is probably roughly proportional to the neutrophil count with the chance of a severe and possibly fatal infection being substantially increased with neutrophil counts below 500 per mm^3. The monocytopenia observed in these patients coupled with their neutropenia contributes substantially to the predisposition to infection.

Agranulocytosis (Schultz syndrome) Severe neutropenia occurs as an occasional or rare reaction to a great variety of drugs (Table 63-4). In most instances the patient is seen by the physician several weeks or months after beginning the offending agent and presents acutely ill with fever, sore throat, and oral or perianal ulceration. The total leukocyte count is often 1,000 to 2,000 per mm^3, and neutrophils are absent from the blood and bone marrow. Marrow examination generally will exclude leukemia as the cause. Marrow recovery is the rule if the patient can be sustained long enough after the drug is discontinued. The pathophysiologic mechanisms for these reactions remain poorly understood. Both toxic effects of drugs on neutrophil formation and immunologic mechanisms causing accelerated cell destruction have been proposed and demonstrated in a few instances.

With some drugs, e.g., chloramphenicol, phenothiazines, carbamazepine (Tegretol), and propylthiouracil, patients may have a gradually declining neutrophil count, probably due to suppressed neutrophil production. It is not absolutely certain that these patients will develop agranulocytosis if the drug is not discontinued. However, as a rule, the presumed offending agent should be discontinued if the neutrophil count falls below 3,000 per mm^3.

Neutropenia and hematotoxic drugs In sufficient doses, a great number of therapeutic agents predictably cause leukopenia and neutropenia. This is particularly true for the agents used in cancer chemotherapy and for immunosuppressive therapy of nonmalignant, inflammatory diseases (Chap. 323). These drugs reduce neutrophil production. If the neutrophil count is not allowed to drop below 1,000 to 2,000 cells per mm^3 or if the period of neutropenia is brief, infectious complications are infrequent.

Neutropenia and nutritional deficiencies Vitamin B_{12} and folic acid deficiency are sometimes accompanied by neutropenia as well as neutrophil hypersegmentation, particularly when folate deficiency is coupled with alcoholism. Copper deficiency, which may occur with chronic hyperalimentation, also reduces blood neutrophils.

Neutropenia with infections Certain infections may be accompanied by neutropenia. These include typhoid and paratyphoid fever (Chap. 140), brucellosis (Chap. 144), tularemia (Chap. 145), infectious mononucleosis (Chap. 209), infectious hepatitis (Chap. 299), yellow fever (Chap. 212), measles (Chap. 201) and many other viral infections, malaria (Chap. 215), kala azar (Chap. 216), and the rickettsial diseases (Chaps. 179 to 187). For the most part, these neutropenias are mild and their precise mechanisms are not known. It is postulated that they are largely due to redistribution of cells out of the circulating pool into an enlarged marginal pool. In certain overwhelming infections, for ex-

TABLE 63-4
Drugs producing neutropenia

INFREQUENTLY CAUSE NEUTROPENIA
Analgesics: Aminopyrine, dipyrone, salicylates
Anticonvulsants: Dilantin, carbamazepine
Anti-inflammatory drugs: Phenylbutazone
Antimicrobial agents: Chloramphenicol, penicillins, sulfonamides, organic arsenicals
Antithyroid agents: Propylthiouracil, methimazole
Phenothiazine: Chlorpromazine, promazine
Tranquilizers: Meprobamate
REGULARLY CAUSE NEUTROPENIA
Alkylating agents: Nitrogen mustard, busulfan, chlorambucil, cyclophosphamide
Antibiotics: Daunomycin
Antimetabolites: Methotrexate, 6-mercaptopurine, 5-fluorocytosine

ample, gram-negative bacteremia, pneumococcal pneumonia, and miliary tuberculosis, the occurrence of neutropenia portends a poor prognosis. This is particularly true in alcoholics, malnourished individuals, and patients with preexisting hematopoietic diseases.

Neutropenia with splenomegaly Neutropenia occurs in Felty's syndrome (Chap. 62), congestive splenomegaly (Chap. 62), Banti's syndrome (Chap. 62), Gaucher's disease (Chap. 113), and sarcoidosis (Chap. 228) as well as the infectious diseases with splenomegaly. There are often an associated mild thrombocytopenia and anemia. Splenic sequestration, as well as increased peripheral utilization, are proposed mechanisms. The predisposition to infection with these disorders is quite variable. Splenectomy to attempt to alter the neutropenia should be reserved for patients with repeated severe infections.

NEUTROPHIL DYSFUNCTION The normal functions of mature neutrophils are chemotaxis, phagocytosis, microbicidal action, and digestion of foreign material. There are a few specific diseases and syndromes in which these functions are abnormal. More commonly, defects in neutrophil function are observed which are secondary to other diseases such as alcoholism, diabetes mellitus, uremia, rheumatoid arthritis, and lupus erythematosus. Other defects occur secondary to abnormalities of complement and immunoglobulin metabolism.

Chemotaxis Accumulation of neutrophils in response to inflammation is most often deficient because of neutropenia. The tissue neutrophil response is also reduced by drugs, such as alcohol and glucocorticosteroids, which impair neutrophil adherence to the vascular endothelium. Chemotactic defects due to complement abnormalities have been observed chiefly in patients with either C3 or C5 deficiency. In general, defects permitting complement activation and C3 generation by the alternate complement pathway, for example, C1r, C2, and C4 deficiency, are associated with only a temporary delay in generation of chemotactic factor, and these patients have comparatively few infections. Defects in chemotaxis also may occur because of complement depletion in essential C3 hypercatabolism and possibly in acute glomerulonephritis and systemic lupus erythematosus. Chemotactic factor inactivators and inhibitors have been described in Hodgkin's disease, cirrhosis, uremia, and a few other circumstances. In patients with these complement-related disorders, the cells are usually normal when tested with normal serum. Cellular defects in chemotaxis have been described in the Chédiak-Higashi syndrome, lazy-leukocyte syndrome, newborn infants, and some patients with congenital ichthyosis, diabetes mellitus, rheumatoid arthritis, burns, hypogammaglobulinemia, and acute infections. In the lazy-leukocyte syndrome, the patients have gingivitis, stomatitis, and otitis with relatively few severe infections. They also have severe neutropenia, but the bone marrow shows ample mature neutrophils. The marrow neutrophils are not mobilized with endotoxin administration, and the cells show defective chemotaxis and random migration in vitro. In *Job's syndrome,* characterized by recurrent staphylococcal abscesses, eczema, and high IgE levels, a cellular defect in chemotaxis is also observed. Abnormal chemotaxis and defective phagocytosis have been recognized with hypophosphatemia and consequently diminished intracellular ATP. A specific chemotactic defect has been described resulting from the lack of the normal cellular contractile proteins necessary for cell movement.

Phagocytosis Reduced serum opsonic activity is the best-known cause for abnormal phagocytosis. This occurs in hypo- and agammaglobulinemia and certain complement disorders, including most of those with reduced chemotaxis, especially if activated C3 is not generated normally. Defective opsonic activity has been documented in premature infants, sickle-cell anemia, lupus erythematosus, and cirrhosis.

Microbicidal defects A few patients have reduced killing mechanisms because of isolated lysozomal enzyme deficiencies. In hereditary and acquired myeloperoxidase deficiency the leukocytes are morphologically normal except that specific staining shows decreased or absent myeloperoxidase. Eosinophil peroxidase is normal. The bactericidal and fungicidal defect is not as severe as in chronic granulomatous disease, and severe infections have been infrequent. Neutrophil lysozyme deficiency and total absence of secondary granules have been described with accompanying subnormal bactericidal activity.

CHRONIC GRANULOMATOUS DISEASE (CGD) This disorder is characterized by severe recurrent infections of the skin, lymph nodes, lungs, liver, and bones. The infections are caused chiefly by staphylococci and certain gram-negative bacteria (particularly *Escherichia coli, Serratia marcescens,* and *Salmonella*). Histologically the tissues usually show a granulomatous reaction, lipid-filled macrophages, and multiple small abscesses. The neutrophils are morphologically normal. Neutrophil production, blood counts, and chemotaxis are also normal. Other measures of host defenses, including delayed hypersensitivity and lymphocyte functions, are normal, but immunoglobulins may be increased. The neutrophils, as well as the monocytes, have a greatly impaired ability to kill the types of microorganisms with which these patients usually become infected. Phagocytosis of bacteria is normal, but the metabolic burst which follows ingestion is markedly blunted, and H_2O_2 is not generated normally. When CGD neutrophils phagocytize streptococci or pneumococci, these bacteria are killed normally because the bacteria contribute H_2O_2 from their own metabolism to the intracellular environment. This observation emphasizes the key role of the H_2O_2 in the intracellular bactericidal mechanism. The cellular defect is most easily measured by determining the amount of nitroblue tetrazolium (NBT) reduction which occurs when the patient's cells are incubated with this dye. Normally NBT is reduced intracellularly to a blue-black substance, blue formazan, which precipitates in the cell and can be seen as black intracellular particles. In CGD cells this reaction does not occur. The diagnosis is confirmed by observing that postphagocytic O_2 consumption, glucose C-1 oxidation, or the iodination reaction is reduced.

Recent studies indicate that NADPH oxidase may be the critically deficient enzyme in CGD. However, deficiencies of NADH oxidase, glutathione peroxidase, and other enzymes have been described in patients having typical

CGD. The genetic heterogeneity indicated by family studies and the variable clinical presentations of CGD suggest that several different molecular lesions may result in this clinical picture. In *familial lipochrome histiocytosis* the neutrophils have a similar defect, but this disorder is described only in women, has a late onset, and presents very striking lipid-laden histiocytes in many tissues. Severe *deficiency of leukocyte glucose 6-phosphate dehydrogenase* with G-6-PD levels less than 5 percent of normal is also accompanied by neutrophil dysfunction similar to CGD. The management of CGD and its variants depends upon careful observation and detection of infections as early as possible. Cultures of affected tissues are critical for the correct diagnosis and selection of the appropriate antibiotic. Prophylactic antibiotics have probably been useful for some cases but may be accompanied by the usual problems of superinfections and emergence of resistant organisms (Chap. 130).

CHÉDIAK-HIGASHI SYNDROME This rare autosomal recessive disease is characterized by partial albinism, giant lysosomal granules in most granule-containing cells (neutrophils, monocytes, hepatocytes, renal tubular cells), and increased susceptibility to infections. The abnormal blood cells are readily seen on routine blood smears. The disease is usually recognized in children. There are several neutrophil abnormalities including moderately severe neutropenia, reduced marrow neutrophil reserves, and reduced neutrophil chemotaxis. In addition, in microbicidal studies, the giant primary granules are observed to degranulate slowly and thereby delay the killing of phagocytized bacteria. The disease is also accompanied by an accelerated phase with lymphohistiocytic infiltration in the liver, spleen, nerves, and other tissues with accompanying dysfunctions. Treatment is limited to prompt antimicrobial therapy of infections which usually resolve slowly. In the accelerated phase, vincristine and prednisone have been used to retard organ infiltration.

Other neutrophil abnormalities Unusual morphologic abnormalities of neutrophils include hereditary hyposegmentation (Pelger-Huet anomaly); hereditary hypersegmentation; retained remnants of endoplasmic reticulum, chiefly composed of RNA (May-Hegglin anomaly and Doehle bodies); and abnormally large azurophilic granules (Alder-Reilly anomaly). These abnormalities apparently do not interfere with neutrophil function.

OTHER LEUKOCYTIC CELLS

LYMPHOCYTES The chief functions of lymphocytes are production of immunoglobulins and expression of cellular immunity. Immunoglobulins react directly with foreign substances, hastening their removal from the body by many mechanisms (Chap. 71). Cellular immunity is involved in delayed hypersensitivity and homograft rejection. Lymphocytes also can directly damage some foreign cells (cellular cytotoxicity).

On the blood smear, lymphocytes are a reasonably homogeneous collection of mononuclear cells with a small amount of blue cytoplasm containing a few granules. Through the analysis of surface receptors and responses to antigenic and mitogenic stimuli, it has been learned that there are two main types of lymphocytes, T and B cells, with strikingly different biological properties (Table 63-5).

There are undoubtedly other subpopulations of lymphocytes in man, and not every lymphocyte fits the scheme shown in the table. Human lymphocytes are formed chiefly in the bone marrow. Normal T cells develop only in the presence of a normally functioning thymus (Chap. 74). Labeling studies indicate that there is a huge overproduction or ineffective production of lymphocytes by the lymphoid organs but that a substantial portion of the cells which reach the blood may live for years. These long-lived cells are principally T cells. They recirculate through the spleen and lymph nodes, thoracic duct, and bone marrow, leaving and reentering the circulation repeatedly. The precise functions of the surface receptors on these cells are not known, but they are probably involved in antigen recognition and cell-to-cell interactions with macrophages and other lymphocytes.

Lymphocytosis An increase in the absolute lymphocyte count occurs in certain infections: infectious mononucleosis, infectious hepatitis, infectious lymphocytosis, pertussis, tuberculosis, brucellosis, syphilis, thyrotoxicosis, and adrenal insufficiency. A lymphocyte count of greater than 10,000 per mm^3 usually indicates chronic lymphocytic leukemia especially in older patients (Chap. 325). The term "relative lymphocytosis" is sometimes used to describe situations where neutrophils are decreased with an increase in the percentage, but not absolute number, of lymphocytes. This term is misleading and should not be used.

Lymphocytopenia An absolute lymphocyte count of less than 1,000 per mm^3 is observed in less than 5 percent of normal individuals but commonly occurs with acute, stressful illnesses such as myocardial infarction, pneumonia, or sepsis. A transient lymphocytopenia regularly occurs even with very small doses of glucocorticosteroids. Chronic lymphocytopenia occurs in a variety of malignancies, uremia, congestive heart failure, lymphomas (especial-

TABLE 63-5
Characteristics of T and B cells

	T	*B*
Origin	Bone marrow (with thymic influence)	Bone marrow
Life span	Long (months to years)	Short (probably days to weeks)
Circulating pattern	Chiefly recirculating	Chiefly nonrecirculating
Major location		
Lymph nodes	Deep cortical Perifollicular	Germinal centers Subcapsular
Spleen	Periarteriolar	Red pulp
Receptors	Sheep erythrocyte (rosettes) Mitogens (phytohemagglutinin)	Immunoglobulin (Fc) Complement (C3)
Functions		
Cellular immunity	4+	±
Antibody synthesis	0	4+

ly Hodgkin's disease), aplastic anemia, lupus erythematosus, intestinal lymphangiectasia, and other immunologic deficiency syndromes (Wiskott-Aldrich syndrome, ataxia telangiectasia, Di George's syndrome, Swiss-type agammaglobulinemia, and thymic alymphoplasia) (Chap. 74). It also occurs following treatment with antilymphocyte globulin and certain chemotherapeutic agents.

MONOCYTES Monocytes are phagocytic cells with bactericidal capacities similar to neutrophils but with distinctive physiologic characteristics. They form in the bone marrow from promonocytes and have lysosomal granules containing myeloperoxidase, lysozyme, and acid phosphatases. They spend less time in the marrow than neutrophils and enter the blood with mitochondria and protein synthetic capacity intact, able to complete their differentiation as the circumstances demand. Monocytes leave the blood more slowly than neutrophils with a half-disappearance time estimated to be 12 to 24 h. They accumulate after neutrophils in acute inflammations in response to monocyte chemotactic factors.

In response to pinocytosis of serum proteins or ingestion of foreign material, monocytes enlarge and synthesize increased amounts of lysosomal enzymes and thereby are transformed to more active phagocytes called "macrophages." Blood monocytes are the precursors of the pulmonary alveolar macrophages, spleen macrophages, and fixed macrophages of the monocyte-macrophage system (sometimes less precisely called the "reticuloendothelial system"). This system serves chiefly to remove foreign matter from the blood, e.g., bacteria, fungi, injected colloidal substances, and damaged or effete blood cells. During differentiation in each tissue site, monocytes acquire unique characteristics for that particular site. For instance, alveolar macrophages utilize chiefly oxidative phosphorylation to meet energy requirements, whereas peritoneal macrophages may chiefly utilize glycolysis. Generally, in all tissue sites these cells maintain the capacity to divide.

Monocytes have surface receptors for IgG, IgM, and complement, form rosettes with antibody-coated (IgG) erythrocytes, and are capable of synthesizing components of the complement system, transferrin, interferon, endogenous pyrogen, and colony-stimulating factor. In chronic inflammation they are probably responsible for the high serum and urine lysozyme concentrations. Monocytes serve a critical role in processing of antigen essential for both cellular and humoral immunity. They respond to lymphocyte-derived chemotactic and immobilizing factors (migration inhibitory factor, MIF). The incompletely catabolized endogenous materials generated in Gaucher's, Niemann-Pick's, and Fabry's diseases also accumulate in monocytes.

Monocytosis Increases in blood monocytes are observed in certain infections: tuberculosis, subacute bacterial endocarditis, brucellosis, Rocky Mountain spotted fever, malaria, and kala azar; in granulomatous diseases: sarcoidosis, regional enteritis; in some collagen vascular diseases and in malignancies. Monocytosis may occur in leukemia and preleukemia, lymphomas, myeloproliferative syndromes, hemolytic anemias, and chronic idiopathic neutropenia.

Monocytopenia Reduced blood monocyte counts are seen acutely with stress and following glucocorticosteroid administration. Monocytopenia is observed in many acute infections, with aplastic anemia and acute leukemia, and as a direct effect of myelotoxic and immunosuppressive drugs.

EOSINOPHILS Many diseases are encountered where blood or tissue eosinophils are increased (Table 63-6). Eosinophils develop in the bone marrow similar to neutrophils. Their characteristic red-staining granules contain a unique peroxidase. Eosinophils have microbicidal capacities, and although these cells are chiefly involved in allergic and immune responses, their precise function in these responses is not known. Eosinophils are selectively attracted by an eosinophilic chemotactic factor elaborated by lymphocytes in response to certain stimuli. Eosinophils also accumulate in the skin in response to the topical application of allergens in allergic individuals. Animal studies indicate that the blood pool of eosinophils is relatively small compared with the number of these cells in various tissues. Significant tissue eosinophilia may occur in many inflammatory states, not necessarily accompanied by marked blood eosinophilia.

Eosinophilia More than 500 eosinophils per mm^3 blood is infrequent in normal individuals. The most common cause for mild eosinophilia in hospitalized patients is probably some form of drug allergy. Parasitic infections, principally helminthic infections, cause eosinophilia, especially during the invasive phase. Some parasites may be difficult to recognize, e.g., strongyloides (Chap. 221), trichinella (Chap. 223), toxocara (Chap. 221), and filariae (Chap. 224). In these diseases the eosinophil count is rarely greater than 25,000 per mm^3 with the highest counts probably occurring in trichinosis. Protozoan infections generally do not cause eosinophilia. Eosinophilia is usually mild and irregularly present in allergic and collagen vascular diseases and malignancies and is not necessarily a clear guide to disease activity. The hypereosinophilic syndromes cause the highest eosinophil counts, occasionally in the 50,000 to 100,000 per mm^3 range or higher. Many tissues become infiltrated by eosinophils, a condition leading to organ dysfunction, particularly congestive heart failure.

Eosinopenia A reduction in eosinophils occurs with any stress or following corticosteroid administration. No known adverse effects result.

TABLE 63-6
Causes of blood eosinophilia

Drug reactions: Iodides, aspirin, sulfonamides, nitrofurantoin (see Chap. 67)
Parasitic infections: Hookworm disease, strongyloidiasis, toxocariasis, trichuriasis, trichinosis, filariasis, schistosomiasis, echinococcosis, cysticercosis
Allergic diseases: Hay fever, asthma, angioedema, serum sickness, allergic vasculitis, eczema, pemphigus
Collagen vascular diseases: Rheumatoid arthritis, dermatomyositis, periarteritis nodosa
Malignancy: Hodgkin's disease, carcinomatosis, mycosis fungoides, chronic myelogenous leukemia
Hypereosinophilic syndromes: Loeffler's syndrome, Loeffler's endocarditis, eosinophilic leukemia

BASOPHILS These are the least common blood leukocytes; usually none are seen in the routine examination of a blood smear. The distinctive deep-blue granules, characteristically obscuring the cell nucleus, are rich in histamine. These cells are thought to be involved in certain acute allergic responses. Basophils are increased in chronic myelogenous leukemia, myelofibrosis, and polycythemia vera. This finding helps to distinguish these diseases from leukemoid reactions. Basophilia may also be observed occasionally in some chronic inflammatory conditions.

REFERENCES

CHUSID MJ et al: The hypereosinophilic syndrome. Medicine 54:1, 1975

CRADDOCK CG et al: Lymphocytes and the immune response. N Engl J Med 285:324, 1971

GOLDE DW, CLINE MJ: Regulation of granulopoiesis. N Engl J Med 291:1388, 1974

KLEBANOFF SJ: Antimicrobial mechanisms in neutrophilic polymorphonuclear leukocytes. Semin Hematol 12:117, 1975

QUIE PG: Pathology of bactericidal power of neutrophils. Semin Hematol 12:143, 1975

ROWLANDS DT, DANIELE RP: Surface receptors in the immune response. N Engl J Med 293:26, 1975

STOSSEL TP: Phagocytosis. N Engl J Med 290:717, 774, 833, 1974

VAN FURTH R (ed): *Mononuclear Phagocytes in Immunity, Infection and Pathology,* Oxford: Blackwell, 1975

WILLIAMS WJ et al: *Hematology,* New York: McGraw-Hill, 1972

WINTROBE MM et al: *Clinical Hematology,* 7th ed., Philadelphia: Lea & Febiger, 1974

PART THREE | BIOLOGICAL CONSIDERATIONS IN THE APPROACH TO CLINICAL MEDICINE

section 1 | Genetics and human disease

64 GENETIC ASPECTS OF HUMAN DISEASE

JOSEPH L. GOLDSTEIN
MICHAEL S. BROWN

GENETIC PRINCIPLES

More than one-third of the proteins (and hence genes) in each human being exist in a form that differs from the one present in the majority of the population. This remarkable degree of genetic variability, or polymorphism, among "normal" people accounts for much of the naturally occurring variation in body traits such as height, intelligence, and blood pressure. Moreover, these genetic differences produce marked variations in the ability of individuals to handle every environmental challenge, including those that produce disease. Thus, every human disease can be considered to occur as a result of an interaction between a given individual's genetic makeup and his environment. In certain diseases, however, the genetic component is so overwhelming that it expresses itself in a predictable manner without a requirement for extraordinary environmental challenges. Such diseases are termed *genetic disorders.*

MOLECULAR BASIS OF GENE EXPRESSION All hereditary information is transmitted from parent to offspring through the inheritance of specific molecules of deoxyribonucleic acid (DNA). DNA is a linear polymer composed of purine and pyrimidine bases whose sequence ultimately determines the sequence of amino acids in every protein molecule made by the body. The four types of bases in DNA are arranged in groups of three, each group forming a code word, or codon, that signifies a particular amino acid. A *gene* represents the total sequence of bases in DNA that specifies the amino acid sequence of a single polypeptide chain of a protein molecule.

In order to be translated into a polypeptide, each DNA region corresponding to a gene must first be transcribed within the cell nucleus into a molecule called *messenger ribonucleic acid* (mRNA). The mRNA represents a sequence of purine and pyrimidine bases that is "complementary" to that of the DNA. Hence, each adenine of DNA becomes a uridine of RNA, each cytosine of DNA becomes a guanine of RNA, each thymine of DNA becomes an adenine of RNA, and each guanine of DNA becomes a cytosine of RNA. Figure 64-1 shows the DNA and mRNA code words for each of the 20 amino acids that are utilized to form proteins.

The mRNA leaves the cell nucleus and enters the cytoplasm where it becomes associated with *ribosomes* and thereby serves as a template for the ribosomal synthesis of proteins. Each of the 20 precursor amino acids for protein synthesis is attached in the cell cytoplasm to specific molecules called *transfer RNA* (tRNA). Each tRNA contains a sequence of purine and pyrimidine bases that is "complementary" to a specific codon in the mRNA. These tRNA molecules with their attached amino acids line up along the mRNA molecule in the precise order dictated by the mRNA code. Under the action of a variety of cytoplasmic enzymes (initiation factors, elongation factors, and termination factors), peptide bonds are formed between the various amino acids, and the completed protein is released from the ribosome. A schematic diagram of the genetic control of protein synthesis is shown in Fig. 64-2.

MAINTENANCE OF GENETIC DIVERSITY THROUGH TRANSMISSION AND SEGREGATION OF GENES It is estimated that the amount of DNA in the nucleus of each human cell is sufficient to code for more than 100,000 genes and hence to specify more than 100,000 polypeptide chains. The genes are arranged in a linear sequence of DNA that together with certain histone proteins form rod-shaped bodies called *chromosomes.* Each human cell contains 46 chromosomes, arranged in 23 pairs, one of each pair derived from each of the individual's parents. Thus, each individual inherits two copies of each chromosome and hence two copies of each gene. The chromosomal location of the two copies of each gene is termed the *genetic locus.* When a gene occupying a genetic locus exists in two

Second nucleotide

First nucleotide	A or *U*			G or *C*			T or *A*			C or *G*			Third nucleotide
A	**AAA**	*UUU*	Phe	**AGA**	*UCU*	Ser	**ATA**	*UAU*	Tyr	**ACA**	*UGU*	Cys	A or *U*
or	**AAG**	*UUC*		**AGG**	*UCC*		**ATG**	*UAC*		**ACG**	*UGC*		G or *C*
U	**AAT**	*UUA*	Leu	**AGT**	*UCA*		**ATT**	*UAA*	Stop	**ACT**	*UGA*	Stop	T or *A*
	AAC	*UUG*		**AGC**	*UCG*		**ATC**	*UAG*		**ACC**	*UGG*	Trp	C or *G*
	GAA	*CUU*	Leu	**GGA**	*CCU*	Pro	**GTA**	*CAU*	His	**GCA**	*CGU*	Arg	A or *U*
G	**GAG**	*CUC*		**GGG**	*CCC*		**GTG**	*CAC*		**GCG**	*CGC*		G or *C*
or	**GAT**	*CUA*		**GGT**	*CCA*		**GTT**	*CAA*	Gln	**GCT**	*CGA*		T or *A*
C	**GAC**	*CUG*		**GGC**	*CCG*		**GTC**	*CAG*		**GCC**	*CGG*		C or *G*
	TAA	*AUU*	Ile	**TGA**	*ACU*	Thr	**TTA**	*AAU*	Asn	**TCA**	*AGU*	Ser	A or *U*
T	**TAG**	*AUC*		**TGG**	*ACC*		**TTG**	*AAC*		**TCG**	*AGC*		G or *C*
or	**TAT**	*AUA*		**TGT**	*ACA*		**TTT**	*AAA*	Lys	**TCT**	*AGA*	Arg	T or *A*
A	**TAC**	*AUG*	Met	**TGC**	*ACG*		**TTC**	*AAG*		**TCC**	*AGG*		C or *G*
	CAA	*GUU*	Val	**CGA**	*GCU*	Ala	**CTA**	*GUA*	Asp	**CCA**	*GGU*	Gly	A or *U*
C	**CAG**	*GUC*		**CGG**	*GCC*		**CTG**	*GAC*		**CCG**	*GGC*		G or *C*
or	**CAT**	*GUA*		**CGT**	*GCA*		**CTT**	*GAA*	Glu	**CCT**	*GGA*		T or *A*
G	**CAC**	*GUG*		**CGC**	*GCG*		**CTC**	*GAG*		**CCC**	*GGG*		C or *G*

Note: The DNA codons appear in boldface type; the complementary RNA codons are in italics. A = adenine, C = cytosine, G = guanine, T = thymine, U = uridine (replaces thymine in RNA). In RNA, adenine is complementary to thymine of DNA; uridine is complementary to adenine of DNA; cytosine is complementary to guanine, and vice versa. "Stop" = termination. The amino acids are abbreviated as follows:

Ala = alanine	*Cys = cysteine*	*His = histidine*	*Met = methionine*	*Thr = threonine*
Arg = arginine	*Gln = glutamine*	*Ile = isoleucine*	*Phe = phenylalanine*	*Trp = tryptophan*
Asn = asparagine	*Glu = glutamic acid*	*Leu = leucine*	*Pro = proline*	*Tyr = tyrosine*
Asp = aspartic acid	*Gly = glycine*	*Lys = lysine*	*Ser = serine*	*Val = valine*

FIGURE 64-1
The genetic code.

or more different forms, these alternate forms of the gene are referred to as *alleles.*

In humans, a given gene resides at a specified genetic locus on one particular chromosome. For example, the genetic locus for the Rh blood group is on chromosome 1; at this chromosomal site there are two Rh genes, one on chromosome 1 derived from the mother and the other on chromosome 1 derived from the father. When two genes at the same genetic locus are identical, the individual is a *homozygote.* When the two genes differ (i.e., two alleles are present at the locus), the individual is a *heterozygote.* Each individual is homozygous at some loci and heterozygous at others. Figure 64-3 shows a map of human chromosome 1, illustrating the location of those genes that have been assigned loci on this chromosome.

FIGURE 64-2
A schematic diagram of the genetic control of protein synthesis, illustrating the flow of genetic information from DNA to messenger RNA (mRNA) to the polypeptide chain of a protein molecule. Although DNA exists in a double-stranded form, only one of the two strands is used as a template for transcribing mRNA.

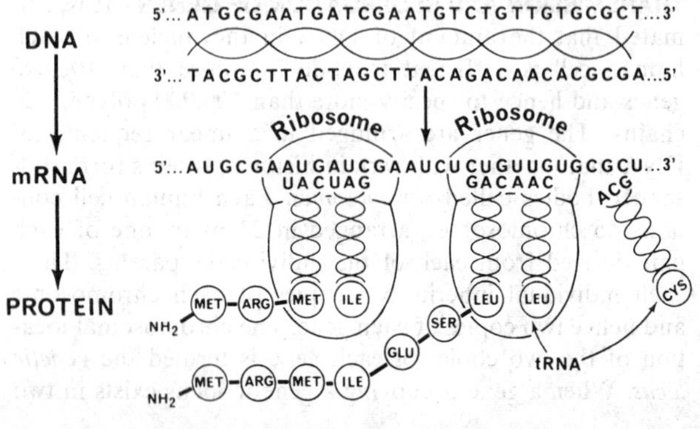

The genetic information carried on chromosomes is transmitted to daughter cells under two different sets of circumstances. One of these occurs whenever a somatic cell (i.e., a nongerm cell) divides. This process, called *mitosis,* functions to transmit identical copies of each gene to each daughter cell, thus maintaining a uniform genetic makeup in all cells of a single organism. The other set of circumstances prevails when genetic information is to be transmitted from one individual to an offspring. This process, called *meiosis,* functions to produce germ cells (i.e., eggs or spermatozoa) that possess only one copy of each parental chromosome, thus allowing for new combinations of chromosomes to occur when egg and sperm cells fuse during fertilization.

During the process of meiosis, the 46 chromosomes of an immature germ cell arrange themselves in 23 pairs at the center of the nucleus, each pair being composed of one chromosome derived from the mother and its homologous chromosome derived from the father. At a specified point in the meiotic process, the two partner chromosomes separate, only one of each pair going into each daughter cell, or gamete. Thus, meiosis produces gametes with a reduction in the number of chromosomes from 46 to 23, each gamete having received one chromosome from each of the 23 pairs. The assortment of the chromosomes within each pair is random so that each germ cell receives a different combination of maternal and paternal chromosomes. During the process of fertilization, the fusion of egg and sperm cells, each of which has 23 chromosomes, results ultimately in an individual with 46 chromosomes.

The independent assortment of chromosomes into gametes during meiosis produces an enormous diversity among the possible genotypes of the progeny. For each 23 pairs of chromosomes, there are 2^{23} different combinations of chromosomes that could occur in a gamete, and the likelihood that one set of parents will produce two offspring with the identical complement of chromosomes is one in $2^{23} \times 2^{23}$ or one in 7×10^{13} (assuming no monozygotic or identical twins).

RECOMBINATION Adding even further to the enormous genetic diversity in humans is the phenomenon of *genetic recombination.* During meiosis, when homologous chromosomes are paired, bridges frequently form between corresponding regions of the chromosome pair. These bridges, or *chiasmata,* are regions in which the two chromosomes break at identical points along their length and subsequently rejoin, the distal segments having been switched from one homologous chromosome to another. This process is designated *crossing over.* Although no net change in the amount of genetic material occurs during crossing over, a recombination of genes does occur. For example, consider a chromosome with two loci, A and B, located at opposite ends of the same chromosome. On this particular chromosome, the A locus has a rare allele x and the B locus also has a rare allele y. Without the phenomenon of recombination every offspring that inherited the x allele at the A locus would also inherit the y allele at the B locus. However, if recombination occurs, the A locus with the x allele would then be on the opposite chromosome from the B locus with the y allele. In this case any offspring that inherited the x allele at the A locus could not inherit the y allele at the B locus.

Crossing over in humans occurs with great frequency in every meiosis, and the resultant recombination of genes may occur at any point on a chromosome. The farther apart two genes are on the same chromosome, the greater is the likelihood that a crossing over will occur in the space between them. When two genes are on the opposite ends of a long chromosome, the probability of recombination is so great that their respective alleles are transmitted to offspring almost independently of one another, just as if the two gene loci were on different chromosomes. On the other hand, gene loci that are close together on the same chromosome are said to be *linked* so that there is a great likelihood that offspring will inherit the same combination of alleles that are present on the parental chromosome.

Several examples of *gene linkage* can be seen from the map of human chromosome 1 (Fig. 64-3). For example, the locus for the gene specifying the Rh blood group factor and the locus for the gene producing one form of the dominant trait, hereditary elliptocytosis, occur in close proximity on this chromosome. Thus, if a subject with hereditary elliptocytosis transmits the disease to an offspring, the offspring will usually inherit the allele that is present at the Rh locus on this chromosome. If the Rh allele happens to be a rare one in the population (such as r'), one can assume that whichever offspring inherits the r' allele at the Rh locus will also inherit the abnormal allele at the elliptocytosis locus. On the other hand, if an offspring does not exhibit the r' allele, he or she will not usually have elliptocytosis. The concept of linkage does not imply an association between any particular set of Rh alleles and the disease state elliptocytosis, but rather between the two genetic loci. Thus, in different families the abnormal elliptocytosis allele may be linked to the R^1, R^0, r_2, or any other allele at the Rh locus, depending on the allele that happened to be at that locus when the elliptocytosis mutation occurred. Stated another way, the elliptocytosis locus is linked to the Rh locus in every family, but the particular Rh allele with which it is associated will differ from family to family.

MUTATION Broadly defined, a *mutation* is a stable, heritable alteration in DNA. Although the causes of mutation in humans are largely unknown, a variety of environmental

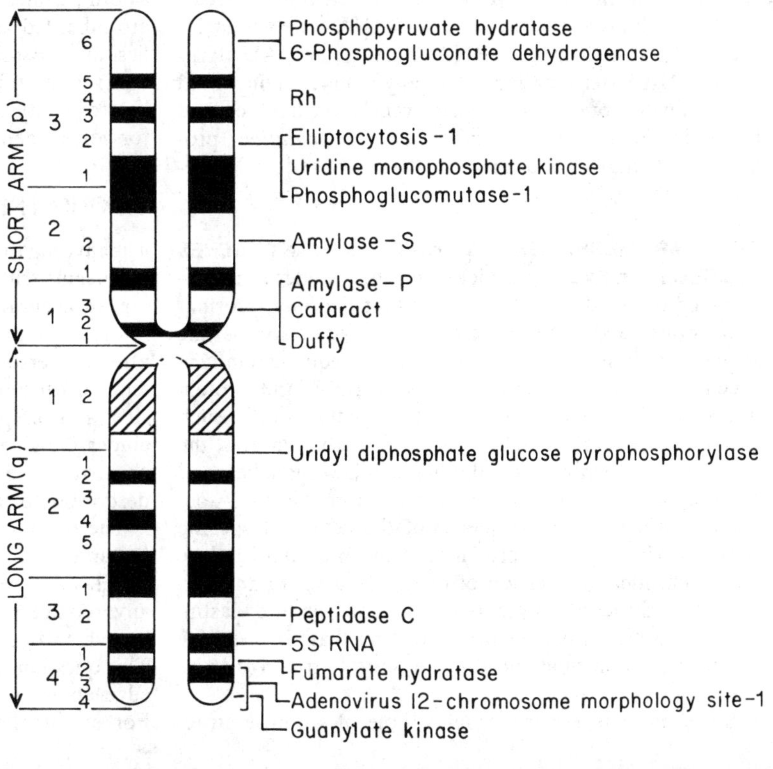

FIGURE 64-3
Gene map of human chromosome 1. This single chromosome is shown as it occurs in the metaphase stage of cell division, having replicated but not yet divided. The unseparated homologous parts are known as chromatids *and remain attached at the centromere. The portions of a chromatid extending above and below the centromere are the* chromosome arms. *The black bands represent those genetic regions of the chromosome that stain brightly by a fluorescent dye such as quinacrine; the white bands are the negatively staining regions; the hatched area is a variable region that stains differently (i.e., either brightly or negatively) in the chromosomes of different individuals. The numbered designations for the various segments of the chromosome are listed on the left. Each gene that has been localized to this chromosome is listed opposite its genetic locus on the right. (Data provided by Frank H. Ruddle and Victor A. McKusick)*

agents, such as radiation, viruses, and chemicals, are among the factors that are implicated.

Mutations can involve a visible alteration in the structure of a chromosome, such as a deletion or translocation of a portion of a chromosome (see below), or they can involve a minute change in one of the purine or pyrimidine bases of a single gene. Most commonly, such "point" mutations consist of the substitution of one base for another, changing the meaning of the codon containing that base, hence their designation as *missense mutations.* For example, in the gene coding for the β-chain of hemoglobin, the sixth position normally contains either the nucleotide triplet CTT or CTC, both of which code for the amino acid glutamic acid (Fig. 64-1). The mutation that gives rise to hemoglobin C produces a change of the first base of this triplet from cytosine to thymine, changing the triplet to TTT or TTC, either of which codes for lysine. On the other hand, the mutation that gives rise to hemoglobin S produces a change in the second base of the same triplet (from thymine to adenine), producing either CAT or CAC, which codes for valine. Thus, in the sixth position of the β-chain of hemoglobin, the normally occurring glutamic acid may be replaced with either lysine (producing hemoglobin C) or valine (producing hemoglobin S). More than 84 such single-base mutations in the hemoglobin β-chain have been identified in different population groups, and many of these mutations produce a different clinical syndrome. Of all the mutations so far elucidated in humans, the vast majority involve such single-base changes.

Besides producing an amino acid substitution, a single-base substitution can also cause another abnormality in protein synthesis—premature chain termination. Three mRNA code words (UAA, UAG, and UGA) normally do not specify an amino acid but constitute the signal that the message has ended and that the protein chain should be released from the ribosome (Fig. 64-1). If a change occurs in DNA that produces one of these mRNA code words [for example, a switch in an mRNA triplet from UAU (tyrosine) to UAA (termination)], the polypeptide chain would be terminated prematurely when translation had reached that point. Such mutations, called *non-sense mutations,* produce short fragments of proteins that have reduced function.

CELLULAR MECHANISM BY WHICH MUTANT GENES PRODUCE DISEASES Critical to the modern understanding of heredity is the concept that the only information transmitted from generation to generation is the sequence of bases in DNA and that these sequences in turn specify only the primary structure of RNA and protein molecules. All other chemical reactions within a cell—such as the synthesis of complex lipids and carbohydrates, the formation of membranes and other cellular organelles, and the accumulation and partitioning of inorganic ions—occur as a secondary consequence of the action of specific proteins. Many of these proteins are enzymes that catalyze the biochemical conversion of one molecule into another. Others are structural proteins such as collagen and elastin, and still others are regulatory proteins that dictate how much of each enzyme and each structural protein is to be made.

Since proteins are the cellular molecules whose structures are encoded by genes, mutations in genes exert their deleterious effects by altering the structure of enzymes, structural proteins, or regulatory proteins. For example, in a disease such as glycogen storage disease, type I (von Gierke's disease), massive accumulation of glycogen in the liver is due not to a primary structural abnormality in the polysaccharide glycogen but to a structural abnormality in a protein, glucose 6-phosphatase, an enzyme that is required to liberate glucose from glycogen. Other examples of the biochemical mechanisms by which mutant genes alter cellular metabolism are discussed below in Simply Inherited Disorders.

GENETIC HETEROGENEITY When two or more mutations can produce a similar clinical syndrome, genetic heterogeneity is said to exist. Hemophilia is one example of such a genetically heterogeneous syndrome. A clinically similar bleeding disorder can be caused by mutations at either of two different loci on the X chromosome, one leading to a deficiency of factor VIII (classic hemophilia) and the other causing a deficiency of factor IX (Christmas disease). It is now generally believed that most, if not all, hereditary diseases, when carefully analyzed, will be shown to be genetically heterogeneous.

Genetic heterogeneity may result from the existence of a series of different mutations at a single genetic locus (allelic mutations) or from mutations at different genetic loci (nonallelic mutations). The hemoglobinopathies (e.g., sickle-cell anemia and sickle-cell hemoglobinopathy) are examples of allelic mutations in the gene encoding the β-chain of hemoglobin that can produce a similar clinical phenotype. Hemophilia is an example of a syndrome in which nonallelic mutations can produce a similar clinical picture (see above).

In some cases of heterogeneity, both the genetic locus and the mode of inheritance will differ, depending on the mutation. For example, spastic paraplegia, Charcot-Marie-Tooth peroneal muscular atrophy, and retinitis pigmentosa are inherited as autosomal dominant traits in some families, as autosomal recessives in others, and as X-linked recessives in still others. The identification of such genetic heterogeneity in these disorders is of obvious importance for correct genetic counseling.

TAKING THE FAMILY HISTORY

The investigation of a patient with a possible genetic disorder begins with the *family history.* The first step in obtaining an accurate family history involves obtaining certain information on the *proband* or *index case* (i.e., the clinically affected person who has brought the family to attention) and on each of the *first-degree relatives* (i.e., the parents, sibs, and offspring of the proband). This information includes the given name, surname, maiden name, birth date or current age, age at death, cause of death, and name or description of any disease or defect.

The second step includes asking six questions designed to survey the family for the presence of disease or defect. (1) Has any relative an identical or similar trait? (2) Has any relative a trait that is absent in the proband but is known to occur in some patients with the same disease? This question requires that the physician have some knowledge about the manifestations of the disease in question. For example, when obtaining the family history from a proband with dissecting aneurysm caused possibly by Marfan's syndrome, one should ask about the occurrence of eye abnormalities, cardiac abnormalities, and skeletal abnormalities in the proband's relatives. (3) Has any relative a trait that is recognized to be genetically determined? The purpose of this question is to ascertain the occurrence of hereditary disease in the family even though the patient himself may not be involved. (4) Has any relative an unusual disease, or has any relative died of a rare condition? The purpose of this question is to identify a condition that might be genetically determined though not recognized as such by the informant. In addition, this question may help to identify conditions in relatives that might be etiologically related to the patient's problem. For example, a patient with pheochromocytoma should be suspected of having von Recklinghausen's disease if he has a brother with scoliosis and mental retardation, both of which can be manifestations of the neurofibromatosis (von Recklinghausen's) gene. (5) Is there any consanguinity in the family? This inquiry should be made directly, but in addition one should ask whether common last names appear in the families of husband-wife pairs. Consanguineous marriage may be the source of a rare autosomal recessive syndrome, and sometimes its presence in the family may not be known by the proband. (6) What is the ethnic origin of the family? Persons of various ethnic origins, such as blacks, Jews, and Greeks, have increased chance of specific genetic diseases. Table 64-1 lists examples of simply inherited disorders that are found with increased frequency in various ethnic groups.

CATEGORIES OF GENETIC DISORDERS

Genetic diseases generally fall into one of three categories: (1) *Chromosomal disorders* involve the lack, excess, or abnormal arrangement of one or more chromosomes, producing excessive or deficient genetic material. (2) *Mendelian or simply inherited disorders* are determined primarily by a single mutant gene. This is indicated by the fact that these disorders display simple (mendelian) inheritance patterns which can be classified into autosomal dominant, autosomal recessive, or X-linked types. (3) *Multifactorial disorders* are caused by an interaction of multiple genes and multiple exogenous or environmental factors. Although many of these multifactorial disorders, such as essential hypertension and cleft lip and palate, are said to run in families, the inheritance pattern is complex and the risk to relatives is much less than that seen in the single-gene (mendelian) disorders. Each of these three categories of genetic disease presents different problems with respect to causation, prevention, diagnosis, genetic counseling, and treatment.

Chromosomal disorders

The karyotype of an individual (i.e., the number and structure of the chromosomes) can be ascertained from readily accessible body tissues, such as peripheral blood lymphocytes or skin, by growing them in tissue culture until active cell proliferation occurs and then preparing single cells for examination of chromosomes by microscopy. Recent developments have made it possible to identify accurately each individual chromosome by special staining of DNA sequences, by the affinity of fluorescent dyes (such as quinacrine hydrochloride) for certain chromosomal segments

that can be visualized by fluorescence microscopy, and by treatment with special dyes (Giemsa) and proteolytic enzymes (trypsin). These techniques produce characteristic *banding patterns* for each chromosome (Fig. 64-4).

The number of chromosomes in normal individuals is 46, of which 44 are the 22 pairs of *autosomes* and the other two are the *sex chromosomes.* Females have two X chromosomes (XX), and males have one X chromosome and one Y chromosome (XY). Each of the 22 pairs of autosomes and the two sex chromosomes can be distinguished on the basis of size, location of the centromere (which divides the chromosome into arms of equal or unequal length), and the unique banding pattern (Fig. 64-4). The relative length of the arms and the position of the centromere are used as further criteria to divide the human chromosomes into seven groups (designated A to G) (Fig. 64-4).

TABLE 64-1
Examples of simply inherited disorders that occur with increased frequency in specific ethnic groups

Ethnic group	*Simply inherited disorder*
African blacks	Hemoglobinopathies, especially HbS, HbC, persistent α- and β-thalassemias Glucose 6-phosphate dehydrogenase deficiency
Armenians	Familial Mediterranean fever
Ashkenazi Jews	Abetalipoproteinemia Bloom's syndrome Dystonia musculorum deformans (recessive form) Factor XI (PTA) deficiency Familial dysautonomia (Riley-Day syndrome) Gaucher's disease (adult form) Neimann-Pick disease Pentosuria Tay-Sachs disease
Chinese	α-Thalassemia Glucose 6-phosphate dehydrogenase deficiency Adult lactase deficiency
Eskimos	Pseudocholinesterase deficiency Adrenogenital syndrome
Finns	Congenital nephrosis
French Canadians	Tyrosinemia
Japanese	Acatalasemia
Lebanese	Homozygous familial hypercholesterolemia
Mediterranean peoples (Italians, Greeks, Sephardic Jews)	β-Thalassemia Glucose 6-phosphate dehydrogenase deficiency Familial Mediterranean fever Glycogen storage disease, type III
Northern Europeans	Cystic fibrosis
Scandinavians	α_1-Antitrypsin deficiency
South African whites	Porphyria variegata

SOURCE: *Data modified from McKusick, pp. xv–lvi, 1975.*

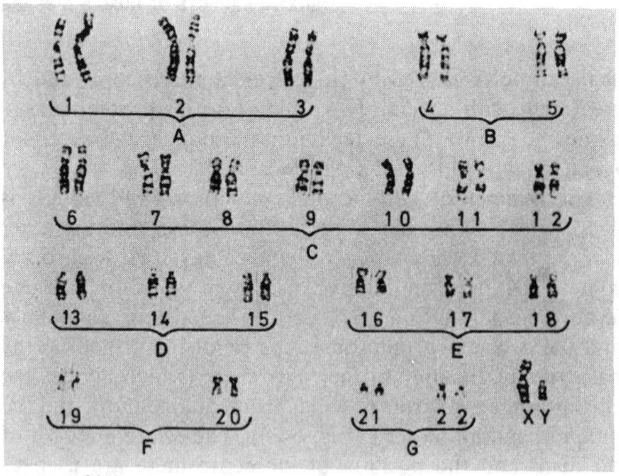

FIGURE 64-4
The karyotype of a normal male showing the chromosomes of a single somatic cell in the metaphase stage of cell division. The photographic images of the chromosomes have been cut out and arranged according to descending length and varying arm ratio. The chromosomes have been stained by the Giemsa technique, which allows each chromosome pair to be identified by its unique banding pattern. Chromosomes 1 to 22 are the autosomes. The sex chromosomes in this normal male are an X and a Y. The normal female has an identical karyotype except for the absence of the Y chromosome and the presence instead of a second X chromosome. (Courtesy of Kurt Hirschhorn)

CHROMOSOMAL SYNDROMES Most chromosomal disorders found in humans can be classified into one of four groups: (1) Excess or loss of one or more chromosomes (*aneuploidy*); (2) breakage and loss of a piece of a chromosome (*deletion*); (3) breakage of two chromosomes with transfer and fusion of parts of the broken fragments onto each other (*translocation*); and (4) abnormal splitting of the centromere during mitosis so that one arm is lost and the other is duplicated to form one symmetrical chromosome with two genetically identical arms (*isochromosome formation*). In addition, chromosomal *mosaicism* may occur such that a single individual may possess two cell lines, or *clones,* each differing in its chromosomal constitution. For example, a large portion of patients with Turner's syndrome have been shown to possess some cells with a 45 XO constitution and other cells with a normal 46 XX. Their karyotype is symbolized 45 XO/46 XX.

The most important of the autosomal syndromes involving a numerical abnormality are those that are due to the presence of three rather than two copies of a particular chromosome. The *autosomal trisomies* responsible for specific clinical syndromes include (1) trisomy 21 (Down's syndrome, or mongolism), characterized by mental retardation, a characteristic facies, and marked hypotonia; (2) trisomy 13, characterized by ocular coloboma, cleft lip and palate, polydactyly, and average life span under one year; and (3) trisomy 18, characterized by micrognathia, severe failure to thrive, multiple malformations, and life span under three months.

The numerical aberrations of the sex chromosomes include three disorders with 47 chromosomes (47 XXY, 47 XYY, and 47 XXX) and one disorder with 45 chromosomes (45 XO). The XXY karyotype is found in the majority of patients with Klinefelter's syndrome, which is characterized by testicular dysgenesis, infertility, gynecomastia, tallness, and behavioral changes. Most men with a 47 XYY karyotype seem to be normal and fertile; however, some may be unusually tall and show tendencies to criminality and other behavioral abnormalities. Women with the 47 XXX karyotype are usually clinically normal but may be mentally retarded and deficient in secondary sexual development. The 45 XO karyotype is found in about one-half of patients with Turner's syndrome, which is characterized by ovarian dysgenesis, failure of secondary sexual development, shortness of stature, renal anomalies, and pterygium coli. The other one-half of patients with Turner's syndrome who do not have a 45 XO karyotype prove to have either mosaicism (45 XO/46 XX or 45 XO/46 XY) or a structural abnormality of the X chromosome, such as an isochromosome-X.

The nuclei of all somatic cells of women (i.e., all body cells except the oogonia) possess a chromatin mass, called the *sex chromatin* or *Barr body.* The Barr body is not present in the somatic cells of men. The Barr body represents the one inactivated X chromosome in each female cell as predicted by the Lyon hypothesis (discussed below). The number of Barr bodies in a nucleus is one less than the number of X chromosomes. Thus, in Turner's syndrome (45 XO) and in normal men (46 XY), no Barr body is seen; in Klinefelter's syndrome (47 XXY) and in normal women (46 XX), a single Barr body occurs; and in 47 XXX women, two Barr bodies are seen. The epithelial cells of the buccal mucosa provide the most convenient source of tissue for determining the number of Barr bodies in a patient with a suspected disorder of the sex chromosomes. Table 64-2 shows a correlation between sex phenotype, sex chromatin, and sex chromosomes in a variety of clinical disorders.

Numerical aberrations of autosomes and sex chromosomes appear to arise through nondisjunction either during meiosis in one parent (i.e., in spermatogenesis or oogenesis) or in the first mitotic cleavage of the zygote. In meiotic nondisjunction, both chromosomes of a given pair pass

TABLE 64-2
Correlations of phenotype, sex chromatin, and sex chromosomes

	Sex phenotype	*Barr bodies (maximum number per cell)*	*Sex-chromosome constitution*
Normal male	Male		XY
Testicular feminization syndrome	Female (with testes)		XY
Double Y (or XYY) male	Male		XYY
Turner's syndrome	Female		XO
Normal female	Female		XX
Klinefelter's syndrome	Male		XXY
Klinefelter's syndrome	Male		XXYY
Triple X syndrome	Female	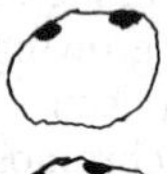	XXX
Triple X-Y syndrome	Male		XXXY
Tetra X syndrome	Female	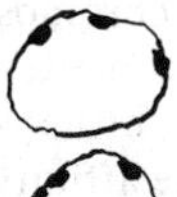	XXXX
Tetra X-Y syndrome	Male		XXXXY
Penta X syndrome	Female	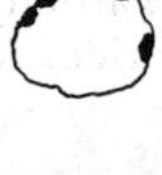	XXXXX

into one gamete rather than separating so that during fertilization when an additional copy is added there are three copies of the same chromosome in the new zygote forming the embryo instead of the pair found in normal persons. The cause of chromosomal nondisjunction is unknown.

Of the chromosomal aberrations due to translocations, the most important clinical syndromes are those due to a rearrangement between chromosomes 14 and 21 (D/G translocations) and those due to a rearrangement between chromosomes 21 and 22 (G/G translocations). Both types of translocations can result in the presence of excess material from chromosome 21 in an individual and can produce Down's syndrome. About 10 percent of patients with Down's syndrome born to women below age thirty have a translocation (either 14/21 or G/G). On karyotype analysis, patients with 14/21 translocation have the normal number of 46 chromosomes, including two normal chromosomes 21, one normal chromosome 14, and an unpaired large chromosome that results from the joining of one chromosome 21 to one chromosome 14 (Fig. 64-5*A*). As in trisomy 21, the genetic material of chromosome 21 is represented in triple dosage (Fig. 64-5*B*). There are no clinical differences between children with the trisomy 21 form of Down's syndrome and those with the translocation form.

Studies of the parents of children with the 14/21 translocation form of Down's syndrome show one of two situations: (1) In about 50 percent of cases both parents have normal karyotypes, a circumstance in which the translocation is assumed to have originated during gametogenesis and involving little risk of recurrence to subsequent children; (2) in the remaining 50 percent of cases one of the parents has a karyotype consisting of 45 chromosomes with one normal chromosome 14, one normal chromosome 21, and a large chromosome that contains fused copies of both the 14 and 21 chromosomes (Fig. 64-5*C*). Because of the presence of a normal amount of genetic material, the "balanced" carrier is clinically normal, but during meiosis the segregation of these chromosomes into the egg or spermatozoon may produce several different kinds of gametes: (1) A normal gamete containing the normal 14 and 21 chromosomes but not the 14/21 translocation chromosome (fusion of this gamete with a normal gamete will produce a normal individual); (2) a gamete containing the 14/21 translocation chromosome, but neither the normal 21 nor 14 chromosome (fusion of this gamete with a normal gamete produces an individual with a normal phenotype who carries a "balanced" translocation just like the parent); (3) a gamete containing the 14/21 translocation chromosome plus one copy of either the normal 14 or 21 chromosome or both (products of fertilization will have excess genetic material and will be clinically abnormal); or (4) a gamete containing no 14/21 translocation but in which the normal 14 or 21 chromosome is absent (products of fertilization will have a deficiency of genetic material and will be eliminated by spontaneous abortion because a deficiency of genetic material is very poorly tolerated by the fetus, in contrast to its reaction to extra genetic material). As a result, offspring of a carrier of a "balanced" translocation may be normal, may be a "balanced" translocation carrier and clinically normal, may be "unbalanced" and have Down's syndrome, or may be aborted early in pregnancy. About 5 to 20 percent of the live-born offspring of an individual who is a "balanced" translocation carrier for the 14/21 chromosome will have Down's syndrome, depending on whether the father (5 percent) or the mother (20 percent) carries the "balanced" translocation.

In contrast to the above situation, studies of the parents of children with the G/G translocation form of Down's syndrome indicate that most G/G translocations occur sporadically.

ETIOLOGY AND FREQUENCY OF CHROMOSOMAL ABNORMALITIES Very little is known about the factors that cause chromosomal disorders in man. The most important finding is the association between increasing maternal age and nondisjunction syndromes such as Down's syndrome (trisomy 21) and Klinefelter's syndrome (47 XXY). Figure 64-6 shows the marked increase in incidence of the trisomy 21 form of Down's syndrome among older mothers. A pos-

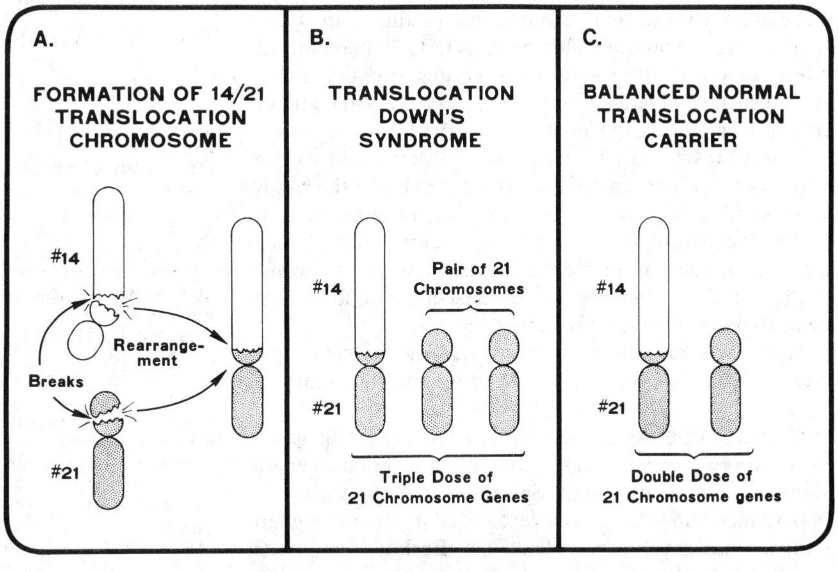

FIGURE 64-5
Abnormal chromosomes involved in the 14/21 translocation form of Down's syndrome. A *Formation of a 14/21 translocation chromosome by breakage and rejoining of the long arms of two chromosomes into a single translocation chromosome (with loss of the broken short arms).* B *When the fertilized egg receives this 14/21 translocation chromosome plus the usual two 21 chromosomes, the result will be a baby with Down's syndrome having a triple dose of 21 chromosomes.* C *When the fertilized egg receives the 14/21 translocation chromosome plus one 21 chromosome, the result will be a normal balanced translocation carrier, who will have a 5 to 20 percent risk of having a child with Down's syndrome.*

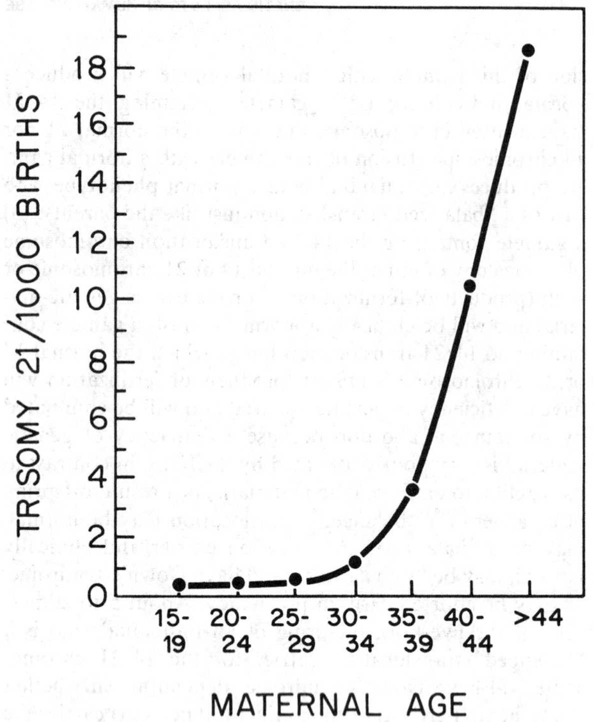

FIGURE 64-6
The relation of maternal age to the risk of having a child with Down's syndrome. (Modified from CO Carter, KA Evans, Lancet 2:785, 1961)

sible etiologic role for other factors, such as genetic predisposition, autoimmune disorders (involving the thyroid gland, in particular), viruses, chemical mutagens, and radiation, has also been suggested.

The detected frequency of chromosomal aberrations in karyotypes of unselected newborn infants is 1 in 200 (0.5 percent), while among first-semester spontaneous abortions the frequency of chromosomal defects is as high as 50 percent. Thus, the vast majority of chromosomal abnormalities are lost in early fetal life. A high frequency of chromosomal aberrations has, however, been observed in association with several clinical abnormalities, including (1) multiple congenital malformations (5 to 20 percent); (2) infertility and sterility in different groups of patients (1 to 10 percent); (3) mental retardation (1 to 3 percent); and (4) certain forms of malignancy.

In most instances chromosomal disorders occur as new mutations. Both parents are usually normal, and the risk of recurrence to relatives is low. However, in those cases in which one parent is the carrier of a chromosomal rearrangement, such as in the translocation form of Down's syndrome, the recurrence risk to subsequent children may be as high as 20 percent (discussed above).

Table 64-3 lists the most frequently encountered chromosomal abnormalities occurring among live-born infants.

CHROMOSOMES AND CANCER Cancer cells display a wide array of chromosomal abnormalities but in general show no consistent pattern. Specific consistent chromosomal abnormalities have been recognized in three malignancies: chronic myelogenous leukemia, Burkitt's lymphoma (a translocation involving chromosomes 8 and 14), and meningioma (a deficiency of all or part of chromosome 22). In most cases of chronic myelogenous leukemia, more than 90 percent of the dividing bone marrow cells have a distinctive abnormal karyotype. In the abnormal karyotype the long arm of chromosome 22 is translocated to one of the larger chromosomes, most often to the long arm of chromosome 9 (Fig. 64-7). The remaining short arm of chromosome 22 is visualized as an abnormally small single chromosome, called the *Philadelphia chromosome.* The Philadelphia chromosome occurs only in the precursor cells of granulocytes, red blood cells, and platelets; it is not found in other somatic cells or in the germ cells. It is likely that the origin of chronic myelogenous leukemia is related to an initial somatic mutation occurring in a single myelocytic precursor cell which results in the Philadelphia chromosome and that this chromosomal rearrangement, in turn, causes a loss of growth control of myelocytic cells.

Chromosomal aberrations such as unrepaired chromosomal breakage, translocations, deletions, and fusion figures are associated with a predisposition to malignancy in three autosomal recessive disorders—Bloom's syndrome, ataxia telangiectasia, and Fanconi's anemia. Since each of these disorders is due to a single mutant gene, it is likely that the abnormal gene product predisposes to chromosomal mutation which in turn predisposes to malignancy.

INDICATIONS FOR OBTAINING A CHROMOSOMAL ANALYSIS A complete chromosome analysis is clinically indicated in the following situations: (1) In children with multiple congenital anomalies, with mental defects of unknown cause, and with failure to grow for unknown reasons; (2) in children with suspected Down's syndrome and in their parents if the possibility of a balanced translocation exists; (3) in couples in whom the wife aborts repeatedly; (4) in families producing many congenitally abnormal children; (5) in women with primary amenorrhea; (6) in men and women with ambiguous external genitalia; and (7) in patients with hematologic malignancies, such as chronic myelogenous leukemia.

Simply inherited disorders

Disorders caused by the transmission of a single mutant gene show one of three simple (or mendelian) patterns of inheritance: (1) Autosomal dominant, (2) autosomal reces-

TABLE 64-3
Frequency of chromosomal disorders among live-born infants

Disorder	*Population frequency*
AUTOSOMAL ABNORMALITIES	
Trisomy 21 (Down's syndrome)	1 in 600
Trisomy 18	1 in 5,000
Trisomy 13	1 in 15,000
SEX CHROMOSOME ABNORMALITIES	
Klinefelter's syndrome (47 XXY)	1 in 450 males
XYY syndrome (47 XYY)	1 in 1,000 males
Triple-X syndrome (47 XXX)	1 in 1,000 females
Turner's syndrome (45 XO, 46 XO/XX, 46 XO/XY, isochromosome-X)	1 in 1,500 females

sive, or (3) X-linked. The distinction between "dominant" and "recessive" is one of convenience in pedigree analysis and does not imply a fundamental difference in genetic mechanism. The term *dominant* implies that a mutation will be clinically manifest when an individual has a single dose of this mutation (or is *heterozygous* for it), while *recessive* implies that a double dose (or *homozygosity*) is required for clinical detection. Genes are never dominant or recessive; their effects, however, produce clinical patterns that are classified as dominant or recessive. Despite their overall clinical "normality," individuals who are heterozygous for "recessive" genes often have biochemical abnormalities that are demonstrable in the laboratory; on the other hand, those who are homozygous for "dominant" genes are usually more severely affected than are the heterozygotes.

With few exceptions, each of the approximately 1,200 or so mendelian diseases is rare. However, as a group these disorders constitute an important cause of morbidity and death, accounting directly for more than 5 percent of all hospital admissions.

The demonstration that a particular disease or syndrome shows one of the three mendelian patterns of inheritance implies that its pathogenesis, no matter how complex, is due to an abnormality in a single protein molecule. For example, in sickle-cell anemia, the entire clinical syndrome, including such seemingly unrelated disturbances as anemia, pain crises, nephropathy, and predisposition to pneumococcal infections, are all the physiologic consequences of having thymine instead of adenine at a specific site in the gene that codes for the β-chain of hemoglobin, producing a substitution of a valine for a glutamic acid in the sixth amino acid position in the protein sequence.

In many mendelian disorders, especially in those with dominant inheritance, it is not possible to demonstrate directly the protein that is primarily altered by the mutation. In such cases (e.g., adult polycystic kidney disease and tuberous sclerosis) only the distal physiologic effects of the mutation are recognizable. Nevertheless, it is safe to assume that a single primary defect exists whenever a disease is transmitted by a single gene mechanism and that the various manifestations of the disease all can be related to the mutational event by a more or less complicated "pedigree of causes." Table 64-4 lists the most commonly encountered mendelian disorders affecting adults.

AUTOSOMAL DOMINANT DISORDERS Dominant diseases are those manifest in the heterozygous state, that is, when only one abnormal gene (*mutant allele*) is present and the corresponding partner allele on the homologous chromosome is normal. The gene responsible for an autosomal

FIGURE 64-7
Karyotype of a mitotic cell obtained from the peripheral blood of a patient with chronic myelogenous leukemia. The chromosomes were stained with quinacrine mustard and examined with a fluorescent microscope. The Philadelphia (Ph^1) chromosome results from the loss of most of the long arm of one chromosome 22. The chromosomal material lost from chromosome 22 is translocated to the long arm of chromosome 9. Note the similar intensity of fluorescence of the normal chromosome 22 and the additional material on the long arm of chromosome 9. (Courtesy of Janet D. Rowley)

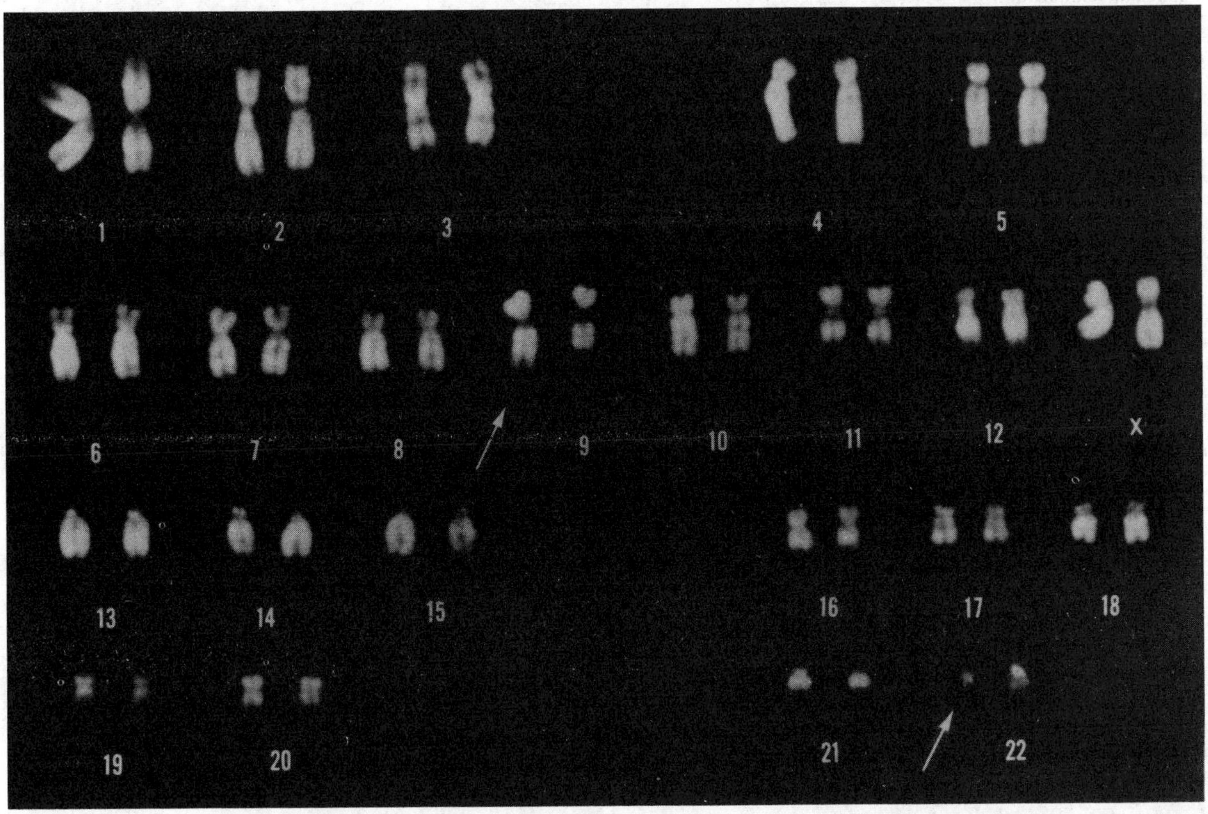

TABLE 64-4
Some relatively frequent mendelian disorders affecting adults

AUTOSOMAL DOMINANT DISORDERS

Familial hypercholesterolemia
Hereditary hemorrhagic telangiectasia
Marfan's syndrome
Hereditary spherocytosis
Adult polycystic kidney disease
Huntington's chorea
Acute intermittent porphyria
Osteogenesis imperfecta tarda
von Willebrand's disease
Myotonic dystrophy
Hemochromatosis
Idiopathic hypertrophic subaortic stenosis (IHSS)
Noonan's syndrome
Neurofibromatosis
Tuberous sclerosis

AUTOSOMAL RECESSIVE DISORDERS

Deafness
Albinism
Wilson's disease
Sickle-cell anemia
β-Thalassemia
Cystic fibrosis
Hereditary emphysema (α_1-antitrypsin deficiency)
Homocystinuria
Familial Mediterranean fever
Friedreich's ataxia
Phenylketonuria

X-LINKED DISORDERS

Hemophilia A
Glucose 6-phosphate dehydrogenase deficiency
Fabry's disease
Ocular albinism
Testicular feminization
Chronic granulomatous disease
Hypophosphatemic rickets
Color blindness

dominant disorder is located on one of the 22 autosomes, and both males and females can be affected. Since alleles segregate independently at meiosis, there is a one-in-two chance that the offspring of an affected heterozygote will inherit the mutant allele and, similarly, a one-in-two chance of the offspring inheriting the normal allele.

FIGURE 64-8
Pedigree pattern of an autosomal dominant trait. Note the vertical *pattern of inheritance.*

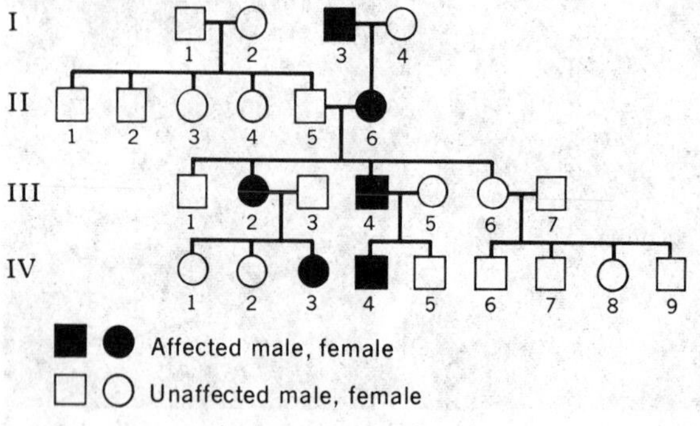

Figure 64-8 shows a typical pedigree involving an autosomal dominant trait. The following features are characteristic: (1) Each affected individual has an affected parent (unless the condition arose by a new mutation in the given individual or is mildly expressed in the affected parent); (2) an affected individual will bear, on the average, both normal and affected offspring in equal proportions; (3) normal children of an affected individual will have only normal offspring; (4) males and females are affected in equal proportions; (5) each sex is equally likely to transmit the condition to male and female offspring, with male-to-male transmission occurring; and (6) vertical transmission of the condition through successive generations occurs, especially when the trait does not impair reproductive capacity.

While half of the offspring of an individual with an autosomal dominant condition will inherit the disease, it is not necessarily true that each affected person must have an affected parent. In every autosomal dominant disease a certain proportion of affected persons owe their disorder to a new mutation rather than to an inherited mutation. Since the estimated frequency of mutation is 5×10^{-6} mutations per gene per generation and since a dominant trait, by definition, requires a mutation in only one of a pair of alleles, one would expect that about 1 in 100,000 newborn persons would possess a new mutation at any given genetic locus. Many of these mutations either will not impair the function of the gene product or will involve a recessive function so that the mutation will be clinically silent. Others, however, will cause a defective gene product that gives rise to a dominant trait. The parent in whose germ cells the mutation arose will be clinically normal. Likewise, the siblings of the affected individual will be normal since the mutation will affect only a single germ cell. However, the affected individual will be able to transmit the disease, and half of his or her children will be affected.

The proportion of patients with dominant disorders who represent new mutations is inversely proportional to the effect of the disease in question on biologic fitness. The term *biologic fitness* refers to the ability of an affected individual to produce children who survive to adult life and reproduce. In the extreme case, if a dominant mutation produced absolute infertility, then all observed cases would of necessity represent new mutations, and it would be impossible to prove the genetic transmission of the trait. In less severe disorders, as in tuberous sclerosis, the severe mental retardation reduces biologic fitness to about 20 percent of normal, and the proportion of cases due to new mutations is about 80 percent. Other examples of the relation between biologic fitness and the proportion of new mutations in dominant disorders are shown in Table 64-5.

Many new mutations appear to occur in the germ cells of fathers who are of relatively advanced age. Such a "paternal age effect" is seen, for example, in Marfan's syndrome in which the average age of fathers of sporadic or "new mutation" cases (thirty-seven years) is in excess of the mean age of fathers generally (thirty years) and also in excess of the age of fathers who transmit Marfan's disease due to an inherited mutation (thirty years).

Before one concludes that a dominant disorder in a given patient with unaffected parents is the result of a new mutation, it is important to consider two other possibilities: (1) That the gene may be carried by one parent in whom the disease is of low expressivity (discussed below), and (2) that extramarital paternity may have occurred,

TABLE 64-5
Approximate proportion of patients affected by new mutations in some autosomal dominant disorders

Disorder	*Percentage*
Achondroplasia	80
Tuberous sclerosis	80
Neurofibromatosis	40
Marfan's syndrome	30
Myotonic dystrophy	25
Huntington's chorea	4
Adult polycystic kidney disease	1
Familial hypercholesterolemia	Very low

since such is found in about 3 to 5 percent of randomly studied children in the United States.

Most autosomal dominant disorders show two characteristic features that are not usually seen in recessive syndromes: (1) *Delayed age of onset* and (2) *variability in clinical expression.* Delayed age of onset is seen in disorders such as Huntington's chorea and adult polycystic kidney disease. These disorders do not manifest clinically until adult life, even though the mutant gene is present from the time of conception. Variability in clinical expression is illustrated dramatically by the multiple endocrine adenoma–peptic ulcer syndrome. Patients in the same family inheriting the same abnormal gene may have hyperplasia or neoplasia of one or all of a wide variety of endocrine tissues such as the pancreas, parathyroid glands, pituitary gland, or adipose tissue. The resulting clinical manifestations are extremely diverse; different members of the same family may develop peptic ulcers, hypoglycemia, kidney stones, multiple lipomas of the skin, or bitemporal hemianopsia. The recognition that each family member suffers from the same genetic abnormality can be very difficult, as illustrated by the family pedigree in Fig. 64-9.

Since dominant mutations involve a type of gene product that in a 50 percent deficiency is capable of producing clinical symptoms in heterozygotes, the responsible mutations are likely to involve abnormalities in two classes of proteins: (1) Those that regulate complex metabolic pathways, such as membrane receptors and rate-limiting enzymes in pathways under feedback control, and (2) key structural proteins, such as hemoglobin or collagen.

The basic biochemical defects have been identified in only a handful of the approximately 600 autosomal dominant disorders. These include familial hypercholesterolemia (abnormal cell surface receptor that binds plasma low-density lipoprotein and thereby regulates cholesterol metabolism); hereditary methemoglobinemia and several hemolytic anemias due to unstable forms of hemoglobin (abnormal hemoglobin molecule); hereditary angioneurotic edema (abnormal protein inhibitor of an enzyme involved in the serum complement system); acute intermittent porphyria (abnormal enzyme that catalyzes a rate-limiting step in the heme biosynthetic pathway); and a rare form of overproduction gout (abnormal enzyme that catalyzes a rate-limiting step in the purine biosynthetic pathway).

AUTOSOMAL RECESSIVE DISORDERS Autosomal recessive conditions are those that are clinically apparent only in the homozygous state, that is, when both alleles at a particular genetic locus are mutant alleles. The gene responsible for an autosomal recessive disorder must be located on one of the 22 autosomes; thus, both males and females can be affected.

Figure 64-10 shows a pedigree in which an autosomal recessive trait is present in the family. The following features are characteristic: (1) The parents are clinically normal; (2) only siblings are affected, and vertical transmission does not occur; and (3) males and females are affected in equal proportions.

The relative infrequency of recessive genes in the population and the requirement for two abnormal genes for

FIGURE 64-9
Pedigree of a family affected with the multiple endocrine adenoma–peptic ulcer syndrome, a disorder inherited as an autosomal dominant trait. Circles *denote females;* squares, *males.* Open *circles and squares denote unaffected relatives;* closed *circles and squares denote affected relatives. Deceased relatives are indicated by the oblique line. The age of each relative is indicated above his or her symbol. Note the marked variation in clinical expression among living affected heterozygotes.*

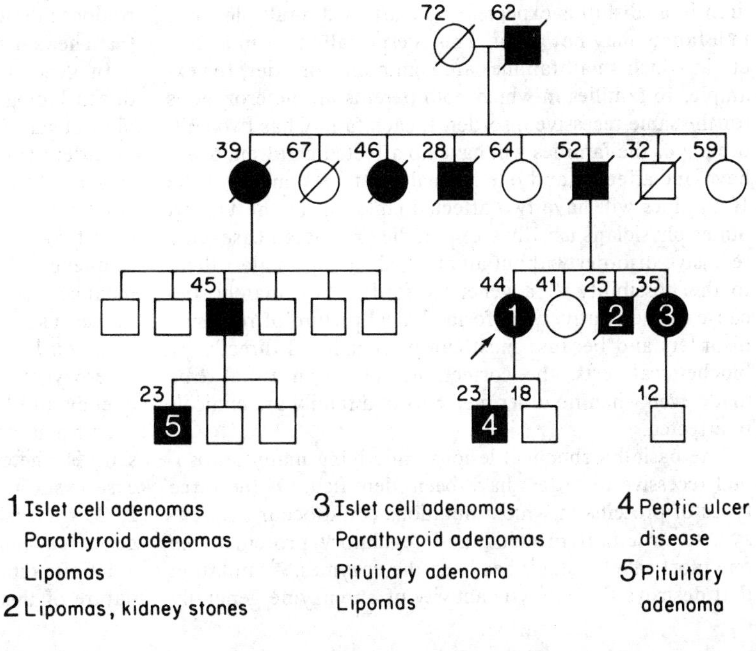

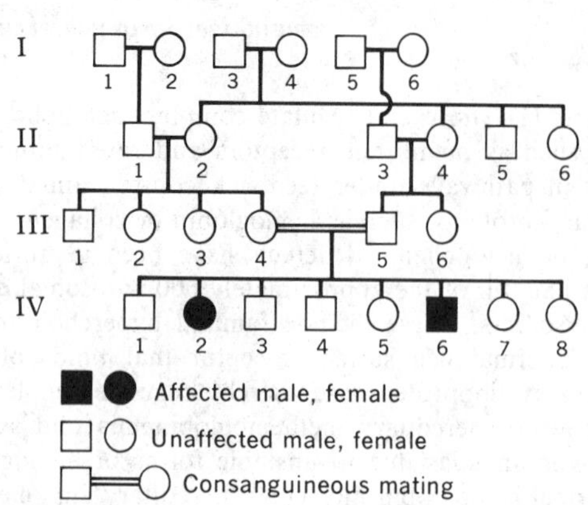

FIGURE 64-10
Pedigree pattern of an autosomal recessive trait. Note the horizontal *pattern of inheritance.*

clinical expression combine to create special conditions for autosomal recessive inheritance: (1) The more infrequent the mutant gene in the population, the stronger the likelihood that affected individuals are the product of consanguineous matings (see below); (2) if a husband and a wife are both carriers for the same autosomal recessive gene, 25 percent of the children will be normal, 50 percent will be heterozygous carriers, and 25 percent will be homozygous and affected with the disease; (3) if an affected individual marries a heterozygote (as may occur with consanguineous marriage), half the children will be affected, and a pedigree simulating dominant inheritance will result; and (4) if two individuals with the same recessive disease marry, all their children will be affected.

The clinical picture in autosomal recessive disorders tends to be more uniform than that of dominant diseases, and the age of onset is often early in life. As a general rule, recessive disorders are more commonly diagnosed in children, while dominant diseases are more frequently encountered in adults.

Since with recessive inheritance only one of four children in a sibship is expected to be affected, multiple cases in a family may not occur. This is especially true in a society in which small families are common. Consider, for example, 16 families in which both parents are heterozygous for the same recessive disorder. If each family has two children, 9 of the families will have no affected children, 6 will have one affected and one normal child, and only 1 of the 16 families will have two affected children. In the United States physicians usually see sporadic or isolated cases of a recessive disorder without an affected sibling to alert them to the possibility of a genetic disorder. Fortunately, because of the relatively uniform clinical picture of recessive disorders and because most can be diagnosed directly by biochemical tests, the correct diagnosis can usually be made even when no other members of a family are clinically affected.

The basic biochemical lesions underlying many autosomal recessive disorders have been identified. Of the three types of proteins in which mutations could occur (i.e., enzymes, structural proteins, and regulatory proteins), the one most easy to study has been the enzymes. A mutation that destroys the catalytic activity of an enzyme generally does not impair the health of a heterozygote (i.e., an individual who has one mutant allele specifying a functionless enzyme and one normal allele on the partner chromosome specifying a normal enzyme). In this situation each cell in the body usually produces about 50 percent of the normal number of active enzyme molecules. However, normal regulatory mechanisms function to avert any clinical consequences of this 50 percent deficiency, and so heterozygotes usually are clinically normal. On the other hand, when an individual inherits functionless alleles at both loci specifying an enzyme, the reduction in enzyme activity is too great for a compensatory mechanism to overcome the deficiency, and a disease results. For example, heterozygotes for phenylketonuria who have half the normal activity of phenylalanine hydroxylase are clinically asymptomatic because the body compensates for the half-normal level of the enzyme by raising the substrate concentration approximately twofold. Under these conditions a normal amount of phenylalanine can be metabolized with no symptoms. On the other hand, the homozygote for phenylketonuria has such a severe reduction in phenylalanine hydroxylase activity that enormous levels of phenylalanine and its derivatives accumulate, causing detrimental brain development. As in the case of phenylketonuria, the majority of enzyme deficiency states produce *simultaneously* both a simple accumulation of one or more metabolites preceding the enzymatic block and a deficient production of other metabolites distal to the block in the metabolic pathway.

Most of the genetic enzyme deficiencies that have been elucidated are not only inherited as recessive traits, but also tend to involve enzymes that participate in catabolic pathways. Frequently these enzymes degrade organic molecules that are ingested in the diet, such as galactose (galactosemia), phenylalanine (phenylketonuria), and phytanic acid (Refsum's syndrome). A special class of such catabolic diseases is that in which the deficiency affects an acid hydrolase that occurs within lysosomes. In these *lysosomal storage disorders* the substrate, usually a complex lipid or polysaccharide, accumulates within swollen lysosomes in specific organs, giving the cells a foamy appearance. Examples of such lysosomal diseases include the mucopolysaccharidoses such as Hurler's syndrome (α-iduronidase deficiency) and the lipid storage diseases such as Gaucher's disease (glucocerebrosidase deficiency).

In general, recessive diseases are rare because the reduced biologic fitness of homozygotes acts to remove the mutant gene from the population. However, a few recessive disorders, such as cystic fibrosis and sickle-cell anemia, are very common. To explain this paradox, it has been postulated that the biologic fitness of heterozygotes is greater than that of noncarriers for these genes. In such a case the frequency of the gene in the population depends on the balance between the increased fitness of the relatively numerous heterozygotes and the reduced fitness of the less common homozygotes. A small selective advantage of the heterozygote over the normal results in a high gene frequency and hence a high birth frequency of homozygotes even when the disease is lethal. Thus, about 1 in 22 Caucasians is a heterozygous carrier for the genetically lethal disease cystic fibrosis, and the disease occurs in about 1 in 2,000 Caucasian births. In order to maintain such a high gene frequency, heterozygotes for cystic fibrosis must have a definite reproductive advantage over noncarriers, but the nature of this advantage is unknown. However, in sickle-cell anemia, another recessive disorder with high frequency among certain populations, heterozygotes appear to have increased resistance to malaria.

Inasmuch as recessive diseases require the inheritance of a mutation at the same genetic locus from each parent, when the genes are rare, the likelihood of any two parents being carriers for the same defect becomes very small. However, if the parents have a common ancestor and if that ancestor was a carrier for the same recessive gene, then the likelihood that two of the descendants would each have inherited the gene becomes relatively great. The rarer the recessive gene, the stronger becomes the likelihood that an affected individual will have resulted from such a consanguineous mating. On the other hand, certain recessive genes are so common in the population that the likelihood of two random parents being carriers is great enough to eliminate the need for consanguinity. For common traits such as sickle-cell anemia, phenylketonuria, cystic fibrosis, and Tay-Sachs disease, all of which have a high carrier frequency in certain populations, consanguinity is usually not present in the parent.

In general, consanguinity is an infrequent finding clinically in families with recessive diseases in the United States. This is because the background rate of consanguinity in the general population is very low. In most of the United States (as opposed to areas with relative geographic isolation such as northern Norway and Switzerland), a disorder must indeed be rare before it is associated with an important frequency of consanguinity. For example, consanguinity is expected in a large proportion of families having children with very rare disorders such as the Laurence-Moon-Biedl syndrome and abetalipoproteinemia.

Genetic compounds represent a special type of recessively inherited disorder in which the affected individual's two mutant genes, although derived from the same genetic locus, are not identical. The mutations in the paternal and maternal alleles presumably involve different alterations in the DNA of the same gene. Sickle-cell-C hemoglobinopathy is an example of such a *heteroallelic* compound state in which individuals have a gene for sickle-cell hemoglobin on one chromosome and a gene for hemoglobin C on the homologous chromosome.

X-LINKED DISORDERS The genes responsible for X-linked disorders are located on the X chromosome; therefore, the clinical risk and severity of the disease are different for the two sexes. Since a female has two X chromosomes, she may be either heterozygous or homozygous for a mutant gene, and the trait may therefore demonstrate either recessive or dominant expression. Males, on the other hand, have only one X chromosome, so they can be expected to display the full syndrome whenever they inherit the gene regardless of whether the gene behaves as a recessive or as a dominant trait in the female. Thus, the terms *X-linked dominant* or *X-linked recessive* refer only to the expression of the gene in women.

An important feature of all X-linked inheritance is the absence of male-to-male (i.e., father-to-son) transmission of the trait. This follows because a male must always contribute his Y chromosome to his sons; hence, he can never contribute his X chromosome. On the other hand, a male contributes his one X chromosome to all his daughters.

The pedigree in Fig. 64-11 illustrates the characteristic features of X-linked recessive inheritance. (1) In contrast to the vertical transmission in dominant traits (parents and children affected) and the horizontal transmission in autosomal recessive traits (siblings affected), the pedigree pattern in X-linked recessive traits tends to be oblique because of the occurrence of the trait in the sons of normal carrier sisters of affected males (uncles and nephews affected) (Fig. 64-11*A*); (2) male offspring of carrier women have a 50 percent chance of being affected; (3) all female offspring of affected males are carriers, and affected males do not transmit the disease to their sons (Fig. 64-11*B*); (4) unaffected males do not transmit the trait to any offspring; and (5) affected homozygous females occur only when an affected male marries a carrier female (Fig. 64-11*C*).

FIGURE 64-11
Pedigree patterns of an X-linked recessive trait. A *Note the* oblique *pattern of inheritance.* B *An affected female can result from the mating of an affected male and a carrier female, as in the consanguineous marriage shown here.* C *An affected male mating with a normal noncarrier female has all normal sons and all carrier daughters. (Courtesy of Victor A. McKusick)*

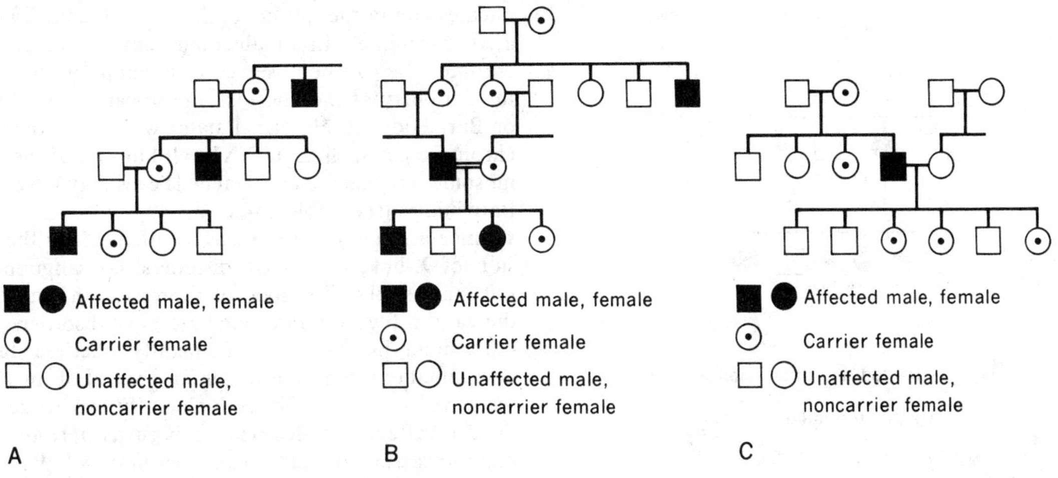

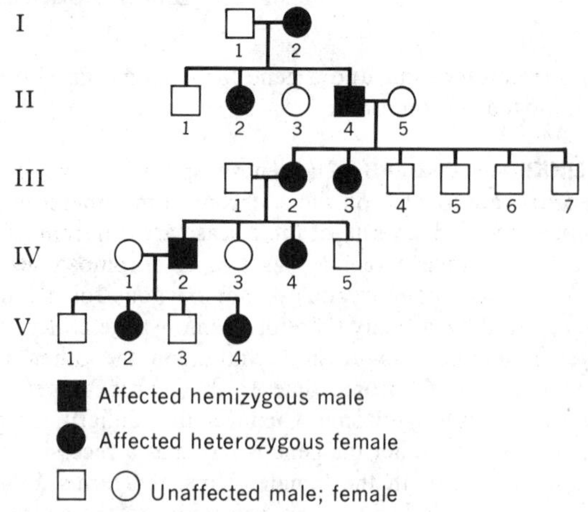

FIGURE 64-12
Pedigree pattern of an X-linked dominant trait.

Examples of X-linked recessive disorders in humans include hemophilia A, nephrogenic diabetes insipidus, the Lesch-Nyhan syndrome, Duchenne form of muscular dystrophy, glucose 6-phosphate dehydrogenase deficiency, testicular feminization, and Fabry's disease. Color blindness is also inherited as an X-linked recessive trait, but it is sufficiently frequent (occurring in about 8 percent of Caucasian males) that the occurrence of homozygous colorblind females is no rarity.

X-linked dominant inheritance is illustrated by the pedigree in Fig. 64-12. Its characteristic features are as follows: (1) Females are affected about twice as often as males; (2) an affected female transmits the disorder to half of her sons and half of her daughters; (3) an affected male transmits the disorder to all his daughters and to none of his sons; and (4) the syndrome is more variable and less severe in heterozygous affected females than in hemizygous affected males. One common trait, the Xg(a+) blood group, is inherited as an X-linked dominant trait, as are diseases such as vitamin D–resistant rickets (hypophosphatemic rickets) and pseudohypoparathyroidism.

FIGURE 64-13
Pedigree pattern of an X-linked dominant trait lethal in the hemizygous male.

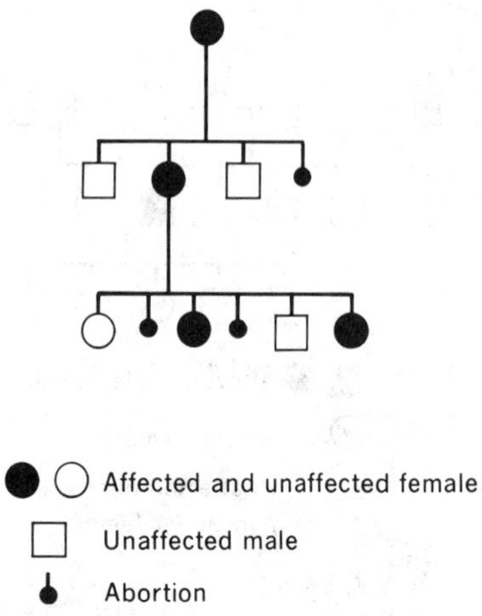

Some rare conditions may be inherited as X-linked dominant traits in which there is lethality in the hemizygous male. The characteristics of this form of inheritance are illustrated by the pedigree in Fig. 64-13: (1) The disorder occurs only in females who are heterozygous for the mutant gene; (2) an affected mother transmits the trait to half of her daughters; (3) an increased frequency of abortions occurs in affected women, the abortions representing affected male fetuses. Conditions that appear to be transmitted by this mode of inheritance include incontinentia pigmenti, focal dermal hypoplasia, orofaciodigital syndrome, and hyperammonemia due to ornithine transcarbamylase deficiency.

Understanding of the mechanisms of gene expression of X-linked traits in females has been greatly advanced by the so-called *Lyon hypothesis* or *X-inactivation hypothesis.* (The term *hypothesis* is used for historical reasons only; Lyon's hypothesis can now be regarded as proved fact.) This hypothesis states that early in embryonic development one of the two X chromosomes in each somatic cell of a female is inactivated. The inactivation process is random, so that for each cell there is an equal probability that the paternally or maternally derived X chromosome will be inactivated. The inactivated X chromosome is rendered permanently nonfunctional, so that all progeny of the initial cell inherit the same active and inactive X chromosomes. Thus, each female is a mosaic; on the average, half of her cells express the X chromosome of the father, and half express the X chromosome of the mother. If a mutation in a gene is carried on one of her X chromosomes, about one-half of the cells in each tissue will be normal and the other half will manifest the mutant phenotype. However, chance or selection of one or the other set of clones of cells may disturb these proportions in any given individual. Depending on the proportions of mutant and normal X chromosomes in each tissue, a genetically heterozygous female may either be clinically normal or have mild or severe manifestations of the disease. To illustrate, mothers of boys with the X-linked recessive Duchenne form of muscular dystrophy may occasionally show mild manifestations of the disease, such as limb girdle weakness or hypertrophied calves.

In each female cell the nonfunctional X chromosome can be visualized by several techniques. By ordinary staining, the inactivated X chromosome in metaphase appears heteropyknotic (very condensed in appearance), and it replicates late in the mitotic cycle ("late-labeling" with tritiated thymidine). In nondividing cells the inactivated X chromosome can be observed as a clump of chromatin at the periphery of the nucleus—the so-called sex chromatin or Barr body. In abnormal states with more than two X chromosomes such as 47 XXX, all but one of the X chromosomes are inactivated, so female cells may have multiple Barr bodies (see Table 64-2).

Since a single mutant allele is sufficient for the expression of X-linked recessive disorders, consanguinity does not increase the likelihood of expression in males, unlike the case in the rare autosomal recessive disorders. On the other hand, just as in the dominantly inherited disorders, new mutations can be a factor. In general, if an X-linked recessive condition reduces biologic fitness to zero, one-third of affected males will be born as a result of new mutations and an additional one-third will be born to mothers who themselves are carriers as a result of a new mutation. Thus, only one-third will come from a classic pedigree manifesting oblique transmission. An example of such a disease is the Duchenne form of muscular dystrophy in which affected hemizygous males are so severely disabled that they never reproduce. In hemophilia A, in which the biologic fitness is greater than zero, about 20 percent of affected males represent new mutations.

In families in which only one male is affected with an X-linked recessive disease and there is no other family history of the trait, it is essential for proper genetic counseling that the mother undergo biochemical tests or other relevant studies to determine whether she is a carrier. If she is a carrier, half of her daughters will be carriers and half of her sons will be affected. On the other hand, if her affected son represents a new mutation, only his daughters will inherit the gene. At present, biochemical tests can identify female carriers for several X-linked diseases including the Lesch-Nyhan syndrome, Fabry's disease, Hunter's syndrome, hemophilia, and the Duchenne form of muscular dystrophy.

The distinction between X-linked inheritance and *sex-influenced autosomal dominant inheritance* is important. Both baldness and hemochromatosis are probably inherited as autosomal dominant traits, yet both disorders occur mainly in men and rarely in women. Heterozygous females rarely manifest the hemochromatosis gene because of menstruation and pregnancy, which mitigate against the overaccumulation of iron, and they express the baldness gene only when a source of testosterone becomes available as occurs with a masculinizing tumor of the ovary.

Multifactorial genetic diseases

The common chronic diseases of adults (such as essential hypertension, coronary heart disease, diabetes mellitus, peptic ulcer disease, and schizophrenia) as well as the common birth defects (such as cleft lip and palate, spina bifida, and congenital heart disease) have been long known to "run in families." They fit best into the category of *multifactorial genetic diseases.* The genetic element in these disorders rarely manifests itself in an all-or-none fashion as it does in the simply inherited (mendelian) disorders and in chromosomal aberrations. Instead, it is the interaction of multiple genes with multiple environmental factors that produces the familial aggregation.

In the multifactorial genetic diseases, there is a *polygenic component* consisting of a series of genes that interact in a cumulative fashion. If an individual inherits just the right combination of these genes, he passes beyond a "threshold of risk," at which point an *environmental component* determines whether and to what extent he is clinically affected. In order that another individual in the same family express the same syndrome, he must inherit the same or a very similar combination of genes. Since the first-degree relatives of an affected individual (i.e., parents, siblings, and offspring) each share half of his genes, they are all at increased risk of exhibiting the same polygenic syndrome. Second-degree relatives (uncles, aunts, and grandparents) share on the average one-fourth of an individual's genes $(1/2)^2$, and third-degree relatives (cousins) share one-eighth $(1/2)^3$. Thus, as the degree of relation becomes more distant, the likelihood of a relative inheriting the same combination of genes becomes less. Moreover, the chances of any relative inheriting the right combination of risk genes decrease as the number of genes required for the expression of a given trait increases.

Since the precise number of genes responsible for polygenic traits is unknown, the risk of inheritance for a relative of an affected individual is difficult to calculate, and the standard is based on empiric risk figures (i.e., a direct tally of the proportion of affected relatives in previously reported families). In contrast to the simply inherited disorders in which 25 or 50 percent of the first-degree relatives of an affected proband are at genetic risk, multifactorial genetic disorders are generally observed empirically to affect no more than 5 to 10 percent of first-degree relatives. Moreover, in contrast to mendelian traits, the recurrence risk of multifactorial conditions varies from family to family, and its estimation is significantly influenced by two factors: (1) The number of affected persons already present in the family, and (2) the severity of the disorder in the index case. The greater the number of affected relatives and the more severe their disease, the higher the risk to other relatives. For example, the risk of cleft lip in the siblings of a child with unilateral cleft lip is about 2.5 percent, but if the lesion in the index case is bilateral, the risk in the siblings rises to 6 percent. Table 64-6 lists the empirical risk figures for the familial recurrence of a number of multifactorial genetic diseases.

The hypothesis of a polygenic component in the inheritance of multifactorial diseases has been given a sound basis in recent years by the demonstration that at least one-third of all gene loci harbor polymorphic alleles that vary among individuals. Such a large degree of variation in normal genes undoubtedly provides the substrate for variations in genetic predisposition with which environmental factors can interact. So far, the genetic loci most strikingly associated with predisposition to specific diseases are those that constitute the HL-A system. The products of these genes are proteins that are found on the surface of body cells and that enable an individual's immune system to distinguish its own cells from those of someone else. Each HL-A locus in the population consists of multiple alleles, each of which produces an immunologically distinct pro-

TABLE 64-6
Empiric risks for some common multifactorial genetic diseases affecting adults

Disorder in index case	*Estimated absolute risk for first-degree relatives, %*
Cleft lip and/or palate	3
Congenital heart disease	4
Coronary heart disease	8 for male relatives 3 for female relatives
Diabetes mellitus	5
Epilepsy	5
Hypertension	10
Manic-depressive psychosis	10–15
Psoriasis	10–15
Schizophrenia	15
Thyroid disease (autoimmune disorders including hyperthyroidism, thyroiditis, primary myxedema, simple goiter)	10

tein. For example, an individual may inherit any 2 of 20 alleles at the HL-AB locus.

An important observation of recent years has been the finding that certain alleles at the HL-A loci predispose individuals to certain specific diseases. For example, if the B27 allele at the HL-AB locus is inherited by an individual, he has a 121-fold greater chance of developing ankylosing spondylitis than an individual who lacks this allele (Table 64-7). Ankylosing spondylitis remains a multifactorial disease, however, because its development clearly requires one or more other factors in addition to the B27 allele. Thus, less than 15 percent of people who inherit this allele develop this disease. Table 64-7 lists some of the diseases associated with alleles at the HL-A loci. Several of them in the past have been suspected to be of viral etiology, suggesting that the HL-A loci may dictate the mode of expression of certain viral diseases.

Multifactorial disorders are heterogeneous in the sense that the relative contribution of the polygenic factors ("risk genes") and environmental factors to the etiology will vary greatly from patient to patient. However, it is important to remember that among common phenotypes which are largely multifactorial, often a small proportion will be created by major mutant genes. For example, although coronary heart disease is usually of multifactorial etiology, about 5 percent of subjects with premature myocardial infarctions are heterozygotes for familial hypercholesterolemia, a single-gene disorder that produces atherosclerosis in

TABLE 64-7
Alleles at the HL-A loci that are associated with multifactorial genetic diseases

Disease	*Genetic locus*	*Specific allele*	*Relative risk**
Ankylosing spondylitis	HL-AB	B27	121
Reiter's syndrome	HL-AB	B27	40
Psoriasis with arthritis	HL-AB	B27	5
Celiac disease	HL-AB	B8	10
Chronic active hepatitis	HL-AB	B8	4
Myasthenia gravis	HL-AB	B8	4
Diabetes mellitus	HL-AB	BW15	3
(insulin-dependent)	HL-AD	DW3 (LD-8a)	3
Hyperthyroidism	HL-AD	DW3 (LD-8a)	4
Addison's disease	HL-AD	DW3 (LD-8a)	10
Multiple sclerosis	HL-AD	DW2 (LD-7a)	5

* Relative risk *is the probability of the disease developing in an individual with the specific allele divided by the probability of its development in an individual who does not possess this specific allele.*

TABLE 64-8
Examples of inherited disorders involving an abnormal response to drugs

Disorder	*Molecular abnormality*	*Mode of inheritance*	*Frequency*	*Clinical effect*	*Drugs producing abnormal response*
Slow inactivation of isoniazid	Isoniazid acetylase in liver	Autosomal recessive	~ 50% of U.S. population	Polyneuritis	Isoniazid, sulfamethazine, sulfamaprine, phenelzine, dapsone, hydralazine
Suxamethonium sensitivity	Pseudocholinesterase in plasma	Autosomal recessive	Several mutant alleles; most common affects 1 in 2,500	Apnea	Suxamethonium, succinylcholine
Coumadin	? Altered receptor or enzyme in liver with increased affinity for vitamin K	Autosomal dominant	Rare	Inability to achieve anticoagulation with usual doses of drug	Coumadin
Glaucoma	Unknown	? Autosomal dominant	Common	Increased intraocular pressure	Corticosteroids
Malignant hyperthermia	Unknown	Autosomal dominant	~ 1 in 20,000 anesthesized patients	Severe hyperpyrexia, muscle rigidity, death	Such anesthetics as halothane, succinylcholine, methoxyfluorane, ether, cyclopropane
Unstable hemoglobins					
Hemoglobin Zurich	Arginine substitution for histidine at sixty-third position of β-chain of hemoglobin	Autosomal dominant	Rare	Hemolysis	Sulfonamides
Hemoglobin M	Hemoglobin composed of 4 β-chains	Autosomal dominant	Rare	Hemolysis	Sulfisoxazole
Glucose 6-phosphate dehydrogenase deficiency	Glucose 6-phosphate dehydrogenase in erythrocytes	X-linked recessive	~ 1×10^8 affected persons in world; common in persons of African, Mediterranean, Asiatic origin; multiple mutant alleles	Hemolysis	Analgesics, sulfonamides, antimalarials, nitrofurantoin, other drugs

SOURCE: *From ES Vesell, Drug therapy, N. Engl J Med 287:904, 1972.*

the absence of any other predisposing factor. Similarly, in a small proportion of patients with other common diseases such as peptic ulcer disease or "essential" hypertension, the condition is not multifactorial but determined by a single gene, as in the multiple endocrine adenoma–peptic ulcer syndrome or the medullary thyroid carcinoma–pheochromocytoma syndrome, respectively.

INTERACTION BETWEEN SINGLE GENETIC AND ENVIRONMENTAL FACTORS

Many diseases are now recognized to result from an interaction between a specific genotype and a specific environmental factor. In particular, inherited single-gene mutations have been shown to produce clinically significant and often life-threatening idiosyncratic responses to certain drugs.

Table 64-8 lists the most important of these *pharmacogenetic disorders,* which encompass all the mendelian modes of inheritance. Perhaps the most common is glucose 6-phosphate dehydrogenase deficiency, an X-linked recessive trait in which a variety of drugs may precipitate a hemolytic anemia. Plasma pseudocholinesterase deficiency and hepatic transacetylase deficiency are examples of autosomal recessive traits which alter drug catabolism so that when the muscle relaxant suxamethonium or the antituberculous drug isoniazid is administered, apnea or peripheral neuropathy, respectively, may ensue. Malignant hyperthermia is an autosomal dominant trait in which acute hyperpyrexia, muscle rigidity, and hyperkalemic cardiac arrest may be induced by administration of any one of several anesthetic agents. Acute intermittent porphyria is another example of a genetic disorder that is exacerbated by drugs, such as barbiturates.

Misinterpretation of adverse drug reactions may result in serious harm to patients. In general, all unusual idiosyncratic reactions should be considered to be genetically determined until proved otherwise. Fortunately, the pharmacogenetic disorders are a group of diseases for which therapy is straightforward: avoidance of the noxious drug by patient and relatives.

In addition to drugs, other factors in the environment may aggravate specific genetic traits. Cigarette smoke may have deleterious effects on persons homozygous and possibly heterozygous for α_1-antitrypsin deficiency, who are predisposed to the development of emphysema. Patients with xeroderma pigmentosa and anhydrotic ectodermal dysplasia are unusually sensitive to sunlight and high temperatures, respectively. Avoidance of milk at an early age prevents many of the complications ordinarily seen in persons with galactosemia.

Genetic-environmental interactions are particularly important in pregnancy. Women who are affected with phenylketonuria may develop high plasma phenylalanine levels during pregnancy, and thus their offspring may suffer from a variety of phenylalanine-induced birth defects even though the offspring may not themselves have phenylketonuria. Other examples of diseases resulting from an adverse genetic relation between the mother and fetus include erythroblastosis caused by Rh incompatibility (Chap. 314) and diabetic embryopathy, a term that refers to a series of major birth defects occurring in about 5 percent of the offspring of women who are clinically diabetic during pregnancy.

REFERENCES

BORGANONKAR DS: *Chromosomal Variation in Man. A Catalog of Variants and Abnormalities,* Baltimore: Johns Hopkins, 1975

BROWN MS, GOLDSTEIN JL: New directions in human biochemical genetics: Understanding the manifestations of receptor deficiency disorders. Prog Med Genet vol. XII (in press)

CARTER CO: Genetics of common disorders. Br Med Bull 25:52, 1972

CAVALLI-SFORZA LL, BODMER WF: *The Genetics of Human Populations,* San Francisco: Freeman, 1971

CHILDS B, DER KALOUSTIAN VM: Genetic heterogeneity. N Engl J Med 279:1205, 1267, 1968

HARRIS H: *The Principles of Human Biochemical Genetics,* 2d ed., New York: American Elsevier, 1975

MCKUSICK VA: *Mendelian Inheritance in Man: Catalogs of Autosomal Dominant, Autosomal Recessive and X-linked Phenotypes,* 4th ed., Baltimore: Johns Hopkins, 1975

——, CLAIBORNE R: *Medical Genetics,* New York: HP Publishing, 1973

NORA JJ, FRASER FC: *Medical Genetics: Principles and Practice,* Philadelphia: Lea & Febiger, 1974

STANBURY JB et al: *The Metabolic Basis of Inherited Disease,* 3d ed., New York: McGraw-Hill, 1972

STEINBERG AG et al: *Progress in Medical Genetics,* vol 1, Philadelphia: Saunders, 1976

WATSON JD: *Molecular Biology of the Gene,* 3d ed., New York: W. A. Benjamin, 1976

65
PREVENTION AND TREATMENT OF GENETIC DISORDERS

JOSEPH L. GOLDSTEIN
MICHAEL S. BROWN

APPROACHES TO PREVENTION

In view of the present trend for couples to have smaller families, there is increasing concern that children should be healthy and free of genetic diseases, and primary-care physicians are called upon to play a more active role in the prevention and treatment of hereditary diseases. In most clinical situations, genetic advice can be given by the primary physician once the relatively simple principles of medical genetics (Chap. 64) and genetic counseling (discussed below) have been mastered.

RETROSPECTIVE GENETIC COUNSELING The prevention of genetic diseases requires the identification of matings that are capable of producing defective genotypes. These may involve matings in which one of the two individuals is carrying a dominant or X-linked gene mutation or a balanced translocation, or matings in which both individuals are carriers of a deleterious recessive gene. Such individuals are usually identified through an affected child or near relative, in which case retrospective genetic counseling can be provided.

When advising family members about the risk of transmitting a disorder that has already affected someone in the family, the counselor's first step is to be certain of the *correct diagnosis*—in particular, to make certain that the problem in question is really of genetic origin. This is especially important in disorders that may have either a genetic or a nongenetic etiology, such as deafness or mental retardation. Second, if the disease has a hereditary element, the possibility of *genetic heterogeneity,* i.e., a situation in which clinically similar genetic disorders show varying patterns of inheritance, must be considered. For example, there are two types of hereditary methemoglobinemia that resemble each other quite closely, but one shows autosomal recessive and the other autosomal dominant inheritance.

To estimate the *recurrence risk,* what is known of the genetic mechanisms controlling the relevant disorder must be determined. When more than one genetic mechanism exists, or when environmental factors can cause clinically indistinguishable traits, the *relative probabilities* of the different mechanisms operating in the particular family are computed. For conditions determined by simple mendelian inheritance, there is no difficulty in predicting the probability of an offspring being affected, provided that the genotypes of the parents can be recognized. Identification of the parental genotype is easiest for autosomal recessive and X-linked disorders since the basic lesions in these two forms of mendelian inheritance usually involve simple enzyme deficiencies for which biochemical tests are now available.

For autosomal dominant disorders, identification of the parental genotype is considerably more difficult since the basic defect is known for only a few of these disorders, and the diagnosis of the heterozygote for a dominant disorder depends almost exclusively on the clinical evaluation and a careful pedigree analysis. In counseling a family in which one relative is affected with a dominant disorder, it is important that appropriate clinical examination of all first-degree relatives and appropriately selected distant relatives be carried out. If relatives appear unaffected, there is the possibility that the clinical symptoms may be masked by *delayed age of onset* and *variability in expression.* When no relatives are affected, the possibility of a new dominant mutation must be entertained. Table 65-1 lists the most commonly encountered dominant disorders affecting adults and the best clinical methods currently available for detection of the heterozygote.

When advising families about multifactorial genetic diseases, such as diabetes mellitus, in which the inheritance pattern is not clear-cut, the physician must resort to empiric risk estimates that have been derived from retrospectively assembled data (Table 64-6).

Once the parental genotypes are determined, the genetic prognosis is usually presented in terms of probability that a given couple will produce an affected offspring. The physician providing genetic counseling must make certain that the couple understands not only the meaning of such absolute risk figures, but also the severity of the disease and the variability in clinical expression. In other words, in dealing with a disorder such as neurofibromatosis, it is important for the parents to realize not only that they have a 50 percent risk of producing a child with this disorder but also that a certain proportion of patients with the disorder have severe disease, a certain proportion have mild disease, etc. They should also have an understanding of the potential impact of the disease on their family; a disease that is lethal at birth might be classified by some as more "severe" than one that is lethal at age 16, but the latter is likely to have a much more profound impact on the family.

Although different families initially react in different ways to the same risk, most couples who seek genetic advice can be expected to take a responsible course of action that is based on the information quoted. Generally, the physician should avoid giving direct advice to the couple as to whether they "should" or "should not" have children. For serious genetic disease, with a recurrence risk equal to or greater than 1 in 10, most parents are usually deterred from planning further children. When the risks are less than 1 in 10, most parents usually continue with additional pregnancies.

PROSPECTIVE GENETIC COUNSELING In contrast to retrospective genetic counseling in which advice is given after the birth of at least one affected family member, in prospective genetic counseling advice is provided to possible carriers of recessive genes before an affected individual is born. As a first step, this requires the identification of heterozygous individuals by a population-screening procedure. Second, unmarried heterozygotes are instructed about the risk of their having affected children if they marry another heterozygote for the same gene. Finally, if two heterozygotes are already married, there is the possibility of interrupting the birth of affected infants if the disease can be diagnosed *in utero* by amniocentesis.

Population screening for heterozygote detection is possible for several autosomal recessive disorders (such as sickle-cell anemia, thalassemia major, and Tay-Sachs disease) that occur in certain populations with high frequency. For example, 8 percent of the American black population are carriers of the sickling gene, and 4 percent of the American Jewish population of Eastern and Central European extraction are carriers of the Tay-Sachs gene.

Screening programs raise many ethical and social problems. Informing a healthy person that he or she is carrying a specific mutant gene that may cause disease in the children if a certain type of mate is chosen differs from counseling parents who have already had an affected child. Very little is known about the social and psychologic effects as well as occupational discrimination that may result from discovering that a person carries a "bad" gene.

PRENATAL DIAGNOSIS The use of transabdominal amniocentesis permits diagnosis of certain genetic diseases at a stage early enough to terminate a pregnancy and to prevent the birth of a defective child. This procedure gives high-risk couples the opportunity to have unaffected children provided they are willing for the pregnancy to be terminated in the event that an abnormal fetus is detected. Amniocentesis consists of the transabdominal aspiration of amniotic fluid from the uterus. The procedure is preferably performed between the fourteenth and sixteenth weeks of pregnancy. When performed by a trained gynecologist, the technique is relatively safe for both mother and fetus.

Direct examination of the amniotic fluid itself may be diagnostic. For example, an elevated level of α-fetoprotein is a relatively good indicator of the presence of spina bifida or some other related neural tube abnormality. More frequently, prenatal diagnosis requires culture of the fetal

TABLE 65-1
Methods for detection of asymptomatic heterozygotes in frequently encountered dominantly inherited disorders

Disorder	*Method of heterozygote detection* Physical findings	Laboratory tests	Therapeutic advantage of early diagnosis
GASTROINTESTINAL, LIVER, AND PANCREAS			
Hemochromatosis		Serum iron	Prevent cirrhosis, heart failure, and diabetes
Gilbert's disease		Serum bilirubin	Avoid confusion with more serious forms of liver disease
Peutz-Jeghers syndrome	Melanin spots on lips, buccal mucosa, and digits	X-ray of small intestine	Clarify cause of gastrointestinal bleeding
Familial polyposis		X-ray of colon; colonoscopy	Prevent colon carcinoma
Gardner's syndrome	Multiple sebaceous cysts; lipomas; fibromas; osteomas; dental abnormalities; desmoid tumors	X-ray of colon and small intestine; colonoscopy	Prevent colon carcinoma
METABOLIC AND ENDOCRINE			
Medullary thyroid carcinoma–pheochromocytoma syndrome		Serum calcitonin; measurement of blood pressure	Prevent thyroid carcinoma and complications of hypertension
Multiple endocrine adenomatosis	Multiple lipomas	Serum calcium, gastrin, blood sugar; x-rays of sella turcica, stomach, and small intestine	Prevent complication of hyperparathyroidism, hypoglycemia, peptic ulcer, metastatic cancer
Familial hyperparathyroidism		Serum calcium, parathyroid hormone	Prevent renal damage and other complications of hypercalcemia
Familial hypercholesterolemia	Tendon xanthomas, xanthelasma, arcus corneae	Serum cholesterol; low-density lipoprotein receptor activity of cultured fibroblasts	Prevent premature coronary heart disease
HEART AND VASCULAR			
Holt-Oram syndrome	Abnormality of thumb and carpals; murmur of atrial septal defect	X-ray of hands; cardiac evaluation	Prevent complications of atrial septal defect
Noonan's syndrome	Hypertelorism; small chin; low-set ears; ptosis; pectus deformity; cryptorchidism; murmur of pulmonic stenosis	Cardiac evaluation; x-ray of skeleton; intravenous pyelogram (renal anomalies)	Prevent heart failure
Idiopathic hypertropic subaortic stenosis (asymmetric septal hypertrophy)	Presystolic gallop; characteristic carotid arterial pulse	EKG; echocardiogram	Prevent sudden death, syncope, angina, heart failure
Dominantly inherited form of atrial septal defect	Heart murmur	EKG showing first degree heart block, right bundle branch block, right axis deviation	Prevent complications of atrial septal defect
HEMATOLOGIC			
Hereditary spherocytosis	Splenomegaly; jaundice	Blood smear; reticulocyte count; hemoglobin; osmotic fragility test	Prevent anemia, cholelithiasis
Hereditary hemorrhagic telangiectasia	Telangiectasia of tongue, lips, conjunctiva, ears, fingers; pulmonary AV fistula	X-ray of lungs	Clarify cause of nosebleeds and gastrointestinal bleeding
von Willebrand's disease		Immunologic and functional assays of plasma antihemophilic globulin levels; bleeding time	Prevent gastrointestinal and urinary bleeding

Table 65-1 (continued)

Disorder	Method of heterozygote detection: Physical findings	Method of heterozygote detection: Laboratory tests	Therapeutic advantage of early diagnosis
CONNECTIVE TISSUE AND BONE			
Ehlers-Danlos syndromes (types I, II, III)	Loose-jointedness; fragile, stretchable, bruisable skin; subcutaneous calcified spherules		
Marfan's syndrome	Ectopic lens; mitral and aortic murmurs; excessive length of extremities	Slit-lamp examination; metacarpal index by x-ray	Reduce risk of aortic dissection; prevent blindness
Osteogenesis imperfecta	Multiple fractures; loose-jointedness; blue scleras; deafness; aortic regurgitation	X-ray of bones	
RENAL			
Alport's syndrome	Nerve deafness; cataracts, lenticonus, spherophakia	Urinalysis, slit-lamp examination	Prevent uremia
Nail-patella syndrome	Dysplastic nails; absent patellas	X-ray of pelvis (iliac horns); urinalysis	Clarify cause of hematuria and azotemia
Polycystic kidney disease		Urinalysis; intravenous pyelogram; renal arteriogram; measurement of blood pressure	Prevent uremia and complications of hypertension
Renal tubular acidosis		X-ray of kidneys (nephrocalcinosis); urine pH, calcium; serum electrolytes, calcium	Prevent acidosis, osteoporosis, kidney stones
RESPIRATORY			
Hereditary angioneurotic edema		Serum level of C1-esterase inhibitor of complement	Reduce risk of sudden death caused by laryngeal edema and clarify cause of acute abdominal pain
DERMATOLOGIC			
Neurofibromatosis	*Café au lait* spots; neurofibromas; scoliosis		Prevent malignant degeneration of neurofibromas
Waardenburg syndrome	Wide bridge of nose; frontal white blaze of hair; heterochromia iridis; white eye lashes; deafness		Clarify cause of deafness
Basal-cell nevus syndrome	Multiple basal-cell carcinomas; jaw cysts; pits on palms and soles; skeletal defects (ribs, spina bifida, scoliosis)	X-rays of skull (calcification of falx cerebri) and skeleton	Removal of cutaneous cancers; provide cosmetic surgery

cells in vitro, a process which usually takes 3 weeks. By this means the karyotype of the fetus can be determined, to ascertain fetal sex and to detect various chromosomal aberrations. Moreover, many inborn errors of metabolism can be detected by suitable assays of specific enzyme activities in the cultured fetal cells. Table 65-2 lists those enzyme deficiency states for which prenatal diagnosis is currently feasible. More disorders are constantly being added to this list.

Prenatal diagnosis by amniocentesis is currently indicated in the following high-risk situations: (1) Couples having a previous child with spina bifida or anencephaly (5 percent recurrence risk); (2) couples having a previous child with a chromosomal aberration such as the trisomy 21 form of Down's syndrome (1 to 2 percent recurrence risk); (3) couples in whom either the husband or wife carries a balanced translocation chromosome for Down's syndrome (5 percent recurrence risk for male carriers and 20

Disorder	Method of heterozygote detection: Physical findings	Method of heterozygote detection: Laboratory tests	Therapeutic advantage of early diagnosis
NEUROLOGIC			
Charcot-Marie-Tooth disease	Pes cavus; atrophy of anterior tibial and calf muscles ("stork legs"); absence of deep tendon reflexes	Biopsy of muscle and of sural cutaneous nerve	Improve walking by corrective shoes and orthopedic measures
Myotonic dystrophy	Myotonia; muscle wasting of temporal and sternocleidomastoid muscles; cataracts; frontal baldness; signs of hypogonadism	Slit-lamp examination; electromyography; measurement of serum immunoglobulins; electrocardiogram	Anticipate complete heart block
Acute intermittent porphyria		Measurement of uroporphyrinogen synthetase activity in red blood cells	Reduce risk of neuropathic attacks by avoidance of aggravating drugs such as barbiturates
Tuberous sclerosis	Adenoma sebaceum; cutaneous white macules; shagreen patch; periungual fibromas		Prevent seizures
Huntington's chorea	Paranoia, other personality changes; choreic movements; dementia		
Periodic paralysis syndromes (hypo-, hyper-, and normokalemic types)	Cold-induced myotonia	Electromyogram; serum potassium	Reduce frequency of attacks by avoidance of aggravating agents such as high-carbohydrate diet and exposure to cold
PHARMACOGENETIC			
Malignant hyperthermia		Serum creatine phosphokinase	Prevent fatal episode of hyperthermia induced by general anesthesia

TABLE 65-2
Inborn errors of metabolism for which prenatal diagnosis is feasible

LIPIDOSES

Cholesteryl ester storage disease
Fabry's disease
Gaucher's disease
Krabbe's disease (globoid cell leukodystrophy)
Metachromatic leukodystrophy
Neimann-Pick disease
Refsum's syndrome
Tay-Sachs disease and other gangliosidoses
Wolman's syndrome

MUCOPOLYSACCHARIDOSES

β-Glucuronidase deficiency
Hunter's syndrome
Hurler's syndrome
Sanfilippo's syndrome
Scheie's syndrome

AMINO ACID AND RELATED DISORDERS

Argininosuccinicaciduria
Citrullinemia
Cystathionine synthetase deficiency (homocystinuria)
Cystinosis
Histidinemia
Maple syrup urine disease
Methylmalonic aciduria

DISORDERS OF CARBOHYDRATE METABOLISM

Fucosidosis
Galactosemia
Glucose 6-phosphate dehydrogenase deficiency
Glycogen storage diseases, types II, III, and IV
Mannosidosis

MISCELLANEOUS DISORDERS

Adenosine deaminase deficiency
Familial hypercholesterolemia, homozygous form
Hypophosphatasia
I-cell disease
Lesch-Nyhan syndrome
Lysosomal acid phosphatase deficiency
Orotic aciduria
Sickle-cell anemia
Testicular feminization
Thalassemia
Xeroderma pigmentosa

SOURCE: *From Milunsky, pp. 239 to 241, 1975.*

percent for female carriers); (4) couples at high risk for having a child with a detectable inborn error of metabolism (Table 65-2) (25 to 50 percent recurrence risk); (5) pregnant women thirty-eight years of age and older who have a greater than 1 to 2 percent chance of carrying babies with Down's syndrome; and (6) women whose *male* fetuses have a 50 percent risk of being affected with a serious X-linked recessive disorder such as the Duchenne form of muscular dystrophy or classic hemophilia. Many such couples would elect to carry through the pregnancy if the fetus were found to be a female, but would abort if it were found to be a male.

APPROACHES TO TREATMENT

The goal of treatment for genetic diseases is to modify the natural history of the genetic trait so that an affected person may live a comfortable and healthy life despite his mutant genotype. Such treatment can be achieved for a number of inherited diseases using a variety of approaches, including (1) exclusion or restriction of toxic foods, (2) metabolic supplementation, (3) removal of toxic products, (4) surgery, and (5) organ transplantation. Table 65-3 lists examples of hereditary diseases affecting adults that can be successfully treated at the present time.

REFERENCES

EPSTEIN CJ: Prenatal diagnosis of genetic disorders. Adv Intern Med 20:325, 1975

MILUNSKY A: *The Prevention of Genetic Disease and Mental Retardation,* Philadelphia: Saunders, 1975

WORLD HEALTH ORGANIZATION: *Genetic Disorders: Prevention, Treatment, and Rehabilitation.* WHO Tech. Rep. 497, 1972

TABLE 65-3
Some treatable hereditary disorders affecting adults

Method of treatment	*Disorder*
REDUCTION OF TOXIC FOOD	
Lactose	Lactase deficiency
Galactose	Galactosemia
Fructose	Fructose intolerance
Neutral fats	Familial lipoprotein lipase deficiency
Cholesterol and saturated fats	Familial hypercholesterolemia
Phytanic acid	Refsum's syndrome
Phenylalanine	Phenylketonuria
METABOLIC SUPPLEMENTATION	
Vitamin D and phosphate	Hypophosphatemic rickets
Gamma-globulin	Agammaglobulinemia
Factor VIII (AHG)	Hemophilia
Cortisol	Adrenogenital syndromes
Thyroxine	Familial goiters
Growth hormone	Pituitary dwarfism
REMOVAL OF TOXIC PRODUCT	
Cystine removal by D-penicillamine	Cystinuria
Copper removal by D-penicillamine	Wilson's disease
Iron removal by phlebotomy	Hemochromatosis
SURGERY	
Splenectomy	Hereditary spherocytosis
Portacaval shunt	Glycogen storage disease, type I
Colectomy	Familial polyposis of the colon
Thyroidectomy	Medullary thyroid carcinoma syndrome
ORGAN TRANSPLANTATION	
Kidney	Fabry's disease
Kidney	Adult polycystic kidney disease

section 2 | Clinical pharmacology

66
PRINCIPLES OF DRUG THERAPY

JOHN A. OATES
GRANT R. WILKINSON

QUANTITATIVE DETERMINANTS OF DRUG ACTION

Safe and effective therapy with drugs requires their delivery to target tissues in concentrations within the narrow range that yields efficacy without toxicity. Optimal precision in achieving concentrations of drug within this therapeutic "window" can be achieved with regimens that are based on the kinetics of the drug's availability to target sites. This chapter deals with the principles of drug elimination and distribution that form the basis for loading and maintenance regimens for the average patient and considers instances in which elimination of the drug is impaired (e.g., renal failure). The kinetic basis for optimal utilization of plasma level data is also discussed.

PLASMA LEVELS AFTER A SINGLE DOSE The levels of lidocaine (Chap. 239) in plasma following intravenous administration decline in two phases as illustrated in Fig. 66-1; such a biphasic decline is typical for most drugs. Immediately following rapid injection, all the drug is in the plasma compartment, and the high initial plasma level reflects its confinement to this small volume. Subsequently, the drug is rapidly distributed from plasma into the extravascular compartment, and the period of time during which this is occurring is referred to as the *distribution phase.* For lidocaine this distribution phase is virtually complete within 30 min; then there is a slower rate of fall, referred to as the *equilibrium phase* or the *elimination phase.* During this phase, the drug levels in plasma and those in the tissues of the body are in equilibrium.

Distribution phase Pharmacologic events during the distribution phase depend on whether the level of drug at the receptor site closely reflects that in the plasma. If this is the case, the pharmacologic effects, whether favorable or adverse, may be inordinately great during this period. For example, following a small bolus dose (25 mg) of lidocaine, antiarrhythmic effects may be evident during the early distribution phase but disappear as levels rapidly fall below those that are minimally effective and even before equilibrium between plasma and tissue is reached. Thus, larger single doses or multiple small doses must be administered in order to achieve an effect that is sustained into the equilibrium phase. The toxicity of high levels of some drugs during the distribution phase precludes administration of a single intravenous loading dose that will achieve therapeutic levels during the equilibrium phase. For example, the administration of a loading dose of the anticonvulsant, phenytoin (diphenylhydantoin) as a single intravenous bolus can cause cardiovascular collapse due to the high levels during the distribution phase. For this reason, if a loading dose of phenytoin is administered intravenously, it must be given in fractions (10 to 15 percent of the total loading amount) at intervals sufficient to permit substantial distribution of the prior dose before the next is given. For similar reasons, the loading dose of many potent drugs that rapidly equilibrate with their receptors is divided into fractional doses for intravenous administration.

After an oral dose that delivers an equivalent amount of drug into the systemic circulation, plasma levels during the distribution phase do not rise nearly as steeply as they do after an intravenous bolus dose. Because the drug is not absorbed instantly after oral administration, it is delivered into the systemic circulation more slowly, and much of the drug is already distributed by the time absorption is complete. Thus, procainamide, which is almost totally absorbed after oral administration, can be given as a single 750-mg loading dose with little risk of hypotension; in contrast, loading of the drug by the intravenous route is more safely accomplished by giving the loading dose in fractions of about 100 mg at 5-min intervals in order to avoid the hypotension that would ensue during the distribution phase in some patients if the entire loading dose were given as a single bolus.

In contrast, other drugs are distributed to their sites of action only slowly during the distribution phase. For example, levels of digoxin at the receptor site (and its pharmacologic effect) do not reflect plasma levels during the distribution phase (Chap. 239). Digoxin is transported (or bound) to its cardiac receptors more slowly by a process that proceeds throughout distribution. Thus, plasma levels during a distribution phase of several hours are falling while levels at the site of action and pharmacologic effect are increasing (Fig. 66-2). Only at the end of the distribution phase when the drug has reached equilibrium with the receptor does the concentration of digoxin in plasma reflect pharmacologic effect. For this reason, there should be a 4-h wait after the distribution phase before samples for plasma levels of digoxin that are to be used as a guide to therapy are obtained.

Equilibrium phase After distribution has proceeded to the point where the concentration of drug in plasma is in equilibrium with that in the tissues outside the vascular compartment, the levels in plasma and tissues fall in parallel as the drug is eliminated from the body. Thus, the equilibrium phase is sometimes also referred to as the *elimination phase.*

Most drugs are eliminated as a first-order process. During the equilibrium phase, a characteristic of the first-order process is that the time required for the level of drug in

FIGURE 66-1
Concentrations of lidocaine in plasma following the administration of 50 mg intravenously. The half-life of 108 min is computed as the time required for levels to fall from any given value during the equilibrium phase ($Cp_{initial}$) to one-half that level. Cp_0 is the hypothetical concentration of lidocaine in plasma at time zero if equilibrium had been achieved instantly.

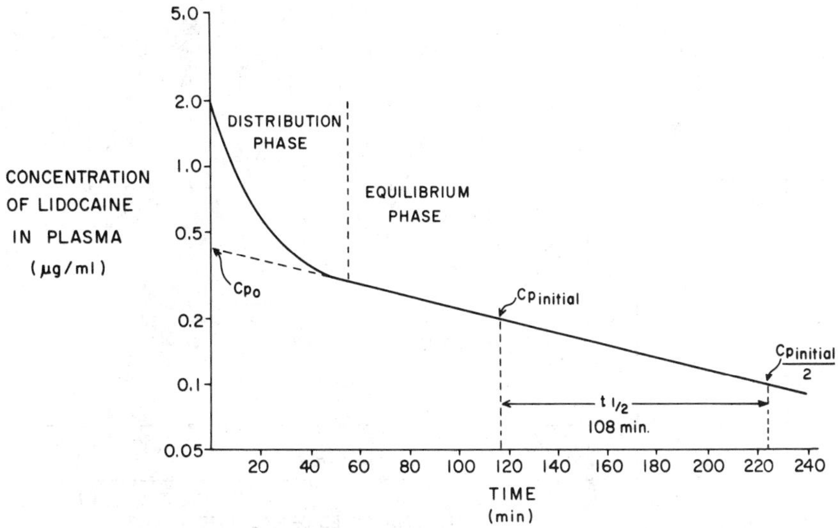

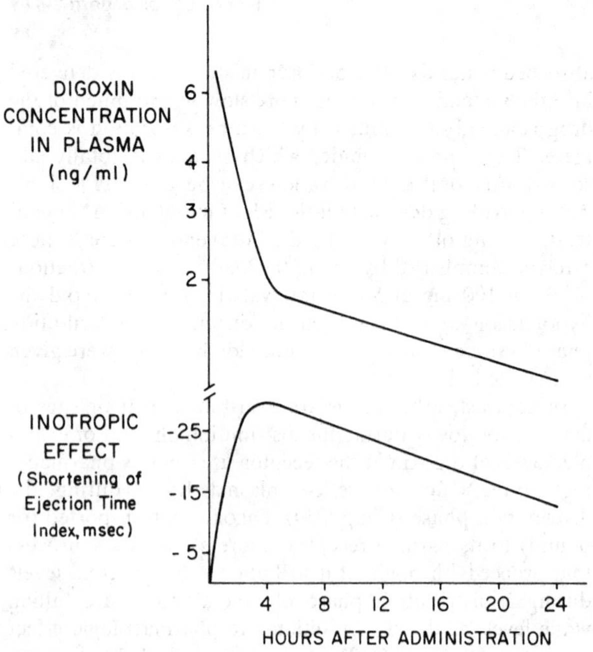

FIGURE 66-2
The time course of concentrations of digoxin in plasma and inotropic effect following intravenous administration of 0.8 mg of the drug.

plasma to fall to one-half the original value (the half-life) will be the same regardless of which point on the plasma level curve is chosen as a starting point for the measurement. Another characteristic of the first-order process is that a plot of the concentrations in plasma versus time during the equilibrium phase are linear on a semilogarithmic graph. From such a plot (Fig. 66-1) it can be seen that the half-life of lidocaine is 108 min.

One can readily calculate what amount of the administered dose remains in the body at any multiple of the half-life interval following administration:

Number of half-lives	*Amount of dose remaining in the body, %*
1	50
2	25
3	12.5
4	6.25
5	3.13

In theory, the elimination process never reaches completion. From a clinical standpoint, however, elimination can be considered as being essentially complete when it has reached 90 percent. Therefore, for practical purposes, *a first-order elimination process can be said to reach completion after 3 to 4 half-lives.*

DRUG ACCUMULATION—LOADING AND MAINTENANCE DOSES With repeated administration of a drug, the amount in the body will accumulate if the elimination of the first dose is incomplete when the second dose is given, and both the amount of drug in the body and its pharmacologic effect will increase with continuing administration until they reach a plateau. The accumulation of digoxin administered in repeated maintenance doses (without a loading dose) is illustrated in Fig. 66-3. As 65 percent of digoxin remains in the body at the end of 1 day in a patient with normal renal function, the second dose will raise the amount of digoxin in the body (and average plasma level) to 165 percent of that following the first dose. Each subsequent dose will result in greater amounts in the body until a plateau is attained. At the plateau, or *steady state,* drug intake per unit of time is the same as the rate of drug elimination. For *all drugs* with first-order kinetics, the time required to accumulate to steady-state levels can be predicted from the half-life because accumulation also is a first-order process with a half-life identical to that for elimination. Hence, accumulation will reach 90 percent of steady-state levels at the end of 3 to 4 half-lives. For digoxin, with a half-life of 1.6 days (with normal renal function), accumulation thus will be practically complete in 5 days (Chap. 239). Continuing infusion of the drug at a constant

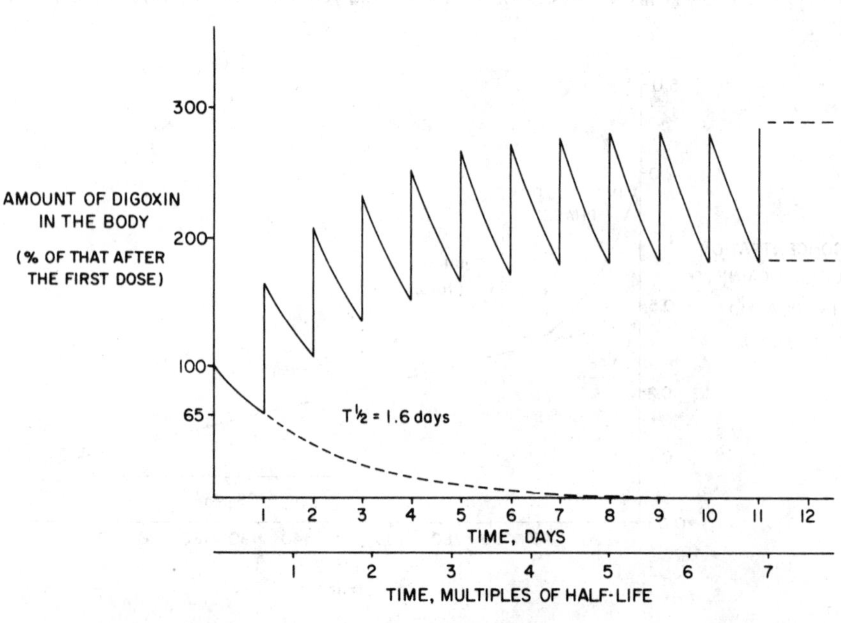

FIGURE 66-3
The time course of digoxin accumulation when a single daily maintenance dose is given (without a loading dose). Note that accumulation is more than 90 percent complete by the end of 4 half-lives.

rate exceeding the rate of elimination also will result in progressive accumulation to steady state over a time course predictable from the elimination curve for that drug (Fig. 66-4).

When the time required to reach steady-state levels is longer than one wishes to wait, plasma levels may be achieved more rapidly by the administration of a *loading dose.* Loading entails the administration of an amount that will bring the concentration in plasma (at equilibrium) to the level present during steady state. This may be accomplished by the administration of the loading amount as a single dose, or in the case of drugs with low therapeutic indexes (the therapeutic index is the ratio of the toxic dose to the therapeutic dose) the loading amount is given in a series of fractions of the total loading amount. As the accumulation of procainamide to 90 percent of steady state by infusion would require approximately 10 h (3.3 × the half-life of 3 h), a loading regimen is almost always desirable. The load required to suppress an arrhythmia, however, varies among individuals from 300 to 1,000 mg, and rapid intravenous administration of the *average loading dose* would cause hypotension during the high plasma levels in the distribution phase in some patients. Therefore, the intravenous loading dose of procainamide is given in fractions (e.g., 100 mg every 5 min) until the arrhythmia is controlled or adverse effects such as hypotension signal that no further drug should be given. Dividing the loading dose into fractions is appropriate for most drugs that, like procainamide, have a low therapeutic index. This permits better individualization of the loading amount and avoids needless adverse effects that might occur during the distribution phase of a single large dose.

The size of loading dose required to achieve the plasma levels present at steady state can be determined from the fraction of drug eliminated during the dosage interval and the maintenance dose (in the case of intermittent drug administration). For example, if the fraction of digoxin eliminated daily is 35 percent and the planned maintenance dose is to be 0.25 mg daily, then the loading dose to achieve steady-state levels should be 100/35 times the maintenance dose, or approximately 0.75 mg. Thus

$$\text{Loading dose} = \frac{100}{\text{\% of drug eliminated per dosage interval}} \times \text{maintenance dose}$$

The fraction of drug eliminated during any dosage interval can be determined from a semilogarithmic graph, in which the total body dose at time zero is set at 100 percent and the fraction remaining at the end of 1 half-life is 50 percent.[1] Conversely, if the loading dose is known, the maintenance dose can be similarly calculated.

Regardless of the size of the loading dose, *after maintenance therapy has been given for 3 to 4 half-lives, the amount of drug in the body is determined only by the maintenance dose.* The independence of the plasma levels at steady state from the load is illustrated in Fig. 66-4, which indicates that the elimination of any drug given at time 0 (elimination curve) would be practically complete after 3 to 4 half-lives.

[1] *The fraction of drug remaining in the body at the end of a dosage interval can be determined nongraphically from the equation*

$$\text{Fraction of drug remaining in body} = e^{-kt}$$

Values for e^{-kt} can be obtained from a table of natural exponential functions where k is the fractional elimination constant (described in the next section) and t is the time interval from drug administration. k is equal to 0.693/t1/2.

FIGURE 66-4

The time course of plasma levels of lidocaine following a single intravenous dose (——) compared with those during a constant intravenous infusion (- - -). This relationship applies to all drugs that rapidly achieve equilibrium between plasma and tissues.

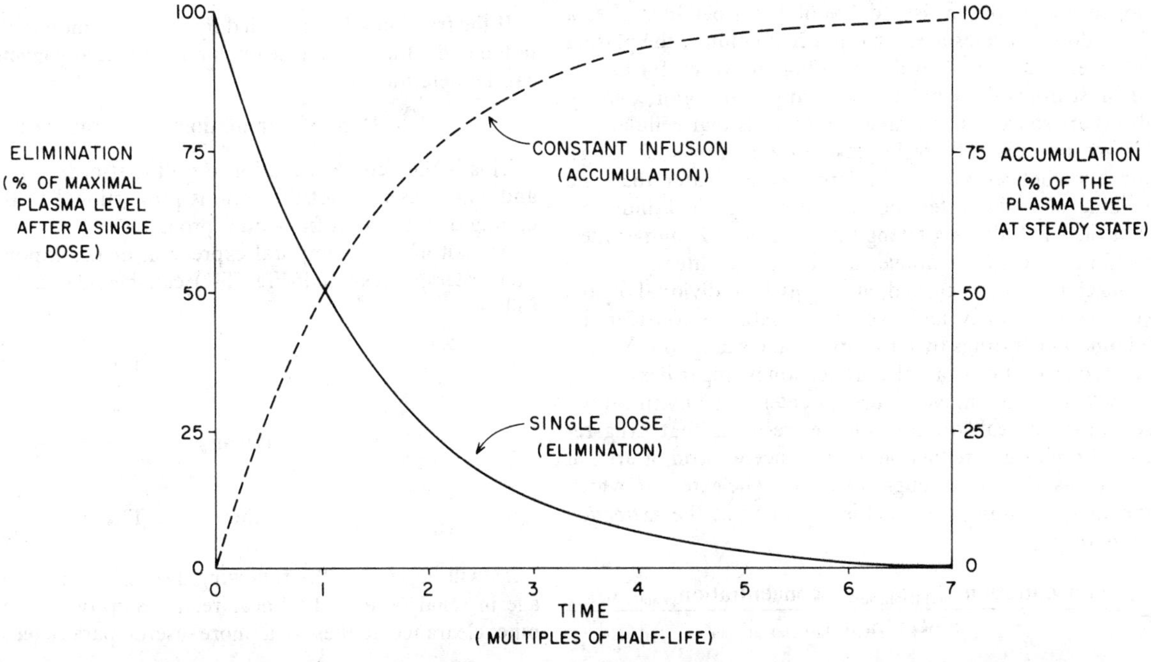

DETERMINANTS OF PLASMA LEVELS DURING THE EQUILIBRIUM PHASE An important determinant of the level of drug in plasma during the equilibrium phase after a single dose is the extent to which the drug has distributed outside the plasma compartment. For example, if the distribution of a 3-mg dose of a large macromolecule is confined to a plasma volume of 3 liters, then the concentration in plasma will be 1 mg per liter. However, if a different drug is distributed so that 90 percent of it leaves the plasma compartment, then only 0.3 mg will remain in the 3-liter plasma volume, and the concentration in plasma will be only 0.1 mg per liter. The extent of extravascular distribution at equilibrium can be expressed by the term *apparent volume of distribution,* or Vd. More precisely, Vd expresses the constant relationship between the amount of drug in the body and the plasma concentration at equilibrium:

$$\text{Vd} = \frac{\text{amount of drug in body}}{\text{plasma concentration}}$$

The amount of drug in the body is expressed as mass (e.g., milligrams), and the plasma concentration is expressed as mass per volume (e.g., milligrams per liter). Thus the Vd is a hypothetical volume into which a quantity of drug would distribute if its concentration in the entire volume were the same as that in plasma. Although it does not represent a real volume, it is an important quantity because it determines the fraction of total drug which is in the plasma and therefore the fraction available to the organs of elimination. An approximation of the Vd in the equilibrium phase can be obtained by estimating the concentration of drug in plasma at time zero (Cp_0) by a back-extrapolation of the equilibrium phase plot to zero time as illustrated in Fig. 66-1. Then, after intravenous administration when the amount in the body at time zero is the dose, we have

$$\text{Vd} = \frac{\text{dose}}{Cp_0}$$

For the administration of the large macromolecule mentioned above, the measured Cp_0 of 1 mg per liter after a 3-mg dose indicates a Vd that is a real volume, the plasma volume. This example is the exception, however, for the Vd of most drugs does not relate to any real volume; many drugs are so extensively taken up by cells that cellular levels greatly exceed those in plasma water. For such drugs, the hypothetical Vd will be large, even greater than the volume of body water. For example, Fig. 66-1 indicates that the Cp_0 following 50 mg lidocaine is 0.42 mg per liter, yielding a Vd by the above equation of 119 liters.

As elimination is carried out largely by individual organs such as the kidney and liver, it is useful to consider the elimination of drugs by these organs according to the *clearance* concept. For example, in the kidney, regardless of the extent to which removal of drug is determined by filtration, secretion, or reabsorption, the net result is that drug removal results in a reduction of the concentration of drug in plasma as it passes through the organ. The extent to which the concentration is reduced is expressed as the *extraction ratio,* or E.

$$E = \frac{\text{concentration}_{\text{arterial plasma}} - \text{concentration}_{\text{venous plasma}}}{\text{concentration}_{\text{arterial plasma}}}$$

If the extraction is complete, E will be 1. If the total plasma flow to the kidneys is Q ml per min, the total volume of plasma from which drug is completely removed in a unit time (clearance) is determined as

$$\text{Clearance}_{\text{renal}} = \frac{\text{Q} \cdot \text{E ml}}{\text{min}}$$

If the extraction ratio of penicillin is 0.5 and renal plasma flow is 680 ml per min, then penicillin's renal clearance will be 340 ml per min. If the extraction ratio of a compound is high, as is the case for renal extraction of para-aminohippuric acid (PAH) or hepatic extraction of propranolol, then clearance becomes entirely a function of organ blood flow.

Clearance from the total body (Cl) is the sum of clearance from all organs of elimination and is the best measure of the efficiency of the elimination processes. If a drug is removed by both renal excretion and hepatic metabolism, then

$$\text{Cl} = \text{Cl}_{\text{renal}} + \text{Cl}_{\text{hepatic}}$$

Thus, if penicillin is eliminated by both renal clearance (340 ml per min) and hepatic clearance (36 ml per min) in a normal individual, total clearance will be 376 ml per min. If renal clearance is reduced to half, total clearance = 170 + 36 = 206 ml per min. In anuria, total clearance will equal hepatic clearance.

Only the drug in the vascular compartment can be cleared during each passage through an organ. To ascertain the effect of a given plasma clearance by one or more organs on the rate of removal of drug from the body, the clearance must be related to the volume of "plasma equivalents" to be cleared, that is, the volume of distribution. If the volume of distribution is 10,000 ml and clearance is 1,000 ml per min, then one-tenth of the drug in the body is eliminated per minute. This fraction, clearance/Vd, is known as a *fractional elimination constant* and is designated as k:

$$\text{Fractional elimination per unit time} = k = \frac{\text{clearance}}{\text{Vd}}$$

If the fraction k is multiplied by the total amount of drug in the body, the actual rate of elimination at any given time can be determined:

$$\text{Rate of elimination} = k \cdot \text{amount in body}$$

This is the general equation for all first-order processes and expresses the fact that rate is proportional to the declining quantity in a first-order process.

As half-life is a temporal expression of the exponential first-order process, half-life ($T\frac{1}{2}$) can be related to k as follows:

$$T^1/_2 = \frac{0.693}{k}$$

$$\text{Because} \quad k = \frac{\text{clearance}}{\text{Vd}}$$

$$\text{then} \quad T^1/_2 = \frac{0.693 \times \text{Vd}}{\text{clearance}}$$

As will be seen in the following discussion on drug dosage in renal failure, the linear relationship of k to creatinine clearance makes k a more useful parameter upon which to base calculations of the changes in drug elimination that occur with a known reduction in creatinine clearance in renal insufficiency. Half-life is not linearly related to clearance.

The important relationship

$$T^1/_2 = \frac{0.693 \times Vd}{\text{clearance}}$$

expresses clearly that half-life is determined by both clearance and volume of distribution. Thus, for example, half-life is shortened when phenobarbital induces the enzymes responsible for hepatic clearance of a drug, and half-life is lengthened when a drug's renal clearance is attenuated in renal failure. Also, the half-life of some drugs is shortened when their volume of distribution is reduced. If, as in the case of cardiac failure, the volume of distribution is reduced at the same time that clearance is reduced, there may be little change in drug half-life to reflect the impaired clearance, but plasma levels will be increased. In treating patients after an overdose, expectations of how hemodialysis will affect the drug's elimination are dependent on its volume of distribution. When the volume of distribution is very large, as is the case with tricyclic antidepressants (Vd of nortriptyline equals more than 2,000 liters), the removal of drug, even with a high-clearance dialyzer, will proceed slowly.

The extent to which a drug is bound to plasma protein also determines the fraction of drug extracted by the organ(s) of elimination. Altered binding will change the extraction ratio significantly, however, only when elimination is limited to the free drug in plasma. The extent to which binding influences elimination depends on the relative affinity of the plasma binding versus the affinity of the drug for the extraction process. The high affinity of the renal tubular anion transport system for many drugs will lead to extraction of both bound and free drug, and the efficient process by which the liver removes propranolol will result in extraction of most of this highly bound drug from blood.

For drugs with high extraction ratios, binding to plasma protein serves as a transport vehicle to enhance delivery of drug to the elimination site. In contrast, when the extraction mechanism is less avid and extraction is limited largely to free drug, the fraction of drug that is bound to plasma protein may be considered as a reservoir that slows elimination and lengthens half-life. This generally occurs when the extraction ratio of the organ of elimination is less than the fraction of free drug and is termed *restrictive elimination.* Glomerular filtration is a process that is restricted to the unbound fraction, as is the metabolism of drugs with low extraction ratios such as phenytoin and warfarin.

For those drugs with restrictive elimination, differences among individuals in binding to plasma proteins can be expected to produce variation in the fraction of drug that is unbound and the elimination rate. Differences in binding may be of genetic origin, or may result from drug interactions, uremia, hypoalbuminemia, or jaundice.

STEADY STATE With a constant infusion of drug, the infusion rate equals elimination rate at steady state. Therefore,

$$\underset{\text{(amt/unit time)}}{\text{Infusion rate}} = \underset{\text{(amt/vol)}}{\text{plasma concentration}} \times \underset{\text{(vol/unit time)}}{\text{Cl}}$$

when the units for amount, volume, and time are consistent.

Thus, if clearance (Cl) is known, the infusion rate required to achieve a given plasma level can be calculated. An approach to estimating the clearance of a number of drugs is discussed below in the section on renal disease.

When the dose is given intermittently instead of by infusion, the above relationship between plasma concentration and the dose administered at each dosage interval can be expressed as

$$\text{Dose} = \text{plasma concentration}_{\text{avg}} \times \text{Cl} \times \text{dosage interval}$$

The average plasma concentration implies that, as seen in Fig. 66-3, levels can be considerably higher and lower than the average during the dosage interval.

When a drug is given orally and is not completely absorbed, the calculated dose must be divided by the fraction (F) of drug that reaches the systemic circulation following oral administration:

$$\text{Oral dose} = \frac{\text{plasma concentration}_{\text{avg}} \times \text{Cl} \times \text{dosage interval}}{\text{F}}$$

DRUG ELIMINATION THAT IS NOT FIRST ORDER The elimination of some important drugs such as phenytoin and salicylate does not follow first-order kinetics when amounts of drug in the body are in the therapeutic range. For these drugs, the clearance is not a constant value but changes as levels in the body fall during elimination or after changes in dose. This pattern of elimination is said to be *dose-dependent.* Accordingly, the time for the concentration to fall to one-half becomes less as plasma levels fall; this halving-time is not truly a half-life, however, because the term *half-life* applies to first-order kinetics and is a constant. The elimination of phenytoin is dose-dependent, and when very high levels are present (in the toxic range) the halving-time may be longer than 72 h, whereas after the concentration in plasma has declined to lower levels, the clearance increases and the concentration in plasma will halve in 20 to 30 h.

When drug is eliminated by first-order kinetics, the plasma level at steady state is directly related to the amount of the maintenance dose, and a doubling of the dose should lead to doubling of the steady-state plasma level. However, for phenytoin and other drugs with dose-dependent kinetics, increases in the dose may be accompanied by disproportionately large increases in plasma level. Thus, if the daily dose of phenytoin is increased from 300 to 400 mg, plasma levels rise by considerably more than 33 percent. Unfortunately, the extent of increase is not predictable because of the wide interpatient variability in the extent to which clearance deviates from first order. Salicylates are eliminated by dose-dependent kinetics at the higher plasma levels, and in children particular caution must be taken with the administration of high doses. Ethanol metabolism also is dose-dependent, with obvious implications. The mechanisms involved in dose-dependent kinetics may include the saturation of the rate-limiting step in metabolism or a feedback inhibition of the rate-limiting enzyme by a product of the reaction.

INDIVIDUALIZATION OF DRUG THERAPY

Recognition of factors modifying drug action is essential for therapy that provides optimal benefit with minimal risk to each individual patient. Certain disease states can modify the delivery of a drug to its site of action.

RENAL DISEASE Where urinary excretion is an important route of elimination, renal failure results in decreased drug clearance and therefore slower removal of the drug from the body, so that administration according to the usual dosage regimen leads to greater accumulation and an increased likelihood of toxicity. A reasonable therapeutic goal in such cases is to modify the dosage schedule so that the average drug concentration in the plasma of the patient with renal insufficiency is the same, and steady state is reached after a similar time interval, as in the patient with normal renal function.

One approach to dosage alteration in renal insufficiency is to calculate the *fraction of the normal dose* that is to be given at the usual dosage interval. This fraction can be determined from data on either drug clearance (Cl) or the fractional rate constant (k), based on the fact that both renal clearance and renal k are directly proportional to creatinine clearance. Thus, the dose in renal insufficiency is

$$\text{Dose}^{ri} = \text{dose} \times \frac{\text{Cl}^{ri}}{\text{Cl}}$$

where ri = renal insufficiency
Cl = clearance from the whole body with normal renal function
Dose = maintenance dose with normal renal function ($\text{Cl}_{cr} \sim 100$ ml per min)

The normal clearance and that in renal impairment (Cl^{ri}) can be obtained by employing the data in Table 66-1 in the following equations:

$$\text{Cl} = \text{Cl}_{renal} + \text{Cl}_{nonrenal}$$

$$\text{Cl}^{ri} = \text{Cl}_{renal} \cdot \frac{\text{measured Cl}_{creatinine}}{100} + \text{Cl}_{nonrenal}$$

As the Cl_{renal} values in Table 66-1 are those found with a $\text{Cl}_{creatinine}$ of 100 ml per min, then the renal clearance of drug in renal insufficiency is obtained by multiplying Cl_{renal} by the ratio of measured $\text{Cl}_{creatinine}$ (in milliliters per minute) to 100 ml per min.

For gentamicin, with a normal Cl_{renal} of 78 ml per min and $\text{Cl}_{nonrenal}$ of 3 ml per min, Cl = 81 ml per min. Therefore, with a creatinine clearance of 12, $\text{Cl}^{ri} = 78 \times {}^{12}/_{100} + 3 = 12.4$ ml per min. If the dose of gentamicin for a given infection should be 1.5 mg/kg/8 h in the presence of normal renal function, then

$$\text{Dose}^{ri} = 1.5 \text{ mg/kg/8 h} \cdot \frac{12.4 \text{ ml/min}}{81 \text{ ml/min}} = 0.23 \text{ mg/kg/8 h}$$

In the patient with renal insufficiency, this computation will yield an average plasma level during a dosage interval that is the same as the average plasma level during the dosage interval with normal renal function; the peaks and troughs, however, will vary less from the average.

All calculation of dosage is most accurately based on the clearance of a drug, because this is a direct measure of the efficiency of drug removal. However, clearance data are not available for some drugs, in which case [if it is assumed that renal disease does not affect the distribution of the drug (Vd)], the dosage fraction can be approximated from the ratio of the fractional rate constant for elimination from the total body in renal failure (k^{ri}) to that with normal renal function (k). The approach is the same as that employed with clearance data:

$$\text{Dose}^{ri} = \text{dose} \times \frac{k^{ri}}{k}$$

By use of values from Table 66-2, k and k^{ri} can be calculated:

$$k = k_{renal} + k_{nonrenal}$$

$$k^{ri} = k_{renal} \cdot \frac{\text{measured Cl}_{creatinine}}{100} + k_{nonrenal}$$

In some instances it may be desirable to calculate a dose that will yield a certain plasma level at steady state. This approach is most appropriate for constant intravenous infusions where 100 percent of the dose is delivered to the systemic circulation. When clearance of a drug in a patient with renal insufficiency is calculated as above, then

$$\text{Dose}^{ri}_{(amt/time)} = \text{Cl}^{ri}_{(vol/time)} \cdot \text{plasma concentration}_{(amt/vol)}$$

where the time, amount, and volume terms are uniform.

If a plasma concentration of carbenicillin of 100 μg per ml is the therapeutic objective in a patient with a creatinine clearance of 25 ml/min, the infusion rate is calculated as follows. Carbenicillin clearance is

$$\text{Cl}^{ri} = 68 \cdot \frac{25}{100} + 10 = 27 \text{ ml/min}$$

Therefore, carbenicillin should be infused at a rate of 2,700 μg per min.

Should the method of calculating dose based on the desired plasma level be applied to intermittent-dose therapy, particular attention should be given to the fact that the calculation is based on an *average* plasma level and that peak plasma levels will obviously be higher. In addition, if a drug is given orally and is not completely absorbed, the computed dose must be divided by the fraction of drug which reaches the systemic circulation following oral administration (F) (see Steady State above).

In all the above calculations, it is assumed that the nonrenal clearance and nonrenal k are constant in renal fail-

TABLE 66-1
Clearances of drugs

Drug	*Renal clearance,* ml/min*	*Nonrenal clearance, ml/min*
Ampicillin†	340	12
Carbenicillin	68	10
Digoxin†	110	36
Gentamicin	78	3
Kanamycin	60	0
Penicillin G‡	340	36

* *The "normal" renal clearances are those associated with a clearance of creatinine of 100 ml per min.*
† *The fraction of digoxin absorbed after an oral dose (F) is approximately 0.6 and F for ampicillin is 0.5.*
‡ *One microgram of penicillin G = 1.6 units.*

TABLE 66-2
Rate constants for renal and nonrenal elimination of drugs

Drug	k_{renal}*, h^{-1}	$k_{nonrenal}$, h^{-1}
Cephalexin	0.67	0.03
Cephaloridine	0.37	0.03
Cephalothin	1.37	0.03
Cephazolin	0.34	0.02
Chloramphenicol	0.00	0.3
Chlortetracycline	0.00	0.1
Colistin	0.28	0.02
Doxycycline	0.00	0.03
Erythromycin	0.37	0.13
Isoniazid (fast inactivators)	0.10	0.3
Isoniazid (slow inactivators)	0.10	0.1
Lincomycin	0.09	0.06
Methicillin	1.23	0.17
Minocycline	0.02	0.04
Oxacillin	1.05	0.35
Polymyxin B	0.14	0.02
Procainamide	0.14	0.07
Rifampin	0.00	0.25
Streptomycin	0.26	0.01
Sulfadiazine	0.05	0.03
Sulfamethoxazole	0.00	0.7
Tetracycline	0.07	0.01
Tobramycin	0.345	0.005
Trimethoprim	0.04	0.02
Vancomycin	0.117	0.003
	day^{-1}	day^{-1}
Digitoxin	0.03	0.07
Ouabain	0.09	0.3

* *The k_{renal} values are those associated with a creatinine clearance of 100 ml per min.*

ure. In fact, when cardiac failure accompanies renal failure, metabolic clearance for many drugs is reduced. Accordingly, when a drug with a narrow therapeutic index, such as digoxin, is used in cardiac failure, an appropriate precaution would be to reduce the value for nonrenal clearance (or k) to about one-half.

In addition to adjusting the maintenance dose in patients with renal failure, consideration must also be given to the necessity of a loading dose. Since this dose is designed to bring the plasma concentration, or more particularly the amount of drug in the body, rapidly to the level that is reached at steady state, there is no need to modify the usual loading dose, if one is normally used. For many drugs, however, their elimination is sufficiently rapid that the time required to reach steady state is not clinically significant and no loading dose is usually used. On the other hand, in renal failure where the half-life may be significantly prolonged, this accumulation period may become unacceptably long. In such a case, for a drug given intermittently, a loading dose may be calculated as described in Drug Accumulation above. For an infusion, the loading dose may be approximated (when all units are consistent) as

$$\text{Loading dose}^{ri} = \frac{\text{infusion rate}^{ri}}{k}$$

Because of the considerable individual differences in volumes of distribution, rates of metabolism, and hepatic blood flow, the above calculations of drug dose for patients in renal failure must be viewed as valuable approximations which prevent the use of doses that are grossly excessive or inadequate for most patients. However, *maintenance dosages are most accurate when plasma level data are employed as a feedback to enable adjustment of the dose where necessary.*

LIVER DISEASE In contrast to the predictable decline in renal clearance of drugs when glomerular filtration is reduced, it is not possible to make a general prediction of the effect of liver disease on hepatic biotransformation of drugs (Chap. 295). Rather, in hepatitis and cirrhosis there is a spectrum of changes ranging from impaired to increased drug clearance. Even when there is advanced hepatocellular disease, the magnitude of impairment in drug clearance usually is only about two- to fivefold. The extent of such changes, however, cannot be predicted by any of the commonly available tests of liver function. Consequently, even though it may be suspected that drug elimination is altered in a patient with liver disease, there is no quantitative base upon which to adjust the dosage regimen. Therefore, the drugs of choice are those which evidence or clinical experience indicates that the body satisfactorily handles despite impaired liver function. Alternatively, the usual drug and dosage regimen may be employed with alertness to the potential for unexpected drug accumulation and exaggerated effects.

Portacaval shunting creates a special situation because the effective hepatic blood flow is substantially reduced. This procedure has its greatest effect on drugs that normally have a high extraction ratio so that their clearance is largely a function of blood flow; thus the clearance of such drugs (e.g., propranolol and lidocaine) will be remarkably reduced by portacaval shunting. In addition, the fraction of an administered oral dose reaching the systemic circulation will be significantly increased, because drug that is shunted around the liver during the absorption process will escape the efficient first-pass metabolism by this organ.

CIRCULATORY INSUFFICIENCY—CARDIAC FAILURE AND SHOCK Under conditions leading to decreased tissue perfusion, redistribution of the cardiac output occurs to preserve blood flow to the heart and brain at the expense of other tissues (Chap. 237). As a result, the drug shifts into a smaller volume of distribution, higher drug concentrations are present in the plasma, and the vital organs are exposed to these higher concentrations. If either the brain or heart are sensitive to the pharmacologic effect of the drug, an alteration in response will occur.

Furthermore, the decreased perfusion of the kidney and liver may impair drug clearance by these organs either directly or indirectly. Thus, in severe congestive heart failure, in hemorrhagic shock, and particularly in cardiogenic shock, the response to the usual dose of the drug may be excessive, and dosage modification may be necessary. For example, the clearance of lidocaine is reduced by about 50 percent in cardiac failure, and consequently therapeutic plasma levels are achieved at infusion rates of only about half of those usually required. In cardiac failure there also is a significant reduction in lidocaine's volume of distribution which results in the requirement of a smaller loading dose. Similar situations are thought to exist for procainamide, theophylline, and possibly quinidine. Unfortunately, predictors of these types of pharmacokinetic alterations are unavailable. Therefore, loading doses should be conservative, and continued therapy should be monitored closely, following clinical indicators of toxicity and plasma levels.

DISEASE-INDUCED CHANGES IN PLASMA BINDING Many drugs circulate in the plasma partly bound to the plasma proteins and other constituents. Since only the unbound or free drug can distribute to the site of pharmacologic action, the therapeutic response should be related to the free rather than the total circulating plasma drug concentration. In most cases the degree of binding is fairly constant across the therapeutic concentration range so that significant error is not caused by individualizing therapy on the basis of measuring levels of total drug in plasma. However, several clinical states such as hypoalbuminemia, liver disease, and renal disease can decrease the extent of drug binding so that at any total plasma level there is a greater concentration of free drug and a risk of increased response and toxicity. The drugs for which such changes are important are those which are normally highly bound in the plasma (> 90 percent) because a small alteration in the extent of binding produces a large relative increase in the fraction of drug in the unbound form.

The binding of phenytoin is altered in patients with chronic renal failure by an unclear mechanism; the percentage of unbound drug increases about fourfold from a normal of approximately 7 percent to as high as 25 to 30 percent. Similar, but less pronounced, changes are also seen in patients with viral hepatitis, jaundice, and the nephrotic syndrome, and with other drugs such as diazoxide, digitoxin, clofibrate, and certain sulfonamides.

The pharmacokinetic consequences of these binding changes, particularly with respect to total drug levels, depend on whether the clearance and distribution are dependent on the unbound or total drug. For many drugs, including those cited above, elimination and distribution are largely restricted to the free fraction, and therefore a decrease in binding leads to an increase in the clearance and distribution of the total drug. The relative magnitudes of thse changes are such that the net effect is to shorten the half-life. For example, in uremia the half-life of phenytoin may be as low as 6 to 8 h compared with a normal value of about 20 to 30 h. However, the clearance of *free* drug is unaffected, and the average steady-state plasma concentration of unbound drug is unaltered. Accordingly, the appropriate modification of the dosage regimen in clinical conditions with reduced drug binding is simply to administer the usual daily dose of the drug, but in divided doses at more frequent intervals. Individualization of therapy can then be based on either the clinical response or the plasma concentration of unbound drug. It is critical that the patient not be titrated into the usual therapeutic range for concentration of *total* drug in plasma since this will inevitably lead to supraeffective response and toxicity.

INTERACTIONS BETWEEN DRUGS

The effect of some drugs can be altered markedly by the administration of other agents. Such interactions can sabotage therapeutic intent by producing excessive drug action (with adverse effects) or decreasing the action of a drug, rendering it ineffective. Drug interactions must be considered in the differential diagnosis of unexpected responses to drugs, taking into account that ambulatory patients often come to the physician with a legacy of drugs acquired during their previous medical experiences. A meticulous drug history will minimize the unknown elements in the patient's therapeutic milieu; it should include examination of the patient's medications and calls to the pharmacist to identify prescriptions, if necessary.

There are two principal types of interactions between drugs. *Pharmacokinetic interactions* result from alteration in the delivery of drugs to their sites of action. *Pharmacodynamic interactions* are those in which the responsiveness of the target organ or system has been modified by other agents.

Pharmacokinetic interactions causing diminished drug delivery

IMPAIRED GASTROINTESTINAL ABSORPTION Aluminum ions, present in antacids, form insoluble chelates with the tetracyclines, thereby preventing absorption of these drugs. Ferrous ions similarly block tetracycline absorption. Cholestyramine, an ionic exchange resin, binds thyroxine, triiodothyronine, and the cardiac glycosides with sufficiently high affinity to impair their absorption from the gastrointestinal tract. This resin probably also interferes with the absorption of other drugs, and it is safest not to give it within 2 h of their administration. Oral administration of para-aminosalicylate interferes with the absorption of rifampin by a mechanism not yet determined.

All the above instances of impaired absorption result in a reduction in the total amount of drug absorption, with reduced area under the plasma level curve and reduced peak plasma levels, as well as lower steady-state concentrations of the drug involved.

INDUCTION OF HEPATIC DRUG-METABOLIZING ENZYMES When the elimination of the drug proceeds largely via biotransformation, an increase in the rate at which it is metabolized reduces its availability to sites of action. The biotransformation of most drugs occurs largely in the liver, because of its mass, high blood flow, and concentration of enzymes that metabolize drugs. The initial step in metabolism of many drugs is executed by the mixed-function oxidase enzymes located in the hepatic endoplasmic reticulum. These enzyme systems containing cytochrome P-450 oxidize the molecule by a variety of reactions including aromatic hydroxylations, *N*-demethylations, *O*-demethylations, and sulfoxidations. The products of these reactions are usually more polar (and more readily excreted by the kidney).

The number of mixed-function oxidase enzyme units in the liver can be increased by treatment with enzyme inducers, of which phenobarbital is the prototype. Almost all the barbiturates in clinical use increase the mixed-function oxidase enzymes. Induction with phenobarbital can occur with doses of as little as 60 mg daily. Mixed-function oxidases are also induced by glutethimide, phenytoin, and rifampin, and by occupational exposure to chlorinated insecticides such as DDT, as well as by alcohol.

The actions of a number of drugs are inhibited by treatment with inducing agents. Phenobarbital and other inducers lower plasma levels of warfarin, bishydroxycoumarin, digitoxin, quinidine, dexamethasone, and metyrapone. These interactions all have obvious clinical significance. With the coumarin anticoagulants, the major risk occurs when an appropriate level of anticoagulation is achieved while the coumarin drug is coadministered with an inducing agent. When the inducer is discontinued, e.g., following discharge from the hospital, plasma levels of the coumarin anticoagulant will rise and lead to excessive anticoagulation. Barbiturates have been shown to lower the plasma levels of phenytoin in some patients, but the clinical effect of reduced phenytoin levels is probably counterbalanced by the anticonvulsant effects of phenobarbital.

There is considerable variation among individuals in the extent to which drug metabolism can be induced. In some patients phenobarbital leads to marked acceleration in the rate of drug metabolism, whereas little induction is seen in others. This variability in the extent of induction of mixed-function oxidases is largely genetically determined.

In addition to inducing the mixed-function oxidase enzymes, phenobarbital has a number of other effects on hepatic function. It increases liver blood flow, bile flow, and the hepatocellular transport of organic anions. The conjugation of drugs and bilirubin is also enhanced by inducing agents.

INHIBITION OF CELLULAR UPTAKE OR BINDING The guanidinium antihypertensives, guanethidine and bethanidine, are transported to their site of action in adrenergic neurons by an energy-requiring membrane transport system for biogenic monoamines. Although the physiologic function of the transport system is re-uptake of the adrenergic neurotransmitter, it also transports a variety of ring-substituted bases, including guanethidine and bethanidine, into the adrenergic neuron against a concentration gradient. Inhibitors of norepinephrine uptake will prevent the uptake of the guanidinium antihypertensives into adrenergic neurons and will thereby block their pharmacologic effects. The tricyclic antidepressants are potent inhibitors of norepinephrine uptake. Consequently, concomitant administration of clinical doses of tricyclic antidepressants including desipramine, protriptyline, nortriptyline, and amitriptyline will almost totally abolish the antihypertensive effects of guanethidine and bethanidine. Although they are less potent inhibitors of norepinephrine uptake, doxepin and chlorpromazine, when given in doses of greater than 100 mg daily, produce dose-related antagonism of the action of the guanidinium antihypertensives. In patients with severe hypertension, the loss of control of blood pressure resulting from these drug interactions can lead to serious clinical complications such as stroke and malignant hypertension.

Amphetamine also antagonizes the antihypertensive effect of guanethidine by displacing it from its site of action within the adrenergic neuron (Chap. 250). Ephedrine, a component of many drug combinations used in asthma, also antagonizes the effect of guanethidine, probably by both inhibition of uptake and displacement from the neuron.

The antihypertensive effect of clonidine in humans is partially antagonized by the tricyclic antidepressants. Clonidine lowers arterial pressure by reducing sympathetic outflow from the blood-pressure-regulating centers in the hindbrain (Chap. 250). This central hypotensive action is antagonized by the tricyclic antidepressants, probably because these antidepressants prevent clonidine's uptake into the neurons in the brain where it must be stored in order to exert its antihypertensive effect.

Pharmacokinetic interactions causing increased drug delivery

INHIBITION OF DRUG METABOLISM If the active form of a drug is cleared largely by biotransformation, inhibition of its metabolism will lead to a prolonged half-life and to accumulation of the drug during maintenance therapy. Excessive accumulation due to inhibited metabolism leads to significant adverse effects in the case of several drugs.

The metabolism of phenytoin is inhibited by a number of drugs. Clofibrate, phenylbutazone, chloramphenicol, disulfiram, bishydroxycoumarin, and isoniazid can raise the steady-state plasma levels of phenytoin by more than twofold. In the case of isoniazid, the extent of inhibition of phenytoin metabolism is a function of the genetically determined rate of isoniazid acetylation; substantial inhibition of phenytoin metabolism and resultant clinical toxicity are seen only in those individuals who are slow acetylators.

Inhibited metabolism may lead to abrupt development of symptoms such as somnolence, mental confusion, and disturbance of gait in patients who have not changed their phenytoin dosage.

Impaired metabolism of tolbutamide with severe hypoglycemia has resulted from coadministration of clofibrate, phenylbutazone, chloramphenicol, and bishydroxycoumarin. Excessive anticoagulation by warfarin may result from inhibition of its metabolism by disulfiram or phenylbutazone, or by concurrent and copious ingestion of ethanol. Warfarin is administered as a racemic mixture, and its S(−) isomer has 5 times the anticoagulant potency of the R(+) isomer. Phenylbutazone selectively inhibits the metabolism of the S(−) isomer, and only when this isomer is examined specifically can the substantial reduction in its metabolism produced by phenylbutazone be unmasked.

Azathioprine is readily converted in the body to an active metabolite, 6-mercaptopurine, which in turn is inactivated in part by xanthine oxidase which sequentially oxidizes it to 6-thiouric acid. When allopurinol, a potent inhibitor of xanthine oxidase, is administered concurrently with standard doses of azathioprine or 6-mercaptopurine, life-threatening toxicity (bone marrow suppression) can result. Therefore, it has been recommended that the doses of azathioprine and 6-mercaptopurine be reduced to one-third or one-fourth the usual amounts when allopurinol is given at the same time. These are rough approximations of the dose modifications, and the quantitative aspects of this interaction have not been determined.

INHIBITION OF RENAL SECRETION A number of drugs are secreted by the organic anion transport system in the renal tubule. Inhibition of this tubular transport system can cause excessive accumulation of a drug when this is the major pathway of its elimination. Several drugs, including phenylbutazone, probenecid, salicylates, and bishydroxycoumarin, will competitively inhibit this transport system. Patients receiving the oral antidiabetic acetohexamide have developed profound hypoglycemia when phenylbutazone was added to their drug regimen. This exaggerated hypoglycemia resulted from the inhibition by phenylbutazone of the tubular secretion of hydroxyacetohexamide, an active metabolite which is responsible for most of the hypoglycemic effect that ensues from acetohexamide administration. Renal tubular secretion contributes substantially to the elimination of penicillin, which can be inhibited by probenecid.

INHIBITION OF PLASMA PROTEIN BINDING When the binding of a drug to plasma protein is reduced by another agent, more unbound drug will be made available to receptor sites for any given level of total drug. Reduction in the binding of a drug does not have significance in vivo unless the drug is very highly bound (more than 90 percent). A drug may alter the binding of another by competitive displacement or by an interaction with protein (usually albumin) to decrease binding affinity. Reduction in the extent of binding also will make more drug available to the organs of clearance, and if the drug normally has a low extraction ratio because binding sequesters the drug in plasma (restrictive elimination), then reduction of binding will increase its clearance. As a result, following a binding displacement interaction, total and free drug levels at steady state will fall until free-drug concentration returns to the previous levels; at steady state, the average unbound warfarin levels should be independent of the degree of binding. Therefore, in most instances, any enhancement of the pharmacologic effect will be transient.

Although reduction of the binding of many drugs by others has been demonstrated in vitro, the only instance where clinical significance clearly has been linked to reduced binding is the potentiation of the anticoagulant effect of warfarin by chloral hydrate in high dosage. Chloral hydrate is converted in the body to trichloroacetic acid, which displaces warfarin from albumin-binding sites. As a result there is a transient increase in the anticoagulant effect of warfarin, persisting for only a few days until the concentration of free warfarin returns to previous levels. Although phenylbutazone also displaces warfarin from plasma protein, this contributes little to the sustained potentiation of warfarin's effect by phenylbutazone. The latter is largely attributable to inhibition of the metabolism of the S(−) isomer of warfarin by phenylbutazone, which produces an increase in levels of both bound and unbound warfarin that persists as long as phenylbutazone is administered (unlike the transient increase in unbound levels that results solely from a binding displacement interaction).

Pharmacodynamic and other interactions between drugs

Therapeutically useful interactions in which the combined effect of two drugs is greater than that of either drug alone are numerous. These favorable drug combinations are covered extensively in specific therapeutic sections in this text, and the following is directed toward those pharmacodynamic interactions that create unwanted effects. Two drugs may act on separate components of a common process and yield effects greater than either drug alone. For example, small doses of aspirin (less than 1 g daily) will not alter the prothrombin time appreciably in patients who are stabilized on warfarin therapy. However, the addition of aspirin to patients therapeutically anticoagulated with warfarin increases the risk of bleeding because aspirin inhibits platelet aggregation. Thus the combination of impaired functions of both the platelets and the fluid-phase clotting system increases the potential for hemorrhagic complications in patients receiving warfarin therapy.

Occasionally, the addition of bacteriostatic antibiotics such as the tetracyclines and chloramphenicol to bactericidal agents (e.g., penicillin) may impair the cure of infections (Chap. 130). In vitro, the combination of bacteriostatic and bactericidal agents yields a combined effect resembling that of the bacteriostatic agent alone. This may have clinical significance in meningitis, and, on the basis of studies in experimental animals, it is suggested that when bactericidal drugs need to be used, the administration of the static drug be delayed 1 h after initiating the bactericidal agent.

VARIABLE ACTIONS OF DRUGS CAUSED BY GENETIC DIFFERENCES IN THEIR METABOLISM

ACETYLATION Isoniazid, hydralazine, procainamide, and a number of other drugs are metabolized by acetylation of a hydrazino or amino group. This reaction is catalyzed by *N*-acetyl transferase, a nonmicrosomal (soluble) enzyme in the liver that transfers an acetyl group from acetyl coenzyme A to the drug. Individuals differ markedly in the rate at which drugs are acetylated, and there is a bimodal distribution of the population into "rapid acetylators" and "slow acetylators." The rate of acetylation is under genetic control; rapid acetylation is an autosomal dominant trait.

The toxic, sometimes fatal, hepatitis that occurs in about 1 percent of patients on isoniazid occurs predominantly in rapid acetylators. The greater hepatotoxicity in rapid acetylators appears to result from the synthesis of more acetylisoniazid which is further metabolized to acetylhydrazine, a potent hepatotoxin. Acetylhydrazine exerts its toxic effect through an active metabolite that binds covalently to macromolecules in the hepatic cells that produce it. Conversely, the lupus erythematosus–like syndrome produced by hydralazine (Chap. 250) occurs only in individuals who are slow acetylators.

Because these important toxic drug effects are largely predictable from the acetylation phenotype, it is of value to determine the rate of acetylation in patients who are to receive isoniazid, or those who would benefit from doses of hydralazine above the 200 mg per day dose that can be safely employed in the population at large. Acetylation phenotype can be determined by measuring the ratio of acetylated to nonacetylated dapsone or sulfamethazine in plasma or urine following administration of a test dose of these acetylation substrates. The ratio of monoacetyldapsone to dapsone in plasma at 6 h after dapsone administration is less than 0.35 for slow acetylators and greater than 0.35 for rapid acetylators. At 6 h following the administration of sulfamethazine, less than 25 percent of the drug in the plasma is in the acetylated form in slow acetylators (rapid acetylators, more than 25 percent); in the urine collected in the 5- to 6-h interval after administration of sulfamethazine, less than 70 percent of the drug is in the acetylated form in the slow acetylator (rapid acetylators, more than 70 percent).

METABOLISM BY MIXED-FUNCTION OXIDASES In healthy individuals taking no other medications, the major determinant of the rate of metabolism of drugs by the hepatic mixed-function oxidases is genetic. In contrast to the bimodal distribution of individuals with respect to acetylation rates, there is a unimodal distribution for most drugs metabolized by enzymes of the hepatic endoplasmic reticulum, indicating control by multiple genes. The genetically controlled variation in hepatic clearance is marked for some of these drugs. Steady-state plasma levels of nortriptyline, propranolol, and chlorpromazine vary by more than tenfold between individuals. This has obvious consequences in attempting to predict effect from a given dose in those individuals who differ markedly from the average.

CONCENTRATION OF DRUGS IN PLASMA AS A GUIDE TO THERAPY

Optimal individualization of therapy is assisted by measuring the concentration of certain drugs in plasma. Genetic variation in elimination rates, interactions with other drugs, disease-induced alterations in elimination and distribution, and other factors combine to yield a wide range of plasma levels in patients given the same dose. Furthermore, the problem of noncompliance with prescribed regimens during continuing therapy is an endemic and elusive cause of therapeutic failure. There are clinical indicators that assist the titration of some drugs into the desired range, and no chemical determination is a substitute for careful observations of the patient's response to treatment. However, the therapeutic and adverse effects are not precisely quantifiable for all drugs, and in complex clinical situations estimates of the action of a drug may be misleading. For example, previously existing neurologic disease may obscure the neurologic consequences of intoxication with phenytoin. Because half-life, accumulation, and steady-state plasma levels are difficult to predict for drugs with dose-dependent kinetics, the measurement of plasma levels is particularly useful as a guide to the dose of this group of drugs.

Particularly when there is a narrow range between the plasma levels yielding therapeutic and adverse effects, the concept of the average dose will not benefit the patient whose levels are inadequate for therapeutic effect or in the toxic range. Adjustment of dosage based on creatinine clearance in renal insufficiency will minimize gross over- and undertreatment, but still is a calculation based on an average and will not yield ideal treatment for all patients.

Data on concentrations of drugs in plasma are utilized most effectively in the framework of the known kinetics of the drug, including consideration of whether the levels are likely to reflect the steady state, whether they represent the equilibrium phase (cf. the distribution phase discussed above), and the extent to which disease-induced changes in the drug binding can influence the concentration of total (bound plus unbound) drug. In addition, the variability among individual responses to given plasma levels must be recognized. This is illustrated by a hypothetical population dose-response curve (Fig. 66-5) and its relationship to the therapeutic range or therapeutic "window" of desired plasma levels. The defined therapeutic window should include the levels at which the majority of patients will achieve the intended pharmacologic effect. However, there are a few people who are quite sensitive to the therapeutic effects of most drugs, responding to lower levels, whereas others are sufficiently refractory as to require levels that impose an increased likelihood of adverse effects as a potential price for therapeutic benefit. For example, a few patients with strong seizure foci will require plasma levels of phenytoin exceeding 20 μg per ml in order to control their seizure disorders. Increments in dosage to achieve this effect may be appropriate. However, with an elevation in dose that yields levels at which adverse effects become more frequent, one must exercise heightened sensitivity for subtle changes in higher integrative function. In addition, because

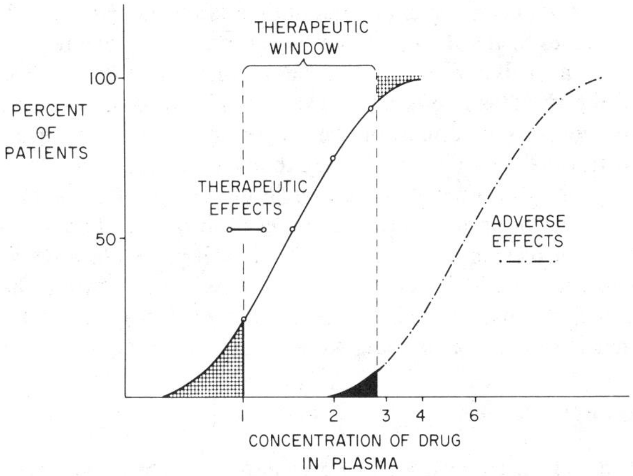

FIGURE 66-5
The cumulative percentage of patients responding to increasing levels of drug in plasma with both therapeutic and adverse effects. The therapeutic "window" defines the range of concentrations of drug that will achieve therapeutic effects in most patients with adverse effects in only a small percentage.

TABLE 66-3
Concentrations of drugs in plasma: relation to efficacy and adverse effects

Drug	*Efficacy**	*Adverse effects†*
Carbenicillin	100 μg/ml‡	300 μg/ml
Digitoxin	12 ng/ml	25–30 ng/ml
Digoxin	0.8 ng/ml	2.0 ng/ml
Gentamicin	4 μg/ml§	12 μg/ml
Lithium	0.5 meq/liter	1.3 meq/liter
Penicillin G	1–25 μg/ml¶	
Phenytoin (diphenylhydantoin)	10 μg/ml	20 μg/ml
Procainamide	4 μg/ml	8 μg/ml
Quinidine	3 μg/ml	7 μg/ml
Theophylline	8 μg/ml	20 μg/ml

* *The therapeutic effect is infrequent or slight at levels below these.*
† *The frequency of adverse effects increases sharply when these levels are exceeded.*
‡ *Minimal inhibitory concentration (MIC) for most strains of Pseudomonas aeruginosa. MIC for other, more sensitive, organisms is less.*
§ *Dependent on the MIC. Higher levels (up to 8 μg per ml) may be desired when host defenses are impaired.*
¶ *There is a wide range of MIC of penicillin for various organisms, and the MIC of all those for which penicillin is used is < 20. "Massive" penicillin therapy with 20 million units daily achieves levels of 20 to 25 μg per ml in patients with clearance of creatinine of 100 ml per min.*

phenytoin has dose-dependent kinetics, it would be essential to monitor carefully the variable and possibly large extent of plasma level increment that can accompany small increases in the dosage as levels exceed 20 μg per ml.

As also illustrated in Fig. 66-5, some patients may be prone to adverse effects at levels which are well tolerated by most of the population, and therefore elevation of levels to those achieving a high probability of therapeutic effect may bring on unwanted actions in the exceptional patient.

Table 66-3 presents for a number of drugs the concentrations in plasma that are associated with probable adverse and therapeutic effects in most patients. Its use within the guidelines discussed should permit more effective and safer therapy for those patients who are not "average."

REFERENCES

DETTLI L: Individualization of drug dosage in patients with renal disease. Med Clin North Am 58(5):977, 1974

SHAND DG et al: Pharmacokinetic drug interactions, in *Handbook of Experimental Pharmacology,* vol. 28, *Concepts in Biochemical Pharmacology,* eds JR Gillette, JR Mitchell, part 3, New York: Springer-Verlag, 1975, p. 272

WILKINSON GR, SHAND DG: A physiological approach to hepatic drug clearance. Clin Pharmacol Ther 18:377, 1975

67 REACTIONS TO DRUGS

LEIGHTON E. CLUFF
JACQUES R. CALDWELL

INTRODUCTION Drugs are the cornerstone of patient management and are used for diagnostic, prophylactic, and therapeutic purposes. In addition, they have increasingly become recognized as causes of disease. There are few diseases which are not managed by drug administration, and the adverse effects of drugs can involve every organ and system of the body.

Major advances in the research, development, and regulation of drugs ensure in most instances their uniformity, claims of effectiveness, and safety, and identify their recognized hazards. However, the extremely large number of different drugs and drug products available over the counter (OTC) or by prescription from a physician makes it impossible for a physician or patient to obtain or retain the knowledge necessary to use all these drugs well. It is understandable, therefore, that many OTC drugs are used unwisely by the public, and that restricted drugs may be prescribed incorrectly by physicians.

Most physicians use no more than 50 drug products in their practice, gaining familiarity with their effectiveness and safety. Most patients probably use only a limited number of over-the-counter drugs. Nevertheless, many patients receive care and drug prescriptions from more than one physician, and surveys have shown that in any 30-day period patients may consume more than three different OTC drug products containing nine or more different chemical agents.

Twenty-five to fifty percent of patients may make errors in self-administration of prescribed medicines, and this can be responsible for adverse drug effects. Elderly patients are most likely to commit such errors. One-third or more of patients also may not take their prescribed medications. It also seems likely that many patients commit similar errors in taking OTC drugs, by not reading or following the directions for use of the medicines provided on the containers. Physicians must recognize that providing directions with prescriptions does not always guarantee their patients' compliance.

Every drug can produce untoward consequences, even when used according to standard or recommended methods of administration. When used incorrectly, the drug's effectiveness may be reduced, or adverse reactions can be expected to occur more frequently. The administration of several drugs during the same period of time also may result in adverse drug-drug interactions.

In the hospital all the drugs a patient is given usually are under the control of a physician, and patient compliance is ensured. Errors may occur, nevertheless, in that the wrong drug or dose may be given, or the drug may be given to the wrong patient, although systems improving drug distribution and administration in hospitals have reduced this problem. On the other hand, there are no means for controlling how appropriately ambulatory patients take prescription or OTC drugs. The potential for adverse drug-drug interactions, both in ambulatory and in hospitalized patients, is great. Avoidance of this problem requires awareness of and familiarity with drug interactions by the physician, nurse, pharmacist, and patient. In addition, a drug history has become increasingly important as an integral part of the evaluation of every patient. Patient drug profiles collected by dispensing pharmacists, used to advise and counsel patients and physicians about possible deleterious administration of different drugs concomitantly, have become increasingly important.

Patients vary widely in the ways in which they absorb, metabolize, and excrete drugs. The bioavailability of a drug, as measured pharmacokinetically, usually varies to a larger degree from patient to patient than from batch to batch or manufacturer to manufacturer. Administration of a standard dose of a drug to reasonably uniform groups of individuals, for example, is characterized by finding a few patients who have high and others who have very low blood levels, or who absorb, metabolize, or excrete the drug slowly or rapidly. Drugs having a wide dose-response curve or a large therapeutic-toxic dose ratio may produce a desired effect with little risk of toxicity when given in standard doses. But drugs having a steep dose-response curve or a narrow therapeutic-toxic ratio are more likely to produce untoward consequences or fail to produce a desired therapeutic effect when given in a standard dose.

Drugs are foreign chemical substances and may act to induce immunologic responses, but vary widely in the frequency with which they cause allergic reactions and in the clinical manifestations of these allergic reactions. Moreover, allergic reactions to drugs account for only about 15 percent of all drug-induced illnesses. The remaining 85 percent are attributable to pharmacologic rather than immunologic mechanisms.

The factors determining the reasons some, but not all, patients receiving a drug develop an adverse reaction are largely unknown. Patients who have experienced one adverse drug reaction have a predisposition to developing others. The probability of patients developing an adverse reaction to a drug is directly related to the number of different drugs taken during the same period of time (e.g., during hospitalization or in the preceding few days). Women, elderly patients, and persons with certain racial characteristics are more likely to experience adverse drug reactions than are others. The presence of renal, hepatic, intestinal, or atopic disease, and some heritable or acquired diseases may predispose to adverse drug reactions. Familiarity with these associations is important in anticipating, recognizing, managing, and preventing drug-induced illness.

Two to five percent of patients admitted to the medical and pediatric services of general hospitals have illnesses attributable to drugs. Five to thirty percent of patients experience adverse reactions to drugs during hospitalization. An unknown proportion of fetal or neonatal abnormalities may be due to medicines taken by the mother during pregnancy or parturition. An undetermined number of illnesses caused by drugs are responsible for visits of patients to physicians' offices. In short, the magnitude of the problem posed by drug-induced disease has become exceedingly large. Increased understanding of the determinants of these reactions is essential if adverse drug effects are to be avoided, corrected, or eliminated.

EPIDEMIOLOGY Epidemiologic studies of adverse drug reactions have been helpful in evaluating the magnitude of the overall problem, in calculating the rate of reactions to individual drugs, and in characterizing some of the determinants of adverse drug effects.

Patients receive on the average 10 different drugs while hospitalized, and this figure may be as high as 60. The sicker the patient, the more drugs are given, but, as expected, there is a corresponding increase in the likelihood of adverse drug reactions. When fewer than six different drugs are given to hospitalized patients, the probability of an adverse reaction is about 5 percent, but if more than 15 drugs are given, the probability is higher than 40 percent. Retrospective analysis of ambulatory patients has revealed a history of some adverse drug effects in 20 percent of them.

Epidemiologic studies revealing the rates of adverse drug reactions are limited by the availability of suitable controls. Hence, both major and minor manifestations of presumed drug-induced illness are difficult to establish. Gastrointestinal signs and symptoms, particularly vomiting and diarrhea, account for approximately one-third; neurologic manifestations account for about one-fifth; cardiovascular, metabolic, and cutaneous manifestations each account for about one-tenth; and hematologic and other manifestations each account for about 5 percent of adverse drug reactions. Women experience twice as many gastrointestinal manifestations of adverse drug effects as do men. The case fatality ratio from drug-induced disease in hospitalized patients varies from 2 to 12 percent.

Most adverse drug effects are caused by well-established drugs such as digitalis preparations, penicillin, and psychotropic agents, but diuretics, anticoagulants, and antihypertensive drugs are also important causes of drug-induced disease.

Patients admitted to the hospital for a drug-induced illness or with a prior history of an untoward effect are three times more likely than other patients to develop another adverse drug reaction. This indicates a predisposition to untoward drug effects possibly related to heritable or metabolic factors, causing abnormal degradation, detoxification, or excretion of drugs, associated with renal, hepatic, or immunologic dysfunction and enzyme defects. Simultaneous administration of different drugs also may inhibit or enhance enzyme production or competition for protein binding, influencing pharmacologic activity and metabolism.

ETIOLOGY Adverse reactions to drugs may be attributable to pharmacologic or immunologic mechanisms, but in many instances the mechanism is not known. Different descriptive terms are used to characterize adverse reactions depending upon their manifestations and presumed mechanisms. Pharmacologic effects other than those for which the drug is usually administered are referred to as *side effects.* Patients showing unusual susceptibility to the pharmacologic actions of a drug are said to have an *idiosyncrasy.* Reactions associated with manifestations typical of immunologic diseases are often called *allergic. Facilitative* reactions are indirect consequences of drug administration, such as development of staphylococcal enteritis following administration of oral antibiotics which have altered the intestinal microflora. Drugs given to parents and responsible for congenital abnormalities in their infants are called *teratogenic* or *mutagenic. Toxic* reactions due to overdosage may be responsible for serious untoward effects, but can be easily differentiated from other adverse reactions developing in persons who have been given a normal dose of a drug.

For practical purposes it is important to differentiate adverse reactions to drugs into only two classes: those attributable to the drugs' pharmacologic action and those unrelated to it. Reduction in dosage of a drug responsible for a pharmacologic reaction will usually prevent or abort the untoward effect. If the reaction is attributable to immunologic mechanisms, reduction in dose of the drug ordinarily will not terminate the reaction, and in the allergic individual even minute doses may result in catastrophic events. In addition, patients predisposed to an idiosyncratic drug reaction may experience this effect with a drug dose significantly lower than that usually given for a therapeutic effect. This predisposition to exaggerated pharmacologic drug action may be related to defective drug metabolism or excretion, to genetic abnormalities, as in patients with erythrocytes deficient in glucose 6-phosphate dehydrogenase, or to drug interactions.

Immunologic mechanisms Most pharmacologic agents are poor immunogens since they consist of small molecules with molecular weights less than 2,000. Stimulation of antibody synthesis or sensitization of lymphocytes by a drug or one of its metabolites usually requires in vivo activation and covalent linkage to protein, carbohydrate, or nucleic acid.

Drug stimulation of antibody production may mediate tissue injury by one of several mechanisms. The antibody may attack the drug affixed to a cell by covalent linkage and thereby destroy the cell, as occurs in penicillin-induced hemolytic anemia. Complexes of antibody-drug-antigen may be passively adsorbed by a bystander cell which is destroyed by activation of complement; this occurs in Sedormid-induced thrombocytopenia. Drugs may alter host tissue, rendering it antigenic, and stimulate autoantibodies; e.g., hydralazine and procainamide can chemically alter nuclear material, stimulate formation of antinuclear antibody, and occasionally cause lupus erythematosus. Autoantibodies may be stimulated by drugs which neither interact with the host antigen nor have any chemical similarity to the host tissue, e.g., alpha methyldopa frequently stimulates formation of antibodies to host erythrocytes, yet the drug does not itself attach to the erythrocyte nor share any chemical similarities with the antigenic determinants on the erythrocyte.

Serum sickness (Chap. 75) results from deposition of circulating drug-antibody complexes on endothelial surfaces. Complement activation occurs, chemotactic factors are generated locally, and an inflammatory response appears at the site of complex entrapment. Arthralgias, lymphadenopathy, glomerulonephritis, or cerebritis may result. Penicillin is the most common cause of serum sickness today. Many drugs, particularly the antimicrobial agents, induce production of IgE which affixes to mast cell membranes. Contact with a drug antigen initiates a series of biochemical events within the mast cell and results in the release of mediators which may produce urticaria, wheezing, rhinorrhea, and occasionally hypotension characteristic of anaphylaxis.

Drugs may also excite cell-mediated immune responses. Topically administered substances may interact with sulfhydryl or amino groups in the skin and react with sensitized lymphocytes to produce the rash characteristic of contact dermatitis. Other types of rashes may also appear from the interaction of serum factors, drugs, and sensitized lymphocytes. The role of drug-activated lymphocytes in the immune mechanisms governing destruction of visceral tissue is unknown.

Drug-drug interaction (Chap. 66)

Diseases predisposing to reactions Some patients have a peculiar predisposition to allergic and other adverse reactions to therapeutic agents. Persons with atopic illness may have an increased risk of developing drug allergies. The maculopapular rash associated with ampicillin therapy occurs much more frequently in patients with infectious mononucleosis, chronic lymphocytic leukemia, and hyperuricemia than in individuals with other illnesses. Patients with latent or quiescent acute intermittent porphyria may have an attack precipitated by the administration of barbiturates. Patients with peptic ulcer disease or gastritis are predisposed to gastroduodenal hemorrhage when they are given aspirin, corticosteroids, indomethacin, and probably anticoagulants. Patients with renal insufficiency are likely to develop drug toxicity when given drugs which are largely excreted by the kidney.

MANIFESTATIONS Adverse effects of drugs attributed to their pharmacologic action are drug-specific. Allergic reactions, however, are often the same irrespective of the incriminated drug. Some presumed allergic reactions, however, are more common with certain drugs than with others.

The commonest manifestations of allergy to drugs are no different from hypersensitivity reactions of other types and include rashes, asthma, and the symptoms of serum sickness. These are easily recognized clinically as allergic in origin. Other features of drug allergy are less easily characterized. Table 67-1 summarizes some common drug reactions which include both allergic and pharmacologic side effects.

Skin Morbilliform, urticarial, and maculopapular rashes are probably the most common skin reactions, but many others including vesicular, bullous, exfoliative, eczematous, and purpuric eruptions have been observed. Pruritus is frequent. Although the type of skin lesion usually will not help identify the causative drug, certain skin reactions are relatively specific. Erythema multiforme or nodosum is seen in allergy to Dilantin, bromides, iodides, trimethadione, and sulfonamides. "Fixed" drug eruptions are most frequently due to aminopyrine, phenolphthalein, or Atabrine. Photosensitization during drug therapy occurs characteristically with chlorpromazine, phenothiazine, sulfonamides, and tetracycline derivatives, particularly demeclocycline.

Fever Fever may be an isolated manifestation of drug allergy, and most pharmaceuticals in common use, including most antibiotics and chemotherapeutic agents, can produce a febrile reaction. However, the tetracycline derivatives are uncommon causes of drug fever, and digitalis has rarely, if ever, been incriminated as the cause of a pyrogenic reaction. Elevation of temperature may appear abruptly after treatment begins, or it may develop in a stepwise fashion during or after the second week of drug administration. Drug fever is often associated with chills and constitutional symptoms and may be accompanied by leukocytosis. High, sustained fevers usually indicate small-vessel vasculitis. Discontinuing therapy usually results in defervescence within a short period, although several days may be required for return of the temperature to normal.

Blood Changes in the formed elements of the blood are common during drug allergy, but severe bone marrow suppression and its associated complications are most characteristic with immunosuppressive or antineoplastic drugs. Some drugs have been found to have limited or no effects on the blood, while others produce specific abnormalities. For example, penicillin has not been incriminated as a cause of serious hematologic abnormalities. In therapeutic doses, acetanilid is probably not a cause of anemia, agranulocytosis, thrombocytopenia, or aplastic anemia; in high dosage, however, it may produce leukocytosis, methemoglobinemia, and acute hemolysis. *Methemoglobinemia* also occurs with antipyrine, nitrites, sulfonamides, primaquine, and pamaquine, but this reaction is probably not allergic in origin. Barbiturates, salicylates and para-aminosalicylic acid rarely, if ever, produce agranulocytosis. *Eosinophilia* may accompany allergic reactions of many types, but it occurs with such frequency as an isolated finding during therapy with streptomycin or Nirvanol that it has no significance. *Lymphocytosis* is common in patients receiving Dilantin and Nirvanol, and *polymorphonuclear leukocytosis* may be found in individuals taking Dilantin or atropine.

The erythrocyte abnormality responsible for the *acute hemolytic anemia* induced by primaquine, sulfonamides, and nitrofurans in certain individuals is attributable to a genetically determined enzyme deficiency. *Jaundice* due to pharmaceutical agents is discussed in Chap. 299.

Nervous system A variety of neurologic manifestations may appear during drug therapy, but in the majority of instances there is little evidence to incriminate allergy as a cause. The commonest reactions consist of psychotic changes or alterations in consciousness and may be seen with digitalis, atropine, thiocyanates, sedatives, and steroids. Among other drugs that produce adverse effects on the nervous system (ranging from paresthesia and peripheral neuritis to deafness) are streptomycin, hydralazine, chlorpromazine, Diamox, isoniazid, polymyxin, neomycin, and kanamycin.

Other reactions Nausea, vomiting, and diarrhea are exceedingly common. Abdominal pain in the absence of other symptoms may be produced by quinine, chlorpromazine, and primaquine. Albuminuria and cylindruria occur particularly with heavy metals, bacitracin, polymyxin, colistin, gentamicin, and some of the cephalosporins. Dilantin, chloral hydrate, sulfonamides, trimethadione, Phenurone, colchicine, thiocyanates, gentamicin, kanamycin, cephaloridine, and amphotericin B occasionally produce renal dysfunction, probably because of their direct toxic action. Amphotericin B may produce tubular necrosis and renal calcification, but this is only occasionally associated with significant evidence of renal insufficiency and nitrogen retention. Hypersensitivity to sulfonamides has resulted in acute hemorrhagic nephritis.

Vasculitis Histologic lesions indistinguishable from those of polyarteritis nodosa have been found in the tissues of patients who have experienced allergic reactions to iodides, Dilantin, sulfonamides, and penicillin. Manifestations of systemic lupus erythematosus have appeared during therapy with isoniazid, hydralazine, procainamide, and a few other drugs but usually have been reversible following discontinuation of the drug (Chaps. 77 and 78).

Anaphylaxis (Chap. 72)

DIAGNOSIS The manifestations of drug-induced diseases, whether attributable to pharmacologic, immunologic, or other mechanisms, resemble those associated with other diseases and may be produced by different and dissimilar drugs. Recognition of the role of a drug or drugs responsible for illness is dependent upon appreciation of the possible implication of adverse reactions to drugs in any disease, identification of a temporal relationship between drug administration and development of illness, and familiarity with the manifestations most often caused by particular drugs. Although specific reactions have been described as resulting from the use of particular drugs, there is always a "first," and any drug should be suspected of causing an adverse effect if the clinical setting is appropriate.

Illness induced by a drug's pharmacologic action may be more easily recognized than illness attributable to immunologic or other mechanisms. For example, side effects such as cardiac arrhythmias in patients receiving digitalis, hypoglycemia in patients given insulin, and bleeding in patients receiving anticoagulants are more easily related to the prescribed drug than are symptoms like fever or rash, which may be caused by many drugs or by other factors.

Once an adverse reaction is suspected, discontinuance of the suspected drug followed by disappearance of the reaction is presumptive evidence of a drug-induced illness. Reappearance of the reaction upon readministration of the drug is confirmatory evidence of the relationship. With pharmacologic adverse reactions, lowering the dosage may also be followed by disappearance of the reaction, and increasing the dose may cause it to reappear. When the reaction is thought to be allergic, however, readministration of the drug may be hazardous, since anaphylactic shock may develop. Readministration is unwise under these conditions unless alternate drugs are not available and treatment is mandatory.

If the patient is receiving many different drugs when an adverse reaction is suspected, the drugs most likely to be incriminated can usually be identified. All drugs may be discontinued at once, or they may be discontinued one at a time at intervals of 1 to 2 days. Depending on the excretion or metabolism of the drug and on the nature of the reaction, the manifestation may or may not disappear promptly. If the drug is eliminated slowly, the reaction may persist, but if it is excreted rapidly, the reaction may disappear quickly. Drug fever usually terminates within 24 to 48 h after administration of a drug is discontinued. Rashes and arteritis may persist for a longer period of time.

Blood and urine levels of a drug may be useful in determining whether toxic levels have been reached or whether the drug is eliminated slowly or rapidly. Investigation of potential drug-drug interactions by determining that such interactions have been previously recognized may be useful under some circumstances when more than one drug appears to be involved in the reaction.

Serum antibody has been demonstrated in some persons with drug allergy involving cellular blood elements, as in agranulocytosis, hemolytic anemia, and thrombocytopenia. In other types of drug allergy, precipitation, hemagglutination, or complement fixation tests with drugs or drug degradation products have only rarely been clearly related to adverse reactions. Skin tests with the drug or its degradation products also are often of little value in identifying the allergic individual. These poor results testify to the inadequacy of present methods of testing and are not an argument against an immunologic basis for allergic drug reactions. Demonstration of derivatives (e.g., penicilloyl) responsible for many penicillin allergic reactions has provided tools for testing persons suspected of having penicillin allergy, but even these tests are not completely reliable.

Eliciting a drug history from patients is important diagnostically. Attention must be directed to nonprescription, or over-the-counter, as well as prescription drugs. Each type can be responsible for adverse drug effects, and frequently adverse interactions occur between drugs purchased by patients over the counter and those prescribed by physicians. In addition, it is common for patients to be cared for by several physicians, and duplicative, additive, counteractive, or synergistic drugs may, therefore, be taken if the physicians are not aware of the patients' histories.

Table 67-1
Clinical manifestations of adverse reactions to some drugs

1 DERMATOLOGIC

a Exfoliative dermatitis
- Penicillin
- Sulfonamides
- Barbiturates
- Hydantoins
- Phenylbutazone

b Toxic epidermal necrolysis
- Phenylbutazone
- Hydantoins
- Sulfonamides
- Tetracycline (demeclocycline)

c Stevens-Johnson syndrome
- Penicillin
- Phenolphthalein
- Sulfonamides

d Acne
- Anabolic steroids
- Corticosteroids
- Androgens
- Bromides

e Erythema nodosum
- Penicillin
- Sulfonamides
- Sulfonylureas

f Fixed drug eruptions
- Phenolphthalein
- Phenacetin
- Barbiturates
- Sulfonamides
- Salicylates

g Photodermatitis
- Demeclocycline
- Griseofulvin
- Sulfonamides
- Sulfonylureas
- Thiazides

h Urticaria
- Penicillin
- Ampicillin
- Sulfonamides
- Aspirin
- Barbiturates
- Opiates

i Pigment changes
- ACTH
- Busulfan
- 6-Mercaptopurine
- Phenothiazines
- Arsenic
- Hypervitaminosis A
- Oral contraceptives
- Gold and silver salts
- Chloroquine
- Quinacrine
- Aldylating agents

j Alopecia
- Cytotoxic drugs
- Heparin
- Clofibrate
- Colchicine

2 HEMATOPOIETIC

a Pancytopenia
- Chloramphenicol
- Phenylbutazone
- Mephenytoin
- Trimethadione
- Organic arsenicals
- Gold salts

b Hemolytic anemia (G-6-PD deficiency)
- 8-Aminoquinoline
- Sulfonamides
- Nitrofurans
- Sulfones
- Cinchona alkaloids
- Phenylhydrazine

c Hemolytic anemia (immune)
- Penicillin
- Quinidine
- Methyldopa
- Levodopa
- Cephalosporins
- Sulfonamides

d Megaloblastic anemia
- Folic acid antagonists
- Diphenylhydantoin
- Barbiturates
- Oral contraceptives

e Methemoglobinuria or sulfhemoglobinuria
- Phenacetin
- Acetanilid
- Nitrites
- Nitroglycerine
- Nitrates
- Chloroquine

f Agranulocytosis
- Antineoplastic drugs
- Aminopyrine
- Chloramphenicol
- Sulfonamides
- Chlorpromazine
- Propylthiouracil
- Phenindione

g Thrombocytopenia
- Analgesics
- Cinchona alkaloids
- Sulfonamides
- Barbiturates
- Thiazides
- Tolbutamide
- Hydantoins

h Pseudolymphoma
- Diphenylhydantoin
- Mephenytoin
- Phensuximide
- Ethotoin
- Primidone

3 CARDIOVASCULAR

a Aortic valve disease
- Methysergide

b Ischemic heart disease
- Vasopressin
- Oxytocin
- Ergot
- Methysergide
- Antihypertensive drugs

c Myocardiopathy
- Emetine
- Allergic drug reactions

d Pericarditis
- Hydralazine (with SLE)
- Anticoagulants (hemorrhage)

e Congestive heart failure
- Propranolol
- Sodium bicarbonate
- Corticosteroids
- Mannitol infusions

f Arrhythmias
- Sympathomimetic amines
- Thyroid hormone
- Digitalis
- Quinidine
- Atropine
- Emetine
- Propranolol
- Guanethidine
- Thioridazine
- Procainamide

4 GASTROINTESTINAL

a Swollen or hairy tongue
- Antibiotics (tetracyclines)
- Oral corticosteroids

b Dental enamel hyperplasia or discoloration
- Tetracyclines

c Gingival hyperplasia
- Diphenylhydantoin
- Bismuth and mercury compounds

d Parotitis
- Phenylbutazone
- Guanethidine
- Isoproterenol
- Vincristine

e Peptic ulceration and hemorrhage
- Aspirin
- Corticosteroids
- Phenylbutazone
- Indomethacin
- Ethacrynic acid
- Anticoagulants

f Pancreatitis
- Corticosteroids
- Thiazides
- Azulfidine
- Azathioprine
- Oral contraceptives

g Cholestatic jaundice
- Phenothiazines
- Chlordiazepoxide
- Meprobamate
- Tricyclic antidepressants
- Androgens
- Anabolic steroids
- Oral contraceptives
- Sulfonylureas
- Erythromycin estolate
- Thiouracil

h Hepatocellular jaundice
- Halothane
- MAO inhibitors
- Isoniazid
- Novobiocin
- Phenylbutazone
- Indomethacin
- Antineoplastic drugs
- Hydantoins
- Propylthiouracil

i Altered liver function without jaundice
- Azathioprine
- Methyldopa
- Erythromycin estolate
- Triacetyloleandomycin
- Ampicillin
- Cephalothin
- Coumarin
- Mithramycin
- Oral contraceptives (Budd-Chiari syndrome)

j Hepatic fibrosis or granulomas
- Halothane
- Iproniazid
- Acetohexamide
- Chlorpromazine
- Tolbutamide
- Methotrexate
- Chlorambucil

5 RESPIRATORY

a Asthma
- Aspirin
- Indomethacin
- Aminopyrine
- Tartrazine
- Propranolol

b Pulmonary infiltrates and fibrosis
- Nitrofurantoin
- Hydrochlorothiazide
- Busulfan
- Cyclophosphamide
- Methotrexate
- Methysergide
- Ganglionic blockers

c Apnea or hypoventilation-neuromuscular blockade
- Aminoglycoside antibiotics
- Polymyxin antibiotics
- Succinylcholine

d Pulmonary infection
- Corticosteroids (activation tuberculosis)
- Antineoplastic-immunosuppressive drugs (aspergillosis, *Pneumocystis carinii,* and cytomegalovirus)

6 ENDOCRINE

a Inappropriate ADH secretion
- Vasopressin
- Oxytocin
- Vincristine
- Cyclophosphamide
- Chlorpropamide
- Thiazides

b Diabetes mellitus, hyperglycemia
- Corticosteroids
- Oral contraceptives
- Thiazides
- Furosemide
- Diazoxide

c Hypoglycemia
- Insulin
- Sulfonylureas
- Phenformin
- Propranolol

d Thyroid gland disorders
- Perphenazine
- Oral contraceptives
- Dimetane
- Phenindione
- Iodides

Tolbutamide
Chlorpropamide
Lithium carbonate
Chlorpromazine
Imipramine

e Adrenal gland disorders
Corticosteroids
Busulfan
Anticoagulants
Laxative abuse (Hyperaldosteronism)

f Gynecomastia
Estrogens
Androgens
Spironolactone
Digitalis
Phenothiazines
Reserpine
Methyldopa

g Galactorrhea
Phenothiazines
Oral contraceptives
Chlorprothixene
Reserpine
Chlordiazepoxide
Imipramine
Amitriptyline
Methyldopa

7 URINARY TRACT

a Renal insufficiency
Heavy metals
Phenacetin
Sulfonamides
Kanamycin
Gentamicin
Polymyxin B
Colistin
Cephaloridine
Amphotericin B

b Nephrotic syndrome
Mercurial diuretics
Gold salts
Trimethodione
Paramethadione
Phenindione
Probenecid
Tolbutamide

c Renal tubular acidosis
Degraded tetracycline
Amphotericin B

d Renal calculi
Acetazolamide
Vitamin D
Allopurinol (xanthine)

e Nephrogenic diabetes insipidus
Lithium carbonate
Demeclocycline

f Hemorrhagic cystitis
Cyclophosphamide

8 GYNECOLOGIC

a Amenorrhea
Oral contraceptives
Cyclophosphamide
Haloperidol
Imipramine
Chlordiazepoxide
Methyldopa

b Vaginal carcinoma
Diethylstilbestrol (maternal use)

9 METABOLIC

a Hyponatremia
Diuretics
Drug-induced inappropriate ADH secretion
Corticosteroid withdrawal
Enemas
Mannitol

b Hyperkalemia
Spironolactone
Triamterene
Antineoplastic drugs
Corticosteroid withdrawal

c Hypokalemia
Diuretics
Laxative abuse
Corticosteroids
Amphotericin B
Alkali-induced alkalosis
Insulin

d Metabolic acidosis
Paraldehyde
Phenformin
Amphotericin B
Ammonium chloride
Acetazolamide

e Hypercalcemia
Milk-alkali syndrome
Vitamin D
Thiazides

f Hypocalcemia
Mithramycin
Drug-induced malabsorption
Drug-induced renal insufficiency

g Hyperuricemia
Thiazides
Chlorthalidone
Ethacrynic acid
Furosemide
Aspirin (small doses)
Antineoplastic drugs

h Porphyria
Barbiturates
Aminopyrine
Chlordiazepoxide
Meprobamate
Sulfonamides
Hydantoins
Tolbutamide

10 MUSCULOSKELETAL

a Myopathy and myalgia
Corticosteroids
Chloroquine
Emetine
Colchicine
Clofibrate
Thiabendazole
Methysergide

b Rheumatic syndrome
Isoniazid
Pyrazinamide
Ethionamide

c Bone disorders
Tetracycline (retarded bone growth)
Corticosteroids (osteoporosis, retarded bone growth)
Heparin (osteoporosis)

11 NEUROLOGIC

a Peripheral neuropathy
Heavy metals
Isoniazid
Hydralazine
Nitrofurans
Kanamycin
Streptomycin
Colistin
Imipramine
Amitriptyline
Vincristine
Chloroquine

b Myasthenia
Quaternary ammonium compounds
Quinine
Quinidine
Procainamide
Chlorpromazine
Streptomycin
Kanamycin
Colistin

c Extrapyramidal syndromes
Haloperidol
Thioxanthenes
Rauwolfia
Prochlorperazine
Phenothiazines
Levodopa

d Seizures
Amphetamines
Phenothiazines
Imipramine
Amitriptyline
Isoniazid
Lidocaine

e Stroke and intracerebral bleeding
Oral contraceptives
Anticoagulants
MAO inhibitors plus tricyclic antidepressants or sympathomimetic amines

f Pseudotumor cerebri
Corticosteroids
Oral contraceptives
Tetracyclines
Hypervitaminosis A
Nalidixic acid

12 MULTISYSTEM

a Fever
Penicillins
Novobiocin
Para-aminosalicylic acid
Amphotericin B
Antihistamines
Cephalosporins
Barbiturates
Hydantoins
Quinidine

b Systemic lupus erythematosus
Hydralazine
Procainamide
Isoniazid
Hydantoins
Sulfonamides
Penicillins

c Vasculitis
Penicillin
Sulfonamides
Propylthiouracil
Iodides
Phenylbutazone

d Serum sickness
Penicillins
Streptomycin
Sulfonamides
Propylthiouracil
Barbiturates
Hydantoin

e Anaphylaxis
Penicillin
Cephalosporins
Streptomycin
Dextrans
Procaine
Insulin

13 INFECTIONS

Antibiotics
Corticosteroids
Immunosuppressive agents

14 OCULAR

a Extraocular muscle disorders
Furaltadone
Polymyxin B
Colistin
Phenothiazines

b Cataracts
Phenothiazines
Corticosteroids
Oral contraceptives

c Glaucoma
Corticosteroids
Mydriatics
Sympathomimetic amines
Phenothiazines

d Retinopathy
Chloroquine
Phenothiazines

e Optic neuritis
Chloramphenicol
Streptomycin
Isoniazid
Ethambutol
Quinine
Oral contraceptives

15 EAR

a Vestibular disorders
Streptomycin
Gentamicin

b Deafness
Neomycin
Kanamycin
Furazolidine
Ethacrynic acid
Furosemide
Quinine
Aspirin

Every physician should determine what drugs a patient has been taking, at least during the preceding 30 days, before prescribing any medications. A history of previous adverse drug effects in patients is common. Since these patients have a predisposition to other drug-induced illnesses, familiarity with such a history should dictate added caution in prescribing drugs.

Some patients have a heritable predisposition to reactions to certain drugs, which may be recognized by specific biochemical study. For example, erythrocyte G-6-PD deficiency can be identified; patients with the defect are usually Negroes. Such patients may have an acute hemolytic crisis when sulfonamides, nitrofurantoins, probenecid, tolbutamide, and aminoquinolines are given. These crises can be avoided by testing for the enzyme defect before administering these drugs. Similarly, persons with an abnormal serum pseudocholinesterase may have apnea when given succinylcholine.

No drug is completely safe and any drug may cause illness. A high index of suspicion is essential for recognizing adverse drug reactions and for identifying reactions not previously described.

TREATMENT AND PROPHYLAXIS Allergic reactions to drugs usually subside promptly when administration of the agent is discontinued. Occasionally, however, the reaction persists for prolonged periods despite withdrawal of the drug. Recurrent urticaria for many months after a penicillin reaction is a common example. In the event of persistent or severe manifestations of drug allergy, the use of adrenocortical steroids is indicated. Adrenal steroids, antihistamines, and epinephrine are usually ineffective in alleviating pharmacologic reactions due to a drug. Reactions of this type are best managed by withdrawing the offending drug or reducing the dose, and administering appropriate pharmacologic antagonists.

A specific history of hypersensitivity to a given drug contraindicates its readministration unless the clinical situation is serious. When such a situation arises, the procedure of choice is to look for an alternative agent which is just as efficacious. In a number of instances, when it has been judged necessary to prescribe a drug to which a patient is known to be allergic, the concomitant administration of adrenal steroids has completely suppressed the manifestations of hypersensitivity. However, adrenal steroids will not prevent or control anaphylactic shock. Desensitization by administering progressively increasing dosages of a drug such as penicillin should be used only as a last resort. Although desensitization is often successful, there are occasional examples of "desensitized" individuals who experienced a fatal anaphylactic reaction upon receiving a large systemic dose of the drug in question.

The Food and Drug Administration and the pharmaceutical manufacturers are accumulating information on adverse drug reactions. They solicit the cooperation of all physicians in reporting reactions to drugs.

REFERENCES

CLUFF LE et al: *Clinical Problems with Drugs,* Philadelphia: Saunders, 1975

——, JOHNSON JE: Drug fever. Progr Allergy 8:149, 1964

——, PETRIE JC: *Clinical Effects of Interaction between Drugs,* New York: American Elsevier, 1974

DOWLING HF: *Medicines for Man,* New York: Knopt, 1970

GARDNER P, CLUFF LE: The epidemiology of adverse drug reactions: A review and perspective. Johns Hopkins Med J 126:77, 1970

HANSTEN PD: *Drug Interactions,* Philadelphia: Lea & Febiger, 1974

HURWITZ N: Predisposing factors in adverse reactions to drugs. Br Med J 1:536, 1969

STEWART RB, CLUFF LE: Studies on the epidemiology of adverse drug reaction VI: Utilization and interactions of prescription and nonprescription drugs in outpatients. Johns Hopkins Med J 129:319, 1971

section 3 | Metabolic considerations

68 INTERMEDIARY METABOLISM OF PROTEIN, FAT, AND CARBOHYDRATE

GEORGE F. CAHILL, JR.

Before discussing specific metabolic pathways and their roles in health and disease, a few general biochemical principles should be outlined. The metabolic system, as a whole, is governed by innumerable control mechanisms in cells and tissues whereby a pathway can be activated as needed, or can be inhibited as products accumulate. The net result is a finely integrated summation of an almost infinite number of chemical reactions occurring in all body cells, coordinated by signal systems such as hormones, levels of circulating substrates, and, not infrequently, the nervous system.

ENZYMES AND CONTROL MECHANISMS All biochemical reactions are controlled by specific proteins, the enzymes. Thus, as true catalysts, the enzymes accelerate molecular transformations, and do so by initially binding with the reactant. Thus enzyme (E) plus substrate (S) form a complex (ES) which then dissociates to form enzyme plus the altered molecule (P) or product. Without the enzyme, substrate would yet be converted to product, but much more slowly, frequently in years instead of seconds. The concentration of substrate needed to saturate one-half the catalytic sites on the enzyme molecule is referred to as the K_m, or Michaelis constant. Thus the conversion of E to P, in the reaction

$$E + S \rightarrow ES \rightarrow E + P + \text{energy}$$

is a function of the concentration of S, the amount of enzyme E, the concentration of product P, and, most importantly, the release of energy. If there is little or no energy exchanged, the overall reaction is readily reversible. This situation is frequently encountered in most enzymatic sequences not subject to regulatory control. On the other hand, if there is a large energy release, the reaction, although theoretically reversible to a limited degree, is, practially speaking, unidirectional. It is at these "committed" steps where checks and balances are exerted by other regulators in order to control the entire pathway. Frequently involved are other participants in the reaction, which may directly contribute reactants and serve as coenzymes, first binding to the enzyme at a site near where the substrate binds and then transferring a part of their molecule to the substrate to form the product. The enzyme also may be altered by agents which bind to it and do not participate directly in the reaction. These factors, by distorting the three-dimensional structure of the enzyme, can alter either the activity of the enzyme itself or the binding affinity of substrate, product, or coenzyme. An enzyme capable of being distorted by such factors is an *allosteric* enzyme and offers a unique mechanism whereby molecules can finely accelerate or decrease the rate of a given enzymatic reaction. The total amount of enzyme available is a function of the genetic code, of its transcription and translation, and of the rate of removal of the enzyme by degradation. Finally, other cofactors, such as metals and inorganic or organic ions, are frequently necessary as part of the enzyme complex and, again, may either inhibit or augment the overall reaction.

Abnormalities resulting in disease have been shown to occur at each of these regulatory sites. The reaction may be altered because of inadequate substrate concentration, or, possibly, similarly structured molecules may competitively displace the substrate from the enzyme. In addition, there can be a lack of necessary coenzymes, or displacement of cofactors by inhibitors, or there may be substances that distort the enzyme (allosteric regulators), thereby increasing or decreasing its activity. Finally, there may be a primary inherited abnormality in the amino acid sequence of the enzyme itself, or in another protein-regulating synthesis of the enzyme. Disease states in man have been demonstrated for each of the possible aberrations described above.

ENERGY Except for organisms capable of using the sun's energy (autotrophs) to drive their metabolic machinery, living matter needs a constant input of fuel not only for growth but for maintenance (homeostasis). The principal storage form of energy in all living matter is the hydrogen-carbon bond. A major part of the metabolic machinery is involved in translating this energy into energy that can be readily used for synthetic reactions, for locomotion, for pumping ions or molecules against concentration gradients, and for many other essential cell processes. The energy requirement for almost all these is provided in the form of the high-energy phosphate bond (Fig. 68-1). The phosphate radical is rich in electrons, and two phosphates adjacent to each other contain much energy, or in biochemical language, a high-energy phosphate bond (~P). Likewise, a phosphate adjacent to other highly negatively charged groups contains much energy (8 to 10 kcal per mole), an example being creatine phosphate. On the other hand, a phosphate in ester linkage to an alcohol contains relatively less energy (2 kcal per mole) and is called a low-energy phosphate bond; it does not participate in energy transfer processes.

The site for most high-energy phosphate formation is in the mitochondria. These intracellular organelles are literally energy transducers which, with the help of enzyme sequences in the cell fluid (the cytosol), prepare and partially degrade the original molecule bearing the hydrogen-carbon bond. The energy from this bond is then converted into an as yet hypothetic high-energy phosphate intermediate (X~P), which, in turn, transfers the ~P to a phosphate on a specific purine (adenine) nucleotide to form adenosine triphosphate (ATP) from adenosine diphosphate (ADP). The ATP is then capable of diffusing from the mitochondria to the site in the cell needing the energy.

In Fig. 68-2 is sketched a single mitochondrion inside a cell. It consists of an aqueous phase containing the enzymes of the tricarboxylic acid cycle (Krebs cycle or citric acid cycle) which receives acetyl CoA and in one turn discharges two molecules of CO_2 and a number of high-energy phosphate bonds (30 ATP). The latter are formed by transfer of the energy of the carbon-hydrogen bond from the original acetyl CoA to specific carriers, nicotinamide-adenine dinucleotide (NAD^+) and flavin adenine dinucleotide (FAD), which enter the solid phase of the mitochondrion, the cristae, where the energy is transformed into high-energy phosphate, and the hydrogen finally meets oxygen to form water. Thus in the presence of oxygen, acetyl CoA, and a need for a high-energy phosphate,

FIGURE 68-1
The structure of adenosine triphosphate. Energy is stored in the two terminal high-energy phosphate bonds (denoted in the text as ~P) and is released or transferred to support reactions requiring energy (endergonic).

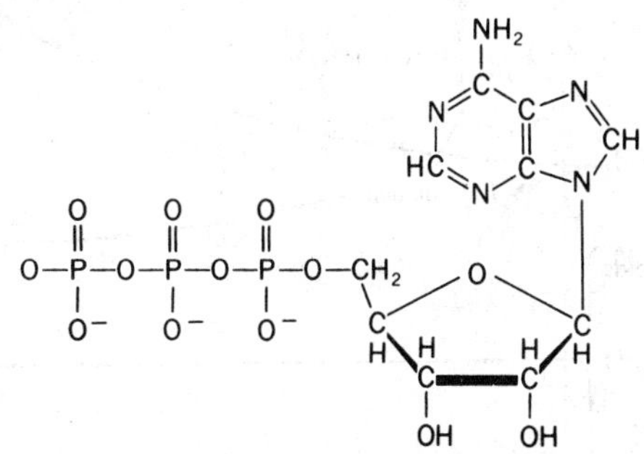

the cycle turns, hydrogen is transferred to the sequence of enzymes (the respiratory chain) in the cristae, and water and $\sim$P are produced. What turns the system on is the need for $\sim$P as signaled by the presence of ADP, and the system runs until the ADP is made into ATP. Thus ADP added to mitochondria initiates oxygen consumption, which continues as long as ADP is available ("respiratory control"). Oxygen consumption not linked to $\sim$P production results in heat alone, or "uncoupled" oxidative phosphorylation. Normally three $\sim$P molecules are produced for each oxygen molecule in a well-coupled respiratory chain.

Not all the cells' high-energy phosphate is derived from mitochondria; Fig. 68-2 shows two sites where $\sim$P is produced in the metabolism of glucose to pyruvate. Nonmitochondrial generation (anaerobic glycolysis) may occur in the absence of oxygen, and, as discussed below, may be crucial to the cell, or even to the survival of the entire organism.

The acetyl CoA which provides the bulk of mitochondrial fuel can be derived from several sources. It is the final common pathway of the breakdown of all carbohydrates, being formed by pyruvate decarboxylation in the mitochondrion itself with thiamine (vitamin B_1) and lipoic acid as cofactors. Acetyl CoA is also formed from long-chain fatty acids which enter the mitochondria esterified to carnitine where they are again reesterified with coenzyme A (a cofactor containing the vitamin pantothenic acid). The fatty acid coenzyme A molecule then undergoes sequential removal of hydrogen, the hydrogen being transferred to the respiratory chain for energy production as NADH or FADH (cofactors containing the vitamins nicotinamide and riboflavin), and cleavage of two carbons at a time to form acetyl CoA, which in turn enters the tricarboxylic acid cycle. Ketone bodies can also directly contribute acetyl CoA to mitochondrial oxidation, as can certain amino acids after deamination and partial degradation. Thus all three metabolic fuels, carbohydrate, fat, and protein, feed acetyl CoA into mitochondrial metabolism for terminal combustion and generation of high-energy phosphate.

FIGURE 68-2

A general scheme of energy and molecular transformations in compartments of the cell. Glucose is transported across the cell membrane, phosphorylated through use of high-energy phosphate bond ($\sim$P), and then transformed either to store its energy content (upward, glycogenesis) or to release its energy content (downward) via (1) breakdown of glycogen by phosphorylase (A)*; (2) oxidation through the glycolytic cycle to form acetyl CoA; (3) hydrogen transfer* (B) *to enter the mitochondrial apparatus; (4) oxidation through the pentose pathway. Energy is transformed into useful form via the consumption of O_2 in mitochondrial membranes* (C) *with concomitant esterification of inorganic phosphate (P_i) to form a (hypothetic) high-energy phosphate intermediate compound (X$\sim$P), which can be used to synthesize ATP (see Fig. 68-1); this mitochondrial process is oxidative phosphorylation. The mitochondrial matrix contains enzymes catalyzing the Krebs (tricarboxylic acid) cycle, transforming the energy released from acetyl CoA produced from glucose, amino acids, ketone bodies, or fatty acids. Further details are discussed in the text.*

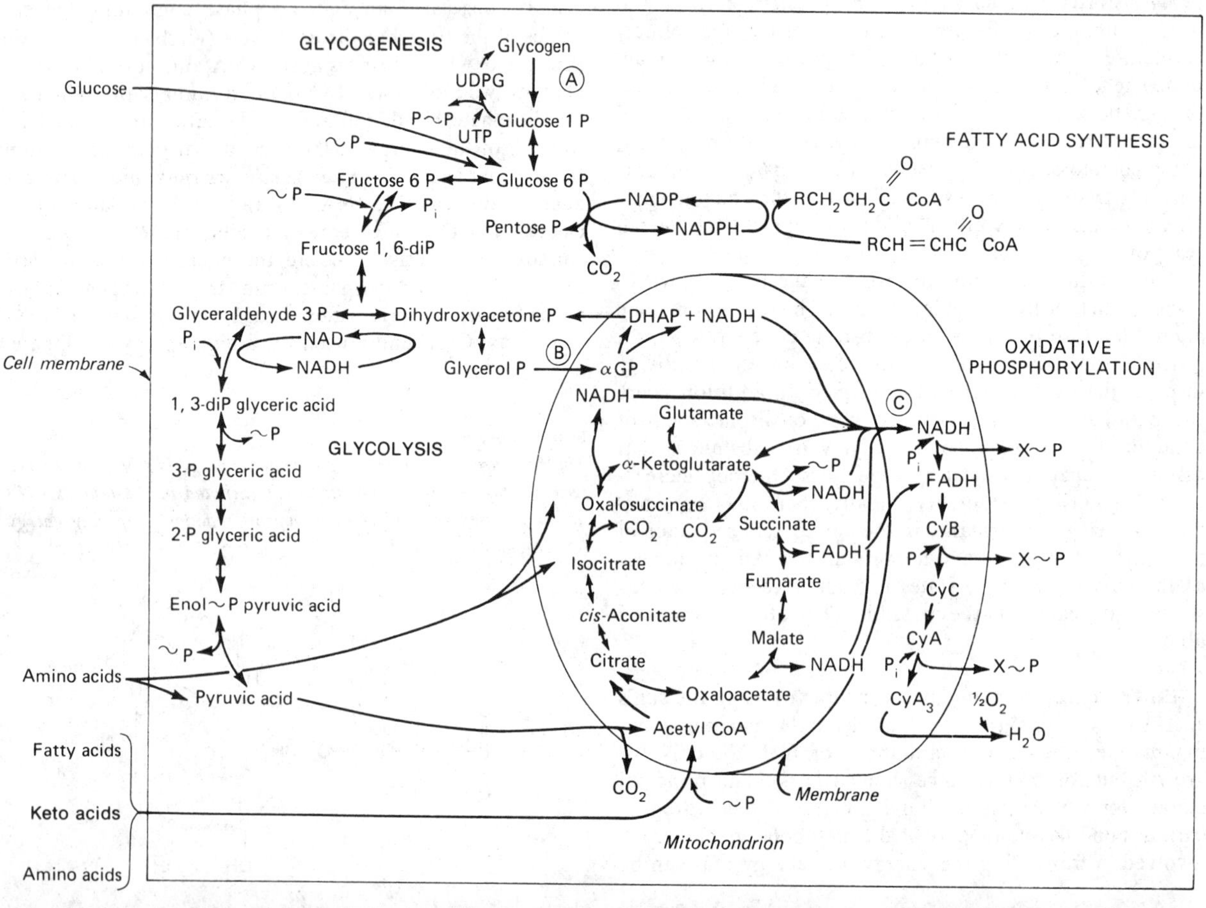

GLUCOSE METABOLISM Mitochondrial generation of ATP, although accounting for more than 90 percent of all energy produced in the cell, is not the only source of utilizable energy. Anaerobic glycolysis in the cytoplasm also produces two ~P molecules per molecule of glucose oxidized, as indicated in Fig. 68-2. The efficiency of energy transformation, the amount of useful energy obtained per molecule of fuel consumed, is much lower in glycolysis than in mitochondrial oxidative phosphorylation; in other words, glycolysis is a very inefficient means of supplying large amounts of energy.

In the utilization of glucose by a cell, it is first phosphorylated to glucose 6-phosphate by the enzyme hexokinase. Adenosine triphosphate is utilized in the process, yielding ADP and glucose 6-phosphate. Thus a high-energy bond is consumed and a low-energy bond generated with loss of heat, which makes the reaction essentially unidirectional and therefore a potential site of metabolic control. Glucose 6-phosphate occupies a strategic position with reference to several biochemical pathways.

Glycolysis This sequence of reactions is the most important route of glucose 6-phosphate metabolism. After the conversion of glucose to glucose 6-phosphate, a step requiring ATP, glucose 6-phosphate is converted to fructose 6-phosphate, to which another high-energy phosphate is added from ATP to form fructose 1,6-diphosphate. This is another step yielding much energy as heat, using a high-energy phosphate, and producing one with low energy, and is therefore essentially unidirectional. It has been suggested that this reaction controls the entire glycolytic pathway. This step is opposed by another enzyme, fructose 1,6-diphosphatase, which converts fructose 1,6-diphosphate back to fructose 6-phosphate. The latter enzyme, as expected, is located in tissues which produce glucose, and therefore is found in liver, where its activity is increased by any one of a group of metabolic stimuli which accelerate gluconeogenesis, e.g., glucocorticoids. Conversely, fructose 1,6-diphosphatase is essentially lacking in tissues such as muscle, adipose tissue, or brain, where the only route of glucose metabolism is via glycolysis to pyruvate and lactate, and then via acetate and the citric acid cycle to CO_2 in the presence of oxygen.

After formation of fructose 1,6-diphosphate, the hexose unit is split into two interconvertible 3-carbon phosphorylated sugars. One of these, glyceraldehyde 3-phosphate, is dehydrogenated and phosphorylated to form NADH and 1,3-diphosphoglyceric acid, which through a series of reactions yields pyruvate and two high-energy phosphate bonds per 3-carbon residue. Thus the overall reaction is:

$$\text{Glucose} + 2 \sim\text{P} + 2\text{P}_i + 2\text{NAD}^+ \rightarrow 2 \text{ pyruvate} + 4 \sim\text{P} + 2\text{NADH} + 2\text{H}^+$$

where P_i is inorganic phosphate. If oxygen is lacking and the NADH cannot be oxidized to NAD^+, its hydrogen atom can be disposed of in the conversion of pyruvate to lactate, and thereby NAD^+ is replenished for further glycolysis. Thus the overall reaction is:

$$\text{Glucose} + 2 \sim\text{P} \rightarrow 2 \text{ lactate} + 4 \sim\text{P}$$

or

$$\text{Glucose} \rightarrow 2 \text{ lactate} + 2 \sim\text{P}$$

This sequence, termed *anaerobic glycolysis,* since it can occur in the absence of oxygen, can provide a small but, in an emergency, significant and necessary amount of energy. Anaerobic glycolysis is limited, however, by the accumulation of lactic acid which eventually lowers the pH to a degree not compatible with cellular function. Certain tissues, such as the red blood cell or renal medulla, which are devoid of, or very low in, mitochondria, normally derive their energy by this process, and the lactic acid so produced is released into the circulation to be metabolized by other tissues.

GLYCOGEN Glycogen is a very large, complex polymer of branching chains of glucose units and serves as a storage form of carbohydrate. Although present in all tissues, it plays its most significant role in liver and in muscle, in the former as the reserve for blood glucose maintenance between meals and in the latter as the principal source of fuel during strenuous activity. Glycogen is synthesized from glucose 1-phosphate by an enzyme sequence whose activity, in turn, is regulated by its interconversion into an active form or into an inactive form, each interconversion being controlled itself by a separate enzyme which can exist in an active or inactive form. This highly complex system is increased in overall activity by insulin and glucose and is decreased by physiologic events stimulating glycogen breakdown. For example, in liver, epinephrine or glucagon react with the cell membrane to generate the formation of cyclic adenosine monophosphate (cAMP) (Fig. 68-3) which in turn activates the turning off of the glycogen-synthesizing system.

Glycogen breakdown occurs via a separate pathway, and, as expected, being essentially unidirectional, is a site of metabolic regulation. The same events that turn on the glycogen-synthesizing system turn off the glycogenolytic system, and vice versa. Cyclic AMP therefore activates enzymes which in turn activate other enzymes to activate the enzyme phosphorylase (by its conversion from an inactive phosphorylase) to cleave glucose units off the terminal glycogen chains. The net effect is a mechanism whereby a few molecules of the initial signal, such as epinephrine acting on the muscle or liver cell, or glucagon on the liver cell, can

FIGURE 68-3
The structure of cyclic 3′,5′-adenosine monophosphate (cyclic 3′,5′-AMP or cyclic adenylate). It is produced in the cell from adenosine triphosphate.

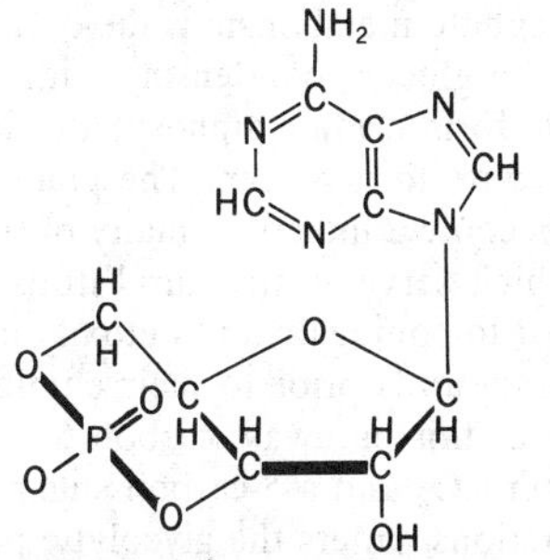

initiate a rapid amplification resulting in an almost instantaneous cessation of glycogen synthesis and a rapid acceleration of glycogen breakdown. In liver, this results in glucose release; in muscle, fuel for aerobic or anaerobic glycolysis.

Not discussed here is the role of the enzymes involved in forming the branch points or in cleaving the branch points; these are discussed in Chap. 111, Disorders of Glycogen Synthesis and Mobilization.

DIRECT OXIDATIVE PATHWAY In several tissues (adipose, liver, adrenal, mammary) reduced $NADP^+$ (NADPH) is required to provide the hydrogen and electrons for synthesis of lipid. Thus a certain proportion of glucose 6-phosphate is oxidized by glucose 6-phosphate dehydrogenase to 6-phosphogluconic acid and NADPH, and the former then is oxidized to a compound which loses carbon 1 as CO_2 and produces another NADPH and a pentose phosphate, ribulose 5-phosphate. Through a complicated series of reactions, the pentose phosphates return to the main glycolytic sequence as fructose 6-phosphate or triose phosphate. This metabolic route is significant in lipid-synthesizing tissues such as developing brain, in adipose tissue where it is involved in the conversion of dietary glucose into stored fatty acid, and in certain endocrine glands active in synthesizing steroid hormones.

GLUCOSE 6-PHOSPHATASE This enzyme provides yet another pathway of glucose 6-phosphate metabolism and is located only in those tissues capable of producing glucose: liver and kidney, and also placenta. In the liver, it is the final common pathway for glucose production and opposes the action of the glucose phosphorylating system. The activity of glucose 6-phosphatase in liver is increased in states associated with increased glucose production (diabetes, excess adrenal glucocorticoids) and is decreased in those associated with increased insulin or carbohydrate intake. Again there are two "unidirectional" enzymes at an important site of metabolic control, one for the production and the other for the uptake of glucose by liver. The role of the enzyme in kidney is apparently different and may be related to the process of reabsorption of metabolic intermediates which are converted to glucose 6-phosphate and then are released into the bloodstream. It is clearly not related to the renal tubular reabsorption of glucose since this process does not involve phosphorylation or dephosphorylation. In type I glycogenosis, this enzyme is deficient in body tissues, particularly liver (see Chap. 111), resulting in severe hypoglycemia.

GLUCURONIC ACID PATHWAY An alternative route of glucose 6-phosphate metabolism is the oxidation of carbon 6 of glucose, the glucose condensing with uridine triphosphate (UTP) to form uridine diphosphate glucose (UDPG), similar to its route to glycogen. The glucuronic acid thus formed may become a moiety in many of the complex carbohydrates which serve as structural units (glycoproteins) or may be used to conjugate and detoxify endogenous and exogenous compounds prior to their elimination from the body. As part of this pathway, carbon 6 of UDPG can be cleaved to form CO_2 and a 5-carbon sugar which, through a series of reactions, enters the glycolytic pathway. One of the intermediates in this sequence, l-xylulose, may accumulate and be excreted in the urine in the benign disease, essential pentosuria, which is due to lack of the enzyme that catalyzes the subsequent step in the sequence (Chap. 96).

SORBITOL PATHWAY Another route of glucose metabolism, not involving prior phosphorylation, is one in which glucose is directly reduced at carbon 1 to a polyalcohol, sorbitol. Much attention has been paid to this metabolic route since the enzyme involved has a high K_m for its substrate, and only in hyperglycemia does much sorbitol accumulate in certain tissues such as the lens of the eye or peripheral nerves. This process has been indicted in certain of the complications of diabetes (Chap. 95).

ACETATE AND PYRUVATE METABOLISM Just as glucose 6-phosphate occupies a position at the crossroads of many metabolic reactions, so do acetate and its closely related products. Pyruvate, the terminus of the previously mentioned pathways, to be further metabolized, must be decarboxylated in the presence of NAD^+ and coenzyme A, thiamine, and lipoic acid to form CO_2 and acetyl CoA (see Chap. 84). Free acetate itself is of only minor importance in nonruminants as a metabolic fuel. It is the acetyl CoA, therefore, which can enter the subsequent metabolic routes.

In the process of fatty acid synthesis, the acetyl CoA accepts CO_2 to form malonyl CoA, and through a series of reactions involving condensations and reductions (NADPH derived from glucose oxidation via the direct oxidative pathway) a 16-carbon, saturated, long-chain fatty acid, palmitic acid, is formed; this can then be extended or unsaturated by other enzyme systems. This sequence takes place primarily in adipose tissue but also in liver and to a lesser extent in other tissues. Another route open to acetyl CoA is the formation of ketone bodies, a reaction which occurs exclusively in liver. There is some question as to whether ketones are formed by direct condensation of two acetyl CoA's or via an intermediate comprising three acetyl CoA's, namely, β-hydroxy-β-methylglutaryl CoA. A third route for acetyl CoA metabolism, via β-hydroxy-β-methylglutaryl CoA, is in the formation of the steroid nucleus and the various compounds derived from it by further metabolic changes, such as cholesterol, steroid hormones, and bile salts. The fourth and perhaps most important route is the condensation of acetyl CoA with oxaloacetate to form citrate, the first step in the sequence of intramitochondrial reactions involving the Krebs (or citric or tricarboxylic acid) cycle, as previously described.

Another pathway of pyruvate metabolism is the direct condensation with CO_2 to form oxaloacetate. This sequence is important in liver and is catalyzed by an enzyme, pyruvic carboxylase. In fasting, or in diabetes mellitus in which fat breakdown to acetyl CoA occurs at a rapid rate, the high level of acetyl CoA accelerates this reaction. Normally oxaloacetate would accept the acetyl CoA to form citrate for oxidation via the citric acid cycle, but this reaction is apparently blocked in the fasting state or in diabetes, and under these conditions the oxaloacetate is phosphorylated and decarboxylated to form phosphoenolpyruvate by another enzyme important in liver, phosphoenolpyruvate carboxykinase. By this sequence, pyruvate is converted to phosphoenolpyruvate and then to glucose, a reaction which cannot proceed directly in this direction because of the energy differential.

USES OF ATP A detailed listing of specific reactions into which ATP enters is found in standard biochemical texts. A selected few are of illustrative interest. Studies indicate that the mitochondrion, a self-sufficient apparatus in many ways, transforms energy and also has the capacity to maintain high internal electrolyte concentrations when it is functioning in its energy-producing role. Mitochondria can accumulate K^+, Ca^{2+}, Mg^{2+}, Mn^{2+}, and phosphate ions while oxidizing and phosphorylating, but not when phosphorylation is uncoupled. The purpose of the accumulation is as yet obscure, for Ca^{2+} ions, for instance, are themselves uncoupling agents. However, demonstrations that parathyroid hormone is capable of affecting phosphate and Ca^{2+} exchanges in mitochondria in vitro are of obvious importance in understanding the mechanism of action of the hormone. The contribution of the osmotic work done by mitochondria toward that of the whole cell is not yet clear.

A major role of ATP in the body is to serve as the ultimate energy source for muscle contraction. The details of the molecular events concerned with this physical process are still a matter for investigation, but ATP is necessary for the relaxation phenomenon, whereby the contracted actomyosin fibrils resume their more elongated form, primed for the next contraction. Indeed, so definite is the association between the use of ATP and muscle contraction that the actomyosin molecule is called an *ATPase*. The dependence of muscle contraction on ATP is reflected in the demands of the myocardium, for instance, for a continued supply of utilizable energy derived from oxidation. The myocardium is supplied with large, intricate mitochondria, and interference with the supply of oxygen by a decrease in blood flow produces noncontracting myocardial areas with differences in electrical potential (see Chap. 233). Such changes probably increase cellular permeability so that enzymes (e.g., lactic dehydrogenase and the transaminases from cytoplasm, and intramitochondrial enzymes such as malic dehydrogenase) leak into the circulation to provide biochemical diagnostic criteria of impaired myocardial function. Biochemical lesions of the myocardium that interfere with the generation of ATP occur in anemia, thyrotoxicosis, and beriberi, and result in a myocardial contractile defect which is not susceptible to the beneficial action of digitalis, ordinarily so effective when the contractile mechanism itself operates at a disadvantage but has an adequate energy supply. Defects in energy transformation in skeletal muscle appear to be present in at least two diseases, as demonstrated by functional and structural changes in muscle mitochondria in patients with thyrotoxicosis and in two reported cases of nonthyrotoxic hypermetabolism.

Another significant use of ATP is the generation of heat to maintain body temperature. In the synthesis of ATP by oxidative phosphorylation, for example, only 60 percent of the energy liberated from oxidation of its substrates is transformed by the mitochondrion to phosphate bond energy. An appreciable portion of the liberated energy is evolved as heat, which assists in maintaining body temperature. When the external environment increases the need for heat production, the body responds with an increased rate of oxygen consumption.

The synthesis of the polymeric compounds that store energy in the body requires ATP, e.g., the condensation of glucose 1-phosphate to form glycogen, of acetyl CoA to form fatty acids, of soluble RNA–amino acid complexes to form polypeptides and proteins, and of nucleosides to form nucleotides.

ENERGY TRANSFORMATION To survive, a species must possess mechanisms whereby it can deposit and store fuel during periods of availability and be able to mobilize this fuel at times of increased need; in addition, it must store and mobilize fuel for the necessary chemical reactions required to maintain the integrity of its structure.

The human body contains numerous organic compounds with energy potential: lipids, carbohydrates, proteins, and nucleic acids. The lipids are by far the most quantitatively important form of storage of fuel, in addition to providing other functions such as insulation of the body as a whole or as essential components in the structure of cell walls, myelin, and other membranes. Carbohydrates serve as a lesser form of fuel storage. Protein serves as the structural basis for all enzymes, contracting elements such as muscle, or supporting structures such as collagen, and in addition as a fuel, or precursor for carbohydrate in the process of gluconeogenesis. Nucleic acids form fundamental components in the hereditary and synthetic mechanisms and are usually not available as fuels. The body can be divided into four main metabolic compartments, adipose tissue, nervous tissue, muscle, and liver.

ADIPOSE TISSUE Adipose tissue is composed of between 60 and 90 percent triglyceride and thus contains 6 to 8 kcal per g total wet tissue. A normal 70-kg male may have 12 kg adipose tissue and thereby a potential fuel reserve of approximately 90,000 kcal, which theoretically could support life for well over 2 months. In obesity, 100 kg adipose tissue may be present—an entire year's supply!

Adipose tissue metabolism (Fig. 68-4) is controlled by many factors, which may be grouped into two general classes, anabolic and catabolic. A rise in blood glucose level following ingestion of carbohydrate stimulates insulin production; insulin directly increases glucose uptake into adipose tissue, where, in the process of lipogenesis, it is metabolized via acetyl CoA into fatty acids, which are then esterified with glycerol to form triglycerides. Thus the individual has converted a less efficient fuel on a weight basis (carbohydrate) to a more efficient form of energy storage (lipid). Some of the ingested glucose may also be converted to glycogen in liver, muscle, and adipose tissue. These carbohydrate stores serve two ancillary purposes: (1) as a temporary storage site during ingestion of large amounts of carbohydrate (until the lipogenetic process can store the energy as fat), and (2) as an emergency store of quickly available glucose for anaerobic glycolysis during periods of stress. The economy of storage of energy as lipid far surpasses that as carbohydrate, since triglyceride is deposited in an extraaqueous phase, whereas glycogen is stored with water and electrolytes; 1 g glycogen-containing tissue yields only 1 to 1½ kcal, and it is therefore one-fourth to one-sixth as efficient for storage of energy as an equivalent unit of lipid-containing tissue (see Chap. 46, Gain in Weight. Obesity).

Insulin appears to exert other effects on adipose tissue. Following a fatty meal, triglycerides enter the bloodstream in the form of lipoproteins—chylomicrons—via the thoracic duct. They may then enter the liver and be chemically modified and released into the circulation, or they may be directly incorporated into adipose tissue where they are hydrolyzed into free fatty acids and reesterified into triglyceride. These many rearrangements of the originally ingested fat may be the animal's mechanism to ensure that the fat which it stores in its adipose tissue contains the correct number and types of fatty acids. Insulin in the fed individual apparently plays an important role in the uptake of circulating triglycerides into adipose tissue, in addition to its role in promoting lipogenesis from glucose.

Fuel stored as adipose tissue triglyceride is released in only one form, free fatty acids. Adipose tissue free fatty acid concentration is in equilibrium with the fatty acid bound to albumin in the circulation; thus, a rise in adipose tissue free fatty acids induces a release of these into the circulation. The level of free acids in adipose tissue is controlled by several factors. Insulin decreases this level by providing increased glucose uptake, which supplies increased glycerol acceptor for esterification of fatty acids in the cell. Insulin also inhibits the breakdown of triglyceride into free fatty acid. Conversely, lack of insulin, as in fasting, increases adipose tissue free fatty acid by a reversal of these processes and thereby augments fatty acid release. Among other substances which increase fatty acid production by adipose tissue are norepinephrine, epinephrine, and growth, thyroid, and adrenal hormones. The action of epinephrine and norepinephrine on free fatty acid mobilization depends on the thyroid status, being increased in hyperthyroidism and decreased or absent in hypothyroidism. The principal physiologic control of free fatty acid release and circulating levels is probably the balance of sympathetic nerve endings producing norepinephrine which causes generation of cyclic AMP (Fig. 68-3) in the adipose cell membrane. Cyclic AMP then activates the intracellular lipolytic system. Insulin, on the other hand, increases the catabolism of cyclic AMP and thus inhibits free fatty acid release.

NERVOUS TISSUE Nervous tissues require a continuous supply of glucose (Fig. 68-5). This glucose utilization is independent of insulin, of glucose concentration (as long as it is adequate), or of the state of nervous activity. Only in severe metabolic derangements producing coma is there a significant decrease in the use of glucose (except for a gradual slight decrease with age probably due to a progressive attrition of neurons). During prolonged starvation, however, and probably in individuals who are consuming a very high fat (ketogenic) diet, the brain may decrease its glucose utilization without loss of function because of its capacity to utilize acetoacetate and β-hydroxybutyrate.

In nervous tissue glucose is totally glycolyzed and then oxidized to CO_2 by the tricarboxylic acid cycle. Thus glu-

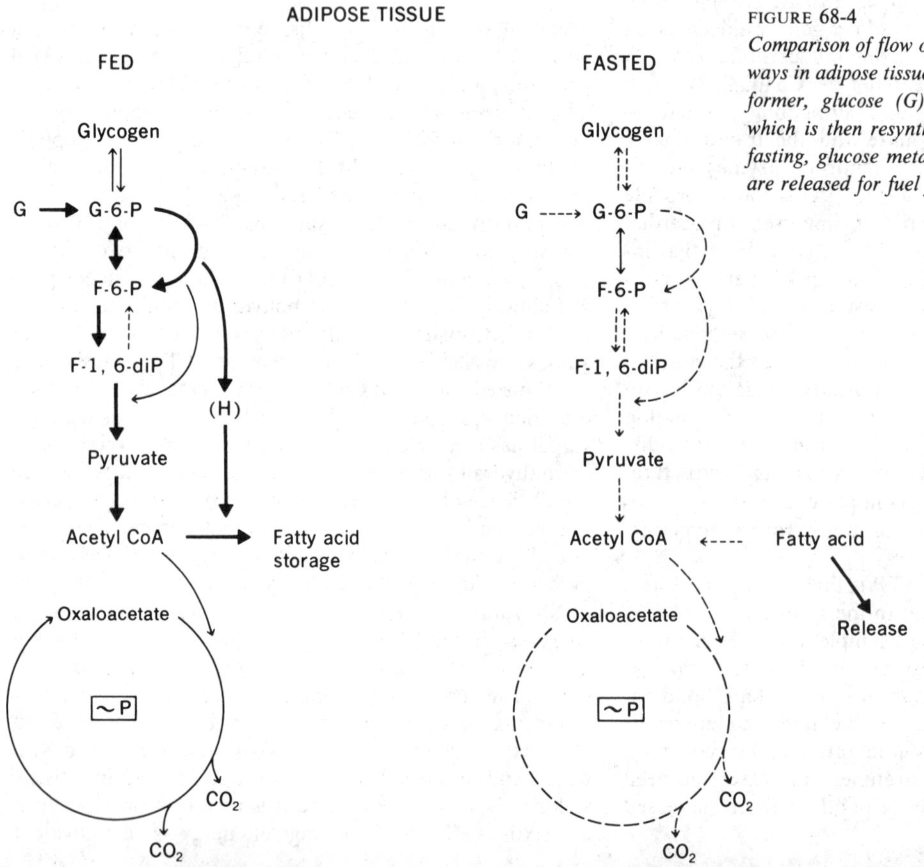

FIGURE 68-4
Comparison of flow of substrate across metabolic pathways in adipose tissue in the fed and fasted state. In the former, glucose (G) is metabolized to acetyl CoA, which is then resynthesized to fat and stored. During fasting, glucose metabolism is limited, and fatty acids are released for fuel for the remainder of the body.

cose and oxygen must always be available: if their supply is interrupted, brain function ceases almost immediately. Brain glycogen levels are extremely low and insignificant as an energy source.

MUSCLE Muscle tissue is versatile in that it can utilize several different fuels to support activity (Fig. 68-5). Glucose is readily removed by muscle from the circulating fluids under the stimulus of insulin, although increased muscular activity or anoxia can also increase glucose uptake. The glucose in muscle is readily glycolyzed to lactic acid, and, if there is adequate oxygen, to CO_2 and water. The glucose may also be stored as glycogen to be used as emergency fuel for glycolysis when oxygen is unavailable or relatively inadequate.

Muscle mitochondria also readily utilize fatty acids as fuel. These can come from several sources, from free fatty acids circulating in the blood, having been released from adipose tissue, from fat stored directly in the muscle itself, or possibly from circulating triglyceride derived from the diet or the liver. Whatever the origin, the fatty acid is oxidized completely to CO_2 and water, and it is fat which serves as the major contributor of energy to muscle metabolism.

A third type of fuel for muscle is derived from the liver as a product of the incomplete combustion of fatty acids, namely, acetoacetic and β-hydroxybutyric acids, which, with acetone, form the ketone bodies. These two acids are also completely metabolized to CO_2 and water in muscle and in certain circumstances can provide a major share of muscle fuel.

By mechanisms not yet clarified, muscle selectively metabolizes ketone bodies, then fatty acids, and, as a last resort, glucose. If ketones are unavailable and free fatty acid concentration is low, as after carbohydrate or insulin administration, muscle will then readily metabolize glucose. Conversely, if ketone or fatty acid concentrations are high, glucose metabolism is minimized, even in the presence of insulin, and the glucose which is taken into the tissue is converted to and stored as glycogen.

One major role of muscle is to serve as a storehouse for amino acids. It is now accepted that a primary site of insulin action is in muscle, where insulin stimulates the incorporation of circulating amino acids into muscle protein. This action is biochemically distinct from the effect on glucose. If insulin is lacking, this process is decreased or even reversed, and amino acids are mobilized by proteolysis and release. Adrenocortical hormones oppose the insulin effect. In fasting, amino acids are mobilized from muscle, and during feeding, when insulin increases, amino acids are incorporated into muscle protein. Removal of both insulin and adrenal hormones achieves a new balance, but one without flexibility in either direction.

LIVER Of the four groups of tissues playing a major role in body fuel economy, the liver (Fig. 68-6) serves as the director of traffic and, as such, is metabolically more complicated than adipose, nervous, and muscle tissues. During

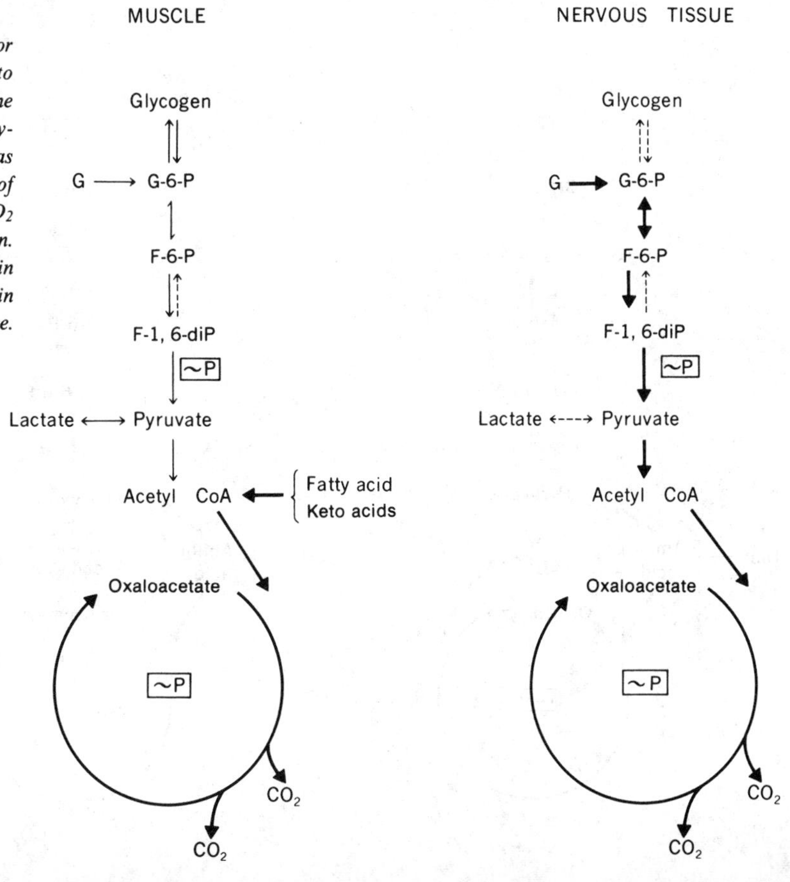

FIGURE 68-5
Muscle tissue utilizes predominantly fatty acid or ketone as a source of fuel, but it is also able to derive limited amounts of energy (~P) from the conversion of glucose to lactate (anaerobic glycolysis). Nervous tissue is able to utilize only glucose as its metabolic fuel, and requires a constant supply of oxygen for total combustion of the glucose to CO_2 in order to derive energy for adequate function. With elevated levels of keto acids (see text) brain can use these in place of glucose. This occurs in prolonged starvation and is not shown in this figure. See Fig. 68-1.

fasting, it must provide glucose for those tissues requiring glucose for survival (mainly the brain). In contrast, during times of carbohydrate ingestion, it stops producing glucose and, instead, removes and stores glucose as glycogen, transiently if the glycogen reserve is already adequate, or more permanently if the glycogen reserve has been previously depleted by prolonged fasting or other stress.

Unlike peripheral cells, the liver cell is very permeable to glucose, and the concentration of glucose in the blood is approximated by the concentration in the liver cell, being slightly greater if glucose is being produced by the liver and slightly less if glucose is being removed. The net flow of glucose inside the liver cell into and out of the metabolically activated pool of glucose, glucose 6-phosphate, is a function of two enzymes present in liver, glucokinase and glucose 6-phosphatase. The activity of the former is increased by insulin or carbohydrate feeding, and that of the latter by fasting, insulin insufficiency, or adrenal steroids. Thus the activities of these two opposing systems direct the net flow of glucose into and out of the liver, and exercise control over the concentration of glucose in the circulating fluids.

Liver is also unique in possessing other enzymes which are located at metabolic control sites in the sequence of reactions between amino acids and glucose. These enzymes increase in activity during times of increased gluconeogenesis, as in association with early fasting, diabetes, or adrenal steroid administration, and are decreased by carbohydrate feeding or insulin administration.

During fasting, the liver must provide glucose for tissues requiring this fuel, primarily brain, but also spinal cord, peripheral nerve, leukoctyes, erythrocytes, renal medulla, and probably others. This it does by synthesizing new glucose (gluconeogenesis) from glycogenic amino acids released into the circulation from muscle, and, to a lesser extent, from lactate or pyruvate returning to the liver from peripheral tissues, as well as from glycerol arising from lipolysis in adipose tissue. Normally liver contains only 80 to 100 g glycogen, about one-half a day's supply of carbohydrate, should gluconeogenesis not be stimulated to provide the glucose needed by the organism. The liver in a briefly fasted normal man produces approximately 180 g glucose daily, of which about 144 g is oxidized by brain to CO_2 and water and 36 g is returned as lactate and pyruvate. The bulk of this glucose is derived from glycogen between meals and during the usual overnight fast. But if man is deprived of food for a more prolonged period, approximately 10 g glycogen is conserved for emergency glycolysis, and blood glucose concentration is then maintained by gluconeogenesis.

The liver in the normally fed individual mainly uses amino acid as its source of fuel. During fasting, the amino acid which is presented to the liver is diverted, for reasons of economy, into glucose synthesis, and the liver now uses to meet for its own needs the energy derived from the partial oxidation of fatty acids to ketone bodies, from which one-third of the total potential energy of the fatty acid is derived. Thus gluconeogenesis, amino acid metabolism (and therefore urea production), and ketone body production are intimately related.

When the animal is fed, liver metabolism is grossly altered through a number of complicated mechanisms. Gluconeogenesis ceases, those amino acids which enter the liver are metabolized, providing the needed energy for the

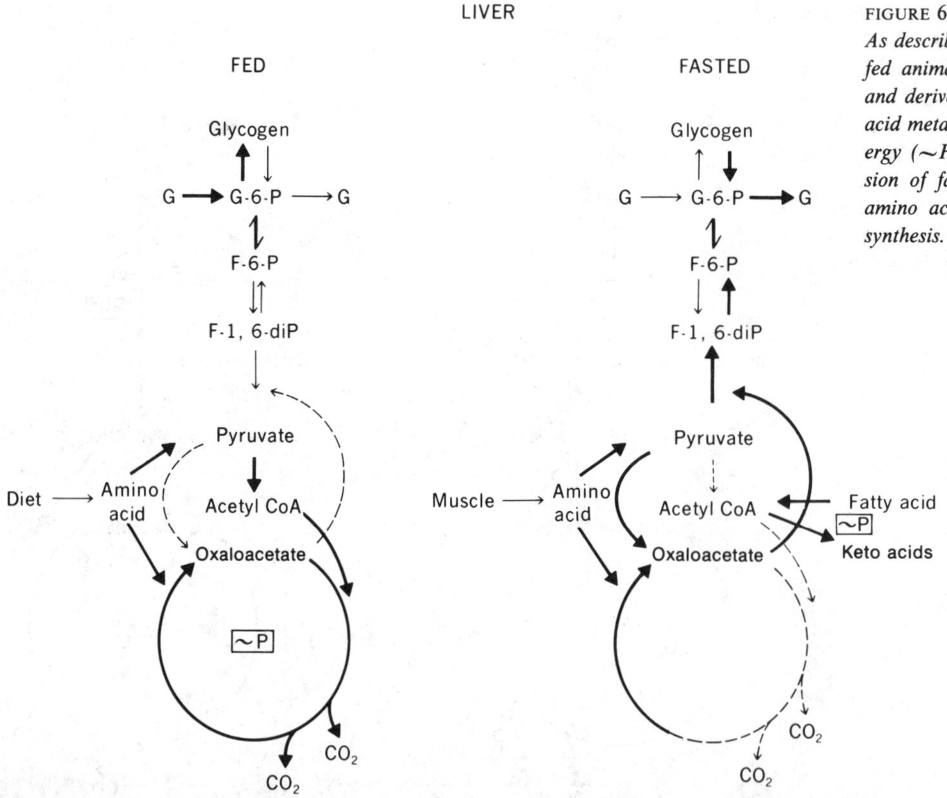

FIGURE 68-6
As described in the text, the liver in the fed animal stores glucose as glycogen and derives its own energy from amino acid metabolism. During fasting, its energy (~P) is derived from the conversion of fatty acids to keto acids, and amino acids are diverted into glucose synthesis.

liver's own metabolic processes, and ketone production ceases. The level of free fatty acids in the circulation falls, since their release from adipose tissue is inhibited by insulin. The liver, however, continues to remove about one-fourth of the total turnover of free fatty acids, but now, since its own energy is adequately provided by amino acid oxidation via its citric acid cycle, the liver esterifies these free fatty acids and returns them as triglyceride to the periphery instead of converting them to ketone bodies. In other words, during fasting, amino acid carbon is diverted into gluconeogenesis, and since the liver's own energy needs are met primarily by ketogenesis, the citric acid cycle of the liver assumes a minor role in the production of energy. During feeding, the citric acid cycle predominates, amino acids are deaminated and their products are oxidized via the cycle, and ketone production essentially ceases.

TOTAL MAN Normal man readily adapts to nutritional and environmental changes by altering hormone levels and responsive metabolic pathways, thereby maintaining a finely regulated "internal environment." Thus homeostasis is closely preserved in the face of diverse nutritional and metabolic alterations such as feeding or fasting, during exercise and acute or chronic stress, whether the stress is physical, as in trauma or infection, or emotional. Several of these states with direct clinical application are discussed below.

THE FASTED STATE In normal postabsorptive humans, blood glucose concentration is maintained at approximately 80 mg per 100 ml, with hepatic production equaling utilization, mainly by brain, which oxidizes 100 mg glucose per minute to CO_2 and H_2O. Interruption of brain substrate metabolism by low glucose concentration, by a decrease in circulation, or by a decrease in available oxygen results in dysfunction within minutes of deprivation and in irreversible damage if the deprivation is prolonged. The highest centers usually reflect the metabolic defect first, as evidenced by bizarre behavior, frequently with signs and symptoms of epinephrine discharge (palpitations, cold skin, sweatiness, and piloerection). Unconsciousness follows, and eventually, if the substrate or oxygen availability becomes more restricted, respiratory arrest and death occur (see Chap. 97).

The maintenance of circulating glucose concentration is a most important homeostatic process. Between meals this regulation is achieved mainly by hepatic glycogenolysis. However, since total liver glycogen amounts to 80 to 100 g, hepatic glycogen synthesis and storage begins soon after a meal has been ingested in order to replete the glycogen used between meals. But after more prolonged fasting, as occurs overnight, glucose levels begin to be directly maintained by gluconeogenesis as glycogen stores become depleted.

Tissues other than brain, such as red cells, renal medulla, and some smooth muscle, also use glucose as fuel, but, lacking mitochondria for terminal oxidation of glucose to CO_2, derive their energy from glycolysis of the glucose to lactate, returning the latter back into the bloodstream for removal by liver (and kidney) and reincorporation into glucose (the Cori cycle). Thus overall glucose production is slightly greater than that needed by brain, but terminal oxidation of glucose to CO_2 is mainly by this organ.

In the postabsorptive state, glucose is largely excluded from tissues other than brain. Muscle and adipose tissue, which, with brain, are the main glucose consumers in the fed state, markedly diminish their glucose utilization. If the fasting continues for more than a day, glucose is almost totally excluded from these tissues. Instead, muscle uses free fatty acids liberated from adipose tissue, and, should the starvation be of several days' duration, uses them both directly and indirectly as keto acids formed by the partial oxidation and degradation of the fatty acids by liver.

The glucose derived from gluconeogenesis is synthesized partly from returning lactate (Cori cycle), partly from glycerol released from the adipose tissue, and mainly from amino acids released from muscle (Fig. 68-7). The overall control appears to be insulin, with glucagon possibly playing a significant secondary role. As glucose levels fall, there is decreased insulin release from the pancreas and, since the half-life of insulin is 10 min, insulin levels fall accordingly. Muscle proteolysis is very sensitive to low levels of insulin, while high levels of insulin slow this process and thereby inhibit amino acid formation and release. As shown in Fig. 68-7, a decrease in insulin as occurs after an overnight fast initiates a release of amino acids from muscle to liver. Liver, in the presence of low levels of insulin and above-normal levels of glucagon, readily converts amino acids into glucose. In fact, early in fasting or simply between meals, it is this bihormonal shift which mobilizes liver glycogen as the first mechanism for the maintenance of blood glucose levels.

STARVATION, MORE PROLONGED Brain in an average-sized individual consumes one-third to one-fourth of the total calories, or about 500 kcal per day. In order to support this rate of glucose consumption by gluconeogenesis from muscle amino acids in prolonged starvation, mobilization of the major share of total body protein over several weeks would be required, an event incompatible with survival. As mentioned above, part of the fatty acids released from adipose tissue are metabolized in liver to keto acids and transported by the blood to muscle. As the levels of acetoacetate and β-hydroxybutyrate, the principal keto acids, rise in the blood, brain progressively oxidizes them as fuel and reduces its glucose consumption accordingly. The net effect is a decreased glucose requirement to 20 to 30 mg instead of 100 mg per min. Thus muscle nitrogen is spared and survival is markedly prolonged. The levels of acetoacetate and β-hydroxybutyrate in blood rise to 1.5 and 6 m*M* respectively, and HCO_3^- is reduced accordingly, resulting in a mild but tolerable metabolic acidosis, in marked contrast to the uncontrolled diabetic in whom these organic acids can result in levels of 15 to 20 m*M* due to overproduction and underutilization.

Starvation and protein-calorie malnutrition are further discussed in Chap. 82.

Small carbohydrate intake If one administers 100 mg glucose per min to normal man, the small increase in glucose concentration provokes increased secretion of insulin, and the resulting elevated level, in turn, suppresses muscle proteolysis and amino acid release, liver gluconeogenesis, and keto acid production. Thus, by providing exogenous substrate for brain, liver glucose production is decreased. The net result is a marked sparing of muscle protein; however, some proteolysis and irreversible metabolism of essential amino acids takes place to a small extent. Nevertheless, the amount of muscle protein spared by this carbohydrate administration may be crucial to preservation of effective coughing and clearing of the tracheobronchial tree, in other words, the difference between survival and death. Thus any patient not eating should receive 100 to 150 g glucose daily in order to minimize muscle catabolism until the patient can again eat.

Large carbohydrate intake Should the influx of carbohydrate surpass that needed by brain, the next priority is the displacement of fatty acid oxidation by glucose, particularly in muscle. This displacement is achieved by the yet higher level of insulin suppressing free fatty acid release from adipose tissue, and circulating levels of free fatty acids decrease accordingly. At the same time glucose forms a greater share of muscle substrate. If the carbohydrate load surpasses the total caloric needs to maintain metabolic processes, the excess glucose has two available metabolic routes. One is to be converted into and stored as glycogen in muscle or liver and the other is to be taken up into adipose tissue, converted into fat, and stored as such. Since the normal person usually eats meals rather than nibbling around the clock, lipogenesis and fat storage occur with each meal, with lipid mobilization occurring between meals. Variations in the concentration of insulin appear to be the message signaling the tissues to either store or mobilize fuel. Inability to achieve a high insulin level postprandially results in delayed uptake of metabolic fuel, i.e., glucose intolerance.

Oral vs. parenteral carbohydrate intake A given amount of carbohydrate, if ingested orally, results in a greater rise in insulin levels when compared with the same amount infused parenterally and, subsequently, in a greater capacity to remove the glucose and other fuels such as amino acid and triglyceride from the circulation. This higher insulin level is probably due to one or more not definitely characterized hormones released from the gut mucosa, which in turn sensitize the beta cells to produce more insulin. Overproduction of these factors may play a role in the postprandial hypoglycemia which may complicate gastric surgery and possibly in other hypoglycemic states (see Chap. 97).

INSULIN DEFICIENCY During fasting, the low insulin level (Fig. 68-7) initiates release of peripheral fuels and augments the capacity for liver gluconeogenesis. The latter is also stimulated by the associated increase in glucagon secretion. Should the insulin be pathologically low, due to defective beta cells, or to resistance to the insulin released, an unopposed release of fuel would occur as well as unopposed gluconeogenesis, hyperglycemia, ketonemia, and all the symptomatology of diabetic ketoacidosis (Fig. 68-8) (Chap. 95). On the other hand, if there is a low but significant amount of insulin, glycogenolysis and inadequate removal of ingested or infused glucose would result in hyperglycemia, glycosuria, and dehydration without a significant degree of ketoacidosis, as demonstrated in the syndrome of nonketotic hyperosmolar coma.

FIGURE 68-7
Quantitative estimation of the flow of metabolic fuels by a normal fasted man for a period of 24 h, utilizing 1800 kcal. With more prolonged fasting of one or more weeks, peripheral tissues such as heart and skeletal muscle decrease ketone utilization, and as the levels of acetoacetate and β-hydroxybutyrate rise in blood, brain draws a major share of its energy from their oxidation, decreasing glucose consumption accordingly. Thus brain glucose utilization decreases from 144 g per day, as shown below, to less than half this amount, sparing protein mobilization for hepatic gluconeogenesis accordingly.

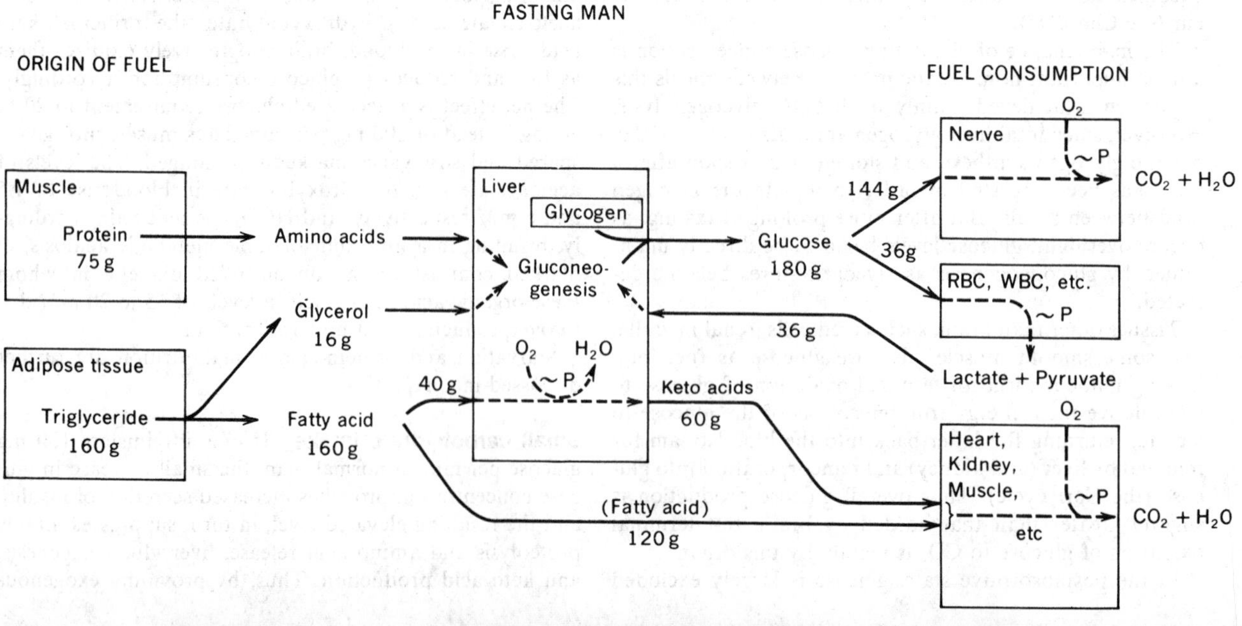

TRAUMA AND INFECTION During stress, be it physical, metabolic, or even emotional, the associated sympathetic activity results in beta cell suppression as well as increased mobilization of fatty acids from adipose tissue and glucose from liver glycogenolysis. Thus a diabetic type of metabolism may occur, resulting in delayed or inadequate removal of circulating fuels and, if severe, in hyperglycemia of sufficient degree to produce hyperosmolar coma. This may be iatrogenically induced in severely ill subjects overenthusiastically given carbohydrate. Another sequela of trauma or severe infection, such as peritonitis or septicemia, is accentuated mobilization of peripheral protein reserves, the "hypercatabolic" state. This process is very resistant to physiologic levels of insulin by an as yet uncharacterized mechanism, and may lead to such severe protein catabolism that the patient dies within several weeks because of ineffective respiratory musculature.

EXERCISE The energy for skeletal muscle during exercise is provided by several metabolic fuels. First there is the expected use of the small intracellular depot of ATP, producing ADP, which is rapidly replenished to ATP by creatine phosphate, until generation of substrate-derived ATP for glycolysis can be initiated. Thus the first few contractions of strong exercise are supported; next there is rapid glycogenolysis due to activation of the phosphorylase system, and ATP and lactic acid are generated from anaerobic glycolysis. Aiding this is augmented glucose uptake from the extracellular fluid which also ends up as lactic acid, later to be made into glucose by liver (Cori cycle) or to be oxidized to CO_2 by other tissues. The brisker the exercise, the more lactate produced and later to be consumed (as part of the "oxygen debt" needed to recharge the entire system back to its prior homeostatic state). In certain animals there are muscles rich in glycogen which can contract rapidly and anaerobically with much force, the so-called white or "twitch" muscles. Chicken breast is an excellent example.

With more sustained exercise, blood flow brings free fatty acids and oxygen to the muscle for aerobic metabolism, and ATP is produced by mitochondria. Glucose uptake and some glycogenolysis may still ensue, but the bulk of ATP is from fatty acid-derived acetyl CoA metabolized over the citric acid cycle. Again, in certain animals, muscles for long-sustained activity are rich in blood supply, myoglobin, and cytochromes, thanks to the numerous mitochondria, and thus the muscles are "red." In human beings, muscles are mixtures of these two types of fibers, again leading to a greater physical versatility as compared with lower animals.

With either brief or sustained exercise, the sympathetic nervous system plays an important role, initiating free fatty acid release from adipose tissue by augmenting generation of cyclic AMP and, in turn, triglyceride lipolysis. There is also an increase in glucagon which stimulates liver glycogenolysis to provide glucose.

FIGURE 68-8
Quantitative estimation of the flow of metabolic fuel for a period of 24 h in a subject with diabetes mellitus; the subject was losing 25 g keto acids and 100 g glucose in the urine. This glucose is in addition to that amount lost in the urine if the subject were eating and spilling the ingested carbohydrate. Thus a net negative carbohydrate balance of this degree is the causative factor which necessitates increased gluconeogenesis and the resultant ketosis. Net energy loss is 2400 kcal.

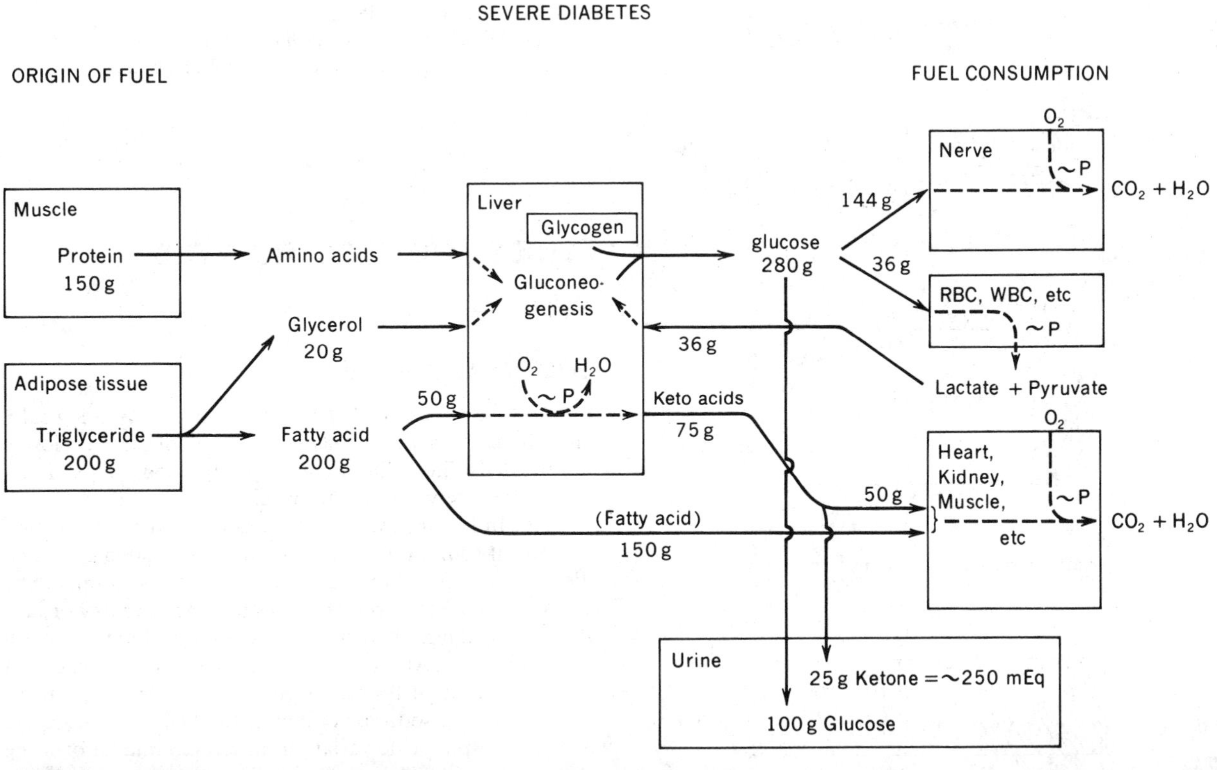

Ineffective exercise can result from a number of lesions, inadequate perfusion being obvious, and results in painful cramping such as is seen in intermittent claudication. Also, defective glycogenolysis due to hereditary muscle phosphorylase deficiency can produce similar symptoms early in brisk exercise, and can even result in muscle damage as reflected by myoglobinemia and myoglobinuria. However, if the exercise is gradually increased, oxygen and free fatty acid utilization can be accelerated, and eventually strong exercise can be done by individuals with this rare disorder in glycogen metabolism. Obviously, there is no lactate accumulation (see Chap. 111) in affected subjects. Finally, there is some evidence that the final cramping and pain of the athlete with exhaustion fatigue may be associated with utilization of the last glycogen reserves in the muscle.

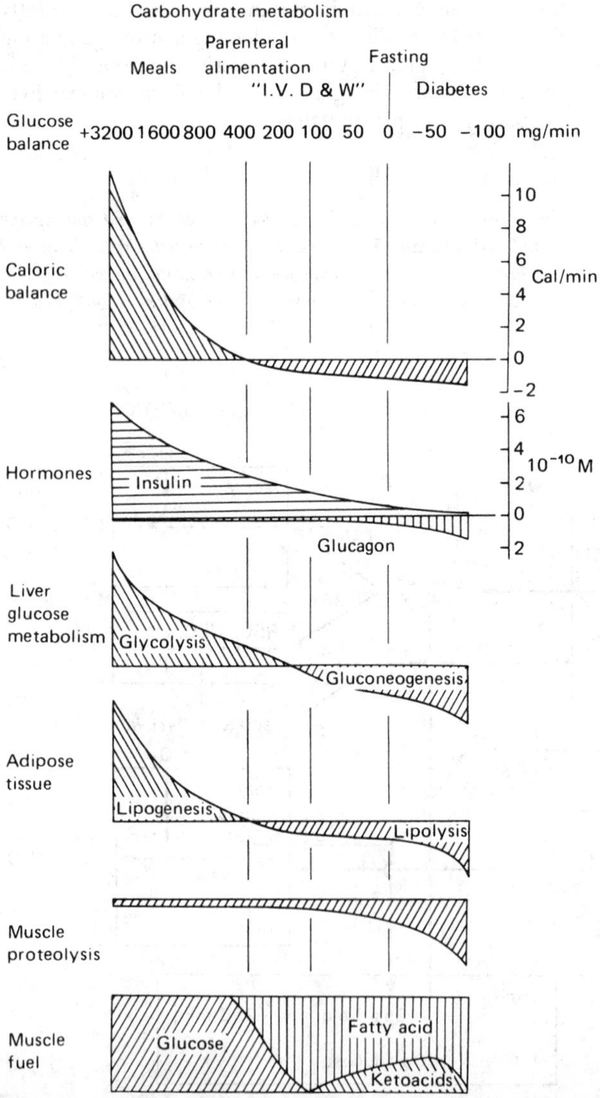

FIGURE 68-9
The spectrum of carbohydrate balance in humans, progressing from a large carbohydrate-containing meal to a net negative carbohydrate loss as occurs in uncontrolled diabetes. Also shown are the interrelations and metabolic states of certain tissues as altered by the hormonal and substrate changes. Glucose balance refers to the rate of glucose entering or leaving the body. Thus with large meals, 3,200 mg per min may be absorbed. In fasting, the net balance is 0. In diabetes, there may be a net negative balance due to glucosuria.

MUSCLE MASS As critical for muscle use as the energy supply is its mass and efficiency. These are a function of muscle cellularity and the amount of contractile protein contained therein. As stated earlier, muscle provides amino acids during fasting for glucogenic fuel, and this process is a function of low insulin levels. During feeding, the higher insulin level promotes resynthesis of the muscle protein catabolized previously. Thus total muscle nitrogen is integrated into the fuel needs of the body as a whole. But for each single muscle, its own content of contractile protein per cell is a function of its use. An unused muscle atrophies in spite of ample insulin and amino acid. This is particularly true of denervated muscle. Conversely, even in the face of overall body catabolism, a given muscle can maintain its mass, or even undergo exercise hypertrophy. The clinical extrapolation is to keep essential muscles, such as the intercostals and diaphragm, active in a debilitated individual by encouraging coughing, even with tracheal suction as a stimulus, and as much other physical exercise as tolerated. Anabolic steroids, as a means of maintaining or augmenting muscle nitrogen, are virtually ineffective as compared with the effect of exercise itself.

The spectrum of carbohydrate balance in humans is presented diagrammatically in Fig. 68-9.

REFERENCES

CAHILL GF JR: Physiology of insulin in man. Diabetes 20:799, 1971

HAVEL RJ: Caloric homeostasis and disorders of fuel transport. N Engl J Med 287:1186, 1972

LARNER J: *Intermediary Metabolism and Its Regulation,* Englewood Cliffs: Prentice-Hall, 1971

RENOLD AE et al: Diabetes mellitus, in *The Metabolic Basis of Inherited Disease,* 4th ed., eds JB Stanbury et al, New York: McGraw-Hill, in press

69
FLUIDS AND ELECTROLYTES

NORMAN G. LEVINSKY

SODIUM AND WATER

PHYSIOLOGIC CONSIDERATIONS Both physiologically and clinically, sodium and water metabolism are closely interrelated. The sodium content of the body depends on the balance between dietary intake and renal excretion of sodium. In health, extrarenal losses of sodium are negligible. Renal sodium excretion is closely regulated to match dietary content. Within 2 to 4 days after sodium intake stops, urinary excretion decreases to 5 meq per day or less. If dietary sodium is abruptly increased, sodium excretion promptly rises. About one-half of the surfeit is excreted within the first 24 h and the remainder over the next few days. Thus, the sodium content of the body remains quite constant despite wide variations in sodium intake; over the range of 0 to 400 meq per day, total body sodium varies only by about 10 percent.

Although detailed knowledge of the mechanism of this renal response is limited, certain general points deserve emphasis because of their clinical relevance. Sodium loads tend to increase glomerular filtration and to depress proximal tubular reabsorption of sodium, while sodium deficits have the opposite effects. Thus, delivery of sodium to the distal segments of the nephron tends to vary in parallel with extracellular sodium. Reabsorption in the loop of Henle and distal convolutions appears to change proportionately with the rate of sodium delivery. This modulates variations in the amount of sodium entering the collecting ducts, where final adjustments are made. Multiple regulatory factors control these tubular adjustments. Of these, only the role of of aldosterone is well established; its principal action is to stimulate sodium transport in the distal nephron. There is some evidence for a "natriuretic hormone" which inhibits sodium reabsorption, perhaps at a distal tubular site such as the collecting duct. Changes in proximal tubular reabsorption in response to altered sodium balance appear to be mediated, at least in part, by changes in hemodynamic factors in the peritubular microcirculation. Undoubtedly, other regulatory mechanisms remain to be defined. The multiplicity of control mechanisms prevents abnormalities of any single mechanism from grossly distorting the regulation of sodium excretion. For example, increased aldosterone secretion leads only to limited and transient sodium retention, because the initial accumulation of sodium stimulates opposing natriuretic factors such as increased glomerular filtration and decreased proximal tubular reabsorption.

All but 2 to 5 percent of the sodium in the body is located in the extracellular fluids. (Approximately 40 percent of total body sodium is located in bone, but this fraction does not participate significantly in most physiologic processes and will not be considered further.) Except for minor differences in concentration due to the Gibbs-Donnan effect of plasma proteins, the electrolyte compositions of plasma and interstitial fluid are essentially equal. For practical purposes, plasma composition can be considered representative of the entire extracellular compartment. Total extracellular volume approximates 20 percent of body weight. Of this, 5 percent represents plasma volume and 15 percent the volume of interstitial fluids. Thus, in a 70-kg individual with a plasma sodium concentration of 140 meq per liter, extracellular sodium content will approximate 2,000 meq. The volume of intracellular fluid is approximately twice as great as that of extracellular fluid, i.e., about 40 percent of body weight. However, since intracellular sodium concentration is less than 5 meq per liter, total intracellular sodium content is only about 100 to 150 meq. The asymmetric distribution of sodium across cell membranes is maintained by expenditure of a large fraction of the energy derived from cell metabolism, which is required constantly to pump sodium out of cells against its electrochemical gradient. All the principal electrolytes are asymmetrically distributed across cell membranes. The principal electrolytes of the extracellular fluids are sodium, chloride, and bicarbonate. The major electrolytes of the intracellular fluids are potassium, magnesium, calcium, and organic anions, including proteins.

Since sodium salts account for more than 90 percent of the total osmolality of the extracellular fluid, variations in plasma sodium concentration are almost always reflected in equivalent changes in plasma osmolality. Exceptions due to accumulation of other solutes in plasma are discussed later. Although the electrolyte compositions of intracellular and extracellular fluids differ markedly, they are always in osmotic equilibrium, since water moves rapidly across cellular membranes to dissipate osmotic gradients. Therefore, although sodium is largely confined to extracellular fluids, plasma sodium concentration is an index not only of the relative proportions of sodium and water in those fluids but also the relation between total body solute and total body water. An example is the effect of shift of sodium from extracellular to intracellular fluid without a change in total body solute. Movement of sodium into cells would not cause hyponatremia, since water would shift into cells with the sodium. On the other hand, a primary decrease in the concentration of osmotically active solute within cells would decrease total body solute; although there would be no change in total body sodium or water, hyponatremia would result from the shift of intracellular water into the extracellular compartment.

A very effective mechanism involving the hypothalamus, the neurohypophysis, and the kidney regulates plasma osmolality. Changes of 2 percent or less in plasma osmolality can be detected by osmoreceptors in the hypothalamus. Small increases in osmolality stimulate the secretion of antidiuretic hormone (ADH) from the neurohypophysis, while small decreases suppress secretion of the hormone. Normal plasma osmolality is approximately 280 to 300 mosm per kg water; the exact level is determined by the "set" of the hypothalamic osmoreceptors in a given individual. When ADH secretion is maximal, urine volume will be about 500 ml per day, and urine osmolality will be 800 to 1,400 mosm per kg. In the absence of ADH, minimal urine osmolality is 40 to 80 mosm per kg, and maximum water diuresis can reach 15 to 20 liters per day or more. The capacity of this receptor-effector system is sufficient to maintain plasma osmolality within narrow limits despite large variations in the volume and concentration of dietary fluids.

The total sodium *content* of the body is determined by renal sodium regulatory mechanisms described earlier. However, the principal determinant of plasma sodium *concentration* is water metabolism rather than total body sodium content. If excess sodium were to be ingested and retained, hypernatremia would be only transient. Water intake would increase because of thirst, and the fluid ingested would be retained because hypernatremia (hyperosmolality) would stimulate ADH secretion. Expanded extracellular volume, not hypernatremia, would be the end result. Conversely, if the osmoregulatory system is functioning normally, loss of sodium without water would not result in permanent reduction of plasma sodium concentration. The initial reduction would shut off secretion of ADH, and a water diuresis would ensue. The final outcome would be contraction of extracellular volume, while plasma sodium concentration would be restored to normal. It should be apparent that changes in total sodium content tend to cause changes in extracellular volume. In this sense, the sodium content of the extracellular fluid determines extracellular volume. On the other hand, changes in plasma sodium concentration reflect altered regulation of water excretion, not changes in total body sodium content alone. Clinically, plasma sodium concentration per se gives no information about the amount of sodium present in the body. Total body sodium content is determined by the volume of extracellular fluids as well as by the concentration of sodium in these fluids. Extracellular volume is usually the dominant factor since changes in volume tend to be greater than changes in sodium concentration. Plasma sodium concentration reflects merely the relative proportions of sodium and water (or, more exactly, of total body solute and water), not the absolute amount of sodium in the body. Either hyponatremia or hypernatremia may occur when total body sodium content is decreased, normal, or increased.

CLINICAL DISORDERS Deficits and excesses of sodium and water occur in a great variety of clinical circumstances. The manifestations of the underlying illness may overshadow the clinical features of the fluid and electrolyte disorder. Theoretically, disturbances of sodium and water metabolism can be classified into four categories, reflecting a primary excess or deficit of water or sodium. Practically, such isolated disturbances are uncommon. A primary excess of sodium leads to edema; it is not ordinarily considered as an electrolyte disorder but as a feature of underlying disease, such as congestive heart failure, hepatic cirrhosis, or nephrotic syndrome. Primary sodium deficits are nearly always accompanied by water depletion, leading to the clinical syndrome of extracellular volume depletion. Pure or disproportionate water excess leads to hyponatremia, relative or absolute water depletion to hypernatremia. A practical clinical classification of disorders of sodium and water metabolism is given in Table 69-1.

Volume depletion

Combined sodium and water deficits are far more frequent than isolated deficits of either constituent. Although the term *dehydration* is often used for combined deficits, this usage is confusing. Dehydration should be used to describe relatively pure water depletion leading to hypernatremia; *volume depletion* or some similar term should be used for combined deficits.

Pathogenesis As noted earlier, elimination of sodium from the diet will not by itself lead to sodium depletion, since urinary sodium excretion will quickly fall to very low levels. Therefore, sodium depletion is always due either to extrarenal losses or to abnormal renal losses.

GASTROINTESTINAL The most common cause of volume depletion is loss of a significant fraction of the 8 to 10 liters of gastrointestinal fluids normally secreted daily. Since the principal secretions contain potassium and hydrogen ion or bicarbonate in large amounts, volume depletion due to gastrointestinal losses is often combined with potassium depletion and acidosis or alkalosis.

Significant volume depletion may be caused by sequestration of secretions within an obstructed gastrointestinal tract or within the peritoneal cavity in peritonitis. Rapid reaccumulation of ascites after paracentesis may cause contraction of the effective circulating blood volume.

SKIN The sodium concentration of sweat varies from 5 to 50 meq per liter; sodium concentration increases with higher rates of sweating and in adrenal insufficiency. Because sweat is always a hypotonic solution, sweating leads to water deficits out of proportion to sodium losses. In burns, capillary damage may lead to sequestration of large amounts of sodium and water in the injured skin.

RENAL Abnormal losses of sodium in the urine may occur in both acute and chronic renal diseases. Early in the recovery (diuretic) phase of *acute renal failure,* urinary sodium concentration tends to be high (50 to 100 meq per liter), and substantial deficits may ensue. With rare exceptions, severe sodium wasting does not persist beyond the first few days. It is important to discriminate between increased sodium excretion which represents elimination of excess salt retained during the oliguric period and true tubular sodium wasting which depletes normal extracellular sodium. Only the latter requires replacement. Acute salt wasting due to tubular damage may also occur immediately after relief of prolonged *obstruction* of the urinary tract. Although such a postobstructive diuresis may be severe, it rarely persists for more than several days as a clinically important phenomenon.

Patients with *chronic renal failure* have limited ability to decrease sodium excretion in response to decreased intake. They will become progressively volume-depleted if their

TABLE 69-1
Disorders of sodium and water metabolism

- *I* Combined sodium and water depletion (volume depletion)
  - *A* Extrarenal losses
    - *1* Gastrointestinal (vomiting, diarrhea, gastrointestinal suction, fistulas)
    - *2* Abdominal sequestration (peritonitis, rapid reaccumulation of ascites)
    - *3* Skin (sweating, burns)
  - *B* Renal losses
    - *1* Renal disease (chronic renal failure, salt-wasting tubular disease, diuretic phase of acute renal failure)
    - *2* Osmotic diuresis (diabetic glycosuria)
    - *3* Adrenal insufficiency (Addison's disease)
- *II* Hyponatremia
  - *A* Associated with sodium and water depletion (volume depletion)
  - *B* Associated with sodium retention and edema
  - *C* Primary dilutional
  - *D* Adrenal insufficiency
  - *E* Syndrome of inappropriate secretion of antidiuretic hormone
    - *1* Spontaneous
    - *2* Drug-induced
  - *F* Essential ("sick-cell syndrome")
  - *G* Osmotic (hyperglycemia, mannitol)
  - *H* Artifactual (hyperlipemia, hyperproteinemia, laboratory error)
- *III* Hypernatremia
  - *A* Extrarenal water loss
    - *1* Skin (insensible losses, burns, sweat)
    - *2* Lungs (insensible)
  - *B* Renal water loss
    - *1* Diabetes insipidus (pituitary, nephrogenic)
    - *2* Osmotic diuresis (glycosuria, urea diuresis)
  - *C* Primary excess of sodium (excessive salt administration without access to water)
  - *D* Adrenal hyperfunction (Cushing's disease, primary hyperaldosteronism)

intake is restricted by the anorexia, nausea, and vomiting characteristic of uremia or because of their physician's instructions. Large deficits may develop insidiously over many days or weeks. A "vicious circle" may result, in that volume depletion will tend further to compromise renal function. Sodium-wasting renal disease, i.e., negative sodium balance when dietary sodium is normal, is very rare. It occurs in occasional patients with tubulointerstitial diseases of the kidney, especially medullary cystic disease.

Renal sodium wasting in the presence of normal intrinsic renal function occurs in three clinical circumstances. Perhaps the most common is sodium depletion due to continued administration of potent *diuretics* after edema has been relieved or to patients whose edema is sequestered and cannot be mobilized. For example, attempted treatment of cirrhotics with ascites may result in depletion of overall extracellular volume rather than mobilization of ascitic fluid. An obligatory *osmotic diuresis* may also cause renal sodium wasting despite normal renal function. Marked glycosuria in uncontrolled diabetes mellitus is the most frequent clinical example. Administration of osmotic diuretics such as mannitol and urea is a common iatrogenic cause. Volume depletion in patients receiving high-protein tube feedings may be due to an osmotic diuresis of urea formed by protein metabolism. Finally, renal sodium wasting despite normal intrinsic function occurs in *adrenal insufficiency* due to a deficiency of mineralocorticoids.

Clinical features and diagnosis The cause of volume depletion can usually be suspected from a history of inadequate salt and water intake together with vomiting, diarrhea, or excessive sweating; the symptoms of poorly controlled diabetes mellitus or of renal or adrenal disease may be elicited. The key findings on physical examination are those of plasma and extracellular volume depletion. Decreased skin turgor is usually present in patients with significant volume contraction. It can be estimated clinically by noting the slow rate of return of skin to its original position when it is raised between the examiner's fingers. An area of skin normally free of wrinkles and not subject to wide variations in the thickness of subcutaneous tissue, such as that over the sternum, should be selected for this maneuver. With moderate volume depletion, blood pressure is usually normal when the patient is recumbent, although resting tachycardia may be present. Postural hypotension, i.e., a drop of 5 to 10 mmHg in the sitting or standing position, is often present. With greater degrees of volume depletion, even recumbent blood pressure is reduced, and frank shock may occur. The patient with moderate or severe degrees of volume contraction is often lethargic, weak, confused, or obtunded. Such patients are usually oliguric, even when recumbent blood pressure is normal.

LABORATORY FINDINGS The hematocrit and plasma protein concentration are increased, but values within the normal range are interpretable only if prior values are known. Plasma sodium concentration may be decreased, normal, or increased, depending upon the proportion between deficits of sodium and of water. Plasma creatinine and urea nitrogen are usually increased, since the glomerular filtration rate is decreased ("prerenal azotemia"). Urinary sodium concentration may be of value in differentiating extrarenal and renal sources of sodium loss if the probable cause is not clear from the history. With extrarenal losses, urinary sodium concentration will be less than 10 meq per liter; the concentration will usually exceed 20 meq per liter if renal or adrenal disorders are at fault. However urinary sodium may ultimately fall below this level even in patients with renal salt-wasting if sodium depletion becomes very severe.

Treatment The principal clinical manifestations of extracellular volume depletion are due to reduction of plasma and interstitial fluid volume. Since there is no convenient clinical method for assessing these volumes, the effect of treatment must be determined by following the clinical response through evaluation of changes in parameters such as blood pressure, urine output, and skin turgor. Modest deficits of sodium and water can often be corrected by increased oral intake in patients not suffering from gastrointestinal disorders. Severe depletion requires therapy with intravenous solutions. Isotonic saline (0.85%) is the infusion of choice in patients whose serum sodium concentration is approximately normal. The amount to be infused can be estimated from the history of prior losses and from the severity of the physical findings of extracellular volume contraction. Patients with clinically moderate volume contraction usually require replacement with 2 to 3 liters of saline, while patients with severe depletion may require much larger volumes. The need for correction of other concurrent electrolyte abnormalities may alter the composition of the required infusion; e.g., some of the sodium may be given as bicarbonate to patients with volume contraction and metabolic acidosis, or potassium may be added in patients with concurrent potassium depletion. In estimating the total amount to be infused, allowance for ongoing losses must be included. Since the amount to be infused cannot be calculated precisely, patients should be monitored carefully to avoid fluid overload and congestive failure.

Hyponatremia

Pathophysiology Hyponatremia indicates that the body fluids are diluted by an excess of water relative to total solute. Hyponatremia is not equivalent to sodium depletion, which is only one of a number of clinical states in which it may occur (see Table 69-1). Most types of hyponatremia can be considered to result from defective urinary dilution. The normal response to dilution of body fluids is a water diuresis, which corrects the hypoosmotic state. Normal water diuresis requires three factors. (1) Secretion of ADH must be suppressed. (2) Sufficient sodium and water must reach the diluting sites of the nephron, in the ascending limb of Henle's loop and the distal convoluted tubule. (3) These nephron segments must function normally, reabsorbing sodium while remaining impermeable to water.

Three general types of mechanisms may cause defective water diuresis in patients with hyponatremia. (1) Secretion of ADH may continue "inappropriately" despite hypotonicity of extracellular fluid, which normally shuts off secretion of the hormone. (2) Insufficient sodium may reach the diluting segments to permit the formation of an adequate amount of dilute urine. Inadequate delivery of tubular fluid to distal sites may be due to reduced glomerular filtration and/or enhanced proximal tubular reabsorption. Even in the absence of ADH, distal tubular segments are not absolutely impermeable to water; small amounts of water continue to leak from the hypotonic tubular fluid into the isotonic cortical and slightly hypertonic medullary interstitial fluid. The amount of water leaking back in this manner becomes an increasingly large fraction of the volume of dilute urine formed, as the diluting process is progressively limited by decreasing delivery. Hence, urine osmolality rises progressively. In some instances, this mechanism may even result in excretion of a urine hypertonic to plasma, despite the absence of ADH. (3) Sodium transport in the diluting segments may be defective or water permeability may be excessive at these sites even in the absence of ADH. One of these three factors can account for most types of hyponatremia. However, it must be recognized that information about actual disease states is incomplete.

Paradoxically, hyponatremia in *volume depletion* and in *edematous states* appears to result from similar mechanisms. Delivery of sodium and water to the diluting segments of the nephron is reduced because of decreased glomerular filtration, increased proximal tubular reabsorption, or both. Volume-mediated secretion of ADH may also be a factor in these conditions. Contraction of plasma or extracellular volume is the stimulus to these changes in renal function and hormone secretion during salt depletion. These volumes appear to be normal or increased in most edematous patients. However, it is believed that the "effective" volume is reduced by decreased cardiac output or sequestration of fluid beyond the central circulation. Essential hyponatremia may be an additional mechanism in some edematous patients (see below).

The normal kidney can excrete 15 to 20 liters of dilute urine per day. Normal water intake, regulated by thirst and habit, is a small fraction of this maximum excretory capacity. Hence, *dilutional hyponatremia* usually occurs only when defective water diuresis or water intake unregulated by thirst is present. Oliguric patients may develop dilutional hyponatremia if the volume of oral and intravenous fluids is not limited appropriately. The ability to excrete a normal volume of dilute urine is progressively limited in advancing chronic renal failure. Hyponatremia may be precipitated in patients with advanced renal failure by instructions to force fluids. In the postoperative state, water diuresis is limited by a number of factors, such as secretion of ADH induced by pain or narcotics and extracellular volume contraction. The administration of excessive volumes of hypotonic solutions to such patients is a common cause of hyponatremia. Very rarely, psychogenic polydipsia may be so severe that the rapid ingestion of huge quantities of fluids may overwhelm normal excretory capacity and produce symptomatic dilutional hyponatremia despite normal renal diluting mechanisms.

Multiple factors appear to play a role in limiting water diuresis in patients with *adrenal insufficiency.* Deficient secretion of mineralocorticoid hormones may lead to sodium depletion, with consequent reduction of glomerular filtration and enhancement of proximal tubular sodium reabsorption. Moreover, glucocorticoid deficiency directly reduces filtration. Therefore, adrenal insufficiency will tend to decrease delivery of sodium to diluting sites. In addition, glucocorticoid deficiency directly or indirectly prevents the maintenance of normal water impermeability in distal diluting segments of the nephron. Some evidence suggests a direct effect of glucocorticoid deficiency on water permeability of distal tubular epithelium, but conflicting data indicate that inappropriate secretion of ADH may occur when glucocorticoids are deficient.

Hyponatremia in patients with chronic *inappropriate secretion* of *antidiuretic hormone* is principally due to water retention, but continued urinary losses of sodium also contribute to producing a mild negative sodium balance. Renal sodium wasting is related to volume expansion, since it can be eliminated by restricting fluid intake. The mechanisms by which extracellular expansion may increase sodium excretion have been discussed above.

A limited number of observations suggest that some patients may be hyponatremic in the absence of a defect in water diuresis. The terms "essential hyponatremia" and "sick-cell syndrome" have been applied to this category. Osmoreceptor cells in the hypothalamus are thought to be "reset" to maintain a decreased level of body fluid osmolality as though it were normal. The genesis of such a syndrome is speculative; it has been suggested that changes in cellular metabolism might lead to a primary reduction in cellular osmolality. Such a reduction in intracellular solute would result in a shift of water out of cells, thereby diluting extracellular fluids and initiating hyponatremia. Once the osmoreceptor was "reset," water and sodium metabolism would behave normally. Urine would become dilute or concentrated if plasma sodium fell or increased slightly from the new "normal" level for that patient.

Hyponatremia due to *accumulation* of *osmotically active solutes* in the plasma is the sole exception to the rule that hyponatremia means decreased plasma osmolality. In this type of hyponatremia, plasma osmolality is increased. Plasma sodium is diluted by movement of water out of cells along the osmotic gradient created by addition to the plasma of the abnormal solute, such as glucose or mannitol. It should be noted that solutes which equilibrate across cell membranes do not induce movement of water from cells. Thus, high plasma urea levels in patients with renal failure do not cause hyponatremia.

Clinical features and diagnosis In *sodium* (volume) *depletion,* hyponatremia per se is usually of little clinical significance. The major features are those of extracellular volume contraction, described above. Reduction of plasma sodium concentration by more than 10 to 15 meq per liter is rare in the absence of obvious decreases in skin turgor, postural or recumbent hypotension, and some degree of azotemia.

In *edematous states* such as congestive heart failure, cirrhosis, and the nephrotic syndrome, the severity and frequency of hyponatremia correlates to some extent with the magnitude of the edema and the seriousness of the underlying condition. Hyponatremia is usually present in patients with advanced disease unless water intake is restricted. The hyponatremia itself is often of little clinical significance. The principal features are those of the underlying disease. However, symptomatic hyponatremia may occur, most often in connection with vigorous diuretic therapy or excessive oral or parenteral intake of dilute fluids.

The diagnosis of *primary dilutional hyponatremia* is usually evident from the history. This diagnosis should be considered in postoperative patients and in patients with acute or chronic renal failure. Since extracellular fluid volume is expanded by water retention, blood pressure and skin turgor are normal. Plasma creatinine and urea are normal unless preexisting renal disease is present.

The *syndrome* of *chronic inappropriate secretion* of *antidiuretic hormone* (SIADH) is defined by a unique group of clinical features. (1) Urine osmolality is not maximally dilute even when marked hyponatremia is induced by water loading. In most cases, urine osmolality exceeds plasma osmolality. (The elaboration of hypertonic urine is presumptive evidence of ADH secretion if the glomerular filtration rate is normal.) (2) Plasma creatinine and urea are normal or low, indicating that the glomerular filtration rate is normal or increased. (3) During fluid loading, hyponatremia increases due to water retention and urinary sodium wasting. During restriction of fluid intake, hyponatremia and urinary sodium wasting are corrected. It should be noted that sodium wasting during volume expansion may be minimal or even absent in patients with extreme degrees of hyponatremia. In clinical testing to demonstrate these features, patients with symptomatic hyponatremia or plasma sodium concentrations below 125 meq per liter should first have their fluid intake restricted to 800 to 1,000 ml per day or less. Infusion of small volumes of hypertonic saline may be appropriate in symptomatic patients. During restriction of fluid intake, hyponatremia should disappear promptly, and urinary sodium excretion should not exceed intake. Thereafter, plasma and urinary parameters should be evaluated during daily administration of 2 to 3 liters of fluids by mouth or intravenously. Urine osmolality will always exceed 100 mosm per liter (urine specific gravity greater than 1.003); in the great majority of instances, it will exceed plasma osmolality, despite progressive dilution of body fluids. Urinary sodium excretion will usually exceed sodium intake during this phase of fluid loading. Two to three days of this regimen are ordinarily sufficient to demonstrate the requisite clinical pattern for SIADH without inducing symptomatic hyponatremia.

SIADH has been found frequently in patients with oat-cell carcinoma of the lung but has also been described in patients with a variety of other neoplasms. In some of these patients there is evidence that the tumor is secreting ADH or a substance with analogous biological activity (see also Chap. 91). The syndrome has also been reported in patients with disorders of the central nervous system, including meningitis and encephalitis. It is assumed that ADH in these patients is secreted in response to direct stimulation of the hypothalamic osmoreceptors. SIADH has also been noted in a number of apparently unrelated disorders such as acute porphyria and hypothyroidism. The stimulus to ADH in these patients is unknown.

An ever-increasing list of pharmacological agents has been reported to induce SIADH. The list includes: (1) the oral hypoglycemic agents, chlorpropamide and tolbutamide; (2) antineoplastic and immunosuppressive agents, vincristine and cyclophosphamide; (3) psychoactive drugs, carbamazepine (Tegretol) and amitriptyline (Elavil). These agents exert their antidiuretic effects either by potentiating the tubular action of small amounts of ADH or by stimulating inappropriate secretion of ADH. In addition, diuretics such as thiazides may induce a syndrome indistinguishable from SIADH, probably by a direct renal action to limit water excretion in patients ingesting moderate to large amounts of dilute fluids.

Since patients with *adrenal insufficiency* may have the combination of defective dilution of the urine and sodium wasting, hyponatremia due to Addison's disease can occasionally be confused with SIADH. Usually, other clinical features of adrenal insufficiency such as hyperkalemia, pigmentation, and hypoglycemia will suggest the correct diagnosis. However, specific tests of adrenal cortical function are indicated whenever the diagnosis is in doubt.

Essential hyponatremia (sick-cell syndrome) may occur in a variety of chronic illnesses, such as pulmonary tuberculosis, congestive heart failure, and hepatic cirrhosis. This type of hyponatremia is asymptomatic; skin turgor, blood pressure, and renal function are normal, unless altered by the primary disease. Definitive diagnosis of essential hyponatremia requires the demonstration of normal urinary dilution in response to water loading, normal urinary concentration during dehydration, and normal renal sodium excretory responses to sodium loading and restriction.

The diagnosis of hyponatremia due to *increased plasma concentrations* of *osmotically active solute* is usually apparent from the history and clinical features of uncontrolled diabetes. Plasma sodium concentration will decrease by about 1.6 meq per liter with every elevation of 100 mg per 100 ml in plasma glucose above normal. This type of hyponatremia should also be considered whenever there is a history of recent administration of mannitol, especially to oliguric patients unable to excrete it promptly. Since plasma osmolality is increased, clinical manifestations of hypotonicity are absent in this type of hyponatremia.

In patients with severe hyperlipemia or, very rarely, with extreme hyperproteinemia, hyponatremia which is clinically *artifactual* may be reported by the laboratory. In severe hyperlipemia part of any unit volume of plasma taken for analysis will be lipid, which is sodium-free. This type of hyponatremia is rarely reported unless the plasma is grossly milky. In patients with extreme hyperproteinemia, proteins occupy more than the normal 7 percent of plasma volume, thereby reducing the proportion of aqueous sodium-containing fluid per unit of plasma taken for analysis. In both cases, hyponatremia will be reported by the laboratory because the sodium concentration will be low in milliequivalents per liter of plasma. However, sodium concentration per liter of plasma water and plasma osmolality are normal; hence, this type of hyponatremia has no clinical significance.

DIFFERENTIAL DIAGNOSIS Although the type of hyponatremia can be defined without difficulty in many patients, differentiation among categories may be very difficult. More than one type of hyponatremia may occur in a specific disease entity. For example, hyponatremia in patients with hepatic cirrhosis is usually associated with edema or is due to excessive administration of diuretics, but essential hyponatremia may also occur in this condition. Moreover, current categories may prove artificial or inaccurate when the pathophysiology of hyponatremia is more completely understood and specific diagnostic tests such as a sensitive assay for ADH are readily available. Despite these limitations, the classification outlined above is a useful framework for diagnosis and treatment.

The history is often the most important factor in differential diagnosis. For example, prolonged vomiting, diarrhea, or nasogastric suction will suggest volume depletion. Primary dilutional hyponatremia or hypernatremia associated with sodium losses should be suspected in the postoperative period. Critical information to be derived from the physical examination includes the presence or absence of edema, signs of volume depletion, and evidence of disordered cerebral function. Initial laboratory studies of value include the plasma creatinine and urinary osmolality (specific gravity) and sodium concentration. The combination of high urine specific gravity (above 1.005), increased urinary sodium concentration, and normal or low plasma urea or creatinine in a hyponatremic patient without clinical evidence of volume depletion suggests the diagnosis of SIADH. A maximally dilute urine in a hyponatremic patient suggests psychogenic polydipsia or essential hyponatremia.

CLINICAL MANIFESTATIONS Neurologic dysfunction is the principal clinical feature of hyponatremia. The severity of symptoms is related to the degree of hyponatremia and the rapidity with which it develops. Patients may be lethargic, confused, stuporous, or comatose. If hyponatremia develops rapidly, signs of hyperexcitability such as muscular twitches, irritability, and convulsions may occur. These are believed due to intracellular movement of water, leading to swelling of brain cells. Hyponatremia rarely causes clinical symptoms when plasma sodium is above 125 meq per liter, although symptoms may occur occasionally at higher levels if the decrease in concentration has been rapid.

Treatment Hyponatremia itself is often of little clinical significance and requires no specific treatment. When hyponatremia is associated with volume depletion, treatment is directed to correction of the volume deficits. In the occasional patient with sodium depletion whose plasma sodium concentration is less than 125 meq per liter, some of the intravenous sodium replacement fluids should be administered as hypertonic saline. Hyponatremia associated with edema responds to effective treatment of the underlying disease. Moderate, nonprogressive hyponatremia in edematous patients usually does not cause symptoms. Attempts to correct such hyponatremia by restriction of fluid intake induce thirst and discomfort without improving the clinical picture or longevity. Patients with severe or progressive hyponatremia may require some restriction of water intake, especially during vigorous treatment with diuretics. However, moderate limitations to the range of 1,000 to 1,500 ml per day will often suffice to avoid symptoms or progressive hyponatremia. More severe restriction should be instituted only if specific clinical or laboratory observations warrant. Since edematous subjects have excess total extracellular sodium, hypertonic saline solution should not be administered, except in rare instances in which clinical manifestations of extreme hyponatremia, such as coma or convulsions, justify emergency measures. Dilutional hyponatremia is treated by water restriction. Only if severe symptoms occur is hypertonic saline infusion required. Hyponatremia due to SIADH responds to limitation of fluid intake; restriction to the range of 1,000 to 1,200 ml per day is ordinarily adequate. Occasional patients with marked hyponatremia due to this syndrome may be symptomatic and require initial therapy with hypertonic saline infusions.

When severe hyponatremia of any type is to be treated intravenously, 5% sodium chloride is the infusion of choice. The amount of sodium to be given should be calculated by multiplying the deficit in plasma sodium concentration (milliequivalents per liter) by total body water (approximately 50 to 60 percent of body weight). Although the administered sodium will remain in the extracellular compartment, the osmotic effect of the hypertonic saline will cause water to shift out of cells. The amount needed to raise plasma sodium concentration to the range of 125 to 130 meq per liter should be calculated and infused over several hours. The patient's symptoms and clinical status, especially with respect to circulatory congestion, should be carefully assessed throughout the infusion. Complete correction of hyponatremia, if clinically indicated, is usually best carried out more slowly, by water restriction or oral sodium supplementation if possible.

Hypernatremia

Pathophysiology Hypernatremia is due to a deficit of body water relative to total body solute or sodium content. Without exception, hypernatremia indicates that the body fluids are hypertonic. Since hypertonicity normally stimulates thirst, severe persistent hypernatremia occurs only in patients who cannot respond to thirst by voluntary ingestion of fluid, e.g., infants or mentally obtunded patients. In such individuals, loss of dilute body fluids will progressively elevate body fluid osmolality. Initial losses of water are from the extracellular compartment, but water deficits are rapidly equilibrated throughout total body water. The rise in extracellular fluid tonicity causes intracellular water to shift into the extracellular compartment. In effect, approximately two-thirds of pure water deficits are derived from intracellular fluid. Hence, the clinical findings of extracellular volume depletion occur in patients with relatively pure deficits of water only when such deficits are very large. The principal clinical features are attributable to decreased intracellular volume, especially dehydration of cells in the central nervous system. Brain cells appear to adapt to chronic hyperosmolality by accumulating increased intracellular solute. When hyperosmolality is rapidly corrected, the increase in total intracellular solute may promote brain swelling even at normal or slightly elevated plasma osmolality. These mechanisms may account for the clinical observation that rapid correction of hypertonicity sometimes causes deterioration of central nervous function. The identity of the excess brain solute is uncertain; experimental data suggest that potassium accumulation may account for part of the excess in chronic hypernatremia.

Minimal persistent hypernatremia may be seen in some patients with Cushing's disease and hyperaldosteronism. Presumably stimulation of renal tubular reabsorption by adrenal steroids initiates the hypernatremia. It is not known why the thirst mechanism fails to maintain normal body fluid osmolality.

Pathogenesis The principal causes of hypernatremia are listed in Table 69-1. The most frequent is unreplaced loss of hypotonic fluid from the skin and lungs. Insensible losses of water from these sources may reach several liters per day, especially in patients with fever or increased respirations. Since sweat is hypotonic fluid, hypernatremia will develop if sweating patients are unable to drink. Major losses of insensible water may occur in patients with extensive burns. Renal losses may lead to hypernatremia in two clinical circumstances, diabetes insipidus and solute diuresis. Alert patients with diabetes insipidus ordinarily maintain normal or only slightly hypertonic body fluids despite massive renal water wasting by increasing fluid intake appropriately. However, diabetes insipidus may develop acutely in patients who suffer cerebral trauma or undergo neurosurgical procedures. In such patients, careful attention to replacement of urinary losses is mandatory to avoid severe hypernatremia. In an osmotic diuresis, urinary sodium concentration is less than plasma concentration; therefore, hypernatremia tends to occur. Hypernatremia due to a urea diuresis may develop when patients unable to complain of thirst are placed on a high-protein tube feeding. Examples include patients with severe cerebrovascular accidents who are unable to swallow and postoperative neurosurgical patients. In the syndrome of hyperosmolar nonketotic diabetic coma, severe hyperosmolality of the body fluids is due to a combination of hyperglycemia and relative or absolute hypernatremia. The hypernatremia is a consequence of an intense glucose osmotic diuresis in patients who are unable to ingest fluids. Since hyperglycemia itself causes hyponatremia by inducing a shift of water from cells, the presence of hypernatremia in the face of extreme hyperglycemia indicates that total body water is severely depleted. Hypernatremia due to an osmotic diuresis is usually accompanied by significant extracellular volume depletion, since both sodium and water are lost.

In rare instances, hypernatremia may result from an absolute excess of sodium rather than from water depletion. Examples are hypernatremia caused by accidental substitution of salt for sugar in infant feeding formulas and administration of excessive amounts of hypertonic saline to comatose adults.

Clinical features and diagnosis The principal clinical manifestations of hypernatremia are observed in the central nervous system. Confusion, obtundation, stupor, or coma may develop, depending on the severity of the hyperosmolality. These symptoms appear to be due to dehydration of brain cells; the clinical features are similar whether hyperosmolality is due to hypernatremia or extreme hyperglycemia. In patients with pure water deficits, manifestations of extracellular volume depletion are minimal because only one-third of the deficit is derived from extracellular fluid. As already noted, combined deficits are common, especially in patients who are undergoing an osmotic diuresis; in such individuals, the signs and symptoms of volume depletion may overshadow those due to hypernatremia.

Treatment Water by mouth or intravenous administration of a dilute solution (5% dextrose or 0.45% saline) is the treatment of hypernatremia. Calculation of water requirements must be based on total body water, since water deficits are drawn from both intracellular and extracellular fluid and both must be repleted. Hypernatremia should be corrected slowly; no more than half the water deficit should be replaced in the first few hours. Excessively rapid correction of hypernatremia may cause clinical deterioration of central nervous function.

POTASSIUM

PHYSIOLOGIC CONSIDERATIONS Potassium is the principal intracellular cation. Active transport maintains a cellular concentration of approximately 160 meq per liter, forty times that in extracellular fluid. All but 2 percent of the 2,500 to 3,000 meq of potassium in the body is within cells. Since potassium is a large fraction of total cellular solute, it is a major determinant of the volume of the cell and the osmolality of the body fluids. Moreover, potassium is an important cofactor in a number of metabolic processes. Extracellular potassium, while a small fraction of the total, greatly influences neuromuscular function. The ratio of intracellular to extracellular potassium concentration is the principal determinant of membrane potential in excitable tissues. Since extracellular potassium concentration is low, small deviations in absolute concentration will produce large variations in this ratio; conversely, only large changes in intracellular potassium will influence the ratio significantly. These relationships have practical consequences. For example, toxic effects of hyperkalemia can be mitigated by inducing movement of potassium from extracellular fluid to cells.

The relation between plasma and cellular potassium is complex and influenced by a number of factors, prominent among them being acid-base balance. Acidosis tends to shift potassium out of cells, and alkalosis favors movement of potassium from extracellular fluid into cells. Thus, a patient with normal total body potassium will tend to be hyperkalemic if acidotic and hypokalemic if alkalotic. During potassium depletion, plasma potassium initially decreases about 1 meq per liter for each 100 to 200 meq lost. However, plasma potassium falls much more slowly after it reaches 2 meq per liter. Thus, a plasma potassium in the range of 2 to 3.5 meq per liter is a reasonably accurate guide to the magnitude of depletion, but plasma potassium concentrations less than 2 meq per liter may reflect a wide range of deficits, from moderate to very severe. Plasma concentration increases about 1 meq per liter after acute administration of 100 to 200 meq potassium. Assuming an extracellular volume of 15 liters, 150 meq would be expected to raise plasma potassium by about 10 meq per liter. Thus, it is evident that the largest fraction of administered potassium rapidly enters cells. Renal excretion also increases promptly. Chronic exposure to high potassium diets enhances both tissue uptake and renal excretion of the ion; the mechanism of these adaptations is uncertain. Sustained hyperkalemia rarely is caused by excess intake, because these mechanisms normally function so efficiently. Impaired renal excretion or cellular transfer are the usual causes of hyperkalemia.

Of the usual potassium intake of 50 to 150 meq per day, all but a few milliequivalents are excreted in the urine. Normally, stool and sweat contain only about 5 meq per day. As already noted, the kidneys respond to acute and chronic changes in potassium intake by corresponding changes in excretion. Excess potassium is excreted promptly; about half of an acute load appears in the urine within 12 h. The renal response to potassium depletion is more sluggish. Excretion does not fall to minimal levels for 7 to 14 days. During this period, a deficit of 200 meq or more may develop in an individual on a potassium-deficient diet. Renal excretory mechanisms for potassium are complex. Potassium in the urine is secreted in the distal convoluted tubule and collecting duct; filtered potassium is nearly quantitatively reabsorbed in more proximal segments. Potassium secretion appears to be determined by the potassium concentration of tubular cells and by an electrochemical gradient favoring diffusion of the ion into tubular fluid. Net excretion is the resultant of secretion and concurrent reabsorption in the distal segments. Among the key influences on this complex system are aldosterone, sodium reabsorption, and acid-base balance. Aldosterone stimulates potassium secretion. Thus, hyperkalemia increases potassium excretion by two mechanisms: it stimulates adrenal secretion of aldosterone, and it directly enhances renal secretion, presumably via increased tubular cell potassium. Sodium reabsorption in the distal tubule creates the electrical gradient which favors potassium secretion. Hence, increased distal sodium reabsorption will favor potassium excretion. For example, administration of diuretics which bring more sodium distally will increase potassium excretion, especially in patients with edema and secondary aldosteronism. Conversely, a low sodium diet decreases potassium excretion even in patients with primary aldosteronism; distal secretion is limited and reabsorption of potassium in collecting ducts is stimulated. Alkalosis enhances and acidosis depresses renal potassium secretion, probably by inducing corresponding changes in cell potassium.

POTASSIUM DEPLETION AND HYPOKALEMIA Pathogenesis The principal causes of potassium depletion are listed in Table 69-2. As noted earlier, renal excretion of potassium falls slowly in persons on potassium-deficient diets. During the 10 to 14 days before balance is achieved, significant deficits may occur. Thus, in contrast to sodium, moderate potassium depletion may result from *poor intake* alone. The most frequent cause of potassium deficiency is *gastrointestinal loss.* The potassium concentration of gastric fluid is approximately 5 to 10 meq per liter; significant deficits may result from direct losses of potassium in *vomitus.* The concomitant alkalosis maintains urinary potassium excretion at levels inappropriately high for the degree of potassium depletion. *Diarrhea* may also lead to large potassium deficits, since the potassium concentration of liquid stool is 40 to 60 meq per liter.

The most frequent *renal* cause of potassium depletion is probably administration of *diuretics* without adequate dietary potassium supplementation. All diuretics in common use except spironolactone, triamterene, and amiloride promote potassium excretion, especially in edematous patients with secondary aldosteronism. Potassium excretion is increased during an *osmotic diuresis.* In patients with diabetic ketoacidosis, potassium depletion due to glycosuria may be masked by the shift of potassium out of tissues caused by acidosis. Failure to recognize potassium depletion may lead to serious cardiotoxicity from sudden hypokalemia when the acidosis is corrected with insulin or alkali. A normal plasma potassium concentration in an acidotic patient strongly suggests potassium depletion.

Urinary potassium loss is often due to *excessive mineralocorticoid activity.* Hypokalemia is characteristic of *primary aldosteronism,* but may be minimal in patients with restricted sodium intake. *Secondary aldosteronism* causes renal potassium-wasting and hypokalemia in malignant hypertension and in patients with renin-secreting renal tumors. *Bartter's syndrome* is characterized by hypersecretion of renin, secondary aldosteronism, hypokalemia, and alkalosis. Blood pressure is normal. Edema is absent; indeed, there is a tendency toward salt wasting and hyponatremia. Juxtaglomerular cell hyperplasia is a prominent feature. The stimulus to hyperplasia is unknown; hypotheses include resistance to angiotensin in blood vessels and subclinical volume depletion due to renal tubular sodium wasting. The syndrome is most frequent in children and adolescents. *Licorice* contains a compound with mineralocorticoid activity; patients who consume huge amounts may become hypokalemic. Excessive levels of *glucocorticoids* stimulate secretion of renal potassium (and hydrogen), leading to hypokalemia and alkalosis in patients with *Cushing's syndrome* and those receiving *therapeutic steroids.*

Renal tubular potassium wasting is a feature of *renal tubular acidosis.* Some patients with monocytic or myelomonocytic *leukemia* have developed hypokalemia. Renal potassium wasting in these patients appears to correlate with lysozymuria, and it has been suggested that the enzyme may interfere with tubular function. In *Liddle's syn-*

TABLE 69-2
Causes of potassium depletion and hypokalemia

I Gastrointestinal
- *A* Deficient dietary intake
- *B* Gastrointestinal losses (vomiting, diarrhea, villous adenoma, fistulas, ureterosigmoidostomy)

II Renal
- *A* Diuretics
- *B* Osmotic diuresis (glycosuria)
- *C* Excessive mineralocorticoid effects
  - *1* Primary aldosteronism
  - *2* Secondary aldosteronism (including malignant hypertension, Bartter's syndrome, juxtaglomerular cell tumor)
  - *3* Licorice ingestion
  - *4* Glucocorticoid excess (Cushing's syndrome, exogenous steroids, ectopic ACTH production)
- *D* Renal tubular diseases
  - *1* Renal tubular acidosis
  - *2* Leukemia with lysozymuria
  - *3* Liddle's syndrome

III Hypokalemia due to shift into cells (no depletion)
- *A* Hypokalemic periodic paralysis
- *B* Insulin effect

drome, a rare familial disorder, renal potassium wasting is an intrinsic tubular abnormality.

Clinical features and diagnosis The most prominent features of hypokalemia and potassium depletion are neuromuscular. Moderate degrees of depletion may be asymptomatic, especially if they develop slowly. Some patients, however, may complain of muscle weakness. With more severe or acute degrees of hypokalemia and potassium deficiency, marked and generalized weakness of skeletal muscles is prominent. Very severe or abrupt development of hypokalemia may lead to virtually total paralysis, including the respiratory muscles. Rhabdomyolysis may occur in patients with potassium depletion. On physical examination, in addition to decreased motor power, the patient may demonstrate decreased or absent tendon reflexes.

Abnormalities in the electrocardiogram are common in patients with hypokalemia and potassium depletion. The characteristic changes include flattening and inversion of the T wave, increased prominence of the U wave, and sagging of the S-T segment. These alterations are not well correlated with the severity of the disturbance in potassium metabolism and cannot be relied on as indexes of the clinical significance of a potassium deficit. Although moderate potassium depletion rarely affects cardiac action, severe or rapid reduction in serum potassium may cause cardiac arrest. Potassium deficiency enhances the cardiac toxicity of digitalis preparations.

Renal tubular function is markedly impaired by potassium depletion. The most prominent abnormality is decreased concentrating ability, which may cause polyuria and polydipsia. Glomerular filtration rate is normal or only slightly reduced; moderate reductions may occur in occasional patients with chronic potassium-depletion nephropathy. Renal regulation of potassium excretion remains normal. The urinalysis is benign: protein excretion is normal or minimally increased, and the urinary sediment is normal or demonstrates only a slight increase in hyaline or granular casts.

DIAGNOSIS The cause of hypokalemia and potassium depletion is usually evident from the history. However, patients whose potassium deficiency is caused by chronic abuse of laxatives or psychogenic, self-induced vomiting will rarely volunteer an accurate history. Patients with villous adenomas of the rectum sometimes report that their feces are formed; careful questioning will reveal the elimination of the characteristic mucous secretion of the tumor.

When the history is obscure, evaluation of urinary potassium excretion may be helpful in determining the origin of the potassium deficit. If gastrointestinal losses have occurred, urinary excretion will usually be less than 20 to 25 meq per liter. Although renal conservation of potassium is slow, excretion will have fallen to these levels by the time that clinically significant deficits of potassium have accumulated. On the other hand, when renal potassium wasting is the cause, urinary concentration will usually exceed 20 meq per liter. However, lower concentrations may be found in severely depleted patients, in those with excessive mineralocorticoid activity while on low sodium intake, and in patients where diuretics have been stopped at the time of examination.

Treatment When possible, potassium depletion should be corrected by increased dietary intake or supplementation with potassium salts. Potassium chloride is the salt of choice, especially in alkalotic patients. Enteric-coated potassium chloride tablets have been responsible for ulceration of the small bowel, due to release of high concentrations of potassium salts. Organic salts such as gluconate or citrate are adequate in patients who are not severely alkalotic.

Intravenous treatment is required for patients with gastrointestinal disorders or when the potassium deficiency is severe. It must be emphasized that the potassium *concentration* in commonly available intravenous solutions of potassium chloride is 2,000 meq per liter. Concentrations in intravenous infusions should not exceed 40 or at the most 60 meq per liter. The rate of infusion should not exceed 20 meq per h or approximately 200 to 250 meq per day, unless the need for more rapid infusion has been demonstrated in the individual patient by evidence of continuing losses large enough to justify more intensive therapy. The results of treatment are best monitored by repeated determinations of plasma potassium and evaluation of clinical symptoms such as muscular weakness or paralysis. Disappearance of electrocardiographic abnormalities correlates only roughly with improvement in total body potassium content. However, during rapid intravenous administration of potassium, the electrocardiogram should be monitored to avoid cardiac toxicity from inadvertent hyperkalemia.

Hypokalemia and hypocalcemia may occur together, for example, in patients with malabsorption syndrome. The neuromuscular effect of each electrolyte abnormality is masked by the other. Treatment of either disorder alone may precipitate symptoms. Thus, treatment of hypokalemia alone may precipitate tetany, and conversely, treatment of hypocalcemia without correcting the hypokalemia may exacerbate the manifestations of potassium deficiency.

HYPERKALEMIA Pathogenesis The causes of hyperkalemia are shown in Table 69-3. *Inadequate renal excretion* is the most frequent cause. When oliguria or anuria is present, as in acute renal failure, progressive hyperkalemia is the rule. Plasma potassium will rise by about 0.5 meq/liter/day if there are no abnormal loads. Chronic renal failure does not cause severe or progressive hyperkalemia unless oliguria supervenes. Adaptive changes of unknown etiology increase potassium excretion per residual nephron as chronic renal failure progresses. However, patients with chronic renal failure are functioning at the limits of their excretory capacity. Hence, hyperkalemia may develop rapidly if the potassium load is increased or excretory capacity is limited, e.g., by administration of spironolactone.

Hyperkalemia is a cardinal feature of *adrenal insufficiency* (Addison's disease) and of selective *hypoaldosteronism.* In the latter condition, cardiac toxicity (heart block) due to hyperkalemia is the principal clinical manifestation.

A kilogram of tissue such as muscle or erythrocytes contains about 80 meq potassium, and damaged cells release potassium into the plasma. Hence hyperkalemia may be seen when there is *muscle-crushing injury, hemolysis,* or *in-*

TABLE 69-3
Causes of hyperkalemia

I Inadequate excretion
- *A* Renal failure
  - *1* Acute renal failure
  - *2* Severe chronic renal failure (especially with marked acidosis or oliguria)
- *B* Adrenal insufficiency
  - *1* Hypoaldosteronism
  - *2* Addison's disease
- *C* Diuretics which inhibit potassium secretion (spironolactone, triamterene, amiloride)

II Shift of potassium from tissues
- *A* Tissue damage (muscle crush, hemolysis, internal bleeding)
- *B* Drugs: succinylcholine, digitalis poisoning
- *C* Acidosis
- *D* Hyperkalemic periodic paralysis

III Excessive intake

IV Pseudohyperkalemia
- *A* Thrombocytosis
- *B* Leukocytosis
- *C* Poor venipuncture technique
- *D* In vitro hemolysis

ternal hemorrhage. Acidosis drives potassium out of cells and leads to hyperkalemia. Severe progressive hyperkalemia is not ordinarily a consequence of increased release of potassium from damaged or acidotic tissues alone. However, acidosis and tissue damage often occur together with acute renal insufficiency; under these circumstances, severe hyperkalemia may develop quickly. In contrast to the increase of 0.5 meq per liter per day typical of uncomplicated anuria, plasma potassium in anuric patients with tissue damage may increase 2 to 4 meq per liter per day. Such rapidly progressive hyperkalemia may be an important cause of death in military casualties. In patients with trauma, burns, or neuromuscular diseases such as paraplegia and multiple sclerosis, the muscle relaxant *succinylcholine* may cause dangerous hyperkalemia. This agent apparently releases potassium from muscle by depolarizing cell membranes. In *hyperkalemic periodic paralysis,* the hyperkalemia is associated with repeated attacks of muscular paralysis. The mechanism of this syndrome is not understood. Ingestion of increased amounts of potassium may precipitate attacks.

Patients with extreme thrombocytosis or, more rarely, extreme leukocytosis in leukemia may demonstrate the phenomenon of pseudohyperkalemia. Platelets or white blood cells release potassium during blood clotting in vitro. While serum potassium may be grossly abnormal, plasma potassium is not increased. Artifactual elevation of plasma potassium may occur if blood is drawn after repeated fist clenching to make veins more prominent during application of a tourniquet. Artifactual hyperkalemia may be suspected when electrocardiographic abnormalities are absent despite apparently marked elevation of serum potassium.

Clinical features and diagnosis The most important toxic effects of hyperkalemia are cardiac arrhythmias. The characteristic sequence of electrocardiographic changes is shown in Fig. 69-1. The earliest manifestation is the development of high peaked T waves, especially prominent in precordial leads. Hyperkalemia does not prolong the QT interval, unlike other disorders which induce peaking of

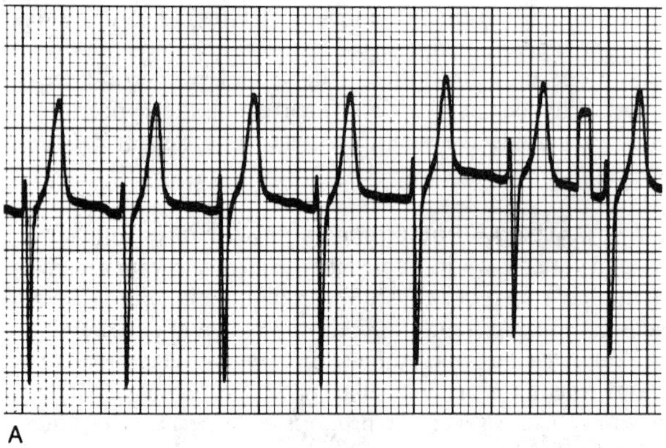

A

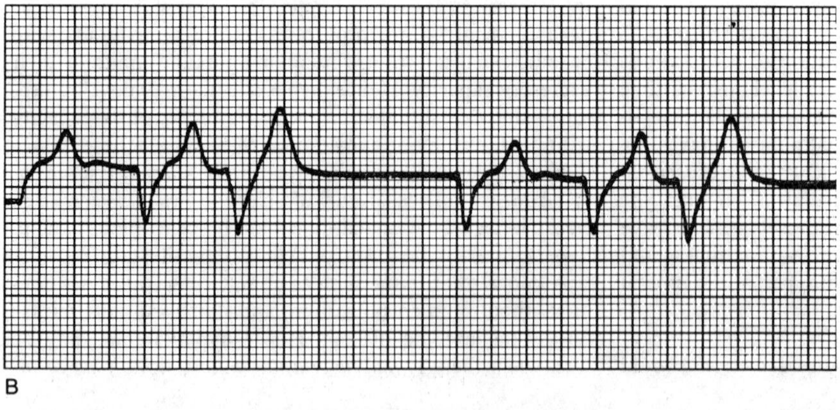

B

FIGURE 69-1
Electrocardiographic changes in hyperkalemia. A *Early toxicity in a patient with plasma potassium of 6.8 meq per liter. Note symmetrical peaking of T waves.* B *Advanced toxicity in a patient with plasma potassium of 8.6 meq per liter. QRS complexes are abnormally widened, P waves have disappeared, and ventricular rhythm is irregular. (From NG Levinsky, Potassium in clinical medicine. Clinician 1973)*

the T waves. Later changes include prolongation of the P-R interval, complete heart block, and atrial asystole. As plasma potassium rises further, ventricular complexes may deteriorate. The QRS becomes progressively prolonged and finally tends to merge with the T wave in a sine wave configuration. Terminally, ventricular fibrillation and standstill may occur.

Occasionally moderate or severe hyperkalemia may have striking effects on peripheral muscles. Ascending muscular weakness can occur, progressing to flaccid quadriplegia and respiratory paralysis. Cerebral and cranial nerve function are normal, as is sensation.

Treatment In considering appropriate therapy, it is helpful to classify hyperkalemia according to degrees of severity. The seriousness of hyperkalemia is best estimated by considering both the plasma potassium and the electrocardiogram. When the plasma potassium is less than 6.5 meq per liter and electrocardiographic changes are limited to peaking of T waves, hyperkalemia can be considered minimal. When the plasma potassium is 6.5 to 8 meq per liter and T-wave peaking is the only electrocardiographic abnormality, hyperkalemia may be considered moderate. Severe hyperkalemia is present if the plasma potassium exceeds 8 meq per liter or if electrocardiographic abnormalities include absent P waves, widened QRS complexes, or ventricular arrhythmias. Minimal hyperkalemia can usually be treated by elimination of a cause, such as potassium-sparing diuretics, or by treatment of accompanying acidosis. More severe or progressive hyperkalemia requires vigorous therapy. Severe cardiac toxicity responds most rapidly to infusion of calcium. Ten to thirty ml of 10% calcium gluconate may be infused intravenously within a period of 1 to 5 min under constant electrocardiographic monitoring. While calcium infusions do not alter plasma potassium, they counteract the adverse effects of potassium on neuromuscular membranes. The effect of calcium infusions, while almost immediate, is relatively transient if the hyperkalemia is not treated directly.

In moderately severe hyperkalemia, infusion of hypertonic glucose solutions will decrease toxicity by shifting potassium into cells. In the first 30 min, 200 to 500 ml of 10% glucose may be given. An additional 500 to 1,000 ml may be infused over the next several hours. Ten units of regular insulin may be given subcutaneously, although this is probably necessary only in insulin-deficient diabetic patients. This treatment may reduce serum potassium by 1 to 2 meq per liter, and effects persist for a number of hours. The infusion of sodium bicarbonate will also help lower serum potassium rapidly by causing potassium to shift into cells. Also, 44 to 132 meq alkali (2 to 3 ampuls) may be added to a liter of glucose. Although this agent is most valuable in acidotic patients, it also is effective in individuals with normal acid-base status. The effect occurs within 1 h and persists for a number of hours thereafter. The infusion of hypertonic sodium solutions may also be effective in reversing cardiac toxicity, especially in hyponatremic or volume-depleted patients. In part the effect depends simply on dilution of plasma potassium, but there may be a direct effect of elevated plasma sodium to antagonize hyperkalemic neuromuscular toxicity as well. Glucose, bicarbonate, and sodium may be combined in a "therapeutic cocktail," formulated by adding an ampul or two of sodium bicarbonate to a liter of 5% dextrose in 0.9% saline.

None of the measures just described removes potassium from the body. Cation exchange resins such as sodium polystyrene sulfonate may be given by retention enema in the treatment of moderate or severe hyperkalemia. Enough potassium may be removed by a single enema to reduce potassium by 0.5 to 2 meq per liter within an hour, and repeated enemas can be given. These resins can also be given repeatedly by mouth to maintain low plasma potassium concentration. Twenty grams are given three or four times a day together with 20 ml of a 70% sorbitol solution, as required to ensure the passage of several loose stools daily. In patients with renal failure, hemodialysis and peritoneal dialysis will effectively control hyperkalemia. However, they are relatively slow techniques, and patients with severe hyperkalemia should be treated first with one of the methods previously discussed.

REFERENCES

Sodium and water

BARTTER FE, SCHWARTZ WB: The syndrome of inappropriate secretion of antidiuretic hormone. Am J Med 42:790, 1967

MOSES AM, MILLER M: Drug-induced dilutional hyponatremia. N Engl J Med 291:1234, 1974

ROSS EJ, CHRISTIE SBM: Hypernatremia. Medicine 48:441, 1969

WEINER M, EPSTEIN FH: Signs and symptoms of electrolyte disorders. Yale J Biol Med 43:76, 1970

Potassium

BRENNER BM, BERLINER RW: Transport of potassium, in *Handbook of Physiology,* sect. 8, *Renal Physiology,* eds J Orloff, RW Berliner, Washington: American Physiological Society, 1973

CANNON PJ et al: Juxtaglomerular cell hyperplasia and secondary aldosteronism (Bartter's syndrome): A reevaluation of the pathophysiology. Medicine 47:107, 1968

LEVINSKY NG: Management of emergencies. VI. Hyperkalemia. N Engl J Med 274:1076, 1966

MICHELIS MF, MURDAUGH HV: Selective hypoaldosteronism. Am J Med 59:1, 1975

SCHWARTZ WB, RELMAN AS: Effects of electrolyte disorders on renal structure and function. N Engl J Med 276:283, 1967

SURAWICZ B: Relationship between the ECG and electrolytes. Am Heart J 73:814, 1967

70
ACIDOSIS AND ALKALOSIS

NORMAN G. LEVINSKY

PHYSIOLOGIC CONSIDERATIONS Normal metabolism continuously produces acids. Despite the addition of some 20,000 m*M* carbonic acid and 80 m*M* of nonvolatile acids to body fluids daily, the free hydrogen ion concentration of these fluids is fixed within a narrow range. The pH of extracellular fluid is normally between 7.35 and 7.45 (hydrogen ion, 45 to 35 n*M* per liter). The pH of intracellular fluids cannot be determined with precision, but most methods suggest a mean intracellular pH in the range of 6.9. It seems likely that hydrogen ion concentration varies among intracellular organelles and cytoplasm even within individual cells. Although the free hydrogen ion concentration of body fluids is exceedingly low, protons are so reactive that even minute changes in concentration significantly influence enzymatic reactions and physiologic processes. Immediate defense against untoward changes in pH is provided by body buffers which can take up or release protons instantaneously in response to changes in acidity of body fluids. Regulation of pH ultimately depends on the lungs and the kidneys.

The principal acid product of metabolism is carbon dioxide, equivalent to potential carbonic acid. The normal concentration of carbon dioxide in body fluids is fixed at 1.2 m*M* per liter (P_{CO_2} 40 mmHg) by the lungs; at this concentration, pulmonary excretion equals metabolic production. Although carbon dioxide reacts with water and body buffers during transport from cells to pulmonary alveoli, no net change in body fluid composition results, since the CO_2 excreted by the lungs is directly equivalent to the CO_2 produced by cells. When a nonvolatile acid is produced by metabolism, the protons are removed instantaneously from body fluids by reaction with buffers. In extracellular fluid, bicarbonate is converted to water and carbon dioxide, which is excreted by the lungs. Although this mechanism effectively minimizes changes in acidity, it destroys bicarbonate and uses up cell buffer capacity. The total buffer capacity of the body fluids is about 15 meq per kg body weight. Thus, the normal rate of production of nonvolatile acids would be sufficient to deplete the body buffers completely in 10 to 20 days, were it not for the unique ability of the kidney to eliminate protons from the body by secretion into the urine, thereby regenerating bicarbonate and cell buffer capacity.

The principal source of nonvolatile acid appears to be metabolism of methionine and cystine in dietary proteins, which produces sulfuric acid. Additional sources include the incomplete combustion of carbohydrates and fats, which produces organic acids; the metabolism of nucleoproteins, which produces uric acid; and the metabolism of organic phosphorus compounds, which releases protons and inorganic phosphates. The diet does not normally contain significant amounts of preformed acids or alkalis, but significant amounts of potential acid (e.g., an excess of cationic acids, such as lysine) or alkali (e.g., citrate) may be present.

The principal functions of the kidney in acid-base metabolism can be viewed as retention of existing bicarbonate and generation of new bicarbonate to replace that used to buffer nonvolatile acids. Bicarbonate is reabsorbed in both proximal and distal segments by secretion of protons into tubular fluid. The bicarbonate concentration of extracellular fluid is, in effect, set by this process. If plasma bicarbonate rises so that filtered load exceeds renal reabsorptive capacity, bicarbonate will be excreted rapidly and normal plasma bicarbonate will be restored promptly. New bicarbonate is generated by secretion of protons onto urinary buffers. Normally, one-third is titrated onto phosphate, converting HPO_4^{2-} to $H_2PO_4^-$, the remainder onto ammonia. The amount of free acid which can be excreted in the urine is negligible, even at the minimum urine pH of 4.8. However, acidification of the urine is essential for titration of acid onto phosphate and ammonia. Changes in the pH of body fluids lead to regulatory responses by the kidney. Acidosis stimulates renal hydrogen ion secretion. Ammonia production increases, and more protons can be excreted as ammonium. In extreme acidosis, ammonia production may increase tenfold or more above the normal rate of 40 to 50 meq per day. The rate of bicarbonate reabsorption and hence plasma bicarbonate is determined, in part, by carbon dioxide concentration. Thus, hypercapnia stimulates renal bicarbonate reabsorption and elevates plasma bicarbonate, presumably because the increased concentration of carbonic acid in tubular cells enhances renal hydrogen ion secretion. Hypocapnia has the opposite effects.

The respiratory response to changes in blood pH is almost instantaneous. Acidosis stimulates and alkalosis depresses ventilation. The respiratory center in the medulla appears to respond to a pH intermediate between those of blood and cerebrospinal fluid.

EVALUATION OF ACID-BASE BALANCE In practice, classification of acid-base disorders is based on measurements of changes in the bicarbonate–carbonic acid system, the principal buffer of extracellular fluid. Because intracellular and extracellular buffers are functionally linked, measurement of the plasma bicarbonate system provides useful information about total body buffers. The relationship among the elements of the bicarbonate system is usually described in terms of the Henderson-Hasselbalch equation:

$$\text{pH} = \text{p}K + \log \frac{HCO_3}{H_2CO_3}$$

(The p*K* of carbonic acid is 6.1. H_2CO_3 is calculated as αP_{CO_2}; α, the solubility factor for carbon dioxide in body fluids, is 0.031 m*M*/liter/mmHg P_{CO_2}. For a normal P_{CO_2} of 40, H_2CO_3 is calculated as $40 \times 0.031 = 1.2$ m*M* per liter.)

Acidosis is defined as a physiologic disturbance which tends to add acid or remove alkali from body fluids, while *alkalosis* is any physiologic disturbance which tends to remove acid or add base. Since compensatory processes may minimize or prevent a change in the hydrogen ion concentration of the plasma, some authors prefer to use the terms *acidemia* and *alkalemia* to indicate those situations in which the pH of the plasma is measurably altered. *Respiratory* disorders are those in which the primary change is in the concentration of carbon dioxide (carbonic acid). As can be seen from the Henderson-Hasselbalch equation, a fall in carbon dioxide concentration will tend to cause alkalemia, while an increase in carbon dioxide concentration will cause acidemia. *Metabolic* disorders are those in which the primary disturbance is in the concentration of bicarbonate. Since bicarbonate appears in the numerator of the buffer salt/acid ratio in the Henderson-Hasselbalch equation, increased bicarbonate concentration causes alkalemia while a decrease in bicarbonate causes acidemia.

A major problem in the clinical assessment of acid-base disorders results from the compensatory responses of the lungs and the kidney. A primary change in carbon dioxide concentration induces a compensatory renal response which alters plasma bicarbonate in the same direction. Conversely, a primary alteration of plasma bicarbonate will induce compensatory changes in plasma carbon dioxide. Consider a patient with chronic respiratory insufficiency who has the following set of acid-base parameters: P_{CO_2}

70 mmHg, HCO_3 33 m*M* per liter, pH 7.30. The clinician needs to know whether the elevation of plasma bicarbonate is merely the appropriate renal response to the primary hypercapnia or a metabolic acid-base disorder is superimposed. No calculations or a priori reasoning will provide the answer to this key question. Such information can be derived only from in vivo observations in which the usual compensatory response to a given degree of chronic hypercapnia is determined.

Appropriate clinical and experimental observations in humans (and animals) have been made in all common primary acid-base disturbances. They are most readily visualized and used for analysis of clinical acid-base disorders by the "confidence band" technique, as shown in Fig. 70-1. Each band represents the mean ± 2 SD, that is, 95 percent of observations, for the compensatory response to each primary disturbance. In the example under discussion, inspection of the confidence band marked *chronic respiratory acidosis* indicates that 95 percent of individuals with chronic elevation of P_{CO_2} to 70 would have bicarbonates between 37 and 44 meq per liter, due to renal compensation. Thus, the bicarbonate of 33 meq per liter in the example cannot be interpreted as solely the result of an appropriate compensatory response to chronic hypercapnia. A second acid-base disorder, presumably metabolic acidosis, must be superimposed. Obviously, the use of this figure is no panacea nor does it obviate the need for common sense clinical evaluation of alternative possibilities. For example, if the patient under discussion had only recently developed hypercapnia, the bicarbonate of 33 meq per liter would be too high for a purely compensatory response to acute respiratory acidosis and would be interpreted as superimposed metabolic alkalosis. The difference between these two interpretations depends entirely on the clinical recognition of the chronicity of the primary respiratory disorder. The use of Fig. 70-1 in each type of acid-base disturbance is described in the appropriate section of this chapter.[1]

METABOLIC ACIDOSIS

PATHOPHYSIOLOGY Metabolic acidosis is caused by one of three mechanisms: (1) Increased production of nonvolatile acids; (2) decreased acid excretion by the kidney; (3) loss of alkali. In intracellular fluid excess protons replace potassium, which shifts out of cells, tending to elevate plasma levels. Extracellular bicarbonate is reduced by reaction with hydrogen ions or, in patients wasting alkali, by loss of bicarbonate in urine or stool. The decrease in pH stimulates respiration, and P_{CO_2} is lowered. Inspection of the confidence band for metabolic acidosis (Fig. 70-1) indicates that a decrease in P_{CO_2} of roughly 1 mmHg can be expected for each decrement of 1 m*M* per liter in plasma bicarbonate. Complete respiratory compensation for primary metabolic acidosis does not occur. Respiratory compensation for acute acidosis tends to be somewhat greater than for chronic metabolic acidosis. The minimum level of P_{CO_2} which can be attained is approximately 10 mmHg; levels below 15 to 20 mmHg are rarely maintained in chronic metabolic acidosis. When kidney function is normal, net acid excretion increases promptly in response to metabolic acidosis. Most of the initial rise is due to increased titration of urinary phosphate as urine pH falls below 5.2. Over several days, ammonia production by the kidney increases and becomes quantitatively by far the most important mechanism for excreting excess protons. Net acid excretion may increase five to ten times above normal, reaching a maximum of several hundred milliequivalents per day.

PATHOGENESIS The major causes of metabolic acidosis are shown in Table 70-1. Renal disease is the most common cause of *chronic* metabolic acidosis. In *chronic renal failure,* the principal defect is decreased ability to excrete ammonium, but some patients also waste bicarbonate, especially at plasma levels of 18 m*M* per liter or above. Acidification of the urine and formation of titratable acidity is usually normal. Plasma bicarbonate tends to fall progressively as renal insufficiency becomes increasingly severe. However, plasma bicarbonate usually stabilizes at levels of 12 to 18 m*M* per liter; it rarely falls below 10 m*M* per liter, even in advanced uremia. The mechanisms of stabilization are thought to be (1) stimulation of acid excretion by advancing acidosis, which occurs to some extent even in the diseased kidney, and (2) buffering of the daily metabolic acid load by carbonate and phosphate in bone. Chronic metabolic acidosis is the hallmark of tubular dysfunction in *renal tubular acidosis,* which may be a primary renal disease, part of the Fanconi syndrome, or associated with a number of nonrenal primary disorders (see Chap. 104). In

FIGURE 70-1
In vivo nomogram, showing bands for uncomplicated respiratory or metabolic acid-base disturbances. Each "confidence" band represents the mean ± 2 SD for the compensatory response of normal subjects or patients to a given primary disorder. (From Arbus, 1973)

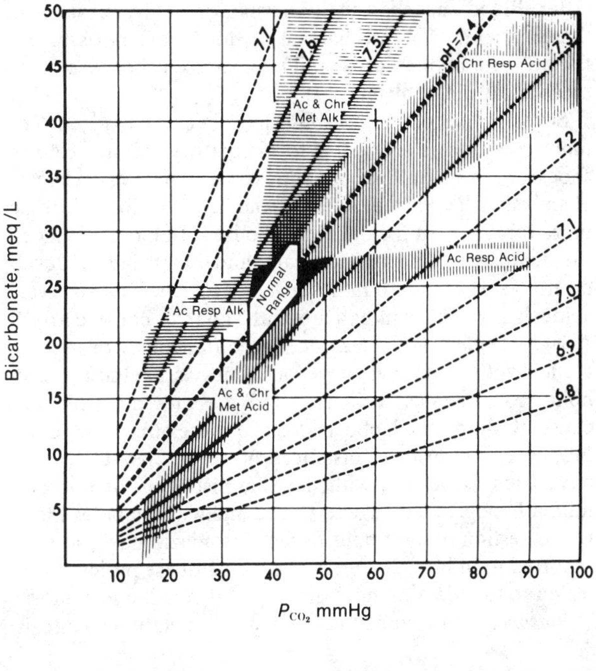

[1] *Although the confidence band method does not permit automatic identification of simple or complicated acid-base disorders, it is much preferable to other techniques such as "buffer base" or "base excess-deficit" for reasons discussed in detail by Schwartz and Relman. These terms are not used in this chapter.*

TABLE 70-1
Causes of metabolic acidosis

I Renal disease
  A Chronic renal failure
  B Renal tubular acidosis
  C Acute renal failure
II Increased acid production
  A Ketoacidosis
    1 Diabetic acidosis
    2 Ketoacidosis associated with alcoholism
    3 Starvation ketosis
  B Lactic acidosis
    1 Secondary to circulatory insufficiency
    2 Primary
    3 Drug-induced: phenformin, poisoning with isoniazid
    4 Total fasting in obese patients
  C Poisoning
    1 High anion gap: salicylates, methanol, ethylene glycol
    2 Normal anion gap: ammonium chloride, lysine, arginine
III Loss of alkali
  A Diarrhea
  B Ureteroenterostomy
  C Acetazolamide

acute renal failure, plasma bicarbonate usually decreases by no more than 1 to 2 m*M* per liter per day; greater rates of fall suggest the presence of some cause of increased acid production, such as damaged tissue or sepsis.

The most common cause of *acute* metabolic acidosis is increased production of nonvolatile acids. In *diabetic ketoacidosis,* acetoacetic and β-hydroxybutyric acids are produced more rapidly than they can be metabolized. Severe ketoacidosis may occur in *association* with *acute* and *chronic alcoholism.* Typically patients have given a history of prolonged abstention from food, protracted vomiting, and appreciable alcohol intake just before development of the ketoacidosis. β-Hydroxybutyrate, acetoacetate, and lactate accumulate in the plasma. The ketosis may be overlooked because the ratio of β-hydroxybutyrate to acetoacetate tends to be unusually high; the nitroprusside test used for clinical detection of plasma ketones responds only to the latter. Blood sugar is usually normal or mildly elevated in these patients. The mechanism of the syndrome is uncertain. *Starvation* may cause mild ketoacidosis because of increased fat metabolism.

Several types of *lactic acidosis* have been recognized. The most common is *secondary* to circulatory failure, e.g., in shock or sepsis. In these patients, tissue hypoxia accelerates glycolysis (the Pasteur effect), and lactic acid is formed more rapidly than it can be metabolized. In most instances, the acidosis is mild or moderate, and blood lactate levels do not exceed 5 to 10 m*M* per liter. However, more severe acidosis may occur in patients with shock or cardiac arrest. *Primary lactic acidosis* may occur spontaneously or in association with a number of serious illnesses, including alcoholic liver disease, leukemia, and diabetes mellitus. The cause of idiopathic lactic acidosis in these circumstances is unknown. Occasional instances of severe lactic acidosis have been associated with the administration of phenformin, a hypoglycemic agent, to patients with diabetes mellitus. Ingestion of enormous doses of isoniazid has also been reported to induce the syndrome. Some obese patients subjected to total fasting have developed severe lactic acidosis.

Poisoning is a frequent cause of acute metabolic acidosis. Among the more common agents are salicylates, ethylene glycol, and methyl alcohol. Each of these intoxicants appears to create a metabolic block, which leads to production of a mixture of endogenous organic acids. The quantities of acid formed far exceed the amount which can be attributed to acidic properties of the drugs or their metabolites. Salicylates have the additional effect of stimulating the respiratory center directly. Respiratory alkalosis is the earliest derangement in salicylate intoxication and may be the only acid-base disorder in some patients. Several medications may induce hyperchloremic acidosis; these include ammonium chloride, lysine and arginine hydrochloride, and diuretics such as acetazolamide, which inhibit carbonic anhydrase.

Loss of *alkali* may be the cause of acute or chronic metabolic acidosis. Severe *diarrhea* or intestinal malabsorption usually causes mild to moderate acidosis due to the loss of bicarbonate in liquid stool, in which concentrations of 40 to 60 m*M* per liter may be present. Ureterosigmoidostomy, i.e., transplantation of the ureters into the sigmoid colon, leads to metabolic acidosis both because of exchange of chloride for bicarbonate by intestinal epithelium and because renal disease (obstructive uropathy and pyelonephritis) often develops. Acidosis has virtually been eliminated as a problem by the more modern technique for urinary diversion, in which a bladder is formed from a small isolated loop of ileum.

CLINICAL FEATURES AND DIAGNOSIS There are few specific symptoms or signs of metabolic acidosis; diagnosis depends on recognition of the clinical setting and appropriate laboratory studies. In acute metabolic acidosis, hyperventilation is usually evident and may be extremely intense (Kussmaul respiration). However, it is ordinarily impossible to detect increased respiration by physical examination in patients with chronic metabolic acidosis, despite substantial reduction of P_{CO_2}. Acute, severe acidosis produces a variety of nonspecific symptoms ranging from fatigue through confusion, stupor, and coma; vascular collapse and shock may occur. Chronic metabolic acidosis may produce no symptoms or may be associated with fatigue and anorexia, although it is usually difficult to determine whether these symptoms reflect the acidosis per se or are related to the underlying disease.

The characteristic laboratory features are reduction of plasma bicarbonate and blood pH, together with a compensatory reduction in P_{CO_2} (see Fig. 70-1). Hyperkalemia is often present. In those instances in which the cause of metabolic acidosis is not evident from the history or clinical setting, calculation of unmeasured anions (anion gap) may help in differential diagnosis. Unmeasured anions are calculated by subtracting the sum of plasma bicarbonate and chloride from plasma sodium concentration; the normal value is 4 to 12 m*M* per liter. In those instances in which acidosis is due to loss of bicarbonate or to administration of acid with chloride, the anion gap will be normal (hyperchloremic acidosis). This category includes diarrhea, loss of upper intestinal fluid, ureterosigmoidostomy, renal tubular acidosis, and administration of ammonium chloride, lysine, or arginine chloride and acetazolamide. When production of nonvolatile acids is increased or renal failure is present, the anions associated with metabolic acids will accumulate in plasma. An increase in unmeasured anions is typical of renal failure, diabetic and alcoholic ketoacidosis, lactic acidosis, and poisoning by salicylates, ethylene glycol, and methyl alcohol.

TREATMENT The treatment of metabolic acidosis depends on its cause and severity. In *chronic renal failure,* mild or moderate metabolic acidosis does not require treatment. When plasma bicarbonate falls below 15 m*M* per liter, it is reasonable to treat patients with oral alkali, such as sodium bicarbonate or sodium citrate. The dose is gradually increased until plasma bicarbonate concentration rises to about 18 to 20 m*M* per liter. Some patients appear to benefit symptomatically from elevation of bicarbonate to this level, and fatigue, anorexia, and malaise tend to be alleviated. Caution must be exerted to avoid excessively rapid alkalination of the plasma, which may precipitate tetany; excess sodium given with alkali may aggravate hypertension or edema. Acidosis should be corrected as completely as possible in patients with *renal tubular acidosis;* this will avoid hypercalciuria, osteomalacia, nephrocalcinosis, and lithiasis. Patients with *acute renal failure* do not ordinarily require specific therapy for acidosis. Dialysis instituted for management of the renal failure should maintain an adequate plasma bicarbonate.

Diabetic *ketoacidosis* responds to insulin, and most patients do not require treatment with alkali. However, when acidosis is extreme (pH less than 7.1 or bicarbonate less than 6 to 8 meq per liter), intravenous bicarbonate therapy is justified. The ketoacidosis associated with alcoholism responds rapidly to infusions of glucose and saline. Insulin is not required, nor should alkali be given unless acidosis is extreme. The ketoacidosis of starvation is mild and requires no specific treatment.

Secondary *lactic acidosis* responds to treatment of the underlying disorder by measures which improve the circulation. Idiopathic lactic acidosis is resistant to treatment because production of lactic acid by metabolism is very rapid. Administration of several hundred milliequivalents of alkali in a few hours may be sufficient to raise plasma bicarbonate in some patients. Even if the acidosis can be corrected, patients with primary lactic acidosis usually die, since no treatment is available for the underlying metabolic disorder.

The acidosis associated with *diarrhea* or loss of alkaline upper-intestinal secretions is usually associated with other electrolyte abnormalities, including volume depletion and potassium deficiency. Treatment with intravenous infusions appropriate for all these abnormalities may be required.

Some general points about therapy with alkali are worth emphasis. Oral treatment with sodium bicarbonate should usually begin with 1 g three times daily and be increased to maintain the desired plasma bicarbonate level. Some patients find that sodium bicarbonate leads to upper gastrointestinal discomfort; a 10% sodium citrate solution may be more palatable. In treatment of acute metabolic acidosis by intravenous administration of alkali, sodium bicarbonate is the agent of choice. The concentration of bicarbonate to be given depends upon the severity of the acidosis and any associated disorders of serum sodium concentration. Typically, concentrations of bicarbonate between 44 and 132 meq per liter are achieved by adding 1 to 3 ampuls sodium bicarbonate to a liter of dextrose in water. The concentration of bicarbonate in these ampuls is 880 meq per liter (44 meq in 50 ml); they should never be given undiluted in the treatment of acidosis, since rapid infusion may induce serious or even fatal cardiac arrhythmias, especially if given as a bolus through a central venous catheter. The total amount of alkali needed to raise plasma bicarbonate can be estimated from the effects of administration of acid loads. In experiments, approximately equal amounts of acid appear to be buffered by extracellular bicarbonate and by intracellular buffers. (In extremely severe acidosis, a greater fraction of the acid load may be buffered within cells.) Therefore, it is appropriate to calculate the amount of alkali needed by assuming that approximately half will accept protons from intracellular buffers and be destroyed; the other half will elevate plasma bicarbonate concentration. Thus, the calculation would be: millimoles of bicarbonate required equals desired increment in plasma concentration (millimoles per liter) times 40 percent of body weight. The 40 percent figure represents twice the extracellular volume. It is rarely desirable to infuse enough alkali to elevate plasma bicarbonate to normal. Possible untoward effects include hypokalemic cardiac toxicity in patients who are substantially potassium-depleted; tetany in patients with renal failure or hypocalcemia; and congestive failure due to excess sodium. Moreover, alkalosis may supervene. Cerebrospinal fluid bicarbonate does not equilibrate rapidly with plasma. Hence the respiratory center, which responds to acidity both of blood and cerebrospinal fluid, maintains some degree of hyperventilation as plasma bicarbonate is increasing. This type of respiratory alkalosis may sometimes persist for several days after correction of metabolic acidosis. In acute acidosis due to overproduction of metabolic acids, successful treatment of the primary disorder will cause rapid metabolic conversion of lactate and ketone bodies to bicarbonate. Thus, excessive administration of bicarbonate early in therapy also may lead to metabolic alkalosis at a later stage of treatment, when endogenous bicarbonate has been reconstituted by improvement in metabolism.

METABOLIC ALKALOSIS

PATHOPHYSIOLOGY Metabolic alkalosis is usually initiated by increased loss of acid from the stomach or the kidney. However, excretion of bicarbonate at high plasma concentrations is normally so rapid that alkalosis will not be sustained unless bicarbonate reabsorption is enhanced or alkali is continuously generated at a great rate. Clinically, maintenance of metabolic alkalosis is most often due to stimulation of bicarbonate reabsorption by a volume (chloride) deficit. During volume depletion, renal conservation of sodium takes precedence over other homeostatic mechanisms, such as correction of alkalosis. Since in alkalosis a large fraction of plasma sodium is paired with bicarbonate, complete reabsorption of filtered sodium requires reabsorption of bicarbonate as well. Alkalosis is sustained until volume depletion is corrected by administration of sodium chloride. This diminishes tubular avidity for sodium and provides chloride as an alternative anion for reabsorption with sodium; excess bicarbonate can then be excreted with sodium.

The mechanism of metabolic alkalosis in patients with

excess mineralocorticoid activity is not fully clarified. Mineralocorticoids stimulate renal hydrogen ion secretion; presumably, elevation of plasma bicarbonate is initiated by increased urinary loss of protons as ammonium and titratable acidity. Stimulation of tubular acid secretion also enhances bicarbonate reabsorption, thereby sustaining the metabolic alkalosis. Patients with excess mineralocorticoid activity are not volume- or chloride-deficient. Hence, this type of metabolic alkalosis does not respond to sodium chloride administration.

The mechanism of alkalosis associated with severe potassium depletion is incompletely understood. To some extent extracellular alkalosis may be initiated by a shift of hydrogen ions into cells as potassium is lost. Renal proton secretion is stimulated by potassium depletion. The older concept that hydrogen and potassium compete for secretion on a transport carrier in the distal nephron has been discarded. Nevertheless, part of the sodium reabsorbed distally does exchange for hydrogen or potassium, although the linkage is now understood to be indirect, in that sodium reabsorption creates a favorable electrical gradient for countermovement of cellular cation into the urine. In potassium depletion cellular potassium concentration falls, and hydrogen ion concentration appears to increase. It seems likely that this change in the intracellular ratio of the two ions in renal epithelial cells promotes hydrogen ion secretion and maintains a high renal threshold for bicarbonate.

Respiratory compensation for metabolic alkalosis is limited. Alveolar ventilation decreases, and $P\text{CO}_2$ is elevated. However, since this response is limited by hypoxia, $P\text{CO}_2$ rarely rises above 50 to 55 mmHg.

PATHOGENESIS The causes of metabolic alkalosis are outlined in Table 70-2. *Vomiting* and *gastric drainage* usually induce only minimal or moderate alkalosis, but occasional patients, especially those with increased gastric acid secretion, e.g., with acid-peptic disease or the Zollinger-Ellison syndrome, may develop very severe alkalosis.

Alkalosis may be present in patients treated with any *diuretic* except those which specifically inhibit bicarbonate reabsorption, such as acetazolamide, or those which inhibit distal cation secretion, such as spironolactone and triamterene. Alkalosis due to oral treatment with diuretics is usually mild. Acute administration of very potent intravenous diuretics such as ethacrynic acid to patients on low salt diets may induce more severe alkalosis due to rapid loss of sodium chloride in the urine. Sudden contraction of extracellular volume elevates plasma bicarbonate; renal excretion of excess bicarbonate is prevented by the mechanism discussed above.

Patients with chronic hypercapnia due to respiratory insufficiency maintain high plasma bicarbonate concentrations (see Respiratory Acidosis below). If respiration improves, $P\text{CO}_2$ will fall promptly. However, urinary excretion of excess bicarbonate previously generated by renal compensatory mechanisms will take a number of days. In patients on low salt diets or diuretics who have a volume (chloride) deficiency, *posthypercapneic* alkalosis of this type may persist indefinitely unless sodium or potassium chloride is added to the diet. The mechanism in this condition is the same as that which causes persistent alkalosis in vomiting, described earlier.

Alkalosis is variable in patients with excess mineralocorticoid activity. Minimal or moderate alkalosis is usually present in patients with *Cushing's syndrome* or *primary aldosteronism.* More marked alkalosis may be seen in patients with extreme adrenal hyperfunction associated with ACTH-secreting tumors, such as bronchogenic carcinoma. Moderate alkalosis is typical of patients with *Bartter's syndrome.*

Although alkalosis and *potassium depletion* are often associated, mild or moderate potassium depletion is rarely the sole cause of sustained metabolic alkalosis. However, extreme degrees of potassium depletion (serum potassium usually 2 meq per liter or less) may cause metabolic alkalosis. This type of alkalosis is not corrected by administration of sodium chloride but does respond to administration of potassium.

For reasons noted earlier, alkalosis due to administration of alkali cannot be sustained unless large amounts are given. When renal function is compromised, alkalosis may be sustained by smaller exogenous loads. This is apparently the mechanism of alkalosis in the milk-alkali syndrome, in which hypercalcemic nephropathy and alkalosis develop in response to excessive intake of absorbable alkali. The nephropathy limits bicarbonate excretion, thus maintaining the alkalosis.

CLINICAL FEATURES AND DIAGNOSIS There are no specific clinical signs or symptoms. Severe alkalosis may cause apathy, confusion, and stupor. If serum calcium is borderline or low, rapid development of alkalosis may lead to tetany. The diagnosis of metabolic alkalosis depends on recognition of the clinical setting and appropriate laboratory studies. Plasma bicarbonate is increased, and elevation of $P\text{CO}_2$ is insufficient to prevent alkalemia (see Fig. 70-1). Plasma potassium concentration is often reduced, and the electrocardiogram may reveal changes in T and U waves typical of hypokalemia; it is uncertain whether these changes are due to alkalosis itself or to associated alterations in potassium metabolism. Despite elevation of plasma bicarbonate, the urine pH is usually less than 7 in patients with sustained metabolic alkalosis. This "paradoxical aciduria" reflects the fact that bicarbonate reabsorption must be increased if metabolic alkalosis is to be sustained.

TREATMENT Mild or moderate metabolic alkalosis rarely requires specific treatment. In patients with gastric alkalosis, infusion of saline solutions is usually sufficient to enhance renal bicarbonate excretion and to correct alkalosis

TABLE 70-2
Causes of metabolic alkalosis

I Associated with volume (chloride) depletion
  A Vomiting or gastric drainage
  B Diuretic therapy
  C Posthypercapneic alkalosis
II Associated with hyperadrenocorticism
  A Cushing's syndrome
  B Primary aldosteronism
  C Bartter's syndrome
III Severe potassium depletion
IV Excessive alkali intake
  A Acute
  B Milk-alkali syndrome

by mechanisms discussed above. Administration of potassium chloride is also helpful in treating or preventing alkalosis in these patients and those with diuretic-induced alkalosis. In patients with adrenal hyperfunction, alkalosis is corrected by specific treatment of the underlying disease. In Bartter's syndrome, which is not subject to specific treatment, large amounts of potassium chloride may be required to correct hypokalemia and alkalosis. Whenever alkalosis and potassium depletion occur together, potassium depletion should be treated with potassium chloride, not with an organic salt of potassium.

Rarely, prolonged gastric losses in patients with metabolic alkalosis may be severe enough to require intravenous therapy with acidifying agents. Ammonium chloride or arginine hydrochloride may be given slowly under such circumstances. In most patients the use of potentially toxic acidifying agents can be avoided by appropriate treatment with saline and potassium chloride.

RESPIRATORY ACIDOSIS

PATHOPHYSIOLOGY Failure of ventilation promptly increases P_{CO_2} (carbonic acid) because metabolic production of carbon dioxide is so rapid. Acute respiratory acidosis is modulated to a limited degree by tissue buffers. As can be seen from the curve labeled *acute respiratory acidosis* in Fig. 70-1, immediate tissue buffering is insufficient to elevate plasma bicarbonate more than a few milliequivalents per liter. If hypercapnia is sustained, renal acid excretion is enhanced, and bicarbonate reabsorption stimulated. Over a period of several days, plasma bicarbonate rises approximately 3 meq per liter for each increase of 10 mmHg in P_{CO_2}, thereby minimizing the degree of acidemia. The increment in plasma bicarbonate attributable to renal activity is represented by the difference between the curves marked *chronic respiratory acidosis* and *acute respiratory acidosis.*

PATHOGENESIS *Acute* respiratory acidosis occurs whenever there is a sudden failure of ventilation. Common causes include depression of the respiratory center by cerebral disease or drugs, neuromuscular disorders, and cardiopulmonary arrest. *Chronic* respiratory acidosis occurs in pulmonary diseases such as chronic emphysema and bronchitis, in which ventilation and perfusion are mismatched and effective alveolar ventilation is decreased. Chronic hypercapnia may also result from primary alveolar hypoventilation or from alveolar hypoventilation related to extreme obesity (Pickwickian syndrome). Acute and chronic diseases characterized principally by interference with alveolar gas exchange, such as chronic pulmonary fibrosis, pneumonia, and pulmonary edema, usually cause hypocapnia rather than hypercapnia. In these conditions, hypoxia stimulates increased ventilation; since carbon dioxide is much more diffusible than oxygen, excretion of carbon dioxide is enhanced despite the barrier to gas exchange. Hypercapnia occurs only with respiratory fatigue or extremely severe disease.

CLINICAL FEATURES AND DIAGNOSIS It is often difficult to separate the manifestations of respiratory acidosis from those of associated hypoxia. Moderate hypercapnia, especially if it develops slowly, probably has no specific clinical features. When P_{CO_2} exceeds 70 mmHg, patients progressively become confused and obtunded. Asterixis may be noted. Papilledema may occur, apparently because intracranial pressure is increased by the cerebral vasodilation characteristic of hypercapnia. Dilatation of conjunctival and superficial facial blood vessels may be noted.

The diagnosis of acute respiratory acidosis is usually evident from the clinical situation, especially if respiration is obviously depressed. Proof requires laboratory confirmation that P_{CO_2} is elevated. Acidemia is always present in patients with acute hypercapnia. Acidosis in acute cardiopulmonary arrest is usually a combination of a lactic metabolic acidosis and acute respiratory acidosis. Patients with chronic hypercapnia are usually acidemic. However, some individuals with minimal or moderate chronic hypercapnia may have normal or even slightly elevated plasma pH, as may be seen from Fig. 70-1. The mechanism of full compensation or of "overcompensation" in such individuals is unknown. However, significant elevation of pH in patients with chronic hypercapnia is almost always due to complicating metabolic alkalosis. Diuretics, low salt diets, and posthypercapneic alkalosis are frequent causes of this type of superimposed acid-base disorder.

Because of the differences between plasma bicarbonate in acute hypercapnia and in chronic hypercapnia, proper interpretation of acid-base parameters in respiratory acidosis depends on clinical information. This is discussed in an earlier section of this chapter.

TREATMENT The only worthwhile approach to treatment of respiratory acidosis is correction of the underlying disorder. Rapid infusion of alkali is justified in cardiopulmonary arrest. In other circumstances, attempted treatment of respiratory acidosis with infusions of alkali or with buffers such as THAM is of transient benefit and has no role in practical management.

RESPIRATORY ALKALOSIS

PATHOPHYSIOLOGY Acute reduction in carbon dioxide concentration releases hydrogen ion from tissue buffers, which minimize alkalemia by reducing plasma bicarbonate. Acute alkalosis also enhances glycolysis; increased production of lactic and pyruvic acids lowers serum bicarbonate and raises plasma concentrations of the corresponding anions by a millimole or two. Reduction in P_{CO_2} through its effect on plasma bicarbonate concentration decreases renal bicarbonate reabsorption. In chronic hypocapnia, serum bicarbonate is maintained at a reduced level because of decreased renal reabsorption.

PATHOGENESIS The causes of respiratory alkalosis are shown in Table 70-3.

CLINICAL FEATURES AND DIAGNOSIS Depending on its severity and acuteness, hyperventilation may or may not be clinically apparent. In acute respiratory alkalosis, the clinical picture is rather characteristic: patients complain of paresthesias, numbness, and tingling; of light-headedness; and, if alkalosis is sufficiently severe, of manifestations of tetany. Alkalosis directly enhances neuromuscular excita-

TABLE 70-3
Causes of respiratory alkalosis

I Acute
  A Hyperventilation due to anxiety
  B Fever
  C Exercise
  D Acute hypoxia (e.g., pneumonia, acute pulmonary edema, asthma)
  E Salicylate intoxication
  F Excessive mechanical ventilation
  G Bacteremia, especially gram-negative
II Chronic
  A Cerebral disease (tumor, encephalitis, etc.)
  B Chronic hepatic insufficiency
  C Pregnancy
  D Chronic hypoxia (lung disease, cyanotic heart disease, adaptation to high altitudes)

bility; this effect, rather than the modest decrease in ionized plasma calcium induced by alkalosis, is probably the major cause of tetany. Severe respiratory alkalosis may cause confusion or loss of consciousness, perhaps due to cerebral vasospasm induced by hypocapnia.

The diagnosis may be suspected from the clinical setting but must be confirmed by analysis of the plasma bicarbonate system. Hypocapnia together with a variable degree of alkalemia is found; plasma bicarbonate is decreased but is rarely below 15 m*M* per liter.

TREATMENT The only successful treatment for respiratory alkalosis is elimination of the underlying disorder. In the acute hyperventilation syndrome, sedation, reassurance, and, if symptoms are sufficiently severe, rebreathing into a bag will usually terminate the attack.

REFERENCES

ARBUS GS: An in vivo acid-base nomogram for clinical use. Can Med Assoc J 109:291, 1973

BRACKETT NC JR et al: Acid-base response to chronic hypercapnia in man. N Engl J Med 280:124, 1969

LEVY LH et al: Ketoacidosis associated with alcoholism in nondiabetic subjects. Ann Intern Med 78:213, 1973

OLIVA PB: Lactic acidosis. Am J Med 48:209, 1970

RELMAN AS: Renal acidosis and renal excretion of acid in health and disease. Adv Intern Med 12:295, 1964

SCHWARTZ WB, RELMAN AS: A critique of the parameters used in the evaluation of acid-base disorders. N Engl J Med 268: 1382, 1963

SELDIN DW, RECTOR FC: The generation and maintenance of metabolic alkalosis. Kidney Int 1:306, 1972

section 4 | Immunologic considerations

71
INTRODUCTION TO CLINICAL IMMUNOLOGY

K. FRANK AUSTEN

The immunologic response not only constitutes the principal means of an individual's defense against pathogenic microorganisms, but also is capable of mediating adverse clinical reactions. Whether an immune response is defined clinically as immunity or hypersensitivity is determined by its effect on the host; the distinction does not necessarily imply different mechanisms of elicitation. The components of the immune system may be considered in terms of the sequential manner in which they contribute to the immune response. The principal features include immunogens capable of initiating the immune response; cellular processing of immunogenic material; products of the immune response; control mechanisms of the response; and consequences, both beneficial and detrimental, of the immune response. Consideration of the immunologic response in terms of these arbitrary divisions affords a basis for a clinical approach to the diagnosis and management of immune deficiency states and hypersensitivity syndromes.

INITIATION OF THE IMMUNE RESPONSE A substance must ordinarily be recognized as foreign in order to elicit an immune response. The ability of a substance to evoke such a response is termed *immunogenicity;* the capacity to react specifically with the antibodies induced is termed *antigenicity.* The distinction is useful because many simple substances of less than 1,000 molecular weight are not immunogenic unless coupled covalently or by large numbers of ionic bonds to macromolecules but can react with antibodies of appropriate specificity; such simple substances are termed *haptens.*

Deliberate initiation of the immune response is accomplished most reliably by injection of the immunogen. Feeding is not usually effective because, being proteins, most immunogens are digested in the gastrointestinal tract. The oral route may, however, be utilized under certain circumstances, such as with attenuated poliomyelitis virus. Natural immunization to environmental substances may occur by such diverse routes as inhalation of plant or tree pollens, ingestion of certain foods or drugs, and skin contact with drugs or natural chemicals such as the catechols of poison ivy plants.

CELLULAR BASIS OF IMMUNE RESPONSES Immunogens that are injected subcutaneously drain into local lymph nodes; those that are administered intravenously localize in the spleen. Within these lymphoid organs, the immunogens are taken up by the macrophages; this step is considered important in most immune responses. Macrophages catabolize most of the immunogen but retain a few molecules in a partially or completely undegraded state for presentation to the lymphocyte for immune recognition. The macrophages are nonspecific handlers of the immunogen and do not determine the specificity of the immune response. The specificity of the immune response depends on the interaction of the immunogen with lymphocytes which, according to selectional theories, are genetically precommitted to interact with a particular antigen.

Two kinds of lymphocytes are present in peripheral lymphoid organs. The so-called *B lymphocytes,* derived from bone marrow stem cells in mammals and cells from the bursa of Fabricius in birds, are situated in the lymphoid follicles and are distinguishable by a large concentration of immunoglobulin molecules on their surface membranes. B lymphocytes can be identified immunocytochemically by the presence of immunoglobulin on the surface. B cells incubated with antibodies to immunoglobulin labeled with a fluorescent dye are shown to have discrete spots of immunoglobulin disseminated throughout their plasma membrane. The surface immunoglobulin molecules are mostly of the IgM class, although a substantial number of cells also have IgD. It is thought, however, on the basis of indirect experimental evidence, that all the surface immunoglobulin molecules are directed against a single antigen determinant. B lymphocytes also have on their surface a receptor for the C3 component of complement (see below) and for aggregated immunoglobulin (Fc receptor). Thus, antigen-antibody-complement complexes will bind to their surfaces. B lymphocytes represent about 20 percent of peripheral blood lymphocytes and about 50 percent of the spleen lymphocytes. The immunoglobulin on the membrane of the B lymphocyte interacts with antigen, and the B lymphocyte then differentiates into a plasma cell. Plasma cells are short-lived cells which actively secrete immunoglobulin. A single plasma cell secretes antibody molecules of a single class and specificity.

The so-called *T lymphocytes,* derived from the thymus, are situated in the areas of recirculation in the lymphoid organs, and do not have demonstrable immunoglobulin molecules on their membranes. Thus the presence or absence of immunoglobulins on lymphocytes can serve to establish whether the cells are T or B in kind. In the human, T lymphocytes can be identified by their ability to bind sheep erythrocytes to their surfaces (E rosette test); this binding is nonimmunologic in nature. About 80 percent of peripheral blood lymphocytes are of the T class. The T lymphocytes react specifically with antigen, proliferate, and participate in a series of essential immunologic reactions. T lymphocytes are the effector cells in cell-mediated immunity in part because of a capacity to secrete a series of protein molecules (lymphokines) which attract and activate host macrophages. Macrophages activated by T-cell products are more microbicidal than others, and T cells are essential in the immune defense against many facultative, intracellular bacteria, viruses, and parasites. Lymphokines produced in cultures of lymphocytes exposed to antigen have been partially purified. T cells are also important cellular components in transplantation immunity, and the interaction of lymphocytes with major histocompatibility antigens of other cells can be studied in vitro in the mixed lymphocyte reaction. When lymphocytes from two different individuals are cultured, the T cells recognize the histocompatibility differences and undergo proliferation which is assessed by pulsing the culture with radioactive DNA precursor (such as tritiated thymidine) and determining its incorporation by the cell. T cells can interact directly with and kill foreign cells such as tumor cells. Finally, the immune response of B cells to many antigens requires the participation of T cells. In these cases, T cells act as "helpers," perhaps by direct contact with the B cells and/or by releasing active stimulatory molecules. It has been shown experimentally that B and T cells need to interact with different determinants in the same antigen molecule for optimal results. In contrast, in some circumstances T cells have been shown to have a negative regulatory effect by inhibiting immune responses, and some forms of unresponsiveness are attributed to the action of "suppressor" T cells.

Following an immunogenic stimulus the regional lymph nodes (or spleen) become hyperplastic and increase severalfold in weight, and the specific antibody levels in the efferent lymph exceed those in the afferent lymph entering the regional node. Net antibody synthesis by isolated lymph node tissue also has been demonstrated in vitro. The evidence that the plasma cell is particularly active in antibody synthesis includes (1) the prominence of plasma cells as lymphoid tissue becomes hyperplastic in response to an immunogenic stimulus; (2) the approximate relationship between the antibody extractable from such tissue with the plasma cell content; (3) the demonstration by immunofluorescent staining procedures of gamma-globulin in the cytoplasm of plasma cells; and (4) the clinical observations of increased numbers of plasma cells in circumstances of gamma-globulin overproduction and the virtual absence of such cells in heritable disorders of antibody production.

Antibody synthesis by spleen lymphoid cells has also been demonstrated in vitro. A suitable method involves the culture of spleen cell suspensions with foreign red blood cells; about 4 to 7 days after culture the spleen cells are embedded in a slide or dish with soft agar containing the foreign red blood cells and complement; if the cell is a plasma cell, it will secrete antibody which will mediate lysis of the neighboring red blood cells and form a visible plaque. With this method the actual number of cells making antibody can be readily determined. This in vitro system has confirmed that T and B lymphocytes and macrophages are necessary to produce an in vitro immune response and that the B lymphocyte proliferates after antigenic stimulation and before its conversion into actively secreting plasma cells.

As shown in Fig. 74-1 the macrophage presents the immunogenic molecules to two types of lymphocytes—B lymphocytes bearing specific immunoglobulin which differentiate into plasma cells, and T lymphocytes involved in cell-mediated immunity and serving a helper function in antibody formation.

PRODUCTS OF THE IMMUNE RESPONSE Structure of immunoglobulins The immunoglobulins (Fig. 71-1) are a group of serum proteins with a distinct electrophoretic mobility and the capacity to behave as antibodies. On the basis of different physicochemical and immunochemical properties, immunoglobulins have been divided into a number of major classes. The fundamental molecular unit of all classes of immunoglobulins, as determined by the employment of reducing and denaturing agents, consists of two heavy (H) and two light (L) polypeptide chains linked by interchain disulfide bonds and non-covalent bonds. Each H chain is usually linked to its respective L chain by a single disulfide bond, and two or more disulfide bonds link the heavy chains. IgM macroglobulin consists of five of these subunits joined by disulfide bonds and J chains. IgA can exist either as a monomer or as a polymer held together by J chains. The non-covalent bonds between the polypeptide chains are predominantly hydrophobic bonds. When the enzyme papain is employed, human IgC is split into three fragments; two, termed Fab, are identical and contain the antigen-combining sites, and the third, Fc, can be crystallized and is responsible for the unique biologic activities of a class. The Fab fragment consists of an L chain and the N-terminal half of the H chain, termed the Fd fragment, joined by their interchain disulfide bond; the Fc fragment consists of the C terminal portions of the two H chains held by their interchain disulfide bonds. The molecular basis of the specificity of bivalent antibody for antigen resides in the Fab fragments. The combining site is probably constructed predominantly from the Fd fragment of the H chain, while the L chain contributes indirectly by interacting with and stabilizing the neighboring Fd fragment. Differing antibody specificities depend on differing primary amino acid sequences in the region of the combining site; these differences exist in both the H and L chains, which vary in the combining site region but are constant in the C-terminal ends of the chains.

For the L chain the constant portion is approximately one-half the chain, whereas in the H chain the invariable portion includes the Fc piece and about one-half the Fd fragment. It is the antigenic differences in the invariable portion of the H chain which permit division of the human immunoglobulins into five major classes (IgG, IgA, IgM, IgD, and IgE). The constant portion of the L chain allows recognition of two types (kappa and lambda), which occur in combination with all five H chains (gamma, alpha, mu, delta, and epsilon). The molecular formulas for the preponderant immunoglobulin class, IgG, would thus be gamma$_2$ lambda$_2$ ($\gamma_2\lambda_2$) and gamma$_2$ kappa$_2$ ($\gamma_2\kappa_2$). IgG is further subdivided into four subclasses, IgG 1 to 4, on the basis of minor intraclass antigenic differences. In addition to the designation of class and subclass by structural differences, there are genetic differences within a class, termed *allotypy*, expressed by additional discrete structural differences. Genetic expression of structural differences in three of the gamma-chain subclasses, 1 to 3, has been related to the Gm loci, while allotypic differences in the kappa chain reside in the Inv locus.

Primary immune response The immune response to the first introduction of an immunogen is termed *primary*. In a primary response, possibly because of the differential sensitivity of the methodology employed, the IgM antibodies are recognized somewhat earlier than those of the IgG class. The IgM antibodies are observed within the first week of immunization and decline thereafter as the titer of IgG antibodies increases. This relationship and the finding that formation of IgM antibodies requires appreciable levels of immunogen have been interpreted to indicate that IgG antibodies inhibit synthesis of antibodies of the IgM class. Lymphocytes lodged in the mucosa of the intestine and along the respiratory tract appear to lead to synthesis of antibodies of the IgA and IgE class in response to local deposition of immunogen by ingestion or inhalation. The view that IgM antibodies represent a primitive product of the immune response is supported by the predominant synthesis of this antibody class in the newborn and by phylogenic observations. In addition to sequential changes in immunoglobulin class, heterogeneity of the primary re-

FIGURE 71-1

Schematic of γG-globulin. Heavy chains (H) consist of an Fc fragment, which is the same in all molecules of given subclasses, and an Fd fragment, part of which is constant and part of which varies in composition in different myeloma proteins. Similarly, light chains L have a constant and a variable half. A light chain and an Fd fragment make up the Fab fragment. S—S is a disulfide bond. N and C are N and C terminal ends. Gm and Inv are genetic factors associated with H and L chains respectively. The solid color denotes the constant region while the dashed boxes represent the variable regions.

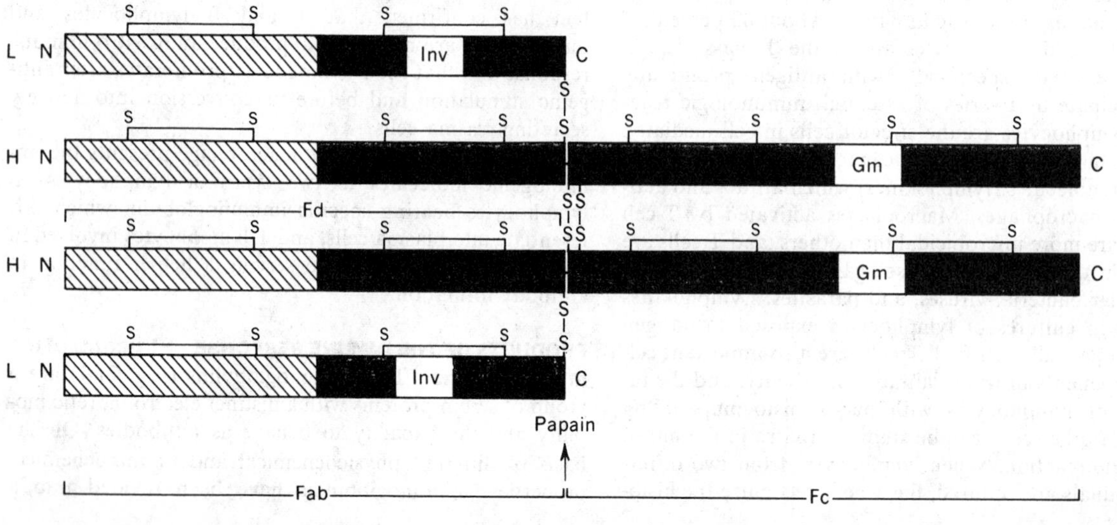

sponse occurs within the IgG class, expressed as an increasing affinity for the antigen. This may be explicable in terms of continued formation of new antibodies capable of interacting with increasing numbers of diverse antigenic determinants on the macromolecular immunogen.

Secondary immune response When the antibody levels have diminished following initial immunogenic exposure, a subsequent encounter will evoke an enhanced response, termed *secondary* or *anamnestic.* The anamnestic response requires a lower threshold dose of immunogen for elicitation and is characterized by a shortened lag phase for appearance of detectable product and a higher and more persistent antibody response. Although the quantity of antibody produced per unit time is usually much greater in the secondary response, the doubling time appears to be about the same as in the primary, which is consistent with the participation of more cells rather than an augmentation in the rate of synthesis per cell. The antibodies formed after the secondary stimulus have a much higher affinity for the corresponding antigenic determinant than those appearing after a comparable time during the primary response. The high-affinity antibodies characteristic of the secondary response are of the IgG class.

Determination of antibody synthesis Studies by immunofluorescent techniques have demonstrated that individual lymph node cells produce only a single class of heavy and light chains at any one time. The preliminary evidence suggests that L chains are made on small polyribosomes and H chains on large ones; it is held that half the immunoglobulin molecules, consisting of single L and H chains, are assembled through attachment of free L chains to the polyribosomal-bound H chains, and that the product then is released for assembly into a bivalent immunoglobulin molecule. Although it has been demonstrated that antibody specificity is determined by amino acid sequence, there is no real insight into the molecular basis by which a flexibility sufficient to recognize the vast array of potential immunogens is maintained. Theories of antibody production continue to be assessed; they range from instructive (in which the immunogen helps shape the corresponding antibody) to selective (in which the immunogen selectively stimulates a cell or portion of the gene already capable of producing the desired product). The latter theory seems most consistent with the data at hand.

The consequences of the immune response grouped as cellular immunity are of great biologic importance but cannot be presented in physicochemical terms. Accordingly, these cellular phenomena, along with the humoral responses, will be examined in the sections dealing with control mechanisms and the biologic consequences of the immune response.

CONTROL MECHANISMS OF THE IMMUNE RESPONSE

Wide variations usually are observed in the amounts of specific antibody formed in different individuals of the same species in response to a similar immunogenic stimulus. Experiments involving inbred strains of mice and guinea pigs have demonstrated genetic control of the immune response to a variety of antigens. The antigens used usually contained few antigenic determinants. While some strains manifested a high immune response to a particular antigen, others responded poorly or not at all. This genetic control follows classic mendelian genetics and in most instances is an autosomal dominant trait. In addition, control of this aspect of the immune response is associated with the histocompatibility genes of the strain and resides at the level of thymic cell function. In man there is evidence that the capacity to make antibodies of the IgE class in response to inhaled pollens is associated with an increased incidence of a similar immunoglobulin response to drugs and other environmental antigens.

Role of the thymus The development of the capacity to respond to an immunogen is dependent on a functioning thymus gland as well as on other lymphoepithelial structures arising embryologically as outpouchings of the gut wall and eventually consisting of lymphocyte populations in close proximity to epithelial cells of endodermal origin. Experimental studies have revealed that neonatal thymectomy interferes with the development of the lymphoid system, profoundly impairs the immunologic capabilities termed "cellular immunity" (such as rejection of foreign-tissue grafts and delayed hypersensitivity), and also under certain circumstances diminishes humoral responses. The manner in which the thymus mediates the development of these aspects of immunologic competence is not entirely clear but may include (1) an environment in which "stem" cells, possibly of bone marrow origin, differentiate to become immunologically competent before being distributed peripherally to populate node tissue; (2) elaboration of humoral factors regulating the maturation of peripheral lymphocytes; and (3) the exertion of "censorship," whereby potentially self-reacting clones are eliminated. It has now been shown principally through experiments in the mouse that some of the cells in the thymus undergo a process of maturation and then enter the recirculating pool of lymphoid cells, mixing with the B type of lymphocytes. The proliferative response of peripheral blood lymphocytes to mitogens like phytohemagglutinin or concanavalin A is attributed to the presence of these functional thymic derived lymphocytes. The consequences of thymectomy are less dramatic in the adult animal, but there is evidence that the thymus continues to provide a mechanism whereby immunologically uncommitted cells acquire the capacity to respond to specific immunogens.

In birds there is an anatomic separation of the central control of the capacity to develop cellular and humoral immunity; the former is regulated by the thymus and the latter by the bursa of Fabricius. In mammals the precise equivalent of the bursa has not been established, but it is assumed to be some portion of the gut-associated lymphoid tissue. The evidence in the human for some division of central control resides in the existence of patients with hereditary lesions expressed predominantly as defects in cellular immunity, humoral immunity, or both.

T lymphocytes are long-lived and abundant in the blood-forming part of the recirculating pool of lymphocytes. From the blood, these cells pass into the deep cortex of lymph node and then into the efferent lymphatics, eventually returning to the blood. Through this recirculation the T lymphocyte is situated to appreciate the entrance of foreign material to which it can react. As was analyzed before, the thymic-derived cells play a central regulatory role, influencing B-cell function in a positive or negative way and mediating the responses of macrophages.

Tolerance The capacity of an individual's immune response to distinguish between self and foreign macromolecules was termed "horror autotoxicus" by Ehrlich and "self-tolerance" by Burnet. An operational definition of tolerance sufficient to include a variety of terms developed from special experimental circumstances is "a state of specific immunologic nonreactivity to an immunogenic stimulus which would be followed by a recognizable response in a normal host." Though moderate doses of an immunogen can initiate the immune response, an excessive dose is followed by a state of tolerance or specific nonreactivity to any subsequent dose of the immunogen, although unrelated immunogens, in appropriate dose, are fully active. The physical state of the antigen is important in inducing or maintaining a state of tolerance; antigens that are soluble and of low molecular weight are highly effective in inducing tolerance, while the same antigen in aggregated forms may trigger an immune response. Tolerance is more easily established in the neonate than in the adult, is maintained by persistence of the immunogen, and can be manifested by impairment of either humoral or cellular immunity. The T lymphocyte is made tolerant with much smaller amounts of antigen than the B lymphocyte, and the tolerance state in the T-cell population is very long-lived in contrast to the short duration of tolerance in the B lymphocytes.

The mechanisms of tolerance are diverse and may involve the following: (1) Deletion of a clone of antigen-committed immunocompetent cells; this event may occur when antigen or an antigen-antibody complex in a large excess bypasses the macrophage and interacts in some deleterious way directly with the lymphocyte; (2) production of active suppressive T cells; in these instances it is possible to show that the cells from a tolerant animal transplanted to a normal animal will not allow a specific normal immune response to develop; and (3) presence of blocking antibodies in cases of transplantation and tumor immunity; in these instances inactivation of the immunocompetent lymphocyte may result from antibody complexed to antigen and/or from some direct blockade of the cellular antigens by the antibody.

FIGURE 71-2

The classic and alternative pathways for mechanisms of complement activation. The derivation of $\bar{D}$ and $\bar{P}$ from their precursor proteins of the alternative pathway, D and P, respectively, is not depicted, and the point(s) at which endotoxins or aggregated IgA initiate the sequence is not indicated, as these issues are not defined.

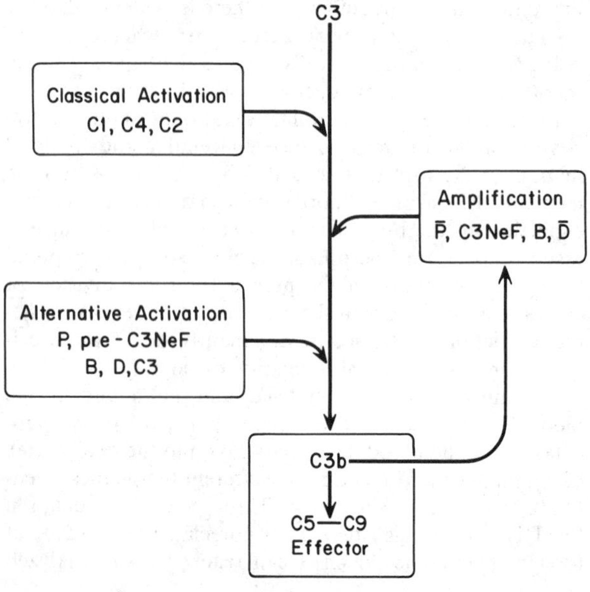

Autoimmunity The appearance of antibodies in the human directed against self represents an autoimmune response. These autoantibodies may reflect a normal response to tissue antigens which are separated anatomically from the immune system during fetal development and appear later as a consequence of tissue breakdown. Autoantibodies also may arise following abrogation of tolerance in a normal immune system by an exogenous antigen cross-reacting with self or because an abnormal immune system has lost the capacity to distinguish self. Autoantibodies do not necessarily indicate an autoimmune disease. The latter term must be restricted to situations in which the autoimmune response, humoral or cellular, is responsible for tissue injury.

CONSEQUENCES OF THE IMMUNE RESPONSE: HOST RESISTANCE The consequences of the immune response are termed *immunity* when beneficial to the host and *hypersensitivity*, or *allergy*, when detrimental. This is a clinical judgment and does not imply that the basic pathways leading to immunity or hypersensitivity are different.

The constituents of host defense in the normal person are both nonimmunologic and immunologic; those developing as a result of deliberate immunization or overt infection are exclusively immunologic. The nonimmunologic lines of defense include the extrinsic barriers to pathogen penetration, both mechanical and enzymatic, and the intrinsic cellular elements—circulating polymorphonuclear leukocytes and monocytes and fixed mononuclear phagocytic cells. Although these cellular elements are effective in the absence of an immune response, they clearly operate much more effectively in its presence. The so-called *natural antibodies* are present in normal persons who have not been subjected to deliberate immunization or overt infection; these natural antibodies would appear to result from the host's subclinical exposure to the specific pathogen or some cross-reacting pathogen. This makes it possible to consider the role of the immune response in host defense without further reference to a subclinical or overt encounter with the immunogen.

Serum complement The humoral immune response participating in host resistance appears to involve a supporting system known as serum complement; hence, it is relevant to examine this system before evaluating the role of the various immunoglobulin classes in host defense. The complement system may be divided into four functional sections: two pathways for activation, namely the classical and alternative (properdin), an amplification mechanism for augmenting the activating pathways, and a final common effector pathway to which the activating sequences are directed and from which are derived the biologic activities (Fig. 71-2). The constituent proteins of the classical complement system are symbolized with a capital C and a number designating the component (e.g., C1, C4, C2, C3, C5 to C9), and the activated state of a component is indicated by a bar over the letter (e.g., $C\bar{1}$). Cleavage fragments are suffixed with lowercase letters (e.g., C5a and C5b) while an inactive fragment is denoted with a lowercase i (as in C5i). A provisional nomenclature for alternative pathway factors uses letters rather than numbers, maintaining the other conventions as described for the classic components.

When an immune aggregate, or a target cell sensitized by interaction with specific antibody of the IgG1, IgG2, IgG3, or IgM class against some cell-surface antigen, interacts with normal serum, the first component of complement (C1) binds to the complex and is converted from an inactive precursor form to an active enzyme of the serine esterase class. Complex-bound active C1 ($C\bar{1}$) then acts on its natural substrates, the fourth and second components of complement, yielding a new cell-bound enzymatic activity consisting of major fragments of C4 and C2; the $C4\bar{2}$ unit is termed C3 convertase and initiates the effector pathway. $C4\bar{2}$ decays by loss of $C\bar{2}$ activity, thereby limiting its functional potential, but can be regenerated by the action of $C\bar{1}$ on additional C2. The action of C3 convertase on C3 results in the release of the lesser fragment (C3a) with anaphylatoxic activity into the fluid phase with the binding of the major portion of the molecule, C3b, to the macromolecular carrier, thereby shifting the activity to that of a C5 convertase. The complex bearing C3b can attach to a specific receptor on primate red blood cells, neutrophilic or eosinophilic polymorphonuclear leukocytes, monocytes, and B lymphocytes, a phenomenon known as *immune adherence* which enhances phagocytosis of appropriate cell types. The cleavage of fifth component (C5) yields another fragment with anaphylatoxic properties (C5a) while interaction of the fifth, sixth and seventh complement components produces a fluid-phase trimolecular complex capable of reacting with unsensitized cells to elicit directed migration or mediate subsequent lysis by C8 and C9. Although the complement reaction is cytolytic at the C8 interaction stage, formation of the pentamolecular complex $C\overline{56789}$ is critically more efficient in completing the reaction by osmotic lysis accompanied by alterations of the cell membrane termed "holes," as seen by electron microscopy. These final steps in the complement reaction do not involve cleavage beyond C5 and occur by covalent assembly of the cytolytic $C\overline{5\text{-}9}$ complex. The system has biologic meaning because it is lethal for some target cells and results in the elaboration of various by-products capable of mediating an inflammatory response (Fig. 71-3). The latter include the anaphylatoxins C3a and C5a, which produce a local increase in vascular permeability by releasing histamine from tissue mast cells, bringing more antibody and complement to the site of the lesion, and also contract smooth muscle; *chemotactic factors,* C3a, C5a, and $C\overline{567}$, which attract polymorphonuclear leukocytes and monocytes; *complex-bound C3b,* which promotes immune adherence and enhanced phagocytosis; and $C\overline{567}$, which prepares unsensitized bystander cells for lysis by C8 and C9. The complement reaction may be beneficial or detrimental to the host, depending on whether the antigens against which the antibody mediating the reaction is directed are foreign or self, and whether their effects are limited or excessive as the result of appreciable release of lysosomal contents from phagocytic cells.

An alternative pathway to complement activation was described some twenty years ago to consist of a group of serum factors which interacted with complex microbial polysaccharides to form a C3-cleaving enzyme distinct from $C\overline{42}$ (Fig. 71-2). $\bar{D}$, whose active site is of the serine esterase class, cleaves B in the presence of C3b, the major cleavage fragment of C3, to form the labile bimolecular complex, $C\overline{3B}$, which is similar to $C\overline{42}$ in its capacity to activate C3 to C9 (Fig. 71-3). $C\overline{3B}$ decays by loss of $\bar{B}$ activity, which limits its potential for cytolytic activity, but can be regenerated by the action of $\bar{D}$ on additional B. Activated properdin, $\bar{P}$, a nonimmunoglobulin gammaglobulin, binds to C3b and retards decay of convertase function, thereby profoundly augmenting activation of C3 to C9 by $C\overline{3B}$. Since this convertase is formed with C3b derived from initiation of either the alternative or classical activating pathways, its formation and amplification function are common to both. Amplification occurs by intense C3 cleavage with recruitment of the terminal effector sequence and the attendant biologically active reaction products (Fig. 71-3). An activity present in the serum of some patients with hypocomplementemic membranoproliferative glomerulonephritis initiates C3 cleavage independently of the classical activating pathway and is termed C3 nephritic factor (C3 NeF); C3 NeF is physicochemically distinct from properdin but functions in a manner analogous to $\bar{P}$ in the amplification sequence by stabilization of $C\overline{3B}$. The proteins involved in the amplification step also participate in the initiating reaction of the alternative pathway, but the mechanisms of P, pre-C3 NeF, and D activation and their interaction with native B and C3 to provide initial C3 cleavage are still being elucidated.

Two general types of control mechanisms limit the extent to which the complement system may be activated: The first type is inherent and is represented by the rapid decay rates of the two C3 convertases, $C\overline{42}$ and $C\overline{3B}$, which restrict activation of the terminal attack sequence, C3 to

FIGURE 71-3
The terminal complement sequence and attendant biologic activities.

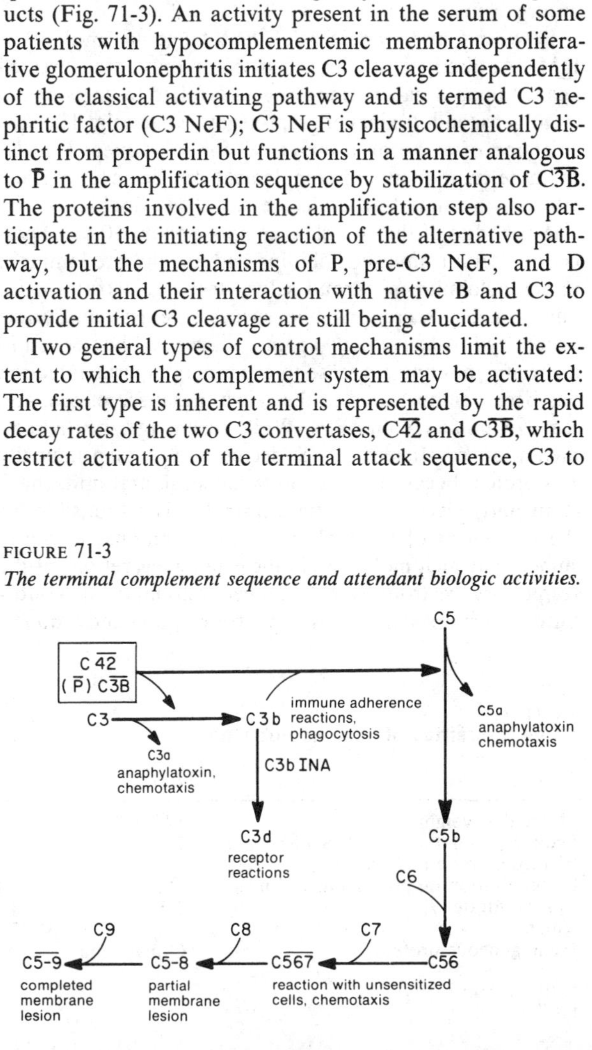

C9, and by the labile binding sites on C$\bar{3}$, C$\bar{4}$, and C$\bar{5}$, which limit potential binding after cleavage activation. The second type is extrinsic and is exemplified by two naturally occurring control proteins: C$\bar{1}$ inhibitor (C$\bar{1}$INH), which inhibits the active site of C$\bar{1}$; and C3b inactivator (C3bINA), which cleaves C3b to destroy cytolytic function in the classical or alternative pathways as well as the amplification reaction, followed by fragmentation into C3c and C3d. An additional type of control is represented by the anaphylatoxin inactivator (AI), which inactivates biologically active products but does not directly restrict activation of complement.

Antibody IgG (Table 71-1) composes 70 to 80 percent of the serum antibodies of the human and is almost exclusively responsible for the antibodies to viruses, toxins, and gram-positive pyogenic bacteria. It is transported across the placenta, while other maternal immunoglobulins mostly are excluded from the fetal circulation. The interaction of IgG with antigen to activate the complement system leads to the development of anaphylatoxins, a release of chemotactic factors, and the capacity of the complex to undergo immune adherence and enhanced phagocytosis; it may be of great importance in controlling pyogenic microorganisms.

Between 5 and 10 percent of the total serum antibody is IgM. Antibodies of this class commonly are directed against lipopolysaccharide antigens typified by the somatic 0 antigens (endotoxins) of gram-negative bacteria. The sensitization of a site on a target cell for subsequent lysis by the nine components of complement can be accomplished either by a single IgM molecule or an IgG doublet.

Antibodies of the IgA class compose about 10 to 20 percent of serum immunoglobulins and are the predominant immunoglobulin in parotid saliva, tears, colostrum, nasal and bronchial secretions, bile, succus entericus, and urine. Secretory IgA has activity against viruses and bacteria, and a specific immune response to experimental virus infection has been demonstrated in the saliva, nasal secretions, and tears of human volunteers. While serum IgA has a sedimentation coefficient of 7S, secretory IgA is principally 11S protein because of an additional structural unit, the T (transport) piece. The T piece probably is responsible for the movement of the molecules into secretions; it is presumed that such molecules in the external secretions of the respiratory, gastrointestinal, and genitourinary tract contribute to host resistance, possibly by mediating activation of the alternative complement pathway. The functions in host resistance of the trace immunoglobulin IgD is unknown. IgE, by activating mast cells in the presence of specific antigen to generate and release diverse chemical mediators of an inflammatory response, may play a role in physiologic host defense by recruitment of proteins and cells from the blood prior to extensive local tissue damage.

Specific cellular immunity Specific cellular immunity to intracellular pathogens has been demonstrated experimentally in several models, the most direct of which has involved *Listeria monocytogenes* infection in the mouse. Mice infected with a sublethal dose of this organism developed resistance to a dose 100 times the LD_{50}. Resistance was not associated with the appearance of antibody because agglutination titers were negligible and protection could not be conferred by passive transfer of serum; resistance was, however, correlated in time with the development of delayed-type skin hypersensitivity to listeria culture filtrate. Furthermore, monolayer cultures of normal mouse peritoneal macrophages are destroyed readily by inoculation with listeria, while cultures obtained from resistant animals, previously infected with sublethal challenge, are capable of eliminating the organism. These peritoneal macrophages are demonstrating specific cellular immunity because their activity is not diminished by repeated washing or enhanced by the addition of normal or immune serum to the culture. Furthermore, these macrophages are capable of destroying intracellular pathogens, other than those used to initiate the immune response such as *Brucella abortus* or *Salmonella typhimurium,* indicating that upon specific activation, cellular immunity may be expressed in a nonspecific fashion. On the other hand, the induction of cellular immunity is specific because recall can be initiated only by an organism which has previously been used to initiate a primary response. The association of cellular immunity with the cutaneous reaction of delayed hypersensitivity suggests that the specificity resides in the sensitized lymphocyte, which then "activates" the macrophage to exhibit a nonspecific increased resistance to intracellular pathogens. This is somewhat analogous to humoral immunity, wherein specificity resides with the antibody produced by the plasma cell while the execution involves the nonspecific complement system.

The experimental data considered above imply that a deficiency of IgG would predispose to pyogenic infection, and a defect in cellular immunity to infection with intracellular pathogens. These generalizations are supported by clinical observations in patients illustrating such heritable or acquired defects (Chap. 74).

TABLE 71-1
Some properties of immunoglobulins

Property	*IgG*	*IgA*	*IgM*	*IgD*	*IgE*
Molecular weight	145,000	±160,000	900,000	±160,000	200,000
Sedimentation coefficient (Svedberg)	7	7(9,11,13,15)	19	7	8
Electrophoretic mobility	γ	γ-β	γ-β	γ-β	γ-β
Concentration (approx.), mg/100 ml	1,200	200	100	3	0.03
Carbohydrate, %	2.5	10	10	10	10
Valence	2	2	5*	2†	2†
Homogeneous protein	G myeloma	A myeloma	Macroglobulin	D myeloma	E myeloma

* *10 potential*
† *Likely*

CONSEQUENCES OF THE IMMUNE RESPONSE: HYPERSENSITIVITY The adverse, or allergic, manifestations of the immune response traditionally have been divided on the basis of their time course following antigen challenge into *immediate, subacute,* and *delayed* hypersensitivity. Clear differences exist in the mechanisms whereby these three broad catogories of clinical responses arise.

Immediate hypersensitivity Immediate hypersensitivity consists of all the allergic responses that begin within minutes of antigen-antibody interaction and may be divided into *cytotoxic* or *anaphylactic* on the basis of the mediation of the clinical response. In a cytotoxic reaction, such as an acute hemolytic transfusion reaction in man, the critical damage is to the primary target cell selected because the responsible complement-fixing antibody is directed against some cell-surface antigen. In an anaphylactic reaction, the interaction of antigen with antibody results in the formation and/or release of chemical mediators which act at secondary sites, namely, smooth muscle and vascular tissue.

The term *anaphylaxis* was introduced to describe the profound shock with subsequent death observed in dogs upon reinjection of the poison of the sea anemone. The occurrence of a fatal response to repeat injection rather than the demonstration of immunity or prophylaxis prompted this designation. The clinical aspects of the anaphylactic reaction can be localized or generalized, depending upon the route of antigen exposure and the rate of absorption, and are due to the action of diverse chemical mediators released with great rapidity by antigen activation of a discrete number of target tissue mast cells previously sensitized by antibody of the IgE class. The primary chemical mediators (Table 257-1) include histamine (β-imidazolylethylamine), which constricts smooth muscle by direct and cholinergic reflex action and augments vascular permeability; eosinophil chemotactic factor of anaphylaxis (ECF-A), an acidic tetrapeptide(s) which preferentially attracts eosinophils as compared with neutrophils; slow-reacting substance of anaphylaxis (SRS-A), an acidic sulfate ester with molecular weight of approximately 400, which constricts smooth muscle and enhances vascular permeability; and platelet-activating factor (PAF), a lipid-like principle with molecular weight of 300 to 500, susceptible to inactivation by phospholipase D, which initiates platelet secretion and aggregation. Additional mediators of much greater molecular weight in a stage of preliminary characterization are a kinin-generating protease and a neutrophil chemotactic factor of anaphylaxis (NCF-A). These primary chemical mediators differ not only in structure and function but also in that histamine, ECF-A, and NCF-A are stored preformed in the cells, while SRS-A and PAF are derived immediately upon immunologic activation.

That the antibody which prepared human tissues for the immediate type of hypersensitivity reactions was of a unique immunoglobulin class, namely IgE, was not established until 1966 and was immediately confirmed by the recognition of a multiple myeloma protein with skin-fixing properties belonging to this same class. The heavy and light chains of immunoglobulins are not only bridged by disulfide bonds but exhibit disulfide bridged loops within chains which divide these structures into domains; IgE manifests an extra fourth domain within the constant region of the H chain as compared with IgG, but the tissue-fixing capacity of IgE has not been shown to reside in a particular domain. As the concentration of IgE in plasma is expressed in nanograms per milliliter, it seems likely that the binding sites for tissue mast cells serve to approximate IgE molecules (sensitization) for bridging by antigen, an event essential to activation of the cell for mediator generation and release. The partial delineation of the biochemical steps involved in the immunologic release of chemical mediators from human lung tissue permits the development of a theoretical model for mechanisms of pharmacologic modulation (Fig. 71-4). The interaction of specific antigen with tissue-fixed IgE antibody results in membrane perturbation with the transport of extracellular calcium ions to the site of a proesterase (E) which is converted to an active chymotrypsin-like serine esterase ($\bar{E}$); the esterase engages in further autocatalytic activation and acts upon its substrate, perhaps removing an inhibitory protein. The influx of calcium ions may be critical to either initial activation or autocatalytic activation of the proesterase to the esterase which then decays (Ei). Whether the subsequent energy-dependent step is related to the function of a "contractile protein" has not been established, but dense bands of microfilaments have been observed around mast cell granules, particularly during degranulation. The cellular accumulation of SRS-A which requires calcium ions and an intracellular esterase occurs during the phase of histamine and ECF-A release. Both the generation of SRS-A and the release of newly formed and preformed mediators are facilitated by cholinergic stimulation to increase intracellular levels of cyclic 3′,5′-guanosine monophosphate (cyclic GMP) and prevented by β-adrenergic agonists or other stimuli which elevate the level of cyclic 3′,5′-adenosine monophosphate (cyclic AMP). The natural fall in intracellular cyclic AMP levels which accompanies anaphylactic histamine release from purified mast cell populations presumably influences the same site in the

FIGURE 71-4
Schematic presentation of the steps in the IgE-dependent generation and release of chemical mediators.

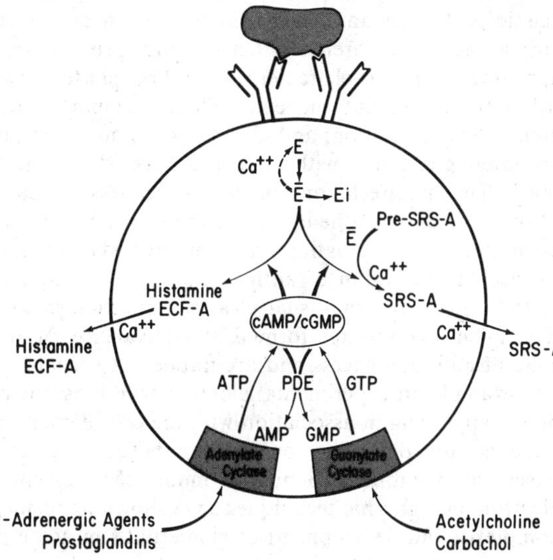

reaction sequence as that subject to pharmacologic manipulation. The findings that agents which chelate calcium ions, alter cyclic nucleotide levels, and inhibit microtubule assembly all influence the later phases of the reaction are compatible with microtubular function being essential to a late secretory step in mediator release. In addition to the intracellular prerequisites and controls of mediator generation and release, there is secondary modulation of the anaphylactic reaction through the influx of eosinophils directed by ECF-A. Eosinophils share with neutrophils the capacity to deliver a histaminase, but in contrast to other peripheral leukocyte types contain arylsulfatase B and a phospholipase D which inactivate SRS-A and PAF, respectively.

Arthus reaction Subacute hypersensitivity reactions, depending on the deposition of immune complexes, activation of the complement system, and infiltration of polymorphonuclear leukocytes, are termed *Arthus lesions* when produced in the skin and *serum sickness* when they occur systemically. In contrast to the immediate clinical wheal of cutaneous anaphylaxis brought about by the release of chemical mediators, the Arthus lesion is a hemorrhagic reaction which develops over 4 to 10 h and is associated with a marked polymorphonuclear leukocyte infiltrate of venules with surrounding edema and hemorrhage with or without secondary thrombosis. The reaction is not elicited by precipitating antibodies which do not activate complement and is depressed in experimentally induced C3 deficiencies or in acquired leukopenia. The mechanism of the Arthus lesion appears to be as follows: (1) Antigen-antibody aggregates are deposited in vessel walls; (2) the complement system is activated, and the chemotactic principles are elaborated; (3) polymorphonuclear leukocytes enter, resulting in (4) enhanced phagocytosis of the aggregates, which, in turn (5) leads to release of lysosomal enzymes with secondary focal necrosis of the vessel wall.

Serum sickness Serum sickness (Chap. 75) may be considered a disseminated form of the Arthus lesion, although the polymorphonuclear leukocytic infiltrate is less striking in the arteritis or glomerulitis of serum sickness than in the classic Arthus lesion. When a human or an experimental animal receives a foreign or heterologous protein, the disappearance curve is characterized by three phases: (1) Distribution throughout the extracellular compartment; (2) metabolic degradation; and (3) immune elimination due to an immune response with the appearance of specific antibody. The manifestations of serum sickness appear just prior to the onset of the immune elimination phase and are attributed to circulating antigen-antibody complexes formed in the region of antigen excess; these complexes apparently escape the usual clearance mechanisms effective against complexes formed at equivalence or in the zone of antibody excess and are trapped at vascular sites. For example, in experimental glomerular lesions, the complexes appearing in association with the complement components are deposited on the epithelial side of the basement membrane. Similarly, immunofluorescent and electronmicrographic techniques have shown deposition of complexes and development of glomerulitis in acute poststreptococcal nephritis and systemic lupus erythematosus in the human. However, this is not the only recognized immunologic mechanism of clinical renal disease; in Goodpasture's syndrome and certain other instances of nephritis an anti-basement membrane antibody is deposited on the endothelial side of the basement membrane and may produce direct cytotoxic injury.

Delayed hypersensitivity These reactions are exemplified in the skin by the tuberculin skin test or contact sensitivity and are implicated in the classic allograft rejection reaction of the unmodified recipient. The cutaneous response of erythema and induration is evident within 12 h and reaches a peak in 24 to 48 h. Granulocytes about small blood vessels are abundant in 12 h, but by 24 h a massive accumulation of mononuclear cells predominates. The delayed hypersensitivity response differs from the cutaneous anaphylactic or Arthus lesion because it is not transferred by serum but requires the transfer of viable lymphocytes in experimental animal models. The lymphocyte plays an essential role because (1) transfer of the delayed reaction can be achieved with thoracic duct cells, (2) the reaction can be suppressed in animals or humans treated with an antiserum against the lymphocyte, and (3) the capacity to show contact sensitivity or allograft rejection in heritable or acquired lymphocyte deficiency states is impaired. In humans, the delayed reaction has been transferred with whole cells or an extract of peripheral blood cells termed *transfer factor,* which has a molecular weight of less than 10,000. Elicitation of the delayed skin reaction requires a larger portion of the antigen than does interaction with humoral antibody; this phenomenon, referred to as *hapten-carrier specificity,* means that the specificity for eliciting a delayed response exceeds that of the reaction requiring humoral antibodies. Although this specificity seems to reside in the sensitized lymphocyte, it is only part of the reaction mechanism. In vitro studies have shown that lymphocytes stimulated by specific antigen or nonspecific mitogens, such as phytohemagglutinin, release soluble mediators or lymphokines whose in vitro effects include chemotaxis, macrophage activation, cytotoxicity, and recruitment of normal lymphocytes into the proliferating lymphocyte pool. Because probably less than 2 percent of the cells at the site of a delayed hypersensitivity reaction are specifically sensitized, it is thought that these mediators, elicited by the stimulation of a relatively small number of sensitive lymphocytes, act as biologic amplifiers of the cellular immune reaction. Consequently, possible causes of anergy in diseases such as sarcoidosis, measles, and Hodgkin's disease include defects in lymphocyte function, in mediator function, and in participation of nonsensitized cells such as macrophages.

CONCLUSION In understanding both heritable and acquired defects in host resistance, it is important to appreciate not only the elements of the immune response contributing specificity, such as the immunoglobulins and the sensitized lymphocytes, but also the role of the nonspecific elements, such as the complement sequence, the polymorphonuclear leukocyte, and the macrophage. These nonspecific elements provide the killing mechanism after a specific immunoglobulin or sensitized lymphocyte has interacted with cell-surface antigens of the pathogen. Defects may occur at any point in the sequential steps in the afferent and efferent arcs of the immune response as well as in the nonspecific humoral and cellular systems which are activated in the final expression of the response. Similarly, in considering hypersensitivity to an exogenous or endogenous immunogen, immunochemical and immunopathologic definition of the lesion will assist materially in understanding its mechanism and in arriving at a rational course of therapy, which then may be directed at any point in the afferent and efferent arcs of the immune response or at the nonspecific participants involved in its expression.

REFERENCES

Austen KF, Becker EL: *Biochemistry of the Acute Allergic Reactions, Second International Symposium,* Oxford: Blackwell Scientific Publications, Ltd., 1971

David JR: Migration inhibitory factor and mediators of cellular hypersensitivity in vitro. Prog Immunol 1:399, 1971

Davis BD et al: Immunology, sec. II in *Microbiology,* New York: Hoeber-Harper, 1967

Fearon DT, Austen KF: The human complement system: Biochemistry, biology, and pathobiology. Essays Med Biochem, II (in press)

Janeway CA et al: *The Gamma Globulins,* Boston: Little, Brown, 1967

Katz DH, Benacerraf B: The regulatory influence of activated T cells on B cell responses to antigen. Adv Immunol 15:2, 1972

Mackaness GB, Blanden RV: Cellular immunity. Prog Allergy 11:89, 1967

Müller-Eberhard HJ: Chemistry and reaction mechanisms of complement. Adv Immunol 8:1, 1968

Pillemer L et al: The properdin system and immunity. I. Demonstration and isolation of a new serum protein, properdin, and its role in immune phenomena. Science 120:279, 1954

Ruddy S et al: The complement system of man. N Engl J Med 287:489, 1972

Schur PH: Gamma G subclasses. Prog Clin Immunol 1:71, 1972

Unanue ER: Regulatory role of macrophages in antigenic stimulation. Adv Immunol 15:64, 1972

Wolstenholme GEW, Porter R: *Ciba Foundation Symposium on the Thymus,* Boston: Little, Brown, 1966

72
DISEASES OF IMMEDIATE TYPE HYPERSENSITIVITY

K. FRANK AUSTEN

INTRODUCTION The capacity of a toxic substance, when injected repeatedly, to elicit an adverse reaction rather than a protected state was recognized and designated *anaphylaxis* by Portier and Richet in 1902. Von Pirquet, perceiving that immunity and hypersensitivity were intimately linked, coined the term *allergy* in 1906 to imply a state of changed reactivity. The inadvertent passive transfer of an acute allergic response to horses by a blood transfusion from an allergic to a nonallergic subject was recognized in 1919 by Ramirez. Passive transfer of serum from a patient allergic to fish to the skin of a normal recipient followed by the antigen-induced appearance of wheal and flare at that site was accomplished by Prausnitz and Küstner in 1921, and this technique became the reference for defining a spe-

cific allergy. The association of allergic rhinitis and asthma in the same patient, often with a familial background, and the presence in serum of passive transfer activity to the clinical allergen led Coca and Cooke in 1923 to introduce the concept of *atopy* to imply a propensity to develop the altered state without an unusual exposure to the relevant allergens. As presently used, the term *atopic allergy* implies a familial tendency to manifest alone or in combination such conditions as asthma, rhinitis, urticaria, and eczematous dermatitis (atopic dermatitis). However, individuals without an atopic background may also develop hypersensitivity reactions, particularly urticaria and anaphylaxis, associated with the same class of antibody found in atopic individuals. Thus, the designation *diseases of immediate type hypersensitivity* presents a more suitable framework than the broad term *allergy* or the restrictive definition of atopy.

The activity in human serum passively transferred in the Prausnitz-Küstner reaction was established in 1966 as belonging to a unique immunoglobulin class, IgE; a myeloma protein with skin-fixing capacity was independently recognized and shown to be of the same class. The fixation of IgE to human basophils has been demonstrated by radioautography and electron microscopy. The presence of IgE on human tissue mast cells is inferred by analogy from radioautographic studies with monkey tissues. The biochemical characteristics of mast-cell activation, mediator generation, and secretion of both preformed and newly derived mediators are considered elsewhere (Chap. 71; Fig. 71-3) utilizing information gained from studies with human lung slices or peripheral blood leukocytes rich in basophils. IgE-dependent mediator generation and release also occur in the mast cells of human nasal polyps or skin and have been related to those tissues most involved in diseases of immediate type hypersensitivity.

The physicochemically and functionally diverse mast-cell-derived mediators, presented elsewhere (Table 257-1), include: histamine, which increases venular permeability and elicits both direct and reflex alterations in pulmonary mechanics; eosinophil chemotactic factor of anaphylaxis (ECF-A) with preferential chemotactic activity for eosinophils; neutrophil chemotactic factor of anaphylaxis (NCF-A), an uncharacterized protein with selective attraction for neutrophils; slow-reacting substance of anaphylaxis (SRS-A) with permeability-enhancing and smooth-muscle-contracting activity; and platelet activating factor (PAF), a lipid capable of initiating platelet secretion and aggregation. Thus the mast cell, bearing a specific recognition unit in the form of IgE, and positioned in tissues, has the capacity to respond to a foreign substance by eliciting a local increase in venular permeability and by initiating the influx of certain cell types from the marginated cell pool; this response allows plasma proteins such as antibody and complement and various phagocytic cells to be recruited to the reaction site without the necessity for extensive local tissue injury. On the other hand, an uncontrolled response could proceed from a physiologic local reaction to a self-perpetuating inflammatory state.

Consideration of the mechanism of immediate type hypersensitivity diseases in the human has focused largely on the IgE-dependent recognition of otherwise nontoxic substances. Support for this thesis has come from the finding that clinical ragweed pollenosis (hay fever) and reaginic antibody (IgE) production in response to the major purified protein antigen from ragweed pollen extract, antigen E, can be correleted with the human lymphocyte histocompatibility antigen (HL-A) haplotypes in successive generations of certain kindreds. A critical haplotype was unique for each family, indicating that the immune response (Ir) gene for antigen E is closely linked to the HL-A system. In another study, reaginic antibody to a minor ragweed pollen antigen, Ra5, was associated with a major histocompatibility antigen of the HL-A7 cross-reacting group in different kindreds. Although under separate genetic control from the specific immune response, IgE levels are elevated in most patients with atopic allergy. It is also likely that diseases of immediate type hypersensitivity may occur because of deficient intracellular controls of mediator generation or release, or both, or that the extracellular controls directed against mediator inactivation are impaired.

ANAPHYLAXIS **Definition** The life-threatening anaphylactic response of a sensitized human appears within minutes after administration of specific antigen and is manifested by respiratory distress often followed by vascular collapse, or shock without antecedent respiratory difficulty. Cutaneous manifestations exemplified by pruritus and urticaria with or without angioedema are characteristic of such systemic anaphylactic reactions.

Predisposing factors and etiology There is no convincing evidence that age, sex, race, occupation, or geographic location predisposes a human being to anaphylaxis except through exposure to some immunogen. According to some studies, atopy predisposes individuals to penicillin anaphylaxis.

The materials capable of eliciting the systemic anaphylactic reaction in the human include the following: heterologous proteins in the form of antiserum, hormones, enzymes, Hymenoptera venom, pollen extracts, and foods; polysaccharides such as iron dextran; and most commonly diagnostic agents and drugs such as antibiotics and even vitamins. The diagnostic and therapeutic agents are generally of low molecular weight and are considered to function as haptens which form immunogenic conjugates with host proteins. The conjugating hapten may be the parent compound, a nonenzymatically derived storage product, or a metabolite formed in the host.

Pathophysiology and manifestations Individuals differ in the time of appearance of perception of symptoms and signs, but the hallmark of the anaphylactic reaction is the onset of some manifestation within seconds to minutes after introduction of the antigen, generally by injection or less commonly by ingestion. There may be upper or lower airway obstruction or both. Laryngeal edema may be experienced as a "lump" in the throat, hoarseness, or stridor, while bronchial obstruction is associated with a feeling of tightness in the chest or audible wheezing. A particularly characteristic feature is the eruption of well-circumscribed, discrete cutaneous wheals with erythematous, raised, serpiginous borders and blanched centers. These urticarial eruptions are intensely pruritic and may be localized or distributed. They may coalesce to form giant hives, and seldom persist beyond 48 h. A localized, nonpitting, deeper edematous cutaneous process, angioedema, may also be present. It may be asymptomatic or cause a burning or stinging sensation.

In fatal cases with clinical bronchial obstruction, the lungs show marked hyperinflation on gross and microscopic examination. The microscopic findings in the bronchi, however, are limited to luminal secretions, peribronchial congestion, submucosal edema, and eosinophilic infiltration, and the acute emphysema is attributed to intractable bronchospasm which subsides with death. The angioedema resulting in death by mechanical obstruction occurs in the epiglottis and larynx, but the process is also evident in the hypopharynx and to some extent the trachea; on microscopic examination there is wide separation of the collagen fibers and the glandular elements; vascular congestion and eosinophilic infiltration are also present. Patients dying of vascular collapse without antecedent hypoxia from respiratory insufficiency have visceral congestion but no major shift in the distribution of blood volume. Whether the associated electrocardiographic abnormalities, with or without infarction, noted in such patients reflect a primary cardiac event or are secondary to a critical reduction in plasma volume has not been established.

The manifestations of the anaphylactic syndrome have been attributed to release of endogenous histamine. The role of SRS-A in altering pulmonary mechanics by causing marked bronchiolar constriction awaits further definition. The mediator(s) of the primary vascular collapse also remains obscure.

Diagnosis The diagnosis of an anaphylactic reaction depends largely upon an accurate history revealing the onset of the appropriate symptoms and signs within minutes after the responsible material is encountered. When only a portion of the full syndrome is present, such as isolated urticaria, sudden bronchospasm in an asthmatic patient, or vascular collapse after intravenous administration of an agent, it is difficult to exclude a nonimmunologic, toxicologic, or idiosyncratic response. For example, intravenous administration of a chemical mast-cell-degranulating agent elicits generalized urticaria, angioedema, and a sensation of retrosternal oppression without clinically detectable bronchoconstriction or hypotension. Furthermore, nonsteroidal anti-inflammatory agents such as indomethacin, aminopyrine, mefenamic acid, and acetylsalicylic acid may precipitate a life-threatening episode of obstruction of upper or lower airways in asthmatic subjects which is clinically reminiscent of anaphylaxis but is not associated with a detectable IgE response.

The presence of a labile reagin (IgE) in the heart blood of a patient dying of systemic anaphylaxis has been demonstrated at postmortem by passive transfer of the serum intradermally into a normal recipient, followed in 24 h by antigen challenge into the same site, with subsequent development of a wheal and flare, the Prausnitz-Küstner reaction. Indeed, such a reagin can be transiently identified in the serum of most patients who develop systemic anaphylaxis to a variety of different agents. In order to avoid the hazards of transferring hepatitis to the recipient in the Prausnitz-Küstner reaction, it is preferable to employ the less sensitive monkey recipient or a human leukocyte suspension enriched with basophils for subsequent antigen challenge.

Treatment and prevention Early recognition of an anaphylactic reaction is mandatory since death occurs within minutes to hours after the first symptoms. Mild symptoms such as pruritus and urticaria can be controlled by administration of 0.2 to 0.5 ml of 1:1000 epinephrine subcutaneously, with repeated doses as required at 3-min intervals for a severe reaction. If the antigenic material was injected into an extremity, the rate of absorption may be reduced by prompt application of a tourniquet proximal to the reaction site, administration of 0.2 ml epinephrine into the site, and removal of an insect stinger, if present, without compression. An intravenous infusion should be initiated to provide for administration of epinephrine, diluted a further fiftyfold, in the event of a vascular collapse, volume expanders, and vasopressive agents for intractable hypotension. Whether epinephrine acts to prevent mediator release, to reverse the action of mediators on target tissues, or both, is not established; but its early administration appears critical. When epinephrine fails to control the situation, hypoxia due to airway obstruction or related to a cardiac arrhythmia, or both, must be considered. Oxygen via a nasal catheter or intermittent positive pressure breathing of oxygen with 0.5 ml isoproterenol diluted 1:200 in saline may be helpful, but either endotracheal intubation or a tracheostomy is mandatory if progressive hypoxia exists (Chaps. 35, 129, and 268). Ancillary agents such as the antihistamine diphenhydramine, 50 to 80 mg intramuscularly or intravenously, and aminophylline, 0.25 to 0.5 g intravenously, are appropriate for urticaria-angioedema and bronchospasm, respectively. Intravenous corticosteroids are not effective for the acute event but may be considered for persistent bronchospasm and hypotension.

Prevention of anaphylaxis must take into account the sensitivity of the recipient, the dose and character of the diagnostic or therapeutic agent, and the effect of the route of administration on the rate of absorption. If there is a definite history of a past anaphylactic reaction, even though mild, it is advisable to select another agent or procedure. A skin test should be performed before the administration of certain materials producing a high incidence of anaphylactic reactions, such as horse serum or allergenic extracts, or when the nature of the past adverse reaction is unknown. Since even a skin or conjunctival test can produce a serious reaction, a scratch test should precede these tests in a high-risk situation. In the event that an agent must be used despite a positive history, a positive skin test, or both, the following precautionary measures should be taken. An intravenous infusion should be started, with intubation equipment and a tracheostomy set at hand; the material should be given intradermally, then subcutaneously, and then intramuscularly in increasing doses at 20 to 30-min intervals so that the initial dose by the next route does not exceed the final dose by the previous route. It is difficult to be certain that the desensitized mediator-containing cells have been accompanied by untoward consequences. It may be critical in this "exhaustion" or "pharmacologic" desensitization to give the therapeutic agent at regular intervals to prevent the reestablishment of a sensitized cell pool of hazardous size. A different form of protection involves the development of antibody of the IgG class which is protective against Hymenoptera venom-induced anaphylaxis by interacting with antigen so that less reaches the sensitized tissue mast cells.

URTICARIA AND ANGIOEDEMA **Definition** Urticaria and angioedema may appear separately or together as cutaneous manifestations of localized nonpitting edema; a similar process may occur at mucosal surfaces of the upper respiratory or gastrointestinal tract. *Urticaria* involves only the superficial portion of the dermis presenting as well-circumscribed wheals with erythematous raised serpiginous borders with blanched centers which may coalesce to become giant wheals. *Angioedema* is a well-demarcated localized edema involving the deeper layers of the skin including the subcutaneous tissue. Recurrent episodes of urticaria and/or angioedema of less than 6 weeks duration are considered acute, while attacks persisting beyond this period are designated chronic. Urticaria and angioedema must be differentiated from contact sensitivity, an acute vesicular eruption that progresses to chronic thickening of the skin with continued allergenic exposure, and from atopic dermatitis, a condition that may present as erythema, edema, papules, vesiculation, and oozing proceeding to a subacute and chronic stage in which vesiculation is less marked or absent, and in which scaling, fissuring, and lichenification predominate in a distribution that characteristically involves the flexor surfaces. The mechanisms and relationships of these conditions to immediate hypersensitivity are unknown.

Predisposing factors and etiology The occurrence of urticaria and angioedema is probably more frequent than usually described because of the evanescent, self-limited nature of such eruptions, which seldom require medical attention when limited to the skin. Although persons in any age group may experience acute or chronic urticaria and/or angioedema, these lesions increase in frequency after adolescence, with the highest incidence occurring in persons in the third decade of life; indeed, one survey of college students indicated that some 15 to 20 percent had experienced a pruritic wheal reaction.

The etiology is established in less than one-quarter of the cases of chronic urticaria. Acute urticaria and/or angioedema are characteristic of the anaphylactic syndrome and are recognized concomitants of subacute immunologic disease classified as "serum sickness" (Chap. 75). Urticaria and/or angioedema occurring during the appropriate season in patients with seasonal respiratory allergy or as a result of exposure to animals or molds is attributed to inhalation of pollens, animal dander, and mold spores, respectively. However, urticaria and angioedema secondary to inhalation are relatively uncommon compared with ingestion of fresh fruits, shellfish, chocolate, nuts, tomatoes, and various drugs, including penicillin-contaminated milk products, which may elicit not only the anaphylactic syndrome with prominent gastrointestinal complaints but also chronic urticaria. Additional etiologies include physical stimuli such as cold, solar rays, exercise, mechanical irritation (dermographism), and sources of specific antigens such as parasitic infestations and other infectious processes and occasionally malignancies.

Pathophysiology and manifestations Urticarial eruptions are distinctly pruritic, involve any area of the body from the scalp to the soles of the feet, and appear in crops of 24- to 72-h duration so that lesions that are fading in one area develop in another. Any area of the body may be involved, but the most common sites are the extremities, external genitalia, and face, particularly the region of the eyes and lips. Although self-limited in duration, angioedema of the upper respiratory tract may be life-threatening due to laryngeal obstruction, while gastrointestinal involvement may present with abdominal colic, with or without nausea and vomiting, and may precipitate unnecessary surgical intervention. No residual discoloration occurs with either urticaria or angioedema unless there is an underlying process leading to superimposed extravasation of erythrocytes.

The pathology of urticaria and angioedema is usually characterized by massive edema of the dermis in urticaria, and the subcutaneous tissue as well as dermis in angioedema. Collagen bundles in affected areas are widely separated, and the venules are sometimes dilated. The perivenular infiltrate may consist of lymphocytes, eosinophils, and neutrophils that are present in varying combination and number throughout the dermis. Allergen-induced wheal and flare reactions are characterized by mast-cell degranulation and an accumulation of eosinophils over hours to days. Although the cellular infiltrate is not a consistent feature of the usual urticarial eruption, urticaria can be a manifestation of necrotizing angiitis, in which case there is marked cellular infiltration, fibrinoid necrosis of the venules, nuclear debris, and erythrocyte extravasation.

The elicitation of a wheal and flare response upon injection of the relevant allergen into a patient with urticaria and/or angioedema, or into a site in a normal recipient prepared with serum from the patient, the Prausnitz-Küstner reaction, indicates an IgE-dependent, mast-cell-mediated reaction. In addition to mast-cell degranulation and eosinophilic infiltration, histamine and an uncharacterized slow-reacting substance are released into the involved tissues. Taken together, these findings are compatible with allergen-induced, IgE-dependent mast-cell degranulation associated with the generation and release of vasopermeability principles such as histamine, SRS-A, and ECF-A (Table 257-1).

Perhaps the best-studied example of mast-cell-mediated urticaria and angioedema is *cold urticaria.* Acquired cold urticaria is a disorder in which patients exposed to cold experience a urticarial eruption that may evolve into angioedema and be associated with syncope. Cryoglobulins, cryofibrinogens, cold agglutinins, or hemolysins may be recognized, but not in the majority of patients. The finding in a number of patients of a serum factor, characterized as being of the IgE class, that is capable of transferring the cold urticaria reaction to a skin site of a normal recipient has focused attention upon the mast cell in this condition. Immersion of an extremity in an ice bath precipitates angioedema of the distal portion with urticaria at the air interface within minutes of the challenge. Both histamine and ECF-A appear in the venous effluent during the immersion period and persist for as long as 30 min, while there is no elevation in the plasma or serum levels of these mast-cell-derived mediators in the venous blood of the contralateral unchallenged extremity.

DIAGNOSIS The rapid onset and self-limited nature of urticarial and angioedematous eruptions are distinguishing features. Additional characteristics are the occurrence of the urticarial crops in various stages of evolution and the asymmetrical distribution of the angioedema. Urticarial and/or angioedema involving IgE-dependent mechanisms are often appreciated by historical considerations implicating specific allergens, by seasonal incidence, by exposure to certain environments, or by physical stimuli such as cold, exercise, sunlight (solar urticaria), or trauma (dermographism).

Direct reproduction of the lesion with physical stimuli is particularly valuable because they so often establish the cause of the lesion. When antibody is involved, the diagnosis can be confirmed by careful testing with the eliciting factor to determine if a local wheal and flare result, and by passive transfer of such a reaction with serum of the patient to a skin site in a normal recipient, the Prausnitz-Küstner phenomenon. Passive transfer to the skin of a nonhuman primate or in vitro to human basophils may also be attempted; however, these procedures are less sensitive than the Prausnitz-Küstner reaction for the detection of allergen-induced responses and are negative to the physical stimuli. IgE-mediated urticaria and/or angioedema may or may not be associated with an elevation of total IgE or with peripheral eosinophilia. Fever, leukocytosis, or an elevated sedimentation rate are characteristically absent.

Urticaria and/or angioedema have also been observed as isolated manifestations of necrotizing angiitis involving the skin. Hypocomplementemia may or may not be present, but the sedimentation rate is usually elevated.

Hereditary angioedema (HAE) is transmitted as an autosomal dominant deficiency in the function of the inhibitor of the first component of complement (C$\bar{1}$INH). Recurrent gastrointestinal attacks with or without cutaneous angioedema are a characteristic feature, and death from laryngeal edema is a substantial hazard especially in certain kindreds. These patients do not have urticaria. An acquired deficiency of C$\bar{1}$INH observed in occasional patients with lymphatic malignancies is clinically identical to HAE but can be distinguished by the lack of a hereditary element, variability in the level of C$\bar{1}$INH, and a deficiency in the serum level of the first complement component.

Although the diagnosis of urticaria and/or angioedema may be clarified by establishing an IgE-mediated, mast-cell-dependent mechanism by demonstrating necrotizing angiitis with or without hypocomplementemia or by showing C$\bar{1}$INH deficiency, there are many instances of this syndrome in which immunopathologic clues are lacking and where the process is termed idiopathic.

Prevention and treatment Identification of the etiologic factor(s) and their elimination provide the most satisfactory therapeutic program; this approach is feasible to varying degrees with IgE-mediated allergens or physical stimuli. Topically applied steroids are of no benefit in the management of urticaria and/or angioedema, and while systemic steroids have no proved value, they are helpful in an occasional patient with necrotizing cutaneous angiitis or even ordinary urticaria/angioedema. Antihistamines and sympathomimetic agents often provide symptomatic relief; cyproheptadine, hydroxyzine, and similar drugs are held to be even more beneficial.

ALLERGIC RHINITIS Definition Allergic rhinitis is characterized by sneezing, rhinorrhea, obstruction of the nasal passages, conjunctival and pharyngeal itching, and lacrimation. Although commonly seasonal owing to its relation to airborne pollens, other patterns and etiologies occur. The use of the term "hay fever" to describe seasonal allergic rhinitis is a common convention but is literally inappropriate because the symptom complex is neither produced by hay nor associated with fever.

Predisposing factors and etiology Allergic rhinitis generally presents in atopic individuals, that is, in persons with a family history of a similar or related symptom complex and a personal history of collateral allergy expressed as eczematous dermatitis, urticaria, and/or asthma (Chap. 257). Symptoms generally appear before the fourth decade of life and tend to diminish gradually with aging, although complete spontaneous remissions are uncommon. A relatively small number of weeds which depend upon wind rather than insects for cross-pollination, as well as certain grasses and trees, produce insufficient quantities of pollen suitable for wide distribution by air currents to elicit seasonal allergic rhinitis. The dates of pollination of these species generally vary little from year to year in a particular locale but may be quite different in another climate. Molds, which are widespread in nature because they occur in soil or decaying organic matter, may propagate spores in a pattern dependent upon climatic conditions. Perennial allergic rhinitis occurs in response to allergens that are present throughout the year such as in desquamating epithelium in animal dander, the plant materials processed or chemicals utilized in an industrial setting, or the dust accumulating at work or at home. Dust has a diverse content including mites, and many patients with allergic rhinitis are sensitive only to house dust. Moreover, in many patients with this disease, no clear-cut allergen can be demonstrated. When present, the ability of allergens to cause rhinitis rather than lower respiratory symptoms may be attributed to their size, 10 to 100 μm. When inhaled, they are retained within the nose without progressing to the lower respiratory tract.

Pathophysiology and manifestations Episodic rhinorrhea, sneezing, and obstruction of the nasal passages with lacrimation and pruritus of the conjunctiva, nasal mucosa, and oropharynx are the hallmarks of allergic rhinitis. The nasal mucosa is pale and boggy, but the nares are not reddened or excoriated. The conjunctiva may be congested and edematous; the pharynx is generally unremarkable but may appear injected. Swelling of the turbinates and mucous membranes with obstruction of the sinus ostia and eustachian tubes precipitates secondary infections of the sinuses and middle ear, respectively, commonly in perennial but rarely in seasonal disease. Nasal polyps often arise concurrently with edema and/or infection within the sinuses and increase obstructive symptoms.

Biopsy specimens of nasal mucosa during an episodic allergic reaction show profound submucosal edema with infiltration predominantly by eosinophils, although some neutrophil polymorphonuclear leukocytes are present. Polyps, a feature in perennial rhinitis, are mucosal protrusions containing chiefly edema fluid with variable degrees of eosinophilic infiltration. Edema, and its clinical counterpart, rhinorrhea, are a consequence of adjustment to external temperature that is mediated by blood flow to the tissues as well as the filtering action of the nasal mucosa. The convoluted nasal passages readily filter out particles above 10 μm in size by impingement in a mucous blanket at bends in their course; ciliary action then moves the entrapped particles toward the pharynx. Entrapment of pollen and digestion of the outer coat by mucosal enzymes such as lysozyme release protein allergens generally of 10,000 to 40,000 molecular weight. Mast cells located beneath and possibly in the respiratory mucosa in close approximation to venules and sensitized with IgE then respond to the allergen(s) derived from the pollen grains.

The mucosal surface fluid contains not only IgA that is present preferentially because of its secretory piece, but also IgE, which apparently arrives by diffusion from plasma cells distributed in proximity to mucosal surfaces. IgE fixes to mucosal and submucosal mast cells, and the intensity of the clinical response to inhaled allergens is quantitatively related to the naturally occurring or experimentally defined pollen dose. Specific IgE is distributed not only to tissue mast cells but also to circulating basophilic leukocytes; patients with more severe clinical disease have basophils which release histamine in response to lesser concentrations of allergen in vitro than do cells from patients with milder disease. Human nasal polyps from ragweed-sensitive patients release histamine, ECF-A, and SRS-A upon challenge with ragweed allergen in vitro. Polyps from nonallergic patients with cystic fibrosis or chronic sinusitis, passively sensitized by interaction with serum of a ragweed-sensitive patient, release the same mediators upon challenge with the allergen. Thus, the mast cells of nasal polyp tissue, and presumably of the nasal mucosa and submucosa, generate and release mediators through IgE-dependent reactions which are capable of producing tissue edema and eosinophilic infiltration. Seasonal or perennial abnormalities of the mucosa may facilitate further the capacity of the allergen to reach the tissue mast cells and might also augment the seasonal booster in specific IgE.

Diagnosis The diagnosis of seasonal allergic rhinitis depends largely upon an accurate history of occurrence coincident with the pollination of the offending weeds, grasses, or trees. The continuous character of perennial allergic rhinitis due to contamination of the home or place of work makes historical analysis difficult, but there may be a variability in symptoms that can be related to animal exposure or work habits. The term *vasomotor rhinitis* designates a symptom complex resembling perennial allergic rhinitis without an established allergic basis. Other entities to be excluded are exposure to irritants, upper respiratory infection, pregnancy with prominent nasal mucosal edema, and the use of certain therapeutic agents such as rauwolfia. Nasal polyps are a characteristic of perennial allergic rhinitis and are often associated with sinus infection.

The nasal secretions of allergic patients are rich in eosinophils, and peripheral eosinophilia with elevations in relation to clinical exacerbations is a common feature. Total serum IgE is frequently elevated, but the demonstration of immunologic specificity for IgE is critical to an etiologic diagnosis. Some normal individuals will exhibit a wheal and flare skin response to intracutaneous inoculation of high concentrations of common airborne allergens. The diagnosis rests not only on the skin test alone, but also on the correlation of the clinical history with skin reactivity to concentrations of allergen selected by controlled testing. This provides the best balance of selectivity with specificity. Scratch tests with food allergens are unreliable but are not dangerous, while intracutaneous testing may be, and elimination diets are the best approach to the diagnosis. Regardless of method of testing, food allergy is uncommon as a significant cause of allergic rhinitis.

Functional immunochemical in vitro tests to demonstrated IgE are available.

Prevention and treatment Avoidance of exposure to the offending allergen is the most effective means of controlling allergic diseases; removal of pets from the home to avoid animal danders, utilization of air filtration devices to minimize the concentrations of airborne pollens, travel to nonpollinating areas during the critical periods, and even a change of domicile to eliminate a mold spore problem may be necessary. *Immunotherapy,* often termed *hyposensitization* consists of repeated subcutaneous injections of gradually increasing concentrations of the allergen(s) considered to be specifically responsible for the symptom complex. Controlled studies in ragweed and grass allergic rhinitis have established that patients are partially relieved of their symptoms by such treatments applied over a period of years. Improvement appears to be dose-related, and the end point is based either on severe adverse local or systemic reactions to the allergen injection or on satisfactory relief of symptoms. The immunologic characteristics of a response include a rise in antibodies of the IgG class and a reduction in the reactivity of the peripheral leukocytes enriched for basophils to a fixed dose of allergen as assessed by histamine release. The antibodies of the IgG class might well reduce or neutralize the quantity of allergen available for interaction with the tissue mast cells but, more importantly, could modify the seasonal booster response in specific IgE synthesis. The increased threshold for response of peripheral basophil leukocytes could relate to "biochemical desensitization" or "exhaustion" from repeated exposure to allergen, possibly presented as an immune complex incapable of fully activating the target cells, or from a fall in cell-bound specific IgE.

Management with pharmacologic agents offers a diverse approach. Antihistamines are the only specific end-organ antagonists available for control of a mast-cell-derived reaction and are limited to competition with but one mediator. Nonetheless, antihistamines are very effective for some patients, and the side effects such as drowsiness and gastrointestinal distress, which limit the dosage of a particular preparation, can sometimes be circumvented by use of an agent of different structure. Local or small doses of systemic corticosteroids used seasonally are highly effective and without appreciable side effects. When required for perennial rhinitis, aerosol preparations of potent steroids sprayed directly into the nostrils may control symptoms without undue systemic effects. Alpha-adrenergic agents may be utilized orally or as nose drops to shrink the nasal mucous membranes and reduce secretions; however, these agents have the disadvantage that rebound vasodilatation and increased secretions are common. Disodium cromoglycate applied to the nasal mucosa by spray or as a powder offers an additional approach since the action is directed solely at preventing generation and release of mast-cell mediators; early studies indicate that it has greater efficacy in seasonal than in perennial allergic rhinitis.

REFERENCES

AUSTEN KF: Systemic anaphylaxis in the human being. N Engl J Med 291:277, 1973

KALINER M et al: Immunologic release of chemical mediators from human nasal polyps. N Engl J Med 289:277, 1973

KAPLAN AP et al: In vivo studies of mediator release in cold urticaria and cholinergic urticaria. J Allergy Clin Immunol 55:394, 1975

LICHTENSTEIN LM, NORMAN PS: Pathogenesis of allergic rhinitis, in *Immunological Diseases,* 2d ed., ed M Samter, Boston: Little, Brown, 1971, p. 825

NORMAN PS, LICHTENSTEIN LM: Allergic rhinitis: Clinical course and treatment, in *Immunological Diseases,* 2d ed., ed M Samter, Boston: Little, Brown, 1971, p. 840

SHEFFER AL, AUSTEN KF: Vascular responses: Urticaria and angioedema, in *Dermatology in General Medicine,* eds T Fitzpatrick et al, New York: McGraw-Hill, 1971, p. 1261

SOTER NA et al: Urticaria and arthralgias as manifestations of necrotizing angiitis (vasculitis). J Invest Dermatol 63:485, 1974

73
MULTIPLE MYELOMA AND OTHER PLASMA CELL AND LYMPHOCYTE DYSCRASIAS

EDWARD C. FRANKLIN

DEFINITION AND CLASSIFICATION The group of plasma cell dyscrasias consists of several disorders generally characterized by the uncontrolled proliferation of cells normally involved in antibody synthesis. In most instances, this is accompanied by the synthesis of a homogeneous immunoglobulin and/or one of its constituent polypeptide chains. Though precise classification of these disorders based on morphology is difficult, characterization of the proteins produced by the neoplastic cells permits their grouping into three major categories: (1) multiple myeloma—IgG, A, D, and E; (2) macroglobulinemia—IgM; (3) heavy-chain diseases—γ, α, and μ. A closely related variant that is being recognized more frequently as a result of widespread use of serum protein electrophoresis is *benign monoclonal gammopathy,* a clinically benign condition in which a serum protein abnormality is noted in the absence of a significant plasma cell abnormality.

ETIOLOGY As is true of most other neoplastic disorders, little is known about etiologic factors. The rare association of chromosomal abnormalities and the occasional familial occurrence do not provide real clues. Viral particles have been demonstrated repeatedly, but in the absence of successful transmission of the disease with cell-free extracts of tissues, it is most likely that these represent superinfections in immunologically debilitated hosts. The available animal models, especially those in mice, have not provided insights into the etiology of the human disease.

MULTIPLE MYELOMA

CLINICAL PICTURE Multiple myeloma is the most common of the plasma cell dyscrasias. It is characterized by the infiltration of the marrow by neoplastic plasma cells which in most instances produce a myeloma protein and/or one of its constituent polypeptide chains. In the advanced phases of the disease, the proliferating plasma cells result in diffuse osteoporosis, characteristic punched-out bony lesions often involving the skull, with no obvious repair on x-ray films, or pathologic fractures, most frequently of the vertebrae and ribs. Dissolution of bone, which may ultimately give rise to hypercalcemia, used to be explained by the erosive action of the invading plasma cells. Recent evidence suggests that the elaboration by the plasmacytes of an osteoclast-stimulating factor may be responsible in most cases. Though painful fractures and bony lesions have long been considered the hallmark of myeloma, it now appears that the majority of patients with myeloma do not have clinically apparent bony lesions at the time of diagnosis, or even later in the disease, and that such lesions are often a late manifestation of the disease. This is probably in part the result of earlier diagnosis of the disorder in the latent period, which may last several years and during which the serum electrophoretic pattern is abnormal in the absence of clinical evidence of disease. In spite of the frequent absence of clinically apparent bony lesions until the tumor cell number reaches 1×10^{12} (about 1 kg) per m^2, virtually every patient with multiple myeloma (with the possible exception of those rare persons with multiple soft-tissue plasmacytomas) has widespread infiltration of the marrow with malignant plasma cells which generally can be detected by bone marrow aspiration (see below).

The presence of nonspecific findings such as weakness, anemia, an elevated sedimentation rate, or an unexplained infection, particularly bacterial pneumonia, is grounds for suspecting this disorder and for attempting its diagnosis. Occasionally attention is directed to myeloma through the discovery of a homogeneous protein in the serum or urine or the gradual onset of the nephrotic syndrome. As the disease progresses, the following manifestations may become prominent: (1) Frequent and recurrent infections, most often bacterial pneumonias, which are often the immediate cause of death. They are usually the result of impaired antibody synthesis, but occasionally defects in cellular immunity and a decrease in polymorphonuclear leukocytes, either as a manifestation of the disease or as a result of therapy, are responsible. (2) Chronic renal dysfunction, with several factors contributing to the development of renal failure. Probably the most common is the tubular damage resulting from the reabsorption of large amounts of Bence Jones proteins filtered by the glomeruli, or the occasional development of proteinaceous casts, which can obstruct and destroy entire nephrons. In the initial phases the so-called myeloma kidney is associated with proteinuria, which may progress to the nephrotic syndrome and uremia. Occasionally specific tubular reabsorption defects, including the Fanconi syndrome of adults, are seen. Somewhat rarer are amyloid deposits in the kidney, which may give rise to nephrosis and occasionally to renal failure. Other factors contributing to renal disease are severe hypercalcemia, recurrent pyelonephritis, and hyperuricemia, due either to rapid cellular turnover or to vigorous cytotoxic therapy. Acute renal failure may be precipitated by severe dehydration or by massive uricosuria following a course of chemotherapy. (3) Damage to other organs, such as the nervous system, especially the cord and nerve roots (which may be damaged by a pathologic fracture of a vertebra), the liver and spleen (which may be injured by the deposition of amyloid), and on rare occasions, the lungs and other structures, in which localized plasmacytomas develop. Clinically apparent involvement by myeloma deposits in the liver, spleen, and lymph nodes is very rare and thus distinguishes multiple myeloma from some of the related disorders, such as macroglobulinemia and heavy-chain disease. In about 5 to 10 percent of the patients symptoms are due to the abnormal protein, which can induce symptoms by a variety of mechanisms (see below).

LABORATORY FEATURES A number of nonspecific laboratory abnormalities is noted. A marked elevation of the sedimentation rate is the rule and often provides the first clue to this illness. Anemia, probably the result of many factors (including marrow replacement, hemolysis, infection, renal failure, and effects of therapy) is common, and the blood smear often shows marked rouleau formation. In addition, hyperuricemia (as a result of rapid cell turnover), uremia, and hypercalcemia without an increase in alkaline phosphatase may be seen.

Though multiple myeloma may be suspected on clinical grounds, the diagnosis requires the demonstration of characteristic changes in the marrow and is usually supported by finding a homogeneous spike on serum and urine electrophoresis. Because of the uneven distribution of the lesions and the importance of histologic documentation, a normal marrow aspirate in a patient clinically suspected of having multiple myeloma should be followed by additional aspirates or marrow biopsies from other sites. Characteristically, in the marrow there is an increase in plasma cells, which make up more than 15 percent and often up to 90 percent of myeloid cells. They frequently occur in sheets, are often binucleate, and may contain one or two nucleoli. The cytoplasm is usually blue with Wright's stain, because of the abundance of ribonucleic acid but may on occasion be acidophilic; the rough endoplasmic reticulum may contain proteinaceous inclusions known as Russell's bodies. The nuclear chromatin is often finer than that of a normal plasma cell, and the nucleus may show some mitotic figures. In rare instances of plasma cell leukemia, plasma cells can be seen in the peripheral blood. Occasionally, the marrow is infiltrated by lymphocytoid plasma cells rather than by the characteristic plasma cells.

A homogeneous protein component ranging in mobility from the slow γ- to the α_2-globulin is seen on serum electrophoresis in about 60 percent of patients, in the urine only in about 20 percent, and in both serum and urine in another 20 percent. Probably fewer than 2 percent of patients, especially those with far-advanced rapidly progressive disease, fail to show a spike; such patients often show a marked depression of all immunoglobulins. The abnormal component is generally first detected on paper or cellulose acetate electrophoresis, and is recognized on the basis of its homogeneity rather than by the absolute concentration. Although in most patients the concentration of γ- or β-globulins is definitely increased, an absolute increase is not required for the diagnosis. Routine electrophoresis alone is incapable of further defining the nature of the protein component; differentiation between the major classes and subclasses of immunoglobulins requires immunoelectrophoretic analyses. Since the frequency of an immunoglobulin class or subclass among myeloma proteins is similar to that of the normal counterpart, IgG myelomas are more common than IgA, IgD myelomas are quite rare, and only a small number of IgE myelomas has been noted. Detection of an abnormal protein in the urine is also best accomplished by electrophoretic and immunoelectrophoretic techniques, since Bence Jones proteins can be missed when Albusticks are used. In the absence of significant renal disease, only a homogeneous component representing light chains, Bence Jones proteins, is seen. With severe renal damage late in the disease, this component may be obliterated by the presence of most of the serum proteins which pass through the damaged glomeruli. As with normal immunoglobulins, κ light chains are about twice as frequent as λ proteins.

DIAGNOSIS The characteristic clinical features coupled with the results of bone marrow aspirates and serum and urine electrophoresis make definitive documentation relatively easy, although on occasion more than one site has to be aspirated to demonstrate the plasma cell abnormality. It is important to attempt to differentiate myeloma from "benign monoclonal gammopathy," metastatic tumors to bone, and on occasion hyperparathyroidism. With a proper index of suspicion, multiple myeloma can be documented in many elderly persons with unexplained infections, bone pain, renal disease, and anemia.

PROGNOSIS When this disease is diagnosed in the clinically obvious state, the prognosis is unfavorable; most patients left untreated are dead within a year or two. With the more frequent discovery of the disease during the latent period between its onset and its clinical perception, more patients now survive for longer periods after diagnosis. In addition, chemotherapy (see below) has significantly improved the prognosis.

The myeloma cell mass, and hence the prognosis, appear to be rather accurately reflected by the extent of the bony lesions on x-ray, the serum calcium and hemoglobin levels, the concentration of a homogeneous immunoglobulin in serum and urine, and the level of serum albumin. In addition, renal dysfunction, regardless of cause, affects the prognosis adversely. Using these criteria, attempts are being made to evaluate clinical staging systems to monitor the course of the disease and the effects of therapy. Renal failure, recurrent infections, and general debilitation are the most common causes of death in this disease.

TREATMENT Proper nutrition, hydration, mobilization, and analgesia are important as supportive measures and help delay the onset of hypercalcemia and some of the renal complications. Allopurinol is of use in preventing hyperuricemia, and steroids aid in the treatment of hypercalcemia. Plasmapheresis is of value when the hyperviscosity syndrome is present (see below). X-ray therapy is used in the treatment of localized lesions, particularly those resulting from the presence of bony lesions, and can be used, together with systemic chemotherapy, under careful supervision.

Chemotherapy with either of two alkylating agents (melphalan and cyclophosphamide) is the treatment of choice and, if properly used, results in clinical improvement and prolongation of survival in more than 50 percent of patients. There are few deleterious side effects. In addition to subjective increase in well-being and a decrease in bone pain, objective signs of improvement include a rise in hematocrit, decrease in the myeloma protein and a concomitant increase in normal immunoglobulin levels, decreased frequency of infections, and lack of progression and sometimes healing of bony lesions. These agents can be given either by continuous therapy (melphalan 2 to 4 mg per day, cyclophosphamide 1 to 4 mg per kg per day), often after an initial loading dose, or by intermittent therapy (melphalan 0.25 mg per kg per day for 4 days every 6 weeks, together with prednisone). Several reports suggest that intermittent therapy with steroids, and perhaps the added use of cycle-active drugs like vincristine, may be more effective. Regardless of the regimen employed, the patients must be carefully followed to prevent severe marrow depression. White blood cell counts between 2,000 to 4,000 per mm^3 are considered safe; if the levels fall lower, therapy must be discontinued temporarily. Perhaps either as a consequence of the longer period of survival of treated patients or the use of alkylating agents, myelomonocytic leukemia is being seen with increased frequency terminally.

BENIGN MONOCLONAL GAMMOPATHY

A closely related disorder which is often difficult to distinguish from multiple myeloma is the entity known as benign monoclonal gammopathy. This has been recognized through the application of electrophoresis as a routine laboratory procedure. In a large study in Sweden about 1 percent of the population was shown to have a homogeneous serum spike, usually an IgG or IgA globulin. In persons over seventy, the incidence increased to 3 percent. Careful study of these asymptomatic individuals usually reveals only a moderate increase of plasma cells in the marrow and no evidence of anemia, bony lesions, or renal disease. Generally, there is less than 2 g per 100 ml γ-globulin, and Bence Jones proteins are rarely noted. Long-term follow-up of such cases has not yet been carried out, but up to now few of them have progressed to overt myeloma. Although it seems possible that some of these persons may have multiple myeloma in the latent period and will later develop the clinical manifestations of the disease, it seems likely that many have a benign disorder, possibly a pronounced immune response to some unknown antigen. Homogeneous antibodies in the absence of myeloma have been induced in genetically predisposed mice and rabbits with pneumococcal and streptococcal antigens and may represent the experimental counterpart to this disorder. Regardless of the ultimate nature of this disorder, most investigators now feel that chemotherapy is not warranted.

Closely related to this disease is the association of a myeloma spike with a variety of neoplasms and certain other diseases. Though it is tempting to speculate that some of these conditions represent an immune response to an underlying disease, there is no evidence to support such a view.

MACROGLOBULINEMIA

Macroglobulinemia includes a spectrum of disorders ranging from a mild, relatively benign, and often slowly progressive lymphocytic infiltration of the marrow and lymphoid organs to malignant and progressive forms of lymphosarcoma or lymphocytic leukemia, always associated with the presence in the serum of a homogeneous macroglobulin spike. Since this entity is defined by the biochemical abnormality in the serum, it may include the IgM equivalent of the benign monoclonal gammopathies.

Clinically, the disease generally occurs in the elderly and resembles a malignant lymphoma in the advanced stages. Many patients seek medical attention because of weakness, weight loss, and mild anemia, and may continue with mild nonspecific complaints for many years. Later they may develop bleeding from mucous membranes, signs and symptoms of the hyperviscosity syndrome (see below), lymphadenopathy, and hepatosplenomegaly. Not infrequently the disease may become more malignant and assume many of the clinical features of lymphosarcoma or lymphatic leukemia. Bone lesions are rare, and amyloid is occasionally seen as a complication. Not infrequently patients with macroglobulinemia develop the cold agglutinin syndrome (see below). Symptoms related to the abnormal proteins are more common in macroglobulinemia than in multiple myeloma.

LABORATORY FINDINGS As in multiple myeloma, anemia, increased sedimentation rate, and hyperuricemia are common. The diagnosis is suspected on clinical grounds and confirmed by electrophoresis, immunoelectrophoresis, and ultracentrifugation, which reveals a homogeneous IgM protein with a sedimentation coefficient of 19S and smaller amounts of more rapidly sedimenting components. Bence Jones proteins are often seen in the urine. The bone marrow may at times contain plasma cells but generally is infiltrated with lymphocytes or lymphocytoid plasma cells. Many mast cells may be seen. When involved, lymph nodes and spleen have the pathologic features of lymphosarcoma. If indicated, serum viscosity should be measured and cold agglutinins should be looked for.

PROGNOSIS AND TREATMENT Depending on when the diagnosis is made, the disease may be slowly progressive or rapidly fatal. In the early stages, no treatment is needed. Later on, the indications for chemotherapy and the type needed are similar to those in chronic lymphocytic leukemia. Occasionally x-ray therapy is indicated for local lesions. If hyperviscosity is symptomatic, vigorous therapy is imperative (see below).

HEAVY-CHAIN DISEASES

As with macroglobulinemia, this disorder is defined by the demonstration of the characteristic immunoglobulin heavy-chain (H-chain) fragment in serum or urine. Three of the five possible types of heavy-chain disease (γ, α, and μ), each with a characteristic clinical picture, have been recognized. Though these diseases may be suspected on clinical grounds, a definitive diagnosis is based on finding the appropriate heavy-chain fragment in the serum and/or urine.

GAMMA HEAVY-CHAIN DISEASE About 40 patients with γ heavy-chain disease have been studied. Most of them were elderly, although one was eighteen years old. Weakness, weight loss, lymphadenopathy (which may wax and wane), hepatosplenomegaly, and recurrent infections are common features. Of particular interest is the frequent involvement of the nodes in Waldeyer's ring, which may give rise to palatal edema and erythema and occasionally to respiratory difficulty. Bony lesions have been noted only once; clinically the disorder resembles a lymphoma more than myeloma.

Anemia, lymphocytosis, eosinophilia, thrombocytopenia, and hyperuricemia are commonly found. Since the marrow and lymph nodes are infiltrated with plasma cells, lymphocytes, or lymphocytoid plasma cells, the diagnosis cannot be made on morphologic grounds. It requires the demonstration in the serum and urine of a broad protein peak, usually with a β-globulin mobility, which is reactive with antiserums to γ chains and unreactive with antiserums to light chains. In some patients the protein may be present in trace amounts; in others it is produced in large amounts. The prognosis of this disorder is rather poor; most of the patients have died within 6 months to 4 years after diagnosis, most frequently of overwhelming infections. Chemotherapy has not proved useful. In several instances the disorder has progressed to a less differentiated form of reticulum cell sarcoma with concomitant decrease in heavy-chain production. Amyloidosis has been reported in two of the patients.

ALPHA-CHAIN DISEASE For unknown reasons, this appears to be the most common form of heavy-chain disease. In general, the disease occurs in the younger age groups and involves organs which normally synthesize IgA. In more than 90 percent of the 80 cases seen to date, a plasmacytic infiltrate of the intestinal tract gives rise to diarrhea, steatorrhea, and severe malabsorption. Since this disorder is most commonly encountered in the Mediterranean area, the intestinal form is often referred to as *Mediterranean lymphoma.* While generally rapidly progressive, the occurrence of remissions on only minimal therapy in several patients has raised the possibility of an infectious etiology. Four patients with involvement limited to the respiratory tract have been reported. As is the case with all types of heavy-chain diseases, the diagnosis can be suspected on clinical grounds, but cannot be proved without finding a protein reactive with antiserums to α chains but not light chains in serum and often in the urine. Because of the not infrequent presence of hidden light chains in IgA myeloma proteins, the absence of light chains must be confirmed chemically in most instances.

MU-CHAIN DISEASE The rarest of these entities is μ-chain disease; most of the 11 reported cases were seen in individuals with long-standing chronic lymphatic leukemia (CLL). Five of these patients also excreted a Bence Jones protein, and one had amyloid. An unusual feature, which should direct attention to the possibility of this entity in patients with CLL, is the finding of plasma cells with large vacuoles in the cytoplasm. This disorder of immunoglobulin synthesis is seen only rarely in CLL, however, since several surveys of large groups of patients failed to uncover additional instances. The diagnosis is difficult to make, since the protein is present in the serum in amounts too small to give rise to a characteristic spike and is not found in the urine. The abnormality is detected on immunoelectrophoresis by finding a component reactive with antisera to μ chains but not to light chains. Although almost all known patients died shortly after the detection of the protein, no statement can be made about the prognosis, since it is not known how long the disease had been present prior to its discovery.

OTHER IMMUNOGLOBULIN DISORDERS

NATURE OF IMMUNOGLOBULINS Correlation of the type of protein produced with several clinical syndromes has permitted a more precise classification of these disorders than was possible on morphologic grounds alone. In order to understand the disorders of protein synthesis, two points concerning normal immunoglobulin synthesis should be considered: (1) under normal conditions, synthesis of heavy and light chains is approximately equal, so that only intact immunoglobulins are secreted (a minimal excess of light chains is always noted however); (2) only one type of immunoglobulin is secreted by a cell at any single point of its existence. Bearing these two assumptions in mind, one may best view the protein components produced in these disorders in the light of the normal immunoglobulins and their structural units (Table 73-1).

Thus if heavy- and light-chain synthesis remains balanced in the markedly expanded cell pool, a patient with myeloma or macroglobulinemia will have a homogeneous myeloma protein or macroglobulin belonging to one of the major classes or subclasses. These proteins resemble normal immunoglobulins, and since many have been shown to possess antibody activity, they may represent no more than a normal component produced in excess. In certain instances, asynchronous production of heavy and light chains occurs. If only light chains are produced, a homogeneous protein spike (often with the thermal properties of a Bence Jones protein) appears in the urine and usually no abnormal protein is found in the serum. Since they represent light polypeptide chains and often fail to demonstrate the characteristic thermal properties of precipitating at 56°C and going back in solution at 100°C, it is preferable to refer to them as light-chain proteins and to rely on electrophoretic and immunologic methods for their identification. These cases cannot be classified as belonging to any of the major classes of plasma cell neoplasms and have on occasion been referred to as light-chain disease. If light-chain synthesis exceeds that of heavy chains, both a serum spike, related to one of the major classes of immunoglobulins, and a light-chain component are found in the urine. Occasionally, because of the existence of larger polymers or decreased catabolism, light chains accumulate in the serum and may give rise to a spike. In a small percentage of patients (1 to 2 percent), often late in the course of the disease, synthesis of heavy and light chains ceases so that no homogeneous component is seen. Such patients are often hypogammaglobulinemic, since background immunoglobulin synthesis is depressed.

Structurally altered proteins and polypeptide chains have been noted with increasing frequency. The most striking examples are seen in patients with "heavy-chain disease." Several γ- and α-chain proteins have been studied in sufficient detail to delineate the nature of the defect. In all instances where proteolytic digestion can be excluded, the proteins represent an incomplete heavy chain having an internal deletion of part of the Fd variable region and all the Fd constant region, with resumption of synthesis either just before or after the hinge region in the Fc fragment. Although determinations vary with the nature of the defect as well as with biosynthetic studies in vitro, in several instances these proteins represent synthetic products, and further proteolytic digestion seems to have occurred in a few. It is of interest that in all instances of γ and α heavy-chain disease, light-chain production has stopped, whereas in most patients with μ-chain disease, free light chains can be found.

While the heavy-chain disease proteins represent extreme examples of defective molecules, it has also been demonstrated that apparently intact myeloma proteins may have smaller deletions of parts of the heavy or light chain. It seems likely that in all these instances, the abnormal protein is the result of a mutation of a structural gene. In patients producing large amounts of intact proteins, regulatory factors ensuring the balanced synthesis of H and L chains persist, although it seems likely that the proliferating cells are no longer subject to feedback regulation. Where there is asynchronous polypeptide chain production, most often a fraction of the tumor cells produces only L chains, although a regulatory defect in some cases seems possible.

TABLE 73-1
Disorders of protein synthesis

*Disorder**	*Serum abnormality*
I Balanced synthesis: H = L	Homogeneous serum protein
II Unbalanced synthesis: L > H	
A Excess L	Homogeneous serum protein + Bence Jones protein
B Only L	Bence Jones protein only
III No synthesis: H + L	Hypogammaglobulinemia
IV Structural mutations:	
A Heavy-chain diseases	Broad serum spike
B Half molecules	Homogeneous serum protein
C Myelomas with deletion	Homogeneous serum protein

* *H = heavy-chain proteins; L = light-chain proteins.*

EFFECTS OF THE ABNORMAL PROTEINS The clinical manifestations of multiple myeloma and macroglobulinemia generally reflect the existence of a malignant disease and not the presence of the abnormal protein. In some patients, however, the existence of large amounts of the abnormal proteins, the synthesis of proteins with unusual solubility or antibody properties, or occasionally the marked depression of normal γ-globulins may be responsible for certain clinical features outlined below.

Hyperviscosity syndrome The presence in serum in high concentrations of a protein, most often a macroglobulin, may cause a marked rise in viscosity, which in turn may interfere with efficient circulation to the brain, digits, kidneys, or eyes. The fundi may show a characteristic appearance, with extremely dilated venules and many hemorrhages. The hyperviscosity often results in the sudden onset of confusion, which frequently progresses to severe organic central nervous system disturbances. Progressive signs of cardiac and peripheral vascular insufficiency result from the impaired circulation in the small capillaries. The diagnosis may be confirmed by demonstration of increased serum viscosity with an Ostwald viscosimeter. Treatment must be instituted immediately, with repeated plasmaphereses until the viscosity is diminished and symptoms subside, following which a maintenance schedule, in conjunction with appropriate chemotherapy, must be worked out to control the underlying disease. Plasmapheresis is particularly successful in patients with macroglobulinemia, because these high molecular weight proteins are confined largely to the intravascular space. Where indicated chemotherapy should be directed at the primary disorder (myeloma or macroglobulinemia).

Cryoglobulinemia Somewhat similar clinical findings may result from the presence of cryoglobulins, which are proteins that precipitate in the cold and redissolve on warming. Although cryoglobulins are often not associated with symptoms, they may on occasion cause peripheral vascular insufficiency and even gangrene after exposure to low temperatures. Cryoglobulins are often associated with multiple myeloma and macroglobulinemia, but they may occur even more commonly in small amounts in systemic lupus erythematosus or other "connective tissue" diseases, or even in the absence of any overt illness. About one-quarter of cryoglobulins are G myeloma proteins, less than 10 percent are macroglobulins, and about two-thirds are mixtures of IgG and IgM molecules. These mixtures are most often found in patients with arthralgia, one of the connective tissue diseases, and are associated with purpura and not infrequently with progressive, often fulminant, renal lesions reminiscent of those seen in nephritis caused by antigen-antibody complexes. In about one-third of these subjects the IgM component is monoclonal, presumably the product of a malignant clone of lymphocytes. The precise mechanism for cryoprecipitation is not known, and in general, there is little correlation between symptoms and the amount of cryoglobulins or the temperature at which precipitation occurs. There is evidence that many cryoglobulins may, in fact, be antibodies to γ-globulins.

Cold agglutinin disease Another disorder directly related to an unusual group of macroglobulins is the hemolytic anemia induced by cold agglutinins. Although antibodies which cause hemolysis after exposure to the cold may be seen transiently in certain infections, such as infectious mononucleosis or atypical pneumonia, they rarely cause severe hemolysis in any disease other than macroglobulinemia or lymphosarcoma. The cold agglutinins are generally directed against the I antigen of the red blood cell and usually possess only κ light chains. Unlike antibodies which interact with red blood cells at body temperature, cold agglutinins usually appear free in the circulation.

Bence Jones proteins Another disorder related to abnormal proteins is the renal disease seen in patients with Bence Jones proteinuria. The filtration of large amounts of these proteins through the glomeruli exposes the tubules to an enormous reabsorptive load, which may cause degeneration of tubular cells, deposition of proteinaceous inclusions in the cells, and the formation of tubular casts. This is often referred to as "myeloma kidney," and may result in renal failure with uremia or in the appearance of the nephrotic syndrome. Severe dehydration preceding certain diagnostic procedures such as intravenous pyelograms may be sufficient to precipitate acute renal failure in these patients. The kidney has been clearly established as the prime site of degradation of small proteins such as light chains. Consequently, the bulk of Bence Jones proteins is catabolized by the normal kidney, and only the excess appears in the urine. When renal function becomes impaired, the degradative function is diminished and the amount of Bence Jones protein in the urine often increases markedly.

Amyloid Amyloid is a fibrillar substance often associated with this group of diseases. It is discussed in detail in Chap. 114. It is likely that amyloid associated with plasma cell dyscrasias consists of fragments of light chains and that amyloid-like fibrils can be produced from certain Bence Jones proteins by proteolysis in vitro.

Miscellaneous On rare occasions paraproteins may interact with other substances, such as calcium and some of the clotting factors, or may coat blood platelets and interfere with the normal mechanisms of blood coagulation and hemostasis.

Hypogammaglobulinemias The recurrent infections often seen in patients with hypogammaglobulinemias (Chap. 74) are not directly caused by the presence of abnormal proteins but are probably attributable to the decrease in the immune response which is caused by the diminished production of immunoglobulins.

REFERENCES

Alexanian R et al: Combination chemotherapy for multiple myeloma. Cancer 30:382, 1972

Axelsson U, Hallen J: A population study on monoclonal gammopathy. Acta Med Scand 191:111, 1972

Brouet JC et al: Biologic and clinical significance of cryoglobulins. Report of 86 cases. Am J Med 57:775, 1974

Cohen JH, Rundles W: Managing the complications of plasma cell myeloma. Arch Intern Med 135:177, 1975

Forte FA et al: Heavy chain disease of the μ (γM) type: Report of the first case. Blood 37:137, 1970

Franklin EC (ed): Immunoglobulin diseases. Semin Hematol, 10, part 1, January, 1973, part 2, April, 1973 (series of reviews on the immunoglobulins and their disorders)

——: μ-Chain disease. Arch Intern Med 135:71, 1975

—— et al: Heavy chain disease—A new disorder of serum gamma globulins. Am J Med 37:332, 1964

HALLEN J: Discrete gammaglobulin (M-) components in serum: Clinical study of 150 subjects without myelomatosis. Acta Med Scand [Suppl] 462, 1966

HAMMACK WJ: Treatment of myeloma. Arch Intern Med 135:157, 1975

KYLE RA et al: Multiple myeloma and acute leukemia associated with alkylating agents. Arch Intern Med 135:185, 1975

MACKENZIE M, FUNDENBERG HH: Macroglobulinemia: An analysis of 40 patients. Blood 39:874, 1972

MELTZER M, FRANKLIN EC: Cryoglobulinemia—A study of 29 patients. I. IgG and IgM cryoglobulins and factors affecting cryoprecipitability. Am J Med 40:828, 1966

—— et al: Cryoglobulinemia—A clinical and laboratory study. II. Cryoglobulins with rheumatoid factor activity. Am J Med 40: 837, 1966

OSSERMAN K, TAKATSUKI K: Plasma cell myeloma—γ-globulin synthesis and structure: A review of biochemical and clinical data with the description of a newly recognized and related syndrome, Hγ2 chain (Franklin's) disease. Medicine 42:357, 1963

RITZMANN SE: Idiopathic (asymptomatic) monoclonal gammopathies. Arch Intern Med 135:95, 1975

SALMON, S, DURIE BGM: Cellular kinetics in multiple myeloma. Arch Intern Med 135:131, 1975

SELIGMANN M: Immunochemical, clinical and pathological features of α chain disease. Arch Intern Med 135:78, 1975

74
IMMUNE DEFICIENCY DISEASES

ALEXANDER R. LAWTON III
MAX D. COOPER

INTRODUCTION Immunologic functions are mediated by two developmentally divergent, but functionally interacting, families of lymphocytes. The activities of B and T lymphocytes, and their products, in host defense are closely integrated with the functions of other cells of the reticuloendothelial system. Fixed and wandering macrophages play an important role in the trapping and processing of antigens and become effector cells, especially when activated by products of T lymphocytes. The scavenger activity of polymorphonuclear leukocytes is directed and made specific by antibodies in concert with products of the complement system (Chap. 71). The interaction of basophils and tissue mast cells with IgE antibodies in causation of immediate hypersensitivity is discussed in Chap. 72. Consideration of these interrelationships is an important part of the analysis of patients with suspected immune deficiency.

CLINICAL DISEASE FEATURES COMMON TO IMMUNE DEFICIENCY Immunodeficiency syndromes, whether congenital, spontaneously acquired, or iatrogenic, are characterized by unusual susceptibility to infection and, sometimes, to autoimmune disease and lymphoreticular malignancies. The types of infection often provide the first clue to the nature of the immunologic defect.

Patients with defects in humoral immunity have recurrent or chronic sinopulmonary infection, meningitis, and bacteremia, most commonly caused by pyogenic bacteria such as *Hemophilus influenzae, Streptococcus pneumoniae,* and staphylococci. This spectrum of infections is similar to that occurring in patients with normal immune responses, but with either neutropenia or a deficiency of the pivotal third component of complement (C3), suggesting that a tripartite collaboration involving antibody, complement, and phagocytes exists as the chief mechanism of host defense against pyogenic organisms. Binding of antibody to the bacterial surface causes activation of the complement system. One cleavage product of activated C3 serves as a chemotactic factor for polymorphonuclear leukocytes. Activated C3b fixed to bacterial surfaces facilitates phagocytosis by interaction with C3b receptors on neutrophils.

The response of agammaglobulinemic patients to systemic virus infections is equally instructive. The clinical course of primary infection with agents such as varicella or rubeola, unless complicated by bacterial infection, does not differ significantly from that of the normal host. Agammaglobulinemic patients rarely manifest failure to produce antibodies by having multiple episodes of the same viral illness. One important exception to the implication that antibodies are needed primarily to provide lasting immunity to virus infections occurs with hepatitis B virus; agammaglobulinemic patients fail to clear the Australia antigen and have a fulminant, often fatal, course.

The occurrence of unusual serious infection, for example, *H. influenzae* meningitis in an older child or adult, warrants consideration of humoral immune deficiency. Bacterial infections in certain sites may also suggest this possibility. Chronic otitis media occurs frequently in patients with hypogammaglobulinemia, and is significant because of its relative rarity in normal adults. Pansinusitis, although almost invariably present in immunoglobulin deficiency, is a less helpful finding because it is not rare in apparently normal people. Bacterial infections of the skin or urinary tract are less frequent problems in hypogammaglobulinemic patients.

Abnormalities of cell-mediated immunity predispose to *disseminated virus infections,* particularly with latent viruses such as herpes simplex (Chap. 206), varicella-zoster (Chap. 205), and cytomegalovirus (Chap. 211). Patients so affected also almost invariably develop mucocutaneous candidiasis, and frequently acquire widely disseminated fungal infections.

Pneumonia caused by the protozoan *Pneumocystis carinii* is also common (Chap. 219).

Infestation with the intestinal parasite *Giardia lamblia* is a frequent enough cause of diarrhea in antibody-deficient patients to warrant diagnostic duodenal aspiration and intestinal biopsy when the organism cannot be demonstrated in the stool.

T-cell deficiency is probably always accompanied by some abnormality of antibody responses, although this may not be reflected by hypogammaglobulinemia. This may explain in part why patients with primary T-cell defects are also subject to overwhelming bacterial infection.

The most severe form of immune deficiency occurs in individuals, usually infants, who lack both cell-mediated and humoral immune functions. They are susceptible to the whole range of infectious agents including organisms not ordinarily considered pathogenic. Multiple infections with viruses, bacteria, and fungi occur, often simultaneously. Because donor lymphocytes cannot be rejected by the recipients, blood transfusions can produce fatal graft-versus-host disease.

DIFFERENTIATION OF T AND B CELLS The functional deficits which occur in both congenital and acquired immunodeficiencies can be most usefully viewed as defects at various points along the differentiation pathways of immunocompetent cells. For this reason certain features of the development and differentiation of T and B cells that are especially relevant to the analysis of immunodeficiency are briefly presented here; Chap. 71 provides a general account of their roles in cellular and humoral immunity.

A subpopulation of hemopoietic stem cells may become restricted to lymphoid differentiation prior to migration to the thymus, where T cells are generated, or to the fetal liver and adult bone marrow, where B-cell development occurs (Fig. 74-1). A major function of central lymphoid tissues is to generate the clonal diversity characteristic of the immune system. Each T or B lymphocyte is induced to express on its surface receptor molecules of a unique specificity for antigen. The receptors of B lymphocytes are immunoglobulins. The nature of T-cell receptors is not yet precisely defined, but they may be similar or identical to the variable regions of immunoglobulins. Proliferation of individual clones of lymphocytes is stimulated in the central lymphoid organs and is determined genetically. This process of clonal development is independent of antigen and reflects a genetically programmed sequence of differentiation analogous to that of primary erythropoiesis or myelopoiesis. This phase, termed *primary differentiation,* begins early in human fetal development but probably continues into adult life.

The developmental sequence for expression of diverse immunoglobulin classes by human B lymphocytes begins with expression of IgM. The expression of IgD on IgM-bearing cells occurs later. Lymphocytes committed to synthesis of IgG, IgA, and IgE are all derived from IgM-bearing precursors through a genetic switch mechanism.

There is increasing evidence suggesting that the diversity of T lymphocyte function is associated with developmentally divergent subpopulations of T-cells. T lymphocytes which, as helpers or suppressors, regulate B-lymphocyte differentiation may not be the same as those capable of becoming killer cells. This developmental heterogeneity may explain some immunodeficiencies in which T-cell functions are impaired selectively.

In addition to generating T cells, the thymus apparently secretes hormonal products which regulate cellular maturation in peripheral lymphoid tissues. These hormones have been called *thymosin* or *thymin;* deficiencies of these factors have been implicated in some immunodeficiencies.

The events designated *secondary differentiation* (Fig. 74-1) follow stimulation of specific clones of lymphocytes by antigen. These processes are synonymous with the immune response (Chap. 71). Particularly important in consideration of immunodeficiencies are the collaborative interactions among macrophages, T cells, and B cells. B lymphocytes can proliferate in response to thymus-dependent antigens without the help of T cells, and may differentiate to IgM-secreting plasma cells when stimulated by thymus-independent antigens such as polysaccharides. However, production of normal quantities of antibodies, particularly those of the IgA and IgG classes, requires the collaboration of T cells.

Differentiation of T or B cells may be arrested at either the primary or secondary stage (Fig. 74-1). Reflecting the complex cellular interactions involved in immune responses and the pivotal role played by T lymphocytes, immune deficiencies primarily involving T cells are usually also associated with abnormal B-cell function. Conversely, immunodeficiencies manifested primarily by inability to produce antibodies may be caused by T-cell defects not associated with abnormal cell-mediated immunity.

EVALUATION OF IMMUNODEFICIENT PATIENTS Many of the laboratory assays used for precise evaluation of immunologic functions in man are available only in specialized centers; nevertheless, most immunodeficiencies may be diagnosed by thoughtful use of tests available in most clinical laboratories. Table 74-1 presents a résumé of laboratory investigations roughly in order of increasing complexity.

A careful history will usually indicate whether the major problem involves the antibody-complement-phagocyte system or cell-mediated immunity. A history of a normal response to smallpox vaccination or of contact dermatitis due to poison ivy suggests intact cellular immunity. Lymphopenia and the absence of palpable lymph nodes may be important findings. However, patients with profound immunodeficiency may have diffuse lymphoid hyperplasia.

Humoral immunity With rare exceptions, deficiency of humoral immunity is accompanied by diminished serum concentration of one or more classes of immunoglobulin. Normal values vary with age, and adult concentrations of IgM (100 mg per 100 ml) are reached at about one year, of

FIGURE 74-1

Sites of defects in lymphoid differentiation that cause immunodeficiencies. When neither T nor B cells develop, the defect presumably involves a common lymphoid precursor. Rarely, other hemopoietic cell lines are also absent, indicating an even more severe abnormality of hemopoietic stem cells. Absence of either T or B cells suggests malfunction or absence of the thymus or the bursa equivalent. However, agammaglobulinemia and deficiencies of some T-cell functions may occur despite the presence of normal numbers of B or T cells in the circulation. Failure of B lymphocytes to differentiate to plasma cells may be due to intrinsic cellular abnormalities or to faulty T-cell regulation.

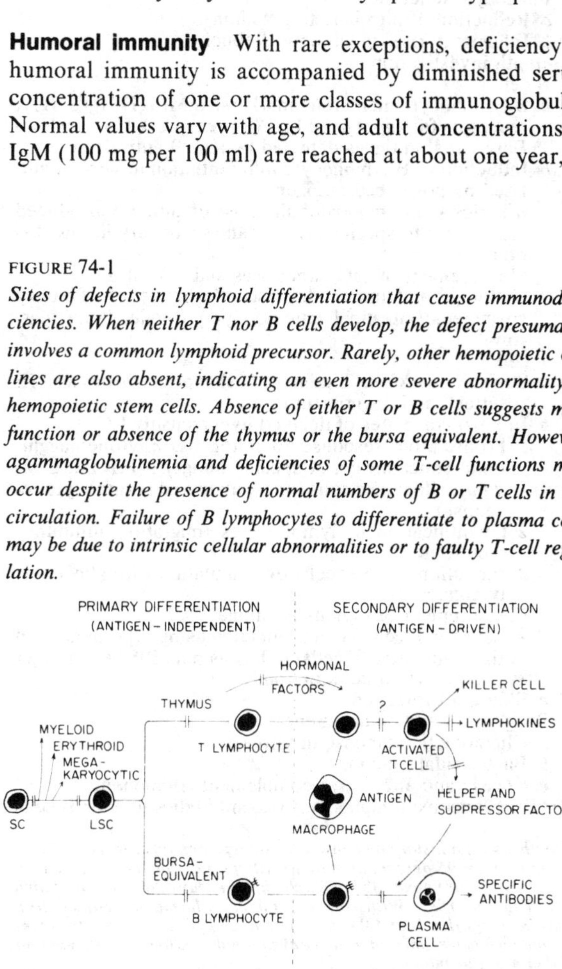

IgG (1,000 mg per 100 ml) at five to six years, and of IgA (200 mg per 100 ml) at puberty (Chaps. 71, 73). Also, the wide range of values among normal adults creates difficulty in defining the lower limits of normal. Reasonable estimates for low normal values are 40 mg per 100 ml for IgM, 500 mg per 100 ml for IgG, and 50 mg per 100 ml for IgA.

TABLE 74-1
Laboratory evaluation of host defense defects

A Preliminary screen*
- *a* Complete blood count with differential smear
- *b* Quantitative immunoglobulin levels

B Readily available studies†
- *1* B-cell function
  - *a* Natural or commonly acquired antibodies: isohemagglutinins, "febrile" agglutinins, antibodies to common viruses (rubella, rubeola, influenza), and toxins (diphtheria, tetanus)
  - *b* Response to immunization (typhoid, polio, diphtheria-tetanus vaccines)
- *2* T-cell function
  - *a* Skin tests (P.P.D., mumps, *Candida, Trichophyton,* histoplasmin), streptokinase-streptodornase (Varidase, 1:200)
  - *b* Contact sensitization with dinitrochlorobenzene
  - *c* Chest x-ray (thymus shadow in infants, thymoma in adults)
- *3* Complement
  - *a* C3 (β_1C globulin)
  - *b* CH_{50} (total hemolytic complement)
- *4* Phagocyte function
  - *a* Reduction of nitroblue tetrazolium
  - *b* Inflammatory skin window (Rebuck)

C In-depth investigation
- *1* B cell
  - *a* B-lymphocyte membrane markers: IgM, IgD, IgG, IgA; receptors for aggregated IgG (Fc receptor), C3, Epstein-Barr virus; antigens detected by anti-B antiserum
  - *b* Induction of B-lymphocyte differentiation in vitro stimulated by pokeweed mitogen
  - *c* Kinetics and immunoglobulin class of antibody produced in response to specific primary and secondary immunization
  - *d* Measurement of IgG subclasses and κ/λ ratio
  - *e* Histologic and immunofluorescent examination of biopsy specimens (intestinal mucosa, lymph node, bone marrow)
- *2* T cell
  - *a* Surface markers: binding of sheep erythrocytes (E rosettes), anti-T antiserum
  - *b* In vitro correlates of delayed hypersensitivity
    - *1* Proliferative response to mitogens: phytohemagglutinin, concanavalin A specific antigens (P.P.D., *Candida*); allogeneic cells (one-way mixed lymphocyte response)
    - *2* Quantification of lymphokines (migration inhibitory factor, etc.)
    - *3* Induction of killer cells by stimulation with allogeneic lymphocytes
  - *c* Measurement of thymus hormones
  - *d* Assays for T-cell "helper" function using supernatants of antigen-activated T cells or T cells plus PWM to trigger B-lymphocyte differentiation
  - *e* Skin graft rejection
- *3* Phagocytes and complement
  - *a* Chemotactic response in vitro
  - *b* Bactericidal function
  - *c* Classic and alternative complement components
- *4* Miscellaneous: lymphocytotoxic antibodies to T or B cells

* *Together with a history and physical examination, these tests will identify more than 95 percent of patients with primary immunodeficiencies.*
† *These assays are generally available in either hospitals or state public health laboratories. With rare exceptions, information gained from tests in categories* A *and* B *is sufficient to diagnose and treat those immunodeficiencies amenable to conventional treatment with gammaglobulin or plasma.*

In the presence of borderline hypogammaglobulinemia assessing the patient's capacity to produce specific antibodies becomes particularly important. Most hospital laboratories can measure isohemagglutinins, antistreptolysin O, and "febrile agglutinins." Typhoid H and O agglutinins can be measured before and after immunization with standard typhoid vaccine. Many state public health laboratories can perform titrations for antibodies to common viral agents.

Since antibody deficiency may be mimicked clinically by deficiency of complement components, measurement of total hemolytic complement (CH_{50}) and C3(β_1C) should be a part of the evaluation of host defense. Estimation of numbers of circulating B lymphocytes has been of great value in determining the pathogenesis of certain types of immune deficiency. B lymphocytes are identified by the presence of membrane-bound immunoglobulins; additional markers include receptors for aggregated IgG (Fc receptor), receptors for the third component of complement (C3 receptor), and receptors which specifically bind the Epstein-Barr virus. Fc receptors and C3 receptors are also found on circulating monocytes. Moreover, not all B lymphocytes bear the C3 receptor. The Epstein-Barr virus receptor appears to be highly specific for B lymphocytes. They can also be identified and enumerated by specific heterologous antiserums, although these are difficult to prepare.

Pokeweed mitogen (PWA), an extract of the plant *Phytolacca americana,* has the capacity to induce B lymphocytes in culture to proliferate and differentiate to plasma cells. This activity requires the presence of T lymphocytes, which also proliferate in response to PWM. Thus, this assay can measure not only the capacity of B lymphocytes to differentiate, but can also assess the "helper" or "suppressor" function of patients' T lymphocytes.

Cellular immunity Human T lymphocytes can be most easily enumerated by their capacity to bind sheep erythrocytes in the cold, forming what are called *E rosettes.* The nature and function of this receptor are unknown, but they are not related to the antigen-specificity of T cells. T cells can also be enumerated by use of specific antiserums.

T-lymphocyte function can be measured in vivo by delayed hypersensitivity skin testing, using a variety of antigens to which the majority of older children and adults have been sensitized. Among the most useful are P.P.D., histoplasmin, *Candida* extract, *Trichophyton* extract, mumps, and streptokinase-streptodornase. The capacity to become sensitized to a new antigen may be tested by application of dinitrochlorobenzene to the skin, followed 2 weeks later by patch testing at a different site.

T-lymphocyte function may be estimated in vitro by the capacity of cells to proliferate in response to antigens to which the patient has been sensitized, to lymphocytes from an unrelated donor, or to the T-cell mitogens, which include phytohemagglutinin, concanavalin A, and pokeweed mitogen. The response is usually quantified by measurement of incorporation of radioactive thymidine into newly synthesized DNA. It is also possible to measure the production of lymphokines, particularly migration inhibition factor, by activated T cells. Finally, the ability of T cells activated in mixed lymphocyte culture to lyse target cells sensitized by phytohemagglutinin can be measured.

The capacity of T lymphocytes from immunologically normal persons to be activated in vitro with antigens or mitogens may be abolished or markedly diminished by acute febrile illness, treatment with corticosteroids, or stress. Except for these situations, there are relatively few instances in which normal numbers of T lymphocytes, as measured by the E rosette test, are not associated with relatively normal function in the aforementioned in vitro assays.

CLASSIFICATION Primary immunodeficiencies may be either congenital or acquired, and are currently classified according to mode of inheritance and whether the defect involves T cells, B cells, or both. Unfortunately, the best current classification, established by an expert committee of the World Health Organization, still places the majority of immunodeficiency diseases in an undefined category called *common variable immunodeficiency.* In general, this classification will be followed in the following discussion, which emphasizes three related concepts; first, that immunodeficiencies are most logically viewed as defects of cellular differentiation; second, that these defects may involve either primary development of T or B cells or the antigen-dependent phase of their differentiation; and third, that defects of secondary B-cell differentiation may in some instances reflect T-cell abnormalities resulting from faulty T-B collaboration.

Secondary immunodeficiencies are those not caused by intrinsic abnormalities in development or function of T and B cells. Examples are immune deficiency associated with malnutrition, protein-losing enteropathy, and intestinal lymphangiectasia. Also considered secondary are immunodeficiencies resulting from hypercatabolic states such as occur in myotonic dystrophy, immunodeficiency associated with lymphoreticular malignancy, and immunodeficiency resulting from treatment with x-rays, antilymphocyte serum, or cytotoxic drugs.

Severe combined immunodeficiency (SCID) This syndrome is characterized by gross functional impairment of both humoral and cell-mediated immunity. It is usually congenital, may be inherited either as an x-linked or autosomal recessive defect, or may occur sporadically. Affected infants rarely survive beyond one year. This syndrome has been associated with a diversity of defects in development of immunocompetent cells, some of which may be related to specific enzymatic abnormalities.

The classic example of SCID, *Swiss-type agammaglobulinemia,* is characterized by severe lymphopenia involving both T and B cells, and is inherited with an autosomal recessive pattern. Rarely, other hemopoietic cell lines fail to develop. The cellular defect in these forms of SCID logically rests with the precursor common to both T and B cells. The immunologic defects in a few of these patients have been repaired following transplantation of fetal liver as a source of stem cells, confirming the hypothesis that they have a thymus and bursa equivalent capable of supporting differentiation of normal stem cells. Some patients with autosomal recessive SCID are deficient in an enzyme involved with nucleic acid metabolism, adenosine deaminase (ADA). The precise role of ADA in lymphoid differentiation is not yet understood, but improvement of both clinical status and immunologic function has been described following treatment of a patient with exogenous enzyme.

Other patients with SCID have normal or only moderately diminished numbers of circulating lymphocytes; this feature has often been associated with the x-linked inheritance pattern. Virtually all the lymphocytes from several patients had surface immunoglobulins characteristic of B lymphocytes, suggesting that this form of SCID may be related to a faulty thymus epithelium.

A number of individuals with SCID have been successfully treated by transplantation of histocompatible bone marrow from sibling donors. The same treatment has been used in children and adults with leukemia or aplastic anemia (Chap. 76) following purposeful destruction of the immune system by irradiation and cytotoxic drugs. Other modes of treatment, including fetal liver transplants, have been successful in restoring immunocompetence, but as yet there are only short-term survivors. Treatment of these patients should probably be attempted only in centers with a strong research interest in this problem. It is crucial that these patients be recognized early and not be given blood transfusions which may cause fatal graft-versus-host disease.

T-cell immunodeficiency Primary T-cell defects are extremely difficult to define. Reflecting the diversity of T-cell functions, abnormalities of T-cell development may be responsible for a wide spectrum of immune deficiencies including severe combined immunodeficiency, apparently isolated defects in cell-mediated immunity, and syndromes presenting as antibody deficiency with apparently normal cell-mediated immunity. These defects may be acquired as well as congenital. Until very recently, laboratory assays of T-lymphocyte function were limited to correlates of cell-mediated immunity; no means were available for studying T-cell regulation of B-cell differentiation. With the development of appropriate methodology it will undoubtedly be found that clinically significant abnormalities of T cells are much more common and heterogeneous than is now appreciated.

DI GEORGE SYNDROME This is the classic example of isolated T-cell deficiency and results from maldevelopment of organs derived embryologically from the third and fourth pharyngeal pouches. Affected infants usually present with congenital cardiac defects, particularly those involving the great vessels, hypocalcemic tetany due to failure of parathyroid development, and absence of the thymus. Other associated abnormalities may include abnormal ears, shortened philtrum, and hypertelorism. Serum immunoglobulin concentrations are usually normal. Lymphocyte counts may be normal, but virtually all the lymphocytes are B cells. Carefully performed autopsies have often revealed a tiny, histologically normal thymus, usually in an ectopic location. With time, a few patients developed functional T cells. Patients with Di George's syndrome have had transplants of fetal thymus and subsequently have developed normal cell-mediated immunity, associated with T cells of host origin.

Children lacking the congenital anomalies associated with the Di George syndrome may present with severe impairment of cell-mediated immunity. Some have normal or even increased immunoglobulin levels, while others have selective deficiencies of one or more immunoglobulin classes. Specific antibody responses are usually impaired even in patients with normal concentrations of immunoglobulins. This ill-defined entity has been called the *Nezelof syndrome.*

In the light of present knowledge, these patients seem closely related to that subgroup of patients with severe combined immunodeficiency in whom failure of T-cell development appears to be the primary abnormality. Two recently reported patients had normal numbers of circulating B lymphocytes but diminished numbers of T cells and absent responses to T-cell mitogens. In one such patient, T-cell deficiency was associated with inherited deficiency of the enzyme nucleotide phosphorylase which functions in the same metabolic pathway as adenosine deaminase.

A few patients with isolated T-cell deficiency have been treated with fetal thymus grafts. Some have shown improvement in numbers of circulating T cells, in vitro reactivity to mitogens, and clinical condition, while others have had no change in status. A patient treated with thymosin developed increased numbers of circulating T cells and delayed hypersensitivity skin reactions associated with clinical improvement. Transfer factor has been reported to benefit a few patients.

ATAXIA-TELANGIECTASIA This is an autosomal recessive genetic disorder characterized by cerebellar ataxia, oculocutaneous telangiectasia, and immunodeficiency. Onset of truncal ataxia usually occurs in infancy and is progressive. Immunodeficiency is clinically manifest by recurrent and chronic sinopulmonary infection leading to bronchiectasis. The two most frequent causes of death are chronic pulmonary disease and malignancy. Lymphomas are most common, although carcinomas have also occurred.

The immunologic abnormalities seem to be related to maldevelopment of the thymus. If found at all, the thymus in autopsied patients has been markedly hypoplastic and similar in appearance to an embryonic thymus. Patients' lymphocytes frequently respond poorly to T-cell mitogens in vitro. Cutaneous anergy and delayed rejection of skin grafts are common. Although the number and class distribution of B lymphocytes are usually normal, most patients are deficient in serum IgE and IgA, and a smaller number have reduced serum levels of IgG. IgM and IgD are usually normal. This suggests a maturational arrest of B lymphocytes secondary to T-cell dysfunction. Indeed, in one IgA-deficient patient, peripheral lymphocytes were triggered by pokeweed mitogen to develop into IgA-synthesizing plasma cells.

There is circumstantial evidence that ataxia-telangiectasia may involve a generalized defect in cellular differentiation. Ovarian agenesis occurs frequently. Persistence of very high levels of oncofetal proteins, including α-fetoprotein and carcinoembryonic antigen, has been found in patients' serum. At the other end of the age spectrum are signs of progeria, including premature graying and early development of senile keratoses and vitiligo. It has been suggested that the telangiectasia is also related to progeria.

Only symptomatic treatment is available. Unless severe deficiency of IgG is present, therapy with gamma-globulin is not indicated. Transplantation with histocompatible bone marrow was followed in one patient by increased synthesis of IgA and transient improvement of cellular immune responsiveness, but chimerism could not be demonstrated.

Immunoglobulin deficiency syndromes X-LINKED AGAMMAGLOBULINEMIA This syndrome represents a central failure of B-lymphocyte differentiation. The majority of affected males have very few immunoglobulin-bearing B lymphocytes in their circulation and lack primary and secondary lymphoid follicles. They usually have a substantial number of small mononuclear cells bearing receptors for aggregated immunoglobulin and C3. Although resembling B lymphocytes, these cells have been shown to have markers characteristic of the monocyte line and to lack the B-lymphocyte specific surface antigen(s) and receptors for Epstein-Barr virus. A few patients with well-documented x-linked agammaglobulinemia have had a normal number of B lymphocytes, suggesting that there may be two distinct forms of this disease.

Agammaglobulinemia is a misnomer, as most patients with this and other forms of severe panhypogammaglobulinemia synthesize some immunoglobulins, primarily of the IgG class. Within the same family some affected males have had substantial levels of IgM, IgG, and IgA, while others have been nearly agammaglobulinemic. All these patients were markedly deficient in circulating B lymphocytes. This observation suggests that the few B lymphocytes which are generated are fully capable of differentiating to plasma cells and secreting immunoglobulins. A form of arthritis with some of the features of rheumatoid disease occurs in some of these patients and may remit following treatment with gamma-globulin.

TRANSIENT HYPOGAMMAGLOBULINEMIA OF INFANCY This is a reversible syndrome in which normal physiologic hypogammaglobulinemia of infancy is unusually prolonged and severe. IgG levels of normal-term infants commonly drop to levels of 300 to 400 mg per 100 ml between three and six months of age as maternally derived IgG is catabolized; levels subsequently rise reflecting the infants' increased synthetic capacity. In transient hypogammaglobulinemia, the rate of synthesis of IgM, IgG, and IgA remains low for long periods. Some of these infants have a reduced number of B lymphocytes while others have a normal number.

ISOLATED DEFICIENCY OF IgA This is by far the most commonly encountered immunodeficiency, occurring with a frequency of approximately 1 in 600 individuals. With rare exceptions, both serum and secretory IgA are involved. Many adults with isolated IgA deficiency do not seem to have unusual problems with infection. Nevertheless, this condition is not benign. A substantial proportion of IgA-deficient individuals develop precipitating antibodies to IgA. These patients may have severe anaphylactic reactions when transfused with normal blood from a blood bank.

As a group, individuals with IgA deficiency have an increased number of respiratory infections of varying severity, and a few have had severe pulmonary disease such as bronchiectasis. Chronic diarrheal disease also occurs. The incidence of asthma and other atopic diseases among IgA-deficient patients is high, and, conversely, the incidence of IgA deficiency among atopic children has been found to be twenty to forty times that in the normal population. In one study it was found that combined deficiency of IgE and IgA (or IgE deficiency alone) did not predispose to recurrent respiratory infections, while IgA-deficient patients with normal or elevated IgE had recurrent sinopulmonary disease. IgA deficiency is also significantly associated with autoimmune diseases such as rheumatoid arthritis and systemic lupus erythematosus.

IgA deficiency may be familial, but no single pattern of inheritance has been encountered consistently. It has occurred in association with congenital intrauterine infections, such as toxoplasmosis, rubella, and cytomegalovirus infection. Several patients with abnormalities of chromosome 18 have had isolated IgA deficiency. Most commonly, the syndrome appears as a sporadic defect. It may be transient or acquired late in life.

The pathogenesis of IgA deficiency, whether genetic or caused by environmental insult, apparently involves a block in terminal differentiation of B lymphocytes. Of more than 60 patients studied, only one has lacked normal numbers of IgA-bearing B lymphocytes in the circulation. Patients' lymphocytes cultured with pokeweed mitogen were induced to become mature cells containing and secreting large amounts of IgA. Although peripheral lymphocytes from IgA-deficient patients generally respond normally to T-cell mitogens, diminished numbers of circulating T cells as detected by the E rosette test and abnormal production of lymphokines by stimulated T cells have been described. Thus, it seems likely that the failure of IgA-bearing B lymphocytes to mature to secretory plasma cells in many patients may reflect a subtle deficiency in T-cell function. A primary T-cell defect, rather than IgA deficiency per se, may help to explain the striking association of IgA deficiency with other immunologically related diseases.

Treatment of IgA deficiency is symptomatic. IgA cannot be effectively replaced by exogenous gamma-globulin or plasma, and use of either would greatly increase the risk of development of antibodies to IgA. IgA-deficient patients in need of transfusion should be screened for the presence of antibodies to IgA, and ideally should be given blood only from IgA-deficient donors. All patients known to be IgA-deficient should be warned of the risk of severe transfusion reactions which may occur following infusion of only a few milliliters of blood.

X-LINKED IMMUNODEFICIENCY WITH INCREASED LEVELS OF IgM This is a specific syndrome only because of its inheritance pattern. IgG levels are usually very low, and IgA low or undetectable, while IgD levels may be high. The clinical patterns of infection are similar to those occurring with other hypogammaglobulinemic states. The number and distribution of B lymphocytes bearing IgM, IgG, and IgA have been normal, suggesting that this type of immunodeficiency may also involve a block in terminal differentiation of B lymphocytes.

ISOLATED DEFICIENCY OF IgM This syndrome has been reported rarely in this country, but was detected frequently in a British population. Approximately 20 percent of these patients were asymptomatic while 60 percent had severe recurrent infections, often with bacteremia. Other associated conditions included gastrointestinal disease, atopy, splenomegaly, and development of malignancy. The condition was frequently familial, and was four times more common in males than females. The number of circulating B lymphocytes has varied from very low to normal.

Common variable immunodeficiency This represents a heterogeneous group of syndromes which may be congenital or acquired, sporadic or familial, and which occur in both males and females. These patients have in common the clinical manifestations of antibody deficiency associated with panhypogammaglobulinemia, with deficiency of IgG and IgA, or rarely, with selective IgG deficiency.

Approximately one-third of these patients have few or no circulating B lymphocytes, suggesting a central failure of development of this cell line. The remainder have B lymphocytes, and more than half have a normal number and class distribution. In the few patients studied, B lymphocytes capable of binding specific antigens were present and increased in frequency following immunization. Consistent with the evidence that B lymphocytes in these patients are able to recognize antigens and proliferate, but fail to differentiate to plasma cells, is the fairly common finding of lymphoid hyperplasia, including splenomegaly and nodular lymphoid hyperplasia of the gut.

In agammaglobulinemic patients having B lymphocytes, the pathogenesis of immune deficiency must involve the failure of these cells to differentiate to plasma cells. By use of assays capable of measuring B lymphocyte differentiation to plasma cells in vitro, three major types of defect have been tentatively identified. First, in some patients there is evidence that T cells, or their products, may actively suppress terminal differentiation of B lymphocytes. Second, the helper function of T cells in the induction of B-cell differentiation may be impaired. A third type is intrinsic to B lymphocytes. Some hypogammaglobulinemic patients' B lymphocytes have failed to differentiate to plasma cells even when cultured with pokeweed mitogen in the presence of normal T cells. In other instances, patients' lymphocytes have been induced to synthesize immunoglobulin but fail to secrete it.

Cells from some agammaglobulinemic patients having normal B-lymphocyte numbers respond normally to pokeweed mitogen in vitro. Studies of their separated T and B lymphocytes have shown no distinctive abnormalities of the types described above.

IMMUNODEFICIENCY WITH THYMOMA Recognition of this condition provided one of the early clues as to the role of the thymus in immunobiology. Remarkably, many patients with this syndrome have a normal number of T cells and normal cell-mediated immunity, but are very deficient in circulating B lymphocytes and are hypogammaglobulinemic. Since patients with thymoma may also have deficiencies of other hemopoietic cells, a stem-cell defect has been suspected.

WISKOTT-ALDRICH SYNDROME This is an x-linked genetic disease characterized by eczema, thrombocytopenia, and repeated infections. Affected boys often present with bleeding in infancy. They rarely survive childhood, dying of complications of bleeding, infection, or lymphoreticular malignancy. The immunologic defects in this disease are well characterized but poorly understood. Serum concentrations of IgM are usually decreased, while IgA and IgG are normal. However, synthetic rates for all three classes may be elevated, indicating a significant element of hypercatabolism. The number and class distribution of B lymphocytes usually have been normal. Some patients acquire a diminished number of T cells as evaluated by the E rossette test and appraisal of lymph node biopsies. Functionally, these boys are unable to make antibodies to polysaccharide antigens normally; responses to protein antigens are often not impaired. They are frequently anergic, and their T cells do not respond normally to challenge with ubiquitous antigens. However, responses to T-cell mitogens, such as phytohemagglutinin, are generally normal. Serial appraisal of affected boys suggests that the defects in T-cell function are secondary. It is possible that the Wiskott-Aldrich syndrome reflects a primary defect in the B lymphocyte.

A number of patients with this syndrome have been treated with transfer factor obtained from leukocytes of normal donors. About half appear clinically improved, as judged by a decreased number of infections, clearing of eczema, and, in a few, increased platelet counts. Clinical improvement has been correlated with transfer of delayed hypersensitivity skin reactions to antigens to which the donor was sensitive. Hemolytic anemia, nephrotic syndrome, and development of lymphoreticular malignancy have all occurred in patients with and without transfer factor treatment.

Miscellaneous immunodeficiency syndromes Infection with *Candida albicans* is the almost universal accompaniment of severe deficiencies in cell-mediated immunity. The syndrome of *chronic mucocutaneous candidiasis* is different because superficial candidiasis is usually the only major manifestation of immunodeficiency. These patients rarely develop systemic infection with *Candida* or other fungal agents and are not unusually susceptible to virus or bacterial disease. The syndrome is often congenital and may be associated with single or multiple endocrinopathies as well as iron deficiency. Treatment of associated conditions may lead to improvement or even cure of *Candida* infection.

No uniformity of immunologic defects has been identified in these patients, although defects of antibody formation have been detected occasionally. Humoral immunity, including ability to make specific anti-*Candida* antibodies, is usually normal. Many patients are anergic, some to a variety of antigens and some only to *Candida;* anergy in some patients has been related to inability of their lymphocytes to produce migration inhibition factor.

Results of treatment with antifungal agents, such as amphotericin B, have been variable, but generally not encouraging. In some patients, clearing of the *Candida* lesions by treatment with antifungal agents has been maintained with periodic administration of transfer factor.

IMMUNODEFICIENCY ASSOCIATED WITH SERUM LYMPHOCYTOTOXINS This syndrome has been reported in a few patients with recurrent bacterial and fungal infections. Most have had fluctuating lymphopenia. Both cellular immunity and specific antibody responses were impaired, although immunoglobulin levels were usually normal.

IMBALANCES OF IgG SUBCLASSES Some patients with repeated infections and only moderately decreased serum IgG levels may have an imbalance of IgG subclasses. A few such patients appeared to benefit from administration of gamma-globulin. *Kappa light-chain deficiency* has also been reported in association with recurrent infections, and doubtless many more subtle gaps in antibody diversity, which may be clinically significant, will be elucidated.

TREATMENT OF IMMUNODEFICIENCIES Experimental therapy for patients with either T-cell or combined immunodeficiencies has been mentioned in discussion of these conditions.

Replacement therapy with human gamma-globulin should be used primarily in patients who have recurrent bacterial infections and are deficient in IgG. Maintenance of serum IgG levels between 100 and 300 mg per 100 ml is sufficient to prevent most overwhelming infections, although chronic sinusitis, otitis media, and bronchitis often persist. These serum levels usually can be achieved by intramuscular injection of IgG, 100 mg per kg, at monthly intervals, following a loading dose of twice this amount given over a period of several days. Forty milliliters of 16% gamma-globulin, given in two or more sites at one time, is about the maximum tolerable in adults. If more is needed, it is probably preferable to increase the frequency of injections. In patients with mild to moderate IgG deficiency (300 to 400 mg per 100 ml) the decision to treat must be based on clinical symptoms and on failure to respond to antigenic challenge, because injection of gamma-globulin at the recommended doses will not significantly elevate serum IgG levels. Gamma-globulin treatment is of no value in patients with deficiencies of immunoglobulins other than IgG.

An alternative method of treatment is infusion of fresh plasma, 10 to 20 ml per kg at intervals of 3 to 4 weeks. Plasma therapy has the advantages of being less painful and of replacing IgM and IgA as well as IgG; however, both IgM and IgA have a half-life of only a few days. The disadvantage of plasma is the risk of transmitting hepatitis, which is particularly devastating in immunodeficient patients. This risk can be minimized by use of selected donors, usually family members, carefully screened for the absence of Australia antigen or antibody.

Therapy with exogenous IgG usually does not prevent chronic sinopulmonary infection and its all too frequent progression to pulmonary fibrosis and bronchiectasis. Therefore, maintenance of good pulmonary toilet with regular postural drainage is an important part of patient management. The principles of antibiotic therapy are not different in these than other patients, except that the index of suspicion of bacterial infection should remain very high.

REFERENCES

AIUTI F et al: Identification, enumeration, and isolation of B and T lymphocytes from human peripheral blood. Scand J Immunol 3:521, 1974

BERGSMA D et al (eds): *Immunodeficiency in Man and Animals, Birth Defects,* Original Article Series, vol. XI, no. 1, The National Foundation–March of Dimes, Sunderland, Mass.: Sinauer Associates, 1975

COOPER MD, LAWTON AR: The development of the immune system. Sci Am 231:58, 1974

—— et al: Meeting Report 2nd International Workshop on Primary Immunodeficiency Diseases in Man. Clin Immunol Immunopathol 2:416, 1974

JOHNSTON RB JR et al: Disorders of host defense against infection: Pathophysiologic and diagnostic considerations. Med Clin North Am 57:421, 1973

MÖLLER G (ed): T and B lymphocytes in humans. Transplant Rev 16, 1973

STIEHM ER, FULGINITI VA (eds): *Immunologic Disorders in Infants and Children,* Philadelphia: Saunders, 1973

75
IMMUNE COMPLEX DISEASES

BRUCE C. GILLILAND
MART MANNIK

DEFINITION Immune complex diseases are characterized by the deposition of antigen-antibody complexes in vascular and glomerular basement membranes and by the presence of these complexes in the circulation and in other body fluid compartments. The localization of immune complexes in tissues initiates immunologically mediated inflammation with resultant tissue damage. Immune complex diseases have a common pathogenic mechanism, but the etiology is variable, and therefore the sources of antigens differ from disease to disease. The immune complex diseases constitute a clinical syndrome which includes glomerulonephritis, arthritis, skin eruptions, pericarditis, pleuritis, and vasculitis at diverse sites.

PATHOGENESIS Upon the first exposure to a foreign substance, the host develops an antibody response after a week or 10 days. The synthesized antibodies result in formation of antigen-antibody complexes, which facilitate removal of the antigen. Normally, the majority of immune complexes are removed by cells in the reticuloendothelial system (also called the mononuclear phagocyte system). However, when complexes are deposited at other sites such as along vascular and glomerular basement membranes, inflammation may develop at these sites, leading to the signs and symptoms of immune complex disease.

The concepts of immune complex disease in humans have been evolved largely in animal models, including both spontaneous and experimentally induced disease. Acute serum sickness can be induced in experimental animals by injection of a foreign protein such as bovine serum albumin. Antigen disappears from the circulation in three phases: the first represents equilibration of the antigen between the intra- and extravascular compartments; the second is produced by catabolism of the antigen; the third involves the immune clearance of the antigen due to newly made specific antibodies. During the initial part of the immune clearance phase, small circulating immune complexes are formed. As more antibody is synthesized, the lattice structure of the immune complexes increases, until the complexes reach a critical lattice structure and then are rapidly removed from the circulation by the reticuloendothelial system in the liver and elsewhere. Once the circulating immune complexes reach a critical size, they also activate the complement sequence and thereby cause a decrease in total hemolytic complement or individual complement components. This event does not ensue if the complexes are formed by antibodies incapable of complement activation (Chap. 71). The overwhelming bulk of the antigen in the form of immune complexes is removed from the circulation by the reticuloendothelial system. For example, in experimental animals less than 1 percent of the circulating immune complexes becomes entrapped in the kidneys as determined in chronic serum sickness models or by intravenous injection of preformed immune complexes. Yet, these small quantities of immune complexes suffice to cause glomerulonephritis. In human diseases no data are available on the total burden of circulating immune complexes or on the amount deposited in kidneys. The exact nature of the complexes that become deposited in the vascular or glomerular basement membranes is not certain, but persistence of complexes in the circulation is a requirement for development of renal disease. In rabbits, the release of vasoactive amines facilitates the deposition of immune complexes in the glomeruli, but in humans this mechanism has not been demonstrated. Coincident with circulating immune complexes and complement utilization, clinical abnormalities develop in experimental animals (Fig. 75-1). These abnormalities include glomerulonephritis, vasculitis, arthritis, skin eruptions, pleuritis, and pericarditis. Once the antigen is completely cleared, the complement levels return to normal, and gradually the lesions in target organs subside. Thus, acute serum sickness is a limited disease and progresses only as long as antigen persists in the recipient.

In experimental animals the acute serum sickness model

FIGURE 75-1
Schematic presentation of events in experimental acute serum sickness. In this experimental animal, antibody production began on the eighth day with the appearance of circulating immune complexes and subsequent decrease in serum complement (C). Vasculitis, glomerulonephritis, and arthritis develop after deposition of immune complexes. With the clearance of immune complexes by the reticuloendothelial system, the pathogenic process ceases, free antibody can be detected, and the inflammatory events run their course and gradually abate.

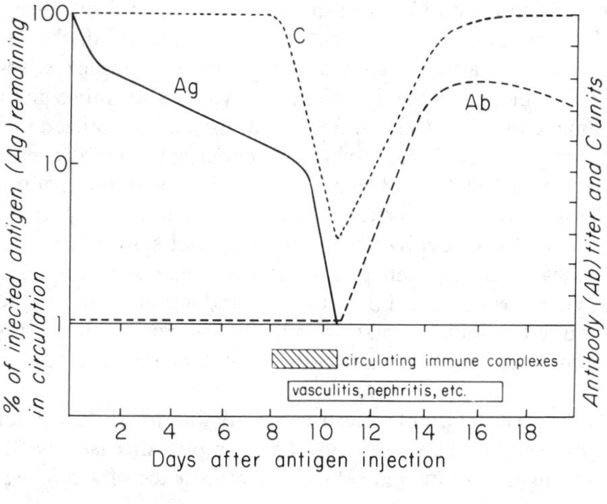

can be converted to a chronic serum sickness or immune complex disease model by repeated administration of antigen. The development of clinical abnormalities in such models can be achieved by frequent (daily or several times a week) administration of an appropriate dose of antigen. For development of maximal lesions the total dose of antigen should result in slight antigen excess in relation to the specific antibody pool. In such a model, renal failure due to chronic proliferative glomerulonephritis can be achieved. These animals also develop vasculitis in other locations, and extensive antigen, antibody, and C3 deposits are identifiable.

A chronic immune complex disease can develop spontaneously in animals with viral or other microbial infection that provides a continued source of antigen for immune complex formation. Glomerulonephritis develops in mice with persistent lymphocytic choriomeningitis virus, Maloney sarcoma virus, or lactic dehydrogenase virus infection, and in Aleutian disease of mink. Immune complexes consisting of antivirus antibody, virus antigen, and complement components (mainly C3) can be identified in the kidney and serum of these animals. Immune complex nephritis resembling closely that of systemic lupus erythematosus occurs in the F_1 hybrid of New Zealand black and New Zealand white mice. Deoxyribonucleic acid (DNA), antibodies to DNA, and C3 deposits are found in the glomerular basement membrane. In addition, C-type RNA viral antigens are present in glomeruli and serum of these mice. The role played by C-type RNA virus infection in this and other autoimmune diseases is currently under investigation.

A localized experimental immune complex disease can be generated by repeated injection of a foreign substance into the same location of an immunized animal. For example, rabbits immunized with killed *Escherichia coli* develop arthritis when the killed microorganism is injected into the joint cavity. The same type of inflammation can be achieved by injection of a foreign protein into the joints of a previously immunized animal. Intense inflammation can be induced in a similar manner in other body cavities such as the pericardial and pleural cavities. Again, the local immunologically induced inflammation progresses as long as antigen is present. The synovitis of rheumatoid arthritis appears to be a local immune complex disease of joints.

Immune complexes activate complement components, leading to formation of vasoactive peptides and to release of chemotactic factors. Neutrophils accumulate in the involved area and phagocytize the immune complexes, resulting in release of lysosomal enzymes and subsequent damage to structural components of tissue. In localized immune complex disease such as rheumatoid synovitis, monocytes, T cells, and B cells subsequently accumulate in the lesion because of specific chemotactic factors. Many newly arrived B cells evolve to plasma cells that synthesize antibodies to the antigen present at the site. For example, if bovine serum albumin is used to induce arthritis in the rabbit, the bulk of plasma cells in the synovium of this animal will synthesize antibodies to bovine serum albumin.

PATHOLOGY Light microscopy of the renal lesion of acute serum sickness or immune complex disease reveals swelling of endothelial cells and the presence of a few leukocytes. In the chronic form, thickening of the basement membrane is accompanied by accumulation of neutrophils and proliferation and swelling of endothelial cells. Epithelial cells proliferate to form crescents with eventual obliteration of Bowman's space. The renal lesions may be classified as showing mesangioproliferative, focal proliferative, diffuse proliferative, or membranous glomerular involvement, depending on the extent of the disease and the characteristics of the inflammatory response (Chap. 274). Immunofluorescent studies of the kidney in both the acute and chronic forms of disease reveal granular deposits of immunoglobulin and complement (C3) in the mesangial matrix or along the glomerular basement membrane. Transmission electron microscopy shows electron-dense deposits in the mesangial matrix, the subendothelial space, the subepithelial space, and the glomerular basement membrane.

The histology of the vascular lesion initially shows accumulation of neutrophils and proliferation of endothelial cells. This is followed by disruption of the internal elastic lamina and fibrinoid necrosis of the vessel wall. Mononuclear cells appear later. The vasculitis may vary from an intense inflammatory lesion consisting mainly of polymorphonuclear cells to one in which only perivascular cuffing with mononuclear cells is seen at the time of biopsy. If the examination is made early in the course, granular deposits of immunoglobulin and complement may be identified by immunofluorescence. However, within hours, these immune deposits are removed by the inflammatory response.

ETIOLOGY For any given immune complex disease the etiology consists of the nature and source of the antigens that form immune complexes as well as the immunogens that incite the immune response. In most immune complex diseases the antigen and immunogen are the same substance, but in certain autoimmune diseases they may differ. Thus, in immune complex diseases the etiologic factors may be drugs, microorganisms, tumors, or the host's own tissues. If strict criteria are employed, the etiology of an immune complex disease is defined when the specific antigens and antibodies causing the tissue inflammation are identified. This has been achieved largely by elution of antigens and antibodies from the target tissues or by immunofluorescent microscopy using specific antigens and antibodies. The list of established immune complex diseases has grown steadily (Table 75-1). A number of diseases, particularly glomerulonephritis and vasculitis, have all the hallmarks of immune complex diseases in terms of the clinical pattern of the disorder and the deposition of immunoglobulins at sites of inflammation, but the involved antigens are not defined—therefore, these disorders are often listed as "probable" immune complex diseases.

Drugs produce immune complex disease either by acting as immunogens or by inducing synthesis of autoantibodies by an unknown mechanism. Numerous drugs and foreign proteins (e.g., penicillins, sulfonamides, horse antitoxin to tetanus, and horse antihuman lymphocyte serum) are potentially immunogenic and cause immune complex disease. Binding of a drug or its metabolite to a serum protein may be necessary for its immunogenicity.

A form of immune complex disease restricted to the destruction of platelets or red blood cells is occasionally observed following administration of stibophen, phenacetin, quinine, or quinidine. Antibodies made in response to one of these drugs combine with the drug to form an immune complex. These complexes are adsorbed to the blood cell surface and activate complement, leading to either hemolytic anemia or thrombocytopenia. Some drug-induced neutropenias may also develop by this mechanism.

Other drugs do not act as immunogens but instead stimulate the synthesis of autoantibodies, especially those with specificity to nuclear antigens. Patients receiving drugs such as procainamide, hydralazine, or hydantoins may form antinuclear antibodies and manifest features of systemic lupus erythematosus. Several months of drug administration may be required before the onset of symptoms. The autoantibodies persist for months after administration of the drug has been discontinued.

Several types of infections are accompanied by immune complex disease, and many have glomerulonephritis as a common feature. Antigens derived from the responsible microorganisms are presumed to be released at the site of bacterial growth and then are deposited as immune complexes in glomeruli; however, the identification of bacterial antigens in glomeruli has been difficult. Examples include poststreptococcal glomerulonephritis, the glomerulonephritis of bacterial endocarditis, infected ventriculoatrial shunt, osteomyelitis, quartan malaria, and hepatitis B infection.

Manifestations of immune complex disease may accompany viral infections. For example, the preicteric phase of hepatitis B infection can be recognized by the appearance of fever, arthritis, and skin eruptions along with low serum complement and circulating hepatitis-associated antigen (Chap. 299). As the arthritis and rash subside and complement levels return to normal, the hepatitis-associated antigen disappears from the circulation, and antibodies to the antigen can then be demonstrated with the onset of clinical manifestations of hepatitis. In this disorder the immune complexes consist of viral surface antigens (HB_sAg) and the specific antibody.

Fungal diseases such as coccidioidomycosis may be accompanied by erythema nodosum and arthritis, most likely due to immune complex deposition.

Patients with malignancies may develop arthritis, arthralgia, and skin eruptions. Renal biopsies in some patients with nephrotic syndrome associated with adenocarcinoma of the colon have shown IgG, complement components, and carcinoembryonic antigen in the glomerular basement membrane. As methods are developed for identifying other tumor antigens, examples of immune complex disease will increase.

The autoimmune group of disorders is characterized by immune complexes composed of autologous antigens and their specific antibodies. The prototype of this group is systemic lupus erythematosus characterized by formation of antinuclear antibodies (Chap. 77). In particular, deposition of immune complexes consisting of native DNA, and antibodies to native DNA, in the glomerular basement membrane and other tissues leads to inflammation at these sites. Another example is mixed cryoglobulinemia in which immune complexes composed of IgG–anti-IgG can be identified in the precipitate. The antibody in these immune complexes consists of IgG, IgA, or IgM, and the antibody specificity is directed to IgG. These complexes are soluble at body temperatures and show progressive insolubility as the temperature is lowered. Upon deposition, they produce glomerulonephritis, arthritis, and vasculitis. Cutaneous lesions may also develop owing to precipitation of complexes at reduced temperatures in the extremities. Immune complexes of IgG–anti-IgG are also found in rheumatoid arthritis and in hypergammaglobulinemic purpura of Waldenström, in which joint inflammation, pleuritis, pericarditis, and vasculitis are not uncommon.

Autologous antigens may be released by prior tissue damage to serve first as immunogens and later as antigens in the generation of immune complex disease. For example, in sickle-cell disease, renal tubular cell antigens are released from damaged tubular cells, antibodies to these antigens are synthesized, and the resultant immune complexes are deposited in the glomerular basement membrane.

Many forms of vasculitis, especially small-vessel vasculitis, are caused by deposition of immune complexes (Chap. 78). Biopsy of an involved site may reveal immunoglobulins along with complement components. The absence of these substances, however, does not exclude an immune complex pathogenesis because immune complexes may be destroyed by the inflammatory process within hours of their deposition. The nature and source of antigens that lead to immune complex-induced vasculitis are largely unknown. In some patients with periarteritis nodosa, hepatitis-associated antigen is found in the serum. Furthermore, the antigen, antibodies, and complement components are present in the involved vessel wall, suggesting a pathogenic role for these specific immune complexes.

A localized form of immune complex disease occurs when antibodies come in contact with their antigens at or near the site where antigen is being released or where it is being absorbed. The gingivitis of periodontal disease is thought to be generated by complexes composed of bacterial antigens from the plaque and the specific antibodies. Studies of experimental thyroiditis indicate that antibodies specific to thyroglobulin react with this antigen as it is released from the follicular cells. Immune complexes are formed between the follicular basement membrane and the follicular cells, leading to interstitial inflammation. Thyroiditis in humans may be produced by a similar mech-

TABLE 75-1
Immune complex diseases in humans

Serum sickness (animal antitoxins and antiserums, drugs)
Systemic lupus erythematosus
Mixed cryoglobulinemia
Poststreptococcal glomerulonephritis
Arthritis, polyarteritis, glomerulonephritis of hepatitis B infection
Rheumatoid arthritis
Hypersensitivity pneumonitis (e.g., farmer's lung)
Drug-induced hemolytic anemia and thrombocytopenia due to stibophen, quinine, quinidine, or phenacetin
Glomerulonephritis associated with:
- Quartan malaria
- Syphilis
- Leprosy
- Infectious mononucleosis
- Typhoid fever
- Bacterial endocarditis
- Infected ventriculoatrial shunts
- Tumors (carcinoembryonic antigen)
- Renal tubular antigens
- Chronic thyroiditis

anism. The synovitis of rheumatoid arthritis also represents a localized immune complex disease, in part attributed to antibodies to IgG (rheumatoid factors) that are produced in the synovium. Hypersensitivity pneumonitis, such as pigeon breeder's lung and farmer's lung, results from antibodies uniting with the respective inhaled antigen in the alveolar wall (Chap. 256).

CLINICAL MANIFESTATIONS Since immune complex diseases have a common pathogenic mechanism, many of the clinical manifestations are similar even though the responsible antigens may be quite different. Glomerulonephritis, arthritis, and skin lesions are frequently observed, either individually or in various combinations. Renal involvement may not be apparent clinically or by urinalysis; however, biopsy may show immune deposits in the mesangium or in the glomerular capillary loop. Pleuritis, pericarditis, and small-vessel vasculitis also occur. The number and severity of clinical manifestations vary among patients even when the disorder is produced by a single etiologic agent. The reasons for this variability are not apparent.

The clinical manifestations and course of the acute, self-limited form of immune complex disease are best exemplified by serum sickness following injection of a foreign protein such as horse antitoxin to diphtheria or tetanus. In the person who has not been previously exposed to the antitoxin, the first manifestation is reddening and swelling at the site of injection, occurring 1 to 2 weeks after antitoxin administration. This is followed within a few days by fever, myalgia, skin lesions, arthralgias or arthritis, gastrointestinal symptoms, and lymphadenopathy including nausea, vomiting, and abdominal pain. The skin lesions are most commonly urticarial, but petechial, erythematous, macular, or morbilliform lesions may be seen. Arthritis usually begins in one or two joints and rapidly progresses to include many joints. The wrists, ankles, knees, and small joints of the hand are most commonly involved. Acute glomerulonephritis with red blood cell casts, proteinuria, and decreasing renal function may develop. Vasculitis of the vasa nervorum produces peripheral neuropathy. Rarely meningoencephalitis may develop. In a person with previous exposure to the antitoxin, the above manifestations may appear 3 to 4 days following exposure. The same syndrome may occur after administration of a drug or in association with infection.

An anaphylactoid reaction may follow administration of a drug or foreign protein in a previously immunized patient who has preformed circulating antibodies to the specific antigen (Chap. 72). This reaction begins minutes after exposure and is characterized by urticaria, bronchospasm, dyspnea, diarrhea, hypotension, and shock. This reaction may be fatal. It is caused by the release of large amounts of vasoactive peptides.

Chronic forms of immune complex disease occur in patients who have prolonged or repeated availability of the antigen. Such conditions are seen when the antigen is released from a persistent microorganism or a persistent tumor, or when the antigen is a normal constituent of the host. Examples include bacterial endocarditis, adenocarcinoma of the colon, and systemic lupus erythematosus.

DIAGNOSIS Immune complex disease should be suspected in a patient presenting with arthritis, skin eruptions, and glomerulonephritis. It should also be considered in patients with pericarditis, pleuritis, vasculitis, and/or neuropathy. When the presence of an immune complex disease is suspected, the offending antigen must be identified by historical or laboratory inquiry. A detailed history of drug exposure is extremely important. The presence of chronic bacterial or viral infections must be sought by history and by physical and laboratory examinations.

Several diseases with diffuse vascular involvement in many organ systems may mimic immune complex disease. Patients with a left atrial myxoma may have showers of skin lesions due to small emboli of myxomatous tissue. Similarly, patients with nonbacterial thrombotic endocarditis have peripheral embolization to small blood vessels. These patients may also have arthralgias. Patients with thrombotic thrombocytopenic purpura develop skin lesions, arthralgias, or arthritis, central nervous system abnormalities, and renal failure. The severity of the thrombocytopenia and absence of an inflammatory component in the purpuric skin lesions help to distinguish this entity from immune complex disease.

LABORATORY FINDINGS The laboratory abnormalities in patients with immune complex disease include an elevated erythrocyte sedimentation rate, anemia, mild leukocytosis, and occasionally eosinophilia. The cerebrospinal fluid often shows pleocytosis. The urine may contain protein, red blood cells, and red blood cell casts. Serum complement may be low. Conduction abnormalities may be present on the electrocardiogram.

In the patient suspected of having immune complex disease, the search for antigen should include blood cultures for detection of bacteria that may release the antigens and serologic tests for viral antigens, such as the hepatitis B antigen. Serologic tests for detection of antibody to microbial antigens may be useful in detecting the underlying etiology. These include heterophil, antistreptolysin O, and fluorescent treponemal antibody absorption tests, to mention just some. Tumor antigens, such as the carcinoembryonic antigen, should be sought. In the autoimmune diseases, antibodies to nuclear antigens (Chap. 77) and antibodies to IgG (rheumatoid factors) point to the underlying disorder. Tests for cryoglobulins should be performed; if they are found, specific antigens and antibodies can be characterized. Measurements of serum complement can be helpful in supporting the diagnosis initially and in following the course of immune complex diseases. Since immune complexes primarily activate the classic complement pathway, both the early and late components of complement will be consumed. A normal complement level does not exclude the presence of immune complex disease because the rate of synthesis may compensate for the degree of complement consumption.

Examination of tissue by immunofluorescence or by electron microscopy may be helpful in establishing the diagnosis of immune complex disease. Demonstration of IgG and complement components in the glomerular basement membrane by immunofluorescence indicates deposition of immune complexes. They stain in a granular or "lumpy" pattern. In contrast, a linear pattern of staining is seen when antibody is directed to antigens of the glomerular basement membrane (e.g., in Goodpasture's syndrome). Also, the detection of immunoglobulin and complement in the wall of involved blood vessels suggests an immune complex etiology. Phagocytosis of these deposited complexes results in the finding of immunoglobulins and complement in the phagolysosomes of neutrophils and macrophages.

The detection and quantification of circulating immune complexes is possible with specialized techniques that are currently investigational. Immune complexes can be identified by analytical ultracentrifugation, but this technique is insensitive. Certain monoclonal rheumatoid factors (anti-IgG antibodies) are effective in combining and precipitating with immune complexes containing IgG. Also, the first component of complement (C1q) can be used to detect complexes containing IgG since this molecule combines firmly with IgG in large-latticed immune complexes. It has also been possible to detect circulating immune complexes by the use of a human lymphoblastoid cell line (called the Raji cell line). This human lymphoblastoid cell line binds complement-fixing immune complexes with the C3b receptor. These techniques are limited by the requirement to form an immune complex lattice of a critical size, in order to facilitate binding of complement or interaction with cell receptors, and by the subclass of antibody. Once these and other techniques become generally available, they may help the clinician to diagnose immune complex disease. The finding of decreased total hemolytic complement, decreased complement components, immunoglobulin and complement tissue deposits, or elevated titers of specific antibodies provides only inferential evidence for the presence of circulating immune complexes.

TREATMENT The principles of therapy for immune complex diseases are to remove the offending antigen and to reduce the inflammation when it threatens to compromise organ function. When a drug is suspected of causing immune complex disease, its administration should be stopped immediately. In patients with immune complex disease associated with an infection, such as bacterial endocarditis, adequate doses of the appropriate antibiotic should be given.

Patients experiencing an anaphylactoid reaction should be given 1 ml epinephrine 1:1,000 and pharmacologic doses of hydrocortisone or dexamethasone intravenously. Tracheostomy or intubation may be necessary in the event of progressing laryngeal edema.

In acute or subacute immune complex disease, anti-inflammatory drugs such as salicylates will usually reduce joint pain. Antihistamines or small doses of epinephrine will relieve urticaria. In some patients the severity of disease warrants the use of corticosteroids which help to minimize clinical manifestations. Prednisone, 40 mg per day, can be given over a 2-week period with gradual tapering. Tissue damage may be slowed in chronic immune complex disease by the use of corticosteroids alone or in combination with immunosuppressive drugs. Treatment of the chronic forms of immune complex disease is discussed in detail in the chapters dealing with the specific disorders.

REFERENCES

COCHRANE CB, KOFFLER D: Immune complex disease in experimental animals and man. Adv Immunol 16:185, 1963

DIXON F: The role of antigen-antibody complexes in disease. Harvey Lect 52:21, 1963

KOHLER P: Clinical immune complex diseases. Medicine 52:419, 1973

MANNIK M et al: The fate and detection of circulating immune complexes, in *Clinical Aspects* II, *Progress in Immunology* II, eds L Brent et al, New York: American Elsevier, 1974

OLDSTONE MBA, DIXON F: Immune complex disease in chronic viral infections. J Exp Med 134:32s, 1971

ROY LP et al: Etiologic agents of immune-deposit disease, in *Progress in Clinical Immunology,* ed RS Schwartz, New York: Grune & Stratton, 1972

SOBEL AT et al: C1q deviation test for the detection of immune complexes, aggregates of IgG, and bacterial products in human serum. J Exp Med 142:139, 1975

THEOFILOPOULOS AN et al: Binding of soluble immune complexes to human lymphoblastoid cells. II. Use of Raji cells to detect circulating immune complexes in animal and human sera. J Exp Med 140:1230, 1974

76
TRANSPLANTATION

CHARLES B. CARPENTER
JOHN P. MERRILL

INTRODUCTION Transplantation of the human kidney is now a justified procedure for the treatment of advanced chronic renal failure. Approximately 17,000 cases have been reported to the Human Transplant Registry as of January, 1975, from 288 institutions, of which 164 are in the United States. In 1974 70 percent of the donors were cadavers, 13 percent parents, and 14 percent siblings. Of the total number of transplants performed, approximately 15,000 were first transplants, 1,500 second transplants, and 130 third. This represents an increasing incidence of second kidney transplants. Table 76-1 shows 1- and 2-year graft and patient survival rates, according to donor category. This represents an increasing philosophy on the part of transplant teams to decrease immunosuppressive therapy so that in the case of severe rejection the kidney rather than the patient may be lost. The incidence of second transplants reflects data showing that a first transplant from a cadaver does not impair the chances of success of a second transplant from a related donor. The figures for graft survival, however, show no improvement from 1970

TABLE 76-1
Functional survival rates of first transplants

Donor source	*Year of transplant*	*1 year, %*	*2 years, %*
Sibling	1970	81.1	78.2
	1971	73.7	69.6
	1972	79.9	73.7
Parent	1970	73.8	68.3
	1971	73.7	66.8
	1972	71.7	61.1
Cadaver	1970	55.3	47.2
	1971	53.1	45.7
	1972	50.6	42.6

to 1972. This suggests that methods of immunosuppressive therapy which have been uniformly utilized from 1970 to 1975 remain inadequate. Human liver, pancreas, bone marrow, heart, and endocrine glands have been transplanted, but with less success. The results of cardiac transplantation in one of the largest and best-studied series in the United States show a 45 percent 1-year survival.

IMMUNOLOGIC CONSIDERATIONS Necessary to the understanding of transplantation immunity are the following terms: *autograft*—the transplantation of tissue from one part of an individual to another part of the same individual; *isograft*—the transplantation of tissues between two individuals of the same inbred strain. Because in these cases the antigens of the donor and recipient are identical, no histocompatibility difference exists and no immune response to the graft occurs. A case in point in man is transplantation between identical twins. In an *allograft,* i.e., a graft of tissues between two individuals of the same species, histocompatibility differences may be strong or weak, depending on the individual and the species. A *xenograft* is a graft between individuals of two different species. The term "heterograft" is still used synonymously with xenograft.

NATURE AND ROLE OF THE MAJOR HISTOCOMPATIBILITY GENE COMPLEX (HL-A) The fate of transplanted tissues and organs depends upon a number of factors, but the recipient's immune response to graft antigens is the central event. Definition of antigenic systems which serve as strong barriers to transplantation has therefore become a major investigative interest, having both practical application in clinical transplantation and theoretical value in understanding the natural role of the histocompatibility antigens in immunobiology.

A single chromosomal complex codes for the major histocompatibility antigens in all vertebrate species investigated so far. The mouse is the most completely studied species because of the availability of numbers of inbred and recombinant strains which can be employed in studies to determine the precise role of each of the gene products of the histocompatibility (H-2) chromosomal segment. Except for some details of the ordering of the genes on the chromosomal segment, the human HL-A system is thus far quite analogous to the H-2. In a general sense, incompatibility for major locus antigens constitutes a strong barrier to transplantation of tissues and organs, and in clinical experience matching for major locus antigens affords excellent transplantation results since the minor mismatches are easily suppressed by immunosuppressive drug therapy. The HL-A gene complex is a portion of the C6 human chromosome and consists of several series of paired alleles which are inherited from generation to generation in a dominant fashion, segregating randomly from other important antigens such as the ABH red cell blood groups.

FIGURE 76-1

HL-A gene complex. A single C6 chromosomal segment is shown with a schematic representation of the relative order and spacing of the major alleles. The A locus (SD-1 or LA), B locus (SD-2 or four), and C locus (SD-3) determine serologically defined cell surface antigens, while the D locus (MLR or LD) is responsible for the proliferative response of lymphocytes in mixed lymphocyte culture (MLC). The entire region encompassing the B and D loci is postulated to contain genes governing immune responses (Ir). Evidence exists for other serologically defined loci near the D locus, and for a second weak MLR locus between the first (A) and second (B) loci.

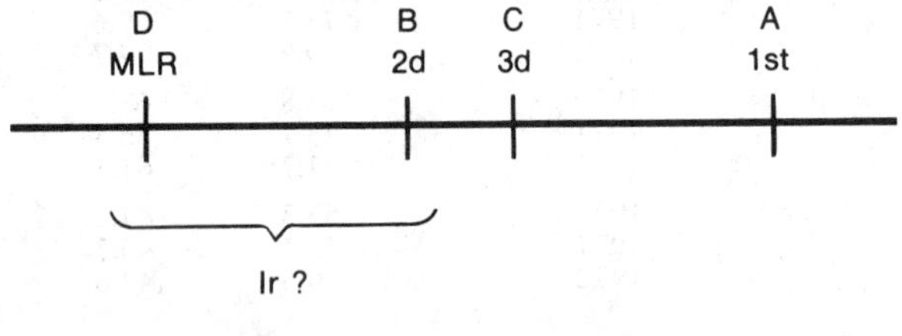

Serologically defined (SD) and lymphocyte defined (LD) antigens The development of antileukocyte antibodies after multiple blood transfusions and as a result of pregnancy was first recognized as involving a series of antigens distinct from red cell blood group antigens. HL-A antigens are defined serologically by serums from human sources, principally multiparous females, and are present in varying densities in most body tissues, including B cells, T cells (see Immunology of Rejection below), and platelets, but not on mature red blood cells (Chap. 71). The number of serologically defined specificities is very large, and the HL-A system is at present the most polymorphic genetic system known in humans. There are known to be three clearly defined loci within the HL-A complex for serologically defined (SD) HL-A antigens. The products of each of the loci are immunochemically distinct from each other, and each is highly polymorphic within the human population (Fig. 76-1). The A locus (SD-1 or LA) and B locus (SD-2 or -4) were recognized as such in 1970, and the C locus (SD-3) shortly thereafter. There are over 35 clearly defined serologic specificities for the first and second series, while over five C-locus specificities are known. Considering the number of variants of these major groups, it is possible to state that there are approximately 90 serologic specificities present in Caucasian leukocytes. Antigens of the major complex are all prefixed by HL-A, but this may be omitted when the context is clear. Antigens tentatively accepted as a result of World Health Organization workshops have a W after the locus designation. The HL-A antigens of African and Oceanic peoples are not as well defined at present, although they include some of the antigens commonly found in Caucasians. The distribution of HL-A antigens is distinctive for certain racial groups and can serve as anthropological markers in the study of migration patterns.

Since chromosomes are paired, each individual has six serologically defined HL-A antigens, three for each parent. Each of these chromosomal sets is termed a *haplotype,* and by simple Mendelian inheritance 25 percent of siblings will have identical haplotypes, 50 percent will share a haplotype, and the remaining 25 percent will be completely incompatible. Evidence that this gene complex plays the major role in the transplantation response comes from the fact that haplotype-matched sibling donor-recipient combinations show excellent results in kidney transplantation, in the vicinity of 95 percent long-term survival.

Linked to the serologically defined antigens, but distinct from them, is another locus which determines the in vitro proliferative response of lymphocytes to mismatched haplotypes. Because haplotype-matched, HL-A–identical siblings have negative mixed lymphocyte culture responses, it was initially assumed that the HL-A antigens were responsible for the proliferative response of lymphocytes mixed in tissue culture. However, a number of recombinants in families have shown clearly that a distinct locus, called D, exists for the mixed lymphocyte response (MLR), and is responsible for a vigorous mixed lymphocyte culture (MLC) proliferative response, even in the presence of HL-A antigen identity (Fig. 76-2). The recombinant rate in human families is around 1 percent between the B and D loci, and it is also approximately 1 percent between the A and B loci.

D-locus antigens, sometimes called MLR-S (stimulating), are not as yet clearly identifiable by serotyping techniques, but only by the MLC response in tissue culture (lymphocyte defined). Serologically defined specificities closely related to the D locus have been discovered and have the special property of not being expressed on platelets or T lymphocytes. These specificities may be useful markers for the closely lined D-locus determinants and certain immune response (Ir) genes. The third locus is much more closely linked to the second series according to presently available data. Recombinant rates among all these loci are low enough in most cases to ensure that within a family the HL-S antigens will serve as markers for the entire haplotype, including the D locus. A recombinant frequency of approximately 1 percent indicates that there is considerable room for a large number of genes within the complex, and a number of undefined antigens may exist; however, they are all inherited en bloc with a family. HL-A serotyping is therefore a valuable system for marking family haplotypes. In the outbred human population, however, HL-A antigens are much less likely to predict compatibility for other genes in the complex.

There are at least two additional major classes of genes within the HL-A complex; one is for complement, with separate genes for C2, C4, and factor B (GBG), and the other involves immune responsiveness to ragweed antigen and possibly to measles virus. The latter findings are of enormous importance in relation to the analogy to mouse H-2 systems where the MLR region is closely linked to a number of genes responsible for certain immune responses (Ir region). There are, therefore, a number of genes in this complex which are related to the immune response, ranging from the immunogenicity of certain antigens to the proliferative response (MLC) to the complex. Furthermore, the serologically defined antigens serve as targets for alloimmune effector mechanisms, while components of the complement mediator system can play a role in the effector phase. It is apparent therefore that the major histocompatibility gene complex has evolved to play a major role in body defense and has a significance far in excess of its relationship to current efforts in clinical transplantation.

Disease associations If the major histocompatibility complex serves a critical natural biological function, what might that be? Hypotheses have been put forth relating to immune surveillance against neoplastic cells which develop in the course of an individual's lifetime. It is apparent also that the system could play an important role in pregnancy because of the histoincompatibility that always exists between the mother and the fetus. Work in inbred mouse models indicates the importance of some of the gene products of this locus during the phase of antigen recognition and cell-to-cell cooperation in initiation of an immune response. It is possible also that the high degree of polymorphism present ensures the survival of the species in relation to the large numbers of microbiological agents present in the environment. Self-tolerance which happens to cross react with microbiological agents would produce a high degree of susceptibility, resulting in lethal infection, whereas the high degree of polymorphism present in the HL-A system provides assurance that segments of the population will recognize the offending agent as foreign and initiate the appropriate response. All these hypotheses relate to the survival value of the system under selective evolutionary pressures, and there is some evidence for each of them.

The most striking circumstantial evidence on the role of the major histocompatibility complex in human immunobiology comes from the finding that a number of disease processes are positively associated with certain HL-A antigens within the population. The search for such associations has been stimulated by the discovery of immune response genes linked to the H-2 complex in the mouse, and also by the H-2 complex–linked susceptibility to murine oncogenic viruses. Although surveys of human malignancies, including leukemias and lymphoproliferative

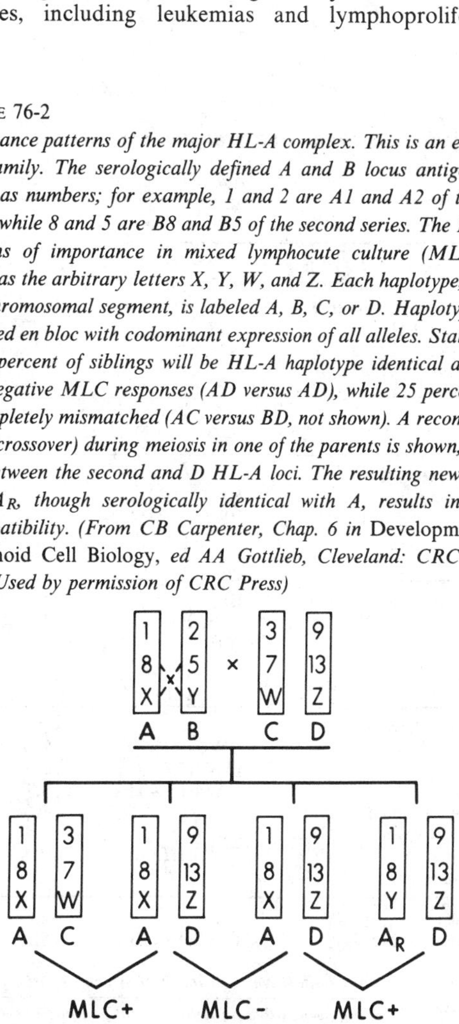

FIGURE 76-2
Inheritance patterns of the major HL-A complex. This is an example of a family. The serologically defined A and B locus antigens are shown as numbers; for example, 1 and 2 are A1 and A2 of the first series, while 8 and 5 are B8 and B5 of the second series. The D-locus antigens of importance in mixed lymphocute culture (MLC) are shown as the arbitrary letters X, Y, W, and Z. Each haplotype, shown as a chromosomal segment, is labeled A, B, C, or D. Haplotypes are inherited en bloc with codominant expression of all alleles. Statistically, 25 percent of siblings will be HL-A haplotype identical and will have negative MLC responses (AD versus AD), while 25 percent will be completely mismatched (AC versus BD, not shown). A recombinant event (crossover) during meiosis in one of the parents is shown, occurring between the second and D HL-A loci. The resulting new haplotype, A_R, though serologically identical with A, results in MLC incompatibility. (From CB Carpenter, Chap. 6 in Developments in Lymphoid Cell Biology, *ed AA Gottlieb, Cleveland: CRC Press, 1974. Used by permission of CRC Press)*

disorders, have not shown consistent associations with serologically defined HL-A phenotypes, some very striking correlations exist between HL-A antigens of the second locus and a number of diseases in which the pathogenesis is unclear (Table 76-2). Most striking is the increased frequency of HL-A-B27 (formerly called W27) in certain rheumatic diseases, particularly ankylosing spondylitis, a condition already known to have a strong familial tendency. B27 is present in about 5 percent of the Caucasian population, while it appears in 87 percent of 286 patients combined from five studies. Expressed as a relative risk, the antigen B27 confers a susceptibility to the development of ankylosing spondylitis which is 127 times that in the general population. Similarly, Reiter's syndrome and reactive arthritis to at least three bacterial infections (yersinia, salmonella, and gonococcus) show a high degree of association with B27. Furthermore, acute anterior uveitis has a similar high association with the same antigen. Since it is well known that significant overlap exists among these three conditions (spondylitis, Reiter's syndrome, and uveitis), it seems likely that B27 is a marker for a clustering of connective tissue responses to a number of infectious agents, or unknown environmental factors. It was suggested initially that juvenile rheumatoid arthritis might also show a similar B27 association, but a larger series with careful exclusion of coexistent spondylitis was not confirmatory, reinforcing, in a negative way, the specificity of B27 for spondylitis. Though less striking, the increased incidence of B27 in cases of psoriatic arthritis is also highly significant, and contrasts with the increased incidence of HL-A-B13 and HL-A-BW17 in psoriasis per se. Patients with rheumatoid arthritis or gout show no alteration in HL-A antigen frequencies.

Gluten-sensitive enteropathy (celiac disease, nontropical sprue) in both children and adults shows a clear-cut association with HL-A-B8. The actual percentage of such patients having this antigen ranges from 66 to 88 percent in five studies in which B8 was present in 16 to 29 percent of controls. The same antigen is also present in increased frequency in patients with chronic active hepatitis or dermatitis herpetiformis. Pemphigus is the only disease in which a first-series antigen, HL-A-A10, has shown an increased incidence.

Three endocrinopathies have been under intensive investigation following initial reports of increases in HL-A-B8 frequency. Juvenile (insulin-dependent) diabetes mellitus has shown an HL-A-BW15 association. With techniques for typing of D-locus antigens by performance of mixed lymphocyte cultures with homozygous stimulating cells in which the paired D-locus antigens are identical, a greater degree of association with the D-locus determinants, HL-A-DW3 (LD-8a) and HL-A-DW4 (LD-15a), has been reported. These antigens are often linked to their respective second-series HL-A antigens, but these results would indicate that the loci related to juvenile diabetes are closer to the D locus than to the second series. Similar results have been obtained with Addison's disease. MLR typing has revealed an association with HL-A-DW2 (LD-7a) and multiple sclerosis, while the frequently linked HL-A-B7 antigen is less frequently associated.

Hence, this summary of the known disease associations with the HL-A gene complex described a spectrum, ranging from an extremely high degree of correlation with a serologically defined B locus HL-A antigen, through diseases in which both B- and D-locus markers correlate, to a disease in which only the D-locus determinant is disease-associated. It is clear that definition of this spectrum is only in its preliminary stages, and there are already some hints that certain D-locus determinants have a higher frequency in patients with rheumatoid arthritis, for example. Also in a small series of gluten-sensitive patients, the frequency of an HL-A-B8 linked, but not identical, serological specificity to non-T cells is very high. It is likely that the development of precise typing systems for identification of products of genes of the "left" of the B locus series, encompassing the D and related regions, will mark susceptibility in a number of diseases, such as leukemia, lymphoma, other malignancies, lupus erythematosus, and rheumatoid arthritis, in which HL-A typing has been inconclusive.

TABLE 76-2
Associations between HLA antigens and disease

Disease	*Antigen*	*Relative risk**
RHEUMATIC		
Ankylosing spondylitis	B27	127
Reiter's syndrome	B27	71
Acute anterior uveitis	B27	31
Psoriatic arthritis	B27	4.7
Reactive arthritis *(yersinia, salmonella, gonococcus)*	B27	150(estimated)
GASTROINTESTINAL		
Gluten-sensitive enteropathy	B8	9.5
Chronic active hepatitis	B8	3.6
SKIN		
Dermatitis herpetiformis	B8	4.3
Psoriasis vulgaris	B13, BW17	4.3
Pemphigus	A10	3.1
ENDOCRINE		
Juvenile diabetes mellitus	B8	2.1
	BW15	3.0
	DW3(LD-8a)	4.5
	DW4(LD-15a)	3.7
Graves' disease	B8	3.6
Addison's disease	B8	6.4
	DW3(LD 8a)	10.5
NEUROLOGIC		
Myasthenia gravis	B8	4.4
Multiple sclerosis	DW2(LD-7a)	5.0

* *Relative risk* = *(% antigen-positive patients) (% antigen-negative controls) / (% antigen-negative patients) (% antigen-positive controls)*

LINKAGE DISEQUILIBRIUM Before reviewing the possible mechanisms of HL-A gene complex influences in disease susceptibility, it is necessary to point to the most salient feature of the population genetics of HL-A antigens, namely, the presence of linkage disequilibria among certain antigens of the A and B, B and C, and B and D loci. A linkage disequilibrium means that antigens of closely linked loci appear together more frequently than predicted by random association. The classic example is the linkage disequilibrium present between the A-locus antigen, HL-A-A1, and B-locus antigen, HL-A-B8, in Caucasian populations of Western Europe and America. One expects the coincidence of A1 and B8 to be the product of their individual frequencies, or 0.17 times 0.11 equals approximately 0.02. The observed frequency of A1 and B8 in Caucasians is 0.06, three times that expected, and an increase of 0.04. The latter value is termed Δ (delta), and is a measure of the disequilibrium. Other first and second series haplotype disequilibria have been recognized, and include (A3, B7), (B2, B12), (A29, B12), and (A11, BW35). Furthermore, some D-locus determinants are now known to be in linkage disequilibrium with second-series antigens (for example, DW3 and B8), and C-locus antigens often have a Δ with B-locus antigens. Just as the serologically defined HL-A antigens can serve as markers for the genes of an entire haplotype within a family, they may also serve as markers within a whole population for specific genes, but only where a linkage disequilibrium exists.

The development of linkage disequilibria is a matter of some importance because such gene associations may have some bearing on their function. For example, it has been proposed that selective pressures during the course of evolution have been the major factor in the survival of certain gene combinations in a haplotype. Such a theory would suggest, for example, that A1 and B8, along with certain D-locus and other determinants, conferred a selective advantage in the face of epidemics such as the plague or smallpox. It would go on to conclude that the descendants of the survivors now display susceptibility to certain diseases because of their unique gene complex which happens to confer an abnormal response to nonlethal environmental agents. The major difficulty with this hypothesis is the assumption that selection would have to work on several genes simultaneously in order to account for the observed deltas; however, the need for complex interactions among the products of the several loci of the major histocompatibility complex is only beginning to be appreciated, and it is possible that selection could force multiple linkage disequilibria.

On the other hand, one does not require the selection hypothesis to establish deltas in a population. With fusion of a population lacking certain antigens with one having a high frequency of antigens in equilibrium, a Δ can develop within a very small number of generations. For example, the increasing Δ value for A1, B8, found as one samples populations from East to West, from India to Western Europe, can be explained on the basis of migration and fusion. In smaller groups, consanguinity, a founder effect, and gene drift may account for disequilibria. Finally, certain linkage disequilibria could occur as a result of a nonrandomness in crossing over during gametic meiosis, because of chromosomal segments which are either more or less likely to break. In any event, the facts strongly suggest that a large number of nonrandom associations exist throughout the HL-A gene complex, and the reasons for their existence, when they are better understood, may relate closely to the mechanism underlying certain disease susceptibilities.

MECHANISMS There are three main hypotheses regarding the mechanisms by which histocompatibility complex genes influence disease susceptibility. The first is termed *molecular mimicry* and would propose that immunochemical similarities between HL-A glycoproteins and microbiological agents result in an impaired immune response because of cross-reacting tolerance of self-antigens. In order to be consistent with the observed facts of the dominance of disease susceptibility in the heterozygous state (e.g., ankylosing spondylitis occurs with B27 on one haplotype only), such a hypothesis would lead to the conclusion that the diseases in question are the result of chronic infection with a depressed immune response. Although cross-reactions between HL-A glycoproteins and streptococcal proteins have been demonstrated, there are no other clearly demonstrated relationships, and direct attempts to show cross-reactivity between yersinia organisms and B27 have been negative. Most telling with regard to B27 and ankylosing spondylitis is the finding that B27 associates with this disease only when it is on a haplotype with the first series antigens, A2 or A9, providing evidence that B27 per se is most likely a marker for a linkage disequilibrium with other HL-A region genes.

The second hypothesis suggests that HL-A antigens may serve as *receptors for specific viruses,* resulting in an increased susceptibility to infection. This hypothesis has problems similar to the first, and direct attempts to show predilections for cell invasion by a variety of known viruses and cells of various HL-A types have been unrewarding.

The third hypothesis, one which is gaining increased acceptance, is that important *immune response (Ir) genes* are present in the HL-A gene complex, and that HL-A antigens are markers for genes in linkage disequilibrium with them. The degree of association would then depend upon the distance between the marker and disease genes on the chromosome, and the degree to which crossing-over between them may be restricted. Clearly, dermal responsiveness to ragweed antigen segregates with HL-A haplotypes in atopic families, although the HL-A antigens themselves may not be the same. A suggestive association with a D-locus gene and ragweed antigen E reactivity now exists, indicating that the gene(s) for a heightened immediate hypersensitivity response is placed far enough into the putative Ir region so that B-locus series HL-A antigens are not good markers. When one considers the association of HL-A-B8 and HL-A-DW3 markers with so many diseases (juvenile diabetes, Addison's disease, Graves' disease, gluten sensitivity, myasthenia gravis), it is tempting to conclude that a control mechanism for immune responsiveness, particularly with regard to autoimmunity, is involved. The observed dominance of susceptibility in heterozygotes suggests the need for a positive response, rather than a deficient one. Since the etiologic agent is known in one of these diseases (gluten), and strongly suspected in another (Coxsackie virus in juvenile diabetes mellitus), carefully designed studies should provide evidence regarding immune responsiveness to the agent versus an exaggerated secondary response to damaged tissue antigens. The numbers of genes involved and the variety of ways in which the final patterns of various diseases present may well be highly variable. Nevertheless, the way is now open to a better understanding of the genetic control of immune responsiveness in disease states.

Tissue typing for transplantation Study of the HL-A gene complex has, at present, limited direct clinical application, but its relationship to transplantation efforts is central. Siblings matched for the major antigens are easily treated with conventional drug therapy, and renal transplant results are in the range of 90 to 95 percent long-term success. A small number of A- and B-locus identical, but D-locus incompatible, transplants have been performed, and although not statistically significant, the majority of these have been rejected. The general experience in bone marrow transplantation also emphasizes the importance of matching for the D-locus region, even when, due to recombination, the serologically defined A- and B-locus antigens are mismatched. Since the degree of linkage disequilibrium between HL-A serologically defined antigens and other genes, including the D locus, is variable, and in many cases absent, matching of HL-A-A and -B antigens for cadaveric renal transplantation is poorly predictive of graft success. Some series in Europe have provided evidence for improved survival with increasing numbers of A- and B-locus antigen matches, but these results have not been completely confirmed in North America, possibly because the greater degree of racial inhomogeneity in the New World reduces the amount of linkage disequilibrium between A, B, D, and other loci of the major histocompatibility gene complex. In contrast, some evidence exists for the importance of D-locus matching as assessed by retrospective results in MLC responses between cadaver and recipient lymphocytes. Since the MLC takes 5 to 7 days for the development of measurable degrees of proliferation (^{3}H-thymidine incorporation), more rapid means (<24 h) of typing for these antigens are needed.

HL-A serologically defined A- and B-locus differences are clearly of major importance once an alloimmune response has been initiated, as these determinants are the major, though not the sole, targets for both humoral and cellular effector mechanisms. Forty to fifty percent of patients exposed to blood products while on chronic hemodialysis develop complement-dependent cytotoxic antibodies to allogenic lymphocytes. The "high responder" sensitized patients may make a selective response against certain HL-A antigens, or may develop such a polyspecific response that they react with 90 to 100 percent of a randomly selected population. Transplants are not performed when the specific cross matches of recipient serums with donor lymphocytes are positive, because of a very high likelihood of an immediate "hyperacute" rejection. Furthermore, sensitized patients receiving cadaveric renal grafts have a high failure rate, even though the specific donor cross match is negative, indicating either a lack of sensitivity in the test or the absence of the relevant antibodies at that particular time. Evidence for the latter comes from the reported improvement in kidney survival rates when additional serums, obtained at monthly intervals while on dialysis, are used at the time of cross match, or if analyses of anti-HL-A specificities in the serums are made. Either way, mismatches can be avoided by assessment of past, as well as present, reactivities. In other words, a profile of the patient's immunologic memory is developed in order to avoid anamnestic responses. Further improvement in practical matching techniques, employing more sensitive cross matches and techniques for assessment of direct and antibody-dependent, cell-mediated cytotoxicity may offer further refinement in solving this major problem in cadaveric renal transplantation. Avoidance of sensitization would appear to offer a logical approach; however, a number of female patients have been sensitized by prior pregnancies, and occasionally the development of such cytotoxins is not explained by either pregnancy or blood transfusion. More important is the absence of data to confirm the notion that patients who never receive blood will have improved graft results; in fact, one such study shows an increased failure rate in nontransfused patients. Taken together, these results at present suggest that genetic control of the alloimmune response also exists in man, although no correlation can be made with HL-A phenotypes. Prior exposure to alloantigens provides a definition of who is a "low responder" and who is a "high responder," and in the latter case it is now possible to avoid, in many instances, the specific mismatches to which a response has already been made, selecting a "new" incompatibility which, as a primary response, is more amenable to conventional drug therapy.

Although minor transplantation antigen incompatibilities may on occasion be of importance in renal transplantation, the only other major antigenic system of proved importance is the ABH red blood cell system, a genetic system which segregates randomly from HL-A; for example, HL-A-identical siblings can be mismatched for ABH. The rules of blood transfusion apply with regard to group O being a universal donor and group AB being a universal recipient. The clinical importance of non-HL-A, non-ABH systems in bone marrow transplantation is greater than with organ grafts because of the graft-versus-host reactivity which commonly occurs in HL-A-matched marrow recipients, and, in fact, has become the major limiting factor in clinical marrow grafting.

Another important application of HL-A typing is in matching for platelet transfusions in individuals sensitized by prior blood component exposure. Platelets express most of the HL-A serologic specificities (A and B loci), but not the D-locus antigens. Matching donor and recipient lymphocyte HL-A serologically defined antigens (A and B loci) is of proved value in improving survival of transfused platelets in sensitized recipients.

IMMUNOLOGY OF REJECTION Knowledge of the immunology of tissue transplantation stems largely from animal experimentation. However, enough evidence has accumulated in man, particularly in kidney transplantation, to indicate that the evidence is similar though not identical for the different species. The following observations describe reasonably accurately the events that transpire during the rejection of most human tissue transplants. Spleen and bone marrow grafts differ because in these instances cells capable of reacting against the recipient (graft-versus-host reaction) are transplanted.

From data derived both from animal and human experience, it appears that the rejection of transplanted tissue results from the antigenic stimulus of a two-component lymphoid system (Fig. 76-3). The lymphocytes involved are the offspring of marrow-derived stem cells. As these stem cells mature under the direct or humoral influence of (1) the thymus or (2) a human equivalent to the cells of the avian bursa, they develop antigen receptors so that they can respond in a cooperative manner to make an immune response when stimulated by antigen. The mature lymphocytes comprising the two distinct populations are for convenience abbreviated as (1) thymus-dependent (T) and (2) bone marrow (bursa)-dependent (B). Cooperative interaction between T and B cells, through the mediation of a substance furnished by the T cells after antigenic stimulation, is necessary for initiation of the immune response. This cell interaction may take place upon the dendrites of tissue macrophages. In the case of the renal allograft, donor antigen may stimulate either T or B cells by way of antigen liberated from the kidney and reaching the lymphocytes by the bloodstream or lymphatics; or by contact between the recipient's lymphocytes and donor antigen as the former circulate through the kidney.

Some T cells are long-lived, circulating in the peripheral blood but "homing" in on lymphoid organs. They are responsible for cell-mediated immunity (CMI) such as graft rejection, delayed hypersensitivity (tuberculin skin test), the immune response to intracellular organisms, and possible "surveillance" which protects against growth of spontaneously occurring neoplasia. B cells are shortlived, noncirculating cells, largely responsible for the production of immune globulins, often referred to as "circulating antibody" or "humoral antibody." Both cell types are involved in immunity to transplants. A third effector system, involving the cooperative effort of graft-specific IgG antibodies and a nonimmune non-T cell, tentatively called a K cell, is now recognized. K cells interact with the Fc portion of the target-cell-bound IgG to mediate antibody-dependent cell-mediated cytotoxicity. Both lymphocytes and monocyte subpopulations may have K-cell activity. Even the polymorphonuclear leukocyte can damage IgG-coated target cells. Allografts to recipients previously unexposed to donor antigen are rejected as a "first-set" graft, largely through the T-cell system. Recipients who have previously been immunized to donor allografts by exposure to donor antigens by blood transfusions or by a previous transplant, or who have been the recipients of xenografts, have circulating preformed humoral antibody, and such grafts undergo "humoral rejection" in which the B-cell mechanism predominates. Because unrelated individuals may share one or more specific HL-A determinants, a recipient may become immunized to the tissues of a donor by previous exposure to transfused white blood cells/or platelets from another individual whose tissues contain the same antigens as the allograft donor. Once a kidney has been in place for several days in a previously unsensitized recipient, humoral immunity may become superimposed upon the cellular rejection; therefore, both types of immune processes may mediate the rejection of an allograft, with one or the other predominating; furthermore, the K-cell mechanism provides a potential link between humoral and cell-mediated immunity.

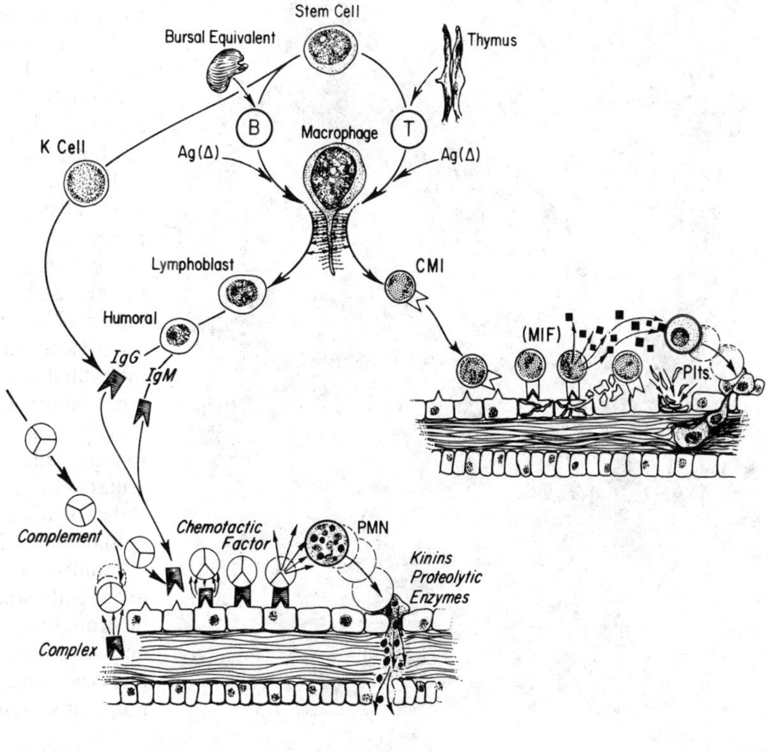

FIGURE 76-3
Overall scheme of the development of effector mechanisms in graft rejection. Bone marrow stem cells differentiate under the influence of the thymus gland into mature thymus-derived (T) lymphocytes, or under the influence of an equivalent to the avian bursa of Fabricius into mature bone-marrow-derived (B) lymphocytes. Exposure to antigen (Δ) results in an interaction between T cells and B cells, and often involves macrophages. The sensitized B cells after mitoses develop into immunoglobulin-secreting cells (e.g., plasma cells), illustrated here by IgG and IgM. Such immunoglobulins may form immune complexes with antigen in the circulation which activate the complement sequence, or they may react directly with antigens on the blood vessel surface. Elaboration of secondary mediators, including the products of complement activation, results in vascular damage as illustrated. Sensitized T lymphocytes are the primary effector cells in cell-mediated immunity (CMI) and may react directly with antigens in the graft to exert a cytotoxic effect. In addition, T cells release factors, such as macrophage migration inhibition factor (MIF) which may accelerate the rate of mononuclear cell infiltration. In addition, it has been shown that unsensitized non-T cells (K cells) can be activated to exert cytotoxic effects by the fixation of IgG to target cells, followed by interaction of the IgG (Fc portion) with a receptor on the K cell. Nonimmune B cells may have K-cell activity, but since other mononuclear cells can react with IgG on target cells, the K cell is shown as having a separate lineage. Finally, platelet aggregation and thrombosis can occur following the endothelial damage induced by any of these mechanisms.

The rejection of an allograft by an individual who has not previously been exposed to donor antigens occurs first by way of the CMI pathways in which the sensitized lymphocytes predominate. In the case of the kidney, the sensitized lymphocyte first combines with an antigen on vascular endothelium. Very early in the rejection process cells can be seen in contact with the small venules. The precise mechanism of the damage induced by the sensitized "killer" T lymphocytes awaits elucidation, but immunoglobulins and complement are not required. Rather, a cyclic nucleotide (cAMP and cGMP)-dependent secretory process which follows direct cell-to-cell contact has been implicated. Similarly, the interaction of sensitized lymphocytes and antigens at the graft site is likely to release migration inhibitory factor (MIF) which may account for the accumulation of mononuclear (histiocytic) cells at the graft site. Some of these cells migrate through the vessel wall and are seen as perivascular accumulations. Intravascular accumulations result in slowing of flow, stasis, and graft ischemia. B lymphocytes, specifically sensitized, or K cells nonspecifically recruited by the prior formation of immune complexes of antibody and histocompatibility antigens, may also appear in the graft along the endothelial lining of vessels. Recovery of infiltrating cells from rejecting organs for study has shown that B cells, T cells, K cells, and monocytes may all be present. Of importance is the fact that donor-specific "killer" cells have been recovered from both animals and human allografts. When significant amounts of circulating antibodies, principally IgG and IgM, appear, the complement sequence is initiated. If intense, such activation may release significant amounts of polymorphonuclear (PMN) chemotactic factors, and PMNs are attracted to the graft, where the release of lysosomal enzymes from the leukocytes may result in damage to the vascular wall. In addition, the deposition of platelets is facilitated, with the release of vasoactive kinins and the deposition of fibrinogen and fibrin. This sequence of events is corroborated by histologic observations of rejection demonstrating interstitial infiltration of cells, and damage to vascular endothelium with the deposition of fibrin, complement, and immune globulins. It can be shown also that the earliest evidence of renal allograft rejection is redistribution of blood flow from the cortex to the corticomedullary area, reflecting the primary role of the influence of vascular damage in the rejection process.

FIGURE 76-4

Biopsy of the renal cadaveric allograft illustrating obliterative endarteritis. Loss of the media is associated with intimal thickening. The elastic tissue shows dissolution of the elastica. The evidence for arteritis with subsequent thrombosis are typically the gaps in the elastica and media. The intimal thickening probably represents organization of a thrombus formed in response to the arteritis. (From GJ Dammin and JP Merrill, Transplantation, tissue rejection and the kidney, Chap. 20 in Structural Basis for Renal Disease, *ed EL Becker, New York: Hoeber-Harper, 1968)*

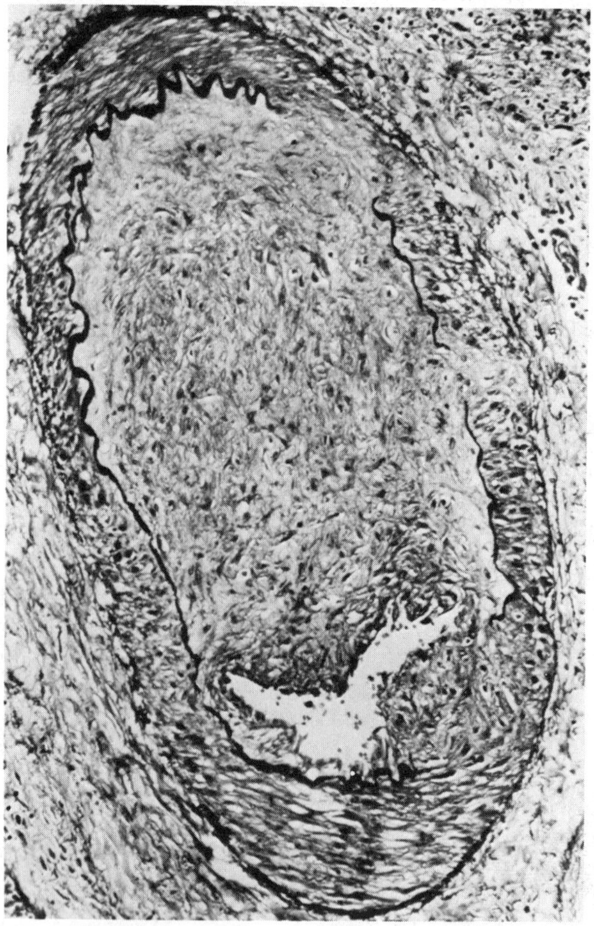

When a kidney is transplanted into a heterologous species or an individual previously sensitized to donor antigen, it is immediately perfused by "preformed" humoral antibody directed specifically against graft antigen. Again, the sequence of events which takes place reflects primarily the vascular site of injury. In such an instance little cellular infiltrate may be seen, but destruction to the vessel wall is violent and immediate, occurring in a matter of minutes in some instances. Platelet thrombi, the deposition of fibrin, and necrosis of vascular endothelium are prominent, and flow through the graft may cease within minutes or hours. Presumably, the same humoral mechanisms discussed above participate, but the sequence of events is accelerated; thus, the term "hyperacute rejection" has been applied.

The failure of transplanted kidneys after 2 or even 3 years of adequate function is due to a form of "chronic rejection." In such kidneys the development of nephrosclerosis, with proliferation of the vascular intima of renal vessels, and intimal fibrosis with marked decrease in the lumen of the vessels take place (Fig. 76-4). The result is renal ischemia, hypertension, widespread tubular atrophy, interstitial fibrosis, and glomerular atrophy with eventual renal failure. Occasionally, lobular or proliferative glomerulonephritis may be the initiating factor and may progress to renal failure. Most long-term vascular lesions and glomerular lesions are probably the result of subclinical episodes of rejection with damage to capillary and vascular epithelium and resultant healing fibrosis and sclerosis.

Finally, there is evidence that humoral antibody, in all probability some fraction of IgG, may actually play a role in promoting the *survival* of the allograft. This enhancing antibody may block the action of cytotoxic "killer" lymphocytes, thus preventing the disastrous effects of the immune onslaught against the graft.

IMMUNOSUPPRESSIVE TREATMENT When histocompatibility differences exist between donor and recipient, it is necessary to modify or suppress the immune response in order to enable the recipient to accept a graft. Immunosuppressive therapy in general suppresses all immune responses, including those to bacteria, fungi, and even malignant tumors. Agents used in man to suppress the immune response are the following:

Drugs *Azathioprine (Imuran),* an analogue of 6-mercaptopurine, is the keystone to immunosuppressive therapy in man. This agent can inhibit synthesis of deoxyribonucleic acid (DNA), ribonucleic acid (RNA), or both. Because cell division and proliferation result as part of the immune response to antigenic stimulation, suppression may be mediated by the inhibition of mitosis of immunologically competent lymphoid cells interfering with synthesis of DNA. Alternatively, inhibition may be brought about by blocking the synthesis of ribonucleic acid (possibly messenger RNA), which is thought to play an immunologic role in the processing of antigens prior to lymphocyte stimulation. Therapy with azathioprine is generally instituted 2 to 5 days prior to transplantation in the recipient of a living donor kidney and on the day of transplantation in the case of a cadaver recipient. The drug is continued at levels of 2 to 3 mg per kg per day, as long as the allograft functions. Because the drug is rapidly metabolized by the liver, its dose need not be varied directly in relation to renal function, even though renal failure results in retention of the metabolites of azathioprine. Some patients are unusually sensitive to this drug, particularly when renal function is compromised, and reduction in dosage is required because of leukopenia and occasionally thrombocytopenia. Excessive amounts of azathioprine may also cause jaundice, anemia, and alopecia. In one series of cadaver allografts the prospective donor was treated with massive doses of cyclophosphamide and methylprednisolone in an attempt to decrease the antigenicity of the graft by eliminating "passenger leukocytes." The preliminary results of this technique are encouraging.

The *corticosteroids,* usually in the form of prednisone, are important adjuncts to immunosuppressive therapy. Of all the agents employed, prednisone has effects that are easiest to assess, and in large doses it is unquestionably the most effective agent for the reversal of rejection. In general, 150 to 200 mg prednisone is given immediately prior to or at the time of transplantation, and the dosage is reduced to maintenance levels over a period of 2 weeks. The well-known side effects of the corticosteroids, particularly impairment of wound healing and predisposition to infection, make it desirable to taper the dose as rapidly as possible in the immediate postoperative period. Customarily methylprednisolone, 1 to 2 g, intravenously, is administered immediately upon diagnosis of beginning rejection. When the drug is effective, the results are usually apparent within 48 to 96 h, and the dose may be subsequently tapered over a 5-day period and oral prednisone resumed. Such "pulse" doses are less effective in the slow rejection process which may not become apparent until 2 to 3 years after transplantation. Although most patients whose renal function is stable after 6 months or a year do not require large doses of prednisone, maintenance doses of 20 mg per day are the rule. Many patients tolerate an alternate-day course of steroids better without an increased risk of rejection.

When jaundice or nephritis appears in patients maintained on azathioprine, *cyclophosphamide* may be substituted. It appears to be as effective in the maintenance of renal allografts as Imuran and somewhat more effective in hepatic allografts. Leukopenia, alopecia, cystitis, ovarian fibrosis, and aspermia may result if the dosage is not carefully regulated.

Antilymphocyte globulin (ALG) When serums from animals made immune to host lymphocytes are injected into the recipient, a marked suppression of cellular immunity to the tissue graft results. The action upon CMI is considerably more effective than upon humoral immunity. A globulin fraction of the serum is the agent generally employed. For use in man peripheral human lymphocytes, thymocytes, lymphocytes from cadaver spleens, or those harvested from thoracic duct fistulas have been utilized. More recently, cultured human lymphoblasts, which can be produced in large quantities, offer the advantage of availability. These cells are injected into horses, rabbits, or goats to produce antilymphocyte serum, from which the globulin fraction is then separated. The globulin is injected intramuscularly, or preferably intravenously, 5 days to a week prior to transplantation and continued for 2 to 3 weeks thereafter. Although ALG is unquestionably effective in prolonging grafts in experimental animals, its efficacy in transplantation of human tissue is somewhat less clear, even though an effective preparation of ALG may result in the disappearance of a previously positive delayed-type of skin reaction. ALG should be used with extreme caution in human beings; it cannot now be considered part of routine immunosuppressive therapy. Possibly further exploration of this preparation, particularly employing larger doses, may result in the development of an effective agent which can be used with relatively little hazard of serum sickness or nephrotoxic nephritis.

Other techniques Of the alternate techniques of immunosuppression, thymectomy and splenectomy have not favorably influenced the course of human kidney transplants. Local irradiation to the transplanted kidney in two or three doses of 350 rd each has also been utilized. Current evidence suggests that this technique may result in fewer early rejection episodes in cadaveric transplants than in nonirradiated controls.

COMPLICATIONS OF RENAL TRANSPLANTATION The complications of human renal transplantation often result from the use of *immunosuppressive therapy.* Wound infection with gram-negative organisms is common, as is breakdown of wounds, particularly the ureteral anastomosis. Pulmonary infections with a variety of unusual organisms, including *Candida* (Chap. 175), *Aspergillus* (Chap. 178), *Nocardia* (Chap. 177), *Pneumocystis* (Chap. 219), and cytomegalovirus (Chap. 211), also occur. Their relationship to a general defect in immunologic integrity is clear. The complications of *corticosteroid* therapy are well known and include gastrointestinal bleeding, hemorrhagic pancreatitis, and impairment of wound-healing. Leukopenia, anemia, and jaundice occur as a result of azathioprine administration.

Even identical twins who do not require immunosuppressive therapy develop complications. In 18 sets of identical twins whose original disease was glomerulonephritis, 11 developed a similar histologic lesion in the transplanted kidney. The glomerular lesion is not, however, limited to the isograft, nor is it necessarily a question of "catching" the disease in the transplant because of continuing antiglomerular activity. A number of patients with true allografts treated with immunosuppressive therapy have developed typical glomerular lesions over a period of years. One patient who received a successful allograft from his mother developed a classic nephrotic syndrome with glomerulonephritis 2½ years after transplantation. Because the reason for transplantation initially was the accidental removal of a single normal ectopic kidney, the development of glomerulonephritis in the transplant cannot be attributed to "continuing activity."

Glomerular lesions occur in some 10 to 15 percent of allografts. In many of these the lesions so resemble those of the patient's own original disease that they must be considered recurrences of the original disease. The recurrence of the nephrotic syndrome with "nil disease" in transplanted kidneys whose recipient's original nil disease had progressed to renal failure, the recurrence in renal allografts of the classic lesions of IgA nephropathy and those of membranoproliferative glomerulonephritis with electron-dense deposit disease are classic examples. In the latter the incidence of recurrence has been reported as high as 30 to 40 percent. In many instances, however, the recurrence of the original renal lesions may represent no threat to the patient's immediate prognosis. Finally, in at least one case, glomerulonephritis has developed apparently *de novo* in a patient who had survived 5 years with a normally functioning allograft.

Sensitization of the human recipient to the antigens of the renal allograft may occur because of exposure to these antigens via blood transfusions or pregnancy. When the cytotoxic antibodies are directed against the antigen of the donor, rapid rejection of the graft occurs, and even when the cytotoxic antibodies in the recipient's serum are not specific for those of the donor, the prognosis for graft survival is poorer than in unsensitized individuals. This is discussed elsewhere in this chapter.

The incidence of *tumors* arising in patients on immunosuppressive therapy in one well-studied group was 5.6 percent, or approximately 100 times greater than that observed in the general population in the same age range. These figures correspond with those in the world experience of approximately 17,000 cases. The most common lesions were cancer of the skin and lips and carcinoma *in situ* of the cervix. These lesions were easily treated. There was a high incidence of lymphomas, particularly reticulum cell sarcoma of the nervous system. The prognosis was poor when these lesions occurred. Two possibilities are suggested for the high incidence of cancer in transplant recipients: (1) Immunosuppressive therapy impairs the "immunologic surveillance" of the lymphoreticular system, in consequence of which potentially malignant cellular mutations are not detected and destroyed; (2) immunosuppressed individuals frequently harbor viruses, some of which may be oncogenic.

Tumor cells have been transplanted inadvertently with kidneys taken from cadaver donors and occasionally from living donors. The immunosuppressive therapy which allows the kidney to be tolerated in the recipients also apparently permits survival and propagation of the malignant tumor. In two instances cessation of immunosuppressive therapy resulted in rejection of both the graft and the tumor with its metastases.

Urinary fistula requiring nephrostomy may be the result of rejection of the ureter, disruption of the ureteral blood supply, infection, or a combination of all three. Wound infection and failure of the wound to heal are not uncommon, particularly when the higher doses of steroids are required.

Hypercalcemia may develop within days or weeks after transplantation and persist for as long as 7 years. In many instances this appears to be due to markedly enlarged parathyroid glands which have developed during the uremic phase and do not spontaneously regress with the resumption of normal renal function. In other instances no elevation of blood levels of parathyroid hormone can be found. Although several instances of renal and vascular calcification have been reported, renal function in general does not appear to suffer. However, when bone disease occurs or persists in the presence of hyperparathyroidism, subtotal parathyroidectomy is indicated. Glucocorticoid administration may contribute to the hypercalcemia. *Aseptic necrosis* of the head of the femur has been reported in 10 to 20 percent of the posttransplant patients. This complication is probably due to preexisting uremic bone disease or hyperparathyroidism, plus the large doses of corticosteroid.

The incidence of death from *myocardial infarction* and *cerebrovascular accidents* is considerably higher in transplant recipients than in the population at large. The contributing factors are preexisting hypertension, vascular disease, and hypertriglyceridemia, which occurs in uremic patients and persists in the posttransplant period. There is possibly a contribution by hypercalcemia. *Gastrointestinal hemorrhage* is also a complication.

SELECTION OF RECIPIENTS FOR KIDNEY TRANSPLANTATION Table 76-3 lists practical considerations in the selection of a recipient for a human renal allograft. Such a procedure should be undertaken only when conservative treatment has failed, when there are no reversible elements in the patient's renal failure, and when he is too sick to be

TABLE 76-3
Contraindications to human kidney transplantation

1 Absolute contraindications:
- *a* Reversible renal involvement
- *b* Ability of conservative measures to maintain useful life
- *c* Major extrarenal complications (cerebrovascular or coronary disease; neoplasia)
- *d* Active infection
- *e* Active glomerulonephritis
- *f* Previous sensitization to human tissue

2 Relative contraindications:
- *a* Age
- *b* Presence of vesical or urethral abnormalities
- *c* Iliofemoral occlusive disease
- *d* Diabetes mellitus
- *e* Inactive lupus erythematosus
- *f* Psychiatric problems

maintained comfortably with the usual methods of treatment. However, the considerable success with kidneys transplanted from blood relatives, reports of success with second or third kidney transplants, and the ability to maintain patients who have had transplant failures on hemodialysis justify consideration of kidney transplantation before the patient is critically ill and possibly even before it is obvious that hemodialysis is the only other course. Transplantation should not be utilized in an attempt to salvage patients from failure to thrive on dialysis. On the other hand, when no well-matched related donor is available, the patient and his physician should carefully consider the relative risks outlined in Table 76-1 against those of continued dialysis. Approximately 15 percent of dialysis patients receiving cadaver transplants cannot be successfully returned to dialysis if the graft fails. The attrition rate in most well-run dialysis programs is about 4 to 7 percent per year. Each case, of course, must be individualized before the statistics have pertinence. The recipient should be free of life-threatening extrarenal complications such as cancer, severe coronary artery disease, and cerebrovascular disease. Provided that diffuse vascular involvement is not present, diabetes itself is not a contraindication. Although age may be a limiting factor, the "physiologic" age rather than the chronologic age contraindicates transplantation. A cadaver transplant into an eighty-two-year-old patient is on record, and adult renal allografts have been transplanted into recipients as young as three. Although abnormalities of the bladder and urethra present additional hazards, successful renal allografts have been placed in individuals with these abnormalities by prior construction of an artificial bladder (i.e., ileal conduit) into which the donor ureter is placed. The demonstration of "preformed antibodies" in the potential recipient prior to transplantation is a contraindication when in the standard lymphocytotoxicity test these antibodies react specifically to donor cells.

DONOR SELECTION Donor sources are cadavers or volunteer blood-related living donors. Living volunteer donors should be found completely normal on physical examination and should be of the same major ABO blood group, because there is good evidence that crossing major blood group barriers prejudices survival of the allograft. It is, however, possible to transplant a kidney of a type O donor into an A or B recipient. Selective renal arteriography should be performed on volunteer donors to rule out the presence of multiple or abnormal renal arteries, because the surgical procedure is inordinately difficult and the ischemic time of the normal kidney prohibitively long when vascular abnormalities exist. Cadaver donors should be free of malignant neoplastic disease because of possible transmission of cancer to the recipient.

Although tissue typing for A- and B-locus HL-A antigens is of limited value for cadaver donors, direct cross matching for the presence of preformed antibodies against specific donor tissue is mandatory. The chances of finding a perfect A- and B-locus 4-antigen match between unrelated donor and recipient are calculated to be between 1 in 300 and 1 in 1,000, varying with the incidence of HL-A antigens in the population. If, in addition, antigens of the D locus are found to be of practical importance, matching will require a large recipient pool, maintained on hemodialysis. A coordinated regional or national system of computerized information sharing and logistical support for the transportation of cadaver kidneys to the suitable recipient is under development. It is now possible to remove cadaver kidneys and to maintain them for up to 48 h on cold pulsatile perfusion or simple flushing and cooling. This should permit adequate time for various typing, cross matching, transportation, and selection problems to be solved.

CLINICAL COURSE AND MANAGEMENT OF THE RECIPIENT Usually, but not invariably, bilateral nephrectomies are performed prior to transplantation, and the recipient is maintained on intermittent hemodialysis. Removal of the patient's own diseased kidneys obviates one source of infection in the postoperative period and facilitates the diagnosis of rejection of the allograft, since variations in renal function and urine sediment are then related only to changes in the allograft. However, bilateral nephrectomy also potentiates the anemia of the patient maintained on dialysis, and therefore ideally the procedure should be performed as close as is feasible to the projected time of transplantation. There is statistical evidence that transplanted kidneys fare better if the recipient has been previously nephrectomized, although the reason for this is unclear. It should be ascertained also that the recipient has a normally functioning bladder and lower outflow tract.

Adequate hemodialysis should be performed within 48 h prior to surgery, and care should be taken that the serum potassium level is not markedly elevated so that intraoperative cardiac arrhythmias can be averted. In patients who have been presensitized to donor tissue, hyperacute rejection may take place on the operating table. Within minutes the kidney will become swollen, tense, and a mottled purple in color, and blood flow may cease soon thereafter. Thrombotic obliterative lesions may be seen by frozen section, and if they are extensive the kidney should be removed. Postoperatively the diuresis that occurs must be carefully monitored; in many instances it may be massive, reflecting the inability of ischemic tubules to regulate sodium and water excretion. Massive potassium losses may occur and occasionally result in cardiac arrhythmias. The chronically uremic patient undoubtedly has some excess of extracellular fluid, and some degree of negative balance should be accomplished provided circulatory hemodynamics remain stable.

Although immunosuppressive regimens vary, a typical program would be the following:

Azathioprine in a dose of 4 mg per kg is given for 2 days preoperatively to recipients of a living donor transplant; on the day of operation it is administered by the intravenous route, and it is continued for about 1 week, depending upon renal function. It is then reduced to 3 mg per kg, and the maintenance dose is 1½ mg per kg by mouth. In recipients of kidneys from living donors the equivalent of 300 to 500 mg cortisone is given on the day of operation; this dose is maintained for 2 days and is decreased gradually to a maintenance dose of 50 to 100 mg cortisone, usually administered as the prednisone equivalent. For rejection episodes, 1 to 2 g soluble corticosteroid in the form of methylprednisolone is administered intravenously daily for a 5-day period. This is decreased to 800, 600, and 400 mg over the next 10-day period while oral prednisone dosage is maintained at 25 to 50 mg.

The rejection episode Early diagnosis of rejection is imperative, because prompt institution of vigorous therapy may reverse renal function and prevent irreversible damage due to fibrosis. Clinical evidence of rejection is characterized by fever, swelling, and tenderness over the allograft, and by significant reduction in urine volume. In patients whose renal function is good initially, oliguria may be accompanied by decreased urinary sodium concentration and increased osmolarity. These changes may not be present in the more chronic stages of rejection or when renal function is impaired at the onset of rejection. A transplanted cadaver kidney frequently undergoes a period of anuria which may last as long as 3 weeks without prejudicing the eventual function of the graft. In this instance, the reversible lesion is presumably due to ischemia, and the diagnosis of rejection becomes more difficult. Renal arteriography and radioactive Hippuran renograms may be useful in ascertaining changes in the renal vasculature and in renal blood flow, even in the absence of urinary flow. When renal function has been good initially, a rise in the blood urea nitrogen level and a decrease in the creatinine clearance may herald the onset of rejection. The serum creatinine or its clearance is more reliable, because fever and the administration of prednisone may influence the concentration of blood urea nitrogen without necessarily reflecting a decrease in urea clearance. Increase in the 24-h excretion of urinary lysozyme has been helpful. Increase in proteinuria may reflect rejection, but when it occurs later in the course of the postoperative period, predominant glomerular disease may be present. Hypertension is also a concomitant of rejection. When hypertension responds to prednisone, it is likely that rejection has been responsible for the elevation of blood pressure, because other forms of hypertension usually do not improve with corticosteroid therapy. A number of tests have been posed for the diagnosis of rejection which depend upon the measurements of variation in expressions of cellular or humoral immunity; none of these, however, are well correlated with the onset of clinical rejection. Others, such as the measurement of lysozyme excretion and that of fibrin-split products reflect nonspecific renal damage, although the latter test may have somewhat more pertinence to the rejection mechanism.

Modification of the usual clinical manifestations of infection by immunosuppressive therapy is a major problem in the posttransplant period. The signs and symptoms of infection may be masked and distorted, and fever without obvious cause is common. Only after days or weeks will it become apparent that it has a viral or fungal origin. The importance of blood cultures in such patients cannot be overemphasized, because systemic infection without obvious external foci is frequent. Particularly important are rapidly occurring pulmonary lesions, which may result in death within 5 days of onset. When these become apparent, immunosuppressive agents should be discontinued except for maintenance doses of prednisone. In the case of *Pneumocystis carinii,* pentamidine seems to be the treatment of choice; amphotericin B has been used effectively in systemic fungal infections. Involvement of the oropharynx with *Candida* may be treated with local Mycostatin. Small doses (a total of 300 mg) of amphotericin given over a period of 2 weeks may be effective in refractory oral candidiasis. The treatment of jaundice in transplant patients should include cessation of Imuran therapy. It is surprising that total cessation of Imuran therapy often does not result in rejection of a graft. In some instances of jaundice, cyclophosphamide may be substituted for Imuran. Antiplatelet agents and anticoagulants, although effective in theory, have not been strikingly successful in the prevention of the chronic vascular lesion.

The condition of patients who have been discharged from the hospital should be closely observed in a specialized outpatient clinic whose physicians are familiar with the problems and complications of the posttransplant patient. When, in spite of repeated efforts to reverse the rejection, renal function progressively fails, the philosophy should be to save the patient, not the graft. Excessive immunosuppressive therapy may lead to fatal infection or bleeding. A biopsy of the graft may establish the irreversibility of the lesion. When such irreversibility is established, the graft should be removed and the patient started again on hemodialysis. Infection and occasionally hemorrhage at the operative sites days and even months following removal of the graft occasionally occur and must be carefully watched. Psychologic complications following transplantation are common. Depression and anxiety may reflect both the difficult, stressful postoperative course and the anxiety and uncertainty of the physician.

In spite of the potential teratogenic effects of immunosuppressive agents 64 women and 68 men have become parents after transplantation. The incidence of congenital abnormalities in the offspring is not unusual.

From the results shown in Table 76-1 and the summary of complications, it is evident that immunosuppressive therapy as currently used in renal transplantation is inadequate. What is badly needed is a solution to the problem of producing specific immunologic unresponsiveness to the antigens of the donor without affecting the recipient's immune potential for infective agents. Such techniques have been successfully developed for the experimental animal, and their safe application to man is eagerly awaited.

TRANSPLANTATION OF OTHER TISSUES Organs other than the kidney which have a potential for clinical transplantation are the liver and heart. Two possible indications for *liver transplantation* are chronic hepatic failure and malignancy which is localized to the liver. Two techniques for liver transplantation have been utilized in man: (1) *Orthotopic*—the recipient's own liver is removed and the transplant is substituted for it in the anatomic position. (2) *Auxiliary*—the recipient's liver is left in place and the allograft is placed in the right paravertebral gutter. The donor's vena cava then is interposed in the recipient terminal inferior vena cava, and the hepatic artery is anastomosed to the right common iliac artery. Finally, the end of the allograft portal vein is anastomosed to the recipient's superior mesenteric vein.

Immunosuppressive regimens are similar to those in kidney transplantation. There is some suggestion that the use of antilymphocyte globulin is more effective in liver allografting. Obviously, the donor source must be a cadaver. Complications of liver transplantation have been strikingly different from those encountered with renal allografts. In many instances an initial hemorrhagic diathesis with fibrinolysis occurs. This is followed by a phase of hypercoagulability in the successfully transplanted recipient, which in one instance resulted in fatal pulmonary emboli. Infections also seem to present a greater problem than with renal allografts. These complications are not insurmountable, however, and there are now a number of liver-transplant recipients who have survived for 2 years or more. Although at this time liver transplantation is not as clinically feasible a procedure as kidney grafting, in a few centers with expertise and experience in this technique liver transplants continue to be performed, it is hoped with steady improvement in the results.

Transplantation of the heart has been accomplished successfully in man in a number of instances. Current results suggest that it is comparable to transplantation of the cadaver kidney and that results probably will improve. Indications for cardiac transplantation are myocardial insufficiency, usually due to severe coronary artery disease and myocardial fibrosis, and failure to respond to the most rigorous medical measures. The donor must be a cadaver and is usually an individual whose death has resulted from trauma or suicide. The question of the ethics and morals raised by the removal of a heart capable of sustaining life in another individual has been discussed by many medical and lay authors. It seems eminently reasonable that if "death" of the brain has occurred, as evidenced by lack of electrical activity in the electroencephalogram over a period of 24 to 36 h, dilated pupils, failure of spontaneous respiration, and lack of peripheral reflexes, the ability to maintain respiration or cardiac output by artificial methods is academic. Nevertheless, the decision as to when to discontinue these efforts should be made independently by the physician caring for the prospective donor in consultation with one or two colleagues. The question of whether the heart is to be used for transplantation should not affect this decision. Once the decision has been made, the donor can be maintained until the recipient is prepared for operation. Recently a human "auxiliary heart" has been transplanted with initial success. The anastomosis of the donor heart to that of the recipient is made in such a way that the normal left ventricle of the donor assists the failing left ventricle of the recipient while the hypertrophied right ventricle of the recipient is allowed to continue to function in the pulmonary circuit, thus eliminating the sudden load imposed upon the normal right ventricle by the preexisting pulmonary hypertension. At present, cardiac transplantation is and should be done only in specialized centers with highly skilled and experienced teams. Its future as an important therapeutic procedure is still unclear.

Human *spleen* and *pancreas* have been transplanted with limited success. If it could be shown that normal spleen can produce a useful amount of antihemophilic globulin (AHG), transplantation of that organ to some patients with hemophilia would provide a distinct advantage over standard substitution therapy. Transplantation of lymphoid tissue (including spleen) for total agammaglobulinemia has resulted in temporary improvement, but eventually the transplanted lymphoid tissue rejects the host (graft versus host reaction). Temporary success in transplanting pancreas in diabetics also has been reported, but substitution therapy seems more feasible.

Various other *endocrines,* including parathyroid, adrenal, and thyroid, have all been transplanted, with only temporary success. A large percentage of *corneal grafts* survive as allografts in man, primarily because the cornea is not vascularized, which excludes immunologically competent cells. Grafts of bone and blood vessels do not survive as living allografts but act as a "scaffolding" over which host tissue may grow.

Transplantation of allogenic bone marrow in man is of particular interest to patients with leukemia and aplastic anemia and has resulted in a number of attempts to modify these diseases by this means. Similarly, the reconstitution of the defect in congenital or acquired agammaglobulinemia or alymphocytosis has been attempted by grafting into such recipients cells competent to produce cell-mediated immunity or humoral immunity. When the recipient and donor are identical twins, no immunosuppressive therapy is necessary, and 50 percent of the recipients transplanted have done well. Aplastic anemia has also been treated by marrow-grafting between siblings who are 4-antigen HL-A matches and MLC-negative. In this case the recipient is prepared with cyclophosphamide and total body irradiation, while methotrexate is given after grafting. Some 50 percent of these patients have also done well. In the treatment of acute leukemia the object is to destroy as many of the malignant cells as possible; therefore, 1,000 rd total body irradiation plus cyclophosphamide is given, and, in addition, to enhance the immune reaction of donor cells against malignant antigens, the recipient is immunized by radiation-killed malignant cells. In the instances where this was accomplished between identical twins, 10 remissions longer than 3 months and 1 greater than 49 months have occurred. The recipients of matched allogenic marrow, similarly prepared, have done increasingly well, with 100 percent survival for greater than 50 days in cases transplanted in the first 6 months of 1974 in Thomas' series. Immune-competent donor cells reacting against the antigens of the host result in a "graft versus host reaction" in some 70 percent of the cases. This may be acute or indolent and is characterized by involvement of the skin, liver, and gastrointestinal tract. Infection, similar to that seen in kidney transplant recipients, is common. Methotrexate, cyclophosphamide, and antithymocyte globulin have been used in the treatment of this syndrome with some success. A striking and unexpected phenomenon has been malignant transformation of donor cells in two instances. Comparison of results of 1974 with those of 1969 show a marked improvement in survival rates and a decreased incidence of complications.

Transplantation of a normal allogenic liver to repair the metabolic defect in Wilson's disease has been reported in two instances with some preliminary success, and the transplantation of the kidney not as a functioning excretory organ but as a source of the congenitally absent enzyme has been attempted in Fabry's disease and oxalosis. The long-term results are disappointing.

ORGAN PRESERVATION If it were possible to remove cadaver organs and to store them for a period of weeks or longer under conditions permitting their successful replantation, one of the difficult problems in organ procurement would be solved. Bone marrow is the only organ that can be stored easily for prolonged periods.

XENOGRAFTS Kidneys, lungs, and hearts have been transplanted to human beings from various primates, including chimpanzees and baboons. Although one chimpanzee kidney graft functioned well for more than 7 months, clinical efforts in this area have been abandoned.

REFERENCES

BRENT L, PINTO M: Induction of specific unresponsiveness by donor antigen and non-specific immunosuppression, in *Immunological Aspects of Transplantation Surgery,* 1974, p. 317

CARPENTER CB et al: The role of antibodies in the rejection and enhancement of organ allografts. Adv Immunol 22 (in press)

DAUSSET J et al: The association of the HL-A antigens with diseases. Clin Immunol Immunopathol 3:127, 1974

DAVID DS et al: Hypercalcemia after renal transplantation: Long-term follow-up data. N Engl J Med 289:398, 1973

DEGOS L, DAUSSET J: Human migrations and linkage disequilibrium of HL-A system. Immunogenetics 3:195, 1974

LOWRIE EG et al: Survival of patients undergoing chronic hemodialysis and renal transplantation. N Engl J Med 288:863, 1973

MCDEVITT HO, BODMER WF: HL-A, immune response genes, and disease. Lancet 1:1269, 1974

MERRILL JP: New perspectives on pathogenesis and treatment of rejection in kidney transplantation. Kidney Int 7:318, 1975

PENN I: The incidence of malignancies in transplantation recipients. Transplant Proc 8:323, 1975

SVEJGAARD A et al: HL-A and disease associations—A survey. Transplant Rev 22:3, 1975

THOMAS ED et al: Medical Progress: Bone-marrow transplantation. N Engl J Med 292:832, 895, 1975

VANROOD JJ et al: Disease predisposition, immune responsiveness and the fine structure of the HL-A supergene. Transplant Rev 22:75, 1975

77

SYSTEMIC LUPUS ERYTHEMATOSUS

MART MANNIK
BRUCE C. GILLILAND

INTRODUCTION Systemic lupus erythematosus (SLE) is a disease of unknown cause. However, abundant evidence shows that immunologic mechanisms of tissue injury are important in its pathogenesis. The clinical presentation and the course of SLE are variable. A hallmark of this disease is the presence of a number of antibodies to nuclear components, but other immunologic abnormalities exist as well. Some patients with SLE have spontaneous remissions, others respond favorably to treatment with corticosteroids, and in some patients the course is unresponsive to available medications. On the basis of detailed studies of animal models that resemble SLE, viral infections and genetic predisposition appear etiologically important.

PATHOGENESIS The serum of patients with SLE contains many antibodies; among them are the antibodies to deoxyribonucleic acid (DNA), nucleoprotein, histones, nuclear ribonucleoprotein, and other nuclear constituents. These antibodies are collectively termed antinuclear antibodies (ANA). The antinuclear antibodies alone are harmless; their presence in vivo or in tissue cultures does not harm living cells, since antibodies do not penetrate the membrane of living cells. However, the antinuclear antibodies participate in the pathogenesis of SLE by forming antigen-antibody complexes with their specific antigens. DNA and antibodies to DNA, nucleoprotein and antibodies to nucleoprotein, as well as complement components, have been demonstrated in the renal glomerular basement membrane and in the vascular basement membrane of patients with SLE. These observations resemble the findings in experimental serum sickness (Chap. 75). In acute and chronic experimental serum sicknesses, antigen-antibody complexes circulate transiently. Though the bulk of these materials is removed by the reticuloendothelial system, small amounts of immune complexes are entrapped by vascular and glomerular basement membranes. During the formation of antigen-antibody complexes, complement is consumed and the serum concentration of complement is decreased. Similarly, during the active phase of SLE, serum complement is decreased and circulating immune complexes can be detected with sensitive techniques. For these reasons SLE has been classified as an immune-complex disease. Even though DNA and nucleoprotein have been identified in tissue lesions, the source of these antigens has not been clarified. Other antigen-antibody systems may also be involved.

In experimental immune-complex diseases of animals and in human serum sickness, inflammation in joints, pleura, and pericardium occurs because of the presence of antigen and subsequent immune-complex formation. Similar mechanisms may well explain the multitude of clinical manifestations in patients with SLE.

ETIOLOGY The reasons for development of the antinuclear and other antibodies in SLE are not clear. Furthermore, the origin of the antigens in tissue lesions has not been elucidated—they may be autologous nuclear components, or they may originate from invading microorganisms. The hypothesis that SLE results from a viral infection in genetically predisposed persons is supported by several observations. The strongest support for this hypothesis comes from studies on the F_1 hybrids of New Zealand black (NZB) and white (NZW) mice that develop a syndrome analogous to SLE. These mice develop among other manifestations renal lesions, antinuclear antibodies, antibodies to DNA, and decreased serum complement. DNA and antibodies to DNA exist in the renal deposits of immune complexes along with viral-coat antigens and specific antibodies to these antigens. In addition, C-type viruses have been identified in these mice. Furthermore, in certain colonies of dogs SLE-like disease can be transmitted with cell-free extracts, and C-type viruses have been identified in these animals in association with the disease. In a very high percentage of patients with SLE, cytoplasmic virus-like tubuloreticular structures are found by electron microscopy in endothelial cells of glomerular and other capillaries. These structures initially were thought to represent viruses, but now are thought to represent an unidentified response to cell injury. Similar inclusions are seen in other disorders, but with lesser frequency.

In humans and mice with SLE, abnormalities exist in the

regulatory mechanisms of the immune response. A suppression of cell-mediated immunity is apparent with an enhanced activity of humoral immunity. These observations suggest a diminution of the T-cell suppressor mechanism on B-cell functions. These abnormalities may account for the multitude of antibodies to intracellular components as mentioned above, but the reasons for the existence of these abnormalities remain obscure.

A genetic predisposition for SLE has been suggested by the subclinical or clinical abnormalities in relatives of patients with SLE and by the high concordance of clinical SLE in monozygotic twins. On the other hand, the finding of a high prevalence of lymphocytotoxic antibodies among household contacts, including but not limited to blood relatives, raises the possibility of nongenetic transmission of SLE. The occurrence of SLE and lupus-like syndromes in patients with several inborn errors of complement (deficiencies of Clr, Cls, C4, C2, and C5) has been noted but not explained.

PATHOLOGY The pathologic changes in SLE are variable and depend on the stage of the disease. Fibrinoid deposits are commonly seen in blood vessels, among collagen fibers, and on serosal surfaces. Hematoxylin bodies are specific for SLE and are defined as hematoxylin-stained round or oblong masses in areas of inflammation. Hematoxylin bodies are thought to represent degenerated nuclei that have interacted with antinuclear antibodies.

The renal lesions in patients with SLE have been classified into *focal glomerulonephritis, diffuse glomerulonephritis,* and *membranous lupus nephritis.* In focal glomerulonephritis some glomeruli show focal hypercellularity, accumulation of inflammatory cells, and thickening of basement membrane. Immunofluorescent microscopy shows the presence of immunoglobulins and the third component of complement (C3) in involved areas as well as in the mesangium of uninvolved areas. In diffuse glomerulonephritis the same changes are present in all glomeruli, but frequently in an uneven manner. The basement membrane may be considerably thickened. Tubular atrophy and interstitial infiltration with lymphocytes and plasma cells are present. On immunofluorescent microscopy, extensive "lumpy-bumpy" deposits of immunoglobulin and C3 are seen along the basement membrane. On electron microscopy, the electron-dense deposits are found on the endothelial side of the basement membrane and in the mesangium.

In membranous lupus nephritis little hypercellularity is present, but the basement membrane is diffusely thickened. Tubular atrophy and interstitial mononuclear cells are present as well. Immunofluorescent microscopy discloses granular deposits of immunoglobulins and C3. By electron microscopy these deposits are localized on the epithelial side of the basement membrane and within the basement membrane. The mechanisms for these differences in renal involvement have not been elucidated.

The biopsy of skin lesions in patients with SLE will show atrophy, epidermal hyperkeratosis, and keratotic plugging. The dermis is edematous and infiltrated variably with lymphocytes, plasma cells, and histiocytes. On immunofluorescent staining the epidermal-dermal junction has IgG and C3 deposits. Similar changes are frequently present in clinically uninvolved skin. The mechanism for development of these deposits has not been clarified.

Widespread small-vessel vasculitis may be present in many organs. Such lesions exist in the synovium and show both mononuclear and polymorphonuclear infiltration. Autopsy studies on SLE patients with central nervous system abnormalities may show necrotizing vasculitis of arterioles and capillaries in many parts of the brain. Microinfarcts of brain tissues may be apparent. In some patients abundant deposits of immunoglobulins and complement components occur at the basement membrane of the choroid plexus analogous to glomerular deposits of immune complexes. The spleen shows marked intimal proliferation of penicillar and central arteries, which gives an "onion skin" appearance to these vessels. The heart valves and chordae tendineae have at times nonbacterial verrucous vegetations (Libman-Sacks endocarditis).

CLINICAL MANIFESTATIONS SLE is predominantly a disease of women (9 women to 1 man) in the second to fifth decades of life, but it spares neither children nor persons of advanced age. The prevalence of SLE is 2 to 3 per 100,000. Most recent estimates indicate that 77 percent of patients with SLE have a 5-year survival and that renal disease and central nervous system involvement decrease this survival. The most frequent causes of death are uremia, heart failure, hemorrhage, central nervous system disease, and intercurrent bacterial infections.

Patients with SLE may present with a variety of abnormalities, including arthritis and arthralgias, cutaneous manifestations, nephritis, fever, central nervous system manifestations. Raynaud's phenomenon, pleurisy, pericarditis, hemolytic anemia, leukopenia, or thrombocytopenia (Table 77-1).

Arthritis and *arthralgias* are the most frequent presenting as well as the most common complaints during the course of the illness. The arthralgias are fleeting; they involve the hands or feet and also large joints. Redness, warmth, tenderness, and synovial effusions are frequently present. However, deformities are rare, and the erosions so characteristic of rheumatoid arthritis are unusual. The synovial fluid white blood cell counts are relatively low (less than 3,000 per mm^3), and mononuclear cells predominate. Aseptic necrosis may occur, in part because of therapy with corticosteroids. Profound muscle weakness and tenderness reflect myositis in some patients.

Fever is frequent during the course of SLE. Fatigue, mal-

TABLE 77-1
Clinical manifestations during the course of systemic lupus erythematosus

Manifestation	*Cumulative percentage of patients*
Arthritis and arthralgias	92
Fever	84
Skin eruptions	72
Lymphadenopathy	59
Renal involvement	53
Anorexia, nausea, vomiting	53
Myalgia	48
Pleuritis	45
Central nervous system abnormalities	26

SOURCE: *Modified from EL Dubois, 1974.*

aise, anorexia, and weight loss also occur. However, systemic complaints may be totally absent in some patients.

Cutaneous manifestations of SLE include a variety of lesions. A facial eruption, with butterfly distribution over the malar areas and bridge of the nose, consists of erythema, atrophy, telangiectasia, and keratotic plugging. This characteristic rash occurs in about 40 percent of patients. Similar eruptions may occur in other parts of the body, particularly in the exposed areas. At times skin eruptions are precipitated or worsened by exposure to ultraviolet rays. Patchy alopecia occurs with similar frequency. Patients with SLE may have short broken hairs above the forehead, the so-called "lupus hairs." Dermal vasculitis can be found in about 20 percent of patients, usually as small infarcts of the digital skin. In some patients only erythema due to excessively large or numerous capillaries around the digits and fingernails is seen. Ulcers may be encountered on nasal or oral mucous membranes. Other cutaneous manifestations include purpura, bullae, hives, and angioneurotic edema. Raynaud's phenomenon is seen in about one-fifth of patients with SLE.

Discoid lupus is a chronic skin ailment with lesions usually confined to face, neck, arms, and scalp. Scaling is prominent, with atrophy, telangiectasia, and keratotic plugging. Deep scars remain when the lesions subside. Only a few of these patients go on to develop systemic lupus erythematosus. On the other hand, some patients with SLE also have discoid lesions.

Renal involvement is one of the most serious manifestations in SLE. Clinically detectable evidence of renal involvement is seen in about one-half of all patients with SLE. These abnormalities extend from minimal proteinuria and few red blood cell casts to massive hematuria, proteinuria, and frank nephrotic syndrome. In some patients renal involvement goes on to total renal failure; in others there is a course of exacerbations and remissions, with eventual renal failure. Some patients respond well to treatment or improve spontaneously, but minimal proteinuria and decreased creatinine clearance may persist as evidence of irreversible damage. In nearly all carefully investigated patients with SLE, electron microscopic or immunofluorescent abnormalities have been observed even when renal function and urinary sediment are normal. In these patients the immune deposits are located primarily in the glomerular mesangium.

The development of superimposed urinary tract infection should always be kept in mind, since these patients seem liable to such infections.

Cardiopulmonary abnormalities are moderately frequent in patients with SLE. Symptoms and signs of pericarditis or other cardiac abnormalities are encountered in almost 50 percent of them. Pericarditis may be the presenting complaint, with the usual physical and electrocardiographic findings. Tamponade due to SLE pericarditis is unusual. Myocarditis may occur. The nonbacterial verrucous endocartitis is rarely diagnosed clinically but should be suspected when new murmurs develop in the absence of bacterial endocarditis. Symptomatic or asymptomatic pleural involvement occurs in nearly half the patients. Patchy and transient parenchymal infiltrates have been noted, and occasionally severe lupus pneumonitis may occur. The cause of these abnormalities is not known, and they are difficult to distinguish from infiltrates caused by infections.

Neurologic manifestations represent another serious aspect of SLE. A variety of central nervous system manifestations has been noted in 20 to 50 percent of patients. Among these are convulsive disorders, followed in frequency by abnormalities in mental functions and cranial nerves. Peripheral neuropathies are infrequent. Occasionally patients present with primarily mental dysfunction, e.g., emotional lability, psychosis, organic brain syndrome, without other significant symptoms. Cerebrospinal fluid of patients with central nervous system involvement may show slight to moderate increase in protein concentration and mild increase in lymphocytes; usually these occur late in the disease. The electroencephalograms are abnormal, with diffuse nonspecific changes. The brain scans may show focal increased uptake of isotope during active central nervous system involvement.

Lymph node enlargement occurs in many patients with SLE. Such abnormalities may be diffuse or local. Characteristically the nodes are not tender. The enlargement of nodes is thought to occur because of increased activity of the immune system. Splenomegaly occurs in about 10 percent of patients and may be associated with hemolytic anemia. *Hepatomegaly* is found in about 25 percent of patients. The cause for hepatomegaly is not fully known. Lupoid hepatitis is a syndrome of chronic active hepatitis associated with positive tests for LE cells or antinuclear antibodies (Chap. 300).

LABORATORY MANIFESTATIONS A variety of abnormalities in *hematologic* and *immunologic* tests may be encountered in SLE (Table 77-2).

A mild, normochromic, normocytic *anemia* is seen frequently. Most likely this is the hypoproliferative anemia that accompanies many inflammatory processes. Less frequently patients have severe immune-hemolytic anemia that requires steroid therapy or splenectomy. *Leukopenia* is seen in over half the patients. The mechanisms for leukopenia and thrombocytopenia are not fully delineated, but intravascular immune complexes as well as antibodies directed to leukocytes and platelets may contribute to these abnormalities. A potentially serious but infrequent prob-

TABLE 77-2
Laboratory abnormalities in systemic lupus erythematosus

Abnormality	*Percent of patients*
HEMATOLOGIC	
Anemia (Hb < 11 g/100 ml)	72
Leukopenia (WBC < 4,500/mm³)	61
Thrombocytopenia (platelets < 100,000/mm³)	15
Positive direct Coombs test	14
Circulating anticoagulants	Rare
IMMUNOLOGIC	
Positive tests for ANA	99
Positive LE cell tests	60–80
Hypocomplementemia	75
Increased γ-globulin (> 1.5 g/100 ml)	60–77
Positive tests for rheumatoid factors	20
Biologic false positive tests for syphilis	15

lem is the occurrence of *clotting defects* due to antibodies to factor VIII, IX, or X or to the presence of an inhibitor to prothrombin. Prior to a renal biopsy, the integrity of the clotting mechanism must be evaluated.

Urinalysis and renal function studies indicate that over half the patients with SLE have mild to severe damage to the kidneys. With early or focal glomerulonephritis the creatinine clearance may be normal, and only mild proteinuria and microscopic hematuria may exist. With more extensive renal involvement proteinuria may become significant (>0.5 g per day), and the urine sediment may contain abundant red and white blood cells and red blood cell casts as indicators of glomerular damage.

The serum albumin/globulin ratio becomes reversed because of an increase in immunoglobulins, particularly IgG. Serum electrophoresis reveals that the major elevation is in γ-globulin. Small amounts of cryoglobulins, composed of immunoglobulins and complement components, may be present. The erythrocyte sedimentation rate (ESR) tends to be high in patients with active disease.

The most characteristic laboratory abnormalities in SLE are the autoantibodies. The presence of ANA in a patient with active SLE is almost a sine qua non for the diagnosis. These tests are now widely available as a diagnostic aid. The ANA are usually detected by rat or mouse liver sections (other tissues with nucleated cells may also be used); the test serum is applied to the tissue section, antibodies to nuclear antigens interact with the nuclei, other proteins are washed away, and the ANA are detected with an antiserum to human immunoglobulins (these antibodies are coupled with fluorescein isothiocyanate that permits their detection with appropriate microscopy). The ANA include antibodies to single-stranded DNA, double-stranded (native) DNA, deoxyribonucleoprotein, histones, nuclear ribonucleoprotein, and an acidic nuclear protein. Patients with SLE also have antibodies to RNA, ribosomes, lysosomes, and other cytoplasmic constituents. The reasons for such a large number of antibodies are not clear. Many of these antibodies persist even when the disease is quiescent, except that the titers of antibodies to native DNA tend to be higher during exacerbations of the disease. The lupus erythematosus cell test (LE cell test) is positive less frequently than the test for ANA because more antibodies are required for positivity. The listed antibodies to nuclear antigens are not specific to SLE, but when three or more of these antibodies are present, the likelihood of SLE in a given patient is very high. In end-stage renal disease due to SLE the tests for ANA may become negative.

During flare-ups of SLE the total serum hemolytic complement (expressed in 50 percent hemolytic units—CH_{50}) or individual components of complement are decreased owing to activation by immune complexes. The most frequently used measurements of complement components are the immunochemically determined C3 and C4 levels. These measurements are useful in following the response to therapy or for detecting exacerbations. Occasionally the complement levels remain low in spite of apparent full clinical remission; the reasons for this are not known. In addition, during clinically active disease, circulating immune complexes can be detected.

About 20 percent of patients with SLE develop positive tests for rheumatoid factors, but the titers tend to be lower than in rhematoid arthritis. False positive tests for syphilis are encountered, at times prior to clinical onset of SLE. Antinuclear antibodies occur in many other diseases (rheumatoid arthritis, 20 percent; Sjögren's syndrome, 60 percent; scleroderma, 40 percent) and are induced by several drugs (see below).

DIAGNOSIS The possibility of SLE should be considered in any young or middle-aged female in the presence of three or four of the symptoms or signs listed in Table 77-1 or in the presence of glomerulonephritis, hemolytic anemia, leukopenia, or thrombocytopenia. A positive test for ANA is essential for diagnosis. Other diseases that cause positive tests for ANA must be considered, and they must often be excluded on the basis of clinical observations alone. Major consideration must be given to rheumatoid arthritis, scleroderma, Sjögren's syndrome, and the history of ingestion of drugs that might have induced a positive test for ANA.

Drug-induced SLE Hydralazine and procainamide clearly induce a syndrome similar to SLE in some patients. This syndrome includes arthralgias, arthritis, myalgias, pleurisy, pericarditis, fever, skin eruptions, lymphadenopathy, and positive tests for ANA. Renal disease and central nervous system involvement are very unusual in drug-induced SLE. Prospective studies have shown that about 70 percent of patients receiving procainamide develop positive tests for ANA within weeks or months. A much smaller proportion become symptomatic. Once the drug is discontinued, the symptoms abate in a few weeks but occasionally may smolder on for months; recovery may be hastened by treatment with corticosteroids. The ANA tests revert to negative in a few months. Isoniazid alone or with *para*-aminosalicylic acid (PAS), several anticonvulsants (Dilantin, Mesantoin), phenothiazine derivatives, alphamethyldopa, and levodopa have also been associated with positive tests for ANA. In some patients the administration of sulfonamides, penicillin, and oral contraceptives has been associated with exacerbations of SLE.

TREATMENT A cure for SLE is not available. However, abundant experience indicates that appropriate therapy may suppress flare-ups and prolong life. The optimal treatment programs for various manifestations of SLE have not been defined. Adequately designed studies have been difficult to perform because of the variability in the manifestations and course of the disease and the lack of adequate prognostic parameters. Cortiocosteroids remain the cornerstone of therapy, even though the "immunosuppressive" drugs seem to be helpful in some patients.

Arthralgias, arthritis, myalgias, and fever may respond adequately to rest and salicylates. Antimalarials have been used successfully for the same symptoms, as well as for control of skin eruptions. Chloroquine was used widely in mild SLE, but potential retinal toxicity has decreased its usage. Hydroxychloroquine in small dosages (200 mg per day) seems safe, but the patient should be cautioned about potential toxicity, and careful examination by the ophthalmologist should be conducted at least twice a year. Exposure to ultraviolet light should be avoided, particularly with active and recurrent skin lesions. If skin involvement becomes debilitating and does not respond to conservative therapy, corticosteroids in small to moderate dosages should provide relief.

Central nervous system involvement, pericarditis, myocarditis, pleurisy, severe myositis, severe hemolytic anemia, clotting problems, significant leukopenia, and thrombocytopenia are indications for use of corticosteroids. In desperate situations, particularly in central nervous system involvement with seizures or psychosis, relatively high doses should be used (even up to 2 mg prednisone or prednisolone per kg body weight). Once improvement has occurred, the dose should be tapered and adjusted to maintain control of symptoms. Many of the above manifestations can be controlled with 10 mg prednisone or less per day as a maintenance dose. If a flare-up occurs and is recognized by the patient and the physician, only a moderate (5 to 10 mg) increase of the prednisone dose may provide control of symptoms. Careful follow-up of patients, with judicious use of laboratory tests, is essential in treatment of the above manifestations of SLE. Psychosis or other mental disturbances may be difficult to evaluate in a patient who is receiving steroids for SLE, since such symptoms may be caused by the steroids or by the SLE. No single laboratory test, including cerebrospinal fluid complement levels, can distinguish between these two possibilities. With further increase of the steroid dosage the symptoms should decrease if they are due to central nervous system involvement by SLE.

Several approaches to the treatment of SLE nephritis have been advocated, but no currently available program is useful in all patients. Renal biopsy is recommended for establishing the nature of glomerular lesions, since those with focal lupus glomerulonephritis respond to treatment well or improve spontaneously. Perhaps the most useful program is to start with 40 to 60 mg prednisone or prednisolone per day until all clinical symptoms have abated. This may take a few weeks; the urinary sediment should improve, and complement should return toward normal. Thereafter the steroid dose should be reduced gradually to the minimal dose to keep the patient free of symptoms. With severe focal involvement and with diffuse lupus glomerulonephritis or membranous glomerulonephritis, higher doses (up to 150 to 200 mg prednisone or prednisolone) have been tried and found helpful for some patients, with subsequent improvement of renal function. However, the diffuse and membranous lesions do not respond well. For these reasons azathioprine (1 to 2 mg per kg body weight) or cyclophosphamide (100 to 150 mg per day) has been added to prednisone. Cyclophosphamide and prednisone appear to be the most effective combination, but many serious side effects are encountered, including marrow toxicity, hemorrhagic cystitis, alopecia and sterility; their long-term risks are not fully known. The search for better combinations of drugs and new medications for treatment of severe SLE continues.

Any intercurrent infections must be recognized and treated with appropriate therapy. Patients with SLE, either because of their disease or as a consequence of treatment, are liable to bacterial infections, which are a leading cause of death among them.

Exacerbations of SLE tend to occur during the third trimester of pregnancy or in the immediate post-partum period. Nevertheless, many patients with SLE can be carried to term and successful delivery with appropriate therapy. Therefore, SLE is not an absolute indication for therapeutic abortion, but the procedure is recommended during life-threatening active disease.

REFERENCES

Block SR et al: Studies of twins with systemic lupus erythematosus. Am J Med 59:533, 1975

Decker JL et al: Cyclophosphamide or azathioprine in lupus glomerulonephritis. A controlled trial: Results at 28 months. Ann Intern Med 83:606, 1975

Dubois EL (ed): *Lupus Erythematosus,* 2d ed., Los Angeles: University of Southern California Press, 1974

Frank MM, Atkinson JP: Complement in clinical medicine. *Disease-a-Month,* Chicago: Year Book, January, 1975, p. 21

Fries JF, Holman HR: *Systemic Lupus Erythematosus: A Clinical Analysis,* vol. 6, LH Smith (ed); *Major Problems in Internal Medicine,* Philadelphia: Saunders, 1975

Hughes GRV: Frequency of anti-DNA antibodies in SLE, RA and other diseases. Scand J Rheumatol [Suppl] 11:42, 1975

Notman DD et al: Profiles of antinuclear antibodies in systemic rheumatic diseases. Ann Intern Med 83:464, 1975

Phillips PE: The virus hypothesis in systemic lupus erythematosus. Ann Intern Med 83:709, 1975

Pollack VE et al: The clinical course of lupus nephritis: Relationship to the renal histological findings, vol. 1, *Perspectives in Nephrology and Hypertension,* eds P Kincaid-Smith et al, New York: Wiley, 1973, p. 1167

Winfield JB et al: Specific concentration of polynucleotide immune complexes in cryoprecipitates of patients with systemic lupus erythematosus. J Clin Invest 56:563, 1975

78 VASCULITIS

MART MANNIK
BRUCE C. GILLILAND

Many clinical syndromes of necrotizing inflammation of blood vessels exist. In most of these conditions the etiology is not known, but several descriptive classifications have been offered, depending on the size of the involved blood vessels, the anatomic sites, the stage of the inflammation, and the histologic characteristics of the lesions. In these conditions cellular infiltration, necrosis and fibrinoid deposits are present in the walls of blood vessels and perivascular areas. The cellular infiltrates are composed of polymorphonuclear leukocytes in acute stages; with progression of the lesion, monocytes, lymphocytes, and plasma cells appear. Giant cells are encountered in some types of vasculitis. Endothelial edema and proliferation, together with hemorrhage, contribute to diminution or occlusion of the vascular lumen and subsequent ischemic symptoms and signs.

Most forms of vasculitis are thought to be caused by immunologic phenomena. Multiple reasons exist for this belief. Necrotizing inflammation of blood vessels is a common finding in experimentally induced immune-complex diseases (Chap. 75). Vasculitis is a known manifestation of human serum sickness and occurs frequently in several known immune-complex diseases. For example, in systemic lupus erythematosus DNA, antibodies to DNA, and complement components have been identified in vascular lesions; in mixed cryoglobulinemia IgG, antibodies to IgG, and complement components have been seen in involved vessels. Furthermore, in some patients with polyarteritis the hepatitis-associated antigen has been implicated as the causative agent with the finding of antigen, immunoglobulins, and complement in the lesions. In other types of necrotizing inflammation, immunoglobulins and complement components have been visualized with immunofluorescent microscopy, but antigens have not been identified. Future work should identify the etiologic factors in many forms of vasculitis. Until then, however, the histologic and clinical features of the vasculitides serve to classify them.

Periarteritis nodosa was delineated by Kussmaul and Maier in the last century. In the early 1950s Zeek's careful descriptive work laid the foundation for most of the classifications of vasculitides. The descriptive classifications of vasculitides have been helpful in predicting the prognosis and response to therapy of individual patients. Upon careful microscopic examination of the lesions, the vasculitides can usually be placed in one of the five categories indicated in Table 78-1. However, at times the clinical problem defies categorization, and even within each of these categories variability from patient to patient is common. The nature of the antigen, the type of antibodies produced, the size of immune complexes formed, and cellular immunity are some of the factors that may play a role in the pleomorphism of the clinical picture in the various vasculitides.

PERIARTERITIS NODOSA

Pathology In periarteritis nodosa, the necrotizing inflammation involves muscular arteries, adjacent veins, occasionally arterioles and venules, but not capillaries. The lesions involve segments of vessels, at times affecting only part of the circumference, and there is a predilection for the bifurcation of arteries. These areas may form small aneurysms, which may rupture. During the active disease each patient has acute lesions that show predominantly polymorphonuclear leukocytic infiltration of the vessel walls and perivascular areas, as well as chronic lesions with mononuclear cell infiltration and partial healing. These observations suggest that the disease process is continuous, with repeated insults, and if it is caused by immune mechanisms, there must be repeated or continuous availability of antigen(s).

The lesions of periarteritis nodosa are widespread throughout the body; they are commonly found in the coronary arteries, mesenteric arteries, kidneys, muscles, vasa nervorum, etc. The extent and location of lesions dictate the severity of clinical symptoms. Central nervous system involvement is unusual. The lungs are usually not involved, but this point has caused controversy and confusion among those contributing to literature in the field. Necrotizing inflammation and granuloma formation in blood vessels accompanied by lung involvement and eosinophilia should be classified as allergic granulomatosis.

Clinical manifestations Periarteritis nodosa is usually a disease of adulthood, but it occurs in childhood and senescence. It affects two to three men for every woman. The onset of the disease is extremely variable. Often an antecedent history of upper respiratory tract infection or reaction to drugs is recorded.

The early complaints of patients with polyarteritis nodosa include fever, weakness, anorexia, weight loss, myalgias, and arthralgias. With the progression of the disease several organs may show involvement. Small, 5- to 10-mm nodules occur along the course of the arteries as a result of aneurysm formation. Vascular occlusion of such vessels leads to ecchymoses, ulceration (often secondarily infected), and

TABLE 78-1
Classification of vasculitis

Periarteritis nodosa	*Allergic granulomatosis*	*Wegener's granulomatosis*	*Hypersensitivity vasculitis*	*Giant-cell arteritis*
SIZE OF INVOLVED BLOOD VESSELS				
Muscular arteries, adjacent veins, occasional arterioles	Muscular arteries, adjacent veins, occasional arterioles	Arteries, arterioles, venules, some capillaries	Arterioles, venules, capillaries	Large and medium arteries
HISTOLOGY AND STAGE OF LESIONS				
Necrotizing inflammation, coexistence of acute and healing lesions, no giant cells	Necrotizing inflammation with granulomas, coexistence of acute and healing lesions, giant cells in granulomas	Necrotizing inflammation with granulomas, coexistence of acute and healing lesions, giant cells in granulomas	Necrotizing inflammation, all lesions in same stage, no giant cells	Inflammation without necrosis, no neutrophils or giant cells present
ANATOMIC PREDILECTIONS				
Widespread, common to branching points of arteries; lungs not involved	Widespread but lungs frequently involved	Upper and lower respiratory tract involved; necrotizing glomerulitis	Widespread but common to skin, serosal surfaces, glomeruli	All large arteries, including aorta, coronary, vertebral, carotid, temporal, mesenteric

gangrene of fingers or toes. Muscle weakness may evolve. Arthralgias are common, but severe and persistent arthritis is uncommon. Mononeuritis multiplex evolves because of involvement of the vasa nervorum. Asymmetric and multiple nerve trunks may be involved. Retinal exudates and hemorrhages may occur.

Pericarditis and pleuritis, with or without effusions, are common. Involvement of coronary arteries may lead to myocardial ischemia or infarction, but electrocardiographic abnormalities may be recorded in the absence of symptoms.

Abdominal complaints are frequent (in 60 to 70 percent of patients) and include abdominal pain, nausea, vomiting, diarrhea, and bleeding. All these symptoms are related to the involvement of the mesenteric arteries as they enter the intestinal wall. The mesenteric vasculitis may lead to mucosal ulceration, with hemorrhage, perforation, and infarction. The acute abdominal symptoms early in the disease lead to erroneous diagnoses of intraabdominal catastrophies of other causes, often resulting in unavoidable but unnecessary laparotomy. The liver may be involved, and massive hepatic infarction has been reported. Periarteritis of the gallbladder may cause cholecystitis and perforation.

Renal involvement occurs in over half the patients, and predominantly large vessels are involved. Glomerulosclerosis occurs, with severe involvement. Hypertension may evolve along with renal failure. However, hypertension may occur early in the disease when renal function is normal. The causes of death in polyarteritis nodosa include renal failure, myocardial infarction, infections, congestive heart failure, and gastrointestinal bleeding.

Laboratory findings and diagnosis No specific chemical or serologic tests exist for periarteritis nodosa. The leukocyte count is elevated in about 80 percent of patients, principally because of neutrophilia. Anemia may be present because of blood loss and the inflammatory process. The erythrocyte sedimentation rate is often elevated. Other abnormalities depend on the organ involvement, e.g., hematuria, proteinuria, and decreased renal function due to kidney involvement; abnormal electrocardiogram (ECG) due to coronary artery vasculitis, etc. Angiography will show multiple small aneurysms at branch points of mesenteric, renal, and other small arteries.

The diagnosis of periarteritis nodosa often causes difficulties. This diagnosis should be suspected in patients with involvement in several of the systems mentioned above, particularly in adult males. Infections, systemic lupus erythematosus, trichinosis, heart failure, Hodgkin's disease, and most other syndromes can be ruled out. Histologic examination of tissue is essential for proper diagnosis and for distinction from other vasculitides. Clinically involved tissue is best for histologic examinations, and tender subcutaneous nodules, tender muscles, and skin infarcts are suitable. Each tissue should be examined thoroughly because of the segmental nature of the lesions. Blind muscle biopsy has yielded positive information only in one-third of patients shown to have periarteritis later. The frequent finding of vasculitis in testes at autopsy has resulted in the recommendation of testicular biopsy.

Hepatitis-associated antigen has been found in the circulation of 30 to 40 percent of patients with periarteritis nodosa. The same substance has been identified in vascular lesions along with immunoglobulins and complement, suggesting that in these patients the vasculitis is caused by immune complexes containing the hepatitis antigen. In this group of patients the disease tends to begin with fever, polyarthralgias, myalgias, rash, and urticaria. A significant proportion of patients with this form of vasculitis develops liver involvement and liver failure. The evaluation of a patient with polyarteritis should include a search for the hepatitis B antigen.

In some patients the necrotizing vasculitis appears to follow a bout of serous otitis media. The basis of this association has not been established.

Treatment The prognosis of periarteritis nodosa with involvement of many organ systems is grim. Hypertension and renal involvement are thought to predict rapid progression of the disease. In untreated patients one-half to two-thirds have died within a year, but these statistics are heavily biased by postmortem studies and selective inclusion of severely ill patients. Treatment with corticosteroids frequently leads to rapid symptomatic improvement (initial dose 40 to 60 mg prednisone or prednisolone per day, tapered subsequently). In one study 5-year survival in untreated patients was estimated at 13 percent. Controlled studies on the use of cytotoxic (immunosuppressive) drugs have not been recorded, but some experiences suggest that these agents may help when other drugs have failed.

ALLERGIC GRANULOMATOSIS Allergic granulomatosis is separated from periarteritis nodosa because of pathologic and clinical differences, but the etiology is unknown in both.

Pathology The organs and the size of vessels that are segmentally involved are the same in allergic granulomatosis as in periarteritis nodosa. However, in allergic granulomatosis, eosinophils tend to be abundant in lesions, epithelioid cells are numerous, giant cells are present, and a marked accumulation of inflammatory cells occurs, thus leading to the granulomatous appearance. Pulmonary involvement is frequent and striking, with granuloma formation in the vessel walls and perivascular areas.

Manifestations Patients with allergic granulomatosis frequently give a history of an antecedent respiratory infection. Many have asthma that precedes evidence of vasculitis. In contrast to polyarteritis nodosa, fever is common. Fifty-four percent of these patients have peripheral eosinophilia, with eosinophils in excess of 1,500 per mm^3. The radiologic examination is not diagnostic, but parenchymal lung lesions include consolidation in small and large areas. Pleural effusions are not common.

Involvement of other organs is quite similar to that in periarteritis nodosa, and includes the heart, kidneys, intestine, and peripheral nerves.

Treatment This has not been evaluated systematically. Sporadic reports and analogy to other forms of necrotizing vasculitis indicate that corticosteroids, in the same doses used for periarteritis, are the drugs of choice. Cytotoxic (immunosuppressive) drugs might be tried in patients unresponsive to corticosteroids.

WEGENER'S GRANULOMATOSIS Wegener's granulomatosis is separable from other vasculitides by clinical and pathologic criteria, but the etiology is unknown. Untreated, the disseminated form of this disease is fatal in most patients, but the use of cyclophosphamide has provided dramatic improvement.

Pathology Typical Wegener's granulomatosis is characterized by (1) necrotizing granulomatous lesions in the upper part of the airway, lower part of the respiratory tract, or both; (2) generalized focal necrotizing inflammation of arteries and veins, almost always in the lungs and frequently in other organs; (3) necrotizing glomerulitis. In the nose, paranasal sinuses, nasopharynx, glottis, and middle ear, accumulation of granulation tissue, ulceration, and even destruction of bony tissue may occur. A severe granulomatous reaction, with giant cells, fibrosis, and necrosis, is seen microscopically. Arteries, arterioles, veins, and venules adjacent to and away from granulomas are involved, with severe necrotizing inflammation in variable stages. The trachea, bronchi, and lung parenchyma develop granulomatous masses; those in the lung may cavitate. Massive accumulation of chronic inflammatory cells and giant cells is seen, together with partial necrosis. In addition, necrotizing vasculitis takes place in pulmonary blood vessels. Focal necrotizing glomerulitis and necrotizing vasculitis of small arteries are seen in the kidneys. Splenic infarcts are not uncommon. Necrotizing vasculitis with granulomas may occur in every organ.

At times typical lesions of Wegener's granulomatosis may be confined to the lungs or other single organs. These limited forms may go on to rapidly progressive lethal disease.

Clinical manifestations This illness affects men and women equally, usually occurring in middle age. The onset may be insidious, with years of nonbacterial rhinorrhea, sinusitis, or chronic otitis media, at times accompanied by abnormal chest x-ray films. In others, the disease first becomes symptomatic with explosive onset of fever, malaise, and weight loss; abnormalities in the upper and lower parts of the respiratory tract and kidneys develop later. The initial upper respiratory symptoms may last for years, but the generalized disease usually runs a short course with survival for less than 1 year.

The upper respiratory tract involvement manifests itself as rhinorrhea, chronic sinusitis, nasal obstruction, hearing loss, hoarseness, dysphagia, or epistaxis. On examination, accumulation of granulation tissue, ulcerations, and infection may be evident. The disease may extend to the orbit. Cough, hemoptysis, dyspnea, and pleurisy may evolve, but bronchospasm does not occur. Hilar enlargement and multiple or single nodules of varying size may be encountered on x-ray films of the chest. Cavitation, with very thin walls, may be seen. The lesions tend to be bilateral and in the lower lung fields. Abnormal chest films without symptoms have at times led to the diagnosis of "limited" Wegener's granulomatosis. These x-ray patterns are not diagnostic and resemble tumors and other granulomatous processes. Patients may complain of myalgias and arthralgias. Pericardial and myocardial involvement are seen, and the central nervous system and peripheral nerves may be affected. Skin lesions include purpuric nodules and skin infarcts that may progress to ulceration. Renal abnormalities tend to progress from microscopic hematuria and proteinuria to renal failure.

No specific serologic or biochemical tests are available for Wegener's granulomatosis. Mild anemia, elevated erythrocyte sedimentation rate, mild leukocytosis without eosinophilia, and urinary abnormalities are common. Tissue examination is essential for proper diagnosis. Infectious granulomas, lethal midline granuloma, sarcoidosis, and other vasculitides should be considered in the differential diagnosis.

Treatment Once patients develop the generalized phase of Wegener's granulomatosis, the clinical course is short, and average survival is 5 to 6 months after the diagnosis is made. Administration of high doses of corticosteroids (prednisone or prednisolone in dosage of 60 mg per day or more) results in some improvement and prolongation of life. Encouraging results have been obtained with the use of cyclophosphamide. Highly active disease has been suppressed, and patients have survived for several years, at times in complete remission. The optimal dose of cyclophosphamide has not been established. In severely ill patients intravenous dosages of 4 to 15 mg per kg body weight have been employed successfully. In patients with smoldering course of the illness, oral dosages of 75 to 150 mg per day have induced a remission. Cyclophosphamide has been discontinued in some patients without recurrence, but others have been maintained on low doses. With severe generalized Wegener's granulomatosis use of cyclophosphamide seems advisable, but in limited forms of the disease the potential benefits must be weighed against the known hazards of this drug.

HYPERSENSITIVITY VASCULITIS (SMALL-VESSEL VASCULITIS) Hypersensitivity vasculitis has been given many names because of its varied clinical picture. The role of immunity in its pathogenesis is inferred by similarity to experimental models, and in some patients with this disorder the involvement of antigen-antibody complexes is documented. Basically, the arterioles, venules, and capillaries of many organs are involved by necrotizing inflammation. In a single patient, all lesions tend to be of the same age. The clinical picture depends on the extent of the disease and on the primary target organ. Systemic lupus erythematosus, rheumatoid arthritis, and mixed cryoglobulinemia are excellent examples of this type of vasculitis in which immune mechanisms have been implicated in the pathogenesis of the blood vessel inflammation. Drugs and microbial infections have also been implicated as the causative agents.

Pathology Hypersensitivity vasculitis (small-vessel vasculitis) is the most frequently encountered vasculitis. The inflammation and necrosis involve arterioles and capillaries; muscular and large arteries are spared. As a result, the clinical symptoms do not evolve from large vessel ischemia and infarction but result from hemorrhagic and exudative lesions and microinfarcts. Many organs may be involved, including skin, mucous membranes, brain, lungs, heart, gastrointestinal tract, kidneys, and muscle. Neutrophils have accumulated in small-vessel walls and in perivascular areas. Necrosis, edema, and extravasation of blood are present. Many neutrophils are fragmented; hence some prefer to call this form of vasculitis "leukocytoclastic angiitis." Healing and hyalinization occur late. Focal or diffuse glomerulonephritis occurs in some patients. Characteristically all vascular lesions are in the same stage of evolution, in contrast to what occurs in periarteritis nodosa. This observation suggests episodic, rather than continuous, exposure to immune complexes, if indeed this is the mechanism of injury. Immunopathologic studies have shown deposits of immunoglobulins and complement components in active vasculitic skin lesions, if examined within 24 h of their development.

Clinical manifestations The clinical manifestations and onset of hypersensitivity vasculitis are variable, and the reasons for this variability are not known. In some patients the skin manifestations are extensive; systemic manifestations and involvement of other organs predominate throughout the course of the illness in others. In some the disease follows a quick course that leads to death, but most patients survive for years and may recover without recurrences.

In youngsters and in some adults hypersensitivity vasculitis may present as the Henoch-Schönlein syndrome, with prodromal headache, anorexia, fever, abdominal pain and bleeding, arthralgias, purpuric eruptions, and evidence of renal involvement. In adults the criteria for the Henoch-Schönlein syndrome are not usually fulfilled; however, in a group of adults with refractory urticaria and arthralgias, small-vessel vasculitis was present in the skin lesions.

The history of an antecedent respiratory infection may be obtained; drugs may have been ingested (the list is long and includes penicillin, sulfonamides, other antibiotics, salicylates, phenylbutazone, phenacetin, propylthiouracil, busulfan, iodides, vaccines, phenothiazines). Fever is a common systemic symptom. The skin lesions include urticaria, purpura, ecchymoses, papules, nodules, vesicles, and necrotic ulcerations. Lesions may occur anywhere, but they tend to have some symmetry, and the lesions predominate in lower extremities—the legs, ankles, and feet. Patients frequently complain of itching, burning, stinging, and pain in the skin lesions. They may have myalgia, arthralgia, and arthritis. The joints may be warm, red, and painful with acute effusions. However, synovitis of long duration with synovial hypertrophy is unusual, and bony erosions do not develop, unless rheumatoid arthritis is present. Pulmonary infiltrates and pleural effusions may be found on chest roentgenograms. Pericarditis and myocarditis may develop, accompanied by electrocardiographic abnormalities. These patients may have peripheral neuropathy and encephalopathy, manifested by confusion, delirium, and coma. Diffuse electroencephalographic abnormalities may be present. Renal involvement becomes apparent, with microscopic hematuria, proteinuria, and decreasing renal function. Abdominal and gastrointestinal bleeding pain occur.

Similar clinical manifestations accompany the vasculitis associated with systemic lupus erythematosus, rheumatoid arthritis, and mixed cryoglobulinemias. Patients with subacute bacterial endocarditis may have small-vessel vasculitis, as manifested by the Osler's nodes, Roth's spots, arthralgias, and glomerulonephritis.

Laboratory studies Elevation of the erythrocyte sedimentation rate is the most common abnormality. Mild anemia and moderate leukocytosis occur. Complement levels may be reduced. If vasculitis occurs in systemic lupus erythematosus, antinuclear antibodies will be found, as will rheumatoid factors in patients with rheumatoid arthritis and in mixed cryoglobulinemia. Examination of the urinary sediment and evaluation of proteinuria and renal function are indicated for initial evaluation and follow-up of these patients. Biopsy of lesions is important.

Treatment The mortality figures for this disorder are variable because many series are based on autopsy findings. Spontaneous improvement occurs in some patients; in others the disease lingers. If drugs, toxins, or other environmental factors are suspected, all these exposures should be eliminated. If this disorder is immunologically mediated, then removal of the antigen would be the best treatment. Uncontrolled observations suggest that corticosteroids favorably influence the course of this disorder. The optimal dosages have not been determined; 40 to 60 mg prednisone or prednisolone seems reasonable at the onset, but the dose should be reduced when symptoms, signs, and laboratory tests show improvement. The dose should be increased when flare-ups occur. By analogy to systemic lupus erythematosus and Wegener's granulomatosis, cytostatic (immunosuppressive) drugs might be used in desperate situations. However, the results of controlled clinical trials with this therapy are not yet available.

GIANT-CELL ARTERITIS Giant-cell arteritis (also called *temporal* or *cranial arteritis*) is an inflammation of arteries in elderly persons. The cause of the disorder is unknown, and the pathogenesis of arterial inflammation has not been elucidated. However, some evidence for both humoral and cellular immunity to elastic arterial tissue has been presented. Any large or medium-sized artery may be involved, including the superficial temporal artery. Giant-cell arteritis responds dramatically to treatment with corticosteroids.

Pathology The inflammatory changes of giant-cell arteritis affect the large and medium-sized arteries without involving the arterioles and capillaries. Histiocytes, epithelioid cells, multinucleated giant cells, lymphocytes, and plasma cells accumulate in the intima and media adjacent to the internal elastic lamina of medium-sized arteries. The elastic lamina is highly fragmented and absent in some areas. In large arteries and the aorta, the media tends to be prominently involved with inflammation and fragmentation of the elastic fibers. The intima is thickened more than expected from age alone. The lesions are spotty and do not involve long stretches of the arteries. Thrombosis may occur at sites of inflammation.

The segmental lesions of giant-cell arteritis may involve any arteries, including the superficial temporal artery. The aorta is frequently involved, and aneurysms and dissection have been recorded. The external and internal carotid arteries and the vertebral artery systems are involved. Inflammation and occlusion of the ophthalmic or central retinal artery lead to blindness. Involvement of iliac, femoral, mesenteric, and coronary arteries may cause ischemia and infarction in the respective sites. The distribution and histopathology of the lesions in giant-cell arteritis resemble the pathology of pulseless disease or Takayasu's syndrome (see Chap. 251).

Clinical and laboratory manifestations Giant-cell arteritis is a disease of the elderly that affects both sexes nearly equally. This illness has rarely been diagnosed before the age of fifty and usually affects those above sixty. The symptomatic involvement of arteries is frequently preceded by systemic symptoms, including fever, sweats, malaise, fatigue, anorexia, and weight loss. The fevers tend to be low grade but may be striking. A fever of unknown origin in an elderly person, accompanied by a very high erythrocyte sedimentation rate, should always raise the diagnostic possibility of giant-cell arteritis.

Patients with giant-cell arteritis often have the *polymyalgia rheumatica* syndrome. This is characterized by an aching pain and stiffness in the neck and shoulders, which may extend to the upper arms and less frequently to the forearms. The hips and thighs may be similarly involved. Aching is increased with motion. Marked morning stiffness may be present. The muscles may be tender, and disuse atrophy may ensue. Joint pain in the shoulders, hips, and, less commonly, peripheral joints is reported, but objectively the joints are usually not inflamed and do not show synovial hypertrophy, even though small effusions may be present. Biopsy of asymptomatic temporal arteries will establish a histologic diagnosis of giant-cell arteritis in some patients with polymyalgia rheumatica. The segmental occurrence of the lesions must be kept in mind in interpreting the results of the biopsies. The frequency of positive temporal artery biopsies varies from series to series, but the true prevalence of giant-cell arteritis in polymyalgia rheumatica remains unknown.

Headache is a frequent symptom, particularly in patients who have clinical temporal arteritis, with tender and thickened temporal arteries. The headache has no typical pattern, but marked scalp tenderness is often prominent. Furthermore, these patients may complain of intermittent claudication of the jaws and tongue upon mastication or talking.

Loss of vision is a serious complication of giant-cell arteritis. Blindness usually develops suddenly without significant warning, but mild visual disturbances may herald total visual loss. Usually for months or weeks these patients will have had other complaints suggestive of giant-cell arteritis or polymyalgia rheumatica. Aortic aneurysms, aortic dissection, mesenteric arteritis, myocardial ischemia, and infarction and claudication of the lower extremities have been attributed to giant-cell arteritis.

Laboratory findings The significant abnormalities in laboratory tests include a very high erythrocyte sedimentation rate (ESR), mild hypoproliferative anemia, and elevation of the α-globulins and fibrinogen. The ESR exceeds 50 mm per h (by Westergren's method) and often reaches values above 100 mm per h. Important negative findings include normal serum levels of muscle enzymes and normal electromyograms even in the presence of severe polymyalgia. Muscle biopsies disclose no characteristic changes.

In the absence of specific diagnostic tests, the diagnosis of giant-cell arteritis or polymyalgia rheumatica has to rest on clinical findings and a positive biopsy. The symptoms discussed above, in the presence of a high ESR in an elderly person should raise the question of giant-cell arteritis or polymyalgia rheumatica. A temporal artery biopsy should be considered early in the evaluation of such patients. Other causes of high ESR must, of course, be considered, including occult neoplasms and chronic infections.

Treatment Though patients with the polymyalgia rheumatica syndrome and giant-cell arteritis may obtain some relief from their symptoms with salicylates, indomethacin, or phenylbutazone, the basic process of arteritis does not seem to improve. Patients with this disorder, however, have a remarkable response to corticosteroid treatment. The clinical symptoms abate in a few days, the ESR and the hypoproliferative anemia return toward normal within 2 weeks, and the reversal of arterial lesions has been documented by arteriography. Several dosage schedules have been recommended. A starting dose of 30 to 40 mg prednisone or prednisolone (or its equivalent) per day has worked well, but the dose should be reduced gradually when symptoms have abated and the ESR has decreased. The maintenance dose is usually less than 10 mg prednisone per day. This drug can be ultimately discontinued altogether in the majority of patients. The hazards of corticosteroids should be considered, and the prolonged use of high doses of corticosteroids should be discouraged.

REFERENCES

Churg J, Strauss L: Allergic granulomatosis, allergic angiitis and periarteritis nodosa. Am J Pathol 27:277, 1951

Fauci AS, Wolff SM: Wegener's granulomatosis: Studies in eighteen patients and a review of the literature. Medicine 52: 535, 1973

Gocke DJ: Extrahepatic manifestations of viral hepatitis. Am J Med Sci 270:49, 1975

Hamilton CR Jr et al: Giant cell arteritis: Including temporal arteritis and polymyalgia rheumatica. Medicine 50:1, 1971

Hamrin B: Polymyalgia arteritica. Acta Med Scand [Suppl]:533, 1973

Klein RG et al: Large artery involvement in giant cell (temporal) arteritis. Ann Intern Med 83:806, 1975

Reza MJ et al: Wegener's granulomatosis. Long-term follow-up of patients treated with cyclophosphamide. Arthritis Rheum 18: 501, 1975

Sams WM Jr et al: Human necrotizing vasculitis: immunoglobulins and complement in vessel walls of cutaneous lesions and normal skin. J Invest Derm 64:441, 1975

Sergent JS, Christian CL: Necrotizing vasculitis after acute serous otitis media. Ann Intern Med 81:195, 1974

Soter NA et al: Urticaria and arthralgias as manifestation of necrotizing angiitis (vasculitis). J Invest Derm 63:485, 1974

Zeek PM: Periarteritis nodosa and other forms of necrotizing angiitis. N Engl J Med 148:764, 1953

PART FOUR NUTRITIONAL, HORMONAL, AND METABOLIC DISORDERS

section 1 Nutritional deficiencies

79
NUTRITIONAL REQUIREMENTS

THEODORE B. VAN ITALLIE
GEORGE V. MANN

Only about 48 of the thousands of substances involved in human metabolism are essential and must be supplied by the diet. All the remaining compounds can be synthesized in the body. Requirements for the essential nutrients vary among and within species, and are influenced by differing physiologic circumstances such as growth, pregnancy, lactation, and level of physical activity. The nature of the diet itself (for example, the relative proportions of fat and carbohydrate) can affect requirements for certain nutrients. Because of these considerations, definitions of nutritional requirements can only be approximations.

The major nutrients, fat, protein, and carbohydrate, were extensively studied during the latter portion of the nineteenth century. Subsequently, certain of the macrominerals indispensable for growth and health were identified. Systematic studies were begun about 1900 by F. G. Hopkins and E. V. McCollum and were extended by H. C. Sherman, H. Steenbock, the Mellanbys, C. Elvehjem, and many others. Laboratory animals or human subjects were fed chemically defined diets; when growth failure or other signs of deficiency appeared, food concentrates or synthetic materials were added to the diet to ascertain which essential nutrient had been lacking. This method made it possible to produce in animals disorders which mimic human disease and to isolate essential organic factors (vitamins). The vitamins were first named alphabetically and then, when they were identified, were given chemical names. One of two or more similar chemical compounds capable of fulfilling a specific vitamin function is known as a *vitamer.*

Since 1943, the Food and Nutrition Board of the National Research Council–National Academy of Sciences has published formulations of daily nutrient intakes that are judged to be adequate for the maintenance of good nutrition in the population of the United States. These formulations have been designated *recommended daily dietary allowances* (RDA) (Table 79-1). With the exception of calories, the RDA allow a margin of safety, often generous, for individual variations. Accordingly, individuals whose diets do not supply the RDA are not necessarily malnourished, nor should diets be judged "poor" simply because they do not precisely meet RDA standards.

The tabulations in the RDA represent value judgments based on the existing knowledge of nutritional science. The physiologic and biochemical bases for the RDA vary for each specific nutrient. In general, the procedure has been to identify the minimum requirement and then provide an additional allowance sufficient to take care of individual variation. In some cases this has entailed adding to the observed mean twice the standard deviation of the distribution of minimal requirement for the subjects measured.

The RDA should not be mistaken for another widely used reference table published, with periodic revisions, since 1941 by the Food and Drug Administration. This is called the *minimum daily requirements* (MDR). It was intended for use in the regulation of food products in commerce. To avoid unnecessary confusion between the RDA and the MDR, the Food and Drug Administration is phasing out MDR in favor of RDA.

The Food and Drug Administration has also proposed a set of standards, the United States recommended daily allowances (USRDA), for use in regulation of food labeling for nutrient content. These standards are derived from the RDA, but of necessity are based on very few broad age groups, rather than on the somewhat larger number of age-sex groups for which the RDA were established. It should be understood that the purposes of the two sets of standards are not the same.

The essential elements and compounds necessary in the human diet are listed in Table 79-2. The essentiality of a nutrient varies according to species, the stage of growth and development, and metabolic circumstances. Ascorbic acid is necessary for primates and certain rodents and birds because they lack the enzyme necessary for one step in the formation of ascorbic acid from glucose. The essential amino acids illustrate the relativity of the term *essential.* For example, glycine and L-cystine are essential for chickens during periods of feather growth but not at other times.

DIET COMPOSITION The energy for resting metabolism,

TABLE 79-1
Recommended daily dietary allowances of Food and Nutrition Board[1]

	Age, years	Weight, kg	Weight, lb	Height, cm	Height, in.	Energy, kcal	Protein, g	Fat-soluble vitamins: Vitamin A activity, RE[2]	Fat-soluble vitamins: Vitamin A activity, IU	Fat-soluble vitamins: Vitamin D, IU	Fat-soluble vitamins: Vitamin E activity,[4] IU
Infants	0.0–0.5	6	14	60	24	kg × 117	kg × 2.2	420[3]	1,400	400	4
	0.5–1.0	9	20	71	28	kg × 108	kg × 2.0	400	2,000	400	5
Children	1–3	13	28	86	34	1,300	23	400	2,000	400	7
	4–6	20	44	110	44	1,800	30	500	2,500	400	9
	7–10	30	66	135	54	2,400	36	700	3,300	400	10
Men	11–14	44	97	158	63	2,800	44	1,000	5,000	400	12
	15–18	61	134	172	69	3,000	54	1,000	5,000	400	15
	19–22	67	147	172	69	3,000	54	1,000	5,000	400	15
	23–50	70	154	172	69	2,700	56	1,000	5,000		15
	51+	70	154	172	69	2,400	56	1,000	5,000		15
Women	11–14	44	97	155	62	2,400	44	800	4,000	400	12
	15–18	54	119	162	65	2,100	48	800	4,000	400	12
	19–22	58	128	162	65	2,100	46	800	4,000	400	12
	23–50	58	128	162	65	2,000	46	800	4,000		12
	51+	58	128	162	65	1,800	46	800	4,000		12
Pregnant						+300	+30	1,000	5,000	400	15
Lactating						+500	+20	1,200	6,000	400	15

[1] *Allowances are intended to provide for individual variations among most normal persons in the United States living under usual environmental stresses. Diets should be based on a variety of common foods in order to provide other nutrients for which human requirements have been less well defined.*
[2] *Retinol equivalents.*
[3] *Assumed to be all as retinol in milk during the first 6 months of life. All subsequent intakes are assumed to be half as retinol and half as β-carotene when calculated from international units. As retinol equivalents, three-fourths are as retinol and one-fourth as β-carotene.*
[4] *Total vitamin E activity, estimated to be 80 percent as α-tocopherol and 20 percent as other tocopherols.*

synthesis of body tissues, physical activity, excretory processes, and for maintenance of thermal balance is supplied by the major foodstuffs, carbohydrate, fat, and protein. In the United States approximately 12 percent of dietary calories is derived from protein, 42 percent from fat, and 46 percent from carbohydrate. A variable portion of dietary protein is used for anabolic purposes; the remainder contributes to the energy pool. The proportion of fat and protein in the American diet has tended to increase since 1900 as the contribution of carbohydrates, especially the polysaccharides from foods such as potatoes and cereal flours, has decreased from 43 percent (1909) to their present 29 percent of dietary food energy. Consumption of sugars and other sweeteners increased during the first part of this century; since about 1925 it has remained fairly stable at 16 to 17 percent of total calories.

The human organism has a remarkable versatility in adapting to different food mixtures. Thus, the hunters and pastoralists of the world subsist on meat or milk diets which contain less than 50 g carbohydrate daily, and many agriculturists and vegetarians maintain reasonable health on diets with only 30 to 40 g protein and 25 g or less fat daily. It is important to recognize that dietary adequacy can be obtained with widely different food mixtures (Fig. 79-1). By *adequacy* is meant the level of nutrition that permits achievement of the genetic potential of the individual.

TABLE 79-2
Essential nutrients for human beings*

Elements	Macro	Na, K, Ca, Mg, P, Cl, S, C, H, O, N
	Micro	Fe, Zn, Cu, Mn, Co, I
	Probable	Cr, Ni, V, Sn, Mo, Se, F
Vitamins	Water-soluble	Thiamine, riboflavin, vitamin B_6, nicotinic acid, folacin, pantothenic acid, cobalamin, biotin, ascorbic acid
	Fat-soluble	Vitamin A-carotene, vitamins D, E, and K, essential fatty acids (linoleic, arachidonic)
Nitrogenous	Essential amino acids	Lysine, threonine, leucine, isoleucine, methionine, tryptophan, valine, phenylalanine, histidine
	Nonessential nitrogen	

* *Choline is not considered a vitamin. When optimal amounts of cobalamin, serine, and methionine are available, choline is synthesized from them.*

CALORIES In the estimation of energy requirements, the RDA use the concept of the *reference man* and the *reference woman.* The reference man weighs 70 kg; the reference woman weighs 58 kg. Both are assumed to be engaged in light occupations, to live in an environment with a mean temperature averaging 20°C (68°F), and to wear clothing compatible with thermal comfort. Allowances are stipulated for two age categories: persons of 23 to 50 years and those over 50. Adjustments to the recommended average allowances must be made for increased physical activity, for body size, and, occasionally, for climate. The energy cost of physical activity is slightly increased in an ambient temperature below 14°C (57°F) or above 30°C (86°F). While the approximate rate of decrease of resting metabolic rate is known to be about 2 percent per decade in adults, it is difficult to estimate the degree of reduction in physical

Water-soluble vitamins							*Minerals*					
Ascorbic acid, mg	*Folacin,*[5] *μg*	*Nicotinic acid,*[6] *mg*	*Riboflavin, mg*	*Thiamine, mg*	*Vitamin B_6, mg*	*Vitamin B_{12}, μg*	*Calcium, mg*	*Phosphorus, mg*	*Iodine, μg*	*Iron, mg*	*Magnesium, mg*	*Zinc, mg*
35	50	5	0.4	0.3	0.3	0.3	360	240	35	10	60	3
35	50	8	0.6	0.5	0.4	0.3	540	400	45	15	70	5
40	100	9	0.8	0.7	0.6	1.0	800	800	60	15	150	10
40	200	12	1.1	0.9	0.9	1.5	800	800	80	10	200	10
40	300	16	1.2	1.2	1.2	2.0	800	800	110	10	250	10
45	400	18	1.5	1.4	1.6	3.0	1,200	1,200	130	18	350	15
45	400	20	1.8	1.5	2.0	3.0	1,200	1,200	150	18	400	15
45	400	20	1.8	1.5	2.0	3.0	800	800	140	10	350	15
45	400	18	1.6	1.4	2.0	3.0	800	800	130	10	350	15
45	400	16	1.5	1.2	2.0	3.0	800	800	110	10	350	15
45	400	16	1.3	1.2	1.6	3.0	1,200	1,200	115	18	300	15
45	400	14	1.4	1.1	2.0	3.0	1,200	1,200	115	18	300	15
45	400	14	1.4	1.1	2.0	3.0	800	800	100	18	300	15
45	400	13	1.2	1.0	2.0	3.0	800	800	100	18	300	15
45	400	12	1.1	1.0	2.0	3.0	800	800	80	10	300	15
60	800	+2	+0.3	+0.3	2.5	4.0	1,200	1,200	125	18+[7]	450	20
80	600		+0.5	+0.3	2.5	4.0	1,200	1,200	150	18	450	25

[5] *Folacin allowances refer to dietary sources as determined by* Lactobacillus casei *assay. Pure forms of folacin may be effective in doses less than one-fourth of the recommended dietary allowance.*
[6] *Although allowances are expressed as nicotinic acid, it is recognized that on the average 1 mg nicotinic acid is derived from each 60 mg dietary tryptophan.*
[7] *This increased requirement cannot be met by ordinary diets; therefore, the use of supplemental iron is recommended.*
Source: Recommended Dietary Allowances, 8th ed., Food and Nutrition Board, National Academy of Sciences–National Research Council, Washington, 1974.

activity that is associated with advancing age. The RDA provide for a reduction in energy allowances for persons above 50 years of age to 90 percent of the amount required during the preceding two decades.

Pregnancy requires an extra allowance of about 80,000 kcal; thus during pregnancy a daily additional intake of 300 kcal is believed adequate. This figure does not take into account the decrease in physical activity that may occur in the third trimester in women who are not required by employment or household responsibilities to maintain their usual work output. During lactation an average milk yield of about 850 ml per day is assumed, an amount which requires expenditure of about 765 kcal per day. However, since women achieving 11 to 12.5 kg gains during pregnancy will have stored 2 to 4 kg fat, this extra energy reserve can be drawn upon to provide about one-third of the cost of milk production. For this reason, the RDA during lactation have been set at 500 additional kcal per day.

The major variable affecting energy needs in adults is physical activity. The cost of physical activity covers a wide range. At very high levels of activity, which are necessarily intermittent, one's energy output may be twelve times that expended while sitting in a chair. Much of the mild to moderate obesity that develops insidiously with advancing age can be accounted for by the decreases in resting metabolic rate and voluntary energy expenditure that occur without a corresponding reduction in calorie intake. Many obese adolescents and adults are relatively inactive physically. Cultural attitudes and technical developments in the Western world have dramatically decreased the energy expenditure associated with most occupations and have reduced the energy output incident to daily living. Thus,

FIGURE 79-1
The range of dietary mixtures compatible with good nutrition encountered in various groups of individuals. Social classes I to V are those designated by the Registrar General of the United Kingdom in accordance with socioeconomic status. Class I refers to professional persons, class V to unskilled laborers.

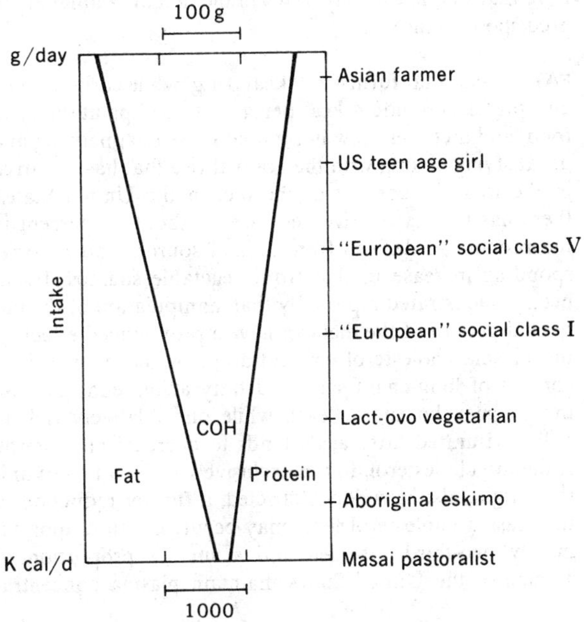

for the average person, an increase in activity level requires a positive effort in a setting which often tends to discourage physical exercise. The consequences of such physical inactivity are obesity and health problems of many kinds, possibly including an increased risk of coronary heart disease (see Chap. 68).

CARBOHYDRATE With the exception of ascorbic acid, there are no carbohydrates known to be essential in the human diet. However, the body requires carbohydrate as an energy source for the brain and for other specialized purposes. If these needs are not met by carbohydrate from the diet, the body must draw first on its very limited stores of liver glycogen and then use protein and glycerol from dietary and endogenous sources to help maintain glucose homeostasis. Although it is not possible to define a precise minimum requirement for carbohydrate, adults accustomed to normal diets tend to exhibit increasing hyperketonemia and ketonuria as the carbohydrate intake is reduced below 75 g per day (see Chap. 68). Nevertheless, adaptation to a diet very low in carbohydrate is possible (Fig. 79-1).

After infancy, a relatively high proportion of nonwhite populations and a considerably smaller proportion of Caucasoids are deficient in the intestinal enzyme lactase and may exhibit a relative intolerance to the lactose in milk. For the most part, such intolerance is not clinically serious and, in children, may be largely circumvented by taking smaller quantities of milk more frequently. There is evidence that a diet high in sucrose, particularly in the form of candy, may promote dental caries. Moreover, certain individuals with endogenous hypertriglyceridemia (type IV) often exhibit a decrease in plasma triglyceride concentrations when the proportion of carbohydrate in the diet is appreciably reduced. Some investigators believe that simple (refined) carbohydrates are more likely to induce hypertriglyceridemia in susceptible individuals than isocaloric amounts of the more complex polysaccharides of cereals, potatoes, flour, rice, and other vegetables. With these possible exceptions, there are no persuasive reasons to believe that simple carbohydrates in the diet are damaging or predispose to disease.

FAT Dietary fat furnishes 9 kcal per g, while carbohydrate and protein provide 4 kcal per g. Fats add palatability to food, and diets very low in fat tend to be unappetizing and unsatisfying. Along with the gradual rise that has occurred in the total fat content of the diet in the United States, there has been a relative decrease of about 10 percent in the proportion derived from animal sources and a corresponding increase in that from vegetable sources. It has been demonstrated repeatedly that manipulation of the fatty acid pattern of the diet can have a pronounced effect on the plasma cholesterol concentration. A diet with a high content of long-chain saturated fatty acids tends to raise the plasma cholesterol level, while one relatively rich in polyunsaturated fatty acids tends to decrease cholesterol. If dietary cholesterol, found exclusively in food fats of animal origin, also is rigidly restricted, a further reduction in the plasma cholesterol level may occur. Because approximately two-thirds of men and a smaller proportion of women in the United States maintain plasma concentrations of cholesterol that are thought to be undesirably high in terms of risk of coronary disease (greater than 200 mg per 100 ml), a number of health agencies have recommended that measurement of the plasma lipid "profile" be a routine part of all health maintenance examinations and that, where indicated, dietary modifications designed to lower plasma levels of cholesterol and triglycerides be instituted (see Chap. 249).

Two polyunsaturated fatty acids, arachidonic acid and its precursor, linoleic acid, have been shown to be essential nutrients for laboratory animals and for infants. Linoleic acid cannot be synthesized by animals and must, therefore, be supplied in the diet, but arachidonic acid can be formed from linoleic acid in the animal body. The prostaglandins appear to derive from the linoleate family of fatty acids. If the ratio of triene to tetraene fatty acids in serum is used as an index of essential fatty acid deficiency, the minimum requirement of infants appears to be near 2 percent of the caloric intake. The possibility that essential fatty acid (EFA) deficiency can occur in adults would seem remote in view of the extensive stores of linoleate normally present in human adipose tissue. Nevertheless, a number of instances of apparent EFA deficiency have been reported in children and adults maintained on fat-free intravenous feeding for prolonged periods.

Food fat serves as the vehicle for absorption of the fat-soluble vitamins, notably, vitamins A, D, E, and K. Thus, when the diet remains very low in fat or when steatorrhea is chronically present, deficiencies of the fat-soluble nutrients are much more likely to occur.

In contrast to the long-chain fatty acids that predominate in nature, fatty acids with eight and ten carbons enter the circulation via the portal system and appear to require only minimal amounts of pancreatic lipase and bile salts for their efficient digestion and absorption. Thus, triglycerides composed of these "medium-chain" fatty acids are useful in the nutritional management of patients with chylous fistulas and a variety of forms of intestinal malabsorption.

PROTEIN **Amino acids** Protein is a dietary essential because of its component amino acids. Food proteins contain various combinations of the 20 natural amino acids, of which at least nine are known to be essential for adults. Infants also require histidine. More information concerning the amino requirements of humans will emerge as further experience is gained with prolonged total parenteral feeding.

After digestion and absorption, the amino acids derived from dietary protein are utilized to meet a variety of needs, depending upon the metabolic circumstances. When sufficient dietary calories are available, amino acids can be used efficiently for anabolic purposes; however, when the caloric intake is grossly insufficient, a large proportion of dietary amino acids may be diverted for the provision of energy. In general, the energy requirements of the body take precedence over its anabolic needs. As described in Chap. 82, there is a spectrum of protein-calorie malnutrition ranging from protein deficiency with sufficient calories (kwashiorkor) to a dietary energy deficiency which is not relieved even by high-quality protein in the diet (marasmus).

Genetic determinants govern the formation of proteins. Protein in the body can be formed only with the simultaneous presence of the amino acids appropriate for the protein. Lacking one or more of the essential amino acids, the body's capacity to make protein is restricted and the subject goes into negative nitrogen balance. Alpha-keto acids derived from tissue proteins and from carbohydrate intermediates are readily aminated to furnish nonessential amino acids. In addition to the nutritional requirement for each of the essential amino acids there is a need for nitrogen which can be used in the synthesis of both essential and nonessential amino acids from the appropriate carbon skeletons. Knowledge of this biochemical transformation has been applied in the nutritional management of uremia (Chap. 273).

Estimates of amino acid needs of adults are largely based on nitrogen balance studies, while requirements for infants and children are characterized as the least amounts compatible with maximum growth. Balance is a statement of the net economy of a substance, positive during retention, negative during loss. Nitrogen is lost from the body mainly in the urine, the amount being highly dependent upon protein intake. Urea nitrogen tends to predominate in the urine with high protein diets and to form a smaller proportion of total nitrogen in the urine on protein-free diets. Fecal nitrogen is relatively constant, averaging about 1 g per day in healthy adults. A small additional quantity of nitrogen is lost through the skin, in the breath, and in various secretions. Recently, the estimates of essential amino acid needs have been supplemented with studies of responses of blood amino acid levels at various intakes.

Nitrogen losses for individual male subjects weighing about 70 kg and consuming proteins of high quality together with sufficient calories to maintain weight average about 5.2 g per day. Because the nitrogen content of protein is about 16 percent, the sum of the excreted nitrogen times 6.25 (derived from 100/16) represents a protein loss of 33 g per day for a 70-kg man, or 0.47 g per kg body weight. This value has been increased by 30 percent to take into account individual variability, resulting in an allowance of 0.6 g/kg/day of high-quality protein to cover the needs of almost all healthy individuals in the population. After a further correction has been made for an estimated 75 percent efficiency of utilization, the allowance for the mixed proteins of the United States diet has been set at 0.8 g/kg/day. Thus the allowance for a 70-kg man is 56 g protein per day and for a 58-kg woman, 46 g. Growing children and pregnant or lactating women are given additional allowances of protein for growth and secretion.

The quality of dietary protein can be critically important, especially in infants who have a far greater need for essential amino acids than do adults. The nutritional quality of a dietary protein can be determined in several ways. A useful experimental method has been measurement of *biologic value,* which is the percent nitrogen absorbed from a given protein that is retained in the body under specified conditions. Another method of estimating protein quality is simply to obtain an analysis of its amino acid composition. The resulting pattern of essential amino acids is then matched with those of several reference proteins, and on the basis of such a comparison a *chemical score* is assigned. Egg protein is generally accepted as having an optimal amino acid composition for the support of growth in the rat and has been assigned a chemical score of 100. Accordingly, this protein, which also has a very high biologic value, is often used as a reference standard. Proteins which are low in biologic value generally are deficient in one or more of the essential amino acids and are designated as having a reduced chemical score. For example, wheat flour, which has a low content of lysine, has a chemical score of 40 or less.

Deficiencies of essential amino acids in human beings are not associated with specific signs or symptoms. However, the so-called "pellagragenic" diet may be deficient in available tryptophan (Chap. 83).

Proteins which are low in one or more of the essential amino acids often must be taken in increased amounts in order to furnish a sufficient quantity of the limiting amino acid or acids to permit synthesis of body protein. Two or more proteins, each deficient in different essential amino acids, can complement one another when eaten together. Between them they may furnish a high-grade protein. This is one reason for advising people to eat a variety of foods to ensure a sound diet. It is also the basis for the search for indigenous food proteins in areas of the world where protein malnutrition is prevalent in order to find a combination of native proteins which will yield an adequate mixture of high biologic value. This usually is a more economic and feasible solution than importing a complete protein or introducing entirely new foods.

Generally, the available amino acid pattern of plant proteins is less like that of human tissues than proteins from animal sources. However, since animal proteins require that time, labor, plant proteins, and other foodstuffs be used to feed livestock for their production, a long-term goal has been to find ways in agriculture, food technology, and cookery to make mixtures of complementary plant proteins which will be as nutritious as most animal proteins.

VITAMINS Except for folic acid and vitamin B_{12} which are discussed in Chap. 310, and vitamin D, which is discussed in Chap. 352, the vitamins known to be important to human health are considered in Chaps. 83 to 86.

ESSENTIAL ELEMENTS The essential elements are listed in Table 79-2. They have been classified as macroelements and trace elements on the basis of their concentrations within the body. Carbon, hydrogen, oxygen, nitrogen, and sulfur are components of the organic compounds of which the major foodstuffs are composed. Specific deficiencies of these macroelements therefore do not occur. On the other hand, deficiencies of the other macroelements and of trace elements do occur in humans and/or animals. The trace elements are discussed in Chap. 87; sodium, chlorine, potassium, and magnesium are discussed in Chap. 69; calcium and phosphorus are discussed in Chap. 352, and iron in Chap. 309.

REFERENCES

Evaluation of Protein Quality, Publication 1100, National Academy of Sciences–National Research Council, Washington, 1963

McCollum EV: *A History of Nutrition,* Boston: Houghton Mifflin, 1962

Recommended Dietary Allowances, 8th ed., Food and Nutrition

Board, National Academy of Sciences–National Research Council, Washington, 1974

SENIOR JR (ed): *Medium Chain Triglycerides,* Philadelphia: University of Pennsylvania Press, 1968

80

MALNUTRITION: CONCEPTS OF PATHOGENESIS AND TREATMENT

THEODORE B. VAN ITALLIE

PATHOGENESIS Human nutritional disease can be divided into two broad etiologic categories, *primary malnutrition* and *secondary,* or *conditioned, malnutrition.* In primary malnutrition, the diet is at fault; in conditioned malnutrition, the diet is potentially adequate but, for a variety of reasons, the affected individual is unable to make use of available foodstuffs properly. Broadly considered, conditioning factors include disorders that affect eating behavior, ingestion, absorption, transport, utilization, metabolic requirements, and excretion (Table 80-1). When a patient exhibits some form of malnutrition of which the cause is not readily evident, it is helpful to examine both the primary (dietary) and conditioning factors that could be responsible.

Primary malnutrition is prevalent in technically underdeveloped areas where the food supply often is uncertain and the nutritional properties of food are not understood. In such areas and among the poor and underprivileged classes of all countries the problems of too little food and too little choice are compounded by lack of judgment in the selection of food or its preparation. The stress of infection and parasitic infestation often exacerbates the effects of undernutrition in these groups. Human beings cannot select an adequate diet from a variety of foods by instinctive reliance upon taste or the other senses, but require some measure of nutrition education. For the most part, culture determines food behavior, and children learn early in life how their culture has dealt with food. The most important teacher of nutrition is the mother. Once food habits are established, they are very difficult to change; however, instruction of mothers concerning diet and other matters pertaining to health ("mothercraft") and the teaching of nutrition in elementary schools offer major opportunities to correct or modify poor food habits.

TABLE 80-1
Categories of conditioned malnutrition (with examples)

1 *Altered eating behavior* Anorexia nervosa Alcoholism Food "faddism" Bulimia 2 *Impaired ingestion* Oropharyngeal disease Myasthenia gravis Esophageal stricture 3 *Defective absorption* Intrinsic factor deficiency Pancreatic insufficiency Gluten enteropathy Obstructive jaundice 4 *Faulty transport* Abetalipoproteinemia Hyperlipoproteinemia	Deficiency of retinol-binding protein (RBP) 5 *Impaired utilization* Diabetes mellitus Insufficient lipoprotein-clearing factor 6 *Increased metabolic requirements* Fever Hyperthyroidism Illness or injury Rapid growth, pregnancy, lactation 7 *Excessive excretion* Protein-losing enteropathy Addison's disease Primary aldosteronism

Dietary deficiencies can result from at least two kinds of changes. The food supply may alter; thus, the change to polished rice in the Orient led to endemic beriberi. Also, a shift may occur from a wide to a narrow assortment of food choices. For example, nutritional deficiencies may occur when fresh vegetables are replaced by a few canned foods.

Certain principles should be kept in mind in relation to the causes and management of primary malnutrition.

1 *Animals, including humans, adapt to the available food.* This adaptation occurs for many nutrients; for example, when the protein supply is low, the adult human organism uses dietary nitrogen with increasing efficiency and eventually can achieve nitrogen equilibrium on as little as 30 g dietary protein a day.
2 *Nutrient deficiencies are often multiple.* An inadequate diet of natural foods rarely will be low in only one essential nutrient. This is important in therapy since treatment with a single nutrient may aggravate coexistent deficiencies of other nutrients.
3 *The nutrient requirements of human beings are known.* There is no foundation for the faddists' argument which advocates unconventional foods for managing ill health because it is contended that "unknown essential nutrients" are supplied by these crude or unprocessed foods.
4 *Frank deficiency disease appearing in a few individuals* often is indicative of subclinical disease in others of the same family or social group.

A type of primary malnutrition can also result from an overabundance of certain dietary constituents. Examples include the dental mottling that results from excess fluoride in the water supply, the hyperlipoproteinemia that may follow a prolonged, excessive intake of foods rich in cholesterol and saturated fats, and the obesity that results from a continuing overgenerous intake of calories.

Despite abundance of food, misguided or misinformed choices can result in dietary imbalance and nutritional deficiency. For example, nutritional surveys have disclosed a surprisingly high incidence of primary malnutrition, clinical and subclinical, among certain population groups in the United States. In a sampling of 10 states during the years 1968 to 1970, the most commonly observed nutrient deficiencies were of iron, vitamin A, vitamin C, and riboflavin. Folic acid deficiency also was found to be relatively common, particularly among pregnant and lactating women. A high prevalence of low hemoglobin and hematocrit values was found throughout all segments of the population that was surveyed. These low levels were associated with low levels of serum iron and serum transferrin saturation and, to a lesser extent, with low levels of serum folic acid. Unexpectedly, many adolescent and adult males had low hemoglobin levels. Apparently, the low levels of hemoglobin in the surveyed population were chiefly due to nutritional iron deficiency. The reported deficiencies of vitamins A and C and riboflavin were largely based on evidence from biochemical measurements and dietary intake data. In these categories, deficiency states rarely reached the florid, clinical level, but it was judged that the affected individuals were at risk with respect to these nutrients. It must be emphasized that the Ten-State Nutrition Survey was not representative of the country as a whole since it was focused principally on low-income families, although some middle- and upper-income families were included in the survey sample. Prevalence of malnutrition or risk of malnutrition was generally inversely related to income.

The conditioned forms of malnutrition are relatively more prevalent in affluent societies and are the nutritional problems most commonly encountered in hospital practice. In addition to the nutritional deficiencies that are secondary to other diseases, nutritional disorders may result from the use of drugs that induce anorexia or interfere with the absorption, utilization, or excretion of one or more nutrients (Table 80-2). Accordingly, when a drug must be administered for a prolonged period, the physician should be aware of its possible effects on nutritional status.

PRINCIPLES OF THERAPY AND SUPPORTIVE CARE Treatment of nutritional disease depends in part on whether the malnutrition is primary or conditioned. In primary malnutrition, therapy is a matter of providing the needed nutrients in appropriate amounts. However, some patients with primary malnutrition are gravely ill and must be treated as medical emergencies. In such instances (for example, in patients severely ill with pellagra, beriberi, or vitamin A deficiency), general supportive care is essential, and vitamin therapy may have to be initiated by the parenteral route (Chaps. 83, 84, and 86). When the malnutrition is conditioned, treatment is often much more complicated and prolonged. In order to overcome or circumvent the conditioning effects of the underlying disorder, a program of compensatory nutritional therapy generally is required. The kind of treatment indicated is determined by the nature of the underlying disorder. Compensatory nutritional therapy may involve (1) either increasing or reducing the daily allowance of one or more nutrients; (2) administration of nutrients by upper gastrointestinal tube or parenterally; and (3) feeding of "tailored" nutrients (like medium-chain triglycerides) to circumvent a block in digestion, absorption, or transport. In patients with certain inborn errors of metabolism, e.g., phenylketonuria or galactosemia, diets that rigidly restrict the improperly metabolized nutrient may be required to prevent serious organic damage (Chaps. 103 and 112).

PARENTERAL NUTRITION The commonest form of parenteral nutrition is *short-term intravenous feeding.* This is the conventional procedure used to correct acute deficits of water, electrolytes, vitamins, and other nutrients, or to prevent ketosis and reduce the excessive tissue breakdown that occurs in response to total or semistarvation, or to help maintain patients nutritionally during self-limited acute illnesses and for several days following surgery. This type of parenteral nutrition is relatively safe and simple since the dextrose and saline solutions that are used are not appreciably hypertonic and can be given via peripheral veins.

Unfortunately, sufficient calories to ensure utilization of parenterally given amino acids for anabolic purposes cannot be provided by short-term intravenous feeding unless excessively large volumes of isotonic or mildly hypertonic solutions are administered. Thus, during conventional intravenous alimentation, nitrogen and energy deficits tend to build up and, if a shift to oral feeding is not possible for a protracted period, the patient gradually suffers progressive debility with its attendant complications (Chap. 82).

Hypertonic glucose solutions providing a more adequate supply of calories cannot be given by the peripheral route because of the high risk of local venous thrombosis. Only by the use of fat emulsions suitable for parenteral administration and providing as much as 1600 kcal per liter is it possible to deliver in isotonic form sufficiently high concentrations of calories. *Total parenteral nutrition* has been employed increasingly in an attempt to meet all the nutri-

TABLE 80-2
Drug-induced nutrient deficiencies (with examples)

Drug	*Nutrient affected*	*Probable mechanism*	*Potential clinical result*
Estrogen and progesterone compounds (oral contraceptive agents)	Folic acid	Impaired tissue uptake and/or conversion to metabolically active coenzyme	Megaloblastic anemia
	Vitamin B_6	Increased requirement for the vitamin	Increased xanthurenic acid excretion after tryptophan loading; "depression, anxiety, hyperirritability"
Isonicotinic hydrazide (INH) (and other hydrazides)	Vitamin B_6	Diversion of vitamin to the inactive INH pyridoxal hydrazone	Peripheral neuritis; hypochromic, microcytic anemia
	Nicotinic acid	Interference with nicotinic acid synthesis from tryptophan by inactivation of vitamin B_6	Pellagra-like syndrome
Diphenylhydantoin	Folic acid	Impaired tissue uptake and/or conversion to metabolically active coenzyme	Megaloblastic anemia
Penicillamine	Vitamin B_6	Binding of vitamin causing inactivation	Peripheral neuritis; convulsions
Cholestyramine	Triglycerides and fat-soluble nutrients	Bile acid binding	Steatorrhea; deficiencies of fat-soluble vitamins
Phenobarbital and phenytoin (long-term anticonvulsant drug therapy)	Vitamin D and 25-OH vitamin D	Increased catabolism of vitamins, decreased formation of 25-OH vitamin D, or both	Osteomalacia

tional needs of certain patients who cannot be fed via the gastrointestinal tract. It is a procedure capable of maintaining patients in good nutritional condition for prolonged periods while the underlying disorder is being treated.

In the absence of fat emulsions which would be safe for parenteral use, it was found feasible to administer hypertonic glucose solutions via an indwelling catheter placed with its tip in the superior vena cava or other central venous sites where the rate of blood flow and intraluminal diameter permit rapid dilution, thereby minimizing the possibility of local phlebitis and thrombosis. In adults, placement is usually accomplished by percutaneous infraclavicular subclavian catheterization, with the tip of the catheter positioned in the lower third of the superior vena cava. This technique permits administration of concentrated nutrient solutions characteristically providing 2500 kcal and as much as 100 g amino acids in 2500 ml water over a 24-h period. Vitamins, macroelements, and trace minerals in appropriate quantities may be added to the intravenous mixture. However, care must be taken to ensure that substances added to such solutions are compatible and suitable for intravenous use.

Although total parenteral nutrition is lifesaving for many patients and can shorten the illness and convalescence of many others, the procedure is potentially hazardous as well as expensive and time-consuming. It should be used only when oral or tube feeding is contraindicated or inadequate, and when conventional parenteral alimentation is unable to provide adequate nutritional support for the patient. Examples of clinical situations in which total parenteral nutrition may be lifesaving include gastrointestinal fistulas with peritonitis, severe burns, severe tetanus, obstructing lesions of the gastrointestinal tract in which surgical intervention must be delayed, renal failure, postoperative massive bowel resection, severe unresolving pancreatitis, acute stages of inflammatory bowel disease, and prolonged coma if hope for recovery of the patient remains.

Although relatively uncommon, a number of technical complications may be associated with catheter placement. These include accidental arterial entry, puncture of the lymphatic ducts, malposition of the catheter, and pneumothorax. More common and potentially more serious is the complication of septicemia which can originate from contaminated solutions or solution lines and from the catheter tract. Patients with chronic infection, inanition, and diseases affecting immune mechanisms are particularly prone to septicemia. In addition, the persistent hyperglycemia associated with administration of a concentrated glucose solution may favor bacterial growth and spread. For these reasons, meticulous attention to the sterility of the nutrient solutions and the delivery system is essential to safe long-term parenteral alimentation.

Serious metabolic complications may occur during prolonged intravenous feeding, particularly if the parenteral solutions are nutritionally inadequate in any important respect. Care must be taken to provide all the essential nutrients in the appropriate amounts; for example, hypophosphatemia with paresthesias, obtundation, and hyperventilation has been noted in patients in whom phosphate administration was neglected. Attention also must be given to the needs of patients for certain trace elements and for linoleic acid during long-term intravenous feeding. Thus, in addition to compulsive care of the delivery system, the patient's metabolic responses to intravenous feeding must be carefully monitored, and the cardiovascular, renal, gastrointestinal, and endocrine status kept in mind. It is essential to test the patient's ability to tolerate and adjust to a large glucose load. In patients with impaired glucose tolerance, insulin administration may be necessary to prevent prolonged severe hyperglycemia with its undesirable consequences. Potentially serious but uncommon complications associated with the administration of hypertonic glucose include coma related to hyperosmolar nonketonic hyperglycemia, acidosis, and osmotic diuresis with electrolyte loss and dehydration. In some patients, symptomatic hypoglycemia has occurred following cessation of intravenous glucose administration, particularly if an infusion that contains insulin is stopped abruptly. Accordingly, care must be taken to avoid inadvertent interruption or reduction of the infusion rate. When the decision is made to discontinue total parenteral feeding, the infusion rate should be decreased gradually so as to permit the patient to adapt to a reduced glucose load.

In addition to frequent measurements of plasma electrolytes and blood and urine glucose concentrations, it is necessary to follow carefully such parameters as the complete blood count, the blood urea nitrogen, serum proteins, and hepatic enzymes. Arterial blood pH and gases also must be determined at appropriate intervals. Attention must be paid to plasma concentrations of calcium, magnesium, and phosphate. Finally, fluid intake and output should be recorded, and patients should be weighed daily.

Apart from providing general nutritional support, total parenteral nutrition is designed to offset abnormal nutrient losses and to maintain or augment calorie stores. Of major importance is the need to maintain nitrogen equilibrium in patients with adequate protein reserves and to promote protein anabolism in individuals who are protein-depleted. To accomplish this objective, a suitable mixture of essential and nonessential amino acids must be given in sufficient amounts to permit protein anabolism or, in catabolic situations, to prevent or minimize nitrogen losses. It has been recommended that at least 150 kcal be supplied for every gram of nitrogen infused. The daily calorie requirement for a patient at bed rest without fever or the presence of a serious catabolic process is about 30 kcal per kg body weight. Where significant tissue losses have occurred or a catabolic process persists, energy intake may have to be increased to 50 kcal/kg/day or more.

Protein anabolism during parenteral alimentation also requires the simultaneous availability of potassium (approximately 3.5 meq per g nitrogen), magnesium, and phosphate. Insufficiency of these macroelements in malnourished patients may impair nitrogen retention. Finally, physical therapy of the patient with active or, if that is not possible, passive exercises is desirable to promote muscle renewal and diminish calcium loss from bones and to avoid other undesirable consequences of prolonged bed rest.

The complexity and hazards of the procedure require that total parenteral nutrition be carried out under the close supervision of a properly trained team that includes physicians, nurses, and a pharmacist.

REFERENCES

DUDRICK SJ et al: Long-term parenteral nutrition with growth, development, and positive nitrogen balance. Surgery 64:134, 1968

ROE DA: Drug-induced deficiency of B vitamins. NY State J Med 71:2770, 1971

SHILS ME: Guidelines for total parenteral nutrition. JAMA 220:1721, 1972

Ten-State Nutrition Survey, 1968–1970. Department of Health, Education, and Welfare Publication no. (HSM) 72:8131, 1972

81
ASSESSMENT OF NUTRITIONAL STATUS

THEODORE B. VAN ITALLIE

Diagnosis of malnutrition requires special attention to the nutritional history (of which the dietary history is part), recognition of physical signs suggestive of nutritional deficiency disease, the use of appropriate laboratory studies, including x-rays, and, on occasion, observation of the patient's response to a therapeutic trial.

NUTRITIONAL HISTORY The nutritional history is not merely concerned with the current and past dietary intake but also takes into consideration the many conditioning factors that may affect nutriture. Examples of such factors are given in Table 80-1.

Although an extensive nutritional history is not routinely required, certain clues in the regular history should alert the physician to the need for further exploration of the patient's nutritional status. In the adult, these include an appreciable change in body weight (5 lb or more), excessive consumption of ethanol, bizarre food practices (e.g., clay eating), "food faddism," use of drugs capable of affecting nutriture (e.g. isoniazid, diuretics), menorrhagia, repeated, closely spaced pregnancies, and chronic anorexia or diarrhea. When appropriate, an attempt should be made to elicit evidence of previous malnutrition, with particular attention to the signs and symptoms of nutrient deficiency states (Table 81-1). It should be kept in mind that the reliability of the dietary history cannot be taken for granted. Some patients, especially alcoholics, are either unwilling or unable to provide accurate information about their dietary intake.

Unless the physician is particularly interested in nutritional problems, the dietary history usually is best obtained from the patient by a trained dietitian or nutritionist; however, the physician should first brief the interviewer concerning the clinical problem to ensure that all pertinent information will be elicited. The most commonly used approaches to the dietary history are the so-called 24-h dietary recall and the food record. In the former procedure, the interviewer makes a detailed listing of the foods consumed by the patient during the previous 24 h, obtaining estimates of the quantity of each food item consumed during this period. Usually the nutritionist will also obtain supplementary information such as how often major foods are eaten, food likes and dislikes, and use of vitamin and mineral supplements. In the latter procedure, the food record, subjects record their own intake for a specified period, in accordance with the instructions of the dietitian. It is of course essential to determine how long a certain type of diet has been consumed, because deficiency states almost always evolve slowly.

Initially, the physician requires only enough information about dietary intake to rule out certain possibilities or to suggest the need for further diagnostic investigation. For example, if the patient is an adolescent girl subsisting principally on a milk diet, primarily riboflavin deficiency can be ruled out; however, iron deficiency should be suspected.

The physician will find it useful to obtain a brief history of food taken in a typical day, using as a reference the five major food groups in Table 81-2. In this way the physician can determine whether there are any apparent problems that require further exploration.

PHYSICAL SIGNS Although very few clinical signs are pathognomonic of specific nutritional deficiency syndromes, many signs strongly suggest nutritional deficiency disease and also provide valuable clues to the nature of the deficiency. When two or more clinical signs characteristic of a deficiency disease are present simultaneously, their diagnostic significance is greatly enhanced. The common suggestive signs associated with a number of deficiency syndromes are listed in Table 81-1 together with pertinent laboratory tests.

Gross obesity and marked emaciation are readily perceived by inspection; however, certain patients appear to be normally nourished until the status of the subcutaneous fat is estimated by measurement of skin-fold thickness, either by means of suitable calipers or by palpation. Such measurements may disclose a marked reduction of subcutaneous fat suggestive of a chronic energy deficit. Or, conversely, an apparently undernourished patient may exhibit adequate fat stores.

BODY COMPOSITION Techniques for the in vivo measurement of body composition have been developed during the last three decades, starting with studies of body density. A variety of methods has been used to estimate total body fat, "lean body mass," and various fluid "compartments," including total body water, extracellular water, and plasma volume. Isotope dilution procedures have been employed to estimate the pool sizes of certain vitamins and minerals in the human body composition that are associated with different kinds of malnutrition; however, the more complex measurements are not readily available and are therefore of little practical value in nutritional diagnosis.

ANTHROPOMETRIC MEASUREMENTS Measurement of height and body weight should never be neglected; they are the two most commonly used measures of growth in children and adolescents. In adults, use of the simple concept of *relative weight* is helpful in quantifying percent deviation from the so-called desirable body weight. One of several definitions of desirable weight is the average weight

TABLE 81-1
Deficiency syndromes

Deficiency	*Common suggestive signs*	*Laboratory tests*
Vitamin A	Bitot's spots Conjunctival xerosis Corneal xerosis Keratomalacia Xerosis of skin Follicular hyperkeratosis (without perifollicular hemorrhage)	Plasma vitamin A Plasma carotene: reflects dietary intake of carotenoids Dark adaptation tests, electroretinogram; electronystagmogram
Thiamine (beriberi)	Calf-muscle tenderness Weakness of legs (squatting test) Loss of ankle and knee jerks Hypesthesia and paresthesia Cardiac enlargement, tachycardia, pulmonary congestion, and peripheral edema	Erythrocyte transketolase (ETK) activity and in vitro effect on ETK activity of thiamine pyrophosphate (TPP) Urinary thiamine (μg/g creatinine): reflects dietary intake Blood pyruvate, alpha-ketoglutarate levels: variably useful Erythrocyte thiamine concentration
Riboflavin (ariboflavinosis)	Angular stomatitis (or angular scars) Cheilosis Magenta tongue Atrophic lingual papillae Corneal vascularization Angular palpebritis (angular blepharitis) Dyssebacia Scrotal (or vulvar) dermatosis	Erythrocyte glutathione reductase (EGR) activity and in vitro effect on EGR activity of flavin adenine dinucleotide (FAD) Urinary riboflavin (μg/g creatinine): reflects dietary intake
Nicotinic acid (pellagra)	Scarlet and raw tongue Atrophic lingual papillae Tongue fissuring Malar and supraorbital pigmentation Pellagrous dermatosis	Urinary N^1-methylnicotinamide (mg/g creatinine)
Vitamin B_6	Nasolabial seborrhea Glossitis Peripheral neuropathy with symmetric sensory and motor deficits, more likely in the lower extremities Drug-resistant convulsions in infants	Erythrocyte glutamic-oxaloacetic transaminase (EGOT) activity and in vitro effect on EGOT activity of pyridoxal phosphate Tryptophan load test (effect on urinary excretion of xanthurenic and quinolinic acids) Urinary vitamin B_6 excretion (μg/g creatinine): reflects dietary intake
Vitamin C (scurvy)	Spongy and bleeding gums Petechiae Ecchymoses Follicular hyperkeratosis with coiled hairs and perifollicular hemorrhage ("pink halo") Intramuscular or subperiosteal hematoma Painful epiphyseal enlargement	Ascorbic acid concentration in (*1*) plasma, (*2*) whole blood, and (*3*) white blood cells Urinary ascorbic acid Vitamin C load test
Protein-calorie malnutrition (kwashiorkor—marasmus) (young children)	Psychomotor change Dyspigmentation of hair Easy pluckability of hair Thin sparse hair Straight hair Moon face Diffuse depigmentation of skin Flaky-paint dermatosis Edema Muscle wasting Hepatomegaly	Serum albumin concentration Serum amino acid ratio (leucine, isoleucine, valine, methionine, glycine, serine, glutamine, taurine) Urinary excretion of hydroxyproline (hydroxyproline index) Urinary excretion of creatinine per 24 h Analysis of anagenic hair roots for volume, protein, or DNA
Semistarvation (older children and adults)	Marked loss of subcutaneous fat Muscle wasting Dirty-brown patchy pigmentation of face, especially malar eminences Parotid enlargement Weakness and physical inactivity Bradycardia at rest	Relative weight Measurement of skin-fold thickness Basal metabolic rate Lean body mass (derived from measurement of body density, ^{40}K-counting, or estimation of total body water)
Vitamin D (rickets)	*Active rickets (in young children):* Epiphyseal enlargement (painless) (over six months of age) Beading of ribs Persistently open anterior fontanelle (after eighteen months of age) Craniotabes (under one year of age) Muscular hypotonia	Serum alkaline phosphatase concentration Plasma assay for 25-hydroxycholecalciferol (25-HCC)

TABLE 81-1
Deficiency syndromes *(continued)*

Deficiency	*Common suggestive signs*	*Laboratory tests*
	Healed rickets (in older children or adults): Frontal or parietal bossing Knock-knees or bowlegs Deformities in thorax (Harrison's sulcus, pigeon chest) *Osteomalacia (in adults)*	
Iron	Pallor Angular stomatitis Atrophic lingual papillae Thin, brittle nails with spooning (koilonychia)	Plasma iron level Plasma iron-binding capacity Status of marrow iron Hematocrit Blood hemoglobin concentration Erythrocyte morphology Erythrocyte protoporphyrin concentration
Folic acid	Pallor Glossitis Aphthous stomatitis	Erythrocyte folate concentration Serum folate concentration Urine formiminoglutamic acid (FIGLU) excretion after histine load Neutrophil and erythrocyte morphology Bone marrow morphology
Vitamin B_{12}	Pallor Mild icterus ("lemon-yellow" color of skin in lightly pigmented subjects) Anorexia, flatulence, diarrhea Paresthesia Ataxia Loss of position and vibratory sense Areflexia with extensor plantar responses Optic neuritis Occasionally dementia, forgetfulness (Each of above can appear as an isolated finding)	Serum vitamin B_{12} concentration Radioactive vitamin B_{12} absorption (Schilling test) Correction of abnormal Schilling test by concomitant administration of intrinsic factor (IF) Urinary methylmalonate excretion Bone marrow morphology Serum bilirubin Tests for circulating IF antibody

SOURCE: *Jelliffe, The Assessment of the Nutritional Status of the Community, World Health Organization, Geneva, 1966*

of individuals of given sex and height at age 22. Relative weight (RW) is calculated by the following formula:

$$RW = 100 \times \text{actual weight/desirable weight}$$

Other anthropometric measurements include determination of skin-fold thickness (mentioned above) to obtain information concerning the amount and distribution of subcutaneous fat and measurements of head, body, and limb circumferences (corrected for subcutaneous fat) at standard sites. The chest/head circumference ratio is useful in detecting protein-calorie malnutrition in early childhood, while poor muscle development or muscle wasting is characteristic of all forms of protein-calorie malnutrition.

BIOCHEMICAL TESTS Biochemical measurements used in assessing nutritional status are listed in Table 81-3. Specimens for analysis should be obtained before the findings are modified by nutritional supplements or by a change in diet.

In addition to the usual measurements of urinary excretion rates of nutrients and their products and of concentrations of nutrients in plasma, erythrocytes, and leukocytes, more sophisticated tests have been devised that are based on the metabolic roles of certain vitamin-dependent cofactors. For example, vitamin B_6 is known to be necessary for the transformation of tryptophan to nicotinic acid. In vitamin B_6 deficiency, this pathway is partly interrupted, and

TABLE 81-2
A synopsis of U.S. basic food groups and their nutrient contribution*

	Essential nutrient contribution											
Food group	*Calories*	*Protein*	*Ca*	*P*	*Fe*	*Vitamin A and carotene*	*Vitamin D*	*Vitamin C*	*Nicotinic acid, thiamine, riboflavin, pyridoxine*	*Folic acid*	*B_{12}*	*Vitamin E*
Dairy	+	+	+	+	−	+	+	−	+	−	+	−
Meat	+	+	−	+	+	−	−	−	+	−	+	+
Cereal and bread	+	±	−	+	−	−	−	−	+	+	−	+
Vegetables	±	±	+	−	+	+	−	+	+	+	−	−
Fruit	±	−	−	−	−	+	−	+	−	±	−	−

* *Some cereal products are enriched with iron. Liver is rich in vitamin A and folic acid. Fresh orange juice contains significant amounts of folic acid. Most vegetable oils and nuts contain abundant amounts of vitamin E.*

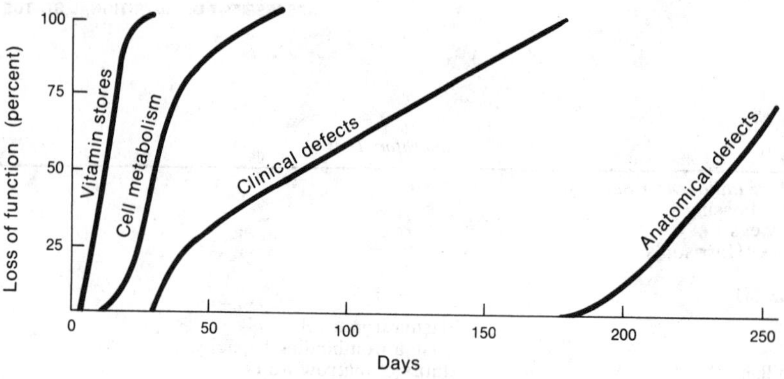

FIGURE 81-1
Stages in the development of a vitamin deficiency (based on thiamine depletion in human volunteers). (Adapted from J. Marks, The Vitamins in Health and Disease, Boston: Little, Brown, 1968, p. 19)

TABLE 81-3
Biochemical aids in diagnosing nutritional deficiency (adult values)

Nutrient	*Test**	*Level suggesting deficiency*	*Usual range†*
Protein	Total protein (S), g/100 ml	<6.0	6.3–8.6
	Total albumin (S), g/100 ml	<2.8	3.5–4.2
Vitamin A and carotene	Vitamin A (S), μg/100 ml	<10	20–49
	Carotene (S), μg/100 ml	<20	40–300
Vitamin D	Total calcium (S), meq/l	<3.5	4.6–5.5
	Phosphorus (S), meq/l	<0.8	1.5–2.2
	Alkaline phosphatase (S), IU/l	>155	35–148
	25-Hydroxycholecalciferol (P), ng/ml	<10	10–40
Vitamin E	Tocopherols (P), mg/100 ml	<0.4	0.6–1.5
Vitamin K	Prothrombin activity (P), % of normal	<70	70–100
Vitamin C	Ascorbate, mg/100 ml		
	Buffy coat (leukocytes, platelets)	<10	25–40
	Whole blood	<0.3	0.4–1.0
	Plasma	<0.1	0.20–0.39
	Urinary ascorbate after administration of 100 mg ascorbic acid intravenously, percent of test dose excreted over subsequent 3 h	<5	>50
Thiamine	Pyruvate (B), mg/100 ml	>1.0	0.3–0.9
	Erythrocyte transketolase (ETK) activity, μg hexose/ml/h	<800	900–1200
	Thiamine pyrophosphate effect on ETK activity, %	>25	<16
	Urinary thiamine, μg/g creatinine	<27	66–129
Riboflavin	Erythrocyte riboflavin, μg/100 ml RBC	<10	15–19.9
Nicotinic acid	Urinary riboflavin, μg/g creatinine	<27	80–269
	Urinary N^1-methylnicotinamide, mg/g creatinine	<0.5	1.6–4.29
Vitamin B_6	Urinary "xanthurenic acid" after 2 gL-tryptophan, μmol/24 h	>50	<50
Pantothenic acid	Pantothenate (S), ng/ml	<50	100
Folic acid	Folate activity (S), ng/ml	<3	6–21
	Folate activity (RBC), ng/ml	<140	160–650
	Urinary formiminoglutamic acid (FIGLU) after 15 g L-histidine, mg/24 h	>35	<17
Vitamin B_{12}	Vitamin B_{12} activity (S), pg/ml (*Euglena gracilis*)	<100	200–960
	Urinary methylmalonate, mg/24 h	>10	<5
Iron	Iron (S), μg/100 ml	<50	60–160
	Iron-binding capacity (S), μg/100 ml	>450	250–410
	Erythrocyte protoporphyrin concentration, μg/100 ml RBC	>90	6–40
Copper	Copper (S), μg/100 ml	<70	81–147
Zinc	Zinc (P), μg/100 ml	<50	55–150
Manganese	Manganese (S), μg/100	<0.08	0.08–0.26
Sodium	Sodium (S), meq/l	<135	136–145
Potassium	Potassium (S), meq/l	<3.6	3.5–5.0
Magnesium	Magnesium (S), meq/l	<1.4	1.5–2.5
Iodine	Urinary iodine, μg/g creatinine	<25	>50

* *P, plasma; S, serum; B, whole blood.*
† *Values falling between the* usual range *and the* level suggesting deficiency *may be considered low or marginal in appropriate instances. Values above the* usual range *are not necessarily undesirably high.*

hence abnormal quantities of intermediate products, such as kynurenine and quinolinic and xanthurenic acids, are excreted in the urine. This is the basis of the tryptophan load test (Chap. 84). Use of tyrosine loading in ascorbic acid deficiency involves a similar principle (Chap. 85). Employment of biochemical tests in therapeutic trials is discussed below.

THERAPEUTIC TRIALS Therapeutic trials can play an important role in the diagnosis of a deficiency syndrome, particularly if the physical signs and laboratory findings are equivocal. For example, the effect of a given nutrient on the reticulocyte count can be helpful in defining the nutritional etiology of an anemia. Rapid improvement of clinical signs after therapy also may be observed in a variety of nutritional deficiencies, with obvious diagnostic implications. Thus, the clinical response to thiamine administration of patients with beriberi or Wernicke's ophthalmoplegia is often sufficiently prompt and dramatic to confirm the diagnosis. When a therapeutic trial is conducted, however, it is essential that only the test nutrient be administered; the patient should receive an appropriate dose of a single vitamin or mineral rather than the mixtures that are so readily available.

At the biochemical level, measurement of the effect of therapy on excretion of an "abnormal" metabolic product (e.g., the effect of vitamin B_6 on xanthurenic acid excretion) can serve as a useful extension of clinical assessment. Finally, in vitro trials have been devised in which, for example, thiamine pyrophosphate or flavin adenine dinucleotide is added to a system containing an erythrocyte hemolysate. The ability of such vitamin-derived coenzymes to correct a specified biochemical defect in vitro provides a valuable index of the extent of deficiency of the vitamin in question.

In general, nutrient stores must be depleted before low plasma levels of the nutrient are found. Biochemical derangements and functional and anatomic defects occur later in the course of a deficiency. In making a nutritional assessment, it is often sufficient to measure the concentration in blood or the excretion rate in urine of a nutrient or its metabolite. If this screening procedure discloses a problem, more definitive biochemical studies may be required.

REFERENCES

BEHNKE AR: Anthropometric evaluation of body composition throughout life. Ann NY Acad Sci 110:450, 1963

JELLIFFE DB: *The Assessment of the Nutritional Status of the Community,* World Health Organization, Geneva, 1966

Manual for Nutrition Surveys, 2d ed., Bethesda, Md.: Interdepartmental Committee on Nutrition for National Defense. National Institutes of Health, 1963

MOORE FD et al: *The Body Cell Mass and Its Supporting Environment: Body Composition in Health and Disease,* Philadelphia: Saunders, 1963

National Center for Health Statistics: *Preliminary Findings of the First Health and Nutrition Examination Survey, United States, 1971–1972, Dietary Intake and Biochemical Findings.* Vital and Health Statistics. U. S. Department of Health, Education, and Welfare Publication (HRA) 74-1219-1, Washington, 1974

82
STARVATION AND PROTEIN-CALORIE MALNUTRITION

THEODORE B. VAN ITALLIE

STARVATION Although modern technology has greatly reduced the risk of mass starvation in many countries, there still are large areas where famine is endemic and sometimes epidemic. But even if mass hunger were not a problem, the subject of starvation would remain of compelling interest to the physician. This is because "conditioned starvation," namely, the sustained calorie deficiency occurring in association with disease, is one of the important problems that must be faced. An informed approach requires that physicians be familiar with the clinical and metabolic consequences of starvation. This will also permit them to distinguish the findings directly attributable to the primary disease from those produced by the superimposed calorie deficiency.

Metabolic changes (see also Chap. 68) The most reliable information about the metabolic changes that occur during prolonged human starvation has been obtained from studies of experimentally induced caloric deprivation such as the Carnegie Nutrition Laboratory Experiment (1919) and the Minnesota Experiment (1950). In general, the changes in body composition observed during starvation, whether primary or conditioned, reflect the body's attempt to adapt to undernutrition. Most conspicuously, the fat stores are utilized in order to spare "structural" protein. Thus, body fat diminishes at a considerably more rapid rate than does muscle. Skeletal muscle, thyroid, and pancreas diminish in mass in roughly the same proportion as the body taken as a whole. More extensive losses occur in other soft tissue organs, notably the liver and the intestine. In contrast, the brain and skeleton show minimal gross changes, while the heart, kidneys, and adrenal glands exhibit proportionately less weight loss than that of the total body. In short, the central nervous system and circulation are maintained whatever the cost to less essential parts of the organism.

The body also conserves calories by reducing its output of energy. Basal metabolism decreases substantially as does voluntary physical activity. It is noteworthy that emaciated patients with anorexia nervosa frequently fail to restrict voluntary activity and, indeed, may exhibit marked physical restlessness. This characteristic should help to identify the individual with undiagnosed anorexia nervosa who, in other respects, may be difficult to distinguish from patients suffering from involuntary starvation.

It is difficult to generalize about the metabolic changes that occur in response to starvation since the picture in total caloric deprivation differs markedly from that in semistarvation in a number of respects. For example, hyperketonemia and hyperuricemia are characteristic of total caloric starvation; they are rarely observed in semistarvation. Semistarved individuals are usually ravenously hungry; those undergoing a total fast often report complete absence of hunger. Endocrine and metabolic changes that occur in fasting human beings are discussed in Chap. 68.

Clinical findings The semistarved patient characteristically complains of feeling weak, tired, irritable, and depressed. He may also describe himself as "feeling old," with loss of libido, lack of ambition, and narrowing of interests. Sitting on any hard surface is uncomfortable, and muscle soreness and muscle cramps often are troublesome. He is frequently harassed by polyuria and nocturia. The nails grow slowly and the hair falls out in increasing amounts. Cuts and other wounds heal very slowly. The extremities too readily become numb, and cold temperatures are poorly tolerated. The hands and feet feel cold even when the ambient temperature is relatively warm.

On inspection, the semistarved individual looks haggard, pale, and emaciated. Clinical manifestations of specific vitamin deficiencies usually are not evident. The hair is dry, and irregular areas of "dirty-brown" pigmentation are often present, particularly around the mouth, under the eyes, and on the malar eminences. The eyes are dull and the scleras seem to lose their vascularity, looking like unglazed porcelain. At times edema, particularly of the eyelids and cheeks, may mask the degree of emaciation and give the face a swollen appearance. In some cases, the parotid glands may be enlarged.

The neck is thin and looks abnormally long; the clavicles, scapulae, ribs, vertebral column, iliac crests, and other bony protuberances are prominent; the buttocks are thin and sagging. When not edematous, the extremities are sticklike, and the nailbeds and lips may show a slight cyanosis. Goosefleshlike changes are often present in certain skin areas, most commonly on the exterior surfaces of the thighs and upper arms. On palpation, the skin is cold, dry, rough, and inelastic. The skin folds show marked loss of subcutaneous fat. Muscle tone is poor and peripheral edema may be present. The pulse is weak, regular, and very slow at rest. The blood pressure usually is low, with the systolic pressure often 100 mmHg or less. The heart is small to percussion, but the heart sounds are readily heard owing to the thinness of the chest wall. The abdomen is scaphoid, and the liver and spleen usually are not enlarged. The deep tendon reflexes are diminished or may be absent.

Systemic changes During severe caloric undernutrition marked changes in cardiovascular function take place. Heart size decreases and marked bradycardia (in the range of 34 to 40 beats per min) usually occurs. Electrocardiographic changes are observed, with reduction in amplitude of the P wave and QRS complex. A marked rightward shift of the QRS and T axes also may occur. These parameters return slowly to normal during nutritional rehabilitation. The arterial blood pressure and the pulse pressure tend to diminish as starvation progresses. Venous blood pressure also is reduced, although the plasma and extracellular fluid volumes increase markedly relative to body weight.

Moderate anemia is commonly found in association with semistarvation, and its severity increases gradually with the degree and duration of calorie restriction. In the Minnesota experiment, the mean hemoglobin concentration decreased from 15.1 to 11.7 g per 100 ml after 24 weeks of semistarvation. Leukopenia also occurred with the mean white blood cell count diminishing from 6,346 to 4,129 per mm^3. No significant change took place during this time in the relative proportions of polymorphonuclear leukocytes and lymphocytes.

Despite an absolute decrease of 27.5 percent in the "active tissue" compartment (body weight minus the sum of fat plus extracellular water plus bone minerals), plasma protein concentrations in the Minnesota subjects diminished only slightly during semistarvation. Indeed, the small reductions that occurred were more than offset by the average increases in plasma volume. Thus, the changes in circulating hemoglobin reflected more accurately the loss of active tissue (body protein "reserves") during calorie deprivation than did the behavior of the plasma proteins. Moreover, electrophoretic analyses of serum samples from these subjects after 24 weeks of reduced food intake showed only a minimal reduction of the gamma-globulins.

Early in starvation, urea is the chief nitrogenous component of the urine. As the body's adaptive mechanisms permit it to conserve protein more efficiently, urinary urea decreases, being replaced by ammonia. Elaboration of this "basic" ion helps the organism to conserve sodium and potassium. In addition, the decreased solute load reduces the obligate urinary volume and thereby conserves body water.

In contrast to the reduced urinary output during total caloric starvation, polyuria of 2 to 3 liters or more per 24 h and nocturia are the most commonly described features of renal dysfunction in semistarved patients. Such individuals appear to have a reversible defect in renal concentrating ability.

Populations subjected to prolonged semistarvation often exhibit an increased prevalence of active tuberculosis, and semistarved individuals tend to tolerate infections poorly. Nevertheless, the evidence that semistarvation affects mechanisms of immunity is equivocal. In any case, susceptibility to infection must be distinguished from the increased severity of response to infection.

Starvation edema The edema that occurs in starved persons usually does not result from either hypoalbuminemia or congestive heart failure; indeed, venous pressure during starvation generally is lower than normal. The edema fluid itself is very low in protein. "Famine edema" occurs gradually, usually after the first month of semistarvation, and at first is transient, occurring late in the day. Initially, the crural areas and the eyes are likely to be involved. As undernutrition continues, the edema becomes more constant and more massive. Keys et al. suggested that in ordinary cases of famine the edema is not due to accumulation of new tissue fluid only but to retention in relative excess of the prestarvation level of extracellular fluid. Loss of elasticity and other changes in tissue structure also are thought to play an important role in the pathogenesis of famine edema.

If the body's adaptative mechanisms fail to protect the semistarved individual from still further loss of weight, particularly lean body mass, a preterminal stage of starvation is entered. In this final phase, often accompanied by persistent diarrhea, marked weakness and apathy reduce further the limited intake of liquids and food. Edema yields to progressive dehydration, followed by coma and death.

Psychologic effects Even a loss of about 10 percent of

body weight can be accompanied by increased irritability and reduced libido in previously lean individuals. As semistarvation progresses and still more weight is lost, the depleted individual tends to become moody, depressed, and, if the starvation is primary, excessively preoccupied with food. Personal appearance and social behavior deteriorate, and the semistarved individual may be apathetic, lose ability to concentrate, and have difficulty in thinking. Nevertheless, in adults, intellectual performance is affected only minimally by semistarvation.

Medical management With rare exceptions, individuals suffering from starvation uncomplicated by other serious disease respond well to small quantities of ordinary food taken by mouth at frequent intervals. Use of "predigested" products has little if any advantage; indeed, simple foods such as skim milk powder appear to be preferable. Intravenous feeding is beneficial only in the occasional subject who cannot tolerate food by mouth; furthermore, parenteral fluids must be administered with extreme caution in order to avoid precipitating heart failure.

During early rehabilitation from semistarvation, if a large increase in food intake is permitted, there is rapid weight gain and a sharp rise in the resting metabolic rate. Concurrently, the plasma and extracellular fluid volumes remain high, while the cardiac output and cardiac index are still reduced. The venous pressure and pulse rate may rise well above normal, cardiac enlargement and peripheral edema may occur, and borderline or even overt heart failure may develop.

An appropriate rehabilitation diet for patients recovering from starvation uncomplicated by other serious illness is approximately 110 percent of the recommended daily allowances (RDA) for that individual, calculated on the basis of his or her "desirable" weight. Initially, feedings should be small, however, and offered frequently until the tolerance of the patient to food is established. Vitamin and protein supplementation are of value only in cases complicated by specific deficiency states. The sodium content of the diet should be limited so as to prevent or minimize edema.

Recovery from starvation moves at a frustratingly slow pace. Weakness, easy fatigability, and muscular aches, as well as irritability and depression, may persist for many weeks or even months after the start of rehabilitation. Polyuria also may continue for several months. Recovery of strength and working capacity is slow and seems to parallel the sluggish rate of return to normal of the lean (active) tissue compartment and the blood hemoglobin concentration. The electrocardiogram may require several months to revert to normal. The habit of conserving energy tends to become ingrained, and during rehabilitation the formerly starved patient often must be hectored to return to a more normal level of physical activity.

During rehabilitation, body fat tends to increase to a point well beyond the prestarvation level, and this extra fat deposition may persist for a year or longer after the end of starvation. Thus, the formerly starved person may take on a paradoxically obese appearance during part of the prolonged convalescence.

PROTEIN-CALORIE MALNUTRITION *Protein-calorie malnutrition of early childhood* is an inclusive designation that has been used to embody a spectrum of nutritional disorders of varying severity which range from the protein deficiency syndrome known as *kwashiorkor* at one extreme to *nutritional marasmus* at the other. Because marasmus appears to be much more prevalent worldwide than kwashiorkor, the suggestion has been made that the term *energy-protein malnutrition* be substituted for *protein-calorie malnutrition.* This form of malnutrition is by far the major cause of infant and childhood mortality and morbidity in the world because of its very high prevalence in many developing countries. It has been estimated that at any given time approximately 400 million preschool children throughout the world suffer from some degree of protein-calorie malnutrition.

The West African term *kwashiorkor* was introduced by Williams in 1933 to describe a syndrome most commonly observed in children between the ages of one and three years. However, the disorder can occur later in childhood and occasionally in adults. The term is said to denote illness in a child displaced from its mother by a subsequent pregnancy. A number of conditioning factors such as parasitism, infectious diarrhea, and childhood exanthems contribute to precipitation of the florid stage of the disease; however, the principal cause is a high carbohydrate diet that provides insufficient protein. A similar syndrome can be induced in pigs and monkeys by feeding a low-protein diet in which the calories are derived principally from carbohydrate. The clinical features of the syndrome are variable, depending on the extent of the dietary imbalance, the age of onset, the duration of the deficiency state, and the severity of the conditioning factors. Characteristically, the child with kwashiorkor is wretched, emotionally unresponsive, and anorexic. He exhibits weakness and retardation of growth and motor development. It is difficult to judge true weight in the child with kwashiorkor because of edema. Although muscle wasting is invariably present, some subcutaneous fat may be retained and, on occasion, as in the case of the frequently cited, but seldom encountered, Jamaican "sugar baby," the child actually may be obese. The status of the subcutaneous fat reflects the child's caloric intake. A "moon-face" appearance is frequently present in kwashiorkor, particularly in obese individuals.

Edema is the principal sign of kwashiorkor and is closely associated with hypoalbuminemia. The edema is of the dependent type, and the presence of pretibial pitting can be readily ascertained. When present, the skin lesions are characteristic; they consist of dyspigmentation, manifested as sharp-edged erythematous patches in white-skinned groups. Desquamation leading to the virtually pathognomonic flaky-paint dermatosis also may be present. Skin changes are most often confined to the perineum in infants and to exposed surfaces in older children. Hair changes are variable and may include dyspigmentation with lightening of color, straightening of curly hair, silkiness of texture, and "easy pluckability." One or more "stripes" of lightened hair color ("flag sign") may attest to alternating intervals of good and poor nutrition in the past.

Although fatty liver is an almost invariable pathologic finding, hepatomegaly occurs inconstantly. Associated disorders include anemia and vitamin deficiency, especially

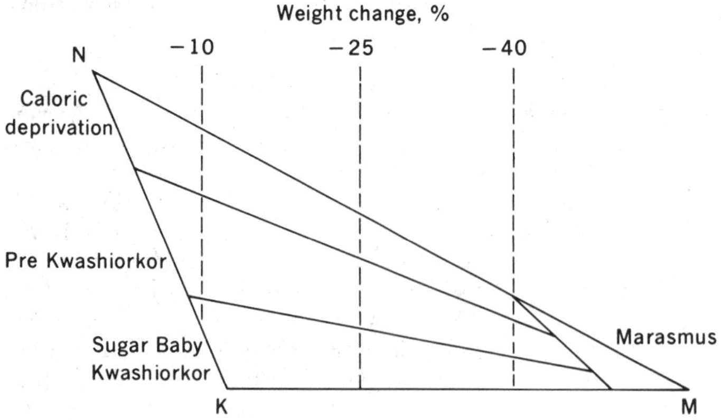

FIGURE 82-1
Relation of marasmus (M) and kwashiorkor (K). The energy depletion is indicated along the abscissa, the extent of protein depletion along the ordinate. The classic example of kwashiorkor, the "sugar baby" fed a pablum of starch, will show but little weight loss because his energy stores are preserved. The child with marasmus is greatly underweight and protein-depleted. Infection may move a child rapidly toward K and M. (Adapted from NS Scrimshaw and M Behar: Malnutrition in underdeveloped countries. N Engl J Med 272:137, 1965)

deficiencies of vitamin A and folic acid, as well as a variety of infections and infestations.

Nutritional marasmus is comparable with severe semistarvation in adults, resulting from a very low intake of all nutrients, including protein. This disorder most commonly affects infants during the first year of life, and its most conspicuous features are marked wasting of muscle and fat and retardation of growth. Infants with nutritional marasmus are tiny and have a typically wizened facies which makes them appear prematurely old. The edema and apathy that characterize kwashiorkor are not present; however, minor dyspigmentation of the hair may occur, and associated vitamin deficiencies have been observed. Between the extremes of advanced kwashiorkor and marked marasmus lies a continuum of intermediate syndromes which, in turn, range from "latent" and marginal to forms of marked severity (Fig. 82-1).

Laboratory findings in protein-calorie malnutrition are highly variable, depending in part on the patient's location in the kwashiorkor–nutritional marasmus spectrum and the severity of the disorder. The plasma protein concentration, notably albumin, is greatly reduced in kwashiorkor. However, hypoalbuminemia is a relatively late complication, and measurement of this parameter is of debatable value in the detection of marginal cases. "Plasma aminograms" show a reduction in most of the essential amino acids and normal or higher values for most of the nonessential group. This observation is not surprising in light of the fact that the need of infants for essential amino acids (in milligrams per kilogram of body weight) is approximately eight times that of adults. A shortened form of the plasma aminogram entails measurement by paper chromatography of four essential amino acids (leucine, isoleucine, valine, methionine) and four that are nonessential (glycine, serine, glutamine, taurine). In kwashiorkor the ratio of dispensable to indispensable amino acids is high (5–10:1) as compared with normally fed controls (2:1).

Although amino acid ratios are usually abnormal in kwashiorkor, they are frequently normal in marasmus. Thus, in recent years somatic measurements, although nonspecific, have gained favor as sensitive indices of protein-calorie malnutrition, including the marasmic portion of the spectrum. The relative usefulness of several simple methods such as measurement of height, weight, head circumference, and midarm circumference is currently under investigation.

Considerable evidence has accumulated that a significant impairment of intellectual performance may be one of the long-term consequences of protein-calorie malnutrition of even a mild to moderate degree.

REFERENCES

BENEDICT FG et al: *Human Vitality and Efficiency under Prolonged Restricted Diet,* Washington: Carnegie Institution, Publication no. 280, 1919

Calorie Deficiencies and Protein Deficiencies: Proceedings of a Colloquium, London: J. & A. Churchill, Ltd., 1968

JELLIFFE DB: Protein-calorie malnutrition in tropical preschool children: A review of recent knowledge. J Pediatr 54:227, 1959

KEYS A et al: *The Biology of Human Starvation,* Minneapolis: University of Minnesota Press, 1950

MÖNCKEBERG F et al: Malnutrition and mental development. Am J Clin Nutr 25:766, 1972

83
PELLAGRA

GEORGE V. MANN
THEODORE B. VAN ITALLIE

HISTORY During the eighteenth century, a new disease began to appear with increasing frequency in northern Spain and Italy. First called *mal de la rosa* by Casal (from the erythematous skin lesions), the malady soon came to be known as *pelle agro* (skin, rough), from which the present-day name, pellagra, is derived. Casal described the prominent features: "a horrible crust" involving the skin, particularly of the hands and neck; "painful burning of the mouth"; "perpetual shaking of the body"; and "mania."

Pellagra emerged in epidemic proportions in the southern United States in the early 1900s. Joseph Goldberger, of the U. S. Public Health Service, soon showed in classic studies that diet alone could cure, prevent, or cause the disease. In 1937, Elvehjem and his coworkers showed that nicotinic acid (niacin) would cure black tongue, a pellagra-like disease, in dogs. Shortly thereafter nicotinic acid proved effective in the therapy of clinical pellagra. When it was found that the essential amino acid, tryptophan, is a precursor of nicotinic acid, it became clear that pellagra results from a deficiency of dietary tryptophan and/or nicotinic acid. Studies of the efficiency of tryptophan conversion to nicotinic acid indicate that an average of 60 mg dietary tryptophan is equivalent to 1 mg nicotinic acid. Deficiency of other nutrients, such as riboflavin, thiamine, folic acid, and vitamin B_{12}, may complicate the disease. The persistent relation of dietary corn to the development of pellagra has been a subject of recurrent investigative interest. Since most of the nicotinic acid in corn is in the "bound" form and may be biologically unavailable, this fact has been invoked to explain the association of corn diets with pellagra. However, other cereals also contain a high proportion of bound nicotinic acid; thus, the role of nicotinic acid binding in pellagragenic diets awaits clarification.

PREVALENCE After 1940, the prevalence of endemic pellagra diminished greatly in the United States, presumably because of some combination of economic improvement, changed food habits, and enrichment of flour with nicotinic acid. The disease is still important in sections of South Africa, Asia, and the Balkans. The greatest prevalence is in women, aged twenty to forty-five years, i.e., the childbearing, lactating group.

Primary pellagra is extremely rare in the United States today. "Secondary" or "conditioned" pellagra may develop in persons who have some other disease such as chronic diarrhea or cancer. Chronic alcoholism is the most common cause, although the chronic alcoholic is more likely to manifest deficiencies of thiamine and folic acid. Polyneuritis, as well as skin changes and other signs characteristic of pellagra, may be observed in the same individual.

CLINICAL FINDINGS Classically, pellagra was considered to be characterized by the four D's: diarrhea, dermatitis, dementia, and death. However, before pellagra becomes clinically manifest and the patient seeks the help of a physician, certain prodromal symptoms may be present. These include loss of appetite leading to weight loss, indigestion, diarrhea or constipation, generalized weakness, lassitude, burning sensations in the mouth, headache, and insomnia. These symptoms are usually followed after varying periods of time by the manifestations of full-blown pellagra, which affect the skin, alimentary tract, nervous system, and to a lesser extent the blood. Pellagra is a seasonal disease with acute exacerbations in the spring and early summer, when a combination of the winter's impairment of diet and a new exposure to sun and heavier work seem to precipitate the acute episodes.

The skin lesions may begin as an erythema that looks very much like sunburn. Burning or itching may be intense. The initial changes may be followed by the formation of vesicles or by peeling. The erythematous skin may assume a dirty-brown color and then becomes rough and scaly. This stage, which may not necessarily be preceded by erythema, may remain for prolonged periods. Characteristically, the skin lesions are symmetrical and tend to be localized over exposed areas: the backs of the hands, the face, neck, elbows, and knees, and the most exposed areas of the feet. In addition, the scrotum, vulva, and perianal region may be involved. Unilateral dermatitis usually is associated with local pressure, trauma, heat, or sunlight. The evolution of the lesions may differ: erythema of the hands may appear while hyperkeratosis of the legs is already present. Seborrhea about the nose with comedo formation (sometimes attributed to riboflavin deficiency) may be conspicuous (Fig. 83-1).

Sore mouth is a common complaint. Changes in the tongue are conspicuous; in fact, glossitis is thought by some to be a more sensitive gage of the disease than skin lesions. The tip and margins of the tongue become hyperemic, a change that may spread to involve the entire surface so that the structure acquires a beet-red appearance. Small ulcers sometimes appear. Inflammatory lesions may be found in the mucous membranes of the mouth. Secondary infection is common, particularly with fusospirochetal organisms. In advanced stages of the disease, the tongue may be pale with complete atrophy of the papillae. Angular lesions, i.e., gray macerated or ulcerated areas at the corners of the mouth, are frequently present. Pain on swal-

FIGURE 83-1
Pellagra in a young girl. (Courtesy of JG Prinsloo and the American Journal of Clinical Nutrition*)*

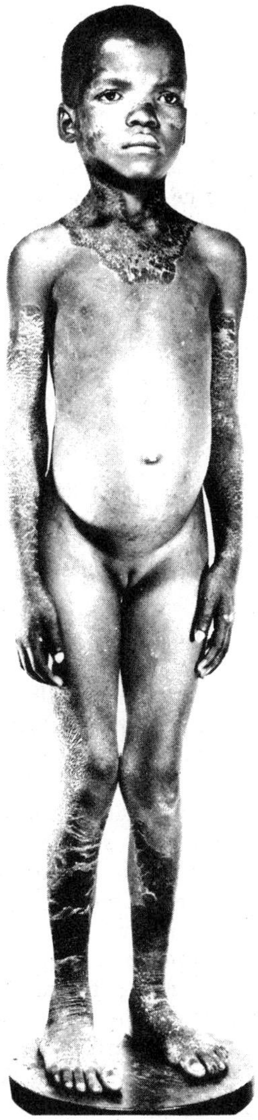

lowing is common. Anorexia, accompanied by epigastric discomfort, is a frequent complaint. Diarrhea has generally been a prominent part of the pellagra syndrome but is not always present. Stools are small, frequent, and watery, and thus quite different from those in sprue. The liver usually is not enlarged.

Neurologic signs and symptoms rarely appear at the beginning of the disease but are common when skin or alimentary manifestations are prominent. Thiamine deficiency may be responsible for a variable proportion of the neurologic findings. Subjectively, the patient may complain of vertigo, weakness, headache, paresthesia, anesthesia, and general aches. Severe pain of the hands and feet may be present. Objectively, tendon reflexes are abnormal, usually diminished. Coarse tremors of the tongue, head, or extremities may be noted on examination. Muscular spasms are sometimes prominent. Mental disturbances are a feature of endemic pellagra; they include "nervousness," confusion, depression, insomnia, apathy, and delirium. The neurologic findings are not specific for pellagra.

LABORATORY FINDINGS Dietary nicotinic acid is required for the formation of two coenzymes, nicotinamide-adenine dinucleotide (NAD) and nicotinamide-adenine dinucleotide phosphate (NADP). Chemical examinations of the blood are of little diagnostic help in pellagra. Gastric analysis reveals achlorhydria in about one-half the cases. The two principal metabolites of nicotinic acid found in the urine are N^1-methylnicotinamide and its 6-pyridone derivative. In pellagra the combined excretion of these two metabolites in the urine is usually less than 2 mg in 24 h. In mild deficiency, slightly larger quantities are excreted. Normal subjects receiving adequate diets excrete 12 to 18 mg of the two metabolites per day.

Anemia is present in approximately one-half the cases of pellagra, but in only about one-quarter is it of any consequence. The anemia may be related to a deficiency of folic acid or vitamin B_{12} with macrocytic anemia developing in some cases.

PATHOLOGY The earliest skin lesions show dilatation of the superficial blood vessels and proliferation of their endothelial cells. The superficial connective tissue elements of the corium assume a spongy appearance. The epidermis, which may already show hyperkeratosis, separates from the corium with the formation of a vesicle. There may be increased pigmentation of the superficial hyperkeratotic layer with decrease in pigment cells in the basal region. Chronic lesions merely show hyperkeratosis. The epithelium of the tongue is atrophic, with loss of papillae; a subacute inflammatory reaction may be present. The esophagus is commonly the site of acute inflammation with loss of epithelium. Alterations in the remainder of the intestinal tract are not particularly noteworthy, except in the colon. Small ulcers may be present in the colon with abscess formation in the submucosa; cystic dilatations of the mucous glands are prominent. The liver may contain excessive fat, which is usually periportal in distribution. The lining of the vagina frequently is acutely inflamed with superficial ulceration. The neurologic changes are variable and consist of atrophy of cerebral neurons, degeneration of peripheral nerves, nerve roots, and tracts in the spinal cord. The bone marrow may show erythroblastic or, rarely, megaloblastic hyperplasia.

PATHOGENESIS When humans subsist on a diet of which the main staple is corn and in which there is little other protein, pellagra is likely to ensue. Corn is nutritionally inferior to other foods in a number of ways, particularly when modern milling procedures are employed. Its protein is low in quantity and, more important, in quality because it is low in two essential amino acids, tryptophan and lysine. Although corn contains appreciable quantities of nicotinic acid when assayed chemically, much of this vitamin is present in "bound" form and appears to be biologically available only if it is hydrolyzed. Nicotinic acid is found in high concentrations in liver, yeast, red muscle meats, fish, coffee, and wheat germ. Vegetables and cereals contain much less.

Meat protein, dairy products, and eggs generally are limited or entirely lacking in the pellagrin's diet. Furthermore, diets that have been associated with pellagra have been deficient not only in protein, but also in available riboflavin, thiamine, and vitamin B_{12}.

The multiple nutrient deficiency aspects of pellagra have been recognized for some time, and they cause one to ask: What is the definition of pellagra? Some workers would be restrictive and define the disease as pure tryptophan–nicotinic acid deficiency. The argument is that since the cardinal symptoms respond to nicotinic acid, pellagra should be regarded as a deficiency of this vitamin. Since, however, some of the classic symptoms and signs are alleviated not by nicotinic acid therapy but by other nutrients, it may be preferable to define pellagra as a multiple deficiency syndrome produced principally by deficiency of tryptophan–nicotinic acid, but usually associated with deficiencies of folic acid, riboflavin, thiamine, and, occasionally, vitamin B_{12}.

DIAGNOSIS Physical signs in endemic pellagra often are suggestive but not absolutely diagnostic. The dietary history is especially important. The diagnosis of incipient pellagra or the recognition of cases without skin manifestations ("pellagra sine pellagra") is more difficult. Here it may be necessary to evaluate the response to therapy with nicotinic acid and other nutrients. Measurement of N^1-methylnicotinamide and its pyridone in a 24-h urine sample may be of help. Fasting plasma concentrations of free tryptophan have been reported to be low in untreated adult pellagrins. The possibility of overt or subclinical pellagra should be considered in every person with a compatible diet history who suffers from gastrointestinal disease or ethanol abuse.

Three forms of disorder with pellagra-like skin lesions, though uncommon, are worthy of mention. The first is a rare hereditary affliction called *Hartnup disease* (Chap. 105). This syndrome consists of a pellagra-like skin rash following exposure to sunlight, intermittent cerebellar ataxia, aminoaciduria, and the excretion of large amounts of indole-3-acetic acid and indican in the urine. Increased quantities of protoporphyrin are found in the stool. Other manifestations of pellagra, such as glossitis, stomatitis, or gastrointestinal symptoms, are not present. The skin lesions respond to therapy with nicotinic acid.

A second form of pellagra-like disease has been reported in patients receiving isoniazid, the tuberculostatic drug which is also a pyridoxine (vitamin B_6) antagonist. Pyridoxine is needed for the conversion of tryptophan to nicotinic acid, and in severe deficiency this conversion may be reduced. In such patients peripheral neuritis and pellagra-like skin lesions appear and may not regress even when the drug is discontinued. Treatment with nicotinic acid often is efficacious in curing the skin lesions. Pyridoxine preparations will usually relieve the neurologic manifestations.

The third condition in which pellagra-like skin lesions have been observed is malignant carcinoid tumors (*malignant argentaffinomas*). These tumors produce such large amounts of 5-hydroxytryptamine (serotonin) from tryptophan that a conditioned form of nicotinic acid deficiency may result in severe cases. In addition to skin lesions, the patients may exhibit other symptoms characteristic of pellagra: mental confusion, diarrhea, and glossitis.

TREATMENT Severely ill pellagrins, particularly those with diarrhea and dementia, should be treated as emergencies. Water and electrolyte deficits must be corrected immediately. Oral administration of niacinamide in doses of 200 mg two or three times a day is recommended until the acute symptoms have subsided and the patient is able to eat properly. Niacinamide is free from the unpleasant vasomotor effects of nicotinic acid. Occasionally it may be necessary to give niacinamide intravenously, but the oral route is preferable and adequate for most patients with pellagra. Riboflavin and thiamine also should be given in therapeutic amounts, since deficiencies of these nutrients are commonly associated with pellagra. A daily maintenance dose of the other vitamins should be a part of the therapeutic regimen, and a high-calorie, high-protein diet is desirable. Frequent small feedings are advocated at first. Stomatitis, diarrhea or constipation, and oozing of ulcerated lesions of the skin will necessitate symptomatic care.

PROGNOSIS Until the advent of vitamin therapy, the prognosis of pellagra was grave, but now it is excellent. The glossitis begins to decrease in 24 h; the papillae of the tongue begin to regenerate by the end of the first week. Lesions of the lips begin to heal in 2 to 3 days. Gastrointestinal symptoms improve in 24 to 48 h, and diarrhea usually ceases by the end of the first week. Demented patients usually become rational after 3 or 4 days, unless irreversible brain damage has occurred. Polyneuritis, if present, may require some time to improve.

REFERENCES

GILLMAN J, GILLMAN T: *Perspectives in Human Malnutrition: A Contribution to the Biology of Disease from a Clinical and Pathological Study of Chronic Malnutrition and Pellagra in the African.* New York: Grune & Stratton, 1951

GOLDSMITH GA: Niacin: Antipellagra factor, hypocholesterolemic agent. Model of nutrition research yesterday and today. JAMA 194:167, 1965

HANKES LV et al: Tryptophan: Abnormal metabolism in pellagra patients. Metabolism 19:465, 1970

MELMON KL et al: Distinctive clinical and therapeutic aspects of syndromes associated with bronchial carcinoid tumors. Am J Med 39:568, 1965

SYDENSTRICKER VP: The history of pellagra, its recognition as a disorder of nutrition and its conquest. Am J Clin Nutr 6:409, 1958

TRUSWELL AS et al: Plasma tryptophan and other amino acids in pellagra. Am J Clin Nutr 21:1314, 1968

84 THIAMINE DEFICIENCY, ARIBOFLAVINOSIS, AND VITAMIN B_6 DEFICIENCY

THEODORE B. VAN ITALLIE

BERIBERI History During the seventeenth, eighteenth, and nineteenth centuries, a disease peculiar to the Far East became known to Western physicians. The principal characteristics of this disease, *"oriental beriberi,"* as described by a nineteenth-century physician, were "a feeling of numbness, sense of weight and weakness in the legs, edema of the feet, unsteady and tottering walk with almost total palsy, rigidity and various affections of the nerves, oppression and weight in the precordium, and, occasionally, sudden death." The disease was endemic throughout South China, Southeast Asia, the Philippines, the East Indies, and parts of India.

Later studies revealed the close relation of rice in the diet to the development of the disease. Beriberi was eradicated from the Japanese Navy by Takaki, who added meat, vegetables, and condensed milk to the rice diet of the common sailor. In Batavia (now Djakarta), Eijkman observed a beriberi-like disease in fowl fed polished rice; the birds could be cured with unpolished grain. By 1912, the therapeutic effectiveness of rice polishings had been demonstrated, particularly in patients with the acute cardiac manifestations of beriberi. This led E. B. Vedder, a U.S. Army physician, to recommend to R. R. Williams, a chemist working in Manila, that the protective substance be isolated. In 1936, Williams and his coworkers announced the chemical structure and synthesis of the active principle, thiamine.

Prevalence Today the prevalence of clinical beriberi in the Far East is greatly reduced. However, cases are still encountered, particularly in infants and pregnant or lactating women. In the United States thiamine deficiency is most commonly found in alcoholics. The presence of thiamine in enriched flour and white bread has virtually eradicated primary beriberi among the urban poor.

Clinical findings Three main types of beriberi have been recognized in the Orient: a chronic form in which neurologic involvement is prominent *(dry beriberi),* an acute form with heart failure, and a less acute state in which edema is the most characteristic manifestation *(wet beriberi).* The onset of the chronic neurologic form is insidious. Over the course of days or weeks, the patient becomes easily fatigued and experiences feelings of heaviness in the legs, together with stiffness and aching in the muscles. In time the muscles become weaker, acutely painful, and then atrophic. The extensors of the foot usually are affected first, then the muscles of the calf and thigh. Pain followed by atrophy occurs in the muscles of the arms; the muscles of the trunk may be affected later. Associated with these signs and symptoms are foot drop and wrist drop, together with loss of ankle and knee reflexes. Paresthesias and anesthesias may be demonstrated, particularly in the lower extremities. Circumoral anesthesia may be present. Aphonia is sometimes a symptom. Walking becomes difficult, and the patient can only shuffle about with a cane or is forced to hold on to objects to keep from falling. The severity of neurologic involvement may fluctuate. In time, however, the patient becomes completely bedridden.

With persistent anorexia, progressive weight loss occurs. Diarrhea may further complicate the nutritional picture. Cardiac changes may accompany these neurologic disturbances or may appear suddenly in the absence of any evidence of involvement of the nervous system. The cardiac manifestations consist of palpitations, precordial pain, and dyspnea, which may come on in paroxysms without warning. The heart is found to be enlarged, and tachycardia is present. Prominent venous pulsations are noted in the neck. Edema of the lower extremities usually is present. The blood pressure is not elevated, but the pulse pressure is increased and venous pressure is elevated. Death may occur suddenly.

In infants beriberi continues to be a health problem in the Far East. In babies the manifestations may be aphonic, in which the child loses its voice; cardiologic, a sudden episode of labored breathing, cyanosis, and, if treatment is not prompt, cardiac arrest leading to death; pseudomeningitic; and gastrointestinal, with failure to gain weight, constipation, and vomiting. These babies are typically born of mothers with low dietary intakes of thiamine and consequently low levels in their milk. The infant seems to flourish until quite suddenly it is stricken, usually at three to six months of age. The disorder is prevented by giving the mother thiamine and treated by the administration of thiamine to the infant. Such treatment will often bring a dramatic cure in a matter of hours.

In the mid-1930s, observers in large urban clinics in the Occident began to recognize instances of cardiac and neurologic disease occurring predominantly in alcoholics. In some areas the prevalence of these forms of occidental beriberi, as these entities came to be called, was high. The clinical aspects of this form of heart disease are described in Chap. 237.

The symptoms and signs relative to neurologic involvement in alcoholics have the characteristics of a progressive polyneuritis with sensory and motor defects (Chaps. 118, 340, and 341). Almost invariably there is a history of excessive consumption of alcohol and poor dietary intake. In addition, such patients frequently exhibit manifestations of delirium tremens or Wernicke's disease. To such examples of neurologic involvement in poorly nourished, chronic alcoholics have been added other syndromes in recent years, such as alcoholic amblyopia, central pontine myelinolysis, and corticocerebellar degeneration. None of these changes, including Wernicke's disease, has been described in beriberi occurring in Asian peoples.

Thiamine is involved in a number of key reactions in the glycolytic and pentose phosphate pathways of glucose metabolism. Consequently, disturbances of lactate and pyruvate oxidation and of pentose phosphate shunt reactions would be expected to reflect alterations of these functions.

Pathology Postmortem examinations performed at the turn of the century in the Orient on patients who died with neurologic manifestations of beriberi revealed myelin degeneration of the peripheral nerves, with loss of axoplasm. Lesions in the brain and spinal cord have not been reported from the Orient. Among the sporadic cases designated as neurologic beriberi encountered in the Occident, usually among alcoholics, lesions of peripheral nerves also have been described. More prominent, however, are changes in the brain. Alterations characteristic of Wernicke's disease include bilateral hemorrhagic necrotic foci in the mammillary bodies, the hypothalamic nuclei, and midline structures, as well as reactions of microglia and astrocytes. Damage to the optic nerve and lesions in the spinal cord have been reported.

The heart is likely to be enlarged, but this increase in size usually is due to dilatation, although hypertrophy of the right ventricle has sometimes been noted. The myocardial fibers do not exhibit necrosis, although swelling and vacuolization may be prominent. No cellular infiltration is present.

Pathogenesis Rice is the principal foodstuff of one-half or more of the inhabitants of the world. The introduction of power milling machinery at the end of the nineteenth century led to a great increase in beriberi in the Far East. When rice is highly milled, most of its vitamin content, such as thiamine, riboflavin, nicotinic acid, pantothenic acid, and pyridoxine, is removed. Lipids and minerals, such as calcium, iron, and iodine, which are present in the outer portions of the grain, are lost as well.

Although the rice eater's diet is deficient in a number of nutrients, the principal manifestations of beriberi—the derangements in cardiac and neurologic function—appear to be related to thiamine deficiency. The therapeutic response of the patient with cardiovascular beriberi, whether infant or adult, to thiamine is good evidence for this relation. The development of anatomic lesions in the hearts of experimental animals deprived of thiamine is further proof for the relation of this vitamin to the integrity of the myocardium.

The precise relation of thiamine to maintenance of the integrity of the peripheral nervous system is uncertain. The predilection of the nervous system for injury in thiamine deficiency suggests that the vitamin is especially crucial for those tissues which depend upon carbohydrate metabolism exclusively for their energy sources. Moreover, the pentose phosphate pathway is needed for lipid synthesis. This is one of the ways in which thiamine deficiency could lead to demyelinization. The clinical response of neurologic defects to thiamine usually is not rapid, but this can be explained if the damage has been severe enough to have caused structural loss. Hence, regeneration is necessary if function is to be restored.

In contrast, the ophthalmoplegia of Wernicke's disease may improve within a few hours after thiamine administration, and lesions similar to those observed in Wernicke's disease have been demonstrated in the brains of thiamine-deficient animals. The enigma of the rarity of Wernicke's disease in the Orient (except among Western prisoners of war) remains.

Diagnosis Patients with neuritic (dry) beriberi exhibit tenderness of the calf muscles and have difficulty in rising from a squatting position. Patellar and Achilles tendon reflexes are usually hypoactive or absent. Paresthesias are common, but loss of vibratory and position sense is less common.

Cardiovascular (wet) beriberi is characterized by edema of the lower extremities and varying grades of congestive heart failure. Cardiomegaly and pulmonary congestion are common, together with evidence of high-output failure, including a relatively shortened circulation time. Low-output failure is occasionally observed. Electrocardiographic changes in cardiovascular beriberi are similar to those of potassium deficiency and may include prolongation of the Q-T interval, low voltage, and flat or inverted T waves.

Urinary thiamine levels are valuable in population surveys but of far less use in the diagnosis of individual cases. Although a urinary thiamine excretion rate of less than 65 μg per g creatinine is considered indicative of a low or deficient thiamine status, many apparently healthy individuals have been found to fall within this "deficient" range. Measurement of blood thiamine concentrations is of limited diagnostic value. Estimation of erythrocyte transketolase (ETK) activity, an enzyme which functions in the pentose phosphate pathway and requires thiamine as a cofactor, and the in vitro response of ETK activity to added thiamine pyrophosphate (TPP) are more helpful. One to two hours after the patient has been treated with thiamine, the ETK activity increases to a level equivalent to or higher than that observed when the initial blood sample was incubated with TPP. An in vitro TPP effect greater than 16 percent strongly suggests thiamine deficiency.

Beriberi usually is readily identified if it is included in the differential diagnosis. In the Occident, beriberi may be overlooked because of a "low index of suspicion" and failure to obtain an adequate dietary history, particularly in patients suspected of alcoholism. All too frequently, cardiovascular beriberi is considered only after the patient in congestive failure fails to respond appropriately to conventional treatment with digitalis and diuretics. When suitable biochemical tests are not available, the best criterion for the diagnosis of beriberi is the response of the patient to thiamine administration. In cardiovascular beriberi, improvement after administration of thiamine may be dramatic; marked diuresis, decrease in heart rate and size, and clearing of pulmonary congestion may occur within 12 to 48 h.

In patients with the Wernicke-Korsakoff syndrome irreversible brain damage occurs rapidly; hence early recognition and treatment are vital. Ophthalmoplegia may respond dramatically to thiamine.

Treatment When there is cardiac or neurologic involvement, beriberi becomes a medical emergency. Prompt administration of thiamine is essential. Initially, 60 mg thiamine should be given intramuscularly, followed by 25 mg per day in divided doses orally for 1 to 2 weeks. Thereafter, 2.5 mg per day should be sufficient. Ordinarily, increments above individual oral doses of 2.5 mg per day are largely unabsorbed. Since patients with beriberi often exhibit multiple deficiencies, they should also receive the other water-soluble vitamins in therapeutic quantities.

Prognosis The response to thiamine of infants and adults with cardiovascular beriberi in the Orient is one of the most dramatic in medicine. In the Occident, such dramatic responses are seen less often. Although the eye signs of Wernicke's disease improve after thiamine administration, the loss of memory for the immediate past and the confabulation (Korsakoff's psychosis) respond only if the disease is treated early.

RIBOFLAVIN DEFICIENCY Ariboflavinosis still is a common nutritional deficiency in many developing countries. In the United States, there appears to be a positive correlation between family income and riboflavin intake. Riboflavin deficiency is found sporadically among the poor and in alcoholics, but its prevalence is not known precisely. Deficiency of riboflavin almost always occurs in association with deficiencies of other B vitamins. Riboflavin requirement is related to "metabolic body size," represented as body weight in kilograms taken to the 0.75 power; riboflavin allowances for adults are approximately 1 to 2 mg per day. Milk, eggs, fish, meat (especially liver), and certain vegetables are good sources of riboflavin; when dietary protein intake is adequate in adults, a deficiency of riboflavin usually does not occur. Exposure of milk to direct sunlight destroys a considerable amount of vitamin content; riboflavin in food also is destroyed by treatment with alkali.

Riboflavin is the precursor of two flavoprotein coenzymes, flavin mononucleotide (FMN) and flavin adenine dinucleotide (FAD), and thereby plays a central role in many important metabolic processes. In the tissues very little of the vitamin is stored as riboflavin; nearly all is in the form of FMN and FAD. Thyroid hormone regulates the conversion of riboflavin to FMN and FAD by increasing the activity of the enzyme flavokinase, which catalyzes the transformation of riboflavin to FMN. Thyroid hormone causes smaller increases in the activities of FAD pyrophosphorylase, which converts FMN to FAD, and of FMN phosphatase, which degrades FMN to riboflavin. In hypothyroidism, flavokinase activity decreases, and tissue levels of FMN and FAD are also diminished.

Riboflavin is absorbed from the upper intestinal tract, and apparently is phosphorylated to FMN in the intestinal mucosa. The presence of food increases the rate of intestinal absorption. Riboflavin and FMN circulate in plasma both free and bound to plasma proteins. The physiological significance of protein binding in plasma is unknown. Riboflavin is excreted predominantly in urine.

Lack of riboflavin in young rats results in cessation of growth and extensive skin changes. Maternal riboflavin deficiency in experimental animals produces prominent congenital malformation in the offspring. In adult animals riboflavin deficiency produces enlarged livers with a high content of triglyceride and glycogen. Electron microscopy in mice discloses giant mitochondria within hepatic cells. Deficient rats exhibit abnormalities of tryptophan metabolism and excrete excessive quantities of anthranilic and xanthurenic acids. Apparently riboflavin is required for the formation of pyridoxal phosphate from pyridoxine phosphate. The former coenzyme, in turn, is needed for normal metabolism of tryptophan. The brain contains a number of riboflavin-requiring enzymes.

In riboflavin-deficient patients, angular stomatitis, cheilosis, and sore throat are early findings. Subsequently, seborrheic dermatitis of the face and scrotum, glossitis, and a generalized dermatitis involving trunk and extremities may occur. The eyes itch and burn, and the patient may complain of photophobia and visual impairment; corneal vascularization may occur. Late findings include neuropathy and mild anemia. Human riboflavin deficiency has been induced experimentally by means of a riboflavin antagonist, galactoflavin. In such individuals clinical symptoms occur more rapidly and are more marked than in patients with dietary restriction of the vitamin alone.

The anemia of experimentally induced riboflavin deficiency in primates is normochromic and normocytic and is associated with red cell hypoplasia and reduced reticulocytosis. The anemia responds promptly to riboflavin administration, an increase in the reticulocyte count occurring within a few days after initiation of treatment. Apparently, normal utilization of folic acid is dependent upon the integrity of certain flavoprotein enzymes; hence, the anemia of riboflavin deficiency may be related in part to an associated disturbance of folic acid metabolism. This finding may have implications for the use of folate antagonists in cancer chemotherapy.

Clinical diagnosis of riboflavin deficiency is often difficult because ariboflavinosis usually occurs in conjunction with other vitamin deficiency states. Moreover, the stomatitis, glossitis, and dermatitis are not specific to riboflavin deficiency. Corneal vascularization, if present, is a useful (but not a pathognomic) sign. A careful dietary history is helpful in suggesting the diagnosis. When suitable laboratory tests are not available, a therapeutic trial is indicated.

In the past, the laboratory diagnosis of riboflavin deficiency has depended on measurement of blood levels of riboflavin and its derivatives. Measurements performed on erythrocytes appear to yield more reliable information about riboflavin nutrition than plasma concentrations. The urinary excretion of riboflavin also has been suggested as providing useful diagnostic information.

An in vitro enzyme assay for glutathione reductase and the increase in its activity induced by FAD (analogous to the TPP-effect for thiamine) gives promise of a specific diagnostic test of human riboflavin deficiency. This test is based on the observation that the magnitude of increase in erythrocyte glutathione reductase activity after ingestion of riboflavin correlates well with the level of dietary intake of this vitamin. In normal subjects fed a riboflavin-free diet for only 1 week, significant changes in erythrocyte glutathione reductase activity occur when FAD is added to the reaction mixture in vitro. The suitability of this determination for large-scale nutritional surveys remains to be established.

The recommended therapeutic dose of riboflavin is about 10 mg orally; treatment at this level should be continued until the manifestations of the deficient state have regressed. Larger doses of riboflavin may be administered safely without untoward effects.

VITAMIN B_6 DEFICIENCY Vitamin B_6 is a collective term for three naturally occurring pyridines: pyridoxine, pyridoxal, and pyridoxamine; pyridoxal phosphate and pyridoxamine phosphate are the metabolically active forms. Pyridoxal and pyridoxamine are found mainly in animal products, and pyridoxine occurs in plant foods. Of these three vitamers, pyridoxine is the main source of vitamin B_6 activity in the average diet.

Pyridoxal phosphate is known to serve as a coenzyme for the decarboxylases, deaminases, transaminases, and a number of other enzymes. It also appears to be incorporated into the glycogen phosphorylase of muscle. In rats, a deficiency of vitamin B_6 causes cachexia, and anemia; in young pigs, scaling of the skin and a profound microcytic, hypochromic anemia, epileptiform convulsions, and sensory neuron degeneration develop. Deficiency of vitamin B_6 causes multiple changes in the metabolism and functioning of the brain. Seizures have occurred in babies fed formulas deficient in vitamin B_6. Nasolabial seborrhea, cheilosis, and angular lesions may reflect a deficiency of vitamin B_6; however, these signs are nonspecific and frequently are not nutritionally related. Rarely, a red, painful tongue with denudation of the epithelium with or without fissures may be associated.

Vitamin B_6 is involved in the reactions by which tryptophan is converted to nicotinic acid. Thus, when this vitamin is deficient, increased quantities of intermediate products and their derivatives are formed and excreted in the urine. Of these, xanthurenic acid appears to reflect most reliably the state of vitamin B_6 nutriture. The quantity of xanthurenic acid excreted following a *tryptophan load* provides a sensitive index of vitamin B_6 deficiency. Use of a 2-g L-tryptophan dose seems least likely to distort the metabolic state through overloading and has been reported to afford the greatest reproducibility of the quantities of tryptophan metabolic intermediates excreted in the urine. By means of tryptophan loading it has been possible to demonstrate disturbances of tryptophan metabolism, presumably reflecting B_6 deficiency, early in pregnancy and in women using oral contraceptives. Large doses of pyridoxine (25 mg per day) were needed to correct the altered vitamin B_6-tryptophan metabolism resulting from oral contraceptive use. Vitamin B_6 also has an important role in the metabolism of methionine.

The major urinary metabolite of pyridoxine is 4-pyridoxic acid. This compound disappears from the urine at an early stage of deprivation; hence its continued presence in the urine would appear to rule out vitamin B_6 deficiency. It also has been suggested that stimulation of erythrocyte glutamic-oxaloacetic transaminase (EGOT) activity by pyridoxal phosphate in vitro can serve as a useful measurement in the evaluation of vitamin B_6 nutritional status.

A number of drugs interfere with vitamin B_6 utilization. Isoniazid and hydralazine form inactive derivatives and increase B_6 requirements. Penicillamine and cycloserine act as antimetabolites of vitamin B_6. Polyneuritis may appear as a complication of therapy with these agents and can be relieved by supplying large amounts of pyridoxine hydrochloride.

A form of sideroblastic anemia with microcytic red cells is responsive to therapy with pyridoxine. The toxicity of pyridoxine and derivatives is extremely low in humans (Chap. 309). In infants receiving normal diets convulsive seizures have been described which could be relieved by administration of pyridoxine. Such observations have led to the concept of pyridoxine dependency due to a genetically determined requirement for unusually large amounts of pyridoxine.

REFERENCES

BRIN M: Erythrocyte transketolase in early thiamine deficiency. Ann NY Acad Sci 98:528, 1962

FRIMPTER GW et al: Vitamin B_6 dependency syndromes. Am J Clin Nutr 22:794, 1969

LANE M et al: The rapid induction of human riboflavin deficiency with galactoflavin. J Clin Invest 43:357, 1964

LUHBY AL et al: Vitamin B_6 metabolism in users of oral contraceptive agents: 1. Abnormal urinary xanthurenic acid excretion and its correction by pyridoxine. Am J Clin Nutr 24:684, 1971

RIVLIN RS: Riboflavin metabolism. N Engl J Med 283:463, 1970

SAUBERLICH EH et al: Thiamine requirements of the adult human. Am J Clin Nutr 23:671, 1970

STURMAN JA, RIVLIN RS: Pathogenesis of brain dysfunction in deficiency of thiamine, riboflavin, pantothenic acid, or vitamin B_6, *Biology of Brain Dysfunction,* ed GE Gaul, New York: Plenum, 1975, p. 425

85
SCURVY

THEODORE B. VAN ITALLIE

HISTORY One of the first clear-cut descriptions of scurvy appears in records of the Crusades. When the long sea voyages of discovery began toward the end of the fifteenth century, scurvy became commonplace and soon ranked first among causes of disability and mortality in sailors. In 1747 James Lind, a British naval surgeon, in a model experiment, studied the effects of several types of treatment, such as one composed of "two oranges and one lemon given every day." The sailors, who were described as having "putrid gums, the spots and lassitude, with weakness of their knees," responded dramatically. Infantile scurvy began to receive attention after 1883, when Barlow described the syndrome as it is recognized today. With increasing use of breast milk substitutes, scurvy became common in the urban areas of Europe and the United States at the turn of the century.

A disease of the growing bones of guinea pigs similar to that seen in children was produced by dietary means in 1907. Twenty-five years later, a biologically active, crystalline material was isolated from lemon juice and from paprika. This compound was later synthesized and shown to be ascorbic acid.

PREVALENCE In previous times scurvy in adults tended to occur in epidemic form. In the United States scurvy now is seen only in occasional individuals, sometimes in alcoholics and food faddists, but more often in men living alone whose diet is grossly unbalanced and is devoid of sources of ascorbic acid ("bachelor scurvy"). Sporadic cases of scurvy continue to appear in pediatric clinics, usually as a result of maternal error or neglect.

CLINICAL FINDINGS The principal manifestations of scurvy in the adult include follicular hyperkeratosis with perifollicular hemorrhage, swollen, bleeding gums, petechiae, aching muscles, fatigue, and emotional changes. These changes appear after 2 or more months of depletion. Subsequently, arthralgias involving the large joints occur, and these may be followed by joint effusion. Fatigue and psychologic disturbances may be early symptoms.

Oral lesions occur almost exclusively in individuals who have retained their own teeth and are most severe in those with preexisting gingivitis. Reddening and swelling of the interdental papillae occur first, soon followed by hemorrhage. Less well-known features of scurvy include the appearance of minute hemorrhages and small aneurysms in the bulbar conjunctivas. The development of a Sjögren-like (sicca) syndrome also has been noted.

The clinical picture in children is very different from that in adults. The peak age incidence is 8 months; few cases are seen after the first year. The most prominent sign on physical examination is tenderness of the lower extremities, which are also usually somewhat swollen. The legs are characteristically partially flexed and guarded. Involvement of the upper extremities is less common. The extremities are obviously painful, and the child may scream when approached. The costochondral junctions may be enlarged, and crepitus of the epiphyseal areas of the ankles and wrists may be felt. The gums are swollen and hemorrhagic when teeth are present, but show little change before teeth erupt. Subcutaneous hemorrhages may be observed; these tend to be in the form of ecchymoses, not the pinpoint hemorrhages seen about the follicles in the adult. Follicular lesions are uncommon in children. Hemorrhages may occur elsewhere: suborbital with proptosis, epistaxis, hematuria, or signs of subdural bleeding.

LABORATORY FINDINGS The concentration of ascorbic acid may be determined in samples of serum (or plasma), whole blood, or in the buffy coat layer. The ascorbate concentration in the buffy coat most faithfully reflects the body pool of L-ascorbic acid (about 1,500 mg in normally nourished adults) and is the preferred measurement; however, this procedure is technically difficult and seldom used in the United States.

Diagnostically, the more conveniently measured serum and plasma concentrations are equivalent to those in whole blood, except when the ascorbate level is low. Thus, when serum levels are in the vicinity of 0.2 mg per 100 ml (a concentration often associated with deficiency), whole blood, because it contains a fraction of the buffy coat, is a somewhat more reliable indicator of vitamin C status. Clinically manifest scurvy is to be expected when the whole blood concentration falls below 0.3 mg per 100 ml.

Saturation or load tests may be of some help in evaluating ascorbic acid nutriture. When tissue stores are filled, 50 percent or more of an oral load (5 mg per lb) of ascorbic acid will be excreted in the urine during the subsequent 24 h. In depleted patients urinary excretion of the vitamin may range from 0 to 20 percent of the test dose.

PATHOLOGY In adults, the most conspicuous finding at autopsy is the presence of generalized hemorrhage. The perifollicular lesions and ecchymoses noted clinically are conspicuous. In addition, extravasations of blood are found in the pericardial or pleural cavities, the walls of the intestinal tract, bladder, and renal pelves. In young adults separation of the epiphyses or costochondral junctions may be present, as well as subperiosteal hemorrhage.

In children the most characteristic changes at autopsy are in the skeleton. The periosteum is found to be separated or may be easily stripped from the shaft of a bone, and the costal or epiphyseal cartilages are separated from the shaft of the rib or a long bone. Microscopic examination at the cartilage-shaft junction shows a dense "lattice" of spicules of calcified cartilaginous matrix, many of which have fractured. Little bone has formed on this lattice which, furthermore, has not been destroyed. In less advanced cases, fractures occur only at the edges or corners of the bone. Hemorrhage may be observed in the marrow or beneath the periosteum. As a result of decreased osteoid formation, the cortex and trabeculae of the shaft are reduced in thickness. Aside from hemorrhages elsewhere—subdural, subpleural, and subcutaneous—little else is found that is specific for scurvy. Rickets frequently coexists in such children.

PATHOGENESIS Scurvy represents the reaction of particular hosts, such as humans, other primates, certain birds and fish, and the guinea pig, to a lack of ascorbic acid in the diet. Most other mammalian species can synthesize the vitamin from D-glucose or D-galactose. Ascorbic acid is found in high concentrations in citrus and other fruits, leafy vegetables, tomatoes, tubers, most grasses, and sprouting plants. The vitamin content of human milk varies, since the mother is dependent on dietary sources. Milk from a well-nourished woman contains 5 to 7 mg ascorbic acid per 100 ml. Fresh cow's milk contains 1.0 to 2.6 mg per 100 ml; however, storage and sterilized infant formulas prepared from cow's milk or proprietary foods may be expected to produce scurvy in infants if the product has not been fortified or the diet is not supplemented with a source of ascorbic acid.

Scurvy, broadly speaking, is a genetic disease in that the tissues of the susceptible species have lost their ability to synthesize ascorbic acid. The chemical steps in the formation of the vitamin are well known:

$$\text{D-glucuronate} + \text{NADPH} + \text{H}^+ \rightarrow \text{L-gulonate} + \text{NADP}^+$$
$$\text{L-gulonate} + \text{NAD}^+ \rightarrow \text{L-gulonolactone} + \text{NAD}^+ + \text{H}^+$$
$$\text{L-gulonolactone} \rightarrow \text{L-ascorbate} + H_2O$$

Liver and kidney tissues of all mammalian species so far studied can carry out the first two reactions above. Animals subject to scurvy do not have an enzyme system which permits the third reaction.

In ascorbic acid–deficient organisms, the connective tissue cells can proliferate. However, their microscopic appearance reveals their functional impotency; their cytoplasm is scanty, and virtually no stainable RNA is present. The basic structural disturbance in scurvy is the failure of various types of connective tissue cells to form their respective collagenous matrices. Fibroblasts are unable to elaborate collagen; osteoblasts and adontoblasts do not synthesize osteoid and dentine. The lack of formation of these matrices explains the failure of wounds to heal, the changes in the growing bone of infants and children, and the alterations in the teeth of experimental animals.

Collagen is characterized chemically by large amounts of glycine, proline, hydroxyproline, and hydroxylysine. The presence of hydroxyamino acids makes collagen unique, since these amino acids are not found in other proteins. Hydroxyproline is not synthesized in the absence of ascorbic acid, which appears to be needed for synthesis of an essential protein enzyme. Since exogenous hydroxyproline is not incorporated into collagen, all the hydroxyproline in the collagen molecule must be derived from the hydroxylation of proline in vivo. The point in collagen synthesis at which hydroxylation of proline takes place has been shown to be following the formation of an initial polypeptide of proline, lysine, and glycine called *protocollagen* or *procollagen*. In this reaction an enzyme called *collagen proline hydroxylase* serves as a catalyst.

The role of ascorbic acid in maintaining the integrity of blood vessels is not clear, but since the integrity of collagen is affected as a result of ascorbic acid deficiency, it is probable that the blood vessels lose the support provided by these fibers and, hence, become more liable to the effects of minor trauma.

Certain other metabolic defects may be observed as a result of ascorbic acid deficiency. One of the most interesting aspects of ascorbic acid function is its nonspecific relation to metabolism of the aromatic amino acids, phenylalanine and tyrosine. Premature infants deficient in ascorbic acid excrete relatively large amounts of homogentisic, parahydroxyphenyllactic, and parahydroxyphenylpyruvic acids in the urine when excess phenylalanine and tyrosine are administered. The defect appears to be an inability to metabolize the extra load of tyrosine. Defective synthesis of norepinephrine and of serotonin may be important components of the scorbutic syndrome. Loss of vasomotor stability occurs in human scurvy and might help to explain the sudden death that can occur in this disease. Ascorbic acid is implicated in the secretion of the aqueous humor. The vitamin also plays a role in the metabolism of folic acid, i.e., in the transformation of this material to folacin (citrovorum factor). Occasionally, scurvy is associated with a macrocytic anemia which responds to vitamin C and folic acid. Ingestion of ascorbic acid in food also aids in the absorption of dietary iron.

DIAGNOSIS The clinical features of full-blown scurvy in adults or infants are characteristic. Also helpful is the feeding history in infants. If an infant four to six months or older has been bottle-fed with boiled milk or milk substitutes from birth or shortly after and has received no supplemental ascorbic acid, the possibility of scurvy should be considered. The dietary history of adults is likewise important because the disease often is observed in individuals subsisting on diets obviously low in ascorbic acid content.

X-ray examination in the adult is of no particular help in diagnosis, except that one may see alterations in the lamina dura of the jaws. In infants, x-ray examination of the skeleton may be helpful. At the junction between the epiphyseal cartilage and shaft of the long bones, there may be a zone of increased density, which represents the area of excess spicules of calcified cartilaginous matrix, some of which may have fractured (Fig. 85-1). There may also be defects, i.e., areas of rarefaction, at the "corners" of the bones, and these result from fractures at the periphery of the junction between cartilage and shaft. The formation of spurs or projections of the periosteum about the margins of the cartilage also is characteristic. In addition, the bone film will show a "ground-glass" appearance, which reflects the decrease in density due to diminished width of the cortices and size of the medullary trabeculae.

TREATMENT Infants should be given fresh orange juice in single or multiple doses each day. This may be sweetened. If orange juice is refused, synthetic ascorbic acid may be employed orally, 100 to 300 mg per day. There is little or no need for parenteral therapy. In view of the skeletal changes, children in whom the disease is in the stage of healing should be handled as little and as gently as possible. It is not necessary to manipulate any bony deformities, nor should splints or casts be applied.

FIGURE 85-1

Four characteristic changes of scurvy. Large subperiosteal hemorrhages are being calcified. The epiphyseal margin shows a translucent line medially, the "corner sign" of Park. The epiphyseal plates are dense, and the bone shaft shows a "ground glass" appearance with lack of trabecular detail. (Courtesy of David Baker, Columbia University.)

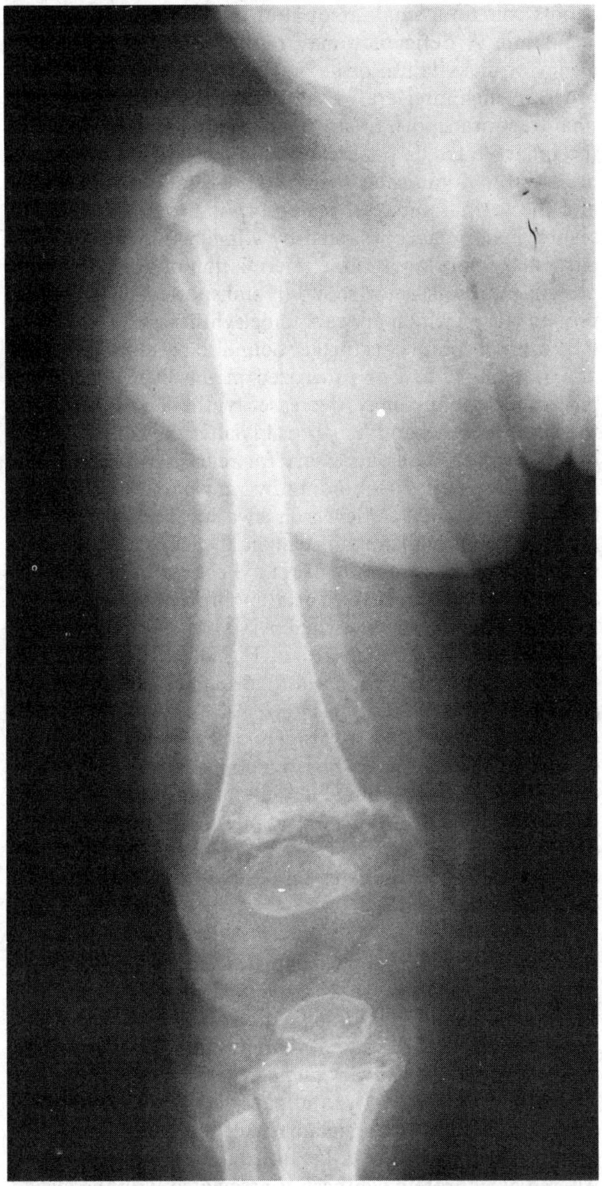

In adults treatment involves administration of orange juice or ascorbic acid in divided doses up to 500 mg per day. Citrus juices generally contain about 40 to 50 mg ascorbate per 100 ml. A diet rich in vitamin C should be initiated and continued in both children and adults.

If scurvy is suspected, samples of blood and urine should be obtained promptly for laboratory analysis. Then ascorbic acid should be administered as outlined above. Scurvy is potentially fatal, and delay in treatment should never be permitted.

About 10 percent of ingested ascorbic acid may be excreted in the urine as oxalate. Acidification of the urine by ingestion of large amounts of ascorbic acid can cause the precipitation of urate, oxalate, or cystine stones in the urinary tract. Large doses of vitamin C also may inactivate vitamin B_{12}, interfere with the action of anticoagulants, and interfere with the accuracy of clinical tests for glycosuria. In the absence of firm evidence for the usefulness of large doses of ascorbic acid in treatment or prevention of colds or other infections, the use of large amounts of vitamin C for such purposes cannot be recommended, and the potential dangers should be appreciated. Because of potentially unfavorable effects on reproduction, high doses of vitamin C should not be taken during pregnancy.

PROGNOSIS Under therapy gum lesions, if present in infants and in adults, begin to regress in 2 to 3 days. Periosteal shadows, resulting from new bone formation, begin to appear in the long bones of infants after approximately a week. Hemorrhages in the skin usually disappear in 2 to 3 weeks.

REFERENCES

ABBOUD FM et al: Autonomic reflexes and vascular reactivity in experimental scurvy in man. J Clin Invest 49:298, 1970

BURNS JJ: Biosynthesis of L-ascorbic acid: Basic defect in scurvy. Am J Med 26:740, 1959

DYKES MHM, MEIER P: Ascorbic acid and the common cold: Evaluation of its efficacy and toxicity. JAMA 231:1073, 1975

GOULD BS: *Collagen Biosynthesis,* London: Academic, 1970, p. 139

HESS AF: *Scurvy, Past and Present,* Philadelphia: Lippincott, 1920

HODGES RE et al: Clinical manifestations of ascorbic acid deficiency in man. Am J Clin Nutr 24:432, 1971

86 DEFICIENCIES OF VITAMINS A, E, AND K. HYPERVITAMINOSIS A

(Vitamin D, see Chap. 352)

THEODORE B. VAN ITALLIE

VITAMIN A History One of the first symptoms of vitamin A deficiency is inability to see in subdued light (night blindness). Treatment of the condition has been known empirically for millennia; Hippocrates recommended the use of ox liver. Over a century ago, Bitot called attention to the simultaneous occurrence of night blindness and lesions of the conjunctiva. At the turn of the century, Mori suggested that ocular lesions seen in Japanese children might be related to a lack of fat in the diet. Early in the twentieth century, two groups of investigators in the United States recognized that a fat-soluble factor was essential for growth, survival, and the prevention of xerophthalmia in rats. In 1924, Bloch reported that xerophthalmia in Danish children could be prevented by feeding them butterfat or cod-liver oil. Somewhat later, the provitamin A status of β-carotene and certain other carotenoids was established. The chemical structures of β-carotene and vitamin A were described in 1930 and 1931, respectively.

The internationally adopted nomenclature for compounds with vitamin A activity is used in this chapter, as follows: *retinol* denotes vitamin A alcohol; *retinyl ester* is vitamin A ester; *retinal* is vitamin A aldehyde, and *retinoic acid* signifies vitamin A acid. The Food and Nutrition Board of the National Research Council–National Academy of Sciences has recommended that vitamin A activity in foods be expressed as the equivalent weight of retinol rather than the traditional units. In terms of international units, 1 retinol equivalent is equal to 3.33 IU retinol or 10 β-carotene. (See Laboratory Findings below.)

Prevalence Today, the areas of greatest prevalence of endemic vitamin A deficiency are found in Indonesia, India, Indochina, Central America, the Middle East, and the Philippines. Vitamin A deficiency is the principal cause of blindness in the world, and yet this occurs mostly in tropical areas where the carotenoids that would prevent it are plentiful. Clinically significant vitamin A deficiency is most likely to develop in young children, and the blindness in adults attributed to vitamin A deficiency usually has its origin in childhood. The real need is to educate mothers to change feeding practices which limit intake by children of foods containing vitamin A activity.

Pathogenesis At least two forms of vitamin A alcohol are known (A_1 or retinol and A_2 or 3-dehydroretinol), together with the acid and aldehyde derivatives, retinoic acid and retinal. The vitamins A are intimately related to provitamins, the carotenes, and certain other pigmented compounds. Of these, only dietary β-carotene is of any real significance as a provitamin A. A part of ingested carotene is absorbed by the cells of the intestinal mucosa and transformed into vitamin A. Bile is important in this process. Vitamin A is usually present as retinyl ester in foods; it is hydrolyzed in the intestinal tract and absorbed as retinol. Within the cells of the intestinal mucosa, retinol is esterified, usually by palmitic acid, and carried in chylomicrons via the thoracic duct to the liver, where it is stored. As needed, retinyl ester is hydrolyzed to the alcohol and transported to the tissues attached to retinol binding protein (RBP), an alpha$_1$-globulin which, in turn, is bound to prealbumin. Retinal is found in the retina and is important in the visual process. The interrelations between alcohol, acid, and ester forms of vitamin A have been greatly clarified. Undoubtedly, there is more than one "active form" of vitamin A. In the eye it is 11-*cis*-retinal, but in support of growth, tissue differentiation, and glycopeptide synthesis, retinoic acid is effective. Since retinoic acid does not substitute for retinal in the eye and biologically cannot be reduced to either the alcohol or the acid, there must be at least two "active forms." Moreover, retinoic acid does not substitute for retinal or retinol in the reproductive system.

The greatest concentration of vitamin A in humans is found in the liver. Appreciable concentrations are also present in the kidneys, adrenals, lungs, and the retina. Fat depots contain a small amount of the vitamin.

Vitamin A deficiency may result from dietary insufficiency of this vitamin or its precursors or because of some process which interferes with its absorption from the intestinal tract, transport, or storage in the liver. Obstruction of the biliary tract or pancreatic ducts in children or adults may lead to diminished absorption of vitamin A. Diarrhea and the various types of malabsorption syndromes, when severe, may be accompanied by vitamin A deficiency. Of particular importance is the interrelation of vitamin A and protein nutrition, since retinol is transported by a specific protein (RBP) which appears to be synthesized in the liver. RBP-retinol complex is further bound to prealbumin which also is thought to be synthesized in the liver. Therefore, protein deficiency may decrease synthesis of these two transport proteins and may possibly alter the activity of the hydrolyzing enzymes necessary for release of retinol from its ester form prior to binding by transport proteins. The low serum vitamin A levels in kwashiorkor may largely reflect a functional impairment in the hepatic release of vitamin A. Small amounts of retinyl ester and carotenoids are present and travel with beta-lipoproteins.

The intricate reactions whereby vitamin A enters the visual process are summarized in Fig. 86-1. Retinal is the prosthetic group of photosensitive pigment in both rods *(rhodopsin)* and cones *(iodopsin)*. All-*trans*-retinol is oxidized to all-*trans*-retinal; this compound isomerizes in the dark to the 11-*cis* form which, combined with *opsin*, forms *rhodopsin*. After absorbing light, the 11-*cis* isomer of retinal is converted back to the corresponding all-*trans* form. Energy to operate this reaction is supplied by light, and the energy exchange stimulates impulses which travel via the optic nerve to the brain.

Pathology The tissues chiefly affected are epithelial in nature, principally those which ordinarily are not keratinized. These include the lining epithelium of the upper and lower respiratory passages, genitourinary tract, eye and paraocular glands, salivary glands, accessory glands of the tongue and buccal cavity, and pancreas. The fundamental change is thought to be metaplasia of the normal nonkeratinized lining cells into a keratinizing type of epithelium. Altered glycoprotein synthesis is associated with the loss of

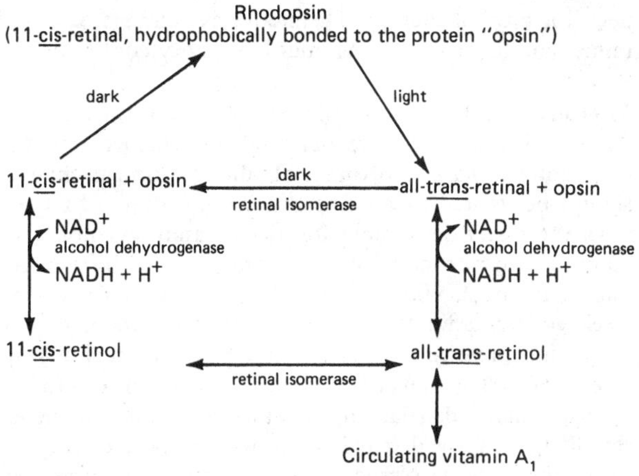

FIGURE 86-1
The reactions whereby vitamin A enters the visual process.

mucous cells. The cornea becomes dry, wrinkled, and hazy owing to intrinsic changes as well as to lack of tears as a result of obstruction of the ducts. The ciliated epithelium of the respiratory tract is replaced by a keratinizing lining so that the important mechanical effects of the cilia are lost. However, the basal cells in all areas retain their potentiality for reverting to normal if their supply of vitamin A is restored.

How vitamin A maintains the integrity of epithelial structures remains a mystery. Vitamin A appears to be implicated in the metabolism of intracellular structures, the lysosomes, in glycoprotein synthesis and in mucopolysaccharide metabolism, and in steroid hormone formation.

Clinical findings The term *xerophthalmia* is used here in an inclusive sense to refer to certain structural abnormalities of the eye resulting from vitamin A deficiency. The lesions usually exhibit a definite sequence of stages in development. The initial change, which is called *xerosis (xerosis epithelialis conjunctivae),* consists of dryness and opacity of the bulbar conjunctiva. Secretion of tears is decreased. At the lateral margin of the cornea a triangular-shaped accumulation of sticky secretion may appear which projects onto the conjunctiva but not over the cornea. This is the Bitot spot, which resembles a plaque or pseudomembrane filled with bubbles (Fig. 86-2). While not pathognomonic, this lesion is highly suggestive of vitamin A deficiency. As the photograph indicates, the Bitot spot has the appearance of a fleck of meringue. This material is difficult to scrape off. Fine pigmentation may also be present throughout the conjunctiva. These alterations are either accompanied or soon followed by haziness and dryness of the cornea *(xerosis corneae).* The tarsal glands along the eyelid frequently are enlarged. Photophobia may be marked. The most serious consequence is the appearance of small, epithelial erosions on the cornea. These soon become infected and enlarged. If this ulceration continues, destruction of the cornea *(keratomalacia)* occurs, a process that may be extremely rapid. Thus a child with conjunctivitis and photophobia may open his eyes one morning to reveal the lens extruded, the bulb collapsed, and vision irrevocably lost (Fig. 86-3). Short of this, the cornea may heal but with a scar that greatly limits vision. In general, the severity of the eye lesions and the rapidity with which they occur are inversely proportional to age.

As already noted, *night blindness* is an early consequence of vitamin A deficiency. Two other terms, *nyctalopia* and *hemeralopia,* have been used to refer to this condition. *Nyctalopia* means an inability to see in subdued light. *Hemeralopia* refers to a decrease in vision that follows exposure to bright light. Defective ability to see in subdued light may be established by certain tests; however, these are difficult to perform under routine conditions and are particularly unsuited for children. The technique of electroretinography can be used to assess nyctalopia objectively in children as well as adults. Vitamin A deficiency is only one cause of night blindness, however; indeed, in the United States and other technically advanced countries diseases involving pigmentary degeneration of the retina remain the principal cause of nyctalopia.

FIGURE 86-2
Bitot's spots showing the characteristic meringue texture. (Courtesy of DS McLaren and the American Journal of Clinical Nutrition*)*

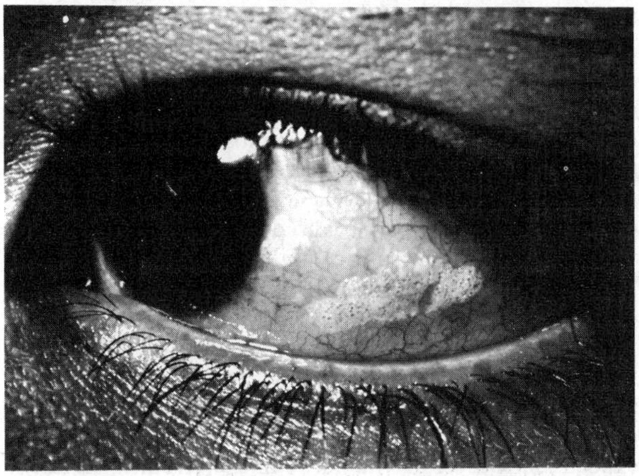

FIGURE 86-3
Destruction of the eye by colliquative necrosis of the cornea. The lens is about to drop out. (Courtesy of DS McLaren)

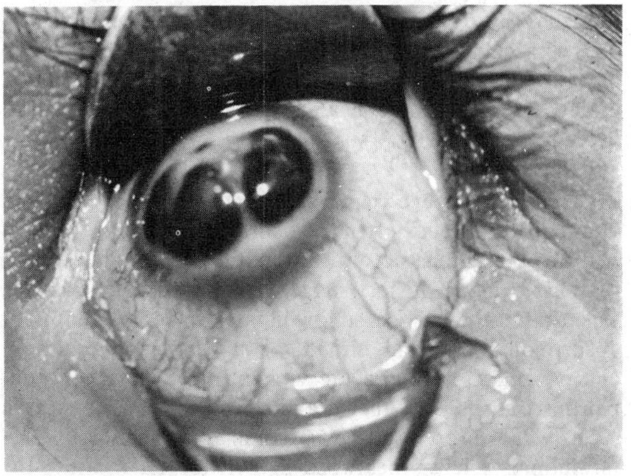

The nonocular manifestations of vitamin A deficiency frequently are obscured by signs of general malnutrition or the presence of some conditioning disturbance, such as chronic obstruction of the pancreatic or biliary ducts, which may lead to poor absorption of the vitamin. Follicular hyperkeratosis often is found in association with vitamin A deficiency. Keratinization of the hair follicles and atrophy of the sebaceous glands result in the formation of dry papules with protruding cornified plugs. Characteristically, the lesions appear on the buttocks and on the extensor aspects of the legs and arms. Other cutaneous changes include dryness (xerosis) of the skin and acne. It must be emphasized that none of these skin manifestations is specific for vitamin A deficiency. Tracheitis, bronchitis, and pneumonia are complications sometimes associated with severe vitamin A deficiency.

Laboratory findings Laboratory values for vitamin A in serum or plasma are expressed in micrograms per 100 ml or, less commonly, in international units (IU) per 100 ml. One IU is equivalent to 0.3 μg vitamin A or 0.6 μg β-carotene. Serum values for vitamin A and carotene are usually considered to be normal if over 20 and 40 μg per 100 ml, respectively. When values for vitamin A and carotene fall to 10 and 20 μg per 100 ml, respectively, the deficient state is probably present. Vitamin A concentrations lower than 10 μg per 100 ml are diagnostic, but only if acute febrile illness, protein malnutrition, and liver disease have been ruled out. Carotene values may be misleading since the usual laboratory procedure nonspecifically measures all carotenoids and some interfering pigments. Also, carotene values tend to reflect the immediate dietary intake and do not necessarily parallel vitamin A status. Serum vitamin A levels in the range of 20 to 50 μg per 100 ml provide little information of value about vitamin A status except to indicate that the storage tissues are not totally depleted.

Valuable information on vitamin A nutriture among population groups has been obtained from postmortem analyses of liver tissue. For instance, among well-nourished groups in Canada, values averaging approximately 100 μg per g have been obtained. Liver reserves of vitamin A in persons living in economically developed countries vary widely, and there is often a lack of correspondence between liver stores of vitamin A and plasma values. In conditions such as liver disease in which synthesis of retinol binding protein is decreased, plasma vitamin A concentration may be decreased while tissue reserves remain adequate. In cirrhosis of the liver, reserves of vitamin A also may be extremely low. Cancer, chronic nephritis, and a variety of infections appear to be associated with rapid depletion of vitamin A reserves.

Diagnosis The eye changes and biochemical findings in vitamin A deficiency often are poorly correlated. Diagnosis and treatment must not wait for all the confirmatory information. A dietary history suggesting a low carotene intake, especially if the diet is also low in fat with consequent poor absorption of carotene, should be suggestive. Protein deficiency appears to aggravate vitamin A deficiency by impairing transport of the vitamin in vivo. Malabsorption states will also predispose to vitamin A deficiency.

Vitamin A levels below 20 μg per 100 ml indicate the need for prompt therapy. Distinctive eye changes demand immediate therapy even without laboratory confirmation.

Therapy Oral administration of 25,000 IU vitamin A daily for 1 or 2 weeks is recommended for the treatment of conjunctival changes or night blindness. Corneal changes should be treated as an emergency, and for the first few days the water-dispersible form of vitamin A should be administered intramuscularly in daily doses of 100,000 IU. Subsequently, 25,000 IU should be given orally for several weeks to build up tissue reserves. When chronic malabsorption is present, a water-miscible preparation should be given orally. The diets of children with vitamin A deficiency are usually also lacking in other nutrients and hence should be improved, particularly with respect to protein. While the integrity of specialized epithelial structures does require vitamin A, it has not been shown that high intakes of vitamin A will prevent infections.

Prognosis The outcome as far as sight is concerned depends on the degree of involvement of the ocular structures before therapy is instituted. If only clouding of the cornea has occurred, prognosis is excellent. However, if perforation and infection of the anterior chamber have taken place, restoration of sight is virtually unknown.

HYPERVITAMINOSIS A The ingestion by infants and adults of large amounts of vitamin A (doses ranging from 50,000 to more than 500,000 IU per day) results in a variety of signs and symptoms that sometimes may be extremely confusing, particularly if a history of ingestion has not been elicited. In adults, excessive amounts of the vitamin often are self-administered in the mistaken belief that such treatment can ward off respiratory infection or improve the appearance of the skin. Because preparations for young children containing vitamin A are usually highly concentrated, accidental overdosage sometimes occurs.

In infants, the effects of acute toxicity are drowsiness, vomiting, and bulging of the fontanels as a result of increased intracranial pressure. More chronic evidences of toxicity include failure to gain weight, alopecia, coarseness of hair texture, hepatomegaly, and bone pain. X-ray examination of the skeleton reveals characteristic areas of periosteal new bone formation, particularly prominent in the shafts of the long bones.

In adults, symptoms of acute hypervitaminosis A appear within 4 to 8 h following ingestion of toxic doses of the vitamin. Headache is the predominant manifestation, but blurred vision or diplopia, nausea, vomiting, vertigo, and drowsiness all may be present. In chronic hypervitaminosis A, bone pain and osseous changes similar to those occurring in children may be observed. In addition, calcification of ligaments, tendons, and subperiosteal tissues may be seen on x-ray examination. Peeling of the skin, neuritis, fissures and sores at the corners of the mouth, coarsening of the skin, alopecia, and localized areas of hyperpigmentation of the epidermis are common. Chronic ingestion of large amounts of vitamin A has been reported to result in a disorder of hepatic function resembling cirrhosis. Hypervitaminosis A also can produce psychiatric side effects that may mimic severe depression or schizophrenia. Finally, the physician should be aware that prolonged ingestion of high doses of vitamin A is potentially teratogenic. As might be expected, the level of vitamin A in the serum is elevated;

values up to 2,000 μg per 100 ml have been reported. However, plasma values of 165 μg per 100 ml and lower may accompany hypervitaminosis A. Plasma values cannot be relied upon to provide the diagnosis of either hypo- or hypervitaminosis A in every instance. Fortunately, the prognosis is good when vitamin A ingestion ceases.

Mention should be made of *carotenemia,* because it may be confused with jaundice. When large amounts of carotene-containing foods are ingested, the blood plasma may contain a high enough concentration of pigment to impart a yellowish color to the skin (especially the palms of the hands and the nasolabial folds) but not the conjunctivas (Chap. 43). *Carotenemia,* in turn, should be distinguished from *lycopenemia,* an analogous condition that results from excessive consumption of tomatoes or tomato juice.

VITAMIN E Vitamin E is the generic name for a group of closely related, naturally occurring, fat-soluble compounds, the tocopherols. Of these, α-tocopherol is biologically the most potent (1 IU = 1 mg *dl*-α-tocopherol acetate). Although they are active as antioxidants, the β, γ, and δ forms of tocopherol appear to be poorly absorbed and are often disregarded in dietary calculations. Vitamin E acts as an antioxidant in food and in animal tissues, inhibiting the peroxidation of unsaturated fatty acids and of such labile compounds as vitamin A. In the absence of vitamin E, rabbits and other herbivorous animals develop a nutritional form of muscular dystrophy, with degeneration and diffuse fibrosis of muscle fibers, deposition of ceroid in smooth muscle, and creatinuria. Rodents appear to require vitamin E for normal reproduction, while vitamin E-deficient chicks develop an exudative diathesis and encephalomalacia. Monkeys rendered vitamin E-deficient exhibit a megaloblastic anemia which is reversed by α-tocopherol treatment. Certain synthetic antioxidants can replace α-tocopherol in preventing reproductive failure in rats, while selenium can substitute in part for vitamin E to prevent some of the manifestations of muscular dystrophy. Thus, it remains unclear whether vitamin E has any specific function beyond its role as a lipid antioxidant.

Erythrocytes from tocopherol-deficient laboratory animals and human subjects exhibit an increased in vitro susceptibility to hemolysis induced by dilute hydrogen peroxide, and this test has been used for the clinical examination of vitamin E status. However, the hemolytic response to peroxide is not specific since it depends not only on the serum tocopherol concentration but on other variables, including the content of peroxidizable lipid in the erythrocyte membrane. Abnormal peroxide hemolysis usually does not occur when the serum tocopherol level exceeds 0.5 mg per 100 ml.

Infants are born with low serum levels of tocopherol and appear to be especially susceptible to vitamin E deficiency, particularly if they are fed diets relatively high in unsaturated vegetable oils that are unsupplemented with tocopherols. The vitamin E-deficiency syndrome that has been observed in premature infants is characterized principally by edema, anemia, thrombocytosis, and an erythematous papular eruption of the skin which is followed by desquamation. Children with cystic fibrosis and other forms of severe, chronic steatorrhea have been reported to have low serum levels of tocopherol, muscular lesions resembling those in experimentally induced nutritional muscular dystrophy, increased serum creatine phosphokinase (CPK) activity, and creatinuria that is reversed by administration of α-tocopherol.

Clinically manifest vitamin E deficiency is extremely rare in adults; however, clinical studies have demonstrated that when the diet contains a high content of polyunsaturated fatty acids, more dietary vitamin E is needed to maintain a "normal" serum tocopherol concentration (usual range 0.6 to 1.4 mg per 100 ml) and a normal erythrocyte life span. Fortunately, most unsaturated margarines, shortenings, and salad oils also contain appreciable quantities of tocopherols, and the apparent absence of vitamin E deficiency in the general population suggests that the quantity of vitamin E in the United States diet is adequate. The recommended dietary allowance for adults is 12 to 15 IU per day.

A regrettable disparity exists between the wishful expectations of many individuals concerning the supposed health benefits of vitamin E and the existence of supporting experimental data. Reliable evidence is lacking that supplementary vitamin E, in whatever dose, can favorably affect physical endurance, cardiac status, potency, fertility, or longevity in individuals with normal serum levels of α-tocopherol.

VITAMIN K Vitamin K occurs in nature in at least two major forms: vitamin K_1 *(phylloquinone)* which is present in most edible vegetables, particularly in green leaves, and vitamin K_2 which is produced by intestinal bacteria. All the many compounds with vitamin K activity are structurally related to the simpler compound, 2-methyl-1,4-naphthoquinone *(menadione).* Menadione may be formed in the gut by the action of intestinal bacteria on vitamins K_1 and K_2. After absorption, menadione is converted in the body to the active *menaquinone.* Vitamin K is required by humans and other animals to maintain prothrombin and clotting factors VII, IX, X, and possibly V. The vitamin appears to act at the ribosomal level, combining with a regulatory protein to control prothrombin synthesis.

Under ordinary circumstances, adequate amounts of vitamin K (judged to be about 0.03 g per kg for adults) are available from the diet and from intestinal bacteria that synthesize the vitamin. Because the naturally occurring forms of vitamin K are fat-soluble and are poorly stored in the body, a conditioned deficiency can occur in association with diseases that interfere with fat absorption. In addition, long-term treatment with certain antimicrobial drugs may temporarily eliminate intestinal bacteria as a vitamin K source. The coumarin anticoagulant drugs appear to induce hypoprothrombinemia by dissociating vitamin K from its regulatory protein. Atypical responses to treatment with coumarin drugs have been attributed to variations in dietary intake of vitamin K or, rarely, to a genetically determined resistance to their anticoagulant action.

Newborn infants tend to be deficient in vitamin K, exhibiting low plasma levels of several coagulation factors in the prothrombin complex. Such deficiencies result from minimal stores of vitamin K at birth, lack of an established intestinal flora, and a very limited dietary intake of the vitamin. The higher concentration of vitamin K in cow's milk (60 μg per liter) as compared with human milk (15 μg per liter) would seem to explain the greater incidence in the past of neonatal hemorrhage among breast-fed infants. Evidence has accumulated that the routine administration of vitamin K to neonates decreases the incidence of hemorrhage. Thus, all newborn infants should receive vitamin K prophylactically. A single intramuscular dose of 0.5 to 1.0 mg of the water-miscible form of vitamin K_1 should suffice for this purpose. Menadione and its water-soluble derivatives have been known to induce kernicterus in premature infants when given in relatively high doses (in excess of 5 mg). This toxic effect has been attributed to increased hemolysis and inhibition of glucuronide formation. Because vitamin K_1 is free of these side effects, its use is clearly preferable during pregnancy and for the neonate. Vitamin K_1 also is more effective than other vitamin K-active compounds in the treatment of coumarin overdosage.

REFERENCES

HASSAN H et al: Syndrome in premature infants associated with low plasma vitamin E levels and high polyunsaturated fatty acid diet. Am J Clin Nutr 19:147, 1966

OOMEN HAPC: Vitamin A deficiency, xerophthalmia and blindness. Nutr Rev 32:161, 1974

RUSSELL RM et al: Hepatic injury from chronic hypervitaminosis A resulting in portal hypertension and ascites. N Engl J Med 291:435, 1974

SMITH FR, LINDENBAUM J: Human serum retinol transport in malabsorption. Am J Clin Nutr 27:700, 1974

Supplementation of Human Diets with Vitamin E. Food and Nutrition Board, National Research Council–National Academy of Sciences, 1973

SUTTIE JW: Vitamin K and prothrombin synthesis. Nutr Rev 31: 105, 1973

87
DISTURBANCES IN TRACE ELEMENT METABOLISM

DAVID D. ULMER

Inorganic ions are crucial to virtually all biochemical and physiologic processes. Some, present in tissues only in minute quantity, micrograms to picograms per gram of wet organ, are arbitrarily designated *trace elements.* Of these, iron, iodine, copper, manganese, molybdenum, selenium, chromium, fluorine, silicon, nickel, zinc, tin, and vanadium are now thought to be essential for animal life.

The functions of trace elements have been defined at levels of biological complexity ranging from isolated enzymes to intact animals. Thus, many metals participate in enzymic catalysis through substrate binding, activation of the enzyme-substrate complex, or by formation of a tight coordination complex with the enzyme such that the two are isolated together as a unit, i.e., *metalloenzyme.* Critical biological functions in animals are disrupted by deprivation of essential metals resulting in discrete deficiency states. Toxic manifestations owing to grossly excessive exposure to metals are also well recognized. The biological effects of metals, both essential and toxic, are often conditioned by *metal-ion antagonism;* i.e., one metal induces a biological effect by altering the requirement for another, usually through competition for the same biochemical sites. As a consequence, such metal-ion *imbalances* are likely among the most common and certainly the most elusive sources of either metal-deficiency or intoxication states. This phenomenon complicates investigative efforts and helps to account for the fact that proved manifestations of trace-element deficiency in human beings, except for those due to iron and iodine, are rare despite extensive documentation of deficiency syndromes in many animal species. Indeed, evidence that tin, vanadium, fluorine, silicon, and nickel may be essential to animal life has been obtained only during the past 5 years.

ZINC The average adult human body contains 1.4 to 2.3 g zinc; highest concentrations are found in liver, voluntary muscle, bone, prostate, and eye. The minimum daily requirement (about 15 mg) is easily attained in most diets since the element is widely distributed in food, particularly meat, shellfish, liver, gelatin, bread, cereals, lentils, peas, beans, and rice. However, *phytic acid* in the diet binds zinc tightly, limits its absorption, and operates as a conditioning factor to induce zinc deficiency. Zinc has been shown to be crucial to growth and development of numerous species. It is an essential component of many enzymes in the liver, pancreas, and other organs, and its importance for protein synthesis may be surmised from recent evidence that both DNA and RNA polymerases are zinc metalloenzymes. While marked changes in the zinc content of tissues, blood, and urine accompany many different human diseases, the relationship of such alterations to the underlying conditions are, for the most part, poorly understood. Experimental zinc deficiency in primates results in retarded growth, loss of hair, and parakeratosis of the tongue. Spontaneous zinc deficiency in animals is also manifested by gonadal atrophy, dermatitis, and diarrhea. A probable human counterpart to animal zinc deficiency has been observed in individuals living in Iran and Egypt and subsisting on diets consisting largely of bread and beans and nearly devoid of animal protein. The victims exhibit short stature owing to retarded growth, testicular atrophy with hypogonadism, and geophagia, and have decreased zinc concentrations in plasma, red blood cells, and hair; they improve after oral supplementation with zinc for several months. Correction of concomitant iron deficiency may also play a role in improvement.

A beneficial action of zinc in repair and healing processes has long been postulated and reexamined in recent years, stimulated by reports of the effectiveness of the metal in promoting healing of surgical wounds and chronic ulcers. The data from numerous studies now appear to indicate that wound-healing is delayed in patients with zinc deficiency and is restored to normal by oral administration of zinc. However, controlled studies suggest that zinc has no effect upon wound-healing in normal persons.

The identification of liver alcohol dehydrogenase as a zinc metalloenzyme generated investigations which showed that patients with severe alcoholic cirrhosis exhibit marked abnormalities in zinc metabolism. However, the therapeutic significance of these observations remains uncertain.

Zinc toxicity may result from excessive ingestion of the

element in food or drink, although the margin of safety is large. Nausea, vomiting, colic, and diarrhea are predominant manifestations. Toxicity also results from inhalation of high concentrations of zinc oxide fumes, leading to *metal-fume fever* or *brass chills.* Once a fairly common industrial hazard, this self-limited, acute illness is accompanied by fever, shaking chills, excessive salivation, headache, cough, malaise, and pronounced leukocytosis.

COPPER Copper is an essential nutrient for animals and is critical to such diverse activities as heme synthesis, connective tissue metabolism, bone development, and nerve function. Experimental copper deficiency is manifested by severe anemia and decreased concentrations of plasma copper and the serum copper protein, *ceruloplasmin (ferroxidase).* Ceruloplasmin catalyzes oxidation of ferrous to ferric ions and is postulated to control the rate of iron uptake by transferrin—hence, availability to reticulocytes of iron from heme synthesis. Copper is also a component of a number of other critical metalloenzymes, e.g., cytochrome oxidase, lysine oxidase, polyphenol oxidases, amine oxidases, and the cupreins—cuprozinc proteins in liver, red cells, and brain which appear to function as superoxide dismutases and may also serve in quenching highly reactive singlet oxygen in cells. Copper is important to mitochondrial function and is found frequently as a component of ribonucleic acid.

The copper concentration in adult human beings averages 1.5 to 2.5 μg per g fat-free tissue; the metal concentrates in liver, heart, brain, kidneys, and hair; for example, to 18 to 45 μg per g dry weight in liver. Balance is maintained on an average intake of 2 to 5 mg copper daily, obtained readily from meats, particularly liver and kidney, shellfish, raisins, whole-grain cereals, dried legumes, and nuts. Bile constitutes a major route of excretion.

Elevated concentrations of copper in serum are observed in a large number of acute and chronic diseases and appear to be a manifestation of response to stress. Hypocupremia is a more specific finding and is associated primarily with hepatolenticular degeneration (Wilson's disease), certain dysproteinemias of infancy, the nephrotic syndrome (secondary to renal loss of copper proteins), intestinal malabsorption, and kwashiorkor. Acute poisoning owing to ingestion of metallic copper manifests as nausea, vomiting, hematemesis, and melena, and may be accompanied by centrilobular liver necrosis. Rapid absorption of copper sulfate through the skin, as employed for therapy of burns, or through use of copper-containing dialysis equipment, has resulted in acute hemolytic anemia. Increased copper accumulation is observed in Wilson's disease (Chap. 110), primary biliary cirrhosis (Chap. 301), and prolonged extrahepatic biliary tract obstruction (Chap. 305).

Frank copper deficiency is rare in human beings, but has been reported in severely malnourished infants and in adults receiving prolonged intravenous hyperalimentation. Anemia, leukopenia, and neutropenia are observed, and the bone marrow is megaloblastoid, contains increased sideroblasts, and shows a predominance of early granulocytes and cytoplasmic vacuolization of erythroid and myeloid elements (maturation arrest). The hematologic abnormalities are reversed by oral copper therapy.

An abnormality in copper transport by intestinal cells has been described in *Menkes' kinky hair disease,* a rare X-chromosome-linked inherited syndrome manifested by cerebral and arterial degeneration, hypothermia, hair changes, and bony lesions.

COBALT Although cobalt deficiency occurs in ruminants, the physiologic significance of cobalt to most other animals and humans is limited to its participation in reactions of vitamin B_{12}, of which it is a component (Chap. 310). Acute cobalt poisoning in humans is manifested by nausea, vomiting, diarrhea, tinnitus, and loss of hearing, while chronic administration of cobalt induces polycythemia and, by blocking iodine uptake, may produce goiter, especially in children. During the last decade, cobalt added to beer as an antifoaming agent produced several localized epidemics of an extraordinary cardiomyopathy, often accompanied by pericardial effusion, frequently with fatal outcome.

SELENIUM Selenium deficiency has not yet been verified in humans; however, in animals deficiency results in liver necrosis, striking pallor, and degeneration of skeletal muscle, *white-muscle disease,* occasionally involving the heart. It has been recognized for many years that these alterations resemble certain of the manifestations of vitamin E deficiency in animals and can be ameliorated by dietary supplementation with sulfur-containing amino acids. The nature of these interrelationships has been partially clarified recently by findings that selenium is a component of glutathione peroxidase in red blood cells and likely other tissues. Hence, selenium, like vitamin E, appears to help protect against damage from complex intracellular peroxides.

MANGANESE Manganese activates a host of critical intracellular enzymes; among these, mitochondrial pyruvate carboxylase has recently been identified as a manganese metalloenzyme. The metal appears to play a role in such important metabolic functions as oxidative phosphorylation, fatty acid metabolism, and the synthesis of proteins, mucopolysaccharides, and cholesterol. Experimental manganese deficiency has been described in animals, but not as yet in humans.

NICKEL Nickel has been found to be firmly bound to RNA from several tissues and may act to stabilize nucleic acid structure. The metal is also postulated to play a general role in the maintenance of membrane structure and function. A nickel-containing α-2-macroglobulin, nickeloplasmin, has been isolated from both human and rabbit serum, but its significance is uncertain at present. Nickel carbonyl, formed from nickel and carbon monoxide, is exceedingly dangerous and produces severe lung inflammation and liver necrosis. Chronic excess industrial exposure to nickel is associated with an increased incidence of lung and nasal carcinoma.

SILICON (and silica) Silicon is a component of many mucopolysaccharides and may contribute to connective tissue structure by bridging polysaccharide chains or linking polysaccharides to proteins. Inhalation of fine particles of free crystalline silica (SiO_2) produces a pulmonary inflammatory response, granuloma formation, and chronic fibrosis (silicosis).

FLUORINE In pharmacologic doses, fluorine exerts anticariogenic effects, promotes stabilization of newly synthesized bone matrix, and inhibits bone resorption, providing a rationale for its use in treatment of osteoporosis. Chronic ingestion of fluorides in moderate amounts produces mottling of dental enamel (fluorosis); in larger amounts, e.g., from ingestion of insect poisons, fluorides cause nausea, vomiting, abdominal pain, diarrhea, and tetany often resulting in death from cardiovascular collapse.

CHROMIUM Chromium, in the form of a low molecular weight organic complex, *glucose tolerance factor,* present in brewer's yeast, animal meats, and grains, is required for normal glucose metabolism in several animal species. The ability of mammals to synthesize glucose tolerance factor appears to be limited, and, in humans, marginal chromium deficiency may possibly accompany protein-caloric malnutrition, pregnancy, and old age. While diabetics often exhibit altered chromium metabolism, the precise relation of this metal to diabetes remains uncertain.

REFERENCES

HOESTRA WG et al (eds): *Trace Element Metabolism in Animals.* Baltimore: University Park Press, 1974

LOURIA DG et al: The human toxicity of certain trace elements. Ann Intern Med 76:307, 1972

NELDNER KH, HAMBRIDGE KM: Zinc therapy of acrodermatitis enteropathica. N Engl J Med 17:879, 1975

SCHWARTZ K: Recent dietary trace element research, exemplified by tin, fluorine, and silicon. Fed Proc 33:1748, 1974

ULMER DD: Metals—from privation to pollution. Fed Proc 32:1958, 1973

VILTER RW et al: Manifestations of copper deficiency in a patient with systemic sclerosis on intravenous hyperalimentation. N Engl J Med 291:188, 1974

section 2 | Hormonal disorders

88
GENERAL CONSIDERATIONS AND MAJOR SYNDROMES

GEORGE W. THORN

INTRODUCTION It is now generally agreed that hormones do not initiate new events in the complicated biochemistry of metabolic processes, but rather produce their effects by regulating enzymatic and other chemical reactions already present. In view of the relatively large number of hormones, their diverse chemical structures, and their multiple sites of action, it may be assumed that scarcely a single important metabolic event can escape the effect of their primary or secondary action. From this, one may conclude that a true understanding of any disease process or physiologic disorder must encompass an appreciation of the possible etiologic role of hormones and the factors regulating their synthesis, release, and degradation. In this regard, one may point to such widely diverse actions as the effect of catecholamines (adrenal medulla) on brain metabolism and psychologic behavior; the effect of adrenal steroids on the inflammatory reaction associated with infection, trauma, surgery, or burns; the effect of insulin on adipose tissue metabolism; and the importance of growth hormone on the fabrication of body proteins.

In this edition, the chapter on diseases of parathyroid function has been moved from the endocrinology section to a later section in which is presented a coordinated discussion on calcium and bone metabolism and diseases involving abnormalities in parathyroid function, vitamin D, and calcitonin (see Chaps. 352 to 357).

MECHANISMS OF ENDOCRINOPATHIES Characteristically, endocrine abnormalities arise as a consequence of increased or decreased hormone secretion. In the majority of patients, the clinical manifestations derive from an excess of or deficiency of the *normally* secreted hormone. However, in certain syndromes, such as some cases of adrenal virilism, the endocrinopathy may result from secretion of an abnormal hormone. In addition, hormonal disorders may result from aberrations in the metabolism or degradation of hormones. For example, a deficiency of plasma proteins may decrease the quantity of hormone-carrying protein in the blood and hence modify significantly the balance between "free" and "bound" thyroid hormone; liver disease may alter the conjugation or degradation of steroid hormones, giving rise to abnormal blood and tissue hormone levels. In such types of abnormalities, however, serious endocrine disorders will result only if the "servo-regulating" mechanism, or feedback response, fails to stimulate the appropriate reaction in the trophic gland. Endocrine abnormalities may also develop when local tissues are unable to respond to normal hormonal level. For example, localized myxedema over the tibia may occur in the presence of thyrotoxicosis or euthyroidism; in cases of pseudohypoparathyroidism, the abnormalities observed in hypoparathyroidism occur despite the presence of normal parathyroid glands. In some endocrinopathies, heightened tissue susceptibility to hormone action is the determining factor in the genesis of the syndrome, e.g., hirsutism in young women with a minimal abnormality in androgenic steroid secretion, or extreme degrees of hyperpigmentation observed in patients with early adrenal insufficiency and increased melanin pigmentation on a racial basis.

Hormonal secretions in general show wide fluctuations

throughout the 24-h period, times of high activity often alternating with times of reduced secretion; e.g., in the early morning the level of adrenal cortical secretory activity is high. Evidence is accumulating that endocrinopathy may result from a loss of cyclic diurnal pattern due to a more or less constant hormonal elaboration throughout the day and night, resulting in only a slight increase, if any, in total secretion. Two important considerations have been derived from these observations: (1) Interpretation of single determinations of hormone content—of blood, tissues, or urine—reflecting instantaneous or relatively short collection periods may be unreliable; for final evaluation, repeated determinations, longer collection periods, or isotopic "turnover" studies may be required. (2) Clinical application of the cyclic method of hormone administration has been quite successful in minimizing undesirable hormone side effects while maintaining control of the underlying disease process.

DIAGNOSTIC APPROACH TO ENDOCRINE ABNORMALITIES The suspicion that an endocrine abnormality may play a role in a patient's illness will often derive initially from the gross physical appearance of the patient, as in myxedema, hyperthyroidism, pituitary dwarfism or gigantism, acromegaly, hypogonadism, carotenemia (diabetes mellitus or hypothyroidism), Addison's disease, Cushing's syndrome, and the adrenogenital syndrome. Although a careful history and physical examination will in most instances provide presumptive evidence of an underlying endocrine disorder, the definitive diagnosis will almost invariably depend upon the values obtained from laboratory examinations. Here, accuracy in diagnosis depends upon the specificity of the laboratory test, its precision and its reproducibility, the care and understanding with which specimens are collected, and the reliability of the laboratory that carries out the procedures. It is essential to realize, however, that a single determination of a specific hormone (in blood, urine, or tissue) does not necessarily establish or exclude an endocrine abnormality. The addition of hormonal "turnover" or "secretory" measurements by means of isotopic techniques represents a great step forward. The use of stressful situations or specific substances such as ACTH (adrenocorticotropin) for the adrenal, thyroid-stimulating hormone (TSH) for the thyroid, and glucose for the detection of early diabetes permits one to test the functional reserve of these endocrine systems and thereby facilitates the diagnosis of potential endocrine deficiency at a time when prophylactic measures may prove effective. In the evaluation of endocrine disorders associated with excessive secretion, suppressive-type tests are of greatest value; in deficiency states stimulatory tests often yield the most information. In the succeeding chapters, particular attention will be devoted to indicating the usefulness and limitations of diagnostic methods and the degree of specificity attached to the procedure. Because of its great practical importance, the source of common errors related to these determinations will also be emphasized.

ENDOCRINE SYNDROMES Although secretions of the endocrine glands govern widespread metabolic activities throughout the body, from the viewpoint of the internist, major endocrine disorders present over and over again as a relatively limited number of syndromes. These will be reviewed briefly in relation to the cardinal manifestations of disease.

Weakness and increased fatigability (see also Chaps. 15 and 16) These are without doubt the most frequent presenting symptoms of adult patients seeking assistance from the internist or general practitioner. Although in the majority of instances these complaints derive primarily from emotional or psychologic disturbances, underlying organic disease must always be considered. When endocrine abnormalities are suspected, one should inquire first whether the symptoms have been accompanied by *weight loss*—if so, adrenal cortical insufficiency, hyperthyroidism, and diabetes mellitus should be considered. Adrenal cortical insufficiency, if present, should be accompanied by some increase in pigmentation, hypotension, gastrointestinal disturbances, and perhaps salt craving. Hyperthyroidism would be suggested by goiter, eye changes, tremor, intolerance for heat, etc., and diabetes mellitus by polyuria and polydipsia.

Without weight loss, but with symptoms of weakness and fatigability, one would consider hypothyroidism, hypopituitarism, hyperparathyroidism, and hyperaldosteronism. The first of these is characteristically associated with delayed reflexes, intolerance to cold, dry skin, and carotenemia. Hypopituitarism is suggested by oligomenorrhea or amenorrhea in the female, impotence in the male, decreased tolerance to cold, hypoglycemic episodes, and hypotension. Hyperparathyroidism is suggested by the association of bone pain, renal calculi, and polyuria. Hyperaldosteronism might be accompanied by significant hypertension, demonstrable muscular weakness, polyuria, and electrocardiographic changes that suggest potassium depletion.

Menstrual irregularities (see also Chaps. 50 and 99) In addition to pregnancy and local disease of the uterus, menstrual irregularities are associated with four major endocrine disturbances: (1) *primary ovarian failure,* prior to natural menopause and characterized by hot flashes, gain in weight, increased emotional instability, and elevated urinary values of follicle-stimulating hormone, for example, polycystic disease of the ovaries or the Stein-Leventhal syndrome; (2) *secondary ovarian failure,* associated with reduced or absent urinary gonadotropins and evidence of other target gland deficiencies, i.e., thyroid and adrenal; (3) *hypothyroidism,* in which menorrhagia as well as oligomenorrhea frequently occurs; (4) *adrenogenital syndrome,* in which oligomenorrhea or amenorrhea is seen in combination with increased muscular development, hirsutism, and other signs of masculinization. *A history of use or discontinuance of "the pill" should always be investigated as a cause of menstrual irregularity.*

Hirsutism (see also Chap. 59) Increased body hair in females and decreased scalp hair in both sexes is a frequent disorder for which patients seek medical attention. Unfortunately, most female patients with increased hair do not have a demonstrable excess of adrenal or ovarian androgens. Increased androgenic secretion should be considered when *hirsutism* is associated with menstrual irregularities and amenorrhea, or with other evidence of virilism, i.e., increased muscular development and increased size of clitoris.

Although loss of scalp hair and baldness is almost never due to a specific endocrinopathy, a receding hair line in female patients associated with *increased* body hair should always suggest excessive androgenic hormone secretion of adrenal or gonadal origin. Thinning of the hair is frequent in patients with Cushing's syndrome, hypothyroidism, or hypopituitarism. It is rare, however, to observe disturbances in hair growth as a manifestation of serious endocrine abnormality in the absence of rather well-defined signs and symptoms of adrenal, pituitary, or gonadal dysfunction.

Impotence and decreased libido (see also Chap. 51) Although these cardinal manifestations of functional disorder are a frequent basis for medical consultation, they are rarely due primarily to endocrinopathies. In addition to primary disease of the generative organs, however, *anterior pituitary deficiency,* especially associated with chromophobe adenomas, should be considered. Evidence of local tumor (changes in vision, headache, etc.) and associated target gland deficiencies (adrenal, thyroid, and gonadal) should be sought. Patients with diabetes mellitus will often exhibit both impotence and decreased libido, but in most instances this occurs after the disease has been present for some time. Patients whose impotence is caused by serious organic disease are less likely to have this as their primary complaint, in contrast to those in whom impotence is a primary manifestation of emotional or psychologic difficulty.

Obesity (see also Chap. 46) Obesity suggests the possibility of an underlying endocrine disturbance, which in practice rarely is causative. However, two serious disorders must be considered in patients with marked, generalized obesity. The first is diabetes mellitus, and this should be investigated with a postprandial glucose determination and a glucose tolerance test, if fasting blood glucose levels are within the normal range and if sugar is not present in the urine. The second serious disorder is insulinoma. Hunger, increased appetite, and weight gain are characteristic of patients with insulinoma as well as of those with "reactive" hypoglycemia. The former experience the greatest degree of hunger and symptoms after prolonged fast, the latter shortly after eating, particularly after a meal of high carbohydrate content. In both instances appetite and food intake are stimulated by absolute or relative hypoglycemia, and the vicious cycle is continued.

Hypothyroidism and mild hypopituitarism may be associated with moderate obesity. The final diagnosis of the former will require laboratory tests of thyroid functions; the latter requires tests for the adequacy of target gland function.

Gross obesity in Cushing's syndrome is rare—what is more common is loss of adipose tissue in the extremities with an increase in abdominal fat pad, striae, and "buffalo hump."

There is no doubt that castration or ovarian failure predisposes to obesity. However, in young women there often occurs a reversal of this cycle; namely, rapid weight gain secondary to excess food intake, stress, and anxieties, which may be *followed* by oligomenorrhea or amenorrhea. Whether the weight gain itself is of primary importance in the genesis of the ovarian dysfunction, or whether weight gain and altered gonadal function are both secondary to changes in the hypothalamic centers is not known. However, it is well established that improvement in emotional status and with weight loss, normal ovulation and menstruation will often ensue.

Gynecomastia and galactorrhea Gynecomastia occurs physiologically in normal males at puberty and may persist through adolescence. Gynecomastia should always raise the suspicion of seminiferous tubule dysgenesis with fibrosis, a variant of Klinefelter's syndrome. Marked degrees of breast development in adolescent males or the onset of gynecomastia in later life may indicate the presence of an estrogen-secreting tumor of the adrenal gland. Choriogenic tumors and more rarely interstitial cell and granulosa cell tumors of the testes may also produce gynecomastia, as can the ectopic secretion of follicle-stimulating hormone (FSH) by a bronchogenic tumor. It regularly follows estrogen therapy in the treatment of carcinoma of the prostate, cirrhosis of the liver, and malnutrition; a variety of drugs, including spironolactone, are nonendocrine causes of the syndrome.

Galactorrhea, or abnormal lactation, is sometimes observed in patients with acromegaly or chromophobe adenomas of the pituitary gland. A condition associated with persistent post-partum lactation and amenorrhea is referred to as the Chiari-Frommel syndrome. In these disorders galactorrhea is very likely related to increased prolactin secretion. Lactation may also be induced by hypothalamic suppression with catecholamine-depleting or -blocking drugs such as reserpine, the phenothiazines, and methyldopa.

Hypertension (see also Chaps. 93, 94, and 250) Hypertension is another frequent disorder that should suggest an underlying endocrine abnormality. The hypertensive patient with minimal abnormalities in urinary constituents but with polyuria and nocturia suggests hypokalemia (hyperaldosteronism) or hypercalcemia (hyperparathyroidism). Clinically the hypokalemic patient with *hyperaldosteronism* rarely presents with the malignant form of hypertension and characteristically exhibits neuromuscular weakness. The electrocardiogram will often reveal changes consistent with potassium depletion, whereas serum sodium concentration is usually *elevated.* The problem is to exclude hypokalemia induced by diuretic administration, especially the thiazides, and the ensuing secondary hyperaldosteronism.

Patients with hypertension, polyuria, and hypercalcemia associated with *hyperparathyroidism* will frequently give a history of urinary calculi or bone pain. They may also present the stigmas of psychoneurosis as a consequence of sustained hypercalcemia. Band keratopathy is rare except with long-continued elevated serum calcium level.

Two characteristic findings in patients with hypertension secondary to *pheochromocytoma* are the cyclic nature of hypertension in the classic syndrome and the absence of obesity. Unfortunately, most tumors secrete predominantly norepinephrine; hence, the textbook picture of tachycardia, nervousness, sweating, and glucosuria is infrequent.

Hypertension and moderate obesity, particularly of the truncal type, suggest *Cushing's syndrome.* This possibility is greatly increased if diabetes mellitus, easy bruisability, and pink abdominal striae are present. Every hypertensive patient with diabetes mellitus should be screened for adrenal overactivity.

Hypertension as an early manifestation of diabetes mellitus is uncommon. However, since hypertensive-vascular disease is such a frequent complication of diabetes mellitus, hypertensive patients—especially those who are obese—should have postprandial blood glucose determined and glucose tolerance test performed.

Hypertension as a manifestation of *adrenogenital syndrome* should be considered in young subjects with associated evidence of virilism.

Polyuria and polydipsia Polydipsia and polyuria should always suggest the possibility of diabetes mellitus and diabetes insipidus. The syndrome can also ensue as a result of severe hypokalemia (primary hyperaldosteronism, Cushing's syndrome, and excessive diuretic therapy) or hypercalcemia (hyperparathyroidism and vitamin D intoxication). "Psychogenic" diabetes insipidus and primary renal disease enter the differential diagnosis.

Abnormalities in growth (see also Chaps. 90 and 92) Abnormalities in growth, particularly in children, are associated with *hyposomatotropism, gonadal dysfunction, hypothyroidism,* and *cretinism.* The latter must be detected within the first few weeks after birth if serious damage to the central nervous system is to be prevented. All babies with *persistent* umbilical hernia should be screened for possible *hypothyroidism.* Untreated diabetes mellitus will result in retarded growth, as will excess cortisol and androgen secretion. Long-standing renal disease will impair skeletal growth and mimic an endocrinopathy because of the frequent coexistence of secondary hyperparathyroidism.

Closely related to abnormalities in growth among adolescent boys is the problem of *undescended testes.* A conservative approach is urged, and the reader is referred to Chap. 98 for details as to the management of this important problem.

Additional manifestations Also suggesting possible endocrine abnormalities are the following signs:

1 Changes in the skin (see also Chaps. 57 to 59). Dryness in hypothyroidism and Addison's disease; thin, atrophic skin with "wrinkles" in pituitary and gonadal failure; easy bruisability in Cushing's syndrome; moist, fine, warm skin in hyperthyroidism; coarse, reduplicated skin in acromegaly; hyperpigmentation in Addison's disease.

2 Arthropathies are not infrequent in acromegaly, gigantism, myxedema, and primary gonadal failure.

3 Tetany and convulsive seizures (see Chap. 24) may indicate hypoglycemia (insulinoma, reactive hypoglycemia, Addison's disease, hypopituitarism), hypocalcemia (hypoparathyroidism), or hypokalemia (hyperaldosteronism, Cushing's syndrome).

4 The presence of edema (see Chap. 32) should suggest hypothyroidism or myxedema as well as secondary hyperaldosteronism and Cushing's syndrome.

5 Psychologic abnormalities (see Chap. 14) are frequently observed in Addison's disease and Cushing's syndrome as well as in hypopituitarism, hypothyroidism, hyperthyroidism, hyperparathyroidism, and acromegaly.

IATROGENIC ENDOCRINOPATHIES With the widespread use of corticosteroids, thyroid, and sex hormones as nonspecific therapeutic agents, new and difficult problems present themselves to the internist and endocrinologist. One may be faced with iatrogenic Cushing's syndrome, hyperthyroidism, or virilism—or severe adrenal insufficiency or hypothyroidism if specific hormone therapy is discontinued rapidly or completely. Special problems relating to these phenomena will, because of their seriousness, be discussed at length in relation to each of the specific hormones so implicated. The use of hormones as nonspecific therapeutic agents, while offering great promise in many serious and often fatal diseases, is fraught with difficulties and requires in addition to a thorough knowledge of the endocrine preparations a comprehension of their physiologic and pharmacologic effects.

89 HYPOTHALAMUS AND RELEASING HORMONES

JOSEPH B. MARTIN

That the hypothalamus is involved in the regulation of the pituitary gland has been recognized since the turn of the century. The mechanism of this control, particularly in the case of the anterior pituitary, resisted precise definition until very recently. It is now known that such control is exerted by a class of specialized neurons called *neurosecretory cells,* the cell bodies of which reside in the basal hypothalamus. Neurosecretory cells function both as neurons and as hormone-secreting cells. Stimulation of the neurosecretory cell results in release of its hormonal product directly into the blood to circulate to the appropriate target site. The neurosecretory cell thus functions as the final link in neuroendocrine control in much the same manner as the anterior horn cell of the spinal cord serves as the final pathway for control of voluntary skeletal muscle.

The classic example of the neurosecretory cell is the hypothalamic supraoptic or paraventricular neuron. The posterior pituitary or *neurohypophysis* develops embryologically as an evagination from the hypothalamus. Axons of the supraoptic and paraventricular cells traverse the pituitary stalk to terminate in the neurohypophysis in direct contact with blood vessels. Depolarization of the cell and its terminal axon results in release of vasopressin (ADH) and oxytocin into the systemic bloodstream. Because of their large size, these neurosecretory cells are called *magnocellular* neurons (Fig. 89-1).

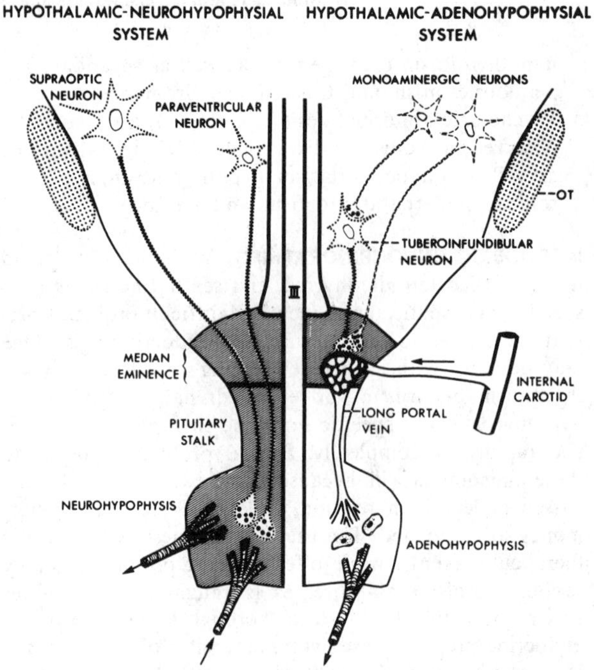

FIGURE 89-1
Diagram of the hypothalamic-pituitary axis. Indicated on the left is the hypothalamic-neurohypophyseal system consisting of supraoptic and paraventricular neurons, axons of which terminate on blood vessels in the posterior pituitary (neurohypophysis). The hypothalamic-adenohypophyseal system is illustrated on the right. Tuberoinfundibular neurons, believed to be the source of the hypothalamic regulatory hormones, terminate on the capillary plexus in the median eminence. The pituitary portal system is derived from branches of the internal carotid which forms a primary capillary bed in the median eminence. The long portal veins drain the capillary plexus into the sinusoids of the anterior pituitary (adenohypophysis). Supraoptic, paraventricular, and tuberoinfundibular neurons are all classed as neurosecretory cells. *The activity of tuberoinfundibular neurons is influenced by monoaminergic cells.*

The anterior lobe of the pituitary or *adenohypophysis* is derived embryologically from the epithelial lining of the primitive mouth cavity and has no direct innervation from the brain. Regulation of the adenohypophysis is achieved by a group of small (*parvicellular* or *tuberoinfundibular*) hypothalamic neurons located around the inferior margin of the third ventricle. The fine, unmyelinated axons of these neurons form the *tuberohypophyseal* or *tuberoinfundibular* tract, which terminates upon capillaries of the pituitary portal system in the outer zone of the basal hypothalamus (Fig. 89-1). The hypothalamus in this area protrudes as the *median eminence,* which consists of the terminations of the tuberohypophyseal tract, the capillary plexus, and the emerging fibers of the supraoptic and paraventricular-hypophyseal tracts. The capillary plexus of the median eminence is formed by branches of the superior hypophyseal arteries which arise directly from the internal carotid artery. Tuberoinfundibular neurons are believed to synthesize, transport, and release small-molecular-weight peptides (hypothalamic regulatory factors or hormones) which enter the capillary bed of the median eminence to be carried to the adenohypophysis via the pituitary portal veins.

The adenohypophysis is the source of seven major hormones: thyroid-stimulating hormone (TSH), adrenocorticotropin (ACTH), prolactin, growth hormone (GH), and the gonadotropins, luteinizing hormone (LH), and follicle-stimulating hormone (FSH); melanocyte-stimulating hormone (MSH) in humans is also produced by the adenohypophysis rather than the intermediate lobe as occurs in lower animals.

From a functional standpoint, therefore, regulation of anterior pituitary hormone secretion is dependent entirely upon the release from the hypothalamus of the hypothalamic regulatory hormones. It is postulated that each anterior pituitary hormone is controlled by an appropriate hypothalamic hormone. Three of these substances, thyrotropin-releasing hormone (TRH), luteinizing-hormone-releasing hormone (LHRH), and somatostatin (growth-hormone-release-inhibiting hormone), have been identified and synthesized. These developments have resulted in a rapid extension of knowledge of neuroendocrine control in human beings and in the emergence of new concepts concerning endocrine disease.

PRINCIPLES OF NEUROENDOCRINE REGULATION

NEUROENDOCRINE REFLEXES Homeostasis and adaptation of the organism to its environment require continual monitoring of the internal and external milieu. In the case of endocrine regulation, it can be shown that certain of these responses occur in a classic reflex fashion. Assumption of an upright posture, for example, triggers ADH release via a baroreceptor reflex that is relayed to the hypothalamus through the brainstem. ADH is released into the blood to stimulate the kidney to preserve water, thereby increasing blood volume. Similar reflex release of anterior pituitary hormones can also be demonstrated. Suckling of the breast stimulates nerve endings which establish an afferent volley of nerve impulses that ascend via the spinal cord and brainstem to the hypothalamus. Release of hypothalamic prolactin-releasing factor activates the pituitary to secrete prolactin which circulates back to the breast to stimulate milk production and secretion. These are examples of neuroendocrine reflexes; the afferent limb consists of a neural pathway, the efferent limb of a hormonal secretion. Abnormalities of release of pituitary hormones may occur as a result of interruption or alteration in such reflex mechanisms.

EPISODIC HORMONE SECRETION AND EFFECTS OF SLEEP Frequent measurements of serum hormone levels throughout the day and night have shown that all anterior pituitary hormones are released in an episodic or pulsatile pattern. Experimental studies have shown that the pulses of secretion are dependent upon hypothalamic influences presumably mediated by intermittent release of the hypothalamic regulatory hormones.

Significant changes in hormone secretion occur during normal sleep. There is a prominent burst of GH secretion during the first 2 h of night sleep, associated with slow-wave sleep. This surge of GH may account for up to 60 percent of the total 24-h secretion of GH during the adolescent period of maximal growth. Other anterior pituitary hormones, such as prolactin, ACTH, and TSH, are secreted in greater amounts during the latter stages of night sleep; the rise in ACTH during this time accounts for the diurnal variation in pituitary-adrenal function. The onset of puberty has recently been shown to be associated with a significant nighttime rise in serum LH levels; it has been suggested that this is the earliest harbinger of puberty.

Activation of pituitary secretion can also result from neural stimuli arising in higher brain centers. Acute stress, either physical or emotional, in addition to its stimulatory effects on ACTH secretion, also elicits a rise in serum prolactin and GH levels. Chronic or recurrent stress may result in severe aberrations of endocrine function. Emotional or maternal deprivation in the young child may cause GH deficiency accompanied by growth failure, a condition that is rapidly reversible by placing the child in a compassionate environment. Stress in the adolescent or young woman may cause transient or prolonged amenorrhea. These various disturbances in endocrine function result from aberrations in neural control of adenohypophyseal secretion.

FEEDBACK CONTROL Neurosecretory neurons of the hypothalamus are not regulated only by neural inputs. The hypothalamus and possibly other regions of the brain are responsive to feedback effects of circulating hormones such as thyroxine, cortisol, testosterone, estrogen, and progesterone. These effects, which include both negative and positive regulatory influences, act to determine the level of hypothalamic activity. Circulating hormones also act at the pituitary level to determine pituitary sensitivity to hypothalamic hormones.

HYPOTHALAMIC REGULATORY HORMONES

THYROTROPIN-RELEASING HORMONE The first hypothalamic hormone to be identified was TRH, so-named because of its potent effects on TSH release. TRH, a tripeptide of molecular weight 362 (Fig. 89-2*A*), is extraordinarily potent. It is estimated that one molecule of the peptide can stimulate release of over 100,000 molecules of TSH. There is a rapid, measurable rise in serum TSH within 2 to 5 min after intravenous injection of TRH, with the peak of the response occurring at 30 to 45 min (Fig. 89-3*A*).

The regulation of TSH secretion is achieved by an interaction between the stimulatory effects of TRH and the negative feedback effects of thyroid hormones. This interaction occurs predominantly at the level of the anterior pituitary. Elevation in circulating thyroid hormone levels, as in thyrotoxicosis, results in pituitary resistance to TRH (Fig. 89-3*B*). Conversely, in hypothyroidism, pituitary responsiveness to TRH is enhanced.

FIGURE 89-2

Structural formulas of the known hypothalamic regulatory hormones. A *Thyrotropin-releasing hormone, TRH.* B *Luteinizing-hormone-releasing hormone, LHRH. This is also termed gonadotropin-releasing hormone, GNRH.* C *Somatostatin, GRIH.*

A pyroGlu-His-Pro amide

B pyroGlu-His-Trp-Ser-Tyr-Gly-Leu-Arg-Pro-Gly amide

C

H-Ala-Gly-Cys-Lys-Asn-Phe-Phe-Trp-Lys-Thr-Phe-Thr-Ser-Cys-OH

To the surprise of most investigators, TRH has also been shown to be equally potent in causing prolactin release. TRH normally has no effect on the release of ACTH, LH, FSH, or GH. However, patients with active acromegaly and some subjects with renal failure show a marked release of GH after administration of TRH.

LUTEINIZING-HORMONE-RELEASING-HORMONE (LHRH) The identification of a hypothalamic peptide with LH-releasing activity was accomplished in 1971. This substance, which consists of 10 amino acids (Fig. 89-2*B*), is also effective in causing FSH release, and current evidence indicates that only one hypothalamic factor is essential for regulation of the gonadotropins. As a result of this dual action, the peptide is increasingly referred to as *gonadotropin-releasing hormone* (GNRH). The peptide is effective in releasing gonadotropins in both men and women. The normal variations in LH and FSH secretion that are the hallmark of the menstrual cycle are attributed to changing feedback effects of the ovarian steroids (estrogen and progesterone) on the hypothalamus and pituitary. Estrogen and progesterone influence the sensitivity of the hypothalamus and pituitary by both positive and negative feedback effects which act both to regulate the release of LHRH and to determine the sensitivity of the pituitary to LHRH. Thus, changes in FSH and LH secretion in the female during the menstrual cycle are brought about by both cyclicity of hypothalamic LHRH release mechanisms and by changes in pituitary responsivity to LHRH.

The effects of LHRH appear to be quite specific for gonadotropin release. Administration to normal subjects has no effect on GH, TSH, prolactin, or ACTH.

SOMATOSTATIN (GROWTH-HORMONE-RELEASE-INHIBITING HORMONE: GRIH) Regulation of GH is achieved by a dual hypothalamic control system consisting of both a releasing factor and an inhibitory factor (Fig. 89-4). The dominant hypothalamic influence is stimulatory since hypothalamic lesions often cause growth failure and loss of normal GH release to various stimuli. In attempting to isolate growth-hormone-releasing factor (GRF), Guillemin and associates were repeatedly impressed by the presence in hypothalamic extracts of potent GH-release-inhibiting activity. They successfully identified this peptide and named it *somatostatin.* It contains 14 amino acids connected by a disulfide bridge (Fig. 89-2*C*). This peptide has been shown to inhibit physiologic GH secretion in humans (such as occurs during sleep) as well as pathologic GH secretion as occurs in acromegaly. In addition to its potent effects on inhibition of GH release, somatostatin also blocks TRH-stimulated TSH release (without affecting TRH-induced prolactin release) and has direct suppressive effects on pancreatic insulin and glucagon secretion. This latter unexpected effect has resulted in the suggestion that somatostatin may be potentially useful in the management of diabetics who manifest excessive glucagon secretion (see Chap. 97). Somatostatin also suppresses gastrin secretion in normal subjects and in patients with gastrin-secreting tumors.

OTHER HYPOTHALAMIC REGULATORY FACTORS The structures of the other hypothalamic regulatory factors, CRF (corticotropin-releasing factor), GRF (growth-hormone-releasing factor), and PIF (prolactin-inhibiting factor), have not been identified. There is also evidence for a PRF (prolactin-releasing factor) separate from TRH. Evidence for the existence of these factors is convincing, and very likely each is a polypeptide. One exception to this generalization is the recent finding that dopamine may function directly at a pituitary level to inhibit prolactin release. MSH, like GH and prolactin, is regulated by both a releasing and an inhibiting hypothalamic factor.

EXTRAHYPOTHALAMIC DISTRIBUTION OF REGULATORY HORMONES TRH, LHRH, and somatostatin have all been shown to be present in significant concentrations in brain regions outside the hypothalamus. Each hormone has also been found in the cerebrospinal fluid. Somatostatin has recently been shown to be present in the gut and pancreas. These findings suggest that these peptides may serve important biologic functions in addition to those associated with anterior pituitary control.

FUNCTION OF MONOAMINES IN NEUROENDOCRINE CONTROL

The hypothalamus contains large concentrations of norepinephrine, dopamine, and serotonin. It is estimated that 10 to 15 percent of hypothalamic tuberoinfundibular neurons contain dopamine, which is concentrated in nerve terminals in the median eminence adjacent to other nerve fibers

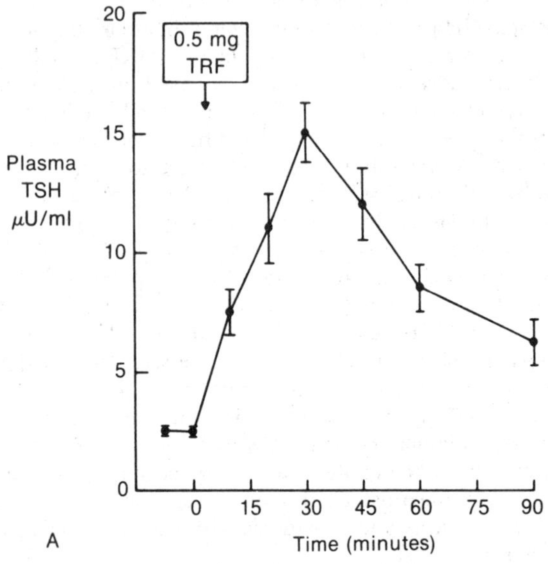

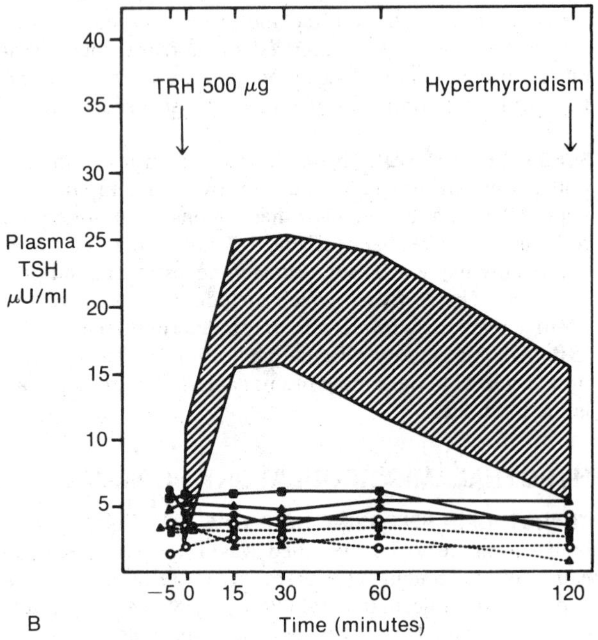

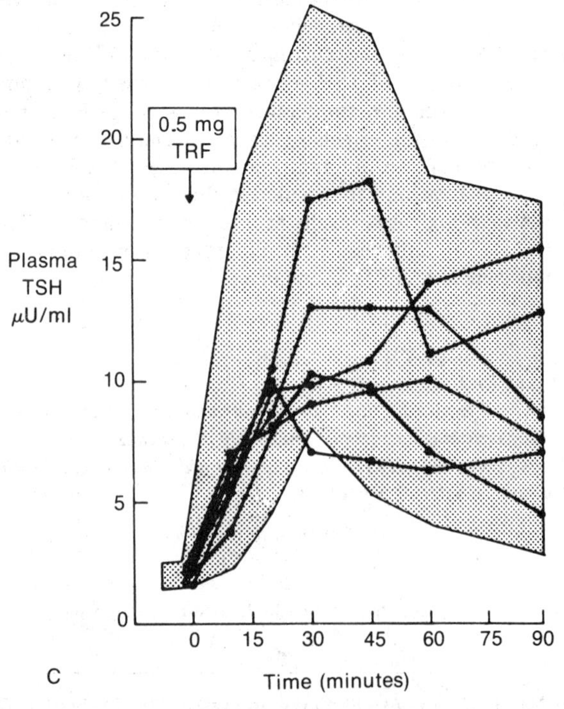

FIGURE 89-3
A *Plasma TSH response to intravenous TRH in 21 normal subjects. An increase in TSH occurs within 10 min. (From Fleischer et al with permission)* B *Plasma TSH responses to TRH in patients with hyperthyroidism. TRH fails to elicit a rise in TSH. The stippled area represents the range of values seen in controls. (From C Gual et al, Administration of synthetic thyrotropin releasing hormone (TRH) as a clinical test for pituitary thyrotropin reserve. Rev Invest Clin 24:35, 1972)* C *Plasma TSH response to TRH in patients with idiopathic panhypopituitarism or isolated TSH deficiency. Base-line TSH levels before TRH are low, but normal TSH responses occur after TRH. (From Fleischer et al with permission)*

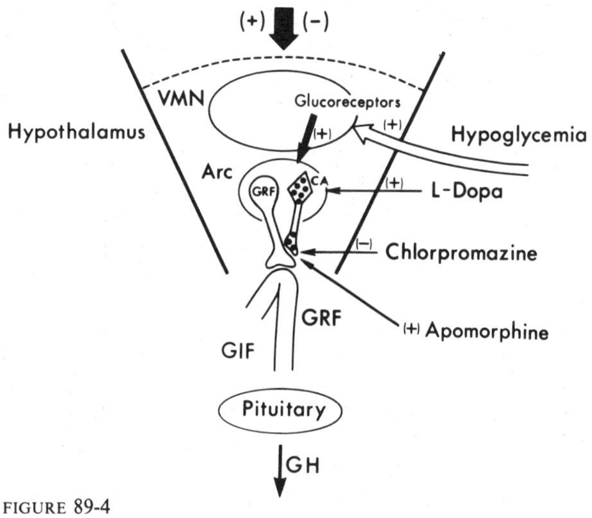

FIGURE 89-4

Hypothetical schematic of hypothalamic GH control to illustrate pharmacologic stimuli that affect GH release. Pituitary GH secretion is regulated by a GH-inhibiting factor (somatostatin) and a GH-releasing factor (GRF). Hypoglycemia induces GH secretion by stimulation of hypothalamic glucoreceptors. L*-dopa triggers GH secretion by increasing substrate for catecholaminergic (? dopaminergic) neurons in the basal hypothalamus. These neurons activate GRF secretion. Chlorpromazine inhibits GH secretion by blocking catecholaminergic receptors. Apomorphine, a dopamine agonist, stimulates GH secretion, probably through release of GRF.*

that are presumed to contain the releasing hormones (Fig. 89-4). In addition to the hypothalamic hormones that regulate the release of GH and prolactin, it appears that catecholamines, in particular dopamine, act to regulate the secretion of GH and prolactin by effects mediated predominantly at a hypothalamic level. The administration of L-dopa, the precursor of norepinephrine and dopamine, causes stimulation of GH release and suppression of prolactin. Evidence suggests that this effect is mediated via dopamine, since apomorphine, a central dopaminergic-receptor stimulating agent also causes GH release and prolactin suppression. Chlorpromazine and other phenothiazine tranquilizers cause a rise in serum prolactin and depression in GH by virtue of their blockade of dopamine receptors. Serotonin has also been implicated in the hypothalamic control of GH and prolactin. Other pituitary hormones in humans do not appear to be affected to any degree by these monoaminergic stimuli.

It is believed that the monoamines act as neurotransmitters in monoaminergic neurons to influence tuberoinfundibular cells either by effects mediated on the cell body or on its terminal in the median eminence (see Fig. 89-1). Dopamine receptors have been identified on pituitary prolactin cells, and it is possible that dopamine suppresses prolactin by a direct pituitary effect.

Aberrations of monoaminergic control have been postulated to play a role in the pathophysiology of certain abnormal GH and prolactin secretory states. In acromegaly, for example, administration of either L-dopa or apomorphine causes a "paradoxical" suppression of GH. Excess prolactin secretion may be treated with dopaminergic agents. These observations have important therapeutic implications as described below.

ABNORMALITIES IN HYPOTHALAMIC-PITUITARY CONTROL

In general, destructive lesions of the hypothalamus or pituitary stalk cause a reduction in secretion of ACTH, TSH, LH, FSH, and GH. Such lesions often result in a rise in serum prolactin due to disruption of normal hypothalamic inhibition. The effects of such lesions on human endocrine function are variable and are not usually as severe as hormone deficiencies secondary to direct pituitary involvement. This may be due to the widespread distribution of releasing-factor neurons in the hypothalamus or possibly to continuing stimulatory effects of releasing factors which in some cases may reach the pituitary via the peripheral blood.

The earliest signs of hypothalamic dysfunction are an absence of diurnal variation in ACTH-cortisol secretion and a loss of GH release from pharmacologic stimuli such as insulin hypoglycemia or arginine. Amenorrhea due to gonadotropin failure is common in the female. TSH secretion is impaired only with massive hypothalamic lesions. Disorders of neuroendocrine function can occur in a variety of pathologic conditions which are summarized in Table 89-1.

Certain cases of pituitary hormone deficiency and of "idiopathic panhypopituitarism" are now believed to be due to hypothalamic absence or deficiency of the appropriate releasing factor.

HYPOTHALAMIC HYPOTHYROIDISM The diagnosis of hypothalamic hypothyroidism is based upon low thyroid function and undetectable TSH levels accompanied by a normal or exaggerated TSH response to exogenous TRH (Fig. 89-3*C*). Although rare, several such cases have now been reported. In most instances, the cause of the deficiency has not been discovered; in a few instances, hypothalamic lesions have been identified.

As such patients present with TSH deficiency but show a normal or exaggerated TSH response to TRH, it has been suggested that the primary pathophysiology in such cases resides in a failure to synthesize and/or release endogenous TRH. These findings indicate that a tertiary (or hypothalamic) form of hypothyroidism exists in addition to the classic primary (thyroid failure) and secondary (pituitary TSH insufficiency) types. The abnormality may be combined with other pituitary hormone deficiencies and be present from birth, suggesting that multiple congenital hypothalamic releasing factor deficiencies may occur.

HYPOTHALAMIC HYPOGONADISM Gonadotropin deficiency secondary to endogenous LHRH deficiency has also been documented. Primary or "isolated gonadotropin-deficiency" is probably usually due to endogenous LHRH deficiency. Patients with Kallmann's syndrome have an association of hypogonadism with anosmia. The majority of these patients have normal LH and FSH responses to administration of LHRH.

Gonadotropin deficiency may occur with suprasellar lesions such as craniopharyngioma or histiocytosis X, or accompany congenital hypothalamic defects. The symptomatology depends on the timing of onset of gonadotropin insufficiency. Occurrence before puberty results in a failure or delay in sexual development. Postpuberal gonadotropin deficiency results in amenorrhea, decreased libido, and atrophy of the gonads.

The term "functional," or psychogenic, amenorrhea is applied to cessation of menstruation in patients who are otherwise healthy and in whom no structural abnormality of hypothalamic-pituitary continuity can be demonstrated. The onset of the amenorrhea frequently coincides with a minor stress such as going away to school and is usually self-limiting. Administration of LHRH results in normal LH and FSH release in such cases, suggesting that the disturbance is secondary to failure of endogenous LHRH release. Female patients with anorexia nervosa frequently present with amenorrhea and often show a normal response to LHRH, indicating the likelihood of a hypothalamic disorder.

HYPOTHALAMIC DISORDERS OF GH SECRETION Idiopathic GH deficiency occurring in isolation or in combination with gonadotropin or TSH deficiency may by analogy be due to a deficit in synthesis or release of GRF. Proof of this possibility must await the identification of GRF.

Growth hormone deficiency and growth failure have been described with hypothalamic lesions due to histiocytosis X, tumors, sarcoidosis, and meningitis. Loss of GH responses to insulin hypoglycemia and L-dopa and absence of sleep-associated GH release commonly occur in such cases. Chronic amphetamine administration may suppress GH release and cause growth failure. In the maternal deprivation syndrome, growth failure and GH insufficiency are reversible with placement of the child in a normal environment.

Paradoxical GH responses, characterized by a rise rather than a fall in serum GH after glucose or by a suppression after L-dopa, have been described in patients with hypothalamic tumors and in acromegaly, malnutrition, carcinoma, Huntington's chorea, and Wilson's disease. These findings imply the existence of a disorder of monoaminergic control of GH in such diseases.

TABLE 89-1
Etiologic classification of hypothalamic–anterior pituitary disorders

CONGENITAL OR HEREDITARY
Hypothalamic hormone deficiency
Hypothalamic hypothyroidism
Hypothalamic hypogonadism
Multiple hormone deficiencies (idiopathic panhypopituitarism)
INFLAMMATORY AND INFECTIOUS
Meningitis
Sarcoidosis
Histoplasmosis X
Tuberculosis
NEOPLASTIC
Hamartoma (infundibuloma)
Teratoma
Ectopic pinealoma
Meningioma
Astrocytoma
Pituitary tumors with suprasellar extension
Adenoma
Craniopharyngioma
Metastatic tumors
Local
Meningeal carcinomatosis
Leukemic or lymphomatous infiltrates
PHYSICAL AGENTS
Stalk section
Surgical
Head injury
Postirradiation
VASCULAR LESIONS
Aneurysm—carotid
Hypothalamic infarction
Vasculitis
Lupus erythematosus
MISCELLANEOUS
Tay-Sachs disease
Acute intermittent porphyria

ABNORMALITIES OF PROLACTIN SECRETION Abnormalities of secretion of prolactin are diagnosed primarily by the appearance of nonpuerperal galactorrhea, i.e., the secretion of milk from the breast at a non-post-partum time. Although this symptom or sign remains the clinical hallmark of abnormal prolactin secretion, the availability of sensitive radioimmunoassays for prolactin has shown that prolactin secretion may be increased in both men and women without any recognizable clinical symptoms. In fact, only one in six women with elevated serum prolactin levels actually develops galactorrhea. Conversely, galactorrhea may occur with normal serum prolactin levels. Galactorrhea is frequently, although not invariably, accompanied by amenorrhea.

Nonpuerperal galactorrhea Galactorrhea may occur in a number of clinical disorders of the hypothalamic-pituitary axis. The basic pathophysiologic mechanism in each case is probably excessive prolactin secretion occurring in a patient whose breasts have been primed by the other hormones which are essential for normal lactation (adrenal corticoids, estrogens, and possibly GH).

The occurrence of post-partum galactorrhea is termed the Chiari-Frommel syndrome which is characterized by persistent lactation, amenorrhea, and gonadal atrophy after pregnancy. A second form of nonpuerperal galactorrhea is recognized in which the disorder occurs spontaneously, with or without menstrual disturbance, and often with no antecedent pregnancy. This disorder is designated the Forbes-Albright syndrome; about half of such subjects have clinical evidence of pituitary tumor, in most instances a chromophobe adenoma. Other patients with the Forbes-Albright syndrome have no clinical evidence of pituitary tumor, although it is probable that many have unrecognized microadenomas of the pituitary.

Documentation of serum prolactin levels has permitted several conclusions concerning these patients. It is now clear that the presence or absence of galactorrhea does not correlate closely with actual serum prolactin levels. Profuse galactorrhea may persist postpartum with a serum prolactin level of 20 to 50 ng per ml (normal less than 25 ng per ml). Contrariwise, pituitary tumors with levels greater than 1,000 ng per ml may not result in galactorrhea unless the breast is primed for milk secretion. Serum prolactin concentration of greater than 150 ng per ml is usually associated with a pituitary tumor.

Other causes of galactorrhea Galactorrhea may occur with any disturbance of hypothalamic-pituitary continuity; the syndrome has been reported in patients with craniopharyngioma, histiocytosis X, sarcoidosis, and other inflammatory or neoplastic disease of the infundibulum or stalk. Surgical or traumatic transection of the stalk causes elevated serum prolactin and may result in galactorrhea. Minimal galactorrhea occurs rather commonly after administration of certain drugs, many of which have in common anticatecholaminergic effects. Thus phenothiazines, alphamethyldopa, and reserpine are thought to induce excessive prolactin secretion by interference with normal hypothalamic dopaminergic inhibitory control mechanisms for prolactin. Hypothyroidism may be associated with galactorrhea and elevated serum prolactin levels. The mechanism of this effect is not entirely clear at the moment but may be due to altered sensitivity of the pituitary to the prolactin-releasing effects of TRH or to interruption of central mechanisms for regulation of PIF secretion.

In addition to disturbances of the hypothalamic-pituitary unit, galactorrhea may result from prolonged irritative lesions of the anterior chest wall, notably postthoracotomy or after herpes zoster involvement of the thoracic nerves. Even prolonged mechanical stimulation of the nipples as by suckling has been known to initiate lactation in nonpregnant or even virgin women. A foster mother may thus be enabled to suckle an adopted child.

Hyperprolactinemia with or without galactorrhea may occur in association with persistent amenorrhea after discontinuation of oral contraceptives. The mechanism of "post-pill" amenorrhea is unknown. A few of these patients have subsequently developed pituitary adenomas.

In most cases of hyperprolactinemia, prolactin secretion does not appear to be autonomous. Thus, prolactin can usually be suppressed in these subjects by L-dopa and by dopaminergic agonists such as bromergocryptine and apomorphine, and further release may be stimulated by TRH or chlorpromazine. Current clinical evidence indicates that suppression of excessive prolactin secretion by L-dopa or bromergocryptine can result in restoration of normal menstruation. These findings suggest that elevated serum prolactin levels inhibit normal ovulatory surges of LH probably by suppression of LHRH release. This is supported by the finding that the majority of such patients respond normally to administration of exogenous LHRH. The recovery of normal cyclic hypothalamic function shortly after suppression of prolactin provides dramatic evidence for this contention.

PITUITARY HYPERSECRETION—A HYPOTHALAMIC DISEASE? The identification of the role of the hypothalamus in control of anterior pituitary hormone secretion has led to the question of whether hypersecretion of anterior pituitary hormones is secondary to hypothalamic oversecretion of releasing factors. A definitive answer to this question is not presently available. Several investigators have reported that the serum of acromegalics contains increased GRF activity as measured by bioassay. A similar pathophysiology, i.e., an abnormal secretion of CRF, has been proposed in certain cases of Cushing's disease.

Refined surgical techniques, in particular transsphenoidal hypophysectomy in which the pituitary fossa is exposed inferiorly through the sphenoid sinus, have resulted in the recognition that excessive pituitary hormone secretion resulting in acromegaly (GH excess), Cushing's disease (ACTH excess), hyperthyroidism (TSH excess), Nelson's syndrome (postadrenalectomy ACTH excess), and galactorrhea (excess prolactin) may be caused by small localized "microadenomata" of the pituitary. Whether these small hypersecretory nodules arise spontaneously or secondary to hypothalamic abnormalities remains to be determined.

Pituitary tumors that secrete excessive LH or FSH are extremely rare. Precocious puberty may, however, result from injury to the hypothalamus. In males, the majority of cases of hypothalamic precocious puberty are due to demonstrable lesions in the hypothalamus, whereas, in females, structural abnormalities are rarely identified.

Diagnosis The basal secretion of most pituitary hormones is normally so low that stimulatory tests are often required to detect an abnormality in secretion. In this respect, the clinical use of the hypothalamic-releasing hormones has been of considerable value. TSH and prolactin reserve can be tested by the administration of TRH (usual dose 100 to 400 μg subcutaneously or intravenously). Administration of LHRH in a dose of 100 μg subcutaneously or intravenously gives an indication of pituitary LH and FSH reserve; the LH response is normally greater than the FSH response. Pharmacologic stimuli provide a means to test ACTH and GH release. Insulin-induced hypoglycemia is a potent stimulant for both ACTH and GH release. L-dopa is effective in stimulating GH release in approximately 80 percent of normal subjects. Physiologic GH release can often be demonstrated 60 to 90 min after onset of night sleep.

Treatment Treatment of hypothalamic-pituitary disorders is directed at the underlying cause. Pituitary tumors are increasingly being managed surgically by the transsphenoidal route, permitting direct access to the sella turcica. The use of synthetic releasing hormones for treatment of primary or secondary hypothalamic hormone failure is presently under investigation. Induction of ovulation and menstruation with subsequent pregnancy has been achieved in patients with amenorrhea after repeated administration of LHRH. Similarily, spermatogenesis has been induced in hypogonadotropic males. Somatostatin has been shown to markedly reduce GH levels in acromegaly and to reduce insulin requirements in diabetics (by suppression of glucagon). A major limiting factor in the clinical use of each synthetic hypothalamic hormone has been its short duration of action. Longer-acting analogues are currently needed for more satisfactory responses.

REFERENCES

BESSER GM, MORTIMER CH: Hypothalamic regulatory hormones: A review. J Clin Pathol 27:173, 1974

BRAZEAU P et al: A hypothalamic polypeptide that inhibits the secretion of immunoreactive pituitary growth hormone. Science 179:77, 1973

FLEISCHER N et al: Synthetic thyrotropin releasing factor as a test of pituitary thyrotropin reserve. J Clin Endocrinol Metab 34: 617, 1972

FRIESEN H: Functional evaluation of prolactin secretion: A guide to therapy. J Clin Invest 51:706, 1972

FROHMAN LA, STACHURA ME: Neuropharmacologic control of neuroendocrine function in man. Metabolism 24:211, 1975

GERICH JE et al: Effects of somatostatin on plasma glucose and glucagon levels in human diabetes mellitus. N Engl J Med 291: 544, 1974

HERSHMAN JM: Clinical application of thyrotropin-releasing hormone. N Engl J Med 290:886, 1974

MARTIN JB: Neural regulation of growth hormone secretion. Medical progress report. N Engl J Med 288:1384, 1973

YEN SSC et al: Variation of pituitary responsiveness to synthetic LRF during different phases of the menstrual cycle. J Clin Endocrinol Metab 35:931, 1972

—— et al: Effect of somatostatin in patients with acromegaly. Suppression of growth hormone, prolactin, insulin and glucose levels. N Engl J Med 290:935, 1974

ZIMMERMAN EA et al: Prolactin and growth hormone in patients with pituitary adenomas: A correlative study of hormone in tumor and plasma by immunoperoxidase technique and radioimmunoassay. J Clin Endocrinol Metab 38:577, 1974

90
DISEASES OF THE ADENOHYPOPHYSIS

DON H. NELSON

The pituitary gland lies at the base of the brain in a bony cavity, the sella turcica, within the sphenoid bone. The normal gland measures 10 by 13 by 6 mm and weighs approximately 0.6 g. Anatomically it is divided into the anterior lobe, which constitutes three-quarters of the weight of the gland, a rudimentary intermediate lobe, and a posterior neural lobe. The classic histology of the anterior lobe divides the cells into three types, depending on the presence and staining characteristics of the intracellular granules. These are the chromophobes, which are agranular, the eosinophils, and the basophils, in the proportions of approximately 52, 37, and 11 percent, respectively. More detailed studies suggest that some of the agranular cells may contain fine acidophilic and basophilic granules; hence the term "amphophils." Such a simplified description of the cells of the anterior pituitary gland does not adequately describe the secretory capacity of the various cells. One cell type can secrete more than one hormone. Chromophobe cells can be either secretory or nonsecretory. Similarly, eosinophils may produce growth hormone or prolactin. Some attempts have been made to localize specific cells which produce specific hormones by histochemical techniques.

According to classic concepts, the chromophobe cells are considered to be nonsecretory, the eosinophilic cells responsible for secretion of growth hormone (HGH, GH), luteinizing hormone (LH), and prolactin (Pr), and the basophilic cells for production of adrenocorticotropin (ACTH), thyroid-stimulating hormone (TSH), and follicle-stimulating hormone (FSH). Such a simple classification, however, does not now seem probable; some pituitary tumors associated with Cushing's syndrome have been found to be composed of chromophobe as well as eosinophilic cells, although the largest number are small basophilic tumors. Similarly, eosinophilic tumors are most often associated with increased production of growth hormone, but tumors of other cell types may occasionally be responsible.

The anterior lobe secretes a variety of peptide hormones, of which six are clearly defined. Growth hormone has a generalized somatic effect on growth; adrenocorticotropin stimulates the secretory activity of the adrenal cortex; thyroid-stimulating hormone (thyrotropin) stimulates the formation and release of thyroid hormones; follicle-stimulating hormone stimulates growth of the graafian follicle and estrogen secretion in the female and spermatogenesis in the male; luteinizing hormone initiates ovulation and luteinization of the mature follicle in the female; in the male, this hormone is the testicular interstitial cell-stimulating hormone (ICSH), responsible for male hormone secretion. Prolactin is responsible for secretion of milk by the properly developed mammary gland. It also is important in maintaining luteal secretion in the rat but does not play an important role in this function in humans. The melanocyte-stimulating hormone (MSH) is secreted by the same cells which produce corticotropin in the adenohypophysis and to a lesser extent by the neurohypophysis.

RELEASING FACTORS The isolation, identification, and synthesis of gonadotropin-releasing hormone, thyrotropin-releasing hormone (TRH), and growth-hormone-release-inhibiting hormone (somatostatin) have added a new dimension to the investigation of patients with hypothalamic pituitary disease. These small polypeptides cause release of the specific pituitary hormone but have also been found to have additional effects. TRH produces an increase in prolactin as well as TSH. It is also of interest that the gonadotropin-releasing factor is effective in releasing both LH and FSH. Other hypothalamic hormones which have been identified include corticotropin-releasing hormone (CRH) and growth hormone–releasing hormone (GRH). (See Chap. 89 for a discussion of these releasing hormones.)

PITUITARY TUMORS

Pituitary tumors account for approximately 10 percent of all intracranial tumors. By far the commonest pituitary tumor is the *chromophobe adenoma,* which is usually nonsecretory in nature. Active pituitary tumors usually secrete only one pituitary hormone in excess. Tumors secreting GH, ACTH, MSH, TSH, and Pr have all been described, although the last three types of tumor are very rare. FSH- or LH-secreting tumors are notable by their absence.

In addition to producing the *signs and symptoms* of hormone excess, discussed in later sections on the specific hormones, these tumors may compress and destroy normal pituitary tissue within the sella turcica and produce hormonal deficiency states, or they may extend out of the sella turcica to compress the optic nerves, hypothalamus, and other nervous structures in the vicinity. Pressure on the optic chiasma most often involves the decussating nerve fibers supplying the nasal retinal fields and leads to loss of the temporal fields of vision and classic bitemporal hemianopsia. Further extension of the tumor may involve one or both optic nerves and result in loss of visual acuity and even in complete blindness. These tumors may also compress the hypothalamus and result in disturbances in sleep, temperature control, appetite, and autonomic nervous functions. Curiously, these tumors are not known to damage the supraopticohypophyseal tract to a degree to cause diabetes insipidus. Involvement of the third, fourth, and sixth cranial nerves is rare but may occur. Headache is a frequent complaint in patients with this condition and has no well-defined pattern.

Clinical evaluation of these patients should include roentgenograms of the skull and visual fields, ophthalmoscopic examination, spinal fluid examination (particularly for increased protein content), and pneumoencephalography, especially in patients with severe optic nerve compression, increased intracranial pressure, or signs of hypothalamic and brain involvement. Carotid angiography may also be useful in delineating any extension of a tumor out of the sella.

Therapy of pituitary tumors generally involves a choice between pituitary irradiation and surgery. Postponement of specific treatment is justifiable in occasional patients with small, localized chromophobe adenomas, in which case specific hormonal replacement therapy should be initiated and the patient carefully observed for signs of tumor growth and extension. Surgical resection of tumor tissue is indicated when there is a rapid deterioration of vision, ventricular obstruction, or significant brain compression. Although surgery provides the greatest opportunity for arrest of tumor growth, it entails calculated morbidity and mortality rates, particularly with the large tumors extending outside the sella turcica. It is important that all patients with pituitary tumors be carefully evaluated for increased or decreased secretion of pituitary hormones. The nonsecretory tumors most commonly produce panhypopituitarism but early in their course may have demonstrable deficiency of only gonadotropins and/or TSH secretion. Those tumors producing specific pituitary hormones in excess should be diagnosed and treated as discussed in specific sections that follow.

Radiotherapy in tissue doses of 3,500 to 4,500 R is often associated with regression of the tumor and relief of local signs and symptoms. In these doses, normal pituitary tissue and surrounding nervous structures are unharmed. Some tumors recur and may require further x-ray therapy or surgery. Techniques such as cryohypophysectomy, proton-beam irradiation, and radioactive implantations have been found useful when applied by specific investigators but should still be considered experimental. Transsphenoidal microsurgery has been successful in some instances in removing well-circumscribed small tumors which are either nonsecretory or secretory of specific hormones such as ACTH or growth hormone.

Hemorrhage into a tumor, so-called "pituitary apoplexy," may result in an acute catastrophe accompanied by severe headache, blindness, hypotension or shock, fever, and signs of meningeal irritation or brain involvement. Emergency treatment is required, which may include surgical aspiration of the sella turcica, use of adrenal steroids, and other supportive measures. Pituitary apoplexy may occur spontaneously and is occasionally observed following irradiation. Although it has been suggested that irradiation may increase the incidence of this condition, there is no clear evidence that this is so.

The craniopharyngioma, which is usually suprasellar in position, is the most common type of tumor involving the pituitary gland in childhood and thus the most common cause of prepuberal hypopituitarism. The tumor represents a secretory vestige of Rathke's pouch cut off from its origin in the roof of the pharynx and carried cephalad by the migrating pituitary anlage. The viscous, cholesterol-containing fluid of such suprasellar cysts is liable to calcification, which provides a useful diagnostic sign on x-ray examination. Although these tumors are more frequent in the younger age group, occasionally they are slow-growing and may not be clinically apparent until adult life. These patients often mature normally and come to the physician with an adult form of hypopituitarism. These tumors usually require surgical intervention. *Other tumors* which may involve the pituitary or the suprasellar area include meningiomas, epidermoid or dermoid tumors, primary or metastatic carcinomas, and granulomatous disorders such as sarcoidosis, gummas, tuberculomas, and Hand-Schüller-Christian disease.

THE EMPTY SELLA SYNDROME It is common to equate enlargement of the sella turcica with an expanding intracranial lesion. At times, however, pneumoencephalography demonstrates that the sella is not occupied by a tumor mass but admits a significant amount of air (Neelon et al). Of 31 patients noted to have air within the sella, 27 were female. Headache was common, but visual field disturbances attributable to lesions of the optic chiasm were absent. The dimensions of the sella were enlarged in 26 of the 31 patients, and endocrine disturbances were noted in eight. The primary empty sella is considered a benign condition probably caused by elevation of intracranial pressure that remodels the anatomy of the sella through a congenital incompleteness of the sella diaphragm.

GROWTH HORMONE

Growth hormone, unlike the other anterior pituitary hormones, does not have a specific "target organ" but has a generalized effect on all tissues and organs. This hormone has a molecular weight of 22,000, although there is some indication that an "active core" may be considerably smaller. Though once thought to be solely concerned with growth in the early years of life, growth hormone has been found to exert significant physiologic functions throughout life. It has been shown to facilitate amino acid transport and incorporation into protein, to mobilize free fatty acids from peripheral fat stores, and to reduce lipid synthesis. Growth hormone also causes renal retention and body storage of calcium, phosphorus, sodium, potassium, and nitrogen as part of its generalized, anabolic action. It has an anti-insulin or diabetogenic action and, in large doses, can produce glucosuria, impaired glucose tolerance, and insulin resistance. Growth hormone is responsible for the elevated level of serum inorganic phosphorus and alkaline phosphatase observed in growing children.

Growth hormone is species-specific, and only primate growth hormone has been found to have significant physiologic effects in humans and to be capable of stimulating growth in pituitary dwarfs.

Plasma growth hormone levels are readily measured by radioimmunoassay, and elevated levels have been found in most patients with acromegaly. Significantly, growth hormone levels have been shown to increase following exercise, prolonged fast, and during hypoglycemia, which suggests a dynamic physiologic role for this hormone throughout life, in addition to its growth-promoting effects in childhood.

Other substances which may produce an increase in plasma growth hormone are arginine, vasopressin, pyrogens, and estrogens. The latter, because of their widespread use in contraceptive preparations, may give falsely high growth hormone values in patients suspected of having acromegaly.

Considerable evidence relates the action of growth hormone on bone to the production of a "plasma sulfation factor," which has been called "somatomedin." This substance, formed in the liver secondary to growth hormone action, has been related also to "plasma insulin-like activity" and has been shown to have antilipolytic and anabolic effects which are similar to those of insulin. Somatomedin mediates the effects of growth hormone to increase synthesis of collagen and other proteins in collagen and has also been shown to increase the synthesis of ribonucleic acids and to promote cell replication (DNA synthesis).

GROWTH HORMONE–SECRETING TUMORS Marie, in 1886, first described the classic clinical manifestations of acromegaly. One year later, Minkowski reported a case with a pituitary tumor, and Benda subsequently showed that such tumors were eosinophilic in nature. In 1895, Brissaud and Meige suggested an association between gigantism and acromegaly, and Hutchinson subsequently reported the pathologic findings in three cases of gigantism associated with pituitary tumors. Acromegaly and gigantism are now recognized as identical disturbances of growth hormone secretion, differing only in the age of onset of the disorder.

GIGANTISM Prior to puberty, excess growth hormone secretion results in a generalized overgrowth of the skeleton and soft tissues with resulting marked increases in height and size. Early in the course of the disorder, these patients are usually physically strong and alert. Later in the disease, however, pituitary insufficiency may develop, with its associated weakness and easy fatigability. Hypogonadism due to gonadotropin deficiency may develop late in the disease.

The underlying lesion is generally an *eosinophilic or mixed cell adenoma of the anterior lobe* which is usually visible radiologically. The condition, although rare, presents no difficulty in diagnosis and needs only to be differentiated clinically from the tall stature of primary gonadal failure. Persons with the latter condition exhibit the characteristic eunuchoid habitus and associated gonadal failure and, unlike the patient with gigantism, have increased titers of plasma LH characteristic of primary hypogonadism. Treatment of pituitary gigantism is similar to that for acromegaly.

ACROMEGALY In adults, the same type of pituitary tumor producing excess growth hormone results in the clinical picture of acromegaly. The disease is usually first manifested by changes in facial features and overgrowth of the head, hands, and feet which may necessitate an increase in hat, glove, or shoe size (Fig. 90-1). In other instances, headache or visual disturbances from local effects of the expanding pituitary tumor may be the first indications of the disorder.

The fully developed syndrome is easily recognized, but in the earlier stages, comparison of serial photographs over a span of years may be extremely helpful in documenting a gradual and progressive change in features. The hands and feet are broad and greatly enlarged, the ends of the digits are square (Fig. 90-2), and prognathism may be so marked as to interfere with mastication. Arthritic manifestations are not unusual, and widespread osteoarthritic-like changes in the bones and joints are often demonstrable. Patients with acromegaly are particularly subject to psychologic disturbances and almost always exhibit considerable emotional instability.

Among the associated endocrine disturbances, enlargement of the thyroid and an increased basal metabolic rate are frequently found. Hyperthyroidism, however, occurs in only a small percentage of cases. Although frank diabetes mellitus is present in only 10 to 15 percent of these patients, glucose tolerance is impaired in the majority of patients during the active phase of the disease. Diabetes mellitus, when present, is typically mild but may be rela-

FIGURE 90-1
A 44-year-old woman with arrested acromegaly. Onset of the disease occurred when patient was twenty-four years of age, when enlargement of the sella turcica was demonstrated. Following x-ray therapy of the pituitary, no further progression of the disease has been observed.

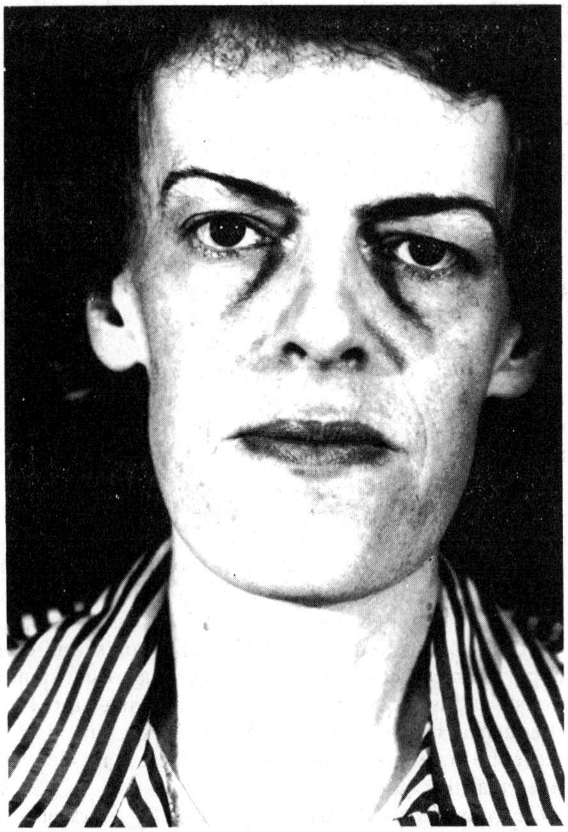

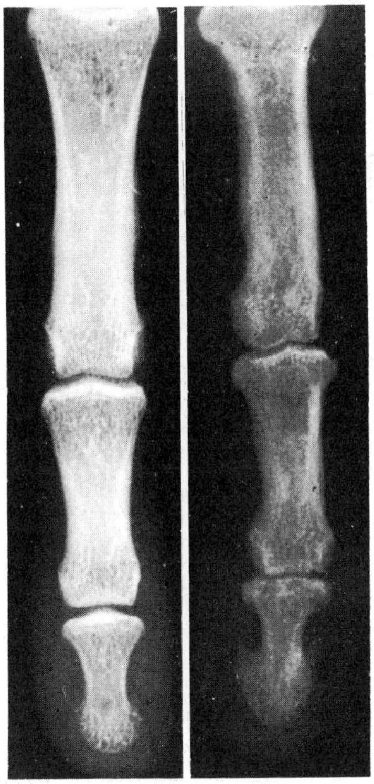

FIGURE 90-2
Characteristic tufting or "arrowhead" appearance of the terminal phalanx in acromegaly (right). Normal phalanx for comparison (left). Note also the thickness of the acromegalic finger.

tively resistant to insulin therapy. Libido may be increased at the onset but is lost subsequently, and gonadal atrophy may occur late in the disease. The course of the disease is usually one of benign chronicity, but fatal termination may occur as a result of cardiac failure, diabetic acidosis, local complications of the tumor, or unrecognized hypopituitarism.

Diagnosis Diagnosis is made by the typical changes in body configuration, possible demonstration of a pituitary tumor by x-ray or visual field defects, and most importantly, by an elevated basal plasma growth hormone level which does not decrease during a standard glucose tolerance test, although in some acromegalic patients a decrease has been seen. Because the skeletal changes are permanent, it is important in the treated as well as the untreated case to determine whether there is continual hypersecretion of growth hormone, or whether a deficiency of growth hormone and perhaps of other hormones has resulted from pituitary destruction from pressure, hemorrhage, or earlier x-ray therapy. Activity of the process is implied by continued skeletal and soft-tissue growth, by the presence of diabetes mellitus or a significantly impaired glucose tolerance test, by elevated levels of serum inorganic phosphorus and alkaline phosphatase, and by increased excretion of hydroxyproline in the urine. The basal plasma growth hormone determination is usually necessary for final determination of activity.

In the determination of levels of plasma growth hormone it is extremely important that initial samples be obtained while the patient is in a basal condition. The growth hormone level is generally less than 3 ng per ml in rested, morning, preprandial state. Moderate exercise, ingestion of a meal, or prolonged fasting will all increase levels of the hormone and thus interfere with proper evaluation. The highest levels of growth hormone are found approximately 1 h after the onset of deep sleep, but other peaks may occur during continued sleep or 2 to 4 h after meals during normal activity (Fig. 90-3). Failure of the growth hormone level to decrease with administration of a normal glucose tolerance test is suggestive that a high basal level is due to sustained secretion of excessive growth hormone not under normal control. The administration of insulin or L-dopa acts as a useful test in stimulating growth hormone secretion as is described further under hypopituitarism. Growth hormone levels may be normally elevated and resistant to suppression during starvation, renal failure, and estrogen therapy, and in patients with severe hepatic disease or diabetic ketoacidosis. A decreased responsiveness to stimulation may be seen in hypothyroidism and during the third trimester of pregnancy. Therapy with thiazines, glucocorticoids, and progesterone may also inhibit secretion of growth hormone. A 100-g glucose load will usually suppress plasma growth hormone to below 5 ng per ml.

There is one familial condition without evidence of increased growth hormone, the Touraine-Solenti-Gole syndrome, in which afflicted individuals present acromegalic features. Particularly suggestive of acromegaly in this condition are the skin changes; thus its common designation, pachydermoperiostitis (idiopathic hypertrophic osteoarthropathy). Although the fingers are often clubbed, the periosteal thickening of the bones is not what one would expect to see in acromegaly. The amount of growth hormone is of course not increased.

Treatment Eosinophilic adenomas may respond to irradiation, but in general this form of therapy is not presently considered to be so effective as an ablative procedure of the pituitary gland. The employment of transsphenoidal microsurgery to specifically remove the hypersecreting adenoma appears promising, but more conventional surgery may be required if the tumor is large and particularly if it extends outside the limits of the sella turcica. The presence of hypopituitarism must be suspected and the appropriate substitution therapy instituted (adrenal, thyroid, and gonadal hormones), particularly if surgery is contemplated. Because of the permanent disfigurement which acromegaly produces, the progress of the disease must be watched closely, particularly in women, and earlier surgical intervention should be considered in an attempt to minimize the cosmetic complications. Although successful therapy will not reverse the bony changes, the decrease in hypertrophy of the skin and subcutaneous tissues may produce an important improvement in appearance.

ADRENOCORTICOTROPIN (ACTH)

This hormone is a polypeptide composed of 39 amino acids with a molecular weight of approximately 4,500. The primary structure has been elucidated, and small quantities have been synthesized (Fig. 90-4).

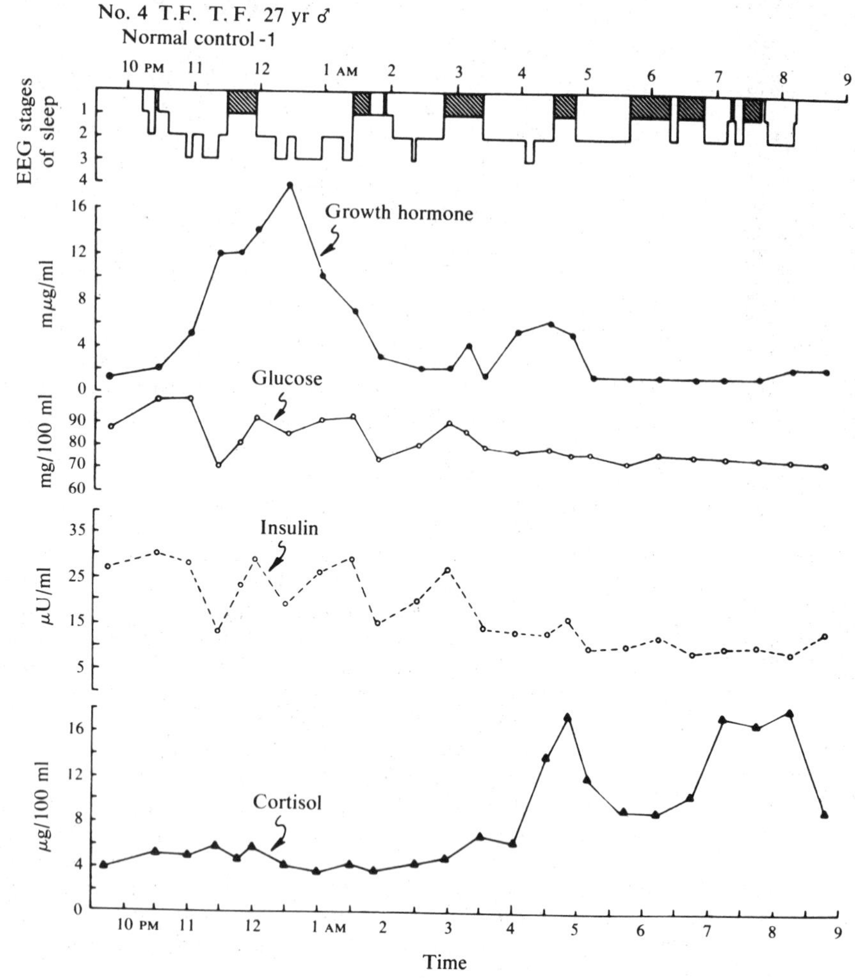

FIGURE 90-3
Plasma growth hormone, glucose, insulin, and cortisol measured simultaneously in a 27-year-old man. Levels of sleep are indicated at the top of the figure with periods of rapid eye movement shown by crosshatched areas. The increase in growth hormone which is characteristic of early sleep and the elevations in plasma cortisol seen in the early morning hours are illustrated. (From Y Takahashi et al, J Clin Invest 47:2079, 1968)

FIGURE 90-4
Amino acid sequences of corticotropin and melanocyte-stimulating hormones. (Modified from I Harris, Nature 184:167, 1959)

Corticotropin
1 2 3 4 5 6 7 8 9 10 11 12 13 39
H—Ser. Tyr. Ser. Met. Glu. His. Phe. Arg. Try. Gly. Lys. Pro. Val.- - - Phe.—OH

α-MSH (pig)
1 2 3 4 5 6 7 8 9 10 11 12 13
CH_3CO-Ser. Tyr. Ser. Met. Glu. His. Phe. Arg. Try. Gly. Lys. Pro. Val.—NH_2

β-MSH (pig)
1 2 3 4 5 6 7 8 9 10 11 12 13 14 15 16 17 18
H—Asp. Glu. Gly. Pro. Tyr. Lys. Met. Glu. His. Phe. Arg. Try. Gly. Ser. Pro. Pro. Lys. Asp.—OH

β-MSH (human)
1 2 3 4 5 6 7 8 9 10 11 12 13 14 15 16 17 18 19 20 21 22
H—Ala. Glu. Lys. Lys. Asp. Glu. Gly. Pro. Tyr. Arg. Met. Glu. His. Phe. Arg. Try. Gly. Ser. Pro. Pro. Lys. Asp.—OH

The principal physiologic effect of this hormone is to stimulate the secretion of hydrocortisone from the adrenal cortex. Under the stimulus of ACTH, the adrenal gland also secretes corticosterone, aldosterone, estrogens, and certain so-called "adrenal androgens." In the case of aldosterone, ACTH is not the chief controlling factor regulating its secretion. As part of its adrenal-stimulating effect, ACTH promotes an increase in adrenal blood flow and hypertrophy of the gland. Certain extraadrenal actions of ACTH of obscure physiologic significance include a lipid-mobilizing effect and a hypoglycemic action. ACTH has intrinsic melanocyte-stimulating activity because of similarities between its *N*-terminal amino acid sequence and the structure of MSH (Fig. 90-4).

Secretion of ACTH is regulated by the concentration of hydrocortisone in plasma and by various parts of the brain, particularly the anterior median eminence of the hypothalamus. Nerve cells in this area are thought to produce one or more peptide neurohormones, termed *corticotropin-releasing hormones* (CRH), which are released into the pituitary portal circulation and stimulate the secretion of ACTH by the anterior pituitary cells. Higher centers of the brain may act to stimulate or inhibit ACTH secretion. It is likely that the effect of corticosteroids to suppress ACTH is directly upon the pituitary gland, whereas the stimulating effect of hypoglycemia, hypoxia, or "stress" acts through the hypothalamus and release of CRH.

Central nervous system activity maintains a diurnal rhythm of ACTH secretion, which results in highest levels in early morning and lowest levels at night. In addition to this diurnal variation, pituitary ACTH is secreted in an episodic manner as is demonstrated in Fig. 90-5. This episodic secretion of ACTH produces a similar episodic secretion of cortisol. In any use of plasma ACTH measurements, therefore, in the determination of adrenal function, it is important to remember that the sample may have been drawn at either a peak or a low point in one of these episodic bursts of secretion. There is a considerable increase in plasma ACTH concentration in adrenal insufficiency. Substantial increases in ACTH secretion occur during stress irrespective of the plasma steroid level. Prolonged administration of corticosteroids depresses the secretion of ACTH and results in adrenal atrophy indistinguishable from that observed in spontaneous hypopituitarism.

CUSHING'S DISEASE (See also Chap. 93)

In 1932, Cushing described the clinical disorder of pituitary basophilism associated with adrenocortical hyperplasia. This concept led to considerable controversy and a voluminous literature on the presence and significance of basophilic adenomas in patients with adrenocortical hyperfunction.

Relatively few patients with adrenocortical hyperfunction first come to the physician with definite enlargement of the pituitary gland; however, the incidence of pituitary tumor is significantly increased in those patients subjected to total adrenalectomy. Since bilateral total adrenalectomy has been widely practiced for less than two decades, it is possible that more patients will develop clinically evident pituitary tumors in due time. Curiously, most of the postadrenalectomy pituitary tumors have proved to be chromophobe adenomas. Eosinophilic and mixed-type tumors have also been found in Cushing's disease, but the largest number are associated with small basophilic tumors or hyalinization of the basophils.

Biologic tests for the measurement of ACTH in plasma, and more recently immunoassay techniques, may be of val-

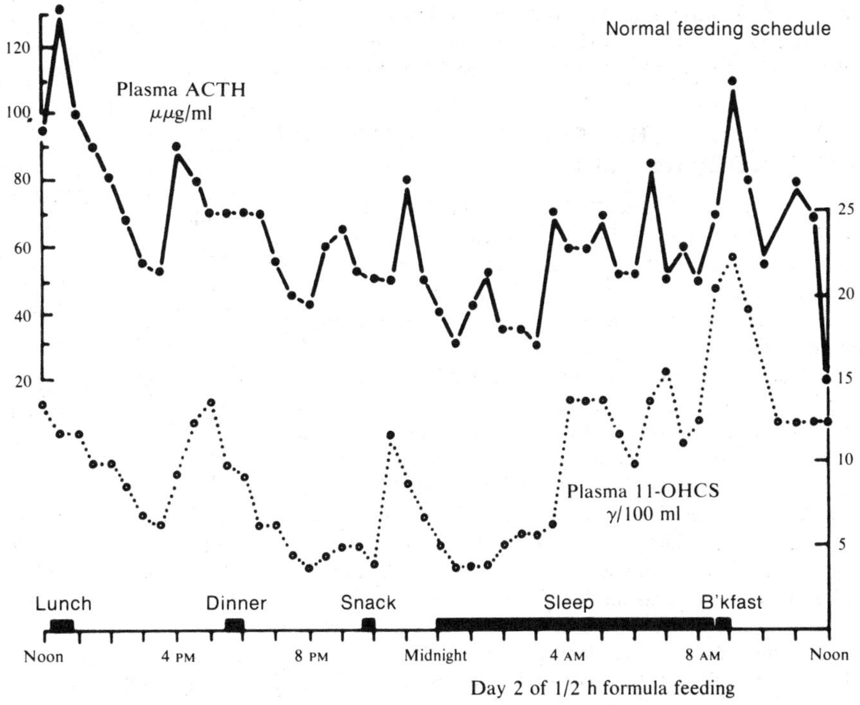

FIGURE 90-5
Levels of plasma ACTH and plasma 11-hydroxycorticosteroids (cortisol) in a normal subject. Determinations were made at half-hourly intervals and illustrate the episodic secretion of ACTH with a relative increase in both ACTH and cortisol in the early morning hours. (From DT Krieger et al, J Clin Endocrinol Metab 32:266, 1971)

ue in establishing the cause of adrenocortical hyperfunction. The finding of an elevated plasma ACTH level suggests a pituitary origin, but such an elevation may also be found in patients who have nonendocrine carcinomas that also secrete ACTH-like substances. A low to absent level of ACTH (<10 pg per ml) suggests adrenal adenoma or carcinoma. A moderately elevated plasma ACTH (200 to 1,000 pg per ml) suggests adrenal hyperplasia secondary to increased pituitary ACTH secretion. A very high plasma ACTH (>1,000 pg per ml) in the absence of signs of a pituitary tumor suggests a nonendocrine or "ectopic" tumor which is producing increased ACTH and adrenal hyperplasia. In a patient who has undergone adrenalectomy for Cushing's disease, an unusually high plasma ACTH (>2,500 pg per ml) is suggestive of an ACTH-secreting pituitary tumor (Nelson's syndrome). These patients usually have intense pigmentation of the skin due to the very high plasma levels of MSH as well as ACTH produced by the secretion of the tumor. The ACTH level is not diagnostic of the specific etiology, however, and other studies are necessary to finalize the diagnosis.

INCREASED PLASMA ACTH IN ADDISON'S DISEASE AND CONGENITAL ADRENAL HYPERPLASIA

Elevated plasma ACTH levels are apparent within 24 h of steroid withdrawal in patients with Addison's disease and fall to normal after a physiologic dose of steroid. This excess production of ACTH is not pathologic and has not been associated with pituitary tumors. It may be, at least in part, responsible for the hyperpigmentation which occurs in this disease, although increased secretion of MSH is probably chiefly responsible.

Patients with congenital adrenal hyperplasia also have elevated plasma ACTH level and, because of a similar mechanism, deficient secretion of hydrocortisone. As far as is known, the pituitary gland is normal in this disease. The excess secretion of ACTH is also easily suppressed by physiologic doses of corticosteroids (see Chap. 93).

INCREASED ACTH SECRETION IN TUMORS OF NONENDOCRINE ORIGIN

A number of patients with Cushing's syndrome secondary to the release of ACTH-like substances from nonendocrine neoplasms have been reported. Carcinoma of the lung is the most frequent type of tumor associated with this syndrome. A number of these tumors have been shown to contain and secrete "big ACTH," a large molecule which is broken down to produce a smaller peptide that is physiologically active ACTH. Of particular interest has been the association of Cushing's syndrome with benign bronchial adenomas as well as malignant tumors. It is possible that neoplastic tumors could also secrete an ACTH-releasing factor which would in turn stimulate the secretion or release of ACTH. The latter could be detected biologically by its effectiveness in the presence of an intact pituitary-adrenal system and its ineffectiveness in the absence of the anterior pituitary gland. To date, there is no evidence that these nonendocrine neoplasms secrete adrenal steroids; hence, removal of both adrenals should result in a cure of the Cushing's syndrome in circumstances which prevent the complete removal of the primary neoplasm.

THYROTROPIN (TSH) (See also Chap. 92)

Thyrotropin is a glycoprotein of approximately 26,000 mol wt. It stimulates the uptake of iodide by the thyroid gland and the synthesis and release of thyroid hormones. Continued stimulation results in hypertrophy of the gland and an increase in the vasculature. Thyrotropin deficiency results in glandular atrophy and depressed thyroid function. The administration of thyroid hormone depresses the secretion of thyrotropin and produces similar changes in thyroid function. There is good evidence that the ventral medial nuclei and paraventricular nuclei of the hypothalamus are involved in the control of TSH secretion, and that destruction of these areas depresses thyroid hormone synthesis.

The role of the anterior pituitary in the causation of primary hyperthyroidism is not clear. Although elevated levels of TSH in the blood of patients with hyperthyroidism have been reported, this is rarely the case, and most patients with hyperthyroidism have low TSH levels. The measurement of plasma TSH is not, therefore, a useful procedure in the evaluation of most patients with hyperthyroidism. A long-acting thyroid stimulator (LATS) has been demonstrated in the plasma of a high proportion of patients with hyperthyroidism. Administration of synthetic thyrotropin-releasing hormone (TRH) with measurement of serum TSH levels is a useful, sophisticated method of demonstrating the functional capacity of the pituitary gland to secrete TSH.

The occurrence of hyperthyroidism following hypophysectomy or pituitary stalk section suggests that TSH may not be essential for the development of hyperthyroidism. It does appear, however, that rare pituitary tumors may secrete excess TSH and result in thyroid hyperplasia and hypersecretion. Since TSH secretion may be increased by stimuli arising in the hypothalamus, it is thought that a mechanism acting through higher central nervous system centers may be related to the not-infrequent development of thyrotoxicosis following major emotional or psychic trauma. It is also probable that increased TSH secretion is involved in the hyperthyroidism associated with acromegaly. Measurement of plasma TSH has considerable usefulness in the investigation of patients with hypothyroidism. Because of the relatively wide variation in thyroxine levels in plasma as well as the influence of binding proteins and substances which interfere with this binding, it has been suggested that an elevated plasma TSH level is the best confirmatory evidence of a diagnosis of hypothyroidism (Fig. 90-6).

GONADOTROPINS (See also Chaps. 98 and 99)

The gonadotropins, FSH and LH, are large protein hormones of approximately 30,000 mol wt. These hormones regulate the development, reproductive functions, and hormonal secretions of the ovary and testicle. Prolactin (Pr) is also classed as a gonadotropin; however, its primary action is on the mammary gland, and though it may be luteotropic (i.e., sustaining the function of the corpus luteum) in lower animal species, this action has not been shown to be of physiologic significance in humans.

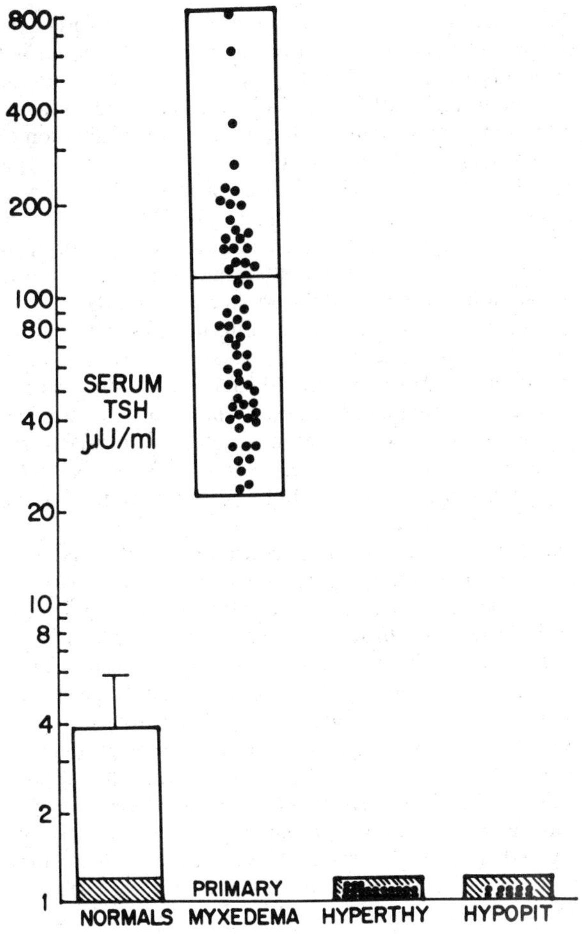

FIGURE 90-6
Serum TSH levels in normal subjects, primary myxedema, hyperthyroidism, and hypopituitarism. The high levels of TSH in primary myxedema indicate the usefulness of this test in diagnosing primary disease of the thyroid, but the relatively low levels in normal subjects make the determination of little value in the diagnosis of hypopituitarism. (From JM Hershman, JA Pitman, Ann Intern Med 74:481, 1971)

The secretion of gonadotropins is influenced by the rate of sex hormone production and by certain areas of the hypothalamus. Castration increases and estrogens decrease the secretion of FSH. The secretion of LH is also increased by castration but is less sensitive to inhibition by estrogens. Progesterone depresses LH secretion in some species. Testosterone is a poor inhibitor of FSH secretion but does block the secretion of LH.

Secretion of LH has been clearly shown to be regulated by the posterior hypothalamus. This area is also important in prolactin secretion, probably by producing a hormone that inhibits the production and release of Pr by the anterior pituitary. Lesions in this area block LH secretion and result in enhanced secretion of prolactin and pathologic lactation.

Gonadotropins are not found in the urine until puberty. Thereafter, they are present in significant quantities throughout life, with peaks of excretion appearing at the time of ovulation and greatly increased levels occurring after the menopause or following castration. Although relatively crude, the bioassay for urinary gonadotropins (FSH assay) is used. The assay is not specific for FSH, since even small quantities of LH appear to be necessary for the biologic action of FSH. Low urinary FSH levels are occasionally found in normal persons, and several determinations are necessary for accurate clinical evaluation. Increasing availability of radioimmunoassay of these and other pituitary hormones makes diagnosis of gonadotropin abnormalities much more reliable. Figure 90-7 illustrates the changes in serum LH and FSH which occur during a normal menstrual cycle. The assay of LH is easier and more reliable than that of FSH. FSH and LH are under the control of a single hypothalamic hormone (LRH). The availability of

FIGURE 90-7
Plasma follicle-stimulating hormone (FSH) and luteinizing hormone (LH) during a normal menstrual cycle in a normal subject. The shadings above and below the solid lines represent 95 percent confidence limits of the means. (From GT Ross et al, Recent Prog Horm Res 26:1, 1970)

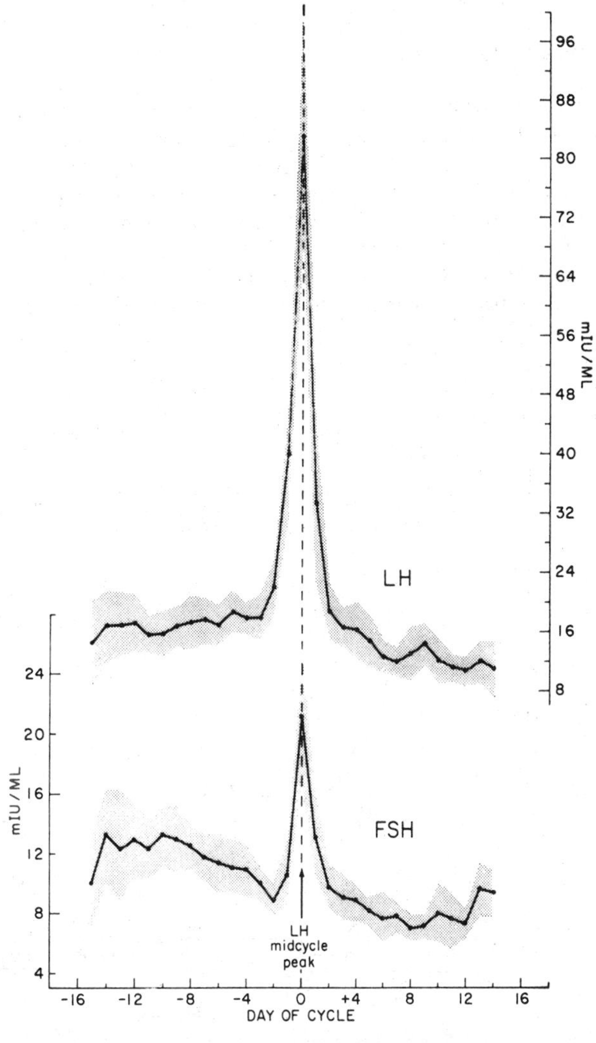

LRH for clinical administration provides the clinician with a simple means of stimulating gonadotropin production. LRH is administered as an intravenous bolus which produces a marked increase in LH with a peak at approximately 30 min following the injection. Clomiphene can also be used to stimulate secretion of LH and FSH. A dosage of 100 to 200 mg is administered daily for 5 to 7 days with repeated serum determination of the gonadotropins. In hypogonadal individuals an elevated serum LH indicates primary gonadal failure, while a low serum LH which does not respond to LRH administration indicates a probable pituitary defect as the etiology of the gonadal failure.

Chorionic gonadotropin (HCG) is derived from the placenta and appears in the urine in large quantities during pregnancy. Preparations from human pregnancy urine are available for clinical use. This hormone has predominantly an LH action and is used clinically to stimulate Leydig cell function and ovulation (Chap. 99).

SEXUAL PRECOCITY No definite pituitary disorders are associated with increased secretion of LH or FSH. There are cases of isosexual precocity, often familial, in which premature but normal sexual development occurs, probably on the basis of early maturation of central nervous system centers regulating gonadotropin formation and release. Lesions of the hypothalamus or pineal gland also may result in premature secretion of gonadotropic hormones and precocious puberty (Chap. 101).

GALACTORRHEA Galactorrhea is a common condition of multiple etiologies which is associated with increased prolactin secretion. Prolactin is the hormone most commonly secreted in excess in patients with pituitary tumors. The association of galactorrhea with a pituitary tumor has been referred to as the Forbes-Albright syndrome, while persistent lactation with amenorrhea following normal pregnancy has been designated the Chiari-Frommel syndrome. Amenorrhea and lactation unassociated with pregnancy are probably secondary to hypothalamic dysfunction. With levels of prolactin of 5 to 15 ng per ml considered normal, elevations above 100 ng per ml have been said to be suggestive of pituitary tumors, but no single determination can be considered to be diagnostic of tumor.

Prolactin is elevated in at least a third of pituitary tumors. It may be increased in patients with acromegaly but is often also increased in patients with "nonsecretory chromophobe tumors" presumably owing to suppression of the secretion of prolactin inhibitory hormone (PIH).

Galactorrhea secondary to drug administration is well known. Tranquilizers, antidepressants, rauwolfia, alpha-methyldopa, spironolactone, digitalis, and estrogens have all been associated with increased prolactin secretion. Hypothyroidism is sometimes associated with galactorrhea probably secondary to increased production of TRH which acts as a stimulus to TSH but also to prolactin secretion. Finally, stimulation of the nipples or irritative lesions to the chest wall may act to produce increased prolactin release. Apomorphine, ergot derivatives, and L-dopa all act to suppress prolactin secretion. Intravenous administration of TRH (250 μg) produces a maximum increment in prolactin 10 to 20 min following injection, while 25 mg chlorpromazine administered intramuscularly gives maximum increases in prolactin 60 to 90 min following injection. Suppression of galactorrhea has been produced by administration of L-dopa, 0.5 g orally every 6 h (Fig. 90-8). Similarly good or even better results have been described with the use of the drug bromocriptin given in doses of 1 mg t.i.d. gradually increased to 2.5 mg t.i.d. It is of interest that elevated levels of prolactin have been observed in the absence of galactorrhea.

PANHYPOPITUITARISM

PREPUBERAL Prepuberal panhypopituitarism, which was first described in 1871 by Lorrain, is a rare condition usually associated with suprasellar cyst or craniopharyngioma.

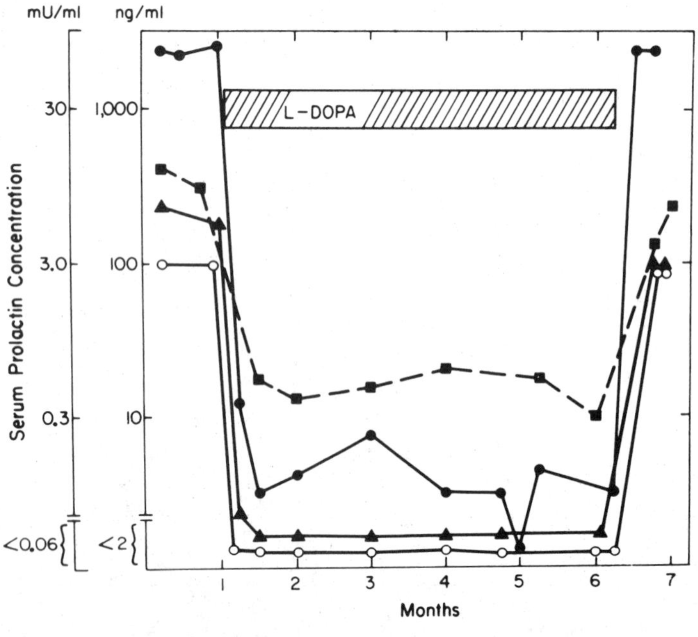

FIGURE 90-8
Effects of L-dopa therapy on serum prolactin levels in four patients treated for a 5-month period. (From Turkington, 1972)

The disease is characterized by dwarfism and subnormal sexual development but normal mentality. The impairment of growth is symmetric, and the body proportions are normal. As in other cases of hypopituitarism, the skin often has a pale yellowish appearance and increased wrinkling. Sexual maturation is delayed, and in rare cases there may be obesity from hypothalamic involvement. Diabetes insipidus is not an infrequent accompaniment.

If the tumor is of sufficient size to affect the optic chiasma, there may be bitemporal hemianopsia or complete blindness. X-ray studies reveal delayed fusion of the epiphyses, suprasellar calcification and, often, destruction of the sella turcica. The condition must be distinguished from genetic dwarfism and from hypothyroidism. Children with a familial type of dwarfism have isolated deficiency of growth hormone secretion but normal production of other pituitary hormones and development of epiphyses consistent with chronologic age. Hypothyroid children have subnormal mentality, infantile body proportions, dwarfism, and the characteristic epiphyseal dysgenesis.

Treatment with cortisone, thyroid, and sex hormones, described in more detail in the next section, should be instituted, with dosage adjusted for body size and age. Although limited by the availability of material, human or monkey growth hormone in doses of 1 to 3 mg weekly is effective in producing growth in these patients. Because of the psychologic and sociologic importance of reaching normal stature, every attempt should be made to obtain such therapy for these patients if the epiphyses have not closed. Growth hormone from nonprimate sources has no effect on growth in humans.

POSTPUBERAL PANHYPOPITUITARISM Panhypopituitarism designates absence of all pituitary secretions and is synonymous with *Simmonds' disease.* Post-partum pituitary necrosis (Sheehan's syndrome) is due to extensive thrombosis of the pituitary circulation during or following delivery, usually associated with blood loss and hypotension. Other causes of panhypopituitarism in the adult include chromophobe adenoma, craniopharyngioma, and the end stages of acromegaly. Less common lesions include gliomas, basilar meningitis, head injuries, and granulomatous disorders such as sarcoid and Hand-Schüller-Christian disease.

Characteristically, patients with Sheehan's syndrome fail to lactate or menstruate. The association of these signs should always suggest this diagnosis. There follows the insidious onset of a host of vague symptoms, including asthenia, lethargy, loss of libido, loss of axillary and pubic hair, and cold intolerance (Fig. 90-9). Some patients appear quite healthy and often are classified as psychoneurotic until the true diagnosis is revealed. Others gradually lapse into a far-advanced state of anterior pituitary insufficiency involving gonadal, thyroid, and adrenal function in approximately that order of development. Physical signs consist of bradycardia, hypotension, loss of axillary, pubic, and scalp hair, premature wrinkling and pallor of the skin, which is fine and atrophic, and a general loss of secondary sex characteristics, with atrophy of the breasts and genitalia.

Irrespective of the cause of panhypopituitarism, the secondary effects on the endocrine glands are similar. There is marked atrophy of the thyroid, adrenals, and gonads. Interference with growth occurs if the lesion appears prior to epiphyseal closure. The pituitary gland has a large reserve, and substantial amounts of pituitary tissue must be damaged before significant hormone deficiency develops. Not all patients develop hypofunction of all three target glands; isolated gonadal failure is relatively common, or gonadal failure may be associated with either thyroid or adrenal insufficiency. Isolated growth hormone, TSH, or ACTH deficiency may also be seen, although the latter is quite rare.

Laboratory findings Laboratory findings reflect decreased function of the target endocrine glands. The serum thyroxine level is almost always low. Serum TSH level is also low in contradistinction to the finding in primary hypothyroidism where the TSH value is elevated. Radioactive iodine uptake is low but is not very useful owing to the difficulty in distinguishing between low normal and low uptakes. Serum testosterone level is low in the male, and estrogens are decreased in the female. Plasma cortisol level will generally be low but may be difficult to interpret because of episodic variations. Hypoglycemia may occur, particularly in the fasting state, as a result of the absence of glucocorticoids and decreased gluconeogenesis. The level of serum cholesterol, unlike that in primary myxedema, is rarely elevated, despite lowered thyroid function. Levels of urinary 17-ketosteroids, 17-hydroxycorticosteroids, and 17-ketogenic steroids are depressed, and urinary gonadotropins are subnormal or absent. Blood levels of ACTH and growth hormone are depressed. A normochromic anemia is often present, and there may be leukopenia and relative lymphocytosis in the presence of adrenal insufficiency. The serum sodium concentration is usually normal, but hyponatremia may occur during periods of stress. The serum potassium level and BUN are usually normal, in contrast to increases seen in the patient with adrenal insufficiency.

Diagnosis The diagnosis of hypopituitarism is generally not difficult to establish once it is suspected, but because of the insidious onset and the variable signs and symptoms,

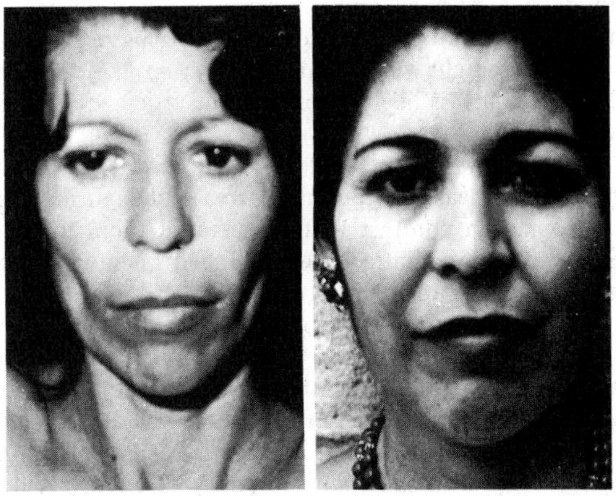

FIGURE 90-9
Photographs of a 40-year-old woman when first seen for hypopituitarism (Simmonds' disease) and after 6 months' therapy.

the disorder may escape detection for many years. These patients often come to the physician with acute medical emergencies associated with infection or trauma and fail to respond normally to the usual therapeutic measures. In such instances, clinical evidence of gonadal, thyroid, or adrenal insufficiency should be sought; if present, it will quickly suggest the diagnosis.

Patients with *pituitary myxedema* must be differentiated from those with primary thyroidal failure. Patients with the pituitary form often do not appear to be so myxedematous as those with primary hypothyroidism. An enlarged thyroid gland is indicative of primary hypothyroidism, since the thyroid is atrophic in hypopituitarism. In the absence of clear evidence of a primary thyroid disorder such as might result from radioiodine therapy, thyroidectomy, or thyroiditis, pituitary insufficiency should be ruled out in every patient with hypothyroidism. This may be done most conveniently by the estimation of serum TSH. A high TSH indicates primary thyroid disorder, a low TSH a possibility of hypopituitarism (Fig. 90-6). If this determination is not available, or not definitive when obtained, studying other parameters of pituitary function such as the ACTH-adrenal axis as described below may be necessary.

Measurement of plasma steroids following the administration of 2-methyl-1,2 bis-(3-pyridyl)-1-propanone (metyrapone) provides a particularly useful index of the ability of the pituitary gland to increase ACTH secretion. This compound inhibits the 11-hydroxylation of the steroid molecule in the adrenal gland and leads to decreased secretion of 17-hydroxycorticosterone (hydrocortisone) and increased secretion of 17-hydroxy-11-deoxycorticosterone (substance S). The hydrocortisone deficiency results in increased ACTH secretion from the anterior pituitary gland, a marked increase in the adrenal secretion of substance S, and a resultant increase in plasma levels of substance S or urinary levels of 17-ketogenic steroids. Patients with normal pituitary-adrenal function will show an increase in these steroids following administration of this drug, but patients with either primary or secondary adrenal insufficiency will fail to demonstrate such an increase (Fig. 90-10). This test is of particular value in assessing pituitary ACTH reserve in patients who have normal or only slightly depressed basal urinary steroid levels. The urinary test, performed by administration of 500 to 700 mg metyrapone orally every 4 h for 48 h with measurement of urinary 17-ketogenic steroids, may produce adrenal insufficiency and should be performed only on hospitalized subjects. The single administration of approximately 30 mg per kg body weight at midnight with estimation of serum 11-deoxycortisol at 8 A.M. is less likely to produce insufficiency and is a useful screening test.

Hypogonadism secondary to pituitary disease is characterized by decreased or absent plasma and/or urinary gonadotropins, in contrast to the increased titers found in primary gonadal failure. The prolonged amenorrhea observed in many patients with chronic illness and especially in those with anorexia nervosa is often confused with that due to panhypopituitarism. Gonadotropin concentration may be low in these patients, but adrenal and thyroid function is usually normal. The most useful single test in ruling out panhypopituitarism is a serum thyroxine determination. Almost all patients with pituitary deficiency will be found to have low values. If thyroid hormone levels are low, it is then necessary to determine the function of other target organs such as the adrenals and gonads. This can be done by estimation of plasma cortisol, plasma or urinary 11-deoxycortisol (substance S) after administration of metyrapone, or adrenal secretory response to ACTH. Ideally, when available, the serum levels of the pituitary hormones are measured after administration of the specific releasing factor of hypothalamic origin or appropriate stimulation of the endogenous hypothalamic hormone.

Other physiologic tests which have been employed in the past in establishing a diagnosis of hypopituitarism, such as the insulin tolerance test and the water test, are less specific and may be life-threatening if not carried out under close supervision.

Patients with pituitary-adrenal insufficiency excrete administered water at a depressed rate, similar to the rate of excretion in patients with primary adrenal failure; however, this test may be falsely positive in the presence of renal, hepatic, or cardiac disease. These patients may develop water intoxication during the test; they should be carefully observed for this complication and treated with intravenously administered cortisol if required.

Treatment The use of pituitary hormones would be true replacement therapy for panhypopituitarism. However, TSH and ACTH must be given daily by intramuscular injection, and pituitary gonadotropins cannot be used suc-

FIGURE 90-10
Response of urinary 17-ketogenic steroids in a hypopituitary patient (M. S.) and a normal subject (G. M.) to Metopirone (750 mg every 6 h for 48 h) and ACTH (40 units intravenously over 8 h on two or three successive days). Note the lack of response to Metopirone (metyrapone) and delayed response to ACTH in the hypopituitary patient.

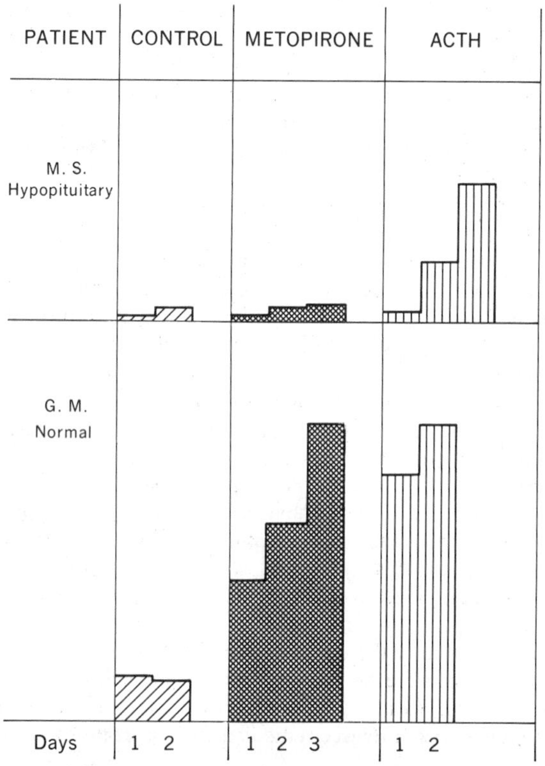

cessfully for any prolonged period because of the tendency to antibody formation. In practice, excellent results are obtained by oral replacement therapy with the target gland hormones. Thyroxine should be given at first in a dose of 0.05 mg a day, with the amount gradually increased over a period of several weeks to a total daily dose of 0.2 to 0.3 mg. Cortisone acetate should be initiated at a level of 5 to 10 mg per day and increased to 15 to 30 mg as needed. Since the administration of thyroid hormone alone in a patient with associated pituitary-adrenal insufficiency may precipitate a serious adrenal crisis, it is important to initiate cortisone therapy prior to or at least simultaneously with thyroxine therapy in these patients. Salt-retaining hormone therapy is not needed.

A long-acting testosterone preparation should be given intramuscularly in doses of 100 to 200 mg every 2 to 4 weeks to male patients; proportionately smaller doses are often beneficial in female patients. In the female patient, estrogens may be given daily by mouth or at intervals of 2 to 4 weeks by injection. If desired, cyclic therapy with estrogens and progesterone may be given to induce artificial menstrual function.

Hormonal therapy is intended only to provide normal replacement of physiologic levels for proper body function. Although the harmful effects of large-dose corticosteroid administration may not be observed with this schedule, psychic disturbances of various kinds are occasionally noted in patients suddenly exposed to full replacement therapy after a long period of adrenal or thyroid hormone deficiency. Another problem often noted is that of excessive appetite in some patients receiving even small doses of cortisone. In this instance, it may be necessary to institute a restrictive diet or to decrease cortisone dosage.

Patients should be given careful instructions concerning their increased cortisol requirements if exposed to stress. They should be told to seek medical attention immediately if they develop fever or other signs of infection, and if traveling to areas in which such care is not available should be instructed on the intramuscular administration of the steroid.

OTHER SYNDROMES OF POSSIBLE PITUITARY ORIGIN

Froehlich's syndrome and the Laurence-Moon-Biedl syndrome are two disorders associated with failure of gonadal development in which disturbances in anterior pituitary gonadotropin secretion are postulated. However, no consistent lesions have been observed in the anterior pituitary, and it is thought that the primary disturbance is in the hypothalamus.

Froehlich's syndrome is associated with adiposity and sexual infantilism. Patients have truncal obesity, the gonads are underdeveloped, and the secondary sex characteristics are absent. The condition may be associated with mental retardation, visual disturbances, diabetes insipidus, and impaired skeletal growth. It is important to differentiate between cases of Froehlich's habitus (obesity and apparently delayed genital development) and true Froehlich's syndrome. The former condition is often observed in normal prepuberal boys who may have normal sex organs hidden in the adipose tissue. With the onset of puberty, these boys develop normally and often lose their adiposity and assume normal adolescent body proportions. Froehlich's

syndrome may be associated with tumors or other disorders of the hypothalamic-pituitary area. The obesity may be caused by damage to hypothalamic centers regulating appetite.

The Laurence-Moon-Biedl syndrome is a hereditary disease characterized by adiposity, genital atrophy, mental retardation, skull deformities, retinitis pigmentosa, and associated congenital malformations such as polydactyly and syndactyly. Fewer than 100 cases have been reported, and there is no evidence of pituitary lesions in these patients. The adiposity and genital atrophy are assumed to be caused by hypothalamic-pituitary dysfunction.

MELANOCYTE-STIMULATING HORMONE (MSH)

MSH appears to be produced chiefly by the same cells of the adenohypophysis which secrete ACTH, although some may be secreted by the neurohypophysis. Two types of MSH have been identified. Alpha-MSH is a polypeptide composed of the same 13 amino acids found in the *N*-terminal position of ACTH (Fig. 90-4). Human β-MSH contains 22 amino acids and is closely related structurally to α-MSH as well as to ACTH. Because of the common *N*-terminal sequence, ACTH preparations have intrinsic melanocyte-stimulating effects; however, pure MSH does not stimulate adrenal cortical secretion. It is of interest that cortisone administration may suppress MSH as well as ACTH secretion from the pituitary gland. Only β-MSH has been detected in human plasma. This substance is present in very low concentrations of approximately 0.1 ng per ml. Increased levels are found in Addison's disease and in Cushing's syndrome. Extremely high levels are present in patients with pituitary tumors occurring after adrenalectomy. High levels have also been demonstrated in patients with ectopic tumors which produce ACTH. An MSH inhibitory factor (MIH) has been demonstrated in the hypothalamus, and it has been suggested that there may also be an MSH-stimulating hormone.

There have been descriptions of MSH-secreting tumors of the pituitary gland. These rare tumors are associated with a generalized increase in pigmentation similar to that observed in patients with pituitary tumors following adrenalectomy for Cushing's syndrome. The hyperpigmentation observed in patients with Addison's disease is due to increased production of MSH as well as ACTH. Increased MSH secretion may also be responsible for the hyperpigmentation observed in some cases of hyperthyroidism, biliary cirrhosis, sprue, and other chronic diseases. Conversely, it is probable that the decreased pigmentation often apparent in patients with panhypopituitarism is due to decreased production of MSH.

REFERENCES

BAIN J, EZRIN C: Immunofluorescent localization of the LH cell of the human adenohypophysis. J Clin Endocrinol Metab 30:181, 1970

BRASEL JA et al: An evaluation of seventy-five patients with hypopituitarism beginning in childhood. Am J Med 38:484, 1965

CRYER PE et al: Diagnosis and therapy of acromegaly. Arch Intern Med 135:338, 1975

DEL POZO E et al: Clinical and hormonal response to bromocriptin (CB-154) in the galactorrhea syndromes. J Clin Endocrinol Metab 39:18, 1974

HARDY J: Transphenoidal hypophysectomy. J Neurosurg 34:581, 1971

LAGERQUIST LG et al: Cushing's disease with cure by resection of a pituitary adenoma. Am J Med 57:826, 1974

NEELON FA et al: The primary empty sella: Clinical and radiographic characteristics and endocrine function. Medicine 52:73, 1973

NELSON DH et al: ACTH-producing pituitary tumors following adrenalectomy for Cushing's syndrome. Ann Intern Med 52: 560, 1960

ONTJES DA, NEY RL: Tests of anterior pituitary function. Metabolism 21:159, 1972

REICHLIN S: Regulation of the hypophysiotropic secretions of the brain. Arch Intern Med 135:1350, 1975

RIMOIN DS et al: Growth hormone deficiency in man: An isolated recessively inherited defect. Science 152:1635, 1966

SNYDER PJ et al: Diagnostic value of thyrotrophin-releasing hormone in pituitary and hypothalamic diseases. Ann Intern Med 81:751, 1974

TOLIS G et al: Prolactin secretion in sixty-five patients with galactorrhea. Am J Obstet Gynecol 118:91, 1974

TURKINGTON RW: Inhibition of prolactin secretion and successful therapy of the Forbes-Albright syndrome with L-dopa. J Clin Endocrinol Metab 34:306, 1972

WILLIAMS RA et al: The treatment of acromegaly with special reference to transsphenoidal hypophysectomy. Q J Med 44:79, 1975

91 DISORDERS OF THE NEUROHYPOPHYSIS

DAVID H. P. STREETEN
ARNOLD M. MOSES
MYRON MILLER

HISTORICAL The first indication of a possible endocrine function of the neurohypophysis came from the observation of Oliver and Schäfer (1895) that an emulsion of whole pituitary gland had pressor effects which were derived, as Howell (1898) showed, from the posterior lobe. In 1906, Dale found evidence of an oxytoxic principle in extracts of the posterior pituitary; it was separated from the pressor substance by Kamm et al (1928). The antidiuretic action of posterior lobe extracts was independently discovered by Farini (1913) and von den Velden (1913), who was also the first to demonstrate this action in patients with diabetes insipidus. Recognition of the relationship between hypothalamic nuclei and the posterior lobe of the pituitary followed demonstration of the anatomic and physiologic basis of the hypothalamoneurohypophyseal system by Fisher, Ingram, and Ranson (1938) and the histologic evidence of the neurosecretory activity of the supraoptic and paraventricular nuclei by Bargmann (1949). The importance of osmolar stimuli to the release of antidiuretic hormone (ADH) was established by the classic studies of Verney (1947). Previously indirect evidence that vasopressin and ADH are identical was confirmed after the synthesis of vasopressin by du Vigneaud et al. This accomplishment followed their synthesis of oxytocin (1953).

HYPOTHALAMONEUROHYPOPHYSEAL SYSTEMS Axons extend from neurons in the supraoptic and paraventricular nuclei of the hypothalamus through the pituitary stalk to the posterior pituitary. Secretory granules formed within the ganglion cells migrate down the axons and are either stored in the neurohypophysis or disrupted with release of the vasopressin or oxytocin which they contain into the bloodstream. There is increasingly convincing evidence that there are two hypothalamoneurohypophyseal systems with largely distinct and independent functions. The first comprises neurons located mainly in the supraoptic nuclei from which axons extend down the supraopticoneurohypophyseal tract to release ADH or vasopressin, a hormone predominantly concerned with the control of water conservation. This system is closely related to the thirst center which regulates fluid intake. The second system originates mainly in the neurons of the paraventricular nuclei from which axons descend into the neurohypophysis and release oxytocin, a hormone which stimulates uterine contraction and milk ejection.

SUPRAOPTICONEUROHYPOPHYSEAL SYSTEM AND ADH

CHEMISTRY Antidiuretic hormone (ADH, vasopressin) is a nonapeptide which comprises six amino acids in a ring and a side chain of three amino acids attached to the cystine (Fig. 91-1). Synthesized in association with ADH is a carrier protein called *neurophysin* which is probably vasopressin-specific. ADH and neurophysin are transported along the axons of the supraopticoneurohypophyseal tract and stored in the neurohypophysis.

PHYSIOLOGY The release of ADH into the circulation is influenced by a number of stimuli (Fig. 91-2). Under normal conditions, ADH release is primarily regulated by osmoreceptors which are probably located in the supraoptic nucleus. Release of ADH is accompanied by neurophysin release but in no consistent quantitative relationship, so

FIGURE 91-1
Structures of vasopressin and oxytocin.

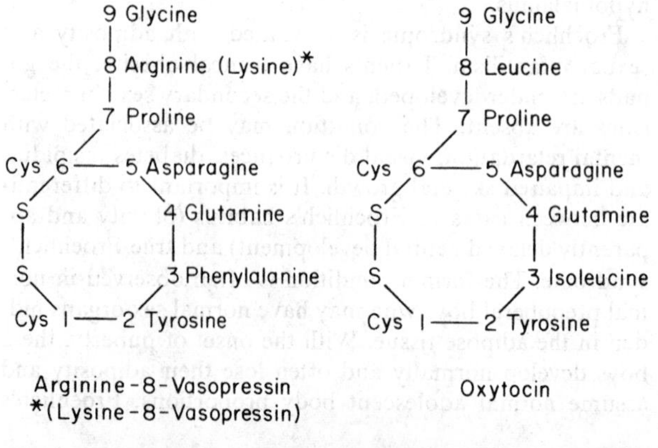

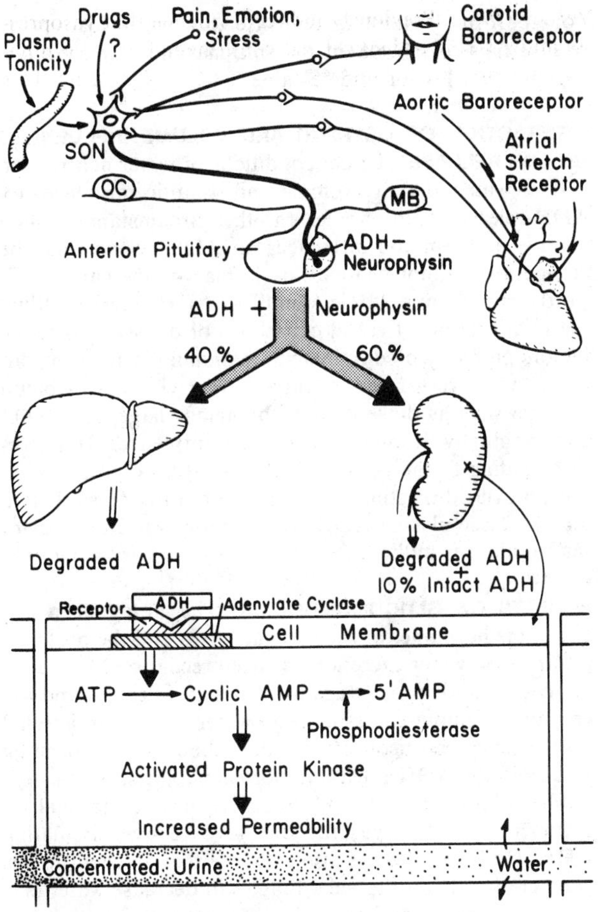

FIGURE 91-2
Schematic representation of control of ADH release and cellular action of ADH.

that neurophysin in the circulation cannot be used as an accurate index of ADH concentration. Other than osmotic influences on ADH release, there are volume receptors in the left atrium and baroreceptors in the aorta and carotid arteries where impulses are perceived and relayed to the hypothalamus, via the vagi, to produce tonic and episodic inhibition of vasopressin release.

ADH acts to conserve water and concentrate urine by enhancing the hydroosmotic flow of water from the luminal fluid through the cells of the collecting tubule of the kidney to the medullary interstitium. This action of ADH assists in maintaining constancy of the osmolality and volume of body fluids. High concentrations of ADH can cause vasoconstriction, as may occur in response to severe hypotension or to infusion of Pitressin for treatment of bleeding esophageal varices.

ADH has been assayed biologically by measuring its antidiuretic or pressor action in experimental animals. More recently ADH has been quantitated in blood and urine by radioimmunoassay. The results may be expressed as units or fractions of units based on pressor activity in the rat, or in terms of weight of purified vasopressin. Arginine vasopressin has a biological activity of approximately 400 U per mg. The human neurohypophysis under conditions of random fluid intake contains approximately 8 U ADH. Under the same conditions peripheral plasma ADH concentration in humans ranges from 1 to 3 μU per ml. The ADH concentration of blood fluctuates, with a maximum concentration late at night and in the early morning, and a minimum in the early afternoon. Under conditions of normal hydration, healthy subjects excrete approximately 10 to 35 μU ADH in 24 h, while releasing 400 to 550 μU from the pituitary. During 24 to 28 h of dehydration the amount released increases three to five times.

Inactivation of ADH occurs largely in liver and kidneys, a major mechanism being the cleavage of the terminal glycinamide to produce a biologically inactive substance. Approximately 10 percent of secreted ADH is excreted in the urine as biologically and immunologically active hormone.

OSMOREGULATION It is thought that ADH is released in proportion to the cellular membrane impermeability of solutes causing osmotic changes. It is generally considered that changes in volume of the osmoreceptor cells caused by changes in plasma osmolality alter the electrical activity of these neurons and the consequent release of ADH. There is evidence from animal studies that osmotic changes which stimulate release also enhance ADH production. The servomechanism between effective plasma osmolality and vasopressin release normally maintains plasma osmolality within a very narrow range. The mean plasma osmolality of normal subjects following a water load of 20 ml per kg body weight is 281.7 milliosmoles per kg, while that which initiates ADH release following infusion of hypertonic saline is 287.3 milliosmoles per kg. Thus the increase in plasma osmolality from full diuresis to the initiation of antidiuresis by hypertonic saline is only 5.6 milliosmoles per kg or 3.0 percent.

The infusion of hypertonic saline at a constant rate into normally hydrated man causes a linear rise in plasma osmolality. After a time interval which depends on the infusion rate and the concentration of the saline, there is an abrupt, progressive fall in free water clearance without a significant change in solute or creatinine excretion. The plasma osmolality at the initiation of antidiuresis under these conditions has been called the osmotic threshold for vasopressin release, and in 73 normal subjects occurred at a mean plasma osmolality of 287.3 milliosmoles per kg.

VOLUME REGULATION Decreases in plasma volume, particularly that moiety which affects the left atrium and perhaps the pulmonary veins, stimulate the release of ADH by reducing the tonic inhibitory impulses from the left atrium to the hypothalamus. The neural impulses travel via the vagi to the reticular formation of the midbrain and diencephalon and thence to the supraoptic nuclei where they are integrated into the other stimuli which affect ADH release. Positive pressure breathing, quiet standing, and vasodilatation due to heat may activate this mechanism which serves to restore plasma volume, even at times overriding osmotic inhibition of ADH release. Circulating ADH concentrations following volume stimulation may reach ten times the levels which are induced by hypertonicity. Increased plasma volume inhibits ADH release by the reverse mechanisms leading to a diuresis and the correction of the hypervolemia. Negative pressure breathing, recumbency, lack of gravitational force as occurs in space travel, submersion in water, and exposure to cold may activate this mechanism.

BARORECEPTOR REGULATION Activation of carotid and aortic baroreceptors causes the release of ADH in response to hypotension. Hypotension due to blood loss is the most potent stimulus to ADH release since it overcomes inhibitory stimuli and causes plasma levels of ADH to approach 1,000 μU per ml at times. These very high concentrations of ADH may cause marked vasoconstriction, which may play a role in the restoration of blood pressure.

NEUROGENIC, PSYCHOGENIC, PHARMACOLOGIC, AND OTHER INFLUENCES Aside from the regulation of ADH release by osmolality, volume, and blood pressure, other factors may exert a major, even overriding, effect on the release of ADH. Cholinergic and beta-adrenergic stimulation release ADH, while atropine and alpha-adrenergic stimulation inhibit ADH release, apparently by actions on the hypothalamus. Emotional stress, emesis, and pain may overcome a diuresis. A diuresis may follow hypnotic suggestion, psychologic conditioning, and inhalation of carbon dioxide. The above observations indicate that higher neural centers may alter ADH release. Pharmacologic agents which may stimulate ADH release include nicotine, morphine, barbiturates, vincristine, cyclophosphamide, clofibrate, chlorpropamide, and some of the tricyclic anticonvulsants and antidepressants. Ethanol has long been recognized to have diuretic properties and to inhibit neurohypophyseal function under a variety of conditions. Recently, some narcotic antagonists have been found to inhibit ADH release. Experimentally chlorpromazine, reserpine, and diphenylhydantoin all diminish the depletion of pituitary vasopressin and the rise in urinary excretion of ADH resulting from water deprivation. In humans, chlorpromazine has rarely caused a syndrome resembling diabetes insipidus, and diphenylhydantoin may be useful in treatment of some patients with centrally mediated SIADH (syndrome of inappropriate ADH secretion).

ADH RESPONSE TO WATER DEPRIVATION AND TO WATER LOAD Water deprivation provides both an osmotic and a volume stimulus to vasopressin release by increasing plasma osmolality and decreasing plasma volume. The maximum osmolality of the urine attained by water deprivation varies considerably, depending on renal medullary osmolality and other intrarenal factors. The administration of water lowers plasma osmolality and expands blood volume, inhibiting the release of ADH via both the osmoreceptor and the atrial volume receptor mechanisms.

An oral water load of 20 ml per kg in normal adults, which results in a fall in plasma osmolality to a mean of 281.7 milliosmoles per kg, causes a maximum diuresis in approximately 1 to 1½ h with the free water clearance rising to approximately 12 ml per min and the urine osmolality falling to 40 to 60 milliosmoles per kg. The delay in attaining a full diuresis is accounted for by the time involved in absorption of water from the gut, in metabolizing previously secreted vasopressin, and for renal recovery from the action of vasopressin. The half-life of vasopressin in the blood of humans is approximately tripled by hydration to 16 to 17 min. In response to a water load ADH release falls to the extent that plasma and urinary ADH become very low or undetectable.

INTERACTION OF OSMOTIC AND VOLUME INFLUENCES ON ADH RELEASE Under conditions of water deprivation and of water loading, volume and osmotic influences on ADH release act in parallel. In other circumstances, when volume and osmotic influences on ADH release may be competitive, minor changes in plasma volume can significantly modify hypertonic stimuli to ADH release. Under the relatively nonstressful conditions of daily life, osmotic factors probably predominate to maintain plasma osmolality within a very narrow range. Larger changes in blood volume, such as those induced by hemorrhage, may blunt and eventually overcome the osmotic influences. Hypotension leading to the activation of arterial baroreceptors exerts an overriding stimulus to the elaboration of ADH and may increase plasma ADH concentrations to hundreds of microunits per milliliter.

EFFECTS OF GLUCOCORTICOIDS The antagonism between the hormones of the adrenal cortex and the posterior pituitary on water excretion has been recognized for years. Glucocorticoids protect against water intoxication and overcome the impaired response to water loading in adrenal insufficiency. Cortisol elevates the saline-induced osmotic threshold for ADH release in normal subjects.

The subnormal ability to dilute the urine in adrenal insufficiency may in part be due to excessive circulating ADH. However, there is also evidence that glucocorticoids can act directly on the renal tubules to decrease water permeability and allow the creation of solute-free water in the absence of ADH. At present it is not clear which mechanism predominates.

CELLULAR MECHANISM OF ADH ACTIVITY Our present understanding of the biochemical basis for the action of ADH on the renal tubule (Fig. 91-2) is that: (1) ADH is attached to specific contraluminal receptor sites; (2) the receptor-hormone complex is coupled to and activates the adenylate cyclase on the same contraluminal membrane; (3) the production of cyclic AMP from ATP is increased; (4) the cyclic AMP is translocated to the luminal cell membrane where it causes the activation of membrane-bound protein kinase; (5) the activated protein kinase causes the phosphorylation of membrane proteins; (6) the phosphorylation of one or more protein constituents of the luminal membrane leads to an increase in its permeability. The ADH-generated cyclic AMP may be inactivated by cytosolic cyclic AMP phosphodiesterase which converts cyclic AMP to 5′-AMP.

The entire sequence of events leading to the transtubular movement of water depends on the integrity of the microtubular system of the epithelial cells. The above biochemical events lead to the passive flow of water along an osmotic gradient across the collecting tubule. The physiologic effect of vasopressin is accompanied by anatomic changes including cell swelling, vacuolization, expansion of the medullary interstitium, and widening of the lateral intercellular spaces of the collecting ducts. The latter changes indicate that fluid resorption during ADH-induced antidiuresis occurs in part by way of lateral intercellular channels.

Various cations and drugs can influence the action of ADH. Calcium, lithium, and prostaglandin E_1 inhibit the adenylate cyclase response to vasopressin. Lithium also interferes with a subsequent biochemical action, as does potassium deficiency. Demethylchlortetracycline inhibits adenylate cyclase stimulation by ADH and also inhibits the cyclic AMP-dependent protein kinase. In contrast, chlorpropamide increases the ADH-induced activation of the adenylate cyclase.

DEFICIENCY OF VASOPRESSIN: DIABETES INSIPIDUS

Diabetes insipidus is a disorder due to impaired renal conservation of water which results from low blood levels of ADH, reflecting deficient vasopressin release in response to normal physiologic stimuli. This uncommon disorder is being recognized more frequently in patients who have undergone pituitary ablation (by hypophysectomy, cryosurgery, or radioactive isotope implants) and in patients with or without known pituitary lesions whose mildly excessive water turnover has been studied appropriately.

PATHOPHYSIOLOGY Deficiency of vasopressin release in response to the appropriate stimuli may result from lesions at a variety of functional sites in the physiologic chain of events which culminates in discharge of the hormone into the bloodstream. There may be a defect in the osmoreceptors where the stimulus to ADH release is normally sensed. Such patients have no antidiuretic response to hypertonic saline, yet develop a good antidiuresis in response to nicotine or acetyl-β-methylcholine (Mecholyl). Occasionally there is an abnormally elevated osmotic threshold for vasopressin release. These patients excrete hypotonic urine in spite of water deprivation until serum sodium rises to chronically elevated levels corresponding to their raised osmotic thresholds for ADH release, above 300 milliosmoles per kg. In other, rare instances elevation of the osmotic threshold has presented with largely asymptomatic hypernatremia associated with loss of thirst and mild or absent evidence of diabetes insipidus. Occasional patients have been reported to show normal antidiuretic responses to osmotic stimuli but impaired responses to such presumably neurogenic influences as nicotine or the smoking of cigarettes. Reduction in the number of supraoptic neurons may be the cause of deficient ADH production in some patients who present clinically with "idiopathic" diabetes insipidus. It is known that removal of the posterior lobe of the pituitary induces permanent diabetes insipidus, but only if the pituitary stalk is sectioned high enough to induce degeneration of most of the neurons of the supraoptic nucleus.

ETIOLOGY Of 51 patients (34 males and 17 females) who satisfied the criteria described under Diagnostic Tests (below) and who had had diabetes insipidus for at least 3 months, findings were as follows. (1) Twenty were shown to have resulted from various types of *neoplastic or infiltrative lesions* of the hypothalamoneurohypophyseal system. In addition to the lesions encountered in this series, other types of malignant metastases (such as carcinoma of the lung and lymphoma), sarcoid, hemorrhage, abscess, meningitis, tuberculosis, and syphilis have been described as occasional causes of diabetes insipidus. (2) An increasingly frequent cause of diabetes insipidus (9 patients) is *surgical procedures in the region of the hypothalamoneurohypophyseal system.* These include hypophysectomy by surgical excision, cryosurgery, implantation of ^{90}yttrium and other radioactive isotopes, and heavy particle irradiation used for known tumors or for other lesions of the system or as a palliative procedure for diabetic retinopathy and metastatic carcinoma of the breast. Experience has confirmed the experimental finding in animals that surgically induced diabetes insipidus usually appears between 1 and 6 days after the operation. It often disappears after being present for a few days, and may remain absent or may recur and become chronic after an "interphase" of 1 to 5 days. (3) A third major group of patients (8 of the 51) developed diabetes insipidus after *severe head injuries,* usually, if not always, associated with fractures of the skull. This type of diabetes insipidus may last indefinitely but frequently lasts only a few days and sometimes (in 2 of our 8 patients) disappears spontaneously after several months or years, presumably because of regeneration of disrupted supraoptic axons within the pituitary stalk. (4) In a fourth group of patients (15 of 51) none of the currently available diagnostic procedures has been successful in revealing the cause. Some of these patients with *idiopathic diabetes insipidus* have other features of hypothalamic and/or pituitary disease such as subnormal stature, hypopituitarism, galactorrhea, and narcolepsy, and they presumably have functional or anatomic lesions of other systems in the hypothalamus or the pituitary, in addition to their dysfunction in the supraopticoneurohypophyseal system. Though no evidence of tumor can be found in these patients, the continued awareness of this possibility is sometimes rewarded by the finding of sellar enlargement after long-term follow-up. Occasional patients with such apparently isolated, idiopathic deficiency of vasopressin have come to autopsy where a striking decrease in the number or virtual absence of ganglion cells has been found in the supraoptic and paraventricular nuclei, associated with loss of Nissl substance in the remaining neurons and obvious gliosis. The neurohypophysis was reduced in size in these patients. It seems likely, therefore, that the reduced number of supraoptic neurons is the cause of the vasopressin deficiency in these patients. In some patients with idiopathic diabetes insipidus the disorder is inherited as a mendelian dominant.

CLINICAL MANIFESTATIONS *Polyuria, excessive thirst,* and *polydipsia* are the only clinical features that are almost invariably present in diabetes insipidus. Characteristically these symptoms are sudden in onset, both when the disorder first presents itself and whenever the effects of administered vasopressin disappear during the long-term therapy of patients with the disorder. In severe cases, the urine is pale in color, and its volume may be immense (up to 16 to 24 liters per day), requiring micturition at intervals of 30 to 60 min throughout the day and night. Much more frequently, however, the urine volume is only mildly to moderately excessive (2.5 to 6 liters per day), and very occasionally it may be less than 2 liters per day, causing no complaints on the part of the patient. Urinary concentration is well below that of the serum (290 milliosmoles per kg, sp gr 1.010) in severe cases but may be higher (290 to

600 milliosmoles per kg) in patients with mild diabetes insipidus (which should not be called "partial" in that most patients can be shown to have small amounts of ADH in their plasma and urine and usually respond to therapy with chlorpropamide).

The slight rise in serum osmolality in consequence of hypotonic polyuria stimulates thirst. Large volumes of fluid are imbibed and cold drinks are preferred, the patients often going to great trouble to secure refrigerated fluids. Although thirst is probably secondary to loss of water in this disorder, the administration of vasopressin often relieves or reduces thirst even in the absence of fluid intake by the patient.

Normal function of the thirst center ensures that polydipsia closely matches polyuria, so that dehydration is seldom detectable except by the frequently observed mild elevation of serum osmolality. However, when adequate replenishment of water lost by excretion is interfered with, dehydration may become severe, causing weakness, fever, psychic disturbances, prostration, and even death. These clinical features are associated with a rising serum osmolality and serum sodium concentration, the latter sometimes exceeding 175 meq per liter. Dehydration may result from impaired function of the hypothalamic thirst center because of extension of the same abnormality that caused the diabetes insipidus. More frequently, dehydration occurs during unconsciousness produced by surgical anesthesia, head trauma, or other causes. It is particularly hazardous to administer large volumes of isotonic saline intravenously or of hyperosmolar protein preparations by nasogastric tube unless adequate amounts of water or hypotonic fluids are administered simultaneously during unconsciousness in patients with untreated diabetes insipidus.

Hydronephrosis is a rare complication of the polyuria, especially in patients who fail to empty their bladders adequately because of uretheral strictures or for other reasons.

DIAGNOSTIC TESTS

1 Dehydration test Comparison of the renal concentrating capacity after dehydration and after vasopressin administration is the simplest and most reliable way of diagnosing diabetes insipidus and of differentiating vasopressin deficiency from other causes of polyuria.

The maximal urinary concentrating capacity is widely variable between individuals, and no absolute lower limits of "normal" can be defined in patients with nonspecific illnesses in whom vasopressin is produced in adequate amounts. It is impossible to distinguish between deficiency and sufficiency of vasopressin release by the absolute level of the urinary osmolality attained after specified periods of water deprivation. On the other hand, if after prolonged dehydration vasopressin administration induces a further rise in urinary osmolality, there is a strong implication that vasopressin deficiency exists. In patients with diabetes insipidus, plasma and urinary levels of ADH are low in relationship to plasma osmolality after dehydration. However, ADH measurements are seldom necessary for the diagnosis of diabetes insipidus.

PROCEDURE

1 Fluids are withheld long enough to accomplish stable hourly urinary osmolalities (with an hourly increase of $<$ 30 milliosmoles per kg in at least three successive hours). This is usually associated with a loss in body weight of at least 1 kg. In patients whose daily urinary volumes exceed 10 liters, the fluid deprivation should begin at 4 A. M. or 6 A. M. so that the patient can be carefully watched and the test terminated if weight loss exceeds 2 kg or the clinical condition deteriorates. In most other polyuric patients whose urinary volumes are less than 10 liters per day, it is preferable to start fluid deprivation at 6 P. M. or midnight and to continue to withhold fluids until noon the following day.

2 Urine specimens are collected hourly for osmolality measurements, from 6 A. M. at least until noon, and preferably until the osmolality has been stable for three hours.

3 At 11 A. M. (if dehydration started at 6 P. M.) or after the 3d hour of stable urinary osmolalities, the patient is given vasopressin as 5 U aqueous Pitressin by subcutaneous injection.

4 Serum osmolality is determined immediately before the injection of vasopressin, and urinary osmolality is measured during the hour after the injection.

Vital signs should be monitored during the dehydration procedure, but when the test has been done as described, adverse effects are extremely rare.

INTERPRETATION In subjects with normal neurohypophyseal function, urinary osmolality never rises by more than 9 percent after the injection of Pitressin, whatever the maximal urinary osmolality might be after dehydration alone (Fig. 91-3). In diabetes insipidus of central origin, the rise in urinary osmolality after Pitressin always exceeds 9 percent (Fig. 91-4). To ensure adequacy of dehydration, plasma osmolality before the vasopressin injection should be

FIGURE 91-3

Dehydration studies in four normal subjects, demonstrating that the maximum urine osmolality varies from approximately 500 to 1,400 milliosmoles per kg, and that the injection of ADH causes no further increase. (From AM Moses and M Miller, Diabetes insipidus, in Current Therapy 3, *eds H Conn and R Conn, Philadelphia: Saunders, 1971, p. 705)*

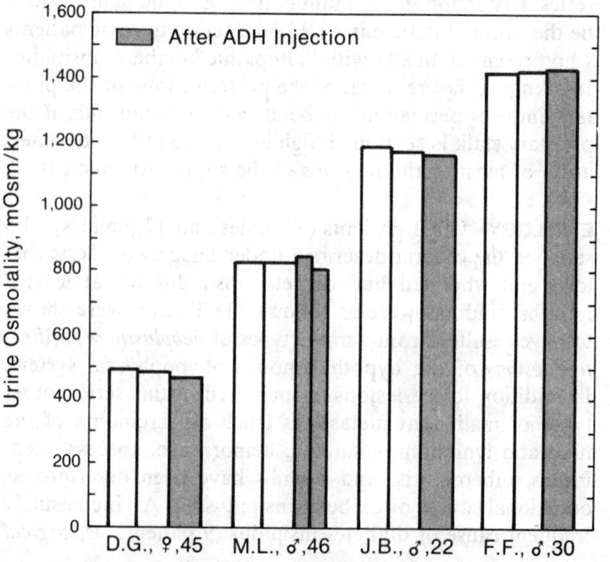

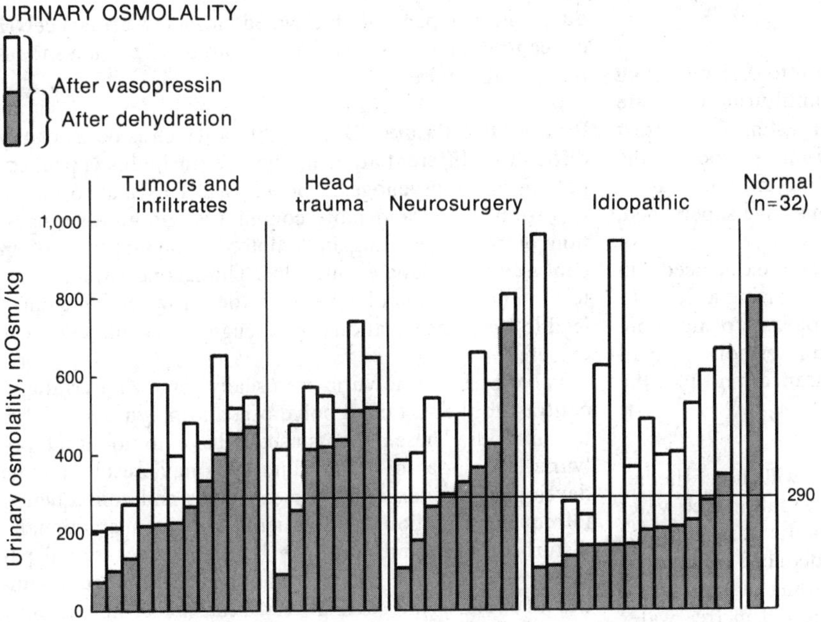

FIGURE 91-4
Changes in urine osmolality following dehydration and vasopressin injection in patients with diabetes mellitus of central origin.

above 288 milliosmoles per kg. Patients with polyuria resulting from renal diseases and potassium depletion usually show little rise in urinary osmolality with dehydration and no further rise after Pitressin injection. Patients with compulsive water drinking (primary polydipsia) often require prolonged water deprivation before serum osmolality reaches 288 milliosmoles per kg and before a plateau in urinary osmolality has been reached. Their urinary osmolality fails to rise by > 9 percent after the administration of exogenous vasopressin.

2 Hypertonic saline infusions Although the dehydration test is the simplest and most conclusive means of demonstrating the presence of diabetes insipidus, the renal response to hypertonic saline infusion may be used and is required to determine whether ADH deficiency is or is not due entirely to a defect in osmoreceptor function. It is important to measure urinary and plasma osmolality in at least one urine specimen before and immediately after the 5% saline infusion, in order to calculate changes in free water clearance so as to obtain conclusive results from this procedure (Fig. 91-5). The test is dangerous in patients who are unable to tolerate a saline load.

PROCEDURE

1. Administer a water load (20 ml per kg by mouth), and replace the urine voided every 15 min by an equal volume of tap water by mouth.
2. Infuse 5% sodium chloride solution intravenously into one arm, preferably by infusion pump, at approximately 0.5 ml per min—to replace solute lost in the urine—until urine flow rate has stabilized, normally at 8 to 20 ml per min, for at least four 15-min periods.

FIGURE 91-5
Effect of 5% saline infusion, 0.125 ml per kg per min, on urinary volume, osmolal clearance and free water clearance in a patient with hypopituitarism treated with hydrocortisone. Note the apparent lack of antidiuretic response when the volume alone is considered. The decrease in free water clearance is masked by the marked increase in osmolal clearance. (From AM Moses and HP Streeten, Am J Med 42:368, 1967)

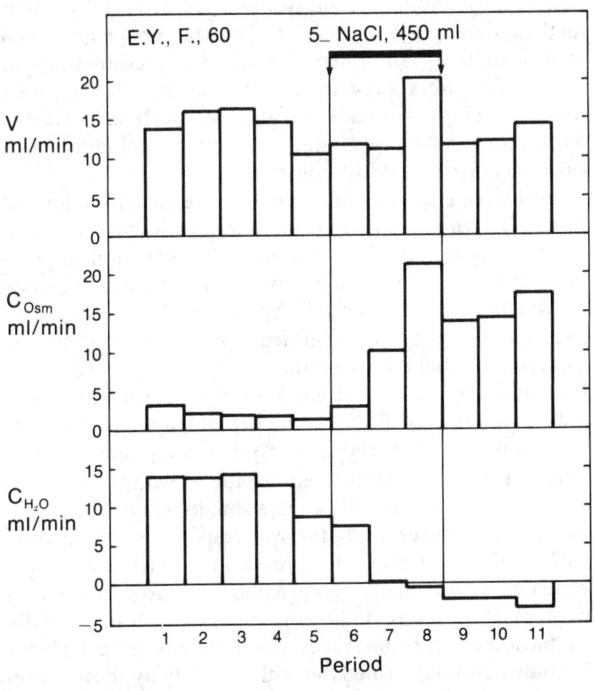

3 Increase the rate of 5% saline infusion to 0.05 ml per kg per min and continue the infusion until urine flow rate has shown an abrupt, sustained fall lasting for at least two 15-min periods, or until ten 15-min periods of the more rapid infusion have elapsed, or until headache, nausea, or other unpleasant symptoms have supervened, whichever comes first.
4 Draw blood through an indwelling cannula or needle in a vein in the other arm every 15 min, starting at least 15 min before the onset of the more rapid rate of infusion.
5 Measure urinary and plasma (or serum) osmolality in all specimens. Calculate free water clearances and plot the data.

INTERPRETATION Inspection of the data will show whether a sudden, clear-cut onset of a progressive fall in free water clearance can be identified. The osmotic threshold for ADH release is the plasma osmolality deduced by interpolation on the best straight line representing plasma osmolality measurements, at the onset of the fall in free water clearance. When defined in this way in water-loaded subjects, the osmotic threshold is normally 287.3 ± 3.3 milliosmoles per kg (mean ± standard deviation). In most patients with diabetes insipidus there is no detectable osmotic threshold, i.e., no fall in free water clearance even after elevating plasma osmolality well above 300 milliosmoles per kg. Occasional patients with diabetes insipidus may have ADH release at an elevated osmotic threshold.

DIFFERENTIAL DIAGNOSIS Diabetes insipidus has to be distinguished from several other types of polyuria (Table 91-1) in all of which there is loss of the renal tubular response to endogenous vasopressin. These other types of polyuria can, therefore, be recognized by failure of response to administered ADH. Among the types of polyuria listed in the table, several are easily distinguishable from spontaneous diabetes insipidus by the history [e.g., recent lithium or mannitol administration, recent surgery under methoxyflurane (Penthrane) anesthesia, or recent renal transplantation]. In others the physical examination or simple laboratory procedures will indicate the diagnosis (evidence of glycosuria, renal disease, sickle-cell anemia, hypercalcemia, or potassium depletion including such causes as primary aldosteronism).

Nephrogenic diabetes insipidus is a rare, usually inherited form of polyuria resulting from unresponsiveness to ADH. It is usually evident from the lack of a reduction in polyuria or rise in urinary osmolality after an injection of vasopressin, as described in the Dehydration Test above. These patients can be distinguished from patients with vasopressin-deficient diabetes insipidus by the usual evidence of inheritance in the renal disorder (very rare in diabetes insipidus) and by lack of the dramatic reduction in daily urine volume which is invariably seen when vasopressin tannate in oil is correctly administered to patients with vasopressin-deficient diabetes insipidus. Occasionally patients with nephrogenic diabetes insipidus will respond to vasopressin with a 40 to 50 percent increase in urinary osmolality, which is intermediate between the responses of patients with mild and severe diabetes insipidus (Miller et al, 1970). In those very rare instances where nephrogenic diabetes insipidus cannot be ruled out with certainty by these procedures, measurement of an elevated plasma or urinary ADH concentration after water deprivation for 12 to 18 h should remove all doubt.

Primary polydipsia One condition which is occasionally difficult to differentiate from diabetes insipidus is primary polydipsia or psychogenic polydipsia. This may occur in two forms. First and more common is chronic overingestion of water resulting in hypotonic polyuria and often confused with diabetes insipidus. The second variant is intermittent ingestion of large quantities of water, which may lead to water intoxication even though a very dilute urine is excreted.

Polydipsia and polyuria are usually somewhat erratic in contrast to the sustained polydipsia and polyuria of diabetes insipidus. These patients usually have no nocturnal polyuria. Polyuria of long duration may result in the development of large bladder capacities and consequently infrequent urination. The patients are often emotionally disturbed. The syndrome may be seen in occasional patients with anorexia nervosa, who may drink huge quantities of water while eating very little. Fluid intake may decrease markedly when food intake increases. Rarely, a patient with chronic fluid overingestion may have a central nervous system lesion, although adipsia or hypodipsia from central nervous system lesions is more common.

The intermittent ingestion of large quantities of fluid may lead to water intoxication and dilutional hyponatremia even though there is normal urinary diluting capacity. This phenomenon is very unusual because normal adults

TABLE 91-1
Major polyuric syndromes due to a decrease in tubular reabsorption of water, solutes, or both

I Water
- *A* Excessive H_2O ingestion
  - *1* Psychogenic polydipsia
  - *2* Postencephalitic polydipsia (rare)
  - *3* In some cases of primary hyperaldosteronism, chronic hypercalcemia, or hypokalemia
- *B* Inability to reabsorb adequate amounts of filtered H_2O
  - *1* Absent vasopressin—diabetes insipidus
  - *2* Renal tubular failure to respond to vasopressin
    - *a* Nephrotic diabetes insipidus (congenital and familial)
    - *b* Nephrotic diabetes insipidus (acquired)
      - *(1)* Usual chronic renal diseases
      - *(2)* Obstructive uropathy
      - *(3)* Multiple myeloma
      - *(4)* Amyloid disease
      - *(5)* Sjögren's syndrome
      - *(6)* Potassium deficiency
      - *(7)* Hyperaldosteronism
      - *(8)* Nephrocalcinosis or renal damage secondary to hypercalcemia, not hypercalciuria
      - *(9)* Unilateral renal artery occlusion
      - *(10)* Postrenal transplantation
      - *(11)* Sickle-cell anemia
      - *(12)* High dose lithium ingestion
      - *(13)* Methoxyflurane anesthesia
      - *(14)* Demethylchlortetracycline therapy

II Solutes: Inability to reabsorb adequate quantities of filtered solutes (osmotic type diuresis)
- *A* Glucose—diabetes mellitus
- *B* Salts—primarily sodium chloride
  - *1* Various types of chronic renal disease, particularly chronic pyelonephritis
  - *2* After various diuretics, including mannitol

Source: Modified from MH Maxwell, CR Kleeman (eds): Clinical Disorders of Fluid and Electrolyte Metabolism, *2d ed., p. 148, New York: McGraw-Hill, 1972. Used by permission.*

can excrete between 10 and 14 ml per min of solute-free water, and it is an unusual circumstance which results in the ingestion of sufficiently more water than this to cause dilutional hyponatremia. The syndrome of water intoxication with normal diluting capacity has been reported in persons who take large enemas, drink excessive amounts of beer, or are given thioridazine (Mellaril). The phenothiazine drugs have parasympathetic effects and may cause dryness of the mouth, which may aggravate tendencies toward compulsive water drinking. It is also possible that thioridazine may directly stimulate the thirst center.

The diagnosis is usually evident from the combination of low plasma and urinary osmolalities. When plasma osmolality is normal, the diagnosis can be made by a normal response to the dehydration test. However, the patients may be so overhydrated that it may require 12 to 18 h of dehydration before hourly urinary osmolalities become constant.

TREATMENT (See Table 91-2.) Diabetes insipidus can be treated by hormone replacement. As is true of most peptides, oral administration of vasopressin is ineffective. Aqueous vasopressin (Pitressin) (20 U per ml) may be administered subcutaneously in doses of 5 to 10 U and usually has a duration of action of 3 to 6 h. The main use of this preparation is in initial management of unconscious patients with acute onset of diabetes insipidus following head trauma or a neurosurgical procedure. The short duration of its action allows recognition of the return of neurohypophyseal function and prevents the development of water intoxication in patients who may be receiving intravenous fluids.

In the past, patients with an established diagnosis of diabetes insipidus have usually been treated with intramuscular injections of vasopressin (Pitressin) tannate in oil (5 U per ml). A single injection of 2.5 or 5 U has an antidiuretic effect for 24 to 72 h. Since this material is a suspension of vasopressin tannate in peanut oil, it is essential that the ampul be warmed and then thoroughly shaken or inverted repeatedly until the brownish deposit of pituitary powder identifiable in the ampul is evenly distributed as a slightly cloudy suspension in the oil. A perfectly dry syringe should always be used. Erratic or poor response to treatment with this agent is usually due to failure to shake the ampul properly.

In recent years, a solution of synthetic 8-lysine vasopressin (lypressin, or Diapid) (50 U per ml) has been available for use by nasal spray. Sprayed deeply into each nostril, a single application may result in an antidiuresis lasting from 4 to 6 h. A 5-ml bottle usually lasts 5 to 7 days when properly used. This form of therapy may be sufficiently effective and long-lasting to obviate the need for vasopressin injections. However, absorption of the vasopressin may be markedly decreased in the presence of an upper respiratory infection or allergic rhinitis with edema of the nasal mucosa. A new synthetic analogue of vasopressin, DDAVP (1-deamino-8-D-arginine vasopressin), may be a superior form of replacement therapy. DDAVP has markedly prolonged antidiuretic activity and is almost completely devoid of pressor activity. When used as a nasal spray, it has an antidiuretic effect for 10 to 12 h, so that the patient may be managed with only a daily morning and evening dose.

Patients with diabetes insipidus who have some residual releasable ADH may respond to oral treatment with several nonhormonal agents. The sulfonylurea, chlorpropamide (Diabinese), has been shown both to stimulate ADH release from the neurohypophysis and to potentiate the action of submaximal amounts of ADH on the renal tubule. These properties of the drug have allowed it to be used successfully in many patients with diabetes insipidus. Doses of 200 to 500 mg, usually taken once daily, are sufficient for an antidiuretic response. Its action usually starts within several hours of administration and lasts for 24 h. Chlorpropamide may restore thirst perception and thus be useful in patients with thirst center defects. Hypoglycemia may occur but can often be avoided by adherence to a regular schedule of meals. The hypolipidemic agent, clofibrate (Atromid), is capable of stimulating ADH release from the neurohypophysis and has been used in the treatment of diabetes insipidus. Doses of 500 mg four times a day often result in a prompt and sustained antidiuresis. In some patients, combined treatment with chlorpropamide and clofibrate results in complete restoration of water regulation to normal. Carbamazepine (Tegretol), used in the treatment of tic douloureux and diabetic neuropathy, has also been observed to produce an antidiuresis in patients with

TABLE 91-2
Agents used in treatment of diabetes insipidus

Drug	*Dose form*	*Usual dose*	*Duration of action, h*
HORMONE REPLACEMENT			
Aqueous vasopressin	20 U/ml ampul	5–10 U subcutaneously	3–6
Vasopressin tannate in oil	5 U/ml ampul	5 U intramuscularly	24–72
Lypressin (LVP)	5-ml bottle, 50 U/ml	10–20 U intranasally	4–6
DDAVP		10–20 U intranasally	10–12
NONHORMONAL AGENTS			
Chlorpropamide	100- and 250-mg tablets	200–500 mg daily	24
Clofibrate	500-mg capsules	500 mg four times daily	24
Carbamazepine	200-mg tablets	400–600 mg daily	24
THIAZIDE DIURETICS			
Hydrochlorothiazide	50-mg tablets	50–100 mg daily	24

diabetes insipidus. This effect is mediated by stimulation of ADH release. Doses of 400 to 600 mg daily are effective, but the drug has not been widely used due to toxicity involving the central nervous system, bone marrow, and liver.

Among 51 patients we have treated for diabetes insipidus over the past 15 years, only five have responded so poorly to lypressin nasal spray or to the oral preparations (chlorpropamide or clofibrate) that they have required continued therapy with vasopressin tannate in oil. Four patients have used this agent to augment the effects of lypressin nasal spray intermittently during upper respiratory infections. Twenty-two patients have been very satisfactorily treated with lypressin nasal spray three to six times daily, for up to 10 years. Fifteen patients have experienced excellent reduction in polyuria and an impressive increase in daily urinary osmolality while receiving chlorpropamide in doses between 100 mg twice daily and 500 mg daily for up to 5 years. There was a fall in plasma glucose concentration in most of these patients which was advantageous in those three patients who had concomitant diabetes mellitus, but caused symptoms which were severe enough to necessitate a change to other forms of treatment in three others. Plasma glucose returned to normal after 1 to 2 weeks in the remaining patients. Three patients were satisfactorily treated with clofibrate alone, and two others responded best to a combination of clofibrate (1.5 to 2 g in divided doses) and chlorpropamide (100 to 150 mg twice daily). Except in the minority of patients who have very severe diabetes insipidus, therefore, a good response can usually be achieved with one or another or a combination of the modalities of treatment which do not require injections.

All the therapeutic agents discussed thus far are effective only in diabetes insipidus and are completely ineffective in nephrogenic diabetes insipidus. In this form of diabetes insipidus, the only agents of clinical value are thiazides and other diuretics. By producing sodium depletion, the diuretics cause a fall in glomerular filtration rate with enhanced reabsorption of fluid in the proximal portion of the nephron. This results in decreased delivery of sodium to the ascending limb of the loop of Henle and consequently reduces capacity to dilute the urine. The therapeutic effect of diuretics in patients with nephrogenic diabetes insipidus is lost unless sodium intake is restricted.

PROGNOSIS The long-term prospects of a patient with diabetes insipidus are dependent primarily upon the underlying cause. In the absence of brain tumor or systemic disease, ready access to water and proper treatment of the polyuria usually lead to a normal life with a virtually normal life expectancy. Early recognition and treatment are important in order to prevent the bladder distention, hydroureter, and hydronephrosis which may develop in patients with long-standing polyuria. The rare patient with adipsia or hypodipsia in association with diabetes insipidus is in danger of developing severe dehydration which may lead to vascular collapse or central nervous system damage. Similarly severe complications may occur in patients with diabetes insipidus who develop impairment of consciousness. For this reason, all patients with diabetes insipidus should carry identification indicating the presence of the disorder and the necessity for treatment and fluid administration.

Syndrome of inappropriate ADH secretion

The syndrome of inappropriate ADH secretion (SIADH) is a disorder in which there is continual release of ADH unrelated to plasma osmolality. Since patients with the syndrome are unable to excrete a dilute urine, ingested fluids are retained, with consequent expansion of the extracellular fluid volume and the development of dilutional hyponatremia. The amount of ADH released and the elevation of urinary osmolality which it produces are considered to be inappropriate only in relationship to the level of plasma osmolality or serum sodium concentration. The hallmark of SIADH is, thus, hyponatremia due to water retention, in the presence of urinary osmolality above plasma osmolality. Rarely, when solute intake is markedly restricted, urine osmolality may be somewhat less than plasma osmolality.

It must be appreciated that water retention can be mediated by ADH as a result of excessive ADH secretion or as a consequence of enhanced renal action of ADH, and that it can also result from mechanisms unrelated to ADH. A fall in renal blood flow or glomerular filtration rate can increase the percentage reabsorption of sodium and water in the proximal portion of the nephron with consequent decrease in delivery of sodium and water to the diluting segment. This leads to impaired ability to dilute the urine and water retention.

ETIOLOGY AND PATHOPHYSIOLOGY SIADH may occur in association with a large number of clinical disorders, especially malignant tumors (Table 91-3). By far the most common malignancy causing SIADH is small-cell or oat-cell carcinoma of the lung, which accounts for more than 80 percent of the cases. The malignant cells are capable of synthesizing, storing, and releasing ADH into the circulation. Chemical and biological analyses of the ADH produced by the neoplasm reveal that the ADH is identical with the arginine-vasopressin produced by the normal neurohypophyseal system. In addition to ADH, neurophysin has been demonstrated in oat-cell carcinomas. Other malignancies which have been associated with SIADH are carcinomas of the pancreas and duodenum, lymphosarcoma, reticulum cell sarcoma, Hodgkin's disease, and thymoma.

Nonmalignant pulmonary tissue also possesses the capability of synthesizing ADH. This may be responsible for the hyponatremia which has long been known to be a common feature of pulmonary tuberculosis, since ADH has been demonstrated in tuberculous lung tissue but not in uninvolved lung or in a suspension of tubercle bacilli. Other pulmonary diseases associated with SIADH are lung abscess and pneumonia, particularly that due to staphylococcus. It would appear that in response to both malignant and infectious diseases lung tissue can acquire biosynthetic capabilities similar to those of the supraoptic nucleus of the hypothalamus.

A number of disorders involving the central nervous system can result in SIADH, presumably by stimulation of the hypothalamic-neurohypophyseal system. These disorders include skull fracture, subdural hematoma, subarachnoid hemorrhage, cerebral vascular thrombosis, and cerebral atrophy. Acute encephalitis may be accompanied by transient SIADH. Other infectious and inflammatory diseases of the central nervous system such as tuberculous meningitis, purulent meningitis, Guillain-Barré syndrome, lupus erythematosus, and acute intermittent porphyria may have hyponatremia due to SIADH as part of the clinical picture. Physical or emotional stress, pain, and positive pressure breathing can cause release of ADH resulting in SIADH.

In recent years, it has become apparent that several drugs used in medical practice may cause water retention and SIADH. Chlorpropamide (Diabinese) stimulates ADH release and enhances the antidiuretic action of submaximal concentrations of ADH. Many cases of chlorpropamide-induced water intoxication have been reported in patients with diabetes mellitus. The antineoplastic drugs, vincristine and cyclophosphamide (Cytoxan), produce the clinical picture of SIADH by causing release of ADH from the neurohypophysis. The tendency to water retention in these patients is aggravated by the common practice of recommending large fluid intake to prevent formation of uric acid calculi and the occurrence of chemical cystitis. Carbamazepine (Tegretol), used in treatment of tic douloureux, has caused water intoxication by stimulating ADH release. There are isolated instances of other drugs, particularly tricyclic compounds, producing SIADH. Clofibrate (Atromid) is capable of stimulating ADH release but has not yet been reported to cause SIADH. Oxytocin possesses inherent antidiuretic activity and, when administered in large amounts to obstetrical patients, may cause water intoxication. Patients who have been exposed to general anesthetics, narcotics, and barbiturates in association with surgical procedures may release excessive amounts of ADH. Thiazide and other diuretics can result in hyponatremia with all the features of SIADH, associated with hypokalemia and decreased exchangeable body potassium. It has been postulated that the severe thiazide-induced potassium loss causes stimulation of the volume receptor mechanism controlling ADH, resulting in persistently high levels of ADH release which may account for impaired water excretion and hyponatremia in these patients.

The excessive ADH released in this syndrome, in combination with water intake in amounts greater than can be excreted at the existing level of urinary osmolality, results in water retention and extra- and intracellular hypotonicity. Sodium excretion is enhanced because of increased glomerular filtration rate and, probably, suppression of aldosterone secretion. Excessive sodium losses aggravate the hypotonicity of body fluids.

TABLE 91-3
Causes of SIADH

1 Malignancy
  - Oat-cell carcinoma of lung
  - Carcinoma of pancreas
  - Lymphosarcoma, reticulum cell sarcoma, Hodgkin's disease
  - Carcinoma of duodenum
  - Thymoma

2 Nonmalignant pulmonary disease
  - Tuberculosis
  - Lung abscess
  - Pneumonia

3 Central nervous system disorders
  - Skull fracture
  - Subdural hematoma
  - Subarachnoid hemorrhage
  - Cerebral vascular thrombosis
  - Cerebral atrophy
  - Acute encephalitis
  - Tuberculous meningitis
  - Purulent meningitis
  - Guillain-Barré syndrome
  - Lupus erythematosus
  - Acute intermittent porphyria
  - Physical or emotional stress
  - Pain

4 Drugs
  - Chlorpropamide
  - Vincristine
  - Cyclophosphamide
  - Carbamazepine
  - Oxytocin
  - General anesthesia
  - Narcotics
  - Barbiturates
  - Thiazide diuretics
  - Tricyclic antidepressants

5 Miscellaneous
  - Hypothyroidism
  - Positive pressure respiration

CLINICAL AND LABORATORY FEATURES Patients with SIADH may present with weight gain, weakness, lethargy, and mental confusion ultimately progressing to convulsions and coma. Rarely do they have signs of edema. Laboratory features suggestive of water retention may be present, including low levels of BUN, serum creatinine, and serum albumin. The serum sodium is generally less than 130 meq per liter, and the plasma osmolality is less than 275 milliosmoles per kg. The urine is almost always hypertonic to plasma. Urinary sodium concentration is usually more than 20 meq per liter.

DIAGNOSIS SIADH should be suspected in any patient with hyponatremia who has evidence of hemodilution and excretes urine which is hypertonic relative to plasma. The finding that urinary sodium concentration is greater than 20 meq per liter is further support for the diagnosis. The possible presence of adrenal insufficiency must be excluded since glucocorticoid deficiency may simulate SIADH. In some patients with adrenal insufficiency, elevated plasma ADH levels have been found and have been attributed to the hypovolemia and hypotension present in these patients. The presence of hypothyroidism must also be excluded since this disorder may be associated with impaired diluting ability. ADH levels are elevated in some patients with hypothyroidism. In a consideration of the diagnosis of SIADH it is also essential to exclude hyponatremia due to sodium depletion, such as that occurring in renal disease, diarrhea, or diabetic acidosis. In contrast to the patients with SIADH, patients with hyponatremia due to sodium depletion usually have clinical features of dehydration with hemoconcentration, elevated BUN, and often urinary sodium concentration less than 20 meq per liter. Other disease states associated with hyponatremia, such as congestive heart failure, renal failure, and liver disease with ascites, must be ruled out. Primary polydipsia can also cause expansion of the plasma volume and dilutional hyponatremia, but can easily be distinguished from SIADH by the invariably dilute urine in patients with primary polydipsia.

In patients with the features of SIADH in whom central nervous system disease and the use of drugs capable of causing water retention can be excluded, the possibility of malignancy must be seriously considered, especially oat-cell carcinoma of the lung. Water retention and hyponatremia may occur before evidence of malignancy can be detected on chest x-ray.

The response to water loading is a useful means of establishing the diagnosis of SIADH. Before water loading is carried out, the serum sodium must be brought to a safe level, generally above 125 meq per liter, by appropriate sodium administration and fluid restriction, and the patient must be free of symptoms of hyponatremia. An oral water load of 20 ml per kg body weight is given over a period of 15 to 20 min, and urine is collected hourly for the next 5 h while the patient is recumbent. In normal individuals given such a water load, more than 80 percent of the water is excreted by the fifth hour and the urinary osmolality falls to less than 100 milliosmoles per kg (sp gr 1.005) during the test. Patients with hyponatremia who excrete the water load normally may be considered to have a low-set osmoreceptor, such as occurs in chronic ill health. In contrast, patients with SIADH excrete less than 40 percent of the water load in 5 h and fail to dilute the urine to hypotonic levels. When a water load has been given to a patient with SIADH, no further water intake should be permitted over the next 24 h until the serum sodium has returned to the pretest value. In this way, production of symptomatic water intoxication can be prevented. Adrenal insufficiency cannot be distinguished from SIADH by the water load test.

Measurement of ADH in plasma and urine by sensitive bioassay or radioimmunoassay has revealed persistence of ADH in both plasma and urine in patients with SIADH at times when the plasma hypoosmolality should have been sufficient to inhibit ADH secretion. In response to further reduction of plasma osmolality after a water load, ADH has remained detectable in plasma and urine, confirming that indeed the ADH secretion is inappropriate relative to plasma osmolality (Miller and Moses, 1972).

It should be emphasized that SIADH cannot be diagnosed with confidence in the presence of severe "stress," pain, hypovolemia, hypotension, and other stimuli which may evoke physiologic release of ADH even in the presence of hypotonicity.

TREATMENT Patients with mild or moderate symptoms related to water intoxication should be treated by restricting fluid intake to about 800 to 1,000 ml daily. If water restriction is adequate, a steady increase in serum sodium or osmolality occurs and body weight decreases. Occasional patients with severe water intoxication must be treated more vigorously. The intravenous administration of 200 to 300 ml 5% saline solution over several hours is usually sufficient to raise the serum sodium to a level where the symptoms will improve. When there is the possibility of congestive heart failure due to the fluid overload, the simultaneous administration of large doses of furosemide usually causes a diuresis sufficient to reduce cardiac overload. When furosemide is given, careful attention must be paid to correction of potassium and other electrolyte losses induced by the drug. If, for any reason, intravenous fluid administration is considered necessary when the serum sodium has been raised to an appropriate level, isotonic saline and not 5% dextrose solution should be infused slowly to maintain stability of the serum sodium concentration.

Once the initial hyponatremia has been improved, careful adherence to a regimen of fluid restriction is necessary to prevent recurrence of water intoxication. Treatment should be directed at the underlying problem. The withdrawal of drugs which might have been causing water retention usually results in prompt clearing of SIADH. The SIADH occurring with central nervous system disorders is usually transient and clears with improvement of the underlying disease. Treatment of pulmonary tuberculosis with appropriate antituberculous therapy results in gradual disappearance of SIADH. Similarly, antibiotic treatment of lung abscess or pneumonia results in resolution of SIADH.

In patients with SIADH due to malignancy, surgical resection, irradiation, or chemotherapy may be successful in alleviating water retention. Sometimes, these measures should be carried out even when there is little likelihood of curing the malignancy since such treatment may correct life-threatening water intoxication and prevent the necessity for rigid fluid restriction. In patients in whom treatment is judged to have been curative, the disappearance of SIADH may be a further indication of the success of treatment. Periodic water load tests may be valuable in following the patients for evidence of recurrence of malignancy.

At present, no drugs are available which are clinically useful in suppressing ADH release from the neurohypophyseal system or from a tumor, or in overcoming a persistent ADH effect on the renal tubules. Diphenylhydantoin inhibits ADH release but is clinically ineffective. Several narcotic antagonists currently undergoing clinical testing are capable of inhibiting ADH release from the neurohypophysis. Their role in the treatment of SIADH remains to be determined. Lithium salts can interfere with the antidiuretic action of ADH on the kidney but are too toxic for use in SIADH. Demethylchlortetracycline can interfere with ADH action and may have a role in treatment of water intoxication, but its usefulness is still unproved.

PROGNOSIS The prognosis of a patient with SIADH depends on the underlying cause of the syndrome. Transient or reversible SIADH such as is seen in central nervous system disorders or following use of water-retaining drugs is usually benign as long as proper treatment of acute water intoxication is effectively carried out. SIADH occurring in association with malignancy has ominous implications since the malignancies most commonly associated are oat-cell carcinoma of the lung and adenocarcinoma of the pancreas, both usually associated with rapid spread and early death. Since SIADH may antedate the clinical appearance of the malignancy, recognition of the syndrome may possibly lead to earlier diagnosis of malignancy at a time when surgical cure is possible. In patients in whom SIADH is not correctable by surgery, irradiation, or chemotherapy, long-term fluid restriction is necessary to prevent symptomatic water intoxication.

PARAVENTRICULAR-NEUROHYPOPHYSEAL SYSTEM AND OXYTOCIN

CHEMISTRY AND PHYSIOLOGY Oxytocin is a nonapeptide which differs by two amino acids from vasopressin (Fig. 91-1). Oxytocin is produced predominantly in the cell bodies of the paraventricular nuclei, and to a lesser extent in those of the supraoptic nuclei. It is synthesized and transported in neurosecretory granules by way of nerve tracts to the neurohypophysis where it is stored or released, in conjunction with an oxytocin-specific neurophysin. Oxytocin release results from nerve impulses originating in the hypothalamus, which cause depolarization of the neurosecretory terminals of the posterior pituitary, and subsequent release of oxytocin through a calcium-dependent process, similar to the mechanism for vasopressin. The secretion of oxytocin, as well as of vasopressin, is inhibited by ethanol. Some stimuli such as pain apparently release oxytocin and vasopressin simultaneously, but most stimuli release the two hormones independently. Oxytocin is primarily liberated during suckling, whereas after an osmotic stimulus or hemorrhage vasopressin is released in much greater quantities than is oxytocin. Manipulation or distention of the female genital tract, artificially or during parturition, appears to be a more effective stimulus to oxytocin release than is suckling.

Oxytocin acts on the excitable membranes surrounding the myometrial and myoepithelial cells and results in an increased force of contraction. Sensitivity of the myometrium to oxytocin increases with the duration of pregnancy, but it is not known if oxytocin per se is responsible for the initiation and maintenance of labor. Oxytocin may have survival value to the offspring since it may hasten the final stages of birth and may lessen the chances of anoxia. Oxytocin continues to exert a contractile action on the myometrium post partum. Circulating oxytocin contracts the myoepithelial cells of the mammary alveoli, causing them to expel preformed milk from the secretory tissue to the nipple. Oxytocin is 100 times more potent than vasopressin in its milk-ejecting activity in the human. In contrast, the antidiuretic potency of oxytocin relative to vasopressin is about 1 to 200. It is unlikely that oxytocin exerts any significant physiologic effect other than on the uterus and breast.

One milligram of purified preparation of oxytocin contains 450 IU of the hormone, and the amount of oxytocin in the posterior pituitary ranges from 10 to 15 units per lobe. In spite of the fact that there is no known role of oxytocin in the male, the male neural lobe stores oxytocin in amounts similar to the female. There is less than 0.75 μU per ml in normal adult male and female plasma, even in the third trimester of pregnancy. During labor, plasma oxytocin concentrations may reach several hundred microunits per milliliter, with a rapid fall to prepartum levels in 5 to 10 minutes after delivery. During suckling, plasma oxytocin levels of the mother vary widely but are usually about 5 to 10 μU per ml. The half-life of oxytocin in the plasma of human beings is about 3 to 5 min. Removal of oxytocin from the circulation is mainly by the kidneys and liver, although the uterus and mammary gland may remove some.

CLINICAL USE OF OXYTOCIN The clinical use of oxytocin is limited to the induction of labor, control of hemorrhage following incomplete abortion and curettage, and treatment of impaired milk ejection. For a detailed discussion of the obstetrical uses of oxytocin, the reader is referred to textbooks on obstetrics. Care must be taken in the use of oxytocin because it may cause uterine rupture and fetal death. The antidiuretic action of oxytocin can be elicited with single intravenous doses of as little as 100 mU. Maximal antidiuresis is reached with 40 to 50 mU per min. Since 10 to 40 U oxytocin per liter of dextrose is often used in obstetrical practice, it is apparent that water intoxication may result. The vasodilatory action of oxytocin may cause sudden deaths of obstetrical patients with heart disease because of hypotension, tachycardia, and arrhythmias. Anesthetics may modify the cardiovascular responses to oxytocin. For instance, in patients under cyclopropane anesthesia, oxytocin produces more hypotension but less tachycardia than in unanesthetized subjects. The vasodilatory effect of oxytocin can be blocked by vasopressin.

REFERENCES

BARTTER FC, SCHWARTZ WB: The syndrome of inappropriate secretion of antidiuretic hormone. Am J Med 42:790, 1967

KNOBIL E, SAWYER WH (eds): The Pituitary Gland—Its Neuroendocrine Control, part I, in *Handbook of Physiology,* sect. 7, Endocrinology, vol. IV, Washington: American Physiological Society, 1974

MILLER M et al: Recognition of partial defects in antidiuretic hormone secretion. Ann Intern Med 73:721, 1970

——, MOSES AM: Urinary antidiuretic hormone in polyuric disorders and in inappropriate ADH syndrome. Ann Intern Med 77:715, 1972

MOSES AM et al: Pathophysiologic and pharmacologic alterations in the release and action of ADH. Metabolism 25:697, 1976

ROBINSON AG: DDAVP in the treatment of central diabetes insipidus. N Engl J Med 294:507, 1976

92 DISEASES OF THE THYROID

SIDNEY H. INGBAR
KENNETH A. WOEBER

The normal function of the thyroid gland is to secrete L-thyroxine (T_4) and 3,5,3′-triiodo-L-thyronine (T_3), iodinated amino acids that are the active thyroid hormones and that influence a diversity of metabolic processes (Fig. 92-1). Diseases of the thyroid gland are manifested by qualitative or quantitative alterations in hormonal secretion, enlargement of the thyroid (goiter), or both. Insufficient hormonal secretion results in the syndrome of *hypothyroidism* or *myxedema,* in which decreased oxygen consumption (hypometabolism) is a classic manifestation. Conversely, excessive secretion of active hormone results in hypermetabolism and other features of a syndrome termed *hyperthyroidism* or *thyrotoxicosis.* Enlargement of the thyroid gland (normally 15 to 25 g in adults) may be generalized or focal. Generalized enlargements may not be absolutely symmetric, however, the right lobe tending to enlarge more than the left. They are associated with increased, normal, or decreased hormone secretion, depending upon the underlying disturbance. Truly focal enlargement usually reflects neoplastic transformation, either benign or malignant, the former sometimes being responsible for hypersecretion of

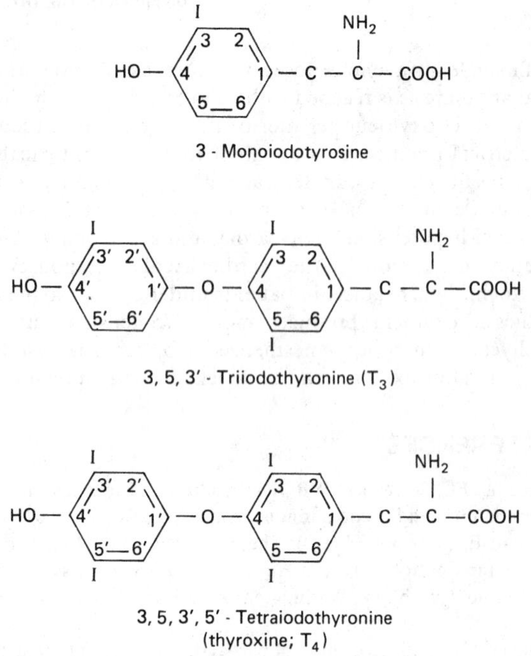

FIGURE 92-1
Structural formulas of the active thyroid hormones, thyroxine and triiodothyronine, and of the inactive precursor, monoiodotyrosine.

hormone and hyperthyroidism, the latter very rarely so. Either type of goiter may result in compression of adjacent structures in the neck or mediastinum.

EMBRYOLOGY, ANATOMY, AND HISTOLOGY

The human thyroid originates embryologically from an evagination of the pharyngeal epithelium with some cellular contributions from the lateral pharyngeal pouches. Progressive descent of the midline thyroid anlage gives rise to the thyroglossal duct, which extends from the foramen cecum near the base of the tongue to the isthmus of the thyroid. Remnants of tissue may persist along the course of this tract as "lingual thyroid," as thyroglossal cysts or nodules, or as a structure contiguous with the thyroid isthmus called the *pyramidal lobe.* The latter is usually not discernible, except when the remainder of the gland is goitrous. In some individuals, lingual thyroid may be the sole functioning thyroid tissue. In such cases, its secretion may or may not be sufficient to maintain a normal metabolic (euthyroid) state.

Knowledge of the ontogenetic sequence in human thyroid development is limited by the availability of specimens for analysis. It is clear, however, that the fetal thyroid acquires the capacity to collect and organify iodine at about 10 weeks gestation. Both T_4 and thyroid-stimulating hormone (thyrotropin, TSH) are detectable in the blood soon thereafter. It is likely that the fetal pituitary-thyroid axis is a distinct functional unit, since little maternal TSH crosses the placenta and transplacental passage of T_4 and T_3 from mother to fetus appears similarly small. A thyroid stimulator termed *human chorionic thyrotropin* (HCT) has been extracted from placenta, but its role in maternal and fetal thyroid physiology is unknown.

The normal adult thyroid is a relatively vascular organ, comprising two lobes joined by an isthmus and lying just anterior and slightly caudad to the cartilages of the larynx. Fibrous septa divide the gland into pseudolobules which, in turn, comprise vesicles, called *follicles* or *acini,* surrounded by a capillary network. Normally, the follicle walls are composed of cuboidal epithelium. Their lumen is filled with a proteinaceous material termed *colloid* which contains a protein peculiar to the thyroid, *thyroglobulin,* within the peptide sequence of which T_4 and T_3 are stored.

HORMONE SYNTHESIS, SECRETION, AND METABOLISM

SYNTHESIS AND SECRETION Thyroid hormone synthesis that is both qualitatively and quantitatively normal depends on entry into the thyroid of adequate quantities of iodine, a constituent of the active hormones, T_4 and T_3; normality of pathways for iodine metabolism within the gland; and concurrent synthesis of a normal receptor protein for iodine, thyroglobulin. Secretion of normal quantities of hormone, in turn, requires both a normal rate of hormone synthesis and the integrity of processes within the gland by which thyroglobulin is hydrolyzed and the hormonally active iodoaminoacids thereby liberated. Iodine enters the thyroid from the bloodstream in the form of inorganic or ionic iodide whose source is twofold: iodide derived either from the deiodination of thyroid hormones or from iodinated agents that the patient may have been given and iodide ingested in food, water, or medication. Formerly, a dietary iodine intake of approximately 200 μg was considered normal within the continental United States, and this was sufficient to sustain a plasma iodide concentration of approximately 0.5 μg per 100 ml. Recently, however, owing largely to enrichment of bread with iodine, the average iodine intake has increased substantially, to values as high as 1,000 μg daily, with corresponding increases in plasma iodide concentration. Iodide is removed from the plasma by the thyroid, kidneys, and salivary and gastrointestinal glands, but since iodide that enters gastrointestinal secretion is reabsorbed, net clearance is effected only by the thyroid and kidneys. In effect, the thyroid and kidneys compete for plasma iodide. However, since renal clearance is largely a function of glomerular filtration rate and is not influenced by humoral factors or plasma iodide concentration, the kidney is normally a passive participant in this competition. Hence, adjustments in the rate of entry of iodide into the thyroid relative to the rate of urinary excretion are mediated by changes in thyroid, rather than renal, avidity.

The reactions involved in the synthesis and secretion of the active thyroid hormones can be divided into four sequential steps (Fig. 92-2). The first involves active inward transport of iodide from the plasma into the thyroid cell and follicular lumen. This occurs at a rate that exceeds passive diffusion of iodide from the gland, with the result that the thyroid is capable of maintaining concentration gradients for iodide (thyroid/plasma concentration ratios) of substantial magnitude (up to 500, or more, under certain physiologic or pathologic conditions). Energy for iodide transport is phosphate bond–derived and therefore depends upon oxidative metabolism within the gland. The

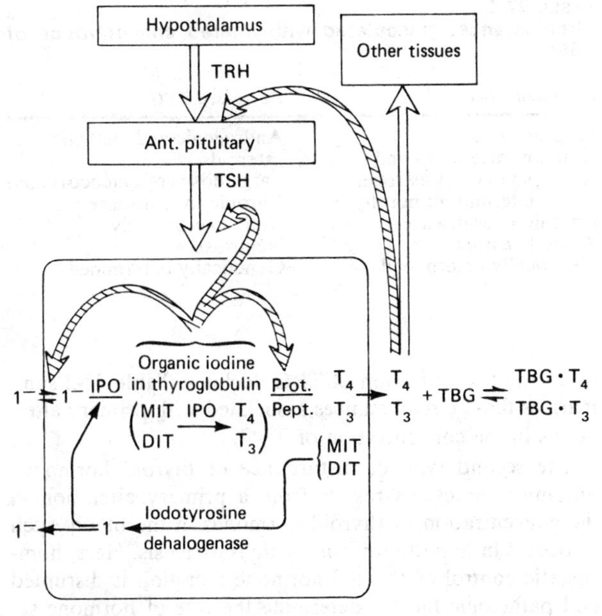

FIGURE 92-2
Schema depicting pathways in the synthesis and secretion of thyroid hormones and mechanisms for the suprathyroidal and intrathyroidal regulation of thyroid function. Small, solid arrows indicate pathways of iodine metabolism; open arrows indicate stimulation; crosshatched arrows indicate inhibitory influences. TRH, thyrotropin-releasing hormone; TSH, thyroid-stimulating hormone; IPO, iodide peroxidase; prot., thyroid protease; peptid., thyroid peptidase; MIT, monoiodotyrosine; DIT, diiodotyrosine; T_4*, thyroxine;* T_3*, 3,5,3′-triiodothyronine.*

second step in hormone biosynthesis involves oxidation of iodide to a higher valence form, as yet undetermined, that is capable of iodinating tyrosyl residues in thyroglobulin, a glycoprotein of approximately 650,000 molecular weight that is synthesized within the follicular epithelium. Oxidation of iodide is effected by an iodide peroxidase, which utilizes hydrogen peroxide generated during the course of oxidative metabolism within the gland. Organic iodinations, which occur at or near the apex of the cell, result in the formation of the peptide-bound, hormonally inactive precursors, monoiodotyrosine (MIT) and diiodotyrosine (DIT). Subsequently, these iodotyrosines undergo oxidative condensation, again through the mediation of peroxidase. This so-called "coupling reaction" occurs within the thyroglobulin molecule and yields a variety of iodothyronines, including T_4 and T_3. Although minute quantities of thyroglobulin are detectable in the blood of normal patients and those with thyroid disease, the vast bulk of thyroglobulin is retained for a time within the gland, serving as a storage form of thyroid hormone, or "prohormone." Liberation of the active hormones into the blood, forming the third step in hormone synthesis and release, involves pinocytosis of follicular colloid at the apical margin of the cells to form colloid droplets. These fuse with thyroid lysosomes to form "phagolysosomes," in which thyroglobulin is hydrolyzed by proteases and peptidases. The final step is release of the now-free iodothyronines, T_4 and T_3, into the blood, while the inactive iodotyrosines are stripped of their iodine by an intrathyroidal enzyme, iodotyrosine dehalogenase. Normally, iodide liberated thereby is largely reutilized in the synthesis of hormone, but a small proportion is normally lost into the blood (iodide leak); this proportion may become very large in abnormal circumstances.

As with iodide, the thyroid is capable of concentrating other monovalent anions. Notable among these is the pertechnetate ion, which is available as the radioactive isotope, sodium pertechnetate Tc 99m. Unlike iodide, little pertechnetate is organically bound; hence, its duration of stay within the thyroid is short. This property, together with its short physical half-life, makes pertechnetate a highly valuable radionuclide for imaging the thyroid with scintillation scanning techniques.

The foregoing reactions are subject to inhibition by a variety of chemical compounds. Such agents are generally termed *goitrogens,* since, by virtue of their ability to inhibit hormone synthesis and indirectly stimulate TSH secretion, they induce goiter formation. Certain inorganic anions, notably perchlorate and thiocyanate, inhibit the iodide transport mechanism and thereby reduce available substrate for hormone formation. The goiter and hypothyroidism that follow, however, can be prevented or relieved by doses of iodide sufficiently large to enable adequate quantities to enter the gland by simple diffusion. The commonly employed antithyroid agents, such as the derivatives of thiourea and mercaptoimidazole, exert more complex actions upon pathways of hormone biosynthesis. These agents, as well as certain aniline derivatives, inhibit the initial oxidation (organic binding) of iodide, decrease the proportion of DIT relative to MIT, and block coupling of iodotyrosines to form the hormonally active iodothyronines. The latter reaction is the most sensitive. Thus, it is possible for the synthesis of hormonally active iodothyronines to be decreased greatly, although the total incorporation of iodine by the thyroid is inhibited but little. In contradistinction to the effect of the monovalent anions, the goitrogenic action of inhibitors of organic binding is not overcome by large quantities of iodine. Indeed, certain weak goitrogens, such as sulfonamides and antipyrine, are rendered more potent when given with iodide, an effect not clearly understood. Iodine itself, when given acutely in large doses, is capable of blocking the organic-binding and coupling reactions. This action (Wolff-Chaikoff effect) is normally transient. In a small proportion of seemingly normal individuals, however, prolonged administration of iodide is associated with continued inhibition of hormone synthesis and development of goiter, with (iodide myxedema) or without hypothyroidism. A large proportion of patients with Graves' disease especially after treatment with radioiodine or surgery and also patients with Hashimoto's disease are inordinately sensitive to the blocking effect of iodide and, when given iodides chronically, develop hypothyroidism. Iodides in large doses are capable of inhibiting proteolysis of thyroglobulin and hormone release, an effect which is most readily demonstrable in hyperfunctioning thyroids and which is responsible for the rapid ameliorative action of iodides in most patients with hyperthyroidism. Lithium, which is administered as the carbonate salt in some patients with depressive states, has a variety of effects on intrathyroidal iodine metabolism. Among these is an action to inhibit hormone release. Thus, like iodides, it can be employed to effect a rapid reduction in the degree of thyrotoxicosis in patients with the hyperthyroidism of Graves' disease.

TRANSPORT AND METABOLISM In the blood, T_4 and T_3 are almost entirely bound to plasma proteins. Electrophoretic analyses indicate that T_4 is bound, in decreasing order of intensity, to an inter-alpha-globulin, termed thyroxine- or thyronine-binding globulin (TBG), to a T_4-binding prealbumin (TBPA), and to albumin. By virtue of its intense affinity for T_4, TBG is by far the major determinant of overall binding intensity. The interaction between T_4 and its binding proteins conforms to a reversible binding equilibrium in which the majority of the hormone is bound and a very small proportion (normally less than 0.05 percent) is free. T_3 is not significantly bound by TBPA and is bound by TBG less firmly than is T_4. As a consequence, the proportion of free T_3 is normally eight to ten times greater than that of T_4. It appears likely that only the free or unbound hormone is available to tissues; therefore, the metabolic state of the patient will correlate more closely with the concentration of free than with the total concentration of hormone in plasma. Furthermore, homeostatic regulation of thyroid function will be directed toward maintenance of a normal concentration of free rather than total hormone. Moreover, the relatively weak binding of T_3 accounts for its failure to contribute materially to the total hormonal iodine concentration in the blood and possibly for its more rapid onset and offset of action. Disturbances of the thyroid hormone–plasma protein interaction are of two general types (see Table 92-1). In the first, the thyroid-pituitary axis is intrinsically normal, and the homeostatic control of thyroid hormone secretion is intact. Under these circumstances, disordered binding interactions result from primary alterations in the concentration of TBG. For example, an increase in TBG will initially lower the concentration of free hormone and thus diminish the quantity of hormone available to tissues. Total hormone concentration in serum will then increase until the concentration of free hormone is restored to normal. At this time, the proportions of T_4 and T_3 that are free will be decreased. The increase in total hormone concentration counterbalances the decrease in the proportion free; as a result, the absolute concentration of free hormone is normal and the metabolic state of the patient is unchanged. Converse changes occur when the concentration of TBG declines. Table 92-2 summarizes those circumstances associated with primary alterations in the concentration of TBG.

TABLE 92-1
Classification of the varieties of disordered thyroid hormone–plasma protein interactions

Type of abnormality	*Serum T_4*	*Percent free T_4 or resin T_3 uptake*	*Free T_4 conc. or T_4-RT_3 index*
1 Primary abnormality in thyroxine-binding proteins			
a Increased binding	↑	↓	N
b Decreased binding	↓	↑	N
2 Primary disorder of thyroid function			
a Hypothyroidism	↓	↓	↓
b Hyperthyroidism	↑	↑	↑

TABLE 92-2
Circumstances associated with altered concentration of TBG

Increased TBG	*Decreased TBG*
Pregnancy	Androgenic and anabolic steroids
Oral contraceptives and other sources of estrogen	Large doses of glucocorticoid
Acute intermittent porphyria	Chronic liver disease
Chronic liver disease	Active acromegaly
Acute hepatitis	Nephrosis
Genetically determined	Genetically determined

The second type of disturbance of thyroid hormone–binding interactions results from a primary alteration in the concentration of thyroid hormones in the blood, such as occurs in hypothyroidism or thyrotoxicosis. Here, homeostatic control of thyroid hormone secretion is disrupted and pathologic factors determine the rate of hormone secretion independent of the thyroid-pituitary axis. Under these circumstances, the concentration of TBG is changed little, if at all, and the concentration of free hormone will vary directly with the total concentration of hormone. Since such changes in circulating hormone usually result from intrinsic disease of the pituitary or thyroid itself, homeostatic mechanisms cannot restore the concentration of free hormone to normal. Primary changes in thyroid function are therefore associated with persistent changes in the concentration of both total and free hormone, and, consequently, with alterations in the metabolic state of the patient. In these disorders, the relative change in the concentration of free hormone is greater than the change in total hormone concentration.

Following their penetration into the cell, T_4 and T_3 undergo a variety of reactions which lead ultimately to their excretion or inactivation. As judged from experiments with isotopically labeled hormones, the major pathway of hormone metabolism is removal of iodine (deiodination). This general pathway is present in all tissues tested, leaves the diphenyl ether link of the thyronine nucleus intact, and accounts for approximately 80 percent of T_4 and T_3 disposal. Approximately 20 percent of labeled T_4 and T_3 is normally lost in the stool, principally in the form of conjugates with glucuronate or sulfate. Substantial quantities of labeled hormones are excreted in the bile and are presumably available for reabsorption, probably after hydrolysis of conjugates. However, the magnitude of the enterohepatic circulation of T_4 and T_3 in humans is unknown. A small proportion of the hormones undergoes oxidative deamination and decarboxylation of the alanine side chain to yield the acetic acid analogues of T_4 and T_3, tetra- and triiodothyroacetic acids. A more important intermediate product of T_4 metabolism is T_3 itself. Since T_3 appears to be approximately three times more potent than T_4 in many metabolic respects, such monodeiodination of T_4, which can occur in many tissues, yields from T_4 a product of enhanced potency. It appears that approximately 30 percent of T_4 is metabolized via conversion to T_3. This would account for almost all the T_3 produced, indicating that only a small proportion of the T_3 in the blood is derived by direct thyroid secretion. A major clinical implication of this is that athyreotic or hypothyroid patients maintained with synthetic L-thyroxine to a normal value of serum T_4 concentration will have, in addition, nearly normal concentrations of T_3 in their blood. Apparently, a variety of physiologic stresses, such as fasting, surgery, or severe illness, inhibits the peripheral conversion of T_4 to T_3, thereby lowering the serum T_3 concentration but leaving the serum T_4 concentration normal or slightly increased. The effect of these changes on the metabolic state of the patient is as yet uncertain.

Under certain circumstances, changes in the activity of cellular processes involved in hormone metabolism may be the major determinant of changes in the rates of metabolic clearance of T_4 and T_3. Both phenobarbital and diphenylhydantoin increase the metabolic clearance of thyroid hormones without increasing the proportion of free hormone in the blood. Indeed, in the case of diphenylhydantoin, both total and free T_4 concentrations are diminished. Nevertheless, a normal metabolic state is maintained, possibly owing to stimulation of the conversion of T_4 to T_3. The effects of these agents are doubtless related to the hypertrophy of smooth endoplasmic reticulum and increased activity of varied microsomal enzymes that they induce.

REGULATION OF THYROID FUNCTION Regulation of thyroid function is effected by two general mechanisms, one suprathyroidal and one intrathyroidal (Fig. 92-2). The proximate mediator of suprathyroidal regulation is thyrotropin or thyroid-stimulating hormone (TSH), a glycopeptide secreted by basophilic cells within the anterior pituitary gland. TSH stimulates thyroid hypertrophy and hyperplasia; accelerates most aspects of glandular intermediary metabolism; enhances synthesis of nucleic acid and protein, including thyroglobulin; and stimulates all steps in thyroid iodine metabolism leading to the synthesis and secretion of thyroid hormones. These actions are thought to be mediated, at least in large part, by increased synthesis of the "second messenger," cyclic 3′5′-adenosine monophosphate.

Regulation of TSH secretion, in turn, is effected by two opposing influences. TRH (thyrotropin-releasing hormone), a tripeptide amide (pyroglutamyl-histidyl-prolineamide) secreted in the ventromedial hypothalamus, reaches the pituitary via the hypophyseal portal capillary system and there stimulates synthesis and secretion of TSH. These effects of TRH are inhibited, however, by the extent of thyroid hormone action within the pituitary, and this is presumed to be closely related to the concentration of free thyroid hormones in the blood. Thus, negative feedback of thyroid hormones on TSH secretion occurs mainly in the pituitary gland itself; in what manner and to what extent thyroid hormones affect the secretion of TRH is unknown.

Intrathyroid regulation of thyroid function is less well understood, but is nevertheless important. In some manner as yet undetermined, changes in glandular organic iodine content are associated with reciprocal changes in thyroidal iodide transport activity, as well as in growth, glucose metabolism, and nucleic acid synthesis. Although these influences are evident in the absence of TSH stimulation, and hence may be termed *autoregulatory,* their most important role is to modify (iodine-enrichment inhibiting, and iodine-depletion enhancing) the response of these functions to TSH.

LABORATORY TESTS The availability of a variety of laboratory tests permits evaluation of many aspects of thyroid hormone economy. Such tests can be divided into five major categories: direct tests of thyroid function; tests related to the concentration and binding of thyroid hormones in blood; metabolic indexes; tests of the homeostatic control of thyroid function; and various tests that do not fit into other categories. A system of abbreviations to designate the various laboratory tests has been adopted by the American Thyroid Association and is used herein.

Direct tests of thyroid function The *thyroid radioactive iodine uptake (RAIU)* is the most commonly used test for assessing glandular function per se. The administered radioiodine (usually ^{131}I) mixes uniformly with the endogenous stable iodide and, in the steady state, indicates what percentage of the iodide entering and leaving the iodide space per unit time is accumulated by the thyroid. The RAIU is usually measured 24 h after ^{131}I administration since it usually has reached a plateau value at this time. The RAIU varies inversely with the pool of endogenous stable iodide and directly with the functional state of the thyroid. Over the last decade, the widespread enrichment of bread and table salt with iodine has led to an increase in the endogenous iodide pool, with the result that the normal range for the 24-h RAIU has declined to approximately 5 to 30 percent of the administered dose. Consequently, this test no longer discriminates between normal and hypothyroid states. Values above the normal range, however, indicate thyroid hyperfunction, and remain useful, therefore, in the diagnosis of hyperthyroidism. The RAIU is also used as part of the thyroid suppression test and the TSH stimulation test.

Tests related to hormone concentration and binding in blood The *serum T_4 concentration* is measured by the ability of stable T_4 extracted from serum, as compared with known quantities of T_4, to displace labeled T_4 from a protein mixture containing TBG. By convention, this test has been designated T_4(D). This test is highly specific and is commonly known by the names of its developers (Murphy-Pattee). The normal range for T_4(D) is 4 to 11 μg per 100 ml. In some laboratories T_4(D) is expressed in terms of its iodine content as T_4I(D). This is derived by multiplying T_4(D) by 0.65, the value for the mole fraction of T_4 that is iodine. Thus, in interpreting values of serum T_4, it is important that one be aware of the manner in which the value is expressed. The *serum protein-bound iodine (PBI) concentration* was, until recently, the only method of estimating serum T_4, and such measurement was possible only by virtue of the iodine content of T_4. This test is much less specific than T_4(D), which has superseded it. It is occasionally useful in detecting the presence of abnormal iodoproteins in the blood arising as a result of an intrathyroidal biosynthetic defect, because here the PBI is disproportionately high in relation to the T_4(D). Normal values for the PBI range from 4 to 8 μg per 100 ml. The *serum T_3 concentration* can be measured by radioimmunoassay, abbreviated T_3(RIA); here, the ability of the stable T_3 in serum to displace labeled T_3 from anti-T_3 antibody is compared with that of known quantities of T_3. Normal values range from about 80 to 160 ng per 100 ml.

As mentioned in the previous section, alterations in the concentration of TBG, as well as alterations in hormone secretion, will influence the total concentration of hormone in the blood. However, only alterations in hormone secretion will lead to steady-state alterations in the concentration of free hormone. The *percent of free hormone (percent FT_4* or *percent FT_3)* can be measured by equilibrium dialysis of serum enriched with a tracer quantity of the labeled hormone, and the product of this value and T_4(D) or T_3(RIA) yields the *concentration of free hormone (FT_4* or *FT_3)*. Measurement of percent FT_4 or percent FT_3 is a cumbersome procedure. Hence, for clinical purposes, the *in vitro uptake test* is employed, as it is simple to perform and yields qualitatively the same information. Here, the serum is enriched with labeled hormone and then incubated with an insoluble, particulate material, such as resin or charcoal, that binds hormone. The percent of labeled hormone taken up by the particulate material varies inversely with the concentration of unoccupied binding sites on TBG. Labeled T_3 is employed in preference to labeled T_4 since it is less strongly bound by the serum and hence yields higher and therefore more accurate uptake values. Normal values for the *resin-T_3 uptake (RT_3U)* range from 25 to 35 percent. Results may also be expressed as the quotient of the RT_3U value in the patient's serum and that obtained in a normal control specimen (*RT_3U ratio*). The product of T_4(D) and RT_3U ratio (*T_4-RT_3 index*) provides an index of FT_4. Primary alterations in the concentration of TBG (Table 92-2) produce *reciprocal* alterations in RT_3U and T_4(D), with the result that the T_4-RT_3 index remains normal. By contrast, primary alterations in T_4 secretion produce changes in RT_3U that are in the same direction as those in T_4(D). Hence, the T_4-RT_3 index affords a better discrimination from normal values than either of its component tests alone.

Metabolic indexes These tests measure the metabolic impact of thyroid hormone in the peripheral tissues. The *basal metabolic rate (BMR)* measures energy expenditure in terms of the amount of O_2 consumed in the basal state. Values are expressed as a percentage difference from the mean value for normal individuals of the same age, sex, and body surface area. The normal range is approximately -15 to $+5$ percent. Owing to the variety of nonthyroidal factors that affect the BMR, however, this test is of limited diagnostic value. Increases in the *serum cholesterol concentration* are suggestive of hypothyroidism of thyroidal origin; however, decreases in serum cholesterol concentration are of little value in the diagnosis of thyrotoxicosis. Prolongation of the *Achilles reflex time* as assessed by kinemometry or photomotography, though not pathognomonic, is suggestive of hypothyroidism, but the test has little discriminatory value in hyperthyroidism.

Tests of homeostatic control The measurement of *serum TSH* has become an important tool in the diagnosis of hypothyroidism and diminished thyroid reserve. The latter state represents a stage in the evolution of hypothyroidism in which a structural or functional abnormality that impairs hormone synthesis is compensated for by hypersecretion of TSH and activation of the thyroid. Serum TSH is measured by radioimmunoassay; here, the ability of TSH in serum to displace labeled human TSH from anti-TSH antibody is compared with that of known quantities of human TSH. The normal range is less than 5 μU per ml; current sensitivity does not generally permit distinction between normal or low values. Measurement of serum TSH affords the best means of distinguishing between untreated hypothyroidism of thyroidal origin, in which the values are invariably increased, and pituitary or hypothalamic hypothyroidism, in which the values are usually undetectable and always within the normal range. In thyrotoxicosis, serum TSH is undetectable, except in rare cases of TSH-secreting tumors.

The *TSH stimulation test* is employed as a means of assessing thyroid reserve. Here, the responses of the RAIU and T_4(D) to an intramuscular injection of bovine TSH are monitored. This test is of major value in the diagnosis of diminished thyroid reserve, in which the gland is under maximum stimulation by endogenous TSH and hence shows no further response to exogenous TSH, and in the differentiation of pituitary hypothyroidism from hypothyroidism of primary thyroidal origin. With the general availability of measurements of serum TSH, however, this test is now less frequently used.

The *thyrotropin-releasing hormone (TRH) stimulation test* is a test which may have value for diverse diagnostic purposes. Following the intravenous injection of TRH in normal subjects, the serum TSH begins to rise at 10 min, peaks between 20 and 45 min, and then falls rapidly. Subnormal response to a standard dose, therefore, may reflect diminished pituitary TSH reserve. The response to TRH within the pituitary is inhibited by thyroid hormone, with the result that a supranormal response occurs in patients with hypothyroidism of thyroidal origin, whereas little or no response occurs in patients with thyrotoxicosis. This lack of response also occurs in some patients with autonomously functioning adenomas and in some with apparently euthyroid Graves' disease. Nevertheless, with these two exceptions, a lack of response serves as an excellent confirmatory test for thyrotoxicosis. This test is also of value in the recognition and differential diagnosis of pituitary and hypothalamic hypothyroidism; in the former, but not the latter, disorder, no response to TRH would be expected.

The *thyroid suppression test* is used to assess whether thyroid function is being controlled by normal homeostatic mechanisms. Normally, exogenous thyroid hormone suppresses pituitary TSH secretion, resulting in a decrease in the RAIU. Since liothyronine is usually employed (100 μg daily for 10 days), the resulting decline in T_4(D), as well as in the RAIU, can serve as an index of suppression. A normal suppressive response is a decrease of the RAIU to less than half of the control value and a decline of the T_4(D) to low normal or subnormal values. In patients with increased TBG, the decline in T_4(D) may be delayed. An abnormal suppression test is always present in hyperthyroidism, irrespective of the underlying cause; this indicates either autonomy of thyroid function, the presence of an abnormal stimulator, or, at least theoretically, unremitting hypersecretion of TSH. A normal suppression test, on the other hand, is incompatible with and excludes the presence of hyperthyroidism. An abnormal suppression test does not necessarily indicate the presence of hyperthyroidism, however, since it is seen after treatment of hyperthyroidism in Graves' disease, in about half of the euthyroid patients with the ophthalmopathy of Graves' disease, and in seemingly euthyroid patients in whom an autonomous hyperfunctioning adenoma has suppressed the remainder of the gland.

Miscellaneous tests Tests for circulating antibodies directed against various glandular components are often of diagnostic value. For example, moderate to high titers of an *antithyroglobulin antibody* are found in the serum of most patients with Hashimoto's disease and in a high proportion of patients with either primary thyroprivic hypothyroidism or Graves' disease. In the active phase of Graves' disease, about half the patients have an abnormal thyroid stimulator in serum that differs from TSH in its longer duration of action in the mouse bioassay system; hence its designation *long-acting thyroid stimulator* (LATS). LATS is an immunoglobulin G of lymphoid origin and appears to be an antibody directed against some component of the thyroid cell plasma membrane.

Imaging by *scintiscanning* permits localization of sites of radioiodine or sodium pertechnetate Tc 99m accumulation. This technique is useful for defining areas of increased or decreased function within the thyroid and for detecting retrosternal goiter, ectopic thyroid tissue, and functioning metastases of thyroid carcinoma.

SIMPLE (NONTOXIC) GOITER

There is considerable confusion concerning the descriptive terms *endemic* and *sporadic* goiter. Endemic implies an etiologic factor or factors common to a particular geographic region. The term has been defined as indicating the presence of generalized or localized thyroid enlargement in over 10 percent of the population. The connotation of sporadic is that goiter arises in nonendemic areas as a result of a stimulus that does not affect the population generally. Since these terms fail to define or distinguish the causes of such goiters and since thyroid enlargement of diverse etiology may exist in both endemic and nonendemic regions, it seems prudent to employ a general term such as simple or nontoxic goiter. This all-inclusive category can be further subdivided into specific etiologic groups as defined by objective procedures. Simple or nontoxic goiter may be defined as any enlargement of the thyroid gland that does not result from an inflammatory or neoplastic process and is not initially associated with thyrotoxicosis or myxedema.

ETIOLOGY Although the causes of simple goiter are manifold, their clinical manifestations are thought to reflect the operation of a common physiopathologic mechanism. Simple goiter results when one or more factors impair the capacity of the thyroid gland in the basal state to secrete quantities of active hormones necessary to meet the needs of the peripheral tissues. Although this has been presumed to lead to increased secretion of TSH, concentrations of TSH in the serum of patients with established simple goiter are usually normal. Hence, some other mechanism of goitrogenesis may be operative. A likely possibility is that depletion of glandular organic iodine accompanying impaired hormone synthesis increases the responsiveness of thyroid structure and function to basal levels of TSH. The resulting increases in both functioning thyroid mass and cellular activity are sufficient to overcome mild or moderate impairment of hormone synthesis; thus, the patient remains metabolically normal, though goitrous. When, however, the underlying disorder is severe, compensatory responses, now including hypersecretion of TSH, are inadequate to overcome the impairment, and the patient is both goitrous and more or less severely hypothyroid. Thus, the entity simple goiter cannot be separated clearly, in the pathogenetic sense, from goitrous hypothyroidism. Specific causes of simple goiter are included in Table 92-3 and may exist with or without hypothyroidism.

PATHOLOGY The histopathology of the thyroid in simple goiter varies with the severity of the etiologic factor and the stage of the disorder at which the examination is made. In its initial stages, the gland reveals a uniform hypertrophy, hyperplasia, and hypervascularity. As the disorder persists or undergoes repeated exacerbations and remissions, uniformity of thyroidal architecture is usually lost. Occasionally, the greater part of the gland may display a reasonably uniform degree of involution or hyperinvolution with colloid accumulation. More often such areas are interspersed with patchy areas of focal hyperplasia. Fibrosis may demarcate a variable number of nodules, which may be hyperplastic or involuted. These may resemble, but do not really represent, true neoplasms (adenomas). Areas of hemorrhage and calcification may be present.

CLINICAL PICTURE In simple goiter, the clinical manifestations arise solely from enlargement of the thyroid since the metabolic state of the patient is normal. In goitrous hypothyroidism, symptoms caused by thyromegaly are similarly present, but are accompanied by signs and symptoms of hormonal insufficiency. Mechanical sequelae include compression and displacement of the trachea or esophagus, occasionally with obstructive symptoms if the goiter becomes sufficiently large. Superior mediastinal obstruction may occur with large retrosternal goiters. Signs of compression can be induced in the case of large retrosternal goiters when the patient's arms are raised above the head (Pemberton's sign); suffusion of the face, giddiness, or syncope may result from this maneuver. Compression of the recurrent laryngeal nerve leading to hoarseness is rare

TABLE 92-3
Classification of the causes of hypothyroidism

- *I* Thyroidal
  - *A* Thyroprivic
    - *1* Congenital development defect
    - *2* Primary idiopathic
    - *3* Postablative (radioiodine, surgery)
  - *B* Goitrous
    - *1* Heritable biosynthetic defects
    - *2* Maternally transmitted (iodides, antithyroid agents)
    - *3* Iodine deficiency
    - *4* Drug-elicited (para-aminosalicylic acid, iodides, phenylbutazone, iodoantipyrine, cobalt)
    - *5* Chronic thyroiditis (Hashimoto's disease)
- *II* Suprathyroidal (trophoprivic)
  - *A* Pituitary
  - *B* Hypothalamic

in simple goiter and suggests neoplasm. Sudden hemorrhage into a nodule may lead to an acute, painful swelling in the neck and may produce or enhance compressive symptoms. Hyperthyroidism not uncommonly supervenes in long-standing multinodular goiter (toxic multinodular goiter). It is not known whether this represents the superimposition of Graves' disease upon a chronic nontoxic goiter or a separate disease entity. In both endemic and sporadic multinodular goiter, the ingestion of excess iodide may result in the development of thyrotoxicosis.

In geographic regions where iodine deficiency is severe, acquired goitrous enlargement may also be associated with varying degrees of hypothyroidism. Cretinism, both goitrous and nongoitrous, occurs with increased frequency in the children of goitrous parents and contributes a significant sector of the socially dependent population in many countries where goiter is common. Although iodine deficiency is doubtless a necessary factor in the etiology of endemic goiter, the frequency of goiter may differ greatly among areas of equally severe iodine deficiency. In such instances, dietary or water-borne goitrogens appear to be important conditioning factors.

DIAGNOSIS The diagnosis of simple goiter requires, first, demonstration of a normal metabolic state and, second, differentiation of the goitrous condition from Hashimoto's disease or thyroid neoplasia. Physical examination alone cannot serve to make the diagnosis. A careful history is important, particularly with respect to the occurrence of thyroid pain or tenderness, rapid change in size, hoarseness, or previous drug ingestion. High titers of circulating antithyroglobulin antibodies (tanned red cell agglutinins > 1/25,000) indicate Hashimoto's disease. Needle biopsy may occasionally be indicated to make or exclude the diagnosis of Hashimoto's disease. In areas where goiter is endemic, high values for the RAIU and low values for urinary iodine excretion are the common pattern. Low normal or subnormal values for T_4(D) are commonly found, even in the absence of hypothyroidism. In such cases, high values for serum T_3(RIA) apparently account for the normal metabolic (eumetabolic) state.

TREATMENT The object of treatment is to remove the thyroidal hyperplasia, either by relieving external encumbrances to hormone formation or by providing sufficient quantities of exogenous hormone to inhibit TSH secretion and thereby put the thyroid gland almost completely at rest. In disorders characterized by decreased thyroidal iodide stores, such as iodine deficiency or impairment of the thyroidal iodide-concentrating mechanism, small doses of iodide may prove effective. Occasionally, a known extrinsic goitrogen can be withdrawn. Most commonly, however, no specific etiologic factor can be detected, and suppressive thyroid therapy is required. For this purpose, sodium L-thyroxine (levothyroxine) in a dose of 200 μg daily is the agent of choice. Suppression of endogenous thyroid function is most readily assessed by serial measurements of the 24-h RAIU. Functional suppression is indicated when the RAIU decreases to very low values. Lesser decreases indicate only partial suppression. In multinodular nontoxic goiter, lack of complete suppression usually indicates the presence of autonomously functioning foci, demonstrable by scanning techniques. RAIU tests can be performed at appropriate intervals, and the dose of exogenous hormone gradually adjusted as needed to achieve maximum suppression. Occasionally, physiologic replacement doses of exogenous hormones will induce mild, but usually transient, symptoms of thyrotoxicity. In such patients, more prolonged intervals between dosage changes will usually permit achievement of full thyroid suppression without inducing symptoms of toxicity.

Reported results of therapy vary widely. There is general agreement that the early diffuse, hyperplastic goiter responds well, with regression or disappearance in 3 to 6 months. In the authors' experience, the later, nodular stage responds less favorably, and significant reduction in gland size is achieved only in about one-third of the cases. Internodular tissue regresses more often than do nodules themselves. The latter may therefore become more prominent during treatment. After maximum regression of the goiter, suppressive medication may be maintained for prolonged periods, reduced to minimal levels, or at times withdrawn. In an unpredictable manner, goiter will in some cases remain relieved while in others it will recur. In the latter instances, suppressive therapy should be reinstituted and should be continued indefinitely. When treatment is initiated in patients of childbearing age, it should probably be continued through the menopause.

In areas of endemic iodine deficiency, the size and prevalence of goiter, and probably the frequency of cretinism, can be reduced by the infrequent injection of iodized oil.

Surgical therapy of simple goiter is physiologically unsound, but it may occasionally be necessary to relieve obstructive symptoms, especially those which persist after a conscientious trial of medical therapy. Surgical exploration of nodular goiter may be indicated in some individuals when evidence suggests carcinoma. However, the suggestion that subtotal resection of multinodular nontoxic goiter affords effective prophylaxis against the development of thyroid carcinoma is unsound. If for some reason subtotal thyroidectomy has been performed, levothyroxine in a dose of 150 to 200 μg daily is recommended to inhibit regenerative hyperplasia and further goitrogenesis.

HYPOTHYROIDISM

Hypothyroidism is a clinical state that may result from any of a wide variety of structural or functional abnormalities that lead to insufficient synthesis of thyroid hormone. Hypothyroidism dating from birth and resulting in developmental abnormalities is termed *cretinism*. The term *myxedema* connotes a severe form of hypothyroidism in which there is accumulation of hydrophilic mucopolysaccharides in the ground substance of the dermis as well as other tissues, leading to thickening of the facial features and doughy induration of the skin.

ETIOLOGY A classification of the causes of hypothyroidism is presented in Table 92-3. In thyroprivic hypothyroidism, loss of thyroid tissue leads to inadequate synthesis of thyroid hormone, despite maximum stimulation of any thyroid remnant by TSH. The most common cause of thyroprivic hypothyroidism is surgical or radioiodine ablation of the thyroid gland in the treatment of Graves' disease. Thyroprivic hypothyroidism may also occur as a primary idiopathic phenomenon. The cause of this disorder is unknown, but the frequency of circulating thyroid antibodies and its coexistence with pernicious anemia and other diseases in which circulating antibodies are found suggest that it may belong to the autoimmune group of diseases. Finally, a developmental defect may result in failure of the gland to gain an adequate size, leading to sporadic nongoitrous cretinism or juvenile hypothyroidism.

Impaired functional ability to synthesize adequate quantities of thyroid hormone leads to hypersecretion of TSH and hence goiter. If this compensatory response is inadequate, goitrous hypothyroidism ensues. The commonest cause in North America is Hashimoto's disease, in which defective organic binding of iodide and abnormal secretion of iodoproteins are frequent biosynthetic abnormalities. Iodide-induced goiter with or without hypothyroidism appears to arise from an intrinsic defect in the organic binding mechanism which permits a persistent Wolff-Chaikoff effect. Patients with Graves' disease, especially after radioiodine treatment, those with Hashimoto's disease, and the normal fetus are particularly susceptible to iodide-induced goiter. In view of the susceptibility of the fetal thyroid to iodide, with resulting goiter and hypothyroidism, women should not be given iodine in large doses during pregnancy. Less common causes of goitrous hypothyroidism are heritable defects in pathways of hormone biosynthesis and ingestion of drugs which induce defects in hormone biosynthesis, such as para-aminosalicylic acid, cobalt, and lithium carbonate. Finally, in many areas of the world where there is environmental iodine deficiency, goitrous cretinism and hypothyroidism occur on an endemic basis. Diminished thyroid reserve occurs as a stage in the evolution of both thyroprivic and goitrous hypothyroidism.

In hypothyroidism of suprathyroidal origin, the thyroid is intrinsically normal, but is deprived of stimulation by TSH. Deprivation of TSH, most commonly the result of post-partum pituitary necrosis or a tumor of the pituitary or adjacent regions, results in pituitary hypothyroidism. Hypothalamic hypothyroidism appears to be less common and results from inadequate secretion of TRH.

CLINICAL PICTURE The general appearance of children with hypothyroidism varies considerably, depending on the age at which the deficiency began and the promptness with which replacement therapy was instituted. Manifestations of cretinism may be present at birth, but are more commonly evident within the first several months, depending upon the extent of thyroid failure. During the neonatal period, the abnormally long persistence of physiologic jaundice, hoarse cry, constipation, somnolence, and feeding problems should call attention to the diagnosis. In later months, delay in reaching the normal milestones of development becomes evident, and the physical characteristics of the cretin appear. These include short stature, coarse features with protruding tongue, broad flat nose, widely set eyes, sparse hair, dry skin, and protuberant abdomen with an umbilical hernia. X-ray examination reveals retarded bone age, epiphyseal dysgenesis, and delayed dental development. Mental development is retarded; eventual intellectual attainment will depend upon how soon full replacement therapy is instituted.

In the older child with hypothyroidism, the clinical manifestations are intermediate between those of infantile and adult hypothyroidism. Retardation of linear growth results in shortness of stature, while retardation of sexual maturation results in delay in the onset of puberty. Poor performance at school may call attention to the diagnosis. The manifestations of adult hypothyroidism are present to a variable degree. X-ray examination reveals delayed union of the epiphyses.

In the adult, early symptoms of hypothyroidism are nonspecific and of insidious onset. They may include lethargy, constipation, cold intolerance, and menorrhagia. Over the succeeding months, slowing of intellectual and motor activity appears, appetite declines, and modest weight gain occurs. The hair becomes dry and tends to fall out. The patient may complain of dry skin and of stiff, aching muscles. The voice becomes deeper and hoarse and auditory acuity may deteriorate. Ultimately, the clinical picture of florid myxedema appears, with dull expressionless face, sparse hair, periorbital puffiness, large tongue, and pale, cool skin which feels rough and doughy. Thyroid tissue is not readily palpable, except in the goitrous variety of hypothyroidism. The heart is enlarged owing to both dilation and pericardial effusion; if the heart is small, pituitary hypothyroidism should be considered. Adynamic ileus may occur, producing the clinical picture of megacolon. Rarely, psychiatric reactions may dominate the clinical picture. The relaxation phase of the deep tendon reflexes is characteristically prolonged, the so-called "hung-up" reflex. If left untreated, the patient with severe long-standing hypothyroidism may pass into a hypothermic, stuporous state (*myxedema coma*), which is frequently fatal. Respiratory depression is an important component of this state, and hence an increased arterial $P\text{CO}_2$ is of premonitory value. Factors which predispose to myxedema coma include cold exposure, trauma, infection, and administration of central nervous system depressants. Dilutional hyponatremia is common in severe hypothyroidism and results from diminished renal perfusion leading to impaired water excretion.

LABORATORY TESTS A decrease in T_4(D) and in the T_4-RT_3 index is common to all varieties of hypothyroidism, as is a decrease in BMR. In the thyroidal varieties, the T_3(RIA) may be decreased to a lesser extent than is the T_4(D), the presumption being that the compensatory hypersecretion of TSH leads to a relative preponderance of T_3 secretion. Because of the decline in the range of normal values, the RAIU is no longer of value in the diagnosis of thyroprivic hypothyroidism, unless it is used as a part of the TSH-stimulation test. In goitrous hypothyroidism, the RAIU may be increased or may display an abnormal pattern of accumulation or retention. The serum TSH is invariably increased in the thyroprivic and goitrous varieties and is normal or undetectable in pituitary or hypothalamic hypothyroidism. In the latter varieties, in addition to possible evidence of intracranial disease, hyposecretion of TSH is accompanied by hyposecretion of other pituitary hormones; this is amenable to laboratory testing (see Chap. 90). A subnormal response of the serum TSH to the administration of TRH will confirm the presence of pituitary hypothyroidism.

Other frequent, but not invariable, manifestations of the hypothyroid state include an increased serum cholesterol in hypothyroidism of thyroidal (but not pituitary) origin, an abnormally prolonged relaxation time of the Achilles reflex, and increased concentrations in serum of creatine phosphokinase, glutamic oxaloacetic transaminase, and lactic dehydrogenase. Electrocardiographic changes are common and include bradycardia, low amplitude, and flattened or inverted T waves. In primary thyroprivic hypothyroidism, overt pernicious anemia reportedly occurs in about 12 percent of patients; histamine-fast achlorhydria and the presence of circulating gastric parietal cell antibodies are even more common.

In addition to patients who are clinically hypothyroid, some patients who appear clinically euthyroid display low values of T_4(D). In such patients, T_3(RIA) is normal or near normal and serum TSH is slightly increased. This phenomenon of T_3-euthyroidism, which is seen most frequently in patients with Hashimoto's or Graves' disease who have been treated with radioiodine, represents in all likelihood a phase in the evolution of frank hypothyroidism. As such, it may be considered as representing a state of diminished reserve in which compensatory hypersecretion of TSH evokes a relative hypersecretion of T_3.

DIFFERENTIAL DIAGNOSIS Little difficulty will be experienced in diagnosing the classic picture of cretinism or juvenile and adult hypothyroidism. Occasionally, a mongoloid infant may be confused with a cretin. However, the characteristic mongoloid eyes, Brushfield's spots in the iris, hyperextensibility of the joints, and normal skin and hair texture distinguish the mongoloid imbecile from the hypothyroid cretin. Chronic nephritis and especially nephrosis may simulate myxedema, particularly because of the facial puffiness and pallor. The nephrotic patient may also display anemia, hypercholesterolemia, and anasarca. Since both the BMR and T_4(D) are often subnormal, the differential diagnosis may be confusing. However, the low T_4(D) is caused by a decrease in plasma protein binding resulting from proteinuria; hence, the T_4-RT_3 index will be normal. Moreover, the RAIU is generally normal or increased.

Treatment Two general types of preparation are available for the treatment of hypothyroidism, synthetic hormone and thyroprotein derived from animal thyroids. Synthetic hormones include L-thyroxine sodium (levothyroxine), L-triiodothyronine sodium (liothyronine), and a combination of the two (liotrix). The preparation of natural origin most commonly used is Thyroid Extract, USP. The approximate therapeutic equivalence of these drugs is presented in Table 92-4. Because of their uniform potency, the authors prefer the synthetic preparations, and of these the authors prefer levothyroxine. Unlike liothyronine, liotrix, and even thyroid extract, its ingestion does not lead to abrupt increases in serum T_3 concentration, which could be dangerous in the older patient or in the patient with coexisting heart disease.

In most instances, restoration of a normal metabolic state should be undertaken gradually, especially in the elderly or the patient with heart disease, since sudden increases in metabolic rate may tax cardiac reserve. In adults, an initial daily dose of 25 μg levothyroxine is recommended, and this can be increased by 25- to 50-μg increments at 2- to 3-week intervals, until a normal metabolic state is attained. The daily dose usually necessary to sustain a normal metabolic state is from 150 to 200 μg, and this is usually accompanied by a T_4(D) at the upper limit of the normal range. Because of its long half-life, levothyroxine is generally administered as a single daily dose. The optimum dose for the individual patient should be based on clinical criteria, the T_4(D) being employed only as a confirmatory test.

In cretinism and juvenile hypothyroidism it is essential that full replacement therapy be begun as soon as possible; otherwise the chances of normal intellectual development and growth are poor. Infants and children require doses of levothyroxine that are disproportionately large in relation to body size. *In pituitary and hypothalamic hypothyroidism, thyroid replacement should not be instituted until treatment with cortisone acetate has been initiated,* since acute adrenocortical insufficiency may be precipitated by an increase in metabolic rate.

In some cases, it is important that hypothyroidism be rapidly treated. These include patients with myxedema coma and, because of the extreme sensitivity to central nervous system depressants, hypothyroid patients being prepared for emergency surgery. Here, intravenous administration of levothyroxine, in conjunction with the use of glucocorticoids, is indicated.

GRAVES' DISEASE

Graves' disease, also known as Parry's or Basedow's disease, is a disorder of unknown etiology with a characteristic triad of major manifestations: hyperthyroidism with diffuse goiter, ophthalmopathy, and dermopathy. Although considered part of the same disease complex, the three major manifestations need not appear together. Indeed, one or two need never appear, and, moreover, the three tend to run a course largely independent of one another. Although hyperthyroidism is the most common manifestation of Graves' disease, it is important to be aware of the fact that this symptom complex, which merely reflects an excessive supply of thyroid hormone to the tissues, can also arise in a variety of other circumstances which are clearly distinct from Graves' disease, as is discussed below.

INCIDENCE Graves' disease is a relatively common disorder which may occur at any age, but occurs especially in the third and fourth decades. The disease is much more frequent in women than in men. In nongoitrous areas the ratio of predominance in women may be as high as 7:1. In endemic goitrous areas the ratio is lower. Hyperthyroidism is comparatively rare in children. When it occurs, there is usually a diffuse goiter free of nodules. There is a distinct

TABLE 92-4
Approximate therapeutic equivalence of various thyroid hormone preparations

Preparation	*Average daily oral maintenance dose*	*Serum T_4*
Thyroid extract, USP	120–180 mg	Normal
Levothyroxine	200 μg	Normal or slightly increased
Liothyronine	50 μg	Decreased
Liotrix ($T_4/T_3 = 4/1$)	2 units	Normal

familial predisposition to Graves' disease; in addition, among family members of patients with Graves' disease, a clinical and immunological overlap exists with respect to Hashimoto's disease, primary thyroprivic hypothyroidism, and pernicious anemia.

ETIOLOGY The cause of Graves' disease is unknown. In view of the varied manifestations of Graves' disease and their differing courses, it is possible, and indeed likely, that no single factor is responsible for the entire syndrome. With respect to hyperthyroidism, it is apparent that central to this disorder is a disruption of homeostatic mechanisms that normally adjust hormone secretion to meet the needs of peripheral tissues; if such were able to operate, hyperthyroidism could not be sustained. In the past, it was suggested that this homeostatic disruption resulted from either overproduction of TSH or development of autonomous hyperfunction within the thyroid itself. More recently, attention has been focused on the etiologic role of a protein that under appropriate bioassay conditions can be demonstrated in the serum of approximately half the thyrotoxic patients with Graves' disease and to date has been convincingly demonstrated to be present only in this disorder and in some euthyroid relatives of patients with this disorder. Like TSH, this protein stimulates hormone release (a property employed in its assay), increases thyroid ^{131}I uptake, stimulates several aspects of thyroid intermediary metabolism, increases the activity of thyroid adenyl cyclase, and is capable of inducing thyroid hyperplasia. As noted above, it is known as the *long-acting thyroid stimulator (LATS),* since, in the bioassay system employed in its measurement, its action is more prolonged than that of TSH. LATS is an immunoglobulin G, the activity of which is retained in the Fab fragment. It can be synthesized by the lymphocytes of patients with Graves' disease. Although the nature of the presumed thyroid antigen is unknown, these findings suggest that LATS is an antibody to some cytologic component of human thyroid. If so, Graves' disease should be included among those disorders associated with, if not necessarily caused by, autoimmune phenomena. Despite its capacity to reproduce in the thyroid of animals many of the features of diffuse toxic goiter, titers of LATS in patients' serums do not correlate well with the presence or absence of thyrotoxicosis or with its degree of severity. Moreover, significant titers of LATS are sometimes associated with normal suppressibility of thyroid function. The latter finding, in particular, makes it unlikely that LATS can alone account for the characteristic features of diffuse toxic goiter in humans. Recent studies have provided evidence that the serums of most patients with Graves' disease contain an immunoglobulin G that is stimulatory for human, but not mouse, thyroid tissue. This material has been termed *LATS protector,* since it appears to prevent the absorption of LATS from serum by thyroid particulates in vitro. Some authorities believe that these humoral antibodies are an epiphenomenon, and that Graves' disease is caused by cell-mediated immunity, but evidence for this view is tentative.

Very little is known of the etiology of the ophthalmopathic component of Graves' disease. In many patients with progressive infiltrative ophthalmopathy, the serum contains one or more factors that cause exophthalmos in the recipient animal (goldfish or Atlantic minnow) or increased uptake of radioactive sulfate in the introrbital Harderian gland of the guinea pig or mouse. Although distinguishable from LATS, the latter factor also may be an immunoglobulin. A product of the peptic digestion of TSH has also been shown to have exophthalmogenic activity in assay systems, but its relation to the pathogenesis of ophthalmopathy is also uncertain. Nothing is known of the etiology of the dermopathy of Graves' disease.

PATHOLOGY In Graves' disease, the *thyroid gland* is diffusely enlarged, soft, and vascular. The essential pathology is that of parenchymatous hypertrophy and hyperplasia, characterized by increased height of the epithelium and redundancy of the follicular wall, giving the picture of papillary infoldings and cytologic evidence of increased activity. Such hyperplasia is usually accompanied by lymphocytic infiltration that may reflect the cell-mediated immune origin of the disease or may merely reflect associated chronic thyroiditis. Following iodine medication, there is colloid storage, which sometimes causes enlargement and increased firmness of the gland. Graves' disease is associated with generalized lymphoid hyperplasia and infiltration, and occasionally with enlargement of the spleen or thymus. Thyrotoxicosis may lead to degeneration of skeletal muscle fibers, enlargement of the heart, fatty infiltration or diffuse fibrosis of the liver, decalcification of the skeleton, and loss of body tissue (including fat deposits, osteoid, and muscle).

The *ophthalmopathy* of Graves' disease is characterized pathologically by an inflammatory infiltrate of the orbital contents, exclusive of the glove, with lymphocytes, mast cells, and plasma cells being the predominant cellular components. The orbital musculature is mainly involved and often is greatly enlarged, largely accounting for the increased volume of the orbital contents that causes the globe to protrude. Muscle fibers show degeneration and loss of striations, with ultimate fibrosis.

The *dermopathy* of Graves' disease is characterized by thickening of the dermis, which is infiltrated with lymphocytes and with hydrophilic, metachromatically staining mucopolysaccharides.

CLINICAL PICTURE The clinical picture of patients with Graves' disease varies according to the type of manifestations present and their individual severity. It is also modified by the age of the patient and the presence of underlying disease in other organs, particularly the heart.

Hyperthyroidism Common manifestations of hyperthyroidism in Graves' disease include goiter, fine tremor (especially of the extended fingers and tongue), increased nervousness, as well as emotional instability, excessive sweating and heat intolerance, palpitations, and hyperkinesis. Loss of weight and of strength usually exist, often despite increased appetite. Weakness is often manifested by difficulty in climbing stairs. When severe wasting of limb-girdle musculature is present, the condition is termed *thyrotoxic myopathy.* Hyperdefecation and occasionally anorexia, nausea, and vomiting may occur. Dyspnea, atrial arrhythmias, and, in individuals over the age of forty, cardiac failure occur not infrequently. Oligomenorrhea and amenorrhea are commoner than menorrhagia. In general, nervous symptoms dominate the clinical picture in younger individuals, whereas cardiovascular and myopathic symptoms predominate in older subjects.

The skin is warm and moist with a velvety texture, and palmar erythema is often found. The hair is fine and silky. Occasionally, increased loss of hair from the temporal aspects of the scalp may be noted. Excessive melanin pigmentation or patches of vitiligo are not uncommon. *Ocular signs* include a characteristic stare with widened palpebral fissures, infrequent blinking, lid lag, failure of convergence, and failure to wrinkle the brow on upward gaze. These signs are thought to result from sympathetic overstimulation and usually subside when the thyrotoxicosis is corrected. The *infiltrative ophthalmopathy* characteristic of Graves' disease is discussed below.

The *diffuse toxic goiter* may be asymmetric and lobular. Often a bruit is heard directly over the gland. When heard, it usually signifies that the patient is thyrotoxic, but it may also rarely be present in association with other disorders in which the thyroid is markedly hyperplastic. Venous hums and carotid souffles should be distinguished from true thyroid bruits. A hyperplastic pyramidal lobe of the thyroid may often be palpable if carefully sought.

Cardiovascular findings include a wide pulse pressure, sinus tachycardia, atrial arrhythmias (especially atrial fibrillation), systolic murmurs, increased intensity of the apical first sound, cardiac enlargement, and at times, overt heart failure. A to-and-fro, high-pitched sound may be audible in the pulmonic area and may simulate a pericardial friction rub.

Ophthalmopathy The clinical signs associated with the ophthalmopathy of Graves' disease may be divided into two components: the spastic and the mechanical. The former includes the stare, lid lag, and lid retraction that accompany thyrotoxicosis and account for the "frightened" facies and classic eye signs previously described. These findings need not be associated with actual proptosis and usually return to normal after appropriate correction of thyrotoxicosis. The mechanical component includes proptosis of varying degrees with ophthalmoplegia and congestive oculopathy characterized by chemosis, conjunctivitis, marked periorbital swelling, and the resultant complications of corneal ulceration, optic neuritis, and optic atrophy. When exophthalmos progresses rapidly and becomes the major concern in Graves' disease, it is usually referred to as *progressive,* and if severe, *malignant exophthalmos.* The term *exophthalmic ophthalmoplegia* refers to the ocular muscle weakness that so commonly accompanies this disorder and results in strabismus with varying degrees of diplopia. Exophthalmos may be unilateral early in the course of the disorder but usually progresses to symmetric involvement.

Dermopathy The dermopathy of Graves' disease usually occurs over the dorsum of the legs or feet and is commonly termed *localized myxedema* or *pretibial myxedema.* It occurs in patients with past or present Graves' disease and is not a manifestation of hypothyroidism per se. About half of the cases occur during the active stage of thyrotoxicosis; in the remainder the lesions develop after treatment. The affected area is usually well demarcated from normal skin by the fact that it is raised, thickened, has a peau d'orange appearance, and may be pruritic and hyperpigmented. The lesions are usually discrete, assuming a plaquelike or nodular configuration, but in some instances the lesions become widely confluent. Clubbing of the fingers and toes with characteristic bony changes differentiable from those of hypertrophic pulmonary osteoarthropathy may accompany the dermal changes (*thyroid acropachy*). Activity of this disorder is usually self-limited.

DIAGNOSIS When severe, Graves' disease presents little difficulty in diagnosis. Florid thyrotoxicosis is manifested by weakness, weight loss despite good appetite, nervous instability, tremor, intolerance to heat, hyperhydrosis, palpitations, and hyperdefecation. When associated with diffuse thyroid enlargement, often accompanied by a bruit, and particularly when associated with ophthalmopathy, Graves' disease presents a clinical picture that is virtually unique. In such instances, laboratory tests, which reveal increased RAIU, T_4(D), T_3(RIA), RT_3U, and T_4-RT_3 index, and increased BMR, serve mainly as base lines for evaluation of therapy, rather than necessary diagnostic aids. Occasionally, laboratory tests reveal a normal RAIU, T_4(D), and RT_3U, the T_3(RIA) alone being increased (T_3-toxicosis).

In less severe cases, particularly when ophthalmopathy is lacking, the diagnosis may be substantially more difficult, since the symptoms of mild hyperthyroidism are similar to those of other disorders (see Differential Diagnosis below). Presence of a goiter makes the diagnosis of hyperthyroidism more likely, but careful palpation is necessary to determine whether toxic multinodular goiter or toxic adenoma is present, since treatment of these disorders may differ from that of diffuse toxic goiter. Absence of thyroid enlargement makes the diagnosis of Graves' disease unlikely, but does not exclude it absolutely. In mild cases, confirmatory laboratory tests assume great importance. Unfortunately, mild hyperthyroidism is often associated with only marginal abnormalities in laboratory tests, and values may, in fact lie within the upper limit of the normal range. In instances like this, the thyroid suppression test or the TRH stimulation test assumes crucial importance.

In a few patients, the clinical picture may be one of apathy, rather than hyperactivity, and evidence of hypermetabolism may be slight. In such patients, myopathic features may be pronounced. More often, cardiovascular manifestations predominate since, in patients with underlying heart disease, even mild hyperthyroidism may produce severe disability. Hence, *all patients with unexplained cardiac failure or irregularities in rhythm, especially if atrial in origin, should be examined for hyperthyroidism.* Clues to the diagnosis include a relatively rapid circulation time and resistance to the usual doses of digitalis, but laboratory confirmation will be required.

DIFFERENTIAL DIAGNOSIS Signs and symptoms in a number of nonthyroidal disorders may simulate certain aspects of the thyrotoxic syndrome. Anxiety is a prominent feature of hyperthyroidism, and there is thus some overlap in the symptomatology of this disorder with that of anxiety states of emotional origin. Such symptoms as tachycardia, tremulousness, irritability, weakness, and fatigue are common to the anxiety of both disorders. In anxiety of emotional origin, however, the peripheral manifestations of excessive thyroid hormones are absent; the skin of the extremities is usually cold and clammy rather than warm and moist. Weight loss, when present in emotional anxiety, is characteristically accompanied by anorexia, whereas in hyperthyroidism it is generally, but not invariably, accompanied by excessive appetite. Hyperthyroidism can occasionally be confused with such disorders as metastatic carcinoma, cirrhosis of the liver, hyperparathyroidism, sprue, and neuromyopathies, such as myasthenia gravis and muscular dystrophy. Hypokalemic periodic paralysis is more common in thyrotoxic patients, especially in the case of Oriental males. Signs and symptoms of hyperthyroidism may overlap with those of pheochromocytoma, which may present with heat intolerance, excessive perspiration, tachycardia with palpitations, and a hypermetabolic state that may often be severe. In all the above disorders, as well as other conditions considered in the differential diagnosis, judiciously applied laboratory tests will usually suffice to differentiate them from hyperthyroidism.

When bilateral ophthalmopathy is accompanied by goiter and thyrotoxicosis, the origin of the ophthalmopathy in the Graves' disease process is virtually assured. The presence of unilateral ophthalmopathy, even when associated with thyrotoxicosis, should alert the physician to the possibility of some other intraorbital or intracranial disease. In the patient who is not thyrotoxic, it is more difficult to ascribe ophthalmopathy to Graves' disease, and other causes must be actively excluded. Among the local causes of unilateral or bilateral exophthalmos are cavernous sinus thrombosis, sphenoidal ridge meningioma, and retrobulbar tumors, including leukemic deposits, as well as the rare granulomatous disorder, pseudotumor oculi. Exophthalmos may also be seen in some patients with certain systemic disorders, such as uremia, accelerated hypertension, chronic alcoholism, chronic obstructive pulmonary disease, superior mediastinal obstruction, and Cushing's syndrome. Ophthalmoplegia in the absence of overt infiltrative manifestations can be confused with that which occurs in diabetes mellitus, myasthenia gravis, and myopathies. When doubt exists concerning the cause of ophthalmopathy, the demonstration of an abnormal thyroid suppression test strongly suggests that the cause is Graves' disease.

When the diagnosis of thyrotoxicosis has been established in a patient lacking the ophthalmopathic manifestations of Graves' disease, other causes of thyrotoxicosis must be considered. Palpation of a symmetric, diffuse goiter, especially if associated with a bruit, excludes the diagnosis of *toxic multinodular goiter* or *toxic adenoma;* both these disorders are discussed in later sections. Absence of a palpable thyroid gland raises the suspicion of ectopic thyroid tissue or, much more commonly, self-administration of thyroid hormone (*thyrotoxicosis factitia*). Ectopic thyroid tissue producing thyrotoxicosis is very rare and is most commonly located in the ovary (*struma ovarii*). RAIU, as measured over the thyroid, is low since TSH secretion is suppressed, but despite this, urinary excretion of the dose of ^{131}I is also low, owing to accumulation of ^{131}I by the ectopic tissue. Functioning ectopic tissue can be located by direct counting or scintillation scanning. Thyrotoxicosis factitia most frequently occurs in medical or paramedical personnel or in those who have easy access to thyroid hormone preparations. Physiologically, it resembles thyrotoxicosis caused by ectopic thyroid tissue in that the patient's thyroid gland is suppressed. By contrast, however, most of an administered dose of ^{131}I will be excreted in the urine. When the disorder is caused by ingestion of preparations containing T_4, such as levothyroxine or thyroid extract, the $T_4(D)$ will be increased. On the other hand, when caused by liothyronine, the $T_4(D)$ will be subnormal. Irrespective of the preparation, the $T_3(RIA)$ will be increased, but more so when liothyronine is the offending agent. Occasionally, thyrotoxicosis may be produced by *tumors of trophoblastic origin,* such as choriocarcinoma of the testis or hydatidiform mole, that elaborate thyroid-stimulating peptides. Very rarely, thyrotoxicosis is due to a TSH-secreting tumor of the pituitary. In these disorders, thyrotoxicosis is associated with hyperfunction of the thyroid gland.

TREATMENT Hyperthyroidism The hyperthyroidism in Graves' disease is a disorder often characterized by cyclic phases of exacerbation and remission, each of unpredictable onset and duration. Moreover, subtle tests of thyroid function indicate that long-standing disease is associated with progressive thyroid failure, probably consequent to chronic thyroiditis, with the result that hypothyroidism or decreased thyroid reserve supervenes. These characteristics of Graves' disease have important implications in the choice of and response to therapy, as is discussed below.

There are two major approaches to the treatment of hyperthyroidism; both are directed to limiting the quantity of thyroid hormones the gland can produce. The first major therapeutic modality, the use of antithyroid agents, interposes a chemical blockade to hormone synthesis, the effect of which is operative only as long as the drug is administered or until a spontaneous remission occurs. Thus, the agents can control successfully a given phase of active thyrotoxicity but probably will not prevent exacerbation at some subsequent period. The second major approach is ablation of thyroid tissue, thereby limiting hormone production. This may be achieved either surgically or by means of radioactive iodine. Since these procedures induce permanent anatomic alterations of the thyroid, they can control the individual active phase and are more likely to prevent recurrence of thyrotoxicity during a later exacerbation. On the other hand, the permanency of the effects of surgery or radiation makes these modes of therapy capable of leading to hypothyroidism, either shortly after treatment or with the passage of years.

Each major mode of therapy has advantages and disadvantages, indications and contraindications. The latter are more often relative than absolute. In general, a trial of long-term antithyroid therapy is desirable in children, adolescents, young adults, and pregnant women, but may also be employed in older patients. Indications for ablative procedures include relapse or recurrence following drug therapy, a large goiter, drug toxicity, and failure of the patient to follow a medical regimen or to return for periodic examinations. Subtotal thyroidectomy is usually elected for patients under the age of forty in whom ablative therapy is required; however, opinions differ, and some authorities employ radioactive iodine in the treatment of patients in the second or third decades. With older patients, radioactive iodine is clearly the ablative procedure of choice, as it is for patients who have had previous thyroid surgery or those in whom serious systemic disease contraindicates elective surgery.

In those patients selected for *long-term antithyroid therapy,* satisfactory control can almost always be achieved if a sufficient dosage of the drug is administered. Most patients can be managed successfully with propylthiouracil, 100 to 150 mg every 6 or 8 h. Methimazole is at least as effective as propylthiouracil when administered in one-tenth the dosage. Once euthyroidism is achieved, the daily dosage may be reduced to the smallest doses that control the thyrotoxicosis fully. In many clinics, however, the initial dose is continued and is supplemented with levothyroxine. By this latter regimen, hypothyroidism resulting from overdosage of antithyroid drugs can be prevented. The undesirable consequences of hypothyroidism, such as enhancement of ophthalmopathy and enlargement of the goiter, may thereby be forestalled. The precise duration of therapy is difficult to predict in the individual patient and may be a function of the spontaneous course of the disease itself. If this is the case, the longer the course of therapy, the more likely it is that the patient will remain well when the drug is discontinued. In general, however, a 12- to 24-month course is usually employed. It had been generally accepted that, following a regimen of this type, approximately half of the patients would remain well for a prolonged period or indefinitely. However, recent experience suggests that the incidence of remission may be much lower currently, possibly as a result of the recent general increase in dietary iodine intake. A normal suppressive response to exogenous thyroid hormone when withdrawal of antithyroid agent is contemplated increases the likelihood that the patient will remain in remission for some time. Decrease in goiter size during treatment has a similar connotation.

The *treatment of hyperthyroidism during pregnancy* is a subject of disagreement. Most physicians believe that antithyroid therapy is preferable to subtotal thyroidectomy, particularly during the first and third trimesters. The major disadvantage of antithyroid therapy is the possibility of inducing goiter and hypothyroidism in the fetus, since antithyroid agents readily traverse the placenta. Hence, a cardinal rule in the use of these agents during pregnancy is that the dosage of antithyroid agent should be the smallest necessary to control hyperthyroidism in the mother. Maintenance of normal values for FT_4 or T_4-RT_3 index will assist in this objective. Some authorities regularly supplement the antithyroid regimen with replacement doses of thyroid hormone. However, available evidence suggests that T_4 and T_3 traverse the human placenta from mother to fetus slowly, if at all. Supplemental thyroid hormone will produce no harm unless a false sense of assurance leads to administration of excessive doses of antithyroid agent or neglect of frequent observation of the patient. From the practical standpoint, pregnancy constitutes the sole indication for the assay of LATS in serum, since high titers in the mother are likely to be associated with thyrotoxicosis in the newborn.

Leukopenia is the principal undesirable side effect of antithyroid drugs. Mild transient leukopenia may occur in approximately 10 percent of patients treated and is not necessarily an indication for discontinuing therapy. When the absolute number of polymorphonuclear leukocytes reaches 1,500 or less, antithyroid medication should be discontinued. Allergic rashes and drug sensitivity develop in a small percentage of patients. These may disappear with antihistamine therapy at the same or reduced dosage of antithyroid agent, but it is probably preferable, when sensitivity reactions occur, to change to another drug. On rare occasions (in less than 0.2 percent), agranulocytosis may occur. This may be sudden in onset. Hepatitis, drug fever, and arthralgias are occasional adverse reactions to antithyroid agents.

Iodide inhibits the release of thyroid hormones from the thyrotoxic gland, and its ameliorative effects occur more rapidly than those of agents that merely inhibit hormone synthesis. Hence, its main use is in patients with actual or impending thyrotoxic crisis or in patients with severe thyrocardiac disease. However, the response to iodide is often incomplete and transient. Furthermore, by expanding the thyroid store of hormone, iodide may prolong greatly the latency of response to subsequently instituted antithyroid therapy. Therefore, iodide should be used in conjunction with the antithyroid agents. If the clinical course of the patient is sufficiently severe to require iodide administration, antithyroid drugs will usually be the primary therapeutic agents and should be given in large doses prior to iodide. Since iodide appears to synergize with radiation in the thyroid, it is also useful in controlling thyrotoxicosis following ^{131}I administration, during the period in which the therapeutic effect of radioiodine has not yet taken place.

Owing to the pronounced adrenergic component in thyrotoxicosis, various *adrenergic antagonists* have been employed in the management of this disorder. Of these, propranolol appears to be the agent of choice because of its relative freedom from side effects. In doses of 40 to 120 mg daily, propranolol alleviates such adrenergic manifestations as sweating, tremor, and tachycardia. However, propranolol should be used only as adjunctive therapy rather than sole therapy, as some have suggested, since the underlying metabolic abnormalities are essentially unaffected. Moreover, although the diminution in heart rate and cardiac work that propranolol induces may be beneficial, the withdrawal of adrenergic support of myocardial contractility contraindicates its use in the patient with coexisting heart disease. As adjunctive therapy, propranolol has its major usefulness in the period during which the response to conventional antithyroid agents or to radioiodine therapy is being awaited and in the management of thyrotoxic crisis. It has also been employed as the sole agent in preparation for thyroidectomy. However, since it does not render the patient euthyroid, with a likely greater risk of surgically induced crisis, its use in this setting is not recommended.

Radioactive iodine (^{131}I) affords a relatively simple, effective, and economical means of treating thyrotoxicosis. Its major advantage is that it can produce the ablative effects of surgery without the immediate operative and postoperative complications. The principal disadvantage of ^{131}I therapy, in the dosage which has usually been employed, is its tendency to produce hypothyroidism with a frequency that increases progressively with time. As many as 40 to 70 percent of patients may develop this complication by 10 years after treatment. Although hypothyroidism is readily treated, once diagnosed, the insidious onset of the disorder may obscure the diagnosis until serious complications have developed. Hence, some recommend that all patients be treated with large doses of ^{131}I to ensure relief of thyrotoxicosis and then be placed on permanent physiologic replacement doses of thyroid hormone.

To date, studies have provided no evidence of significant carcinogenic or leukemogenic effect of radioiodine in those doses commonly used in treating hyperthyroidism. Nevertheless, many physicians prefer to reserve radioiodine therapy for patients over forty years of age, thinking that it is currently not justifiable to administer an agent of undetermined radiation potentialities to younger persons, particularly those of childbearing potential. Patients with recurrent thyrotoxicosis following surgery, those who refuse surgery, or those who have complicating illnesses contraindicating surgery are excellent candidates for radioiodine therapy.

The usual therapeutic dose of ^{131}I (approximately 160 μCi per g estimated gland weight) is the dose that has led to the disturbingly high frequency of hypothyroidism. As a result, though continuing to use this dose, some authorities regularly administer prophylactic replacement doses of thyroid hormone. On the other hand, others have been led to administer smaller doses (approximately 80 μCi per g). Although this may diminish the frequency of late hypothyroidism, or merely delay its onset, such is by no means certain. The smaller dose is less likely to relieve thyrotoxicosis within a relatively short period. Antithyroid agents can be employed, however, to speed the attainment of a eumetabolic state while the effect of the ^{131}I is taking hold. There is general agreement that patients with thyrocardiac disease should receive ^{131}I in large doses in view of the hazard of recurrent thyrotoxicosis.

Radiation thyroiditis is an occasional immediate complication of ^{131}I therapy. When present, it commonly appears within 7 to 10 days and is associated with excessive release of hormone into the blood. For this reason, patients with severe hyperthyroidism or underlying heart disease should be rendered eumetabolic with antithyroid agents before ^{131}I is administered. Interruption of antithyroid therapy for several days before and after ^{131}I treatment will suffice to permit adequate accumulation and retention of administered ^{131}I. The swelling that accompanies radiation thyroiditis may contraindicate the use of large doses of ^{131}I in patients with large retrosternal goiters.

Before radioactive iodine was introduced, *subtotal thyroidectomy* was the classic form of ablative therapy, and it is still widely employed in younger patients in whom antithyroid therapy is unsuccessful. Although precise preoperative programs differ, several general principles should be emphasized. Patients should first be rendered fully euthyroid by means of antithyroid agents. Only then should iodide (5 drops Lugol's solution a day for approximately 10 days) be administered concomitantly to effect an involutional response in the gland. Antithyroid drugs should not be discontinued merely because treatment with iodide is instituted.

Hazards of subtotal thyroidectomy include immediate operative complications, such as anesthetic accidents, hemorrhage sometimes leading to respiratory obstruction, and damage to the recurrent laryngeal nerve leading to vocal cord paralysis. Later complications include wound infection, hemorrhage, hypoparathyroidism or hypothyroidism. In experienced hands, surgery is an effective and relatively safe mode of therapy. Postoperative recurrences are quite uncommon. However, carefully conducted follow-up studies reveal that hypothyroidism follows surgery more frequently than previously suspected, although not as commonly as following treatment with ^{131}I.

Ophthalmopathy, dermopathy When severe and progressive, ophthalmopathy is the most difficult component of Graves' disease to treat satisfactorily. Fortunately, however, in most patients the disorder runs a benign course that is largely independent of the course of the hyperthyroid component. In most instances, the activity of even moderately severe disease declines and disappears with time, although some exophthalmos and ophthalmoplegia may persist. In mild disease, considerable benefit may be obtained from simple measures, such as elevating the head at night, administering diuretics to reduce edema, and providing tinted glasses for protection from sun, wind, and foreign bodies. A 1% solution of methylcellulose or plastic shields may help to prevent corneal drying in patients unable to oppose the lids during sleep. In more severe cases, as evidenced by progressive exophthalmos, chemosis, ophthalmoplegia, or loss of vision, large doses of prednisone (120 to 140 mg daily) should be administered, since this is usually effective in reducing the edematous and infiltrative components. With improvement, the dosage is reduced to the lowest effective level, since prolonged administration of large doses will lead to adverse accompaniments of glucocorticoid excess. In those cases that progress despite these measures, orbital decompression, i.e., removal of part of the bony orbit to relieve intraorbital pressure, will usually halt progression of the disease. The management of the patient must always be conducted in concert with an ophthalmologist.

In general, treatment of associated hyperthyroidism should be carried out much as would be the case were ophthalmopathy not present, since there is no convincing evidence that the mode of treatment of the hyperthyroidism influences the course of the ocular disease. The suggestion that total thyroid ablation by surgery and large doses of ^{131}I are beneficial to the ophthalmic disease has not been borne out. It is agreed, however, that hyperthyroidism should be treated, but that hypothyroidism be avoided.

Severe dermopathy can be alleviated by the topical application of glucocorticoids.

TOXIC MULTINODULAR GOITER

Toxic multinodular goiter is a not infrequent consequence of long-standing simple goiter, although the exact proportion of cases in which this complication arises is uncertain. In areas of nonendemicity, the specific etiology of nontoxic multinodular goiter is usually indeterminate. Hence, it is unclear whether a specific etiologic factor underlies those cases of nontoxic multinodular goiter that progress to a thyrotoxic phase. Common to many nontoxic multinodular goiters, even in areas of iodine sufficiency, is a decrease in the iodine content of thyroglobulin, suggesting either a conditioned deficiency of iodine or an impairment of pathways for its normal incorporation into iodinated amino acids. Pathologically, there is nothing which serves clearly to distinguish the nontoxic from the toxic multinodular goiter. However, as judged from radioautographic and scintillation scanning studies, functional patterns may be of two types. In the first and most common, iodine accumulation occurs diffusely, but in patchy foci throughout the gland. Histologically, associated areas reveal cellular hyperplasia. Whether autonomy of function, a prerequisite for development of thyrotoxicosis, resides in these areas per se, or whether they are responding to an extrathyroidal stimulus, as is thought to be the case in Graves' disease, is uncertain. The second, less common, pattern is that of iodine accumulation in one or more discrete nodules within the gland, the remainder being essentially nonfunctional. Whether the former represent true adenomas or are merely colloid nodules that have developed functional autonomy is also uncertain. In both endemic and sporadic nontoxic multinodular goiter, administration of iodides may lead to the development of thyrotoxicosis, implying that areas of potentially autonomous function had been present.

Because it arises in long-standing simple goiter, toxic multinodular goiter is a disease of the aging or elderly. At least partly for this reason, and perhaps because of the nature of the underlying disease, the clinical presentation differs from that in the thyrotoxicosis of Graves' disease. Ophthalmopathy is rare, and would signal the emergence of Graves' disease superimposed on simple goiter. Some patients may present with quite typical thyrotoxicosis. Often, however, the degree of thyrotoxicosis is less severe than that seen in Graves' disease, although its physiologic impact upon specific organ systems may be great. Notable among these is the cardiovascular system, in which arrhythmias or congestive failure may be precipitated or accentuated by thyrotoxicosis that not infrequently is manifested by only subtle findings in other areas (apathetic hyperthyroidism). Weakness and wasting may often predominate, frequently with loss of appetite, rather than hyperphagia, suggesting the presence of a carcinoma.

A nodular goiter that is readily visible or palpable will establish the diagnosis of thyroid disease. In some instances, however, the thyroid gland is not detectably enlarged. Nevertheless, if suggestive clinical findings are present, the physician is obligated to carry out those measures necessary to establish or to exclude the presence of thyrotoxicosis. This is often difficult, since results of conventional laboratory tests are frequently in the borderline range, consistent with the mild degree of thyrotoxicity. However, a value for T_3(RIA) that would be considered normal for a young adult may represent an increase in the elderly patient, since values for T_3(RIA) normally decline with age. Despite their great value in situations such as this, thyroid suppression tests should not be undertaken in the elderly patient because of the hazard of adverse cardiovascular responses. The TRH stimulation test, however, is quite safe, and an abnormal result would confirm the diagnosis of thyrotoxicosis. When laboratory findings do not permit a clear diagnosis of thyrotoxicosis, but suggestive clinical findings are present, a therapeutic trial of antithyroid drugs is indicated.

Radioactive iodine is the treatment of choice for toxic multinodular goiter, once the diagnosis has been established. Large doses (20 to 30 mCi) are usually required, owing in part to the generally lower RAIU, and in part to the variable degree of function throughout the gland. Moreover, the physiologic instability of the elderly patient makes definitive treatment desirable. For the same reason, it is usually wise to initiate therapy with antithyroid agents, withholding radioiodine until a euthyroid state has been achieved, and thereby forestalling an exacerbation of thyrotoxicosis, should radiation thyroiditis occur. Hypothyroidism is only an uncommon consequence of radioiodine treatment of toxic multinodular goiter, owing to the variable activity of differing portions of the gland, which permits previously quiescent areas to replace functionally those that have been destroyed by ^{131}I.

T_3-TOXICOSIS T_3-toxicosis is a term employed to designate thyrotoxicosis in which T_4(D) is normal or low in the absence of a deficiency of TBG, while the T_3(RIA) is increased. Although the production rate of T_3 is disproportionately increased relative to that of T_4 in all patients with hyperthyroidism, in some this discrepancy is greatly exaggerated. This may occur in association with Graves' disease, multinodular goiter, or hyperfunctioning adenoma. The diagnosis should be suspected in a patient with clinical manifestations of thyrotoxicosis in whom the T_4(D) and FT_4 are normal or low and the RAIU is normal or increased. This, together with the frequently palpable goiter, serves to differentiate this disorder from liothyronine-induced thyrotoxicosis factitia. In contradistinction from patients with nonthyroidal disorders mimicking thyrotoxicosis, patients with this disorder, as would be expected, demonstrate nonsuppressibility of thyroid function in response to exogenous T_3 and blunted or absent responses to TRH. In some patients, thyrotoxicosis with increased T_3(RIA) and normal T_4(D) antecedes emergence of typical increases in both, either during an initial episode of hyperthyroidism or during recurrence after previous treatment.

JOD-BASEDOW PHENOMENON This term refers to the induction by iodine of thyrotoxicosis in a patient with endemic goiter and is seen in areas of environmental iodine deficiency when measures to increase dietary iodine intake have been implemented. The presumption here is that iodine deficiency protects some patients with endemic goiter from developing thyrotoxicosis. A similar phenomenon has been reported to occur in areas of environmental iodine sufficiency in patients with nontoxic multinodular goiter who have received large doses of iodide. Since such patients tend to be elderly with the danger of serious cardiovascular manifestations should thyrotoxicosis ensue, large doses of iodine should not be given to those with multinodular goiter. Similarly, in such patients, pharmaceuticals containing iodine, such as x-ray contrast media, should be used only when indicated and with consideration of the possible hazard of inducing the Jod-Basedow phenomenon.

MAJOR COMPLICATIONS OF THYROTOXICOSIS

THYROCARDIAC DISEASE Thyrotoxicosis imposes a variety of burdens upon the heart. Hypermetabolism of the peripheral tissues increases both the metabolic and nonmetabolic (heat-loss) circulatory load, while direct effects of thyroid hormone on the myocardium increase the force, velocity, and rate of ventricular contraction. As a result, cardiac work and cardiac output are increased. Moreover, atrial irritability is enhanced, leading to tachydysrhythmias, most importantly atrial fibrillation. In the patient with a normal heart, these burdens are usually, but not invariably, tolerated. In the patient with underlying heart disease, however, cardiac insufficiency may be precipitated or aggravated. As would be expected, this complication is more common in the elderly patient and is therefore usually seen in the patient with toxic multinodular goiter, not infrequently as the preponderant manifestation of thyrotoxicosis.

In patients with cardiac insufficiency, clues to the presence of thyrotoxicosis include atrial fibrillation, relatively rapid circulation time, increased cardiac output (high-output failure), and resistance to the usual therapeutic doses of digitalis.

Treatment is directed at both rapid alleviation of thyrotoxicosis and restoration of cardiac compensation. The former objective is best met by initiation of treatment with large doses of an antithyroid agent, followed by iodine if the clinical situation is urgent. Radioiodine, which is the ultimate therapy of choice, is withheld until a eumetabolic state has been achieved and the RAIU has returned to a satisfactory level as the stable iodine is excreted. In less severe cases, radioiodine treatment is anteceded by antithyroid drug treatment alone. Management of the cardiac decompensation is carried out in the usual manner, employing larger than usual doses of digitalis, but with care to avoid digitalis intoxication as the thyrotoxicosis is alleviated. Adrenergic antagonists should not be employed in the presence of cardiac failure.

THYROTOXIC CRISIS The clinical picture of thyrotoxic crisis or storm is that of a fulminating increase in all the signs and symptoms of thyrotoxicosis. In the past, this disturbance was most often observed postoperatively in patients poorly prepared for surgery. However, with the preoperative use of antithyroid drugs and iodide and with appropriate measures directed to control of metabolic factors, weight, and nutritional status, postoperative thyrotoxic crisis should not occur. At present, so-called "medical storm" is more common and occurs in untreated or inadequately treated patients. It is precipitated by surgical emergency or complicating medical illness, usually sepsis. The syndrome is characterized by extreme irritability, delirium, or coma, fever to 106°F or more, tachycardia, restlessness, hypotension, vomiting, and diarrhea. Rarely, the clinical picture may be more subtle, with apathy, severe prostration and coma, but with only slight elevation of temperature. Such postoperative complications as sepsis, septicemia, hemorrhage, and transfusion or drug reactions may mimic thyrotoxic crisis. It is thought that in some patients thyrotoxic crisis is associated with or precipitated by adrenocortical insufficiency. The possibility of this complication gains support from evidence indicating increased adrenocortical hormone requirements in thyrotoxicosis and from evidence of reduced adrenocortical reserve in this disorder.

Treatment of this most serious disorder consists in providing general supportive therapy while undertaking measures for the most rapid alleviation of thyrotoxicosis possible. Supportive therapy includes treatment of dehydration and provision of calories through the intravenous administration of glucose and saline, vitamin B complex, and glucocorticoids. Patients should be placed in a cooled, humidified oxygen tent, and, if hyperpyrexia is present, a cooling blanket should be used. Digitalization is required only in the presence of cardiac failure. If shock exists, intravenous pressor agents should be employed. Therapy of the hyperthyroidism consists of induction of blockade of hormone synthesis by the immediate and continued administration of large doses of an antithyroid agent (e.g., 100 mg propylthiouracil every 2 h). If the patient is unable to swallow the medication, the tablets should be triturated and given by nasogastric tube, as parenteral preparations are unavailable. Following initiation of antithyroid therapy, inhibition of hormone release is sought through the administration of large doses of iodine intravenously or by mouth. To alleviate some of the peripheral effects of thyrotoxicosis, adrenergic antagonists may be used. Propranolol given intravenously or orally appears to be the agent of choice in the absence of cardiac insufficiency. Antithyroid therapy and iodine must be continued until a normal metabolic state is restored, at which time iodine is progressively withdrawn and plans for a definitive regimen of treatment made.

NEOPLASMS

THYROID ADENOMAS True adenomas, as contrasted with localized adenomatous areas, are encapsulated and usually compress contiguous tissue. Adenomas vary greatly in size and histologic characteristics, and are often classified into three major types: Papillary, follicular, and Hürthle cell. The follicular adenomas can be subdivided according to the size of the follicles into colloid or macrofollicular, fetal or microfollicular, and embryonal varieties. There is considerable variation in physiologic differentiation, as judged by their ability to concentrate radioiodine. The more highly differentiated adenomas (follicular) are by far the most common and are also the most likely to mimic the function of normal thyroid tissue. Unlike normal thyroid tissue, however, their function is independent of TSH stimulation (autonomous). They are usually unifocal, presenting as a solitary nodule. Often the patient reports that the nodule has been slowly growing over many years. Initially, their function is insufficient to disturb hormonal equilibrium, although their capacity to accumulate ^{131}I is apparent on scintiscanning (*"warm" nodule*). With the passage of time, the nodule grows larger, and its function increases until it is sufficient to suppress TSH secretion. Consequently, the remainder of the gland undergoes atrophy and loss of function, and the scintiscan then reveals ^{131}I accumulation only in the region of the nodule (*"hot" nodule*). At this time, the patient may or may not appear overtly thyrotoxic, but frank thyrotoxicosis will usually supervene in time (*toxic adenoma*). Relative to its overall rate of occurrence, hyperfunctioning adenoma is a frequent cause of T_3-toxicosis. Not infrequently, hyperfunctioning adenomas undergo hemorrhagic necrosis, resulting in loss of function and the appearance of a *"cold" nodule* on scintiscanning, since the remainder of the thyroid will have resumed function. Only very rarely are hyperfunctioning adenomas carcinomatous. Hyperfunctioning adenomas are readily amenable to ablation by surgery or ^{131}I; large doses of the latter are usually required (10 mCi or greater). Prior to such treatment, it is desirable to administer exogenous TSH and repeat the scintiscan in order to demonstrate the capacity for function in the remaining tissue.

THYROID CARCINOMAS Thyroid carcinoma may be classified into two varieties, depending upon whether the lesion arises in thyroid follicular epithelium or whether it arises from the parafollicular or "C" cells. Since the latter disorder has distinctive physiologic and clinical characteristics, it is discussed separately (see Chap. 354, Medullary Carcinoma).

Carcinomas of follicular epithelium These are of three general histologic types which differ in their clinical course. The least common is *anaplastic carcinoma,* which is histologically undifferentiated, usually afflicts the elderly, and is highly malignant. Usually the lesion is rapidly fatal, owing to extensive local invasion which is refractory to radiation. The second type of tumor, *follicular carcinoma,* is also uncommon and histologically mimics closely normal thyroid tissue. This lesion usually undergoes early hematogenous spread, and hence the patient may present with a distant metastasis, usually in lung or bone. Follicular carcinoma or follicular elements in papillary carcinoma are responsible for those instances in which thyroid carcinoma, *in situ* or in metastases, accumulates significant quantities of ^{131}I. The third and most common type of tumor, *papillary carcinoma,* has a bimodal frequency, peaks occurring in the second or third decades and again in later life. This lesion is usually slowly growing and typically spreads to the regional lymph nodes, where it may remain indolent for many years. Although more common in the older patient, acceleration of the disease may take place at any time. Follicular elements are usually present in both the primary lesion and its metastases, accounting for those instances in which papillary tumors accumulate ^{131}I.

DIAGNOSIS AND MANAGEMENT The diagnosis and management of thyroid carcinoma is closely interwoven with the management of the nodular goiter. In the past, this subject has been one which evoked a wide disparity of views among authorities, stemming largely from seemingly contradictory data. On the one hand, surgically excised specimens of thyroid nodules, particularly solitary nodules, revealed a very high frequency of carcinoma (as much as 20 percent in some series). On the other hand, despite the frequency of nodular goiter in the general population (approximately 4 percent), the frequency of thyroid carcinoma, either newly diagnosed or as a cause of death, is very low. These respective data led to either very vigorous or very conservative approaches with respect to the management of nodular goiter. It now appears that this discordance can be explained, however, by the ability of the physician to select for surgery those patients who are at high risk of harboring thyroid carcinoma, with consequent weighting of statistics derived from surgical series.

The features which lead to a presumptive diagnosis of thyroid carcinoma are rather well defined. They include recent growth, especially if rapid and unaccompanied by tenderness, firm or hard consistency, and diminished or absent function on scintiscan. The presence of finely stippled calcification on x-ray examination suggests the presence of psammoma bodies within a papillary carcinoma. Hoarseness, fixation to adjacent structures, and regional lymphadenopathy are late features. Of particular importance is a history of x-ray irradiation to the head or neck in childhood, since this has been shown to be associated with a high incidence of thyroid carcinoma in later life. A nodule that is present in an otherwise normal gland (solitary nodule) is far more suspicious of thyroid tumor, while one nodule among many is much more likely to be part of a diffuse process, such as simple goiter.

The foregoing features permit the development of general guidelines for the management of nodular goiter. A solitary nodule, especially if nonfunctioning, should be promptly excised, particularly if it occurs in a young woman or in a man of any age, except the most elderly. This is true because multinodular goiter is a disease of older age and predominantly of women. Obviously, the presence of other features described above increase the likelihood of thyroid carcinoma. A prominent but functioning nodule within a multinodular goiter is of little concern. A nonfunctioning nodule within a multinodular goiter should be observed during suppressive therapy. Failure to regress, or particularly an increase in size, over a 3- to 6-month period strongly suggests that surgery is desirable.

At surgery, the nodule should be widely excised and subjected to frozen section examination. A diagnosis of carcinoma is an indication for near-total thyroidectomy in view of the evidence of frequent seeding of carcinoma throughout the gland as a result of transglandular lymphatic spread. Regional lymph nodes should be explored and removed if there is evidence of involvement. Radical neck dissection is no longer felt justified. If permanent sections reveal carcinoma when frozen sections had failed to do so, secondary surgery should be undertaken to remove residual thyroid tissue. Several weeks after surgery, a large scanning dose of ^{131}I is administered (approximately 2 mCi), and a whole-body scan and measurement of urinary ^{131}I excretion obtained. This serves to ablate any residual thyroid tissue and to demonstrate any functioning metastases. If functioning metastases are seen, a therapeutic dose of ^{131}I (approximately 50 mCi) is administered. Thereafter, the patient is given levothyroxine in fully suppressive dosage. At approximately yearly intervals, levothyroxine is replaced by liothyronine for approximately 3 weeks; this is then withdrawn to permit rapid resumption of TSH secretion and stimulation of any functioning residual tissue. If such is found, a further therapeutic dose of ^{131}I is administered. Discrete palpable lymph nodes which have emerged during suppressive therapy can often best be treated by surgical excision. The foregoing procedures are repeated during ensuing years until the disease appears to have been eradicated. Although suppressive therapy is physiologically sound and sometimes spectacularly successful, its general efficacy in the management of thyroid carcinoma is uncertain. Nevertheless, patients who have had carcinoma of the thyroid should be kept on suppressive therapy for the remainder of their lives, except for the brief interruptions described above.

THYROIDITIS

Thyroiditis is a generic term embracing several disorders of differing etiology. There are four general types, of which two are exceedingly uncommon, *pyogenic thyroiditis* and *chronic fibrosing (Riedel's) thyroiditis*. Pyogenic thyroiditis is usually anteceded by a pyogenic infection elsewhere and is characterized by tenderness and swelling of the thyroid, redness and warmth of the overlying skin, and constitutional signs of infection. Treatment consists of antibiotic therapy, along with incisional drainage if a fluctuant area within the thyroid should occur. Riedel's thyroiditis is a rare disorder in which intense fibrosis of the thyroid and surrounding structures, leading to induration of the tissues of the neck, may be associated with mediastinal and retroperitoneal fibrosis. The principal importance of this disorder is that it requires differentiation from thyroid neoplasia.

SUBACUTE THYROIDITIS This disorder, which is also termed *granulomatous, giant-cell,* or *de Quervain's thyroiditis,* is a distinct disorder of the thyroid that appears to be viral in origin.

Symptoms of thyroiditis usually follow those of an upper respiratory infection and most commonly comprise pronounced asthenia, malaise, and symptoms referable to stretching of the thyroid capsule, principally pain over the thyroid or pain referred to the lower jaw, ear, or occiput. Referred, rather than local, pain may predominate. These symptoms may smolder for many weeks before the correct diagnosis is suspected. Less commonly, the onset is acute, with severe pain over the thyroid, accompanied by fever and occasionally symptoms of thyrotoxicosis. Cardinal physical findings include exquisite tenderness and nodularity over the thyroid, which may be predominantly unilateral, but which usually migrates to other areas of the gland. Laboratory tests usually reveal an inordinately increased erythrocyte sedimentation rate and markedly depressed RAIU. Early in the disease, the PBI is usually increased, mainly as a result of iodoprotein release, although the $T_4(D)$ may be increased as well in some patients. Although local or referred pain is the commonest symptom of subacute thyroiditis, occasional patients manifest other typical features of the disease, but have no pain.

If left untreated, the disorder may smolder for months, but eventually will subside with a return of normal thyroid function. In mild cases, aspirin suffices to control the symptoms. In more severe cases, glucocorticoid (prednisone, 20 to 40 mg daily) is generally effective. Return of the RAIU to normal indicates the time at which therapy can be withdrawn without recurrence of symptoms.

HASHIMOTO'S DISEASE This disorder, which is also termed *lymphadenoid goiter,* is a chronic inflammatory disease of the thyroid in which autoimmune factors are thought to play a prominent role. It is a common disorder, occurring most frequently in women of middle age. In all likelihood, it is, in addition, the most common cause of sporadic goiter in children. Evidence of the participation of autoimmune factors includes the lymphocytic infiltration of the gland, as well as the presence in the serum of increased concentrations of immunoglobulins and of antibodies directed against several components of thyroid tissue. Of these, the most important from the clinical standpoint are the antithyroglobulin antibody detected by the tanned red cell agglutination technique and the antimicrosomal antibody detected by immunofluorescence or complement fixation techniques. This disorder also coexists with inordinate frequency with other diseases of a presumed autoimmune nature, including pernicious anemia, Sjögren's syndrome, progressive hepatitis, systemic lupus erythematosus, rheumatoid arthritis, nontuberculous Addison's disease, and Graves' disease itself. These disorders, as well as Hashimoto's disease itself, also appear with unusual frequency in family members of patients with Hashimoto's disease.

Goiter is the outstanding feature of the disease. The enlargement involves the entire gland, but not necessarily symmetrically. Typically, the consistency is rubbery, the margins are scalloped, and the general outline of the gland is preserved. The pyramidal lobe may be prominent. Early in the disease the patient is metabolically normal; however, even then decreased thyroid reserve is often manifest in an increase in serum TSH. With the passage of time, hypothyroidism of increasing severity supervenes, owing to progressive replacement of thyroid parenchyma by lymphocytes or fibrous tissue. Early in the disease, the RAIU and PBI may be increased, reflecting the secretion of iodoproteins, but the $T_4(D)$ is normal. With time, the RAIU, PBI, and $T_4(D)$ decline as clinical hypothyroidism supervenes. Increased $T_3(RIA)$ may herald the development of this sequence. High titers of antithyroglobulin antibody are usually, but not invariably, present. High titers may also occur in other thyroid disorders, particularly primary thyroprivic hypothyroidism and Graves' disease, but with lesser frequency. Patients lacking antithyroglobulin antibody almost always display antimicrosomal antibody. Although the foregoing findings usually suffice to permit a diagnosis, histologic confirmation by needle biopsy is occasionally required. In view of the frequency with which hypothyroidism is either present or eventually develops, treatment with replacement doses of levothyroxine is indicated. In some patients, such therapy is associated with regression of goiter.

REFERENCES

ADAMS DD et al: Stimulation of the human thyroid by infusions of plasma containing LATS protector. J Clin Endocrinol Metab 39:826, 1974

BRAVERMAN LE et al: Effects of replacement doses of sodium L-thyroxine on the peripheral metabolism of thyroxine and triiodothyronine in man. J Clin Invest 52:1010, 1973

INGBAR SH, WOEBER KA: The thyroid gland, in *Textbook of Endocrinology,* 5th ed., ed RH Williams, Philadelphia: Saunders, 1974

ROYCE PC: Severely impaired consciousness in myxedema—A review. Am J Med Sci 261:46, 1971

UCLA CONFERENCE: Thyroid physiology in health and disease. Ann Intern Med 81:68, 1974

UTIGER RD: Serum triiodothyronine in man. Annu Rev Med 25: 289, 1974

93
DISEASES OF THE ADRENAL CORTEX

GORDON H. WILLIAMS
ROBERT G. DLUHY
GEORGE W. THORN

INTRODUCTION Thomas Addison's description in 1849 of a clinical syndrome resulting from destruction of the adrenal glands first attracted attention to these organs. Seven years later Brown-Séquard demonstrated that removal of both adrenals from experimental animals caused death soon after operation, whereas control animals subjected to a sham operation survived. Subsequent investigations established that the life-maintaining hormone was elaborated by cells in the cortex, since destruction of all medullary tissue was not accompanied by the classic signs and symptoms of adrenal insufficiency noted after complete removal of the glands.

Between 1927 and 1930, Hartman and his associates, Rogoff and Stewart, and Pfiffner and Swingle all independently described methods for preparing potent adrenocortical extracts. During the following decade, crystalline steroid substances were isolated from these extracts by Kendall, by Grollman, and by Reichstein. In 1937, Steiger and Reichstein synthesized the first natural corticosteroid, 11-deoxycorticosterone, a year before it was identified in adrenal extracts. From 1940 to 1950, the synthesis of several 11-oxygenated compounds was achieved, including cortisone and hydrocortisone. The contributions of Sarett and his collaborators, Reichstein et al, and Kendall and his coworkers were outstanding in this regard. In 1954 aldosterone, the principal salt-retaining hormone of the adrenal, was identified by Simpson and Tait in collaboration with the Swiss group under Reichstein.

Since 1954, a number of remarkable advances have occurred. ACTH has been isolated, its amino acid sequence determined, and the complete molecule synthesized. A number of substances which interfere with the action of adrenal steroids have also been synthesized. For example, amphenone and 2-methyl-1,2-bis-(3-pyridyl)-1-propanone (metyrapone) interfere with the synthesis of hydrocortisone. Spironolactone and 2,4,7-tri-amino-6-phenylpteridine (triamterene) block the physiologic effects of aldosterone. Among the most significant advancements have been the refinements in the ease and accuracy with which steroids and their metabolic products may be measured, e.g., by double isotope derivative, competitive protein-binding radioassay, and radioimmunoassay techniques.

BIOCHEMISTRY AND PHYSIOLOGY

STEROID NOMENCLATURE The adrenal steroids contain as their basic structure a cyclopentenoperhydrophenanthrane nucleus consisting of three 6-carbon hexane rings and a single 5-carbon pentane ring (D). The carbon atoms are numbered in a predetermined sequence beginning with ring A (Fig. 93-1). The Greek letter Δ indicates a double bond, as does the suffix -ene. The position of a substituent below or above the plane of the steroid molecule is indicated by the letters α and β, respectively. The α-substituent is drawn with a broken line (- -OH), and the β-substituent is drawn with a solid line (—OH). The C_{19} steroids are those which have substituent methyl groups at positions C-18 and C-19. C_{19} steroids that also have a ketone group at C-17 are termed *17-ketosteroids.* These C_{19} steroids have predominant androgenic activity. The C_{21} steroids are those which have a 2-carbon side chain (C-20 and C-21) attached at position 17 of the D ring and, in addition, have substituent methyl groups at C-18 and C-19. C_{21} steroids that also possess a hydroxyl group at position 17 are termed *17-hydroxycorticosteroids* or *17-hydroxycorticoids.* The C_{21} steroids may have either predominant glucocorticoid or mineralocorticoid properties. *Glucocorticoid* signifies a C_{21} steroid with predominant action on intermediary metabolism, and *mineralocorticoid* indicates a C_{21} steroid with predominant action on the metabolism of the body minerals, sodium and potassium.

BIOSYNTHESIS OF ADRENAL STEROIDS Cholesterol, derived from the diet and from endogenous synthesis via acetate, is the principal starting compound in steroidogenesis. The three major adrenal biosynthetic pathways lead to the production of glucocorticoids (cortisol), mineralocorticoids (aldosterone), and adrenal androgens (dehydroepiandrosterone) (Fig. 93-2). Separate zones of the adrenal cortex have differing capacity to synthesize specific hormones. The outer (glomerulosa) zone is mainly involved in aldosterone biosynthesis, and the inner (fasciculata-reticularis) zone, mainly involved in cortisol and androgen biosynthesis.

Glucocorticoid pathway Δ5-Pregnenolone is formed after cleavage of the side chain of cholesterol. Δ5-Pregnenolone is converted to progesterone by the action of the enzymes 3β-hydroxydehydrogenase and Δ5,Δ4-isomerase.

FIGURE 93-1
Basic steroid structure and nomenclature.

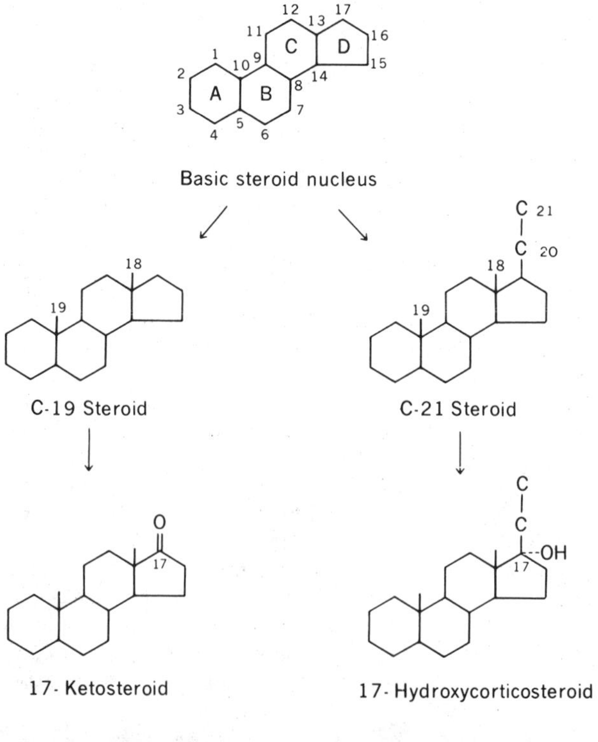

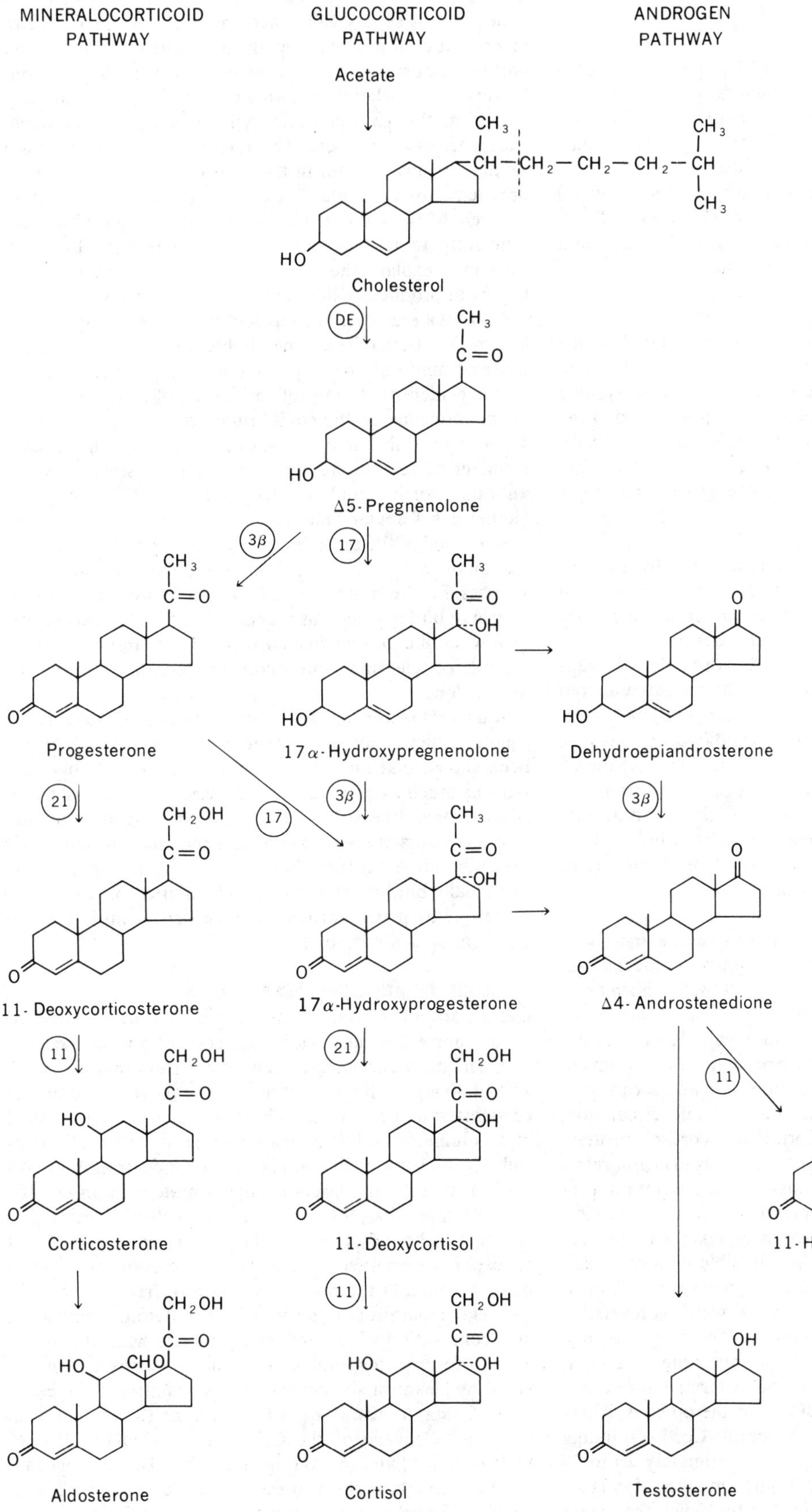

FIGURE 93-2
Biosynthetic pathways for adrenal steroid production. Major pathways to mineralocorticoids, glucocorticoids, and androgens. Circled letters and numbers denote specific enzymes: DE = *debranching enzyme; 3β = 3β-ol-dehydrogenase with Δ4-Δ5 isomerase; 11 = C-11 hydroxylase; 17 = C-17 hydroxylase; 21 = C-21 hydroxylase.*

A series of hydroxylations mediated by specific hydroxylating enzymes then occurs in sequential fashion at C-17, then at C-21, and finally at C-11. Hydroxylation at position C-17 of progesterone produces 17α-hydroxyprogesterone, which in turn has a hydroxyl group introduced at C-21 by the enzyme C-21 hydroxylase, producing 11-deoxycortisol (compound S). Finally, a third hydroxyl group is introduced at the C-11 position to produce cortisol (compound F, hydrocortisone), the major glucocorticoid.

Mineralocorticoid pathway Progesterone, after transformation from Δ5-pregnenolone, is hydroxylated at the C-21 position to form 11-deoxycorticosterone. This is then hydroxylated at the 11 position to form corticosterone (compound B). A hydroxyl group is then introduced at the 18 position to form 18-hydroxycorticosterone, the immediate precursor of aldosterone. With conversion of the hydroxyl group at C-18 to an aldehyde group, the major mineralocorticoid, *aldosterone,* is formed.

Androgen pathway Δ5-Pregnenolone is 17α-hydroxylated and then cleaved of its C-20:C-21 side chain to form dehydroepiandrosterone, the main precursor of the urinary 17-ketosteroids. Dehydroepiandrosterone is transformed to androstenedione by the enzymes 3β-hydroxydehydrogenase and Δ5,Δ4 isomerase. Androstenedione can undergo direct transformation to testosterone as a result of hydrogenation at position C-17. Androstenedione can also be hydroxylated at position C-11, producing 11-oxygenated 17-ketosteroids which are exclusively of adrenal origin.

It is unlikely that the normal adrenal gland can aromatize testosterone or androstenedione to estradiol and estrone; these conversions probably take place in the liver or in fat cells from adrenal precursors.

STEROID TRANSPORT In the analysis of the metabolic actions of steroids, an important feature is the mechanism of transport from origin to site of action. Many hormones, including some of the steroid hormones, e.g., testosterone and cortisol, appear to circulate to a considerable extent bound to plasma proteins. Aldosterone, however, seems to have a relatively poor binding affinity for any serum protein. Cortisol, after release into the systemic circulation, occurs in the plasma in three forms: free cortisol, protein-bound cortisol, and cortisol metabolites. *Free cortisol* refers to that quantity which is physiologically active but not protein bound and, therefore, represents a form of cortisol acting directly on tissue sites. Normally, less than 5 percent of circulating cortisol is free. The diffusible fraction is estimated to range between 0.7 and 1.0 μg per 100 ml. *Protein-bound cortisol* is that portion of cortisol which is reversibly bound to circulating plasma proteins. There are two distinct cortisol-binding systems of plasma. One is a high-affinity, low-capacity alpha 2-globulin termed *transcortin* or *cortisol-binding globulin* (CBG), and the other is a low-affinity, high-capacity protein, albumin. Cortisol-binding globulin in normal man can bind approximately 20 to 25 μg cortisol per 100 ml plasma. As the amounts of cortisol released by the adrenal gland exceed this level, the excess becomes bound in part to albumin and a greater proportion circulates unbound. The CBG level may be increased by administration of natural or synthetic estrogens. This endogenous rise in CBG is accompanied by a parallel rise in protein-bound cortisol, with the result that the plasma cortisol concentration is elevated. However, there is controversy as to whether the free-cortisol levels remain normal even though signs and symptoms of glucocorticoid excess are usually absent. This effect of estrogen on steroid binding is most evident in the third trimester of pregnancy or when estrogen-containing oral contraceptive medication is taken. Most synthetic glucocorticoid analogues bind less efficiently to CBG (approximately 70 percent binding). This may explain the propensity of some synthetic analogues to produce cushingoid side effects at low dosage.

Cortisol metabolites such as tetrahydrocortisol also circulate in the plasma. These metabolites are biologically inactive and bind only weakly to circulating plasma proteins.

It is evident that the protein binding of steroids exerts a major influence on the equilibrium concentration of cortisol across membrane barriers. For example, by this mechanism, urine loss of steroids is minimized, since only the unbound cortisol and its metabolites are filtrable at the glomerulus. Greater than normal quantities of free steroid are excreted in the urine in states characterized by hypersecretion of cortisol, as the unbound fraction of plasma cortisol rises. Furthermore, cortisol binding to proteins serves as a reserve buffer mechanism capable of binding excess cortisol when the plasma-free cortisol is high, and conversely, capable of releasing bound cortisol when the free-cortisol level is low.

Aldosterone appears to be bound to proteins to a much smaller extent than either testosterone or cortisol. It has been shown that an ultrafiltrate of plasma probably contains as much as 50 percent of the circulating aldosterone. Aldosterone, like other steroids, is bound to albumin. There is also some evidence that a separate protein, other than albumin- or cortisol-binding globulin, may participate in partially binding aldosterone. The limited binding of aldosterone by plasma protein may be significant in the metabolism of this hormone.

STEROID METABOLISM AND EXCRETION

Glucocorticoids The principal glucocorticoids secreted by the normal adrenal gland are cortisol and corticosterone. The daily adrenal secretion of cortisol ranges between 15 and 30 mg, with a pronounced diurnal cycle, and that of corticosterone between 2 and 4 mg. Cortisol is distributed in a volume of body fluids approximating the total extracellular fluid space. The total plasma concentration of cortisol in the morning hours is approximately 15 μg per 100 ml, with more than 90 percent of this cortisol appearing in the protein-bound fraction. The plasma concentration of cortisol is determined by the rate of secretion, the rate of inactivation, and the rate of excretion of free cortisol. The liver is the major organ responsible for steroid inactivation and conjugation of the reduced products with glucuronic acid to form water-soluble compounds. Cortisol is inactivated by means of six major biotransformations: (1) reduction of ring A; (2) 11-dehydrogenation; (3) reduction at C-20; (4) cleavage of the C-20:C-21 side chain; (5) 6β-hydroxylation; and (6) conjugation. The 11-dehydrogenase system converts cortisol to the inactive cortisone. This reversible system is an important factor in regulating the level of circulating cortisol under normal circumstances. The enzyme is strongly influenced by the level of circulating thyroid hormone, with hyperthyroidism markedly accelerating the oxidative reaction. The major mechanism for steroid inactivation is the reduction of ring A by the liver. The initial saturation of the C-4:C-5 double bond in ring A by the introduction of two hydrogen ions produces *dihydrocortisol.* Next the C-3 ketonic group of dihydrocortisol is reduced by further addition of two hydrogen atoms to form *tetrahydrocortisol* (THF). Furthermore, cortisone may go through a similar reduction process to produce tetrahydrocortisone (THE). The third mechanism of inactivation, C-20 hydroxylation, is brought into play by the addition of two hydrogen atoms at C-20. Further reduction elsewhere in the molecule is possible, and the products are the cortols and the cortolones. From 5 to 10 percent of the secreted cortisol is metabolized in the liver by cleavage of the C-20: C-21 side chain to form the corresponding 11-oxyketosteroid. Finally, in normal man, 6β-hydroxylation of cortisol represents a relatively minor metabolic transformation. However, under certain circumstances, in infancy and toxemia of pregnancy and with certain drugs, the formation of this product becomes important. The first four transformations produce compounds which are not water-soluble. These compounds are conjugated in the liver with glucuronic acid at position C-3 to produce water-soluble products. Sulfation appears to be a relatively minor process, except perhaps in infancy. The 6β-hydroxycortisol is sufficiently water-soluble that it can clear the kidney without conjugation.

Mineralocorticoids In normal subjects on a normal salt intake, the average daily secretion of aldosterone ranges between 50 and 250 μg, and the plasma concentration ranges between 5 and 15 ng per 100 ml. Since aldosterone is only weakly bound to proteins, its volume of distribution is larger than that of cortisol and approximates 35 liters. Under normal circumstances, greater than 75 percent of circulating aldosterone is inactivated during a single passage through the liver. However, under certain conditions, such as congestive failure, this percentage is markedly reduced.

Under steady-state conditions, aldosterone exists as the 11-18-hemiacetal form rather than the 18-aldehyde form. Most transformations of this compound are reductive in nature. There has been no substantial evidence of oxidative reactions involving aldosterone, in contrast to cortisol metabolism. Of the numerous reductive metabolites that may be formed, 50 percent of aldosterone is transformed into the tetrahydro derivative produced by ring A reduction. This reaction appears to occur only in the liver, and because this metabolite is water-insoluble, it is conjugated with glucuronic acid before it is excreted in the urine. From 7 to 15 percent of aldosterone appears in the urine as a glucuronide conjugate, from which free aldosterone is released on standing at pH 1. This *acid-labile conjugate* appears to be formed both in the liver and in the kidney. The relative proportions appear to be related to relative blood flow to the two organs and the state of general circulation. The acid-labile conjugate is also referred to as the *3-oxo conjugate,* because the 3-oxo grouping is not irreversibly reduced, as it is in tetrahydroaldosterone. Ninety percent of the acid-labile conjugate is excreted within 6 h, whereas comparable tetrahydroaldosterone excretion requires 24 to 36 h. For average salt intake, the 24-h urine excretion of the acid-labile conjugate ranges from 2 to 20 μg, that of the tetrahydro derivative from 25 to 35 μg, and that of the nonconjugated, nonreduced free aldosterone from 0.2 to 0.6 μg.

Adrenal androgens The major androgenic compound secreted by the adrenal gland is dehydroepiandrosterone (DHEA) and its C-3 sulfuric acid ester. From 15 to 30 mg of these compounds is secreted daily. Much smaller amounts of Δ4-androstenedione and 11β-hydroxyandrostenedione and testosterone are secreted. DHEA serves as the major precursor of the urinary 17-ketosteroids after metabolic alterations. The first step, which is irreversible, is the conversion to Δ4-androstenedione (Fig. 93-3). This compound is then interconvertible with testosterone and shares with testosterone a common group of metabolites, formed by the tetrahydro reduction of ring A (androsterone, epiandrosterone, and etiocholanolone). The second major route of transformation is the formation of the 16α-hydroxyl derivative of either dehydroepiandrosterone or its

FIGURE 93-3
Adrenal androgens. Δ-4 Androstenedione and testosterone contribute to the same metabolites.

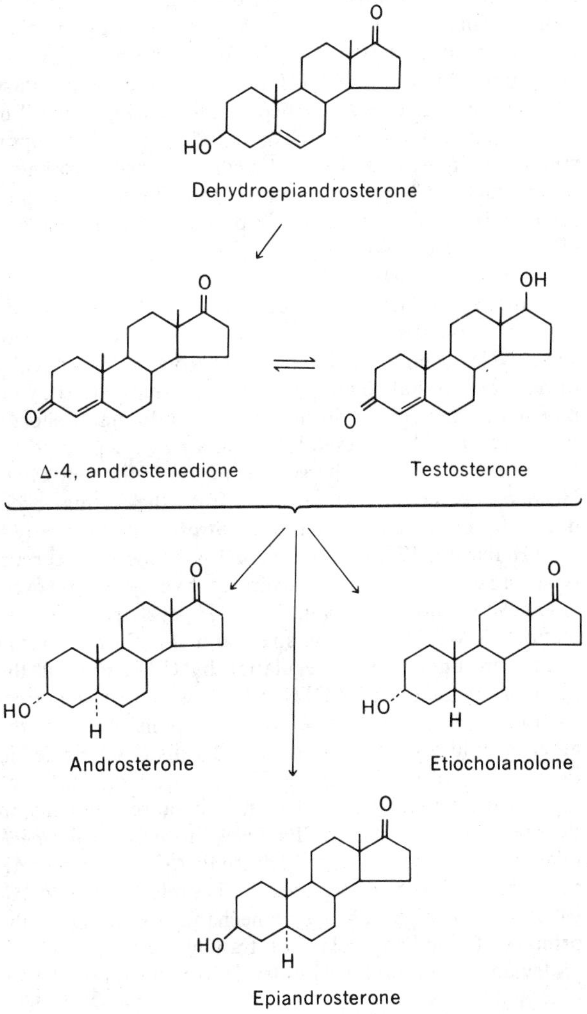

sulfate. In pregnancy, this compound performs a vital role as a precursor in the placental production of estriol.

Two-thirds of the urine 17-ketosteroids in the male are derived from adrenal metabolites, and the remaining one-third comes from testicular androgens. In the female, almost all urine 17-ketosteroids are derived from the adrenal gland. It is improbable that estrogens are synthesized by the normal adrenal gland. There has been no substantial proof of aromatic enzymes being present in adrenal tissue. The increased secretion of estrogens in ovariectomized patients and in feminizing adrenal tumors is probably secondary to the action of liver enzymes on androgenic precursors secreted by the adrenal gland.

ACTH PHYSIOLOGY The adrenocorticotropin hormone (ACTH) (see Chap. 90) is an unbranched long-chain polypeptide containing 39 amino acids. It is stored in and released from the anterior pituitary gland, where histologically it appears to be localized to basophil cells. Only 50 units, or roughly 0.25 mg, of the active peptide are stored in the anterior pituitary. Much of the potential for producing the corticotropic actions of ACTH is present in smaller polypeptide fragments. It appears that the *N*-terminal 24-amino-acid structure retains full biologic potency, while shorter *N*-terminal fragments exhibit reduced biologic activity. The biologic half-life of ACTH is less than 10 min; enzymatic cleavage at the 16–17 position by the plasmin-plasminogen system is probably the mechanism of inactivation. Release of ACTH from the anterior pituitary gland is governed by a "corticotropin-releasing center" in the median eminence of the hypothalamus, which upon stimulation releases a chemical mediator (corticotropin-releasing factor, CRF) that travels via the pituitary-stalk portal bloodstream to the anterior pituitary gland, where it effects the release of stored ACTH (Fig. 93-4; see also Chap. 89).

Three major factors control CRF and ACTH release: plasma free-cortisol concentration, stress, and the sleep-wake cycle. The plasma level of ACTH varies sporadically during the day but roughly follows a diurnal pattern, with a peak occurring just prior to awaking and a nadir shortly before retiring. After several days on a new sleep-wake cycle, the pattern will be altered to conform to the new cycle. However, an occasional deviation from the normal cycle does not produce an alteration. Stress can also affect ACTH release. When an individual is exposed to certain types of stress, e.g., pyrogens, surgery, hypoglycemia, exercise, severe emotional trauma, ACTH levels rise. The secretion of ACTH following stress and the diurnal ACTH release are under neural regulation by CRF. Finally, the principal regulator of ACTH release is the plasma free-cortisol level. Cortisol decreases the responsiveness of the anterior pituitary adrenocorticotropic cells to CRF; i.e., in the presence of cortisol, more CRF is required to produce a given increment of ACTH than in its absence. Thus, in the presence of a constant CRF level, this *negative feedback* relationship causes increased release of ACTH when cortisol levels are low but decreased ACTH release when cortisol levels are high. This servomechanism establishes the primacy of blood cortisol concentration and serves to buffer deviations in blood cortisol levels from a supposed optimal level. It also appears that cortisol feeds back on the hypothalamus (CRF), higher brain centers (hippocampus, septum), and perhaps even on the adrenal cortex as well.

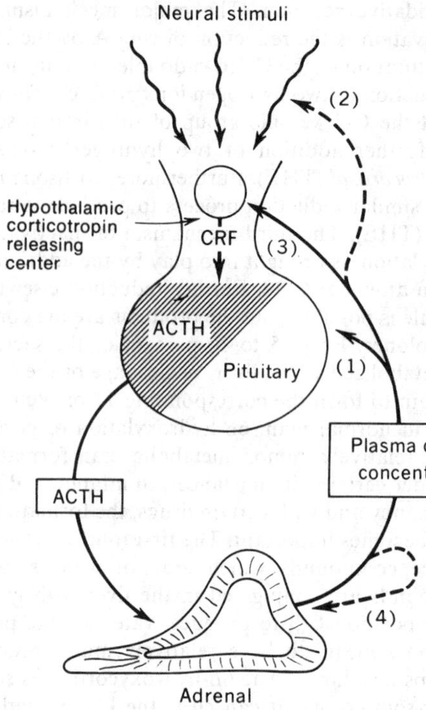

FIGURE 93-4
Hypothalamic-pituitary-adrenal axis. CRF = *corticotropin-releasing factor. (1) Dominant feedback control on the pituitary gland; (2) possible feedback of plasma cortisol on higher nerve centers; (3) on the hypothalamus; (4) and/or the adrenal gland itself.*

Besides its major action in stimulation of the biogenesis and release of steroid hormones by the adrenal gland, ACTH can stimulate melanocytes of amphibians and can increase adipokinetic activity in a number of species. Both these extraadrenal actions have been verified with synthetic ACTH molecules.

The action of ACTH on the adrenal gland itself is rapid; within minutes of its release, there is an increased concentration of steroids in the adrenal venous blood. It produces a number of biochemical changes: (1) an increase in adrenal weight; (2) a decrease in the amount of adrenal lipids, cholesterol, and ascorbic acid; (3) increase in adenyl cyclase activity and in adenosine-3′,5′-monophosphate (cyclic AMP concentration); (4) increase in protein synthesis and oxidative phosphorylation; (5) an accelerated rate of glycogenolysis; and (6) increase in adrenal blood flow. The most likely mechanism by which ACTH stimulates steroidogenesis is via activation of the membrane-bound adenyl cyclase. This would increase the level of adenosine-3′,5′-monophosphate (cyclic AMP), which then activates adrenocortical protein kinase enzymes. This results in the phosphorylation of proteins which in some way activate steroid biosynthesis. Evidence has been obtained which suggests that activation of protein biosynthesis is an important if not an essential part of the action of ACTH. Apparently ACTH increases protein biosynthesis either by stimulation of messenger ribonucleic acid or by enzyme activation.

RENIN-ANGIOTENSIN PHYSIOLOGY (see also Chap. 250) Renin is a proteolytic enzyme with an approximate molecular weight of 35,000 to 40,000. It has been semipurified. It is produced and stored in the granules of the juxtaglomerular cells surrounding the afferent arterioles of the cortical glomeruli. The juxtaglomerular apparatus consists of both the juxtaglomerular cells and the cells of the macula densa. The latter area also contains some renin. Renin acts on the basic substrate angiotensinogen (a circulating alpha$_2$-globulin), made in the liver, to form the decapeptide angiotensin-I. Various inhibitors of intrarenal renin formation are believed to exist (Fig. 93-5). Angiotensin-I is then enzymatically converted by converting enzyme to the octapeptide angiotensin-II by the splitting off of the two C-terminal amino acids. Angiotensin-II is the most potent pressor compound (on a mole for mole basis) made in the body, and it exerts this pressor action by a direct effect on arteriolar smooth muscle. In addition, angiotensin-II is a potent direct stimulus to the production of aldosterone by the zona glomerulosa of the adrenal cortex. Various peptidases, collectively termed "angiotensinases," in organ tissue, vessel walls, and circulating plasma are responsible for the ultimate biochemical degradation of circulating angiotensin-II. Angiotensinases rapidly destroy angiotensin-II (half-life approximately 1 min), while the half-life of renin is more prolonged (10 to 20 min). Finally, a number of studies have documented that other tissues, such as uterus, vascular tissue, brain, and salivary glands, also produce renin-like substances. The significance of these so-called "isorenins" is not understood.

Renin release is controlled by four major factors. For the most part, these are interdependent, and the amount of renin released is a composite of the input of all four. The *juxtaglomerular cells,* which are specialized myoepithelial cells cuffing the afferent arterioles, act as miniature pressure transducers, sensing renal perfusion pressure and corresponding changes in afferent arteriolar perfusion pressures. The changes in pressure are perceived as distortions in the existing stretch on the arteriolar walls. For example, under conditions of a reduction in circulating blood volume, there will be a corresponding reduction in renal perfusion pressure and, therefore, in afferent arteriolar pressure (Fig. 93-5). This will be perceived by the juxtaglomerular cells as a decreased stretch exerted on the afferent arteriolar walls. The juxtaglomerular cells will then release increasing quantities of renin within the kidney circulation, leading to the formation of angiotensin-I. Angiotensin-I leaves the kidney both by renal lymphatic and renal venous outflow. It is converted into angiotensin-II and directly stimulates the adrenal cortex to release increasing quantities of aldosterone. Increasing plasma levels of aldosterone lead to increasing renal sodium retention and thus result in expansion of extracellular fluid volume, which, as it is completed, dampens the initiating signal for renin release. Within this context, the renin-angiotensin-aldosterone system is subserving volume control by appropriate modifications of renal tubular sodium transport.

FIGURE 93-5
Renin-angiotensin-aldosterone volume regulation in normal man.

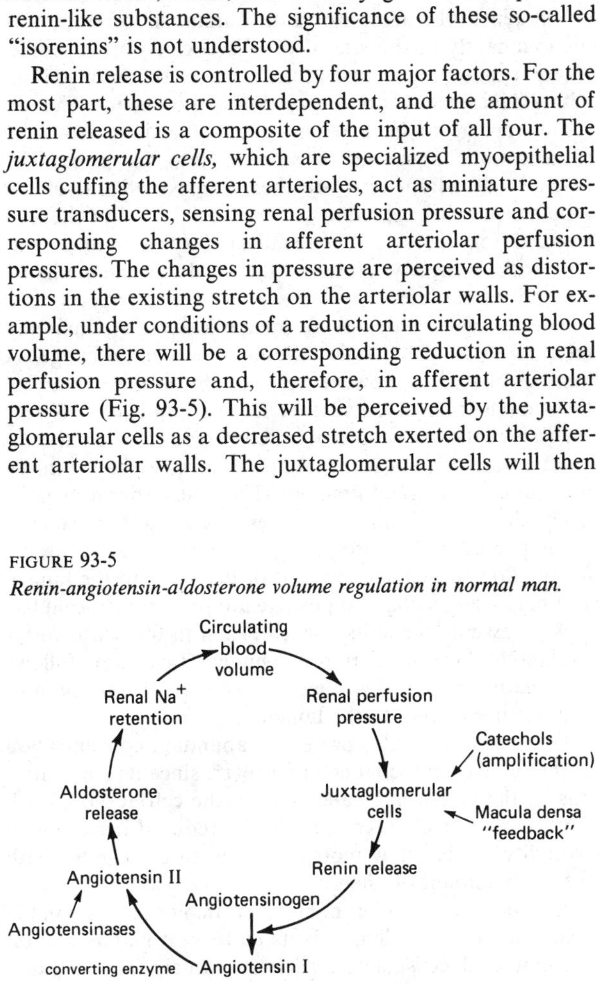

A second control mechanism for renin release centers in the *macula densa* cells. These are a group of special-staining distal convoluted tubular epithelial cells found in direct opposition to the juxtaglomerular cells. It has been suggested that they may function as chemoreceptors, monitoring the sodium load presented to the distal tubule, and that such information, while it is being monitored, is directly fed back to the juxtaglomerular cells, where appropriate modifications in renin release take place. Such an intrarenal renin-release mechanism is said to be capable of operating independently of changes in renal perfusion pressure. Under conditions of increased delivery of filtered sodium to the macula densa, feedback would occur to the juxtaglomerular apparatus, resulting in a release of increasing quantities of renin, which could then be capable of decreasing glomerular filtration rate, thereby reducing the filtered load of sodium. The evidence for this hypothesis is conflicting.

The *sympathetic nervous system* is also a significant factor regulating the release of renin. Infusion of catecholamines directly into the renal artery or electrical stimulation of renal nerves can increase renin release. Conversely, α- or β-adrenergic blockade can block the renin response to upright posture or acute volume depletion. The mechanism by which sympathetic activity alters renin secretion is not known. It may have a direct effect on the juxtaglomerular cell to increase adenyl cyclase activity, or it may act indirectly on either the juxtaglomerular or the macula densa cells by way of a vasoconstrictive action on the afferent arteriole.

Finally, a number of circulating factors may alter renin release. Increasing dietary *potassium* can decrease renin release; decreasing potassium intake increases renin release. These effects are not secondary to a direct effect of potassium on aldosterone secretion with an alteration in sodium balance, since similar renin responses occur with subjects on a low sodium intake. In addition, direct infusion of potassium into the renal artery also decreases renin release. The significance of this potassium effect is unclear. *Angiotensin* itself can exert a negative feedback control on renin release independent of alterations in renal blood flow, pressure, or aldosterone secretion. There is also some evidence that both ACTH and vasopressin can increase renin release. Thus, the control of renin release is complex, consisting of both *intrarenal* (pressoreceptor and macula densa) and *extrarenal* (sympathetic nervous system, potassium, angiotensin, etc.) mechanisms. A given level of renin secretion probably reflects all these factors, with the intrarenal mechanism predominating.

GLUCOCORTICOID PHYSIOLOGY The division of adrenal steroids into glucocorticoids and mineralocorticoids is somewhat arbitrary in that most glucocorticoids have some mineralocorticoid-like properties, and vice versa. The descriptive term *glucocorticoid* is applied to those adrenal steroids having a predominant action on intermediary metabolism. The principal glucocorticoid is cortisol (hydrocortisone). The actions of the glucocorticoids on intermediary metabolism are predominantly anti-insulin and include the regulation of protein, carbohydrate, lipid, and nucleic acid metabolism. Their actions appear mainly to be catabolic in effect, with an increased protein breakdown and nitrogen excretion. Glucocorticoids increase hepatic glycogen content and promote the hepatic synthesis of glucose (gluconeogenesis). These actions of glucocorticoids are in large part explained by the mobilization of glycogenic amino acid precursors from peripheral supporting structures, such as bone, skin, muscle, and connective tissue due to protein breakdown as well as to the inhibition of protein synthesis and amino acid uptake. Glucocorticoid-induced hyperaminoacidemia also indirectly facilitates gluconeogenesis by stimulating glucagon secretion. In addition, glucocorticoids have a direct action on the liver to stimulate the synthesis of hepatic enzymes, such as tyrosine amino transferase and tryptophan pyrrolase. Inhibition of extrahepatic protein synthesis and stimulation of hepatic enzyme synthesis is reflected in the actions of glucocorticoids on nucleic acid metabolism. Corticoids inhibit the synthesis of nucleic acids in most body tissues, but in the liver ribonucleic acid (RNA) synthesis is stimulated. It is postulated that cortisol probably enters the target cell by diffusion, combines with a specific high-affinity cytoplasmic receptor protein, and is transferred to a specific acceptor site on the chromatin tissue of the nucleus, which then produces an increase in RNA synthesis and later in protein synthesis. Glucocorticoids are necessary for fatty acid mobilization by permitting and enhancing activation of cellular lipase by lipid-mobilizing hormones (e.g., catecholamines and pituitary peptides).

The action of cortisol on structural protein and adipose tissue varies considerably in different parts of the body. For example, depletion of protein matrix of the vertebral column may be affected only minimally; peripheral adipose tissue may diminish, whereas abdominal and interscapular fat may accumulate. Glucocorticoids have anti-inflammatory properties, which are probably related to their actions on the microvasculature as well as to cellular effects. Cortisol maintains normal vascular responsiveness to circulating vasoconstrictor factors and opposes the increase in capillary permeability characteristic of acute inflammation. Glucocorticoids also impede endothelial sticking of leukocytes and diapedesis through the capillary wall. Reduced cellular adherence to vascular endothelium is probably secondary to antagonism to the action of migration-inhibiting factor (MIF) by glucocorticoids. Glucocorticoids produce lysis of lymphoid tissue, specifically, T cells or the small lymphocytes derived from the thymus, and diminish the number of circulating eosinophils. Thus, cortisol impairs cellular-mediated immunity, but antibody production is not altered. Glucocorticoids also stabilize lysosomal membranes, thereby suppressing the release of proteolytic acid hydrolases stored in these cytoplasmic organelles. Cortisol has a major effect on body water, in both its distribution and its excretion. It subserves the extracellular fluid volume by a retarding action on the inward migration of water into cells. It affects renal water excretion in a dual manner, by increasing the rate of glomerular filtration and by a direct action on the renal tubule, which actions summate to increase solute-free water clearance. Glucocorticoids, in general, will increase renal tubular sodium reabsorption and cause an increased urine potassium excretion. The integrity of personality is enhanced by cortisol, and emotional disorders are common with either excesses or deficits of cortisol. Lastly, another major action of cortisol is to directly suppress pituitary ACTH secretion.

MINERALOCORTICOID PHYSIOLOGY The major mineralocorticoid produced by the human adrenal cortex is aldosterone. Other mineralocorticoids are produced, i.e., 11-deoxycorticosterone and 18-hydroxy-11-deoxycorticosterone, but because of differences in potency they are far less important than aldosterone. Under normal circumstances, aldosterone has two important "mineralocorticoid" activities: (1) it is a major regulator of extracellular fluid volume, and (2) it is a major determinant of potassium metabolism. It regulates volume through a direct effect on the renal tubular transport of sodium. Aldosterone acts predominantly at the site of the distal convoluted tubule, where it causes a decrease in the urine excretion of sodium with an increase in urine excretion of potassium. The net result appears to be a reabsorption of sodium from the filtrate, while potassium is secreted into the urine. The reabsorbed sodium ions are then transported out of the tubular epithelial cells into the interstitial fluid of the kidney and from there into the renal capillary circulation. Water will passively follow the aldosterone-mediated transported sodium.

The action of aldosterone on the kidney is commonly referred to as the distal sodium-potassium exchange. A number of studies, however, cast doubt on the validity of this simplistic theory. Evidence from a number of sources suggests that potassium is not actively secreted by the tubular epithelium but rather simply follows a change in the transtubular electrical gradient. The reabsorption of positively charged sodium ions causes a fall in the transmembrane potential, thus producing an environment favorable for the flow of positive ions out of the cell into the lumen. The major singly charged positive ion present intracellularly is potassium. Since its concentration in the cell is forty- to eightyfold greater than in the lumen, it passively follows this relative electrical gradient in order to restore the normal positive charge to the lumen.

Hydrogen ion is also present in abundant concentration in the tubular epithelial cell. However, since its concentration in the lumen is greater than in the cell, it would still have to be actively secreted, but the reduced intraluminal positivity would allow more hydrogen to be secreted with the same amount of energy.

Aldosterone and other mineralocorticoids also act on the epithelium of the salivary ducts and sweat glands and on the epithelial cells of the gastrointestinal tract to cause reabsorption of sodium in "exchange" for potassium ions. The subcellular mechanism of action of aldosterone is like that described earlier for cortisol.

When normal individuals are given a long-term course of aldosterone (or a comparable mineralocorticoid, such as parenteral deoxycorticosterone acetate), an initial period of sodium retention is followed by a natriuresis, and sodium balance is reestablished after 3 to 5 days. As a result, clinical edema formation does not develop. This phenomenon is referred to as the "escape phenomenon," signifying an "escape" by the renal tubules from the sodium-retaining action of chronically administered aldosterone. The mechanism responsible for the escape phenomenon has remained elusive. Such an "escape" phenomenon is exhibited by patients with hypertension but is characteristically absent in patients with edema disorders.

There are three well-defined *control* mechanisms for aldosterone release—the renin-angiotensin system, potassium, and ACTH. The renin-angiotensin system is the major system for control of extracellular fluid volume, via regulation of aldosterone secretion. In effect, the renin-angiotensin system attempts to maintain the circulating blood volume constant by causing aldsterone-induced sodium retention during periods registered as volume deficiencies, and by decreasing aldosterone-dependent sodium retention under conditions in which volume is registered as being ample.

Potassium ions can regulate aldosterone secretion independently of the renin-angiotensin system. In normal man, oral potassium loading increases aldosterone excretion, secretion, and plasma levels. In addition, systemic infusion of potassium ions under certain circumstances significantly increases plasma aldosterone levels with as small as a 0.1 meq per liter increase in serum potassium. That this effect is secondary to a direct action of the potassium ion is supported by a number of facts: potassium suppresses renin secretion; the effect of potassium on aldosterone excretion is independent of reciprocal changes in intravascular volume; the infusion of potassium ions directly into the adrenal artery produces an immediate increase in adrenal venous plasma levels; and finally, increasing the potassium content of incubation medium containing adrenal tissue results in an increase in aldosterone production. How potassium alters aldosterone secretion is not known. It may be related to small changes in serum potassium levels, to changes in intracellular potassium concentration, or to a change in the flux of potassium across the adrenal cortical cell membrane.

A number of facts support a role for ACTH in the control of aldosterone secretion. In supine normal man, plasma aldosterone has a rhythm parallel to that of cortisol and presumably ACTH. Physiologic levels of ACTH can also acutely stimulate aldosterone secretion, but this action is not sustained if ACTH is continuously infused for periods greater than 10 to 12 h. However, other studies seem to relegate ACTH to a minor role in the control of aldosterone in normal man. For example, subjects on high-dose steroid therapy for several years and with presumably complete suppression of ACTH have normal aldosterone-secretory responses to sodium restriction. Therefore, chronic ACTH deficiency per se does not alter glomerulosa cell responsiveness.

Finally, the prior dietary intake of both potassium and sodium can alter the magnitude of the aldosterone response to acute stimulation. Increasing potassium intake or decreasing sodium intake will sensitize the response of the glomerulosa cells to acute stimulation by ACTH, angiotensin-II, and/or potassium. In vitro studies in animals indicate that aldosterone-stimulating substances may act on the late (corticosterone to aldosterone) as well as the early (cholesterol to pregnenolone) pathways for aldosterone biosynthesis. Since all acute stimuli increase the activity of the early pathway, an attractive unifying hypothesis that could explain the sensitizing effects of dietary sodium restriction and potassium loading is an increased activity of the final step of aldosterone biosynthesis.

In summary, while physiologic levels of ACTH under certain circumstances may stimulate aldosterone secretion, ACTH seems to be less important than potassium and the renin-angiotensin system in the control of aldosterone production. On the other hand, the renin-angiotensin system and potassium may be of equal importance in the regulation of aldosterone secretion in man (Fig. 93-6). Moreover, the interaction of dietary sodium and potassium can sensitize the response of aldosterone secretion following acute stimulation. Although the existence of early and late pathways for the control of aldosterone biosynthesis in man is speculative, evidence that diet can sensitize aldosterone secretion is consistent with this hypothesis. How dietary changes alter the late pathway, and whether sodium and potassium manipulations are acting on the same cells and/or receptor sites are not clear from the information presently available.

ANDROGEN PHYSIOLOGY Androgens are defined biologically as substances that stimulate male secondary sexual characteristics. The secondary sexual characteristics are affected through inhibition of the female characteristics (defeminization) and accentuation of the male characteristics (masculinization). These are seen clinically as hirsutism and virilization in the female with amenhorrhea, atrophy of the breasts and uterus, enlargement of the clitoris, deepening of the voice, acne, increased muscle mass, increased

FIGURE 93-6
The interrelationship of the volume and potassium feedback loops on aldosterone secretion. Integration of signals from each loop determines the level of aldosterone secretion.

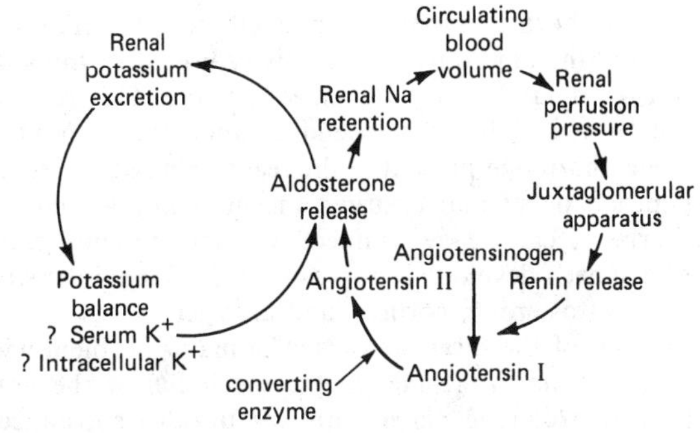

heterosexual drive, and receding hairline. In the male there are increased body and sexual hair and enlargement of the sexual organs. Androgens also increase the synthesis of protein from amino acids, and this anabolic action leads to increased muscle mass and strength. Increased nitrogen retention may be used to assess androgenic biologic potency.

Steroids with predominant androgenic activity have 19 carbon atoms (Fig. 93-1). The principal adrenal androgens secreted are dehydroepiandrosterone (DHEA), androstenedione, and 11-hydroxyandrostenedione. DHEA and its sulfate are *quantitatively* the major androgens secreted by the adrenal cortex. The secretion of DHEA sulfate is approximately 10 mg per day; that of free DHEA is 2 mg per day. In the normal female, approximately 50 percent of the total secreted adrenal androgens are measured in the urine as 17-ketosteroids. DHEA, androstenedione, and 11-hydroxyandrostenedione, when assayed *biologically,* are weak androgens, but all are peripherally interconvertible with the potent androgen, testosterone. In normal women, only 40 percent of testosterone is directly secreted; 60 percent arises from androstenedione.

The release of adrenal androgens is stimulated by ACTH, not by gonadotropins. With ACTH stimulation, 17-ketosteroids increase but to a much lesser extent than do urine 17-hydroxycorticosteroids. Part of this increment in 17-ketosteroid excretion is due to the metabolism of increasing 17-hydroxycorticosteroids by the mechanism of C-20:C-21 side-chain cleavage, producing 11-oxy-17-ketosteroids. Adrenal androgens are suppressed by exogenous glucocorticoid administration, as judged by decrements in urine 17-ketosteroid excretion.

LABORATORY EVALUATION OF ADRENOCORTICAL FUNCTION

Studies of adrenal function have been greatly facilitated by the development of sensitive radioimmunoassay procedures for a variety of steroid and polypeptide hormones. The essential elements of these procedures are (1) the development of a specific antibody which binds the hormone, and (2) competition between isotopically labeled and unlabeled hormone for the binding sites on the antibody. In practice, known amounts of *antiserum* specific for the hormone, *labeled* hormone, and plasma unknown are incubated together. At the completion of the incubation period, an equilibrium has occurred between labeled (H^*) and unlabeled hormone (H) and the specific antibody (Ab):

$$H + H^* + Ab \rightleftharpoons AbH^* + AbH$$

The bound hormone is then separated from the free hormone, and the amount of radioactivity bound to the antibody is compared with that remaining free. This ratio of bound to free is directly dependent upon the amount of unlabeled hormone present in the reaction mixture. By the preparation of standard curves, the unknown amount of the hormone can be determined. By such techniques, assays have been developed for plasma ACTH, angiotensin-I and -II, testosterone, cortisol, and aldosterone, as well as urine levels of the three steroids. The major problem with these assay systems resides in the specificity of the antibody. If it cross-reacts significantly with other substances, then a reliable answer will be achieved only if the plasma or urine is first processed to eliminate the cross-reacting substance.

A second major advance has been the clarification of the interrelation of plasma levels, secretion rates, and clearance rates of steroids. The basic assumption in the measurement of plasma levels or the urinary excretion of steroid metabolites is that they accurately reflect adrenal *secretory* rates of that steroid. A disadvantage of urine *excretion* values is that they may not truly reflect the secretion rate because of improper collection or altered metabolism. Measurement of the actual adrenal secretory rate of a given steroid would be preferable, and such methods are finding increasing clinical application. The adrenal secretory rate is calculated by the dilution that an administered radioactive steroid undergoes as a consequence of the admixture of endogenously secreted nonradioactive steroid hormone with the exogenous radioactive steroid. In practice, a major unique metabolite of the steroid is isolated and purified by chromatography; from a determination of its specific activity (counts per minute per microgram of steroid) and knowledge of the specific activity of the administered steroid one may calculate by the dilution principle the actual amount of the steroid secreted by the adrenal gland during the period of urine collection (usually 24 h). In general, aldosterone and probably cortisol urine secretory rates closely reflect adrenal secretion of these hormones.

Plasma levels reflect the level of secretion only at the time of measurement. The plasma level (*PL*) is dependent on two factors: the secretion rate (*SR*) of the hormone and the rate at which it is metabolized, i.e., its metabolic clearance rate (*MCR*). These three factors can be related mathematically as follows:

$$PL = \frac{SR}{MCR} \quad \text{or} \quad SR = MCR \times PL$$

The secretion rate can also be estimated by determining the MCR and plasma levels of the steroid. When secretion is determined this way, it is called a *blood production rate.* Its accuracy is dependent on how closely the measured plasma levels and metabolic clearance rates reflect a 24-h mean value. When no unique urine metabolite of the hormone exists or when there is significant peripheral interconversion of steroids (such as androgens in the female), then blood production rates more accurately reflect adrenal secretion than do urine secretion rates.

BLOOD LEVELS (See Table 93-1) **Peptides** ACTH and angiotensin-II can be measured by radioimmunoassay. There are still technical difficulties with both assays, related mainly to nonspecificity of the antibodies employed. ACTH is probably secreted episodically during the day, with a general trend for plasma levels to vary diurnally, with lower levels in the early evening than in the morning. Angiotensin-II levels also vary diurnally but are further influenced by dietary sodium intake and posture. Both upright posture and sodium restriction elevate angiotensin-II levels.

Measurements of the enzyme renin are made by several laboratories, utilizing a purified renin substrate. The majority of clinical determinations of the renin-angiotensin system, however, involve measurements of peripheral "plasma renin activity" (PRA) in which the renin activity is gauged by the generation of angiotensin during a standardized incubation period. This method depends on the presence of sufficient angiotensinogen in the patient's plasma as substrate. The generated angiotensin is then measured by radioimmunoassay. Plasma renin activity levels will depend on dietary sodium intake of the patient and whether the patient is ambulatory. In normal recumbent or upright man, a diurnal rhythm for plasma renin activity is characterized by peak values occurring in the morning, with decreases in activity in the afternoon.

Steroids The more cumbersome double-isotope derivative assay and less specific fluorometric method for adrenal steroids are being replaced by radioimmunoassay methods. Cortisol and aldosterone are both secreted episodically, but levels generally decline during the day, with peak values in the morning and low levels in the evening. In addition, the plasma level of aldosterone, but not of cortisol, is increased by dietary potassium loading, sodium restriction, or assuming the upright posture. In the male, circadian and day-to-day variations in plasma testosterone levels have also been reported. In the female, plasma testosterone is higher in the luteal than in the follicular phase of the menstrual cycle.

URINE LEVELS The principal determinations are of urine 17-hydroxycorticoids, 17-ketosteroids, 17-ketogenic steroids, free cortisol, and aldosterone. The urine *17-hydroxycorticoids* are determined as Porter-Silber chromogens, i.e., these steroids react with the reagent phenylhydrazine to produce a characteristic color. This reaction is specific for steroids with a "dihydroxy acetone" C-17 side chain, i.e., with hydroxyl groups on C-17 and C-21 and a ketone group on C-20 (Fig. 93-7). Therefore, this determination will include cortisol, cortisone, tetrahydrocortisol, tetrahydrocortisone, and 11-deoxycortisol but not cortols, cortolones, and pregnanetriol. Normally, daytime (7 A.M. to 7 P.M.) excretion exceeds night values (7 P.M. to 7 A.M.). It is of extreme importance that the completeness of any and all urine steroid collections be checked by urine creatinine determinations.

TABLE 93-1
Range of normal values for tests of adrenal function

Test	*Normal value, range*
Plasma cortisol, μg/100 ml 8 A.M.	9–24
4 P.M.	3–12
Cortisol secretory rate, mg/24 h	5–25
Urine free cortisol, μg/24 h	20–100
17-hydroxycorticoids, mg/24 h	2–10
17-ketogenic steroids, mg/24 h:	
Males	5–23
Females	3–15
Plasma testosterone, μg/100 ml:	
Males	0.3–1.0
Females	0.01–0.1
17-ketosteroids, mg/24 h:	
Males	7–25
Females	4–15
Plasma 11-deoxycortisol (S), μg/100 ml	<1.0
Urine tetrahydro 11-deoxycortisol (THS), mg/24 h	0.1–1.0
Pregnanetriol, mg/24 h:	
0–6 yr	< .2
7–15 yr	<1.2
Over 16 yr	0.5–2.5
Pregnanediol, mg/24 h:	
Males	<1.0
Females	1.1–4.0
Plasma aldosterone, ng/100 ml (100 meq Na, 60–100 meq K, supine)	1–5
Aldosterone secretion, μg/24 h (100 meq Na, 60–100 meq K)	50–250
Aldosterone excretion, μg/24 h (100 meq Na, 60–100 meq K)	2–10
Plasma renin activity, ng/ml/h (100 meq Na, 60–100 meq K, supine)	1–2.5
Plasma angiotensin II, pg/ml (100 meq Na, 60–100 meq K, supine)	10–30
Plasma ACTH (pg/ml) 8 A.M.	5–50

The urine *17-ketosteroids* are those containing a ketone group at C-17; they originate either in the adrenal gland or the gonad. In the normal female, 90 percent or more of total urinary 17-ketosteroids is derived from the adrenal gland, while in the male, only 60 to 70 percent is of adrenal origin. Measurement depends on the Zimmermann reaction, whereby color is produced when 17-ketosteroids are condensed with *m*-dinitrobenzene. This reaction is specific for steroids with a ketone substituent with an adjacent unsubstituted carbon atom (Fig. 93-7). Urine 17-ketosteroid values are highest in young adults and decline with age.

The total urine 17-ketosteroids may be subdivided into those having either an oxygen or hydroxyl substituent at position C-11 (11-oxy-17-ketosteroids) and those having no such groups (11-deoxy-17-ketosteroids). These 11-oxy-17-ketosteroids are uniquely derived from the adrenal gland, since other tissues do not possess the enzymes for active C-11 hydroxylation, whereas the 11-deoxy-17-ketosteroids may arise from adrenal, testicular or ovarian tissue.

Ketogenic steroids is a descriptive term for those C-21 hydroxycorticoids potentially capable of transformation into 17-ketosteroids in vitro. After the excreted 17-ketosteroids are reduced to noninterfering compounds, the side chains of C-21 hydroxycorticosteroids are oxidized to 17-ketonic groups, which then can be measured by the Zimmermann reaction as 17-ketosteroids. The Norymberski technique for ketogenic steroid analysis measures all steroids determined as 17-hydroxysteroids by the Porter-Silber method and, in addition, includes the cortols, cortolones, and pregnanetriol (Fig. 93-7).

The determination of either urine *free cortisol* or *aldosterone* excretion is more difficult, usually requiring radioimmunoassay. Aldosterone excretion is measured by determining the excretion of a major metabolite, usually the acid-labile conjugate. A carefully timed urine collection is a prerequisite for all excretory determinations.

STIMULATION TESTS Stimulation tests are useful in documenting the existence of a hormonal deficiency state. A standardized and specific stimulus for the production and release of a given hormone is applied, and the quantity of the released hormone can then be measured.

Glucocorticoid stimulation tests Within minutes after initiation of an infusion of ACTH, increased cortisol levels are noted in adrenal venous blood. This responsiveness of the adrenal gland to ACTH is utilized as an index of the "functional reserve" of the gland to produce cortisol. Under maximal ACTH stimulation the cortisol secretion increases tenfold to 300 mg per day. Such maximal stimulation is obtainable only with prolonged ACTH infusions. For clinical purposes, the functional adrenal reserve for cortisol production is standardized with a shorter infusion time (8 h). The standard intravenous ACTH test is performed by administering 40 units aqueous ACTH in 500 ml normal saline solution intravenously over an exact 8-h interval (from 8 A.M. to 4 P.M.) on two successive days and collecting the complete 24-h urine output for analysis of creatinine, 17-hydroxycorticoids, or 17-ketogenic steroids. The patient may be ambulatory during this period. With such a method of testing, an average increment of 15 mg (range, 10 to 25) has been noted in urine 17-hydroxysteroids on the first day of testing and an average increment of 25 mg (range, 15 to 35) on the second infusion day, by one commonly used method. Alternatively, the increment in blood cortisol levels may be used to assess adrenal reserve. The cortisol increment above control should be 10 to 20 μg per 100 ml by the first hour and 20 to 40 μg per 100 ml by the eighth hour. In the performance of the test the duration of the infusion must be strictly adhered to. Synthetic α1–24 ACTH has become available as an alternative preparation. Because of its greater purity it has generally replaced the natural ACTH preparation. The standard infusion test would then be 25 units of the α1–24 ACTH in 500 ml normal saline solution. A screening test for adrenal insufficiency utilizes the intramuscular administration of 0.25 mg (25 units) α1–24 ACTH with measurement of the rise in plasma cortisol levels. Normally, there will be a doubling of basal levels within 30 to 60 min or an increment above basal levels of 7 to 11 μg per 100 ml. The test can give a false positive result for adrenal insufficiency, however, because of irregular absorption of the ACTH from the injection site.

Occasionally, it is necessary to prolong the ACTH infusion in order to separate primary from secondary adrenal insufficiency. This can be accomplished by using an 8-h infusion on four or five consecutive days or by a continuous 24- or 48-h infusion. The 48-h test employs an infusion of 50 units of synthetic ACTH in 1,000 ml 5 percent dextrose in water or dextrose in normal saline solution over 24 h for two consecutive days.

Mineralocorticoid and renin-angiotensin stimulation tests Stimulation tests have been devised utilizing a protocol of programmed volume depletion, such as sodium restriction, diuretic administration, or upright posture. A simple potent stimulation test consists of severe sodium restriction and upright posture. After 3 to 5 days of a 10 meq sodium intake, aldosterone secretion or excretion rates should exhibit a two- to threefold increase over control. Supine morning plasma aldosterone levels usually increase three- to sixfold. In addition, plasma levels increase two- to fourfold in response to 2 to 3 h of upright posture. Recumbent plasma renin activity following sodium restriction to 10 meq per day ranges from 2.5 to 8 ng/ml/h and rises to 3 to 20 ng/ml/h following 3 h of ambulation.

Stimulation tests on normal dietary sodium intake may also be carried out by the administration of a potent diuretic, such as 40 to 80 mg furosemide, followed by 2 to 3 h of upright posture. The normal response is a two- to fourfold rise in plasma aldosterone levels. Plasma renin activity usually rises to 8 to 15 ng/ml/h.

The infusion of angiotensin-II (3 to 10 ng/kg/min) is also a potent test of aldosterone responsiveness. However, arterial blood pressure must be continuously monitored and the infusion terminated for pressor responses greater than 10 mmHg. Also, aldosterone responses must be related to specified dietary sodium intakes since sodium restriction markedly enhances aldosterone responsiveness to angiotensin-II.

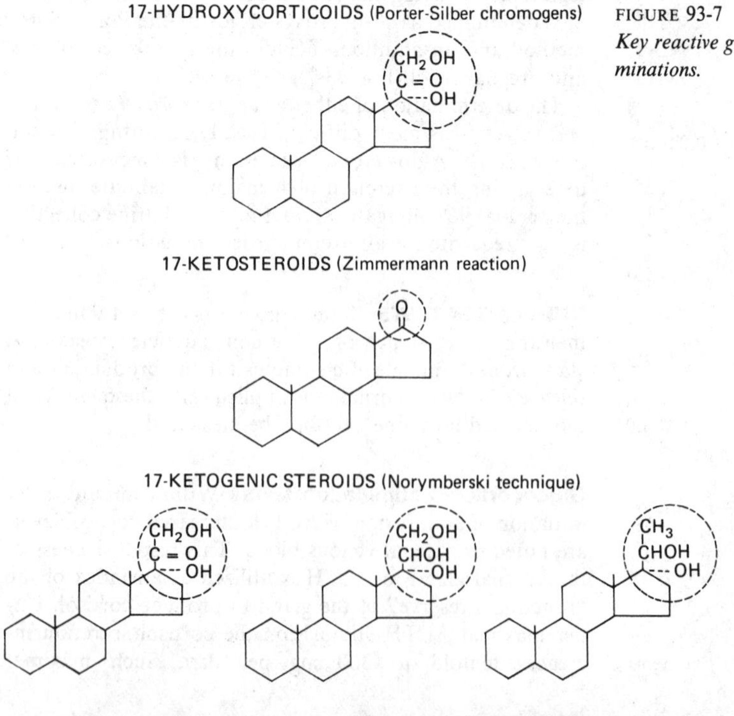

FIGURE 93-7
Key reactive groups (enclosed by dashed circle) in urine steroid determinations.

SUPPRESSION TESTS Suppression tests are used to document hypersecretion of adrenocortical hormones and are based on the demonstration of a decrease in the target hormone following standardized suppression of its tropic hormone. Thus, suppression testing for cortisol hypersecretion would involve suppression of ACTH release, with documentation of an appropriately normal decrease in cortisol production, while suppression testing of aldosterone would involve demonstration of a decrease in aldosterone secondary to suppression of the renin-angiotensin system.

Glucocorticoid suppression tests The hypothalamic-pituitary ACTH release mechanism is sensitive to the circulating blood level of glucocorticoids. When such blood levels are increased in the normal individual, less ACTH is released from the anterior pituitary, and secondarily, less steroid is produced by the adrenal gland. The integrity of this feedback mechanism can be tested clinically by giving a potent glucocorticoid and judging suppression of ACTH secretion by analysis of urine steroid excretory values. A potent glucocorticoid such as dexamethasone is utilized in order that the administered compound may be given in such small amounts that it will not contribute significantly to the steroids to be analyzed.

One or more of the three standard tests are usually employed. The simplest is the overnight dexamethasone suppression test. This involves the measurement of plasma-corticoid levels at 8 A.M. and/or the urine 17-hydroxycorticoid and creatinine excretion between 7 A.M. and 12 noon following the oral administration of 1 mg dexamethasone the previous midnight. The 8 A. M. value for plasma corticoids in normal subjects should be less than 5 μg per 100 ml, and the ratio of urine Porter-Silber chromogens per milligram of creatinine in the 5-h urine specimen should be less than 0.004.

The usual method of testing adrenal suppressibility is to administer 0.5 mg dexamethasone every 6 h for two successive days while collecting urine over a 24-h period for the determination of creatinine, 17-hydroxysteroids, and 17-17-ketosteroids. In patients with a normal hypothalamic-pituitary ACTH release mechanism, a fall in the urine 17-hydroxycorticoids to less than 3 mg a day on the second day of dexamethasone administration is seen.

An intravenous dexamethasone suppression test is used less often. One milligram of dexamethasone is administered intravenously per hour for a total of 3 h, and blood is collected for plasma glucocorticoid determinations. A 50 percent fall in plasma cortisol at the end of 3 h of infusion is normally expected. Normal response to any of the suppression tests implies that the ACTH control of the adrenal glands is physiologically normal. However, an isolated abnormal result, particularly when the overnight suppression test is being used, does not in itself imply pituitary and/or adrenal disease.

Mineralocorticoid suppression tests Mineralocorticoid suppression testing procedures have been devised using saline infusions, oral salt loading, or DOCA administration as the means for expansion of the extracellular fluid volume. With expansion of extracellular fluid volume, there will be a decrease in renal renin release, a decrease in circulating plasma renin activity, and a decrease in aldosterone secretion and/or excretion. This would be the appropriate "normal" response. Varied tests differ in the rate at which extracellular fluid volume is expanded. The "normal saline suppression test" involves the intravenous administration of 2 liters normal saline solution over a 4-h period from 9 A.M. until 1 P.M. on two consecutive days. Aldosterone secretion or excretion rate is measured the day before and on the second day of saline loading; plasma aldosterone levels are measured before and at the end of each saline infusion day. The patient previously has been permitted to come into equilibration on a 10 meq sodium and 100 meq potassium constant diet. Normal response of suppression of aldosterone secretion by this maneuver is a value less than 200 μg per day (excretion < 15 μg per day and supine postinfusion plasma levels < 5 ng per 100 ml). The "oral salt-loading suppression test" is conveniently carried out by abruptly increasing the patient's sodium intake from a constant level of 10 meq per day to 200 meq per day for a period of 3 to 5 days, with measurement of aldosterone levels on the fourth or fifth day, at which time they should be similar to that for the saline suppression test. Potassium intake is held constant throughout the test, since potassium will cause aldosterone secretion to vary independently of the renin-angiotensin system. The "DOCA suppression test" is carried out by placing the patient on a normal (100 meq) or high (200 meq) sodium intake. After the patient is in sodium balance, deoxycorticosterone acetate is administered intramuscularly (10 mg every 12 h) for a period of 3 to 5 days. Normal subjects on a sodium intake of 100 meq daily demonstrate a 70 percent decrease in aldosterone levels when compared with control levels, which means that the aldosterone secretory value should be less than 250 μg per day (excretion $<$ 15 μg per day and supine morning plasma levels < 5 ng per 100 ml).

TEST OF PITUITARY RESPONSIVENESS A number of stimuli, such as insulin hypoglycemia, arginine vasopressin, and pyrogen, will cause release of ACTH from the pituitary by an action on higher nerve centers, the hypothalamus, or the pituitary gland itself. By measuring plasma ACTH, or blood glucocorticoids, the status of pituitary ACTH can be evaluated. Insulin-induced hypoglycemia is a particularly useful test since the release of growth hormone as well as ACTH is stimulated. In this test 0.05 to 0.1 units crystalline insulin per kg body weight is administered intravenously as a bolus to reduce fasting glucose levels at least 50 percent below basal. The normal cortisol response is a doubling above control levels within 30 to 60 min.

Metyrapone (SU4885; Metopirone) is a drug that selectively inhibits the enzyme action of 11-beta-hydroxylase in the adrenal gland. As a result, the conversion of 11-deoxycortisol (compound S) to cortisol is interfered with, and increased amounts of 11-deoxycortisol accumulate while blood levels of cortisol decrease (Fig. 93-2). Since 11-deoxycortisol is a weak suppressor of the hypothalamic-pituitary axis, the anterior pituitary responds to the declining cortisol blood levels by releasing larger quantities of ACTH in an attempt to stimulate the adrenal gland to release additional cortisol, which attempt, however, is thwarted by the metyrapone-induced enzymatic blockade. The metabolites of 11-deoxycortisol are excreted in increasing amounts in the urine, where they are measured as 17-hydroxycorticoids. *Note that the adrenal glands must be capable of being stimulated by ACTH, since assessment of the response depends on adrenal steroid production.*

The metyrapone response has been standardized for clinical evaluation of the reserve capacity of the anterior pituitary gland to release ACTH. Every 4 h over a 24- to 48-h period 750 mg metyrapone is administered orally, and daily urine collections for 17-hydroxycorticosteroids are obtained the day before testing, during the 2 days of testing, and the day after the last dose of metyrapone. The peak response of increased urine 17-hydroxysteroid excretion may be seen on the day after completion of metyrapone administration, and normal individuals will respond with at least a doubling of their basal 17-hydroxysteroid excretion. The metyrapone test will not accurately reflect ACTH reserve if subjects are ingesting exogenous glucocorticoids or drugs that accelerate the metabolism of metyrapone (e.g., Dilantin).

HYPERFUNCTION OF THE ADRENAL CORTEX

Distinct clinical syndromes are produced when excess amounts of the principal adrenocortical hormones are secreted. Thus, excess production of the principal glucocorticoid cortisol is associated with Cushing's syndrome; excess production of the principal mineralocorticoid aldosterone with clinical and chemical signs of aldosteronism; excess production of adrenal androgens with adrenal virilism. As would be expected, these syndromes do not always occur in the "pure" form but may have overlapping features.

CUSHING'S SYNDROME

ETIOLOGY From an analysis of the clinical and pathologic findings in a series of 12 patients, Harvey Cushing, in 1932, established a syndrome characterized by truncal obesity, hypertension, fatigability and weakness, amenorrhea, hirsutism, purplish abdominal striae, edema, glucosuria, and osteoporosis. As knowledge of this syndrome increased and as clinical tests of adrenocortical function became standardized and readily available, the diagnosis of Cushing's syndrome has been broadened into the classification shown in Table 93-2. It is apparent that, regardless of etiology, all cases of Cushing's syndrome are due to increased production of cortisol by the adrenal gland. The majority of cases are due to *bilateral adrenal hyperplasia,* in which the adrenal gland weight usually exceeds the normal combined total weight of 8 to 10 g. Cushing originally postulated that the adrenal hyperplasia in these patients was attributable to the presence of pituitary basophilic adenomas. However, many cases are found without basophilic adenomas. Some are due to ACTH-producing chromophobe adenomas, but these cases represent a small fraction of the total. In the remaining cases attention has focused also on the elaboration of increased amounts of ACTH in the presence of a radiographically normal sella turcica, possibly as a result of pituitary-hypothalamic dysfunction, whereby ACTH secretion is reset to respond to a higher level of circulating cortisol. Measured plasma ACTH levels are usually normal or modestly elevated *or* fail to exhibit a normal decrease late in the day. However, normal plasma ACTH levels should be considered "inappropriately" high in the presence of hypercortisolism. In such cases of Cushing's syndrome due to adrenal hyperplasia, presumably due to excessive ACTH stimulation, both adrenal glands are always affected.

Adrenal adenomas are usually unilateral but on occasion may occur bilaterally. These adenomas may or may not function in autonomous manner; i.e., they may or may not be independent of ACTH stimulation and control. In addition, approximately 10 percent of cases of Cushing's syndrome are associated with *adrenal carcinomas,* most often unilateral and most often functioning autonomously. In those cases of Cushing's syndrome due to unilateral adrenal adenomas or carcinomas functioning independently of ACTH, atrophy of the contralateral gland is often found, attributable to suppression of ACTH release by the high levels of cortisol secreted by the tumors. A small number of patients with Cushing's syndrome are found to have *adrenal rest tumors,* i.e., aberrant adrenocortical tissue occurring outside the adrenal gland. These embryologic remnants may be in the perirenal area, ovaries, or testes and exhibit histologic features of hyperplastic or adenomatous changes.

Nonendocrine tumors secreting polypeptides biologically, chemically, and immunologically indistinguishable from ACTH are also responsible for Cushing's syndrome secondary to bilateral adrenal hyperplasia. These neoplasms also synthesize α and more importantly β melanocyte-stimulating hormones (MSH), with the result that patients frequently are hyperpigmented. The major association of a nonendocrine tumor has been with primitive "oat-cell" carcinomas of the lung; other ACTH-secreting tumors include malignant thymoma, pancreatic carcinoma, and bronchial adenoma. Hypokalemic alkalosis is often prominent in such cases, whereas many of the distinctive physical findings usually associated with Cushing's syndrome may be absent.

TABLE 93-2
Causes of Cushing's syndrome

- *I* Adrenal hyperplasia
  - *A* Secondary to pituitary-hypothalamic dysfunction
  - *B* Secondary to ACTH-producing tumors
    - *1* Pituitary tumors
    - *2* Nonendocrine tumors (bronchogenic carcinoma, thymoma, pancreatic carcinoma, bronchial adenoma)
- *II* Adrenal nodular hyperplasia
- *III* Adrenal neoplasia
  - *A* Adenoma
  - *B* Carcinoma
- *IV* Exogenous, iatrogenic
  - *A* Prolonged use of glucocorticoids
  - *B* Prolonged use of ACTH

INCIDENCE Increasing numbers of patients with Cushing's syndrome are being detected among persons undergoing evaluation for such diverse entities as diabetes mellitus, hypertension, obesity, and osteoporosis. Many of these patients exhibit mild degrees of adrenal hyperfunction. The incidence of nontumorous adrenal hyperplasia in the female is three times that in the male, with the most frequent age of onset being the third or fourth decade. The incidence of Cushing's syndrome secondary to ACTH-secreting tumors will probably rise because of increased awareness of this syndrome.

CLINICAL SIGNS AND SYMPTOMS The frequency of clinical findings is listed in Table 93-3. Knowledge of the physiologic effects of glucocorticoids shows that many of the signs and symptoms logically follow. As a result of mobilization of peripheral supportive tissue, there are muscle weakness and fatigability, osteoporosis, and cutaneous striae. The latter involve a weakening and rupture of collagenous fibers in the dermis, so that the heavily vascularized subcutaneous tissues are exposed. Likewise, because of the loss of perivascular supporting tissue, there is easy bruisability, and ecchymoses often appear at sites of mild trauma. The osteoporosis may be so severe that collapse of vertebral bodies and pathologic fractures of other bones are frequently encountered. As a result of increased hepatic gluconeogenesis and insulin resistance, impaired glucose tolerance following a standard glucose load is common, occurring in 90 percent of patients. Frank diabetes occurs in less than 20 percent of patients, probably in individuals with a familial predisposition to this disorder. Hypercortisolism promotes the deposition of adipose tissue in characteristic sites. This is observed most notably in the upper part of the face, the classic "moon" facies; in the interscapular area, the "buffalo" hump; and in the mesenteric bed, where it produces the classic "truncal" obesity (Fig. 93-8). Rarely, there may be episternal fatty tumors and mediastinal widening secondary to fat accumulation. The reason for this peculiar distribution of lipid is not known. The face also appears plethoric, even in the absence of any increase in red blood cell concentration. Hypertension is most always present, and frequently there are profound emotional changes, ranging from irritability or emotional lability to severe depression, confusion, or even frank psychosis. Acne and hirsutism are frequent in female patients, hirsutism often appearing as a fine "downy" coat over the face, forehead, and upper part of the trunk. Likewise in female patients, oligomenorrhea or amenorrhea is a frequent disturbance.

LABORATORY FINDINGS With rare exceptions, plasma and urinary 17-hydroxycorticoid levels are elevated. Circulating eosinophils are below 100 cells per mm^3 in 90 percent of cases, and patients characteristically show a mild neutrophilic leukocytosis. In spite of markedly plethoric facies, the hematocrit is usually within the normal range, but occasionally erythema with higher hematocrits is encountered, particularly when the syndrome is associated with excessive production of 17-ketosteroids. Serum sodium concentration is usually normal; however, with marked excess secretion of cortisol, there may be hypokalemia, hypochloremia, and metabolic alkalosis. More than three-fourths of patients exhibit intermittent glucosuria, and nearly all have a decreased rate of disappearance of infused glucose from the circulation. Some patients may have frank diabetes, necessitating insulin therapy. X-ray studies usually reveal generalized osteoporosis, most marked in the spine and pelvis, but also frequently found in the skull, with disappearance of the lamina dura, and fractures are often seen in the ribs and vertebrae. Intravenous pyelography and laminograms with or without retroperitoneal insufflation may demonstrate adrenal enlargement, particularly when a carcinoma is the pathologic cause of the disease. More sophisticated x-ray techniques, such as selective adrenal arteriography or venography, may make the localization and diagnosis more specific but are not without risk. The increased friability of the adrenal veins in Cushing's syndrome makes retrograde venography potentially hazardous. The use of ^{131}I-tagged 19-iodocholesterol and sonar scanning techniques may be of considerable value in localizing adrenal tumors and differentiating them from bilateral hyperplasia.

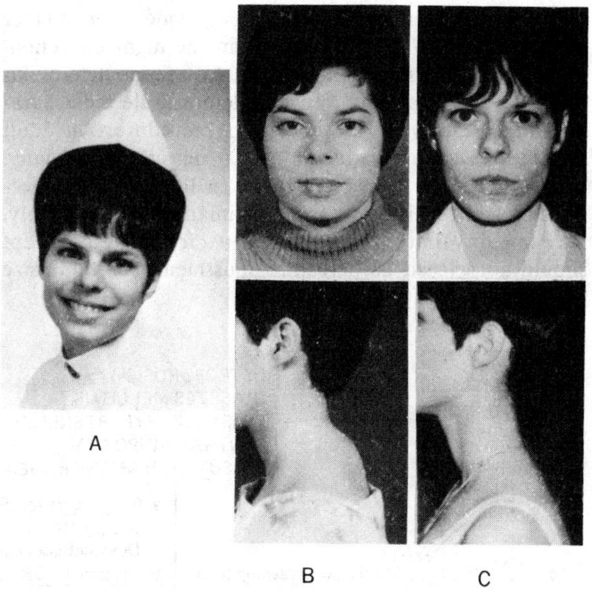

FIGURE 93-8
A twenty-year-old female with Cushing's syndrome due to a right adrenal cortical adenoma: A *Two years prior to surgery, age eighteen.* B *One month prior to surgery, age twenty.* C *One year after surgery, age twenty-one.*

TABLE 93-3
Incidence of signs and symptoms in 35 cases of Cushing's syndrome, percent

Typical habitus	97	Amenorrhea	77
Increased body weight	94	Cutaneous striae	67
Fatigability and weakness	87	Personality changes	66
Hypertension (above 150/90)	82	Ecchymoses	65
Hirsutism	80	Edema	62
		Polyuria, polydipsia	23
		Hypertrophy of clitoris	19

DIAGNOSIS The diagnosis of Cushing's syndrome depends on the direct or indirect demonstration of increased cortisol production in the absence of stress. Once this is established, further testing is carried out to determine whether the excess cortisol is being produced in an autonomous manner, since such knowledge will permit a more specific etiologic diagnosis (see Fig. 93-9, Table 93-4).

For initial screening purposes, the rapid *overnight dexamethasone suppression test* is recommended. Base-line 24-h urine 17-hydroxysteroid and 17-ketosteroid determinations may also be carried out, since values in excess of 10 mg per day for urine 17-hydroxysteroids (Porter-Silber) justify further evaluation. An ancillary screening procedure is to determine the diurnal excretion pattern for urine

17-hydroxysteroids by collecting urine between 7 A.M. and 7 P.M. and 7 P.M. to 7 A.M. The patient with Cushing's syndrome will generally excrete an equivalent or greater amount of the 17-hydroxysteroids in the night collection, in contrast to most normal subjects. Creatinine determinations are of critical importance to demonstrate the accuracy and adequacy of the collection procedure. An adult female excretes approximately 1,000 mg creatinine daily, with about 50 to 60 percent found in the daytime collection; an adult male excretes approximately 1,800 mg daily. Day-to-day variation in creatinine excretion by a patient should not exceed 20 percent. Adjustments for body size can be made; normal subjects excrete 3 to 7 mg 17-hydroxycorticosteroids per g creatinine. If it is demonstrated that the diurnal cycle for steroid excretion is "reversed," i.e., night urine 17-hydroxysteroids are almost equal to or greater than daytime excretion, one then knows that excessive cortisol is being released continuously "around the clock." These urine steroid determinations, which reflect the metabolites of cortisol, are indirect but adequate proof of excessive cortisol production. A direct method is available utilizing radioisotopic cortisol to determine the actual cortisol secretory rate, which in cases of Cushing's syndrome is in excess of 30 mg per day. Another method of direct confirmation of excess cortisol is the determination of the free cortisol in the urine, which reflects

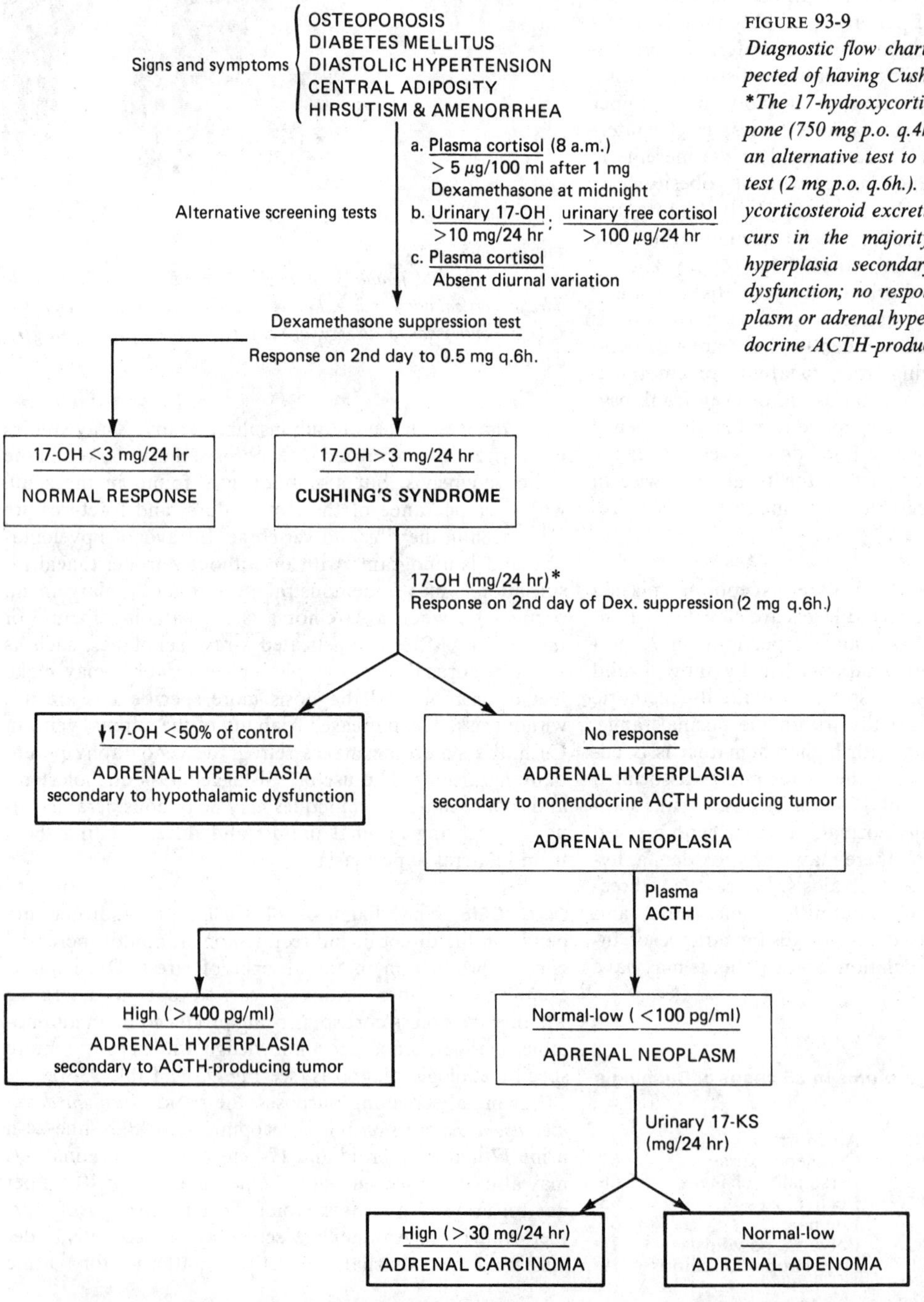

FIGURE 93-9

Diagnostic flow chart for evaluating patients suspected of having Cushing's syndrome.

**The 17-hydroxycorticosteroid response to metyrapone (750 mg p.o. q.4h. × 6 doses) may be used as an alternative test to the high-dose dexamethasone test (2 mg p.o. q.6h.). Increased urinary 17-hydroxycorticosteroid excretion following metyrapone occurs in the majority of patients with adrenal hyperplasia secondary to pituitary-hypothalamic dysfunction; no response suggests an adrenal neoplasm or adrenal hyperplasia secondary to a nonendocrine ACTH-producing tumor.*

the biologically active, unbound cortisol in the blood. Normal persons excrete less than 100 μg free cortisol daily. The sensitivity of this urine free cortisol test resides in the fact that only free cortisol of the plasma is freely filtrable at the glomerulus, and thus increments in the plasma level of this biologically active form are magnified in terms of urine excretory values.

Owing to a marked diurnal variability, plasma 17-hydroxycorticoid determinations are not meaningful when performed in isolated fashion, but demonstration that the expected normal fall in late afternoon or bedtime blood levels does not occur is increasingly used as a diagnostic measure. Normally, late afternoon plasma levels decline by half or more; late evening levels are under 8 μg per 100 ml. If such decreases are not noted, one assumes that continuous hypersecretion of cortisol is occurring.

Specific diagnosis of the type of lesion causing Cushing's syndrome can usually be made by the combined use of ACTH stimulation and dexamethasone-suppression tests. Adrenal hyperplasia, whether caused by hypothalamic dysfunction or by an ACTH-producing tumor, is characterized by hyperreactivity to exogenous ACTH. The continuous stimulation of the hyperplastic glands by endogenous ACTH appears to "prime" the adrenals to this hyperactive response to exogenous ACTH testing. This hyperactive response is evidenced in the parallel rise of both urine 17-hydroxy- and urine 17-ketosteroids. Whereas adrenal cortisol production is suppressed in normal subjects given dexamethasone 0.5 mg every 6 h for 48 h, no suppression occurs in patients with bilateral adrenal hyperplasia given this dosage. Suppression of cortisol production in normal subjects is judged by a decrease in urine 17-hydroxysteroids to less than 3 mg per day, demonstrating that the hypothalamic-pituitary axis is appropriately responsive to increases in blood glucocorticoid levels, with a resultant decline in ACTH release. Lack of suppression in patients with adrenal hyperplasia secondary to "inappropriate" pituitary ACTH secretion given 2 mg daily of dexamethasone suggests that their hypothalamic-pituitary axis is "reset" to a higher blood level of glucocorticoids. When these patients are given higher doses of dexamethasone (2 mg every 6 h) suppression of urine 17-hydroxysteroid levels to values less than half the base-line levels can be demonstrated, consistent with the view that the hypothalamic-pituitary axis is reset upward and is responsive only to higher blood levels of glucocorticoids, at which point an appropriate decline in ACTH release does occur. The finding of a normal plasma ACTH level in these patients is an abnormal sign, since with the elevated blood cortisol levels one would expect a decreased blood ACTH level. On metyrapone testing, patients with adrenal hyperplasia due to pituitary-hypothalamic dysfunction will again demonstrate a hyperactive response. In patients with adrenal hyperplasia secondary to an *ACTH-producing tumor,* such as an oat-cell bronchogenic carcinoma, no suppression will occur after dexamethasone administration and an abnormally depressed metyrapone test result, since pituitary ACTH secretion is suppressed and ACTH production by the tumor functions in an autonomous manner.

In patients with Cushing's syndrome secondary to an

TABLE 93-4
Laboratory evaluation and testing of adrenocortical function in normal subjects and in patients with Cushing's syndrome*

	Plasma Values		*Urine Values*					
	Control		*Control*		*17-OH response to*			
	ACTH 8a pg/ml	*Cortisol 8a/4p μg/100 ml*	*17-OH mg/24 h*	*17-KS mg/24 h*	*25 units synthetic ACTH IV over 8 h*	*Dexamethasone day 2, mg q.6h. 0.5*	*2.0*	*Metyrapone 750 mg q.4h. × 6 doses*
Normal values	<150	17/8	2–10	♀5–15 ♂10–25	↑3–5×	<3.0	<3.0	↑2×
Cushing's syndrome:								
I Hyperplasia with increased ACTH secretion								
A Secondary to hypothalamic dysfunction	50–400	30/25	15–25	20–35	↑4–7×	NR–↓	↓50%	↑3×
B Secondary to tumor secretion								
1 Pituitary	50–400	30/25	15–25	20–35	↑4–7×	NR	NR–↓50%	NR–↑
2 Nonendocrine	400–1,000	50/50	25–40	30–60	NR–↑	NR–↓	NR–↓	NR–↑
II Nodular hyperplasia	<150	30/25	15–25	20–35	NR–↑4–7×	NR	NR–↓	NR–↑
III Neoplasia								
A Adenoma								
1 Complete autonomy	<50	35/35	20–30	5–15	NR	NR	NR	NR
2 Incomplete autonomy	<50	35/25	15–20	5–15	↑3–5×	NR–↓	NR–↓	NR–↑
B Carcinoma	<50	35/35	20–40	50–80	NR	NR	NR	NR
IV Exogenous steroids (iatrogenic)	<50	2/2†	1–5†	5–10†	↑1–2×	NR	NR	NR

* *Abbreviations: NR = no response; ↑ = significant increase above control excretion; ↓ = significant decrease below control excretion;* NR–↑ *= no response or increase; ↓50% = decrease to 50% or more of control excretion value; ↑2 × = increase 2 × control excretion value.*
† *Absolute level dependent on steroid preparation.*

adrenal adenoma, hyperreactivity to exogenous ACTH testing may or may not occur, depending on whether the adenoma is functioning in an autonomous manner; if it is, it will be found ACTH-insensitive and thus fail to demonstrate a brisk rise in urine 17-hydroxycorticoids on ACTH stimulation. The diagnosis of cortisol-producing adrenal adenoma is suggested by the disproportionate elevation in base-line urine 17-hydroxycorticoids with only a modest rise in 17-ketosteroids. Another entity in the differential diagnosis is multinodular ("adenomatous") adrenal hyperplasia, which is an uncommon condition characteristically having features of both hyperplasia and of adenomas. Response to ACTH stimulation is variable, but patients with multinodular adrenal hyperplasia most often do not show suppression with the standard doses of dexamethasone. However, with large doses, such as 4 to 8 mg every 6 h, suppression often occurs.

Metyrapone testing is useful in differentiating adrenal tumors (adenoma or carcinoma) from adrenal hyperplasia, since the adrenal tumors by their autonomy suppress the ACTH-releasing capacity of the pituitary, with the result that on metyrapone challenge testing the pituitary fails to release ACTH in an appropriate manner and the usual rise in urine 17-hydroxycorticoids fails to occur. This finding of impaired response to metyrapone challenge separates adrenal tumors from adrenal hyperplasia, in which normal or hyperactive responses occur.

The diagnosis of *adrenal carcinoma* as a cause of Cushing's syndrome is suggested by *markedly* elevated base-line values of *both* urine 17-hydroxycorticoids and urine 17-ketosteroids. Adrenal carcinoma is usually resistant to both ACTH stimulation and dexamethasone suppression because of the autonomy of the tumor tissue itself and because of extreme atrophy of the normal remaining adrenal tissue. Markedly elevated 17-ketosteroid excretion often leads to virilization in the female. Feminizing estrogen-producing adrenocortical carcinoma in the male usually presents with gynecomastia. Functioning adrenal carcinomas that produce Cushing's syndrome are most often associated with elevated urine excretory values for the metabolites of the intermediates of steroid biosynthesis (such as tetrahydro-11-deoxycortisol and pregnanetriol) in in addition to the cortisol metabolites, suggesting inefficient conversion of the intermediates to the final product. This is in contrast to Cushing's syndrome associated with adrenocortical hyperplasia, in which the elevation of urine steroids is largely accounted for by cortisol metabolites.

Cushing's syndrome is being reported with increasing frequency in association with the autonomous production of ACTH by *nonendocrine tumors,* with the resultant development of adrenal hyperplasia. The majority of these cases have been associated with the primitive small-cell type of bronchogenic carcinoma, and the remainder have been reported chiefly with tumors of thymus, pancreas, or ovary or with bronchial adenomas. The onset of Cushing's syndrome is distinctively sudden in these patients, and this partly accounts for their failure to exhibit all the classic physical findings of the syndrome. Extracts of some of these nonendocrine tumors have produced a compound that is biologically, physiochemically, and immunologically identical to pituitary ACTH. However, studies indicate that the secretion of ACTH by nonendocrine tumors is accompanied by the production of biologically inactive ACTH fragments as well as large ACTH-like peptides ("big ACTH"). Since such tumors often produce large amounts of ACTH and MSH, base-line urine steroid values are usually markedly elevated, and increased skin pigmentation is usually present. A CRF-like material produced by the tumor has also been reported to cause hypercortisolism. Hypokalemic alkalosis, edema, and hypertension are much more common in these patients than in patients with Cushing's syndrome from other causes, and are attributed to extremely high levels of cortisol secretion. These patients will demonstrate a variable response to exogenous ACTH stimulation. A hyperactive adrenal response is seen unless endogenous ACTH levels have produced maximal adrenocortical activation. Similarly *no suppression with dexamethasone* and no increment in urine 17-hydroxycorticoid excretion after metyrapone administration are the rule unless the endogenous secretion of cortisol is not sufficient to suppress pituitary ACTH secretion. Plasma ACTH levels are most often markedly elevated in these patients, a helpful diagnostic finding, since plasma ACTH levels in other categories of Cushing's syndrome are at most modestly elevated.

Hyperpigmentation in patients with Cushing's syndrome always points to an extraadrenal tumor, either in an extracranial location, as discussed in the previous paragraph, or within the cranium. Approximately one-tenth of patients undergoing bilateral adrenalectomy for Cushing's syndrome over subsequent months or years develop chromophobe adenomas with progressive cutaneous hyperpigmentation and erosion of the sella turcica. This suggests that the loss of adrenal tissue, and consequent loss of the usual negative cortisol feedback on ACTH release, may be instrumental in the genesis of such tumors. ACTH and MSH levels in these patients are extremely high. These tumors are usually locally invasive and may impinge on the optic chiasm or extend into the cavernous or sphenoid sinuses. Since intrasellar tumors may be present at an early stage in many patients *without* sellar enlargement, a decisive opinion as to their role in the genesis of Cushing's syndrome or in the sequelae of its surgical therapy must be withheld for further investigation. Clinically, all patients suspected of having Cushing's syndrome must be carefully examined for visual field defects and enlargement of the sella turcica; if defects are found, further diagnostic procedures may be warranted, such as sellar tomography, pneumoencephalography, and angiography. Following bilateral adrenalectomy, patients should also be followed clinically for evidence of progressive hyperpigmentation. Periodic x-ray evaluation of the sella turcica and serial ACTH-MSH levels are also important parameters to follow. A diagnostic flow chart for evaluation of patients suspected of having Cushing's syndrome is presented in Fig. 93-9.

DIFFERENTIAL DIAGNOSIS Patients with exogenous obesity, hypertension, and diabetes mellitus, occurring singly or in combination, present major problems in diagnosis. Extreme *obesity* is uncommon in Cushing's syndrome; furthermore, with exogenous obesity, the adiposity is generalized, not truncal. On adrenocortical testing, abnormalities, if noted in patients with exogenous obesity, are found never to be extensive but only modest. Basal urine steroid excretion levels in obese patients are either normal or slightly elevated, a finding similar to their cortisol secretory values.

Some patients demonstrate an increased percentage of conversion of secreted cortisol into excreted metabolites. Urinary free and blood cortisol levels are normal, and, of greater importance, a normal diurnal pattern in blood and urine levels is seen. On ACTH stimulation some of the patients will demonstrate a brisk response; however, in most cases this response is suppressed easily with dexamethasone. It would appear that exogenous obesity may *cause* alterations in the secretion and metabolism of steroids, pointing up the secondary nature of altered steroid testing patterns sometimes encountered. These patients are best treated by a concerted weight reduction program with periodic retesting of adrenal function.

Iatrogenic Cushing's syndrome, induced by the administration of either glucocorticoids or ACTH, is indistinguishable by physical findings from the endogenous forms of adrenocortical hyperfunction. On occasion one may wish to rule out an underlying endogenous form of Cushing's syndrome that may be clinically magnified by exogenous therapy. This is accomplished by changing the patient's therapy to 1 mg dexamethasone daily while collecting base-line and diurnal split urine output for corticosteroid analysis. Patients with a pure exogenous form of Cushing's syndrome due to prolonged suppression of their hypothalamic-pituitary axis by administered steroid will demonstrate low base-line steroid excretion, predominantly in the daytime, a finding in distinct contrast to that in patients with endogenous Cushing's syndrome. Patients receiving long-term ACTH therapy, in addition to the features of Cushing's syndrome, may also have melanodermia. The production of iatrogenic Cushing's syndrome is related both to the total steroid dose and to the duration of therapy. Also, patients on afternoon and evening doses of steroid develop Cushing's syndrome more readily on smaller daily steroid doses than do patients on a steroid program limited to morning doses only. In addition, there appears to be a marked difference among patients in the enzymatic disposition of administered steroid. Several cases have been reported in which a spontaneous remission of Cushing's syndrome occurred; some have been characterized by intermittent abnormalities in adrenal testing. It is difficult to know whether such abnormalities are functional in nature or true pathophysiologic processes.

THERAPY When an adenoma or carcinoma is suspected, adrenal exploration is performed, with excision of the tumor. Since cortisol production by the tumor generally causes atrophy of the contralateral gland, if an atrophied gland is noted on the initial side of exploration, the tumor must be on the opposite side. Because of this probable atrophy of the contralateral adrenal, the patient is prepared and treated pre- and postoperatively for total adrenalectomy even when a unilateral lesion is suspected, the routine being similar to that for an Addisonian patient undergoing elective surgery (Table 93-9).

The principal antitumor drug used to chemically inhibit adrenal cortical function due to carcinoma is *o,p'*-DDD [2,2-bis-(2-chlorophenyl, 4-chlorophenyl)-1,1-dichloroethane], an isomer of the insecticide DDT. This drug suppresses cortisol production and decreases plasma and urine steroid levels. Although its cytotoxic action is reported to be specific for the glucocorticoid-secreting zone of the adrenal cortex, the zona glomerulosa (site of aldosterone biosynthesis) may also be inhibited. *o,p'*-DDD also alters the extraadrenal metabolism of cortisol, resulting in a smaller percentage being excreted in the urine as 17-OHCS. Therefore, *plasma or urinary free-cortisol* levels must be followed to determine the effect of *o,p'*-DDD on the patient's hypercortisolism. *o,p'*-DDD is given in divided doses three to four times daily. The dose is gradually increased to 8 to 10 g daily or the highest dose tolerated by the patient. Almost all patients experience gastrointestinal (anorexia, diarrhea, or vomiting) or neuromuscular (lethargy, somnolence, dizziness) side effects. All patients should be placed on long-term maintenance glucocorticoid; in some instances mineralocorticoid replacement therapy should also be instituted. In approximately one-third of patients regressions of both tumor and metastases occur, but long-term survival remains discouragingly limited. The mean duration of life from onset of treatment is approximately 8 months. In many patients, *o,p'*-DDD only inhibits steroidogenesis and does not produce regression of tumor metastases. Osseous metastases are usually refractory to *o,p'*-DDD; radiation should be used to treat these lesions.

In patients with a severe form of Cushing's syndrome due to adrenal hyperplasia, with features of hypertension, overt diabetes, psychosis, and osteoporosis with pathologic fractures and in the absence of an enlarged sella turcica, a complete total bilateral adrenalectomy is preferred. Since, as mentioned earlier, one-tenth of these patients develop pituitary tumors after surgery, pituitary irradiation is also indicated in any patient who develops increased pigmentation or in whom the sella turcica size increases postoperatively. In patients past the reproductive years, pituitary irradiation may be carried out prophylactically in conjunction with complete adrenalectomy. It cannot be stressed too strongly that the status of all patients with bilateral adrenalectomy must be followed diligently with periodic reexaminations for evidence of increasing sellar size or pigmentary changes.

In some centers, pituitary irradiation is the primary treatment for bilateral hyperplasia. There are three major methods of directing radiotherapy at the pituitary gland. (1) The classic approach is the use of conventional external radiation at a dose of 3,000 to 5,000 R delivered over several weeks. The total dosage is limited by possible damage to surrounding neural structures and by the loss of additional pituitary tropic function. Treatment has been successful in fewer than one-third of the patients with Cushing's syndrome who were treated solely by this method. (2) The second method is internal pituitary irradiation by the stereotactic implantation of ^{90}Y pellets in the pituitary via the transnasosphenoid route. Possible limitation of this form of therapy may be found once long-term evaluation on the effects of the radiation on perisellar structures (such as the internal carotid artery) has been made. (3) The most recent development has been the use of the alpha particle or proton beam as a source of external radiation. By this method as much as 12,000 R can be directed at the pituitary gland without evident damage to surrounding structures. This is because the beam can be focused more sharply than the more commonly used gamma radiation and because multiple portals of entry can be used. However, with this therapy there is a significant incidence of ocular motor palsies and hypopituitarism. Successful remission of bilateral hyperplasia has also been reported with conventional doses of the serotonin antagonist, cyproheptadine. It is speculated that cyproheptadine blocks the stimulating effect of hypothalamic serotonin on the release of CRF.

Patients with a severe form of Cushing's syndrome are not candidates for therapies such as external pituitary irradiation. The lag time between treatment and remission and a remission rate less than 50 percent contraindicate the use of external pituitary irradiation in the presence of rapidly progressing disease. In severely debilitated patients who are not candidates for bilateral adrenalectomy, a chemical remission can be obtained from *o,p′*-DDD (2 to 10 g per day).

If patients with adrenal hyperplasia are noted to have signs of pituitary tumor (melanodermia, increased sellar size, visual field defects), specific therapy directed at the pituitary gland must be undertaken. In general, the type of therapy is either surgery or some form of radiation. Complications of surgical therapy include cerebrospinal fluid rhinorrhea and optic nerve and posterior pituitary injury, as well as removal of all tropic hormones. The morbidity and mortality rates are greater than with radiotherapy, and therefore surgery is often reserved for those cases not amenable to treatment with radiation.

Treatment of nonendocrine ACTH-producing tumors is surgical removal of the neoplasm. If the neoplastic disease is far advanced, bilateral total adrenalectomy, metyrapone, or *o,p′*-DDD may be indicated to correct the hypercortisolism.

If Cushing's syndrome redevelops after bilateral adrenalectomy, excessive stimulation of a remnant of adrenocortical tissue may be occurring. In very rare instances an embryologic extraadrenal remnant may be stimulated to produce excess cortisol. Surgical exploration is difficult because adrenocortical remnants are small. Measurement of cortisol levels preoperatively from various points along the inferior vena cava may locate the remnant tissue. The use of ^{131}I-tagged 19-iodocholesterol scintillation scanning offers interesting possibilities.

ALDOSTERONISM

Aldosteronism is a syndrome associated with hypersecretion of the major adrenal mineralocorticoid aldosterone. *Primary* aldosteronism signifies that the stimulus for the excessive aldosterone production resides within the adrenal gland; in *secondary* aldosteronism the stimulus is of extraadrenal origin.

PRIMARY ALDOSTERONISM Introduction The constellation of signs and symptoms of excessive inappropriate aldosterone production was first summarized by Conn in 1956. In the original case and in the majority of the subsequent cases, the disease was the result of an *aldosterone-producing adrenal adenoma* (Conn's syndrome). The majority of cases (75 percent) involved a unilateral adenoma, usually small and occurring with equal frequency on either side. Rarely primary aldosteronism has been reported in association with adrenal carcinoma. It is twice as common in women as in men, presenting between the ages of thirty and fifty. In recent years, a number of cases have been reported with clinical and biochemical characteristics previously considered diagnostic of primary aldosteronism, but a solitary adenoma was not found at surgery. Instead, these patients have *bilateral cortical nodular hyperplasia.* The cause of this hyperplasia is unknown. In the literature this disease has been alternatively termed "pseudo" primary aldosteronism (PPA), idiopathic hyperaldosteronism (IHA), or nodular hyperplasia.

Incidence Primary aldosteronism is an uncommon disease. The incidence in unselected hypertensive patients is between 0.5 and 2 percent. Because of special diagnostic procedures involved, diagnosis has been largely restricted to symptomatic patients. With greater availability of these procedures an increased incidence may be seen.

Signs and symptoms The continual hypersecretion of aldosterone increases the renal distal tubular exchange of intratubular sodium for secreted potassium and hydrogen ions, with progressive depletion of body potassium and development of hypokalemia. Almost all patients have diastolic hypertension, usually not of marked severity, and complain of headaches. The hypertension is related in some unknown manner to the increased sodium reabsorption and extracellular volume expansion. *Potassium depletion* is responsible for the major complaints of muscle weakness and fatigue and is related to the effect of intra- and extracellular potassium ion depletion on muscle membrane. The muscle weakness is most striking in the legs and may progress to transient paralysis. Muscles innervated by cranial nerves are usually spared. The polyuria results from impairment of concentrating ability and is often associated with polydipsia. These patients may have electrocardiographic and roentgenographic signs of left ventricular enlargement which is secondary to their hypertension, and hypertensive retinopathy is often seen but papilledema is absent. Electrocardiographic signs of potassium depletion such as prominent U waves are often present and cardiac arrhythmias and premature contractions are not uncommon. In the absence of associated congestive heart failure, renal disease, or preexisting abnormalities (such as thrombophlebitis), edema is characteristically absent in these patients.

In cases of long duration, potassium-depletion nephropathy becomes manifest, with azotemia, often with superimposed bacilluria, and in some instances with congestive heart failure and edema.

Laboratory findings Laboratory findings are dependent on both the duration and the severity of the potassium depletion. On examination of the urine, negative to trace amounts of protein are found, sometimes with superimposed pyuria and bacilluria, presumably because of the predilection of potassium-depleted kidneys for infection. Urine specific gravity is low (less than 1.015), and an overnight concentration test with simultaneous vasopressin administration reveals impaired ability to concentrate the urine. Urine pH is often neutral to alkaline, because of excessive secretion of ammonium and bicarbonate ions; potassium depletion may lower the maximal tubular transfer rate for bicarbonate. Urine 17-hydroxycorticosteroid and 17-ketosteroid excretion levels are always within the normal range in patients with aldosteronomas but may occasionally be elevated in those rare instances of primary aldosteronism due to adrenal carcinoma. Mild azotemia is an inconstant finding.

Serial blood sampling usually reveals *hypokalemia* and sometimes hypernatremia. Serial blood sampling is stressed. The hypokalemia may be severe (less than 3 meq potassium per liter) and reflects significant body potassium depletion, usually in excess of 300 meq. *Hypernatremia* is due to both sodium retention and a concomitant water loss from polyuria. The serum bicarbonate level may be elevated as a result of hydrogen ion loss into the urine and migration into potassium-depleted cells, with alkalosis then developing. The alkalosis is perpetuated with potassium deficiency, since such deficiency increases the capacity of the proximal convoluted tubule to reabsorb filtered bicarbonate. This alkalosis predisposes to signs and symptoms of tetany. If hypokalemia is severe, serum magnesium levels will be reduced. In the absence of azotemia, serum uric acid concentration is normal.

Salivary sodium potassium ratios are reduced in the majority of cases, as is thermal sweat sodium concentration.

Total body sodium content is increased, but not to the degree seen in edematous states. Total exchangeable sodium is moderately elevated, and total exchangeable body potassium is usually, but not invariably, reduced. The volume of extracellular fluid is expanded in most cases, with expansion of plasma volume in many. The expanded extracellular fluid volume is thought to be responsible for the reversed diurnal excretory pattern for salt and water that many of these patients exhibit, with predominant salt and water excretion occurring during the night.

Diagnosis of primary aldosteronism The major criteria which permit the clinician to derive an unequivocal diagnosis of primary aldosteronism are (1) diastolic hypertension without edema; (2) hypersecretion of aldosterone which fails to be suppressed appropriately during volume expansion (salt loading); (3) hyposecretion of renin (as judged by low plasma renin activity levels) which fails to increase appropriately during volume depletion (upright posture); (4) hypokalemia and/or inappropriate urine potassium loss.

Diastolic hypertension is a prerequisite for the diagnosis of primary aldosteronism, even though transient periods of relative normotension may be observed during long-term evaluation. Diastolic hypertension exhibited by patients with primary aldosteronism does not differ from the labile variety of essential hypertension. Blood pressure readings characteristically become reduced after hospitalization, but moderate to severe rises may occur in hospital and are often related to emotional situations. Accelerated (sustained) diastolic hypertension is uncommon but has been reported.

Patients with primary aldosteronism characteristically *do not have edema,* since they are exhibiting a perpetuated "escape" phenomenon. Since they are in a chronic state of escape from the sodium-retaining aspects of mineralocorticoids, they characteristically excrete an administered salt load with a greater rapidity than do normotensive subjects, a characteristic which is shared by patients having essential hypertension. Only a limited sodium retention occurs when patients with primary aldosteronism are given sodium-retaining hormones parenterally. Rarely in patients with associated potassium-depletion nephropathy and azotemia, pretibial edema may be present.

Estimation of plasma renin activity has been valuable in separating patients with primary aldosteronism from those with other causes of hypertension. The failure of plasma renin activity to rise normally during volume-depletion maneuvers (e.g., sodium depletion, diuretic administration, hemorrhage, and/or ambulation) has been a major diagnostic criterion for primary aldosteronism. This is in contrast to what occurs in some hypertensive patients in whom hyperaldosteronism is secondary to *increased* renin levels. However, suppressed renin activity is not diagnostic of primary aldosteronism, as it occurs in about 25 percent of patients with essential hypertension, in patients with hyperaldosteronism secondary to idiopathic bilateral nodular adrenal hyperplasia, and in other mineralocorticoid excess syndromes, including deoxycorticosterone-secreting adrenal tumors.

Since the determination of plasma renin responsiveness is not sufficient, measurement of lack of suppression of aldosterone secretion is necessary to diagnose primary aldosteronism properly. The autonomy exhibited by aldosterone tumors in these patients refers only to their resistance to suppression of hypersecretion during volume expansion; such tumors can and do respond either in normal or supernormal fashion to the stimuli of potassium loading or ACTH infusion. Patients with primary aldosteronism do not respond to volume expansion since their renin-angiotensin system is already suppressed. Appropriate suppression testing may be carried out by saline loading, oral salt loading, or DOCA administration (see Mineralocorticoid Suppression Tests, earlier in this chapter). The autonomy of these tumors to volume expansion is not necessarily complete; many patients with primary aldosteronism will demonstrate some decrease of hypersecretion of aldosterone during volume expansion maneuvers, but such decreases are significantly less than the expected normal response. In some patients apparent suppression of plasma or urinary levels of aldosterone in response to saline loading may be produced by the associated kaliuresis and hypokalemia.

A major criterion for the diagnosis of primary aldosteronism is the demonstration of *hypokalemia* associated with an inappropriately high urine potassium excretion. Judgments as to the significance of a given degree of hypokalemia for a given rate of urine potassium excretion must take into account the patient's potassium and sodium intake. Patients with hypokalemia secondary to diuretics, laxatives, etc., will generally have a 24-h urine potassium excretion of less than 40 meq per day, and often the value is markedly less than this. Most patients with primary aldosteronism, on the other hand, with a potassium intake of 100 meq per day will have a 24-h urine potassium excretion of greater than 40 meq per day. Since potassium excretion can be modified by manipulations in sodium intake, this latter factor must be taken into consideration. During periods of high sodium intake, delivery of sodium ions to the distal tubular sodium-potassium exchange site will be increased, resulting in a rise in potassium excretion over control values. Contrariwise, potassium excretion can be minimized for any degree of hypokalemia by restriction of sodium intake, which limits the amount of sodium reaching the distal tubular exchange site. Patients with primary aldosteronism will always exhibit inappropriate urine potassium losses during either saline or oral salt loading procedures.

Precise localization of aldosterone-producing adenomas may be determined preoperatively in many cases by the technique of percutaneous transfemoral bilateral adrenal vein catheterization with simultaneous adrenal arteriography and venography. Such a technique permits radiologic localization, and, in addition, the adrenal vein sampling may demonstrate a two- to threefold increase in plasma aldosterone concentration on the involved side compared with the uninvolved side. A flow chart for evaluation of patients with suspected primary aldosteronism is presented in Fig. 93-10.

Differential diagnosis All patients with *accelerated hypertension* and hypokalemia must be evaluated for unilateral renal disease. If such a diagnosis is confirmed, an additional diagnosis of primary aldosteronism is unlikely, although in rare instances both have been recorded to occur simultaneously. A useful maneuver in distinguishing between secondary aldosteronism due to accelerated hypertension and primary aldosteronism is to monitor serum potassium levels and aldosterone secretion (or excretory rates) prior to and following therapeutic correction of the hypertension. In patients with accelerated hypertension and secondary aldosteronism, the aldosteronism will subside with successful antihypertensive therapy, i.e., aldosterone parameters will return to normal and the hypokalemia and/or alkalosis will disappear. In distinct contrast, patients with primary aldosteronism in whom successful blood pressure reduction is undertaken will continue to exhibit hypokalemic alkalosis with hypersecretion of aldosterone. An additional maneuver is sometimes useful. This is based on the observation of Melby that the majority of patients with primary aldosteronism become normotensive and normokalemic when treated with the aldosterone antagonist, spironolactone, when given in a dose of 50 to 100 mg every 6 to 8 h daily over a period of 2 to 5 weeks. Some patients with essential hypertension also become normotensive, so a positive response to spironolactone is not diagnostic of primary aldosteronism. Most of these responsive patients with essential hypertension have "low-renin hypertension" (see Chap. 250). Spironolactone therapy in patients with accelerated hypertension and secondary aldosteronism often will correct the electrolyte abnormalities, but hypertension will persist. It is of interest that patients with primary aldosteronism have been successfully managed medically for years through the chronic use of

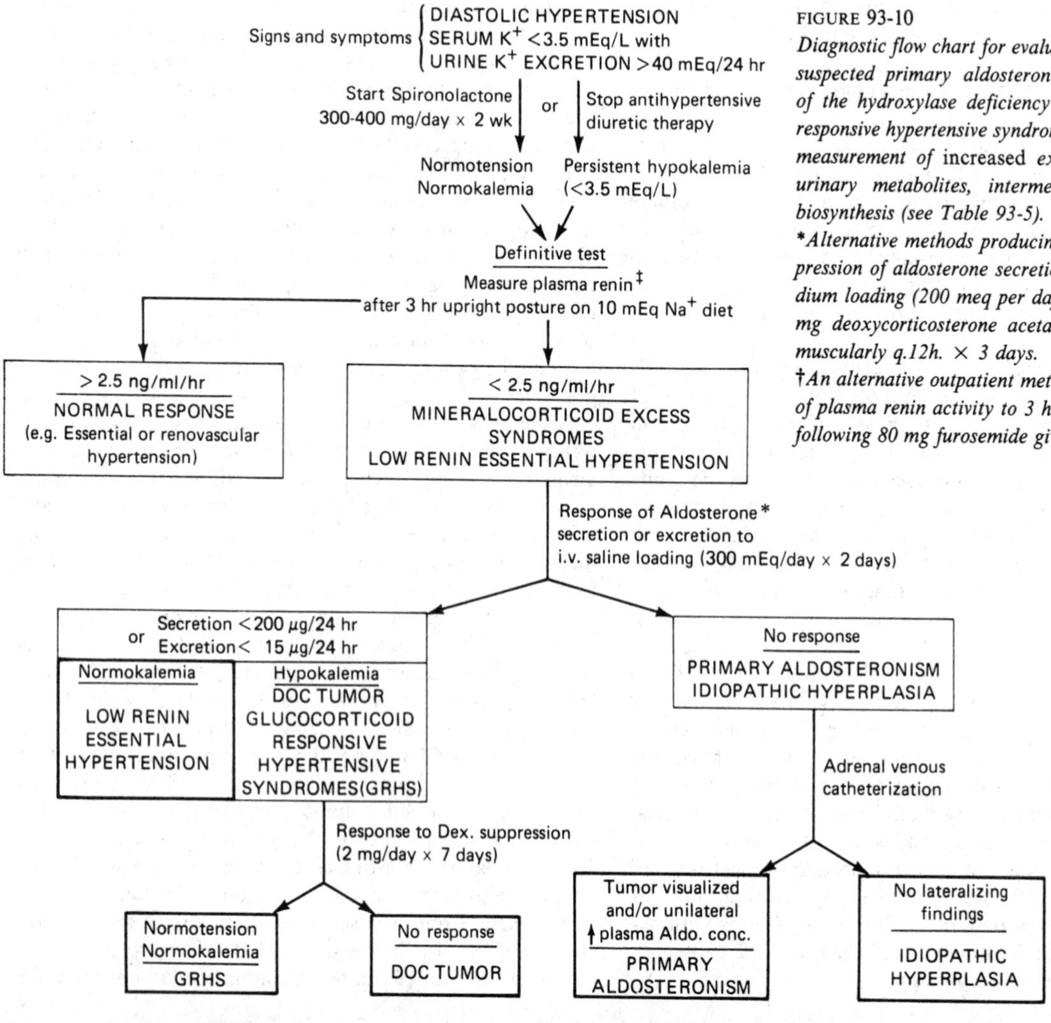

FIGURE 93-10

Diagnostic flow chart for evaluating patients with suspected primary aldosteronism. Identification of the hydroxylase deficiency in glucocorticoid-responsive hypertensive syndromes (GRHS) is the measurement of increased *excretion of certain urinary metabolites, intermediates of cortisol biosynthesis (see Table 93-5).*

**Alternative methods producing comparable suppression of aldosterone secretion include oral sodium loading (200 meq per day × 5 days) or 10 mg deoxycorticosterone acetate (DOCA) intramuscularly q.12h. × 3 days.*

†An alternative outpatient method is the response of plasma renin activity to 3 h of upright activity following 80 mg furosemide given the day before.

spironolactone therapy, but chronic therapy with spironolactone is limited in male patients by the common occurrence of gynecomastia, decreased libido, and impotency.

Primary aldosteronism must also be distinguished from other *hypermineralocorticoid states.* The most common problem is to distinguish between hyperaldosteronism due to an adenoma and that due to idiopathic bilateral nodular hyperplasia. This is of considerable importance, since it is now generally agreed that the hypertension associated with idiopathic hyperplasia is often not benefited by bilateral adrenalectomy. In contrast, the hypertension associated with aldosterone-producing tumors is usually improved or cured following removal of the adenoma. Although patients with idiopathic bilateral nodular hyperplasia tend to have less severe hypokalemia, lower aldosterone secretion, and higher plasma renin activity than patients with primary aldosteronism, differentiation is difficult, if not impossible, solely on clinical and/or biochemical grounds. A significant postural rise in reduced plasma renin levels has been reported to distinguish patients with idiopathic hyperplasia from subjects with primary aldosteronism. Sometimes a definitive diagnosis can be made only at laparotomy, but preoperative cannulation of the adrenal veins may be diagnostic. Cases of primary aldosteronism will demonstrate unilateral increments in plasma aldosterone concentration and/or tumor visualization on the involved site.

In a few instances, hypertensive patients with hypokalemic alkalosis have been found to have deoxycorticosterone (DOC)-secreting adenomas. Such patients will have reduced plasma renin activity levels, but aldosterone measurements will be either normal or reduced, suggesting the diagnosis of mineralocorticoid excess due to a hormone other than aldosterone. Rare cases of hypermineralocorticoidism due to a defect in cortisol biosynthesis, specifically 11- or 17-hydroxylation, have also been reported. ACTH levels are increased, with a resultant increase in the production of the mineralocorticoid 11-deoxycorticosterone. *Hypertension and hypokalemia can be corrected by glucocorticoid administration.* The definitive diagnosis is made by demonstrating an elevation of urinary metabolites of precursors of cortisol biosynthesis (Table 93-5). Occasionally, glucocorticoid administration will produce normotension and normokalemia although a hydroxylase deficiency cannot be identified (Fig. 93-10).

Licorice ingestion produces a syndrome mimicking primary aldosteronism. Licorice contains a sodium-retaining principle, glycyrrhizinic acid, which causes sodium retention, expansion of the extracellular fluid volume, hypertension, depressed plasma renin levels, and suppressed aldosterone levels. The diagnosis is excluded by a careful history.

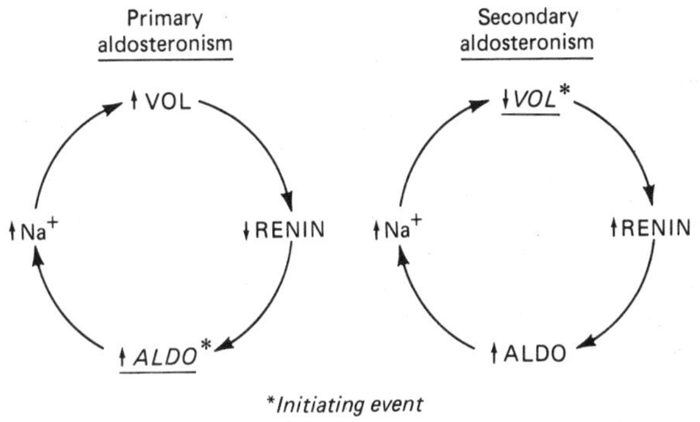

FIGURE 93-11
Responses of the renin-aldosterone volume control loop in primary versus secondary aldosteronism.

SECONDARY ALDOSTERONISM Secondary aldosteronism refers to an appropriately increased production of aldosterone by the adrenal gland in response to stimuli originating outside the gland (Fig. 93-11). In all reported cases, the stimulus has been the renin-angiotensin system. The adrenal production rates of aldosterone are often higher in patients with secondary aldosteronism than in those with primary aldosteronism. Most patients with secondary aldosteronism exhibit this syndrome either as an associated feature of the accelerated phase of hypertension (regardless of the primary disease) or on the basis of an underlying edema disorder. On the other hand, secondary aldosteronism in pregnancy is a normal physiologic response to estrogen-induced increases in circulating levels of renin substrate and plasma renin activity, as well as the antialdosterone actions of the progestins.

Secondary aldosteronism found in hypertensive states

TABLE 93-5
Urine excretory products in congenital adrenal hyperplasia*

Deficiency	*17-KS*	*17-OH*	*THS*	*Pregnanetriol*	*Pregnanediol*	*THDOC*	*THB*	*Aldosterone*
C-21 hydroxylase deficiency:								
Salt-losing	I	N–D	N–D	I	I	D	D	D
Non-salt-losing	I	N–D	N–D	I	N–I	N–I	N–I	N–I
C-11 hydroxylase deficiency	I	I	I	I	N–I	I	D	D
C-17 hydroxylase deficiency	N–D	N–D	N–D	N–D	I	I	I	D–I
C-17 and C-18 hydroxylase deficiency	N–D	N–D	N–D	N–D	I	I	I	D
3β-ol-Dehydrogenase deficiency	I	N–D	N–D	N–D	N–D	N–D	N–D	N–D

* *THS, tetrahydro 11-deoxycortisol; THDOC, tetrahydro 11-deoxycorticosterone; THB, tetrahydrocorticosterone; I, increased; N, normal; D, decreased.*

either is secondary to a primary overproduction of renin (primary reninism) or is caused by an overproduction of renin which is secondary to a decrease in renal blood flow and/or perfusion pressure (Fig. 93-5). Secondary hypersecretion of renin could be due to a narrowing of one or both of the major renal arteries either by an atherosclerotic plaque or by fibromuscular hyperplasia. Over-production of renin from both kidneys also occurs in association with severe arteriolar nephrosclerosis (malignant hypertension) or secondary to profound renal vasoconstriction (accelerated phase of hypertensive disease). These patients exhibit a secondary aldosteronism characterized by hypokalemic alkalosis, absence of edema, moderate to severe increases in plasma renin activity, and moderate to marked increases in aldosterone secretion/excretion rates (see Chap. 250).

Secondary aldosteronism with hypertension is also associated with the rare renin-producing tumor, so-called primary reninism. These patients have all the biochemical characteristics of renal vascular hypertension; however, the primary defect is not a decrease in renal blood flow and/or perfusion pressure but renin secretion by a juxtaglomerular-cell tumor. The diagnosis can be made by the absence of changes in renal vasculature and/or the presence of a space-occupying lesion seen by renal arteriography, with unilateral increases in renal vein renin activity. A second differential test is the change in renin activity when the patient assumes the upright posture. Patients with primary reninism characteristically have a very brisk increase in renin activity in contrast to patients with other forms of secondary aldosteronism.

Secondary aldosteronism is present in most *edema* disorders. Edema may be said to be the cardinal finding on physical examination for the presence of secondary aldosteronism. Hypersecretion of aldosterone in such clinical states correlates best with the phases of rapid accumulation of edema fluid. During phases of stable body weight, aldosterone measurements are often reported to be within the normal range.

Increased aldosterone secretion rates have been amply documented in patients who form edema as a result of either cirrhosis or the nephrotic syndrome. In congestive heart failure, however, elevated aldosterone secretion is a variable finding. The stimulus for aldosterone release in these clinical conditions appears to be *arterial hypovolemia.* Arterial blood volume may be depleted in cirrhosis as a result of decreased hepatic protein synthesis and protein loss into ascitic fluid; likewise, urine protein losses in the nephrotic syndrome may lead to arterial hypovolemia. Despite venous congestion, arterial hypovolemia may occur in congestive heart failure as a result of a failing cardiac output. The finding of normal aldosterone secretory rates in some patients with congestive heart failure requires explanation. It has been shown that approximately 95 percent of the circulating blood aldosterone is removed from the plasma and metabolized or extracted by the liver during a single passage. The rate of removal of aldosterone from plasma is termed its *metabolic clearance rate,* and since aldosterone is almost exclusively "cleared" by the liver, hepatic blood flow will approximate the aldosterone clearance rate. Since the blood level of circulating aldosterone is presumed to be the critical factor in its biologic activity, it is to be appreciated that the blood level will be determined by both the aldosterone secretion rate and the rate of hepatic inactivation. Thus, in clinical states characterized by reduced hepatic blood flow, such as congestive heart failure, an increased blood circulating aldosterone level can occur and result in sodium retention, even though the secretion rate of the hormone is within the normal range. Patients with secondary aldosteronism due to edema disorders differ qualitatively from normal subjects and from patients with primary aldosteronism, in that they fail to exhibit a normal "escape" pattern in response to the chronic administration of DOC. These patients are exquisitely sensitive to the sodium-retaining properties of the mineralocorticoids and will exhibit a profound decrease in urine excretion, often to barely detectable levels. They retain excess salt and water, but this retained fluid is ineffective in terms of reexpanding what is registered by the renin-angiotensin system as a deficient circulating blood volume. Instead, the excess salt and water that are retained accumulate in increasing quantities as edema fluid. Diuretic therapy often exaggerates the features of secondary aldosteronism via the mechanism of acute volume depletion; when this happens hypokalemia and on occasion alkalosis become prominent features.

Secondary hyperaldosteronism may rarely occur without edema or hypertension (Bartter's syndrome). This syndrome is characterized by the signs of severe hyperaldosteronism (hypokalemic alkalosis) with moderate to marked increases in renin activity but normal blood pressure and absence of edema. Renal biopsy shows juxtaglomerular hyperplasia. The pathogenesis of this syndrome is obscure, but many patients have a defect in the renal conservation of sodium. The renal loss of sodium is thought to stimulate renin secretion and subsequently aldosterone production. Hyperaldosteronism produces potassium depletion, with the hypokalemia further elevating plasma renin activity. In some cases, the hypokalemia may be potentiated by a defect in renal conservation of potassium. It has also been proposed that in some of these patients the lack of hypertension is due to vascular unresponsiveness to angiotensin. Whether this is a primary event or simply secondary to the altered metabolic state is unclear.

ADRENAL VIRILISM

INTRODUCTION The adrenal virilizing syndromes result from excessive productions of adrenal androgens, such as dehydroepiandrosterone and Δ4-androstenedione, which are converted to testosterone; the elevated testosterone levels account for most of the virilization. As in other states of adrenocortical hyperfunction, the syndrome may result from hyperplasia, adenoma, or carcinoma. It also may arise in a congenital form, termed *adrenogenital hyperplasia,* due to enzymatic deficits. The adrenal virilizing syndromes may be associated with secretions of greater or smaller amounts of other adrenal hormones and may, therefore, present as "pure" syndromes of virilization or as "mixed" syndromes associated with excessive production of glucocorticoid and some of the characteristics of Cushing's syndrome. In *congenital* adrenal hyperplasia the virilizing syndrome may be associated with either excessive or decreased secretion of mineralocorticoid or decreased production of glucocorticoid.

Since in man hydrocortisone is the principal adrenal steroid regulating ACTH elaboration, and since ACTH stimulates both hydrocortisone and adrenal androgen production, it stands to reason that an enzymatic interference with hydrocortisone synthesis may result in the enhanced secretion of adrenal androgens. In severe congenital virilizing hyperplasia, the adrenal output of hydrocortisone may be so compromised as to cause clinical evidence of glucocorticoid deficiency despite anatomic adrenal hyperplasia. Conversely, a high hydrocortisone output as the result of primary adrenal disease (adenoma) may inhibit ACTH secretion and thus result in a low adrenal androgen output.

INCIDENCE Congenital bilateral adrenocortical hyperplasia is by far the most common adrenal disorder of infancy and childhood. It has also been described later in life, predominantly in women. Its appearance in postpubertal men would obviously not be as clinically apparent; nevertheless, it has been reported. In its various forms, adrenogenital hyperplasia is thought to be related to a defective autosomal recessive gene. Affected family members have similar patterns of steroid excretion and severity of enzymatic deficiencies. The most common form of significant "noncongenital" adrenal virilization is that seen with bilateral adrenocortical hyperplasia and is most frequently associated with various degrees of excessive production of glucocorticoid hormone and the clinical signs and symptoms of Cushing's syndrome.

CLINICAL SIGNS AND SYMPTOMS The congenital form of adrenal hyperplasia is secondary to a defect in steroid enzymatic activity. To date, defects have been described in the C-21, C-18, C-17, and C-11 hydroxylase enzymes, as well as in the 3β-ol-dehydrogenase enzyme. These enzyme deficits usually occur singly. The clinical expression of these enzyme deficiencies is variable, ranging from virilization of the female (C-21 deficiency) to feminization of the male (3β-ol-dehydrogenase deficiency).

Adrenal virilization in the female at birth is associated with ambiguous external genitalia (*female pseudohermaphroditism*). Adrenal virilism due to congenital adrenal hyperplasia in the male is manifested by premature virilization (*isosexual precocity*). The age of onset of virilization is most probably prenatal, after the fifth month of embryonic development. At birth there may be macrogenitosomia in the male infant, and in the female, enlargement of the clitoris, partial or complete fusion of the labia, and sometimes a urogenital sinus. If the labial fusion is nearly complete, the female infant will have external genitalia resembling a penis with hypospadias, changes consistent with female pseudohermaphroditism. Chromosomal sex can be determined by examination of oral mucosal smears or leukocyte cultures. In the *postnatal* period from infancy to adolescence, congenital adrenal hyperplasia will be associated with virilization in the female and isosexual precocity in the male. The excessive androgens produced will result in accelerated growth, with height age exceeding chronologic age. Since epiphyseal closure is hastened by excessive androgens, growth stops but truncal development continues, giving the characteristic appearance of a child of short stature with well-developed trunk. Incomplete variants of congenital adrenal hyperplasia sometimes become manifest only in adult life, with virilization or hirsutism occurring in the female.

In the adult female, regardless of the cause of the condition, the clinical signs and symptoms are those anticipated from excessive androgen production. These include hirsutism, acne, increased sebum production, temporal baldness, deepening of voice, increased muscle mass and strength, decreased breast size, atrophy of uterus, amenorrhea, enlargement of the clitoris, increased heterosexual drive, and development of a male habitus. The clinical distinction between excessive hair growth (hirsutism) and virilization is useful. Virilization signifies that multiple signs of androgen excess are present in addition to hirsutism; one of the more easily recognized of these signs is hypertrophy of the clitoris. Hirsutism in the absence of other signs of virilization is uncommon in these patients. The virilizing syndromes are difficult to document in the *adult* male, for obvious reasons.

The most common form of congenital adrenal hyperplasia (95 percent of cases) is a result of impairment of *C-21 hydroxylation.* There is reduced conversion of 17-hydroxyprogesterone to 11-deoxycortisol and thus reduced formation of cortisol from 11-deoxycortisol (Fig. 93-2). In addition to cortisol deficiency, in approximately one-third of the patients, there is an associated reduction in aldosterone secretion as a result of impaired C-21 hydroxylation of progesterone to 11-deoxycorticosterone, a precursor of aldosterone. Thus, with congenital adrenal hyperplasia secondary to C-21 hydroxylase deficiency, adrenal virilization will be present with or without an associated salt-losing tendency due to aldosterone deficiency. The accumulation of progesterone may also exaggerate any salt-losing tendency, since progesterone has an antialdosterone effect on renal tubular salt conservation. Since a cortisol deficiency exists, the adrenal glands become hyperplastic because of excessive ACTH stimulation. It is probable that the C-21 hydroxylase enzymes, rather than being identical, are isoenzymes. Rather than representing the severity of the enzyme deficiency, the difference between the salt-losing variety and the non-salt losing variety may reside in whether the genetic abnormality involves one or both of these isoenzymes. As a result of the C-21 hydroxylase deficit, precursor products accumulate and are shunted into alternate pathways of metabolism, chiefly the androgen pathways, accounting for the hypersecretion of dehydroepiandrosterone and androstenedione and its 11 β-hydroxylated derivatives. The conversion peripherally of androstenedione to testosterone produces high levels of this potent androgen (Table 93-5).

With a *C-11 hydroxylase* deficiency a "hypertensive" variant of congenital adrenal hyperplasia develops with cortisol deficiency, since there is impaired conversion of 11-deoxycortisol to cortisol. Hypertension and hypokalemia occur because of the impaired conversion of 11-deoxycorticosterone to corticosterone, resulting in the accumulation of 11-deoxycorticosterone, a potent mineralocorticoid. Increased shunting again occurs into the androgen pathway with overproduction of 11-deoxy-17-ketosteroids.

The *C-17 hydroxylase* syndrome is characterized by hypogonadism and hypertension. In patients with this deficiency there is decreased production of cortisol with increased production of progesterone and its metabolite pregnanediol. There is shunting into the mineralocorticoid pathway with hypokalemic alkalosis, hypertension, and suppressed plasma renin activity. In most patients, 11-deoxycorticosterone and corticosterone productions are elevated, while aldosterone secretion is low. The subnormal production of aldosterone in some but not all patients with this syndrome may be related to an associated C-18 hydroxylase deficiency. However, in most patients, it is probably secondary to hypokalemia, intraadrenal regulation of aldosterone biosynthesis by precursor products, or the suppressed renin activity, since treatment restores aldosterone secretion to normal. Because C-17 hydroxylation is required for biosynthesis of adrenal androgens as well as gonadal testosterone and estrogen, this defect is associated with sexual immaturity, high urinary gonadotropin levels, and low urinary 17-ketosteroid excretion. Female patients have primary amenorrhea and lack of development of secondary sexual characteristics. Because of deficient androgen production, male patients have ambiguous external genitalia (male pseudohermaphroditism). Exogenous glucocorticoids can correct the hypertensive syndrome, but sex hormones are necessary to produce sexual maturation.

With the rare 3β-ol-dehydrogenase deficiency, there is impaired conversion of pregnenolone to progesterone, with the result that pathways to both cortisol and aldosterone are "blocked," with shunting then occurring into the adrenal androgen pathway via 17α-hydroxypregnenolone to dehydroepiandrosterone. Since dehydroepiandrosterone is a weak androgen and because this enzyme deficiency is also present in the gonad, the genitalia of the male fetus may be ambiguous or feminized. Conversely, in the female, overproduction of dehydroepiandrosterone may produce virilization.

DIAGNOSIS The diagnosis of adrenal virilism due to *congenital adrenal hyperplasia* should be considered in all infants exhibiting "failure to thrive," particularly those having episodes of acute adrenal insufficiency or salt-wasting, or showing sustained hypertension. The diagnosis is further suggested by the finding of hypertrophy of the clitoris, fused labia, or urogenital sinus in the female and isosexual precocity in the male infant. In infants and children with a *C-21 hydroxylation block,* increased urine 17-ketosteroid excretion is typically associated with an increase in the excretion of pregnanetriol, which is a metabolite of 17α-hydroxyprogesterone. These children will show low urine 17-hydroxycorticoid excretion levels and elevated levels of plasma ACTH. Ketogenic steroid excretion will be elevated, since the depressed 17-hydroxycorticoid excretion is more than offset by increments in pregnanetriol excretion, which metabolite is included in the analysis. On testing with ACTH, the altered metabolic pathways are exaggerated, with sharp rises occurring in 17-ketosteroid excretion and little or no rise in 17-hydroxycorticoid excretion (Table 93-5).

The diagnosis of a *salt-losing form of congenital* adrenal hyperplasia due to defects in both C-21 hydroxylase enzymes is suggested by episodes of acute adrenal insufficiency with hyponatremia, hyperkalemia, dehydration, and vomiting. These infants and children often "crave" salt and exhibit laboratory signs of concomitant deficits in both cortisol and aldosterone secretion.

With the *hypertensive form* of congenital adrenal hyperplasia due to impaired C-11 hydroxylation, the precursor 11-deoxycortisol will accumulate. As a result, both urine 17-keto and 17-hydroxycorticoid excretion may be elevated since 11-deoxycortisol would be included in the analysis of Porter-Silber chromogens. The diagnosis is secured by demonstrating increased amounts of tetrahydro-11-deoxycortisol in the urine with decreased amounts of tetrahydro metabolites of cortisol.

The finding of very high levels of urine dehydroepiandrosterone with low levels of pregnanetriol and of cortisol metabolites is characteristic of patients with congenital adrenal hyperplasia due to 3β-ol-dehydrogenase deficiency. These patients also exhibit marked salt wasting.

The *C-17 hydroxylase* deficiency results in the accumulation of progesterone and its metabolite, pregnanediol. The excretion of deoxycorticosterone and of corticosterone is increased, while aldosterone production is usually subnormal. In some patients aldosterone secretion is elevated.

The adrenal virilizing syndrome in adults is most often due to congenital causes—namely, tumor or adrenal hyperplasia. *Adrenal adenomas* and *carcinomas* may cause a pure or mixed virilizing syndrome. Since adrenal androgens are weak compared with gonadal androgens, adrenal virilization is characterized by *large increments in urine 17-ketosteroid excretion,* often with less impressive clinical signs of virilism. Virilizing adrenocortical adenomas are rare. They produce very high levels of urinary 17-ketosteroids, often greater than 200 mg per day, and are associated with no rise or only a slight rise in urine 17-hydroxysteroids. They may or may not be sensitive to ACTH stimulation and likewise may or may not be sensitive to dexamethasone suppression. *Virilizing adrenal carcinomas* are the most common adrenal tumor causing virilization. They are associated with high urinary 17-ketosteroid excretion, reaching 100 mg or more per 24 h, and may have normal or a moderate rise in 17-hydroxycorticosteroid excretion. They characteristically show no increase in steroid excretion upon stimulation with ACTH, and also characteristically fail to be suppressed with dexamethasone administration. These tumors are often associated with marked virilization of sudden onset. The very high ketosteroid excretion of both virilizing adenomas and carcinomas is made up in large part of the weak androgen dehydroepiandrosterone, which has approximately 5 percent of the androgenicity of testosterone. Functioning adrenocortical carcinomas are characteristically associated with elevated urinary excretion of metabolites of precursors of steroid biosynthesis (such as pregnanetriol and tetrahydro-11-deoxycortisol), probably representing inefficient conversion of intermediate compounds to the final product. The clinical differentiation between virilizing adrenal adenoma and carcinoma is tenuous and cannot be made with certainty preoperatively.

In adrenocortical hyperfunction of Cushing's syndrome, both urinary 17-ketosteroid and 17-hydroxycorticosteroid base-line values will be elevated. Adrenal hyperactivity associated with hirsutism but with normal 17-hydroxycorticosteroid base-line excretion (sometimes termed benign androgenic hyperplasia) represents an ill-defined, controversial, heterogeneous group of patients. Mild hirsutism usually appears after puberty and is characterized by normal or moderately elevated urinary 17-ketosteroids. With ACTH stimulation there is a brisk rise in the urinary 17-ketosteroids when compared with the 17-hydroxycorticosteroids. Base-line 17-ketosteroids are easily suppressed by

TABLE 93-6
Causes of hirsutism in females

I Familial
II Idiopathic
III Ovarian
  A Polycystic ovaries; hilus cell hyperplasia
  B Tumor: arrhenoblastoma, hilus cell, adrenal rest
IV Adrenal
  A Congenital adrenal hyperplasia
  B Noncongenital adrenal hyperplasia (Cushing's)
  C Tumor: virilizing carcinoma or adenoma

daily administration of 2 mg dexamethasone. Some of if not all these patients may have a mild form of congenital adrenal hyperplasia. A flow chart for evaluation of patients with excessive androgen production is presented in Fig. 93-12.

DIFFERENTIAL DIAGNOSIS In the female, the differential diagnosis of hirsutism and virilization is between adrenal and ovarian etiologies (Table 93-6; Fig. 93-12). *Sudden onset of progressive hirsutism and virilization* suggests an adrenal or ovarian neoplasm. Since adrenal tumors secrete weak androgens (such as DHEA), virilizing adrenal neoplasms are characterized by high urine 17-ketosteroid excretion, usually in excess of 30 to 40 mg per 24 h. Failure to reduce 17-ketosteroid levels to normal following dexamethasone suppression (0.5 mg p.o. q.6h. × 7 days) supports a diagnosis of virilizing adrenal tumor and excludes congenital adrenal hyperplasia. The most common *ovarian tumor* causing virilization is the arrhenoblastoma, but other ovarian tumors, such as adrenal rest tumor, granulosa-cell tumor, hilar-cell tumors, and Brenner tumors have been associated with virilization. Virilization due to ovarian tumors is characterized by normal or moderate elevations of urinary 17-ketosteroids, since the neoplasm usually secretes the potent androgen testosterone. Moderate increases in 17-ketosteroid excretion occur in some patients with ovarian neoplasm, but base-line 17-ketosteroid excretion in excess of 30 mg per day is rare with the exception of adrenal rest tumors. Like adrenal neoplasms, ovarian tumors fail to be suppressed by dexamethasone. With the exception of adrenal rest tumors, they are largely independent of ACTH stimulation. Elevations of plasma testosterone or urinary testosterone excretion do not localize the neoplasm to the ovary, since testosterone can be elevated subsequent to pe-

FIGURE 93-12
Diagnostic flow chart for evaluating the status of patients with suspected excess androgen production. Identification of the hydroxylase deficiency in congenital adrenal hyperplasia is the measurement of increased *excretion of certain urinary metabolites of intermediates of cortisol biosynthesis (see Table 93-5).*

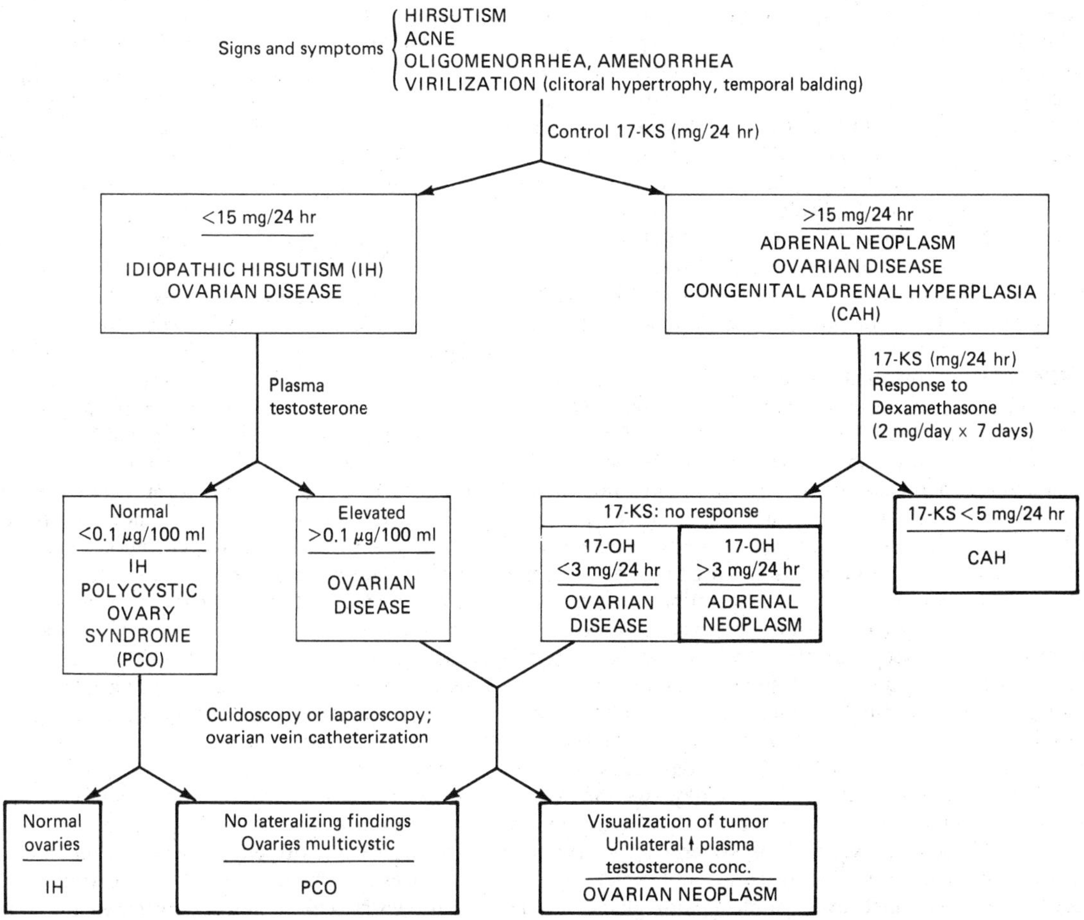

ripheral conversion of adrenal precursors, such as DHEA (see Chap. 99).

Hirsutism without virilization beginning after puberty and associated with normal ovarian histology is diagnostic of idiopathic or familial hirsutism. In a second group of patients, hirsutism is seen in association with sclerocystic or polycystic ovaries. Oligomenorrhea, anovulatory bleeding, and/or amenorrhea commonly occur in these patients. The ovaries may be palpably enlarged bilaterally; unilateral enlargement suggests an ovarian neoplasm. Direct inspection of the ovaries by culdoscopy or laparoscopy is a valuable means of differentiating between ovarian and adrenal causes of hirsutism. If normal ovaries are found, an adrenal origin for the virilization is favored. Alternatively, the discovery of polycystic ovaries does not establish an ovarian causation since polycystic ovaries have been described in association with adrenal virilization. 17-ketosteroid excretion values in hirsute females with polycystic ovary disease or idiopathic hirsutism are usually normal or slightly elevated. *Plasma testosterone* levels tend to be higher in females with polycystic ovary disease than in normal females, and in 20 percent of cases testosterone levels are greater than normal. Studies indicate that some women with idiopathic hirsutism or polycystic ovaries probably have increased blood production rates of testosterone. Studies also indicate that luteinizing hormone (LH) levels are tonically elevated in some patients with polycystic ovary disease.

The differential diagnosis of isosexual precocity in young boys includes pineal tumors (Chap. 101), congenital adrenal hyperplasia, testicular neoplasia, hypothalamic-pituitary dysfunction, and hyperplasia of adrenal rest tissue occurring in the epididymis or testis. Testicular adrenal rests secrete high quantities of 17-ketosteroids and operate under ACTH control. Bilateral testicular enlargement occurs in association with hypothalamic-pituitary lesions (because of stimulation of gonadotropin secretion), as well as with aberrant adrenal rest tissue. Unilateral testicular enlargement with contralateral atrophy usually is seen with true interstitial tumors. In congenital adrenal hyperplasia, the testes remain infantile although the patient is virilized.

TREATMENT Treatment of adrenal virilism is dictated by the type of lesion suspected. Patients with *congenital adrenal hyperplasia* have the fundamental defect of cortisol deficiency with resultant excessive ACTH stimulation, producing hyperplasia of the adrenal glands and causing additional "shunting" into the adrenal androgen pathway. Therapy in these patients consists of daily administration of glucocorticoids (dexamethasone, prednisone, cortisone, etc.) to suppress pituitary ACTH secretion. Because of its cost and intermediate half-life, prednisone has been the drug of choice except in infants, when hydrocortisone is usually used. The amount of steroid required to manage patients with congenital adrenal hyperplasia effectively is approximately 1.5 times the normal cortisol production rate of 12 to 13 mg cortisol per m^2 per day and is given in divided doses two or three times a day. As the patient grows, the maintenance dose obviously should be increased. The dosage schedule is governed by repetitive analysis of the urinary 17-ketosteroids and skeletal growth and maturation, since overtreatment with glucocorticoid replacement therapy retards linear growth. In children, glucocorticoids not only suppress urinary ketosteroid excretion but also end virilization and the associated problems of hyperandrogenicity. Some infants and children with the associated defect of salt wasting require vigorous correction of salt deficits in conjunction with small doses of a potent mineralocorticoid such as 9α-fluorohydrocortisone. Children born with abnormalities of external genitalia may require surgical correction of labial fusion, urogenital sinus, etc. Diagnosis of the adrenogenital syndrome in the newborn with ambiguous external genitalia is crucial to avoid errors in the assignment of sex. Response of these children to steroid therapy is gratifying in that normal growth and development occur and the menarche and onset of spermatogenesis occur at the appropriate age. Many females with this disorder have married and have borne children. Steroid therapy is indicated throughout life, and dosages should be periodically adjusted for major stress as in the Addisonian patient.

In patients with adrenal virilization due to adrenal tumors, prompt surgical intervention with complete excision of the tumor is indicated. One cannot postpone surgical intervention in patients suspected of having virilizing adrenal adenomas, since such adenomas are practically indistinguishable from adrenal carcinomas, both clinically and biochemically. Preoperative localization of adrenal tumors can be attempted by renal tomography or adrenal angiography. Since "pure" virilizing adrenal tumors do *not* cause contralateral adrenal atrophy, thorough inspection and exploration of both suprarenal areas is mandatory. If metastases have occurred, one may consider the use of antitumor drugs, such as *o,p'*-DDD with or without local irradiation. *o,p'*-DDD in one-third of patients has been associated with a regression in peripheral metastases, paralleled by a decrease in urinary 17-ketosteroid and 17-hydroxycorticosteroid excretion; however, long-term survival is rare. In some patients given a trial of *o,p'*-DDD, regression of metastases is not seen, but a fall in steroid biosynthesis occurs.

ADRENAL FEMINIZATION

Adrenal feminization is an exceedingly rare entity and, when present, is almost always due to adrenal tumor. These adrenal tumors will cause feminization in the male, with development of gynecomastia (often with breast tenderness), and change in body habitus, testicular atrophy, feminizing hair changes, and loss of libido. They may occur in "pure" form, i.e., with normal levels of urine 17-ketosteroids, or in "mixed" form, with feminization despite high 17-ketosteroid excretion. They are always associated in the male with increased excretion of estrogen metabolites, such as estrone and estradiol, and subnormal gonadotropin levels. These adrenal tumors secrete increased amounts of androstenedione, which is peripherally converted into the estrogens, estrone and estradiol. Some patients have had elevated urinary values of tetrahydro-11-deoxycortisol, suggesting that 11β-hydroxylation may be impaired.

The majority of adrenal tumors causing feminization are *carcinomas.* They are most common in the age group twenty-five to forty-five. These tumors are almost always unilateral and occur with equal frequency on either side. In rare instances they have occurred in an extraadrenal locus such as the testis. The feminizing adrenal carcinomas are large tumors (weighing several hundred grams) and often are easily palpable on physical examination, whereas feminizing adrenal adenomas are characteristically small tumors. Metastases occur most often to the liver and lungs. Feminizing adrenal tumors do not cause contralateral adrenal atrophy, which makes bilateral exploration mandatory if the initial adrenal explored is normal. *Almost all cases of feminizing adrenal carcinoma are evident on suprarenal tomography studies.* Patients with feminizing adrenal tumors usually have normal to moderately elevated 17-ketosteroid excretion levels. If the urine 17-ketosteroid excretion is greater than 100 mg per day, the diagnosis of a feminizing adrenal carcinoma is almost certain. Urine 17-hydroxycorticoid excretion is usually within the normal range or slightly elevated. Associated Cushing's syndrome is rare. ACTH stimulation causes little change in 17-ketosteroid excretion. The chemical determination of urine estrogen titers always demonstrates an elevated value. The elevated urine estrogen excretion level is principally due to increased estriol and also to increments in estradiol and estrone. Since the estrogens produced by adrenal feminizing tumors are conversion products from androgen precursors, the amount of estrogens elaborated will depend both on the amount of androgen precursors formed and on the efficiency of the androgen-to-estrogen conversion process. Feminizing adrenocortical carcinomas have also been reported to produce gonadotropins (follicle-stimulating hormone and chorionic gonadotropin).

Radiotherapy has not been helpful in treatment. Despite operative intervention, most patients with adrenal feminizing carcinoma die within 3 years of diagnosis. With successful operative removal of feminizing tumors, the urine estrogen titer falls; a failure of the titer to fall or a recurrence of elevated urine titers indicates functioning tumor tissue.

The *diagnosis* of adrenal feminization in the male is strongly suggested by the onset of gynecomastia associated with a flank mass. The additional finding of increased urine estrogen titers confirms the diagnosis. Gynecomastia may also be seen with *testicular tumors* (chorioepithelioma, Sertoli cell, seminoma, interstitial-cell tumor). Estrogen may be secreted by testicular neoplasms, or the tumor may produce chorionic gonadotropins, with an associated elaboration of estrogens by the testes. The course of feminizing adrenal and testicular neoplasms that also synthesize gonadotropins should be followed by estrogen titers and β subunit chorionic gonadotropin titers. Adrenal feminization in the female is more difficult to detect, but it has been reported.

TABLE 93-7
Classification of causes of adrenal insufficiency

- *I* Primary adrenal insufficiency
  - *A* Anatomic destruction of gland (chronic and acute)
    - *1* Infection
    - *2* Invasion: metastatic, fungal, etc.
    - *3* Hemorrhage
    - *4* "Idiopathic" atrophy, autoimmune
    - *5* Surgical removal
  - *B* Metabolic failure in hormone production
    - *1* Virilizing hyperplasia, congenital (certain types)
    - *2* Enzyme inhibitors (metyrapone)
    - *3* Cytotoxic agents (*o,p'*-DDD)
- *II* Secondary adrenal insufficiency
  - *A* Hypopituitarism due to pituitary disease
  - *B* Suppression of hypothalamic-pituitary axis
    - *1* Exogenous steroid
    - *2* Endogenous steroid from tumors

HYPOFUNCTION OF ADRENAL CORTEX

Adrenocortical hypofunction includes all conditions in which the secretion of adrenal steroid hormones falls below the requirements of the body. Various types of adrenal insufficiency are encountered and may be divided into two general categories: (1) those associated with primary inability of the adrenal to elaborate sufficient quantities of hormone and (2) those associated with a secondary failure due to a primary failure in the elaboration of ACTH (Table 93-7).

PRIMARY ADRENOCORTICAL DEFICIENCY (ADDISON'S DISEASE)

This disorder is also called Addison's disease or chronic glucocorticoid deficiency. Addison's classic description in 1855, namely, "general languor and debility, remarkable feebleness of the heart's action, irritability of the stomach, and a peculiar change of the color of the skin," summarizes the dominant clinical features of the disease. Advanced cases usually cause little difficulty in diagnosis, but recognition of the disease in its earlier phases may present a real challenge. The disease, when unrecognized and untreated, carries an almost uniformly poor and frequently fatal prognosis. Early diagnosis is important, since present-day therapy provides complete correction of the metabolic derangement.

INCIDENCE Primary adrenocortical insufficiency is relatively rare. It may occur at any age in life and affects both sexes with equal frequency. Because of increasing therapeutic use of exogenous steroids, secondary adrenal insufficiency is seen with increasing frequency.

ETIOLOGY AND PATHOGENESIS Addison's disease results from progressive adrenocortical destruction, which must involve more than 90 percent of the glands before clinical signs of adrenal insufficiency appear. The adrenal is a frequent site for chronic infectious diseases of the granulomatous variety, predominately tuberculosis but also including fungal infections, such as histoplasmosis, coccidioidomycosis, and cryptococcosis. In previous years, tuberculosis was found at postmortem examination in 70 to 90 percent of cases; however, the most frequent finding at present is *idiopathic* atrophy, and it has been suggested that an autoimmune mechanism may be responsible for this process. Rarely, other lesions are encountered, such as bilateral tumor metastases, amyloidosis, or sarcoidosis.

The possibility that some patients may have primary adrenal insufficiency on an *autoimmune basis* has been strengthened by the finding that one-half of patients with Addison's disease have complement-fixing and/or circulating adrenal antibodies, as tested by the indirect Coons' method. Certain of these patients also have additional circulating antibodies to thyroid or parathyroid tissue, a finding of interest because of the increased incidence of hypothyroidism and hypoparathyroidism in Addison's disease. It is not clear whether these antibodies cause adrenal atrophy or are secondary to the destruction of adrenal tissue.

In 1926, Schmidt described two patients with nontuberculous Addison's disease and chronic lymphocytic thyroiditis. Subsequent reports have documented association of thyroid insufficiency and Addison's disease, and the possibility of a common autoimmune process has been raised as the etiologic factor responsible for *Schmidt's syndrome.* Concomitant parathyroid and adrenal insufficiency and mucocutaneous moniliasis have also been recognized as a familial, autosomal recessive syndrome. Diabetes mellitus, ovarian failure, and pernicious anemia are also seen in association with idiopathic Addison's disease and thyroiditis. Again, what role genetic predisposition and/or autoimmunity may play in the occurrence of these diseases in the same individual is unknown. For example, recent reports indicate a many-fold greater incidence of these endocrine deficiency states in patients with specific human leucocyte antigens. Between 3 and 4 percent of patients with Addison's disease have coexistent hyperthyroidism. The presence of both disorders in the same individual poses a difficult diagnostic problem, since many of the clinical manifestations are similar. Furthermore, the hyperthyroid state may change a subclinical insufficiency to complete adrenal insufficiency, because of the effect, mentioned above, of thyroid hormone on cortisol metabolism.

Further study of patients with combined endocrine dysfunction may prove valuable in revealing the cause of spontaneous adrenal destruction.

CLINICAL SIGNS AND SYMPTOMS Adrenocortical insufficiency is most frequently characterized by an insidious onset of slowly progressive fatigability, weakness, anorexia, nausea and vomiting, weight loss, cutaneous and mucosal pigmentation, hypotension, and occasionally hypoglycemia. These signs and symptoms compose the classic syndrome of Addison's disease; however, the spectrum may vary, depending on the duration and degree of adrenal hypofunction, from a complaint of mild chronic fatigue to the fulminating shock associated with acute massive destruction of the glands in the type of syndrome described by Waterhouse and Friderichsen. Table 93-8 lists the incidence of symptoms and signs noted in cases of Addison's disease.

Asthenia is the cardinal symptom of Addison's disease. Early it may be sporadic, usually most evident at times of stress; as adrenal function becomes more impaired, the weakness progresses until the patient is continuously fatigued, necessitating bed rest. Even the voice may fail, so the speech finally becomes listless and indistinct.

TABLE 93-8
Incidence of symptoms and signs in 125 cases of Addison's disease, percent

Weakness	99	Hypotension (below 110/70)	87
Pigmentation of skin	98	Abdominal pain	34
Pigmentation of mucous membranes	82	Salt craving	22
Weight loss	97	Diarrhea	20
Anorexia, nausea, and vomiting	90	Constipation	19
		Syncope	16
		Vitiligo	9

Hyperpigmentation may be a striking sign of the disease, but its absence does not exclude this diagnosis. It commonly appears as a diffuse brown, tan, or bronze darkening of both exposed and unexposed points such as elbows or creases of the hand and in areas normally pigmented such as the areolas about the nipples. In many patients, bluish-black patches appear on the mucous membranes. Some patients develop dark freckles, and occasionally irregular areas of vitiligo may appear paradoxically. As an early sign, patients may notice an unusually persistent tanning following exposure to the sun.

Arterial hypotension is also extremely frequent, and in severe cases blood pressures may be in the range of 80/50 or less. Postural accentuation is common, and syncope may occur.

Abnormalities of gastrointestinal function are not only extremely frequent but often are the presenting complaint. Symptoms may vary from mild anorexia with weight loss to fulminating nausea, vomiting, diarrhea, and various types of ill-defined abdominal pain, which at times may be so severe as to be confused with an acute condition of the abdomen requiring surgery. Rarely a Landry's type of ascending paralysis with flaccid quadriplegia and mixed sensory defects accompanied by ascending muscular weakness has been noted in conjunction with a higher serum potassium level. In these instances, the electrocardiogram may reflect the hyperkalemia. In addition, patients with adrenal insufficiency frequently have marked personality changes, usually in the form of excessive irritability and restlessness. Enhancement of the sensory modalities of taste, olfaction, and hearing is often present and is reversible with therapy. A decrease in axillary and pubic hair is common in female patients due to loss of adrenal androgen production.

LABORATORY FINDINGS In the milder forms, sometimes called *partial* or *incomplete* Addison's disease, there may be no demonstrable abnormalities in any of the parameters measured in the routine laboratory, and even plasma and urinary steroid determinations may indicate values relatively low yet within normal range. However, definitive studies of adrenal stimulation with ACTH show abnormalities even in this stage of the disease. In the more advanced stages, levels of serum sodium, chloride, and bicarbonate are reduced while serum potassium is elevated. The hyponatremia is due to extravascular loss of sodium both into the urine (due to aldosterone deficiency) and from the vascular compartment into tendons, cartilage, and bone. This extravascular sodium loss depletes extracellular fluid volume and accentuates hypotension. Elevated plasma levels of vasopressin and angiotensin have been reported, and these may be contributing factors to hyponatremia through impairment of free-water clearance. The hyperkalemia is due to a combination of factors, including aldosterone deficiency, impaired glomerular filtration rate, and acidosis. These patients may show marked reduction in heart size, and in about one-quarter of the patients suprarenal calcification is seen but is unfortunately not pathognomonic. The electrocardiogram may show nonspecific changes, and the electroencephalogram a striking reduction and slowing of the predominant activity. The basal metabolic rate may be low, but other thyroid indexes are usually normal. There may be a normocytic anemia, a relative lymphocytosis, and usually a moderate eosinophilia.

DIAGNOSIS The diagnosis of adrenal insufficiency requires demonstration either directly or indirectly of decreased cortisol production by the adrenal in the basal state (*complete* adrenal insufficiency) or the unmasking of decreased cortisol production only in the stimulated state (*incomplete* adrenal insufficiency) (Fig. 93-13).

In all cases of *complete adrenal insufficiency* the cortisol secretory rate is markedly decreased, and this may be ascertained indirectly by the finding of low to absent 24-h urine 17-hydroxycorticoids and urine 17-ketosteroids. Because of the contribution of the male gonads to urine 17-ketosteroids, basal excretory values in complete adrenal insufficiency will be higher for males than females. With incomplete adrenal insufficiency, urine steroid excretion values overlap into the normal range; because of this, a diagnosis of adrenal insufficiency cannot be made solely on the values of basal urine steroid determinations. Plasma cortisol values are from zero to the lower range of normal. Aldosterone secretion is very low, resulting in salt-wasting and secondary rises in plasma renin levels. In patients with primary adrenal insufficiency, plasma ACTH and MSH levels are elevated because of loss of the usual cortisol-hypothalamic-pituitary feedback relationship, whereas in secondary adrenal insufficiency, plasma ACTH values are low, a finding consistent with the absence of increased pigmentation in patients having the latter condition.

The specific and definitive diagnosis of adrenal insufficiency can be made only with the ACTH stimulation test to assay the adrenal reserve capacity for steroid production. In addition, ACTH testing is helpful in establishing whether adrenal insufficiency is primary or secondary. A simple *outpatient* screening test is the measurement of blood cortisol and aldosterone levels 30 to 60 min after the intramuscular administration of 25 units (0.25 mg) α-24 corticotropin. In normal subjects, the blood cortisol level usually doubles, and the absolute increment above control is greater than 7 to 10 μg per 100 ml. Blood aldosterone levels usually increase 5 to 15 ng per 100 ml above control at 30 min. In patients undergoing intravenous ACTH test-

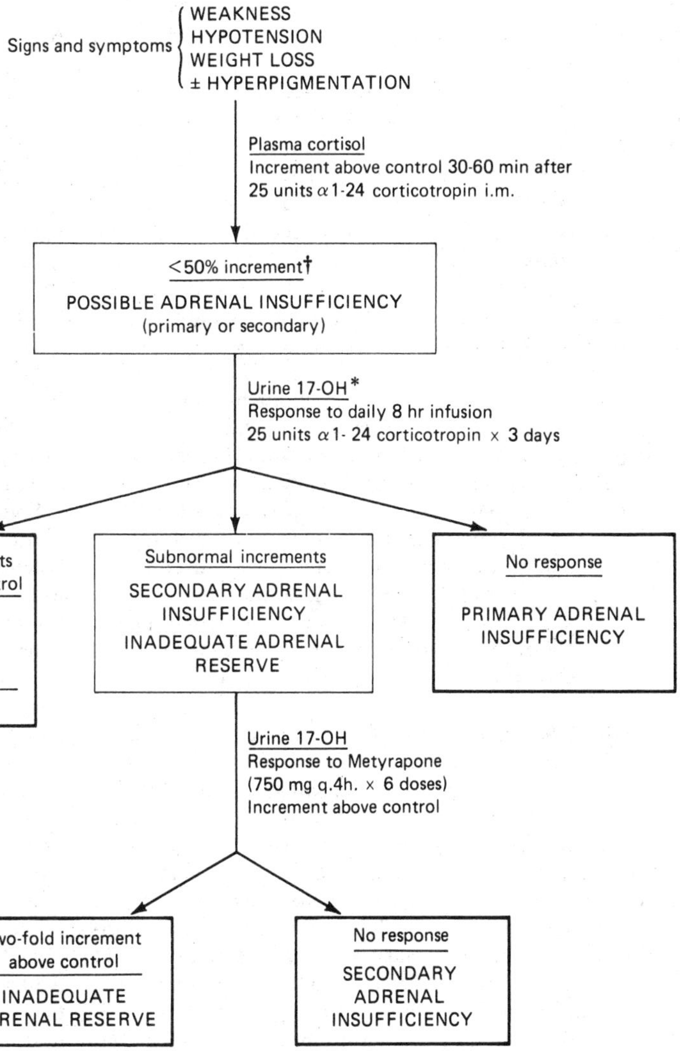

FIGURE 93-13
Diagnostic flow chart for evaluating the status of patients with suspected adrenal insufficiency. Plasma ACTH (and MSH) levels will be low in secondary adrenal insufficiency. In adrenal insufficiency secondary to pituitary tumors or idiopathic panhypopituitarism, other pituitary hormone deficiencies will be present. On the other hand, ACTH deficiency may be isolated, as seen following prolonged use of exogenous glucocorticoids.

†In normal subjects, blood cortisol levels usually double or rise greater than 7 to 10 µg per ml above control at 30 to 60 min following 25 units α1–24 corticotropin I. M. Blood aldosterone levels usually increase 5 to 15 ng per 100 ml above control at 30 min.

**An alternative test to the 8-h infusion of ACTH for 3 to 4 days is a continuous infusion of 25 units of α1–24 corticotropin q.12h for 24 to 48 h.*

ing as a diagnostic method for adrenal insufficiency, saline solution should be utilized as the diluent for the ACTH to be infused, since on occasion patients may experience water intoxication if a diluent of only glucose and water is used. An additional advantage of using saline diluent is that a clinical estimate of adrenal responsiveness may be made by the presence or absence of weight gain during the infusion period, weight gain commonly occurring when adrenocortical function is intact, because of the associated stimulation of aldosterone secretion. The potential dangers of ACTH testing in patients with limited adrenal reserves may be minimized by the prior administration of 1 mg of a potent steroid such as dexamethasone. The excretory products of 1 mg of this compound will not add appreciably to the amount of 17-hydroxycorticoids measured in the urine and therefore will not interfere with the test. For testing purposes, 40 units of ACTH (or 25 units α1–24 corticotropin) is infused daily over 8 h for 4 to 5 successive days, with daily urine collections tested for creatinine, 17-hydroxycorticoid, and 17-ketosteroid levels. Alternatively, a continuous 48-h ACTH infusion may be used by giving 40 units of ACTH (or 25 units α1–24 corticotropin) in 500 ml of 5 percent dextrose in normal saline solution every 12 h for four consecutive 12-h periods. In patients with complete primary adrenal insufficiency, ACTH stimulation by either method will cause a rise in steroid excretion of less than 2 mg per day.

In *incomplete adrenal insufficiency,* ACTH testing carried out by either method will result in subnormal increments in urinary 17-hydroxycorticoids. A variant of this response is sometimes seen in which small increments in steroid excretion occur on the first 3 days of the 5-day infusion test, while on the last 2 days, there is an actual decline in the level of steroids. Alternately, the last 12 h of the continuous 48-h infusion will show a decline in 17-hydroxycorticoid excretion. These results suggest that the limited adrenal tissue has been maximally stimulated and has insufficient steroid reserve capacity.

Indirect tests of adrenocortical hypofunction include (1) a delay in water excretion following an acute water load; (2) defective renal conservation of sodium when a low sodium diet is imposed; and (3) a tendency toward hypoglycemia during fasting. Since ACTH is available for direct evaluation of adrenocortical function, these procedures are not indicated; furthermore, in a patient with adrenocortical insufficiency, water intoxication, sodium deprivation, or hypoglycemia may all be life-threatening situations. A flow chart for evaluation of patients with suspected adrenal insufficiency is presented in Fig. 93-13.

DIFFERENTIAL DIAGNOSIS Since weakness and fatigue are such common complaints, clinical diagnosis of early adrenocortical insufficiency is frequently difficult (Fig. 93-13). However, mild gastrointestinal distress with weight loss, anorexia, and a suggestion of increased pigmentation make mandatory ACTH stimulation testing to rule out adrenal insufficiency, particularly before steroid treatment is begun. Weight loss is useful in evaluating the significance of weakness and malaise. Weight gain associated with lassitude is more characteristic of depressive syndromes. Racial pigmentation in Negroes, Orientals, Indians, Spanish Americans, and Latins may be a problem, but a *recent* and progressive *increase* is usually reported by the Addisonian patient. Hyperpigmentation in other diseases may also present a problem, but the appearance and distribution of pigment in Addison's disease are usually characteristic. Other diseases presenting with hyperpigmentation include hemochromatosis, acanthosis nigricans, porphyria, thyrotoxicosis, polyostotic fibrous dysplasia, chronic metal poisoning (bismuth, lead, arsenic, silver), chronic malnutrition (starvation, anorexia nervosa, sprue syndrome, pellagra), progressive malignancy, chronic anemia, salt-losing nephritis with hypotension, renal tubular acidosis, scleroderma, excess nicotinic acid, and hepatic cirrhosis. In most cases, differentiation from Addison's disease is not difficult, but when doubt exists, ACTH administration ordinarily provides clear-cut differentiation.

TREATMENT All patients with Addison's disease should receive specific hormone replacement therapy. Like diabetics, these patients require careful and persistent education in regard to their disease. Since the adrenal gland elaborates three general classes of hormone, of which two, glucocorticoids and mineralocorticoids, are of primary clinical importance, replacement therapy should correct both deficiencies. Cortisone (or hydrocortisone) is the mainstay of treatment; however, its mineralocorticoid effect, when it is given in sufficient dosage to replace the endogenous hydrocortisone deficiency, is inadequate for complete electrolyte balance; therefore, the patient usually requires other supplementary hormone. Cortisone dosage varies from 12.5 to 50 mg daily, with the majority of patients taking 25 to 37.5 mg in divided doses. Hydrocortisone (30 mg daily) or prednisone (7.5 mg daily) in divided doses may also be given for substitution therapy. Because of its direct local effect on gastric mucosa, patients are advised to take their cortisone with meals or, if this is impractical, with milk or an antacid preparation. In addition, the larger proportion of the dose (25 mg) is taken in the morning and the remainder (12.5 mg) in the late afternoon, to simulate somewhat the normal diurnal adrenal rhythm. Some patients may exhibit insomnia, irritability, mental excitement, and even frank psychosis soon after initiation of therapy; in these the dosage should obviously be reduced. Other indications for maintaining the patient on smaller amounts are hypertension, diabetes, or active tuberculosis.

Since, as mentioned earlier, this amount of cortisone or hydrocortisone fails to replace the mineralocorticoid component of the adrenal gland, supplementary hormone is usually needed. The simplest means is daily oral administration of 0.1 to 0.2 mg of 9α-fluorohydrocortisone. If parenteral administration is indicated, a dosage of 2 to 5 mg deoxycorticosterone acetate in oil may be given every day intramuscularly. An alternative method of therapy is an injection of 25 to 50 mg deoxycorticosterone trimethylacetate in oil intramuscularly every 3 to 4 weeks, but as with the previous use of subcutaneous implantation of pellets of deoxycorticosterone which lasted for 8 to 10 months, most patients prefer the simplicity of daily oral administration of the 9α-fluorohydrocortisone.

Complications of cortisone therapy, with the exception of peptic disease, particularly ulcer or gastritis, are *extremely rare* in the dosage used in the treatment of Addison's disease. However, overtreatment with deoxycorticosterone preparations or 9α-fluorohydrocortisone is more frequent and may present as edema, hypertension, cardiac enlargement, or even congestive failure due to sodium retention. Overtreatment may also present as weakness, progressing to total paralysis, due to hypokalemia. In the management of patients with Addison's disease, periodic measurements of body weight, serum potassium, heart size, blood pressure, and serial electrocardiograms are useful.

Some female patients with Addison's disease experience a persistent decline in libido possibly related to subnormal adrenal androgen production. Small doses of intramuscular depo-testosterone (e.g., 50 mg monthly) may be used to advantage, but overtreatment leading to masculinizing side effects must be avoided.

All patients with adrenal insufficiency, including bilaterally adrenalectomized patients, should carry medical identification, should be instructed in the parenteral self-administration of steroids, and should be registered with a national medical alerting system.

SPECIAL THERAPEUTIC PROBLEMS During periods of intercurrent illness, the dose of cortisone or hydrocortisone should be increased to levels of 75 to 150 mg per day. When oral administration is not possible, parenteral routes should be employed. Likewise, before surgery or dental extractions, excess steroid should be administered. For a representative program of steroid therapy for an Addisonian patient or an adrenalectomized patient undergoing a major operation, see Table 93-9. This schedule is designed to mimic the maximal output of cortisol in normal individuals undergoing prolonged major stress with presumed continuous ACTH stimulation (10 mg per h, 250 to 300 mg per 24 h). The patients should all be advised of these facts and should carry an identification card bearing detailed instructions for the administration of steroid in case of acute illness or injury. Patients should also be advised to increase the dose of 9α-fluorohydrocortisone and add excess salt to their otherwise normal diet during periods of excessive exercise with sweating, during extremely hot weather, or during periods of gastrointestinal upsets. In spite of animal studies demonstrating an increased susceptibility to tubercular spread associated with excess steroid administration, patients with Addison's disease and tuberculosis may be treated safely with maintenance daily doses of cortisone.

COURSE AND PROGNOSIS Untreated Addison's disease characteristically runs a chronic and relentless course. In some patients, its advance is relatively slow, but in all patients the condition may rapidly deteriorate into adrenal crisis. With treatment, the prognosis of the disease is extremely favorable. In fact, some of the degenerative vascular problems such as hypertension or congestive failure are more easily handled in an Addisonian patient than in one with intact adrenal glands.

SECONDARY ADRENOCORTICAL INSUFFICIENCY

Pituitary ACTH deficiency will produce *secondary* adrenocortical insufficiency. ACTH deficiency may be selective, as is seen following prolonged administration of excess glucocorticoids, or may occur in association with multiple pituitary tropic hormone deficiencies (panhypopituitarism) (see Chap. 90). Patients with secondary adrenocortical hypofunction may have many symptoms and signs in common with Addisonian patients but are *characteristically not hyperpigmented* since ACTH and MSH levels are characteristically low. Patients with total pituitary insufficiency will also have signs and symptoms suggestive of multiple hormone deficiencies. An additional feature distinguishing primary from secondary adrenocortical insufficiency is the *near-normal levels of aldosterone secretion* seen in the presence of pituitary and/or isolated ACTH deficiencies. Patients with pituitary insufficiency may present with hyponatremia, which may be dilutional or secondary to subnormal increments in aldosterone secretion in response to sodium restriction. However, the findings of severe dehydration, *hyponatremia,* and *hyperkalemia* are characteristic of severe mineralocorticoid insufficiency and favor a diagnosis of primary adrenocortical insufficiency.

Patients receiving long-term steroid therapy, despite physical findings of Cushing's syndrome, develop adrenal insufficiency both because of prolonged pituitary-hypo-

TABLE 93-9
Steroid therapy schedule for Addisonian patient undergoing a major operation*

	Cortisone acetate (intramuscularly)		*Hydrocortisone infusion*	*Cortisone acetate (orally)*				*Fluorohydrocortisone (orally)*
	7 A.M.	*7* P.M.	*Continuous*	*8* A.M.	*12 Noon*	*4* P.M.	*8* P.M.	*8* A.M.
Routine daily medication				25		12.5		0.1
Day before operation		50		25		12.5		0.1
Day of operation	100	50	200					
Postoperative day 1	50	50	100–150					
" 2	50	50	50–100					
" 3	50	50		25			25	
" 4	50			25	25	25		0.1
" 5				25	25	25	25	0.1
" 6				25	25	25		0.1
" 7				25	12.5	25		0.1
" 8				25	12.5	25		0.1
" 9–13				25		25		0.1
" 14				25		12.5		0.1

* *All steroid doses are given in milligrams.*

thalamic suppression and because of actual adrenal atrophy. Adrenal atrophy results from the loss of endogenous ACTH stimulation, which stimulus is prerequisite for maintaining normal adrenal size. Thus, these patients acquire two deficits, a loss of adrenal responsiveness to ACTH and a failure of pituitary ACTH release. These patients are characterized by low blood cortisol and ACTH levels, low base-line steroid excretion, and abnormal ACTH and metyrapone test results. On testing these patients with ACTH, one looks for the "staircase" response, with successive daily increments in steroid excretion; however, *prolonged ACTH testing* may be needed to elicit such a response. The urine steroid pattern, when adrenal reactivation does occur, often reveals increments in 17-hydroxycorticoids without parallel increments in 17-ketosteroids. Practically all patients with steroid-induced adrenal insufficiency will eventually respond to ACTH testing, but individual response time is most variable, ranging from days to months. Once such patients are shown to have reacquired adrenal sensitivity to exogenous ACTH, their ability to release endogenous pituitary ACTH must be determined. The standard metyrapone test is utilized for this purpose. For a valid metyrapone test, the fact must be previously documented that the patient's adrenal glands are sensitive to ACTH, since the metyrapone test response depends on adrenal responsiveness to released ACTH. For this reason the test is *contraindicated* in patients with suspected or proved adrenal insufficiency. In patients with steroid-induced adrenal insufficiency, abnormal metyrapone tests usually continue for several months after the adrenal glands have regained responsiveness to ACTH. In interpreting the metyrapone test, it is useful to consider it as an endogenous ACTH stimulation test and compare the peak urine 17-hydroxycorticoid excretion with the maximal values previously obtained with exogenous ACTH stimulation.

Plasma ACTH levels help distinguish between primary and secondary adrenal insufficiency, since they are elevated in the former and decreased to absent in the latter.

Substitution glucocorticoid therapy in patients with secondary adrenocortical insufficiency does not differ from that outlined for Addisonian patients. Mineralocorticoid replacement therapy is usually not necessary, since aldosterone secretion is preserved. Otherwise, it is stressed that the basic principles outlined for replacement should be applied to patients with secondary adrenocortical insufficiency.

ACUTE ADRENOCORTICAL INSUFFICIENCY

Acute adrenocortical insufficiency may result from several processes. One of these, usually termed *adrenal crisis,* is a rapid and overwhelming intensification of chronic adrenal insufficiency. Another process involves an acute hemorrhagic destruction of both adrenal glands, usually associated with an overwhelming septicemia. Adrenal hemorrhage associated with anticoagulant therapy in severely stressed patients with increased adrenocortical activity has also been reported. A third, and probably the most frequent, cause of acute insufficiency results from the rapid withdrawal of steroids from patients with adrenal atrophy secondary to chronic steroid administration. In the presence of severe stress, acute adrenocortical insufficiency may also occur in patients with congenital adrenal hyperplasia and those receiving pharmacologic agents which are capable of inhibiting steroid synthesis by the gland (such as *o,p′*-DDD).

ADRENAL CRISIS The long-term survival of patients with Addison's disease largely depends upon prevention and treatment of adrenal crisis. Consequently, the occurrence of infection, trauma (including surgery), gastrointestinal upsets, or other forms of stress requires an immediate increase in hormone. In previously untreated patients, preexisting symptoms are intensified. Nausea, vomiting, and abdominal pain may become intractable. Fever is frequently severe but may be absent. Lethargy deepens into somnolence, and the blood pressure and pulse fail as hypovolemic vascular shock ensues. In contrast, patients previously maintained on chronic glucocorticoid therapy may not exhibit severe dehydration or hypotension until preterminally, since mineralocorticoid secretion is usually preserved.

In all patients presenting in crisis, a precipitating cause should be sought. Intercurrent infection associated with omission or failure to increase maintenance therapy is a common setting.

Treatment is primarily directed toward the rapid elevation of circulating adrenocortical hormone, in addition to the replacement of the sodium and water deficit. Hence, an intravenous infusion of 1,000 ml 5 percent glucose in normal saline solution containing 100 to 200 mg of any of several soluble hydrocortisone preparations is begun rapidly, with the first 250 ml infused in the first ½ to 1 h and the remainder over the ensuing 4 to 8 h. If the condition is extreme, immediate intravenous infusion of 100 mg hydrocortisone in the first few minutes is suggested, followed by a rapid infusion as described above. Epinephrine, 0.2 mg intravenously, may also be indicated. In any case, it is also advisable to administer 100 mg cortisone acetate intramuscularly in case the infusion becomes infiltrated or inadvertently stopped. If the crisis was preceded by prolonged nausea, vomiting, and dehydration, several liters of saline may be required within the first few hours. With large doses of steroid, as, for example, 200 mg cortisone or hydrocortisone, the patient receives a maximal mineralocorticoid effect, and supplementary deoxycorticosterone is superfluous. After the initial infusion, depending on the patient's condition, a second similar infusion may be given; if there has been marked improvement, the patient may be offered oral fluids and be given 50 mg cortisone acetate intramuscularly every 12 h until gastrointestinal absorption is guaranteed, at which time the steroid can be given orally. Steroid dosage is then tapered over the next few days to maintenance levels, with reinstitution of supplementary mineralocorticoid if needed.

ADRENAL HEMORRHAGE Adrenal hemorrhage (adrenal apoplexy) is usually associated with overwhelming septicemia (Waterhouse-Friderichsen syndrome); however, it may also occur in the absence of sepsis. Occasionally, massive bilateral adrenal hemorrhage results from birth trauma. The infant may either be stillborn or die soon after birth of shock and hyperpyrexia. Adrenal hemorrhage also occurs during pregnancy, following idiopathic adrenal vein thrombosis, during convulsions in epilepsy or during electroconvulsive therapy, with excessive anticoagulant therapy, after trauma or surgery, and as a complication of adrenal venography (e.g., infarction of an adenoma). Pain in the flank and epigastrium is frequent, and if the hemorrhagic process ruptures into the abdomen, signs of peritoneal inflammation are present. Acute adrenal insufficiency should also be considered in the differential diagnosis of hypotension in patients maintained on anticoagulant therapy in the period immediately following a myocardial infarction.

The adrenal hemorrhage associated with septicemia is most frequent with meningococcemia but is also seen with overwhelming infections due to pneumococcus, staphylococcus, or *Hemophilus influenzae.* The onset is often explosive, with a shaking chill, violent headache, vertigo, vomiting, and prostration. A petechial rash appears on the skin and mucous membranes and progresses rapidly to a confluent, extensive purpura. Large areas of skin may become grossly hemorrhagic. Body temperature may be subnormal but is usually markedly elevated. Circulatory collapse rapidly ensues, and death may occur within 6 to 48 h. Specific diagnosis requires immediate identification of the organism. Frequently, the septicemia is so massive that organisms may be seen in peripheral blood smears or petechial scrapings. Time is not sufficient for determination of adrenal function; however, a plasma sample for later determination of 17-hydroxysteroid level may be of academic interest.

Treatment must be immediate and intensive. Control of the infection by vigorous administration of parenteral, preferably intravenous, antibiotics is indicated in addition to the steroid schedule delineated for adrenal crisis. Intravenous norepinephrine (4 to 8 mg per liter) may also be required to maintain vascular tone. Since shock may also be associated with massive septicemia without adrenal hemorrhage, one is never completely certain whether adrenal insufficiency is contributing to the patient's decompensation; however, the authors think that because of the increasing frequency of survival of patients treated with steroid, some degree of adrenal insufficiency, whether relative or absolute, is present and that steroid treatment is therefore indicated in all patients in whom fulminating septicemia is associated with shock. The dose range administered in such patients is usually massive (e.g., 1,000 mg hydrocortisone daily).

HYPOALDOSTERONISM

Isolated aldosterone deficiency accompanied by normal cortisol production has been reported in association with hyporeninism; as a congenital biosynthetic defect; postoperatively, following removal of aldosteronoma; during protracted heparin or heparinoid administration; in pretectal disease of the nervous system; in severe postural hypotension; and in association with complete heart block.

In severe cases urine sodium wastage is present on a normal salt intake, whereas in milder forms excessive urine sodium losses occur only during salt restriction. The patients always develop hyponatremia and hyperkalemia, the latter often to a severe degree.

Isolated aldosterone deficiency is most commonly seen in adult subjects in association with hyporeninism, abnormal renal function, and hyperkalemia. Plasma renin and aldosterone levels fail to rise normally following sodium restriction, and biosynthetic defects in the secretion of aldosterone cannot be demonstrated. Aldosterone secretion fails to rise following ACTH stimulation, but cortisol secretion increases normally.

A biosynthetic defect has been noted in some patients who are unable to transform the angular C-18 methyl group of corticosterone to the C-18 aldehyde grouping of aldosterone due to a deficiency of the enzyme 18-hydroxysteroid dehydrogenase. This C-18 transformation requires first the formation of 18-hydroxycorticosterone from corticosterone, and then, secondly, dehydrogenation of the C-18 hydroxyl group to form the characteristic C-18 aldehyde group of aldosterone. These patients will manifest low to absent aldosterone secretion and excretion, elevated plasma renin levels, and elevated secretion and excretion values for corticosterone and 18-hydroxycorticosterone.

The feature common to all patients with hypoaldosteronism has been their inability to *increase* aldosterone secretion appropriately during severe salt restriction. An additional feature has been the reversal of the signs of salt wasting (hyponatremia and hyperkalemia) with the administration of potent mineralocorticoids. For practical purposes the oral administration of 9α-fluorohydrocortisone in a dose of 0.1 to 0.3 mg daily restores electrolyte balance.

NONSPECIFIC USE OF ADRENAL STEROIDS AND ACTH IN CLINICAL PRACTICE

The widespread utilization of glucocorticoids and ACTH in clinical practice emphasizes the need for a thorough understanding of the metabolic effects of these agents when used nonspecifically, if optimum effectiveness is to be obtained and if undesirable side reactions are to be minimized. Before instituting adrenal hormone therapy, a physician should weigh carefully the gains that can reasonably be expected versus the potentially undesirable metabolic actions of pharmacologic doses of hormone. Accurate appraisal will require familiarity with current medical literature, a critical evaluation of the significance of such reports, as well as a clear understanding of the chemical, physiologic, and psychologic changes that hormone preparations of this type are known to induce when used in pharmacologic dosage.

HOW SERIOUS IS THE DISORDER? Clearly, in the case of a patient whose life is threatened by unexplained shock, or in whom other measures have failed, the physician need not hesitate to employ large-dosage steroid therapy. On the other hand, one should exercise restraint in administering pharmacologic doses of steroids to a patient with early rheumatoid arthritis who as yet has not been exposed to the possible benefits of physiotherapy, analgesics, and a well-organized program of general medical care.

HOW LONG WILL GLUCOCORTICOID THERAPY BE REQUIRED? The use of intravenously administered steroids for a period of 24 to 48 h in the treatment of such life-threatening situations as status asthmaticus or pseudotumor cerebri has little or no contraindication, in contrast to the initiation of a program of steroid therapy for chronic asthma, arthritis, or psoriasis. In the latter instances, the almost certain complication of a Cushing's syndrome of some degree must be weighed against the potential benefit to the patient. The need for minimizing these side effects by the use of shorter-acting steroid preparations, alternate-day or interrupted therapy programs, and the judicious use of supplementary adjuvants is evident. The markedly depressed adrenal androgen secretion which accompanies long-continued pharmacologic doses of glucocorticoids in all probability increases the risk of muscle atrophy and osteopenia in female patients.

WHICH ADRENAL PREPARATION IS PREFERABLE? Five considerations need to be taken into account in deciding which steroid preparation to use: (1) the biologic half-life of the particular compound. The rationale behind every-other-day therapy is to decrease the metabolic effects of the steroids for a significant amount of time over the 2-day period, yet at the same time to produce pharmacologic suppression of sufficient duration to maintain the disease in remission. Too long a half-life would defeat the first purpose, and too short a half-life would defeat the second. In general, the more potent the steroid, the longer its biologic half-life tends to be. (2) The importance of the mineralocorticoid effects of the steroid. The newer synthetic steroids have much less mineralocorticoid effect relative to their glucocorticoid effect than cortisol or cortisone (Table 93-10). This may be an important consideration in certain disease states. (3) The fact that cortisone and prednisone, in contrast to the other glucocorticoids, have to be converted to their biologically active equivalents before any anti-inflammatory effects can occur. Because of this, in a clinical condition in which steroids are known to be effective and in which an adequate dose has been given without any response, one should consider substituting hydrocortisone or prednisolone for cortisone or prednisone. (4) The cost of the medication; this is a serious consideration if chronic administration is to be undertaken. Prednisone is the least expensive of available steroid preparations. (5) The appreciable variation among commercial preparations of glucosteroids in the manner in which the tablets are formulated. This factor may significantly modify absorption. Thus it is advisable for a patient whose steroid dosage has been standardized to continue to utilize the same pharmaceutical preparation to avoid relapse or overdosage.

TABLE 93-10
Adrenal preparations*

Commonly used name	Estimated potency† Glucocorticoid	Mineralocorticoid
SHORT-ACTING		
Hydrocortisone	1	1
Cortisone	0.8	0.8
INTERMEDIATE-ACTING		
Prednisone	4	0.25
Prednisolone	4	0.25
Methylprednisolone	5	±
Triamcinolone	5	±
LONG-ACTING		
Paramethasone	10	±
Betamethasone	25	±
Dexamethasone	30–40	±

* *The steroids are divided into three groups according to the duration of biologic activity. Short-acting preparations have a biologic half-life of less than 12 h; long-acting, greater than 48 h; and intermediate, between 12 and 36 h. Triamcinolone has the longest half-life of the intermediate-acting preparations.*

† *Relative milligram comparisons with cortisol, setting the glucocorticoid and mineralocorticoid properties of cortisol as 1. Sodium retention is insignificant in usual doses employed of methylprednisolone, triamcinolone, paramethasone, betamethasone, and dexamethasone.*

ACTH VERSUS STEROIDS In most cases, the only decision of major consequence is whether to use ACTH rather than one of the adrenal steroid preparations. In general, adrenal steroid therapy is effective by mouth and can be regulated more accurately than ACTH therapy. The latter will fluctuate considerably in the amount of steroid produced from day to day, depending on the rate and extent of absorption of ACTH and on the state of the adrenal cortex. ACTH therapy does stimulate the secretion of adrenal androgens as well as hydroxysteroids. The former may have advantages in certain diseases, such as dermatomyositis, in which the adrenal androgens may prove helpful in maintaining the muscle mass while the inflammatory reaction is being suppressed by the 17-hydroxycorticosteroids. Combined androgen and corticoid therapy may, of course, attain the same objective. Sodium retention with ACTH has often been more marked than with cortisone or, particularly, with prednisone therapy.

ACTH therapy has proved useful in the treatment of neuromuscular disorders such as dermatomyositis and multiple sclerosis, particularly in female patients in whom the androgenic stimulation of ACTH may minimize the "muscle-wasting action" of glucocorticoids. Both ACTH and steroid therapy induce hypothalamic-pituitary suppression; however, in ACTH therapy adrenal gland size and activity are maintained, in contrast to the adrenal atrophy usually associated with steroid therapy. ACTH is often used, in small doses, to activate the adrenal cortex before steroid therapy is completely discontinued; however, this is rarely necessary when "every-other-day" intermediate-acting steroid therapy has been utilized.

EVALUATION OF PATIENT PRIOR TO INITIATING STEROID THERAPY (Table 93-11)

Chronic infection Three problems demand attention. (1) Any active infection, particularly tuberculosis, should be identified. If tuberculosis is present, steroid therapy can be employed, if indicated, in conjunction with antituberculous chemotherapy. (2) The chest film and tuberculin test will provide base-line information for future comparison. High-dosage steroids will minimize the tuberculin reaction. For this reason a chest roentgenogram should be carried out at 6- to 12-month intervals, or with evidence of unexplained fever or weight loss, in patients on long-continued steroid therapy. (3) Infection due to "opportunistic" low virulence pathogens should be constantly considered in patients on high steroid dosage, especially when steroid therapy is combined with other immunosuppressive agents.

Diabetes mellitus Prolonged ACTH or cortisone-like steroid therapy may unmask latent diabetes mellitus and aggravate preexisting disease. For this reason a careful history is important to exclude familial incidence of diabetes. It is more valuable to carry out examinations of blood and

TABLE 93-11
A "checklist" for use prior to the administration of steroids in pharmacologic dosages

1 Presence of tuberculosis or other chronic infection (chest x-ray, tuberculin test)
2 History of diabetes mellitus in family (postprandial blood glucose test, preferably after 100-g carbohydrate meal)
3 Evidence of preexisting osteoporosis (spinal x-ray in postmenopausal patients)
4 History of peptic ulcer, gastritis, or esophagitis (stool guaiac test)
5 Evidence of hypertension or cardiovascular disease
6 History of evidence of psychologic disorders
7 Base-line 24 h urinary steroid excretion. (This measurement of the level of endogenous adrenal secretion may prove helpful in estimating the response to exogenous steroid therapy, as well as the dose which may be required. Thus, patients with chronic illness and low endogenous steroid level may be expected to respond more favorably and to a lower steroid dosage than those with high endogenous levels of hormone.)

urine following a test load of carbohydrate. A convenient method consists in measuring blood and urine glucose 2 to 3 h after the ingestion of a breakfast containing approximately 100 g carbohydrate (see Chap. 95). Obviously the presence of frank diabetes mellitus or the demonstration of impaired glucose tolerance will affect the physician's decision to institute adrenal hormone therapy. However, if such therapy appears necessary or desirable in the presence of latent diabetes, the judicious use of supplementary insulin therapy may be added to the therapeutic program. The insulin requirement of known diabetics will usually need to be increased with ACTH or cortisone-like therapy, except in those rare instances in which the diabetic patient is suffering from some degree of insulin resistance in which the anti-inflammatory or antiallergic effect of cortisone enhances the metabolic effectiveness of the insulin sufficiently to balance off the diabetogenic action of the former.

Osteoporosis All patients receiving long-continued steroid therapy are likely to develop some degree of osteoporosis. Obviously, considerable change in bone structure must occur before significant radiologic changes can be demonstrated. For patients at high risk (postmenopausal females, elderly individuals, and patients whose basic disease process results in restricted physical activity) initial films of the thoracolumbar segment of the spine are mandatory. Glucocorticoids decrease intestinal absorption of calcium, are collagenolytic, and may decrease growth hormone secretion. These combined actions make the vertebral column extremely vulnerable. Osteoporosis, with vertebral fractures or compression, is one of the most serious potential hazards of long-term steroid therapy. For this reason, it is urged that a program which includes large doses of vitamin D, fluoride, calcium, and anabolic hormones be prescribed in conjunction with "alternate-day" or interrupted steroid therapy (see below). Serum calcium levels should be monitored at monthly intervals to prevent hypercalcemia.

Peptic ulcer, gastric hypersecretion, or esophagitis Patients with a history of gastric hypersecretion or peptic ulcer are likely to experience aggravation of their symptoms while receiving adrenal hormone therapy. It is not known for certain whether aggravation of peptic ulceration and complicating gastrointestinal hemorrhage reflect the increased gastric secretory activity so frequently associated with adrenal hormone therapy or whether the nitrogen-depleting effect of these hormones accelerates the process of ulceration and perforation. Prophylactic antacid therapy and an ulcer diet are useful precautions in susceptible patients. *The development of anemia in a patient receiving ACTH or cortisone therapy should immediately suggest gastrointestinal bleeding,* and patients should be cautioned to note black or tarry stools. A clear-cut history of peptic ulcer constitutes a contraindication to ACTH and cortisone therapy, and steroid therapy, if required as a life-saving measure, should be accompanied by a vigorous "ulcer-combating" program.

Hypertension or cardiovascular disease In general, the sodium-retaining propensity of most adrenal steroid preparations requires that caution be used when they are given to patients with preexisting hypertension or cardiovascular or renal disease. Use of the now-available preparations in which sodium-retaining activity is minimal (triamcinolone and dexamethasone), restriction of dietary sodium intake, and the use of diuretic agents and supplementary potassium salts, will permit the safe use of steroid therapy where important indications exist. Sodium retention and edema are more marked with ACTH therapy than with glucocorticoid preparations. In some patients with congestive failure or pericardial effusion, steroid therapy may initiate a diuresis.

For all patients in whom prolonged steroid therapy is contemplated cardiovascular-renal status should be carefully evaluated, with a chest x-ray for *heart size* and an electrocardiogram included.

Psychologic difficulties From time to time steroid therapy may be complicated by severe psychologic disturbances; less severe abnormalities are relatively frequent. In general, serious psychologic disturbances are more closely related to the patient's personality structure than to the actual dose of hormone, although, as might be anticipated, larger doses of hormone will be associated with more frequent serious reactions. At present there is no reliable method of determining beforehand a patient's psychologic reaction to steroid therapy. Patients with known psychologic difficulties undoubtedly experience more frequent and more severe disturbances. Further difficulty arises because previous tolerance of steroids does not necessarily ensure immunity to subsequent courses of therapy, and untoward psychologic reactions on one occasion do not invariably mean that the patient will respond unfavorably to a second course of treatment. The physician must follow the course of the patient's condition carefully during the early period of steroid therapy and must take a responsible member of the patient's family into his confidence.

Sleeplessness is a well-known complication of glucosteroid therapy. This can be minimized by using the shorter-acting steroids and by prescribing the total dose as a single early-morning medication (Table 93-12).

"ALTERNATE-DAY" STEROID THERAPY Undoubtedly the single most effective measure in minimizing the cushingoid effects of glucosteroid therapy is to administer the total

TABLE 93-12
Supplementary measures designed to minimize undesirable metabolic effects of glucocorticoids

1 Monitor caloric intake to prevent weight gain.
2 Restrict sodium intake to prevent edema, minimize hypertension and potassium loss.
3 Potassium supplement—a diet high in potassium and supplementary potassium as KCl elixir, 2–3 tsp three times daily with meals
4 Antacid therapy—most patients will do well to receive regular antacid therapy between meals and at night. The antacid should be of the low-sodium variety.
5 Sodium fluoride, 6–9 mg daily (Luride tablets contain 2.2 mg NaF).
Calcium, 600 mg daily.
Vitamin D, 50,000 units twice weekly.
6 Estrogen and androgen therapy for postmenopausal women receiving steroid therapy; not necessary if ACTH is being used. 1.25–2.50 mg conjugated estrogens equine (Premarin) may be given "cyclically."
Oxandrolone (Anavar), 10–20 mg daily in divided doses.
7 "Alternate-day" steroid schedule if possible; if not, a single morning total-steroid dosage; in all instances use an "intermediate-acting" steroid preparation if possible (Table 93-10).
8 Patients maintained on steroid therapy over a prolonged period should be protected by an appropriate increase in hormone level during periods of acute stress. A rule of thumb is to *double* the maintenance dose.

dose for 48 h as a *single* dose, of *intermediate-acting steroid* in the morning, *every other day!* If symptoms of the underlying disorder can be controlled by this technique, the physician can be assured that the therapeutic program is offering a distinct advantage to the patient. Three special considerations deserve mention. (1) The alternate-day schedule may be approached through a series of transition dose schedules which permit the patient an opportunity to adjust more successfully to the ultimate program. (2) The physician should make a conscientious effort to provide the patient with supplementary nonsteroid medications, if required, on the "off day" to minimize symptoms of the underlying disorder. (3) The physician and the patient should recognize that many of the symptoms which may be noted during the off day are really those of relative adrenal insufficiency, rather than an exacerbation of his underlying disease. Fatigue, joint pain, muscle stiffness or tenderness, and even fever, can be accounted for by the rapid fall in plasma cortisol level. Knowing this is of vital importance, since the physician can reassure the patient and will avoid giving up the program on the basis of a misconception.

The alternate-day concept capitalizes on the fact that normally cortisol secretion and plasma levels are highest in the early morning and lowest in the evening. The normal pattern is mimicked by administering steroid in the morning (7 to 8 A.M.), and preferably an intermediate-acting steroid, i.e., one whose hypothalamic-pituitary-suppressing effect lasts less than 1½ days (Table 93-10).

Initially the steroid program will usually require daily or more frequent doses of steroid in order to accomplish the desired anti-inflammatory or immunity-suppressing action. *Only after this desired effect has been achieved is an attempt made to switch over to an alternate-day program!* There are a number of programs which may be employed for transferring a patient from a daily to an alternate-day program. The key points to be considered are flexibility in arranging a program, and the use of supportive measures on the off day. One may attempt a transition by a series of gradations (Table 93-13), rather than by an abrupt complete changeover. In either case it is important to anticipate that the patient will experience some increase in pain or discomfort between the 36 to 48 h following the last dose of steroid.

The general principles advocated in the long-term use of steroids and in implementing an alternate-day schedule are as follows:

1 Utilize intermediate-acting steroids such as prednisone or prednisolone.
2 As soon as possible give the total daily steroid dose as a single morning dose.
3 Begin a transition program just as soon as the clinical manifestations of the diseases are under reasonable control.
4 If possible, ultimately eliminate entirely steroid medication on the alternate day.

WITHDRAWAL OF CORTICOSTEROIDS FOLLOWING THEIR LONG-TERM USE AS PHARMACOLOGIC AGENTS Complete withdrawal of steroids should not be contemplated until an Addisonian or normal replacement dosage has been reached, e.g., equivalent of 25.0 to 37.5 mg cortisone daily or 5.0 to 7.5 mg prednisone. Patients on an alternate-day program for a month or more will experience little difficulty as far as pituitary adrenal function is concerned when the dosage is gradually reduced and finally discontinued. Complications rarely ensue unless undue stress is experienced, and patients should understand that for 1 year or longer, after the complete withdrawal from long-term high-dosage steroid therapy, they should receive supplementary hormone in the presence of serious infection, operation, or injury.

If a patient in the final stage of steroid reduction cannot tolerate an alternate-day program, it is debatable as to whether complete discontinuance should be considered. Under these circumstances a daily dose of steroid could be continued, and at some future date another trial of gradual transition to the alternate-day schedule should be attempted. In patients with life-threatening disorders such as disseminated lupus erythematosus, or widespread skin disorders in which exfoliative dermatitis may complicate complete withdrawal of steroids, it may be desirable to consider life-long maintenance therapy at an Addisonian replacement dosage. These patients will not require mineralocorticoid therapy, as aldosterone secretion, in the absence of severe stress, is usually adequate.

TABLE 93-13
An outline of a schedule to taper patients off pharmacologic doses of glucocorticoids

Day	*Prednisone, mg*	*Day*	*Prednisone, mg*
1	60	13	90
2	40	14	5
3	70	15	90
4	30	16	0
5	80	17	85
6	20	18	0
7	90	19	85
8	10	20	0
9	95	21	85
10	5	22	0
11	90	23	80
12	5	24	0

REFERENCES

AZARNOFF DL: Symposium on steroid therapy. Med Clin North Am 57:1153, 1973

BENNETT AH et al: Twenty years experience in the surgical treatment of adrenocortical hyperplasia. Am Assoc Genito-Urinary Surgeons 64:90, 1972

BIGLIERI EG et al: Adrenal mineralocorticoids causing hypertension. Am J Med 52:623, 1972

BLIZZARD RM et al: Adrenal antibodies in Addison's disease. Lancet II:901, 1972

CAIN JP et al: The regulation of aldosterone secretion in primary aldosteronism. Am J Med 53:627, 1972

DAVIS WW et al: Bilateral adrenal hyperplasia as a cause of primary aldosteronism with hypertension, hypokalemia and suppressed renin activity. Am J Med 42:642, 1967

DLUHY RG et al: Rapid ACTH test with plasma aldosterone levels. Ann Intern Med 80:693, 1974

GRABER A et al: Natural history of pituitary adrenal recovery following long-term suppression with corticosteroid. Trans Assoc Am Physicians 77:296, 1964

LIEBERMAN LM et al: Diagnosis of adrenal disease by visualization of human adrenal glands with ^{131}I-19-iodocholesterol. N Engl J Med 285:1387, 1971

LUBITZ JA et al: Mitotane use in inoperable adrenal cortical carcinoma. JAMA 223:1109, 1973

ORTH DN, LIDDLE GW: Results of treatment in 108 patients with Cushing's syndrome. N Engl J Med 285:243, 1971

SCHAMBELAN M et al: Isolated hypoaldosteronism in adults. A renin deficiency syndrome. N Engl J Med 287:573, 1972

WILLIAMS GH, DLUHY RG: Aldosterone biosynthesis: interrelationship of regulatory factors. Am J Med 53:595, 1972

94 PHEOCHROMOCYTOMA

ROGER B. HICKLER
GEORGE W. THORN

The first pheochromocytoma was described by Frankel in 1886, and this name for the tumor was subsequently designed by Pick to describe its selective coloring by chromium salts. The syndrome of paroxysmal hypertension due to a pheochromocytoma was first clearly described by Labbe, Tinel, and Coumier in 1922. In 1926 Roux and in 1927 Mayo performed the first successful surgical removals of the tumor. In 1936 Beer, King, and Prinzmetal determined that the characteristic paroxysmal rise in blood pressure was associated with the release of hormone from the tumor into the blood. *Persistent* hypertension was first attributed to the tumor in the same year by Kremer.

INCIDENCE It is a rare disorder, but the frequency of its antemortem detection has increased progressively owing to improved diagnostic techniques. Anatomic statistics from the Mayo Clinic showed 15 of these tumors in 15,984 autopsies, an overall frequency of 0.1 percent. Smithwick estimated the frequency in a hypertensive population explored for sympathectomy to be 0.5 percent.

ANATOMY Embryologically two cell types differentiate from a common stem cell, the sympathogonia of the primitive neuroectoderm, to form the adrenal medulla: the chromaffinoblast and the neuroblast, which mature into the chromaffin cell and the sympathetic ganglion cell, respectively. These medullary cells are richly supplied with preganglionic fibers from the splanchnic nerves.

The chromaffin cell is so named because of its capacity to show brown intracytoplasmic granules on treatment with chromium salts, a result of oxidation and polymerization of the catecholamine stored in the granules. Chromaffin cells are found in widely dispersed sites at birth: the adrenal medulla, the paraganglia (along the retropleural and retroperitoneal sympathetic chains), the organs of Zuckerkandl (paired structures lying anterior to the bifurcation of the abdominal aorta), chemoreceptor areas ("glomic tissue" at the carotid bifurcation, along the aortic arch, and at the jugular bulb), and the human dermis. Many of the extraadrenal sites undergo progressive involution until puberty, but remnants account for the extraadrenal occurrences of pheochromocytomas, reported in all the areas cited with the exception of the skin.

PATHOLOGY Over 50 percent of pheochromocytomas occur in the region of the adrenals, sometimes bilaterally, and over 90 percent lie between the diaphragm and pelvic floor. As indicated by metastases, 6 percent are malignant, and 7 percent occur simultaneously in more than one focus. Metastases may be functional and have occurred in liver, lungs, and central skeleton, as well as paraaortic lymph glands. The tumor weight may vary from a gram to several thousand grams (averaging about 100) and correlates poorly with the severity of the symptomatology. The tumors are round, frequently lobulated, and highly vascular. They may show hemorrhagic and necrotic areas with cystic degeneration, particularly in large tumors. On section they appear brown or gray. Histologically they resemble the adrenal medulla; the nuclei are often multiple, cytoplasmic vacuolization is common, and dark staining with chromium salts is characteristic. Benign tumors may invade the capsule and are difficult if not impossible to distinguish from malignant forms on purely histologic grounds. Individual tumor cells usually contain both epinephrine and norepinephrine storage granules. After glutaraldehyde fixation, electron microscopic analysis shows the epinephrine granules as the gray core of round vesicles and the norepinephrine as the black core of oval vesicles. Cells from predominantly epinephrine-secreting tumors show mainly the former and norepinephrine-secreting tumors the latter, the concentration of each correlating with its granular density. There is no ultrastructural distinction between tumors from patients with differing symptoms, e.g., sustained versus paroxysmal hypertension, or a high versus a low rate of catecholamine turnover. There are rare but well-documented case reports of unilateral and bilateral adrenomedullary hyperplasia producing the clinical features of pheochromocytoma.

PHYSIOLOGY The sympathetic nerve terminals and the chromaffin cells of the adrenal medulla and pheochromocytomas synthesize norepinephrine according to the following enzymatic steps: hydroxylation of tyrosine to form dopa (3,4-dihydroxyphenylalanine), decarboxylation of dopa to form dopamine (3,4-dihydroxyphenylethylamine), the latter entering storage vesicles to undergo beta oxidation to form norepinephrine (Fig. 94-1). In the adrenal medulla and most pheochromocytomas a proportion of the norepinephrine undergoes N-methylation to form epinephrine. In the brain, dopamine as well as norepinephrine is stored, both serving as catecholamine neurotransmitters. Epinephrine is the major hormone of the adrenal medulla, constituting 80 percent of its stored content of catecholamine; the major source of norepinephrine is the postganglionic sympathetic neuron, where it acts as the neurotransmitter.

Adrenomedullary and presumably pheochromocytoma catecholamines are released in the process of *exocytosis*, the storage vesicle discharging its entire soluble contents (catecholamines, specific proteins such as dopamine-β-hydroxylase, and ATP) through the cell membrane (Fig. 94-2). However, in pheochromocytomas there is a dissociation between catecholamine and dopamine-β-hydroxylase secretion, probably reflecting an abnormal release mechanism. In the adrenal medulla this release is in response to cholinergic preganglionic sympathetic nerve stimulation and requires calcium ion. A number of agents can directly stimulate chromaffin cells or the adrenergic neurons to release catecholamines; these agents include acetylcholine, nicotine, histamine, 5-hydroxytryptamine, tyramine, and reserpine. An increase in the release of both epinephrine and norepinephrine is caused by a number of physiologic stimuli such as severe muscular work, asphyxia and hypoxia, and hemorrhagic hypotension. Insulin hypoglycemia causes a selective release of epinephrine alone, favoring the concept of separate control of the release of adrenomedullary epinephrine and norepinephrine.

The physiologic effects of the adrenomedullary hormones may be characterized as preparing the organism to meet an emergency situation. Both epinephrine and norepinephrine have a comparable direct beta-adrenergic (inotropic and chronotropic) cardiac effect. However, the predominant alpha-adrenergic (vasoconstrictor) peripheral effect of circulating norepinephrine results in diastolic and systolic hypertension, producing reflex slowing of the heart, so that cardiac output is generally unchanged or reduced. The net peripheral vasodilator (beta-adrenergic) ef-

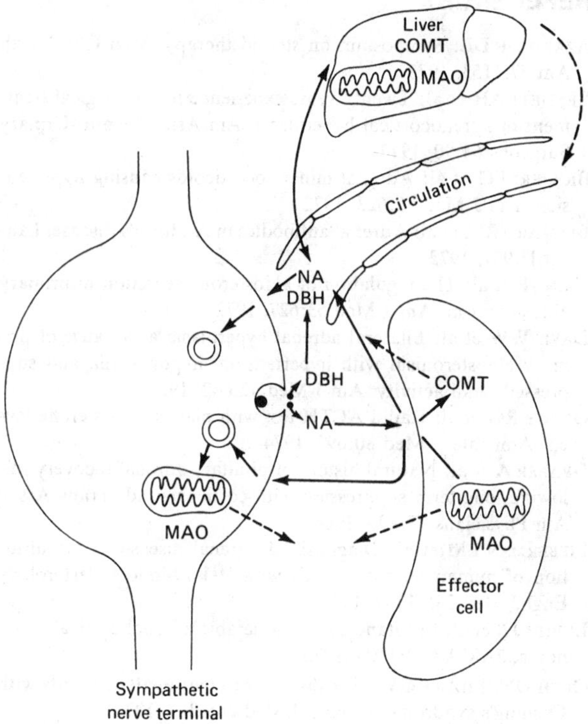

FIGURE 94-2

Fate of norepinephrine at a varicosity of the sympathetic nerve terminal. Norepinephrine (NA) is stored in dense core vesicles together with the norepinephrine-forming enzyme dopamine β-hydroxylase (DBH). When the nerve is depolarized, the vesicle discharges norepinephrine and the soluble portion of dopamine β-hydroxylase into the synaptic cleft, by a process of exocytosis. Norepinephrine acts at the effector cell, and its actions are terminated by reuptake into the neuron, removal by circulation, and subsequent metabolism in the liver or by metabolism in the effector cell by catechol O-methyltransferase (COMT) and mitochondrial monoamine oxidase (MAO). Norepinephrine that leaks out of the vesicle is inactivated by intraneuronal monoamine oxidase. (By permission, from J Axelrod and R Weinshilboum: Physiology in medicine: Catecholamines. N Engl J Med 287: 238, 1972)

FIGURE 94-1

Biosynthesis of norepinephrine in the sympathetic neuron. NA, noradrenaline (norepinephrine); dopa, dihydroxyphenylalanine; MAO, monoamine oxidase. (Adapted from J Axelrod and IJ Kopin, The uptake, storage, release and metabolism of noradrenaline in sympathetic nerves. Prog Brain Res 31:21, 1969. By permission, from J Axelrod and R Weinshilboum: Physiology in medicine: Catecholamines. N Engl J Med 287:238, 1972)

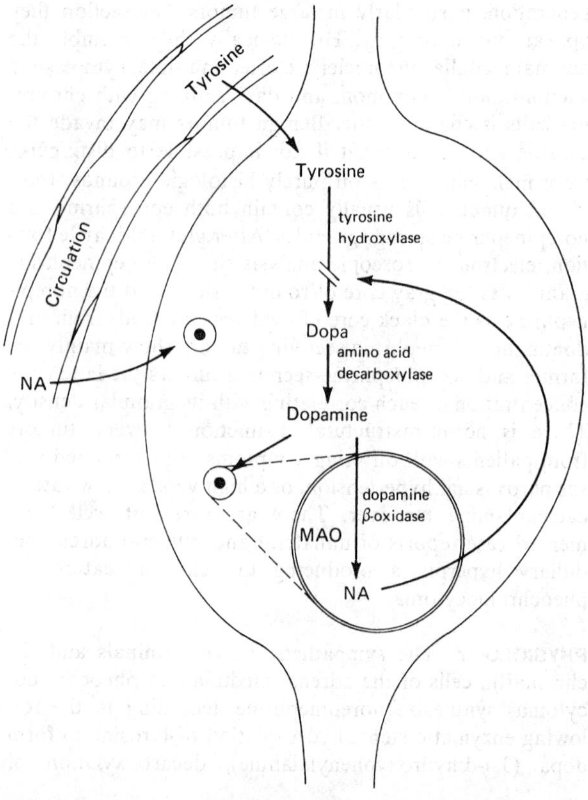

fect of physiological doses of epinephrine (due primarily to vasodilatation of the resistance vessels of skeletal muscle), associated with its beta-adrenergic cardiac effects, produces a rise in cardiac output, with widening of pulse pressure through a rise in systolic pressure; diastolic pressure may fall slightly. Cutaneous and renal vasoconstriction is common to both hormones. Both increase the rate and depth of respiration and stimulate the release into plasma of nonesterified fatty acids from neutral fat depots. Another metabolic effect of epinephrine (and of norepinephrine in large doses), leading to an increased oxygen consumption and respiratory quotient, is the activation of hepatic and skeletal muscle phosphorylase by stimulating adenyl cyclase to increase the formation of cyclic AMP from ATP. This produces an accelerated glycogenolysis. The hepatic release of glucose 1-phosphate elevates blood glucose, and the release of glucose 6-phosphate from muscle elevates blood lactic acid.

CATECHOLAMINE METABOLISM Figure 94-2 shows the metabolic paths of norepinephrine derived from sympathetic nerve endings. The corresponding molecular transformation of released catecholamines of neural and adrenomedullary origin is detailed in Fig. 94-3. The major portion of neurally released norepinephrine is restored in neuronal vesicles in an economical process called "reuptake." Catecholamines released by the adrenal medulla (and pheochromocytomas) and part of the neurally released norepinephrine circulate to the liver. Hepatic catechol O-methyltransferase (COMT) inactivates the catecholamines by converting norepinephrine to normetanephrine and epinephrine to metanephrine. The subsequent action of hepatic monamine oxidase (MAO) converts both these compounds into vanillylmandelic acid and 3-methoxy-4-hydroxyphenylglycol. The latter are the major urinary metabolites, although the metanephrines (normetanephrine and metanephrine) and unmodified catecholamine are also excreted. The effector cell also contains COMT and MAO, contributing to the pool of these inactive methoxylated metabolites of norepinephrine of neural origin. Finally, neuronal monamine oxidase inactivates excess norepinephrine that is outside the storage vesicles, contributing to the circulating pool of metabolites. The concentration of the metanephrines in pheochromocy-

FIGURE 94-3
Metabolism of free catecholamines. Urinary excretion products appear on the lowest line. Excretion products may be conjugated with glucuronide or sulfate. COMT, catechol O-methyltransferase; VMA, 3-methoxy-4-hydroxymandelic acid; MHPG, methoxyhydroxyphenylglycol; MAO, monoamine oxidase. (By permission, from FH Myers et al: Review of Medical Pharmacology, Los Altos, Calif.: Lange, 1971, p. 81)

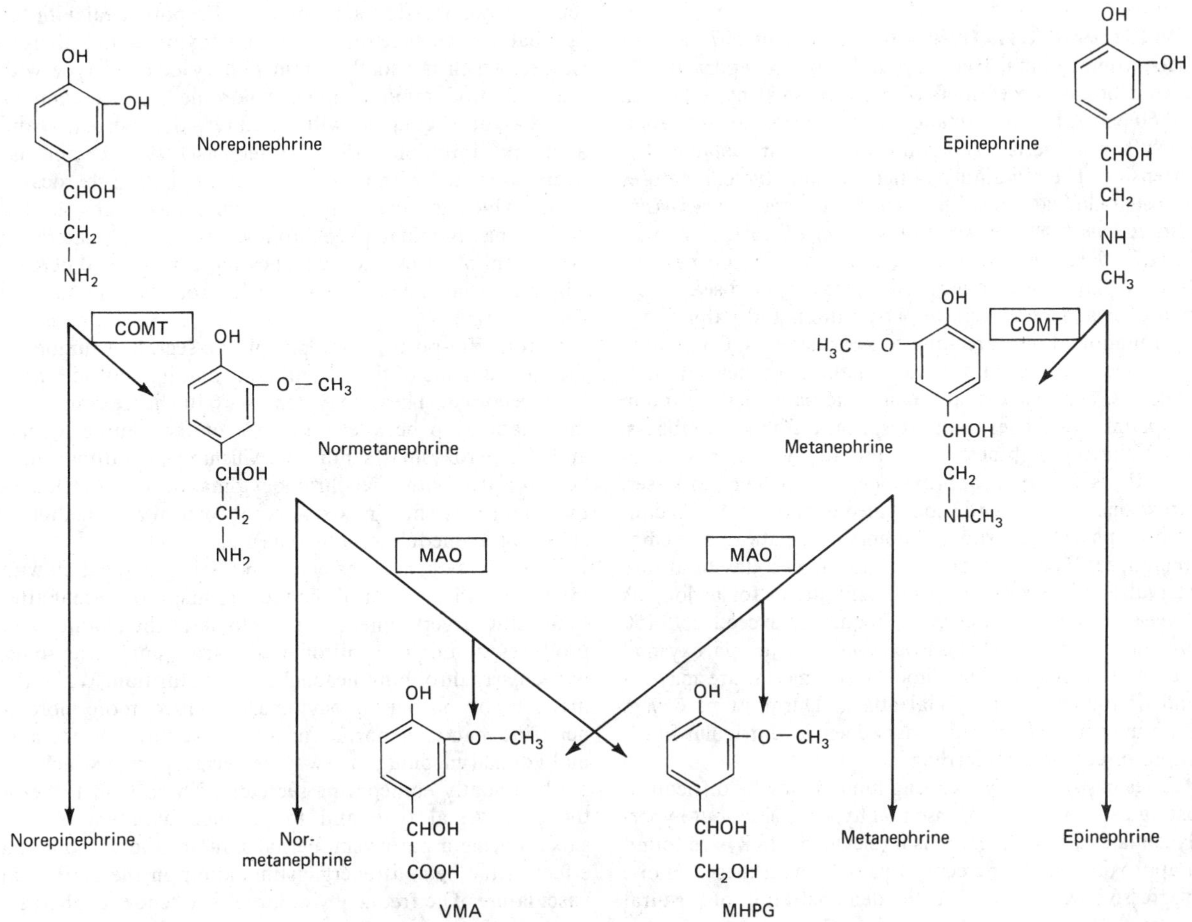

tomas tends to be low, and constant over a wide range of active catecholamine concentration. This suggests that the rate of hormone turnover by the tumor is not modulated by variations in its content of catecholamine-metabolizing enzymes. Bilateral adrenalectomy results in only a minor depression of urinary catecholamines, since 80 percent is normally norepinephrine, largely derived from sympathetic nerve endings. The high activity of these two enzyme systems (MAO and COMT) is indicated by the fact that the daily urinary content, by weight, of the metanephrines (after hydrolyzing the major conjugated fraction free of its glucuronide or sulfate) is approximately seven times, and of vanillylmandelic acid (VMA) approximately thirty times, that of the total catecholamines. Half of the catecholamine is in the "free" form, and half is found as glucuronide or sulfate conjugates.

Increased sympathetic tone increases catecholamine synthesis and turnover, the rate-limiting step being the conversion of tyrosine to dopa by tyrosine hydroxylase. Tissue levels of catecholamines are kept fairly constant, since tyrosine hydroxylase is stimulated by low and inhibited by high catecholamine concentrations. Increased sympathetic nerve activity augments the activity of tyrosine hydroxylase and dopamine β-hydroxylase (Fig. 94-1), both of which enzymes require adrenocorticotropic hormone for functional integrity. Glucocorticoid activity has a potent stimulating effect on the adrenomedullary conversion of norepinephrine to epinephrine by phenylethanolamine-N-methyltransferase.

CLINICAL MANIFESTATIONS In a review of 507 cases of pheochromocytoma, Hermann and Mornex report that 26 percent of cases presented with paroxysmal hypertension and 60 percent with permanent hypertension; of the latter, nearly half had crises superimposed on their sustained hypertension. The remaining 14 percent had atypical features or absent clinical signs. Thus, *the characteristic hypertensive crisis is found in only about one-half of all cases.* Thomas, Rook, and Kvale reviewed the symptoms in 100 patients with the paroxysmal hypertensive form of the disease. The triad of headache, excessive perspiration, and palpitations was found in about three-quarters of instances. Commonly associated manifestations were pallor, nausea, tremor, weakness, nervousness, and epigastric pain. Less common complaints were chest pain, dyspnea, flushing, numbness, visual blurring, tightness of the throat, and dizziness. Bradycardia is found in approximately 20 percent of cases. Paroxysms are frequently spontaneous but may be precipitated by physical exertion, abdominal palpation, and emotional upset. They may occur several times a day or at rare intervals, and may last for only a minute or for as long as a week. Blood pressure levels frequently exceed 250/150 mm during an attack in association with the paroxysmal release of catecholamine. Shock and renal failure may attend or follow a paroxysmal attack. During a paroxysm death may occur from pulmonary edema, ventricular fibrillation, or cerebral hemorrhage.

Cases of *persistently* secreting tumors may be difficult to distinguish from cases of essential hypertension, but hyperglycemia and hypermetabolism (elevated BMR) are found in approximately 50 percent of patients with these tumors. Progressive weight loss and the demonstration of postural hypotension are further suggestive clinical evidence of sustained catecholamine secretion by a tumor. Frank retinopathy (grades 3 to 4 funduscopic changes) is found in more than half of these patients, an appreciably higher incidence than is found in the purely paroxysmal variety. This underscores the gravity of this form of hypertension and the importance of early clinical detection. Notable clinical features of the disorder that have been reported include intermittent claudication associated with tissue necrosis in the presence of palpable pulses, extensive necrosis of the tumor leading to shock, and a paralytic ileus that is frequently fatal associated with massive catecholamine discharge. Renal artery compression has been caused by the tumor. Renal ischemia as a complication of surgical resection of a pheochromocytoma may develop and account for a recurrence of hypertension.

Transient cortical blindness and other transient neurologic deficits have been observed during a hypertensive crisis from pheochromocytomas.

Special features Several unique aspects of the disease deserve emphasis. The tumor may first appear in early childhood or old age, but the average age of onset is during the fourth decade. In childhood pheochromocytoma, the hypertension is almost always of the sustained variety, and the tumor is bilateral in 20 percent of cases and shows a higher incidence of malignancy than in the adult. Distinct genetic factors are implicated in some instances by the prevalence of the tumor in certain families, sometimes in association with other congenital disorders of the neuroectoderm such as neurofibromatosis and central nervous system hemangioblastoma. A number of reports deal with the familial coincidence of pheochromocytoma and thyroid cancer, which is usually the medullary or solid type with amyloid production ("sipple syndrome"). This complex also has been coupled with parathyroid hyperplasia and adenomas (multiple endocrine neoplasia, type 2), and has been associated with a high level of circulating thyrocalcitonin, which is invariably found with medullary thyroid carcinoma. Familial pheochromocytomas are bilateral in 40 percent of cases, the frequency increasing to 70 percent when associated with medullary thyroid carcinoma (see Chap. 354).

Chromaffin-positive norepinephrine-secreting tumors of the glomic tissue of the carotid body and jugular bulb have been reported. These may represent further examples of the relationship between dysplasia of the neuroectoderm and the paroxysmal syndrome. Cushing's syndrome may be associated with pheochromocytoma, in which instances the tumor may show mixed adrenal cortical and medullary cells (corticomedullary adenoma).

True polycythemia has been reported in association with the tumor, with return of the red cell mass to normal after successful surgery. Pheochromocytoma of the bladder wall produces a unique syndrome of paroxysmal symptoms, particularly throbbing headache, or micturition. While the majority of pheochromocytomas produce more norepinephrine than epinephrine (in contradistinction to the normal adrenal medulla), a few have been reported which are predominantly epinephrine secretors. These tend to be of the paroxysmal type and to produce hypotension and shock during a paroxysm, perhaps due to the vasodilating effect of the beta-adrenergic stimulation on the peripheral vasculature. The frequency of a diabetic tendency increases with the ratio of the epinephrine to the total catecholamine content of the tumor, perhaps because of the greater glycogenolytic activity of epinephrine. However, impaired carbohydrate tolerance has been found in pure norepinephrine secretors, and recent evidence indicates that the associated excessive alpha-adrenergic stimulation will inhibit insulin release to account for the impairment.

Over 50 percent of patients dying with a pheochromocytoma have an active myocarditis at autopsy. In the majority of these instances there was prior clinical evidence of left ventricular failure. In all probability this is a direct, "toxic" effect of the high levels of catecholamines on the myocardium.

Finally, a hypertensive response to smoking, to anesthesia, or to therapy with ganglionic blocking agents and guanethidine should raise the strong suspicion of a pheochromocytoma. Complete absence of symptoms and cardiovascular findings has been reported in a patient with an actively secreting pheochromocytoma.

DIAGNOSIS The clinical picture of essential hypertension with marked vasomotor lability strongly suggests pheochromocytoma, but pheochromocytoma with sustained hypertension in the absence of paroxysms may be indistinguishable from essential hypertension. Thus, routine laboratory screening of all patients with significant hypertension is desirable for this potentially curable form of hypertension.

Urinary assay for catecholamines and their methoxy derivatives Modern chemical methods for the determination of 24-h urinary catecholamines and their methoxy derivatives have largely replaced the older pharmacologic tests in routine screening because of their safety and greater accuracy. Current chemical methods for determining urinary free catecholamines involve modifications of the trihydroxyindole (THI) method of Lund. The urinary free catecholamines are adsorbed on an alumina or resin column, eluted with acid, oxidized to form "chromes," which, in turn, are tautomerized in alkali to form strongly fluorescent trihydroxyindoles. Free epinephrine and norepinephrine may be measured separately from fluorometric readings at different wavelengths. After acid hydrolysis to free the conjugated fractions, metanephrine (MN) and normetanephrine (NMN) may be isolated on resin and converted to trihydroxyindoles for fluorometric assay or oxidized to vanillin and read photometrically. VMA is measured by isolation and oxidation to vanillin, which may be read photometrically directly or after color development with added indole.

With these techniques Sjoerdsma and associates determined, simultaneously, the 24-h urinary free catecholamines, metanephrines, and vanillylmandelic acid on 64 patients with proved pheochromocytoma. The results are shown in Fig. 94-4 and indicate that the values obtained for all three assays were above the upper limit of normal in all but a few instances, giving an overall diagnostic reliability in the range of 90 percent. The upper limits of normal are (1) free catecholamines (epinephrine plus norepinephrine), 100 μg; (2) metanephrine plus normetanephrine, 1.3 mg; (3) VMA, 6.5 mg. Therapy with alphamethyldopa will produce false elevation in the free catecholamines and, potentially, in the metanephrines. Monoamine oxidase inhibitors increase the metanephrine and decrease the VMA urinary excretion. With methods that convert VMA to vanillin, dietary considerations may be disregarded in the determination of urinary VMA, but nonspecific chromatographic screening methods should be avoided. In general, *it is important to discontinue sympathomimetic agents and monamine oxidase inhibitors when performing these assays.* The relative diagnostic merits of the three different indexes are debated, and it is probable that any one of them, carefully done, will serve as well as another.

The reliable measurement of plasma catecholamine levels requires highly sophisticated methodology and is not a practical approach. However, using an enzymatic double-labeled isotope assay, Engelman, Portnoy, and Sjoerdsma found the mean plasma catecholamine level in 10 patients with pheochromocytoma to be 5.0 μg per liter as compared with a mean of 0.24 μg per liter in 32 normal patients, with no overlap.

Pharmacologic tests for pheochromocytoma In the absence of facilities for these chemical determinations, reliance may be placed on the various intravenous pharmacologic tests. Along with the phentolamine (Regitine) test, which produces a precipitous fall in blood pressure in pheochromocytomas, there are now in use three "provocative" tests: the older histamine and the newer tyramine and glucagon tests. Unfortunately, deaths have occurred after both phentolamine and histamine in pheochromocytomas, and the pharmacologic approach probably fails to detect as many as 25 percent of cases. The matter is further complicated by the prevalence of false positive responses with these agents. This occurs frequently with phentolamine, occasionally with histamine (up to 11 percent) and tyramine (3 percent), and rarely, if at all, with glucagon. Other advantages of glucagon administration over histamine provocation are the absence of significant side effects, fewer false negative responses, and probable greater safety. The intravenous tyramine test has a higher incidence of false negatives in patients with *familial* pheochromocytoma than in sporadic cases. It has the advantage over histamine and glucagon of causing a milder rise in blood pressure in the presence of a pheochromocytoma, but, by the same token, the end point of a positive reaction is less succinct. It is strongly contraindicated in any patient receiving amine oxidase inhibitor therapy, where the administration of tyramine may precipitate a hypertensive crisis. Histamine and probably glucagon should not be used if the control pressure is 170/110 mm or above, and phentolamine should be ready for immediate administration in the advent of a precipitous rise in blood pressure when these tests are performed. With pressures in the range of 170/110 mm or above, the tyramine and phentolamine tests are the ones of choice.

In a small percentage of patients, particularly during a normotensive period in those with intermittently secreting tumors, 24-h urinary assay for catecholamines (or derivatives thereof) may not be clearly elevated into a diagnostic range. If suspicion is still strong on clinical grounds, the tumor may be provoked to secrete with 0.01 to 0.025 mg histamine base, given intravenously. This should be followed by the rapid injection of 5 mg phentolamine intravenously, should an alarming rise in blood pressure ensue. Blood may be drawn during the control period and at intervals of 2 min in the immediate posthistamine period for plasma assay for catecholamines, or a timed urine specimen (after prior emptying of the bladder) may be collected for a period of 6 h for analysis for catecholamines or methoxy derivatives, which may be expressed as amount excreted per milligram of creatinine.

The upper limit of normal for plasma epinephrine and norepinephrine varies with the method employed and must be established in a given laboratory to determine a diagnostic rise following histamine administration. The upper limit of normal for urinary catecholamines (epinephrine plus norepinephrine) is 0.05 μg per mg creatinine; for metanephrine plus normetanephrine, it is 2.1 μg per mg creatinine; for VMA, it is 9.5 μg per mg creatinine. Levels above these following histamine administration are diagnostic. If a spontaneous attack should occur while a patient is under observation, blood and urinary determinations should be made immediately. The plasma ethylenediamine condensation method for plasma catecholamines is invalid in the presence of uremia.

Localization of tumor While rarely palpable, a tumor mass may be detected on a plain film of the abdomen. A more specialized technique is an intravenous pyelogram with laminography, detecting *adrenal* pheochromocytomas in approximately 50 percent of cases. Another is abdominal filming of the contrast afforded by the presacral injection of carbon dioxide or nitrous oxide, which may detect relatively small tumors. However, variations in the suprarenal fat accumulation may render interpretation difficult. The advent of selective renal and adrenal angiography has afforded superb information in this regard; in some hands, these radiologic procedures are proving to be the ones of choice. Selective retrograde adrenal venography is the most sensitive approach, detecting tumors as small as 1 cm in diameter. The hazards attending these contrast techniques (including the potential for direct tumor stimulation) are apparent, and phentolamine should be ready for immediate administration during their performance. The analysis of catecholamines in plasma obtained by catheter at different levels in the venous system under fluoroscopic control has also been useful. Thoracic tumors, while rare, may be seen on a plain chest film. Overexposure of the film enhances the chance of visualizing posterior masses along the sympathetic chains.

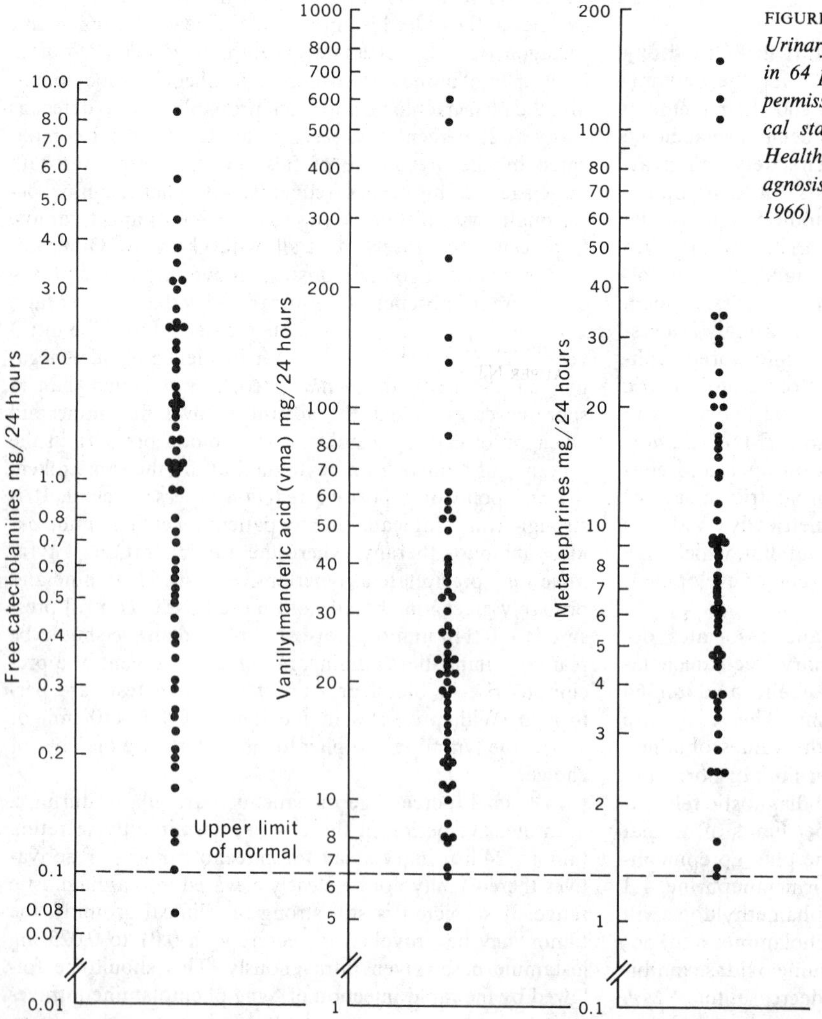

FIGURE 94-4
Urinary excretion of catecholamines and metabolites in 64 patients with proved pheochromocytoma. (By permission, from A Sjoerdsma et al: Combined clinical staff conference at the National Institutes of Health. Pheochromocytoma: Current concepts of diagnosis and treatment. Ann Intern Med 65:1306, 1966)

Crout and Sjoerdsma report that the separate determination of urinary epinephrine and norepinephrine is of predictive value in tumor localization. If there is a significant elevation of epinephrine as well as norepinephrine (42 percent of all cases), the tumor may be expected to lie in or adjacent to one of the adrenal glands or, rarely, in the organs of Zuckerkandl. If the urine contains elevated norepinephrine alone (58 percent of all cases), the tumor, of course, may still be found in one of the adrenal areas. Less than 10 percent of tumors are extraabdominal, and these will generally show only an elevation of urinary norepinephrine and probably reflect a deficiency of N-methylating enzyme, present in the normal adrenal medulla and necessary for the conversion of norepinephrine into epinephrine.

DIFFERENTIAL DIAGNOSIS False positive responses with pharmacologic testing and elevations in urinary levels of catecholamines and derivatives due to interfering substances and laboratory errors have led to unnecessary surgical exploration in many hypertensive patients. This problem is compounded by the elevated plasma levels (or excretion) of catecholamines frequently identifiable in essential hypertension, and in hypertension associated with such states as Guillain-Barré syndrome and intracranial tumors in the region of the posterior hypothalamus and medulla oblongata. Incorrect diagnoses in the presence of a pheochromocytoma have included diabetes mellitus, thyrotoxicosis, anxiety neurosis, "vascular" headache, epilepsy, and hypertensive crises due to lead poisoning and porphyria. A syndrome resembling pheochromocytoma following a stroke, including elevated VMA and catecholamine excretion, has been reported. Caution is recommended in making the diagnosis within several months of a cerebrovascular accident.

Patients with "nonchromaffin" sympathetic tumors, i.e., ganglioneuromas and, particularly, neuroblastomas, have shown elevated levels of norepinephrine in the urine as well as increased excretion of its precursors (dopa and dopamine) and of its methoxy metabolites (metanephrines and VMA). Since some of these patients have associated hypertension, these tumors are to be distinguished from true "chromaffinomas." Serum dopamine β-hydroxylase activity has been found to be elevated in over 50 percent of patients with neuroblastoma and may prove useful in the diagnosis of this disorder.

TREATMENT In patients in whom surgical resection of the tumor cannot be performed, as with functioning metastases, the regular oral administration of the alpha-adrenergic blocking agent phenoxybenzamine (Dibenzyline) has been reported to have controlled most of the disturbing signs and symptoms for a period of many months. This approach has also been recommended routinely for a period of several weeks in order to get patients into an optimum condition in preparation for surgery, as in the presence of malignant hypertension with congestive heart failure. The use of beta-adrenergic blockers, such as propranolol, may also be useful in protecting against beta-adrenergic-mediated cardiac arrhythmias from high circulating levels of catecholamines. An alpha-blocking agent must be used first to obviate the danger of greater hypertension from blocking the vasodilator effect of a predominantly epinephrine-secreting tumor. The use of inhibitors of catecholamine synthesis is another approach to the pharmacologic treatment and preoperative control of patients with pheochromocytoma; preliminary reports of the use of alpha-methyl-paratyrosine in this regard are very encouraging.

Surgical removal of the tumor is the treatment of choice for this potentially lethal disease. Since over 90 percent of all such tumors are located in the abdomen, a careful abdominal incision may be undertaken, even without the certain exclusion of a rare extraabdominal site. Halothane and fluroxene have been recommended as anesthetic agents of choice because of their relative lack of effect on stimulating sympathoadrenal activity, in contradistinction to ether and cyclopropane. To avoid extremes of hypertension during induction of anesthesia and surgical manipulation, an intravenous drip of phentolamine should be ready at all times. To avoid extremes of hypotension on clamping the blood supply of the tumor and following its removal, an intravenous drip of norepinephrine or other pressor amine should also be prepared in advance. *Administration of whole blood or plasma on removal of the tumor may be of paramount importance in preventing postoperative shock,* since the sudden relief of the prolonged vasoconstriction attending the disease produces a state of disparity between the vascular capacity and effective blood volume.

REFERENCES

Axelrod J, Weinshilboum R: Physiology in medicine: catecholamines. N Engl J Med 287:237, 1972

Carney JR et al: Bilateral adrenal medullary hyperplasia in multiple endocrine neoplasia, type 2: The precursor of bilateral pheochromocytoma. Mayo Clin Proc 50:3, 1975

Hermann H, Mornex R: *Human Tumours Secreting Catecholamines: Clinical and Physiopathological Study of the Pheochromocytomas,* New York: Pergamon Press, 1964

Himathongkam T et al: Medical emergency management—Pheochromocytoma. JAMA 230:1692, 1974

Lauper NT et al: Pheochromocytoma: Fine structural, biochemical and clinical observations. Am J Cardiol 30:197, 1972

Marks A, Channick B: Extra-adrenal pheochromocytoma and medullary thyroid carcinoma with pheochromocytoma. Arch Intern Med 134:1106, 1974

Miller S et al: Parathyroid function in patients with pheochromocytoma. Ann Intern Med 82:372, 1975

Radtke W et al: Cardiovascular complications of pheochromocytoma crisis. Am J Cardiol 35:701, 1975

Thomas JD et al: The neurologist's experience with pheochromocytoma: A review of 100 cases. JAMA 197:754, 1966

95
DIABETES MELLITUS

JURGEN STEINKE
J. STUART SOELDNER

Knowledge of diabetes is important because of its high prevalence. It has been estimated that there are 200 million diabetics in the world. After obesity and thyroid disorders, it is the third most common metabolic disorder. Diabetes consists of a metabolic and a vascular component, which are probably interrelated. The metabolic syndrome is characterized by an inappropriate elevation of blood glucose level, associated with alterations in lipid and protein metabolism, for which a relative or absolute lack of insulin is responsible. Its most severe manifestation is diabetic ketoacidosis. The vascular syndrome consists of accelerated nonspecific atherosclerosis (premature aging) and a more specific microangiopathy, particularly affecting the eye and kidney. Thus gangrene of the foot, arteriosclerotic heart disease, blindness, and uremia are the most frequent manifestations of the vascular syndrome. For this reason the long-term prognosis of severe diabetes is not bright, particularly if it is of juvenile-onset type. Statistically the diabetic is faced not only with a decrease in life expectancy but also with the ever-present possibility of disabling complications. Nevertheless, some patients with diabetes do very well for many decades.

HISTORY

Diabetes has been recognized from antiquity. Chinese medical writings mentioned a syndrome of polyphagia, polydipsia, and polyuria. Aretaeus (ca. A.D. 70) described the disease and, referring to the polyuria, gave it its name which comes from a Greek root meaning "To run through."

The study of the chemistry of diabetic urine was initiated by Paracelsus in the sixteenth century. Some 100 years later, Thomas Willis described the sweetness of the diabetic urine, "as if imbued with honey" ("mellitus"), which Dobson proved to be sugar. This led to a rational dietary approach, introduced by Rollo 29 years later. Morton (1686) noted the hereditary character of diabetes. In 1859, Claude Bernard demonstrated the increased glucose content of diabetic blood and recognized hyperglycemia as the cardinal sign of the disease. In 1869, Langerhans, still a medical student, described the islets in the pancreas, which now bear his name. Kussmaul characterized the air hunger and labored breathing of the patient in diabetic coma in 1874. The careful work by clinicians such as Bouchardat, Naunyn, von Noorden, Allen, and Joslin led to a significant therapeutic success with diet. Von Mering and Minkowski carried out their studies in 1889, demonstrating that dogs could be made diabetic by pancreatectomy. However, it took more than 30 years before Banting and Best were able to prepare an extract from dog pancreas capable of reducing an elevated blood glucose level. In 1939, the first long-acting insulin was introduced by Hagedorn. The chemical structure of ox insulin was established by Sanger in 1953; Nicol and Smith described the chemical structure of human insulin in 1960. The basic unit contains two polypeptide chains united by disulfide bridges. In 1964, Katsoyannis in the United States and Zahn in Germany completed the synthesis of both the A and B chains of insulin and were able to combine both chains into biologically active material. In 1967 Steiner described a large "proinsulin" molecule which exhibits only little biologic activity. It is converted by enzymatic cleavage into the smaller biologically active insulin (Fig. 95-1). The experimental work of Loubatieres in France and the accidental discovery of the hypoglycemic action of carbutamide by Franke and Fuchs in Germany, in 1955, initiated the use of oral hypoglycemic agents of the sulfonylurea type. Recently the long-term safety of these oral agents has been questioned.

FIGURE 95-1

Synthesis of insulin from the single-chain, biologically less active precursor, proinsulin. Proteolytic enzymes within the beta cell split off the connecting peptide portion of proinsulin, resulting in the formation of double-chain insulin proper. The A and B chains are bound by disulfide bridges. (Reproduced with permission of W. B. Saunders Company)

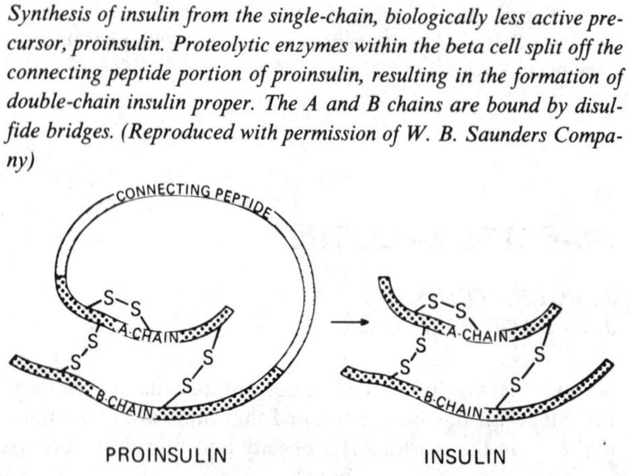

PREVALENCE

Diabetes mellitus is a disease of worldwide distribution. If it is more frequent in some countries than in others, that will have to be established when diagnostic criteria are agreed upon and uniformly controlled detection drives are executed. In the United States there are approximately 4.2 million persons with diabetes. Diabetes is more frequent in older people. The U.S. Public Health Service estimates that there are 1.3 diabetics for every 1,000 persons up to age seventeen, 17 between the ages of twenty-five and forty-four, 43 in the age group forty-five to sixty-four, and 79 over sixty-five years of age. Unless a cure or some preventive measure is found for diabetes, this number will continue to increase for the following reasons: (1) The population grows and becomes older; (2) the life expectancy of the treated diabetic is steadily increasing; (3) since more diabetics live long enough to have children, an increasing number of children will inherit the diabetic gene; (4) obesity, which appears to precipitate diabetes among those predisposed to it, is also on the rise, thus allowing more potential diabetics to emerge; and (5) diabetes detection drives are becoming widespread.

Undiagnosed adult diabetes with few or no symptoms presents a major challenge to the practicing physician. Because diabetic symptoms may be minimal, the patient does not seek medical advice. In the United States for every known diabetic, there probably exists one unknown diabetic. As it is not feasible to test the entire population, it is advisable to concentrate on those individuals with predisposition for the disease. They are (1) relatives of known diabetics, among whom diabetes is 2½ times more frequent than in the general population; (2) obese persons, since 85 percent of diabetic patients are, or were at one time, overweight; (3) persons in the older age groups, as four out of five diabetics are over forty-five; and (4) mothers delivered of large babies, since the birth of a large infant may be an indication of maternal potential diabetes.

Apart from these high-risk groups, routine testing for

diabetes should be performed whenever patients are admitted to a hospital for elective surgery or seen for an annual checkup. Furthermore, it would be desirable to include testing for diabetes in preemployment examinations.

INHERITANCE

It is well established that, in part, diabetes mellitus is inherited. The precise mode of inheritance is still under discussion. The acceptance of heredity for diabetes is based on the greater frequency of diabetes among blood relatives of known diabetics. The pattern of inheritance is characterized by (1) a more frequent occurrence in twin siblings of identical than nonidentical twins; and (2) the equilateral transmission of the trait by either affected parent (i.e., autosomal, non-sex-linked). However, genetic study is complicated by the fact that though susceptibility to diabetes is inherited, the disease itself may not become apparent clinically for years. Genetic studies are based on occurrence of clinical diabetes (phenotype), not on the presence of the genetic predisposition (genotype), for the latter cannot be detected at the present time. It is possible that the diabetic trait may be dominant and the manifest diabetic disease recessive. There is further confusion because diabetes is a syndrome; e.g., chronic pancreatitis may be associated with hyperglycemia indistinguishable from that observed in genetic diabetes. This could lead to false designation of a person as affected with genetic diabetes. Diabetes has a variable age of onset (juvenile-onset and maturity-onset), each with a characteristic clinical pattern. This has led, on the one hand, to the hypothesis of multifactorial (polygenic) inheritance. There is also the hypothesis that the mode of inheritance in juvenile diabetes is homozygous, whereas the hereditary factor in maturity-onset diabetes is heterozygous. On the other hand, Rimoin has reviewed all available genetic data and expressed the belief that no simple hypothesis can explain all of them. It must be remembered that it is still not known what exactly is the genetic marker. Extensive studies in offspring of two diabetic parents have shown that no consistent abnormality could be detected at a time when glucose tolerance was still normal. Therefore an important role must be attributed to precipitating factors such as obesity, infections, and possibly even drugs. Studies have shown an association between certain histocompatibility antigen groups (HL-A-B8 and BW15) and insulin-dependent or juvenile-onset type diabetes. This was not noted in maturity-onset type diabetics. Concordance for diabetes in monozygotic twins is lower for the juvenile-onset type than the maturity-onset type. This suggests that a greater susceptibility for diabetes (perhaps precipitated by a virus) exists in those with certain histeocompatibility antigens (particularly HLA-B8). For these reasons accurate genetic counseling is impossible.

CLASSIFICATION

It is helpful to classify diabetic patients not only according to type of diabetes but also according to present stage of carbohydrate decompensation. The latter implies that progression or regression from one stage to the next occurs and may be very rapid, may proceed slowly, or may never take place. The following states of diabetes are almost universally accepted (Table 95-1): (1) Overt or clinical diabetes: this is frank diabetes either of the ketosis-prone (juvenile) or ketosis-resistant (adult) type. Fasting and random blood glucose levels are definitely elevated; symptoms related to hyperglycemia and glycosuria can usually be elicited. (2) Chemical or asymptomatic diabetes: the fasting blood glucose level is usually normal, but the postprandial level is frequently elevated. The result of an oral or intravenous glucose tolerance test performed in the absence of stress is clearly abnormal. There are no frank diabetic symptoms. If observed in children, this stage is usually of short duration, as the disease progresses rapidly to overt diabetes. There is however, a small group of asymptomatic, young, nonobese diabetic children whose condition appears to remain stationary for years. In adults this chemical stage may be present for years, and some patients never progress beyond it. Despite this, diabetic angiopathy may be present. (3) Latent or stress diabetes: present in a person who at the present time has a normal glucose tolerance but who is known to have been a diabetic at some previous time, i.e., during pregnancy (gestational diabetes), during infection, when obese, or when under stress, such as cerebrovascular accident, myocardial infarction, extensive burns, or endocrinopathies. The status of patients with such temporary carbohydrate intolerance should be watched closely, particularly when there is a family history of diabetes. (4) Prediabetes or potential diabetes: this is a conceptual term, a retrospective diagnosis, applied to the period of time preceding any glucose intolerance. By definition this state cannot be diagnosed with certainty in the current state of our knowledge. The term has been used in reference to the nondiabetic identical twin of a diabetic patient and in the offspring of two diabetic parents.

As to the *types* of diabetes, the following etiologic classification may be applied:

1. *Genetic (hereditary, idiopathic, primary, essential) diabetes,* subdivided according to the age of onset and/or severity into juvenile and adult diabetes types.
2. *Pancreatic diabetes,* in which the carbohydrate intolerance may be attributed directly to destruction of the pancreatic islets by chronic inflammation, carcinoma, hemochromatosis, or surgical removal.
3. *Endocrine diabetes,* in which the diabetes is associated with endocrinopathies such as hyperpituitarism (acromegaly, basophilism), hyperthyroidism, hyperadrenalism (Cushing's syndrome, primary aldosteronism, pheochromocytoma), and pancreatic islet-cell tumor of the A-cell type. Under this category may also be included gestational diabetes and the various forms of stress diabetes listed above.
4. *Iatrogenic diabetes,* precipitated by administration of corticosteroids, certain diuretics of the benzothiadiazine

TABLE 95-1
Stages of diabetes mellitus

1 Clinical = overt = decompensated diabetes
2 Chemical = asymptomatic diabetes
3 Latent = stress diabetes
4 Prediabetes = potential diabetes

type, and possibly also by estrogen-progesterone combinations, etc.

PATHOLOGY

PANCREAS With the use of special stains with the light microscope and with the availability of the electron microscope, it now appears very likely that almost all diabetic patients exhibit a correlation between severity of their diabetes, on the one hand, and reduced total mass of beta cells and degree of beta-cell degranulation, on the other. These two factors correlate with the amount of extractable pancreatic insulin. In general, after several years of established clinical diabetes, the patient with juvenile-onset diabetes shows essentially no extractable pancreatic insulin, whereas the pancreas of the patient with adult-onset diabetes still contains some insulin, approximately half that found in control pancreases. Patients with maturity-onset diabetes studied at autopsy reveal a significant incidence of hyalinization of pancreatic islets.

Of special interest is the finding that some juvenile diabetics who come to autopsy shortly after clinical onset of diabetes show large islets of Langerhans. This would support the concept that the *initial* lesion is not necessarily decreased insulin production by the pancreas.

There is also the rare patient with recent onset of diabetes whose pancreatic islets show lymphocytic infiltration (insulinitis), a lesion again found almost exclusively in young diabetics. This raises the possibility of an autoimmune mechanism or a specific infection restricted to the islets. Recently viruses of the picorna group have been implicated in such a role.

BLOOD VESSELS Atherosclerosis in the diabetic patient is not different from that commonly observed, but it is equally present in both sexes and occurs earlier in life. Coronary artery disease is a frequent cause of death, and cerebrovascular accidents are significantly more common. In addition, these patients usually have small-vessel disease, or microangiopathy, which has been found not only in the capillaries of the renal glomeruli and eye but also in skin and muscle. The initial lesion is a thickened basement membrane, which represents excess glycoprotein and which reacts with periodic acid Schiff (PAS) stain. It is likely that its biosynthesis is related to glucose metabolism.

Retina (See also Chap. 20) Microaneurysms, small hemorrhages, and exudates are often seen in patients after 10 to 15 years of diabetes. Frequently, there is also a striking dilatation of venules. If hypertension is present, its typical retinopathy may be superimposed, particularly segmental arterial constriction. Proliferative retinopathy is found frequently in juvenile diabetes of long duration. There is formation of new blood vessels around the optic disk. Hemorrhage into the vitreous may be the cause of sudden temporary loss of vision. If, in response to repeated extensive hemorrhages, scar tissue forms, it may upon retracting produce retinal detachment. In proliferative retinopathy, a secondary hemorrhagic glaucoma is often the final step leading to total blindness. At the present time, in the United States, diabetic retinopathy is the second most frequent cause of blindness.

A better understanding of the mechanism of early vascular changes has been made possible by the introduction of the in vitro trypsin digestion of the flattened retina. Two types of vascular cells have been described, the endothelial and the mural cell called *pericyte.* In diabetics, there is a specific loss of mural cells, resulting eventually in formation of microaneurysms, the specific diabetic eye lesion. In addition there is shunting of arterial blood, with consequent ischemia of adjacent areas. Finally there may be increased permeability of the blood vessel wall. These findings are supported by in vivo studies employing fluorescein, injected intravenously into the general circulation, followed by serial photographs of the fundus. In diabetics, one finds not only delayed emptying but also leakage of the dye from blood vessels in areas where exudates and hemorrhages are occurring. The earliest lesions are small areas of nonperfusion which can be visualized in life by fluorescence angiography.

KIDNEY The specific diabetic lesion is the nodular glomerulosclerosis described by Kimmelstiel and Wilson. The lesions consist of discrete ball-like masses of PAS-positive material in the mesangial regions of the capillary tufts or lobules. In addition to this Kimmelstiel-Wilson lesion, a diffuse glomerulosclerosis exists which in fact may be commoner than the nodular lesion. This diffuse lesion consists of PAS-positive deposits in the mesangium, consisting mainly of fibrils of a "basement membranelike" material. The diffuse lesion is more often associated with hypertension, proteinuria and nephrotic syndrome.

Exudative-type lesions are also seen. A *fibrinoid* type and a *capsular-drop* type have been distinguished. Also, the tubules often show a thick basement membrane and glycogen deposits. The question has been raised whether this is excess normally structured basement membrane or an abnormal glycoprotein. Experimental data support the latter, since the glycoprotein of diabetic human glomerular basement membrane contains less lysine but more OH-lysine. In addition, the diabetic tissue contains more glucosyl-galactose disaccharide units, which could contribute to increased permeability despite an anatomically thicker basement membrane. Pyelonephritis, a frequent complication, is a local manifestation of the generalized increased susceptibility to infection. Associated with pyelonephritis, a necrotizing papillitis is sometimes seen. It is generally accepted that the nodular lesions, the capsular drop, and the tubular glycogen are specific for diabetes, although the term diabetic nephropathy includes most of the renal pathology.

LINK BETWEEN METABOLIC AND VASCULAR CHANGES

Some of the pathologic changes observed in diabetic patients are obviously secondary to hyperglycemia, such as deposition of glycogen in the loop of Henle, where it is directly correlated to the glucose concentration in the urine. Hyperglycemia also results in deposition of glycogen in non-insulin-dependent organs, such as skin, heart muscle, iris, and ciliary bodies of the eye. The liver of the diabetic patient, except in the terminal stages, contains normal amounts of glycogen; however, the distribution may be abnormal within the nuclei of the hepatic parenchymal cells. Occasionally the liver is enlarged and infiltrated with fat, mainly in untreated or poorly treated diabetics.

The relationship between derangement of intermediary carbohydrate metabolism and microangiopathy has not been clarified and is still the subject of controversy. A series of studies in a variety of animal models tends to reinforce the concept that hyperglycemia and/or the attendant dysinsulinemia are related to a number of secondary pathologic changes that appear in diabetes.

Biochemically the glycoprotein nature of the basement membrane has been established. It contains about 7 percent carbohydrate, and thus there is the possibility that excessive glucose, via an insulin-independent pathway, leads to derangement of the basement membrane, with secondary infiltration by material from the bloodstream. It has been questioned whether such a derangement is necessarily the consequence of only an abnormal glucose metabolism or whether both the level of blood glucose and the state of the basement membrane could be influenced by a third factor. On the other hand, it is now well documented that all the complications of genetic diabetes may occur in secondary forms of diabetes in man and furthermore that they can be reproduced in animals with experimentally induced diabetes.

These considerations have practical consequences in the daily management of diabetes, as they determine how well the blood sugar of the diabetic should be controlled. If one believes that the microangiopathy presents a true complication of the chronic hyperglycemia, then it is reasonable to aim at as close to normal blood sugars as possible. If on the other hand one believes that hyperglycemia is unrelated to the occurrence of the vascular syndrome, then one will reduce blood sugar only to such a level as to minimize signs and symptoms attributable to hyperglycemia.

It is obvious and does not need to be elaborated here that other factors also play a role, as they do in the general nondiabetic population, i.e., hypertension, obesity, fat content of diets, smoking.

PATHOPHYSIOLOGY

The diabetic syndrome is characterized by an absolute or relative lack of circulating insulin. It develops as a consequence of an imbalance between insulin production and release, on the one hand, and hormonal or tissue factors modifying the insulin requirement, on the other.

Insulin is absolutely lacking in those forms of secondary diabetes in which destruction or removal of the pancreas has taken place. Similarly overt juvenile-onset diabetes is characterized by insulin deficiency. One finds essentially no extractable pancreatic insulin, no response to oral hypoglycemic agents of the sulfonylurea type, a marked tendency to ketoacidosis, and therefore dependence on exogenous insulin for survival. It is assumed that diabetes in the child begins when the pancreatic production of insulin declines. However, this is not always irreversible, as at least one-third of all juvenile diabetics will develop a phase of remission, usually within 3 months after the acute onset of the disease. If present, the remission may last from several days to several months; it rarely exceeds 1 year. Often during such a remission no insulin treatment is necessary, and a glucose tolerance test result may be normal. Nevertheless, after this remission the juvenile diabetic progresses rapidly to a state of total insulin deficiency.

The patient with maturity-onset diabetes develops his disease considerably more slowly. At the early stage no symptoms may be present, and diagnosis is suspected by discovery of elevated blood glucose levels 1 or 2 h postprandially. Measurement of serum insulin may indicate close to normal fasting levels; however, the insulin response to administered glucose is abnormal in that it is delayed. This is responsible for the elevated blood glucose level 1 to 2 h postprandially. As insulin release increases with the rising blood glucose, the blood glucose declines; with a delayed but excessive amount of insulin, the blood glucose level may fall precipitously, provoking the symptoms of reactive hypoglycemia between the *third and fifth hour* postprandially. As the disease progresses further, the insulin release becomes less pronounced and the episodes of reactive hypoglycemia tend to disappear; finally the amount of circulating insulin is insufficient to return the blood glucose to normal levels between meals. In maturity-onset diabetes the pancreatic insulin reserve is decreased but rarely totally absent. Thus the occurrence of diabetic ketoacidosis is uncommon.

Although in many patients the contrast between juvenile- and maturity-onset type diabetes is, initially at least, quite sharp, there are crossovers between these two types, and the above comments must be considered only as generalizations.

Regardless of the type of diabetes, by definition, the cardinal sign is hyperglycemia, frequently associated with glycosuria. The hyperglycemia has two components: hepatic overproduction and peripheral underutilization. The source of the glucose released from the liver is dietary carbohydrate, liver glycogen, and gluconeogenesis from amino acids and glycerol. Underutilization of glucose in the peripheral tissue takes place mainly in adipose tissue and muscle, both of which are insulin-sensitive, and is attributed to a lack of circulating insulin. Impaired glucose uptake by muscle leads to loss of muscle glycogen and release of amino acids for gluconeogenesis. Impaired glucose uptake by adipose tissue causes impaired triglyceride synthesis. In addition, with lack of insulin, free fatty acids are released from adipose tissue into the bloodstream. In the liver, part of the fatty acids are metabolized to ketone bodies. Although the latter can be utilized by certain tissues such as muscle, they are formed in excess in the diabetic. They accumulate in the blood and will spill over into the urine. As they are strong acids, it is necessary for the kidney to excrete a fixed base with them, leading to both sodium and potassium loss. Therefore, the diabetic organism loses glucose, water, ketone bodies, and base. This will result in dehydration, ketoacidosis, and weight loss, and in extreme cases may proceed to diabetic coma and death (Fig. 95-2).

The exact mechanism by which insulin acts remains unknown. However, it is well established that tissues vary widely in sensitivity and responsiveness to insulin. For example, in muscle and adipose tissue, insulin probably acts on cell membrane permeability and so facilitates the entry of glucose into the cell. On the other hand, liver cells exhibit no demonstrable permeability barrier to glucose. The insulin effect on liver appears to be on glycogen synthesis and on the phosphorylating mechanism. It has been shown that the liver contains two enzymes for phosphorylation of glucose: hexokinase and glucokinase. Hexokinase is insulin-*independent,* and glucokinase is insulin-*dependent.* The effect of insulin on fatty acids has been mentioned above. It is noteworthy that this antilipolytic action requires a lower level of insulin than that for glucose uptake. Therefore an absolute deficiency of circulating insulin, as in juvenile-onset diabetes, will lead to hyperglycemia and marked lipolysis with resultant ketosis, whereas only a moderate decrease of circulating insulin, as in maturity-onset diabetes, will lead to hyperglycemia without ketosis.

In diabetes the primary inherited defect responsible for the failing insulin production remains unknown. The discovery of *proinsulin* may be a step forward. Proinsulin is a larger molecule than insulin (molecular weight 9,000, versus 6,000) because of some 30 additional amino acids, but it exhibits considerably less biologic activity. It is converted into insulin by cleavage of the connecting peptide chain at the level of arginine (Fig. 95-1). The theory has been presented that in some diabetic patients there is a failure to activate proinsulin. As large quantities of proinsulin would be required to meet the body's insulin demand, this failure could eventually lead to pancreatic exhaustion and thus to frank diabetes. However, despite careful search, this mechanism has not been found to take place in human diabetes.

Polyol *sorbitol* has received much attention, as its formation from glucose could be directly implicated in some of the diabetic complications. A new pathway of glucose has been discovered whereby it is not phosphorylated but rather is directly reduced by aldose reductase to sorbitol in the presence of a high NADPH/NADP ratio. Accumulation of sorbitol within the cells equipped to handle such an enzymatic process will lead to osmotic swelling. This reaction seems to be favored by a high concentration of blood glucose and is currently accepted as biochemical explanation for the occurrence of cataracts and neuropathy in poorly controlled diabetes.

PRECIPITATION OF DIABETES BY EXTRAPANCREATIC FACTORS

OBESITY Though it should not be inferred that all obese individuals are potential diabetics, obesity is frequently associated with diabetes. Biopsy studies have shown that adult-onset obesity is associated with hypertrophy of adipose cells and that the larger the cell, the less responsive to insulin it becomes. As less glucose can be disposed of, the resulting hyperglycemia will lead to hyperinsulinemia. In patients with a genetically predetermined susceptibility, this may lead to pancreatic exhaustion or at least to a relative insulin deficiency.

PREGNANCY In women so predisposed, pregnancy also exerts a definite diabetogenic action. Diabetes may become apparent only during pregnancy and disappear following delivery (gestational diabetes); rarely it remains; frequently, years or decades later, permanent diabetes develops. There is evidence that hormonal factors, such as placental lactogen and marked destruction of endogenous insulin by the placenta, may play a role in precipitating diabetes. It is speculated that the higher frequency of diabetes in adult females may be due to pregnancies and obesity. Contra-

FIGURE 95-2
Pathophysiology of diabetic ketoacidosis.

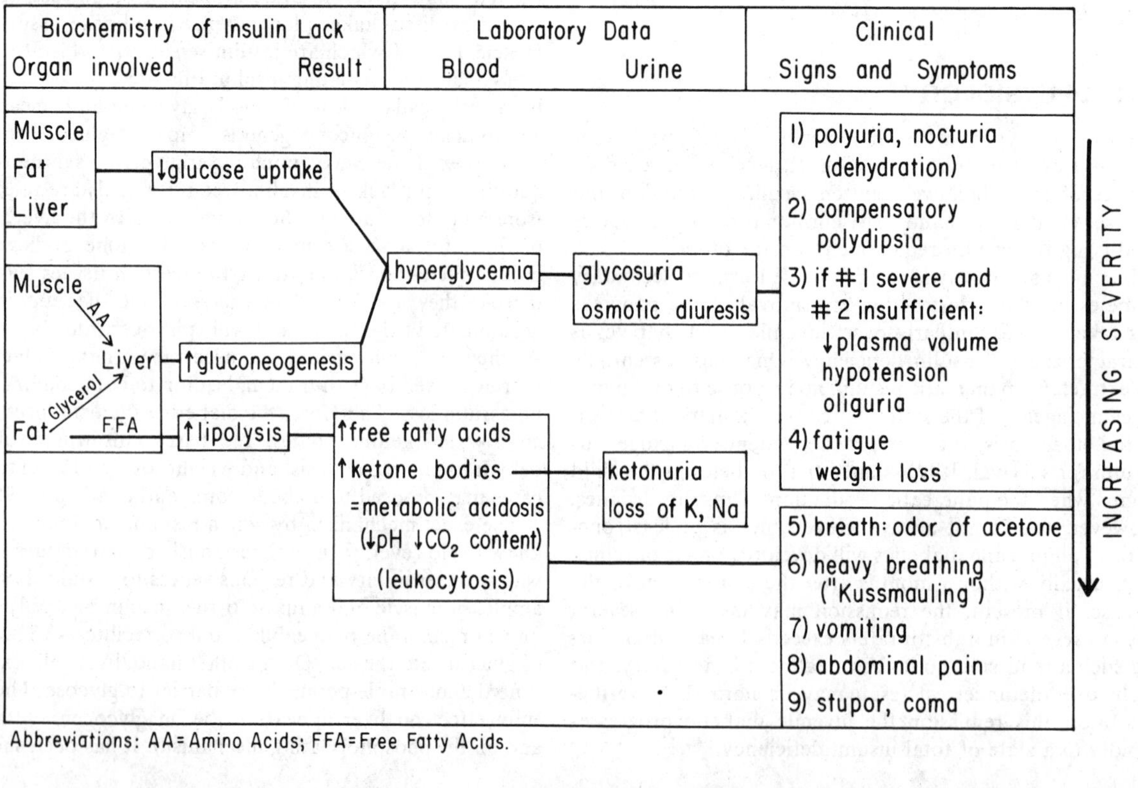

Abbreviations: AA = Amino Acids; FFA = Free Fatty Acids.

ceptive pills which contain estrogen may induce hyperglycemia in susceptible persons.

The diabetogenic action of certain *diuretics of the benzothiadiazine* type has been noted. There is evidence that these drugs mediate such a mechanism by inhibiting pancreatic insulin release. Diazoxide belongs to this group and is currently used for treatment of hypoglycemia due to excess insulin. *Growth hormone* is diabetogenic by decreasing peripheral glucose utilization and by increasing release of free fatty acids. Excessive *epinephrine* causes increased hepatic glycogenolysis and, in addition, inhibits pancreatic insulin release (diabetes in pheochromocytoma). The *steroids* act by increasing hepatic gluconeogenesis and decreasing glucose uptake by adipose tissue. *Thyroxine* increases hunger and food intake and generally heightens the level of metabolic activity. *Infection* of any sort will impair glucose tolerance and may unmask the tendency to diabetes. The diabetogenic mechanism of infection is nonspecific and probably relates to elevated levels of corticosteroids and glucagon, fever that increases the general metabolic load, and possibly catecholamine release, all of which decrease the effectiveness of circulating insulin. In rare instances inflammation of the pancreatic islets takes place.

DIAGNOSIS

The diagnosis of diabetes mellitus is frequently suggested by a history of polydipsia, polyuria, and polyphagia, associated with weight loss. A clinical suggestion of diabetes is confirmed by finding glucose in the urine and by detecting an abnormally elevated blood glucose level. (See Table 95-2 for an outline of the work-up for a patient who has diabetes.)

In the patient without any obvious symptoms suggestive of diabetes, the following procedures are recommended as screening tests for diabetes. By far the simplest test is to obtain a urine specimen 1 to 2 h after a heavy carbohydrate meal. However, in older persons with an elevated renal threshold, the blood glucose level may be elevated without being associated with glycosuria; furthermore, the finding of urinary sugar alone is not diagnostic of diabetes; it may indicate renal glycosuria. Therefore, determination of blood glucose level not only is preferable as a screening procedure but is mandatory to establish the diagnosis of diabetes. Unfortunately much confusion exists as to what represents an abnormal blood glucose value. Whereas there is general agreement that a 1-h postprandial blood glucose level of 200 mg per 100 ml or higher indicates diabetes, there is considerable discussion as to whether abnormality starts above a value of 160, 170, or 180 mg per 100 ml. It has become apparent that clinical information and follow-up studies as well as the method of the blood glucose determination have to be taken into account. In general terms, the upper limits of normalcy increase with age and during pregnancy. As to method, the physician needs to know (1) if capillary or venous blood was used (the capillary blood glucose level will be higher); (2) if the blood glucose was determined on whole blood or plasma (plasma or serum will render higher values than whole blood; on the other hand, severe anemia will give falsely elevated values with whole blood); (3) which particular technique for measuring blood glucose was employed. A rather less specific method such as Folin-Wu will give the highest values, as it measures in addition to glucose also fructose, lactate, pyruvate, etc. The glucose oxidase method will reflect the "true" glucose content and therefore yield the lowest value. The ferricyanide method gives results slightly higher than the glucose oxidase technique. It is apparent that the possible variations are many; therefore the best advice is to be familiar with the methods and normal range in a given hospital. When blood glucose values are reported to outlying institutions or life insurance companies, the type of blood and the technique employed should be noted.

FASTING AND POSTPRANDIAL BLOOD GLUCOSE

The normal range for fasting blood glucose as measured by the autoanalyzer ferricyanide method is between 60 and 100 mg per 100 ml whole blood. An elevated fasting blood sugar level is highly suggestive of diabetes; on the other hand, diabetes can never be ruled out by the presence of a normal fasting blood sugar level. Therefore, it is advisable to obtain a blood sugar determination 1 or 2 h after a meal which contains approximately 100 g carbohydrate, as indicated in Table 95-3 or a regular breakfast to which 50 g glucose has been added. A 1-h value of 170 mg per 100 ml or higher is highly suggestive of diabetes, as is a 2-h value above 120 mg per 100 ml. If the level is borderline, or especially if one wishes definitely to rule out diabetes, then a formal 3-h glucose tolerance test is indicated.

ORAL GLUCOSE TOLERANCE TEST It is mandatory that the patient be on a preparatory diet containing 250 to 300 g carbohydrate for 3 days before testing; otherwise a decreased carbohydrate tolerance may be observed, known as *starvation diabetes.* Physical inactivity also decreases carbohydrate tolerance, and therefore prolonged bed rest may give false positive results. Following a fasting blood glucose determination, 100 g glucose (available commercially in solution) is given and the blood glucose measured at ½ h, 1 h, 2 h, and 3 h; the urine is examined for the presence of sugar. The following are considered upper-normal values with venous blood measured by the autoanalyzer ferricyanide method: fasting, 100 mg per 100 ml; ½ h (or peak value), 170 mg; 1 h, 170 mg; 2 h, 120 mg; and 3 h, 110 mg per 100 ml. There should be no glucose in the urine at any time. The result of the glucose tolerance test in an apparently healthy subject is influenced by at least three factors: diet, physical activity, and age. Age exerts an effect on glucose tolerance. Although standards are not available for individuals of different decades, especially over the age of fifty, it is suggested that between the ages of fifty and fifty-nine the 2-h level may be considered normal up to 130; between the ages of sixty and sixty-nine, up to 140; between the ages of seventy and seventy-nine, up to 150; and above age eighty, above 160 mg per 100 ml. For the 1-h value similar adjustments need to be made. As young healthy people rarely exceed 150 mg per 100 ml, one can allow 10 mg for each decade above fifty years of age. Additional factors known to affect glucose tolerance are fever, infection, endocrinopathies, liver disease, myocardial infarction, cerebrovascular accident, and certain medications such as diuretics of the benzothiodiazine type.

INTRAVENOUS GLUCOSE TOLERANCE TEST As variations of intestinal absorption of glucose may alter a glucose tolerance test, it is occasionally desirable to perform an intravenous glucose tolerance test. This is especially indicated if there is a history of gastrointestinal surgery. Accelerated intestinal absorption of glucose, as in the "dumping syndrome," may result in a diabetic-type oral glucose tolerance curve; however, the intravenous glucose tolerance may be well within normal limits.

The dose of glucose is 0.5 g per kg body weight as a 25% solution. It is administered intravenously within 2 to 4 min, and blood is collected every 10 min for 1 h. Under these conditions, the rate of blood glucose decreases in an exponential manner, and the glucose disappearance can be calculated. Disappearance rate = $70/t\frac{1}{2}$, where $t\frac{1}{2}$ = number of minutes it takes for the blood glucose level to fall 50 percent. In normal individuals the disappearance rate usually exceeds 1.3 percent per min, and values below 1.0 percent are clearly diabetic.

If glucose tolerance tests are performed routinely in a large hospital population, many patients afflicted with chronic diseases such as rheumatoid arthritis or cancer

TABLE 95-2
Work-up of the diabetic patient

HISTORY

Age onset of symptoms diagnosis established present age		*Laboratory* glycosuria blood sugar: fasting postprandial glucose tolerance test			
General polyuria polydipsia polyphagia fatigue ketoacidosis hypoglycemia	*Weight* present usual maximal marital or age 20	*Cardiovascular* angina infarction hypertension stroke	*Feet* claudication ulcer gangrene surgery amputation	*Neurologic* paresthesia pain numbness dizziness	*Vision* blurriness hemorrhage cataract glaucoma
Sexual Male: impotence balanitis Female: birth weight of children abortions vulvar pruritus			*Drug intake* steroids diuretics anticoagulants "the pill"		*Kidney* proteinuria infection neurogenic bladder
Previous treatment Diet: calories weighted measured free	Tablets: type dose duration	Insulin: type dose duration	*Urine testing* daily weekly or less never results		
Complication of diabetic treatment hypoglycemia: insulin tablet	insulin allergy insulin resistance insulin dystrophy	*Heredity* parents other relatives siblings none offspring			

PHYSICAL EXAMINATION—SPECIAL REFERENCE TO

Peripheral vessels	*Neurology*	*Eye grounds*	*Foot*
carotid femoral popliteal dorsalis pedis posterior tibial edema	knee jerks ankle jerks Babinski's reflex pinprick touch vibration	microaneurysm hemorrhages exudates segmental constriction neovascularization fibrous strands	muscle atrophy temperature hair growth pulses blanching on elevation rubor on dependency nails ulcer

CLASSIFICATION OF DIABETES

Stage	*Etiologic*
clinical chemical latent prediabetic	primary genetic secondary: endocrine: obesity, pituitary, thyroid, adrenal pancreatic: surgical removal, carcinoma, pancreatitis, hemochromatosis iatrogenic: steroids, diuretics, other
Concomitant: vascular disease: cardiac, cerebral, peripheral retinal disease neuropathy renal disease	

may exhibit an impaired glucose tolerance curve without any clinical evidence of diabetes. Because many of these cases of "chemical diabetes" will not progress to overt clinical diabetes, one has to be careful not to overdiagnose diabetes.

DIFFERENTIAL DIAGNOSIS OF GLYCOSURIA

(See Chap. 96)

The presence of glucose in the urine should be considered to indicate diabetes until an alternate diagnosis can be definitely established. Glycosuria may indicate a low renal threshold, which is present in pregnancy, in some patients with chronic renal disease, and in patients with idiopathic renal glycosuria. In the latter, glucose is present in most urine specimens, including a second voided specimen after an overnight fast, but the glucose tolerance test result is normal. The transient glycosuria that occurs occasionally in apparently healthy persons under conditions of stress or infection or following ingestion of a high-carbohydrate meal is usually associated with an abnormal glucose tolerance test and, therefore, indicates chemical diabetes.

CLINICAL PICTURE

JUVENILE-ONSET TYPE The juvenile-onset type of diabetes is characterized by a rapid onset, with symptoms such as polydipsia, polyuria, polyphagia, loss of weight and strength, marked irritability, and in children frequently, recurrence of bedwetting. The diabetes is apt to be of the unstable or brittle type, being quite sensitive to the administration of exogenous insulin and easily influenced by physical activity. The patient is liable to ketoacidosis. For adequate treatment, diet and insulin therapy are mandatory. Since the introduction of insulin therapy, diabetic ketoacidosis has been markedly reduced as a major cause of death; the primary causes of early death in diabetic patients are now cardiovascular and renal. Diagnosis of diabetes in this type of patient is usually not difficult. However, occasional children and adolescents have asymptomatic diabetes demonstrable only by postprandial hyperglycemia or glucose tolerance test. In these patients the disease appears to progress very slowly.

MATURITY-ONSET TYPE Maturity-onset diabetes has a less stormy beginning; frequently symptoms are minimal or absent. The chief complaint may be moderate weight loss, or occasionally, weight gain. There may be some nocturia. A female patient might consult her gynecologist because of vulvar pruritus. Frequently, however, the patient seeks medical attention because of vascular complications. As a consequence of blurred or decreased vision, the patient may see an ophthalmologist first, who may diagnose diabetic retinopathy. Fatigue and anemia may be caused by fairly advanced diabetic nephropathy. Diabetic neuropathy may present as paresthesias, loss of sensation, impotence, nocturnal diarrhea, postural hypotension, or a neurogenic bladder. Not infrequently, the patient comes to the physician with an ulcer or gangrene of his toes or heel and on examination is found to have a pulseless or painless foot. Thus the patient with maturity-onset diabetes usually does not present the dramatic, acute metabolic syndrome observed in the juvenile-onset patient but rather a chronic vascular syndrome. It is therefore important to suspect diabetes as an underlying disease under a wide variety of circumstances.

TABLE 95-3
100-g carbohydrate breakfast

Food	*Quantity*	*Carbohydrate, g*
Orange juice	8 oz	24
Cooked cereal or Dry cereal	4 oz or 1 oz	16
Bread	2 slices	32
Egg	1	
Butter	2 pats	
Milk	6 oz	9
Cream	3 oz	4
Sugar	3 tsp	15
Coffee or tea	ad lib.	
Total		100

TREATMENT

GENERAL PRINCIPLES The aims in managing diabetes are (1) to correct the underlying metabolic abnormalities in order to reduce diabetic symptoms; (2) to attain and maintain ideal body weight; (3) to prevent, or at least delay, specific complications commonly associated with the disease (disorders of eye, kidney, nerves); and (4) to stem the nonspecific accelerated atherosclerosis to which the diabetic is particularly liable.

Successful therapy will depend upon the thoroughness with which the physician understands the particular problems in each case, upon how well the patient has been instructed, and upon how conscientious he is about following instructions.

On initiating and during treatment of a patient with diabetes, it is essential to be certain that there is no active focus of infection, as it will aggravate the diabetic state. Infection of the urinary tract should be looked for particularly, and a chest x-ray is imperative. It is also advisable to obtain careful base-line evaluations of the state of the cardiovascular, nervous, and renal systems and of the eye grounds to serve as subsequent points of reference.

General advice should include regular exercise (as it lowers the blood sugar) and avoidance of cigarette smoking. Parameters to be monitored at regular intervals are urine and blood sugars, serum cholesterol and triglycerides, as well as renal function, blood pressure, and body weight.

DIET Dietary treatment of diabetes still constitutes the basis for management, although very often it is difficult to achieve adherence by the patient. The principal points to bear in mind in designing diabetic diets are the facts that the basic nutritional requirements of a patient with diabetes are the same as those of a nondiabetic patient, and that the diet should be varied and palatable.

Purpose The chief aims of a diabetic diet are:

1 Prevent excessive postprandial hyperglycemia and thus symptoms of diabetes

TABLE 95-4
Food exchanges

Food	Approx. meas. 1 exchange	Weight, g
BREAD: carbohydrate 15 g, protein 2 g, fat negligible		
Bread, baker's	1 slice	25
Biscuit, roll	2″ diameter	35
Muffin	2″ diameter	35
Cornbread	1 1/2″ cube	35
Cereals, cooked	1/2 cup, cooked	100
Cereals, dry (flakes, puffed, and shredded varieties)	3/4 cup, scant	20
Rice, macaroni, noodles, spaghetti	1/2 cup, cooked	100
Crackers:		
Graham	2 (2 1/2 × 2 3/4″)	20
Oyster	20 (1/2 cup)	20
Saltines	5 (2″ square)	20
Soda	3 (2 1/2 × 2 1/2″)	20
Round, thin varieties	6–8 (1/2″ diameter)	20
Vegetables:		
Beans, peas, dried (cooked) Includes limas, navy, kidney beans, black-eyed peas, cowpeas, split peas, etc.	1/2 cup, scant	100
Corn	1/3 cup or 1/2 ear	80
Parsnips	1/2 cup	125
Potatoes:		
White, baked	2″ diameter	100
White, boiled, mashed	1/2 cup	100
Sweet or yam	1/4 cup	50
Ice cream, vanilla (omit 2 fat exchanges)	1/8 qt	70
Sponge cake, no icing	1 1/2″ cube	25

Food	Approx. meas. 1 exchange	Weight, g
FRUITS: fresh, cooked, canned, or frozen unsweetened: carbohydrate 10 g per exchange; protein and fat negligible		
Apple, 1 small	2″ diameter	80
Applesauce	1/2 cup	100
Apricots, dry	4 halves	20
Apricots, fresh	2 medium	100
Banana	1/2 small	50
Berries (blackberries, raspberries, and strawberries)	1 cup	150
Blueberries	2/3 cup	100
Cantaloupe	1/2 (6″ diameter)	200
Cherries	10 large or 15 small	75
Dates	2	15
Figs, dried	1 small	15
Figs, fresh	2 large	50
Grapefruit	1/2 small	125
Grapefruit juice	1/2 cup	100
Grapes	12	75
Grape juice	1/2 cup	60
Honeydew melon	1/8 (7″ diameter)	150
Mango	1/2 small	70
Nectarines	1 medium	100
Orange	1 small	100
Orange juice	1/2 cup	100
Papaya	1/3 medium	100
Peach	1 medium	100
Pear	1 small	100
Pineapple	1/2 cup, cubed	80
Pineapple juice	1/3 cup	80
Plums	2 medium	100
Prunes, dried	2 medium	25
Raisins	2 tbsp level	25
Tangerine	1 large	100
Watermelon	1 cup diced 1 slice 3″ × 1 1/2″	175

2 Prevent hypoglycemia if the patient is on exogenous insulin
3 Obtain ideal body weight
4 Normalize serum cholesterol and triglycerides
5 Prevent or delay premature atherosclerosis

Basic caloric requirement This is dictated by ideal weight, physical activity, and occupation of the patient. If he is obese, and most adult diabetics are, the diet should be restricted in total calories, yet be nutritionally adequate. With return to normal weight a marked improvement often will take place of hyperglycemia and glycosuria, frequently associated with a decline in serum triglyceride level. If the patient is undernourished, the initial diet has to exceed the basic caloric requirement. Particularly in children it should be sufficient to achieve desirable growth and development. The desired weight is calculated from the height, taking frame size into consideration. For an approximate calculation of the basic caloric requirement, the ideal weight in pounds is multiplied by 10, or 20 kcal per kg. Example: If a patient's ideal weight is 180 lb, his *basal* caloric requirement will be 1800 kcal. Additional calories are allowed according to the patient's occupation and activities. Calories may be reduced for patients over fifty years of age who are less active. Meals and snacks should be spaced to avoid intermittent hyper- or hypoglycemia, particularly if the patient receives exogenous insulin.

Partition of calories The average American diet consists of carbohydrate, 40 to 50 percent; protein, 15 to 20 percent; and fat, 35 to 40 percent. The diabetic diet can approximate this distribution. The caloric value of carbohydrate and protein is approximately 4 kcal per g, and of fat, 9 kcal per g. Alcohol contains 7 kcal per g, or 168 kcal per oz.

Carbohydrate Carbohydrate is contained in starches (polymer of glucose), milk (glucose, galactose), fruits, and refined sugar (glucose, fructose). To prevent acetonuria and protein catabolism, a minimum of 1 g per lb body weight is necessary, or in the example of the patient weighing 180 lb, 180 g. If more carbohydrates are indicated, concentrated sugars should be avoided to prevent wide swings of blood glucose. Rarely should the total amount of carbohydrates exceed 250 g per day.

Protein Protein is contained in meat, fish, cheese, eggs, etc. A *minimum* of 0.5 g per lb body weight is indicated. This is further increased during pregnancy and during childhood.

Fat Fat is contained in butter, margarine, mayonnaise, cream, bacon, nuts, olives, avocado, and meats in general.

Dietary fats, particularly those of animal origin, together with other factors, such as obesity, hypertension, smoking, and decreased physical activity, seem to play an important

TABLE 95-4 *(continued)*

Food	*Approx. meas. 1 exchange*	*Weight, g*
FAT: carbohydrate and protein negligible; fat, 5 g per serving. Fat exchanges used in cooking must be accounted for.		
Avocado	1/8 (4″ diam.)	24
Butter or margarine	1 tsp level	5
Bacon, crisp	1 slice	10
Cream, light, sweet, or sour—20%	2 tbsp level	30
Cream, heavy—40%	1 tbsp level	15
Cream cheese	1 tbsp level	15
French dressing	1 tbsp level	15
Mayonnaise	1 tsp level	5
Nuts	6 small	10
Oil or cooking fat	1 tsp level	5
Olives	5 small	50

VEGETABLES: carbohydrate 7 g, protein 2 g, fat negligible. One exchange equals 1/2 cup.

Beets	Peas, green	Squash, winter
Carrots	Pumpkin	Turnip
Onions	Rutabaga	

Note: One or more fat exchanges from the diet allowance may be used to season the vegetables. All other vegetables, except those listed under Bread, contain negligible amounts of carbohydrate, protein, and fat. They may be used as desired.

Food	*Approx. meas. 1 exchange*	*Weight, g*
MILK: 170 kcal, carbohydrate 12 g, protein 8 g, fat 10 g per serving		
Milk, plain	1 cup (8 oz)	240
Milk, evaporated	1/2 cup	120
Milk, powder, skim*	1/3 cup (5 1/3 tbsp level)	48
Milk, powder, whole	1/2 cup (8 tbsp level)	35
Buttermilk*	1 cup	240
Milk, skim*	1 cup	240

Food	*Approx. meas. 1 exchange*	*Weight, g*
MEAT (cooked weight): carbohydrate negligible, protein 7 g, fat 5 g per serving		
Meat: beef, fowl, lamb, veal (medium fat), liver, pork, ham (lean)	1 oz	30
Cold cuts: salami, minced ham, bologna, cervelat, liver sausage, luncheon loaf	1 slice 4 1/2″ diam. × 1/8″	45
Frankfurters (8 to 9 per lb)	1	50
Fish:		
Cod, haddock, halibut, herring, etc.	1 oz	30
Salmon, tuna, crabmeat, lobster	1/4 cup	30
Shrimp, clams, oysters (medium)	5	45
Sardines	3 medium	30
Cheese:		
Cheddar type	1 oz	30
Cottage	3 tbsp level	45
Peanut butter (limit to one serving per day unless adjustment is made to balance carbohydrate content)	2 tbsp scant	30
Egg	1	50

* *Add 10 g fat (two fat exchanges). Most commercial buttermilk is skimmed. Check local supplies.*
SOURCE: *Modified from* Meal Planning with Exchange Lists, *obtainable from the American Diabetes Association, Inc., New York, N.Y.*

role in the pathogenesis of atherosclerosis. Therefore fat intake should be kept to a minimum. The amount prescribed is calculated by subtracting calories allowed for carbohydrate and protein from the total caloric requirement. For example: Total calories based on an ideal weight of 180 lb = 1800. Assigned for carbohydrate: 180 × 4 = 720; for protein: 90 × 4 = 360; there remain 1800 − 720 − 360 = 720. These calories given as fat: 720 divided by 9 = 80 g fat. The final diet consists of carbohydrate 180 g, protein 90 g, and fat 80 g. It is advisable to reduce the total amount of cholesterol by avoiding eggs and to supply some of the fat as unsaturated fatty acids. Recently the American Diabetes Association has recommended decreasing fat further and making up calories by increasing carbohydrate. If fat is decreased by 20 g, 180 kcal carbohydrate (= 45 g) have to be added. In the above example, it would be changed to 235 carbohydrate, 60 fat, protein remaining at 90 g.

The American Diabetes Association and the American Dietetic Association have published a booklet on meal planning with exchange lists. In it all the available foods are divided into six types. Foods cannot be switched between the lists but can be interchanged within each list. Food is subdivided into (1) milk exchanges; (2) (*a*) essentially unlimited vegetables, (*b*) somewhat limited vegetables; (3) fruits; (4) bread exchanges which include apart from bread also cereal, rice, spaghetti, potato, etc.; (5) meat exchanges which include meat, cold cuts, egg, fish, cheese, and (6) fat exchanges. In Tables 95-4 and 95-5 these exchange lists are presented in more detail. Food can be weighed or measured with a standard 8-oz measuring cup, a teaspoon, and a tablespoon.

TABLE 95-5
An 1800-kilocalorie diabetic diet order (carbohydrate 180 g, protein 90 g, fat 80 g)

Exchange	*Breakfast*	*Lunch*	*Snack*	*Supper*	*Snack*
Milk	1/2	1			1/2
Bread	2	2	1	2	1
Meat	1	2	1	3	1
Fat	1	1		2	
Fruit	1	1		1	
Vegetable		1		1	
PARTITION IN GRAMS:					
Carbohydrate	46	52	15	47	21
Protein	15	26	9	27	13
Fat	15	25	5	25	10

ORAL HYPOGLYCEMIC AGENTS They appear to have a place in the treatment of maturity-onset diabetes, provided it is of the nonketotic type and that dietary treatment alone is unsuccessful in achieving adequate control. The oral hypoglycemic agents are not related to insulin, nor can they replace it in conditions such as diabetic ketoacidosis. The agents presently in use are of two types: the sulfonylureas and the biguanides. However, the long-term cardiovascular safety of both types of oral hypoglycemic agents has been questioned [University Group Diabetes Program (UGDP)]. The results of this study have stirred much controversy. The comments of rival clinicians and statisticians have become so complex that any practitioner may be excused for being uncertain as how to manage a particular case of diabetes. It must be stated, however, that the American Diabetes Association and the American Medical Association have endorsed the results of the UGDP study. Therefore, caution is urged in prescription of oral agents. At the moment they are recommended without reservation only if (1) dietary measures have failed, (2) the use of insulin is unacceptable to the patient, or (3) only a short-term use of an oral hypoglycemic agent is considered.

The patient with maturity-onset diabetes can often be controlled by diet alone, and this should be given an *adequate* trial for several weeks, unless clinical circumstances such as acute infection dictate otherwise. The multitude of oral agents available, each with somewhat different dosage and duration of action, makes it difficult to master them all; therefore it is recommended that the physician become familiar with one or two. A summary of all the available agents is given in Table 95-6. Potentiation of their actions by other drugs, such as sulfisoxazole (Gantrisin), phenylbutazone (Butazolidin), and bishydroxycoumarin (Dicumarol), has been reported; therefore, the physician should be aware of such possibilities.

Sulfonylureas The sulfonylureas available by prescription are tolbutamide (Orinase), acetohexamide (Dymelor), chlorpropamide (Diabinase), and tolazamide (Tolinase). Although there is some evidence that they directly decrease hepatic glucose output, they act primarily by enhancing the secretion of endogenous insulin. Thus, for these drugs to be effective, at least residual function of the beta cells is necessary.

A patient can be started on sulfonylureas without the prior use of insulin, or he can be transferred from insulin to sulfonylureas. The chance of therapeutic success with these agents is better when clinical diabetes has been present for a relatively short period of time, if the patient is over the age of forty, and if he or she is overweight. A large initial loading dose is not now considered necessary for the sulfonylureas. Side effects include an alleged increased chance of cardiovascular death of unknown mechanism; except for chlorpropamide in high doses, these agents have a good record with respect to hepatic function. Chlorpropamide has also been implicated in an occasional patient in the production of a state of water intoxication with hyponatremia. Thus it should be used with caution in patients with borderline heart failure. Alcohol intolerance has been observed under treatment with sulfonylureas. Occasionally, in elderly undernourished patients, severe hypoglycemia may follow their administration. Apart from this, prolonged hypoglycemia is frequently observed when a sulfonylurea is administered to a patient with uremia, as renal excretion of the drug will be delayed. This is the case particularly with chlorpropamide and acetohexamide, as the former is not metabolized to any significant extent and the latter is transformed by the liver to hydroxyhexamide, which also exhibits a potent hypoglycemic property. In both instances, elevated blood levels of the respective drug will lead to severe and protracted hypoglycemia. If this occurs, prolonged and intensive treatment with intravenous glucose (that is, 200 g within 24 h) and close medical supervision for at least 48 to 72 h are mandatory.

From 20 to 30 percent of diabetic patients initially responding to treatment with sulfonylurea will fail to do so after several months or years. This *secondary failure* can often be attributed to poor adherence to a prescribed diet, the presence of infection, or the gradual progression of the diabetes to a more insulin-deficient state having the anatomic equivalent of further decrease in the number of functioning pancreatic islets.

Tolbutamide This is the most widely used oral hypoglycemic agent. Each tablet contains 500 mg. The biologic half-life is approximately 6 h. It is administered before breakfast *and* before supper, the total daily dose ranging from 1 to 3 g. The excretory product in the urine may give a false positive test for albumin, since it is precipitated by acidifying the urine.

Acetohexamide Tablets are available in strengths of 250 and 500 mg. Its half-life is longer, and therefore a *single* dose may be effective.

Chlorpropamide Tablets are available containing 100 or 250 mg. The biologic half-life is approximately 36 h, and daily administration may result in a cumulative effect. It is not metabolized and thus is almost completely excreted in the urine. The recommended daily dose is 100 to 250 mg before breakfast; it should not exceed 750 mg. Because of its long action, a bedtime snack containing carbohydrate, protein, and fat, e.g., milk with crackers, is advisable. As it has occasionally a slightly greater toxic effect on the liver than has tolbutamide or acetohexamide, and since its long half-life may occasionally result in hypoglycemia in the early morning, it is advisable to keep the daily dose as low as possible.

Tolazamide This is available in 100- and 250-mg tablets with a half-life of approximately 12 h. It is administered in a single or divided dose, not exceeding 1,000 mg per day.

TABLE 95-6
Oral hypoglycemic agents

Generic name	*Available form, mg*	*Average dose, mg*	*Duration of action, h*
Tolbutamide	500	500–1,000 b.i.d.	6–12
Acetohexamide	250 500	250–1,000 A.M.	12–24
Tolazamide	100 250	100–1,000 A.M.	16-24
Chlorpropamide	100 250	100–750 A.M.	24–36
Phenformin	25 (tablet) 50 (capsule) 100 (capsule)	25 b.i.d. 50 b.i.d. 100 b.i.d.	4–6 8–12

BIGUANIDES Phenformin Of the biguanides, phenformin, a phenethyl biguanide (DBI; Meltrol), is commercially available as a 25-mg tablet, with a biologic half-life of 3 to 4 h, and as a 50-mg or 100-mg time-disintegration capsule of longer half-life. The mechanism of action differs fundamentally from that of the sulfonylureas in that phenformin can correct hyperglycemia in the pancreatectomized animal and the hypoglycemic effect cannot be produced in nondiabetic fed subjects. The mechanism of action is still poorly understood, but it appears that phenformin influences the anaerobic pathway of glucose and inhibits hepatic gluconeogenesis. As phenformin makes a diabetic patient occasionally more sensitive to exogenous insulin, it has been suggested that phenformin inhibits an insulin antagonist. Evidence indicates that phenformin decreases glucose uptake by the intestinal mucosa. It is likely that phenformin also interferes with absorption of some vitamins.

The sole use of phenformin as an antidiabetic agent is limited because the effective dose is frequently associated with gastrointestinal side effects such as anorexia, nausea, vomiting, and diarrhea. Furthermore, phenformin may contribute to excessive lactic acid; it should not be used in those circumstances in which marked tissue hypoxia might be expected to occur, i.e., myocardial infarction, hypotension, low arterial blood oxygen saturation. Fatalities have been reported in which severe lactic acidosis, apparently facilitated by the administration of phenformin, constituted an important contributory effect. A recent detailed analysis of the UGDP study showed an increased mortality from all causes due to the increase in cardiovascular deaths in those treated with phenformin. Also noted was an increase in both systolic and diastolic blood pressures, heart rate, use of cardiac glycosides, diuretics, and antihypertensive agents. With these findings in mind, its use might be limited to (1) the very rare patient with maturity-onset diabetes who is allergic to the sulfonylureas (the daily recommended dose of phenformin ranges from 50 to 200 mg, to be given either as tablets t.i.d. or as capsules b.i.d.); (2) combination with sulfonylurea in the elderly patient who fails to respond to a maximum dose of a sulfonylurea; (3) the patient with brittle diabetes on insulin with frequent hypoglycemic reactions, in whom the addition of phenformin might result in reduction of the insulin requirement and thus facilitate control (use of phenformin in this type of patient is often disappointing); (4) the obese overeating diabetic in whom diet and the sulfonylureas have failed and insulin is unacceptable.

INSULIN The use of insulin is clearly indicated in the juvenile-onset diabetic and in those patients with maturity-onset diabetes in whom diet has failed to maintain satisfactory levels of blood glucose in both the fasting and the postprandial state. Furthèrmore, the use of insulin is mandatory in diabetic ketoacidosis. Insulin is a potent hormone of short endogenous half-life once it is absorbed from its subcutaneous injection site.

Types of insulin In the United States the animal sources for insulin are beef and pork. As human insulin has a structure similar to that of pork insulin, the use of pure pork insulin rather than a beef-pork mixture may be preferred. Apart from the species difference, seven types of insulin are commercially available. They may be divided into insulins of fast, intermediate, and long action. Their properties are summarized in Table 95-7.

Each of the insulins is available in three different strengths, namely, 40, 80, and 100 units per ml. The more recently introduced U 100 in conjunction with suitable syringes for relatively small doses (i.e., under 30 units) should eventually lead to the phasing out of U 40 and U 80 with consequently less chance of error of insulin dose. A *unit of insulin* (25 units per mg) has the same potency regardless of whether its *concentration* is 40, 80, or 100 units per ml (that is, U 40, U 80, or U 100). Regardless of the concentration desired, *it should always be measured in a corresponding syringe calibrated for that potency* (U 80 insulin with a U 80 syringe labeled in green, U 40 insulin with a U 40 syringe labeled in red, and U 100 insulin with a U 100 syringe labeled in black). All insulin preparations available since 1972 and 1973 are more pure than previous preparations and are termed *single-peak.* On special request, single-component or monocomponent insulin preparations are available for treatment of patients with insulin allergy or insulin atrophy.

Choice of insulin *Crystalline insulin* is best for emergencies, such as the treatment of diabetic ketoacidosis or the achievement of fast control in the patient with marked hyperglycemia; it is also employed for daily use in combination with an intermediate insulin to bring on earlier action.

Intermediate insulins in a single dose injected before breakfast will control many diabetics. The dosage will be gauged by the prelunch, midafternoon, and fasting blood sugar values. The midafternoon blood glucose level corresponds to the peak of insulin action and will dictate the maximum morning dose. It is advisable that all patients receiving an intermediate insulin be given a midafternoon snack. If the midafternoon blood glucose level is between 80 and 120 mg per 100 ml, and the prelunch value is still unduly elevated, the addition of a small amount of crystalline insulin at breakfast time is indicated. It can be mixed with neutral protamine Hagedorn (NPH) or lente insulin in the same syringe. Almost all maturity-onset diabetes can be adequately controlled by intermediate insulins alone or in combination with crystalline insulin administered before breakfast.

TABLE 95-7
Insulin, types and action curves

Action	*Insulin*	*Modifier*	*Duration of action, hr*	*Peak effect, hr postinjection*
Fast	Crystalline zinc = clear = (regular) = soluble	None	6	2–3
	Semilente	Zinc	12	3–6
Intermediate	Globin	Globin	18	6–8
	NPH	Protamine	24	8–12
	Lente	Zinc	24	8–12
Long	Ultralente	Zinc	36	20–30
	Protamine zinc	Protamine	36	16–24

The patient with juvenile-onset diabetes often develops nocturnal hyperglycemia because of very active gluconeogenesis and, consequently, will exhibit a high fasting blood glucose level associated with glycosuria. Further increase in the morning dose of intermediate insulin will often lead to hypoglycemia in the midafternoon. To reduce the fasting blood glucose to normal levels, a long-acting insulin can be tried, but often a second small dose of the intermediate insulin before supper or at bedtime is preferable. The latter regimen is eminently satisfactory in the 24-h control of juvenile diabetes, and usually patients do not complain about the second injection because they feel so much better. Very rarely, sugar is spilled at bedtime but none before supper. Then the addition of a small amount of crystalline insulin to the evening dose of NPH is indicated, and both are given before supper. As a general rule, whenever insulin is given in the evening in addition to the morning dose, the latter should be reduced.

The use of *long-acting insulin* with the hope of establishing control with a single morning injection, in general, has been disappointing. The basic four insulin treatment patterns are summarized in Table 95-8.

Initiation of insulin therapy If the patient has massive glycosuria and elevated blood glucose level, insulin therapy is begun immediately with crystalline insulin. The following schedule is recommended: 20 units for a blood sugar above 300 mg per 100 ml or 4+ urine test; 10 units for a blood sugar between 200 to 300 mg per 100 ml or a 3+ or 2+ urine sugar. Once the acute syndrome is under reasonable control, or if the metabolic derangement is less dramatic, use of a longer-acting insulin can be started. It is best to start with 10 to 15 units of NPH or lente insulin and increase this by 5 units per day, as indicated by urine tests and blood glucose levels. Most diabetic patients will require between 30 and 50 units of insulin daily.

Complications of insulin therapy INSULIN REACTIONS These are commonly caused by excessive insulin dosage, delayed food intake, or unusual physical activity. Very rarely, an increased sensitivity to insulin is due to early adrenal or pituitary hypofunction. Occasional insulin reactions are almost unavoidable, especially in the juvenile insulin-sensitive diabetic, but they are harmless if recognized and treated early. To reduce them to a minimum, it is essential that the patient know how to test his urine for glucose and, provided he does not have an elevated renal threshold for glucose, how to reduce his insulin dose when his urine tests indicate absence of glucose for several days.

TABLE 95-8
Basic insulin treatment patterns

Pattern no.	*Before breakfast*	*Before supper*	*At bedtime*
1	NPH*		
2	NPH + CZI†		
3	NPH + CZI		NPH
4	NPH + CZI	NPH + CZI	

* *Exchangeable with lente insulin.*
† *CZI = crystalline zinc = regular insulin.*

The patient also must be instructed to eat his meals on time and when unusual physical activity is anticipated, either to reduce his morning insulin dose or to ingest extra calories to compensate for the blood-sugar-lowering effect of exercise.

The signs and symptoms of an insulin reaction vary with the type of insulin used. *Crystalline insulin* produces a rapid fall in blood glucose level which is detected by the glucoreceptors in the hypothalamus and transmitted via neural pathways to induce release of epinephrine, with the purpose of elevating blood sugar level by glycogenolysis and inhibiting pancreatic insulin release. In the insulin-dependent diabetic person, insulin release from the injection site cannot be inhibited, and thus if untreated, the hypoglycemia will continue to persist. The patient will be aware of symptoms of hyperepinephrinemia which enable him to diagnose his condition. It is a *characteristic reaction* of rapid onset consisting of hunger, a peculiar abdominal sensation, sweating, palpitation, tremor, tachycardia, weakness, irritability, and pallor. Patients usually recognize these symptoms early, and they are relieved within 10 to 20 min by ingestion of carbohydrate: sugar, orange juice, candy, etc. For protection, diabetic patients receiving insulin should carry several lumps of sugar with them at all times. A patient in insulin reaction may act as though he were intoxicated, and therefore *it is further recommended that everyone with diabetes carry a card identifying him as a diabetic.* This is especially important for patients with a long history of diabetes. Because of neuropathy, sympathetic nervous system signs may gradually be lost; the patient then lacks indications of impending reaction and may exhibit only impaired cerebral functions. *The intermediate and long-acting insulins produce a more gradual decline in blood glucose level,* with consequently less release of epinephrine; symptoms are produced by deficient glucose metabolism of the higher nervous centers. They consist of headache, blurred or double vision, fine tremor, uncontrollable yawning, hypothermia, mental confusion, incoordination, and eventually, unconsciousness. In elderly persons an insulin reaction may mimic a cerebrovascular accident. Treatment is administration of glucose by mouth or vein, or of glucagon if no vein can be found. Relatives of diabetic patients liable to severe insulin reactions, and especially parents of diabetic children, should be instructed in the use of glucagon. It can be injected subcutaneously, just as insulin is, and will lead to a transient rise in blood glucose level that is long enough to wake the patient up and enable him to receive some carbohydrate by mouth. Whereas the normal beta cell regulates insulin release according to the body's need on a minute-to-minute basis, the condition of the diabetic patient receiving subcutaneous administration of insulin mimics that produced by an autonomous "insulinoma" which does not respond to the patient's need but rather requires the patient to adjust to it with spaced meals and preplanned exercise. Recurrent hypoglycemic attacks, with their attendant anxiety, headache, loss of concentration power, etc., constitute a nuisance to the diabetic patient, but only *severe and prolonged* attacks of hypoglycemia will lead to intellectual deterioration as a result of irreversible damage to cortical neurons. It is unfortunate that the margin between the effective dose of insulin which produces euglycemia and an excessive dose which produces hypoglycemia is so small. However, there is hope of improving this situation in the future with the development of mechanical "beta-cell implants," which would consist of a glucosensor coupled to an insulin reservoir that would release insulin only in response to rising blood sugar level and would shut it off before hypoglycemia develops, or perhaps with an implant of surviving islets of Langerhans or cultured beta cells.

An insulin reaction initiates a counterregulatory mechanism characterized by release of epinephrine, adrenal corticosteroids, and growth hormone. This will result in a *rebound hyperglycemia,* for "hypoglycemia begets hyperglycemia." Knowledge of this physiologic defense mechanism will prevent the physician from administering extra insulin to combat this hyperglycemia. If the insulin reaction is due to excessive insulin, the patient will benefit from a reduced insulin dosage.

REACTIONS AT THE SITE OF INSULIN INJECTION Such reactions are not uncommon at the beginning of treatment. They are characterized by redness, swelling, pain, and nodule formation. As they usually disappear within a few days or weeks, the patient can be reassured, and no treatment is indicated. If the local reaction persists, it can be improved by changing to an insulin of the lente type, which does not contain protamine, or by switching to a pure pork insulin. Occasionally the simultaneous injection of an antihistamine in the same syringe is very helpful. Very rarely systemic allergic reactions occur, mediated by gammaglobulin (IgE); desensitization may be necessary. Skin infections at the site of injection are extremely rare.

INSULIN LIPODYSTROPHY This reaction is characterized by either hypertrophy or atrophy of the subcutaneous adipose tissue at the site of insulin injection. This is frequent and affects children and women more than men. If the patient is bothered by the esthetic aspect of this complication, injection of insulin into other sites is recommended until the lesion improves; then the atrophic area may again be used in the hope of inducing lipogenesis. Single-component insulin injections into the base and/or edge of the atrophic area are of significant benefit.

INSULIN RESISTANCE Almost all diabetic patients treated with insulin for several months will develop circulating antibodies to insulin. However, only a few (approximately 1 in 1,000 insulin-treated diabetics) will develop insulin resistance. By definition it is present if the daily insulin requirement in the absence of ketoacidosis exceeds 200 units. Patients with insulin resistance may require several thousand units daily. When insulin resistance is associated with hemochromatosis, severe infections, Cushing's syndrome, acromegaly, or hyperthyroidism, it is secondary. Frequently, no obvious cause can be detected. Examination of serum will demonstrate the presence of large quantities of antibodies to insulin and an increased insulin-binding capacity. In such patients a trial with pure pork insulin is always justified, and very often a sizable reduction in insulin requirement can be achieved. Single-component insulin has been used with good results. If such measures fail, the use of steroids is indicated, for their anti-insulin effect is outweighed by their anti-immune effect. Rarely the addition of phenformin or sulfonylureas is helpful. The natural course of idiopathic insulin resistance is characterized by spontaneous remission within several weeks or months. Frequently, the resistance breaks abruptly, and the patient exhibits episodes of severe hypoglycemia as the antibody-bound insulin is released and becomes suddenly available.

COMPLICATIONS OF DIABETES

DIABETIC KETOACIDOSIS AND COMA Lack of insulin is the cause of diabetic ketoacidosis. The patient may have (1) undiagnosed diabetes, (2) known diabetes but fail to increase his insulin dose despite poor urine tests, or (3) known diabetes and suffer from nausea and vomiting but reason that he does not need his daily insulin because he does not eat. Omission of insulin probably constitutes the single largest cause of diabetic acidosis. Other common causes are infections and myocardial infarctions.

Diagnosis Among clinical signs and symptoms, vomiting is present in approximately two-thirds of patients with acidosis. Abdominal pain and tenderness may be related to nausea and vomiting or sodium depletion and may be so severe as to mimic an abdominal emergency ("pseudoappendicitis" of diabetic acidosis). Air hunger and heavy labored breathing as described by Kussmaul are expressions of the acidosis and correlate with the reduction in serum CO_2 content. There is dehydration as evidenced by soft eyeballs, dry skin, poor urinary output, and hypotension. Laboratory findings include the following: the urine usually contains massive amounts of glucose and acetone; frequently there is also transient albuminuria. The diagnosis of diabetic ketoacidosis is made, however, by finding hyperglycemia (usually between 300 and 600 mg per 100 ml), ketonemia, and reduction of serum CO_2 content (below 9 meq per liter). The acidosis is metabolic and is caused by accumulation of ketone bodies associated with loss of sodium and potassium. The azotemia is due partly to dehydration and partly to tissue protein breakdown. Serum lipids are generally increased. The rise in hematocrit indicates dehydration; usually there is leukocytosis.

Differential diagnosis On clinical grounds alone it is sometimes difficult to distinguish between diabetic acidosis and an insulin reaction. If any doubt exists, blood should be drawn for laboratory tests and 50 ml of 50% glucose injected intravenously. If the coma is due to insulin reaction, the patient will wake up immediately; if he is in diabetic coma, no harm has been done. Among diagnoses to be considered are salicylate poisoning; lactic acidosis; hyperglycemic hyperosmolar nonketotic coma; and far-advanced renal failure—all conditions which may occur in a diabetic patient.

Treatment Treatment will vary greatly from patient to patient; however, the general principles are as follows:

1 Through a large needle blood is withdrawn for laboratory tests (blood glucose, BUN, Na, K, C1, CO_2 content, pH, hematocrit, white blood cell count, and plasma acetone), and the vein is kept open with an infusion of normal saline solution. The rationale for this rests on the observation that patients in diabetic coma may decompensate very rapidly, and precious time will be lost in finding a vein and performing a venous cutdown. As in other acute emergencies, always ensure an adequate airway and circulation. An ECG should be done to rule out myocardial infarction and as a check upon serum potassium changes. If the patient is comatose or anuric, catheterization is valuable so that urine volume, urine glucose, and ketones can be evaluated. Gastric lavage might be required (using warm saline), especially in more severe cases. Vital signs should be monitored frequently until definite clinical and metabolic improvement is seen, i.e., until the patient is conscious and reasonably alert.

2 Crystalline insulin is administered both subcutaneously and intravenously. The average total dosage of insulin required for patients in diabetic coma within the first 24 h is 200 units. The dosage, of course, will vary from patient to patient; it may have to be larger for an obese diabetic and less in a frail, elderly diabetic. If the patient has been in diabetic coma previously and required 300 units to respond, chances are he may require a similar dose again. The initial dose of insulin will depend primarily on laboratory tests such as blood sugar and plasma ketone. An average initial dose of insulin will depend primarily on laboratory tests such as blood sugar and plasma ketone. An average initial dose would be 50 units intravenously and 50 units subcutaneously. A widely used set of guidelines has been based upon estimations of blood glucose (Table 95-9). Generally of value is reassessment of the clinical condition and at least the blood glucose, plasma acetone, CO_2, pH, and K at the second hour after the immediate initial treatment program and insulin has been instituted. If the blood glucose shows a decline, no further insulin should be given until the clinical and laboratory evaluations are repeated at the fourth hour after initial treatment has been given. If the blood glucose shows an increase at the second 1-h interval, additional insulin should be given at a dose equal to or double the amount given initially. Total reassessment should be repeated hourly in this situation. An occasional patient may require 5,000 or 10,000 units within the first 24 h of treatment.

Recently, there has been a great deal of interest in administering insulin by either continuous intravenous infusion or frequent intramuscular injection. Smooth achievement of control, less hypoglycemia, and a smaller total insulin dose have been demonstrated in various studies. However, not all studies have found equal or improved metabolic responses in their patients. Thus, until additional studies come forth, it is probably best to use the older standard regimens.

3 All patients in diabetic acidosis are severely dehydrated and depleted of sodium and potassium. They will require a large amount of fluid, usually a total of 4 to 8 liters during the first 24 h. Many electrolyte formulas have been proposed for adequate replacement; though their value is not doubted, it is important to start fluid therapy *immediately,* which is best done with the universally available normal (0.9 percent) saline solution. Once treatment is under way and the laboratory has reported values for blood glucose, serum CO_2, and electrolytes, finer adjustments can be made. Part of the fluid may be given as ½*N* saline, particularly in older persons, in whom the central venous pressure should be monitored. The addition of bicarbonate is indicated only if the acidosis is very severe (pH less than 7.0 or 7.1) or the serum bicarbonate is exceptionally depressed (5 mM per liter or less). Bicarbonate, if used, should be administered slowly, and both pH and serum K should be evaluated frequently, and bicarbonate should be immediately discontinued if pH reaches 7.15. A paradoxical CSF acidosis occurs in relationship to the bicarbonate administration. Also, as the systemic acidosis is corrected, it may unmask low red blood cell 2,3-diphosphoglycerate levels. Whereas the acidosis shifts the hemoglobin-oxygen dissociation curve to the right, the reduced 2,3-diphosphoglycerate levels shift the curve to the left, resulting in a compensation. When the acidosis alone is corrected, the shift to the left of the curve due to reduced 2,3-diphosphoglycerate levels may produce tissue hypoxia. Since both phosphate and potassium depletion tend to parallel each other, potassium phosphate can readily be administered (a concentrated IV addition containing 60 meq of both potassium and phosphate in 30 ml is available). Potassium solutions are best administered at a rate not exceeding 20 meq per h; rarely is

TABLE 95-9
Guidelines for insulin dose schedule*

	At 1 h after immediate treatment; blood glucose value of...			
Immediate insulin† *(diagnosis certain)*	*< 300 mg per 100 ml*	*> 300 mg per 100 ml*	*> 600 mg per 100 ml*	*> 1,000 mg per 100 ml*
Adult or mature adolescent				
10 to 25 U IV 10 to 25 U s.c.	0	10 to 25 U IV 10 to 25 U s.c.	50 to 75 U IV 50 to 75 U s.c.	75 to 100 U IV 75 to 100 U s.c.
Adult or mature adolescent (no insulin for many hours or unconscious)				
25 to 50 U IV 25 to 50 U s.c.	0	25 to 50 U IV 25 to 50 U s.c.	75 to 100 U IV 75 to 100 U s.c.	100 to 150 U IV 100 to 150 U s.c.
Children: age ten years or more but not fully grown				
5 to 10 U IV 5 to 10 U s.c.	0	5 to 10 U IV 5 to 10 U s.c.	25 to 35 U IV 25 to 35 U s.c.	40 to 50 U IV 40 to 50 U s.c.
Children: under age ten years				
3 to 5 U IV 3 to 5 U s.c.	0	3 to 5 U IV 3 to 5 U s.c.	15 to 20 U IV 15 to 20 U s.c.	20 to 25 U IV 20 to 25 U s.c.

* *If CO_2 content is 9 mM/liter or less, give the larger insulin dose; if it is 10 to 15 mM/liter and clinical assessment warrants, give lower insulin dose.*
† *All insulin is regular.*

there a need to administer more than 100 to 200 meq during the initial 24 h of treatment. It is best to commence phosphate administration about 2 to 3 h after the treatment program has been started, at a time when the extracellular fluid compartment has been somewhat repleted. (A commonly used additive to IV saline is potassium chloride, 2 meq per ml.) It has been suggested that 50 to 70 meq phosphate should be administered (calcium solutions should never be given along with phosphate). The need for and administration of potassium can be monitored with the ECG. Signs of hypokalemia are flattening or inversion of T waves, depressed S-T segments, prolongation of the Q-T interval, and appearance of U waves. Hyperkalemia produces a high-peaked T wave, wide QRS, disappearance of P waves, AV dissociation, and, at high levels, disorganization of the ECG. Once the blood glucose approaches 200 mg per 100 ml, intravenous fluid should be changed to 5% glucose in saline in order to avoid hypoglycemia and possible cerebral edema, as the patient responding to treatment will suddenly become more sensitive to insulin.

4 There are useful accessory procedures in the treatment of diabetic acidosis. If the patient is unconscious, gastric lavage should be performed to prevent aspiration pneumonia. If the patient is in obvious circulatory collapse, blood, plasma, or a plasma volume expander should be given. Finally, the precipitating cause for the development of diabetic acidosis has to be established for each patient so that specific treatment can be initiated. Errors frequently made are (*a*) not providing enough insulin soon enough, (*b*) not providing enough fluids, (*c*) not providing enough potassium, (*d*) providing too much bicarbonate.

5 The acute phase of diabetic acidosis is considered to be ended once the patient is completely responsive, the blood glucose level is below 200 mg per 100 ml, the serum diluted 1:1 shows no evidence of acetone, serum CO_2 is normal, and the urine shows minimal glycosuria. Ketonuria may persist for 24 to 48 h. Now is the time to start the patient on intermediate insulin in a small dose to prevent a relapse into ketosis, and also, if needed, to give crystalline insulin in amounts dictated by urine sugar levels. A soft diet should be started. It is essential to begin with frequent small feedings. Intravenous fluid administration may be discontinued as soon as the patient is able to retain liquids by mouth. The overall mortality rate of patients with diabetic ketoacidosis is approximately 5 percent. It may be 10 to 20 percent in a city or county hospital because patients arrive late. A very rare but serious complication of diabetic ketoacidosis is facial mucormycosis (see Chap. 176). Also, cerebral edema with irreversible coma should be kept in mind.

HYPERGLYCEMIC HYPEROSMOLAR NONKETOTIC COMA

This entity is characterized by extreme elevation of blood glucose levels (values of 1,000 mg per 100 ml or higher are not rare; "syrupy" blood), and absent or only minimal ketonemia. The marked hyperglycemia and the associated hypernatremia secondary to water loss lead to an increase in extracellular fluid osmolarity with consequent intracellular dehydration, the effect of which on the central nervous system accounts for the neurologic symptoms and coma. This syndrome is probably more widespread than has been estimated in the past. It is usually seen in middle age but more commonly in older subjects, frequently in nursing homes. In two-thirds of cases, prodromal symptoms of polydipsia, polyuria, and glycosuria have been present, and some degree of renal impairment can be demonstrated in the majority of patients. An acute illness often is a precipitating event (i.e., pneumonia, uremia, pyelonephritis, pancreatitis, or acute myocardial infarction). In other instances, there may be a precipitating procedure such as peritoneal dialysis, hemodialysis, severe burn, or hyperalimentation. A number of drugs have been thought to trigger this syndrome, among them corticosteroids, diuretics (thiazides and furosemide), propranolol, diphenylhydantoin, and immunosuppressive agents. The clinical picture is one of shock, hyperpyrexia, tachycardia, postural hypotension, and hyperventilation, occasionally with Kussmaul-type respiration. The skin shows decreased turgor, the mucous membranes are dry, the eyes are sunken and soft. Neurologic disorders are many and may include hyperreflexia, mild disorientation, and coma. One-third of the patients may have seizures, usually focal in nature, and Kernig's sign has been seen.

Laboratory findings are an elevated blood glucose, generally greater than 600 mg per 100 ml, absent or mild elevations of plasma acetone, an elevated BUN (that is, <50 mg per 100 ml), an elevated creatinine, normal to elevated electrolytes, normal to slightly depressed pH, and a distinctly elevated serum osmolarity. Serum osmolarity can be estimated by multiplying the Na concentration times 2 and adding 5.5 for each 100 mg glucose (molecular weight of glucose is 180, therefore $100/18 = 5.5$) and 3.6 for each 10 mg per 100 ml BUN. Normal values range between 290 and 310 milliosmoles per liter. A patient with values of Na of 160 meq per liter, blood glucose of 1,000 mg per 100 ml, and a BUN of 40 mg per 100 ml exhibits an approximate serum osmolarity of $320 + 55 + 14 = 389$ milliosmoles per liter. The highest level recorded is 458 milliosmoles per liter.

Why these patients show minimal ketosis is not clear. It is plausible that insulin levels sufficient to minimize ketosis but insufficient to reduce the hyperglycemia might be the basis for this syndrome. The extreme hyperosmolarity itself could have an important metabolic effect upon intermediary metabolism. Current studies have suggested that the profound hyperosmolarity may have an inhibitory effect upon adipose tissue lipolysis, reducing free fatty acid flux to the liver, and thus preventing increased ketogenesis.

Treatment should be instituted rapidly. Because of the fragile condition of these patients and the many uncertainties regarding the nature of this syndrome, guidelines have been difficult to establish regarding fluid, electrolyte, and insulin treatment programs. Throughout treatment, constant observations and frequent blood chemistry studies are required. Intravenous fluid, preferably hypotonic saline (one-half normal) should be administered at a rate of 0.5 to 1.0 liter per h, particularly if the serum sodium is greater than 130 meq per liter and the patient is normotensive. If the serum sodium is less than 130 meq per liter, and the patient is hypotensive, normal saline should probably be given and plasma expanders considered. Some evidence suggests that initially, normal saline should be given, followed an hour or so later by one-half normal saline. The basic objective is to gradually rehydrate both the intracellular and extracellular fluid compartments without overloading the cardiovascular system, producing disparities of the distribution of water and electrolytes among body fluid compartments, or, on the other hand, producing circulatory collapse by too-rapid a shift of fluid from the vascular space to the extravascular (intracellular) space.

Insulin must be given intravenously. Caution initially must be maintained until the effect of the initial dose upon blood glucose and electrolytes has been observed. A dose of 10 to 40 U regular (crystalline) insulin appears appropriate. Some patients are markedly sensitive to insulin. Within 2 to 3 h after initiation of therapy, trends will emerge both clinically and biochemically that will influence the next stage of treatment. Fluid infusion rates can then be adjusted, potassium and phosphate can be added to the infusion fluid, and additional insulin (20 to 50 U) can be given intravenously. A too-rapid fluid replacement rate or a too-rapid decline of blood glucose is to be avoided. The blood glucose level should not be less than 250 mg per 100 ml during the first 24 to 48 h. Assessments of the clinical picture and the blood glucose levels should be determined every 2 to 3 h, and additional insulin given if required. Some patients may require a total amount of insulin of only 25 U, whereas others may require 200 U or more. Mortality rates have been as high as 40 to 75 percent. Approximately one-third expire within the first 24 h of treatment. The main causes of death are associated illnesses, shock, electrolyte abnormalities, and cerebral edema. In those who recover, later control of diabetes may not necessitate insulin therapy.

LACTIC ACIDOSIS This is a frequent concomitant of shock (cardiogenic, hemorrhagic, septic, etc.). It can also be seen associated with leukemia, diabetes, and following ethanol and phenformin ingestion. States producing tissue hypoxia can produce this syndrome characterized by acidosis (pH less than 7.3) and an increase in blood lactate (greater than 2.0 meq per liter). The plasma bicarbonate levels are low and an anion gap produced by the excess lactate is present. To be remembered is the fact that the Acetest test for ketosis may be spuriously low in lactic acidosis (acetoacetate relatively low but β-hydroxybutyric acid relatively high).

Therapy is to be focused upon reduction of lactate production and the acidosis. First, the aim should be to increase tissue perfusion, reduce hypoxia, and combat shock. Sodium bicarbonate administration, sometimes in large doses, is usually required. Attention to blood sugar levels and serum electrolytes is mandatory.

DIABETIC RETINOPATHY This can be detected in varying degrees in more than 90 percent of diabetic patients after 20 years of clinical diabetes.

The earliest recognizable lesions on fundoscopy are dilatation of veins and "microaneurysms," which actually consist of small punctate hemorrhages. Unless they occur within the macula, the vision will not be impaired. Capillary degeneration leads to fluid leakage from the vessels and patches of edema occur which appear to be the site of exudate formation. This stage of the retinopathy can remain stationary for many years. It is the patient with long-term juvenile diabetes whose condition may progress to a more malignant stage, that of neovascularization and proliferative retinopathy. The new blood vessels usually emanate from the disk and grow toward the vitreous. If a preretinal hemorrhage occurs, organization takes place with formation of fibrous and collagenous tissue. Shrinkage of the scar tissue will produce retinal detachment (see Color Plate 8). Advanced diabetic retinopathy is frequently associated with retinal lesions caused by atherosclerosis, arterial hypertension, and renal insufficiency.

The appearance of retinopathy is fundamentally related to duration of diabetes. Controversy exists over whether strict chemical control of the metabolic component of diabetes will delay its onset or make it less severe. Photocoagulation is considered when the process has proceeded to the stage of edema and exudates. The earlier stages of venous dilatation, microaneurysms, and hemorrhages are usually not treated. Proliferative retinopathy (neovascularization) is another indication for photocoagulation. Newer forms of treatment are directed toward the affected eyes themselves and include various green and red laser treatments of the retina. Preliminary results indicate that these procedures may be applied to *early* retinal lesions, and the results obtained are encouraging. Although various types of pituitary ablation procedures have been employed as a treatment for diabetic retinopathy, enthusiasm for them has diminished.

A large-scale collaborative study of various retinal photoablative procedures is underway which may provide the answers to many questions concerning these procedures. A recent report from this study shows that photocoagulation treatment is beneficial in patients whose eyes have extensive new vessels on or near the optic disk. Treatment also appears to be beneficial when vitreous hemorrhage is present and when early new vessels on or near the optic disk are present, and also in patients with extensive new vessels away from the optic disk in the presence of vitreous hemorrhage. Also encouraging are various new types of vitreous surgery to remove fibrinous membranes, blood clots, etc. These permit retinal examination, photocoagulation of abnormal bleeding vessels, and improvement of vision.

DIABETIC NEPHROPATHY See Chap. 283.

DIABETIC NEUROPATHY This is a common, distressing complication of diabetes which is difficult to treat at any stage. Although it most frequently involves peripheral nerves, it may involve any portion of the nervous system and, thus, has an almost unlimited range of manifestations (Table 95-10). The peripheral neuropathy is characterized by a nonsegmental distribution. An interesting differential diagnosis is presented by the patient with severe headache and ocular palsy. If an intracranial aneurysm can be ruled out by angiogram, diabetic neuropathy may be the underlying cause. The neuropathy may be primarily metabolic (sorbitol pathway), which is potentially reversible, or primarily vascular, which is less amenable to treatment.

Neuropathy related to sexual function (retrograde ejaculation, impotence) has been identified as a most disturbing complication of diabetes in men. One study has found lesions of the autonomic nerves in the corpora cavernosa. Libido persists despite the impotency (see Chap. 51).

Treatment of diabetic neuropathy consists of careful

control of the diabetes; unfortunately, it is not specific, and weeks or months may pass before improvement, if any, takes place. Diphenylhydantoin (Dilantin), 100 mg three or four times daily, has provided some patients with relief. If improvement is not noted in 3 to 4 days, therapy should be discontinued.

GANGRENE OF THE FEET This is a serious and frequent complication of diabetes, especially in the older age group. It may be due to vascular lesions ("pulseless" foot) or to neuropathy ("painless" foot), usually with a superimposed infection or injury. Gangrene may also be associated with small-vessel disease in which pedal pulses are not decreased. Arterial insufficiency is diagnosed by a history of claudication, nocturnal cramps, or night pain. On examining the patient, one finds weak or absent pedal pulses, blanching of the foot when it is raised above a 45° angle, cyanosis, and delayed venous filling when the foot is dependent. There may be lack of hair growth and muscle atrophy. Diagnostic aids include oscillometry, arteriography, and ultrasonic flowmeter (Doppler). If arterial bypass operation fails or cannot be done, amputation is the treatment; unfortunately, in one-third of the patients amputation of one leg is followed by loss of the other leg within 3 years. Hence, prevention or at least delay of onset, of gangrene is of paramount importance. Education of the patient to prevent injuries and infections is of the utmost importance. Simple rules for prevention include (1) washing the feet with warm but *never hot* water each evening; (2) applying lanolin two or three times weekly if the skin is dry; (3) inserting lamb's wool between overlapping toes; (4) avoiding injuries to feet (the patient should never go barefoot); (5) not cutting toenails if vision is poor; (6) treating of corns and calluses by a qualified podiatrist or surgeon; (7) stopping smoking.

SURGERY AND DIABETES MELLITUS

Patients with diabetes mellitus may be affected by any surgical disease and on rare occasion may even be the object of spectacular surgical triumphs; the first successful heart transplant was performed in a diabetic. In addition, in the diabetic population-at-large conditions requiring surgery, such as peripheral vascular disease, gallbladder disease, and cancer of the pancreas, are more frequent.

The present surgical mortality in diabetics is approximately that of the general population. The surgical risk is increased in diabetics in the presence of poor metabolic control, obesity, arteriosclerosis, and cardiovascular-renal disease. However, even for the patient with uncomplicated diabetes, operation and anesthesia constitute an additional metabolic stress, which will accentuate the predisposition to hyperglycemia and ketosis. Nevertheless, diabetes constitutes no contraindication to surgery; if the case is an emergency, only a few hours are generally needed to evaluate and prepare such a patient for operation.

On admission for elective or emergency surgery, the patient with diabetes presents either of two situations: he is a known diabetic under treatment with varying degree of metabolic control, or the diagnosis of diabetes is suggested by routine preoperative testing. If the scheduled surgery is elective in nature and the diabetes requires further regulation, surgery should be postponed until glycosuria is minimal, acetonuria absent, and the preprandial blood glucose level close to normal. If, on the other hand, surgery is urgent and marked hyperglycemia and ketosis are present, vigorous treatment is started immediately with intravenous fluid and insulin. The majority of diabetic patients will not present this dramatic problem. Their management during surgery will vary according to the severity of their condition. As a general principle, one should aim to prevent acetonuria and excessive protein breakdown by providing an adequate carbohydrate intake. This is done on the day of surgery by replacing the oral feedings with intravenous 5% or 10% glucose in water or saline solution, the volume being dictated by the cardiac state and fear of overhydration. Usually, 1,000 to 1,500 ml of 5% glucose in saline solution is sufficient. By history and laboratory evaluation three types of diabetes are encountered: (1) Patients with mild diabetes, treated with diet alone; only close surveillance with frequent urine testing and daily blood glucose is required. (2) Patients on oral hypoglycemic agents. As oral intake is usually impossible on the day of surgery, these patients are best changed to a small amount of intermediate-acting (lente or NPH) insulin, for example, 10 to 20 units. Once oral feedings are resumed in the postoperative period, insulin is discontinued and the respective tablets are restarted at the former dose. (3) Patients previously on insulin and with well-controlled diabetes receive on the day of surgery two-thirds of their usual *total* dose, preferably divided into a preoperative and postoperative dose, and with crystalline insulin omitted. Example: Preoperative insulin dose = 10 units crystalline insulin 35 units NPH, total dose 45 units. Therefore, on the day of surgery, one-third, or 15 units, NPH is given preoperatively, and 15 units NPH is given postoperatively. It is customary in some centers not to give any preoperative insulin, presumably because of fear of hypoglycemia, and only to administer crystalline insulin according to urine test in the postoperative period. In our experience, hypoglycemia occurs rarely if the preoperative insulin is only NPH or lente, provided the total dose is reduced by one-third and, furthermore, if glucose is administered intravenously throughout the operative period. The benefits of this regimen are that the patient does not escape into severe hyperglycemia or ketosis with resultant electrolyte imbalance during surgery or the

TABLE 95-10
Diabetic neuropathies

PERIPHERAL
Sensory: loss of vibratory sense, paresthesias, pain, loss of pain, usually subacute, symmetric, and distal
Neuromuscular: weakness, paralysis, absent tendon reflexes, diabetic amyotrophy (thighs), extraocular muscle palsies
AUTONOMIC
Eye: pupillary changes
Gastrointestinal: delayed gastric emptying, gallbladder dysfunction, nocturnal diarrhea
Genitourinary: sexual impotence, atonic urinary bladder, retrograde ejaculation
Vascular: orthostatic hypotension
Bones and joints: neuropathic joint (Charcot)
Skin: neurogenic ulcer, absent sweating, dependent edema

immediate postoperative period. In summary, treatment of the diabetic during surgery will depend on previous diabetic management and on the extent of the surgical procedure, as outlined in Table 95-11.

PREGNANCY AND DIABETES MELLITUS

The problem of management during pregnancy has assumed increasing importance, as young diabetic patients now survive longer and are thus capable of procreation. Infertility in female diabetic patients, common before insulin therapy, is rarely seen with good control of the diabetes. The problems engendered by pregnancy in diabetics concern maternal survival, fetal salvage, and prevention of diabetes in the offspring.

Today pregnancy carries but slightly added risk to the mother with well-managed diabetes; the maternal survival is 99.7 percent (White). In contrast, fetal mortality is still high. Stillbirths among diabetics are six times as common as among nondiabetics. Fetal salvage ranges between 90 to 95 percent and will depend on the duration of the mother's disease and presence or absence of vascular lesions such as nephropathy.

DIAGNOSIS In patients not previously known to be diabetic, pregnancy may induce a temporary state of diabetes. The diagnosis may offer some difficulty, since with the lowered renal threshold of pregnancy, glycosuria is not uncommon even among nondiabetic pregnant women. If urinary glucose is found during pregnancy and there is, in addition, a history of frequent miscarriages, of babies with a birth weight exceeding 9 lb, or a family history of diabetes, diabetes should be suspected. The diagnosis can be firmly established only by abnormal blood glucose levels, whether fasting or postprandial. If they are borderline, performance of a glucose tolerance test is definitely indicated. Diagnostic criteria are slightly different during pregnancy. The upper limit of normal at the second hour is 145 rather than 120 mg per 100 ml.

TREATMENT The best results are obtained by close cooperation between the patient, the internist, and the obstetrician. The treatment of pregnant diabetic patients entails the same general health measures as those recommended for nondiabetic pregnant women. It is desirable to maintain a high intake of protein (i.e., at least 2 g/kg body weight/day) with a total caloric intake of 30 kcal per kg body weight and an adequate intake of calcium and iron. To prevent edema and minimize hydramnios, a low-salt diet is indicated, and the liberal use of diuretics is advisable. In most women, diabetes is regulated throughout pregnancy with insulin. Because of the lowered renal threshold for glucose one should not attempt to keep the urine sugar-free. It is admittedly often difficult to avoid excessive weight gain, but at least 200 g carbohydrate must be utilized to prevent ketosis.

Care of a diabetic patient through the first trimester may be difficult because of nausea and vomiting. In the last trimester the insulin requirement usually increases concurrently with a rise in adrenal cortical activity, the presence of placental lactogen, and placental destruction of insulin. It is of utmost importance to detect preeclamptic toxemia and hydramnios, since treatment will reduce fetal mortality. Timing of delivery is also important. The more advanced the diabetic state of the mother, the earlier the delivery should be attempted. Fetal viability can be monitored by determining estradiol levels in maternal urine. Patients with only chemical diabetes can be delivered at term; patients with vascular complications should be delivered at the thirty-sixth week. The child may be delivered vaginally or by section. Early delivery has the advantage of removing the infant before it becomes too large and before placental circulation is impaired. The latter may be either the cause or the effect of the tendency of toxemia. A sudden decrease of insulin requirement to prepregnancy level or even lower usually follows delivery, presumably because of removal of placental lactogen or possibly a temporary state of hypopituitarism. Thus, it is advisable to omit insulin altogether on the day of delivery and to administer only one-half the prepregnancy dose for 3 to 5 days following delivery. Similarly, any coverage with regular insulin should be reduced, that is, 10 units for 4+ urine sugar, 5 units for 3+, and no coverage for 2+, 1+, or trace.

TABLE 95-11
Management of diabetes on the day of surgery

	Previous diabetic treatment		
Surgical procedure	*Diet only*	*Oral hypoglycemic agent*	*Insulin*
Minor	Observe	Withhold until after procedure	Withhold until after procedure
Major	Observe	Change to insulin (10–20 units NPH)	One-third of total dose preoperatively; one-third postoperatively; crystalline insulin only if needed

REFERENCES

ALBERTI KGMM et al: 2,3-Diphosphoglycerate and tissue oxygenation in uncontrolled diabetes mellitus. Lancet 2:391, 1972

BEIGELMAN PM: Severe diabetic ketoacidosis, 482 episodes in 257 patients. Diabetes 20:490, 1971

BIERMAN EL: Principles of nutrition and dietary recommendations for patients with diabetes mellitus. Diabetes 20:633, 1971

LUNDBECK K, KEEN H: *Blood Vessel Disease in Diabetes Mellitus,* Milano, Italy: Il Ponti, 1971

MCGARRY J, FOSTER DW: Regulation of ketogenesis and clinical aspects of the ketotic state. Metabolism 21:471, 1972

MARBLE A et al (eds): *Joslin's Diabetes Mellitus,* 11th ed., Philadelphia: Lea & Febiger, 1971

NELSON PG et al: Histocompatibility antigens in diabetic identical twins. Lancet 2:193, 1975

Proceedings Fiftieth Anniversary Insulin Symposium (Indianapolis, Ind., Oct. 18–20, 1971). Diabetes 21:385, 1972

Report of the National Commission on Diabetes to the Congress of the United States. U.S. Department of Health, Education and Welfare, Public Health Service, National Institutes of Health. DHEW Publication No. (NIH) 76-1018 to 76-1024, 76-1031 to 76-1033, 1976

SOLER NG et al: Comparative study of different regimens in management of diabetic ketoacidosis. Lancet 2:1221, 1975

SPIRO RG: Search for a biochemical basis for diabetic microangi-

ography. Diabetologia 12:1, 1976
SUSSMAN K: *Juvenile-onset Diabetes,* Springfield, Ill.: Charles C Thomas, 1971
University Group Diabetes Program: A study of the effects of hypoglycemia agents on vascular complications in patients with adult-onset diabetes. Diabetes 19 (Suppl 2):474, 1970
——: A study of the effects of hypoglycemic agents on vascular complications in patients with adult-onset diabetes. V. Evaluation of phenformin therapy. Diabetes 24 (Suppl 1):65, 1975

96
NONDIABETIC MELITURIAS

J. STUART SOELDNER

DEFINITION The nondiabetic meliturias comprise a group of diverse conditions in which sugar is detected in the urine by usual clinical testing in patients in whom diabetes mellitus is not suspected on other clinical grounds. In all cases of melituria, the clinical and laboratory work-up of the patient must include studies that rule out diabetes mellitus (see Chap. 95).

CLASSIFICATION The major distinction to make among meliturias is whether they are glucosurias or nonglucosurias. The readily available copper reduction type of tests (such as Clinitest, Ames Company), which detect any reducing sugar, and glucose-specific tests (such as Clinistix, Ames Company, or Tes-Tape, Eli Lilly and Company) permit easy and rapid differentiation of glucosuric from nonglucosuric meliturias. The general classification of the meliturias is outlined in Table 96-1. Of all the other types of meliturias, *only sucrosuria* will not be detected by the copper reduction type of tests.

There are certain situations in which the conventional tests for melituria will be adversely affected. Some conditions, disease states, drugs, or poisons which might influence the conventional urine tests are outlined in Table 96-2. It is of more than passing interest that many situations result in both a false positive copper reduction test and a false negative (or delayed positive) glucose oxidase enzyme test.

TABLE 96-1
The meliturias

Group	*Compounds*
Pentosurias	L-Xylulose, L-arabinose, D-ribose
Hexosurias	Glucose*, galactose, fructose
Heptosurias	Mannoheptulose
Dissaccharidurias	Lactose, sucrose†, maltose

* *The only sugar which produces a positive glucose oxidase test*
† *Will* not *produce positive copper reduction test*

PHYSIOLOGY The renal glomerular filtrate contains glucose in a concentration which equals that in plasma water. Glucose is reabsorbed in the proximal convoluted tubules by an energy-requiring active transport process. As the concentration of glucose in plasma water increases, the amount of glucose actively absorbed by the tubules reaches a transfer maximum (Tm) which in the normal adult is about 300 to 350 mg per min. When arterial blood glucose levels reach 150 to 180 mg per 100 ml, the amount of glucose presented to the tubules usually exceeds the Tm, and glucose begins to appear in the urine. Theoretically, as the glucose load delivered to the nephron increases, the amount reabsorbed by the tubules approaches a maximum Tm. In man, this theoretic situation is never quite achieved. Deviations from this ideal (or splay) occur in which glucose is excreted by the kidney before the Tm is reached. It is suspected that as the glucose load increases toward the Tm, some individual nephrons will achieve their Tm and excrete glucose. The blood glucose concentration which results in glucosuria is usually termed the *renal threshold.* Among the important factors that can vary this threshold are the glomerular filtration rate, variations in renal blood

TABLE 96-2
Factors responsible for deviant urine tests for melituria

I False positive copper reduction type tests	
Condition:	*Compound:*
A Unclean glassware	Some dentifrices, cleansers, and bleaches
B Antibiotic therapy	Penicillin, streptomycin, cephalosporins, nalidixic acid, isoniazid, para-aminosalicylic acid, chloramphenicol, tetracyclines
C Renal tubule transport blockers	Carinamide, probenecid
D L-Dopa therapy	3,4-Dihydroxyphenylacetic acid
E Alkaptonuria	Homogentisic acid
F Miscellaneous drugs/poisons	Salicylates, ascorbic acid, chloral hydrate, chloroform, hippuric acid, amino acids, formaldehyde, oxalic acid, phenols, menthol, and turpentine
G Certain x-ray contrast media	Sodium diatrizoate (Hypaque), meglumine iothalamate (Conray), diatrizoate meglucamine (Renovist)
II False negative copper reduction type tests	
A Outdated reagents	
III False positive glucose oxidase enzyme strips	
A Unclean glassware	Certain cleansers and detergents (hypochlorite, chlorine, and peroxides)
IV False negative (or delayed positive) glucose oxidase enzyme strips	
A Conditions above (*ID to IF*)	
B Carcinoid syndrome	5-Hydroxyindoleacetic acid
C Hepatic disease	Bilirubin glucuronide
D Uremia	Indoles

distribution, and minor alterations in the ratio of glomerular filtering surface to tubular absorptive capacity resulting in a normal distribution of slight glomerulo-tubular imbalances, physiologically expressed as splay about the mean Tm.

Some patients with diabetes mellitus may have a renal threshold lower than normal. Parallel studies of blood glucose and urine glucose will furnish a practical guide as to the significance of glucosuria in such patients.

GLUCOSURIC MELITURIAS

It should be assumed that any glucosuric melituria represents diabetes mellitus until proved otherwise. Following the detection of glucosuria (a positive glucose oxidase urine test), it is of prime importance to document the blood sugar level and the corresponding degree of glucosuria. A large number of conditions, some relatively infrequent, can produce both glucosuria and hyperglycemia in the absence of true idiopathic diabetes mellitus (Table 96-3). In many situations, the glucosuria may be present when only mild carbohydrate or glucose intolerance is present. Disease of the pancreas (or the islet of Langerhans) resulting in a functional deficiency of beta cells are sometimes obvious (such as in pancreatitis), but may be geographically localized and/or rare (scorpion bite).

The relation between various hyperendocrinopathies and hyperglycemia, with resultant glucosuria, should be kept in mind as causes of *secondary diabetes mellitus.* In addition, a number of diseases involving the central nervous system have been shown to be related to hyperglycemia and/or glucosuria. Many varieties of gastrointestinal disease have also been implicated. Renal diseases, especially the uremic state, appear to be associated with glucosuria. A relatively large number of metabolic diseases and chronic diseases are also implicated as causes of nondiabetic glucosuria, again usually associated with hyperglycemia or carbohydrate intolerance.

Those conditions associated with clear-cut hyperglycemia or variable hyperglycemia are discussed in detail in Chap. 95. Those conditions mentioned in Sec. II of Table 96-3 represent a group in which care must be taken to document the presence of hyperglycemia. Temporary renal glucosuria may occur in pregnancy, especially in the latter half. If screening blood glucose tests (such as a blood glucose level determined 1 h after a breakfast liberal in carbohydrate) are suspicious, then an oral glucose tolerance should be done. If this is not normal, repeat tests should be performed (see Chap. 95). Much the same approach should be used to exclude diabetes in chronic disease states. In these situations, however, the deleterious effect of age, poor nutrition, and inactivity per se upon the glucose tolerance test should be kept in mind. The following discussion deals primarily with those glucosurias not associated with hyperglycemia (Table 96-3).

RENAL GLUCOSURIA This is a benign condition characterized by the excretion of glucose in the urine in the pres-

TABLE 96-3
Nondiabetic glucosurias

- *I* Usually not associated with hyperglycemia
  - *A* Renal
    - *1* Renal glycosuria
    - *2* Fanconi syndrome
  - *B* Drugs/chemical agents/poisons
    - *1* Phlorizin
    - *2* Heavy metal salts (chromium, mercury, uranium, ferric compounds, lead, cadmium, lithium)
    - *3* Curare
    - *4* Carbon monoxide
    - *5* Caffeine
    - *6* Morphine
    - *7* Strychnine
    - *8* Chloroform
  - *C* Metabolic
    - *1* Glucoglycinuria (rare)
    - *2* Glucose-galactose malabsorbtion (rare)
- *II* Relation to hyperglycemia uncertain or variable
  - *A* Metabolic
    - *1* Pregnancy
  - *B* Chronic disease
    - *1* Rheumatoid arthritis
    - *2* Malignant disease
    - *3* Vascular hypertension
    - *4* Chronic nephritis and nephrosis
  - *C* Chemical
    - *1* Organophosphorous compounds
    - *2* Pimozide
- *III* Usually associated with hyperglycemia
  - *A* Ablation of islets of Langerhans
    - *1* Surgical removal
    - *2* Pancreatitis, acute or chronic
    - *3* Carcinoma of pancreas
    - *4* Hemochromatosis
    - *5* Cystic fibrosis
    - *6* Scorpion bite pancreatitis
  - *B* Endocrine hyperfunction
    - *1* Acromegaly
    - *2* Hyperthyroidism
    - *3* Hyperadrenocorticism
    - *4* Pheochromocytoma
    - *5* Functioning beta-cell tumor
    - *6* Functioning alpha-cell tumor
  - *C* Nervous system diseases
    - *1* Hypothalamic damage
    - *2* Amyotrophic lateral sclerosis
    - *3* Severe emotional stress
    - *4* Brain tumors
    - *5* Brain trauma
    - *6* Cerebral hemorrhage
  - *D* Gastrointestinal disease
    - *1* Severe hepatic disease
    - *2* Glycogen storage diseases
    - *3* Postgastrectomy syndrome
  - *E* Renal disease
    - *1* Uremia
  - *F* Metabolic disease
    - *1* Obesity
    - *2* Infections
    - *3* Poststarvation feeding
    - *4* Burns
    - *5* Physical inactivity
    - *6* Potassium deficiency
    - *7* Lipoatrophic diabetes
    - *8* Fractures
    - *9* Asphyxia
  - *G* Drugs
    - *1* Oral antiovulatory steroids (progestational-estrogenic)
    - *2* Benzothiadiazine compounds (chlorothiazides, hydrochlorothiazides, diazoxide)
    - *3* Adrenocorticosteroids/adrenocorticotropic hormone
  - *H* Miscellaneous/mixed
    - *1* Postmyocardial infarction

ence of a normal concentration of blood glucose. The "true" type of renal glucosuria is rare. This is defined as persistent and constant glucosuria even in the fasting state with blood glucose levels below 100 mg per 100 ml. There are, however, other types of renal glucosuria in which the renal threshold is somewhat reduced so that glucosuria occurs after meals or glucose loads but not in the fasting state. A renal glucose titration test has been devised to quantify the Tm and to estimate the minimum threshold (F_{min}). By means of this technique, two types of abnormal curves have been described: type A in which there is a low threshold and a low Tm, and type B with a low threshold, an exaggerated splay to the curve, and a normal Tm.

Studies of families exhibiting renal glucosuria have shown that mild and severe types A and B can occur in the same pedigree, suggesting that familial renal glucosuria can be inherited as an autosomal recessive trait. Renal biopsy studies, few in number, have not revealed any specific anatomic defect. Thorough evaluation of these patients by multiple blood glucose determinations, fasting or following meals, and oral glucose tolerance tests clearly rules out diabetes. Ketosis develops only during starvation rather than following dietary excess. Although this disease appears not to be related to diabetes, some studies have suggested that it may progress to true diabetes; however, the greater bulk of evidence suggests that the prevalence of diabetes in these patients is no greater than in the general population. Renal glucosuria, particularly the more severe type, appears to be a lifelong condition. Its severity may be reduced as the subject ages, probably because of arteriosclerosis. Hypertension or renal disease may also minimize the degree of glucosuria. In contrast to the frequent urinary tract infections seen in diabetic glucosuria, urinary tract infections appear not increased. Care must be taken at the time of diagnosis to identify those persons with borderline oral glucose tolerance tests. A regular follow-up program for at least the first few years should establish effectively the diagnosis of a benign condition.

FANCONI SYNDROME In addition to renal glucosuria, various other entities are related to glucosuria without hyperglycemia. The Fanconi syndrome with defective absorption of amino acids, phosphate, bicarbonate, and glucose is described in greater detail elsewhere (see Chaps. 104 and 105). This syndrome secondary to ingestion of outdated tetracyclines and multiple myeloma has also been described.

CHEMICAL AGENTS An increasing number of drugs, chemicals, poisons, and toxins have been related to defects of renal tubular absorption of glucose, particularly heavy metal salts.

METABOLIC A combined glucosuria/glycinuria has been described, but is quite rare.

NONGLUCOSURIC MELITURIA

In patients with persistent normoglycemic melituria, identification of the type of sugar excreted is important. The vast majority prove to be glucose, but the number of nonglucosurias is sufficiently frequent to warrant special study. These nonglucosurias are for the most part benign and have no relation to diabetes. Their recognition may have important ramifications in regard to employment, military service, life insurance, etc. By the use of readily available testing materials, a preliminary diagnosis can often be made.

TEST PROCEDURES

1 Benedict's test, or a modification (Clinitest). This test is positive for all sugars found in urine, except sucrose. Fructose, L-xylulose, and mannoheptulose produce a positive reaction somewhat easier than does glucose (10 min at 55°C, or 3 h at room temperature using Benedict's test).
2 Glucose oxidase test (glucose specific). Paper strips (Tes-Tape and Clinistix) are available for quick testing. False negative or delayed positive results can occur (see Table 96-2).
3 Bial (orcinol hydrochloride) reaction. It is positive for pentose.
4 Seliwanoff (resorcinol hydrochloride) reaction. It is positive for fructose.
5 Paper chromatography systems can readily identify the sugar.
6 Osazone crystals. Characteristic crystals can be produced with phenylhydrazine (methylphenylhydrazine for fructose). In addition, glucose and fructose produce the same osazone but at slightly different rates. Melting point determinations show a characteristic 205°C for glucosazone and 157 to 160°C for pentosazone.
7 Fermentation with baker's yeast. Glucose and fructose are always, galactose usually, lactose occasionally, and pentose and mannoheptulose never, fermented.

PENTOSURIA Essential pentosuria, or chronic essential pentosuria, is a rare benign condition inherited as an autosomal recessive trait. Only 1 in 40,000 to 50,000 applicants for life insurance in the United States were found to have this condition. Most reported cases have been in Jewish or Lebanese families. It is characterized by the excretion of L-xylulose in the urine, 1 to 4 g per day. The Benedict's test usually shows a green end point. Paper chromatography easily demonstrates the L-xylulose. Current evidence suggests that this condition is produced by a deficiency of NADP-linked xylitol dehydrogenase, which is involved in the xylitol step in the glucuronic acid pathway (glucuronic acid to gulonic acid to L-xylulose to xylitol to D-xylulose to pentose phosphate pathway to hexose phosphate). The condition is harmless, asymptomatic, and unrelated to diabetes. It requires no treatment. The heterozygote can be identified by a glucuronolactone loading test.

Alimentary pentosuria in which the urine may contain small amounts (less than 0.1 g) of L-arabinose or L-xylose may follow the ingestion of large amounts of plums, cherries, fruit juices, or grapes. Ribosuria (D-ribose) in very small amounts may be found in the urine of some patients with muscular dystrophy.

FRUCTOSURIA **Essential fructosuria** This is a benign asymptomatic metabolic defect which is rare and appears to be confined to Jewish people. Males and females are equally affected. Less than 100 cases appear in the world literature. Following fructose ingestion in these persons, blood fructose levels reach higher values and remain higher for a longer period of time than in normal subjects. About 10 to 20 percent of a fructose load may appear in the urine. It is thought that there is a primary deficiency of hepatic fructokinase in these subjects. reducing the conversion of fructose to fructose 1-phosphate. No treatment is required in this condition.

Hereditary fructose intolerance This condition is a rare error of metabolism in which ingestion of fructose or foods high in fructose leads to symptomatic hypoglycemia and vomiting. In the very young, failure to thrive, hepatomegaly, jaundice, ascites, and plasma electrolyte imbalance may be seen. Occasionally, some degree of renal tubular dysfunction is noted. The metabolic defect is a deficiency of hepatic fructose 1-phosphate aldolase usually associated with a deficiency of hepatic fructose 1,6-diphosphate aldolase. It is thought to be inherited as an autosomal recessive trait. The mechanism responsible for the hypoglycemia is thought to be due to reduced gluconeogenesis and/or glycogenolysis rather than increased peripheral glucose utilization. Hepatic levels of adenosine triphosphate (ATP) and inorganic phosphorus are reduced, which may explain the defective hepatic glucose output.

Early recognition and treatment is mandatory if liver damage, renal dysfunction, and death are to be avoided. If fructose-containing foods are eliminated from the diet, the outlook is excellent. Interestingly, these patients usually have few or no dental caries, owing to their avoidance of foods containing fructose or sucrose.

GALACTOSURIA Galactosemia is a congenital and hereditary disease characterized by an inability to utilize ingested galactose or galactose-containing foods. Galactosuria is seen only when galactose is part of the diet (see Chap. 112).

HEPTOSURIA Mannoheptulose may appear in the urine after one eats large amounts of avocado. Although it is of no clinical importance, it is of interest that mannoheptulose inhibits insulin secretion by the beta cell.

DISACCHARIDURIA

Lactosuria Lactose may appear in the urine toward the end of pregnancy and during lactation. During pregnancy, the finding of sugar in the urine should be followed up by a glucose tolerance test. Lactosuria can, of course, be a presumptive diagnosis on the basis of a positive copper reduction test but a negative glucose oxidase enzyme test. Lactosuria can be seen in patients with severe intestinal damage (celiac sprue) and in children with lactose intolerance without lactase deficiency. Lesser and variable lactosuria occurs in the syndrome of lactose intolerance with lactase deficiency.

Maltosuria Maltosuria and isomaltosuria are rare, but have been reported in the urine of severely injured patients.

Sucrosuria Alimentary sucrosuria has been noted in normal individuals ingesting large amounts of cane sugar. Small amounts of sucrose have been described in the urine of patients with cystic fibrosis. Endogenous sucrosuria, difficult to explain, has been noted rarely. In reported cases, specific gravity of the urine has been as high as 1.070, and up to 200 g sucrose has been detected in a 24-h urine collection. One must keep in mind *cases of deception* in which patients bring in a urine sample to which they have added cane sugar, not realizing that sucrose will not produce a positive copper reduction test or a positive glucose oxidase enzyme test. *An unusually high specific gravity leads one to think of factitious sucrosuria.* A more difficult case of deception is the urine sample to which a reducing sugar has been added.

REFERENCES

ELSAS LJ, ROSENBERG LE: Familial renal glycosuria: A genetic reappraisal of hexose transport by kidney and intestine. J Clin Invest 48:1845, 1969

LEVIN B et al: Fructosaemia: Observations on seven cases. Am J Med 45:826, 1968

MARBLE A: Nondiabetic melituria, in *Joslin's Diabetes Mellitus,* 11th ed., eds A Marble et al, Philadelphia: Lea & Febiger, 1971, p. 818

STANBURY JB et al (eds): *The Metabolic Basis of Inherited Disease,* 4th ed., Pentosuria, HH Hiatt; Fructosuria, ER Froesch; Cystinosis and the Fanconi Syndrome, JE Seegmiller et al; Renal Glycosuria, SM Krane; New York: McGraw-Hill, in press

WANG YM, VAN EYS J: The enzymatic defect in essential pentosuria. N Engl J Med 282:892, 1970

97 HYPERINSULINISM, HYPOGLYCEMIA, AND GLUCAGON SECRETION

STEFAN S. FAJANS

The maintenance of a constant blood glucose level is an essential part of homeostasis. A blood glucose level below the lower limits of normal reflects a defect in one or more of two kinds of homeostatic processes: (1) those which add glucose to the blood by (1) mobilization of glucose from glycogen stores, (b) formation of carbohydrate from nonglucose sources (gluconeogenesis), and (c) absorption of ingested carbohydrate; and (2) those which remove glucose from the blood through utilization of glucose by liver, adipose tissue, muscle, brain, and other tissues.

Spontaneous hypoglycemia is a symptom complex caused by or associated with a variety of diseases. A precise classification of hypoglycemia based on etiology and pathologic physiology that is both complete and logical is difficult to establish, since in some entities the mechanism is still poorly understood while in others the cause of hypoglycemia may be multifactorial. From the clinical view, patients with hypoglycemia can be grouped according to the usual relation of hypoglycemia to the fasting or postprandial (fed) state as listed in Table 97-1. This scheme facilitates an approach to diagnosis. The table and text indicate the conditions which cause hypoglycemia primarily in infancy and childhood. Interference with the homeostatic mechanisms that regulate the blood glucose level may take place at different steps of metabolism or in different tissues, even if the underlying cause of hypoglycemia is a single one. For example, in patients with hyperinsulinism, hypoglycemia may be the result of inhibition of hepatic glucose production, of increased glucose uptake in insulin-sensitive tissues, and of decreased inflow to the liver of substrates needed for gluconeogenesis, such as reduced mobilization of amino acids from muscle and of glycerol from fat. As another example, impaired hepatic glucose output due to reduced gluconeogenesis may be the result of a number of causes, such as : (1) hormonal excess [insulin or nonsuppressible insulin-like activity (NSILA)], (2) deficiency of hormones, such as cortisol or glucagon, which cause acute activation of hepatic enzymes or chronic induction of enzyme synthesis, (3) decreased supply of substrates, such as amino acids, glycerol, or lactate, due to a variety of causes (cortisol or growth hormone deficiency, or of idiopathic origin), (4) decrease in substrate oxidation, (5) genetic deficiency of a rate-limiting hepatic enzyme, or (6) diffuse hepatic disease.

The clinical symptoms and signs of hypoglycemia are the same regardless of the underlying cause. The symptoms which occur in any given patient vary with the degree and the rate of decline of blood glucose levels and with the variable and individual susceptibility of the underlying state of the central and autonomic nervous systems. Symptoms associated with a rapid decline in blood glucose levels are due in part to activation of the autonomic nervous system and the ensuing release of epinephrine. The symptoms are sweating, shakiness, trembling, tachycardia, palpitation, piloerection, anxiety, nervousness, weakness, fatigue, hunger, nausea, and vomiting. Other symptoms of hypoglycemia result from decreased uptake of glucose and decreased utilization of oxygen by the brain. They usually occur when the decline in blood glucose to low levels is slow and/or when hypoglycemia is severe or prolonged. These symptoms are headache, lightheadedness, disturbance of vision, lethargy, yawning, faintness, restlessness, sense of unreality, and difficulty with speech and thinking. Other manifestations may be agitation, mental confusion, outbursts of temper or queer, bizarre, and psychotic behavior, somnolence, stupor, prolonged sleep, loss of consciousness, coma, fever, and hypothermia. Twitching, convulsions, "epilepsy," and bizarre neurologic signs, motor as well as sensory in nature, may occur. Prominent signs observed in patients with alcohol-induced hypoglycemia are hypothermia, conjugate deviation of eyes, extensor rigidity of extremities, positive Babinski signs, and trismus. Repeated hypoglycemic episodes may lead to loss of intellectual ability. Extensive and permanent mental or neurologic damage may result from frequent and prolonged episodes of hypoglycemia, particularly in children.

TABLE 97-1
Classification of spontaneous hypoglycemia

- *I* Fasting hypoglycemia
  - *A* Organic hypoglycemia: recognizable anatomic lesion
    - *1* Pancreatic islet beta-cell disease with hyperinsulinism in the adult*
      - *a* Adenoma, single or multiple
      - *b* Microadenomatosis, with or without macroscopic islet-cell adenomas
      - *c* Carcinoma, with metastases
      - *d* Adenoma(s) or carcinoma, associated with adenomas or hyperplasia of other endocrine glands (familial multiple endocrine adenomatosis)
      - *e* Hyperplasia (rare)
    - *2* Pancreatic islet beta-cell disease with hyperinsulinism in infancy and childhood*
      - *a* Hyperplasia (leucine-sensitive or -insensitive)
      - *b* Nesidioblastosis
      - *c* Adenoma
    - *3* Nonpancreatic tumors associated with hypoglycemia
    - *4* Anterior pituitary hypofunction
    - *5* Adrenocortical hypofunction
    - *6* Acquired diffuse hepatic disease
    - *7* Severe congestive heart failure
    - *8* Severe renal insufficiency in non-insulin-dependent diabetic patients
  - *B* Hypoglycemia due to specific hepatic enzyme deficiency (infancy and childhood)
    - *1* Glycogen storage diseases
    - *2* Glycogen synthase deficiency
    - *3* Fructose 1,6-diphosphatase deficiency
  - *C* Functional hypoglycemia: no recognizable or persistent anatomic lesion
    - *1* Ethanol and poor nutrition
    - *2* Deficiency of glucagon†
    - *3* Severe inanition
    - *4* Ketotic hypoglycemia (infancy and childhood)
    - *5* Transient hypoglycemia in the newborn of low birth weight
    - *6* Transient hyperinsulinism of the newborn (hyperplasia of pancreatic islet cells reported)
      - *a* Infant of diabetic mother
      - *b* Erythroblastosis fetalis
    - *7* Insulin autoimmunity without previous insulin administration (?)
  - *D* Exogenous hypoglycemia
    - *1* Insulin administration
    - *2* Sulfonylurea administration
    - *3* Ingestion of ackee fruit (hypoglycin)
    - *4* Miscellaneous drugs
- *II* Reactive (postabsorptive) hypoglycemia
  - *A* Functional hypoglycemia: no recognizable anatomic lesion
    - *1* Reactive functional: idiopathic
    - *2* Reactive secondary to mild diabetes
    - *3* Alimentary hyperinsulinism
  - *B* Hypoglycemia due to specific hepatic enzyme deficiency
    - *1* Hereditary fructose intolerance (fructose 1-phosphate aldolase deficiency): infancy and childhood
    - *2* Galactosemia: infancy and childhood
    - *3* Familial fructose and galactose intolerance

* *May manifest also as reactive (postabsorptive) hypoglycemia which is glucose- or leucine-induced.*
† *May manifest also as reactive (postabsorptive) hypoglycemia, which is amino acid-induced.*

PANCREATIC ISLET-CELL DISEASE

Pathology Approximately 90 percent of functioning islet-cell tumors are benign; approximately 10 percent are definitely malignant with identified metastases. Scattered microadenomatosis interspersed with normal islets, with or without macroscopic adenomas, occurs in about 10 percent of patients with benign tumors. The author is aware of only a few patients with proved diffuse hyperplasia of the islet cells as a cause of hyperinsulinism and hypoglycemia in the adult. Functioning islet-cell tumors may be diagnosed at any age, with a majority of cases occurring between thirty and sixty years. Benign islet-cell adenomas vary in size from 0.15 to 15 cm in diameter, but the majority are between 0.5 and 3.0 cm. They are usually encapsulated, firmer than the normal pancreas, highly vascular, purplish and occasionally whitish in color, and they may present a smooth or irregular surface. They are found to be equally distributed throughout the head, body, and tail of the pancreas. Benign adenomas of islet-cell tissue rarely occur outside the pancreas. Multiple adenomas are found in approximately 10 percent of cases. Multiple adenomas of islet cells may be associated with adenomas or hyperplasia of the parathyroids and other endocrine glands (familial multiple endocrine adenomatosis) and with peptic ulceration (ulcerogenic Zollinger-Ellison syndrome). Insulin-secreting malignant islet-cell tumors and islet tumors of patients with microadenomatosis or familial multiple endocrine adenomatosis may also secrete other polypeptide hormones such as glucagon, gastrin, adrenocorticotropic hormone (ACTH), and melanocyte-stimulating hormone (MSH). Some tumors, including heterotopic pancreatic islet-cell tumors, may produce 5-hydroxytryptophan and/or serotonin and are associated with the carcinoid syndrome. A family history of diabetes has been found in 25 to 30 percent of patients with functioning islet-cell tumors.

Clinical picture Symptoms of hypoglycemia due to islet-cell adenoma may develop insidiously, with periodic hypoglycemic attacks becoming more frequent and more severe. Fasting and exercise precipitate attacks. Attacks usually occur in the early morning hours before breakfast, when the patient would have been fasting the longest, or they may occur in the late afternoon, especially if the noon meal is missed. Symptoms may also occur 2 to 5 h after meals. Symptoms and signs secondary to decreased cerebral oxygen utilization usually predominate over symptoms secondary to hyperepinephrinemia. The pattern of symptoms is usually repetitive in the same patient, but it may differ from patient to patient. Many patients learn to avert symptoms by taking frequent feedings, including a feeding at night. Obesity may thereby result but is not seen in the majority of patients. In patients with malignant, metastatic tumors, symptoms are rapidly progressive or may arise from hepatic metastases.

FIGURE 97-1

A *Abnormal levels of plasma insulin and blood glucose and abnormal IRI/G during last 4 h of a 14-h fast in a patient with proved islet-cell adenoma (I.H.).* B *Normal levels of plasma insulin and blood glucose and normal IRI/G during a 72-h fast in an 18-year old female patient (C. C.) with functional reactive hypoglycemia.*

Diagnosis A typical symptomatic attack with demonstrated hypoglycemia and relief of symptoms and signs by administration of glucose constitute the diagnostic criteria outlined by Whipple. This "triad of Whipple" is not specific for patients with hyperinsulinism due to pancreatic islet-cell disease, as it may occur in patients with other types of hypoglycemia. The level of plasma glucose after an overnight fast (10 h) is usually below 60 mg per 100 ml, but it may be normal in some patients. There may be fluctuation from normal to subnormal from day to day. In seven (18 percent) of our last 38 patients with proved islet-cell disease all overnight fasting plasma glucose levels were above 60 mg per 100 ml on seven consecutive days. More prolonged fasting is the most helpful diagnostic procedure to document fasting hypoglycemia. Prolongation of the overnight fast for 4 h usually will cause a fall in plasma glucose to below 50 mg per 100 ml. In the majority of patients more severe fasting hypoglycemia (plasma glucose below 35 mg per 100 ml) can be induced within the first 12 to 24 h of fasting. In subjects without fasting hypoglycemia, plasma glucose will not decline below 60 mg per 100 ml during the first 24 h of fasting. If hypoglycemia and typical symptoms are not induced, fasting should be prolonged for up to 72 h, at which time the patient should be exercised vigorously. In patients with insulinomas, or other types of fasting hypoglycemia, exercise produces a further fall in blood glucose levels, but it produces a rise in blood glucose in patients with functional hypoglycemia. On clinical grounds, other types of organic hypoglycemia and the exogenous hypoglycemias can usually be ruled out.

Assays of plasma insulin (Chap. 95) performed in conjunction with fasting plasma glucose levels provide the most reliable data with which to confirm or establish a diagnosis of insulinoma. In our laboratory, the upper limit of normal for a fasting plasma concentration of insulin in nonobese subjects (below 116 percent of ideal body weight) is 24 μU per ml (mean + 2 SD). Elevated fasting levels of plasma insulin in peripheral blood (in absolute terms) are not found in all patients with functioning islet-cell tumors. Thus, while a diagnosis of insulinoma is confirmed by an elevated fasting insulin level, a "normal" level does not rule out this diagnosis. When fasting insulin levels are measured daily for several days in the same patient, an elevated level can frequently be found in at least one specimen. Nevertheless, even when measurements were made on 7

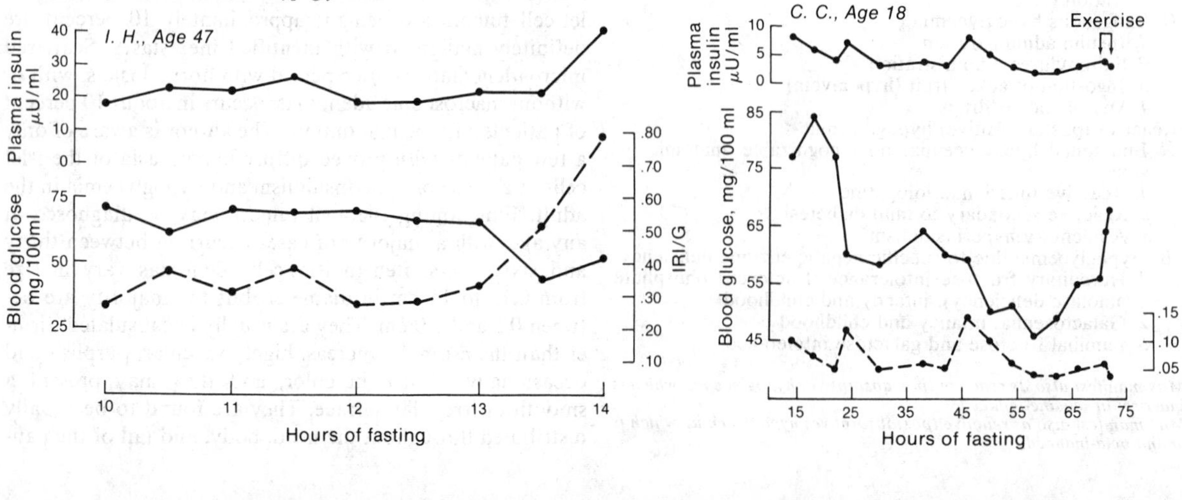

consecutive days, fasting plasma levels of insulin were not found to be elevated in 6 (16 percent) of 38 patients. However, a plasma insulin level in the "normal range" associated with a fasting blood sugar level in the hypoglycemic range is also significant, as it is inappropriately high for the existing level of blood glucose. In addition, when the overnight fast is prolonged for 4 h or more in patients with pancreatic islet-cell disease and with fasting plasma glucose levels in the borderline range, the plasma glucose level may fall into the hypoglycemic range while the level of serum insulin remains constant or rises. This demonstrates an abnormal glucose-insulin homeostatic relation (Fig. 97-1) and is good evidence for the presence of autonomous insulin-producing tissue. An abnormal insulin-glucose relationship in the fasting state can be expressed as the ratio of the plasma concentration of immunoreactive insulin (in microunits per milliliter) to the concentration of plasma glucose (in milligrams per 100 ml), (IRI/G). The use of an "amended IRI/G" may provide even greater discrimination between inappropriately elevated levels of serum IRI and normal levels (see Table 97-2). During the 72-h fast the decreases in blood glucose are greater in females than in males, but there is a proportional fall in plasma insulin, so that the IRI/G or "amended IRI/G" ratio is the same for males and females. Utilizing the IRI/G or amended IRI/G ratio, 68 or 79 percent, respectively, of our 38 patients with islet-cell disease had abnormal ratios after the first overnight fast. On the basis of fasting plasma specimens collected after five consecutive overnight fasts, all patients had abnormal ratios. When a single overnight fast was prolonged for up to 14 h, all but two of these 38 patients had abnormal ratios. In normal subjects and in those patients whose hypoglycemia is not caused by hyperinsulinism, fasting is associated with a progressive fall in plasma insulin concentration and maintenance of a normal IRI/G or amended IRI/G ratio.

An elevated fasting level of plasma insulin after an overnight fast is not specific for insulinoma. It is also seen in obese patients (without fasting hypoglycemia) and has been reported in patients with galactosemia and familial fructose and galactose intolerance. The IRI/G ratio would be expected to be normal in these patients.

The estimation of fasting plasma levels of proinsulin and "proinsulin-like components" may be helpful in the diagnosis of islet-cell tumors particularly when one cannot demonstrate definite increases in plasma levels of total immunoreactive insulin (IRI). In 82 percent of patients with islet-cell tumors the proinsulin component was clearly elevated and exceeded 25 percent of fasting total IRI.

Provocative tests of insulin secretion are rarely necessary in the differential diagnosis of hypoglycemia, but they may be useful in some insulinoma patients who have levels of serum insulin in the borderline range and who can tolerate prolonged fasts without symptoms. The tumors may secrete excessive amounts of insulin on stimulation. The intravenous tolbutamide test is one such test. After blood for a fasting blood glucose determination is obtained, 1 g sodium tolbutamide dissolved in 20 ml distilled water is injected intravenously over 2 min. Subsequently blood levels of glucose are determined every 15 min for the first hour and every 30 min during the second and third hours of the test. Plasma levels of insulin are obtained during the test at the same time intervals, and, in addition, at least every 5 min during the first 15 min after administration of tolbutamide.

TABLE 97-2
Work-up of adult patient with suspected hypoglycemia

I Careful history and physical examination
II Laboratory tests and procedures
- *A* Patient with suspected "reactive" or functional hypoglycemia
  - *1* Glucose tolerance test to differentiate between:
    - *a* Reactive functional hypoglycemia
    - *b* Reactive hypoglycemia secondary to mild diabetes mellitus
    - *c* Alimentary hyperinsulinism
    - *d* "Pseudohypoglycemia" or "nonhypoglycemia"
  - *2* If fasting hypoglycemia needs to be ruled out, proceed with *B1*. Fast up to 72 h with exercise at end
- *B* Patient with suspected fasting hypoglycemia
  - *1* Fasting plasma glucose and insulin levels
    - *a* After overnight fast, multiple daily determinations
    - *b* During 4-h prolongation of overnight fast
    - *c* During 12- to 72-h fast, if fasting plasma glucose level is not diagnostic after *(a)* and *(b)*, use multiple determinations
    - *d* After exercise during last 2 h of 72-h fast, blood specimens before and after exercise
    - *e* Determine: $\frac{\text{IRI}}{\text{G}}\left(\frac{\text{plasma insulin } \mu\text{U/ml}}{\text{plasma glucose mg/dl}}\right)^*$

      "amended" $\frac{\text{IRI}}{\text{G}}\left(\frac{\text{plasma insulin } \mu\text{U/ml} \times 100}{\text{plasma glucose mg/dl} - 30}\right)^\dagger$
  - *2* Provocative tests of insulin secretion. (Pancreatic islet-cell disease suspected or to be ruled out; insulin levels with *B1* not yet available or not diagnostic. Islet-cell tumor suspected because entities given in *4* to *7* have been ruled out; no, minimal, or moderate hypoglycemia after overnight fast)
    - *a* Tolbutamide test
    - *b* Leucine test
    - *c* Glucagon test

      } serial plasma glucose and insulin determinations
  - *3* Islet-cell tumor diagnosed
    - *a* Celiac and mesenteric angiography for localization
    - *b* Liver scan if carcinoma suspected in view of rapid course, severe hypoglycemia, and hyperinsulinemia
    - *c* X-ray of skull, serum calcium, and phosphorus to rule out multiple endocrine adenomatosis
  - *4* In older patient consider extrapancreatic neoplasm within thorax, liver, abdomen, retroperitoneal space, pelvis
    - *a* X-ray of chest
    - *b* Flat film of abdomen
    - *c* Gastrointestinal series
    - *d* Intravenous pyelogram
  - *5* If pituitary, adrenal, or pancreatic alpha-cell insufficiency suspected:
    - *a* Growth hormone levels after arginine infusion, insulin-induced hypoglycemia, L-dopa, or exercise
    - *b* Adrenal cortical function tests: metyrapone test
    - *c* Glucagon levels after arginine infusion
  - *6* Diffuse liver disease: liver function tests, response to glucagon
  - *7* Rule out factitious hypoglycemia
    - *a* Insulin antibodies are usually a sign of recent insulin administration; measurement of serum-connecting peptide.
    - *b* Check for sulfonylurea blood levels; urinary tolbutamide excretion product; leucine sensitivity
  - *8* Test for gluconeogenetic reserve if alcohol hypoglycemia suspected, alcohol infusion, pituitary and adrenal function tests

* $\frac{IRI}{G}$ *abnormal:* > *0.30 in nonobese patients*
> *0.30* and *plasma glucose below 60 mg per dl in obese patients*

† "Amended" $\frac{\text{IRI}}{\text{G}}$ *abnormal:* > *50 in nonobese patients*
> *50* and *plasma glucose below 60 mg per dl in obese patients*

A normal response to tolbutamide consists of a return of blood glucose to 70 percent or more of fasting levels after an initial drop in blood glucose. In patients with islet-cell tumors tolbutamide induces a greater reduction in blood glucose and prolonged hypoglycemia. Tolbutamide-induced hypoglycemia persisted for 3 h in 50 of 55 patients subsequently proved to have insulinomas. In these 55 patients fasting blood glucose levels were 50 mg per 100 ml or above. The lower the fasting blood glucose, the more frequently will the test have to be terminated early because of severe neurologic symptoms. False positive blood glucose responses can occur in association with severe liver disease, alcoholic hypoglycemia, idiopathic hypoglycemia of infancy, severe undernutrition, and azotemia. They also may occur in some patients with nonpancreatic tumors and associated hypoglycemia, particularly in those patients in whom blood glucose levels decrease rapidly with fasting. In contrast, no false positive glucose responses have occurred in patients with functional hypoglycemia or diabetes mellitus with reactive hypoglycemia, or in patients without spontaneous hypoglycemia.

Assays of plasma insulin in conjunction with the intravenous tolbutamide test are essential for the interpretation of an abnormal serum glucose response and allow termination of the test when necessary. The finding of excessive increases in plasma insulin levels (above 195 μU per ml within the first 15 min after intravenous administration of tolbutamide and/or, more significantly, prolonged elevation thereafter of plasma insulin, with increments above basal levels of 50 μU per ml at 30 min and/or of 25 μU per ml at 45 min and of 15 μU per ml at 60 min) differentiates insulinoma patients from patients with false positive blood glucose responses. Approximately 85 percent of patients with islet-cell tumors exhibit an abnormal insulin response to intravenously administered tolbutamide. However, an increase in levels of insulin in the normal range after intravenous tolbutamide does not rule out the existence of hyperinsulinism due to pancreatic islet-cell disease.

Sensitivity to leucine may be useful diagnostically. In adolescent or adult patients, a decrease in blood glucose over 25 mg per 100 ml *and* a maximum increase in plasma insulin over 30 μU per ml or a sustained increase in plasma insulin of more than 20, 15, and 10 μU per ml at 30, 60, and 90 min after administration of leucine (200 mg per kg over 30 min) strongly suggest diagnosis of an insulinoma. Approximately 80 percent of patients with functioning islet-cell tumors exhibit an exaggerated response to leucine. In childhood, sensitivity to leucine does not differentiate between islet-cell hyperplasia and insulinoma. Severe leucine-induced hyperinsulinemia and hypoglycemia will also be obtained in factitious hypoglycemia due to surreptitious administration of sulfonylureas, since profound sensitivity to leucine-hypoglycemia can be induced in normal subjects by pretreatment with such compounds. A negative response to leucine does not rule out the existence of an insulinoma.

After the intravenous administration of 1 mg glucagon, an exaggerated increase in serum levels of insulin over 160 μU per ml and/or increases above 60, 40, and 20 μU per ml at 30, 40, or 60 min, respectively, is seen in 50 to 75 percent of patients with islet-cell tumors. When this occurs, the hyperglycemic effect of glucagon may be subnormal and may be followed by a profound fall in blood glucose.

If provocative tests are to be employed in patients with suspected islet-cell disease, all three tests should be used, since an abnormal response may be obtained with one but not another of these tests. Obese patients may have an exaggerated rise in plasma insulin with any of these stimuli to insulin secretion, but the hyperinsulinemia is not accompanied by abnormal levels of plasma glucose.

The oral glucose tolerance test (Chap. 95) may give a relatively flat curve with a fall of plasma glucose into the hypoglycemic range without a rebound elevation due to excessive insulin release from the tumor. In contrast to its indispensability for the differentiation of the common causes of the reactive (postabsorptive) hypoglycemias of the functional type, this test is not useful in the differential diagnosis of the fasting hypoglycemias.

A suppression test has been described for the diagnosis of insulinomas. When fish insulin was used to induce hypoglycemia in 12 patients with insulinomas, suppression of endogenous insulin secretion (measured with antiserum specific to human insulin) was impaired in all, in contrast to normal or obese subjects. Unfortunately, fish insulin is not available in most countries.

Inappropriate elevation of the concentration of plasma insulin in the presence of hypoglycemia after an overnight fast or after more prolonged fasting remains the cornerstone of the diagnosis of pancreatic islet-cell disease in the adult. For a brief discussion of islet-cell disease in infancy and childhood, refer to Other Causes of Fasting Hypoglycemia below.

Treatment When the diagnosis of functioning islet-cell disease with hyperinsulinemia is made, early surgery is indicated to relieve hypoglycemia and distressing symptoms, to prevent possible damage to the central nervous system, and to prevent obesity, which makes surgical management more difficult. Identification of a tumor at the time of surgery may present a problem. Selective pancreatic (celiac and mesenteric) arteriography has made it possible to localize some of these tumors preoperatively. It was successful in locating a tumor radiographically in 15 of 28 patients with proved islet-cell tumors. Of these 15 tumors, several were located in the head of the pancreas and could not be palpated by the surgeon at the time of laparotomy.

The benzothiadiazine compound, diazoxide, particularly when used in conjunction with one of the diuretic thiazides, such as trichlormethiazide, has been useful to elevate blood levels of glucose into the normoglycemic range if operation must be delayed for weeks or months. Diazoxide causes increase in blood glucose by decreasing the secretion of insulin. In addition, diazoxide and the diuretic thiazides elevate blood glucose by one or more extrapancreatic mechanisms. Effective combination dosages range between 150 and 450 mg for diazoxide and 1 and 3 mg for trichlormethiazide per day. The drugs should be discontinued 2 days before surgery.

The surgical approach to insulinomas may be complicated by difficulty in identifying the tumor, particularly when the tumors are small, located deep within the pancreatic parenchyma, and not detected by angiography. Moreover, multiple tumors are not uncommon. If a tumor is not identified, meticulous and extensive exploration of the pancreas including the head and uncinate process should be carried out using multiple capsulotomies, if necessary, after the pancreas has been mobilized and its entire length has been palpated. In the absence of finding a definite insulinoma, resection of first the tail and then the body of the pancreas, up to the great vessels, is justified, since a significant proportion of tumors are located in these areas. After excision of the adenoma or a 70 to 80 percent pancreatectomy, the patient is usually cured, except in cases of unlocated tumors in the head of the pancreas or in some patients with microadenomatosis. In the latter case, treatment with diazoxide and trichlormethiazide has been successful for up to 8 years. Diphenylhydantoin, another suppressor of insulin release, has not been shown to be as useful as a palliative agent in such patients.

In approximately 20 percent of cases diagnosed histologically as carcinoma, follow-up observations have failed to reveal a recurrence of symptoms or tumor for several years. Lethal hyperpyrexia has been reported in the first few postoperative days; a temperature of over 104°F warrants the intravenous administration of glucocorticoids.

Patients with nonresectable metastatic islet-cell tumors present a management problem, since their hypoglycemia may be so severe as to respond only poorly to oral and even intravenous glucose administration. Diazoxide has proved to be an effective agent for the alleviation of symptomatic and biochemical hypoglycemia in some of these patients. To counteract the sodium-retaining effect of diazoxide administered in a dose of 600 to 1,000 mg per day, a natriuretic thiazide should be used.

In patients with metastatic islet-cell carcinoma, the careful use of streptozotocin is indicated. This antibiotic, experimental antitumor agent is a highly effective cytotoxic agent for pancreatic beta cells, although it can cause renal and hepatic toxicity. Some patients with metastatic islet-cell carcinoma who were treated with streptozotocin have had complete relief from hypoglycemia and regression of tumor mass for months or years.

The use of glucocorticoids may also be valuable.

NONPANCREATIC TUMORS ASSOCIATED WITH HYPOGLYCEMIA Severe hypoglycemia has been reported in more than 200 patients harboring nonpancreatic tumors of mesothelial, epithelial, or endothelial origin. Most of these tumors are mesothelial in type and are classified as fibromas, sarcomas, or fibrosarcomas. They are usually situated in the thorax, the retroperitoneal space, or the pelvis. They may be attached to the diaphragm or found within the liver. Other cases of nonpancreatic tumors associated with severe hypoglycemia include more than 40 patients with primary hepatic carcinoma, 14 with carcinoma of the adrenal cortex, 5 with gastrointestinal carcinomas, 2 with pseudomyxoma peritonei, 2 with bronchogenic carcinoma, and 1 with a bronchial carcinoid tumor. The common clinical characteristics of these tumors, particularly of the fibrosarcomas, are their slow growth and their massive size (up to 10 kg). Hypoglycemia disappears after resection or occasionally after irradiation of the tumor. Many theories have been advanced to explain the mechanism by which these tumors cause hypoglycemia, but none of these is applicable to all patients. A block in hepatic glucose output, excessive glucose consumption by tumor tissue with a high rate of anaerobic glycolysis, and inhibition of lipolysis have been reported in some of these patients. In the majority of patients immunoreactive insulin and insulin-like activity in serum or extract of tumor tissue have been normal or subnormal. High levels of serum insulin have been reported in one patient with severe hypoglycemia due to a large fibrosarcoma and in another patient with a bronchial carcinoid tumor with metastases. Only rarely have tumor extracts contained immunologically recognizable insulin. Twelve reports indicate that extracts of tumors from some of these patients contain an insulin-like substance stimulatory in either isolated rat diaphragm or epididymal fat pad systems. It is possible that some of these tumors synthesize a polypeptide closely related to insulin, but which, in the majority of instances, is not recognized immunologically as insulin. It may suppress hepatic glucose output. Recently, by the use of a new radioreceptor assay, elevation in the circulating concentration of the insulin-like peptide, NSILA-S (nonsuppressible insulin-like activity soluble in acid alcohol) was detected in five of seven hypoglycemic patients with nonislet-cell tumors.

OTHER CAUSES OF FASTING HYPOGLYCEMIA Although it is infrequent, fasting hypoglycemia may occur in patients with *hypofunction of the anterior pituitary* (Chap. 90) or *hypofunction of the adrenal cortex* (Chap. 93) when associated with poor nutrition. Usually, other stigmata of these disorders enable one to make a diagnosis. In infants and children, hypoglycemia due to isolated growth hormone deficiency has been reported. Occasionally, diffuse and extensive *hepatic disease* may be associated with hypoglycemia. Fasting hypoglycemia has been observed in patients with *severe congestive heart failure* and in diabetic patients with *severe renal insufficiency* at a time when the need for insulin or hypoglycemic agents has disappeared. Reduced delivery of gluconeogenetic substrates to the liver may be responsible for the hypoglycemia.

Hypoglycemia due to a genetic defect in a specific *hepatic enzyme* involved in glycogenolysis or gluconeogenesis is infrequent and occurs primarily in children. Occasionally fasting hypoglycemia can be traced to a glycogen storage disease (Chap. 111). A syndrome consisting of hypoglycemia and lactic acidosis in infancy due to a defect in hepatic fructose 1,6-diphosphatase activity has been described.

Alcohol ingestion superimposed upon an inadequate dietary intake can precipitate acute hypoglycemia. Blood glucose levels as low as 10 or 20 mg per 100 ml have been observed. Inhibition of gluconeogenesis is primarily responsible for the hypoglycemia in conjunction with depletion of liver glycogen stores. In healthy subjects alcohol may precipitate hypoglycemia after fasting for 48 to 72 h. In certain susceptible individuals (such as patients with ACTH deficiency) alcohol may precipitate hypoglycemia without prior deprivation of food intake. The blood glucose response to infused ethanol has been used as a test for gluconeogenetic reserve in patients in whom a susceptibility to alcohol hypoglycemia is suspected.

A young male has been reported who developed hypoglycemia on prolonged fasting (28 h) as well as after protein meals. *Glucagon deficiency* was documented during fasting and after ingestion of protein meals and infusion of arginine. Also, *severe inanition* may lead to fasting hypoglycemia, presumably due to failure of delivery of an adequate supply of substrates for gluconeogenesis.

In infancy and childhood the most common type of fasting hypoglycemia is that classified as *ketotic hypoglycemia.* Usually by nine years of age these children "outgrow" the occurrence of hypoglycemia. In susceptible children, "ketotic hypoglycemia" (onset usually after eighteen months of age) is precipitated by caloric deprivation. Such children are thought to have a deficiency of the gluconeogenetic precursor, alanine. Plasma levels of insulin are appropriate for the prevailing level of plasma glucose.

Infants with hyperinsulinemic hypoglycemia (pancreatic islet-cell disease), whether leucine-insensitive, have more persistent fasting hypoglycemia. In these children with either islet-cell hyperplasia or nesidioblastosis, preoperative differentiation from functioning islet-cell tumors is impossible at present, although the occurrence of insulinoma is uncommon in this age group. Transient fasting hypoglycemia and hyperinsulinemia have also been reported in newborn infants of diabetic mothers, and in infants with erythroblastosis fetalis. Fasting hypoglycemia also occurs in infants with visceromegaly, gigantism, microcephaly, macroglossia, and omphalocele.

In the leucine-sensitive and leucine-insensitive types of hyperinsulinemic hypoglycemia, plasma levels of insulin are usually elevated. In these infants and in the transient neonatal hypoglycemia in infants of diabetic mothers or of erythroblastosis fetalis, plasma levels of insulin, when in the normal range in absolute terms, are inappropriately high in the presence of hypoglycemia.

EXOGENOUS HYPOGLYCEMIA The possibility of factitious hypoglycemia as a result of surreptitious administration of insulin or sulfonylureas should always be considered, particularly in nurses, other medical personnel, and relatives of diabetic patients. The clinical features may be indistinguishable from those of patients with functioning islet-cell tumors, and some patients have undergone pancreatic resection during which no abnormality was found before the correct diagnosis was made. If self-administration of insulin is suspected, the presence of insulin antibodies in serum may suggest it. Determination of insulin antibodies in the serum should be part of the evaluation of every patient with the clinical features of an insulinoma. (See determination of serum-connecting peptide below.)

Several patients with spontaneous hypoglycemia have been reported whose serum contained insulin-binding antibodies without previous *known* immunization to exogenous insulin. These patients have been thought to have a form of "insulin autoimmunity." During the periods of hypoglycemia, large amounts of immunoreactive insulin were extracted from the serum. If such a syndrome exists, specifically differentiated from factitious hypoglycemia due to self-administration of insulin, hypoglycemia may occur when insulin secretion from beta cells continues after saturation of the insulin-binding capacity has been approached, or when insulin becomes disassociated from the antigen-antibody complex containing excessive insulin. The latter phenomenon may occur in some diabetic patients in whom larger than usual amounts of insulin-binding antibodies are produced by administration and immunization with exogenous insulin. It may be difficult to distinguish between spontaneous hypoglycemia produced by possible "insulin autoimmunity" and factitious hypoglycemia due to surreptitious administration of insulin. Measurement of serum-connecting peptide may be of help in determining whether the insulin measured in plasma is of endogenous or exogenous origin.

In the case of ingestion of tolbutamide (Orinase) in large amounts, acidification of the urine will disclose a white precipitate which is a crystallization of the carboxylated excretion product of tolbutamide. In addition, plasma concentrations of sulfonylurea drugs may be determined. In Jamaica, profound hypoglycemia has occurred in individuals who have ingested the unripened ackee fruit containing the amino acid, hypoglycin. It leads to interference with oxidation of long-chained fatty acids, thus limiting energy for gluconeogenesis.

REACTIVE (POSTABSORPTIVE) HYPOGLYCEMIA

REACTIVE FUNCTIONAL HYPOGLYCEMIA The most frequently encountered hypoglycemic disorder in the adult in whom no demonstrable anatomic lesion can be demonstrated is "functional" or "reactive" hypoglycemia. These patients have normal fasting blood glucose levels. Reactive functional hypoglycemia occurs almost uniformly in tense, striving individuals with some emotional problems. Excessive secretion of insulin in response to the normal rise of blood glucose following meals is seldom found. The mechanism involved in this type of hypoglycemia remains unclear. The diagnosis is suspected by a history of intermittent hypoglycemic symptoms occurring 2 to 3 h after ingestion of a meal rich in carbohydrates, and it is confirmed by an oral glucose tolerance test extended for 4 to 5 h, blood samples being obtained at half-hour intervals. Additional samples should be drawn at the time of onset of symptoms of hypoglycemia. After an initial normal rise in blood glucose, it is not unusual in such patients to find blood glucose levels of 30 to 40 mg per 100 ml between the second and fourth hour of the test associated with reproduction of the patient's postprandial symptoms and with a spontaneous return of the blood glucose level toward fasting levels shortly thereafter.

The usual symptoms produced by reactive hypoglycemia are transitory and often subside spontaneously in 15 to 30 min. Weakness, hunger, inward trembling, sweating, palpitations, and tachycardia are the most common symptoms in these patients. Severe central nervous system dysfunction, especially loss of consciousness or convulsions, does not occur, and the severity of symptoms is not progressive. In patients with functional hypoglycemia attacks are more frequent when emotional stress and anxiety are greater. A prolonged or 72-h fast is well tolerated, and the concentration of blood glucose rarely drops below 45 mg per 100 ml and the IRI/G ratio remains normal. A 72-h fast is required only if there is a questionable history of fasting hypoglycemia or if fasting levels of plasma glucose are borderline or low. A family history of diabetes mellitus is usually absent. Recent publicity in the popular press and in books by some medical authors has led the public and some segments of the medical profession to believe that spontaneous hypoglycemia is a widespread and unrecognized cause of many physical and psychic ills. Promoting such a notion is a mistake. Persistent symptoms such as *chronic* fatigue, depression, lethargy, loss of vitality, or anxiety that affect the population of the United States are not due to hypoglycemia ("nonhypoglycemia"). Furthermore, during a routine oral glucose tolerance test many normal subjects will exhibit plasma glucose levels below 50 mg per 100 ml and occasionally below 40 mg per 100 ml without the occurrence of symptoms. A definite diagnosis of functional hypoglycemia is justified only in the patient who has a history of transient symptoms typical of hypoglycemia occurring 2 to 4 h after meals and in whom the glucose tolerance test reproduces both hypoglycemia and synchronous symptoms.

Treatment The distressing symptoms experienced by patients with functional hypoglycemia may be prevented by a diet low in carbohydrate (75 to 100 g), and high in protein, with adequate fat to maintain caloric requirements. The diet is divided into three to six feedings, with protein and carbohydrate proportions divided equally among the meals. In patients with a history suggestive of reactive hypoglycemia but in whom the diagnosis cannot be substantiated by a glucose tolerance test, diet therapy may be tried. An important approach is to improve the psychologic and emotional status of the patient with functional hypoglycemia. Counseling by the physician and tranquilizers may prove useful. Some patients resistant to diet therapy may be helped by anticholinergic drugs that delay gastrointestinal absorption. The prognosis is good, as usually the disease is self-limiting within a few months or years.

REACTIVE HYPOGLYCEMIA SECONDARY TO MILD DIABETES The reactive hypoglycemia secondary to mild diabetes has a different underlying mechanism than reactive functional hypoglycemia, and the prognosis is different. Whereas in patients with reactive functional hypoglycemia the pancreatic insulin release is well-timed in response to the rising postprandial blood glucose, in patients with mild diabetes the insulin release is delayed. It is not until the blood glucose rises to frankly diabetic levels that insulin is secreted in excess. Measurements of serum insulin during glucose tolerance tests in such patients have demonstrated that relatively large amounts of insulin are released, albeit late; the blood glucose then decreases from diabetic to normal levels and further to hypoglycemic levels. This type of hypoglycemic response is most likely to occur between the third and the fifth hours. It is apparent that these patients have only mild diabetes, since endogenous insulin is available, and their fasting blood glucose is within normal limits. Their carbohydrate intolerance can be detected by a postprandial blood glucose determination or an oral glucose tolerance test. Frequently there is a family history of diabetes mellitus.

Treatment consists of a diabetic diet with limitation of carbohydrate intake and frequent feedings. Weight reduction in the obese patient may normalize glucose tolerance, with disappearance of reactive hypoglycemia. Unlike the relatively benign prognosis of reactive functional hypoglycemia, this disorder is not self-limiting, and some patients may eventually progress to a more advanced state of insulin deficiency and the clinical syndrome of diabetes mellitus (Chap. 95).

ALIMENTARY HYPOGLYCEMIA In patients with gastroenterostomy or subtotal gastrectomy, hypoglycemia is due to excessive insulin release in response to excessive postprandial hyperglycemia facilitated by accelerated absorption of glucose (alimentary hyperinsulinism). In addition, excessive release of insulin may also be secondary to excessive release of gastrointestinal factors subsequent to the rapid passage of food into the small intestine. The diagnosis is made by history of abdominal surgery, and an abnormal oral glucose tolerance test characterized by elevation of the peak blood glucose level but not the 2-h level. In some patients alimentary hyperinsulinism and hypoglycemia are observed in the absence of gastric surgery. Treatment also consists of the prescription of a diet with reduced carbohydrate intake and multiple feedings.

OTHER CAUSES OF POSTPRANDIAL HYPOGLYCEMIA
Some patients with organic islet-cell disease may have hypoglycemia postprandially due to excessive insulin release stimulated by ingestion of carbohydrate. Approximately 80 percent of adult patients and 30 percent of children with pancreatic islet-cell disease will demonstrate excessive insulin release after administration of leucine. In only the latter group of patients will the ingestion of protein high in leucine content precipitate symptomatic hypoglycemia. Hypoglycemia following the ingestion of fructose occurs in patients with hereditary fructose intolerance, because of an inborn error of metabolism in which there is a deficiency of the enzyme hepatic fructose 1-phosphate aldolase. In patients with galactosemia, ingestion of galactose will precipitate hypoglycemia.

Table 97-2 suggests a sequence of diagnostic studies to be followed in an adult patient with suspected spontaneous hypoglycemia.

REGULATION OF GLUCAGON SECRETION AND EFFECTS OF GLUCAGON

SOURCE AND CHARACTERISTICS Glucagon is a polypeptide hormone secreted by the alpha cells of the islets of Langerhans. A glucagon identical to pancreatic glucagon is also believed to be secreted by alpha cells in the gastric fundus and duodenum which are ultrastructurally indistinguishable from pancreatic alpha cells. The hormone is made up of 29 amino acids in a straight chain and has a molecular weight of 3,485. With a sensitive radioimmunoassay employing an antiserum specific for glucagon, its concentration can be assayed in pancreatic tissue and in blood. The plasma concentration of glucagon in peripheral blood is approximately 80 pg per ml in the basal state. From different portions of the gastrointestinal mucosa (stomach, but particularly small intestine) extracts have been prepared which have immunologic characteristics similar to but not identical with pancreatic glucagon. This immunoreactive material, called *gut glucagon, enteroglucagon, or glucagon-like immunoreactive material,* has been found to be separable into two fractions, one of molecular weight of approximately 7,000 and the other with a molecular weight of 3,500. The former differs from glucagon in biologic activity (see the following).

FACTORS INFLUENCING SECRETION OF GLUCAGON Unger and associates have demonstrated that insulin-induced hypoglycemia is followed by increases in the concentration of glucagon in pancreatic and peripheral blood. Starvation is another stimulus to increased secretion of glucagon. The ingestion of protein meals and the intravenous or oral administration of certain amino acids (arginine or alanine) are other potent stimuli to the secretion of pancreatic glucagon. Administration of pancreozymin and gastroinhibitory polypeptide (GIP), gastrointestinal hormones released after protein ingestion, has also been found to increase plasma levels of glucagon and to augment the effect of amino acids on glucagon secretion. Exercise and any form of stress are other factors stimulating increased glucagon secretion. On the other hand, hyperglycemia due to orally or intravenously administered glucose causes suppression of glucagon secretion.

The oral, but not the intravenous, administration of glucose is followed by a significant increase in immunoreactive glucagon in peripheral blood which is due to release of gut glucagon.

METABOLIC EFFECTS OF GLUCAGON Glucagon exhibits a marked effect on carbohydrate, protein, and lipid metabolism in vivo and in vitro. Glucagon stimulates hepatic glycogenolysis by increasing cyclic 3′,5′-adenosine monophosphate (AMP) which leads to increased phosphorylase activity. Increased glycogenolysis and inhibition by glucagon of hepatic glycogen synthase (also via cyclic AMP) cause hyperglycemia. Glucagon stimulates gluconeogenesis by promoting the hepatic uptake of amino acids. It inhibits the incorporation of amino acids into liver protein and increases excretion of nitrogen. Glucagon, by activating the adenyl cyclase systems, also promotes lipolysis in liver and adipose tissues. The resulting increased hepatic concentration and oxidation of free fatty acids stimulate hepatic gluconeogenesis and ketogenesis.

In addition to these effects of glucagon on hepatic and adipose tissues, glucagon has a direct effect on stimulating increased release of insulin from the pancreatic beta cells independent of the increases in blood glucose. Glucagon's effect on pancreatic beta cells may also be mediated by activation of the adenyl cyclase system. Gut glucagon of molecular weight 7,000 also increases the secretion of insulin but does not have the hepatic effects of pancreatic glucagon.

Other extrahepatic effects of glucagon are a positive inotropic effect upon cardiac muscle, a stimulation of adrenal medullary secretion, and a slight lowering of serum levels of calcium and phosphate.

PHYSIOLOGIC ROLE OF GLUCAGON The extreme sensitivity of hepatic and adipose tissues to glucagon and the fact that increased secretion of glucagon is stimulated by fasting and hypoglycemia suggest that glucagon is released in order to provide for increased distribution of energy substrates during periods of glucose need. Glycogenolysis and gluconeogenesis will lead to increased levels of blood glucose, and increased lipolysis will furnish free fatty acids for energy and will stimulate gluconeogenesis. In contrast to the effects of fasting and hypoglycemia, rapid increases in blood glucose inhibit the secretion of glucagon. Amino acid-induced glucagon release after protein feeding may be an important factor in preventing hypoglycemia which might otherwise occur during amino acid-induced insulin release. Thus the maintenance of a normal blood glucose concentration depends on the coordinated biological action of both insulin and glucagon.

Whether pancreatic glucagon plays a physiologic role in mediating increased release of insulin is still to be demonstrated.

ABNORMALITIES OF GLUCAGON SECRETION A glucagonoma syndrome which may be the specific result of hypersecretion of pancreatic glucagon has been described. These patients have harbored islet-cell tumors of the alpha-cell type containing glucagon, most tumors being malignant. The clinical syndrome has included elevation in plasma concentration of glucagon, hyperglycemia, depressed plasma amino acid concentration, weight loss, bullous or eczematoid dermatitis, anemia, and stomatitis. Most patients were postmenopausal women. In patients in whom a glucagonoma was completely or partially resected, there was complete or partial recovery.

Abnormalities of glucagon secretion have also been reported in patients with diabetes of genetic origin. High postprandial plasma levels of glucagon have been noted in overtly diabetic patients, and, in contrast with normal subjects, plasma levels of glucagon did not decrease after carbohydrate ingestion or glucose infusion. Protein ingestion or arginine infusion induced exaggerated increases in plasma glucagon. Although fasting levels of glucagon were in the normal range, or only elevated slightly, they were inappropriately high for the degree of hyperglycemia. It was suggested that overt diabetes is characterized by a continuous state of relative or absolute hyperglucagonemia and that excess glucagon may exaggerate the metabolic consequences of insulin insufficiency. Somatostatin (a hypothalamic polypeptide that inhibits the release of human growth hormone and glucagon) lowered fasting plasma glucagon and glucose levels and also abolished the glucagon response to arginine. These effects were independent of suppression of growth hormone secretion. Unger and associates have postulated that human diabetes mellitus may be a bihormonal disorder characterized by a pancreatic alpha-cell dysfunction with excessive glucagon secretion as well as by diminished insulin release.

Patients with familial multiple endocrine adenomatosis have been shown to have elevated levels of plasma glucagon in addition to evidence of hyperinsulinism, hyperparathyroidism, and other hormonal hypersecretions. Patients with hyperinsulinism due to pancreatic microadenomatosis and carcinoma have also had elevated levels of plasma glucagon.

A syndrome associated with decreased secretion of glucagon and hypoglycemia accentuated by a high-protein, low-carbohydrate diet has been observed (Bleicher et al). Some infants and children with so-called "idiopathic hypoglycemia" may be found to be deficient in glucagon. Decreased plasma levels of glucagon and decreased glucagon reserve have been reported in some patients with severe chronic pancreatitis and associated diabetes. The plasma glucagon response to intravenously administered arginine should prove to be a valuable test for pancreatic glucagon reserve.

CLINICAL USEFULNESS OF GLUCAGON ADMINISTRATION In the presence of normal glycogen stores, glucagon produces a hyperglycemic effect when given subcutaneously, intramuscularly, or intravenously. The acute administration of glucagon has been used clinically most frequently in the treatment of severe insulin-induced hypoglycemia of labile diabetic patients when oral or intravenous administration of glucose was not possible. Large amounts of glucagon have been administered to selected patients with severe heart failure and cardiogenic shock. Some patients appear to have been benefited from the positive inotropic effect of glucagon.

GLUCAGON TESTS Several types of glucagon tests have been employed. One test takes advantage of the glycogenolytic properties of glucagon as a means for assessing adequacy of hepatic glycogen stores and the competency of enzymes in producing glycogenolysis. One milligram glucagon is injected intravenously over 4 min, and blood specimens are obtained at 0, 20, 30, 45, 60, 90, and 120 min. In healthy subjects the blood glucose level rises from 30 to 90 mg per 100 ml, 20 to 30 min after injection of glucagon. In patients with cirrhosis or glycogen storage disease there is a subnormal or no increase in blood glucose.

Another glucagon test takes advantage of the insulin-releasing property of glucagon. In patients with functioning pancreatic islet-cell disease, injection of 1 mg glucagon may be followed by excessive increases in plasma insulin. Blood samples are obtained at −15 min and 0 time, and again, 3, 5, 10, 15, 30, 45, 60, 90, 120, 150, and 180 min after injection of glucagon. Excessive increases in plasma insulin (maximal over 160 μU per ml and above 60, 40, and 20 μU per ml after 30, 40, or 60 min, respectively) after injection of glucagon occur in 50 to 75 percent of patients with insulin-secreting tumors. Such a finding may be associated with a subnormal rise in blood glucose but may be followed by an excessive secondary decrease in blood glucose. The test may have to be interrupted if severe hypoglycemic symptoms develop. Such patients should be treated with intravenous glucose.

Intravenous administration of 0.5 to 1.0 mg glucagon has been used in the past as a provocative test in patients suspected of harboring pheochromocytoma. In patients with pheochromocytoma, glucagon may evoke release of excessive quantities of pressor amines, resulting in a hypertensive paroxysm.

REFERENCES

Black J: Diazoxide and the treatment of hypoglycemia. Ann NY Acad Sci 150:194, 1968

Bleicher SJ: Hypoglycemia, in *Diabetes Mellitus, Theory and Practice,* eds M Ellenberg, H Rifkin, New York: McGraw-Hill, 1970, p. 972

Broder LE, Carter SK: Pancreatic islet cell carcinoma. II. Results of therapy with streptozotocin in 52 patients. Ann Intern Med 79:108, 1973

Fajans SS et al: Differential diagnosis of spontaneous hypoglycemia, Chap. 44 in *Endocrinology and Diabetes,* eds LJ Kryston, RA Shaw, New York: Grune & Stratton, 1975, p. 453

Fajans SS: Fasting hypoglycemia in adults. N Engl J Med 294: 766, 1976

Harrison TS et al: Current surgical management of functioning islet cell tumors of the pancreas. Ann Surg 178:485, 1973

Mallinson CN et al: A glucagonoma syndrome. Lancet 2:1, 1974

Muller WA et al: Abnormal alpha-cell function in diabetes: Response to carbohydrate and protein ingestion. N Engl J Med 283:109, 1970

Rolins JM et al: Selective angiopathy in localizing islet-cell tumors of the pancreas. A further appraisal. Radiology 100:525, 1973

Schein PS et al: Islet cell tumors: Current concepts and management. Ann Intern Med 79:239, 1973

Sherman BM et al: Plasma proinsulin in patients with functioning pancreatic islet cell tumors. J Clin Endocrinol Metab 35:271, 1972

Yager Y, Young RT: Non-hypoglycemia is an epidemic condition. N Engl J Med 291:907, 1974

98 DISEASES OF THE TESTES

JOHN F. CRIGLER, JR.
LESLIE I. ROSE
EUGENIA ROSEMBERG

HISTORY Androgen deficiency resulting from loss of testicular tissue was undoubtedly recognized by prehistoric man, as was the associated sterility; indeed, testicular tissue was recommended for impotence over 30 centuries ago. This dual function of the testes, as both the site of spermatogenesis and the primary site of male hormone production, was clearly defined in the middle of the nineteenth century when Berthold returned to the capon the characteristics, both physical and behavioral, of the cockerel by testicular grafts, and when his contemporaries, the anatomists von Kolliker, Leydig, Sertoli, and Schweigger-Seidel, defined the morphologic characteristics of the gland. They recognized the spermatogonia, spermatids, the Sertoli (or sustentacular) cells, and cells located interstitially between the tubules (the Leydig or interstitial cells).

The tropic role played by the anterior pituitary gland in the development and maintenance of testicular function was demonstrated by Smith and Engle in 1927, and several years later Butenandt isolated androsterone from male urine. By 1935, testosterone had been synthesized from cholesterol and isolated in crystalline form from bull testes. In addition, it was conclusively shown to be the most significant natural androgenic material.

Early in the present century, experimental studies in certain animals indicated a role of the central nervous system in coitus-stimulated ovulation. Thus, luteinizing hormone was the first hormone of the anterior pituitary shown to be under hypothalamic control. In 1930, Popa and Fielding described the hypophyseal portal vessels, which subsequently were shown by Harris (1950) to be involved in mediating hypothalamic regulation of anterior pituitary-gonadal function in rats. Schally and coworkers (1971) have reported the structure and laboratory synthesis of the porcine LH- (luteinizing hormone) and FSH- (follicle stimulating hormone) releasing hormone (LH-RH/FSH-RH or GnRH), a neurohumoral decapeptide active in humans which was originally postulated to exist by Hinsey and Markee (1933), Friedgood (1936), Harris (1937), and Brooks (1938).

Embryologists had debated for many years the relative importance of sex chromosomal pattern, hormones, or "determiners" secreted by the embryonic gonads, and maternal hormones on sex differentiation. In 1917, Lillie described the role of sex hormones in the development of freemartins. Wiesner proposed in 1935 that there is an autonomous tendency which results in female development unless opposed by male hormone. However, it was not until the late 1940s and early 1950s that Alfred Jost (1947) and other experimental embryologists clearly demonstrated that secretions of the fetal testes are necessary for development of male genital ducts and external genitals and regression of female genital ducts and that female development occurs in the absence of gonads. About the same time, Barr and Bertram (1949) described sex chromatin masses at the periphery of the nucleus in resting ganglion cells of female cats, a distinguishing characteristic of the female sex subsequently shown to be present in the peripheral cells of most mammalian species. The application of this simple cytologic means of assessing the number of X chromosomes and of more sophisticated cytogenetic techniques to the study of patients with sexual abnormalities has enhanced significantly our understanding of the role of genetic factors in gonadal and other somatic development, information which has been of great importance in elucidating the pathophysiology of testicular disorders.

DEVELOPMENT Embryogenic In the fourth to sixth weeks of fetal development, the primitive genital ridge differentiates into cortical and medullary components capable of becoming either a testis or an ovary. If the primordial germ cells which migrate from the dorsal endoderm of the yolk sac to the urogenital ridge have a Y chromosome, they become incorporated into testicular cords which differentiate *in situ* from the blastema of the indifferent genital ridge. The primary sex cords undergo proliferation to form seminiferous tubules which subsequently link with convoluted tubules of mesonephric origin (rete testis and epididymis) and channel into the Wolffian duct. The cortex of the primitive gonad becomes isolated by the tunica albuginea and involutes. The histogenesis of testicular tunica albuginea and the regression of the Müllerian ducts are closely related, the latter shown by Josso and others to result from the local production of a nonsteroidal "inhibitory substance" probably secreted by the fetal Sertoli cells. At approximately eight weeks, characteristic fetal Leydig cells appear and subsequently secrete fetal masculinizing hormones (androgens) necessary for the development of Wolffian duct structures (vas deferens, seminal vesicles), enlargement of the genital tubercle, and fusion of the labioscrotal and urethral folds to form male external genitalia. If the primordial germ cells have two X chromosomes and no Y chromosome, the cortical component and primordial germ cells proliferate and persist as the future ovary with subsequent involution of the medullary component of the undifferentiated gonad. In the absence of masculinizing factors of the fetal testis (development presumably evoked by the presence of a Y chromosome), normal female development of genital ducts and external genitalia takes place, with the formation of the fallopian tubes, uterus, and upper vagina from the Müllerian ducts, regression of the Wolffian system, and persistence of the small genital tubercle and unfused urethral and labioscrotal folds.

Postnatal Shortly after birth the testes measure 1.5 to 2.0 cm in length and 0.7 to 1.0 cm in width and weigh approximately 0.5 g each. The interstitial cells, active during uterine life as a result of chorionic and fetal pituitary gonadotropins, undergo dedifferentiation and remain quiescent or semiquiescent until puberty. However, with current sensitive techniques, both gonadotropic and sex steroid hormones in blood have been demonstrated at all ages. It is recognized, also, that infants and children with primary gonadal disorders (e.g., gonadal dysgenesis) may have increased levels of gonadotropins in serum and urine, indicating a restraining influence of the prepuberal gonad upon the gonadotropic production of the pituitary. At birth, 10 percent of male infants have incompletely descended testes, but after the first year, this figure drops to 2 to 3 percent. Late prepuberal descent further decreases the number, so that only 0.3 to 0.4 percent of males have either unilateral or bilateral undescended testes, postpuberally, unilateral undescended testes being four to five times more frequent than bilateral.

During adolescence, each testis increases in size, as a result chiefly of changes in the seminiferous tubules under the stimulation of pituitary FSH and androgens produced locally by developing interstitial cells. The fully developed testis measures 3.5 to 5.5 cm in length and 2.1 to 3.2 cm in width, and weighs 15 to 20 g. Interstitial cell–stimulating hormone (ICSH or LH) induces interstitial cell differentiation, with the production of male sex hormones, genital enlargement, and the development of secondary sexual characteristics.

Aberrations in embryonic development It is currently postulated that sex-determining genes on the X and Y chromosomes are responsible, through their effects on cellular function of the primitive gonad, for differentiation of these tissues into either a testis or an ovary. Embryologic studies have indicated that normally functioning fetal testes are required for male differentiation of genital ducts and external genitalia. The fetal testis appears to produce at least two types of substances: (1) a Müllerian duct–inhibiting substance which causes involution of the Müllerian duct and may have a role in development of the Wolffian system, and (2) an androgen(s) which appears to be necessary for Wolffian duct development and is required for masculinization of the external genitalia. The correlation between chromosomal patterns, gonadal differentiation, and subsequent genital development in human beings has been quite consistent. Some cases, however, remain unexplained by the above-stated concepts, although they do not disprove the hypothesis, since current techniques do not detect all chromosomal anomalies (mosaicism, interchange of sex-determining factors between X and Y chromosomes, etc.) or measure directly fetal gonadal function.

If gonadal tissue does not develop (gonadal dysgenesis, genotypic XO, X isochromosome X, X deleted X, etc.) or fetal testicular cells are nonfunctioning before differentiation of genital ducts in a genotypic male (XY), *both internal and external genitalia are entirely female.* Partial failure in testicular development or in the elaboration of fetal masculinizing hormones (genotypic XY or mosaics having a cell line with a Y chromosome) results in ambiguous internal and external genital development, the type of abnormality reflecting the age of onset and degree of fetal gonadal dysfunction. Patients who had abnormal fetal testes, therefore, may have genital development ranging from almost complete feminization through incomplete fusion of the labioscrotal and urethral folds with some enlargement of the genital tubercle and various degrees of development of the Müllerian ducts to mild degrees of hypospadias. In addition, if testicular tissue exists unilaterally (true hermaphrodite, mixed gonadal dysgenesis), male development of genital ducts occurs on the side of the testes and Müllerian duct structures develop on the side with the ovary or missing gonad. These findings are consistent with observations in other animal species which demonstrate a local effect by diffusion of fetal masculinizing hormones (Chap. 64).

Some genotypic males (XY) who have histologically normal-appearing testes before puberty show *total feminization of external genitalia although internal genitals are masculinized* (syndrome of testicular feminization). This abnormality is inherited as either an X-linked recessive or a male-limited autosomal dominant mutant gene, as half the genotypic males are affected. The lack of masculinization of external genitals (but not of internal genitalia), the absence of sexual hair (found in approximately one-third of the patients), and the occurrence of feminization at adolescence with normal plasma and urine testosterone concentrations for males indicate an abnormality in the response of tissues to androgens. Decreased reduction of testosterone to 17β-hydroxyandrostane urinary metabolites and activity of the steroid Δ^4-3-keto-5α-oxidoreductase of skin, which catalyzes the transformation of testosterone to 17β-hydroxy-5α-androstan-3-one (dihydrotestosterone), a metabolite with biologic activity comparable to testosterone, has been demonstrated in these patients. Intramuscular administration of dihydrotestosterone to a patient with testicular feminization, however, failed to produce the changes in urinary nitrogen, phosphorus, and citric acid excretion observed in a control individual. More recently, the lack of response to androgens has been shown also to result from a deficiency in a cytosol-binding protein required for transport of the active hormone to the nucleus of the cell. These new biochemical observations now provide an explanation for the inability of end organ tissue to show the expected response to testosterone. Feminization of the external genitals of these patients may be so complete that the abnormality is discovered only later in life when primary amenorrhea, the absence of sexual hair, or the appearance of inguinal masses makes the diagnosis apparent. Surgical exploration of these patients reveals the presence of vas deferens, epididymis, and testes, the latter showing variation in histologic findings with age and the completeness of the defect. After adolescence, tubular adenomas and hyperplasia of Leydig cells (often adenomatous) are common, and malignant degeneration has been reported. For this reason, surgical removal of testes is recommended.

Occasionally, genotypic males (XY) and individuals with a mosaic cell line containing a Y chromosome and ambiguous external genitals (slight enlargement of the genital tubercle with or without partially fused labioscrotal folds) have fallopian tubes, uterus, and vagina. These patients have either unilateral or bilateral dysgenetic testes which presumably do not produce the "Müllerian inhibitory substance" or sufficient fetal androgens to totally masculinize the external genitals. Androgen insensitivity has not been demonstrated in these individuals. As in patients with the androgen-insensitive type of male pseudohermaphroditism, abnormal gonadal tissue should be removed surgically since dysgerminomas, embryonal dysgerminomas, and gonadoblastomas commonly arise from dysgenic testis.

Finally, *masculinization of external genital development of a genotypic female* fetus (XX) may be induced by excessive fetal adrenal androgens (patients with congenital adrenocortical hyperplasia) or by excess androgens produced or taken (usually synthetic progestational steroid hormones) by the mother during pregnancy. Defects induced by these extragonadal androgens are limited to the external genitalia (hypertrophy of the genital tubercle with various degrees of fusion of the labioscrotal and urethral folds), so that if the condition is recognized, an appropriate female sex assignment can be made and the genital abnormality surgically corrected. The external genitals should be surgically corrected as soon after birth as possible.

PHYSIOLOGY The role of fetal testicular function on genital development has been described above. The precise interrelationships of hypothalamic-pituitary and testicular functions (Fig. 98-1) (see also Chap. 89) at adolescence and

FIGURE 98-1
Scheme showing hypothalamic-anterior pituitary-testes relationship.

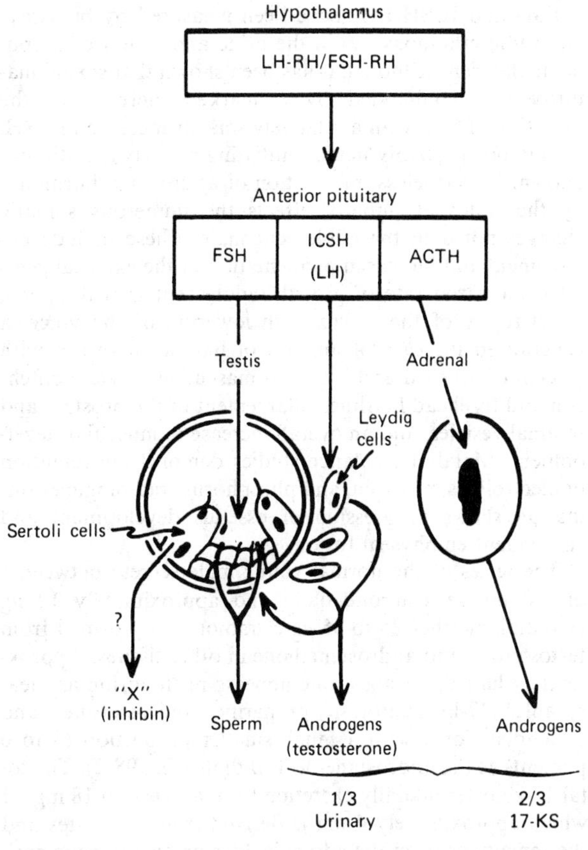

in adult life are not completely defined. A hypothalamic-releasing substance (GnRH) which stimulates secretion of pituitary gonadotropins has been isolated from porcine sources and found to be a decapeptide with the following amino acid sequence: (pyro)glu-his-trp-ser-tyr-gly-leu-arg-pro-gly-NH_2. Parenteral administration of the synthesized polypeptide to preadolescent boys and men increases serum ICSH(LH) and FSH levels. ICSH, reportedly identical to luteinizing hormone (LH) of females elaborated by the anterior pituitary gland, induces development and subsequently functional maintenance of the testicular interstitial (Leydig) cells. Pituitary FSH stimulates development of the seminiferous tubules. The role of ICSH(LH) and testosterone in seminiferous tubular development and spermatogenesis is not well defined, but significant local concentration of testosterone is necessary for spermatogenesis. It is generally accepted that the Leydig cell is the principle site of synthesis of steroid hormones (testosterone, estrogens, and others), although testosterone can be synthesized from precursors or transformed to various metabolites by other tissues including seminiferous tubules and epididymis. Steroidogenic activity in the latter tissues may be important in providing increased local concentrations. The probable role of ICSH(LH) and the Leydig cell in hormonal production in human beings is illustrated by observations on so-called "fertile eunuchs," patients who show spermatogenesis but lack masculine secondary changes and in whom testicular biopsies show a decrease in the number of mature Leydig cells. These patients have a relative ICSH(LH) deficiency and respond well to therapy with human chorionic gonadotropin (HCG).

FSH and ICSH(LH) have been measured by bioassays and radioimmunoassays in the urine and serum of prepuberal children. Although it has been shown that sexual maturity is accompanied by a marked increase in the excretion of LH, with a relatively smaller increase in FSH, the factors, probably neural, initiating puberty are still unknown. Nevertheless, production of androgenic hormones by the testes at puberty effects the numerous somatic changes noted in the adolescent male. These include enlargement and increased pigmentation of the external genitalia, increased rate of growth (adolescent growth spurt), hypertrophy of the larynx with lowering of the voice, a generalized increase of amount of hair to hirsutism with growth of a beard and a typical masculine pelvic escutcheon and forehead hairline, enlargement of the prostate and seminal vesicles, and an overall increase in muscular development. Metabolic balance studies demonstrate retention of electrolytes, nitrogen, and phosphorus; radiologic examination shows progression of osseous development and subsequent epiphyseal fusion.

The testes of the normal young male secrete between 4 and 8 mg testosterone daily and approximately 10 μg estradiol, another 25 to 35 μg estradiol being formed from testosterone and androstenedione in other tissues. Approximately half the testosterone appears in the urine as measurable 17-ketosteroids, primarily androsterone and etiocholanolone, with a much smaller proportion (3 to 6 percent) as the androstane-$3\alpha,17\beta$-diols (Fig. 98-2). The total 17-ketosteroid daily excretion for males is 8 to 18 mg, of which approximately 4 mg is derived from the testes and the remainder from the adrenals. Plasma testosterone concentrations in young adult males vary from 0.3 to 1.2 μg per 100 ml (mean 0.6 μg per 100 ml), whereas normal females of similar age have plasma concentrations between 0.02 and 0.07 μg per 100 ml. Studies of testosterone metabolism in normal men above sixty years of age indicate that with advancing years, there is a significant decrease in both total and free serum testosterone levels and metabolic clearance rate (thus a decrease in blood production rate) and a change in the extraglandular and extrahepatic metabolism similar to that observed in hypogonadal males. It is well known that urinary 17-ketosteroid excretion diminishes with increasing age. Rarely, however, is sudden cessation in gonadal function, analogous to the process in the female, observed in the male.

Studies have demonstrated that in some tissues the hormonal activity of testosterone is mediated by the intracellular reduction of testosterone to 17β-hydroxy-5α-androstan-3-one (dihydrotestosterone, DHT) (Fig. 98-2). The enzyme, Δ^4-3-keto-5α-oxidoreductase, required for this reaction has been demonstrated in male accessory sex tissues, skin, hair follicles, brain, and testes. This enzyme is located in the cytoplasm and nuclear membrane of androgen target cells. The DHT formed in the cytoplasm is bound to a specific binding protein which aids in transporting DHT to the nucleus. In the nucleus, DHT binds strongly to nuclear protein and is thought by this mechanism to influence RNA synthesis and cellular function. Some patients with testicular feminization lack 5α-reductase activity, whereas others have a deficiency of the cytoplasmic binding protein. These biochemical defects are responsible for the lack of masculinization of these genetic males with normal testosterone secretion (see previous paragraph).

The principal abnormalities of testicular function, listed according to their effects on both interstitial and seminiferous tubular activity, are summarized in Table 98-1.

HYPOGONADISM

The clinical term *hypogonadism* as most often used refers to failure in interstitial cell function which results in decreased or absent production of male sex hormones. Seminiferous tubular failure, however, often is associated and, indeed, may occur without significant changes in testicular hormonal production (Sertoli-cell-only syndrome and postpuberal abnormalities). Both testicular functions may be decreased either primarily by a developmental or destructive lesion of the testes or secondarily by failure in production of pituitary gonadotropins or the hypothalamic releasing hormone, GnRH.

PREPUBERAL HYPOGONADISM The clinical picture of hypogonadism is directly related to the time of development of androgen deficiency. Prepuberal deficiency results in an absence of the adolescent growth spurt and varying degrees of failure to develop the expected secondary sexual characteristics associated with maturity. Absence of androgen production by the testes is associated with persistent infantile genitalia, a barely palpable prostate, female distribution of pubic and axillary hair, absence of seborrhea and acne, a partial to total lack of facial and body hair, and the absence of a deepening of voice. Although growth rate is decreased, it continues, and in the absence of epiphyseal closure results in a tall "eunuchoid"

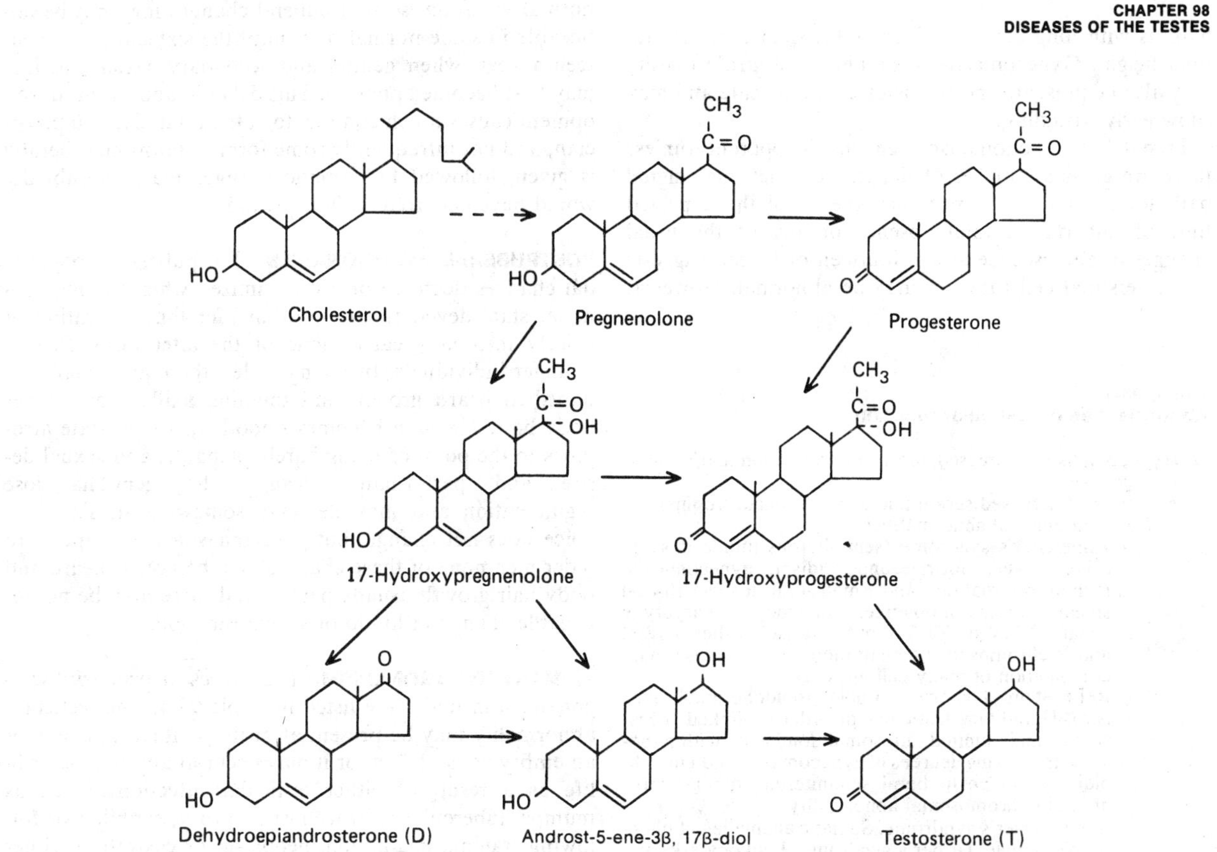

FIGURE 98-2

Synthesis and metabolism of androgens. The broken line between cholesterol and pregnenolone signifies a series of reactions. The latter reactions and the conversion of pregnenolone to progesterone, 17-OH pregnenolone, 17-OH progesterone, dehydroepiandrosterone (D), androst-5-ene-3β,17β-diol, androst-4-ene-3,17-dione (Δ), and testosterone (T) occur in the testis. In addition, it is well recognized that D is irreversibly converted to Δ and that Δ and T are interconverted in peripheral tissue, a fact which permits the formation of small amounts of T from D, a major adrenal secretory product. Approximately 40 percent of T is metabolized to the major urinary 11-deoxy-17-ketosteroids, D, androsterone (A), and 5β-androsterone (E), and only 2 to 6 percent to 5α- and 5β-diols. The latter pathway of T metabolism, specifically, the conversion of T to 17β-hydroxy-5α-androstan-3-one (DHT), is recognized to be essential for the expression of androgen activity in certain androgen-sensitive tissues. The major T metabolites, A, E, 5α- and 5β-androstane-3α,17β-diols, are conjugated as glucuronides and sulfates, principally, by the liver, before excretion into the urine by the kidney.

habitus with long arms and legs and a span 2 in. greater than height. Gynecomastia, wide hips, and girdle obesity may also be present. The skin is pale and delicate and may show early wrinkling.

Prepuberal hypogonadism remains inapparent (unless there are gross anomalies of the testes, which may signal pathologic changes at an earlier age) until the expected time of puberty. A total absence of any of the usual changes of adolescence at age fourteen or fifteen suggests that interstitial cell function may be abnormal. However, as in other developmental states, there is a wide range of normal variation, so that puberal changes may not be noticeable in some normal boys until the sixteenth or seventeenth year, when genital and secondary sexual changes may first become apparent. This delay in adolescent development causes much concern to patient, family, and physician, and not infrequently some form of hormonal therapy is given, followed by somatic changes that undoubtedly would have occurred without treatment.

TABLE 98-1
Abnormalities of testicular function

- *I* Hypogonadism (decreased androgen production and/or spermatogenesis)
  - *A* Primary (increased serum and urinary gonadotropins)
    - *1* Developmental abnormalities
      - *a* Klinefelter's syndrome (seminiferous tubule dysgenesis). Classic form—eunuchoidism, gynecomastia, mental retardation, and small firm testes. Buccal smear—chromatin-positive. Leukocyte karyotype usually XXY or XXYY but may have other poly X and Y chromosomal constitution and mosaicism with combination of many cell lines
      - *b* Reifenstein's syndrome (male pseudohermaphroditism). Hereditary testicular disorder (X-linked recessive or male-limited autosomal dominant) with hypospadias, varying degrees of gynecomastia and eunuchoidism, and postpuberal seminiferous tubular atrophy. No chromosomal abnormality
      - *c* Male Turner's syndrome. Somatic anomalies of phenotypic female Turner's syndrome. Leukocyte karyotype usually XY, but occasional abnormal chromosomes of mosaicism. Variable testicular histology and function
      - *d* Sertoli-cell-only syndrome (germinal aplasia). Normal development. Infertility. No chromosomal abnormality. Normal serum testosterone. Etiology unknown
      - *e* Anorchia. Cryptorchid with no somatic anomalies. Usually, no testicular tissue present. No chromosomal abnormality. Etiology unknown
    - *2* Postpuberal abnormalities
      - *a* Seminiferous tubule failure
        - *1* Orchitis (mumps, tuberculosis, leprosy, gonorrheal infection, brucellosis, syphilis, etc.), hyperpyrexia, irradiation, trauma, neoplasm, or surgical castration
        - *2* Congenital disorders—myotonia dystrophica, cystic fibrosis, Laurence-Moon-Biedl syndrome
        - *3* Idiopathic
      - *b* Leydig-cell failure (male climacteric)
  - *B* Secondary (decreased serum and urinary gonadotropins)
    - *1* Isolated gonadotropin deficiency. Often associated with congenital anomalies, including anosmia or hyposmia, harelip, cleft palate, etc. May be inherited as an X-linked recessive or male-limited autosomal dominant trait
    - *2* Isolated ICSH deficiency (fertile eunuch)
    - *3* Multiple pituitary deficiencies (panhypopituitarism)
      - *a* Idiopathic prepuberal
      - *b* Secondary to neurohypophyseal lesions—neoplasm (chromophobe, astrocytoma, hamartoma, teratoma), cyst (craniopharyngioma), or granulomatous process (sarcoid, etc.)
      - *c* Congenital disorders—Laurence-Moon-Biedl syndrome
- *II* Hypergonadism (excessive androgen production)
  - *A* Primary (functioning interstitial cell tumor)
  - *B* Secondary (increased serum or urinary gonadotropins for age)
    - *1* Familial
    - *2* Tumor in region of third ventricle (pinealoma, astrocytoma, hamartoma, teratoma, and craniopharyngioma)

POSTPUBERAL HYPOGONADISM Postpuberal hypogonadal changes decrease or are minimized when the hypogonadal state develops late in adult life; thus castration of elderly men may cause none of the alterations seen in younger individuals. In young males, there are usually diminished beard growth and thinning axillary and other body hair. The skin becomes smoother, the prostate atrophies to the point of being barely palpable, and sexual desire and performance wane. The genitalia lose pigmentation and may decrease somewhat in size. The voice does not change, but gynecomastia may appear. In older men none of these changes may be noted; beard and body hair growth usually persist, and there may be no noticeable change in libido or sexual function.

PRIMARY HYPOGONADISM The causes of primary hypogonadism in males are listed in Table 98-1. The testicular abnormality may be present at birth as either a genetic or an embryologic defect, or it may occur at any time later in life as a result of either testicular infections (such as mumps, tuberculosis, brucellosis, leprosy, syphilis) or following trauma, irradiation, neoplasm or castration, either surgical or accidental. Beginning in early adolescence, even before the appearance of the obvious physical characteristics of hypogonadism, the patient may have increased serum concentrations of pituitary gonadotropic hormones (measured by radioimmunoassay) and may excrete excessive quantities in the urine. The immature mouse uterine weight assay, which measures both ICSH(LH) and FSH, is used most frequently for determination of total urinary gonadotropin content. In addition, because of lack of testosterone synthesis, plasma testosterone concentrations as well as urinary 17-ketosteroid excretion of adult patients are significantly decreased. It should be stated here with emphasis, however, that the patient's own tissues clinically observed frequently provide the most significant assay of androgen production. The following syndrome is an example of primary hypogonadism.

KLINEFELTER'S SYNDROME (SEMINIFEROUS TUBULE DYSGENESIS) Klinefelter, Reifenstein, and Albright described in 1942 a clinical syndrome of hypogonadism that includes gynecomastia, eunuchoidism, elevated levels of serum and urinary gonadotropins, and decreased testicular size associated with hyalinization of the tubules. Barr demonstrated that many of these patients were *chromatin-positive,* exhibiting nuclei similar to those seen in females (see Chap. 64). Culture of leukocytes in vitro in the presence of colchicine has permitted direct chromosomal counting and classification; and, indeed, many patients with the triad described by Klinefelter et al. have been shown to possess an extra sex chromosome, resulting in a karyotypic classification of 22 autosomes plus 2 X chromosomes and 1 Y chromosome (see Chap. 64). Thus, they have 47 instead of

46 chromosomes, and it is therefore not surprising that many of these patients also have various degrees of mental deficiency. A clue to the diagnosis of this disorder, which has an incidence of approximately 1 in 400 males from studies performed in newborns, often lies in the behavior and personality of the Klinefelter patient. Talkativeness with little substance to the content is an outstanding behavioral trait. Klinefelter's syndrome in some patients who lack the classic clinical findings of gynecomastia, eunuchoidism, and small testes may be discovered only when they appear in an infertility clinic. In addition, Klinefelter's syndrome is not infrequently discovered when the patient seeks medical care for chronic pulmonary disease, obesity, diabetes mellitus, varicose veins, and thrombophlebitis, disorders which appear to be more prevalent in these patients; thus, the spectrum of Klinefelter's syndrome is broad, including obviously feminized males on one end and, on the other end, normally virilized men with only abnormal microscopic testicular anatomy but often with the associated diseases listed above.

SECONDARY HYPOGONADISM Secondary hypogonadism results from failure of pituitary elaboration of the necessary tropic hormones, specifically ICSH and FSH (Table 98-1, *I-B*). Isolated deficiencies of gonadotropic hormones without demonstrable loss of other pituitary hormones have been described in males in association with anosmia or hyposmia by Kallman. The condition may be inherited either as an X-linked recessive or as a male-limited autosomal dominant trait. Very rarely, an isolated ICSH deficiency occurs. In most cases, however, there is an associated loss of other pituitary tropic hormones, resulting in growth failure before adolescence and in decreased thyroid, adrenal, and gonadal function at all ages. When there is a progressive loss of hypothalamic-pituitary function because of a neoplasm (chromophobe adenoma, astrocytoma, hamartoma, teratoma), cyst (craniopharyngioma) or granulomatous process (sarcoid), a decrease of gonadotropins is at times the first deficiency observed, and the patient, therefore, may appear in the clinic with isolated hypogonadism. Prepuberal hypopituitarism is usually recognized because of the short stature that results from growth hormone deficiency. Occasionally, however, testes of preadolescent boys with other evidences of pituitary dysfunction are significantly small. Froehlich in 1901 described such an obese hypogonadal boy with signs of a tumor in the hypothalamic area. Since then, Froehlich's name has been inappropriately applied to the condition of a large group of overweight boys with slightly retarded maturation but with normal linear growth and no demonstrated hypothalamic lesion; in such cases the delay in maturation is without any real clinical significance. Patients with the Laurence-Moon-Biedl syndrome have been described with both primary (germinal aplasia) and secondary (hypogonadotropic) hypogonadism.

The absence of serum and urinary gonadotropins after the age of adolescence in patients with diminished gonadal function is diagnostic of secondary hypogonadism. Studies of growth, thyroid, adrenal, and antidiuretic hormones may reveal clinically unsuspected deficiencies. Skull roentgenogram may also show intracranial calcification, enlargement of the sella turcica, or erosion of the clinoid processes, and visual field examination may demonstrate early involvement of the optic nerves.

EVALUATION OF HYPOGONADAL STATES An outline of principal clinical and laboratory information required for the diagnosis of the various hypogonadal states of males (Table 98-1) is listed in Table 98-2. A careful history and physical examination are of obvious importance, as they describe the biologic abnormality. The measurement of serum and urinary gonadotropins most often differentiates between the primary disorders of the testis and testicular deficiencies resulting from neuroendocrine dysfunctions, the latter due primarily to decreased production of either

TABLE 98-2
Clinical and laboratory diagnosis of hypogonadism in adolescent and adult males

I Clinical manifestations of hypogonadism in males
- *A* Adolescence. Androgen deficiency–decreased rate of physical growth (absent growth spurt), eunuchoid body proportions, immature facies without change in voice or appearance of acne and seborrhea, small penis with or without small testes, decreased or absent (if also adrenal androgen deficiency) pubic and axillary hair, occasionally gynecomastia. Seminiferous tubules—lack of development resulting in small and, with tubular fibrosis firm, testes
- *B* Adult. Androgen deficiency–decreased libido and sexual performance, diminished beard growth and decreased axillary and pubic hair, decreased pigmentation and size of penis and scrotum, atrophy of prostate, occasionally gynecomastia. Seminiferous tubular failure—infertility, decreased testicular size

II Primary testicular disorders (characterized by increased serum and urinary gonadotropin levels)
- *A* History. Presence of development anomalies; behavior or personality disorder; associated illness (mumps, tuberculosis, venereal disease, chronic pulmonary disease, liver dysfunction, diabetes mellitus, etc.); decreased or absent sense of smell; family history of similar disorder
- *B* Physical examination. Height, body proportions (span; U/L, U = height minus L, L = symphysis pubis to floor), weight, amount and distribution of sexual hair, presence of gynecomastia, size and pigmentation of penis and scrotum, size and consistency of testes (small, hard testes seen with tubular fibrosis), specific testing of Ist cranial nerve
- *C* Laboratory
  - *1* Serum LH, FSH, testosterone (T), and 17β-estradiol (E_2) and urinary gonadotropin levels and their response to clomiphene citrate, GnRH, and human gonadotropins.
  - *2* Evaluation of other neuroendocrine functions—thyrotropin (TSH), adrenocorticotropin (ACTH), growth hormone (GH), and vasopressin (ADH) production—either by direct measurement in serum before, during, and after appropriate stimuli (thyrotropin-releasing hormone, metyrapone, insulin-induced hypoglycemia, sleep, hypertonic saline solution, etc.) or by indirect measurement of thyroid (*l*-thyroxine and *l*-triiodothyronine levels, resin T_3-binding, etc.) and adrenal (serum cortisol response to insulin-hypoglycemia; serum cortisol and 11-deoxycortisol and urinary 17-KS and 17-OHCS response to metyrapone, excretion of water load, etc.) function and changes in serum osmolality and in urine specific gravity or osmolality after an appropriate tolerated water fast
  - *3* X-ray—skull and hand and wrist (bone age)
  - *4* Ophthalmologic examination with visual field determinations
  - *5* Semen analysis and testicular biopsy (isolated LH or GnRH deficiencies, the so-called fertile eunuch; Klinefelter's syndrome)
  - *6* Other neurologic studies (lumbar puncture, pneumoencephalogram, brain scans, electroencephalogram, etc.) as indicated

hypothalamic GnRH or pituitary ICSH(LH) and FSH. As synthetic releasing hormones become more available, differentiation between central nervous system (usually hypothalamic) and pituitary lesions will be possible. More readily available, specific techniques for measuring testosterone, 17β-estradiol, and other sex steroid hormones and their binding protein in serum make it possible now to diagnose significant abnormalities of hormone production more easily and to monitor the patient's response to therapeutic regimens.

TREATMENT OF HYPOGONADISM Patients with primary hypogonadism (increased serum and urinary gonadotropins) require testosterone replacement therapy. Preparations commonly used are listed in Table 98-3. The usual method of therapy is to start with relatively small doses of the long-acting depot preparations of testosterone, giving 50 mg every 2 weeks and increasing it by 25- to 50-mg increments at 6- to 12-month intervals according to the patient's response. The dosage subsequently (after epiphyseal fusion in adolescent boys) is increased to 200 mg every 2 weeks to obtain full androgen effect, including deepening of the voice and increased facial hair. Final adult maintenance requirements are usually satisfied by 100 mg of the depot preparation every 2 weeks or 200 mg every 3 to 5 weeks. Excessive acne formation, edema from retention of sodium, and undesirable personality changes all indicate overtreatment, and the dosage should be diminished appropriately.

In patients with secondary hypogonadism, a trial on HCG may be indicated. Usually HCG, 1,000 to 4,000 IU, every 5 days for 6 to 9 months, is given as a single course. If regression to a hypogonadal state occurs when HCG is discontinued, either HCG may be reinstituted and continued (especially in patients with isolated LH deficiency who have normal testicular function—hormone production and spermatogenesis—on treatment) or testosterone therapy as outlined above may be begun. A gonadotropin preparation rich in FSH has been obtained from human menopausal urine. Experience with this preparation in gonadotropin-deficient postpuberal males indicates that it can restore spermatogenesis to normal. Both the prepuberal and adult testes seem to require stimulation with ICSH(LH) before spermatogenesis can be induced by administration of the human menopausal gonadotropin preparation.

Early studies of patients with hypogonadotropic hypogonadism using synthetic GnRH have provided evidence that this hormone may be of great therapeutic importance in those individuals who respond with the production and release of pituitary gonadotropins. Until the present, however, multiple daily injections of GnRH have been required for therapeutic effect.

TABLE 98-3
Hormonal therapy for hypogonadism

Preparations	*Route and dosage*
Methyltestosterone (Linguet)	Sublingual 5–10 mg, 4 times daily
Testosterone propionate	Intramuscular 25–50 mg, 3 times weekly
Testosterone enanthate, testosterone cyclopentylpropionate, testosterone phenylacetate	Intramuscular 100–200 mg every 1–2 weeks for maximum effect—and every 2–5 weeks for maintenance
Human chorionic gonadotropin	Intramuscular 1,000–4,000 IU every 5 days for 6–9 months, with response monitored by measurement of serum testosterone levels Repeated courses as required

HYPERGONADISM

The production of excessive quantities of androgenic hormones in the adult male results in little, if any, morphologic or functional change. However, in the child, the somatic changes associated with puberty may be induced at an early age and therefore become clinically apparent (precocious puberty). The causes of hypergonadism and isosexual precocity in the male are listed in Table 98-1. Hypergonadism may be due to excessive androgen production from a functioning testicular tumor, the Leydig cell, or interstitial cell, carcinoma. Children with these tumors show all the changes associated with puberty, such as increased hair growth and phallic enlargement, and usually have a palpable testicular tumor. However, the presence of the tumor may be difficult to determine if the testes are undescended, or if the tumor is extremely active in producing hormone but is very small. Plasma testosterone concentrations are increased. Urinary 17-ketosteroids, however, may be normal or only slightly increased, because of the marked potency of testosterone. Serum and urinary gonadotropin levels are usually suppressed. Hypergonadism may also result from an early onset of puberty due to altered hypothalamic-pituitary function. The sequence of development is similar to that observed in adolescence, with enlargement of genitalia, appearance of pubic and axillary hair, deepening of the voice, and appearance of acne and seborrhea occurring in that order and beginning as early as one to two years of age. The testes are large for the patient's chronologic age but are in accord with the size expected for the degree of maturity exhibited by the remainder of his somatic development. Gonadotropins may be present in the urine but are not invariably measurable by routine assay procedures. In the early stages, the level of 17-ketosteroids may not be significantly elevated for the patient's chronologic age (in contrast to virilism produced by adrenal abnormalities), but subsequently it rises to a degree appropriate for his developmental age. Isosexual precocity of this type in males, although uncommon, is often familial, in contrast to the more frequently occurring true precocity in females, from whom a family history of early puberty is seldom obtained. When true precocity occurs in males without a family history, it is almost always associated with space-occupying lesions in the region of the third ventricle (pinealoma, astrocytoma, hamartoma, and rarely a craniopharyngioma). The continued production of androgens excessive for their age in these patients results in accelerated skeletal growth and, especially, maturation during childhood, followed by early closure of the epiphyses, ending in an adult who frequently is smaller than his contemporaries.

Isosexual precocity in the male may also result from excessive quantities of adrenal androgens. The pattern of accelerated growth and development is similar to that produced by testicular hormones. The testes remain, however, prepuberal in size; gonadotropins are invariably low for the stage of development. The diagnosis is made on the basis of a markedly elevated level of urinary 17-ketosteroids. For further discussion, see Chap. 93.

NEOPLASMS OF THE TESTES

Neoplasms of the testes are the most common tumors of men twenty-nine to thirty-five years of age but may appear at any age. They occur more often in cryptorchid testis (1 in 2,000) than in descended testis (1 in 100,000), even when the cryptorchid testis is surgically placed in the scrotum. For this reason, frequent examination of the surgically corrected cryptorchid testis is recommended. The following classification of testicular neoplasms is given in their relative order of frequency:

1 Seminoma (germinoma)
2 Teratocarcinoma
3 Embryonal carcinoma
  a Chorioepithelioma
  b Others
4 Teratoma
5 Interstitial cell tumor
6 Fibroma, lipoma, adrenoma, myxoma
7 Unclassified varieties

In addition, lymphoma, plasmacytoma, leukemia, and carcinoma of other tissues occasionally produce secondary tumors in the testes. The incidence of teratocarcinoma is roughly constant throughout life, whereas the incidence of seminoma tends to rise with age. One-year survival is rare for patients with embryonal carcinomas and chorioepitheliomas, not uncommon for those with teratocarcinomas and teratomas, and the rule for those with seminomas.

Endocrine changes (such as hyperestrogenism with gynecomastia and increased secretion of gonadotropins with a positive test for chorionic gonadotropin) are occasionally seen with chorioepitheliomas, as well as with other embryonal carcinomas and teratocarcinomas. The endocrine effects of interstitial cell tumors have been discussed.

Diagnosis The diagnosis is made by palpating a mass, usually firm, smooth, and painless. Neoplasms must be distinguished from the changes induced by tuberculosis or gonorrheal epididymitis, from syphilis (usually accompanied by a positive serologic test and a response to specific therapy), and from the various fluid-containing cysts (hydrocele, spermatocele), which may be transilluminated. The diagnosis may be aided also by increased urinary excretion of 17-ketosteroids, estrogens, or gonadotropins; the latter give a positive Aschheim-Zondek test result. When no testicular tumor can be palpated and adrenocortical disease has been excluded in a patient with a possible functioning testicular tumor, it may be necessary to catheterize selectively the spermatic veins and the inferior vena cava to obtain venous samples for determination of plasma estrogen and androgen concentrations in order to locate the tumorous testis. Rarely, tumor cells may be identified in the semen. Serum alpha fetoprotein has been found to be elevated in many patients with testicular tumors.

Treatment Surgical removal is indicated in any tumor of the testes; in seminomas, when surgery is accompanied by irradiation of the lymphatic drainage, a 10-year survival rate of 90 percent may be achieved. In metastatic seminoma, the addition of an alkylating agent such as chlorambucil, 4{-*p*-bis [(2-chloroethyl) amino]-phenyl}butyric acid, to surgical and x-ray therapy has proved useful. A combined surgical and medical approach is often productive in the treatment of other malignant testicular tumors. The nature of the chemotherapy is dictated in part by the stage and the cell type of the tumor. In terato- and embryonal carcinomas, a combination of chlorambucil and dactinomycin, methotrexate and vincristine, or vinblastine with bleomycin may be tried. In chorioepithelioma, methotrexate (4-amino-N^{10}-methylpteroylglutamic acid) alone or with actinomycin D has been used.

DISEASES OF THE PROSTATE

BENIGN PROSTATIC HYPERTROPHY This pathophysiologic disorder, which affects a high proportion of elderly men, is a significant cause of dysuria and incontinence (see Chap. 47) and urinary tract obstruction (see Chap. 278). It has also been considered a potentially precancerous lesion. Hormonally, the prostate is significant as a clinical indicator of androgen secretion, since appreciable reduction in prostatic size accompanies either primary or secondary hypogonadism as well as those disorders of liver function characterized by excessive estrogen activity. Tissue from hypertrophic prostates has been found to have an increased content of the biologically active testosterone metabolite, 5α-dihydrotestosterone.

CARCINOMA OF THE PROSTATE Adenocarcinoma of the prostate is one of the most common tumors of men. It is rare before the age of forty; the incidence rises rapidly with advancing age, with the condition occurring microscopically in 10 to 15 percent of men in the fifth decade and in as many as 60 percent of those in the eighth decade. However, only one-fourth of these cases may become clinically apparent before death. Three-fourths of these tumors arise in the posterior lobe. The majority are easily palpable; hence, frequent routine rectal examinations are indicated to demonstrate early, operable tumors. Although the whole gland need not be enlarged, the presence of stony, hard, indurated nodules or masses strongly suggests adenocarcinoma. Frequently, there may be an elevation in the "prostatic" fraction of serum acid phosphatase while the tumor is still located within the prostatic capsule, and elevation of this enzyme may serve to differentiate a benign hypertropic nodule from a malignancy. Once the tumor has spread locally from the gland, particularly after it has metastasized, total serum acid and alkaline phosphatase levels may be greatly elevated.

Therapy consists of radical prostatectomy; irradiation by x-ray, radium, or radioactive isotopes (colloidal gold); and estrogen hormonal treatment (especially when metastatic disease develops). Androgens are decreased by orchidectomy and by adrenalectomy or adrenocortical suppression following dexamethasone administration (1 to 2 mg given orally in divded doses); estrogen levels are increased by administering diethylstilbestrol, 10 to 15 mg daily, or the equivalent dosage of other estrogenic products. Currently, antiandrogens (cyproterone acetate, etc.) are being evaluated also for their effectiveness in the treatment of this disorder.

REFERENCES

ALBERT A: Bioassay and radioimmunoassay of human gonadotropins. J Clin Endocrinol Metab 28:1683, 1968

BARDIN CW et al: Androgen metabolism and mechanism of action in male pseudohermaphroditism: A study of testicular feminization, in *Recent Progress in Hormone Research,* vol. 29, ed RO Greep, New York: Academic, 1975, p. 65

BESSER G: Hypothalamus as an endocrine organ. Br Med 3:560, 1974

GRUMBACH MM, VAN WYK JJ: Disorders of sex differentiation, in *Textbook of Endocrinology,* ed RH Williams, Philadelphia: Saunders, 1974, p. 423

JIRASEK JE: *Development of the Genital System and Male Pseudohermaphroditism,* Baltimore: Johns Hopkins, 1971

LIPSETT MD, SHERINS RJ: The testis, in *Duncan's Diseases of Metabolism,* eds PK Bondy, LE Rosenberg, Philadelphia: Saunders, 1974, p. 1553

PAULSEN CA: The testes, in *Textbook of Endocrinology,* ed RH Williams, Philadelphia: Saunders, 1974, p. 323

RUBIN P (ed): Current concepts in cancer. No 29. Cancer of the urogenital tract: Testicular tumors. JAMA 213:89, 1970

99
DISEASES OF THE OVARY

JANET W. McARTHUR

HISTORY The ovulatory function of the ovaries was first described by a Dutch physician, Renier de Graaf, in 1673. He recognized small fluid blisters, now known as *graafian follicles,* which had succeeded in reaching the surface of the ovaries before ovulation. The hormonal function of the ovaries was first demonstrated in 1896, by the German biologist Knauer, who showed that ovarian grafts in the dog would prevent the uterine atrophy that follows castration. It was next observed, by Marshall and Jolly, that the ovarian secretion which produced estrus differed from that which was formed by the corpus luteum. The presence of estrogens in the follicles was proved by R. T. Frank, and their occurrence in urine was established by Allen and Doisy, who demonstrated the effectiveness of potent urinary extracts in producing estrus in the vaginal mucosa of rodents. This relatively simple biologic assay method became of incomparable help in the isolation and synthesis of estrogenic compounds.

In 1929, Butenandt and Doisy and associates isolated estrone in a crystalline form from the urine of pregnant women. In 1930, estriol was identified by Browne in human placentas, and in 1936, MacCorquodale obtained estradiol, the most potent natural estrogen, from ovarian follicular fluid. The progestational activity of the corpus luteum hormone was first demonstrated by Corner and Allen in 1929. Five years later progesterone was isolated and identified simultaneously and independently by Butenandt, Allen, Slotta, and Harmann. The chemical structure of the pituitary gonadotropic hormones, follicle-stimulating hormone (FSH) and luteinizing hormone (LH), is not yet known in comparable detail but is undergoing rapid elucidation. Like pituitary thyroid-stimulating hormone and human chorionic gonadotropin (HCG), both are glycoprotein in nature and are composed of two similar but nonidentical subunits. The release (and perhaps also the synthesis) of the pituitary gonadotropins appears to be controlled by a single hypothalamic hormone, the FSH- and LH-releasing factor (FSH-LH-RF), a decapeptide which was isolated and synthesized by Schally in 1971 (Fig. 99-1).

INTRODUCTION The ovary is a specialized organ of reproduction which serves (1) as an exocrine gland which liberates gametes for fertilization, and (2) as a complex of endocrine glands which secretes hormones responsible for (*a*) the growth and cyclic function of the reproductive tract, and (*b*) a variety of metabolic effects in nongenital tissues.

FIGURE 99-1
The structural formula of FSH-LH-RF.

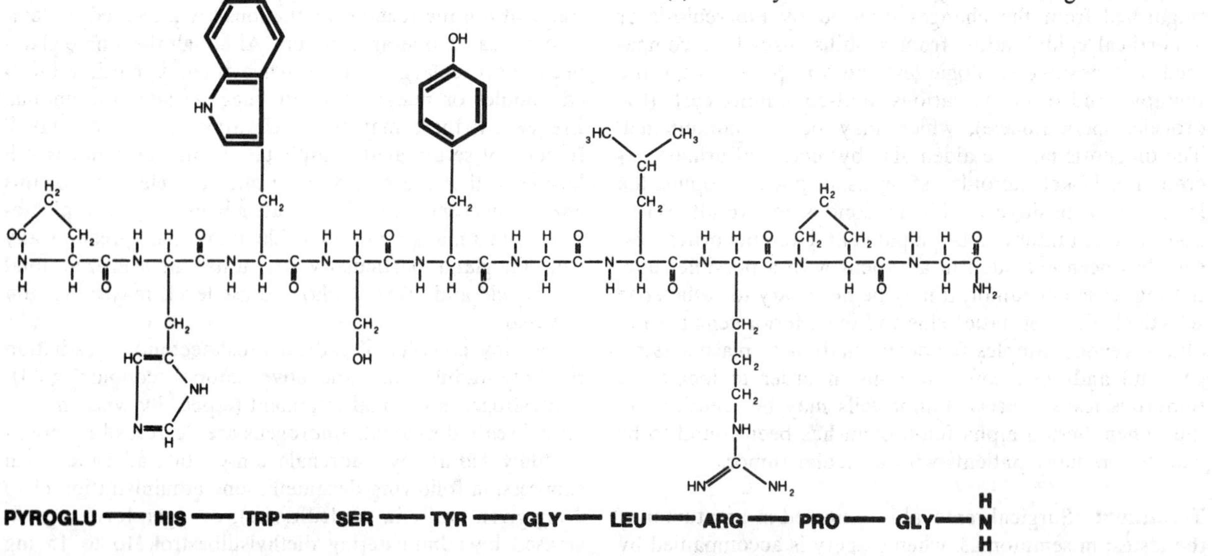

During mature reproductive life a new endocrine gland, the follicle, is activated each month. After ovulation the follicle undergoes transformation into a second gland of internal secretion, the corpus luteum. To the extent that the formation of the corpus luteum requires the prior existence of a follicle, the two structures are interdependent. Nevertheless, differences of fundamental significance obtain between their secretory products. Both structures are embedded in an interstitium, or stroma, which constitutes a third endocrine gland.

A major difference between the ovary and the testis is that the former is endowed with a finite stock of germ cells, whereas the latter proliferates gametes continuously. The number of ova reaches a maximum 5 months before birth. Thereafter the number declines, mainly as the result of atresia, until by the end of the fifth decade the original complement of germ cells is exhausted. An inexorable, though less-rapid, decline in follicular hormone secretion begins in the fifth decade. In addition, the secretion of luteal hormones becomes more and more erratic as the incidence of anovulatory cycles increases. By old age, only the ovarian stroma retains any semblance of functioning tissue.

DEVELOPMENT The formation of the gonads begins at a very early stage, when the embryo has attained a crown-rump length of 5 mm (twenty-one to twenty-eight days of age). The genetic sex of the conceptus is identifiable even earlier, at the age of fifteen days, by the presence of nuclear sex chromatin in the female. During the seventh week, the ovarian destiny of the "indifferent gonad" can be inferred histologically by the absence of the epithelial cords which characterize the developing testis.

Four major phases in the development of the ovary are recognized: (1) migration of primordial germ cells from their site of origin in the endoderm of the primitive gut to bilateral thickenings (the "germinal ridges") of the coelomic epithelium ventral to the developing mesonephros, (2) proliferation of the germinal and nongerminal cells in the genital ridges, (3) division of the gonads into a peripheral cortex and a central medulla, and (4) sex differentiation, consisting of proliferation of the cortex and involution of the medulla in the female, and the reverse process in the male. A complex sex-determining mechanism, the details of which are obscure, is responsible for the conversion of the "indifferent gonad" into an ovary or testis. The cortical germ cells (oogonia) increase rapidly in number as a result of mitotic division, whereupon they enter the meiotic prophase, to become, by definition, oocytes. Each is soon invested by a single layer of smaller supporting cells to form the primordial follicles. In this resting phase the oocytes remain throughout childhood and adult life until either preovulatory maturation or pseudomaturation with atresia occurs. The oocytes appear to exert an inductive influence upon the surrounding granulosa cells, since follicles fail to develop in ovaries which lack oocytes, and oocyte atresia is followed by granulosal degeneration.

COMPARTMENTS The complexity of the tasks devolving upon the ovary is reflected in the heterogeneity of its structure. Throughout active reproductive life, morphologic and biochemical events are occurring simultaneously in the follicular, luteal, and interstitial compartments. Anatomic specialization in the ovary is paralleled by a degree of biochemical specialization. Thus, although in vitro studies reveal that upon incubation with acetate, each of the compartments is capable of synthesizing all the major categories of gonadal steroids, in vivo there is a preferential formation of estrogen by the follicle, of progestogens by the corpus luteum, and of androgens by the stroma.

Follicle Follicular growth comprises two phases. During the first, the oocyte enlarges rapidly to virtually adult dimensions while the investing cortical cells (the membrana granulosa), which convert the germ cell into a primordial follicle, grow very slowly. During the second phase, further growth of the oocyte is minimal but the follicle enlarges rapidly and develops an antrum, which fills with fluid secreted by the granulosa cells. The antrum first appears when the follicle attains a diameter two or three times that of the contained oocyte. Once a follicle has acquired an antrum it becomes, by definition, a graafian follicle.

Maturation falls short of completion in all but that minute proportion of graafian follicles destined to ovulate. Periodically, in response to gonadotropin stimulation (see below), the elected follicle exhibits an intense preovulatory growth spurt, accompanied by the increasing antral distention, the loosening of the cumulus oophorus (those granulosa cells which hold the egg in the suspension), and the hypertrophy and hyperemia of the theca interna. As the follicle enlarges, its wall thins and presently ruptures, releasing the ovum into the peritoneal cavity. A complex of satellite follicles enlarges concomitantly, but to a lesser extent, and after ovulation they undergo rapid atresia.

Growth of the follicle is paralleled by biochemical processes resulting in the secretion of estrogen and, during the immediately preovulatory phase, of small amounts of progesterone. At the peak of follicular activity, the secretion rate of estradiol varies from 0.2 to 0.5 mg per 24 h. The prime locus of estrogen synthesis has not been directly identified but is believed to be the theca interna.

Corpus luteum Following ovulation, the ruptured follicle is converted into a corpus luteum, which likewise has a limited anatomic and biochemical life span. This is divisible into stages of proliferation and hyperemia, vascularization, maturity, and retrogression. The secretion of estrogen is continued and is supplemented by the secretion of progesterone. Biosynthetic activity increases steadily and becomes maximal on days 21 to 22 of the menstrual cycle, when implantation of the fertilized ovum occurs. Estimates of the progesterone secretion rate, though discrepant, agree qualitatively in that they reveal a phenomenal increase in the biosynthetic capacity of the transformed follicle, to the vicinity of 20 to 40 mg progesterone per day.

How the follicular-to-luteal change in the pattern of hormone synthesis is effected is the subject of much speculation. One view is embodied in the so-called "two-cell" theory. This postulates that the cells of the theca interna are endowed with the full enzyme complement required for the synthesis of estradiol-17β, whereas the cells of the granulosa possess little or no 17-desmolase activity and only weak 17-hydroxylase activity. During the follicular phase, the well-vascularized theca interna cells synthesize estrogens, which have ready access either to the follicular fluid or the systemic circulation, whereas the granulosa cells, lacking a blood supply, are presumably deprived of the nutrients required for hormone synthesis. After ovulation, the granulosa cells become richly vascularized, undergo enlargement, and form the corpus luteum. However, in consequence of their enzymic endowment, they are ill equipped to synthesize estrogen in quantity and secrete mainly progesterone.

Interstitium The interstitium, or stroma, acts as a supporting matrix for the follicles, corpora lutea, and corpora albicantia, and, in addition, it secretes steroids. Qualitative and quantitative changes in its structure occur in association with various reproductive processes. During pregnancy there is increasing luteinization of the stroma, and during the postmenopausal years stromal proliferation and luteinization are frequent. In extreme old age, the stroma tends to lose its stimulated appearance. The higher grades of stromal luteinization are sometimes associated with clinical indications of androgen hypersecretion.

The hilus may come eventually to be regarded as a fourth ovarian compartment, but at present it is generally treated as a specialized portion of the interstitium. It contains elements resembling testicular Leydig cells, which occur in nests, the size of which varies at different ages. Hyperplasia of these cells may occur during pregnancy, and the larger hilus cell complexes are more frequent in elderly women.

FIGURE 99-2

Plasma levels of FSH, LH, estradiol, and progesterone during the human menstrual cycle. The day of the midcycle LH peak is utilized as the central reference point for all data, and is designated as Day 0. (Adapted from L Speroff and R Vande Wiele, Am J Obstet Gynecol 109:234, 1971)

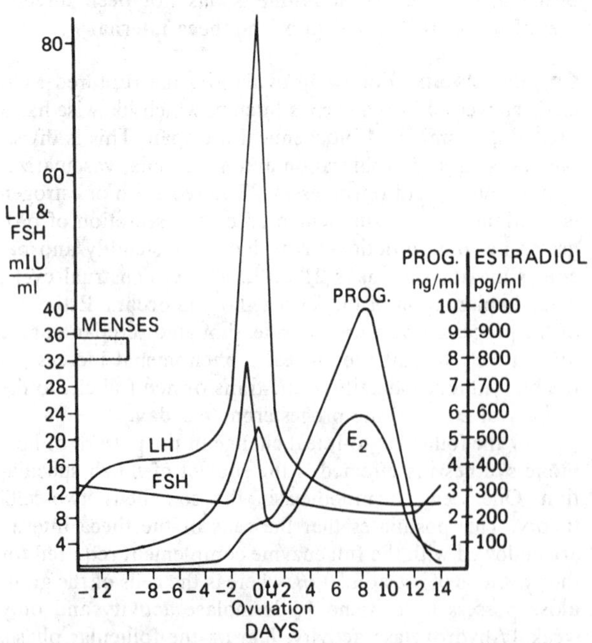

Androstenedione and dehydroepiandrosterone can be extracted from normal ovarian stroma, the highest concentrations being found in the hilus.

PHYSIOLOGIC CONTROL OF THE OVARY The *follicles* of the ovary are generally believed to be capable of development to the antrum stage in the absence of pituitary function. However, evidence suggests that more immature follicles may be responsive to gonadotropins and that their progression is contingent upon gonadotropic stimulation. Further maturation of the follicles and the sequential changes which characterize the normal menstrual cycle are clearly dependent upon the release of gonadotropins from the anterior lobe of the pituitary gland (Fig. 99-2). Follicular growth is stimulated by FSH, while follicular fluid production, steroidogenesis, and luteinization appear to be stimulated by LH. The growth of the ovulatory complex of follicles for a given cycle begins during the luteal phase of the preceding cycle and continues in response to the high FSH levels which are attained during the early follicular phase. As the complex matures, the rate of estrogen secretion, initially minimal, becomes more rapid. The increasing plasma concentration of estradiol presently exceeds a threshold level, triggering a surge of LH and FSH, which causes further enlargement of the preovulatory follicle, enhanced estrogen secretion, ovulation, and corpus luteum formation. After cessation of the gonadotropin surge, the continued presence of low levels of LH in the circulation permits the *corpus luteum* to develop and to attain maximal capacity to synthesize estrogen and progesterone. However, unless supplementary luteotropic stimulation in the form of HCG secreted by the trophoblast of a conceptus embedded during the midluteal phase is delivered, the corpus luteum begins to regress within 9 to 11 days after ovulation, and its secretory capacity rapidly diminishes. No uterine luteolytic factor such as that demonstrated in the sheep has as yet been isolated in the human being, and the mechanism responsible for the decline remains obscure. The in vitro synthesis of steroids by the *stroma* is increased by LH and HCG which, in the female as in the male, are interstitial cell-stimulating hormones.

The control of gonadotropin secretion is vested in the central nervous system. Regulation is effected by means of a vascular link between the hypothalamus and the pituitary, the hypothalamic-hypophyseal portal system. The neurohormone which regulates pituitary gonadotropin secretion is synthesized in the so-called hypophysiotropic area. This area occupies a medial position in the ventral hypothalamus, and extends from the median eminence to the optic chiasm. Neural inputs from other regions of the central nervous system (CNS) are received by the hypophysiotropic area, which translates them into neurohormonal signals to the pituitary. Biogenic amines acting as synaptic transmitters have the capacity to alter the level of activity of the FSH-LH-RF-secreting neurons in the hypophysiotropic area. In animals, dopamine exerts a stimulatory effect and serotonin an inhibitory effect upon the release of FSH-LH-RF. The areas of the human brain which are critically involved in reproduction are not yet accurately delineated. However, in rats a region of the medial basal hypothalamus which is responsive to the negative feedback action of estrogen and progesterone sustains acyclic gonadotropin release. A more rostral region which includes the suprachiasmatic area is responsive to the positive feedback action of estrogen. Under proper hormonal and environmental conditions, this region activates the terminal infundibular region and evokes the ovulatory gonadotropin surge.

HORMONES OF THE OVARY

The ovary secretes a water-soluble nonsteroid hormone or hormone complex known as relaxin and three types of steroid hormones: estrogens, progestogens, and androgens.

NONSTEROID (RELAXIN) Relaxin has not been isolated as a chemical entity, but its activity is associated with a water-soluble polypeptide structure. In conjunction with estrogens and progestogens, it facilitates parturition in certain mammals by loosening the symphysis pubis and sacroiliac joints. Relaxin has also been reported to soften the cervix, increase the uterine responsiveness to oxytocin, and promote tubuloalveolar growth of the mammary gland. In human pregnancy, blood relaxin values reach a maximum during the thirty-sixth week and remain high until delivery, whereupon a precipitous fall occurs. The cellular source in the ovary is unknown, and since the hormone can apparently be formed in other organs of the reproductive tract, its specificity as an ovarian secretion is in doubt.

STEROIDS The ovarian steroids are synthesized from acetate via cholesterol and pregnenolone by essentially the same pathways as exist in other steroid-producing organs—the testis, adrenal cortex, and placenta (Fig. 99-3).

Estrogens The term *estrogen* refers strictly to substances capable of inducing estrus, or sexual receptivity, in female mammals. However, it has been extended to include compounds which produce certain uterine changes and to the steroid metabolites of true estrogens, whether or not these possess biologic activity. In the nonpregnant female, the ovary is the principal site of estrogen formation; during pregnancy, estrogen formation by the fetoplacental unit gradually increases until, by the third trimester, it may exceed ovarian production by a thousandfold.

Estradiol-17β is believed to be the primary secretory product of the human ovary and to be interconvertible with estrone by dehydrogenases which are present in the ovary and in many other tissues. Estrone and estradiol are in turn, irreversibly converted to estriol, an estrogen of human urine that is quantitatively important, especially during pregnancy. Additional estrogenic metabolites of low biologic activity have been isolated in great number from human tissues and from the urine of pregnant and nonpregnant women.

The natural estrogens are all 18- or 19-carbon steroids which are characterized by the aromatic nature of ring A, the oxygen substituent at C-17, and the phenolic hydroxyl group at C-3. Many nonsteroidal estrogens have been synthesized for clinical use; they produce biologic effects resembling those of the natural estrogens. Representative examples from both the natural and synthetic categories are depicted in Fig. 99-4.

The liver is the principal site of the interconversion of estradiol and estrone, and is largely responsible for the inactivation of estrogen in the body. Protein-bound estrogen is abstracted from the plasma and excreted into the bile, from which it returns to the liver via the enterohepatic circulation. Degradation of estrogen is accomplished by (1) conversion to relatively inactive estrogenic compounds, (2) conjugation with glucuronic and sulfuric acids for excretion in the urine as water-soluble complexes, and (3) oxidation to unknown nonestrogenic substances.

Progestogens The term *progestogen* refers to substances which serve to prepare the uterus for the reception and development of the fertilized ovum. It has been extended to include compounds capable of duplicating, in whole or in part, the effects produced by the corpus luteum secretions.

Progesterone is synthesized by all the steroid-producing glands. When secreted by the corpus luteum and placenta it exerts powerful physiologic effects in its own right; in addition, it is thought to serve as the key intermediate from which the androgens, estrogens, and corticosteroids are ultimately derived.

The ovarian progestogens consist of progesterone (the most important and abundant compound) and at least two other steroids: 20α- and 20β-dihydroprogesterone. Both these partially reduced compounds have been detected in human follicular fluid and in the corpus luteum and placenta, the 20α isomer in higher concentration than the 20β. The basic molecule consists of 21 carbon atoms, two of which are contained in the side chain at C-17. These compounds are secreted by the follicle just prior to ovulation and are produced in much larger amounts by the corpus luteum. The quantity of progesterone which can be isolated from the corpus luteum is small compared with the amounts of progesterone secreted during the luteal phase

FIGURE 99-3
Biosynthetic pathways for the synthesis of ovarian estrogen in the human female. (Adapted from OW Smith and KJ Ryan, Am J Obstet Gynecol 84:141, 1962)

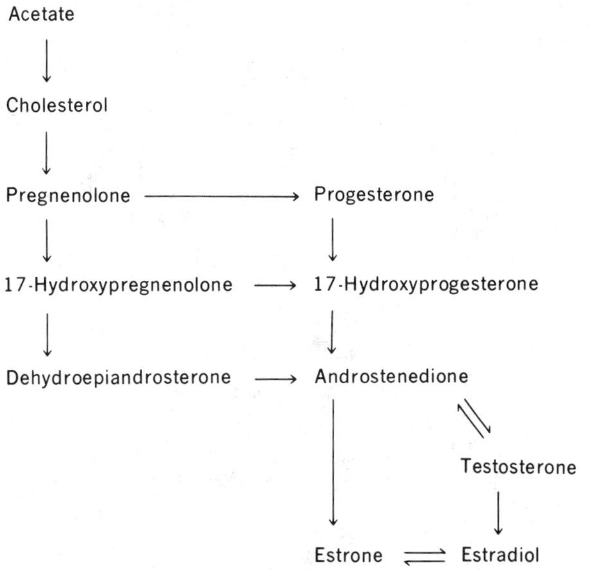

of the cycle, indicating that progesterone is secreted almost as rapidly as it is produced.

A number of progestational steroids which mimic various facets of natural progesterone action have been synthesized. Many exhibit androgenic or estrogenic as well as progestational properties and, in these qualitative differences from the natural hormone, differ materially from the synthetic estrogen compounds. The short half-life of progesterone and the large doses consequently required to elicit biologic effects have prompted efforts to alter the progesterone molecule so as to increase its potency. Two groups of progestogens far surpassing the natural hormone in oral activity have been synthesized: (1) derivatives of testosterone (e.g., ethiosterone) and of 19-nortestosterone (e.g., norethynodrel and norethindrone), the latter exhibiting the marked enhancement of oral potency which results from the removal of the angle methyl group C-19 attached to C-10 and (2) compounds derived from 17-hydroxyprogesterone [e.g., medroxyprogesterone (Provera), chlormadinone]. Esterification of 17α-hydroxyprogesterone by caproic or other long-chain fatty acids yields long-acting preparations useful for parenteral administration.

The structural formulas of some representative synthetic progestational steroids are shown in Fig. 99-5 together with allied natural compounds.

The liver is largely responsible for the inactivation of progesterone, which it first reduces to pregnanediol and then conjugates with glucuronic acid for excretion in the urine. These processes are aided by an enterohepatic circulation which differs from that of the estrogens in that approximately 30 percent of progesterone or its metabolites is lost in the feces, whereas the estrogens are almost completely absorbed from the intestine. Some 10 to 15 percent of exogenously administered progesterone can be accounted for by urinary pregnanediol, and a small additional percentage by several isomers and closely related pregnane derivatives. The major degradation products of progesterone are unknown.

Androgens That the ovary possesses the biochemical potential for androgen production has long been evident from physiologic and clinical observation. In vitro incubations reveal, moreover, that testosterone is a product of the stroma and of no other ovarian compartment. However, in vivo studies are bringing to light an exceedingly complex situation.

Although *testosterone* is present in measurable amounts in the circulation of the human female, the ovarian contribution, as measured in the venous effluent, is negligible. It would appear that such androgen precursors as androstenedione and dehydroepiandrosterone, which are secreted to a small extent by the ovaries and to a greater extent by the adrenal cortex, are converted to active androgens in the peripheral tissues. According to one view, the function of androstenedione and dehydroepiandrosterone may be to serve as prehormones (endocrine secretions which possess little or no inherent biologic activity but which, after peripheral conversion to more active compounds, contribute significantly to the overall biologic effect). Peripheral conversion could be by any tissues, including those of the target organs. This arrangement would enable effective concentrations of an active product (e.g., testosterone or dihydrotestosterone) to be achieved locally in regions such as the clitoris without the high circulating levels of androgen which would virilize a female subject.

Androstenedione is thought to be converted in the liver to testosterone and to undergo intrahepatic conjugation with glucuronic acid without mixing with the plasma testosterone. Thus, testosterone glucosiduronate is not a unique metabolite of testosterone. A proportion of plasma testosterone is reduced by the liver to the weakly androgenic compound, androsterone, and its inactive isomer, 5β-androsterone, and these compounds are rendered water-soluble by conjugation with glucuronic and sulfuric acid.

LEVELS IN BODY FLUIDS Estrogens Plasma levels of estradiol are measurable by fluorometric, isotopic, and immunologic methods. During the normal cycle, the range extends from 75 to 1,000 pg per ml.

FIGURE 99-4
The structural formulas of some important estrogens, natural and synthetic.

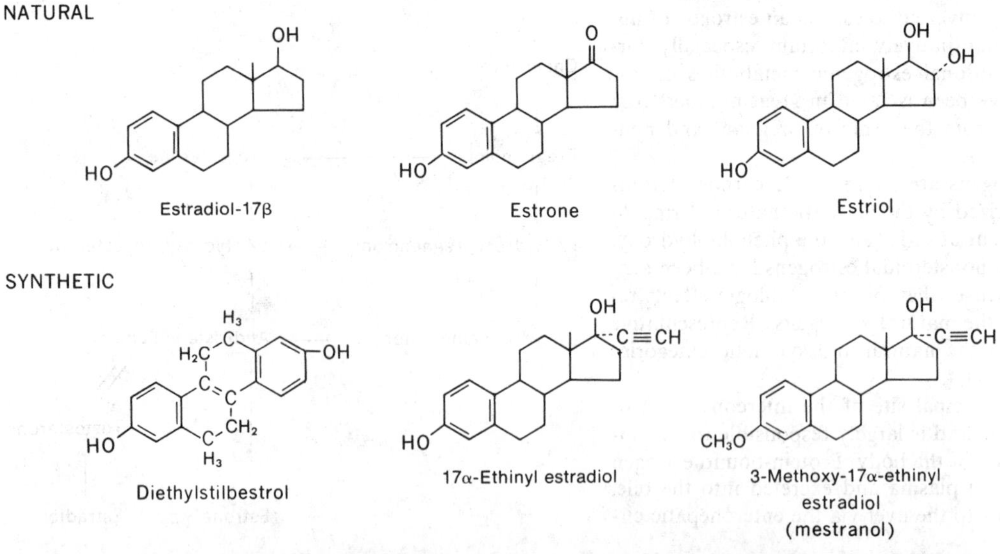

The natural estrogens are measurable in urine by colorimetric and fluorometric methods. During the menstrual cycle, two peaks of estrogen excretion are generally noted, one in midcycle immediately prior to ovulation, and the other during the midluteal phase. During the midcycle peak, the "total" estrogen excretion (estradiol plus estrone and estriol) does not normally exceed 100 μg per 24 h. In the fifth decade of life, the urinary estrogen levels of women commence a steady decline. The urinary estrogen level of postmenopausal women is low and is derived, in large part, from androstenedione secreted by the adrenal cortex.

Urinary levels of endogenous estrogen in patients with liver disease are variable, with only a portion displaying the increased levels that might be anticipated.

Urinary estrogen determinations are sometimes helpful in detecting granulosa cell or theca cell tumors in postmenopausal women. The adrenogenital syndrome and occasional adrenocortical tumors are also associated with elevated levels of urinary estrogen.

FIGURE 99-5

The structural formulas of some important progestogens and allied compounds.

NATURAL

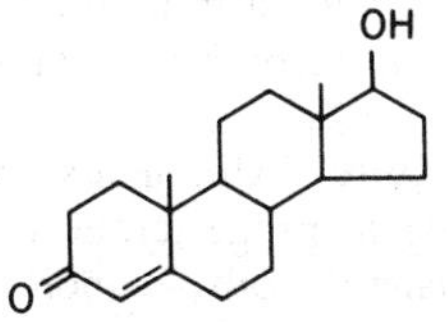

Testosterone

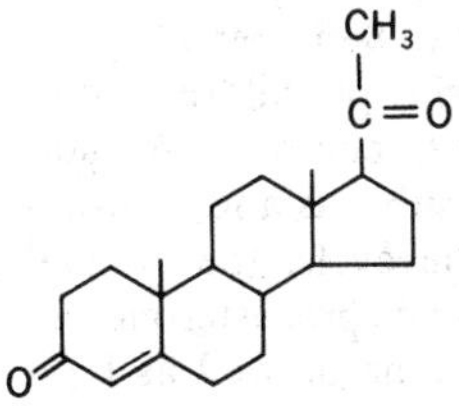

Progesterone

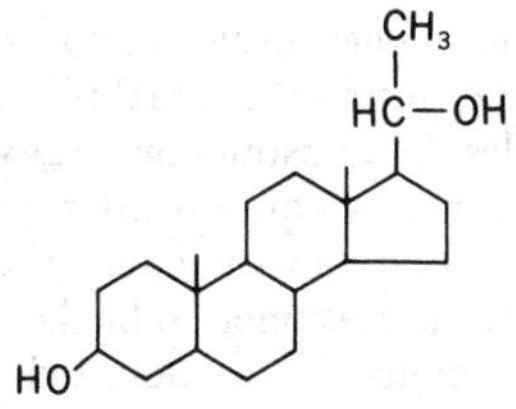

Pregnandiol

SYNTHETIC

17-Hydroxyprogesterone derivatives

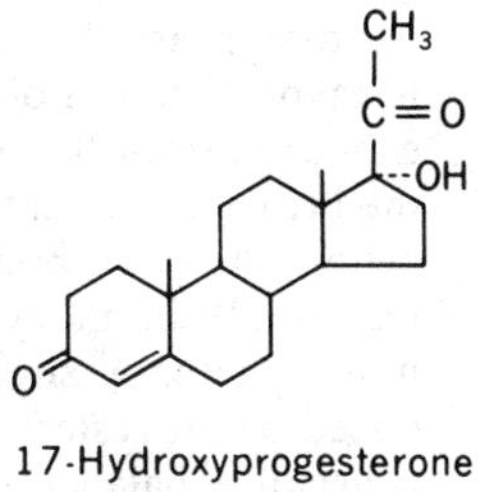

17-Hydroxyprogesterone

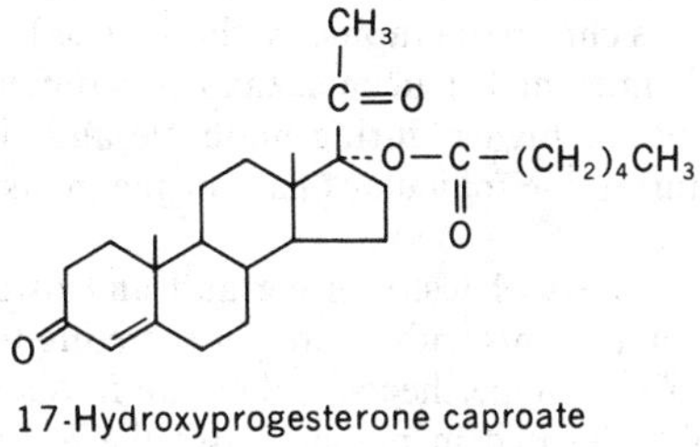

17-Hydroxyprogesterone caproate
(delalutin)

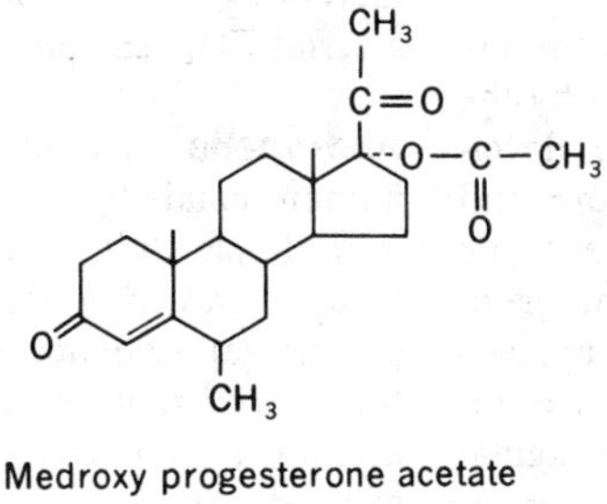

Medroxy progesterone acetate
(provera)

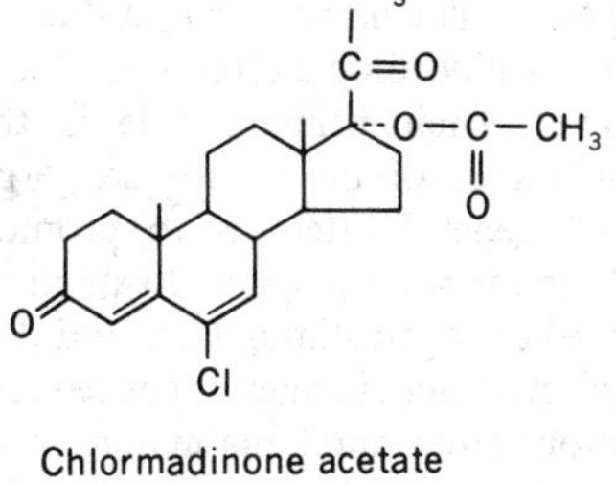

Chlormadinone acetate
(lormin)

Testosterone and 19-Nortestosterone derivatives

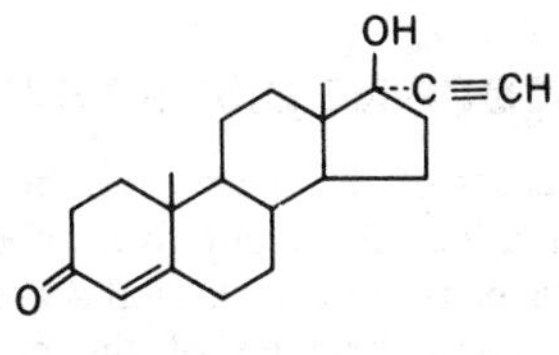

Ethisterone
(pranone, lutocylol)

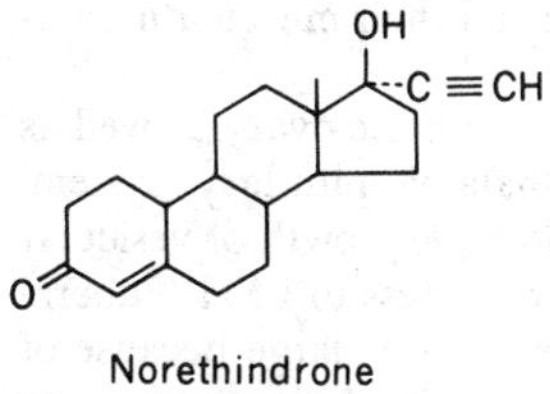

Norethindrone
(norlutin)

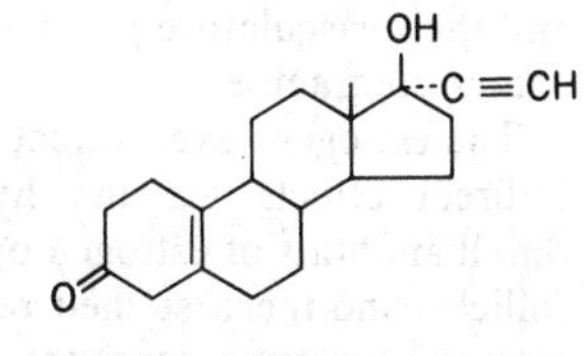

Norethynodrel

Progestogens *Progesterone* plasma levels are measurable by isotopic and immunologic methods. During the normal menstrual cycle, the range extends from 0.5 to 20 ng per ml.

Pregnanediol, the most important reduction product of progesterone, is excreted in the urine as the glucosiduronate and is measurable by gravimetric, colorimetric, and gas chromatographic techniques. Although pregnanediol is not a unique metabolite of progesterone, there is a rough correlation between the rate of pregnanediol excretion and the rate of progesterone secretion. Low and relatively constant levels of urinary pregnanediol (in the vicinity of 1 mg per 24 h) are detected during the follicular phase of the cycle; higher levels, with a range of 2 to 8 mg per 24 h, are found during the luteal phase. The urine of children, adult males, and postmenopausal women also contains pregnanediol in low concentrations; in these subjects and in women during the follicular phase of the cycle, the adrenal cortex is presumed to be the source. Since progesterone can be secreted by a luteinized theca interna as well as by a corpus luteum, elevated levels of urinary pregnanediol do not necessarily connote the prior occurrence of ovulation.

Androgens *Testosterone, androstenedione,* and *dehydroepiandrosterone* are measurable in the plasma by double isotope dilution and by immunologic methods. In normal women the plasma testosterone level is below 0.1 μg per ml. *Testosterone glucosiduronate* is measurable in the urine by isotopic and gas chromatographic methods. The levels tend to be several times higher in men than in women, and in the latter they are higher during midcycle and the luteal phase than during the follicular phase of the menstrual cycle.

The plasma levels of testosterone and androstenedione are increased in patients with androgen-secreting tumors of the ovary and with hyperthecosis; they are frequently, but not invariably, elevated in patients with the Stein-Leventhal syndrome.

ACTIONS Estrogens The name estrogen does scant justice to the diversity of physiologic effects produced by the estrogenic hormones. Their primary role is the development and maintenance of the female sex organs, and perhaps their most general effect is to promote tissue growth. At puberty the tubes, uterus, and vagina enlarge in response to increased estrogen stimulation, and the appearance of the external genitalia changes in consequence of fat deposition in the mons pubis and labia majora. The vaginal epithelium thickens during the follicular phase of the menstrual cycle, with shedding of a large number of cornified epithelial cells containing pyknotic nuclei. The cervix is stimulated to secrete mucus of low viscosity and high permeability to spermatozoa. The uterine and tubal mucosa and their vasculature proliferate, and their musculature becomes contractile.

The estrogens exert direct effects on the ovary as well as indirect effects via the hypothalamic-pituitary system. Small amounts of estrogen promote the growth of vesicular follicles and increase their responsiveness to FSH. Puberal estrogen secretion causes the breasts to enlarge because of increased fat deposition, development of the supporting stroma, and ductal growth. The increased melanin pigmentation of the nipples and perineum is due, at least in part, to estrogen. There is a widespread deposition of fat in the subcutaneous tissues, particularly in the buttocks and thighs, leading to the characteristic rounding of the female figure.

The estrogens stimulate cell division in the deeper layers of the skin and gingivae, and in the mucosae of the oral cavity, nose, and urethra, causing a more rapid replacement of the outer cornified layers. Bone metabolism is significantly affected, with increased osteoblastic activity, a positive calcium and phosphorus balance, widening of the pelvic outlet, and accelerated epiphyseal closure. The composition of the circulating lipids is altered, with a fall in total cholesterol level and an increase in the α-lipoprotein fraction over the β fraction. Estrogens increase the levels of serum thyroxine-binding globulin, corticosteroid-binding globulin, ceruloplasmin, total copper, prothrombin, and factor V. Antithrombin activity is decreased by estrogens.

Progestogens Although secreted in far greater amounts than estrogen, progesterone exerts only negligible effects on the general body economy. It produces few specific changes when present alone, acting ordinarily in conjunction with estrogen. Progesterone tends to encourage tissue differentiation, rather than growth. Its most important function is to induce secretory changes in the lining of the tubes and uterus, the endometrium being thereby adapted for the implantation of the fertilized ovum. The viscosity of the cervical mucus is increased during the postovulatory phase, rendering it impermeable to spermatozoa, and ferning disappears. Tubal and uterine contractility are altered to favor transport of the fertilized ovum and to prevent its expulsion from the uterus. Lobuloalveolar proliferation of the breast is stimulated. Progesterone exerts a thermogenic action, the basal body temperature increasing by approximately 1°F in midcycle and remaining elevated during the luteal phase. A slightly negative nitrogen balance is induced by progesterone, and by antagonism to aldosterone, a negative balance of sodium, chloride, and water is favored. Progesterone acts as a mild respiratory stimulant, increasing minute ventilation while decreasing alveolar and arterial CO_2 tension and the respiratory quotient.

Androgens The physiologic role of the androgens in the human female has not been clearly delineated. However, it is probable that they act to promote a positive nitrogen balance and to increase libido and muscular strength. Experimental evidence suggests that by local action within the ovary small amounts of androgen hasten antrum formation by separating the granulosa cells; larger amounts cause destruction of ova and granulosa cell atrophy. It may be that atresia of those follicles not destined to ovulate is promoted by androgens. In excess, these compounds may blight the follicles of the ovary in the Stein-Leventhal syndrome, contributing to its polycystic structure.

ENDOCRINE DISORDERS OF THE OVARY

Diseases of the ovary may be classified as endocrine and nonendocrine, depending on the presence or absence of disturbances in hormonal secretion. Endocrine diseases of the ovary, because of the prominence of their systemic manifestations, are of concern to the internist as well as the gynecologist and are considered here. Nonendocrine diseases, which comprise such entities as endometriosis, infections, and nonfunctioning tumors of the ovary, tend to produce localized effects and are not treated in this chapter. The endocrine disorders of the ovary may be classified as (1) hypo-, hyper-, or dysfunctional, (2) primarily ovarian in origin, or secondary to disturbances elsewhere, and (3) congenital or acquired. Some disorders, particularly those secondary to disturbances of hypothalamic or pituitary secretion, are general in that they affect follicular, luteal, and interstitial functions. Others are compartmental in that they involve only one or two of the major subunits of the ovary (Table 99-1). Methodologic difficulties are responsible for the meager documentation of many ovarian syndromes. However, as these are overcome, a rational biochemical schema for classification is emerging.

Because of the specialized role of the ovary as an *organ of reproduction,* its disturbances tend to give rise to more restricted symptoms than do those of many other endocrine organs. Unless the influence of a feminizing tumor, for example, is projected against the barren sexual background of childhood or the postmenopausal years, the manifestations may be so inconspicuous as to escape notice. Disorders heralded by infrequent menstruation, staining, or the disappearance of cramps may be trivial in systemic terms and yet have profound reproductive consequences. This is attributable to the fact that except during periods of temporary dissociation, such as adolescence and lactation, the exocrine and endocrine activities of the ovary are firmly integrated. Any deficiency in either results in impaired reproductive function.

OVARIAN HYPOFUNCTION

Although the suspension of established ovarian function is readily recognizable as pathologic, it may be less easy to determine whether delayed sexual maturation in a child reflects hypofunction of clinical significance. The *menarche* presently occurs at a mean age of 12.6 years; since its timing is significantly influenced by genetic factors, the family history as regards menarcheal age should be investigated. The menarche is ordinarily preceded by breast development, a spurt in skeletal growth, and the appearance of pubic hair (axillary hair tends to appear almost simultaneously with the menarche). The presence of any of the secondary sex characteristics, or of superficial cells in the vaginal smear or urinary sediment, constitutes presumptive evidence of incipient ovarian activation.

TABLE 99-1
Classification of the endocrine disorders of the ovary

- *I* Ovarian hypofunction
  - *A* Primary
    - *1* General
      - *a* Gonadal dysgenesis (Turner's syndrome)
      - *b* Menopause
  - *B* Secondary
    - *1* General
      - *a* Hypothalamic disorders
      - *b* Hypopituitarism
      - *c* Constitutional and metabolic disturbances
    - *2* Compartmental
      - *a* Anovulatory bleeding
      - *b* Inadequate luteal phase
- *II* Ovarian hyperfunction
  - *A* Primary
    - *1* Feminizing tumors
    - *2* Masculinizing tumors
  - *B* Secondary
    - *1* General: true precocious puberty
    - *2* Compartmental
      - *a* Persistent follicle cyst
      - *b* Corpus luteum cyst
      - *c* Stein-Leventhal syndrome and hyperthecosis
- *III* Ovarian dysfunction
  - *A* Choriocarcinoma
  - *B* Struma ovarii
  - *C* Carcinoid

Primary ovarian hypofunction

GONADAL DYSGENESIS (TURNER'S SYNDROME) Upon gaining the germinal ridges, the primordial germ cells may, for obscure reasons, degenerate without undergoing transformation into primordial follicles. A "streak gonad," incapable not only of ovulation but also of estrogen secretion, is thereby formed. In rare instances, the medullary stroma and hilus cells of such gonads secrete sufficient androgen to induce mild virilization.

In patients with this genetic disorder, the breasts fail to develop, sex hair growth is sparse, and the titers of FSH and LH early rise to menopausal levels. Although amenorrhea is the rule, the germ cell endowment is occasionally sufficient to permit menstruation for a few years, and one well-documented instance of pregnancy has been reported. The key genetic defect is an abnormality of the second X chromosome in some of or all the cells of the patient. Approximately one-half of the patients have a 45-X chromosome constitution, one-third have mosaicism (most frequently 45-X-46-XX), and a small proportion have a structural defect of the 1-X chromosome with the loss of a proportion of its genetic material. The presence of other congenital anomalies such as short stature, webbing of the neck, short metacarpals, and coarctation of the aorta often suggests the diagnosis during the prepuberal years.

Cyclic replacement therapy is indicated to prevent osteoporosis, premature aging of the skin, and other consequences of estrogen deficiency. Natural estrogens may be combined with progestational agents in the manner described for the treatment of the menopause (see below), and a similar schema for periodic surveillance followed.

MENOPAUSE The menopause, or final cessation of menses, is the consequence of a form of ovarian hypofunction that is experienced by all women who survive to middle life. Fertility diminishes considerably before the menopause, apparently because the uterus becomes less efficient in supporting young embryos. The current median age of the menopause, which is 50 years, seems to be unrelated either to an early or a late menarche. An interval of approximately 2 years generally supervenes between the first symptoms of the climacteric and the cessation of menses. The manner in which menstruation ceases is variable (Table 99-2).

Hot flashes occur in 80 to 85 percent of menopausal women and constitute the most troublesome symptom. They generally begin before the periods cease and may continue, though with diminishing frequency and intensity, for many years. Their pathologic physiology is obscure. Subjective sensations of warmth are confined to the chest, neck, and face and may be accompanied by diffuse or patchy flushing of the skin and sweating. Hot flashes are characteristically brief, lasting only a few minutes, and occur most frequently when heat production is increased (e.g., after emotional stress or, less frequently, after meals) or when the dissipation of heat is impaired by bedclothes or by high ambient temperatures and humidity. The severity of menopausal symptoms is affected by the rate at which involution of the ovary takes place. In women experiencing a sudden (not necessarily surgical) loss of ovarian function, hot flashes are likely to be severe, and dyspareunia due to atrophy of the vagina may be troublesome. In women experiencing a gradual decline of ovarian activity, amenorrhea may be the sole symptom.

Mild depression is not uncommon in menopausal women, its frequency tending to be inversely proportional to the patient's understanding of menopausal physiology. A "menopausal syndrome" in a psychiatric sense appears to be nonexistent. Women with anxiety neurosis, hysteria, phobic states, hypochondriasis, or obsessive-compulsive neurosis during the menopause are generally found to have had the illness in earlier life. Psychological problems unrelated to the menopause per se are common in the 40- to 55-year-old group and relate to the "empty nest" syndrome; responsibility for the care of adolescent children and aging parents; ungratified sexuality; fears of obesity, cancer, and the loss of sexual attractiveness; and the fear of having ultimately to depend upon children or charity.

Termination of menstrual function before the age of 40 may be considered premature. A small proportion of patients experiencing a precocious menopause exhibit an unusual propensity to autoimmune disease, which may affect the ovaries. A few additional patients have sex chromosome mosaicism. In the majority of instances, no explanation can be found. The cause of the naturally timed climacteric is likewise somewhat obscure. It appears to reflect the progressive depletion of oocytes and the loss of their inductive effect upon the granulosa and theca cells. With a diminution of the steroid-feedback influence upon the hypothalamus and/or pituitary, the gonadotropin titer rises, and the release of FSH and LH is no longer coordinated. Eventually the stroma remains as the only functional compartment of the ovary. Particularly in instances where the occurrence of a precocious menopause is suspected, the increased circulating levels of pituitary gonadotropins are useful diagnostically. The finding of one, or preferably two, elevated plasma levels of FSH (which rises earlier and higher in the climacteric than does LH) is virtually pathognomonic of ovarian failure.

Treatment of the menopause comprises: (1) the exclusion of organic causes of any associated menorrhagia, (2) detailed explanation of the physiologic consequences of the climacteric, ventilation of the patient's anxieties, and reassurance, and (3) hormonal replacement. Estrogen treatment suppresses hot flashes and prevents or relieves dyspareunia. Moreover, by decreasing the rate of bone resorption, estrogens appear to delay the onset of osteoporosis. Whether estrogens can exert a prophylactic effect upon coronary artery disease in women remains to be determined.

The fear that estrogen treatment increases the expected incidence of carcinoma of the breast and uterus appears to be unfounded. However, mastalgia in estrogen-treated women may cause concern, vaginal bleeding sometimes necessitates a diagnostic curettage, and fluid retention occasionally requires concomitant diuretic therapy. In consequence, the attitude of many physicians as well as patients toward hormonal treatment is ambivalent.

In the case of patients in whom chronic cystic mastitis or prior cancer of the breast or uterus has been excluded, a convenient practice is to give estrone sulfate (or the equivalent dosage of another natural estrogen) in the daily dose required to suppress hot flashes (1.25 to 2.5 mg) during the first 3 weeks of each month. During days 17 to 21 inclusive of estrogen treatment, medroxyprogesterone acetate 5 to 10 mg, or the equivalent dosage of another progestational agent, is added to effect secretory differentiation of the endometrium, thereby preventing cumulative hyperplasia and dysfunctional bleeding. Sex steroid treatment can be continued indefinitely, and when, in later years, withdrawal flow no longer occurs, the program can be simplified by omission of the progestational component. Tension can be more effectively diminished by supplementing the hormonal program with mild sedatives or tranquilizers, such as phenobarbital 15 mg or chlordiazepoxide 5 mg, several times daily, than by increasing the estrogen dosage. Regular periodic examinations of the breasts and pelvis are essential, as are vaginal smears. A maturation index obtained on the latter is helpful in regulating the estrogen dosage and serves as a screening test for malignancy, particularly of the cervix. However, smears are less reliable for the detection of carcinoma of the endometrium, the more prevalent uterine lesion in the menopausal age group. Therefore, the Papanicolaou smear should be supplemented with an endometrial biopsy before estrogen treatment is instituted. At yearly intervals thereafter an endometrial biopsy, Gravlee jet washing, or other endometrial monitoring procedure should be performed as a precautionary measure. In the event of bleeding which is abnormal in timing or quantity, a dilatation and curettage is indicated.

TABLE 99-2
First menstrual indication of impending natural menopause

Symptom	*Percentage*
Irregularity	34
Periods farther apart	23
Scanty periods	20
"Flooding"	16
Sudden cessation	8

SOURCE: *M Newton and PL Odom, The menopause and its symptoms. South Med J 57:1309, 1964*

Secondary ovarian hypofunction

HYPOTHALAMIC DISORDERS Ovarian hypofunction associated with congenital disorders affecting the hypothalamus, such as the *Laurence-Moon-Biedl syndrome,* is described elsewhere (Chap. 90). A different congenital disorder is believed to be responsible for the rare association of primary amenorrhea with anosmia or hyposmia.

Destructive lesions of the hypothalamus, such as those resulting from the expansion of tumors and cysts, may induce ovarian hypofunction. The *Frommel-Chiari syndrome* of continued lactation and genital atrophy following childbirth appears to be due to a lesion which somehow impairs the secretion of the prolactin-inhibiting factor and that of the FSH- and LH-releasing factor. In a high proportion of such patients, ovulation can be induced by treatment with clomiphene citrate (Clomid) in 5-day courses at a dosage of 50 to 100 mg per day (Fig. 99-6). This agent blocks the negative feedback action of estrogen at the hypothalamic level and evokes the release of FSH and LH from the pituitary.

Emotional strain which alters the afferent neural input to the hypothalamic centers controlling the secretion of the FSH-LH-RF is perhaps the commonest cause of amenorrhea, apart from pregnancy. The vulnerability of girls in the ten- to twenty-year age group to such stresses as attending school away from home has given rise to the term "boarding school amenorrhea." In older women the menstrual cycle is more resistant to disturbance, and either exceptional stress or frank emotional illness, such as depression, is required to suspend ovarian function. Treatment with Clomid will sometimes bring about ovulation, but in severe cases, psychotherapy may be needed to restore normal cyclicity.

HYPOPITUITARISM In early life, the commonest pituitary cause of sexual infantilism is a *craniopharyngioma;* in adult life, *chromophobe* or *eosinophil adenomas of the pituitary* and *necrosis resulting from post-partum hemorrhage (Sheehan's syndrome)* are the most frequent pituitary lesions resulting in ovarian insufficiency (Chap. 90). *Granulomatous diseases* (Hand-Schüller-Christian syndrome, sarcoid) and metastatic tumors or neoplasms arising in surrounding structures (meningioma) may diminish pituitary function at any age.

Headache, visual disturbances, or impaired growth suggest the possibility of a pituitary disorder in prepuberal girls, although failure of the menses to begin (primary amenorrhea) may be the sole manifestation. In adults, the cessation of menses previously present (secondary amenorrhea) and the coupling of lactation with amenorrhea should suggest the possibility of a chromophobe or acidophil tumor of the pituitary. X-ray visualization of the sella turcica and determination of the plasma prolactin level are essential components of the investigation of all patients with obscure amenorrheas. Sequential treatment with preparations of human menopausal urinary gonadotropin (as a source of FSH) and of human chorionic gonadotropin (as a source of LH-like activity) has, in occasional cases, resulted in ovulation and pregnancy. Pituitary enlargement sufficient to impair vision has occurred during the third trimester in some gonadotropin-treated patients with infertility due to pituitary tumor; such enlargement requires emergency measures.

CONSTITUTIONAL AND METABOLIC DISTURBANCES Severe constitutional illnesses such as *congenital heart disease, chronic renal disease,* or *rheumatoid arthritis* may delay the menarche and, in adult life, may cause amenorrhea and sterility. Injudicious dieting with too-rapid weight loss, anorexia nervosa, poorly controlled diabetes mellitus, and hyperthyroidism may also impair reproductive function. The point of impact of these different disorders upon the hypothalamic-pituitary-ovarian chain is poorly defined. A recovery of ovarian function generally follows successful treatment of the primary condition.

The adrenogenital syndrome (Chap. 93), a severe metabolic disorder commonly due to adrenocortical hyperplasia, is associated with pseudohermaphroditism and sexual infantilism. The adrenal cortex secretes estrogens as well as the "adrenal androgens" in greatly increased amounts, and the former, in particular, impair the hypothalamic control of FSH and LH release. Suppression of adrenal estrogen secretion by the administration of corticosteroids is speedily followed by sexual maturation and menstruation.

Postcontraceptive amenorrhea (i.e., that ensuing upon the suspension of a program of cyclic sex steroid treatment) is a not-uncommon iatrogenic state, which may or may not be accompanied by lactation. Omission of oral contraceptive preparations is generally followed by a prompt return of menstrual function. However, in some instances, prolonged and even seemingly permanent amenorrhea has followed omission. Anxiety and depression, sometimes associated with a significant loss of weight, may compound the problem. Women with previously irregular menses appear to be especially susceptible to this complication, and should be advised to employ nonhormonal means of contraception. In a proportion of the less severely affected patients, the amenorrhea can be terminated by means of Clomid treatment.

ANOVULATORY (DYSFUNCTIONAL) BLEEDING Puberty and the premenopausal years are epochs during which the sluggish waxing and waning of the ovarian follicles, with an abnormally prolonged secretion of estrogen and an absence of ovulation, are particularly likely to occur. A teetering level of circulating estrogen results and is likely to be accompanied by painless menorrhagia (excessive menstrual bleeding), metrorrhagia (intermenstrual bleeding), or both, interspersed with long periods of amenorrhea. Anovulatory (dysfunctional) uterine bleeding, or *metropathia hemorrhagica,* is so common at the two extremes of reproductive life as to be virtually physiologic. During the postmenarcheal and adult years, the condition is traceable to an absence of the midcycle LH surge with abnormally low levels of estrogen in the circulation and a deficiency of progesterone.

On rare occasions, a persistent follicle cyst is large enough to be outlined on bimanual examination. However, the diagnosis must ordinarily be made by exclusion. The

FIGURE 99-6
The structural formula of Clomid.

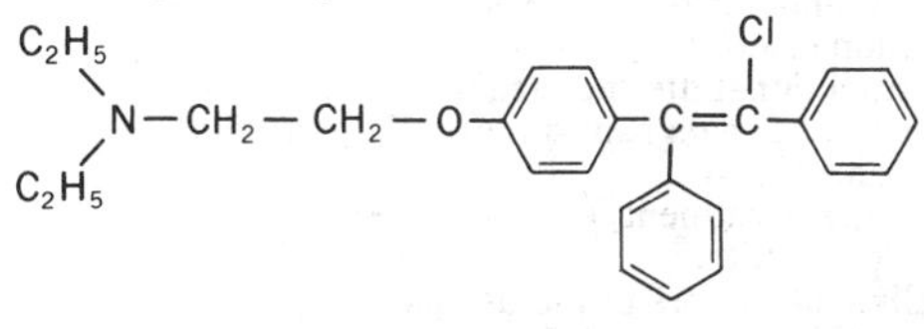

disorders requiring differentiation vary according to the age of the patient (Table 99-3).

Dysfunctional uterine bleeding is rarely fatal, but anemia is frequent and requires replacement treatment with iron. In younger patients, the oral progestational agents, fortified with estrogen, are exceedingly effective hemostatic agents. Doses of, for example, 2.5 to 10 mg daily of norethynodrel with mestranol (Enovid) may be given for a period of 3 weeks and then withdrawn to permit a "medical curettage." When the bleeding has been checked and the hemoglobin level restored, normal ovulatory menstrual function may resume spontaneously. If this does not occur, intermittent treatment with Clomid may establish a normal feedback mechanism, with cyclic release of the gonadotropic hormones.

The rare but grave occurrence of bleeding from carcinoma of the vagina in puberal girls whose mothers were treated with diethylstilbestrol during pregnancy may be confused with dysfunctional bleeding. Inquiry concerning this possibility should be made routinely, and where a positive history is elicited, gynecologic consultation for detailed inspection of the vagina (if necessary, under anesthesia), complemented if indicated with Schiller's staining and biopsy, should be obtained. Because of the frequent occurrence of necrosis in such tumors, a negative Papanicolaou smear cannot be relied upon to exclude the diagnosis of vaginal cancer. In older patients with bleeding which is seemingly dysfunctional in origin, pelvic examination under anesthesia and curettage to exclude organic lesions is mandatory.

INADEQUATE LUTEAL PHASE A clinically inconspicuous syndrome characterized by somewhat abbreviated menstrual cycles, infertility, and tendency to abortion is the so-called "inadequate luteal phase." In this disorder, the secretory activity of the corpus luteum is deficient and its term of activity is abbreviated.

A short luteal phase is physiologic (1) in the later phases of the postmenarcheal period, when it is an important cause of "adolescent sterility" (anovulation is the proximate cause of infertility during the immediately postmenarcheal years), and (2) in the puerperium, when menstrual periodicity is gradually being regained. At other times it is pathologic.

The diagnosis may be suspected from the character of the basal body temperature record, which is characterized by a slow rise to the luteal level and abbreviation of the luteal plateau. Confirmatory evidence may be obtained by histologic dating of appropriately timed endometrial biopsies or by demonstration of subnormal levels of plasma progesterone during the luteal phase. The cause of the condition is uncertain. However, there is evidence suggestive of a relative deficiency of FSH during the follicular phase, with impaired development of the follicle and subsequent inadequacy in corpus luteum formation or function.

TABLE 99-3
Some important causes of vaginal bleeding during different epochs of reproductive life

1 Adolescence
- *a* Dysfunctional uterine bleeding
- *b* Blood dyscrasias
- *c* Malignant tumors of the vagina

2 Maturity
- *a* Complications of pregnancy
- *b* Benign tumors (fibromyomas of the uterus, polyps of the endometrium and cervix)
- *c* Malignant tumors of the cervix and corpus of the uterus
- *d* Pelvic inflammatory disease

3 Premenopause
- *a* Dysfunctional uterine bleeding
- *b* Benign and malignant tumors of the uterus

4 Senescence
- *a* Estrogen treatment
- *b* Senile vaginitis
- *c* Malignant tumors of the uterus
- *d* Feminizing tumors of the ovary

OVARIAN HYPERFUNCTION

Ovarian hyperfunction may be relative or absolute. Thus, the elaboration of estrogen in amounts which are supraphysiologic for the reproductive age of the subject constitutes hyperfunction, even though the quantity secreted is less than that characteristic of mature reproductive life.

Primary ovarian hyperfunction

FEMINIZING TUMORS *Granulosa and theca cell tumors* and, on occasion, certain other ovarian neoplasms may secrete estrogen. The stromal elements of tumors in the latter category (e.g., cystadenofibroma and primary adenocarcinoma of the ovary) may resemble those of the thecoma or may contain elements resembling theca-lutein or stroma-lutein cells. The histogenesis of these tumors is uncertain. However, it would appear that granulosa and theca cell tumors arise from the stroma or its follicular wall derivatives and recapitulate the elements of the follicular wall. Approximately 5 percent of the reported granulosa cell tumors arise before puberty, 55 percent during the period of reproductive life, and 40 percent after the menopause. Theca cell tumors tend to occur in a slightly older age group.

The *symptoms* depend on the age of the patient. Precocious pseudopuberty and intermittent uterine bleeding result from the function of such tumors during the premenarcheal years; irregular uterine bleeding, frequently alternating with periods of amenorrhea, is common during active reproductive life; bleeding is the characteristic manifestation of these tumors during the postmenopausal years.

Granulosa cell tumors compose approximately 10 percent of all primary ovarian carcinomas and are the most common hormone-secreting tumors of the ovary. From 10 to 15 percent of granulosa cell tumors exhibit a low degree of malignancy, in contradistinction to theca cell tumors, which are rarely, if ever malignant. Both are almost invariably unilateral and tend at times to produce ascites. The Meigs syndrome of ascites and hydrothorax has been observed, especially with the theca cell tumor. Endometrial hyperplasia is a frequent concomitant, and the incidence of uterine leiomyoma, adenomyosis, and adenocarcinoma is increased.

The *diagnosis* is sometimes suggested by an unexpectedly high proportion of superficial cells in the vaginal smear. Urinary estrogen levels tend to be somewhat increased, and gonadotropin levels are occasionally depressed for a given age. Surgical removal is the treatment of choice.

MASCULINIZING TUMORS The *arrhenoblastoma* and the

hilus cell tumor of the ovary are rare androgen-secreting lesions, the histogenesis of which is uncertain. The majority of arrhenoblastomas tend to occur in comparatively young women, while the hilus cell tumor is characteristically a neoplasm of the late reproductive or postmenopausal years. Both are ordinarily unilateral and benign. The clinical course is one of defeminization followed by masculinization. The 17-ketosteroid excretion tends to be normal or only slightly increased and to be refractory to dexamethasone suppression. Plasma testosterone levels are often elevated. The treatment is surgical.

The so-called *"lipoid cell tumor" of the ovary* is a lesion with an uncertain histogenesis, although in certain instances it appears to arise from the ovarian stroma. The large rounded polyhedral cells of which the tumor consists lack the pathognomonic crystalloids of Reinke but are otherwise identical with Leydig cells. The syndrome of masculinization resulting from the secretion of this tumor may be clinically indistinguishable from that produced by the arrhenoblastoma. The 17-ketosteroid excretion may assist in the differentiation in that it is generally elevated, sometimes to a marked degree. Both premenarcheal and postmenopausal cases have been reported, but twice as many tumors have occurred in premenopausal as in postmenopausal women.

Secondary ovarian hyperfunction

TRUE PRECOCIOUS PUBERTY *Sexual precocity* associated with pituitary activation of graafian follicles is generally idiopathic or "constitutional" in origin. Constitutional precocity is presumed to be due to preternaturally early maturation of the hypothalamus, which escapes from the inhibition exerted by the small but physiologically significant amounts of estrogen secreted by the infantile ovary. Gonadotropin secretion can be materially reduced, with regression of the secondary sexual characteristics and protection from the hazard of pregnancy, by intramuscular injections of medroxyprogesterone acetate. The dosage is easily monitored by periodic determinations of the maturation index, either from vaginal smears or from the sediment of freshly voided urine.

Sexual precocity is a cardinal feature of *Albright's syndrome of polyostotic fibrous dysplasia* (Chap. 357). There is no clear indication of the pathogenesis, and a genetic basis for the precocity has been postulated. In rare instances, the ovary is activated prematurely by gonadotropic hormones released in consequence of hypothalamic stimulation by cysts or tumors, and by postencephalitic or postmeningitic lesions.

An unusual form of precocity is that associated with *hypothyroidism,* which increases ovarian sensitivity to endogenous gonadotropins. The precocity can be reversed by the administration of desiccated thyroid in doses sufficient to provide physiologic replacement. These observations contrast with the effects of hypothyroidism on adult women, who commonly experience a failure of ovulation, with a tendency to dysfunctional bleeding.

PERSISTENT FOLLICLE CYSTS Follicle cysts which persist during the climacteric tend to differ from those of puberty and the reproductive years in that, because of the hypersecretion of FSH and LH, they are likely to secrete estrogen in amounts exceeding those which are physiologic during mature reproductive life. Massive estrogen treatment designed to inhibit the gonadotropic support of a palpable mass presumed to be a cystic follicle is warranted and is sometimes successful. However, because of the impossibility of distinguishing benign cysts from malignant tumors by palpation, the length of such trials should be carefully limited.

CORPUS LUTEUM CYSTS The classic instance of physiologic luteal hyperfunction is the first trimester of pregnancy. In response to stimulation by chorionic gonadotropin, the corpus luteum of pregnancy secretes estrogen and, to a lesser extent, progesterone in amounts which exceed those characteristic of the luteal phase of the menstrual cycle.

A biochemically similar, but pathologic, state results from the formation of corpus luteum cysts. These may arise spontaneously or iatrogenically as a result of the *administration of Clomid.* Those occurring in Clomid-treated patients may be multiple, giving rise to a severalfold enlargement of the ovary; those occurring spontaneously tend to be single, seldom exceeding a walnut in size.

The presenting complaint of patients with spontaneous cysts is often that of *sudden amenorrhea.* Such cases are frequently mistaken for ectopic pregnancy because of the adnexal enlargement, hyperemia of the vagina and cervix, and the swelling and tenderness of the breasts. The cysts are sensitive to touch, with fragile walls which are likely to rupture. The suspicion of ectopic pregnancy is therefore likely to be compounded by the occurrence of acute abdominal pain. So difficult is the clinical diagnosis that many patients are, in fact, operated upon to exclude the possibility of ectopic pregnancy.

The cysts resulting from Clomid treatment may enlarge with sufficient rapidity to induce lower abdominal discomfort. They are less fragile than the spontaneous variety and ordinarily regress spontaneously after the drug is discontinued.

STEIN-LEVENTHAL SYNDROME AND HYPERTHECOSIS OF THE OVARY These uncommon but important conditions reflect hypersecretion of androgens by the ovarian stroma and perhaps by the hyperplastic and luteinized theca interna enveloping the subcapsular cysts and atretic follicles. *Plasma levels of androstenedione and dehydroepiandrosterone,* which may be converted peripherally to *testosterone,* are elevated, as, on occasion, are plasma levels of testosterone itself. The history is one of *irregular menstrual cycles,* generally experienced from puberty onward, and sometimes interspersed with long periods of amenorrhea and abnormal bleeding. There is hypersecretion of LH which tends to be released in erratic bursts (with an absence of the normal midcycle surge). The ovaries become polycystic, and, since ovulation occurs only rarely, there is associated sterility. Over a period of time the patients tend to develop hirsutism and, in occasional cases, frank virilism.

If the stroma contains nests of lipid-laden lutein cells, the term *hyperthecosis* is applied. Whether the Stein-Leventhal syndrome and hyperthecosis represent a pathologic continuum or distinct entities is uncertain. Hyperthecosis generally evolves in a manner similar to that described for the Stein-Leventhal syndrome. Occasionally, however, there is an abrupt onset in older women (sometimes after pregnancy), and there may be associated hypertension and impaired glucose tolerance.

There is much to suggest that an abnormal hypothalamic-ovarian feedback mechanism is responsible for the disorder. Prior to the introduction of Clomid treatment, *wedge resection of a substantial amount of ovarian tissue* was the treatment of choice for the induction of ovulation. It is still of value in those patients who prove to be refractory to Clomid. Because of the characteristic hyperresponsiveness of the polycystic ovary, *Clomid is best administered initially* in a dose of 25 to 50 mg daily for 3 to 5 days, which is somewhat lower than that ordinarily effective in patients with persistent anovulation due to other causes. Neither Clomid treatment nor wedge resection ameliorates the hirsutism, except in rare instances.

In a proportion of patients with menstrual irregularities, hirsutism, and a high-normal or slightly elevated 17-ketosteroid excretion, differentiation of mild adrenocortical hyperplasia from the Stein-Leventhal syndrome may be difficult (Chap. 93). Patients with this complex of findings should be given the benefit of a suppression test with small doses of a glucocorticoid, such as prednisone 2.5 mg three times a day.

OVARIAN DYSFUNCTION

In rare instances, bizarre dysfunction results from the presence of *ovarian teratomas. Choriocarcinoma,* a highly malignant tumor which secretes chorionic gonadotropin, may arise in the ovary of a prepuberal girl and induce sexual precocity. *Struma ovarii,* which is generally a benign neoplasm, may secrete thyroid hormone at any age. Occasionally, the rate of secretion is so rapid as to induce thyrotoxicosis. *Carcinoid tumors* are sometimes found in dermoid cysts containing intestinal or bronchial epithelium. They may induce the characteristic "carcinoid flush," together with cyanosis and diarrhea, and may, in rare instances, exhibit metastatic spread.

REFERENCES

GUAL C, ROSEMBERG E (eds): *Hypothalamic Hypophysiotropic Hormones. Physiological and Clinical Studies,* Amsterdam: Excerpta Medica, 1973

MARX JL: Estrogen drugs: Do they increase the risk of cancer? Science 191:838–882, 1976

MORRIS JM, SCULLY RE: *Endocrine Pathology of the Ovary,* St. Louis: Mosby, 1958

ROSS GT et al: Pituitary and gonadal hormones in women during spontaneous and induced ovulatory cycles. Recent Prog Horm Res 26:1, 1970

RYAN KJ, GIBSON DC (eds): *Menopause and Aging,* U. S. Department of Health, Education, and Welfare Publication (N.I.H.) 73–319, Bethesda, Md: Public Health Service, 1973

SAVARD K et al: Gonadotropins and ovarian steroidogenesis. Recent Prog Horm Res 21:285, 1965

VANDE WIELE RL et al: Mechanisms regulating the menstrual cycle in women. Recent Prog Horm Res 26:63, 1970

100 DISEASES OF THE BREAST

KENDALL EMERSON, JR.

APPROACH TO DISEASES OF THE BREAST For any physician providing primary care to adult women the examination of the organs of reproduction is most important, because they are the commonest source of fatal and preventable disease to which womankind is heir. Too often in this age of specialization the internist is apt to refer this task to a gynecologist, forgetting that the routine services of two doctors are a rare luxury today. This is not to say that every physician must be an expert in gynecology. It is a duty and responsibility, however, to be able to distinguish the abnormal from the normal in the breasts and pelvic organs, to be competent and thorough in examining them, and *never* to hesitate to call for assistance if there is the slightest doubt concerning the normality of the findings.

HISTORY The earliest description of cancer of the breast, and probably of cancer in any form, is credited to the Egyptian physician Imhotep in 3000 B.C. and is recorded in the Edwin Smith Surgical Papyrus under Case Number 39, "Bulging Tumor of the Breast." The studies of Sir Astley Cooper in 1845 provided an adequate morphologic description of the breast and the first suggestion of its possible relationship to menstrual dysfunction. In the latter half of the nineteenth century German investigators discovered that normal breast development in animals depended upon intact ovarian function, and in 1896 Sir George Beatson first demonstrated the inhibition of the growth of mammary cancer by oophorectomy in human beings. The role of the corpus luteum and pituitary in the development of the breasts has been brought to light during the present century by the works of L. Loeb, Gardner, Riddle, Corner, Turner, and many others.

CONGENITAL ANOMALIES The occurrence of aberrant breast tissue (polymastia) and supernumerary nipples (polythelia) situated along the so-called "milk line" extending from the midclavicle to the inguinal ligament has been noted in art and legend since recorded time. Absence of one or both breasts (amastia) occurs very rarely.

ENDOCRINE RELATIONSHIPS The growth of the normal nonlactating breast is directly dependent upon the synergistic action of three hormones: estrogens, cortisol, and prolactin, not on growth hormone, as previously thought; normal reproduction and lactation can occur in women with congenital isolated growth hormone deficiency. Progesterone, in addition to prolactin, is essential for the complete functional development of the alveolar lobules and the secretion of milk, whereas estrogens suppress lactation, apparently by end organ inhibition. This accounts for the absence of lactation during pregnancy, in spite of elevated prolactin blood levels, and for its onset with the withdrawal of placental estrogens after delivery. Prolactin can induce lactation in the absence of progesterone, if other adrenal steroid precursors are present. In pregnancy a polypeptide hormone which has both lactogenic and growth-promoting activity is secreted in large amounts by the placenta (chorionic somatomammotropin or placental lactogen) and may play an important role in preparing the breast, as well as maternal metabolism, for milk production.

Prolactin, unlike the other hypophyseal hormones, is secreted autonomously by the anterior pituitary, as first demonstrated by the spontaneous occurrence of lactation in women whose pituitaries had been isolated from hypothalamic control by stalk section for the treatment of breast cancer, a procedure which was often successful in controlling the disease. Prolactin secretion can be increased by the thyrotropin-releasing factor (TRF), but it normally appears to be under the negative control of a specific prolactin-inhibitory factor (PIF), actively produced by the hypothalamus. Both PIF and the gonadotropin-releasing factor, LRF, are stimulated by dopaminergic neurotransmitters, possibly dopamine itself. This results in an inverse relationship between the rate of release of prolactin and the gonadotropins, FSH (follicle-stimulating hormone) and LH (luteinizing hormone). Thus the persistent lactation associated with amenorrhea and low FSH level which occasionally follows pregnancy (Chiari-Frommel syndrome), or the withdrawal after prolonged use of estrogen-containing contraceptives, may result from interference with a single neurotransmitter. In some instances the augmenting effect of TRF on prolactin release may play a role, since the lactation may sometimes be interrupted by thyroid administration. Lactation may also be induced occasionally by hypothalamic suppression with catecholamine-depleting or blocking drugs such as reserpine, the phenothiazines, and methyldopa, which results in high circulating levels of prolactin. This effect can be counteracted by the administration of L-dopamine or the ergot alkaloid, 2-Br-alpha-ergocryptine (CB 154). Finally, lactation may result directly from the excessive production of prolactin in eosinophilic or chromophobe adenomas of the pituitary with growth hormone (acromegaly) or without it (Forbes-Albright syndrome), or it may be without any demonstrable cause (Argonex-del Castillo syndrome), in which case it usually turns out ultimately to be due to an adenoma (see Chap. 90).

The hormones of greatest clinical importance in relation to the breast are the estrogens. Engorgement of the breasts may be seen as a transient phenomenon in newborn infants because of the high level of circulating estrogens of placental origin. The normal development of the female breast at puberty, which is sometimes accompanied by intermittent tenderness and edema, results from the rising levels of circulating estrogens secreted by the maturing ovarian follicles just prior to the menarche. Precocious breast development may occur as a result of inherited or constitutional factors; of abnormal pituitary, ovarian, or adrenal activity associated with functional tumors or hyperplasia of these organs; or of locally irritating lesions such as tumors of the pineal or fourth ventricle, fibrous dysplasia of the bones of the base of the skull, as in Albright's disease (polyostotic fibrous dysplasia), or rarely following viral encephalitis.

GYNECOMASTIA Gynecomastia occurs physiologically in normal males at puberty and may persist through adolescence. This breast enlargement usually subsides spontaneously, but if it presents a sufficiently serious psychologic problem, simple mastectomy with preservation of the nipples is justified, since any reasonable hormonal treatment is ineffective. Gynecomastia should always raise the suspicion of seminiferous tubule dysgenesis with fibrosis, a variant of Klinefelter's syndrome, in which there is usually an elevated urinary excretion of follicle-stimulating hormone and a female pattern of sex chromatin (see Chap. 98).

Marked degrees of breast development in adolescent males or the onset of gynecomastia in later life may indicate the presence of an estrogen-secreting tumor of the adrenal gland. These tumors are usually associated with an elevation in level of the urinary 17-ketosteroids, the excretion of which is not further stimulated by ACTH (adrenocorticotropic hormone) or suppressed by adrenal steroids. Every effort should be made to locate such tumors by radiographic means and to remove them surgically because, though they are rare, a high percentage, if not all, are malignant.

Choriogenic tumors and, more rarely, interstitial cell and granulosa cell tumors of the testes may produce gynecomastia. This condition is also seen in males with cirrhosis of the liver and in states of severe malnutrition, presumably in both instances because of failure of inactivation of circulating estrogens. It regularly follows administration of estrogenic compounds in the treatment of carcinoma of the prostate and even occasionally occurs during testosterone therapy in eunuchoidism. Transient gynecomastia occurs as a normal physiologic phenomenon in elderly men and may be associated with the administration of common therapeutic agents having a basic steroid structure such as digitalis and spironolactone. Very rarely, gynecomastia may result from the ectopic secretion of FSH by a bronchogenic carcinoma.

GALACTORRHEA See Chaps. 89 and 90.

INFECTIONS OF THE BREAST Acute pyogenic infections of the breast are largely confined to the first 2 months of lactation and usually involve the staphylococcus, less often a beta-streptococcus. They should be prevented by proper hygiene and treated with appropriate antibiotics. Very rarely an acute mastitis unassociated with lactation may occur during the course of paratyphoid or typhoid fever, brucellosis, or mumps.

Chronic tuberculous mastitis is a rarity today. It usually results from the extension of tuberculosis of the underlying bone into the breast tissue and should be suspected from the presence of multiple sinus tracts and the finding of active tuberculosis elsewhere.

INFLAMMATORY LESIONS Mammary duct ectasia is a benign condition, usually seen in elderly women with atrophic breasts, in which the mammary ducts in or just beneath the nipple become dilated and filled with cellular debris and lipid-containing material. Intermittent pain and local inflammatory changes may be present, and because a discharge, at times bloody, and retraction of the nipple may occur, this condition must be differentiated from carcinoma. Excision of the nipple is usually indicated.

Fat necrosis is a common occurrence following trauma which may be so slight as not to have been noticed. It presents as a painful lump usually associated with some ecchymosis and may be followed by local atrophy and dimpling of the skin, at which stage biopsy must be performed to distinguish it from carcinoma.

Thrombosis of the thoracoepigastric veins and sclerosing subcutaneous phlebitis (Mondor's disease) occur after trauma or for no apparent reason and are manifest by the appearance of long cordlike structures, initially tender, in the outer half of the breast, frequently extending up into the axilla or down toward the epigastrium. They may persist up to a year, but no treatment is indicated.

Sarcoid may very rarely involve the skin of the chest, and secondary amyloidosis may involve the breast tissue itself. Eosinophilic granuloma may occur in the submammary folds.

It must not be forgotten that carcinoma of the breast may rarely present as a subacute red, warm, indurated mass, resembling a bacterial cellulitis, the so-called "inflammatory carcinoma." This lesion may be suspected when the skin over it presents the characteristic *peau d'orange* appearance.

FIBROCYSTIC DISEASE With each menstrual cycle there is a recurring biphasic stimulation first of proliferation of breast tissue by estrogens, then of alveolar secretory activity by progesterone, followed by a period of involution. In most women these changes are of such slight degree as to cause few if any clinical symptoms. Not infrequently, however, well-marked inflammatory changes may occur preceding each menses, with tenderness, engorgement, and increasing nodularity of the breasts. This is more often seen in nulliparous women and may subside after childbearing and lactation. Methyltestosterone, 5 mg daily for 7 to 10 days before each menstrual period, will often provide relief. Suspected cysts in the breast may be aspirated safely in the office with local anesthesia if biopsy is done promptly in any of the following circumstances: (1) no fluid is obtained; (2) the cyst fluid is grossly bloody; (3) the mass does not completely disappear with aspiration; and (4) the fluid reaccumulates during succeeding days. Cytologic examinations of cyst aspirates have been shown repeatedly to be of no value.

In the later years of reproductive life the continued recurrent stimulation and involution of the breasts in the course of each menstrual cycle may result in diffuse and nodular fibrosis and the formation of cysts of varying sizes, so-called "chronic cystic mastitis." This condition may simulate carcinoma but is usually distinguishable by the fact that it is intermittently painful and may subside to some extent following menstruation. Nevertheless, carcinoma may coexist and be masked by the diffuse nodularity of the cystic disease. Moreover, the incidence of mammary carcinoma is greater in patients with fibrocystic disease of the breasts, and it is unwise to delay biopsy of suspicious areas in the hope that they may subside by the end of the next menstrual cycle. In severe cases simple mastectomy is fully justified. Subcutaneous mastectomies with preservation of the nipples may be done in some cases, and the breasts may be reconstructed with silastic implants.

TUMORS OF THE BREAST Benign fibroadenomas of the breast may occur at any age but are more common in women under the age of thirty. They may be distinguished from carcinomas by their mobility and well-defined margins, but biopsy is nonetheless imperative.

Benign intraductal papillomas may occur and cause a bloody discharge from the nipple. They are usually small and difficult to feel but may be located by noting that area of the breast on which pressure causes the bleeding. Excision is always advisable.

Sarcomas of all types make up less than 3 percent of all breast tumors. Fibrosarcomas are the most frequent; lymphosarcomas occasionally originate in the breast. Liposarcomas and hemangiosarcomas have been reported rarely. Cystosarcoma phylloides is a curious, very large, relatively rapidly appearing tumor arising usually from a preexisting fibroadenoma. It presents as a tender, warm, cystic mass often replacing the whole breast. The skin over it is thinned, and the superficial veins are dilated. The tumor consists of fibrous cords covered with epithelium arising from the duct system. The cords are separated by cystic areas which become filled with leaflike (phylloides) projections of epithelial tissue. Although these tumors are usually benign, blood-borne metastases have been reported and surgical removal of the tumor is always indicated.

CARCINOMA OF THE BREAST In Western civilization carcinoma of the breast is the most frequent malignant tumor to which the human female is subject and accounts for a greater number of deaths than any other single form of cancer in women. It occurs with increasing frequency from the age of twenty up to the menopause, when its incidence levels off until a second rise in frequency occurs after the age of sixty-five. For reasons as yet not entirely clear, breast cancer is very much less common in Japan and other Oriental countries.

Etiology The cause of breast cancer, like that of most other forms of malignant disease, is unknown. A few factors affecting its incidence are, however, reasonably well established. The very strong hereditary influence seen in mice may be carried over, though in a much smaller degree, to human beings. A two- to sevenfold increase in the familial incidence of the disease is reported. In this connection renewed interest in a milk-borne virus, first proposed by Bittner in 1936, has been aroused by the finding of alleged virus particles and of virus-related information in the DNA (deoxyribonucleic acid) of human breast cancer cells. Antigens have been extracted from human tumors which cross-react with antigens obtained from the milk-borne murine mammary tumor virus (MuMTV), as well as with other human breast tumors from males and females alike. Moreover, serum from human breast cancer patients is capable of rendering the MuMTV noninfectious in mice, suggesting the real possibility of prophylactic immunization in humans, which has already been successful in mice. It must be emphasized that there is not a shred of evidence for the transmission of human mammary cancer through nursing.

The role of the *estrogenic hormones* in the genesis of breast cancer in human beings is still controversial. The conservative view at the present time is that estrogens do not initiate the cancer but may hasten its development in genetically susceptible individuals, in whom their prolonged use should be discouraged. Estrogenic substances can clearly be shown to stimulate the growth of breast cancer, once it is manifest, in a high proportion of women. The risk of breast cancer increases directly with the total duration of ovarian activity and is significantly diminished in women undergoing surgical castration before the age of forty. On the other hand, it is a remarkable fact that the vast increase in the use of estrogens for contraception during the past 15 years has not increased the incidence of breast cancer, but may even have had a protective effect. Conversely, it has been demonstrated statistically that women who excrete a subnormal proportion of androgen metabolites in their urine, and, therefore, of estrogens as well, are more likely to develop cancer of the breast and have a poorer prognosis when they do so. There is some evidence that estriol may have a protective effect in humans: for example, Oriental women excrete more estriol than Caucasian women under similar conditions. Oriental women also show a greater degree of host resistance, however, as demonstrated by a much more pronounced lymphocytic response to the presence of a mammary tumor.

It has also been shown that the risk of breast cancer is reduced as much as 70 percent in women completing their first pregnancy and lactation by the age of eighteen, as compared to the general population at risk. The extent of this reduction in risk decreases progressively with age, and a first pregnancy above the age of thirty may actually increase the cancer risk. The number of pregnancies after the first has no further protective effect, nor do abortions. Similar observations have been made in other mammalian species. These findings suggest that the initiating carcinogenic factors begin to operate at puberty but are somehow inhibited by the normal processes of pregnancy and lactation; the earlier this occurs, the more complete the inhibition.

Preliminary epidemiologic studies from several sources indicate that the prolonged ingestion of reserpine, a prolactin secretagogue, increases the incidence of human breast cancer, thus tending to implicate prolactin rather than estrogens in an etiologic role. Definite though transient remissions of the disseminated disease have been obtained in a few human trials of prolactin suppression with L-dopa. Since removal of estrogens by pituitary stalk section may induce a remission even while lactation is occurring, however, both hormones may well be involved in different phases of the human disease.

Observations on the epidemiology of breast cancer suggest that environmental influences may play a role. The disease is more common in Japanese women living in the United States than in Japan, in the women of Denmark than in their Scandinavian sisters in Finland, and in fat women than in thin. Wynder has gone so far as to speculate that one common variable, the quantity of saturated fat in the diet, might affect the growth of mammary cancer directly by providing precursors for the synthesis and/or a vehicle for the storage of the fat-soluble estrogens. Of particular interest is the high incidence of both breast cancer and polycystic ovaries among the Parsis in Bombay, more than twice that of the general population in India. This ancient religious sect comprises a closely interrelated and affluent community having access to a relatively rich diet, thus combining both genetic and environmental factors which might favor the growth of mammary cancer.

Pathology The primary site is usually in the ducts, less often in the alveoli. Multicentric origins are a frequent occurrence, and all gradations of differentiation may be observed. It is common to see a marked proliferation of dense connective tissue surrounding groups of malignant cells, whether primary or metastatic, the so-called "scirrhous carcinoma." Unfortunately all degrees of differentiation may be found in different portions of the same tumor and little prognostic value can be attached to the histologic appearance of any one area of such a malignancy.

Mammary carcinoma is likely to metastasize relatively early to the regional lymph nodes—axillary and supraclavicular if the primary site is in the outer half of the breast, the internal mammary chain if the disease arises in the inner quadrants of breast tissue. From there spread occurs primarily to bone, lungs, liver, skin, and subcutaneous tissues generally, less frequently to the brain. Blood-borne metastases may occur even before lymphatic spread is clinically evident. It is interesting that there is a predilection for metastases to occur in the ovaries, adrenals, and pituitary—areas rich in the hormones stimulating the growth of this type of epithelial cell.

Diagnosis The diagnosis of breast cancer is facilitated by the fact that it is possible to palpate directly this type of neoplasm. Unfortunately, the diffuse nodularity of the adult female breast makes it difficult to detect early lesions. As a rule the physician must depend on such evidence as hardness, fixation to underlying structures, or dimpling of the overlying skin to distinguish a malignant mass from a benign nodule of breast tissue, and by the time these distinguishing signs have become apparent the cancer has all too often metastasized. Direct exposure of the breasts to irradiation with low-voltage x-rays in order to bring out contrasts in soft-tissue densities, so-called "mammography" or "xeroradiography," has been of great value in screening for breast cancer and in discovering small lesions in large, fatty breasts. When secretions are obtainable from the nipple, cytologic examination may be helpful. The majority of patients with breast cancer suggest the diagnosis themselves because of their ready detection of abnormal lumps or masses during self-examination. Although the procedure of self-examination of the breast may be decried as tending to encourage neuroticism and cancerphobia, it is the only practical way by which we can succeed in reducing the death rate from cancer of the breast until a final cure for cancer has been found.

Treatment Total *surgical excision* provides the only permanent cure for carcinoma of the breast, and x-ray therapy the best palliation for localized disease. The technical details of the surgical and radiologic treatment of breast cancer are beyond the scope of this chapter, as is the controversy over radical versus simple mastectomy with extensive local irradiation. Because of the susceptibility of breast cancer to changes in its endocrine environment, however, every physician should be cognizant of the remarkable palliative effect which can be achieved in patients with inoperable mammary cancer by intelligent hormonal manipulations.

The two most important factors governing the prognosis of disseminated breast cancer and the success of its treatment or palliation are (1) the age of the patient and (2) the length of the free interval between the discovery of the primary tumor and the appearance of metastases. As with neoplasia in general, the younger the age at which it occurs, the more rapid and malignant is its growth. The only exceptions to this rule are the rare cases of *juvenile breast cancer* reported in patients from three to fifteen years of age, which appear to have a more benign course. The length of the free interval is a rough measure of the balance between the biologic activity, or turnover rate, of tumor cells and the poorly understood factors of host resistance.

The rationale of the *endocrine treatment of breast cancer* is predicated on the assumption that in the total population of malignant cells some retain their metabolic dependency for growth upon estrogens for variable lengths of time before ultimately becoming autonomous. The first aim of therapy, therefore, is to remove all sources of estrogen from the afflicted subject. It is possible to determine the extent to which any given breast cancer is estrogen-dependent by measuring its content of 17-beta-estradiol receptors, a technique which has become well established and should be available to any laboratory with facilities for performing radioimmunoassays. Current data indicate that about 60 percent of all breast cancers contain such estrogen receptors and that the majority of these will respond favorably to endocrine ablation, whereas the reverse is true when estrogen receptors are absent. It has been strongly recommended that the measurement of estrogen receptors be made a routine procedure when the initial pathologic diagnosis is made.

There is increasing evidence, but not universal agreement, that prophylactic oophorectomy and prednisone suppression of adrenal estrogen precursors at the time of initial mastectomy may significantly prolong the free interval, if not the total survival time, of those patients with metastases ostensibly confined to axillary lymph nodes (stage II). In patients with symptomatic or remote metastases (stages III and IV), oophorectomy alone will induce a remission in 40 percent before the menopause and in 50 percent or more if combined with bilateral adrenalectomy. Since the adrenal cortex takes over the role of estrogen production after the menopause, it seems logical to combine both these procedures at one time. The remissions so produced last from 6 months to 5 years or longer and provide a normal quality of life for most of this time. The frequency of these favorable responses should be materially increased by the proper selection of patients according to the estradiol receptor content of their tumors.

FIGURE 100-1
Pathways of influence on mammary tumor cell growth. Substances such as estriol and nafoxidine may compete for estradiol receptors in the tumor cell without stimulating its growth. One pathway not depicted is suppression of estrogen production by progesterone.

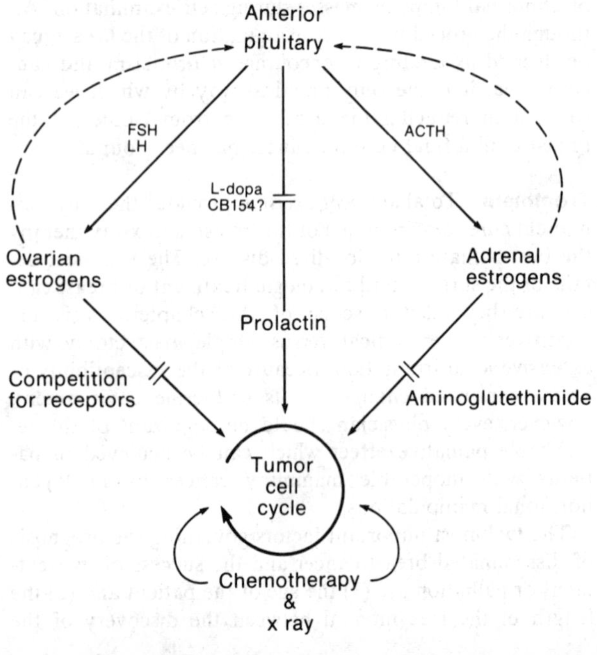

Surgical *hypophysectomy,* or *pituitary stalk* section, induces a functional ovarian and adrenal ablation and results in a remission rate equal to but no greater than that brought about by the surgical extirpation of these target organs. The technical problems involved in total removal of the hypophysis and the degree of morbidity arising therefrom have tended to discourage this procedure. It has the theoretic advantage of eliminating the potential stimulating effect of prolactin on the tumor cells, and the longest reported remissions (10 years or more) have followed hypophysectomy. Pituitary ablation by roentgen or nuclear bombardment is too gradual to be of value in retarding the progress of a rapidly growing neoplasm.

Functional suppression of estrogen production by the ovaries may be achieved by the administration of depot progesterone, 200 mg intramuscularly, at monthly intervals, and simultaneously, the production of adrenal estrogen precursors can be inhibited by amino-glutethimide, 1 to 2 g, and dexamethasone, 1.5 mg daily. Such measures may be successful in retarding mammary cancer growth when surgical procedures are unavailable or unwarranted, but they are less certain and suppression is rarely as complete.

The rapid advances in the development of cytotoxic chemicals with varying cell cycle specificities and larger margins of safety have added greatly to the therapeutic armamentarium for the treatment of breast cancer. Current evidence indicates that prompt and prolonged administration of these agents in patients with axillary metastases will lengthen significantly their free interval. The addition of chemotherapy to endocrine ablative procedures in stage III disease with distant metastases appears to prolong the remission in patients with estrogen-dependent tumors and may even induce a remission in a substantial number of those without estrogen receptors who would otherwise not benefit from the surgery. Many patients too sick for surgical procedures may show striking improvement for 1 to 2 years following administration of prednisone, 15 to 30 mg daily, with chemotherapy. Among the agents of proved value at present are Adriamycin, cyclophosphamide, and L-phenylalanine mustard to reduce total cell mass, and vincristine, methotrexate, and 5-fluorouracil used serially or in various combinations to provide cell cycle specificity. Careful supervision of therapy is essential to avoid unnecessary toxicity, with which the physician should be familiar (see Chap. 323).

In older patients, 15 years or more past the menopause, *large doses of estrogens* may provide remarkable palliation. This paradoxic effect of estrogens has never been fully explained.

The place of *androgens and estrogens* in the treatment of

metastatic breast cancer has been well defined by a report of the American Medical Association's Council on Drugs, based on a 10-year nationwide cooperative study. In summary, androgens produced objective remissions in approximately 20 percent of patients both before and after the menopause. Estrogens, which should not be used before the menopause, will induce remissions in about 36 percent of patients during the first 8 postmenopausal years and in more than 38 percent in later years. Estrogens have a greater relative effect on soft tissue and visceral metastases than on bone but equal or exceed the effect of androgens on all types of tissue. Estrogens must be employed in large doses to achieve these results, e.g., stilbestrol, 15 mg, or ethynyl estradiol, 3 mg daily. Smaller amounts may adversely affect the tumor. Nausea and vomiting may occur at the onset of treatment but can be controlled by antiemetic agents and will disappear in time. Uterine bleeding may be troublesome but can usually be controlled by the cyclic administration of progesterone or methyltestosterone.

The optimum dose of *androgens* has been found to be equivalent to 100 mg testosterone propionate given intramuscularly three times weekly. Recent experience indicates that the newer anabolic androgens, such as 17-beta, 17-alpha dimethyltestosterone in oral doses of 50 mg four times daily, may be equally effective, with much less tendency to produce the undesirable masculinizing side effects of testosterone. The major pathways by which mammary tumor cell growth may be influenced are summarized in Fig. 100-1.

All patients, but especially those within the first 8 postmenopausal years, should be observed carefully during the first few days and weeks of treatment because both androgens and estrogens may cause an exacerbation of their disease, estrogens by a direct stimulating effect and androgens presumably by being converted in small but effective amounts to estrogens. One of the most serious complications produced by administration of these hormones in patients who exhibit extensive skeletal metastases is calcium intoxication. This is presumed to result from the sudden stimulation of growth of the bony metastases by the hormone, with correspondingly rapid destruction of bone and flooding of the circulation with calcium. There is a marked increase in urinary calcium excretion, the serum calcium level may rise to as high as 15 to 20 mg per 100 ml, and drowsiness, coma, convulsions, and death from renal failure may ensue. It is important to distinguish this condition from cerebral or liver metastases or the terminal effects of widespread cancer because it can be reversed by forcing fluids, withdrawal of the offending hormone, the administration of large amounts of hydrocortisone, 200 mg daily by slow intravenous drip or in divided oral doses daily, until symptoms subside. The administration of neutral phosphate salts, in doses equivalent to 1.5 g phosphorus daily, may be of great value, presumably by redirecting the flow of calcium away from the kidneys back into bone.

Because of this and other serious complications, estrogen and androgen therapy is being replaced more and more by chemotherapy and by endocrine ablative procedures whenever possible. Current trends in the therapy of breast cancer are shown in Table 100-1.

Hypercalcemia may, of course, occur spontaneously in far advanced autonomously growing malignancy with widespread skeletal metastases but can still usually be controlled with the above measures plus the addition of a chemotherapeutic agent. Occasionally hypercalcemia may be found in the absence of demonstrable bony involvement. It has also been reported that a "calcium-mobilizing" steroid may be elaborated by breast tumors.

Carcinoma occurs in the male breast at least 100 times less frequently than in the female. Otherwise it behaves in exactly the same manner. The treatment is the same except that orchiectomy replaces oophorectomy. Prednisone and hypophysectomy have both been shown to induce remissions when the primary disease has metastasized, and progestational compounds may be of value.

The best treatment for localized bony and soft-tissue metastases is irradiation, since the local control rate is in the range of 75 to 80 percent. Painful bony lesions are especially susceptible to this modality. Irradiation may be used in conjunction with systemic therapy, and at times may postpone the need for major ablation or chemotherapy, especially when only one or two metastases are evident or are symptomatic.

Metastases to weight-bearing bones should be treated prophylactically to avoid incapacity associated with pathologic fractures, especially femoral lesions. It is frequently worthwhile to perform operative reduction of pathologic femoral fractures, in conjunction with radiotherapy, to keep the patient ambulatory and to avoid the general deterioration that often occurs when such patients become bedridden. Many patients with slow-growing metastases may survive for prolonged periods in surprising comfort with carefully planned palliation.

Psychologic support for patients with carcinoma of the breast is extremely important. It has been noted by many observers that these patients fear death less than they fear abandonment, especially by their primary-care physician. Because of the frustration and sense of professional failure that patients with diffuse metastases may engender in the physician, there should be a deliberate effort to see these patients at regular intervals to give supportive care even when the major modalities of therapy are no longer producing significant improvement.

TABLE 100-1
Treatment of breast cancer: alternative methods following surgery

Stage I-no apparent metastasis	Observe
Stage II-axillary metastasis only	Chemotherapy (more aggressive therapy would add prednisone treatment or oophorectomy and adrenalectomy)
Stage III-distant metastasis (skin, bone, lung parenchyma)	Chemotherapy plus oophorectomy and adrenalectomy; androgens for premenopausal patients and estrogens for postmenopausal patients (when ablative procedures are unavailable or unacceptable)
Stage IV-visceral metastasis (brain, liver, pulmonary lymphatics	Chemotherapy plus prednisone; estrogens (when ablative procedures are unavailable or unacceptable); surgery if patient's condition allows

REFERENCES

HAAGENSEN CD: *Diseases of the Breast,* 2d ed., Philadelphia, Saunders, 1971

JENSEN EB, POLLEY TZ, SMITH S, BLOCK GW, FERGUSON DJ, DESOMBRE ER: Prediction of hormone dependency in human breast cancer, in *Estrogen Receptors in Human Breast Cancer,* eds WL McGuire, EP Vollmer, PP Carbone, New York: Raven Press, 1975, pp. 37–56

MACMAHON B, COLE P, BROWN J: Etiology of human breast cancer: A review. J Natl Cancer Inst 50:21–42, 1973

MOORE DH, CHARNEY J: Breast cancer: Etiology and possible prevention. Am Sci 63:161–168, 1975

MOORE FD, VANDEVANTER S, BOYDEN C, LOKICH J: Adrenalectomy with chemotherapy in the treatment of advanced breast cancer: Objective and subjective response rates; duration and quality of life. Surgery 76:376–390, 1974

SMITHLINE F, SHERMAN L, KOLODNY HD: Prolactin and breast carcinoma. N Engl J Med 292:784–791, 1975

101
DISEASES OF THE PINEAL GLAND

RICHARD J. WURTMAN

INTRODUCTION Since the discovery of melatonin in 1958, compelling evidence has accumulated that the mammalian pineal is not a vestige but an important component of a neuroendocrine control system. This organ has been shown to function as a neuroendocrine transducer: it receives a cyclic input of sympathetic nervous "information" which is generated by retinal effects of environmental lighting. In response to this input, the pineal secretes a hormone, melatonin, into the bloodstream, much as the adrenal medulla releases epinephrine in response to cholinergic nervous stimulation. The synthesis and secretion of melatonin vary with a 24-h periodicity, thereby providing the body with a circulating "clock" apparatus. Until very recently, no assay was available to permit measurement of melatonin in human blood or urine. Largely as a consequence, human pineal physiology remained conjectural, and the only disease states that could clearly be associated with pineal malfunction were those caused by pineal neoplasms. Now urinary melatonin can be measured, and it is apparent that the same factors that control the synthesis and secretion of this hormone in experimental animals also do so in humans. There is thus reason for optimism that our understanding of pineal physiology and pathophysiology, and of the possible medical uses of pineal compounds, will soon expand.

ANATOMY AND BIOCHEMISTRY OF THE PINEAL The human pineal gland is a flattened, conical organ which lies beneath the posterior border of the corpus callosum and between the superior colliculi. It originates embryologically as an evagination of the ependyma which lines the roof of the third ventricle, and remains connected to this region by the pineal stalk. The adult gland weighs about 120 mg; its dimensions are 5 to 9 mm in length, 3 to 6 mm in width, and 3 to 5 mm in thickness. Most of the pineal is enveloped by pia mater, from which blood vessels, unmyelinated nerve fibers, and septa of connective tissue penetrate the gland, thereby dividing it into lobules. The pineal glandular or parenchymal cells on the periphery of the lobule are elongated; those in the central zone are ovoid. They contain numerous granular bodies (which might represent a stored secretion), and give rise to processes that terminate adjacent to the capillary endothelium.

In 1960, Kappers made the important discovery that the primary innervation of the mammalian pineal originates not within the brain but rather from sympathetic cell bodies in the superior cervical ganglia. Subsequent studies using the electron microscope revealed that the sympathetic nerve endings terminate directly on pineal parenchymal cells in an anatomic relationship that resembles the synapse. The sympathetic innervation of pineal glandular cells appears to be a new evolutionary adaptation. Such a parenchymal innervation may be unique in the body, and itself invalidates the vestige theory of pineal function.

In 1917, McCord and Allen showed that the pineal gland of the cow contained a factor which causes amphibian skin to blanch. When pineal homogenates were fed to tadpoles, the melanin granules within dermal melanophores aggregated around the cell nuclei, thereby lightening the skin. (This effect is opposite to that produced by the melanocyte-stimulating hormone, MSH, which is secreted by the pars intermedia of the pituitary gland.) Four decades later, Lerner and his colleagues identified this pineal factor as melatonin (5-methoxy-*N*-acetyltryptamine) (Fig. 101-1). Melatonin appears to have no effect on the melanocytes which are responsible for normal skin pigmentation in human beings.

Melatonin was shown to be a derivative of serotonin (Fig. 101-1), a widely distributed indole stored in very large quantities in mammalian pineals. It differs from all indoles previously identified in mammals in that it contains a methoxy group. The enzyme which catalyzes this methoxylation reaction (hydroxyindole-O-methyl transferase, HIOMT) was shown to be concentrated within the pineal gland in mammals. The high degree of localization of HIOMT has sometimes been used as a "marker" to differentiate true pinealomas from pineal tumors of glial or other origin.

PHYSIOLOGY OF THE MAMMALIAN PINEAL Environmental lighting conditions exert several important effects on the mammalian neuroendocrine apparatus. Light acts as an "inducer" that modifies the rate of sexual maturation; girls who have been deprived of light from birth may show early pubescence. The sequence of day and night also acts to generate some 24-h biologic rhythms and to synchronize other rhythms which are produced by signals arising from within the body. There is evidence that one function of the mammalian pineal might be to mediate some of these endocrine effects of light. The "information" about light travels to the pineal by a route which involves (1) the inferior accessory optic tract, (2) centers in the brain and spinal cord that regulate the sympathetic nervous system, and (3) the sympathetic nerves to the pineal which originate in the superior cervical ganglia. The diurnal variation in pineal melatonin secretion, recently demonstrated for the first time in humans, provides the body with a circulating "clock" which is under the direct control of the lighting environment.

Less is known about which organs take cues from the

pineal "clock" than about the mechanism responsible for its rhythmic changes. It seems likely that melatonin exerts physiologic inhibitory effects on gonadal and thyroid function and also modifies behavior and electroencephalographic activity. When tiny amounts of melatonin are implanted in the median eminence of the hypothalamus or the midbrain reticular formation, the increase in pituitary luteinizing hormone (LH) content which normally follows castration is blocked. Melatonin placed in the cerebrospinal fluid suppresses the secretion of pituitary LH and enhances the secretion of prolactin. Melatonin administration also changes the levels of serotonin in the brain.

PINEAL PATHOLOGY Two pineal lesions have been of interest to the clinician: pineal calcification, which is a universal autopsy finding, and pineal tumors, which are best known for their endocrine sequelae. In rare instances, pineal glands have also contained cancer metastases, gummas, tuberculous granulomas, or isolated segments of skeletal muscle.

Pineal calcification often first becomes visible on skull roentgenograms around the time of puberty, and it has been suggested that the gland degenerates at this time of life, and then becomes calcified. However, recent studies have not supported this hypothesis. If pineals are examined by appropriate microscopic techniques, evidence of calcification often is seen in patients who died long before the age of puberty. A ground substance believed to serve as the matrix for calcification was seen in 8 of 28 pineals taken from children under one year of age. Moreover, studies of pineal function have failed to show any differences between heavily calcified glands taken from aged subjects and pineals from young subjects with no gross evidence of calcification. The functional significance of pineal calcification remains entirely unexplained. The chemical identity of the calcified material appears to be hydroxyapatite; crystals of this compound taken from human pineals are similar to those prepared from bone or tooth.

Pineal tumors may be divided into several distinct categories by their microscopic appearance. Somewhat more than half of all pineal tumors may be classified as true pinealomas. These tumors contain clusters of two distinct types of cells: large spheroidal epithelial cells, and small dark-staining cells with little cytoplasm and an ultrastructure indistinguishable from that of the lymphocyte. About 10 to 15 percent of all reported pineal tumors have been teratomas; these may contain mucus-secreting columnar epithelial cells, adenocarcinoma tissue, and areas resembling thyroid, muscle, cartilage, bone, and nerve. Like other midline teratomas, they are often malignant. The remainder of pineal tumors have been of vascular or glial origin.

Confirmation of pineal origin of the large pinealoma cells has been hampered by the lack of specific pineal function which could be measured in these cells (such as the uptake of ^{131}I by thyroidal cells in follicular adenomas). However, studies suggest that assays for the melatonin-forming enzyme (HIOMT) may provide such a "marker." Two pineal tumors containing this enzyme have been described; one was a metastasis from a parenchymal pinealoma, and the other, a specimen from an ectopic pinealoma. Both tumors had the characteristic histologic appearance of the parenchymal pinealoma. No data are yet available on blood or urinary melatonin levels in subjects with pineal tumors.

The natural history of a pineal tumor is related to its size and its histologic appearance. Tumors which originate within the pineal gland usually become clinically manifest because of symptoms which arise from their location (e.g., internal hydrocephalus, elevated cerebrospinal fluid pressure, and oculomotor signs such as paralysis of upward gaze, or Parinaud's syndrome); less frequently, the

FIGURE 101-1

Synthesis of melatonin in the pineal gland. The pineal takes up tryptophan from the circulation; the amino acid is hydroxylated to form 5-hydroxytryptophan; this is then converted to the amine serotonin (5-hydroxytryptamine) by the enzyme aromatic L-amino acid decarboxylase. Some of the serotonin synthesized in the pineal is destroyed by oxidative deamination, forming 5-hydroxyindole acetic acid. However, the major fraction of pineal serotonin is N-acetylated and O-methylated to form the hormone melatonin.

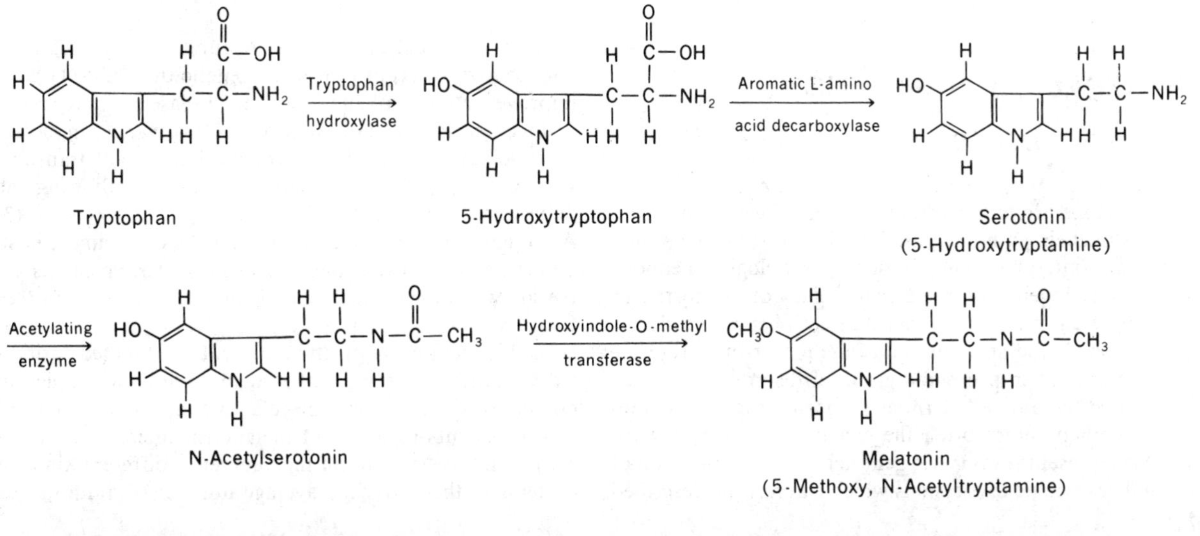

patient's family initially seeks medical attention because of the development of precocious puberty. About one-third of all boys below the normal age of sexual maturation who have pineal tumors develop precocious puberty. This neoplasm accounts for about 10 to 15 percent of all precocious sexual development in males. For unexplained reasons, pineal tumors are much less common among girls and are not associated with precocious menarche. Some investigators have suggested that the precocious sexual development in pinealoma patients is a nonspecific consequence of the pressure that these tumors exert on surrounding brain tissue. Kitay and others have summarized the evidence against this "pressure hypothesis": (1) Pineal tumors may produce precocious puberty, no gonadal signs, or even delayed pubescence. The endocrine effects of a particular tumor appear to be unrelated to its size. (2) Most cases of precocious puberty develop in patients with nonparenchymal tumors (frequently teratomas). An occasional parenchymal tumor leads to gonadal enlargement, but more commonly these neoplasms are associated with delayed pubescence or with secondary gonadal failure. (3) Gonadal abnormalities have been observed in a large number of pinealoma patients whose tumors had neither produced signs of a chronic elevation in cerebrospinal fluid pressure nor invaded other brain areas. The demonstration that a pineal hormone, melatonin, influences normal sexual maturation in rats supports the hypothesis that precocious puberty develops in pinealoma patients because the damaged pineal fails to release an inhibitory hormone. It has not been possible to test this hypothesis directly, because no assay is available which can be used to measure the level of melatonin or its metabolic products in blood or urine. It is noteworthy, perhaps, that both patients described above whose tumors contained melatonin-forming activity showed evidence of depressed sexual function.

Parenchymal pinealomas frequently show a good, if temporary, clinical remission following irradiation. Patients generally receive 3,000 to 5,000 R; radiation is administered over a wide portal because pinealomas not infrequently metastasize throughout the ventricles and the subdural space. Japanese surgeons have reported encouraging results following the surgical extirpation of pinealomas; however, this method is complicated by the relative inaccessibility of the pineal, and consequently is used rarely in the United States. A patient with metastatic parenchymal pinealoma has been repeatedly treated during a 10-year period with x-ray and chemotherapeutic agents; each time an objective decrease in tumor mass occurred.

A small number of tumors with histologic appearance of pinealomas originate elsewhere in the brain at some distance from the normal pineal gland. These "ectopic pinealomas" generally arise in the hypothalamus in the region of the infundibulum. Hence, patients usually present a picture similar to that seen with craniopharyngioma with a clinical triad of bitemporal hemianopsia, hypopituitarism, and diabetes insipidus. Most ectopic pinealomas show a good clinical response to irradiation.

REFERENCES

LYNCH JH et al: Daily rhythm in human urinary melatonin. Science 187:169, 1975

RAMSEY HJ: Ultrastructure of a pineal tumor. Cancer 18:1014, 1965

WOLSTENHOLME GEW, KNIGHT J (eds): *The Pineal Gland,* Edinburgh: Churchill-Livingstone, 1971, p. 401

WURTMAN RJ, CARDINALI DP: The pineal organ, in *Textbook of Endocrinology,* ed RH Williams, Philadelphia: Saunders, 1974, p. 832

section 3 | Errors of metabolism

102 GENERAL CONSIDERATIONS

LLOYD H. SMITH, JR.

Few diseases are either wholly genetic or wholly environmental in their pathogenesis. The degree to which "environment" (microbiologic, physical, psychologic, chemical) is injurious depends on the genetic legacy of the host. This may represent a specific genetic defect phenotypically expressed as altered structure and function or inappropriate amount of a given protein, a group of disorders still often designated by Garrod's term as "inborn errors of metabolism." Perhaps more often the genetic propensity toward disease represents polymeric gene action, the summation of a number of genic expressions which can now be described only by statistical approaches. A number of factors have contributed to recent interest in genetic diseases: (1) With improved control of environment, disease is increasingly endogenous rather than exogenous. (2) Advances in molecular biology have elucidated the mechanisms of transmission and expression of genetic information, allowing the definition of certain diseases with increased precision. (3) Although genetic diseases cannot now be cured in the host, knowledge of the resulting biochemical derangements often allows rational means of treatment to be devised (see Chap. 64).

In this section major attention will be directed to individual genetic diseases rather than to broader topics in population genetics or molecular biology. It is not clear how many inborn errors of metabolism there are. By the use of current estimates of the number of different kinds of proteins in the body, the average number of amino acids per protein, and the possibility that at a given point any one of 20 amino acids might be substituted, it may be estimated that the possibilities for variation in structural genes alone are $>10^{10}$. Many factors reduce the number of diseases which are recognized. Certain variations are trivial, lead to no biologic disadvantage, and merely constitute the chemical basis of individuality. Other defects are intrinsically lethal and contribute to the high incidence of spontaneous abortions. Variations may occur not only among diseases but also within diseases, depending on the site of alteration in the protein and the degree of resulting dysfunction. More than 100 abnormal hemoglobins have been described. It may well be, by analogy, that there are more than 100 types of galactosemia or phenylketonuria. Individual genetic diseases vary widely in frequency, from diabetes mellitus (3 to 5 percent of the population) to sulfituria (a single case description). The variables in frequency—mutation rate and the balance of biologic advantage and disadvantage—are now the subject of considerable interest in human genetics.

The usual *inborn error of metabolism* results from the absence or severe reduction in catalytic activity of an enzyme, whether the protein is physically missing or is present but altered in a fashion which impairs its function. In microorganisms genetic disorders of too much enzyme activity occur. No examples of genetic diseases due directly to excessive enzyme activity have been found in humans, although enzyme activities may be secondarily increased because of failure of control mechanisms (e.g., Δ-aminolevulinic acid synthetase in acute intermittent porphyria). *Genetic disorders* usually produce disease by the *accumulation of substrate of the abnormal enzyme or* by *absence or reduced availability of its product.* This concept is illustrated simply in diagrammatic form first introduced by Charles Dent:

Normal		Disease	
Gene	Gene	Gene	Gene
↓	↓	⇣	⇣
E	E	E	e

Normal: A ⟶ B ⟶ C

Disease: A ---→ B ---→ c (with B accumulated above and below)

The accumulation of substrate B is the most frequently encountered abnormality productive of disease. This may be related to the fact that most genetic disorders so far discovered are in degradative pathways of metabolism. Some examples of substrate (and substrate by-product) toxicity are described in greater detail in subsequent chapters: phenylalanine and its by-products in phenylketonuria, galatose 1-phosphate in galactosemia, oxalate in primary hyperoxaluria, homogentisic acid and its pigment polymer in alkaptonuria. Such defects may result in storage diseases such as the lipidoses, cystinosis, and the glycogen storage diseases. The accumulated precursor may inhibit other metabolic pathways or interfere with amino acid transport into cells. Often the biochemical mechanism of injury is obscure.

Genetic disorders may lead to disease because of *absence* or *reduced availability of the product* rather than through accumulation of the precursor. Most of the recognized examples lie in defects in plasma protein synthesis or in the sequence of hormone synthesis, described elsewhere in this book. For example, deficiency of circulating thyroxine and triiodothyronine is the major defect in the various specific genetic forms of familial cretinism (Chap. 92), producing damage to the developing central nervous system, delayed maturation of the skeleton, hypometabolism, and failure of inhibition of TSH (thyroid-stimulating hormone) release, with resulting goiter. Similarly, deficiency of hydrocortisone in congenital adrenal virilism (Chap. 93) is the ultimate cause of adrenocortical hyperplasia (via ACTH) and of the excessive synthesis of steroidal precursors into adrenal androgens. A large number of genetic disorders of the synthesis of circulating proteins which participate in hemostasis have been described. In fact these proteins have been largely discovered in the study of patients with a hemorrhagic diathesis. The ultimate deficiency common to these disorders is that of appropriate formation of cross-linked fibrin polymer. The multiple types of genetic blocks in glycolysis associated with chronic nonspherocytic hemolytic anemia probably share a common deficiency of erythrocytic ATP (adenosine triphosphate). The defect in albinism is absence of melanin; and a major defect in the von Gierke form of glycogen storage disease is deficiency of circulating glucose secondary to loss of glucose 1-phosphatase activity. In hereditary orotic aciduria, uridine becomes an essential metabolite. In a sense these disorders represent analogues of auxotrophism in bacteria.

A number of *genetic diseases* have now been described in which there is a *defect* in the *active transport of metabolites across membranes,* as summarized in Chap. 105. Occasionally the physical properties of the abnormal protein may constitute the mechanism of disease, as in the propensity toward stacking and tactoid formation in sickle-cell anemia and the heritable disorders of connective tissue. Pharmacogenetics refers to inherited alterations in drug metabolism, sensitivity of response, and toxicity. As an example, pseudocholinesterase deficiency is innocuous except during the use of certain muscle relaxants in anesthesia, when prolonged paralysis may result. Immunogenetics refers not only to immunologic markers in gamma-globulins but also to the inherited basis of antigenic (chemical) individuality. It is apparent that genetic alterations may be productive of disease through a variety of mechanisms, both subtle and direct.

Genetic diseases cannot now be "cured" in the host, although current advances in molecular biology suggest that this limitation may eventually be removed. Knowledge of the mechanism of disease, however, often allows effective palliative measures to be instituted. Many of these are illustrated in the discussion of specific diseases in the chapters of this section. See Table 65-3 for specific therapeutic procedures.

Garrod wrote in 1908, "The existence of chemical individuality follows of necessity from chemical specificity, but we should expect the differences between individuals to be still more subtle and difficult of detection." The molecular biology of genetic transmission and expression is perhaps the most important area of scientific advance in the past two decades. Application of these advances in humans has elucidated a large number of genetic errors of metabolism, some of which are described in specific detail in the following chapters.

REFERENCES

HARRIS H: *Garrod's Inborn Errors of Metabolism,* New York: Oxford, 1963

ROSENBERG LE: Inborn errors of metabolism, in *Duncan's Diseases of Metabolism,* 7th ed., eds PK Bondy, LE Rosenberg, Philadelphia: Saunders, 1974, p. 31

STANBURY JB et al (eds): *The Metabolic Basis of Inherited Disease,* 4th ed., New York: McGraw-Hill, in press

103 GENETIC DISORDERS OF AMINO ACID METABOLISM

LLOYD H. SMITH, JR.

In a sense, all genetic diseases represent disorders of amino acid metabolism in their phenotypic expression as protein synthesis. A large number of disorders represent specific defects in the synthesis, degradation, or membrane transport of individual amino acids. Three of Garrod's four original "inborn errors of metabolism" were those of amino acid metabolism (albinism, alcaptonuria, and cystinuria). The study of these disorders has greatly enhanced our understanding of normal pathways of amino acid metabolism and transport. In this chapter, only phenylketonuria, homocystinuria, and disorders of branched-chain amino acids are reviewed. Others have been classified as storage diseases (Chap. 104) or as errors in membrane transport (Chap. 105). In Table 103-1, a summary of genetic disorders of amino acid metabolism is presented with references for further information. The inclusion or omission of certain diseases is arbitrary in that they may represent defects in metabolism several steps removed from the parent amino acid.

PHENYLKETONURIA

DEFINITION Phenylketonuria, first described by Folling in 1934, is a metabolic disorder secondary to an inherited deficiency of phenylalanine hydroxylase. This results in the accumulation of phenylalanine and some of its metabolites (notably phenylpyruvate, phenyllactate, phenylacetate, and *O*-hydroxyphenylacetate) and a syndrome of mental deficiency. Other neurologic deficits, epileptic seizures, and reduced pigmentation may also occur.

GENETICS AND PATHOGENESIS Phenylketonuria is transmitted as an autosomal recessive trait, occurring in its clinical (homozygous) form with a frequency of about 1 in 15,000 to 20,000 births in the United States. About 0.64 percent of the inmates in institutions for the mentally defective are patients with homozygous phenylketonuria. Heterozygotes usually exhibit slightly elevated fasting levels of plasma phenylalanine and reduced rates of plasma clearance of phenylalanine after its oral administration. Although some studies have suggested an increased incidence

TABLE 103-1
Genetic disorders of amino acid metabolism (partial listing)*

Disease	*Enzyme deficiency*
Albinism:	
Ocular	Unknown
Oculocutaneous	Tyrosinase; tyrosine permease (?)
Alcaptonuria‡	Homogentisic acid oxidase
Argininosuccinic aciduria	Argininosuccinase
Carnosinemia	Carnosinase
Citrullinemia	Argininosuccinic acid synthetase
Cystathioninuria	Cystathionase (pyridoxine dependency in most patients)
Cystinosis‡	Not established
Histidinemia	Histidase (L-histidine ammonia lysase)
Homocystinuria‡	Cystathionine synthetase
Hydroxyprolinemia	Hydroxyproline oxidase
Hyper-β-alaninemia	β-Alanyl-α-ketoglutaric amino transferase (not established)
Hyperammonemia (congenital):	
Type I	Carbamyl phosphate synthetase
Type II	Ornithine transcarbamylase
Hyperglycinemia (nonketotic)	Glycine decarboxylase
Hyperlysinemia:	
Periodic	L-Lysine NAD oxidoreductase

Signs and symptoms	*Laboratory abnormalities*	*Transmission*	*References*
Absence or marked reduction of pigmentation in the eye, defects in vision	No changes in blood or urine	X-linked recessive	Fitzpatrick TB, Quevedo WC, Jr.†
Hypopigmentation of eye and skin, defects in vision, sensitivity to actinic radiation in both tyrosinase-positive and -negative types	No changes in blood or urine	Autosomal recessive; two types are not allelic	
Pigmentation of cartilage and other connective tissues (ochronosis), degenerative arthritis, calcification of intervertebral disks	Homogentisic acid elevated in urine; serves as a reducing agent and also forms a dark pigment on standing, especially after alkalinization	Autosomal recessive	La Du BN†
Severe mental retardation, ataxia, seizures, hepatic dysfunction, abnormally friable hair	Elevated plasma and CSF argininosuccinate, citrulline, and sometimes ammonia; argininosuccinate in urine	Autosomal recessive	Shih VE†
Mental retardation, seizures, spasticity, myoclonic jerks	Excessive plasma and urine carnosine and anserine	Probably autosomal recessive	Scriver CR†
Mental retardation, nausea, vomiting, tremors, hypotonicity, intermittent hyperammonemia	Citrulline elevated in blood and urine; blood NH_3 elevated postprandially; urea normal	Probably autosomal recessive	Shih VE†
Mental deficiency may or may not be present; no other specific clinical picture has emerged	Excessive excretion of cystathionine in urine	Probably autosomal recessive	Mudd SH, Levy H†
Dwarfism, rickets, symptoms of acidosis and advancing renal failure, opacities from cystine deposits in corneas; a few patients have ocular cystinosis only	Renal tubular defects of the de Toni-Fanconi syndrome, uremia, cystine crystals in leukocytes	Autosomal recessive	Seegmiller JE et al
Variable mental retardation, possibly in a special tendency toward speech and language disorders	Increased histidine in blood and urine; increased excretion of imidazolepyruvate, imidazolelactate, and imidazoleacetate; low plasma glutamate; high blood and urine alanine	Autosomal recessive	La Du BN†
Mild mental deficiency (sometimes absent), ectopia lentis, osteoporosis, thromboembolic complications, skeletal deformities resembling Marfan's syndrome	Elevated plasma and urine methionine and homocystine	Autosomal recessive	Mudd SH, Levy H†
Variable mental retardation	Free L-hydroxyproline elevated in plasma and urine; bound hydroxyproline normal	Probably autosomal recessive	Scriver CR†
Failure of normal growth and development, seizures, somnolence	Increased plasma β-alanine and γ-aminobutyric acid (GABA); increased urine β-alanine, GABA, taurine, γ-aminoisobutyric acid	Not established	Scriver CR†
Vomiting, lethargy, flaccidity	Hyperammonemia, metabolic acidosis, mild elevation of plasma and urinary glycine, cyclic neutropenia	Not established	Freeman JM et al, J Pediatr 65:1039, 1964
Vomiting, lethargy, coma, especially after high protein ingestion; muscular rigidity, hepatomegaly, mental retardation	Hyperammonemia, increased plasma glutamine, increased urinary orotic acid and uridine	Probably X-linked dominant	Shih VE†
Mental retardation, seizures, spastic paraplegia	Increased plasma and urinary glycine	Probably autosomal recessive	Nyhan WL†
Vomiting, spasticity, coma, mental retardation, exacerbation by protein ingestion	Hyperlysinemia and hyperargininemia with increase in blood ammonia intermittently, related to protein ingestion	Probably autosomal recessive	Ghadimi H†

* *In addition to the references listed, excellent reviews are: WL Nyhan (ed), Heritable Disorders of Amino Acid Metabolism, New York: Wiley, 1974; LE Rosenberg, CR Scriver, Disorders of amino acid metabolism, in Duncan's Diseases of Metabolism, 7th ed., eds PK Bondy, LE Rosenberg, Philadelphia: Saunders, 1974, p. 465.*

† *From JB Stanbury et al (eds), The Metabolic Basis of Inherited Disease, 4th ed., New York: McGraw-Hill, in press.*

‡ *This disease is discussed in more detail in the text.*

of mental deficiency or psychiatric disturbances in families of patients with phenylketonuria, the heterozygous state has not been demonstrated to be injurious.

In addition to classic phenylketonuria, there are several other disorders associated with elevation of serum phenylalanine during the neonatal period. These disorders may represent milder forms of phenylketonuria, transient forms due to delayed development of the phenylalanine transaminase, tyrosinemia, or tyrosinosis. Children born of mothers with phenylketonuria may also exhibit brain damage from intrauterine exposure to the deranged maternal metabolism of phenylalanine.

Phenylalanine is normally hydroxylated in the para position to form tyrosine, involving a complex biochemical reaction catalyzed by phenylalanine hydroxylase with an unconjugated pteridine, 7,8-dihydrobiopterin, as a cofactor. There may be three isozymes of phenylalanine hydroxylase, which may explain some of the variability found in the disease. The isozymes are restricted to liver where enzyme activity increases in the first few weeks after birth. Active enzyme fails to appear in the phenylketonuric infant. This results in accumulation of dietary phenylalanine in the plasma and presumably in cells, with secondary diversion (by transamination) into phenylpyruvate, phenyllactate, phenylacetate, and *O*-hydroxyphenylacetate, all four of these phenyl acids being excreted together with phenylalanine in the urine. Phenylalanine is a competitive inhibitor of tyrosinase on the pathway of melanin synthesis, which explains the decreased pigmentation of hair, eyes, and skin. High levels of phenylalanine in body fluids inhibit transport of amino acids into cells. The resulting deprivation of essential amino acids in the developing brain may be the immediate cause of cerebral damage, although this has not been established. Other explanations relate to altered patterns of synthesis of pharmacodynamic amines (serotonin, norepinephrine, phenylethylamine, etc.). There is decreased myelinization in the brains of patients with phenylketonuria.

CLINICAL PRESENTATION AND DIAGNOSIS Retardation of mental development, usually of severe degree, is the major manifestation of phenylketonuria. Since the mental defect is stationary and not progressive in older children or adults, the brain injury appears to be limited to a particularly sensitive stage in brain development. Other neurologic abnormalities sometimes found are tremors, seizures, muscular hypertonicity, hyperkinesis, and EEG abnormalities. As noted, there tends to be reduced pigmentation of skin, hair, and eyes. Eczema and growth retardation have been described.

Early diagnosis is essential for successful treatment since the neurologic abnormalities, once established, are largely irreversible. Diagnosis before one month of age requires the demonstration of grossly elevated levels of plasma phenylalanine. The excretion of the associated metabolites may not be remarkable at this time. Testing by screening for phenylketonuria of all newborn infants and of all infants of thirty days and under when admitted to a hospital is now mandatory in the majority of states. This routine blood testing can be carried out quite simply using the bacterial inhibition assay (Guthrie) or a fluorometric procedure. Positive tests must be carefully followed up with

TABLE 103-1
Genetic disorders of amino acid metabolism (partial listing) *(conti*

Disease	*Enzyme deficiency*
Hyperlysinemia: Persistent	Lysine: α-ketoglutarate reductase
Hyperoxaluria (primary):‡	
Type I	2-Oxo-glutarate: glyoxylate carboligase
Type II	D-Glyceric dehydrogenase
Hyperprolinemia:	
Type I	Proline oxidase
Type II	Δ′-Pyrroline-5-carboxylate-dehydrogenase
Hypersarcosinemia	Sarcosine dehydrogenase (not established)
Hypervalinemia‡	Valine-α-ketoglutarate transaminase (not established)
Isovaleric acidemia‡	Probably isovaleryl-CoA dehydrogenase
Maple syrup urine disease (branched-chain ketoaciduria)‡	Oxidases of α-ketoisocaproic acid, α-ketoisovaleric acid, α-keto-β-methylvaleric acid
β-Mercaptolactate cysteine disulfiduria	Not established
Methylmalonic aciduria:	
Vitamin B_{12}-responsive	Synthesis of 5′-deoxyadenosylcobalamin
Vitamin B_{12}-unresponsive	Methylmalonyl CoA racemase, or methymalonyl CoA carbonylmutase
Phenylketonuria‡	Phenylalanine hydroxylase
Propionic acidemia	Propionyl CoA carboxylase
Sulfituria	Sulfite oxidase
Tyrosinemia	ρ-Hydroxyphenylpyruvic acid oxidase (?–not established)
Tyrosinosis	Tyrosine transaminase (?) ρ-Hydroxyphenylpyruvic acid oxidase (?–not proved)

Signs and symptoms	*Laboratory abnormalities*	*Transmission*	*References*
Vomiting, spasticity, coma, mental retardation, exacerbation by protein ingestion. May be clinically normal	Hyperlysinemia and hyperlysinuria; no elevation of blood ammonia	Probably autosomal recessive	Ghadimi H†
Symptoms and signs of kidney stones and advancing renal failure	Increase in urinary oxalate, glycolate, and glyoxylate	Autosomal recessive	Williams HE, Smith LH, Jr.†
Symptoms and signs of kidney stones and advancing renal failure	Increase in urinary oxalate and L-glyceric acid	Autosomal recessive	Williams HE, Smith LH, Jr.†
Often no signs or symptoms; some increased linkage with renal disease	Hyperprolinemia, excess urinary excretion of proline, hydroxyproline, and glycine	Probably autosomal recessive	Scriver CR†
Usually associated with mental retardation and a convulsive disorder	Same as in type I, but also excess excretion of Δ′-pyrroline-5-carboxylic acid	Probably autosomal recessive	Scriver CR†
Often a benign trait. Rarely associated with mental deficiency	Increase in plasma and urinary sarcosine	Autosomal recessive	Gerritsen T, Waisman HA†
Mental and somatic retardation, nystagmus, hypotonicity, unresponsiveness, vomiting	Valine elevated in plasma and urine	Presumed autosomal recessive	Dancis J, Levitz M†
Mild psychomotor retardation, intention tremor, attacks of acidosis, stupor, and coma; "sweaty-foot smell" of breath	Elevated plasma isovaleric acid	Not established; probably autosomal recessive	Budd MA et al, N Engl J Med 277:321, 1967
Progressive deterioration of central nervous system function usually beginning shortly after birth and leading to early death; sweet, maple syrup-like odor to urine and sweat	Elevated levels of leucine, isoleucine, valine, and their corresponding keto acids in blood and urine	Autosomal recessive	Dancis J, Levitz M†
May have no clinical abnormalities or be associated with mental deficiency	Excessive urinary excretion of the mixed disulfide of β-mercaptolactate and cysteine	Not established	Crawhall JC†
Signs and symptoms of recurrent ketoacidosis	Metabolic acidosis, hyperglycinemia and hyperglycinuria, hypoglycemia during attacks; marked methylmalonic aciduria	Probably autosomal recessive	Rosenberg LE†
Signs and symptoms of recurrent ketoacidosis	Metabolic acidosis, hyperglycinemia and hyperglycinuria, hypoglycemia during attacks; marked methylmalonic aciduria	Probably autosomal recessive	Rosenberg LE†
Severe mental deficiency, tremors, seizures, muscular hypertonicity, hyperkinesis, reduced pigmentation	Plasma phenylalanine elevated; phenylalanine, phenylpyruvate, phenyllactate, phenylacetate, and *O*-hydroxyphenylacetate elevated in urine	Autosomal recessive	Sidbury JB, Tourian A†
Developmental retardation, dehydration, lethargy, coma precipitated by high protein ingestion	Recurrent ketoacidosis, elevation of serum glycine and propionic acid; intermittent elevations of serum valine, leucine, and isoleucine	Autosomal recessive	Rosenberg LE†
Severe neurologic abnormalities at birth, deteriorating to an almost decorticate state; ectopia lentis in single described case	Excessive urinary excretion of sulfite, thiosulfate, and *S*-sulfo-L-cysteine; reduced urine sulfate	Not established	Laster L et al, J Clin Invest, 46: 1082, 1967
Vomiting, diarrhea, rickets, failure to thrive, hepatosplenomegaly, sometimes mental retardation	Proximal tubular dysfunction with laboratory findings of Fanconi's syndrome; elevation of serum tyrosine and sometimes methionine; marked elevation of urinary excretion of *p*-hydroxyphenyllactic acid	Autosomal recessive	La Du BN†
Single patient had myasthenia gravis	Excessive urinary excretion of *p*-hydroxyphenylpyruvic acid	Not established	La Du BN†

quantitative measurements of plasma phenylalanine and study of urinary metabolites to differentiate the disease from transient hyperphenylalaninemia related to prematurity, tyrosinemia, heterozygosity, or other disorders with elevation of serum phenylalanine. This is important because restrictive diets may be injurious in patients other than those with phenylketonuria. The ferric chloride test, a transient blue or olive-green color appearing on the addition of a few drops of 5% $FeCl_3$ to 5 ml urine, is still useful for screening older children or adults and is usually positive in infants.

TREATMENT The biochemical abnormalities can be corrected by preventing the accumulation of phenylalanine. This is done by a special diet in which protein is replaced by an amino acid mixture low in phenylalanine (Ketonil, Lofenolac). Supplementary foods are given to supply only the amount of L-phenylalanine needed for body growth. The program should attempt to maintain normal weight gain and plasma phenylalanine levels between 3 and 10 mg per 100 ml. The restrictive diet should be started as soon as possible and continued for at least 6 to 8 years. Some patients treated from early infancy have developed normal intelligence. Little permanent improvement can be achieved by treatment begun later, the main effect being that of prevention of further intellectual deterioration.

HOMOCYSTINURIA

DEFINITION Homocystinuria is a genetic disease resulting from markedly reduced activity of cystathionine synthase, an enzyme which catalyzes an important step in the transsulfuration pathway converting methionine to cysteine. It is characterized clinically by ectopia lentis, osteoporosis, thromboembolic phenomena, skeletal changes suggestive of Marfan's syndrome, and mental retardation (in approximately 50 percent of patients). There is excessive urinary excretion of homocystine and several other sulfur-containing compounds. Of the genetic disorders of amino acid metabolism, homocystinuria may rank second in frequency, following phenylketonuria. It occurs once in every 20,000 to 40,000 births (see also Chap. 64). Excessive excretion of homocystine has also been found in three other rare genetic disorders which create blocks in the enzymatic conversion of homocystine to methionine. A nongenetic form of homocystinuria may be produced pharmacologically by the pyrimidine analogue 6-azauridine triacetate.

GENETICS AND PATHOGENESIS Homocystinuria is transmitted as an autosomal recessive trait. Heterozygotes have no stigmata of the disease, no detectable plasma homocystine, and no elevation of plasma methionine. They sometimes exhibit delayed plasma clearance of methionine loads given orally or intravenously. Assays of liver biopsy specimens, fibroblast cultures, and phytohemagglutinin-stimulated lymphocytes from parents of homocystinurics (presumed heterozygotes) have revealed cystathionine synthase activities intermediate between those of patients and controls. Homozygotes exhibit virtual absence of this enzyme activity in liver, brain, fibroblasts, and transformed lymphocytes. Approximately one-half of the patients have responded to large doses of pyridoxine with marked biochemical improvement. In vitro studies in homocystinuric fibroblasts suggest an impaired binding of pyridoxal 5-phosphate by the synthase apoenzyme.

In the absence of cystathionine synthase, homocystine and methionine accumulate, and cysteine (or cystine) becomes an essential amino acid. The connective tissue disorder may result from an interference with the normal cross-linkage of collagen by homocystine. There is important new evidence that the thrombogenic mechanism of homocystinuria may result from homocystine-induced endothelial injury, leading to patch desquamation and subsequent platelet adherence and clotting. It has been suggested that the ability of homocystine to form mixed disulfides may inactivate critical sulfhydryl groups of enzymes. No role of cysteine deficiency has been established. Other sulfur-containing metabolites such as 5-amino-4-imidazole-carboxamide-5′-S-ribonucleoside, S-adenosylhomocysteine, and homolanthionine are found in excess in urine of patients with homocystinuria and may contribute to the diverse structural and functional manifestations of the disease.

CLINICAL PRESENTATION AND DIAGNOSIS Patients with homocystinuria often exhibit a superficial resemblance to those with Marfan's syndrome (Chap. 367). Some of the skeletal and connective tissue abnormalities which have been described are ectopia lentis, severe juvenile osteoporosis, kyphosis, scoliosis, genu valgum, deformities of the sternum such as pectus excavatum and pectus carinatum, abnormalities of the palate, and arachnodactyly. Mental deficiency is common, being found in approximately half of these patients, and psychotic behavior suggestive of schizophrenia has been observed. When mental deficiency is present, it is not usually as severe as that of phenylketonuria. Recurrent arterial and venous thromboses may complicate the course and lead to early death from pulmonary embolism or coronary or carotid occlusion. Patients with homocystinuria tend to resemble one another, with their skeletal deformities, light-colored hair, and coarse skin with malar flush and livido reticularis. Diagnosis is established by finding homocystine in the urine using paper or ion exchange column chromatography and should be confirmed by analysis of the amino acid pattern of plasma. As a disulfide, homocystine will also give a positive nitroprusside reaction in urine, but must then be differentiated from cystine by chromatographic techniques. Plasma methionine is elevated but plasma cystine is reduced.

TREATMENT All patients should receive a trial with pyridoxine (250 to 500 mg per day). If biochemical improvement occurs, this form of treatment should be continued. If there is no response to pyridoxine, beneficial results may be obtained from the use of a diet low in methionine (20 to 40 mg per kg per day), supplemented by L-cystine. These programs may lead to improvement in the chemical derangements. There is accumulating evidence that they may reduce the severity of the clinical manifestations of the disease as well.

MAPLE SYRUP URINE DISEASE (BRANCHED-CHAIN KETOACIDURIA)

DEFINITION Maple syrup urine disease, so named because of the characteristic odor of the urine and sweat of affected patients, is a rare genetic disorder of the metabolism of branched-chain amino acids and their corresponding keto acids. It is associated with severe neurologic damage and mental retardation occurring in the early neonatal period, usually leading to early death. In two large surveys of newborn infants, the incidence was found to be between 1 in 100,000 and 1 in 250,000 births. The disorder may occur as a milder variant with episodic or intermittent symptoms and biochemical abnormalities. A third variant with response to large doses of thiamine has been found in a single child.

Six other disorders of branched-chain amino acid metabolism have been discovered. One child with severe mental and physical retardation has exhibited persistent hypervalinemia in the absence of any abnormality of leucine or isoleucine metabolism. Sixteen patients have been found with isovaleric acidemia associated with recurrent episodes of vomiting, acidosis, and coma and with mild mental retardation. Other disorders of branched-chain amino acid metabolism, which are not described further here, include propionic acidemia, ketotic hyperglycinemia, methylalonic acidemia, β-hydroxyisovaleric aciduria, β-methylcrotonyl glycinuria, and α-methyl-β-hydroxybutyric aciduria.

GENETICS AND PATHOGENESIS Leucine, isoleucine, and valine are normally metabolized to their corresponding keto acids (α-ketoisocaproic acid, α-keto-β-methylvaleric acid, and α-ketoisovaleric acid, respectively) by transamination. Previous biochemical studies suggested that a common enzyme catalyzed the transamination of all three amino acids, but the transamination defect for valine in leukocytes from the patient with hypervalinemia was specific for this amino acid alone. The branched-chain keto acids formed from the corresponding amino acids then undergo oxidative decarboxylation in complex reactions comparable to those catalyzed by pyruvate and α-ketoglutarate oxidases. It is not clear whether there are two or three specific enzymes which catalyze these reactions. In maple syrup urine disease the activities of all three keto acid oxidases are markedly reduced in brain, kidney, liver, and peripheral leukocytes. The loss of activity of two or three analogous but seemingly distinct enzymes is unexplained. One postulate is that of a genetic defect in the synthesis of a common enzyme subunit. The disease is transmitted as an autosomal mendelian recessive trait. Some, but not all, presumed heterozygotes have reduced activities of the keto acid oxidases in their leukocytes, but otherwise exhibit no clinical or chemical stigmata of the disease. The metabolic block in these parallel degradative pathways leads to the accumulation of three branched-chain keto acids and the corresponding amino acids in blood and their excessive excretion in urine. The mechanism of neurologic damage has not been established, although several hypotheses have been advanced. The keto acid derivatives of leucine and valine inhibit the activity of L-glutamic dehydrogenase in brain homogenates. Another suggestion relates to the inhibition of transfer of other essential amino acids into the central nervous system in the presence of elevated plasma levels of the branched-chain amino acids.

In isovaleric acidemia there is deficient activity of isovaleryl CoA dehydrogenase, which normally converts this compound to β-methylcrotonyl CoA in the pathway of leucine metabolism. It is probably inherited as a rare autosomal recessive trait.

CLINICAL PRESENTATION AND DIAGNOSIS Infants with maple syrup urine disease are normal at birth but begin within a few days to exhibit progressive deterioration, with lethargy, poor feeding, diminished awareness, hypertonicity alternating with flaccidity, and convulsions. The characteristic urine odor from which the name derives is present. Death generally occurs within the first few weeks of life from severe neurologic damage with respiratory disturbances. If death is delayed, mental retardation becomes apparent. A few patients exhibit a milder form of the disease, with intermittent branched-chain ketonuria. The diagnosis is usually first suggested from the odor of the urine, described as sweet, caramel-like, or like maple syrup. The urine gives a positive ferric chloride test and dinitrophenylhydrazine reaction for keto acids. The diagnosis is best established by ion exchange column chromatography of plasma to demonstrate elevated levels of leucine, isoleucine, and valine. Methods for demonstrating the enzyme defect in circulating leukocytes have been described.

The single Japanese child with hypervalinemia had vomiting, lethargy, and failure to thrive beginning soon after birth. There was severe retardation of physical and mental development at age three. The diagnosis was established by the finding of isolated elevation of valine in plasma and urine. Patients with isovaleric acidemia have recurrent episodes of vomiting and acidosis, mental retardation, and a variety of neurologic manifestations (ataxia, intention tremor, lethargy, coma). Acute episodes are accompanied by a characteristic offensive odor (which led to the discovery of the disorder), described as being like cheese or sweaty feet.

TREATMENT The treatment of maple syrup urine disease, like that of phenylketonuria, is based on the use of a diet restricted in the corresponding amino acids beginning early in life before the onset of permanent neurologic damage. In practice this has been very difficult because of the necessity to balance three different amino acids, the ubiquitous distribution of the branched-chain amino acids in foods, and the large number of plasma chromatographic analyses required. A few encouraging results have been reported using strict dietary therapy. It is not clear whether such treatment can be omitted in later life. A selective restriction of valine and leucine should offer a rational approach to hypervalinemia and isovaleric acidemia, respectively.

REFERENCES

DANCIS J, LEVITZ M: Abnormalities of branched-chain amino acid metabolism [hypervalinemia, branched-chain ketonuria (maple syrup disease), isovaleric acidemia], in *The Metabolic Basis of Inherited Disease,* 4th ed., eds JB Stanbury et al, New York: McGraw-Hill, in press

HARKER LA et al: Homocystinemia, vascular injury and arterial thrombosis. New Engl J Med 291:537, 1974

KOCH R et al: Phenylalaninemia and phenylketonuria, in *Heritable Disorders of Amino Acid Metabolism,* ed WL Nyhan, New York: Wiley, 1974, p. 109

MCKUSICK VA: Homocystinuria, in *Heritable Disorders of Connective Tissue,* ed VA McKusick, St. Louis: Mosby, 1972

MUDD SH, LEVY H: Disorders of methionine metabolism, in *The Metabolic Basis of Inherited Disease,* 4th ed., eds JB Stanbury et al, New York: McGraw-Hill, in press

PERRY TL: Homocystinuria, in *Heritable Disorders of Amino Acid Metabolism,* ed WL Nyhan, New York: Wiley, 1974, p. 395

SIDBURY JB, TOURIAN A: Phenylketonuria, in *The Metabolic Basis of Inherited Disease,* 4th ed., eds JB Stanbury et al, New York: McGraw-Hill, in press

SNYDERMAN SE: Maple syrup urine disease, in *Heritable Disorders of Amino Acid Metabolism,* ed WL Nyhan, New York: Wiley, 1974, p. 17

WADA Y et al: Idiopathic hypervalinemia: Probably a new entity of inborn error of valine metabolism. Tohoku J Exp Med 81:46, 1963

104
STORAGE DISEASES

Alcaptonuria and Ochronosis
Primary Hyperoxaluria with Oxalosis
Cystine Storage Disease

LLOYD H. SMITH, JR.

A number of genetic diseases are characterized by excessive storage of metabolites in the host. Most often these represent blocks in degradative pathways. Examples may be cited in the glycogen storage diseases (Chap. 111), the lipidoses (Gaucher's disease, Fabry's disease, Niemann-Pick disease, Tay-Sachs disease, Tangier disease, metachromatic leukodystrophy) (Chap. 113), certain amino acid degradative diseases (primary hyperoxaluria with oxalosis, alcaptonuria with ochronosis, possible cystine storage disease), and possibly in some of the mucopolysaccharidoses (e.g., Hurler's syndrome) (Chap. 367). In addition excessive retention of dietary minerals may occur, as in hemochromatosis (Chap. 108) and Wilson's disease (Chap. 110). Tophaceous gout represents a special case, with excessive production and/or renal retention of a metabolic end product, uric acid (Chap. 107). Most of the above disorders are described elsewhere in this book. This chapter is concerned only with certain storage diseases of amino acid metabolism.

ALCAPTONURIA AND OCHRONOSIS

DEFINITION Alcaptonuria, one of the original inborn errors of metabolism studied by Garrod, is a rare disorder in the degradative pathway of phenylalanine and tyrosine metabolism. The genetic defect in the activity of the enzyme homogentisic acid oxidase leads to the accumulation and excessive urinary excretion of homogentisic acid. There is an associated deposition of dark pigment in connective tissues (ochronosis) and a particular form of degenerative arthritis. Over 600 cases have been reported.

GENETICS AND PATHOGENESIS Homogentisic acid, a normal intermediate in the metabolism of phenylalanine and tyrosine, is oxidized with opening of the phenyl ring to form maleylacetoacetic acid. The enzyme homogentisic acid oxidase, which catalyzes this step, has been found to be missing in activity in liver and kidney from patients with alcaptonuria. This disease seems to be transmitted as an autosomal mendelian trait, with a frequency of about one in 200,000 births. No biochemical method for detection of presumed heterozygotes has been devised, nor do they exhibit any of the clinical features of the disease. The renal excretion of excessive homogentisic acid (3 to 7 g per day) fully accounts for the reducing properties of urine, gentisic acid being the only other metabolite excreted in excess. At neutral pH or above, homogentisic acid is rapidly oxidized to a brown or black polymer, with darkening of the urine on standing and with staining of wet diapers or linen. The melanin-like polymer of homogentisic acid binds irreversibly to collagen, and this interaction is the presumed cause of cartilaginous degeneration and the resulting arthritis.

CLINICAL PRESENTATION AND DIAGNOSIS Alcaptonuria is a benign disorder until middle life, when degenerative joint changes begin in the majority of cases. Prior to this time the darkening of urine may be unnoticed. With the onset of arthritis, the large joints and the spine are affected with pain and stiffness, interspersed with periods of acute inflammation, which may resemble rheumatoid arthritis. In contrast to rheumatoid arthritis, small joints tend to be spared. Limitation of motion of the joints and ankylosis of the lumbosacral spine often occur later in the course of the disease. The roentgenogram of the spine is often almost pathognomonic, with degeneration and dense calcification of the intervertebral disks and resulting narrowing of the spaces. Ochronotic pigmentation may often be seen in the transmitted blueness of cartilages of the ear, nose, and costochondral junctions, and in brown areas in the sclerae, most frequently located at the intersections of the lateral rectus muscles. Pigment also occurs in heart valves, larynx, tympanic membranes, sweat glands, and skin. There may be an increased frequency of pigmented prostatic stones. A high incidence of degenerative cardiovascular disease has been described in older ochronotic patients, but a cause-and-effect relationship has not been firmly established. The diagnosis is usually made from the triad of *arthritis, ochronotic pigmentation,* and *urine which darkens* on the addition of strong alkali. On treatment with ferric chloride, alcaptonuric urine turns purple-black. Homogentisic acid may be conclusively demonstrated by chemical tests, chromatographic characteristics, or a specific enzymatic assay. Reversible acquired ochronosis has been described in the past after the prolonged use of carbolic acid dressings for cutaneous ulcers.

TREATMENT Alcaptonuria carries with it no metabolic disadvantage other than the deposition of polymerized pigment in connective tissues and the associated degenerative changes. Ascorbic acid, as a strong reducing agent, will impede the oxidation and polymerization of homogentisic acid in vitro. Its use in large doses has been suggested as a possible means of preventing pigment formation and deposition in ochronotics, but its efficacy has not been demonstrated. The long and relatively benign course of the illness discourages attempts at rigid control of phenylalanine or tyrosine in the diet. Symptomatic treatment is similar to that of osteoarthritis (Chap. 358).

PRIMARY HYPEROXALURIA AND OXALOSIS

DEFINITION Primary hyperoxaluria is a genetic disorder characterized biochemically by continued excessive urinary excretion of oxalic acid and clinically by calcium oxalate nephrolithiasis and nephrocalcinosis. At postmortem examination calcium oxalate is usually found to be widely deposited in the tissues, a condition called *oxalosis.* In its typical form primary hyperoxaluria generally leads to uremia and early death. A few milder cases have been described in adult life with recurrent calcium oxalate kidney stones.

GENETICS AND PATHOGENESIS Primary hyperoxaluria has been shown to represent two distinct genetic disorders, associated with glycolic aciduria (type I) and L-glyceric aciduria (type II), respectively. They are described here together, since they have similar levels of urinary oxalate and are indistinguishable clinically. The excessive synthesis of oxalate in glycolic aciduria results from a block in an alternate route of metabolism of its precursor, glyoxylic acid. The activity of the enzyme α-ketoglutarate:glyoxylate carboligase, which catalyzes the synthesis of α-hydroxy-β-keto adipic acid, has been found to be markedly reduced in liver, spleen, and kidney preparations. The resulting expansion of the glyoxylate pool behind the site of the metabolic block leads to its excessive oxidation to oxalic acid and reduction to glycolic acid. All three of these 2-carbon acids are excreted in increased amounts in the urine. The disease seems most likely to be transmitted as an autosomal mendelian recessive trait, but no means of detecting presumed heterozygotes has been found. In L-glyceric aciduria there is absent activity of D-glyceric dehydrogenase (demonstrated in leukocytes), an enzyme which catalyzes the reduction of hydroxypyruvic acid in the catabolic pathway of serine metabolism. The accumulated hydroxypyruvate is reduced by lactic dehydrogenase to the unnatural L isomer of glyceric acid, which is excreted in the urine. The reduction of hydroxypyruvate is coupled enzymatically to the oxidation of glyoxylate to oxalate, catalyzed by lactic dehydrogenase, as the probable explanation of the resulting hyperoxaluria. L-Glyceric aciduria is transmitted as an autosomal recessive trait, and partial reductions in D-glyceric dehydrogenase activity are found in heterozygotes. The pathogenesis of stone formation, nephrocalcinosis, and oxalosis seems to relate directly to the insolubility of calcium oxalate. The disease can be simulated in animals, and humans, by pyridoxine deficiency, which presumably inhibits the transamination of glyoxylate to glycine. In addition to pyridoxine deficiency, another acquired form of hyperoxaluria is that associated with ileal disease and malabsorption. These patients have a continuing excessive absorption of dietary oxalate, perhaps because of intraluminal calcium. In this disorder, known as enteric or absorptive hyperoxaluria, patients have normal or low urinary glycolate and no detectable urinary L-glycerate.

CLINICAL PRESENTATION AND DIAGNOSIS Primary hyperoxaluria usually presents in childhood with recurrent kidney stones, with or without radiographically demonstrable nephrocalcinosis (Chap. 279). Rarely renal failure secondary to nephrocalcinosis may be the initial finding. The course of the childhood form of the disease is usually that of progressive renal failure leading to death from uremia. With the onset of uremia patients may exhibit severe peripheral arterial spasm and necrosis with resulting vascular insufficiency. In adults kidney stones are frequent, and occasionally mild nephrocalcinosis is found, but renal function is usually well preserved. The diagnosis is established by demonstrating excessive excretion of oxalic acid in the absence of pyridoxine deficiency or ileal disease. The normal child or adult excretes less than 60 mg oxalic acid/1.73 m^2/24 h. Patients with primary hyperoxaluria usually excrete at least two or three times that amount. The differential diagnosis of the glycolic aciduria (most frequent) and L-glyceric aciduria subvariants depends on specific measurements of those metabolites in urine.

TREATMENT There is no specific treatment for primary hyperoxaluria at this time. Large doses of pyridoxine (100 mg per day) may reduce urine oxalate, but the effect is not striking. Measures which may reduce the risk of stone formation are of use, such as forcing fluids, the use of a high phosphate regimen, and oral magnesium oxide (Chap. 279). Because of the seriousness of the disorder, attempts are being made to develop an inhibitor of oxalate synthesis, comparable to the use of allopurinol in gout. Renal transplantation has been invariably followed by rapid deposition of calcium oxalate in the transplanted kidney with early loss of function. The hyperoxaluria of pyridoxine deficiency responds promptly to vitamin replacement. Enteric hyperoxaluria is now treated with a low oxalate diet together with measures which may be indicated for the associated malabsorption. Studies suggest that the aluminum antacids may be effective in reducing oxalate hyperabsorption.

CYSTINOSIS AND FANCONI'S SYNDROME

DEFINITION Cystine storage disease, or cystinosis (Lignac-de Toni-Fanconi syndrome), is a rare genetic disorder, usually found in childhood in association with Fanconi's syndrome. Rarely, ocular and systemic cystine storage occurs in an adult form in the absence of renal disease. Fanconi's syndrome is a descriptive phrase for a group of physiologic abnormalities which occur with proximal renal tubular dysfunction, notably glucosuria, generalized amino aciduria, phosphaturia, and renal tubular acidosis. Cystinosis is only one of many diseases which may be associated with Fanconi's syndrome, a classification of which is given in Table 104-1.

GENETICS AND PATHOGENESIS The metabolic defect resulting in cystine storage has not yet been discovered. A number of enzymes in cystine metabolism have been assayed without finding any consistent abnormality, and earlier claims of reduced levels of blood cystine reductase have not been confirmed. Marked increases in cystine have been found in circulating leukocytes and in fibroblasts grown in tissue culture from patients with cystinosis. The free cystine is compartmentalized within the lysosomes of the cell. The disease seems to be transmitted as an autosomal recessive trait, with heterozygotes demonstrating intermediate levels of intracellular cystine. Plasma cystine levels are usually normal or slightly elevated only. The biochemical link between cystine storage and proximal renal tubular dysfunction is obscure in the childhood form of the disease. In the benign adult form of the disease there is no renal dysfunction. Cystine has the ability to form mixed disulfides with sulfhydryl groups. It has been suggested that the injurious effect of cystine storage may result from inhibition of sulfhydryl-containing enzymes by the formation of half-cystine residues on the proteins. A number of the other agents which cause the tubular dysfunction of Fanconi's syndrome are known inhibitors of sulfhydryl-requiring enzymes. A common biochemical mechanism of Fanconi's syndrome may be interference with the energy-yielding processes necessary for active transport in the proximal tubule. Patients with nephropathic cystinosis eventually develop severe glomerular damage as well.

As outlined in Table 104-1, Fanconi's syndrome may be of diverse origins, both inherited and acquired. It represents a nonspecific pattern of failure of proximal renal tubular absorptive function, varying greatly in the degree of severity and the spectrum of functions impaired. The individual disease processes are not discussed here. In idiopathic Fanconi's syndrome and that associated with cystinosis, microdissection studies have demonstrated a consistent structural change in the proximal tubule, the so-called "swan neck deformity." The proximal tubule is shortened and exhibits atrophy with flattened epithelium in the region adjacent to a normal-appearing glomerulus. These epithelial changes are not specific, however, and may merely represent the structural manifestations of injury.

CLINICAL PRESENTATION AND DIAGNOSIS Cystine storage disease with Fanconi's syndrome is a serious disorder which usually leads to death from uremia by the age of ten.

TABLE 104-1
Classifications of Fanconi's syndrome

- *I* Idiopathic
  - *A* Sporadic
  - *B* Familial
- *II* As part of a genetic disease
  - *A* Cystinosis
  - *B* Wilson's disease
  - *C* Tyrosinemia
  - *D* Lowe's syndrome
  - *E* Hereditary fructose intolerance (with fructose)
  - *F* Galactosemia (with galactose)
- *III* Medullary cystic disease
- *IV* Acquired
  - *A* Abnormality of protein metabolism
    - *1* Nephrotic syndrome
    - *2* Multiple myeloma
    - *3* Sjögren's syndrome
    - *4* Amyloidosis
  - *B* Drugs
    - *1* Outdated tetracycline
    - *2* 6-Mercaptopurine
    - *3* Isophthalanilide
  - *C* Heavy metals
    - *1* Mercury
    - *2* Uranium
    - *3* Cadmium
  - *D* Malignancy
- *V* Experimental (animals)
  - *A* Maleic acid
  - *B* Malonic acid

Failure to thrive and severe resistant rickets with stunting of growth develop in the first few months of life. Rickets results from several derangements: (1) failure of tubular reabsorption of phosphate with hypophosphatemia, (2) proximal renal tubular acidosis with bicarbonate wastage and chronic systemic acidosis, (3) hypercalciuria secondary to acidosis, and (4) the inhibition of osteoid calcification (vitamin D resistance) produced by azotemia. A more complete description of rickets and osteomalacia is presented elsewhere (Chaps. 352 and 353). Secondary hyperparathyroidism is a frequent complication and may exacerbate tubular dysfunction. Glucosuria may be scanty and intermittent or profuse and constant at a normal blood glucose level; it is sometimes sufficient to produce ketosis and contribute to further exacerbation of acidosis. Excessive urinary loss of potassium associated with renal tubular acidosis may lead to hypokalemia with muscle weakness or paralysis. Potassium depletion may produce "clear-cell nephropathy" with further deterioration of renal tubular function, especially a renal tubular concentration defect productive of polyuria. Generalized amino aciduria occurs, with a nonspecific pattern. Although cystine is usually excreted in excess, the urinary concentration is not sufficient to lead to cystine kidney stones. Hypouricemia may result from failure of reabsorption of uric acid. It has been found that patients with Fanconi's syndrome excrete lysozyme and light chains of gamma-globulins in the urine as well. Pyelonephritis is frequent and may contribute, along with interstitial fibrosis, to the onset of renal failure. The idiopathic Fanconi's syndrome may occur in an identical clinical and pathologic combination except for the absence of cystine storage. The clinical presentation may be dominated by other manifestations of the primary disease productive of Fanconi's syndrome (Table 104-1). Rarely, cystinosis may occur in the adult in the absence of renal dysfunction (Cogan's syndrome). Crystalline rods or plates of cystine are found in the cornea and conjunctiva as the only manifestation of adult cystinosis. Similar ocular cystinosis occurs in the infantile form of cystinosis, together with peripheral retinopathy characterized by patchy areas of depigmentation and pigment clumps.

The *diagnosis* of Fanconi's syndrome depends on the demonstration of the characteristic pattern of proximal renal tubular defects, of which the most important are phosphaturia, generalized amino aciduria, glucosuria, and renal tubular acidosis of the proximal (bicarbonate flooding) type. All these defects may be found individually or in various combinations, and may even vary with time in a given patient. It is therefore most useful to describe the actual physiologic derangements rather than to take refuge in the eponym. In cystinosis cystine crystals may be demonstrated by slit-lamp examination of the eye, or may be found in bone marrow or circulating leukocytes. Cystinotic leukocytes have very high levels of cystine by chemical analysis, even in the absence of demonstrable crystals. The characteristic retinopathy may be one of the earliest manifestations.

TREATMENT Treatment would logically be directed toward the disease resulting in Fanconi's syndrome and toward replacement therapy to compensate for renal dysfunction. Some of the diseases listed in Table 104-1 can be treated (Wilson's disease, hereditary fructose intolerance, etc.); others cannot. In the absence of specific information about its biochemical defect, attempts to treat cystinosis have generally been unrewarding. The use of D-penicillamine or dithiothreitol has been advocated in an attempt to regenerate active sulfhydryl groups on enzymes (see Wilson's disease, Chap. 110). The use of these agents has not resulted in objective evidence of improvement. Cystine is synthesized from the essential amino acid methionine, so that specific dietary treatment has not been vigorously pursued. Renal transplantation has been carried out successfully in a number of children with cystinotic renal failure. Renal biopsies have demonstrated cystine accumulation in the donor kidneys but the excess cystine appears to occur only in interstitial inflammatory cells of recipient origin. No cystine crystals have as yet been found in the epithelial cells of the proximal tubules of the transplanted kidneys. Treatment of the secondary physiologic derangements has been directed toward replacement of calcium, phosphate, sodium, and potassium to reverse chronic acidosis, rickets (osteomalacia in the adult), and hypokalemia. Large amounts of vitamin D are required (usually 50,000 to 400,000 IU daily) to promote normal calcification of bone. It has been reported that vitamin D may improve certain parameters of tubular function as well, reducing amino aciduria, glucosuria, and bicarbonate wasting, possibly through reduction of the associated secondary hyperparathyroidism. Shohl's solution (98 g sodium citrate and 140 g citric acid per liter) is a suitable source of buffer base for chronic acidosis. Chronic potassium supplementation is not usually required after its initial repletion and the correction of acidosis. Improved healing of rickets may occur with supplemental phosphate if phosphaturia is severe. Despite considerable symptomatic improvement and healing of rickets, progressive renal damage in cystinosis leads to early death from uremia. Adult cystinosis is a benign disorder which does not require treatment. The treatment of adult Fanconi's syndrome is similar to that described for the infantile form, but the prognosis is much better.

REFERENCES

BOQUIST L et al: Primary oxalosis. Am J Med 54:673, 1973

LA DU BN: Alcaptonuria, in *The Metabolic Basis of Inherited Disease,* 4th ed., eds JB Stanbury et al, New York: McGraw-Hill, in press

MORRIS RC, JR., et al: Genetic and metabolic injuries of the kidney, in *The Kidney,* eds BM Brenner, FC Rector, Jr, Philadelphia: Saunders, 1976

O'BRIEN W et al: Biochemical, pathologic and clinical aspects of alcaptonuria, ochronosis, and ochronotic arthropathy. Am J Med 34:813, 1963

SCHNEIDER JA: Clinical aspects of cystinosis, in *Cystinosis,* ed JD Schulman, U.S. Department of Health, Education, and Welfare Publication (NIH) 72–249, Government Printing Office, 1972, p. 11

——: Recent advances in cystinosis, in *Heritable Disorders of Amino Acid Metabolism,* ed WL Nyhan, New York: Wiley, 1974, p. 618

SEEGMILLER JE et al: Cystinosis and the Fanconi syndrome, in *The Metabolic Basis of Inherited Disease,* 4th ed., eds JB Stanbury et al, New York: McGraw-Hill, in press

WILLIAMS HE, SMITH LH, JR.: Primary hyperoxaluria, in *The Metabolic Basis of Inherited Disease,* 4th ed., eds JB Stanbury et al, New York: McGraw-Hill, in press

105
ERRORS IN MEMBRANE TRANSPORT

Cystinuria
Hartnup Disease
Renal Glycosuria
Renal Tubular Acidosis

LLOYD H. SMITH, JR.

The transfer of metabolites across cell membranes is usually an active energy-requiring process of considerable specificity. The enzymology of these processes and the required structural characteristics of cell membranes are poorly understood, although this now represents an important area of biochemical and biophysical investigation. A number of human diseases are best described as genetic defects in active transport of specific substances across epithelial cell membranes. In none of them has a specific enzymatic or structural defect been identified, other than in the description of the functional derangement. It is possible that defects may occur in the active transport of metabolites among the specific compartments or organelles within cells.

Some of the genetic diseases which might be classified as errors in membrane transport are cystinuria; Hartnup disease; hereditary renal tubular acidosis, renal glycosuria, familial renal gout; vasopressin-resistant diabetes insipidus; congenital hemolytic anemia with high sodium, low potassium in the red cells; familial goiter with iodide transport defect; methionine malabsorption syndrome; isolated tryptophan malabsorption (blue diaper syndrome); glucose and galactose malabsorption disease; congenital alkalosis with diarrhea (chloridorrhea); and hereditary intestinal malabsorption of vitamin B_{12}. Hemochromatosis might qualify in this category as an error in excessive transport of iron. This section will be limited to brief presentations of cystinuria, Hartnup disease, renal glycosuria, and hereditary renal tubular acidosis.

CYSTINURIA

DEFINITION Cystinuria is a genetic disorder (or group of closely related disorders) characterized by continued excessive excretion of the dibasic amino acids cystine, lysine, arginine, and ornithine. This results from a transport defect for these amino acids in the renal tubule. Similar transport defects occur in the intestinal mucosa. The sole clinical manifestations are those of recurrent cystine kidney stones and their sequelae. Patients tend to be of short stature, which has been attributed, without supporting evidence, to lysine deficiency.

GENETICS AND PATHOGENESIS Cystinuria has been known to be a familial disease for almost a century. It was one of the four original "inborn errors of metabolism" studied by Sir Archibald Garrod, who demonstrated its transmission in a pattern consistent with autosomal recessive inheritance. Further advances awaited the application of modern methods of amino acid analysis and the study of tubular transport in the kidney in vivo and in intestinal mucosal biopsies in vitro. In approximately two-thirds of the families of affected patients the presumed heterozygotes have normal levels of urinary dibasic amino acids. In the remaining families heterozygotes excrete increased amounts of cystine and lysine. At least one additional phenotype can be identified on the basis of intestinal transport studies. Several families have been studied with different genetic types in conjugal heterozygotes of cystinuria. The resulting patterns of double heterozygote defects have been interpreted as evidence for multiple allelic mutations. The incidence of homozygous cystinuria is approximately 1:40,000.

For many years cystinuria was attributed to a defect in cystine metabolism and was often confused with cystine storage disease (cystinosis). Dent and Rose first demonstrated by clearance techniques that impaired renal tubular reabsorption of the specific amino acids cystine, lysine, and arginine was the explanation of aminoaciduria. Subsequent studies indicated similar defects in tubular reabsorption of ornithine and of the mixed disulfide cysteine-homocysteine. Clearance of cystine may significantly exceed glomerular filtration rate, indicating net tubular secretion of this amino acid. Plasma levels of the involved amino acids are reduced. A common renal tubular mechanism has been confirmed by competition of lysine, arginine, and ornithine for transport during infusion studies. A common transport mechanism for these three amino acids has been found in tissue-slice preparations of kidney in vitro. It has not been possible to demonstrate a defect in cystine transport in vitro in renal biopsies from patients with cystinuria. Rarely, excretion of cystine or the other dibasic amino acids may occur as isolated defects. The interrelation of these transport defects at the level of the renal tubule remains to be clarified.

The transport defect for dibasic amino acids in cystinuria is also found in the intestine. This was first demonstrated by oral tolerance tests. It has been clearly confirmed in studies of active transport in jejunal mucosal biopsy specimens in vitro. At least three patterns of mucosal transport can be identified. With impaired absorption, lysine and ornithine are decarboxylated by intestinal bacteria to cadaverine and putrecine, respectively. These diamines are partially metabolized to pyrrolidine and piperidine, and all these compounds are excreted in increased amounts in cystinuric urine. No impairment of amino acid transport has been found in tissues other than the renal tubule and the intestinal mucosa in cystinuria.

Normal urinary excretion of cystine varies with size and diet, but has an upper normal range of about 18 mg per g creatinine. In homozygous cystinuria cystine excretion usually varies between 0.4 to 1.0 g per day, although values as high as 3.0 g per day have been found. The solubility of cystine in urine is approximately 350 to 400 mg per liter. Supersaturation and crystallization readily occur, particularly during nocturnal concentration of the urine. The accretion of such crystals as stones, with the resulting complications of obstruction and infection, is the direct cause of disability in cystinuria. Patients with mental retardation may have a higher incidence of cystinuria. Cystinuria has also been reported as associated with hereditary hypocalcemia in infancy, celiac disease, and hyperuricemia.

DIAGNOSIS The clinical manifestations of cystine kidney stones are indistinguishable from those of other kidney stones: flank pain, colic, hematuria, obstructive uropathy, infection. Cystine stones are as densely radiopaque as calcium-containing kidney stones. In overall incidence they constitute approximately 1 to 2 percent of all kidney stones. It is important to establish the composition of kidney stones in order to institute rational programs of stone prophylaxis (Chap. 279).

The most direct diagnostic procedure is that of stone analysis because cystine stones occur only in the genetic disorder cystinuria. The appearance of cystine crystals in the sediment of concentrated, acidified (addition of glacial acetic acid to pH 4.5), chilled urine specimens usually indicates a cystine concentration of greater than 200 to 250 mg per liter. The crystals are hexagonal plates resembling the formula of a benzene ring. The nitroprusside test for cystine is a nonspecific reaction for sulfhydryl groups after reduction of disulfides by sodium cyanide. It can be made semiquantitative for cystine in the absence of other sulfhydryl compounds.

The specific aminoaciduria of cystine, lysine, arginine, and ornithine can be directly demonstrated by paper or ion exchange column chromatography of urine. This pattern is diagnostic of genetic cystinuria. Several clinical disorders of hyperdibasicaminoaciduria have been described in the absence of cystinuria.

TREATMENT As a genetic disease cystinuria cannot be "cured" in the host (except by renal homotransplantation). In order to prevent formation and growth of stones, attempts are made to reduce the concentration of cystine in urine and to increase the solubility of cystine at a given urine concentration. Urinary excretion of cystine can sometimes be reduced by a diet low in methionine, the most important cystine precursor. Of greater practicality, cystine concentration can be reduced by increasing urine volume by forcing fluids, especially at night. Some increase in cystine solubility is obtained by alkalinizing the urine, but the solubility curve rises steeply only at pHs higher than 7.2.

A more direct approach is that of forming mixed disulfides of cysteine with other sulfhydryl compounds with enhancement of solubility. The use of D-penicillamine (1 to 2 g daily) leads to the excretion of a soluble cysteine-penicillamine disulfide (solubility fifty times greater than cystine) with reduction of cystine excretion below saturation concentrations. Pyridoxine supplementation (50 to 100 mg) should be given to prevent secondary deficiency of the vitamin, which forms a complex with penicillamine. Unfortunately, D-penicillamine is frequently toxic (causing fever, rash, arthralgias, nephrotic syndrome, pancytopenia), so that its use should be reserved for those patients who cannot be treated successfully by other means. Newer compounds, such as *N*-acetyl-D-penicillamine, are being developed in the search for a less toxic agent capable of forming a relatively soluble disulfide with cysteine in vivo.

HARTNUP DISEASE

Hartnup disease (also called H disease) is a genetic disorder of the transport of a group of monoaminomonocarboxylic acids which share a common transport mechanism in the renal tubule and in the intestinal mucosa. The disease, which may occur in 1 per 16,000 live births, seems to be the homozygous manifestation of an autosomal recessive trait; the heterozygous state is not detectable by current techniques. Hartnup disease is characterized by massive aminoaciduria of alanine, serine, threonine, asparagine, glutamine, valine, leucine, isoleucine, phenylalanine, tyrosine, tryptophan, histidine, and citrulline. In contrast to what occurs in cystinuria, the associated intestinal defect is more important in producing the symptoms of the disease—intermittent pellagra-like rash appearing after exposure to sunlight, attacks of cerebellar ataxia often accompanying the skin manifestations, and psychiatric changes varying from emotional instability to dementia. The disease may often be asymptomatic, especially if there is good nutrition. Impaired absorption allows for bacterial degradation of amino acids which may (1) lead to nicotinamide deficiency from loss of precursor tryptophan, thereby producing pellagra, and (2) allow for the production and absorption of toxic metabolic products injurious to the central nervous system. The specific amino acid metabolites responsible for the signs and symptoms of cerebral and cerebellar dysfunction have not been identified. An isolated defect in tryptophan absorption, the blue diaper syndrome, does not result in a rash or in cerebellar dysfunction. The diagnosis can be established by the pattern of urinary amino acids, measured by paper or ion exchange chromatography. Most patients respond well to maintenance treatment with oral nicotinamide (50 to 200 mg per day). A high-protein diet is also recommended to counter the amino acid loss in the intestine and in the urine.

RENAL GLYCOSURIA

DEFINITION Renal glycosuria is a genetic disorder in which glucose is excreted in the urine at normal concentrations of blood glucose. In order to avoid confusion with other conditions associated with melituria, Marble's strict criteria should be followed (Chap. 96): (1) glycosuria occurs in the absence of hyperglycemia; (2) all specimens of urine should contain glucose with relatively little fluctuation in glycosuria related to diet; (3) the oral glucose tolerance test result is normal (sometimes slightly flat); (4) the reducing substance is specifically identified as glucose, ruling out other meliturias such as pentosuria, fructosuria, galactosuria, sucrosuria, maltosuria, mannoheptulosuria; (5) the storage and utilization of carbohydrates are normal. By these criteria, including the absence of other disorders of proximal renal tubular function, renal glycosuria can be identified as a rare (94 cases in 50,000 cases of melituria at the Joslin Clinic), isolated transport defect. Use of the more liberal criteria proposed by Lawrence, i.e., glycosuria which occurs with a normal glucose tolerance test result, will permit detection of many more abnormalities.

GENETICS AND PATHOGENESIS Current information is most consistent with the transmission of renal glycosuria as a mendelian dominant characteristic, although the suggestion has been made that the defect may be expressed in heterozygotes with homozygotes representing severer forms of the disease. Diabetes mellitus is frequently found in the families of patients with renal glycosuria. Whether renal glycosuria defined by the strict Marble criteria is a precursor of diabetes is disputed. Many patients with renal glycosuria by the Lawrence criteria will develop clinical diabetes mellitus within a few years of diagnosis.

No consistent structural alteration has been demonstrated in the renal tubule by light or electron microscopy. Most studies of the renal defect have been carried out by classic clearance techniques. Plasma glucose is completely filtrable in the glomerulus and is reabsorbed by an active process in the proximal tubule. The biochemical basis of active reabsorption of glucose has not been demonstrated; specifically, no intermediary product has been found. Reabsorption exhibits saturation kinetics with a transfer maximum (Tm) of about 325 ± 36 mg per min per 1.73 m^2 in the normal adult. Clearance studies in renal glycosuria have failed to yield a consistent pattern. In some patients a low Tm for glucose has been found; in others the Tm has been normal but there has been an increased splay in the curve describing the relationship of glucose reabsorbed to that filtered. Renal glycosuria could result from any one of the following defects: decrease in the anatomic mass of the proximal tubule in relation to its glomerulus (glomerulotubular imbalance), abnormal distribution of the transport system relative to glomerular filtration whether on a functional or anatomic basis, an abnormality in the presumed enzymatic step or steps (permeability, hypothetical membrane carrier, energy-yielding reactions) which constitute the active transport process. It is likely that there may be different genetic and pathogenetic forms of the disease.

DIAGNOSIS AND CLINICAL IMPLICATIONS The criteria for diagnosis have been included in the definition. It is important to identify the reducing substance as glucose (by glucose oxidase, for example) and also to rule out other primary or secondary renal tubular defects (e.g., aminoaciduria, phosphaturia, renal tubular acidosis). Most patients with renal glycosuria have no defect in intestinal transport of sugars. The related disorder of glucose and galactose malabsorption is characterized by impaired intestinal absorption of these monosaccharides and by renal glycosuria. In one Swiss family, renal glycosuria was coupled with hyperglycinuria (glucoglycinuria), transmitted as an autosomal dominant trait. The prognosis of renal glycosuria appears to be excellent except insofar as it may herald subsequent clinical diabetes. No treatment is required.

RENAL TUBULAR ACIDOSIS

DEFINITION Renal tubular acidosis (RTA) is a clinical disorder or group of disorders characterized by inability of the kidney to excrete an appropriately acid urine. This results in a persistent metabolic acidosis with hyperchloremia, and may be complicated by potassium depletion, hypercalciuria, or both. RTA may occur as an isolated tubular defect (sporadic or familial) or in association with dysproteinemic states, hyperthyroidism, vitamin D intoxication, and amphotericin B toxicity. In addition to this "classic" or "distal RTA," impaired acidification can also be caused by "proximal RTA" due to bicarbonate wasting. The syndrome of RTA may be closely simulated by the chronic administration of potent carbonic anhydrase inhibitors. Its extracellular fluid pattern of hyperchloremic acidosis may be found following bilateral ureterosigmoid transplantations, during the ingestion of large amounts of ammonium chloride, or in some patients with chronic pyelonephritis.

GENETICS AND PATHOGENESIS Although often secondary to other metabolic disorders, RTA may occur with otherwise normal or nearly normal renal function and in the absence of associated diseases. Some of these cases have appeared to be sporadic; others have exhibited definite familial aggregation. The pattern of inheritance, including transmission in three successive generations, is consistent with a mendelian dominant trait. It seems unlikely that the transient infantile form of RTA, with a negative family history, represents the same disorder.

A complete discussion of the pathogenesis of RTA would demand a full treatment of the role of the kidney in the defense of acid-base balance. In brief, the kidney serves this homeostatic function in several closely related ways: by excretion of certain anionic products of metabolism (phosphate, sulfate), by conservation of filtered bicarbonate, by tubular secretion of hydrogen ions in exchange for sodium, and by tubular synthesis and excretion of ammonia. In RTA phosphate and sulfate excretions are not impaired in the absence of secondary renal failure. Normally, filtered bicarbonate is largely reclaimed in the proximal renal tubule by hydrogen ion exchange for sodium. This mechanism (as measured by the Tm for bicarbonate reabsorption) is usually unimpaired in RTA. The excretion of ammonia is often reduced, but only in proportion to the reduced urine acidity and glomular filtration rate (GFR). The most plausible mechanism for RTA is that of inability of the distal renal tubule to develop a steep H^+ gradient between extracellular fluid and tubular urine. This transport defect or "gradient defect" for H^+ in the distal tubule results in reduced urine titratable acidity and ammonia, increased urinary loss of sodium and potassium (due to increased tubular exchange of potassium in lieu of H^+ for sodium), and systemic acidosis. Sustained acidosis results in mobilization of calcium from bone and hypercalciuria. There is also a reduction in urinary citrate which may contribute along with hypercalciuria to the kidney stone diathesis.

A second form of RTA has been described which is due to a defect in proximal tubular reabsorption of bicarbonate. In "proximal RTA," bicarbonate floods the normal distal H^+ secretory mechanism leading to impaired acidification. In contrast to what occurs in classic RTA, the Tm for bicarbonate is reduced. This disorder may occur as an isolated tubular defect or as part of the Fanconi syndrome. It has been described with heavy metal poisoning (cadmium, mercury), Wilson's disease, Lowe's syndrome, hereditary fructose intolerance, galactosemia, hyperparathyroidism, during rejection reactions following renal transplantation, with use of outdated tetracycline, and also in some patients with dysproteinemic states.

DIAGNOSIS AND CLINICAL IMPLICATIONS The diagnosis of RTA depends upon demonstration of impaired acidification of the urine in the face of systemic acidosis and in the absence of uremia. In mild cases this may require a further acid challenge (0.1 g ammonium chloride per kg body weight). The serum chloride is usually elevated commensurate with the reduction in serum bicarbonate. Other disorders noted above which may lead to secondary impairment of renal tubular acidification must be excluded. The most important complications of RTA are potassium depletion (weakness, paralysis, secondary renal tubular dysfunction) hypercalciuria (nephrocalcinosis, nephrolithiasis, osteomalacia, or rickets), pyelonephritis, and renal failure secondary to these factors. Proximal RTA may be difficult to distinguish from the classic or distal type. A bicarbonate titration curve shows gross impairment of reabsorption in proximal RTA, and other features of the Fanconi syndrome may be present. Urine pH may fall to normal acidic levels when the plasma bicarbonate is sufficiently low so that flooding of the distal acidification mechanism no longer occurs.

TREATMENT In distal RTA acidosis, hypercalciuria, and potassium wasting are usually corrected by the oral administration of 1.0 to 1.5 meq per kg per day of sodium bicarbonate, given in three divided doses. Alkali replacement may be better tolerated as Shohl's solution (140 g citric acid and 98 g hydrated crystals of sodium citrate per liter), given in a dosage of 50 to 100 ml per day in divided doses. The amount of alkali given should be sufficient to return the serum bicarbonate and pH to a normal range. Supplementary potassium and/or calcium and vitamin D may be required temporarily until body stores of these minerals have been repleted. In proximal RTA, larger amounts of sodium bicarbonate or citrate are required to return extracellular fluid bicarbonate toward normal because of continued excessive urinary bicarbonate wastage.

REFERENCES

CRAWHALL JC: Cystinuria—diagnosis and treatment, in *Heritable Disorders of Amino Acid Metabolism,* ed WL Nyhan, New York: Wiley, 1974, p. 17

JEPSON JB: Hartnup disease, in *The Metabolic Basis of Inherited Disease,* 4th ed., eds JB Stanbury et al, New York: McGraw-Hill, in press

KRANE SM: Renal glycosuria, in *The Metabolic Basis of Inherited Disease,* 4th ed., eds JB Stanbury et al, New York: McGraw-Hill, in press

MARBLE A: Non-diabetic melituria, in *The Treatment of Diabetes Mellitus,* eds EP Joslin et al, Philadelphia: Lea & Febiger, 1959

SEBASTIAN A et al: Metabolic acidosis with special reference to renal acidosis, in *The Kidney,* eds BM Brenner, FC Rector, Jr., Philadelphia: Saunders, 1976

SELDIN DW: Renal tubular acidosis, in *The Metabolic Basis of Inherited Disease,* 4th ed., eds JB Stanbury et al, New York: McGraw-Hill, in press

THIER SO, SEGAL S: Cystinuria, in *The Metabolic Basis of Inherited Disease,* 4th ed., eds JB Stanbury et al, New York: McGraw-Hill, in press

106
THE CARCINOID SYNDROME

JOHN A. OATES

The association of carcinoid tumors with cutaneous flushes, telangiectasia, diarrhea, cardiac valvular lesions, and bronchial constriction eluded recognition until 1953. Once this connection was established by Thorson, Biörk, Björkman, and Waldenström, and independently by Isler and Hedinger, it was clear that the syndrome was mediated by release of one or more biologically active agents by the tumor. Serotonin was the first such agent to be discovered, and overproduction of this amine is the most consistent biochemical indicator of the carcinoid syndrome. Serotonin, however, is not the sole mediator of the clinical syndrome. These tumors vary in their synthesis of indoles and may elaborate chemically unrelated agents such as bradykinin, histamine, and adrenocorticotropic hormone (ACTH). Furthermore, evidence suggests that an additional unidentified substance participates in the production of flushing. Within the broad classification of carcinoid tumors there is great diversity in the production of biologically active substances and in the mechanisms for their storage and release. Accordingly, there is a varied spectrum of clinical manifestations.

PATHOLOGIC ANATOMY OF THE TUMOR Carcinoid tumors are slowly growing neoplasms of enterochromaffin cells. The metastatic tumors associated with carcinoid syndrome usually arise from small primary tumors in the ileum. The syndrome is also produced by neoplasms arising from the remainder of the small intestine, from organs derived from the embryonic foregut (e.g., bronchus, stomach, pancreas, and thyroid), and from ovarian or testicular teratomas.

Carcinoid tumors have an unusual proclivity for metastasis to the liver and may involve this organ extensively, with minimal metastatic disease elsewhere. Extrahepatic metastases occur in bone, where they are often osteoblastic, and in lung, pancreas, spleen, ovaries, adrenals, and other organs.

Primary carcinoid tumors of the appendix are common, but they rarely metastasize. Those from the large intestine may metastasize but almost never exhibit endocrine effects.

The usual carcinoid tumor arising from the ileum has the classical histologic pattern of dense nests of cells with uniform size and nuclear appearance. Histochemically, they typically exhibit an argentaffin reaction in which the cells convert a silver salt to metallic silver. A positive argentaffin reaction is not required for the diagnosis, however, and carcinoid tumors arising from organs of the embryonic foregut are usually argyrophyllic, containing few if any argentaffin cells. Tumors from these organs also have a broad histologic spectrum, which in the lung ranges from typical bronchial carcinoid to a form indistinguishable from oat-cell carcinoma.

Neoplasms of foregut origin with histologic features resembling carcinoids may produce excessive amounts of polypeptide hormones such as gastrin, insulin, calcitonin, glucagon, corticotropin, and vasoactive intestinal polypeptide without exhibiting the usual features of carcinoid syndrome. These carcinoid tumors probably share a common embryologic origin with those producing carcinoid syndrome, arising from the neuroectodermal cells of the neural crest.

CLINICAL FEATURES Unlike most metastatic neoplasms, carcinoid tumors have an unusually slow rate of growth; most patients survive for 5 to 10 years after the disease is recognized. For much of the duration of the illness, morbidity may result largely from the endocrine function of the tumor. Death results from cardiac or hepatic failure and from complications associated with tumor growth.

Vasomotor paroxysms The most common clinical feature is cutaneous *flushing.* The typical flush is erythematous and involves the head and neck (blush area). Some patients exhibit vivid color changes from red to violaceous to pallor during its course. Prolonged flushing attacks may be associated with lacrimation and periorbital edema. The systemic effects of the flush are variable. It may be accompanied by tachycardia, and the blood pressure usually falls or does not change. A rise in blood pressure during flushing is rare, and carcinoid syndrome is not a cause of sustained hypertension.

Flushing may be provoked by excitement, exertion, eating, ethanol ingestion, and epinephrine administration.

Telangiectasia In addition to paroxysms of cutaneous vasodilatation, some patients also develop purple telangiectasia, primarily on the face and neck and most marked in the malar area.

Gastrointestinal symptoms Intestinal hypermotility with borborygmi, cramping, and explosive diarrhea may accompany the episodic flushes. Chronic hypermotility with diarrhea is more common. When this is severe, malabsorption may occur.

Cardiac manifestations There is a unique deposition of fibrous tissue on the endocardium of the valvular cusps and cardiac chambers. It occurs primarily in the right side of the heart, but may involve the left side to a minimal degree. The fibrous deposition does not penetrate the internal elastic membrane. Distortion of the valve cusps, chordae tendineae, and papillary muscles interferes with valvular function in the right side of the heart and may lead to regurgitation, stenosis, or combined functional lesions. There is, however, a tendency for the fibrosing process to produce incompetence at the tricuspid valve and stenosis of the smaller pulmonary orifice, a deleterious hemodynamic combination. A high cardiac output, with its attendant imposition on cardiac function, may be found in some patients with carcinoid syndrome; this is due either to a continuing release of a vasodilator or to excessive flow in the metastatic tumors.

Pulmonary symptoms Bronchoconstriction is a less common feature of the syndrome, but it may be severe. It is usually most pronounced during flushing attacks.

General In addition to the endocrine effects, the tumors themselves may cause intestinal obstruction or bleeding. Necrosis of intestinal or hepatic tumor masses may produce abdominal pain, tenderness, fever, and leukocytosis. Hepatomegaly from the metastatic disease is usually present with the syndrome. Extensive metastatic involvement of the liver by these slowly growing tumors may occur before the liver function test results become abnormal.

ENDOCRINE FUNCTION OF THE TUMORS **Serotonin** The most constant biochemical characteristic of carcinoid tumors is the presence of tryptophan hydroxylase, which catalyzes the formation of 5-hydroxytryptophan (5-HTP) from tryptophan (Fig. 106-1). Most tumors also contain the enzyme aromatic L-amino acid decarboxylase, which catalyzes the formation of 5-hydroxytryptamine (serotonin). Carcinoids from the stomach and from other organs derived from the embryonic foregut, however, are frequently deficient in this decarboxylase and release 5-HTP from the tumor.

FIGURE 106-1
Metabolic pathway of serotonin.

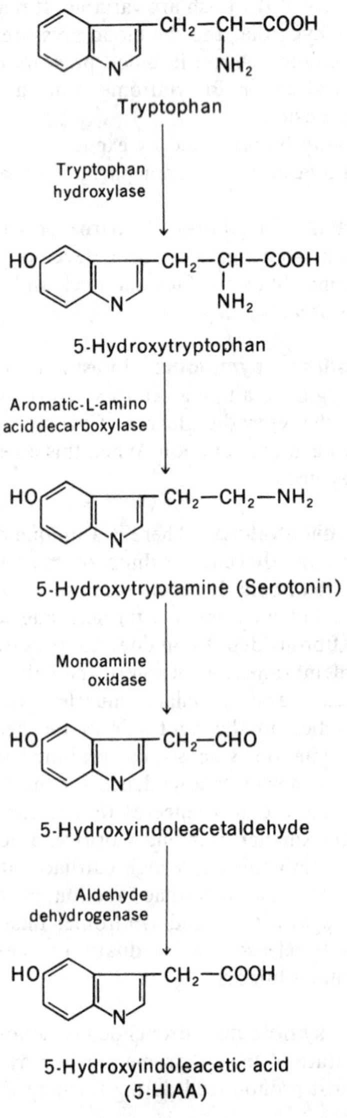

Following its release from the tumor, serotonin is inactivated primarily by the enzyme monoamine oxidase; uptake into platelets also contributes to removal of free serotonin from blood. Monoamine oxidase oxidizes serotonin to 5-hydroxyindoleacetaldehyde, which is rapidly converted to 5-hydroxyindoleacetic acid (5-HIAA) by aldehyde dehydrogenase. This acid is rapidly excreted in the urine, and almost all circulating serotonin can be accounted for as urinary 5-HIAA.

Carcinoid tumors vary widely in their capacity to store serotonin, with concentrations of the amine in tumors ranging from a few micrograms per gram to 3 mg per g. The concentration in the tumor appears unrelated to the rate of synthesis of serotonin as reflected by urinary 5-HIAA. Generally, tumors from the ileum have a much higher storage capacity for serotonin than do tumors from organs of the embryonic foregut.

Bradykinin A potent vasodilator peptide, bradykinin is released during flushes in some cases of carcinoid syndrome. In a few of these, excessive amounts continue to be released between flushes. Bradykinin and related kinins are formed by the action of a group of enzymes (kallikreins) which split these peptides from kininogen, a plasma globulin. It is thought that catecholamines and other stimuli initiate bradykinin formation, either by release of kallikrein from the tumor or by initiation of a sequence that leads to activation of the kallikrein normally present in plasma.

Other biologically active substances Some carcinoid tumors, particularly those of gastric origin, produce and release excessive amounts of histamine. This can be detected by an increased excretion of this amine in the urine.

Carcinoid syndrome has been associated with hyperadrenocorticism in a number of instances. This results from ectopic production of an adrenocorticotropic hormone by the tumors, which usually originate from sites other than the ileum (bronchus, pancreas, ovary, and stomach).

In a few cases, "multiple endocrine adenomas" have been seen in conjunction with carcinoids arising from organs of the embryonic foregut. The associated tumors have included parathyroid adenomas and pancreatic tumors, producing Zollinger-Ellison syndrome.

PATHOPHYSIOLOGY Serotonin contributes to those aspects of the syndrome related to intestinal hypermotility, and there is evidence that the fibrous deposits on the endocardium also result from increased levels of circulating serotonin.

A secondary effect of serotonin overproduction occurs when a large fraction of dietary tryptophan is shunted into the hydroxylation pathway (Fig. 106-2), leaving less tryptophan available for the formation of nicotinic acid and protein. When urinary excretion of 5-HIAA exceeds 200 to 300 mg daily, low levels of plasma tryptophan and evidence of nicotinamide deficiency are seen.

Mechanism of the flush The mechanism of the flush is unclear. Release of the flush-provoking substance(s) can be triggered by the catecholamines, and this probably accounts for the association of flushing with excitement and emotional stimuli. For experimental induction of flushing, injection of isoproterenol in amounts as little as 0.5 μg may be effective. Serotonin was originally thought to be the mediator of flushes, but injection of this amine does not produce a mimicking of the carcinoid flush, and patients may exhibit flushes without increased levels of plasma serotonin. Bradykinin is a potent vasodilator, and its injection will stimulate one type of carcinoid flush which is characterized by erythema in association with tachycardia and hypotension. Release of this peptide, however, could not be detected in a number of patients during flushing. While bradykinin, serotonin, and histamine may contribute to the varied types of flushes observed in the carcinoid syndrome, there appears to be an additional flush substance which has not yet been identified.

DIAGNOSIS With its full constellation of clinical features, carcinoid syndrome is easily recognized. The diagnosis also must be considered when any one of its features is present.

The diagnostic hallmark of carcinoid syndrome is *overproduction of 5-hydroxyindoles* with *increased urinary excretion of 5-hydroxyindoleacetic acid.* Normally, excretion of 5-HIAA does not exceed 9 mg daily. Ingestion of foods containing serotonin may complicate the biochemical diagnosis of carcinoid syndrome; both walnuts and bananas contain enough serotonin to produce abnormally elevated urinary excretion of 5-HIAA after their ingestion. Some drugs also interfere with the analysis of urinary 5-HIAA; cough syrups containing guaiacolate cause falsely elevated values, and phenothiazines interfere with the colorimetric test. When dietary 5-hydroxyindoles are excluded, a urinary excretion of more than 25 mg of 5-HIAA daily is diagnostic of carcinoid. Elevations in the range of 9 to 25 mg may be seen with carcinoid syndrome, nontropical sprue, or acute intestinal obstruction.

Measurement of *serotonin in blood* or platelets is of interest but has less diagnostic value than assay of the major metabolite of serotonin in the urine.

Measurement of an increased concentration of *serotonin in tumor tissue* is a useful and sometimes necessary supplement to histologic examination. A portion of suspected tumor should always be frozen for serotonin analysis (see Table 106-1).

VARIANTS OF THE SYNDROME: RELATION TO SITE OF TUMOR ORIGIN The origin of the tumor influences the biologically active substances produced and their storage and release. Carcinoid tumors arising from organs derived from the embryonic foregut (bronchus, stomach, and pancreas) tend to differ from those arising distal to the mid-duodenum (midgut). The typical carcinoid syndrome usually results from tumors of midgut origin, which almost invariably secrete serotonin with little or no 5-HTP. Tumor serotonin content is likely to be high, and the tumor usually contains dense nests of argentaffin-positive cells. Metastasis to bone and skin is infrequent.

In contrast, tumors arising from the embryonic foregut contain fewer argentaffin cells, have lower serotonin content, and may secrete 5-HTP. Hyperadrenocorticism and multiple endocrine adenomas are more likely to be associated with this group, and metastasis to bone and skin is more frequent.

In addition to the general characteristics of the foregut group, certain clinical and biochemical features have been associated with gastric and bronchial carcinoids. Patients with gastric carcinoids frequently exhibit unique flushing which begins as a bright-red patchy erythema with sharply delineated serpentine borders; these patches tend to coalesce as the blush heightens. Food ingestion is especially likely to produce flushes. The tumors usually are deficient in decarboxylase enzyme and secrete 5-HTP; histamine secretion is also common, as is a high incidence of peptic ulceration. Diarrhea and heart lesions are not prominent features in the patients who secrete largely 5-HTP from the tumor without much preformed serotonin.

When the carcinoid tumor arises from the bronchus, attacks of flushing tend to be prolonged and severe and may

FIGURE 106-2
Metabolic pathways of tryptophan.

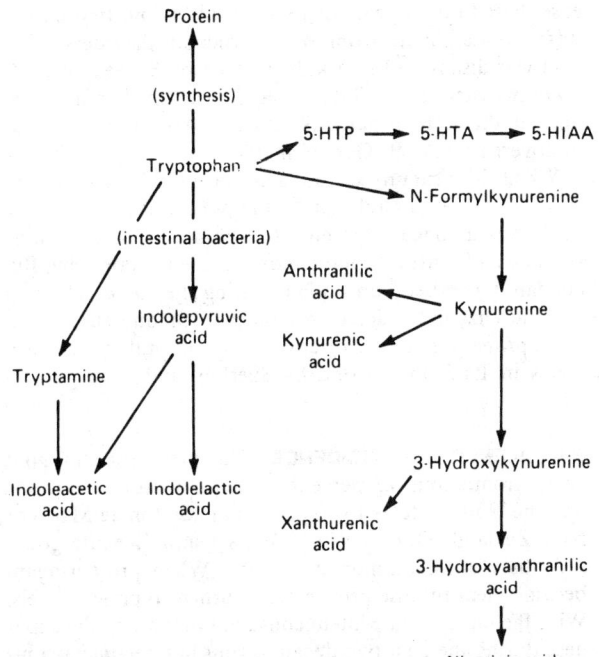

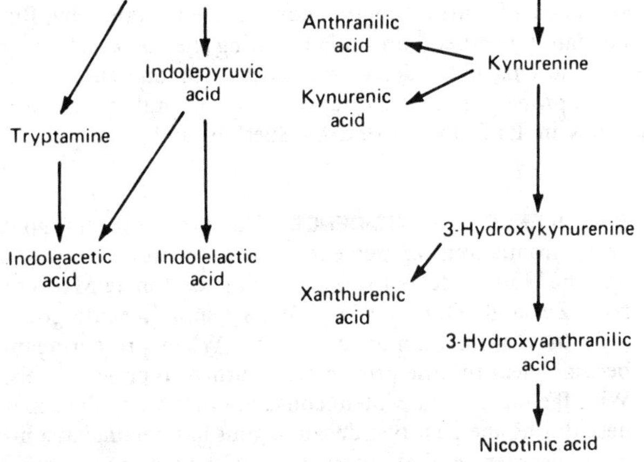

TABLE 106-1
Outline of diagnostic approach to a patient with suspected carcinoid syndrome

I Quantitative determination of 24-h urinary excretion of 5-HIAA (5-hydroxyindoleacetic acid).
II When elevated 5-HIAA confirms clinical evidence for carcinoid syndrome, curable ovarian, testicular, or bronchial primary tumors should be sought.
III Consideration of possible treatment of the syndrome by surgical resection of hepatic metastases or hepatic arterial perfusion of chemotherapeutic agents requires:
- *A* Assessment of the location and character of hepatic metastases with arteriography and scintillation scanning of the liver.
- *B* Evaluation of hepatic and cardiac function.
- *C* A search for extrahepatic metastases in bone and other sites.

IV In patients with substantial diarrhea, possible malabsorption of nutrients should be investigated.

be associated with periorbital edema, excessive lacrimation and salivation, hypotension, tachycardia, anxiety, and tremulousness. Nausea, vomiting, explosive diarrhea, and bronchoconstriction may progress to a severe degree. This group is therapeutically unique in that the severe flushes often can be prevented by corticosteroids, and chlorpromazine may be helpful in relieving the symptoms.

TREATMENT Recognition of the carcinoid syndrome has led to complete surgical cure of a few patients with tumors arising in ovarian or testicular teratomas or in the bronchus; by releasing their secretions directly into the systemic circulation, tumors from these locations can produce the syndrome before metastatic disease occurs. As the humoral substances released by tumors draining into the portal circulation are largely metabolized by the liver, tumors arising in this location produce the syndrome only after hepatic metastasis. Because of the relatively slow growth of carcinoid tumors, palliative resection of hepatic metastases is beneficial in carefully selected cases. Resection of large isolated hepatic metastases has led to relief of the symptoms of carcinoid syndrome and marked reductions in urinary 5-HIAA excretion for periods of several years. In some cases with multiple metastases, removal of as much as a hepatic lobe may be considered when the metastases are located primarily in the portion of the liver to be resected, as determined by arteriography, scintillation scanning of gamma-emitting colloidal particles taken up by the liver, and inspection of the hepatic surface at surgical exploration.

Chemotherapy of carcinoid tumors has not yielded the extent or duration of palliation achieved with selective removal of hepatic metastases. Hepatic arterial perfusion with agents such as 5-fluorouracil has been the most successful of the chemotherapeutic approaches.

Pharmacologic therapy directed at the humoral mediators of the syndrome is useful in some cases. Methysergide, a serotonin antagonist, will improve the diarrhea, but prolonged therapy with this agent can produce retroperitoneal fibrosis. Blockade of serotonin synthesis with the tryptophan hydroxylase inhibitor *p*-chlorophenylalanine also ameliorates the diarrhea. The prevention of severe flushing by corticosteroids and amelioration of the syndrome by phenothiazines are limited largely to patients with tumors arising from the bronchus and other organs derived from the embryonic foregut.

Nicotinamide should be given to those patients who shunt a large fraction of dietary tryptophan into the hydroxyindole pathway.

Hypotensive episodes should not be treated with catecholamines; by stimulating the release of vasoactive substances from the tumor, norepinephrine, epinephrine, and other agents with adrenergic activity can exaggerate and prolong the circulatory disturbance. If hypotension requires therapy, volume expansion or methoxamine infusion is the preferred approach.

REFERENCES

OATES JA, BUTLER TC: Pharmacologic and endocrine aspects of carcinoid syndrome. Adv Pharmacol 5:109, 1967

ROBERTSON JIS et al: The mechanism of facial flushing in the carcinoid syndrome. Q J Med 31:103, 1962

SJOERDSMA A et al: A clinical, physiologic and biochemical study of patients with malignant carcinoid. Am J Med 20:520, 1956

VAN SICKLE DG: Carcinoid tumors; analysis of 61 cases, including 11 cases of carcinoid syndrome. Cleve Clin Q 39:79, 1972

107
GOUT AND OTHER DISORDERS OF URIC ACID METABOLISM

JAMES B. WYNGAARDEN

Primary gout represents a group of inborn metabolic disorders leading to hyperuricemia, recurrent attacks of a characteristic acute arthritis, and tophaceous deposits of sodium urate. Nephrolithiasis and parenchymatous renal disease commonly develop during the course of the illness. Secondary gout is an acquired form of the disease which supervenes in the course of a number of disorders in which hyperuricemia occurs.

A classification of gout is presented in Table 107-1.

HISTORY In the fifth century B.C., gout was described as podagra, cheiagra, or gonagra by Hippocrates, depending on whether the big toe, wrist, or knee was involved. Tophi were first described by Galen. The term *gout* is derived from the Latin *gutta,* a drop, and reflects an early belief that the disease was caused by a poison, falling drop by drop into the joint. A drug used in treating gout, probably identical with colchicine, was described in the Ebers Papyrus (1500 B.C.). The agent was known to Byzantine physicians in the fifth century A.D., and was brought to this country from Europe by Benjamin Franklin, who himself suffered from gout. Many men of royalty and genius have been afflicted with this disease.

The modern clinical history of gout began in 1683 with Thomas Sydenham, whose superb description of the disease, based on 34 years of personal affliction, first clearly differentiated gout from other articular disorders. Uric acid was discovered in a kidney stone by Scheele in 1776. Twenty years later Wollaston and Pearson demonstrated urate in the tophi of patients with gout. Hyperuricemia was discovered by A. B. Garrod in 1848.

When the structure of uric acid was established by Emil Fischer in 1898, its relation to the purine bases of nucleic acids was at once apparent. The pathways of enzymatic synthesis of purine compounds were elucidated by Buchanan, Greenberg, and others during the 1950s. The first specific enzymatic defect responsible for one subtype of adult primary gout was discovered by Seegmiller and associates in 1966, the second by Sperling and colleagues in 1971.

PREVALENCE AND INCIDENCE The prevalence of gout varies from about 0.3 percent in the population of Europe and the United States to 10 percent in adult male Maori of New Zealand. During World Wars I and II acute gouty arthritis was uncommon in Europe. When protein again became plentiful, the prevalence returned to prewar levels. With the increase in protein consumption among the Japanese during the past two decades, gout has become a common disorder in that population. Although traditionally considered a disease of middle and upper social classes, gout involves all nationalities and income groups.

Primarily gout is a disease of the adult male. In large series, only 3 to 7 percent of cases are found in women, and these are chiefly in the postmenopausal group. Gout is very rare in prepuberal children and, when it occurs, may represent a specific form of gout associated with choreoathetosis, self-mutilation, and mental deficiency (Lesch-Nyhan syndrome), or with glycogen storage disease, type I (von Gierke's disease, Chap. 111).

Secondary gout generally constitutes 5 to 10 percent of cases of gout, and, especially in those instances complicating myeloproliferative disorders or hypertensive cardiovascular disease may involve women in as many as 25 percent of cases. In special circumstances secondary gout may be more common. In a 14-year period, one-half of new cases of gout in Framingham, Massachusetts, occurred in subjects taking thiazide diuretics. In regions of the United States where bootleg whiskey is consumed, lead nephropathy is an important antecedent of gout. In one Southern Veterans' Administration hospital 37 of 43 male patients admitted with gout in 1 year showed evidence of lead intoxication.

INHERITANCE The familial incidence of gout is generally reported as 6 to 18 percent in the United States, but may be much higher, as reflected in figures ranging up to 75 percent in English series. The incidence of hyperuricemia

TABLE 107-1
Classification of gout

Type	*Metabolic disturbance*	*Specific defect*	*Inheritance*
PRIMARY GOUT			
Adult primary gout			
Normal excreter of uric acid (75–80% of primary gout)	Overproduction of uric acid and/or underexcretion of uric acid (often both in same subject)	Undefined	Polygenic ?Autosomal dominant forms
Overexcreter of uric acid (20–25% of primary gout)	Overproduction of uric acid	Undefined	Unknown
Gout associated with specific protein defects:			
Associated with glycogen storage disease, type I (von Gierke's disease) (juvenile gout)	Overproduction of uric acid, plus underexcretion of uric acid; excessive deposition of glycogen and lipids; hypoglycemia	Glucose 6-phosphatase: deficiency or absence	Autosomal recessive
Associated with cerebral palsy, mental deficiency, and self-mutilation (Lesch-Nyhan syndrome) (childhood)	Overproduction of uric acid	Hypoxanthine-guanine phosphoribosyltransferase (HGPRT): deficiency (virtually complete)	X-linked
Associated with onset in early adult life, renal stone, occasionally with neurologic disease (<1% of primary gout)	Overproduction of uric acid	HGPRT: deficiency (partial)	X-linked
Associated with marked uric aciduria, stones in early adult life (rare)	Overproduction of uric acid	PP-ribose-P synthetase mutant: excessive activity	Unknown
Associated with tophaceous gout and minimally elevated plasma urate levels (rare)	Reduced binding of urate to plasma protein	α_1-α_2-Globulin: partial deficiency of urate-binding protein	Autosomal recessive
SECONDARY GOUT			
Hematologic disorders			
Myeloproliferative diseases; chronic hemolytic anemia	Excessive production of uric acid	Accelerated turnover of nucleic acids	
Chronic renal diseases			
Glomerulonephritis, pyelonephritis, polycystic kidney disease	Reduced excretion of uric acid	Reduced renal functional mass	
Lead nephropathy	Reduced excretion of uric acid	?Acquired tubular lesion	
Hypertensive cardiovascular disease	Reduced excretion of uric acid	?Role of hyperlacticacidemia in suppression of tubular secretion of urate	
Hyperuricacidemogenic drugs	Reduced excretion of uric acid	?Suppression of tubular secretion of urate by drug or metabolite	
Starvation, especially in treatment of obesity	Reduced excretion of uric acid	Suppression of renal tubular secretion of urate by β-hydroxybutyric acid and other ketone bodies	

among asymptomatic blood relatives of gouty subjects is about 25 percent. The genetic determinants of hyperuricemia are multifactorial. Population studies suggest that some are autosomal dominant and others are sex-linked dominant factors. The metabolic and genetic heterogeneity of gout underscores the need for definition of specific subtypes so that patterns of transmission of each may be determined. In addition, serum urate values are positively correlated with surface area, obesity, and "ponderal index." Environmental factors, such as diet, alcohol, and drugs, operate in conjunction with genetic factors in determining hyperuricemia.

PATHOGENESIS OF HYPERURICEMIA The concentration of uric acid in body fluids is determined by the balance between rates of production and elimination of urate. Uric acid is formed by oxidation of purine bases, which are of both exogenous (dietary) and endogenous (biosynthetic) origins. After several days of reduced purine intake, the body contains about 1,200 mg uric acid and turns over about 700 mg per day. Two-thirds of this amount is excreted in the urine; one-third is excreted in bile, gastric, and intestinal secretions and is destroyed by colonic bacteria. The accumulation of excessive quantities of urate in the gouty subject could theoretically result from increased absorption of dietary purines, endogenous overproduction, diminished renal or gastrointestinal excretion, diminished endogenous destruction of urate, or a combination of these factors. Abnormalities of absorption or of intestinal uricolysis have been excluded, and endogenous uricolysis is not a significant process in human tissues because they lack uricase. In contrast, *abnormalities of endogenous purine production* and of *uric acid excretion* are important in the pathogenesis of hyperuricemia of both primary and secondary gout.

The normal range of uric acid excretion in American males is 250 to 600 mg per day on a restricted purine diet. About 20 or 25 percent of gouty subjects consistently excrete excessive amounts of uric acid. Tracer studies of the rate of turnover of the urate pool or of incorporation of labeled precursors, such as glycine, into urinary uric acid, indicate that these subjects synthesize abnormal amounts of purines. Such studies also disclose excessive purine production in about two-thirds of gouty subjects who excrete normal amounts of uric acid in the urine. A significant minority remains in whom present methods of study do not disclose excessive purine synthesis.

FIGURE 107-1
Metabolic donors of atoms of the purine ring.

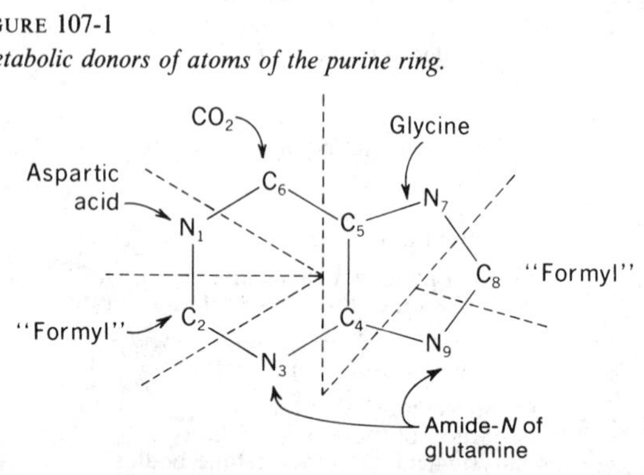

The structure of the purine ring and the metabolic precursors of individual atoms are shown in Fig. 107-1, and the major intermediates of nucleotide synthesis and uric acid production in Fig. 107-2. The key reaction is as follows:

L-Glutamine + α-phosphoribosylpyrophosphate + H_2O → β-phosphoribosylamine + L-glutamic acid + PP

This reaction is the site of a feedback regulatory process operated by the nucleotide products of the pathway. The amidophosphoribosyltransferase catalyzing this first reaction has special inhibitor sites that are sensitive to adenylic and guanylic acids. Accelerated purine biosynthesis must involve an accelerated rate of this and subsequent reactions. The rate of purine biosynthesis will depend upon (1) the availability of the key substrates, glutamine and phosphoribosylpyrophosphate (PP-ribose-P), (2) the activity of amidophosphoribosyltransferase and the integrity of its regulatory mechanisms, and (3) the concentrations of regulatory nucleotides at the feedback control sites on the enzyme.

It is likely that examples of defects of each of these three classes of controls will be found in patients presently classified as having primary gout, and thus allow more precise definitions of metabolic defects and subtypes of gout. In a few patients an understanding of the molecular defect leading to excessive purine biosynthesis has already been achieved.

Hypoxanthine-guanine phosphoribosyltransferase deficiency In 1 or 2 percent of adult gouty subjects with overproduction of uric acid, the responsible metabolic defect is a remarkable deficiency of activity of the enzyme which catalyzes the reconversion of hypoxanthine and guanine to their respective ribonucleotide form by condensation with phosphoribosylpyrophosphate.

Hypoxanthine + PP-ribose-P → inosinic acid + PP
Guanine + PP-ribose-P → guanylic acid + PP

Hypoxanthine-guanine phosphoribosyltransferase is the same enzyme in which activity is even more severely reduced in children with the Lesch-Nyhan syndrome. A number of different types of abnormality of the enzyme have been demonstrated in different families with juvenile or adult forms of the deficiency.

Phosphoribosylpyrophosphate synthetase variants Mutant forms of PP-ribose-P synthetase have been identified in several gouty families. The enzyme is normally activated by inorganic phosphate and inhibited by nucleotides. The mutant enzymes, of which three different types have been described, all exhibit markedly increased activity, resulting in increased intracellular concentrations of PP-ribose-P, accelerated purine biosynthesis, exceptionally high daily excretion values of urinary uric acid, and recurrent renal lithiasis as well as articular gout.

Other defects Two other enzymatic abnormalities have been described in gout which may result in increased synthesis of PP-ribose-P and of purines. These are *glucose 6-phosphatase deficiency* [von Gierke's (type I) glycogen storage disease] and *glutathione reductase variants* (with increased activity), both of which are thought to result in increased synthesis of ribose phosphate esters. A defect of glutamine metabolism has been proposed as the driving force of excessive purine biosynthesis in primary gout. Plasma glutamate concentrations may be above normal; a decreased activity of glutamic acid dehydrogenase has been suggested as diverting glutamate toward glutamine and purine production. In addition, increased hepatic activity of *xanthine oxidase* has been reported in gouty overproducers of uric acid; this may represent secondary enzyme induction rather than a primary lesion. A partial deficiency of a *urate-binding* α_1-α_2-*globulin* has been described in a few gouty families without other known defects of purine metabolism. It is suggested that such a deficiency would favor tissue deposition of urate at lower than usual plasma values.

Renal handling of urate Excretion of urate is dependent on glomerular filtration, tubular reabsorption, and tubular secretion. A small percentage (5 to 8 percent) of plasma urate may be bound to nondiffusible elements, but the bulk of plasma urate is thought to be freely filtrable. Most (98 percent) is reabsorbed, and the largest part of *excreted* urate (80 to 85 percent) derives from tubular secretion.

As pointed out above, evidence for overproduction of uric acid is equivocal or lacking in a substantial percentage of "normal-excreter" gouty subjects. These are subjects whose urate excretion data often suggest most strongly the existence of a specific tubular defect in handling of urate. Figure 107-3 illustrates the tendency of gouty subjects to require a plasma urate value of 2 or 3 mg per 100 ml greater than the nongouty subject in order to achieve a given rate of urate excretion. This tendency is least evident, if at all, in the patient who overexcretes flamboyantly, and is most prominent in the gouty subject with normal turnover of the urate pool or normal values of incorporation of purine precursors into uric acid.

The pathophysiologic basis of this putative tubular defect is unknown. Among the possibilities are changes in renal tubular blood flow, changes in rate of transfer of urate into renal cells, or abnormalities of the secretory transport system itself. The latter mechanism presumably requires both a specific carrier and an energy-generating system. A number of chemical substances are known to

FIGURE 107-2
Purine biosynthesis and catabolism. The first reaction of the pathway is under inhibitory control of adenosine and guanosine 5′-phosphates. Key enzymes are indicated in parentheses.

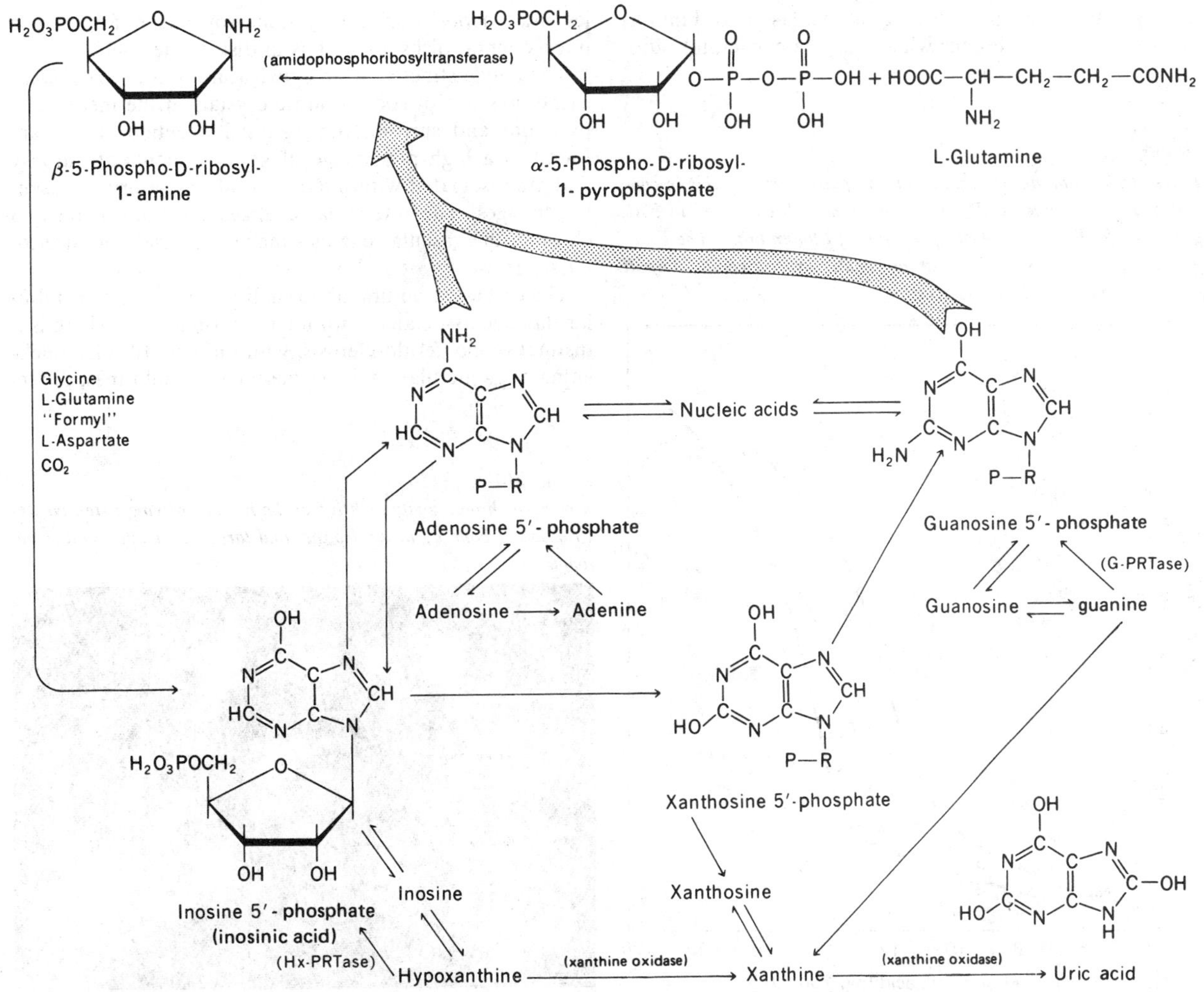

inhibit urate excretion, presumably by blocking tubular secretion of urate. Some gouty patients with normal uric acid excretion and apparently reduced tubular secretion of urate may have gout secondary to unrecognized tubular damage, e.g., lead poisoning, rather than primary gout.

HYPERURICEMIA A satisfactory definition of hyperuricemia is difficult to offer, as serum urate values form a continuous distribution from low to high. Statistical definitions depend on the populations examined and methods employed. In the United States the central 95 percent segments of the distributions are approximately 2.2 to 7.5 mg per 100 ml in males and 2.1 to 6.6 mg per 100 ml in females, by automated colorimetric methods. Such methods overestimate true serum urate values, as determined by uricase methods, by about 1 mg per 100 ml. The physicochemical solubility of uric acid in solutions having the sodium composition of body fluids is about 6.4 mg per 100 ml at pH 7.4. Protein binding of urate may account for an additional 0.4 mg per 100 ml of plasma at 37°C. Only a rare gouty subject will have serum urate values of less than 7 mg per 100 ml when reliable methods, such as the uricase differential spectrophotometric method, are employed.

HYPOURICEMIA Plasma urate values of < 2 mg per 100 ml, unrelated to drug action, are rare. They may be due to a congenital deficiency of xanthine oxidase (xanthinuria) or to renal tubular lesions which may be congenital (idiopathic reabsorptive defect), or acquired (Wilson's disease, Fanconi's syndrome, liver disease with jaundice, Hodgkin's disease, carcinoma).

FIGURE 107-3
Rates of excretion of uric acid at various plasma urate levels in control and gouty subjects. The urate levels have been raised in both groups by feeding of RNA or by infusion of lithium urate. The gouty group (open symbols) includes asymptomatic hyperuricemic, normal excreter, and overexcreter subjects.

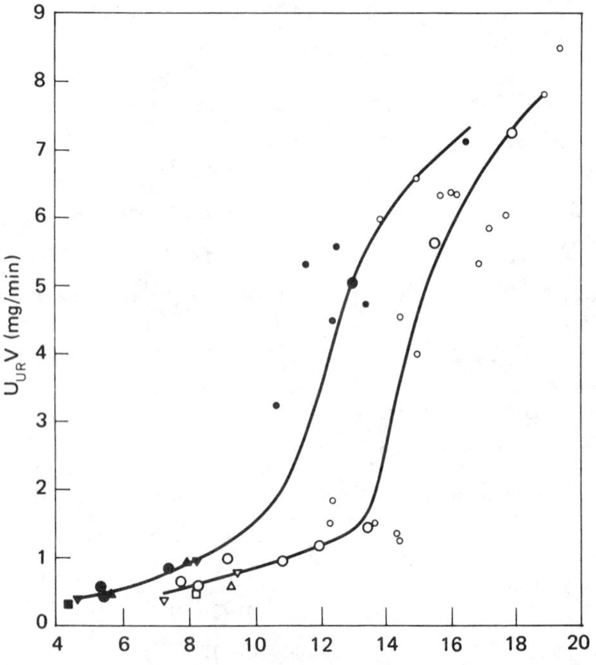

PATHOLOGY The pathognomonic lesion of gout is the *tophus,* a urate deposit surrounded by an inflammatory and foreign-body reaction. Because urate crystals are water-soluble, nonaqueous fixatives are necessary to preserve urate deposits in histologic sections. Urate crystals are brilliantly anisotropic when viewed with polarized light under the microscope. In gout, urates tend to deposit in cartilage, epiphyseal bone, periarticular structures, and kidneys.

Tophi commonly occur in the helix or antihelix of the ear, the olecranon and patellar bursas, and tendons. Less commonly, they occur in skin of fingertips, palms, or soles, the tarsal plates of the eyelids, the nasal cartilages, in the cornea or sclerotic coats of the eye, or along nerves, causing carpal-tunnel or tarsal-tunnel syndromes. Rarely they develop in the myocardium, aortic or mitral valves, vocal cords, and arytenoid cartilages.

In the joint, cartilaginous degeneration, synovial proliferation and pannus, destruction of subchondral bone, proliferation of marginal bone, and sometimes fibrous or bony ankylosis develop. The punched-out lesions of bone commonly seen in roentgenograms of gouty patients represent marrow tophus deposits, which may communicate with the urate crust on the articular surface through erosions and defects in articular cartilage (Fig. 107-4). In vertebral bodies, urate deposits are found in marrow spaces adjacent to intervertebral disks, as well as in disk tissue itself.

The only distinctive histologic feature of the *gouty kidney* is the presence of sodium urate crystals in the medulla or pyramids and surrounding giant-cell reaction. These are found in a high percentage of gouty patients at autopsy and are associated with interstitial inflammatory or vascular changes. The interstitial changes are both acute and chronic; the vascular changes include arterial and arteriolar sclerosis.

The earliest structural abnormality in the kidney is tubular damage associated with interstitial reaction. There is a distinctive glomerulosclerosis, with uniform fibrillar thickening of glomerular capillary basement membranes, differ-

FIGURE 107-4
Advanced chronic gouty arthritis of the hands, showing extensive destruction of bone by urate deposits and large asymmetric soft-tissue tophi.

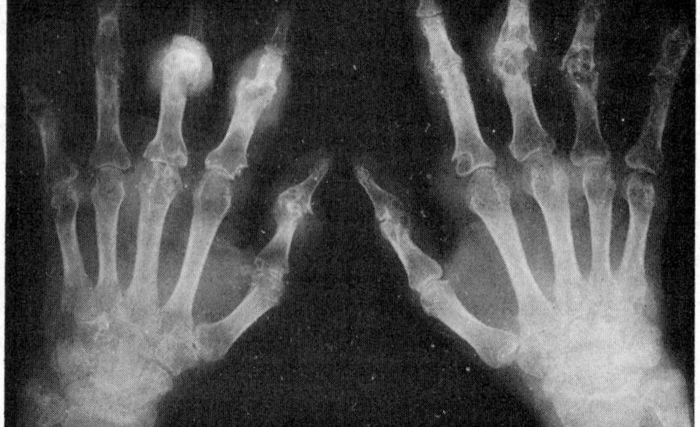

ent from that of nephrosclerosis or diabetic glomerulosclerosis. The Henle's loops show early atrophy and dilatation, occasionally associated with brown-pigment degeneration of epithelium. The interstitial reaction is maximal near the changes in the Henle's loops. In kidneys without tophi this reaction tends to spare the medulla and juxtamedullary cortex. The inflammatory changes do not appear to be of infectious origin. The vessels, both arteries and arterioles, show increased basophilia and degenerative changes which are out of proportion to the parenchymal changes.

CLINICAL MANIFESTATIONS The natural history of primary gout consists of three phases: asymptomatic hyperuricemia, acute gouty arthritis (characteristically recurrent with asymptomatic intervals), and chronic gouty arthritis.

Asymptomatic hyperuricemia In idiopathic gout this phase begins as an accentuation of the normal rise in serum urate value that occurs at puberty in the male and at the menopause in the female. Only a limited number of hyperuricemic subjects develop symptomatic gout, urolithiasis, or renal or vascular injury. The majority live their lives with no detectable ill effects of this biochemical abnormality.

In the population study in Framingham, Massachusetts, the likelihood of developing gout increased with the degree of hyperuricemia, and with age. Nevertheless, at mean age fifty-eight, only 17 percent of subjects with serum urate values between 7 and 7.9 mg per 100 ml had developed gout. In those with values between 8 and 8.9 mg per 100 ml the figure was 23 percent, but in those above 9 mg per 100 the figure had increased to 82 percent. The peak age of onset of acute gout is about forty-five years, although first attacks have occurred in men of eighty years or more.

Acute gouty arthritis When gout becomes clinically manifest, it usually appears abruptly, as fulminating arthritis of a peripheral joint. It is difficult to improve on Sydenham's description of the acute attack:

The victim goes to bed and sleeps in good health. About two o'clock in the morning he is awakened by a severe pain in the great toe; more rarely in the heel, ankle or instep. This pain is like that of a dislocation, and yet the parts feel as if cold water were poured over them. Then follow chills and shivers, and a little fever. The pain, which was at first moderate, becomes more intense. With its intensity the chills and shivers increase. After a time this comes to its height, accommodating itself to the bones and ligaments of the tarsus and metatarsus. Now it is a violent stretching and tearing of the ligaments—now it is a gnawing pain and now a pressure and tightening. So exquisite and lively meanwhile is the feeling of the part affected, that it cannot bear the weight of the bedclothes nor the jar of a person walking in the room. The night is passed in torture, sleeplessness, turning of the part affected, and perpetual change of posture; the tossing about of the body being worse as the fit comes on. Hence the vain effort, by change of posture, both in the body and the limb affected, to obtain an abatement of the pain.

The initial attack usually subsides spontaneously in a few days to a few weeks, and recovery is generally complete. About 50 percent of initial attacks involve the great toe (podagra), and occasionally the initial attack is bilateral. Ninety percent of gouty patients experience podagra during the course of their disease. Next as sites of initial involvement are the instep, ankle, heel, knee, and wrist. Recurring bursitis of shoulder or elbow may be a manifestation of gout, but 83 percent of involved joints are of the lower extremity. The more distal the site of involvement, the more typical is the character of the attack.

There are no characteristic changes of plasma urate levels that precede, accompany, or follow an acute attack of gouty arthritis. In some patients there may be an elevation of urinary uric acid excretion values during the acute attack, perhaps mediated by the uricosuric action of corticosteroids secreted during the stress of gouty inflammation. This sequence could explain the normal serum urate values occasionally observed during acute attacks. Garrod proposed in 1859 that the acute gouty paroxysm was triggered by precipitation of sodium urate crystals in the joint or neighboring tissues. In 1899, Freudweiler reproduced acute gouty attacks by injection of microcrystals of sodium urate, hypoxanthine, or xanthine. These observations have been confirmed by others with both purine and nonpurine microcrystals. A proposed pathogenetic mechanism involves crystallization of sodium urate from supersaturated body fluids, activation of the complement system and of Hageman factor by crystal surfaces, production of vasoactive kinin-like peptides in synovial fluid, induction of an inflammatory response involving leukotaxic factors, leukocytosis, ingestion of microcrystals by leukoctyes, destruction of leukocytes, and release of lysosomal enzymes, with potential destruction of mucoproteins of cartilage (Fig. 107-5).

The events leading to the initial crystallization of monosodium urate, after an average of 30 years of asymptomatic hyperuricemia, are poorly understood. Attacks may be precipitated by stress of many kinds, dietary, physical, and emotional. One patient may indict fatiguing travel, another unusual walking or hiking (e.g., "pheasant hunter's gout"), or celebrations such as holiday dinners or alcoholic sprees. Ethanol intoxication may exacerbate hyperuricemia. Ethanol oxidation is coupled to pyruvate reduction (NAD-NADH-linked enzyme systems), and the lactate produced interferes with uric acid secretion in the renal tubule. Operative procedures are particularly likely to induce acute gout in hyperuricemic individuals, generally on the third to seventh postoperative day.

Interval gout The asymptomatic phase following the acute attack may last from a few weeks to many years. Generally in 6 months to 2 years the patient will suffer another episode in the same or another joint. With time, attacks tend to recur with increasing frequency. Later attacks are often polyarticular, more severe, longer, and accompanied by fever. Roentgenographic changes may develop, and the attacks may abate more gradually than before, but the joints may recover complete function.

Chronic gouty arthritis Before effective control of hyperuricemia became possible, 50 to 60 percent of gouty patients developed visible tophi, permanent joint changes, or chronicity of symptoms. The incidence of tophi now ranges from 13 to 25 percent. Development of tophi is correlated with height of serum urate concentration, severity of renal involvement, and duration of the disease. The time from initial attack to the beginning of chronic symptomatic or visible tophaceous involvement is usually many years, and ranged from 3 to 42 years in one large series, with an average of 11.6 years.

Chronic gouty arthritis is a consequence of the progressive inability to dispose of urate as rapidly as it is produced. The urate pool expands and crystalline deposits of urate appear in cartilage, synovial membranes, tendons, soft tissues, and elsewhere. In 1 or 2 percent of patients, tophi of the helix of the ear may be present at the time of the initial acute attack. Tophaceous deposits may produce irregular, asymmetric, moderately discrete tumescences over joints, requiring larger shoes or gloves. The classic gouty shoe is one with a window cut to accommodate an irregularly prominent joint, usually the first metatarsophalangeal. At later stages, tophaceous enlargements of Achilles tendons, or saccular distentions of olecranon bursas, are common and characteristic.

The process of tophaceous deposition advances insidiously, and although the tophi themselves are relatively painless, there are often progressive stiffness and persistent aching of affected joints. Eventually extensive destruction of joints and large subcutaneous tophi may lead to grotesque deformities, particularly of hands and feet, and to progressive crippling (Fig. 107-4). The tense, shiny, thin skin overlying the tophus may ulcerate and extrude white chalky or pasty material composed of myriads of fine, needlelike crystals.

As chronic gouty changes and renal disease advance, acute attacks occur less frequently and are milder; those that appear may be superimposed upon the indolent soreness of an involved joint, or may seek out new locations of previously uninvolved sites.

No joint is exempt from chronic gouty involvement, although those of the lower extremity and hand are most commonly involved. The hip and spinal joints are rarely affected by tophaceous changes in the absence of extensive disease elsewhere. Radiographic changes of the sacroiliac joint and aseptic necrosis of the hip are sometimes attributable to gout.

Urolithiasis The incidence of renal stones is about a thousandfold higher in gouty subjects than in the general population. Approximately 20 percent of gouty patients with normal urinary uric acid excretion values and 40 percent of those with elevated excretion values develop stones. Of those who pass stones, about 20 percent have had their first episode of urolithiasis before the onset of gouty arthritis. In 84 percent of gouty subjects the stones are pure uric acid (not sodium urate); in 4 percent, uric acid and calcium oxalate; in 12 percent, calcium oxalate or phosphate alone. Pure uric acid stones are radiolucent. Some gouty subjects pass uric acid sludge, gravel, or sand, occasionally almost daily.

Several factors have been implicated in the pathogenesis of stones. In 20 to 25 percent of gouty patients, urinary uric acid excretion values are excessive. Also, as a group, gouty subjects tend to produce acid urines, and do not show normal postprandial alkaline tides. Renal ammonia production is subnormal in response to a given acid load. The deficit in ammonia is compensated by an increase in titratable acidity.

Renal disease in gout Many gouty subjects show evidence of renal disease. Twenty to forty percent show albuminuria, which is rarely heavy in quantity and is often intermittent. Hypertension is present in one-third and is usually benign. Concentrating ability may be impaired. Mild degrees of nitrogen retention are common and often stable or only slowly progressive. Renal dysfunction does not shorten life expectancy in the average gouty subject, even though uremia is reported to be the eventual cause of death in 17 to 25 percent of gouty subjects. The majority of gouty patients die of cardiac or cerebral vascular disease (60 percent) or malignancies, which occur in about the same incidence and at about the same time of life as in nongouty American males.

Obesity and hypertriglyceridemia in gout In population studies serum urate values are correlated with body weight and ponderal index. Patients with primary gout average 18 to 30 percent overweight in various series. Seventy-five percent or more of patients with primary gout have hypertriglyceridemia which is an associate of the obesity. Serum triglyceride values are not elevated in lean gouty subjects. In hyperuricemia and gout secondary to lead poisoning (saturnine gout) plasma triglyceride values are normal. Ethanol consumption may be excessive in both types of patients.

Gout associated with specific enzymatic defects Patients with virtually complete deficiency of hypoxanthine-guanine phosphoribosyltransferase (HGPRT) exhibit features of cerebral palsy, plus self-mutilation, mental deficiency, and marked hyperuricemia and uric aciduria (Lesch-Nyhan syndrome). The onset is within the first year of life. Renal stones and gout may supervene. Death occurs from renal failure, usually by age ten. Patients with partial deficiencies of HGPRT activity usually develop gout within the first two or three decades of life, show very high urinary uric acid values, and commonly develop stones. In about 20 percent of cases there is some neurologic abnormality, ranging from mild spinocerebellar ataxia to typical cerebral palsy.

All reported patients are males, although some abnormalities of purine metabolism may be present in the mothers. Phosphoribosyltransferase (PRT) deficiency obeys the laws of X-linked transmission, with full expression only in hemizygous males. Patients with mutant form of PP-ribose-P synthetase share the features of early onset of renal stones or gout and marked uric aciduria, but have not shown neurologic lesions.

Secondary gout Any acquired hyperuricemic state may be complicated by secondary gout. This disorder occurs in 5 to 9 percent of patients with polycythemia vera, especially those cases merging into the phase of myeloid metaplasia, occasionally in secondary polycythemia complicating congenital heart disease or chronic pulmonary disease, in chronic myelogenous leukemia, multiple myeloma, or chronic hemolytic anemias. In such instances the mean age of onset is later, women are more commonly involved, and both serum and urinary uric acid values tend to be higher than in idiopathic primary gout. Acute gouty arthritis may occasionally antedate evidence of the myeloproliferative disorder by many months, or even by several years.

In all the instances mentioned above, hyperuricemia appears to result from an increased turnover of nucleic acid. Hyperuricemia may also result from reduced renal excretion of urate, either because of chemical interference with tubular secretion of urate or because of reduced renal mass due to parenchymal disease.

Typical gouty attacks may occur in patients receiving such drugs as hydrochlorothiazide or pyrazinamide, which interfere with urate excretion. Extreme obesity may be associated with renal hyperuricemia. Total caloric restriction may result in extreme hyperuricemia, which is correlated with serum levels of β-hydroxybutyric acid and is not infrequently associated with severe attacks of acute gouty arthritis involving especially the knees and ankles.

Chronic renal disease is a frequent cause of hyperuricemia, but apparently few patients with glomerulonephritis, pyelonephritis, or polycystic renal disease live long enough to develop gout. The number may increase with chronic dialysis programs, and acute gouty arthritis has complicated the course of patients so managed. Gout continues to be found in patients who survive lead exposure early in life and go on to develop the slowly progressive nephritis of plumbism.

Hyperuricemia complicates untreated benign essential and renal hypertension in 20 percent of cases and malignant hypertension in 65 percent of cases; it has been attributed provisionally to renal anoxia and local lactic acid excess. Gout occurs in 10 percent or more of patients previously subjected to sympathectomy or adrenalectomy for hypertension. In the absence of family data it may be difficult to distinguish between sporadic primary gout and gout secondary to hypertensive renal disease, or chronic lead intoxication.

DIAGNOSIS Acute gouty arthritis is readily diagnosed by its typical explosive onset, the characteristic severity of involvement of the peripheral joint, the presence of hyperuricemia, and the rapid response to treatment with colchicine. Less typical presentations may be difficult to distinguish from other arthritides on clinical grounds. If present, tophi or typical roentgenologic findings of punched-out, destructive lesions will suggest the correct diagnosis. In patients lacking such lesions, the only pathognomonic finding is the presence, in the leukocytes of synovial fluid, of urate crystals which are needlelike and birefringent under polarized light (Fig. 107-5). Valuable clues in the diagnosis are a history of renal stones or of antecedent mild trauma or surgery in the patient or a history of gout, arthritis, or renal stones in the family (see Table 107-2).

FIGURE 107-5
Crystals of sodium urate monohydrate in leukocytes of synovial fluid in acute gouty arthritis, as viewed under partially polarized light. (Courtesy of Daniel J. McCarty, Jr.)

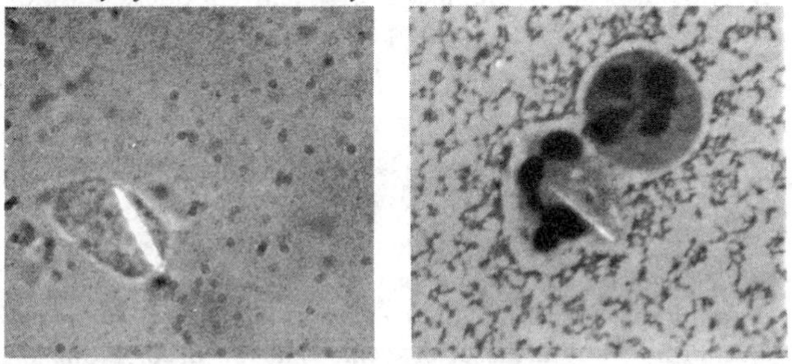

Chronic gouty arthritis may be diagnosed by the presence of urate deposits in or near the affected joints or bursas or of soft-tissue deposits in the helix of the ear, the fingertips, the Achilles tendon, or other locations. The diagnosis may be confirmed by removal of the chalky contents of a tophus, microscopic identification of sodium urate crystals by optical means, or chemical identification by the murexide test or, preferably, by ultraviolet spectrophotometry and degradation by uricase.

DIFFERENTIAL DIAGNOSIS Acute gout must be differentiated from acute rheumatic fever, rheumatoid arthritis, traumatic arthritis, osteoarthritis, pyogenic arthritis, sarcoid arthritis, cellulitis, bursitis, tendonitis, and thrombo-

TABLE 107-2
Outline of work-up of patient with suspected gout

HISTORY

Previous typical acute arthritic attacks or kidney stones, or family history of same or chronic tophaceous gout; history of use of diuretics (especially thiazide) or of unbonded alcohol.

PHYSICAL EXAMINATION

Presence of acute monarticular arthritis, especially of first metatarsal phalangeal joint; or of asymmetric but polyarticular arthritis; or of tophi especially of helix of ear. Vascular status, especially blood pressure. Obesity.

X-RAYS

Of afflicted joints; of hands and feet; intravenous pyelogram for renal function and possibility of stones.

ELECTROCARDIOGRAM

CHEMISTRIES

Serum urate (several), blood urea nitrogen (BUN) or creatinine, plasma cholesterol and triglycerides. Twenty-four-hour urinary uric acid × 2-3, after 3 to 5 days of low-purine diet (of questionable value during acute attack or if patient receiving drugs which affect uric acid levels). Creatinine clearance.

If urinary uric acid values normal or low, and BUN normal or moderately elevated, check for lead intoxication: urinary lead determination after infusion of disodium-dicalcium EDTA (ethylenediaminetetraacetic acid); assay of erythrocyte δ-ALA-dehydratase activity.

If urinary uric acid values increased, check for occult myeloproliferative syndrome or chronic hemolysis; or for specific enzymatic subtype, by assay of erythrocyte enzymes (HGPRT activity: PP-ribose-P synthetase activation as function of inorganic phosphate concentration).

DIAGNOSTIC PROCEDURES

Arthrocentesis, examination of synovial fluid, especially for needlelike intracellular (WBC) crystals which are anisotropic under polarized light. With a first-order red compensator, urate crystals are yellow when oriented in parallel, blue when perpendicular to axis of compensator.

Aspiration or biopsy of tophi, and examination for urate crystals, as above.

Analysis of urinary stone. Uric acid stone (pure or mixed) in a hyperuricemic individual has same metabolic significance as articular gout.

phlebitis. *Reiter's syndrome* in men and *palindromic arthritis* in women may present similar clinical manifestations of episodes of acute arthritis followed by periods of complete remission, but hyperuricemia will not generally be present, joint fluid will not contain urate crystals, and colchicine is ineffective. *Pseudogout,* which is chiefly a disorder of elderly persons and is manifested by acute attacks of arthritis of knees and other joints, is always accompanied by calcification of joint cartilage; the synovial fluid contains nonurate crystals of calcium pyrophosphate or apatite. The patients are not usually hyperuricemic.

Chronic gouty arthritis must be differentiated from all other chronic arthritides which cause deformities of joints, chiefly rheumatoid arthritis, osteoarthritis, traumatic arthritis, and residua of pyogenic arthritis. The history of onset, progression, response to colchicine, and demonstration of hyperuricemia, asymmetric tumescences, typical roentgenographic changes, and tophi or crystals of urate in synovial fluid and leukocytes should establish the diagnosis.

TREATMENT The therapeutic aims in gout are (1) to terminate the acute gouty attack as promptly as possible; (2) to prevent recurrences of acute gouty arthritis; (3) to prevent or reverse complications of the disease resulting from deposition of sodium urate in joints and kidneys; and (4) to prevent formation of uric acid kidney stones. Treatment depends on the stage at which the patient is seen.

Acute attack *Colchicine* is the only therapeutic agent for acute gout of specific diagnostic value. It should be given as soon as the diagnosis is suspected. The initial dose of 0.5 to 1.2 mg colchicine is followed by 0.5 or 0.6 mg every hour for 8 h, then every 2 h until pain is relieved or until nausea, vomiting, cramping, or diarrhea develops. Maximum tolerated doses range from 4 to 10 mg. In most patients dramatic relief of pain and gastrointestinal side effects occur simultaneously. The diarrhea may be treated with paregoric, 4 ml, or Kaopectate, 30 ml, after each loose stool. Colchicine should be discontinued until gastrointestinal symptoms subside. Since the effective dose of colchicine varies, each patient should learn his own tolerance dose and stop just short of this in treatment of subsequent attacks. Colchicine affords relief in 90 percent of patients within 24 to 48 h; a second full therapeutic dose should not be repeated sooner than 72 h.

Colchicine may also be given intravenously. The usual initial dose is 1 to 3 mg in 20 ml saline solution given slowly, and if a single dose is not effective, the injection may be repeated once in 4 to 5 h (maximum intravenous dose, 3 to 5 mg). Gastrointestinal symptoms are uncommon with intravenous administration.

Indomethacin is equally effective in acute gout. It is given orally in initial doses of 50 mg three or four times a day. When pain is relieved, doses are tapered over another 48 to 72 h. Larger doses may cause severe headache, gastric distress, or a transient depersonalization reaction in some patients, but these side effects have been noted only rarely in gouty patients receiving short courses of the drug.

Phenylbutazone is also effective in acute gouty arthritis, and may be preferred when the gouty attack has proceeded for some time, or when the attack does not abate completely with colchicine or indomethacin. The initial dose is 400 mg orally, followed by 100 mg every 4 to 8 h for 2 to 3 days. Oxyphenbutazone, a metabolite of phenylbutazone, is also effective in acute gout. The dose is the same as that of phenylbutazone, and the same precautions should be taken.

Patients who recognize prodromal symptoms may abort acute attacks by prompt institution of colchicine or phenylbutazone therapy; they frequently require only a few tablets to achieve success.

If full doses of colchicine, indomethacin, or phenylbutazone are contraindicated, or ineffective, ACTH gel may be employed. Doses of 40 to 80 USP units are given intramuscularly every 6 to 8 h for 2 to 3 days, rarely longer, following which the doses are reduced in stepwise fashion and discontinued. To avoid rebound attacks of gout after ACTH therapy, 0.6 mg colchicine should be given two or three times daily during and after administration of ACTH for at least 7 days.

Hydrocortisone in a dose of 25 to 50 mg injected intraarticularly into the involved joint is useful in treating acute gout limited to a single joint or bursa, and relief from pain is usually prompt and complete within 24 to 36 h. Steroid hormones are not recommended for parenteral use in acute gout, as the effects are inconsistent and rebound attacks frequent.

During the acute attack, bearing weight on the involved joints should be avoided. In severe attacks the patient will invariably immobilize himself voluntarily, but in milder attacks it is necessary for the physician to insist on this. Mobilization is permitted as soon as the joint is no longer painful.

Interval phase The patient with gout should avoid high purine foods so as to lessen the burden of uric acid excretion. A severe limitation of purine-containing foods is rarely indicated, unless renal function is poor. Gradual weight reduction is indicated if the patient is overweight, and may of itself reduce hyperuricemia and the tendency to develop attacks of gout. Sudden weight reduction may precipitate gouty attacks and should be avoided. In general, diets of moderate protein content, somewhat low in fat, are preferred.

A high fluid intake is advisable to maintain a urinary output of 2,000 ml per day. Uric acid excretion is thus promoted, and the dangers of crystal formation in the kidney or ureter are reduced. Alcoholic beverages, especially beer, ale, and wine, should be avoided if possible, as they may precipitate attacks. Distilled alcoholic beverages, in moderation, generally have little influence on the gouty process.

The daily ingestion of 0.6 to 1.8 mg colchicine is generally effective in reducing the number of acute gouty attacks in patients who are subject to frequent episodes. Maintenance colchicine therapy is particularly important during the first year or two after institution of uricosuric drugs, or of allopurinol.

Chronic gouty arthritis Use of a drug to lower the serum level of uric acid to 6 mg per 100 ml or less is indicated in all gouty patients with visible tophi, with roentgenographic evidence of urate deposits, or with a history of two or more major attacks of acute gouty arthritis. The drug of choice is allopurinol, but uricosuric agents may be used. None of these agents is of any value in the immediate treatment of the acute attack. With both types the number of acute gouty attacks may be increased during the first 6 months unless maintenance colchicine therapy is given, whereas after 12 to 18 months the number may be decidedly reduced. Uricosuric drugs block tubular reabsorption of filtered urate. Those of use in gout are probenecid, sulfinpyrazone, and salicylates.

Probenecid is given in doses of 0.5 to 3 g daily in two or three evenly spaced doses (average dose, 1 to 1.5 g). This drug may produce gastrointestinal upsets, headaches, or skin rash.

Sulfinpyrazone may be given in doses of 100 to 600 mg daily in three or four divided doses (average dose, 300 mg). This drug is related to phenylbutazone and may cause untoward reactions, but is generally somewhat better tolerated than probenecid.

Salicylates block the uricosuric action of both probenecid and sulfinpyrazone and must not be used concurrently. Salicylates are uricosuric when given in high doses (4 to 6 g daily), but few patients can tolerate these quantities.

With all uricosuric agents the doses should be low initially, so as to avoid sudden excretion of large quantities of urate. Fluids should be forced so as to prevent formation of concentrated urine, especially during the late hours of the night. During the first days or weeks of therapy the urine should be kept at pH 6 or above, by administration of sodium bicarbonate or sodium citrate–citric acid (Shohl's solution); this may be difficult to achieve, as gouty patients tend to produce acid urine. In patients who are mobilizing urate, and especially those who form uric acid gravel, alkalinization during the night, when fluid intake is reduced, is important. A single 250-mg tablet of acetazolamide (Diamox) taken at bedtime will serve to keep the urine alkaline and dilute throughout the night.

A second approach toward controlling serum urate levels is that of regulating production of uric acid, rather than (or in addition to) augmenting its excretion. This is achieved by use of *allopurinol*, a potent inhibitor of xanthine oxidase. Allopurinol is converted to oxipurinol in the body, and the latter compound has a longer biologic half-life (28 h), ultimately being largely excreted in the urine. Inhibition of conversion of hypoxanthine and xanthine to uric acid permits these uric acid precursors to be excreted instead. Use of allopurinol results in reduction of levels of uric acid in serum *and in urine*. The drug is effective even in the presence of renal failure, when uricosuric agents generally are not. Its action is not blocked by salicylates. The usual dose is 300 mg, given orally once a day. In the presence of moderate nitrogen retention the dose of allopurinol should be reduced as the biologic half-life of the active metabolite, oxipurinol, is prolonged. Allopurinol is usually well tolerated, but may cause gastric irritation, diarrhea, or skin rash, or induce an attack of gout. Uricosuric agents may be used concurrently to hasten mobilization of urate deposits. Since allopurinol decreases uric acid excretion, it is also very useful in controlling uric acid stone formation, especially in patients who are overproducers of uric acid.

In selected patients *surgical removal* of large extraarticular *urate deposits*, such as those in olecranon bursas, may be advisable. Occasionally amputation of irreparably damaged digits, especially those containing draining sinuses, is indicated. Physical therapy and appropriate self-help devices are valuable in patients who are partially disabled.

Asymptomatic hyperuricemia Asymptomatic hyperuricemia is frequent in family members of patients with gout and in the general population. One must exclude hyperuricemia as a manifestation of reduced renal function or of action of certain drugs. Asymptomatic hyperuricemia generally requires no therapy, as only about one-third of patients will ever develop articular attacks, and adequate therapy can be instituted when these supervene. Exceptions exist in patients with serum levels of uric acid above 9 mg per 100 ml by phosphotungstic acid methods, especially if the urinary excretion levels are low and there is a family history of tophaceous involvement. In such circumstances the asymptomatic subject should be treated with allopurinol before articular or renal complications develop. It is essential that the physician maintain frequent close observation of the patient.

The role of diet It is not necessary to restrict purine intake severely in most gouty patients. However, weight reduction of the overweight patient and abstinence from alcohol may be markedly beneficial. In some patients who have achieved ideal weight and ceased use of alcohol, all clinical manifestations of gout have disappeared, and normal plasma and urinary urate levels, as well as normal values of the miscible urate pool and of glycine incorporation into urate have been reestablished. The analogy with dietary control of hyperglycemia and adult-onset diabetes is obvious, but the physiologic mechanisms of response are equally obscure.

Secondary gout Treatment of gouty arthritis occurring secondary to hematopoietic disturbances is the same as for primary gout except that one must be especially alert to potential complications. The basal uric acid excretion may be high, and use of uricosuric agents may intensify the risk of crystalluria and of tubular or ureteral blockage (uric acid nephropathy). High fluid intake and alkalinization are of great importance. The drug of choice for control of hyperuricemia for these patients is allopurinol.

XANTHINURIA

This is a rare genetic disorder, caused by a marked deficiency or absence of xanthine oxidase activity in liver and small-intestine mucosa. In the lactating female enzyme activity is deficient in breast milk or colostrum as well. Xanthinuria is probably transmitted as an autosomal recessive trait, but the heterozygote cannot be identified by present methods of study. A phenocopy of the genetic disorder is produced by allopurinol. Xanthine oxidase catalyzes the oxidation of hypoxanthine to xanthine, and of xanthine to uric acid. The disorder is characterized by the replacement of urinary uric acid by hypoxanthine and xanthine. When dietary purines are restricted, serum urate values are less than 1 mg per 100 ml, and urinary urate usually less than 30 mg per day. Twenty-five well-documented cases have been reported. In seventeen the patients had no symptoms referable to the metabolic defect, and were diagnosed during study of hypouricemia. Three adult patients had muscle cramps on exercise, and a myopathy associated with crystalline deposits of hypoxanthine and xanthine in muscle. In seven patients urinary xanthine stones developed at ages ranging from two to forty-eight years. Xanthine stones, like urate, are radiolucent. They can be identified by spectrophotometric, chromatographic, or crystallographic methods. Urinary oxypurine (xanthine plus hypoxanthine) excretion values range from 100 to 600 mg per day, of which 70 to 95 percent is xanthine, whose solubility in urine is less than that of uric acid at pH 5, and is increased very little in neutral or mildly alkaline urine. The lack of larger excretion values of hypoxanthine is attributed to its active reutilization by reconversion to inosinic acid. Xanthinuria must be differentiated from other causes of hypouricemia, in almost all of which serum urate values are above 1 mg per 100 ml, and the urine contains considerably more uric acid than in patients with xanthinuria.

Treatment is nonspecific. Maintenance of a high fluid intake and large urine volume is advised. Alkalinization is not indicated, as the high pK_{a1} value of xanthine (7.7) allows only minimal increases in xanthine solubility at pH values that can safely be achieved and maintained. In three patients allopurinol resulted in a reduction in xanthine and increase in hypoxanthine excretion. Its use is logical in patients with low residual activity of xanthine oxidase, particularly if they have formed xanthine stones.

REFERENCES

Gout

KELLEY WN et al: Hypoxanthineguanine phosphoribosyltransferase deficiency in gout. Ann Intern Med 70:155, 1969

——, WYNGAARDEN JB: The drug therapy of gout, in *Seminars in Drug Treatment,* vol. 1, eds JR DiPalma, B Calesnick, New York: Henry M. Stratton, 1971, p. 119

RUNDLES RW et al: Effects of xanthine oxidase inhibitor on clinical manifestations and purine metabolism in gout. Ann Intern Med 60:717, 1964

WYNGAARDEN JB: Gout, in *The Metabolic Basis of Inherited Disease,* 4th ed., eds JB Stanbury et al, New York: McGraw-Hill, in press

——: Metabolic defects of primary hyperuricemia and gout. Am J Med 56:651, 1974

YU TF, GUTMAN AB: Uric acid nephrolithiasis in gout: Predisposing factors. Ann Intern Med 67:1133, 1967

Xanthinuria

SEEGMILLER JE: Hereditary xanthinuria, in *Duncan's Diseases of Metabolism,* 7th ed., ed PK Bondy, Philadelphia: Saunders, 1973, p. 739

WYNGAARDEN JB: Xanthinuria, in *The Metabolic Basis of Inherited Disease,* 4th ed., eds JB Stanbury et al, New York: McGraw-Hill, in press

108 HEMOCHROMATOSIS

GEORGE E. CARTWRIGHT

DEFINITION Hemochromatosis (bronze diabetes) is an iron-storage disease, characterized pathologically by excessive deposition of iron in parenchymal tissues, and clinically by hepatomegaly and eventual liver insufficiency, skin pigmentation, diabetes, arthropathy, cardiac disease, and hypogonadism. The first clinical description of the disease was given by Trousseau in 1865. In 1889 von Recklinghausen named the disease *hemochromatosis* and described the iron-containing pigment, hemosiderin. The articular manifestations of hemochromatosis were first described by Schumacher in 1964.

INCIDENCE Hemochromatosis is a rare disease, recognized in approximately 1 in 20,000 hospital admissions, and 1 in 7,000 hospital deaths. It is observed ten times as frequently in males as in females. Nearly 70 percent of all patients develop their first symptoms between the ages of forty and sixty years. Hemochromatosis is rarely clinically manifested below the age of twenty years.

PATHOGENESIS Hemochromatosis (a *parenchymal* cell iron overload) is observed in the following types of patients: (1) those with idiopathic (primary, familial, hereditary) hemochromatosis; (2) those with a defect in hemoglobin synthesis associated with a high degree of ineffective erythropoiesis (erythropoietic hemochromatosis); (3) those with chronic liver disease (alcoholic hemochromatosis); and (4) those with excessive oral intake of iron over many years (Bantu siderosis, medicinal hemochromatosis, dietary hemochromatosis).

Idiopathic hemochromatosis is the consequence of an abnormality in the regulatory mechanism for iron absorption. The resulting progressive accumulation of iron is reflected in an early increase in the plasma iron and saturation of transferrin with iron. In advanced disease, the tissues contain over 20 g iron; total body iron in normal persons is in the range of 3 to 5 g. The excess iron is deposited primarily in parenchymal tissues, especially those in which there is organ dysfunction. Iron in the liver increases fifty to one hundred times; in the heart ten to fifteen times; in the spleen, kidney, and skin about five times. The mode of inheritance of idiopathic hemochromatosis has been disputed. Earlier investigators favored the dominant mode of transmission. Evidence for an autosomal recessive inheritance with decreased penetrance in the female has been submitted recently. According to this concept homozygotes have large iron stores and manifest the disease. Heterozygotes have normal or slightly elevated iron stores and develop the disease only when added factors such as alcohol, anemia, or increased oral iron intake contribute to an accumulation of iron in excess of their usual stores.

Erythropoietic hemochromatosis is observed in association with chronic disorders of erythropoiesis, particularly in those with a defect in hemoglobin biosynthesis and ineffective erythropoiesis. Also in this group of disorders the absorption of iron is increased. In addition, such patients are frequently treated with medicinal iron and transfusions.

Erythropoietic hemochromatosis has been observed in particular in patients with sideroblastic anemia and thalassemia. Porphyria cutanea tarda, a disorder characterized by a defect in porphyrin biosynthesis, is also associated with excessive parenchymal iron deposits. However, the magnitude of the iron loading is insufficient to produce tissue damage.

Hemochromatosis is observed not infrequently in *alcoholic subjects with chronic liver disease.* The differential diagnosis between alcoholic hemochromatosis and idiopathic hemochromatosis may be difficult. The cause of the excessive parenchymal deposition of iron is poorly understood. There is some evidence that alcohol may enhance the absorption of iron. Ineffective erythropoiesis in association with folate deficiency or an abnormality in pyridoxal phosphate metabolism may be a complicating factor in some patients; alcoholic beverages, particularly wines, may contain appreciable quantities of iron; and finally these individuals may be heterozygous for the hemochromatosis gene.

The *excessive ingestion of iron* over many years may result in hemochromatosis. Under the term *Bantu siderosis,* hemochromatosis has been observed in malnourished Bantu subjects with long-term excessive oral iron intake because of their practice of brewing fermented beverages in vessels made of iron. There are a few isolated reports of the development of hemochromatosis in normal subjects taking medicinal iron over many years.

The common denominator in all patients with hemochromatosis is the presence of excessive iron in parenchymal tissues with resultant tissue damage. Parenteral administration of iron in the form of transfusions or iron preparations results in reticuloendothelial cell iron overload. Only in patients with an abnormality in erythropoiesis does the *parenteral administration of iron* result in deposition of iron in parenchymal tissues.

PATHOLOGY At autopsy the enlarged, nodular liver and pancreas present a striking ochre color. Histologically iron is deposited in many organs but particularly in the liver and pancreas. The epidermis of the skin is thin, and melanin pigment is found in the cells of the basal layer. Hemosiderin is deposited almost entirely in the corium. There are hemosiderin deposits in the myocardium, and they may be associated with myocardial edema, necrosis, and fibrosis. Testicular atrophy is frequently present, both grossly and histologically. Deposits of iron may be observed in the pituitary gland and around the synovial lining cells of the joints. Calcium pyrophosphate crystals may be seen to lie within deposits of calcium embedded in the synovial tissue.

The deposition of iron in the liver of patients with idiopathic hemochromatosis is almost exclusively in the parenchymal cells. In the early stage, iron is deposited predominantly in the lobular periphery and fibrosis is absent. This stage progresses to periportal septum formation with perilobular fibrosis and deposition of iron in septa. Inflammatory cells are few in contrast to prominent proliferation of bile ductules. In the moderately advanced stage, nodules of even size are observed. In the advanced stage, an irregular multilobular cirrhosis of postnecrotic type develops.

CLINICAL MANIFESTATIONS The symptoms and signs of hemochromatosis are related to liver impairment, skin pigmentation, diabetes, cardiac disease, arthropathy, and hypogonadism.

The initial symptoms most frequently encountered are related to the onset of diabetes. Weakness, lassitude, weight loss, change in skin color, abdominal pain, dyspnea, edema, ascites, loss of libido, and peripheral neuritis are also frequent initial symptoms.

Hepatomegaly, pigmentation, spider angiomas, splenomegaly, arthropathy, ascites, cardiac arrhythmias, congestive heart failure, loss of body hair, testicular atrophy, and jaundice are the most prominent physical signs.

The *liver* is usually the first tissue known to be damaged, and hepatomegaly is present in more than 95 percent of symptomatic cases. Hepatic enlargement may exist in the absence of symptoms or in the presence of normal liver function tests. Indeed, over half the patients with symptomatic hemochromatosis have little or no laboratory evidence of functional impairment of the liver, in spite of hepatomegaly and proved fibrosis. Loss of body hair, palmar erythema, testicular atrophy, and gynecomastia are often seen. Manifestations of portal hypertension and esophageal varices may occur but are less commonly observed than in Laennec's cirrhosis. Splenomegaly is present in approximately half the cases. Hepatoma develops in about 35 percent. The incidence of this last complication increases with age and is the most common cause of death in treated patients.

Excessive *skin pigmentation* is present in about 90 percent of the patients at the time the diagnosis is established. Pigmentation may be due to deposition of melanin or iron or both. In general, melanin deposition gives rise to bronzing, iron deposition to a metallic-gray hue. Pigmentation usually is diffuse and generalized, but frequently it is deeper on the face, neck, extensor aspects of the lower forearms, dorsa of the hands, lower legs, genital regions, and in scars. In only 10 to 15 percent of cases is there demonstrable pigmentation of the oral mucosa.

Diabetes and symptoms therefrom develop in about 65 percent of all patients. Diabetes is more likely to develop in patients with a family history of diabetes than in those without such a history. The presence of a family history of diabetes, the existence of liver disease, and direct damage to the pancreas by iron deposition may all contribute to the development of diabetes in hemochromatosis. The management of the diabetes is similar to that of diabetes mellitus except for a higher incidence of insulin resistance and of insulin fat atrophy. Late degenerative sequelae are the same as in diabetes mellitus.

Arthropathy, which differs from osteoarthritis and rheumatoid arthritis, develops in about 50 percent of patients. It most commonly occurs after the age of fifty years but may occur at any time in the course of the disease, even as a first manifestation or long after therapy. The small joints of the hands, especially the second and third metacarpophalangeal joints, are the earliest and usually the first joints to be involved. A progressive polyarthritis involving wrists, hips, and knees may ensue. Acute, brief attacks of synovitis associated with chondrocalcinosis (pseudogout), chiefly in the knees, may occur. Roentgenologic manifestations consist of cystic changes and sclerosis in the subchondral bones, loss of articular cartilage with narrowing of the joint space, diffuse demineralization, and hypertrophic bone proliferation. Chondrocalcinosis is seen frequently, and the presence of calcium pyrophosphate deposits has been documented. The mechanism of these abnormalities and their relationship to iron metabolism is not known.

Cardiac involvement is the presenting manifestation in about 15 percent of patients with hemochromatosis. The most common cardiac manifestation is congestive heart failure. It is observed not infrequently in young adults, and symptoms of congestive failure may develop suddenly, with rapid progression to death if untreated. The heart is diffusely enlarged, and such cases may be misdiagnosed as idiopathic cardiomyopathy if other overt manifestations are absent. A great variety of cardiac arrhythmias may be present, particularly supraventricular beats and paroxysmal tachyarrhythmias. Atrial flutter, atrial fibrillation, and varying degrees of atrioventricular block have also been described.

Loss of libido and *testicular atrophy* are common in hemochromatosis. The former may antedate the other clinical manifestations of the disease. The testicular atrophy is probably due to the loss of gonadotropins associated with a generalized depression of the pituitary gland as a result of the destruction of the gland by the deposition of iron. A depression in plasma-luteinizing hormone has been demonstrated.

DIAGNOSIS The association of (1) hepatomegaly, (2) skin pigmentation, (3) diabetes, (4) heart disease, (5) arthritis, and (6) evidences of hypogonadism should suggest the diagnosis of hemochromatosis. However, a parenchymal iron overload of insufficient duration or modest degree may exist without any of the six clinical manifestations, with only one and any one of the six, with any combination of the six, or with all six clinical manifestations. Therefore, the diagnosis should be considered in siblings of a patient with hemochromatosis and in any patient with unexplained hepatomegaly, idiopathic cardiomyopathy, or loss of libido.

The history should be particularly detailed in regard to disease in other members of the family, alcohol ingestion, and iron intake. The blood should be examined for anemia and evidences of abnormal erythropoiesis to rule out iron loading secondary to a hematologic disease such as thalassemia or sideroblastic anemia. Confirmation of the presence of liver, pancreatic, cardiac, and joint disease should be obtained by physical examination, roentgenologic examination, and routine function tests of these organs. It then remains to demonstrate that there is a parenchymal iron overload.

The simplest and most readily available screening test for the diagnosis of the disease is measurement of plasma iron, plasma iron–binding capacity, and calculation of the percentage of saturation of the iron-binding protein with iron. Early in the course of the disease and long before organ dysfunction can be detected, the plasma iron increases, the plasma iron–binding capacity decreases, and the plasma iron–binding protein saturates with iron (Table 108-1). These changes may also occur in patients with acute hepatic damage, severe hypoplasia of the erythroid marrow, or ineffective erythropoiesis, but from whatever cause they indicate parenchymal iron overload. These changes will be present in all patients with hemochromatosis except in the presence of a complicating severe infection or malignancy such as hepatoma.

In untreated patients with hemochromatosis, the serum ferritin level is greatly increased (Table 108-1) and the serum ferritin concentration correlates with the magnitude of body iron stores. The serum ferritin concentration is also increased, and increased to a degree disproportionate to iron stores, in patients with infection, liver disease, and hemolytic anemia. However, this determination, if available, is helpful in establishing the presence of iron overload.

Excessive hepatic parenchymal iron deposits may be demonstrated by injecting 0.5 g desferrioxamine intramuscularly. Normal subjects excrete less than 2 mg iron in the urine in the subsequent 24 h. When the value exceeds more than 4 mg, the patient has an excessive load of parenchymal iron. Patients with untreated idiopathic hemochromatosis usually excrete more than 10 mg chelate iron in the urine in 24 h (Table 108-1).

The definitive test for the diagnosis of hemochromatosis is the demonstration of parenchymal iron overload by needle biopsy of the liver. The degree of parenchymal iron loading can be estimated by examination of a histologic section stained for iron; the degree of cirrhosis can be estimated in routine histologic sections; and micromethods are available for the chemical measurement of the liver iron concentration (Table 108-1).

It is of particular importance to examine family members when the diagnosis of idiopathic hemochromatosis is established. Asymptomatic as well as symptomatic family members with the disease will have an increase in plasma iron, a decrease in total iron-binding capacity, and saturation of transferrin with iron. These changes occur even before the iron stores are greatly increased, as determined by chelatable iron excretion or by serum ferritin concentration. A liver biopsy should then be performed, since it is imperative to establish the diagnosis and begin therapy before tissue damage occurs.

The differential diagnosis between parenchymal iron overload and reticuloendothelial iron overload is usually not difficult. Reticuloendothelial iron overload is not associated with tissue damage; the plasma iron is not increased; and the urinary excretion of iron after desferrioxamine administration does not exceed 4 mg. The relative degrees of

TABLE 108-1
Representative iron values in normal subjects and in patients with idiopathic hemochromatosis

Determination	*Normal subjects*	*Patients with idiopathic hemochromatosis*
Plasma iron, μg/100 ml	50–150	180–300
Total iron-binding capacity, μg/100 ml	250–370	200–300
% transferrin saturation, μg/100 ml	22–46	80–100
Serum ferritin, ng/ml	3–180	900–6,000
Urinary iron,* mg/24 h	0–2	9–23
Liver iron, μg/100 mg dry wt	30–140	600–1,800

* *After intramuscular administration of 0.5 g desferrioxamine.*

parenchymal iron overload and reticuloendothelial iron overload can be determined definitively by liver biopsy.

The distinction between idiopathic hemochromatosis and alcoholic cirrhosis associated with an iron overload is a relative one which is frequently not easily made. In general, patients with alcoholic cirrhosis of the liver have a lesser degree of iron overload, as determined by the plasma iron concentration, serum ferritin concentration, and urinary iron excretion after desferrioxamine administration. The degree of parenchymal iron deposition in liver biopsy specimens from patients with alcoholic cirrhosis is usually mild in comparison with the degree of fibrosis. The deposition of iron is out of proportion to the degree of fibrosis in idiopathic hemochromatosis. Iron deposition in septa occurs more commonly in idiopathic hemochromatosis than in alcoholic cirrhosis.

TREATMENT The therapy of idiopathic hemochromatosis involves the removal of the excess body iron and supportive treatment of damaged organs.

Iron is best removed from the body by weekly or twice weekly phlebotomy of 500 ml. Although there is an initial modest decline in the volume of packed red blood cells to about 35 ml per 100 ml, the anemia stabilizes after several weeks. The plasma iron concentration remains increased until the available iron stores are depleted. Since one 500-ml unit of blood contains from 200 to 250 mg iron and about 25 g iron must be removed, 2 or 3 years of weekly phlebotomy are usually required. When the plasma iron level becomes normal, phlebotomies are performed at such time intervals as are required to maintain a plasma iron concentration of less than 150 μg per 100 ml. Usually one phlebotomy every 3 months will suffice. The adequacy of the therapy may be evaluated at any time by measuring the plasma iron, the percentage of saturation of transferrin with iron, or the urinary iron excretion after desferrioxamine administration. These measurements become abnormal promptly with iron reaccumulation and precede the increase in serum ferritin concentration.

Chelating agents such as desferrioxamine, when given parenterally, remove 10 to 20 mg iron per day, about half that mobilized by a weekly phlebotomy. Phlebotomy is not only a more effective but also a less expensive, more convenient, and safer treatment for patients with idiopathic hemochromatosis. Chelating agents may be used as a substitute method for iron removal when anemia or hypoproteinemia is severe enough to preclude phlebotomy.

The management of the hepatic failure, cardiac failure, and diabetes differs little from conventional management of these conditions. Loss of libido and change in secondary sex characteristics are partially relieved by testosterone therapy.

PROGNOSIS The life expectancy of untreated patients with idiopathic hemochromatosis after the disease has become clinically manifest averages 4.4 years, but several instances have been recorded of patients living up to 20 or 30 years. The average duration of life after diabetes has developed is 3 years. The principal causes of death in untreated patients are cardiac failure (30 percent), hepatic coma (15 percent), hematemesis (14 percent), hepatoma (14 percent), and pneumonia (12 percent).

Life expectancy is extended to an average of more than 8

years by removal of the excessive stores of iron and maintenance of these stores at near-normal levels. The 5-year survival rate with therapy is increased from 33 to 89 percent.

With removal of iron by repeated phlebotomy, the liver and spleen decrease in size, liver function studies return to normal, pigmentation of skin decreases, and cardiac failure is reversed. Carbohydrate tolerance improves in about 40 percent of cases. The fibrosis in the liver may decrease but is usually unchanged. Removal of excess iron has little or no effect on the hypogonadism or arthropathy. Hepatoma occurs as a late sequela in about one-third of the patients despite adequate iron removal.

REFERENCES

BEAMISH MR et al: Transferrin iron, chelatable iron and ferritin in idiopathic hemochromatosis. Br J Haematol 27:219, 1974

DYMOCK IW et al: Arthropathy of haemochromatosis. Ann Rheum Dis 29:469, 1970

——: Observations on the pathogenesis, complications and treatment of diabetes in 115 cases of haemochromatosis. Am J Med 52:203, 1972

GRACE ND, POWELL LW: Iron storage disorders of the liver. Gastroenterology 67:1257, 1974

HARKER LA, FUNK DD, FINCH CA: Evaluation of storage iron by chelates. Am J Med 45:105, 1968

SADDI R, FEINGOLD J: Idiopathic haemochromatosis: An autosomal recessive disease. Clin Genet 5:234, 1974

109
DISORDERS OF PORPHYRIN METABOLISM

GEORGE E. CARTWRIGHT

DEFINITIONS *Porphyrins* are fluorescent pigments that possess a basic structure of four pyrrole rings linked by methene (—CH—) bridges (Fig. 109-1). The individual porphyrins differ from each other according to the nature of the eight possible side chains. Each porphyrin has a number of stereoisomers. *Porphyrinogens* are colorless compounds (reduced porphyrins) with a basic structure of four pyrrole rings linked by methane (—CH_2—) bridges.

Porphyrin pigments are widely distributed throughout the plant and animal worlds in chlorophyll, hemoglobin, catalase, and a number of cytochrome and peroxidase enzymes.

The term *porphyrinuria* refers to excessive excretion of porphyrins in the urine. *Coproporphyrinuria,* the excretion of increased amounts of coproporphyrin, is not uncommon and occurs in a variety of conditions. The term *porphyria* embraces a group of diseases, each with unusual and characteristic manifestations, which have in common the excessive excretion of one or more porphyrins, porphyrinogens, and/or porphyrin precursors (Δ-aminolevulinic acid and porphobilinogen) in the urine and/or feces.

HISTORY Congenital porphyria was first described by Günther in 1911. Much of the knowledge of the chemistry of the porphyrins came from Hans Fischer and his school in Munich. In 1915, these workers described, named, and isolated in crystalline form the uroporphyrins and coproporphyrins from the urine of a patient (Petry) with congenital porphyria. Shemin and Granick and their groups in New York have made substantial contributions to knowledge of the biosynthesis of the porphyrins. Contributions to the understanding of the types and manifestations of porphyria have come from Waldenström in Sweden, Rimington in England, Barnes and Dean in South Africa, and Watson, Schwartz, and Schmid in the United States.

FIGURE 109-1
The structural formulas of the porphyrin and porphyrinogen nuclei and diagrammatic formulas of the important naturally occurring porphyrins.

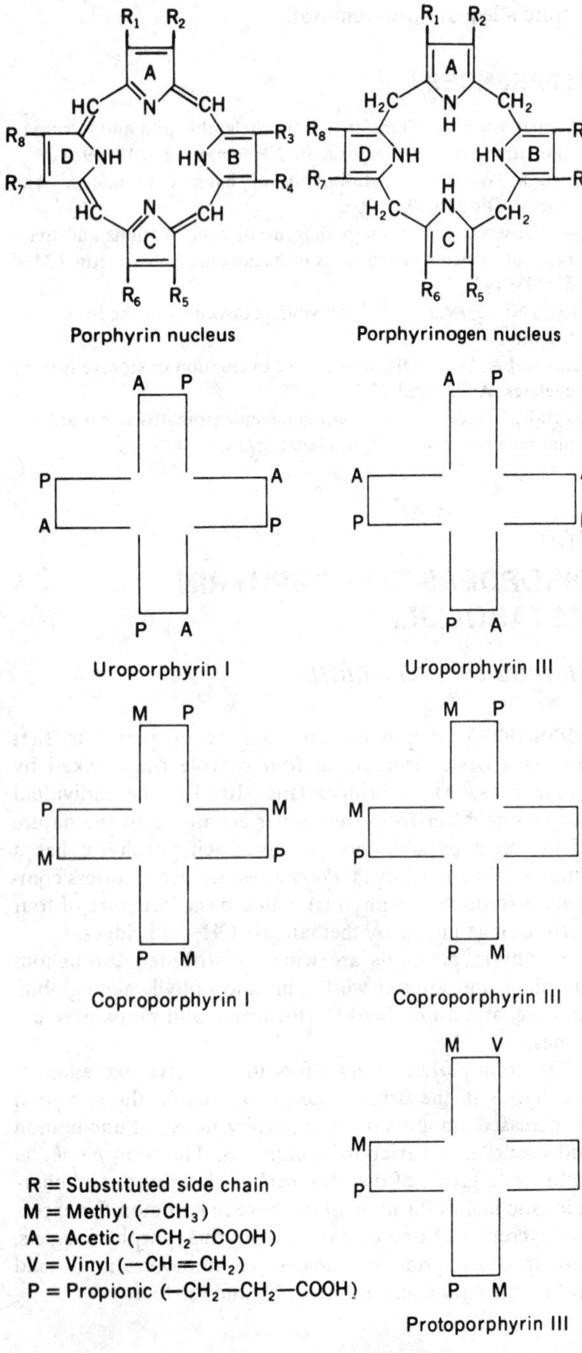

BIOSYNTHESIS The complex porphyrin molecule is synthesized in the body from two simple precursors, acetate and glycine (Fig. 109-2). Acetate enters the Krebs tricarboxylic acid cycle (Chap. 68) and is converted into succinate. Succinyl CoA (active succinate) is then formed in the presence of Mg^{2+} ion, adenosine triphosphate (ATP), and coenzyme A (CoA). The activated form of succinate condenses with glycine in the presence of the enzyme Δ-aminolevulinic acid synthetase (ALA-S) to form the five-carbon compound, Δ-aminolevulinic acid (ALA) and carbon dioxide by the decarboxylation of glycine. This step occurs within mitochondria and is the rate-limiting step in heme biosynthesis. A series of cytoplasmic reactions then takes place. Two molecules of ALA, in the presence of glutathione (GSH) and an enzyme, Δ-aminolevulinic acid dehydrase (ALA-DH), condense to form the monopyrrole, porphobilinogen, which contains acetic acid (A) and propionic acid (P) side chains. In the next step in heme synthesis, four molecules of porphobilinogen condense to form the reduced tetrapyrrolic structure, uroporphyrinogen. This step is catalyzed by at least two enzymes, uroporphyrinogen I synthetase (US) and uroporphyrinogen III cosynthetase (UC). Although these enzymatic steps have been studied in detail, the precise sequence of reactions leading to the asymmetric uroporphyrinogen III molecule is not known. The oxidized molecule, uroporphyrin III, is not in the direct pathway of heme synthesis but is a by-product. Uroporphyrinogen III (reduced uroporphyrin) is converted to coproporphyrinogen by the enzyme uroporphyrinogen decarboxylase (UD). Coproporphyrinogen III is then converted to protoporphyrinogen III in the presence of coproporphyrinogenase (C), an enzyme associated with the outer mitochondrial membrane. Recent evidence suggests that a second enzyme, protoporphyrinogen oxidase (PO), may be required for the oxidation of protoporphyrinogen IX to protoporphyrin IX. Protoporphyrin IX is converted to heme in the presence of iron, glutathione, and the intramitochondrial enzyme, heme synthetase (HS). The final steps in the assembly of the hemoglobin molecules occur in the cytoplasm where the heme molecules attach to globin chains.

METABOLISM The most important of the naturally occurring porphyrins are uroporphyrin (isomer types I and III), coproporphyrin (types I and III), and protoporphyrin (type III).

Protoporphyrin III is present in hemoglobin and is, therefore, the most important of the porphyrins from the physiologic standpoint. It is absent from urine. The concentration of fecal protoporphyrin is related to the amount of blood in the gastrointestinal tract, the rate of liberation of protoporphyrin from hemoglobin by fecal bacteria, and the excretion of protoporphyrin by the liver.

Coproporphyrin is the predominant porphyrin in urine and feces under normal circumstances. Coproporphyrinuria of a modest degree occurs in a variety of clinical conditions which are not associated with demonstrable enzymatic defects in porphyrin metabolism, such as infections, liver disease, acute alcoholism, myocardial infarction, Hodgkin's disease, and hemolytic anemia. In lead poisoning, more marked coproporphyrinuria may occur in association with several enzymatic defects in the porphyrin biosynthetic pathway. Coproporphyrinuria is also found in patients with certain types of porphyria. Abnormally high fecal coproporphyrin values are found in patients with certain types of porphyria, as well as in patients with hemolytic anemia.

Uroporphyrin is normally excreted in urine in only trace amounts. The urinary excretion of this porphyrin is moderately increased in lead poisoning and is greatly increased in patients with certain types of porphyria.

PORPHYRIA

Porphyria may be divided into two general groups (Table 109-1). In erythropoietic porphyria, excessive quantities of porphyrins accumulate in the normoblasts and erythrocytes. Under these circumstances, red fluorescence may be observed when the cells are exposed to ultraviolet light. The predominant porphyrin synthesized in erythropoietic uroporphyria (congenital porphyria) is uroporphyrin; in erythropoietic protoporphyria, protoporphyrin. In porphyria hepatica, excessive porphyrin production occurs in the liver. Hepatic porphyria may be subdivided further into at least four different types: acute intermittent porphyria, porphyria variegata (porphyria cutanea tarda hereditaria, mixed porphyria, South African Caucasian porphyria, protocoproporphyria), porphyria cutanea tarda, and hereditary coproporphyria.

This classification, although clinically useful, is not entirely satisfactory. Specific inherited enzymatic defects have now been identified in three of the porphyrias (erythropoietic uroporphyria, acute intermittent porphyria, and porphyria cutanea tarda). The enzymatic defects are present in many tissues, although the resulting metabolic derangements are most prominent in either erythroid tissue or liver. There is some overlap between the erythropoietic and hepatic groups, particularly in erythropoietic protoporphyria. Finally, not all patients with hepatic porphyria can be classified clearly into one of the four subgroups.

Porphyria erythropoietica

ERYTHROPOIETIC UROPORPHYRIA This is a very rare disorder, inherited probably as a recessive mendelian characteristic. The clinical manifestations occur very early in life, sometimes even a few days after birth, but often they are not observed until after an interval of a year or two. The disease is characterized by the excessive deposition of porphyrin in the tissues, leading to pronounced photosensitization. The early lesions of photodynamic origin are the blisters of the hydroa estivale (hydroa vacciniforme) on skin surfaces exposed to light, especially of the face and hands. In time, scarring and mutilation occur. After years of continued photosensitivity, the mutilation becomes extensive, with loss of fingers and portions of the nose and

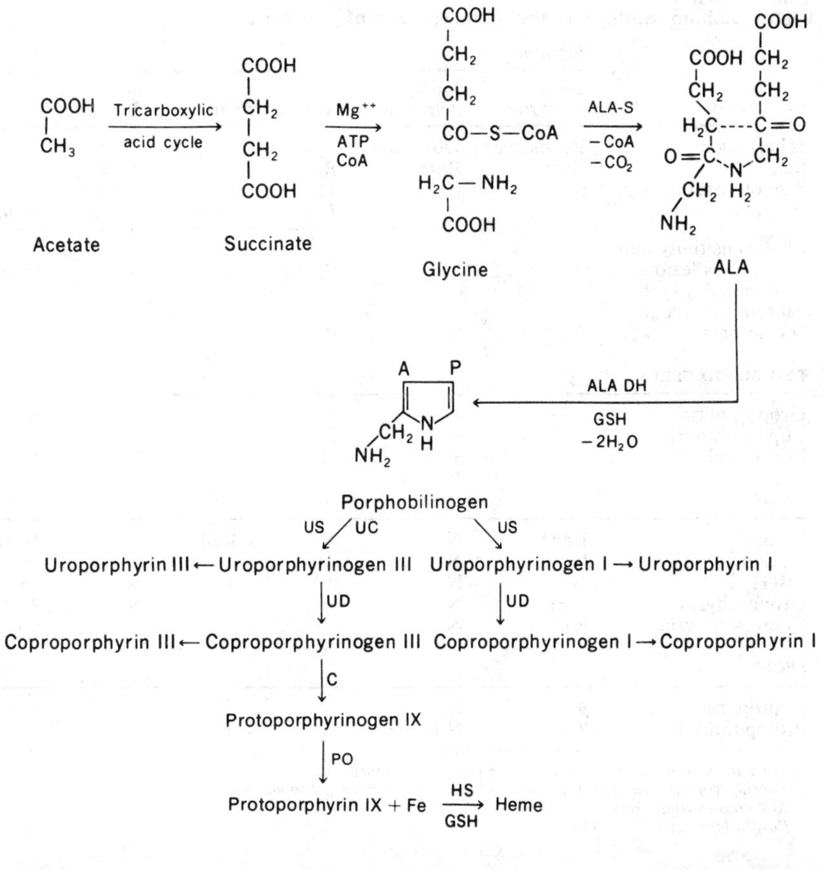

FIGURE 109-2
The biosynthesis of the porphyrins from acetate and glycine and the biosynthetic pathway of heme. CoA, *coenzyme A;* ATP, *adenosine triphosphate;* ALA-S, *Δ-aminolevulinic acid synthetase;* ALA, *Δ-aminolevulinic acid;* ALA-DH, *Δ-aminolevulinic acid dehydrase;* GSH, *glutathione;* US, *uroporphyrinogen I synthetase;* UC, *uroporphyrinogen III cosynthetase;* UD, *uroporphyrinogen decarboxylase;* C, *coproporphyrinogenase;* PO, *protoporphyrinogen oxidase;* HS, *heme synthetase;* A, *acetate;* P, *propionic acid.*

ears, scarring of the cheeks and about the mouth, ectropion, or symblepharon. Skin not exposed to light remains unaffected. Hemolytic anemia and splenomegaly are an integral part of the disease. Erythrodontia may be observed in those cases in which sufficient porphyrin has been deposited in the teeth to make them grossly red or reddish brown. Teeth which do not show erythrodontia in ordinary light may exhibit red fluorescence in Wood's light. Red fluorescence may be seen in the phalangeal bones if a strong source of ultraviolet light is allowed to shine through the fingers. There is no marked disturbance of the nervous system, nor is there abdominal colic.

Normoblasts in the bone marrow are the source of the excessive porphyrins formed in this disease. The predominant porphyrin formed in the normoblasts and excreted in the urine is uroporphyrin I. For this reason, the disease has been called *erythropoietic uroporphyria,* rather than congenital porphyria. The activity of uroporphyrinogen III cosynthetase (Fig. 109-2) is reduced in both erythrocytes and fibroblasts. The activity of the enzyme in heterozygotes is intermediate between that in normal subjects and that in homozygotes with the disease.

The color of the urine varies from pink to red. Uroporphyrin I is the predominant porphyrin excreted, although the excretion of coproporphyrin I and 7, 6, 5, and 3 carboxyl porphyrins is also increased. If the pH of the urine is adjusted to 3 to 4 with dilute hydrochloric acid, the uroporphyrin is adsorbed onto talc. The talc will be tinted deep red-brown and will fluoresce a brilliant red under ultraviolet light. The excretion of porphyrin precursors, Δ-aminolevulinic acid and porphobilinogen, is not increased.

The disease is slowly progressive, and death is usually due to intercurrent infection or severe hemolytic anemia. At autopsy there is extensive deposition of porphyrins in the skeleton and tissues. This may be so pronounced as to color the bones red. Erythroid hyperplasia of the bone marrow and splenomegaly are additional pathologic features.

Treatment Exposure to sunlight should be avoided. The harmful and disfiguring effects of light may be ameliorated by the use of an appropriate sunscreen preparation. Splenectomy is indicated if there is evidence of increased erythrocyte destruction. Splenectomy may be associated not only with amelioration of the hemolytic anemia but also with a reduction in photosensitivity and porphyrin excretion. Suppression of erythropoiesis by hypertransfusion also reduces both photosensitivity and porphyrin excretion.

ERYTHROPOIETIC PROTOPORPHYRIA Erythropoietic protoporphyria, the most common form of erythropoietic porphyria, is transmitted as an autosomal dominant characteristic. The disease usually becomes manifest in childhood and is characterized clinically by *skin photosensitivity with intense, painful itching, edema, and erythema of the exposed parts.* Chronic skin changes may develop on the dorsa of the hands, especially over the knuckles, but may also be observed on the nose, cheeks, and lips. Biochemically, the disorder is characterized by an increase in the *protoporphyrin content of the normoblasts and erythrocytes,* an increased

TABLE 109-1
Distinguishing features of the several types of porphyria

	Erythropoietic		*Hepatic*						
Characteristics	*Uro-porphyria*	*Proto-porphyria*	*Acute intermittent*		*Variegata*		*Cutanea tarda*	*Hereditary coproporphyria*	
Inheritance	Recessive	Dominant	Dominant		Dominant		Dominant	Dominant	
Sex	Both	Both	Both		Both		Both	Both	
Age of onset, years	0–5	0–5	15–40		10–30		Any age	Any age	
Phase of disease			*Latent*	*Acute*	*Latent*	*Acute*		*Latent*	*Acute*
Photosensitivity and cutaneous lesions	++++	++	0	0	0	+ or 0	++	0	0 or +
Abdominal, psychic, and/or neurologic symptoms	0	0	0	++	0	+	0	0	+
RED BLOOD CELLS									
Uroporphyrin	++++	++	N	N	N	N	N	N	N
Coproporphyrin	+++	++	N	N	N	N	N	N	N
Protoporphyrin	++	++++	N	N	N	N	N	N	N
URINE,									
Color*	Red*	N*	N*	Red*	N*	N or red*	Red*	N*	N or red*
Δ-ALA†	N	N	+	++	N	++	N	+	++
PBG‡	N	N	++	++++	N	++	N	+	++
Uroporphyrin	++++	N	++	++	N	+++	++++	N	++
Coproporphyrin	++	N	++	++	N	+++	++	N or +	+++
FECES									
Coproporphyrin	++	N	N	+	++++	+++	N	++	++++
Protoporphyrin	++	N to ++	N	+	++++	+++	N	N	+

0, absent; N, normal; +, increased; ++++, greatly increased.
* *Freshly voided. On standing, the urine may become deep brownish-red or black.*
† *Δ-Aminolevulinic acid.*
‡ *Porphobilinogen.*

level of plasma protoporphyrin, and an increased excretion of protoporphyrin in the feces. The urinary excretion of Δ-ALA, porphobilinogen, coproporphyrin, and uroporphyrin is not increased. However, several patterns of chemical abnormality have been demonstrated in patients with the disease and in members of their families. Elevation of free erythrocyte protoporphyrin may occur with no increase in plasma or fecal protoporphyrin. Fecal protoporphyrin may be increased with no abnormalities of plasma or erythrocyte protoporphyrin. The complete biochemical stigmata of the disease have been observed in the absence of skin photosensitivity.

The course of the disease is usually benign, with symptoms related only to the skin. However, a mild hemolytic anemia may develop, and liver disease may be a more common feature of this porphyria than previously recognized. The livers of such patients contain large deposits of protoporphyrin, and the accumulation of pigment is accompanied by bile stasis and varying degrees of portal inflammation, ductal proliferation, and fibrosis. In recent years, an increasing number of patients have been reported who have developed cirrhosis of the liver. In some cases, the liver disease has progressed rapidly and terminated in hepatic failure.

A modest decrease in the activity of heme synthetase (HS, Fig. 109-2) has been demonstrated in fibroblasts, hepatocytes, and normoblasts from patients with the disease. This deficiency may explain the accumulation of protoporphyrin and hence the biochemical and clinical features of the disease.

Beta-carotene, 30 mg daily orally, may be of value in reducing dermal photosensitivity to sunlight. Cholestyramine resin, 4 g t.i.d. before meals, may facilitate the removal of protoporphyrin from the liver and be of some value in preventing the progression of the hepatic lesions.

Porphyria hepatica

ACUTE INTERMITTENT PORPHYRIA This is an uncommon disease which affects both sexes, with a slight predilection for the female. Young adults or the middle-aged are most frequently affected. Acute porphyria is extremely rare below the age of fifteen and after the age of sixty. The familial occurrence of the disease is marked. It is probably transmitted as a mendelian dominant characteristic. The disease is characterized clinically by (1) periodic attacks of intense abdominal colic, usually accompanied by nausea and vomiting; (2) obstinate constipation; (3) neurotic or even psychotic behavior; and (4) neuromuscular disturbances. The mortality rate is high.

Abdominal pain is frequently the presenting complaint. The pain is usually colicky in nature and may be extremely severe and associated with spasm without localizing signs but with fever, tachycardia, and leukocytosis. The abdominal signs may be, and frequently are, mistaken for manifestations of renal colic, acute appendicitis, cholelithiasis, or pancreatitis. It is not uncommon for patients with porphyria to have multiple surgical scars on the abdomen. The neurologic manifestations are quite varied and may include neuritic pain in the extremities, areas of hypesthesia and paresthesia, and foot and wrist drop. Paraplegia or a complete flaccid quadriplegia may ensue and may be followed by bulbar paralysis and death. Except for pain in the extremities, sensory changes are usually not prominent, and signs of upper motor neuron changes are usually absent. The neurologic manifestations may simulate a wide variety of conditions, including poliomyelitis, encephalitis, and arsenic or lead poisoning. A true ascending paralysis of the Landry type is not observed.

The patients frequently have many vague "neurotic" complaints, even when in remission from an attack. With an attack they may become confused or even psychotic. Hypertension may accompany an attack, there may be temporary loss of vision, and convulsions have been described.

The course of the disease is extraordinarily variable. Recurrent abdominal crises may be present for years, or the patient may die in the first attack. It is not at all uncommon to find in one parent or in several siblings of a patient with porphyria that porphobilinogen, the diagnostic feature of porphyria, is increased in the urine, even though they have never had active symptoms of the disease. This condition is called *latent porphyria.* In general, the neuromuscular and psychotic symptoms are late manifestations, and with their appearance the prognosis becomes grave. Between attacks there may be no symptoms. The mechanism by which the latent disease is converted to manifest disease, i.e., an attack of acute porphyria, is unknown. However, it is clear that drugs, such as barbiturates, which induce Δ-ALA synthetase and thereby enhance the synthesis of porphobilinogen are capable of provoking attacks. Acute attacks have been precipitated by exposure to many different drugs, particularly barbiturates and sulfonamides. Menstruation, low carbohydrate intake, pregnancy, infection, alcohol, or lead may be the precipitating factor in some patients. In others, no precipitating factor may be elicited.

Acute intermittent porphyria is characterized by the excessive excretion in the urine of the porphyrin precursors, Δ-aminolevulinic acid and porphobilinogen. Examination of the tissues of such patients, in contrast to the findings in erythropoietic porphyria, reveals that the porphyrin content of the bone marrow is normal. The liver, on the contrary, regularly exhibits increased quantities of the porphyrin precursors. The freshly voided urine is normal in color; on standing in the sunlight it turns to a burgundy wine color or even black. This color change can be hastened by adding a small amount of acid to the urine and boiling for 30 min. The explanation for these color changes is that porphobilinogen (colorless), not uroporphyrin (red), is excreted in the urine. Heating of porphobilinogen in an acid medium results in the nonenzymatic formation of uroporphyrin, together with a dark brown or reddish-brown nonporphyrin pigment.

The inherited metabolic defect in acute intermittent porphyria is a partial deficiency of the enzyme uroporphyrinogen I synthetase (US, Fig. 109-2). The liver and erythrocytes contain reduced levels of this enzyme. Individuals with latent porphyria may be detected by assay of erythrocyte uroporphyrinogen I synthetase even at times when urinary excretion of porphobilinogen and Δ-aminolevulinic acid are normal. The partial deficiency of uroporphyrinogen I synthetase results in a secondary enzymatic aberration in the heme biosynthetic pathway. Induction of the first enzyme in the heme biosynthetic pathway, ALA synthetase, is regulated by feedback inhibition and repression exerted by heme, the end product in the pathway. Thus, the partial block in the heme biosynthetic pathway resulting from the decreased activity of uroporphyrinogen I synthetase leads to induction of ALA synthetase. This in turn results in the overproduction of Δ-aminolevulinic acid and porphobilinogen. The relationship between the metabolic abnormalities and the symptoms remains unknown. However, agents which further induce ALA synthetase, such as barbiturates, certain steroid metabolites, and a variety of other drugs, may precipitate acute attacks.

The qualitative determination of porphobilinogen in the urine by the Watson-Schwartz modification of the Ehrlich reaction is a simple and valuable screening test for the diagnosis of symptomatic patients with this disorder. The test is unreliable in asymptomatic patients. In this test 5 ml freshly voided urine is mixed with 5 ml Ehrlich's reagent (0.7 g paradimethylaminobenzaldehyde, 150 ml concentrated hydrochloric acid, 100 ml water). After mixing, 10 ml aqueous saturated sodium acetate is added. The solution is then extracted successively with 10 ml chloroform and 10 ml *n*-butanol. A positive test for porphobilinogen gives an intense red color remaining in the aqueous layer. This test is also positive in patients with porphyria variegata during acute attacks. It is negative in patients with erythropoietic porphyria and in patients with porphyria cutanea tarda.

The urinary excretion of Δ-aminolevulinic acid and porphobilinogen may be measured quantitatively by means of a simple, commercially available chromatographic method. Normally, less than 3 mg of either Δ-aminolevulinic acid or porphobilinogen is excreted in 24 h. Symptomatic patients excrete 30 to 200 mg porphobilinogen per 24 h and 8 to 150 mg Δ-aminolevulinic acid. During remissions the excretion of porphobilinogen is usually 12 to 60 mg and the excretion of Δ-aminolevulinic acid is 6 to 18 mg. In a few asymptomatic patients the values may fall within the normal range.

The most reliable and specific method for the diagnosis of acute intermittent porphyria, particularly in the asymptomatic latent stage, is the measurement of the activity of uroporphyrinogen I synthetase in erythrocytes.

Treatment The most effective treatment of the acute attack is to provide a liberal intake of glucose, either orally or intravenously. A low carbohydrate intake enhances ALA synthetase induction, and a high intake suppresses the induction of this enzyme, the so-called "glucose effect." Rapid remissions may be induced by a high carbohydrate intake. Symptomatic therapy consists of opiates such as meperidine (Demerol) for relief of severe pain, phenothiazines for control of mild pain and mental symptoms, paraldehyde for sedation, and neostigmine for severe constipation. Hyponatremia and hypochloremia secondary to inappropriate antidiuretic hormone secretion may occur in some patients during acute attacks and require therapy. Respiratory support may be required in patients with progressive neuropathy.

Prevention of acute attacks is most important. Drugs and toxins which precipitate acute attacks should be avoided, as well as periods of low carbohydrate intake. In women whose attacks are related to the menstrual cycle, suppression of ovulation with progesterone-estrogen contraceptive pills may be helpful in reducing the frequency of attacks.

PORPHYRIA VARIEGATA Porphyria variegata is characterized clinically by cutaneous lesions or acute attacks of abdominal colic and not infrequently by both. The disease is inherited as a non-sex-linked mendelian dominant. The onset of symptoms is usually between the ages of ten and thirty years. The outstanding biochemical feature of the disorder is the increased excretion of coproporphyrin and protoporphyrin in the feces *at all times* in the course of the disease.

During the latent phase of the disease the patients are entirely asymptomatic. Porphyrinuria is usually absent, and the porphyrin precursors, Δ-aminolevulinic acid and porphobilinogen, are not excreted in increased amounts. The disease can be diagnosed only during the latent phase by examination of the stools for porphyrins. A simple screening test can be done by obtaining a small specimen of stool on a glove. The specimen is extracted with about 2 ml of solvent containing equal parts of glacial acetic acid, amyl alcohol, and ether. The supernatant solution is then extracted with 1.5 *N* HCl and viewed in a Wood's lamp. Red fluorescence in the acid layer is proportional to the porphyrin content.

In a number of patients, particularly males, the skin is unusually sensitive to light and blisters and abrades easily. Healed depigmented scars may be present over the exposed surfaces, particularly the hands. Hyperpigmentation of the skin may occur, and hirsutism has been observed in females. The photosensitivity and cutaneous deformities are not so great as in erythropoietic porphyria.

Acute attacks of jaundice and abdominal colic, accompanied in some cases by psychotic manifestations and motor paralysis, may intervene in the course of the disease. Indeed, any of or all the manifestations of acute intermittent porphyria may make their appearance. As in acute intermittent porphyria, death or recovery may occur. During the acute attacks the excretion of porphyrins in the feces frequently decreases, and the excretion of coproporphyrin and uroporphyrin in the urine increases. Both Δ-aminolevulinic acid and porphobilinogen are usually excreted in increased amounts in the urine during acute attacks. It has been suggested that the disease remains asymptomatic as long as the liver is capable of excreting the porphyrins in the bile (latent phase); when this capacity is impaired, bilirubinemia, porphyrinemia, porphyrinuria, and cutaneous lesions appear (cutaneous phase); and finally when porphyrin metabolism is greatly disturbed, Δ-aminolevulinic acid and porphobilinogen appear in the urine, and all the manifestations of acute intermittent porphyria may develop (acute phase). This disorder was formerly called porphyria cutanea tarda hereditaria, but the name was not entirely suitable, since not all patients develop cutaneous lesions.

The treatment for this type of porphyria is the same as for acute intermittent porphyria. The "glucose effect" has been shown to operate in porphyria variegata as well as in acute intermittent porphyria.

PORPHYRIA CUTANEA TARDA Porphyria cutanea tarda is the most commonly occurring form of porphyria. The disease is characterized clinically by photosensitive dermatitis, hyperpigmentation of the skin, liver disease, and hypertrichosis. The skin is usually sensitive both to light and to mechanical trauma. Blisters appear on the exposed skin areas, frequently ulcerate, and finally lead to scar formation. The skin lesions are indistinguishable from those observed in porphyria variegata, but abdominal pain and neurologic complications are absent. The photosensitivity is similar to that in erythropoietic uroporphyria but not as marked.

Porphyria cutanea tarda is characterized biochemically by excessive hepatic synthesis and urinary excretion of uroporphyrin I. The urine does not contain increased quantities of Δ-aminolevulinic acid or porphobilinogen. The excretion of porphyrins in the feces is usually normal or only slightly increased.

This disorder has been described (1) in male subjects, forty to seventy years of age, with alcoholic cirrhosis; (2) in Bantu subjects in South Africa with cirrhosis of the liver; (3) in subjects exposed to hexachlorobenzene; (4) in subjects exposed to polychlorinated phenols; (5) in rare subjects exposed to certain drugs such as estrogens, busulfan, sulfonal, phenobarbitone, tolbutamide, chlorpropamide, or Dilantin; (6) in a few patients with hemolytic anemia and a high degree of ineffective erythropoiesis; and (7) in a few patients with hepatic adenoma or systemic lupus erythematosus. Hepatic parenchymal iron overload is present in virtually all patients and is manifest by an increased serum iron concentration and an increased saturation of the iron-binding protein with iron.

Porphyria cutanea tarda was once considered to be an acquired disease. It is now known to be inherited as an autosomal dominant trait and to be due to a partial deficiency of the enzyme uroporphyrinogen decarboxylase (Fig. 109-2). The disease remains latent until precipitated by a hepatic parenchymal iron overload. Subjects with latent porphyria cutanea tarda can be detected by demonstrating decreased activity of uroporphyrinogen decarboxylase in circulating erythrocytes.

The enzyme uroporphyrinogen III cosynthetase is inhibited in vitro by both ferrous iron and uroporphyrinogen III. It has been suggested that the excretion of uroporphyrin I is due to the inhibition of the uroporphyrinogen III cosynthetase by iron and by the accumulation of uroporphyrinogen III that occurs because of the partial deficiency of uroporphyrinogen decarboxylase.

Phlebotomy is an effective treatment for porphyria cutanea tarda. The beneficial effect is related to the removal of excess iron from the liver. The administration of chloroquine has been successfully employed in the treatment of porphyria cutanea tarda, but significant risks are involved in its use.

HEREDITARY COPROPORPHYRIA The unique feature of this disease is an increased excretion of coproporphyrin, isomer type III. In the latent phase, the patients are asymptomatic, and the only abnormality usually detectable is an increased excretion of coproporphyrin III in the urine and feces, particularly the latter. Urinary Δ-ALA and porphobilinogen may be normal or slightly increased. Acute attacks, similar to those which occur in acute intermittent porphyria, can be provoked by the ingestion of barbiturates and possibly by certain tranquilizers and anticonvulsants. During these attacks there is an excessive excretion of Δ-ALA and porphobilinogen in the urine, in addition to a massive excretion of coproporphyrin in both urine and stool. About forty cases of this disorder have been reported. Psychiatric symptoms may be present without other clinical manifestations of porphyria. Skin photosensitivity has been described in a few patients. The disease is inherited as a dominant characteristic and occurs in both sexes. A high glucose intake is the most effective form of therapy.

The neurologic and psychiatric aspects of porphyria are discussed further in Chaps. 331 and 26, respectively.

REFERENCES

ELDER GH et al: The porphyrias: A review. J Clin Pathol 25:1013, 1972

MAGNUSSEN CR et al: A red cell enzyme method for the diagnosis of acute intermittent porphyria. Blood 44:857, 1974

MARVER HS, SCHMID R: The porphyrias, in *The Metabolic Basis of Inherited Disease,* 3d ed., eds JB Stanbury et al, New York: McGraw-Hill, 1972, p. 1087

MEYER, UA: Hepatic porphyrias, in *Progress in Liver Diseases,* vol V, eds H Popper and F. Schaffner, New York: Grune & Stratton, 1975

WINTROBE MM et al: The porphyrias, in *Clinical Hematology,* 7th ed., Philadelphia: Lea & Febiger, 1974, p. 1021

110 HEPATOLENTICULAR DEGENERATION (WILSON'S DISEASE)

GEORGE E. CARTWRIGHT

DEFINITION Wilson's disease (hepatolenticular degeneration, progressive lenticular degeneration, pseudosclerosis of Westphal and Strümpell, tetanoid chorea of Gowers) is a rare, autosomal recessively inherited disorder, characterized by excess copper storage, particularly in the liver, kidneys, brain, and cornea, leading eventually to liver disease, proximal renal tubular reabsorption abnormalities, basal ganglion disease, and the characteristic rusty-brown corneal ring known as the *Kayser-Fleischer ring.*

HISTORY Kinnier Wilson, in 1912, in his classic monograph, "Progressive Lenticular Degeneration," defined this disease entity. A similar condition had previously been described in 1883 by Westphal and later by Strümpell. The symptoms resembled those of multiple sclerosis, but no demyelinative plaques were observed. For that reason it was called *pseudosclerosis.* The cirrhosis of the liver was overlooked until Spielmeyer reexamined the cases many years later. His studies and the clinical observations of Hall left little doubt that hepatolenticular degeneration and pseudosclerosis were the same disease. The corneal ring was described in 1902 by Kayser in a case diagnosed as "multiple sclerosis," but to Fleischer is due the credit for appreciating its significance in relation to the disease as it is now known.

A marked increase in the copper content of both the

brain and the liver was demonstrated by Haurowitz in 1930 and was later confirmed by Glazebrook and Cummings. Mandelbrote and his associates in 1948 observed by chance that the urinary output of copper was high and that this output is increased by the administration of BAL (British anti-lewisite). In the same year Uzman and Denny-Brown found that a persistent aminoaciduria is associated with the disease. Ceruloplasmin deficiency was recognized as a feature of the disease by Scheinberg and Gitlin in 1952. An effective treatment of the disease was introduced by Walshe in 1956.

INHERITANCE The condition is inherited as an autosomal recessive trait. The occurrence of Wilson's disease in the general population is about 1 in 200,000 persons. Heterozygotes are clinically well, although they may exhibit some of the biochemical abnormalities of the abnormal homozygotes. Since only about 1 in 200 persons in the general population is heterozygous for the Wilson's disease gene, most affected individuals are the products of consanguineous marriages.

PATHOGENESIS The clinical and pathologic manifestations are due to the toxic effects of the excessive amounts of copper on the tissues. Thus, Wilson's disease may be viewed as a copper storage disease. Patients with this disease ingest a normal amount of copper in the diet, but copper is retained in the liver, possibly because of an inability to excrete it at the normal rate in the bile.

During the first years after birth, copper accumulates progressively and primarily in the cytoplasm of hepatocytes. After some years the concentration of copper in the liver reaches values of 500 to 2,000 μg per g dry weight, necrosis of liver cells occurs, and copper is released into the serum and is deposited in other tissues. The copper which remains in the liver is sequestered in lysosomes in order to protect the cells from the toxic effects of the metal. In many patients this period of hepatic copper release and redistribution takes place slowly and in an orderly manner. In others the release of copper from the liver to the serum is more abrupt. Copper is then taken up by erythrocytes, and hemolytic anemia may occur as a consequence of oxidative damage to the red blood cells by the copper. In still others, the shift in copper is made with greater difficulty, and overt hepatic failure may ensue. If the patients survive this period of hepatic copper release and redistribution, they may again become asymptomatic while copper is accumulating in other tissues, particularly the kidneys, brain, and cornea. Accumulation of copper in the kidneys leads to damage to the proximal renal tubules. Neurologic disease results from the toxic effects of the copper on the brain. The deposition of copper in the cornea produces the characteristic Kayser-Fleischer ring.

Normally about 95 percent of the copper in serum is firmly bound to the serum enzyme ceruloplasmin. A deficiency of ceruloplasmin is one of the most characteristic biochemical abnormalities in this disease. The remainder of the copper in serum is bound to albumin and represents copper in the process of transport from the gastrointestinal tract and from one tissue to another. The amount of copper bound to albumin is increased in Wilson's disease, and since this copper is easily dissociable from the albumin, a portion is filtered by the kidneys, and this accounts for the hypercupriuria which is a feature of the disease. Since there is a greater reduction in ceruloplasmin than there is increase in albumin-bound copper, the total serum copper concentration is usually reduced.

It has been postulated that the inherited defect is an inability to synthesize ceruloplasmin. However, a mechanism whereby a deficiency of ceruloplasmin can lead to excessive tissue deposits of copper is not known. It would seem more likely that there is an intrahepatic defect in the metabolism of copper which leads to both impaired excretion of copper in the bile and impaired ceruloplasmin synthesis.

PATHOLOGY The histology of the liver varies considerably upon the stage of the disease. In the early, asymptomatic years, the liver appears grossly and histologically normal despite an increase in hepatic copper, or it may be enlarged by fatty infiltration. During the active hepatic stage, the changes are those of chronic active hepatitis: necrosis, erosion of the marginal plate, Councilman bodies, parenchymal collapse, polymorphonuclear and round-cell infiltration, proliferation of bile ducts, and Mallory's cytoplasmic hyalin. In patients with neurologic disease, the histology is that of postnecrotic cirrhosis with finely or coarsely nodular cirrhosis, bands of fibrous tissue of variable widths, round-cell infiltration, proliferation of small bile ducts, and glycogen-filled nuclei. Splenomegaly is a common finding.

The most striking gross finding in the brain is cavitation of the putamen on each side and rarely of cerebral cortex and white matter. In many cases, probably more than half, the putamen and caudate nuclei are atrophic and of light grayish-brown color, and there is no evidence of cavitation. Microscopic examination almost invariably reveals a remarkable hyperplasia of protoplasmic astrocytes in the cerebral cortex, lenticular and caudate nuclei, subthalamic nuclei of Luys, substantia nigra, and dentate and red nuclei. Nerve-cell loss is widespread but is most pronounced in the lenticular and dentate nuclei and cerebral cortex. The protoplasmic astrocytosis does not differ from that observed in hepatic coma.

CLINICAL MANIFESTATIONS The clinical manifestations of Wilson's disease usually first appear between the ages of six and twenty years. Rarely do they occur before the age of six years, but may be first noted as late as forty years of age. The mode of onset is extremely variable. Patients may present with symptoms and signs associated with liver disease, hemolytic anemia, or neurologic disease, less commonly with psychiatric, renal, or bone disease.

Liver disease is the most frequent mode of presentation, and it is usually noted between six and fifteen years of age. Clinically, the liver disease closely resembles chronic active hepatitis. The hepatic disease is frequently severe and progressive and accompanied by all the usual signs of liver insufficiency such as spider angiomas, jaundice, hepatomegaly, splenomegaly, ascites, hematemesis, anemia, leukopenia, and thrombocytopenia. Death may supervene from either hemorrhage or hepatic failure if the diagnosis is not established and appropriate specific therapy instituted.

The first clinical manifestation may be in the form of a Coombs-negative hemolytic anemia in the absence of overt hepatic disease. The hemolytic episodes may be severe and recurrent but are usually transient and self-limited. Jaundice in some patients is due to concomitant hepatic failure and hemolytic anemia.

Neurologic disease appears at a somewhat later age than the hepatic and hematologic manifestations. A deteriorating performance at school, particularly in handwriting, and difficulty in speech are usually first noted. Tremor of one or of both the upper extremities, or of the head and trunk, may be an early as well as a prominent neurologic sign. The tremor is accentuated by excitement or attention being drawn to it. Abnormal movements of choreic or choreoathetoid type are present in some patients. Rigidity may be intermittent or constant. A mixture of parkinsonism and cerebellar ataxia is characteristic of the disease.

An occasional patient may present with psychiatric disturbances, renal disease, or bone disease. The proximal renal tubular defect may lead to aminoaciduria, peptidiuria, proteinuria, glycosuria, uricosuria, and phosphaturia. The uricosuria is associated with a diminished level of uric acid in the serum. The phosphaturia may result in hypophosphatemia and eventually in osseous change. Skeletal abnormality, manifested by osteomalacia, cartilage injury, or bone fragmentation, is a frequent finding in the disease. Azure lunulae, bluish crescent areas at the nail bases, have been observed in several patients.

The most remarkable and unique feature of the disease is the Kayser-Fleischer ring, a rusty-brown ring of pigment, located at the periphery of the cornea in Descemet's membrane. The pigment extends to the limbus and usually goes completely around the cornea; occasionally there may be only a crescent-shaped distribution. Although well-formed rings are easily visible in ordinary light, in the early stages of the disease or in patients in whom the color of the iris is brown, it may be necessary to use a slit lamp to visualize the rings. Under slit-lamp examination, the ring is seen to be composed of a multitude of granular specks. The rings are pathognomonic of the disease and are present in all patients with neurologic manifestations. Failure of an experienced observer to demonstrate rings by slit-lamp examination of a patient with neurologic abnormalities virtually rules out Wilson's disease. The rings may not be present in the early stages of the disease. They may be absent in children during the stage of acute hepatic disease and/or hemolytic anemia.

CLINICAL COURSE The course of the disease is extremely variable. Death occurs in about one-half of the patients who develop the severe, acute type of liver disease. The disease is frequently undiagnosed and untreated at this stage. The chronic active hepatitis may persist for months, or the jaundice and ascites may subside completely, never to recur during the course of the disease. A period in which the patients are asymptomatic not infrequently follows the acute hepatic or hemolytic anemia stage. About 40 percent of the patients enter the neurologic stage without a history of recognized acute hepatic decompensation or hemolytic anemia. Once the neurologic stage begins, it is usually progressive and invariably fatal if untreated. In the terminal stage, the facial muscles become set in a stiff, vacuous smile, permanent contractures and deformities are prominent, the neck and trunk become rigid, the upper extremities are held rigidly in flexion at the elbow, wrist, and metacarpal joints, and the lower extremities are held in a position of extension. Dysarthria or even anarthria is an almost constant finding in advanced cases. Cachexia and muscular wasting may be extreme. Terminally, marked mental deterioration may be present. The sensory system is intact and the reflexes are normal. Pyramidal signs are usually absent. This terminal stage is now rarely observed because of earlier diagnosis and effective therapy.

DIAGNOSIS The triad of Kayser-Fleischer rings, cirrhosis of the liver, and signs of basal ganglion disease is pathognomonic of this condition.

During the neurologic stage, the disease is relatively easy to diagnose. Kayser-Fleischer rings are present. Signs of liver disease may be established by liver function studies and/or by liver biopsy. The neurologic disorder may be confused with Parkinson's syndrome. Occasionally cerebellar ataxia, chorea, choreoathetosis, dystonia, or psychiatric disturbance predominates.

The diagnosis of Wilson's disease may be confirmed by finding one or more of the following four abnormalities in copper metabolism: (1) a serum copper concentration of less than 80 μg per 100 ml; (2) a serum ceruloplasmin concentration of less than 20 mg per 100 ml; (3) a urinary excretion of more than 100 μg of copper in 24 h; or (4) a liver copper concentration of more than 250 μg per g of dried weight (see Table 110-1).

In the early asymptomatic stage during which copper is accumulating in the liver, neurologic signs are absent and Kayser-Fleischer rings are frequently not present. Liver function studies may be normal. The serum copper and ceruloplasmin concentrations are most commonly decreased. The urinary excretion of copper is usually increased, and the concentration of copper in the liver is increased (250 to 2,000 μg per g). The disease may be difficult to distinguish from the heterozygous conditions. In some heterozygotes the serum copper may be decreased (60 to 80 μg per 100 ml), the serum ceruloplasmin decreased (5 to 20 mg per 100 ml), and the liver copper concentration increased (40 to 200 μg per g).

During the period of active liver disease, the disorder may be extremely difficult to diagnose. Kayser-Fleischer rings may or may not be present. Neurologic signs are usually absent. The diagnosis of Wilson's disease should be considered in all patients under the age of thirty years with a diagnosis of chronic active hepatitis. The serum copper and ceruloplasmin concentrations may be decreased, nor-

TABLE 110-1
Alterations in copper metabolism in Wilson's disease

Determination	*Normal subjects**	*Wilson's disease†*
Serum copper, μg/100 ml	114 81–147	10–110
Ceruloplasmin, mg/100 ml	33 25–43	1–20
Urine copper, μg/24 h	15 5–25	100–4,000
Liver copper, μg/g, dry weight	31 18–45	250–2,000

* *Mean and range ±2 standard deviations.*
† *Expected range.*

mal, or even increased during the period of active necrosis. The urinary excretion of copper is usually greatly increased and may be of the order of 1,000 to 4,000 μg in 24 h. The concentration of copper in the liver is greater than 250 μg per g of dried weight and may be as much as 2,000 μg.

During the stage of hemolytic anemia, Kayser-Fleischer rings may not be present and the neurologic examination is usually normal. The serum copper is normal or increased, although the ceruloplasmin concentration is usually decreased. The concentration of copper in the liver is increased, as is the excretion of copper in the urine.

Hypocupremia and hypoceruloplasminemia are not specific for Wilson's disease. These two abnormalities are present in all normal newborn infants up to the age of four to six months and in some patients with kwashiorkor, sprue, celiac disease, and the nephrotic syndrome. Hypercupriuria may be observed in the nephrotic syndrome, in patients with alcoholic cirrhosis of the liver, and in patients with biliary cirrhosis. However, in the last two diseases mentioned, the serum copper and ceruloplasmin concentrations are normal or increased. In patients with biliary cirrhosis, the concentration of copper in the liver may be as great as in Wilson's disease.

TREATMENT The therapy of Wilson's disease is directed toward (1) the prevention of the continued accumulation of copper in the body and (2) the removal of copper already deposited.

Sulfurated potash, technical, 20 mg three times daily with meals, prevents the absorption of copper by the formation of insoluble unabsorbable copper sulfide in the gut. This therapy is continued for 6 to 12 months and then discontinued. No undesirable side effects have been observed from such therapy.

The administration of the copper chelating agent, D-penicillamine (β,β-dimethylcysteine), results in the mobilization of copper from the tissues and an increase in its excretion in the urine. Therapy consists of 0.5 g of the D isomer given orally three times daily for the lifetime of the patient. Acute "sensitivity" reactions manifested by fever, skin rash, adenopathy, arthralgia, severe leukopenia, or thrombocytopenia develop in about one-third of patients. Desensitization and therapy with corticosteroids are required in such cases. The chronic administration of less than 2 g D-penicillamine daily is rarely associated with toxicity other than minor skin changes or diminution in taste. The most troublesome complication of therapy is the development of proteinuria. This may be mild in degree and may improve spontaneously despite continuation of the drug. In a few patients the proteinuria may be associated with a lupus-like syndrome, the nephrotic syndrome, and/or immune-complex glomerulitis requiring discontinuation of D-penicillamine. Triethylenetetramine dihydrochloride has been used in such patients as a substitute for penicillamine.

PROGNOSIS The disease is progressive and invariably fatal if untreated. Therapy is dramatically effective except in some patients with active liver disease in whom treatment is not begun sufficiently soon. After prolonged therapy, Kayser-Fleischer rings fade away, neurologic signs disappear, and liver function abnormalities revert to normal, even though hypocupremia, hypoceruloplasminemia, and hypercupriuria persist or become even more pronounced.

REFERENCES

CARTWRIGHT GE, LEE GR: The pathogenesis and evolution of Wilson's disease. Epatologia 20:51, 1974

DEISS A et al: Long-term therapy of Wilson's disease. Ann Intern Med 75:57, 1971

STERNLIEB I: Evolution of the hepatic lesion in Wilson's disease (hepatolenticular degeneration). Prog Liver Dis 4:511, 1972

——, SCHEINBERG IH: Chronic hepatitis as a first manifestation of Wilson's disease. Ann Intern Med 76:59, 1972

——, ——: Prevention of Wilson's disease in asymptomatic patients. N Engl J Med 278:352, 1968

111

DISORDERS OF GLYCOGEN SYNTHESIS AND MOBILIZATION

RICHARD A. FIELD

The glycogen deposition diseases occupy a noteworthy place in the evolution of the conceptual approaches to the modern methods of study of disease. In 1952, Dr. Gerty T. Cori demonstrated by specific enzymatic studies of tissue from patients that von Gierke's disease is due to the loss of activity of a single tissue enzyme, and thus she provided a prototype for the study of genetically determined metabolic aberrations. Since the points of enzymatic abnormality of most of the syndromes to be discussed in this chapter concern the steps of synthesis and degradation between glucose 6-phosphate and glycogen, a working schema of these pathways is presented in Fig. 111-1. The Cori classification of glycogen deposition diseases is shown in Table 111-1.

GLUCOSE 6-PHOSPHATASE DEFICIENCY (HEPATORENAL GLYCOGENOSIS) First described pathologically by von Gierke in 1929, this condition, characterized by enlargement of liver and kidneys and bouts of severe hypoglycemia, is probably the most frequent form of glycogenosis. Symptoms and recognizable clinical signs usually appear in the first year of life, and hepatomegaly may be detectable at birth. The disorder is transmitted as an autosomal mendelian recessive characteristic.

Pathologic physiology Under normal conditions hepatic glycogen serves as the main reservoir compound in the overall economy of blood glucose homeostasis. During and after ingestion of carbohydrate foods, a major portion of the glucose arriving in the liver via the portal system is phosphorylated and, by several intermediary steps, is stored as the regularly branched polysaccharide, glycogen (Chap. 68). During the postcibal period, peripheral utilization of glucose depletes circulating glucose, with the result that liver glycogen is depolymerized and free glucose is released into the hepatic vein (Chap. 68). The overall intracellular reactions in this process are called glycogenolyses, and the final enzymatic step is the hydrolytic dephosphorylation by the specific enzyme hepatic glucose 6-phosphatase (Fig. 111-1). Absence or marked reduction of this enzyme activity can be demonstrated by direct tissue assay in hepatorenal glycogenosis and accounts for most of, if not all, the metabolic disturbances noted in patients with this condition. The central feature of this limitation of hepatic glucose release is hypoglycemia, and it follows that little or no elevation of blood glucose concentration occurs after the injection of glucagon or epinephrine. Likewise, the normal expected rise in blood glucose level is not observed in patients with this hepatic enzyme deficiency following the intravenous administration of fructose or galactose. For all intents and purposes, these hexoses are metabolized solely by the liver, and ultimately are converted intracellularly to glucose 6-phosphate, which, like the molecules of the same compound derived from glycogen depolymerization, cannot be dephosphorylated in the absence of glucose 6-phosphatase so as to appear in the bloodstream as free glucose. The administration of glycerol, another glucogenic substance, has been advocated in that it can be administered either parenterally or orally. As with fructose or galactose, there is no rise of blood glucose after glycerol. Apparently large quantities of glucose 6-phosphate are disposed of by increasing the amounts carried through the steps of anaerobic glycolysis resulting in an increased production and release of lactic and pyruvic acids; thus, hyperlacticacidemia is a characteristic finding in the syndrome and can be strikingly augmented by the administration of glucagon or other stimuli of hepatic glycogenolysis. Although ketonemia, lipemia, and ketonuria are frequently observed, because of the relative unavailability of glycogen stores and the resultant hypoglycemia which triggers mobilization of fat to meet energy requirements, marked and dangerous lactic acidosis is also frequent and may supervene precipitously. It is believed that

FIGURE 111-1
Pathways of glycogen synthesis and breakdown.

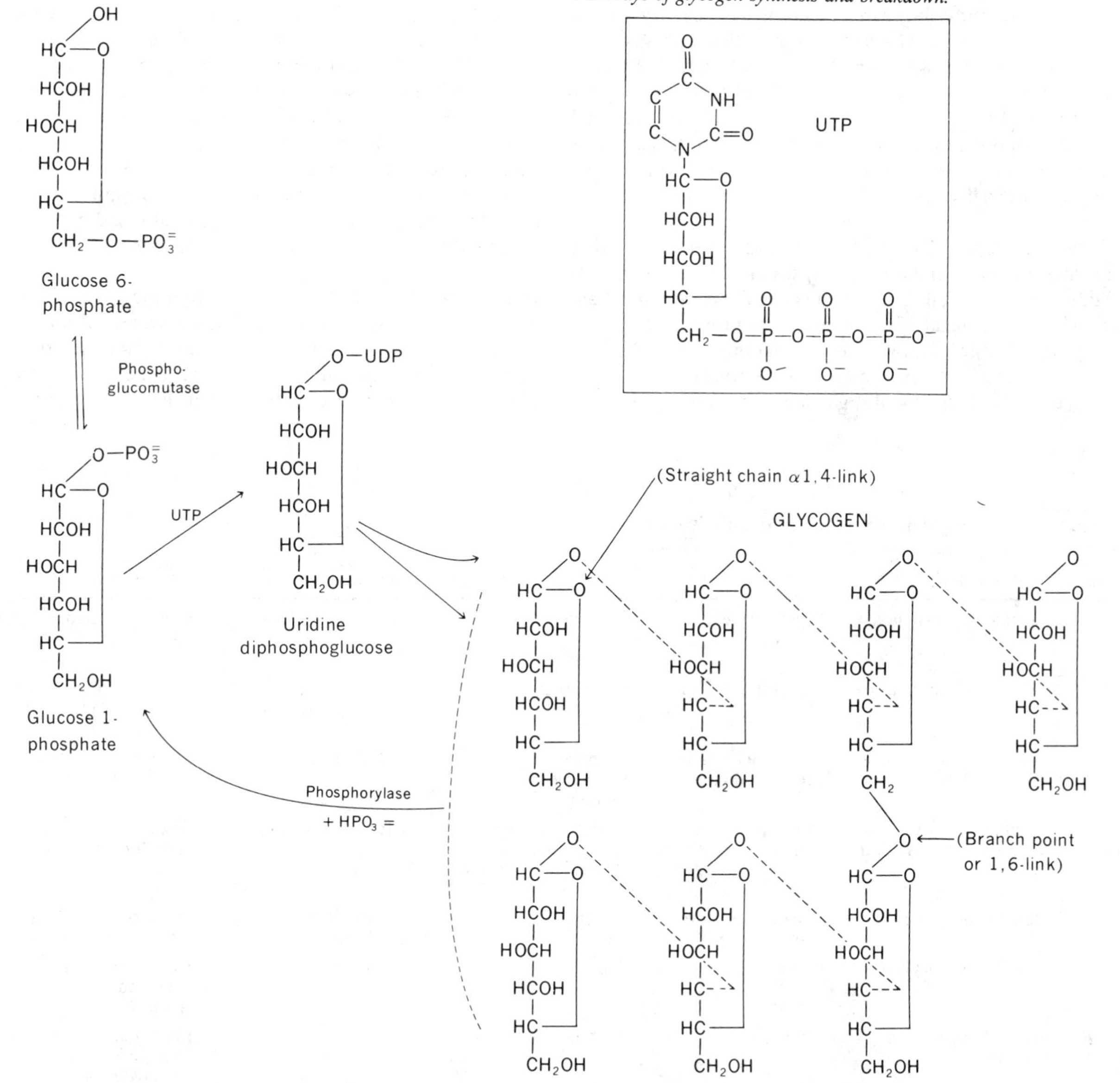

the chronic hyperlacticacidemia is responsible for disturbance in renal clearance of water and accounts for the hyperuricemia seen in this condition. Chronic acidosis on a cellular level may play a role in the generally retarded growth, mild normochromic unresponsive anemia, hypophosphatemia, and generalized decreased bone density with mushrooming of the metaphyses and frequent fractures observed in these patients. Glycosuria and nonspecific aminoaciduria without aminoacidemia also occur and may be striking. It has been suggested that these findings correlate with the severity of glycogen infiltration and the hypothetically intracellular accumulation of phosphorylated hexoses in the renal tubular cells; but other impairments of renal function are not prominent.

Pathology In some cases a marked hemorrhagic diathesis occurs, characterized by prolonged bleeding time and an abnormal deficiency in platelet adhesiveness, perhaps related to the accumulation of glycogen platelets. The liver is markedly enlarged, smooth, firm, and brownish in color. Microscopic study shows the liver cells to be enlarged up to three times the normal size and to be filled with glycogen and at times excessive amounts of fat. In the kidneys, which are usually at least double normal size, intracellular excess of glycogen is found in the cells of the proximal tubules. That the excess of glycogen persists in these organs long after death is not surprising when the nature of the biochemical defect is recalled.

Clinical picture The child is pale and undersized, with a fat face and neck and a markedly distended abdomen containing a huge, easily palpable liver without associated ascites or splenomegaly. Xanthomas with prominent lipemia may be a feature. Occasionally, epileptiform seizures and vomiting occur; however, more often the gravity and prevalence of the low blood sugar level are not appreciated until serious central nervous system deterioration has resulted. Remission of the hypoglycemia occurs in some patients after puberty. The pathogenesis of this change has not been fully explained, although an attractive theory has been the increased cycling of glycogen with release of increasing numbers of glucose molecules at branch points by the action of branching enzyme.

Laboratory examinations These examinations reveal fasting hypoglycemia, hyperlipidemia, hyperlacticacidemia, anemia, and, at times, ketonemia, and ketonuria. After glucose ingestion or infusion, the fall of blood levels may be delayed, yielding a pseudodiabetic curve. This may be explained as impaired capacity to increase the already superabundant stores of liver glycogen, rather than as a failure to utilize glucose at a normal rate in peripheral tissues. There is hypersensitivity to insulin, and severe prolonged hypoglycemia may follow its administration. Suspicion of this disorder is warranted when typical clinical characteristics are present and consonant results with glucagon or epinephrine challenge tests and of galactose, fructose, or glycerol infusion have been obtained. Final diagnosis, as with all glycogenoses, rests on biochemical assay of enzyme activity in biopsy material, in this instance, liver. In typical cases, glucose 6-phosphatase activity is found to be absent or reduced to less than 10 percent of normal in the liver and absent in the mucosa of the small intestine. There is no ready explanation for the three cases reported in which glucose 6-phosphatase activity was either normal or only moderately reduced despite the careful characterization of the cases as clinically and pathophysiologically entirely consistent with the diagnosis.

Differential diagnosis The sporadic reports of cases of liver glycogenosis in which multiple enzymatic abnormalities in the glycogen pathways can be demonstrated and other cases in which members of the same kinship have distinctly different enzymatic lesions have given rise to

TABLE 111-1
Disorders of glycogen deposition and mobilization

Cori type	*Enzyme defect*	*Organ*	*Glycogen structure*	*Eponymic name*	*Suggested clinical name*
1	Glucose 6-phosphatase	Liver, kidney, intestine (?)	Normal	von Gierke's disease	Glucose 6-phosphatase deficiency hepatorenal glycogenosis
2	α-Glucosidase (maltase)	Generalized	Normal	Pompe's disease	α-Glucosidase deficiency generalized glycogenosis
3	Amylo-1,6-glucosidase (debrancher)	Liver, heart, muscle, leukocytes	Abnormal; missing or very short outer chains	Forbes' disease	Debrancher deficiency limit dextrinosis
4	Amylo-(1,4:1,6) transglucosidase (brancher)	Liver, probably other organs	Abnormal; very long inner and outer unbranched chains	Andersen's disease	Brancher deficiency amylopectinosis
5	Muscle phosphorylase	Skeletal and cardiac muscle	Normal	McArdle-Schmid-Pearson disease	Myophosphorylase deficiency glycogenosis
6 *A*	Liver phosphorylase	Liver	Normal	Hers' disease	Hepatophosphorylase deficiency glycogenosis
B	Liver phosphorylase kinase	Liver	Normal		Phosphorylase kinase deficiency glycogenosis

both diagnostic and conceptual confusion. At present, it is not clear whether such cases result from secondarily induced adaptations, a close relation of chromosomal genetic loci for determining and controlling the formation of the different enzymes, or from the influences of environmental factors. Until further investigations clarify these situations or augment the details of pathways of glycogen metabolism, the nonrestrictive labeling of cases that do not fit, either biochemically or functionally, into the classic groupings as simply "liver glycogen disease" seems wise.

Treatment Although no means of increasing tissue activity levels of glucose 6-phosphatase in typical cases is available, earlier diagnosis, combined with recognition of hypoglycemia, acidosis, and intercurrent infection as the causes of morbidity and mortality, has markedly improved the life expectancy in this disease. The observation that the disturbances in metabolism and function in patients who survive beyond the fifth year tend to ameliorate provokes inquiry into the biochemical mechanisms by which such could occur and points to the necessity for assiduous care of the afflicted infant. It appears that in cases with prolonged survival the hyperuricemia and urate deposition which result, especially in the kidneys, become the major causes of difficulties. For this the daily administration of 0.5 to 2.0 g probenecid (Benemid) may be employed (Chap. 107). The use of allopurinol, an inhibitor of urate formation, can also be recommended when secondary complications of hyperuricemia are manifested.

In a small number of cases, surgical transposition of the vena cava and the portal vein has been performed with clinical improvement in hypoglycemia. Diazoxide, a thiazide compound with capability of inhibiting insulin release, has been shown to improve hypoglycemia in some cases.

α-GLUCOSIDASE DEFICIENCY GENERALIZED GLYCOGENOSIS This disorder, the most devastating form of glycogenosis, causes death within the first two years of life. It is marked by a generalized deposition of glycogen and by striking cardiomegaly. Symptoms and signs appear within one or two months after birth and quickly produce an infant with marked muscular hypotonia, enlarged tongue, cretinoid appearance, cardiomegaly, and neurologic deficits. Increased susceptibility to recurrent respiratory infections is based on poor ventilative and tussive efforts.

The structure of isolated glycogen is normal, and hyperglycemia promptly follows glucagon or epinephrine administration or the infusion of galactose or fructose. Glycogen accumulation in vacuoles located in the cytoplasm of almost all body cells occurs to a variable degree and is a process in which the leukocytes participate. The principal mechanisms of death are cardiac failure and pneumonitis. The disease is familial in occurrence, and the mode of inheritance appears to be through a single recessive autosomal gene.

Hers has demonstrated in the tissues of five affected infants the absence of a normally ubiquitous α-(1 → 4) glucosidase which has optimum activity in the acid range. The enzyme characteristically hydrolyzes maltose and glycogen to glucose and can catalyze the transglucosylation from maltose to glycogen. Present hypotheses regarding glycogen metabolism do not provide a locus of influence at which this enzyme could effect glycogen deposition. Furthermore, spontaneous glycogenolysis occurs in excised tissues. Hers emphasizes the possible lysosomal nature of the enzyme and suggests that the polysaccharide accumulation is the result of a failure of physiologic digestion of areas of cytoplasm by the defective lysosomes. This interpretation is in agreement with the clinical observations of an absence of hypoglycemia, ketosis, and hyperlipidemia and the concept that the manifestations are the result of disruption of muscle fibers by the progressive glycogen accumulation. Although the clinical picture is highly characteristic, diagnosis depends on the demonstration of the absence of the acid α-(1 → 4)glucosidase in biopsy material.

Electron microscopic studies have demonstrated two forms of cytoplasmic glycogen aggregates, a monogranular and a multigranular. The ensacculated membrane-limited vacuoles found only in this condition probably represent lysosomes which have autophaged large amounts of monogranular glycogen and are unable to digest it because of their deficiency of acid maltase.

Treatment is unavailing, although chemotherapy of intercurrent bacterial respiratory infections appears to prolong life.

DEBRANCHER ENZYME DEFICIENCY (LIMIT DEXTRINOSIS) AND BRANCHER ENZYME DEFICIENCY (AMYLOPECTINOSIS) These two conditions are the result of defects of the enzymes concerned with the formation and the disengagement of the branch points of the typically arborized glycogen molecule (types 3 and 4 in Table 111-1). In the first instance, there is a deficiency of the specific enzyme required for cleavage of the branch point bond, and therefore glycogenolysis is interrupted as the first branch point is reached and a glycogen of abnormal structure with excessively frequent branch points and shortened inner and outer chains results. When the branching enzyme is deficient, an unusually structured glycogen which possesses excessively lengthened inner and outer chains and a paucity of branch points is produced. Apparently, this structure formation, which resembles that of plant starch, gives the polysaccharide the physical characteristics which lead to its sequestration within the cells, where it acts as an irritative nidus, producing a characteristic increase in periportal connective tissue and inflammatory cell infiltration.

Limit dextrinosis is a relatively frequent type of glycogenosis; amylopectinosis is exceedingly rare, only a few cases having been recognized. Since the clinical picture of the debrancher deficiency disturbance (limit dextrinosis) so closely resembles a mild form of the glucose 6-phosphatase deficiency, many cases of the former were mistakenly diagnosed as the latter before precise enzymatic assay techniques were available. The confusion need no longer arise even on clinical grounds or on the basis of functional tests, for in limit dextrinosis infusions of galactose lead to prompt intrahepatic conversion to glucose, with prompt hyperglycemia, there being no impediment to dephosphorylation and release. In the differential diagnosis in cases with equivocal hyperglycemic responses to glucagon or epinephrine and in which hepatomegaly, growth retardation, and a tendency to hypoglycemia and ketonuria contribute uncertainty, a liver biopsy need not be done, since it has been demonstrated that the debrancher enzyme is also absent in leukocytes, muscle, and erythrocytes. Furthermore, fasting levels of lactate and pyruvate are likely to be normal, in contrast to the situation with the type 1 case (glucose 6-phosphatase deficiency), where they are distinctly elevated. In the type 3 case, erythrocyte glycogen content is elevated, but again this is not so in the type 1 individual.

Prognosis for the type 3 defect appears to be relatively good, and at least two patients with this condition have reached the fifth decade of life. Logical treatment consists of a high-protein, relatively low fat diet, with frequent feedings, prompt treatment of intercurrent infections, and prohibition of strenuous exercise, cardiodepressant drugs, and anesthetics, since the myocardium may be involved.

GLYCOGEN DEPOSITION SYNDROMES DUE TO DEFICIENCIES OF GLYCOGEN PHOSPHORYLASES Glycogen phosphorylase (type 5, Table 111-1) catalyzes glycogen depolymerization by phosphorylytic cleavage to yield glucose 1-phosphate and thus mediates the major initiating step in making the glucose moieties available for metabolism. In the liver the bulk of the glucose derived from the action of this enzyme ultimately defends the level of blood sugar and maintains an adequate supply for the peripheral tissues, while in the muscle the phosphorylase-produced hexose phosphate provides an immediate fuel source for the energy demanded by quick, sharp increases in contractile activity. Muscle and liver phosphorylase are distinctly different proteins immunologically, structurally, and functionally, and it appears that each has its own genetic determinant. Both enzyme activities are enhanced by epinephrine, while only liver phosphorylase responds in vivo to injections of glucagon.

MYOPHOSPHORYLASE DEFICIENCY GLYCOGENOSIS (McARDLE) A group of patients consisting of members of several unrelated families have been shown to be lacking in muscle phosphorylase activity. None has any growth retardation, disturbance in carbohydrate economy, or abnormality of response to glucagon or epinephrine administration. However, they have in common an incapacity to perform prolonged or strenuous muscle work and are excessively sensitive to ischemic conditions in this regard because of the occurrence of weakness, pain, and spasm of the exercised muscle. An interesting "second-wind" phenomenon in which muscle pain abates as exercise is continued has been observed in some patients. The demonstration of the isolated absence of muscle phosphorylase adequately explains the clinical phenomena when the importance of brisk glycogenolysis in supplying substrate for anaerobic glycolysis during ischemic muscle work is recalled. The impediment limiting the acceleration and augmentation of anaerobic glycolysis thus curtails increased lactate production. The failure to detect a significant rise in lactate concentration in the venous return from a muscle working under imposed ischemic conditions is a useful diagnostic test. A modest excess of glycogen in the muscles has been described, and in some cases prolonged exercise may cause breakdown of muscle cells and myoglobinuria. Although it has been shown that cardiac muscle shares the defect, no cardiac disturbance on this account has been described.

Since liver phosphorylase is normal in amount and activity, patients do quite well provided they accept limitations in exertion, protect themselves from tight garments that produce muscle ischemia, and fortify themselves with exogenous carbohydrates before attempting unusual physical tasks.

Patients with a clinical picture similar to that of myophosphorylase deficiency who have normal muscle phosphorylase activity but markedly reduced muscle phosphofructokinase activity have been described. Myoglobinuria and defective response of serum lactate to ischemic exercise have also been observed in these patients. An autosomal recessive mode of inheritance has been suggested.

HEPATOPHOSPHORYLASE DEFICIENCY GLYCOGENOSIS (HERS) Isolated development of hepatomegaly in infancy or childhood with a tendency to fasting hypoglycemia due to excessive accumulation of hepatic glycogen of normal structure characterizes this condition. Little in the way of other metabolic or developmental disturbance accrues as a consequence of the sluggish glycogenolysis which results from the partial reduction of hepatophosphorylase activity. The deficiency of the enzyme can be demonstrated biochemically in hepatic tissue or in leukocytes. No therapy beyond avoidance of prolonged fasting and the administration of a high-protein diet with frequent feedings appears to be necessary. The mechanism of failure of hyperglycemic response to glucagon or epinephrine is obvious, and the normal response to galactose infusion as well as the normal serum lactate level and lack of hyperlipemia allows easy differentiation of this disease from the more devastating glucose 6-phosphatase deficiency. Transmission appears to be by means of an autosomal recessive gene.

An interesting variant of this form of glycogenosis has been observed in a number of patients with this same mild clinical picture. Absence of hepatic phosphorylase kinase activity leading to an inability to activate hepatic phosphorylase has been documented in biopsied material from several of these patients. This form of glycogenosis is inherited as an X-linked recessive trait, the only form of glycogen storage disease with this mode of inheritance. No specific treatment is known.

A number of patients with apparent hepatic glycogen storage disease do not have the enzyme deficiencies described above and, therefore, do not fit into this classification. Further studies of glycogen and carbohydrate metabolism in these patients will be necessary before a complete classification of the glycogenoses can be made.

REFERENCES

DRASH A, FIELD JB: The glycogen storage diseases. DM October, 1971

HOWELL RR: The glycogen storage diseases, in *The Metabolic Basis of Inherited Disease,* eds JB Stanbury et al, 4th ed., New York: McGraw-Hill (in press)

MCADAMS JA et al: Glycogen storage disease types I to X. Criteria for morphologic diagnosis. Hum Pathol 5:463, 1974

112 GALACTOSEMIA

KURT J. ISSELBACHER

DEFINITION Galactosemia refers to an inborn error of metabolism associated with an impairment in the metabolism of galactose. Two disorders are currently recognized. "Classic" galactosemia is due to the deficiency of the enzyme galactose 1-phosphate uridyl transferase; it is typically associated with cataract formation, mental retardation, and cirrhosis. The second disorder, first described in 1965, is due to galactokinase deficiency and leads primarily to cataract formation.

PATHOGENESIS Lactose, the main carbohydrate in milk, is a disaccharide containing galactose and glucose; when ingested it is hydrolyzed by intestinal lactase. Normally the absorbed galactose is converted in the liver to glucose. The first reaction in this pathway involves the phosphorylation of galactose to galactose 1-phosphate by galactokinase:

$$\text{Galactose} + \text{ATP} \xrightarrow{\text{galactokinase}} \text{galactose 1-phosphate}$$

The gene for galactokinase has been assigned to chromosome 17. The next step involves the conversion of galactose 1-phosphate to glucose 1-phosphate. This involves the participation of uridine diphosphate (UDP) sugars and the enzyme galactose 1-phosphate uridyl transferase as follows:

$$\text{Galactose 1-phosphate} + \text{UDP-glucose} \xrightarrow{\text{transferase}} \text{UDP-galactose} + \text{glucose 1-phosphate}$$

The UDP sugars can be reversibly interconverted by an epimerase reaction:

$$\text{UDP-galactose} \underset{}{\overset{\text{epimerase}}{\rightleftharpoons}} \text{UDP-glucose}$$

Several alternate pathways of galactose metabolism appear to exist. Galactose can be converted (reduced) in the presence of NADPH (or NADH) to galactitol (dulcitol) by aldose reductase, an enzyme which occurs especially in the lens. Galactose can be oxidized to a limited extent by galactose dehydrogenase leading eventually to the formation of galactonic acid, xylulose, and CO_2. There is also a pyrophosphorylase reaction involving the interaction of galactose 1-phosphate with uridine triphosphate to form UDP-galactose. One or more of these pathways may account for a limited galactose metabolism in some patients with galactosemia.

In galactokinase deficiency, galactose accumulates in the blood and tissues. In the lens galactose is converted by aldose reductase to galactitol, a sugar to which the lens is impermeable. As a consequence, excessive hydration occurs which, together with a decrease in lenticular glutathione, leads to cataract formation.

In classic galactosemia, transferase deficiency leads to tissue accumulation of galactose 1-phosphate and galactose. As in galactokinase deficiency, cataracts develop secondary to galactitol accumulation in the lens. It is assumed but not proved that the cirrhosis and mental retardation of classic galactosemia are in some manner related to increased amounts of galactose 1-phosphate in these tissues. Elevated blood galactose levels may lead to a decreased hepatic output of glucose and hypoglycemia. In the kidney and intestine, accumulation of galactose and galactose 1-phosphate appears to lead to an inhibition of amino acid transport.

Both galactokinase- and transferase-deficiency galactosemia are transmitted as autosomal recessive traits. Heterozygotes for these disorders have half-normal enzyme levels but are asymptomatic. Maternal deficiency of galactokinase, together with a significant lactose intake during pregnancy, may contribute to cataract formation during fetal development. However, not all persons with half-normal transferase enzymes in their cells are carriers of galactosemia. Some individuals homozygous for another gene, called the Duarte variant, normally have only half-normal transferase levels. This group can be differentiated from galactosemia heterozygotes on the basis of the electrophoretic properties of the mutant enzyme. In both types of galactosemia, the disorder is due either to the functional deficiency or absence of the involved enzyme. In the classic type of galactosemia there is evidence that the disorder is due to a structural gene mutation and that the enzyme (transferase) protein is present but structurally altered and not functioning normally.

The exact incidence of classic galactosemia is still unclear. Estimates range from 1 in 18,000 to 1 in 100,000 births. Population studies indicate that 0.8 to 1.3 percent of the population are heterozygous for the galactosemia gene and about 10 percent carry the Duarte variant.

CLINICAL FEATURES Symptoms of classic galactosemia usually begin within days to several weeks after birth. The infant usually is reluctant to ingest breast milk or milk formulas, develops vomiting, shows poor nutrition, and fails to thrive. Jaundice, hepatomegaly, and evidence of liver disease may then develop. Cataracts are usually not present at birth but occur gradually over a period of weeks to months. Mental retardation may be difficult to detect but becomes evident after 6 or 12 months. The only recognized complication of galactokinase deficiency is cataract formation.

DIAGNOSIS Galactokinase deficiency should be suspected in infants or children with cataract formation who have non-glucose-reducing substances in their urine. The diagnosis is made by demonstrating the deficiency of galactokinase in red blood cells.

Classic galactosemia must be considered when one or more of the clinical features described above are found. If the patient is ingesting milk, reducing sugar may be found in the urine, which gives a negative glucose oxidase reaction (i.e., is not glucose) and is identified as galactose by other techniques, such as chromatography. If the child is vomiting, has a poor food intake, or is on intravenous glucose feedings, galactose may not be present in the urine. The definitive diagnosis consists of demonstrating a lack or deficiency of red cell galactose 1-phosphate uridyl transferase. A variety of assay techniques have been described. The disease can also be diagnosed prenatally by enzyme studies on cultured cells obtained by amniocentesis.

In the neonatal period galactosemia needs to be differentiated from primary liver disease. With liver damage, galactose removal from the blood is impaired, and elevated blood galactose levels as well as galactosuria may occur. However, in hepatitis or cirrhosis the transferase levels will be normal.

TREATMENT The treatment of galactosemia consists of the removal of galactose-containing foods from the diet, especially milk. In infants, milk substitutes such as Dextri-Maltose and Nutramigen are often used. Soybean preparations have also been used in the past, but their polysaccharides contain some galactose and they should be avoided.

The institution of a galactose-free diet usually leads to a dramatic improvement in the patient; in fact, all clinical features except for mental retardation may improve or disappear. In general, patients are kept on galactose-free diets indefinitely or at least until they have reached adequate physical and neurologic development.

REFERENCES

GITZELMANN R et al: Galactose metabolism in a patient with hereditary galactokinase deficiency. Eur J Clin Invest 4:79, 1974

SEGAL S: Disorders of galactose metabolism, in *The Metabolic Basis of Inherited Disease,* 3d ed., eds JB Stanbury et al, New York: McGraw Hill, 1972, p. 174

TEDESCO TA et al: The genetic defect in galactosemia. N Engl J Med 292:737, 1975

113 DISORDERS OF LIPID METABOLISM AND XANTHOMATOSES

DONALD S. FREDRICKSON

Lipidosis is a general term applied to disorders characterized by abnormal concentrations of lipids in tissues or in extracellular fluid. Sometimes it is restricted to only those abnormalities of lipid metabolism that are inheritable. *Xanthomatosis* is a morphologic term referring to lipid accumulation in tissues in association with large *foam cells.* The list of lipidoses and xanthomatoses in Table 113-1 encompasses most of the *primary* disturbances in lipid metabolism and includes some disorders in which secondary lipid storage is prominent and some of the disorders of adipose tissue. Omitted are several disorders in which lipids accumulate concomitantly with primary abnormalities in metabolism of other substances. Noteworthy among these are mucopolysaccharidoses and the glycogen storage diseases.

PLASMA LIPOPROTEIN ABNORMALITIES

The commonest of the lipidoses are those that feature alterations in concentrations of the plasma lipids. These can usually be detected and diagnosed by measurements of cholesterol and triglyceride concentrations in plasma. It is easier to understand these disorders, however, when they are considered in terms of lipoproteins, the form in which nearly all lipids, except free fatty acids, are present in plasma. Both selective increases and severe deficiency or absence of some of the groups or classes of lipoproteins can occur. Abnormalities in the lipoproteins themselves characterize very few disorders. Usually the lipoproteins are simply markers for intracellular abnormalities in lipid or carbohydrate metabolism that are reflected in abnormal plasma concentrations of lipids.

HYPERLIPOPROTEINEMIA

Increased concentrations of plasma lipids and lipoproteins represent metabolic problems that are difficult both to classify and to treat. Diagnosis proceeds in the following manner:

1. Measurement of plasma cholesterol *and* triglyceride concentrations after an overnight fast. For at least 2 weeks prior to the sampling, the patient should be maintaining steady weight, eating the diet usual for the population, and not taking drugs known to affect plasma lipid concentrations. As a rule, *hyperlipidemia* is present in any individual below the age of 50 years whose cholesterol concentration exceeds 240 mg per 100 ml or triglyceride exceeds 200 mg per 100 ml.
2. Screening for diseases to which hyperlipidemia may be *secondary* (such as hypothyroidism, obstructive liver disease, poorly controlled insulinopenic diabetes mellitus, plasma protein abnormalities. Treatment of secondary hyperlipidemia is directed at the underlying disease.
3. Translation of *primary hyperlipidemia* to a particular lipoprotein pattern. For this purpose the essential tests are the cholesterol and triglyceride determinations, observation of plasma after it stands overnight at 4°C for a *chylomicron* layer at the top, and an estimation of low-density lipoprotein (LDL, beta-lipoprotein) concentration (Table 113-2). Lipoprotein electrophoresis is not essential, and preparative ultracentrifugation is necessary only for a certain diagnosis of type III hyperlipoproteinemia.
4. Careful examination for xanthomas.
5. Examination of first-degree relatives. The last step is necessary to establish genetically determined hyperlipoproteinemia.

Classification of primary hyperlipidemia or hyperlipoproteinemia (HLP) continues to evolve. Nearly all hyperlipidemia can be converted to one of six abnormal lipoprotein patterns by arbitrary guides shown in Table 113-2. As Table 113-1 indicates, a given type of HLP does not signify a single disease. It also does not indicate whether the disorder is familial; and, in some familial disorders, a single abnormal genotype may be expressed in more than one lipoprotein or lipid pattern. For the practicing physician, the value of determining the type of hyperlipoproteinemia is its frequent association with certain clinical manifestations and its tendency to respond to relatively specific forms of therapy.

HYPERCHYLOMICRONEMIA (TYPE I HLP) This lipoprotein pattern reflects severe disability in removal of dietary triglycerides (in chylomicrons) from plasma without any marked increase in endogenous glycerides (pre-beta-lipoproteins). Normally, chylomicrons are not visible upon gross inspection or by electrophoresis of plasma drawn in the postabsorptive state. In type I HLP there is marked hyperchylomicronemia and a decrease in all other lipopro-

TABLE 113-1
Lipidoses and xanthomatoses

I Abnormal plasma lipoprotein concentrations
- *A* Hyperlipoproteinemia (HLP) or hyperlipidemia
  - *1* Hyperchylomicronemia (exogenous hyperglyceridemia; type I HLP)
    - *a* Primary
      - *(1)* Familial lipoprotein lipase deficiency
      - *(2)* Other
    - *b* Secondary, to
      - *(1)* Paraproteinemia
      - *(2)* Uncontrolled diabetes mellitus
  - *2* Hyperbetalipoproteinemia (hypercholesterolemia; type IIa HLP)
    - *a* Primary
      - *(1)* Familial monogenic disorders
        - *(a)* Familial hypercholesterolemia
        - *(b)* Familial combined hyperlipidemia, phenotypic variant of
      - *(2)* Other familial disorders
      - *(3)* Dietary-induced and other sporadic forms
    - *b* Secondary to other diseases
  - *3* Hyperbeta- and hyperprebetalipoproteinemia (mixed hypercholesterolemia and hyperglyceridemia; type IIb HLP)
    - *a* Primary
      - *(1)* Familial combined hyperlipidemia, phenotypic variant of
      - *(2)* Familial hypercholesterolemia, phenotypic variant of
      - *(3)* Other familial disorders
      - *(4)* Sporadic forms
    - *b* Secondary to other diseases
  - *4* Type III HLP ("floating-beta" or "broad-beta" disorder; dysbetalipoproteinemia)
    - *a* Primary (usually familial)
    - *b* Secondary to hypothyroidism, uncontrolled diabetes mellitus, or paraproteinemia
  - *5* Hyperprebetalipoproteinemia (endogenous hyperglyceridemia; type IV HLP)
    - *a* Primary
      - *(1)* Monogenic familial disorders
        - *(a)* Familial combined hyperlipidemia, phenotypic variant of
        - *(b)* "Pure" endogenous hyperglyceridemia
      - *(2)* Other familial forms
      - *(3)* Sporadic forms
    - *b* Secondary to other diseases
  - *6* Hyperchylomicronemia and hyperprebetalipoproteinemia (mixed hyperglyceridemia; type V HLP: sometimes a variant expression of severe hyperprebetalipoproteinemia)
    - *a* Primary
      - *(1)* Familial form(s)
      - *(2)* Sporadic
    - *b* Secondary to paraproteinemia, uncontrolled diabetes mellitus, nephrotic syndrome, and other diseases
- *B* Dyslipoproteinemia (circulation of abnormally lipidated lipoproteins)
  - *1* Hyperlipidemia of obstructive jaundice
  - *2* Familial lecithin: cholesterol acyltransferase (LCAT) deficiency
  - *3* Type III HLP (see above)
- *C* Hypolipoproteinemia
  - *1* Primary
    - *a* Familial diseases
      - *(1)* Abetalipoproteinemia
      - *(2)* Hypobetalipoproteinemia
      - *(3)* Tangier disease (alpha-lipoprotein deficiency)
    - *b* Sporadic or subtle genetic variations?
  - *2* Secondary to malabsorption, paraproteinemias, and possibly other diseases

II Lipid storage diseases due to deficient activity of a lysosomal enzyme
- *A* Beta-galactosidase deficiencies
  - *1* G_{M_1} gangliosidosis
    - *a* Generalized gangliosidosis (type I)
    - *b* Juvenile G_{M_1} gangliosidosis (type II)
  - *2* Krabbe's globoid cell leukodystrophy
  - *3* Lactosyl ceramidosis
- *B* Alpha-galactosidase deficiency (Fabry's disease; angiokeratoma corporis diffusum universale)
- *C* Beta-glucosidase deficiency (Gaucher's disease)
  - *1* Nonneuronopathic ("adult")
  - *2* Acute neuronopathic ("infantile")
  - *3* Chronic neuronopathic ("juvenile")
- *D* Cerebroside sulfatase deficiency (metachromatic leukodystrophy)
  - *1* Late infantile form
  - *2* Adult form
  - *3* Variant with multiple sulfatase deficiencies
- *E* Ganglioside G_{M_2}-hexosaminidase deficiencies
  - *1* Type 1, Tay-Sachs disease (hexosaminidase A deficiency)
  - *2* Type 2 (hexosaminidases A and B deficiency)
  - *3* Type 3 (lesser hexosaminidase A deficiency)
- *F* Sphingomyelinase deficiencies
  - *1* Clear-cut enzyme deficiency (massive sphingomyelin storage)
    - *a* Acute neuronopathic form (type A; classic Niemann-Pick disease)
    - *b* Nonneuronopathic form (type B)
  - *2* Possible deficiency (mild sphingomyelin excess)
    - *a* Juvenile or delayed neuronopathic form (type C)
    - *b* Nova Scotia variant (type D)
- *G* Ceramidase deficiency (Farber's disease; disseminated lipogranulomatosis)
- *H* Acid cholesteryl ester hydrolase and triglyceride lipase deficiencies
  - *1* Wolman's disease
  - *2* Cholesteryl ester storage disease

III Phytanic oxidase deficiency (storage of 3,7,11,15-tetramethyl hexadecanoic acid; Refsum's disease; heredopathia atactica polyneuritiformis)

IV Granulomatous diseases with lipid storage
- *A* Histiocytosis X (xanthoma disseminatum, eosinophilic granuloma, Hand-Schüller-Christian disease, Letterer-Siwe disease)
- *B* Lipoid proteinosis (Urbach-Wiethe disease)
- *C* Lipoid dermatoarthritis

V Other xanthomatoses
- *A* Secondary to paraproteinemias (with macroglobulinemia, multiple myeloma, other paraproteinemias)
- *B* With normolipoproteinemia
  - *1* Cerebrotendinous xanthomatosis (cholestanol storage disease)
  - *2* β-sitosterolemia and xanthomatosis
  - *3* Simple xanthomas
  - *4* Associated with trauma and chronic infections

VI Adipose tissue disorders
- *A* Relapsing panniculitis (Weber-Christian disease)
- *B* Lipodystrophy
  - *1* Lipomas
  - *2* Adiposis dolorosa (Dercum's disease)
  - *3* Insulin lipodystrophy
- *C* Lipoatrophy
  - *1* Partial (progressive lipodystrophy)
  - *2* Total (lipoatrophic diabetes mellitus)

teins. The plasma is milky, and the triglyceride concentration ranges from 1,500 to 15,000 mg per 100 ml. Within 3 to 5 days of institution of a fat-free diet, chylomicrons disappear, a modest increase in pre-beta-lipoproteins occurs, and beta- and alpha-lipoproteins increase but remain low; the plasma clears, glycerides are in the range of 200 to 500, and cholesterol is lower than 200. Such "pure" hyperchylomicronemia usually occurs in a rare familial syndrome.

Familial forms Hyperlipemia (lactescent plasma or serum due to hyperglyceridemia) dependent upon dietary fat intake was first reported in a child by Burger and Grutz in

1932; familial incidence was recorded by Hold, Aylward, and Timbres shortly thereafter. About 100 cases have since been discovered. The metabolic defect is believed to be deficient activity of the enzyme lipoprotein lipase. This enzyme facilitates removal of triglycerides at the capillary endothelial wall by promoting hydrolysis of the glyceride esters. The enzyme is "released" into plasma by heparin, and patients with this syndrome have uniquely low postheparin lipoprotein lipase activity.

CLINICAL PICTURE The disease is usually detected within the first decade, although sometimes not until early adulthood, usually when marked hyperlipemia is discovered during work-up for either sudden appearance of eruptive xanthomas, moderate hepatosplenomegaly, or bouts of severe abdominal pain. The latter usually follow a period of high fat intake. The pain is usually epigastric or midabdominal and rarely radiates to the back; it may be associated with signs of peritoneal irritation and fever and can mimic a number of acute abdominal emergencies. Recurrent pancreatitis is common and has been the cause of premature death in several patients. There is no evidence that familial hyperchylomicronemia is associated with accelerated vascular disease.

DIAGNOSIS In the untreated state, the triglyceride is greater than 1,000 mg per 100 ml, the chylomicron test is positive, and the heavy cream layer overlies a clear infranatant layer. The typical lipid and lipoprotein pattern and other manifestations in an otherwise healthy child or young adult provide a presumptive diagnosis if the acquired (secondary) form has been excluded. A fat-free diet should be administered for 1 week; the predicted changes in lipoproteins should occur rapidly. Familial hyperchylomicronemia is rare and sometimes is confused with more common mixed hyperglyceridemia (type V HLP). Patients with primary type V HLP differ in that (1) removal of fat from the diet is followed by rapid disappearance of chylomicrons from plasma, but pre-beta-lipoproteins tend to increase greatly, usually leaving plasma triglyceride concentrations well above 500 mg per 100 ml; (2) the protamine-sensitive (lipoprotein lipase) component of postheparin lipolytic activity is vanishingly small in familial hyperchylomicronemia, but usually normal in type V HLP; (3) the glucose intolerance and hyperinsulinemia that are very common in type V HLP are not characteristic of familial hyperchylomicronemia.

GENETICS The full-blown disorder appears in either sex. Vertical transmission has not been observed. The disorder(s) now perceived as familial hyperchylomicronemia usually appear to require a double dose of an abnormal allele for expression.

TABLE 113-2
Type of hyperlipoproteinemia as suggested by cholesterol (C) and triglyceride (TG) concentrations

C high; TG < 150	IIa
C high; TG 150–400	IIb, III*, or IV
C high; TG 400–1,000	III*, IV, or V†
C high; TG > 1,000	I†, or V†
C normal; TG > 150	IV

* *Suggested by broad beta band on electrophoresis, but positive diagnosis requires demonstration of abnormally high cholesterol content of very low density lipoproteins.*
† *Positive chylomicron tests.*

TREATMENT To avoid the crippling attacks of abdominal pain, pancreatitis, and foam-cell accumulation in liver, spleen, and bone marrow seen in most cases, it is recommended that the daily intake of fat be kept to 20 to 25 percent of calories or a maximum of 50 g fat per day. Both saturated and unsaturated fats are cleared poorly. Commercial preparations of medium-chain glycerides offer means of satisfying craving for fat without inducing chylomicronemia, since these glycerides go directly to the liver in the portal vein.

Secondary type I HLP Phenocopies of familial hyperchylomicronemia are produced by systemic lupus erythematosus or other diseases in which there are abnormal circulating globulins or other proteins. In such patients, heparin resistance, possibly due to heparin binding by the abnormal protein, is present and manifested by decreased prolongation of thrombin time. The hyperlipoproteinemia fluctuates with changes in the plasma protein abnormality. Depression of postheparin lipolytic activity also occurs in uncontrolled diabetes mellitus and may be associated with type I HLP. Treatment is directed toward the underlying diseases.

HYPERBETALIPOPROTEINEMIA (TYPE II HLP) Occasionally the concentration of alpha- or high-density lipoproteins may be uniquely elevated and produce plasma cholesterol concentrations of 250 to 300 mg per 100 ml. This hypercholesterolemia is not considered pathologic. It is perhaps most commonly seen in women receiving estrogens and can usually be detected from marked increase in staining of the alpha-lipoproteins on electrophoresis. Nearly always, however, hypercholesterolemia in the presence of a normal or modestly elevated triglyceride concentration means hyperbetalipoproteinemia (an increase in LDL concentrations). In the World Health Organization (WHO) classification, hyperbetalipoproteinemia alone is called type IIa HLP; when there is associated hyperglyceridemia, due to increased concentration of pre-beta- or very low density lipoproteins (VLDL), the pattern of hyperlipoproteinemia is called type IIb.

Mechanisms regulating the synthesis of cholesterol, its removal from plasma and conversion to bile acids, which are the principal excretion products of cholesterol, are among some of the important determinants of LDL concentrations. "Pure" hyperbetalipoproteinemia is likely due to alterations in such regulators and tends to be responsive to reduced dietary intake of sterol or saturated fats or to administration of bile acid sequestering resins. One of the major sources of plasma LDL is provided by catabolism of VLDL, the principal carriers of endogenous glycerides. Changes in VLDL turnover may lead to hyperbetalipoproteinemia and hyperglyceridemia. When VLDL metabolism is unstable, the VLDL and LDL concentrations may vary considerably over short periods of time. When this happens, the lipid pattern may shift variably between type IIa and type IIb HLP and simple endogenous hyperglyceridemia. Hyperbetalipoproteinemia is usually not present when triglycerides are greater than 400 mg per 100 ml. In the presence of lesser glyceride concentrations, one may estimate LDL concentrations in terms of their cholesterol content (C_{LDL}) by the formula

$$C_{LDL} = C - \left(\frac{TG}{5} + 45\right)$$

where C = plasma cholesterol
TG = plasma triglyceride concentration
45 = average for the cholesterol in high-density lipoprotein (HDL)

A C_{LDL} exceeding 170 may be considered as hyperbetalipoproteinemia.

Mild primary hyperbetalipoproteinemia is most commonly sporadic and usually is ameliorated by reducing the amount of cholesterol and saturated fat ingested. It is very rarely associated with xanthomas. Familial hyperbetalipoproteinemia can be recognized reliably only by family screening. There are at least two forms, which are expressed when a single abnormal (dominant) allele is present: *familial hypercholesterolemia* and *familial combined hyperlipidemia.*

Familial hypercholesterolemia (hypercholesterolemic xanthomatosis) This is the oldest known form of familial HLP. The presence of one abnormal gene causes hyperbetalipoproteinemia that is easily detectable by one year of age, and often at birth. Type II HLP may be the only abnormality throughout life, but subcutaneous xanthomas, particularly in the Achilles and extensor tendons of the hands, the elbows, and over the tibial tuberosities, and cutaneous xanthomas begin to appear at about age twenty. This is often accompanied by early evidence of atherosclerosis, particularly involving the coronary arteries. By age fifty, the risk of premature ischemic heart disease is three to ten times normal. Corneal arcus is common. Diabetes, hyperuricemia, or other abnormalities seen in other forms of hyperlipoproteinemia do not seem to be unusually frequent. Offspring of two affected parents (homozygotes) have more severe hyperbetalipoproteinemia; they may have cutaneous xanthomas at birth, and atherosclerosis is particularly severe, often leading to acquired aortic stenosis and death from ischemic heart disease between ages one and thirty. Familial hypercholesterolemia affects both sexes and occurs in Caucasoids and black and Oriental races. The gene prevalence in the United States is of the order of 1:1000. Normally LDL binds to cell membranes. This promotes LDL catabolism and regulates intracellular synthesis of cholesterol by depressing activity of hydroxymethyl glutaryl (HMG)-CoA reductase. LDL binding is partially defective in heterozygotes and nearly totally so in homozygotes. In the latter some of the excess cholesterol in tissues may be due to unbridled synthesis *in situ.* Several genetic variants of this defect are likely.

DIAGNOSIS On the usual American diet, children with familial hypercholesterolemia nearly always have a C_{LDL} greater than 165 mg per 100 ml. This cutoff point corresponds to a plasma cholesterol of between 220 and 240. The cholesterol in heterozygotes is usually between 250 and 500, the mean value being slightly higher in adults than children. Triglyceride concentrations are normal in 95 percent of children below age ten (type IIa HLP). The frequency of modest elevations up to 500 mg per 100 ml increases with age, and about one-third of adults have type IIb HLP. Homozygotes have cholesterol levels of 500 to 1,000. Demonstration of abnormal binding of LDL or excessive cholesterol synthesis is possible in tissue culture of skin fibroblasts. The diagnosis is otherwise presumptively based on the presence of hyperbetalipoproteinemia *and* tendon xanthomas in at least one parent (or both, for homozygotes) or other first-degree relatives. When the parental phenotypes are known, affected offspring can usually be diagnosed from values of C_{LDL} in cord blood.

TREATMENT Because tissue culture studies suggest that heterozygotes require higher LDL levels to regulate cell synthesis of cholesterol, arguments have been advanced against lowering plasma LDL. Imbibation of cholesterol by vascular intima is likely enhanced at high LDL concentrations, however, and the general practice is to reduce the dietary content of cholesterol and saturated fat as soon as diagnosis is made. This will nearly always reduce the hyperlipidemia by 10 to 20 percent, often more dramatically in younger children. Cholestyramine, in two to four divided doses totaling 16 to 24 g per day, will further lower plasma cholesterol by 15 to 30 percent. Present practice dictates use of the drug in heterozygotes who are between fifteen and fifty-five years of age and whose plasma cholesterol remains above 300 mg per 100 ml despite stringent diet. Homozygotes sometimes respond to cholestyramine alone, or in combination with nicotinic acid. Xanthomas will soften and disappear if hyperlipidemia is successfully suppressed.

Combined hyperlipidemia (multiple lipoprotein types) This is a much more common form of familial HLP. Either hypercholesterolemia (type IIa HLP), hyperglyceridemia (type IV), or the two in combination (type IIb) occurs in different first-degree relatives. Among adults, about half of such relatives are affected, children less frequently. The patients with type II HLP usually have cholesterol levels of 250 to 350 mg per 100 ml, rarely have xanthomatosis, tend to have much more variable lipid elevations, and may often convert from one abnormal lipoprotein pattern to another. These features help distinguish this abnormality from familial hypercholesterolemia. The hazard of premature ischemic heart disease is increased. There are no specific biochemical tests for diagnosis, and family screening is necessary for a presumptive diagnosis. The liability of the hyperlipidemia implies that triglyceride or VLDL metabolism is primarily affected. Therapy should first concentrate upon a diet that maintains ideal body weight and is prudent in content of cholesterol, saturated fats, and alcohol. When dietary measurements fail to lower cholesterol below 300 or triglycerides below 250, therapeutic trial of clofibrate, nicotinic acid, or possibly *d*-thyroxine should be considered. The usefulness of cholestyramine is not yet established.

Other familial or sporadic forms Neither of these syndromes may be considered to represent single mutants. There also probably are polygenic forms of hyperbetalipoproteinemia. Familial involvement must always be sought in the absence of specific biochemical tests for phenotypes.

The management of hyperbetalipoproteinemia of obscure origin proceeds empirically on the basis of distinctions already discussed for *familial hypercholesterolemia* and *combined hyperlipidemia.* It is also predicated on an unproved assumption that reduction in hyperlipidemia reduces the hazard of premature vascular disease, a premise that includes greater emphasis on younger patients.

TYPE III HYPERLIPOPROTEINEMIA This pattern is characterized by the presence of lipoproteins of density less than 1.006 that usually are beta-migrating ("floating beta"). The definitive test is the presence of an increased content of cholesterol in these cases of VLDL, a test which requires preparative ultracentrifugation. There are usually increased pre-beta-lipoproteins and often a positive visual test for chylomicrons. Half of patients have a broad beta band on electrophoresis, hence the synonym *broad-beta disease.* The cholesterol and glyceride concentrations tend to be similar, and fluctuate considerably between 200 and 1,000 mg per 100 ml. Type III hyperlipoproteinemia appears to be due to a marked increase in VLDL production; the usual catabolic pathways are overwhelmed, and "intermediate" lipoproteins accumulate that are otherwise never seen in quantity. The anomalous lipoproteins may be seen transiently with severe hypothyroidism or uncontrolled diabetes mellitus. They are most strikingly evident in a rare familial disorder.

Familial type III HLP CLINICAL PICTURE The disorder is rarely detected before age twenty, and manifests later in women unless the menopause has been hastened or severe obesity is present. In addition to the typical lipoprotein pattern, two-thirds of patients have peculiar raised yellow plaques (plane xanthomas) in the palmar creases or on the fingers. Most of them also have soft, reddish-yellow, single or confluent xanthomas on the elbows. Some have pedunculated xanthomas on the buttocks and elsewhere on the limbs; a few have tendon xanthomas. The majority of patients have intermittent claudication and evidence of decreased blood flow in the lower extremities; some have premature ischemic heart and cerebrovascular disease. Most have glucose intolerance, many are hypersecretors of insulin. Practically all are abnormally "carbohydrate-inducible," in terms of an exaggerated rise of plasma glycerides on high carbohydrate feeding. Hyperuricemia is common.

DIAGNOSIS The ascertainment of the characteristic lipoprotein pattern is necessary for absolute diagnosis. The VLDL have anomalous composition that persists at any level of hyperlipidemia. The usual pattern of severe mixed hyperlipidemia, when combined with palmar xanthomas and severe vascular disease, allows a presumptive diagnosis. On the average, half of adult first-degree relatives will have hyperlipidemia, which may be type III or type IV HLP. Abnormality rarely appears in children of propositi before they become adults.

TREATMENT The hyperlipidemia in type III HLP nearly always can be returned to normal with appropriate treatment. The skin xanthomas also disappear, lending encouragement that treatment may desirably affect the hazard for premature vascular disease. Treatment consists sequentially of (1) reduction to ideal weight; (2) institution of a rigorous diet, with special attention to keeping carbohydrate intake below 5 g/kg/day by increasing the intake of polyunsaturated fat, if necessary, and elimination of alcohol; and (3) clofibrate, 2 g per day. The therapeutic effect of these steps is additive. Lipids should be monitored at least every 3 months. Nicotinic acid, 3 g per day, may be used in place of clofibrate.

HYPERPREBETALIPOPROTEINEMIA (ENDOGENOUS HYPERGLYCERIDEMIA: TYPE IV HLP) The plasma triglyceride concentration reflects mainly the transport of glycerides that come directly from the diet (in chylomicrons) and others that are secreted from the liver, intestine, and perhaps other tissues (in VLDL or pre-beta-lipoproteins). When chylomicrons are not visible—and the anomalous lipoproteins of type III HLP are not present—increased plasma triglycerides are equated with endogenous hyperglyceridemia (type IV HLP). The diagnosis is thus not difficult (Table 113-2), but this belies the many possible causes of endogenous hyperglyceridemia. The secretion of VLDL is influenced by many emotional and hormonal factors controlling release into plasma of free fatty acids, the major precursors of endogenous glycerides, their uptake by liver, oxidation or conversion to glycerides, and secretion as VLDL. The hydrolysis of VLDL glycerides and their uptake and reesterification in adipose tissue are also important regulators of the triglyceride concentration.

Among determinants acting on these metabolic pathways are caloric balance, supply and utilization of carbohydrate, insulin activity, alcohol intake, estrogen administration, physical activity, and stress. Moderate hyperglyceridemia may therefore be secondary to many diseases and have many primary causes. Evidence is accumulating that hyperglyceridemia in the presence of normal cholesterol concentrations increases risk of premature ischemic heart disease.

Familial type IV HLP Endogenous hyperglyceridemia occurs in families in several disorders. These include the *familial combined hyperlipidemia* where it is one of the variant phenotypic expressions of a single gene. Hyperglyceridemia will be associated with significant hyperbetalipoproteinemia in some affected relatives. In *type III HLP* simple hyperglyceridemia also occurs in some relatives at a greater than expected frequency. The presence of anomalous lipoproteins in one or more relatives provides the diagnosis. There is also a *monogenic endogenous hyperglyceridemia* in which half of relatives have type IV HLP; expression is less frequent in children. This syndrome is one of the most common of all genetic disorders, the frequency of the responsible gene(s) being of the order of 1:500 in Americans. It is frequently accompanied by glucose intolerance and hyperuricemia and is worsened by obesity. There are no specific biochemical tests to establish any of the above phenotypes in a given patient with endogenous hyperglyceridemia. It is desirable to have as much information about the family as possible.

TREATMENT Management of *primary* endogenous hyperglyceridemia is presently the same regardless of the cause. It consists of (1) maintenance of ideal weight; (2) avoidance of an excess contribution of carbohydrate to total calories (less than 45 percent); (3) restriction of alcohol intake; (4) in patients where the above measures fail to lower glycerides below 250 to 300 mg per 100 ml, a therapeutic trial of clofibrate or nicotinic acid may be justified. Avoid use of nicotinic acid in diabetes. Because triglycerides tend to be variable, their concentration should be followed weekly during any trial of therapy.

Secondary forms Endogenous hyperglyceridemia occurs in many other diseases such as poorly controlled diabetes mellitus, hypothyroidism, dysproteinemias, the nephrotic syndrome, idiopathic hypercalcemia, Werner's syndrome, Tangier disease, LCAT deficiency (see below), and other lipidoses. Oral contraceptives and other estrogen-containing drugs may provoke hyperglyceridemia.

MIXED HYPERGLYCERIDEMIA (TYPE V HLP) Severe hyperglyceridemia, especially when the triglyceride concentration exceeds 1,000 (Table 113-2), usually implies chylomicronemia in addition to endogenous hyperglyceridemia. Upon standing, the turbid plasma separates into a cream layer overlying a turbid infranatant (VLDL). In some patients the plasma VLDL pool may be initially increased because of oversecretion of endogenous glycerides. This taxes the normal glyceride removal mechanisms, and chylomicrons also accumulate. Alternatively, triglyceride clearance itself may be defective. It is difficult to distinguish between these situations by any widely applicable clinical tests. Postheparin lipoprotein lipase activity is, at best, an indirect measure of the functional capacity for triglyceride removal. While the type V HLP secondary to uncontrolled diabetes mellitus is related to deficient maintenance of lipoprotein lipase activity by insulin, most instances of primary type V HLP are not associated with obvious deficiency in this enzyme activity.

Familial forms Patients with primary type V often come from families in which more than half of adult first-degree relatives have hyperglyceridemia, some with chylomicrons in the fasting state, others without them. It is probable that there are genetic differences between some of these families and many of the more common ones in which only lesser endogenous (type IV) hyperlipoproteinemia is present. There are no unique biochemical tests which segregate such families, however, or which allow one to determine whether primary type V HLP in a given patient is sporadic or familial. Most affected patients are adults.

CLINICAL FEATURES The majority of patients with primary type V HLP have glucose intolerance; many have hyperinsulinemia, and some complain of paresthesias ("diabetic neuropathy"?). Hyperuricemia and obesity are common, as is a history of excess ethanol intake. Bouts of abdominal pain, sometimes associated with chemical signs of pancreatitis, are typical and make this form of hyperlipoproteinemia potentially lethal. Hepatosplenomegaly, foam cells in bone marrow aspirates, lipemia retinalis, and eruptive xanthomas also may be present. There is probably an increased hazard of premature vascular disease.

TREATMENT All patients are benefited by some restriction in fat intake, but very severe restriction (below 40 g fat per day) is difficult to maintain, and the resultant increase in carbohydrate content of the diet sometimes causes marked increases in VLDL. Maintenance of ideal weight is usually helpful in suppressing the plasma glyceride elevations. Nicotinic acid (1.5 to 3.0 g per day) is sometimes very effective and may keep patients free of abdominal pain for years. Alcohol and estrogens are to be avoided.

Secondary type V HLP All the diseases which may cause type IV HLP may sometimes give rise to this more severe form of hyperglyceridemia. The patient's fat intake may often determine whether chylomicronemia complicates lesser degrees of endogenous hyperglyceridemia. It is not known how often pancreatitis produces hyperglyceridemia; the reverse definitely occurs.

OTHER HYPERLIPOPROTEINEMIAS

All hyperlipidemia is not encompassed in these major lipoprotein patterns. Notable exceptions are hypercholesterolemia and hyperphospholipidemia associated with obstructive liver disease. This is accompanied by the presence of abnormal lipoproteins (Lp-X). It is detected by the combination of jaundice, hypercholesterolemia, and a great increase in *unesterified* plasma cholesterol, or by use of antiserums to Lp-X. Abnormally lipidated lipoproteins also accompany hyperlipidemia in familial LCAT deficiency, and possibly other lipidoses described below. *Autoimmune hyperlipoproteinemia* refers to hyperlipidemia due to interactions of various gamma-globulins with lipoproteins and consequent interference with their metabolism. This is included in secondary hyperlipidemia due to paraproteinemia.

HYPOLIPOPROTEINEMIA

Beta- (low-density) lipoprotein deficiency

ABETALIPOPROTEINEMIA Abetalipoproteinemia is a rare familial disease, uniquely characterized by complete absence from plasma of apolipoprotein B and of the lipoproteins of which it is a constituent. The plasma contains only alpha-lipoproteins. The syndrome follows a fairly uniform course, beginning before the age of one year, with *malnutrition* and growth retardation, lordosis, abdominal distention, and steatorrhea. *Ataxia,* nystagmus, weakness and areflexia, and other signs of progressive neurologic dysfunction, particularly involving the posterolateral columns and spinocerebellar tracts, then appear. *Pigmentary retinal degeneration* develops during adolescence. The erythrocytes have a crenated appearance (*acanthocytosis*). The esterified lipids of these cells and of the plasma are deficient in both lecithin and lineoleic acid. Dietary fat is assimilated but is held up in the intestinal mucosal cells, creating a pathognomonic picture detectable by peroral biopsy. Some fat is absorbed, possibly by direct passage through the portal system into the liver.

The disease appears to be the homozygous state for one of several defective genes controlling triglyceride secretion from cells. One gene does not affect lipoprotein concentrations in the heterozygote. Another gene produces hypobetalipoproteinemia in the heterozygote. The life span in homozygotes is limited. One cause of death is cardiac arrhythmia possibly related to ceroid deposition in the heart. Familial instances of acanthocytosis and neurologic abnormalities without abetalipoproteinemia have also been reported.

Diagnosis The diagnosis is suspected when a plasma cholesterol concentration less than 100 mg per 100 ml is associated with the above clinical picture. It must be confirmed by immunochemical evidence of the absence of apo-LDL from plasma.

Treatment There is no definitive therapy. Medium-chain triglycerides may help provide some fat intake in the absence of chylomicron formation, and low vitamin A levels have been increased with supplements.

HYPOBETALIPOPROTEINEMIA Abnormally low cholesterol and glyceride concentrations with decreased, but not absent, beta- and very low density lipoproteins are common in malnutrition or malabsorption due to a variety of causes. Remissions are promptly associated with a rise in cholesterol and beta-lipoproteins. Rarely, patients with paraproteinemia may have severe hypolipoproteinemia, possibly due to autoantibodies to lipoproteins. There are also *heritable* forms of hypobetalipoproteinemia including the heterozygous form of abetalipoproteinemia. Beta-lipoprotein levels down to 10 percent of normal occur, usually with no disability.

Alpha- (high-density) lipoprotein deficiency

Tangier disease is a rare recessive inheritable disorder characterized in the homozygote by absence of normal alpha- or high-density lipoproteins and storage of cholesteryl esters throughout the body, particularly in reticuloendothelial cells and Schwann cells of peripheral nerves. This storage leads to peculiar orange discoloration of the tonsils and pharyngeal and rectal mucosa, corneal infiltration, and recurrent peripheral neuropathy. Splenomegaly and hypersplenism may occur. The basic defect is suspected to affect the synthesis of a major apoprotein of high-density lipoproteins (apo-A-I). Other lipoproteins are also affected, however, LDL levels being very low and VLDL levels increased. The plasma cholesterol is between 50 and 125 mg per 100 ml, and triglycerides usually are over 200 mg per 100 ml. Diagnosis is based on immunochemical evidence that apo-A-I is present in only trace amounts coupled with the typical tonsillar changes or other evidence of cholesteryl ester accumulation. Heterozygotes have HDL concentrations that are lower than normal. There is no treatment.

Plasma HDL deficiency as severe as that in Tangier disease but without tonsillar involvement has been observed in a few other adults. Whether this represents other mutations or dyslipoproteinemia secondary to other occult disease has not been determined.

PLASMA LECITHIN: CHOLESTEROL ACYLTRANSFERASE (LCAT) DEFICIENCY This is a rare familial disorder seen mainly in Scandinavians. The clinical manifestations include proteinuria, anemia with target-cell formation, and corneal infiltration. Plasma-esterified cholesterol and alpha-lipoproteins are markedly reduced, and unesterified cholesterol and lecithin are greatly increased. LCAT enzyme normally esterifies the plasma cholesterol, and activity of the enzyme is severely deficient in this disorder. Renal failure may occur, and kidney transplantation has been employed as therapy.

LIPID STORAGE DISEASES

THE SPHINGOLIPIDOSES Many lipidoses are characterized by tissue rather than plasma lipid abnormalities. *In all it is exceedingly important that specimens of tissues obtained for diagnostic purposes be retained frozen without fixatives for chemical and enzymatic analyses. Histochemical diagnosis is usually not definitive.* The sphingolipidoses represent one group of these disorders; each member of this group is characterized by the accumulation of a specific (and different) derivative (−R) of ceramide (acylsphingosine).

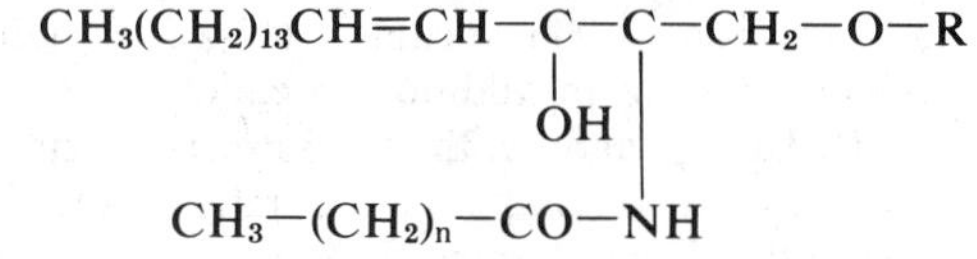

Ceramide

These are all inheritable disorders; each may involve the nervous system. Most occur in several clinical forms or syndromes, possibly reflecting mutations at different loci. The underlying defect in each is deficiency of a specific lysosomal enzyme in the pathway of lipid catabolism (Table 113-1). They may also be grouped according to chemical similarities in the particular lipids that abnormally accumulate in the tissues.

GANGLIOSIDOSES (see also Chap. 340) *Gangliosidosis* is a generic term for several familial neurologic disorders associated with varying degrees of blindness and dementia. An older and somewhat misleading term for them is *amaurotic family idiocy.* Three of these diseases have been identified as characterized by defective metabolism and accumulation of different gangliosides, the major lipids in gray matter. *G_{M1} gangliosidosis, generalized gangliosidosis,* or *pseudo-Hurler's disease,* involves both brain and viscera. The tissues contain abnormal amounts of galactosylgalactosaminyl(*N*-acetylneuraminido)galactosylglucosyl ceramide. A galactosidase attacking the terminal glycosidic bond is deficient. *G_{M2} gangliosidosis* includes *Tay-Sachs disease,* which fatally involves only the central nervous system. The excess ganglioside is *N*-acetylgalactosaminyl(*N*-acetylneuraminido)galactosylglucosyl ceramide. Different phenotypic variants of G_{M1} and G_{M2} gangliosidoses are recognized (Table 113-1). A G_{M3} gangliosidosis has also recently been identified.

GAUCHER'S DISEASE This designation is applied to several syndromes due to deficient activity of a β-glucosidase, known more specifically as glucocerebrosidase. This enzyme catalyzes the cleavage of glucose from glucocerebrosides (glucosyl ceramide), compounds which arise from more complex glycolipids and gangliosides found in the formed elements in blood and in many other tissues. Deficient glucocerebrosidase activity occurs as the result of at least two different mutations which result in clinical disease in the homozygous state. The commonest phenotype is called type 1, or the *nonneuronopathic* type. This is the most common of all the sphingolipid storage diseases. An *infantile* or *acute neuronopathic* form (type 2) and a *juvenile* or *subacute neuronopathic* form (type 3) are also recognized. All forms are associated with glucocerebroside accumulations in reticuloendothelial cells that take on a characteristic appearance (Gaucher cells), with hepatosplenomegaly of varying degrees and bone lesions. Types 2 and 3 are also accompanied by devastating neuronal changes which are apparently due to decrease in enzyme activity below some critical level. The different nature of the mutations causing Gaucher's disease is emphasized by the appearance of only one phenotype in affected members of the same family and disparate ethnic distributions. Type 1 is about 30 times more frequent in Ashkenazi Jews than in any other ethnic group. Type 2, though rare, is more common in non-Jews. It is possible that some type 3 patients represent genetic compounds, i.e., bear an abnormal allele for type 1 and type 2.

Etiology, morbid anatomy, and pathogenesis The normal destruction of leukocytes and erythrocytes liberates large amounts of ceramide lactoside (galactosylglucosyl ceramide), globoside (*N*-acetylgalactosaminyl-galactosylgalactosylglucosyl ceramide), and similar compounds which give rise to glucosyl ceramide. Limited catabolism of this substance leads to formations of Gaucher's cells. Their appearance is sufficiently distinctive to be diagnostic. They are 20 to 80 μm in diameter, round, oval, or spindle-shaped, and possess one or more small, eccentrically placed, nuclei. The cytoplasm has the appearance of crinkled tissue paper showing numerous wavy fibrillae. These are visible in ordinary Wright's stain smears, but are best seen in supravital preparations or with electron microscopy. On electron microscopy these fibrillae are seen to be tubular structures with diameters of 120 to 750 Å which are up to 5 μm in length. Each structure contains 10 to 12 fibrils twisted around the long axis of the tubule with a distance between fibrils of about 80 Å.

Gaucher cells are found throughout the body, but are present in greatest concentration in the spleen, liver, bone marrow, and lymph nodes of the paraaortic and thoracic chain. They are found in significant concentration in the alveolar capillaries of the lung. All tissues so involved show an increase in content of glucocerebroside, which can rise higher than 200 times the normal.

In the acute neuronal form, ganglion cell destruction, glial proliferation, and demyelinization may be found in the brain, particularly in the region of the cranial nerve nuclei. Yet evidence of storage of glycolipid is minimal in neuroneurons and is restricted mainly to perivascular cells.

Clinical manifestations The typical patient with the acute neuronopathic form appears normal at birth, but by three months of age has developed problems with feeding, has a cough with frequent pulmonary infections, and is found to have an enlarged liver and spleen. Neurologic signs usually appear by six months and most commonly involve cranial nerves and extrapyramidal tracts. The usual patient dies from either pulmonary infection, progressive neurologic disease, or thrombocytopenic bleeding by age nine months; few survive beyond their second year.

The chronic nonneuronopathic form may begin in childhood; most patients have signs and symptoms by age 15 to 20 years, but the diagnosis has been made in old age. The disease varies markedly in its severity from patient to patient, and a normal life expectancy is possible. The most common life-threatening problem is bleeding secondary to thrombocytopenia. That this is due to increased sequestration and destruction of platelets in a markedly enlarged spleen is suggested by the observation that splenectomy leads to a marked decrease of thrombocytopenia. Repeated pulmonary infections may also be a problem, particularly when the disease begins in childhood. Although the liver is often enlarged and liver function tests may be abnormal, liver failure is not common, but portal hypertension may occur. Pain in the limbs associated with expanding bone lesions is common. Pathologic fractures may occur. Of the roentgenographic abnormalities of bone, the development of a radiolucent area in the lower end of the femur in the contour of an Erlenmeyer flask is the typical lesion. Yellow-brown pingueculae may be seen on the conjunctiva on either side of the cornea, and similar pigmentation may be found on the exposed areas of the skin.

The subacute neuronopathic variety begins in childhood, and both visceral and bone involvement may be fairly advanced before progressive central nervous system changes begin, often first as seizures or behavioral disorders.

Diagnosis When a typical clinical syndrome is associated with finding of characteristic cells in marrow aspirates, the diagnosis is reasonably certain and further assured when the plasma acid phosphatase activity is markedly increased. It should be kept in mind that in leukemia there may be sufficient overload of the catabolic pathways for leukocyte glycolipids to cause Gaucher cells to appear in tissues and occasionally lead to a false diagnosis. Definitive diagnosis of Gaucher's disease should be obtained by measurement of glucocerebrosidase activity in leukocytes, cultured skin fibroblasts, liver biopsy, or other tissue. Heterozygous carriers can be detected by measurement of glucocerebrosidase activity in fresh leukocyte preparations or cultured fibroblasts. The affected homozygote can also be identified in amniotic cell cultures.

Treatment and prognosis There is no established therapy in this disease with the exception of splenectomy for correction of thrombocytopenia. The decision as to when to perform the splenectomy must be individualized. Most would not recommend splenectomy unless severe thrombocytopenia associated with significant hemorrhage has developed. Relief of bone pain has been reported following steroid therapy or irradiation, but this is not a consistent finding. Replacement of the missing glucocerebrosidase by infusion of purified enzyme from the human placenta has been performed experimentally with some temporary success.

GLUCOSYL CERAMIDE TRIHEXOSIDOSIS (FABRY'S DISEASE) (see Chap. 318) In this sex-linked disorder the manifestations are usually seen only in males and are due to deposition of glycolipids, mainly a trihexoside (galactosylgalactosylglucosyl ceramide), in blood vessels and nerves. Galactosylgalactosyl ceramide also accumulates. Because of its unusual skin lesions, this disease is also known as *angiokeratoma corporis diffusum universale.* The activity of an α-galactosidase is deficient.

GALACTOSYLSULFATIDOSIS (see also Chap. 340) *Metachromatic leukodystrophy* is a disorder that usually develops between 1 and 2 years of age. Abnormal amounts of sulfuric acid esters of galactosylceramide accumulate in the brain and kidney. The sulfatides are excreted in urine, making possible a provisional diagnosis. The disease is due to deficient cerebroside sulfatase activity.

GALACTOSYLCEREBROSIDOSIS (see Chap. 340) *Krabbe's globoid cell leukodystrophy* is a rapidly fatal, demyelinating disease of infants. Diagnosis is made by the finding of deficient activity of a β-galactosidase in leukocytes or serum.

NIEMANN-PICK DISEASE This is a rare group of familial disorders, first described in 1914, in which sphingomyelin, the phosphorylcholine ester of *N*-acylsphingosine, accumulates in foamy-appearing reticuloendothelial cells throughout the body. Increased cholesterol is also stored in some cases. The activity of the lysosomal hydrolase, sphingomyelinase, which catalyzes liberation of phosphoryl choline from sphingomyelin, is decreased in some but not all forms. On the basis of differences in age of onset, presence or absence of neurologic disease, and levels of sphingomyelinase activity, it has been suggested that at least four phenotypic expressions exist, based on an unknown number of mutants. All are associated with hepatosplenomegaly and marrow foam cells. Type A becomes evident within a few months of birth and is accompanied by progressive neuronal dysfunction, leading to death within 3 years. Type B begins as early and has visceral involvement as severe as type A, yet neuronal involvement is absent. Types C and D develop later and feature more protracted neuronal dysfunction. Sphingomyelinase activity is very low in types A and B, and somewhat decreased in type C. The level of activity has not been firmly established in type D.

Etiology and pathogenesis Each syndrome is apparently inherited as a simple mendelian recessive trait, both sexes being equally involved. No case has been observed in more than one generation in a single pedigree. Over half the reported cases of type A have been in Ashkenazi Jews, but many other ethnic groups have been involved. Type D has so far been restricted to patients from a Nova Scotian population.

The *foam cells* in Niemann-Pick disease are reticuloendothelial cells, 20 to 90 μm in diameter, and are so filled with vacuoles that they have a mulberry appearance. The nucleus is small and is placed eccentrically but may be multiple. The vacuoles have a faint bluish hue with Wright's stain, are positive to Baker's stain, and may also stain with Sudan III and other fat stains. These cells may be found everywhere but are essentially prominent in the spleen, liver, lymph nodes, lung, and bone marrow.

In forms of the disease except type B, swelling, vacuolization, and degeneration of Nissl substance are found in the ganglion cells of the nervous system. There are also demyelination, scarring and fibrosis, and proliferation of glial cells which become converted to foam cells. In the retina, destruction of ganglion cells in the surrounding area may leave a grayish background, against which the macula stands out as a cherry-red spot.

Diagnosis Definitive diagnosis of type A or B is best made by demonstration of low sphingomyelinase activity in leukocytes, cultured skin fibroblasts, or tissue samples. These two phenotypic forms can be distinguished only by the manifestations observed in a previously affected sibling. This is extremely important since presumably cultured amniotic cells from an affected homozygote of either type will have equally low enzyme activities. Diagnosis of type C requires a combination of clinical picture, increased sphingomyelin content of liver or spleen, and somewhat decreased sphingomyelinase assays. Heterozygote carriers for type A can be diagnosed by enzyme assay in fresh leukocytes or, preferably, cultured skin fibroblasts.

Treatment There is no specific therapy. Splenectomy is of little value unless severe thrombocytopenia has developed.

DISSEMINATED LIPOGRANULOMATOSIS (FARBER'S DISEASE) This is a rare disease that appears in infancy as generalized nodular periarticular swelling and dysphonia. There is progressive systemic involvement with widespread proliferation of histiocytes and neuronal abnormalities. Storage cells appear containing both mucopolysaccharide and lipids. The basic disorder appears to involve the metabolism of both ceramide and acid mucopolysaccharides. Deficient activity of ceramidase has been reported.

CHOLESTERYL ESTER AND TRIGLYCERIDE HYDROLASE DEFICIENCIES

There are two inheritable disorders in which massive amounts of cholesteryl esters and triglycerides are stored in liver, spleen, lymph nodes, bone marrow reticulocytes (foam cells), intestine, and other tissues. Associated with this storage is severe deficiency in lysosomal enzyme activity catalyzing hydrolysis of cholesteryl esters and triglycerides at acid pH. Diagnosis is made from enzyme assays on cultured skin fibroblasts or lipid measurements on a biopsy of the liver, coupled with the clinical picture.

WOLMAN'S DISEASE This disorder is manifested in infancy by failure to thrive associated with hepatosplenomegaly, gastrointestinal symptoms, and adrenal calcification demonstrable by x-ray. There is no treatment, and death usually occurs by six months of age.

CHOLESTERYL ESTER STORAGE DISEASE This disease has a more benign course, being compatible with adult life. Massive hepatomegaly, with or without splenomegaly, and hypercholesterolemia are common features. Hypertriglyceridemia and accelerated atherosclerosis also may occur. Much of the lipid stored in tissues is converted to insoluble ceroid pigment. There is no treatment.

PHYTANIC OXIDASE DEFICIENCY

REFSUM'S DISEASE In this condition there is accumulation of phytanic acid (3,7,11,15-tetramethyl hexadecanoic acid) in the esterified lipids present in both tissues and plasma. This familial disease is characterized by ataxic neuropathy, anosmia, retinitis pigmentosa, dry skin, skeletal deformities, and ichthyosis and is commonest in children or young adults of Scandinavian ancestry. Parents may have high levels of phytanic acid in plasma without other abnormalities. The prognosis is guarded, with the symptoms sometimes progressing to complete blindness and deafness, but often waxing and waning. Relapses are somewhat irregular, being correlated with the degree of increase in cerebrospinal protein. Phytanic acid, which is normally present only in trace quantities, constitutes 10 to 30 percent of total plasma fatty acids. The inherited defect is a block in the alpha oxidation of the phytanic acid derived from dietary phytols. The relation of phytanate accumulation to the nervous disorders is unknown. Diagnosis is usually made by chromatographic analysis of plasma. Therapy consists of a low-phytol diet.

CEROID STORAGE Ceroid and lipofuscin are insoluble pigments believed to arise from peroxidation of unsaturated fatty acids. They are identified histochemically by the combination of red periodic acid-Schiff stain, acid-fastness, and autofluorescence in ultraviolet light. Ceroid deposition is a feature of abetalipoproteinemia and many lipid-storage diseases and does not represent a specific disorder. The *syndrome of the sea-blue histiocyte* pertains to a diverse group of patients who have foam cells in bone marrow that appear light blue with Giemsa's stain. Identical-appearing cells occur in many of the known lipid-storage diseases, and their presence does not define a clear-cut or specific disease.

GRANULOMATOUS DISEASES WITH LIPID STORAGE

Frequently considered among the lipid storage diseases are certain tissue proliferative disorders sometimes accompanied by lipid deposition.

HISTIOCYTOSIS X (see also Chap. 320) This is the generic term for a group of disorders that affect the reticuloendothelial system and which may be either different stages or forms of the same disease. *Letterer-Siwe disease* and *xanthoma disseminatum* may be the two extremes of such abnormalities, with *eosinophilic granuloma* and *Hand-Schüller-Christian disease* representing intermediate and special forms. The usual order of progression of the pathologic lesions is reticuloendothelial cell proliferation and hyperplasia, granulomatous changes featuring eosinophils and giant cells, conversion of reticulum cells and histiocytes to foam cells or xanthomas, and finally, fibrosis. These disorders do not appear to be hereditary.

LIPOID PROTEINOSIS In *lipoid proteinosis* (cutaneous-mucosal hyalinosis; Urbach-Wiethe disease) the lesions share enough histologic features of *histiocytosis X* to suggest an etiologic relation. The skin and mucous membranes of the pharynx and larynx are infiltrated by extracellular deposits of hyalin material. Clinical manifestations include hoarseness or aphonia, widely distributed skin papules, dental anomalies, and symmetric calcifications in the region of the sella turcica as seen by x-ray. The disease is not incompatible with long life. This disorder may be heritable.

LIPOID DERMATOARTHRITIS In *lipoid dermatoarthritis* polyarthritis is associated with multiple nodular or papular skin lesions. In both skin and synovial tissues there is an infiltration of histiocytes, eosinophils, lymphocytes, red blood cells, and multinucleated giant cells. The joint changes may be extremely destructive, producing *arthritis mutilans,* or the "opera-glass hand." Serologic reactions for rheumatoid arthritis are negative. Familial occurrence has not been reported.

OTHER XANTHOMATOSES

NORMOLIPOPROTEINEMIC XANTHOMATOSES Many chronic infections, particularly accompanied by exudates, and other proliferative processes, such as osteitis fibrosa cystica or traumatic lesions, may be associated with collections of foam cells (*xanthomas*) and sometimes crystals of cholesterol. Most skin xanthomas are secondary to hyperlipoproteinemia, but *juvenile xanthomas* (nevoxanthoepithelioma) are benign skin lesions that can appear without abnormal plasma lipids. *Xanthelasmas* need not always be associated with hyperlipoproteinemia; very rarely they occur, along with Achilles tendon xanthomas, in family members who are normolipoproteinemic.

CEREBROTENDINOUS XANTHOMATOSIS An unusual example of normolipoproteinemic xanthomatosis is a familial disease in which large nodules appear on the upper portions of the Achilles tendons, often followed by pulmonary insufficiency and neurologic dysfunction, including dementia and progressive spastic ataxia. These signs are due to xanthomatous deposits in tendons, lung, and brain, which contain cholesterol and cholestanol (5α-cholestan-3β-ol). Cholestanol and other neutral and acidic sterols also appear in bile in abnormal amounts. The metabolic defect has not been established.

β-SITOSTEROLEMIA AND XANTHOMATOSIS Normally, vegetable sterols in the diet, such as β-sitosterol and stigmasterol, are little absorbed, and only traces appear in the blood. In an unusual genetically determined disease absorption of vegetable sterols is demonstrably increased. These sterols may compose 10 percent of plasma sterol. The abnormality is associated with tendinous xanthomas. The prognosis is unknown. Although plasma sitosterol levels can be controlled by restriction of ingestion of vegetable sterols, the value of such arduous therapy has not been established.

ADIPOSE TISSUE DISORDERS

Adipose tissue can be a site of expression of many disorders including those of connective tissue, lipid, and carbohydrate metabolism. There is therefore no simple classification of the adipose tissue diseases.

RELAPSING PANNICULITIS (WEBER-CHRISTIAN DISEASE) This classification may represent several diseases that share similar but rather nonspecific histologic changes (see Chap. 55).

LIPODYSTROPHY Although the term *lipodystrophy* is sometimes used to describe *lipotrophy,* it also has a generic meaning that allows it to encompass several disorders in which adipose tissue is abnormal but not necessarily absent. Several abnormalities may properly be considered forms of lipodystrophy.

Lipomas These are benign mesenchymal tumors consisting of circumscribed masses of adipose tissue. There is usually a capsule, but the cells are histologically indistinguishable from ordinary fat. They may occur nearly anywhere in the body, singly or as multiple fatty growths (lipomatosis), most commonly in subcutaneous tissues. They also arise in retroperitoneal or peritoneal areas, in breast, mesentery, and mediastinum, and in other body cavities and organs. Lipomas have caused intestinal obstruction or dyspnea by superior mediastinal obstruction and may embarrass the function of other vital tissues. Rarely they may calcify, and it has been presumed that they may on occasion give rise to liposarcomas or other malignant tumors, but there is no general agreement on this. Multiple lipomas may be symmetrically placed and may run in families. The therapy is surgical excision; occasionally they will recur in the same site.

Adiposis dolorosa (Dercum's disease) *Adiposis dolorosa* refers to a poorly defined disorder in which painful subcutaneous lipomas, often widely and symmetrically situated, are sometimes associated with asthenia, decreased cutaneous sensation, motor weakness, or other evidence of peripheral neuropathy. Some patients have also had adenomas in the pituitary, thyroid, or adrenal glands. There may or may not be accompanying generalized obesity. Siblings may be similarly involved. The interstitial neuritis observed in the original adipose tissue nodules by Dercum has not been seen in many subsequent cases. There is no specific therapy.

Insulin lipodystrophy This term refers to changes in subcutaneous fat at the site of insulin injection (see Chap. 95) and may involve either localized hypertrophy or atrophy of adipose tissue.

LIPOATROPHY Lipoatrophy may be partial or complete.

Partial Also called *progressive lipodystrophy* or *Barraquer-Simons disease,* partial lipoatrophy is characterized by the absence of subcutaneous fat over wide, symmetric areas of the body. The remaining parts of the body have normal or sometimes increased subcutaneous fat deposits. It occurs predominantly in females and often begins in childhood. The onset is usually insidious; the disease may begin with loss of subcutaneous fat in the face and subsequently involve that of the upper extremities and upper trunk. In other instances, the disorder may begin at the level of the iliac crest and extend downward. There are no subjective symptoms. The cause is unknown. There is no known therapy.

Total The rarer total or generalized lipoatrophy (also called *Seip-Lawrence syndrome* or *lipoatrophic diabetes mellitus*) occurs with equal frequency in males and females. Early in life the subcutaneous fat deposits begin to disappear until only those in the breasts may be retained. Diabetes mellitus is usually, but not always, present and is associated with high plasma insulin levels. Often hypertrichosis, acanthosis nigricans, hyperglyceridemia, hepatomegaly, sometimes portal cirrhosis, and serious nephropathy occur. Sometimes there is penile or clitoral hypertrophy, hypermetabolism, and gigantism. The urine may contain an insulin antagonist. The cause(s) of the disorder are not understood. The course of the disease may be either indolent or rapidly progressive. No therapy is known.

REFERENCES

BHATTACHARYYA AK, CONNOR WE: β-Sitosterolemia and xanthomatosis. J Clin Invest 53:1033, 1974

BRADY RO: The lipid storage diseases: New concepts and control. Ann Intern Med 82:257, 1975

—— et al: Identification of heterozygous carriers of lipid storage diseases. Am J Med 51:423, 1971

—— et al: Replacement therapy for inherited enzyme deficiency: Use of purified glucocerebrosidase in Gaucher's disease. N Engl J Med 291:989, 1974

BROWN MS, GOLDSTEIN JL: Familial hypercholesterolemia: Genetic, biochemical, and pathophysiological considerations. Adv Intern Med 20:273, 1975

FREDRICKSON DS: It's time to be practical. Circulation 51:209, 1975

GOLDSTEIN JL et al: Hyperlipidemia in coronary heart disease II, Genetic analysis of lipid levels in 176 families and delineation of a new inherited disorder, combined hyperlipidemia. J Clin Invest 52:1569, 1973

STANBURY JB et al (eds): *The Metabolic Basis of Inherited Disease,* 3d ed, Chaps. 26–35, New York: McGraw-Hill, 1972

114 AMYLOIDOSIS

EVAN CALKINS

Amyloid is an eosinophilic hyaline material which, because of its structural features, exhibits a striking affinity to certain dyes, such as Congo red.

Amyloidosis, a disease resulting from the infiltration of organs by amyloid, has been recognized as a clinical and pathologic entity for over 130 years. However, the chemical composition of amyloid remained a mystery until recently. The development of new methods of solubilization and isolation and the availability of improved analytical techniques have now permitted investigators to identify and characterize the basic components of amyloid. The main amyloid protein is a microfiber which possesses properties distinct from those of any other known mammalian protein. These include a characteristic appearance on electron microscopy, and an antiparallel beta-pleated sheet conformation as seen by x-ray diffraction. This fibrillar ultrastructure is not specific for a single protein but is shared by several amyloid proteins that possess strikingly different amino acid sequences.

A systematic correlation of the specific composition of the major fibril protein and the clinical situations and patterns in which amyloidosis occurs has not yet been accomplished. Most of the data assembled to date support the validity of distinguishing between the broad classes of amyloid cited in Table 114-1 under the headings *A* and *B*. A true appreciation of the nature and classification of amyloidosis (or, more properly, the amyloid diseases) must await further analytical data, especially on the forms of amyloid referred to under *C* in Table 114-1.

Amino acid sequencing of the major amyloid protein derived from patients with multiple myeloma and from patients with so-called "primary" amyloidosis (Table 114-1, *B*) indicates the presence, in high concentration, of a subunit having a sequence homologous with the amino terminal portion of immunoglobulin light chains. The possibility that this form of amyloid is derived from immunoglobulin light chains is further supported by two observations: (1) over the past decade immunoglobulin abnormalities have been observed in the serum and/or urine of an increasing percentage of patients with sporadic "primary" amyloidosis; (2) Glenner and his colleagues have shown that Bence Jones proteins isolated from the urine of some patients with multiple myeloma can be enzymatically degraded to form, in vitro, amyloid fibers with typical staining characteristics and x-ray diffraction pattern.

A second amyloid fibril protein (amyloid A) has been isolated from patients with amyloidosis accompanying prolonged inflammatory diseases and familial Mediterranean fever, and from experimentally induced amyloid in monkey, duck, and guinea pig. This protein is composed of polypeptide subunits with a molecular weight of 8,500 daltons. Immunologic and chemical data, including amino acid sequence, have shown that samples of this protein extracted from different individuals are virtually identical and are unlike any other known protein. A close antigenic relationship has, however, been demonstrated with a serum protein (an α 1-globulin) present in low concentration in normal persons and in progressively increasing concentration with advancing age. Increased concentrations of this substance have also been noted in the serum of most but not all patients with amyloidosis, especially the secondary form, and in many patients with chronic inflammatory diseases of the sort known to predispose to amyloidosis. The precise nature of the relationship between this serum protein and the antigenically related subunit of type A amyloid fibril protein is still unknown. While it is tempting to postulate that this serum component may bear a relationship to the types of amyloid known to accumulate, in trace amounts, in the brain, heart, aorta, and other organs of most elderly patients, these forms of amyloid have not yet been characterized with sufficient clarity to justify this conclusion. Data are also not yet available on the chemical characteristics of the many forms of hereditary amyloidosis other than that accompanying familial Mediterranean fever.

It has been proposed that the type of amyloid which may be seen adjacent to certain tumors of neuroectodermal origin (i.e., medullary carcinoma of the thyroid, gastrinoma, pheochromocytoma, and insulinoma) is probably different, chemically, from other forms of amyloid. Utilizing histochemical techniques it has been shown that these particular amyloid accumulations lack tryptophan and tyrosine, while containing increased amounts of aspartic and glutamic acids. It has been suggested that this type of amyloid may be formed from the complexing of precursors of polypeptide hormones secreted by these cells in a manner paralleling the postulated complexing of nonimmunoglobulin subunits or immunoglobulin light-chain components in other forms of amyloid. A similar mechanism may explain the amyloid infiltration of the islets of Langerhans seen in many patients with diabetes mellitus.

TABLE 114-1
Types of amyloid

A Secondary type (type A amyloid, of unknown origin)
- *1* Prolonged inflammatory disease
- *2* Amyloid with familial Mediterranean fever

B Primary type (type B amyloid, of immunoglobulin origin)
- *1* Multiple myeloma or macroglobulinemia
- *2* Sporadic primary amyloidosis

C Other forms (type C amyloid)
- *1* Amyloid of aging
- *2* Amyloid adjacent to tumors of neuroectodermal origin*
- *3* Localized amyloidosis
- *4* Specific genetic forms

* *This form of amyloid has been referred to as APUD amyloid, because of the cytochemical characteristics of the polypeptide hormone-secreting cells with which it is associated. These characteristics are as follows:* (A) *fluorogenic amine content (catecholamine, 5-hydroxytryptamine, dihydroxyphenylalanine, and related compounds);* (P *and* U) *amine precursor uptake;* (D) *amino acid decarboxylase and related properties.*

CLINICAL ASPECTS Clinical manifestations of amyloidosis are numerous and varied and so closely mimic other conditions that the diagnosis is frequently missed. Functional disturbances due to amyloid infiltration occur primarily in three organs, the kidney, heart, and gastrointestinal tract, including the tongue.

Renal involvement is the preponderant manifestation in most cases of secondary amyloidosis, in amyloidosis accompanying familial Mediterranean fever, in the majority of patients with amyloidosis accompanying multiple myeloma, and in approximately one-half the patients with sporadic "primary" amyloidosis.

Initially amyloid appears in the renal glomeruli and, frequently, arteriolar walls. Later, the intertubular connective tissue may be involved. The chief clinical manifestation is proteinuria, leading to the nephrotic syndrome. Later renal failure ensues. Hypertension is not, in our experience, a characteristic concomitant of renal amyloidosis, unless the patient also suffers from a coexistent renal disorder such as pyelonephritis or unless the amyloid infiltration is sufficiently extensive to involve the papillae. The amyloid-laden kidney is apt to be of normal or slightly increased size. With the development of renal failure, the extent of proteinuria may decrease.

Amyloid infiltration of the heart is present in nearly all patients with sporadic "primary" amyloidosis, amyloidosis accompanying multiple myeloma, and in certain familial forms of amyloid as well. It is occasionally encountered in patients of advanced age, in whom it is referred to as "senile amyloidosis." In our experience, cardiac involvement in secondary amyloidosis is minimal or absent. The amyloid-infiltrated heart is characterized by a striking increase in weight, frequently reaching values of 600 g or more. Clinically, the heart is usually slightly or moderately enlarged. Approximately half the patients with cardiac amyloidosis have congestive heart failure, often accompanied by pleural effusion. Heart sounds may be faint; murmurs are infrequent. Electrocardiogram frequently shows low voltage and conduction or rhythm disturbances. In some cases, ECG changes closely resemble those of myocardial infarction, although this diagnosis is infrequently confirmed at autopsy. Digitalis therapy is usually ineffective and may be very hazardous. A large number, in one series as many as half, of patients with cardiac amyloidosis die suddenly and unexpectedly, presumably of arrhythmia. Sudden death is especially likely to occur following administration of digitalis.

Amyloid may involve any portion of the gastrointestinal tract, from the tongue to the anus. Infiltration of the tongue, not infrequently encountered in the immunoglobulin-related forms of amyloidosis (type B), is rarely seen in secondary amyloidosis. Although the tongue may be enlarged, it is most characteristically stiff, leading to serious problems in deglutition and phonation. Amyloid infiltration of the stomach and small or large intestine may lead to decreased motility, bleeding, and, rarely obstruction. More frequently, the infiltration is lesser in extent, and may be manifested by malabsorbtion syndrome. Diarrhea is especially characteristic of so-called "primary familial amyloidosis" of the type which sometimes occurs in people of Portuguese ancestry. Diarrhea in these patients is largely due to amyloid infiltration of the splanchnic nerves.

Amyloid infiltration may also be seen in nearly every other tissue of the body, especially the liver, spleen, lung, adrenal, thyroid, skeletal muscles, peripheral nerves, skin, synovium, and vitreous humor. The involvement of these organs is often limited to the walls of the small blood vessels and may not result in any clinical manifestations. In other patients, the vascular involvement is accompanied by parenchymal infiltration, sometimes extensive, resulting in enlargement and stiffening of the organ. Amyloid infiltration of these organs is rarely associated with interference with function, except through pressure on adjacent tissues—i.e., nerve involvement secondary to amyloid infiltration of nerve sheaths or carpal ligaments. Amyloid infiltration of the small blood vessels of the skin, particularly in primary or myeloma-related amyloidosis, is frequently manifested by purpura occurring, chiefly, in or near the folds of the skin in the inguinal area, axilla, etc.

Although insufficient data are available to permit clear association between the chemical types of amyloid fibril-protein and the clinical manifestations, certain general patterns emerge. Secondary amyloidosis is manifested predominantly by renal disease. Primary and myeloma-related amyloidosis is manifested predominantly by cardiac involvement, with renal manifestations present in approximately one-half the patients. Widespread involvement of the small blood vessels appears to be more characteristic of primary and myeloma-related amyloid than of the secondary form. Patients with multiple myeloma (and, probably Waldenström's macroglobulinemia as well) have a somewhat greater tendency to exhibit parenchymal organ infiltration than do patients with sporadic "primary" amyloidosis. One manifestation, carpal-tunnel syndrome, appears to be especially characteristic of amyloidosis accompanying multiple myeloma.

In aged patients, amyloid tends to be confined to small traces in the aorta, brain (senile plaques), and other tissues. Occasionally, however, elderly patients (seventy years of age or more) may develop diffuse amyloid infiltration of the heart.

DIAGNOSIS The one factor, aside from a high index of suspicion, on which the diagnosis depends is demonstration of the presence of amyloid in properly stained biopsy material or by electron microscopy. If renal manifestations are present, biopsy of this organ usually leads to the definitive diagnosis. Biopsy of appropriate tissues in carpal-tunnel syndrome, peripheral neuropathy, or small-intestine involvement entails little hazard and should provide histologic confirmation if the clinical diagnosis is correct. When clinical involvement centers in organs which are, themselves, inaccessible to biopsy, rectal biopsy may prove helpful. This should be obtained so as to include submucosal blood vessels (a rectal valve provides a propitious site). Liver biopsy is, in our opinion, hazardous in amyloidosis because of the possibility of hemorrhage.

Patients suspected of having amyloidosis should be studied carefully to identify possible underlying inflammatory disease, multiple myeloma, or other disorders of immunoglobulins. Workup should include bone marrow examination, protein electrophoresis, and immunoelectrophoresis of serum and urine. Prior to assay, urine should be concentrated twenty to thirty times to enhance the detectability of Bence Jones proteins. Amyloidosis should be considered in patients with intractable heart failure, especially if there is association of purpura, proteinuria, or other manifestations which might be due to amyloidosis. Cardiac catheterization may yield hemodynamic values similar to those encountered in constrictive pericarditis.

PREVALENCE Though *traces* of amyloid will be seen at autopsy in 90 percent of patients ninety years of age or over, very few of these patients exhibit sufficient degrees of amyloid accumulation to become symptomatic. In a recent series, amyloidosis was diagnosed in 0.5 percent of cases studied at autopsy in a major urban medical center (yielding a total of eight cases a year). Less than one-half of these had been diagnosed clinically. Thus, amyloidosis as a clinical entity is still a rare disease in this country.

COURSE When secondary amyloidosis develops, it usually does so after many (7 to 15) years of continued inflammatory stimulus. A few diseases, such as juvenile rheumatoid arthritis and regional enteritis, show an unusual propensity for the development of amyloidosis, occasionally in as short a time as 3 years. Once established, the course of secondary amyloidosis is variable; mean survival at present is 3 to 5 years. In a number of reported cases, treatment of the underlying inflammatory disease has been followed by slowing of the progression of the disorder and, occasionally, by decrease in the size of spleen or liver. Once the renal involvement progresses to the point of renal failure, however, death usually ensues within approximately 1 year—a figure which may be improved by renal transplantation. When the amyloidosis occurs as a manifestation of multiple myeloma, the prognosis is especially grave. Primary amyloidosis not accompanied by multiple myeloma carries a much more hopeful prognosis.

TREATMENT In patients with secondary amyloidosis, vigorous efforts should be directed toward treatment of removal of the underlying inflammatory stimulus. In patients with amyloidosis accompanying multiple myeloma or Waldenström's macroglobulinemia, treatment with an agent such as melphalan has seemed eminently logical. On the other hand, the results, so far as amyloidosis is concerned, have been variable and not particularly encouraging. An excellent clinical remission has been reported in a single case of widespread primary amyloidosis, with nephrosis, following simultaneous treatment with melphalan, prednisone, fluoxymesterone and, initially, D-penicillamine.

Renal transplantation has been employed in an increasing number of patients with end stage renal disease due to amyloidosis. A recent review indicated successful well-functioning transplants in 11 of 21 amyloid patients in whom this procedure was attempted. Five patients have survived for more than 3 years since transplantation—two for 10 years and one for 7. As a rule, the transplanted kidneys have not shown evidence of amyloid infiltration, despite, in a number of instances, slow but continued progression of amyloidosis of other organs.

Patients with cardiac amyloidosis should be given the benefit of a well-planned conservative regime. If digitalis administration is indicated, it should be carried out under continuous monitoring; anticoagulant therapy should be avoided because of the high frequency of hemorrhagic complications.

Colchicine treatment has been found to inhibit the formation of experimental amyloidosis in mice, but its possible value in human amyloidosis has not yet been proved. Though colchicine has been shown to prevent the febrile attacks in familial Mediterranean fever (FMF), the possible effects of colchicine therapy on FMF-related amyloidosis has not, to our knowledge, been examined.

In summary, the availability of new methods for isolation and characterization of amyloid has led to a new understanding of its nature, its possible origin, and the diseases it produces. It is hoped that, as this new knowledge expands, it will lead to better modes of prevention and therapy of this discouraging but fascinating disease.

REFERENCES

ADVISORY COMMITTEE TO THE RENAL TRANSPLANT REGISTRY: Renal transplantation in congenital and metabolic diseases. A report from the ASC/NIH Renal Transplant Registry. JAMA 232:148, 1975

BRANDT K et al: A clinical analysis of the course and prognosis of 47 patients with amyloidosis. Am J Med 44:955, 1968

COHEN A et al: Resolution of primary amyloidosis during chemotherapy. Ann Intern Med 82:466, 1975

FRANKLIN EC: Amyloidosis. Bull Rheum Dis 26:832–836, 1975

GLENNER GG et al: The immunoglobulin origin of amyloid. Am J Med 52:141, 1972

ISBOE T et al: Amyloidosis, plasma-cell dyscrasia, monoclonal immunoglobulins and Bence-Jones proteins. N Engl J Med 290: 473, 1974

KYLE RA AND BAYRD ED: Amyloidosis: Review of 236 cases. Medicine 54:271, 1975

PEARSE AG et al: The genesis of apudamyloid in endocrine polypeptide tumors: Histochemical distinction from immunoamyloid. Virchows Arch (Zellpathof) 10:93, 1972

ROSENTHAL CJ et al: Variation with age and disease of an amyloid A protein–related serum component. J Clin Invest 55:746, 1975

WRIGHT JR et al: Relationship of amyloid to aging. Medicine 48:39, 1969

PART FIVE | DISORDERS DUE TO CHEMICAL AND PHYSICAL AGENTS

section 1 | Chemical intoxications

115 GENERAL CONSIDERATIONS AND PRINCIPLES OF MANAGEMENT

JAN KOCH-WESER

Poisoning by chemical agents is a common and serious medical problem. In the United States accidental poisonings cause about 5,000 deaths each year. Suicides by chemical agents annually number more than 6,000. Malicious poisoning has become less common since the development of scientific toxicology, but toxic chemicals administered by homicides and abortionists are responsible for more deaths than is generally appreciated. In addition to fatal poisonings there is a much greater number of persons who are made seriously ill by chemical agents but recover after appropriate therapy. Unfortunately, some such victims are left with permanent sequelae of their intoxication. Finally, chemical agents impair the health of very many people by mechanisms not generally thought of as intoxications. Chemical carcinogenesis and mutagenesis, chronic alcoholic liver disease, allergic reactions, and chemical addiction and withdrawal syndromes are the most important examples.

Accidental poisonings may occur in the home or through industrial exposure. The former are far more frequent and usually acute; industrial intoxication is ordinarily the result of chronic exposure. Accidental poisoning is most commonly due to ingestion of toxic substances and involves children in the majority of cases. Each year 1 to 2 million American children accidentally swallow toxic materials, and approximately 1 ingestion in 1,000 is fatal. Aspirin is involved in 25 percent of all ingestions, other medicines in another 25 percent. Cleaning and polishing agents are ingested by 15 percent, while cosmetics, pesticides, petroleum products, and turpentine paints account for 6 percent each. Younger children tend to ingest household products, older children are more likely to choose drugs.

The frequency of accidental poisonings reflects the enormous number of toxic substances found in the American home. Many such accidents could be avoided by simple preventive measures. Physicians can play an effective role in safety education. All toxic substances must be kept out of the reach of small children. Household chemicals and medicines should be kept in the original containers, and all such containers should be labeled. Before taking or administering any medicine, one should check the label carefully.

Despite all precautions, accidental, suicidal, and criminal poisonings will remain an important problem which every physician must be prepared to treat promptly and effectively. Besides their immediate therapeutic responsibilities, physicians have legal obligations in cases of attempted suicide, homicide, criminal abortion, and industrial exposure. The physician should also obtain psychiatric care for any patient who has attempted suicide by poison.

DIAGNOSIS OF CHEMICAL POISONING

Optimal management of the poisoned patient requires a correct diagnosis. Unfortunately, in many such patients poisoning is initially not even considered as a possible cause of the clinical picture. The patient may be unaware of exposure to poison or, as after attempted suicide or abortion, he may be unwilling to admit it. Although the toxic effects of some chemical substances are quite characteristic, most poisoning syndromes can simulate other diseases.

Poisoning is usually included in the differential diagnosis of coma, convulsions, acute psychosis, acute hepatic or renal insufficiency, and bone marrow depression. It may not be considered when the major manifestation is a mild psychiatric disturbance or neurologic disorder, abdominal pain, bleeding, fever, hypotension, pulmonary congestion, or skin eruption. Chronic, insidious intoxications are much more frequently missed than acute poisonings whose symptoms appear suddenly and may be immediately related to a specific event. Physicians should always remember the variegated manifestations of poisoning and maintain a high index of suspicion.

In every case of poisoning, identification of the toxic agent should be attempted. Specific antidotal therapy is obviously impossible without such identification. In cases of homicide, suicide, or criminal abortion the identity of the poison may be of legal importance. When poisoning results from industrial exposure or therapeutic mishap, accurate knowledge of the responsible agents is essential for future prevention.

In acute accidental poisoning the offending substance may be known to the patient. In many other cases information can be obtained from relatives or acquaintances, by a search for containers at the scene of the poisoning, or by questioning the patient's physician or pharmacist. Frequently such procedures yield only the trade name of a product, which gives no clue to its component chemicals. A number of books which identify the active ingredients of household products, agricultural compounds, proprietary medicines, and poisonous plants are listed in the references to this chapter. A small handbook of this type should be carried in every physician's bag. Poison control centers and manufacturers' representatives are other useful sources of such information. When poisoning is chronic, rapid identification of the toxic agent from the history is frequently impossible. It is therefore fortunate that the lesser therapeutic urgency of such cases usually permits the required painstaking exploration of the patient's habits and environment.

Some poisons can produce clinical features characteristic enough to strongly suggest the diagnosis. Careful examination of the patient may reveal the unmistakable odor of cyanide; the cherry-colored flush of carboxyhemoglobin in skin and mucous membranes; the pupillary constriction, salivation, and gastrointestinal hyperactivity produced by cholinesterase-inhibitor insecticides; or the lead line and extensor paralyses of chronic lead poisoning. Unfortunately, these features are not always present, and in any case telltales are the exception in chemical poisonings.

Chemical analysis of body fluids provides the most definite identification of the intoxicating agent. Some common poisons, such as aspirin, bromides, and barbiturates, can be identified and even quantitated by relatively simple laboratory procedures. Others require more complex toxicologic techniques, such as gas chromatography or bioassay, which are performed only in specialized laboratories. Furthermore, the results of toxicologic determinations are rarely available in time to guide the initial treatment of acute poisoning. Nevertheless, specimens of vomitus, gastric aspirate, blood, urine, and feces should always be saved for toxicologic study if diagnostic or legal questions are likely to arise. Chemical analyses of body fluids or tissues are of particular value in the diagnosis and evaluation of chronic intoxications. Finally, they are useful in following the success of some forms of therapy.

TREATMENT OF CHEMICAL POISONING

Although the physician should always try to identify the poison, such attempts must never delay vital therapeutic measures. Most poisons do not have specific antidotes. Essential supportive care must be given as indicated by the patient's clinical state and does not require knowledge of the toxic agent. Symptomatic treatment of circulatory, respiratory, neurologic, and renal function should be immediately administered as to any other seriously ill patient.

Correct treatment of the poisoned patients thus requires knowledge of both the general principles of management and the details of therapy for specific poisons. Treatment involves four steps: (1) prevention of further absorption of the poison, (2) removal of absorbed poison from the body, (3) symptomatic or supportive therapy, and (4) administration of systemic antidotes (Table 115-1). The first three are applicable to most types of poisoning, the fourth can be used only when the toxic agent is known and a specific antidote is available. Success often depends upon speed of treatment, and, when indicated by the clinical situation, several approaches should be used simultaneously.

PREVENTION OF ABSORPTION OF INGESTED POISONS If appreciable amounts of a poison have been ingested, one should always attempt to minimize its absorption from the gastrointestinal tract. The success of such endeavors depends upon the time elapsed since ingestion and upon the site and speed of absorption of the poison. Prompt action is essential, and it is better to proceed with makeshifts than to waste time while waiting for special equipment or drugs. Conversely, it is unwise to temporize with unpredictable remedies when reliable and effective methods for removal of poison from the gastrointestinal tract are available. When skillfully applied, these methods do not lead to such complications as pulmonary aspiration, gastrointestinal perforation, or convulsions.

Evacuation of the stomach Attempts to empty the stomach are always worthwhile unless specifically contraindicated. They may be highly successful if made soon after ingestion. Significant amounts of poison may be recovered from the stomach hours after ingestion because gastric emptying may be delayed by gastric atony or pylorospasm.

Emesis occurs spontaneously after the ingestion of many poisons. It may be induced in the home by mechanical stimulation of the posterior pharynx or by administration of gastric irritants such as a strong solution of salt or mustard. The emetic action of syrup of ipecac (not the fourteen times more concentrated fluid extract) in 10- to 20-ml dosage is more effective and is safe enough for home use. Regrettably its action has an average latent period of 20 min and depends in part on gastrointestinal absorption, so that

TABLE 115-1
Treatment of acute chemical poisoning

I Prevention of further absorption of poison
- *A* Poisoning by ingestion
  - *1* Emptying the stomach
    - *a* Induction of vomiting
    - *b* Gastric lavage
  - *2* Minimizing gastrointestinal absorption
    - *a* Neutralization and precipitation
    - *b* Adsorption
    - *c* Catharsis
- *B* Poisoning by other routes

II Removal of absorbed poisons from body
- *A* Detoxification—enzyme induction?
- *B* Biliary excretion—interruption of enterohepatic circulation
- *C* Urinary excretion
  - *1* Forced diuresis
  - *2* Alteration of urinary pH
- *D* Dialysis
  - *1* Peritoneal dialysis
  - *2* Hemodialysis
- *E* Charcoal or resin hemoperfusion
- *F* Exchange transfusion
- *G* Chelation and chemical binding

III Supportive therapy

IV Administration of systemic antidotes
- *A* Chemical agents
- *B* Pharmacologic antagonists

it cannot be used in conjunction with other measures intended to minimize absorption of the poison. Apomorphine, 0.06 mg per kg intramuscularly, acts within 5 min but may cause prolonged vomiting. When given intravenously in doses of 0.01 mg per kg, apomorphine tends to produce almost immediate vomiting which is not followed by any other central nervous system effects. All attempts to induce emesis are more often successful if large amounts of fluid have been administered, but these may also hasten passage of the poison through the pylorus. Fluids with high fat content are preferable, since they enter the duodenum more slowly. Not uncommonly it is impossible to induce vomiting, and valuable time should not be lost with hopeful waiting. Induction of vomiting should not be attempted after ingestion of antiemetic drugs, in severely depressed or convulsing patients, or (because of the danger of gastroesophageal perforation or tracheal aspiration of vomitus) in patients who have ingested strong caustics or liquid hydrocarbons which are potent lung irritants (e.g., kerosene, furniture polish).

In comparison with emesis, *gastric lavage* is more predictably and immediately active but usually no more effective in removing poison from the stomach. It can be employed in unconscious patients, and removal of gastric contents reduces the risk of aspiration of vomitus in such patients. It is, however, contraindicated after the ingestion of strong corrosives because of danger of perforating injured tissues. When properly performed, gastric lavage carries little risk of aspiration of gastric contents into the lungs. The patient should be prone, with head and shoulders lowered. A mouth gag is placed and a gastric tube of sufficient diameter to permit withdrawal of particulate matter (size 30) is passed into the stomach. If central nervous system function is depressed and introduction of the tube produces retching, or if pulmonary irritants have been ingested, it is wise to place a *cuffed endotracheal tube* before lavaging. Gastric contents are withdrawn with a large syringe and usually contain most of the poison that will be removed. Thereafter 200 ml (less in children) of warm water or other lavaging solution is alternately instilled and withdrawn until the aspirate becomes clear.

Interference with gastrointestinal absorption Since neither emesis nor gastric lavage empties the stomach completely, one should also minimize absorption by administering substances which inactivate or trap ingested poisons. If mineral acids, alkalies, or other corrosives have been swallowed, water, milk, or a neutralizer (aluminum hydroxide, milk of magnesia, dilute vinegar) is given. Some toxic alkaloids can be precipitated and rendered insoluble by the administration of sulfate. Many other poisons are effectively adsorbed by powdered, activated charcoal. A good grade of activated charcoal can rapidly adsorb as much as half its weight of many common poisons. It is more effective than the so-called "universal antidote," which should be relegated to oblivion. Administration of 100 to 200 ml of a slurry of activated charcoal should be alternated with evacuation of the stomach.

Adsorption by charcoal is reversible, and the effectiveness of adsorption of many poisons varies with the pH. Acidic substances are adsorbed better in acid solutions and may therefore be released in the small intestine. It is desirable to speed the charcoal with its adsorbed poison through the intestine as quickly as possible. This will also decrease intestinal absorption of any unabsorbed poison which has passed beyond the pylorus. It is best accomplished by oral or gastric administration of an osmotic cathartic. Sodium sulfate in 10 to 30 g dosage is the cathartic of choice, since, unlike magnesium sulfate, it produces no symptoms after systemic absorption. Cathartics are generally contraindicated after the ingestion of strong corrosives.

PREVENTION OF ABSORPTION OF POISON FROM OTHER SITES Most topically applied poisons can be removed by copious flushing with water. In certain instances weak acids or bases or appropriate organic solvents are more effective, but rapid and voluminous washing with water should always proceed while they are being obtained. Chemical antidotes can be hazardous because tissue injury may result from the heat of the chemical reaction.

The systemic distribution of injected poisons can be slowed by the application of cold to the injection site or by the proximal application of a tourniquet. Cruciate incision and suction is generally ineffective except after poisonous bites.

Following inhalation of toxic gases, vapors, or dusts, the victim should be removed into clean air and adequate ventilation maintained. If the patient cannot be moved, a protective mask should be applied.

REMOVAL OF ABSORBED POISON FROM THE BODY Unlike prevention or retardation of absorption, measures to speed removal of the toxic agent from the body rarely have much influence on the peak poison concentration. However, they can significantly abbreviate the time during which the concentration of many poisons remains above any given level and may thereby reduce morbidity, avoid complications, and save lives. In judging the need for such measures one must consider the patient's clinical state, the properties and metabolic fate of the poison, and the amount absorbed as judged by the history and the blood level. Removal of some poisons can be accelerated by several methods; selection depends on the clinical urgency, the amount in the body, and the skills and equipment available.

Detoxification Since many poisons are metabolically inactivated in the body, it is regrettable that no clinically effective measures to accelerate detoxification are known. Induction of hepatic enzymes would seem to hold some promise in the treatment of poisonings by certain long-acting drugs whose inactivation depends on the activity of inducible enzymes. The clinical usefulness of this approach remains to be shown. At present, therefore, one must rely on measures capable of accelerating excretion of the poison.

Biliary excretion Certain organic acids and active drugs are secreted into the bile against large concentration gradients. Again, this process cannot presently be accelerated. However, the intestinal resorption of substances already secreted into the bile can be decreased by duodenal suction or osmotic catharsis. These procedures may be useful in poisonings by substances such as glutethimide and chlortetracycline, the action of which is significantly prolonged by their enterohepatic circulation.

Urinary excretion Acceleration of renal excretion is applicable to a much larger number of poisons. Renal excretion of toxic substances depends on glomerular filtration, active tubular secretion, and passive tubular resorption. The first two processes should be protected by maintenance of adequate circulation and renal function, but for practical purposes they cannot be accelerated. On the other hand, passive tubular resorption of many poisons plays an important role in the prolongation of their action and can frequently be decreased by readily available methods.

Passive resorption of most filtered poisons occurs largely in the proximal tubules, because their concentration in the filtrate increases as salt and water are reabsorbed. It can be partly prevented by inhibiting water resorption at this site. This is best accomplished by the administration of osmotic diuretics such as mannitol or urea. By infusing 10 to 20 g per h of mannitol or urea after a loading dose of 25 to 50 g, urine volumes up to 1 liter per h can be achieved. Intravenous administration of 40 mg furosemide further increases urine flow. Great care must be used to supply water and electrolyte needs at the same time. Osmotic diuretics should not be used in the presence of congestive heart failure, shock, or renal failure. The effectiveness of forced diuresis in increasing renal excretion has been demonstrated for salicylates, barbiturates, meprobamate, and glutethimide but is potentially applicable to all ultrafiltered poisons which are passively reabsorbed.

Alteration of the urinary pH can also inhibit passive back-diffusion of some poisons and increase their renal clearance. The renal tubular epithelium is more permeable to uncharged molecules than to ionized solutes. Weak organic acids and bases readily diffuse out of the tubular fluid in their un-ionized form but are trapped in it when ionized. Acidic poisons are largely ionized only at pHs above their pK_a. Alkalinization of the urine greatly increases the ionization in the tubular fluid of such organic acids as phenobarbital and salicylate. In contrast, the pK_a of pentobarbital (8.1) and secobarbital (8.0) is so high that renal clearance is not greatly increased by raising the urinary pH into the physiologic alkaline range. Alkalinization of the urine is achieved by the infusion of sodium bicarbonate, sodium lactate, or tromethamine (which also acts as an osmotic diuretic) at a rate determined by the urinary and blood pH. Excessive systemic alkalosis or electrolyte disturbances must be carefully prevented. A combination of forced diuresis and alkalinization of the urine can raise the renal clearance of some acidic poisons tenfold or more and has been found highly effective in poisoning by salicylate and phenobarbital. The full range of its clinical applicability is undoubtedly much wider but remains to be established. Depression of the urinary pH beyond its usual range may increase the renal clearance of some weakly basic poisons, but clinical data are lacking.

Finally, the renal excretion of certain poisons can be increased in a highly specific fashion. An example is the removal of bromide by administration of chloride and chloriuretics. Such methods are discussed with the individual poisons.

Dialysis The relative effectiveness of forced diuresis at favorable urinary pH and of dialysis must differ widely among drugs but has been established for very few. For barbiturates and some other poisons which are not actively secreted by the renal tubules, maximal clearance rates during extracorporeal dialysis are considerably greater than during peritoneal dialysis or forced diuresis. The latter two maneuvers appear about equally effective. Of course, a skilled team can proceed simultaneously with dialysis and solute diuresis. Dialysis has been found effective in the removal of barbiturates, borate, bromide, chlorate, dimercaprol, diphenylhydantoin, ethanol, ethchlorvynol, ethinamate, glutethimide, glycols, isoniazid, methanol, salicylate, sulfonamides, and thiocyanate. Beyond these, it would theoretically accelerate the removal from the body of any dialyzable toxin which is not irreversibly bound to tissues.

Peritoneal dialysis can be easily performed in any hospital and may be continued for long periods. It is particularly valuable for the removal of poisons if renal function is impaired. Obviously, its effectiveness does not extend to large-molecule, nondialyzable poisons and is decreased by a high degree of protein binding or lipid solubility of the toxic substance. Peritoneal clearance can be increased if the dialyzed poison can be trapped chemically in the dialysis fluid so that a high gradient of the dialyzable portion is maintained from blood to peritoneal cavity between fluid changes. A 5% concentration of albumin in the dialysis solution acts as an effective ligand during the dialysis of salicylate and should be similarly useful for the removal of other albumin-bound poisons. Another approach to prevent back-diffusion consists of making the pH of dialysis fluid sufficiently greater or less than 7.4 to ionize poisons which are dialyzable only in the undissociated form. Finally, the addition of various drugs to the dialysis fluid can increase peritoneal dialysis, presumably by increasing peritoneal blood flow or mesothelial permeability. The clinical value of this approach has not yet been defined.

Hemodialysis is unquestionably the most effective procedure for removing large amounts of dialyzable poisons. For barbiturates dialysance rates of 50 to 100 ml per min have been achieved, a removal rate two to ten times faster than during peritoneal dialysis or forced diuresis. Dialysis against solutions containing albumin or lipids can further speed removal of certain poisons. Extracorporeal dialysis is clearly the procedure of choice for the rapid removal of dialyzable poisons from patients who have absorbed amounts which make survival unlikely even under the best supportive care. Since the required equipment and skilled personnel are available only in a few hospitals, the possibility of transfer of such patients to one of these institutions should be considered.

Charcoal or resin hemoperfusion Perfusion of blood through activated charcoal or exchange resin columns achieves higher clearance rates for some poisons than hemodialysis. However, significant reductions in the formed elements of the blood may occur during the use of these techniques.

Exchange transfusion Withdrawal and replacement of blood is an effective procedure for the removal of those poisons which are not highly tissue-bound or lipid-soluble and therefore remain in the blood in appreciable concentration. It has obvious advantages in poisoning by nondiffusible and particularly by highly albumin-bound toxins. Though it requires little specialized equipment, its applicability to adults is limited by the requirement of large amounts of blood.

Chelation and chemical binding The removal of some poisons is accelerated by chemical interaction with other substances followed by renal excretion. These substances are usually considered specific antidotes and are discussed with the individual poisons.

SUPPORTIVE THERAPY Most chemical poisonings are reversible, self-limited disease states. Skillful supportive therapy can keep many seriously poisoned patients alive and their detoxifying and excretory mechanisms functioning until the concentration of poison in the body has fallen to safe levels. Symptomatic measures are especially important when the poison is one of the many compounds for which no specific antidote is known. Even when an antidote is available, disturbances of vital functions must be prevented or controlled by appropriate supportive care.

The poisoned patient may suffer a variety of physiologic disturbances. Most of these are not peculiar to chemical intoxications, and their therapeutic management is described elsewhere in this text. Only those aspects of supportive therapy specially relevant to poisonings are briefly discussed here.

Central nervous system depression Specific therapy directed against the depressant effects of poisons on the central nervous system is usually both unnecessary and difficult. Most poisoned patients will emerge from coma as from a prolonged anesthesia. During the period of unconsciousness meticulous nursing care and close observation are essential. If depression of medullary centers results in circulatory or respiratory failure, these vital functions must be immediately and vigorously supported by chemical or mechanical means.

The use of analeptics in the treatment of poison-induced central nervous system depression has been largely abandoned, for the following reasons: (1) Their effect is unpredictable, and their use in intoxicated patients produces an abnormal pattern of nervous activity in which paroxysmal excitation and convulsions may be superimposed on depression. (2) The availability of artificial ventilation and of effective measures to support the circulation has lessened the need for rapid restoration of normal medullary function. (3) It is doubtful that analeptics shorten the duration of coma sufficiently to justify their risks, and they have not been shown to improve prognosis. Certainly these agents should never be employed to restore consciousness, and it is doubtful whether their use to hasten the restoration of spontaneous breathing and active reflexes is ever justified. Picrotoxin, pentylenetetrazol, bemegride, and ethamivan are available analeptics.

Convulsions Many poisons (e.g., chlorinated hydrocarbons, insecticides, strychnine) cause convulsions by their specific excitatory effects. Poisoned patients may also have convulsions because of hypoxia, hypoglycemia, cerebral edema, or metabolic disturbances. In such cases these abnormalities should be corrected as far as possible. Regardless of the cause of the convulsions, anticonvulsant drugs are often required. Short-acting compounds, such as intravenously administered thiopental, may be preferable, because in poisoned patients profound depression may accompany or quickly follow convulsions. Intravenously administered diazepam has also been effective.

Cerebral edema Intracranial hypertension due to cerebral edema is also a characteristic effect of some poisons and a nonspecific result of other chemical intoxications. Cerebral edema is characteristically seen in poisoning by lead, carbon monoxide, and methanol. Symptomatic treatment consists of use of adrenocortical steroids and, when necessary, the intravenous administration of hypertonic solutions of mannitol or urea.

Hypotension The causes of hypotension and shock in the poisoned patient are legion, and often several of them coexist. Poisons can depress the medullary vasomotor centers, block autonomic ganglia or adrenergic receptors, directly depress the tone of arterial or venous smooth muscle, reduce myocardial contractility, or induce cardiac arrhythmias. Less specifically, the poisoned patient may be in shock because of tissue hypoxia, extensive tissue destruction from corrosives, loss of blood or fluids, or metabolic disturbances. When possible, these abnormalities should be promptly corrected. If the central venous pressure is low, fluid replacement should be the first therapeutic approach. Vasoactive drugs are often helpful and sometimes essential in the hypotensive poisoned patient, particularly in shock resulting from central depression. As in shock from other causes, choice of the most appropriate agent requires an analysis of the hemodynamic disturbance which goes beyond determination of the arterial pressure.

Cardiac arrhythmias Disturbances of cardiac impulse generation or conduction in the poisoned patient arise from the effects of certain poisons on the electrical properties of cardiac fibers or from myocardial hypoxia or metabolic disturbances. The latter should be corrected and antiarrhythmic agents administered as indicated by the nature of the arrhythmia (Chap. 238).

Pulmonary edema The poisoned patient may develop pulmonary edema because of depressed myocardial contractility or because of alveolar injury from irritant gases or aspirated fluids. The latter type of edema is less responsive to treatment and may be associated with laryngeal edema. Therapeutic measures include suctioning, administration of high concentrations of oxygen under positive pressure, aerosols of surface-active agents, bronchodilators, and adrenocortical steroids.

Hypoxia Poisoning may cause tissue hypoxia by various mechanisms, and several of these may operate in one patient. Inadequate ventilation can result from central respiratory depression, from muscular paralysis, or from airway obstruction by retained secretions, laryngeal edema, or bronchospasm. Alveolar-capillary diffusion may be impaired by pulmonary edema. Anemia, methemoglobinemia, carboxyhemoglobinemia, or shock can interfere with oxygen transport. Cellular oxidation may be inhibited by cyanide, fluoroacetate, or general protoplasmic poisons. The highest priority in treatment must be given to maintenance of an adequate airway. The clinical situation and the site of obstruction may indicate frequent suctioning, insertion of an oropharyngeal airway or of an endotracheal tube, or a tracheotomy. If despite a clear airway ventilation remains inadequate, as judged by clinical appearance or by measurement of minute volume or blood gases, artificial ventilation by appropriate mechanical means is imperative. Administration of high concentrations of oxygen is indicated whenever tissue hypoxia occurs. When the central nervous system is severely depressed, oxygen administration often results in apnea and must be combined with artificial ventilation. Hyperbaric oxygen may be helpful in some situations. The treatment of methemoglobinemia, carboxyhemoglobinemia, and inhibition of cellular oxidation is discussed under the specific poisons which produce these changes.

Acute renal insufficiency Renal failure with oliguria or anuria may occur in the poisoned patient because of shock, dehydration, or electrolyte disturbances. More specifically, it may be due to the nephrotoxic potential of some poisons (e.g., mercury, phosphorus, carbon tetrachloride, bromate), many of which are concentrated and excreted by the kidney. Renal damage due to poisons is usually reversible. The management of acute renal insufficiency is outlined in Chap. 272.

Electrolyte and water disturbances Imbalances of fluid and electrolytes are common features of chemical poisoning. They may result from vomiting, diarrhea, renal insufficiency, or therapeutic maneuvers such as catharsis, forced diuresis, or dialysis. These disturbances are corrected or, ideally, prevented by appropriate therapy. Certain poisons produce more specific defects, such as metabolic acidosis (e.g., methanol, phenol, salicylate) or hypocalcemia (e.g., fluoride, oxalate). These abnormalities and any specific treatment are described under the individual poisons.

Acute hepatic insufficiency The primary manifestation of some poisonings (e.g., chlorinated hydrocarbons, phosphorus, cinchophen, certain mushrooms) is acute hepatic failure. Its management is described in Chap. 299.

ADMINISTRATION OF SYSTEMIC ANTIDOTES Specific antidotal therapy is available for only a few poisons. Some systemic antidotes are chemicals which exert their therapeutic effect by reducing the concentration of the toxic substance. They may do this by combining with the poison (e.g., ethylene diaminetetraacetate with lead, dimercaprol with mercury) or by increasing its excretion (e.g., chloride or mercurial diuretics in bromide poisoning). Other systemic antidotes compete with the poison for its receptor site (e.g., atropine with muscarine, nallorphine and naloxone with morphine, vitamin K_1 with Coumadin). Specific antidotes are discussed with the individual poisons.

REFERENCES

ARENA JM: Current status—The management and treatment of poisoning. General principles and specific antidotes. Mod Treat 8:461, 1971

——: *Poisoning,* 3d ed., Springfield, Ill.: Charles C Thomas, 1974

ARLEFF AI et al: Coma following nonnarcotic drug overdosage—Management of 208 adult patients. Am J Med Sci 266:405, 1973

COLEMAN AB: Accidental poisoning. N Engl J Med 277:1135, 1967

CORBY DG et al: The efficiency of methods used to evacuate the stomach after acute ingestions. Pediatrics 40:871, 1967

——: Management of acute poisoning with activated charcoal. Pediatrics 54:324, 1974

DEICHMAN WB, GERARDE HW: *Toxicology of Drugs and Chemicals,* New York: Academic, 1969

DREISBACH RH: *Handbook of Poisoning: Diagnosis and Treatment,* 8th ed., Los Altos, Calif.: Lange, 1974

GOSSELIN RE, SMITH RP: Trends in the therapy of acute poisonings. Clin Pharmacol Ther 7:279, 1966

KAY S: *Handbook of Emergency Toxicology,* 3d ed., Springfield, Ill.: Charles C Thomas, 1973

KNEPSHIELD JH et al: Dialysis of poisons and drugs—Annual review. Trans Am Soc Artif Intern Organs 19:590, 1973

LAWRENCE RA: Household agents and their potential toxicity. Mod Treat 8:511, 1971

LOCKET S: Haemodialysis in the treatment of acute poisoning. Proc R Soc Med 63:427, 1970

MATTHEW H, LAWSON AAH: *Treatment of Common Acute Poisonings,* 2d ed., Baltimore: Williams & Wilkins, 1970

MOFENSON HC, GREENSHER J: The unknown poison. Pediatrics 54:336, 1974

POLSON CJ, TATTERSALL RN: *Clinical Toxicology,* 2d ed., Philadelphia: Lippincott, 1969

ROSENBAUM JL et al: Resin hemoperfusion: a new treatment for acute drug intoxication. N Engl J Med 284:874, 1971

STOLMAN A: The absorption, distribution, and excretion of drugs and poisons and their metabolites. Prog Chem Toxicol 5:1, 1974

THIENES CH, HALEY TJ: *Clinical Toxicology,* 5th ed., Philadelphia: Lea & Febiger, 1972

VERHULST HL, CROTTY JJ: Childhood poisoning accidents. JAMA 203:1049, 1968

Toxic product information

ADAMS WC: Poison control centers: their purpose and operation. Clin Pharmacol Ther 4:293, 1963

BROWN RL: *Pesticides in Clinical Practice,* Springfield, Ill.: Charles C Thomas, 1966

Drug Identification Guide, Oradell, N.J.: Medical Economics, Inc., 1975

GLEASON MN et al: *Clinical Toxicology of Commercial Products,* 3d ed., Baltimore: Williams & Wilkins, 1969

GOODMAN LS, GILMAN A: *The Pharmacological Basis of Therapeutics,* 4th ed., New York: Macmillan, 1970

KINGSBURY JM: *Poisonous Plants of the United States and Canada,* 3d ed., Englewood Cliffs, N.J.: Prentice-Hall, 1964

The Merck Index, 8th ed., Rahway, N.J.: Merck & Co., Inc., 1968

NATIONAL ACADEMY OF SCIENCES: *Toxicants Occurring Naturally in Foods,* publ. 1354, Washington: 1966

SAX NI: *Dangerous Properties of Industrial Materials,* 3d ed., New York: Reinhold, 1968

WILSON CO, JONES TE: *American Drug Index,* Philadelphia: Lippincott, 1975

116
COMMON POISONS

JAN KOCH-WESER

The poisons discussed in this chapter are those encountered by the general population such as commonly used drugs, household products, solvents, pesticides, and poisonous plants. It has been necessary to disregard many uncommon toxic materials as well as products to which exposure occurs only in specialized industrial environments. Details concerning poisoning by such compounds may be found in some of the references following Chap. 115. Toxic effects of many drugs are considered throughout this text in conjunction with their therapeutic use. Manifestations of hypersensitivity to chemicals are described in Chap. 67. The following discussions of specific poisons stress those details of their action which are pertinent to the recognition or treatment of clinical poisoning.

ACIDS Corrosive acids are used widely in industry and laboratories. Ingestion is almost always with suicidal intent. Death has occurred after an oral dose of 1 ml of a corrosive acid.

Toxic effects of corrosive acids are largely due to their direct chemical action. They convert tissue protein to acid proteinate which is soluble in the acid. Irritation, bleeding, sloughing, and perforation of the esophagus and stomach are common. Mouth and pharynx are brownish-black and may have a charred appearance. Yellow staining is seen after ingestion of nitric and picric acids. Severe pain in mouth, pharynx, chest, and abdomen is the rule and is soon followed by vomiting and diarrhea of coffee grounds appearance. Frequently profound shock develops. About half of those who ingest significant amounts of acid die from its immediate effects. The survivors often develop mediastinitis or peritonitis from esophageal or gastric perforation. Delayed perforation of the esophagus or stomach also occurs. Recovery from acid ingestion is often associated with esophageal stricture.

Ingested acid must be immediately diluted a hundredfold by water or milk or neutralized with weak alkali. Milk of magnesia or magnesium and aluminum antacids are excellent for the purpose. Sodium bicarbonate should be avoided because the evolved carbon dioxide may rupture an eroded viscus. The danger of perforation also contraindicates the use of emesis or gastric lavage except during the first 30 min after ingestion. Following the emergency measures, appropriate supportive therapy is administered for the relief of pain and the treatment of shock, perforation, and infection.

Certain gases found in industry may combine with water in the lungs to form corrosive acids. During rapid decomposition of plant material in silos, oxides of nitrogen are released which form nitric acid in the lungs. Inhalation of such gases causes coughing and choking sensations which are followed after a latent period of 6 to 8 h by pulmonary edema. Treatment is supportive. Symptoms of dyspnea and hemoptysis may be prolonged, and frequent relapses may occur.

ALKALIES Strong alkalies such as ammonium hydroxide, potassium hydroxide (potash), potassium carbonate, sodium hydroxide (lye), and sodium carbonate (washing soda) are widely used in industry and in cleansers and drain cleaners. Sodium and potassium phosphates find use as water softeners. Strong alkalies form soaps with fats and proteinates with proteins, resulting in penetrating necrosis of tissues. Fatalities have occurred from the ingestion of 5 to 30 g of such compounds.

The toxic effects of alkalies are almost entirely due to irritation and destruction of local tissues. Ingestion is followed by severe pain in mouth, pharynx, chest, and abdomen. Vomiting of blood and sloughed mucosa and diarrhea are common. Reflex loss of vascular tone frequently leads to profound shock. Perforation of the esophagus or stomach may be immediate or delayed for several days. Mouth and pharynx show erythema and gelatinous necrotic areas. After ingestion of water softeners profound reduction in serum calcium may be seen and lead to tetany and hypotension. Ingestion of strong alkali is rapidly fatal in about 25 percent of cases. Survivors usually suffer from esophageal strictures.

Treatment consists of immediate administration of large amounts of water, milk, fruit juices, or 10 percent vinegar. The volume of liquids should exceed that of the ingested alkali a hundredfold. Vomiting should be allowed to occur, and gastric lavage may be performed during the first half-hour after ingestion. Because of the danger of perforation, both are contraindicated thereafter. After the ingestion of water softeners (phosphates), calcium gluconate should be administered intravenously as needed. Treatment is otherwise symptomatic and directed at the relief of pain, respiratory obstruction due to edema of the hypopharynx, fluid loss, and shock.

Inhalation of ammonia, which is used as a refrigerant, results in irritation of the upper and lower parts of the respiratory tract. Laryngeal and pulmonary edema may occur and must be treated symptomatically.

ANILINE This substance is used in printing and cloth-marking inks, crayons, paints, and paint removers. Both aniline and its derivatives, such as toluidine, nitroaniline, and nitrobenzene, are widely used in industrial synthesis. Aniline is absorbed from the gastrointestinal tract and through the lungs or skin. Ingestion of 1 g aniline has been fatal. Methemoglobinemia is the most important manifestation. Headache, dizziness, hypotension, convulsions, and coma may occur. If the acute period is survived, jaundice and anemia may appear. Treatment consists of correction of methemoglobinemia (see Chap. 316) and supportive measures.

ANTIHISTAMINES The common and unprescribed use of antihistamines makes them readily available for accidental overdosage and suicidal attempts. There is wide variation from patient to patient in tolerance to these drugs and in the manifestations of poisoning. A dose of 200 mg diphenhydramine has been fatal in one adult, whereas another tolerated 2 g. Manifestations of poisoning are central nervous system excitement or depression. In children the usual toxic manifestations are excitement, hyperthermia, hyperreflexia, tremors, and convulsions, followed by central nervous system depression. In adults depressive manifestations with drowsiness, stupor, and coma predominate, but convulsions followed by further depression may occur.

Treatment is supportive and directed toward removal of the unabsorbed drug and maintenance of vital functions. Stimulants should be avoided. Convulsions may be controlled with short-acting barbiturates, ether, or succinylcholine. Some antihistamines have prominent atropine-like properties. Patients poisoned with these drugs may show manifestations of atropine poisoning and are treated correspondingly.

ANTIMUSCARINIC COMPOUNDS Atropine, related belladonna alkaloids (hyoscyamine and scopolamine), and synthetic substitutes (e.g., benztropine, cyclopentolate, homatropine, methantheline, propantheline) are widely prescribed drugs and occur in many proprietary mixtures used in the treatment of gastrointestinal and upper respiratory diseases, asthma, and parkinsonism. Poisoning, especially in children, may also occur from the excessive use of ophthalmic solutions containing such compounds. Finally, children may be intoxicated by eating plants containing up to 0.5 percent of atropine or related alkaloids. Such plants are *Atropa belladonna* (deadly nightshade), *Hyoscyamus niger* (henbane), and *Datura stramonium* (Jamestown or Jimson weed).

Individual sensitivity to the toxic effects of belladonna alkaloids varies widely; fatalities have occurred from as little as 10 mg atropine, but doses of 500 mg have been survived. Young children are particularly susceptible to poisoning with belladonna alkaloids. Older persons appear to be more sensitive to the central nervous system effects of these drugs. Since atropine is both hydrolyzed in the liver and excreted unchanged in the urine, insufficiency of hepatic or renal function may lead to poisoning on therapeutic dosage.

The most characteristic manifestations of atropine poisoning are those of parasympathetic blockade: dryness of mucous membranes, thirst, dysphagia, hoarseness, xerophthalmia, dilated pupils, blurring of vision, rise in intraocular tension, flushing, dryness and increased temperature of the skin, fever, tachycardia, hypertension, urinary retention, and abdominal distention. This widespread parasympatholysis is almost diagnostic of belladonna poisoning, but the diagnosis can be further confirmed by the absence of any parasympathomimetic effects following the intramuscular injection of 10 mg methacholine.

Central nervous system symptoms are also very common during belladonna intoxication. Atropine and scopolamine produce similar toxic psychoses. Restlessness, excitation, confusion, and incoordination precede mania, hallucinations, and delirium. Patients intoxicated by scopolamine not infrequently show lethargy and somnolence rather than excitement. In severe intoxication with belladonna alkaloids, central nervous system depression and coma are the rule. When death results it is because of circulatory collapse and respiratory failure.

In the treatment of belladonna poisoning, gastric lavage with an aqueous slurry of activated charcoal should be initiated quickly. Symptomatic treatment is directed at the reduction of body temperature, the moistening of mucous membranes, and, when necessary, urethral catheterization. Excitement, convulsions, or depression may require appropriate pharmacotherapy. Parasympathomimetic agents, such as methacholine or pilocarpine, are of little value, since they cannot be given in concentrations sufficient to overcome the peripheral cholinergic blockade. Furthermore, they have no effect on the potentially lethal central nervous system toxicity of the belladonna alkaloids.

Death occurs in fewer than 1 percent of cases of atropine or scopolamine poisoning. No permanent sequelae have been observed, but manifestations may persist for several days.

BARIUM Poisoning may be due to the ingestion of rodenticides which contain soluble barium salts or of depilatories that contain barium sulfide. Intoxication may also occur in industry or from the accidental use of a soluble barium salt as a radiopaque contrast medium. Barium is extremely toxic, producing intense stimulation of muscles of all types. Its action on the gastrointestinal musculature causes vomiting, colic, and diarrhea. Skeletal muscle tremors and spasm are commonly seen. Arteriolar spasm results in marked hypertension. Cardiac arrhythmias may proceed to ventricular fibrillation. Anxiety, weakness, and convulsions may occur. Death is usually due to cardiac arrhythmia or respiratory arrest.

Treatment consists of the oral administration of 250 ml 10% sodium sulfate or 5% magnesium sulfate. This will precipitate and remove any unabsorbed barium in the gastrointestinal tract. A dose of 10 ml of a 10% solution of sodium sulfate should be slowly administered intravenously every 30 min until symptoms subside. Procainamide may be used to reduce the danger of fatal cardiac arrhythmias. If necessary, pain should be relieved and artificial ventilation with oxygen administered.

BENZENE, TOLUENE These solvents are used in paint removers, dry-cleaning solutions, and rubber or plastic cements. Benzene is also present, to some extent, in most gasolines. Poisoning may result from ingestion or from the breathing of concentrated vapors. Toluene is the major ingredient in the cement used by teen-age glue sniffers.

Acute poisoning by these compounds causes central nervous system manifestations. With sufficient exposure, symptoms progress from an initial period of restlessness, excitement, euphoria, and dizziness to coma, convulsions, and respiratory failure. Ventricular arrhythmias may occur.

Chronic poisoning by benzene or toluene results from repeated exposure to their vapors in low concentration. Central nervous system symptoms include irritability, insomnia, headache, tremors, and paresthesias. Anorexia and nausea are also common. Fatty degeneration of the heart, liver, and kidneys may occur. By far the most important manifestation of chronic exposure to benzene is bone marrow depression, which may progress to aplastic anemia and complete aplasia of the bone marrow. Individual susceptibility to this effect varies greatly and may not become apparent for months after the initial exposure to the poison.

Treatment of both acute and chronic poisoning is symptomatic. After ingestion, emesis must not be induced, and gastric lavage should await placement of an endotracheal tube with an inflatable cuff. Neurologic, pulmonary, or cardiovascular problems are treated as in poisoning by petroleum distillates.

BLEACHES Clorox, Purex, Sanichlor, and other bleaching solutions contain 3 to 6% sodium hypochlorite. Their corrosive action in mouth, pharynx, and esophagus is similar to that of sodium hydroxide. Acid gastric juice releases hypochlorous acid from such solutions. This compound is very irritating to mucous membranes, and inhalation of its fumes causes severe pulmonary irritation and pulmonary edema. However, the systemic toxicity of hypochlorous acid is low. Perforation and stricture formation are rare after the ingestion of bleaching solutions. The fatal dose is approximately 30 ml.

Treatment consists of emesis or gastric lavage with water, milk, milk of magnesia, aluminum hydroxide, or sodium bicarbonate solution. Acid antidotes should not be used. If available, 200 ml of a 5% solution of sodium thiosulfate should be administered by mouth, since this will immediately reduce hypochlorite to nontoxic products. Supportive measures may be needed as in alkali poisoning.

BORIC ACID This compound is a very weak germicide and has been widely employed in powders, lotions, solutions, and ointments. Though not highly toxic, boric acid is not nearly as benign as widely assumed. The lethal dose is approximately 15 g in adults and 5 g in infants. Such amounts can be easily absorbed through abraded skin, from serous cavities, and after ingestion. Furthermore, accumulation of the compound occurs because of slow renal excretion.

Regardless of the route of administration, the first symptoms of poisoning are nausea, vomiting, and diarrhea. These are followed by headache, weakness, restlessness, and an erythematous rash which may progress to desquamation of skin and mucous membranes. Renal toxicity and shock are common, and more than 100 fatalities have occurred. Treatment is entirely supportive. Boric acid should always be labeled as a poison and must not be applied to extensive skin lesions.

BROMATES These compounds are used as neutralizers in cold wave preparations. They produce widespread tissue injury, particularly in central nervous system and kidneys. The fatal oral dose of bromates is approximately 5 g. On contact of bromate with gastric acid, hydrogen bromate, an irritating acid, is formed. Ingestion of bromates is followed by vomiting, diarrhea, abdominal pain, drowsiness, coma, convulsions, hypotension, hematuria, oliguria, anuria, and hemolysis.

Treatment consists of emesis or gastric lavage with sodium bicarbonate solution followed by catharsis. A dose of 250 ml of a 1% sodium thiosulfate solution should be administered intravenously. Peritoneal dialysis or hemodialysis effectively removes bromate from the body. Appropriate supportive therapy should be given.

CANTHARIDIN This active principle of *Cantharis vesicatoria* (Spanish fly) is not a useful therapeutic agent. Poisoning is due to the unfortunate and wishful reputation of cantharidin as an abortifacient or aphrodisiac. The compound is a very potent irritant to all tissues, and ingestion of 10 mg may be fatal. Initial symptoms after ingestion are severe burning pain in the upper part of the gastrointestinal tract, hematemesis, and bloody diarrhea. These are rapidly followed by burning urethral pain, priapism, hematuria, oliguria, anuria, uremia, hepatic failure, myocarditis, shock, delirium, and coma. Death may occur within a few hours or up to 1 week after poisoning. Treatment is entirely symptomatic and supportive.

CARBON MONOXIDE Carbon monoxide is a colorless, odorless, tasteless, and nonirritating gas produced by the incomplete combustion of carbonaceous materials. Almost any flame or combustion device emits carbon monoxide. The gas is present in the exhaust of internal combustion engines in a concentration of 3 to 7 percent. Much higher concentrations are present in most illuminating and heating gases, but not in natural gas. Carbon monoxide is annually responsible for hundreds of accidental and suicidal deaths.

The toxic effects of carbon monoxide are the result of tissue hypoxia. Carbon monoxide combines with hemoglobin to form carboxyhemoglobin. Since carbon monoxide and oxygen react with the same group in the hemoglobin molecule, carboxyhemoglobin is incapable of carrying oxygen. The affinity of hemoglobin for carbon monoxide is two hundred times greater than for oxygen, and at equilibrium 1 part of carbon monoxide in 1,500 parts of air will result in 50 percent conversion of hemoglobin to carboxyhemoglobin. Carboxyhemoglobin also interferes with the release of oxygen from oxyhemoglobin. This further reduces the amount of oxygen available to the tissues and explains why tissue anoxia appears in the carbon monoxide-poisoned person at levels of arterial oxyhemoglobin concentration well tolerated by the anemic patient.

The extent of saturation of hemoglobin with carbon monoxide depends on the concentration of the gas in inspired air and on the time of exposure. The severity of hypoxic symptoms depends further on the state of activity of the individual, his tissue oxygen needs, and his hemoglobin concentration. As a general rule, no symptoms will develop at a concentration of 0.01 percent carbon monoxide in inspired air, since this will not raise blood saturation above 10 percent. Exposure to 0.05 percent for 1 h during light activity will produce a blood concentration of 20 percent carboxyhemoglobin and result in a mild or throbbing headache. Greater activity or longer exposure to the same concentration causes a blood saturation of 30 to 50 percent. At this point headache, irritability, confusion, dizziness, visual disturbances, nausea, vomiting, and fainting on exertion may be observed. After exposure for 1 h to concentrations of 0.1 percent in inspired air, the blood will contain 50 to 80 percent carboxyhemoglobin, which results in coma, convulsions, respiratory failure, and death. On inhalation of high concentrations of carbon monoxide, saturation of the blood proceeds so rapidly that unconsciousness may occur suddenly and without warning. When poisoning is more gradual, the individual may notice decreased exercise tolerance and dyspnea on exertion or even at rest. Excessive sweating, fever, hepatomegaly, skin lesions, leukocytosis, bleeding diathesis, albuminuria, and glycosuria have also been described. Cerebral edema and intracranial hypertension may result from the increased permeability of hypoxic capillaries. Myocardial hypoxia is reflected by electrocardiographic abnormalities.

The most characteristic sign of carbon monoxide poisoning is the cherry color of skin and mucous membranes, which is due to the bright red carboxyhemoglobin. If the characteristic flush is not present, 5 ml of 40% sodium hydroxide may be added to 5 ml of a 5% solution of blood in water. An oxyhemoglobin solution will turn brown, but a carboxyhemoglobin solution remains red.

Treatment of carbon monoxide poisoning requires effective ventilation in the presence of high oxygen tensions and in the absence of carbon monoxide. If necessary, ventilation should be supported artificially. Pure oxygen should be administered. This will result not only in the replacement of carbon monoxide by oxygen in the hemoglobin molecule but also in the partial relief of tissue hypoxia by oxygen dissolved in the plasma. For the same reasons hyperbaric oxygen is helpful in seriously poisoned patients. Transfusion of blood or packed cells is also of value. In order to reduce tissue needs for oxygen, the patient must be kept absolutely quiet. The induction of hypothermia may further reduce oxygen requirements.

During the recovery from carbon monoxide poisoning symptoms regress gradually. If severe tissue hypoxia has obtained too long, neurologic symptoms such as tremors, mental deterioration, and psychotic behavior may persist. Histologic changes characteristic of hypoxia may be observed in cerebral cortex, medulla, myocardium, and other organs.

CASTOR BEANS The castor bean plant (*Ricinus communis*) is grown for commercial and ornamental purposes. The beans contain ricin, an extremely toxic albumin, which causes agglutination and hemolysis of red blood cells and injury to all other cells. After a delay of several hours to 2 days following ingestion, abdominal pain, vomiting, and profuse diarrhea appear and produce severe dehydration. Extreme weakness, drowsiness, disorientation, stupor, coma, convulsions, respiratory depression, and circulatory collapse may develop. Intravascular clotting and hemolysis have been observed. If the patient survives the acute symptoms, oliguria may progress to anuria and uremia, with death after several days. Treatment consists of fluid replacement, alkalinization of the urine with sodium bicarbonate to prevent precipitation of hemoglobin in the kidneys, and supportive measures.

CATHARTIC RESINS Colocynth, croton oil, gamboge, and podophyllum are drastic cathartics because of their content of highly irritating plant resins. These compounds have no therapeutic use; poisoning is usually the work of ignorant pranksters. Oral administration of 1 g of these substances has been fatal. Symptoms are burning pain in mouth, esophagus, and stomach, hematemesis, watery or bloody diarrhea, dehydration, shock, coma, and death. Treatment consists of removal of the irritant from the gastrointestinal tract and supportive measures. Large amounts of parenteral fluids, blood replacement, and morphine and atropine to quiet the intestinal tract may be required.

CHLORATES Sodium and potassium chlorates are strong oxidizing agents and are found in gargles, mouthwashes, matches, and weed killers. After oral ingestion, 2 g has been fatal for children and 10 g for adults. Chlorate ion acts as a catalyst in the production of methemoglobinemia, and absorption of a small amount can result in a high methemoglobin concentration. The symptoms of chlorate ingestion are those of local mucosal irritation and of methemoglobinemia (see Chap. 60 and 316). Renal toxicity is common. Treatment is directed at the methemoglobinemia and is otherwise supportive.

CHLORINATED INSECTICIDES These compounds are common ingredients of dusts, sprays, and solutions used as insecticides. The great majority of these compounds are chlorinated diphenyls (e.g., DDT, TDE, DFDT, DMC, Neotran) or chlorinated polycyclic compounds (e.g., aldrin, chlordane, dieldrin, endrin, heptachlor). Lindane is a hexachlorobenzene. The toxic effects of all these agents are similar. The chlorinated insecticides are soluble in lipid and organic solvents but not in water. They are poorly absorbed unless dissolved in a vehicle such as kerosene, petroleum distillates, or other organic solvents. Under these circumstances they readily enter the body through the skin, lungs, or gastrointestinal tract. These compounds vary considerably in toxicity, and the toxicity of the dissolving vehicle must also be considered. The effects of the solvent may overshadow or modify those of the insecticide.

The initial symptoms of acute poisoning are nausea, vomiting, headache, dizziness, apprehension, excitement, and muscular tremors and weakness. These symptoms progress to generalized central nervous system hyperexcitability and delirium and clonic or tonic convulsions. This stage is in turn followed by progressive depression with paralysis, coma, and death. In chronically poisoned patients cerebellar symptoms and evidence of liver damage may develop. Hepatic toxicity is particularly prominent in poisoning by a hexachlorobenzene. Treatment consists of gastric lavage and catharsis, anticonvulsive therapy with short-acting barbiturates, artificial ventilation, and other supportive measures. Sympathomimetic compounds should be avoided, since chlorinated insecticides apparently increase susceptibility to ventricular fibrillation.

CHOLINESTERASE INHIBITOR INSECTICIDES Many substances used in agriculture for control of soft-bodied insects are potent inhibitors of cholinesterase. Most of these compounds are organic phosphates (e.g., Parathion, Malathion, Systox, TEPP, HETP, OMPA), others are carbamates (e.g., Dimetan, Mactacil). The toxicity of these compounds varies widely. They are usually prepared for use by dilution with powders, organic solvents, or water. Formulations containing 1 to 95 percent of the active ingredient are available. The cholinesterase inhibitor insecticides are rapidly absorbed through the intact skin and after inhalation or ingestion.

The organic phosphate esters act by combining with and inactivating acetylcholinesterase. Since this enzyme normally breaks down the acetylcholine liberated by the central nervous system, autonomic ganglia, parasympathetic nerve endings, and motor nerve endings, its inactivation allows the accumulation of large amounts of acetylcholine at these sites. In the central nervous system initial stimulation is followed by depression of cells, resulting in convulsions followed by coma and respiratory depression. Initial stimulation and later blockade of autonomic ganglia results in multiple and variable dysfunctions of structures innervated by the autonomic nervous system. Accumulation of acetylcholine at parasympathetic nerve endings produces pupillary constriction and blurring of vision; stimulation of intestinal muscle resulting in abdominal cramps, vomiting, and diarrhea; stimulation of secretory glands causing rhinorrhea, salivation, sweating, and bronchorrhea; constriction of the bronchial musculature with symptoms of respiratory distress; depression of the cardiac sinus pacemaker activity; and impairment of atrioventricular conduction. Persistence of acetylcholine at the neuromuscular junction results in muscular tremors, cramps, and fasciculations which are followed by neuromuscular block and flaccid paralysis. Other important clinical manifestations of these poisons are cyanosis and pulmonary edema.

Management consists of emesis or lavage, catharsis, and washing of contaminated skin with soap and water. Atropine should be given immediately to block the parasympathetic and central nervous system effects. A dose of 2 mg is injected intramuscularly and repeated every 10 min until parasympathetic manifestations are controlled and signs of atropinization appear. The same dosage must be repeated frequently to maintain xerostomia and mild tachycardia. Fatal respiratory failure or pulmonary edema may occur quickly upon cessation of atropine therapy. Atropine is virtually ineffective against the autonomic ganglionic actions of acetycholine and against the peripheral neuromuscular paralysis. Certain oximes act as cholinesterase reactivators. Pralidoxime is useful in the treatment of organic phosphate cholinesterase inhibition but should not be used if the inhibition is due to a carbamate. A dose of 1 g pralidoxime in aqueous solution is administered intravenously over a 5-min period and may be repeated twice each day. Supportive therapy includes administration of oxygen with artificial ventilation if necessary, removal of pulmonary secretions by suction, and treatment of convulsions with short-acting barbiturates. Energetic therapy with artificial ventilation, atropine, and pralidoxime allows survival after doses of organic phospate esters vastly exceeding the usual fatal dose.

CYANIDE The cyanide ion is an exceedingly potent and rapid-acting poison, but one for which specific and effective antidotal therapy is available. Cyanide poisoning may result from the inhalation of hydrocyanic acid or from the ingestion of soluble inorganic cyanide salts or cyanide-releasing substances such as cyanamide, cyanogen chloride, and nitroprusside. Parts of many plants also contain substances such as amygdalin which release cyanide on digestion. Among these are the seeds of certain stone fruits (chokecherry, pin cherry, wild black cherry, peach, apricot, bitter almond), cassava roots, the berries of the jet berry bush, the leaves and shoots of elderberry, and all parts of hydrangea. Cyanides are widely used in industry and for fumigation and may reach the home in photographic chemicals or silver polishes. As little as 300 mg potassium cyanide may cause death.

The extreme toxicity of cyanide is due to its ready reaction with the trivalent iron of cytochrome oxidase. The role of the enzyme in cellular oxygen utilization is inhibited by the formation of the cytochrome oxidase–cyanide complex. The resultant cytotoxic hypoxia leads to cellular dysfunction and death.

Inhalation of hydrogen cyanide may cause death within a minute. Oral doses act more slowly, requiring several minutes for the appearance of symptoms and up to several hours for death. The first effect is an increase in ventilation because of the blockade of oxidative metabolism in the chemoreceptor cells. As more cyanide is absorbed, there are headache, dizziness, nausea, drowsiness, hypotension, profound dyspnea, characteristic electrocardiographic changes, coma, and convulsions. Death always occurs within 4 h.

Cyanide poisoning is a true medical emergency. Treatment is highly effective if given rapidly. The chemical antidotes should be immediately available wherever emergency medical care is dispensed. The diagnosis may be made by the characteristic "bitter almond" odor on the breath of the victim, and physicians should familiarize themselves with this smell. Since the saturation of hemoglobin is not disturbed by cyanide, cyanosis is not seen until respiratory depression supervenes. The objective of treatment is the production of methemoglobin by the administration of nitrite. The trivalent iron of methemoglobin competes with cytochrome oxidase for the cyanide ion. The cytochrome oxidase–cyanide complex dissociates, and enzymatic function and cell respiration are restored. Further detoxification is then achieved by the administration of thiosulfate. Under the influence of the tissue enzyme rhodanese, thiosulfate reacts with cyanide liberated by the dissociation of cyanmethemoglobin to form thiocyanate. This substance is relatively nontoxic and readily excreted in the urine.

Since speed is of the essence, nitrite should be immediately administered by inhalation of amyl nitrite perles, one every 2 min unless blood pressure is below 80 mmHg. This is followed as soon as possible by the intravenous injection of 10 ml of 3% sodium nitrite over a 3-min period. An intravenous infusion of norepinephrine may be necessary to maintain blood pressure during this injection period. After the administration of sodium nitrite, 50 ml of 25% sodium thiosulfate should be administered intravenously over a 10-min period. Supportive measures, especially artificial respiration with 100% oxygen, should be instituted as soon as possible, but, unless methemoglobinemia is produced promptly, other forms of treatment are of no value. Administration of sodium nitrite and sodium thiosulfate may have to be repeated. If the patient survives 4 h, recovery is likely but residual cerebral symptoms may persist.

DETERGENTS AND SOAPS These substances fall into the three groups of anionic, nonionic, and cationic detergents. The first group contains common soaps and household detergents. They may cause vomiting and diarrhea but have no serious effects, and no treatment is required. However, some laundry compounds contain phosphate water softeners whose ingestion may cause hypocalcemia. The ingestion of nonionic detergents is harmless and requires no treatment.

Cationic detergents, such as benzalkonium chloride (Zephiran) and many others, are commonly used for bactericidal purposes in hospitals and homes. These compounds are well absorbed from the gastrointestinal tract and interfere with cellular functions. The fatal oral dose is approximately 3 g. Ingestion produces nausea and vomiting, and shock, coma, convulsions, and death may occur in a few hours. Treatment consists of minimizing gastrointestinal absorption by emesis or gastric lavage with ordinary soap solution, which rapidly inactivates cationic detergents. If significant absorption has occurred, intensive supportive therapy may be required.

ERGOT This fungus (*Claviceps purpurea*) grows on rye and contains a number of highly toxic alkaloids (e.g., ergotamine, ergonovine) which are used in the treatment of migraine or as uterine stimulants. Poisoning may be due to therapeutic overdosage, particularly in patients with severe infections or liver disease, but more commonly results from the use of ergot as an abortifacient. The epidemic form of chronic ergot poisoning due to the ingestion of contaminated grain is now rarely seen. Ingestion of 1 g ergot has been fatal; ergotamine has caused gangrene in doses of 10 mg per day. Symptoms of acute or chronic ergot poisoning are vomiting, diarrhea, burning abdominal pain, severe muscle pains, ischemic peripheral gangrene, headache, psychotic behavior, muscle tremors, convulsions, and coma. Circulatory disturbances are due both to prolonged vasoconstriction and to intimal hyperplasia and thrombosis. Treatment of ergot poisoning is symptomatic. Vigorous vasodilator and analgesic therapy should be employed.

FLUORIDES Fluoride salts are widely used in insecticides. The gases fluorine and hydrogen fluoride are used in industry. The latter is a strong corrosive. Fluorine and fluorides are cellular poisons which block the glycolytic degradation of glucose. Fluorides also form an insoluble precipitate with calcium and cause hypocalcemia. Finally, in an acid medium fluorides form the corrosive hydrofluoric acid. Ingestion of 1 to 2 g sodium fluoride may be fatal.

Inhalation of fluorine or hydrogen fluoride produces coughing and choking. After an asymptomatic period of a day or two, fever, cough, cyanosis, and pulmonary edema may develop. Ingestion of fluoride salts is followed by nausea, vomiting productive of corroded tissues, diarrhea, and abdominal pain. Consequent to the decrease in serum calcium the victim develops muscular hyperirritability, fasciculations, tremors, spasms, and convulsions. Death is due to respiratory paralysis or circulatory collapse. If the patient survives the acute period, jaundice and oliguria may appear. Chronic fluoride poisoning (fluorosis) is characterized by weight loss, weakness, anemia, brittle bones, and stiff joints. Mottling of teeth is seen when exposure occurs during enamel formation.

Acute fluoride poisoning is treated by immediate administration of milk, lime water, calcium gluconate, or calcium lactate solution. Following lavage or emesis 10 g calcium gluconate and 30 g sodium sulfate should be administered to precipitate and remove fluoride from the intestine. Then 10% calcium gluconate or 1% calcium chloride should be slowly injected intravenously and repeated as needed to prevent a positive Chvostek's sign. Symptomatic and supportive therapy is administered as indicated.

FORMALDEHYDE This gas is available as 40% solution (Formalin) which is used as a disinfectant, fumigant, or deodorant. Poisoning by Formalin may be diagnosed by the characteristic odor of formaldehyde. Formaldehyde reacts chemically with cellular constituents, depresses cellular functions, and causes cell death. The fatal dose of Formalin is about 60 ml.

Ingestion of Formalin immediately causes severe abdominal pain, nausea, vomiting, and diarrhea. This may be followed by collapse, coma, severe metabolic acidosis, and anuria. Death is usually due to circulatory failure.

Treatment consists of immediate administration of activated charcoal followed by emesis and gastric lavage with a solution containing 1% ammonium carbonate and 2% sodium bicarbonate. Parenteral administration of sodium bicarbonate is indicated to combat acidosis. The treatment is otherwise supportive.

GLYCOLS Ethylene glycol and diethylene glycol are commonly used in antifreeze solutions. The more than 50 annual deaths from these compounds usually result from intentional drinking of antifreeze by alcoholics. The fatal dose of ethylene glycol is about 100 g, that of diethylene glycol somewhat lower. Both compounds are metabolized to oxalate in the body.

The initial symptoms of acute poisoning by these glycols resemble those of alcoholic intoxication. They may progress to vomiting, stupor, coma with absent reflexes and anisocoria, and convulsions. Tachypnea, bradycardia, and hypothermia are commonly seen. After massive ingestion death may occur from respiratory failure within a few hours or from pulmonary edema within a day or two. If the patient survives the acute stage, hepatic and renal necroses manifest themselves with jaundice, anuria, and uremia.

Treatment is largely supportive. The administration of ethyl alcohol and of intravenous calcium gluconate may be helpful by slowing the oxidation to oxalic acid and by precipitating the acid. However, the effectiveness of these procedures has not been definitely established. Dialysis is highly successful in the removal of ethylene and diethylene glycol from the body.

HALOGENATED HYDROCARBONS Halogenated hydrocarbons (carbon tetrachloride, ethylene chlorohydrin, ethylene dichloride, methyl halides, tetrachloroethane, trichloroethylene) find wide industrial use as solvents, refrigerants, fumigants, and in chemical synthesis. They enter the home in household cleaners, floor waxes, fire extinguishers, and rubber or plastic cements. These compounds are highly fat-soluble and produce cell damage either directly or after conversion in the body to other compounds. Individual halogenated hydrocarbons differ considerably in the degree and the exact manifestations of their toxicity, but in sufficient concentration all these compounds are capable of inducing central nervous system depression and varying amounts of hepatic and renal toxicity. Myocardial depression, vascular damage, and pulmonary edema may also occur.

The most important halogenated hydrocarbon is carbon tetrachloride, widely employed as a nonflammable solvent and fire extinguisher fluid. Poisoning may occur from inhalation of the vapor, ingestion, or, rarely, percutaneous absorption. An oral dose of as little as 4 ml may be fatal. Absorption from the gastrointestinal tract is slow and unpredictable but is increased by the presence of fats and alcohol. Abdominal pain, hematemesis, and hepatic damage are more common and severe after ingestion than when the poison is inhaled. Inhalation may lead to irritation of the upper part of the respiratory tract.

Acute systemic absorption of carbon tetrachloride results in nausea, dizziness, confusion, and headache within a few minutes. Depending upon the quantity absorbed, the symptoms may quickly progress to stupor, coma, convulsions, respiratory failure, hypotension, or ventricular fibrillation. The patient may recover from these immediate manifestations until evidence of hepatic or renal toxicity appears several hours to several days after the exposure. Liver and kidney damage may also occur in the absence of any severe early central nervous system effects. Initially tender hepatomegaly may be present, jaundice may be rapidly progressive, and death due to severe centrilobular necrosis may occur within days. The renal lesion has the characteristics of acute tubular necrosis, and manifests itself by proteinuria, hematuria, oliguria, or anuria. Uremia, acidosis, hypertension, and pulmonary edema may develop as complications of renal failure. Optic neuritis, pancreatitis, and adrenal cortical necrosis are less common manifestations of carbon tetrachloride intoxication.

Chronic poisoning may occur after repeated exposures to low concentrations of carbon tetrachloride and may also lead to liver or kidney damage. More usually it manifests itself by vague symptoms of fatigue, weakness, mental confusion, abdominal pain, anorexia, nausea, blurring of vision, and paresthesias.

Treatment of acute poisoning by halogenated hydrocarbons includes vigorous effects at minimizing gastrointestinal absorption by lavage or emesis and catharsis. Treatment is otherwise symptomatic. Sympathomimetic drugs should be avoided because of the danger of inducing ventricular arrhythmias in the sensitized myocardium. Acute renal and hepatic failure must be carefully managed. Hemodialysis is often required and may be lifesaving until kidney function returns three or more weeks after poisoning.

IODINE The traditional antiseptic iodine tincture is an alcoholic solution of 2% iodine and 2% sodium iodide. Strong iodine solution (Lugol's solution) is an aqueous solution of 5% iodine and 10% potassium iodide. Tincture of iodine is approximately 2 g. Iodides are very much less toxic, and no fatalities have been reported.

The diagnosis of iodine poisoning is suggested by the brown staining of the oral mucous membranes. The effects are largely due to the corrosive effects of the compound on the gastrointestinal tract. Burning abdominal pain, nausea, vomiting, and bloody diarrhea may occur soon after ingestion. If the stomach contained starch, the vomitus is blue or black. Tissue trauma from corrosive gastroenteritis and fluid loss by vomiting and diarrhea may result in shock. Severe edema of the glottis, fever, delirium, stupor, and anuria have also been observed.

Treatment consists of gastric lavage with a starch solution made by adding 15 g flour or cornstarch to 500 ml water. Thereafter, catharsis should be induced, and milk should be given orally to relieve gastric irritation. Sodium thiosulfate will reduce iodine to less toxic iodide; 100 ml of a 5% solution should be given orally and 10 ml of a 10% solution intravenously every 4 h. With appropriate treatment most patients poisoned by iodine survive, but esophageal strictures may complicate their recovery.

IPECAC, EMETINE Emetine is the major alkaloid of ipecac (dried roots or rhizomes of *Cephaelis ipecacuanha*) and is used for the treatment of amebiasis. Syrup of ipecac is used as an emetic or expectorant. Poisoning may be accidental or suicidal but most commonly results from overdosage during therapy, at times because of the erroneous substitution of the much more potent fluid extract of ipecac for syrup of ipecac. Emetine and other alkaloids of ipecac have serious toxic gastrointestinal, central nervous, and myocardial effects. The fatal oral dose of emetine is about 1 g.

Manifestations of poisoning begin with nausea, vomiting, diarrhea, and abdominal pain. Cardiac effects are heralded by electrocardiographic changes, and the depression of myocardial contractility leads to dyspnea, tachycardia, shock, and congestive heart failure. Coma and convulsions may occur, but death is usually due to heart failure. Treatment is symptomatic. Administration of digitalis may be of value.

IRON SALTS Ferrous or ferric salts produce gastrointestinal corrosive damage. Following mucosal damage, large amounts of iron may be absorbed, particularly in children. The fatal oral dose in children is 5 to 10 g.

Very soon after ingestion, nausea, vomiting, diarrhea, and abdominal pain appear. Systemic effects include acidosis, shock, drowsiness, coma, and respiratory failure. These initial symptoms may partially clear but then recur with increased severity. In the later stages signs of hepatic and renal toxicity may appear.

The absorption of ingested iron should be minimized by the usual measures. Gastric lavage with a 10% sodium bicarbonate solution will precipitate the ferrous ion. Edetate calcium disodium 30 mg per kg daily in divided doses should be administered intravenously or orally. Deferoxamine methane sulfonate (Desferal) is even more effective as an iron-chelating agent than edetate. Use of chelating agents is guided by determinations of serum iron and iron-binding capacity. Peritoneal dialysis and hemodialysis effectively remove iron from the body. Acidosis, shock, and renal or hepatic toxicity must be treated supportively.

ISOPROPYL ALCOHOL This compound is used as a sterilizing agent or as rubbing alcohol. Ingestion produces gastric irritation and raises the danger of vomiting with aspiration. The systemic effects of isopropyl alcohol are similar to those of ethyl alcohol, but it is approximately twice as potent as the latter. Coma is readily produced but rarely lasts longer than 12 h. Isopropyl alcohol is oxidized to acetone in the body, and transient acetonuria is common, but significant acidosis does not occur. Gastric lavage should always be performed to minimize the danger of aspiration following vomiting in the unconscious patient. Supportive therapy is required only after ingestion of massive amounts, and there are no sequelae other than transient gastritis.

MAGNESIUM Magnesium sulfate is used intravenously as a hypotensive agent and orally as a cathartic. The magnesium ion is a profound depressant of the central nervous system and of neuromuscular transmission. Poisoning after oral or rectal administration is unlikely in the presence of normal renal function, because the kidney removes magnesium more rapidly than it is absorbed by the gastrointestinal tract. In the presence of impaired renal function an oral dose of 30 g may be fatal. Symptoms begin at a serum magnesium level of 4 meq per liter, and concentrations of over 12 meq per liter may be fatal. Oral ingestion of concentrated solutions may cause gastrointestinal irritation. Manifestations of systemic poisoning are depression of reflexes, flaccid paralysis, hypotension, hypothermia, coma, and respiratory failure. Respiratory death usually precedes significant myocardial depression. The actions of magnesium on neurologic and neuromuscular function are antagonized by calcium. Treatment of magnesium poisoning therefore includes the intravenous administration of 10 ml of a 10% solution of calcium gluconate, which may be repeated as necessary.

METHYL ALCOHOL This simplest of alcohols, also called wood alcohol or methanol, is used as a solvent, antifreeze, paint remover, and as a denaturant in ethyl alcohol. Denatured ethyl alcohol preparations, such as Sterno or Solox, contain 5 to 15 percent methyl alcohol as well as other denaturants. Methyl alcohol poisoning is due almost entirely to its ingestion as a substitute for ethanol or to the drinking of denatured ethyl alcohol. The toxic dose is very variable: death has occurred after a dose of 20 ml, but 250 ml has been ingested with survival. As little as 15 ml methanol has caused permanent blindness.

Methanol is less inebriating than ethyl alcohol, and inebriation is not a prominent symptom of methyl alcohol intoxication. Methanol is oxidized in the body to formaldehyde and to formic acid. The rate of its metabolism is independent of the concentration in the body and is only 15 percent that of ethanol. The enzyme alcohol dehydrogenase appears to be responsible for the first step in oxidation. The enzyme system will preferentially utilize ethyl alcohol if this compound is also available. Thus ethyl alcohol may depress the rate of metabolism of methanol. The manifestations of methanol poisoning are largely due to the accumulation of its toxic metabolites. These products, especially formaldehyde, have toxic actions on many cells, and the retina and optic nerve are specifically damaged. The toxic metabolites of methyl alcohol are also responsible for the severe acidosis, which is the most prominent feature of methyl alcohol poisoning. This acidosis is partly due to the accumulation of formic acid, but formate also appears to exert an inhibitory effect upon enzymes involved in the oxidation of carbohydrate with consequent accumulation of acid intermediates.

Symptoms of methanol poisoning usually do not appear until 12 to 24 h after ingestion, when sufficient toxic metabolites have accumulated. Manifestations consist of headache, dizziness, nausea, vomiting, severe abdominal and back pain probably due to pancreatitis, vasomotor disturbances, central nervous system depression, and respiratory failure. Visual disturbance is almost universal and ranges from mild blurring of vision to total blindness. Impairment of vision may be transient, but permanent blindness may follow survival of the acute intoxication. The pupils are dilated and nonreactive, and there is hyperemia of the optic disk and retinal edema. Severe abdominal tenderness and spasm or nuchal rigidity may be present. Acidosis is commonly severe, but Kussmaul's respiration is absent in many severely acidotic patients (plasma, carbon dioxide-combining power below 20 meq liter).

In the treatment of methyl alcohol intoxication gastric lavage is of use only during the first hour or two. The mainstay of treatment is intravenous administration of large amounts of sodium bicarbonate. Return of acidosis is frequent after initial correction, and additional alkali must be administered as indicated by close observation of the patient and laboratory determinations. Peritoneal dialysis and hemodialysis effectively remove methanol from the body and are useful in view of its slow oxidation. The administration of 0.5 ml per kg ethyl alcohol every 2 h may inhibit the metabolism of methyl alcohol and is useful in conjunction with dialysis. Supportive therapy must be administered as required by the patient's clinical state.

MUSHROOMS There are many species of poisonous mushrooms, but in the United States most poisoning is due to *Amanita muscaria* (fly agaric) or *Amanita phalloides* (destroying angel). More than 100 deaths result each year from consumption of wild poisonous mushrooms, 90 percent being due to *A. phalloides.* Fatalities have occurred after ingestion of only part of one mushroom.

Amanita muscaria contains the parasympathomimetic alkaloid muscarine, as well as variable amounts of a substance active on the central nervous system and a parasympatholytic alkaloid. Symptoms are largely those of parasympathetic stimulation: lacrimation, pupillary constriction, perspiration, salivation, nausea, vomiting, diarrhea, abdominal pain, bronchorrhea, wheezing, dyspnea, bradycardia, and hypotension. Muscular tremors, confusion, excitement, and delirium are common in severe poisoning. Very rarely symptoms of atropine poisoning have predominated. After ingestion of *A. muscaria* symptoms appear within minutes to 2 h. The patient may die within a few hours, but with appropriate therapy complete recovery in 24 h is the rule.

Amanita phalloides, some other *Amanita* species, and *Galerina venenata* contain heat-stable polypeptide cytotoxins which are rapidly bound to tissues. Severe cell damage and fatty degeneration may occur in liver, kidneys, striated muscle, and brain. Ingestion of these dangerous mushrooms is followed by a latent period of 6 to 20 h. Manifestations of cytotoxicity may then appear suddenly and consist of severe nausea, violent abdominal pain, bloody vomiting and diarrhea, and cardiovascular collapse. Headache, mental confusion, coma, or convulsions are common. Painful and tender hepatomegaly, jaundice, hypoglycemia, dehydration, and oliguria or anuria frequently appear on the first or second day after ingestion. The victim may die from acute hepatic necrosis (yellow atrophy) within 4 days. About one-half of all poisonings with *A. phalloides* have a fatal outcome in 5 to 8 days. Recovery tends to be slow.

Ingestion of other poisonous mushrooms may cause gastrointestinal symptoms, visual disturbances, ataxia, disorientation, convulsions, coma, fever, hemolysis, and methemoglobinemia.

Treatment of mushroom poisoning depends upon the species ingested. If parasympathomimetic manifestations are prominent, atropine in doses of 1 to 2 mg is given intramuscularly and repeated every 30 min until symptoms are controlled. Poisoning by cytotoxic mushrooms can be treated only symptomatically. Fluid and electrolyte balance must be carefully maintained. Hypoglycemia should be avoided; large quantities of carbohydrate may exert some protective effect on the liver. Excitement, convulsions, pain, hypotension, and fever may need symptomatic therapy. Hemodialysis is of no value in removing the toxin but may be required to maintain renal function until recovery occurs.

NAPHTHALENE Poisoning by this substance is almost always due to ingestion of moth repellents. An oral dose of 2 g has been fatal. Nausea, vomiting, and diarrhea are the initial symptoms. Larger doses may produce hepatic damage with jaundice and renal toxicity which may progress to hematuria, oliguria, or anuria. Depending upon the amount ingested, central nervous system manifestations may range from headache, mental confusion, and excitement to coma and convulsions. In persons with glucose 6-phosphate dehydrogenase-deficient red blood cells the ingestion of naphthalene will produce hemolysis. Treatment consists of emesis or gastric lavage and catharsis and supportive measures.

NICOTINE This alkaloid is an exceedingly potent and rapidly acting poison. It is a component of many insecticides. Nicotine is readily absorbed from the oral and gastrointestinal mucosa, from the respiratory tract, and through the skin. The lethal dose for an adult is approximately 50 mg, the quantity contained in two cigarettes. However, tobacco is much less toxic than would be anticipated on the basis of its nicotine content. Nicotine is poorly absorbed from ingested tobacco, and on smoking, most of the nicotine is burned. Nicotine acts on chemoreceptors, on synapses in the central nervous system and in autonomic ganglia, on the adrenal medulla, and on neuroeffector junctions. Furthermore, its initial stimulant effects are followed by a depressant phase of action. It is not surprising that the manifestations of nicotine poisoning are highly complex and somewhat unpredictable.

Small doses of nicotine produce nausea, vomiting, diarrhea, headache, dizziness, and neurologic stimulation manifested by tachycardia, hypertension, hyperpnea, tachypnea, sweating, and salivation. Larger doses also cause cortical irritability, progressing to convulsions, and myocardial arrhythmias. Finally coma, respiratory depression and arrest, and cardiac arrest or fibrillation may supervene. Severe poisoning may cause death within a few minutes.

Treatment consists of gastric lavage with activated charcoal or with a 1:10,000 solution of potassium permanganate, which oxidizes nicotine. Atropine, 2 mg, and phentolamine, 5 mg, may be given intramuscularly or intravenously and repeated as often as required to control signs and symptoms of parasympathetic or sympathetic hyperactivity. These compounds are ineffective in preventing paralysis of the respiratory muscles and disturbances in cardiac rhythm. Careful attention must be given to artificial ventilation with oxygen and to therapy of catecholamine-induced cardiac tachyarrhythmias. Propranolol is the drug of choice for the latter purpose. Nicotine is rapidly detoxified in the liver, and recovery will be prompt if the patient can be tided over the initial period.

NITRITES Poisoning by the nitrite ion may result from the ingestion of large amounts of drugs such as amyl nitrite or sodium nitrite. Nitrites are also used to preserve the color of meat, and amounts in excess of the allowable residue of 0.01 percent may appear in food. Ingested nitrates may be reduced to nitrite by intestinal bacteria, especially *Escherichia coli.* Except after the ingestion of very large amounts, adults usually absorb all nitrate before this reduction takes place. However, in children nitrite poisoning may result from the ingestion of nitrates or nitrate-containing well water. Fatalities have occurred from the oral ingestion of 2 to 4 g nitrites.

Acute nitrite poisoning may lead to severe headache, flushing, dizziness, hypotension, and syncope. Usually the patient need only be positioned to facilitate venous return to the heart. Pressor agents are seldom required. The most important toxic effect of the nitrite ion is its ability to oxidize hemoglobin to methemoglobin (Chaps. 60 and 316).

OXALIC ACID This acid is found in ink eradicators and stain removers. It is corrosive and combines with calcium to form insoluble calcium oxalate. Ingestion causes irritation and corrosion of mouth, esophagus, and stomach, followed by vomiting and abdominal pain. After absorption the reduction in serum calcium leads to muscular tremors, tetany, convulsions, and cardiovascular collapse. Ingestion of 5 g may cause death within minutes. Following recovery from the acute episode there may be renal failure due to blockage of renal tubules by calcium oxalate crystals.

Treatment consists of induction of emesis or gastric lavage with milk, limewater, chalk, or calcium salts. A dose of 10 ml of 10% calcium gluconate should be given intravenously and repeated as required to maintain normal serum calcium and prevent tetany. In supportive therapy the maintenance of a high urine output is essential.

PARAQUAT Paraquat is a dipyridilium compound which is used in 5 to 20% aqueous solutions as a herbicide. It is rapidly inactivated on contact with soil. It has been responsible for more than 20 accidental and suicidal deaths in recent years. An oral dose of 5 mg per kg may be fatal. Ingestion causes a burning sensation and vomiting. After a delay of 2 to 5 days ulcerations in the mouth and esophagus, oliguria, and hemoptysis appear. These may be followed in severe cases by jaundice, fever, respiratory distress, cardiovascular collapse, and death. Pathologic findings include characteristic pulmonary lesions, focal myocardial necrosis, and renal tubular necrosis.

Early administration of activated charcoal and gastric lavage with diluted bentonite magma can decrease absorption. Forced diuresis and hemodialysis are effective and should be started early. Treatment is otherwise supportive since no antidote is known.

PETROLEUM DISTILLATES Petroleum distillates (diesel oil, gasoline, kerosene, paint thinner, solvent distillate) are liquids with a boiling point between 50 and 325°C. They contain variable amounts of branched or straight-chain aliphatic and aromatic hydrocarbons. Kerosene is widely used as a fuel and as a vehicle for cleaning agents, furniture polishes, insecticides, and paint thinners. Not surprisingly, each year petroleum distillates cause about 100 accidental deaths in the United States, 90 percent of these in young children. Furthermore, these products are annually responsible for almost 20,000 hospitalizations. Ingestion of

10 ml kerosene has been fatal, but adults have recovered from as much as 250 ml. Petroleum distillates are central nervous system depressants; they damage cells by dissolving cellular lipids. Pulmonary damage manifested by pulmonary edema or pneumonitis is a common and serious complication.

Inhalation of gasoline or kerosene vapors induces a state resembling alcoholic intoxication. Headache, nausea, tinnitus, and a burning sensation in the chest may also be present. When aliphatic hydrocarbons are inhaled, these symptoms may progress to profound drowsiness or coma with absence of deep reflexes. If the distillate contains a high proportion of aromatic hydrocarbons, the coma is characterized by tremors, muscle jactitations, hyperactive reflexes, and convulsions. Death is usually due to respiratory depression, rarely to ventricular fibrillation.

The oral ingestion of petroleum distillates causes irritation of the mucous membranes of the upper part of the intestinal tract. When large amounts have been ingested, the same manifestations as after inhalation may appear. Frequently eructation or vomiting results in aspiration of petroleum distillates into the trachea. Because of their low surface tension, minute amounts of these substances may then spread widely throughout the lungs and produce pulmonary edema and pneumonitis. Pulmonary damage may also arise because of absorption of ingested petroleum distillates from the gastrointestinal tract. However, kerosene is at least one hundred times more toxic by the intratracheal route than when ingested.

In the treatment of poisoning by petroleum distillates extreme care must be used to prevent aspiration. When large amounts have been ingested, gastric lavage should be performed but only after insertion of an endotracheal tube with an inflatable cuff. A vegetable oil and a saline cathartic may be administered to decrease the absorption of the poison. All victims of kerosene poisoning should be hospitalized for at least 24 h for observation. If signs or symptoms of pulmonary irritation appear, adrenal steroids, oxygen under positive pressure, and antibiotics to prevent bacterial pneumonia are often of value. Symptomatic therapy for central nervous system depression or convulsions may be necessary. Sympathomimetic amines should be avoided because of the danger of inducing ventricular fibrillation in the hydrocarbon-sensitized heart.

PHENOL Phenol and related compounds (creosote, cresols, hexachlorophene, hydroquinone, Lysol, resorcinol, tannic acid) are widely used as antiseptics, caustics, and preservatives. These substances poison all cells by denaturing and precipitating cellular proteins. The approximate fatal oral dose ranges from 2 ml for phenol and cresols to 20 ml for tannic acid.

Ingestion of phenolic compounds produces erosion of mucosa from mouth to stomach. The corroded areas may have a characteristic dead-white appearance. Hematemesis and bloody diarrhea may occur. After an initial phase of hyperpnea due to stimulation of the respiratory center, stupor, coma, convulsions, pulmonary edema, and shock are seen. The initial respiratory alkalosis is soon followed by a profound acidosis. The latter results from the renal excretion of base during the alkalotic stage, from the acidic nature of the phenolic radical, and from disturbances in carbohydrate metabolism presumably due to defects in enzymatic function. If the patient survives the acute stage, acute tubular necrosis may lead to oliguria or anuria and hepatic toxicity to jaundice.

Poisoning by phenolic compounds may often be diagnosed by their characteristic odor. Development of a violet or blue color of the urine after addition of a few drops of ferric chloride indicates the presence of a phenolic compound.

Treatment is directed at decreasing the absorption of ingested poison by administration of water, milk, or activated charcoal slurry and their removal by emesis or gastric lavage. Olive oil or castor oil dissolves phenol and retards its absorption. Supportive therapy consists of correction of the acidosis, the control of shock and convulsions, and the maintenance of a patent airway in the face of glottal edema by intubation or tracheotomy.

PHOSPHORUS Phosphorus occurs in two forms: a red, nonpoisonous form and a yellow, fat-soluble, highly toxic form. The latter is used in rodent and insect poisons and in fireworks. Yellow phosphorus and phosphides cause fatty degeneration and necrosis of tissues, particularly of the liver. The lethal ingested dose of yellow phosphorus is approximately 50 mg.

Ingestion of yellow phosphorus is followed within 1 h by burning pain in the upper part of the gastrointestinal tract, vomiting, diarrhea, and a garlic odor of the breath and excreta. The patient may die in coma during the first day or two, or symptoms may subside after a few hours. Then, 1 to 2 days later, the victim may develop tender hepatomegaly, jaundice, hypocalcemia, hypotension, and oliguria, and may die following convulsions and coma. Death from acute hepatic necrosis may occur in a few days.

Treatment consists of vigorous and repeated induction of emesis or gastric lavage. Calcium gluconate is given intravenously to maintain serum calcium level. Treatment is otherwise supportive, and a protective regimen for the liver should be instituted.

SALICYLATES Each year 30 million lb aspirin is consumed in the United States, and salicylates can probably be found in every American household. It is therefore not surprising that salicylates (aspirin, methyl salicylate, salicylic acid, sodium salicylate) are more commonly involved in poisonings than any other agent. Aspirin is found in almost all compound analgesic tablets. Methyl salicylate (oil of wintergreen) is present in most skin liniments, and salicylic acid is used in ointments and corn plasters. The ingestion of 10 to 30 g aspirin or sodium salicylate may be fatal to adults, but survival has been reported after an oral dose of 130 g aspirin. On the other hand 3 g salicylate in a teaspoon of methyl salicylate has been fatal in children.

Salicylate intoxication may result from the cumulative effect of therapeutic administration of high doses. There is considerable individual variation: toxic symptoms may begin at dosages of 3 g per day or may not appear when 10 g per day is given. Toxic symptoms are also poorly correlated with the serum salicylate concentration, but few patients become intoxicated at levels less than 15 mg per 100 ml and most at levels over 35 mg per 100 ml. Therapeutic salicylate intoxication is usually mild and is called "salicylism." The earliest symptoms are vertigo, tinnitus, and impairment of hearing. Further overdosage causes nausea, vomiting, sweating, diarrhea, fever, drowsiness, headache, dimness of vision, and mental aberrations. The latter may be characterized by confusion, excitement, restlessness, and talkativeness; this "salicylate jag" resembles alcoholic intoxication without the euphoria. The central nervous system effects may progress to hallucinations, convulsions, and coma. Toxic doses of salicylates also have a direct stimulant effect on the respiratory center, resulting in hyperventilation, loss of carbon dioxide, and respiratory alkalosis. Renal excretion of bicarbonate may partially compensate for this.

In acute salicylate poisoning due to accidental or suicidal ingestion of massive amounts, the same manifestations may be seen in more rapid succession. However, they are usually overshadowed by severe disturbances in the acid-base balance which follow a definite sequence. Early in the course of intoxication there may be only hyperpnea, and the seriousness of the poisoning may not be appreciated at that time. The hyperventilation causes a fall in blood P_{CO_2} and an increase in pH. Renal excretion of bicarbonate, sodium, and potassium will bring the pH back toward normal and produce a compensated respiratory alkalosis. At that point the buffering capacity of the extracellular fluid will have been significantly decreased. In young children and after large doses in adults further developments may then produce a combination of respiratory acidosis and metabolic acidosis which stems from a number of factors. High concentrations of salicylate depress the respiratory center and cause CO_2 retention. Renal function becomes impaired because of dehydration and hypotension, and inorganic, metabolic acids accumulate. Furthermore, salicylic acid derivatives may displace several milliequivalents of blood bicarbonate. Finally, salicylates impair carbohydrate metabolism and cause accumulation of acetoacetic, lactic, and pyruvic acids. Severe acidosis and disturbances in electrolyte balance are most commonly seen in febrile young children.

Blood salicylate levels are of value in the estimation of the severity of poisoning. Serious poisoning is rare at levels less than 50 mg per 100 ml but usual at levels between 50 and 100 mg per 100 ml. Levels above 100 mg per 100 ml during the first 6 h after poisoning signify severe intoxication and may be fatal. Excretion of salicylates is renal, and in the presence of normal renal function about 50 percent will be excreted in 24 h. Addition of a few drops of ferric chloride solution to 5 ml boiled acidified urine containing salicylate yields a violet color and may aid in diagnosis.

Treatment of salicylate poisoning is largely supportive. In order to decrease absorption, activated charcoal is administered and emesis is induced, or lavage with sodium bicarbonate solution is performed. Disturbances of acid-base or electrolyte balance and hypoglycemia are corrected by the intravenous administration of appropriate solutions. Respiratory depression may require artificial ventilation with oxygen. Convulsions may best be treated by the administration of succinylcholine and artificial ventilation with oxygen. Central nervous system-depressant agents should not be used. In order to increase renal excretion of salicylate, osmotic diuresis is induced and the urine is alkalinized. Peritoneal dialysis and hemodialysis are also highly effective in removing salicylate from seriously poisoned patients.

SMOKE Poisoning by smoke is usually due to carbon monoxide inhalation. However, burning material may also release irritant fumes. Many irritant gases combine with water to form corrosive acids or alkalies and cause chemical burns of exposed skin and of the upper part of the respiratory tract. Such gases (and the corrosives formed) are ammonia (ammonium hydroxide), nitrogen oxide (nitric acid), sulfur dioxide (sulfurous acid), and sulfur trioxide (sulfuric acid). These irritating gases as well as hydrogen sulfide may also be present in smog. Another highly toxic gas which may be inhaled by firefighters or victims is phosgene. This compound is formed by the high-temperature decomposition of chlorinated hydrocarbons and is released when carbon tetrachloride from fire extinguishers comes into contact with hot surfaces.

After inhalation of irritant gases the victim may notice burning pain in throat and chest and severe coughing. These symptoms may subside completely, but from several hours to a day after exposure dyspnea and cyanosis may appear and progress rapidly to severe pulmonary edema and death from respiratory and circulatory failure. Treatment consists of administration of oxygen and adrenal steroids and appropriate therapy of pulmonary edema, should that develop.

In many localities the term *smoke* is used to describe paint removers, lacquer thinners, antifreezes, and other solvent mixtures which are ingested for their supposed alcohol content. The toxicity of these compounds depends on their ingredients. Some such materials have caused profound hypoglycemia by a poorly understood mechanism. This possibility should be considered in the differential diagnosis of what appears to be alcoholic coma. The intravenous administration of glucose as a therapeutic test may be indicated.

SULFIDES Hydrogen sulfide is a gas released by the decomposition of organic sulfur compounds and is widely used in industry. Carbon disulfide is an industrial solvent. Other sulfides have industrial uses and release hydrogen sulfide in contact with water or acids. Significant concentrations of hydrogen sulfide may be present in smoke or smog. Inhalation of hydrogen sulfide in concentrations above 50 ppm (fifty times the minimum detectable by smell) causes conjunctivitis, headache, nausea, soreness of the upper respiratory passages, pulmonary edema, and drowsiness. Concentrations in excess of 300 ppm may cause coma, respiratory depression, and death. Ingestion of carbon disulfide or soluble sulfides is followed by vomiting, headache, hypotension, respiratory depression, tremors, coma, convulsions, and death. The fatal oral dose of carbon disulfide is approximately 1 g. Treatment of sulfide intoxication is supportive. Administration of sodium nitrite may promote the binding of sulfide in sulfmethemoglobin.

VOLATILE OILS The volatile or essential oils (citronella oil, eucalyptus oil, menthol, pine oil turpentine) are colorless liquids which irritate all tissues. Poisoning may result from occupational exposure (painters) and accidental or suicidal ingestion. Unfortunately, some volatile oils also have an undeserved reputation as abortifacients. Absorption occurs from skin, intestine, or lungs; the less volatile oils are more slowly absorbed. Ingestion of 15 g turpentine has been fatal.

Ingestion is rapidly followed by abdominal burning, nausea, vomiting, and diarrhea. Inhalation produces severe bronchial irritation and may be followed by delirium, coma, and convulsions. If the patient survives the acute stage of poisoning, evidence of renal damage may appear and progress to acute tubular necrosis with anuria.

Treatment is entirely supportive. When gastric lavage is undertaken, aspiration must be prevented with extreme care. Since the renal lesion is reversible, treatment for renal failure should be vigorous and include dialysis if necessary.

REFERENCES

Antimuscarinic compounds

HOEFNAGEL D: Toxic effects of atropine and homatropine eyedrops in children. N Engl J Med 264:168, 1961

WEINTRAUB S: Stramonium poisoning. Postgrad Med 28:364, 1960

Barium

DEAN G: Seven cases of barium carbonate poisoning. Br Med J 2:817, 1950

Benzene, toluene

BROWNING E: Toxic solvents: a review. Br J Ind Med 16:23, 1959

BROZOVSKY M, WINKLER EM: Glue sniffing in children and adolescents. NY State J Med 65:1984, 1965

GLASER HH, MASSENGALE ON: "Glue-sniffing" in children. Deliberate inhalation of vaporized plastic cements. JAMA 181: 300, 1962

Boric acid

VALDES-DAPENA MA, AREY JB: Boric acid poisoning. J Pediatr 61:531, 1962

WONG LC et al: Boric acid poisoning: report of 11 cases. Can Med Assoc J 90:1018, 1964

Cantharidin

OAKS WW et al: Cantharidin poisoning. AMA Arch Intern Med 105:574, 1960

Carbon monoxide

ANDERSON RF et al: Myocardial toxicity from carbon monoxide poisoning. Ann Intern Med 67:1172, 1967

COSBY RS AND BERGERON M: Electrocardiographic changes in carbon monoxide poisoning. Am J Cardiol 11:93, 1963

CRAIG TV et al: Hypothermia. Its use in severe carbon monoxide poisoning. N Engl J Med 261:854, 1959

LILIENTHAL JL JR: Carbon monoxide. Pharmacol Rev 2:324, 1950

MEIGS JW, HUGHES JPW: Acute carbon monoxide poisoning; an analysis of 105 cases. AMA Arch Ind Hyg 1:90, 1950

SMITH G et al: Treatment of coal gas poisoning with oxygen at 2 atmospheres pressure. Lancet 1:816, 1962

Castor bean

BRUGSCH HG: The castor bean. N Engl J Med 262:1039, 1960

Caustics

HALLER JA, BACHMAN K: The comparative effect of current therapy on experimental caustic burns of the esophagus. Pediatrics 34:236, 1964

YARINGTON CT JR: Ingestion of caustic; a pediatric problem. J Pediatr 67:674, 1965

Chlorate

KNIGHT RK et al: Suicidal chlorate poisoning treated with peritoneal dialysis. Br Med J 3:601, 1967

Chlorinated insecticides

FINLEY AH, HAGGERTY RJ: Toxic hazards, insecticides. Chlorinated hydrocarbons. N Engl J Med 258:812, 1958

ZAVON MR: Chlorinated hydrocarbon insecticides. JAMA 190: 595, 1964

Cholinesterase inhibitor insecticides

HEATH DF: *Organophosphorus Poisons,* Oxford: Pergamon, 1961

HOBBIGER F: Reactivation of phosphorylated acetylcholinesterase, in *Cholinesterases and Anticholinesterase Agents,* Handb Exp Pharmak Suppl 15:921, 1963

MANN JB: Diagnostic aids in organophosphate poisoning. Ann Intern Med 67:905, 1967

QUINBY GE: Further therapeutic experience with pralidoximes in organic phosphorus poisoning. JAMA 187:202, 1964

WYCKOFF DW et al: Diagnostic and therapeutic problems of parathion poisonings. Ann Intern Med 68:875, 1968

Cyanide

CHEN KK, ROSE CL: Treatment of acute cyanide poisoning JAMA 162:1154, 1956

COPE C: The importance of oxygen in the treatment of cyanide poisoning JAMA 175:1061, 1961

PHOAN M: Cyanide poisoning from choke cherry seed. Am J Med Sci 204:550, 1942

Detergents

ARENA JM: Poisonings and other health hazards associated with use of detergents. JAMA 190:56, 1964

CANN HM, VERHULST HL: Toxicity of household soap and detergents and treatment of their ingestion. Am J Dis Child 100:287, 1960

Fluorides

PETERS JH: Therapy of acute fluoride poisoning. Am J Med Sci 216:278, 1948

Glycols

HAGGERTY, RJ: Toxic hazards, deaths from permanent antifreeze ingestion. N Engl J Med 261:1296, 1959

HAGSTAM KE et al: Ethylene glycol poisoning treated by haemodialysis. Acta Med Scand 178:599, 1965

PETERSON DI et al: Experimental treatment of ethylene glycol poisoning JAMA 186:965, 1963

PONS CA, CUSTER RP: Acute ethylene glycol poisoning: a clinicopathologic report of eighteen fatal cases. Am J Med Sci 211:544, 1946

Halogenated hydrocarbons

BAERG RD, KIMBERG DV: Centrilobular hepatic necrosis and acute renal failure in "solvent sniffers." Ann Intern Med 73:713, 1970

BROWNING E: Toxicology of organic compounds of industrial importance. Ann Rev Pharmacol 1:397, 1961

MYATT AV, SALMONS JA: Carbon tetrachloride poisoning. Arch Ind Hyg Occup Med 6:74, 1952

OETTINGEN WF von: *The Halogenated Hydrocarbons of Industrial and Toxicological Importance,* Amsterdam: Elsevier, 1964

Ipecac, emetine

SMITH RP, SMITH DM: Acute ipecac poisoning. N Engl J Med 265:523, 1961

WELCHMAN JM: The cardiac toxicity of emetine. J Trop Med Hyg 60:296, 1957

Iron salts

COVEY TJ: Ferrous sulfate poisoning: review, case summaries and therapeutic regimen. J Pediatr 64:218, 1964

JACOBS J et al: Acute iron intoxication. N Engl J Med 273:1124, 1965

LEIKIN S: Deferoxamine as a chelating agent. J Pediatr 72:148, 1968

Isopropyl alcohol

FREIREICH AW et al: Hemodialysis for isopropanol poisoning. N Engl J Med 277:699, 1967

Methyl alcohol

BENNETT IL JR et al: Acute methyl alcohol poisoning: a review based on experiences in an outbreak of 323 cases. Medicine 32:431, 1953

COOPER JR, KINI MM: Biochemical aspects of methanol poisoning. Biochem Pharmacol 11:405, 1962

SETTER JG et al: Studies on the dialysis of methanol. Trans Am Soc Artif Intern Organs 13:178, 1967

SMITH ME: Interrelations in ethanol and methanol metabolism. J Pharmacol 134:233, 1961

Mushrooms

BUCK RW: Mushroom toxins—a brief review of the literature. N Engl J Med 265:681, 1961

PAASO B, HARRISON DC: A new look at an old problem: Mushroom poisoning. Am J Med 58:505, 1975

Naphthalene

HAGGERTY RJ: Naphthalene poisoning. N Engl J Med 255:919, 1956

Nicotine

OBERST BB, MCINTYRE RA: Acute nicotine poisoning. Pediatrics 11:338, 1953

Nitrites

BUCKLIN R, MYINT MK: Fatal methemoglobinemia due to well water nitrates. Ann Intern Med 52:703, 1960

Paraquat

HARGREAVE TB et al: Paraquat poisoning. Postgrad Med J 45:633, 1969

MCDONAGH BJ, MARTIN J: Paraquat poisoning in children. Arch Dis Child 45:425, 1970

Petroleum distillates

BROWNING E: *Toxicity and Metabolism of Industrial Solvents,* Amsterdam: Elsevier, 1965

JACOBZINER H, RAYBIN HW: Kerosene and other petroleum distillate poisonings. N Y State J Med 63:3428, 1963

LAWTON JJ JR, MALMQUIST CP: Gasoline addiction in children. Psychiatr Q 35:555, 1961

MAYOCK RL et al: Kerosene pneumonitis treated with adrenal steroids. Ann Intern Med 54:559, 1961

SUBCOMMITTEE ON ACCIDENTAL POISONING: Cooperative kerosene poisoning study. Pediatrics 29:648, 1962

Phosphorus

ARENA JM: Phosphorus poisoning. Clin Pediatr (Phila) 2:132, 1963

DIAZ-RIVERA RS et al: Acute phosphorus poisoning in man; a study of 56 cases. Medicine 29:269, 1950

FLETCHER GF, GALAMBOS JT: Phosphorus poisoning in humans. Arch Intern Med 112:846, 1963

Salicylates

DONE AK: Salicylate intoxication; significance of measurements of salicylate in blood in cases of acute ingestions. Pediatrics 26:800, 1960

——: Salicylate poisoning. JAMA 192:770, 1965

——: Treatment of salicylate poisoning. Mod Treatment 4:648, 1967

HILL JB: Salicylate intoxication. N Engl J Med 288:1110, 1973

LEVY G, TSUCHIYA T: Effect of activated charcoal on aspirin absorption in man. Clin Pharmacol Ther 13:317, 1972

MORGAN AG, POLAK A: Acetazolamide and sodium bicarbonate in treatment of salicylate poisoning in adults. Br Med J 1:16, 1969

PROUDFOTT AT, BROWN SS: Acidaemia and salicylate poisoning in adults. Br Med J 2:547, 1969

SEGAR WE, HOLLIDAY MA: Physiologic abnormalities of salicylate intoxication. N Engl J Med 259:1191, 1958

117
HEAVY METALS

DAVID C. POSKANZER

Three highly effective chemicals, BAL, Versene, and penicillamine, are available for treatment of systemic poisoning with heavy metals by forming nontoxic, stable cyclic compounds with polyvalent metallic ions, thus permitting the offending material to be excreted safely in the urine.

The first to be developed was BAL (British antilewisite, 2,3-dimercaptopropanol, dimercaprol), which was originally intended as an antidote against the arsenical war gas, lewisite. Its tendency to combine with certain metallic ions such as arsenic, mercury, cobalt, nickel, antimony, and gold is so great that it can remove them from combination with the enzymes whose function they impair in the body. By itself BAL is not useful in treating lead poisoning. Because the effectiveness of BAL depends to some extent upon the speed with which its administration is begun, every attempt should be made to avoid delay in its use. For serious systemic intoxications, BAL should be given in doses of 5 mg per kg body weight intramuscularly as a 10% solution in oil and 20% benzyl benzoate. No single dose should exceed 300 mg. This dose should be repeated every 4 h on the first day and every 6 h on the second day. Thereafter, it should be given three times daily for several days; doses should then be tapered and discontinued about 10 days after acute poisoning. When the dose of poison has been relatively small, the schedule of BAL administration may be reduced by one-third. Because BAL is excreted in part by the kidneys, it can accumulate to toxic concentrations in anuric patients. Overdosage results in nervousness, hyperactivity, muscle twitching, and hyperreflexia. Large doses may produce convulsions. The presence of the material in tears sometimes causes blepharospasm. In patients with anuria or oliguria, therefore, BAL should be administered with caution and at a lower dosage than outlined above. If symptoms of overdosage occur, sedatives should be administered.

The second antidote to metal poisons is the chelating agent Versene (ethylenediaminetetraacetate, EDTA), which forms cyclic, stable, soluble, nontoxic compounds with most metals. Because Versene reacts with calcium in the same way as with other metals, it must be given as the calcium salt (Calcium Disodium Versenate; calcium disodiumedetate) to avoid hypocalcemia. The material has been used with notable success in the treatment of lead poisoning. It is given in a dosage of 1.0 g in 250 ml of 5% glucose intravenously every 12 h for 5 days. After a pause to allow for further solution of metal from body stores a second and even a third course may be given.

Penicillamine (Cuprimine; β,β-dimethylcysteine) is an excellent chelating agent for copper, mercury, and lead, promotes their excretion in the urine, and has the additional advantage of being well absorbed from the gastrointestinal tract. It may be given orally, while BAL and Versene require systemic injection. N-Acetyl-*dl*-penicillamine is even more effective than penicillamine in protecting against the effects of mercury, probably because it is more resistant to metabolic degradation, and it has the advantage of being less toxic. Penicillamine is administered orally in a dose of 1 to 4 g daily on an empty stomach to avoid chelation of dietary metals. It has much lower toxicity than BAL, the only other agent which is effective in the treatment of Wilson's disease (hepatolenticular degeneration), in which toxic amounts of copper are deposited in various tissues, but has the disadvantage of acute sensitivity reactions. It has also been shown to be useful in lead poisoning, but the excretion of urinary lead may not be as high after oral penicillamine as after intravenous Calcium Disodium Versenate.

N-Acetyl-*dl*-penicillamine, available as an investigational drug, has been demonstrated to be effective in mercury poisoning and has the advantage of allowing much higher doses with fewer toxic effects. It has less effect on copper levels than penicillamine and is therefore used in the treatment of mercury poisoning when one would wish to maintain copper levels. The administration of 1 to 2 g daily in divided doses for 10 days gives good results.

ANTIMONY Symptoms of poisoning after the ingestion of antimony may occur when an acid food is allowed to stand in cheap enamelware or "graniteware" for a sufficient time to allow solution of antimony, which is used in the manufacture of these products. Certain parasiticidal drugs also contain this metal. The symptoms are similar to those produced by arsenic, except that antimony causes a more rapid onset of gastrointestinal symptoms. Treatment is the same as for arsenic, including use of BAL. Circulatory collapse occurs early and requires vigorous supportive treatment.

ARSENIC Arsenic poisoning is usually the result of accidental or suicidal ingestion of insecticides or rodenticides containing Paris green (copper acetoarsenate) or calcium or lead arsenate. Pesticides containing arsenic are a frequent source of poisoning in rural areas of the United States. Medications such as Fowler's solution (potassium arsenite) and the organic arsenicals (arsphenamines and arsenoxides) were once common causes of intoxication.

The toxic dose of inorganic arsenic varies considerably and seems to depend upon individual susceptibility. Orchardists have been found to ingest as much as 6.8 mg arsenic a day without any signs of intoxication. On the other hand, as little as 30 mg arsenic trioxide has been fatal. Arsenic has a predilection for keratin, and the concentration of arsenic in the hair and nails is higher than that in other tissues. Arsenic reacts with the —SH groups in certain tissue proteins and thus interferes with a number of enzyme systems essential to cellular metabolism. Pathologic changes in fatal inorganic arsenical poisoning are fatty degeneration of the liver, hyperemia and hemorrhages of the intestine, and renal tubular necrosis. The peripheral nerves often show fragmentation and resorption of myelin, with disintegration of axis cylinders.

The symptoms of acute poisoning by the oral route are nausea, vomiting, diarrhea, severe burning of the mouth and throat, and agonizing abdominal pains. The vomitus often contains blood. Circulatory collapse is frequent, and death may ensue within a few hours. With chronic exposure, the first signs of poisoning are usually weakness, prostration, muscular aching, or nervous system involvement; gastrointestinal symptoms are minimal. In patients exposed to arsine gas (hydrogen arsenide), the outstanding features are hemolysis, chills, fever, and hemoglobinuria.

Patients who recover from acute poisoning and those with chronic intoxication usually develop skin and mucosal changes, peripheral neuropathy, and linear pigmentations in the fingernails (see Chap. 331). The *cutaneous manifestations* appear within 1 to 4 weeks and consist of a diffuse, dry, scaly desquamation, occasionally with hyperpigmentation, over the trunk and extremities. Hyperkeratoses of the palms and soles and edema of the face and extremities may also occur. The mucous membranes also show evidence of irritation, with conjunctivitis, photophobia, pharyngitis, or irritating cough. About 5 weeks after exposure to arsenic, a transverse white stria, 1 to 2 mm in width, appears above the lunula of each fingernail *(Mees line)*. Patients with more than one exposure to arsenic may show double lines several millimeters apart.

Symptoms of headache, drowsiness, confusion, and convulsions are seen in both acute and chronic intoxication. Evidence of peripheral neuropathy usually appears 1 to 3 weeks after exposure. There are numbness, tingling, and burning of the feet and hands, followed by muscular weakness. The extremities show a decrease in touch, pain, and temperature sensations, in a symmetrical "stocking-glove" distribution, and distal weakness with inability to walk or stand, weakness of grip, and wrist drop. Tendon reflexes are absent or diminished, and atrophy of the affected muscles develops rapidly.

The laboratory findings usually consist of moderate anemia and a leukopenia of 2,000 to 5,000 white blood cells per mm^3 with mild eosinophilia. There is slight proteinuria, and liver function tests show mild abnormalities. The spinal fluid is normal.

None of the clinical or laboratory manifestations of arsenic poisoning is specific, and the diagnosis depends upon analysis of the urine for arsenic. Because arsenic is found widely in nature, and hence in water and food, its discovery in hair and nails may not be diagnostic. Normal persons have an average concentration of 0.05 mg arsenic per 100 mg hair. Concentrations of arsenic greater than 0.1 mg per 100 mg hair are considered indicative of poisoning. The minimal level of arsenic in the urine indicating intoxication is difficult to establish. Normal persons have been found to excrete between 0.01 and 0.06 mg arsenic per liter, and a few individuals as much as 0.2 mg per liter. Although there is considerable overlap, most patients with evidence of arsenic intoxication will be found to excrete more than 0.1 mg per liter; soon after acute exposure, many will show levels greater than 1 mg per liter.

The treatment for acute ingestion is gastric lavage (see Chap. 115). Replacement of lost fluids and elevation of blood pressure by vasopressor agents is often indicated. Immediate treatment with BAL should be instituted. Patients with peripheral neuropathy rarely show significant improvement with BAL and continue to have sensory disturbances and weakness for many months. Dramatic responses, however, have been observed with the use of BAL in the treatment of exfoliative dermatitis, bone marrow depression, and encephalopathy caused by the arsphenamines and the organic arsenicals. BAL is of little value in the treatment of the hemolysis caused by inhalation of arsine.

BISMUTH Poisoning by bismuth was formerly almost entirely a complication of antisyphilitic therapy. Now it rarely complicates Bi salts taken for intestinal disorder. Toxic manifestations may appear in the mouth (gingivitis, followed by stomatitis), the kidneys (albuminuria and nephrotic syndrome), or the skin (exfoliative dermatitis), requiring immediate interruption of bismuth injections. The development of a bluish stippled line of pigmentation just at the margin of the gums is not dangerous but suggests that oral hygiene should be improved. Bismuth subnitrate occasionally gives rise to methemoglobinemia (Chap. 316).

CADMIUM Poisoning is likely to occur after ingestion of an acid food prepared in a cadmium-lined vessel. The classic example is lemonade served from metal cans. Symptoms of nausea, vomiting, diarrhea, and prostration usually develop within 10 min after ingestion. Treatment is symptomatic, and symptoms ordinarily subside within 24 h. The short length of time after ingestion and the typical circumstances suggest the diagnosis. Inhalation of cadmium fumes in industry produces an acute, extremely severe pneumonitis. The use of BAL is not recommended for cadmium intoxication, as the BAL-cadmium complex dissociates in the kidneys and cadmium is nephrotoxic.

COPPER See Chap. 87 for discussion of Disturbances in Trace Element Metabolism, including copper, zinc, cobalt, nickel, silicon, and fluorine.

GOLD Because practically all cases of poisoning by gold are associated with its use in the treatment of arthritis, diagnosis is usually easy. Manifestations are skin rashes of various types, bone marrow depression, icterus, oliguria, nausea, vomiting, and gastrointestinal bleeding. Treatment consists of symptomatic relief of discomfort and the use of BAL, an effective antidote.

LEAD Poisoning results from inhalation of fumes as from burning storage batteries, from solder, paint spraying, or processes requiring the remelting of metallic lead. Ingestion of lead-containing materials such as paint, or water which has stood in lead pipes, is less important in adults. Illicit whiskey contaminated by lead solder in the pipes of stills has been responsible for cases of poisoning. Bullets or buckshot containing lead can cause poisoning years after becoming embedded in a serous cavity. The most common form of lead poisoning today is that encountered in children who ingest lead-containing outdoor paint, often used indoors in older houses. It has a sweetish, apparently attractive taste. Absorption is slow by any route, and prolonged exposure is required for the development of symptoms. Lead is a cumulative poison, excreted slowly. Acute poisoning is virtually nonexistent. Symptoms may develop suddenly after chronic exposure. Most of the absorbed lead is deposited in the bones; blood, urine, and feces contain only small amounts.

Manifestations of poisoning are colic, encephalopathy, peripheral neuritis, and anemia.

Lead colic, or painter's cramps, is characterized by agonizing, wandering, poorly localized abdominal pain, often with spasm and rigidity of the musculature of the abdominal wall. There is no fever or leukocytosis. Needless surgery has been carried out in these patients for supposed perforation of peptic ulcer or other catastrophe. Morphine has surprisingly little effect upon the pain; intravenous injection of calcium salts affords relief within a short time, although pain may recur. Attacks of colic seem to be brought on by intercurrent infection or alcoholic overindulgence.

Encephalopathy occurs chiefly in children and is manifested by convulsions, somnolence, mania, delirium, or coma. The mortality rate is high when convulsive seizures and coma occur. In an unexplained acute encephalopathy of childhood, increased intracranial pressure associated with high protein and the absence of cells should suggest the possibility of lead poisoning.

Peripheral neuritis with paralysis, characteristically involving the muscles most used (e.g., wrist drop in painters, etc.), occurs in patients exposed to lead, often in the absence of other symptoms. It is rare in children. (See Chap. 331.)

Mild anemia, probably the result of increased brittleness of the erythrocytes as well as a defect in cell maturation, is common. Pallor is out of proportion to anemia in patients with chronic plumbism and is attributed to spasm of small vessels in the skin. Anemia is almost never severe and is characterized by the presence of large numbers of erythrocytes with basophilic stippling. This is seen in other hematologic disorders, but a smear showing stippling should arouse suspicion of lead poisoning. In patients with poor oral hygiene a "lead line" of black lead sulfide may develop along the gingival margins. This is not seen in edentulous persons and is rare in children.

Patients with lead poisoning excrete increased amounts of coproporphyrin III in the urine (see Chap. 109). This is so consistent that examination of a urine specimen for porphyrin is the best screening test in suspected cases. A few milliliters of urine should be acidified with acetic acid and shaken with an equal volume of ether. Exposure of a specimen prepared in this manner under a Wood's lamp will reveal reddish fluorescence of the ether layer if coproporphyrin is present. A positive test result is strongly in favor of lead intoxication. Urinary lead determinations are of aid in confirming the diagnosis; a level of 0.2 mg per liter or more is usually regarded as significant, although interpretations vary. Diagnosis can be confirmed by promoting lead excretion with three doses of Calcium Disodium Versenate (25 mg per kg) at 8-h intervals. Excretion of over 500 μg in 24 h is indicative of excessive lead burden. A single blood lead level is rarely of help in diagnosis in adults because blood is cleared promptly of circulating lead.

Lead encephalopathy occurs chiefly in children, has a significant mortality rate, and causes severe permanent brain damage in 25 percent of survivors. Encephalopathy in adults is rare and usually results from consumption of lead-contaminated illicit liquor. Once minor symptoms of poisoning are present, acute encephalopathy can develop with unpredictable rapidity. Any child with symptoms suggestive of lead poisoning should be considered to have a medical emergency and should be hospitalized immediately. The onset of encephalopathy is signaled by the development of gross ataxia, persistent vomiting, and intermittent lethargy and stupor. These symptoms are followed by convulsions, mania, and coma.

The most important single feature of treatment is removal of the patient from further exposure to lead. Once abnormal absorption is terminated, virtually all the lead in the body is shifted into bone. Chelating agents do not remove significant quantities of lead from bone. It takes approximately twice as long to excrete a given burden of lead as it does to accumulate it. As long as significant quantities of lead remain in bone, any intercurrent illness which causes demineralization can cause mobilization of toxic quantities of lead into soft tissues and exacerbate plumbism.

The treatment of lead encephalopathy is begun once adequate urine flow is established. A combination of BAL and Calcium Disodium Versenate is employed, and the Versene therapy continued for 5 to 7 days. If Calcium Disodium Versenate is given alone in the presence of very high tissue concentrations of lead, some of the toxic effects may be intensified. Acute symptoms usually subside within 48 to 72 h after Versene is begun. Within 2 weeks urinary excretion of coproporphyrin ceases, and there is sometimes a dramatic improvement in neuritis.

Symptoms of acute increased intracranial pressure are best treated with repeated doses of mannitol given intravenously. High-potency corticosteroids are also useful in relieving cerebral edema in patients with lead encephalopathy.

The problem of lead poisoning in children is so significant that many health departments are carrying out extensive programs for removal of lead-containing paints in old low-income housing areas.

In adults combined therapy with BAL and Calcium Disodium Versenate followed by oral penicillamine is probably indicated whenever blood levels exceed 100 mg lead per 100 g blood, even in the absence of symptoms. Evidence of lead toxicity is usually present at this level, and the risk of symptomatic episodes is considerable. The use of oral penicillamine alone in a dose of 1 to 1.5 g daily for 3 to 5 days in mildly symptomatic cases has been suggested and has the advantage of easy administration and the avoidance of painful injections.

MERCURY Poisoning occurs chiefly as a result of the acute ingestion of a soluble salt, usually mercuric chloride (bichloride of mercury). Toxic symptoms may occur with 0.1 g, and 0.5 g is almost always fatal unless immediate treatment is instituted. The mercuric ion is corrosive and produces severe local inflammation. Oral, pharyngeal, and laryngeal pain are severe; abdominal cramps with nausea and vomiting occur within 15 min. As mercury is absorbed, it is concentrated in the kidneys, where it poisons the tubular cells, producing a tendency to diuresis within the first 2 to 3 h. The combination of vomiting, dehydration, shock, and progressive tubular damage, however, soon leads to anuria and uremia. The poison is also excreted into the colon and produces severe enteritis, with bloody diarrhea and tenesmus. Death is usually from uremia. The chief objectives of treatment are to prevent the shock of dehydration and to remove mercury from the body. Early in treatment, copious quantities of fluid should be infused intravenously to prevent dehydration and to reduce the concentration of mercuric ion in the renal tubules. That the patient is anuric early is often simply the result of dehydration and shock. In such instances, forcing fluids is advisable. However, the gradual development of oliguria and anuria in a hydrated patient indicates renal damage by mercury, and at this stage a regimen for acute renal shutdown should be instituted (Chap. 272).

Chronic poisoning from metallic mercury vapor occurs in persons exposed to large amounts of the metal in laboratories or in industry and occasionally as a result of prolonged therapeutic use, as in vaginal douches. Manifestations may be those of subacute poisoning, with salivation, stomatitis, and diarrhea or primary neurologic signs, including tremors of the extremities, tongue, and lips, ataxia and dysarthria, erethism, a state of easy embarrassment, irritability, apprehension, withdrawal, and depression.

Some poison can be removed from the body by gastric lavage, but more important in treatment is the binding of the mercuric ion in a harmless compound by BAL. The therapeutic usefulness of BAL depends on its immediate administration. In chronic mercury poisoning, N-acetyl-*dl*-penicillamine may well be the drug of choice. It can be administered orally and appears to chelate mercury selectively, with considerably less effect on copper, which is essential to many metabolic processes.

SILVER Most poisoning by silver involves silver nitrate, a caustic salt. There are intense nausea, vomiting, and diarrhea after swallowing nitrate (lunar caustic), and death from shock may occur within a few hours. The mouth is usually deeply stained by silver nitrate. Treatment is entirely supportive, with fluid replacement and control of pain.

Chronic exposure (usually to nose drops) produces a peculiar bluish skin discoloration (argyria).

THALLIUM Thallium is a component of certain rodenticides and depilatories, and clinical poisoning is usually a result of accidental ingestion of these materials. The fatal dose is approximately 1.0 g. Manifestations are vomiting, diarrhea, and leg pains, followed by weakness. About 3 weeks after poisoning, the patient's hair falls out, providing a strong diagnostic clue if the cause has not previously been determined. Treatment is symptomatic. The alopecia is temporary if the patient recovers.

REFERENCES

ARENA JM: Treatment of mercury poisoning. Mod Treat 4:734, 1967

AUB JC et al: Lead poisoning. Medicine 4:1, 1925

BANK WJ et al: Thallium poisoning. Arch Neurol 26:456, 1974

CHISHOLM JJ JR: Poisoning due to heavy metals. Pediatr Clin North Am 17:591, 1970

DOOLAN PD et al: Acute renal insufficiency due to dichloride of mercury: Observations of gastrointestinal hemorrhage and BAL therapy. N Engl J Med 249:273, 1953

HAMILTON A, HARDY HL: *Industrial Toxicology,* 3d ed. Acton, England: Publishing Sciences Group, Inc., 1974

HEYMAN A: Systemic manifestations of bismuth toxicity: Observations on 4 patients with pre-existent kidney disease. Am J Syph Gonor Vener Dis 28:721, 1944

JENKINS RB: Inorganic arsenic and the nervous system. Brain 89: 479, 1966

KARK RAP et al: Mercury poisoning and its treatment with *N*-acetyl-D,L-penicillamine. N Engl J Med 285:10, 1971

KENDREY G, ROE FJC: Cadmium toxicology. Lancet 1:1206, 1969
KEUSLER CJ et al: Arsine poisoning, mode of action and treatment. J Pharmacol Exp Ther 88:99, 1946
LEVINE WG: Heavy-metal antagonists, in *The Pharmacological Basis of Therapeutics,* 5th ed., eds LS Goodman, A Gilman, New York: Macmillan, 1975, p. 912
LONGCOPE WT, LUETSCHER JA: The use of BAL (British antilewisite) in the treatment of the injurious effects of arsenic, mercury, and other metallic poisons. Ann Intern Med 31:545, 1949

118 ALCOHOL

MAURICE VICTOR
RAYMOND D. ADAMS

Intemperance in the use of alcohol creates many problems in modern society, the importance of which can be judged by the repeated emphasis they receive in contemporary writings, both literary and scientific. These problems may be divided into three categories—psychologic, medical, and sociologic. The main psychologic problem is why a person drinks excessively, often with full knowledge that such action will result in physical injury to himself and irreparable harm to his family. The medical problem embraces all aspects of alcoholic habituation as well as the diseases which result from overindulgence in alcohol. The sociologic problem comprises the effects of sustained inebriety on the family and community.

The various problems raised by excessive drinking cannot be separated from one another, and physicians must therefore be conversant with all sides of the subject. They may be asked to help a patient conquer his alcoholic tendency or to diagnose and to treat the numerous diseases to which he is subject; often they must admit or commit the patient to a general or mental hospital, according to the nature of the presenting clinical disorder; and lastly, they may be required to enlist the aid of available social agencies when such services are needed by either the patient or his family.

Alcoholism has been defined as both a chronic disease and a disorder of behavior, characterized in either context by drinking of alcohol to an extent that surpasses the social drinking customs of the community and that interferes with the drinker's health, interpersonal relations, or means of livelihood. Reduced to pharmacologic terms, it is addiction to alcohol. The precise number of such persons, commonly called alcoholics, in the United States is not known. In 1971, the Department of Health, Education, and Welfare estimated that about 9 million men and women (7 percent of the adult population) "manifested the behavior of alcohol abuse and alcoholism." It requires little projection of the imagination to conceive of the havoc wrought by alcohol in terms of decreased productivity, accidents, crime, mental and physical disease, and disruption of family life.

PHARMACOLOGY AND METABOLISM OF ALCOHOL Ethyl alcohol, or ethanol, is the active ingredient in beer, wine, whiskey, gin, brandy, and other less common alcoholic beverages. In addition, the stronger spirits contain enanthic ethers, which give the flavor but have no important pharmacologic properties, and small amounts of impurities such as amyl alcohol and acetaldehyde, which act like alcohol but are more toxic. Contrary to prevailing opinion, the content of B vitamins in American beer and other liquors is so low as to have little nutritional value.

Alcohol is absorbed from both the stomach and the small intestine. Its presence may be detected in the blood within 5 min after ingestion, and the maximum concentration is reached in 30 to 90 min. The ingestion of milk and fatty foods impedes and water facilitates its absorption. The rate of absorption increases after Billroth I and II gastrectomies, and in these individuals maximum blood alcohol concentrations are higher and attained faster than in subjects with intact stomachs.

After entering the bloodstream, alcohol enters the various organs of the body, as well as the spinal fluid, urine, and pulmonary alveolar air, in concentrations which bear a constant relationship to that in the blood. It is eliminated chiefly by oxidation to carbon dioxide, less than 10 percent being excreted chemically unchanged in the urine, sweat, and breath. The energy liberated by the oxidation of alcohol is equivalent to 7 kcal per g.

Alcohol is metabolized primarily in the liver via the cytoplasmic enzyme alcohol dehydrogenase to generate acetaldehyde. It can also be oxidized by catalase and a microsomal oxidase, but the physiologic and quantitative roles of these pathways is not clear. Acetaldehyde is further oxidized to acetate by acetaldehyde dehydrogenase of liver mitochondria and subsequently to acetyl coenzyme A and CO_2.

For all practical purposes it may be accepted that once absorption is ended and an equilibrium established with the tissues, ethyl alcohol is oxidized at a constant rate, independent of its concentration in the blood (about 150 mg alcohol per kilogram of body weight per hour, or about 1 oz 90-proof whiskey per hour). Actually, slightly more alcohol is burned per hour when the initial concentrations are very high, but this increment is of little clinical significance. On the other hand, the rate of oxidation of acetaldehyde does depend on its concentration in the tissues. This fact is of importance in connection with the drug disulfiram (Antabuse), which raises the tissue concentration necessary for the metabolism of a certain amount of acetaldehyde per unit of time. The patient taking both Antabuse and alcohol will accumulate an inordinate amount of acetaldehyde, resulting in nausea, vomiting, and hypotension, sometimes pronounced and even fatal in degree. This pharmacologic principle underlies the treatment of alcoholism with Antabuse.

Very few factors are capable of increasing the rate of alcohol metabolism. However, it seems well established that chronic alcoholics metabolize alcohol faster than normal individuals. Amino acids (especially alanine) and fructose also enhance ethanol metabolism, but their use clinically to speed oxidation is limited. Alcohol also reduces the intestinal absorption of nutrients such as glucose, amino acids, calcium, folate, and vitamin B_{12}. This inhibition of absorption may contribute to the malnutrition frequently found in alcoholic subjects. Starvation slows the rate of alcohol metabolism in the liver, although this varies greatly in degree from one person to another.

PHYSIOLOGIC AND PSYCHOLOGIC EFFECTS OF ALCOHOL There appears to be a direct action of alcohol on the excitability and contractility of heart muscle. With intoxicating doses there is a rise in cardiac rate and output and in systolic and pulse pressures, and a cutaneous vasodilatation at the expense of splanchnic constriction. Some authors have stated that prolonged intoxication may have a damaging effect on cardiac and skeletal muscle, a degeneration of fibers supposedly due to suppression of myophosphorylase activity. Increased sweating and vasodilatation cause a loss of body heat and a fall in body temperature.

In low concentrations, by whatever route it is administered, alcohol stimulates the gastric glands to produce acid, apparently by antral activation of gastrin release, and possibly by causing the tissues to form or release histamine. With the ingestion of alcohol in concentrations of over 10 to 15 percent, the secretion of mucus is increased, the stomach mucosa becomes congested and hyperemic, and the secretion of acid may then become depressed. This is a state of acute gastritis, from which recovery may be relatively rapid. The increase in appetite following ingestion of alcohol is due to the stimulation of the end organs of taste and to a general sense of well-being. Similarly, the reviving effect of alcohol in fatigue states is a cerebral one, not due to a direct stimulating effect on muscle or other organs.

Alcohol has a number of other metabolic effects. In the area of *lipid metabolism* it can cause hypertriglyceridemia as well as lead to a fatty liver. It interferes with *carbohydrate metabolism* and can produce hypoglycemia by impairing gluconeogenesis; however, a significant degree of hypoglycemia will occur only if hepatic glycogen stores are depleted. Under certain conditions alcohol can also interfere with the peripheral utilization of glucose and produce hyperglycemia. When ethanol is oxidized, there is a simultaneous generation of reduced nicotinamideadenine dinucleotide (NAD); as a result pyruvate is converted to lactate. Thus alcoholism may result in increased levels of serum lactate, occasionally *lactic acidosis* and also *hyperuricemia* secondary to the inhibitory action of lactic acid on the renal excretion of uric acid.

Alcohol has other *renal effects.* Patients frequently exhibit low serum levels of phosphate and magnesium presumably because of increased renal excretion of these ions. There are also well-recognized effects on water excretion; thus the ingestion of 4 oz of 100-proof bourbon whiskey may result in a diuresis comparable with that which follows the drinking of large amounts of water. This diuresis is most likely due to the transient suppression of the release of antidiuretic hormone (ADH) from the supraopticohypophyseal system, since a relatively small amount of alcohol injected directly into a carotid artery evokes a prompt diuresis without a detectable rise in the concentration of alcohol in the systemic blood. Alcohol does not alter the sensitivity of the kidney tubules to endogenous or exogenous ADH (Pitressin) and has no discernible effect on renal hemodynamic function in normal persons. The degree of diuresis seems to be more closely related to the duration of the rising blood alcohol level than to the rate of increase or the absolute level attained if the period of alcohol intoxication is sustained. Diuresis occurs only during the initial phase of alcohol administration and does not persist during prolonged drinking. There are also an increased urinary excretion of ammonium and a titratable acidity following alcohol ingestion, owing to a mild degree of both metabolic and respiratory acidosis. The former is presumably due to an accumulation of acid metabolites and the latter to the direct action of alcohol on the respiratory center.

Apart from the derangements noted above, the obvious actions of acute, nonlethal doses of alcohol are those exerted on the nervous system, constituting the characteristic symptoms and signs of alcohol intoxication. It is now generally accepted that alcohol is not a stimulant of the central nervous system, but a depressant. Some of the early effects of alcohol, manifested by garrulousness, aggressiveness, and excessive activity and increased electrical excitability of the cerebral cortex, all of which suggest stimulation, are due to the inhibition of certain subcortical structures (high brainstem reticular formation?) which ordinarily modulate cerebral cortical activity. Similarly, the initial hyperactivity of tendon reflexes may represent a transitory escape of spinal motor neurons from higher inhibitory centers. With increasing amounts of alcohol, however, the depressant action spreads to involve the cerebral cortical neurons as well as other brainstem and spinal neurons.

All manner of motor performance, whether the simple maintenance of a standing posture, the control of speech and eye movements, or highly organized and complex motor skills, is adversely affected by alcohol. The movements involved in these acts are not only slower than normal but also more inaccurate and random in character and therefore less adapted to the accomplishment of specific ends.

Alcohol also impairs the efficiency of mental function by interfering with the learning process, which is slowed and rendered less effective. The facility of forming associations, whether of words or of figures, tends to be hampered, and the power of attention and concentration is reduced. The person is not as versatile as usual in directing thought along new lines appropriate to the problems at hand. Finally, alcohol impairs the faculties of judgment and discrimination and, all in all, the ability to think and reason clearly.

A scale relating the various degrees of clinical intoxication to the blood alcohol levels in nonhabituated persons has been constructed. At blood alcohol levels of 30 mg per 100 ml, a mild euphoria was detectable, and at 50 mg per 100 ml, a mild incoordination. At 100 mg per 100 ml, ataxia was obvious; at 300 mg per 100 ml, the patient was stuporous; and a level of 400 mg per 100 ml was accompanied by deep anesthesia and could prove fatal. These figures are valid, provided that the alcohol content rises steadily over a 2 h period.

It should be emphasized, however, that such a scale has no value in the chronic alcoholic patient. It does not take into account two adaptive changes that every organism makes to alcohol, which are an increased rate of alcohol metabolism by the liver and also development of tolerance. Thus it is common knowledge that a habituated individual can drink more alcohol and show fewer of its nervous system effects than a moderate drinker or abstainer. In the chronic alcoholic subject the ingestion of a given amount of alcohol will result in a lower blood alcohol level than in a nonalcoholic individual; furthermore for a given blood alcohol level one will observe lesser degrees of "drunkenness" or inebriation. The organism is capable of adapting to alcohol after a very short exposure. If the alcohol concentration in the blood is raised very slowly, no symptoms appear, even at quite high levels. It would appear that the important factor in this rapid adaptability is not so much the rate of increment or the height of the blood alcohol level, but the length of time the alcohol had been present in the body. It has also been shown that if the dosage of alcohol which causes blood levels to reach a certain height is held constant, the blood alcohol concentration falls and clinical evidence of intoxication disappears. The cause of this fall in alcohol concentration is not clear. This type of tolerance has been termed "metabolic" and refers to the adjustments made by the nervous system to long-continued exposure to alcohol. There must be a subtle alteration in the metabolism of the neurons such that they can function in the face of high tissue alcohol levels. This alteration requires some time for its establishment. Removal of alcohol from the habituated nervous system results in another disturbance in neuronal function, presumably an overactivity.

CLINICAL MANIFESTATIONS OF ALCOHOLISM Although alcohol may alter the function of practically every organ system, the important clinical effects are mainly on the digestive organs and on the nervous system.

Effect on digestive organs Symptoms of disordered gastrointestinal function are particularly common in alcoholics; of these the most distinctive are *morning nausea and vomiting.* Characteristically, the patient can suppress these symptoms by taking a drink or two, after which he is able to consume large quantities of alcohol without their recurrence until the following morning. Since sufficient alcohol actually relieves these symptoms, they are probably not due to the local effects of alcohol on the stomach, but have a "central" origin and represent the mildest manifestations of the withdrawal syndrome (see below).

Other complaints referable to the gastrointestinal system are abdominal distention, epigastric distress, belching, typical or atypical ulcer symptoms, and hematemesis. The most common pathologic basis for these symptoms is a superficial *gastritis,* which is an almost invariable sequel to prolonged drinking. Most instances of gastritis are benign, and the symptoms subside after a few days of abstinence, but more severe forms are associated with mucosal erosions or ulcerations and may be the source of serious bleeding. The incidence of *peptic ulcer* is exceptionally high in alcoholics. A less frequent but serious cause of hematemesis is the so-called *Mallory-Weiss syndrome,* which is characterized by lacerations of the mucosa at or just below the gastroesophageal junction. In many of these cases bleeding is preceded by an episode of forceful vomiting or protracted retching. The typical lesions appear to depend upon raising the intragastric pressure to 100 to 150 mmHg, i.e., to the range of pressure attained by normal subjects during a period of induced straining and retching.

Patients admitted to the hospital following a period of prolonged drinking and severe dietary depletion almost invariably show enlargement of the liver because of infiltration of the parenchymal cells with fat (see Chap. 296). This fatty liver is essentially reversible provided that the patient remains abstinent and receives a nutritious diet. A form of hepatocellular necrosis or *alcoholic hepatitis* is observed frequently in chronic alcoholics, especially following a severe drinking bout. About 8 percent of patients with severe alcoholism develop a permanent form of liver disease, i.e., *cirrhosis,* in which a diffuse proliferation of fibrous tissue replaces the normal lobular architecture of the organ. The alcoholic forms of liver disease are discussed in Chap. 301.

The excessive use of alcohol is also a significant factor in the causation of pancreatitis. The mildest form of this disorder may be attributed to gastritis or may go unnoticed, unless erroneously suspected by elevations of the serum amylase level. In more severe form pancreatitis presents as an acute abdominal catastrophe, i.e., with epigastric pain, vomiting, and rigidity of the upper abdominal muscles. In these circumstances the pancreas appears tense and edematous, often with a serosanguineous exudation of fluid on its surface. The most severe form is that of hemorrhagic pancreatitis (Chap. 307). Alcoholics may also develop a chronic relapsing form of pancreatitis. This type is often associated with irregular calcification of the pancreas.

[The *management* of the various gastrointestinal complications of alcoholism is considered in the section dealing with these diseases (Chaps. 284 and 288).]

Effect on nervous system A large number of neurologic disorders are associated with alcoholism. The factor common to all of them, of course, is the abuse of alcohol, but the mechanism by which alcohol produces its effects varies widely from one group of disorders to another. The classification which follows is based for the most part on known mechanisms.

I Alcohol intoxication—drunkenness, coma, excitement ("pathologic intoxication")
II The abstinence or withdrawal syndrome—tremulousness, hallucinosis, "rum fits," delirium tremens
III Nutritional diseases of the nervous system secondary to alcoholism
  A Wernicke-Korsakoff syndrome
  B Polyneuropathy
  C Optic neuropathy ("tobacco-alcohol amblyopia")
  D Pellagra
IV Diseases of uncertain pathogenesis, associated with alcoholism
  A Cerebellar degeneration
  B Marchiafava-Bignami disease
  C Central pontine myelinolysis
  D Cerebral atrophy
  E "Alcoholic" cardiomyopathy and myopathy
V Neurologic disorders consequent upon Laennec's cirrhosis and portal-systemic shunts
  A Hepatic stupor and coma
  B Chronic hepatocerebral degeneration

ALCOHOL INTOXICATION Drunkenness is such a common phenomenon that its psychologic and physical manifestations require little elaboration. The signs consist of varying degrees of exhilaration and excitement, loss of restraint, irregularity of behavior, loquacity, slurred speech, incoordination of movement and gait, irritability, drowsiness, and, in advanced cases, stupor and coma. On rare occasions acute intoxication is characterized by an outburst of irrational, combative, and destructive behavior, which terminates when the patient falls into a deep stupor and for which he may later have no memory. This state has been referred to as "pathologic intoxication" or "acute alcoholic paranoid state." Allegedly this reaction may follow the ingestion of relatively small amounts of alcohol, and it has been variously ascribed to constitutional differences in susceptibility to alcohol, previous cerebral injury, and "an underlying epileptic predisposition." However, there are no critical data to support any of these contentions. An analogy may be drawn between this state of alcoholic excitement and a similar reaction which occasionally complicates the administration of barbiturates.

Alcohol acts on nerve cells in a manner akin to the general anesthetics. Unlike the latter, however, the margin between the dose of alcohol that produces surgical anesthesia and that which dangerously depresses respiration is a very narrow one, a fact which accounts for the occasional fatality in cases of alcoholic narcosis.

The signs of alcohol intoxication are distinctive, and most forms present no problem in diagnosis or management. On the other hand, coma due to alcohol may present difficulties in differential diagnosis. It should be stressed that the diagnosis of alcoholic coma is made not merely on the basis of a flushed face, stupor, and the odor of alcohol, but only after the careful exclusion of all other causes of coma (see Chap. 22). Furthermore, alcoholic coma is not always benign, as are the more common manifestations of intoxication. Serious depression of respiration, heralded by a loss of corneal and pupillary reflexes, calls for intensive respiratory care and the treatment of peripheral vascular collapse, if this should supervene.

Treatment of alcohol intoxication Mild to moderate degrees of intoxication require no special treatment. Certain time-honored remedies such as a cold shower, strong coffee, forced activity, or induction of vomiting may be helpful, but there is no evidence that any of these methods influences the rate of disappearance of alcohol from the blood. *Alcoholic stupor* is also a short, self-limited state, and if the vital signs are normal no special therapeutic measures are necessary. *Pathologic intoxication* may require the use of restraints and the parenteral administration of phenobarbital sodium (200 mg subcutaneously) or amobarbital sodium (500 mg intramuscularly), repeated once in 30 to 40 min if necessary.

Coma due to alcohol intoxication is a medical emergency. The main object of treatment is to prevent respiratory suppression and the complications which it engenders. The management of the comatose patient is described in Chap. 22. One should like to be able to lower the blood alcohol level as rapidly as possible. The administration of insulin and glucose or fructose for this purpose is of little practical value. Analeptic drugs such as amphetamine, pentylenetetrazole (Metrazol), and various mixtures of caffeine and picrotoxin are antagonistic to alcohol only insofar as they are powerful cerebral cortical stimulants and overall nervous system excitants; they do not hasten the combustion of alcohol.

THE ABSTINENCE OR WITHDRAWAL SYNDROME A second category of alcoholic neurologic disease comprises the tremulous, hallucinatory, epileptic, and delirious states. Although a sustained period of chronic intoxication is the underlying factor in each of these disorders, the symptoms become manifest only *after a period of relative or absolute abstinence* from alcohol—hence the designation *abstinence* or *withdrawal syndrome.* Each of the major manifestations of the withdrawal syndrome may occur distinct from the others and will be so described; more frequently, however, they occur in various combinations. The prototype of the patients afflicted with these symptoms is the spree or periodic drinker, although the steady drinker is not immune if, for some reason, he or she stops drinking.

Tremulousness By far the most common manifestation of the abstinence syndrome is a state of tremulousness, commonly referred to as "the shakes" or "the jitters," combined with general irritability and gastrointestinal symptoms, particularly nausea and vomiting. The symptoms first show themselves after several days of drinking, usually in the morning, after the short period of abstinence that occurs during sleep. The patient then needs to "quiet his nerves" with a few drinks. Indeed his symptoms are relieved by alcohol, only to return on successive mornings with increasing severity. The usual spree lasts about 2 weeks, but the duration varies greatly. It is terminated not only because of recurrent tremor and vomiting, but for one or more other reasons such as lack of funds, weakness, self-disgust, injury, illness, or collapse. The symptoms then become greatly augmented, reaching their peak intensity 24 to 36 h after the complete cessation of drinking.

At this stage, the patient presents a distinctive clinical picture. He is alert and startles easily. His face is deeply flushed, the conjunctivas are injected, and there is usually a tachycardia, anorexia, nausea, and retching. He may complain of insomnia and craves rest and sleep. Preoccupied with his misery, he is inattentive and disinclined to answer questions, and may respond in a rude or perfunctory manner. The patient may be mildly disoriented in time and have a poor memory for events of the last few days of his drinking spree but shows no serious confusion, being generally aware of his surroundings and the nature of his illness.

Generalized tremor is an outstanding feature of this illness. It is of fast frequency (6 to 8 oscillations per s), slightly irregular, and variable in its severity, tending to diminish when the patient is in quiet surroundings and to increase with motor activity or emotional stress. The tremor may be so violent that the patient cannot stand without help, speak clearly, or feed himself. Sometimes there is little objective evidence of tremor, and the patient complains only of being "shaky inside."

Although the flushed facies, anorexia, tachycardia, and tremor subside to a large extent within a few days, the patient does not regain his full composure for a much longer time. The overalertness, tendency to startle easily, and jerkiness of movement may persist for a week or longer; the feeling of uneasiness may not leave the patient completely for 10 to 14 days, and only at the end of this time is he able to sleep undisturbed, without sedation. An attempt should be made to keep the patient in the hospital for this length of time. To discharge him after a few days increases the likelihood that he will turn to alcohol to suppress his still-present tenseness and sleeplessness.

Hallucinosis Symptoms of disordered perception occur in about one-quarter of the tremulous patients. The patient may complain of "bad dreams"—nightmarish episodes associated with disturbed sleep, which are difficult to separate from real experience. Sounds and shadows may be misinterpreted, or familiar objects may be distorted and assume unreal forms. Although these are not hallucinations in the strict sense of the term, they represent the most common forms of disordered sense perception in the alcoholic. Hallucinations may be purely visual or auditory in type, mixed visual and auditory, and occasionally tactile or olfactory. There is little evidence to support the popular belief that certain visual hallucinations are specific to alcoholism. They are more commonly animate than inanimate and may comprise various forms of human, animal, or insect life. They may occur singly or in panoramas; they may appear shrunken or enlarged; they may be natural in appearance or take distorted and hideous forms (see also Chap. 26).

ACUTE AND CHRONIC AUDITORY HALLUCINOSIS This phenomenon merits separate consideration. For many years, an alcoholic psychosis has been recognized in which vivid auditory hallucinations are the major abnormality. Kraepelin referred to this as the *hallucinatory insanity of drunkards or alcoholic mania.* The central feature of the illness, in the beginning, is the occurrence of auditory hallucinations despite an otherwise clear sensorium, i.e., the patients are not confused, disoriented, or obtunded and have an intact memory. The hallucinations may be musical or take the form of unstructured sounds such as buzzing, ringing, shots, or clicking. More often they are formed (vocal) in nature. When the voices can be identified, they are attributed to the patient's family, friends, or neighbors, rarely to God, radio, or radar. The voices may be addressed directly to the patient, but more frequently they discuss him in the third person. In the majority of cases the voices are maligning, reproachful, or threatening in nature and are disturbing to the patient; a significant proportion, however, are not unpleasant and leave the patient undisturbed. The voices are intensely real and vivid, and they tend to be exteriorized; i.e., they come from behind the door, from the corridor, or through the floor. Another quality of these formed hallucinations (and of visual ones) is the appropriateness of the patient's emotional response to them. He may call on the police for protection or barricade himself against invaders; he may even attempt suicide to avoid what the voices threaten. The hallucinations are most prominent during the night, and their duration varies greatly—they may be momentary, or they may recur intermittently for days on end and, in exceptional instances, for weeks or months.

Most patients, while hallucinating, have no appreciation of the unreality of their hallucinations. As improvement occurs, the patient begins to doubt their reality, is reluctant to talk about them, and may even question whether he had been sane during the episode. Full recovery is characterized by the realization that the voices were imaginary and by the ability to recall, sometimes with remarkable clarity, the abnormal thought content of parts of the psychotic episode.

A unique feature of this psychosis is the evolution of a chronic auditory hallucinosis in a small proportion of the patients. The patient becomes quiet and resigned, even though the hallucinations remain threatening and derogatory. Ideas of reference and influence and other poorly systematized paranoid delusions become prominent. At this stage these patients show many of the symptoms of schizophrenia—illogical thinking, vagueness, tangential associations, and a dissociation of affect and of thought content. There is some evidence that repeated attacks of acute auditory hallucinosis render the patient more vulnerable to this paranoid schizophrenic-like syndrome.

Withdrawal seizures ("rum fits") In this particular setting (i.e., where relative or absolute abstinence follows a period of chronic inebriation) there is a marked tendency to develop convulsive seizures. Over 90 percent of seizures occur during the 7- to 48-h period following the cessation of drinking, with a peak incidence between 13 to 24 h. During the period of seizure activity the electroencephalogram may be abnormal, but it reverts to normal in a matter of days, even though the patient may go on to develop delirium tremens. Also during the period of seizure activity the patient is unusually sensitive to stroboscopic stimulation. About half these patients respond to this activating procedure with generalized myoclonus (photomyoclonus) or a convulsive seizure (photoconvulsion). In contrast, patients with idiopathic epilepsy rarely show this type of response to photic stimulation.

Seizures occurring in the abstinence period have a number of other distinctive features. There may be only a single seizure, but in the majority of cases they occur in short bursts of two to six, or even more, and an occasional patient develops status epilepticus. The seizures are grand mal in type, i.e., major generalized convulsions with loss of consciousness. A focal seizure or seizures should always suggest the presence of a focal lesion (usually traumatic) in addition to the effects of alcohol. Almost one-third of the patients with generalized seizure activity go on to develop delirium tremens, in which case the seizures invariably precede the delirium. The postictal confusional state may blend imperceptibly with the onset of the delirium, or there may be a clearing of the postictal state, over several hours or even a day or two, before the delirium sets in. Seizures of this type occur in patients who have been drinking for many years, so that they have to be distinguished from other forms of epilepsy beginning in adult life.

It is suggested that the term *rum fits,* i.e., the words used by the alcoholic himself, be reserved for seizures which possess the attributes described above. This would serve to distinguish this form of seizure activity, which occurs only in the immediate abstinence period, from that which occurs in the interdrinking period, long after withdrawal has been accomplished. It is also important to note that the "idiopathic" or posttraumatic forms of epilepsy may be influenced by alcohol. In patients with these types of epilepsy, a seizure or seizures may be precipitated by only a short period of drinking (e.g., a weekend, or even one evening of heavy social drinking); interestingly, in these circumstances, the seizures occur not when the patient is intoxicated, but usually the morning after, in the "sobering-up" period.

Electroencephalographic findings in alcoholic subjects

with "rum fits" do not support the notion that the seizures merely represent latent epilepsy made manifest by alcohol. Instead, the electroencephalogram (EEG) reflects a sequence of changes induced by alcohol itself—a decrease in the frequency of brain waves during the period of chronic intoxication; a rapid return of the EEG to normal immediately after cessation of drinking; the occurrence of a brief period of dysrhythmia (sharp waves and paroxysmal changes) which coincides with the flurry of convulsive activity; and again, a rapid return of the EEG to normal. Except for the transient dysrhythmia in the withdrawal period, the incidence of EEG abnormalities in patients who have had "rum fits" is not greater than in the normal population, in sharp contrast to patients who are indeed subject to seizures (see Chap. 330).

Delirium tremens This is the most dramatic and grave of all the alcoholic complications. It is characterized by profound confusion, delusions, vivid hallucinations, tremor, agitation, and sleeplessness, as well as by increased activity of the autonomic nervous system, i.e., dilated pupils, fever, tachycardia, and profuse perspiration. The clinical features of delirium have been presented in detail in Chap. 26.

Delirium tremens develops in one of several settings. The patient, an excessive and steady drinker of many years' duration, may have been admitted to the hospital for an unrelated illness, accident, or operation, and 3 to 4 days later becomes delirious. Or, following a prolonged spree, he may have already experienced several days of tremulousness and hallucinosis, or one or more seizures, and may even be recovering from these symptoms, when he suddenly develops delirium tremens.

In the majority of cases delirium tremens is benign and short-lived, ending as abruptly as it begins. Consumed by the relentless activity and wakefulness of several days' duration, the patient falls into a deep sleep; he awakens lucid, quiet, and exhausted, with virtually no memory for the events of the delirious period. Less commonly, the delirious state subsides gradually; more rarely still, there may be one or more relapses, several discrete episodes of delirium being separated by lucidity, the entire process lasting for as little as several days or as long as 4 to 5 weeks. When the delirium occurs as a single episode, the duration is 72 h or less in over 80 percent of the cases.

About 15 percent of cases of delirium tremens, as defined above, end fatally. In many of these there is an associated infectious illness or injury, but in a few no complicating illness is discernible. Patients frequently die in a state of hyperthermia or peripheral circulatory collapse; in some, death comes so suddenly that the nature of the terminal events cannot be determined.

Closely related to typical delirium tremens and about as common are the *atypical delirious-hallucinatory* or *confusional states,* in which one facet of the delirium tremens complex assumes prominence to the practical exclusion of the other symptoms. The patient may simply exhibit a transient state of quiet confusion, agitation, and peculiar behavior lasting several days or weeks. Other patients present a vivid hallucinatory-delusional state and abnormal behavior, consistent with their false beliefs. Unlike typical delirium tremens, the atypical states always present as a single circumscribed episode without recurrences, are only rarely preceded by epilepsy, and do not end fatally. This may be another way of saying that they are a partial or less severe form of the disease.

Pathologic examination is singularly unrevealing in patients with delirium tremens. Edema and brain swelling have been absent in the authors' pathologic material except when there was shock, terminal hypoxia, or electrolyte imbalance, and there have not been any significant microscopic changes in the brain. Abnormalities of the blood nonprotein nitrogen, carbon dioxide, spinal fluid, serum sodium, chloride, sugar, potassium, and calcium occur unpredictably. The electroencephalographic findings have been discussed in relation to alcoholic epilepsy.

The *pathogenesis* of the tremulous-hallucinatory-delirious state has been a matter of considerable controversy. The idea that it simply represents the most severe form of alcohol intoxication is not tenable. The symptoms of toxicity, consisting of slurred speech, uninhibited behavior, staggering gait, stupor, and coma, are distinctive and different from the symptom complex of tremor, hallucinations, fits, and delirium. The former symptoms are associated with an elevated blood alcohol level, whereas the latter become evident only when the blood alcohol is reduced. Finally, the toxic symptoms increase in severity as more alcohol is consumed, whereas tremor and hallucinosis and even full-blown delirium tremens may be nullified by the administration of alcohol.

Although much discussed in the past, there is no evidence that endocrine abnormality or nutritional deficiency plays a role in the genesis of delirium tremens and related symptoms. Instead, they are of neural origin—the parts of the nervous system which became habituated to alcohol appear to overreact when it is withdrawn. The duration of the illness seems to correspond to the time required for neuronal excitability to return to normal. The lesion is a biochemical one, of obscure nature, still.

It is evident, from observations in both man and experimental animals, that the one indispensable factor in the genesis of delirium tremens and related disorders is the withdrawal of alcohol, following a period of chronic intoxication. Further, these observations indicate that the emergence of withdrawal symptoms depends upon a decline in the blood alcohol level from a previously higher level and not necessarily upon the complete disappearance of alcohol from the blood. The mechanism(s) by which the withdrawal of alcohol produces symptoms are only beginning to be understood. It has been shown that the early phase of alcohol withdrawal (beginning 7 to 8 h after cessation of drinking) is regularly attended by a drop in serum magnesium levels and a rise in arterial pH values, on the basis of respiratory alkalosis. Indeed it is possible that the compounded effect of these two factors, both of which are associated with hyperexcitability of the nervous system, might be responsible for seizures and perhaps for other symptoms which characterize the early phase of withdrawal. The elevation in pH is explained as withdrawal release of the neurons of the "respiratory center," which had been previously rendered insensitive to circulating CO_2. In the "rebound" phase these cells become more sensitive than normal to CO_2, with resultant hyperventilation and respiratory alkalosis. But as an explanation of delirium tremens, hypomagnesemia is probably not important, since the serum magnesium level has frequently been restored to normal before the onset of the delirium.

Treatment of alcoholic withdrawal syndrome The general aspects of management of the delirious and confused patient have been described in Chap. 26.

More specifically the treatment of delirium tremens begins with a careful search, followed by appropriate treatment, for associated injuries (particularly head injury with cerebral lacerations or subdural hematoma), infections (pneumonia or meningitis), pancreatitis, and liver disease. Because of the frequency and seriousness of these complications, skull and chest roentgenograms should be obtained and lumbar puncture should be performed routinely. In severe forms of delirium tremens, the temperature, pulse, and blood pressure should be recorded at 30-min intervals in anticipation of peripheral circulatory collapse and hyperthermia, which, added to the effects of injury and infection, are the usual causes of death in this disease. In the case of shock, one must act quickly, utilizing whole-blood transfusions, fluids, and vasopressor drugs. The occurrence of hyperthermia demands the use of a cooling mattress in addition to specific treatment for any infection that may be present.

A very important element in treatment is the correction of fluid and electrolyte imbalance. Severe degrees of agitation and perspiration may require the administration of 6,000 ml fluid daily, of which 1,500 ml should be normal saline solution. The specific electrolytes and the amounts in which they are added are governed by the laboratory values for these electrolytes. Occasionally, the withdrawal syndrome is characterized by hypoglycemia, in which case the administration of glucose becomes of prime importance. Rarely, alcoholic patients present with severe ketoacidosis and normal or only slightly elevated blood glucose concentrations. Usually such patients recover promptly, without the use of insulin.

A special danger attends the use of glucose solutions in alcoholic patients. Usually these persons have subsisted on a diet disproportionately high in carbohydrate (alcohol is metabolized almost entirely as carbohydrate) and low in thiamine, and their reserves of B vitamins may have been further reduced by gastroenteritis and diarrhea. The administration of intravenous glucose may serve to consume the last available stores of thiamine and precipitate Wernicke's disease. For this reason it is good practice to add B vitamins in all cases requiring parenterally administered glucose, even though the alcoholic disorder under treatment, i.e., delirium tremens, is not primarily due to vitamin deficiency.

In respect to the use of drugs, it is important to distinguish between mild withdrawal symptoms, which are essentially benign and responsive to practically all sedative drugs, and delirium tremens, which has a serious mortality and is relatively unresponsive to drugs. In the case of minor withdrawal symptoms, the purpose of medication is to ensure rest and sleep. In delirium tremens, the object of drug therapy is to blunt agitation, prevent exhaustion, and facilitate the administration of parenteral fluid and nursing care; one does not attempt to suppress agitation at all costs, since to accomplish this requires an amount of drug that might seriously depress respiratory function.

A wide variety of drugs is effective in controlling withdrawal symptoms. Some of the more popular are prochlorperazine (Compazine), chlorpromazine (Thorazine), meprobamate, chlordiazepoxide (Librium), hydroxyzine (Vistaril), and diazepam (Valium). There is little difference in the therapeutic efficacy of these drugs, and it is not certain that any of them can prevent hallucinosis or delirium tremens; however some studies suggest that intravenous diazepam may shorten the duration and decrease the mortality rate of the latter disorder. In general, phenothiazine drugs should be avoided because of their epileptigenic properties. Furthermore, the advantages of the oral administration of these drugs over paraldehyde have not been proved by controlled studies; in fact, there is some evidence that in the more severe forms of the withdrawal syndrome paraldehyde is superior to both chlorpromazine and promazine. Paraldehyde has the additional advantage of being extremely safe provided it is freshly prepared and kept in brown, tightly stoppered bottles to prevent deterioration and the accumulation of acetaldehyde. If the patient can take medication orally, doses of 8 to 12 ml in orange juice should be given. It may also be administered rectally, but the intramuscular route should be avoided if possible, since it may damage nerves, and it should be given intravenously only with great caution because of the danger of respiratory depression. If parenteral medication is necessary, sodium phenobarbital or sodium amytal in doses of 120 mg, repeated at 3- to 4-h intervals, may be given, provided there is no serious liver disease. Some physicians prefer to use intravenous diazepam, giving 10 mg initially and repeating this dose at 20- to 30-min intervals until the patient is calm but awake. Such treatment is effective but requires careful monitoring to avoid hypotension and hypoventilation.

Treatment of "rum fits" In most cases the type of convulsive seizure that occurs in the withdrawal period ("rum fits") does not require the use of anticonvulsant drugs. In this setting there may be only a single seizure or a brief flurry of seizures which usually have ceased by the time that certain medicines, such as diphenylhydantoin (Dilantin), become effective. The parenteral administration of sodium phenobarbital early in the withdrawal period could conceivably prevent "rum fits" in patients with a previous history of this disorder or in those who might be expected to develop seizures on withdrawal. Also, the long-term administration of anticonvulsants is not practical; if the patient remains abstinent, he will be free of seizures, and if he resumes drinking he usually abandons his medicines. In rare instances, withdrawal seizures take the form of status epilepticus; such cases should be managed like status of any other type (see Chap. 24). Alcoholics with a history of idiopathic or posttraumatic epilepsy should drink only in moderation or not at all, because of the deleterious effects of relatively short periods of drinking on their epilepsy, and they should be maintained on anticonvulsant drugs.

NUTRITIONAL DISEASES OF THE NERVOUS SYSTEM

These diseases compose a relatively small but serious group of illnesses in chronic alcoholics. In contrast to the role of alcohol in intoxication and abstinence syndromes, its role in these nutritional diseases is purely secondary, serving mainly to displace food in the diet. These illnesses, the role of alcohol in their production, and their treatment, are discussed in Chap. 340, Metabolic and Nutritional Diseases of the Nervous System, and Chap. 331, Diseases of the Peripheral Nervous System.

ALCOHOLIC DISEASES OF UNCERTAIN PATHOGENESIS Included in this category are several diverse disorders which are practically always encountered in alcoholic patients. Their relationship to the excessive use of alcohol is not fully understood and probably is not crucial, since all of them have been described in nonalcoholic patients. There is a considerable amount of indirect evidence that these disorders are nutritional in origin, but as yet this relationship must be regarded as unproved.

Alcoholic cerebellar degeneration This term is applied to a nonfamilial type of cerebellar ataxia which occurs in adult life against a background of prolonged ingestion of alcohol. The symptoms may progress slowly over a long period, but more frequently they evolve in a subacute fashion (several weeks or months), after which they remain stationary for many years. Often they are present in mild form and worsen considerably after an attack of pneumonia or delirium tremens. The signs are those of cerebellar dysfunction, affecting stance and gait predominantly. The legs are involved more frequently and severely than the arms, and nystagmus and speech disturbances are rare. Once established, the signs change very little, although some improvement of gait (due mainly to recovery from complicating polyneuropathy) may follow cessation of drinking. The essential pathologic changes consist of degeneration of varying severity of all the neurocellular elements of the cerebellar cortex, particularly of the Purkinje cells, with a striking topographic restriction to the anterior and superior aspects of the vermis and hemispheres. The disorder of stance and gait seems to be related to the lesion in the vermis, and the ataxia of the limbs to the anterior lobe of the cerebellum. A similar clinical syndrome has been observed in a few nutritionally depleted nonalcoholic patients.

It is likely that the cerebellar lesions in this disorder and in Wernicke's disease represent the same disease process. The latter designation is used when the cerebellar abnormalities are associated with the characteristic ocular and mental disorders, and the term "alcoholic" cerebellar degeneration when only the cerebellar signs are clinically manifest.

Marchiafava-Bignami disease (primary degeneration of the corpus callosum) This is a rare complication of alcoholism originally described in Italian men addicted to crude red wine. The symptoms are diverse and include psychic and emotional disorders, delirium and intellectual deterioration, convulsive seizures, and varying degrees of tremor, rigidity, paralysis, apraxia, aphasia, and sucking and grasping reflexes. The duration is variable, from several weeks to months, and recovery is possible. The pathologic picture is more constant than the clinical one. It consists of symmetrically placed areas of demyelination in the corpus callosum, particularly the middle lamina, and less consistently of the anterior commissure and other parts of the white matter. Axis cylinders are better preserved than medullated fibers in these areas, and there are appropriate reactions in the macrophages and astrocytes. Various degrees of recovery may occur if abstinence from alcohol and good nutrition are established and maintained.

Pontine myelinolysis This term refers to a unique pathologic change affecting the center of the basis pontis, in which the medullated fibers are destroyed in a single symmetric focus of varying size. In contrast, the axis cylinders, nerve cells, and blood vessels are relatively well preserved. The disease may manifest itself by pseudobulbar palsy and quadriplegia, but usually the lesion is so small that it causes no symptoms and is found only at postmortem examination. The relationship of this condition to either alcoholism or malnutrition is obscure, but most of the cases have occurred in patients with prolonged and severe nutritional depletion.

Cerebral atrophy The pathologic examination of relatively young alcoholic patients not infrequently discloses an unexpected degree of convolutional atrophy, most prominent in the frontal lobes, and a symmetric enlargement of the lateral and third ventricles. The ventricular enlargement may also be found on pneumoencephalography. In some patients these findings are associated with overt complications of alcoholism, such as the Wernicke-Korsakoff syndrome, but in many of them no other abnormalities can be found, and the history discloses no symptoms of neurologic disease. The nature of this disorder is quite unclear.

"Alcoholic" myopathy Attention has been drawn to several disorders of skeletal and cardiac muscle, apparently primary in nature, in association with chronic alcoholism. One type of myopathic syndrome, which may be generalized or focal, is characterized by the acute onset of severe pain, tenderness, and edema of muscles, accompanied by myoglobinuria, renal damage, and hyperpotassemia in severe cases. In other cases, diffuse muscle weakness is associated with hypopotassemia and vascular necrosis of muscle. It will be recognized, of course, that these acute forms of muscle weakness are not confined to alcoholics. Yet another type is characterized by the subacute development of weakness and atrophy of the proximal limb and girdle muscles, with "myopathic" changes in the electromyogram and elevated creatine phosphokinase levels in serum, but without local pain or edema. Muscle power is slowly restored in these patients following abstinence from alcohol and improvement in nutrition. That this disorder represents a primary affection of muscle has not been established beyond doubt. Muscle biopsies that we have examined from such patients suggest that it may represent a proximal form of polyneuropathy, despite relatively mild clinical signs of peripheral nerve disease. "Alcoholic cardiomyopathy" is the name given to a nonspecific affection of cardiac muscle which has a higher incidence in patients with chronic alcoholism than in the nonalcoholic population. The role of alcohol, malnutrition, or some hitherto unsuspected factor in the genesis of these disorders is not known, and their structural and biochemical basis requires further study (see Chap. 345).

NEUROLOGIC DISORDERS CONSEQUENT UPON CIRRHOSIS AND PORTAL-SYSTEM SHUNTS *Hepatic coma* refers to an episodic disorder of consciousness which frequently complicates (or terminates) advanced liver disease and/or portal-system shunts. It is associated with typical electroencephalographic abnormalities and intermittency of sustained muscular contraction which presents as an irregular flapping movement of the outstretched limbs (asterixis). Patients dying in hepatic coma consistently show an increase in the number and size of the protoplasmic astrocytes throughout the central nervous system, particularly in the deep layers of the cerebral and cerebellar cortex, the basal ganglia, and the dentate nuclei.

Less frequently, cirrhosis is complicated by a chronic and largely irreversible form of hepatocerebral disease, the main symptoms of which are dementia, dysarthria, ataxia, and athetosis. The brain in such cases shows not only an astrocytic hyperplasia but also a degeneration of nerve cells and fibers, the distribution of the destructive lesions following closely that of the astrocytic changes. Both hepatic coma and the chronic form of hepatocerebral disease are characterized by hyperammonemia, which is probably important in their pathogenesis. Ammonium is derived from the bacterial action on intestinal proteins and normally is converted to urea in the liver. A failure to metabolize ammonium, or perhaps some other substance absorbed from the bowel, may be the result of either hepatocellular disease or of shunting of blood around the liver. Presumably, the acute and rapidly developing effect of this toxin on the brain is episodic stupor or coma, which is reflected pathologically by a diffuse astrocytic hyperplasia; a prolongation of this effect may lead to irreversible neurologic symptoms and parenchymal lesions.

The treatment of recurrent hepatic stupor and coma is discussed in Chap. 301. Therapy consists essentially of the use of low-protein diets, cleansing of the lower colon, sterilization of the colon by administration of a drug such as neomycin, and acidification of its content with lactulose. Intractable cases of coma and protein intolerance, as well as the chronic form of hepatocerebral disease which cannot be controlled by these medical means, have also been treated by colectomy or by exclusion of the colon, but these operations have been largely abandoned because of their high mortality. The neurologic complications of liver disease are considered further in Chaps. 296, 301, and 340.

TREATMENT OF ALCOHOL ADDICTION Following recovery from the acute medical and neurologic complications of alcoholism, the underlying problem—that of alcohol dependence—remains. To treat only the medical complications and to leave the management of the drinking problem to the patient himself is indeed shortsighted. Almost always drinking is resumed, with a predictable recurrence of medical illness. For this reason the physician must be prepared to deal with the addiction or at least to initiate treatment.

The problem of excessive drinking is formidable but not necessarily as hopeless as it is made out to be. A common misconception among physicians is that specialized training in psychiatry and an inordinately large amount of time are required to deal with the addictive drinker. Actually, a successful program of treatment can be initiated by any interested physician, using the standard techniques of history taking, establishing rapport with the patient, and seeing him frequently, though not necessarily for prolonged periods. A useful point at which to undertake this task is during convalescence from a serious medical or neurologic complication of alcoholism or in relation to loss of employment, arrest, or threatened divorce. Such a crisis may help convince the patient, better than any argument presented by family or physician, that his drinking has reached serious proportions.

The requisite for successful treatment is total abstinence from alcohol, and for all practical purposes, this represents the only permanent solution. It is generally agreed that any attempt to curb the drinking habit will fail if the patient continues to drink. There are said to be cases in which the patient has been able to reduce his intake of alcohol and eventually to drink in moderation, but they must be extremely rare. Also, it is frequently stated that the patient must recognize that he is an alcoholic, i.e., that his drinking is beyond his control, and he must express willingness to be helped. Undoubtedly there is truth in both these statements, but they should not be interpreted to mean that the patient must gain this recognition and willingness entirely on his own initiative and that he will be helped only after he does so. The physician can do a great deal to help the patient understand the nature of his problem and thus to motivate him to accept treatment. Logic and reasoning must be used to convince the patient that abstinence is preferable to chronic inebriety. The patient must be made fully aware of the medical and social consequences of continued drinking and must also be made to understand that because of some constitutional peculiarity (like that of the diabetic, who cannot handle sugar) he is incapable of drinking in moderation. These facts should be presented in much the same way as one would explain the essential features of any other disease. There is nothing to be gained from adopting a punitive or moralizing attitude; nor should the patient be given the idea that he is in no way blameworthy for his illness. There appears to be an advantage in making the patient feel that he is responsible for doing something about his drinking.

The prevalent belief that an alcoholic will not stop drinking under duress also requires qualification. In fact, one of the few careful studies of this matter disclosed that relatively few patients would have sought help unless pressure had been exerted by family or employer; furthermore, patients who came to the clinic under duress of this sort did just as well as those who came voluntarily.

If an earnest and sustained effort by the physician fails to convince the patient that alcohol offers a problem, it is usually impossible to modify his alcoholic tendency. The only way to make such an individual discontinue drinking is to commit him to a psychiatric hospital or special institution for the management of alcoholism in the hope that with forced abstinence and improvement in his physical state he will gain insight and later accept psychiatric or other forms of therapy.

On the other hand, if the patient comes to realize that his drinking is beyond control and that he needs to do something about it, his chances of being helped are raised considerably. Indeed, under these circumstances, many persons stop drinking of their own volition. Some of these patients, despite the best of intentions, will relapse. This should not serve as an excuse to abandon treatment; many patients have attained a state of prolonged sobriety after several false starts. A number of methods have proved valuable in the long-term management of patients. The most important of these are the use of Antabuse, aversion treatment, psychotherapy, and the participation in social organizations for combating alcoholism.

Antabuse (tetraethylthiuram disulfide, disulfiram) interferes with the metabolism of alcohol, so that a patient who takes both alcohol and Antabuse accumulates an inordinate amount of acetaldehyde in the tissues, resulting in nausea, vomiting, and hypotension, sometimes pronounced in degree. It is no longer considered necessary to demonstrate these effects to the patient; it is sufficient to warn him of the severe reactions that may result if he drinks while he has the drug in his body. Treatment with Antabuse is instituted only after the patient has been sober for several days, preferably longer. It should never be given to patients with cardiac or liver disease. The drug is taken each morning, or at another suitable time daily, in a dosage of 0.5 g, preferably under supervision. This form of treatment is of particular value in the spree or periodical drinker, in whom relapse from abstinence usually represents an impulsive rather than a carefully planned or premeditated act. The patient taking Antabuse, aware of the dangers of mixing liquor and the drug, is "protected" against the impulse to drink, and this protection may be renewed every 24 h by the simple expedient of taking a pill. The willingness with which the patient accepts this form of treatment also serves as a rough index of his motivation. Should the patient drink when he is taking Antabuse, the ensuing reaction is usually severe enough to require medical attention, and a protracted spree can thus be prevented. Antabuse may in rare instances lead to a mild polyneuropathy if continued over a period of months or years. It must then be discontinued.

The aversion treatment consists of the simultaneous administration of a drink of alcohol and an injection of emetin. The violent nausea and vomiting which ensue are intended to create in the patient a strong revulsion for alcohol. This form of treatment, as well as other types of conditioned reflex treatment, has been successfully employed in special clinics but has not gained widespread popularity.

Alcoholics Anonymous (AA), an informal fellowship of former alcoholics, has proved to be the single most effective force in the rehabilitation of alcoholic patients. The philosophy of this organization is embodied in their so-called "twelve steps," a series of propositions about alcohol and alcoholism which guide the patient to recovery. The AA philosophy stresses in particular the practice of making restitution, the necessity to help other alcoholics, trust in God, the group confessional, and the belief that the alcoholic is powerless over alcohol. AA philosophy also embodies the 24-h plan, in which the alcoholic strives for just 24 h of abstinence (a concept inspired by the Sermon on the Mount) as a means of facilitating the maintenance of sobriety. Although accurate statistics are lacking, it is stated that about half the members who express more than a passing interest in the program have no relapses, and that a significant additional number relapse but eventually recover.

The methods used by AA are not suited to every patient; some prefer the more personalized approach offered by special clinics and centers for the treatment of alcoholism. The physician should, therefore, be fully aware of all the community resources which are available for the management of this problem, and should be prepared to take advantage of them in appropriate cases.

Finally, it should be noted that alcoholism is frequently associated with psychiatric disease of some other type. There is among alcoholics an increased frequency of schizophrenia, psychoneurosis, sociopathy, and particularly manic-depressive disease. In the latter case, the prevailing mood is far more often one of depression than of mania, and is more often encountered in the female who is more apt to drink under these conditions than the male. The presence of concomitant psychiatric disease complicates the management of the alcoholism, and in these circumstances expert psychiatric help should be sought.

REFERENCES

Alcohol and Health. U.S. Department of Health, Education, and Welfare Publication (HSM) 72-9099, 1971

RUBIN E, LIEVER CS: Alcoholism, alcohol and drugs. Science 172: 1097, 1972

THOMPSON WL et al: Diazepam and paraldehyde treatment of severe delirium tremens. A controlled trial. Ann Intern Med 82: 175, 1975

VICTOR M: The pathophysiology of alcoholic epilepsy, in "The Addictive States." Res Publ Assoc Res Nerv Ment Dis 46:431, 1968

——: Treatment of alcoholic intoxication and the withdrawal syndrome. A critical analysis of the use of drugs and other forms of therapy. Psychosom Med 28 (4, pt. 2):636, 1966

——, HOPE J: The phenomenon of auditory hallucinations in chronic alcoholism. J Nerv Ment Dis 126 (5,6):451, 1958

—— et al: A restricted form of cerebellar cortical degeneration occurring in alcoholic patients. AMA Arch Neurol 1:577, 1959

WOLFE SM, VICTOR M: The relationship of hypomagnesemia and alkalosis to alcohol withdrawal symptoms. Ann NY Acad Sci 162:973, 1969

—— et al: Respiratory alkalosis and alcohol withdrawal. Trans Assoc Am Physicians 81:344, 1969

119
OPIATES AND OTHER SYNTHETIC ANALGESIC DRUGS

MAURICE VICTOR
RAYMOND D. ADAMS

The drugs included in this category are morphine, opium, heroin (diacetylmorphine), dihydromorphinone (Dilaudid), codeine (methylmorphine), Pantopon, dihydrocodeinone (Hycodan), dihydroxycodeinone (Eucodal), and 14-hydroxydihydromorphinone (Numorphan). The synthetic analgesics meperidine (Demerol), the meperidine derivatives, anileridine and alphaprodine (Nisentil), methadone (Dolophine or amidone), metopon (6-methyldihydromorphinone), racemorphan (Dromoran), levorphan, (*l*-Dromoran), *d*-propoxyphene (Darvon), diphenoxylate (the main component of Lomotil), and phenazocine (Prinadol) possess properties similar to those of the opiates, both in their pharmacologic effects and in the patterns of abuse, the differences being mainly quantitative. In fact, *d*-propoxyphene has such low addictive liabilities that it is not controlled by the federal narcotic laws. The same statement applies to the synthetic analgesic pentazocine (Talwin), and although its overall addictive quality is low, cases of physical dependency have been reported.

As with alcohol and the barbiturates, the opiates will be considered from two points of view: (1) acute poisoning, and (2) addiction.

OPIATE POISONING Because of the high incidence of addiction, which leads to irregular and nonmedical usage of opiates, poisoning is not an infrequent accident. This may happen as a result of ingestion with suicidal intent, errors in the calculation of dosage, variations in drug potency, or unusual sensitivity. Children may exhibit an increased susceptibility to opiates, so that relatively small doses prove toxic. This is true also in adults who have myxedema, Addison's disease, chronic liver disease, or pneumonia. Acute poisoning may also occur in addicts who are unaware that tolerance for opiates declines quickly after the withdrawal of the drug: upon resuming the habit a formerly well-tolerated dose can be fatal.

Varying degrees of unresponsiveness, shallow respirations, slow respiratory rate (e.g., two to four per minute), or periodic breathing, miosis, bradycardia, and hypothermia are the well-recognized clinical manifestations of acute poisoning. In the most advanced stage the pupils dilate, the skin and mucous membranes become cyanotic, and the circulation fails. The immediate cause of death is usually respiratory depression, with consequent asphyxia. Patients who have a cardiorespiratory arrest are sometimes left with a residuum of anoxic encephalopathy. Others who recover from coma may occasionally reveal a hemiplegia, presumably due to vascular occlusion. In the stage of mild intoxication, anorexia, nausea, vomiting, constipation, and loss of sexual interest are the only symptoms.

Treatment consists of gastric lavage (after oral ingestion) with a cuffed endotracheal tube in place should the patient be comatose. This procedure may be efficacious many hours after ingestion, since one of the toxic effects of opiates is severe pylorospasm, which may cause much of the drug to be retained in the stomach. Other measures must be directed toward the maintenance of an adequate airway and oxygenation, as described in the following chapter. If the patient does not respond rapidly to these measures, naloxone (Narcan) should be administered. This is a specific antidote to the opiates and also to the synthetic analgesics. It is now preferred to *N*-allylnormorphine (Nalline) because naloxone has no agonistic properties; hence, naloxone will not depress respiration further if the diagnosis of opiate poisoning is mistaken. For opiate poisoning, the dose of naloxone is 0.7 mg per 70 kg *intravenously*, repeated once or twice if necessary at 5-min intervals for an adequate respiratory response. The improvement in circulation and respiration is usually dramatic. In fact, failure of naloxone to produce such a response should cast doubt on the diagnosis of opiate intoxication. If an adequate respiratory response to naloxone is obtained, the patient should be observed carefully for 24 h, and further doses of naloxone (50 percent higher than previously found effective) may be given *intramuscularly* as often as necessary. Naloxone has little direct effect on consciousness, however, and the patient may remain drowsy for many hours. This is not harmful, provided respiration is well maintained.

Once the patient regains consciousness, usually in about 8 h, other complaints such as severe pruritus, sneezing, persistent obstipation, and urinary retention may necessitate symptomatic treatment. Nausea and severe abdominal pain, due presumably to pancreatitis (from spasm of the sphincter of Oddi), are other troublesome symptoms. The antidote must be used with great caution in an addict who has taken an overdose of opiate, because in this circumstance it may precipitate withdrawal phenomena.

In addition to the toxic effects of opiate itself, the addict is exposed to a variety of neurologic and infectious complications, resulting mainly from the injection of crude adulterants (mainly quinine, lactose, powdered milk, fruit sugars) and various infectious agents (injections often administered by unsterile methods). Amblyopia, due probably to the toxic effects of quinine in the heroin mixtures, has been reported, as well as transverse myelopathy and several types of peripheral neuropathy. The spinal cord disorder expresses itself clinically by the abrupt onset of paraplegia with a sensory level on the trunk. Pathologically, there is an acute necrotizing lesion involving both grey and white matter over a considerable vertical extent of the thoracic and occasionally the cervical region. In some cases the myelopathy has followed the first intravenous injection of heroin after a prolonged period of abstinence. Involvement of single peripheral nerves, particularly of the radial nerve, and painful affection of the brachial plexus, independent of compression and remote from the site of injection, have been observed.

An acute generalized myopathy with myoglobinuria and renal failure has been ascribed to the intravenous injection of adulterated heroin. Brawny edema and fibrosing myopathy are the sequelae common to venous obliteration resulting from the administration of heroin, and its adulterants by the intramuscular and subcutaneous routes. Occasionally there may be an inexplicable swelling of an extremity (sometimes massive) into which heroin had been injected subcutaneously or intramuscularly. Infection and venous thrombosis appear to be involved in its causation.

The diagnosis of drug addiction or the suspicion of this diagnosis should always encourage surveillance for infectious complications, particularly abscesses and cellulitis at injection sites, septic thrombophlebitis, hepatitis, and periarteritis. Tetanus, endocarditis (due mainly to *Staphylococcus aureus*), spinal epidural abscess, meningitis and brain abscess, and tuberculosis are found less frequently.

OPIATE ADDICTION Just over a decade ago there were about 60,000 persons addicted to narcotic drugs in the United States, not including those who were receiving drugs because of hopeless medical diseases. This represented a relatively small public health problem, in comparison with the large numbers of patients that abused barbiturates and alcohol; and the addiction problem was of serious proportions in only a few cities—New York, Chicago, Los Angeles, Washington, and Detroit. In the past ten to fifteen years a remarkable increase in opiate (principally heroin) addiction has taken place. The number of addicts in the United States has risen tenfold, and in New York City alone it is estimated that there are more than 300,000 (although these figures are subjects of controversy).

Etiology and pathogenesis A number of factors, socioeconomic, psychologic, and pharmacologic, all contribute to the genesis of opiate addiction. In our culture, the most susceptible subjects are young men or delinquent youths living in the economically depressed areas of large cities, but a significant number are now found in the suburbs and in small cities. The onset of opiate use is usually in adolescence, with a peak at seventeen to eighteen years. Fully two-thirds of addicts start using the drug before the age of twenty-one. A disproportionately large number are American Negroes and persons of Puerto Rican or Mexican descent. Almost 90 percent of addicts engage in criminal activity, often necessary to obtain their daily ration of drug, but most of these have had arrests or convictions prior to addiction. Also, many of them show psychiatric disorders, psychoneurosis and psychopathy being the most common. However, the precise "personality" factor which renders them vulnerable to addiction has not been defined. Association with addicts is the chief reason for beginning addiction. A small, almost insignificant, proportion of addicts are introduced to drugs by physicians in the course of an illness.

The abuse of opiate drugs evolves in three successive phases: (1) episodic intoxication, or euphoria, (2) pharmacogenic dependence, or addiction, and (3) the propensity to "relapse after cure."

Some of the symptoms of opiate intoxication have already been considered. Of equal importance are the symptoms designated as *"morphine euphoria,"* a term which refers to the pain- and anxiety-reducing abilities of this drug, as well as to the state of elation or sense of unusual well-being which it produces and which is much sought after by psychopathic thrill-seekers. Individuals who take opiates for their euphoria-producing effects quickly discover the need to increase the dose in order to obtain an effect which approaches that of the original dose. Although the intensity of the initial euphoria is not fully recaptured, the progressively increasing dose of drug does abate the discomforts which arise as the effects of each injection wear off. In this way the use of opiates becomes self-perpetuating. At the same time a marked degree of tolerance is produced, so that enormous amounts of drugs, e.g., 5,000 mg of morphine daily, have been administered without the development of toxic symptoms. The mechanism of tolerance is still not understood fully, although it is a subject of much interest and speculation. The various theories related to physical dependence have been discussed fully by Wikler (see references).

The altered physiologic state that develops with continued use of the drug is manifested in another dramatic way at the time of withdrawal. This constitutes a specific illness, termed the *abstinence syndrome.* Strictly speaking, addiction is defined as physical or pharmacologic dependence. This definition distinguishes between *addicting drugs* (opiates, alcohol, barbiturates) and *habit-forming drugs* (bromides, cocaine, and marihuana), since no consistent abstinence symptoms follow the discontinuation of the latter group, even after prolonged exposure. Stated in another way, all addicting drugs are habit-forming, but the opposite is not true. The place of amphetamines in this scheme is uncertain. Undoubtedly they are habit-forming drugs. Withdrawal of *d*-amphetamine, following prolonged oral or intravenous use, is regularly followed by prolonged sleep [of which a high percentage is rapid eye movement (REM) sleep], from which the patient awakens with a ravenous appetite. The deep sleep can be reversed by administration of *d*-amphetamine.

The intensity of the opiate abstinence syndrome depends mainly on the dose of the drug and duration of addiction, but also on individual factors. In respect to morphine it has been found that the majority of individuals receiving 240 mg daily for 30 days or more will show moderately severe abstinence symptoms following withdrawal, whereas mild grades of opiate abstinence signs can be precipitated by the opiate antagonist, nalorphine, as early as after 2 days of administration of 15 mg morphine four times daily, or of equivalent doses of methadone or heroin.

The abstinence syndrome which occurs in the morphine addict may be taken as the prototype of the opiate group. The first 8 to 16 h of abstinence usually pass asymptomatically. At the end of this period yawning, rhinorrhea, sweating, and lacrimation become manifest. At first mild, these symptoms increase in severity over a period of several hours and then remain constant for several days. The patient may be able to sleep during the early period but is restless, and thereafter insomnia remains a prominent feature. Dilatation of the pupils, recurring waves of gooseflesh, and twitchings of the muscles appear. The patient complains of severe aches in the back, abdomen, and legs and of hot and cold "flashes" so that he covers himself with blankets. By the end of about 36 h the restlessness becomes more extreme, and nausea, vomiting, and diarrhea usually develop. The temperature, respiration, and blood pressure are slightly elevated. All these symptoms reach their peak intensity 48 to 72 h after withdrawal, and then gradually decline. The abstinence syndrome is rarely fatal. After 7 to 10 days, all clinical signs of abstinence have disappeared, although the patient may complain of insomnia, nervousness, weakness, and muscle aches for several more weeks, and a small deviation of a number of physiologic variables can be detected with refined techniques for up to 10 months (protracted abstinence).

There are two types of abstinence changes—*nonpurposive* and *purposive.* The former comprise the various autonomic and neuromuscular signs and are relatively transient in nature. That these symptoms represent an altered physiologic state and are not psychic in origin has been clearly demonstrated experimentally. Physical dependence on morphine and other opiate drugs develops even in the lower limbs of dogs whose spinal cords have been transected; the flexor and crossed extensor spinal reflexes that are depressed or abolished by the opiate become remarkably exaggerated when the drug is withdrawn. The purposive changes refer to the patient's craving for the drug and the manipulative activity directed toward obtaining it. These symptoms may persist indefinitely and are important in relation to that characteristic of addiction referred to as *habituation, emotional dependence,* or *psychologic dependence.* These terms are used interchangeably and refer to the substitution of drug-seeking activities for all other aims and objects in life.

Habituation is regarded as the most important quality of

addiction, since it is this feature which governs the initial use of the drug and relapse following apparent cure of addiction. An individual takes a drug initially not because he needs the drug to prevent withdrawal symptoms but because of its euphoria-producing effect, i.e., the relief of pain and emotional discomfort. Similarly, relapse to the use of the drug may occur long after the nonpurposive abstinence changes seem to have disappeared. The cause of relapse is imperfectly understood. It has been theorized that fragments of the abstinence syndrome may remain as a conditioned response, and that these abstinence signs may be evoked by the appropriate environmental stimuli. Thus, when a "cured" addict finds himself in a situation where narcotic drugs are readily available, or in circumstances that were responsible for the initial use of drugs, the incompletely extinguished drug-seeking behavior reasserts itself.

The characteristics of addiction and of abstinence are qualitatively similar with all the drugs of the opiate group as well as the related synthetic analgesics. The differences are mainly quantitative and are related to the differences in dosage, potency, and length of action. Heroin is two to three times more potent than morphine but otherwise the same; nevertheless, the heroin withdrawal syndrome encountered in hospital practice is usually mild in degree because of the low dosage of this drug in the street product. Dilaudid and metopon are more potent than morphine and have a shorter duration of action; hence the addict requires more doses per day, and the abstinence syndrome comes on and subsides more rapidly. The length of action of Dromoran is somewhat longer than that of morphine, but withdrawal phenomena are similar to those of morphine in temporal course and intensity. Abstinence symptoms from codeine, while very definite, are less than those from morphine. The addiction liabilities of Darvon are even less than those of codeine. Abstinence symptoms from methadone are less intense than those from morphine and do not become evident until 3 to 4 days after withdrawal; furthermore, this drug is qualitatively different from morphine insofar as autonomic signs are less severe in the abstinence period. For these reasons methadone is used in the treatment of morphine addiction. Demerol addiction is of particular importance because of the high incidence among doctors and nurses and because there is still a widespread belief that this drug is nonaddicting. Tolerance to the toxic effects of Demerol is not complete, so that the addict may show tremors, twitching of the muscles, confusion, hallucinations, and at times convulsions. Signs of abstinence appear in 3 to 4 h after the last dose and reach maximum intensity in 8 to 12 h, at which time they may be worse than those of morphine abstinence.

Diagnosis of addiction This is usually made by the patient's statement that he is using and needs drugs. Should he decide to conceal this fact, one must rely on collateral evidence such as miosis, needle marks, emaciation, or abscess scars. Demerol addicts are likely to have dilated pupils and twitching muscles. A method for the testing of the urine for opiates is now generally available. The finding of morphine or other opiates (heroin is excreted as morphine) in the urine would confirm the suspicion that the patient has taken or has been given a dose of such drugs within 24 h of the test.

Formerly it was necessary to isolate questionable cases and to observe the patient over a period of at least 2 days for signs of abstinence. Through use of the specific morphine antagonist *N*-allylnormorphine (nalorphine, Nalline) and naloxone (Narcan), a diagnosis of addiction to opiates and related analgesic drugs can be made within an hour. Naloxone, which is now preferred for this purpose, should be administered only in the presence of another physician or nurse, with the full understanding and permission of the patient. The drug is given intravenously, slowly, using a syringe containing 1 ampul (0.4 mg). The injection is stopped when pupillary dilatation, increased respiratory rate, lacrimation, rhinorrhea, sweating, and yawning appear. If, after 5 to 10 min, no such signs appear, a second injection may be given in the same way. If again the patient shows no abstinence signs, it may be assumed that he is not physically dependent upon opiates. Naloxone may be injected *subcutaneously,* in the same dosage as intravenously. Again, if the patient has taken more than occasional doses of the drug within a week of the test, the administration of naloxone will precipitate symptoms of abstinence. These become evident within 5 min of the first injection, reach their peak intensity in 20 min, begin to decline in 60 min, and disappear after 3 h. Nalline and Narcan do not precipitate abstinence symptoms in Demerol addiction, unless the patient has been taking more than 1,600 mg daily.

Management and avoidance of addiction The ambulatory treatment of addiction never succeeds and should therefore not be undertaken, except in special settings, such as a carefully supervised methadone treatment program (see below). Addicts who are refused opiates may ask for methadone, Demerol, or Dromoran, on the ground that these drugs are synthetic and nonaddicting. These drugs are addicting and have been legally defined as opiates. The physician should also be aware that he is breaking both the letter and the spirit of the regulations if he prescribes narcotics for an addict merely for the purpose of preventing abstinence changes. Occasional exceptions may be made in cases of seriously ill addicts who are awaiting treatment in a hospital or methadone program, or of patients who are suffering from incurable, painful disease.

An alternate method, and one that is used now almost exclusively, is to substitute methadone for opiate, in the ratio of 1 mg methadone for 3 mg morphine, 1 mg heroin, or 20 mg meperidine. Since methadone is long-acting and effective orally, it need be given only twice daily by mouth—10 to 20 mg per dose being sufficient to suppress abstinence symptoms. After a stabilization period of 3 to 5 days on this dosage of methadone alone, the drug may be reduced rapidly and withdrawn over a similar period of time. Regardless of the method of drug withdrawal employed, treatment is best carried out in an institution with proper facilities for postwithdrawal rehabilitation in a drug-free environment or where methadone or an antagonist may be administered. Such institutions, private or municipal, are available in most large communities.

The physician must be constantly alert to the dangers of

addiction, particularly in susceptible individuals, i.e., in those with psychoneurosis, psychopathic personality, or alcoholism. The use of opiates should be limited to cases where pain is the chief problem; they should not be used primarily as sedatives, for the relief of asthma, or even in patients with chronic pain until all other measures have been exhausted. It follows that it is most important to make a precise diagnosis of the cause of pain, since in some cases measures other than opiates will suffice, while in others, such as hysteria and depression, narcotics are contraindicated.

If narcotics have to be used for the relief of pain, consideration should be given to the choice of the appropriate drug and to the mode of administration. Morphine is still the drug of choice for most patients requiring relief of severe pain for short periods. Demerol may be useful in patients who cannot tolerate morphine. Patients with chronic pain should be managed with the least potent and smallest dosage of drug that will relieve them; doses should be spaced as far apart as possible and discontinued as soon as the need for pain relief has passed. In general, the opiates should be administered orally whenever possible, and the intravenous route should be avoided, since this method produces maximum euphoria and, hence, the greatest danger of addiction. The oral administration of codeine and aspirin is a useful way to begin treatment of the patient with chronic pain. If these drugs fail to control the pain, the parenteral administration of codeine should be tried. If the more potent opiates are needed, methadone and levorphan should be used, because of their effectiveness by the oral route and the relatively slow development of tolerance. Should long-continued injections of morphine or meperidine become necessary, maximum analgesic effect is obtained with 10 mg morphine rather than with 15 mg, as is often prescribed, and with 60 to 70 mg rather than with 100 mg meperidine. In these cases, use of the narcotic antagonist pentazocine (Talwin) might be considered. It is claimed that this drug, administered parenterally in doses of 40 to 60 mg, has analgesic effects comparable to those of morphine and other opiates, but has less addicting properties. The respiratory depression produced by pentazocine, as by opiates, can be counteracted by naloxone.

Ambulatory treatment of opiate addiction The most significant development in the treatment of opiate (almost exclusively heroin) addiction has been the establishment and growth of ambulatory methadone maintenance clinics. The scope of this activity, like the incidence of addiction, cannot be stated precisely, but can be judged roughly by the fact that about 40,000 addicts were participating in such programs in 1973 in New York City alone.

The method of treatment consists of the oral administration of methadone, twice daily, in doses sufficient to suppress the craving for heroin and to abolish the euphoria-producing effects of that drug given intravenously (heroin blockade). The daily dosage of methadone required to achieve these effects varies between 60 and 100 mg; some patients can be maintained on as little as 40 mg per day, and with higher dosage they need take the drug only once in 48 h. In principle, these effects could be achieved by multiple daily injections of heroin or morphine, but the effectiveness of methadone orally, its prolonged duration of action, and the fact that it precludes the desire and need for taking other opiates make methadone far more practical.

Methadone is no longer dispensed in tablet form but only as a liquid (dissolved in fruit juice), which is taken under supervision. (N.B.: Soon a mixed methadone-naloxone tablet and a long-acting form of methadone to cover weekends will become available.) The collection of urine samples is also supervised, and these are analyzed for opiates and other drugs, to monitor the patient's adherence to the program. Once this has been established, the patient is allowed to take home a 1- to 3-day supply. These measures are designed to prevent the diversion of methadone into illicit channels. Various forms of individual psychotherapy, group psychotherapy, social service counseling, and vocational guidance are included in most programs. The use of former heroin addicts (who are themselves on methadone treatment) as counselors is considered to be a particularly important adjunct to methadone treatment.

The results of methadone treatment are difficult to assess and vary considerably from one program to another. Even the best programs suffer an attrition rate of about 25 percent after several years. Of the patients who remain, between 75 and 85 percent achieve a high degree of social rehabilitation, i.e., they are gainfully employed and no longer engage in criminal behavior or prostitution. This has been the very notable achievement of the methadone maintenance programs.

Although the effectiveness of methadone treatment in the social rehabilitation of many addicts cannot be doubted, a number of questions about this method remain. The usual practice of methadone programs is to accept only adult addicts with a history of heroin addiction for several years. This leaves unanswered the problem of the adolescent addict. Although some individuals have been withdrawn from methadone, this has been accomplished so far in a relatively small number, and their capacity to maintain a drug-free existence remains to be determined. This means that the large majority of addicts now enrolled in methadone programs are committed to an indefinite period of methadone maintenance, and the effects of such a regimen are uncertain.

An alternate method of ambulatory treatment of the opiate addict involves the use of narcotic antagonists. Cyclazocine is the best known of these. After withdrawal of the opiate, cyclazocine is administered orally, in increasing amounts over a period of 2 to 6 weeks, until a dosage of 2 mg per 70 kg is being taken twice daily. The cyclazocine-stabilized individual is highly refractory to the euphoria-producing and pharmacologic effects of opiates. The idea of treatment is to continue the administration of cyclazocine until all drug-seeking behavior is extinguished, after which it is withdrawn. More recently, interest has centered about the opiate antagonist naltuexone which is virtually devoid of agonistic activity and twice as potent as naloxone; it has the added advantages of being effective orally and in much smaller doses than naloxone. The value of this kind of "extinction therapy" has not yet been determined, but the results in some patients have been encouraging, and the search for improved methods of using opiate antagonists continues.

Obviously none of these methods promise lasting success unless combined with reeducation, vocational habilitation, and social adjustment.

REFERENCES

BALL JC, CHAMBERS CK (eds): *The Epidemiology of Opiate Addiction in the United States,* Springfield, Ill.: Charles C Thomas, 1970

DOLE VP, NYSWANDER ME: Methadone maintenance and its implication for theories of narcotic addiction. Res Publ Assoc Res Nerv Ment Dis 46:359, 1968

MARTIN WR: The basis and possible utility of the use of opioid antagonists in the ambulatory treatment of the addict. Res Publ Assoc Res Nerv Ment Dis 46:367, 1968

——: Theories related to physical dependence, in *The Chemical and Biological Aspects of Drug Dependence,* eds SJ Mule, H Brill, Cleveland: Chemical Rubber Press, 1972, p. 359

——et al: Naltrexone, an antagonist for the treatment of heroin dependence. Effects in man. Arch Gen Psychiatry 28:784, 1973

RICHTER RW et al: Neurological complications of heroin addiction. Bull NY Acad Med 49:3, 1972

WIKLER A: Drug dependence, p. 1, in *Clinical Neurology,* eds AB Baker, LH Baker, Hagerstown, Md.: Harper & Row, 1971

120 BARBITURATES

MAURICE VICTOR
RAYMOND D. ADAMS

The high incidence of addiction, suicides, and accidental deaths attributable to the improper use of the barbiturate drugs is a matter of continuing concern to the medical profession. The production of barbiturates greatly exceeds the amount needed for therapeutic purposes; almost 500,000 kg is produced each year in the United States, enough to supply thirty 60-mg barbiturate capsules for every person in the country. It is estimated that barbiturates account for 20 percent of acute poisonings admitted to general hospitals and that they are responsible for 6 percent of suicides and 18 percent of accidental deaths, figures exceeded by no other single poison. Despite an estimated mortality rate of only 8 percent of hospitalized cases, barbiturates reportedly cause about 1,500 deaths annually in the United States. This figure is probably a gross underestimation, since in 1964 there were over 2,200 registered deaths in Great Britain due to barbiturate poisoning and for the period 1957 to 1963, an average of 166 fatalities occurred yearly in New York City alone.

About 50 barbiturates have been marketed for clinical use, but only seven or eight are encountered with any frequency: These are now classified under the federal drug control laws as follows:

Schedule II:	pentobarbital (Nembutal)
	secobarbital (Seconal)
	amobarbital (Amytal)
Schedule III:	aprobarbital (Alurate)
	thiopental (Pentothal)
Schedule IV:	barbital (Veronal)
	phenobarbital (Luminal)

In the United States, pentobarbital, secobarbital, and amobarbital are the most commonly abused barbiturates. All the barbiturates are similar pharmacologically and differ only in their speed of onset and duration of action. The clinical problems posed by the barbiturates are different, however, depending on whether the intoxication is acute or chronic, and these two types will be considered separately.

In addition to the barbiturates, a number of nonbarbiturate sedative and hypnotic drugs have to be considered, since they have been shown to possess very much the same intoxicating and addicting properties as the barbiturates.

ACUTE BARBITURATE INTOXICATION Acute barbiturate intoxication results from the ingestion of large amounts of the drug either accidentally or with suicidal intent. Another form of accidental poisoning occurs in individuals who are intoxicated with barbiturates or with alcohol and who, being confused, ingest more of the drug than was intended. This type of poisoning has been termed *involuntary suicide.*

The ingestion of barbiturates with suicidal intent is most frequently the act of a depressed person. The hysteric or psychopath may take an overdose as a suicidal gesture and sometimes become seriously intoxicated because of a miscalculation or ignorance of the toxic dosage. At times, no psychiatric disease is present, the drug being taken impulsively or while the individual is inebriated. The combination of alcohol and barbiturate intoxication is frequent and particularly dangerous, since these drugs have an additive effect.

Site and mode of action of barbiturates Barbiturates decrease the excitability of nerve cells, although the mechanism is not fully understood. Attempts have been made to localize the action of barbiturates to certain anatomic regions, or even to specific nuclei within the nervous system, but it would appear that all parts are to some extent sensitive to the drug. Nevertheless, the reticular formation of the thalami and midbrain are particularly susceptible. There is little experimental evidence to support the notion that the administration of barbiturates first depresses cerebral cortical activity and then sequentially affects the anatomically lower centers. Reflex and other activity of the nervous system are probably depressed simultaneously, although in some cases the spinal reflexes appear to be accentuated in the early stages of poisoning.

Symptoms and signs The symptoms and signs of acute barbiturate intoxication vary with the type and the amount of drug, as well as with the length of time that has elapsed since it was ingested. Pentobarbital and secobarbital produce their effects quickly, and recovery is relatively rapid. Phenobarbital induces coma more slowly, and its effects tend to be prolonged. The duration of action of these drugs can be judged from the hypnotic effect of an average oral dose. In the case of the long-acting barbiturates, such as phenobarbital, barbital, and diallylbarbituric acid, it lasts 6 h or more; with the intermediate-acting drugs, amobarbital and aprobarbital, 3 to 6 h; with the short-acting drugs, secobarbital and pentobarbital, less than 3 h.

In general, much larger doses of long-acting barbiturates are required to produce a depth of unconsciousness comparable with that produced by the short-acting ones. The ingestion by adults of more than 3.0 g secobarbital, pentobarbital, amobarbital, or diallylbarbituric acid at one time may be fatal unless intensive and skillful treatment is applied promptly; it has been estimated that to produce a comparable effect, the following amounts of long-acting barbiturates would have to be ingested: 6.0 to 9.0 g phenobarbital, 5.0 to 20.0 g barbital, and 15.0 g aprobarbital. Because of the serious complications of prolonged coma, the fatalities are greater with the long-acting than with the short-acting drugs.

Clinically, it is useful to recognize three grades of severity of acute barbiturate intoxication, particularly in regard to prognosis and treatment. Mild intoxication follows the ingestion of approximately 0.6 g pentobarbital or its equivalent. The patient is drowsy or asleep, a state from which he is readily roused by calling his name loudly or by shaking him. The symptoms resemble those of alcohol intoxication, except that the face is not flushed, the conjunctivas are not suffused, and there is no odor of alcohol. The patient thinks slowly, and there may be mild disorientation, lability of mood, impairment of judgment, slurred speech, drunken gait, and nystagmus. Reflex activity and vital signs are not affected.

Moderate intoxication follows the ingestion of five to ten times the oral hypnotic dose. Here the state of consciousness is more severely depressed and is usually accompanied by depressed or absent deep reflexes and slow but not shallow respiration. Corneal reflexes are retained, with occasional exceptions. At times the patient can be roused by vigorous manual stimulation; when awakened, he is confused and dysarthric, and after a few moments he drifts back into coma. At other times the patient cannot be roused by any means. In the latter case the depth of coma and seriousness of the respiratory depression may be roughly judged by the response of respiration to the inhalation of 10% carbon dioxide or to painful stimulation such as the application of firm pressure to the sternum or supraorbital ridge. If these stimuli cause an increase in the depth and rate of respiration, the outlook for recovery is good, and only symptomatic treatment is indicated.

Severe intoxication occurs with the ingestion of fifteen to twenty times the oral hypnotic dose. The patient cannot be roused by any of the means indicated. Respiration is slow and shallow or irregular, and pulmonary edema and cyanosis may be present. The deep tendon reflexes are usually but not invariably absent. Most often, the patients show no response to plantar stimulation, but in those who do the plantar responses are extensor. In the most advanced cases the corneal and gag reflexes may also be abolished. Ordinarily the pupillary light reflex is retained in severe intoxication and is lost only if the patient is asphyxiated. In the early hours of coma, there may be a phase of rigidity of the limbs, hyperactive reflexes, ankle clonus, extensor plantar signs, and decerebrate posturing; persistence of these signs indicates a severe degree of anoxia. The temperature may be subnormal, the pulse thready and rapid, and the blood pressure at shock levels.

Diagnosis The diagnosis of barbiturate intoxication is made from the history and physical findings. If a reasonable suspicion of the diagnosis exists, a careful search for drugs or their containers may be rewarding. One should also examine the mouth and gastric contents for any characteristically colored capsules. Acute barbiturate intoxication which presents as a state of coma must be distinguished from other forms of coma by the method outlined in Chap. 22, Coma and Related Disturbances of Consciousness. Actually there are few conditions other than barbiturate intoxication which cause a flaccid coma with reactive pupils, hypothermia, and hypotension. Glutethimide poisoning may produce an identical clinical picture, excepting that the pupils are always fixed (a parasympathomimetic action). Laryngeal spasm and sudden apnea also characterize glutethimide intoxication. In the differential diagnosis, hysteria presents the main problem.

The use of gas chromatography has provided a reliable means of identifying the type and amount of barbiturate in the blood. The major virtue of this method is in determining the precise cause of coma when this is in question. The blood level also helps to identify the drug as long- or short-acting, thus giving information as to whether the therapeutic problem will be short or prolonged. A blood barbiturate level of 2 mg per 100 ml in a *comatose* patient is usually due to poisoning with secobarbital or pentobarbital; although the immediate mortality is high in such instances, the therapeutic problem will be short. A level of 11.5 to 12.0 mg per 100 ml is usually due to poisoning with barbital or phenobarbital, and the comatose state will be prolonged. Because of the potentiating effects of alcohol, a patient who has ingested both drugs may be comatose with relatively low blood barbiturate levels. For this reason, and also because of differences in individual tolerance, the correlation between blood barbiturate levels and depth of coma is not entirely dependable.

The *electroencephalogram* may also be useful in diagnosis, since characteristic patterns accompany barbiturate intoxication. In mild intoxication, the normal activity is replaced by fast activity, in the range of 20 to 30 Hz, and is most prominent in the frontal regions. In more severe intoxication, the fast waves become less regular and interspersed with 3- to 4-Hz slow activity. In the most advanced cases, there are short periods of suppression of all activity, separated by bursts of slow (delta) waves of variable frequency.

Management The management of acute barbiturate intoxication depends on its severity. In mild or moderate intoxication, recovery is the rule, and no vigorous treatment is required. The mildly intoxicated patient should be watched closely for signs of deepening coma, and analeptics such as coffee or parenteral caffeine sodium benzoate may be used. If the patient is unresponsive, special attention should be given to maintaining respiration and urinary excretion and to the prevention of infection. It is most important to maintain a patent airway, at first by the insertion of an endotracheal tube; suctioning should be used when necessary, and the patient should be turned frequently. Tracheotomy and bronchoscopic suctioning usually become necessary if atelectasis becomes manifest, or if intubation must be maintained for longer than 48 h. If there is any risk of respiratory depression or underventilation, it is advisable to support respiration, so as to provide adequate oxygenation and minimize the risk of atelectasis.

Cases of severe respiratory depression, with cyanosis and pupillary dilatation, represent a serious medical emergency. A clear airway should be secured immediately and some form of assisted respiration begun with an automatic intermittent positive-pressure respirator. If the patient is in shock, the foot of the bed should be elevated, and norepinephrine and whole blood or plasma administered. Catheterization is required to determine the adequacy of urinary output, to obtain samples for laboratory examination, and to prevent distention of the bladder. Since the amount of barbiturate cleared by the kidney is directly proportional to the amount of urine formed, 8 to 10 liters of 5% glucose in saline solution should be given daily. Forced diuresis is also important because toxic amounts of barbiturate have an antidiuretic effect. Coma of any significant duration requires the administration of other electrolytes as well, the amounts being governed by their serum and urinary values. The occurrence of pulmonary and urinary infections calls for the use of appropriate antibiotic treatment.

If ingestion has been recent, gastric lavage may be a useful therapeutic as well as a diagnostic measure. It must be performed within several hours of ingestion of the drug, since barbiturates are absorbed rapidly and completely. Laryngospasm may complicate this procedure but can be avoided by preliminary endotracheal intubation; the stomach must be entirely emptied to prevent aspiration.

Dialysis of the blood by means of the artificial kidney has proved to be an effective form of therapy. This measure should be reserved for cases of profound intoxication due to long-acting barbiturates, in which a trial of symptomatic measures has failed, and in which uremia or anuria develops.

The treatment of severe barbiturate intoxication with analeptic drugs (Metrazol, picrotoxin, Megimide), which enjoyed a brief period of popularity, has been generally abandoned. These drugs are antagonistic to barbiturates only insofar as they are powerful cortical stimulants as well as overall nervous system excitants; they do not affect the rate of metabolism of excretion of barbiturate. Recent reports have stressed the value of alkalinization of the blood, by the use of large amounts of bicarbonate solution, as a means of mobilizing the barbiturate and increasing its rate of excretion. This method of therapy does seem to be useful, particularly where phenobarbital is the responsible agent.

Occasionally, in the case of a barbiturate addict who has taken an overdose of the drug, recovery from coma is followed by the development of abstinence symptoms, which have to be managed by the methods outlined below.

CHRONIC BARBITURATE INTOXICATION Barbiturate addiction The problem of chronic barbiturate intoxication is quite different from that of acute intoxication, because of the phenomena of tolerance and addiction as well as the effects of withdrawal of drugs. In these respects there is a close similarity to the problem of chronic alcoholism.

Chronic barbiturate intoxication, like other addictions, tends to develop on a background of some psychiatric disorder, most commonly depression or psychoneurosis with symptoms of anxiety and insomnia, or so-called "character disorder." The drug is usually prescribed for nervousness and insomnia; as the desired effects are lost, the patient increases the dose gradually until he is taking an amount sufficient to produce symptoms when it is withdrawn. Individuals with character disorders are usually introduced to the drug by associates; since the drug is taken for its intoxicating effect, the dose tends to be increased rapidly. Addiction to alcohol or to opiates may predispose to barbiturate addiction. Alcoholics find that barbiturates effectively relieve their nervousness and tremor; then they may continue to take both alcohol and barbiturates, or the barbiturate may replace the alcohol. Heroin and morphine addicts may turn to barbiturates when they are unable to obtain opiates. As with other addicting drugs, the incidence of barbiturism is particularly high in individuals with ready access to drugs, such as physicians, pharmacists, and nurses.

The symptoms and signs of chronic barbiturate intoxication may be described in relation to (1) the toxic effects of the drug, (2) the development of tolerance, and (3) the effects of sudden withdrawal of the drug after a period of prolonged intoxication.

The toxic manifestations of chronic barbiturism are much the same as those of mild acute barbiturate or alcohol intoxication. The barbiturate addict thinks slowly, shows an increased emotional lability, and becomes untidy in his dress and personal habits. The neurologic signs are quite characteristic and include dysarthria, nystagmus, and cerebellar incoordination. Both the mental and neurologic signs fluctuate greatly, being more severe if the drug is taken in the fasting state and tending to increase during the day as more of the drug is ingested. If the dosage is elevated rapidly, the signs of moderate or severe intoxication become manifest.

A characteristic feature of chronic barbiturate intoxication is the development of tolerance, sometimes striking in degree. The average addict will ingest about 1.5 g daily of a potent barbiturate and will not develop signs of severe intoxication unless this amount is exceeded. Tolerance to barbiturates does not develop as rapidly as to opiates. Daily doses of 2 g have been reached, but this takes many months. Individual variations in the degree of tolerance make it difficult to state precisely the minimal amount of drug which must be ingested before the resulting condition is designated as chronic barbiturate intoxication. Most persons can ingest 0.4 g daily for as long as 3 months without developing major withdrawal signs (seizures or delirium). With a dosage of 0.8 g daily, the efficiency at all tasks is greatly reduced, and after a period of 2 months on this dosage, abrupt withdrawal will result in serious symptoms in the majority of patients. Even after 2 weeks of this dosage, some patients will show mild withdrawal symptoms and paroxysmal electroencephalographic changes with photic stimulation. Individuals taking 0.4 to 0.7 g daily fall into an intermediate category; practically all show some mental dulling, and episodes of forgetfulness and occasionally severe withdrawal symptoms may occur.

Abstinence or withdrawal syndrome Following the withdrawal of barbiturates from chronically intoxicated individuals, a characteristic sequence of symptoms occurs. Immediately following withdrawal the patient seemingly improves over a period of 8 to 12 h as he loses the symptoms of intoxication. After this short period a new group of symptoms appears, consisting of nervousness, tremor, postural hypotension, and weakness. Generalized seizures, with loss of consciousness, may then occur, usually between the second and fourth days of abstinence, occasionally as long as 6 or 7 days after withdrawal. There may be a single seizure, several, or rarely status epilepticus. The convulsive phase may be followed directly by a delusional-hallucinatory state or a full-blown delirium, indistinguishable from delirium tremens, or a varying degree of improvement may follow the seizures, before the delirium becomes manifest. Death has been reported under these circumstances. The abstinence syndrome may occur in varying degrees of completeness; some patients have seizures and recover without developing delirium, and others have a delirium without preceding seizures. The abrupt onset of seizures or an acute psychosis in adult life should always raise the suspicion of addiction to barbiturates or other sedative-hypnotic drugs and withdrawal effects.

The electroencephalogram (EEG) shows a number of changes during chronic barbiturate intoxication and following withdrawal. During chronic intoxication, the predominant pattern is that of fast activity of moderate voltage, interspersed with some 6- to 8-Hz activity chiefly in the frontal and parietal regions. The EEG findings do not correlate closely with the degree of intoxication, but some subjects do develop "EEG tolerance," i.e., a disappearance of the rapid pattern described above, while receiving moderate doses of barbiturate (400 mg daily for 90 days). On withdrawal of barbiturates the fast activity diminishes. Also in the first few days of abstinence, paroxysmal bursts of mixed spike and slow waves or 4-Hz "spike and dome" paroxysmal discharges may not be associated with seizures. Characteristically, in the withdrawal period, there is a greatly heightened sensitivity to photic stimulation, to which the patient responds with myoclonus or a seizure, accompanied by paroxysmal changes in the EEG. Most of these abnormalities disappear after 4 or 5 days, and the EEG pattern is usually completely normal in 2 weeks.

INTOXICATING AND ADDICTING EFFECTS OF OTHER SEDATIVE-HYPNOTIC DRUGS In recent years a large number of nonbarbiturate sedative-hypnotic drugs have been introduced into medical practice. At least eight of them have the same intoxicating and addicting effects as barbiturates. These drugs are meprobamate (Miltown, Equanil), glutethimide (Doriden), ethinamate (Valmid), ethchlorvynol (Placidyl), methyprylon (Noludar), chlordiazepoxide (Librium), diazepam (Valium), methaqualone (Quaalude), and perhaps oxazepam (Serax). Like the barbiturates, the toxic effects of these drugs consist of slurred speech, nystagmus, ataxic gait, drowsiness, confusion, and coma. Furthermore, if the daily dose exceeds a minimal safe range, a state of physical dependence develops, so that abstinence symptoms appear upon withdrawal of the drug. These include hallucinations, seizures, and delirium, symptoms indistinguishable from those of the barbiturate and alcohol withdrawal syndrome. The seriousness of the abstinence syndrome in these cases is emphasized by reports of death following withdrawal of meprobamate, methyprylon, and diazepam. In view of these observations, physicians must exercise caution in prescribing new sedative drugs which are continually being introduced and which are said to possess no addicting or habit-forming properties. Treatment of the symptoms which result from withdrawal of the nonbarbiturate sedative drugs requires barbiturate substitution, followed by its gradual withdrawal at a rate not to exceed 0.1 g daily. It should be noted that diphenylhydantoin (Dilantin) and phenothiazine derivatives are not effective against abstinence convulsions.

TREATMENT OF CHRONIC BARBITURATE INTOXICATION

This should always be carried out in the hospital. If the diagnosis of addiction is made before signs of abstinence have appeared, the first step in treatment should be the determination of the "stabilization dosage." This is the amount of short-acting barbiturate required to produce mild symptoms of intoxication (nystagmus, slight ataxia, and dysarthria). Usually 0.2 g pentobarbital given orally every 6 h is sufficient for this purpose. The patient is examined 1 h after each dose. If the signs of intoxication are severe, the next scheduled dose is reduced or omitted. If, instead, tremulousness and postural tachycardia appear, an additional 0.1 g pentobarbital is given and the next scheduled dose is increased. This method is preferable to a blind reduction of dosage, since patients frequently underestimate the amount of drug taken. In such patients, establishment of the "stabilization dosage" may have diagnostic as well as therapeutic value. A patient who can take 0.8 g or more pentobarbital daily, without developing signs of intoxication, is probably physically dependent on drugs of this type. Then a gradual withdrawal of the drug is undertaken, 0.1 daily, the reduction being stopped for several days if abstinence symptoms appear. Recently withdrawal has been facilitated by a substitution of phenobarbital for the pentobarbital and then the withdrawal from phenobarbital. In this way a severely addicted person can be withdrawn in 14 to 21 days. Patients undergoing withdrawal treatment require careful observation for symptoms of abstinence, and special precautions have to be taken to prevent the smuggling or concealment of drugs.

If the patient presents with severe withdrawal symptoms, such as seizures, he should be given 0.3 to 0.5 g Luminal Sodium intramuscularly and then enough to maintain a state of mild intoxication. Most anticonvulsant medicines have been shown to be ineffective against barbiturate withdrawal convulsions. Withdrawal should then be carried out as indicated above. If the abstinence symptoms are not severe, it is not necessary to reintoxicate the patient, but treatment can proceed along the lines laid down for the delirious and confused patient (Chap. 26).

The same principles of treatment apply to patients who are addicted to nonbarbiturate hypnotic-sedative drugs. Thus, if the drug and its dosage can be determined, it should be withdrawn at the rate of one therapeutic dose per day. Should abstinence symptoms appear, the reduction in dosage is stopped for several days. If the offending drug cannot be identified, a barbiturate such as Seconal can be administered to the point of mild intoxication and then withdrawn, in the manner indicated above.

After recovery has taken place, whether from symptoms of chronic intoxication or withdrawal or from acute intoxication due to attempted suicide, the psychiatric problem requires evaluation and an appropriate plan of therapy. Many of the considerations in the management of alcoholism are equally applicable to the patient addicted to barbiturate or nonbarbiturate hypnotic drugs (Chap. 113, Alcohol).

BARBITURATE PROVOCATION OF OTHER DISEASES At

times the administration of one of the barbiturates may induce an attack of another disease. The most striking example of this is in hereditary porphyria where a severe and sometimes fatal outbreak of abdominal pain, psychosis, and polyneuropathy may follow the ingestion of a few capsules of Seconal (see Chap. 109). With severe liver disease, detoxification of barbiturates may be impaired, as is discussed in Chap. 296.

REFERENCES

CLEMMESEN C, NILSSON E: Therapeutic trends in the treatment of barbiturate poisoning: The Scandinavian method. Clin Pharmacol Ther 2:220, 1961

ESSIG C: Chronic abuse of sedative-hypnotic drugs, in *Drug Abuse* (Proc Int Conf), ed CJD Zarafonetis, Philadelphia: Lea & Febiger, 1972, p. 205

FRASER HF et al: Degree of physical dependence induced by secobarbital or pentobarbital. JAMA 166:127, 1958

ISBELL H et al: Chronic barbiturate intoxication: An experimental study. Arch Neurol Psychiatr 64:1, 1950

PLUM F, SWANSON AC: Barbiturate poisoning treated by physiological methods. JAMA 163:827, 1957

WULFF MH: The barbiturate withdrawal syndrome: A clinical and electroencephalographic study. Electroencephalogr Clin Neurophysiol (suppl) 14:173, 1959

121 SEDATIVE-HYPNOTIC, PSYCHOTHERAPEUTIC, STIMULANT, AND PSYCHOTOGENIC DRUGS

MAURICE VICTOR
RAYMOND D. ADAMS

SEDATIVE-HYPNOTIC DRUGS

This class of drugs, also referred to as *depressants*, may be divided into two main groups. The first includes the barbiturates, the bromides, chloral hydrate, and paraldehyde. In the past decade, a second group of drugs comprising meprobamate and other glycerol derivates, and chlordiazepoxide (Librium), diazepam (Valium), and related benzodiazepine drugs, have become far more important than any other sedatives. Indeed, the benzodiazepines are the most commonly prescribed drugs in the world today. Their advantages over the older sedative-hypnotic drugs are their *relatively* low toxicity and addictive potential and their minimal interactions with other drugs.

BROMIDES At the present, bromides are seldom prescribed by physicians, but are contained in certain "nerve tonics" and proprietary remedies (Nervine, Neurosine), and so cases of bromide intoxication are encountered with some regularity. Acute poisoning with bromide is rare because large doses of the drug are irritating to the gastric mucosa, and vomiting prevents the attainment of significant blood levels. Taken in smaller doses, however, bromide tends to accumulate in the body because of its slow excretion by the kidney, and toxic symptoms may appear in a matter of weeks. These symptoms are caused by the bromide ion itself and are not simply a reflection of a de-

crease in chloride due to the displacement of the chloride by the bromide ion.

The symptoms of chronic bromide intoxication are predominantly in the mental sphere and range from dizziness, drowsiness, irritability, and emotional lability to a quiet confusional state, with impairment of thinking and memory and, in severe cases, to delirium and mania or stupor and coma. Skin manifestations are associated in many cases, taking the form usually of an acne-like eruption and less frequently of proliferative nodular lesions, resembling those of tertiary syphilis. Headache, mild conjunctivitis, gastric distress, anorexia, and constipation may be associated as well. The blood bromide levels and the severity of toxic symptoms do not necessarily correspond. As a general rule, levels of 75 mg per 100 ml (9 meq per liter) or more are considered abnormal and diagnostic of bromism, if the clinical picture suggests it. However, higher levels are sometimes well tolerated, and symptoms of bromism may persist for some days even after the blood levels have been reduced to normal or near-normal levels.

Treatment consists of removing the source of bromide and administering sodium chloride (at least 6 g daily, in divided doses). Ammonium chloride may be substituted if an accumulation of sodium is to be avoided and if there is no danger of an uncompensated acidosis or hepatic failure. Confused or delirious patients require sedation, and anorectic and emaciated patients need careful nursing care and special attention to diet. The administration of a mercurial or thiazide diuretic serves to promote a bromide diuresis. Hemodialysis is an effective means of removing bromide and should be utilized in the most severe cases of intoxication.

CHLORAL HYDRATE This is the oldest and at the same time one of the safest, most effective, and cheapest of the sedative-hypnotic drugs. After oral administration, chloral hydrate is reduced rapidly to trichloroethanol, which is the agent responsible for the depressant effects on the central nervous system. A significant portion of the trichloroethanol is excreted in the urine as the glucuronide, which may give a false positive test for glucose.

In large doses, chloral hydrate is toxic to the heart, kidneys, and liver, but only in the presence of preexisting disease in these organs. Chloral hydrate is a strong gastric irritant, so that it requires dilution and should not be taken on an empty stomach. Tolerance and addiction to chloral hydrate develop only rarely, and for these reasons it is an appropriate medication for the management of insomnia, particularly the type which is associated with depression. Poisoning with chloral hydrate is a rare occurrence and resembles acute barbiturate intoxication, except for the finding of miosis, which is said to characterize the former. In combination with alcohol, the well-known "Mickey Finn" or "knockout drops," its effects are additive, leading to a rapid onset of coma. Death from poisoning is due to respiratory depression and hypotension; patients who survive these events may show signs of liver and kidney disease.

PARALDEHYDE This hypnotic is also effective and safe,

providing that certain precautions are taken in its preparation and administration. On exposure to light, paraldehyde decomposes to acetaldehyde, which is very toxic, and oxidizes to acetic acid. It must be freshly prepared, therefore, and stored in tightly stoppered, amber-colored bottles. Paraldehyde is unique in that a significant proportion is excreted unchanged through the lungs; the remainder is detoxified in the liver, so that it should be used cautiously in patients with liver disease.

Paraldehyde has a wide margin of safety when administered orally (or rectally), and even three or four times the usual dose (8 to 10 ml) causes no more than prolonged sleep or mild stupor. Intramuscular use of the drug should be avoided because of its propensity to produce sterile abscesses and to damage the sciatic nerve if injected too close to it. Intravenous injections should be made with caution and only in a hospital, because of their unpredictable effects on respiration. The main objections to this drug are its bitter taste (this can be obviated by diluting in fruit juice) and its lingering, unpleasant odor.

Paraldehyde is very effective in suppressing the tremulousness, restlessness, and insomnia that characterize the early phase (6 to 60 h) of the alcohol withdrawal period. Patients with these symptoms make repeated demands for paraldehyde, which is not surprising in view of the pharmacologic similarities between this drug and alcohol and the effectiveness of both drugs in suppressing withdrawal symptoms. This should not present a problem in management, however, if the need for the drug is determined before each dose is given and the drug is withdrawn as soon as the agitation and tremor are under control. Should a relapse from abstinence then occur, substitution of paraldehyde for alcohol rarely if ever occurs.

BENZODIAZEPINE GROUP The foregoing drugs have been replaced to a large extent by two drugs, chlordiazepoxide (Librium) and diazepam (Valium). These latter drugs have been used extensively to control anxiety, and they are probably more effective than the barbiturates in this respect. They have also been used to control overactivity and destructive behavior in children and the symptoms of alcohol withdrawal. Diazepam is particularly useful in the treatment of delirious patients who require parenteral medication. The benzodiazepines possess anticonvulsant properties, and the intravenous use of diazepam is an effective means of controlling status epilepticus, as indicated in Chap. 14. In addition, diazepam has been used with moderate success in the treatment of certain extrapyramidal movement disorders and dystonic spasms.

Other widely used benzodiazepine drugs are flurazepam (Dalmane), which is useful in the treatment of insomnia (see Chap. 16), and carbamazepine (Tegretol), which now has a definite place in the treatment of seizures and tic douloureux (Chap. 14). Two newer members of this group, clonazepam and nitrazepam, may also prove to have utility in the management of seizure disorders.

The benzodiazepine drugs, while comparatively safe in the recommended dosages, are far from ideal. They frequently cause unsteadiness of gait and drowsiness and at times hypotension and syncope, particularly in the elderly. In severely disturbed schizophrenic patients, rage, hostility, uncontrollable excitement, confusion, and depersonalization may develop. Nausea, diminished libido, headache, skin rashes, leukopenia, eosinophilia, agranulocytosis, and enhancement of the effects of alcohol have all been reported but are rare. Additional central nervous effects are slurred speech, dysphagia, ataxia, confusion, and faulty memory.

CARBONIC ACID DERIVATIVES These drugs are capable of modest depressant action and are appropriate for relieving mild degrees of nervousness, anxiety, and muscle tension, although they provide no advantage over the barbiturates. Maximal action occurs with relatively small doses of these drugs. Meprobamate (Equanil, Miltown) is the best-known member of this group. With average doses (400 mg, three or four times a day) the patient is able to function quite effectively; large doses cause ataxia, drowsiness, stupor, coma, and vasomotor collapse. Hypersensitivity reactions in the form of fever, pruritis, and erythematous, maculopapular, and occasionally urticarial or bullous eruptions have been reported. Cutaneous petechiae or ecchymoses may also occur, without thrombocytopenia. Diplopia, syncope, menstrual irregularities, angioneurotic edema, peripheral edema, leukopenia, thrombocytopenia, and pancytopenia are other rare complications.

It should be reiterated that addiction to meprobamate does occur and if four or more times the daily recommended dose is administered over a period of weeks to months, withdrawal symptoms (including convulsions) may appear, resembling those which follow withdrawal of barbiturate in a chronically intoxicated patient. Several other nonbarbiturate sedative-hypnotic drugs, described earlier in this section, have the same liability.

ANTIPSYCHOTIC DRUGS

Since the mid-1950s, a large new series of pharmacologic agents, loosely referred to as *tranquilizers,* has come into prominent use, mainly for the control of schizophrenia, psychotic states associated with "organic brain syndromes," and certain instances of manic-depressive disease. The mechanism by which these drugs ameliorate disturbances of thought and affect in these psychotic states is poorly understood, but has been attributed to their ability to inhibit or partially block dopamine receptors in the brain; probably their parkinsonian side effects can also be attributed to this mechanism.

There are a large number of antipsychotic drugs on the market, and no attempt will be made here to describe or even list all of them. Some have had only an evanescent popularity, and others have yet to prove their value. Chemically these compounds form a heterogeneous group, four categories being of particular clinical importance: (1) the phenothiazines, (2) the thioxanthines, (3) the butyrophenones, and (4) the *Rauwolfia* alkaloids. Two new antipsychotic drugs of promise are just now being introduced. These are molindone (Moban), an indole derivative, and loxapine (Loxitane), a dibenzoxazepine derivative. They represent new classes of chemical compounds, and it is predicted that they will be used increasingly in patients not responsive to the other antipsychotic drugs or who suffer intolerable side effects from them.

PHENOTHIAZINES This group comprises some of the

most widely used tranquilizers such as chlorpromazine (Thorazine, Largactil), promazine (Sparine), triflupromazine (Vesprin), prochlorperazine (Compazine), perphenazine (Trilafon), fluphenazine (Permitil, Prolixin), thioridazine (Mellaril), and trifluoperazine (Stelazine). In addition to their psychotherapeutic effects, these drugs have a number of other actions, so that certain members of this group are used as antiemetics (prochlorperazine) and antihistaminics (promethazine).

The phenothiazines have had their widest application in the treatment of the psychoses (schizophrenia and to a lesser extent manic-depressive psychosis). Their use outside psychiatry should be discouraged. Under the influence of these drugs, many patients who would otherwise be hospitalized are able to live at home and even work productively; the hospital care of hyperactive and combative patients has been greatly facilitated.

Side effects of the phenothiazines are frequent and often serious. All of them may cause a cholestatic type of jaundice, agranulocytosis, convulsive seizures, orthostatic hypotension, skin sensitivity reactions, mental depression, and disorders of the extrapyramidal motor system. Jaundice and blood dyscrasias have occurred less often with prochlorperazine, perphenazine, and fluphenazine than with other members of the group, but the extrapyramidal side effects have been relatively more pronounced. Several types of extrapyramidal symptoms have been noted. (1) A parkinsonian syndrome—masked facies, tremor, generalized rigidity, shuffling gait, and slowness of movement; these symptoms appear after several weeks of drug therapy. (2) Muscle spasms and dystonia, taking the form of involuntary movements of facial muscles and protrusion of the tongue (so-called buccolingual or oral masticatory syndrome), dysphagia, torticollis and retrocollis, oculogyric crises, and tonic spasms of a limb (dyskinesias); these complications usually occur early in the administration of the drug, sometimes after the initial dose, and often can be improved dramatically by the intravenous administration of diphenhydramine hydrochloride (Benadryl). (3) An inability to sit still and an inner restlessness, so that the patient paces the floor constantly (akathisia). (4) Lingual-facial-buccal dyskinesia as well as choreoathetotic movements of the trunk and limbs may occur as a late and persistent complication (tardive dyskinesia) of long-term therapy with phenothiazines or haloperidol.

These extrapyramidal reactions must be recognized at once and the medication discontinued, but even then the disorder may persist for weeks or months, and often permanently. Administration of antiparkinsonian drugs of the anticholinergic type (trihexyphenidyl, procyclidine, benztropine) may hasten the recovery from some of the symptoms. Oral, lingual, and laryngeal dyskinesias are affected relatively little by any antiparkinsonian drugs. Sometimes, however, one such medication has a better effect than another. Amantadine (Symmetrel) in doses of 50 to 100 mg t.i.d. has been useful in some cases of postphenothiazine dyskinesia. Chlorprothixene (Taractan), a *thioxanthene* drug with effects similar to the phenothiazines, and thioridazine (Mellaril), although not the best tranquilizing agents, are favored by some because of their lesser tendency to produce symptoms of extrapyramidal motor disorder. The latter drug, however, if given in large doses over a period of time, may cause deposits in the macula of the retina with resulting visual impairment.

BUTYROPHENONES These drugs (haloperidol, trifluperidol) have much the same antipsychotic effects as the phenothiazines, as well as the same side effects. Unlike the phenothiazines, they have little or no adrenergic blocking action. The butyrophenones are effective substitutes for the phenothiazines in patients who are intolerant to the latter drugs, particularly to their autonomic effects.

RESERPINE This is the prototype of the *Rauwolfia* alkaloids. It was in relation to the sedative effects of these drugs that the term *tranquilization* was used for the first time. These drugs, so effective in controlling hypertension, are no longer recommended for the treatment of mental disorders, except perhaps in patients who cannot tolerate phenothiazines. When given in therapeutic doses, the *Rauwolfia* alkaloids often provoke a parkinsonian syndrome or a serious depression of mood, which may prove more troublesome than the disorder for which they were prescribed.

Meprobamate, chlordiazepoxide, and diazepam are often referred to as "minor tranquilizers," the implication being that these drugs share the antipsychotic properties of the phenothiazines. This is not the case. In fact, the minor tranquilizers resemble the barbiturates in their pharmacologic (depressant) effects (including the ability to produce tolerance and physical dependence) and are more appropriately referred to clinically as *antianxiety* drugs (see above).

It hardly need be pointed out that the tranquilizing drugs have been much abused. This would be suspected just from the frequency with which they are being prescribed. It is stated that in the decade 1955 to 1965, 50 million patients in the United States received chlorpromazine alone. These powerful medications have specific indications, noted above, and the physician should be certain of the diagnosis before using them. They are far too frequently and improperly used for nervousness, apprehension, anxiety, mild depression, and the many normal psychologic reactions to trying environmental circumstances. These drugs are not curative, but only suppress or partially alleviate symptoms, and they should not serve as a substitute for, or divert the physician from, the use of other measures for the relief of the abnormal mental state.

ANTIDEPRESSANT DRUGS

Two classes of drugs—the monoamine oxidase (MAO) inhibitors and dibenzazepine derivatives—are particularly useful in the treatment of depression. The adjective *antidepressant,* used to describe these drugs, refers to their therapeutic effect and is used here in deference to common clinical practice. *Antidepressive* or *antidepression* drugs would be preferable, since the term *depressant* still has a pharmacologic connotation which does not necessarily equate with the therapeutic effect. For example, barbiturates and chloral hydrate, which still have a certain usefulness in the treatment of depression, are in fact depressants in the pharmacologic sense; in this case depressants act as mood elevators or antidepressants. These commonly used terms must not be confused—one refers to a drug that reduces nervous system excitability and the other to the capacity of the drug to ameliorate the symptoms of mental depression.

MONOAMINE OXIDASE INHIBITORS The observation that iproniazid, an inhibitor of MAO, has a mood-elevating effect in tuberculous patients initiated a great deal of interest in compounds of this type and led quickly to their exploitation in the treatment of depression. Iproniazid (Marsilid) proved exceedingly toxic and was soon taken off the market, as have several more recently developed MAO inhibitors; but other drugs, much better tolerated, have become available. These include isocarboxizid (Marplan), nialamide (Niamid), phenelzine (Nardil), and tranylcypromine (Parnate), the latter two being the most frequently used. Tranylcypromine has proved to be the most potent of these agents, but it has also produced the most serious toxic effects.

The exact mode of action of the MAO inhibitors has not been determined. They have in common the ability to block the oxidative deamination of naturally occurring amines (norepinephrine, epinephrine, and serotonin), and it has been suggested that the accumulation of these neurohormonal substances is responsible for the antidepressant effect. However, these drugs inhibit many enzymes other than monoamine oxidases and have numerous actions unrelated to enzyme inhibition. Furthermore, many agents with antidepressant effects like those of the monoamine oxidase inhibitors do not inhibit this enzyme. At the present time, one cannot assume that the therapeutic effect of these drugs has a direct relation to the property of MAO inhibition.

These drugs must be dispensed with great caution and a constant awareness of their potentially serious side effects. They may at times cause excitement, restlessness, agitation, insomnia, and anxiety; occasionally, with the usual dose and more often with an overdose, mania and convulsions may occur (especially in epileptic patients). Other side effects are increased neuromuscular activity in the form of muscle twitching and involuntary movement of an extremity, urinary retention, skin rashes, tachycardia, hepatic disturbance, jaundice, visual impairment, enhancement of glaucoma, impotence, sweating, muscle spasms, and a variety of paresthesias. Orthostatic hypotension of a serious degree may develop.

Patients taking MAO inhibitors must be warned against the use of dibenzazepine derivatives (Tofranil and Elavil) and also sympathomimetic amines and tyramine, for they may induce a severe hypertensive episode and cerebral vascular accident, headache, atrial and ventricular arrhythmia, pulmonary edema, and even death. Sympathomimetic amines are contained in some of the commonly used nasal sprays, nose drops, and in so-called coryza tablets and tyramine-containing cheeses, yogurt, beer, and wine.

The MAO inhibitors have widespread possibilities of potentiating the effect of other drugs. In particular, the phenothiazines and other powerful central nervous system stimulants should not be given with the MAO inhibitors, since severe reactions and occasional fatalities have followed their concomitant use. Exaggerated responses to the usual dose of meperidine (Demerol) and other narcotic drugs have also been observed; respiratory function may be depressed to a serious degree, and hyperpyrexia, agitation, and pronounced hypotension may occur as well, sometimes with fatal issue. Unpredictable side effects may also accompany the simultaneous administration of barbiturates.

DIBENZAZEPINE DERIVATIVES (TRICYCLIC ANTIDEPRESSANTS) Soon after the first convincing successes in the treatment of depression with MAO inhibitors, a new class of tricyclic compounds appeared. The first of this group was imipramine (Tofranil), which was soon followed by amitriptyline (Elavil), and then by desipramine (Norpramin) and nortriptyline (Aventyl). The first two members of this group have proved to be the most popular.

The exact mode of action of these agents is unknown, but there is evidence that these agents inhibit re-uptake of monoamine neurotransmitter substances, and their antidepressant effect has been attributed to this action. In the absence of other considerations, they are presently the most effective drugs for the treatment of patients with depressive illnesses, particularly those with retarded depressions, that are associated with insomnia (early morning awakening), decreased appetite, weight loss, and decreased libido. Persistence of their pharmacologic effects after the drug is stopped is very short in comparison with the MAO inhibitors, and their side effects are far less frequent and serious.

The tricyclic or dibenzazepine compounds are potent anticholinergic agents, and their most prominent and serious side effects (orthostatic hypotension, urinary bladder weakness) are due to peripheral anticholinergic action. They may also produce central nervous system excitement, leading to insomnia, agitation, and restlessness, but usually these effects are controlled readily by the use of phenothiazines or chlordiazepoxide given concurrently or in the evenings. Occasionally they may cause ataxia and blood dyscrasias. The dibenzazepine drugs should never be given with an MAO inhibitor, since the reactions which may occur are frequently serious; hypertensive crises and lethal hyperpyrexia have been reported. These reactions have allegedly occurred when small doses of imipramine were given to patients who had discontinued the MAO inhibitor one week previously.

STIMULANTS

These drugs, which act primarily as stimulants of the central nervous system, have a relatively limited therapeutic use but assume clinical importance for other reasons. Some members of the group, e.g., the amphetamines, are much abused, and others are not infrequent causes of poisoning.

AMPHETAMINES Amphetamine (Benzedrine) and its *d*-isomer, dextroamphetamine, are powerful analeptics and in addition have significant hypertensive, respiratory-stimulant, and appetite-depressant effects. These drugs are useful in the management of narcolepsy, but they are much more widely and indiscriminately used for the control of obesity and the abolition of fatigue. Undoubtedly, they are able to reverse fatigue, postpone the need for sleep, and elevate mood, but these effects are not entirely predictable and certainly not indefinite, and the user must pay for the period of wakefulness with even greater fatigue and often with depression. Because of the popularity of the amphetamines and ease with which they can be procured, instances of acute and chronic intoxication are observed frequently. Nonetheless, dextroamphetamine in doses of 5 mg morning and noon is a useful agent in the treatment of certain reactive depressions, such as the ones which follow myocardial infarction or stroke. The toxic signs are essentially an exaggeration of the analeptic effects—restlessness, excessive speech and motor activity, tremor, and insomnia. In severe cases, hallucinations, delusions, and changes in affect and thought processes may occur, a state that may be indistinguishable from paranoid schizophrenia. Treatment consists of removal of the offending drug and the administration of antipsychotic drugs. Nitrites may be useful if the blood pressure is markedly elevated.

METHYLPHENIDATE Having much the same type of action as amphetamine, this drug (Ritalin) is useful in the treatment of narcolepsy and, paradoxically, in the management of overactive children.

PICROTOXIN A powerful nervous system excitant, the main effects of this drug are to produce convulsive seizures and to reverse respiratory depression induced by drugs, particularly by barbiturates. However, the modern treatment of barbiturate intoxication does not include the use of picrotoxin or other analeptics, because of their epileptogenic properties and because barbiturate intoxication can be managed successfully by other means (see preceding section). It has been shown by Eccles and his colleagues that picrotoxin increases neuronal activity by blocking presynaptic inhibition, i.e., blocking the action of inhibitory fibers that synapse with the presynaptic terminals of excitatory fibers.

STRYCHNINE The action of strychnine is to increase neuronal excitability by interfering with postsynaptic inhibition; the therapeutic value is negligible. In children accidental poisoning may occur from ingestion of "A.S. & B." cathartic pills or "rat biscuits." Very rarely, strychnine is taken with suicidal intent. After a period of heightened irritability and muscle twitching, tonic seizures occur, characterized by opisthotonus, rigid extension of the legs, facial tetanus, and apnea due to spasm of the muscles of respiration. Death from anoxia may follow several seizures. The immediate need, in the treatment of strychnine poisoning, is to control the convulsions. This calls for the intravenous administration of a short-acting barbiturate or the application of inhalation anesthesia if the appropriate drug is not immediately available; endotracheal intubation is an important safeguard. The patient must then be observed carefully, and if any signs of irritability recur, more sedative should be given. During this period, supportive care is indicated, as for any comatose patient. Morphine, which is principally a medullary depressant, is contraindicated.

PENTYLENETETRAZOL This drug (Metrazol, Cardiazol) is a potent stimulant of all parts of the nervous system. For a number of years it served as the convulsive agent in shock treatment of depression and schizophrenia but was abandoned in favor of less dangerous and more effective forms of convulsive therapy. The use of this drug to activate latent epileptogenic foci or to reproduce convulsions, with the purpose of studying the underlying cerebral mechanisms, although once a common test method, has been virtually discontinued.

BEMEGRIDE, NIKETHAMIDE These two drugs, the latter with the trade name Coramine, act much like pentylenetetrazol. For many years common clinical practice was to administer nikethamide as a final therapeutic gesture in patients dying of cardiac and respiratory failure, but there is little evidence that this drug has a significant stimulant effect on either heart or respiration. Poisoning with these drugs, which is usually due to parenteral overdosage, is best treated with barbiturates.

CAFFEINE The therapeutic value of caffeine and other xanthine derivatives stems from their diuretic effects and their ability to stimulate the heart and nervous system. The major use of these agents is to abolish fatigue and maintain wakefulness, and the usual mode of administration is in coffee, a cup of which contains 100 to 150 mg caffeine. Overdosage leads to insomnia, mild delirium, tinnitus, tachycardia, prominent diuresis, and cardiac arrhythmias. The excitatory effects are easily controlled with barbiturates, and fatalities due to caffeine poisoning are extremely rare.

CAMPHOR Formerly a popular stimulant, camphor is now rarely used therapeutically; however, occasional cases of poisoning are still seen as a result of ingestion of liniment (camphorated oil) or moth flakes. The manifestations of poisoning are headache, sensation of warmth, confusion, clonic convulsions, and terminal respiratory depression; the characteristic odor of camphor facilitates the diagnosis. Treatment consists of supportive care and the cautious use of barbiturates to combat convulsions.

PSYCHOTOGENIC DRUGS

Included in this category are a heterogeneous group of drugs, the primary effect of which is to alter perception, mood, and thinking out of proportion to other aspects of cognitive function and consciousness. This group of drugs comprises lysergic acid derivatives, e.g., lysergic acid diethylamide (LSD); phenylethylamine derivatives (mescaline and peyote); psilocybin; certain indolic derivatives, *Cannabis* (marijuana), and a number of less important compounds. They are also referred to as psychotomimetic drugs, hallucinogens, illusinogens, and psychedelics, but none of these names is entirely suitable.

Tolerance to LSD, mescaline, psilocybin, and other psychotogenic drugs develops rapidly, even on a once-daily dosage. Furthermore, subjects tolerant to any one of these three specific drugs are cross-tolerant to the other two. Tolerance is lost rapidly when these drugs are discontinued abruptly, but no abstinence syndromes ensue. In this sense, addiction does not develop, although users may become dependent upon them for emotional support. In the case of marihuana, reverse tolerance (i.e., increasing sensitization) may be observed initially, but on continued use, tolerance to the euphoriant effects of the drug has been observed in one of the few chronic experimental studies that have been made, and the subjects reported jitteriness during the first 24 h after abrupt cessation of marijuana smoking, although no objective withdrawal signs could be detected.

LSD, MESCALINE, PSILOCYBIN These drugs produce much the same clinical effects if given in comparable amounts. The perceptual changes are the most dramatic—the user describes vivid visual hallucinations, alterations in the shape and color of objects, unusual dreams, and feelings of depersonalization. An increase in auditory acuity has been described, but auditory hallucinations are rare. Cognitive functions are difficult to assess because of inattention, drowsiness, and inability to concentrate and to cooperate in mental testing. The somatic symptoms consist of dizziness, nausea, drowsiness, paresthesias, and blurring of vision. Sympathomimetic effects—pupillary dilatation, piloerection, hyperthermia, and tachycardia—are prominent, and the user may also show hyperreflexia, incoordination of the limbs, and ataxia.

MARIJUANA When taken by inhaling the smoke from cigarettes, marijuana produces effects which are prompt in onset and evanescent. In low doses the symptoms are like those of mild intoxication with alcohol. With increasing amounts of drug, the effects are similar to those of LSD, mescaline, and psilocybin, and they may be quite disabling for many hours. Very large doses result in severe depression and stupor, but death is unusual.

The fact that small quantities of these drugs can produce gross mental aberrations has stimulated the search for similar but endogenous substances that may be responsible for schizophrenia and other psychoses. The mechanisms involved in producing and antagonizing the psychotomimetic effects are also being studied intensively, in the hope of elucidating the mechanisms of the psychoses and finding improved psychotherapeutic agents. Doubtless these studies are adding greatly to our knowledge of abnormal behavior, but the fundamental problems remain to be solved.

Numerous claims have been made that LSD and related drugs are effective in the treatment of mental disease and a wide variety of social ills and that they have the capacity to increase one's intellectual performance, creativity, and self-understanding. At this time, there are no acceptable studies that validate any of these claims.

LSD is not yet an approved drug, and use of marijuana is governed by the federal narcotic laws. Nevertheless, these drugs are very widely used. They are taken by narcotic addicts as a temporary substitute for more potent drugs, by "drug heads," i.e., individuals who use literally any agent that alters consciousness, and by many troubled, unhappy college and high-school students, often for reasons that they cannot ascertain. The unsupervised use of these drugs is attended by a number of serious adverse reactions, taking the form of acute panic attacks, long-lasting psychotic states resembling paranoid schizophrenia, "flashbacks" (spontaneous recurrences of the original LSD experience, often precipitated by smoking marijuana and accompanied by panic attacks), or by serious physical injury, consequent upon impairment of the user's critical faculties. Whether prolonged usage leads to permanent damage to the nervous system is not certain; there are some data suggesting that this may happen. The reports claiming that LSD may cause chromosomal damage remain to be validated. A discussion of the legal implications of the illicit use of these drugs and their social impact is beyond the scope of this chapter but can be found in the references cited below.

REFERENCES

DIMASCIO A, SHADER RI (eds): *Clinical Handbook of Psychopharmacology,* New York: Science House, 1970

DIPALMA JR (ed): *Drill's Pharmacology in Medicine,* New York: McGraw-Hill, 1971

HOLLISTER LE: *Chemical Psychoses: LSD and Related Drugs,* Springfield, Ill.: Charles C Thomas, 1968

——: Mental disorders—Antianxiety and antidepressant drugs. N Engl J Med 286:1195, 1972

——: *The Clinical Use of Psychotherapeutic Drugs,* Springfield, Ill.: Charles C Thomas, 1973

IVERSEN SD, IVERSEN LL: *Behavioral Pharmacology,* New York: Oxford, 1975

JARVIK MD: Drugs used in the treatment of psychiatric disorders, in *Pharmacological Basis of Therapeutics,* 4th ed., eds LS Goodman, A Gilman, New York: Macmillan, 1970, p. 151

WIKLER A: Drug dependence, in *Clinical Neurology,* eds AB Baker, LH Baker, New York: Harper & Row, 1971

section 2 | Emergencies due to environmental and physical agents

EMERGENCY MEDICINE

ROBERT G. PETERSDORF

EXPANDING SCOPE OF EMERGENCY MEDICINE One of the expanding areas of medicine is the diagnosis and management of acute emergencies. This is a consequence of a number of developments. Firstly, technical advances have given physicians the ability to treat some conditions that were almost invariably fatal in the past. Apparatus for electroconversion of the heart, respiratory assistance devices, potent drugs, fiberoptic endoscopes, and improved techniques of blood banking are just some of these advances. Secondly, in the past decade the public has come to depend on the emergency room as an entry point into the health care system to an increasingly greater extent, not

TABLE 1
Chapters dealing with medical emergencies

Category	*Title*	*Chapter no.*
Cardiovascular-pulmonary	Pain in the Chest	7
	Faintness, Syncope, and Episodic Weakness	16
	Cough and Hemoptysis	29
	Dyspnea and Pulmonary Edema	30
	Palpitation	33
	Hypotension and the Shock Syndrome	34
	Sudden Cardiovascular Collapse and Death	36
	Heart Failure	237
	Cardiac Dysrhythmias	238
	Pharmacologic Treatment of Cardiovascular Disorders	239
	Electrical Reversion of Cardiac Arrhythmias	240
	Acute Myocardial Infarction	245
	Pericardial Disease	246
	Diseases of the Aorta	251
	Asthma	257
	Pulmonary Thromboembolism	266
	Adult Respiratory Distress Syndrome	268
Endocrine	Diseases of the Neurohypophysis	91
	Diseases of the Thyroid	92
	Diseases of the Adrenal Cortex	93
	Diabetes Mellitus	95
	Hyperinsulinism, Hypoglycemia, and Glucagon Secretion	97
	Gout and Other Disorders of Uric Acid Metabolism	107
	Disorders of the Parathyroid Gland	353
Gastrointestinal-liver	Abdominal Pain	8
	Hematemesis and Melena	42
	Disorders of Porphyrin Metabolism	109
	Familial Mediterranean Fever	229
	Gastrointestinal Endoscopy	285
	Acute Intestinal Obstruction	292
	Acute Appendicitis	293
	Cirrhosis	301
	Diseases of the Pancreas	307
Renal-acid base	Fluid and Electrolytes	69
	Acidosis and Alkalosis	70
	Acute Renal Failure	272
Blood and blood-forming organs	Bleeding	61
	Hemolytic Anemias	313
	Methemoglobinemia and Sulfhemoglobinemia	316
	Bleeding Disorders Caused by Vascular Abnormalities	318
	Disorders of Blood Coagulation	319
Central nervous system	Coma and Related Disturbances of Consciousness	22
	The Convulsive State and Idiopathic Epilepsy	24
	Delirium and Other Acute Confusional States	26
	Cerebrovascular Diseases	334
	Traumatic Diseases of the Brain	335
	Pyogenic Infections of the Central Nervous System	337
	Myasthenia Gravis and Episodic Muscular Weakness	350
Environmental and physical disturbances	Disturbances of Heat Regulation	11
	Disorders Caused by Venoms, Bites, and Stings	122
	Disorders Due to Alterations of Barometric Pressure	123
	Problems of Air and Space Travel	124
	Radiation and Electrical Injuries	125
	Immersion Injury and Drowning	126
Chemical intoxications	Common Poisons	116
	Heavy Metals	117
	Alcohol	118
	Opiates and Other Synthetic Analgesic Drugs	119
	Barbiturates	120
	Sedative-Hypnotic, Psychotherapeutic, Stimulant, and Psychotogenic Drugs	121
Infectious and immunological	Diseases of Immediate Type Hypersensitivity	72
	Septic Shock	129
	Chemotherapy of Infection	130
	Meningococcal Infections	136
	Tetanus	156
	Botulism	157
	Other Clostridial Infections	158

only in city-county and other public hospitals but also in community hospitals. This, in turn, has led to the development of a new type of health professional—the emergency room physician; it is estimated that there are approximately 15,000 full-time emergency physicians in practice in community hospitals. Thirdly, residency programs in emergency medicine have been established in some 35 teaching centers. Fourthly, improved prehospital care achieved in some localities by trained paramedical personnel has emphasized the need for better first-line care in emergency rooms. Fifthly, the trend toward regionalization in emergency care has made it incumbent upon communities to provide a network of up-to-date emergency facilities. Finally, the interest on the part of charitable foundations and the federal government has provided a potent impetus for upgrading emergency facilities and for training the staff to man them. The federal interest culminated in the Emergency Medical Services Systems Act of 1973 (PL 93-154) which adds a section to the Public Health Services Act of 1944 (PL 78-410) "to provide assistance and encouragement for the development of comprehensive area-wide emergency medical systems." This law emphasizes local planning for emergency services; consumer participation; availability of emergency medical services to all irrespective of ability to pay; the development of training programs for physicians, nurses, and technologists in emergency medicine; improvement of the physical facilities in emergency departments of hospitals; standards of quality for emergency room personnel, and much more. Most importantly, this law does not differentiate between an emergency defined by the patient and by the health professional. Clearly, this legislation will provide the stimulus and resources to place increasing emphasis on the emergency room in the provision of health care.

CONTENT OF EMERGENCY MEDICINE Emergency medicine is defined as a broad-based specialty that takes responsibility for the immediate care of the patient. In a few instances, the problem which is considered an emergency can be resolved by the emergency physician alone; in most circumstances, following emergency treatment, the patient is referred to the primary physician for follow-up care, or is admitted to a hospital to be cared for by the primary physician and whatever consultants are appropriate. Emergency medicine borrows its skills from the traditional specialties of medicine. Examples include the management of epistaxis by the otorhinolaryngologist; the removal of a foreign body from the eye by the ophthalmologist; the initial assessment of acute trauma by the surgeon; the stopping of vaginal hemorrhage by the gynecologist; and the reversion of ventricular tachycardia with drugs by the cardiologist. The practice of emergency medicine should be measured in terms of an hour or two rather than days or weeks. It is obvious that the correct handling of an emergency will often be lifesaving; conversely, failure to make the correct diagnosis and to institute appropriate treatment may result in a fatal outcome.

EMERGENCY MEDICINE AS PART OF INTERNAL MEDICINE While trauma, burns, and lodgment of foreign bodies make up a significant part of the problems that present as medical emergencies, it is clear that many acute emergencies fall within the province of the internist and should be included in a textbook of medicine. These comprise not only the "classic" medical emergencies such as acute cardiac arrhythmias, status asthmaticus, coma from drug overdosage or diabetic ketoacidosis, but also problems that may come to the internist less frequently such as acute alcoholism, heat stroke (Chap. 11), anaphylaxis (Chap. 72), bee sting, or drowning. Indeed, the well-trained internist should be familiar with and capable of treating the majority of acute emergencies described in this textbook.

In the accompanying table are listed the chapters dealing with topics in emergency medicine. This list is by no means complete, and acute emergencies may be covered to a limited extent in chapters not listed. For example, while pneumococcal meningitis is certainly a medical emergency, its discussion makes up only a small portion of the chapter on pneumococcal infections, and its management is covered in the chapter on pyogenic infections of the nervous system. Conversely, only portions of chapters listed in the table deal with emergencies. For example, the recognition and treatment of thyroid storm make up only part of the chapter on thyroid diseases but it is the only place in the book where this subject is covered. Despite some shortcomings, it is hoped that the listing will provide a ready reference to readers who deal with acute and emergent situations in internal medicine.

REFERENCES

HARVEY JC: The Emergency Medical Services Systems Act of 1973. JAMA 230:1139, 1974

MILLS JD: Introduction: Overview of the field of emergency medicine, in *Emergency Department Organization and Management,* ed AL Jenkins, St. Louis: Mosby, 1975, p. 1

SPROWAL CW, MULLANY PJ (eds): *Emergency Care: Assessment and Intervention,* St. Louis: Mosby, 1974

122 DISORDERS CAUSED BY VENOMS, BITES, AND STINGS

JAMES F. WALLACE

INTRODUCTION Humans have the propensity to come into contact with a great variety of venomous animals. These contacts occur with many zoologic classes including snakes, lizards, sea animals, spiders, scorpions, and numerous species of insects. In general two types of injuries result: those due to the direct effect of venom on the victim, as exemplified in snakebite, and those due to indirect effects of the poison, of which hypersensitivity reaction to bee stings is an example. Each year in the United States at least 50 persons die as the result of venomous injuries. Three groups of animals—hymenopterous insects, snakes, and spiders—account for over 90 percent of the fatalities. Of even greater public health significance is the loss in economic productivity and human potential resulting from the many serious, nonfatal envenomations which occur annually in otherwise healthy children or working adults.

SNAKE BITE **Epidemiology** Fewer than one-tenth of the nearly 3,500 known species of snakes are venomous. These poisonous varieties belong to five families or subfamilies: Elapidae (cobras, kraits, mambas, and coral snakes) found in all parts of the world except Europe; Viperidae (true vipers) found in all parts of the world except the Americas; Hydrophidae (sea snakes); Crotalidae (pit vipers) found in Asia and the Americas; and Colubridae (boomslangs, bird snakes) of the African continent. The poisonous varieties of the United States, with the single exception of the coral snake, are pit vipers and include rattlesnakes, the water moccasin, and the copperhead. Although this discussion centers around these species, the therapeutic measures outlined are applicable to snakes in all parts of the world.

The number of individuals bitten by poisonous snakes in the United States is estimated to be about 8,000 per year, with a relatively large number occurring in the Southeastern and Gulf states, particularly Texas. Deaths are not reported separately but are undoubtedly rare, numbering fewer than 20 per year, and most are due to bites of various species of rattlesnake. In many European countries deaths from snakebite have averaged only one every 3 to 5 years for the last half-century. In contrast, the estimate of annual deaths from snakebite throughout the world is between 30,000 and 40,000 with the largest number occurring in the countries of Burma and Brazil, where 2,000 deaths are estimated to occur each year.

Etiology The *coral snake* is found in the Southern states from Florida to Arizona. It is usually marked by alternating red and black bands separated by yellow rings; however, black and albino forms exist. Coral snakes are generally nocturnal in their activities, shy and elusive, and rarely bite humans. Their fangs are short and permanently erect; the highly toxic venom is injected into multiple puncture wounds produced by a series of chewing movements.

The *pit vipers* are so named because of a small pit between the eye and the nostril. Large venom glands in the temporal regions give the head a triangular appearance. They are generally aggressive and likely to strike if disturbed. The fangs are long and hinged, folding posteriorly when the mouth is closed. Pit vipers strike suddenly with a forward thrust of the head. The instant that the erect fangs make contact, venom is expressed by sudden muscular contraction.

The *rattlesnakes,* recognized by the horny rattle on the tail which buzzes when the snake is disturbed, are widely distributed. The diamondbacks (*Crotalus adamanteus* in the Southeast and *C. atrox* in the Southwest) are the largest and most dangerous snakes in this country. Others include the prairie rattler (*C. confluentus*), the timber rattler (*C. horridus*), and the pigmy rattlers.

The *water moccasin,* or cottonmouth (*Agkistrodon piscivorus*), is found in swampy areas or along the banks of streams. It is a strong swimmer and can bite under water. This snake is notorious for inflicting severe facial bites when disturbed in the branches of small trees. The copperhead, or highland moccasin (*A. mokasen*), is a closely related species. Its bite is painful but rarely fatal.

Pathogenesis SNAKE VENOMS The venoms of most species which have been analyzed have been found to be mixtures of several toxic proteins and enzymes with diversified and complicated pharmacologic effects. As an example, the venom of the Indian cobra (*Naja naja*) contains these distinct and separate substances: a neurotoxin, a hemolysin, a cardiotoxin, a cholinesterase, at least three phosphatases, a nucleotidase, and a potent inhibitor of cytochrome oxidase. Several venoms, including those of the pit vipers, contain hyaluronidase and numerous proteolytic enzymes. Although the exact roles of these components in toxicity are incompletely understood, the venom of a given species is usually predominantly neurotoxic or necrotizing, and frequently associated with hemolysis, abnormalities of blood coagulation, changes in cardiac dynamics, and alterations in vascular resistance. The venom of elapids, including the coral snake, is neurotoxic, with death resulting from respiratory paralysis probably caused by damage to brain centers and a curariform interference with transmission at the neuromuscular junction. The venom of crotalid snakes produces local tissue injury, hemorrhage, and hemolysis; death is often preceded by circulatory collapse associated with a marked fall in circulating blood volume resulting from pooling of blood in the microcirculation, and loss of plasma due to increased capillary permeability. Systemic absorption of venom occurs through the lymphatics, and therapeutic measures designed to reduce lymphatic function are helpful in controlling symptoms.

FACTORS AFFECTING SEVERITY OF SNAKE BITE Several factors affect the outcome of snake bite:

1 The age, size, and health of the patient. Envenomation in children is usually serious, and a fatal outcome more likely, since a relatively large dose of poison is injected into a small victim.
2 Location of bite. Bites on extremities or into adipose tissue are less dangerous than those on the trunk, face, or directly into a blood vessel. A direct strike of the fangs is more dangerous than a scratch, a glancing blow, or one hitting a bone. The discharge orifice of a fang is well above its tip so that the point of the fang can penetrate the skin without envenomation; even a thin layer of clothing may afford great protection. Because of the superficial nature of the wound as many as one-fifth of patients bitten by venomous snakes will have no evidence of envenomation, even though the fangs have penetrated the skin.
3 The size of the snake (a large pit viper can inject over 1,000 mg venom, six times a lethal dose for an adult), the extent of its anger or fear (if hurt it may inject a larger amount of venom), the condition of the fangs (broken or recently renewed), and the condition of the venom glands (recently discharged or full). All these factors are important. Contrary to popular belief, the bite of a snake which has recently killed and fed is not necessarily less venomous for humans; the snake usually does not exhaust its venom in a single bite.
4 The presence of various bacteria, particularly clostridia and other anaerobic organisms, in the mouth of the snake or on the skin of the victim. This may lead to serious infection in the necrotic tissues at the local site.
5 Exercise or exertion, such as running, immediately after the bite. This speeds systemic absorption of toxin.

Manifestations Following the bite of a pit viper, severe burning pain develops within a few minutes at the site of the wound. Local swelling rapidly develops and spreads in all directions, accompanied by the appearance of ecchymoses and bullae over the involved area. As the edema spreads, serosanguinous fluid oozes from the puncture wounds. Later gangrene of the skin and subcutaneous tissues may develop. Systemic effects resulting from the absorption of venom and local tissue destruction may include fever, nausea and vomiting, circulatory collapse, bleeding into the skin and from all body orifices, low-grade jaundice, neuropathic muscle cramping, pupillary constriction, disorientation, delirium, and convulsions. Death may occur after 6 to 48 h. Survival may be attended by massive local tissue loss from gangrene or secondary infection, or may be complicated by acute renal failure, secondary to disseminated intravascular clotting and cortical necrosis, or by tubular necrosis following circulatory collapse.

The bite of the coral snake causes little pain and local swelling. There are usually multiple fang marks. Within 10 to 15 min numbness and weakness begin in the region of the bite followed by ataxia, ptosis, pupillary dilatation, palatal and pharyngeal paralysis, slurring of speech, salivation, and occasionally nausea and vomiting. The patient becomes comatose, develops respiratory paralysis and seizures, and dies within 8 to 72 h.

Cobra bites are painful and are often accompanied by severe hemolysis, local necrosis, and sloughing in addition to their neurotoxic effects. There is little pain and no edema at the site of a sea snake bite. Symptoms of systemic envenomation follow a latent period which may vary from 15 min to 8 h. Although the venom is both myotoxic and neurotoxic, the injury to skeletal muscle is most prominent and is characterized by generalized muscle pain, weakness, and myoglobinuria. Hemorrhagic manifestations predominate following envenomation by colubrids (boomslangs and bird snakes) and many pit vipers including certain species of rattlesnake.

Laboratory abnormalities In severe cases, laboratory abnormalities may include progressive anemia, polymorphonuclear leukocytosis of 20,000 to 30,000 cells per mm^3, thrombocytopenia, hypofibrinogenemia, disordered tests of coagulation, proteinuria, and azotemia.

Treatment An attempt should be made to determine with certainty that the patient has been bitten by a poisonous snake. Absence of distinct fang punctures and failure of local pain, edema, numbness, or weakness to appear within 20 min are strong evidence against snake venom poisoning. It has been estimated that at least one-fifth of all bites by poisonous snakes in the United States show no evidence of envenomation.

FIRST AID This consists of reassuring and calming the victim and instituting measures to retard the absorption of venom and to remove it from the tissues as quickly as possible after the bite. The patient should be promptly placed at rest and the bitten extremity immobilized to reduce the rate of spread of the venom. If anatomically feasible, a wide tourniquet should be placed a few centimeters above the bite and made tight enough to allow one finger to pass beneath with difficulty. The purpose is to impede lymph flow; it is not necessary to obstruct venous return. The tourniquet should be loosened and moved proximally at hourly intervals when local swelling causes it to tighten. Unless the victim can be transported to a hospital within less than 15 min, incision and suction of the wound should be started prior to evacuation. By use of whatever antisepsis is available, 1.0 cm *linear* (not cruciate) incisions about 0.5 cm deep should be carefully made through each fang mark and suction applied. A rubber bulb, breast pump, or heated jar are all preferable to mouth suction, but if other means are not available and no oral lesions are present, this method may be employed. Suction should be continued for at least 1 h following the bite. The practice of making multiple incisions along the advancing edge of edema as swelling progresses has not been found to be beneficial and is no longer advised. *Incision and suction are extremely important and should be diligently carried out in every poisonous snake bite.* When begun promptly, they may result in the removal of up to 50 percent of subcutaneously injected venom.

As soon as possible, the patient should be transferred to a hospital. Immobilization of the affected part during transportation is important in controlling lymph flow and is best achieved by splinting. Although ice packs relieve pain and slow lymphatic drainage, they do not neutralize venom, and their use can result in irreparable damage to already injured tissue through freezing.

IMMEDIATE HOSPITAL CARE This should include appropriate treatment for shock and respiratory difficulty, antivenin, measures to combat infection, and general supportive care.

Antivenin is the only specific treatment of snake venom poisoning, and its use in severe bites is vital. In the United States polyvalent crotaline antivenin effective against all American pit vipers and antivenin for North American coral snake poisoning are commercially available. Both products are a lyophylized powder of refined horse serum. Kits are available containing antivenin powder (reconstituted by diluting with water to 10 ml per ampul), syringe, normal horse serum for prior sensitivity testing of the patient, and detailed instructions. Intravenously administered antivenin leads to the most rapid and effective response. It is not advisable to infiltrate antivenin at the local site. The initial dose should depend upon the amount of envenomation; for severe bites 10 to 15 vials (100 to 150 ml) may be required. When progressive swelling in the bitten part ceases, an adequate dose has generally been achieved; improvement in the victim's clinical signs is often extremely rapid.

In the patient with severe envenomation who is allergic to horse serum, the relative risks of death from anaphylaxis rather than from venom poisoning should be carefully weighed before undertaking desensitization with small doses of diluted horse serum.

No antivenin for other snakes is manufactured in the United States, but antiserum for various types is usually kept on hand at large zoos all over the world. A national antivenin index is maintained by the Oklahoma City Zoo [(405)424-3344], and telephone consultation service for physicians is also available at the Los Angeles County/University of Southern California Medical Center.

Maintaining *respiration* by mechanical or other means is important. In patients bitten by elapid snakes, respiratory failure is usually reversible. *Tetanus toxoid* or *tetanus immune globulin* of human origin should be given. If wound infections appear, antibiotics should be used with the knowledge that the predominant microorganisms in the mouths of snakes are gram-negative pathogens. Treatment should be preceded by appropriate aerobic and anaerobic cultures. *Fasciotomy* may be necessary to prevent further ischemic injury to a massively swollen limb. *Surgical debridement* of vesicles and superficial necrotic tissue should be done near the end of the first week following the bite. *Relief of pain* with salicylates or meperidine, moderate sedation, maintenance of fluid balance, measures to combat shock and hemorrhagic diathesis, and appropriate management of coma or convulsions are all important.

The usefulness of corticosteroids to prevent tissue damage or systemic intoxication has not been convincingly demonstrated. However, these drugs may be of value in the management of severe shock associated with envenomation and for allergic reactions following the administration of antivenin.

Prevention In snake-infested regions long trousers, high shoes, boots or leggings, and gloves should be worn. Most important of all is to look where one steps or reaches. A sharp knife or lancet, tourniquet, suction bulb, and antiseptic suffice for an emergency kit, and in inaccessible areas, antivenin should also be carried.

POISONOUS LIZARD BITE Of the nearly 3,000 species of lizard in the world, only two are venomous: the Gila monster (*Heloderma suspectum*) of the arid southwestern United States and the closely related Mexican beaded lizard (*H. horridum*) which inhabits the lowland forests of Western Mexico. These reptiles are not aggressive, and virtually every instance of their attacking a human has involved teasing or handling the animals in captivity. The venom is elaborated in eight glands in the floor of the mouth and secreted directly into the oral cavity, where it bathes the teeth, which are grooved posteriorly. The lizard clings tenaciously and is often dislodged only after considerable effort; envenomation occurs by contamination of the wound. The venom contains a potent neurotoxin which is undoubtedly responsible for its lethal effect on experimental animals. Death in humans following a bite is extremely rare. Most often, human envenomation results in tissue injury, excruciating pain, massive edema, and patchy erythema. Acute systemic symptoms may last for 3 to 4 days and include nausea, vomiting, hematemesis, blurred vision, dyspnea, dysphonia, and profound weakness. Intense hyperesthesia of the bitten extremity may persist for several weeks. There is no antivenin available. Treatment should consist of tourniquet, incision, suction, cooling of the bitten area, measures to prevent or combat infection, including tetanus, and supportive measures. Parenteral meperidine (Demerol) or infiltration of local anesthetic around the bite should be used to relieve pain.

ENVENOMATION BY SPIDERS, SCORPIONS, INSECTS, AND OTHER ARTHROPODS The bite of many spiders is locally irritating, and several species can cause severe, even fatal systemic poisoning in man. The most numerous and important of the venomous spiders are members of the genus *Latrodectus,* widely distributed throughout the world. In the United States and Canada, *Lat. mactans,* the black widow or shoe-button spider, causes a majority of clinically significant arachnidism. In Florida, *Lat. bishopi,* the red-legged widow spider, has been reported to produce human poisoning resembling mild black widow bite. From the Southern and Midwestern states, there are increasing numbers of reports of poisoning from the bite of common brown spiders, including *Loxosceles reclusa* and *Lox. unicolor.* These bites are characterized by intense local pain and ischemic necrosis at the site, often followed by deep ulceration. Hemolysis occasionally is seen, and in severe cases hemoglobinuria and acute renal failure may occur.

The symptoms and mortality from bites of large, hairy spiders, the tarantulas, such as *Lycosa raptoria* and *Phoneutria fera* in Brazil or *Glyptocranium gastereanthoides* in Peru, and of such spiders as *Loxosceles laeta* in Chile are similar, with severe ulceration, necrosis, and hemolysis. Neurotoxic manifestations of the type produced by *Latrodectus* are sometimes admixed with local necrosis and hemolysis.

It is the female *Lat. mactans,* the black widow, that bites man. She is glossy black with a body 1 cm in diameter, a leg span of 5 cm, and a characteristic red hourglass mark on her abdomen. She spins her web in woodpiles, sheds, basements, or outdoor privies, is very aggressive, and will bite on slight provocation. The venom produces diffuse central and peripheral nervous excitement, autonomic activity, muscle spasm, hypertension, and vasoconstriction.

In the United States, most black widow bites occur between April and October, and many patients are males bitten on the genitalia or buttocks while using a privy. After a momentary sharp pain at the site, there is cramping pain that begins locally within 15 to 60 min and gradually spreads. It may involve all extremities and the trunk. The abdomen is boardlike, and the waves of pain become excruciating, causing the patient to turn, toss, and cry out. Respirations are often labored and grunting. There are also nausea, vomiting, headache, sweating, salivation, hyperactive reflexes, twitching, tremor, paresthesias of hands and feet, and occasionally, systolic hypertension. A mild polymorphonuclear leukocytosis is usual, and many patients have slight fever. After several hours, the pains subside, although mild recurrences for 2 or 3 days are common. It may be a week before well-being is restored. Deaths due to cardiac or respiratory failure have occurred, mostly in children and the aged.

Because the bite itself is not prominent, patients are often thought to have some abdominal catastrophe such as perforated ulcer, pancreatitis, or volvulus. Renal colic, coronary occlusion, tetanus, strychnine poisoning, tabetic crisis, lead colic, and porphyria are other conditions to be ruled out. The abdomen is not tender to palpation in arachnidism, and pains in the extremities are not typical of most of these other disorders.

Treatment For *Latrodectus* poisoning, treatment consists of measures to relieve pain and administration of antiserum. Initial treatment should include a hot tub bath which affords prompt, although temporary, relief. An intravenous injection of calcium gluconate or magnesium sulfate usually produces dramatic, but transient, cessation of cramps.

Opiates are sometimes necessary. When available, a single intramuscular injection of 1 ampul (2.5 ml) reconstituted antiserum usually is quite effective within a few hours. If the cramps return, administration of antiserum can be repeated.

Treatment of *Loxosceles* bites consists mainly of local wound management and treatment of secondary infection if it occurs. The parenteral use of corticosteroids within the first 24 h following a bite has been advocated in order to prevent progression of the lesion, but convincing evidence that this is efficacious is lacking. The ulcer usually heals spontaneously, although skin grafting may be required on occasion. Renal failure should be treated as advised in Chap. 272.

SCORPION STING Scorpions are eight-legged arthropods. Glands in the terminal segment produce venom, which is injected into the victim by a stinger located on the tip of the tail. Scorpions often enter dwellings. During the day they retreat into crevices; emerging at night, they often get into shoes and clothing and even into bedding. They do not deliberately attack humans, but accidental contact results in a sting.

Of about 650 species, roughly 40 occur in the United States, distributed over three-fourths of the nation. They are most numerous in the South from Florida to California, but the only two lethal species, *Centruroides sculpturatus* and *C. gertschi,* are limited to Arizona and portions of neighboring states.

Dangerous species found in the United States, *C. sculpturatus* and *C. gertschi,* reach a maximal length of about 7 cm. Their sting may be fatal to young children or old people, but seldom to a healthy adult.

Most of the nonlethal species of scorpions in the United States cause only minor reactions, like a bee sting. Some in the Southwest, however, produce local edema and ecchymosis, with burning pain. In contrast, many species whose venom has potentially dangerous systemic effects, including the Arizona *Centruroides,* evoke little or no visible reaction at the site of the sting. There is an immediate burning sensation followed by local paresthesia ("pins and needles"), hyperesthesia, or numbness. These sensations spread to involve the whole extremity, and within an hour or two, malaise, restlessness, lacrimation, rhinorrhea, salivation, perspiration, nausea, and vomiting appear.

The patient passes from an agitated state with hyperactive reflexes into coma; convulsions follow. In addition to these neurotoxic symptoms, cardiovascular effects due to myocarditis may be seen and include various arrhythmias and intractable heart failure. Death usually occurs within 12 h, but sometimes as late as 2 days after the sting.

Treatment This consists of immediately placing a tourniquet on the extremity just proximal to the sting in order to delay the absorption of venom. If available, ice packs may be applied to the wound and to the affected limb, with care not to create additional tissue injury through freezing. The tourniquet must be removed in 5 to 10 min, but the limb is kept cool for at least 2 h. After this time, if treatment has been applied promptly, no serious effects are experienced following the sting of *C. sculpturatus* or *C. gertschi.* If the sting is on the head, trunk, or genitalia, of course, a tourniquet cannot be used, but the area may be cooled.

Although tourniquet, incision, and suction as in the treatment of snake bite have been recommended, the amount of venom is minute; it produces no local necrotizing effect and is absorbed very rapidly.

Specific antivenin, reconstituted from lyophilized cat serum, is available in some areas and should be employed if the victim develops signs of central nervous system or cardiac involvement. Supportive therapy is directed at combating shock and dehydration. Barbiturates in large doses are useful in reducing restlessness.

Prevention This depends upon alertness in avoiding contact with scorpions in infested areas. Clothing and shoes should be well shaken before being put on in the morning. Towels and bedclothes should be inspected. A house infested with scorpions can in time be rid of them by closing all obvious ways of ingress; picking up debris in the environment, such as piles of brush, logs, stones; introducing a mixture of fuel oil or kerosene, containing a small amount of creosote, between the earth and the house foundation; and spraying with a mixture of 2% chlordane, 10% DDT, and 0.2% pyrethrins in an oil base.

HYMENOPTERA STINGS Each year in the United States, nearly twice as many people die as a result of bites by hymenopterous insects (including bees, wasps, hornets, and fire ants) as from poisonous snake bites. Occasionally, multiple stings in enormous numbers (500 to 1,000) are the cause of death. However, the majority of systemic reactions and deaths are due to allergic reactions to the venoms of these insects.

Hymenopteran venoms contain histamine, various kinins, and other vasoactive substances, phospholipases, and hyaluronidase. They are hemolytic and neurotoxic in addition to being effective hypersensitizing agents. The usual reaction to a single wasp sting or bee sting is sharp pain, local wheal and erythema, intense itching, and in loose tissues, such as the eyelid or genitalia, considerable edema which subsides in a few hours. Only in the rare case when a bee is swallowed or inhaled and edema of the laryngopharynx or glottis develops is there danger. A sting directly into a peripheral nerve can destroy its function for a time, much as does an injection of alcohol. Bell's palsy has followed a sting into the trunk of the facial nerve.

In hypersensitive individuals, a single sting may produce serious anaphylaxis with urticaria, nausea, abdominal cramps, asthma, massive edema of the face and glottis, dyspnea, cyanosis, hypotension, coma, and death. Sensitization is usually the result of previous stings. Beekeepers who develop allergic rhinitis followed by asthma when near bees or objects that have been in contact with bees are likely to have serious reactions to stings. It has been estimated that nearly 1 percent of the general population in this country has hymenoptera allergy.

Many species of ant can produce stinging bites with local redness and swelling. The most notorious of these is the fire ant (*Solenopsis saevissima*), whose bite may result in extensive vesiculation and skin necrosis similar to that caused by the brown recluse spider.

Treatment The usual sting is treated by local cool application and antipruritic lotions or oral antihistamines. Epinephrine, 0.3 to 0.5 ml of a 1:1,000 aqueous solution subcutaneously repeated every 20 to 30 min, may be lifesaving in patients with an allergic reaction to a bee sting or wasp sting. Ice packs can slow the absorption of venom and also relieve pain. Oxygen, endotracheal intubation, vasopressors, and other supportive measures should be used as needed. In addition, corticosteroids should be employed in severe cases, although their maximum effect is not achieved until several hours after administration.

Prevention Desensitization by injection of whole-body extract of bees, wasps, hornets, and yellowjackets currently is recommended for any patient who has had a systemic or generalized reaction to hymenopterous insect stings. Immunotherapy with purified Hymenoptera venom antigen, still undergoing clinical investigation, appears to be much more protective than whole-body extracts and likely will soon be the preferred material for desensitization. In addition, allergic patients should make every effort to avoid contact with these insects. If exposure seems likely, they should carry a kit containing a syringe of epinephrine for immediate use in case of a sting, without waiting for symptoms to develop.

TICK BITE The local reaction to the bite of a tick may be nothing more than an itching papule which subsides within a few days unless there is secondary bacterial infection. However, incomplete removal of a tick, with retention of the mouthparts, may result in the local formation of a nodule which continues to grow and is sometimes annoyingly pruritic. The definitive treatment is surgical excision of the nodule. Histologically, the nodule is a granuloma, but the inflammatory response is sometimes so bizarre and changes in the overlying epithelium are so striking that, in the absence of a history of tick bite, a mistaken diagnosis of malignant tumor may be made.

Removal of a tick by steady pulling is preferable to crushing. Touching with a hot object such as a glowing cigarette, freezing, or applying a drop of oil or nail polish facilitates removal without leaving embedded remnants.

Tick paralysis A progressive, ascending, flaccid paralysis which is reversible sometimes develops in humans and certain other mammals while a tick is engorging upon them. Human cases have most frequently been reported from the northwestern United States and Western Canada, where the wood tick, *Dermacentor andersoni* Stiles, is responsible. The dog tick, *D. variabilis* Say, has been identified in a number of cases occurring in the Southeastern states. *Amblyomma americanum,* the lone star tick, and *A. maculatum,* the Gulf Coast tick, have also been incriminated.

This disorder is caused by a neurotoxin apparently injected by the engorging tick. This toxin acts upon spinal and bulbar nuclei, slowing motor nerve conduction without affecting neuromuscular transmission. The toxin appears to be destroyed or excreted rapidly, for when the tick is removed the nerve cells soon regain normal function.

The tick must feed for several days before symptoms develop. Paralysis is seen in experimental animals after 5 to 6 days of engorgement. Male ticks feed for a shorter period than female ticks, a fact which may explain why they are less likely to cause paralysis.

Most human cases occur in children, generally in young girls. The tick is usually attached to the scalp and hidden by the hair, but may be found on any part of the body, especially the ear, axilla, groin, vulva, or popliteal region.

The patient may be irritable and have mild diarrhea for 24 h before frank motor involvement appears. There are weakness and poor control of the legs, the tendon reflexes in the legs are diminished or absent, and the Romberg sign is positive. Temporary improvement may occur, and if the tick is removed at this stage, true paralysis may never develop. Otherwise the symptoms recur within 24 h, with flaccid paralysis which extends in 24 to 48 h to involve the trunk, arms, neck, tongue, and pharynx. Sensory changes are usually absent, but there may be paresthesia and hyperesthesia in the affected extremities. Nystagmus, strabismus, and facial paralysis are sometimes noted. The respirations become shallow, rapid, and irregular. The patient sinks into stupor, cyanosis appears, and death results from respiratory paralysis or from obstruction of the airway by aspirated material. There is little or no fever unless a secondary infection is present. The leukocyte count is usually not elevated, but moderate leukocytosis may occur. The spinal fluid is almost always normal.

Tick paralysis is apt to be confused with poliomyelitis, the more so because ticks are active in warm weather when poliomyelitis is most prevalent.

Among other diseases which might be considered in differential diagnosis are polyneuritis, transverse myelitis, the Guillain-Barré syndrome, myasthenia gravis, the Eaton-Lambert myasthenic syndrome, and botulism.

Definitive treatment is removal of the tick. Mouthparts retained in the skin should be promptly excised. The patients's body should be searched for other ticks. There is striking improvement within a few hours after removal of ticks.

If the tick is removed before bulbar involvement develops, the paralysis subsides and recovery is complete in a few days, sometimes within 24 h. The patient should be observed until the recovery trend is established, because if other ticks or retained mouthparts have been overlooked, the paralysis may progress. When bulbar or respiratory paralysis is present, death may occur if the tick is not removed in time. Other treatment is supportive.

OTHER ARTHROPOD BITES Flea bite There are many fleas that attack man, including *Pulex irritans* and chicken fleas. In sensitive individuals, the salivary secretion of these bloodsuckers produces large, itching papules. Treatment is symptomatic only. Elimination of fleas from the environment may be very difficult, but persistent treatment of animals and of premises with appropriate insecticides is usually successful.

Centipede bite Local irritation is the usual reaction to centipede venom, although extensive necrosis and systemic illness have followed severe poisoning by tropical species. Treatment is purely symptomatic.

Caterpillar urticaria Contact with hairy caterpillars of many species produces irritation of skin or mucous membranes. The type of venom involved is not known, but severe pain, erythema, urticaria, and even blister formation may come on rapidly after direct contact with caterpillars, after handling cocoons, or on being exposed to windblown fuzz. There are often a regional lymphangitis and transient eosinophilic leukocytosis. The discomfort subsides within 24 h, but local soaks, oral antihistaminics, and, when pain is severe, oral codeine are often indicated.

Bedbug bite Members of the genus *Cimex* inflict bites that leave reactions varying from a simple puncture to large urticarial lesions, apparently depending on the sensitivity of the bitten individual. There is no specific treatment.

Chiggers or redbugs These are tiny mites which are commonly found in foliage, grass, etc., in many parts of the world. In the United States, the larval form of *Eutrobicula alfreddugesi* attacks the skin by secreting a substance which digests tissue, creating a red papule that itches intensely. The tiny reddish larva can be seen in the center of the lesion. Treatment is palliative and consists of antipruritic applications. The use of insect repellents, appropriate protective clothing, and prompt bathing after exposure reduce the risk of infestation considerably.

Bloodsucking-fly bite Many species of flies, particularly the horsefly and the deerfly, viciously attack and feed upon warm-blooded animals, including humans. Occasionally, transmission of diseases such an anthrax, tularemia, loiasis, and trypanosomiasis has been attributed to horseflies and deerflies. More commonly in North America, however, their bites are responsible for painful, intensely pruritic cutaneous lesions which may be followed by delayed localized allergic reactions characterized by erythema, edema, and urticaria. Treatment should include thorough cleaning of the bite sites, topical corticosteroids, and oral antihistaminics for severe itching. Antibiotics may be necessary if the wounds become secondarily infected.

Myiasis There are, generally speaking, three ways in which human tissues may become infested by maggots. Species of flies which usually deposit eggs in carrion, feces, or garbage may lay eggs in an open wound or ulcer, usually a lesion that is necrotic and suppurating. When the larvae hatch, they feed upon the dead tissue; despite the unesthetic aspects, the deliberate introduction of maggots has been used to supplement surgical debridement.

Occasionally, food containing fly eggs will be ingested, and when the larvae hatch, *intestinal myiasis* can result in nausea, cramps, and diarrhea. The larvae are passed in the feces.

Finally the larvae of many flies, including the sheep fly and horsefly, will attack living, viable tissue. If eggs are laid in the eyes, nose, ears, mouth, or vagina, an event that usually occurs in sleeping infants, the larvae hatch out and can produce extensive destructive lesions; indeed, fatalities have been reported.

The treatment for maggot infestation is surgical removal by irrigation and mechanical extraction. Obviously, control of fly populations by appropriate sanitary precautions is the important step in prevention. Protection of infants by screening and of wounds by bandaging is indicated in infested areas.

MARINE ANIMAL VENOM DISEASES The venoms of certain marine animals are known to cause illness in humans after injection or inoculation under naturally occurring conditions. Information concerning these toxins is limited; most appear to be composed of proteins and peptides as well as other substances that are pharmacologically active. Although probably less complex than the venoms of reptiles, many marine animal venoms are capable of causing several pathologic effects including neurotoxicity as well as local necrosis.

Portuguese man-of-war and jellyfish stings The burning discomfort induced by contact with sea nettles or jellyfish is familiar to most surf bathers. Contact with the tentacles of the colorful Portuguese man-of-war (*Physalia* species), which is found mainly in or near the Gulf of Mexico, or the more toxic jellyfish (*Chiropsalmus* of the Indian Ocean and *Rhizostoma* of the Atlantic) is followed by burning pain, swelling, and erythema. Severe, generalized muscular cramps, nausea, vomiting, and pulmonary edema may occur. Victims have died as a result of jellyfish stings, sometimes within minutes after contact. In nonfatal cases, systemic symptoms usually subside within several hours.

Treatment consists of removing any tentacles still clinging to the skin after first inactivating the toxins in their nematocysts with local application of alcohol, ammonia, or even dry sand. Analgesics should be used for pain control, and antihistaminics if there is an accompanying pruritic rash. Corticosteroids may be helpful in severe cases.

Sea anemone sting ("sponge diver's disease") Contact with certain sea anemones (especially *Sargatia elegans*) in Mediterranean and African waters produces extensive dermatitis with chronic ulceration. Occasionally, especially during August and September, systemic symptoms of headache, sneezing, nausea, chills, fever, and collapse are noted. Rare fatalities have occurred. No specific therapy is known; symptomatic treatment with topical steroids or oral antihistaminics may provide temporary relief.

Cone shell poisoning The colorful cone shells are highly prized by collectors. However, many species in the Pacific are venomous, a great danger to unwary hobbyists who pick them up. The poison, a neurotoxin, is delivered into a wound inflicted by pointed hollow teeth resembling darts in the long proboscis of the animal. Local manifestations include sudden intense pain, followed by swelling and numbness which may persist for several days. Symptoms of serious poisoning include muscular incoordination and weakness progressing to respiratory paralysis. Death may occur within 3 to 6 h, but recovery within 24 h is the rule. There is no specific therapy; recommended treatment is the use of tourniquet, incision, and suction (as for snake bite), and supportive measures which may include artificial respiration and administration of oxygen.

Sponge dermatitis Direct contact with several species of sponge results in a painful dermatitis, which may persist for several weeks. The lesions appear to be caused by mechanical irritation from the exoskeleton of the sponge as well as by toxins within its tissues. Delayed hypersensitivity reactions may also occur. Antihistaminics provide relief from the pruritus; dilute acetic acid ameliorates local pain strikingly, while alkali will intensify it. The lesions are self-limited.

Sea urchin sting Contact with the spines of some species of sea urchin results in painful erythema and ulceration, occasionally accompanied by neurotoxic symptoms of weakness and frank paralysis of lips, tongue, and face lasting for several hours. Treatment is purely symptomatic and supportive. The toxins isolated from sea urchins have produced paralysis in animals and are notably resistant to heat. Deaths from paralysis and drowning have been reported.

Neurotoxic shellfish poisoning Certain dinoflagellates, which compose part of the marine phytoplankton, elaborate a potent neurotoxin. Occasionally, conditions in coastal waters become favorable for the growth of excessive numbers of these organisms, causing the water to develop an amber appearance termed the "red tide" and killing massive numbers of fish by exhausting their oxygen supply. When humans ingest shellfish which have themselves ingested toxic dinoflagellates, an illness characterized by circumoral paresthesias, generalized muscular weakness, dysphonia, and occasionally respiratory arrest may occur. Treatment should include induced emesis and purgation and whatever additional supportive measures are necessary. Spontaneous recovery usually takes place within 24 h.

Venomous fish stings The dorsal fins or spines of bullhead sharks, dogfish, and ratfish and the dorsal and other fins of the scorpion fish, weeverfish, toadfish, and catfish are grooved, and at their bases are found venom glands. Injury by these spines results in severe pain and swelling and, in some instances, neurotoxic manifestations. Local gangrene with extensive tissue loss is a complication of catfish stings that may prolong convalescence. Little or nothing is known of the venoms involved. Suction and hot applications are advocated immediately after injury. Tetanus toxoid or antitoxin should be given also. Narcotics are often required to control the pain. Secondary pyogenic infection is a frequent complication.

Probably the most frequent type of venomous fish injury in the United States is that produced by the lashing tail of the stingray of the California coast (*Urobatis halleri*). The bony spine is encased in a sheath of epithelial cells containing venom which is expressed into the puncture wound. The wound may be several centimeters deep; portions of the bony spine may break off in it, or, more often, the integumentary sheath remains in the wound. The venom is a circulatory depressant in animals, but local injury predominates in humans. There are immediately severe pain and blanching followed by erythema and edema. Symptoms due to systemic absorption of venom are infrequent but may include salivation, muscle cramps and weakness, cardiac arrhythmias, seizures, and death. Treatment consists of application of a tourniquet (the vast majority of these injuries occur on the legs) and copious syringing of the wound with saltwater to remove fragments of sheath followed by immersion in water as hot as the patient can stand for 1 h. The venom is heat-labile, and extensive trials have indicated the usefulness of this last procedure. Tetanus toxoid or antiserum is indicated; as with other fish stings, pyogenic infection is a frequent complication.

REFERENCES

Hymenoptera stings

BARNARD JH: Studies of 400 hymenoptera sting deaths in the United States. J Allergy Clin Immunol 52:259, 1973

BROWN LL: Fire ant allergy. South Med J 65:273, 1972

BUSSE WW et al: Immunotherapy in bee sting anaphylaxis: Use of honeybee venom. JAMA 231:1154, 1975

MCLEAN JA: Management of insect sting reactions. Mod Treat 5:814, 1968

MARKS MB: Stinging insects: Allergy implications. Pediatr Clin North Am 16:177, 1969

Marine animal venoms

HALSTEAD BW: Poisonous and venomous marine animals of the World. Washington: U.S. Government Printing Office, vol. I, 1965, vol. III, 1970

KEEGAN HL, MACFARLANE WV (eds): *Venomous and Poisonous Animals and Noxious Plants of the Pacific Region,* Oxford: Pergamon, 1965

RUSSELL FE: Marine toxins and venomous and poisonous marine animals. Adv Marine Biol 3:255, 1965

SOUTHCOTT RV: Notes on stings of some venomous Australian fishes. Med J Aust 2:722, 1970

Other arthropod bites

FRAZIER CA: *Insect Allergy: Allergic and Toxic Reactions to Insects and Other Arthropods,* St. Louis: Warren H. Green, 1969

HANEVELD GT: Centipede bites. Br Med J 2:592, 1952

MCMILLAN CW, PURCELL WR: Health hazard from caterpillars. N Engl J Med 271:147, 1964

Scorpion stings

BARTHOLOMEW C: Acute scorpion pancreatitis in Trinidad. Br Med J 1:666, 1970

HOREN WP: Insect and scorpion sting. JAMA 221:894, 1972

SITA DEVI S et al: Defibrination syndrome due to scorpion venom poisoning. Br Med J 1:345, 1970

STAHNKE HL: Arizona's lethal scorpion. Ariz Med 29:490, 1972

Snake and lizard bites

ALBRITTON DC et al: Venenation by the Mexican beaded lizard (*Heloderma horridum*). Report of a case. S Dak J Med 23:9, 1970

MCCULLOUGH NC, GENNARD JF: Treatment of venomous snake bite in the United States. Clin Toxicol 3:483, 1970

MINTON SA JR: *Venom Diseases,* Springfield, Ill.: Charles C Thomas, 1974

RUSSELL FE: Pharmacology of animal venoms. Clin Pharmacol Ther 8:849, 1967

—— et al: Snake venom poisoning in the United States: Experience with 550 cases. JAMA 233:341, 1975

STAHNKE HL et al: Bite of the Gila monster. Rocky Mt Med J 67:25, 1970

Spider bites

BERGER RS: A critical look at therapy for the brown recluse spider. Arch Dermatol 107:288, 1973

EDITORIAL: Spider bites. Lancet 2:509, 1969

GORHAM JR: The brown recluse spider, loxosceles reclusa and necrotic spider bite—A new public health problem in the United States. J Environ Health 31:138, 1968

HOREN WP: Arachnidism in the United States. JAMA 185:839, 1963

Tick paralysis

CHERINGTON M, SNYDER RD: Tick paralysis: Neurophysiologic studies. N Engl J Med 278:95, 1968

EDITORIAL: Tick paralysis. Br Med J 3:314, 1969

SCHMITT N et al: Tick paralysis in British Columbia. Can Med Assoc J 100:417, 1969

123 DISORDERS DUE TO ALTERATIONS OF BAROMETRIC PRESSURE

HERBERT A. SALTZMAN

INTRODUCTION The biologic requirement for a breathing gas containing sufficient oxygen and the geography of the earth limit long-term habitation by human beings to a relatively narrow band of barometric pressure (P_B) ranging from that prevailing slightly below sea level (1 atm abs) in the deeper valleys to the reduced pressure encountered at an altitude of 18,000 ft (0.5 atm abs) on a mountain. Sojourns of less than 10 days are possible at altitudes above 25,000 ft with proper acclimatization, motivation, and equipment. In order to survive and perform efficiently beyond these boundaries, a well-tolerated breathing gas must be provided continuously. This is accomplished at the increased barometric, i.e., hyperbaric, pressures encountered in diving by lowering the fractional concentration of inspired O_2 [$F(IO_2)$] so that the inspired tension [$P(IO_2) \cong F(IO_2) \times P_B$] is below that known to cause toxicity (less than 0.4 to 0.5 atm abs). At pressures greater than 7 atm abs, helium is usually substituted for nitrogen in the breathing gas in order to prevent the narcosis associated with exposure to hyperbaric concentrations of certain inert gases. In the virtual vacuum of extraterrestrial space, humans must be contained within an envelope of pressure so that dissolved gases in tissues remain in solution and so that the $P(IO_2)$ is greater than 0.2 atm abs. By use of these principles, specially trained persons have performed efficiently for many days while orbiting earth and while exposed to increased pressures, as great as 61.6 atm abs, in an environmental chamber. In the open sea, humans have descended to a depth of 1,000 ft (31 atm abs).

Exposures to altered barometric pressures under less severe conditions are commonplace in today's world, however. Each day, many persons travel comfortably at very high altitudes in modern airplanes, protected from the external uninhabitable environment by partial restoration of normal air pressure within the cabin. Each year millions of enthusiasts dive in water to considerable depths, wearing diverse kinds of underwater breathing apparatus. Some of these individuals make their living at the sea bottom seeking minerals such as oil. Others, working in pressurized air, construct tunnels, underground transit systems, conduits, and bridges. Smaller numbers exposed to simulated altitude and depth in environmental chambers perform experiments. Also, many patients suffering from decompression sickness, air embolism, carbon monoxide poisoning, gas gangrene, and certain other conditions are treated with hyperbaric O_2 in pressure chambers. In all these circumstances, serious and even lethal injury can occur acutely after exposure to an altered barometric pressure. Successful therapy depends upon accurate assessment and appropriate intervention by the physician.

Injuries to human beings may occur during pressurization, continuous exposure to a constant pressure, or decompression. In most instances the injuries appear mediated by concurrent obligatory changes in pressures of ambient gases. Decompression sickness and toxicity from oxygen are the most important examples. The former is thought to occur principally during excessively rapid decompression when dissolved inert gases in the body, no longer in equilibrium with a falling pressure, undergo a change of physical state and bubbles form; this gas phase within blood vessels and tissue leads presumably to the clinical presentation of pain and organ malfunction. Toxicity from O_2 occurs after exposure to an excessive dose. The pulmonary manifestations become evident after continuous exposures of approximately 24 h to pure O_2 at sea level (1 atm abs) and after as short a time as 6 h at 2 atm abs. Concentrations greater than 2.5 atm abs will produce neurologic toxicity, with convulsions, before overt pulmonary problems become evident. In some instances, injuries may be due to altered barometric pressure alone. Some authorities regard the recently described high-pressure nervous syndrome, occurring at extreme depths of water, as an example of a phenomenon induced by pressure alone. The special environment in which altered pressure is encountered can lead to serious and even lethal injury also. Divers face imminent death from drowning should they become detached from a functioning breathing apparatus. Mechanical failure of an environmental chamber or aircraft cabin leading to accidental explosive decompression may cause lethal injury due to decompression sickness or air embolism. Also, human beings can be and have been incinerated by fire during confinement. When a high concentration of O_2 is present in a confined environment, quenching measures lag far behind the mercurial spread of fire.

The application of preventive measures has been successful in reducing injuries. Gradual decompression, after hyperbaric exposure, affords high (95 percent) but not complete protection from symptomatic decompression sickness. Inhalation of pure O_2 will accelerate elimination of inert gases from body tissues by lowering the partial pressure of inert gases in the blood; this is the only satisfactory means for preventing the occurrence of decompression sickness during a rapid ascent to high altitudes. Toxicity from O_2 can be prevented in most instances by prudent selection of proper breathing gases during hyperbaric exposures. Proper training of divers can substantially reduce the risk from drowning and loss of consciousness following breath holding or hyperventilation. The mechanical failure of essential equipment can be reduced by careful design and improved operational procedures. Among measures recommended to minimize the risk of fire are avoidance of flammable gases, elimination of equipment capable of causing ignition, and selective administration of oxygen via individual breathing assemblies, thereby avoiding the requirement to fill large environmental chambers with O_2.

Once injury has occurred, the effectiveness of treatment

depends upon the nature of the problem. In general, prompt implementation of therapy is associated with satisfactory results in most dysbaric injuries. Decompression sickness is a good example. Recompression therapy is remarkably effective in both mild and severe cases. Moribund victims have recovered dramatically following prompt treatment. Even after substantial delays in implementing therapy, reversal of major neurologic deficits has occurred. Use of recently developed special treatment tables, employing O_2 at less than 3 atm abs, has been associated with further improvement of overall results.

In order to achieve the best possible results from treatment, dysbaric injury must be recognized promptly and the victim should be transported immediately to a facility providing a technologic and human capability for implementing recompression therapy. In cooperation with divers and other lay groups, the physician bears responsibility for organizing an effective total system for retrieval and therapy. Recruitment and training of lay persons is an essential part of this responsibility.

EFFECTS OF PRESSURIZATION AND EXPOSURE TO INCREASED BAROMETRIC PRESSURE **Barotrauma** Human beings tolerate huge increases in ambient pressure provided hydraulic forces are distributed evenly. Small gradients of hydrostatic pressure may cause severe discomfort, however. Characteristic loci are occluded rigid-walled, gas-containing pockets within the body, such as the paranasal sinuses, carious teeth, and middle ear. In response to the relatively negative pressure within the closed space, transudation and hemorrhage occur until the pressure gradient no longer exists. If the middle ear is affected (barotitis), the accumulation of fluid can be visualized readily. The course is benign, and treatment beyond decongestants and analgesics is seldom necessary.

Compression arthralgia Rapid pressurization, in excess of 3 atm abs per min, to pressures greater than 10 atm abs, will be associated frequently with arthralgia. This occasionally disabling phenomenon does not occur during relatively slow pressurization. The cause is obscure; speculation concerning it has centered about osmotic shifts of fluid away from involved joints because tissue gas tensions are temporarily less than in blood. Compression arthralgia subsides generally within a few hours after terminating pressurization.

High-pressure nervous syndrome In recent years, a new phenomenon, designated as the "high-pressure nervous syndrome," has been observed in persons at approximately 34 atm abs. Manifestations, which involve the central nervous system principally, include neuromuscular disturbances (incoordination, fasciculations, and tremors) and impaired function of higher centers (disorientation, transient somnolence, and impaired balance). In other mammalian species, exposures to substantially greater pressures have led to convulsions and death. If the rate of pressurization is very rapid, manifestations may occur at a lesser depth. The severity varies remarkably among different individuals, and amelioration occurs spontaneously within a few hours after interrupting further pressurization. Experimental evidence suggests the possibility that neural membranes are compressed by surrounding increased hydrostatic forces. Attendant clinical disability in humans can be minimized by slowed rates of compression, by scheduled brief interruptions of pressurization, and by use of a ternary gas mixture in which nitrogen is added to the customary helium-O_2 mixture.

Increased density of the breathing gas Inhaled gas density increases linearly with pressure. As a result, the calculated work of breathing increases greatly. If the breathing gas density is seven or more times that of air at sea level, maximal ventilation will be reduced so that the capacity for performing work is severely constrained. Substitution of helium, a very light gas, for nitrogen in the breathing medium reduces the inspired gas density greatly and ventilatory limitations to sustained heavy physical activity can be avoided until the barometric pressure is greater than 31 atm abs.

Inert gas narcosis Persons breathing air at pressures greater than 3 atm abs demonstrate psychomotor impairment similar to that induced by intoxicants, such as alcohol. Perturbations of mood, judgment, and motor performance become more severe as pressure increases; prompt reversal of symptoms occurs during decompression. Experienced divers perform better than neophytes under comparable conditions, but at 10 atm abs disability is uniformly severe. This phenomenon, termed nitrogen narcosis, is caused by the increased pressure of this so-called inert component in air. Multiple inert gases have a narcotic action, seemingly in proportion to solubility in oil. For example, zenon is much more potent than nitrogen. Relatively insoluble gases such as neon and helium have little if any narcotic action. Though the cause of narcosis is not yet established, one plausible explanation—swelling of neural membranes due to absorption of inert gas in lipid—is supported by the antagonistic effects of increased hydrostatic pressure in experimental models. Extraordinary diving feats to extreme depths in recent years have been made possible by the substitution of a nonnarcotic inert gas, helium, for nitrogen in the breathing medium. The risks associated with narcosis can be reduced further by limiting descents by air-breathing divers to less than 150 to 200 ft (less than 7.5 atm abs). Helium-O_2 breathing gases should be employed for deeper dives.

Counterdiffusion phenomena Recently, a remarkable phenomenon akin to decompression sickness has been observed in those exposed to a constant increased barometric pressure. The manifestations have been primarily cutaneous, with occurrence of pruritic raised lesions during immersion in a helium-O_2 medium, while breathing a gas containing a different inert component. Experimental studies provide good support for the thesis that the cause is diffusion of inert gases in opposite directions between subcutaneous tissues and the external environment. This counterdiffusion of gases, differing in physical characteristics of diffusivity and solubility, leads to supersaturation in involved tissues and formation of gas bubbles at lipid-aqueous interfaces. The ultimate significance of this phenomenon has yet to be elucidated. Substitution of one inert gas for another is common diving practice, however, and as a consequence, extreme caution is recommended presently at pressures greater than 6 to 7 atm abs.

Hyperbaric O_2 effects If pulmonary gas exchange is efficient, breathing O_2 in a hyperbaric environment will lead to significantly increased oxygenation of arterial blood. The increase in content of O_2 is less striking than the increase in the partial pressure of O_2 because of its low solubility coefficient. A twentyfold rise in Pa_{O_2} to 2,000 mmHg, at 3 atm of O_2 abs is not unusual. Under these conditions, vasoconstriction and reduced systemic blood flow occur. Evidence for increased O_2 uptake by tissues has been obtained also, although the storage capacity is very small compared to the rate of metabolic O_2 utilization. Since hypoxia is a common feature in many severe human illnesses, hyperbaric oxygen has been tested as a therapeutic modality. Accumulated experience provides evidence of benefit and strong support for use of this modality in the treatment of decompression sickness, air embolism, carbon monoxide poisoning, and clostridial myonecrosis. Controversy persists concerning clostridial infection, however. Proponents report dramatic improvement in patients and controlled animal models, while opponents find no significant differences in comparing published uncontrolled results in patients with series treated by conventional means only. Failure to utilize available hyperbaric facilities in the treatment of these several clinical problems has led to legal challenge in the courts, however. A number of other clinical problems such as osteomyelitis, osteoradionecrosis, cutaneous burns, severe anemia, and both acute and chronic ischemic processes have been reported also as benefiting from treatment with hyperbaric oxygen; observations are scant or results vary in this latter group, and no general consensus regarding therapeutic merit is yet available. The early hopes for wide therapeutic application of hyperbaric oxygen have remained unfulfilled. In part this is so because hyperbaric oxygenation of arterial blood fails to relieve hypoxia distal to an occluded artery in the absence of an effective microcirculation. Also, the occurrence of overt toxicity after comparatively short exposures to hyperbaric oxygen has prevented continuous employment, as would be desirable in treatment of sustained hypoxia.

O_2 toxicity Overt O_2 toxicity in human beings has two characteristic forms, pulmonary and neural. Pulmonary O_2 toxicity occurs after exposure to 0.5 atm abs or more of O_2. The tolerated latent period may be a few days at sea level and decreases rapidly under hyperbaric conditions, with overt symptoms occurring in humans between the sixth and eighth hours at 2 atm abs. Continuous exposure leads inevitably to irreversible impairment of gas exchange. Pulmonary pathologic findings are those of pneumonia, hemorrhage, edema, changes in the morphology of alveolar cells, and hyalin membrane formation. With exposure to O_2 pressures in excess of 2.5 atm abs, signs of neural toxicity occur before overt pulmonary damage is discernible. The tolerated latent period decreases as the P_{O_2} increases. Twitching, pallor, nausea, and finally convulsions are observed. After interruption of the hyperoxic exposure, prompt improvement ensues, and no lasting damage has been observed in human beings. In experimental animals, continuation of the hyperoxic exposure leads to unconsciousness and death, however.

The mechanism of oxygen toxicity is not known fully, but the mystery has been elucidated in part. Biologic oxidations, enzymatic and otherwise, generate formation of free radicals. These reactive intermediates participate readily in chemical reactions that are inimical to cellular integrity. These destructive reactions are prevented or minimized by elaborate and specific defense mechanisms. Tolerance to O_2 correlates well with the level of one enzymatic component of the protectant system, superoxide dismutase. Some observers believe that these defenses are overwhelmed by the increased concentration of O_2. Others believe that inactivation of key enzymes or inadequate repletion of high-energy intermediates within the cell are principal causes of O_2 toxicity.

Intermittent exposure is by far the most utilized approach to prevention of O_2 toxicity. Both the hyperbaric therapist and the diving medical officer have learned to limit the dose of O_2 to 3 atm abs or less, with each treatment period constrained, in general, to less than 3 h. Simple sedative compounds such as chloral hydrate are used also to prevent convulsive seizures in circumstances where these are anticipated, as in acutely ill febrile patients.

Other helium effects Helium, an essential component of the breathing gas during deep dives, imposes significant functional burdens by distorting speech patterns so that essential communication from the diver is impaired. Speech unscramblers ameliorate this problem to some extent, but other special means of communication are generally necessary in order for adequate communication to be maintained. Also body heat loss is excessively rapid in helium; as a consequence, the comfort zone of temperature is relatively narrow and individuals so exposed complain frequently of being too cold or too warm. Careful selection of garments and sophisticated environmental control systems are partially effective preventive measures.

Intercurrent illness After prolonged exposure to increased atmospheric pressure, the risk of decompression sickness precludes a safe rapid return to sea level. With exposures to very greatly increased atmospheric pressures, a rapid reduction in ambient pressure would be fatal. Therefore, any intercurrent illness requires assessment and treatment in the hyperbaric environment. Anticipation of potential problems, adequate provision of necessary supplies, and special medical training of exposed personnel may be of the utmost therapeutic importance in managing inevitable medical casualties successfully.

EFFECTS OF DECOMPRESSION Decompression sickness The most important injury associated with decompression is decompression sickness. Evolution of a gas phase in tissues and blood due to excessively rapid elimination of stored inert gas is known to be the principal cause. This may occur either during decompression after a hyperbaric exposure to more than 2 atm abs or during a simulated ascent from sea level (decompression) to less than 0.5 atm abs. Excessive body weight, prolonged exposure, and exercise are aggravating factors, presumably because of increased tissue uptake of inert gas. Increasing age, fatigue, and past injury are among known aggravating factors that are presumed to be associated with relative impairment of gas transport from tissues to the external environment. A well-known phenomenon affecting the likelihood of decompression sickness is acclimatization. After regular exposure to increased pressure, individuals become less susceptible to overt decompression sickness. Acclimatization is lost when regular hyperbaric exposures terminate. Diverse secondary effects complicate the pathophysiologic evolution of decompression sickness. Intravascular fluid volume is depleted, and platelet–red blood cell aggregates form, with release of active intermediate compounds such as serotonin and adenosine compounds.

The clinical manifestations of decompression sickness are diverse, presumably reflecting sequestration of gas bubbles in the various vascular beds and extravascular spaces. Overt consequences may ensue only after bubbles lodge in regions where they produce ischemia and lead to pain or disturbed function. Separate classification of minor (type 1) and serious (type 2) clinical manifestations as tabulated in Table 123-1 facilitates recognition of diverse clinical patterns and formulation of treatment plans appropriate to severity in the individual patient. Minor and severe manifestations of decompression sickness may be present in the same individual in more than 30 percent of the cases, however, and a careful search for subtle type 2 involvement is mandatory in all instances.

Mild (type 1) decompression sickness is characterized by pain and cutaneous or lymphatic involvement. Pain is the most common manifestation, with limb localization in or near joints. After excursion dives in which compressed air is breathed, pain occurs three times more often in the upper as compared to lower limbs. After deep oxygen-helium diving, or after prolonged exposure to compressed air, as is the case for caisson workers, pain occurs three to four times more often in lower than in upper limbs. Initially, the victim may be aware only of numbness. Characteristically, the discomfort becomes more severe with the passage of time and may be so intense as to require therapy with potent analgesic medications. Local edema may occur over the site of pain. During prompt recompression, the pain subsides completely or lessens. Untreated limb pain will subside gradually over a period of days. Cutaneous manifestations of decompression sickness include pruritus and cutaneous circulatory manifestations in which pruritus is followed within an hour by patchy cutaneous vasodilatation, associated at times with evidence of vascular stasis, i.e., central cyanotic areas giving a mottled appearance. No treatment is required for pruritus alone. Recompression is rapidly effective for cutaneous lesions. Untreated symptoms regress gradually over a 2- to 3-day interval. A less common manifestation of mild (type 1) decompression sickness is localized edema. Lymphatic obstruction is a significant etiologic factor in many of these cases. Again, recompression provides prompt relief. Inappropriate fatigue, after decompression, is also common. Although the cause is obscure, excessive malaise is regarded as an integral part of the clinical picture associated with decompression sickness.

Serious (type 2) decompression sickness is characterized by neural or cardiorespiratory involvement. Manifestations are diverse, multifocal, and unpredictable. In the absence of recompression therapy, the natural history of type 2 decompression sickness is also variable. More fulminant cases may terminate in cardiorespiratory collapse and death. Permanent serious neurologic deficits including paraplegia may occur. In other instances, severe neurologic deficits resolve gradually over periods of weeks and months.

Neurologic lesions in type 2 decompression sickness involve the spinal cord far more commonly than the central nervous system. The onset may be insidious, with a sequence of limb paresthesia or weakness followed within some minutes by paralysis. One useful premonitory manifestation is the occurrence of girdle pains in the trunk. Central nervous system manifestations include visual aberrations, headaches, abnormal behavior, and disturbed labyrinthine function with vertigo, nystagmus, nausea, and vomiting. Migraine-like symptoms also occur, particularly in individuals with histories of true migraine headaches.

Type 2 decompression sickness involving the cardiorespiratory systems is characterized by substernal discomfort, cough, dyspnea, tachypnea, and malaise. During inhalation, a sharp "catch" sensation is characteristic ("chokes"). In instances of serious (type 2) decompression sickness, particularly when more than one recompression is required, manifestations of hemoconcentration and hypovolemic shock are noted occasionally. Postural hypotension, oliguria, and very high hematocrits have been reported. In these clinical situations, ancillary therapy, including fluid repletion, colloid infusions, glucocorticoid, and heparin administration, may be particularly important.

Under circumstances in which decompression sickness is a valid consideration, the most important differential diag-

TABLE 123-1
Signs and symptoms of decompression sickness

Type 1 (mild)		*Type 2 (severe)*		*Types 1 and 2*
Extremities	*Skin*	*Central nervous system*	*Cardiorespiratory*	*Systemic*
Pain (bends), paresthesia, numbness, edema	Pruritus, mottling, rash, pallor	Loss of consciousness, scintillating scotomas, Ménière's syndrome, vertigo, aphasia, staggering gait, spastic paralysis, sensory loss, bladder and bowel paralysis	Substernal distress, paroxysmal coughing, tachypnea, asphyxia (chokes), shock, hemoconcentration, platelet-RBC aggregates	Malaise, altered body temperature,* sweating

* *Not clearly associated with type 1 category.*

nostic consideration is pulmonary barotrauma resulting in one or more of three characteristic complications: intraarterial air embolism, mediastinal emphysema, and pneumothorax. In the former instance, neurologic sequelae, including loss of consciousness, are characteristically prompt and severe. Less severe cases may not permit differentiation on a clinical basis, however. Penetration of air into the mediastinum or pleural compartment is associated with complaints of chest pain, dyspnea, hemoptysis, and at times, subcutaneous crepitation. The problem of recognition is simplified somewhat in practice by the requirement for prompt recompression both for severe decompression sickness and for intraarterial air embolism.

Bone necrosis Repetitive prolonged exposure to air at pressure is associated with the occurrence of infarcts in long bones. Lesions may become evident after many months or years have elapsed. If the infarct occurs at an articular surface, subsequent destruction of the joint surface can be disabling; but if the lesion is elsewhere than at a joint surface, there are no symptoms. Caisson workers exposed repeatedly for more than 3 h to pressures greater than 3 atm abs are particularly vulnerable, and careful medical supervision is mandatory. Rigorous conservative decompression schedules appear to reduce the frequency of bone infarcts. This potentially serious medical problem is assessed best by periodic radiologic survey of the long bones. Special radiographic techniques and assessment by observers with experience or special training in interpretation increase the reliability of these diagnostic procedures.

Prevention of decompression sickness Acute decompression sickness can be prevented or the incidence minimized by gradual decompression after a hyperbaric exposure or by breathing pure O_2 prior to exposure to less than normal atmospheric pressure. In the former instance, increased body stores of inert gas, accumulated during the hyperbaric exposure, are eliminated from the body during gradual decompression without development of overt symptoms. In the latter circumstance, the breathing of pure O_2 will reduce body stores of inert gas dramatically. The likelihood of subsequent serious aerial decompression sickness is reduced dramatically as a consequence. Schedules for safe decompression have, for the most part, been derived from empiric testing and are approximately 95 percent effective.

Treatment of decompression sickness Acute decompression sickness is treated with recompression. Recently developed special tables, employing intermittent periods of pure oxygen and air breathing at slightly less than 3 atm abs are convenient, safe, and effective. In cases where severe central nervous system involvement is present, these tables are being used with increasing frequency and considerable success. Some experts prefer immediate recompression to greater pressures, however, and this is the universal recommendation when relief is not obtained by breathing O_2 at shallow depths. Criteria and details of treatment schedules are outlined fully in the *U.S. Navy Diving Manual.* Of particular interest is the common observation that serious disability will respond to recompression therapy even after some days have elapsed. The prognosis for full recovery is good even when the initial response is partial, rather than complete. Ultimate full restoration of function may occur over as long a period as 2 years. In addition to recompression therapy, general supportive measures, fluid repletion, anticoagulants, low molecular weight dextran infusions, and resuscitation measures have been reported to be beneficial. Though extensive multiple-treatment measures are seldom necessary in uncomplicated cases, the occasional victim presenting with severe cardiorespiratory and neurologic dysfunction may require intensive management in an acute care unit of a modern hospital.

Pulmonary barotrauma Failure to exhale during rapid decompression, as in the case of a free ascent in water to the surface, causes a positive gradient of pressure to develop between the intrapulmonary compartment and the external environment. An occasional consequence is rupture of intrapulmonary blood vessels and entrance of free gas into pulmonary venous blood, the pleural compartment, or the mediastinum. Dissemination of free gas, in relatively large quantities, to the central nervous system is associated with profound impairment of function, including loss of consciousness and motor paralysis. This very serious and acute illness is termed *air embolism.* Instances have been reported following a too-rapid ascent from depths of less than 15 ft. Scuba diving and submarine escape training are two circumstances in which the occurrence of air embolism, shortly after ascent to the surface, is not uncommon. Characteristically, the central nervous system deficit is severe, and recompression treatment must commence within a very few minutes if a satisfactory outcome is to be attained. Occasionally, manifestations are less severe and, if the circumstances are such that decompression sickness is possible, a reliable diagnostic separation may be impossible. The manifestations of pneumothorax and mediastinal emphysema differ from spontaneous occurrences of these entities only in the clinical setting of prior rapid surfacing from a dive.

Prevention of air embolism by proper training of divers and by elimination of especially susceptible populations is the most effective form of management. Individuals with structural pulmonary abnormalities, particularly with cystic changes, are regarded as particularly vulnerable. The importance of preventive training is magnified by the poor results that follow delayed recompression treatment.

EFFECTS OF EXPOSURE TO HIGH ALTITUDE **Acclimatization** Millions of persons live permanently at high altitude, more than 1 mile above sea level. The number at the extreme upper limit of approximately 18,000 ft is small, however. These hardy individuals work hard and rear their families successfully despite an inspired $P\text{O}_2$ that approximates half the sea level value. Intensive study of Andean natives, living under these severe conditions, has revealed characteristic adaptations, including a decreased body weight relative to height, an increased vital capacity and ventilatory capacity, increased red blood cell mass and myoglobin, elevated pulmonary arterial pressures, hypertrophy of muscle both in the right ventricle and in smaller pulmonary vessels, vasoconstriction, and a shift of the hemoglobin dissociation curve to the right, facilitating unloading of oxygen at a higher relative Po_2.

A newcomer to altitude undergoes acclimatization over an extended interval. Initial acute symptoms include dyspnea, tachycardia, malaise, headache, and insomnia. Physical activity and ascent to a higher altitude exacerbate these symptoms, reflecting hypoxia, compensatory hyperventilation, and associated respiratory alkalosis. The more acute symptoms usually subside within a few days. During a subsequent interval, lasting up to 1 month, increased pulmonary ventilatory capacity and cardiac output, a gradual increase in red blood cell mass and hemoglobin, increased myoglobin, and altered perfusion of certain tissues are among the observed compensatory changes that tend to restore a more normal aerobic capability.

High-altitude pulmonary edema A unique syndrome of pulmonary edema occurs in some unacclimatized healthy persons who travel within a day or so from their homes in a sea level environment to an elevation of over 9,000 ft. Residents at high altitude, living for a time at sea level, also may develop acute pulmonary edema on returning to altitude. Characteristic manifestations include tachycardia, rapid respirations, cyanosis, rales, x-ray changes of confluent or nodular alveolar densities, and a prompt response to rational management. Removal to a lower elevation, O_2 inhalation, and conventional measures for treatment of pulmonary edema are beneficial. This syndrome can be prevented in large part by gradual acclimatization with adequate staging of the ascent to a high altitude.

Chronic mountain sickness Occasionally long-term dwellers at high altitude lose tolerance to this environment. Erythrocytosis occurs, with a hematocrit usually in excess of 70 percent. The classic findings of cor pulmonale ensue, including fatigue, dyspnea, somnolence, cyanosis, plethora, clubbing, and pulmonary hypertension. Treatment with O_2 is associated with prompt improvement, and this syndrome resolves upon removal to a sea level environment. Hypoventilation appears to be a key element in the etiologic chain. As a consequence, this syndrome of chronic mountain sickness, or Monge's disease, has much in common with the idiopathic hypoventilation syndrome observed at sea level. The reason for the apparent diminished respiratory response to hypoxia is obscure.

REFERENCES

BEHNKE AR: Decompression sickness: Advances and interpretations. Aerosp Med 42:255, 1971

BENNETT PB, ELLIOTT DH (eds): *Physiology and Medicine in Diving and Compressed Air Work,* Baltimore: Williams and Wilkins, 1975

CLARK JM: The toxicity of oxygen. Am Rev Resp Dis 110(6):40, part 2, 1974

GREGORY EM, FRIDOVICH I: Oxygen toxicity and the superoxide dismutase. J Bacteriol 114:1193, 1973

HOLLAND JA et al: Experimental and clinical experience with hyperbaric oxygen in the treatment of clostridial myonecrosis. Surgery 77:75, 1975

NATIONAL ACADEMY OF SCIENCE, NATIONAL RESEARCH COUNCIL: *Fundamentals of Hyperbaric Medicine,* Washington: Federation of American Scientists for Experimental Biology, 1966

PRATT PC: Pathology of pulmonary oxygen toxicity. Am Rev Resp Dis 110(6):51, part 2, 1974

SALTZMAN HA et al: Effects of pressure on ventilation and gas exchange in man. J Appl Physiol 30:43, 1971

U.S. NAVY DIVING MANUAL, Nav. Ships 0994-001-9010, Washington: Navy Department, 1973

124
PROBLEMS OF AIR AND SPACE TRAVEL

STUART BONDURANT

Ordinary air travel imposes so little physiologic stress that most patients who can be moved at all can be moved by air if proper equipment and attendants are available. Medical problems unique to air travel may be caused by unusual environmental conditions which may be encountered because of limitations of equipment or abnormal operating circumstances.

Many modern aircraft fly at altitudes of 20,000 to 40,000 ft, with cabins pressurized to maintain an effective cabin altitude of less than 7,500 ft (jets) or 9,000 ft (reciprocating engines). Unusual accelerations may be encountered, and the normal metabolic diurnal rhythm may be disturbed by rapid movement between time zones.

ALTITUDE An increase in altitude is equivalent to a decrease in barometric pressure. There is a consequent reduction in the partial pressure of oxygen and an increase in the volume of any gas trapped within the body (Table 124-1). The normal person acclimatized to sea level can tolerate oxygen tension equivalent to that at altitudes of 10,000 to 12,000 ft with little change in arterial oxygen saturation. At altitudes above 12,000 ft, hypoxia becomes more marked and supplementary oxygen is usually used. By breathing 100 percent oxygen, one can maintain normal oxygen saturation at altitudes of 30,000 to 35,000 ft.

TABLE 124-1
Representative values of arterial oxygen and the relative volume of gas at various altitudes

		Arterial blood		
Altitude, ft	*Pressure, mmHg*	*Oxygen tension, mmHg*	*Oxygen saturation, %*	*Relative volume of gas*
0	760	94	98	1.0
5,000	632	66	92	1.2
8,000	564	60	89	1.25
10,000	523	53	86	1.5
14,000	446	44	79	1.7
18,000	379	36	71	2.0
37,500 with 100% O_2	159	74	94	4.8
44,000 with 100% O_2	116	36	72	6.5

A second consequence of decreased barometric pressure is expansion of gas trapped in body cavities. In the normal person, intestinal gas is passed as it expands, and middle-ear and sinus air escapes without difficulty during ascent. Gas which cannot escape (as in the case of pneumothorax or pneumoperitoneum) may cause pain, injury, or death. Patients with intracranial gas from wounds or diagnostic procedures in body cavities should not be exposed to a significant decrease in barometric pressure.

ACCELERATION Acceleration is the instantaneous rate of change of velocity. The unit of acceleration, *g*, is the acceleration of a body which is falling freely *in vacuo* due to earth's gravity. It represents a change in velocity of 32.2 ft per s each second. Most of the physiologic consequences of acceleration are due to the force (inertia) which is equal in magnitude but opposite in direction to that causing the acceleration. Thus, headward acceleration causes footward displacement of soft tissues and blood. Duration, magnitude, direction, and rate of onset of acceleration determine the physiologic effects. In general, the longer and greater the acceleration, the less well it is tolerated. Prolonged forward or backward acceleration is tolerated better (approximately 14 to 20*g*, limited by apnea) than headward acceleration (4 to 7*g*, limited by blackout and cerebral ischemia); footward acceleration (3 to 5*g*, limited by asystole and conjunctival and mucous membrane bleeding) is tolerated least well. Brief headward accelerations of 25*g* and backward accelerations of 40*g* are tolerated by normal subjects when well positioned and supported. In ordinary flight, linear accelerations greater than 1*g* are not encountered. Turbulent flight may cause brief linear accelerations of 10 to 12*g*, which are great enough to cause fractures in persons who are not restrained. Angular accelerations of turn and the linear-angular accelerations of turbulent flight are important causes of motion sickness.

DIURNAL RHYTHMS A dissociation between metabolic diurnal rhythms and actual local time may occur following longitudinal flight or flight over the poles. From 3 to 5 days may be required for diurnal metabolic rhythms to come into phase with the new local time. There are no proved adverse clinical or physiologic effects of changing the diurnal rhythm. However, the management of diseases with diurnal manifestations, such as peptic ulcer, and the scheduling of important medications, such as insulin, should be carefully planned in preparation for a trip to another time zone.

MISCELLANEOUS Some fuels and lubricants and their combustion products are toxic and may, with equipment failure, become concentrated in closed cabins. Reciprocating engines produce large quantities of carbon monoxide. Jet engines use fuels which are vesicants, with fumes that may cause nausea, vomiting, and headache. Pyrolysis of lubricating oils produces fumes which cause conjunctival irritation. Ozone has not accumulated in toxic quantities.

Flight line personnel develop hearing loss after prolonged exposure to jet noise unless protected by position or by mechanical devices. Noise levels inside aircraft are very low, and those in terminals and around airfields are apparently insufficient to cause hearing loss.

SUPERSONIC TRANSPORT Supersonic transports cruise at speeds of Mach 2 to Mach 3 (1,300 to 1,800 mi per h) at altitudes of 50,000 to 70,000 ft. Cabin pressure, oxygen content, and temperature are similar to those of current jet aircraft. There are two potential environmental hazards which are not present in ordinary subsonic air travel: ozone and radiation.

Ozone is present in the toxic concentration of 6 to 9 ppm at the operational altitude of the supersonic transport. For this reason, the cabin atmosphere control system includes thermal or catalytic devices for the dissociation of ozone to maintain concentrations below 0.2 ppm.

Passengers and crew can be exposed to galactic cosmic radiation and to solar flare radiation. Under the most adverse ordinary circumstances galactic cosmic radiation, composed of protons, alpha particles, and a few heavy nuclei, can be less than 2 millirem (mrem) per h or approximately 6 mrem for a single intercontinental flight. The aircrew may receive 2 rem per year from this source. Solar flares produce protons and heavy nuclei. During a major solar flare, the dose rate for a passenger may reach 2 millirads (mrd) per h. For this reason, the aircraft carry radiation monitoring equipment and descend to lower altitudes when major solar flares occur.

The supersonic transport causes a sonic boom, or wave of overpressure, of approximately 2.0 lb per ft^2 at ground level along a corridor of 25 mi on each side of the flight path. Overpressure of this magnitude does not cause physical or physiologic damage but does cause psychologic reactions.

AIRCREW SELECTION Physical requirements for aircrews are described in appropriate governmental and airlines literature. Absence of circulatory, pulmonary, neurologic, visual, and auditory defects is of particular importance.

AIR TRANSPORTATION OF PATIENTS Since it is now possible to fly without experiencing physiologically significant departure from the usual environmental conditions, there are no absolute medical contraindications to moving patients by air. However, in many instances patients should not be moved at all, and in others, adequate aircraft with pressurized cabin and attending personnel may not be available. Commercial airlines will carry many patients subject to the discretion of the airline medical director. In addition to the condition of the patient, the comfort and convenience of other passengers must be a major factor in the decision of the commercial airlines. The following points apply to air transportation in general. Specific advice concerning commercial air transportation should be obtained from the appropriate airline medical director.

Circulatory disease The lower partial pressure of oxygen which may be encountered constitutes the major deterrent to flight for patients with circulatory diseases. With oxygen breathing, normal arterial oxygen saturation can be maintained at all altitudes encountered in routine flight (Table 124-1). There is no evidence that ordinary flying is associated with an increased incidence of angina, myocardial infarction, or cerebral vascular accidents.

Coronary artery disease manifested by occasional angina or old myocardial infarction, minimal cerebral or peripheral vascular disease, hypertension, and compensated congenital or rheumatic heart disease appears to entail no added risk in flying. Patients with angina related to emotional stress may benefit from preflight sedation.

Patients with severe or frequent angina, severe hypertension, recent vascular accidents, or cardiac decompensation at rest or with moderate exercise should fly only when a pressurized aircraft or supplementary oxygen is available to maintain ambient oxygen tension at levels of 150 mmHg (sea level equivalent) or more. It is generally considered preferable to forego unnecessary flying for 6 weeks after a myocardial infarction or a cerebral infarction or hemorrhage.

Pulmonary disease Persons with pulmonary decompensation at rest or with very mild exercise should fly only if ambient oxygen tension is maintained at levels of 150 mmHg or more and facilities and personnel are available to treat acute ventilatory decompensation. Persons with pulmonary decompensation with moderate (two flights of stairs) or severe exercise usually fly without difficulty to altitudes of 10,000 ft. Asthmatic patients who do not respond well to self-administered treatment should not fly unattended during acute episodes. The likelihood of rupture of an emphysematous bleb does not appear to be increased by ordinary flight. Because of the increase in volume of bullae as altitude increases (Table 124-1), patients with marked bullous emphysema are advised not to fly above 6,000 ft. Individuals with pneumothorax should not fly unless the cabin pressure is maintained at ground-level equivalent. Expansion of the trapped gas causes, in effect, a tension pneumothorax. Several patients with therapeutic pneumothorax have died in flight.

Hematologic disease In the absence of cardiopulmonary disease, patients with a hemoglobin of 7 to 9 g per 100 ml usually tolerate flight at 4,000 to 6,000 ft without difficulty. If greater cabin altitudes are to be encountered, hemoglobin should be above 10 g per 100 ml.

Hypoxia causes increased sickling of erythrocytes containing hemoglobin S. There have been many well-documented reports of splenic infarction in patients with hemoglobin S during flights which usually exceeded 10,000 ft and lasted for several hours. Two patients with SC hemoglobin have had splenic infarctions during flights which did not exceed 6,000 ft. If ambient oxygen tension cannot be maintained at 150 mmHg, flying is contraindicated for patients with SS (sickle-cell anemia) and SC hemoglobin and for those with SA (sickle-cell trait) who have large quantities of hemoglobin S. Others with hemoglobin S should be restricted to cabin altitudes below 10,000 ft. Symptoms of splenic infarction, nausea, vomiting, left upper quadrant pain, and shock should be treated with supplemental oxygen and immediate return to ground level.

Pregnancy A large amount of experience has accumulated which suggests that ordinary flying has no adverse effects on the normal pregnant woman or fetus. Pregnant women should sit, when possible, facing the rear of the plane and should place the seat belt over the upper thighs and hips rather than around the abdomen. When pregnancy is complicated by preeclampsia or cardiopulmonary or hematologic disease, considerations similar to those discussed above for the nonpregnant patient apply.

Ear, nose, and throat disease Acute infections of the upper respiratory tract and chronic sinusitis may obstruct the eustachian tubes or sinus ducts, with barotitis or barosinusitis resulting when external pressure is increased during descent. If it is necessary for a person with acute upper respiratory infection to fly, use of a nasal spray containing ½% phenylephrine (Neo-Synephrine) 6, 3, and ½ h before flight and ½ h before descent may help to maintain patency of the ducts. A swallow or a Valsalva maneuver with the nose occluded will usually open the ducts. Children may be fed during descent to encourage swallowing. The treatment of barotrauma depends on its severity and the underlying cause. Intubation of the eustachian tubes is not advised. In most instances, conservative treatment with decongestants will suffice. Severe barotitis may be associated with hemorrhage into the middle ear, requiring myringotomy and aspiration of blood to prevent ossicular ankylosis. Plastic repair of the ducts may be required to prevent recurrence.

Metabolic disease Control of diabetes may be complicated by rapid movement from one time zone to another and by motion sickness. Careful planning of the flight in terms of elapsed rather than local time, with consideration of the meals to be served and appropriate management of motion sickness, should enable the patient with well-controlled diabetes to fly without difficulty. Patients in diabetic acidosis may be transported after treatment is started if in-flight medical facilities are adequate.

Communicable disease Persons known to have a communicable disease may not enter a state or nation without the consent of the local health department.

Postoperative conditions Because of the expansion of abdominal gas with decrease in barometric pressure, it is generally considered preferable to forego flying for 10 days after abdominal or other major surgery. However, experience with air evacuation of military casualties suggests that, with proper facilities and personnel, practically all patients whose condition is stable can be moved by air if necessary. Most persons with fractures are flown without difficulty. Fracture of the mandible, particularly when the mandible is immoblized, constitutes a special problem because of the possibility of vomiting and aspiration. A quick-release wire support has been designed for in-flight use.

Epilepsy Most patients with well-controlled epilepsy fly to altitudes of 10,000 ft without difficulty. Flight to greater altitude in unpressurized aircraft may precipitate seizures.

MOTION SICKNESS The use of modern aircraft has considerably reduced the incidence of motion sickness. The problem remains because of occasional turbulent flights and persons who are extremely susceptible to motion sickness. Such persons should sit over the wings of the aircraft, where motion is least. Cyclizine (Marezine) 50 mg, meclizine (Bonine) 25 mg, and dimenhydrinate (Dramamine) 50 mg are effective prophylactic agents.

SPACE TRAVEL The medical problems of space flight relate in part to the design of spacecraft and propulsion systems and in part to the characteristics of the space environment.

With design and engineering improvements it will be possible to build spacecraft which require only a small departure from our ordinary environment. For example, the accelerations of launch and reentry which are of the order of 4 to 8*g* in present systems could be reduced to a fraction of a *g* by prolonging the time of acceleration. Present Soviet manned space systems operate with a cabin atmosphere which is very near that at sea level on earth. To avoid the effects of weightlessness, an acceleration equivalent to that of the earth's gravity can be produced by rotating the spacecraft, if this should prove necessary. Radiation shielding can be provided, albeit with a weight penalty. Present space systems represent a series of engineering compromises which are necessary largely because of the limitations of the propulsion systems.

During space flight several adaptations have been observed. Human performance, eating, drinking, urination and defecation, respiration, heart rate, and blood pressure have showed no important changes. Weight loss may occur during the first few days of orbital flight. It is related in part, at least, to negative water balance associated with decreased fluid intake. Several astronauts have had leukocytosis, that is, 20,000 to 30,000 leukocytes per cubic millimeter of blood, upon return to earth, presumably due to stress and immobilization. There is evidence of a reduction in red blood cell mass during orbital flight, possibly related in part to the high ambient oxygen tension. Astronauts may manifest orthostatic hypotension after return to gravitational field. This may be due to reduced blood volume as well as impaired cardiovascular response to gravity. Weightlessness is associated with a negative calcium balance, but the effect has not been important in flights of less than 2 months' duration.

REFERENCES

GIBBONS HL, FROMHAGEN C: Aeromedical transportation and general aviation. Aerosp Med 42(7):773, 1971

MCFARLAND RA: Air travel across time zones. Am Sci 63:23, 1975

MOYLAN JA, PRUITT BA: Aeromedical transportation. JAMA 224:1271, 1973

OXER HF: Aeromedical evacuation of the seriously ill. Br Med J: 3:692, 1975

PRESTON FS: Medical aspects of aerospace travel. Proc R Soc Med 65:187, 1972

SHAEFER HJ: Radiation exposure in air travel. Science 172:780, 1971

YANOWITCH RE, SIRKIS JA: Air travel and the handicapped. Aerosp Med 45(8):879, 1974

125 RADIATION AND ELECTRICAL INJURIES

EUGENE P. CRONKITE
JAMES F. WALLACE

RADIATION INJURY Types of radiation The types of ionizing radiation most often causing injury are x-rays, gamma rays, alpha and beta rays, protons, and neutrons. X-rays and gamma rays are identical; a separate name was given because of their difference in origin. The former are produced by x-ray machines and as secondary emissions from particle accelerators or electron tubes. The latter are produced by radioactive decay. In general, gamma radiations are more energetic than x-rays; however, the energy spectrum of x-rays is continuous. Beta rays are electrons. Ordinary electrons originate from the shells surrounding the atomic nucleus, and beta rays originate only from within the nucleus. Alpha rays are the stripped nuclei of the helium atom with a mass of 4 and a charge of 2+. Protons are stripped nuclei of hydrogen atoms with a mass of 1 and a charge of 1+. Protons are becoming of more interest because of their common use as primary particles in accelerators and their prevalence as an extraterrestial space radiation as described by Van Allen. Protons are of additional interest since they are usually the secondary damaging particle produced by neutron interaction with tissue or other materials. Neutrons have a mass of 1 and charge of 0. Biologic injury is produced primarily by ionization from secondary charged particles in diverse ways. Fast neutrons react principally with the hydrogen atoms, and as a result of the collision a portion of the energy is imparted to the hydrogen atom and a proton is ejected which does the damage. With thermal or slow neutrons the damage is done by actual capture of the neutrons and a secondary emission of ionizing radiation as the transmuted hydrogen, nitrogen, or other substance in tissue decays and emits radioactivity. These are the basic types of radiation with which a physician may be concerned.

Mechanism of action The most acceptable current view to account for a major part of the biologic effects of radiation may be divided into three interlinked steps. First, photons, or particles, penetrate the protoplasm, interacting to produce ion pairs. This reaction takes of the order of 10^{-13} s. The second step is a primary radiochemical reaction of these ions primarily with water, producing free radicals such as H and OH. These reactions take about 10^{-9} s. These free radicals produce a further chain of reactions with themselves and tissue water to produce further reactive forms such as H_2O_2 and HO_2. These products persist for microseconds or in part a few seconds. The last reaction is between these products and critical protoplasmic molecules. The nature of this last reaction is not known, but since the actual amount of energy imparted to the system is small, it is generally thought that the damage must involve substances of low concentration but major importance to the living system, for example, nucleic acids or enzymes.

Dose units Two dose units are essential for the understanding of the quantitative effects of radiation. The *roent-*

gen (R), a measure of total dose in air, is defined as the quantity of x-ray or gamma radiation such that the associated corpuscular emission per 0.001293 g air at standard conditions produces in air ions carrying one electrostatic unit of either sign. For energy to be deposited, there must be an interaction with matter. Hence, with x-rays passing through a vacuum, no radiation dose is delivered. In practice we are interested in the energy imparted to various tissues from a number of different types of radiation, and it is therefore essential to have a second unit of radiation which overcomes the limitation of the roentgen. This second unit, the *rad* (rd), is a unit of absorbed dose equal to 100 ergs per g of absorbed energy which applies to any type of radiation in any tissue. For small pieces of tissue in an x-ray beam of 1 R per min, the absorbed dose is very close to 1 rd per min. However, as irradiated objects become larger and change in composition, one must consider the diminution in intensity due to the interaction of radiation with matter (buildup and then exponential attenuation) and the changing types of interaction (photoelectric effect, Compton effect, etc.). In tissue of uniform density this leads to a decreasing absorbed dose at successive levels after equilibrium is attained. However, at interfaces such as soft tissue and bone, the absorbed dose may sharply increase. Thus, in addition to the exposure dose in roentgens and the absorbed dose in rads, one must be concerned with the distribution of the absorbed dose in the areas of interest. For example, if there is sufficient protection of bone marrow by shielding of one's own tissues to permit marrow regeneration and survival from what is considered an otherwise fatal *exposure dose,* one may ascribe incorrectly some great benefit to a procedure used therapeutically.

The *density of ionization* in tissue varies with the energy and type of radiation as well as the tissue composition. The density of ionization is referred to as *specific ionization* (ions per unit track length) or as *linear energy transfer* (LET, kiloelectron volts deposited per unit track length). Among other factors, the density of ionization influences the biologic effect for equivalent amounts of energy deposited, in general the effect being greater with more densely ionizing radiation. This leads to consideration of the relative biologic effectiveness (RBE), which is defined as the ratio of the dose in rads of standard radiation (usually x-ray or gamma radiation of 250 to 400 kV energy) to produce a given degree of biologic effect, to the dose in rads of an unknown radiation to produce the same degree of biologic effect. For example, if the median lethal dose (LD_{50}) of x-rays is 600 rd and for neutrons 300 rd, the RBE will be 2. The RBE may vary with the biologic response or the conditions of irradiation. For example, when the same radiations are used, a different value may be obtained for mortality, cataract, or tumor development. Another useful unit is the rem, which stands for roentgen equivalent mammal. Numerically, rem = rads × RBE.

Also of importance is the *dose rate.* In general, the lower the dose rate, the less will be the acute somatic effect. In a crude sense, dose rates in excess of approximately 5 R per min give essentially the same result. However, as the dose rate falls below 5 R per min, the effect per unit of radiation becomes less. In the past, genetic effects were believed independent of dose rate. This implies that all increments of radiation received by the gonads, irrespective of when or how, would add up directly as mutations, to give a total effect ultimately to be measured as detectable effects in succeeding generations. However, it is now known that there is a dose-rate dependence in respect to the production of mutations by irradiation of spermatogonia in mice and also for leukemogenesis in mice, which is considered to be a somatic genetic effect of bone marrow irradiation.

If the dose of radiation is sufficiently high, actual death of any living cell can be observed promptly in terms of classic pathologic criteria of cell necrosis. However, after lower doses of radiation (precise values vary with the tissue), only disturbances in cell proliferation are seen. The rate at which cells divide is decreased. DNA synthesis is impaired in two manners: (1) the rate of synthesis is slower; (2) cells may continue DNA synthesis and become polyploid. It is reasonably certain that radiation has effects other than the outright killing of cells and the interference with mitosis and DNA synthesis.

The diminution in the production of new cells in these tissues that are undergoing continual renewal (mucosa, blood, gonads, etc.) results in a progressive hypoplasia to total atrophy, depending on dose. Some cells still capable of mitosis that are not killed outright may be so injured that they will go through one or two generative cycles, producing abnormal progeny, such as giant metamyelocytes and hypersegmented neutrophils, before dying. The atrophy of these steady-state cell renewal systems and direct injury of other tissues produce clearly defined clinical syndromes.

Clinical phenomena in relation to dose and time after exposure Human experience is based on the effects of atomic bombs; accidental exposure to fallout from a hydrogen bomb; laboratory and reactor accidents in the United States, U.S.S.R., and Yugoslavia; and on *whole-body* clinical radiotherapy. After any radiation accident close cooperation of the physician and health physicist is essential to obtain the best estimate of the radiation dose and to evaluate its probable effect in terms of the likely *distribution of the absorbed dose* in rads. However, clinical signs and symptoms remain paramount in the management of human disease and injury. Physical estimates of dose never substitute for clinical judgment and experience.

Three acute radiation syndromes may be classified generally as *cerebral, gastrointestinal,* and *hematopoietic.*

The *cerebral* syndrome is produced by extremely high doses of radiation, i.e., following exposure to several thousand roentgens. It is always fatal, whether the radiation is delivered to the brain alone or to the whole body. Three processes have been described: a prodromal phase of nausea and vomiting; then listlessness and drowsiness ranging from apathy to prostration (probably traceable to nonbacterial inflammatory foci in the brain); and finally, a more generalized component characterized by tremors, convulsions, ataxia, and death. This sequence was observed in an industrial accident, death occurring 36 h after exposure.

The *gastrointestinal* syndrome occurs when the dose of radiation is lower, in the range of 600 to 1,500 R. It is characterized by intractable nausea, vomiting, and diarrhea; these lead to severe dehydration, diminished plasma volume, vascular collapse, and death. The syndrome is initiated by a pronounced "intoxication," arising presumably from diffuse necrosis of tissue throughout the body; it is extended by severe injury to the gastrointestinal tract. The latter development is caused by two factors: direct killing of a fraction of the crypt cells and inhibition of mitosis. The mature epithelial cells continue to migrate out onto the villus in an orderly fashion, eventually being lost from the tip of the villi; this produces a progressive diminution in the number of cells covering the villi. The epithelial cells progressively become cuboidal and then squamous in appearance, and ultimately the intestinal villi become denuded, with massive loss of bloody plasma into the intestine. The usual 3- to 4-day death from the gastrointestinal syndrome can be prevented by massive plasma replacement during the first 4 to 6 days after irradiation. After doses greater than circa 1,300 R regeneration is poor and slow. After doses below roughly 1,300 R, regeneration commences around the sixth day with complete restoration of the gastrointestinal epithelium. However, the respite is only temporary, since hematopoietic failure will ensue, commencing within 2 to 3 weeks.

The *hematopoietic syndrome* which occurs following whole-body exposure in the midlethal range is accompanied by temporary anorexia, nausea, and vomiting which is maximal between 6 and 12 h after exposure to doses of radiation between 600 and 800 R. Thereafter, the gastrointestinal symptoms rapidly subside so that within 24 to 36 h after exposure the subject is usually asymptomatic. These symptoms have been correlated with a period of rapid necrosis of radiosensitive tissues. The prodromes must be distinguished from the gastrointestinal syndrome described earlier and from that which occurs later on. After subsidence of the prodromes, a period of relative well-being is experienced, during which atrophy of lymph nodes, spleen, and bone marrow progresses, leading to a pancytopenia. This atrophy is the result of two clearly defined processes—direct killing of radiosensitive cells and inhibition of new cell productuion. In the peripheral blood, lymphopenia commences immediately, becoming maximal within 24 to 36 h. Thereafter, the lymphocytes remain at low levels for weeks and recover over several months. Within a few hours after irradiation a neutrophilic leukocytosis appears. Following this an oscillation in the neutrophil count occurs, the rate at which it falls to the minimum being a function of the dose of radiation. After sublethal and low lethal doses, the minimal values occur in 4 to 6 weeks; after high lethal doses granulocytes diminish more rapidly, and minimal values approaching zero appear within 7 to 10 days.

Thrombopenia and its relation to radiation bleeding have been studied exhaustively. After single doses of radiation a close correlation with the decrease in the platelet count and the tendency to bleed is evident. In animals and after various accidents, significant purpura was seen only when the platelet counts fell below 20,000 per mm^3. The platelets remain steady or increase for 2 to 3 days after irradiation and thereafter diminish more or less linearly with time, the ultimate minimum and the rate attained being dose-dependent. After about 200 rd, it takes about 30 days for minimum platelet levels to develop. After 600 to 800 rd, minimal levels were observed within 10 to 12 days. Earlier observations in which bleeding in radiation injury was attributed primarily to hyperheparinemia have been refuted. Today there is no evidence of hyperheparinemia; consequently the use of antiheparin agents in the therapy of bleeding induced by radiation is not indicated. Fresh viable platelet transfusions will stop bleeding, and maintenance of platelet levels by platelet transfusions will prevent development of bleeding in animals.

Decreases in the red blood cell count are prominent only after large doses of radiation that significantly interfere with new cell production and produce bleeding.

Studies of *decreased resistance to infection* have resulted in the conclusion that there are (1) a dose-dependent decrease in circulating granulocytes and lymphocytes; (2) a dose-dependent impairment of antibody production; (3) impairment of granulocyte migration and phagocytosis; (4) decreased ability of the reticuloendothelial system to kill phagocytized bacteria; (5) diminished resistance to diffusion in subcutaneous tissues; and (6) hemorrhagic areas of the skin and bowel that present foci for entrance and growth of bacteria. Obviously an increased susceptibility to infection by both commensals and pathogens must be present.

Inhomogeneous exposure to radiation The preceding description of radiation injury was based primarily on human clinical experience and animal experimentation in which the distribution of dose absorbed by tissues was relatively uniform. However, in actuality, conditions of exposure may be such that there are marked inhomogeneities in absorbed dose. For example, the geometry of an exposure may result in almost no exposure to the lower part of the body and very heavy exposure to the abdomen and hands, resulting in extensive necrosis of the skin of these areas in addition to the fatal injury to deeper tissues. In one accident, the direction of the beam resulted in severe exposure to the head, but the low energy permitted marked attenuation of the beam within the head, so that the absorbed dose through the brain decreased markedly from the side closest to the beam to the side farthest from it. The superficial layers of the brain were injured badly, but death did not ensue because vital centers were not destroyed. In evaluating any radiation accident, one must reconstruct the geometry and consider the probable distribution of absorbed dose within the body. What may initially appear as a fatal accident in terms of air exposure dose may turn out to be sublethal when effects of distribution of the absorbed dose are considered.

Management of acute human radiation injury Presumptive evidence of exposure to radiation and signs or symptoms described earlier must be recognized before there need be cause for concern. No therapy is available for the cerebral form of radiation injury after uniform brain exposure. Whereas a small percentage of persons with the gastrointestinal syndrome may be kept alive until the affected tract regenerates, they must also face the hematopoietic syndrome; hence that is the real therapeutic problem. Therapy rests on the control of the sequelae of marrow aplasia and thus is similar to management of drug-induced and idiopathic marrow aplasia, suggesting that combined use of antibacterials and transfusions would be useful. The spontaneous course of human radiation injury has clearly shown that signs and symptoms develop at different times in different subjects after identical doses of radiation. Accordingly, the time of institution and type of therapy should be individualized. The following general therapeutic regimen is outlined.

1 Prevention and/or control of infection is of major importance since the most common cause of death is infection from gram-negative bacteria. Although not of proved value, ultraisolation techniques should be used if available. Medical staff carrying nasopharyngeal pathogens or with respiratory infections are forbidden entrance to rooms of patients who have suffered potentially fatal irradiation.
2 Observe *fluid* and *electrolyte* balance closely and restore as necessary with appropriate replacement solutions.
3 Provide bland diet.
4 Administer antibiotics as described in Chap. 128 in an attempt to achieve a "sterile" patient and minimize fatal sepsis from gram-negative commensal organisms during the period when blood granulocytes are below 750 per mm^3.
5 *Treat infection* when it develops or relapses. Commence with antibiotics that are effective against a wide spectrum of gram-negative and -positive organisms, for example, cephalothin, gentamicin, ampicillin in maximal dosage (see Chap. 130, Chemotherapy of Infection). One is fighting for additional time to allow spontaneous marrow regeneration. Granulocyte transfusions, although not commonly available, may be lifesaving.
6 *Use fresh whole blood* to control bleeding and/or to restore adequate red blood cell levels. When the hematocrit is returned to normal range, control bleeding by fresh platelet concentrates to keep platelet count above 25,000 per mm^3.

The preceding therapy has increased the survival rate of animals. Unless infection or serious hemorrhage develops, therapy is not needed. Many human beings with epilation, severe pancytopenia, and purpura have recovered without therapy from doses of radiation ranging from 200 to 300 R. Recently individuals who received 400 to 500 R inhomogeneous irradiation have recovered when treated in accordance with this therapeutic regimen despite near-zero granulocyte and platelet counts.

Syngeneic and autologous bone marrow transplantation will prevent death in almost all otherwise fatally irradiated animals up to doses of about 1,200 R. Allogeneic bone marrow transplantation, when successful, may be complicated by a graft-versus-host (GVH) immunologic reaction. This can be minimized but not eliminated by using only donors that are perfectly matched for human lymphocyte histocompatibility antigens (HL-A). In addition GVH disease can be induced by fresh blood, platelet, and granulocyte transfusions containing viable HL-A incompatible lymphocytes in immunosuppressed recipients. The probability of a GVH disease can be reduced by irradiation of the blood, platelets, or granulocytes by 1,500 rd prior to transfusion. Whereas GVH disease may be acutely fatal in some instances, it may assume a chronic form involving degenerative processes particularly in skin, kidneys, and liver.

Although marrow transplantation has been acclaimed as the solution to fatal whole-body radiation, the results in human beings so far do not warrant optimism. This author believes it should be reserved for patients in whom there is a progressive deterioration of the hematopoietic system with granulocytes falling below 500 per mm^3 in the first 2 weeks after exposure and an early rapid decline in the platelet count. In the rare case in which there is an identical twin, bone marrow transplantation should be lifesaving following fatal radiation injury up to a maximum exposure of about 1,200 R. Rigid rules cannot be formulated in advance. Decisions can be made only at the bedside.

Prevention Nothing can substitute for prevention. Shielding, distance, and limiting of exposure time are the only effective preventive measures against exposures from radiation sources, whether in industry, medical practice, military action, or civil defense. A series of drugs, primarily sulfhydryl groups, that will protect against radiation by an effective dose reduction up to 50 percent are available. However, these must be administered within minutes preceding exposure. Accidents and warfare are not predictable. The severe toxic effects of these drugs prevent continuous prophylactic administration.

Long-term effects Radiation alters the "information system" of proliferating somatic and germ cells. Thus the perpetuating cells of the blood, gastrointestinal tract, skin, lens, gonads, and other areas pass on either "bad or inadequate information," presumably in altered DNA, to their progeny, resulting in late somatic disease, e.g., cancer, cataracts, degenerative disorders, or nonspecific shortening of life. Leukemia yield from radiation in human groups has been quantified. It is asserted, but not proved, that there is no threshold and that the yield of leukemia increases with dose. However, the greatest exposure of the American public comes from the medical use of diverse types of radiation (predominantly diagnostic x-rays). If the assumption of no threshold dose for leukemia is correct, the medical uses of radiation are producing their small toll in an additional burden of leukemia and probably other disease also. Therefore, it behooves the practitioner to be exceedingly cautious and to expose patients to radiation only when it is clearly indicated and needed for diagnosis.

Radiation can produce mutation of genes, the information and transmission centers for heredity. Of this there is no doubt. Not all mutations are harmful, but the chances are overwhelming that a change will be detrimental to the species. Not all mutations produce visible, immediately detectable effects. The concern is not only with an increase in the number of obvious freaks or cripples but with changes that will lead to such undesirable characteristics as lowered life expectancy, decreased fertility, a general increase in physical and mental disease, and an increase in fetal or neonatal death rates. It is the less obvious changes that are of the greatest importance. The more obvious changes usually lead to early death in the individual and reduced fertility in those that survive. Thus the harmful mutant is relatively quickly deleted from the population. The more subtle changes, however, are propagated longer and affect a very large number of persons. The mutation may be dominant or recessive. Most dominant mutations are also lethal, and many such mutations may be missed because the fertilized egg never develops far enough to be recognized as a new individual. If the mutation is recessive, the mutant will not become evident unless both parents of the individual have the same mutant genes and transfer these to the individual concerned. It is extremely difficult to quantify these considerations. If the mutation rate were increased by a single exposure of the population to radiation, the effects would be spread through many generations. Half the total damage produced would not be observed until some 30 to 50 generations had been born. These are the practical considerations that make the problem particularly difficult to analyze. Damage that is inflicted now cannot be detected now and will only become evident many generations hence. These considerations also indicate why it is not possible to take negative evidence in populations that have been exposed to date as an indication that the degree of genetic damage is small. If, for instance, an effect were already obvious in the children born of individuals irradiated in Japan by the atom bombs, it would mean that the total genetic effect would be great indeed. These are sobering considerations for thoughtful persons. Since exposure to irradiation cannot be avoided in our modern industrial society and in the practice of medicine and because of the uncertainty about the quantitative effect in producing somatic or genetic effects, it is mandatory that exposure be minimal and rigidly controlled in order to protect the present generations from somatic effects and future generations from genetic effects.

ELECTRICAL INJURIES **Epidemiology** Electrical injury has become progressively more common since the first human fatality from accidental electrocution was reported in 1879. In the United States, approximately 1,000 deaths occur annually from electric current accidents, while another 200 persons die as a result of being struck by lightning. In addition, major electrical burns presently constitute nearly 5 percent of all admissions to burn centers in this country. Electrical injuries occur most commonly among utility pole linemen and construction workers who come into contact with high-tension current, but nearly a third result from accidents in the home or other settings including the hospital with its many electrically powered instruments and appliances.

Pathogenesis In understanding the fundamental aspects of electric current injury, it is helpful to consider some electrophysical principles. For an electric current to flow, there must be a closed pathway or circuit, and a difference in potential or voltage must exist between two points in this completed circuit. The flow of current is directly related to the voltage difference and inversely proportional to the electrical resistance between two points in the circuit (Ohm's law). High-resistance paths allow relatively small currents to flow, while low resistances permit large currents to flow. When voltage is very high, flow of current will likewise be relatively great, unless the resistance is increased proportionally to the voltage; however, if the potential difference between the two points can be minimized, the current flow can also be minimized regardless of resistance.

Although the end result of passage of an electric current through the human body is unpredictable in the individual case, many factors are known to influence the nature and severity of electrical injuries. Body tissues vary considerably in their *resistance* to the flow of current, with conductivity being roughly proportional to water content. Bone and skin offer relatively high resistance, while blood, muscle, and nerve are good conductors. The resistance of normal skin can be lowered by *moisture,* and this factor alone can convert what might ordinarily be a mild injury to a fatal shock. Of importance at the time of contact is *grounding* which, if effective, can minimize the voltage difference between two points in the electric circuit and thus lower the intensity of current passing through the body. The *pathway of the current through the body* is also crucial. An accident involving passage of a current between a point of contact on the leg and the ground is less likely to be injurious than one between the head and the foot, in which the heart lies between the two poles of the circuit. Similarly, a small current leak which would be innocuous when applied to the surface of the intact body may result in a fatal arrhythmia when conducted directly to the heart via a low-resistance intracardiac catheter. *Duration of contact* also influences the outcome of electrical injury. Alternating current is much more dangerous than direct current, partly because of its ability to produce tetanic muscular contractions which prevent the victim from being able to release contact with the circuit. This is usually accompanied by sweating, which lowers skin resistance, allowing current of still greater intensity to pass into the body until fatal cardiac arrhythmia results.

While the effects of electricity upon the body are incompletely understood, many pathophysiologic features of severe electrical injury have been described. In general, when sudden death occurs following low-voltage shock, it is due to the direct effect of relatively small amounts of current upon the myocardium resulting in ventricular fibrillation. With high-tension injury (greater than 1,000 V) cardiac asystole and respiratory arrest occur probably as a result of injury to the medullary centers of the brain.

In addition, contact with high-intensity current may cause three types of thermal injuries. Current coursing externally to the body from the contact point to the ground may generate temperatures as high as 10,000°C and cause extensive carbonification of skin and immediately underlying tissues termed *arc* or *flash burns.* Such burns often ignite surrounding clothing or nearby objects which result in *flame burns.* Finally, there is injury due to the *direct heating* of tissues by electric current. As it traverses the skin, energy from current is converted into heat-producing coagulation necrosis at the points where it enters and exits from the skin as well as in striated muscle and blood vessels through which it passes. The associated vascular injury results in thromboses, often at sites distant from the body surface, and accounts for the observation that a greater amount of tissue destruction characteristically occurs in an electrical injury than is apparent on first inspection.

Pathology In patients who die immediately, autopsy findings are limited to burns and generalized petechial hemorrhages. If patients survive for a period of days or longer, postmortem examination reveals focal necrosis of bone, large blood vessels, muscle, peripheral nerves, spinal cord, or brain. Renal tubular necrosis may also be seen when acute renal failure follows extensive tissue destruction.

Clinical manifestations Immediately after a severe electrical shock, patients are usually comatose, apneic, and in circulatory collapse from ventricular fibrillation or cardiac standstill. Surviving this stage, they often are disoriented, combative, and frequently may have seizures. Often they will be found to have fractures of bone caused either by convulsive muscular contractions accompanying the shock or from falls at the time of the accident. Hypovolemic shock often appears soon after high-tension electrical injury and is due to the rapid loss of fluid into areas of tissue damage, and from body surface burns. Hypotension, along with renal tubular damage from myoglobin and hemoglobin pigments liberated during massive muscle necrosis and hemolysis, may lead to acute renal failure.

Besides the extensive destruction of tissue occurring instantly in electrical burns, additional injury from ischemia produced by swelling of damaged tissues may appear later, often accompanied by severe metabolic acidosis. Other serious complications which may be seen are gastrointestinal hemorrhage from preexisting or acute ulcers, and both anaerobic and aerobic infections originating in inadequately debrided necrotic muscle masses.

Late effects include various neurologic disabilities, visual disturbances, and the residual damage left by burns. Nervous system injuries are frequent and include peripheral neuropathies, incomplete transection of the spinal cord, and reflex sympathetic dystrophies, as well as late convulsive disorders and intractable headache. The development of cataracts of one or both eyes has been reported to occur up to 3 years following electrical injury.

Laboratory findings Immediately following major electrical injury the hematocrit is commonly elevated and the plasma volume reduced, reflecting sequestration of fluid in the wound. Unless extensive flame burns are also present, serial determinations of either of these parameters provide a good means of monitoring the adequacy of fluid replacement therapy. Myoglobinuria is seen frequently in association with severe shocks, and when it persists following establishment of urine flow, usually indicates massive muscle injury. In many patients arterial blood pH determinations will indicate the presence of metabolic acidosis. Lumbar puncture may show elevated pressure associated with cerebral edema or bloody spinal fluid as a result of intracerebral hemorrhage. The electrocardiogram not infrequently shows tachycardia and minor S-T segment alterations which can persist for several weeks following injury. Unexplained acute hypokalemia leading to respiratory arrest and cardiac arrhythmias has developed in some patients between the second and fourth weeks following injury.

Treatment Removal of victims from contact with the current should be accomplished immediately without touching them directly. Rescuers should use a rubber sheet, wooden pole, or other nonconductive material to detach them, and this should be preceded by cutting off the source of current when possible. If the victim is not breathing, mouth-to-mouth ventilation should be instituted at once. Although most cases who survive develop spontaneous respiration within half an hour, complete recovery after longer periods occurs often enough so that respiratory support should be continued for at least 4 h. If there is no evidence of heartbeat, external cardiac massage should accompany ventilatory resuscitation. Persons struck by lightning frequently have cardiac asystole which responds to a manual blow to the chest, while victims of low-voltage shocks will usually require defibrillation to restore heart action. During cardiopulmonary resuscitation and evacuation to the hospital, attention should be paid to possible broken bones and spinal cord injuries incurred at the time of the accident.

Subsequent hospital management of patients with electrothermal injuries requires considerable specialized care; whenever feasible, they should be referred to an appropriate burn or trauma unit.

Rapid institution of fluid and electrolyte therapy for hypovolemic shock and acidosis is essential, with guidelines being the patient's urine output, hematocrit, osmolality, central venous pressure, and arterial blood gases. Standard burn formulas should not be used to estimate fluid therapy since these are based only upon extent of body surface area injury and do not take into account the additional tissue damage usually present. If myoglobinuria persists after adequate urine flow has been established, the use of furosemide or an osmotic diuretic such as mannitol along with alkalinization of the urine is frequently indicated. Management of the electrical wound should include adequate debridement of necrotic tissue and often will require fasciotomy to prevent further ischemic injury. Tetanus prophylaxis should be administered to all burned patients, while topical antimicrobial chemotherapy with Sulfamylon or silver nitrate may be useful in preventing or delaying infections in extensive surface burns. Survivors of the acute episode often require extensive treatment for infection, cerebral edema, and delayed hemorrhage as devitalized tissues slough. If acute renal failure occurs, it should be managed as described in Chap. 272.

Prevention Proper installation of appliances, grounding of telephone lines and radio and television aerials, and the use of rubber gloves and dry shoes when working with electric circuits should be routine. Unused wall sockets should be kept plugged and live extension cords not left unattended, particularly in households where there are young children. During a severe thunderstorm, refuge near hilltops, riverbanks, hedges, telephone poles, and trees should be avoided. The safest shelter is the closed house, while an automobile, cave, ditch, or even lying flat on the ground are relatively secure. In hospitalized patients, the hazard of ventricular fibrillation precipitated by minute current leaks conducted directly to the myocardium from monitoring equipment via pacemakers or intravascular manometric catheters should be more widely appreciated. Hospital personnel should be aware that in addition to medical instruments, patient contact with two or more other power line–operated devices such as television sets, radios, electric razors, lamps, and especially electric beds can also result in electrocution if the heart lies within the current path through the patient. These hazards can be minimized by proper grounding of equipment *before* a patient is connected to the instrument, periodic measurement for leakage of current supplied by each device, and by instruction in the principles of electrical safety for hospital personnel who use the complex and dangerous equipment that is so much a part of modern medical practice.

REFERENCES

Radiation injuries

Bond VP et al: *Mammalian Radiation Lethality,* New York: Academic, 1965

Casarett AP: *Radiation Biology,* Englewood Cliffs, N.J.: Prentice-Hall, 1968

Cronkite EP, Bond VP: *Radiation Injury in Man,* Springfield, Ill.: Charles C Thomas, 1960

Graw RG, Yankee RA: Principles of hematologic supportive care. Med Clin North Am 57:441, 1973

Hempelmann LH: The acute radiation syndrome: A study of 9 cases and a review. Ann Intern Med 36:279, 1952

Higby DJ et al: Filtration leukopheresis for granulocyte transfusion therapy. Clinical and laboratory studies. N Engl J Med 292:761, 1975

Lea DE: *Actions of Radiation on Living Cells,* New York: Macmillan, 1947

Levine AS et al: Protected environments and prophylactic antibiotics. A prospective controlled study of their utility in the therapy of acute leukemia. N Engl J Med 228:477, 1973

Radiation carcinogenesis in man, report of 19th session of U.N. Scientific Committee on the Effects of Atomic Radiation, suppl. 14 (A/5814), chap. 3, 1964

Rubin PR, Casarett GW: *Clinical Radiation Pathology,* Philadelphia: Saunders, 1968

Electrical injuries

Apfelberg DB et al: Pathophysiology and treatment of lightning injuries. J Trauma 14:453, 1974

Artz CP: Changing concepts of electrical injury. Am J Surg 128: 600, 1974

Baxter CR: Present concepts in the management of major electrical injury. Surg Clin North Am 50:1401, 1970

DiVincenti FC et al: Electrical injuries: A review of 65 cases. J Trauma 9:497, 1969

Kay NRM et al: The management of electrical injuries of the extremities. Surg Clin North Am 53:1459, 1973

Kilpatrick DG: The electrical environment. Med Clin North Am 55:1095, 1971

Taussig HB: Death from lightning—and the possibility of living again. Ann Intern Med 68:1345, 1968

126
IMMERSION INJURY AND DROWNING

RUSSELL S. FISHER

About 7,000 deaths by drowning occur in the United States each year. This is the fourth leading cause of accidental death and represents about one-fifteenth of the total number of fatal accidents.

DIAGNOSIS The term *drowning* is used to categorize a series of related phenomena resulting from submersion in a liquid medium that is per se innocuous. It, therefore, includes asphyxial changes as well as complex acute hemodynamic alterations and disturbances of the biochemical equilibrium of the blood.

PATHOGENESIS Knowledge of the sequence of phenomena that occur in drowning is based upon a number of observations on humans and on experimental drowning in animals. Submersion is usually followed by an intensive and panicky struggle in an effort to reach the surface. Breath holding for varying lengths of time has been recorded to occur in the next stage, possibly lasting until the accumulating CO_2 in blood and tissues stimulates the respiratory center sufficiently to lead to an inevitable inhalation of considerable volumes of water. Swallowing of water, coughing and vomiting, loss of consciousness, and terminal gasping with flooding of the lungs and death then take place in rapid succession. When the process is interrupted before terminal gasping has set in, spontaneous recovery sometimes occurs. It has commonly been asserted that drowning essentially involves asphyxia resulting from obstruction of the airway by the drowning fluid. More recent investigations, however, show that the mechanism of death by drowning is far more involved than mere deprivation of air. Asphyxial death in drowning is said to occur in between 10 and 15 percent of all cases and is supposedly due to laryngospasm and closure of the glottis. It is not quite understood why 10 to 15 percent of drowning deaths are, apparently, associated with this mechanism, considering that laryngospasm is not detectable at autopsy and the finding of dry lungs does not indicate whether water was or was not inhaled. Moreover comparative enzymologic studies in rats of fresh- and saltwater drowning and asphyxia by exclusion of air indicate significant statistical differences between test and control groups. This seems to stress further the distinction between the mode of death in asphyxia versus that of drowning. In the majority of fatalities, death results from complex pathophysiologic events differing widely according to the chemical composition of the submersion liquid. For purposes of illustration, drowning in freshwater and seawater may be considered as separate entities.

Drowning in freshwater Large amounts of water enter the lungs, and because of the hypotonicity of freshwater, rapid absorption into the circulating bloodstream takes place. This results in a sudden and violent increase in blood volume, with hemodilution and hypervolemia. Using deuterium oxide in the water as a tracer, Swann and Spafford have demonstrated that after a dog has been submerged 2 min, its blood may be diluted by as much as 51 percent of its original volume. This hemodilution is associated with massive hemolysis and an inevitable upset of the normal balance of the blood constituents. Sodium, chloride, calcium, proteins, and hemoglobin are all diluted, and the level of potassium rises. Ventricular fibrillation is often considered to be a characteristic feature of freshwater drowning. When it occurs, expulsive heartbeats are arrested at once. Ventricular fibrillation is believed to be directly related to the dilution of the blood electrolytes, in particular sodium. It cannot, however, be produced experimentally by injecting large volumes of water intravenously. The precedent condition is anoxia; the animal must be anoxic for an experimental hydremic plethora to cause fibrillation. The original hypothesis, based upon animal experiments, of "potassium intoxication" secondary to massive hemolysis as the underlying factor causing ventricular fibrillation has proved erroneous. The main intracellular cation in dog erythrocytes is not potassium as in humans, but sodium, and freshwater drowning and hemolysis in the dog do not release a flood of potassium ions. The slight increase observed in plasma potassium after freshwater drowning may be accounted for by prolonged anoxia. These speculations do not answer the question of whether ventricular fibrillation occurs in freshwater drowning in humans, but it would appear desirable to include defibrillation in the emergency treatment of a drowning victim. It is interesting to note that dilution of the blood in freshwater drowning is associated with up to a 33 percent decrease in the blood alcohol concentration, i.e., a drowning victim with a blood alcohol level of 0.18 percent may have had up to 0.24 percent before submersion.

Drowning in seawater Seawater is strongly hypertonic. Its salt concentration, mainly sodium chloride, is over 3 percent. Submersion in seawater results in a rapid diffusion of salts into the bloodstream. The concentration of sodium, chloride, magnesium, etc., in the plasma rises conspicuously, while water moves from the circulation into the pulmonary alveoli—thus reestablishing the osmotic equilibrium. The consequences are marked hemoconcentration and fulminant pulmonary edema. Hypotension and hypovolemia accompanied by considerable bradycardia develop, and death supervenes within a few minutes. Ventricular fibrillation is not usually observed in experimental saltwater drowning in spite of the adverse prevailing electrolyte environment, probably because the plasma sodium level is elevated rather than low.

Death associated with diving (see also Chap. 123) In the case of divers, death is often the result of underwater asphyxia following hyperventilation; the latter leads to a sharp fall in blood carbon dioxide and to vasoconstriction, which in turn brings about a decrease of the cerebral circulation. Diminished cerebral blood flow is followed by loss of consciousness, which leads to inhalation of water. Involuntary exhalation against a closed glottis results in hypotension and diminished cardiac output, further aggravating the condition. In diving with a scuba (self-contained underwater breathing apparatus), the cause of death is usually closely associated with the overconfidence of the diver in the breathing machine. Nitrogen narcosis occurs commonly, resulting from the increase of nitrogen concentration in the tissues as evident from Henry's law, according to which the solubility of a gas is directly proportional to the absolute pressure upon it. There is an increase of 1 atmosphere (atm) of pressure for each 33 ft of water depth. Barotrauma and air embolism are second in frequency and occur during the ascent of the diver, when the air inhaled from the scuba expands proportionately as the pressure decreases (Boyle's law). An ascent, for instance, from 33 ft results in a twofold increase in volume because of the decrease in pressure from 2 to 1 atm. At this point any interference with expiration prevents release of this increased volume and results in acute pulmonary emphysema with tears in the lungs, hemoptysis, hemothorax, air embolism, and often death.

Careful investigation of the circumstances of submersion is mandatory to rule out cervical spinal trauma in those cases where the victim dove into the water and impacted the bottom.

RESUSCITATION FROM DROWNING The main objective of adequate resuscitation in drowning is to institute such measures before circulatory failure sets in. Resuscitative procedures currently employed consist of clearing the airway by postural drainage, suction, etc., and giving artificial respiration, supplemented by closed-chest cardiac massage if no heart sounds are obtainable and the pulse is absent. Intermittent positive-pressure breathing with air, or preferably with oxygen, should be employed when such is available, and external electrical defibrillation should be carried out as soon as feasible after the condition arises. Plasma infusion to correct hemoconcentration is often thought to be of great value in saltwater drowning, while in freshwater drowning it may be expected that an exchange transfusion, which in itself is a relatively harmless procedure, will be effective in reestablishing a normal circulating blood volume and in correcting an upset electrolyte balance. So-called "semi-" or "near drowning" in which death occurs suddenly several hours or longer after submersion has been repeatedly reported, but the mechanism of death in such cases remains obscure. Treatment should be directed to maintaining high cerebral oxygen supply and preventing pneumonia. Lower nephron nephrosis may also be anticipated in survivors of freshwater submersion, because of hemoglobinemia; if oliguria or anuria develops, appropriate therapy should be initiated. Methylprednisolone therapy has been suggested for pulmonary edema following near drowning (Sladen and Zauder).

REFERENCES

DENNY MK, READ RC: Scuba-diving deaths in Michigan. JAMA 192:220, 1965

KVITTINGEN TD, NAESS A: Recovery from drowning in fresh water. Br Med J 1:1315, 1963

SLADEN A, ZAUDER HL: Methylprednisolone therapy for pulmonary edema following near drowning. JAMA 215:1793, 1971

SPITZ WU: Drowning. Hosp Med 5:8, 1969

——: Drowning, in *Medicolegal Investigation of Death,* eds WU Spitz, RS Fisher, Springfield, Ill.: Charles C Thomas, 1973, pp. 296–310

SWANN HG: Mechanism of circulatory failure in fresh and sea water drowning. Circ Res 4:241, 1956

PART SIX | DISORDERS CAUSED BY BIOLOGIC AGENTS

section 1 | Basic considerations

127 AN APPROACH TO INFECTIOUS DISEASES

ROBERT G. PETERSDORF

INTRODUCTION The vast majority of human and animal diseases of known etiology are produced by biologic agents: viruses, rickettsias, bacteria, mycoplasma, fungi, protozoa, or nematodes. No small part of the past and present importance of infectious diseases in medical practice is attributable to their enormous frequency and the public health implications of the contagiousness of many of them. However, developments in sanitary engineering, vector control, techniques of immunization, and specific chemotherapy have modified the situation favorably. Although important exceptions remain, infectious diseases as a class are more easily prevented and more easily cured than any other major group of disorders. Despite the virtual elimination of certain infectious diseases and profound reduction in the morbidity and mortality of many, man is by no means free of infection. In fact, the total human load of disease produced by microbial parasites has decreased only modestly, primarily through smallpox and malaria control and better health care in developing countries. As certain specific microbial infections have been controlled, others have emerged as troublesome therapeutic and epidemiologic problems. With the introduction of cytotoxic drugs, massive x-ray irradiation in the treatment of malignant diseases, and immunosuppressive agents to control the rejection of transplanted organs, the insertion of prosthetic devices into the bloodstream, and the progressive longevity of people with chronic degenerative diseases, infections due to organisms previously considered saprophytic or commensal have increased. These infections have also been termed *opportunistic*. As Dubos has pointed out, microbial infections appear to form an inherent part of human life.

Because of better environmental sanitation and other measures that now prevent contact with many microbial agents, and the development of acquired immunity early in childhood, certain infections have been seen more frequently in adults. For example, as contact with poliomyelitis virus in childhood declined in many countries, paralytic poliomyelitis became more common in young adults. *Hemophilus influenzae* meningitis is being reported more frequently in adults than heretofore, and decreasing infection with the tubercle bacillus raises questions about the status of antituberculous immunity in adults.

As antimicrobial agents reduce the mortality associated with certain common infections, other microbes emerge as important causes of human disease. If an infection occurs during or immediately following a course of chemotherapy, it is often caused by a microorganism that is resistant to the drug that was given; such an infection is termed a *superinfection*. While it is relatively unusual nowadays for patients to die of uncomplicated pneumococcal pneumonia, a disease readily handled with available antimicrobials, it is common to see serious disease produced by microorganisms which are much more resistant even though they are often part of man's normal microbial flora. These include staphylococci, gram-negative enteric bacilli, and a variety of anaerobes and fungi (Chap. 128).

THE PARASITE AND THE HOST The interaction between microorganism and man that results in infection and disease is complex. Much has been learned about the way in which microbes enter the body, the ways in which they produce tissue injury, the influence of specific immunity and "nonspecific" resistance of the host, and the mechanisms of recovery. Unfortunately, it is not yet possible to transfer in any specific way much of the information that has been acquired to the individual patient with an infection. In this presentation those general aspects of the host-parasite relationship that form the basis for diagnostic procedures, that are of importance in deriving therapeutic principles, or that help explain the epidemiology of infection are stressed.

Infection and clinical disease It is well known that microorganisms of different species or different strains of the same species vary widely in their capacity to produce disease and that human beings are not equally susceptible to the disease caused by a given bacterium or virus. Furthermore, while a specific infectious disease will not occur in the absence of the causative organism, the mere presence of the organism in the body does not lead invariably to clinical illness. Indeed, the production of symptoms in man by many parasites is the exception rather than the rule, and the *subclinical infection* or the "carrier state" is the usual host-parasite relationship. *Disease* in a clinical sense is not synonymous with the presence of the organism or *infection* in a microbiologic sense. In fact, for most organisms the number of subclinical infections far exceeds that of clinical disease. Even rabies virus infection, which was at one time believed to nearly always cause progressive fatal disease in nearly all instances, has been shown to produce a significant number of subclinical infections in both animals and man.

Mechanisms of injury It is customary to refer to bacteria or other microorganisms that are capable of producing disease as *pathogenic. Virulence*, the *degree* of pathogenicity, should be distinguished from *invasiveness*, the ability to spread and disseminate in the body. For example, *Clostridium tetani* is pathogenic and, by virtue of its exotoxin, highly virulent, but it is almost completely lacking in invasiveness. These distinctions are valuable in microbiology and experimental pathology, but they often mean relatively little at a clinical level. Under certain circumstances and in certain anatomic locations, mildly "pathogenic" organisms can produce fatal disease, or highly "pathogenic" species can multiply without producing any harmful effect.

A few parasites produce *toxins* that account for the tissue damage and physiologic alterations of infection. *Hypersensitivity* to components of the parasite is demonstrable in several infections to account for the manifestations of disease. For many pathogenic agents, an explanation of their damaging effects upon the host is incomplete or wholly lacking. Generally, therefore, the aim of therapy is to stop multiplication or to kill the parasites with appropriate drugs; in diseases caused by toxin-producing organisms, the use of antiserum (as in tetanus or diphtheria) is the definitive procedure, and chemotherapy is of secondary importance.

The tendency of certain pathogenic organisms to *localize in certain cells or organs* and to produce damage is also unexplained. Clinically, however, the presence of disease in a specific anatomic site or a combination of symptoms referable to certain organs often suggests the identity of the causative organism. For example, the pneumococcus usually causes infection in the lung but almost never in the kidney, and *H. influenzae* infections are confined almost solely to the respiratory tract and meninges. Similarly, in the presence of disease known to be caused by a given agent, complicating involvement of other tissues can be anticipated or predicted. Examples include the multiple lung abscesses which are so characteristic of hematogenously disseminated staphylococcal disease and metastatic skin lesions which complicate *Pseudomonas* bacteremia.

Frequently, the proper management of infectious disease involves the use of techniques completely unrelated to microbiology or chemotherapy, in an effort to support the function of damaged organs. Survival in poliomyelitis may depend upon treatment of respiratory failure, the management of heart failure in endocarditis is sometimes a greater problem than the eradication of the causative organism, and in epidemic hemorrhagic fever, or Weil's disease, maintenance of fluid and electrolyte balance, with peritoneal dialysis or hemodialysis during the stage of acute renal failure, is the important therapeutic objective.

Resistance and susceptibility Many so-called "host factors" are known to influence the likelihood that disease will occur if organisms enter the tissues, or to play a determining role in the outcome once the infection has become established. These include natural or acquired antibodies, interferon, properdin, phagocytic activity, and the level of the general inflammatory response, which is generally manifested by cellular activity such as chemotaxis, phagocytosis, and release of lysozomal enzymes (Chap. 63).

In experimental animals, sex, microbial strain, age, route of infection, the presence of specific antibody, other diseases, nutritional state, and the use of such procedures as exposure to ionizing radiation or high environmental temperature or administration of mucin, nitrogen mustard, adrenal steroids, epinephrine, xerosin, and metabolic analogues can be shown to exert a profound effect upon infection by bacteria, viruses, and other agents.

In man, these factors are no less important, although controlled studies are lacking for many. Alcoholism; diabetes; deficiency or absence of immunoglobulins (Chap. 74); defects in cellular immunity (Chaps. 63 and 74); malnutrition; chronic administration of adrenal hormones; chronic lymphedema; ischemia; the presence of foreign bodies such as bullets, calculi, or bone fragments; obstruction of a bronchus, the urethra, or any hollow tube; agranulocytosis or congenital defects in bactericidal or virucidal activity (Chap. 63); various blood dyscrasias, and many other circumstances influence susceptibility to systemic or local infection. Furthermore, in those instances where the extenuating condition is remediable, the probability of recovery is enhanced.

Racial differences in susceptibility, such as the poor resistance of dark-skinned people to tuberculosis, their predilection for developing disseminated coccidioidomycosis, and the resistance of Negroes to malaria caused by *Plasmodium vivax* are well established. Resistance to infection may be determined genetically. The relation of sickle-cell trait to malaria is one example. The increased frequency and severity of some infections in children, of others in pregnant women, and still others in the aged are familiar.

Prior contact with an organism or its products, whether by active infection or by artificial immunization, increases resistance to some infections, such as measles, diphtheria, and pertussis by stimulating antibody production, but seems to have little influence on resistance to others, such as gonorrhea.

Present knowledge of the factors involved in human resistance and susceptibility is incomplete. Explanations such as changes in physical or chemical activity of phagocytes; antibacterial substances such as lysozyme, phagocytin, or lysozomal enzymes; qualitative or quantitative alterations in serum proteins; disordered metabolism at the cellular level, "products of tissue injury" that influence vascular permeability, and the effects of tissue pressure remain to a considerable extent in the realm of hypothesis.

The profound influence of host factors upon the infectious process makes it clear, however, that their understanding is probably essential for the control of infections in predictable fashion.

PATHOGENESIS OF INFECTION With relatively minor variations, the development of an infectious disease follows a consistent pattern. The parasites enter the body through the skin, nasopharynx, lung, intestine, urethra, or other portal. A number of microorganisms adhere to their site of primary attack through fimbriae, pili, and surface antigens; the adherence of *Bordetella pertussis* to respiratory epithelium, the gonococcus to urethral epithelium, and possibly some gram-negative urinary pathogens to the epithelium of the renal pelvis are some examples. Once established in the host, the organisms can multiply and, in so doing, establish a local or primary lesion. From this site, there may be local spread along fascial planes or tubular structures, such as a bronchus or ureter. The next step may be systemic spread of the microorganisms via the circulating blood. Bacteria can enter the bloodstream by direct invasion of vessels, a relatively unusual occurrence, or more commonly by traversing peripheral lymph nodes to enter the thoracic duct lymph and thence the venous system. In the bloodstream, they spread to other tissues and can produce distant or secondary lesions. In infections such as tetanus and diphtheria, distant lesions are produced by toxins elaborated at the primary site without systemic spread of the parasites. The infectious process may terminate in recovery or death at any stage: the local lesion, systemic spread, or distant lesion.

The apparent inconsistency of this pattern in clinical medicine is attributable to the fact that the infection is recognized as a clinical entity only at the stage when symptoms are most likely to appear. For example, pneumococcal pneumonia is a local lesion, and the distant lesion, pneumococcal meningitis, is referred to clinically as a complication. In the meningococcal infections, the local lesion, a nasopharyngitis, is rarely symptomatic and has no status as a clinical entity, but the stage of spread, meningococcemia, and the commonest distant lesion, meningitis, are clinical entities. A rarer distant lesion, arthritis, is called a complication. In a patient who has osteomyelitis, a clinical entity, a recent furuncle may be referred to as a predisposing factor. In another patient with extensive furunculosis who develops osteomyelitis, the infection in bone may be regarded as a complication of the superficial infection. The stages mentioned are in no way limited to bacterial diseases; the primary lesion of poliomyelitis is intestinal, viremia may occur without neurologic involvement, or a distant lesion, the classic "infantile paralysis," may be established.

Because of established clinical usage and terminology based upon the symptomatic illness that leads patients to seek medical aid, the consistency of this general sequence in the pathogenesis of infection is often not recognized. However, the concept is useful and offers some basis for systematizing what may otherwise seem to be a miscellaneous collection of unrelated clinical signs and symptoms.

CLINICAL MANIFESTATIONS OF INFECTIONS So varied are the disorders attributable to infection or infestation of man by lower organisms that generalizations about them are difficult. The clinical manifestations of infection can duplicate those of diseases of any other etiology. However, certain clinical features are highly suggestive of infection, including abrupt onset, fever, chills, myalgia, photophobia, pharyngitis, acute lymphadenopathy and splenomegaly, gastrointestinal upset, and leukocytosis or leukopenia. It is obvious that the presence of one, several, or all of these features does not constitute proof of the microbial origin of illness in a given patient. Conversely, serious, even fatal, infectious disease may exist in the absence of fever or other signs and symptoms.

Although there is no infallible clinical criterion of infection, it is still possible to recognize accurately many specific infectious diseases from information obtained by *history, physical examination, blood count, and urinalysis*. The importance of interrogation about past illness, predisposing factors such as alcoholism, familial disease, exposure to ill persons, contact with animals or insects, ingestion of contaminated food, type and order of onset of symptoms, and recent or remote residence in endemic areas is discussed in subsequent chapters for specific diseases and etiologic agents. Cardinal physical signs are also described for each entity.

The mechanisms that produce most of the signs and symptoms of human infection are unknown. The pathogenesis of fever is discussed in Chap. 12. The physiologic alterations underlying "malaise," "postinfectious asthenia," "toxicity," and other common complaints are completely mysterious. The factors responsible for leukocytosis or leukopenia are only partially understood (Chap. 63). Why the rash of typhus begins on the trunk while that of another rickettsiosis, Rocky Mountain spotted fever, begins on the extremities is unanswered. Failure to understand these manifestations does not impair their clinical usefulness, although it is probable that understanding them might lead to more accurate diagnosis and better management.

DIAGNOSTIC PROCEDURES When dealing with diseases produced by living agents, it is evident that confirmation of a presumptive diagnosis, or sometimes the first suggestion of the etiology of illness, depends upon laboratory procedures. The availability of a multitude of laboratory tests in the modern hospital has not made it possible to substitute a "routine laboratory work-up" for history, physical examination, and observation of a patient's course. Indeed, the information derived from these procedures is the only reasonable basis for selecting the tests to be performed by the laboratory.

The importance of roentgenographic changes, alterations in chemical constituents of the blood, and tests of the functional capacity of organs such as the liver and kidney is as great in infectious disease as in illnesses of other etiologies and needs no discussion here.

The specific procedures for the diagnosis of infectious disease involve *direct demonstration of the causative organism or proof of its presence by indirect means.*

Demonstration of the organism In bacterial disease, it is often possible to find the causative organism by *microscopic examination of properly stained preparations of sputum, spinal fluid, and other body fluids*. This simple procedure is often neglected as an unnecessary bother when material is being sent for bacteriologic culture, but it is a most valuable source of immediate information. In some diseases, the etiologic agent cannot be cultured easily, e.g., *Borrelia*, and in others isolation is time-consuming (tuberculosis, blastomycosis). In some patients with systemic candidiasis, an increasingly important problem in patients with compromised host resistance, *Candida* blastospores and pseudohyphae have been found in blood smears several days before the blood culture became positive. The discovery of pneumococci, meningococci, and *H. influenzae* in stained smears of cerebro-spinal fluid permits the initiation of specific chemotherapy immediately with the assurance that the regimen is the proper one.

Direct examination of bone marrow is a useful method for demonstrating organisms in some diseases such as kala azar, histoplasmosis, and tuberculosis. In protozoan (amebiasis, malaria) and parasitic diseases (schistosomiasis, filariasis), *direct examination of blood, feces, or urine* is the only feasible method for establishing a diagnosis.

There are also infections in which the detection of characteristic cytologic changes or the causative organism itself in smears or histologic sections of biopsy material may be the quickest method for diagnosis. Tubercles and tubercle bacilli in lymph nodes or liver biopsies, *Mycobacterium leprae* in skin or nasal scrapings, inclusion bodies in the skin lesions of varicella or variola and the exudate of inclusion conjunctivitis, "Warthin" cells from the nasal or pharyngeal mucosa in measles, schistosome ova in punch biopsies of rectal mucosa, and the Councilman bodies of yellow fever in the liver are examples. In addition, characteristic histologic changes make it feasible to identify the lesions of chancroid, syphilis, lymphogranuloma venereum, or viral hepatitis in biopsy specimens. Indeed, even in diseases where other reliable tests are available, diagnosis by histologic examination is sometimes the most rapid method available; the characteristic muscle lesion of Weil's disease is an example (Chap. 166).

Special microscopic techniques *Dark-field examination* of material from genital lesions for the spirochete of syphilis is a well-known but often neglected procedure. In several other spirochetal diseases, including leptospirosis, the dark-field technique can be useful, but experience in recognition of the organisms is necessary for correct interpretation of findings.

Fluorescence microscopy in which the causative organisms can be recognized and identified rapidly by the use of fluorescent antibody preparations (Coons' technique) is being used in the diagnosis of syphilis, gonorrhea, pertussis, streptococcal pharyngitis, and a number of other bacterial, viral, fungal, and parasitic infections. The final role of this procedure remains to be established, but with increasing availability of specific serums and continuing technical refinement, it will certainly be of increasing value in the future. A promising but as yet experimental technique involves the use of enzymatic labeling to localize antigens and antibodies. The immunoperoxidase method may gain wide acceptance, because it can be performed with a simple light microscope rather than the more expensive and technically difficult fluorescence microscope.

The nitroblue tetrazolium (NBT) test is based on the increased intracytoplasmic reduction of NBT by actively phagocytic segmented neutrophils. Although initially thought to be important in distinguishing pyogenic (bacterial) from nonpyogenic infections, there have been too many false positive and false negative tests to make this a practical tool. The NBT test is of value in screening for chronic granulomatous disease (CGD) (Chap. 63).

Culture and animal inoculation Specimens for bacteriologic culture should be collected *before the initiation of chemotherapy*. The material to be cultured—sputum, pus, blood, or bone marrow—should be selected on the basis of the suspected infections, and the precise cultural techniques employed—media, CO_2 incubation, anaerobic incubation—must be determined in similar fashion. Gas chromatography as a means for rapidly differentiating bacterial species may turn out to be an important new diagnostic technique. There are new developments in identification of a wide range of viruses in tissue culture, and refinements in these techniques are increasing the value of tissue culture in clinical diagnosis.

In several infections, including Weil's disease, rat-bite fever, certain mycoses, tuberculosis, and the rickettsioses, the etiologic organism can be isolated by *inoculation of appropriate material into mice or guinea pigs*. This is a cumbersome and potentially dangerous procedure for routine use, but may need to be employed with appropriate precautions in selected instances. Many viruses can also be isolated by inoculation of appropriate animals. This is rarely feasible for ordinary clinical diagnosis and, for several agents, is hazardous.

Blood cultures and bacteremia Because of the peculiar clinical importance of demonstrating bacteria in the bloodstream and because there are varying opinions about optimal timing and sites of sampling for blood cultures, it is of practical importance to understand something about the mechanisms of bacteremia.

Excepting intravascular infections (bacterial endocarditis or endarteritis, mycotic aneurysm, suppurative thrombophlebitis), bacteria usually enter the circulation through the lymphatic system. Consequently, when bacteria multiply at a site of local infection in the tissues, the likelihood of bacteremia parallels the occurrence of local conditions that favor drainage of lymph from the infected area to the thoracic duct and eventually to the venous blood. These factors include the number and anatomic arrangement of local lymph vessels, accumulation of fluid, increase in tissue pressure, and manipulation of the part.

Once bacteria enter the blood, they are removed rapidly by the fixed phagocytes of the reticuloendothelial system in the liver, spleen, and bone marrow and by engulfment in polymorphonuclear leukocytes in capillaries, especially those of the lung.

Clinically, bacteremia can be transient, intermittent, or continuous. Many transient bacteremias result from manipulation of infected or contaminated tissues, common examples being instrumentation of the genitourinary tract, tonsillectomy, dental procedures, and massage or surgical incision of furuncles or abscesses. In the vast majority of instances, the sudden discharge of bacteria into the blood produces no symptoms or, at most, a rigor and brief fever, and the organisms are promptly removed. The great danger of these "man-made" bacteremias is their role in producing bacterial endocarditis in patients with endocardial damage or intracardiac prostheses.

Transient bacteremia accompanies the early phase of many infections. In pneumococcal pneumonia, the typical rigor at the onset is a result of transient bacteremia. In most cases, with localization of the pulmonary lesion, blood cultures rapidly revert to negative. The poor prognosis of patients with pneumonia who continue to have positive blood cultures is not due to the presence of organisms in the blood but reflects spreading infection in the lung itself.

A sudden single influx of microorganisms into the bloodstream may be followed by a shaking chill and fever. However, there is a "lag period" of 30 to 90 min before the febrile response (Chap. 12). During this delay, the bacteria are usually promptly removed from the circulation by phagocytosis; consequently, a blood culture taken at the time of the rigor may be negative.

Continuous bacteremia is a feature of the first several days of typhoid fever, of brucellosis, and of intravascular infections such as endocarditis or endarteritis.

Blood cultures should be taken at frequent intervals in patients with febrile disease of unknown cause; in general, an attempt should be made to obtain blood *before* an expected rise in fever or chill. When a patient is suspected of subacute bacterial endocarditis, or another of the diseases in which bacteremia is constant and is not too ill, two to four cultures daily for 2 to 3 days are more than sufficient to establish the diagnosis, and treatment in such cases should not be withheld for a longer period. However, when there are manifestations of acute endocarditis, with severe systemic symptoms and evidence of embolization, several cultures should be obtained over the course of a few (3 to 6) h, and treatment should then be instituted promptly. In no case are more than a total of six blood cultures required. The number of positive cultures falls off rapidly if the initial six are negative.

There is no evidence that arterial blood cultures possess any advantage over venous cultures. Suspected bacteremia is sometimes mentioned as a contraindication to diagnostic lumbar puncture because of the possible development of meningitis, but clinical evidence does not support this idea. Culture of bone marrow is occasionally superior to peripheral blood for recovery of organisms in typhoid, brucellosis, and rare cases of subacute bacterial endocarditis. It is common practice to make pour plates of blood and to quantify bacteremia in terms of a certain number of colonies per milliliter of blood. Although this procedure may seem cumbersome, colony counts are of value in distinguishing contaminating organisms. Colony counts may also be of prognostic value because a large number of organisms in the absence of severe clinical disease almost always means that bacteria are entering the bloodstream from a contaminated extracorporeal focus such as an infusion or an arteriovenous shunt. When blood cultures are taken for diagnostic purposes, some should be incubated in carbon dioxide, and a sample of blood should also be cultured in thioglycollate broth or some other anaerobic medium. Anaerobic cultures are especially important in women with puerperal or postabortal infections.

Immunologic methods These diagnostic methods are intended to supply evidence of past or present infection by demonstrating antibodies in serum or other body fluids, by indicating changed reactivity of the host (hypersensitivity, allergy) to products of the organism, or rarely to detect components of the causative organism in the body.

SEROLOGIC TESTS The finding on a single occasion that a patient's serum contains antibody that reacts with a certain antigen merely indicates that the patient has had previous contact with the antigen or a closely related substance. For this reason, with rare exceptions, the clinical interpretation of serologic tests depends on serial determinations. If the antibody titer is found to *rise or fall significantly*, it is likely that the response is a result of recent contact with the antigen. In subsequent chapters, the need for serologic testing of acute phase and convalescent serum is emphasized repeatedly. *In any patient with a puzzling illness, a sterile specimen of serum should be preserved in a frozen state so that it can, if necessary, be studied and compared with serum collected at a later date.*

Prior contact with an antigen may be the result of past immunization with vaccines; interpretation of serum agglutinin titers for typhoid bacilli is often made difficult by prior immunization. The so-called "anamnestic reaction," a nonspecific stimulation of antibody formation by an acute illness (e.g., a rise in *Brucella* agglutinins in a patient with acute tularemia), occurs only when the two organisms are antigenically related, and rarely presents a serious problem.

The methods employed for detecting antibody rises in various infections have been selected empirically on the basis of the ease with which the test can be performed and careful study to correlate the results of the test with other diagnostic criteria in patients. Therefore, the fact that antibodies against one agent are detected by a precipitin technique, another by agglutination of whole organisms or the production of capsular swelling, another by indirect fluorescent-antibody methods, and still another by complement fixation is a practical matter and bears no necessary relation to the agent, the type of infection, or its pathogenesis. By coating some particulate material, such as erythrocytes or latex, with antigen derived from a certain organism, antibody can sometimes be demonstrated by an agglutination test rather than by some more complex method.

Particular properties of the causative organism can sometimes be utilized to devise a simplified clinical test for antibody. Two striking instances of this are widely used. The ability of influenza and related viruses to clump erythrocytes makes possible the demonstration of antibody to virus by merely testing the capacity of a patient's serum to prevent the agglutination of red blood cells by suspensions of virus, the so-called "hemagglutination-inhibition" reaction. Similarly, because many microorganisms possess hemolytic components or toxins, the assay of a patient's serum for capacity to prevent lysis of red blood cells is a convenient and simple clinical test for antibody. The antistreptolysin O test in group A *Streptococcus pyogenes* infections is an example of this.

In a few infections, predominantly those caused by viruses, the only reliable serologic test is a *neutralization or protection* test, an assay of the protection afforded by the patient's serum against active infection in tissue culture or in experimental animals. This technique is time-consuming and is usually performed only in diagnostic virology laboratories.

Some mention of "nonspecific" serologic changes may serve to emphasize again that clinical laboratory tests have come into use *only because they have been found to correlate reasonably well with clinical findings*. In several diseases, it has been found, often accidentally, that serum antibody develops that will react with antigens derived from sources other than the etiologic agent (which may actually be unknown). Common examples are heterophil agglutinins in infectious mononucleosis, cold agglutinins in mycoplasma pneumonia, and the agglutination of certain strains of *Proteus* bacilli by serum of patients with rickettsial diseases. The Wassermann test for syphilis and related flocculation tests are performed with antigens derived from sources completely unrelated to *Treponema pallidum*.

The results of serologic tests must be interpreted in the light of other information about the patient, including such factors as previous immunizations and illnesses, the possibility of exposure to chemically but etiologically unrelated antigens, and the importance of a changing titer in serial tests as opposed to a single isolated observation.

SKIN TESTS Exposure to antigens of certain types, by various routes, and under circumstances not completely understood often results in the development of immediate (anaphylactic, atopic) hypersensitivity or delayed (bacterial, tuberculin) hypersensitivity.

Active infection with some, but not all, bacteria and viruses results in delayed hypersensitivity to the infecting agent in some, but not all, individuals. Clinically, this allergic state is detected by intradermal injection of the organism or one of its components; in a sensitive individual, induration and erythema will appear at the local site within 24 to 48 h. If an individual is highly "sensitive" or if the amount of antigen injected is excessive, there may be extensive local inflammation with necrosis, vesicle formation, edema, regional lymphadenopathy, and even malaise and fever. Antigens prepared in concentrations unlikely to provoke severe reactions are generally available for intradermal testing for tuberculosis, leprosy, mumps, lymphogranuloma, venereum, cat-scratch disease, chancroid, brucellosis, tularemia, glanders, toxoplasmosis, blastomycosis, histoplasmosis, coccidioidomycosis, and many other infections. The immune reaction to vaccination (Chap. 204) is also an example of delayed dermal hypersensitivity.

The reliability, specificity, and usefulness of the individual tests differ and are discussed in the chapters on specific infections. However, certain general principles apply to their use and interpretation:

1 They are highly useful in epidemiologic surveys as indicators of the incidence of infection in a population.
2 In most individuals, dermal reactivity persists for many years or for life. A single positive test means only that at some past time the individual was infected with the organism (or a closely related one). Unless supplementary information in the form of clinical findings, cultural studies, or more specific serologic data bear out the presence of active infection, a diagnosis of the disease is not justified.
3 The appearance of a positive dermal reaction in an individual known to have been nonreactive a short time before is good evidence of recent infection; this is a useful method for detecting tuberculosis.
4 *A negative intradermal test does not rule out past or present infection.* For unknown reasons, patients with measles, Hodgkin's disease, or sarcoidosis often develop a state of *anergy*, or inability to react to intradermally injected antigens. In several diseases, dermal sensitivity develops after weeks or months of infection; an important example is acute histoplasmosis, in which patients can be ill for many weeks without showing a positive skin test. The skin test to coccidiodin is always negative in disseminated coccidioidomycosis; in far-advanced or miliary tuberculosis in elderly patients, failure to react to intradermal tuberculin in the usual amounts employed for testing occurs in as many as 10 to 15 percent of the cases.

Intradermal injection of antigens derived from sources other than microorganisms usually produces an immediate *wheal and erythema* reaction which subsides promptly. The greatest clinical usefulness of this type of reaction is in the detection of allergy to foreign serums, pollens, and animal dander (Chap. 72). The skin tests for demonstrating infestation with helminths (trichinosis, filariasis) produce reactions of the immediate type in allergic individuals, but many of the antigens employed are so nonspecific that they are of little use in diagnosis.

IMPORTANCE OF SPECIFIC DIAGNOSIS IN INFECTIOUS DISEASES

Medicine and microbiology The diagnostic procedures employed for infectious diseases are no more absolute than those in other diseases; they cannot be blindly equated with the science of microbiology. The responsibility for interpreting the facts supplied by the bacteriologist, immunologist, and virologist in the total context of a patient's illness remains that of the physician. A positive tuberculin skin test certainly does not indicate that a patient has active tuberculosis. The finding of *Candida albicans* (*Monilia*) in a stool culture does not necessarily mean that a patient's diarrhea is caused by intestinal moniliasis. The presence of staphylococci in nasal cultures from a patient with headaches does not establish a diagnosis of staphylococcal sinusitis. A throat culture containing group A beta-hemolytic streptococci does not rule out diphtheria, nor does such a culture establish that a febrile illness in a patient with mitral stenosis is a recurrence of acute rheumatic fever rather than bacterial endocarditis. A positive serologic test for syphilis, which measures Wassermann-type antibodies, may be the first sign of lupus erythematosus.

The etiologic agent From a practical point of view, two important steps are vital to the correct diagnosis of infection: (1) The organ(s) or organ systems involved must be found; (2) the etiologic agents causing the infections must be identified precisely. A previous section has dealt with the diagnostic approaches that are available, and the following three chapters describe some important problems in infectious diseases, namely infections that occur in the compromised host, gram-negative bacteremia and shock, and antimicrobial therapy. The remaining chapters take up the specific bacteria, spirochetes, fungi, rickettsias, viruses, mycoplasma, and protozoa which cause infections. The common syndromes caused by these agents are described in the individual chapters. For example, bacterial pneumonia is discussed in detail in the chapter on pneumococcal infections (Chap. 133), osteomyelitis is described with staphylococcal infections (Chap. 134), the manifestations of bacteriuria are described in Chaps. 138 and 277, and those of meningitis in Chaps. 133, 136, and 337. Nevertheless, when confronted with specific organ involvement, it is important to know the most common pathogens which cause disease in the involved organ. Table 127-1 provides a listing of those pathogens. Used in conjunction with the individual chapters dealing with specific agents and the summary of chemotherapy (Chap. 130), the table should provide a rational guide to treatment which often must be instituted before the results of antimicrobial sensitivity tests are available.

Chemotherapy The impact of chemotherapy upon mortality and morbidity from infection and upon epidemic disease is now a matter of record. These therapeutic agents, however, have in no way lessened the importance of specific diagnosis; indeed, their availability has increased the need for obtaining exact etiologic information. It requires but a moment's reflection to realize that the substitution of a prescription for a broad-spectrum antibiotic or a quick injection of penicillin for the systematic collection of facts and thoughtful consideration of diagnostic possibilities is a fallacious, unwise, and dangerous practice. Numerous antibiotics with overlapping spectra are now available, dosages for different infections vary widely, the drugs themselves are potentially dangerous, and their administration entails considerable expense. They should never be prescribed as placebos, antipyretics, or substitutes for diagnosis. In the vast majority of instances in which this is done, patients

TABLE 127-1
The syndromic approach to infection

	Etiologic agents		
Type of infection	*Common*	*Relatively common*	*Unusual but important*
Skin and subcutaneous tissue	*Staphylococcus aureus*	*Streptococcus pyogenes, Candida,* and superficial fungi	Gram-negative bacilli (burns, wounds)
Sinusitis	*Strep. pneumoniae* *Staph. aureus*	*Strep. pyogenes, H. influenzae*	Mucorales
Pharyngitis	Respiratory viruses, *Strep. pyogenes*	Gonococcus	*Corynebacterium diphtheriae*
Epiglottitis	*Hemophilus influenzae*		
Otitis, mastoiditis	*Strep. pneumoniae, H. influenzae* (children)	*Staph. aureus, Strep. pyogenes*	*Pseudomonas, Proteus*
Pneumonitis	*Strep. pneumoniae, Mycoplasma pneumoniae, Mycobacterium tuberculosis*	*Staph. aureus, Klebsiella-Enterobacter,* respiratory viruses	*Strep. pyogenes,* gram-negative enteric bacilli, psittacosis, systemic fungi, *pneumocystis, H. influenzae, Pasteurella multocida*
Empyema and lung abscess	*Staph. aureus,* anaerobic streptococcus, *Bacteroides, Fusobacterium*	*Klebsiella* (abscess)	
Bacterial endocarditis	*Strep. viridans, Staph. aureus,* enterococcus	*Strep. pneumoniae,* anaerobic streptococcus	*Pseudomonas, Candida*
Gastroenteritis	*Salmonella, Shigella,* enteric viruses	*Staph. aureus, Escherichia coli* (enterotoxic), clostridia	*Pseudomonas, Entamoeba histolytica, Vibrio cholerae, V. parahemolyticus*
Peritonitis, cholangitis, intraabdominal abscess	*E. coli,* enterococcus, *Bacteroides,* anaerobic streptococcus, *Fusobacterium*	*Klebsiella-Enterobacter, Proteus* species	Clostridia, *Staph. aureus*
Urinary infection (cystitis, pyelonephritis)	*E. coli, Klebsiella-Enterobacter,* paracolon, *Proteus,* enterococcus	*Pseudomonas*	*Staph. aureus*
Urethritis	Gonococcus, ?*Mycoplasma, Chlamydia,* ?*Acinetobacter (Mima-herellea)*	*Treponema pallidum*	
Pelvic inflammatory disease	Gonococcus, *E. coli Bacteroides,* anaerobic streptococcus	*Klebsiella-Enterobacter,* enterococcus, *Fusobacterium*	Clostridia, *Staph. aureus*
Bones (osteomyelitis)	*Staph. aureus*	*Salmonella*	*Strep. pyogenes*
Joints	*Staph. aureus,* gonococcus, *Strep. pneumoniae, H. influenzae*	*Strep. pyogenes, Neisseria meningitidis*	
Meninges	*Strep. pneumoniae, H. influenzae, N. meningitidis;* echo; coxsackie and mumps viruses	*E. coli, Klebsiella-Enterobacter, Proteus, Pseudomonas*	*Strep. pyogenes, M. tuberculosis, Cryptococcus, Staph. aureus, Listeria monocytogenes*

recover just as they would if no "therapy" had been given, and the drugs are wasted. More importantly, an inadequate dosage of a drug or the wrong agent may suppress symptoms temporarily without achieving cure and may make isolation of the etiologic agent difficult, delay recognition of the true nature of an illness, and postpone the institution of curative treatment. Furthermore, antibiotics may select out resistant variants or facilitate the transfer of R factors between both pathogenic and commensal enterobacteria. Resistant variants can then replace sensitive strains and pose the additional hazard of spread to others. Finally, to expose a patient to the risk of drug reaction without proper indication is inexcusable, whether the drug is an antibiotic, a sedative, a laxative, or a narcotic.

Epidemiologic and other considerations Just as the decision to administer antibiotics to a patient with a febrile illness of presumed infectious etiology must be made on an individual basis, the selection of cases in which extensive cultural and serologic testing is required is a matter of judgment. The majority of common grippe-like illnesses subsides spontaneously, and symptomatic treatment is sufficient. However, because of this tendency toward spontaneous recovery and also because the results of serologic tests may not be available until after recovery has taken place, the effort to determine the specific etiology of illness is often considered an impractical, "academic" procedure. Such an attitude fails to recognize that in addition to the individual patient, the welfare of the community must be considered. For example, a clinical diagnosis of "virus pneumonia" may turn out, following serologic tests, to be psittacosis. Although the "index" patient may have recovered completely, others in the community may be at risk until the "pet parakeet" which was the source of the illness has been eliminated.

Pursuing the diagnosis of obscure, often self-limited, illnesses may be academic, but this approach has led to clarification of some important etiologic relations. For example, the syndrome of infectious mononucleosis has been linked with development of antibody to a herpes-like virus, the EB virus (Chap. 209); some cases of erythema multiforme may be due to herpes simplex virus; several patients with encephalitis have been found to have central nervous system infections with myxoviruses. Some congenital anomalies have been related to prenatal viral infections; this relationship is well known for rubella (Chap. 202), but a number of other viruses (CMV, varicella, herpes simplex) have been implicated, although with less certainty. The finding of bacteria-like bodies in the intestinal mucosa of patients with Whipple's disease and the improvement of these patients with tetracycline therapy provides another example of an entity of unknown etiology entering the realm of infectious diseases. Patients with sarcoidosis have been shown to have high titers against herpes-like virus, similar to patients with infectious mononucleosis, Burkitt's lymphoma, and carcinoma of the posterior nasal space. The relation of these viruses to these diseases is not clear; suffice it to say, these associations raise some interesting possibilities concerning the lymphocytic system and virus infections. Along the same vein, the possibility has been raised that the Chédiak-Higashi syndrome, a rare familial disorder characterized by albinism, photophobia, nystagmus, anomalous cellular granules, marked susceptibility to infection, and development of lymphoma, is caused by a virus. This association, among others, relates the field of infection to that of oncogenesis.

These discoveries clearly are the result of academic procedures which might have little immediate applicability to infection in a particular patient; yet few can question their fundamental biologic importance. Moreover, it is conceivable that they will assume practical importance in the future.

REFERENCES

AVRAMEAS S: Immunoenzymatic techniques: Enzymes as markers for the localization of antigens and antibodies. Int Rev Cytol 27:349, 1970

BENNETT IL JR, BEESON PB: Bacteremia: A consideration of some experimental and clinical aspects. Yale J Biol Med 26:241, 1954

BROOKS JB et al: Gas chromatography as a potential means of diagnosing arthritis. I. Differentiation between staphylococcal, streptococcal, gonococcal, and traumatic arthritis. J Infect Dis 129:660, 1974

BURNET M: *Natural History of Infectious Disease*, New York: Cambridge, 1953

CLUFF LE, JOHNSON JE III: *Clinical Concepts of Infectious Diseases*, Baltimore: Williams & Wilkins, 1972

DAVIS BD et al: *Microbiology*, New York: Harper & Row, 1968

DUBOS RJ: *Biochemical Determinants of Microbial Disease*, Cambridge: Harvard, 1954

——: *The Evolution of Microbial Diseases: Bacterial and Mycotic Diseases of Man*, 4th ed., Philadelphia: Lippincott, 1965, p. 20

HIRSHAUT Y et al: Sarcoidosis, another disease associated with serologic evidence for herpes-like virus infection. N Engl J Med 283:502, 1970

HORSFALL FL JR: Cancer and viruses. Bull NY Acad Med 42:167, 1966

——, TAMM I: *Viral and Rickettsial Diseases of Man*, 4th ed., Philadelphia: Lippincott, 1965

MACLEOD CM, CLUFF LE: Symposium on non-specific resistance to infection. Bacteriol Rev 24:1, 1960

SEGAL AW: Nitroblue-tetrazolium tests. Lancet 2:1248, 1974

WHITE JG: Virus-like particles in the peripheral blood cells of two patients with Chédiak-Higashi syndrome. Cancer 19:877, 1966

WILSON GA, MILES AA: *Topley and Wilson's Principles of Bacteriology and Immunity*, 6th ed., Baltimore: Williams & Wilkens, 1975

WOOD WB JR: Studies on the cellular immunology of acute bacterial infections. Harvey Lect 47:72, 1951-1952

128 INFECTIONS IN THE COMPROMISED HOST

ROBERT G. PETERSDORF
DAVID C. DALE

DEFINITION An individual who is abnormally susceptible to infections is called a *compromised host*. This heightened susceptibility may occur because of some alteration in host-defense mechanisms (e.g., leukocytes, immunoglobulins, complement, mucosal and epithelial barriers, tissue vascular supply), because the normal surface bacteria have been changed by antibiotics, or because a foreign body (e.g., artificial heart valve, shunt, catheter) has been implanted. A *nosocomial infection* is an infection acquired during hospitalization, usually in a compromised host.

EPIDEMIOLOGY With the increased use of aggressive immunosuppressive chemotherapy, corticosteroids, and antimicrobial drugs, iatrogenic alterations in host defenses are being more frequently encountered, particularly in hospitalized patients. Hospital-acquired infections occur in approximately 5 percent of all patients admitted to a general hospital. The prevalence of hospital infection is approximately 12 percent in large tertiary-care hospitals and 6 percent in community hospitals, and the incidence figures are 6 percent and 3.5 percent, respectively. In numerical terms, there are approximately 1.5 million hospital infections in the United States annually. The most common nosocomial infections encountered are urinary tract infections (40 percent), surgical wound infections (25 percent), respiratory infections (15 percent), and infections in skin and subcutaneous tissues, septic thrombophlebitis, and bacteremia.

PREDISPOSING FACTORS Defects in host resistance Infections occur with increased frequency in a wide variety of disease states (Table 128-1). Leukemic and severely granulocytopenic patients have reduced inflammatory responses and frequently develop pneumonia and sepsis because of tissue invasion by a wide variety of indigenous microorganisms. With burns, uremia, diabetes, and glucocorticosteroid therapy, numerous components of host defenses are abnormal, and consequently many types of infections occur. In certain diseases there are more specific patterns of susceptibility to infections. For example, the defective H_2O_2 production by neutrophils and monocytes in chronic granulomatous disease markedly impairs bactericidal function for only certain bacteria (Chap. 63). Opsonic defects occur in patients with agammaglobulinemia, multiple myeloma, and other disorders affecting immunoglobulins and predispose to infections by encapsulated bacteria, e.g., pneumococci and *Hemophilus influenza*.

Many associations of diseases and susceptibility to infection are recognized. For many of these mechanisms of enhanced susceptibility are incompletely understood. These include hypoparathyroidism and candidiasis, alveolar proteinosis and nocardiosis, sickle-cell disease and salmonellosis, splenectomy and pneumococcal bacteremia, Hodgkin's disease and cryptococcal meningitis, and cystic fibrosis and *Pseudomonas* pulmonary infections. In clinical practice, these associations are of far less importance than the susceptibility to infection caused by the use of glucocorticosteroids, immunosuppressive drugs, and antibiotics. Chronic therapy with corticosteroids not only favors acquisition of new infections but may also result in reactivation and dissemination of latent diseases such as tuberculosis. These agents cause monocytopenia and lymphopenia, decrease neutrophil and monocyte chemotaxis, impair monocyte bactericidal activity, suppress delayed hypersensitivity, and, if given in sufficient doses, may decrease antibody formation. Steroids also mask the signs and symptoms of infections. The cytotoxic and immunosuppressive drugs (e.g., cyclophosphamide, azathioprine, methotrexate, chlorambucil) enhance susceptibility to infection chiefly by causing granulocytopenia, monocytopenia, and lymphopenia. In transplant patients with certain inflammatory diseases (e.g., systemic lupus erythematosus, vasculitis, and glomerulonephritis), the conjoint use of corticosteroids and immunosuppressive drugs greatly enhances the risk of infection. It is the corticosteroids which are chiefly responsible for this heightened susceptibility, except when the granulocyte count has been severely reduced by cytotoxic drugs (absolute neutrophils less than 1,000 per mm^3).

Superinfections Superinfections may be defined as infections which occur while a course of antimicrobial therapy is administered for either therapeutic or prophylactic purposes. They are seen in approximately 2 percent of all patients treated with antibiotics, and are more common when antimicrobials are given in large doses, when several antimicrobials are administered concurrently, or when broad-spectrum agents are employed.

Clinical superinfections must be distinguished from the normal ecologic change in bacterial flora which accompanies all antimicrobial therapy. Most antibiotics lower the number of resident microorganisms and occasionally eradicate them entirely; the normal flora is then replaced by resistant exogenous or more commonly endogenous bacteria. In the vast majority of instances the number of bacteria replacing those eradicated by the drug is small, and clinical disease does not take place. However, when the concentration of the superinfecting organisms is high, and anatomic conditions are favorable, clinical superinfection is likely to occur.

Superinfections are particularly common following administration of certain drugs; the tendency for *Pseudomonas* to colonize and infect patients receiving one of the cephalosporins is a notable example. Clinically significant superinfections usually appear 4 to 5 days after chemotherapy is instituted and must be watched for, especially in patients being treated for pneumonia, chronic obstructive lung disease, otitis, and urinary tract infection, or when a urethral catheter is in place. They often complicate the course of patients with respiratory viral diseases, particularly influenza, who are given antibiotics to prevent bacterial complications. As a rule, superinfections are caused by organisms that are resistant to the drug the patient is receiving; penicillinase-producing staphylococci were in the past the most common offenders, but gram-negative enteric bacilli and fungi are now the most common superinfecting microorganisms. The usual clinical manifestations include recrudescence of fever and other signs and symptoms at the site of the initial infection.

Other diagnostic and therapeutic measures resulting in infections The hospitalized patient is subjected to a variety of diagnostic and therapeutic procedures which predispose to infection. These include insertion of intravenous catheters and urethral catheterization, particularly if an indwelling catheter is left in place; less commonly, injections, thoracenteses, paracenteses, aspiration of joints, lumbar punctures, and tissue biopsies may be incriminated. At least 2 to 3 percent of operative procedures are complicated by infections; the rates vary with the type of operation. Large surgical wounds associated with prolonged

TABLE 128-1
Infections in the compromised host

Conditions	*Major defects*	*Etiologic agents*	*Infections*
ABNORMALITIES OF LEUKOCYTES			
Leukemia, aplastic anemia, agranulocytosis	Neutropenia, monocytopenia	*Staphylococcus aureus, E. coli, Klebsiella, Pseudomonas, Candida, Pneumocystis, Aspergillus*	Pneumonia, bacteremia, ulcers and abscesses of oropharynx, anus, and skin
Chronic granulomatous disease	Decreased bactericidal activity	*Staph. aureus, E. coli, Serratia, Salmonella*	Lymphadenitis, abscesses in lung, liver, bone
Chediak-Higashi syndrome	Neutropenia, decreased chemotaxis and bactericidal activity	*Staph. aureus, Strep. Pyogenes, E. coli*	Cellulitis, abscesses
Hodgkin's disease—lymphoma	Lymphocytopenia, reduced delayed hypersensitivity, decreased chemotaxis	*M. tuberculosis, Listeria, E. coli, Salmonella, Candida, Cryptococcus, Toxoplasma, Pneumocystis,* herpes zoster, herpes simplex, cytomegalovirus	Pneumonia, bacteremia, hepatitis
Di George syndrome	Defective cellular immunity	*Staph. aureus, Strep. pneumoniae,* varicella-herpes zoster, cytomegalovirus	Otitis, pneumonia
HUMORAL DEFECTS			
Agammaglobulinemia, dysgammaglobulinemias, intestinal lymphangectasia, multiple myeloma, chronic lymphocytic leukemia, splenectomized patients	Decreased opsonization	*Strep. pneumoniae, H. influenza,* rubella, *Giardia lamblia*	Sinusitis, pneumonia, bacteremia
Complement deficiencies: C3, C5	Decreased chemotaxis and opsonization	*Staph. aureus, Proteus, Pseudomonas*	Otitis, sinusitis, pneumonia, septicemia
OTHER DISEASE STATES			
Ataxia telangectasia	Reduced IgA and IgE, decreased cellular immunity	*Staph. aureus, Strep. pneumoniae, Strep. pyogenes,* gram-negative enteric bacilli, *Pneumocystis*	Sinusitis, bronchitis, pneumonia
Wiskott-Aldrich syndrome	Defective antibody response to polysaccharides, defective cellular immunity	*Staph. aureus,* gram-negative bacilli, herpes simplex	Otitis, abscesses, pneumonia
Burns	Tissue necrosis, loss of epithelial barrier, lymphocytopenia	*Strep. pyogenes, Staph. aureus,* gram-negative enteric bacilli, particularly *Pseudomonas, Candida,* herpes simplex	Cellulitis, bacteremia, pneumonia
Diabetes	Reduced neurovascular supply, decreased leukocyte chemotaxis and bactericidal activity	*Staph. aureus, Candida,* gram-negative enteric bacilli, *M. tuberculosis, Mucoraceae*	Cellulitis, urinary tract infection, bacteremia
Hemolytic disease	Reduced monocyte-macrophage function (RES clearance)	*Salmonella, Bartonella, Strep. pneumoniae*	Bacteremia, pneumonia, osteomyelitis, meningitis
Uremia	Lymphocytopenia, impaired delayed hypersensitivity, decreased chemotaxis	*E. coli, Klebsiella, Staph. aureus, Pseudomonas*	Urinary tract infection, pneumonia, bacteremia
Cystic fibrosis	Bronchial obstruction by hyperviscous mucus	*Staph. aureus, Pseudomonas*	Bronchitis, pneumonia
IATROGENIC			
Glucocorticosteroids	Decreased cellular immunity, decreased chemotaxis	*Staph. aureus,* gram-negative enteric bacilli, *Candida, Toxoplasma,* herpes zoster, herpes simplex, *Pneumocystis*	Cellulitis, bacteremia, pneumonia
Cytotoxic drugs	Neutropenia, monocytopenia, lymphopenia, loss of mucosal barriers	Gram-negative enteric bacilli, *Candida, Pseudomonas*	Bacteremia
Antibiotics	Colonization by resistant bacteria	*Staph. aureus,* resistant gram-negative bacilli, especially *Pseudomonas, Serratia, Mima-Herellea*	Superinfections
Prosthetic devices	Foreign body	*Staph. aureus,* gram-negative enteric bacilli, *Candida*	Abscesses, bacteremia

operative procedures are the most likely to become infected. Infections are common in association with the use of equipment for inhalation therapy, and may be spread in the hospital by a variety of inanimate vehicles. The risk of a nosocomial infection depends on the underlying disease as well as on the number and complexity of therapeutic or diagnostic manipulations, and is enhanced by the concomitant indiscriminate use of antibiotics.

ETIOLOGY The bacteria usually responsible for infections in the compromised host are staphylococci (Chap. 134), *Escherichia coli, Klebsiella-Enterobacter* and *Proteus* (Chap. 138), *Pseudomonas* and *Mima-Herellea* (Chap. 139), *Serratia* (Chap. 139), *Salmonella* (Chap. 140), *Mycobacterium tuberculosis* (Chap. 161), and *Listeria* (Chap. 153). Among the fungi, *Candida* (*Monilia*) (Chap. 175), *Cryptococcus* (Chap. 170), *Mucoraceae* (*Mucormycosis*) (Chap. 178), *Nocardia* (Chap. 177), and *Aspergillus* (Chap. 178) are frequent pathogens implicated in secondary infections. *Cytomegalovirus* (Chap. 211), hepatitis viruses (Chap. 299), *herpes zoster* (Chap. 205), *Pneumocystis* (Chap. 219), and *Toxoplasma* (Chap. 218) are also encountered as causes of infection in patients with depressed resistance.

MANIFESTATIONS The clinical picture of an infection in the compromised host will vary with its site and, to a lesser extent, the microorganism causing it. In most instances, the major sign is fever. In patients with hospital-acquired infections, signs of infection usually occur after 4 to 5 days in the hospital. In these patients, the diagnosis may rest only on signs of local inflammation such as phlebitis, cellulitis, or evidence of a deep-seated infection. Sometimes a hospital-acquired infection may be heralded by no more than unexplained hyperventilation, confusion, or disorientation, early manifestations of septic shock (Chap. 129).

Postoperative infections These consist primarily of wound infections or collections of pus which form in and around the operative site. Although urinary tract infections and pneumonia are common in patients who have undergone surgery, postoperative infections are usually related to the surgical locus rather than an unrelated site. The majority of wound infections are caused by only a relatively few surgical procedures; these infections are particularly likely to occur when operations are long or require extensive resection and when contamination is unavoidable. Abdominal perineal resections, wounds involving arterial bypass grafts, insertion of cardiac prostheses, and portacaval shunts are associated with a relatively high rate of complicating infections. Most postoperative wound infections are caused by staphylococci and gram-negative enteric bacteria. Although group A *Strep. pyogenes* infections are averted with most chemoprophylactic regimens, wound infections which develop in patients receiving postoperative chemoprophylaxis usually are caused by organisms resistant to the drug being given. In general, chemoprophylaxis has not been successful in preventing wound infections in "clean" surgical procedures. In contaminated or "dirty" surgical cases, especially with open wounds or abdominal trauma, early administration of antibiotics has been shown to reduce postoperative wound infections.

Cutaneous, subcutaneous, and soft-tissue infections While wound sepsis constitutes the major part of superficial infections, other sites are involved. These include abscesses in the skin, subcutaneous tissues and muscle, cellulitis, decubitus ulcers, vascular stasis ulcers, and lesions secondary to diminished arterial blood supply. Most often staphylococci are the causative organisms, but group A and anaerobic streptococci, gram-negative bacilli, and even clostridia may be pathogenic under these circumstances. These infections may follow subcutaneous or intramuscular injections or extravasation of intravenous infusions. Soft tissue infections involving the perineal and perianal areas are common in acute leukemias. Although the infections usually remain localized, they may involve contiguous structures and may produce bacteremia. Gas in soft tissues should call to mind infection with *E. coli* as well as anerobic organisms. Antimicrobial therapy should be directed at the specific organism. Staphylococcal infections should be treated with penicillinase-resistant penicillin unless the organism is shown to be sensitive to penicillin G. Surgical drainage and debridement are often essential to recovery.

Burns regularly become infected secondarily. Most of these patients are receiving systemic or local chemoprophylaxis, and usually infection develops after the gram-positive flora has been replaced by gram-negative organisms, particularly *Pseudomonas*. These organisms are usually acquired from the environment and have been shown to survive on the floors, walls, and equipment used in burn wards. The sudden development of shock in a patient with a burn is almost certain evidence that *Pseudomonas* bacteremia is present. Treatment is discussed in Chaps. 129 and 139.

Urinary tract infections Urinary tract infections usually are associated with instrumentation of the urethra, bladder, or ureters and most often are due to insertion of an indwelling urethral catheter which permits entry of bacteria from the external environment to the bladder. Nosocomial urinary infections do not occur without predisposing instrumentation. The organisms are usually *E. coli, Klebsiella-Enterobacter, Serratia, Proteus, Pseudomonas,* and enterococci and tend to be resistant to one or several antibiotics. Epidemics of *Klebsiella-Enterobacter* and *Pseudomonas* urinary infections following spread of bacteria from contaminated equipment have been reported. Most patients with hospital-acquired bacteriuria are asymptomatic, some have cystitis, and others have clear-cut evidence of pyelonephritis which may be associated with bacteremia. Treatment should be reserved for patients with symptoms and for those suspected of bacteremia. Patients with indwelling catheters who have asymptomatic bacteriuria should not receive antibiotics since it is unlikely that the organisms will be eradicated; instead, superinfections will develop.

Considerable progress has been made in preventing hospital-acquired urinary infections by maintaining a system of closed drainage accompanied by an antibacterial rinse. In this fashion, the urine can be kept sterile for 5 to 7 days after insertion of the catheter. Failure to maintain closed drainage will result in infection in almost all patients within 48 h after catheter drainage is instituted.

skin, is a rare but well-documented complication of chronic hemodialysis.

Pneumonia Pulmonary infections are common in hospitalized patients with a variety of severe medical or surgical diseases. They may follow aspiration from any cause, atelectasis, heart failure, tracheostomy, and therapy with drugs that depress respiration. In a general hospital, pneumonia occurs commonly as a complication of cardiac or neurosurgery, but these infections are also seen in debilitated general medical patients, particularly when respiratory assistance devices have been employed. Mainstream reservoir nebulizers containing saline solutions are often heavily contaminated with *Pseudomonas*, flavobacteria, *Acinetobacter* (*Herellea*), and *Achromobacter* and are capable of producing severe pulmonary infections when nebulized directly into the tracheobronchial tree. This risk can be reduced sharply by bubbling a 0.25% acetic acid solution through the nebulizing equipment for 5 min prior to use. Gram-negative enteric bacteria usually are implicated in nosocomial pulmonary infections, particularly when patients have received antimicrobials. Although tracheostomies are sometimes necessary to maintain adequate ventilation, they are almost invariably associated with infections. Pulmonary infections are less common in association with tracheal intubation, which is preferable to tracheostomy. However, when tracheostomy is necessary, infection can be prevented only by meticulous aseptic technique during suctioning and the use of sterile suction catheters. The major therapeutic problem in many patients with complicating infections of the lung is mechanical; positive pressure breathing, postural drainage, frequent suctioning, and sometimes bronchoscopy are at least as important in the treatment of these infections as appropriate antibiotics.

Bacterial endocarditis Patients undergoing open-heart surgery have a relatively high incidence of wound, urinary, and pulmonary infections, but the most dreaded complication of open-heart surgery is endocarditis on a prosthetic valve. It occurs predominantly in patients whose operation is conducted on cardiopulmonary bypass, and surgery on the aortic valve is complicated by endocarditis much more frequently than surgery on the mitral valve. *Staphylococcus aureus* and *S. albus* are the most common pathogens. Clinical signs of endocarditis are often absent, and fever during the first four postoperative weeks provides the best clue to infections which follow in the wake of surgery. However, in some instances the prosthetic valve becomes infected years after its insertion, emphasizing the importance of preventing bacteremia in these patients. The prophylactic regimens for preventing endocarditis are detailed in Chap. 132. The diagnosis depends upon isolation of the organism from blood cultures. Treatment of endocarditis on intracardiac prostheses has been notoriously unsuccessful, and although the infection may be suppressed with antibiotics, reoperation, which often has a fatal outcome, may be necessary. Therefore, to prevent endocarditis, antimicrobial administration to patients undergoing open-heart surgery has become routine practice. It is clear that administration of a penicillinase-resistant penicillin or a cephalosporin will prevent postoperative pneumococcal endocarditis, but the efficacy of these drugs in preventing endocarditis with other organisms, including staphylococci, is less certain. Bacterial endocarditis, usually with organisms found in the

Bacteremia Invasion of the bloodstream can occur in any nosocomial infection, and among the various foci, the urinary tract predominates. However, the *indwelling venous catheter* is fast becoming the most common source of bacteremia in hospitalized patients, particularly when it is left in place longer than 48 h. Many of these patients develop phlebitis before bacteremia, and the catheter should be removed from all patients with inflammation at the catheter site. Staphylococci are implicated most often in catheter-associated infections, but *Acinetobacter* (*Mima-Herellea*) and other gram-negative organisms have been cultured from both the local site and the bloodstream.

Treatment of catheter-induced bacteremia requires removal of the catheter and systemic antimicrobial therapy; the treatment of staphylococcal bacteremia is discussed in Chap. 134 and that of gram-negative sepsis in Chap. 129. These infections can be prevented by (1) use of the catheter only when absolutely necessary; (2) strict aseptic technique during placement of the catheter; (3) application of bacitracin-neomycin-polymyxin ointment at the catheter site; and (4) removal of the catheter within 48 h, or sooner if phlebitis or cellulitis is present.

Patients receiving parenteral *hyperalimentation* appear to be at particular risk for developing *Candida* septicemia. The reason for this complication is not clear, but prolonged intravenous catheterization is probably the most important factor in the pathogenesis of this syndrome.

A number of cases of bacteremia emanating from *intravenous infusion* sets have been reported. Usually contamination occurs after the set has been placed into use, and the screw cap appears to be the most vulnerable site for introducing exogenous bacteria. The organisms that have been incriminated in clinical bacteremia usually have been *Escherichia* or *Klebsiella-Enterobacter*, but in addition to these, other gram-negative enteric organisms, staphylococci, and corynebacteria have been cultured from infusion sets. In most instances, contamination could be traced to faulty technique involved in changing bottles, adding medications, adjusting air filters, etc., and attention to the details of handling these materials by *all hospital personnel* is essential if this complication is to be prevented. Finally, the storage of blood products at room temperature has also been implicated in bacteremia. *Enterobacter* sepsis was induced in several patients transfused with pooled platelets, and a significant number of other bacteria including staphylococci, streptococci, *Sarcina, Herellea, Pseudomonas*, and flavobacter have been recovered from packed pooled platelets.

Miscellaneous nosocomial infections *Staphylococcal parotitis* is common in debilitated patients with a variety of medical diseases; it often follows in the wake of dehydration. *Septic arthritis* is not uncommon in patients with antecedent rheumatoid or degenerative joint disease who are subjected to diagnostic aspiration of the joint or who are treated with intraarticular drugs, usually corticosteroids. Pneumococcus, group A *Strep. pyogenes*, and staphylococcus are the most common pathogens. Septic arthritis of the sternoclavicular joint has also been described following placement of an intravenous catheter into the subclavian vein. *Iatrogenic meningitis* is a rare complication of spinal anesthesia, epidural block, injection of the stellate ganglion, diagnostic lumbar puncture, and myelography. Pneumococcus, staphylococcus, and *Pseudomonas* have been cultured from these patients. *Staphylococcal enterocolitis* occurs primarily in patients who have had gastrointestinal surgery who were given antibiotics preoperatively. It is also common in patients with liver disease who are treated with neomycin to reduce ammonia production by the bowel flora. Oral vancomycin (0.5 g every 6 to 12 h for four doses), systemic penicillinase-resistant penicillins, or cephalosporins are all effective modes of treatment.

Infections occurring during organ transplantation

Aside from host-versus-graft reactions (Chap. 76), infections pose the most serious threat to patients undergoing organ transplantation. These patients all receive immunosuppressive drugs and large quantities of adrenal cortical hormones and have readily available portals of entry for a variety of microorganisms. Multiple infections are common. Coagulase-positive staphylococci, *Pseudomonas*, gram-negative enteric bacilli, and enteric (non-group A) streptococci are the usual offending bacteria. These organisms are often present in the nasopharynx or on the skin of patients prior to transplantation, and for this reason it is recommended by some authorities that all staphylococcal carriers be treated with a penicillinase-resistant penicillin for several days prior to the procedure and afterward until the wound has healed. Likewise, bacteriuria should be eradicated before surgery. When transplantation is performed for pyelonephritis, the ureters should be excised in their entirety along with kidneys.

Patients who have undergone transplantation are particularly susceptible to fatal pulmonary infections which may produce few symptoms and signs. In addition to the bacteria mentioned above, cytomegalovirus, *Candida, Aspergillus*, and *Pneumocystis* are found at autopsy. These infections are characterized by little in the way of an inflammatory response, and the fungi, in particular, tend to produce a necrotizing reaction. Although no definitive information is available, it is likely that pulmonary superinfections with fungi or cytomegalovirus in these patients have an almost uniformly fatal prognosis.

LABORATORY FINDINGS Cultures of pus, appropriate body fluids, and blood form the cornerstone of treatment and always should be obtained even in patients receiving chemotherapy. Antimicrobial sensitivity tests should be performed when indicated. Gram stains of pus or secretions are helpful when only one or two types of bacteria are present in large numbers, but may be misleading and should be interpreted with caution. Superinfections usually are accompanied by leukocytosis, but granulocytopenia may be seen because of previous drug therapy or underlying disease. Moreover, many patients have a leukocytosis to begin with, and an elevated leukocyte count is of value as a clue to a complicating infection only if the count was normal previously.

THERAPEUTIC CONSIDERATIONS Because most nosocomial infections are caused by bacteria, treatment depends upon identification of the organism but must not be delayed until the results of cultures and sensitivity tests are at hand. Hence, the antibiotic must be chosen on the basis of previous cultures, the gram-stained smear, and the clinical

picture. For example, patients with subcutaneous and soft-tissue infections should be treated with a penicillinase-resistant penicillin and those with bacteriuria with a drug active against gram-negative enteric bacteria or enterococci. Patients with pneumonia or sepsis may require treatment with several drugs pending identification of the pathogen. The appropriate regimens are found in chapters dealing with the specific organisms and in the chapter on chemotherapy (Chap. 130). A general approach to therapy of undiagnosed bacteremia is provided in Chap. 129. Removal of the mechanical factors which are often the basis for complicating infections is as important as chemotherapy. This may involve withdrawing intravenous or urethral catheters, drainage of pus, debridement of a burn eschar, removal of sutures, aspiration of bronchial secretions, a change in inhalation equipment, and even, occasionally, removal of a cardiac prosthesis.

PREVENTION A number of steps can be taken to diminish the prevalence of hospital infections, and to eliminate some altogether. These include the following:

Surveillance Many hospitals have found a full-time or part-time nurse-epidemiologist useful in monitoring the prevalence of hospital infections, their relation to antibiotic usage, the location of infection, etc. In addition to providing early clues about the presence of infections, the epidemiologist can maintain a high index of awareness among hospital personnel, and perhaps indirectly reduce the prevalence of infection.

Isolation of infected patients Patients with untreated staphylococcal wound or pulmonary infections, pulmonary tuberculosis, and hepatitis should be isolated. However, it is important not to maintain isolation after it is no longer required. Too rigid adherence to isolation procedures may interfere with essential patient care.

Control of personnel Hospital personnel with purulent draining lesions should be removed from patient contact, but those with minor infections should not. Routine screening of hospital personnel for carriage of staphylococci is not useful. It is important to maintain the immune status of hospital workers against smallpox, poliomyelitis, diphtheria, and tetanus. Early detection of tuberculosis is essential, and periodic chest x-rays and tuberculin skin tests need to be encouraged. Tuberculosis poses a serious hazard to hospital workers as well as patient contacts. Likewise, hospital personnel must guard closely against infection with hepatitis B virus; dialysis units and blood processing areas pose particular risks.

Control of the environment Needless to say, cleanliness should be the hallmark of every hospital. Particular care needs to be observed in certain patient care areas in which the prevalence of nosocomial infections is high—nurseries, operating rooms, and intensive care units. All these must have ample facilities for hand-washing, and hand-washing must be enforced rigidly. Routine sampling of air or fomites in patient care areas is wasteful, although this procedure is useful for spot-testing air nebulizers, fluids for soaking surgical instruments, and ethylene oxide sterilizers, and for monitoring potential common source outbreaks of infection.

Control of patient care procedures Indwelling intravenous and urethral catheters, respiratory assistance devices, and intravenous infusion sets are probably the four procedures that are employed in all patients at risk of developing nosocomial infections. In them the appropriate measures for preventing these infections described above are absolutely essential.

Antimicrobial prophylaxis While prophylactic antibiotics have been useful when aimed at a single organism such as the group A *Strep. pyogenes* to prevent rheumatic fever, the meningococcus, and occasionally other pathogens, nosocomial infections are usually caused by one or more of several strains, species, and genera of microorganisms. In this situation, the attempt to place an "antibiotic umbrella" over the infection-prone patient has been futile; in fact, the use of antibiotics prophylactically has generally resulted in superinfection with endogenous or exogenous organisms resistant to the drug being administered.

PROGNOSIS Most nosocomial infections occur in patients being treated for another disease which is often chronic, disabling, and potentially fatal. While these secondary infections demand vigorous treatment, they may be only incidental to the patient's primary problem. For example, a patient with disseminated carcinomatosis will die even if his complicating infection is contained; and conversely a complicating infection often will not respond to therapy unless a remission is produced in the underlying disease. However, in many instances, nosocomial infections could have been prevented by more attention to meticulous technique or by greater restraint in the use of manipulative procedures, antibiotics, and other potent drugs.

REFERENCES

BENNETT JE: Diagnosis and therapy of systemic mycoses in the immunosuppressed host. Transplant Proc 5:1255, 1973

BERNARD HR, COLE WR: The prophylaxis of surgical infection: The effect of prophylactic antimicrobial drugs on the incidence of infection following potentially contaminated operations. Surgery 56:151, 1964

BRIGGS WA et al: Severe pneumonia in renal transplant patients. Ann Intern Med 75:887, 1971

BUCHHOLZ DH et al: Bacterial proliferation in platelet products stored at room temperature. N Engl J Med 285:429, 1971

COLLINS RN et al: Risk of local and systemic infection with polyethylene intravenous catheters. N Engl J Med 279:340, 1968

CURRY CR, QUIE PG: Fungal septicemia in patients receiving parenteral hyperalimentation. N Engl J Med 285:1221, 1971

DALE DC, PETERSDORF RG: Corticosteroids and infectious diseases. Med Clin North Am 57:1277, 1973

DUMA RJ et al: Septicemia from intravenous infusions. N Engl J Med 284:257, 1971

EICKHOFF TC: Infectious complications in renal transplant recipients. Transplant Proc 5:1233, 1973

FEINGOLD DS: Hospital-acquired infections. N Engl J Med 283:1384, 1970

LEVINE AS et al: Hematologic malignancies and other marrow failure states: Progress in management of complicating infections. Semin Hematol 11:141, 1974

MYERS BR et al: Current patterns of infection in multiple myeloma. Am J Med 52:87, 1972

NEIMAN P et al: Interstitial pneumonia and cytomegalovirus infection as complications of human marrow transplantation. Transplantation 15:478, 1973

REMINGTON JS: The compromised host. Hosp Pract 4:59, 1972

SHUCK JM: Infection control in burns. Surg Clin North Am 52:1425, 1972

SICKLES EA et al: Clinical presentation of infection in granulocytopenic patients. Arch Intern Med 135:715, 1975

TAN JS et al: Neutrophil dysfunction in diabetes. J Lab Clin Med 85:26, 1975

THORNTON GF, ANDRIOLE VT: Bacteriuria during indwelling catheter drainage: II. Effect of a closed sterile drainage system. JAMA 214:339, 1970

YOUNG RC et al: Fungemia with compromised host resistance. Ann Intern Med 80:605, 1974

129
SEPTIC SHOCK

ROBERT G. PETERSDORF

DEFINITION Septic shock is characterized by inadequate tissue perfusion, usually following bacteremia with gram-negative enteric bacilli. This circulatory insufficiency is a consequence of increased peripheral vascular resistance, pooling of blood in the microcirculation, diminished cardiac output, and tissue anoxia.

ETIOLOGY Septic shock may be associated with gram-positive infections, notably those due to pneumococci and streptococci, although it is more common following bacteremia with gram-negative bacilli: the *Enterobacteriaceae* (Chap. 138) and *Pseudomonas* and related organisms (Chap. 139). Gram-negative anaerobic bacteremia with *Bacteroides* species is also a precursor of septic shock, although in this situation the syndrome is less fulminating than with aerobic gram-negative bacilli. The shock syndrome is not due to bloodstream invasion with bacteria per se, but is related to release of endotoxin, the lipopolysaccharide moiety of the organisms' cell walls, into the circulation.

EPIDEMIOLOGY Gram-negative bacteremia and septic shock occur primarily in hospitalized patients who usually have an underlying disease which renders them susceptible to bloodstream invasion. Predisposing factors include diabetes mellitus; cirrhosis; leukemia, lymphoma, or disseminated carcinoma; transplantation and its associated immunosuppression; childbirth; a variety of surgical procedures and antecedent infections in the urinary, biliary, or gastrointestinal tracts. Most adults with gram-negative sepsis are elderly males, but neonates and child-bearing women are also prone to develop this syndrome. There has been an appreciable increase in the prevalence of serious gram-negative infections among hospitalized patients since 1935. For example, in 1958, the diagnosis of gram-negative sepsis was 0.8 per 1,000 hospital admissions; in 1968, this had risen to 8.0 per 1,000, and in one recent series it was 10 per 1,000. In addition to the predisposing factors mentioned above, the widespread use of antibiotics, immunosuppressive and cytotoxic agents, adrenal steroids, intravenous catheters, humidifiers, and other hospital equipment (Chap. 128), and the increasing longevity of patients with chronic diseases has given momentum to this upward trend.

PATHOGENESIS AND PATHOLOGY With the exception of *Pseudomonas* and *Mima-Herellea,* which are ubiquitous in the hospital environment, most of the bacteria causing gram-negative sepsis are normal commensals in the gastrointestinal tract. From there they may spread to contiguous structures as in peritonitis following appendiceal perforation, or migrate from the perineum into the urethra or bladder. Gram-negative bacteremia follows infection in a primary focus, usually the genitourinary tract, biliary tree, gastrointestinal tract and adjoining structures or lungs, and, less commonly, the skin, bones, and joints. In patients with leukemia, the skin and subcutaneous tissues or the lungs are often portals of entry, as is also the case in burn patients. In many instances, however, notably in patients with debilitating diseases, cirrhosis, and cancer, no primary focus is apparent. When bacteremia is followed by metastatic lesions in distant sites, classic abscess formation occurs. More often, however, the autopsy findings in gram-negative sepsis reflect primarily the infection at the primary locus and show involvement of target organs: pulmonary edema; hemorrhage and hyaline membrane formation in the lungs; tubular or cortical necrosis in the kidney; patchy necrosis in the myocardium; superficial ulceration in the gastrointestinal tract; and generalized thrombi in the capillaries.

PATHOPHYSIOLOGY General considerations Endotoxin exerts its major effects on small blood vessels with sympathetic (alpha-receptor) innervation. The toxin causes intense arteriolar and venospasm leading to significant immobilization of blood in the pulmonary, splanchnic, and renal capillaries, and to stagnant anoxia in these tissues. Local acidosis develops and promotes relaxation of the arteriolar sphincters while the venules remain constricted. Blood pools in the capillary bed, and the increased hydrostatic pressure results in leakage of plasma into the interstitial fluid. This, in turn, results in a sharp decrease in effective circulating blood volume and lowered cardiac output and systemic arterial hypotension, which stimulates the baroreceptors and results in further sympathetic activity, vasoconstriction, and selective reduction of blood flow to visceral organs and skin. If ineffective perfusion of vital organs is permitted to continue, metabolic acidosis and severe parenchymal damage ensue, and shock is then irreversible. In man, the kidneys and lungs are the organs particularly susceptible to endotoxin; oliguria as well as tachypnea and, in some instances, pulmonary edema develop early. In general, the heart and brain are spared early in shock, and myocardial failure and coma are late and often terminal manifestations of the shock syndrome. There is also experimental evidence that, following the administration of live gram-negative bacteria, significant arteriovenous shunting occurs around the capillary beds of susceptible organs. This intensifies tissue anoxia. Finally, in some instances the cells seem unable to utilize available oxygen. The net result of defective tissue perfusion is a sharp decrease in AV oxygen difference and lactic acidemia.

Inflammatory phenomena in shock The probable active substance in endotoxin, lipid A, is responsible for a variety of complex reactions, which profoundly affect host resistance. Firstly, it activates complement, and patients with fatal gram-negative shock show a decrease in C3 complement. Secondly, lipid A activates factor XII (Hageman factor) which, in turn, leads to activation of kallikrein from its inactive precursors. Kallikrein then activates bradykinin, a potent local vasodilator which promotes the pooling of blood in peripheral tissues as well as increased capillary permeability and localized tissue damage. In addition, endotoxin per se, by a mechanism analogous to the generalized Shwartzman reaction, produces fibrin thrombi in capillaries, and these form the nidi of the fibrin-platelet aggregates which are typical of the pathologic picture in advanced shock.

Hemodynamic alterations in man Many of the observations dealing with the pathophysiology of endotoxin shock were made in animals, and the hemodynamic data often varied according to the species studied and the dose of endotoxin administered. The establishment of centers for the study of shock has permitted detailed pathophysiologic studies in man. The results of these studies may vary with the time at which they are performed. For example, early in septic shock, the picture is one primarily of vasodilatation with an increase in cardiac output, a decrease in systemic vascular resistance, a decrease in central venous pressure, and an increase in stroke volume. In contrast, later in septic shock, the predominant picture is one of vasoconstriction with an increase in systemic vascular resistance, a decrease in cardiac output, a decrease in central venous pressure, and a decrease in stroke volume. Despite these differences, certain patterns of septic shock have emerged when large groups of patients have been studied. These may be summarized as follows:

1 Shock characterized by a normal cardiac output, normal blood volume, normal circulation time, normal or high central venous pressure, normal or high pH, and *reduced* peripheral resistance. These patients have warm, dry skin. While hypotension, oliguria, and lactic acidemia are present, the prognosis is generally good. Shock in this group has been attributed to shunting of blood through arteriovenous communications, making it unavailable for perfusion of vital organs.

2 Shock characterized by normal blood volume, high central venous pressure, normal or high cardiac output, reduced peripheral resistance but *marked metabolic acidosis,* oliguria, and very high blood lactate indicating ineffective tissue perfusion or impaired oxygen utilization. Despite the presence of warm, dry extremities in these patients, the prognosis is extremely poor.

3 Patients with low blood volume, low central venous pressure, high hematocrit, increased peripheral resistance, low cardiac output, hypotension, oliguria, but only a moderate elevation of blood lactate and normal or slightly high pH. These patients may be hypovolemic prior to bacteremia, and their prognosis is reasonably good provided intravascular volume is restored, bacteremia is treated with appropriate antibiotics, septic foci are removed or drained, and vasoactive drugs are given.
4 Shock characterized by low blood volume, low central venous pressure, low cardiac output, marked decompensated metabolic acidosis, and severe lactic acidemia. In these patients the extremities are cool and cyanotic. The prognosis is very poor.

These observations suggest that there are various stages of septic shock, from hyperventilation, respiratory alkalosis, vasodilatation, and high or normal cardiac output in early shock, to perfusion failure characterized by high-grade lactic acidemia, metabolic acidosis, low cardiac output, and small AV oxygen difference in irreversible, late shock. Moreover, in some patients there is little correlation between the outcome and the hemodynamic abnormalities.

COMPLICATIONS OF SEPTIC SHOCK **Coagulation defects** In most patients with septic shock there is a deficiency in several clotting factors, due to consumption of these factors, a syndrome termed *disseminated intravascular coagulation* (DIC). The pathogenesis of this syndrome involves the activation of the intrinsic clotting system by factor XII (Hageman factor) followed by deposition of fibrin-platelet aggregates on the capillary thrombi that have formed as a result of the generalized Shwartzman reaction. The fibrin-platelet aggregates are typical of DIC, which is characterized by a decrease in factors II, V, and VIII, fibrinogen, and platelets. There may be some degree of fibrinolysis, with appearance of split products (positive Fi test). These clotting abnormalities are present to some degree in most patients with septic shock, but usually there is no clinical bleeding, although hemorrhagic phenomena due to thrombocytopenia or deficiency in clotting factors occur occasionally. A more important effect of further disseminated intravascular coagulation is development of capillary thrombi, particularly in the lung. Unless there is bleeding, the coagulopathy requires no therapy and disappears spontaneously as shock is treated.

Respiratory failure Respiratory failure is the most important cause of death in patients with shock, particularly after the hemodynamic aberrations have been corrected. The respiratory lesion has been called the "shock lung" and is characterized by pulmonary edema, hemorrhage, atelectasis, hyaline membrane formation, and formation of capillary thrombi. The severe pulmonary edema may be a consequence of a marked increase in capillary permeability resulting in a "pulmonary leak." It may occur in the absence of heart failure. Respiratory failure may develop and progress even as other abnormalities return to normal. Pulmonary surfactant decreases, and pulmonary compliance becomes progressively compromised.

Renal failure Oliguria occurs early in shock and is probably due to low intravascular volume and inadequate renal perfusion. If renal perfusion remains inadequate, acute tubular necrosis develops. In an occasional patient, renal cortical necrosis, as occurs in the generalized Shwartzman reaction, is seen.

Cardiac failure Many patients with septic shock develop myocardial failure even though they were free of heart disease prior to development of shock. On the basis of experimental data, heart failure has been attributed to a product of lysosomal enzyme activity in the ischemic splanchnic region. This product has been termed myocardial depressant factor (MDF). Functionally, there is left ventricular failure as indicated by an increase in left ventricular end-diastolic pressure.

Other organs Superficial ulcerations of the gastrointestinal tract manifested by hemorrhage are common, as are abnormalities in liver function, characterized by hypoprothombinemia, hypoalbuminemia, and mild jaundice.

CLINICAL MANIFESTATIONS Usually gram-negative bacteremia begins abruptly with chills, fever, nausea, vomiting, diarrhea, and prostration. When septic shock develops, there are, in addition, tachycardia; tachypnea; hypotension; cool, pale extremities, often with peripheral cyanosis; mental obtundation, and oliguria. When present in its full-blown form, gram-negative shock is detected readily, but occasionally the findings are quite subtle, particularly in old, debilitated patients or in infants. Unexplained hypotension, increasing confusion, and disorientation or hyperventilation may be the only clues to septic shock. Some patients are hypothermic, and in the absence of fever the diagnosis is often missed. Jaundice occurs occasionally and signifies infection in the biliary tree, intravascular hemolysis, or "toxic" hepatitis. As shock progresses, oliguria persists, and heart failure, respiratory insufficiency, and coma supervene. Death usually occurs from pulmonary edema, generalized anoxemia secondary to respiratory insufficiency, cardiac arrythmias, disseminated intravascular coagulation with bleeding, cerebral anoxia, or a combination of these factors.

LABORATORY FINDINGS The laboratory data in septic shock vary greatly and depend in many instances on the cause of the shock syndrome and on the stage of shock. The volume of packed red blood cells is often elevated and falls to below normal as the volume deficit is repaired. There usually is *leukocytosis* between 15,000 and 30,000 per mm^3 with a shift to the left. However, the white blood cell count may be normal, and some patients have leukopenia. The *platelet count* is usually decreased, and the prothrombin consumption and partial thromboplastin times may be abnormal, reflecting a deficiency of *clotting factors.*

The *urinalysis* shows no specific abnormalities. Initially, the specific gravity is high; as oliguria persists, isosthenuria develops. The *blood urea nitrogen* and *creatinine* are elevated, and creatinine clearance is reduced.

Simultaneous measurements of urine and plasma osmolalities are a useful clue to impending renal failure. If the urinary osmolality is greater than 400 milliosmoles and the ratio of urine to plasma osmolality is greater than 1.5, renal function is preserved and oliguria is probably due to volume depletion. On the other hand, a urine osmolality of less than 400 and a urine/plasma ratio less than 1.5 signify renal failure. Electrolyte patterns vary considerably, but there is a tendency to *hyponatremia* and hypochloremia. The serum potassium may be high, low, or normal. The *bicarbonate concentration* is usually low and *blood lactate* is elevated. A high level of blood lactate is the most reliable clue to poor tissue perfusion.

Early in endotoxin shock there is *respiratory alkalosis* manifested by a low P_{CO_2} and high arterial pH, probably an attempt to blow off CO_2 to compensate for developing lactic acidemia and because of progressive anoxemia. As shock progresses, *metabolic acidosis* develops. There often is striking *anoxemia,* and P_{O_2} values below 70 mmHg are common. Hemodynamic measurements usually show a low *central venous pressure,* low *pulmonary artery and wedge pressures,* low *cardiac output* and cardiac index, high *peripheral resistance,* and slow circulation time. Occasionally cardiac output is hypernormal, and systemic vascular resistance low. *Blood volume* is usually low, but this determination is notoriously unreliable in septic shock and should not be trusted. The *electrocardiogram* generally shows depression of the S-T segment, inversion of the T waves, and a variety of arrhythmias, and may mistakenly suggest the diagnosis of myocardial infarction.

In untreated septic shock, the blood cultures should reveal the causative pathogens, but bacteremia is often intermittent and the blood cultures may be negative. Furthermore, many patients will have received antimicrobial agents when they are first seen, masking the bacteriologic diagnosis. *A negative blood culture does not exclude the diagnosis of septic shock.* Culture of the primary septic focus may aid in the diagnosis, but the bacteriology may have been altered by prior chemotherapy. The ability of endotoxin to coagulate the blood of the horseshoe crab *Limulus* is the basis of a test for endotoxemia, but this test has often been unreliable.

DIAGNOSIS The diagnosis of septic shock is not difficult in the presence of chills, fever, and an overt focus of infection. However, none of the obvious clues may be present. Elderly, debilitated patients, in particular, may have severe infections in the absence of fever. Unexplained confusion and disorientation and hyperventilation without abnormal chest x-rays should call the diagnosis to mind. Pulmonary embolism, myocardial infarction, cardiac tamponade, aortic dissection, and silent hemorrhage are entities often confused with septic shock.

COURSE The rational treatment of septic shock depends upon careful monitoring of patients. Specifically four parameters need to be followed at the bedside:

1 The status of the pulmonary circulation and, to a lesser extent, of left ventricular function should be monitored by insertion of a Swan-Ganz catheter. A pulmonary wedge pressure in excess of 15 to 18 cm H_2O signifies fluid overload. When a Swan-Ganz catheter is not available, the *central venous pressure* (CVP) should be measured. Insertion of a catheter into the great veins or right atrium provides an accurate index of the relation between right ventricular competence and effective blood volume and should be used as a guide to fluid replacement therapy. When the CVP exceeds 12 to 14 cm water, there is some danger of overloading the circulation and precipitating pulmonary edema. It is important to be sure that the flow through the catheter is free and that the catheter is not in the right ventricle. Either a Swan-Ganz catheter or a CVP line should be placed in every patient with septic shock.
2 The *pulse pressure* serves as an estimate of stroke volume.
3 *Cutaneous vasoconstriction* provides a clue to peripheral resistance, although it does not reflect accurately blood flow to kidney, brain, or gut.
4 Hourly *urine output* should be used to monitor splanchnic blood flow and visceral perfusion. Usually this requires placement of an indwelling urethral catheter.

By means of these four measurements the patient with shock can be followed carefully and managed intelligently. Indirect arterial blood pressure does not provide an accurate picture of the hemodynamic situation, and perfusion of vital organs may be adequate in patients with hypotension; conversely, some patients with normal blood pressures may have marked pooling and inadequate visceral blood flow. Direct measurement of arterial pressure is helpful but usually not necessary.

Where possible, these patients should be treated in intensive care units in hospitals that have laboratories available for measurement of arterial and venous pH, blood gases, blood lactate, renal function, and electrolytes.

TREATMENT **Support of respiration** In many patients with septic shock arterial P_{O_2} is markedly depressed. It is essential to establish an airway at the outset and to administer oxygen nasally or by mask. Tracheal intubation usually suffices; tracheostomy is rarely necessary. However, a positive pressure-volume cycled respirator should be employed early to achieve proper ventilation and to overcome the severe hypoxia.

Volume replacement With the CVP or pulmonary wedge pressure as a guide, blood volume should be replaced with blood (if anemia is present), plasma, dextran (molecular weight 70,000 or 40,000), human serum albumin, and appropriate electrolyte solutions, primarily dextrose-saline and bicarbonate (which is preferable to lactate for treating the acidosis). The quantity of fluid required may be considerably in excess of "normal" blood volume and may amount to 8 to 12 liters in only a few hours. Large quantities may be required even when the cardiac index is normal. *Oliguria in the presence of hypotension is not a contraindication to continued vigorous fluid therapy.* In order to guard against pulmonary edema, diuresis with furosemide should be attempted when the CVP reaches a level of approximately 10 to 12 cm and the pulmonary artery pressure 16 to 18 cm of water.

Antibiotics Blood cultures and cultures of relevant body fluids or exudates should be taken before instituting antimicrobial therapy. Drugs should be given intravenously, and bactericidal agents used when possible. When the results of blood cultures and sensitivities are known, one of the appropriate drugs recommended in the chapters dealing with the specific infections and discussed in Chap. 130 should be given. Usually cultures and sensitivities are not at hand at the onset of shock, and the etiologic diagnosis entails an educated guess based upon culture from the primary focus—urine, bile, pus, or sputum, or on the setting in which the infection occurs. For example, a young woman with dysuria, chills, and flank pain and septic shock is likely to have *Escherichia coli* bacteremia, while gram-negative sepsis in a burn patient is probably caused by *Pseudomonas.* The drugs of choice for gram-negative bacteremia are:

E. coli:	Ampicillin or cephalothin
Klebsiella-Enterobacter:	Gentamicin
Proteus mirabilis:	Ampicillin or cephalothin
Pr. rettgeri, morganii, or *vulgaris:*	Gentamicin and/or carbenicillin
Mima-Herellea:	Gentamicin and/or carbenicillin
Pseudomonas:	Gentamicin and/or carbenicillin

The dosages and routes of administration for these agents are detailed in Chap. 130. Cephalothin can be substituted for ampicillin in patients with a history of penicillin allergy. Because of its toxic effect on the vestibular portion of the eighth nerve, gentamicin must be given cautiously to oliguric patients; a single dose of 80 mg achieves blood levels which should suffice throughout the period of oliguria. Similar precautions should be taken with kanamycin, where the loading dose is 1.0 g.

When the cause of septic shock is unknown, therapy should be initiated with both gentamicin and cephalothin or a penicillinase-resistant penicillin; many investigators add carbenicillin to this regimen. If *Bacteroides* is suspected, chloramphenicol or 7-chlorlincomycin (clindamycin) can be added. As soon as culture results become available, the unnecessary drugs can be deleted.

Surgical intervention Many patients with septic shock have an abscess, infarcted or necrotic bowel, an inflamed gallbladder, infected uterus, pyonephrosis, or other local situations which lend themselves to surgical drainage or excision. As a rule, successful treatment of shock requires surgical intervention even if the patient is desperately ill. Operations should not be postponed "to get the patient in shape" because these patients' condition will continue to deteriorate unless the septic focus is removed or drained.

Vasoactive drugs Usually, septic shock is accompanied by maximal stimulation of alpha-adrenergic receptors, and pressor agents which act by stimulating these receptors such as norepinephrine, levarterenol, and metaraminol are contraindicated. The two groups of drugs which have been of value in septic shock are alpha-receptor blocking agents exemplified by phenoxybenzamine and phentolamine (Regitine) and beta-receptor stimulants, notably isoproterenol and dopamine.

Phenoxybenzamine (Dibenzylene), an adrenolytic agent, effects a central phlebotomy by reducing resistance and increasing intravascular capacity. Hence there is a redistribution of blood. Blood leaves the lungs, relieving pulmonary edema and enhancing gas exchange. Central venous pressure and left ventricular end-diastolic pressure fall, cardiac output rises, and peripheral venous constriction regresses. The recommended dose is 0.2 to 2.0 mg per kg intravenously. Small doses can be injected instantaneously and large doses over a period of 40 to 60 min. Fluids must be given simultaneously to compensate for the increment in venous capacitance; failure to do so aggravates shock. Dibenzylene is not available for general use, and experience with phentolamine has not been great enough to recommend it.

Chlorpromazine in multiple small doses of 2.5 to 5 mg also relieves vasoconstriction through its direct adrenolytic effect and by ganglionic blockage.

Isoproterenol (Isuprel) counteracts arteriolar and venous constriction in the microcirculation by its direct vasodilating effect. In addition, the drug exerts a direct inotropic effect on the heart. Cardiac output is increased by stimulation of the myocardium and by reduction of cardiac work as peripheral resistance decreases. The dose of isoproterenol is 2 to 8 μg per min for the average adult. Ventricular arrhythmias may result from this drug, and shock may be made worse if fluid administration does not keep pace with relieved vasoconstriction.

Dopamine hydrochloride is used widely for treatment of shock. Unlike other vasoactive agents, this drug increases renal blood flow and with it glomerular filtration, sodium excretion, and urine flow. This effect is seen at low doses (1 to 2 μg/kg/min). At a dose of 2 to 10 μg/kg/min, the beta receptors in the heart are stimulated with a resulting increase in cardiac output but without increase in heart rate or blood pressure. Between 10 and 20 μg/kg/min there is some effect on the alpha receptors with a rise in blood pressure. Above 20 μg/kg/min, alpha stimulation predominates, and vasoconstriction may reverse the dopaminergic effects on the renal and splanchnic circulations. Treatment should be started at 2 to 5 μg/kg/min and the dose increased until urine flow and blood pressure respond. Most patients respond to doses of 20 μg/kg/min or less. Side effects include ectopic beats, nausea and vomiting, and occasionally tachyarrythmias. They usually disappear with reduction in dosage.

Digitalis and diuretics A rapidly acting preparation of digoxin or Cedilanid should be given when the CVP or pulmonary artery pressure remains high in the face of systemic hypotension. In addition, the urine output of these patients should be increased, preferably with intravenous furosemide.

Adrenal cortical hormones In very large doses these agents may overcome increased peripheral resistance, mitigate the cellular injury evoked by endotoxin, perhaps by stabilizing lysozomes, prevent platelet aggregation, and have a variety of other actions which may be beneficial to the host. The only way that these hormones are effective in septic shock is in dosages of 30 mg methylprednisolone per kg given as a single dose and repeated for two or three doses. Usually by that time the issue has been decided and the drug can be discontinued without tapering. While these high-dose steroid regimens have been controversial, the evidence that they are effective is mounting.

Other measures Hemorrhage must be controlled with

whole blood, fresh-frozen plasma, cryoprecipitate, or platelet transfusion, depending on the clotting abnormality. Treatment of disseminated intravascular coagulation with heparin remains a controversial and hazardous procedure but is sometimes necessary. Hyperbaric oxygen has been tried in gram-negative bacteremia with indifferent results.

PROGNOSIS The measures described above usually will resuscitate most patients, at least temporarily. Indicators of a favorable response are:

1 Improved sensorium and general appearance
2 Decreased peripheral cyanosis
3 Warming of the skin over the extremities
4 Urine output of 40 to 50 ml per h
5 Increased pulse pressure
6 Return of CVP and pulmonary artery pressure to normal
7 Increased blood pressure

The ultimate outcome, however, is dependent upon several other factors:

1 Ability to eliminate the source of infection with surgery or antibiotics. The prognosis of urinary tract infections, septic abortions, abdominal abscesses, gastrointestinal or biliary fistulas, and subcutaneous or anorectal abscesses is better than that of primary foci in the skin or lungs. However, extensive abdominal surgery, even if necessary, is associated with a poor prognosis.
2 Previous contact with the organism. Patients with chronic urinary tract infections who develop bacteremia rarely have severe gram-negative shock, perhaps because they have become tolerant to the endotoxin.
3 Underlying disease. Patients with lymphoma or leukemia who develop septic shock while their hematologic disease is out of control rarely recover; conversely, if hematologic remission is achieved, the shock is more likely to respond to therapy. Patients with antecedent heart disease and with diabetes mellitus also have a poor prognosis.
4 Metabolic status. The development of severe metabolic acidosis and lactic acidemia—irrespective of cardiac output—is associated with a poor prognosis.
5 Development of pulmonary insufficiency even after the hemodynamic abnormalities have been corrected.

The overall mortality of septic shock remains 50 percent; however, with better monitoring and more physiologic treatment, the outcome should improve.

PREVENTION The poor results in the treatment of septic shock are not due to lack of potent antibiotics or vasoactive agents. Rather, failure to institute therapy sufficiently early is a major roadblock to success. Septic shock usually is recognized too late, all too often after irreversible changes have taken place. Because 70 percent of patients who are likely to develop septic shock are in the hospital *before* signs and symptoms of shock appear, it is essential to watch patients who are candidates for development of shock assiduously, to treat their infections vigorously and early, and to perform appropriate surgery before catastrophic complications occur. There is some preliminary evidence that early therapy of septic shock improves the ultimate outcome. Finally, the protective effect of antiserum in experimental animals may, at some time in the future, be applicable to man.

REFERENCES

BRYANT RE et al: Factors affecting mortality of gram-negative rod bacteremia. Arch Intern Med 127:120, 1971
CHRISTY JH: Treatment of gram-negative shock. Am J Med 50:77, 1971
CORRIGAN JJ JR et al: Changes in the blood coagulation system associated with septicemia. N Engl J Med 279:851, 1968
GOLDBERG LI: Dopamine—Clinical uses of an endogenous catecholamine. N Engl J Med 291:707, 1974
HARDAWAY RM et al: Intensive study and treatment of shock in man. JAMA 199:799, 1967
JONES LW, WEIL MH: Water, creatinine and sodium excretion following circulatory shock with renal failure. Am J Med 51: 314, 1971
MACLEAN LD et al: Patterns of septic shock in man—A detailed study of 56 patients. Ann Surg 166:543, 1967
MCHENRY MC, HANK WA: Bacteremia caused by gram-negative bacilli. Med Clin North Am 58:623, 1974
MILLER RI et al: Biochemical mechanisms of generation of bradykinin by endotoxin. J Infect Dis 128:S 144, 1973
MYEROWITZ RL et al: Recent experience with bacillemia due to gram-negative organisms. J Infect Dis 124:239, 1971
NISHIJIMA H et al: Hemodynamic and metabolic studies in shock associated with gram-negative bacteremia. Medicine 52:287, 1973
ROBIN ED et al: Capillary leak syndrome with pulmonary edema. Arch Intern Med 130:66, 1972
TARAZI RC: Sympathomimetic agents in the treatment of shock. Ann Intern Med 81:364, 1974
WINSLOW EJ et al: Hemodynamic studies and results of therapy in 50 patients with bacteremic shock. Am J Med 54:421, 1973

130
CHEMOTHERAPY OF INFECTION

WILLIAM M. M. KIRBY
ROBERT G. PETERSDORF

INTRODUCTION From the standpoint of overall reduction in morbidity and mortality rates, the greatest impact of drug therapy has been in the field of infectious diseases. Modern chemotherapy of infectious diseases dates from the mid-1930s when the sulfonamides were introduced. Penicillin G, the first of the antibiotics to be used systemically, came into widespread use in the early 1940s, and since then several dozen chemotherapeutic agents have appeared that are effective in a wide variety of bacterial, rickettsial, fungal, and parasitic infections. The efficacy of antimicrobial agents is due to their action in inhibiting growth of the parasite rather than to an enhancement of defense mechanisms, and it is remarkable that such a large number of substances can interfere effectively with multiplication of invading organisms without seriously damaging the cells of the host. Effective new agents continue to appear in surprising numbers, both from large-scale screening programs in which samples of organic matter are tested for antimicrobial activity and from chemical modifications of the known chemotherapeutic drugs. Specific recommendations for therapy are made in chapters dealing with individual diseases; this section is devoted to general principles of chemotherapy and to a consideration of individual therapeutic agents.

FACTORS INFLUENCING SELECTION OF ANTIMICROBIAL AGENTS AND THE OUTCOME OF THERAPY

SUSCEPTIBILITY OF THE INFECTING MICROORGANISMS

No antimicrobial agent is effective against all pathogenic microorganisms; each has its own spectrum of activity against one or a variety of species, within which the majority of strains have been found to be susceptible. There are a few instances, such as the susceptibility of group A streptococci and pneumococci to penicillin G, in which resistant strains occur rarely if at all, and where treatment with penicillin can be given without concern about resistance. With the majority of chemotherapeutic agents, however, a variable percentage of strains of each susceptible species is resistant, i.e., they are not inhibited by concentrations of the drug attainable in the patient's blood and tissues with the usual dosage schedules. It is customary, therefore, in serious infections to determine the susceptibility of most pathogens to a variety of chemotherapeutic agents, and this has become one of the most important functions of clinical microbiology laboratories. *Dilution methods* of susceptibility testing, considered to be the most accurate, involve making serial dilutions of each agent to be tested in agar or broth, adding a standardized inoculum of the infecting organisms, and determining the smallest amount (the minimal inhibitory concentration, MIC) of the drug that inhibits growth after overnight incubation. *Agar dilution tests* are used routinely in some laboratories with sufficient volume to justify them, and mechanized or preprepared *broth dilution methods* are available. Automated methods are also being developed commercially. Although expensive, they are becoming simpler and more accurate, and at least one provides a result within 3 h. For the majority of laboratories, however, the simpler *agar diffusion method,* which is accurate and reliable when properly performed, remains the one usually used. With this technique, zones of inhibition of growth of a standardized inoculum of the infecting organism around filter paper disks impregnated with antibiotics are measured, and the zone sizes reflect the inhibitory concentrations of drug, which are in turn related to the blood levels usually attained. Susceptibility of 8 to 10 chemotherapeutic agents can be tested on a single large agar plate, and a report of *susceptible, intermediate,* or *resistant* can be made. Disk testing has a number of limitations; it is applicable chiefly to rapidly growing pathogens, and the results are usually not reported until 24 h after the pathogen is isolated.

BACTERICIDAL VERSUS BACTERIOSTATIC AGENTS Although these are relative terms, some chemotherapeutic drugs can be clearly shown to have a killing (bactericidal) action at or near the minimal inhibitory concentration, while others simply inhibit bacterial growth (bacteriostatic), leaving the host to strike the *coup de grâce.* Bactericidal agents include the penicillins, cephalosporins, aminoglycosides, polymyxins, and vancomycin, while examples of bacteriostatic agents are the tetracyclines, sulfonamides, chloramphenicol, erythromycin, and lincomycin. Bactericidal agents give definitely superior results in diseases such as bacterial endocarditis and are more likely to give a favorable response in life-threatening infections, particularly when there is impairment of the host's defense mechanisms. In mild infections in otherwise healthy individuals, on the other hand, there is little to choose between "-cidal" and "-static" agents. In uncomplicated urinary tract infections, due to *Escherichia coli,* for example, the clinical results are as good with sulfonamides as with broad-spectrum penicillins or cephalosporins.

CLINICAL PHARMACOLOGY Knowledge of the clinical pharmacology of antimicrobial agents is helpful in prescribing therapy that is both safe and effective. Important information includes details of absorption and excretion, blood and urine levels with various routes of administration, protein binding, renal clearance, half-lives of drugs, stability in solutions and within the body, and the conversion to metabolic breakdown products. With some agents, such as ampicillin, much higher blood levels are obtained with the same doses given parenterally than orally, whereas with others such as dicloxacillin and doxycycline, where there is complete absorption from the intestinal tract, the oral and parenteral doses are the same. Because of possible incompatibilities, *it is advisable never to administer more than one agent at a time by the intravenous route.* Absorption from the intestinal tract is impaired by a variety of foods and chemicals, and, in general, antimicrobials should be administered temporally as far removed from food and other drugs, such as antacids, as possible.

Antimicrobials are bound to a varying extent to serum proteins, especially albumin. Although the significance of protein binding is uncertain and controversial, it is clear that the bound antibiotic has no antimicrobial activity, and it is probable that the concentration of free, unbound antibiotic in the tissues, at any one time, is no greater than the peak level of free antibiotic in the blood. All other features being equal, antimicrobials with relatively low binding should be preferable to those with a high degree of binding. In general, this point of view is reflected in the dosages of antimicrobial agents that are commonly recommended.

Renal clearance is one of the most important determinants of antibiotic blood levels and is mainly responsible, for example, for the much higher levels attained with the same dose of cephaloridine than of cephalothin, and of carbenicillin than of ampicillin. Antibiotics with a high renal clearance such as penicillin G and cephalothin have a large component of tubular secretion, and their blood levels are elevated to a greater degree by probenecid than those of ampicillin and cephaloridine, where the tubular contribution is less important. Plasma half-life, the time required for a blood level to fall by one-half, is also determined primarily by renal clearance mechanisms and is much shorter for those penicillins and cephalosporins that are secreted by the renal tubules than for antibiotics such as the aminoglycosides with little or no tubular component. Protein binding also has an important influence on the half-life of antibiotics, particularly those that are excreted mainly or entirely by glomerular filtration. Thus, the plasma half-life of gentamicin, which is not bound by proteins, is 2 h, whereas that of doxycycline, which is over 90 percent protein-bound, is about 16 h. Antibiotics with little or no protein binding have a much larger apparent volume of distribution (AVD) than those with a high degree of binding, i.e., the AVD of gentamicin is 30 percent of body weight compared with 14 percent for cefazolin. Cephalothin has a high plasma clearance with a high rate of nonrenal clearance due to its partial conversion in the body to a less active metabolic breakdown product. These are a few examples of the pharmacologic features of individual antimicrobial agents; others will be mentioned as the individual drugs are considered.

DOSE, ROUTE, AND DURATION OF THERAPY In prescribing dosages of antimicrobial agents, the objective is to deliver a concentration in excess of that needed to inhibit and/or kill the infecting organism at the site of infection. Since it is difficult to measure tissue concentrations, a blood level that exceeds the MIC two- to eightfold is a commonly accepted guideline. This is an arbitrary concentration of drug and obviously does not take into account all the variations in penetration into different tissues, or the role of host defense mechanisms. These variations may be very important because in many instances, infections have been cured with antibiotics such as the tetracyclines where the concentration of free, active drug in the blood is not much greater than the MIC. The relation between blood levels and MIC does not hold in urinary tract infection, where the concentration of drug cleared by the kidney usually far exceeds the MIC. In this situation, an excess of drug in the urine is obviously important.

The route of administration, as well as the dose, is important in achieving appropriate drug levels. In general, parenteral therapy should usually be given in severe infections to be certain that high, effective blood levels are attained. The *intravenous route* is especially indicated initially in meningitis, endocarditis, and osteomyelitis, where barriers to penetration of the antimicrobial agent can be overcome by high blood levels. Intravenous therapy is also indicated when there is hypotension, and when bleeding diatheses are present. For milder infections, *intramuscular administration* is often an acceptable or preferable alternative, particularly with antibiotics such as procaine penicillin that cause relatively little pain and produce prolonged, effective blood levels. With gentamicin, blood levels are the same with an intramuscular injection as with an intravenous infusion given over a period of 60 min, so that the route can be chosen on the basis of comfort for the patient and the need for other intravenous medications. The *oral route* is used chiefly for mild to moderate infections, and for completion of therapy of severe infections after they have been brought under control with parenteral therapy. Absorption from the intestinal tract is variable even in the fasting state, and all oral antibiotics should be taken at least 1 h before and 3 h after food and other medications. This presents difficulties with drugs such as antacids that need to be taken frequently and that are especially likely to interfere with absorption of antimicrobial agents. Parenteral administration is often the only solution to this problem.

The optimal duration of antimicrobial treatment is unknown for many infections, and there is considerable variation from one medical center to another in the length of time antimicrobial therapy is given. In bacterial endocarditis, for example, the usual course of parenteral therapy may vary from 2 to 8 weeks with an average of about four weeks. For most acute infections a good general rule is to continue therapy for 2 to 3 days after the temperature has returned to normal and all signs of infection have subsided. However, fever can continue for weeks from sterile effusions complicating pneumonia, and cerebrospinal fluid abnormalities can persist for considerable periods in bacterial meningitis, leading to a continuation of chemotherapy for much longer than is necessary. Empiricism needs to be tempered with reason and experience, and in actual practice the guidelines for duration of therapy must be sufficiently flexible to be appropriate for the patient being treated.

ALLERGY AND TOXICITY The patient's allergic history should always be explored before prescribing antimicrobial agents. In addition to allergic manifestations in general, a report of previous drug allergies is of particular importance, and agents that have caused clear-cut reactions should be avoided. Unfortunately, no reliable test is available to determine the presence of allergy to the penicillins, and they may or may not be well tolerated by patients with a history of a previous reaction. The possibility of a severe anaphylactic reaction can be reliably excluded by skin tests containing major and minor determinant mixtures, but only the major mixture is commercially available. When administration of a penicillin is considered essential, one approach is to begin with a very small dose intravenously and increase the amount every few minutes until it is learned whether the patient can tolerate the antibiotic. Specifically, with an intravenous infusion running 1 unit penicillin diluted in 3 to 5 ml saline or glucose solution is injected slowly into the tubing, and 5 min is allowed to elapse to see if an untoward reaction occurs. A solution of epinephrine is available in another syringe to be injected if needed. If no reaction occurs, 2, 5, 10, 25, and 50 units, etc., are injected at 5-min intervals, and within an hour or so it either becomes apparent that the patient can tolerate a full therapeutic dose, or he develops a reaction that is readily controlled by epinephrine. If a reaction occurs, administering another antibiotic is usually best, although in mild reactions, continuing the penicillin along with antihistamines and/or steroids is possible in some instances. Such a program can be quite troublesome as well as risky, requiring frequent adjustments to suppress urticaria and itching. The number of alternative antibiotics available is large enough that switching to another agent is usually the best course to follow.

Drug toxicity related to renal function is of particular importance. Some antimicrobials, such as the penicillins, cephalothin, chloramphenicol, erythromycin, and lincomycin, are relatively safe at normal or only slightly reduced dosage in the presence of impaired renal function. Other agents, such as the aminoglycosides, are potentially quite toxic but can be administered at reduced dosage if proper guidelines, based on serial determinations of the serum creatinine, are followed, and particularly if blood levels can be monitored. Certain toxic agents should be avoided if at all possible in the presence of renal insufficiency. These include most of the tetracyclines, streptomycin, cephaloridine, the sulfonamides, the nitrofurans, and nalidixic acid. One of the long-acting tetracyclines, doxycycline, has the same half-life in healthy and uremic subjects, and can be administered to patients with impaired renal function either orally or intravenously. A number of patients with chronic renal failure are being maintained on dialysis programs, and may require antimicrobials for a variety of infections. Table 130-1 summarizes adult dosage schedules for various antibiotics for patients with renal failure, on or off dialysis.

SITE OF INFECTION Soft-tissue infections in sites with a good blood supply and a minimum of tissue necrosis are, in general, easily treated. In meningitis and endocarditis, on the other hand, penetration into the site of the infection presents formidable problems and is not infrequently reponsible for treatment failures. Penetration across the blood-brain barrier is a complex phenomenon involving protein binding, lipid solubility, and ionization of the drug being administered. In addition, the permeability of this barrier to drugs depends on the degree of inflammation. Because of their low toxicity the penicillins can be administered in doses large enough to provide therapeutic concentrations in the spinal fluid, whereas more toxic drugs such as the aminoglycosides and polymyxins must be injected intrathecally to be effective clinically in meningitis. On the other hand, agents such as the sulfonamides, chloramphenicol, and the tetracyclines appear in the spinal fluid in amounts adequate for the treatment of some types of meningitis when they are given in doses appropriate for the treatment of systemic infections.

Other examples of problems of penetration, and of the influence of localized physiologic conditions, may be cited. The sulfonamides are excreted in the saliva in amounts adequate to eradicate the meningococcal carrier state, whereas most penicillins and tetracyclines are not. However, most of the strains of meningococci encountered at the present time are sulfonamide-resistant. In urinary infections, erythromycin and the aminoglycosides are relatively ineffective at an acid pH, whereas a pH of less than 5.5 is essential for the activity of methenamine mandelate (Mandelamine). The lack of efficacy of sulfonamides in the presence of pus, due to the competition for binding sites by the large amounts of *p*-aminobenzoic acid present, greatly limits the usefulness of this class of drugs.

Foreign bodies, abscesses, and obstruction to normal pathways of drainage almost always interfere with the response to chemotherapy and usually prevent cure until they are removed, drained, or relieved. Suture materials, prostheses, sequestrations, and calculi are examples of foreign bodies that interfere with drug therapy and usually, but not always, need to be removed. In many abscesses, bacteria tend to be in a metabolically inactive state in which they are not actively synthesizing cell wall and are not susceptible to the damaging effects of some antimicrobial drugs; hence drainage plus chemotherapy is necessary to eradicate the infection. Obstruction to bronchial, biliary, and renal drainage interferes seriously with the response of bacterial infections to antibiotics, and these infections generally cannot be cured with these drugs until the obstruction is relieved. A thorough knowledge of the mechanical, metabolic, and physiologic factors is essential in planning therapy that will bring about optimal results in infections located in different parts of the body.

COMBINATION THERAPY, SYNERGISM, ANTAGONISM Once the etiologic agent is known or can be anticipated, most bacterial infections can be treated successfully with a *single* antimicrobial agent. Combination therapy is used frequently, however, to broaden the antibacterial spectrum while awaiting the results of cultures, and also to cover the

TABLE 130-1
Recommended dosages of antimicrobials in oliguric patients (creatinine clearance less than 10 percent of normal)

		Dosage significantly affected by dialysis	
Agent	*Dosage off dialysis**	*Hemodialysis*	*Peritoneal dialysis*
Penicillin G	0.5–2 million units q.6–8h.		No
Ampicillin	1 g; then 0.5 g q.8h.	Yes (0.5–1 g q.6h.)	No
Methicillin	1 g q.8–12h.	No	No
Oxacillin	1 g q.8–12h.	No	No
Dicloxacillin	0.5 g q.8h.	No	Yes (25 μg/ml)†
Carbenicillin	2 g; then 1 g q.8–12h.	Yes (1 g q.4h.)*	Yes (100 μg/ml)†
Cephalothin	1 g q.8–12h.	Yes (1 g q.6h.)*	Yes (20 μg/ml)†
Cephaloridine‡	1 g q.24h.	Yes (0.5g q.4h.)*	Yes (20 μg/ml)†
Chloramphenicol	0.5 g q.6h.	No	No
Erythromycin	0.5 g q.6h	No	No
Lincomycin	250 mg q.12h.	No	No
Kanamycin	0.5 to 1 g; then 0.5 g q.3–4d. (or 7 mg/kg body weight q. third half-life)§	Yes (250 mg after each dialysis)*	Yes (20 μg/ml)†
Gentamicin	80 mg; then 40 mg q.2d.	No	
Colistin (polymyxin E)	200–300 mg; then 100–150 mg q.2–4d.	No	No
Polymyxin B	100–150 mg; then 50–100 mg q.2–4d.	No	No
Vancomycin	1 g q.10–14d.	No	

* *Dosages for intramuscular or intravenous administration.*
† *When antibiotic blood levels are affected significantly by peritoneal dialysis, the agents should be added to the dialysate at the desired serum concentration, with continuation of the usual intramuscular or intravenous administration. Figures in parentheses represent suitable concentrations when adding to peritoneal dialysis fluid.*
‡ *Not used because of nephrotoxicity; may prove useful in patients on chronic dialysis programs to whom nephrotoxicity is of no significance.*
§ *Plasma half-life (hours)* $= \dfrac{(3.6)\ (\text{body weight in kilograms})}{\text{creatinine clearance (milliliter/minute)}}$ *This formula may be applied to patients with normal renal function as well as to patients with renal insufficiency. Thus a man weighing 50 kg whose kanamycin plasma half-life is calculated as 12 h would receive 350 mg every 36 h.*
SOURCE: *Bulger RJ, Petersdorf RG, Postgrad Med 47:160, 1970*

possibility that a mixed infection might be present. For example, in a hospitalized patient who suddenly becomes ill with presumed sepsis, cephalothin and gentamicin may be given empirically to provide antibacterial activity against a variety of gram-positive and -negative pathogens that might be fatal if therapy were delayed (Chap. 129). Over 100 fixed-dose combinations were once available commercially in the United States for oral or parenteral therapy, but virtually all have been ordered off the market by the Food and Drug Administration on the grounds that it has not been shown in controlled studies that both agents contribute to the claimed therapeutic effects, that the amounts of each agent present were often not appropriate, and that patients were often being exposed to the potential hazards of two drugs when only one was needed. When combination therapy is indicated, it is most rational to prescribe separately the indicated drugs in doses that take into the account the patient's age, weight, and physiologic status.

Another indication for giving two antimicrobial agents simultaneously is to prevent the emergence of resistant mutants. An example is the administration of ethambutol in conjunction with isoniazid in tuberculosis. In some instances, a second agent is given to avoid superinfections; the use of nystatin together with tetracycline to prevent an overgrowth of *Candida albicans* that causes disorders such as thrush and vaginitis is an example. In general, this is a questionable practice.

A clinically significant enhancement of antibacterial activity from exposing microorganisms to two or more drugs is rare. Usually the two drugs have an indifferent effect, but sometimes additive action can be demonstrated. True synergism occurs with penicillin and streptomycin and other aminoglycosides against many strains of enterococci, and with gentamicin and carbenicillin against *Pseudomonas* and some other gram-negative bacilli. In severe *Pseudomonas* infections, it should be theoretically possible to reduce the dose and thus the cost and toxicity of gentamicin and carbenicillin because of their synergistic action, but in actual practice the extent of the reduction that would be compatible with maximal efficacy is unpredictable, and it is safer to administer full doses and not risk compromising the therapeutic result. With enterococci, penicillin disrupts the cell wall and permits streptomycin to gain access to the ribosomes, to which it is lethal. Strains with ribosomes that are resistant to streptomycin do not manifest synergism in vitro between penicillin and streptomycin, and treating infections by these strains with a penicillin-streptomycin combination is probably no better than using penicillin alone. Penicillin or ampicillin plus kanamycin or gentamicin also has shown significant synergism against enterococci. Clinically significant antagonism between antimicrobial agents is also rare, a prime example being a higher mortality rate in pneumococcal meningitis treated with penicillin and tetracycline compared with penicillin alone. The rate of killing by penicillin is decreased by the presence of the bacteriostatic agent, tetracycline, and this can alter the outcome when survival depends on rapid killing of the pneumococci.

SUPERINFECTION AND RESISTANCE DURING ANTIMICROBIAL THERAPY A number of microorganisms are genetically resistant to clinically feasible levels of one or more antimicrobials, and they obviously will not be affected by antibiotic therapy. Most antibiotics will alter the host's normal flora by removing those organisms which are sensitive to the drug. In most cases this ecologic change is of little consequence, but occasionally the commensal bacteria of the host set up infection in the same location as the original infection, a state termed *superinfection* (Chap. 128). The superinfecting organism is resistant to the drug being administered, and determining its susceptibility is helpful in selecting the most appropriate antimicrobial drug. Some superinfecting organisms, particularly gram-negatives, acquire resistance to multiple drugs by an episomal transfer mechanism (R factors). For example, multiple-resistant *E. coli* and *Klebsiella-Enterobacter* pose a particular hazard to hospitalized patients.

Comparatively few organisms become resistant to the antibiotic being given during therapy. Some that do develop resistance are *E. coli* to streptomycin and nalidixic acid, occasional strains of staphylococci to erythromycin, and *Pseudomonas* to carbenicillin. In general, however, sensitive organisms are supplanted by resistant ones, rather than acquiring resistance themselves. From a practical point of view, it is important to know which agents are likely to induce resistance, and to look for this phenomenon clinically.

SPECIFIC ANTIMICROBIALS

PENICILLINS Penicillinase-susceptible The prototype, *Penicillin G* (benzyl penicillin), is still widely used, especially parenterally, when high blood levels are desirable as in meningitis and endocarditis. Large doses are necessary either continuously or at 3- to 4-h intervals because of problems of penetration into vegetations and across the blood-brain barrier, and also because of its high renal clearance, which is due chiefly to rapid tubular excretion. Blood levels can be doubled by the concomitant administration of probenecid, 0.5 g every 6 h, but since penicillin G is now quite inexpensive and the optimal blood levels are not precisely known, it is customary in most instances simply to give more penicillin. *Procaine penicillin* is well tolerated intramuscularly and is quite slowly absorbed, so that injections need to be given only every 12 to 24 h for the treatment of many infections due to susceptible bacteria. In dosage of 300,000 to 600,000 units every 12 h, it is the drug of choice for most patients with pneumococcal pneumonia. *Benzathine penicillin* provides a depot in the muscle that releases penicillin so slowly that low blood levels are present for 2 to 3 weeks. These low levels are adequate for the therapy and prevention of streptococcal pharyngitis, for the treatment of some forms of syphilis, and for the prevention of recurrences of rheumatic fever.

Penicillin G given orally in doses of 250,000 units once or twice daily is also effective in preventing streptococcal sore throats, but less so than benzathine penicillin (Chap. 242). Because of its instability in the presence of acid, however, it is less reliable for therapy than the acid-stable penicillin V (phenoxymethyl penicillin), and attempts to overcome this disadvantage by giving larger amounts of penicillin G are associated with an increased incidence of nausea and diarrhea. A number of dosage forms of penicillin G are available; an important feature of their continued usefulness is the fact that very little resistance has developed among penicillin G-susceptible microorganisms.

Broad-spectrum penicillins *Ampicillin* differs from penicillin G only in the presence of an amino group in the side chain, but this minor chemical difference is responsible for some unique features that have led to the widespread use of this antibiotic. Ampicillin is active in low concentrations against a number of gram-negative bacteria causing respiratory *(Hemophilus influenzae),* intestinal *(Shigella, Salmonella),* and urinary *(E. coli, Proteus mirabilis)* infections. When it is given orally, the peak blood level occurs later (2 to 3 h versus ½ to 1 h) and is lower than with penicillin V, and the ampicillin blood level then declines more slowly. This more prolonged blood level, along with its greater in vitro activity, is probably responsible for the greater efficacy of ampicillin, compared with penicillin V, in the oral therapy of gonococcal urethritis.

When given in an intravenous infusion, blood levels are more than 80 percent higher with ampicillin than with penicillin G chiefly because of its much higher rate of renal clearance (390 versus 210 ml per min per 1.73 m^2). When the in vitro activity of the infecting organisms is the same for the two antibiotics, this difference can mean equal efficacy with smaller doses of ampicillin, or higher blood levels with the same dose when maximum serum concentrations are considered necessary. Ampicillin is also more stable in the body, with a serum half-life twice as long as penicillin G, due chiefly to slower breakdown by the liver. Serum protein binding of ampicillin is approximately 20 percent compared with 60 percent for penicillin G and 80 percent for penicillin V; this may mean that with ampicillin there is a higher concentration of free, active antibiotic at the site of infection. All these features contribute to the efficacy and widespread use of ampicillin, and in the United States, competition has led to a marked decrease in the cost in the last few years. Although ampicillin has remained an effective drug against most organisms, increasing resistance has developed among a significant number of strains of *E. coli* and a few of *H. influenzae.*

Hypersensitivity reactions occur with about the same frequency with ampicillin as with penicillin G and V, and with all three are much more frequent and severe when the drug is given parenterally and topically than by the oral route. About 5 to 10 percent of patients develop skin rashes with oral ampicillin, but the incidence is as high as 90 percent when patients with infectious mononucleosis take this drug. This remarkably high incidence, which does not occur with penicillins G and V, does not represent true penicillin allergy, and its exact nature is not known. Although acid-stable, ampicillin is not very well absorbed when taken orally, giving peak blood levels only one-sixth as high as dicloxacillin and cephalexin. *Amoxicillin,* a derivative with a hydroxyl group on the benzene ring, is much better absorbed orally, with blood levels and urinary excretion more than twice as great on the average as ampicillin. Blood levels are roughly equivalent to those of ampicillin given intramuscularly, and amoxicillin has a lower incidence of intestinal side effects when given in half the dose orally. *Pivampicillin,* an ester that is also absorbed better than ampicillin orally, has not been approved for marketing in the United States because of potential hepatotoxicity. *Hetacillin,* a penicillin with a complex side chain, is hydrolyzed rapidly in the body to ampicillin, and for practical therapeutic purposes can be regarded as the same as ampicillin.

Carbenicillin is a broad-spectrum penicillin similar chemically to ampicillin, except that the amino group in the side chain is replaced by a carboxyl group. As a result, carbenicillin is active in vitro against *Pseudomonas,* indole-positive *Proteus,* and some strains of *Enterobacter,* in addition to the other gram-negatives that are susceptible to ampicillin. The MIC for *Pseudomonas* is much higher than that usually considered within the therapeutic range for other antibiotics, i.e., about 75 to 100 μg per ml for most strains and as high as 500 μg per ml for a few. However, extraordinarily high blood levels can be readily attained, in the range of 200 to 400 μg per ml., so that carbenicillin provides the safety and bactericidal activity of a penicillin for some organisms that have been notably refractory to most other antibiotics. The much higher blood levels that can be readily attained with carbenicillin as compared with ampicillin are due chiefly to its much lower renal clearance (100 versus 210 ml per min per 1.73 m^2). In addition, carbenicillin is much more stable in the body, so that blood levels obtained with 30 g a day in patients with normal renal function can be achieved with only 3 or 4 g a day in patients with no renal function. Since many patients with severe gram-negative infections have considerable renal impairment, reduced doses can be administered with the knowledge that full therapeutic blood levels will be achieved. To give 30 g daily for the therapy of severe *Pseudomonas* infections in patients with normal renal function, it is customary to administer 5 g intravenously every 4 h, diluting each dose in 100 to 200 ml fluid and allowing it to drip into the vein within 1 to 2 h. Except for severe *Pseudomonas* infections, 30 g daily is not necessary, and much smaller doses, 10 or 15 g daily, are adequate for the therapy of other gram-negative infections, including those caused by indole-positive *Proteus* and *Enterobacter.* Urinary concentrations in excess of 1,000 μg per ml are attained with 0.5- or 1.0-g doses intramuscularly, so that doses comparable to those used with ampicillin are appropriate for urinary tract infections, including those due to *Pseudomonas.* An oral form of carbenicillin, the indanyl salt of the sodium ester, has become available, and one or two 0.5-g tablets (each equivalent to 382 mg carbenicillin) every 6 h produce urinary concentrations well in excess of MICs for susceptible gram-negative bacilli, including *Pseudomonas.*

An increase in bacterial resistance has been noted in some patients with severe gram-negative infections treated with carbenicillin, but the frequency and extent of the resistance has varied in different reports. The concomitant administration of gentamicin has tended to delay the development of resistance to carbenicillin, and in addition a synergistic action has been found to occur with these two antibiotics against many gram-negative bacilli. It has therefore become customary in severe infections to give both these antibiotics, to enhance antibacterial activity and to delay the emergence of resistance as well. Since there is inactivation of the antibiotics, especially gentamicin, when the two are present in the same solution for several hours, it is preferable to administer them separately, either intramuscularly or intravenously, and under these circumstances the blood levels of each are the same as if they were being given alone. Ticarcillin, a newer semisynthetic penicillin, has pharmacokinetic properties very similar to those of carbenicillin but is two to four times as active in vitro against *Pseudomonas.* However, variability in patients has made it difficult to show clear-cut clinical superiority.

Penicillinase-resistant penicillins The advent of these antibiotics in the early 1960s greatly enhanced the ability to cope with severe staphylococcal infections, because at that time over three-fourths of strains causing infections in hospitals were penicillinase producers, and this high incidence has persisted. Furthermore, the number of strains resistant to these new penicillins has remained very small, especially in the United States. This is probably due to the low incidence of naturally occurring methicillin-resistant strains, and the fact that only a small proportion of the cells in a "resistant" culture are actually lacking in susceptibility. In contrast, certain European hospitals now report that over 20 percent of strains of *Staph. aureus* are methicillin-resistant; the reason for the difference is unknown.

Five penicillinase-resistant penicillins are currently marketed in the United States: *methicillin, oxacillin, nafcillin, cloxacillin,* and *dicloxacillin.* The first three are available for parenteral administration. Methicillin is less active when tested in broth cultures than are oxacillin and nafcillin, but this is probably offset by its much lower protein binding, 40 percent as compared with 90 percent or more for the other two. Clinical studies do not provide convincing evidence of superiority of any of these three penicillins for the parenteral therapy of severe staphylococcal infections. Methicillin is given in the same dose as, or in twice the dose of, the other two because of its lower in vitro activity, i.e., 1 or 2 g every 4 to 6 h in adults. For intravenous administration, each dose is diluted in 50 to 100 ml fluid, and is infused over a period of 30 min to minimize phlebitis. Intramuscular injections are painful and are poorly tolerated for more than a few days. Methicillin nephritis, an uncommon but important allergic reaction, has been reported rarely with oxacillin and nafcillin; it is not known whether this is due simply to the fact that methicillin is more widely used. Nafcillin has been found by many observers to give lower blood levels than equal doses of oxacillin; this appears to be due to sequestration of nafcillin in the liver and possibly in other tissues so that less is available to circulate in the blood. The therapeutic implications of this phenomenon are unknown.

With oral administration, both nafcillin and oxacillin give low blood levels, and for this reason their use is avoided by some. Cloxacillin gives blood levels twice as high and dicloxacillin four times as high as oxacillin when the same doses are given orally. However, there is also a progressive increase in serum protein binding (92 percent for oxacillin, 94 percent for cloxacillin, and 96 percent for dicloxacillin), so that the differences in free, active antibiotic may offset the blood level differences. In general cloxacillin or dicloxacillin in doses of 0.5 g and 0.25 g four times daily, respectively, is preferred for oral administration. The efficacy of these antibiotics, either initially in mild to moderate soft-tissue infections, or for completion of therapy following administration of one of the three parenteral preparations described above, is well established by clinical experience.

The chief indication for the penicillinase-resistant penicillins is the therapy of infections caused by penicillinase-producing staphylococci, but they are often administered empirically before the etiologic organism is known. Pneumococci and most streptococci are more susceptible to penicillin G and ampicillin, but blood levels are sufficiently high with the penicillinase-resistant penicillins, especially when given parenterally, so that it is not necessary to give both types of penicillins to provide coverage for these organisms. However, infections caused by enterococci and *Neisseria* cannot be expected to respond to therapy with a penicillinase-resistant penicillin given alone, and if these organisms are suspected, penicillin G or ampicillin should be used.

CEPHALOSPORINS The cephalosporins differ from the penicillins in having a six-membered dihydrothiazine ring, instead of a five-membered thiazolidine ring, fused to the beta-lactam ring. As a result of this chemical difference there is no true cross-allergenicity, and most patients who are allergic to penicillins can be treated with cephalosporins without hypersensitivity reactions. The small number in whom this is not possible seem to be highly allergic individuals who react separately to the two groups of antibiotics.

Most bacteria susceptible to the penicillins are also susceptible to the cephalosporins, including group A and viridans streptococci, pneumococci, penicillin G-sensitive and resistant *Staphylococcus aureus, Neisseria, clostridia, Actinomyces,* and *Corynebacterium diphtheriae.* Among the gram-negatives most strains of *E. coli, P. mirabilis, Klebsiella* but not *Enterobacter, Shigella, Salmonella,* and most strains of *H. influenzae,* are susceptible. The cephalosporins act on the cell wall in a manner similar to the penicillins, and are bactericidal. As with the penicillins, there has been little tendency for susceptible species to become resistant despite widespread use of the cephalosporins for more than a decade.

Among the cephalosporins marketed in the United States, the experience has been greatest with four: cephalothin, cephaloridine, cephaloglycin, and cephalexin. The first two are effective only when given parenterally, and the last two are available only as oral preparations. Because of its broad spectrum of activity, *cephalothin* is used widely in hospitals, often in conjunction with other antibiotics, for initial therapy in seriously ill patients while awaiting the results of cultures. It is usually administered intravenously in doses of 1 or 2 g every 4 or 6 h; each dose is diluted in 50 to 100 ml fluid and infused over a period of 20 to 30 min to minimize the phlebitis that occurs frequently with more concentrated solutions. Convincing evidence of nephrotoxicity is lacking, and only a moderate reduction in dosage is necessary in the presence of uremia. Cephalothin is partially converted in the body to a metabolic breakdown product, desacetylcephalothin, that is less active than the parent compound, particularly against gram-negative bacteria. This partial breakdown is relatively small in extent, usually not more than 25 percent, and for the most part is of no importance clinically because of the large quantity of the parent compound present. Meningococcal meningitis may be a possible exception; in this disease relapses and failures to eradicate the infecting organism have been described. Meningococci have been observed to be only about one-fifteenth as susceptible to desacetylcephalothin, which has been found to be present in the spinal fluid in significant amounts. *Cephaloridine* has three potential advantages over cephalothin because it is less painful on intramuscular injection, is less avidly bound to protein (15 versus 70 percent), and achieves much higher and more prolonged blood levels with the same dose. The blood level differences favoring cephaloridine are due to lower renal clearance and greater stability in the body. However, cephaloridine is nephrotoxic, causing renal tubular damage when blood levels are excessive, and the recommended dose is limited to no more than 4 g daily in adults with normal renal function. Reduced doses are necessary in patients with impaired renal function; precise recommendations are available in the labeling that accompanies the antibiotic. Because of its nephrotoxicity, cephaloridine should be restricted for the most part to patients in whom it is necessary to administer a cephalosporin intramuscularly. However, intravenous administration is warranted in a few patients with meningitis or endocarditis who are allergic to the penicillins and in whom high blood levels are considered important. Cephaloridine is less stable in the presence of staphylococcal penicillinase than cephalothin, but it has not been possible clearly to relate this characteristic to inferior clinical results. Cephalothin, on the other hand, has definitely been shown to be as effective as the penicillinase-resistant penicillins for the treatment of severe infections due to penicillinase-producing staphylococci.

Cephaloglycin is poorly absorbed orally, giving low blood levels, but provides urinary concentrations adequate for the therapy of some urinary infections. However, its usefulness has practically disappeared with the advent of *cephalexin,* a well-absorbed oral cephalosporin that gives high blood levels, has low serum protein binding, is over 90 percent excreted in the urine without nephrotoxicity, and has no adverse metabolic breakdown product. A 0.5g dose of cephalexin orally gives an average peak blood level in adults of about 18 μg per ml, six times as high as that produced by the same dose of ampicillin. Cephalexin has the same antibacterial spectrum as the other cephalosporins, although it is somewhat less active against some organisms in vitro. Its efficacy in infections caused by *H. influenzae* has been questioned but is now accepted in the official labeling.

Cephapirin is almost identical in antibacterial spectrum and pharmacologic characteristics to cephalothin, and *cephradine* has a similar relationship to cephalexin. The parenteral form of cephradine gives low, prolonged blood levels intramuscularly, and its efficacy with intravenous administration is being evaluated. *Cefazolin,* although quite highly protein-bound (about 85 percent), produces high blood levels because of its low renal clearance and has a longer half-life than cephalothin and cephaloridine. Parenterally, 0.5 g cefazolin is probably equivalent to 1.0 g cephalothin and cephapirin for most infections. However, cephalothin is the only one of these cephalosporins that is not inactivated by large inocula of some strains of *Staph. aureus;* it has not been established whether this is of any significance clinically. Other cephalosporins, including *cefoxitin, cefamandole,* and *cephacetrile,* are still in the investigative stage, and selection of the most favorable members of this group will remain a lively subject for the next few years.

AMINOGLYCOSIDES *Streptomycin,* one of the first antibiotics available for systemic administration, was widely used during the late 1940s and the 1950s. For a number of years it was given almost routinely in conjunction with penicillin in surgical cases for the prophylaxis and treatment of postoperative infections. Because of the tendency for highly resistant organisms to appear within 2 or 3 days, and its potential for causing vestibular damage and deafness, streptomycin has been largely supplanted by kanamycin and gentamicin, although it is still in use for certain specific purposes. Tuberculosis is still treated with streptomycin, particularly when triple drug regimens are used for the first few weeks. Streptomycin is also used in conjunction with penicillin to treat *Strep. viridans* endocarditis and some enterococcal infections and for the treatment of certain less common infections such as brucellosis and tularemia. In addition to vestibular nerve toxicity, other adverse reactions of streptomycin include rashes, fever, contact dermatitis, pancytopenia, anaphylaxis, and renal irritation.

Neomycin, another aminoglycoside that appeared in the 1940s, is no longer used parenterally because of its nephro- and neurotoxicity. Respiratory arrest is a serious adverse reaction that has occurred when neomycin is instilled topically in the peritoneal cavity in anesthetized patients, and deafness has resulted from the topical application of neomycin soaks injudiciously in burns and wounds. Neomycin is useful and relatively safe when given orally in doses of 4 to 6 g daily to "prepare" the bowel preoperatively, and in patients with hepatic insufficiency where inhibition of bacterial growth in the intestine is necessary to reduce the absorption of nitrogenous substances. However, the amount of neomycin absorbed from the intestine is variable, and toxic levels have been demonstrated in some patients. Neomycin is also used as a spray and an ointment to decrease the bacterial count in individuals who are nasal carriers of staphylococci.

Kanamycin is similar in structure to neomycin but is sufficiently less toxic that it is widely used parenterally for the therapy of infections caused by most of the commonly encountered gram-negative bacilli except *Pseudomonas.* It is also active against staphylococci, but not against the other common gram-positive pathogens such as streptococci and pneumococci. Kanamycin should be administered intramuscularly or by slow intravenous infusion in doses not larger than 7.5 mg per kg every 12 h, and the total dose should not exceed 15 g in patients with normal renal function. Kanamycin is not protein-bound, and is excreted by glomerular filtration; over 80 percent of a dose appears in the urine within 24 h. In contrast to the penicillins, the toxic blood level is not greatly above the therapeutic blood level, and the dose needs to be decreased when there is impaired renal function. The best way to accomplish this is by measuring blood levels once or twice a day; this can be done by bioassay within 3 or 4 h. Blood level determinations are not widely available, however, and dosage is usually adjusted on the basis of the serum creatinine. The full therapeutic dose is given every three half-lives, and the serum half-life has been shown to be about three times the serum creatinine. Thus, if the serum creatinine is 7, the half-life is 21, and this means that the usual dose of 7.5 mg per kg should be administered every 63 h. An alternative plan is to administer half the usual dose every half-life; this has the advantage that the drug concentration in the blood does not reach as low a level prior to each succeeding dose. There has been little tendency for pathogens to become resistant to kanamycin despite its widespread use in hospitals. Kanamycin is administered alone to treat specific infections, and is used even more widely in conjunction with other antibiotics in seriously ill patients where the exact etiologic diagnosis is pending, or remains indeterminate. *Amikacin* is similar to kanamycin in antibacterial spectrum and pharmacologic characteristics, except that it is also active against *Pseudomonas,* and is less susceptible than gentamicin to inactivation by bacterial enzymes. Its relative efficacy and toxicity in relation to kanamycin, gentamicin, and tobramycin will become apparent only after widespread use over a period of several years.

Gentamicin is similar to kanamycin in its antibacterial spectrum, and in addition is active against *Pseudomonas.* Its toxicity is similar to that of kanamycin except that it is more likely to cause *vestibular* damage rather than deafness. Most gram-negative pathogens are highly susceptible to gentamicin, although MICs vary considerably depending on the medium used for in vitro testing. Human serum potentiates the action of gentamicin against most gram-negative organisms but inhibits its action against *Pseudomonas;* this is related to the presence of calcium and magnesium. Gentamicin is given in much smaller doses than kanamycin, i.e., 80 versus 500 mg every 8 h, and a representative peak blood level is 3 to 4 μg per ml, both with intramuscular injections and with slow intravenous infusions. Its basic pharmacology is nearly the same as for kanamycin, and the same principles and detailed procedures that were described above for modifying dosage in the presence of impaired renal function are applicable. For many infections 3 mg/kg/day is adequate, but for the more severe ones the doses should be increased to 5 mg/kg/day.

Tobramycin is very similar to gentamicin in all respects except that it is two to four times more active against most strains of *Pseudomonas,* and is also active in vitro against some of the gram-negatives that are now resistant to gentamicin. Conversely, some tobramycin-resistant strains are susceptible to gentamicin. Extensive clinical usage will be required to establish the relative merits of these two antibiotics.

TETRACYCLINES Since they first appeared in the late 1940s, the tetracycline antibiotics have been very widely used because of their broad spectrum of activity against many gram-positive and gram-negative bacteria, and also other microorganisms such as *Mycoplasma, Rickettsia,* and *Chlamydia.* They have been effective, although not necessarily the drugs of choice, in the treatment of common venereal diseases including gonorrhea, syphilis, lymphogranuloma venereum, and granuloma inguinale. Their use has become more restricted during the last decade because of the advent of bactericidal antibiotics such as the cephalosporins, the penicillinase-resistant penicillins, and gentamicin, and increasing awareness of the limitations of the tetracyclines. These limitations include the appearance of resistant strains of commonly encountered pathogens such as group A streptococci and pneumococci, the primarily bacteriostatic action of the tetracyclines, the occurrence of hepatotoxicity with high blood levels, the relatively high incidence of superinfections, and the common occurrence of side effects such as nausea, diarrhea, and photosensitivity reactions. Despite these limitations, the tetracyclines are still widely used for respiratory, urinary, soft tissue, and venereal infections.

Chlortetracycline (Aureomycin) and *oxytetracycline* (Terramycin), the two original compounds, have been largely replaced by *tetracycline,* which is marketed by a number of companies, and competition has led to a marked reduction in its price. The usual adult dose is 1 to 2 g daily in two to four equally divided doses. Intramuscular preparations are not very satisfactory, but the intravenous form is well-tolerated and gives relatively high blood levels with doses of 0.5 g every 12 h. Excessive blood levels occur with renal insufficiency unless the dose is decreased, and can cause fatty degeneration of the liver, which may be fatal because tetracycline persists in the body for many days when its normal route of excretion through the kidneys is blocked.

Four long-acting tetracyclines are available: *demeclocycline, methacycline, doxycycline,* and *minocycline.* They have high protein binding (over 90 versus 70 percent for tetracycline) and a prolonged plasma half-life, so that blood levels are well maintained when they are administered orally only every 12 to 24 h. However, the half-life of tetracycline is sufficiently prolonged so that blood levels with administration only every 12 h are similar to those of the smaller doses recommended for the long-acting tetracyclines. Unfortunately, the reduction in dose is not matched by a proportional decrease in price. The potential advantages for the long-active tetracyclines, i.e., greater convenience from less frequent administration and decreased cost from lower doses, have not been entirely realized, and these preparations cannot be recommended as possessing clear-cut advantages over tetracycline. Doxycycline is the single exception to this because it does not give excessive blood levels in the presence of renal insufficiency following either oral or intravenous administration. This provides a safety feature when the exact status of the patient's renal function is uncertain or unknown.

ERYTHROMYCIN, LINCOMYCIN, CLINDAMYCIN *Erythromycin* is primarily a bacteriostatic antibiotic that is active against the commonly encountered gram-positive bacteria, and is used chiefly for the oral therapy of respiratory and soft-tissue infections, particularly in patients thought to be allergic to penicillin. The susceptibility of *Mycoplasma pneumoniae* to erythromycin enhances its usefulness in respiratory infections. Erythromycin base is absorbed in an erratic manner and cannot be relied upon. Erythromycin estolate has been thought to give much higher blood levels than erythromycin stearate, but the difference may be not as great as was once postulated because the estolate needs to be hydrolyzed in the body to the active form, and the hydrolysis is not as complete as during the blood level assay procedure. The estolate salt is associated with a low incidence of cholestatic hepatitis, which is readily reversible and rarely serious. The usual oral dose is 1 or 2 g daily. Intramuscular preparations are irritating, and intravenous administration is not used widely, partly because the preparations are not entirely satisfactory but chiefly because oral therapy is adequate for most infections treated with erythromycin.

Lincomycin and *clindamycin* are similar in antibacterial activity and clinical usefulness to erythromycin. Clindamycin gives somewhat higher blood levels and has less gastrointestinal side effects than lincomycin. An excellent parenteral preparation of both is available. Clindamycin is considerably more active against *Bacteroides fragilis,* and intravenous administration of this antibiotic in abdominal and pelvic infections is widely advocated for this reason. However, pseudomembranous colitis is a fairly frequent and at times serious side effect which has led to recommendations that these antibiotics be used chiefly for hospitalized patients with significant infections, and that they be discontinued at once if diarrhea occurs.

Chloramphenicol This antibiotic has a broad spectrum of activity similar to the tetracyclines and during the 1950s was very widely used. However, the occurrence of aplastic anemia, even though quite uncommon (about 1 in 25,000 persons exposed) has led to a restriction of chloramphenicol to those serious infections in which it is quite clearly the drug of choice. Typhoid fever is the principal example, and there are occasionally other severe gram-negative infections where the etiologic agent is susceptible only to chloramphenicol. With increasing interest in anaerobic infections, it is now realized that *B. fragilis* is the commonest of the anaerobic pathogens and that over half the strains are resistant to the penicillins and tetracyclines. This has led to an increase in the use of chloramphenicol since almost all *Bacteroides* strains are susceptible to it. However, clindamycin is also very active against *B. fragilis,* and since a parenteral preparation has become available, it has partially replaced chloramphenicol for the treatment of patients with proved or presumed *Bacteroides* infections. Clindamycin lacks the broad gram-negative spectrum of chloramphenicol, and for this reason, the latter may be preferred under certain circumstances. In addition, clindamycin's propensity to producing colitis should restrict its use.

Chloramphenicol is well absorbed by the oral route, and the usual adult dose is 0.5 g every 6 h. The parenteral preparation, chloramphenicol succinate, is hydrolyzed in the body to the active form, and this conversion is incomplete so that the blood levels with intravenous administration are not much higher than when the antibiotic is taken by mouth. With intramuscular administration, blood levels are considerably lower than with the oral route, and although the drug was widely used by this route for a number of years, the present labeling does not authorize intramuscular injections.

In addition to aplastic anemia, which may be an allergic or "idiosyncratic" reaction that usually occurs with prolonged and repeated administration, chloramphenicol inhibits protein synthesis, especially with doses larger than 2 g a day, an effect that is reversible. Clinically this is manifested by leukopenia, inadequate erythropoiesis (anemia), and thrombocytopenia as well as absence of reticulocytosis, high serum iron, and full saturation of transferrin. To monitor toxicity, blood counts should be performed at least twice weekly and the antibiotic should be stopped if there is significant hematologic toxicity. The gray syndrome, consisting of pallor, listlessness, and often death, occurs in neonates who have inadequately developed hepatic and renal mechanisms for metabolizing chloramphenicol; this can be prevented by restricting the dose to 25 mg/kg/day.

POLYMYXINS Polymyxin B and E (colistin) are polypeptide antibiotics that are active against most gram-negative bacteria except for the *Proteus* group. They have been of importance chiefly because of their action against *Pseudomonas aeruginosa.* However, their use systemically has decreased markedly since the advent of gentamicin and carbenicillin, which appear to be superior.

Polymyxin B is administered intramuscularly every 8 h, or as a continuous intravenous infusion, in doses no larger than 2.0 mg/kg/day. It is effective in treating urinary infections, but its efficacy in systemic infections is uncertain. Polymyxin B is also administered topically for eye and ear infections, and intrathecally for *Pseudomonas* meningitis. Colistin is available as the sodium salt of colistimethate and is administered in doses of 3.0 to 5.0 mg/kg/day intramuscularly or intravenously as described for polymyxin B.

Polymyxin B and colistimethate both cause perioral paresthesias and other neurotoxic manifestations with excessive blood levels; of these, apnea is the most life-threatening. Renal irritation and azotemia, which are usually reversible, may also occur. It is important to monitor renal function and to decrease the dose in the presence of renal insufficiency.

VANCOMYCIN Vancomycin is a relatively toxic but highly effective antibiotic that warrants special consideration because of its occasional usefulness in treating certain specific infections. Vancomycin is bactericidal and is effective against gram-positive bacteria including penicillinase-producing staphylococci and enterococci. It is particularly useful in treating severe staphylococcal infections when penicillins and cephalosporins cannot be given, and in the treatment of *S. viridans* and enterococcal endocarditis under the same circumstances. It can be given only by the intravenous route, and 0.5 g every 6 h for 2 or 3 weeks is the usual dose. Thrombophlebitis is the principal side effect; it can be minimized by diluting each dose in 100 ml fluid and administering it over a period of at least 1 h. Chills, fever, renal irritation, and deafness are other adverse reactions that have been described, and these can be minimized by slow administration and by reduction of the dose if renal function is impaired.

SULFONAMIDES The sulfonamides have been used clinically since 1937, and were the principal drugs administered for systemic antibacterial chemotherapy before penicillin and the other antibiotics became generally available. Their role has declined steadily, and they now occupy an important although relatively small place in clinical therapy since they are less active than the antibiotics, they are primarily bacteriostatic, resistant organisms occur frequently, and adverse reactions are common. Uncomplicated urinary tract infections due to *E. coli* are the principal indication for sulfonamides because of their efficacy, relative safety, and low cost. In addition, sulfonamides are drugs of choice for the therapy of nocardiosis. They are no longer the preferred agents for the treatment of bacillary dysentery, meningococcal infections, and *H. influenzae* meningitis.

Sulfonamides are still prescribed on a large scale for upper respiratory infections, but their efficacy in these situations is highly questionable since the majority of such infections is caused by viruses.

Sulfadiazine, once widely used as an all-purpose sulfonamide, tends to produce crystalluria and has been largely replaced by the more soluble *sulfisoxazole* (Gantrisin) and its close congener, *sulfamethoxazole* (Gantanol). Mixtures of three sulfonamides (trisulfapyrimidines) are also widely used since they are associated with a low incidence of crystalluria. The sulfonamides are usually administered orally, although very satisfactory intravenous preparations of the sodium salts are available. Orally, an initial dose of 2 to 4 g is followed by 1 g every 4 to 6 h.

Long-acting sulfonamides have also been used widely, and their only advantage is that they can be administered orally only once or twice daily. Examples are sulfamethoxypyridazine and sulfadimethoxine. The primary clinical indication for these long-acting compounds has been urinary tract infections, in instances where the convenience of taking only one dose a day has been considered important. However, it is undesirable to use a drug that leaves the body slowly, because this may prolong adverse reactions. Moreover, certain severe toxic reactions such as erythema multiforme or myocarditis have been reported to occur more commonly with long-acting sulfonamides. It is probably best not to use this class of compounds at all.

There are also some poorly absorbed sulfonamides, succinylsulfathiazole (Sulfasuxidine) and phthalysulfathiazole (Sulfathalidine), that are used principally to decrease the number of bacteria in the colon prior to certain types of abdominal surgery. These agents are of doubtful value. The drug Azulfidine (Chap. 291) is of value in ulcerative colitis.

Adverse reactions caused by the sulfonamides include erythema multiforme, serum sickness, hemolytic and aplastic anemias, arthralgias, hepatitis, nausea, vertigo, and lesions resembling those of polyarteritis nodosa.

ANTIFUNGAL AGENTS *Amphotericin B* is a highly toxic antibiotic that is effective in the treatment of deep-seated mycotic infections. It produces marked improvement and occasional cures in cryptococcosis, histoplasmosis, blastomycosis, disseminated candidiasis, and coccidioidomycosis, and it has a beneficial effect in at least some cases of aspergillosis and mucormycosis. It is administered intravenously in 5% dextrose solution over a period of 5 or 6 h. The safest procedure is to administer 1 mg on the first day, 5 mg on the second, and 10 mg on the third. The dose is then increased by 5 to 10 mg each day until 1 mg per kg is being administered daily. The dose may then be changed to 1.5 mg per kg every other day; treatment is continued for 2 to 4 months, depending on the severity of the infection and upon the patient's response. In patients with severe infections where intensive therapy is considered essential, it may be necessary to assume the risk of administering 15 mg very cautiously as the initial dose, with the addition of antihistamines and/or steroids to help ameliorate the chills and fever, which are quite variable from patient to patient. In some debilitated patients who develop *Candida* infections with oral or esophageal lesions, or bacteremias secondary to intravenous catheters, 10 or 15 mg amphotericin B daily for only 3 or 4 days may be adequate to bring the infection under control.

Some degree of renal impairment invariably occurs when amphotericin B is administered for several weeks; this is manifested during therapy by a rise in the blood urea nitrogen (BUN) and serum creatinine. Renal function may return to normal following therapy if attention is devoted to giving the minimum amount of drug that is compatible with a satisfactory therapeutic response, and if particular care is exercised in lowering the dose and frequency of administration when the creatinine becomes markedly elevated. Many patients have permanent renal damage; this poses special problems when relapses occur and subsequent courses of therapy are needed. Other adverse effects of amphotericin B include anemia, hypokalemia, thrombocytopenia, and hepatitis.

Nystatin (Mycostatin) is another antifungal antibiotic that is less potent than amphotericin B and is too toxic for systemic administration. It is applied topically in ointments, tablets, and suspension. It is used particularly for oral, intestinal, skin, and vaginal lesions due to *Candida,* and the best results are obtained when applications are made several times a day. The individual dose varies from 100,000 to 1 million units, depending on the location of the lesion.

Flucytosine is an oral antifungal agent that is relatively nontoxic and has been used successfully in cryptococcal, *Candida,* and *Torulopsis* infections. The dose is 150 mg/kg/day administered in divided doses at 6-h intervals. Some cases of cryptococcal meningitis and pulmonary disease have seemed to respond as well as to amphotericin B, but flucytosine is, in general, less potent than amphotericin. An appreciable percentage of initial isolates of *Candida* are resistant to the drug, and resistance also occurs during therapy. Adverse effects have consisted chiefly of nausea, vomiting, diarrhea, and rashes, but pancytopenia and abnormal liver function tests have also been reported.

Flucytosine is not effective in histoplasmosis, blastomycosis, and coccidioidomycosis. It is indicated chiefly in patients with severe cryptococcal, *Candida,* and *Torulopsis* infections who cannot tolerate amphotericin B. It can also be used for *Candida* infections of the bladder and for superficial lesions that do not respond to topical therapy. There is in vitro evidence of synergism between flucytosine and amphotericin B, and clinical results in some severe systemic infections appear to have been improved by administering these two antifungal agents together.

ANTITUBERCULOSIS DRUGS *Isoniazid* remains the most important single agent for the treatment of tuberculosis. After years of being considered virtually free from adverse reactions, hepatotoxicity has been reported on a number of occasions, although not sufficiently frequently to make routine liver function tests in individuals receiving prolonged therapy mandatory. *Ethambutol* is replacing aminosalicylic acid (PAS) as the usual companion drug for isoniazid because it avoids the necessity of taking large numbers of tablets and also avoids the gastrointestinal side effects associated with PAS. *Rifampin* is another important drug that is comparable with isoniazid in activity against tuberculosis; it should be used in combination with other drugs to prevent the emergence of rifampin-resistant tubercle bacilli. Streptomycin is still used to some extent, particularly for triple drug therapy in seriously ill, hospitalized patients. The secondary drugs, used chiefly in cases that have failed to respond to initial therapy, are cycloserine, pyrazinamide, ethionamide, and viomycin. These drugs are all associated with significant toxic side effects and should be administered and monitored by experts who are familiar with their use. A more detailed consideration of the antituberculosis drugs and the present treatment regimens are given in Chap. 161.

MISCELLANEOUS ANTIBACTERIAL AGENTS *Spectinomycin* is an antibiotic that is effective in single 2- to 4-g doses intramuscularly for the treatment of gonorrhea. Side effects are minimal, and it is useful to have an agent similar in effectiveness to penicillin available for the treatment of patients who are allergic to penicillin or who have failed to be cured by penicillin.

Nitrofurantoin is an antibacterial agent that is effective in treating urinary tract infections although susceptibility of the *Proteus* group is variable and *Pseudomonas* is resistant. It is usually administered orally in doses of 100 mg four times a day. In addition to treating acute uncomplicated urinary tract infections, it is widely used to suppress symptoms of infection in patients with prostatism and other chronic obstructive uropathies. Nausea is sometimes troublesome, and pulmonary hypersensitivity and peripheral neuropathy may occur. The latter is especially likely to occur with renal insufficiency, and nitrofurantoin should be used very cautiously in the presence of uremia.

Nalidixic acid is another drug used orally for urinary tract infections. Its principal defect lies in the rapidity with which bacteria become resistant to it. This means that cultures should be made during, as well as following, therapy to be sure that bacteria are being cleared from the urinary tract. The usual dose is 4 g daily in divided doses for 1 to 2 weeks. Nausea, vomiting, and rashes are the chief adverse reactions.

Co-trimoxazole, a fixed-dose combination of trimethoprim (80 mg) and sulfamethoxazole (400 mg), is synergistic in this ratio against most gram-negatives causing urinary tract infections except for *Pseudomonas.* It is also active in vitro against a variety of other pathogens and is used in other countries for many types of infections. In the United States it is approved so far only for urinary infections. Because of its cost it should be used chiefly when the infecting organisms are not susceptible to other antimicrobials. It may be of particular value, however, in preventing recurrent bouts of bacteriuria.

Troleandomycin (TAO) is an antibiotic similar to, although less active than, the erythromycins. It is an ester and occasionally causes cholestatic jaundice. In general, erythromycin, lincomycin, and clindamycin are preferable to troleandomycin because of their greater antibacterial activity.

DRUGS OF CHOICE

It is quite clear from reading about the pharmacology of individual agents, as well as about their indications and uses in individual diseases, that many agents are available for the treatment of these diseases. Table 130-2 presents a summary of drugs, indications, dosage schedules, routes of administration, and duration of therapy. The table presents only a limited number of drugs, and many equally acceptable regimens are available. Moreover, while these treatment programs are appropriate for the present, changes in them should be expected as new drugs come on the market and as more experience with the newer agents is gathered.

CHEMOPROPHYLAXIS OF INFECTION

Much of the time antimicrobial agents are directed at *preventing* infection rather than treating it. Prophylaxis fell into disrepute a number of years ago when penicillin and streptomycin, given for 7 to 10 days, led to a high incidence of superinfections. More recently, however, well-controlled studies have shown a lower infection rate, particularly in potentially contaminated or dirty sites where surgery is performed, with only 1 or 2 days of an appropriate antibiotic, usually a cephalosporin. Examples include abdominal surgery, caesarean sections with ruptured membranes, compound fractures, and the placement of prostheses. Furthermore, when prophylaxis is directed at a single sensitive pathogen, it may be effective; an example is penicillin G in the prevention of streptococcal pharyngitis. Table 130-3 summarizes situations in which the efficacy of antimicrobial prophylaxis has been examined. This table is by no means complete; in addition, antibiotics are used prophylactically "by custom"; examples include in skull fractures to prevent meningitis, arterial grafting, lung surgery, major osseous trauma, etc. In these situations the effectiveness of prophylaxis is based on hearsay and "clinical impressions."

DISADVANTAGES OF ANTIBIOTIC PROPHYLAXIS Even if it is not effective, antimicrobial prophylaxis is unlikely to be harmful if it is maintained for only a short period of time, less than 5 days, and if only a single drug is used in comparatively low doses. On the other hand, prophylaxis with multiple drugs, administered in high doses and for relatively prolonged periods, is much more likely to be harmful. Adverse effects include: (1) superinfections (see above and Chap. 128); (2) increased incidence of toxic or allergic reactions to drugs (Chap. 67); (3) increased cost; and (4) last, but not least, a sense of false security on the part of some physicians. In some instances, antimicrobial prophylaxis tends to promote laxity in the careful observation of the patient. However, many of the patients who are given antibiotics prophylactically are precisely the ones who are susceptible to complicating infections, and in them particular care must be taken to watch assiduously for the development of infection and to treat it promptly when it occurs. Such policy is often superior to the use of antimicrobial prophylaxis.

REASONS FOR FAILURE OF CHEMOTHERAPY

This chapter as well as others dealing with specific disease entities has documented that there are few organisms not sensitive to some antibiotic. Despite this seemingly salutary observation, a large number of patients develop infections and many continue to die from them. In these patients antibiotics appear to have failed. Often this failure of chemotherapy is more apparent than real and may be attributed to one of several reasons.

TABLE 130-2
Conventional antibiotic regimens for adults with normal renal and hepatic function

Organism	*Disease*	*Drug*	*Dosage*	*Route*	*Duration*
Pneumococcus	Lung	Penicillin G (procaine)	600,000 U q.12h	IM	5–10 days[1]
	Meningitis	Penicillin G (aqueous)	20 million U/day	IV	7–10 days
	Joints	Penicillin G (aqueous)	20 million U/day	IV	7–10 days
	Endocarditis	Penicillin G (aqueous)	20 million U/day	IV	4–6 weeks[2]
Group A *Streptococcus*	Pharyngitis	Penicillin G (procaine)	600,000 U/day	IM	10 days[3]
	Erysipelas	Penicillin G (procaine)	600,000 U/day	IM	10 days[3]
	Other sites	See Pneumococcus			
Coagulase-positive *Staphylococcus*[4]	Furunculosis, cellulitis, abscess	Erythromycin	500 mg q.6h	PO	7–10 days
		or cloxacillin	500 mg q.6h	PO	7–10 days
		or cephalexin	500 mg q.6h	PO	7–10 days
	Pneumonia	Methicillin	1.0 g q.4h	IM,IV	10–14 days
		or cloxacillin	500 mg q.6h	PO	10–14 days
		or dicloxacillin	250 mg q.6h	PO	10–14 days
		or cephalothin	1.0 g q.4h	IV	10–14 days
	Arthritis	Methicillin	1.0 g q.4h	IV	10–14 days
		or cephalothin	1.0 g q.4h	IV	10–14 days
	Meningitis, endocarditis	Methicillin	1.0 g q.2h	IV	4 weeks
		or cephalothin	1.0 g q.2h	IV	4 weeks
	Enterocolitis	Vancomycin	500 mg q.6h	PO	Until diarrhea ceases
Streptococcus viridans	Endocarditis	Penicillin G,	6–12 million U/day	IV	14 days
		then penicillin V	500 mg q.4h.	PO	14 days
		Penicillin G	6–12 million U/day	IV	14 days
		plus Streptomycin	500 mg q.12h	IM	14 days
Strep. fecalis (enterococcus)	Genitourinary infection	Ampicillin	500 mg q.6h.	PO	10–14 days
		plus gentamicin	3 mg/kg/day	IM,IV	10–14 days
	Surgical wound	Ampicillin	1 g q.6h	IM or IV	7–10 days
		plus gentamicin	3–5 mg/kg/day	IM,IV	7–10 days
	Endocarditis	Ampicillin	8–12 g/day	IV	4 weeks
		or penicillin G	20 million U/day	IV	4 weeks
		plus gentamicin,	3–5 mg/kg/day	IM,IV	2 weeks
		or kanamycin	7.5 mg/kg q.12h	IM	2 weeks
		or streptomycin	500 mg q.12h	IM,IV	2 weeks
Neisseria meningitidis	Meningitis, meningococcemia	Penicillin G	20 million U/day	IV	7–10 days
N. gonorrheae	Urethritis	Penicillin G (procaine)	4.8 million U/day	IM	1 dose
		or spectinomycin[5]	2 g/day	IM	1 dose
	Arthritis	Penicillin G (aqueous)	6 million U/day	IV	7–10 days
Hemophilus influenzae	Bronchitis and pneumonia	Ampicillin	500 mg q.4h.	PO	5–7 days
		or tetracycline	500 mg q.6h.	PO	5–7 days
	Meningitis	Ampicillin	8–12 g/day	IV	7–10 days
		or chloramphenicol	50–100 mg/kg/day (given q.6h)	IV	7–10 days
Brucella	Brucellosis	Tetracycline	500 mg q.6h.	PO	14 days
		and streptomycin	500 mg q.12h.	IM	14 days
Salmonella typhosa	Typhoid fever	Chloramphenicol[6]	1.0 g q.8h.	IV,PO	14 days
		or ampicillin[6]	1.0 g q.6h.	PO,IM IV	14 days
Salmonella	Abscess, bacteremia	Ampicillin	1.0 g q.4h.	IV	2–4 weeks
Shigella	Shigellosis	Ampicillin	500 mg q.4–6h.	PO,IM IV	7 days
Klebsiella	Genitourinary infection	Gentamicin	3 mg/kg/q.8h	IM,IV	10–14 days
		or cephalothin	500 mg q.6h	IM,IV	10–14 days
		or cefazolin	500 mg q.6h	IM,IV	10–14 days
		or kanamycin	7.5 mg/kg/q.12h	IM	

[1] *Last 3–4 days can be given orally as penicillin V 2 g/day in many cases.*
[2] *Last 2 weeks can be given as penicillin V 4–6 g/day orally.*
[3] *Penicillin V 1-2 g/day for 10 days or a single shot of 1.2 × 10^6 U benzathine penicillin is an acceptable alternate.*
[4] *Appropriate doses (see Pneumococcus and Streptococcus) of penicillin G (parenteral) or penicillin V (oral) if organism is sensitive to penicillin G.*
[5] *For patients allergic to penicillin.*
[6] *Start with parenteral but switch to oral as soon as possible.*
[7] *Early follow-up cultures are essential to be sure resistance has not developed.*
[8] *Uncomplicated infections only.*

FAILURE TO ADJUST THE DOSE OF THE ANTIBIOTIC Different doses of antibiotics are required in different locations. For example, 600,000 units penicillin G is more than adequate to cure pneumococcal pneumonia, but as much as 20 million units may be required to cure pneumococcal meningitis and more than 50 million units to treat pneumococcal endocarditis. The pneumococcus in each of these locations remains exquisitely sensitive to penicillin, nor is the penetration of the drug inadequate. However, the host's environment is such that higher doses are required to cure the infections in different locations. Failure to appreciate this phenomenon may lead to inadequate doses.

TREATMENT OF NONBACTERIAL INFECTIONS Viral infections do not respond to the drugs generally considered as antibiotic agents, and these drugs must not be expected to exact a therapeutic effect in these situations. Similarly, antibiotics do not prevent bacterial complications of viral infections.

FAILURE TO DRAIN PURULENT MATERIAL OR TO REMOVE OBSTRUCTION Antimicrobial drugs work well only in an

TABLE 130-2 *(continued)*

Organism	*Disease*	*Drug*	*Dosage*	*Route*	*Duration*
K. pneumoniae	Pneumonia, bacteremia	Cephalothin	1.0 g q.4h	IV	7 days
		or cefazolin	1.0 g q.4h	IV	7 days
		or kanamycin	7.5 mg/kg q.12h	IM	7 days
		or gentamicin	5 mg/kg/day	IM,IV	7 days
Pasturella tularensis	Tularemia	Streptomycin	1.0 g q.12h.	IM	10–14 days
Enterobacter aerogenes	Genitourinary infection	Nalidixic acid[7]	1.0 mg q.6h	PO	10–14 days
		or kanamycin	7.5 mg/kg q.12h	IM	7 days
		or gentamicin	3 mg/kg/day	IM,IV	7 days
	Bacteremia	Kanamycin	7.5 mg/kg q.12h	IM	7 days
		or gentamicin	3–5 mg/kg/day	IM,IV	7 days
		and/or carbenicillin	30 g/day	IV	7 days
Escherichia coli	Genitourinary infection	Sulfisoxazole[8]	1 g q.6h	PO	10–14 days
		or tetracycline	500 mg q.6h	PO	10–14 days
		or ampicillin	500 mg q.6h	PO	10–14 days
		or nitrofurantoin	100 mg q.6h	PO	10–14 days
	Bacteremia, arthritis, peritonitis	Ampicillin	6–12 g/day	IV	7–10 days
		or kanamycin	7.5 mg/kg q.12h	IM	7–10 days
		or gentamicin	3–5 mg/kg/day	IM,IV	7–10 days
		or cephalothin	1–2 g q.4h	IV	7–10 days
	Meningitis	Ampicillin	8–12 g q.4h	IV	7–10 days
		or chloramphenicol	50–100 mg/kg/day (q.6h)	IV	7–10 days
Proteus mirabilis	Urine	Ampicillin	500 mg q.6h	PO	10–14 days
		or cephalexin	500 mg q.6h	PO	10–14 days
	Blood	Ampicillin	6.0 g/day	IV	7–10 days
		or kanamycin	7.5 mg/kg q.12h	IM	7–10 days
		or cephalothin	6.0 g/day	IV	7–10 days
		or gentamicin	5 mg/kg/day	IM,IV	7–10 days
Indole-positive *Proteus*	Urine	Kanamycin	7.5 mg/kg q.12h	IM	10–14 days
		or carbenicillin[9]	1 g q.6h	IV	10–14 days
		or nalidixic acid	1 g q.6h	PO	10–14 days
		or gentamicin	3–5 mg/kg/day	IM,IV	10–14 days
	Blood	Kanamycin	7.5 mg/kg q.12h	IM	7–10 days
		or carbenicillin	4 g q.4h	IV	7–10 days
		or gentamicin	5 mg/kg/day	IM	7–10 days
Pseudomonas	Blood, joint	Gentamicin	5 mg/kg/day	IM,IV	7 days
		plus carbenicillin	5–6 g q.4h	IV	7 days
	Meningitis, brain abscess	Gentamicin	5 mg/kg/day	IV,IM	5–7 days
		plus carbenicillin	5–6 g q.4h	IV	5–7 days
		and gentamicin	4 mg q.12–18h	Intra-thecally	7 days
	Urine	Colistin	75 mg q.6h	IM	10–14 days
		or carbenicillin[9]	2 g q.6h	IM,IV	10–14 days
		or polymyxin B	30 mg q.6h	IM,IV	10–14 days
		or oxytetracycline	500 mg q.6h	PO	10–14 days
		or gentamicin	3 mg/kg/day	IM,IV	10–14 days
Bacteroides	Abscess, bacteremia	Chloramphenicol	0.5 g q.4h	IV,PO	10–14 days
		or Clindamycin	0.6 g q.6–8h	IV	10–14 days
			then 0.3 g q.6h	PO as long as necessary	
Mycoplasma	Sputum	Erythromycin	250–500 mg q.6h	PO	7 days
		or tetracycline	500 mg q.6h	PO	7 days

[9] *The indanyl ester of carbenicillin 1 g q.6h may be given orally.*

environment free of obstruction. Infections will not respond optimally unless obstructions such as a plug of mucus or an enlarged prostate, or a foreign body such as a suture or splinter, are removed, or unless purulent material is drained. It is particularly important to drain an abscess cavity because antibiotics do not kill bacteria enmeshed in pus.

SUPERINFECTIONS The role of antibiotics in promoting superinfections is mentioned above and in Chap. 128. In 2 to 3 percent of patients seeming failure of antimicrobials is a consequence of superinfection.

DRUG REACTION The development of drug fever without rash or any other manifestation of hypersensitivity may make it appear as if the infection were not responding to therapy, when instead the fever is due to the very drug being given to cure the infection. Drug fever is extremely common with certain antimicrobials, particularly penicillin. The best way to make the diagnosis is simply to discontinue therapy. If fever disappears, the diagnosis is established. A second challenge with the suspected drug is neither necessary nor safe.

INCORRECT DRUG Only rarely does chemotherapy fail because the incorrect drug has been administered. Most drugs have a sufficiently broad spectrum, and combinations of drugs are administered with sufficient frequency, whether indicated or not, to make it highly unlikely that the patient is not given an agent active against the etiologic pathogen. One of the most common errors, when the patient is not responding, is to add more antimicrobials indiscriminately, when the correct course should be to discontinue therapy and to watch the patient.

DEFECTS IN HOST RESISTANCE The type of patient requiring antimicrobial therapy has changed from a young or middle-aged individual to an elderly one with degenerative and debilitating disease or one whose host defenses have been compromised by neoplastic disease, large doses of antimicrobials, antineoplastic or immunosuppressive drugs, x-ray therapy, major surgical procedures, or transplants. For a variety of reasons, this type of patient does not, and should not be expected to, respond to antimicrobials as does a normal individual. This factor is often ignored in gauging the results of chemotherapy. It does not mean that antibiotics should not be used when indicated; rather, no miraculous results should be expected in patients with severe associated disease of noninfectious origin.

TABLE 130-3
Chemoprophylaxis of infections

DRUGS THAT ARE USUALLY EFFECTIVE FOR:	
Group A streptococcus (rheumatic fever)	Penicillin G, sulfonamides
Neisseria meningitidis	Rifampin, minocycline
N. gonorrheae (ophthalmia)	Penicillin, silver nitrate
Enteropathic *Escherichia coli* diarrhea	Neomycin, kanamycin
Streptococcus viridans (SBE)	Procaine penicillin G, vancomycin, procaine penicillin G + streptomycin
Congenital syphilis	Penicillin
Tuberculin contacts	Isoniazid
DRUGS THAT ARE SOMETIMES EFFECTIVE FOR:	
Shigellosis	Ampicillin, neomycin
Gonococcal urethritis	Penicillin
Chronic bronchitis *(Hemophilus influenzae* or *Diplococcus pneumoniae)*	Ampicillin, tetracycline
Infections encountered during	
Prolonged labor	Ampicillin, tetracycline
Short-term urethral catheterization (< 24 h)	Ampicillin, tetracycline, nitrofurantoin
Cardiac surgery	Methicillin
Large-bowel surgery (preoperative prophylaxis)	Neomycin, kanamycin
Cystic fibrosis	Tetracycline
Contaminated surgical wounds	Cephalothin
ALL DRUGS ARE USUALLY INEFFECTIVE FOR:	
Viral respiratory disease	
Viral exanthems	
Infections encountered during:	
Clean abdominal surgery	
Gynecologic surgery	
Burns	
Coma	
Shock	
Congestive heart failure	
Prematurity	
Prolonged urethral catheterization (> 24 h)	
Prolonged intravenous catheterization	
High-dose steroid therapy	

REFERENCES

BENNETT JE: Chemotherapy of systemic mycoses. N Engl J Med 290:30, 1974

BENNETT WM et al: A guide to drug therapy in renal failure. JAMA 230:1544, 1974

CLUFF LE, JOHNSON JE (eds): *Clinical Concepts of Infectious Diseases,* Baltimore: Williams & Wilkins, 1972

GARROD LP, O'GRADY F: *Antibiotic and Chemotherapy,* 4th ed., Baltimore: Williams & Wilkins, 1973

Handbook of Antimicrobial Therapy, New Rochelle, N.Y.: Medical Letter, 1974

HOEPRICH PD: *Infectious Diseases,* 1st ed. New York: Harper & Row, 1972

KABINS SA: Interactions among antibiotics and other drugs. JAMA 219:206, 1972

SYMPOSIUM ON AMIKACIN. J Infect Dis (in press)

SYMPOSIUM ON AMOXICILLIN. J Infect Dis 129:S121–274, 1974

WEINSTEIN L: Chemotherapy of microbial diseases, in *The Pharmacological Basis of Therapeutics,* eds LS Goodman, A Gilman, New York: Macmillan, 1975, p. 1090

section 2 | Infections of specific tissues and anatomic sites

131 LOCALIZED INFECTIONS AND ABSCESSES

ROBERT G. PETERSDORF

GENERAL CONSIDERATIONS

INTRODUCTION In contrast to most bacterial diseases, which can be conveniently described in terms of their specific etiologic pathogens, there are some in which the clinical picture is determined primarily by their location. Examples of such infections include abscesses, soft-tissue infections, bacterial endocarditis (Chap. 132), pyogenic infections of the central nervous system (Chap. 337), urinary tract infections (Chap. 277), lung abscess (Chap. 259), mediastinitis (Chap. 264), liver abscess (Chap. 303), appendicitis and appendiceal abscess (Chap. 293), diverticulitis (Chap. 291), osteomyelitis (Chap. 134), and infections of the pericardium (Chap. 246). Infections in these sites can be caused by many pathogens, and although their bacteriologic identification may be time-consuming, knowledge of the usual flora causing infection in certain anatomic loci should permit institution of therapy before the results of cultures are available. Although treatment of these infections is usually surgical, the internist may be the first one to see these patients and may also be the one to prescribe chemotherapy on the basis of the presumed pathogen.

ETIOLOGY Localized pyogenic infection can develop in any region or organ of the body, and may be initiated by *trauma* and secondary bacterial contamination, by some *alteration in local conditions* that renders a tissue susceptible to infection with organisms already present as part of the "normal flora" to which it is ordinarily resistant, by *contiguous spread* from a nearby lesion, or by *metastatic implantation* of microorganisms carried in blood or lymph.

Under appropriate conditions of lowered tissue resistance, almost any of the common bacteria can initiate an infectious process. Cultures from open lesions such as those of the skin or from intraabdominal foci arising from perforations of the gastrointestinal tract frequently contain several bacterial species; as might be expected, the organisms found most frequently are the "normal flora" of these regions.

Infection in some areas is more likely to be caused by certain organisms, staphylococci in the skin and coliform bacteria in the urinary tract, and special features of the tissue reaction produced by some bacterial species make it possible to recognize infection by them with considerable accuracy. The *staphylococci* produce rapid necrosis and early suppuration with large amounts of creamy yellow pus (Chap. 134). Group A beta-hemolytic streptococcal infections (Chap. 135) tend to spread rapidly through tissues, causing intense edema and erythema but relatively little necrosis and thin, serumlike exudate; anaerobic streptococci (Chap. 135) produce necrosis and profuse, brownish, foul-smelling pus. *Pseudomonas* infections (Chap. 139) are often rather indolent, with thick, bluish-green exudate; the *pneumococcus* (Chap. 133) stimulates the production of viscid greenish pus containing large plaques of fibrin and denatured protein.

The causative agents of many other diseases are capable of producing localized infection in tissues that are not usually involved in the specific "clinical entities" ascribed to them. An example is the cutaneous ulcer caused by *Corynebacterium diphtheriae* (Chap. 154).

The identification of infecting organisms is important in the choice of local or systemic chemotherapy. However, when infection occurs in a certain area, as in paranasal sinuses or cutaneous ulcers, or shows up in sputum, it is unlikely that sterility can ever be achieved. In these locations, serial cultures during therapy must be interpreted in this light.

PATHOGENESIS Factors predisposing to the initiation and persistence of infection in a tissue include trauma, obstruction of normal drainage (sweat glands, biliary tract, bronchial tree, urinary tract), ischemia (infarction, gangrene), chemical irritation (by gastric contents, bile, or intramuscularly injected drugs), hematoma formation, accumulation of fluid (lymphatic obstruction, cardiac edema), foreign bodies (bullets, splinters, sutures), and others such as the occurrence of stasis or turbulence in the vascular system.

Infection in soft tissue usually begins as a *cellulitis,* a diffuse acute inflammation with hyperemia, edema, and leukocytic infiltration but little or no necrosis and suppuration. With some organisms, this is followed by necrosis, liquefaction, accumulation of leukocytes and debris, suppuration, loculation and walling off of the pus, and formation of one or more *abscesses.* Abscess formation is particularly likely to follow infection in a preexisting space or cavity, examples being the fallopian tubes or lung cysts.

The local spread of infection generally follows the path of least resistance along fascial planes; proper surgical treatment is based upon a knowledge of these routes, which will be described for specific infections later in this chapter. Lymphatic spread may lead to lymphangitis, lymphadenitis, or, if the regional nodes suppurate, to the formation of a *bubo.* Involvement of local venules or large veins may lead to infective thrombophlebitis with resulting bacteremia, septic embolization, and systemic dissemination of infection. Staphylococci, streptococci, and bacteroides are notorious for the frequency with which they produce vascular lesions of this type.

Depending upon the infecting organism and the anatomy of the affected region, a small abscess may subside completely; there may be gradual encapsulation of the accumulated pus and persistence of the focus in a quiescent state; or the lesion may "point" and rupture into adjacent tissues or to the outside surface of the body, as usually happens with furuncles. Spontaneous drainage ordinarily leads to subsidence and healing of a superficially situated suppurative focus. However, if the abscess is deeply situated and well encapsulated, there are often persistence of a fistulous tract and the formation of a chronic, draining sinus. *The development of persistent sinuses over an area of suppuration produced by ordinary pyogenic bacteria should always suggest involvement of underlying bone or the presence of a foreign body.* Fistulas that open onto the skin are, of course, soon colonized by microorganisms from the external environment. Ordinary bacterial cultures of drainage fluid almost invariably show a mixed flora and should not be relied upon for the etiologic diagnosis of the underlying disease. This is particularly important in disorders that characteristically lead to persistent sinus formation: tuberculosis, actinomycosis, blastomycosis, melioidosis and glanders, tularemia, and, rarely, amebic abscess of the liver or cecum. In these situations, superficial organisms about the opening of the sinus tract may mask the true nature of the lesion by obscuring the real pathogen.

MANIFESTATIONS Secondary infection of wounds and cutaneous ulcers is usually recognizable by inspection. Infections of the skin and subcutaneous tissues almost invariably produce the classic manifestations: *redness, tenderness, heat,* and *swelling.* Reddish streaks extending proximally and associated with tender enlargement of regional lymph nodes indicate lymphangitis. Systemic symptoms may be absent or mild, or there may be fever, malaise, prostration, and leukocytosis.

Infection and suppuration in deeper tissues or in body cavities are often manifested by local pain and tenderness, but the task of locating and determining the exact nature of the lesion may be difficult. The palpation of a tender mass is helpful, but muscle spasm and intervening structures often interfere. Abdominal or pelvic examination under anesthesia is sometimes useful in these circumstances.

Auscultation may reveal a friction rub over an abdominal viscus, the pleura, or the pericardium. The rapid development of an effusion in the pericardium, pleura, abdomen, or a joint should suggest infection. Similarly, fluid detected by transillumination of paranasal sinuses or inspection of the tympanic membrane may be the first sign of infection.

Depending on the location of an abscess, symptoms and signs referable to encroachment upon adjacent structures may dominate the picture. Respiratory obstruction may be the first sign of mediastinal abscess; dysphagia often first calls attention to peritonsillar or retropharyngeal abscesses; and tamponade is sometimes the initial clue to pericardial infection. Localizing signs of dysfunction are especially striking and important with brain and spinal cord abscesses, although brain abscesses may be clinically silent (Chap. 337). In some patients local pain and tenderness or signs of dysfunction are mild or equivocal, and fever, prostration, and weight loss dominate the picture. The fever may be low-grade but is often hectic, with repeated rigors and drenching night sweats. Fatigue and anemia are frequent, and weight loss may be so rapid as to result in emaciation within a few weeks. A patient with these symptoms and signs may have chronic subphrenic, perinephric, or other abscess in the complete absence of any detectable physical sign pointing to the location of a large accumulation of pus. With the advent of antibiotics some deep-seated abscesses present the picture of a chronic illness manifested by no more than malaise, easy fatigability, low-grade fever, mild anemia, and an elevated sedimentation rate because of prior treatment with antimicrobials.

Fluctuation of a mass on palpation is a reliable sign that it contains fluid, perhaps pus, but failure to detect this sign when deeper structures are examined is no guarantee that suppuration is absent and should not be taken by itself to indicate that the mass is noninfectious in origin or that drainage is not required.

LABORATORY FINDINGS Peripheral polymorphonuclear leukocytosis is frequent with abscesses, and significant unexplained elevation of the white blood cell count in any patient should lead to a search for localized suppuration. Depending on the severity and duration of infection, there may be a chronic normocytic, normochromic anemia. The sedimentation rate is almost always rapid. Mild albuminuria, occasionally noted in febrile patients, has no diagnostic import.

Pus or fluid obtained by needle aspiration or incision of a suspected lesion should *always* be stained and examined directly in addition to being cultured aerobically and anaerobically. Pus is a poor metabolic substrate, and bacteria may fail to grow in cultures from an abscess of long standing. In such instances, the findings on microscopic examination may be the only guide in choosing proper chemotherapy. *Failure to examine exudates with Gram's stain is the single greatest deterrent to appropiate antimicrobial therapy;* it is the responsibility of the internist as well as the surgeon to see that this procedure is performed.

Blood cultures are often positive in intravascular infections such as septic thrombophlebitis and endocarditis (Chap. 132) and in pyogenic infections in which localized abscesses are metastatic, as in staphylococcal, streptococcal, and *Salmonella* bacteremias. Moreover, manipulation, including surgical incision, of any localized infection may be followed by transient bacteremia.

Noninvasive techniques are often helpful in the diagnosis of abscess. X-ray examinations may be of considerable help in detecting localized collections of pus when they show atypical collections of gas, displacement of organs, and tissue densities in abnormal locations. Scintiscans are also most helpful. The isotope ^{67}gallium citrate is localized selectively in abscesses, although neoplasms may give false positive results. Of even more potential value is the technique of diagnostic ultrasound, which is not only useful in localizing abscess but also may provide clues to the size of the abscess and to the presence of multiple abscesses or loculation. Angiography is useful in detecting abscesses in highly vascular organs such as the spleen.

THERAPEUTIC CONSIDERATIONS Recognition of the striking symptomatic improvement that follows spontaneous evacuation of a suppurative focus led long ago to the adoption of *surgical incision* for the treatment of abscesses. The exact reasons for the amelioration of local and constitutional manifestations that results from drainage of pus are unknown, but, clinically, the benefits of adequate incision and drainage are unequivocal.

Incision of infected tissue before the stage of liquefaction and accumulation of pus is often deleterious and fails to relieve discomfort. Premature incision may even at times facilitate spread of infection. For this reason, it is sometimes necessary to wait until an abscess "ripens," i.e., localizes and "comes to a head." The *application of heat* to an area of inflammation will relieve pain and often speed the subsidence of cellulitis without suppuration. If necrosis of tissue is already under way, hot applications appear to facilitate localization of the process and accumulation of pus, making incision and drainage feasible at an earlier time. Another procedure that aids in reduction of swelling and relief of pain is *elevation of the affected part.*

The availability of specific chemotherapeutic drugs has modified the need for heat, elevation, and incision surprisingly little. The early administration of chemotherapeutics has reduced the incidence of suppurative complications in many disorders, but once suppuration has appeared, antimicrobial drugs become remarkably incapable of eradicating the infecting organisms, although they may mask the classical clinical features of abscess formation.

Some antimicrobials, notably the penicillins, appear to retain their antibacterial activity in the presence of pus, while others, exemplified by the aminoglycosides and the polymyxins, are at least partially inactivated in purulent exudates. However, inability of the drug to penetrate into an area of suppuration is rarely the reason for therapeutic failure. Although this possibility exists in some infections, such as osteomyelitis, it is usually overcome by increasing dosage. Because direct instillation of the antibiotic into an infected area is not, by itself, a curative procedure, other factors are probably more important than faulty diffusion of the agent into the purulent focus. Nevertheless, in some infections, such as empyema or pyarthrosis, and with some agents which provide poor tissue levels, such as the polymyxins and gentamicin, direct instillation of an antimicrobial into an area of suppuration is distinctly worthwhile.

It has been shown clearly that an established inflammatory exudate is a relatively poor environment for bacterial multiplication. Because the bactericidal action of the penicillins and the cephalosporins is exerted only against multiplying organisms, it is believed that failure of these antibiotics to eradicate bacteria in an abscess is related to the organisms' inactive metabolic state. Although the mechanism of their antibacterial action differs from that of the penicillins, bacteriostatic agents such as tetracycline or chloramphenicol also are incapable of eradicating bacteria in the static phase of growth. Furthermore, by definition, these drugs are capable only of inhibiting multiplication of bacteria and usually exert no direct lethal action; the death of organisms in any infection treated with bacteriostatic agents is dependent on other mechanisms. For most pyogenic bacteria, phagocytosis is one of the most important of these mechanisms (although there must be others that have not been studied so carefully), and it is known that, in the absence of phagocytes or in circumstances which inhibit their activity, bacteriostatic drugs are relatively ineffective. In fluid-filled cavities, particularly in the metabolically unfavorable milieu of an abscess, phagocytosis is greatly reduced. Consequently, despite inhibition of bacterial multiplication, organisms can remain dormant and survive for long periods of time. It is probably a combination of these two circumstances, decreased multiplication of bacteria and decreased phagocytosis, that makes infection on the heart valves, in the kidney, or in the meninges so relatively resistant to antimicrobial therapy. Relatively large doses of bactericidal drugs for long periods are needed to achieve cure.

Antimicrobial drugs may be expected to prevent suppuration if given early or to prevent spread of an existing abscess, but cannot be substituted for surgical drainage. Indeed, their use in the face of a lesion requiring evacuation of pus is one of the most common serious errors in treating pyogenic infections.

In empyema, suppurative pericarditis, or pyarthrosis, excellent therapeutic results are sometimes achieved by aspiration of pus and instillation of antibiotics into the infected area. The success of this procedure, however, is fully as dependent on the adequacy of drainage as it is upon the instillation of the antibiotic, and if there is loculation or if the exudate becomes too viscid to allow removal, surgical incision and drainage through a large-bore tube become mandatory.

In the presence of infective thrombophlebitis, surgical interruption of the veins by ligation or, in some cases, by total excision of an infected segment is sometimes indicated to prevent seeding of other organs by infected emboli.

CLINICAL FEATURES OF INFECTIONS IN VARIOUS REGIONS

Superficial abscesses

SKIN AND SUBCUTANEOUS TISSUES *Impetigo* is a superficial infection caused by hemolytic staphylococci and group A hemolytic streptococci. It is primarily a disease of children, common in warm weather, characterized by multiple erythematous lesions which vesiculate and are intensely pruritic. Local spread occurs through scratching and release of infected vesicle fluid. Serious complications are metastatic abscesses and hemorrhagic nephritis. Treatment consists of local and general cleansing of the skin, application of bacitracin-neomycin ointment, covering with a loose dressing to prevent further contamination, and appropriate systemic antibiotics.

Deeper infections of the skin are almost invariably staphylococcal in origin and are described in Chap. 134. Erysipelas, a characteristic dermal lesion produced by group A streptococci, is described in Chap. 135.

Lymphadenitis with or without suppuration may complicate any pyogenic skin lesion and is often striking with superficial streptococcal infections. Specific diseases characterized by suppurative regional lymphadenitis include lymphogranuloma venereum (Chap. 190), cat-scratch disease (Chap. 208), tularemia (Chap. 145), and bubonic plague (Chap. 146).

INFECTIONS OF THE HAND These are almost invariably secondary to trauma and are very common. Because of the rapidity with which infection can spread through the complex fascial spaces of the hand, wrist, and forearm, with the production of irreparable functional damage, *any deep infection in this area should receive expert surgical attention immediately*. The importance of such care has in no way been lessened by the availability of antibiotics.

The ordinary *paronychia*, or "run-around," is a superficial infection of the epithelium lateral to a nail, usually a result of tearing a hangnail and most frequently caused by staphylococcus. Hot applications will lead to subsidence of paronychial cellulitis, but often a superficial blister of pus appears or the infection burrows beneath the nail to form a painful *subungual abscess*. Incision and drainage with partial or complete removal of the nail are then necessary. Recurrence is common, especially in nail biters, and this seemingly trivial infection can cause painful disability. Chronic paronychial inflammation produced by various fungi occurs in diabetics, and a similar lesion is seen in psoriasis and some types of pemphigus.

What appears to be a small furuncle of the webs of the fingers sometimes produces a *collar-button abscess*, consisting of a superficial and deep compartment connected by a narrow tract. Evacuation of the shallow pocket without emptying the deeper abscess can lead to puzzling persistence of infection. Sometimes a foreign-body granuloma forms in the skin of the digital webs. This is most common in barbers, in whom a hair is the core of the foreign-body granuloma, the "barber's interdigital pilonidal sinus."

Infection of the distal phalanx of a finger, usually acquired by pinprick, thorn prick, etc., may lead to the formation of a *felon*, or *whitlow*. This is a suppurative infection in the tightly enclosed fibrous compartments of the finger pulp, the "anterior closed space," which can compromise the distal blood supply by compression of the digital arteries, with consequent necrosis of bone and the development of osteomyelitis. The manifestations are swelling, extreme pain, and tenderness of the palmar surface of the finger tip. The treatment is immediate incision directly over the lesion, sometimes by the use of a trephine, and cutting all the fibrous septa that radiate from the periosteum to the subcutaneous fascia.

Suppurative tenosynovitis, usually a complication of a puncture wound, is an even more serious infection of the hand from the point of view of functional damage; early diagnosis and treatment are mandatory to prevent permanent disability from destruction of the tendon or its sheath. The three cardinal manifestations of tenosynovitis are (1) exquisite tenderness limited to the course of the sheath; (2) the fingers held in flexion; and (3) extension of the involved finger, producing excruciating pain, most marked at the base of the digit. *Immediate incision* of the sheath is indicated, not only to prevent damage to the tendon itself but to avoid proximal extension of the process into the major fascial spaces of the hand or forearm. Vigorous antibiotic treatment should accompany surgery. The definitive treatment of any serious infection of the hand is a matter for a skilled surgeon, but the early recognition of the need for surgery often falls to other physicians.

Human bites lead to very important hand infections, which, if neglected, almost invariably produce a highly destructive, necrotizing lesion contaminated by a mixture of aerobic and anaerobic organisms. A deliberately inflicted bite on the hand or elsewhere is usually recognized as dangerously contaminated, but wounds on the knuckles produced by striking an opponent's teeth with the fists may not be recognized as potentially dangerous. In general, bite wounds should be cleaned thoroughly and not sutured. Patients should be given prophylaxis for tetanus and antibiotics, preferably both a penicillinase-resistant penicillin and ampicillin.

CHRONIC CUTANEOUS ULCERS A partial list of the causes of chronic ulcers of the skin includes circulatory disturbances, such as varicose veins and obliterative arterial disease, extensive injury from frostbite or burns, trophic changes accompanying many neurologic disorders, bedsores or decubiti, systemic diseases such as sickle-cell disease and myxedema, neoplasms, and various infections. No matter what the underlying disease, secondary infection is very likely to occur and to interfere with healing, complicate grafting or other restorative procedures, or produce extension of the process.

The management of secondary bacterial infection in skin ulcers associated with obliterative arterial disease, a common problem in diabetics, is especially important, because infection is frequently the factor that precipitates spreading gangrene and makes amputation necessary.

Studies of the microflora of chronic cutaneous ulcers have almost invariably shown bacteria of many species, including staphylococci, aerobic and anaerobic streptococci, coliform bacilli, and members of the *Proteus* and *Pseudomonas* groups. Depending on the patient's environment and on systemically or locally administered antimicrobial drugs, the predominating bacterial species show great variation when lesions are cultured serially. Particularly noteworthy is the replacement of sensitive organisms by resistant strains or species during the course of chemotherapy.

Treatment of chronic dermal ulcers should be directed toward the underlying disorder but should also include *local debridement* and *chemotherapy*. Debridement by surgical excision is often needed, but the local application of proteolytic enzymes such as Varidase, a mixture of streptokinase and streptodornase, or trypsin, so-called "chemical or medical debridement," is sometimes sufficient. Intensive systemic administration of antibiotics should be carried out only in conjunction with definitive surgical procedures or when infection can be controlled in no other way. The prevention of infection by "prophylactic" administration of antimicrobial drugs is futile because it results in the development of a flora resistant to the drugs being used. The *local application of antibiotics* is sometimes highly effective, and it is in the management of chronic mixed infections of this type that several potent but toxic antibiotics have great value. An ointment or solution containing neomycin, bacitracin, and polymyxin exerts a bactericidal effect against a wide variety of organisms and will sometimes temporarily sterilize a chronic lesion. Other useful topical medications are furacin and 3 percent acetic acid, which is especially helpful in *Pseudomonas* infections.

Diphtheritic ulcer of the skin is discussed in Chap. 154.

INFECTIONS OF THE HEAD AND NECK Pustules of the nose and upper lip may be particularly dangerous, because they are likely to extend intracranially through the angular vein to the cavernous sinus. These lesions should be treated conservatively, manipulation or incision should be avoided if possible, and systemic antibiotics should be used if local swelling or redness appears.

Suppurative parotitis, which is usually a complication of chronic debilitating disease or blockage of Stensen's duct by a calculus, is largely avoidable by maintenance of hydration and oral hygiene. Its onset is heralded by local pain and swelling; fever and chills are frequent. Frank pus can sometimes be expressed from the duct, and the gland itself is firm and tender, often with pitting edema of the overlying skin and facial palsy. Most cases of suppurative parotitis are caused by hemolytic *Staphylococcus aureus.* Treatment consists of removal of obstructing calculi, but its mainstay is antimicrobial therapy with a penicillinase-resistant penicillin, cephalothin, or vancomycin. Incision and drainage of a septate gland such as the parotid has not been particularly effective. Despite chemotherapy and drainage, the mortality rate of suppurative parotitis is 30 to 50 percent, perhaps because this infection occurs in patients with debilitating disease.

The use of penicillin and other antibiotics has reduced the incidence of many formerly common suppurative complications of streptococcal pharyngitis. However, as a result of streptococcal sore throat, *Bacteroides* infections of the pharynx, or introduction of infection by trauma to the floor of the mouth or the pharyngeal wall, abscesses of the deep cervical structures still occur. *Suppurative cervical adenitis,* once an all-too-common sequel to streptococcal pharyngitis in children, is now rare. *Peritonsillar abscess (quinsy)* is manifested by fever, sore throat, unilateral pain radiating to the ear on swallowing, and enlargement of the tonsil with redness and swelling of the adjacent soft palate. Treatment with penicillin and irrigations of warm saline solution sometimes lead to subsidence of the process, but if digital palpation reveals fluctuation, surgical drainage with or without tonsillectomy is indicated. Organisms associated with peritonsillar abscess include *Streptococcus pyogenes, Strep. pneumoniae, Staph. aureus, Klebsiella-Enterobacter,* and, most commonly, *Bacteroides* species.

The course of *deep cervical infections* is fully as dependent upon the anatomic arrangement of fascial planes as is that of infections of the hand. Infection in this area is serious and is attended by fever, prostration, and leukocytosis. A tender mass may be palpated, but *surgical evacuation of such an infection should not be delayed because of failure to detect fluctuation,* which is usually absent because of the dense fascial layers.

Infection of the *sublingual space,* so-called "Ludwig's angina," is characterized by brawny induration of the submaxillary region, edema of the floor of the mouth, and elevation of the tongue. There are severe pain, dysphagia, and, within hours, dyspnea from respiratory obstruction. The causative organisms of this and other neck abscesses, in addition to those mentioned above, include *Hemophilus influenzae* and *Escherichia coli.* Mortality was formerly about 50 percent. *Treatment* consists of large doses of penicillin and careful observation. If there is significant progression of obstruction during the 4 to 6 h after treatment is instituted, wide incision is indicated and tracheostomy may need to be performed.

The retropharyngeal space lies between the muscles anterior to the cervical vertebrae and the pharyngeal mucosa. *Retropharyngeal abscess,* formerly common in children, is manifested by dysphagia, progressive stridor, pain, and fever. The bulging mass is easily seen and can completely occlude the airway within hours. Incision and drainage are mandatory; spontaneous rupture may lead to death by aspiration. Esophageal perforation during endoscopy may result in abscess as a late complication. Tuberculous abscess, secondary to spinal disease, occasionally appears in the retropharyngeal space; it is painless, and relief of obstruction follows surgical incision.

Submastoid abscess, or suppuration in the submastoid space, known as *Bezold's abscess,* is usually secondary to otitis and produces nuchal rigidity, which may lead to a mistaken diagnosis of otogenous meningitis. Infection can extend down the carotid sheath to the mediastinum. A suppurative thrombophlebitis of the jugular vein usually accompanies this infection, and the vessel is easily felt as a tender cord. Bacteremia and systemic spread of infection are common, and the involved venous segment may need to be excised. Spontaneous rupture of the carotid artery with rapid death from exsanguination is a rare complication.

Therapy of head and neck abscesses includes surgical incision and drainage, open treatment of infected wounds, and systemic antibiotics, which should include agents active against *Bacteroides,* particularly if there is foul-smelling pus.

DEEP-SEATED INFECTIONS

SPLENIC ABSCESS Splenic abscess occurs by several mechanisms: (1) dissemination via the bloodstream during bacteremia; primary foci include the endocardium, lung (lung abscess or pneumonia), pleural cavity (empyema), skin and soft tissues, ear and nasopharyngeal structures, and pelvis (pelvic inflammatory disease and septic abortion); (2) infection in a spleen damaged by bland infarcts (sickle-cell disease, leukemia) or more rarely, by other diseases such as malaria, typhoid, hydatid or dermoid cysts, and ameboma or by trauma (following subcapsular hematoma formation); (3) extension from a perforated or diseased stomach, colon, or tail of the pancreas, as in carcinoma; and (4) rarely, without apparent cause. The most common causative organisms are Enterobacteriaceae, *Pseudomonas, Serratia,* and *Bacteroides.* It is important to differentiate single from multiple abscesses; the former are more readily diagnosed and respond to surgical therapy. The latter are usually the result of generalized sepsis, often occur in debilitated or immunosuppressed patients, are diagnosed only with difficulty, and respond poorly to therapy because the patient has either infection elsewhere or concomitant lethal disease. The onset is sudden, with chills, fever, and left upper quadrant pain. There are tenderness and muscle spasm, and the skin and subcutaneous tissues overlying the spleen may be edematous. Involvement of the upper pole commonly leads to left pleuritic pain, radiating to the shoulder, with elevation of the diaphragm or left pleural effusion. Lower pole abscess gives signs of tender splenomegaly and peritoneal inflammation. Splenic friction rub is often audible. Disorders to be considered in differential diagnosis are subphrenic abscess, infection or infarction of the left lower lobe of the lung, bland infarction of the spleen, pancreatic pseudocyst, pyelonephritis, and abscess secondary to perforation of the transverse colon. X-ray examinations are an important adjunct in the diagnosis. Abnormal radiographic findings include (1) soft-tissue mass in left upper quadrant; (2) extraintestinal gas, which may occur even in the absence of gas-forming bacteria but which is probably due to perforation of an adjacent hollow viscus; (3) downward displacement of the splenic flexure of the colon; (4) inferior displacement of the left kidney, best visualized on an intravenous pyelogram; (5) displacement of the stomach bubble medially; (6) elevation of the left hemidiaphragm; and (7) left pleural effusion. Spleen scan is of great value in delineating solitary abscesses but does not readily localize multiple lesions which tend to be smaller. Sometimes combined spleen-lung scan provides clues to perisplenic (or left subdiaphragmatic) lesions. Angiography with selective catheterization of the splenic artery is most helpful in detecting multiple as well as single abscesses.

Treatment consists of administering antibiotics and performing splenectomy. The splenic artery and vein should be ligated prior to splenectomy. An abscess in a very ill patient may require splenotomy and drainage, with more definitive surgery at a later time. Splenic abscess is particularly common in patients with sickle-cell disease, but splenic infarction in subacute bacterial endocarditis caused by *Strep. viridans* almost never suppurates. Infected splenic infarcts are a rare cause of continued bacteremia in acute bacterial endocarditis, even in the face of massive chemotherapy, and splenectomy may then be necessary to achieve the final eradication of the organism.

SUBPHRENIC ABSCESS Peritoneal infections show a striking tendency to localize in the upper part of the abdomen between the transverse colon and the diaphragm. True subphrenic abscesses are located between the liver and diaphragm on the left or right, and many so-called "subphrenic infections" are, in fact, subhepatic. Most of these infections are related to perforations in the gastrointestinal or biliary tracts, and over half of them follow operations on the gallbladder, duodenum, or stomach. Subphrenic abscesses following perforated appendicitis occur rarely nowadays. Closed blunt trauma following laceration of the liver is an important cause, and a few abscesses occur without predisposing neighborhood infection. These may occur on the left and may be caused by *Salmonella.* The most common organisms are *E. coli,* non-group A streptococci, staphylococci, and *Klebsiella-Enterobacter;* mixed infections are common. As with other intraabdominal infections, *Bacteroides* sp. is playing a progressively greater role. About 60 percent of abscesses occur on the right, 25 percent on left, and 15 percent are bilateral. They are more common in males and elderly patients, who often have a debilitating disease such as cancer. *Any patient with persistent fever and a history of recent intraabdominal sepsis should be suspected of having a subphrenic abscess.*

Manifestations include fever, upper abdominal pain, and tenderness, usually along the costal margin. Shoulder pain, dyspnea, dullness, and rales at the lung base are more common than abdominal signs and symptoms, and emphasize the location of a true abscess between the liver and the diaphragm. Foul sputum connotes perforation of the abscess into the lung. The localizing signs are by no means striking in all cases, however. The widespread practice of "covering" postoperative patients with antibiotics prophylactically can attenuate subphrenic infection without eradicating it and may result in an insidiously progressive illness with weight loss, malaise, fatigue, and low-grade fever beginning weeks or months after a laparotomy, a syndrome termed *chronic subphrenic abscess.* Roentgenograms may show gas, sometimes with an air-fluid level beneath the diaphragm. The gas is usually from a perforated viscus or enters through an external sinus; it is only rarely the result of bacterial multiplication.

Other radiographic findings include pleural effusion, which is usually sterile, basilar infiltrates, and elevation—but not necessarily fixation—of the diaphragm. Barium meal with the patient in the head-down position may show indentation of the gastric fundus in left subphrenic abscess, a lesion that is often notoriously difficult to localize. Combined lung-liver scintiscan is a considerable advance in the diagnosis of subphrenic abscess. The use of gallium-technetium subtraction scanning for the localization of subphrenic abscess seems particularly useful.

The outlook in subphrenic abscess is poor because so many patients have cancer as an underlying cause. Among benign predisposing causes, patients who develop subphrenic abscess in the wake of a perforated gastric ulcer seem to do poorly. Even with surgical drainage, the mortality rate approaches 30 to 35 percent; without it, nearly 75 percent of patients die. Drainage should be extraperitoneal, usually through the bed of the twelfth rib. Appropriate antibiotics should be given, both locally and systemically, keeping in mind the possibility that the infection may be caused by an anaerobe.

RETROPERITONEAL INFECTIONS Strictly speaking, all perinephric, most pancreatic, and many subphrenic abscesses are located outside the peritoneum, but the term *retroperitoneal abscess* usually refers to infection in the lumbar and iliac regions. Suppuration in these areas is relatively rare, but the importance of recognizing its existence in patients with fever and pain in the lower part of the back is great. In one series, the average duration of illness in 65 patients before diagnosis was approximately 1 month.

Infection in the retroperitoneal space usually reflects extension from posterior perforations of the appendix, small bowel or colon, pancreatic, renal, or spinal infections, and occasionally suppurative lymphadenitis in the iliac area, usually secondary to streptococcal infections of the lower extremities in children.

Lumbar abscess is characterized by tenderness and spasm of the back muscles on the affected side, and a mass is usually palpable in the lumbar region; or there may be a prominent, tender abdominal mass without lumbar pain or spasm. Infection in the wall of the abdominal aneurysm, often with *Salmonella,* may present as a lumbar abscess. Flexion of the hip (psoas sign) occurs in a few cases but is more often present with infections lower in the retroperitoneal area. *Fever, leukocytosis,* and *lumbar spasm* should suggest the diagnosis. The absence of a palpable mass may lead to protracted observation, and it is in these instances that palpation under anesthesia is often helpful.

Psoas (iliac) abscess is typically attended by abdominal pain in the iliac or inguinal region, and, particularly when the psoas muscle is involved, severe pain may be referred to the hip, thigh, or knee. Careful palpation of the lower part of the abdomen or groin usually reveals a mass, and fullness and tenderness on rectal examination are common. Hip spasm (psoas sign) is often present. Although psoas abscesses characteristically occur in association with tuberculosis of the spine, the acute bacterial form has been reported in perforation or fistula formation of the bowel in Crohn's disease (regional enteritis). Roentgenograms may delineate the inflammatory mass; pyelography shows displacement of the kidney or ureter in some cases, scoliosis with concavity on the side of the infection, and blurring of the psoas shadow. When regional enteritis is suspected, a small-bowel x-ray and barium enema should be performed. Treatment consists of surgical drainage and appropriate antibiotic therapy.

PANCREATIC ABSCESS Pancreatic abscess usually occurs in a site of pancreatic necrosis following acute pancreatitis. It should be suspected in patients who develop fever and who have persistent ileus, abdominal pain and tenderness, nausea, vomiting, and general deterioration following acute pancreatitis. A mass is palpable in half the patients. The amylase is elevated only irregularly, but there is usually leukocytosis (15,000 to 20,000 cells per mm^3), a low serum albumin, and an elevated alkaline phosphatase. Blood cultures may be positive and usually contain coliform bacteria. The diagnosis can be suspected by displacement of adjacent structures on contrast radiography, and ultrasound echocardiography has been helpful in delineating the mass.

The definitive diagnosis can be made only by drainage, which is mandatory. Multiple drains should be used along with appropriate antibiotics which should include agents active against Enterobacteriaceae as well as anaerobes. Failure to drain the abscess may result in one of several lethal complications such as perforation into adjacent structures, erosion of the left gastric, splenic, and gastroduodenal arteries with exsanguination, and the development of further abscesses in the pancreas and peritoneal and retroperitoneal spaces.

RENAL ABSCESS Single or multiple abscesses of the renal *cortex* are almost invariably the result of metastatic implantation of staphylococci from another focus. There is no relationship to previous renal disease; the infection occurs in younger individuals, is usually unilateral, and occurs on the right side oftener than on the left. Many patients give a history of recent skin infection such as furuncle. Although acute pyelonephritis is a diffuse disease with foci of cellular infiltrates in the interstitium of the renal medulla, these inflammatory foci may coalesce to form a distinct abscess cavity. This situation probably ensues more frequently than is generally appreciated.

The onset of renal abscess is abrupt, with chill and fever, followed by costovertebral pain and tenderness. If the abscess is cortical, the urine contains *no white blood cells;* medullary abscesses are usually accompanied by pyuria. The stained urinary sediment will show myriads of gram-positive cocci in cortical abscesses and gram-negative organisms in medullary abscesses. Transient gross or microscopic hematuria may occur at the onset. The white blood cell count is usually elevated and may exceed 30,000 cells per mm^3. Physical signs are usually localized to the region of the kidney, but abdominal spasm may lead to confusion with appendicitis, cholecystitis, or pancreatitis. Early in the disease, ureteral calculus or acute hydronephrosis may be considered as possible diagnoses. Sudden onset of *fever, leukocytosis, and renal pain in the absence of pyuria* should suggest the diagnosis of renal abscess, especially in a patient with infection elsewhere. Obstruction of the ureter by pus or cellular debris may also yield a urine sediment sparse in white blood cells and bacteria. *Treatment* consists of appropriate antibiotics, adequate fluids, and relief of pain. An abscess may suddenly discharge into the renal pelvis, with relief of pain and the passage of cloudy urine containing enormous numbers of leukocytes and bacteria. *Complications* include formation of a thick-walled chronic renal "carbuncle," requiring surgical removal, rupture into the perirenal space, and secondary pyelonephritis, usually produced by coliform bacilli. Recovery is ordinarily prompt, and chronic sequelae are rare.

Perinephric abscess in the past was most often due to hematogenous dissemination during streptococcal or staphylococcal infection, but at present it more often follows calculi in the ureter and hydronephrosis, noncalculous renal infection, tuberculosis, and actinomycosis. Diabetics are particularly susceptible. The causative organisms are those which are primarily responsible in acute pyelonephritis—*E. coli, Proteus* species, and *Klebsiella-Enterobacter.* Flank pain with radiation to the upper part of the abdomen, back, or even the shoulder, nausea, vomiting, fever, malaise, leukocytosis, tenderness with spasm of flank and upper abdominal muscles, and a palpable mass which moves with respiration are the main manifestations. Symptoms referable to the urinary tract are present when perinephric abscess is associated with pyelonephritis or stone. In a few patients, elevation of the diaphragm on the diseased side occurs and leads to confusion with subphrenic infection. The psoas muscle is involved by the inflammatory process, and patients are frequently more comfortable with the thigh held in flexion. The roentgenogram occasionally will reveal a mass; there is usually blurring of the renal silhouette; and the psoas shadow is indistinct on the involved side. There may also be scoliosis to the side of the lesion, fixation of the kidney, anterior displacement of the organ on lateral pyelograms, and gas formation within the perinephric mass, or total nonvisualization of the kidney. Chest roentgenograms often show basal infiltrates and pleural effusions. Complications include perforation into adjacent organs, particularly the colon. *Treatment* by surgical drainage and systemic administration of antibiotics (*not* urinary antiseptics) is usually followed by dramatic subsidence of pain and fever, and unless intrinsic renal disease is present, recovery is complete. Nevertheless, the overall outcome is poor, in part because the diagnosis is often made too late or is missed altogether, and also because of the generally poor condition of many of these patients. Among adverse prognostic factors are: (1) delay in diagnosis; on medical records these patients are often designated as having F.U.O.; (2) concomitant diabetes mellitus; (3) azotemia (BUN ≥ 50); (4) leukocytosis ($\geq 25{,}000$ cells per mm^3); (5) bacteremia; (6) history of urinary tract obstruction or infection. In general, patients admitted to urologic services have done better, perhaps because the diagnosis was more obvious and treatment could be instituted earlier.

RECTAL ABSCESS Most of these infections are superficial and involve the perirectal region, and many are associated with fistulas. Infection in the apocrine glands (hidradenitis) or folliculitis in the perianal region, extension of cryptitis or obstructions in the "anal glands" which open into the crypts of Morgagni, and contamination of submucosal hematomas, sclerosed hemorrhoids, or anal fissures may lead to abscess formation. These are usually painful, easily palpable, often visible on inspection. Superficial rectal abscesses may be confused with Bartholin's cysts, sebaceous cysts, tuberculosis, actinomycosis, urethroperineal fistulas, carcinoma of the anus, foreign body, pilonidal sinus, and lymphogranuloma venereum, gonorrhea, and syphilis in homosexuals. Treatment is application of heat and appropriate drainage or excision. Antibiotics may be indicated in some instances.

Difficulties in diagnosis are likely to arise with infections higher in the rectum. Most are in the ischiorectal area, but those above the pelvic diaphragm, the so-called *supralevator abscess,* are particularly elusive. Patients with this type of infection often have fever, malaise, and leukocytosis for several days or even weeks before any symptoms referable to the rectum develop. There is vague pelvic discomfort, relieved by defecation, and constipation punctuated by short episodes of diarrhea is common. In males, the inflammation often involves the base of the bladder, and urinary urgency or retention is not infrequent, falsely centering attention on the urinary tract as the source of fever and malaise. Eventually, the abscess produces severe pain, chills, and fever; palpation and instrumentation will reveal the swelling in the rectal ampulla. Such an abscess may surround the rectum and produce narrowing that is differentiated from that caused by neoplasm by the fact that the mucosa remains intact. A useful sign of deep rectal abscess is eliciting of severe pain by pressure in the region between the anus and the coccyx. The supralevator space is continuous with the ischiorectal space, with both the gluteal and obturator regions, and with the retroperitoneal space. In neglected cases, the abscess may drain through the skin of the perineum, the groin, or the buttock or may extend as high as the perirenal areas. Rectal abscesses are not uncommon in patients with preexisting anorectal disease, diabetes, alcoholism, and neurologic disease; infections in this area are also peculiarly frequent in patients with acute leukemia, especially when the white blood cell count is severely depressed. Because the clinical picture may be that of "fever of unknown origin" for a long period, it is important that thorough digital and endoscopic examination of the rectum be carried out in febrile patients. A rectal examination should be made in all patients with diabetes, especially if ketosis is present; failure to observe this rule has more than once led to delay in detecting the infection responsible for diabetic ketosis or coma.

A rectal abscess may be a forerunner of both ulcerative colitis and regional enteritis, and may occur months and even years before other overt manifestations of these diseases. For this reason, proctosigmoidoscopy, colonoscopy, barium enema, and, often, upper gastrointestinal roentgenograms are indicated in nonhealing rectal lesions.

Treatment of high rectal abscesses consists of incision and drainage, hot sitz baths, analgesics, and antibiotics directed at *E. coli,* paracolon, *Klebsiella-Enterobacter, Bacteroides,* and a variety of streptococci, which make up the polymicrobial flora of these lesions.

REFERENCES

BARNHILL JF: Deep abscess of the neck: Surgical treatment. Am J Surg 42:207, 1938

BLAIR DC et al: Localization of infectious processes with gallium citrate Ga^{67}. JAMA 230:82, 1974

CURRERI WP et al: Subphrenic abscess secondary to salmonellosis. Arch Surg 95:189, 1967

EISENHAMMER S: The internal anal sphincter and the anorectal abscess. Surg Gynecol Obstet 103:501, 1956

FRIDAY RO et al: Detection and localization of intraabdominal abscesses by diagnostic ultrasound. Arch Surg 110:335, 1975

GADACZ T et al: Changing clinical spectrum of splenic abscess. Am J Surg 128:182, 1974

GASTON EA, WARREN LO: Supralevator abscess. N Engl J Med 229:613, 1943

JANKE WH, BLOCK MA: Chronic retroperitoneal pelvic abscesses. Arch Surg 90:389, 1965

JOHNSON TH JR: The subdiaphragmatic abscess in the antibiotic era. South Med J 61:455, 1968

KYLE J: Psoas abscess in Crohn's disease. Gastroenterology 61: 149, 1971

LIDDELL TD et al: Anorectal suppurative disease. Am J Surg 125: 189, 1973

MAGILLIGAN DJ JR: Suprahepatic abscess. Arch Surg 96:14, 1968

OZERAN RS: Subdiaphragmatic abscess. Am Surg 33:64, 1967

PETERSDORF RG et al: Staphylococcal parotitis. N Engl J Med 259:1259, 1958

RICHARDS L: Retropharyngeal abscess. N Engl J Med 215:1120, 1936

ROSENBERG M: Chronic subphrenic abscess. Lancet II:379, 1968

SALVATIERRA O JR et al: Perinephric abscess. J Urol 98:296, 1967

THORLEY JD et al: Perinephric abscess. Medicine 53:441, 1974

WARSHAW AL: Pancreatic abscesses. N Engl J Med 287:1234, 1972

Superficial abscesses

BUNNELL S: *Surgery of the Hand,* 4th ed., ed TH Boyes, Philadelphia, Lippincott, 1964

132 INFECTIVE ENDOCARDITIS

LAWRENCE L. PELLETIER, JR.
ROBERT G. PETERSDORF

DEFINITION Infective endocarditis is a microbial infection of the heart valves or of the endocardium in proximity to congenital or acquired cardiac defects. A similar clinical illness develops when there is infection of arteriovenous fistulas or aneurysms. The infection may develop abruptly or insidiously, may pursue a fulminant or prolonged course, and is fatal unless treated. The infection caused by indigenous microorganisms with low pathogenicity is ordinarily subacute, whereas infection by microorganisms with high pathogenicity is often acute. Fever, cardiac murmurs, splenomegaly, anemia, hematuria, mucocutaneous petechiae, and embolic manifestations are characteristic of the disease. Viridans streptococci are the commonest cause of bacterial endocarditis when superimposed upon congenital or rheumatic endocardial lesions and are usually associated with a subacute course.

ETIOLOGY AND EPIDEMIOLOGY Acute bacterial endocarditis is caused by relatively pathogenic microorganisms, exemplified by *Staphylococcus aureus*, pneumococcus, group A streptococcus, and less often gonococcus, *Histoplasma capsulatum*, *Brucella*, and *Listeria*. Endocarditis attributed to these organisms usually follows dissemination from an infected focus, which is often undetectable. Endocarditis caused by staphylococci, coliform bacilli, and *Candida* has been described frequently among intravenous drug users. Infection of the heart due to staphylococci, *Candida*, *Aspergillus*, or coliform bacillus and resembling endocarditis is a rare but serious complication of surgery in which sutures or prostheses have been placed in the heart or peripheral arteries. Primarily in alcoholics, endocarditis is sometimes observed in association with pneumococcal meningitis and bacteremia (Chap. 133). Staphylococcal endocarditis can result from bacteremia associated with septic thrombophlebitis or a cutaneous, bone, or pulmonary infection. Group A streptococcal endocarditis is probably never a complication of streptococcal pharyngitis, but may follow the bacteremia of streptococcal skin or puerperal infection.

Subacute bacterial endocarditis usually develops in persons with rheumatic valvular or congenital cardiac lesions. It is most commonly caused by the viridans streptococci, which are part of the normal upper respiratory bacterial flora. *Streptococcus faecalis* (enterococcus), indigenous to the fecal and perineal flora, is an increasingly important cause of subacute bacterial endocarditis, particularly in elderly men with prostatism or women with genitourinary tract infections. *Staphylococcus aureus* may produce subacute as well as acute bacterial endocarditis. Suppuration, cellulitis, or other infected foci may precede subacute bacterial endocarditis but are recognized infrequently. Viridans streptococci are commonly found in the blood immediately after dental manipulation or extraction. Tonsillectomy and bronchoscopy are also occasionally associated with transient bacteremia. Chewing of food or use of a water jet may result in bacteremia in patients with gingival disease or dental infection. Transient bacteremia of this sort is probably an important initiating factor in subacute bacterial endocarditis.

PATHOGENESIS Subacute bacterial endocarditis occurs most frequently in persons with preexisting heart disease in the absence of congestive cardiac failure or chronic atrial fibrillation. Valvular stenosis without insufficiency is infrequently associated with bacterial endocarditis. Infection most commonly involves the left side of the heart. The mitral, aortic, tricuspid, and pulmonary valves may be involved, in the order of frequency listed. Valves damaged by rheumatic fever are most commonly involved, but valves damaged by syphilis and arteriosclerosis are also susceptible to bacterial endocarditis. Enterococcal endocarditis in elderly men is associated with involvement of the aortic valve, and frequently results in marked valvular damage. Subacute bacterial endocarditis rarely involves interatrial septal defects. Mitral valve leaflet prolapse or idiopathic hypertrophic subaortic stenosis may predispose to endocarditis. Infection in patients with interventricular septal defects often involves the endocardium opposite the septal defect in the direction of the shunt. Infection associated with patent ductus arteriosus develops on the pulmonary side of the ductus. Drug addicts frequently develop right-sided endocarditis involving the tricuspid valve. Valvular infection in association with rheumatic heart disease is usually on the valve edge along the line of closure.

Hemodynamic events are important in the pathogenesis of the disease. Alterations in blood flow can cause marked changes in vascular endothelium. It has been demonstrated experimentally that bacteria are deposited on the endothelium in areas of high flow with decreased lateral pressure. These factors are undoubtedly important in determining the situations and location where bacterial endocarditis develops. Infection in the heart is most often at a site of a structural change or abnormality. Thrombi that develop on endocardial irregularities have been implicated as foci for bacterial implantation, and it seems likely that a sterile vegetation consisting of platelets and fibrin is the nidus on which bacteria become implanted.

Serum antibodies in high titer against the infecting microorganisms are often found in patients with bacterial endocarditis. The presence of opsonizing antibodies to bacteria may facilitate localization of organisms on the endocardium during transient bacteremias. However, the role of immunity in the development of bacterial endocarditis is not known.

Infective endocarditis leads to deposition of fibrin and platelets about the site of infection, producing a vegetation. Highly pathogenic microorganisms often cause rapid valvular destruction and ulceration. Less pathogenic microorganisms usually cause less valvular destruction or ulceration but can lead to development of large polypoid vegetations. The infection may extend from the valve to the surrounding mural endocardium or penetrate the valve ring to produce a mycotic aneurysm or myocardial abscess. Involvement of chordae tendineae may lead to rupture and valvular insufficiency. Acute bacterial endocarditis, particularly when caused by *Staph. aureus*, often is associated with abscesses in the valve ring. Vascularization of involved valves may increase during endocarditis but rarely extends into the area of infection. Phagocytes are not prominent in the area of bacterial growth, which may explain why infection by microorganisms of low pathogenicity progresses uncontrolled without bactericidal antimicrobial therapy. The lack of vascularization of the granulation tissue in the vegetation also may account for ineffectiveness of host defenses and the requirement for intensive treatment.

The bacteremia of intravascular infections is ordinarily continuous. For this reason few blood cultures are required to demonstrate the microorganisms. The microorganisms are primarily cleared from the blood by the reticuloendothelial cells of liver and spleen. There is no obvious reduction in the number of bacteria in the blood during circulation through the extremities. Arterial blood cultures, therefore, are no more likely to show bacteremia than are venous blood cultures.

Embolization is a characteristic feature of infective endocarditis. The friable fibrin vegetations may separate from the site of infection and be propelled as emboli into the systemic or pulmonary circulation, depending on whether the endocarditis involves the left or right side of the heart. Emboli vary in size and most often involve the brain, spleen, kidney, gastrointestinal tract, heart, or extremities. Emboli in fungal endocarditis tend to be large and occlude major vessels. Pulmonary infarction or abscess is common in right-sided endocarditis. Septic infarction is uncommon in subacute bacterial endocarditis caused by microorganisms of low pathogenicity, and suppurative complications are rarely seen at these sites when viridans streptococci are the offending agents. Osteomyelitis has been described, however, as an embolic complication of endocarditis due to viridans streptococci and enterococci. Septic infarction is common in acute bacterial endocarditis attributable to bacteria of high pathogenicity, as are metastatic abscesses. Involvement of major arteries by emboli produces mycotic aneurysms, which may rupture. Myocardial infarction may develop after coronary embolization. In addition, focal myocarditis is common in subacute bacterial endocarditis and may be embolic.

The spleen is frequently enlarged, particularly in subacute cases. Three types of renal lesions may be produced. When large emboli find their way into the kidney, infarction may develop. Small emboli may produce a focal glomerulitis. In many instances, there is a diffuse glomerulonephritis that is indistinguishable from other types of immune complex glomerulonephritis. Petechial skin lesions, characterized histologically by acute vasculitis, are probably not embolic and may be immunologic in origin. Other skin lesions associated with pain, tenderness, and cellulitis, however, may be embolic.

MANIFESTATIONS Subacute bacterial endocarditis Patients ordinarily cannot date the onset of the infection. Symptoms begin insidiously, and gradually the illness becomes apparent. In some individuals, however, the onset of infection can be related to a recent dental extraction, urethral instrumentation, tonsillectomy, acute respiratory infection, or abortion.

Weakness, fatigability, weight loss, feverishness, night sweats, anorexia, and arthralgia are the usual symptoms of subacute bacterial endocarditis. Emboli may produce paralysis, chest pain, acute vascular insufficiency with pain in the extremities, hematuria, acute abdominal pain, or sudden blindness. Painful fingers or toes and painful skin lesions may also be important symptoms. Chills are not common.

Physical examination may reveal a variety of findings, none of which alone is pathognomonic of subacute bacterial endocarditis. The association of the different manifestations, however, usually provides a characteristic picture of the disease. The patient usually appears chronically ill and pale and has an elevated temperature. The fever is most often remittent, with afternoon or evening peaks. The pulse is usually rapid, and if cardiac failure complicates the infection, it may be greater than expected with the degree of fever.

Mucocutaneous lesions are common and vary in type. Petechiae are most frequent and may be found in the mucosa of the mouth, pharynx, or conjunctivas. These small, red, hemorrhagic-appearing lesions do not blanch on pressure and are not tender or painful. On the mucous membranes or conjunctivas these petechiae may have a pale center. Small, occasionally flame-shaped hemorrhages are found in the retina, and may also have pale centers (Roth's spots). Petechiae may be found anywhere on the skin but are most common over the upper part of the trunk anteriorly. They are frequently difficult to distinguish from angiomas, but they gradually become brownish and disappear. Frequently, petechiae continue to appear, even during convalescence. Linear hemorrhages (splinter hemorrhages) may be found under the nails, but these are difficult to differentiate from traumatic lesions, particularly in manual laborers. These mucocutaneous lesions are not specific for bacterial endocarditis but may be found in patients with other diseases such as profound anemia, leukemia, trichinosis, and sepsis without endocarditis.

The pulp of the fingers may show tender subcutaneous papules which are purplish or erythematous (Osler's nodes). Larger erythematous, painful, and tender nodules may develop on the palms of the hands or soles of the feet. These are probably embolic lesions. Emboli to larger peripheral arteries may result in gangrene of fingers, toes, or larger portions of the extremities.

Clubbing of the fingers is observed in long-standing or prolonged bacterial endocarditis. Mild jaundice is found occasionally.

Findings in the heart are usually those of underlying heart disease. Major changes in cardiac murmurs, primarily development of a new diastolic murmur, may be attributable to ulceration of a valve, dilatation of the heart or valve ring, rupture of chordae tendineae, or development of a very large vegetation. Minor changes in systolic bruits are usually of little significance. In rare instances, no cardiac murmurs are detected. In this situation, right-sided endocarditis or an infected pulmonary or peripheral arteriovenous fistula should be suspected.

Splenomegaly is common in subacute bacterial endocarditis. Rarely is the spleen tender, but a friction rub may be heard over it when there is infarction. Hepatomegaly is not characteristic unless heart failure develops.

Arthralgia is relatively common, and arthritis resembling acute rheumatic fever may occur.

Embolic phenomena may precipitate awareness of the infection. Sudden development of hemiplegia, flank pain with hematuria, abdominal pain with melena, pleuritic pain and hemoptysis, left upper abdominal pain with splenic friction rub, blindness, or monoplegia in a patient with fever and cardiac murmurs makes bacterial endocarditis suspect. Pulmonary emboli in right-sided endocarditis may be confused with pneumonia.

Acute bacterial endocarditis Infectious endocarditis caused by highly pathogenic microorganisms usually begins abruptly. Suppurative infection commonly antedates the onset of endocarditis. For example, infection of the heart may develop as a complication of pneumococcal meningitis, septic thrombophlebitis, group A streptococcal cellulitis, or staphylococcal abscesses. The source of cardiovascular infection, therefore, is often evident.

Acute bacterial endocarditis often involves the normal heart, in contrast to the subacute infection, which almost invariably involves the abnormal heart. It is particularly common in intravenous drug users. The acute infection is fulminant and pursues a rapid course. Fever is often greater, may be intermittent, and in certain instances (as in gonococcal endocarditis) may be characterized by a double quotidian temperature curve. Chills are common. Petechiae may be numerous, and embolic phenomena are prominent. Osler's nodes and painful erythematous nodules of the palms and soles are uncommon. Hematuria is seen with embolic lesions of the kidney, and diffuse glomerulonephritis may occur. Destruction of the cardiac valves can be complicated by rupture of chordae tendineae or perforation of cusps, leading to rapidly progressing cardiac failure. Metastatic abscesses are frequent following septic emboli.

Prosthetic valve endocarditis Intracardiac infection may develop about a suture or prosthesis following cardiac surgery. Symptoms and signs may be indistinguishable from those of bacterial endocarditis, but they may be sparse and consist only of fever or valve dysfunction. A change in prosthetic sounds detected by auscultation, phonocardiogram, or ultrasonogram (echocardiogram) may indicate impaired excursion of the valve due to vegetations. A postoperative regurgitant murmur, or abnormal position or movement of the valve on fluoroscopic examination may indicate partial dehiscence of the prosthesis from the valve annulus due to infection. "Nonpathogenic" organisms such as *Staph. epidermidis*, diphtheroids, and other micrococci may be cultured from blood and should not be dismissed as possible contaminants in this situation. *Staph. epidermidis, Staph. aureus*, coliform bacillus, and fungous infections tend to develop soon after surgery and are associated with a poor prognosis and a high incidence of antibiotic resistance. After the immediate postoperative period, organisms such as the viridans streptococci, enterococcus, and *Staph. epidermidis* are the usual cause of infection. These infections, occurring weeks or months after surgery, may have a better prognosis and may be controlled by antibiotics alone, although surgical removal of the foreign body may be necessary.

LABORATORY FINDINGS Leukocytosis with neutrophilia is the rule but is by no means an invariable finding. Macrophages (histiocytes) may be found in the blood, particularly in the first drop of blood obtained from the earlobe. Normocytic, normochromic anemia is almost always found in subacute bacterial endocarditis but may not be present early in acute bacterial endocarditis. The erythrocyte sedimentation rate is increased. Serum immunoglobulins are increased but return to normal during convalescence. The result of the anti-gamma-globulin latex fixation test is commonly positive, and that of the Rose-Waaler test is negative. Mild bilirubinemia is detected occasionally. Proteinuria is common, and microscopic hematuria is frequent. Serum total hemolytic complement and the third component of complement may be decreased. An ultrasonogram of the heart may demonstrate valvular vegetations.

Blood cultures are positive in the majority of cases. Three to five cultures of 10 ml of blood taken at intervals, determined by the patient's clinical status, are usually adequate to demonstrate the bacteremia, if it is demonstrable at all. Blood cultures may not become positive for several days, if at all, in patients who have received antibiotics prior to the time when cultures are obtained. Failure to demonstrate bacteremia or delayed growth in blood cultures also may be due to infection by unusual microorganisms such as *Histoplasma capsulatum, Brucella, Pasteurella, Hemophilus parainfluenzae*, or anaerobic streptococci which require special nutrient media or prolonged periods of incubation. Endocarditis of the right side of the heart is as likely to produce bacteremia as endocarditis involving the left side of the heart. Aspergillus endocarditis is seldom associated with positive blood cultures. *Coxiella burnetii* endocarditis is diagnosed by serologic tests, since blood cultures are always negative.

DIFFERENTIAL DIAGNOSIS When several of the manifestations of infective endocarditis occur together, the diagnosis is not difficult. In particular, the presence of fever, petechiae, splenomegaly, microscopic hematuria, and anemia in a patient with cardiac murmurs is most suggestive of infection. When only a few manifestations are present, however, the diagnosis is not simple. Prolonged fever in a patient with rheumatic heart disease is particularly troublesome, but the diagnosis of bacterial endocarditis should be considered in every patient with fever and a heart murmur. The diagnosis becomes even more difficult when blood cultures show no growth.

Acute rheumatic fever with carditis is often difficult to distinguish from bacterial endocarditis, and in a few instances, active rheumatic fever has been found to coexist with the valvular infection. The diagnosis of rheumatic carditis hinges on a combination of clinical and laboratory criteria (Chap. 242).

Subacute bacterial endocarditis is a common cause of "fever of undetermined origin" (Chap. 12). It may be mistaken for a hidden neoplasm, systemic lupus erythematosus, periarteritis nodosa, poststreptococcal glomerulonephritis, and intracardiac tumors such as myxoma of the atrium. Dissecting aneurysms with acute aortic regurgitation also may mimic bacterial endocarditis. Drug fever may be erroneously diagnosed as bacterial endocarditis. Postoperative endocarditis should be suspected in patients who develop fever, anemia, and leukocytosis after cardiovascular surgery. In these postoperative patients, the various postthoracotomy and postcardiotomy syndromes must also be considered.

PROGNOSIS Recovery from untreated bacterial endocarditis is rare. With appropriate antibiotic therapy, however, over 70 percent of the patients survive the infection. Intravenous drug users with right-sided staphylococcal endocarditis generally have a good prognosis. The infection has a poor prognosis under the following circumstances: (1) when congestive heart failure is present; (2) when bacteremia is not demonstrable; (3) when the organisms are resistant to multiple antimicrobials; (4) when therapy is delayed; (5) when infection develops on a prosthetic valve. Prosthetic valve, gram-negative bacillus, fungal and acute bacterial types of endocarditis are associated with the poorest prognosis.

The commonest cause of death in treated endocarditis is congestive heart failure, attributable either to valve destruction or to myocardial damage. Additionally, death may be precipitated by embolization to vital organs, by renal insufficiency, by rupture of a mycotic aneurysm, or by complications following cardiac surgery. Many patients recover completely without apparent worsening of the underlying cardiovascular disease. When recurrent endocarditis develops, it usually involves the same valve and is due to failure to kill microorganisms in an environment of suboptimal host resistance.

Further reduction in the mortality rate of infective endocarditis will depend primarily on the increased use of cardiac surgery in combination with antimicrobial therapy to eliminate refractory infections, and the early replacement of damaged valves in patients with congestive heart failure.

PROPHYLAXIS Patients with suspected congenital or acquired valvular heart disease should be given antibiotics immediately before dental manipulation, obstetric delivery, urethral catheterization, or other forms of intubation. The rationale for this practice is that when these patients develop bacteremia, they are more likely to develop endocarditis. The best experimental evidence available holds that for prevention of endocarditis caused by viridans streptococci with penicillin, both a high concentration and prolonged duration of action are necessary. It has been shown that penicillin and streptomycin act synergistically in killing viridans streptococci. These data suggest that the best practical regimen is a single dose of 1.2 million units of aqueous procaine penicillin administered with 1 g streptomycin within 30 min of dental surgery. A loading dose of 2 g penicillin V followed by 0.5 g of the drug at 6-h intervals for 48 h is probably equally effective. Patients who are allergic to penicillin should receive 2 g cefazolin plus 1 g streptomycin intramuscularly or 1 g vancomycin intravenously. The best regimen for preventing enterococcal endocarditis is ampicillin plus gentamicin. No firm dosage schedules have been established, but 2 g ampicillin followed by 0.5 g every 6 h plus 3 to 5 mg per kg gentamicin in three divided doses for a total of 48 h given simultaneously should be adequate. *The prophylactic doses of penicillin used to prevent group A streptococcal infection and recurrent rheumatic fever will not prevent bacterial endocarditis*, although these doses of penicillin (200,000 units once or twice daily) rarely predispose to bacterial endocarditis caused by penicillin-resistant microorganisms.

TREATMENT Successful therapy of bacterial endocarditis is ensured when treatment is begun early in the illness, when an effective *bactericidal* antimicrobial is selected, and when treatment is continued over a relatively long period of time.

Selection of the most effective antibiotic for treatment of bacterial endocarditis depends on the sensitivity of the infecting microorganism. When bacteremia is not demonstrated, selection of the therapeutic agent depends on understanding the probable infecting bacteria and their probable antibiotic sensitivity.

Bacterial endocarditis in young persons with rheumatic or congenital disease is most often due to the viridans streptococci. These microorganisms are usually very sensitive to penicillin G. Administration of 2.4 to 6 million units of penicillin daily to these patients is usually effective in eliminating the infection when therapy is continued for 4 weeks. The penicillin should be given parenterally for 2 weeks, but for the second 2 weeks may be oral (phenethicillin or V-cillin). There is a synergistic effect of streptomycin with penicillin on *Strep. viridans*, and streptomycin in a dose of 0.5 g twice a day may be administered in addition to penicillin. Streptomycin should be given for no longer than 2 weeks.

Bacterial endocarditis in older men and women after abortion or endometritis is often due to *Strep. faecalis* (enterococci). These microorganisms are relatively resistant to penicillin alone. The combination of penicillin with gentamicin is synergistic against these bacteria, however, and administration of these two antibiotics together is the treatment of choice in the infection. Penicillin G should be given parenterally in a dose of 12 to 24 million units a day, together with gentamicin in a dose of 3 to 5 mg per kg a day divided into three doses. Ampicillin in dosage of 6 to 12 g per day may be substituted for penicillin G. Treatment must be continued for a minimum of 4 weeks.

Penicillin G, 6 to 12 million units a day given parenterally, is satisfactory for treatment of pneumococcal and group A streptococcal endocarditis. Treatment should be continued for 4 weeks. Penicillinase-resistant penicillin analogues should be used in the initial treatment of staphylococcal endocarditis, because of the possibility that the infection is due to a penicillin-resistant organism. Methicillin should be given intravenously in a dose of 12 g per day in divided doses in 50-ml volumes injected over 20 to 30 min. Oxacillin, nafcillin, cephalothin, cefazolin, and vancomycin may be administered in lieu of methicillin. If the staphylococcus is found to be sensitive to penicillin G, this antibiotic should be given rather than methicillin, in a dose of 16 to 24 million units per day. Treatment should be continued for at least 4 weeks. In staphylococcal endocarditis, in particular, attention must be given to possible metastatic abscesses requiring surgical drainage.

In patients allergic to penicillin, cephalothin, cefazolin, and vancomycin are alternative drugs. If an allergic reaction to penicillin develops during the course of therapy, antihistamines or corticosteroids may be used to alleviate the manifestations of the reaction.

Usually fever begins to disappear within 3 to 7 days after the start of treatment of bacterial endocarditis. Embolic complications of the disease, heart failure, and infection by insusceptible microorganisms, however, may delay defervescence. Drug fever may occasionally supervene and complicate the febrile course. Cessation of all therapy for 72 h is not hazardous and may identify such a drug reaction readily. Sterile emboli or late valve rupture occasionally occurs up to 12 months after cessation of therapy.

Some patients with arteriovenous fistulas, endocarditis produced by resistant organisms, and infected cardiac prostheses may require surgical intervention before the infection can be controlled. In addition, early valve replacement should be considered in patients who develop marked valvular damage (particularly aortic or mitral regurgitation) as a consequence of bacterial endocarditis. Valve replacement has been lifesaving and must be effected before intractable heart failure ensues.

Fungal endocarditis is usually fatal. However, a few survivors have been reported after surgical debridement or replacement of the infected valve combined with amphotericin B therapy.

When bacterial endocarditis recurs, it usually develops within 4 weeks after treatment is terminated. Reinstitution of antibiotic therapy will be required, but the sensitivity of the microorganism to the antibiotic must be reevaluated. Relapse may indicate inadequate or inappropriate therapy.

If bacterial endocarditis develops more than 6 weeks after cessation of treatment, it usually is a new infection.

REFERENCES

CHERUBIN CD, NEU HC: Infective endocarditis at the Presbyterian Hospital in New York City from 1938–1967. Am J Med 51:83, 1971

GOODMAN JS et al: Infection after cardiovascular surgery: Clinical study including examination of antimicrobial prophylaxis. N. Engl J Med 278:117, 1968

GUTMAN RA et al: The immune complex glomerulonephritis of bacterial endocarditis. Medicine 51:1, 1972

HOOK EW, KAYE D: Prophylaxis of bacterial endocarditis. J Chronic Dis 15:635, 1962

KERR AJ JR: *Subacute Bacterial Endocarditis*, Springfield, Ill.: Charles C Thomas, 1955

LERNER PI, WEINSTEIN L: Infective endocarditis in the antibiotic era. N Engl J Med 274:199, 1966

——: Infective endocarditis: A review of selected topics. Med Clin North Am 58:605, 1974

MENDA KB, GORBACH SL: Favorable experience with bacterial endocarditis in heroin addicts. Ann Intern Med 78:25, 1973

REYES MP et al: *Pseudomonas* endocarditis in the Detroit Medical Center 1969–72. Medicine 52:173, 1973

SLAUGHTER L et al: Prosthetic valvular endocarditis. Circulation 47:1319, 1973

WILSON WR et al: Prosthetic valve endocarditis. Ann Intern Med 82:751, 1975

section 3 | Diseases caused by gram-positive cocci

133 PNEUMOCOCCAL INFECTIONS

ROBERT AUSTRIAN

ETIOLOGY The pneumococcus is a gram-positive encapsulated coccus that usually grows in pairs or short chains. In the diplococcal form, the adjacent margins are rounded and the opposite ends slightly pointed, giving the organisms a "lancet" shape. In stained preparations of exudate, gram-negative forms are sometimes present. Because pneumococci produce greenish discoloration of blood agar, they are sometimes confused with alpha-hemolytic streptococci, to which they are closely related. The two organisms can be distinguished by the bile solubility and mouse virulence of the pneumococcus or by serologic typing. Another method, utilizing inhibition of pneumococci by Optochin-impregnated paper disks, is less cumbersome and very effective, but standard zones of inhibition determined for aerobic cultures cannot be applied to cultures grown under 5 percent carbon dioxide for the identification of pneumococcus.

The capsular substances are complex polysaccharides and are the basis for dividing pneumococci into serotypes. Organisms exposed to type-specific antiserum show a positive capsular precipitin reaction, the *Neufeld quellung reaction;* by this means, 84 serotypes have been identified. All are pathogenic for human beings, but types 1, 3, 4, 7, 8, and 12 are encountered most frequently in clinical practice. Types 6, 14, 19, and 23 often cause pneumonia in children but are less common in adults.

Specific typing of pneumococci remains of great clinical importance if pneumococcus is to be identified with regularity, but has been largely abandoned since the introduction of sulfonamides and antibiotics which are effective against pneumococci of all types. Recognition of pneumococcus has decreased significantly since the abandonment of pneumococcal typing by many clinical laboratories.

EPIDEMIOLOGY Pneumococci are normal inhabitants of the human upper respiratory tract in 5 to 60 percent of the population, depending upon the season. Pneumococcal infection occurs predominantly during the winter and early spring; the ratio of infection in males and females is 3:2, and morbidity and mortality are higher for blacks than whites. Person-to-person transmission by droplets is undoubtedly common, but true epidemics of pneumococcal pneumonia are rare, even in closed populations. Patients with pneumococcal infection need not be isolated because the risk of cross infection is relatively small, but they should not be placed close to patients with other respiratory or cardiac disease.

PATHOGENESIS The mechanism by which pneumococci damage tissue is obscure. It is conceivable that toxic substances may be elaborated, but no such toxin has been demonstrated. The capsular substances, though nontoxic, are known to be necessary factors in virulence, and protect the organism to a certain extent from engulfment by phagocytes.

Invasion of the tissues of the nasopharynx rarely, if ever, occurs, and "pneumococcal pharyngitis" is a doubtful entity. The organisms multiply readily in vivo, however, and may produce acute inflammation in the lungs, serous cavities, and endocardium.

The normal human respiratory tract is provided with a variety of mechanisms which act to guard the lungs from infection. The lower respiratory tract is protected by the glottis and larynx, and material passing these barriers stimulates the expulsive cough reflex. Removal of small particles impinging on the walls of the trachea and bronchi is facilitated by their mucociliary lining; and growth of bacteria reaching normal alveoli is inhibited by their relative dryness and by the phagocytic activity of alveolar macrophages. Any anatomic or physiologic derangement of these coordinated defenses tends to augment the susceptibility of the lungs to infection. Anesthesia, alcoholic intoxication, convulsions, and disturbed innervation of the larynx depress the cough reflex and may permit aspiration of infected material. Alterations in the tracheobronchial tree leading to anatomic changes in the epithelial lining or to localized obstruction increase the vulnerability of the lungs to infection. Pulmonary edema, local or generalized, resulting from viral infection, inhalation of irritant gases, cardiac failure, or contusion of the chest wall, provides a fluid menstruum in the alveoli for the growth of bacteria and their spread to adjacent areas of the lung. Viral infection of the respiratory epithelium with concomitant disruption of its component cells interferes significantly with the clearance of bacteria from the lungs, an observation in accord with the high incidence of pneumococcal pneumonia during epidemics of viral influenza and its frequent clinical association with sporadic viral respiratory infections.

Pneumonia begins usually in the right lower, right middle, or left lower lobe, those areas to which gravity is most likely to carry upper respiratory secretions aspirated during sleep. Bronchial embolization with infected mucinous secretions during the course of an upper respiratory infection appears to be the initiating factor in many cases of pneumococcal pneumonia. Protected initially from phagocytosis by mucinous material, the bacteria multiply and, in infected alveoli, evoke the outpouring of proteinaceous fluid which serves both as a nutrient and as a vehicle for spread to adjacent alveoli. Soon thereafter, polymorphonuclear leukocytes migrate from the pneumococcal population before the appearance of detectable antibody. Delay in the polymorphonuclear leukocytic response occurs during alcoholic intoxication and certain forms of anesthesia, permitting spread of infection. Adrenocortical steroids and their congeners may also interfere with leukocyte migration. Later, as the pneumonic lesion evolves, macrophages appear in the exudate and remove the debris of fibrin and cells. It is probable that antibody to the capsular polysaccharide of the invading pneumococcus makes its appearance locally in the lung before being detectable in the circulation. Such antibody increases the efficiency of phagocytosis approximately twofold and causes agglutination of the organisms and their adherence to alveolar walls, thereby slowing their dissemination in the lung. The outcome of infection depends, therefore, on the rate at which bacteria can multiply in the edema fluid and spread, and on the host's ability to immobilize and destroy them by phagocytosis. Individuals with hypogammaglobulinemia and patients with multiple myeloma incapable of producing anticapsular antibody are liable to recurrent attacks of pneumococcal pneumonia. Repeated infection with the same pneumococcal type should always prompt a search for dysgammaglobulinemia.

Failure of local defense mechanisms in the lung results in lymphatic spread of pneumococci to the hilar lymph nodes. In the sinusoids of these organs, a sequence of events not unlike that in the lung ensues. If infection is not checked in this secondary line of defense, organisms find their way into the thoracic duct and then into the circulation. Although transient bacteremia may occur at the onset of many cases of pneumococcal pneumonia, it is detectable in only 25 to 30 percent of cases. Bacteremia, which reflects the body's inability to localize the pulmonary infection, is a poor prognostic sign and carries with it the danger of metastatic infection. The mortality of treated or untreated bacteremic pneumococcal pneumonia is four times that resulting from comparably managed nonbacteremic infections. Metastatic infection secondary to bacteremia may occur in the meninges, joints, or peritoneum or on the endocardium. Direct spread from the infected lung may give rise to pleural empyema or to pericarditis.

Natural recovery from pneumococcal infection coincides usually, but not invariably, with the appearance of detectable type-specific antibody in the circulation and is often accompanied by a dramatic and abrupt fall in temperature, the so-called "crisis." Antibody aids recovery by increasing the efficiency of phagocytosis and by limiting dissemination of the organisms. Bacteriostatic drugs, such as sulfonamides, facilitate control of the infection by limiting the size of the pneumococcal population, but the host's defense mechanisms are still required for the elimination of the bacteria. Bactericidal agents, such as penicillin, cause the death of pneumococci in the lung and are effective when some of the host's defense mechanisms are compromised. With the arrest of infection, the alveolar exudate undergoes liquefaction, the inflammatory debris is removed by expectoration and via the lymphatic channels, and the lung is restored to its normal state. Necrosis of pulmonary tissue as a result of pneumococcal infection is distinctly uncommon. Primary pneumococcal lung abscess is a rare clinical entity, although the diagnosis is mistakenly made at times when pneumococcal infection complicates lung abscess of other origins.

In addition to causing pneumonia and its metastatic sequelae, pneumococcus can extend from the nasopharynx to its adjacent structures, giving rise to otitis media, mastoiditis, paranasal sinusitis, or conjunctivitis. Soft-tissue abscesses are rare but may occur.

PNEUMOCOCCAL PNEUMONIA

Pneumococcal pneumonia is a disease remarkable for its uniformity, in contrast to other infections such as typhoid fever and tuberculosis. The diseases produced by different pneumococcal serotypes show little variation in severity or in clinical manifestations. The prognosis in type 3 pneumococcal pneumonia is usually regarded as poor, probably because type 3 infections occur frequently in the aged and in patients with other debilitating diseases such as diabetes and congestive heart failure. The usual lesion in adults is segmental or lobar in distribution, but in children and the aged, bronchopneumonia, characterized by patchy involvement, is frequent.

MANIFESTATIONS Pneumonia is often preceded for a few days by coryza or some other form of common respiratory disease. The onset is usually so abrupt that patients frequently can state the exact hour that illness began. There is a sudden *shaking chill* in more than 80 percent of the cases and a rapid rise in temperature, with corresponding tachycardia and an increase in respiratory rate (tachypnea).

Most patients with pneumococcal pneumonia have a single rigor unless antipyretic drugs are administered, and repeated chills should suggest another etiologic agent.

About 75 percent of patients develop severe *pleuritic pain* and *cough,* productive of pinkish or "rusty" mucoid sputum within a few hours. The chest pain is agonizing, and respirations become rapid, shallow, and grunting as the patient tries to splint the affected side. Many patients are mildly cyanotic as a result of reduced alveolar ventilation, which accompanies altered respiration, and show dilatation of the alae nasi when first seen. Patients appear acutely ill; but nausea, headache, and malaise are not prominent, and most individuals are alert. Pleuritic pain and dyspnea are the dominant complaints.

In the untreated disease, there are sustained fever of 102.5 to 105°F, continued pleuritic pain, cough, and expectoration; and *abdominal distention* is frequent. *Herpes labialis* is a common complication. After 7 to 10 days, there are diaphoresis, abrupt defervescence, and dramatic improvement in well-being, the "crisis."

In cases which terminate fatally, there is usually extensive pulmonary involvement, and dyspnea, cyanosis, and tachycardia are prominent. Circulatory collapse or a picture resembling heart failure is common. Death in a few patients is associated with empyema or some other suppurative complication such as meningitis or endocarditis.

Physical examination reveals restricted motion of the affected hemithorax. Tactile fremitus may be decreased during the initial day of illness but is usually increased when consolidation is fully established. Deviation of the trachea away from the affected lung suggests pleural effusion or empyema. The percussion note is dull, and if the lesion is in an upper lobe, impaired motion of the diaphragm can be detected on the affected side. Very early in the course of infection, breath sounds are diminished, but as the lesion evolves, they become tubular or bronchial in quality, and bronchophony and whispered pectoriloquy can be elicited. These findings are accompanied by fine crepitant rales.

EFFECT OF SPECIFIC CHEMOTHERAPY Pneumococcal pneumonia usually improves promptly when an appropriate antimicrobial drug is given. Within 12 to 36 h after initiation of treatment with penicillin, temperature, pulse, and respiration begin to fall and may reach normal values, pleuritic pain subsides, and the spread of the inflammatory process is halted. The temperature of approximately half the patients, however, requires 4 days or longer to become normal, and failure of the patient's temperature to reach normal in 24 to 48 h should not prompt a change in antibacterial therapy in the absence of other indications.

COMPLICATIONS The typical course of pneumococcal pneumonia can be modified by the development of one or more local or distant complications:

In the lung ATELECTASIS Atelectasis of all or part of a lobe may occur during the active stage of pneumonia or after treatment has been instituted. The patient may complain of sudden recurrence of pleuritic pain and show rapid respirations. Small areas of atelectasis are often detected by x-ray in the absence of symptoms. These areas usually clear with coughing and deep breathing, but bronchoscopic aspiration is occasionally necessary. If atelectasis is allowed to persist, the affected area becomes fibrotic and functionless.

DELAYED RESOLUTION The removal of exudate from the lung following pneumococcal infection is usually complete within 2 to 3 weeks, at which time the x-ray of the chest appears normal; but occasionally, especially in elderly individuals and in alcoholics, consolidation persists for longer periods. Sometimes the involved area never becomes reaerated, and fibrosis results.

ABSCESS Lung abscess is a rare sequel to pneumococcal infection, although pneumococcal pneumonia is a not uncommon complication of lung abscess of other origins. It is manifested by continued fever and profuse expectoration of purulent sputum. X-ray shows one or more cavities. This complication is exceedingly rare in patients who receive penicillin therapy and is most likely to follow infection with pneumococcus type 3.

In adjacent structures PLEURAL EFFUSION Pleural effusion occurs in about 5 percent of patients with pneumococcal pneumonia, even with specific therapy. The amount of fluid is usually not sufficient to cause obvious displacement of mediastinal structures. Usually the effusion is sterile and is reabsorbed spontaneously within a week or two. Sometimes, however, the effusion is large and requires aspiration.

EMPYEMA Prior to the introduction of effective chemotherapy, empyema occurred in 5 to 8 percent of patients with pneumococcal pneumonia; it is now observed in less than 1 percent of treated cases. It is manifested by persistent fever or pleuritic pain, together with signs of pleural effusion. In the early stages, the gross appearance of infected fluid may not differ from that of a sterile pleural effusion; later, there is a profuse outpouring of polymorphonuclear leukocytes and fibrin, resulting in an exudate of thick greenish pus containing large clots of fibrin. The quantity of exudate may become large enough to displace mediastinal structures. In neglected cases, this process leads to extensive pleural scarring, with limitation of thoracic movement. Rupture and drainage through the chest wall *(empyema necessitatis)* occurs but is rare. Metastatic *brain abscess* is an occasional complication of chronic empyema.

PERICARDITIS A particularly serious complication is spread of infection to the pericardial sac. This lesion is characterized by pain in the precordial region, a friction rub synchronous with the heartbeat, and distention of cervical veins, although one or all of these findings may be absent. The possibility of coexisting purulent pericarditis should be considered whenever a very ill patient with pneumonia develops empyema.

Metastatic infections *Arthritis* occurs more often in children than in adults. The affected joint is swollen, red, and painful, with a purulent effusion. It usually subsides promptly with systemic administration of penicillin, although aspiration and intraarticular injection of penicillin may be necessary in adults.

Acute bacterial endocarditis complicates pneumococcal

pneumonia in fewer than 0.5 percent of cases. Its manifestations and treatment are discussed below. *Meningitis,* another complication of pneumococcal pneumonia, is also discussed subsequently.

Paralytic ileus Gaseous abdominal distention is commonly present and in severely ill patients may assume such serious proportions that the term *paralytic ileus* is justified. This complication further impairs respiratory movement by elevation of the diaphragm and constitutes a difficult problem in management. A rarer and more serious gastrointestinal complication is acute gastric dilatation.

Impaired liver function Alterations in liver function are very common during the course of pneumococcal pneumonia, and mild jaundice is not at all rare. The pathogenesis of the jaundice is not entirely clear.

LABORATORY FINDINGS *X-ray of the chest* reveals a homogeneous density in the affected area of lung. In well-established cases, the density may occupy one or more entire lobes. The white blood count usually shows a polymorphonuclear *leukocytosis* ranging from 12,000 to 25, 000 cells per mm^3. A normal leukocyte count or leukopenia is sometimes observed in patients with overwhelming infection and bacteremia, in the aged, and in alcoholics. The *blood culture* is positive for pneumococci during the first 3 or 4 days of untreated illness in 20 to 25 percent of cases. The *sputum,* when stained by Gram's method, shows polymorphonuclear leukocytes and variable numbers of gram-positive cocci, singly and in pairs. These can be typed directly, by the Neufeld quellung or capsular precipitin reaction technique, and this procedure should be employed to facilitate diagnosis whenever possible. Occasionally, pneumococci may be seen directly in granulocytes in patients with bacteremia by examining the buffy coat after staining with Wright's stain. These patients often have asplenia.

DIFFERENTIAL DIAGNOSIS OF PNEUMONIA Fever, cough, and pulmonary consolidation form a symptom complex that can be produced by many diseases of infectious, toxic, or other origin.

Staphylococcal pneumonia (Chap. 134) is encountered most often in infants, in adults during an epidemic of influenza, and in debilitated individuals as a nosocomial infection. The clinical picture is less uniform than that of pneumococcal pneumonia. Multiple chills, early formation of lung abscess or pneumatoceles, and empyema suggest the diagnosis. Stained smears of sputum contain myriad staphylococci.

Hemolytic streptococcal pneumonia (Chap. 135) may occur in association with influenza or measles or following streptococcal sore throat. Toxemia is often profound, and empyema is a common complication. The diagnosis is confirmed by cultures of sputum, blood, and pleural fluid.

Friedländer's (Klebsiella) pneumonia (Chap. 138) is commonest in adults, and about half such infections occur in alcoholics. Sputum is tenacious and contains large numbers of gram-negative bacilli. Recovery may be accompanied by residual pulmonary scarring and cavitation, and relapses are not uncommon.

Tularemia (Chap. 145) is often accompanied by pulmonary lesions of varying clinical prominence. A cutaneous

lesion or a history of contact with the vectors of the disease assist in making the diagnosis.

Other bacterial pneumonias: Other bacteria can produce pneumonia. Pneumonia caused by enterobacteria *(Escherichia coli, Proteus* species, *Pseudomonas)* occurs usually in the debilitated and aged, in alcoholics, in those with deranged defenses against infection, and following the administration of antimicrobials (Chap. 128). Of infections caused by salmonellas, those with *Salmonella chloraesuis* are most often complicated by pneumonia. *Bacteroides* species may give rise to necrotizing pneumonia (Chap. 159). *Hemophilus influenzae* is a common cause of pulmonary infection in children and may be an occasional cause of pneumonia in adults (Chap. 142). Pulmonary lesions occur in melioidosis (Chap. 147) and predominate in pneumonic plague (Chap. 146).

Mycoplasma pneumoniae infection (Chap. 188) is usually more insidious in onset than bacterial pneumonia and affects primarily children and young adults. It is rarely fatal.

Viral pneumonias (Chaps. 194, 195) may result from infection with a variety of agents including myxoviruses, respiratory syncytial virus, adenoviruses, rhinoviruses, Coxsackie, echo, and rheoviruses, and the viruses of measles and varicella. Although many of the illnesses are mild and resemble that caused by *Mycoplasma pneumoniae,* occasional infections caused by influenza virus may be difficult to distinguish from bacterial pneumonia. Secondary bacterial pneumonia may complicate viral pneumonia, especially in influenza and measles.

Psittacosis (ornithosis) (Chap. 191) may follow contact with an infected avian species.

Differential diagnosis of *Q fever* is discussed in Chap. 186.

Acute tuberculous pneumonia (Chap. 161) may be difficult to recognize because tubercle bacilli may not be demonstrable in the sputum early in the disease. Many patients with tuberculous pneumonia feel surprisingly well, despite consolidation of an entire lobe. *Pleurisy with effusion* is seldom abrupt on onset, cough (when present) is nonproductive, and the physical and x-ray findings are those of pleural fluid rather than of consolidation.

Mycotic infections: Histoplasmosis (Chap. 173), blastomycosis (Chap. 171), and coccidioidomycosis (Chap. 172) may present initially as acute pneumonic processes. Infections with actinomycetes (Chap. 169) are more likely to be confused with tuberculosis or lung tumor.

Lung abscess (Chap. 259) may have an abrupt onset resembling that of pneumonia. A history of epilepsy, alcoholic intoxication, tonsillectomy, or aspiration of a foreign body suggests the diagnosis. The development of cavitation accompanied by expectoration of large amounts of foul-smelling sputum makes the diagnosis clear. Pneumococcal pneumonia at the site of the lesion may complicate the illness at any stage prior to treatment.

Atelectasis (Chap. 259) may occur in bedridden patients or following surgery when respiratory motion is limited and when the cough reflex is depressed. Infection of the collapsed pulmonary segment may lead to pneumonia. Diagnosis is facilitated when the mediastinum is shifted toward the affected side.

Neoplasms are considered in Chap. 263.

Pulmonary adenomatosis (Chap. 263) is an uncommon neoplasm that may at first be mistaken for bacterial pneumonia.

Pulmonary infarction (Chap. 266) is especially frequent in patients with congestive heart failure and surgical procedures. It may be asymptomatic or may present many of the features of pneumonia, though true chills are rare. Septic pulmonary infarcts may be complicated by abscess and cavitation and, in women, suggest the diagnosis of septic abortion or puerperal sepsis.

Other points in differential diagnosis Pulmonary infiltrates may be seen in the lungs of patients with *uremia* and of those with *acute pulmonary edema* and *heart failure.*

The inhalation of noxious materials, irritants, allergenic substances, or lipids can lead to pulmonary infiltrates and clinical symptoms that may at times be mistaken for bacterial pneumonia. The diagnosis rests on an accurate history of occupation, habits, and exposure.

Pneumonitis may occur as a feature of erythema multiforme, lupus erythematosus, rheumatic fever, vasculitis, or intestinal helminthiasis. Infectious mononucleosis and lymphocytic choriomeningitis are sometimes accompanied by pulmonary infiltrations. Pulmonary lesions of viral origin occur in a small proportion of patients with smallpox, chickenpox, or measles. Rupture of an amebic liver abscess into the pleural cavity can be mistaken for acute pneumonia; and, in a patient with estivoautumnal malaria, blockage of pulmonary capillaries by parasites can lead to confusion with respiratory infection.

EXTRAPULMONARY PNEUMOCOCCAL INFECTION

Pneumococcal meningitis The pneumococcus is second only to the meningococcus as a cause of purulent meningitis in adults; in children, meningitis caused by *H. influenzae* is also more frequent than pneumococcal infection.

Pneumococcal meningitis can develop as a "primary" disease without preceding signs of infection elsewhere; as a complication of pneumococcal pneumonia; by extension from otitis, mastoiditis, or sinusitis; or following a skull fracture which creates an opening between the subarachnoid space and the nasal cavity or paranasal sinuses. Patients with pneumococcal endocarditis frequently develop meningeal infection. Patients with multiple myeloma and with sickle-cell disease seem to be liable to pneumococcal infection of the meninges, just as they are to pneumonia.

The *manifestations* are of those of any acute pyogenic meningitis (Chap. 337) and include chills, fever, headache, nuchal rigidity, Kernig's and Brudzinski's signs, delirium, and cranial nerve palsies. Evidence of otitis, sinusitis, or pneumonia should be carefully sought by physical and roentgenographic examination in all patients.

The *spinal fluid* is under increased pressure, appears cloudy, often with a greenish tint, and shows a high protein and low glucose content. Stained smears usually reveal gram-positive diplococci and polymorphonuclear leukocytes; in some patients, the number of cells in the spinal fluid is surprisingly small, and much of the cloudiness is produced by the bacterial content. The diagnosis can be established rapidly by identification of pneumococci in the spinal fluid by Gram's stain and by direct typing with the Neufeld quellung reaction.

With appropriate chemotherapy, recovery can be expected in 70 percent of cases; the prognosis is better in children than in infants or in adults. Relapse may occur but is unusual if adequate treatment is carried out. Subarachnoid block, the result of accumulation of large amounts of thick exudate in the meningeal space and at the base of the brain, is now an unusual complication.

Pneumococcal endocarditis Endocarditis is usually a complication of pneumonia or meningitis. The clinical picture is that of acute bacterial endocarditis (Chap. 132), with remittent fever, splenomegaly, and metastatic infection of the lungs, meninges, joints, eye, and other tissues. Petechiae are uncommon. The infection can attack normal valves and is particularly likely to occur in the aortic valve. The valvular infection is destructive, and loud murmurs and heart failure develop rapidly. Rupture or perforation of cusps or even rupture of the aorta may occur. The blood culture is consistently positive for the pneumococcus in the absence of treatment with antimicrobial drugs; yet at the same time antibodies to the infecting organism may be demonstrable in the blood, a combination of findings seldom observed except in endocarditis or brucellosis. Although the infection is relatively easy to cure with penicillin, damage to valve leaflets, especially to the cusps of the aortic valve, may be followed by rapidly progressive heart failure. Surgical repair or replacement of damaged valvular structures should be carried out early, before heart failure becomes intractable.

Pneumococcal peritonitis Pneumococcal peritonitis is a rare disease which occurs in young girls; presumably the vagina and fallopian tubes are the portal of entry. Symptoms are fever, pain, abdominal distention, vomiting, and accumulation of peritoneal fluid. The diagnosis is made by examination of the purulent ascitic fluid; blood cultures are often positive, and a polymorphonuclear leukocytosis is the rule. In adults, the disease may occur in association with cirrhosis or with carcinoma of the liver. Peritonitis used to be a common complication of the nephrotic syndrome, particularly in children, but is rare nowadays.

TREATMENT Specific antimicrobial therapy Penicillin G (benzyl penicillin) is the drug of choice for all manifestations of pneumococcal infection. Although mutants of pneumococcus resistant to this drug can be selected in the laboratory, evidence that they may occur in the respiratory flora of human beings has been lacking until recently. Strains of pneumococcus manifesting a modest increase in resistance to penicillin have now been recovered infrequently from humans; and although the level of such resistance does not preclude treatment with this antibiotic, awareness of the phenomenon is necessary. The minimum curative dose for *pneumonia* caused by strains of usual sensitivity to penicillin G is less than 60,000 units daily, and a total dose of 600,000 units daily provides a good margin of safety for bacteremic and nonbacteremic pulmonary infection in adults in the absence of an extrapulmonary focus. Treatment may be administered at 12-h intervals in doses of 300,000 units aqueous crystalline penicillin G or procaine penicillin. Therapy should be continued until the patient has been afebrile for 48 to 72 h. The response is usually dramatic, and relapse is extremely uncommon. Pneumococcal pneumonia can be treated adequately with oral penicillin, preferably one of the drugs resistant to gastric acid (Chap. 130), in dosage of 1.2 to 2.4 million units daily. *Peritonitis* usually responds within 36 to 48 h to 2 to 4 million units of penicillin daily.

Pneumococcal *meningitis* should be treated with 12 to 20 million units aqueous penicillin G daily intravenously in adults. In many clinics, even larger amounts are used, though care must be taken to avoid neurotoxicity from excessive dosage. Intrathecal administration of penicillin is not necessary. The addition of sulfadiazine to this regimen affords no advantage, and supplementary administration of chlortetracycline (and presumably, of other broad-spectrum drugs) may exert a deleterious effect. In the presence of sinusitis, otitis, or mastoiditis, surgical drainage should be carried out as soon as is feasible. The response of meningitis is usually less dramatic than that of pneumonia; patients often remain febrile and disoriented, and signs of meningeal irritation may persist for several days, but improvement becomes gradually evident with continued treatment.

Large doses are required in pneumococcal endocarditis also—12 to 20 million units daily by intravenous injection. Rapidly developing heart failure in these patients and the tendency to form myocardial abscess, however, often lead to a fatal outcome despite large doses of antibiotics. Surgical repair or replacement of damaged heart valves should be considered when cardiac failure develops.

Cephalosporins in parenteral doses of 1 to 2 g daily are effective in pneumoccal pneumonia but must be administered with caution to those hypersensitive to penicillin. These drugs should not be used in the treatment of pneumococcal meningitis because of their poor ability to penetrate the blood-cerebrospinal fluid barrier. The *tetracyclines* in doses of 1 to 2 g daily, *erythromycin* in doses of 1.6 g daily, or *lincomycin* in doses of 1.2 g daily are effective treatment for pneumococcal pneumonia but are recommended only for patients who have had untoward reactions to penicillins or cephalosporins. Mutants of pneumococcus resistant to each of these antibiotics have been isolated from humans; if one of these drugs is to be employed, it is essential to ascertain that the organism is sensitive to it. Despite its efficacy, chloramphenicol should not be used to treat pneumococcal infections other than meningitis in the patient hypersensitive to penicillin. *Sulfonamides* have little place in the present-day treatment of pneumonia and are useless in endocarditis and meningitis. Aminoglycosides, such as gentamicin, kanamycin, and streptomycin, should not be employed to treat pneumococcal infections.

Pneumococcal arthritis responds to systemic penicillin, but aspiration and intraarticular instillation of the drug may be necessary.

Empyema should be detected and treated as early as possible. When an effusion is found, the fluid should be examined for organisms; and if they are present, 50,000 to 200,000 units of penicillin G should be injected intrapleurally. In addition the same antibiotic should be administered systemically in doses of 6 to 8 million units a day. Aspiration of fluid and instillation of penicillin should be carried out at 1- to 2-day intervals until cultures are persistently negative and fever disappears. Fluoroscopic guidance may be needed for aspiration of small empyema pockets. If the exudate is especially thick or viscid, streptokinase-streptodornase (Varidase) may facilitate its withdrawal. When definite improvement is not evident in 4 to 6 days or when the empyema is of long duration, a large-lumen intercostal tube should be placed in the pleural cavity to facilitate drainage. Failure to effect prompt cure of empyema may be followed by pleural fibrosis and necessitate subsequent surgical decortication of the lung to restore pulmonary function.

Other measures Oxygen administered through a face mask should be used to treat significant cyanosis, cardiac failure, and delirium. Codeine, 32 to 64 mg every 4 h, will usually control pleuritic pain. When pain is severe, it may require intercostal nerve block with 1 to 2 percent procaine for relief.

Prognosis and prevention Although the mortality from pneumococcal pneumonia has diminished significantly since the advent of antimicrobial drugs, available evidence indicates that the incidence of the disease has changed little, if at all. The fatality rate in patients over the age of twelve years with bacteremic pneumococcal pneumonia treated with an antibiotic is 18 percent; and, in patients over the age of fifty and in those with underlying systemic illness, it is significantly higher.

Signs of poor prognosis in pneumonia include leukopenia, bacteremia, multilobar involvement, any extrapulmonary focus of pneumococcal infection, presence of preexisting systemic disease, circulatory collapse, and occurrence of the infection in the first year of life or after the age of fifty-five. Infection with pneumococcus type 3 has a higher mortality rate than that caused by other pneumococcal types. Death is most likely to occur in individuals sustaining irreversible physiologic damage early in the course which is unaltered by antimicrobial therapy. Until the nature of the injury produced by pneumococcus is understood and ways devised to repair it, vaccination will remain the only means of protecting those at high risk of a fatal outcome.

Despite the large number of pneumococcal serotypes, most of the serious infections are caused by a limited number; organisms of capsular types 1 through 8 account for 60 percent of such infections in adults. The efficacy of prophylactic vaccination with 50 μg each of the capsular polysaccharides of pneumococcal types 1, 2, 5, and 7 was demonstrated convincingly by MacLeod et al in 1946, and the properties of hexavalent vaccines were studied later by MacLeod, Heidelberger, and their associates. Most individuals receiving such vaccines showed an antibody response to all six antigens, and half maximal levels of antibody persisted for 5 to 8 years following a single injection of vaccine. Preparations of pneumococcal vaccines were available commercially for a short period but were removed from the market because their use was considered unnecessary by most physicians. This view has been challenged by more recent clinical and epidemiologic studies that have shown vaccines containing 12 to 14 capsular polysaccharides to be 85 percent effective in preventing type-specific pneumococcal infection in adults. Where pneumococcus is the predominant cause of pneumonia, such vaccines have brought about a 50 percent reduction in the total incidence of pneumonia. Re-licensure of such vaccines by 1977 is probable. The potential utility of similar vaccines in the prevention of pneumococcal otitis media in infancy and early childhood remains to be determined. Should they prove effective in preventing this pediatric disorder, they would be of significant value in lessening the impairment of hearing in certain segments of the population.

REFERENCES

AUSTRIAN R: Pneumococcal endocarditis, meningitis, and rupture of aortic valve. AMA Arch Intern Med 99:539, 1957

——, GOLD J: Pneumococcal bacteremia with especial reference to bacteremic pneumococcal pneumonia. Ann Intern Med 60: 759, 1964

HANSMAN D et al: Increased resistance to penicillin of pneumococci isolated from man. N Engl J Med 284:175, 1971

HEFFRON R: Pneumonia with Special Reference to Pneumococcus Lobar Pneumonia, New York: Commonwealth Fund, 1939

KAUFFMAN CA et al: Purulent pneumococcic pericarditis: Continuing problem in antibiotic era. Am J Med 54:743, 1973

LEPPER MH, DOWLING HF: Treatment of pneumococci meningitis with penicillin compared with penicillin plus aureomycin. AMA Arch Intern Med 88:489, 1951

MACLEOD CM et al: Prevention of pneumococcal pneumonia by immunization with specific capsular polysaccharides. J Exp Med 82:445, 1945

MERRILL CW et al: Rapid identification of pneumococci: Gram stain vs. quellung reaction. N Engl J Med 288:510, 1973

RAGSDALE AR, SANFORD JP: Interfering effect of incubation in carbon dioxide on the identification of pneumococci by optochin discs. Appl Microbiol 22:854, 1971

SHULMAN JA et al: Errors and hazards in the diagnosis and treatment of bacterial pneumonias. Ann Intern Med 62:41, 1965

TORRES J, BISNO AL: Hyposplenism and pneumococcemia. Am J Med 55:851, 1973

WOOD WB JR: Studies on the mechanism of recovery in pneumococcal pneumonia: 1. The action of type specific antibody upon the pulmonary lesion of experimental pneumonia. J Exp Med 73:201, 1941

ZINNEMAN HW, HALL WH: Recurrent pneumonia in multiple myeloma. Ann Intern Med 41:1152, 1954

134
STAPHYLOCOCCAL INFECTIONS

MARVIN TURCK

INTRODUCTION Staphylococci most commonly produce relatively harmless superficial suppurative infections in human beings. They also produce serious infections of the lungs, pleural space, endocardium, myocardium, long bones, kidneys, and surgical wounds.

The majority of life-threatening staphyloccal infections arise within hospitals, and these infections are considered among the "diseases of medical progress." Although staphylococcal cross infection in hospitals may be less frequent now than 10 to 15 years ago and although various gram-negative rods and fungi challenge the staphylococcus as the most common nosocomial pathogens, there is good evidence that the problem has not disappeared.

ETIOLOGY Staphylococci are members of the genus *Micrococcus.* The genus includes many morphologically similar saprophytic microorganisms which do not cause human infection. The parasitic micrococci of primary concern in medicine are grouped in the species *M. pyogenes.* Through established usage, these pathogenic micrococci are termed *staphylococci.*

Staphylococci are spherical gram-positive cells. On solid agar media, staphylococcal colonies develop characteristic pigmentation by which three species can be differentiated: *M. pyogenes* var. *aureus (Staphylococcus aureus),* golden yellow; *M. pyogenes* var. *albus (S. albus),* ivory white; and *M. citreus,* lemon yellow. Most human infections are caused by *S. aureus,* a few by *S. albus.* The name "staphylococcus" derives from the characteristic grapelike clusters of organisms seen in stained smears prepared from colonies on solid media. In stained smears obtained from pus, smaller clusters, diploids, and short chains are seen. In such preparations, staphylococci characteristically retain their uniform round shape, in contrast to the boatlike forms assumed by pneumococci. Staphylococci may be seen within the cytoplasm of polymorphonuclear cells in pus, a rare finding in other gram-positive coccal infections.

In general, pathogenic strains possess a broader complement of biochemical activity than do nonpathogenic strains. Most staphylococci isolated from human infections produce yellow pigment and hemolyze blood cells. The ability to produce coagulase, a substance which clots the plasma of certain animals and human beings, the elaboration of *alpha toxin,* and the fermentation of *mannite* are characteristic of infection-producing strains. The ability of a given strain to produce coagulase is generally considered the best single evidence of pathogenicity. Staphylococci that are coagulase-positive and ferment mannitol are classified by bacterial taxonomists as *S. aureus,* whether they produce the "aureus" pigment or not.

Different strains of pathogenic staphylococci can be recognized by the patterns of lysis produced by staphylococcal bacteriophages. Although the technique is cumbersome, phage typing of staphylococci has allowed more precise strain characterization and is commonly used in studies of intrahospital disease and epidemics of staphylococcal infection.

PATHOGENESIS Little is known of the events which allow staphylococci to invade host tissues. Though strains of staphylococci capable of producing infection are common skin and mucous membrane inhabitants, an enormous number of bacteria must be used to establish experimental infections in animals or humans, and more than a million organisms are necessary to produce serious infection in most laboratory animals. Over 50 percent of serious staphylococcal infections of deep tissues arise from cutaneous foci, and a smaller number originate in the respiratory or genitourinary tract. Direct inoculation of staphylococci into the bloodstream also is a route of infection amongst drug addicts. The integument and mucous membranes of heroin addicts appear to have a unique susceptibility to colonization by *S. aureus.*

Staphylococcal disease is more common in patients with *diabetes, liver disease, renal failure,* severe *debilitation* and/or *malnutrition,* or when skin continuity is broken. *Abrasions, wounds, burns,* and skin areas denuded by *exfoliative dermatitis* are commonly infected with staphylococci. *Influenza, measles,* and *mucoviscidosis* appear to predispose to primary staphylococcal invasion of the lung. Patients receiving *broad-spectrum antimicrobial therapy* also appear to have a higher incidence of staphylococcal disease.

Staphylococci invade the integument via hair follicles and sebaceous glands. When skin continuity has been breached, local microbial multiplication is accompanied by inflammation and tissue necrosis at the site of infection. Polymorphonuclear leukocytes rapidly enter the area and ingest large numbers of staphylococci. Thrombosis of surrounding capillaries occurs; fibrin is deposited about the periphery; and, later, fibroblasts create a relatively avascular wall about the area. The fully developed staphylococcal lesion consists of a central core of dead and dying leukocytes and bacteria which gradually liquefies to form characteristic thick, creamy pus, surrounded by a fibroblastic wall.

When host mechanisms fail to contain the cutaneous or subcutaneous infection, staphylococci may enter the bloodstream. Common sites of metastatic seeding are the diaphyseal ends of long bones in children, lungs, kidneys, endocardium, myocardium, liver, spleen, and brain.

Certain biologic properties of staphylococci appear to contribute to pathogenicity. Many pathogenic strains elaborate an *exotoxin* (alpha toxin) capable of causing dermal necrosis in animals. Fever, tachycardia, cyanosis, shock, and death ensue when exotoxin is administered to experimental animals, a picture similar to that seen occasionally in certain fulminating cases of staphylococcal bacteremia in human beings. A delta toxin also has been incriminated in pathogenesis of severe staphylococcal infection. However, it is conjectural that any of these toxins has any role in the circulatory disturbances seen prior to death.

The high correlation between *coagulase* production and virulence suggests that this substance is important in the pathogenesis of staphylococcal infections. Coagulase has been said to protect staphylococci from phagocytosis by polymorphonuclear leukocytes, to promote abscess formation in humans and in animal species which have coagulable plasmas, or to protect staphylococci from bacteriostatic substances present in normal serum. However, none of these postulates has shown that coagulase per se is a determinant of pathogenicity, and its precise role has not been established.

Certain pathogenic staphylococci produce a *leukocidin* which destroys human and rabbit leukocytes in vitro. Some strains elaborate *hyaluronidase.* Many staphylococci produce an *enterotoxin* which produces nausea, vomiting, and diarrhea in certain experimental animals and in humans.

In vitro and in vivo studies have indicated that pathogenic staphylococci can survive within human leukocytes, whereas nonpathogenic strains do not. Such intracellular survival may be a means of transporting staphylococci and spreading them to distant tissues. This intracellular survival may also account for the relative refractoriness of staphylococcal infection to antibiotic treatment.

IMMUNITY Some degree of resistance to staphylococcal infections develops with age. For example primary staphylococcal pneumonia is common in infants but rare in adults. Acute staphylococcal osteomyelitis is almost exclusively a disease of children. Abscess formation appears less common and bacteremia more frequent in infants than in adults.

Coagulase-positive staphylococci have a characteristic cell wall teichoic acid, which may be antiphagocytic. Certain unusual strains possess a definite mucopolysaccharide capsular structure which impedes phagocytosis, and specific opsonizing antibody is required for the ingestion of these unusual strains. A number of antistaphylococcal antibodies have been shown to pass from mother to fetus, and the incidence of a variety of antibodies rapidly rises with age. Virtually 100 percent of adults possess antibodies to several staphylococcal antigens in their serum. Nevertheless, the role of humoral immunity in modifying or protecting against staphylococcal infection is uncertain. Immunization of animals with alpha toxin, toxoids, coagulase, or whole staphylococci may prolong experimental staphylococcal infection, but does not protect against eventual death. There has been no satisfactory demonstration that human staphylococcal disease is followed by immunity or that infection can be modified significantly by vaccination.

EPIDEMIOLOGY Pathogenic strains of staphylococci reside in the anterior nares and upon the skin of a significant number of people. Hospital patients and personnel have significantly higher staphylococcal carrier rates than the general population.

While staphylococci remain viable for long periods in dust, blankets, or clothing, and viable staphylococci are often demonstrable in the environment by air-sampling techniques, the significance of airborne transmission remains uncertain, and the best evidence suggests that direct person-to-person contact is the most important means of transmission of staphylococci. Active staphylococcal infections are probably a more serious source of cross infection than the simple carrier state. For example, discontinuation of the use of hexachlorophene in hospital nurseries has been associated with an increase in infection in some hospitals, and it is apparent that continued surveillance in hospitals is necessary to thwart the development of epidemics of staphylococcal infection.

Certain phage types of staphylococci have been associated with a majority of intrahospital infections. Some strains, particularly antibiotic-resistant strains in phage group III, appear to have greater "epidemic virulence" than other staphylococci. In specific hospitals, one phage type often emerges to prominence and may cause most of the serious intrahospital infections. Such "epidemic strains" have shifted from time to time and vary from hospital to hospital. The high incidence of active staphylococcal disease in carriers of certain strains (e.g., the 80/81 strains) suggests that some staphylococci may possess higher virulence for humans than others. Some of the decrease in the frequency of staphylococcal infection in hospitals has been attributed to the disappearance of 80/81 strains.

ANTIMICROBIAL RESISTANCE In the past, the introduction of new antibiotics active against staphylococci has generally been followed by the appearance of staphylococci specifically resistant to that agent. When penicillin was first introduced, fewer than 10 percent of staphylococcal strains isolated from patients or carriers were resistant to penicillin. Now 60 to 90 percent of staphylococci isolated from hospitalized patients throughout the Western world are resistant to penicillin G, and the incidence of infection due to penicillinase-producing strains in nonhospitalized individuals is almost as high as in hospitalized patients. The incidence of resistance to a specific antimicrobial has correlated closely with the frequency of its administration, and the emergence of resistant strains has followed the use of most antibiotics. Vancomycin, first employed in 1958, and the penicillinase-resistant penicillins and the cephalosporins, both introduced in the 1960s, have been exceptions to this rule. Although some strains of *S. aureus* resistant to the penicillinase-resistant penicillins, such as methicillin, have produced infections in England, France, and the United States, such strains have been unusual in this country, and, in general, these agents have retained a high degree of activity against both penicillin-sensitive and penicillin-resistant staphylococci. However, methicillin resistance may emerge as a problem in the future.

Most observations on the incidence of antimicrobial-resistant strains have been made within hospitals where antimicrobial use is heaviest. It has been shown that drug-susceptible strains carried by patients may be replaced by drug-resistant phage group III staphylococci present in the hospital environment during antimicrobial treatment. These strains are in turn acquired by hospital personnel who serve as reservoirs of potentially pathogenic, antimicrobial-resistant strains. Staphylococci isolated from population groups outside the hospital have shown a slower increase in the incidence of antimicrobial-resistant strains, but in some communities the incidence of extrahospital infections caused by penicillin-resistant strains is similar to that found in hospitalized patients.

MANIFESTATIONS Superficial infections Simple infection of hair follicles manifested by a minute erythematous nodule without involvement of the surrounding skin or deeper tissues is termed *folliculitis.* A more extensive and invasive follicular or sebaceous gland infection with some involvement of subcutaneous tissues is termed a *furuncle,* or *boil.* Itching and mild pain are followed by progressive local swelling and erythema, and the overlying skin becomes exquisitely painful on pressure or motion. Relief of pain occurs promptly after spontaneous or surgical drainage.

Furuncles occur most commonly on the face, neck, axillas, forearms, buttocks, thighs, breast, upper back, and labia. The acne of adolescence is frequently complicated by secondary furunculosis. Staphylococcal infection may involve the sweat glands in the axillas *(hidradenitis suppurativa).* These infections may be deep-seated, slow to localize and drain, and are liable to recurrence and scarring.

Staphylococcal infections within the thick, fibrous, inelastic skin of the back of the neck and upper part of the back lead to formation of a *carbuncle.* The relative thickness and impermeability of the overlying skin lead to lateral extension and loculation, and a large, indurated, painful lesion with multiple ineffective drainage sites results. These extensive lesions appear more frequently among diabetics. Carbuncles produce fever, leukocytosis, extreme pain, and prostration. Bacteremia is common.

Osteomyelitis Staphylococci are responsible for the majority of cases of *acute osteomyelitis.* This infection occurs most commonly in children under the age of twelve, but adults also are susceptible to acute osteomyelitis, especially of the spine. There appears to have been a sharp decrease in the incidence of acute osteomyelitis since the introduction of antibiotics. Approximately 50 percent of patients give a history of a furuncle or superficial staphylococcal infection preceding osteomyelitis. Bone involvement follows hematogenous dissemination of bacteria. The frequent localization in the diaphyseal end of long bones is thought to be due to the endarterial circulation of the diaphysis. Many patients give a history of preceding trauma to the involved area.

Once established, infection spreads through the newly formed juxtaepiphyseal bone to the periosteum or along the marrow cavity. If the infection reaches the subperiosteal space, the periosteum is lifted, a subperiosteal abscess forms, and rupture with infection of the subcutaneous tissues may occur. Rarely, the joint capsule is penetrated, producing a pyogenic arthritis. There is death of bone, producing a *sequestrum,* followed by new bone formation, the *involucrum.*

Occasionally indolent staphylococcal infections of bone remain localized within dense granulation tissue about a central necrotic cavity. Such a local infection may persist for years as a so-called "Brodie's abscess."

Osteomyelitis in children usually begins abruptly with chills, high fever, nausea, vomiting, and progressive pain at the site of bony involvement. Muscle spasm about the affected bone is a common early sign of osteomyelitis, and the child may refuse to move the affected limb. Leukocytosis is the rule. Blood cultures are positive for staphylococci in 50 to 60 percent of cases early in the disease. The tissues overlying the involved bone become edematous and warm, and the skin becomes erythematous and shiny. Anemia develops during the course of untreated disease. Roentgenograms are usually normal during the first week. Bony rarefaction, local periosteal elevation, and new bone formation can frequently be seen during the second week.

Staphylococcal spinal infection in the adult differs considerably from acute osteomyelitis in the child. The onset is less abrupt, and there is a greater tendency for bony fusion with obliteration of the disk space.

DIAGNOSIS Osteomyelitis should be suspected in any child with fever, limb pain, and leukocytosis. Similarly, neck or back pain in an adult, when accompanied by fever, should raise the possibility of acute osteomyelitis or a disk space infection. History of a preceding cutaneous infection, local tenderness over the bone, and the finding of *S. aureus* in blood cultures are confirmatory. In early stages, osteomyelitis must be differentiated from acute rheumatic fever and pyogenic arthritis.

PROGNOSIS Prior to the advent of antimicrobials, the overall mortality was approximately 25 percent. Death was more common in individuals with demonstrable bacteremia. Chronic osteomyelitis with recurrent activation and metastatic foci in other bones was common. However, acute staphylococcal osteomyelitis is declining in incidence, death is rare, and chronic osteomyelitis is also becoming less frequent.

Staphylococcal pneumonia Staphylococci are the cause of approximately 1 percent of bacterial pneumonias. This disease occurs sporadically except during epidemics of influenza, when staphylococcal pneumonia is more common, although even then it is not as frequent as pneumococcal infection.

Primary staphylococcal pneumonia in infants and young children is a frequent cause of pyopneumothorax and pneumatocele. This complication occurs early and should suggest *S. aureus* infection. In older children and adults, primary staphylococcal pneumonia may be secondary to influenza or measles. In addition, staphylococcal pneumonia has been seen in hospitalized patients with mucoviscidosis, leukemia, collagen disease, or other chronic debilitating disease.

In healthy adults, staphylococcal pneumonia is generally preceded by an influenza-like respiratory infection. Onset of staphylococcal involvement is abrupt, with chills, high fever, progressive dyspnea, cyanosis, cough, and pleural pain. Early peripheral vascular collapse is common, and examination frequently reveals a patient who seems sicker than his physical findings would suggest. Sputum in the early phases is not characteristic, but may be bloody or frankly purulent. Admixture with blood may produce a thick, creamy pink sputum.

Staphylococcal pneumonia in hospitalized patients usually begins more insidiously. Increasing fever, tachycardia, and an elevated respiratory rate may be the only indications of infection. Typical pneumonic symptoms may be absent. The disease is also less abrupt when pulmonary involvement occurs during the course of staphylococcal bacteremia, as may be the case in drug addicts or in patients with endocarditis. Staphylococci generally produce patchy, centrally located areas of pneumonia. Pleural involvement and empyema are common.

Because of the central pulmonary involvement, chest findings are variable. Signs of frank consolidation are rare. Scattered fine to coarse rales and rhonchi may be heard over the involved areas. Empyema produces typical signs of pleural fluid. Signs of abscess may appear late in the course of the disease. Bacteremia is unusual in primary staphylococcal pneumonia (less than 20 percent of patients), and *its presence should suggest that the pneumonic involvement is metastatic and secondary to foci of infection elsewhere.*

The course of staphylococcal pneumonia may be stormy despite adequate antimicrobial therapy. Gradual defervescence starting 48 to 72 h after the initiation of therapy is the rule. Pulmonary abscesses or empyema cavities may require surgical treatment.

DIAGNOSIS Staphylococcal pneumonia must be differentiated from other pneumonias. The preceding influenza-like illness, rapid onset of pleural pain, cyanosis, and prostration out of proportion to physical findings should suggest primary staphylococcal pneumonia. The finding of masses of polymorphonuclear leukocytes and gram-positive intraleukocytic cocci strongly suggests the diagnosis. The blood leukocyte count is generally above 15,000. Pneumonia developing suddenly or insidiously, with higher fever, tachycardia, and leukocytosis, in debilitated hospitalized patients receiving antimicrobials should be considered to be staphylococcal in origin.

PROGNOSIS Prior to 1942, mortality ranged from 50 to 95 percent. The presence of bacteremia was almost invariably associated with a fatal outcome. The prognosis has improved with the use of antimicrobials, but some patients continue to die with staphylococcal pneumonia, especially debilitated individuals acquiring staphylococcal pneumonia in the hospital. Abscess formation and pleural involvement often prolong convalescence.

Staphylococcal bacteremia Staphylococcal bacteremia may arise from any local staphylococcal infection. Infections of the skin (including infections about inlying venous cutdowns or catheters), respiratory tract, bones, or genitourinary tract precede bacteremia. Trauma to local lesions, such as pinching, or surgical drainage before adequate localization may precipitate bacteremia.

Rarely, patients with bacteremia die in 12 to 24 h, with high fever, tachycardia, cyanosis, gastrointestinal symptoms, and vascular collapse. Commonly, the disease progresses more slowly, with hectic fever and metastatic abscess formation in the skin, bones, kidneys, brain, lungs, myocardium, spleen, or other tissues. *Meningitis* is an occasional complication.

Endocarditis may occur in patients with protracted bacteremia. Normal heart valves are frequently involved, the aortic being the most frequent. Typically, staphylococcal endocarditis runs an acute course with high fever, progressive anemia, and metastatic abscesses in the skin and deeper structures. Rupture of the valve leaflets and valve ring abscesses are common. Specific diagnosis of endocardial involvement is difficult; because of its frequency, it should be assumed to be present in patients with staphylococcal bacteremia with demonstrable cutaneous lesions (petechiae or cutaneous pustules) and a significant heart murmur. At times, especially among addicts with right-sided valvular lesions, a significant heart murmur may not be demonstrable. Both coagulase-positive and coagulase-negative staphylococci have been a major cause of endocarditis in patients undergoing cardiac surgical procedures, particularly valve replacement (Chap. 132), and both coagulase-positive and coagulase-negative staphylococci occasionally produce a subacute endocarditis indistinguishable from that produced by *Streptococcus viridans.* Persistent *Staphylococcus albus* bacteremia has also been common after ventriculoatriostomy.

Staphylococcal bacteremia is generally accompanied by a polymorphonuclear leukocytosis of 12,000 to 20,000, but a normal leukocyte count or leukopenia is occasionally seen. Diagnosis of bacteremia can be facilitated by doing a Gram stain of the buffy coat, which may show staphylococci within the cytoplasm of polymorphonuclear cells. Anemia develops rapidly during the course of the illness. Cyanosis and hypoxemia may be seen with staphylococcal bacteremia, even in the absence of significant pulmonary lesions on chest roentgenogram.

PROGNOSIS Staphylococcal bacteremia is an extremely serious disease. Prior to the development of antimicrobials, over 80 percent of individuals died, the majority within 10 days of the onset of illness. The development of endocarditis or meningitis during bacteremia was almost invariably fatal. The sulfonamides produced little alteration in this mortality rate. With the administration of effective antibiotics and appropriate surgical treatment of local sites of infection, 50 to 70 percent of patients survive. However, when staphylococcal endocarditis has occurred on a prosthetic cardiac valve, the outcome has been almost invariably fatal unless reconstructive surgery can be performed.

Staphylococcal food poisoning Certain strains of staphylococci produce an enterotoxin which is responsible for many outbreaks of acute gastroenteritis. The enterotoxin is heat-stable and not readily destroyed at ordinary cooking temperatures. Foods are commonly contaminated from superficial infections in food handlers or by nasal droplets containing pathogenic staphylococci. Cream-filled pastries, custards, cottage cheese, milk products, or meats which have been improperly refrigerated, thus allowing staphylococcal multiplication, are the common offenders.

Symptoms typically appear 1 to 6 h after ingestion of enterotoxin-contaminated food. Onset is usually abrupt, with severe nausea, vomiting, cramping abdominal pain, diarrhea, and prostration. The disease is brief and requires only rest and sedation. Rare fatalities have occurred in the aged. The diagnosis is based on the short incubation period, the epidemic nature of the disease, the short duration of symptoms, and the lack of fever. The etiology can be established only if specimens of ingested food can be shown to contain large numbers of enterotoxin-producing staphylococci. Staphylococal food poisoning should not be confused with staphylococcal enterocolitis, an illness associated with actual proliferation and overgrowth of viable staphylococci in the gut (Chap. 128).

Miscellaneous infections Staphylococci may cause otitis, sinusitis, or mastoid infections as well as infection in and around the orbit. Certain strains elaborate an erythrogenic toxin that results in a rash indistinguishable from that of streptococcal scarlet fever. Epidemics of staphylococcal pyoderma in newborn infants and maternal breast abscesses are a recurring problem in maternity units, but appear to be decreasing in frequency.

TREATMENT Features of staphylococcal infection which influence therapy While the development of penicillinase-resistant penicillins and cephalosporins has simplified treatment, certain characteristics of staphylococcal disease should be borne in mind in designing therapy.

1 The host setting in which infection occurs. Acute staphylococcal infections arising outside the hospital in otherwise healthy adults have a better prognosis than intrahospital infections arising in sick individuals with compromised host defense mechanisms.

2 The rapid necrosis of tissues produced by staphylococci. Delays in effective therapy may allow a progressing infection to advance to frank abscess formation. While many antimicrobials reach abscess cavities in adequate concentrations, the physiologic insusceptibility of microorganisms residing in the areas of extensive necrosis or suppuration renders antibiotic therapy quite ineffective in this situation. Surgical drainage of such lesions is often required.

3 The sluggish response to therapy. Staphylococci are killed slowly by antimicrobials, and relapses are frequent. Hence antimicrobial therapy must be continued longer than in many bacterial infections.

4 The problem of antimicrobial resistance. While treatment must be initiated empirically when serious staphylococcal infection is suspected, rational therapy requires that the antibiotic susceptibility of the infecting strain be known.

Treatment of serious staphylococcal infections The effectiveness of the penicillinase-resistant penicillins has simplified the approach to life-threatening staphylococcal disease. However, two methods of initiating treatment when serious staphylococcal disease is suspected have been proposed.

In the *first method,* following appropriate cultures, treatment with large doses of both aqueous penicillin *and* methicillin (or parenteral oxacillin or nafcillin) should be instituted immediately. In adults, aqueous penicillin, 20 million units, should be given by continuous intravenous drip. The companion penicillinase-resistant penicillin can be given intravenously or intramuscularly. Methicillin is rapidly eliminated from the body, and initial doses of 2 g every 4 h are indicated. Parenteral oxacillin or nafcillin in doses of 1 or 2 g every 4 h can be substituted for methicillin.

If in vitro sensitivity studies show the infecting strain to be sensitive to penicillin G, therapy with methicillin can be discontinued and treatment maintained with aqueous penicillin alone. If the strain is penicillin-resistant, the penicillinase-resistant penicillins alone should be continued.

The above regimen may be theoretically advantageous because penicillin-sensitive strains of staphylococci are twenty- to fiftyfold more susceptible to penicillin G than to methicillin. However, in fact, there is little clinical proof that this regimen is necessary even in patients with severe life-threatening staphylococcal infection.

In the *second method* a penicillinase-resistant penicillin is used alone. Nearly all strains of staphylococci are susceptible to penicillinase-resistant penicillins, and because of the high incidence of penicillinase-producing staphylococci as causes of infection, some authorities initiate treatment with methicillin, oxacillin, or nafcillin alone, shifting to aqueous penicillin G if the strain is subsequently proved to be susceptible to that drug.

Despite differences in structure, the major allergenic properties of the penicillins reside in the 6-aminopenicillanic acid molecule. There is significant cross allergenicity between penicillins, and patients who have had well-established allergic reactions to penicillin G should not receive penicillinase-resistant penicillins. Further, there is increasing evidence that a significant number of these individuals may react to the cephalosporin derivatives as well. These agents, which are good antistaphylococcal drugs, have a 7-aminocephalosporanic acid nucleus quite similar to that of penicillins and should be used with caution in patients with prior reactions to penicillin.

Cephalothin and *cephaloridine* are semisynthetic derivatives of cephalosporin C. Cephalothin is highly active against both penicillin-sensitive and penicillin-resistant strains. Cephaloridine appears more susceptible to staphylococcal penicillinase and should not be used in treatment of severe infections by penicillin-resistant strains unless the organism is shown to be sensitive to it. Intramuscular or intravenous doses of 1 to 2 g cephalothin every 4 h are recommended; the dose of cephaloridine is limited to 1 g every 6 h by regulation because of its potential for nephrotoxicity. Two cephalosporin preparations are cefazolin and cephapirin. The usual dose of cefazolin for severe staphylococcal infection is 1 g every 6 h intramuscularly or intravenously. The dose and route of administration for cephapirin are similar.

Vancomycin is uniformly active against coagulase-positive staphylococci regardless of their sensitivity to penicillin. It should be given intravenously in doses of 1 to 1.5 g over a 30- to 40-min period every 12 h.

The development of these new agents has relegated several antibiotics formerly used in treatment to minor or secondary roles. Lincomycin, clindamycin, and erythromycin are still useful in certain circumstances, but are not frontline agents in staphylococcal bacteremia. They are used primarily in patients allergic to penicillin.

Changes in therapy Established staphylococcal infections respond slowly even to the most effective antimicrobial regimens, making it difficult to know when therapy should be considered inadequate. Characteristically, 24 to 48 h elapse before a decline in fever is noted, and recovery is accompanied by slow return of the temperature to normal in 7 to 10 days. Treatment should be continued for a minimum of 4 to 6 weeks if endocarditis is suspected.

Special therapeutic situations ASYMPTOMATIC NASAL CARRIER STATE The role of asymptomatic carriers in hospital transmission of infection remains controversial. Hospital personnel are carriers if they harbor, in their anterior nares, coagulase-positive staphylococci which are producing intrahospital disease, and it is generally agreed that they must be removed from nursery units, operating theaters, delivery rooms, and surgical floors. Although no method of treatment has been uniformly satisfactory, the following regimens have had limited success in treatment of nasal carriers.

1 Simple removal from the hospital environment for 3 to 4 weeks
2 Frequent baths with germicidal soaps
3 The use of topical antibiotics of low sensitizing potential in a water-soluble base (i.e., bacitracin, neomycin, or a combination of these agents) four to five times daily for 2 weeks

If the carrier state returns, a second course of treatment is indicated. In infants, colonization with disease-producing strains may be prevented by deliberate implantation of a staphylococccal strain of low virulence. This approach has been applied to adult carriers in a limited way, but evidence regarding its efficacy is not yet available.

SUPERFICIAL INFECTIONS Superficial infections frequently do not require the use of antibiotics. There is no adequate therapy for recurrent furunculosis, but if the disease is severe, antimicrobial treatment may be attempted. Antibiotics to which the strain is susceptible should be administered systemically for a minimum of 10 to 14 days. Local moist heat, immobilization of the infected part, and incision and drainage should be utilized. The surrounding skin should be protected with a coating of zinc oxide to prevent maceration. Treatment of the nasal carrier state by the local application of topical antibiotics (see above) may be advisable. Careful daily baths with germicidal soaps, attention to personal and family hygiene, and the passage of time appear to be measures most likely to interrupt the process. Attempts to prevent recurrence by autogenous or other vaccines have not been effective.

EMPYEMA Empyema should be treated by aspiration, generally with a large-bore tube since loculation and thick exudate may prevent adequate needle drainage. Direct instillation of penicillin or methicillin into the pleural space may be beneficial, and this procedure is employed in some instances. Similarly, while the local instillation of proteolytic enzymes may occasionally aid in liquefying the exudate, surgical drainage is generally necessary and should be performed promptly.

OSTEOMYELITIS The initial regimen already outlined for other serious infections is recommended, and treatment should be continued for 14 to 28 days in acute osteomyelitis. Local drainage of abscess cavities in soft tissues or bones should be considered in all patients in whom severe pain persists or when response to antimicrobials is inadequate. If sequestration occurs, devitalized bone should be removed. Lincomycin has been reported to be superior to other agents in the treatment of chronic osteomyelitis, but the evidence for this is not convincing. The optimal duration of treatment in established chronic infection is not known, but frequently several months of antimicrobial therapy are recommended.

NURSERY EPIDEMICS The hazards of epidemic staphylococcal disease in newborn nurseries are well recognized. Pediatric texts should be consulted for full discussion of the special techniques employed in prevention and management of nursery infections. The use of deliberate colonization of newborns with a staphylococcus of low disease potential to prevent colonization with more pathogenic strains has important biologic implications.

REFERENCES

EICKHOFF TE: Hospital infections. Disease-a-Month (Chicago), September, 1972

JESSEN O et al: Changing staphylococci and staphylococcal infections. N Engl J Med 281:627, 1969

KOENIG MG: Staphylococcal infections: Treatment and control. Disease-a-Month (Chicago), April, 1968

NAHMIAS AJ, EICKHOFF TC: Staphylococcal infections in hospitals. N Engl J Med 265:74, 120, 177, 1962

WATANAKUNAKORN C et al: Some salient features of *Staphylococcus aureus* endocarditis. Am J Med 54:473, 1973

WISE RI: Modern management of severe staphylococcal disease. Medicine 52:295, 1973

135 HEMOLYTIC STREPTOCOCCAL INFECTIONS

CHARLES H. RAMMELKAMP, JR.

INTRODUCTION

Streptococci are probably the most important bacterial pathogens of human beings. They can invade any tissue, and depending on the site of invasion and the host-parasite relationship, produce different clinical syndromes. They cause such common, dramatic, acute septic illnesses as sore throat, scarlet fever, lymphangitis, puerperal fever, and erysipelas. In addition, certain serologic strains are capable of producing serious late complications, including acute rheumatic fever and acute glomerulonephritis.

ETIOLOGY

Streptococci are gram-positive and tend to form chains. Cultured on sheep blood agar they produce three types of reactions. *Alpha* colonies exhibit a zone of incomplete hemolysis with greenish discoloration; they are termed *viridans* streptococci. *Beta*-hemolytic colonies exhibit complete clearing of sheep red blood cells because of the action of hemolysins, including streptolysins O and S. *Gamma* colonies are nonhemolytic.

On the basis of specific carbohydrates, 13 serologic groups of streptococci have been identified; they are designated A through O. All groups may infect human beings, but respiratory infections are caused by group A and only rarely by groups C and G streptococci. Groups A and B cause neonatal and post-partum sepsis. Group D, or enterococci, both hemolytic and nonhemolytic varieties, are found in the intestine and are responsible for infections of the urinary tract and abdominal cavity. There are over 50 specific types of group A streptococci which are identified by a precipitin test for M protein or by an agglutination reaction to the T antigen. The M protein is responsible for type-specific immunity in humans and is probably responsible for the virulence of group A organisms. Glossy forms of group A which contain no M protein are avirulent.

Several extracellular products are produced by streptococci. *Streptolysin O* is produced by groups A, C, and G, and antibody develops following infection. Approximately 85 percent of group A respiratory infections result in a measurable increase in antistreptolysin O. *Streptolysin S* is nonantigenic.

Scarlatinal or *erythrogenic toxin* is responsible for the rash of scarlet fever. Toxigenic strains are lysogenic and vary in the amount of toxin produced. There are three immunologically distinct toxins which may account for second attacks of scarlet fever.

Streptokinase is an enzyme that catalyzes the conversion of plasminogen to plasmin causing the lysis of fibrin. It is produced by strains of groups A, C, and G and occasionally in small amounts by groups B and F streptococci. Group A strains vary in the amount produced. Two distinct streptokinases, A and B, are produced by group A streptococci, and antibodies develop following infection; however, this antibody is not widely employed as a diagnostic test. *Diphosphopyridine nucleotidase* is produced by certain strains of group A streptococci, especially type 12, a nephritogenic strain. When leukocytes ingest such strains, a leukocytotoxic effect is immediately apparent. Antibody develops which inhibits the action of the enzyme.

Four specific immunologic *deoxyribonucleases,* A, B, C, and D, are produced by group A streptococci. These enzymes depolymerize the viscous deoxyribonucleoprotein present in thick pus and have been used clinically to liquefy exudates.

Hyaluronidase, or spreading factor, attacks the polysaccharide gel of the capsule of the streptococcus and the ground substance of connective tissue. It is produced by group A streptococci and in large amounts by types 4 and 22. Antibodies develop following infection. Whether or not hyaluronidase is responsible for the tendency of streptococci to spread rapidly in tissues is not known. Other substances produced by streptococci include *leukocidin, proteinase,* and *amylase.*

EPIDEMIOLOGY

Aerobic streptococcal infections are observed in all races, in both sexes, and at all ages and occur during any season of the year throughout the world. Streptococcal respiratory infections, including scarlet fever, are encountered especially during the colder months of the year. Under the age of three months, streptococcal infections are rare. Between the ages of six months and ten years, scarlet fever occurs frequently. Tonsillitis and pharyngitis are especially prevalent throughout childhood and early adult life. In women during the childbearing period, puerperal infections caused by streptococci occur occasionally. Finally, erysipelas, which may occur at any age, appears to be more prevalent in infants and elderly persons.

Soon after birth, alpha streptococci appear in the upper part of the respiratory tract and may be isolated therefrom throughout life. Streptococci of Lancefield groups C and G and, more rarely, organisms of groups other than A may be isolated from the oropharynx of 5 percent or more of the normal population.

The group A flora of the oropharynx is made up of many different specific types, but usually several types predominate. In general, at least 5 percent of the people of any community harbor group A streptococci. The prevalence varies and depends upon the cultural methods used as well as upon environmental, host, and bacterial factors. Persons under twenty years of age are most likely to harbor group A streptococci, especially if the tonsils are present.

Following either apparent or inapparent infection, the carrier state usually persists for several months and occasionally for longer periods. Throat cultures inoculated directly on blood agar plates during the first, fourth, eighth, and eleventh weeks following infection show 10 or more colonies of streptococci in 90, 65, 25, and 10 percent of patients, respectively. Carriers of non-group A streptococci usually show only a few colonies on culture. In addition, as the carrier state progresses, the streptococci lose their ability to produce M protein, so that by the eleventh week, about 40 percent of strains cannot be typed. Quantitative examination of cultures and typing provide important data regarding the possible duration of the carrier state, and this information is valuable in determining whether or not therapy should be instituted.

Ability to spread disease appears to be an attribute of individuals who have been infected recently. Whether this is due to the large number of streptococci in the nose and oropharynx or whether such organisms are especially capable of parasitizing another person cannot be determined from the available evidence. It is established that nasal carriers of group A streptococci are likely to spread disease. The spread of streptococci in any population group is related to the degree of exposure, and during the winter months when people are confined to enclosed areas, and under crowded conditions, dissemination of bacteria is especially likely to occur.

Group A streptococci naturally deposited in dust and on blankets will not produce respiratory infections in human beings. The evidence implicates the direct mode of transfer as primarily responsible for dissemination of such infections.

Outbreaks of streptococcal infection occasionally occur following the contamination of food. These outbreaks are dramatic because a large number of persons are affected almost simultaneously.

Primary infection of the upper part of the respiratory tract is undoubtedly the most common form of streptococcal infection in humans. It is doubtful whether anyone in the United States escapes one or more of these infections. In most areas the disease is endemic. Epidemics are usually due to one or, at the most, several types of group A streptococci, while many different types are responsible for cases of pharyngitis and tonsillitis occurring sporadically.

Tonsillitis and pharyngitis are characterized by an acute sore throat which may or may not be accompanied by a cutaneous rash. If a rash is observed, a diagnosis of *scarlet fever* is made. The severity and frequency of scarlet fever are decreasing; the reason for this is not entirely clear.

Bacterial pneumonia caused by aerobic streptococci accounts for less than 5 percent of all cases of pneumonia. The disease is almost invariably caused by group A streptococci and may arise secondarily to an infection of the upper part of the respiratory tract such as influenza and measles.

Formerly it was thought that *erysipelas* was caused by a specific strain of beta-hemolytic streptococcus, but it is now known that group A, C, or G streptococci may be isolated from the skin lesions. Group A organisms are responsible for the majority of infections, and the organisms may belong to any of the various types of this group. Erysipelas tends to occur in the older age groups, especially in those individuals with chronic disabling diseases. Immunity does not develop; in fact, individuals who have had one attack are more susceptible than the normal population. In some of the recurrences, however, the organisms cannot be isolated from the skin lesions but may be found in the oropharynx. In these instances the disease may be due to absorption of some streptococcal toxin, which, in turn, causes the local inflammatory lesion in the skin that has altered its reactivity.

Wounds may be infected by droplet contamination at the time of dressing. *Lymphangitis* may arise from a minute abrasion.

Numerous studies have indicated that either aerobic or anaerobic streptococci cause *puerperal sepsis,* but approximately 70 percent of fatal cases are due to beta-hemolytic streptococci. Because the group A streptococcus is rarely isolated from the genital tract either before or after labor, infection probably is contracted from an outside source and occasionally from the respiratory tract of the patient herself.

In contrast to streptococcal pharyngitis, *impetigo* occurs most frequently during the summer and early fall months and in most tropical climates. Minor skin trauma, insect bites, and poor personal hygiene predispose to infection, especially in infants and young children. Modes of infection are not well defined, but physical contact with infected children, deposits in the environment, or transfer by flies probably play a role. Primary respiratory spread is not required. Impetigo is especially likely to be caused by M types 8, 11, 22, 33, 41, 43, 52 to 54, 56, 59, 61 and in addition by the nephritogenic skin M types 2, 49, 55, 57, and 60. Rheumatic fever, rarely, if ever, follows such skin infections.

PATHOGENESIS

Streptococci gain entrance into the body through inhalation and are usually cleared away rapidly by normal defense mechanisms. Multiple factors determine whether or not infection occurs. The *dosage* of streptococci is important; infection usually results when there is exposure to large numbers of group A streptococci, as occurs in foodborne outbreaks. The *virulence* of streptococci is decisive, since non-group A streptococci and nontypable group A organisms rarely produce recognizable respiratory disease. Rapid passage of typable group A organisms in a human being is thought to increase virulence, but there is no good evidence to support this hypothesis.

Perhaps as important as the organism itself is the susceptibility of the host. Immunity to group A infection is type-specific and, once acquired, lasts for years. In the absence of type-specific antibody, phagocytosis is markedly suppressed, and invasion and spread of organisms can occur rapidly. Recovery in 5 to 7 days is assumed to be due to the development of type-specific antibodies, with attending phagocytosis and killing of the bacteria. Little is known concerning immunity in group A skin infections or infections with other groups of streptococci. Indeed, streptococci of groups A, B, C, and D, as well as anaerobic streptococci and viridans streptococci, are opportunistic, invading the uterus after abortion, infecting wounds, causing endocarditis, peritonitis, urinary tract infections, meningitis, and metastatic abscesses. In addition to these suppurative complications, immediate and delayed allergy to group A streptococcal products develops in early life, which may be responsible for the pathogenesis of some cases of *erythema nodosum. Rheumatic fever* and *glomerulonephritis* are extremely unique complications of only group A infections. Evidence is accumulating to support the concept of the possible role of cross-reactive antigen-antibody systems in the pathogenesis of rheumatic fever and rheumatic valvular disease. Less clearly defined immune mechanisms appear to be important in acute poststreptococcal glomerulonephritis. Why only certain types of group A streptococci cause nephritis is unknown, nor is there an explanation for the clinical observation that rheumatic fever seldom, if ever, follows a skin infection.

MANIFESTATIONS

ACUTE TONSILLITIS, PHARYNGITIS, AND SCARLET FEVER Symptoms The incubation period is usually 3 to 5 days. The illness begins abruptly with symptoms of feverishness, chilliness, headache, and sore throat. Nausea and vomiting are especially common in children. A few patients complain of diarrhea. Within a period of 24 to 48 h the disease reaches its maximum intensity. Chilliness is a constant symptom, but true rigors are rare. Approximately 75 percent or more of the patients complain of headache, malaise, and loss of appetite.

Sore throat is almost constantly present within 24 h of onset. The soreness is aggravated by swallowing and may be referred to the neck, so that even turning of the head is accompanied by pain. Nasal obstruction and discharge are minor complaints but occur in 60 percent of patients. About half the patients develop very mild symptoms referable to the lower part of the respiratory tract, including cough and hoarseness. The cough is not productive and is rarely associated with chest pain. Loss of voice due to laryngitis does not occur. Earache is common amd may last a few hours to several days. Occasionally, epistaxis is observed.

During the period of maximum temperature there may be a diffuse blush of the skin. In some cases it becomes more pronounced, and a diagnosis of *scarlet fever* is made. The rash appears 1 to 5 days after onset of illness and is first noticed over the neck and upper part of the chest. It spreads rapidly to include the skin over the abdomen and upper and lower extremities. The face appears flushed, and circumoral pallor is prominent. Itching occasionally occurs but is rarely severe.

Physical signs The degree of prostration varies, but the majority of patients appear mildly or moderately ill. The temperature is usually elevated to 102 to 104°F; occasionally it may be as high as 106°F. A few patients have no fever. In children the pulse rate is between 140 and 160, in adults between 120 and 140 per min.

Various degrees of diffuse redness of the mucous membranes of the posterior pharynx, faucial tonsils, and soft palate are invariably present. The uvula is frequently edematous, as are the tonsils and pharynx. Lymphoid hyperplasia and edema give the posterior pharynx a cobblestone appearance. Characteristically there is discrete to confluent exudate on the tonsils, and variable numbers of pinhead-size areas of exudate appear on the pharynx. In severely ill patients these are seldom seen, because nasal secretions cover the posterior wall. The exudate is often yellow, sometimes gray or white, and is relatively easily removed by swabbing. In about 20 percent of adults, and more frequently in infants, exudative lesions on the mucous membranes do not develop. If sinusitis and rhinitis are present there is a thick mucopurulent nasal discharge which may be tinged with blood. In children the nares may be excoriated. The cervical lymph nodes just below the angle of the jaw are the first to enlarge; rarely they attain such size that the head is thrown back. Marked adenopathy is frequently followed by suppuration.

In those patients with *scarlet fever* the signs include both an enanthem and an exanthem. The appearance of the throat is similar to that seen in tonsillitis and pharyngitis without rash, except that diffuse redness is more intense and has been described as "boiled-lobster" red. There may be punctate redness of the soft and hard palate. The buccal mucous membranes appear red and swollen, as do the lips. About the second to fifth day, small mild-white patches may be seen on the buccal mucous membranes. They represent desquamation of the epithelium and are easily peeled off.

Early in the course of the infection the tongue is heavily coated and grayish. Soon the tip and edges become an angry red. Fungiform papillae become swollen and emerge through the gray surface of the tongue. By the fourth to fifth day there is complete lingual desquamation, which leaves multiple papillary elevations, the so-called "strawberry tongue."

The color of the exanthem varies and has been described as scarlet, bright red, rose-colored, or dull, dusky red. At a distance there appears to be a uniform blush, but upon close inspection innumerable small reddish points are seen. Because of pinpoint elevations at the site of the hair follicles, the skin may feel like sandpaper. This sign is of special importance in races where the skin is heavily pigmented. When the eruption is intense, there may be many small miliary vesicles over the chest and abdomen. A mild degree of jaundice is common in individuals with extensive exanthem. The face may be free of rash, but ordinarily the temples and cheeks are deep red, leaving an area of pallor around the mouth and nose. The rash is due to hyperemia, and pressure causes it to fade. In some areas there may be punctate hemorrhages which do not fade; these are commonly seen in the creases at the elbow flexure (Pastia's sign), groin, and axillary folds.

Course of illness The majority of upper respiratory illnesses caused by group A streptococci are self-limited. In adults the temperature usually returns to normal by the third to fourth day; in children fever may persist for 5 to 9 days. The temperature curve is not characteristic, although there is usually a slight morning remission. In patients with scarlet fever the temperature remains elevated until the rash has reached its maximum intensity. Fever may last for several weeks, but in such instances it is well to search for some suppurative complications. The constitutional symptoms, as well as the localizing symptom of sore throat, usually disappear shortly after the fever subsides.

The edema, redness, and exudate disappear rapidly, and except for a few small isolated spots of exudate and a slight degree of redness, the throat appears normal shortly after the fever subsides. The lymphoid tissues of the posterior pharynx as well as the tonsils decrease in size and by the third to sixth week appear to be normal. The lymph nodes may not return to normal size for 6 weeks.

When rash does occur, it usually makes its appearance

on the second day, reaches its maximum intensity shortly thereafter, and then begins to fade. The exfoliation of the epithelium begins during the decline of the eruption and is seen first in those areas where the rash originally appeared. By the sixth to seventh day it is more or less generalized. On the hands and feet the skin sheds in flakes or, more rarely, as an entire cast of the hand or foot. The skin in these areas becomes dry, hard, and wrinkled. The most typical form of desquamation is seen beneath the free edge of the fingernails. A fissure appears under the edge of the nail and then widens, revealing the soft, pinkish underlying skin.

Laboratory findings In 80 percent of patients the total leukocyte count is increased. During the first 2 days of disease the average count is 14,000, and as the illness progresses, it returns to normal values. If the number of leukocytes remains elevated after 1 week, evidence of a complication may be found. During the first 2 days of illness eosinophils are rarely seen, but convalescence is characterized by an increase in number of these cells. Patients with scarlet fever are especially likely to have eosinophilia. Frequently a trace of albumin may be found in the urine during the acute phase of the illness, and rarely, such specimens show a few red blood cells or casts. Proteinuria during the first 5 days of illness is transient and is not attended by serious sequelae.

Diagnosis Important features in the diagnosis of streptococcal pharyngitis and tonsillitis are the history of an acute onset of soreness on swallowing, associated with feverishness and other constitutional symptoms. The physical signs of diffuse redness and edema of the mucous membranes of the oropharynx, tonsils, and soft palate, the presence of discrete to confluent exudate, and the enlargement and tenderness of the lymph nodes at the angle of the jaw are especially helpful. These findings, together with a leukocyte count of at least 12,000, suggest a streptococcal infection. If the culture of the local lesion shows a predominant growth of beta streptococci, the diagnosis is established with certainty. When only a few colonies grow on the blood agar plate, it is impossible to be sure whether the patient is a carrier or actually has an infection due to the streptococcus. In such cases it is of considerable help to obtain acute and convalescent blood specimens for determination of antistreptolysin titers.

When a rash is associated with the above clinical and laboratory findings, the diagnosis is scarlet fever. Confirmation is obtained if the skin desquamates.

Differential diagnosis of sore throat *Nonbacterial exudative tonsillitis and pharyngitis* must be differentiated from streptococcal infections of the oropharynx (Chap. 195). Adenoviruses will produce respiratory infections associated with exudative lesions, and in some outbreaks the conjunctiva is involved. In general the onset of illness is not rapid, sore throat is seldom marked, and constitutional symptoms are mild. Hoarseness and cough are likely to occur several days after the onset. The exudate is rarely confluent. The lymph nodes may be slightly enlarged but are not remarkably tender. The leukocyte count is usually normal, although in a few cases it may be slightly elevated. Cultures of the throat fail to show beta-hemolytic streptococci. Occasionally a few streptococci are recovered, but these organisms usually belong to groups other than A and occur only in small numbers.

Infectious mononucleosis is most frequently observed in young adults and, because of the local reaction in the throat, is likely to be confused with streptococcal pharyngitis (Chap. 209). The onset may be insidious, and malaise is prominent. Sore throat with exudative lesions of the tonsils is observed in over half the cases. Fever is more prolonged than is usual in streptococcal infections. Lymph node enlargement is more generalized, but suppuration is not observed. The spleen may be palpable. In 10 to 15 percent of cases a fleeting skin rash occurs, which may be identical with that seen in scarlet fever. The blood changes are characteristic, and a positive heterophil antibody test is usually obtained.

Vincent's angina (Chap. 160) is not easily confused with streptococcal infections. The disease is characterized by insidious onset without constitutional symptoms. Fever is rare. The area surrounding the exudate shows little inflammatory reaction, generally only one tonsil is involved, and cervical adenopathy is usually unilateral.

In contrast to streptococcal pharyngitis, the onset of *diphtheria* is rarely sudden and the symptoms are not severe (Chap. 154). Sore throat is not a constant feature of the disease. The exudate is smooth and cream-colored and appears to be incorporated in the mucous membranes. The membrane is removed with difficulty, leaving a bleeding bed. Cutaneous rashes are absent. Cultures show *Corynebacterium diphtheriae.*

In patients with a rash, the disease must be differentiated from *rubella* (Chap. 202) and *rubeola* (Chap. 201). In German measles the posterior cervical lymph node enlargement is helpful, as well as the fact that the rash tends to be macular and discrete. The tongue never peels, and a leukopenia is characteristic. In measles there are prodromal respiratory symptoms, and the maculopapular rash occurs chiefly on the face and neck. The presence of Koplik's spots aids in establishing the diagnosis.

Streptococcal infections without exudate or a cutaneous rash must be differentiated from *influenza virus infection* (Chap. 196) and *common respiratory diseases* (Chap. 195). In general, this differentiation cannot be made on clinical evidence alone, and the leukocyte count, culture studies, and serologic tests must be employed.

Primary *herpes simplex pharyngitis* (Chap. 206) and *herpangina* (Chap. 195) are characterized by vesicles which rupture and produce small ulcers covered with exudate. Herpetic lesions are scattered over all mucous membranes of the mouth, and the kissing ulcer under the tip of the tongue is typical. The ulcers of herpangina, caused by Coxsackie A viruses, are observed on the anterior pillars and the soft palate. In both diseases the leukocyte count is usually normal.

Sinusitis, otitis media, mastoiditis, and peritonsillar abscess Infection of the paranasal sinuses probably occurs to a minor degree in all patients with streptococcal respiratory infections. Sinusitis and otitis media presenting overt clinical signs develop in approximately 3 percent of patients whose tonsils and adenoids are intact. Mastoiditis is observed in less than 1 percent of patients. Peritonsillar cellulitis is observed in 2.5 percent of patients with tonsils, but it rarely occurs in those whose tonsils have been removed or in those patients who receive proper therapy with antibiotics. The diagnosis and management of these suppurative complications are described in Chap. 28.

PNEUMONIA AND EMPYEMA Primary group A streptococcal pneumonia is rare in the absence of influenza, but many cases may occur during an influenza epidemic. The onset of pneumonia tends to be abrupt, with symptoms of chills, fever, anorexia, and vomiting. Cough, sputum that is pink and thin, and chest pain are characteristic. The temperature is usually high (104°F), and fever is intermittent. Examination reveals scattered fine rales, but signs of lobar consolidation are rare.

The leukocyte count is high (20,000 to 30,000), and large numbers of group A organisms are cultured from the sputum. Usually the blood cultures are sterile. With proper therapy with penicillin, recovery is rapid. Empyema is a frequent complication in patients who receive no therapy. The pleural fluid is pink and thin; it thickens only when infected with other organisms.

PERICARDITIS, ARTHRITIS, PERITONITIS, AND MENINGITIS Streptococcal infections of the various body cavities result from bacteremia or from extension from a local lesion. *Pericarditis,* a rare complication, is especially likely to occur during the course of pneumonia or empyema. The diagnosis is difficult, because the symptoms arising from pericarditis are overshadowed by the primary disease. The first sign may be a sudden increase in pulse rate and the development of an audible pericardial friction rub.

Suppurative arthritis is secondary to bacteremia or to extension of a local cellulitis. It is a rare complication of streptococcal sore throat. Pain is the most common symptom, and usually only one joint is involved. The pain is first noticed on motion, but within a short period redness, swelling, and tenderness develop and the pain becomes intense. Aspiration reveals a fluid containing polymorphonuclear leukocytes and streptococci. Nonsuppurative arthritis seen in patients with scarlet fever during the first week of illness indicates the onset of rheumatic fever and should not be considered a manifestation of erythrogenic toxin.

Infection of the peritoneum with the hemolytic streptococcus is rare but is especially apt to be associated with such local infections as erysipelas and scarlet fever. In these cases the organism belongs to Lancefield group A. Symptoms develop rapidly, and in addition to fever and other constitutional symptoms, prostration, abdominal pain, and vomiting are prominent. The pulse is rapid and weak. The abdomen is distended, tender, and rigid to palpation.

Streptococcal *meningitis* is usually caused by group A organisms, but occasionally members of other groups may be isolated from the spinal fluid. In most instances the meningitis arises by extension from otitis media, mastoiditis, or petrositis, which are especially likely to develop following infection of the respiratory tract and are seen most frequently in the young. Prior to the introduction of specific therapy these infections were always fatal. The symptoms are not distinguishable from those of other types of bacterial meningitis. All patients, especially infants, with infections of the middle ear should be watched for signs of meningeal irritation.

WOUND AND SKIN INFECTIONS, LYMPHANGITIS, PUERPERAL FEVER, AND ERYSIPELAS Wounds, small abrasions, and children with chickenpox and other skin lesions may become infected with group A or C streptococci. *Impetigo* in children caused by group A streptococci is common. The initial lesion is a papule which then becomes vesicular with a small surrounding area of erythema. The vesicles rupture early so that they may not be observed by the physician, who sees instead small crusted lesions. Regional adenopathy is usually present. Pure cultures of streptococci are obtained from the vesicle, but, in addition, staphylococci may be present in the crusted stages. Bullous impetigo is primarily staphylococcal in origin.

Hemolytic streptococci are responsible for the majority of cases of *lymphangitis,* characterized by the rapid development of one or more fine red streaks extending upward from the hand or foot. Usually the process continues up to the axilla or groin, and the lymph nodes in these areas become enlarged and tender. Associated with the spread of the infection in the lymphatics, such symptoms as rigor, fever, malaise, headache, and vomiting occur. Occasionally the bloodstream is invaded. The original site of infection in these cases of lymphangitis may not be apparent. Although these infections may be serious, the course of the illness is usually short, and suppuration along the course of the lymphatics seldom occurs. Within 2 weeks after a streptococcal respiratory infection, some children develop persistent *lymphadenitis.* In children with enlarged cervical nodes 75 percent of the cases are secondary to a streptococcal infection. In these patients aspiration of the node will usually reveal the organism.

Puerperal infection may be caused by group A streptococci, but group B has assumed the predominant role in both puerperal infection in the mother and neonatal sepsis and meningitis in the infant. In the mother, the streptococci invade the endometrium and lymphatics and may result in bacteremia. A high, irregular fever, rapid pulse, leukocytosis, and a foul-smelling discharge yielding group B streptococci are characteristic. In the infant almost all infections occur in the first 60 days of life. Sepsis develops acutely within 48 h of birth and is manifested by respiratory distress. In this instance the same group B serotype is found in the vagina and in the child. When onset of infection occurs later, it is characterized by meningitis, and in this case fewer than 25 percent of the maternal vaginal cultures grow the infecting organism.

Erysipelas is an acute streptococcal infection of the skin and, to a lesser extent, of the mucous membranes. Group A streptococci are the usual cause, but other streptococci may cause this syndrome. The onset is usually abrupt, after an incubation period of 1 to 4 days. A history of preceding respiratory infection is sometimes obtained. The initial symptoms include chilliness, feverishness, headache, malaise, anorexia, and vomiting. At the onset the local cutaneous lesions may not be apparent. The skin may itch and feel sore around the point of entry of the organisms. Within a few hours, the cutaneous lesion becomes obvious.

The face is most commonly involved, but any area of the body may be infected. The point of entry may be just anterior to the ear, at the inner canthus of the eye, around the lips and nose, or over the cheeks. From these points the lesion spreads rapidly, reaching its maximum extent within 3 to 6 days. Erysipelas frequently involves the butterfly area of the cheeks and nose. The lesion consists of an advancing border which is raised from the surrounding normal skin and may be purple. Within this border the skin is tense and usually a dark dull red. If the infection occurs in areas where the skin is lax, such as around the eyes, edema is pronounced. The eyelids frequently become so swollen that they cannot be opened. Blebs or necrotic areas may appear as the disease progresses.

At the height of the infection the temperature is usually high (104 to 105°F), although occasionally the febrile response is slight. The bloodstream is not uncommonly invaded during this period. In most instances recovery is apparent by the sixth to seventh day. The local lesion begins to fade in the center, with some desquamation and pigmentation. No scarring results unless abscesses develop.

Before the introduction of chemotherapy, the fatality rate was about 15 percent. During the first 6 months of life approximately 65 percent of patients die, while in older children and young adults the death rate is low. In patients with fatal infections the lesion is likely to involve the trunk.

BACTEREMIA Streptococci are a common cause of bacteremia, but in uncomplicated tonsillitis and pharyngitis the organisms rarely invade the bloodstream. Bacteremia occurring under the age of twenty usually is secondary to otitis media, mastoiditis, or thrombosis of the lateral or cavernous sinuses. In adults, invasion of the bloodstream is especially likely to occur in puerperal infections, whereas after the age of forty bacteremia is usually secondary to cellulitis and erysipelas. Metastatic abscesses are infrequent.

The diagnosis of bacteremia is difficult and can be made only by culturing the organisms from the blood. The sudden development of chills and high fever suggests invasion of the bloodstream. There may be arthritis, signs of pneumonia, petechiae, or skin eruptions. In fulminating cases, anemia develops rapidly and jaundice may occur. Without specific therapy the mortality rate is 70 percent.

OTHER STREPTOCOCCAL INFECTIONS Non-group A and anaerobic streptococci as well as viridans streptococci cause a wide variety of infections in human beings. Since these organisms are carried in the upper respiratory and the gastrointestinal tracts, they are opportunistic, invading tissues when resistance is lowered.

Group D streptococci, or enterococci, are a frequent cause of urinary tract infections and peritonitis; less frequently they cause bacterial endocarditis. In this instance, small metastatic abscesses may be observed which rarely develop when the endocarditis is caused by viridans streptococci. Group D organisms cause some urinary tract infections in women and in men with prostatic obstruction. Treatment with ampicillin is effective, but in treating endocarditis penicillin combined with streptomycin, kanamycin, or gentamicin is usually employed (Chap. 132).

Group C streptococci may infect burns and wounds, but they rarely cause pharyngitis or endocarditis. Streptococci of most groups have been isolated from such infections as endocarditis, meningitis, and abscesses in various tissues.

Anaerobic streptococci along with bacteroides (Chap. 159) may be cultured from the mouth, intestinal tract, and vagina, and therefore one or both of these organisms are frequently cultured from septic foci. The majority of infections occur in the perineal and inguinal regions. Thus perirectal, pilonidal, and sebaceous cyst abscesses are commonly associated with this organism. Aspiration of oral debris may result in an abscess in the lung and empyema. Brain abscess arises secondary to infections of the lungs or nasal sinuses. The fact that the brain is relatively avascular may predispose to infections with anaerobic bacteria.

A number of characteristic infections caused by anaerobic streptococci have been described. *Streptococcal myositis* develops slowly and is characterized by marked edema, crepitant myositis, and pain. Many leukocytes and chains of gram-positive cocci are seen in the seropurulent exudate. *Chronic burrowing ulcers* and *progressive synergistic gangrene* are two primarily surgical infections. The former usually develops following surgery and progresses over several months; sinus tracts develop, but pain and systemic reactions are minimal. *Synergistic gangrene,* in contrast, is painful. It develops around stay sutures and gradually spreads, presenting as an ulcer surrounded by gangrenous skin.

TREATMENT

There are now several agents which may be employed in the therapy of aerobic streptococcal infections. The sulfonamides exert a bacteriostatic effect against all Lancefield groups except D. However, some strains of group A streptococci have acquired resistance. Most antibiotics have some antistreptococcal activity, but penicillin clearly is the best antistreptococcal drug because it kills group A organisms. If it is administered for at least 10 days, in most instances all streptococci are eliminated. Therapeutic measures which do not result in the eradication of the infecting organism do not alter the attack rate of rheumatic fever.

The administration of penicillin or other antibiotics within 24 h of the onset of streptococcal respiratory infections results in definite improvement of the symptoms and signs. When therapy is instituted after 48 h, a favorable effect is difficult to demonstrate, but suppurative complications, including sinusitis, otitis media, and peritonsillar cellulitis are prevented. The time that treatment is started is not decisive in the reduction of rheumatic fever; however, early therapy may be important in the prevention of nephritis. In general, proper therapy instituted during the first 24 h of illness will reduce the predicted rheumatic fever attack rate by 95 to 98 percent. If therapy is started 1, 2, or 3 weeks after the onset of sore throat, the reduction in attack rates is 90, 67, and 42 percent, respectively. Therefore, to prevent rheumatic fever, a full course of therapy should be given to those who have recovered from acute-phase symptoms and receive no therapy even though the onset was 3 weeks previously.

In the average case of streptococcal infection, whether scarlet fever, tonsillitis, or erysipelas, sufficient concentration of antibiotic can be maintained readily by a single injection of 600,000 to 1,200,000 units of benzathine penicillin. In patients with rheumatic heart disease who develop a streptococcal infection, it is advisable to administer 600,000 units of procaine penicillin twice daily for 2 weeks.

Oral therapy may be prescribed, but many patients discontinue the medication when the acute symptoms subside. Under these circumstances, the organism frequently invades the tissues again, and a clinical relapse occurs. More important, the attack rate of the nonsuppurative complications is not altered. All forms of oral medication must be taken in full doses for at least 10 days and preferably for 2 weeks. Oral penicillin G should be given in doses of at least 250,000 units four times daily. Penicillin V in dosage of 1 to 2 g daily or phenethicillin may be preferable, because these agents resist degradation by gastric acid. Patients sensitive to penicillin may be given erythromycin in doses of 0.25 g every 6 h. Tetracycline drugs should not be employed because of the high prevalence of resistant strains.

The *sulfonamides* should never be employed in the treatment of streptococcal infections, because they fail to eliminate the infecting organism and do not alter the subsequent attack rate of rheumatic fever. Penicillin decreases the incidence of suppurative complication of tonsillitis and pharyngitis.

Infections of the mastoid and paranasal sinuses should be treated by the parenteral administration of 1.2 to 2.4 million units penicillin G every day. Streptococcal pneumonia should be treated with somewhat larger amounts of penicillin. Empyema, purulent pericarditis, and arthritis are treated best by local instillation of 10,000 to 50,000 units penicillin G every 48 to 72 h until cultures are sterile. In addition, full doses of parenteral penicillin should be administered. In these infections early treatment is required if surgical drainage is to be avoided.

Treatment of streptococcal infections caused by groups other than A with penicillin is usually effective, although some strains of groups D and F are relatively resistant. In treating anaerobic infections, drainage of the abscesses, debridement, and supportive measures are important. Cultures and smears of exudate or aspirate from patients with cellulitis or streptococcal myonecrosis will assist in the selection of the proper antibiotics to be used in addition to penicillin.

PREVENTION

There is no completely adequate method for the prevention of streptococcal infections. A number of procedures will limit the spread of the organism. The problem is exceedingly complicated because group A streptococci occur in the upper part of the respiratory tract of many individuals.

In the past it was customary to isolate all patients with scarlet fever, but this seems unwarranted, particularly because no precautions are taken for sore throat without a rash caused by the same bacterium. Any patient with a streptococcal infection of the upper part of the respiratory tract may be a source of infection. During the acute stage of all such illnesses the patient should be advised against intimate contact with others.

Approximately 90 percent of patients with untreated streptococcal infections continue to carry the organism in the pharynx 3 months after the acute infection. Usually the number of organisms is small. Individuals with suppurative sinusitis are likely to harbor large numbers of streptococci and are a dangerous source of infection. Proper therapy of acute infections with penicillin prevents the development of the carrier state and promptly eliminates the organism.

Individuals or groups can be protected from streptococcal infections by the prophylactic use of sulfonamides. For this purpose 1 g sulfadiazine or sulfisoxazole is administered daily. When given to populations already experiencing an epidemic, this prophylactic measure will control the outbreak as long as the drug is administered. When therapy is discontinued, streptococcal infections again occur because of the failure of sulfonamides to eliminate the infecting organism. For this reason, oral penicillin in doses of 250,000 units two or three times daily for 10 days or a single injection of 1,200,000 units of benzathine penicillin is a preferred form of prophylaxis in large groups. Benzathine penicillin in doses of 600,000 and 1,200,000 units will protect the individual from new infections for 3 or 4 to 6 weeks, respectively.

Tonsillectomy has been employed widely as a prophylactic measure against streptococcal infections because tonsillitis cannot occur if the organ is removed. However, no protection is afforded against streptococcal pharyngitis. Indeed, tonsillectomy makes subsequent recognition of the cause of the respiratory illness more difficult.

REFERENCES

BORNSTEIN DL et al: Anaerobic infections—review of current experience. Medicine 43:207, 1964

DAJANI AS et al: Etiology of cervical lymphadenitis in children. N Engl J Med 268:1329, 1963

HORN KA et al: Group B streptococcal neonatal infection. JAMA 230:1165, 1974

REINARZ JA, SANFORD JP: Human infections caused by non-group A or D streptococci. Medicine 44:81, 1965

STOLLERMAN GH: Nephritogenic and rheumatogenic group A streptococci. J Infect Dis 120:258, 1969

WANNAMAKER LW: Differences between streptococcal infections of the throat and of the skin. N Engl J Med 282:23, 1970

——, MATSEN JM: *Streptococci and Streptococcal Diseases: Recognition, Understanding and Management,* New York: Academic, 1972

section 4 | Diseases caused by gram-negative cocci

136
MENINGOCOCCAL INFECTIONS

HARRY N. BEATY

DEFINITION The meningococcus *Neisseria meningitidis* is the causative organism of a variety of infections, notably meningitis and bacteremia.

ETIOLOGY The organism responsible for "cerebrospinal fever" was first described by Weichselbaum in 1887. It was subsequently assigned to the genus *Neisseria,* and is now designated by the binominal *Neisseria meningitidis* and the common name meningococcus. In stained smears, meningococci are gram-negative and characteristically appear as single cocci or diplococci with flattened adjacent sides. They grow well on solid or semisolid media containing blood, serum, or ascitic fluid, and thrive best at temperatures between 35 and 37°C in an atmosphere reduced in oxygen and containing 5 to 10 percent CO_2. The organism is recovered readily from biologic fluids when fresh specimens are inoculated on warm chocolate agar plates which are incubated 18 to 24 h in a candle jar or in a more sophisticated apparatus that provides a suitable environment.

The biochemical reactions of the *Neisseria* are relatively limited, but they contain cytochrome oxidase, which is responsible for the positive "oxidase" test, and clinically significant species usually are differentiated by their ability to produce acid in glucose, maltose, or sucrose. Typically the meningococcus ferments both glucose and maltose, but on occasion maltose-negative strains have been isolated.

Meningococci can be divided into serologic groups on the basis of agglutination reactions with immune serum. The present classification into groups A, B, C, and D was agreed upon in 1950, but since 1960, new groups including X, Y, and Z have been identified. The major groups are remarkably heterogeneous, but subclassification with bacteriocin typing or additional serologic markers has been possible.

EPIDEMIOLOGY The natural habitat of meningococci is the nasopharynx of man, and no other reservoir or vector has been recognized. The principal means of spread is through inhalation of droplets of infected nasopharyngeal secretions, and it is unlikely that the disease is spread by contact with contaminated fomites. Meningococci cause either epidemic or sporadic disease, and there is a cyclic variation in the prevalence of meningococcal infection with peaks of increased frequency occurring every 8 to 12 years and lasting 4 to 6 years. A minor upward trend in this cycle began in the United States in 1962 and reached a peak in 1965. For the epidemic years 1967 through 1971, the attack rate of meningococcal disease was lower and constant, but subsequently it has declined further. The prevalence of meningococcal infection is also subject to seasonal influences; the lowest attack rate occurs in midsummer and the highest in late winter and early spring. This seasonal variation follows that of other bacterial and viral respiratory infections and may reflect crowded indoor living conditions encountered during the winter months.

The attack rate of meningococcal disease is highest for children between six months and one year of age. A second, much lower, peak in incidence occurs among adolescents, and the lowest attack rate occurs in individuals over twenty-five. There is no clear-cut tendency for racial or sexual predominance, but presumably because of an increased opportunity to acquire infection, males develop meningitis and meningococcemia more frequently than females. Military recruits are particularly susceptible, and worldwide epidemics of meningococcal outbreaks usually parallel less apparent trends in the civilian population.

Since 1915, most epidemics of meningococcal disease have been caused by group A meningococci, and strains of groups B and C have been associated with sporadic, interepidemic infections. However, in the outbreaks of 1963 and 1964 a major shift in the pattern of meningococcal infection became apparent as group B meningococci were isolated from the majority of clinical infections in both civilian and military populations. In 1967, over 70 percent of meningococci isolated were group B. However, early in 1968, another shift began, and in the epidemic years 1969 through 1972, the majority of meningococcal strains submitted to the Center for Disease Control were group C. More recently, group B has again become the most prevalent serogroup isolated in the United States, and group Y is increasing in importance. Group A isolates continue to be encountered infrequently. Coincident with these epidemiologic shifts has been a waxing and waning of the proportion of isolates which are resistant to sulfadiazine. When the majority of meningococci causing disease were group B, most strains were resistant to sulfadiazine. Today, approximately 80 percent are sensitive. Similarly, as group C emerged as the predominant serogroup, sulfadiazine resistance was the rule, but in the epidemic year 1974, about one-third of group C isolates were sensitive. Sulfadiazine resistance has been recognized among isolates of all major serogroups, and future major shifts may occur.

The potential for the meningococcus to produce serious outbreaks of disease has been reemphasized by recent events in Brazil. A large urban epidemic was first recognized in São Paulo in 1971, and it increased in intensity over the next several years. In 1974, the predominant strain of meningococcus producing disease changed abruptly from group C to group A, and the epidemic spread to other major cities in Brazil. In July and August, 1974, about 6,000 confirmed cases of meningococcal disease were admitted to hospitals in São Paulo alone. Massive immunization programs have been implemented, but their effect is still being evaluated.

Carriers Between epidemics, 2 to 15 percent of the individuals in urban centers harbor meningococci in the nasopharynx. When sporadic cases of meningococcal disease occur, the carrier rate in close contacts may rise to 40 percent, and in closed populations or during epidemics, may approach 100 percent. Although some individuals harbor meningococci for months or years, nasopharyngeal infection is usually transient, and in 75 percent of carriers the organism disappears within a few weeks. The relation between the proportion of carriers in a population and the occurrence of meningococcal disease is unclear. Case-to-case transmission of infection is documented rarely, and carriers, not patients, are the foci from which disease is spread. It appears that the prevalence of meningococcal disease can be attributed to the prevailing carrier rate only in a general way, and that the occurrence of clinical disease is most dependent on unknown circumstances within the host which lead to spread of infection beyond the nasopharynx.

Immunity The fact that meningococcal meningitis is primarily a disease of childhood has long suggested that natural immunity develops in most individuals within the first two decades of life. There is a correlation between susceptibility to meningococcal disease and absence of bactericidal antibody in the serum, and the serum of most adults contains antibodies to pathogenic strains of meningococci. Natural immunization appears to result from asymptomatic carriage of meningococci in the nasopharynx. Not only does the carrier state produce antibodies to the infecting strain, but cross-reacting antibodies may develop, even after colonization with avirulent nongroupable organisms. The immunity conferred by meningococcal meningitis or meningococcemia is usually group-specific, and second episodes of meningococcal disease have been encountered only infrequently.

PATHOGENESIS The primary focus of meningococcal infection is the nasopharynx. In most instances, this infection is subclinical, but occasionally localized inflammation occurs and mild symptoms develop. Dissemination of meningococci from the nasopharynx occurs via the bloodstream, and generally is followed by clinical manifestations of meningococcal disease. *Purulent meningitis* is the most common form of metastatic infection encountered and is either associated with signs and symptoms of meningococcemia or constitutes the predominant clinical expression of illness. Organisms in the meninges induce an acute inflammatory reaction, and purulent exudate spreads across the surface of the brain. Rarely, a more extensive inflammatory reaction is responsible for an acute diffuse encephalitis.

Although the mechanisms responsible for the pathologic changes associated with meningococcal infection have not been explained entirely, the tissue injury observed in laboratory animals appears to be caused by an endotoxin which is biochemically and biologically similar to endotoxins of enteric bacilli. It may be responsible for hypotension and vascular collapse observed in fulminant meningococcemia and may also play a role in the pathogenesis of the purpura and visceral hemorrhages associated with meningococcal bacteremia. Thrombosis of dermal venules, adrenal sinusoids, and renal glomerular capillaries is most commonly seen in patients who die of fulminant meningococcemia and is strikingly similar to the pathologic changes observed in the experimental Shwartzman reaction. It is postulated that endotoxin either induces a Shwartzman reaction directly or effects the release of clotting factors which initiate intravascular coagulation and produce these characteristic pathologic changes.

CLINICAL MANIFESTATIONS Ninety to ninety-five percent of patients with meningococcal disease have meningococcemia and/or meningitis.

Meningococcemia Thirty to fifty percent of patients who develop overt disease have meningococcemia without meningitis. The onset of clinical illness may be abrupt, but patients usually have nonspecific prodromal symptoms of cough, headache, and sore throat followed by the sudden development of spiking fever, chills, arthralgia, and muscle pains which may be particularly severe in the lower extremities and back. Patients usually appear acutely ill with an inordinate degree of prostration. In addition to high fever, tachycardia, and tachypnea, mild hypotension may be present. However, clinical shock does not occur unless fulminant meningococcemia supervenes. In the course of meningococcal bacteremia, about three-fourths of the patients develop a characteristic petechial rash. Lesions are frequently sparse, and the axillae, flanks, wrists, and ankles are the most commonly involved sites. Often petechiae are located in the center of lighter-colored macules, and they may become nodular as the disease progresses. The diagnosis of meningococcemia occasionally can be established by demonstrating gram-negative diplococci in scrapings from these nodular lesions. In severe cases, purpuric spots or large ecchymoses develop, and a widespread petechial or purpuric eruption suggests fulminating disease. However, the absence of rash does not necessarily indicate that the illness will be mild.

Fulminant meningococcemia, or the Waterhouse-Friderichsen syndrome, is meningococcemia associated with vasomotor collapse and shock. It occurs in 10 to 20 percent of patients with generalized meningococcal infection, and is associated with a high fatality rate. The onset is abrupt, and profound prostration frequently occurs within a few hours. Petechiae and purpuric lesions enlarge rapidly, and hemorrhage into the skin may be extensive. Early in the preshock stage, there is generalized vasoconstriction; patients are alert and pale, with circumoral cyanosis and cold extremities. Upon entering the shock stage, however, coma develops, the cardiac output decreases, and the blood pressure drops. Unless incipient shock is recognized and appropriate therapy instituted early, death from cardiac and/or respiratory failure almost invariably occurs. Patients who recover may have extensive sloughing of skin lesions and even loss of digits because of gangrene.

Chronic meningococcemia is a rare form of meningococcal infection which lasts for weeks or months and is characterized by fever, rash, and arthritis or arthralgia.

Typically, the fever is intermittent, and during afebrile periods, which may last several days, patients appear remarkably well. The usual rash is a maculopapular or polymorphous eruption which waxes and wanes with the fever, but petechial or nodular lesions may be seen. Joint involvement is present in two-thirds of the patients, and splenomegaly is detected in about 20 percent. If the diagnosis is not suspected or treatment is otherwise delayed, complications such as meningitis, carditis, or nephritis may occur.

Meningitis Meningitis is a common form of meningococcal disease which occurs primarily in children over six months of age and in adolescents. Fever, vomiting, headache, and confusion or lethargy are the commonest symptoms; in about one-fourth of the patients, symptoms begin abruptly and rapidly increase in severity. The more typical patient, however, has symptoms of an upper respiratory tract infection followed by an illness which progresses over several days. Twenty to forty percent of patients have meningitis without clinical evidence of meningococcemia, and the diagnosis depends upon bacteriologic examination of the cerebrospinal fluid. However, when meningitis occurs in association with a petechial or purpuric rash, a presumptive diagnosis of meningococcal disease is warranted, because this pattern of illness is seen only rarely in other infections.

Rarer manifestations The meningococcus is a rare cause of purulent conjunctivitis or sinusitis. Primary pneumonia previously was considered a rare manifestation of meningococcal infection, but increasing numbers of cases are being reported. In one study of military recruits, 69 cases of clinical pneumonia due to group Y meningococci were reported. Bacterial endocarditis also has been reported. On rare occasion, meningococci have produced genital infections clinically indistinguishable from gonococcal disease.

LABORATORY FINDINGS

Aside from bacteriologic data, laboratory studies are of little value in establishing the diagnosis of meningococcal infection. Polymorphonuclear leukocyte counts usually range from 12,000 to 40,000 cells per mm^3, but in meningococcemia, normal or low leukocyte counts may be encountered. Anemia is uncommon, and levels of serum electrolytes and blood urea nitrogen are normal unless shock develops. Patients with prominent hemorrhagic manifestations may have low platelet counts and decreased levels of circulating clotting factors as a result of intravascular coagulation. In meningitis, the cerebrospinal fluid pressure is increased, and the fluid usually contains from 100 to 40,000 polymorphonuclear leukocytes per mm^3. The protein content is increased, and the concentration of glucose is almost always less than 35 mg per 100 ml and often is between 0 and 10 mg per 100 ml.

Meningococci can be recovered readily from cultures of blood or spinal fluid, and, on occasion, material aspirated from skin lesions or joints yields the organism. In addition, gram-negative diplococci may be seen in stains of nodular petechiae or the buffy coat of blood from patients with meningococcemia. In meningococcal meningitis, a smear of the spinal fluid is diagnostic in about half the patients but often shows only a few intracellular bacteria which are located with difficulty.

COMPLICATIONS

Herpes labialis occurs in 5 to 20 percent of patients with meningococcal disease. Other complications, which result from neurologic damage or secondary foci of infection, are uncommon following appropriate treatment and are often transient. Seizures or deafness occur in 10 to 20 percent of patients during the acute stages of meningitis, but postmeningitic epilepsy is rare, and the frequency of permanent eighth nerve damage is probably less than 5 percent. Peripheral neuropathy, cranial nerve palsies, and hemiplegia are seen occasionally, but usually clear completely within 2 to 4 months. Hydrocephalus and thrombosis of venous sinuses, once frequent sequelae of meningococcal meningitis, are encountered rarely. A number of patients complain of recurrent headache, emotional lability, insomnia, backache, memory loss, and difficulty in concentrating for months after an episode of meningitis. The organic basis for these symptoms is obscure, but they usually disappear a year or two after the infection.

Arthritis is a common metastatic complication of meningococcemia and occurs in 2 to 10 percent of patients. As a rule, multiple joints are involved, and signs and symptoms may not appear until after treatment of meningitis or meningococcemia has been instituted. Joint fluid usually contains many granulocytes, but meningococci are recovered infrequently. Antibiotic therapy does not appear to influence the course of the arthritis, and permanent joint changes are rare. Other purulent complications have become extremely uncommon since antibiotics have gained widespread use. Pneumonia occurs occasionally, but it is uncertain whether it is caused by the meningococcus or coincident infection with other bacteria. Bacterial endocarditis is quite rare, but *a high proportion of patients who die of meningococcal infection have myocarditis.* The etiology of these myocardial changes is uncertain, but cardiac failure may be an important factor in the pathogenesis of the shock syndrome in meningococcemia. A pericardial friction rub or electrocardiographic change of pericarditis is seen in about 5 percent of patients, and rarely purulent pericarditis may develop.

DIAGNOSIS

The diagnosis of meningococcal disease depends upon recovering *N. meningitidis* from cultures of blood, spinal fluid, or petechial scrapings from patients with a typical clinical picture. Where available, counterimmunoelectrophoresis of serum or spinal fluid to detect meningococcal antigen may be helpful. Recovery of meningococci from the nasopharynx does not, in itself, establish the diagnosis.

Few diseases need to be considered seriously in the differential diagnosis of meningococcal disease. If meningococcal meningitis is not accompanied by manifestations of bacteremia, it is indistinguishable from meningitis caused by other common pathogens. Occasionally, the common viral exanthems, Rocky Mountain spotted fever (Chap. 180), and vascular purpuras may be confused with meningococcemia, and their differentiation depends upon demonstration of the organism and knowledge of the epidemiology and clinical manifestations of each disease.

TREATMENT Antimicrobial therapy of suspected or documented meningococcal disease should be instituted as early as possible. Penicillin G is the drug of choice, and should be administered intravenously. The dosage for the treatment of meningitis in adults is 12 to 24 million units per day, and in the pediatric age group, 16 million units per square meter (day). Meningococcemia can be treated with 5 to 10 million units a day, because it is not necessary to achieve high levels of antibiotic in the spinal fluid. If treatment with these doses is continued for a minimum of 7 days, or 4 to 5 days after the patient becomes afebrile, relapse is extremely rare. Ampicillin in doses of 200 to 400 mg per kg (day) is as effective as penicillin G, and has been recommended for initial treatment of meningitis in children because it is effective against most *Hemophilus influenzae.* When bacteriologic confirmation of meningococcal disease is available, however, treatment should be switched to penicillin G because it is less costly. Meningococci are susceptible to other antimicrobial agents such as chloramphenicol and tetracycline, but they should not be used unless a patient is allergic to penicillin. Under these circumstances, chloramphenicol hemisuccinate 4.0 to 6.0 g per day in divided doses (in adults) is an acceptable alternate. Sensitivity tests usually indicate that cephalothin could be a suitable alternative to penicillin, but treatment failures with this drug have been reported. *Because a significant proportion of meningococci isolated are resistant to sulfonamides, these drugs should not be used alone in the treatment of meningococcal infections,* and their use in combination with penicillin offers no advantage.

Patients with meningococcal infections require supportive treatment as well as antimicrobial therapy. Maintenance of fluid and electrolyte balance and prevention of respiratory complications in comatose patients are of primary concern. When shock occurs, visceral perfusion must be improved by maintenance of an adequate intravascular volume, treatment of heart failure, and support of the blood pressure. Vasoactive drugs should be employed according to the pathophysiologic derangement in each individual case. These derangements can be determined best by carefully monitoring the blood pressure, pulse, arterial blood gases, cardiac output, peripheral resistance, pulmonary artery wedge pressures, and arteriovenous oxygen differences. When blood pressure must be raised immediately, norepinephrine may be indicated. However, if improved tissue perfusion is the primary goal, an agent such as dopamine is likely to be more effective. When heart failure is present, diuretics and digitalis should be given. When intravascular coagulation is recognized, treatment with heparin, whole blood, or fibrinogen can be tried, but dramatic results should not be expected. Massive doses of adrenal cortical steroids as used in the treatment of septic shock (Chap. 129) may be helpful, but lower "replacement" doses are of uncertain value.

PREVENTION With the widespread emergence of sulfonamide-resistant meningococci, alternate methods of preventing meningococcal disease in closed populations were sought. High molecular weight polysaccharide antigens from organisms of serogroups A and C have been shown to induce a group-specific bactericidal antibody response after subcutaneous injection. Large-scale field trials with the group C vaccine led to a 90 percent reduction in group C disease among vaccinated recruits. Similar results are expected with the group A vaccine, and when a suitable antigen from group B organisms is available, it is likely that a highly effective polyvalent vaccine can be developed.

For intimate contacts of sporadic cases of meningococcal disease, chemoprophylaxis should be considered. If the organism isolated from the patient is sensitive to sulfonamides, these drugs are preferred for prophylaxis. When sensitivities are not known or the organism is resistant to sulfonamides, rifampin in dosage of 600 mg a day for 4 days or minocycline in dosage of 100 mg every 12 h for 5 days can be expected to temporarily eradicate the carrier state and minimize spread of meningococci. Because of some reports of a high incidence of vestibular symptoms with minocycline, rifampin is considered by some to be the drug of choice. However, in large populations, rifampin may not be effective because of rapid appearance of rifampin resistance.

PROGNOSIS Before the introduction of antibiotics, meningococcal meningitis, and meningococcemia were almost invariably fatal. With prompt and appropriate chemotherapy, the mortality rate of meningitis without fulminant meningococcemia has dropped to less than 10 percent in the United States, and neurologic sequelae are rare. The mortality of fulminant infection remains high primarily because patients are often in irreversible shock when treatment is instituted. Most deaths occur within 24 to 48 h of admission, and the capacity of the meningococcus to kill a perfectly healthy individual within a few hours remains one of the most awesome characteristics of this disease.

REFERENCES

ARTENSTEIN MS et al: Prevention of meningococcal disease by group C polysaccharide vaccine. N Engl J Med 282:417, 1970

DAVIS CE, ARNOLD K: Role of meningococcal endotoxin in meningococcal purpura. J Exp Med 140:159, 1974

DEMORAIS JS et al: Epidemic disease due to serogroup C *Neisseria meningitidis* in São Paulo, Brazil. J Infect Dis 129:468, 1974

GOLDSCHNEIDER I et al: Human immunity to the meningococcus: I. The role of humoral antibodies. J Exp Med 129:1307, 1969

MANIOS SG et al: Fulminant meningococcemia. Scand J Infect Dis 3:127, 1971

MCCORMICK JB et al: Trends in disease caused by *Neisseria meningitidis:* 1972 and 1973. J Infect Dis 130:212, 1974

137 GONOCOCCAL INFECTIONS

KING K. HOLMES

DEFINITION Gonorrhea, an infection of columnar and transitional epithelium caused by *Neisseria gonorrhoeae,* is the most common reportable communicable disease in the United States. Anatomic sites which can be infected directly by the gonococcus include the urethra, anal canal, conjunctivas, pharynx, and endocervix. Local complications include endometritis, salpingitis, peritonitis, and bartholinitis in the female, and periurethral abscess and epididymitis in the male. Systemic manifestations of gonococcemia include arthritis, dermatitis, endocarditis, and meningitis as well as myopericarditis and hepatitis.

ETIOLOGY *Neisseria gonorrhoeae* is a gram-negative diplococcus which forms oxidase-positive colonies and is differentiated from other *Neisseria* by its ability to ferment glucose, but not maltose, sucrose, or lactose. Occasionally, fastidious strains of *N. gonorrhoeae* repeatedly fail to ferment glucose but can be identified by specific immunofluorescent staining.

At least four morphologically distinct forms of colonies occur when gonococci are passed in vitro. Colony forms T_1 and T_2 retain virulence during repeated selective subculture in vitro and are covered by surface projections called *pili,* which are visible on electron microscopy. Spontaneous transition to colony forms T_3 and T_4 results in some loss of virulence, together with disappearance of pili. Gonococcal strains cannot be differentiated by colonial morphology since each strain gives rise to all colony forms. However, gonococcal strains now can be typed on the basis of nutritional auxotrophic requirements (auxotyping) or surface antigenic variation.

EPIDEMIOLOGY The only natural host for *N. gonorrhoeae* is man, although chimpanzees have been inoculated experimentally and have subsequently transmitted the infection during intercourse. An estimated 3 million cases of gonorrhea were treated in the United States in 1975. Teenagers compose nearly 25 percent of cases, while 90 percent are age thirty or under. The annual incidence rate of reported gonorrhea in the United States began to increase dramatically in 1964 and more than tripled between 1963 and 1975. The main contributing factor was probably the introduction of oral contraceptives and the intrauterine contraceptive device in the early sixties. The incidence rate of gonorrhea in the early seventies has stabilized in the United Kingdom and fallen in Scandinavian countries but continues to climb in the United States. The reported incidence rate in the United States is now three times higher than in England and Wales. The true incidence rate is probably nearly 10 times higher in the United States, since reporting of gonorrhea is far more complete in the United Kingdom, where most patients with gonorrhea are seen in public clinics for sexually transmitted diseases. Suboptimal clinical practice, including use of subcurative therapy and especially failure to trace infected contacts, probably contributes to the higher incidence rate in the United States.

Gonorrhea incidence and prevalence rates are known to be related to age, sex, race, socioeconomic status, and marital status—risk factors which influence sexual behavior, illness behavior, and accessibility of health care. The highest rates occur at ages eighteen to nineteen, in noncaucasians, in the poor, in large cities, and in unmarried persons—particularly those who live alone. The incidence is perceived as highest in men, while the prevalence is perceived as highest in women. The prevalence rate is so high among women in the United States that endocervical cultures are advocated for gonorrhea case detection in asymptomatic women age thirty or under. Approximately 2 to 3 percent of women routinely tested by private physicians have gonorrhea. Unfortunately, there is now greater reliance in the United States upon routine endocervical culturing than upon contact tracing, which is far more efficient for control of gonorrhea. The single most important axiom about the epidemiology of this disease is that *gonorrhea is usually spread by carriers who have no symptoms or have ignored symptoms.* Symptomatic patients, male or female, have usually been recently infected by such carriers, who must in turn be traced and treated to prevent reinfection. *Men and women with symptomatic gonorrhea should always be interviewed to identify their recent sex contacts, who should be examined and treated if infected.*

There are interesting regional differences in the antibiotic resistance of *N. gonorrhoeae.* Resistance is greatest in Southeast Asia and Africa where prophylactic or low-dose therapy is common; intermediate in the United States and Australia; and least in Scandinavia, the United Kingdom, and Western Europe. Increasing levels of gonococcal resistance to penicillin G and tetracycline were noted during the 1960s in the United States, where subcurative therapy was common and importation of resistant strains occurred during the Vietnam war. From 1970 through 1975, no further increase in resistance to these antibiotics has been noted in the United States.

CLINICAL MANIFESTATIONS The clinical spectrum of gonococcal infections depends upon the site of inoculation, the duration of infection, and the presence or absence of local or systemic spread of the organism.

Gonorrhea in the male The usual incubation period of gonococcal urethritis ("clap") in the male is 2 to 6 days following exposure, although longer intervals are not infrequent, and some men never develop symptoms. Symptoms include a purulent urethral discharge, usually associated with dysuria and frequent urination. Although approximately 90 to 95 percent of men who acquire urethral gonococcal infection develop urethral discharge, most symptomatic men seek treatment and are removed from the infectious pool. The remaining men who never develop symptoms or who ignore their symptoms constitute about two-thirds of the infected men at any point in time, and they serve as the source of spread of infection to women. Before antibiotic treatment became available, symptoms of urethritis persisted for an average of 8 weeks, and unilateral epididymitis occurred in 5 to 10 percent of untreated men. Epididymitis is now an uncommon complication, and gonococcal prostatitis occurs rarely, if at all. Most cases of epididymitis and virtually all cases of prostatitis in young men are not gonococcal, and the specific etiology is not known. Other local complications of gonorrhea which are now unusual include inguinal lymphadenitis, edema of the penis due to dorsal lymphangitis or thrombophlebitis, submucous inflammatory "soft" infiltration of the urethral wall, paraurethral abscess or fistula, unilateral inflammation or abscess of Cowper's gland (which lies between the thumb and forefinger when the forefinger is in the anal canal and the thumb is positioned anteriorly on the perineum), abscess of Tyson's gland(s) (which open on either side of the frenulum), and, rarely, seminal vesiculitis.

In homosexual men, anorectal and pharyngeal gonococcal infection are common. Anorectal infection may be asymptomatic from the outset or may produce anorectal burning or pruritus, tenesmus, and a bloody, mucopurulent rectal discharge. Proctoscopy is essential to exclude syphilis, lymphogranuloma venereum, granuloma inguinale, and other conditions which cause similar symptoms. These symptoms may subside without treatment, leaving a chronic asymptomatic carrier state. Pharyngeal gonococcal infection occurs in approximately 20 percent of homosexual men or heterosexual women who engage in fellatio with men who have urethral infection. Pharyngeal infection may produce exudative tonsillitis but frequently is asymptomatic.

Gonorrhea in the female Acute uncomplicated gonorrhea in the female often causes dysuria, frequent urination, increased vaginal discharge due to exudative endocervicitis, abnormal menstrual bleeding, and anorectal discomfort. While dysuria and frequency in young men arouse the suspicion of gonococcal urethritis, the same symptoms in a young woman are often automatically attributed to "cystitis." Actually, only about one-half of young women with these symptoms are found to have at least 10^5 coliform bacteria per ml of clean voided midstream urine, while many of those without significant bacteriuria have gonococcal infection of the urethra and of Skene's glands. Young women with dysuria should have a pelvic examination and endocervical culture for gonorrhea. Compression of the urethra through the anterior vaginal wall against the symphysis pubis may express urethral exudate which can be examined by Gram's stain and culture. Acute symptoms of gonococcal urethritis in the female may subside spontaneously or following subcurative therapy with sulfonamides or urinary antiseptics. The proportion of women with gonorrhea who never develop symptoms is undefined.

Asymptomatic gonococcal infection in the female involves the endocervix, urethra, anal canal, and pharynx, in decreasing order of frequency. Extension of infection from the endocervix to the fallopian tubes occurs in at least 15 percent of women with gonorrhea. This tends to occur soon after acquisition of infection or during menstruation and results in *acute salpingitis,* the major complication of gonorrhea. Extension of infection to the pelvis may produce signs of pelvic peritonitis, accompanied by nausea and vomiting, and may lead to pelvic abscess. Early antibiotic treatment, before development of adnexal masses, restores normal tubal function and fertility in nearly all cases of salpingitis. However, if prominent adnexal swelling has occurred before treatment is begun, bilateral tubal dysfunction occurs in 15 to 25 percent.

Spread of gonococci into the upper abdomen may cause *gonococcal perihepatitis* (Fitz-Hugh–Curtis syndrome) manifested by right upper quadrant or bilateral upper abdominal pain and tenderness, and occasionally by a hepatic friction rub.

Acute inflammation of Bartholin's gland is usually unilateral and frequently is due to gonococcal infection. The acutely infected duct is surrounded by a red halo and exudes pus at the posterior third of the labium majus. Occlusion of the duct results in formation of a Bartholin's abscess. Chronic Bartholin cysts are rarely caused by active gonococcal infection.

There is suggestive evidence that endocervical gonococcal infection is associated with prematurity and prolonged labor following rupture of membranes, both of which may produce increased perinatal morbidity.

Gonorrhea in children During childbirth, the gonococcus may infect the conjunctivas, pharynx, respiratory tract, or anal canal of the newborn. The risk of contamination increases with prolonged rupture of membranes. Prevention of gonococcal ophthalmia by prophylactic use of 1% silver nitrate eyedrops has led to the emergence of inclusion conjunctivitis caused by *Chlamydia* as a more common form of ophthalmia neonatorum. During the first year of life, infection of the infant usually results from accidental contamination of the eye or vagina by an adult. Between one year of age and puberty, most cases of gonorrhea involve vulvovaginitis in females who have been molested by a relative, and medicolegal considerations necessitate a complete bacteriologic diagnosis.

Disseminated gonococcal infection In some areas of the world, from 1 to 3 percent of adults with gonococcal infection develop gonococcemia. Approximately two-thirds of such patients are women. The majority of men and women with gonococcemia do not have symptoms of urogenital, anorectal, or pharyngeal gonococcal infection. Gonococcemia may occur soon after acquisition of new infection or later, during menstruation. There is suggestive evidence that gonococci which cause disseminated infection are uniquely resistant to the complement-mediated bactericidal activity of normal human serum. These organisms tend to be fastidious strains with distinctive nutritional requirements. Patients with deficiency in the sixth and eighth components of complement have been reported to have increased susceptibility to gonococcemia and meningococcemia, but not to other infections.

The onset of gonococcemia is characterized by fever, polyarthralgias, and papular, petechial, pustular, hemorrhagic, or necrotic skin lesions. Approximately 3 to 20 such lesions appear, usually on the distal extremities. Gonococci are demonstrable by immunofluorescent staining or culture in about two-thirds of gonococcal skin lesions. The initial joint involvement is characteristically limited to tenosynovitis involving several joints asymmetrically. The wrists, fingers, knees, and ankles are most often involved. Without treatment, the duration of gonococcemia is variable; the systemic manifestations of bacteremia may subside spontaneously within a week. (It is possible that many such cases go undiagnosed and the actual risk of gonococcemia exceeds current estimates.) Alternatively, septic arthritis ensues, often without prior symptoms of bacteremia. Pain and swelling then increase in one or more joints, with accumulation of purulent synovial fluid, leading to progressive destruction of the joint if treatment is delayed. A continuum exists from the manifestations of bacteremia (polyarthralgias, new skin lesions) to septic arthritis, but the probability of positive blood cultures decreases sharply after 48 h of illness, and the probability of recovery of gonococci from synovial fluid increases with increasing duration of illness. Gonococci are infrequently recovered from early effusions containing $< 20,000$ leukocytes per mm^3, but are usually recovered from effusions containing $> 80,000$ leukocytes per mm^3. In the individual patient, gonococci are seldom recovered from blood and synovial fluid simultaneously.

Other common manifestations of disseminated gonococcal infection include mild myopericarditis and "toxic" hepatitis. Endocarditis and meningitis are infrequent but severe complications. Endocarditis is suggested by pathologic or changing heart murmurs, major embolic phenomena, severe myocarditis, deterioration of renal function, or an unusually large number of skin lesions.

DIFFERENTIAL DIAGNOSIS Gonococcal infection produces several common clinical syndromes which have multiple etiologies or which mimic other conditions. An approach to the differential diagnosis and management of these syndromes is presented below.

Urethritis in men At the present time in the United States only about one-third of all cases of urethritis in men are caused by *N. gonorrhoeae.* Approximately 40 percent of nongonococcal urethritis (NGU) is caused by *Chlamydia trachomatis.* Some evidence suggests that *Ureaplasma urealyticum* (T-mycoplasma) causes many of the remaining cases of NGU, although this organism often colonizes the urethra of men without urethritis. The urethral discharge produced by *N. gonorrhoeae* is usually profuse, yellow or yellowish-green, and associated with dysuria, whereas nongonococcal urethral exudate is usually demonstrable only by "stripping" the urethra, is white or clear and mucoid, and is less often associated with dysuria. In the individual patient, however, confirmation of gonorrhea by Gram's stain of urethral exudate is required. The Gram's stain is positive for gonorrhea if typical gram-negative diplococci are seen within a neutrophil, equivocal if only extracellular gram-negative diplococci are seen, and negative if no gram-negative diplococci are seen. Culture is most helpful in following up equivocal smears. Patients with equivocal or negative smears should be treated with tetracycline hydrochloride 0.5 g four times daily for 10 days. This is usually adequate for gonorrhea if present.

The sex partner(s) of men with NGU should probably also receive tetracycline in the same dose, since cervical *Chlamydia* infection is demonstrable in most sex partners of men with chlamydial NGU. Men with positive urethral Gram's stain should be treated for gonorrhea as described below.

Vaginitis and cervicitis *Trichomonas vaginalis* produces profuse purulent malodorous vaginal discharge, usually without vulvar pruritus. *Candida albicans* produces vulvar pruritus, vulvovaginitis, and a whitish curd-like discharge comprising mycelia, vaginal epithelial cells, and neutrophils. *Neisseria gonorrhoeae, Herpes simplex,* and probably *Chlamydia trachomatis* produce true cervicitis, which is manifested clinically as increased purulent vaginal discharge. *Herpes simplex* produces ulcerative lesions on the exocervix, while *N. gonorrhoeae* causes capillary dilatation and friability of the endocervix and junctional epithelium. Compression of the cervix between speculum blades expresses purulent exudate and often causes slight bleeding in the acute stages of gonorrhea. This exudate is suitable for examination by Gram's stain if the exocervix has first been thoroughly wiped clean, before the exudate is expressed. *Chlamydia trachomatis* and *T. vaginalis* have been recovered from as many as 60 percent of women with gonorrhea. Thus, in women with abnormal vaginal discharge, *T. vaginalis* should always be excluded by wet-mount examination, and *N. gonorrhoeae* should be excluded by endocervical culture.

Many cases of so-called "cervicitis" in women actually represent cervical ectropion, produced by outward migration of the junctional zone onto the exocervix. This occurs commonly during pregnancy or in women taking oral contraceptives and may cause a clear vaginal discharge. It is often unnecessarily treated by cautery.

The term *nonspecific vaginitis* is applied to abnormal vaginal discharge in the absence of gonorrhea, trichomoniasis, candidiasis, or genital herpes. Inflammation of the vaginal mucosa is seldom demonstrable by colposcopy, and the greyish discharge is usually composed predominantly of vaginal epithelial cells rather than leukocytes. The etiology of this entity is unknown and therapy is empirical.

Pelvic inflammatory disease (PID) The incidence of acute, spontaneous PID, unrelated to obstetrical complications or surgery, can be estimated as about a half-million cases per year in the United States. About 50 percent of these are caused by *N. gonorrhoeae,* alone or in combination with cervicovaginal commensal bacteria. Nongonococcal PID is usually caused by cervicovaginal bacteria, including *Bacteroides fragilis* and anaerobic gram-positive cocci. The peak incidence of gonorrhea occurs in the late summer and autumn each year, and the proportion of cases of PID which are associated with gonococcal infection is also highest during these months.

PID should always be considered in young women with lower abdominal pain and tenderness. Pelvic examination discloses maximal tenderness in the adnexal area, which is usually bilateral and is reproduced by cervical motion. Recent onset of abnormal vaginal discharge or abnormal menstrual bleeding in a patient with abdominal pain strongly suggests PID. Fever, chills, nausea, vomiting, adnexal mass, leukocytosis, and elevation of the erythroctye sedimentation rate are common but are *not always* present. Purulent cervical exudate, onset of pain during menstruation, dysuria, proctitis, and history of recent exposure to a male with urethritis all are more common in gonococcal PID than in nongonococcal PID. The risk of PID is increased two- to ninefold in women wearing an intrauterine contraceptive device (IUD). The risk is maximal during the first 2 months after insertion, but persists as long as the device is in place. IUD-associated salpingitis usually is nongonococcal. There is no fever, and the major manifestation is indolent progression of minimally symptomatic adnexal masses.

Gonococcal perihepatitis may mimic acute cholecystitis, with transient nonvisualization of the gallbladder and mild liver function abnormalities. Perihepatitis should be distinguished from the hepatitis which occurs during gonococcemia. Perihepatitis also occurs as a complication of nongonococcal PID, presumably resulting from spread of other bacteria from the pelvis to the upper abdomen. Bacteremia and suppurative pelvic thrombophlebitis are unusual in acute spontaneously occurring PID.

The clinical diagnosis of PID is imprecise, and failure to

respond to appropriate antibiotic therapy should always lead to reevaluation of the diagnosis before consideration of a change in antibiotics. Laparoscopy may disclose other diagnoses, such as ectopic pregnancy, acute appendicitis, pelvic endometriosis, corpus luteum hematoma, ovarian tumor, mesenteric lymphadenitis, or occasional complications such as tuboovarian abscess.

Acute arthritis The gonococcal arthritis-dermatitis syndrome is probably the commonest form of acute arthritis in young adults, and must be differentiated in particular from Reiter's syndrome, other forms of septic arthritis, acute rheumatoid arthritis, and systemic lupus erythematosus. Gonococcemia may be complicated by myocarditis, which mimics acute rheumatic fever or bacterial endocarditis, and by "toxic" hepatitis, which must be differentiated from hepatitis B viremia. Meningococcemia and *Yersinia* infection are less common causes of acute polyarthritis.

Demonstration of *N. gonorrhoeae* by culture or specific immunofluorescent antibody stain in synovial fluid, blood, cerebrospinal fluid, or skin lesions is diagnostic of acute gonococcal arthritis. Failing this, the diagnosis of gonococcal arthritis is virtually certain if (1) *N. gonorrhoeae* is recovered from the urethra, cervix, pharynx, anal canal, or conjunctiva, or from the patient's sex partner; (2) pustular, hemorrhagic, or necrotic skin lesions are distributed on the extremities; and (3) a therapeutic antibiotic trial produces subjective improvement and normal temperature within 48 h, and loss of all objective signs of arthritis within 2 weeks. Patients with gonococcal arthritis who have highly purulent synovial effusions may, however, have persistent fever and progressive arthritis despite adequate antimicrobial therapy, and may require repeated closed joint irrigations with saline before improvement occurs.

If only two of the above three criteria are met, the diagnosis of gonococcal arthritis remains probable, particularly if other diagnoses listed above are excluded. Conjunctivitis rarely occurs in gonococcal arthritis and suggests the diagnosis of Reiter's syndrome in men with acute arthritis. HL-A histocompatibility haplotype W27 is associated with Reiter's syndrome but not with gonococcal arthritis. Gonococcal arthritis has been reported in several women with active lupus erythematosus, in whom hypocomplementemia may predispose to gonococcemia.

LABORATORY DIAGNOSIS The Gram's stain of urethral or endocervical exudate is considered diagnostic of gonorrhea when typical gram-negative diplococci are seen within leukocytes, is equivocal if only extracellular gram-negative diplococci are seen, and is negative if no gram-negative diplococci are seen. When these criteria are employed by experienced microbiologists, the sensitivity and specificity of Gram's stain of the urethral exudate approach 100 percent. The specificity of Gram's stain of purulent cervical exudate also is high, but the sensitivity is only 60 percent or less. Thayer-Martin (TM) medium, which contains antibiotics to inhibit most other organisms selectively, is most useful for recovering the gonococcus from the endocervix, anal canal, and pharynx, which are colonized by a mixed bacterial flora. After inoculation, the TM medium should be placed in an atmosphere containing 3 to 10 percent carbon dioxide to permit growth of the gonococcus. This can be accomplished in a candle jar, by packaging the TM medium in sealed vials to which carbon dioxide was added before sealing (Transgrow medium), or by generation of carbon dioxide chemically within tubes of media which are sealed after inoculation. Inoculated media should be incubated at 36°C for 48 h, and putative gonococcal colonies should be confirmed by oxidase reaction, Gram's stain, and sugar fermentation tests. The latter are especially important for isolates from the pharynx and anal canal and for cultures obtained from populations which have a low prevalence of gonorrhea, such as prenatal patients.

In men with incubating or chronic asymptomatic urethral infection without exudate, or as a test of cure following treatment, a very thin cotton swab or wire bacteriologic loop should be inserted 2 cm into the anterior urethra and used to inoculate TM medium. Cultures of the pharynx and anal canal should be obtained from all homosexual men with suspected gonorrhea.

The most efficient test for gonorrhea in women is the endocervical culture, which is positive on a single examination in approximately 80 percent of those with gonorrhea. This diagnostic yield can be increased by performing a second endocervical culture on enriched chocolate agar medium which does not contain antibiotics and by performing cultures of the anal canal, urethra, and pharynx.

Standard blood culture broth medium containing 3 to 10 percent carbon dioxide should be used in culturing blood and is also recommended for culturing synovial fluid. In pus from skin lesions, *N. gonorrhoeae* is more often demonstrable by Gram's stain or immunofluorescent staining than by culture. A fourfold or greater rise in gonococcal antibody can be demonstrated in paired serums from many patients with gonococcal arthritis, using complement fixation, immunofluorescent, or gonococcal pili antigen-binding assays, but such tests are not generally available. Techniques designed to detect gonococcal infection by testing of a single serum have been limited thus far by inability to differentiate antibody due to past gonorrhea from antibody due to current infection.

TREATMENT The preferred drugs for gonococcal infection are penicillin G, ampicillin, and amoxicillin. As shown in Table 137-1, the regimen recommended by the Communicable Disease Center (CDC) for uncomplicated urethral, cervical, rectal, or pharyngeal gonococcal infection for both men and women is aqueous procaine penicillin G given with oral probenecid. The recommended dose cures incubating syphilis, and was found to be 97 percent effective for gonorrhea in a national cooperative study from 1972 to 1974. With parenteral penicillin G, the risk of anaphylaxis in patients who deny previous penicillin allergy has been shown to be 0.04 percent. The risk of procaine reaction due to transient neurotoxic serum concentrations of procaine is probably between 0.1 and 1 percent with the currently recommended dosage. Ampicillin 3.5 g (or amoxicillin 3.0 g) can be given orally with probenecid with nearly equal efficacy and less toxicity. A single intramuscular dose of 2 g spectinomycin is adequate for gonorrhea in both sexes and is recommended for treatment failures, because gonococci which demonstrate increased resistance to penicillin, ampicillin, or tetracycline show no cross-resistance to spectinomycin. For pharyngeal gonococcal infection spectinomycin and the ampicillin-probenecid regimen are much less effective than the procaine penicillin or tetracycline regimens.

Either spectinomycin or tetracycline can be used for penicillin-allergic patients. Tetracycline is no longer effective for gonorrhea as a single dose, and hence should be used only for reliable patients. Other tetracyclines are not more effective than tetracycline hydrochloride. Tetracycline has the significant advantage of curing simultaneously acquired *Chlamydia* and *Ureaplasma* infections, thus preventing postgonococcal urethritis (PGU). Usually appearing 2 or 3 weeks after treatment, PGU occurs in up to 50 percent of men treated for gonorrhea with penicillin or ampicillin.

About half of the cases of PGU appear to be caused by *Chlamydia trachomatis* which was probably acquired at the same time as gonorrhea but did not become clinically apparent until later because of the longer incubation period of chlamydial infection. When PGU occurs, it can be managed, like NGU, with tetracycline, 0.5 g four times a day for at least 7 days.

All patients with gonorrhea should have a serologic test for syphilis at the time of diagnosis. Those treated with the recommended procaine penicillin G regimen need not have later follow-up tests for syphilis, since this regimen cures incubating syphilis. In geographic areas where syphilis is endemic, and in all homosexual males, a follow-up serologic test for syphilis is recommended 6 weeks and 3 months after treatment of gonorrhea if ampicillin, spectinomycin, or tetracycline was used. As a test of cure of gonorrhea, follow-up cervical, anal canal, and other appropriate cultures should be obtained from women, and urethral and other appropriate cultures from men, 7 to 14 days after completion of therapy.

Hospitalization is recommended for women with suspected salpingitis if the diagnosis is uncertain and surgical emergencies must be excluded, if there is suspicion of pelvic abscess, if the patient is pregnant or unable to follow an outpatient regimen of oral medication because of nausea and vomiting, or if she is not responding to outpatient therapy. The treatment schedules recommended in Table 137-1 for PID have given satisfactory short-term results in both gonococcal and nongonococcal PID in limited trials, but additional data are needed. It is clear, however, that the single-dose procaine penicillin G–probenecid regimen recommended for uncomplicated gonorrhea is inadequate for the treatment of PID, even for gonococcal PID. In severe cases of PID, especially when pelvic abscess is suspected, treatment must be individualized, and alternative antibiotics and surgical drainage may be needed.

Treatment of gonococcal arthritis, on the other hand, can be accomplished satisfactorily with several regimens. Gonococci recovered from patients with gonococcal arthritis have been significantly less resistant to penicillin or tetracycline than isolates from patients with uncomplicated gonorrhea. However, because of the threat of endocarditis, meningitis, and joint sepsis, all patients with disseminated infection should preferably be hospitalized and treated with aqueous crystalline penicillin G intravenously, 10 million units per day until clinical improvement occurs. Treatment can then be completed on an outpatient basis with

TABLE 137-1
Recommended treatment for gonococcal infection

	Treatment of choice	*Alternative regimens*
Uncomplicated gonorrhea in men and women	Aqueous procaine penicillin G, 4.8 million units, divided and given in two intramuscular injections at one visit, *plus* 1 g probenecid given orally just prior to the injections	Oral, less toxic: Ampicillin 3.5 g orally plus 1.0 g probenecid Treatment failure: Spectinomycin 2 g single intramuscular injection Penicillin allergy: (1) Spectinomycin 2 g intramuscularly, (2) tetracycline 1.5 g orally, followed by 0.5 g orally four times a day for 4 days
Pharyngeal infection	Same as above	Tetracycline 1.5 g orally followed by 0.5 g orally four times a day for 4 days
Gonorrhea in pregnancy	Same as above	Penicillin allergy: (1) Erythromycin 1 g orally followed by 0.5 g four times daily for 4 days (? suboptimal efficacy), (2) cefazolin 2 g intramuscularly plus 1 g probenecid (? cross-allergenic with penicillin), (3) spectinomycin 2 g IM (? fetal ototoxicity)
Acute PID, outpatient	Tetracycline 1.5 g orally followed by 0.5 g four times a day for 10 days	Ampicillin 3.5 g orally plus 1.0 g probenecid followed by ampicillin 0.5 g orally four times daily for 10 days
Acute PID, hospitalized	Aqueous crystalline penicillin G, 20 million units intravenously each day until improved, then 0.5 g ampicillin four times a day to complete 10 days of therapy	The need for additional or alternative antibiotics requires further study. Gentamicin plus clindamycin, or chloramphenicol, is often used for severe nongonococcal PID
Disseminated gonococcal infection	Aqueous crystalline penicillin G, 10 million units intravenously each day until improved, then 0.5 g ampicillin four times a day to complete 7 days of therapy	Penicillin allergy: Tetracycline 1.5 g orally followed by 0.5 g orally four times a day for 7 days
Pediatric gonococcal infection	See "Gonorrhea—CDC recommended treatment schedules," in References.	

ampicillin, 2 g per day orally to complete a 7- to 10-day course of therapy. As summarized in the CDC recommendation, a 3-day course of high-dose intravenous penicillin therapy alone, or treatment with ampicillin, 3.5 g daily orally with 1 g probenecid, followed by 0.5 g four times a day for 7 days, also probably represents adequate therapy for disseminated gonococcal infection. Failure to improve with one of these regimens strongly suggests a diagnosis other than disseminated gonococcal infection. Repeated joint aspiration or closed irrigation of the joint with sterile saline may be required to reduce inflammation in patients with high synovial fluid leukocyte counts. Open drainage is seldom if ever required for gonococcal arthritis. Temporary immobilization of the joint may reduce discomfort for the patient and may be useful during initial ambulation in patients with persistent effusions of the knee or ankle. Antibiotics should not be injected directly into the joint.

Gonococcal conjunctivitis in the adult or newborn should be managed as a medical emergency by irrigation of the conjunctiva with penicillin, together with penicillin G given intravenously.

PREVENTION AND CONTROL There is probably no more striking illustration than gonorrhea of the failure of a specific treatment alone to eradicate a communicable disease. Vaccination is not available, and there is some doubt as to whether any resistance to reinfection occurs during natural infection, although humoral, local, and cellular immune responses have all been demonstrated during acute or recurrent gonococcal infection. Use of the condom can prevent transmission. Prophylactic antibiotics are also effective but are not recommended for general use. The efficacy of local vaginal antiseptic and spermicidal preparations for prevention of venereal disease requires further study. The most effective additional measure now available for control of gonorrhea is tracing sexual contacts of infected patients. Experienced interviewers are able to identify and bring to treatment an average of one additional case for every patient interviewed.

REFERENCES

ESCHENBACH DA et al: Polymicrobial etiology of acute pelvic inflammatory disease. N Engl J Med 293:166, 1975

FALK V: Treatment of acute nontuberculous salpingitis alone and in combination with glucocorticoids. Acta Obstet Gynecol Scan XLIV [Suppl 6]:1965

Gonorrhea—CDC recommended treatment schedules. Morbidity Mortality 23:341, 1974

HOLMES KK et al: Disseminated gonococcal infection. Ann Intern Med 74:979, 1971

——: Gonococcal infections: Clinical, epidemiologic, and laboratory perspectives, in *Advances in Internal Medicine,* vol. 19, ed GH Stollerman, Chicago: Year Book, 1974, p. 259

——: Etiology of nongonococcal urethritis. N Engl J Med 292:1199, 1975

JACOBSEN L, WESTROM L: Objectivized diagnosis of acute pelvic inflammatory disease. Am J Obstet Gynecol 105:1088, 1969

KAUFMAN RE et al: National gonorrhea therapy monitoring study: Treatment results. N Engl J Med 294:1, 1976

TRONCA E et al: Demonstration of *Neisseria gonorrhoeae* with fluorescent antibody in patients with disseminated gonococcal infection. J Infect Dis 129:583, 1974

section 5 | Diseases caused by enteric gram-negative bacilli

138 INFECTIONS DUE TO ENTEROBACTERIACEAE

MARVIN TURCK

ESCHERICHIA COLI INFECTIONS

ETIOLOGY *Escherichia coli* is a group of gram-negative nonsporing rods which belong to the tribe Enterobacteriaceae. They generally ferment lactose, as opposed to the medically significant non-lactose-fermenting organisms, such as *Salmonella, Shigella,* and *Proteus.* The so-called "paracolon" bacilli are organisms which ferment lactose late, irregularly, or not at all, and on more careful biochemical and antigenic testing are found to belong to one or another of the genera of the Enterobacteriaceae, which comprise *Salmonella, Arizona, Citrobacter, Shigella, Escherichia, Klebsiella, Enterobacter, Hafnia, Serratia, Proteus,* and *Providencia.* All these organisms are readily culturable on ordinary media and are aerobic and facultatively anaerobic. All species ferment glucose, reduce nitrates to nitrites, and are oxidase-negative and catalase-positive. They are differentiated among members of their own tribe by biochemical and serologic tests. It is important to make this differentiation, not only taxonomically, but also because of epidemiologic and therapeutic implications.

PATHOGENESIS *Escherichia coli* is regarded generally as a normal commensal in the gastrointestinal tract, from which it may spread to infect contiguous structures if normal anatomic barriers are interrupted, as occurs in appendiceal perforation. It is believed that the urinary tract is infected from without via urethral contamination, but direct hematogenous spread may also account for renal infection. Once infection has occurred in a primary focus, further spread to distant organs may occur via the bloodstream. There is experimental and clinical evidence that *E. coli* tends to settle in avascular or necrotic tissue. In more than

50 percent of *E. coli* infections the urinary tract is the portal of entry; infections of the hepatobiliary tree, peritoneal cavity, skin, and lung are not uncommon. A number of patients with *E. coli* bacteremia have no demonstrable portal of entry; they often have neoplastic and hematologic diseases, and *E. coli* is considered an "opportunistic" invader. There may be other defects in host resistance, including diabetes mellitus, cirrhosis, and sickle-cell anemia, or recent administration of irradiation, cytotoxic drugs, adrenal steroids, or antibiotics. There also is epidemiologic evidence that *E. coli* and other Enterobacteriaceae tend to avidly colonize the skin and mucous membranes of debilitated patients, possibly accounting for the increased frequency of these infections in patients with advanced illness. Morphologically the lesions produced in various tissues show typical acute inflammation with pus and abscess formation. There is a common misconception that *E. coli* bacterial infections are characterized by a foul-smelling, feculent exudate. Such an odor is caused by anaerobic streptococci or *Bacteroides* species, which are often associated with coliform bacteria in mixed infection. In fact, organisms of the genus *Bacteroides* frequently far outnumber *E. coli* as the most prevalent gram-negative flora in the intestine.

EPIDEMIOLOGY Strains of *E. coli* are characterized by their somatic (O), flagellar (H), and capsular (K or B) antigens, and there are hundreds of different serologic varieties. Any of the strains is capable of causing disease. Clinical and epidemiologic studies have demonstrated that certain specific *E. coli* serotypes are more frequently incriminated in diarrheal disease of the infant and newborn, that is, 026:B6, 055:B5, 0111:B4, and 0127:B8. Strains incriminated in infantile diarrhea probably are disseminated within nurseries by symptomatic or asymptomatic infant carriers, mothers, and nurses. Although fecal contamination is the usual mode of spread, airborne contamination and fomite spread may also occur.

Some epidemiologic studies have suggested that *E. coli* 04, 06, and 075 are responsible for most *E. coli* infections other than infantile diarrhea. It is unclear whether these strains actually are more virulent or merely are more prevalent than other somatic types. In fact, virulence factors may be associated more closely with the K than with the somatic antigen, and may account for the frequency in which certain strains cause parenchymal infection.

MANIFESTATIONS Urinary tract infections *Escherichia coli* accounts for well over 75 percent of urinary tract infections, including cystitis, pyelitis, pyelonephritis, and asymptomatic bacteriuria. Strains cultured from patients with acute, uncomplicated urinary tract infections are almost invariably *E. coli,* whereas other Enterobacteriaceae and strains of *Pseudomonas* become prevalent among patients with chronic infection. Urinary tract infections are discussed in Chap. 277.

Peritoneal and biliary infections *Escherichia coli* can usually be cultured from a perforated or inflamed appendix or from abscesses secondary to perforated diverticula, peptic ulcers, subphrenic or lesser sac abscesses, mesenteric infarction, etc. Often, other organisms, including anaerobic streptococci, clostridia, and bacteroides, are found along with *E. coli.* Acute cholecystitis with gangrene and perforation is often associated with *E. coli* infection. An air-fluid level associated with stones or a circumferential layer of gas in the wall of the gallbladder may be detectable by x-ray and is characteristic of acute emphysematous cholecystitis. From the gallbladder, infection may ascend via the biliary tree to produce cholangitis and multiple liver abscesses. More rarely *E. coli* infection in the peritoneal cavity may produce a septic thrombophlebitis of the portal vein (pylephlebitis), which in turn is followed by liver abscesses.

Bacteremia Invasion of the bloodstream is the most serious manifestation of *E. coli* infection; it is characterized usually by the sudden onset of fever and chills, but sometimes only by mental confusion, dyspnea, or unexplained hypotension. It is most common in patients with urinary tract infection and biliary or intraperitoneal sepsis, and following abortions or pelvic surgery. In some patients no portal of entry is evident. Most cases occur in elderly males, presumably because of the high incidence of urethral instrumentation and catheterization in this group. Fever ranges between 100 and 106°F and is higher in younger patients. Hyperventilation may be an early sign. Hypotension may be present from the onset but usually occurs within 12 to 16 h after bacteremia; if it is persistent, it is accompanied by oliguria and often by mental confusion, stupor, and coma. The skin is warm and dry initially, but most patients develop some evidence of peripheral vasoconstriction characterized by cold and cyanotic extremities. Fortunately hypotension is transient and self-limited in most patients with *E. coli* bacteremia and is absent altogether in some. However, about 25 percent of patients with bacteremia develop more prolonged hypotension, a syndrome known as *gram-negative* or *endotoxin shock,* which is discussed in Chap. 129.

Occasionally *E. coli* bacteremia develops in patients with cirrhosis without an overt portal of entry. This has been variably attributed to portosystemic shunts both in and around the liver, impaired reticuloendothelial function, and diminution in humoral and cellular defense mechanisms.

Other manifestations *Escherichia coli* may produce abscesses anywhere in the body. Subcutaneous infections are found at the site of insulin administration in diabetics, in extremities with ischemic gangrene, or in surgical wounds. Perirectal phlegmons are not uncommon in patients with leukemia. Subcutaneous abscesses are often characterized by formation of gas in tissue, especially among diabetics, which may be detected by crepitation or by x-ray and which must be differentiated from clostridial infection. From 5 to 10 percent of patients with *E. coli* bacteremia develop metastatic infection in bone, brain, liver, and lung. *Escherichia coli* may cause pneumonia *de novo;* also, *E. coli* bacilli are often cultured from sputum in pulmonary superinfections.

Neonatal infection Neonates, particularly premature infants, often develop *E. coli* bacteremia associated with meningitis and bloodborne pyelonephritis. Fecal soiling and absence of maternal gamma-G-globulin (IgM) antibody are two of the factors which render this group particularly susceptible to *E. coli* infections.

Gastroenteritis Children under two years of age develop gastroenteritis, typified by nausea, vomiting, and diarrhea. Most outbreaks have occurred in nurseries and have been due to specific strains of enteropathogenic *E. coli* (EPEC). These particular strains may produce a toxin similar to the toxin elaborated by *Vibrio cholerae.* Fluorescent antibody techniques have been most useful in the rapid identification of these organisms. The rapid dehydration, with its attendant high mortality, demands prompt recognition of this condition, isolation of the infants, and treatment of both patients and contacts with the appropriate antibiotic. *Escherichia coli* is also being recognized as a cause of acute diarrheal disease in adults. Diarrhea presumably is mediated through production of an enterotoxin by some strains (Chap. 155). Occasionally, these organisms may invade the mucosa, a form of disease akin to shigella dysentery.

LABORATORY FINDINGS There are no characteristic laboratory abnormalities. The white blood cell count is usually elevated, and there is a preponderance of granulocytes. At times, however, the white count is normal or low. When *E. coli* infection occurs in previously healthy individuals, anemia is absent, but more commonly there is anemia which is usually related to the patient's underlying disease. *Escherichia coli* grows readily in a variety of bacteriologic media and should be cultured from appropriate secretions and blood. In the presence of gram-negative shock, there are often profound metabolic derangements, including azotemia, metabolic acidosis, hypokalemia, and hyperkalemia, as well as a variety of coagulation defects (Chap. 129).

DIAGNOSIS *Escherichia coli* cannot be differentiated from most other gram-negative bacteria on gram stain, and culture followed by appropriate biochemical characterization is necessary to identify the organism precisely. Fluorescent antibody techniques are valuable for identifying EPEC. In addition, serologic typing of *E. coli* may be useful in individual patients with recurrent urinary tract infections in order to help differentiate between relapse and reinfection.

TREATMENT As with other infections, drainage of pus and removal of foreign bodies are essential. If *E. coli* is suspected as the etiologic agent in a particular infection, choice of an appropriate antimicrobial will depend upon the site and type of infection as well as upon its severity. Often the outcome of the infection depends upon the status of the associated disease, rather than on eradication of bacteria. For example, in acute, uncomplicated urinary tract infection in females, the disease is frequently self-limited even without antimicrobial therapy, and there is no evidence that antibiotics are superior to sulfonamides. Conversely, *E. coli* bacteremia in a patient with leukemia may not respond to antimicrobials unless a hematologic remission is achieved simultaneously.

In most situations, antibiotics should be selected, when possible, on the basis of their in vitro sensitivity tests. Although no drug is uniformly active against all strains of *E. coli,* a number of agents are effective against the majority of clinical isolates. If average obtainable plasma concentrations become the criteria for in vitro susceptibility, approximately 75 percent of *E. coli* strains are likely to be sensitive to the tetracyclines, 85 to 90 percent to chloramphenicol or ampicillin, and 90 percent to gentamicin, kanamycin, polymyxin B, or colistin; 50 percent of *E. coli* isolated from hospitalized patients will be inhibited by streptomycin, and 75 to 90 percent by one of the cephalosporin antibiotics. Many strains of *E. coli* are sensitive to high concentrations of penicillin G (50 to 100 μg per ml), and this drug may be used in dosage of 10 to 40 million units intravenously daily, particularly if probenecid is given concomitantly. This regimen has been largely superseded by ampicillin, 2 to 4 g per day intravenously or intramuscularly; for severe infections the dose can be raised to 6 to 12 g per day. The antibacterial spectrum of ampicillin against *E. coli* is probably identical to that achieved with very high concentrations of penicillin G, and to the spectrum covered by the tetracyclines or chloramphenicol. However, the bactericidal properties of ampicillin may be a distinct advantage over these two drugs, particularly in deep-seated infections. Kanamycin sulfate is useful for the initial treatment of serious *E. coli* infections. Severe urinary tract infections refractory to other antimicrobials have responded to 15 mg per kg per day, intramuscularly, in divided doses every 6 to 8 h. In life-threatening infections, kanamycin can probably be used for 24 to 48 h with little hazard of ototoxicity or nephrotoxicity, even in patients with concomitant renal impairment, pending results of in vitro sensitivity tests. However, some isolates of specific serologic strains of hospital-derived *E. coli* from newborns with diarrheal disease have been resistant to kanamycin and neomycin. Gentamicin has been employed effectively in the initial treatment of severe *E. coli* infections in doses of 3 to 5 mg per kg per day in divided doses every 8 h. This drug has superseded kanamycin in the treatment of many patients. Cephalosporins in concentration of 25 μg per ml or less are effective against many *E. coli* strains. This serum concentration can be obtained only with 1.5- to 2.0-g dosages at 3- to 4-h intervals. Although cephalothin and cefazolin are highly effective against many common pathogens, peak serum concentrations after standard doses barely reach or may fall short of requirements for *E. coli.* Tetracyclines and chloramphenicol are still widely used in the treatment of *E. coli* infection, but better drugs are now available. Polymyxin B and colistin are also effective in vitro against the majority of *E. coli.* However, it is difficult to obtain adequate tissue and serum concentrations with these agents, and they should probably not be used for treatment of systemic *E. coli* infections. Although combinations of antimicrobials, i.e., streptomycin and tetracycline or streptomycin and chloramphenicol, have been recommended, there is little need to employ more than one agent in most situations. Nitrofurantoin (400 mg) and nalidixic acid (2 to 4 g) are reserved for treating patients with *E. coli* bacteriuria, and should not be employed when infection is suspected outside the urinary tract.

PREVENTION Isolation and antimicrobial therapy of infants and contacts are essential to abort epidemic infantile diarrhea. In adults, many *E. coli* infections are hospital-associated, and their incidence can be reduced by limiting use of indwelling urinary catheters, by careful surgical aseptic technique, by appropriate isolation of infection-prone patients, and by judicious use of antibiotics, steroids, and cytotoxic agents. There is mounting evidence that the promiscuous use of antibiotics may propagate the transfer of resistance factors among intestinal *E. coli.* These organisms may in turn transmit their resistance to other virulent Enterobacteriaceae, such as *Salmonella.*

KLEBSIELLA-ENTEROBACTER-SERRATIA INFECTIONS

ETIOLOGY Next to *E. coli,* strains of *Klebsiella, Enterobacter,* and *Serratia* are the most important enteric organisms infecting man. In many laboratories *Klebsiella* are, in general, more resistant to antibiotics, and their isolation from blood, purulent exudates, and urine is of more serious epidemiologic and prognostic significance. The Friedlä nder bacilli (*K. pneumoniae*) are encapsulated gram-negative bacilli, found among the normal flora of the mouth and intestinal tracts. *Klebsiella pneumoniae* has been considered to be a virulent respiratory pathogen since first described by Friedländer in 1882. *Klebsiella* is closely related to the genera *Enterobacter* and *Serratia* and may be differentiated only by certain amino acid decarboxylase tests. In addition to differentiation by these biochemical tests, which group *Klebsiella, Enterobacter,* and *Serratia,* strains of *Klebsiella* usually are nonmotile and form large mucoid colonies on solid media, whereas the other species are typically motile. Klebsiellas also are usually sensitive to concentrations of cephalosporin antibiotics, to which *Enterobacter* and *Serratia* are resistant. These characteristics, however, are not invariable enough to differentiate various isolates from clinical sources. Strains of *Klebsiella* can be further distinguished on the basis of type-specific capsular antigens; more than 75 known capsular types have been identified. There is little evidence that certain types are more virulent than others, and the main role of capsular typing of *Klebsiella* is as an epidemiologic tool in nosocomial outbreaks of infection. The significance of *Enterobacter* and *Serratia* in human infections has been less well clarified than of infections secondary to *Klebsiella,* but all are potential pathogens, especially as opportunistic invaders in the compromised host.

Klebsiella rhinoscleromatis is probably the causative agent of rhinoscleroma, and *K. ozenae* has been isolated occasionally from the nose of patients with ozena, a chronic severe rhinitis associated with turbinate atrophy and progressive anosmia.

PATHOGENESIS *Klebsiella, Enterobacter,* and *Serratia* are all capable of causing disease in diverse anatomic sites. However, results of clinical and epidemiologic studies suggest that differences in pathogenicity may exist among these genera and that precise taxonomic identification is of value. Although infections of the respiratory tract with *K. pneumoniae* have been emphasized most in the past, the urinary tract presently accounts for the majority of clinical isolates. In this site clinical manifestations and pathogenesis are similar to infections produced by *E. coli,* but klebsiellas are more frequently found in patients with complicated and obstructive urinary tract disease. Infections of the biliary tract, the peritoneal cavity, the middle ear, mastoids, paranasal sinuses, and meninges also are not uncommon. In these locations, *Klebsiella* is more frequent than either *Enterobacter* or *Serratia* and is more likely to produce an illness of greater severity. The apparent increased frequency of infection by serratias represents an increase primarily due to nosocomial spread of this organism.

MANIFESTATIONS Symptoms and signs of common infections caused by *Klebsiella*—namely, those involving the urinary tract, biliary tree, and peritoneal cavity—are indistinguishable from those caused by *E. coli.* These infections commonly occur in diabetics and in the form of superinfections in patients who have received antimicrobials to which these organisms are resistant. *Klebsiella* infection is also an important etiologic factor in septic shock (Chap. 129).

Pneumonia *Klebsiella* is well recognized as a pulmonary pathogen, but probably accounts for less than 1 percent of all cases of bacterial pneumonia. The disease is most common in men over forty years of age and is more frequently found in alcoholics. Other factors associated with increased susceptibility include diabetes mellitus and chronic bronchopulmonary disease. Aspiration of oropharyngeal secretions containing *Klebsiella* organisms is the likely inciting factor among alcoholic patients. The clinical manifestations are indistinguishable from those of pneumococcal pneumonia (Chap. 133), with sudden onset of chills, fever, productive cough, and severe pleuritic chest pain. Patients are frequently delirious and prostrated, but this may also occur with pneumococcal infection. A "characteristic" clinical feature, which occurs in only 25 to 50 percent of patients, is the dark-brown or red-currant-jelly sputum which may be so tenacious that the patient has difficulty in expelling it from his mouth and lips. The pulmonary lesion is most frequent in the right upper lobe but often rapidly progresses and, if untreated, may spread from lobe to lobe. Cyanosis and dyspnea develop rapidly, and jaundice, vomiting, and diarrhea may be present. Physical findings consist primarily of signs of consolidation unless pleural effusion or necrotizing pneumonitis with rapid cavitation has intervened. The blood leukocyte count may be elevated but is often low, which probably is merely a reflection of severe infection in an alcoholic patient with poor bone marrow reserve and folate deficiency. Lung abscess and empyema are much more frequent than in pneumococcal pneumonia and are related to the destructive capabilities of this organism. So-called "characteristic" and radiographic features such as bulging fissures and loss of lung volume occur only occasionally, and also may be found in pneumococcal infection, as well as in necrotizing pneumonia caused by other gram-negative species.

Chronic infection of the lung Rarely, infection with *Klebsiella* may progress, often in indolent fashion, to a chronic necrotizing pneumonitis resembling tuberculosis. It may follow acute *Klebsiella* pneumonia but is also seen in patients who give no history of an acute onset. The principal symptoms are productive cough, weakness, and anemia. Hemoptysis, chronic empyema, or sterile serous effusions are also encountered. Cavitation, frequently with thin walls, occurs primarily in the upper lobes.

DIAGNOSIS Diagnosis is established by an awareness of the clinical setting in which *Klebsiella* infections occur and by isolation of the organism. A presumptive diagnosis of *Klebsiella* pneumonia should be made on the basis of gram stain of the sputum which shows a predominance of short, plump, gram-negative bacilli, frequently surrounded by a clear space because of the capsule. Often these gram-negative organisms occur together with gram-positive cocci, and because the gram-positives are easier to see, the gram-negative bacteria may be ignored and the diagnosis may be missed, which, in turn, may lead to potentially serious delays in instituting therapy. Additional proof of *Klebsiella* infection in the lung is afforded by isolation of the organisms from blood and pleural exudate. In extrapulmonary infections, the organisms are readily seen in and cultured from pus or secretions of involved organs.

TREATMENT *Klebsiella, Enterobacter,* and *Serratia* have variable susceptibility to antimicrobial drugs, and cultures of these organisms need to be tested in vitro. Frequently, however, antimicrobial therapy needs to be instituted before results of antibiotic susceptibility tests become available. In general, the majority of strains of *Klebsiella* is susceptible to gentamicin, kanamycin, cephalosporins, chloramphenicol, and polymyxin B or colistin. *Klebsiella* isolates do not respond to penicillin and its analogues, although many isolates of *Enterobacter* are inhibited by 25 μg per ml carbenicillin. The antimicrobial regimen of choice in the treatment of *Klebsiella, Enterobacter,* and *Serratia* infection will vary from one institution to another and will depend upon the degree of clinical severity of infection. In severely ill patients, the combination of an aminoglycoside such as gentamicin (5 mg per kg per day) or kanamycin (15 mg per kg per day) with cephalothin, cephapirin, or cefazolin (6 to 12 g per day) is usually preferred. Because of the relatively poor blood and tissue levels obtained with the polymyxins, they should not be employed as first-line agents in the treatment of severe *Klebsiella* infections despite apparent in vitro susceptibility. Regardless of the antimicrobial regimen employed, treatment should be continued for a minimum of 10 to 14 days and prolonged if there is extensive cavitation. Pleural effusions must be drained; antibiotic therapy alone is not sufficient treatment for closed-space infections of the pleural cavity. At times, rib resection with open drainage may be necessary, and should be considered if effusions recur.

PROGNOSIS Prior to the introduction of antimicrobials, the fatality rate reported in different clinics varied from 50 to 80 percent, and death within 48 h was not infrequent. Even with antimicrobial treatment the course of the disease is quite variable and the prognosis must be guarded. For the most part, this prognosis reflects the age group involved and the frequent association of *Klebsiella* infection with alcoholism, malnutrition, and severe underlying disease.

PROTEUS INFECTIONS

ETIOLOGY The genus *Proteus* consists of gram-negative bacilli which do not ferment lactose and are characterized by their active motility and spreading growth on solid media. There are four pathogenic species: *P. mirabilis, P. vulgaris, P. morganii,* and *P. rettgeri. Proteus mirabilis* causes 75 to 90 percent of human infections and is distinguishable from the other three species by its inability to form indole. All four split urea, with production of ammonia. Some strains of *P. vulgaris* share a common antigen with certain rickettsia, accounting for the appearance of antibodies against *Proteus* organisms (Weil-Felix reaction) in typhus, scrub typhus, and Rocky Mountain spotted fever. The *Providence* group of organisms resembles those of the genus *Proteus* closely except that it fails to produce a urease.

EPIDEMIOLOGY AND PATHOGENESIS Members of the genus *Proteus* are normally found in soil, water, and sewage and are part of the normal fecal flora. Occasionally, they have been implicated as a cause of epidemic diarrhea in infants, but the evidence of this is inconclusive. The organism is frequently cultured from superficial wounds, draining ears, and sputum, particularly in patients who have received antibiotics, and replaces the more susceptible flora eradicated by these drugs. *Proteus* organisms often localize in already damaged tissues, where they produce a typical exudative inflammatory reaction.

MANIFESTATIONS *Proteus* organisms are rarely primary invaders but produce disease in locations previously infected by other organisms. These locations include the skin, ears and mastoid sinuses, eyes, peritoneal cavity, bone, urinary tract, meninges, lung, and bloodstream.

Cutaneous infections *Proteus* organisms are frequently isolated from surgical wounds, particularly following antimicrobial therapy, but they do not interfere with normal wound healing provided that the tissues are viable and foreign bodies are not present. Burns, varicose ulcers, and decubiti may become contaminated with *Proteus* organisms, often in company with other gram-negative organisms or staphylococci.

Infections of the ears and mastoid sinuses Otitis media and mastoiditis in which *Proteus* organisms are present can result in extensive destruction of the middle ear and mastoid sinuses. Fetid otorrhea, cholesteatoma, and granulation tissue constitute a chronic focus of infection in the middle and inner ears and mastoid, and deafness ensues. Paralysis of the facial nerve is an occasional complication. The great danger of these infections lies in intracranial extension, leading to thrombosis of the lateral sinus, meningitis, brain abscess, and bacteremia.

Ocular infections *Proteus* infection may cause corneal ulcers, usually following trauma to the eye, which occasionally terminate in panophthalmitis and destruction of the eyeball.

Peritonitis Being part of the normal intestinal flora, *Proteus* organisms may be isolated from the peritoneal cavity following perforation of viscera or mesenteric infarction.

Urinary tract infections *Proteus* organisms are a common cause of urinary tract infections, usually in patients with chronic bacteriuria, many of whom have had obstructive uropathy, a history of instrumentation of the bladder, and repeated courses of chemotherapy. The organism is rarely a pathogen in anatomically normal urinary tracts except occasionally in patients with diabetes mellitus. *Proteus* organisms are also often cultured from bacteriuric patients with renal or bladder calculi. This fact may be related to the urease activity of this organism, which renders the urine alkaline and provides a fertile medium for formation of ammonium-magnesium-phosphate stones.

Bacteremia Bloodstream invasion is the most serious manifestation of infection with this organism. In 75 percent of cases, the urinary tract serves as the portal of entry; in the remainder, the biliary tree, gastrointestinal tract, ears and sinuses, and skin are the primary foci. *Proteus* bacteremia is frequently preceded by cystoscopy, urethral catheterization, transurethral prostatic resection, or other operative procedures. Clinically, the signs, symptoms, and laboratory findings of *Proteus* sepsis—high fever, chills, shock, metastatic abscesses, leukocytosis, and rarely thrombocytopenia—are indistinguishable from those of bloodstream infections with other gram-negative bacteria.

DIAGNOSIS The diagnosis of *Proteus* infection depends on culture of the organism from blood, urine, or exudate and its identification by appropriate biochemical tests. It is especially important to separate *P. mirabilis,* the indole-negative species, from *P. morganii, rettgeri,* and *vulgaris,* which are indole-positive, because only *P. mirabilis* is susceptible to the action of penicillin and many other antibiotics. *Proteus* organisms are often present in mixed infections with other pathogens. Particular care should be exercised in the isolation of other organisms growing in the same medium with members of the genus *Proteus* lest they be masked by its spreading growth. The spreading character of this organism may also make antibiotic sensitivity tests difficult to interpret.

TREATMENT Most strains of *P. mirabilis* are sensitive to penicillin in high concentration (10 units per ml or greater), ampicillin, carbenicillin, kanamycin, gentamicin, the cephalosporin antibiotics, and chloramphenicol. *Proteus* bacteriuria can be readily eradicated with any of these drugs during treatment; ampicillin in dosage of 0.5 g every 4 to 6 h is highly effective. In severe infection, therapy should be parenteral: 6 to 12 g ampicillin or 20 million units of penicillin G plus kanamycin or gentamicin in divided doses of 15 mg per kg per day and 5 mg per kg per day, respectively, if renal function is adequate. There is good evidence that kanamycin is synergistic with ampicillin and penicillin G in *Proteus* infections, and that chloramphenicol may be ineffective despite the results of in vitro tests. In view of the numerous more effective agents, there is no reason to use chloramphenicol in *Proteus* infections. In general, all strains of *P. mirabilis* are resistant to tetracycline. Most strains other than *P. mirabilis* and *Providence* bacilli are sensitive only to kanamycin or gentamicin. Gentamicin in particular appears to be effective against indole-positive *Proteus.* In addition, although ampicillin and penicillin G alone are ineffective against indole-positive *Proteus,* a combination of either drug and kanamycin or gentamicin may be synergistic. Carbenicillin, a semisynthetic penicillin, is also effective against the majority of indole-positive *Proteus* species. As with all other gram-negative infections, appropriate attention must be given to drainage of pus, maintenance of fluid and electrolyte status, and treatment of circulatory collapse.

REFERENCES

Escherichia coli infections

CONN HO, FESSEL JM: Spontaneous bacterial peritonitis in cirrhosis. Medicine 50:161, 1971

FIELDS BN et al: The so-called paracolon bacteria. Am J Med 42:89, 1967

TILLOTSON JR, LERNER AM: Characteristics of pneumonia caused by *Escherichia coli.* N Engl J Med 277:115, 1967

TULLOCH EF JR. et al: Invasive enteropathic *Escherichia coli* dysentery: Outbreak in 28 adults. Ann Intern Med 79:13, 1973

TURCK M et al: Studies on the epidemiology of *Escherichia coli* 1960–1968. J Infect Dis 120:13, 1969

Klebsiella-Enterobacter-Serratia infections

EDMONDSON EG, SANFORD JP: The *Klebsiella-enterobacter* (aerobacter)-*Serratia* group. Medicine 46:323, 1967

EICKHOFF TC et al: The *Klebsiella-Enterobacter-Serratia* divisions: Biochemical and serologic characteristics and susceptibility to antibiotics. Ann Intern Med 65:1163, 1966

MANFREDI F et al: Clinical observations of acute Friedländer pneumonia. Ann Intern Med 58:642, 1963

PIERCE AK et al: An analysis of factors predisposing to gram-negative bacillary necrotizing pneumonia. Am Rev Resp Dis 94:309, 1966

PRICE DJE, SLEIGH JD: Control of infection due to *Klebsiella* aerogenes in neurosurgical unit by withdrawal of all antibiotics. Lancet 2:213, 1970

Proteus infections

LEWIS J, FEKETY FR: *Proteus* bacteremia. Johns Hopkins Med J 124:151, 1969

MUSHER DM et al: Role of urease in pyelonephritis resulting from urinary tract infection with *Proteus.* J Infect Dis 131:177, 1975

SERIFF NS: Lobar pneumonia due to *Proteus* infection in a previously healthy adult. Am J Med 46:480, 1969

TILLOTSON JR, LERNER AM: Characteristics of pneumonia caused by bacillus *Proteus.* Ann Intern Med 68:287, 1968

TURCK M et al: The role of carbenicillin in treatment of infections of the urinary tract. J Infect Dis 122:529, 1970

139
PSEUDOMONAS AND MIMA-HERELLEA INFECTIONS

MARVIN TURCK

PSEUDOMONAS INFECTIONS

ETIOLOGY *Pseudomonas aeruginosa* is a gram-negative motile rod which generally is not encapsulated and forms no spores. It grows readily in all ordinary culture media, and on agar it forms irregular, soft, iridescent colonies which usually have a fluorescent yellow-green color because of diffusion into the medium of two pigments, pyocyanin and fluorescin. *Pseudomonas* produces acid but no gas in glucose, and it is proteolytic. It is oxidase-positive and produces ammonia from arginine. A number of different strains have been identified by immunofluorescent techniques or bacteriophage typing. There is no evidence that these strains vary in their virulence for man. Other *Pseudomonas* species *(P. maltophilia, P. cepacia, P. fluorescens, P. testosteroni,* and *P. putida)* also may cause infection in man. For the most part, these organisms have been associated with several common-source nosocomial outbreaks; in addition, they have been incriminated in bacteremia, endocarditis, and osteomyelitis in narcotic addicts.

EPIDEMIOLOGY *Pseudomonas* organisms are present on the skin of some normal persons, particularly in the axilla and anogenital regions. They are uncommon in the stools of adults not receiving antibiotics. In the majority of instances, *Pseudomonas* organisms are cultured as avirulent secondary contaminants in superficial wounds, or from the sputum of patients treated with antibiotics. Ordinarily this is of little consequence because the organisms merely fill the bacteriologic vacuum left by the elimination of more sensitive bacteria. Occasionally, however, superinfections with *Pseudomonas* organisms occur in the ear, lung, skin, or urinary tract of patients whose primary pathogen has been eradicated by antibiotics. Serious infections are almost invariably associated with damage to local tissue or with diminished host resistance. Premature infants; children with congenital anomalies and patients with leukemia, usually receiving antibiotics, adrenal steroids, or antineoplastic drugs; patients with burns; and geriatric patients with debilitating diseases are likely to develop *Pseudomonas* infections. Most often these infections occur in the hospital environment, and the organisms have been cultured from a variety of sources in hospitals, including water from laboratory sinks and washbasins, antiseptic solutions, including benzalkonium chloride (Zephiran) and hexachlorophene soap, ophthalmic fluorescein and contact lens solution, saline, penicillin, procaine, and a variety of other medications. Other sources are incubators, humidifying equipment, air-cooling systems, forceps, syringes, and contaminated pressure transducers employed in hospital critical care units. The organism is prevalent in urine receptacles and catheters, and on the hands of orderlies, nurses, and surgeons on urologic wards; in several outbreaks, *Pseudomonas* urinary tract infections have presumably been transmitted from patient to patient by human carriers. Similar epidemics have been reported in nurseries among premature infants, and cross infection on burn wards is also common.

PATHOGENESIS The portal of entry of *Pseudomonas* organisms varies with the patient's age and underlying disease. In infancy and childhood, the skin, umbilical cord, and gastrointestinal tract predominate; in old age, the urinary tract is more often the primary focus. Often the infections remain localized in the skin or subcutaneous tissues. In burns the region below the eschar may become massively infiltrated with bacteria and inflammatory cells, and usually serves as the focus for bacteremia, the single most lethal complication. Hematogenous dissemination is characterized by hemorrhagic nodules in many areas, including the skin, heart, lungs, kidneys, and meninges. The histologic picture is one of necrosis and hemorrhage. Typically the walls of arterioles are heavily infiltrated with bacteria, and the vessels are partially or wholly thrombosed.

MANIFESTATIONS *Pseudomonas* infections occur in many locations, including the skin, subcutaneous tissue, bone and joints, eyes, ears, mastoid and paranasal sinuses, meninges, and heart valves. Bacteremia without a detectable primary focus may also occur.

Infections of the skin and subcutaneous tissues *Pseudomonas* organisms are frequently cultured from surgical wounds, varicose and decubitus ulcers, and burns, particularly following antibiotic therapy. Draining tuberculous or osteomyelitic sinuses may become secondarily infected. The mere presence of *Pseudomonas* in these sites is of little significance provided that bacterial multiplication deep in subcutaneous tissues does not occur and bacteremia does not ensue. Cutaneous infections usually heal after removal or slough of devitalized tissue. *Pseudomonas* organisms may be responsible for green nails in persons whose hands are excessively exposed to water, soap, and detergents, who have onychomycosis, or whose hands are subject to mechanical trauma. The organism can usually be cultured from the nail plate.

Infections of the ear, mastoid, and paranasal sinuses Otitis externa is the most common form of *Pseudomonas* infection which involves the ear. It is particularly troublesome in tropical climates and is characterized by chronic serosanguineous and purulent drainage from the external auditory canal. Otitis media or mastoiditis usually occurs as a superinfection following eradication of pneumococci, streptococci, or staphylococci by antimicrobial agents. Frequently *Pseudomonas* organisms are present in association with other gram-negative or gram-positive organisms.

Infection of the eye Corneal ulceration is the most severe form of ocular *Pseudomonas* infection. It usually follows a traumatic abrasion and may terminate in panophthalmitis and destruction of the globe. Purulent conjunctivitis occurs as a manifestation of *Pseudomonas* infection in premature infants. Contamination of contact lenses or lens fluid may be an important means of infecting the eyes with *Pseudomonas* organisms.

Urinary tract infections *Pseudomonas* organisms are common pathogens in the urinary tract and are usually found in patients with obstructive uropathy who have been subjected to repeated urethral manipulations or to urologic surgery. They are rarely cultured from the urine of patients who have not seen a urologist. At times *Pseudomonas* is one of several pathogenic bacteria in the urine, the others being *Escherichia coli, Klebsiella, Proteus,* and enterococci. *Pseudomonas* bacteriuria is in no way unique and cannot be distinguished from infection with other organisms on clinical grounds.

Gastrointestinal tract *Pseudomonas* organisms have been implicated as a cause of epidemic diarrhea of infancy. In addition, a number of infants dying from neonatal sepsis have the classic necrotic, avascular ulcers of *Pseudomonas* bacteremia in the bowel at autopsy. A "typhoidal" form of *Pseudomonas* infection characterized by fever, myalgia, and diarrhea occurs predominantly in the tropics. This illness, also called 13-day fever or Shanghai fever, is self-limited, and the prognosis is good.

Respiratory tract Primary *Pseudomonas* pneumonia is infrequent, and culture of this organism from the sputum usually is indicative of aspiration of oropharyngeal contents with secondary infection or of superinfection following eradication of a more sensitive flora with antibiotics. Pulmonary infection is often associated with microabscesses. The organism is often isolated from the sputum of patients with bronchiectasis, chronic bronchitis, or cystic fibrosis who have lingering infections punctuated by multiple courses of chemotherapy and is recovered frequently from the stomata of tracheostomy sites. *Pseudomonas* bronchitis and bronchiolitis may be the terminal event in cystic fibrosis.

Meningitis Spontaneous *Pseudomonas* meningitis is most unusual, but the bacilli may be introduced into the subarachnoid space by lumbar puncture, spinal anesthesia, intrathecal medication, or head trauma. Ventriculomastoid or ventriculoatrial shunts performed for hydrocephalus may become contaminated with *Pseudomonas* organisms. Usually revision or removal of the shunt offers the best hope of cure. Meningitis may be a terminal phenomenon in *Pseudomonas* bacteremia and in this instance represents a metastatic infection in the meninges.

Bacteremia Bloodstream invasion tends to occur in debilitated patients, premature infants, children with congenital defects, patients with lymphomas, leukemias, or other malignant tumors, and elderly patients who have undergone surgery or instrumentation of the biliary or urinary tract. *Pseudomonas* bacteremia is an important cause of death in patients with severe burns. In adults, *Pseudomonas* bacteremia is indistinguishable from bloodstream infection with other bacterial species except for two findings: (1) Ecthyma gangrenosum, the classic skin lesion, often located in the anogenital or axillary region as a round, indurated, purple-black area about 1 cm in diameter with an ulcerated center and a surrounding zone of erythema; and (2) the passage rarely of green urine, presumably due to the hemoglobin pigment, verdoglobin. Other features of *Pseudomonas* sepsis include hectic fever, shaking chills, hyperventilation, confusion, delirium, and circulatory collapse. Hypothermia, leukopenia, and thrombocytopenia are more common in *Pseudomonas* bacteremia than in other gram-negative bacteremias but are often related to an underlying blood dyscrasia. In addition to ecthyma gangrenosum, other skin lesions consist of hemorrhagic cellulitis and macular lesions on the trunk similar to "rose spots." Organisms usually can be cultured from cutaneous lesions and may provide an early clue to the diagnosis. *Pseudomonas* organisms may be in the bloodstream concomitantly with other organisms, notably Enterobacteriaceae or staphylococci. More often, however, *Pseudomonas* bacteremia follows staphylococcal sepsis in patients with burns.

Bacterial endocarditis A number of cases of *Pseudomonas* subacute bacterial endocarditis have followed open-heart surgery. Usually the organisms become implanted on a silk suture or a synthetic patch employed for closure of septal defects. Reoperation with removal of the vegetation and foreign bodies offers the best hope of cure. *Pseudomonas* endocarditis has been found on normal heart valves in patients with burns or in drug addicts; it has been postulated that staphylococcal endocarditis develops first and that the vegetation is secondarily infected with *Pseudomonas* organisms. Metastatic abscesses in bone, joints, brain, adrenal glands, and lungs are frequent consequences of *Pseudomonas* endocarditis.

TREATMENT Localized infections should be treated by irrigation with 1% acetic acid or topical therapy with colistin or polymyxin B. The administration of colistin subconjunctivally has been of value in ocular infections. Drainage of purulent material and removal of devitalized tissues are essential. The outcome of *Pseudomonas* bacteremia is more dependent on the underlying disease than on the chemotherapy. For example, in patients with leukemia, remission generally must be attained before sepsis can be controlled. In burns, wound infection must be eradicated before the bloodstream can be cleared of organisms. Most strains of *Pseudomonas* are sensitive to polymyxin B and colistin, and a number of strains respond to oxytetracycline. These drugs should be used in full dosage of 30 to 50 mg every 6 h for polymyxin B (in adults) and 75 to 100 mg every 6 h (in adults) for colistin in life-threatening *Pseudomonas* bacteremia. Both drugs are excellent for eradicating bacteriuria, but because blood levels exceed minimal inhibitory concentrations only two- or threefold, the results in bacteremia and deep-seated tissue infection are inconsistent. Gentamicin, an aminoglycoside antibiotic, inhibits most strains of *Pseudomonas* and has superseded the polymyxin-type antibiotics for systemic infection with *Pseudomonas*. The dose of gentamicin for severe infection in patients with normal renal function is 5 mg/kg/day in divided doses. Carbenicillin is also active against many isolates; however, it must be used in doses of 24 to 30 g per day for control of severe infection. The combination of gentamicin and carbenicillin is frequently employed to delay emergence of resistance during therapy. Asymptomatic bacteriuria, particularly when confined to the bladder, should be treated with the least toxic and least painful agent, which, at times, may be a sulfonamide or a tetracycline. The antimicrobial susceptibility of strains of *Pseudomonas* other than *P. aeruginosa* is quite variable, and each isolate must be tested individually. For example, many of these isolates may be sensitive to chloramphenicol and resistant to gentamicin and carbenicillin.

The prognosis has been improved in burned patients with *Pseudomonas* sepsis as well as in a few other patients with endocarditis and with necrotizing papillitis by the use of large doses of hyperimmune γ-globulin in addition to antimicrobials.

PROPHYLAXIS *Pseudomonas* cross infections in hospitals can be reduced by careful attention to aseptic techniques, particularly in nurseries for premature infants, operating rooms, and urologic wards; avoidance of cold sterilization procedures wherever possible; and scrupulous attention to clean plumbing fixtures, humidifying equipment, etc. Judicious use of antibiotics, steroids, and cytotoxic agents should also diminish the incidence of *Pseudomonas* infections. Systemic antibiotic prophylaxis aimed at preventing colonization and infection with *Pseudomonas* organisms has been notoriously unsuccessful and should be interdicted.

PROGNOSIS The mortality rate in *Pseudomonas* bacteremia is 75 percent and is highest in patients with shock or severe associated disease such as massive third-degree burns, leukemia, or prematurity. When bacteremia originates in the urinary tract and is not accompanied by shock, the prognosis is considerably better. Localized *Pseudomonas* infections do not present a threat to life unless hematogenous dissemination occurs.

MIMA-HERELLEA INFECTIONS

DEFINITION Organisms of the tribe Mimae are pleomorphic, gram-negative bacilli which are easily confused with members of the genus *Neisseria.* Severe infections with these organisms, including meningitis, bacterial endocarditis, pneumonia, and bacteremia, are being described with increasing frequency.

ETIOLOGY *Mima polymorpha,* described by DeBord in 1939, is one of two well-characterized species within the tribe Mimae, the other being *Herellea vaginicola.* Organisms formerly described as *Bacterium anitratum* and B5W are synonymous with *H. vaginicola.* These organisms are pleomorphic, gram-negative, encapsulated, and nonmotile. They grow well on ordinary media, forming white, convex, smooth colonies. Diplococcal forms predominate in colonies grown on solid media; rods and filamentous forms are more common in liquid media. The species can be differentiated from the Enterobacteriaceae by their negative nitrate reaction and from members of the genus *Neisseria,* which they may resemble morphologically, by their simple growth requirements, their bacillary form in liquid media, and their usually negative oxidase reaction. *Herellea vaginicola* may be distinguished from *M. polymorpha* by its capacity to ferment 10 percent lactose.

EPIDEMIOLOGY AND PATHOGENESIS Mimae are ubiquitous and have been cultured from a variety of human sources, including urethral, vaginal, and conjunctival secretions, sputum, pleural fluid, blood, cerebrospinal fluid, feces, cutaneous ulcers, abscesses, chancroid lesions, joint fluid, ascitic fluid, and bone marrow. In addition, these organisms have been found in river water, humidifiers, and oxygen tents. Recent observations indicate that 25 percent of normal subjects are skin carriers of *H. vaginicola,* and 10 percent of *M. polymorpha.* The striking association of mima-herellea bacteremia with cutdowns or indwelling intravenous catheters favors the skin as a major portal of entry in man. The increasing incidence of mima-herellea pneumonia, both as a primary infection and as a superinfection, also points to the respiratory tract as an important portal of entry. It is most likely that the *Mima* organisms are normal human commensals of relatively low virulence which produce serious infections under conditions of decreased host resistance, or in the presence of local tissue trauma, and in this way resemble the Enterobacteriaceae. Although members of the Mimae tribe have been implicated as an important cause of penicillin-resistant venereal urethritis, the evidence for this relation is not convincing. Similarly, the role of these organisms as a cause of conjunctivitis and vaginitis requires documentation.

MANIFESTATIONS Serious infections caused by *Mima* organisms include (1) meningitis, (2) subacute and acute bacterial endocarditis, (3) pneumonia, (4) urinary tract infections, and (5) bacteremia. Usually, the signs and symptoms associated with infections in these sites are no different from those produced by other pathogens. For example, subacute bacterial endocarditis has usually been reported in patients with congenital or rheumatic heart disease and pursues an indolent course, while urinary tract infections may be manifested by asymptomatic bacteriuria, cystitis, or pyelonephritis. Pneumonia often occurs in the form of a superinfection in patients who have received antibiotics, but occasionally herelleae may be primary pathogens in the lung. Occasionally, *M. polymorpha* may be the cause of a fulminating bacteremia, with high fever, vascular collapse, petechiae, and ecchymoses, indistinguishable from fulminant meningococcemia. More often, however, bacteremia is associated with an overt portal of entry, such as infected cutdowns or indwelling intravenous catheters, surgical wounds, or burns, or it may follow urethral or other surgical instrumentation. These patients usually have severe debilitating disease or have undergone surgery. Many times they have received antibiotics, adrenal cortical hormones, irradiation, or tumor chemotherapy and have had infections with other organisms, usually gram-positive, prior to development of sepsis with Mimae. The clinical picture presented by these patients is dominated by endotoxemia, and the prognosis is very poor.

DIAGNOSIS The diagnosis of herelliosis is usually missed because the clinical bacteriology laboratory is unfamiliar with these organisms and reports them incorrectly or because they are considered contaminants. The confusion attending the taxonomic classification of these organisms has not simplified matters. For practical purposes, isolation of mimae-herelleae (or their synonyms, *B. anitratum,* B5W, *Diplococcus mucosus,* or *Neisseria winogradskyi*) from blood, spinal fluid, sputum, urine, or pus should be considered significant unless there is no evidence of infection on clinical grounds. Since Mimae are resistant to penicillin and members of the genus *Neisseria* are sensitive, differentiation of these organisms is of obvious importance.

TREATMENT Antibiotic sensitivities of *Mima* and *Herellea* strains vary, but most strains are inhibited by kanamycin, gentamicin, colistin, or polymyxin B. Sensitivity to the tetracyclines is unpredictable, and most strains are also resistant to penicillin, ampicillin, cephalothin, erythromycin, and chloramphenicol. For serious systemic infections, kanamycin should be administered in doses of 0.5 g intramuscularly every 8 to 12 h (in adults). Since these organisms may produce localized abscesses, surgical drainage may be necessary.

REFERENCES

Mima-Herellea infections

INCLAN AP et al: Organisms of the tribe mimeae: Incidence of isolation and clinical correlation. South Med J 58:1261, 1965

REYNOLDS RC, CLUFF LE: Infections of man with mimae. Ann Intern Med 58:759, 1963

Pseudomonas infections

ALEXANDER JW et al: Immunologic control of pseudomonas infection in burn patients: Clinical evaluation. Arch Surg 102:31, 1971

BODEY GP: Epidemiologic studies of pseudomonas species in patients with leukemia. Am J Med Sci 260:82, 1970

CURTIN JA et al: Pseudomonas bacteremia: Review of 91 cases. Ann Intern Med 54:1077, 1961

FIERER J et al: Pseudomonas aeruginosa epidemic traced to delivery room resuscitators. N Engl J Med 276:991, 1967

GRIEBLE HG et al: Fine particle humidifiers: Source of pseudomonas aeruginosa infections in a respiratory disease unit. N Engl J Med 282:531, 1970

PENNINGTON JE et al: *Pseudomonas pneumonia:* A retrospective study of 36 cases. Am J Med 55:155, 1973

PHILLIPS I et al: Control of respirator-associated infection due to *Pseudomonas aeruginosa.* Lancet 2:871, 1974

STONE HH: Review of pseudomonas sepsis in thermal injury. Ann Surg 163:297, 1966

TILLOTSON JR, LERNER AM: Characteristics of non-bacteremic pseudomonas pneumonia. Ann Intern Med 68:295, 1968

140 SALMONELLA INFECTIONS

EDWARD W. HOOK
RICHARD L. GUERRANT

INTRODUCTION The genus *Salmonella* consists of three species which include more than 1,700 different serologic types. Striking variation in pathogenicity of serotypes occurs, but almost all are pathogenic for animals and man. Specific host preferences characterize certain serotypes, such as *S. typhi,* which under natural conditions of transmission produces disease only in man. *Salmonella* infections in man present a spectrum of clinical syndromes, which sometimes overlap. The syndromes are (1) enteric fever (typhoid or paratyphoid fever), (2) acute gastroenteritis, (3) bacteremia, and (4) localized infection which may occur at almost any site. In addition, *asymptomatic intestinal infections* and *transient convalescent intestinal carrier* states are common. Occasionally, a focus of infection persists in the gallbladder or urinary tract to produce a *chronic carrier* state.

ETIOLOGY Salmonellae are motile gram-negative bacilli that do not ferment lactose or sucrose but ferment glucose. Almost all serotypes produce gas, although *S. typhi* is a notable exception. Salmonellae are divided into three species by biochemical means: *S. typhi, S. cholera-suis,* and *S. enteritidis.* The species are further subdivided into serotypes, which are identified by highly specific O (somatic and H (flagellar) antigens. A given serotype will contain a specific combination of multiple O and H antigens. Identification by serotype is accomplished routinely only in large salmonella typing centers, which have the necessary collection of antiserums required for such work. Salmonellae are also divided into groups on the basis of O antigen composition. Most isolates from natural sources fall into five groups, A to E.

The species *S. typhi* and *S. cholera-suis* consist of only one serotype each (in groups D and C, respectively), whereas the species *S. enteritidis* comprises over 1,700 serotypes (in all groups, including C and D). Considerable overlap in antigenic composition is responsible for the cross-reactivity which is commonly seen in serologic tests with salmonellae.

The Salmonella Surveillance Unit of the Center for Disease Control reports 20,000 to 25,000 isolations of salmonellae annually from human beings in the United States. This number has been consistent over the decade from 1965 to 1974. In descending order, the most frequently isolated serotypes are *S. typhimurium, S. enteritidis, S. newport, S. heidelberg, S. infantis, S. saint-paul, S. thompson, S. typhi, S. derby,* and *S. javiana.* The 10 most frequently isolated serotypes account for about 70 percent of the total isolates from man over this period. *Salmonella typhimurium* perennially accounts for 25 to 30 percent of the isolates. A significant recent change in serotypes isolated from human sources in the United States is the rapidly increasing rate of isolation of *S. agona,* an organism apparently introduced in Peruvian fish meal in 1971. Concern has also arisen over the multiple-drug-resistant *S. wein,* which was the most frequent *Salmonella* isolate in France in 1974 and which is now being isolated in the United States; *S. wein* is resistant to chloramphenicol, ampicillin, sulfonamides, and tetracyclines.

In the subsequent section, typhoid fever, the classic example of enteric fever, is considered separately from other *Salmonella* infections because of its historical importance, the host specificity of *S. typhi,* and the extensive clinical experience with the disease.

TYPHOID FEVER

DEFINITION Typhoid fever is an acute systemic disease resulting from infection with *S. typhi.* The disease is unique to man. It is characterized by malaise, fever, abdominal discomfort, transient rash, splenomegaly, and leukopenia. The most prominent major complications are intestinal hemorrhage and perforation. The disease is the classic example of enteric fever caused by salmonellae. However, enteric fever, similar to typhoid, can also be caused by other *Salmonella* serotypes and is termed *paratyphoid fever.*

EPIDEMIOLOGY *Salmonella typhi* gains access to the body by the oral route in almost all cases as a consequence of the ingestion of contaminated food, water, or milk. Man is the only true reservoir of *S. typhi* in nature, and persons with typhoid fever or convalescent or chronic carriers always serve as the ultimate source of infection. Infected individuals can excrete millions of viable typhoid bacilli in the feces, which are the usual source of contamination of food, or drink. Patients with active disease also occasionally have organisms in respiratory secretions, vomitus, or other body fluids. Flies or other insects can carry organisms from feces or other infected material to food or drink and have been implicated in a few outbreaks. The fact that *S. typhi* may survive freezing or drying enhances the possibility of spread by contaminated ice, dust, foods, and sewage. Oysters or other shellfish are contaminated at times in polluted waters and occasionally serve as sources of typhoid.

The incidence of typhoid fever has steadily decreased in the United States during the past century to the present relatively low level of less than 400 cases per annum. The decrease in incidence has been coincident with improvement in socioeconomic conditions and is specifically related to development of pure water supplies, effective sewage disposal, pasteurization of milk, and methods to detect and control spread of organisms from persons with active disease or from carriers. Typhoid continues to occur on a large scale in countries where sanitation is suboptimal. About 40 percent of the patients with typhoid fever in the United States appear to have acquired the infection in another area of the world.

Typhoid can be eradicated ultimately because the infection is confined to man and both the disease and the carrier state can be controlled by appropriate therapy. The importance of sewage disposal, a pure water supply, and control of carriers is highlighted repeatedly by the occurrence of outbreaks which develop when defects in sanitation occur during natural disasters such as flood.

The sex distribution of patients with typhoid fever in the United States shows no significant predilection. In recent years, about 75 percent of cases have occurred in persons less than 30 years of age. In contrast, the chronic carrier state is much more common in females than males (the female/male ratio is 3:1) and in older individuals (88 percent over 50 years of age).

There is no seasonal variation in incidence of typhoid fever in the United States. However, in areas of the world where the disease is endemic, the incidence increases in the summer months.

PATHOGENESIS The outcome of the interaction between the typhoid bacillus and man is determined during the early hours after ingestion of the organisms. Typhoid bacilli reach the small intestine shortly after ingestion and may multiply there. The organisms may then penetrate the mucosa with minimal epithelial destruction and enter intestinal lymphatics, perhaps via the Peyer's patches, to be carried to the bloodstream. This initial early bacteremia apparently occurs within 24 to 72 h after ingestion of organisms and is rarely detected in natural infections because patients are usually asymptomatic at this early stage. The bacteremia is transient and is rapidly terminated as bacilli are phagocytized by cells of the reticuloendothelial system. Nevertheless, viable bacilli are disseminated throughout the body and apparently persist within reticuloendothelial cells. If multiplication at the intracellular site takes place, organisms reenter the bloodstream, producing a continuous bacteremia for days or weeks. The reappearance of bacteremia corresponds with the onset of manifestations of the disease. The intracellular organisms are eventually destroyed as manifestations of disease subside and recovery ensues. Enhanced intracellular killing and recovery appear to be related to the onset of delayed hypersensitivity. Recovery is unrelated to the appearance, even in high titer, of agglutinins against the somatic, flagellar, or Vi antigens of the typhoid bacillus.

The number of organisms ingested is of obvious importance in determining whether typhoid fever results from exposure to *S. typhi*. Studies in volunteers have shown that about 10^7 typhoid bacilli of the Quarles strain must be taken orally to produce typhoid fever in 50 percent of normal volunteers. The number of organisms ingested also influences the incubation period, and short incubation periods, in general, correspond to large doses of organisms. The volunteer studies have also demonstrated that different strains of typhoid bacilli vary considerably in their capacity to produce disease in man.

The normal flora of the upper intestinal tract is an important protective mechanism against invasion by *S. typhi*. Volunteer studies have demonstrated that antimicrobial therapy a day or so before oral challenge with *S. typhi* markedly decreases the number of viable bacilli required to produce disease. It is possible that certain factors known to be associated with typhoid outbreaks, such as malnutrition, enhance susceptibility to typhoid infection by alterations in the intestinal flora.

During the phase of persistent bacteremia, all organs are repeatedly exposed to typhoid bacilli. Abscess formation may occur but is unusual. However, localization does occur in the gallbladder in almost all cases. Organisms multiply in the bile to high titer, usually without manifestations of cholecystitis, and are excreted with bile into the intestinal tract. Stool cultures, which are usually negative for *S. typhi* during the incubation period and early phases of the disease, become positive in a large proportion of cases during the third or fourth week of the disease, when excretion of organisms multiplying in the bile reaches a peak.

The factors responsible for the fever, leukopenia, and other manifestations of typhoid fever have been inadequately defined. Typhoid bacilli contain biologically active lipopolysaccharides or endotoxins which produce fever, leukopenia, thrombocytopenia, and hyperplasia of reticuloendothelial cells when injected into animals or man. It has been assumed for years that these materials play an important role in the pathogenesis of the signs and symptoms of typhoid fever. However, the evidence regarding the role of endotoxin in the genesis of the manifestations of typhoid is inconclusive. For example, tolerance to the pyrogenic effects of endotoxins can be demonstrated during convalescence from typhoid fever, which suggests release of endotoxins during infection. Nevertheless, other studies show that typhoid fever follows a normal course in volunteers rendered tolerant to endotoxins prior to challenge, indicating that more complex mechanisms than endotoxemia alone are responsible for the sustained fever and toxemia.

PATHOLOGY The most prominent microscopic lesion in typhoid fever is proliferation of large mononuclear cells in many different tissues. Mononuclear hyperplasia leads to lymphadenopathy, splenomegaly, and impressive enlargement of lymphoid tissues in the intestines, especially in the terminal ileum (Peyer's patches). Proliferating mononuclear cells may also be observed in bone marrow, liver, and lung. Studies in volunteers using ^{131}I-tagged aggregated albumin have shown increased phagocytic activity of the reticuloendothelial system by the third to fifth days after onset of symptoms. Necrosis in hyperplastic Peyer's patches may be associated with erosion of blood vessels in the lesions in the intestinal tract, which leads to oozing of blood or massive hemorrhage. Lesions may extend deep into the intestinal wall and cause perforation of the bowel, an event which characteristically occurs late in the disease, most often in the third febrile week. The site of perforation is usually in the distal 24 in. of the ileum.

The gallbladder and bile ducts are routinely infected during the disease. As a rule, this biliary infection is asymptomatic, although acute cholecystitis may occur occasionally. Biliary infection terminates spontaneously during convalescence in the vast majority of patients within 12 months, but about 3 percent of adults continue to harbor organisms in the gallbladder and become chronic carriers of the typhoid bacillus.

MANIFESTATIONS The incubation period averages about 10 days but may vary from extremes of 3 to 60 days depending on the infecting dose.

The clinical manifestations and duration of illness vary markedly from one patient to another. Mild forms of the disease, characterized primarily by fever, may last only a week, or illness may be prolonged, lasting 8 weeks or more if untreated.

In a typical patient not treated with antimicrobials, the illness lasts about 4 weeks. The onset is insidious with headache, malaise, anorexia, and fever. Headache may be the first manifestation of disease and is usually generalized and severe. Chilly sensations are common, and frank chills may be observed. The fever is remittent, frequently increasing in a steplike manner from day to day as the illness develops. Abdominal discomfort, bloating, and constipation are common during the early phase of illness. A dry cough is observed in about two-thirds of the patients and occasionally may be so prominent as to direct attention away from the generalized nature of the infectious process. Nosebleeds may occur during the early phase of illness.

The temperature gradually increases for 5 to 7 days and then plateaus as a continuous or mildly remittent fever in the range of 39 to 40°C. The temperature may be sustained at these levels with little variation for 2 or 3 weeks. A relative bradycardia occurs in 30 to 40 percent of the patients. The prolonged persistent fever leads to general debility; patients are weak and anorectic. Mental dullness is common and delirium may occur. Abdominal pain and marked distention are usual. Constipation, so common during the early phase of illness, may give way to frank diarrhea which occurs in about one-fifth of the patients.

The characteristic rash (rose spots) is most often observed during the second week of the disease. The lesions are small, 2- to 4-mm, erythematous macules which occur in small numbers on the upper abdomen and anterior thorax. The lesions blanch on pressure and last only 2 to 3 days. Some reports describe rose spots in as many as 90 percent of patients, whereas other reports indicate a frequency of only 10 percent or even less. The evasive nature of the rash and the difficulties encountered in detecting lesions in highly pigmented individuals probably account for the marked variation in incidence reported in the literature.

The liver and spleen are frequently enlarged and palpable from the end of the first week of illness. The spleen is palpable in about three-quarters of the patients. The liver may be tender, and occasionally a friction rub is audible over the spleen.

Abdominal tenderness is frequent and distention occurs in the majority of cases. Marked abdominal pain with signs of peritonitis should call attention to the possibility of perforation of the bowel.

After the third week, the symptoms slowly abate, and the temperature returns to normal over a period of days.

Jaundice secondary to extensive mononuclear cell infiltration in the liver and hepatic cell necrosis is a rare complication of typhoid. Acute renal failure also is observed rarely; the pathogenesis of this so-called "typhoid nephritis" has not been adequately defined. Disseminated intravascular coagulation may develop in severe typhoid and lead to additional clinical manifestations secondary to thrombosis or hemorrhage.

Complications Prior to the introduction of chloramphenicol, the prolonged febrile course of typhoid often led to profound debility, weight loss, and multiple nutritional deficiencies. Intestinal hemorrhage and bowel perforation, the most feared complications, were common causes of death. The frequency of complications in typhoid fever has been reduced since the advent of effective chemotherapy.

INTESTINAL HEMORRHAGE Erosion of blood vessels in hyperplastic and necrotic Peyer's patches or in other mononuclear cell accumulations in the wall of the intestine leads to bleeding into the intestinal tract. Occult blood in feces is quite common during the course of the disease, occurring in 20 percent or more of patients. Gross blood is present in feces in about 10 percent of patients, and massive hemorrhage occurs occasionally. Major hemorrhage is usually a late complication, occurring most often during the second or third week of disease. A sudden drop in blood pressure or temperature may be the first manifestation of hemorrhage.

INTESTINAL PERFORATION The pathologic process in the lymphoid tissues of the intestine may also involve the muscular and serosal layers of the bowel and lead to perforation. Prior to the advent of chloramphenicol, perforation occurred in about 3 percent of patients with typhoid. The incidence has been reduced by antimicrobial therapy to about 1 percent. Perforation is most common in the distal 24 in. of ileum and is observed most frequently during the third week of the disease. The onset of perforation may be quite unexpected during an otherwise uncomplicated convalescence. Pain in the right lower quadrant of the abdomen is the most frequent initial manifestation, but signs of localized or generalized peritonitis develop rapidly.

OTHER COMPLICATIONS Typhoid bacilli may localize in any tissue in the body with the production of localized suppurative infection. Meningitis, chondritis, periostitis, osteomyelitis, arthritis, and pyelonephritis are examples of localized infections that may be observed occasionally. Pneumonia is not unusual and may be related to the typhoid bacillus or to a secondary bacterial invader, such as the pneumococcus. Severe deep thrombophlebitis may occur during the febrile period. Late complications also include peripheral neuritis, deafness, and alopecia. Hemolytic anemia may be observed, especially in infected individuals deficient in glucose 6-phosphate dehydrogenase.

Relapse After illness has subsided for a variable period, usually about two weeks, all the manifestations which characterized the initial infection may recur. Blood cultures, negative during convalescence, may become positive again. Although relapse may be severe, it is usually milder and of shorter duration than the original illness. The incidence of relapse was about 5 to 10 percent prior to the introduction of effective chemotherapy. Chloramphenicol has not decreased the frequency of relapse; in fact, the relapse rate in chloramphenicol-treated patients is higher than in patients not receiving the drug. Periods of antimicrobial therapy longer than 2 weeks do not seem to alter the incidence of relapse. Relapse cannot be correlated with the titer of agglutinins against the flagellar, somatic, or Vi antigens of the typhoid bacillus.

Chronic carriers Although the vast majority of patients with typhoid fever eradicate the site of infection in the gallbladder during convalescence, about 3 percent of adults do not, and these individuals become chronic typhoid carriers who continue to excrete organisms in feces for years, usually for life. A chronic carrier is defined as a person documented to have been excreting typhoid bacilli in the stool for a period of at least 1 year. In the United States, almost all chronic carriers have a persistent site of infection in the gallbladder from which organisms reach the intestinal tract in bile. Chronic carriers may be detected by follow-up of patients with typhoid fever, but many carriers give no history of typhoid. In these patients, it is assumed that the initial illness was so mild as to go unrecognized or undiagnosed. Once organisms have been demonstrated in the stools for as long as a year, it is quite unlikely that the focus of infection in the gallbladder will terminate spontaneously. The chronic carrier state is rare in children and occurs more commonly with increasing age and is about three times more common in women than men. It is possible that these age and sex characteristics are related to the greater prevalence of gallbladder disease in older women, a factor which would favor persistence of organisms in the biliary tract.

The chronic biliary carrier is usually asymptomatic. Despite millions of organisms entering the intestine in each milliliter of bile, patients show no systemic manifestations. Gallstones and dysfunction of the gallbladder on cholecystogram can be demonstrated in a large proportion of chronic carriers, and carriers occasionally develop acute cholecystitis.

In areas of the world where *Schistosoma haematobium* infections are common, a chronic urinary carrier state results from localization of typhoid bacilli or other *Salmonella* serotypes in the obstructed urinary tract or adjacent lesions resulting from the schistosomiasis. These chronic urinary carriers not only excrete *Salmonella* in the urine but also may have intermittent bacteremic episodes which are not necessarily accompanied by fever.

LABORATORY FINDINGS Leukopenia of 3,000 to 4,000 cells per mm^3 is characteristic of the febrile phase of typhoid fever. A sudden increase in leukocyte count to 10, 000 cells per mm^3 or higher should suggest the possibility of intestinal perforation, hemorrhage, or a pyogenic complication, but these complications may occur in the absence of leukocytosis. A normocytic normochromic anemia develops during the course of the disease and may be aggravated by blood loss from intestinal lesions. Occult blood and a mononuclear leukocytosis in feces is common from the second week of disease. Urine is usually normal except for transient albuminuria during the febrile period.

The most dependable way to establish a definitive diagnosis of typhoid fever is by blood culture. Organisms can be recovered by culture of blood in 70 to 90 percent of patients during the first week of disease. Bacteremia is continuous and prolonged. Positive blood cultures are obtained in as many as 30 or 40 percent of patients during the third week of disease, but the incidence of bacteremia rapidly decreases after this time. Blood cultures frequently are positive during relapse. Recent evidence in partially treated cases suggests that culture of bone marrow may yield the organism when other cultures are negative.

Only about 10 to 15 percent of patients have positive stool cultures during the first week of disease. However, the frequency of positive stool cultures increases as the disease progresses, reaching a maximum of about 75 percent during the third or fourth week of illness. The frequency of positive cultures then begins to decline so that only about 10 percent of patients have positive stool cultures by 8 weeks after onset of illness. Most of these patients' cultures become negative over the next several weeks or months, but about 3 percent of adults continue to excrete organisms even after 1 year. Persistent excretion in these chronic carriers is secondary to infection in the gallbladder and biliary tract.

The incidence of positive urine cultures varies markedly during the course of typhoid fever and parallels the frequency of positive stool cultures. At least some of the positive cultures represent contamination of urine with feces harboring typhoid bacilli.

The majority of patients, but by no means all, develop a fourfold or greater rise in agglutinins against the somatic or O antigens of the typhoid bacillus during the course of the disease. A fourfold or greater increase in titer in the absence of recent typhoid immunization is compatible with infection with *S. typhi* but is by no means specific. All the group D organisms, one of which is *S. typhi,* as well as organisms in groups A and B, have certain common antigens which can evoke the formation of antibodies reactive with the O antigen used in the Widal test. Agglutinins against flagellar or H antigens also appear, frequently in higher titer than agglutinins against the O antigens. However, the H agglutinins are even more subject to nonspecific variation than O agglutinins and are of no value in diagnosis. Agglutinins begin to appear after about one week of illness and reach a peak titer during the fifth or sixth week. Early antimicrobial therapy may dampen the immunologic response in patients with typhoid fever. Relapse bears no relation to agglutinin titer. Rheumatoid factor activity in high titer can be detected in a large proportion of patients with typhoid or paratyphoid fever.

DIFFERENTIAL DIAGNOSIS The clinical features of typhoid fever, while characteristic and suggestive of the diagnosis, are certainly not pathognomonic. Many other diseases give a clinical picture which may be confused with typhoid; these include the rickettsioses, brucellosis, tularemia, leptospirosis, psittacosis, infectious hepatitis, infectious mononucleosis, primary atypical pneumonia, miliary tuberculosis, malaria, lymphoma, and rheumatic fever. Typhoid should be considered in any patient with unexplained fever, especially if there is a history of recent foreign travel to endemic areas.

TREATMENT Antimicrobial therapy Chloramphenicol is the antibiotic of choice for the treatment of typhoid fever. Despite the fact that a number of antimicrobial agents show excellent in vitro activity against *S. typhi,* chloramphenicol has consistently been shown to be more effective in terminating the febrile toxic course of the disease in the greatest proportion of patients in the shortest period of time. Nevertheless, the response to chloramphenicol is not dramatic or rapid. Subjective improvement usually occurs within about 48 h after beginning therapy, but the temperature usually does not return to normal for 2 to 5 days after initiating treatment. Bacteremia usually clears within hours after therapy is instituted, but occasionally organisms can be recovered from the blood 24 to 48 h after beginning treatment. The dose of chloramphenicol should be 50 mg per kg body weight per day divided into three or four equal doses given orally at intervals of 6 to 8 h. After the patient has become afebrile, the dose may be reduced to 30 mg/kg/day. Therapy should be continued for 2 weeks. If chloramphenicol cannot be given by the oral route, comparable doses should be given parenterally.

Ampicillin in doses of 80 mg/kg/day or 6 g per day for adults divided into four or six doses given parenterally or a combination of trimethoprim and sulfamethoxazole is effective in the treatment of typhoid, but the response is not as predictable or as prompt as with chloramphenicol. If there is a contraindication to therapy with chloramphenicol, ampicillin, amoxicillin, or trimethoprim and sulfamethoxazole are recommended.

Occasional patients with typhoid without evidence of suppurative complications do not respond clinically even after 4 or 5 days of antimicrobial therapy, even though blood cultures become negative. Delayed responses of this type occur in only about 1 percent of patients treated with chloramphenicol, in contrast to 5 or 10 percent of patients treated with ampicillin.

Chloramphenicol-resistant strains have been reported since 1972 from Mexico, Southeast Asia, and India. Resistance is due to a transferable R factor which also codes for resistance to sulfonamides, tetracycline, and streptomycin. *Salmonella typhi* resistant to both chloramphenicol and ampicillin have been isolated from a few patients. If chloramphenicol resistance is encountered, then ampicillin, amoxicillin, or trimethoprim and sulfamethoxazole should be used.

Adrenal hormones The administration of prednisone or steroids with similar activity can terminate within a matter of hours the severe febrile toxemic state seen in some patients. Because of the lag in time between institution of antimicrobial therapy and evidence of response, patients with life-threatening toxemia should be treated with a brief course of adrenal corticosteroids in addition to chloramphenicol. An appropriate regimen is 60 mg prednisone the first day; no additional steroid therapy should be administered. Hypothermia and hypotension occasionally occur within hours after initiation of steroids.

Supportive treatment Nursing care and attention to nutritional requirements are important. Laxatives and enemas should be avoided despite constipation because of the danger of precipitating hemorrhage or perforation. Salicylates should not be used, because in addition to their effects on blood platelets and irritating action on the bowel, these compounds can induce wide swings in temperature with very uncomfortable chills and sweats. Hypothermia and hypotension occur in some patients after administration of salicylates.

Hemorrhage and perforation Patients should be observed carefully to detect these complications at an early stage. Typing and cross matching should be carried out at the time of initial diagnosis of typhoid, and transfusion is indicated in the event of significant hemorrhage. Patients with typhoid are poor surgical risks. If perforation is suspected, emphasis should be placed on efforts to combat shock and decompress the bowel. Additional antimicrobials may have to be added to control peritonitis. Small perforations may localize and can be managed without surgical intervention. However, if evidence of localization does not develop, surgical intervention may be required.

Relapse The therapy of relapse is identical to that for the primary episode.

Chronic carriers Chronic carriers should be investigated for the presence of gallstones or a nonfunctioning gallbladder. Carriers without evidence of gallstones or gallbladder disease on cholecystogram usually can be cured with a prolonged course of ampicillin. One program which has been found to be effective consists of 6 g ampicillin divided into four equal oral doses each day with probenecid for a period of 6 weeks. If gallstones or a nonfunctioning gallbladder are demonstrated on cholecystogram, antimicrobial therapy is unlikely to be effective in terminating the carrier state. These patients should have cholecystectomy, which cures the chronic carrier state in about 85 percent of patients. Ampicillin may be used in conjunction with cholecystectomy. Therapy should be started a few days prior to the procedure and continued for 2 or 3 weeks.

PREVENTION AND CONTROL Although immunization with typhoid vaccine affords significant protection against typhoid infection, the degree of immunity is not great and can be readily overcome with a large dose of organisms. Nevertheless, immunization is recommended for individuals living or traveling in areas where the disease is endemic and for persons working with the organism in laboratories. Adults should receive 0.5 ml vaccine on two occasions separated by a period of 1 or 2 weeks. A yearly booster is required to maintain immunity. Immunization with typhoid vaccine causes a transient elevation for several months in titer of agglutinins against typhoid O antigens and a persistently elevated titer for H antigens.

All typhoid patients should be reported to local health authorities, and stool specimens should be cultured during convalescence. Three consecutively negative stool cultures obtained at weekly intervals indicate that a carrier state has not developed.

Caution should be observed to prevent spread of infection from persons with active disease or from carriers. Chronic or convalescent carriers should not be allowed to prepare food until clear documentation shows that at least three or more stool cultures are negative for typhoid bacilli. Carriers should be cautioned regarding routine sanitary techniques.

PROGNOSIS The mortality rate of typhoid fever prior to the introduction of chloramphenicol was about 12 percent. Death was associated with toxemia, inanition, pneumonia, bowel perforation, and intestinal hemorrhage. The mortality rate is still 2 or 3 percent; deaths are observed primarily in infants, the aged, or individuals with malnutrition or other underlying diseases.

OTHER SALMONELLA INFECTIONS

DEFINITION Bacteria of the genus *Salmonella* may produce asymptomatic infection of the intestinal tract in man or several different clinical syndromes including acute gastroenteritis (or enterocolitis), bacteremia, paratyphoid fever, or localized infections ranging from osteomyelitis to endocarditis. The clinical syndromes resulting from infection with *Salmonella* cannot always be sharply differentiated and sometimes overlap.

Salmonella infections are among the most prevalent communicable diseases caused by bacteria in the United States today. These infections are transmitted in the vast majority of cases from animals to man and occasionally from man to man and are usually brief, self-limited, and mild.

EPIDEMIOLOGY Salmonellas can be isolated from the intestinal tracts of man and many lower animals. The prevalence of asymptomatic excretors of these organisms in the general population is about 0.2 percent, but the most important reservoir of salmonellas is in domestic and wild animal species in which infection rates vary from less than 1 to more than 20 percent. An incomplete list of animals from which *Salmonella* species have been isolated includes chickens, turkeys, ducks, pigs, cows, dogs, cats, rats, parakeets, as well as certain cold-blooded animals and insects. Animals sold as pets, especially baby chicks, ducks, and turtles, may also harbor *Salmonella* and serve as sources of infection.

Salmonella infection is almost always acquired by the oral route, usually by ingestion of contaminated food or drink. Any food product is a potential source of human infection. The source of contamination of food or drink may be asymptomatic human carriers or persons with active clinical disease, but the greatest single source of human infection in the United States is the vast reservoir of *Salmonella* in lower animals. The high incidence of infection in domestic animals used as a source of food for man and present methods of processing foods and food products in bulk result in the availability of foods for human consumption with a potentially high incidence of contamination with *Salmonella.* For example, a significant proportion varying from 1 to more than 50 percent of raw meats purchased in retail markets is contaminated with *Salmonella.* Meat is contaminated by many routes, but the most common are natural infection of the animal used as a source of meat and contamination of the carcass during slaughter and processing. Eggs or egg products, including dried or frozen eggs, are also common sources of *Salmonella* infection. Of the various animal species, domestic fowl, including chickens, turkeys, ducks, and eggs and egg products, constitute the single largest reservoir of infection and the source most often responsible for infection of man. Cooking of food prior to human consumption serves to decrease the possibility of infection. However, salmonellas may survive cooking at low temperature, or food may be recontaminated after cooking by organisms from kitchen equipment or personnel.

Food or drink may also be contaminated by rats, mice, insects, or other vermin harboring these organisms. Cross infection occurs occasionally by the airborne route from dried foods such as egg whites or dust which contain viable *Salmonella. Salmonella* contamination of a large variety of processed foods has also been documented. Some of these foods contain ingredients of animal origin such as eggs, whereas others contain contaminated products of vegetable origin such as coconut or yeast. A variety of pharmaceutical products of animal origin have been shown to be responsible for *Salmonella* infections of man; these products include carmine dye, pancreatin, bile salts, and extracts of various organs such as thyroid, adrenal, and stomach.

Pet turtles may be an important source of *Salmonella* infection in man, especially in children, accounting for perhaps as many as 10 to 20 percent of reported *Salmonella* infections in certain areas. Turtles are infected on breeding farms and continue to excrete organisms in feces into tank water for long periods of time. Although knowledge of the manner of transmission to man is incomplete, it is likely that turtle feces or tank water harboring salmonellas contaminate hands of handlers, from which organisms are passed to the mouth or to food or drink.

Salmonella species may also be transmitted directly or via fomites from man to man or from animals to man without the intervention of contaminated food or drink, but this method of spread is not common. However, cross infection of this type has been shown to be responsible for a number of outbreaks of salmonellosis among patients in nurseries and hospitals. Nosocomial salmonellosis poses a particular threat to newborns, immunosuppressed patients, and those receiving multiple broad-spectrum antibiotics, who may be infected by relatively few organisms. Nursery outbreaks have been traced to newborn infants from mothers with recent *salmonella* infections. Multiple-drug-resistant salmonellae have been found in burn units.

Fish meal, meat meal, bone meal, and other by-products of the meat-packing industry are often contaminated with *Salmonella* organisms. These products are incorporated in animal and poultry feeds and apparently play an important role in the perpetuation of infection among domestic animals.

The true incidence of *Salmonella* infection is difficult to determine. The reported isolations of salmonellas from humans in the United States represent about 10 cases per 100,000 population per annum. However, reported cases represent only a small proportion of the actual number because bacteriologic studies are usually performed only on patients with severe or protracted diarrhea, and many outbreaks are not investigated. Although *Salmonella* infection occurs throughout the year, the Salmonella Surveillance Unit of the National Communicable Disease Center has observed a distinct seasonal pattern with the greatest number of isolations reported from July through October for each year.

A close correlation exists between the *Salmonella* serotypes most often responsible for human infection and those isolated from animals in any specific geographic area. The similarities document the importance of nonhuman reservoirs of *Salmonella* in the epidemiology of *Salmonella* infection in man.

PATHOGENESIS The course of events after salmonellae have gained access to the gastrointestinal tract is determined by the dose, serotype, and invasive potential of the organism, and by the resistance of the host. Different *Salmonella* serotypes show marked variation in invasive potential and capacity to produce disease in man. For example, *S. anatum* characteristically produces asymptomatic intestinal infection and rarely invades the bloodstream. In contrast, *S. cholera-suis,* the most invasive serotype, frequently produces bacteremia and metastatic infection. Bloodstream invasion may occur as a complication of gastroenteritis but usually develops without preceding intestinal symptoms. Bacteremia with any serotype may be transient or prolonged, and may be accompanied by recurrent chills and fever or manifestations of paratyphoid fever. Bloodborne bacteria may localize at any site and lead to suppuration in bone, joints, meninges, pleura, or other tissues.

Multiplication of ingested organisms in the intestinal tract may be followed by symptoms of gastroenteritis. The intestinal irritation and inflammation are produced by a true infection deep in the mucosa as evidenced by polymorphonuclear leukocytes typically found in the diarrheal stool. However, studies in animals have shown that mucosal invasion alone is not sufficient to account for the intestinal fluid observed in experimental infections. The secretory effects of certain strains of *S. typhimurium* can be abolished in animals by indomethicin without altering the invasive process. This has led to the hypothesis of a possible enterotoxin-like effect on upper intestinal transport. However, studies in several experimental models show that salmonellae do not appear to produce an enterotoxin that is comparable with cholera and *E. coli* enterotoxins.

Studies in human volunteers indicate that large numbers of viable organisms must be ingested to produce clinically apparent disease. However, a transient carrier state can be produced with doses 10 or 100 times smaller than those required to evoke symptoms of infection. The minimal infectious dose varies markedly among different serotypes.

Many host factors influence the frequency and nature of *Salmonella* infections. The minimal infectious dose varies considerably among different individual hosts and can be reduced by antacids, antimotility drugs, or antimicrobial agents in experimental animals. Some have reported the precipitation of severe systemic disease following antimotility therapy for mild gastroenteritis.

The bacterial flora of the intestine is important in determining the fate of ingested salmonellas. Administration of certain antibiotics by the oral route to mice results in a 10,000-fold increase in susceptibility to infection with *S. enteritidis.* Somewhat similar observations have been made in experimental typhoid fever in volunteers. In these studies the dose of *S. typhi* required to initiate infection by the oral route in man can be reduced sharply by giving certain antimicrobials orally prior to challenge. Epidemiologic studies have also shown that prior antimicrobial therapy alters the capacity of the human intestinal tract to eradicate *Salmonella* acquired naturally. The effect of antibiotic therapy may be related to a marked diminution in number of bacteroides or other organisms which produce antimicrobial substances such as short-chain fatty acids that are active against *Salmonella.* Alteration in intestinal flora also has been suggested as a mechanism of the increased susceptibility of patients with previous major gastric surgery, especially gastrectomy and gastroenterostomy, to intestinal infection with salmonellas. However, reduced acidity or rapid emptying time consequent to gastric surgery also appear to play a role by increasing the number of viable organisms reaching the small intestine.

Cell-mediated immune mechanisms appear to be important in host resistance to infection with salmonellae. About one-third of patients who are hospitalized because of salmonellosis have some type of major underlying disease, such as leukemia, lymphoma, lupus erythematosus, or aplastic anemia. This may be coincidence but more often reflects a decrease in resistance to bacterial infection in general. In a few diseases there is evidence to indicate an almost specific predisposition to infection by salmonellas that exceeds susceptibility to other bacterial species. Patients with sickle-cell anemia and other hemolytic processes are unusually susceptible to bloodstream invasion by salmonellae. In patients with sickle hemoglobinopathies there is a strong tendency for localization in bone, and salmonellas, not staphylococci, are the most common cause of osteomyelitis in patients with sickle-cell diseases. *Salmonella* bacteremia is also an unusually frequent complication of the acute hemolytic phase of bartonellosis (Chap. 150).

Infants are more susceptible to *Salmonella* infection and remain convalescent carriers for a longer period of time than adults. The mortality rate from the disease is also higher in infants and in the elderly than in young adults.

CLINICAL MANIFESTATIONS Gastroenteritis Although gastroenteritis often occurs in large epidemics among individuals who have eaten the same contaminated food, family outbreaks and sporadic cases are even more common. After an incubation period of 8 to 48 h, there is sudden onset of colicky abdominal pain and loose, watery diarrhea, occasionally with mucus or blood. Nausea and vomiting are frequent but are rarely severe or protracted. Fever of 38 to 39°C is common, and there may be an initial chill. Patients usually have mild to moderate abdominal tenderness on palpation, but severe tenderness, even with rebound, occurs in occasional patients. Peristalsis is usually hyperactive. Abdominal findings may be prominent in some patients and lead to confusion with certain intraabdominal emergencies, such as acute appendicitis or acute cholecystitis. Symptoms usually subside promptly within 2 to 5 days and recovery is uneventful. However, the illness is occasionally more protracted, with persistence of diarrhea and low-grade fever for 10 to 14 days. Fatalities rarely exceed 1 percent of the affected population and are limited almost entirely to infants, the aged, and debilitated patients.

The causative organism can often be isolated from the suspected food and from feces during the acute illness. Stool cultures usually become negative for salmonellae within 1 to 4 weeks, but occasional patients continue to excrete organisms for months. Organisms tend to persist in the stools of infants and young children for longer periods than in older children or adults. The blood leukocyte count is usually normal. The blood culture is usually negative.

Enteric or paratyphoid fever Certain species can produce an illness clinically indistinguishable from typhoid fever, with prolonged fever, rose spots, splenomegaly, leukopenia, gastrointestinal symptoms, and positive blood and stool cultures. The organisms most likely to produce this picture are *S. cholera-suis* and *S. enteritidis,* serotypes *paratyphi A* and *paratyphi B.* Occasionally a typical attack of food poisoning is followed in a few days by manifestations of paratyphoid fever. Generally, paratyphoid fevers tend to be milder than *S. typhi* infections, but differentiation on clinical grounds is not possible in the individual case. Recovery may be followed by continued excretion of the causative organism in the stools for several months, but the chronic carrier state is less frequent than in typhoid fever.

Bacteremia *Salmonella* species may produce a syndrome characterized primarily by prolonged fever and positive blood cultures. Although symptoms of gastroenteritis can precede bacteremia, they are usually lacking, and most cases arise sporadically. In many instances, the only manifestations are prolonged fever, which is usually spiking and is accompanied by repeated rigors, sweats, aching, anorexia, and weight loss. The characteristic features of typhoid and paratyphoid fever, such as rose spots, persistent leukopenia, and sustained fever, are absent. Stool cultures are usually negative. In contrast to the constant bacteremia of typhoid fever, discharge of organisms into the bloodstream is intermittent, and repeated blood cultures may be required to demonstrate the causative organism. At some time in the course of the illness, localizing signs of infection appear in about one-fourth of the cases. Pulmonary infection in the form of bronchopneumonia or abscess, pleurisy, empyema, pericarditis, endocarditis, pyelonephritis, meningitis, osteomyelitis, and arthritis are relatively common. The blood leukocyte count is usually normal, but with the development of focal lesions, polymorphonuclear leukocytosis as high as 20,000 to 25,000 cells per mm^3 occurs. *Salmonella* bacteremia can be a very puzzling disorder, especially before localization takes place, and should be considered in cases of fever of unknown origin.

A prolonged febrile illness lasting weeks or months and characterized by weight loss, marked anemia, hepatosplenomegaly, and bacteremia with *Salmonella* has been described in Brazil and other areas of the world in patients with hepatosplenic schistosomiasis due to *Schistosoma mansoni.* Intermittent bacteremia with *Salmonella* also occurs in patients with *Schistosoma haematobium* infection who are also urinary carriers of *Salmonella.*

Local pyogenic infections *Salmonella* organisms can produce abscesses in almost any anatomic site, and these can occur independently of previous symptoms of gastroenteritis or other systemic illness, or as complications of bacteremias. There is nothing characteristic about the suppurative lesions, and the correct etiologic diagnosis is rarely made on the basis of clinical findings alone. There is a strong tendency for salmonellae to localize in tissues that are the site of preexisting disease. Localization has been described in aneurysms, bone adjacent to aortic aneurysms, hematomas, and many different tumors, including hypernephroma, ovarian cyst, and pheochromocytoma. Meningeal localization of infection is common in newborns and infants, and occasional small outbreaks of *Salmonella* infection in nurseries have consisted almost entirely of meningitis. In addition to suppurative joint disease, a chronic aseptic polyarthritis has been described.

DIAGNOSIS Febrile gastroenteritis produced by presumed viral agents and shigellosis can be distinguished from *Salmonella* gastroenteritis only by appropriate stool cultures, especially in sporadic cases. Polymorphonuclear fecal leukocytes are frequently present in *Salmonella* gastroenteritis and in bacillary dysentery (shigellosis), but not in viral, giardial, or enterotoxin-induced gastroenteritis. Staphylococcal food poisoning usually is not associated with fever, and vomiting is a more prominent feature than in most *Salmonella* infections. Systemic manifestations are usually absent in patients with gastroenteritis caused by enterotoxigenic *E. coli* and *Clostridium perfringens.* Many toxic agents and drugs can produce diarrhea, nausea, and abdominal pain, but fever is rarely a feature of these disorders, and the diagnosis depends upon a history of exposure or ingestion. The diagnosis of paratyphoid fever or *Salmonella* bacteremia depends upon isolation of the causative organism. Agglutination tests with acute and convalescent serums as performed in the usual clinical laboratory are not very helpful. The possibility of an underlying disease should be considered in every patient with a severe *Salmonella* infection.

TREATMENT The treatment of *Salmonella* gastroenteritis is supportive. Dehydration should be corrected by parenteral administration of fluids and electrolytes. Abdominal cramps and diarrhea often are much improved if the patient takes nothing by mouth for 8 to 12 h. Antimicrobial therapy, irrespective of type, does not appear to exert a beneficial effect on the clinical course of *Salmonella* gastroenteritis or decrease the duration of excretion of organisms in the stools. In fact, recent studies show that the period of excretion of *Salmonella* in stools during convalescence is actually longer in patients who have been treated with antimicrobial drugs during the acute illness than in patients who received no antimicrobial therapy. Unless there is documented bacteremia or a protracted febrile course suggesting the diagnosis of enteric fever, antibiotics are *not* indicated in uncomplicated *Salmonella* gastroenteritis.

Chloramphenicol in doses of 3 g daily in adults is the antibiotic of choice in systemic infections including *Salmonella* bacteremia, metastatic infection, and paratyphoid fever. The response is characteristically slow, and the temperature rarely returns to normal until 3 to 4 days after beginning therapy. Therapy should be continued for at least 2 weeks, but in certain infections, such as osteomyelitis or meningitis, the duration may have to be extended. Resistance to multiple antibiotics, including chloramphenicol and ampicillin, occurs, particularly in salmonellae acquired outside the United States. Therefore, antibiotic sensitivity of the organism should be tested in cases of bacteremia, metastatic infection, or enteric fever.

Ampicillin is also effective in systemic infections caused by *Salmonella* strains sensitive to the action of this antibiotic. However, a significant proportion of *Salmonella* strains are highly resistant to ampicillin in vitro. For this reason, ampicillin should not be used in therapy of serious infections unless it is known that the causative organism is sensitive. As in cases of typhoid fever, the combination of trimethoprim and sulfamethoxazole may hold promise in the therapy of salmonella infection when the organism is resistant to chloramphenicol and ampicillin. The tetracycline derivatives have sometimes appeared to exert a beneficial effect, but streptomycin, polymyxin, neomycin, kanamycin, and the sulfonamides are generally ineffective. Antimicrobial resistance is usually related to transferable resistance factors.

Antimicrobial therapy is usually not indicated in convalescent or asymptomatic transient carriers of *Salmonella* species. The carrier state will spontaneously cease in 1 to 3 months in the vast majority of individuals.

The chronic carrier state with localization of infection in the gallbladder and positive stool cultures for a period of time exceeding 1 year is rarely caused by *Salmonella* serotypes other than *S. typhi* and *S. paratyphi* A and B. Its treatment has been discussed. Surgically accessible suppurative lesions should be drained.

PREVENTION AND CONTROL Continuous surveillance and careful reporting of all *Salmonella* isolates improve awareness of new strains, common sources, antibiotic resistance, and the carrier state. Because of the great number of specific serotypes, surveillance and serotyping have occasionally brought attention to widespread occurrence of relatively rare serotypes traced to single sources. Central surveillance of all reported serotypes led to the discovery of an international outbreak in 1974 of *S. eastbourne,* an otherwise rare serotype that was traced to Canadian chocolates. Adequate cooking of meat and egg products and careful surveillance of poultry products and persons who handle food have been only moderately successful in controlling salmonellosis. Probably most important, besides food surveillance, is personal hygiene, including handwashing. Transient or permanent carriers should be warned to take these precautions and, as much as possible, to avoid food preparation. Minimizing the time that foods are allowed to stand at room temperature (as between cooking and refrigeration) should reduce the chances of bacterial growth to infectious inocula.

Careful obstetrical histories for any diarrheal illness at the time a woman enters for delivery should always be

obtained, and mothers and infants so affected should be isolated until cultures rule out *Salmonella* carriage. Finally, because of the increasing antibiotic resistance and the enhanced susceptibility of patients receiving antibiotics, the indiscriminate use of unnecessary or "prophylactic" antimicrobial agents should be avoided.

REFERENCES

BAINE WB et al: Institutional salmonellosis. J Infect Dis 128:357, 1973

BENNETT IL JR, HOOK EW: Some aspects of salmonellosis. Annu Rev Med 10:1, 1959

BLACK PH et al: Salmonellosis—A review of some unusual aspects. N Engl J Med 262:811, 864, 921, 1960

DINBAR A et al: The treatment of chronic biliary salmonella carriers. Am J Med 47:236, 1969

FELDMAN RE et al: Epidemiology of *Salmonella typhi* infection in a migrant labor camp in Dade County, Florida. J Infect Dis 130:354, 1974

FREITAG JL: Treatment of chronic typhoid carriers by cholecystectomy. Public Health Rept US 79:7, 1964

HORNICK RB et al: Typhoid fever: Pathogenesis and immunologic control. N Engl J Med 283:686, 739, 1970

KAYE D et al: Treatment of chronic enteric carriers of Salmonella typhosa with ampicillin. Ann NY Acad Sci 145:429, 1967

MCHUGH GL et al: Salmonella typhimurium resistant to silver nitrate, chloramphenicol, and ampicillin: A new threat to burn units? Lancet 1:235, 1975

OLARTE J, GALINDO E: *Salmonella typhi* resistant to chloramphenicol, ampicillin, and other antimicrobial agents: Strains isolated during an extensive typhoid fever epidemic in Mexico. Antimicrob Agents Chemother 4:597, 1973

REYNOLDS EW et al: Diagnostic specificity of Widal's reaction for typhoid fever. JAMA 214:2192, 1970

ROBERTSON RP et al: Chloramphenicol and ampicillin in salmonella enteric fever. N Engl J Med 278:171, 1968

Salmonella surveillance—Annual summary 1974. Atlanta: Center for Disease Control, 1975

WICKS ACP et al: Endemic typhoid fever. A diagnostic pitfall. Q J Med 40:341, 1971

141 SHIGELLOSIS

HARRY N. BEATY

DEFINITION Shigellosis is an acute, self-limited infection of the intestinal tract of man which is characterized by diarrhea, fever, and abdominal pain. The disease is frequently called *bacillary dysentery,* but the term *shigellosis* is preferred.

ETIOLOGY The genus *Shigella* of the family Enterobacteriaceae includes a group of closely related species which are nonmotile, nonencapsulated, slender, gram-negative rods. They are aerobes or facultative anaerobes and grow best at 37°C. Nutritional requirements are relatively simple, and the ability of these organisms to grow in the presence of bile salts is used in devising selective media which facilitate their isolation. However, *S. dysenteriae* type 1 may be inhibited by these media, and growth may not be apparent for several days. Fermentation of carbohydrates differs according to species, but all strains produce acid in glucose and either fail to ferment lactose or do so only slowly. The shigellas are classified into subgroups A, B, C, or D on the basis of biochemical and antigenic characteristics. The clinically important species within the respective groups are *S. dysenteriae, S. flexneri, S. boydii,* and *S. sonnei.* While these shigellas share antigens among themselves and with other enteric bacilli, serologic classification is not difficult, and with the exception of *S. sonnei* a number of serotypes of each species has been recognized.

The somatic antigen of the shigellas is an endotoxin which is chemically and biologically similar to the endotoxins of other gram-negative bacilli. *Shigella dysenteriae* type 1 (Shiga bacillus) also produces an exotoxin(s) which has neurotoxic and enterotoxic properties. The role of this exotoxin in the pathogenesis of shigellosis is unknown, and there is no evidence that other species of *Shigella* produce a similar substance.

EPIDEMIOLOGY The principal habitat of the shigellas is the gastrointestinal tract of higher primates. Natural disease is limited almost entirely to man, and the convalescent or asymptomatic carrier is the only recognized reservoir. In 1972 a family outbreak of the disease was attributed to a pet monkey. Spread of infection from person to person occurs primarily when organisms on hands and inanimate objects contaminated with infected feces are ingested. In the United States, common source outbreaks usually involve food which has been contaminated by careless handlers. Outbreaks associated with drinking water are rare, but swimming in contaminated rivers or pools can be a cause of infection. In regions where sanitation is poor, flies which have been in contact with infected human feces may serve as an important vector in the transmission of this disease.

Shigellosis is worldwide in distribution, and is particularly common in countries where effective sanitation is lacking. Around ten thousand cases are reported annually in the United States, but many more undoubtedly occur. *Shigella sonnei* is responsible for about three-fourths of the infections encountered in this country; *S. flexneri* is isolated from all but a small percentage of the rest. *Shigella dysenteriae* type 1, which formerly produced disease predominantly in Asia, has been responsible for large outbreaks of diarrhea in Central America. Cases encountered in the United States have occurred almost exclusively among foreign travelers or their contacts, but a few have been encountered in individuals with no known exposure. Major epidemics of shigellosis are uncommon in the United States, but high-risk groups do exist in the inner cities, in mental or penal institutions, and on Indian reservations. Poor sanitation, low standards of personal hygiene, crowded conditions, and a high proportion of children in a population favor spread of the infection. Infected persons may excrete organisms intermittently during convalescence, but the carrier state infrequently persists longer than 3 months.

Humoral antibodies frequently develop in response to clinical infection, but there is no evidence that they influence the course of the disease or protect against reinfection. However, persons living in endemic areas seem to develop immunity to recurrent episodes of clinical disease, and volunteers infected with a specific strain are resistant to rechallenge with that strain for weeks to months. This immunity may be mediated by coproantibody, which has been identified in the stool of patients with shigellosis, or by cellular defense mechanisms in the wall of the bowel. In any event, it has led to the development of live, attenuated vaccines which, given orally, induce the same degree of immunity as natural infection. Parenteral vaccines are of no value.

PATHOGENESIS AND PATHOLOGY The major pathologic feature of shigellosis is mucosal inflammation which usually involves the entire colon and may extend into the terminal ileum. A fibrinous exudate often develops, and necrosis of the mucosa produces shallow ulcers which bleed readily. Microscopic examination shows that the submucosa and muscularis are infiltrated with bacteria and polymorphonuclear leukocytes. Ulcers are sharply demarcated and are not undermined. These lesions are produced only by organisms which penetrate intestinal epithelial cells and multiply in the intestinal mucosa. Avirulent strains multiply in the lumen of the bowel, elaborate endotoxin, and induce intestinal immunity, but without the capability of penetrating the mucosa, they cannot produce disease. Unlike members of the genus *Salmonella* which require a large inoculum to produce infection, as few as 10 to 100 virulent *Shigella* can cause disease. This probably explains why person-to-person spread of this infection is so common.

The systemic manifestations of shigellosis are primarily due to the fluid and electrolyte disturbances consequent to the diarrhea. Bacteremia is rare, except when infection is due to the Shiga bacillus, and fever is often attributed to "toxins" which presumably are absorbed from the intestinal tract.

CLINICAL MANIFESTATIONS *Shigella* infections are characterized by fever, abdominal pain, and diarrhea. However, mild diarrhea alone or asymptomatic infection occurs in a significant proportion of individuals infected. The incubation period is usually 24 to 48 h, and the first symptom is often colicky abdominal pain which is folllowed within an hour by high fever and diarrhea, often accompanied by tenesmus. Other symptoms include nausea, vomiting, headache, myalgia, and convulsions in children. The stools are liquid, greenish in color, contain shreds of mucus, and in 20 to 30 percent of cases various amounts of gross blood. Depending upon the severity of diarrhea and the height of fever, patients may become profoundly dehydrated, and circulatory collapse can occur. Lower abdominal tenderness and hyperactive bowel sounds are common, but there is no peritoneal irritation. Splenomegaly has been reported, but is rare. Sigmoidoscopic examination reveals diffuse mucosal inflammation, often with multiple ulcerations.

LABORATORY FINDINGS Blood leukocyte counts usually range between 5,000 and 15,000 per mm^3, and anemia is uncommon. Microscopic examination of the stool reveals shreds of mucus, erythrocytes, and many polymorphonuclear leukocytes. Stool culture is positive, but blood cultures rarely are. Electrolyte abnormalities depend upon the degree of vomiting and diarrhea.

COURSE Shigellosis is generally a self-limited disease, and patients usually become afebrile in about four days. Diarrhea and abdominal cramps may continue a few days longer, but within a week most patients have recovered. However, a significant proportion of untreated patients continue to shed organisms in the stool for two or more weeks. In about 10 percent of cases a clinical or bacteriologic relapse occurs unless antibiotics are given. In the United States, the overall mortality rate associated with shigellosis is less than 0.1 percent. However, among young children and elderly patients, the illness is often more severe and the prognosis poorer. *Shigella dysenteriae* type 1 produces particularly severe infections, and mortality rates of 25 to 50 percent have been recorded in epidemics produced by this species.

Complications of *Shigella* infections are encountered infrequently. An uncommon but significant problem is perforation of the colon. Hematogenous dissemination of the shigellas is also rare, but these organisms have been encountered in metastatic foci of infection such as abscesses and meningitis. In some series, bacteremia due to other gram-negative bacilli has been seen in association with shigellosis. An acute, nonsuppurative arthritis involving large, weight-bearing joints may occur during convalescence, but in patients given chemotherapy this complication is unusual. Conjunctivitis, iritis, and peripheral neuropathy accompany shigellosis on rare occasions.

DIAGNOSIS A definitive diagnosis can be established when pathogenic members of the genus *Shigella* are isolated from cultures. These organisms survive for only a short time in feces, and fresh stool specimens or rectal swabs should be cultured promptly. Recovery of the shigellas is facilitated if saline suspensions of stool are streaked directly onto selective media such as SS agar or desoxycholate citrate agar. Agglutinating antibodies can be detected in the serum of the majority of patients with positive cultures and may occasionally be of value in establishing the diagnosis of shigellosis. Immunofluorescent techniques which allow rapid detection of organisms in the stool have been developed.

Shigellosis infection should be considered in every febrile illness associated with diarrhea. Occasionally, children with infections such as tonsillitis or otitis have diarrhea, but the major differential diagnosis of shigellosis includes acute ulcerative colitis, viral enteritis, amebic dysentery, salmonellosis, and clostridial or staphylococcal food poisoning. Shigellosis can closely mimic acute ulcerative colitis, and should be excluded with cultures in patients thought to have this disease. In viral infections, fever is uncommon, and the stool usually does not contain gross blood or pus. The onset of amebic colitis is gradual, and the diarrhea is relatively mild. Staphylococcal food poisoning is associated with more nausea and vomiting, and usually is not associated with fever. *Salmonella* infections can be differentiated with certainty only by bacteriologic studies.

TREATMENT The treatment of shigellosis is primarily supportive, and the major goal is correction of fluid and electrolyte abnormalities. Antibiotics are of secondary importance, and are used chiefly to shorten the duration of illness and to prevent relapse. Sulfonamides formerly were effective in the treatment of bacillary dysentery, but almost 90 percent of *S. sonnei* isolated in the United States are resistant to these drugs. More significantly, since 1955 epidemics of shigellosis in various parts of the world, including the United States, have been caused by organisms resistant to multiple antibiotics. The molecular basis for multiple drug resistance involves the episomal transfer (R factor) of drug-resistant determinants between enteric bacilli.

Currently, increasing numbers of isolates in the United States are resistant to a number of antimicrobials. Ampicillin and tetracycline are still the drugs of choice for shigellosis, but widespread resistance to these agents makes it advisable to determine the antibiotic susceptibility of all *Shigella* isolates before chemotherapy is instituted. The decision of whether to treat patients with antimicrobials should be based on several factors such as the nature of the organism (e.g., *S. dysenteriae* infections should be treated), the severity of the illness, the availability of safe and effective drugs, and the patient's social and physical environment.

Lomotil and antispasmodics such as paregoric should not be used in individuals with shigellosis, because these agents have an adverse effect on the course of infection caused by invasive pathogens.

PREVENTION The most important prophylactic measures are the maintenance of proper sanitation and adequate sewage disposal. The detection and elimination of carriers are difficult and rarely practical. Methods for increasing resistance with oral vaccines may be useful in preventing outbreaks among susceptible populations.

REFERENCES

DuPont HL et al: Immunity in shigellosis: I. Response of man to attenuated strains of *Shigella.* J Infect Dis 125:5, 1972

—— et al: Immunity in shigellosis: II, Protection induced by oral live vaccine or primary infection. J Infect Dis 125:12, 1972

——, Hornick RB: Clinical approach to infectious diarrheas. Medicine 52:265, 1973

Weissman JB et al: Impact in the United States of the Shiga dysentery pandemic of Central America and Mexico: A review of surveillance data through 1972. J Infect Dis 129:218, 1974

section 6 | Diseases caused by other gram-negative bacilli

142 HEMOPHILUS INFECTIONS

LOUIS WEINSTEIN

The genus *Hemophilus* consists of nonmotile, gram-negative rods or coccobacilli which require specific growth factors (X and V) for multiplication. The organisms of importance in human disease are *H. influenzae, H. pertussis, H. ducreyi, H. aphrophilus,* the Koch-Weeks bacillus, and *Moraxella lacunata.* Two other species are found in the pharynges of normal individuals and, rarely, may produce pharyngitis *(H. hemolyticus)* or endocarditis *(H. parainfluenzae).* The site invaded most frequently is the respiratory tract, and the organism responsible for the bulk of infections is *H. influenzae.*

HEMOPHILUS INFLUENZAE INFECTIONS

Hemophilus influenzae produces a wide variety of diseases in many organ systems. The organism was first isolated by Pfeiffer during a pandemic of influenza in 1890 and was thought to be the causative agent of this disease. During the 1918 influenza pandemic, extensive bacteriologic investigations revealed a high incidence of *H. influenzae* in the nasopharynges and lungs of patients in many parts of the world.

ETIOLOGY *Hemophilus influenzae* is a gram-negative, nonsporulating, pleomorphic rod. In exudates, the organisms are usually predominantly coccobacillary and can be mistaken for pneumococci or meningococci. Some strains demonstrate bipolar staining and bacillary forms that vary from short rods to long filamentous ones.

Hemophilus influenzae grows well on chocolate agar and Levinthal's medium, which has the advantage of being transparent. On Levinthal's agar, typical colonies are iridescent when viewed by obliquely transmitted light when they are about 4 to 6 h old; this property disappears after 24 h.

Although it had been thought that strains without capsules were nonpathogenic, such strains have been implicated in infections of the respiratory tract. On the basis of specific capsular polysaccharides, *H. influenzae* may be classified into six types. Type B produces about 95 percent of human infections.

EPIDEMIOLOGY *Hemophilus influenzae* infects only human beings naturally. It is not ordinarily invasive for any of the other species, although monkeys can be infected experimentally.

The incidence of *H. influenzae* infections is greatest in the winter and early spring. Nose and throat cultures during these seasons reveal the organisms in many asymptomatic individuals. Penicillin therapy increases the incidence of positive throat cultures.

Children in the first 2 months of life have a high level of passively transferred bactericidal antibody. Between the ages of two months and three years, most children show little antibody, but with aging the levels increase.

PATHOLOGY The characteristic tissue response to *H. influenzae* is acute suppurative inflammation. Infections of the larynx, trachea, and bronchial tree are characterized by edema of the mucosa and thick exudate, and invasion of the lungs results in a bronchopneumonia. A severe, diffuse bronchiolitis may develop in young children. In influenzal meningitis, the brain is covered with thick greenish-yellow exudate.

Microscopic examination of the lesions produced by *H. influenzae* reveals an exudate consisting primarily of polymorphonuclear leukocytes and large numbers of organisms enmeshed in fibrin.

CLINICAL MANIFESTATIONS Severe *H. influenzae* infections are usually accompanied by high fever, usually without rigors, and generalized malaise. In milder infections, fever is inconstant. The commonest diseases produced by this organism are pharyngitis, epiglottitis, laryngotracheitis, pneumonia, bronchitis and bronchiolitis, otitis media, and meningitis. The symptoms and signs of invasion of the respiratory tract or meninges are similar to those of infection of these areas by other organisms, and differential etiologic diagnosis depends upon epidemiologic background, the age of the patient, and demonstration of the causative agent.

Pharyngitis *Hemophilus influenzae* is a relatively common cause of pharyngitis in children; acute influenzal pharyngitis is now being observed more often in adults, where it may develop as a complication of chemotherapy for other infections. Examination of the throat often reveals no remarkable findings. Rarely, however, the pharyngeal mucosa is reddened; patchy, soft, yellow exudate may be present. The pharyngitis tends to persist for many days unless properly treated. Dissociation between the appearance of the pharynx and the intensity of local discomfort is common in adults. The pharyngeal mucosa frequently appears normal or shows only slight diffuse redness at the same time that pain is so severe that swallowing of saliva is difficult and eating impossible.

Epiglottitis Disease of the upper part of the respiratory tract produced by *H. influenzae* is sometimes limited to the epiglottis, which becomes reddened, swollen, and stiff. Discomfort in the hypopharynx and "croupy" breathing may progress to a point at which tracheostomy becomes necessary. This disease is rare in adults.

Laryngotracheobronchitis This is most common in young children. The entire laryngotracheobronchial tree may be infected, with resulting rapidly progressive obstruction of the airway. "Croupy" cough is accompanied by increasing signs of respiratory embarrassment, and tracheostomy is sometimes necessary. Influenzal laryngotracheitis is very rare in adults. The disease can lead to death in children within 18 to 24 h.

Pneumonia Primary pneumonia due to *H. influenzae,* with rare exceptions, is a disease of children. In adults, it is usually secondary to viral influenza, measles, or bacterial pneumonitis. It may complicate rubeola or pertussis in the young. Bacteremia occurs in approximately one-third of the cases.

Bronchitis and bronchiolitis Severe, diffuse bronchiolitis characterized by persistent nonproductive cough, wheezing, and dyspnea occurs primarily in children. Physical examination usually reveals depression and fixation of the diaphragm, prolonged expiration, and typical asthmatic breathing. Roentgenographic examination of the chest discloses increased radiolucence and flattening of the diaphragm consistent with emphysema. This is an extremely serious illness and unless promptly recognized and treated may be rapidly fatal.

Superimposed bacterial infection contributes significantly to the clinical manifestations and progressive deterioration in established chronic bronchitis or "senile emphysema" in adults. Among the bacteria involved, the pneumococcus and *H. influenzae* are the commonest; the latter has been isolated from the respiratory tracts of 80 to 90 percent of patients in Europe. It is recovered much less frequently in the United States.

Otitis media *Hemophilus influenzae* is a common cause of suppurative otitis media in children; the infection is uncommon in adults. In many instances, middle ear disease due to this species is indistinguishable from that produced by *Staphylococcus aureus, Diplococcus pneumoniae,* or group A *Streptococcus pyogenes.* In many cases, however, the appearance is that of serous otitis media and leads to a misdiagnosis of nonbacterial disease. Paracentesis, or aspiration of fluid from the middle ear, and culture are required in such cases to establish the presence of *H. influenzae* and to guide appropriate chemotherapy.

Meningitis *Hemophilus influenzae,* type B, is the commonest cause of meningitis between the ages of six months and two years and is frequent in later childhood. There has been a recent increase in the frequency of this disease in otherwise healthy adults of any age. Next to the pneumococcus, *H. influenzae* is the organism most likely to cause recurrent bacterial meningitis. Ninety-five percent of the cases are produced by type B organisms, a few by type A, and a rare one by nonencapsulated strains. About two-thirds of patients have a preceding infection of the upper part of the respiratory tract or otitis media, and about one-third have bronchopneumonia. Signs of meningeal irritation are usually prominent, except in very young babies, in whom bulging of the fontanels may be the only indication. The diagnosis should be suspected because of the age of the patient and the frequent prodrome of respiratory infection.

Other diseases Subacute and acute bacterial endocarditis may be produced by *H. influenzae* or *H. parainfluenzae.* The influenza bacillus is a rare cause of suppurative pericarditis. In the winter, acute conjunctivitis may be due to *H. influenzae.* No clinical features distinguish this from "pinkeye" produced by the Koch-Weeks bacillus; however, epidemics of conjunctivitis due to the latter are most common in the summer. Although it has been suggested that *H. influenzae* and the Koch-Weeks bacillus are identical, studies indicate that although antigenically related, they are distinct species. *Moraxella lacunata* is also an occasional cause of acute purulent conjunctivitis. Acute pyogenic arthritis due to *H. influenzae* has been reported. Among other diseases produced by this organism are osteomyelitis, paranasal sinusitis, appendicitis, cellulitis, and infections of the liver, genital tract, and skin.

LABORATORY FINDINGS As a rule, infections due to *H. influenzae* are accompanied by polymorphonuclear leukocytosis ranging from 15,000 to 30,000 per mm^3. In young children with severe disease, leukopenia (2,000 to 3,000 leukocytes per mm^3) with a deficiency of polymorphonuclear leukocytes can occur. Bacteremia occurs irregularly in influenzal infections of the respiratory tract but is demonstrable in about 50 percent of cases of meningitis.

COURSE AND COMPLICATIONS The course of *H. influenzae* infections is influenced completely by the location of the disease. Epiglottitis, laryngotracheobronchitis, bronchiolitis, or pneumonia may be fulminating. Some patients succumb to the uncontrolled infection, but in many the cause of death is obstruction of the airway. This cannot always be relieved by surgical methods, because impediment to flow of air is most marked in the smaller radicles of the bronchial tree. Virtually 100 percent of untreated cases of influenzal meningitis terminate fatally. Internal and external hydrocephalus, brain abscess, subdural empyema, diffuse cortical necrosis, and, rarely, shock (the Waterhouse-Friderichsen syndrome) are possible complications. With specific therapy, the incidence of complications is generally sharply reduced. However, if subdural aspiration is carried out routinely in children with influenzal meningitis which is responding to antibiotics, sterile fluid is demonstrable in about half the cases. Neurologic disturbances from subdural effusions are uncommon. Epileptiform seizures due to discrete thrombosis of cerebral veins may occur while the disease is responding favorably to chemotherapy.

TREATMENT *Hemophilus influenzae* is susceptible in vitro to several antimicrobial agents including streptomycin, the tetracyclines, chloramphenicol, and the sulfonamides.

Most strains are inhibited by penicillin G in concentrations of 0.6 μg per ml or less.

Although many strains are still highly sensitive to ampicillin, there has been a recent increase in the frequency of strains resistant to this agent. This has become a sufficiently important problem so that it is now recommended that, after the necessary cultures have been carried out, the initial therapeutic agent of serious infections due to *H. influenzae* be chloramphenicol, as described below. If the organism proves to be resistant to ampicillin, treatment is completed with chloramphenicol. However, if the isolated strain is sensitive to ampicillin, administration of chloramphenicol is discontinued and ampicillin is substituted. For less serious forms of disease due to *H. influenzae* (otitis media, acute pharyngitis) resistant to ampicillin, a tetracycline compound may be effective initially; if the recovered strain proves to be sensitive to ampicillin, treatment is changed to this drug.

The dose of ampicillin in *H. influenzae* meningitis is 300 to 400 mg per kg per day, given in quantities of equal size and equally spaced. The management of otitis media or pharyngitis often requires no more than 100 to 150 mg per kg per day given by mouth. For adults with these infections, 2 to 4 g per day orally for 7 to 10 days usually suffices. Diarrhea is not infrequent in patients treated with ampicillin. Ampicillin therapy may fail in influenzal meningitis when complications, e.g., subdural empyema, supervene.

Although practically all strains of *H. influenzae* are sensitive to very small quantities of penicillin G, the therapeutic effects of this antibiotic are poor, and it must not be used as the sole agent for the treatment of meningitis due to this organism. The results with the tetracyclines are too variable to permit them to be recommended. An alternate regimen useful in influenzal meningitis is chloramphenicol (1 g intravenously every 6 h for adults; for children, 50 mg per kg per day in intravenous doses of equal size and equally spaced) plus sulfisoxazole or sulfadiazine (100 mg per kg per day). Regardless of the drug used, therapy should be continued for 2 weeks. Chloramphenicol or tetracycline is usually sufficient to treat upper respiratory tract infections, pneumonia, or otitis media in patients who are "sensitive" to penicillin.

HEMOPHILUS PERTUSSIS

Whooping cough (pertussis) occurs in about 85 percent of all unimmunized children. It is characterized by an inflammation of the entire respiratory tract which produces paroxysmal cough and the typical inspiratory stridor, or "whoop."

ETIOLOGY The causative agent is *Hemophilus pertussis (Bordetella pertussis),* a short or ovoid, gram-negative, nonmotile, nonsporulating, facultatively anaerobic bacillus. Bipolar staining is frequent, and encapsulation can be demonstrated by special stains.

The organism multiplies best on Bordet-Gengou medium. It contains two antigens. The heat-stable O antigen is common to all strains. Five varieties of a heat-labile specific agglutinogen K (1,2,3,4,5) are also present. All strains contain two or more of these antigens. This is of clinical importance because, in some areas of the world, the infecting strain has been found to have different K agglutinogens than those present in the vaccine being used to prevent the disease, resulting in failure of immunization.

Other infectious agents may rarely produce the syndrome of whooping cough. Among these are *B. parapertussis* and *B. bronchiseptica.* Several types of adenovirus (1,2,3,5,12) have been reported to produce a syndrome identical in all respects to that due to *B. pertussis.*

EPIDEMIOLOGY Pertussis is worldwide. Where the disease has not been present for several years, it tends to assume epidemic proportions when it reappears. In some areas, it is most common during the winter; in others it is seen with greatest frequency in the late summer and fall. The index of contagion is 80 to 100 percent; about 200,000 cases occur in the United States each year.

Approximately 40 percent of episodes of pertussis occur in the first 2 years of life; the same number is observed between the ages of two and five. At least 50 percent of all unvaccinated children have had whooping cough before they reach the age of five and 75 percent by the age of seventeen.

Pertussis is spread by droplets from the respiratory tract. Rarely, the organisms may be transmitted by fomites. Infectivity during the incubation period is questionable; the disease is most contagious during the catarrhal stage. Healthy carriers play no role in dissemination, but mild or missed cases are of great importance.

PATHOLOGY The initial lesion in whooping cough is hyperplasia of the peribronchial and tracheobronchial lymphoid tissue. The bronchi, trachea, larynx, and nasopharynx are soon involved in a necrotizing inflammatory reaction. The organisms are present in large numbers between the cilia of the trachea and following desquamation of the alveolar epithelium.

CLINICAL MANIFESTATIONS The incubation period of whooping cough averages 12 to 15 days but may be as long as 20 days. The first clinical manifestations (catarrhal stage) are slight nasal discharge, conjunctivitis, and mild cough without fever; these persist for 7 to 14 days.

The paroxysmal phase of pertussis follows and is characterized by paroxysms of coughing ending in a loud, crowing inspiratory noise (the whoop), the expulsion of varying quantities of thick, mucoid sputum from the respiratory tract, and vomiting. Episodes of cough may vary from 1 to 2 to 40 to 50 per day. Children under the age of six months frequently do not whoop. The mere presence of a whoop is in itself not diagnostic of pertussis. Rarely, the paroxysms of coughing are preceded by or replaced completely by sneezing.

Fever does not occur in the paroxysmal phase unless complications are present. Soreness over the trachea and main bronchi is common. Spasm, ulcer, or edema of the glottis sometimes occurs. In cases with severe vomiting and inability to retain food, serious inanition, wasting, and tetany may appear.

There is a bleeding tendency in pertussis. This is not associated with detectable defects in the clotting mechanisms; it has been suggested that it may be related to increased fragility of small blood vessels. Hemoptysis, epistaxis, purpura, and subconjunctival or intestinal hemorrhages occur but are usually of little clinical significance.

Findings on physical examination in pertussis are often entirely normal, but there may be injection of the blood vessels of the nose and pharynx. Although there are usually no abnormal findings in the lungs, fine, crackling, "sticky" rales are sometimes present. There are ulcers of the frenum of the tongue in about 20 percent of cases; these occur only in children in whom the lower central incisor teeth are present.

The paroxysmal stage of pertussis usually lasts from 1 to 6 weeks. When coughing persists beyond 6 weeks, it is usually due to the development of a so-called "habit whoop," not to continuation of the disease.

LABORATORY FINDINGS The total peripheral leukocyte count may be over 100,000 cells per mm^3, and mature lymphocytes may constitute 90 percent of the cells. This helps to distinguish the blood picture from that of acute lymphocytosis. The lymphocytosis appears to be induced by an intracellular product of the organism, most of the cells being released from lymphoid tissue including the thymus. Blood cultures are sterile. Nasopharyngeal cultures or "cough plates" on Bordet-Gengou agar are helpful in recovering the organism. X-ray study of the lungs in the uncomplicated case usually reveals only hilar lymphadenopathy and increase in the density of the bronchovascular markings.

COMPLICATIONS Bronchopneumonia occurs in from 1 to 10 percent of cases of pertussis; the organisms most frequently involved are group A *Strep. pyogenes, D. pneumoniae, Staph. aureus, H. influenzae,* and *B. pertussis.* Pneumonitis appearing during the course of chemotherapy is most often due to *Escherichia coli, Proteus* strains, *Klebsiella enterobacter,* or *Pseudomonas aeruginosa.* Another important complication is atelectasis; small areas of collapse are an almost constant finding, but major portions or a whole lung may be involved. Pneumothorax is rare.

The severe coughing of pertussis may lead to several complications. Hemorrhage may appear in the anterior chamber of the eye or in the retina. Detachment of the retina and blindness develop in rare cases. Prolapse of the rectum and inguinal or umbilical hernias have been noted.

Nervous system manifestations are not rare in pertussis. The commonest is convulsions; these often appear as fever develops rapidly during secondary bacterial infection. Other causes of seizures are encephalopathy (1 to 14 percent of cases), multiple petechial or gross hemorrhages of the brain, and cerebral hypoxia. The encephalopathy is characterized by an increase in the protein and cell content of the spinal fluid. Its etiology is unknown. Hyperreflexia, nuchal rigidity, cranial nerve palsies, areflexia, extensor plantar responses, flaccid hemiplegia, spasticity of the extremities, opisthotonus, difficulty in speaking, twitching, papilledema, nystagmus, blindness, strabismus, and dysphagia may occur. Some of the more important residua are mental retardation, recurrent convulsions, personality disorders, amnesia, aphasia, diffuse cerebral atrophy, chorea, and athetosis.

DIAGNOSIS The diagnosis of pertussis can frequently be made on clinical grounds alone. Knowledge of contact is helpful, but the appearance of paroxysms of typical coughing and whooping, after a short period of upper respiratory symptoms, is strongly suggestive of pertussis. It must be stressed, however, that in babies under the age of six months there is usually only paroxysmal coughing, without the characteristic whoop. An increased number of circulating lymphocytes is characteristic.

Isolation of *B. pertussis* from the respiratory tract establishes the diagnosis. Using "cough plates," nasopharyngeal swabs, and Bordet-Gengou medium, positive cultures can be obtained in 90 percent of patients in the catarrhal stage of the disease. The incidence of positive cultures is lower after paroxysmal coughing appears, and decreases with the duration of symptoms. The incidence of positive cultures in the catarrhal stage is about 90 percent. In the first week of the paroxysmal phase it is 75 percent; in the second week, 60 percent; in the third week, 45 percent; in the fourth week, 40 percent; in the fifth week, 10 percent.

Serologic studies are of little or no help in establishing the presence of pertussis.

PREVENTION Active immunization is effective in preventing pertussis in the majority of individuals. This may be started at the age of three months; both antibody production and protection against invasion by *B. pertussis* result. If the procedure is carried out at this early age, a "booster" injection should be administered at the end of the first year of life, and again just before the child starts school. Vaccine should not be given in the presence of the active disease; not only is it useless, but it may provoke serious neurologic reactions. There is evidence that the administration of "quadruple" vaccine—poliomyelitis virus, tetanus and diptheria toxoids, and *H. pertussis*—leads to some degree of suppression of the response to the pertussis bacillus. For this reason, when poliomyelitis vaccine (formalinized) is used, it should be given separately from the "triple" vaccine.

In children who have been exposed to pertussis but have not been actively immunized, passive protection may be given by the injection of 20 to 30 ml of human hyperimmune pertussis antiserum or 2 ml of immune γ-globulin as soon as possible after exposure, and again 1 week later. Such prophylaxis is 75 to 85 percent effective. The use of hyperimmune serum should be avoided if possible because it has been associated with the subsequent development of infectious hepatitis.

TREATMENT Although most of the antimicrobial drugs have been employed in the treatment of pertussis, there is no good evidence that they are beneficial. Chlortetracycline, chloramphenicol, oxytetracycline, erythromycin, and other antibiotics have been used, but the results obtained in controlled studies are not convincing.

There are few controlled studies of serum therapy in whooping cough, but in many clinics it is the practice to administer human hyperimmune serum (20 ml every 48 h for three doses), or immune γ-globulin (2 ml every 48 h for three doses) to all children with pertussis under the age of two.

Most important in therapy of pertussis is repair of the water and salt loss which follows severe and frequent vomiting. If failure to retain food is combated by prompt refeeding, patients can be made to maintain or gain weight.

Early detection of complications is one of the most important factors in the reduction of mortality. The prompt recognition of secondary bacterial infections of the lungs or middle ear, and therapy with a properly selected antibiotic agent lead to cure in practically all cases. When gross atelectasis occurs, correction by tracheal catheter suction or bronchoscopy may be lifesaving. Little can be done to influence the course or outcome of such complications as cerebral hemorrhage or encephalopathy.

Proper management of whooping cough has made the outlook for complete recovery excellent.

HEMOPHILUS APHROPHILUS

Human infections due to *H. aphrophilus,* although uncommon, are being reported with increasing frequency. This species differs from *H. influenzae* in some biochemical characteristics and requires the X but not the V factor for growth in an atmosphere containing 10 percent CO_2, but needs neither factor, in most instances, when incubated in moist air. The diseases produced by *H. aphrophilus* include endocarditis, brain abscess, bacteremia, acute and chronic sinusitis, otitis media, cervical abscess, pneumonia, meningitis, wound infection, and septic arthritis. Most strains of the organism appear to be fairly sensitive to penicillin G, cephalothin, gentamicin, chloramphenicol, and rifampin.

HEMOPHILUS PARAINFLUENZAE

This member of the genus *Hemophilus* differs from *H. influenzae* by requiring the V but not the X factor for growth. The infections in which it has been involved are acute pharyngitis, upper respiratory tract syndromes, acute suppurative otitis media, pneumonia, subacute bacterial endocarditis, meningitis, and brain abscess. Disease produced by this organism responds to treatment with ampicillin, tetracyclines, or chloramphenicol.

HEMOPHILUS VAGINALIS

This organism grows in the absence of both X and V factors. *Hemophilus vaginalis* is present in the vagina of about 30 percent of normal women; it is more common in individuals under forty years of age. Although it is a member of the indigenous vaginal microflora, evidence that it may produce a vaginitis has been presented; about 50 percent of normal volunteers developed acute vaginitis when *H. vaginalis* was introduced locally. The disease is characterized by a gray, malodorous discharge; failure to demonstrate trichomonads and culture of the fluid establish the etiologic diagnosis. The organism is often sensitive to ampicillin and the cephalosporins but may be resistant to the tetracyclines and penicillin G. Some strains may be inhibited by chloramphenicol.

REFERENCES

Hemophilus influenzae

COLLIER AM et al: Systemic infection with *Hemophilus influenzae* in very young infants. J Pediatr 70:539, 1967

FEINGOLD M, GELLIS SS: Cellulitis due to *Hemophilus influenzae* type B. N Engl J Med 272:788, 1965

GOLDSTEIN E et al: *Haemophilus influenzae* as a cause of adult pneumonia. Ann Intern Med 66:35, 1967

HOLDAWAY MD, TURK DC: Capsulated *Haemophilus influenzae* and respiratory tract disease. Lancet 1:358, 1967

NORDEN CW et al: Immunologic responses to *Hemophilus influenzae* meningitis. J Pediatr 80:209, 1972

PATTERSON RL JR, LEVINE DB: *Hemophilus influenzae* pyarthrosis in an adult. J Bone Joint Surg [Am] 47A: 1250, 1965

TURK DC, MAY JR: *Hemophilus influenzae. Its Clinical Importance,* London: English Universities Press, 1967

Hemophilus pertussis

BROOKSALER F, NELSON JD: Pertussis. A reappraisal and report of 190 confirmed cases. Am J Dis Child 114:389, 1967

CONNOR JD: Evidence for an etiologic role of adenoviral infection in pertussis. N Engl J Med 283:390, 1970

MORSE SI, BRAY KK: The occurrence and properties of leukocytosis and lymphocytosis-stimulating material in the supernatant fluid of *Bordetella* cultures. N Engl J Med 129:523, 1970

PEREIRA MS, CANDEIAS JAN: The association of viruses with clinical pertussis. J Hyg (Camb) 69:399, 1971

PRESTON NW: Type-specific immunity against whooping cough. Br Med J 2:724, 1963

WHITE R et al: The modern morbidity of pertussis in infants. Pediatrics 33:705, 1964

WILSON AT et al: Whooping cough: Difficulties in diagnosis and ineffectiveness of immunization. Lancet 2:623, 1965

Hemophilus aphrophilus

SUTTER VL, FEINGOLD SM: *Haemophilus aphrophilus* infections: Clinical and bacteriologic studies. Ann NY Acad Sci 174:468, 1970

Hemophilus parainfluenzae

HABLE KA et al: Three *Hemophilus* species. Am J Dis Child 121:35, 1971

Hemophilus vaginalis

LEWIS JF, O'BRIEN SM: Incidence of *Haemophilus vaginalis.* Am J Obstet Gynecol 103:103, 1969

REGAMEY C, SCHOENKNECHT FD: Puerperal fever with *Haemophilus vaginalis* septicemia. JAMA 225:1621, 1973

143 CHANCROID

KING K. HOLMES

DEFINITION Chancroid, or soft chancre, is an acute, sexually transmitted infection characterized by painful genital ulcerations usually associated with inflammatory, often suppurative, inguinal adenopathy. A presumptive diagnosis is supported by exclusion of syphilis, genital herpes, and other specific causes of genital ulceration, together with improvement following sulfonamide therapy. A specific diagnosis is proved only when *Hemophilus ducreyi* is isolated from the lesion or suppurative node.

ETIOLOGY The specific microbial etiology of chancroid has repeatedly been supported by isolation of Ducrey's bacterium, *H. ducreyi,* in mixed culture from chancroidal ulcers and in pure culture from buboes. However, anaerobic bacteria, particularly *Bacteroides fragilis, B. melaninogenicus,* and anaerobic gram-positive cocci, are often present in genital ulcers, and anaerobic spirochetes which can be confused with *Treponema pallidum* are occasionally seen as well. The role of such organisms as synergistic or independent pathogens remains undefined. The reported frequency of recovery of *H. ducreyi* from typical chancroid ulcers ranges from 15 to 90 percent. *Hemophilus ducreyi* is one of the most poorly characterized of all aerobic pathogens, and isolates from suspect lesions are identified principally by the requirement for whole blood for optimal growth, and by the formation of chains of small gram-negative rods in blood. Organisms possessing these nonspecific properties have also been recovered from smegma of normal men and the vagina of normal women.

EPIDEMIOLOGY The incidence of chancroid is unknown, since bacteriologic diagnosis is difficult, clinical diagnosis inaccurate, and reporting incomplete. Chancroid is most common in Southeast Asia, Africa, and South and Central America, but is becoming rare in developed countries. During 1975 only 811 cases of chancroid were reported in the United States, where the incidence is highest in the Southeast. The sex ratio of reported cases in the United States is five males to one female. Uncircumcised men are more susceptible to chancroid than circumcised men. Prostitution plays a significant role in transmission, and among merchant seamen and military troops whose sexual contacts are prostitutes, chancroid appears to be far more common than syphilis.

CLINICAL MANIFESTATIONS After an incubation period of 3 to 5 days, a small inflammatory papule appears, which becomes pustular or occasionally vesiculopustular and ulcerative within 2 to 3 days. The classic chancroid (Fig. 143-1) is superficial and shallow, ranging from a few millimeters to 2 cm in diameter. The edge usually appears ragged or scalloped and is surrounded by an inflammatory red halo. The base is covered by a necrotic exudate and bleeds easily when the exudate is removed. In contrast with syphilitic chancre, the chancroidal ulcer is extremely painful and tender and is not indurated. In men, the most frequent locations are the preputial orifice or internal surface of the prepuce, and the frenulum; in women, the labia and fourchette. Multiple ulcers are more common than single ulcers.

Acute, painful, tender, inflammatory inguinal adenopathy accompanies over 50 percent of cases, and is unilateral in about two-thirds. In untreated patients, the involved nodes become matted, forming a unilocular suppurative bubo. The overlying skin becomes erythematous, tense, thinned, and finally ruptures, forming a large single ulcer.

DIAGNOSIS Other diseases which may be confused with chancroid, in decreasing order of frequency, are genital herpes, primary syphilis, and lymphogranuloma venereum (LGV). One United States study of 100 consecutive men with penile ulceration disclosed genital herpes in 22, syphilis in 17, and traumatic lesions in 8. Classic chancroid ulcers were noted in 12, only 2 of which yielded *H. ducreyi* on culture. Most of the remaining ulcers were of uncertain etiology. The great majority of lesions diagnosed as chancroid in clinical practice probably actually represent genital herpes, syphilis, or traumatic lesions. The clinical diagnosis of chancroid usually depends upon exclusion of genital herpes and syphilis together with response to sulfonamide therapy.

Primary genital infection with *Herpes virus hominis* type 2 produces tender inguinal adenopathy in approximately 50 percent of cases, but primary genital herpes can usually be readily distinguished by the history of onset with vesicular lesions. Primary genital herpes often produces dysuria and symptoms suggestive of viremia, such as fever, myalgia, and arthralgia, whereas chancroid rarely causes systemic symptoms. Over 80 percent of women with primary herpes have cervical transient ulcerations. A localized cluster of vesicles and a past history of similar lesions characterize recurrent genital herpes.

If viral isolation cannot be attempted, a simple means of diagnosis of genital herpes is by cytology (Papanicolaou) smear obtained from the base of the genital lesion. Multinucleated cells and/or intranuclear inclusions can be seen in about two-thirds of vesicular or pustular herpetic lesions and about 50 percent of ulcerative lesions. In primary syphilis, the chancre is indurated, and the associated adenopathy is bilateral, nontender, and nonsuppurative. However, at least three dark-field examinations should be performed on separate days together with monthly serologic tests for syphilis for 3 months, to exclude syphilis.

The inguinal adenopathy of LGV differs from that of chancroid. The adenopathy of LGV develops after the genital lesion is healed, is indolent, often bilateral and nontender, and develops multilocular suppuration and fistulas. Chancroidal adenopathy appears rapidly, nearly always

FIGURE 143-1
The classic chancroid.

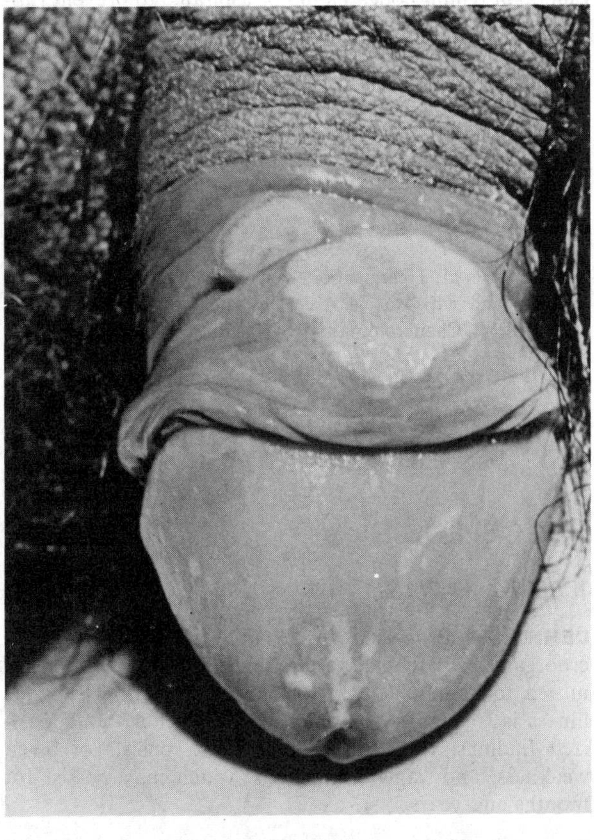

before the ulcer has healed, is more often unilateral, is more painful, and develops unilocular suppuration. A negative LGV complement fixation test provides evidence against LGV.

The only reliable method for laboratory diagnosis of chancroid consists of isolation of *H. ducreyi* from the ulcer or bubo. One recommended method of culture consists of inoculation of pus into tubes containing slants of 1.5 percent nutrient agar, overlain with 2 ml coagulated or defibrinated rabbit blood. The stained smear of exudate from lesions and the histologic appearance of biopsy material may suggest chancroid but are not specific. Immunodiagnostic tests for chancroid are needed.

TREATMENT Comparisons of various antibiotics for treatment of chancroid have been inconclusive, because treated cases have seldom been confirmed by isolation of *H. ducreyi.* Genital herpes usually begins to improve spontaneously about 10 days after onset of primary lesions and 4 days after onset of recurrent lesions, while primary syphilis usually heals 4 to 6 weeks after onset. Nonetheless, sulfonamides are considered more effective than tetracycline or streptomycin for chancroid, and sulfonamide therapy will not interfere with dark-field examination for *T. pallidum* or with development of a positive serologic test for syphilis. If initial dark-field examination of a chancroidal lesion is negative, sulfonamide therapy can be started and the dark-field examination can be repeated on subsequent days. Sulfisoxazole (Gantrisin) is usually effective in a dose of 4 g daily and should be continued until the lesion and adenopathy have healed, which usually requires about 2 weeks. Fluctuant lymph nodes should be aspirated to prevent rupture, since suppuration may progress despite therapy. After three successive dark-field examinations have been negative, if the response to sulfisoxazole is unsatisfactory, tetracycline hydrochloride should be added in a dose of 2 g daily. Alternative antibiotics include streptomycin, erythromycin, and chloramphenicol.

REFERENCES

KERFER RE et al: Treatment of chancroid. A comparison of tetracycline and sulfisoxazole. Arch Dermatol 100:604, 1969

SULLIVAN M: Chancroid. Am J Syph Gonor Vener Dis 24:482, 1940

144 BRUCELLOSIS

WESLEY W. SPINK

DEFINITION Brucellosis (undulant fever) is caused by microorganisms belonging to the genus *Brucella* and is transmitted to human beings from lower animals. The acute illness is frequently characterized by fever without localized findings, while the chronic form consists of fever, weakness, and vague complaints, which may persist for months and years.

HISTORY The first clear-cut picture of the disease was presented in 1863 by Marston, and the etiologic agent *(Brucella melitensis)* was discovered by Bruce in 1886. In 1897, Bang reported that *Br. abortus* was the cause of contagious abortion in cattle in Denmark. In 1911 brucellosis was found to be endemic in the goats of Texas, and Gentry and Ferenbaugh traced human cases to this source. Traum first identified *Brucella* organisms *(Br. suis)* from aborting sows in 1914. New species include *Br. canis,* which causes abortions in dogs, especially the beagle breed, and *Br. ovis,* which causes epidemics that result in sterility in rams.

ETIOLOGY Human brucellosis is primarily due to one of three species: *Br. melitensis* (goats), *Br. suis* (hogs), and *Br. abortus* (cattle). Several subtypes have been described under each of these three main categories. Brucellae are small, nonmotile, non-spore-forming, gram-negative rods. Growth is best at 37°C in trypticase soy broth or tryptose phosphate broth having a pH of 6.6 to 6.8, under conditions in which 10 percent of the air is displaced by carbon dioxide. The differentiation of the three species is dependent upon biochemical and serologic reaction. Strain 19, *Br. abortus,* is a viable attenuated strain used widely for vaccinating cattle. Accidental injection through the skin in veterinarians causes an acute febrile illness, which should be treated with tetracycline.

EPIDEMIOLOGY The natural reservoir of brucellosis is in domestic animals, particularly cattle, swine, goats, and sheep. The disease is very rarely transmitted from person to person.

Studies in the United States and elsewhere indicate that the majority of cases are acquired through contact, and fewer cases are caused by the ingestion of milk or milk products. This trend is due to the enactment of local and state ordinances requiring all milk sold for human consumption to be pasteurized. There is some evidence that brucellosis may be airborne, with the disease resulting from the inhalation of *Brucella.* Infections caused by *Br. abortus* are spread through cow's milk or through dermal contact with *Brucella.* Contact with infected porcine tissue is a common cause of infections due to *Br. suis.* Thus, brucellosis is primarily an occupational disease of rural areas, involving primarily meat-packing plant employees, farmers, veterinarians, and livestock producers. Disease due to *Br. melitensis* is the most common type of brucellosis on a worldwide basis. It occurs in local areas in the United States and is due to the ingestion of goat's milk cheese.

PATHOGENESIS Following invasion of the body by brucellae through the oropharynx or through the skin, the organisms tend to localize in tissues of the reticuloendothelial system, such as the bone marrow, lymph nodes, liver, spleen and also the kidneys. A characteristic but nonspecific reaction of these tissues to the brucellae is the appearance of epithelioid cells, giant cells of the foreign body and Langhans' types, and lymphocytes and plasma cells. Necrosis and caseation rarely occur in these granulomatous areas. When caseation is encountered, it is usually caused by *Br. suis.* The granulomas are similar to those of sarcoidosis and tuberculosis. Other, less frequent, sites of localization of *Brucella* organisms are the bones (especially the spine), the endocardium, and the testes. Although the central nervous system and peripheral nerves are commonly affected deleteriously by brucellae, the mechanism whereby this takes place is not known. Like other blood-borne bacilli, brucellae may on occasion localize in any tissue or organ in the body. Though brucellosis is a common cause of abortions in cattle, swine, and goats, authentic human abortions occur no more frequently with this disease than with other bacteremias. Orchitis in the male is rarely the cause of subsequent sterility.

MANIFESTATIONS The incubation period varies between 5 and 21 days, though many months may elapse between the time of infection and the first appearance of symptoms. The onset in many instances may be insidious; patients have a low-grade fever with no localized findings and complain of headache, weakness, insomnia, sweats, anorexia, constipation, pain over the spine, and generalized aches and pains. Less frequently, the disease may be ushered in by chills, high fever, and prostration, but, again, localizing abnormal physical findings may be absent. An enlarged and tender spleen is usually associated with the more severe cases. Pain on pressure over the vertebrae occurs occasionally, and pain along the course of peripheral nerves, particularly the sciatic nerve, is encountered. Orchitis appears after several days of illness and, like the orchitis of mumps, is ushered in with a chill or chilliness, high fever, and tender and enlarged testes. Painful and swollen joints are seen occasionally, but persistent and deforming arthritis is rare. Signs and symptoms referable to the lungs and pleurae are uncommon. A rare but serious complication is subacute bacterial endocarditis. Ocular disorders are associated with the more chronic forms of the disease.

The initial febrile stage of the illness may last from a few days up to several weeks. The persistence of fever and symptoms is definitely related to physical activity. Rest in bed during the acute illness is frequently associated with prompt improvement. The natural course of the disease in the majority of patients is marked by a permanent remission of fever and symptoms within 3 to 6 months, or sooner. A small number of patients with bacteriologically proved cases may have an illness that persists for a year or more.

The status of *chronic brucellosis* is extremely difficult to assess. There is no doubt that the infection may persist in a relatively small number of individuals for months and years. Such patients are in a state of ill health manifested by weakness, fatigue, mental depression, vague aches and pains, and no abnormal physical findings. Intermittent fever may occur. Of considerable importance in the suspected chronic case is the investigation of possible sites of chronic suppuration manifested by calcified caseating areas in the liver and spleen that can be detected by careful x-ray films of the abdomen. Abacteriuric pyuria should suggest, among other causes, renal suppuration due to brucellae.

LABORATORY FINDINGS A precise diagnosis of brucellosis is dependent upon the results of laboratory procedures.

Blood The total leukocyte count is usually normal, or slightly reduced, but is rarely over 10,000 cells per mm^3. The differential count reveals a relative lymphocytosis. The erythrocyte sedimentation rate is of no specific diagnostic aid, being normal or accelerated.

The most practical method for screening suspected cases of brucellosis is the agglutination reaction. Agglutinins usually appear during the second or third week of illness. If proper techniques and antigens are employed, agglutinins are demonstrated in the vast majority of bacteriologically proved cases. Active brucellosis is usually associated with titers of 1:100 or above. On rare occasions, the titer may be depressed by "blocking antibodies" in chronic illness. Only very rarely are agglutinins absent in patients with bacteriologically proved disease. Agglutinins for brucellosis are not always specific, since cross-reactions occur with the cholera vibrio and with *Pasteurella tularensis.* Agglutinins may persist in the blood long after the patient has recovered. One of the most critical diagnostic problems in the sporadic case of brucellosis is the interpretation of an agglutination titer of 1 to 100 or lower in the absence of definitive bacteriologic data and localizing signs. *Brucella*-agglutinating immunoglobulins in serum consist of both 7S and 19S globulins, but only 7S globulins have been associated with active disease in acute and chronic cases, providing a stimulating dose of antigen (skin test) has not been given prior to obtaining blood from the patient.

At least one, and preferably more, cultures of blood should be carried out in every suspected case of brucellosis. Brucellae have been isolated from aspirated sternal bone marrow when simultaneous blood cultures were sterile. It is too impractical for routine purposes to attempt to isolate brucellae from the urine, bile, or feces.

Intradermal tests A positive reaction to *Brucella* antigen has no more significance than that obtained with tuberculin in suspected cases of tuberculosis. A positive reaction indicates previous invasion of the body by brucellae and does not mean that active disease is present. When agglutinins are absent and cultures remain sterile, considerable caution must be exercised before making a diagnosis of brucellosis, even though the skin test is positive.

DIFFERENTIAL DIAGNOSIS Brucellosis must be differentiated from other acute febrile illnesses such as influenza and other upper respiratory diseases of doubtful etiology. Other diseases from which it must be differentiated include malaria and typhoid fever. Brucellosis may be confused with infectious mononucleosis.

Chronic brucellosis simulates psychoneurosis, anxiety states, and chronic nervous exhaustion. Indeed, a patient with brucellosis may also have these nervous disorders.

TREATMENT Patients with acute brucellosis should be reassured that a large majority of those with the disease recover spontaneously. Rest and psychotherapy are important during the febrile illness.

The course of acute brucellosis can be shortened and complications prevented by the prompt use of tetracycline, in dosage of 0.5 g four times daily orally for at least 3 weeks. In case of a relapse, this dose schedule can be repeated. Except in rare instances there is no advantage in more than two courses of tetracycline therapy. For more seriously ill patients streptomycin in dosage of 0.5 g twice daily may be used in addition to tetracycline. Tetracycline therapy, with and without streptomycin, is also effective in proved chronic brucellosis.

Febrile patients with either acute or chronic brucellosis sometimes have severe anorexia, depression, and generalized debilitation. Such individuals should receive an adrenocorticoid steroid preparation in addition to antibiotic therapy. Prednisone in oral dosage of 20 mg can be given twice daily for 72 to 96 h, or 100 mg hydrocortisone can be administered intravenously, followed by 50 mg orally twice daily.

The therapeutic use of brucella vaccine in chronic brucellosis is of very questionable value and is not recommended.

For the relief of headache and the generalized aches and pains, salicylates may be prescribed; the occasional use of barbiturates is desirable for the insomnia which is so commonly a part of the disease.

PROGNOSIS Although brucellosis may be a chronic and disabling disease, the overall mortality rate is very small. Even without the aid of effective drug therapy, only 15 percent of patients have an illness exceeding 3 months.

Cases of bacteriologically proved brucellosis in which the disease has continued for up to 25 years have been studied at the University of Minnesota Hospitals, but such cases are rare. So-called "chronic brucellosis" is diagnosed all too often on the basis of procedures of doubtful value, especially the intradermal test with *Brucella* antigen.

Relapses can occur in some chronic cases of brucellosis. These recurrences are not common and are manifested by fever, mental and physical disability, and generalized aches and pains. Too little attention has been given to the problem of reinfections. Clinical observations in meat-packing plant employees have confirmed studies made in experimentally infected animals, showing that the immunity induced by one attack of brucellosis is only relative and that second and third infections do take place. In individuals who continue to be exposed to the disease, it may be quite difficult to differentiate between relapses and reinfections. Furthermore, patients who have recovered from brucellosis have an acquired *Brucella* hypersensitivity that may render them extremely susceptible to the effects of contact with *Brucella* antigen. This is particularly applicable to veterinarians who have accidentally injected viable *Brucella* antigen into their skin while immunizing animals. Violent local and systemic febrile reactions follow such an incident within a few hours.

PREVENTION As long as a reservoir of brucellosis persists in domestic animals, human brucellosis will occur. The only practical means of eliminating the disease in human beings is to eradicate the disease from cattle, hogs, sheep, and goats. Control measures in animals have been worked out in the United States, especially for cattle, but porcine brucellosis remains a serious problem in pork-processing plants. Since human brucellosis may be contracted through the ingestion of contaminated milk and milk products, it is essential that only properly pasteurized milk be utilized for human consumption. Brucellosis is an occupational disease involving farmers, livestock workers, veterinarians, and those working in meat-packing plants, and there is no entirely safe means for immunizing these groups against the disease.

REFERENCES

BUCHANAN TM et al: Brucellosis in the United States, 1960–1972. An abattoir-associated disease. Medicine 53:403, 1974

Center for Disease Control: Brucellosis surveillance, annual summary 1973. Issued March 1975

MUNFORD RS et al: Human disease caused by *Brucella canis:* A clinical and epidemiologic study of two cases. JAMA 231:1267, 1975

SPINK WW: *The Nature of Brucellosis,* Minneapolis: University of Minnesota Press, 1956

——: The significance of bacterial hypersensitivity in human brucellosis: Studies on infections due to strain 19, *Brucella abortus.* Ann Intern Med 47:861, 1957

YOUNG EJ, SUVANNOPARRAT U: Brucellosis outbreak attributed to ingestion of unpasteurized goat cheese. Arch Intern Med 135: 240, 1975

145 TULAREMIA

LEIGHTON E. CLUFF

DEFINITION Tularemia (rabbit fever, deer-fly fever, Ohara's disease) is an infectious disease of animals transmitted to human beings by direct contact or by insect vectors. A cutaneous or mucous membrane lesion at the site of inoculation and regional lymph node enlargement are the characteristic manifestations of the disease in humans. Pneumonia or fever without regional manifestations also is a feature of tularemia.

HISTORY The microorganism responsible for tularemia was identified by McCoy and Chapin in 1912 among infected ground squirrels in Tulare County, California. The first description of tularemia in man was by Wherry and Lamb in 1914.

ETIOLOGY *Pasteurella (Francisella) tularensis* is a pleomorphic, nonsporulating, gram-negative bacillus. It can be cultured only on media containing glucose, cystine, and serum. Thorough cooking renders meat from infected animals safe for consumption, but tularemia can develop in persons handling carcasses that have been frozen for many days. *Pasteurella tularensis* is related antigenically to the causative organisms of brucellosis and plague and possesses an endotoxin similar to those of many other gram-negative bacteria.

EPIDEMIOLOGY AND PATHOGENESIS Contact with infected animals is the commonest source of tularemia in humans, but the disease also may be acquired from insects or by exposure to the organism in the laboratory. A variety of rodents, carnivores, ungulates, birds, and arthropods is naturally infected by *P. tularensis,* including rabbits, squirrels, woodchucks, muskrats, skunks, coyotes, foxes, opossums, mice, rats, quail, chickens, pheasants, snakes, ticks, and flies. The Rocky Mountain tick, western wood tick, eastern dog tick, and the Lone Star tick (*Dermacentor andersoni, D. variabilis, D. occidentalis,* and *Amblyomma amer-*

icanum) may act as reservoirs of infection. One species of deer fly (*Chrysops discalis*) and, in Sweden, a mosquito (*Aëdes cinereus*) can transmit tularemia to humans. Ticks are an important reservoir of the disease because the microorganism is transferred transovarially from the female to her progeny. Sporadic episodes and epidemic tularemia have occurred among humans following contact with water and fish contaminated by infected animal carcasses. However, human-to-human transmission of infection does not occur. Wild cottontail rabbits are the principal source of tularemia in the United States. A large-scale epidemic, presumably transmitted by infected muskrats, occurred in Vermont in 1968.

Human beings are highly susceptible to tularemia; the organism usually invades through the skin, mucous membrane, gastrointestinal tract, or respiratory tract. Hunters, butchers, and housewives are most often affected.

PATHOLOGY Microscopically, the primary cutaneous lesion shows neutrophilic infiltration, granulomatous reaction, and necrosis. The regional lymph nodes develop similar changes and often suppurate. The granulomatous reaction in tularemia resembles tubercles in liver, spleen, lung, and kidney. *Pasteurella tularensis* has been recovered from lymph nodes many days after apparent subsidence of the disease.

MANIFESTATIONS The incubation period is 3 to 7 days. Because a typical lesion of skin or mucous membranes is not invariably present, tularemia classically has been separated into several clinical types.

More than 80 percent of infections by *P. tularensis* produce a lesion of the skin or mucous membranes which begins as a reddened papule that may be pruritic and soon ulcerates. The primary lesion in this *ulceroglandular* form of the disease is rarely very painful, is usually present before onset of systemic symptoms, and may not heal until convalescence is well under way. Frequently it is overlooked, or its relation to severe systemic symptoms is not recognized. Regional lymph node enlargement is usually more prominent than that accompanying infections of similar severity produced by other microorganisms. The involved nodes are often exquisitely tender, fluctuant, hot, and reddened. Drainage can occur spontaneously. Generalized lymphadenopathy is present in some cases, but the regional nodes are most prominently involved. There is considerable variation in the intensity of the systemic symptoms of ulceroglandular tularemia; the patient may be almost asymptomatic or severely prostrated. Clinical and roentgenographic evidence of pneumonitis may accompany this form of the disease, illustrating its disseminated character, but bacteremia is rarely demonstrable.

Localized lymph node enlargement without a detectable skin lesion is referred to as *glandular* tularemia. The pathogenesis of this form of the disease is probably identical with that of ulceroglandular tularemia, and the features of the illness are also the same.

Rarely, the portal of entry of the organism is the conjunctiva, where there develops an ulcer, with edema, congestion, lacrimation, photophobia, and pain. In this *oculoglandular* type of tularemia the preauricular, submaxillary, and anterior cervical lymph nodes may enlarge. Corneal ulceration and scarring or perforation of the globe may occur.

Ingestion of contaminated meat or water may result in primary lesions in the gastrointestinal tract. This rare form of the disease produces diarrhea, abdominal pain, nausea, vomiting, melena, and hematemesis, but otherwise differs little from tularemia introduced through other portals. Ulcerative lesions are often found in the buccal mucosa, pharynx, or intestine, and the mesenteric or cervical lymph nodes are involved early in the disease.

Tularemia without obvious primary ulcer or localized lymphadenitis is referred to as *typhoidal*. Constitutional symptoms in typhoidal tularemia differ in no way from those in other types of the disease, although there is usually more prostration. In the absence of localized manifestations, the diagnosis of tularemia is more difficult and depends on serologic tests, isolation of the organism, or a strong epidemiologic history.

Pneumonia may accompany tularemia. Involvement of the lung is secondary to hematogenous dissemination, even when infection is acquired by inhalation of the organism (as in bacteriology laboratories). Pneumonitis in tularemia may cause cough, mucoid sputum, hemoptysis, pleuritic pain, dyspnea, and cyanosis, but extensive x-ray evidence of pneumonitis is sometimes present in the absence of any symptoms of pulmonary disease. Physical findings often correlate poorly with the roentgenologic changes, which consist of diffuse patchy or lobar infiltrations and inconstant hilar adenopathy. Pleural effusion may occur, but lung abscess is rare.

Rarely *P. tularensis* causes endocarditis, pericarditis, peritonitis, appendicitis, osteomyelitis, or meningitis.

Fever in tularemia develops abruptly, often with rigors, and in untreated patients may persist with temperatures of 104 to 106°F for as long as 4 weeks. The fever is sustained or mildly remittent, and defervescence is by lysis.

Splenomegaly is detectable in many patients. An evanescent macular or papular rash is sometimes present on the trunk and extremities early in the disease.

Convalescence in untreated tularemia is prolonged, and fever, lassitude, fatigability, myalgia, irritability, or anorexia may persist or recur for many months. Recovery is usually prompt if acute tularemia is treated with antibiotics. When therapy is delayed, however, patients are more likely to be left with mild debilitation that is unresponsive to further administration of antimicrobial drugs.

Recovery from tularemia is usually followed by immunity to recurrence of disease. However, immunity is not complete, and several instances of second, even third, attacks of tularemia have been recorded. Almost invariably, they have consisted of the development of a local lesion and mild regional adenopathy without systemic symptoms and with little or no fever.

LABORATORY FINDINGS Serum agglutinins for *P. tularensis* are present after the second week of illness. Cross agglutination may occur with antigens of *Brucella*, but this is not a constant finding.

Pasteurella tularensis can be recovered by appropriate cultures or animal inoculation. It is rarely found in blood but can be isolated from the mucocutaneous ulcer or regional lymph nodes with regularity. The organism has been cultured from the sputum and gastric washings even in patients without roentgenographic evidence of pneumonitis. Accidental infection of personnel in diagnostic laboratories may occur.

The skin test with a diluted suspension of killed *P. tularensis,* or purified antigen, becomes positive during the first week of disease. The cutaneous hypersensitivity response is "delayed" and resembles the tuberculin reaction. The skin test may become positive earlier and may remain so longer than the agglutination test.

The total blood leukocyte count is usually normal. The erythrocyte sedimentation rate is normal in ulceroglandular or mild disease but is frequently elevated in severe typhoidal tularemia.

DIFFERENTIAL DIAGNOSIS Brucellosis, typhoid fever, disseminated tuberculosis, the early stage of several rickettsial diseases, and infectious mononucleosis may closely resemble typhoidal tularemia. History of possible contacts is important, and appropriate serologic and cultural studies are usually successful in differentiating these infections. Pneumonic tularemia must be distinguished from viral, mycotic, and other bacterial infections of the lung. The differential diagnosis of pneumonia is discussed in Chap. 133. Oculoglandular syndromes likely to be confused with tularemia are described in Chap. 208.

Ulceroglandular tularemia must be distinguished from a variety of infections in which a *local cutaneous ulcer with regional lymphadenopathy* may occur. Besides pyoderma caused by streptococci or staphylococci, these infections include lymphogranuloma venereum, cat-scratch fever, ratbite fever, bubonic plague, anthrax, glanders, several rickettsioses of which the important one in this country is rickettsialpox, several viral infections of the skin such as orf and cowpox, and inoculation syphilis or tuberculosis. In all these, with the exception of lymphogranuloma venereum and cat-scratch fever, the regional lymph node involvement is usually proportional to the size of the cutaneous ulcer. Extragenital lymphogranuloma is rare; fever and systemic symptoms in cat-scratch fever are rarely severe for more than a few days.

TREATMENT Streptomycin is the antibiotic of choice for tularemia. The dosage is 0.5 to 1 g every 12 h for 10 days. *Pasteurella tularensis* cannot be recovered from lymph nodes or skin lesions after 24 to 48 h of therapy. However, the regional lymph nodes may continue to enlarge and suppurate for several days. Pulmonary lesions usually subside rapidly, although the evolution of the cutaneous lesion is not interrupted. The tetracycline antibiotics and chloramphenicol also are effective, although fever and other manifestations may recur 7 to 14 days after cessation of therapy. Recrudescent illness, however, responds rapidly to readministration of the antibiotic. Aspiration of pus from suppurating nodes rarely is necessary; but if fistulas persist, total surgical removal of the involved tissue can be carried out. Surgery may be followed by transient recurrence of fever despite failure to demonstrate the organism in excised tissues.

PROPHYLAXIS A killed bacterial vaccine developed by Foshay has been shown to stimulate serum agglutinins and induces positive skin reactions to the bacterial antigens, but it produces little immunity to infection with *P. tularensis.* An attenuated live bacterial vaccine has been developed, however, and is effective in inducing protection against infection.

Antibiotic prophylaxis with streptomycin following exposure to tularemia will protect against infection. Chloramphenicol and tetracycline, however, only prolong the incubation period of the disease and do not prevent its occurrence.

Avoidance of contact with possible sources of infection is important in prevention, and the incidence of tularemia in several localities has fallen sharply with the introduction of laws prohibiting the sale of wild rabbits by butchers.

PROGNOSIS The mortality rate in untreated tularemia is 6 to 7 percent. With antimicrobial therapy, death is rare.

REFERENCES

BUCHANAN TM et al: The tularemia skin test. 325 skin tests in 210 persons: Serologic correlation and review of the literature. Ann Intern Med 74:336, 1971

CENTER FOR DISEASE CONTROL: Weekly Rep. 23:299, Aug 24, 1974

MCCRUMB FR JR et al: Studies on human infection with *Pasteurella tularensis*: Comparison of streptomycin and chloramphenicol in the prophylaxis of clinical disease. Trans Assoc Am Physicians 70:74, 1957

STUART BM, PULLEN RL: Tularemic pneumonia: Review of American literature and report of fifteen additional cases. Am J Med Sci 210:233, 1945

YOUNG LS et al: Tularemia epidemic: Vermont 1968. Forty-seven cases linked to contact with muskrats. N Engl J Med 280:1253, 1969

146 YERSINIA (PASTEURELLA) INFECTIONS INCLUDING PLAGUE

JOSEPH E. JOHNSON

Gram-negative bacilli of the genus *Pasteurella* have been reclassified recently in accordance with increasing knowledge about the characteristics of the bacteria. *Pasteurella pestis* (the plague bacillus) and *P. pseudotuberculosis* are now included in the genus *Yersinia* along with a third closely related organism, *Y. enterocolitica. Pasteurella multocida* (formerly *P. septica*) initially included a group of several closely related species producing hemorrhagic septicemia in animals and man. Related species with at least potential pathogenicity for humans include *P. urae, P. haemolytica,* and *P. pneumotropica.*

PLAGUE Definition Plague is an infectious disease of animals (principally wild and domestic rodents) which is transmitted to man through the bite of infected ectoparasites (especially the rat flea). Disease in man is usually characterized by the abrupt onset of high fever, lymphadenopathy and suppuration of regional lymph nodes draining the exposure site, bacteremia, and prostration. This clinical form of the disease is known as *bubonic* plague because of the presence of enlarged suppurating lymph nodes, or *buboes.* Secondary pneumonia may occur and lead to direct respiratory transmission by infectious aerosols from man to man. This primary *pneumonic* type of human disease is highly fatal.

History Plague was known and feared in ancient times and has been the subject of dread as well as a source of literary stimulation to authors from Dionysius in the third century to Camus in the present. At least three major pandemics have occurred in which large segments of the population were destroyed. The first authentic pandemic was recorded in the sixth century A. D.; the second great pandemic occurred in the fourteenth century and was known as the "Black Death," and the last major pandemic originated in China in 1894, spread eventually to all continents, and was first recognized in the United States in 1900. It is likely, however, that the disease was present in the wild rodent population (sylvatic plague) in California long before this. The disease is now well established in wild rodents in many parts of the world, including the western United States. It is present on every continent except Australia. Human disease is endemic in parts of Asia, Africa, and South America, and sporadic human cases still occur in the United States.

Etiology The causative agent, *Yersinia pestis,* is a gram-negative, nonmotile, and non-spore-forming bacillus which grows both aerobically and anaerobically. It is pleomorphic in exudate or sputum, and may appear bacillary, ovoid, or coccal. When stained with Giemsa's or Wayson's stain, it displays a bipolar "safety pin" structure. *Yersinia pestis* grows readily although somewhat slowly on ordinary culture media, forming small, round, transparent colonies which assume a "beaten-copper" appearance after 48 h. At least two types of toxins have been identified, including a soluble exotoxinlike protein and an insoluble endotoxic lipopolysaccharide. Although readily killed by sunlight, organisms have been shown to survive in sterile soil for 16 months and in nonsterile soil for as long as 7 months, and it is likely that organisms may be present in rodent burrows in the absence of fleas and rats for long periods.

Epidemiology Plague is firmly entrenched as an enzootic among approximately 200 species of rodents in many parts of the world. While the disease in wild rodents (sylvatic plague) is not usually a direct threat to man, it nevertheless serves as a vast reservoir for infection of domestic rats (murine or rat plague) which, along with their ectoparasites, live in close association with man. The endemic reservoir of sylvatic plague includes wild rats, ground squirrels, mice, marmots, owls, gophers, badgers, rabbits, prairie dogs, and chipmunks; in the Western Hemisphere the disease is firmly entrenched in the wild rodent population of California, Oregon, Washington, Utah, Idaho, Nevada, New Mexico, Texas, Louisiana, Florida, Michigan, Arizona, Colorado, Montana, Wyoming, Kansas, North Dakota, Hawaii, western Mexico, and western Canada. The principal murine hosts are the domestic rats, *Rattus rattus* and *R. norvegicus,* which are found throughout the world. Although ticks, lice, and bedbugs may occasionally serve as vectors, the principal ectoparasite vector is the oriental rat flea, *Xenopsylla cheopis.*

Between epidemics the infection persists as a chronic disease of wild rodents which is maintained by the insect vector. Although occasionally acquired through contact with wild rodents and their parasites, human disease is usually a result of association with domestic rats and occurs in urban areas in the wake of rat epizootics. When the concentration of people and of rats under circumstances of poor sanitation provides opportunity for the migration of fleas from rats to man, an outbreak is likely to occur. Because sylvatic plague appears virtually impossible to eradicate, it will continue to pose a constant threat of extension into urban rat populations and thence to man. Infection of the flea takes place through ingestion of blood of a bacteremic animal. After multiplication in the intestinal tract of the flea, the organisms are regurgitated when the flea attempts to ingest another blood meal. Because rat fleas will attack man if rats are not immediately available, the infection is likely to be transmitted as the rat population decreases and the fleas transfer from dead hosts to human beings. Plague can be acquired by direct contact with the tissues of an infected animal, by its bite, or by scratching of infected material into the skin.

The bubonic form of the disease rarely results in transmission from man to man because bacteremia in human disease is rarely of a level sufficient to allow infection of fleas. The principal mode of spread from man to man is by the pulmonary route, which occurs when a patient with bubonic disease develops secondary plague pneumonia and thereafter excretes large quantities of organisms in the sputum. Airborne infection by droplet nuclei is highly contagious, and primary pneumonic plague is common among those attending such a patient. Although asymptomatic oropharyngeal carriers have been identified among healthy family contacts of bubonic plague patients in Vietnam, the role of these carriers in the transmission of the disease has not been determined.

Pathogenesis In the more common bubonic form of disease, *Y. pestis* gains entry into the human host through the bite of an infected flea. Organisms are carried to the local lymphatics, then to the bloodstream and finally are disseminated. The prominent clinical manifestations are usually in the lymphatic system. In bubonic plague, a hemorrhagic zone of edema surrounds an inflamed and suppurating group of regional lymph nodes. The glands are hyperplastic and show multiple areas of necrosis, in which there are swarms of organisms. Metastatic lesions sometimes develop in other lymphatics or in the viscera. Particularly likely is the occurrence of secondary pneumonia, which constitutes a potential source of pneumonic spread. Hemorrhages are numerous, probably as a result of a toxin produced by *Y. pestis,* and it is not unusual for individuals given chemotherapy at a late date to die of toxemia when plague bacilli can no longer be cultured from any organ. Primary pneumonic spread occurs through the inhalation of infectious aerosols emanating from another case or, rarely, from infected fomites. It is apparent that the tonsils and/or oropharyngeal mucous membranes may occasionally serve as portals of entry resulting in a cervical bubonic-septicemic form of the disease. Rarely a skin papule forms at the site of entry of the bacillus, and may develop into a pustule or a carbuncle.

Bacteremia is a constant feature of bubonic and pneumonic plague. The precise mechanisms by which the plague bacillus and its toxic factors produce severe tissue injury are not understood completely.

Manifestations After an incubation period of 1 to 12 days (usually 2 to 4 days), the patient develops an acute and often fulminant illness. In the more common *bubonic* variety, symptoms begin abruptly with chills, a rise in temperature to 102 to 105°F, tachycardia, headache, vomiting, uncertain gait, marked prostration, and delirium. The spleen is sometimes palpable. The fleabite at the portal of entry rarely can be seen; if present, it is marked by a papule or vesicle which ultimately becomes pustular. Pain and tenderness are present in the infected regional lymph nodes. Of the buboes, 60 to 75 percent are in the inguinal or femoral regions because the lower extremities are more commonly the site of the initial fleabite. Less often, especially in children, buboes are found in the axillary or cervical regions. Infection may extend to other superficial or deeply situated groups of glands. The bubo consists of a firm, matted group of glands measuring 2 to 5 cm in diameter and is surrounded by a boggy and frequently hemorrhagic zone of edema. It usually suppurates and drains spontaneously after 1 or 2 weeks, although in some instances there is complete resorption.

There is a marked hemorrhagic tendency, presumably because of the effect of plague toxin on blood vessels, and the development of an intravascular coagulopathy (DIC). Petechiae or ecchymoses occur often. Bleeding may occur into a viscus or a serous cavity, or from the nose and alimentary, respiratory, or urinary tracts.

The course of bubonic plague is marked by an irregular or remittent fever, which often drops at the time of appearance of the bubo, only to rise again. In favorable cases, the temperature falls gradually during the second week concomitant with improvement in the general clinical condition. A rise to hyperpyrexic levels or a precipitous fall to normal or to subnormal frequently heralds approaching death. Most fatalities occur during the first week of illness. Although bubonic plague is usually severe, mild cases called *pestis minor* are sometimes seen during epidemics.

The "primary septicemic" form of plague is actually a variant of bubonic disease. The patient experiences a sudden and overwhelming systemic illness. There is a marked constitutional reaction, with chills, fever, rapid pulse, severe headache, nausea, vomiting, and delirium. Death ensues within a few days, before localizing lesions become clinically apparent. Nevertheless, autopsy usually reveals inflammation in some part of the lymphatic system.

Plague also may take the form of pneumonia. The initial cases appear in patients with bubonic plague, of whom as many as 5 percent develop secondary lesions in the lungs. These individuals may provide the starting point for a man-to-man epidemiologic cycle of airborne primary pneumonic plague. It is a fulminating infection accompanied by great prostration, cough, dyspnea, and in the later stages, cyanosis. The sputum is abundant, blood-stained, and teeming with *Y. pestis.* Often there are no clear-cut pulmonary signs, though scattered rales or areas of dullness may be found. In the absence of specific therapy, plague pneumonia invariably ends fatally within 1 to 5 days.

Infection may localize in other regions of the body. Subcutaneous abscesses and cutaneous ulcerations sometimes occur, and occasionally the meninges are involved.

Laboratory findings Laboratory confirmation of plague is relatively simple, although the disease is often misdiagnosed in the United States because of its rarity. Consideration of epidemiologic and clinical features provide highly characteristic leads, and once a suspicion of plague is entertained, it can readily be verified by smear, culture, and animal inoculation of appropriate specimens. The technique of staining a suspected specimen with fluorescent specific antiserum provides an elegant method for rapid identification of *Y. pestis.* If a bubo is present, a small quantity of interstitial fluid should be aspirated from its center. Large numbers of morphologically characteristic bacilli are usually seen in a stained smear. Infected sputum likewise contains many organisms. Bacteremia of varying degrees occurs at some time during the course of the disease in nearly all cases, and methylene-blue staining of venous blood may be useful. Pus and sputum should be cultured on blood agar plates, while blood is inoculated into nutrient broth. Organisms are identified by their morphologic and colonial characteristics and by agglutination with specific antiserum. Guinea pig inoculation is the final step in identification. In this animal the gross and microscopic lesions are highly characteristic. Caution should be observed in handling infected materials or animals, because of the great danger of infection to laboratory workers.

Specific antibodies appear in the serum of patients convalescing from the disease and can usually be detected early in the second week by complement fixation, agglutination, passive hemagglutination, or immunoelectrophoretic agar-gel precipitation methods. A passive mouse-protective test serves to indicate the immune status of a convalescent or vaccinated individual.

The white blood cell count is elevated to levels often above 20,000 cells per mm^3, and there is a predominance of polymorphonuclear leukocytes. The red blood cell count usually is normal.

Diagnosis Early in the acute phase of illness, before the appearance of localizing signs, plague may be confused with severe systemic illnesses such as typhoid, typhus, or malaria. The presence of buboes may suggest other forms of infectious lymphadenitis, including tularemia, syphilis, and lymphogranuloma venereum, as well as lymphadenitis of staphylococcal or streptococcal origin. Pneumonic plague must be distinguished from tularemic, pneumococcal, and other gram-negative pneumonias as well as from anthrax, psittacosis, and mycoplasma pneumonia. The consideration of epidemiologic factors, plus bacteriologic studies, will aid in the differentiation. Serologic diagnosis is of aid only for retrospective confirmation. When plague is suspected, it is imperative to begin treatment as soon as adequate specimens have been taken for culture because early institution of therapy is essential to ensure recovery. To delay treatment may risk toxemic death in the face of a bacteriologic cure.

Treatment When antibiotic treatment is instituted early in the course of the disease, the response is usually dramatic and complete. Even patients with pneumonic or septicemic disease can be cured if treatment is initiated within the first 15 to 20 h after onset. Streptomycin and tetracycline are the drugs of choice. Streptomycin is given intramuscularly in doses of 0.5 g every 4 h for 48 h followed by 0.5 g every 6 h for a total of 7 to 10 days or until the patient has been afebrile at least 3 days. Kanamycin is also effective and may be particularly useful if streptomycin resistance increases. Tetracyclines are given in initial doses of 2 to 3 g daily intravenously, and the dose is reduced to 2 g daily orally when improvement occurs. Chloramphenicol is also a potent antiplague agent and should be given in initial doses of 6 to 8 g daily intravenously (100 mg per kg) and the dose reduced to 3 g (50 to 75 mg per kg) daily orally for a total dose of 20 to 25 g. Sulfonamides are less effective, especially in pneumonic plague, and should be used only when the other agents are not available. Trimethoprim-sulfamethoxazole (co-trimoxazole) has been used successfully. Buboes are treated with hot, moist applications. Incision and drainage should be postponed until the lesion becomes well localized and the patient has been treated with antibiotics.

Control Prevention of plague must be directed toward elimination of endemic rodent foci, and in endemic urban areas constant vigilance is required in detecting and combating rodent epizootics. Prevention includes extermination of rats, eradication of ectoparasite vectors, and sometimes the immunization of the human population. Rats are attacked by poisoning and trapping, by elimination of harborage areas, and by separating them from their food supplies. Unfortunately, rodent control has proved to be most difficult in the endemic areas because of generally poor living standards. Vector control with DDT has been used with brilliant success in diminishing the flea population infecting both rodents and human beings, but studies in Southeast Asia show a significant incidence of DDT-resistant fleas; however, these may yield to other insecticides such as aldrin, dieldrin, and chlordane. The complete elimination of sylvatic plague appears to be impossible in the foreseeable future, and the control program must be aimed at eradicating foci of wild rodent infection around areas of human habitation. In these peripheral zones, the wild and the domestic rodents live commensally, exchange fleas, and threaten the human community.

Patients must be disinfested and carefully isolated, while other intimately exposed persons should be quarantined. Prophylaxis has been achieved effectively in the past by administering sulfadiazine in a dose of 3 g per day for 1 week. However, there is now significant in vitro resistance to sulfadiazine. Alternatively, prophylaxis with streptomycin in a dose of 1 g per day or with tetracycline is often effective.

Vaccines have been used for many years and apparently provide limited and transitory immunity. Three types of vaccines have been available. A formalin-killed vaccine approved for use in the United States has been advised for all persons traveling to Vietnam, Cambodia, and Laos, for those whose vocations bring them into frequent and regular contact with wild rodents in plague enzootic areas, and for all laboratory personnel working with *Y. pestis* or with plague-infected rodents. Although the precise effectiveness of this vaccine has not been measured satisfactorily, it appears to reduce the incidence and severity of the disease. A second promising vaccine is a living attenuated strain of the organism which may be particularly suitable for endemic areas in Asia. Studies in the U. S. S. R. indicate that the attenuated vaccine administered by the aerosol route may be especially valuable in prevention of pneumonic plague. A third vaccine consisting of a chemical extract has been effective in experimental laboratory infections. Immunity is relative, and protection is not always conferred by the active disease, since a number of reinfections have been described. Although general vaccination may be worthwhile in an area threatened by an epidemic, the results are too slow for immediate prophylaxis. In such epidemic situations, combined use of all available control measures is indicated.

Prognosis The availability of effective antibiotic therapy has improved the prognosis in this formerly highly fatal disease. In the past the mortality rate of bubonic plague varied from 50 to 90 percent, and the pneumonic, septicemic, and meningitic forms were almost invariably fatal. In treated cases the mortality is 5 to 10 percent, and even the gravest varieties of infection respond to chemotherapy if treated early enough.

OTHER YERSINIA INFECTIONS (Y. PSEUDOTUBERCULOSIS AND Y. ENTEROCOLITICA) **Etiology** *Yersinia pseudotuberculosis* is a gram-negative, aerobic, facultatively anaerobic, non-spore-forming bacillus, which is coccobacillary when virulent and bacillary when avirulent. It is easily confused with other non-lactose-fermenting *Enterobacteriaceae.* It is nonmotile at 37°C but usually motile at 22°C. *Yersinia enterocolitica,* a closely related organism, has similar characteristics but is distinguished on the basis of biochemical reactions.

Manifestations *Yersinia pseudotuberculosis* is a ubiquitous animal pathogen, worldwide in distribution but identified only in the last decade as a potentially significant human pathogen. Several hundred cases of human infection have now been identified in Europe (especially Scandinavia) and increasingly from Canada and the United States. *Yersinia enterocolitica,* isolated less frequently from animals in the United States, has also now been recognized as a potential cause of a variety of human disease syndromes. Both organisms have been associated with diarrheal diseases, both acute and chronic, and also a usually benign and self-limited form of mesenteric adenitis, clinically simulating appendicitis. Cervical adenitis has also been seen. Rarely, potentially fatal typhoidal and septicemic forms of infection have been described, especially in patients with underlying debilitating diseases. Increasingly, polyarthritis with and without associated erythema nodosum has been associated with *Yersinia* infection.

Reported cases have indicated a 3:1 male predominance especially in older children and young adults infected with *Y. pseudotuberculosis,* while equal sex distribution and a greater incidence in young children and infants has been observed with *Y. enterocolitica.* In addition, *Y. enterocoliti-*

ca has been incriminated in institutional and multiple-family outbreaks.

Transmission has usually been traced to contact with infected animals or contaminated food or water, although person-to-person, hand-to-mouth transmission appears also to be a significant possibility.

Diagnosis Diagnosis may be confirmed by culture of lymph nodes, occasionally of stools, or by serologic titers. Cross reactions with salmonella, *Brucella,* and *E. coli* antigens occur, and serums must be cross-absorbed. With use of both agglutination and hemagglutination methods, titers up to 1:10,240 have been found. Titers lower than 1:160 are not considered significant. The highest antibody titers usually occur during the acute phase of illness, rapidly disappearing by the fourth or fifth month of convalescence, probably reflecting the elicitation of IgM-type antibodies.

Although both species are easily grown on standard laboratory media, identification is more difficult, and routine methods for pathogenic Enterobacteriaceae are inadequate.

The variety of clinical syndromes which have been observed in association with *Y. pseudotuberculosis* and *Y. enterocolitica* may also be confusing. Acute or subacute yersinial enteritis may mimic salmonellosis, shigellosis, and other common enteropathogenic syndromes. Fever, diarrhea, and vomiting are the most common findings in infants and younger children. Fecal leukocytosis has been found in yersinial enteritis indicating ulceration of the intestinal mucosa. Ulcerative colitis may be simulated. Acute septicemic yersiniosis may resemble systemic salmonellosis and other "typhoidal" syndromes. Subacute localizing yersiniosis with hepatic or splenic abscesses may resemble amebic hepatitis. Patients with mesenteric adenitis (usually children) may present the clinical picture of acute appendicitis with mid- or right-lower quadrant abdominal pain, fever, and leukocytosis. At laparotomy the appendix is usually normal, but large inflamed mesenteric lymph nodes are found, sometimes with associated terminal ileitis. Histologic examination of inflamed nodes has revealed reticulogranulocytic infiltration with or without small abscess formation. Polyarthritis of varying severity and duration has been observed, and most often mimics rheumatic fever or juvenile rheumatoid arthritis. Reiter's syndrome may also be simulated. Erythema nodosum has also been increasingly identified in patients with agglutinin rises to *Yersinia,* with or without associated arthritis. Common features in adults have been abdominal pain and fever, with or without arthritis or erythema nodosum.

Treatment Antibiotic treatment is indicated in the more severe cases, especially the septicemic and subacute localizing forms of disease. *Yersinia pseudotuberculosis* is usually susceptible to the aminoglycoside antibiotics (gentamicin, streptomycin, or kanamycin) as well as to tetracycline, chloramphenicol, ampicillin, and the cephalosporins. *Yersinia enterocolitica* is resistant to penicillin G and only variably sensitive to ampicillin and the cephalosporins. In vitro studies indicate a potential role for trimethoprim-sulfamethoxazole.

PASTEURELLA MULTOCIDA INFECTION **Definition** *Pasteurella multocida* (formerly *P. septica*) is a gram-negative nonsporulating bacillus which differs from *Yersinia* organisms in cultural characteristics, antibiotic sensitivity, and pattern of animal parasitism. For example, all strains of *P. multocida* are sensitive to penicillin. *Pasteurella multocida* is frequently identified as a commensal in cattle, horses, swine, sheep, fowl, dogs, cats, and rats, and on occasion causes hemorrhagic septicemia, or chronic pulmonary infiltrates, in these species. Human infection with *P. multocida* is uncommon and usually related to animal contact. Related species which have occasionally been identified as human pathogens include *P. urae, P. haemolytica,* and *P. pneumotropica.*

Manifestations Human disease due to *P. multocida* is usually a consequence of a dog or cat bite and appears as a localized wound infection with cellulitis, suppuration, and adenitis. Osteomyelitis sometimes ensues. Rarely, in patients with bronchiectasis, *P. multocida* is isolated from sputum, and animal handlers are sometimes identified as asymptomatic respiratory carriers. Empyema has occasionally been associated with the organisms. Bacteremia with fever and chills may develop after an animal bite, occasionally without an apparent local lesion. Meningitis, brain abscess, pyogenic arthritis, endocarditis, and pyelonephritis may occasionally complicate the bacteremia.

Not all *P. multocida* infections follow documented animal bites or animal contact.

Diagnosis Except for the association with animal (especially cat) bites, local infections with *P. multocida* show no unique characteristics, and may resemble cat-scratch fever, tularemia, or staphylococcal or streptococcal infection. Leukocytosis, uncommon in tularemia and cat-scratch fever, is the rule in *P. multocida* infection.

Gram's stain of infected material shows pleomorphic gram-negative bacilli, usually extracellular. The bacteria may have bipolar staining and may be mistaken for gram-negative diplococci prior to cultural identification.

Treatment Penicillin in a dosage of 600,000 to 1,200,000 units daily is the preferred antibiotic, but a variety of other antibiotics may be effective.

REFERENCES

Plague

CANTEY JR: Plague in Vietnam, clinical observations and treatment with kanamycin. Arch Intern Med 133:280, 1974

CAVANAUGH DC et al: Some observations on the current plague outbreak in the Republic of Vietnam. Am J Public Health 58: 742, 1968

GIRARD G: Plague. Annu Rev Microbiol 69:253, 1955

HIRST LF: *The Conquest of Plague: A Study of the Evolution of Epidemiology.* Fair Lawn, N. J.: Oxford, 1953

MEYER KF et al: Plague immunization I, past and present trends. J Infect Dis 129:513, 1974

REED WB et al: Bubonic plague in the southwestern United States. Medicine 49:465, 1970

WHO EXPERT COMMITTEE ON PLAGUE: Fourth report. WHO Tech. Rept. Ser. 447, Geneva, 1970

P. Multocida

BEARN AG et al: *Pasteurella multocida* septicemia in man. Am J Med 18:167, 1955

MORRIS AJ et al: *Pasteurella multocida* and bronchiectasis. Bull Johns Hopkins Hosp 91:174, 1952

SWARTZ MN, KUNZ LJ: *Pasteurella multocida* infections in man: Report of two cases—meningitis and infected cat bite. N Engl J Med 261:888, 1959

Yersinia

ARVASTON B et al: Clinical symptoms of infection with *Yersinia enterocolitica.* Scand J Infect Dis 3:37, 1971

GUTMAN LT et al: An inter-familial outbreak of *Yersinia enterocolitica* enteritis. N Engl J Med 288:1372, 1974

HUBERT WT et al: *Yersinia pseudotuberculosis* infection in the United States: Septicemia, appendicitis and mesenteric lymphadenitis. Am J Trop Med 20:679, 1971

LEINO R, KALLIOMAKI JL: Yersiniosis as an internal disease. Ann Intern Med 81:458, 1974

RABSON AR et al: Generalized *Yersinia enterocolitica* infection. J Infect Dis 131:447, 1975

SAARI TN, TRIPLETT DA: *Yersinia pseudotuberculosis,* mesenteric adenitis. J Pediatr 85:656, 1974

147
MELIOIDOSIS AND GLANDERS

JAY P. SANFORD

MELIOIDOSIS Definition Melioidosis is a glanders-like infection of human beings and animals with a protean clinical spectrum. Melioidosis, which means "a resemblance to distemper of asses," bears a striking resemblance to glanders both clinically and pathologically, but is epidemiologically dissimilar.

Etiology Melioidosis is caused by a gram-negative motile bacillus, *Pseudomonas pseudomallei,* which can be differentiated from *Pseudomonas mallei* by bacteriologic and serologic means. *Pseudomonas pseudomallei* (also known as Whitmore's bacillus, or *Pfeifferella whitmori*) is a small, gram-negative, motile, aerobic bacillus. When it is stained with methylene blue, Wayson's, or Wright's stain, marked irregularities with a bipolar "safety pin" pattern are observed. It grows well on standard bacteriologic media, with a characteristic wrinkling of colony surfaces after 48 to 72 h of incubation.

Epidemiology The disease is endemic in Southeast Asia, with the greatest concentration of cases reported from Vietnam, Cambodia, Laos, Thailand, Malaysia, and Burma. Cases in human beings have also been reported from adjacent areas including India, Borneo, the Philippines, Guam, Indonesia, Ceylon, New Guinea, and North Queensland. Cases in humans or animals have been reported from Madagascar, Chad, and Turkey. Human melioidosis has been described only rarely in the Western Hemisphere (Panama, Ecuador), and confirmed melioidosis has occurred in United States or European residents only when they have traveled in endemic areas. From April 1965 through December 1969 there were 187 cases with 13 deaths reported in United States Army personnel who were

or had been in Vietnam. The majority of these cases occurred in individuals without intercurrent illness, although patients who sustained burn injuries in Vietnam accounted for a disproportionately high number of the cases.

Pseudomonas pseudomallei is a saprophyte which can be isolated from soil, stagnant streams, ponds, rice paddies, and market produce in endemic areas. Its ubiquitous nature is illustrated by its isolation as a laboratory contaminant. *Pseudomonas pseudomallei* is capable of causing disease in epizootic form among sheep, goats, swine, and horses. Occasional isolates have also been reported from cows, rodents, dogs, and cats. Although animals are susceptible to the disease, they apparently do not represent a reservoir for human disease. Attempts to culture *P. pseudomallei* from the urine and feces of a large variety of healthy animals have been unsuccessful. Arthropod-borne infection does not occur naturally. Human beings contract melioidosis by soil contamination of skin abrasions. Ingestion, nasal instillation, and inhalation are other probable methods of spread. In contrast to glanders, infections have been uncommon in laboratory workers. Person-to-person transmission of melioidosis is rare. Venereal transmission from a patient with chronic prostatitis with *P. pseudomallei* isolated from prostatic secretions to his wife, who had never been in an endemic area and who had a hemagglutination titer of 1:10,240, has been recorded. Also, the development of melioidosis in a 2-day-old newborn in Hawaii and demonstration of a significant antibody titer in a nurse who had never been in an endemic area but who had worked on wards with melioidosis patients raise the question of spread from person-to-person within a hospital.

Pathology In acute infections, the majority of lesions occur in the lungs, with occasional abscesses in other organs. In subacute infections, lung abscesses tend to be more extensive, and lesions are found throughout the body, in the skin, subcutaneous tissue, meninges, brain, eye, heart, liver, kidney, spleen, bone, prostate, synovial membranes, and lymph nodes. The acute abscesses are characterized by an outer border of hemorrhage, a medial zone heavily infiltrated with polymorphonuclear leukocytes, and an inner core of necrotic debris containing large histiocytes with two or three nuclei that have been termed *giant cells.* A striking histologic feature has been the marked karyorrhexis. In chronic infections, the lesion consists of a central area of caseation necrosis, mononuclear and plasma cells, and granulation tissue. Calcification does not occur.

Clinical manifestations The clinical manifestations of melioidosis are variable. The illness can present as an acute, subacute, or chronic process. The incubation period has not been defined; however, judging by the lapse of time between injury and the development of infection, it may be as short as 2 days. Following a laboratory accident, an incubation period of 3 days ensued. Clinically inapparent infections may remain latent for a number of years after an individual leaves an endemic area, with an interval of 9 years reported in one patient. Men are more often affected than women, a finding which is thought to represent occupational exposure. Melioidosis may be recognized as inapparent infection, asymptomatic pulmonary infiltration, acute localized suppurative infection, acute pulmonary infection, acute septicemic infection, or chronic suppurative infection.

INAPPARENT INFECTION In Thailand, Vietnam, and Malaysia, 6 to 8 percent of healthy adult men have significant antibody titers against *P. pseudomallei,* with the prevalence reaching 20 percent in a group of Army recruits from the rice-growing states of Western Malaysia. Only 1 percent of Thai women had positive reactions. None of the serums from a control group from the United States was positive. The prevalence of significant antibody titers has been reported as 2 percent for Europeans living in Vietnam and 1 to 9 percent in unselected patients in United States Army hospitals and in a group of normal uninjured soldiers who had served in Vietnam. Occasionally, asymptomatic infections have been discovered by routine chest x-ray.

ACUTE LOCALIZED SUPPURATIVE INFECTION Infection by inoculation of a break in the skin usually results in a nodule with an area of acute lymphangitis and regional lymphadenitis. There are usually fever and generalized malaise. This form of infection may rapidly progress to the acute septicemic form.

ACUTE PULMONARY INFECTION The most common form of the disease has been pulmonary infection, which may represent a primary pneumonitis or hematogenous spread. The acute pulmonary infection can vary in severity from a mild bronchitis to overwhelming necrotizing pneumonia. The onset may be abrupt without prodromal symptoms or more gradual, with headache, anorexia, and generalized myalgia. Fever occurs in almost all patients, is often in excess of 102°F, and may be associated with rigors. Dull or pleuritic chest pain is common. Cough, with or without sputum, occurs. There may be mild pharyngitis. Tachypnea may be out of proportion to the fever and findings on physical or x-ray examination. Chest findings may be minimal but usually consist of rales in the area of pneumonitis. In the absence of dissemination, the spleen and liver are not palpable. Laboratory findings include total leukocyte counts ranging from normal to 20,000 per mm^3. Mild normochromic, normocytic anemia may appear during the illness. The pneumonia usually involves the upper lobes with the radiographic appearance of consolidation. Thin-walled cavities, usually 2 to 7 cm in diameter, frequently occur. Without specific therapy, the temperature may become normal within a few days; however, the upper lobe cavitation persists, resulting in a radiographic appearance of tuberculosis. Progressive pulmonary spread or hematogenous dissemination with the development of septicemic manifestations may ensue.

ACUTE SEPTICEMIC INFECTION This is the form originally described primarily among narcotics addicts. Subsequent reports, however, have not shown a predilection for debilitated patients. The onset may be abrupt, with the dominant symptoms depending upon site of major involvement. In individuals with bacteremia complicating pneumonitis, symptoms may include disorientation, extreme dyspnea, severe headache, pharyngitis, watery diarrhea, and development of cutaneous pustular lesions on the head, trunk, or extremities. There is high fever, extreme tachypnea, a flushed skin, and cyanosis. Muscle tenderness may be striking. On examination of the chest, signs may be absent or rales, rhonchi, and pleural rubs may be heard. The liver and spleen may be palpable. Signs of arthritis or meningitis may appear. Patients with the septicemic form usually have a rapidly progressive fatal course, which in some instances may be too fulminant to be altered by therapy. The leukocyte count may be normal or slightly increased. Chest radiographs most commonly show irregular nodular densities 4 to 10 mm in diameter disseminated throughout the lungs. These enlarge, coalesce, and often undergo cavitation as the disease progresses. Pleural effusion is rare. Other radiographic patterns include unilateral irregular mottled densities which become confluent.

CHRONIC SUPPURATIVE INFECTION In some patients secondary abscesses develop which dominate the clinical picture. Organs involved include skin, brain, lung, myocardium, liver, spleen, bones, joints, lymph nodes, and even the eye. These patients may be afebrile.

RECRUDESCENT INFECTION Disease may present as acute localized suppurative, acute pulmonary, acute septicemic, or chronic suppurative infection remote from the probable time of exposure (up to 9 years having been reported). In 6 of 10 reported cases, surgery, trauma, or intercurrent illness appeared to act as triggering events.

Diagnosis Melioidosis should be considered in the differential diagnosis of any febrile illness in an individual who has been in an endemic area, especially if the presenting features are those of fulminant respiratory failure, if multiple pustular or necrotic skin or subcutaneous lesions develop, or if there is a radiographic pattern of tuberculosis in a patient from whom tubercle bacilli cannot be isolated.

Microscopic examination of exudates will reveal poorly staining, small, gram-negative bacilli which show the characteristic staining irregularities and "safety pin" bipolar staining with methylene blue. *Pseudomonas pseudomallei* will grow on most laboratory media, including eosin-methylene blue agar (EMB) or MacConkey's agar, in 24 to 48 h. The organisms can be readily differentiated from *P. mallei* and *P. aeruginosa* by standard bacteriologic procedures. The characteristic wrinkling of the colonies may require 72 h or longer. The hemagglutination, direct agglutination test, and complement fixation test are aids in diagnosis if a fourfold or greater rise in titer is demonstrated in paired serums. Single low titers are difficult to interpret because of nonspecific responses. The complement fixation test is said to be specific with titers above 1:8 during the acute illness, but may cross-react with *P. mallei.* A negative complement fixation test does not exclude disease. The hemagglutination and agglutination tests show more cross-reactions. Titers of 1:40 or more suggest infection.

Treatment The treatment regimen should vary with the form of the disease. Individuals with low-titer positive serologic tests but with no clinical evidence of infection do not require therapy. The choice of antibiotics in active infection should be based upon sensitivity studies, and therapy should be given for a minimum of 30 days. *Pseudomonas pseudomallei* is usually sensitive in vitro to the tetracyclines, chloramphenicol, novobiocin, kanamycin, sulfadiazine or sulfisoxazole, and trimethoprimsulfamethoxazole, and in most instances is resistant to penicillin G, ampicillin, carbenicillin, dicloxacillin, streptomycin, gentamicin, tobramycin, cephalosporins, vancomycin, lincomycin, rifampin, nalidixic acid, and colistin. In patients with pneumonitis who are not too ill, effective therapy has included tetracycline, 2 to 3 g daily (40 mg per kg); chloramphenicol, 3 g daily (40 mg per kg); or sulfisoxazole, 4 g daily (70 mg per kg) for 60 to 150 days. If the patient is severely ill, two of these antimicrobials in combination have been recommended for 30 days followed by another 30 to 120 days of tetracycline alone. The mean interval for sputum cultures to become negative has been 6 weeks. If sputum cultures remain positive for 6 months, surgery with lobectomy should be considered. In patients with extrapulmonary suppurative lesions, therapy should be continued for 6 months to 1 year. The usual principles of surgical drainage should be followed. In desperately ill patients with severe pneumonitis or the septicemic form, multiple antibiotics should be administered by the parenteral route. One such regimen has included the use of chloramphenicol, 12 g per day; novobiocin, 6 g per day; and kanamycin, 4 g per day. In view of the severe potential toxicity of this regimen, its use should be considered only in extremely ill patients, and then only on a short-term basis. Current recommendations for antibiotics in the septicemic form of melioidosis are tetracycline, 4 to 6 g per day (80 mg per kg); chloramphenicol, 4 to 6 g per day (80 mg per kg); and one of the following: sulfisoxazole (140 mg per kg), kanamycin (30 mg per kg), or novobiocin (60 mg per kg). In vitro studies have revealed antagonism between the following pairs of drugs: chloramphenicol-kanamycin; tetracycline-kanamycin; and sulfadiazine-chloramphenicol. Though the significance of such antagonism in clinical therapy has not been assessed, the data would favor selection of novobiocin as the third drug. The dosage should be tapered rapidly as clinical improvement occurs.

Prognosis Prior to antimicrobials, the mortality rate of apparent infection was 95 percent. With better diagnosis and more prolonged appropriate therapy, the mortality rate in all except the septicemic form is low. Even with vigorous appropriate antibiotics and supportive therapy, the mortality rate in patients with melioidosis septicemia is greater than 50 percent. Very few patients have had long-term follow-up, and the incidence of late relapses cannot be predicted.

Prevention There is no means of active immunization. In endemic areas, vigorous cleansing of abrasions and lacerations is recommended.

GLANDERS

Definition Glanders is a serious infection of equine animals caused by *P. mallei,* which is transmitted occasionally to other domestic animals and to human beings.

Etiology *Pseudomonas mallei* is a small, slender, nonmotile, gram-negative bacillus. When it is stained with methylene blue, marked irregularities in staining are observed. Organisms grow on most common meat infusion media, but require glycerol for optimum growth.

Epidemiology Glanders was at one time widespread throughout Europe, but owing to the introduction of control measures, its incidence has decreased steadily in most countries. The disease still occurs in Asia, Africa, and South America, but not in the United States. Glanders has never been common in human beings; the occasional infection, however, may be very serious. There have been no naturally acquired infections in the United States since 1938.

Glanders is primarily a disease of horses, mules, and donkeys, although goats, sheep, cats, and dogs sometimes naturally contract the disease. Pigs and cattle are resistant. In horses, the disease may be systemic, with prominent pulmonary involvement (*glanders*) or may be characterized by subcutaneous ulcerative lesions, and lymphatic thickening with nodules (*farcy*). Inhalation, ingestion, and inoculation through breaks in the skin have been suggested as routes of infection in animals. In human beings, the disease occurs primarily in individuals with close contact with horses, mules, or donkeys through inoculation of or a break in the skin or by exposing the nasal mucosa to contaminated discharges. A number of instances of airborne infection have been reported in laboratory workers.

Pathology The acute lesion is characterized by nodules consisting of polymorphonuclear leukocytes surrounded by a zone of congestion. A characteristic histologic feature is a peculiar nuclear degeneration known as *chromatotexis* which occurs early and is extensive. Small foci of deeply staining detritus within the abscess result from this degeneration. In older nodules, the reaction is characterized by epithelioid cells surrounding an area of central necrosis. Giant cells may be present. Virtually any organ may be involved.

Clinical manifestations The manifestations which frequently overlap may be categorized as (1) acute localized suppurative infection, (2) acute pulmonary infection, (3) acute septicemic infection, and (4) chronic suppurative infection. Nearly 60 percent of patients have been between the ages of twenty and forty years. The disease has been rare in women, probably because of less opportunity for contact.

Infection acquired by inoculation through an abrasion in the skin usually results in a nodule with an area of acute lymphangitis. The incubation period is probably 1 to 5 days. In all types of acute glanders, there are usually fever, generalized malaise, and prostration.

Infection of the mucous membranes may result in a mucopurulent discharge involving the eye, nose, or lips followed by extensive ulcerating granulomatous lesions which may or may not be associated with systemic reactions. With systemic invasion, a generalized papular eruption which may become pustular is frequent. This septicemic form of disease is usually fatal in 7 to 10 days.

Infection by inhalation is followed by an incubation period of 10 to 14 days. The more common symptoms include fever, occasionally associated with rigors, generalized myalgia, fatigue, headache, and pleuritic chest pain. Other symptoms consist of photophobia, lacrimation, and diarrhea. Findings on physical examination are usually normal except for fever and occasional lymphadenopathy, especially in the cervical chain, and splenomegaly. Laboratory findings include mild leukocytosis with 60 to 80 percent neutrophilic leukocytes, but leukopenia with relative lymphocytosis has been recorded. In the acute pulmonary form, chest radiographs characteristically reveal circumscribed densities which suggest early lung abscesses. Other findings may include lobar or bronchopneumonia. In the chronic suppurative form of the disease, the most frequent finding consists of multiple subcutaneous and intramuscular abscesses which most often involve the arms or legs. Approximately one-half the patients will have associated fever, lymphadenopathy, and nasal discharge or ulceration. Visceral involvement including pulmonary or pleural, ocular, skeletal, hepatic, splenic, and meningeal or intracranial involvement occurred in some patients.

Diagnosis Microscopic examination of exudates may reveal small gram-negative bacilli which stain irregularly with methylene blue; however, organisms generally are very scanty, and it is often difficult to find them even in acute abscesses. Giemsa or other modifications of the Romanowski stain may be the best way to identify organisms. *Pseudomonas mallei* and *P. pseudomallei* cannot be distinguished morphologically. Culturing is often avoided because of the hazard to laboratory personnel; however, if cultures are made, growth occurs on most meat infusion nutrient media. The material is often contaminated with other microorganisms, and incubation with penicillin G (1,000 units per ml) prior to culturing may be helpful. Subcutaneous inoculation of material into a guinea pig or hamster affords an alternative means of isolation. Blood cultures are usually negative except in the terminal stages of disease. Serologic tests show a rapidly rising agglutination titer, which reaches levels of 1:640 within 2 weeks. Serum from normal persons has been reported to show agglutination titers in dilutions up to 1:320. The complement fixation test is less sensitive but more specific and usually becomes positive during the third week; it is considered positive in dilutions of 1:20 or greater. The mallein skin test is of help diagnostically; 0.1 ml of a 1:10,000 dilution of commercial mallein is injected intradermally. Erythema exceeding 10 mm in 48 h is considered to represent a specific test. The test becomes positive in most patients by the third or fourth week of disease and remains positive for years.

Treatment The limited number of recent infections in human beings has precluded evaluation of most of the antibiotic agents. Sulfadiazine has been found to be an effective agent in experimental animals and in humans. The dosage utilized has been approximately 100 mg per kg administered in divided doses. In experimental infections, 3 weeks of therapy gave better results than 1 week. Benzyl penicillin is ineffective in vitro and in experimental infections. Streptomycin is bacteriostatic in vitro but was ineffective in experimental infections in hamsters. Antibiotics such as tetracycline, chloramphenicol, and kanamycin have not been evaluated. In the acute infections, appropriate supportive measures are essential, and in chronic suppurative infections, the usual principles of surgical drainage should be followed.

Prognosis The prognosis depends upon the type of infection. The acute septicemic form has been uniformly fatal. The localized or chronic forms have a much better prognosis.

Prevention Next to acquisition from diseased horses, the commonest source of natural disease in human beings has been contact with human glanders. Isolation is indicated.

REFERENCES

EICKHOFF TC et al: *Pseudomonas pseudomallei*: Susceptibility to chemotherapeutic agents. J Infect Dis 121:95, 1970
EVERETT ED, NELSON R: Pulmonary melioidosis, observations in 39 cases. Am Rev Resp Dis 112:331, 1975
HOWE C, MILLER WR: Human glanders: Report of six cases. Ann Intern Med 26:93, 1947
—— et al: The pseudomallei: A review. J Infect Dis 124:598, 1971
JACKSON AE et al: Recrudescent melioidosis associated with diabetic ketoacidosis. Arch Intern Med 130:268, 1972
MCCORMICK JB et al: Human to human transmission of *Pseudomonas pseudomallei.* Ann Intern Med 83:512, 1975
SPOTNITZ M et al: Melioidosis pneumonitis. JAMA 202:950, 1967
ZAJTCHUK R et al: Surgical treatment of melioidosis. J Thorac Cardiovasc Surg 66:838, 1973

148 VIBRIO FETUS INFECTIONS

MARVIN TURCK

DEFINITION *Vibrio fetus* infection is economically the most important cause of infectious abortion in cattle. In human beings, this organism may be associated with obscure febrile illnesses, subacute bacterial endocarditis, meningoencephalitis, and perhaps abortion.

ETIOLOGY *Vibrio fetus* is a motile, comma-shaped or spirillar, gram-negative rod with a single unipolar flagellum. It is best identified by its appearance in smears made from cultured material. The organism is slow-growing and microaerophilic, and grows best in liquid media incubated under increased CO_2 tension. Several serotypes have been isolated by agglutination with antiserums from human and bovine strains. Cross-agglutination reactions occur with other bacterial species, particularly *Brucella abortus.*

EPIDEMIOLOGY AND PATHOGENESIS Vibriosis is a venereal infection of cattle, sheep, and goats; when transmitted to gravid heifers or ewes, it results in abortion. The male acts as an asymptomatic carrier of the infection, and the organism has been isolated from the genitalia and semen of bulls. Although vibriosis has been thought to occur only rarely in humans, reports of this disease are appearing with increasing frequency. Vibriosis in human beings may result from direct contact with the organism, as happens in laboratory-acquired infection, or from direct contact with infected cattle. Food and water have been implicated, without convincing evidence, as vehicles for infection. The mouth has been postulated as a portal of entry because cases of *V. fetus* endocarditis have followed dental extractions. Because *V. fetus* has been isolated from several aborted fetuses and has been the cause of neonatal meningitis, a venereal route of infection has been postulated. It is presumed that, as in cattle, the male acts as an asymptomatic carrier who transmits the infection to a pregnant partner. The relation of *V. fetus* to prematurity, abortion, and neonatal meningitis requires further documentation. In most instances of vibriosis, the portal of entry is not known.

MANIFESTATIONS Fever is the only characteristic sign of vibriosis in adults, and may be relapsing in character. Thrombophlebitis involving both arms and legs is not uncommon. The disease may also present as classic subacute bacterial endocarditis; septic arthritis or osteomyelitis; chronic, indolent meningoencephalitis; and fever and abortion in pregnant women. A number of patients have had coexisting disease, including cirrhosis, cardiac amyloidosis, and chronic lymphatic leukemia, or antecedent gastric surgery. Several neonates with fulminating, lethal meningoencephalitis have been reported. It has been postulated that infection was transmitted to these infants via the placenta. A mild, self-limited diarrheal disease in which vibrios closely related but not identical to *V. fetus* have been isolated from the stool has also been reported in infants.

DIAGNOSIS Lack of awareness of vibriosis by both the bacteriologist and the clinician has resulted in mistaken diagnosis in most instances. The organisms have been erroneously described as "fastidious strains of *Hemophilus.*" Recovery of spirillar organisms in blood cultures should suggest the diagnosis because other spirochetes causing relapsing fever usually do not grow in artificial media. Failure to incubate blood cultures under increased CO_2 tensions may delay growth. Identification of the organisms in smears of cultures is the only definitive method of making the diagnosis, which should then be confirmed by agglutinating the vibrios with specific antiserums. Complement-fixing antibody may be present in high titers in the active phase of the disease. Clinically, vibriosis should be suspected in obscure febrile illnesses associated with thrombophlebitis or abortion and premature delivery in pregnant women.

TREATMENT There are few reports of antibiotic sensitivity of the organisms, and various antibiotics, alone or in combination, have been used. A 10-day course of tetracycline or chloramphenicol in dosage of 2 g per day, alone or coupled with streptomycin, 1 g per day, should eradicate the organisms in most instances. In cases of endocarditis, antimicrobial therapy should be extended to 6 weeks. Kanamycin and erythromycin have also been effective in vitro. Penicillin, novobiocin, vancomycin, and polymyxin B are ineffective.

REFERENCES

KILO C et al: Septic arthritis and bacteremia due to *Vibrio fetus:* Report of unusual case and review of literature. Am J Med 38:962, 1965

LAWRENCE GD et al: Infection caused by *Vibrio fetus.* Arch Intern Med 120:459, 1967

RUBEN FL, WOLINSKY E: Human infection with *Vibrio fetus.* Antimicrob Agents Chemother 1967–1968, p. 143

WHITE WD: Human vibriosis: Indigenous cases in England. Br Med J 2:283, 1967

149 STREPTOBACILLUS MONILIFORMIS INFECTION

ROGER BULGER

DEFINITION *Streptobacillus moniliformis* is a gram-negative organism which can produce an acute febrile disease, characterized by skin and joint manifestations, and, rarely, leading to endocarditis. Most recently cases of *Strep. moniliformis* infection have been associated with the bite of a rat and may be designated as "rat-bite fever," a term which also refers to infections with *Spirillum minus* (Chap. 168).

ETIOLOGY AND EPIDEMIOLOGY *Streptobacillus moniliformis* is a pleomorphic, microaerophilic, gram-negative bacterium, which may yield long, filamentous forms or chains of beaded or fusiform bacilli when grown on artificial media. Although primary isolation is best achieved in specialized fluid media, precise bacteriologic diagnosis is often delayed because isolation from routine blood cultures may require from 2 to 7 days of incubation.

This organism has an unusual capacity to produce stable L-forms during routine growth of the bacterial phase; these L-forms can be maintained in pure culture indefinitely and then may revert to the bacterial phase. The L-form has been isolated from the blood of a human being as long as 10 weeks after the onset of infection.

In some studies, *Strep. moniliformis* has been isolated from the nasopharynx of as many as half the rats investigated, and rats are presumed to be the primary natural reservoir. Human infection most often follows exposure to wild rats, but cases have also been reported following bites by a variety of other rodents. Three cases have been traced to bites by laboratory rats in a single institution within a 6-month period, making this disease an important consideration in febrile illnesses among laboratory workers.

Strep. moniliformis infection has occurred in epidemic proportions in association with ingestion of contaminated food or milk. The outbreak which occurred in 1926 at Haverhill, Massachusetts, is the most famous of these; it involved 86 persons, was related to contamination of raw milk or ice cream with streptobacilli, and led to the disease becoming known as *Haverhill fever* when it is not associated with a rodent bite. Turkeys are also widely infested with streptobacilli, presumably secondary to rat bites, suggesting other potential sources for human infection.

CLINICAL MANIFESTATIONS The incubation period is short, usually 1 to 2 days, although extremes have been described ranging from a few hours to 22 days. The onset of disease is sudden, and may resemble a viral syndrome, with fever, headache, myalgia, malaise, and occasionally vomiting. Chills occur in more than half the patients. Usually the local puncture site will be healed, but it may be ulcerated with associated regional lymphadenopathy.

A discrete macular rash which fades on pressure develops in 75 to 80 percent of the patients 1 to 3 days after the onset of symptoms. This rash is most marked on the extremities, often involving the palms and soles, but may become generalized. In some patients, the cutaneous lesions become purpuric and may become pustular, confluent, or papular.

Involvement of multiple joints appears in about half the patients during the first week. Large joints are usually involved, asymmetrically, but fingers and toes may also be affected. The joint involvement may simply be an arthralgia, but arthritis is also common and it particularly affects the knees; swelling, heat, redness, and effusion may be present.

Clinical signs and symptoms usually regress after 1 to 2 weeks, although without appropriate antimicrobial therapy convalescence may be prolonged because of recurrent fever and arthritis. Abscesses in the brain or other tissues have been rare but serious complications. Bacterial endocarditis is the most feared and potentially fatal complication. Fortunately, it is rare; only 1 of the 337 cases of bacterial endocarditis at the Boston City Hospital during 12 selected years between 1933 and 1965 was due to streptobacillus.

When the infection is food-borne, its clinical manifestations are the same except for the absence of the local lesions.

LABORATORY FINDINGS The blood leukocyte count ranges from 6,000 to 30,000 per mm^3, with an average of only 12,000. Although the total count may be below 10,000, there is usually an increase in the proportion of polymorphonuclear neutrophils with a shift to the left. The organism can usually be isolated from the blood, joint fluid, or pus during the acute febrile phase, but often only after prolonged incubation and occasionally for 1 to 2 weeks after subsidence of fever. Agglutinins against the organism develop during the second or third week and are of diagnostic importance if an increase in titer is demonstrated.

DIFFERENTIAL DIAGNOSIS Infection due to *Strep. moniliformis* must be differentiated from that due to *Spirillum minus* because both occur following rat bites (Chap. 168). Although the manifestations of these two infections can be remarkably similar, the clinical presentations are fairly characteristic of one or the other. The characteristics of *Strep. moniliformis* infections are as follows: latent period usually less than 10 days; prompt healing of the bite site without flare-up at the onset of systemic symptoms; sudden onset of chills and fever followed by a macular rash on the palms and soles; and a high incidence of arthralgias and arthritis. A relapsing febrile course is uncommon. Infections caused by *Spirillum minus* tend to have the following characteristics: prolonged latent period (from 1 to 4 weeks); recurrence of a marked inflammatory response at the site of the rat bite and lymphangitis accompanying the onset of systemic symptoms; sudden onset of fever usually without joint symptoms and often without skin lesions; commonly, a relapsing febrile course.

A clinical picture of sudden onset of fever, nausea, vomiting, myalgias, arthralgias, macular purpuric rash, minimal leukocyte response, and a lack of a focus of infection should also suggest infection with *Rickettsia rickettsii* or Coxsackie B virus.

Streptobacillus moniliformis infection must also be differentiated from other forms of acute infectious arthritis, rheumatic fever, and meningococcemia.

TREATMENT AND PROGNOSIS Before effective antimicrobial therapy was available, the mortality rate in cases of *Strep. moniliformis* infection was approximately 10 percent; death usually was associated with the development of bacterial endocarditis. Prompt treatment with an effective antimicrobial agent should prevent fatalities due to this infection.

A suitable dosage schedule for most infections is 1,200,000 units procaine penicillin intramuscularly or 2 g per day penicillin V orally in divided doses for 7 to 10 days. Erythromycin is acceptable as an alternative in patients with penicillin allergy.

REFERENCES

COLE JS et al: Rat-bite fever. Ann Inter Med 71:979, 1969

HUBBERT WT, MCCULLOCH WF, SCHNURRENBERGER, PR: *Diseases Transmitted from Animals to Man*, Springfield, Ill.: Charles C Thomas, 1975, p 186

MCCORMACK RC et al: Endocarditis due to *Streptobacillus moniliformis*. JAMA 200:77, 1967

ROUGHGARDEN JW: Antimicrobial therapy of rat-bite fever: A review. Arch Intern Med 116:39, 1965

WILSON GS, MILES AA: *Topley and Wilson's Principles of Bacteriology and Immunity*, Baltimore: Williams & Wilkins, 1964, p. 1128

150
BARTONELLOSIS

JAMES J. PLORDE

DEFINITION Bartonellosis (Carrión's disease) is an infection with *Bartonella bacilliformis.* Two well-defined clinical stages occur: an acute febrile anemia of rapid onset and high mortality, designated *Oroya fever,* and a benign eruptive form with chronic cutaneous lesions, called *verruga peruana.* Either of these types may be mild, and asymptomatic cases constitute the greatest epidemiologic hazard.

ETIOLOGY *Bartonella bacilliformis* is a small, motile, aerobic, pleomorphic, gram-negative bacillus which stains reddish violet with Giemsa's stain. It can be cultured on enriched media and does not produce a hemolysin. The organisms are sensitive to several antibiotics in vitro.

EPIDEMIOLOGY The disease is limited to certain valleys in the Andes Mountains comprising parts of Peru, Ecuador, and Colombia. It occurs in regions between the altitudes of 2,400 and 8,000 ft where the sandfly vector, *Phlebotomus,* propagates. Although only *P. verrucarum* has been shown to transmit the disease, other species are undoubtedly involved. Asymptomatic cases and convalescent carriers are the only known reservoir of infection. A low-grade bacteremia may persist for years following resolution of symptoms, and *B. bacilliformis* can be recovered from the blood of 5 to 10 percent of the apparently normal population in an endemic area. Epidemics often coincide with immigration of workers from uninfected areas.

PATHOLOGY AND PATHOGENESIS The manifestations of the disease are thought to reflect the immune status of the host. In nonimmune individuals Oroya fever develops. Large numbers of the *Bartonella* bacteria enter the bloodstream, adhere to erythrocytes, and invade the endothelial cells of the capillaries and lymphatics. The presence of the organisms on the surface of the red blood cell results in their phagocytosis and destruction by the liver and spleen. The red blood cell life span is greatly shortened, and anemia develops. This is accentuated by a defective erythropoietic response early in the course of infection. The pathogenesis of the hemolytic anemia remains unknown. Agglutinins and hemolysins have not been found, and tests for mechanical fragility of red blood cells have given variable results. Invasion and swelling of capillary endothelial cells may lead to vascular occlusion and tissue infarcts. It is possible that an impairment of reticuloendothelial function secondary to massive phagocytosis of red blood cells is responsible for the frequency with which *Salmonella* and other coliform bacteremias are seen in Oroya fever.

With developing immunity, the bacteria nearly disappear from the peripheral blood and capillary endothelium. After a latent period they reappear in the skin and subcutaneous tissue where they are apparently responsible for the development of the hemangioid lesions of verruga peruana. Second attacks of Carrión's disease are unusual. When they occur, they almost invariably present as verruga.

CLINICAL MANIFESTATIONS The incubation period is approximately 3 weeks but may be longer. The initial symptoms are fever and pains in the bones, joints, and muscles. At this point the disease often resembles influenza or malaria, but blood cultures are positive. After these prodromes, the patient usually develops one of the two classic forms of the infection.

Oroya fever This form is characterized by sudden onset of high fever, extreme pallor, weakness, and a precipitous drop in the number of red blood cells. The count may fall from normal to 1 million per mm^3 within 4 or 5 days. The anemia is characterized by normochromic macrocytes in the peripheral blood, striking polychromasia and polychromatophilia, nucleated red blood cells, Howell-Jolly bodies, Cabot rings, and basophilic stippling. There may also be a mild leukocytosis with a shift to the left. Organisms are numerous in the blood, and stained smears may show 90 percent of the erythrocytes heavily invaded. Salmonellosis, malaria, amebiasis, tuberculosis, and other intercurrent infections may occur and are an important factor in fatal cases.

Muscle and joint pain and headache are severe, and insomnia, delirium, and coma are the terminal manifestations. In untreated patients, the mortality rate may exceed 50 percent; death occurs within 10 days to 4 weeks. With treatment, or sometimes spontaneously, recovery results if

the organisms decrease and fever abates. The red blood cell count stabilizes and approaches normal values in about 6 weeks, when convalescence begins.

Verruga peruana This form of the disease, characterized by a profuse skin eruption, may follow the anemic form or may occur in patients without previous symptoms. The verrugas vary in color from red to purple. They may be miliary, nodular, or eroding, and they range in size from 2 to 10 mm up to 3 or 4 cm in diameter. The three types of verruga may occur together; since eruption takes place in successive crops, verrugas of all types and in all stages of development may be found on the same patient. The chief sites involved are the limbs and face, and less frequently the genitalia, scalp, and mucosa of the mouth and pharynx. They may persist for 1 month to 2 years. The eruption is accompanied by pain, fever, and moderate anemia. Bartonellas may be demonstrated in the lesions and cultured from the blood.

DIAGNOSIS A clinical diagnosis can be made with accuracy in endemic areas. During Oroya fever the organism is easily seen on peripheral blood smears. It may be recovered from blood cultures in all stages of the disease.

TREATMENT Oroya fever responds dramatically to a number of antibiotics including tetracycline and chloramphenicol. The latter in a dose of 2 g per day for 7 days is often preferred because of the frequency with which *Salmonella* infections complicate this disease. Fever disappears within 48 h, and the patient recovers rapidly. Transfusions may be required when the anemia is severe. Antibiotic therapy of the verrugal stage may hasten the involution of these lesions. The use of DDT in both the interior and exterior of human dwellings is highly effective in controlling the night-biting sandflies. Insect repellents and bed netting afford personal protection.

REFERENCES

CAUDRA MC: Salmonellosis complication in human bartonellosis. Tex Rep Biol Med 14:97, 1956

KAYE D et al: Factors influencing host resistance to *Salmonella* infections: The effects of hemolysis and erythrophagocytosis. Am J Med Sci 254:205, 1967

RICKETTS WE: Clinical manifestations of Carrión's disease. AMA Arch Intern Med 84:751, 1949

SCHULTZ MG: Daniel Carrión's experiment. N Engl J Med 278:1323, 1968

URETEAGA OB, PAYNE EH: Treatment of the acute febrile phase of Carrión's disease with chloramphenicol. Am J Trop Med 4:507, 1955

WEINMAN D: The bartonella group, in *Bacterial and Mycotic Infections of Man,* 4th ed., eds RJ Dubos, JG Hirsch, Philadelphia: Lippincott, 1965, p. 775

151
GRANULOMA INGUINALE

KING K. HOLMES

DEFINITION Granuloma inguinale is a mildly contagious, chronic, indolent, progressive, autoinoculable, ulcerative disease involving the skin and lymphatics of the genital or perianal areas. The disease may be sexually transmitted and is associated with the presence in affected tissues of an intracellular microorganism, identified morphologically as the Donovan body.

ETIOLOGY Granuloma inguinale was described by McLeod in India in 1882, and in 1905 Donovan described the intracellular bodies which are thought to cause the disease. Granuloma inguinale has been reproduced in humans by inoculation of pus containing Donovan bodies. Similar attempts to reproduce the disease in experimental animals have been unsuccessful. Encapsulated bacteria resembling Donovan bodies have been recovered from lesions and pseudobuboes of granuloma inguinale by inoculation of chick embryo yolk sacs or yolk-agar medium. These bacteria, which are known as *Calymmatobacterium granulomatis,* are antigenically related to *Klebsiella* species but do not reproduce the disease when inoculated intradermally in humans. It is uncertain whether these isolates are responsible for the disease. Similar bacteria have been isolated from feces. Recent electron microscopic studies of Donovan bodies confirm their morphologic resemblance to gram-negative bacteria.

EPIDEMIOLOGY Granuloma inguinale is endemic in the tropics, particularly in New Guinea and among Hindus in India. In the United States, only 54 cases were reported in 1975. Most cases occur in the southeastern states and involve male homosexuals. In reported cases the sex ratio of males to females is nearly 10:1. The disease is uncommon in Caucasians. The reported frequency of granuloma inguinale in conjugal partners of chronically infected patients ranges from 1 to 64 percent. Evidence for sexual transmission includes the age-specific incidence, which corresponds to that of other sexually transmitted diseases, the frequent concomitant presence of syphilis, and the predilection for genital involvement in heterosexuals and for anorectal infection in male homosexuals.

CLINICAL MANIFESTATIONS The incubation period ranges from 8 days to 12 weeks, but most lesions appear within 30 days after sexual exposure.

Granuloma inguinale begins as a papule, which ulcerates and develops into a painless elevated zone of clean, beefy-red, friable granulation tissue. The edges are irregular and spread by continuity or by autoinoculation of approximated skin surfaces. Secondary anaerobic infection may produce pain and a foul-smelling exudate. Less common complications of the disease include deep ulcerations, chronic cicatricial lesions, and exuberant epithelial proliferation which grossly resembles carcinoma. In men, the lesions are usually located on the glans, prepuce, or shaft of the penis, or the perianal area, while infection of the labia is most common in women. Lesions in women often arise at the fourchette and progress anteriorly in a V shape along the vulva. Extragenital lesions may occur, involving the face, neck, mouth, and other sites. The chronicity of the disease is of diagnostic importance, since several months often elapse before patients seek treatment. Extension to the inguinal region by autoinoculation or via the lymphatics results in diffuse intradermal and subcutaneous swelling or suppuration, known as "pseudobubo," because involvement of the underlying lymph nodes is minimal. Locally destructive lesions and secondary infection may produce severe morbidity or death. Fatal disseminated disease, involving the bones or joints, has been reported after several years of chronic local infection. The relationship of granuloma inguinale to subsequent carcinoma of the genitalia is uncertain.

DIAGNOSIS Early granuloma inguinale may be mistaken for the primary chancre or condyloma lata of syphilis. Epithelial proliferation resembling neoplasia in the genital or perianal region in a young subject should always raise the suspicion of granuloma inguinale if unnecessary destructive surgery is to be avoided. Chronic ulcerative or cicatricial changes may resemble lymphogranuloma venereum. Histologic studies in granuloma inguinale reveal marked acanthosis and pseudoepitheliomatous hyperplasia. Because Donovan bodies are seldom detectable in sections stained with hematoxylin and eosin, these changes may lead to an erroneous diagnosis of carcinoma and to unnecessary, destructive surgery. Although silver impregnation techniques are useful for demonstration of Donovan bodies in sections, the diagnosis is best made by examination of impression smears prepared from specimens obtained by punch biopsy from the periphery of a lesion; the deep portion of the specimen is removed, crushed between two slides which are air-dried and fixed in methanol, and stained with Wright-Giemsa stain. With this method, Donovan bodies appear as very rounded coccobacilli, 1 by 2 μm in size, which lie within cystic spaces in the cytoplasm of large mononuclear cells. The capsule stains as a dense acidophilic zone surrounding the bipolar basophilic bacterium, which resembles a closed safety pin. The pathognomonic mononuclear cell is 25 to 90 μm in diameter and has many cystic areas containing Donovan bodies.

Perianal granuloma inguinale may resemble condylomata lata of secondary syphilis. Other venereal diseases, particularly syphilis, very frequently coexist with granuloma inguinale. Repeated dark-field examinations of lesions before treatment and a serologic test for syphilis should therefore be performed.

TREATMENT The treatment of choice is tetracycline, 2 g daily, continued for at least 10 days. The risk of relapse is reduced if treatment is continued until healing is complete. Healing is usually apparent within 3 weeks, as the lesions become pale, flatter, and develop peripheral reepithelialization. Donovan bodies disappear from lesions within a few days after onset of therapy. If tetracycline cannot be given, streptomycin may be used in a dose of 1 g intramuscularly every 12 h for 10 to 15 days. In New Guinea, chloramphenicol or gentamicin are used for cases which appear resistant to tetracycline.

REFERENCES

BEERMAN H, SONCK CE: The epithelial changes in granuloma inguinale. Am J Syph Gonor Vener Dis 36:501, 1952

DAVIS CM: Granuloma inguinale. A clinical, histological, and ultrastructural study. JAMA 211:632, 1970

GOLDBERG J: Studies on granuloma inguinale. Br J Vener Dis 40: 140, 1964

LAL S: Continued efficacy of streptomycin in the treatment of granuloma inguinale. Br J Vener Dis 47:454, 1971

——, NICHOLAS C: Epidemiological and clinical features in 165 cases of granuloma inguinale. Br J Vener Dis 46:461, 1970

RIBEIRO J: Granuloma inguinale. Practitioner 209:628, 1972

U.S. PUBLIC HEALTH SERVICE: Management of chancroid, granuloma inguinale, lymphogranuloma venereum in general practice. USPHS Publ. 255:15, 1964

section 7 | Miscellaneous bacterial diseases

152 ANTHRAX

LEIGHTON E. CLUFF

DEFINITION Anthrax (also called malignant pustule, charbon, splenic fever, milzbrand, woolsorters' disease) is a disease of wild and domesticated animals that is transmitted to human beings by contact with infected animals or their products and, rarely, by insect vectors which act as mechanical carriers of the etiologic organism. The characteristic lesion of human anthrax is a necrotic cutaneous ulcer, the *malignant pustule.* The disease also may be associated with disseminated infection and mediastinitis without mucous membrane involvement or cutaneous ulcer.

HISTORY The classic studies of Robert Koch in 1877, showing that *Bacillus anthracis* was the cause of anthrax, serve as the prototype for the establishment of causation of infectious diseases.

ETIOLOGY *Bacillus anthracis* is a large, encapsulated, gram-positive, aerobic, spore-forming microorganism that grows well in most nutrient media. Its pathogenicity for laboratory animals differentiates it from *Bacillus subtilis,* which it closely resembles. The spores are killed by boiling for 10 min but can survive for many years in soil and animal products, an important factor in persistence and spread of the disease. The anthrax bacillus possesses a capsule of glutamyl polypeptide, which interferes with phagocytosis of the microorganism. In addition, it contains an anticomplementary substance and elaborates a "protective" antigen and a toxin which is probably of importance in determining virulence.

EPIDEMIOLOGY Anthrax is worldwide; repeated outbreaks have occurred in Southern Europe, Africa, Australia, Asia, and on both American continents.

Cattle, horses, sheep, goats, and swine are most commonly infected. There have been outbreaks of anthrax among animals in the United States, centering mostly in South Dakota, Nebraska, Arkansas, Mississippi, Louisiana, Texas, and California. The disease tends to occur in animals in late summer and early fall. An outbreak of anthrax, acquired from goatskin bongo drum heads and goatskin rugs, occurred in Haiti in 1973. In 1974, an epidemic of anthrax developed in cattle in Texas, and in the state of Washington in horses infected from contaminated saddle packs containing goat hair imported from Pakistan.

The disease in human beings is acquired by butchering, skinning, or dissecting infected carcasses or by handling contaminated hides, wool, hair, or other materials. It is seen principally in agricultural and industrial employees. The majority of cases of human anthrax involve workers handling imported and unprocessed wool, hair, or hides. The disease usually follows inoculation of bacilli or spores into the skin, often through a wound or abrasion. Intestinal infection has followed ingestion of contaminated meat, and anthrax may develop after inhalation of spores.

PATHOGENESIS The malignant pustule which follows cutaneous inoculation of anthrax organisms is characterized by vesiculation, neutrophilic infiltration, gelatinous edema, and necrosis. Suppuration is rare in the absence of secondary pyogenic infection. Spread of the bacilli to the regional lymph nodes may be followed by systemic dissemination. Examination of tissues from fatal human cases reveals masses of the bacteria in blood vessels, lymph nodes, and the parenchyma of various organs. There is scanty or no cellular exudation at these foci, but hemorrhage and edema are widespread. So-called "anthrax pneumonia" and "anthrax meningitis" are, in all probability, an expression of this generalized hemorrhage and edema.

The blood of fatally infected experimental animals contains a lethal toxin, which can be neutralized by specific antiserum. This toxin has been isolated in vitro and is important in the pathogenesis of some of the manifestations of the disease.

MANIFESTATIONS The malignant pustule of human anthrax begins usually on an exposed body surface, as a painless, pruritic, erythematous papule, which vesiculates and ulcerates to form a black eschar. Tiny satellite vesicles are frequent. The ulcer may be surrounded by extensive edematous swelling, which is nontender, nonpitting, and so characteristic of anthrax that it is a valuable diagnostic sign. After about 5 days the ulcer begins to subside, but edema may persist for many days or weeks. Mild tenderness and enlargement of regional lymph nodes are frequently present. Constitutional symptoms are often absent despite extensive local changes, but there may be mild fever, headache, and malaise. In disseminated anthrax, high fever, prostration, and a rapidly fatal course are seen. So-called "woolsorters' disease," a highly fatal disseminated infection, is characterized by cyanosis, dyspnea, mediastinitis, and hemoptysis and is probably dependent on the pulmonary route of inoculation. Human infection may occur from ingestion of the uncooked meat of infected animals; however, enormous numbers of organisms are probably necessary to produce disease by this route.

LABORATORY FINDINGS The fluid from the cutaneous lesion frequently contains many bacilli, demonstrable by Gram's stain and culture. Bacilli may be found on direct examination or culture of the blood of patients with bacteremia. The blood leukocyte count is normal in mild cases, but there is polymorphonuclear leukocytosis in severe disease. Similarly, the erythrocyte sedimentation rate may be increased. Patients with meningeal involvement show bloody spinal fluid in which the organisms are easily found by direct examination or culture.

DIAGNOSIS A serologic agar-gel precipitin inhibition test has been devised which has proved useful in epidemiologic studies of anthrax, showing that subclinical infection may occur in persons exposed to the microorganism in industry and demonstrating increasing serum antibody titers following vaccination. A positive diagnosis of anthrax can be made by isolation of the organism in culture. A history of occupational exposure and characteristic eschar and edema should suggest the proper diagnosis. Pyogenic infections of the skin are usually painful; the malignant pustule is not. In addition, cutaneous anthrax is rarely purulent. The differential diagnosis of other diseases characterized by local ulceration at the portal of entry is discussed in Chap. 145.

TREATMENT AND PROPHYLAXIS Many antibiotics are effective in the treatment of human anthrax, including penicillin, chloramphenicol, tetracycline, erythromycin, and streptomycin. A dosage of 600,000 units of penicillin should be given once or twice daily until the local edema subsides. The eschar goes through its natural evolution in spite of treatment, and lymph node enlargement may persist for several days. *Bacillus anthracis* cannot be recovered from the skin lesion after 24 to 48 h of penicillin therapy, but it may persist for a longer period when chloramphenicol or tetracycline is used.

Infection of personnel in industrial plants where contaminated animal products are handled still occurs. An outbreak of inhalation anthrax with a high mortality rate was reported in a goat hair processing mill in the United States in the late 1950s. Sterilization of all raw wool, mohair, etc., would probably remove this hazard but has had only limited use. A vaccine prepared from the "protective" antigen of *B. anthracis* is available and is effective in reducing the incidence of infection in an exposed population. Spore vaccines of various types are used with good effect in domestic animals in endemic areas but are not suitable for use in human beings.

Transmission of anthrax from one human being to another has never been recognized. The cutaneous disease was fatal in 20 to 30 percent of cases before antimicrobial drugs were available. The mortality now is less than 1 percent with proper treatment.

REFERENCES

BRACHMAN PS: *Anthrax,* in *Tice's Practice of Medicine,* vol. III, Hagerstown, Md.: Harper & Row, 1970

CENTER FOR DISEASE CONTROL: Morbidity & Mortality Weekly Rep 24:339, Sept. 28, 1974

GOLD H: Anthrax: Report of 117 cases. Arch Intern Med 96:387, 1955

NORMAN PS et al: Serologic testing for anthrax antibodies in workers in a goat hair processing mill. Am J Hyg 72:32, 1960

SMITH H, KEPPIE J: Observations on experimental anthrax: Demonstrations of a specific lethal factor produced in vivo, by *Bacillus anthracis.* Nature 173:869, 1954

153

INFECTIONS CAUSED BY LISTERIA AND ERYSIPELOTHRIX

PAUL D. HOEPRICH

LISTERIA MONOCYTOGENES INFECTIONS

DEFINITION Listeriosis—disease caused by *L. monocytogenes*—consists of many clinical syndromes. Perinatal infection, acquired either transplacentally or during parturition, is the most nearly unique form of listeriosis.

ETIOLOGY *Listeria monocytogenes* are gram-positive microaerophilic, motile bacilli that form smooth colonies. Seven serotypes have been defined on the basis of O and H antigens. The epidemiologically essential aid of typing is available from the Center for Disease Control in Atlanta, Georgia. Types 1b and 4b are most commonly isolated from humans in the United States. Weakly hemolytic gram-positive bacilli are presumed to be listerias if they are motile (when grown at 20 to 25°C), reduce 2,3,5-triphenyltetrazolium chloride, and display characteristic animal pathogenicity. The Anton test is classical: 3 to 5 days after inoculation into the conjunctival sac of a rabbit or a guinea pig, *L. monocytogenes* causes a keratoconjunctivitis. Also, general listeriosis in the rabbit typically provokes a monocytosis, and focal hepatic necrosis is usual in lethal murine listeriosis.

EPIDEMIOLOGY AND PATHOGENESIS Found on every continent save the Antarctic, *L. monocytogenes* bacilli appear to be primarily saprophytic residents of the soil, mud, stream water, and dry vegetation. Although the bacilli have been isolated from silage and sewage, human infection is uncommon and occurs sporadically; moreover, listeriosis is actually more common in urban than rural dwellers. The reservoir from which human beings become infected is frequently occult and the mode of transmission often obscure. Direct transmission from an infected nonhuman animal via contaminated secretions has been documented only rarely. On the other hand, transmission from the infected pregnant female to her offspring is well established as a route of infection.

Transplacental perinatal infection results in disseminated fetal listeriosis. The fetus is usually stillborn or is prematurely ejected, virtually always with lethal listeriosis. Fetal listeriosis that is acquired during delivery is typically not clinically evident for 1 or 2 weeks post partum and usually presents as a meningitis.

Listeriosis is preponderantly a disease of persons under one month (about 27 percent) and over forty years (about 56 percent) in age.

Although persons in apparent good health may contract listeriosis, infection appears to be facilitated by neoplasia (particularly of the lymphoreticular system), alcoholism, cardiovascular disease, diabetes mellitus, tuberculosis, and any condition requiring treatment with pharmacologic doses of glucosteroids, irradiation, or cytotoxic agents.

MANIFESTATIONS *Meningitis* accounts for about three-fourths of the cases verified by culture and is the predominant clinical form of listeriosis in the United States. Clinically, meningitis caused by *L. monocytogenes* cannot be distinguished from meningitis caused by other kinds of bacteria.

Listeriosis of the newborn, the most nearly unique clinical form of listeriosis, ranges from meningitis that is clinically apparent within 1 month post partum to diffuse disseminated disease in aborted, premature, and stillborn infants and neonates who die within minutes to days after birth. In newborns listeriosis becomes overt 1 to 4 weeks post partum. In these infants, as in children one month to six years of age, listeriosis is generally localized in the central nervous system.

Infants born alive with listeriosis may or may not have fever; yet these babies are critically ill, with cardiorespiratory distress, vomiting, and diarrhea. Dark-red skin papules are frequent, particularly on the lower extremities. Hepatosplenomegaly may be present. This form of listeriosis is also known as septic or miliary granulomatosis, granulomatosis infantiseptica, argentophil-rod infection, or pseudotuberculosis. The findings at postmortem examination are characteristic and mimic those seen in listeriosis of rodents: widely disseminated abscesses varying in size from grossly visible to microscopic, involving, in order of decreasing frequency, liver, spleen, adrenal glands, lungs, pharynx, gastrointestinal tract, central nervous system, and skin. Typically, the lesions are abscesses, but classic granuloma formation may be seen, depending principally on the duration of infection before death. Microscopic examination of a gram-stained smear of meconium from the normal newborn infant does not disclose bacteria; fetal listeriosis results in meconium laden with gram-positive bacilli. For this reason, examination of meconium by Gram's stain and by culture should be carried out whenever there is gross soiling of the amniotic liquid with meconium, prematurity, or unexplained fever in the mother before or at the onset of labor. This is particularly important because listeriosis in the pregnant woman may be asymptomatic or may cause a nonspecific illness. Thus, a week to a month prepartum, there may have been malaise, a chill, diarrhea, pain in the back or flanks, and itching of the skin. Even when symptomatic, the disease is benign and self-limited in the mother; however, as symptoms subside, a decrease or cessation of fetal movement may be noted. Infection of the fetus may occur as early as the fifth month of gestation. Following delivery of infants with proved fetal listeriosis, cervical cultures are, or soon become, negative for *Listeria;* subsequently, conception, gestation, and delivery of normal offspring are usual.

Oculoglandular listeriosis is the rare human analogue of the illness initiated in the rabbit by conjunctival inoculation of *Listeria.* There is a purulent conjunctivitis, which may lead to corneal ulceration. Regional-node involvement usually limits the spread from the eye. However, listerial meningitis has been reported as a complication of oculoglandular listeriosis.

Other rare syndromes caused by *Listeria* include general illness with bacteremia and high fever, endocarditis, polyserositis, and cutaneous infection.

LABORATORY FINDINGS Although *L. monocytogenes* bacilli grow well on the usual culture media, etiologic diagnosis by isolation and identification may be hampered by failure of differentiation from *Corynebacterium* sp., *Erysipelothrix insidiosa,* and *Streptococcus* sp. Recognition of listerial colonies in a mixed culture, as may result with vaginal or cervical specimens, is difficult and may be aided by using selective media and/or enrichment procedures.

Serodiagnosis by assay for agglutinins has not been useful because of the common finding of so-called natural antibodies. Such nonspecific reactions may reflect the known antigenic relationship between *Staphylococcus aureus* and several listerial serotypes. The humoral antibody response to listeriosis in humans is almost exclusively IgM throughout the disease, whereas staphylococci elicit IgG as well as IgM; i.e., treatment of serums with 2-mercaptoethanol may not eliminate nonspecific reactivity.

Monocytosis is not common in human listeriosis. Leukocytosis with neutrophilia, as in any acute bacterial infection, is seen in listerial meningitis, oculoglandular infection, bacteremia, and endocarditis. The cerebrospinal fluid in meningitis is compatible with that in other purulent meningitides.

DIFFERENTIAL DIAGNOSIS Abortion, premature delivery, stillbirth, and neonatal death are more often due to causes other than listeriosis: Rh incompatibility, syphilis, or toxoplasmosis.

In patients with leptomeningitis, conjunctivitis, endocarditis, bacteremia, or polyserositis, reports of isolation of "diphtheroids" or "nonpathogens" must always be challenged. A statement that *L. monocytogenes* has been excluded should be required.

TREATMENT *Listeria monocytogenes* bacilli are susceptible to several antimicrobials in vitro, including penicillin G, tetracyclines, and erythromycin. Dosage and duration of therapy should vary according to the kind of listerial infection under treatment.

In fetal listeriosis, therapy must be rapidly effective and should be bactericidal to be of value. A regimen of proved value has yet to be devised. Penicillin G in a dose of 100 mg (160,000 units) per kg body weight per day given by continuous intravenous injection along with erythromycin (25 to 30 mg per kg body weight per day, also by intravenous injection) merits trial.

Listeria meningitis will usually respond to treatment with penicillin G in a dose of 150 mg (240,000 units) per kg of body weight per day, given by continuous intravenous infusion. Cephalothin is not an acceptable alternative. Erythromycin as the gluceptate or lactobionate can be given in a dose of 60 to 75 mg per kg body weight per day as four equal portions given intravenously every 6 h. Tetracycline is effective—15 mg per kg body weight per day as four equal portions given intravenously every 6 h. Treatment should be continued in full dosage by intravenous injection for 7 days after defervesence.

Listeriosis in the pregnant female and oculoglandular listeriosis can be treated with a 2-week course of either erythromycin (25 to 30 mg per kg body weight per day given as four equal portions, every 6 h by mouth) or tetracycline, in the same dosage as erythromycin.

Endocarditis and bacteremia from an unknown site require vigorous therapy: penicillin G 150 mg (240,000 units) per kg body weight per day by continuous intravenous injection. The addition of erythromycin (dose as given for meningitis) should be evaluated by assay of serum bactericidal activity against the patient's isolate.

PROGNOSIS Prompt, vigorous antimicrobial treatment of the acute forms of listeriosis, excepting fetal listeriosis, is usually curative. On the basis of agglutinin titers (IgG), specific antibody disappears during the months following cure. However, reinfection has not been reported.

ERYSIPELOTHRIX INFECTIONS

DEFINITION Erysipeloid is the commonest and most nearly unique form of human *Erysipelothrix* infection. Infective endocarditis and arthritis are rare forms of *Erysipelothrix* in human beings.

ETIOLOGY As gram-positive, microaerophilic bacilli, *E. insidiosa* may be confused with nontoxinogenic *Corynebacterium* sp. and *Listeria monocytogenes.* However, *E. insidiosa* is nonmotile and fails to grow on media selective for *Corynebacterium* sp. Also, unlike *L. monocytogenes, E. insidiosa* only rarely causes conjunctivitis, following conjunctival inoculation, or monocytosis, after intravenous inoculation, in the rabbit. Because α-hemolysis is commonly evident after 48 h of incubation of *E. insidiosa,* confusion with streptococci may also occur. Isolates of *E. insidiosa* appear to be serologically homogeneous. Although serodifferentiation from other gram-positive bacilli is possible, few laboratories are capable of definitive serodiagnosis.

EPIDEMIOLOGY AND PATHOGENESIS Primarily a saprophyte, *E. insidiosa* is worldwide in distribution. Human beings are virtually always infected by traumatic dermal inoculation; erysipeloid is the usual result. The disease is almost wholly restricted to persons who in their occupations handle edible or nonedible dead animal products. If the bacilli are not successfully confined to the skin, bacteremia may result and may lead to infective endocarditis; in about one-half the reported cases, there was no evidence of preexisting valvular heart disease.

The seasonal incidence of erysipeloid parallels that of swine erysipelas, being highest in summer and early fall. Yet persons who tend pigs, even pigs ill with porcine erysipelas, do not commonly develop erysipeloid.

MANIFESTATIONS Erysipeloid begins 2 to 7 days after injury, often after the initial lesion has healed. An itching, burning, painful irritation may precede and always accompanies the appearance of the maculopapular, nonvesiculated, sharply defined, raised, purplish-red zone surrounding the site of entry. There is local swelling, and when, as is usual, a finger or the hand is involved, nearby joints may become stiff and painful. Centrifugal spread from the site of inoculation is apparent in a day or so. Movement is slow, 1 to 2 cm per 24 h maximally, and more rapid proximally than distally; involvement of the terminal phalanx of a finger is rare, while spread to other fingers and the hand below the wrist is common. With extension, the original center subsides without desquamation or suppuration. There are usually no systemic signs or symptoms; regional lymphangitis and lymphadenitis are rare. Untreated, the disease heals within 3 weeks in most patients, although relapse has been observed.

The manifestations of *Erysipelothrix* endocarditis may be either acute or chronic, depending on the virulence of the infecting strain and on the state of resistance of the host. Usually, there are no classic erysipeloid skin lesions to suggest the disease at the time that endocarditis is clinically evident. However, a history of recent erysipeloid may be helpful.

Erysipelothrix arthritis is not clinically characteristic but usually can be related to erysipeloid or *Erysipelothrix* bacteremia. Isolation of *Erysipelothrix* from synovial fluid has not been reported.

LABORATORY FINDINGS The usual culture media are adequate for the growth of *E. insidiosa.* However, differentiation from diphtheroids, listerias, and streptococci depends primarily on the clinician's alerting the laboratory to the possibility of erysipelothrix.

In erysipeloid, *E. insidiosa* are best recovered by incubating, in broth containing glucose, a full-thickness biopsy of skin removed from the advancing edge of a lesion. Culture of an aspirate obtained after injection of sterile, 0.9% NaCl solution into the periphery of a lesion is less likely to yield *Erysipelothrix.*

With endocarditis and arthritis, the findings are in keeping with the respective clinical syndromes and are in no way characteristic for *E. insidiosa.*

DIFFERENTIAL DIAGNOSIS The appearance and location of erysipeloid, its slow and limited spread, the lack of constitutional reaction, the history of occupation and injury, all serve to identify this disease. The afflicted skin in *erysipelas* is very erythematous, and the face and scalp are affected; there are regional lymphangitis and lymphadenitis, leukocytosis, fever, and malaise. Eczematous lesions may itch, but they display vesicles and little abnormal color. The various erythemas have a different location and do not usually itch or burn; they are more apt to be chronic and nonmigratory.

TREATMENT The penicillins, the cephalosporins, erythromycin, clindamycin, the tetracyclines, and chloramphenicol inhibit *E. insidiosa* in vitro at concentrations practical in therapy. Penicillin G is the agent of choice. Erysipeloid is adequately treated by injection of 1,200,000 units of benzathine penicillin G. Erythromycin (15 mg per kg body weight per day, as four equal portions taken orally for 5 to 7 days) is an alternative. Cure of *Erysipelothrix* endocarditis has been effected by the daily injection of 2,000,000 to 20,000,000 units of penicillin per day for 4 to 6 weeks; the dose should be monitored by determination of the bactericidal activity of serum from the patient against his infecting strain. Intractable cardiac failure may oblige surgical excision of an infected valve and insertion of a prosthesis.

PROGNOSIS Penicillin therapy is highly effective in curing *Erysipelothrix* infections. As with infective endocarditis from any cause, the prognosis is primarily a function of the severity of the valvular damage. Of reported cases, approximately one-half have been fatal; earlier diagnosis, and, perhaps, earlier resort to surgical excision and replacement of infected valves, may improve the outcome.

REFERENCES

GRAY ML (ed): Second Symposium on Listeria Infection. Aug 29–31, 1962, Bozeman, Mont.: Montana State College

HOEPRICH PD: Listeriosis, chap. 46, and Erysipeloid, chap. 79, in *Infectious Diseases,* ed PD Hoeprich, New York: Harper & Row, 1972

MOORE RM, ZEHMER RB: Listeriosis in the United States—1971. J Infect Dis 127:610, 1973

NELSON E: Five hundred cases of erysipeloid. Rocky Mt Med J 52:40, 1955

SEELIGER HPR: *Listeriosis,* Basel: Karger, 1961

154 DIPHTHERIA

LOUIS WEINSTEIN

DEFINITION Diphtheria is an acute infectious disease produced by *Corynebacterium diphtheriae.* It is characterized by a local inflammatory lesion, usually in the upper part of the respiratory tract, and by remote effects resulting from toxin, which affects particularly the heart and peripheral nerves.

ETIOLOGY *Corynebacterium diphtheriae* is a gram-positive, nonsporulating, nonmotile rod. There is a characteristic swelling at one end of the bacillus, which gives it a club shape. Diphtheria bacilli have been classified into *mitis, gravis,* and *intermedius* groups on the basis of colonial morphology, appearance on tellurite medium, fermentation reactions, and ability to produce hemolysis. European workers have suggested that there is a significant difference in the clinical manifestations and in the severity of disease

related to the strain; gravis and intermedius infections are thought to be accompanied by more severe toxic manifestations and a higher death rate. In the United States, the gravis strain is comparatively uncommon, and less significance is attached to the relationship of the type of organism and the clinical form of the disease.

Corynebacterium diphtheriae produces a protein exotoxin which is responsible for many of the clinical manifestations; as little as 0.0001 mg is lethal for guinea pigs. Strains of diphtheria bacilli which elaborate exotoxin are lysogenic. Absence of lysogeny generally is associated with lack of toxin formation and virulence. However, diphtheria may also follow invasion by strains of *C. diphtheriae* that cannot be shown to produce toxin.

EPIDEMIOLOGY Diphtheria occurs primarily in the Temperate Zone and is still very common in some parts of the world. Since 1966, there has been an irregular increase in the number of cases of diphtheria in the United States. Two outbreaks in Texas early in this decade accounted for most of the cases. However, in 1973 to 1975, more than 75 percent of the cases were reported from the Pacific Northwest and the Southwest. The Western Provinces of Canada experienced a similar increase in diphtheria. Until this new geographical trend was recognized, the highest frequency had been in children between one and nine years of age. The attack rate for unimmunized children was seventy times higher than the rate for children who had received primary immunization. In the Pacific Northwest, 77 percent of isolates have been from adults with symptomatic skin lesions. Another striking change has been a decrease in the incidence of laryngeal involvement. In general, diphtheria is acquired by droplet transmission from active cases or carriers, but fomites may play a role in the spread of cutaneous infection.

PATHOGENESIS AND PATHOLOGY The commonest portal of entry for the diphtheria bacillus is the upper respiratory tract. The skin, genitalia, eye, and middle ear may also be sites of invasion. Growth of the organism is superficial in most cases, and there is little tendency to invade the lymphatics or bloodstream except in the terminal stages. The exotoxin elaborated in the local lesion is absorbed and carried by the blood to all parts of the body. The intensity of the toxic effects is greatest when the primary lesion is in the pharynx, less when it is in the larynx, and least when it is on the nasal mucosa or skin. Simultaneous involvement of the pharynx, larynx, trachea, and bronchial tree is associated with most severe intoxication.

The *membrane,* the primary lesion of diphtheria, is thick, leathery, and blue-white and is composed of bacteria, necrotic epithelium, phagocytes, and fibrin. It is surrounded by a narrow zone of inflammation and is firmly adherent to the underlying tissues; bleeding follows its forcible removal. Ulceration is not a regular feature. Regional lymphadenitis is frequent.

The *toxic manifestations* involve primarily the heart, kidneys, and peripheral nerves. The brain is rarely affected. Cardiac enlargement is frequent; this appears to be related to myocarditis rather than hypertrophy. The kidneys may be enlarged and reveal cloudy swelling and interstitial changes. Bronchopneumonia due to *C. diphtheriae* or to secondary invading organisms occurs in some patients, especially those with laryngeal involvement. Membrane is present throughout the bronchial tree when the diphtheria bacillus is responsible for the pulmonary infection. The peripheral nerves may reveal fatty degeneration, disintegration of the medullary sheaths, and involvement of the axis cylinder. Both motor and sensory fibers are affected, but the main impact is on motor innervation. The anterior horn cells and the posterior columns of the spinal cord may be damaged. Other central nervous system involvement includes cerebral hemorrhage, meningitis, and encephalitis. Petechial and purpuric lesions are occasionally present in the kidneys, skin, or adrenals. Endocarditis due to *C. diphtheriae* is rare.

Death results from respiratory obstruction by membrane or edema, or from the effects of toxin on the heart, nervous system, or other organs.

IMMUNITY Susceptibility to the complications of diphtheria is related to the presence or absence of circulating antibody to exotoxin. The Schick test yields a rough estimate of the quantity of antitoxin in the circulation. This test is carried out in the following manner: 0.1 ml purified diphtheria toxin (one-fiftieth the minimum lethal dose) dissolved in buffered human serum albumin is injected intradermally on the volar surface of the forearm; 0.1 ml purified diphtheria toxoid is injected into the other arm as a control. These areas are examined at 24 and 48 h and between the fourth and seventh days and interpreted in the following way:

1 *Positive reaction:* The site of injection of toxin begins to redden in 24 h; this increases and reaches a maximum in about a week, at which time the lesion may be as large as 3 cm in diameter and moderately swollen and tender. There is usually a small (1 to 1.5 cm) dark-red central zone which gradually turns brown, desquamates, and leaves a pigmented area. The area of toxoid injection shows no reaction. A positive test indicates little or no circulating antitoxin and no immunity.
2 *Negative reaction:* There is no reaction at the site of injection of either toxoid or toxin. This is consistent with a blood antitoxin level of 1/30 to 1/100 unit and immunity to ordinary exposure.
3 *Pseudoreaction:* Inflammation at both sites of injection within 12 to 14 h, which reaches a maximum in 48 to 72 h and then fades. This usually indicates immunity plus hypersensitivity to the toxin or other materials in the solution.
4 *Combined reaction:* This begins like the pseudoreaction, but the inflammatory response at the toxin site persists after that in the area of toxoid injection has faded. It indicates delayed sensitivity to toxin or other proteins and either low levels or no antitoxin. The incidence of combined reactions increases with age and is highest in unimmunized groups living in areas where diphtheria is prevalent.

Individuals with negative Schick tests occasionally contract diphtheria, and some persons with positive Schick reactions do not develop the disease after exposure. In some parts of the United States fewer than 50 percent of adults have "protective" levels of circulating antitoxin. The Schick test is not used routinely in the United States, and the ability to perform it should not delay the treatment of asymptomatic contacts of diphtheria.

Second attacks of respiratory diphtheria are rare despite the fact that about 10 percent of patients who have had the disease remain Schick-positive. This suggests that factors other than antitoxin may play a role in protection against infection. In general, immunized patients have a milder illness than unimmunized ones when the initial clinical picture and level of circulating antitoxin are the same. Early therapy of diphtheria with antibiotics may lead to recurrence of the disease if exposure to fresh infections occurs shortly after discontinuation of treatment, suggesting that the development of antitoxic immunity is suppressed in these cases. Full immunization with diphtheria toxoid does not prevent nasopharyngeal carriage of the organism but significantly reduces the case fatality ratio. It also ameliorates the symptoms of active disease.

CLINICAL MANIFESTATIONS The incubation period of diphtheria is 1 to 7 days. The local symptoms vary with the site of the primary lesion. A membrane is not always present. Constitutional reactions usually are of only minor to moderate severity in uncomplicated disease. Fever is usually low (100 to 101°F), unless infection with another organism (often group A *Streptococcus pyogenes*) supervenes. When toxic manifestations are absent, patients feel well except for a varying degree of discomfort at the site of the local lesion. Pallor, listlessness, tachycardia, and weakness are common in more severe cases. Peripheral vascular collapse often develops in the terminal stages of the disease.

Nasal diphtheria Diphtheria is occasionally restricted to the nasal mucosa. It is usually localized to the septum or turbinates in the anterior portion of one side of the nose, does not extend, and may persist for a long time. A foreign body is frequently present. A unilateral serosanguineous discharge is characteristic. When the disease is located in the posterior nasal areas, it commonly extends to the pharynx, from which toxin is absorbed.

Pharyngeal diphtheria The early diphtheritic membrane in the pharynx consists of small areas of soft exudate which wipe off easily and leave no bleeding points. As the disease progresses, the discrete exudate coalesces to form an easily removable thin sheet which spreads to cover tonsils or pharynx, or both. Later, it becomes thicker, bluish-white, gray, or black, depending on the degree of hemorrhage, and is so firmly attached to the underlying tissues that attempts to remove it result in bleeding. If infection with group A *Strep. pyogenes* is superimposed, the pharynx is diffusely red and edematous. Pharyngeal discomfort may occur in up to 25 percent of the cases and in some patients may be severe. There is usually a moderate leukocytosis with 15,000 or fewer white blood cells per mm^3.

Local spread of the pharyngeal membrane may occur, and the throat, tonsils, and soft and hard palates become completely covered. Patients with severe disease may develop so-called "malignant" diphtheria, characterized by marked edema of the submandibular areas and the anterior neck, giving the characteristic "bullneck" appearance. Respiration is noisy, the tongue protrudes, the breath is foul, and the speech thick. The pharyngeal tissues are red and edematous, and the cervical lymph nodes are enlarged. The skin is pale and cool. The patient complains of overwhelming weakness. Purpuric eruptions of the skin, particularly on the neck and anterior chest wall, may appear occasionally. Drowsiness and delirium are common.

Laryngeal diphtheria Involvement of the larynx is usually the result of extension of the diphtheritic membrane from the pharynx. The infection may rarely be limited to the larynx or trachea. This possibility must be considered in the differential diagnosis of all cases of "croup"; it can be ruled out only by direct examination of the airway. The clinical features of this type of disease are described below.

Cutaneous diphtheria Until recently, diphtheria of the skin was a problem primarily in tropical areas where it is responsible for some cases of "jungle sore." However, since 1972, there has been a significant increase in skin diphtheria in the Pacific Northwest and the Southwest. A high attack rate has occurred in native Americans and in indigent males living in "skid row" areas where crowding and poor personal and community hygiene abound. *Corynebacterium diphtheriae,* being unable to penetrate unbroken skin, invades wounds, burns, abrasions, etc. Any break in the skin may be colonized with *C. diphtheriae.* Coagulase-positive *Staphylococcus aureus* and/or beta-hemolytic streptococci frequently are recovered concomitantly. Although the lesions develop most often on the extremities, they may appear at any site including the perianal area. In tropical zones, the typical lesion appears as a round, deep "punched out" ulcer, 0.5 cm to several centimeters in diameter. In the early stages, it is covered by a gray-yellow or gray-brown membrane which strips off early to reveal a clean hemorrhagic base that dries quickly and becomes covered by a thin, leathery, dark-brown or black, adherent membrane. In the untreated case, this separates spontaneously 1 to 3 weeks after infection. The margin of the fully developed ulcer is usually slightly undermined, purple, rolled, and sharply defined. When lesions are infected with a toxigenic strain, anesthesia over the lesion develops within a few weeks. In temperate climates, the lesions are not sufficiently specific to permit visual diagnosis. Cutaneous diphtheria should be suspected in any adult with skin lesions, particularly in the proper epidemiologic setting. Antibiotic therapy will change the character of the skin lesions. Twenty percent of patients with cutaneous diphtheria also have infections in the nasopharynx with the same biotype. Myocarditis or neuropathy occurs in about 3 to 5 percent of patients with cutaneous diphtheria. The Landry-Guillain-Barré syndrome develops occasionally.

Diphtheritic lesions in other areas Diphtheria may involve the uterine cervix, vagina, vulva, bladder, urethra, or penis (after circumcision). Toxic manifestations are common. The tongue, buccal mucous membrane, gums, and esophagus may also be affected. Infection of the conjunctiva occurs rarely. Otitis media may occur as an isolated syndrome or secondary to diphtheria in the upper part of the respiratory tract; the aural infection may become chronic; virulent organisms may be isolated from the discharge for many months.

COMPLICATIONS OF DIPHTHERIA The complications of

diphtheria are of two types: (1) those that result from spread of the membrane in the respiratory tract, and (2) those due to the effects of the toxin.

Extension and spread of membrane The membrane of diphtheria may spread from the fauces over the posterior pharyngeal wall into the larynx, trachea, and, uncommonly, the bronchial tree, leading to severe illness and a high incidence of toxic manifestations. Occlusion of the airway is manifested by tachypnea and, as obstruction increases, restlessness, use of accessory muscles of respiration, cyanosis, and finally death. In some cases, the membrane extends diffusely into the bronchial tree and produces clinical manifestations of pneumonia. Bronchopulmonary diphtheria is very serious, not only because of obstruction but also because of the large surface from which toxin can be absorbed; the death rate is very high. When the pulmonary lesion regresses, pieces of membrane may break off and produce sudden occlusion of the airway; a cast of the bronchial tree may be coughed up. On occasion, pharyngeal membrane has extended into the esophagus and cardia of the stomach.

Toxic complications of diphtheria Studies of the mechanisms of action of diphtheria toxin suggest that it inhibits the transfer of amino acids from soluble RNA to growing polypeptide chains, resulting in failure of the amino acids to be incorporated into the polypeptide; a cofactor, nicotinamide-adenine dinucleotide, is required for activity of the toxin. The effects of the toxin on the myocardium are thought to result from its ability to decrease the rate of oxidation of long-chain fatty acids by interfering with the metabolism of carnitine. Because of this, triglycerides accumulate in the myocardium and cause fatty degeneration of muscle.

Myocarditis develops in about two-thirds of patients with diphtheria. However, it is clinically evident in only about 10 percent of cases; alterations in the intensity of the heart sounds, systolic murmurs, bundle branch block, incomplete or complete heart block, atrial fibrillation, ventricular premature beats or tachycardia, or both, are common. Ventricular fibrillation is a constant threat and is frequently responsible for sudden death. Ninety percent of patients with atrial fibrillation, ventricular tachycardia, or complete heart block die. Overt congestive cardiac failure is uncommon. Evidence of decompensation of the right side of the heart usually develops first; the most common symptom is pain in the right upper quadrant of the abdomen due to rapid engorgement of the liver. Failure of the left side of the heart may appear later. Diphtheritic heart disease is not necessarily "benign" in survivors of the disease; permanent cardiac damage may occur. Fibrosis of the myocardium has been observed in patients who have expired several weeks after "mild" myocarditis was detected electrocardiographically. The degree and extent of fibrotic change has often been greater than could have been predicted on the basis of the type of abnormality present in the ECG.

Peripheral neuritis may occur in the course of diphtheria. Paralysis of the soft palate and posterior pharyngeal wall occasionally appears very early in the disease (2 to 3 days).

A more common neuritis (10 percent of cases) usually develops 2 to 6 weeks after onset of the disease. It is characterized by cranial nerve dysfunction; the third, sixth, seventh, ninth, and tenth nerves are most commonly involved. Loss of accommodation, nasal voice, and difficulty in swallowing are the most frequent manifestations. However, any of the peripheral nerves may be affected, with resulting paralysis of the extremities, diaphragm, or intercostal muscles; death may occur from failure of respiration. The peripheral neuritides which appear in the second to the sixth week of the disease are characterized primarily by motor loss; sensory changes are uncommon and, when present, are minor. Peripheral neuritis may not appear until 2 to 3 months after the onset of diphtheria. In these cases, the clinical picture and course resemble infectious polyneuritis. The outstanding findings are loss of sensation in the "glove-and-stocking" distribution and albuminocytologic dissociation in the cerebrospinal fluid identical with that observed in the Landry-Guillain-Barré syndrome. Motor weakness and areflexia may develop with progression of involvement. Facial diplegia may accompany the other neurologic manifestation. A fatal, rapidly ascending paralysis of the Landry type may develop rarely. Complete recovery is the rule in this late peripheral neuritis, although it may require as long as a year. Encephalitis is a rare toxic complication of diphtheria.

Shock, which develops suddenly and without warning, is an occasional cause of sudden death in this disease. In some instances, this may be a consequence of myocarditis; in others, no cause can be discovered.

Other complications Cerebral infarction with hemiplegia occurs rarely; it is probably due to embolization from atrial thrombi in patients with myocarditis and cardiac dilatation. Superinfection of the lungs is a risk in all patients with diphtheria who are given antimicrobial agents. Purpuric skin eruptions may be seen in severe, malignant cases; thrombocytopenia occurs rarely. A mild morbilliform rash may be present during the early stage of diphtheria. Secondary invasion of the pharynx by group A *Strep. pyogenes* may take place in patients who have not received an antibiotic. Serum sickness occasionally follows the use of antitoxin. Relapses of diphtheria may occur when patients given antimicrobial agents are exposed to fresh cases soon after therapy has been discontinued. Bacteremia, endocarditis, and meningitis are rare complications.

COURSE AND PROGNOSIS The diphtheritic membrane may be present for only 3 to 4 days in mild cases, even when no antitoxin is given; it usually lasts for about a week in cases of moderate severity. Commonly, the pharyngeal lesion increases in extent and thickness during the first 24 h after the administration of antitoxin. As the disease begins to recede, the exudate softens, wipes off easily, leaving no bleeding areas, becomes patchy so that it resembles the picture of "follicular" tonsillitis, and finally disappears, leaving normal underlying mucous membrane.

The fatality rate of diphtheria prior to the use of specific antitoxin was about 35 percent in average cases and 90 percent in those with laryngeal involvement. Since specific serotherapy has been employed, this has been reduced to a range of 3.5 to 22 percent, but it is still highest when the larynx is affected. The overall death rate in the United States is about 10 percent. Death is most frequent in the very young and the old. Immunization is a factor of great importance in prognosis. The fatality rate in immunized individuals is one-tenth that in the unimmunized population. Paralysis is five times and "malignant" disease fifteen times less common in immune than in nonimmune individuals. As a rule, the longer the delay in the administration of antitoxin, the greater the incidence of complications and death. However, antitoxin is ineffective in reducing risks of complications and death if it is given much later than 48 h after diphtheria begins.

A white blood cell count higher than 25,000 per mm^3 is associated with a higher risk of complications and death.

DIAGNOSIS The clinical features of the fully developed diphtheritic membrane, especially in the pharynx, are sufficiently characteristic to suggest the possibility of the disease in most instances. However, the appearance of the pharyngeal exudate alone does not clinch the diagnosis. There are a number of other infections in which pseudomembranes resembling those of diphtheria are present; among these are infectious mononucleosis, streptococcal pharyngitis, viral exudative pharyngitis, fusospirochetal infection, and acute pharyngeal candidiasis.

The specific diagnosis of diphtheria depends completely on demonstration of the organism in stained smears and their recovery by culture. Methylene blue-stained preparations are positive, in experienced hands, in 75 to 85 percent of cases. Diphtheria bacilli can be recovered by culture on Loeffler's medium in 8 to 12 h if patients have not been receiving antimicrobial agents. *Corynebacterium diphtheriae* also multiplies, but more slowly, on ordinary blood agar. If an antibiotic, especially penicillin or erythromycin, has been administered prior to obtaining cultures, the organisms may not grow for as long as 5 days, or may fail to grow at all.

Staining of suspected material with fluorescein-labeled diphtheria antitoxin may allow rapid diagnosis.

TREATMENT Patients with diphtheria should be isolated and kept at strict bed rest; physical effort should be reduced during the early convalescent stages. Local therapy of the diphtheritic lesion is useless. The only specific treatment for diphtheria is antitoxin. Antiserum must never be given until the patient's sensitivity to horse serum, using the eye and skin tests, has been determined. There are several regimens for the administration of antitoxin, and the amount given is often based on an empiric decision. In general, the more severe the disease or the more extensive the membrane formation, the greater is the amount of antitoxin required. A useful schedule is: when exudate is present on only one tonsil, 5,000 units; for lesions covering both tonsils, 10,000 units; when the entire pharyngeal wall and the tonsils are involved, 20,000 to 50,000 units; for laryngeal disease, 50,000 to 100,000 units. Because of the length of time required for antibody to reach maximal levels in the blood after intramuscular injection, no more than one-half the calculated dose is given by this route. If no reaction occurs, the remainder of the antitoxin is infused slowly by vein. Alternatively, after appropriate testing for sensitivity, the entire amount of antitoxin may be given intravenously in 100 to 200 ml isotonic saline over a 30-min period. Desensitization should be attempted if the initial skin or eye test is positive. A rare patient may be sensitive to such a high degree that the antiserum cannot be administered without the risk of death.

Antitoxin should be given as early in the course of diphtheria as possible. The history of military service is not reliable proof of adequate immunization. From World War II until 1956, immunization for diphtheria in the United States military was inconsistent. Since 1957, all branches of the Armed Forces have routinely immunized their personnel. Antimicrobial agents do not alter the course, incidence of complications, or outcome of diphtheria.

Patients with laryngeal obstruction should be watched very carefully. In mild cases, inhalation of warm or cool steam may be beneficial. If advancing signs of airway obstruction develop, intubation or tracheostomy is indicated. These procedures must never be delayed until cyanosis appears, because, at this point, stimulation of the pharynx or trachea may produce cardiac standstill and death. Sedative or hypnotic agents should never be given because they may obscure increasing respiratory difficulty.

The pulse and blood pressure should be measured frequently. Little can be done to alter the course of the myocarditis. Quinidine has been tried to prevent and treat arrhythmias, but appears to be of no value; there is some suspicion that it may produce deleterious effects. The use of procainamide when ventricular premature beats or tachycardia supervene has been suggested, but no documented observations of its effect have been recorded. The administration of digitalis for cardiac failure in diphtheria is controversial. Some consider this drug to be completely contraindicated; others feel, however, that, used carefully, digitalis may be given safely and with beneficial effects. Shock should be treated, depending on its etiology (Chaps. 35 and 129). There is no evidence that corticosteroids or corticotropin are of any value in the treatment of diphtheria or any of its complications.

Treatment of carriers *Corynebacterium diphtheriae* usually disappears from the upper part of the respiratory tract after 2 to 4 weeks in patients who do not receive antimicrobial drugs; in a small number of individuals the organism may persist for a long time or be present permanently. The most effective treatment of the acute and chronic carrier state is erythromycin. A dose of 2 g per day orally in divided doses for 7 days appears to be adequate. Alternative microbials include procaine penicillin G, 600,000 units intramuscularly every 12 h for 10 days; clindamycin, 150 mg four times a day orally for 7 days; rifampin, 600 mg as a single oral dose for 7 days. Tetracyclines, semisynthetic penicillins, and oral cephalosporins are inadequate for the eradication of *C. diphtheriae.* Retreatment is indicated for carriers whose organisms do not disappear on the first trial. This is preferable to tonsillectomy, which may be considered as a last resort should the carrier state persist despite repeated courses of antibiotic.

PREVENTION Diphtheria is, for the most part, a preventable disease. Immunization at the age of three months should be routine. Diphtheria toxoid is best given together with tetanus toxoid and pertussis vaccine (DPT), because antibody titers are higher with combined immunization than with either agent alone. "Booster" doses should be administered at the age of one year and again just before a child goes to school. Although it has been suggested that Schick testing is not necessary in those who have been immunized, many physicians still carry this out to determine the status of antitoxic immunity. A Schick test acts as a "booster." A negative reaction does not indicate absolute protection. The development of highly purified toxoid has made it possible to protect adults with little or no risk of untoward sequelae. In this situation, adult T.d. toxoid containing 1 to 2 L.f. units per ml should be used. With this preparation severe reactions can be avoided. The Moloney test need not be carried out.

Treatment of unimmunized persons exposed to an active case of diphtheria remains controversial. One approach has been to administer 3,000 units antitoxin intramuscularly, after appropriate skin and eye tests. Alternatively, cultures for *C. diphtheriae* can be taken, and a primary series of immunizations initiated. The exposed individual then can be observed closely for signs of active disease. If symptoms occur, antitoxin can be given immediately. In those who have been previously immunized, a "booster" dose of toxoid is usually sufficient. Patients with diphtheria should be quarantined until two successive cultures of the nose, throat, or other infected areas, taken at 24-h intervals, are negative. If antibiotics have been administered, cultural studies should not be initiated until at least 24 h after cessation of therapy.

REFERENCES

BELSER MA, LEBLANC DR: Skin infections and the epidemiology of diphtheria: Acquisition and persistence of *C. diphtheriae* infections. Am J Epidemiol 102:179, 1975

BROOKS ER et al: Diphtheria in the United States 1959–1970. J Infect Dis 129:172, 1974

GOOD I: Myocardial changes in fatal diphtheria: A summary of observations in 221 cases. Am J Med Sci 219:257, 1948

GOOR RS, PAPPENHEIMER AM JR.: Studies on the mode of action of diphtheria toxin. J Exp Med 126:899, 913, 923, 1967

IPSEN J: Circulating antitoxin at the onset of diphtheria in 425 patients. Medicine (Baltimore) 251:459, 1954

——: Immunization of adults against diphtheria and tetanus. N Engl J Med 251:459, 1954

LIVINGOOD CS et al: Cutaneous diphtheria: A report of 140 cases. J Invest Dermatol 7:341, 1946

MCCLUSKEY RV et al: The 1970 epidemic of diphtheria in San Antonio. Ann Intern Med 75:495, 1971

NAIDITCH MJ, BOWER AG: Diphtheria: A study of 1,433 cases observed during a ten-year period at the Los Angeles County Hospital. Am J Med 17:229, 1954

SCHEID W: Diphtherial paralysis: An analysis of 2,292 cases of diphtheria in adults which include 174 cases of polyneuritis. J Nerv Ment Dis 116:1095, 1952

WITTELS B, BRESSLER R: Biochemical lesion of diphtheria toxin on the heart. J Clin Invest 43:630, 1964

155
CHOLERA AND OTHER ENTEROTOXIC INFECTIONS

CHARLES C. J. CARPENTER

DEFINITION Cholera is an acute illness which results from colonization of the small intestine by *Vibrio cholerae.* The disease is characterized by its epidemic occurrence and the production in the more severe cases of massive diarrhea with rapid depletion of extracellular fluid and electrolytes.

ETIOLOGY AND EPIDEMIOLOGY *Vibrio cholerae* is a curved, aerobic, gram-negative bacillus with a single polar flagellum. It is rapidly motile and possesses both O and H antigens. Serologic identification is based on differences in the polysaccharide O antigens.

Cholera has been endemic for a century and a half in the Gangetic Delta of West Bengal and Bangladesh and is often epidemic throughout South and Southeast Asia. The seventh and most recent pandemic spread of this disease, from 1961 to 1975, extended from the Celebes northward to Korea and westward to the whole of Africa and Southern Europe. The last major epidemic of cholera in the Western Hemisphere occurred during 1866–1867.

The majority of major epidemics have clearly been water-borne, but direct contamination of food by infected feces probably contributes to spread during major outbreaks. Poor sanitation appears to be primarily responsible for the continuing presence of cholera, but host factors, such as relative or absolute achlorhydria, also play an important role in the susceptibility of the individual to infection. In endemic areas, cholera is predominantly a disease of children; in rural Bangladesh attack rates are ten times greater in the one- to five-age group than in those above fourteen years of age. However, when the disease spreads to previously uninvolved areas, the attack rates are initially at least as high in adults as in children.

A chronic gallbladder carrier state has been observed in a small percentage of elderly convalescent cholera patients. These chronic *Vibrio* carriers may provide a vehicle for spread outside of endemic areas. The basis for the annual cholera epidemics throughout the Gangetic Delta, for the periodic outbreaks throughout the remainder of South and Southeast Asia, and for the occasional global pandemics has, however, not been clearly delineated.

PATHOGENESIS *Vibrio cholerae* produces a protein enterotoxin which appears to be responsible for all known pathophysiologic aberrations in cholera. This enterotoxin, which has a molecular weight of 84,000, stimulates adenyl cyclase in the intestine epithelial cells, and the resultant increase in intracellular cyclic adenosine 3′,5′-monophosphate leads to secretion of isotonic fluid by all segments of the small intestine. The enterotoxin-induced electrolyte secretion occurs in the absence of any demonstrable histologic damage to intestine epithelial cells or to the capillary endothelial cells of the lamina propria. Precise studies have demonstrated that the stool of the adult cholera patient is nearly isotonic, with sodium and chloride concentrations slightly less than those of plasma, a bicarbonate concentration approximately twice that of plasma, and a potassium concentration three to five times that of plasma. Disease caused by all known strains of *V. cholerae* results in the same stool electrolyte pattern. The pathophysiologic defect in cholera is extracellular fluid depletion with resultant hypovolemic shock, base-deficit acidosis, and progressive potassium depletion. There is no evidence that the cholera *Vibrio* invades any tissue, nor has the enterotoxin been shown, in human disease, to have any direct effect on any organ other than the small intestine.

MANIFESTATIONS The incubation period is generally from 6 to 48 h. This is followed by the abrupt onset of watery, generally painless diarrhea. In the more severe cases, the initial diarrheal stool may be in excess of 1,000 ml, and several liters of isotonic fluid may be lost within hours, leading rapidly to profound shock. Vomiting generally follows, but occasionally precedes, the onset of diarrhea; the vomiting is characteristically effortless and not preceded by nausea. As saline depletion progresses, severe muscle cramps, commonly involving the calves, occur.

When first seen, the typical severely ill cholera patient is cyanotic, with pinched facies, scaphoid abdomen, poor skin turgor, and thready or absent peripheral pulses. The voice is faint, high-pitched, and often inaudible, and there are tachycardia, hypotension, and varying degrees of tachypnea. In all epidemics there are many subclinical or mild cases in which gastrointestinal fluid loss is not severe enough to require hospitalization. With the *el tor* strain of *V. cholerae,* which has been responsible for the most recent pandemic, the ratio of subclinical infections to clinical cholera cases is greater than 10:1.

The disease runs its course in 2 to 7 days, and subsequent manifestations depend on the adequacy of electrolyte repletion therapy. With prompt fluid and electrolyte repletion, physiologic recovery is remarkably rapid, and mortality exceptionally rare. The important causes of death, in inadequately treated patients, are hypovolemic shock, metabolic acidosis, and uremia resulting from acute tubular necrosis.

LABORATORY FINDINGS In epidemics or in endemic areas, the clinical picture should arouse strong suspicion immediately. The most reliable technique for identification of *V. cholerae* consists of direct plating of a sample of cholera stool on bile salt, gelatin-tellurite-taurocholate (GTT), or thiosulfate-citrate-bile salt-sucrose (TCBS) agar. On bile salt or GTT agar the organisms appear as typical translucent colonies within 24 h. On TCBS agar, *V. cholerae* appear at 24 h as distinct, large, yellow colonies. Further classification requires agglutination with type-specific antiserums. In mild or convalescent cases, recovery of vibrios may be enhanced by initial enrichment for 6 h in alkaline peptone water followed by subculture on bile salt, GTT, or TCBS agar. Rapid diagnosis is possible either by directly observing immobilization of vibrios by type-specific antiserums, using dark-field or phase microscopy, or identifying the organisms by immunofluorescent methods.

TREATMENT Successful therapy requires only prompt and adequate replacement of gastrointestinal losses of saline and alkali. A uniformly satisfactory solution for intravenous fluid therapy can be simply prepared by the addition of 5 g sodium chloride, 4 g sodium bicarbonate, and 1 g potassium chloride to 1 liter of pyrogen-free distilled water. If commercially prepared fluids are available, a combination of isotonic sodium bicarbonate (or acetate or lactate) and isotonic sodium chloride, infused in a 2:1 ratio, may be employed. The intravenous fluids are initially infused at 50 to 100 ml per min, until a strong pulse has been restored. The same fluids should subsequently be infused in quantities equal to the gastrointestinal losses. If losses cannot be measured accurately, intravenous fluids should be given at a rate sufficient to maintain a normal radial pulse and normal skin turgor. Overhydration can be avoided by careful observation of neck venous filling and auscultation of the lungs. Close observation is mandatory during the acute phase of the illness, because the cholera patient can lose as much as 1 liter of isotonic fluid per hour during the first 24 h of the disease. Inadequate or delayed restoration of fecal fluid losses may result in a high incidence of acute renal failure. Serious hypokalemic symptoms are rare in adults, and potassium repletion can be carried out orally if potassium-containing intravenous fluids are not available. Hypokalemia contributes significantly, however, to the morbidity in inadequately treated pediatric cholera, and potassium, 10 to 13 meq per liter, should be included in the intravenous fluids administered to pediatric patients.

Although adequate intravenous saline and alkali repletion alone results in rapid recovery of virtually all cholera patients, a dramatic reduction in the duration and volume of the diarrhea and early eradication of vibrios from the stool may be effected by antibiotic therapy. Oral tetracycline, 500 mg every 6 h for the first 48 h of treatment, has been most successful. Other antibiotics, including chloramphenicol and furazolidone, are also of value, but both appear to be slightly less effective than tetracycline.

Oral therapy Since the cholera enterotoxin does not alter glucose-facilitated sodium absorption, fluid repletion can be effected by the oral administration of glucose-containing electrolyte solutions. Since the limiting factor in treatment of cholera in both epidemic and endemic situations is often the lack of adequate quantities of intravenous fluids, the availability of an oral treatment regimen has greatly reduced the mortality from cholera outbreaks during the most recent pandemic spread of this disease. A solution containing glucose 20 g per liter, sodium bicarbonate 4 g per liter, sodium chloride 4 g per liter, and potassium chloride 1 g per liter can be readily prepared and should be satisfactory for treatment of all age groups. This solution, administered orally at a rate equal to the stool losses, can be given to patients with milder cholera cases throughout the course of illness and is satisfactory in the more severe cases, once the hypovolemic shock has been corrected by intravenous fluid therapy. Oral therapy does not decrease the rate of intestinal fluid loss but provides an electrolyte solution which can be absorbed at a rate sufficient, in most cases, to counterbalance the continuing fluid losses. Therefore, successful management of the cholera patient with oral therapy requires just as close supervision, with careful monitoring of pulse volume, skin turgor, and neck veins, as does management with intravenous solutions. Supplemental intravenous fluids must be administered whenever clinical signs of saline depletion recur.

PROGNOSIS Under ideal conditions and with prompt and adequate fluid replacement, mortality approaches zero, and significant sequelae are rare. Unfortunately, death rates as high as 60 percent still occur, especially during the initial phases of certain outbreaks. This high mortality reflects lack of pyrogen-free intravenous fluids in remote areas, the difficulties of initiating treatment promptly when large numbers of cases are occurring in poverty-stricken populations, and the compromises which may have to be made under emergency conditions.

PREVENTION Immunization by standard commercial vaccine, containing 10 billion killed organisms per milliliter, provides significant protection for a limited (4- to 6-month) period. Standard vaccination consists of two 0.5-ml doses separated by a 1-month interval; for Americans traveling in countries in which cholera is endemic, a single dose of 0.5 ml prior to departure is recommended. Immunization with toxoid, which is not yet commercially available, also provides only limited protection for a relatively short period of time. Careful hygiene provides the only sure protection against cholera.

ENTEROTOXIGENIC ESCHERICHIA COLI

DEFINITION Enterotoxin-producing *E. coli* may cause a wide spectrum of diarrheal illnesses, ranging from a severe cholera-like illness, seen in both adults and children in the Indian subcontinent, to the less severe, but troublesome, "turista," frequently seen in North American travelers to Mexico.

ETIOLOGY AND EPIDEMIOLOGY The ability to produce enterotoxin is not restricted to any specific *E. coli* serotype, but results from the presence of a specific plasmid on the surface of the *E. coli.* Since current techniques for demonstrating toxigenicity are cumbersome, the epidemiology of disease caused by enterotoxigenic *E. coli* is poorly understood. Recent investigations suggest that toxigenic *E. coli* may be responsible for a large proportion of cases of "travelers' diarrhea" in visitors to Mexico, as well as a significant number of cases of childhood diarrhea in disadvantaged populations, both urban and rural, in North America. There is, as yet, no adequate explanation for the observation that enterotoxigenic *E. coli* have been implicated in fulminant, cholera-like diarrheal disease in adult patients only in South and Southeast Asia.

PATHOGENESIS Enterotoxigenic *E. coli* produces a heat-labile protein enterotoxin which appears to be responsible for the intestinal fluid loss. This toxin, like the cholera enterotoxin, stimulates adenyl cyclase in the intestinal epithelial cells, resulting in outpouring of a nearly isotonic fluid similar to that observed in cholera. The effect of the *E. coli* enterotoxin is, however, of shorter duration than that of cholera enterotoxin, and the *E. coli* also characteristically colonize the small intestine for a shorter time period than *V. cholerae;* both these factors contribute to the short duration of symptoms in enterotoxigenic *E. coli* infection.

MANIFESTATIONS The incubation period is short, probably 24 to 48 h. The illness which follows is quite variable, ranging from the fulminant, cholera-like disease often seen in Southeast Asia to the much milder "turista," commonly seen in travelers to Central and South America, in which the symptoms of mild diarrhea, abdominal cramps, and occasional low-grade fever are more troublesome than life-threatening.

In fulminant cases, the severe diarrhea seldom lasts longer than 36 h, and the response to fluid and electrolyte repletion is predictable and dramatic. With milder disease, the symptoms are self-limited, ceasing within 48 h in the majority of cases.

LABORATORY FINDINGS As with cholera, the stool contains no blood and few, if any, polymorphonuclear leukocytes. Since *E. coli* are constituents of normal stool flora, and since the ability to produce enterotoxin is not related to any specific serotype, there is no rapid means of laboratory diagnosis of enterotoxigenic *E. coli.* Bioassays, based on ability of *E. coli* isolates to produce fluid in ligated intestinal loops of experimental animals, or to stimulate adenyl cyclase in cells in tissue culture, are reliable but of little practical value under field conditions.

TREATMENT Successful therapy of the more severe cases requires intravenous or oral replacement of intestinal fluid losses, employing the same principles outlined for the treatment of cholera. Antimicrobial therapy has not been shown to be of significant value, probably because of the relatively short duration of the illness. It is not clear that any medications are helpful in the symptomatic treatment of patients with the milder forms of "travelers' diarrhea."

PROGNOSIS Even with the more fulminant cases of disease caused by enterotoxigenic *E. coli,* the prognosis is excellent with adequate fluid replacement.

PREVENTION Careful hygienic practices, with especial attention to ingestion of clean water and adequately cooked foods when living in a generally unsanitary environment, provide the only reasonable protection against toxigenic *E. coli.*

VIBRIO PARAHEMOLYTICUS INFECTION

DEFINITION *Vibrio parahemolyticus,* a halophilic vibrio which is found in coastal waters throughout the world, is the leading cause of acute diarrheal disease in Japan, and has recently been responsible for several outbreaks of acute illness in the Eastern and Southeastern United States as well as on American cruise ships.

ETIOLOGY AND EPIDEMIOLOGY *Vibrio parahemolyticus* is a curved, aerobic, nonmotile, gram-negative bacillus. Although present in coastal waters throughout the temperate zone, it has most commonly been associated with acute diarrheal illness in Japan, presumably because of the frequency of ingestion of raw seafood. It has recently been implicated in several outbreaks of acute diarrheal disease in the coastal United States, always as a common-source outbreak related to ingestion of inadequately cooked seafood, usually shrimp. Secondary cases caused by person-to-person transmission occur rarely, if at all.

PATHOGENESIS Although *V. parahemolyticus* produces a toxin capable of causing intestinal fluid accumulation in the experimental animal, the role of this toxin in human disease is less clear-cut than is that of the cholera enterotoxin. The volume of fluid lost with *V. parahemolyticus* infection is relatively small, and intravenous fluids are seldom required. Like *Shigella, V. parahemolyticus* damages the intestinal mucosa: stools may be bloody and usually contain numerous polymorphonuclear leukocytes. The illness is almost always self-limited, with a median duration of just under 2 days.

MANIFESTATIONS Within 12 to 48 h after ingestion of raw or inadequately cooked seafood, the patient develops an acute diarrheal illness. The volume of fluid lost is generally not great, moderately severe abdominal cramps are a prominent feature, and chills and fever are observed in over half the cases. The illness is almost invariably self-limited, and no deaths have been reported in outbreaks involving over a thousand patients in the United States.

LABORATORY FINDINGS When a common-source outbreak of acute diarrheal disease occurs in a group exposed to fresh or frozen seafood, the index of suspicion should be high and the diagnosis should be confirmed by plating a rectal swab on thiosulfate-citrate-bile salt-sucrose (TCBS) agar, on which typical colonies of *V. parahemolyticus* appear at 24 h. (This organism is easily overlooked on deoxycholate culture plates, as it ferments lactose and would therefore be classified as "no enteric pathogen" in most standard laboratories.) The stool generally has large numbers of polymorphonuclear leukocytes and smaller numbers of erythrocytes, as is the case with other invasive enteric bacterial pathogens.

TREATMENT No therapy is required by the large majority of patients. The disease is self-limited, and antimicrobial therapy shortens neither the course nor the duration of pathogen excretion. Antiperistaltic agents are not of clear-cut benefit. An occasional patient may lose sufficient quantities of intestinal fluid to require oral or intravenous therapy, guided by the same principles employed in the treatment of cholera.

PROGNOSIS The outcome is almost always good. Fatal cases, occasionally reported from Japan, appear to have occurred in rare instances in patients with serious underlying disease.

PREVENTION Since *V. parahemolyticus* is widely distributed in coastal waters, the only effective preventive measure is avoidance of ingestion of inadequately cooked shellfish.

REFERENCES

Cholera

CARPENTER CCJ et al: Clinical studies in Asiatic cholera, I–VI. Bull Johns Hopkins Hosp 118:165, 1966

GANGAROSA EF et al: The nature of the gastrointestinal lesion in Asiatic cholera and its relation to pathogenesis: A biopsy study. Am J Trop Med Hyg 9:125, 1960

HIRSCHHORN N et al: The treatment of cholera, in *Cholera,* eds D. Barua, W. Burrows, Philadelphia: Saunders, 1974, p. 235

MAHALANOBIS D et al: Oral fluid therapy of cholera among Bangladesh refugees. Johns Hopkins Med J 132:197, 1973

WALLACE CK et al: Optimal antibiotic therapy in cholera. Bull WHO 39:239, 1968
WATTEN RH et al: Water and electrolyte studies in cholera. J Clin Invest 38:1879, 1959

Enterotoxigenic E. coli
GORBACH SL et al: Acute undifferentiated human diarrhea in the tropics. I. Alteration in intestinal microflora. J Clin Invest 50: 881, 1971
—— et al: Travelers diarrhea and toxigenic *Escherichia coli.* N Engl J Med 292:933, 1975
SACK RB et al: Enterotoxigenic *Escherichia coli* isolated from patients with severe cholera-like disease. J Infect Dis 123:378, 1971

Vibrio parahemolyticus
BARKER et al: *Vibrio parahemolyticus* outbreak in Covington, Louisiana in August, 1972. Am J Epidemiol 100:316, 1974
THATCHER FS, CLARK DS (eds): *Microorganisms in Foods: Their Significance and Methods of Enumeration,* Toronto: University of Toronto Press, 1968, p. 14

section 8 | Diseases caused by anaerobic bacteria

INTRODUCTION AND GENERAL CONSIDERATIONS

LAWRENCE L. PELLETIER, JR.

Improved culture techniques permit routine isolation and identification of anaerobic bacteria that require conditions of reduced oxygen tension and low redox potential for growth. Anaerobic bacteria are found as normal flora on the skin and mucous membranes of humans, outnumbering aerobic bacteria 1000:1 in the colon and 10:1 in the skin, mouth, and vagina. These bacteria exist in a poorly understood symbiotic relationship in which they protect against colonization and invasion by pathogenic bacteria and contribute to normal digestive function. However, exogenously acquired or endogenous anaerobic organisms may invade and destroy tissue when skin and mucous membrane barriers are compromised by surgery, trauma, or tumor; and when local tissue redox potentials are reduced by ischemia, necrosis, or infection.

Formerly anaerobic infections were recognized by characteristic clinical syndromes such as botulism (Chap. 157), tetanus (Chap. 156), gas gangrene (Chap. 158), lumpy jaw or necrotizing gingivitis. If contamination of specimens by normal anaerobic flora can be avoided, current technology permits isolation of clinically significant anaerobic organisms from as many as 10 percent of specimens submitted to a clinical microbiology laboratory. Approximately two-thirds of these cultures contain more than one organism. Not infrequently, four or five different bacteria may be isolated, and often both aerobic and anaerobic organisms are present simultaneously. Anaerobic infections should be suspected in lesions with foul-smelling discharge, tissue necrosis, gas in tissues, in septic thrombophlebitis, or when organisms are seen on Gram's stain of clinical specimens and aerobic cultures yield negative results.

Any site potentially may be infected but locations adjacent to mucosal surfaces are more commonly associated with anaerobic infection. Infections frequently caused by anaerobes include: chronic otitis media and sinusitis; brain abscess, subdural empyema, and otogenic meningitis; dental abscess, necrotizing gingivitis, and Ludwig's angina; aspiration pneumonia, thoracic empyema and lung abscess; liver abscess; pylephlebitis; peritonitis and intraabdominal abscesses from fecal spillage; endometritis, tuboovarian abscess, pelvic inflammatory disease, puerperal and postabortal sepsis; gas-forming cellulitis and gangrene; postsurgical wound infection, perirectal abscess, and human bite infections.

BACTERIOLOGY The taxonomy of anaerobic bacteria is frequently revised as knowledge about these organisms accumulates. Obligate anaerobic bacteria important in human infections include: (1) gram-positive spore-forming rods—*Clostridium* sp., (2) gram-positive rods—*Lactobacillus* sp., (3) gram-positive branching rods—*Actinomyces, Arachnia,* and *Bifidobacterium* sp., (4) gram-negative bacilli—*Bacteroides, Fusobacterium,* and *Leptotrichia* sp., (5) gram-positive cocci—*Peptococcus* and *Peptostreptococcus* sp., (6) gram-negative cocci—*Veillonella* sp., and (7) gram-positive coryniform bacilli—*Propionibacterium* and *Eubacterium* sp.

TREATMENT Treatment of anaerobic infection consists of surgical drainage, debridement, and antibiotics. The selection of appropriate antibiotic therapy is often complicated by the presence of multiple organisms, delays in isolation and identification of bacteria, and the lack of standardized antibiotic susceptibility tests for anaerobic bacteria. Except for *Bacteroides fragilis* and strains of *Fusobacterium* resistant to penicillin, penicillin G remains the drug of choice for anaerobic infections. Chloramphenicol is effective against *B. fragilis* and should be used in serious anaerobic infection when the etiologic agent is not known with certainty. Clindamycin is effective against most anaerobic bacteria, but many non-*C. perfringens* clostridia and *Fusobacterium* sp. are resistant. The emergence of drug-resistant strains of *Bacteroides, Clostridia, Fusobacterium,* anaerobic cocci, and *Eubacterium* sp. has severely limited the usefulness of tetracycline in anaerobic infection. Anaerobic bacteria are almost uniformly resistant to the aminoglycosides. Metronidazole is bactericidal in vitro against many anaerobic organisms, and favorable preliminary reports of its clinical effectiveness suggest that this drug may play a future role in the treatment of anaerobic infections.

REFERENCES

BALOWS A et al (eds): *Anaerobic Bacteria: Role in Disease.* Springfield, Ill.: Charles C Thomas, 1974

BUCHANAN RE, GIBBONS NE (eds): *Bergey's Manual of Determinative Bacteriology,* 8th ed., Baltimore: Williams and Wilkins, 1974

FINEGOLD SM, ROSENBLATT JE: Practical aspects of anaerobic sepsis. Medicine 52:311, 1973

GORBACH SL, BARTLETT JG: Anaerobic infections. New Engl J Med 290:1177, 1237, 1289, 1974

MEDEIROS AA: Once, all the world was anaerobic. New Engl J Med 287:1041, 1972

156 TETANUS

HARRY N. BEATY

DEFINITION Tetanus is an acute, often fatal, disease caused by an exotoxin produced in a wound by *Clostridium tetani.* It is characterized by generalized increased rigidity and convulsive spasms of skeletal muscles.

ETIOLOGY *Clostridium tetani* is a strictly anaerobic, gram-positive rod which is motile and readily forms endospores. In stained preparations, organisms may occur singly, in pairs, or in long chains. Spore-bearing bacilli usually contain a single, spheric, terminal endospore which swells the end of the organism and produces a characteristic "clubbed" appearance.

The organism grows well on blood agar at 37°C under anaerobic conditions. Slight hemolysis is usually apparent, but isolated colonies are rare because the organism tends to swarm. *Clostridium tetani* is relatively inert biochemically, with no proteolytic activity and no fermentation of carbohydrates. Vegetative forms of the tetanus bacillus are no more resistant to adverse conditions than other bacteria, but spores are highly resistant to antiseptics and moderately resistant to heat.

Ten distinct types of *C. tetani* can be distinguished on the basis of flagellar antigens. All these types have one or more common somatic antigens, and are capable of producing at least two exotoxins. One, a hemolysin, is relatively unimportant clinically. The other, tetanospasmin, generally referred to as tetanus toxin, is a protein with a molecular weight of approximately 145,000 in its dimer form, and is responsible for the clinical manifestations of tetanus. The tetanospasmins produced by the various types of *C. tetani* are essentially identical antigenically, and only one antitoxin is needed to neutralize the tetanus toxins produced by all strains.

EPIDEMIOLOGY The tetanus bacillus is found in the superficial layers of soil and as a saprophyte in the intestinal tract of man and certain animals. It is most frequently encountered in densely populated regions in hot, damp climates and in soil which is rich in organic matter. This explains, in part, why the disease is rare in the polar regions and relatively uncommon in the U.S.S.R., North America, and most of Europe. Urbanization, mechanization of agriculture, and socioeconomic factors such as poverty and lack of availability of health services also significantly influence the occurrence of this disease.

Worldwide, there are probably 300,000 to 500,000 cases of tetanus each year with a mortality rate of roughly 45 percent. There is no racial predilection, but the male-to-female ratio is 2.5:1, even among neonates where the opportunity for infection is presumably equal. In the United States, there are less than 200 reported cases each year, and these occur almost exclusively in nonimmunized or only partially immunized individuals. The highest incidence of disease is among nonwhites in the southern states. However, spores of *C. tetani* are distributed widely throughout urban centers and rural areas of the entire country, and are found commonly on clothing and in house dust, placing the nonimmune individual at risk following relatively minor household injuries. Tetanus has been known to follow surgery and innocuous procedures such as skin testing or intramuscular injection of medication. The disease is inordinately common in narcotics addicts, perhaps because heroin is frequently "cut" with quinine which drastically lowers the redox potential at the site of injection and favors the growth of *C. tetani.*

Tetanus neonatorum is a major cause of infant mortality in developing countries and is directly related to poor obstetric conditions and lack of maternal immunization programs.

PATHOGENESIS AND PATHOLOGY *Clostridium tetani* is a noninvasive organism. Therefore, tetanus can occur only after spores or vegetative bacteria gain access to tissues and produce toxin locally. The usual mode of entry is through a puncture wound or laceration on the hand, foot, or leg. However, tetanus may follow elective surgery, burn wounds, otitis media, dental infection, abortion, and pregnancy. Neonatal tetanus usually follows infection of the umbilical stump. The disease not infrequently follows injuries too trivial to be seen by a physician, and in 20 percent of cases there is neither a history of injury nor a detectable lesion.

Wounds are undoubtedly contaminated frequently with spores of *C. tetani,* but tetanus develops rarely because germination of spores occurs only when the oxygen tension is much lower than that of normal tissue. Spores may survive in the body for months to years and finally produce disease at some later date after minor trauma which alters local conditions. Toxin production in wounds is favored by necrotic tissue, foreign bodies, calcium salts, and associated infections which establish low oxidation-reduction potentials. Infection caused by the tetanus bacillus remains strictly localized, but the toxin produced is transported to the central nervous system via neural pathways. Toxin entering the circulation persists for days, and probably must enter peripheral nerves to spread centrally and cause disease.

The typical clinical manifestations of tetanus are caused

by the effect of tetanospasmin on the central nervous system. The toxin attacks synaptic functions to produce disinhibition of both the alpha and gamma motor systems. Generalized muscle rigidity arises from uninhibited afferent stimuli entering the central nervous system from the periphery. When the stimuli become more vigorous, spasms occur. Emotional and, to a lesser extent, visual stimuli can also cause muscle spasm. Tetanus toxin also has other effects. Peripherally it produces neuromuscular blockade similar to that of botulinum toxin, and it acts directly on muscle to produce contraction which is unaccompanied by an action potential in nerves. Certain clinical observations have raised the possibility that tetanus toxin also has an effect on the sympathetic nervous system.

All the effects of tetanus toxin appear to be self-limited and completely reversible, because patients who recover from the disease have no residual defect. Although there are no distinguishable pathologic changes which are characteristic of tetanus, brainstem lesions have been reported in patients dying from tetanus, and toxic myocarditis has been recognized.

CLINICAL MANIFESTATIONS The incubation period of tetanus, i.e., the time between injury and the appearance of unmistakable symptoms, ranges from 2 to 56 days. However, over 80 percent of patients become symptomatic within 14 days. A short incubation period indicates severe disease, and when symptoms occur within 2 or 3 days of injury, the mortality rate approaches 100 percent.

Nonspecific premonitory symptoms such as restlessness, irritability, and headache are encountered occasionally, but the commonest presenting complaints are pain and stiffness in the jaw, abdomen, or back and difficulty in swallowing. As the disease progresses, stiffness gives way to rigidity, and patients often complain of difficulty in opening their mouths. In fact, trismus is the commonest manifestation of tetanus and is responsible for the familiar descriptive name of *lockjaw.* As more muscles are involved, rigidity becomes generalized, and sustained contractions of facial muscles produce a characteristic expression called *risus sardonicus.* The intensity and sequence of muscle involvement is quite variable. In a small proportion of patients, only local signs and symptoms develop in the region of the injury. In the vast majority, however, most muscles are involved to some degree, and the signs and symptoms encountered depend upon the major muscle groups affected.

Reflex spasms usually occur within 24 to 72 h of the first symptoms, an interval referred to as the *onset time.* As in the case of the incubation period, a short onset time is associated with a poor prognosis. Spasms are caused by sudden intensification of afferent stimuli arising in the periphery, which increases rigidity and causes simultaneous and excessive contraction of muscles and their antagonists. Spasms may be both painful and dangerous. As the disease progresses, minimal or inapparent stimuli produce more intense and longer-lasting spasms with increasing frequency. Respiration may be impaired by laryngospasm or tonic contraction of respiratory muscles which prevents adequate ventilation. Hypoxia may then lead to irreversible central nervous system damage and death.

Patients are almost invariably conscious and mentally alert at the time of admission. Low-grade fever, profuse sweating and tachycardia are common. Deep tendon reflexes are hyperactive, and there may be labile hypertension. The physical examination should be undertaken with care, because reflex convulsive spasms may be precipitated easily. The wound through which *C. tetani* was introduced should be evaluated, and the examination should determine the extent of rigidity; the severity of trismus; the presence or absence of dysphagia and respiratory embarrassment; the frequency, intensity, and duration of convulsive spasms; and the presence of complications such as respiratory infection.

Characteristically, the manifestations of tetanus increase in severity for about 3 days after the first sign, and then remain stable for the next 5 to 7 days. After about 10 days, spasms begin to occur less frequently, and by the end of 2 weeks, they disappear altogether. Although residual stiffness may persist for a prolonged period, most survivors recover completely in 4 weeks.

Tetanus neonatorum is a severe form of the disease which usually occurs within 10 days of birth. Early signs include difficulty in sucking, irritability, and excessive crying associated with peculiar grimacing. Intense rigidity characteristically produces opisthotonus, flexion of the arms, clenched fists, extension of the legs, and plantar flexion of the toes. Typical spasms occur with minimal stimuli.

Complications Complications contribute significantly to the morbidity and mortality of tetanus. Some result from overly vigorous therapy and prolonged bed rest, while others are attributed to the action of tetanus toxin. Inadequate ventilation, either from laryngospasm or spasm of respiratory muscles, is a constant threat. In addition to hypoxia, atelectasis is a common consequence of impaired respiration. Difficulty in swallowing leads to aspiration of secretions, which may also cause atelectasis and initiate pulmonary infection. Thrombophlebitis is occasionally encountered, but bland venous thrombosis is more common and may lead to pulmonary embolization. Cardiovascular complications thought to be due to hyperactivity of the sympathetic nervous system include vasomotor instability, hypertension, tachycardia, arrhythmias, and severe vasoconstriction. Pulmonary edema and hypotension may occur as a consequence of myocarditis. High fever usually signifies secondary infection. Pneumonia is a common late complication of tetanus, and is found in 50 to 70 percent of autopsied cases. Other frequent sites of secondary infections include the original wound, decubitus ulcers, and the urinary tract of patients with indwelling bladder catheters. Fractures of midthoracic vertebrae are probably due to severe spasms, and are particularly common among children and adolescents. Gastrointestinal complications include acute peptic ulceration, paralytic ileus, and constipation. Hemolysis is seen in a small proportion of patients.

Pneumonia is a major cause of death. Other autopsy findings in early deaths include intense congestion of viscera and, occasionally, intracranial hemorrhage or thrombosis. In about 20 percent of cases, no obvious pathology is identified, and death is attributed to the direct effects of tetanus toxin.

LABORATORY FINDINGS There are no laboratory findings characteristic of tetanus. Granulocytosis is seen in about one-third of patients, but anemia is rare. Blood chemistries are almost always normal initially, but various fluid and electrolyte disturbances may arise in the course of the disease. The electrocardiogram usually shows only sinus tachycardia, but occasionally T-wave inversion is seen. Roentgenograms are not helpful except in the evaluation of complications.

The diagnosis of tetanus is entirely clinical and does not depend upon bacteriologic confirmation. *Clostridium tetani* is recovered from the wound in only 30 percent of cases, and not infrequently it is isolated from patients who do not have tetanus. Laboratory identification depends on cultural and morphologic characteristics, absence of fermentative activity, and, most importantly, demonstration of toxin production in mice.

DIFFERENTIAL DIAGNOSIS With the exception of strychnine poisoning, no disease resembles fully developed tetanus. Early on, excluding local causes of jaw pain may be difficult, and the combination of neck stiffness and fever may suggest meningitis. However, this can be excluded by lumbar puncture, because in tetanus the spinal fluid is normal. When there is doubt about the diagnosis, clinical observation usually settles the issue within a matter of hours.

TREATMENT In order to formulate a rational plan of therapy, it is useful to assess the severity of tetanus. *Mild tetanus* is characterized by an incubation period of at least 14 days and an onset time of more than 6 days. Trismus is usually present, but dysphagia is absent, and generalized spasms are brief and mild. *Moderately severe tetanus* has a somewhat shorter incubation period and onset time; trismus is marked, dysphagia and generalized rigidity are present, but ventilation remains adequate even during spasms. The criteria for *severe tetanus* include a short incubation time, an onset time of 72 h or less, severe trismus, dysphagia and rigidity, and frequent, prolonged, generalized convulsive spasms. Because of the poor prognosis of tetanus in older individuals, the disease should be considered moderate to severe in all patients over fifty.

General measures Patients should be hospitalized in an *intensive care unit.* After initial evaluation, necrotic tissue and foreign bodies should be removed from the infected wound, and abscesses should be drained. Patients should be placed in a quiet room and observed closely for development of complications or unexpected changes in the course of the disease. While it is a good general principle to disturb patients as little as possible, vital signs must be monitored and aspiration must be averted by positioning the patient carefully and by aspirating nasopharyngeal secretions frequently. Care must be taken to prevent development of decubitus ulcers or contractures, but many routine nursing procedures should be omitted because they may precipitate uncomfortable or dangerous spasms. Initially, nutrition is not a major consideration, and fluid and electrolyte balance should be maintained over the first several days by administration of appropriate solutions intravenously, accompanied by careful recording of intake and output. After the patient's condition has been stabilized and the threat of aspiration has been minimized, adequate nutrition can be given through a nasogastric tube. Intravenous hyperalimentation may be used in patients with an unusually severe and prolonged illness.

Antiserum Antiserum does not neutralize tetanus toxin fixed in the central nervous system, and does little to ameliorate symptoms already present at the time of admission. However, it has been the practice for many years to give antitoxin to patients with tetanus, and it is likely that the case-fatality ratio in mild to moderately severe disease is reduced significantly when antiserum is administered early. Human tetanus immune globulin (TIG) is generally available in the United States, and is far superior to equine antiserum. Because its half-life is about 25 days, only one dose of 3,000 to 6,000 units intramuscularly is recommended. Local infiltration at the site of the wound is of no proved value, but intrathecal injections may prove to be effective after more careful study. Hypersensitivity reactions do not occur with TIG, obviating the need for pretreatment testing.

If human antitoxin is not available, a single dose of equine antiserum should be given after the patient has been tested for hypersensitivity to horse serum. Although the dosage of heterologous antitoxin often recommended for adults is 100,000 to 200,000 units, studies have shown that 10,000 units is probably optimal. Anaphylaxis can occur despite negative sensitivity tests, and patients must be observed carefully to institute treatment at the first sign of an anaphylactic reaction. Up to 25 percent of patients develop delayed reactions including serum sickness after equine antitoxin. Occasionally, serious neurologic complications accompany other manifestations of serum sickness (Chap. 75).

Active immunization of patients with tetanus is necessary, because the disease does not confer natural immunity. However, there is no need to begin primary immunization until the patient has recovered.

Management of muscle spasms Muscle relaxation is the key to therapy, but mild sedation is desirable also because it reduces the effect of sensory stimuli. Ideally, this should be accomplished without significantly affecting respiration. Although a variety of agents have been used in the treatment of tetanus, none has achieved universal acceptance. However, two groups of drugs, barbiturates and phenothiazines, have been particularly useful. Among the barbiturates, phenobarbital, in adult doses of 50 to 100 mg every 3 to 6 h, produces adequate sedation which may suffice in the management of mild tetanus. When rapid action is required, amylbarbital or pentobarbital, 50 to 200 mg intravenously, may be used. Frequent and severe spasms cannot be managed with barbiturates alone, because the dosage required for control leads to unconsciousness and suppressed respiration. For this reason, muscle relaxants usually are used, either alone or in combination with barbiturates, in the treatment of moderate or severe tetanus. Electromyographic studies have shown that the phenothiazines effectively produce relaxation while sparing the sensorium and respirations. Chlorpromazine, in doses of 200 to 300 mg a day, minimizes rigidity and decreases the frequency of spasms. Diazepam, in adult dosages of 40 to 120 mg a day, is also useful; it acts quickly, relieves rigidity, and has significant sedative effect without depressing respiration. Other drugs which have been employed extensively in the past include mephenesin, meprobamate, paraldehyde, and chloral hydrate.

Another approach to the management of muscle spasms involves the use of neuromuscular blocking agents such as tubocurare. This method can be used only where facilities and personnel are available to provide controlled mechanical ventilation for the paralyzed patient. This limits its application and increases the possibility of pulmonary complications.

Tracheostomy Tracheostomy has an important role in the management of tetanus. It protects against suffocation due to laryngospasm, reduces the risk of aspiration, and facilitates mechanical assistance of ventilation. While most patients with mild tetanus and some with more severe disease can be managed without it, all patients should be considered candidates for tracheostomy, and the necessary equipment should be at the bedside. Where secretions are copious or respiration has been compromised, the need for tracheostomy should be recognized early, and whenever possible it should be performed electively rather than as an emergency.

Other measures Although antibiotics are frequently prescribed to treat the infected wound and prevent toxin production, there is no indication that they influence the disease favorably. If antibiotics are used, penicillin G is the drug of choice because it is highly effective against the tetanus bacillus, and its limited spectrum is less likely to predispose patients to superinfections. Appropriate cultures to detect complicating infections should be obtained periodically throughout the course of the disease, and specific antibiotics prescribed when indicated. Adrenocortical steroids have been used empirically in the treatment of tetanus, but there is no experimental or clinical evidence to support their effectiveness. Likewise, beneficial results have been claimed for hyperbaric oxygen, but insufficient information is available to evaluate its potential.

PREVENTION *Clostridium tetani* is so ubiquitous in nature that the only hope for prevention of tetanus lies in massive immunization programs. Effective active immunization is possible, and if applied universally, according to recommendations, tetanus could be virtually eliminated. Even tetanus neonatorum could be prevented, because infants are protected by antibody which passes the placental barrier. Two types of tetanus toxoids are available for immunization, a fluid and an adsorbed form. The adsorbed toxoid is preferred because it produces higher antitoxin titers and longer-lasting immunity. Immunization failures are exceedingly rare.

According to current recommendations, children two months to six years of age should be immunized with diphtheria and tetanus toxoids and pertussis vaccine (DPT). Ideally, the first dose should be administered within 2 or 3 months of birth, the second and third should follow at 4- to 6-week intervals, and the fourth dose should be given 1 year after the third. Schoolchildren and adults should be immunized with three doses of adult type tetanus and diphtheria toxoids (Td). The second dose should be given 4 to 6 weeks after the first, and the third 6 months to 1 year after the second. A booster of DPT is recommended for children at the time of entrance into kindergarten or elementary school. Thereafter and for everyone else who has received a primary immunization series, routine boosters of Td should be given every 10 years. Side effects are uncommon after the primary series, but occur more frequently in persons who have received an excessive number of booster injections. Reactions usually take the form of local swelling, erythema, lymphadenopathy, and fever, but on rare occasions more severe hypersensitivity reactions occur.

In the management of wounds, the question of prophylaxis against tetanus frequently arises. Because active immunization is so effective, a reliable immunization history can greatly simplify the problem. If a patient has received three or more doses of toxoid, antiserum need not be given, and a toxoid booster is required only if more than 5 to 10 years has elapsed since the last dose. The shorter interval pertains for all but clean, minor wounds. With a history of two previous doses of tetanus toxoid, a booster is indicated, but antitoxin should be used only if a significant wound is more than 24 h old. For patients who have received fewer than two doses of toxoid or have an uncertain immunization history, a dose of Td is required for all wounds, and the primary immunization series should be completed in the succeeding weeks to months. Antiserum is also indicated for these patients unless the wound is clean and minor.

When passive immunization is contemplated, TIG is preferred to horse serum because it offers longer protection and freedom from serious reactions. The currently recommended prophylactic dose for adults is 250 to 1,000 units intramuscularly. If TIG is not available, equine antitoxin in doses of 3,000 to 6,000 units should be administered after careful screening for sensitivity to horse serum. When both toxoid and antitoxin are indicated, they can be given simultaneously, but separate syringes and separate injection sites should be used.

Prompt and adequate care of wounds is also important in preventing tetanus. They should be cleaned carefully, and foreign bodies or necrotic, devitalized tissue should be removed. Administration of tetracycline or penicillin is advocated by some to prevent multiplication of *C. tetani,* but tetanus may occur in spite of prophylactic antibiotics, and their role in the prevention of tetanus has not been established. However, severe wounds should be examined regularly and treated promptly with antimicrobials if infection develops.

PROGNOSIS The overall case-fatality ratio of tetanus is variable, but in the United States it ranges between 50 to 60 percent. This reflects the fact that the incidence of tetanus is eight to ten times greater among people over sixty compared with people ten to twenty years of age, and the mortality rate is twenty-five to fifty times greater in the elderly. Neonatal tetanus is uncommon in this country but is fatal in more than 60 percent of cases. The shorter the incubation period and onset time, the poorer the prognosis in tetanus. Three-fourths of the deaths occur within the first week, primarily from pulmonary infection or aspiration. Survivors recover completely, but remain susceptible to the disease unless actively immunized with tetanus toxoid.

REFERENCES

Brooks GF et al: Tetanus toxoid immunization of adults: A continuing need. Ann Intern Med 73:603, 1970

Furste W, Wheeler W: Tetanus: A team disease, in *Current Problems in Surgery*, Chicago: Year Book, 1972

Habermann E, Wellhöner H: Advances in tetanus research. Klin Wochenschr 52:255, 1974

Tsueda K et al: Cardiovascular manifestations of tetanus. Anesthesiology 40:588, 1974

Young LS et al: An evaluation of serologic and antimicrobial therapy in the treatment of tetanus in the United States. J Infect Dis 120:153, 1969

157 BOTULISM

HARRY N. BEATY
ROBERT W. GRAEBNER

DEFINITION Botulism is an acute form of poisoning which results from ingestion of a toxin produced by *Clostridium botulinum.* The illness is characterized by progressive descending bulbar and skeletal muscle paralysis, and is often fatal.

HISTORY The disease was first recognized over 200 years ago by South German physicians who adopted the term *botulismus* for the often fatal syndrome which sometimes followed the consumption of spoiled sausage (*botulus* is Latin for sausage). Botulism was rare in the United States prior to World War I. The growth of commercial and home canning at this time led to a great increase in cases. A series of studies by K. F. Meyer and his associates in the early 1920s defined the habitat of *Cl. botulinum,* the foods often incriminated, and the conditions necessary for the destruction of *Cl. botulinum* spores. This knowledge led to the virtual elimination of botulism from the commercial canning industry, and most cases of clinical botulism now follow consumption of improperly canned, home-preserved foods. However, the need for constant surveillance is emphasized by periodic outbreaks of botulism caused by commercially processed foods.

ETIOLOGY *Clostridium botulinum* is a strictly anaerobic, spore-forming, gram-positive rod which elaborates a potent exotoxin during growth and autolysis. Morphologically and culturally similar strains are differentiated into types A, B, C, D, E, or F on the basis of antigenic characteristics of the toxin each produces. Type A, B, and E toxins have been implicated most frequently in human disease in the United States. Only two outbreaks of type F botulism have been reported. Types C and D produce disease almost exclusively in animals, including wild waterfowl, cattle, horses, and mink.

Type A and B spores are widely distributed in soil throughout the world. Type A spores are most common in the United States, especially along the Pacific Coast and the Rocky Mountain states. Type B spores have been found more frequently in the Eastern states and in Europe. Type E spores have been demonstrated in lakeshore mud, coastal sand, and sea-bottom silt in northern latitudes. Fish apparently contaminate their intestinal tracts with these spores, which accounts for the high incidence of type E strains in fish-borne botulism. Type F spores have been found in marine sediments collected off the coast of California and Oregon and in salmon taken from the Columbia River.

Botulinum toxins are the most potent poisons known. Types A through F have been purified and identified as simple proteins. Although they differ in terms of antigenicity, molecular size, electrophoretic mobility, and amino acid content, they appear to have an identical effect on neuromuscular transmission. Pharmacologic differences are manifested by the variable susceptibility of specific animal species to the different toxins.

Spores of *Cl. botulinum* can withstand 100°C for several hours. Moist heat at 120°C for 30 min will destroy spores of all types, but the toxins are considerably more heat-labile. All varieties of toxin are destroyed by boiling for 10 min, or by temperatures of 80°C for 30 min.

PATHOGENESIS Most human botulism follows the ingestion of foodstuffs contaminated with preformed botulinus toxin. Rarely, wounds infected with *Cl. botulinum* have been the portal of entry of the toxin. There is no convincing evidence that the botulinus bacillus produces toxin in the human gastrointestinal tract, and no cases of disease have been recognized following the ingestion of fresh food. Clinical botulism can occur only when the following conditions are met: (1) a food product is contaminated with viable *Cl. botulinum* bacilli or spores; (2) proper conditions for germination of the spores exist; (3) time and conditions permit production of toxin prior to eating; (4) the food is not heated or is heated insufficiently to destroy botulinus toxin, (5) the toxin-containing food is ingested by a susceptible host (Table 157-1). Though a relatively anaerobic environment and temperatures above 80°F are optimal for toxin production, strict anaerobic conditions are not necessary and toxin production by some type E strains has been observed at temperatures as low as 6°C (42.8°F).

Although a variety of home-processed foods have been sources of botulism in the United States, certain foods seem to be safer than others. This may be because low pH (acidity) inhibits germination of spores and, therefore, toxin production. Commercially processed smoked fish, tuna,

TABLE 157-1
Important factors in the pathogenesis of botulism

SPORES	
1	Survive at 6°C (42.8°F) for several months
2	Can withstand boiling for several hours
3	Destroyed at 120°C (248°F) after 30 min
TOXIN PRODUCTION	
1	Strict anaerobic conditions not always required
2	Can occur at 6°C (42.8°F)
3	Optimal temperature 30°C (86°F)
4	Reduced at low pH
TOXIN	
1	Destroyed at 80°C (176°F) after 30 min or 100°C for 10 min
2	Unstable at high pH
3	Type E toxin activated by trypsin

peppers, and soup (vichyssoise) have been implicated in outbreaks of botulism. Contaminated foods may appear putrefied, but frequently look and taste perfectly normal, regardless of toxin type.

Botulinus toxins are absorbed primarily in the stomach and upper part of the small intestine. The toxins are large protein molecules which are absorbed after they have been reduced in size by proteolytic enzymes which do not destroy activity. In fact, the toxicity of type E toxin may be enhanced by tryptic digestion. Either absorption is incomplete or toxins are inactivated partially by digestion, because the amount of toxin which appears in the bloodstream is variable, and in animals the lethal dose orally is 1,000 times greater than the lethal dose intravenously. Toxin which reaches the lower part of the small intestine and colon may be absorbed slowly, which probably accounts for the delayed onset and the prolonged symptoms observed in many patients.

Botulinus toxins exert their major effect by blocking neuromuscular transmission in cholinergic nerve fibers. They either inhibit the release of acetylcholine or bind with it at or near its site of release within presynaptic clefts. Muscle reactivity to acetylcholine applied directly to the motor end plate is unimpaired. Central nervous system cholinergic pathways do not appear to be affected significantly in human beings.

CLINICAL MANIFESTATIONS Botulism may vary from a mild illness for which patients seek no medical advice to a fulminant disease which ends in death within 24 h. Symptoms usually begin 12 to 36 h after ingestion of toxin, although extremes of 3 h to 14 days are recorded. In general, the earlier the symptoms appear, the more serious the disease.

The commonest symptoms are ocular; diplopia, blurred vision, and photophobia are frequently the first to appear. Bulbar weakness is manifested by dysphonia, dysarthria, dysphagia, and weakness of the tongue. Symmetric paralysis of the extremities appears, and may progress rapidly in a descending or ascending manner. Weakness of the respiratory muscles may occur early, but this is often asymptomatic until function is moderately impaired.

Impairment of cholinergic autonomic transmission may result in constipation, urinary retention, and reduced salivation and lacrimation. Nausea and vomiting are early symptoms in half the patients, but the absence of these symptoms does not rule out botulism. Gastrointestinal symptoms are more common in type B and E disease than in type A. Some patients with type B disease may have minimal weakness but marked constipation and decreased secretions.

On examination patients are usually alert, oriented, and afebrile, even with severe disease. Ocular signs include ptosis, weakness of extraocular motion, and in some patients failure of accommodation. The pupils are normal in many patients, but in some cases may react sluggishly or may be dilated and unreactive to light. Widespread neuromuscular block results in symmetric flaccid weakness of the palate, tongue, larynx, respiratory muscles, and extremities. Severe paralytic ileus and bladder distention may be present. Deep-tendon reflexes are intact in milder cases, but if significant paralysis is present they are reduced or absent. No pathologic reflexes are detectable. Findings on sensory examination are always entirely normal. Some patients have apparent gait disturbances and incoordination, but this is due to generalized weakness.

Once symptoms are noted, the disease may progress rapidly over several days, with significant changes in status occurring at hourly intervals. A period of stabilization is then followed by gradual recovery over a period of days to months, depending on the severity of intoxication. The mechanism of recovery is not well understood. In wound botulism the patient may be febrile, but the clinical manifestations are otherwise similar. A 10- to 14-day incubation period is common from the time of infection to the onset of toxic symptoms.

LABORATORY FINDINGS Routine laboratory studies do not aid in diagnosing botulism. When it is suspected, public health authorities should be consulted to assist in special studies needed to confirm the diagnosis. Specimens of blood, feces, and gastric contents, as well as suspect foods and their containers should be obtained. These materials should be cultured anaerobically, and extracts of the potentially toxin-containing substances should be injected intraperitoneally into mice. If toxin is present, the animals will develop botulism and usually die within 24 h. Mice protected with the type-specific antiserum will survive. Because of the extreme potency of botulinus toxin, careful collection and laboratory precautions should be used. If wound botulism is suspected, the wound exudate should be submitted for anaerobic culture.

The spinal fluid is always normal. Electrocardiographic abnormalities, including minor disturbances in conduction, nonspecific T-wave and S-T segment changes, and various disorders of rhythm, have been described. Recently, electrodiagnostic studies have been shown to be of value in differentiating botulism from other paralytic diseases, although the findings are not always present throughout the course of the illness. On repetitive supramaximal stimulation of a nerve at rapid rates, the evoked motor action potential may progressively augment in amplitude. This is similar to the response seen in the Eaton-Lambert syndrome. Fibrillations and other electromyographic changes consistent with denervation may be detected after 3 or 4 weeks.

DIFFERENTIAL DIAGNOSIS Botulism must be differentiated from other conditions that produce generalized paralysis. In the Guillain-Barré syndrome, mild sensory abnormalities are nearly always present, and the spinal fluid protein is often elevated. The variant of the Guillain-Barré syndrome with ophthalmoplegia, areflexia, and ataxia may prove particularly confusing. The course of myasthenia gravis is seldom so acute, and the deep tendon reflexes and pupils are normal. Some patients with botulism may show mild improvement after injection of edrophonium (Tensilon), but this improvement is not of the magnitude seen in myasthenia gravis. In tick paralysis the weakness is generally of an ascending pattern, patients may have paresthesias, and a tick is found. In diphtheria, palatal weakness is frequently the first symptom, and a history of prior pharyngitis may be obtained. Cutaneous diphtheria can be differentiated from wound botulism by appropriate cultures. In poliomyelitis the spinal fluid is abnormal and the weakness is often asymmetric and spares the ocular muscles. Vascular accidents of the brainstem can be recognized by associated neurologic signs. Belladonna poisoning presents with markedly dilated pupils and delirium. In organophosphate poisoning the pupils are markedly miotic. Shellfish poisoning, aminoglycoside antibiotic paralysis, and familial periodic paralysis might also prove confusing.

Patients with marked dry mouth may develop a picture simulating pharyngitis. Patients with gastrointestinal complaints and ileus may appear to have other forms of food poisoning or intestinal obstruction.

TREATMENT The most immediate threat to the survival of patients with botulism is respiratory failure. Patients with symptoms or known exposure should be hospitalized. Close observation is essential, and vital capacity should be measured frequently. If respiratory insufficiency develops, the patient may require assisted ventilation with a respirator. Respiratory difficulties may develop rapidly; elective tracheostomy should be performed before onset of respiratory failure, and may be needed to manage secretions even if ventilation is otherwise adequate. Some milder cases may be managed with endotracheal intubation.

If there is no ileus, cathartics and enemas should be given to remove unabsorbed toxin from the intestine, but magnesium citrate and magnesium sulfate should not be given, as the magnesium may potentiate the neuromuscular block produced by botulinus toxin. Nasogastric suction and intravenous hyperalimentation may be needed if ileus is severe. If the bladder is atonic a catheter will be required. Meticulous nursing care and physical therapy are essential to prevent complications.

As soon as the diagnosis of botulism is suspected, the patient should be tested for hypersensitivity to horse serum and treated with trivalent ABE antitoxin (Connaught), which is available from public health authorities. Type-specific antitoxin has been shown to be of benefit in several outbreaks of type E intoxication, but the value in type A and B outbreaks is less certain. Nonfatal hypersensitivity reactions occur in 15 to 20 percent of patients receiving the equine antitoxin, and those that react to a test dose must be desensitized prior to further treatment.

Wound botulism should be treated by careful debridement and irrigation of the wound in addition to systemic antitoxin therapy. The value of antibiotic therapy for wound botulism is not determined. Because there is no evidence that *Cl. botulinum* can multiply in the gastrointestinal tract of the human being, antibiotics should be reserved for specific infectious complications. It is essential that public health officials be notified so that toxin-containing foods can be confiscated, and so that those with possible exposure can be notified.

A number of reports have appeared since 1967 describing the use of guanidine hydrochloride in the treatment of botulism. This drug presumably acts by enhancing the release of acetylcholine from terminal nerve fibers. About half the reported cases have shown some improvement with oral doses of 36 to 50 mg per kg per day, but the drug seems ineffective in those patients with severe respiratory impairment. Dose-related side effects include gastrointestinal upset, paresthesias, and fasciculations. Idiosyncratic reactions include cardiac arrhythmias and blood dyscrasias.

PROGNOSIS The current mortality rate of botulism in the United States is about 25 percent, with type A outbreaks having somewhat higher mortality than types B and E. Death is due to complications such as respiratory failure and pneumonia. With rapid diagnosis and aggressive supportive care, even severely involved patients can recover fully. Artificial respiratory support may be required for many months, and clinical weakness and autonomic symptoms may be noted for as long as 1 year after the onset of disease.

REFERENCES

CENTER FOR DISEASE CONTROL: Botulism in the United States, 1899–1973: Handbook for Epidemiologists, Clinicians, and Laboratory Workers, issued June 1974

CHERINGTON M: Botulism: Ten-year experience. Arch Neurol 30: 432, 1974

FAICH GA et al: Failure of guanidine therapy in botulism A. N Engl J Med 285:773, 1971

KOENIG MC et al: Type B botulism in man. Am J Med 42:208, 1967

MERSON MH, DOWELL VR: Epidemiologic, clinical and laboratory aspects of wound botulism. N Engl J Med 289:1005, 1973

WERNER SB, CHIN J: Botulism—diagnosis, management and public health considerations. Calif Med 118:84, 1973

158
OTHER CLOSTRIDIAL INFECTIONS

EDWARD W. HOOK
GERALD L. MANDELL

INTRODUCTION Bacteria of the genus *Clostridium* are normal inhabitants of soil and the gastrointestinal tracts of man and animals. Most of the species that have been described are saprophytic, but some are pathogenic for man and animals, usually under conditions of lowered host and tissue resistance. Infections with these organisms are often associated with profound systemic manifestations, and all pathogenic clostridia, except *C. tetani* and *C. botulinum*, are capable of causing extensive tissue destruction. Diseases caused by these other clostridia are gas gangrene, cellulitis, postabortal and puerperal sepsis, and on occasion pneumonia, pleurisy, peritonitis, meningitis, endocarditis, cystitis, and bursitis. In addition, ingestion of food contaminated with *C. perfringens* type A is a common cause of enterocolitis.

ETIOLOGY Wounds complicated by gas gangrene usually contain a mixture of pathogenic and saprophytic clostridia, often including *C. tetani*, as well as a variety of other bacteria. *Clostridium perfringens*, the most common, *C. novyi*, or *C. septicum* can be cultured from most cases of gas gangrene and clostridial cellulitis, and *C. perfringens* causes virtually all clostridial infections of the uterus. *Clostridium bifermentans*, *C. histolyticum*, and *C. fallax* are less virulent organisms that occasionally cause gas gangrene but are more commonly associated with localized cellulitis. Proliferation of *C. botulinum* in wounds occasionally leads to clinical manifestations of botulism (Chap. 157).

The clostridia of gas gangrene and related infections are anaerobic or microaerophilic gram-positive bacilli that produce abundant gas in artificial media and form subterminal endospores. *Clostridium perfringens* is encapsulated and nonmotile, rarely sporulates in artificial media, and produces spores that can usually be destroyed by boiling.

EPIDEMIOLOGY AND PATHOGENESIS Clostridia do not penetrate abdominal viscera. Although these organisms can be cultured from one-third to two-thirds of severe traumatic wounds, gas gangrene develops in only an occasional case. The most important prerequisite for the conversion of clostridial contamination of a wound to a progressive infection is an environment with low oxidation-reduction potential, which permits spore germination and anaerobic growth. Local oxidation-reduction potential can be reduced by failure of the blood supply to a contaminated area, by the presence of foreign bodies such as clothing, soil, or fragments of metal or wood, or by the multiplication of other bacteria in the wound. Once multiplication and toxin production are established, rapid invasion and destruction of healthy tissue follow.

The pathogenicity of clostridia is related to the capacity of these organisms to form exotoxins which destroy tissue cells. The nature and amount of toxins vary considerably for different species and strains. For example, at least 12 different extracellular *toxins* are produced by *C. perfringens.* Alpha toxin, a lecithinase, is clearly the most important and is the principal tissue-destroying, hemolytic, and lethal toxin. Other *C. perfringens* products include collagenase, hyaluronidase, hemolytic theta toxin, leukocidin, deoxyribonuclease, and fibrinolysin.

Gas gangrene is characterized by marked systemic symptoms and a local reaction with extensive necrotizing myositis, edema, thrombosis of small vessels, interstitial gas bubbles, and minimal infiltration of leukocytes. The local reaction in infected tissue can be explained by the action of clostridial toxins, especially alpha toxin, but the factors responsible for the systemic reaction are unknown. Alpha toxin, or other clostridial toxins, have not been demonstrated in circulating blood during the course of severe clostridial myonecrosis.

CLINICAL MANIFESTATIONS Clostridial myonecrosis (gas gangrene, clostridial myositis) Gas gangrene develops in anoxic devitalized tissues in which the arterial circulation has been compromised by trauma, constricting tourniquets or casts, or obliterative arterial disease. Infection is most frequent after extensive injury to skeletal muscle, particularly of the thigh and buttock, and is more common in wounds complicated by compound fractures or lodgment of foreign bodies. Once infection is established, it rapidly spreads to involve healthy muscle undamaged by previous trauma or ischemia.

The incubation period is usually 1 to 4 days but may vary from 3 h to 6 weeks or longer. The earliest symptom is sudden, severe pain in the injured part. The distal portion of an involved limb becomes cold and edematous within a few hours, and eventually pulseless and gangrenous. The wound drains a watery, brown or hemorrhagic material which may have a peculiar sweet odor. The appearance of the wound is usually not that of a pyogenic inflammatory lesion. Depending on the duration of the process, the surrounding skin may be normal, white, and tense, or dusky brown and reddish. Vesicles or hemorrhagic bullae may develop, particularly in *C. septicum* infections. Gas is usually not detectable in the tissues by palpation except in advanced lesions, although it may be visible easily by x-ray. Occasionally, tiny bubbles may be seen in the discharge from the wound; rarely, crepitation can be detected at an early stage by auscultation. The involved muscle appears dark red or black, may herniate through the wound, and is noncontractile when stimulated.

Systemic manifestations developing shortly after onset of severe pain and swelling of an injured extremity strongly suggest gas gangrene. The patient is prostrated, pale, and motionless but is usually well oriented, alert, and extremely apprehensive. The temperature usually does not exceed 101°F and may be normal. As the illness progresses, there may be anorexia, vomiting, profuse watery or bloody diarrhea, and eventually circulatory collapse. The pulse rate usually exceeds 120 beats per min and is elevated out of proportion to the temperature. Massive intravascular hemolysis is rare in patients with clostridial myositis. Pericardial effusion is sometimes noted. Delirium and coma may precede death, but more commonly the patient dies suddenly several days after onset of illness, often during surgery or anesthesia. Acute renal failure is occasionally a late complication.

Gas gangrene has been described after hypodermic injection, especially injection of epinephrine. Minor trauma also occasionally activates clostridial spores dormant in scar tissue and leads to development of myonecrosis years after original injury.

Gas gangrene must be differentiated from nonclostridial infections of gangrenous limbs caused by anaerobic streptococci, aerobic gas-forming coliform bacilli (most commonly *Escherichia coli*), *Bacteroides* species, and group A streptococci.

Clostridial cellulitis This is a relatively benign infection of skin and subcutaneous tissues that occurs in a small proportion of wounds contaminated with pathogenic clostridia. The disease is characterized by spreading necrosis of superficial tissues and a profuse, foul-smelling, brown, seropurulent exudate. Gas, which crepitates on palpation, invariably forms in the subcutaneous tissues and may involve an entire limb or form a localized gas pocket. In clostridial cellulitis, the underlying skeletal muscle is not involved, pain is not severe, and the only systemic manifestations are slight fever and moderate tachycardia. It can usually be differentiated from group A streptococcal cellulitis by the presence of subcutaneous gas and the absence of erythema.

Postabortal and puerperal sepsis Uterine infections with *C. perfringens* usually occur after incomplete abortions induced under unsterile conditions and occasionally after spontaneous abortions, prolonged labor at term, ruptured membranes, or operative interference with pregnancy. The organisms presumably invade the damaged endometrium through the retained products of conception. The earliest symptoms may be related to instrumentation and consist of metrorrhagia, suprapubic and back pain, chills, and fever. Fever of 100 to 103°F, often with chills, usually recurs several days after abortion, but the incubation period can be as short as 6 h. Vaginal bleeding is almost invariably present, and there is often a brown, foul-smelling, vaginal discharge containing necrotic tissue. The cervix is soft and patulous, and the uterus and adnexae are usually very tender. The lower abdominal wall is often tense, or signs of generalized peritonitis may be present, secondary to perforation of the uterus or parametrial extension of infection. Nausea, vomiting, and profuse diarrhea are often prominent.

Systemic manifestations may appear with dramatic suddenness. Massive intravascular hemolysis, accompanied by hemoglobinemia, hemoglobinuria, and jaundice, may be the most striking feature of the disease. Icterus may appear within hours after onset of illness. As in gas gangrene, the clinical picture may be dominated by circulatory collapse with hypotension, extreme tachycardia, cyanosis, hyperpnea, and pulmonary edema. Despite severe prostration, the patient is frequently well oriented, alert, and apprehensive. The mortality rate in postabortal or puerperal sepsis caused by *C. perfringens* and associated with intense hemolysis is 40 to 70 percent. Death may occur a few hours after onset or may be delayed for days. Acute renal failure secondary to shock, dehydration, or hemolysis occurs frequently.

Unusual local complications of the uterine infection are gas gangrene of the vagina and rectum and clostridial cellulitis of the anterior abdominal wall following cesarean section or hysterectomy. At times, the infectious process is confined to the endometrium and myometrium with intrauterine gas formation (physometra).

Septic abortion with *C. perfringens* bacteremia without overt hemolysis is a more common occurrence than bacteremia with gross hemolysis, as described above. Death is unusual in the absence of hemolysis.

Diseases to be considered in the *differential diagnosis* include perforated uterus, ruptured ectopic pregnancy, ingestion of toxic abortifacients, streptococcal or staphylococcal puerperal sepsis, pelvic thrombophlebitis with septic pulmonary emboli, acute hepatic necrosis of pregnancy, and sickle-cell crisis.

Clostridium perfringens food poisoning Meat and meat products contaminated with *C. perfringens* type A are frequently responsible for outbreaks of acute gastroenteritis. In 1973 in the United States, *C. perfringens* accounted for 18.5 percent of cases in reported foodborne outbreaks.

Most outbreaks of *C. perfringens* food poisoning have been associated with the ingestion of meat or poultry dishes. Most market meats and poultry are heavily contaminated, and the organism can be isolated with ease from soil, water, air, and human or animal feces. The usual story is that the food has been prepared and cooked 24 h or more before consumption, allowed to cool slowly at room temperature, and then served either cold or warmed. During this period of incubation, contaminating spores which have survived cooking germinate, and clostridia grow to large numbers sufficient to constitute an infectious inoculum. *Clostridium perfringens* food poisoning can be reproduced experimentally in man by feeding the actively growing organisms which apparently multiply and sporulate in the small intestine. Sporulation is associated with the production of an enterotoxin *in situ.*

Typical symptoms of diarrhea with abdominal pain and cramps develop 6 to 24 h after ingestion of meat, stew, or soup which has been stored at a warm temperature for several hours after cooking. Nausea occurs occasionally, but vomiting is rare. Systemic manifestations are usually absent, and recovery is uneventful after 12 to 24 h.

A severe form of clostridial infection termed *enteritis necrotans* was observed in Germany after World War II. This disease was characterized by hemorrhagic necrosis of the small intestine, bloody diarrhea, severe dehydration, shock, and death. A similar infection termed *necrotizing jejunitis* has been described in natives of New Guinea who had eaten inadequately cooked pork.

Miscellaneous clostridial infections Clostridia can be isolated from bile obtained at elective cholecystectomy in patients without symptoms of clostridial infection. Clostridial cellulitis or myonecrosis may occasionally follow surgical procedures, particularly surgery on the gastrointestinal tract or gallbladder. Pathogenic clostridia are occasionally introduced into the abdomen, thoracic cavity, or cranium through penetrating wounds. Primary pneumonia in the absence of a penetrating wound or distant focus has been described. Clostridial pleurisy may involve the underlying lung but is usually an indolent localized infection with minimal systemic manifestations. Meningitis is usually secondary to a puncture wound of the skull and is often associated with a necrotizing cerebritis. Clostridial peritonitis may follow perforation of the gallbladder, appendix, or other viscus and is usually rapidly fatal.

Clostridial septicemia also develops occasionally in patients with far-advanced neoplastic disease, including leukemias, lymphomas, and metastatic solid tumors. Over two-thirds of these patients have been receiving antineoplastic chemotherapy or radiation therapy. The primary site of invasion is usually the gastrointestinal tract which is frequently extensively involved by the neoplastic process. Abdominal surgical procedures, endoscopy, small bowel series, and paracentesis have been reported to predispose to sepsis in these patients. The course of the disease is rapid, death often occurring within 24 h after onset of recognizable infection. Hypotension, hyperpyrexia, and dyspnea are the most common clinical manifestations of infection. Jaundice and hemolysis occur occasionally. Cellulitis, with or without crepitation, may appear in the flanks and should suggest the diagnosis, especially in patients with leukemia or lymphoma.

Cystitis with pneumaturia, gaseous cholecystitis, endocarditis, and bursitis after needle aspiration are other examples of rare clostridial infections.

LABORATORY FINDINGS The diagnosis of gas gangrene, clostridial cellulitis, postabortal sepsis, or other clostridial infections is based primarily on clinical criteria. Smears of wound exudate, uterine scrapings, or cervical discharge may show abundant large gram-positive rods, as well as other organisms. Spores are rarely observed in smears of exudates. Thioglycollate broth, deep meat broth, and blood-agar plates incubated in an anaerobic jar should be inoculated for definitive identification of specific clostridia. However, interpretation of positive wound cultures is difficult because clostridia are frequent contaminants. *Clostridium perfringens* bacteremia is common in postabortal infections but rare in gas gangrene.

Polymorphonuclear leukocytosis occurs frequently in gas gangrene and invariably in postabortal sepsis; total blood leukocyte counts range from 15,000 to 40,000 cells per mm^3 and occasionally exceed 60,000 cells per mm^3. Marked thrombocytopenia develops in about 50 percent of patients with clostridial sepsis. The urine frequently contains protein and casts. Renal insufficiency may lead to severe uremia.

X-ray examination sometimes provides the first clue leading to the correct diagnosis by revealing the presence of gas in muscle, subcutaneous tissue, or uterus; however, demonstration of gas in tissues is not diagnostic of clostridial infection. Other bacteria, especially *Enterobacter* or *Escherichia*, may be responsible for gas production, and occasionally air is sucked into a wound at the time of penetrating injury.

Profound alterations of circulating erythrocytes are common in postabortal sepsis but are much less frequent in other clostridial infection. Hemolytic anemia may develop with almost unbelievable rapidity; the red blood cell count occasionally decreases by 2 million cells per mm^3 in less than 24 h and is associated with hemoglobinemia, hemoglobinuria, and elevated levels of serum bilirubin. Spherocytosis, increased osmotic and mechanical red blood cell fragility, erythrophagocytosis, and methemoglobinemia have also been described. Abnormalities of the clotting mechanism characteristic of intravascular coagulation may be observed in patients with severe clostridial infections.

TREATMENT The traditional therapeutic approach to serious clostridial infection, such as diffuse, spreading myositis, is immediate surgical intervention with wide radical debridement followed by open drainage without closure or open amputation when necessary. Early surgery not only aids diagnosis, but permits decompression of fascial compartments and excision of devitalized muscle and may obviate amputation. A number of authorities feel that hyperbaric oxygen therapy has modified this traditional approach to gas gangrene by assuming priority over radical surgical debridement. Proponents report that hyperbaric oxygenation produces impressive, almost immediate improvement in patients with gas gangrene, with rapid disappearance of systemic toxicity and prompt arrest of local spread of the gangrenous infection. Opinion differs about whether conservative debridement should be carried out before or after hyperbaric oxygen therapy, but no one advocates hyperbaric oxygen alone for gas gangrene. Oxygen toxicity consequent to hyperbaric oxygenation may lead to convulsions in some patients.

Curettage of the uterus should be performed for diagnosis and treatment of postabortal clostridial infections. In the absence of hemolysis, standard therapy for septic abortion with antibiotics and uterine curettage usually produces rapid improvement, even in patients with bacteremia. The mortality rate in patients with abortion, *C. perfringens* bacteremia, and intense hemolysis is high irrespective of the therapeutic approach. The role of hysterectomy is controversial and ill-defined; some surgeons strongly advocate hysterectomy, whereas others feel that the potential benefits of the procedure do not outweigh the risks. Heparinization, exchange transfusion, and hyperbaric oxygen have been utilized but are not of established benefit.

Simple excision and adequate drainage usually suffice for treating clostridial cellulitis.

Penicillin is the antibiotic of choice for all clostridial infections and should be administered in doses of 20 million units a day by continuous intravenous infusion. Cephalosporins and chloramphenicol are also active against most strains of *Clostridium,* and either may be used as an alternative to penicillin in patients with hypersensitivity. Clostridia are also generally, but not universally, susceptible in vitro to tetracycline, clindamycin, and carbenicillin.

The efficacy of polyvalent gas gangrene antitoxin is controversial. Many centers have discontinued the use of antitoxin in the management of patients with suspected gas gangrene or clostridial postabortal sepsis because of questionable efficacy and the risk of hypersensitivity reactions.

Intravenous infusions of blood, plasma volume expanders, fluids, and electrolytes are required to combat shock, anemia, and dehydration. Renal insufficiency should be treated in the same manner as acute tubular necrosis from other causes.

The most reliable protection against gas gangrene is early and adequate wound debridement. Antitoxin is ineffective as a prophylactic agent. The use of clostridial toxoids for prophylactic immunization of individuals in hazardous occupations awaits evaluation.

REFERENCES

Foodborne outbreaks—Annual summary 1973. Atlanta: Center for Disease Control, 1974

HOLLAND JA et al: Experimental and clinical experience with hyperbaric oxygen in the treatment of clostridial myonecrosis. Surgery 77:75, 1975

MACLENNAN JD: The histotoxic clostridial infections of man. Bacteriol Rev 26:177, 1962

MAHN E, DANTUONO LM: Postabortal septicotoxemia due to *Clostridium welchii*: Seventy-five cases from the maternity hospital, Santiago, Chile 1948–1952. Am J Obstet Gynecol 70:604, 1955

MURRELL TGC et al: Pig-bel: Enteritis necroticans: A study in diagnosis and management. Lancet 1:217, 1966

NAKAMURA M, SCHULZE JA: Clostridium perfringens food poisoning. Ann Rev Microbiol 24:359, 1970

PRITCHARD JA, WHALLEY PJ: Abortion complicated by Clostridium perfringens infection. Am J Obstet Gynecol 111:484, 1971

WEINSTEIN L, BARZA MA: Gas Gangrene. New Engl J Med 289:1129, 1973

WYNE JW, ARMSTRONG D: Clostridial septicemia. Cancer 29:215, 1972

159
BACTEROIDES INFECTIONS

EDWARD W. HOOK
MERLE A. SANDE

ETIOLOGY The family Bacteroidaceae consists of all of the gram-negative, non-spore-forming, strictly anaerobic bacilli. Three genera, *Bacteroides, Fusobacterium,* and *Leptotrichia,* are differentiated on the basis of the production of short-chain fatty acids detected by gas liquid chromatography. Members of the genus *Bacteroides* do not produce significant quantities of butyric acid, in contrast to members of the genus *Fusobacterium,* which form butyric acid as a major fermentation product. The genera can be further divided into a number of species and subspecies.

Members of the genus *Bacteroides* are normal inhabitants of the mouth, intestinal tract, and vagina. These organisms are found in human feces in an average concentration of about 10^{11} viable units per gram, outnumbering other bacteria by a hundredfold or more.

Bacteroides are the anaerobes most frequently isolated from clinical specimens, and *B. fragilis* and *B. melaninogenicus* are the species most often responsible for infections in man.

PATHOGENESIS Species of *Bacteroides* are not highly invasive, and infection is usually secondary to an underlying disease, surgical procedure, or therapy which impairs the normal defenses of the host. These organisms utilize substances other than oxygen as the final electron acceptor in reactions which generate energy, and thus will grow only in an environment with a low reduction-oxidation (redox) potential. Healthy, well-vascularized tissue has a relatively high redox potential and will not support growth of anaerobes. Conditions that significantly lower redox potential, such as impairment of blood supply, tissue necrosis, or growth of aerobic bacteria, are necessary to create an environment conducive to proliferation of *Bacteroides.* Infection, therefore, frequently occurs secondary to vascular disease, trauma, surgery, perforated viscus, shock, or malignancy.

Bacteroides are frequently involved in local infections originating from mucosal surfaces in the mouth, intestinal tract, or vagina. The initial reaction is a localized suppurative lesion characterized by formation of fetid pus. The characteristic odor is caused by certain metabolic end products of bacterial origin, primarily short-chain fatty acids and volatile amines. Many species of *Bacteroides* produce collagenases and proteinases which may account for the propensity for abscess formation. In addition, some species produce a heparinase which may account for the localized septic thrombophlebitis frequently seen adjacent to areas of infection. Infection characteristically remains localized, but bloodstream invasion or direct extension to other areas may occur. Localization of bloodborne organisms at distant sites is not unusual and may result in abscess formation in brain, lung, liver, joints, kidneys, or other organs.

Although *Bacteroides* may be isolated in pure culture from infected tissue or pus, other organisms are usually present, particularly streptococci, coliform species, or other anaerobes. *Bacteroides* and anaerobic streptococci have been shown to act synergistically in the induction of abscesses in mice.

MANIFESTATIONS **Nose and mouth infections** *Bacteroides* species, especially *B. melaninogenicus,* are frequently isolated from local suppurative lesions of any tissue liable to contamination with the flora of the mouth. *Bacteroides* are almost always cultured from the foul-smelling pus in gingival or dental abscesses, necrotizing gingivitis (Vincent's), gingival cellulitis after oral surgery, and acute infections of the facial region with external drainage. *Bacteroides* species have also been isolated from mandibular osteomyelitis and may produce a syndrome that includes putrid peritonsillar abscess and thrombophlebitis of the jugular vein.

Various strains of *Bacteroides* and other anaerobic bacteria have been implicated as a cause of about 10 percent of cases of acute bacterial sinusitis. These organisms are particularly common when infections develop after manipulation or extraction of teeth whose roots are adjacent to the floor of the maxillary sinus. A foul-smelling and foul-tasting discharge is characteristic. Anaerobes can also be isolated from about one-half of the patients undergoing surgery for chronic or recurrent maxillary sinusitis; in these patients *Bacteroides* species are commonly isolated. Anaerobic organisms also occasionally produce otitis media and mastoiditis.

Brain abscess Anaerobic bacteria, particularly *Bacteroides* and anaerobic streptococci, have been isolated from 30 to 80 percent of brain abscesses in adults. In one study, 16 of 18 nontraumatic brain abscesses contained anaerobes, and half of these were *Bacteroides* species, including both *B. fragilis* and *B. melaninogenicus.* These lesions may result from either direct extension of suppurative infection involving the sinuses, middle ear, or mastoids, or from hematogenous dissemination from infections elsewhere, particularly the lungs. There is an increased incidence of brain abscess in patients with cyanotic heart disease. Signs and symptoms are mainly those of a space-occupying intracranial lesion with headache followed by changes in mentation, focal neurologic signs, or papilledema. The course may be indolent, and fever is frequently absent. Cerebrospinal fluid findings are variable but may mimic those of aseptic meningitis.

Pleuropulmonary infection Aspiration of oral secretions leads to production of mixed anaerobic infection of the lungs and pleura. *Bacteroides, Fusobacterium* species, and anaerobic streptococci are isolated alone or in combination in a majority of cases of lung abscess and necrotizing pneumonia. These anaerobes are second only to the pneumococcus as a cause of acute bacterial infection of the lungs. Although *B. melaninogenicus* is the most frequent *Bacteroides* species isolated in anaerobic pulmonary infections, *B. fragilis* can be found in 15 to 25 percent of cases. These infections occur primarily in patients with conditions that predispose to aspiration such as altered consciousness, particularly alcoholism, major motor seizure disorders, general anesthesia, oral surgical procedures, and esophageal dysfunction. *Bacteroides* may also produce infection distal to obstructive lesions of the bronchus. These infections are characterized by tissue necrosis, abscess formation, and the production of foul-smelling and foul-tasting sputum. Empyema is not an unusual complication of lung abscess or necrotizing pneumonia. Empyema with anaerobes may also occur as an extension from subdiaphragmatic infection.

The bacterial flora of bronchiectatic cavities frequently includes *Bacteroides* species and other anaerobes.

Abdominal infection Intraabdominal abscesses and generalized peritonitis almost always contain *B. fragilis,* especially when secondary to perforation or leakage from the gastrointestinal tract. These infections are uniformly polymicrobial, with an average of five microbial species. Symptoms include fever with chills, localized or generalized abdominal pain with peritoneal signs, and nausea and vomiting. The abscess cavity may be large enough to be palpable on abdominal or pelvic examination. *Bacteroides fragilis* is isolated from approximately 50 percent of abdominal surgical wounds after trauma involving perforation of the gut and in greater than 50 percent of wound infections following elective colon resection.

Intrahepatic infection Anaerobic bacteria have rarely been implicated in infections of the gallbladder, but they may produce ascending cholangitis and are isolated from 20 to 45 percent of pyogenic intrahepatic abscesses. *Bacteroides* species account for approximately half of these isolates. They may reach the intrahepatic tissue by direct extension from an ascending infection or by embolization from septic portal vein thrombosis. The disease is manifest by fever, chills, abdominal pain, particularly in the right upper quadrant, hepatomegaly, and liver tenderness in most cases. The presence of jaundice usually indicates multiple abscesses.

Pelvic infection The predominant organisms isolated in greater than 75 percent of nongonococcal gynecologic infections are anaerobic. *Bacteroides* species are the major cause of Bartholin's abscess, endometritis, parametritis, parametrial abscess, and pelvic peritonitis, and together with anaerobic streptococci account for the majority of isolates from nongonococcal tuboovarian abscesses. These infections often complicate malignancy or recent surgery and commonly develop within necrotic tissue or products of conception. They are characterized by drainage of foul-smelling pus or blood from the uterus, generalized uterine or localized pelvic tenderness, and continued fever and chills. Suppurative thrombophlebitis of the pelvic veins may complicate these infections and lead to repeated episodes of small septic pulmonary emboli.

Nonclostridial anaerobes, principally *Bacteroides* species and anaerobic streptococci, are also the major invasive pathogens in septic abortions. Bacteremia, often transient and frequently polymicrobic, can be demonstrated in 50 to 60 percent of these patients.

Other local infections Ischemic ulcerations and osteomyelitis of the extremities may be associated with *Bacteroides* invasions especially in patients with peripheral vascular disease. These are characterized by a foul-smelling exudate and may demonstrate gas formation. Severe synergistic gangrene of the abdominal wall has been associated with mixed *Bacteroides* and streptococcal infections.

Hematogenous dissemination Invasion of the bloodstream by these organisms is usually secondary to local infection, particularly those involving the abdominal cavity and pelvis. The initial manifestations are determined by the portal of entry and may be those of endometritis, appendicitis, intraabdominal abscess, or others. When bloodstream invasion occurs, the patient may become extremely ill with chills and hectic fevers ranging from 101 to 106°F. Shock and disseminated intravascular coagulation may develop. The clinical picture may be quite similar to that seen in sepsis with other gram-negative bacilli except for the occasional association of thrombophlebitis. When bacteremia complicates facial or oral infection, the internal jugular vein may be the site of suppurative thrombophlebitis, and in pelvic infections the iliac and femoral veins may be involved. Palpation along the course of the involved veins may disclose a firm, tender cord, indicating the presence of a thrombus. Emboli may be dislodged from peripheral sites of thrombophlebitis, resulting in multiple septic pulmonary infarcts. The pulmonary abscesses or empyema may be the main focus of clinical attention rather than the initial site of infection.

A diffuse hepatitis has been reported with *Bacteroides* bacteremia leading to enlargement and tenderness of the liver with jaundice. Bacterial endocarditis has been reported occasionally. This complication should be considered when classic features of endocarditis are present but when aerobic blood cultures are negative.

LABORATORY FINDINGS Leukocytosis of 12,000 to 25,000 cells per mm^3 may occur in localized *Bacteroides* infections and is almost always present in systemic infection. Patients with liver abscesses or hepatitis may have elevated serum bilirubin values and other aberrations of hepatic function. Gas formation at sites of infection occasionally results in air-fluid levels detectable by roentgenography.

Bacteroides infections should be considered whenever pus with an extremely foul odor is encountered. A smear of the pus will reveal slightly pale, irregularly staining, elongated gram-negative bacilli. *Bacteroides fragilis* frequently demonstrate bipolar staining and resemble safety pins; fusobacteria are thin, delicate, pale-staining gram-negative rods with tapered ends and resemble needlelike crystals; *B. melaninogenicus* may have a coccobacillary appearance. There is usually considerable pleomorphism, and the material will often also contain other gram-positive or gram-negative organisms. The gram stain is of the utmost importance in presumptive diagnosis of *Bacteroides* infections since the organisms are fastidious and cultures may be negative. Definitive diagnosis depends on isolation and identification of the organism. *Bacteroides* grow slowly and may be difficult to detect since organisms that grow more rapidly frequently obscure their isolation and detection. Cultures in liquid medium should be held for a minimum of 14 days.

Correct specimen collection is critical in isolating anaerobic organisms. Even brief exposure to oxygen may kill the more fastidious species. Abscess cavities should be aspirated directly with a syringe, the air expelled, and the needle capped with a sterile rubber stopper. The specimen can then be injected into a carrier bottle containing a reduced environment or transported directly to the laboratory for direct culture on anaerobic media. Such a technique is preferred over the use of cotton swabs or other techniques of open culture.

Only certain specimens should be cultured for *Bacteroides* or other anaerobic bacteria. Since all mucosal surfaces contain anaerobes, it is of no value and, in fact, may be misleading to culture specimens "contaminated" with mucosal bacteria such as expectorated sputum, bronchoscopic aspirates, feces, vaginal secretions, or secretions from mucosal surfaces which normally harbor anaerobes. Acceptable materials for culture include blood, pleural fluid, transtracheal aspirates, pus obtained by direct aspiration into an abscess cavity, and other tissues or fluids which are sterile under normal conditions.

TREATMENT Surgery is of prime importance in the management of patients with *Bacteroides* infections. Drainage of abscess cavities should be carried out as soon as fluctuation and localization occur; perforations must be closed promptly, devitalized tissues or foreign bodies removed, and an adequate blood supply established. Drainage of local suppurative lesions is all that is required for cure in many cases. However, antimicrobial therapy may be indicated in certain infections involving vital organs or when systemic manifestations are present. In patients proved or suspected to have a severe systemic infection caused by *B. fragilis,* either chloramphenicol, 3 g per day divided into three equal doses in adults, or clindamycin, 1.2 to 1.8 g per day divided into three equal doses in adults, is the antimicrobial drug of choice. Chloramphenicol is preferred for patients with infections of the central nervous system because clindamycin does not effectively penetrate the blood-brain barrier. Both antibiotics can be administered orally, but parenteral therapy is advisable for patients with severe infection. Almost all *Bacteroides* strains are susceptible in vitro to concentrations of clindamycin or chloramphenicol readily obtainable in the blood of patients treated with full doses of the antibiotics. Both drugs have well-defined toxicity—chloramphenicol may produce a fatal aplastic anemia, the incidence of this being 1:40,000 to 1:100,000, and will predictably but reversibly depress bone marrow function during long-term high-dose administration. Clindamycin has been associated with diarrhea in up to 20 percent of cases and with proctoscopic evidence of pseudomembranous colitis in up to 10 percent. Although clinically significant colitis occurs with a much lower frequency, this complication can impair medical management of the already seriously ill patient with infection. Clindamycin should be discontinued with the first sign of diarrhea.

Penicillin G is effective for treatment of *Bacteroides* infections caused by organisms other than *B. fragilis.* Many strains of *Bacteroides* are highly resistant to the penicillinase-resistant penicillins, cephalothin, carbenicillin, or ampicillin, and the vast majority of isolates are resistant to streptomycin, kanamycin, neomycin, and gentamicin.

Bacteroides species frequently coexist at infected sites with other anaerobic or aerobic bacteria. Although clindamycin or chloramphenicol shows excellent activity against almost all anaerobes of clinical importance, the occurrence of polymicrobic infection may necessitate administration of another antibiotic in some patients.

Anticoagulant therapy and venous ligation should be considered in patients with thrombophlebitis and multiple septic pulmonary infarctions.

REFERENCES

ALTEMEIER WA et al: Intra-abdominal abscesses. Am J Surg 125:70, 1973

BALOWS A et al (eds): *Anaerobic Bacteria: Role in Disease,* Springfield, Ill.: Charles C Thomas, 1974

BARTLETT JG, FINEGOLD SM: Anaerobic infections of the lung and pleural space. Am Rev Resp Dis 110:56, 1974

CHOW AW, GUZE LB: *Bacteroidaceae* bacteremia: Clinical experience with 112 patients. Medicine 53:93, 1974

EVANS FO et al: *Sinusitis* of the maxillary antrum. N Engl J Med 293:735, 1975

FREDERICK J, BRAUDE AI: Anaerobic infection of the paranasal sinuses. N Engl J Med 290:135, 1974

HEINEMAN HS, BRAUDE AI: Anaerobic infection of the brain. Am J Med 35:682, 1963

LEVISON ME: The importance of anaerobic bacteria in infectious diseases. Med Clin North Am 57:1015, 1973

QUAYLE AA: Bacteroides infections in oral surgery. J Oral Surg 32:91, 1974

RUBIN RH et al: Hepatic abscess: Changes in clinical, bacteriologic and therapeutic aspects. Am J Med 57:601, 1974

SABBAJ J et al: Anaerobic pyogenic liver abscess. Ann Intern Med 77:629, 1972

TEDESCO FJ et al: Clindamycin-associated colitis. Ann Intern Med 81:429, 1974

THADEPALLI H et al: Abdominal trauma, anaerobes, and antibiotics. Surg Gynecol Obstet 137:270, 1973

—— et al: Anaerobic infections of the female genital tract: Bacteriologic and therapeutic aspects. Am J Obstet Gynecol 117:1034, 1973

160
ANAEROBIC MUCOCUTANEOUS INFECTIONS

LAWRENCE L. PELLETIER, JR.

Anaerobic mucocutaneous infections are characterized by gangrenous, foul-smelling ulcers containing large numbers of bacteria and spirochetes. The lesions are usually located in the mouth and pharynx but may occur in the respiratory tract, genitalia, surgical wounds, or human bites.

ETIOLOGY Formerly, these were termed *fusospirochetal infections* owing to the number of fusobacteria and spirochetes present. However, other common mouth bacteria such as viridans streptococci, bacteroides species, anaerobic cocci, anaerobic diphtheroids, and vibrios are also found. The bacteria and spirochetes associated with anaerobic mucocutaneous ulcers are normal flora in the mouths of most adults. These endogenous organisms grow best under anaerobic conditions. In clinical disease the number of organisms increases greatly. It is probable that tissue destruction results from the synergistic interaction of several different species of bacteria under anaerobic conditions.

The precise nature of this interaction, the bacterial species involved, and the triggering host environmental conditions are not yet established. However, the pathogenic role of spirochetes appears minor, and the term *fusospirochetal infection* is no longer appropriate.

CLINICAL MANIFESTATIONS **Acute necrotizing ulcerative gingivitis (trench mouth, Vincent's stomatitis)** The onset of disease is usually sudden and is associated with tender bleeding gums, fetid breath, and a bad taste. The gingival mucosa, especially the papillae between the teeth, becomes ulcerated and may be covered with gray exudate which is removable with gentle pressure. Although involvement of the gums is usually patchy, the process may extend to most of the gingival tissue. If the ulceration is extensive, there are fever, cervical lymphadenopathy, and leukocytosis. The disease may spread to involve other tissues of the oropharynx; it may become less severe and chronic; or it may subside spontaneously. Recurrent ulceration has been described. Most patients who develop ulcerative gingivitis are young adults with poor oral hygiene. Tartar deposits and eruption or extraction of teeth may damage the gums and allow for bacterial invasion. Edentulous persons almost never develop the disease. Ulcerative gingivitis is prevalent in wartime when nutritional deficiency, crowding, and emotional upsets are common. The role of these factors in pathogenesis is not known.

Acute necrotizing ulcerative mucositis (cancrum oris, noma) Occasionally, ulcerative gingivitis spreads to involve the buccal mucosa, the cheek, and the mandible or maxilla, resulting in widespread destruction of bone and soft tissue. The first indication of cancrum oris is usually slight inflammation of the skin of the cheek. The destruction of tissue proceeds very rapidly. The teeth may fall out, and large areas of bone, even the whole mandible, may be sloughed. A strong putrid odor is present. The lesions are not usually painful. The gangrenous lesions eventually heal, but large disfiguring defects are left. Cancrum oris is seen most commonly in severely malnourished children in underdeveloped areas of the world following a debilitating illness. Cancrum oris may complicate acute leukemia or develop in individuals with a genetic deficiency of catalase.

Gangrenous pharyngitis (Vincent's angina) Necrotizing infections of the pharynx may occur alone or in association with ulcerative gingivitis. The main complaints are an extremely sore throat, foul breath, bad taste in the mouth, sensation of choking, and fever. The pharynx in the area of the tonsillar pillars is swollen, red, and ulcerated and is covered with a grayish membrane which peels easily. Lymphadenopathy and leukocytosis are common. The disease may last for only a few days or may persist for weeks if not treated. The lesion begins unilaterally but may spread to the other side of the pharynx or to the larynx. Aspiration of infected material may result in lung abscess.

Infections of human bites Gangrenous lesions resulting from human bites commonly contain mixed oral flora, and fusobacterial septicemia following an infected human bite has been reported. Human bites are much more likely to become infected than dog bites.

Infection of genitalia Gangrenous balanitis and ulcers

and gangrene of the vulva have been associated with mixed anaerobic flora.

DIAGNOSIS The diagnosis can be made with certainty only by demonstrating the typical bacteria and spirochetes in sections of necrotic lesions. In clinical practice the diagnosis is made by the appearance and putrid odor of the lesions. Smears of material from mouth ulcers are not usually helpful because fusospirochetal flora are found in the mouths of healthy persons. Ulcerative gingivitis can be distinguished from herpetic gingivostomatitis by the absence of vesicles and the tendency to involve mainly the gingival papillae. In suspected cases of gangrenous pharyngitis, diphtheria, and streptococcal and infectious mononucleosis, pharyngitis must be excluded by appropriate tests.

TREATMENT Treatment of ulcerative gingivitis consists of local measures and antibacterial therapy if the disease is severe and painful. During the acute phase the patient should avoid brushing his teeth or causing trauma to the gums. A 3% solution of hydrogen peroxide diluted with equal amounts of warm water should be used as a mouthwash several times a day. Tartar and necrotic debris should be removed from the gum margins by a dentist. In severe painful cases of gingivitis penicillin V, 250 mg four times a day, 600,000 units procaine penicillin twice a day, or 1.0 g tetracycline a day should be used until improvement is evident. Metronidazole, a drug with some activity against most anaerobic bacteria, administered in dosage of 250 mg three times a day for 3 to 7 days is as effective as penicillin in promoting healing of gingival lesions and is considered by some to be the most satisfactory drug for the treatment of ulcerative gingivitis. Patients with gangrenous pharyngitis or infections of the genitalia should receive 600,000 units procaine penicillin twice a day or 1.0 g per day of tetracycline. The treatment of cancrum oris consists of antibiotic therapy with penicillin or tetracycline, debridement of necrotic tissue, and eventual repair of damaged structures. Human bites should be cleansed thoroughly, and obviously necrotic tissue should be removed. The wounds should not be sutured but should be left open and irrigated frequently. Antibiotic therapy should be given to all patients with human bites.

REFERENCES

Barnes GP et al: Acute necrotizing ulcerative gingivitis: A survey of 218 cases. J Periodontol 44:35, 1973

Enwonwu CO: Epidemiological and biochemical studies of necrotizing ulcerative gingivitis and noma (cancrum oris) in Nigerian children. Arch Oral Biol 17:1357, 1972

Klotz H: Differentiation between necrotic ulcerative gingivitis and primary herpetic gingivostomatitis. NY State Dent J 39: 283, 1973

Proctor DB, Baker CG: Treatment of acute necrotizing ulcerative gingivitis with metronidazole. J Can Dent Assoc 10:376, 1971

Weinstein RA et al: Cancrum oris-like lesion associated with acute myelogenous leukemia. Oral Surg 38:10, 1974

section 9 | Mycobacterial diseases

161
TUBERCULOSIS

WILLIAM W. STEAD
JOSEPH BATES

DEFINITION Tuberculosis is a necrotizing bacterial infection with protean manifestations and wide distribution. The lungs are most commonly affected, but lesions may occur also in the kidneys, bones, lymph nodes, or meninges or be disseminated throughout the body. The infection may cause clinical disease either (1) shortly after inoculation (sometimes called "primary" tuberculosis) or (2) after a period of months or decades of dormancy (often erroneously referred to as "reinfection tuberculosis"). In the Western world where bovine tuberculosis has been controlled, the portal of entry in man is almost exclusively the lung.

HISTORY Some of the races of man (Caucasian, Mongolian) have lived with tubercle bacilli throughout much of their history, and the infection produces a more chronic disease, only rarely being fulminant. African, American Indian, and Eskimo peoples have had contact with tuberculosis over a much shorter period, and the infection is more prone to produce fulminant disease. Tuberculosis was named to indicate its formation of firm nodules, or *tubercles.* For many years the chronic form (then often called *phthisis* or *consumption*) was considered a degenerative or hereditary disease, quite unrelated to the tuberculosis of childhood which was obviously infectious. Laennec (1819) was the first to recognize the chronic form as merely a later development in the same infection. Koch (1882) identified the causative organism. There has been a great drop in prevalence of tuberculosis in the economically developed countries. The death rate from tuberculosis had already begun to fall by 1900, coincident with improvement in nutrition and standard of living. For the person with clinical tuberculosis, however, the most important development occurred in 1944 with the discovery of streptomycin. With the introduction of para-aminosalicylic acid (PAS) in 1947, isoniazid (INH) in 1952, ethambutol in 1967, and rifampin in 1971, specific therapy became progressively better and easier to administer.

ETIOLOGY *Mycobacterium tuberculosis* is a rod 2 to 4 μm in length and 0.3 μm in thickness. Its distinguishing staining property, i.e., resistance to decolorization by acid alcohol when stained with basic fuchsin, is related to the waxy component of the cell wall. This "acid-fastness" is dependent in some way upon the structural integrity of the bacillus; it is lost when the organisms are damaged by grinding but is not affected by prolonged extraction with fat solvents.

Tubercle bacilli are strict aerobes and thrive best at a P_{O_2} of about 140 mmHg. The organs most commonly affected by tuberculosis are those with relatively high oxygen tension; metastatic foci are most common in the apexes of the lungs where the P_{O_2} is in the range of 120 to 130 mmHg in the upright position, followed by the kidney and the growing ends of bones, where P_{O_2} approaches 100 mmHg. The liver and spleen, where the P_{O_2} is quite low, are rarely affected, except in overwhelming disseminated infection.

Two species of tubercle bacilli affect man: *M. tuberculosis* and *M. bovis.* By far the greatest number of cases in the United States are caused by the former strain. Programs for eradication of bovine tuberculosis have been so effective that the disease now appears only sporadically in this country. Avian bacilli have little invasiveness for man.

Several other species of mycobacteria have been noted to cause chronic pulmonary infection (Chap. 163). The most common are the avian-Battey group (*M. intracellulare* and *M. kansasii*). Clinical infection due to other atypical mycobacteria is rare. These mycobacteria appear not to be transmissible, and the epidemiology of the infections they cause remains obscure. They tend to infect lungs that have been damaged by silicosis or chronic obstructive lung disease. *Mycobacterium kansasii* responds well to antituberculous drugs in high dosage, but *M. intracellulare* is resistant to all drugs presently in use, and a favorable clinical response is less common.

TRANSMISSION Most cases of communicable tuberculosis among adults develop because of a late recrudescence of dormant infection with no history of recent exposure. The liquid caseum from a cavity in such a case abounds in tubercle bacilli which are excreted in aerosolized droplets during coughing, sneezing, and speaking. Droplets larger than 10 μm are usually caught on the mucociliary blanket and cleared from the lung without harm, but droplets of smaller size may reach the respiratory bronchiole and deposit bacilli beyond the protective mucus blanket. There, in a susceptible host, the organisms may invade tissue and establish an infection. Persons who have been infected previously are largely protected from reinfection by specific immunity, which is mediated by T lymphocytes. Teachers, school bus drivers, and nursery workers with infectious tuberculosis are of particular epidemiologic significance because of the great susceptibility of children.

Infection in a susceptible host is caused by inhalation of tubercle bacilli in *fresh* droplet nuclei expelled by a person with cavitary tuberculosis. Transmission can be blocked effectively by ultraviolet light and adequate ventilation and by chemotherapy of the source case. Even though tubercle bacilli can be cultured from dust in a room of a tuberculous person, they constitute no hazard to others in this state because the irregular shape and electrostatic charge of the attached dust particles prevent them from being carried beyond the mucociliary protective mechanism. Early in the course of tuberculous infection, persons are rarely infectious because they expel very few organisms. Tuberculosis cannot be spread on hands, dishes, glasses, utensils, or fomites.

Patients who are on an effective regimen of chemotherapy lose their ability to transmit infection within a short time (probably 2 weeks or less), despite the continued presence of tubercle bacilli on smear and culture of the sputum.

PREVALENCE AND INCIDENCE There has been a great fall in prevalence of tuberculosis in the United States since 1900. Early in this century over 80 percent of the population was infected *before* the age of twenty years. In an autopsy study in 1946, there was evidence of tuberculosis in 80 percent of the persons over the age of fifty. In 1972, only 2 to 5 percent of young adults reacted to tuberculin (except in some urban areas), whereas about 25 percent of persons over the age of fifty reacted. The decline in incidence of the infection is most apparent among children and young adults and is due to a reduction in the number of infectious cases, which in turn is attributable to an improved standard of living, reduced risk of late progression of infection, and prompter recognition and treatment of infectious cases.

The great majority of persons who harbor tubercle bacilli have latent or dormant ("healed") tuberculosis. Apical scars containing viable organisms may remain dormant for many years and then reactivate and produce clinical tuberculosis. Other sites in which tubercle bacilli may lie dormant for years and then recrudesce include the kidney (from which bacilli may spread to the genital tract in the male), spine, long bones, fallopian tubes, brain, and lymph nodes in the hilum and in the neck.

In 1974 there were about 30,000 new cases of clinical tuberculosis in the United States, an incidence of 14 per 100,000, down from 24 in 1966 and 53 in 1953. There were about 15,000,000 tuberculin reactors, indicating a prevalence of infection of 7,000 per 100,000. Of these, 60,000 were under therapy for tuberculosis and 500,000 had healed or dormant tuberculosis. The remainder had never developed clinical tuberculosis but simply harbored foci of latent infection. It is toward the latter group that programs of prophylactic therapy with INH are directed.

Of new tuberculous infections revealed by conversion of tuberculin reaction from negative to positive, 5 to 15 percent progress to serious disease within 5 years if left untreated. The risk of direct progression varies with age: it is greatest when infection begins in the first years of life and next greatest in young adults and adolescents. Among those remaining well for 5 years, a further 3 to 5 percent may develop late recrudescence at some time during life. Thus, the total morbidity rate in persons infected with *M. tuberculosis* is 8 to 20 percent. Both the early and late appearance of tuberculosis can be prevented in 80 percent of individuals if prompt treatment with INH is given when tuberculin "conversion" is discovered.

Mortality has fallen steadily over the past 70 years. Tuberculosis has ceased being the leading cause of death, with over 200 deaths per 100,000 in 1906 but only 1.7 per 100,000 in 1974. This figure may be somewhat low, because residual pulmonary scarring may lead to cor pulmonale and cause death secondarily.

IMMUNITY Natural resistance The Caucasian and Mongolian races have a distinct natural resistance to tuberculosis consisting of an ability to develop an immune response to the infection which enables spontaneous recovery from initial infection. However, late recrudescence may result in chronic disease characterized by cavitation and scarring. Africans, American Indians, and Eskimos were spared tuberculous infection until extensive contact began with members of the white race in which chronic tuberculosis was common. These peoples have less ability to develop an effective immune response to new infection, and in them the infection tends to be more rapidly progressive.

Specific (acquired) immunity Immunity to tuberculosis is mediated largely by T lymphocytes, which, in response to specific antigenic stimulation, liberate several lymphokines which prompt phagocytosis and lysis of mycobacteria. The role of immunoglobulins in the process is less clear, although IgA is often increased in patients with active tuberculosis and drops as the infection is controlled by therapy.

The mechanism by which latent infection recrudesces is not completely understood. From the fact that it occurs more commonly in old age and during other forms of illness, recrudescence appears likely to be due to reduced immunologic surveillance by T lymphocytes.

Tuberculin hypersensitivity The most readily obtained evidence of a past or present infection with tubercle bacilli is the finding of hypersensitivity to tuberculin, a protein derivative of the broth in which tubercle bacilli have been grown. Epidemiologic evidence strongly suggests that tuberculin hypersensitivity indicates the presence of living tubercle bacilli. The larger the skin reaction, the greater the chance that the infection is of clinical significance.

PATHOGENESIS AND PATHOLOGIC ANATOMY Initial infection ("primary" tuberculosis) In the nonimmune subject tubercle bacilli can gain entrance to the body by several routes: lung, gastrointestinal tract, and by direct cutaneous or percutaneous inoculation (as in an accident at the autopsy table). For practical purposes, the only route that is of importance in the United States is the lung. The majority of lesions in the early phase of infection are in the lower two-thirds of the lungs, where ventilation is best and deposition of droplet nuclei more likely. Because they produce no toxins and no tissue reaction, tubercle bacilli initially are free to multiply without deterrence. They reach regional (hilar) nodes and even the bloodstream before their progress is inhibited by the gradual development of specific immunity over a period of several weeks. At this time, the characteristic tissue reaction develops, with epithelioid cell granulomas and caseation necrosis in the pulmonary lesion, regional lymph nodes, and any site to which the bacilli have spread. The number of bacilli drops drastically with the appearance of caseation necrosis, indicating that caseation is associated with the release of cytotoxic material from T lymphocytes which destroys host tissues as well as tubercle bacilli. Thereafter, the infection in the primary site usually heals by a combination of resolution, fibrosis, and calcification. Occasionally defenses fail and the infection may overwhelm the host or proceed directly to a chronic stage.

Silent dissemination Early in the course of a new infection tubercle bacilli reach the general circulation in varying numbers. This event is marked only by fever and mild symptoms and is recognized as tuberculosis only when a patient is being observed closely because of recent exposure to tuberculosis. This stage is important in the pathogenesis of tuberculosis, because it is the time when bacilli reach distant sites to establish metastatic foci of infection that are the seeds from which clinical tuberculosis may develop much later.

While bacilli presumably reach all organs during this silent bacillemia, they establish lesions with frequency in only a limited number of sites, which have one feature in common: high tissue oxygen tension. Despite a paucity of ventilation, the apexes of the lungs in the upright position have the highest oxygen tension in the body (130 mmHg) due to a high ventilation-to-perfusion ratio. Probably for this reason they are the most frequent sites in which viable bacilli persist in a dormant state in metastatic (Simon's) foci and produce clinical disease at a later time.

Latent (dormant) infection When a tuberculosis lesion regresses and heals, the infection enters a latent phase in which it may persist without producing illness. Though the infection may remain dormant for life, it may develop into clinical tuberculosis at any time.

Clinical tuberculosis Fibrocaseous tuberculosis may develop from either direct progression of the initial infection or recrudescence of a dormant lesion, most commonly in the apical portion of the lung. An old caseous hilar lymph node occasionally liquefies and spills its contents into a bronchus, to produce a segmental or lobar tuberculous pneumonia. Massive bloodstream invasion (miliary tuberculosis) may also occur at any stage. Tuberculosis is characterized by localized nodular infiltrations, fibrosis, and cavitation.

MANIFESTATIONS

Recent infection

Uncomplicated initial tuberculous infection often produces no significant clinical illness. It is usually diagnosed only when contacts of an infectious case are examined or when it progresses to a serious form of disease. The incubation period is 4 to 8 weeks from inoculation to appearance of mild fever, malaise, and tuberculin hypersensitivity. Symptoms usually subside without specific therapy because of the appearance of adequate specific immunity. Occasionally, however, the infection progresses, either in the lung or by dissemination through the bloodstream. This turn of events is extremely serious unless detected promptly and treated adequately.

Massive hematogenous dissemination is most likely to occur in a recently infected child of three years or younger. In older children infection only rarely progresses to a fatal form and often passes completely unnoticed. The principal danger arises later during adolescence or early adulthood when the infection may undergo late progression.

Initial tuberculous infection occasionally produces pleurisy with effusion, cervical lymphadenitis, miliary tuberculosis, or meningitis. In addition, allergic manifestations occasionally develop, e.g., erythema nodosum and phlyctenular conjunctivitis.

In the United States, 90 to 98 percent of young adults have never been infected with tuberculosis. There have been several "epidemics" of tuberculosis among such susceptible young persons. For example, sailors aboard ship were infected when infectious tuberculosis developed in a shipmate who had been infected years before. Persons working in the Peace Corps, Armed Forces, or State Department who are assigned to countries where the prevalence of tuberculosis is high may be heavily exposed to tuberculosis. As in children, recent tuberculous infection usually produces only mild and nonspecific symptoms, but in the young adult it has a greater tendency to progress to clinical disease. There may be an area of pneumonitis in any portion of the lung, but obvious hilar adenopathy is not common. When a young adult has a pleural effusion or a parenchymal infiltrate in the lung, a tuberculin test should be performed. If the skin test is positive, the possibility of tuberculosis should be considered strongly. The source of infection is usually an adult with cavitary tuberculosis.

Pulmonary tuberculosis

Pulmonary tuberculosis may follow the initial infection directly or after a short or long period of dormancy. Progressive disease has been observed to develop after 60 years of clinical dormancy. The most striking features of late recrudescent tuberculosis are (1) absence of recent exposure to tuberculosis, (2) tendency to chronicity and cavitation, and (3) production of fibrous tissue of repair. The last two phenomena are characteristic of the responses in persons sensitized to tubercle bacilli. While the solid caseation necrosis of the initial stage contains few bacilli, the *liquid* caseum in a tuberculous cavity contains abundant bacilli and may spread infection via bronchi to other portions of the lungs and into the environment.

SYMPTOMS In most instances, the onset of pulmonary tuberculosis is insidious, and the patient may be entirely asymptomatic. Many cases are discovered because a routine roentgenogram is taken upon admission to the hospital for some other illness.

The earliest symptoms are constitutional and probably result chiefly from liberation of lymphokines stimulated by absorption of tuberculoprotein from numerous bacilli in a hypersensitive host. Abdominal symptoms may dominate the clinical picture. Fever is often present in the late afternoon or evening; its only manifestation may be profuse sweating during sleep ("night sweats"). It is common for a patient with tuberculosis to be unaware of a fever as high as 40°C. General malaise may be present, but often there is nothing more than irritability, depression, and excessive fatigue at the end of the day.

Weight loss may precede symptoms but is often passed off as being due to overwork or to voluntary caloric restriction. Often weight is well maintained until late in the course of the illness. When abdominal symptoms predominate, loss of weight may be rapid.

Headache may be noted occasionally, especially in the evening. Palpitation may occur during mild exertion. Menstruation is usually not disturbed until the disease is advanced, when amenorrhea may develop.

Cough is frequent but not invariable and is often passed off as a "cigarette cough." When sputum is produced, it is usually odorless, green or yellow in color, and raised principally upon arising in the morning. Hemoptysis may accompany the cough and usually consists of streaking of the sputum with small amounts of blood. In some patients the onset of pulmonary tuberculosis is relatively sudden, with fever, productive cough, or pleuritic pain suggestive of bacterial pneumonia.

PHYSICAL AND ROENTGEN EXAMINATIONS Early asymptomatic infiltrations due to tuberculosis are usually undetectable by physical examination, even though obvious by x-ray. Crepitant rales may be present, especially when inspiration is preceded by full expiration and a small cough (posttussive rales).

Long-standing tuberculosis with extensive fibrosis causes contraction and distortion of pulmonary tissue and of bronchi. In such instances, a wide variety of physical signs may be present, such as apical dullness and bronchial breath sounds, coarse rales, deviation of the trachea, and diminished mobility of one hemithorax.

Because findings on examination of the lungs in the early stages are so frequently unremarkable, the importance of the chest roentgenogram in the diagnosis of tuberculosis cannot be overemphasized. Of particular importance is the comparison of the x-ray film with one made months or years earlier, so that subtle changes can be detected in clinically dormant lesions. Because fibrous tissue does not change appreciably with time, any change in the lesions on serial films must be interpreted as indicating pathologic activity of some disease. Among 90 patients over the age of fifty with recently developed pulmonary tuberculosis, over 70 percent showed evidence of preexisting tuberculous scars. Comparison of abnormal films with those taken in previous examinations makes it possible to detect and treat tuberculosis before liquefaction has occurred with spread of bacilli to other portions of the lungs or to other persons.

COMPLICATIONS OF PULMONARY TUBERCULOSIS

Cavitation When defense mechanisms fail, tuberculosis produces liquefaction necrosis and cavitation. The liquid material abounds with tubercle bacilli, making the disease highly infectious.

Hemoptysis In the majority of instances of bleeding from the lungs in tuberculosis, the blood arises from ulceration of the bronchial mucosa and presents as streaks of bright red blood on the sputum. Bleeding usually subsides spontaneously if the patient lies quietly. Bleeding from the pulmonary artery is much more serious. While the branches of the pulmonary artery within a tuberculous lesion usually thrombose, occasionally one may remain open, may be eroded by the liquefaction, and form a mycotic (Rasmussen's) aneurysm. This may rupture and cause death from exsanguination or obstruction of airways. The blood expectorated is copious and dark because of unsaturation of hemoglobin.

Pleurisy with effusion A superficial tuberculous lesion may involve the overlying pleura and give rise to "dry" pleurisy, attended by localized pleuritic pain on deep inspiration. Or a small caseous pulmonary focus may actually erode through the visceral pleura and extrude a small amount of liquid caseum. The immune response to such pleural contamination is a vigorous inflammatory reaction with formation of considerable pleural exudate. Although a pleural effusion may develop at any stage of tuberculosis, it is most common within a few months of the initial infection, particularly in young adults (age fifteen to thirty-five years). The fluid is usually clear and light yellow. Its exudative nature is identified by a high protein content (> 3 g per 100 ml), an elevated LDH, a lymphocytic-cell response, and pH <7.20.

The importance of recognizing the tuberculous nature of such a pleural exudate in a young adult is reinforced by the finding that 65 percent of untreated patients sooner or later develop active tuberculosis. The diagnosis must often be clinical, because smears of the pleural fluid rarely reveal tubercle bacilli, and even the culture is positive in only 20 to 25 percent of cases. Percutaneous needle biopsy may reveal granulomatous pleuritis, but organisms are often not demonstrable. Thus, in most instances, proof of tuberculosis is lacking at the time the antituberculous treatment must be given if development of manifest tuberculosis is to be prevented. Fortunately, the intermediate tuberculin skin test is so regularly negative in healthy young adults that a positive reaction in a patient with a lymphocytic pleural exudate constitutes adequate evidence of tuberculous etiology to warrant initiation of two-drug therapy. However, it is not uncommon for the intermediate-strength purified protein derivative (PPD) test to be negative in patients with large tuberculous effusions, probably because of mobilization of the available T lymphocytes in the pleural exudate, leaving too few in the circulation to produce a positive skin reaction. A second-strength PPD will almost always be positive if the effusion is of tuberculous etiology.

Tuberculous pneumonia The onset of tuberculosis occasionally is quite acute, resembling that of bacterial pneumonia. This picture is seen most often in Negroes, persons with diabetes, children with overwhelming infection, and elderly persons in whom the lungs are flooded with bacilli discharged from an area of liquid necrosis in the lung or hilar nodes. Chills, fever, productive cough, pleuritic chest pain, and leukocytosis may be noted. A stained smear of the sputum usually reveals numerous tubercle bacilli.

Bronchopleural fistula and empyema Though minimal pleural contamination from a small superficial caseous focus produces only a clear exudate, massive contamination from rupture of a large caseous lesion produces pneumothorax (bronchopleural fistula) and tuberculous empyema.

This is one of the most dreaded complications of pulmonary tuberculosis. Tubercle bacilli are usually easily found in the purulent exudate. Management is largely surgical and consists of establishing adequate drainage, in combination with the administration of effective antituberculosis drugs.

Tuberculosis of bronchi, trachea, and larynx These organs are all protected from implantation of *M. tuberculosis* by a covering of secreted mucus but may become involved in advanced cavitary pulmonary tuberculosis with excretion of numerous tubercle bacilli. Bronchial ulceration may result in hemoptysis and a localized wheeze during respiration. The bronchial lumen also may be compromised by pressure of enlarged hilar lymph nodes early in the course of infection.

In a patient with cavitary pulmonary tuberculosis, hoarseness and pain in the throat accentuated by swallowing suggest tuberculous laryngitis. The diagnosis can be confirmed by indirect laryngoscopy. It is important to exclude cavitary tuberculosis before a laryngectomy is performed for carcinoma of the larynx, because tuberculous laryngitis is occasionally mistaken for carcinoma, even on histologic examination. Antituberculous chemotherapy is highly effective for tuberculosis of the mucous membranes.

Bronchi which lie within tuberculous lesions are regularly weakened by the inflammatory process and dilated by contraction of fibrous tissue in healing. In the upper lobes this is rarely clinically significant, but in portions of the lung which are dependent when the patient is upright, it may lead to secondary infection, producing chronic productive cough and sporadic hemoptysis (see bronchiectasis, below).

Gastrointestinal tuberculosis The normal gastrointestinal tract is resistant to penetration by tubercle bacilli, but in cavitary pulmonary tuberculosis associated with excretion of large numbers of bacilli, the mucosa may be penetrated in the ileocecal region. The symptoms consist chiefly of intermittent abdominal pain, cramping, and diarrhea. Occasionally the infection spreads through the wall of the intestine, to produce tuberculous peritonitis (see Peritoneum, below).

DIFFERENTIAL DIAGNOSIS The clinical picture presented by pulmonary tuberculosis varies widely and may simulate a great number of other diseases.

Carcinoma of the lung (Chap. 263) Tuberculosis is commonly confused with carcinoma of the lung because the highest incidence of both diseases is in the upper lobes and in older men. Both cause loss of weight, chronic cough, blood-streaked sputum, and mild fever. In addition to bacteriologic studies for tubercle bacilli, sputum cytology, bronchial brushing, and bronchoscopy should be employed to aid in the differentiation. Comparison of prior roentgenograms may be of considerable help, but in many instances nothing short of a diagnostic thoracotomy will serve to make the distinction. When tuberculosis is considered among the diagnostic possibilities, therapy with two antituberculous drugs should be instituted a few days before thoracotomy in order to minimize complications in the event the lesion is tuberculous.

Mycotic infections (Chaps. 169 to 178). Whenever tubercle bacilli cannot be isolated from a patient suspected of having tuberculosis, appropriate tests should be made for the various fungus infections, which may present with a clinical picture indistinguishable from pulmonary tuberculosis. Helpful skin and serologic tests are available for coccidioidomycosis, histoplasmosis and aspergillosis, but blastomycosis, mucormycosis, cryptococcosis, and sporotrichosis can be diagnosed only by demonstrating the organisms in a biopsy specimen or on culture.

Actinomycosis and nocardiosis Although usually referred to as fungus diseases, these infections are actually caused by bacteria. Diagnosis is made by culture.

Sarcoidosis (Chap. 228) The typical patient with sarcoidosis is afebrile and has a negative tuberculin test and a roentgen picture of diffuse pulmonary infiltrations and hilar adenopathy, but the disease is protean in its manifestations and may mimic tuberculosis. Mediastinoscopy with biopsy of lymph nodes or lung biopsy is of greatest value in establishing this diagnosis. The Kveim test may be helpful when the antigen can be obtained.

Aspiration pneumonia, lung abscess (Chap. 259) Pulmonary infection which is introduced by the drainage of contaminated saliva during sleep from a focus of pyorrhea occurs predominantly in the upper and midposterior portions of the lung and can mimic tuberculosis. The distinction can usually be made eventually, but much valuable time may be lost while the patient is treated for the wrong disease. The presence of putrid sputum, hemoptysis, fever, and leukocytosis in a patient who has pyorrhea and has recently undergone surgery or who drinks to excess strongly suggests a pyogenic abscess. If the differentiation cannot be made readily it may be advisable to treat with antimicrobials in addition to antituberculosis medications.

Other forms of pneumonia Bacterial or mycoplasma infection (Chap. 188) may present with clinical and roentgen appearances which at first may be indistinguishable from pulmonary tuberculosis. Cultures, cold agglutinins, precipitin, and complement fixation tests often establish the correct diagnosis. Cavitation is rare, and sputum examination does not yield tubercle bacilli. Early in the course of infection, tuberculosis may present with a localized infiltrate in the lung and slowly subside spontaneously or coincidentally with tetracycline therapy, similar to mycoplasma pneumonia. If clearing is incomplete, tuberculosis should be strongly considered. A tuberculin skin test should be performed in all patients with "viral pneumonia," particularly if a pleural effusion is present, because of its rarity in viral pneumonia. A positive tuberculin skin test in an adolescent or young adult with pneumonitis strongly suggests tuberculosis because of the infrequency of dormant infection in this age group.

Pneumoconiosis Pulmonary infiltrations associated with exposure to silicon dioxide, asbestos, ferrous oxide, and beryllium as well as hypersensitivity reactions to various organic inhalants may present a roentgenographic appearance suggestive of tuberculosis (Chap. 256). Silicosis may present great difficulty in diagnosis because it may produce conglomerate masses and even cavitation that mimic tuberculosis. When the tuberculin skin test is positive in a patient with silicosis, smoldering tuberculosis is so likely that two-drug therapy is indicated if activity is suggested by x-ray, and prophylaxis with isoniazid is justified if there is no evidence of activity.

Bronchiectasis (Chap. 259) A productive cough due to chronic infection in dilated bronchi occurs much less frequently than formerly because of more effective antibiotic therapy for necrotizing pneumonias of childhood and the reduction in the number of children whose bronchi have been damaged by tuberculosis. The lower and middle lobes (or lingula on the left) are most often involved, and a bronchogram effectively demonstrates the pathologic condition. If the tuberculin skin test is positive, isoniazid should be administered prophylactically to prevent late progression of tuberculosis from coexistent foci in apexes, whether or not they are visible radiographically.

Confusion caused by systemic effects of tuberculous infection Because of the insidious nature of tuberculosis, the clinical picture may be mistaken for that produced by several other disorders. Malaise, easy fatigability, inability to concentrate, anorexia, and loss of weight may be mistaken for psychoneurosis. The symptoms may suggest hyperthyroidism or diabetes mellitus, but with a little care the distinction can be made. Tuberculosis should always be considered in the differential diagnosis of fever of unknown origin (Chap. 12). If the roentgenogram reveals a pulmonary infiltrate, the possibility of tuberculosis is increased, but in cases of disseminated or extrapulmonary tuberculosis, the chest roentgenogram may be normal. In these cases biopsy of an enlarged lymph node, bone marrow, or liver may be of help. Formerly, tuberculosis was overdiagnosed in patients presenting with general systemic symptoms. Today, however, because of a lessening awareness of tuberculosis, the principal danger is that tuberculosis will be overlooked. Furthermore, it is important to realize that tuberculosis may appear without reexposure in anyone who has ever been infected in the past.

Tuberculosis of other organs

Localized tuberculous infection may occur in a number of other organs, notably, the lymph nodes, kidney, long bones, genital tract, brain, and meninges. Organisms reach these sites during the silent bacillemia which often occurs early in the infection.

LYMPH NODES The most common involvement of lymph nodes occurs in the hilus draining the pulmonary site of initial infection. The enlargement is usually modest but may be massive and give rise to obstruction and even ulceration of a major bronchus. The prognosis is good with proper chemotherapy, but the nodes may continue to enlarge for a few weeks after therapy is started and then resolve slowly.

CERVICAL ADENITIS (SCROFULA) This disease has become uncommon in the United States as a result of the elimination of tuberculous cattle and pasteurization of milk, but it occasionally occurs early in the course of infection. Cervical lymphadenitis may also appear as a late manifestation, especially in Negroes. The nodes may be large (several centimeters in diameter) and matted together in a mass with an area of soft fluctuation. Signs of acute inflammation are rarely present. Swelling begins insidiously without systemic symptoms. Spontaneous rupture may occur, with drainage of caseous material. In some cases the offending organism is *M. scrofulaceum* or *M. kansasii,* and for this reason culture of the pus is necessary for accurate diagnosis.

KIDNEY Second to the upper lobes of the lungs, the kidney is the most common site for the late appearance of localized tuberculous infection. The mechanism of implantation is the same as that in the pulmonary apexes, namely, by hematogenous spread early in the infection. The oxygen tension in the cortical portion of the kidney approaches that in arterial blood, which enhances the growth and persistence of tubercle bacilli. As in the lungs, foci of tuberculosis may remain dormant for many years and produce clinical disease late in life. The pathologic process is the same as in the lung: inflammation, followed by caseation, liquefaction, and discharge of contaminated material into the collecting system and down the ureter to the bladder and, in the male, to the genital tract.

Symptoms of renal tuberculosis are usually insidious and may be overlooked completely until the appearance of cystitis or epididymitis. Gross or microscopic hematuria and pyuria with a "sterile" urine on culture for bacteria should always call tuberculosis to mind and lead to the performance of a tuberculin skin test and culture of urine for tubercle bacilli. Intravenous pyelography may reveal a cortical cavity communicating with the calyceal system. Therapy consists of a multiple-drug regimen and should be continued for 18 to 24 months. Symptoms usually subside promptly with chemotherapy. Resection of residual areas of destruction is only rarely necessary.

MALE GENITALS Infection of the genital tract in the male is secondary to renal tuberculosis. Bacilli discharged from a caseous lesion in the kidney may reach the seminal vesicles, prostate gland, and epididymis through their connections with the excretory tract. Symptoms begin insidiously, most commonly with scrotal pain due to inflammation of the epididymis and vas deferens. Tenderness and swelling may be found in the vas, seminal vesicles, and/or the prostate gland.

FEMALE GENITALS When tuberculosis infection occurs after puberty, tuberculosis occasionally spreads hematogenously to the highly vascular fallopian tube. Infection may then spread into the uterus and give rise to endometritis. Symptoms are usually mild and of insidious onset, with abdominal pain, white vaginal discharge, metromenorrhagia, and dyspareunia. Systemic symptoms and signs are uncommon, probably because the infection is indolent and localized. The most common manifestation is sterility, but tubal scarring may cause pregnancy to be ectopic. Tuberculosis of the fallopian tube may also spread to the peritoneum and produce either a tuberculous pelvic abscess or generalized peritonitis.

OSSEOUS TUBERCULOSIS Hematogenous spread of tuberculosis to the long bones and vertebrae is most common when infection occurs in childhood, because of the high Po_2 associated with the vascularity at the epiphyseal plates during active bone growth. It usually occurs within 3 years of infection, but dormant lesions may be reactivated by trauma years later. Infection begins in the ends of the long bones but becomes obvious when it involves the adjacent joint: hip, knee, elbow, or wrist. Tenosynovitis is most common at the wrist.

TUBERCULOUS SPONDYLITIS (POTT'S DISEASE) This disease may result from hematogenous seeding or from spread of infection from paravertebral lymph nodes draining a tuberculous pleurisy. Spondylitis may develop in childhood or be delayed until later in life. Localized pain in the back may be present for months before x-rays reveal an abnormality. Though infection begins in the body of a vertebra, the first radiographic sign is usually destruction and narrowing of an intervertebral disk. A paravertebral abscess may be seen as a fusiform density extending the length of several vertebrae and occasionally dissects downward to the inguinal area. Appropriate drainage and orthopedic management must be combined with prolonged multiple-drug chemotherapy.

PERITONEUM The peritoneum may be implanted with tubercle bacilli when they spread by any of at least four routes: (1) through the wall of infected intestine; (2) from a mesenteric lymph node; (3) from an infected fallopian tube; or (4) from hematogenous seeding in the course of disseminated tuberculosis. Symptoms are insidious, with increasing abdominal girth, but ultimately the patient has fever, night sweats, weakness, diarrhea, and abdominal pain. As with other forms of tuberculosis, there is an increased frequency among alcoholics. Tuberculosis should be strongly considered whenever ascitic fluid contains protein in excess of 3 g per 100 ml, elevated LDH, and abundant lymphocytes. Diagnosis may be made by open or percutaneous needle biopsy.

PERICARDIUM Tuberculous infection may spread from the mediastinal lymph nodes or contiguous segments of lung to the pericardium in the same manner as to the pleura. The pathologic process is the same as in tuberculous pleurisy, with outpouring of a clear exudate, formation of granulomas, and subsequent fibrosis. The clinical picture may be that of chronic pericardial tamponade, with hepatomegaly, edema, friction rub, and enlargement of the cardiac shadow during the active phase, and constriction during the phase of fibrosis. When such an illness is accompanied by afternoon fever or night sweats and a positive tuberculin reaction, tuberculosis should be strongly considered. The diagnosis is usually made by study of aspirated fluid or by open pericardial biopsy. A tuberculous effusion contains more than 3 g per 100 ml protein, an elevated LDH, and lymphocytes. Early in the disease, multiple-drug chemotherapy accompanied by corticosteroids is usually sufficient, but surgical resection of the pericardium is occasionally necessary when the process is well established before therapy is begun.

If tuberculous pericarditis has undergone spontaneous healing, the patient may present years later with the picture of constrictive pericarditis (Chap. 246). Pericardiectomy is often desirable at this stage to improve cardiac function but may be technically difficult because of extensive calcification extending into the myocardium.

ADRENALS Occasionally hematogenous tuberculosis localizes in the adrenal glands and may result in their total destruction, giving rise to adrenal cortical insufficiency (Addison's disease, Chap. 93). This must be differentiated from adrenal cortical atrophy, which is more common, and from other causes of adrenal destruction, such as histoplasmosis. Therapy consists of prolonged administration of antituberculosis agents plus physiologic doses of adrenal steroids.

MENINGES Tuberculosis may involve the meninges, either as a part of miliary tuberculosis or as extension of infection from a focus within the brain. In areas with a high incidence of tuberculosis, tuberculous meningitis is seen most commonly in young children during the first year of infection. In areas of low incidence such as the United States, meningitis is more common among older adults as a result of late reactivation of dormant infection. Pathologically, the meninges contain small tubercles and a fibrinous exudate over the base of the brain.

Symptoms consist of headache, restlessness, and irritability, usually accompanied by fever, malaise, night sweats, and loss of weight. Nausea and vomiting may be prominent. Stiffness of the neck and Brudzinski's sign are usually present. Spinal puncture usually reveals increased pressure, clear fluid containing an increased amount of protein, reduced glucose (less than half the blood glucose), and 100 to 1,000 white blood cells per ml, 80 to 95 percent of which are lymphocytes.

The differential diagnosis includes partially treated pyogenic meningitis, fungal meningitis, carcinomatosis or sarcoidosis of the meninges, and subarachnoid hemorrhage. There is considerable urgency in establishing the correct diagnosis because specific therapy is most effective when instituted early in the course of the illness. Irreversible brain damage may result from waiting 6 to 8 weeks for cultural proof of diagnosis. For this reason it is frequently necessary to begin therapy for tuberculosis on the basis of a presumptive clinical diagnosis while awaiting results of bacteriologic studies. Therapy should include isoniazid and rifampin. Steroids are indicated only when there is an impending subarachnoid block or cerebral edema. Intrathecal therapy is not indicated.

INAPPROPRIATE SECRETION OF ANTIDIURETIC HORMONE (ADH) Older persons with tuberculous meningitis or overwhelming pulmonary tuberculosis occasionally present with somnolence or coma associated with a very low serum sodium concentration (110 to 125 meq per liter), because of inappropriate secretion of ADH. This must be distinguished from adrenal insufficiency, in which the sodium serum concentration is also depressed in concert with an elevated serum potassium level. In addition to use of antituberculosis agents, adequate sodium chloride should be administered and water intake restricted.

Disseminated tuberculosis

SILENT BACILLEMIA Hematogenous dissemination of a small number of tubercle bacilli is common early in the course of infection but usually produces little clinical illness. The principal importance of the event is the seeding of bacilli in sites far removed from the pulmonary site of inoculation.

MASSIVE DISSEMINATION (MILIARY TUBERCULOSIS) When a liquid caseous focus empties its contents into a vein, there is a massive dissemination of tubercle bacilli throughout the body. Defense mechanisms are overwhelmed, and tubercles become established in all organs of the body. Without specific therapy, death is almost a certainty.

Miliary tuberculosis is the most dreaded manifestation of tuberculosis. It may arise shortly after infection or from recrudescence of a dormant focus years or decades later. Because the resistance of the body is overwhelmed, lesions are not limited to those organs with an elevated P_{O_2} but are often found in the liver, spleen, bone marrow, and meninges. The best way to make the diagnosis of miliary tuberculosis is to perform a biopsy of the liver, lymph node, or bone marrow in search of caseating granulomas and tubercle bacilli.

Symptoms are usually nonspecific and consist of weight loss, weakness, gastrointestinal disturbance, fever, and sweats. The patient has usually had a course of penicillin or broad-spectrum antibiotics without control of the fever before the diagnosis comes to mind. Cough is not a prominent feature, but dyspnea may be. The correct diagnosis is often not suspected until the typical "miliary" pattern is noted on the chest roentgenogram. The white blood count may be normal or low, or may show a leukemoid pattern suggesting leukemia. There may be a monocytosis. An identical clinical picture can be presented by histoplasmosis, coccidioidomycosis, blastomycosis, cryptococcosis, and other chronic infections. Therefore, it is imperative to obtain any material possible by biopsy or aspiration to establish a correct diagnosis on which to base therapy.

SUBACUTE AND CHRONIC DISSEMINATION Instead of a single massive invasion of the bloodstream, smaller numbers of tubercle bacilli may escape into the circulation intermittently and give rise to a variety of clinical manifestations, including myelophthisic anemia, low-grade fever, lymphadenopathy, effusion into pleural and peritoneal cavities, and splenomegaly. There may be destructive lesions of bones, kidneys, subcutaneous tissue, or skin. Such a clinical picture is most common in elderly persons with recrudescent infection.

The protean manifestations and bizarre clinical picture caused by subacute and chronic forms of hematogenous tuberculosis provide a tremendous diagnostic challenge. To add to the confusion, the tuberculin reaction is often suppressed in persons with overwhelming infection. The intermediate-strength tuberculin test is often negative, and the PPD no. 2 (see Diagnosis, below) occasionally so. The solution to the clinical problem most commonly comes when the possibility of tuberculosis is belatedly considered. Confirmation must be sought from appropriate histologic and bacteriologic studies. Prognosis is uniformly bad without specific therapy, but good with a multiple-drug regimen including INH.

DIAGNOSIS

TUBERCULIN SKIN TEST Tuberculin is a protein fraction of tubercle bacilli. When introduced into the skin of a person with tuberculous infection, whether clinically apparent or dormant, it triggers release of several lymphokines which over the next 24 to 72 h cause a localized thickening of the skin due to edema and accumulation of sensitized lymphocytes. Although there are several methods for testing healthy populations with tuberculin for evidence of unsuspected infection, the method preferred in clinical practice is to inject 0.1 ml of a solution containing 5 tuberculin units (TU) of purified protein derivative stabilized with Tween 80 (5 TU of PPD-T) into the skin of the volar aspect of the forearm with a small needle—an "intermediate-strength tuberculin test." The test is read 48 to 72 h later and is considered positive if the diameter of skin thickening measures 10 mm or more, doubtful if it is 5 to 10 mm, and negative if it is less than 5 mm.

Intermediate-strength PPD produces a positive reaction in the majority of persons infected with tubercle bacilli. However, it is a biologic test which is dependent upon the presence of an adequate number of circulating sensitized T lymphocytes. False negative results may occur in 15 to 20 percent of persons with clinical tuberculosis if sensitized T lymphocytes are temporarily depleted, as in persons who are clinically ill, febrile, or have a large pleural effusion. If the intermediate PPD is negative in a patient in whom tuberculosis is suspected, the test should be repeated using "second-strength" PPD (100 or 250 TU). If this is also negative, tuberculosis can be dismissed with considerable certainty, although persons who are moribund from tuberculosis may fail to react even to PPD no. 2.

A positive reaction to intermediate-strength PPD indicates the presence of a tuberculous infection but does not help in distinguishing clinical from dormant infection. This distinction must be made on clinical, bacteriologic, and radiographic grounds. A positive reaction which is elicited only by PPD no. 2 in a patient who is clinically ill means that active tuberculosis cannot be dismissed as a diagnostic possibility. In healthy persons, however, it usually signifies only healed tuberculosis or infection with one of the other mycobacteria.

RADIOGRAPHY While never providing an etiologic diagnosis, x-rays of the chest provide extremely valuable information. The abnormality which is most suggestive of tuberculosis is a multinodular infiltrate with cavitation in one or both of the upper lobes of the lung. Because of the propensity of tuberculosis to spread via bronchi to other parts of the lungs, the basilar areas may also be involved. Occasionally, especially in the elderly, the lesions are limited to the lower lobe(s). Multiple infiltrates, especially if bilateral, are most suggestive of tuberculosis, because pyogenic pneumonia and primary carcinoma are much more likely to produce single lesions. Carcinoma usually produces a solid lesion, in contrast to the multinodular infiltrate of tuberculosis. Planigrams (laminograms) are particularly valuable in making such distinctions and in detecting cavitation. Lateral, lordotic, and oblique films are also of value in defining the location and character of lesions. Initially tuberculous infection is not usually apical in location but may involve any other segment of the lungs. Hilar adenopathy is common early in the course of infection in children, but may not be obvious by x-ray in adults. Large pleural effusions are easily detected, but for small ones it may be necessary to place the patient on the *involved* side to permit the fluid to be seen along the lateral chest wall (lateral decubitus film).

BACTERIOLOGIC DIAGNOSIS The only absolute proof of active tuberculosis is the cultural identification of *M. tuberculosis* from tissue or body fluid: sputum, gastric washing, urine, cerebrospinal fluid (CSF), serous effusion, or pus from an abscess or sinus. A useful preliminary examination, however, is to make a smear of the material and stain it for standard microscopy or auromine-rhodamine stain for easier detection by fluorescence microscopy. The smear is not a very sensitive method, but it has the virtue of quickly identifying the patient who is discharging great numbers of organisms into the environment. For positive identification, cultures must be made either on solid egg medium (Löwenstein-Jensen) or Middlebrook 7H-11 medium using 20 to 40 mmHg CO_2 to speed growth.

The most commonly examined material is sputum. When it can be produced spontaneously (usually in the early morning), it makes the most satisfactory material for both smear and culture. If none can be produced spontaneously, the patient may be asked to inhale ultrasonically aerosolized water to stimulate production of bronchial secretions. Bacteriologic specimens may also be collected by bronchial washing, bronchial brushing, or tracheal aspiration. Sputum should never be collected over a 24-h period because this increases the frequency of contamination. Guinea pig inoculation is no longer widely used for identification of *M. tuberculosis* because of the economic and technical advantages of the biochemical methods.

When no sputum can be collected, as in young children or senile or psychotic persons, fasting morning gastric contents may be aspirated and cultured. Diagnosis by smear of this material is less reliable than examination of sputum because of the frequency of saprophytic acid-fast bacteria in the stomach, but the presence of large numbers of acid-fast bacilli strongly suggests that they are significant.

Multiple specimens may be needed before the organisms are recovered. This is particularly true early in the course of tuberculous infection, tuberculous pleurisy with effusion, and when the pulmonary lesions are small and noncavitary. Patients with old chronic tuberculous lesions may shed organisms only intermittently.

HEMATOLOGY The white blood cell count is usually not significantly elevated, except in tuberculous pneumonia (when it may suggest a pyogenic infection) and in miliary tuberculosis (when a leukemoid reaction may be mistaken for leukemia). Hemoglobin and hematocrit are usually normal unless a prolonged period of illness has produced anemia of infection.

URINALYSIS There are no specific changes except when a urinary lesion is present. Renal tuberculosis is not rare in older persons; it most often presents with microscopic hematuria and pyuria with negative cultures for pyogens. Two or three early morning specimens should be submitted for culture. About 10 percent of persons with pulmonary tuberculosis excrete bacilli in their urine, even without detectable urinary tract lesions.

OTHER TESTS Despite great efforts to develop one, there is no specific serologic test to distinguish clinical from dormant tuberculosis. Biopsy of the liver, bone marrow, or lymph node can be of great aid in reaching a presumptive diagnosis of disseminated tuberculosis by revealing caseating granulomas and acid-fast bacilli. Such a finding may be lifesaving by permitting initiation of specific therapy without allowing the disease to progress while awaiting culture confirmation.

TREATMENT

Treatment of tuberculosis is based upon intensive and prolonged use of specific bacterial antagonists. If properly managed, tuberculosis can be cured in more than 95 percent of patients, but accompanying diseases often are the limiting factor. Because healing depends upon body defenses aided by specific drug therapy, the total period of therapy is prolonged, i.e., from 18 to 24 months, although a shorter period of very intensive therapy is presently being investigated. With excellent oral drugs, most of the therapy may be accomplished while the patient is ambulatory and even at work.

Principles of therapy

Chemotherapeutic agents owe their effectiveness to specific interference with various vital functions of the microorganisms without harming the host: isoniazid inhibits DNA (deoxyribonucleic acid) synthesis and intermediary metabolism of *M. tuberculosis,* and ethambutol and rifampin interfere with RNA (ribonucleic acid) synthesis. The first principle of therapy is to choose drugs to which the organisms are susceptible. Fortunately, this presents little difficulty in the United States, where the vast majority of new cases are caused by *M. tuberculosis,* which is susceptible to all the major drugs. In a patient who has never been treated before, therapy with two or three drugs may be initiated without awaiting the results of susceptibility studies.

The second principle is always to *inflict multiple "biochemical lesions"* on the bacilli simultaneously at the outset. Even in a population of organisms that is susceptible to a given drug, a naturally resistant mutant occurs in about 100,000 organisms. Cavitary tuberculous lesions frequently contain many times this number of organisms, and thus enough naturally resistant mutants to permit the emergence of clinical resistance to *any single drug.* This can be avoided only by using several drugs in concert at the onset.

The third principle is never simply to add a single drug to a regimen if the regimen appears to be failing.

The fourth is that therapy must be continued long enough to eradicate virtually all the bacilli; with regimens in use at present, this appears to require 18 to 24 months. If therapy is discontinued before this simply because the patient feels well, bacteriologic tests are negative, and the x-ray has shown improvement, the likelihood of treatment failure is great, because of the lag of anatomic healing and eradication of organisms despite these favorable clinical signs.

Lastly, a single peak concentration of drugs is preferred over an attempt to maintain a blood level throughout the day. Where possible, drugs should be given simultaneously in the full daily dose, preferably before breakfast when intestinal absorption is the most rapid.

Major drugs

ISONIAZID This drug is bactericidal and is the most effective antituberculosis drug to date. It is relatively nontoxic and is well accepted by patients because of ease of administration and freedom from annoying side effects. It acts through interference with DNA synthesis and intermediary metabolism of tubercle bacilli. It is acetylated in the liver and excreted by the kidney. Because of its great effectiveness, it should always be included in the original treatment regimen.

Dose The usual dose for adults is 5 mg/kg/day, usually 300 mg, given as a single dose. In children the dosage is higher: 10 to 15 mg/kg/day, because of more rapid excretion. It is safe to use in pregnancy. In infections with *M. kansasii* a dose of 10 mg/kg/day is often recommended because of the incomplete susceptibility of this organism. Although some persons inactivate INH more rapidly than others, this has proved to be of little clinical significance.

Toxicity Although not common, three types of toxicity from INH occur: (1) Direct toxicity consists of peripheral neuropathy and anemia due to competition of INH with pyridoxine. Pyridoxine in a dose of 30 mg per day effectively combats this problem, which is most common when a large dose is used and in alcoholics whose nutrition is impaired. (2) Allergic reactions consist of skin rash, swelling of the tongue and fever and may require withdrawal of the drug. (3) Hepatocellular toxicity is the most serious toxic effect of INH. Contrary to earlier thought, hepatitis is not due to allergy but to a reaction to a metabolic product of INH degradation in the liver. Symptoms consist of malaise and anorexia followed by nausea, vomiting, fever, and finally jaundice. The best way to detect INH hepatitis is to acquaint each patient with the symptoms for which to be alert and ask him to report them without delay. No more than a 1-month supply of INH should be given, and inquiry about symptoms made each time the patient is seen. A suspected reaction must be confirmed by the following procedure: *discontinue INH at once and draw blood for determination of SGOT, alkaline phosphatase, and serum bilirubin.* If these tests are normal or SGOT only mildly elevated, symptoms are likely due to an intercurrent viral infection, and INH therapy may be reinstituted cautiously. If any of the tests show a threefold elevation, INH hepatitis is very likely and the drug should not be restarted. For minor elevations, one should repeat the studies; if they are normal, restart INH, beginning with 50 mg (one-sixth of a 300-mg tablet) and recheck the laboratory results. If the SGOT is again definitely elevated, INH should not be continued. If INH is continued in the face of symptoms of hepatitis, it may prove fatal. The only therapy required is the withdrawal of the drug.

RIFAMPIN (RIFAMPICIN) This bactericidal drug acts by inhibiting RNA polymerase. Emergence of resistance is rapid when the drug is used alone. The dose is about 10 mg/kg/day, or 600 mg, for adults and about 15 mg/kg/day for children, It is not recommended during pregnancy. Toxicity and side effects are mild, although hypersensitivity with thrombocytopenia may develop when it is administered intermittently or resumed after an interruption. It regularly colors the urine and other body fluids a bright orange, and the patient should be told of this in advance. It may suppress immune mechanisms experimentally, but no clinical application for this effect has been found.

ETHAMBUTOL This bacteriostatic drug acts by inhibiting RNA synthesis in *M. tuberculosis.* It has largely replaced PAS in routine treatment because of better acceptance by patients and fewer toxic reactions. Dosage in original treatment should be 15 mg per kg in a single daily dose, but in retreatment the more reliable dose of 25 mg per kg should always be used. It is not recommended for use in pregnancy or in children who are too young to report changes in vision. Toxicity consists of occasional reduction of visual acuity and temporary reduction of color vision (green). Periodic examination of the visual field and acuity along with asking the patient to report any reduction in visual acuity when reading newsprint are recommended when the larger dose is used.

STREPTOMYCIN An aminoglycoside, this drug inhibits protein synthesis in tubercle bacilli. Toxic effects are hearing loss, ataxia, and allergic reactions. Dosage is 1 g per day for adults, but this should be reduced to 0.5 g per day in persons who are over the age of sixty or of very small stature, or when renal impairment is present. In children the dosage is 20 mg/kg/day. Streptomycin is safe during pregnancy. After daily administration or use for 5 days each week, for 2 months, injections may be reduced to twice a week for an additional period of 2 to 4 months if necessary. Slight dizziness and circumoral paresthesias are common immediately after injections but are usually harmless.

CAPREOMYCIN This cyclic peptide is active against *M. tuberculosis.* It is administered intramuscularly in the same dose as streptomycin. Toxic effects are hearing loss, tinnitus, and pain on injection. There is cross-resistance with kanamycin and viomycin but not with streptomycin.

PYRAZINAMIDE The mechanism of action of this drug is unknown, and there is no simple way to determine susceptibility to it in vitro. Nevertheless, pyrazinamide is an effective drug and in combination with streptomycin is considered bactericidal. It is particularly valuable in retreating patients in whom previous therapy has failed and in whom resistance to some of the major drugs has developed. Its toxicity is to the liver, and it regularly causes an elevation of serum uric acid level. It may be given in a single dose of 30 mg per kg daily.

Minor drugs

PARA-AMINOSALICYLIC ACID (PAS OR PAS-C) Although there has been a wide and favorable experience in treatment of tuberculosis with this drug, it has lost favor because other effective agents which produce fewer side effects and allergic reactions are now available. However, it remains a valuable drug in young children and in pregnancy, where there is limited experience with the new drugs. It acts by interfering with intermediary metabolism of the organisms; it potentiates the effects of INH. Side effects consist of anorexia, nausea, vomiting, and diarrhea. Allergic reactions are common, with chills, fever, skin rash, and general malaise, and may preclude continuation of therapy.

CYCLOSERINE This is a drug of modest efficacy as an inhibitor of cell wall synthesis, again principally for use in retreatment problems. Dosage is 500 to 750 mg per day for adults. Neurotoxicity may result in psychotic behavior or generalized seizures, both of which are largely prevented by pyridoxine in a dosage of 100 to 200 mg per day in divided doses.

ETHIONAMIDE This drug inhibits protein synthesis and is of value in retreatment cases. Its use is limited by its gastric irritation. Dosage is 750 to 1,000 mg per day in adults and should be given in divided doses.

AMINOGLYCOSIDES Kanamycin and viomycin are injectable agents of limited effectiveness but useful in retreatment of resistant cases.

THIOCETAZONE, ISOXYL These drugs are in common use in developing countries, because of moderate effectiveness and low cost, but are not available for use in the United States because of excessive toxicity.

Choice of therapy for clinical tuberculosis

Chemotherapy of tuberculosis is the same regardless of the organ involved. The immediate goal is to halt replication of all tubercle bacilli simultaneously. In cavitary tuberculosis or tuberculous pneumonia, where tubercle bacilli may number 1×10^6 to 10^9, a significant number of naturally resistant mutants to any antituberculosis drug can be assumed to be present. Doubly resistant mutants are very unlikely, however. Therefore, therapy should be given with two bactericidal drugs or a combination of one bactericidal and two bacteriostatic drugs to ensure that no resistant mutants will be permitted to multiply. The long-term goal is to eradicate the tubercle bacilli from the host. Because antituberculous drugs are effective against only replicating bacilli, and tubercle bacilli may replicate quite infrequently, prolonged therapy is necessary to achieve this goal. While the exact time to achieve this end is not known, it appears that 18 to 24 months of uninterrupted therapy is necessary with regimens currently in use.

When the immediate goal of sharp reduction in the bacillary population has been achieved, the risk from drug-resistant mutants is markedly reduced. This point in clinically effective chemotherapy usually occurs within 6 to 12 months and can be recognized by consistently negative cultures and achievement of stability in the radiographic appearance. At that time it is safe to withdraw one or two of the drugs, continuing therapy with isoniazid alone for a total of 18 to 24 months.

Other modalities, once stressed in the treatment of tuberculosis, are of little importance. Bed rest or reduced activity is required only during the period of clinical illness. Thereafter the patient should be encouraged to return quickly to full activity, unless contraindicated by other conditions. Surgery is almost never necessary if the patient cooperates with chemotherapy, except when there is massive hemoptysis, empyema, bronchopleural fistula, or, rarely, a persistent cavity associated with organisms which are resistant to several of the most effective drugs. Surgery in tuberculosis today is largely limited to lung biopsy or resection for undiagnosed pulmonary lesions.

ORIGINAL TREATMENT Isoniazid and rifampin are the most potent bactericidal drugs available against tuberculosis and together constitute the most effective therapeutic regimen for initial treatment. The combination of isoniazid, ethambutol, and streptomycin, followed by isoniazid and ethambutol when sputum smears are negative, is also highly effective. If streptomycin and pyrazinamide are given together, they should be considered as equivalent to one bactericidal drug, and another drug, such as INH or rifampin, should also be given. With any of these regimens one can expect 95 percent of patients to become culture-negative within 3 to 12 months. After 6 to 8 months of negative cultures therapy may be continued for the total of 18 to 24 months with a single drug, such as isoniazid. However, if a patient is slow to convert to a negative culture or has other diseases which may compromise his immune system, two drugs should be continued for the entire period. Results of several short-course regimens of therapy using rifampin-isoniazid were reported at the International Tuberculosis Conference in Mexico City (September 1975). By utilizing these two bactericidal agents simultaneously, it was possible to eliminate the bacterial population from the host more quickly, and 6 to 9 months of therapy appeared adequate to cure 95 percent of even advanced cases of tuberculosis. Furthermore, after a short period of daily administration of RIF 600 mg and INH 300 mg (2 to 4 weeks), effective therapy could be achieved by continuing with twice-weekly administration of RIF 600 mg and INH 900 mg for a like period, thus reducing the expense of rifampin therapy considerably. While experience with this regimen has been extensive in Asia, South America, and Africa, it is just being put into use in the United States.

It is no longer necessary to hospitalize most patients with tuberculosis, and those who are hospitalized may be discharged as soon as clinical illness has abated, a response to treatment is evident, and provisions for outpatient care have been assured. Effective chemotherapy reduces infectiousness promptly even though the sputum smear is still positive for tubercle bacilli. For home therapy to be successful, the patient must comprehend enough of the nature of his disease and the importance of chemotherapy to assure his cooperation. Irregularity in taking medication and premature discontinuance when symptoms subside are the major dangers. The booklet *Understanding Tuberculosis Today,* by W. W. Stead, Central Press, Milwaukee, 1975, available from most local affiliates of the American Lung Association, explains tuberculosis and its therapy in terms most patients can comprehend.

It is imperative that ambulatory treatment not result in inferior medical care. Patients on chemotherapy should be seen weekly for bacteriologic examination until the smears are negative and monthly thereafter at least until cultures are negative. Thereafter, the interval can usually be lengthened to every 4 to 6 weeks during the first 6 months and less often thereafter. Such a program of supervision will ensure early detection of treatment failure, permitting a change in therapy to achieve a favorable result. After the course of chemotherapy has been completed, the patient should be asked to submit two bacteriologic specimens at 6-month intervals for a year and can be released from supervision if they are negative.

RETREATMENT OF "RESISTANT CASES" Failure of initial treatment may result from an inadequate use of drugs at the outset or from premature discontinuance of medication. The skill required to manage a retreatment case is much greater than for initial therapy, and advice should always be sought from a physician who is skilled in this aspect of tuberculosis. *Retreatment does not mean the addition of a drug to a regimen that has failed.* It must always involve the use of three or more drugs which the patient has not received before. Where the patient has received several drugs in the past, it may be necessary to await the results of in vitro susceptibility tests before instituting therapy. The drugs employed must be given in maximum tolerated dosage, and for this reason it is advisable for therapy to be supervised closely.

CORTICOSTEROIDS The use of cortisone and its derivatives has been shown to increase the chance of recrudescence of dormant tuberculosis. Despite this, in patients who are very seriously ill with tuberculosis, these agents may be lifesaving. They should be used only when there is an immediate threat to life, such as hypotension, debilitating fever, dyspnea, or an impending blockage of the subarachnoid space in tuberculous meningitis. Prednisone may be used in a dosage of 40 mg per day for 1 to 2 weeks, then 20 mg for another 8 weeks, and then gradually withdrawn over a period of 3 to 4 weeks in order to prevent a "steroid rebound." The effect upon the temperature and the general well-being of the patient may be dramatic, but there is no decrease in residual fibrosis. In general, the frequency of side effects makes the routine use of steroids in conjunction with chemotherapy unwise.

PREVENTION OF TUBERCULOSIS

Chemoprophylaxis

Clinically inapparent tuberculous infection can be prevented from developing into tuberculosis by judicious use of isoniazid therapy both in recently infected persons and in those with a dormant infection.

RECENTLY INFECTED PERSONS Close contacts of an infectious case of tuberculosis should be tested with tuberculin. Hospital and nursing home personnel should be tested at the time of employment and after each identified exposure, but no less frequently than annually. Any reactor with detectable disease or symptoms should be examined bacteriologically and given treatment with two drugs as outlined earlier. Newly infected persons with normal chest x-rays should be given preventive treatment with isoniazid. The risk of development of clinical tuberculosis in such persons is appreciable (see Prevalence and Incidence above) and greatly exceeds the risk of toxicity from isoniazid.

Close contacts of an infectious case who are under the age of four years are at special risk and should be started on therapy even though the tuberculin test is negative and they appear well. If in 3 months the skin test is still negative, therapy may be discontinued; if positive, it should be continued for a full year.

PERSONS WITH DORMANT INFECTIONS Dormant tuberculous infection may be prevented from developing into clinical disease by treatment with isoniazid. Treatment is generally recommended for reactors under the age of 35 years and especially for those under 25. Over the age of 35 the risk of hepatitis from isoniazid is increased, and preventive therapy is recommended for reactors of unknown duration only if one of the following factors that increases the risk of tuberculosis is present: (1) radiographically detectable apical scars (Simon's foci) suggestive of healed tuberculosis, (2) diabetes mellitus, (3) prolonged steroid therapy, (4) history of gastrectomy, (5) silicosis, (6) any chronic malignancy, such as Hodgkin's disease.

Preventive therapy consists of isoniazid, 300 mg for adults and 5 to 10 mg per kg for children given in a single daily dose for 12 months. Preventive therapy reduces the risk of clinical tuberculosis by about 80 percent, and protection appears to be lasting. While no other drug has been demonstrated effective in prevention of tuberculosis, it seems likely that rifampin would be.

Toxic reactions to isoniazid are uncommon below age thirty-five, but thereafter may be as high as 2.3 percent. They need not be serious if early symptoms are heeded and the medication stopped promptly, as outlined earlier. The booklet *Understanding Tuberculosis Today,* mentioned above can help patients understand the risk of tuberculosis and the rationale for prophylactic chemotherapy.

Biologic prophylaxis

BCG VACCINE BCG, or bacillus Calmette-Guerin, is a live, attenuated strain of bovine tubercle bacilli which has been used widely in many countries to induce specific immunity against tuberculosis. Although it does not reduce the chance of natural infection, it does prevent the development of serious forms of tuberculosis when natural infection occurs. There has been controversy on the effectiveness of BCG, but most authorities agree that it affords about 80 percent protection against the development of clinical tuberculosis. Its greatest value is in infants in countries with high prevalence where exposure of children is common. In the United States vaccination is indicated only for nonreactors who cannot avoid exposure, as when assigned to countries of high prevalence in the Peace Corps, State Department, Armed Forces, etc.

Eradication of tuberculosis

The decline in mortality rates from tuberculosis early in the century led some to predict the eradication of the disease in the United States by 1945. This prediction was based on the idea that infection with tubercle bacilli was harmless and that only reinfections were dangerous. It was reasoned that tuberculosis would disappear when reinfections could be prevented by isolating all infectious cases. It is now clear, however, that clinical tuberculosis developed largely from reactivation of dormant infections and that eradication must await the natural disappearance of tubercle bacilli from the population. It is hoped that this process can be accelerated by the judicious use of INH as prophylactic therapy, but clinical tuberculosis will continue to occur for many years.

Implications of a positive tuberculin reaction

In the United States, the chance of a tuberculin reactor developing clinical tuberculosis from a dormant infection is greater than that of a nonreactor acquiring an infection. Therefore, it is preferable to be tuberculin-negative, unless the positive reaction is induced by vaccination. On the other hand, a non-reactor exposed to tuberculosis in a country of high prevalence would be more likely to become infected than a healthy reactor, and it would be preferable then to be tuberculin-positive, particularly if the positive reaction was induced by vaccination.

REFERENCES

BATES JS: Treatment of tuberculosis. Adv Intern Med 20:1, 1975

——, STEAD WW: Effect of chemotherapy on infectiousness of tuberculosis. Editorial. N Engl J Med 290:459, 1974

COMSTOCK GW, EDWARDS PQ: The competing risks of tuberculosis and hepatitis for adult tuberculin reactors. Am Rev Resp Dis 111:573, 1975

FOX W, MITCHISON DA: Short-course chemotherapy for pulmonary tuberculosis. Am Rev Resp Dis 111:325, 1975

JOHNSTON RF, WILDRICK KH: The impact of chemotherapy on the care of patients with tuberculosis. Am Rev Resp Dis 109: 636, 1974

PAGEL W et al: *Pulmonary Tuberculosis,* London: Oxford, 1964

SINGAPORE TUBERCULOSIS SERVICE/BRITISH MEDICAL RESEARCH COUNCIL: Controlled trial of intermittent regimens of Rifampicin plus Isoniazid for pulmonary tuberculosis in Singapore. Lancet 2:1105, 1975

STEAD WW: Pathogenesis of the sporadic case of tuberculosis. N Engl J Med 277:1008, 1967

——: *Tuberculosis and Atypical Mycobacterioses, Current Therapy,* 25th ed., ed H Conn, Philadelphia: Saunders, 1973, p. 146

——, BATES JH: Evidence of "silent" bacillemia in primary tuberculosis. Ann Intern Med 74:559, 1971

——, ——: Isoniazid hepatitis. A backlash of progress. Ann Intern Med 79:125, 1973

—— et al: The clinical spectrum of primary tuberculosis in adults: Confusion with reinfection in the pathogenesis of chronic tuberculosis. Ann Intern Med 68:731, 1968

YOUMANS GP: Relationship between delayed hypersensitivity and immunity in tuberculosis. Am Rev Dis 111:109, 1975

162 LEPROSY

CHARLES C. SHEPARD

DEFINITION Leprosy (Hansen's disease) is a chronic granulomatous infection of man, which, in its various clinical forms, attacks superficial tissues, especially the skin, peripheral nerves, and nasal mucosa. The two major clinical types are *lepromatous* and *tuberculoid*; when the disease has features of both these types, it is called *borderline*. In addition, an early indeterminate form is seen, which may later develop into one of the three types mentioned.

ETIOLOGY *Mycobacterium leprae*, or Hansen's bacillus, is the causal agent of leprosy. It is an acid-fast rod, found in enormous numbers in lepromatous lesions. Although it has not been cultivated in artificial media, nor convincingly in tissue cultures, it can be propagated in cooler tissues of small rodents, very consistently in the foot pads of mice. The bacillus will also produce heavy systemic infections in a proportion of nine-banded armadillos; armadillos have a lower body temperature. The bacillus multiplies very slowly, so mouse experiments take 6 to 12 months and armadillo experiments take several years. The mouse model has been used much for the study of antileprosy drugs, and the high bacterial yield from armadillos will make many immunologic studies possible. Estimates of bacillary viability can be made microscopically by determination of the "solid ratio" or "morphologic index"; only viable bacilli are thought to stain solidly.

Lepromin is a suspension of killed *M. leprae* prepared from the tissues of lepromatous patients. Intradermal injection elicits, somewhat irregularly, a tuberculin-like reaction at 48 h (Fernandez' reaction) and more consistently, a papular reaction at 4 weeks (Mitsuda's reaction). The Mitsuda reaction is usually positive in tuberculoid patients and negative in lepromatous patients and is therefore an aid in clinical classification. However, because it is also positive in nearly all normal adults, it has no diagnostic value.

EPIDEMIOLOGY At present, there are probably 10 to 20 million persons affected with leprosy in the world. The disease is more common in tropical countries, in many of which 1 to 2 percent or more of the population is affected. It is also common in certain regions with cooler climates, such as Korea, China, and central Mexico. In the United States the chief leprosy areas are Texas, California, Hawaii, Louisiana, Florida, and New York. Some of the cases are acquired domestically, some are acquired abroad.

Leprosy is frequently a family infection. Many patients give a history of prolonged exposure, and in close family contacts (spouse-spouse) of untreated lepromatous patients the attack rate is 5 to 10 percent. Among young children of untreated lepromatous parents, 30 to 50 percent develop a mild, single-lesion type of leprosy which heals spontaneously. After the index case is under treatment, spread within the family apparently does not occur. Transmission from patients with tuberculoid leprosy is uncommon. The portal of entry is a matter of conjecture, but it is probably either the skin or the nasal mucosa. The chief portal of exit is thought to be the nasal mucosa of lepromatous patients.

The incubation period is frequently 3 to 5 years, but it has been reported to range from 6 months to several decades.

CLINICOPATHOLOGIC CLASSIFICATION As is true of other chronic infections, such as syphilis and tuberculosis, the manifestations of leprosy are many and variable. The classification now in general use is based on clinical findings, histopathologic changes, and the lepromin test.

Lepromatous leprosy is one of the polar forms. The involvement is extensive, diffuse, and bilaterally symmetrical. Histologically, there is a diffuse granulomatous reaction with macrophages, large foam (Virchow's) cells, and many intracellular bacilli, frequently in spheroidal masses (globi). The lepromin reaction is negative.

Tuberculoid leprosy is the other polar type. Skin lesions are single or few and are sharply demarcated. Neurologic involvement is relatively pronounced and may be severe. The histologic picture consists of lymphocytes, epithelioid cells, and perhaps giant cells, and bacilli are few and sometimes difficult to demonstrate. The lepromin reaction is usually positive.

Borderline, or *dimorphous*, leprosy is a form in which the clinical features and histologic changes are a combination of the two polar types. The disease may shift toward the lepromatous or the tuberculoid form. Change of either polar type to the other is exceedingly rare.

In all forms of leprosy peripheral nerve involvement is a constant feature. In any histologic section involvement of nerves will tend to be more severe than involvement of other tissues, and in some sections the nerves may be the only tissues involved.

PATHOGENESIS *Mycobacterium leprae* probably enters the body through the skin or nasal mucosa. The early stages of infection have not been described accurately. In lepromatous leprosy bacillemia is frequent and often so profuse that the organisms can be seen in stained smears of peripheral blood. Even in the most advanced lepromatous cases, destructive lesions are limited to the skin, peripheral nerves, anterior portion of the eye, upper respiratory passages above the larynx, testes, and structures of the hands and feet. The probable reason for the predilection of the disease for these tissues is that they are all usually several degrees cooler than 37°C. Two sites of preferential involvement are the ulnar nerves near the elbow and the peroneal nerves where they pass around the head of the fibula; above and below these levels where these nerves take deeper courses, they are much less severely involved. In mice that have been experimentally infected in the foot pads, bacillary multiplication is maximal when the mice are kept at air temperatures at which the foot pad tissues are about 30°C; this is also the usual temperature of the most severely involved tissues of human beings. In patients with lepromatous leprosy, collections of bacilli are also found in the liver, spleen, and bone marrow, but these are probably scavenged from the blood.

A profound lack of cellular immunity for *M. leprae* in lepromatous leprosy is indicated by the histology and by the negative lepromin reaction. Further evidence comes from observations that lepromatous patients' lymphocytes fail to react in vitro to *M. leprae* antigens either with a mitogenic response or by the formation of migration inhibitory factor (MIF). Under the same in vitro conditions the lymphocytes of tuberculoid patients react positively. Moreover, many normal persons exposed to leprosy give positive reactions, indicating the presence of subclinical infections. In addition to this depressed specific cellular immunity for *M. leprae*, lepromatous patients frequently have a partial depression of cellular immunity in general. They have been shown to be deficient in the ability to develop delayed hypersensitivity, their lymphocyte transformation response is weak, and the paracortical areas of their lymph nodes are deficient in lymphocytes. Furthermore, mice that have been rendered T-cell deficient by thymectomy and irradiation followed by bone marrow replacement respond to inoculations of *M. leprae* by developing heavier infections. For these reasons, lepromatous leprosy is thought to be the result of a poor immune response, and tuberculoid leprosy the result of a stronger immune response, but whether these differences in immune state precede the infection or are caused by it is not clear.

CLINICAL MANIFESTATIONS Early leprosy The first signs of leprosy are usually cutaneous. One or more hypopigmented or hyperpigmented macules or plaques may be seen. Often an anesthetic or paresthetic patch is the first symptom noted by the patient, but on careful examination skin involvement can also be found. When contacts are being examined, a single skin lesion is often noted, especially in children; usually, this is a hypesthetic macule that may clear in a year or two without treatment, but specific treatment is usually recommended.

Tuberculoid leprosy Early tuberculoid leprosy is frequently manifested by a hypopigmented macule, sharply demarcated and hypesthetic. Later the lesions are larger, and the margins are elevated and circinate or gyrate. There is peripheral spread and central healing. The lesions appear singly or are few in number and are not symmetrical. Nerve involvement occurs early, and the nerves leading from the lesions may be enlarged. The larger peripheral nerves may be palpably and visibly enlarged, especially the ulnar, peroneal, and greater auricular nerves. There may be severe neuritic pain. Neural involvement leads to muscle atrophy, especially of the small muscles of the hand. Contractures of the hand and foot drop are frequent. Trauma, especially from burns and splinters and from excessive pressure, leads to secondary infection of the hands and to plantar ulcers. Later, resorption and loss of phalanges is frequent. When the facial nerves are involved, there may be lagophthalmos, exposure keratitis, and corneal ulceration leading to blindness.

Lepromatous leprosy The skin lesions are macules, nodules, or papules. The macules are often hypopigmented. The borders of the lesions are not sharp, and the centers of raised lesions are convex (rather than concave as in tuberculoid disease). There is also diffuse infiltration between the lesions. The sites of predilection are the face (cheeks, nose, brows), ears, wrists, elbows, buttocks, and knees. Involvement with infiltration and little or no nodulation may progress so subtly that the disease goes unnoticed. Loss of the eyebrows, especially the lateral portions, is common. Much later the skin of the face and forehead becomes thickened and corrugated (leonine facies), and the earlobes become pendulous.

Nasal symptoms (nasal "stuffiness," epistaxis, and obstructed breathing) are common early symptoms. Complete nasal obstruction, then laryngitis and hoarseness, are also frequent. Septal perforation and nasal collapse lead to saddlenose.

In adult males infiltration and scarring of the testes lead to sterility. Gynecomastia is common. Invasion of the anterior portion of the eye leads to keratitis and iridocyclitis. Painless inguinal and axillary lymphadenopathy occurs.

Neurologic involvement, of the same type as that seen in tuberculoid disease, is less prominent in the lepromatous form. A diffuse hypesthesia involving the peripheral portions of the extremities is common in advanced lepromatous disease.

Reactional states The general course of leprosy is indolent but it may be interrupted by two types of reaction, which tend to complicate chemotherapy.

Erythema nodosum leprosum (ENL) occurs in lepromatous patients, most frequently toward the end of the first year of treatment. Tender, inflamed subcutaneous nodules develop, usually in crops. Each nodule lasts a week or two, but more develop. ENL may last only a week or two, or it may continue for long periods. Low-grade fever accompanies severe ENL, and lymphadenopathy and arthralgias may appear. Even in untreated patients with ENL the bacilli have greatly reduced viability, as indicated by low infectivity for mice and by low "solid ratios." Histologically, ENL is characterized by polymorphonuclear infiltration and deposits of IgG and complement; hence, it resembles an Arthus reaction.

Borderline reaction is seen in borderline patients, more often during treatment. Existing skin lesions develop erythema and swelling, and new lesions may appear. An early influx of lymphocytes is followed by edema and a shift toward tuberculoid histology. Cellular immunity increases. Borderline reactions can be differentiated from frank progression, such as occurs when drug-resistant bacilli appear, by mouse inoculations to test bacillary viability and by histologic studies.

The *Lucio phenomenon* is limited to patients with a diffuse nonnodular lepromatous disease; it is seen more often in Mexico and Central America. Arteritis leads to ulceration of the skin, in a characteristic angular shape, and subsequently to angular thin scars.

Complications The crippling that follows involvement of the peripheral nerves has been mentioned. Leprosy is probably the most frequent cause of crippling of the hand in the world. Blindness also is common.

Amyloidosis is a complication of severe lepromatous disease in the United States but is less common in many other countries.

Patients with leprosy are said to be likely to develop other chronic infections. Tuberculosis is the chief cause of death in many leprosariums.

DIAGNOSIS The demonstration of acid-fast bacilli in the skin smears made by the scraped-incision method is strong evidence for leprosy, but in tuberculoid disease bacilli may be too few for demonstration. Wherever possible, a skin biopsy specimen confined to the affected area should be sent to a dermatopathologist knowledgeable in leprosy. The histologic involvement of peripheral nerves is pathognomonic.

The lepromin reaction has no diagnostic value. No diagnostic blood changes occur. Lepromatous patients frequently have mild anemia, elevated erythrocyte sedimentation rate, and hyperglobulinemia. From 10 to 40 percent of lepromatous patients have false positive serologic tests for syphilis.

The combination of a chronic skin disease and peripheral nerve involvement should always lead to the consideration of leprosy.

The differential diagnosis includes conditions such as lupus erythematosus, lupus vulgaris, sarcoidosis, yaws, dermal leishmaniasis, and a host of banal skin diseases. The skin lesions of leprosy, especially of tuberculoid disease, are characterized by hypesthesia, however, and peripheral nerve involvement can always be demonstrated. Peripheral neuropathy from other causes and syringomyelia may be confused with leprosy.

TREATMENT The treatment of leprosy is largely in the hands of specialists, and hospitalization is advantageous for the first few months while the treatment is being established.

Specific chemotherapy Dapsone (4,4′-diaminodiphenylsulfone, DDS, diaphenylsulfone) is effective and inexpensive. Oral treatment is begun with small doses that are raised during the first few weeks to a maintenance dose of about 50 mg a day in adults. In a few months enough bacilli are killed to render mouse inoculations negative. However, in lepromatous disease nonviable bacilli in large numbers (and a few viable bacilli) persist for many years, and treatment should be continued for 6 to 10 years after the bacilli are no longer demonstrable in skin smears. In tuberculoid disease, especially in the milder cases, treatment is often discontinued after the disease has been rendered clinically inactive for 1 to 3 years. Regularly scheduled follow-up is needed to detect possible relapses of lepromatous cases.

If dapsone is given in the dosage mentioned, toxicity is rare. Dermatitis and hepatitis occur. With higher doses, anemia and methemoglobinemia are seen regularly.

Other sulfones, such as sulfoxone or Sulphetrone, are still used occasionally. Use of acedapsone (DADDS), a repository sulfone given only five times a year, is under extensive study.

Sulfone resistance has been demonstrated in mice on isolates from patients who are unresponsive after many years of sulfone therapy. In these patients the initial response was apparently favorable, but in many of them treatment was interrupted or irregular. After 5 to 20 or more years there is clinical and bacteriological relapse in spite of adequate therapy. The frequency of sulfone resistance is 2 to 8 percent, depending on the initial sulfone given. It is lowest with initial dapsone therapy. Patients with sulfone-resistant bacilli are best treated with rifampin or clofazimine (B663).

The clinical response to adequate therapy is gradual, and the picture may be confused by reactional conditions. However, the basic disease ceases to progress and the skin lesions gradually improve. Recovery from neurologic impairment is limited.

Among nonsulfone drugs that have been recommended in leprosy are thiambutosine, Etisul, and ethionamide. When used alone, they are less effective than dapsone. Rifampin has recently been found to be much more rapidly bactericidal than dapsone, at least initially. Because of its cost, it will probably not be used continuously for years, in the way dapsone has. Combinations of short courses of rifampin with continuous dapsone or acedapsone for as long as is needed, as described above, are under trial.

Treatment of reactional states Moderate ENL is managed by antipyretics and analgesics. If severe, it can be treated with corticosteroids or ACTH; the dosage is adjusted to alleviate severe distress but not to eliminate all signs of reaction. Sulfone therapy should be continued, if necessary in reduced dosage. In the past some leprologists have discontinued sulfone therapy at the first signs of ENL, but most now feel that such action is not warranted because it allows bacillary multiplication. Corticosteroid therapy promotes the viability of *M. leprae* in mice not given antileprosy drugs. Thalidomide is the most effective drug and in appropriate dosage can completely suppress ENL. Because of its teratogenicity, however, its use is severely restricted, and it can be used only when its administration can be strictly controlled.

Borderline reactions, if severe, can be controlled with corticosteroids. They do not respond to thalidomide.

Other measures Many of the deformities and disabilities of leprosy are preventable through proper attention from the beginning of treatment. Plantar ulcers, which are very common, may be prevented by rigid-soled footwear or walking plaster casts, and contractures of the hand may be prevented by physical therapy and application of casts. Reconstructive surgery is frequently necessary. Nerve and tendon transplants and release of contractures can give patients much more functional ability. Vocational retraining is often necessary for those with permanent disability. Plastic repair of facial deformities assists acceptance of patients in society. The psychologic trauma which resulted from prolonged segregation is now minimized by permitting patients to continue therapy at home as soon as possible.

CONTROL Early detection and treatment of the disease, which prevent the further development of deformities and simplify sulfone therapy, can be aided by education of physicians and laity in endemic areas. Because the disease is best treated by specialists, the establishment of clinics is helpful. Regular and complete skin examination of family contacts is essential. Field trials of BCG vaccination in endemic areas have shown contradictory results. Chemoprophylaxis with low dosages of dapsone or with acedapsone injections should be considered for family contacts and groups with high attack rates. Removal of patients from their families and normal environment is probably not necessary, unless the patient fails to cooperate with his therapeutic program.

REFERENCES

COCHRANE RG, DAVEY TF (eds): *Leprosy in Theory and Practice*, 2d ed., Baltimore: Williams & Wilkins, 1964

FASAL P: A primer in leprosy. Cutis 7:525, 1971

Immunological problems in leprosy research. 1. Bull WHO 48:345, and 483, 1973

Morbidity and Mortality Weekly Report: Leprosy—United States, Puerto Rico, May 28, 1976

RIDLEY DS, JOPLING WH: Classification of leprosy according to immunity. A five-group system. Int J Lepr 34:255, 1966

SHEPARD CC: The first decade in experimental leprosy. Bull WHO 44:821, 1971

WHO Expert Committee on Leprosy: Fourth report. WHO Tech. Rept. Ser. 459, 1970

163
OTHER MYCOBACTERIAL INFECTIONS

CHARLES C. SHEPARD

The two most important human mycobacterial pathogens are *Mycobacterium tuberculosis* and *M. leprae*, but morphologically similar acid-fast bacteria are widely distributed in nature as saprophytes and as pathogens of lower animals. In addition, a number of other mycobacteria are known to cause human disease, chiefly chronic cutaneous disease, pulmonary disease, or lymphadenitis. Sometimes in the past, these other human mycobacterial pathogens have been called "atypical mycobacteria" or other confusing terms, but numerical taxonomic studies now show that, as is the case with other microbial pathogens, individual species cause particular diseases and that sometimes several species cause very similar diseases (Table 163-1).

SKIN INFECTIONS Mycobacterium marinum (balnei, "swimming pool" or "fishtank" bacillus) This acid-fast organism inhabits swimming pools, aquaria (saltwater and freshwater), and natural bodies of water that are usually brackish or saline. From contaminated swimming pools, it gains entry through human epidermis through cutaneous abrasions from rough concrete; from aquaria, through cuts; and from fish, through cuts and wounds. A few weeks later nodules develop at the site; they may become verrucous, or they may ulcerate and enlarge to form superficial granulation tissue. The involved area is usually not extensive. In another form, new lesions form centrally from the initial site. The lesions usually remain minor and regress after a year or two, but they may last for years. *Mycobacterium marinum* grows optimally at 25 to 35°C and poorly, if at all, at 37°. This temperature range probably accounts for the lack of systemic spread; regional lymph nodes remain uninvolved unless secondary pyogenic infection occurs.

The diagnosis is made by culturing the organism, usually from biopsy material, at appropriate temperatures. Although it grows slowly on primary isolation, on transfer it grows more rapidly. Histologically, a chronic granuloma with epithelioid and giant cells and sometimes with caseous necrosis is seen. Acid-fast bacteria may be difficult to observe. Many, but not all, patients become tuberculin-positive.

If chemotherapy is needed, ethambutol and rifampin are indicated. Tests for antibiotic sensitivity are helpful.

Prevention of swimming pool outbreaks requires disinfection of the pool. The pool may need to be reconstructed to eliminate rough concrete surfaces.

Mycobacterium ulcerans The ulcers caused by the organism are known by several local names, such as Bairnsdale, Kaferiku, and Buruli, but they are best designated by the name of the organism, since local differences are trivial. The characteristic disease is extensive granulomatous ulceration that destroys subcutaneous tissue down to the muscle or fascia and extends peripherally under an undermined edge. The extensor surfaces of arms or legs are most often affected, but the trunk may be involved. Histologically, necrosis is prominent, and epithelialization extends under the overhanging margins. Systemic invasion does not occur, although new lesions may develop at distant sites. In its natural course, the lesion starts as a local swelling which then ulcerates; it may heal spontaneously or persist for many years with extensive ulceration and contractures. Originally observed in Southern Australia, the disease has since been described in Central Africa, Southeast Asia, and tropical America. Recently, large outbreaks have been described near swamps in Uganda. While a soil habitat is the suspected source, the organism has not been isolated from soil.

Mycobacterium ulcerans grows optimally at 30 to 33°C and poorly, if at all, at 37°C. It grows very slowly even at optimal temperature, and colonies require 7 weeks to grow. Inoculation of mouse foot pads may be helpful in isolation.

Treatment is best carried out with surgical extirpation of necrotic tissue and overlapping margins of the ulcer, followed by skin grafting. Although experimental results indicate that clofazimine and rifampin are active against the organism, chemotherapy seems not to be beneficial in human disease.

PULMONARY INFECTIONS Several mycobacterial species other than *M. tuberculosis* can cause chronic progressive pulmonary disease with cavitation and fibrosis closely resembling pulmonary tuberculosis.

Etiology The species are listed in Table 163-1. *Mycobacterium avium* and *M. intracellulare* are closely related organisms, sometimes difficult to differentiate, and best spoken of as a complex. Cultures have been isolated from soil and from animals, especially chickens, but the source of infection is not established. Cultures of *M. kansasii* have been isolated from the environment. *Mycobacterium xenopi* was first isolated from a toad. *Mycobacterium szulgai* is the most recently recognized species, and all cultures have originated from human disease. *Mycobacterium scrofulaceum* needs to be differentiated from *M. gordonae*, also scotochromogenic and commonly found in soil and water. The *M. fortuitum-chelonei* complex includes *M. abscessus* as a subspecies of *M. chelonei*.

Since similar species may be isolated from normal sputum and the identification of the several species is often carried out in reference laboratories, the etiologic diagnosis may be delayed. However, isolation of the suspect culture from repeated specimens and the presence of multiple (more than 10) colonies in the primary cultures are strong evidence that the organism has an etiologic role.

Epidemiology The mode of transmission of all these pulmonary infections is unsettled. There is cross-sensitization between antigens of the tubercle bacillus and other mycobacteria, but sensitization to the etiologic organism is greater. Comparative tests with antigens from *M. avium-intracellulare* and tuberculin indicate that many healthy individuals in the southeastern United States have been infected by organisms of this group, and in this area chronic pulmonary disease that is not caused by *M. tuberculosis* is often caused by *M. avium-intracellulare*. In Texas and Chicago *M. kansasii* is a more frequent causative agent than *M. avium-intracellulare*. The proportion of new cases caused by mycobacteria other than *M. tuberculosis* varies from 2 to 15 percent and is expected to increase as the number of infections due to *M. tuberculosis* decreases. In contrast to tuberculosis, multiple cases in the same family are very rare, and isolation of the patient is not necessary. In terms of frequency *M. avium-intracellulare* and *M. kansasii* are much the most important, followed by *M. scrofulaceum*. Infections with other species are rare.

Manifestations The symptoms and signs are those of pulmonary tuberculosis (Chap. 161), although there is some tendency for most of the infections to be more indolent. Infections with *M. avium-intracellulare* are more frequent in older adults and in men. Underlying chronic obstructive pulmonary disease is often present in infections due to *M. avium-intracellulare, M. scrofulaceum*, and *M.*

TABLE 163-1
Human mycobacterial pathogens other than *M. tuberculosis* and *M. leprae*

Mycobacterium	*Pigmentation of culture**	*Usual site of disease*	*Usual source of infection*	*Response to drugs*
M. marinum	P	Skin	Swimming pools, aquaria, fish	Good
M. ulcerans	N	Skin	Tropical environment	Variable
M. avium-intracellulare	N	Lungs	Environment, animals?	Poor
M. kansasii	P	Lungs	Environment?	Good
M. xenopi	S	Lungs	Water, animals?	Variable
M. szulgai	S†	Lungs	?	Good
M. scrofulaceum	S	Lungs, lymph nodes	Water, soil	Poor
M. fortuitum-chelonei	N	Lungs, skin (abscesses)	Soil, dirt	Poor

* *P = photochromogenic (develops yellow-orange pigment only when exposed to light). N = nonpigmented. S = scotochromogenic (develops yellow-orange pigment in dark light).*
† *Scotochromogenic at 37°, photochromogenic at 25°C.*

fortuitum-chelonei, and is sometimes present with the other mycobacteria. Extrapulmonary lesions are rare.

Treatment Rational chemotherapy depends upon identification of the etiologic mycobacterium and determination of its drug sensitivity. *Mycobacterium kansasii* infections usually respond well to intensive triple drug therapy with rifampin and a pair selected from isoniazid, ethambutol, and streptomycin. *Mycobacterium avium-intracellulare* infections are often resistant to chemotherapy. Treatment with four drugs chosen from isoniazid, rifampin, ethambutol, ethionamide, and streptomycin (or capreomycin or kanamycin) is recommended, along with appropriate surgery for unclosed cavities. Infections with *M. scrofulaceum* also are often resistant to drugs, and therapy is the same as for *M. avium-intracellulare*. Infections with *M. szulgai* have responded well to chemotherapy, but the others have been difficult to treat.

OTHER INFECTIONS *Mycobacterium scrofulaceum* causes lymphadenitis in children, especially of the nodes draining the buccal mucous membrane. Excision of the node before it has ruptured or drained is the treatment of choice. The *M. fortuitum-chelonei* complex causes local abscesses, particularly from injections given with contaminated needles or syringes; cervical cellulitis also occurs, with the site of entry probably the mouth. *M. fortuitum* has also been incriminated in infections of the sternum following open heart surgery. *Mycobacterium kansasii* and *M. scrofulaceum* can cause disease of bones and joints. Widely disseminated, usually fatal infections with any of these mycobacteria can occur, especially in immunosuppressed patients.

REFERENCES

Barker DJP: Epidemiology of *Mycobacterium ulcerans* infections. Trans R Soc Trop Med Hyg 67:43, 1973

Jolly HW Jr., Seabury JH: Infections with *Mycobacterium marinum*. Arch Dermatol 106:32, 1972

Kubica GP: Differential identification of mycobacteria. VII. Key features for identification of clinically significant mycobacteria. Am Rev Resp Dis 107:9, 1973

Lincoln EM, Gilbert LA: Disease in children due to mycobacteria other than *Mycobacterium tuberculosis*. Am Rev Resp Dis 105:683, 1972

Wolinsky E: Nontuberculous mycobacterial infections of man. Med Clin N Am 58:639, 1974

Zeligman I: *Mycobacterium marinum* granuloma. Arch Dermatol 106:26, 1972

section 10 | Spirochetal diseases

164 SYPHILIS

KING K. HOLMES

The great ailment of modern syphilological practice is a lack of comprehension of the why and wherefore, rather than the what to do.
J. H. Stokes

DEFINITION Syphilis is a chronic systemic infection caused by *Treponema pallidum*, is usually sexually transmitted, and is characterized by an incubation period averaging 3 weeks, followed by a primary lesion associated with regional lymphadenopathy; a secondary bacteremic stage associated with generalized mucocutaneous lesions and generalized lymphadenopathy; a latent period of subclinical infection lasting many years; and, in 30 to 50 percent of untreated cases, a tertiary stage characterized by progressive destructive mucocutaneous musculoskeletal or parenchymal lesions, aortitis, or central nervous system disease.

ETIOLOGY The discovery of *Treponema pallidum* in syphilitic material was made by Schaudinn and Hoffman in 1905. *Treponema pallidum* is one of the many spiral-shaped microorganisms which propel themselves by spinning around their longitudinal axis. The spiral organisms of medical significance, the Treponemataceae, includes three groups which are pathogenic for man and for a variety of other animals: the *Leptospira*, which cause human leptospirosis; the *Borrelia*, including *B. recurrentis* and *B. vincentii*, which cause relapsing fever and Vincent's angina, respectively; and the *Treponema*, responsible for the diseases known as treponematoses. The *Treponema* include *T. pallidum; T. pertenue*, and *T. carateum*, the organisms which cause yaws and pinta (Chap. 165); and *T. cuniculi*, the cause of rabbit syphilis. Other treponema include nonpathogenic species found in the human mouth and several species of anaerobic saprophytic genital treponemes of low pathogenicity which often coexist with anaerobic gram-negative rods in ulcerative genital lesions (so-called "fusospirochetal" infections). These can also be confused with *T. pallidum* on dark-field examination by inexperienced individuals.

Treponema pallidum is a thin, delicate organism with 6 to 14 spirals and tapered ends, measuring 6 to 15 μm in total length and 0.2 μm in width. The cytoplasm is surrounded by a trilaminar cytoplasmic membrane, which in turn is surrounded by a delicate inner mucopeptide layer, the periplast, thought to be composed of alternating molecules of *N*-acetyl glucosamine and *N*-acetyl muramic acid, and which provides some structural rigidity, while an outer lipoprotein membrane is selectively permeable and osmotically sensitive. The unique spiral structure of *T. pallidum* is maintained by six fibrils, three arising at each end of the organism, which wind around the cell body in a groove between the inner cell wall and the outer cell membrane, and may be the contractile elements responsible for motility. None of the four pathogenic treponemes has yet been cultured in vitro, and no convincing morphologic, antigenic, or metabolic differences between them have been discerned. They are distinguished primarily according to the clinical syndrome they produce. Limited animal inoculation studies also indicate some differences in host range and virulence. However, variation in virulence even among different strains of *T. pallidum* has also been noted. The only known natural hosts for pathogenic treponema are man, higher apes, and rabbits, but all warm-blooded animals so far tested can be successfully infected with *T. pallidum*. Lesions can be regularly produced in rabbits, and virulent strains of *T. pallidum* are usually maintained in that species.

HISTORY The first clear descriptions of syphilis were recorded at the end of the fifteenth century, when a pandemic known as the great pox, as distinguished from smallpox, swept over Europe and Asia. Severe morbidity or death often occurred during the secondary stage, indicating an unexplained virulence then which is almost unknown today, except in congenital syphilis. The source of the European pandemic 500 years ago is controversial. The sudden appearance and high morbidity of syphilis in 1494 led to the theory of the importation of a highly virulent strain of *Treponema pallidum* from America. However, many historians discern earlier references to syphilis in various writings dating from Hippocrates.

The sexual mode of transmission of syphilis was recognized early during the European pandemic, and description of the three cutaneous stages of the disease followed. The major cardiovascular and neurologic complications of late syphilis were recognized during the eighteenth and nineteenth centuries. However, the erroneous concept that gonorrhea, chancroid, and syphilis were produced by the same organism was strengthened by John Hunter, who developed syphilis following self-inoculation with gonorrheal pus in 1767. These three diseases were finally distinguished by Ricord and his students in the mid-1800s.

A rapid series of important advances began in 1903 with the successful inoculation of syphilis into primates by Metchnikoff and Rowe. The discovery of *Treponema pallidum* in serum from secondary lesions was made by Schaudinn in 1905 and was confirmed by Landsteiner by dark-field microscopy in 1906. In 1910, Wasserman introduced the complement fixation test for the diagnosis of syphilis, and in the same year, Ehrlich and Hata introduced an arsenic derivative, arsphenamine (Compound 606, Salvarsan), which was effective in treatment.

EPIDEMIOLOGY Nearly all cases of syphilis are now acquired by sexual contact with infectious lesions (i.e., the chancre, mucous patch, or condyloma latum). Uncommon modes of transmission include nonsexual personal contact, contact with contaminated fomites, or infection *in utero* or following blood transfusions.

In the United States, infant deaths due to syphilis, and new admissions of patients with syphilitic psychoses, have fallen by 98 to 99 percent since 1940. The total reported number of cases of late and late latent syphilis has fallen almost every year since 1943. The 40 cases per 100,000 population reported in 1974 represent a decrease of 91 percent since 1943. Only 1,334 cases of congenital syphilis were reported in 1974—a decrease of 92 percent since 1941. The number of new cases of infectious syphilis reached a peak in 1947, then fell steadily to about 6,000 in 1957, but then began to increase again.

Although the reported incidence of syphilis is nearly 20 times as great in nonwhites as in whites, and is higher in urban than in rural areas, these differences partly reflect the fact that indigent urban nonwhites are treated at public clinics, where case reporting is complete. The case rates of early syphilis are highest in the South and in the Coastal states, and in those Central states with large urban populations. The peak incidence of syphilis, like that of gonorrhea, occurs in the age group twenty to twenty-four, followed by ages twenty-five to twenty-nine, then fifteen to nineteen years. In the United States, the male/female ratio of reported early cases (<1 year) has increased from 0.8:1 in 1950 to 2:1 in 1975. In England the ratio is 6:1.

Of all men with primary, secondary, or early latent syphilis interviewed in the United States during 1974, 38 percent were homosexual or bisexual. Primary syphilis is usually not diagnosed in women or in homosexual men. For example, during 1974 in the United States, 42 percent of cases of early syphilis in heterosexual men were detected in the primary stage, whereas only 23 percent of early cases in homosexual men and 11 percent of early cases in women were detected in the primary stage. Anorectal chancres make up over 50 percent of primary syphilis among homosexuals examined in venereology clinics in the United Kingdom, but only 15 percent of primary syphilis among homosexuals examined in the United States. This remarkable difference suggests either a greater reticence of physicians in the United States to examine the anal canal or failure to consider syphilis in the evaluation of anal lesions in men.

In 1975, there were 25,746 cases of primary and secondary syphilis and 26,166 cases of early latent syphilis reported, and the number of unreported cases was several times greater. Comparison of reported case rates of primary and secondary syphilis in the United States with those in England shows that the rates per 100,000 persons between ages twenty and twenty-four were 3.6 times higher for males and 6.1 times higher for females in the United States than in England. The actual difference in case rates between the United States and England is undoubtedly greater, because most cases of syphilis in England are treated by venereologists and reported, whereas most cases in the United States are seen by physicians in private practice and many are not reported. The higher case rates in the United States may be partly attributable to inadequate tracing of sexual contacts of unreported cases.

Interviews of patients with early syphilis disclose an average of three sexual contacts at risk per patient, and "cluster" tracing of additional associates of the patient or his contacts discloses others who are also at risk. Approximately one of two individuals named as contacts of infectious syphilis becomes infected. Many contacts will have already developed manifestations of syphilis when they are first seen, and about 30 percent of apparently uninfected contacts of infectious syphilis who are examined within 30 days of exposure will actually be in the incubation stage and will themselves go on to develop infectious syphilis if not treated. Because of this, the identification and "epidemiologic" treatment of all recently exposed contacts has become an important aspect of syphilis control. Also important is the identification of syphilitics by routine serologic testing of premarital applicants, pregnant females, blood donors, hospital admissions, military inductees, and persons undergoing examination in physicians' offices. Of 40,000,000 blood specimens examined during 1974 in the United States, 1,200,000 tests were reactive, representing untreated syphilis, previously treated syphilis, or false positive tests. Of all reported early syphilis cases of less than 1 year's duration, 57 percent of cases in men and 79 percent of cases in women were detected as a direct result of either contact tracing or serologic testing. Syphilis is under control in some states in which new cases are limited to sporadic outbreaks which tend to involve homosexual men and are contained by aggressive contact tracing.

NATURAL COURSE AND PATHOGENESIS OF UNTREATED SYPHILIS *Treponema pallidum* can rapidly penetrate intact mucous membranes or abraded skin and within a few hours enters the lymphatics and blood to produce systemic infection and metastatic foci long before the appearance of a primary lesion. Thus, blood from a patient with incubating syphilis is infectious. The median incubation period is 21 days but may vary from 10 to 90 days. The generation time of *T. pallidum* in man is 30 to 33 h, and the incubation period of syphilis is inversely proportional to the number of organisms inoculated. The concentration of treponemes generally reaches 10^7 per g tissue before the appearance of a clinical lesion. In experimental infection in rabbits or man, a single treponeme can initiate infection which leads to a discernible lesion only after many weeks, although histopathologic changes are evident earlier, while intradermal injection of 10^7 organisms usually produces a lesion within 72 h.

The primary lesion appears at the site of inoculation, persists for 2 to 6 weeks, and then heals spontaneously. Histopathology of primary lesions shows perivascular infiltration, chiefly by plasma cells and histiocytes, capillary proliferation, and eventually obliteration of small blood vessels. At this time *T. pallidum* is demonstrable in the chancre in spaces between epithelial cells as well as within invaginations or phagosomes of epithelial cells, fibroblasts, plasma cells, and the endothelial cells of small capillaries, within lymphatic channels, and in the regional lymph nodes. Macrophages and polymorphonuclear leukocytes can be seen taking up treponemes into phagocytic vacuoles where the organisms are destroyed.

The generalized parenchymal, constitutional, and mucocutaneous manifestations of secondary syphilis usually appear about 6 weeks after healing of the chancre, although the secondary rash may appear while the chancre is still present, or only after several months have passed. Secondary maculopapular skin lesions show histopathologic features of hyperkeratosis of the epidermis, capillary proliferation with endothelial swelling in the superficial corium, and dermal papillae with transmigration of polymorphonuclear leukocytes, and in the deeper corium, perivascular infiltration by plasma cells. Treponemes are found in many tissues including the aqueous humor of the eye and the cerebrospinal fluid. Cerebrospinal fluid abnormalities are detected in as many as 40 to 50 percent of patients during the secondary stage. Immune complex-induced glomerulonephritis occurs. Generalized lymphadenopathy is present and is characterized by marked follicular hyperplasia, with histiocytic infiltration and lymphocyte depletion of the paracortical areas, where treponema are present in greatest numbers. The reason for the paradoxical appearance of secondary manifestations in the face of high titers of humoral antibody (including immobilizing antibody) to *T. pallidum* is unknown. The secondary rash subsides within 2 to 6 weeks, and the patient enters the latent stage, which is detectable only by serologic testing. Approximately 25 percent of untreated patients experience one or more subsequent generalized or localized mucocutaneous relapses at some time during the first two to four years after infection. Since 90 percent of such infectious relapses occur during the first year, identification and examination of sexual contacts is most important for patients with syphilis of less than 1 year's duration. However, in the International Classification of Diseases, latent syphilis is arbitrarily divided into early latent (less than 2 years' duration) and late latent (over 2 years' duration) stages. About one-third of patients with untreated latent syphilis develop clinically apparent tertiary disease. The most common type of tertiary disease is the gumma, a usually benign granulomatous lesion. The remaining tertiary lesions are caused by obliterative small-vessel endarteritis which usually involves the vasa vasorum of the ascending aorta and less often the central nervous system. Factors which determine development of tertiary disease are unknown, except that trauma may predispose to gumma.

The course of untreated syphilis has been studied retrospectively in a group of nearly 2,000 patients with primary or secondary syphilis diagnosed clinically, before the darkfield and Wasserman tests came into use (the *Oslo Study*, 1891–1951); and prospectively in 431 Negro men with seropositive latent syphilis of three or more year's duration (the *Tuskegee Study*, 1932–1972).

In the Oslo Study, 24 percent of the patients developed relapsing secondary lesions within 4 years, and 28 percent eventually developed one or more manifestations of late syphilis. Cardiovascular syphilis, including aortitis, was detected in 10.4 percent, with no cases occurring in those infected before age 15; symptomatic neurosyphilis occurred in 6.5 percent, and 16 percent developed benign tertiary syphilis (gumma of the skin, mucous membranes, and skeleton). Syphilis was the primary cause of death in 15.1 percent of males and 8.3 percent of the females. However, many patients alive when the Oslo Study was completed remained at risk for developing complications, while tuberculosis and other infections prematurely eliminated others before complications of syphilis occurred, so the Oslo figures probably represent minimum estimates of the risk of late complications. Cardiovascular syphilis was found in 35 percent of men and 22 percent of women who eventually underwent autopsy. In general, serious late complications were nearly twice as common in men as in women.

The Tuskegee Study showed that the death rate of syphilitic Negro men, 25 to 50 years of age, was 17 percent greater than in nonsyphilitics, and 30 percent of all deaths were attributable to cardiovascular or central nervous system syphilis. By far the most important factor in increased mortality was cardiovascular syphilis. Anatomic evidence of aortitis was found in 40 to 60 percent of autopsied syphilitics (versus 15 percent of controls), while central nervous system lues was found in only 4 percent. Hypertension was also increased in the syphilitics. Thus, the incidence of cardiovascular syphilis was higher and central nervous system syphilis lower in the prospective Tuskegee Study, as compared with the Oslo Study.

MANIFESTATIONS Primary syphilis The typical primary chancre usually begins as a single painless papule which rapidly becomes eroded and usually, but not always, is indurated, with a characteristic cartilaginous consistency on palpation of the edge and base of the ulcer. Histologic examination of the ulcer shows mononuclear and histocytic infiltrates with obliterative endarteritis and periarteritis of small vessels. *Treponema pallidum* is seen by electron microscopy to lie in interstitial perivascular spaces and within invaginations or phagosomes of neutrophils, macrophages, endothelial cells, and plasma cells.

The chancre is usually located on the anal canal, usually within view if the buttocks are spread, or on the external genitalia, but it may occur on any site on the body. Primary sites which are commonly overlooked include the cervix and mouth of the female and the perianal area, anal canal, and mouth of the male homosexual. Regional lymphadenopathy accompanies the primary lesion, appearing within 1 week of the onset of the lesion. The nodes are firm, nonsuppurative, and painless. Inguinal lymphadenopathy is bilateral. The chancre heals within 4 to 6 weeks (range 2 to 12 weeks), but the lymphadenopathy may persist for months.

Atypical primary lesions are common. The clinical appearance depends upon the number of treponemes inoculated and upon the preinfection immune status of the patient. A large inoculum produces a dark-field positive ulcerative lesion in nonimmune human volunteers, but in individuals with a previous history of syphilis produces either a small dark-field negative papule, an asymptomatic but seropositive latent infection, or no response at all. A small inoculum usually produces only a papular lesion, even in nonimmune humans. Thus, syphilis should be considered even in the evaluation of trivial or atypical, dark-field negative, genital lesions. The most common genital lesions which must be differentiated from primary syphilis include traumatic, superinfected lesions, genital *Herpesvirus hominis* type II infection (Chap. 206), and chancroid (Chap. 143). *Primary genital herpes* may produce inguinal adenopathy but is initially characterized by multiple painful vesicles which later ulcerate, and with systemic symptoms including fever; *recurrent genital herpes* typically begins with a cluster of painful vesicles without associated adenopathy. *Chancroid* produces painful, superficial exudative, nonindurated, usually multiple ulcers; adenopathy is either unilateral or bilateral, tender, and may suppurate.

Secondary syphilis The manifestations of the secondary stage are protean but usually include symmetric mucocutaneous lesions and generalized nontender lymphadenopathy. The remnant of the healing primary chancre is still present in many cases. The skin rash consists of macular, papular, papulosquamous, and occasionally pustular syphilides, often with one or more forms present simultaneously. Initial lesions are bilaterally symmetric, pale red or pink, nonpruritic, discrete, round macules, 5 to 10 mm in diameter, distributed on the trunk and proximal extremities. After 1 to 2 months, red, papular lesions 3 to 10 mm in diameter also appear. These may progress to necrotic (pustular) lesions in association with increasing endarteritis and perivascular mononuclear infiltration. These lesions are distributed widely and may occur on the palms, soles, face, and scalp. Tiny papular *follicular syphilides* involving hair follicles may result in patchy alopecia and loss of eyebrows or beard. Progressive endarteritis obliterans and ischemia result in superficial scaling of papules (*papulosquamous syphilides*) and eventually may lead to central necrosis (*pustular syphilide*). In warm, moist, intertriginous areas, including the perianal area, vulva, scrotum, and inner thighs, axillas, and the skin under pendulous breasts, papules enlarge and become eroded, to produce broad, moist, pink or gray-white highly infectious lesions called *condyloma lata.* Superficial mucosal erosions, called *mucous patches,* occur in about a third of patients and may involve lips, oral mucosa, tongue, palate, pharynx, vulva and vagina, glans penis, or inner prepuce. The typical mucous patch is a silver-gray erosion surrounded by a red periphery and is usually painless.

During relapses of secondary syphilis, condyloma lata are particularly common, and skin lesions tend to be asymmetrically distributed and more infiltrated, resembling skin lesions of late syphilis, perhaps reflecting increasing cellular immunity.

Constitutional symptoms which may accompany secondary syphilis include fever, weight loss, malaise, and anorexia. Headache and meningismus are common. Acute meningitis occurs in only 1 to 2 percent of patients, but increased cells and protein have been found in the cerebrospinal fluid in 5 percent or more of patients. *Treponema pallidum* has also been recovered by rabbit inoculation from cerebrospinal fluid during secondary syphilis even in the absence of other cerebrospinal fluid abnormalities.

Other less common complications described in secondary syphilis include hepatitis, nephropathy, arthritis and periostitis, and iridocyclitis. It is uncertain whether the association between secondary syphilis and hepatitis is causal or coincidental. *Syphilitic hepatitis* is distinguished by an unusually high serum alkaline phosphatase and by a nonspecific histologic appearance which is unlike viral hepatitis and includes moderate inflammation with polymorphonuclear leukocytes and lymphocytes, some hepatocellular damage, and no cholestasis. The *renal involvement* is associated with proteinuria, an acute nephrotic syndrome, or rarely with hemorrhagic glomerulonephritis, and which is characterized by subepithelial electron-dense deposits and glomerular immune complexes, suggesting that this complication is a form of immune complex glomerulonephritis. Anterior uveitis has been reported in 5 to 10 percent of patients with secondary syphilis, and *T. pallidum* can be demonstrated in the aqueous humor in such cases. Posterior uveitis occurs rarely.

Latent syphilis A diagnosis of latent syphilis is established by the finding of a positive specific treponemal antibody test for syphilis, together with a normal cerebrospinal fluid examination, the absence of clinical manifestations of syphilis on physical examination and chest films, and a history of primary or secondary lesions, history of exposure to syphilis, or delivery of an infant with congenital syphilis. *Early latent* syphilis encompasses the first 2 years after infection, during which relapse of mucocutaneous lesions may occur, while *late latent* syphilis, beginning 2 years after infection, in the untreated patient, is associated with immunity to infectious relapse and with resistance to reinfection. *Treponema pallidum* may still intermittently seed the bloodstream during this stage, pregnant women with latent syphilis may infect the fetus in utero, and transfusion syphilis has been transmitted from patients with latent syphilis of many years' duration. Until recently it was thought that untreated late latent syphilis had three possible outcomes: (1) It could persist throughout the life of the infected individual; (2) it could end in development of late syphilis; (3) it could end with spontaneous cure of infection, with reversion of serologic tests to negative. It is now apparent, however, that the more sensitive antitreponemal antibody tests rarely if ever become negative. Thus, 50 to 70 percent of untreated patients with latent syphilis never develop clinically evident late syphilis, but the occurrence of spontaneous cure is in doubt.

Late syphilis The onset of slowly progressive inflammatory disease of the aorta or central nervous system begins early during latent syphilis. Pathogenic studies have shown evidence of early syphilitic aortitis soon after the secondary lesions subside, while asymptomatic neurosyphilis can be detected readily during life by CSF examination.

ASYMPTOMATIC NEUROSYPHILIS In patients with untreated latent syphilis, if the cerebrospinal fluid (CSF) is normal 2 years or more after infection, there is probably no future risk of subsequent development of neurosyphilis, except for the purely vascular type. The diagnosis of asymptomatic neurosyphilis is made in patients with no clinical manifestations of neurosyphilis who have cerebrospinal fluid abnormalities, including pleocytosis, elevated protein, or positive cerebrospinal fluid Wasserman or Venereal Disease Research Laboratory (VDRL) test. One or more of these findings are present in 20 to 30 percent of patients with untreated syphilis after 2 years. The risk of progression to symptomatic neurosyphilis is two or three times greater in Caucasians than in Negroes and is twice as common in men as in women. The risk of parenchymal neurosyphilis (tabes dorsalis or general paresis) is five times greater in men than in women, supposedly because pregnancy after the initial infection somehow protects women from parenchymal neurosyphilis. In patients with untreated asymptomatic neurosyphilis, the overall cumulative probability of progression to clinical neurosyphilis is about 20 percent in the first 10 years, but increases with passing time, and is highest in those who show the greatest degree of pleocytosis or protein elevation. The fluorescent treponemal antibody (FTA) test on undiluted cerebrospinal fluid has been found to be reactive far more often than the VDRL test in cases of latent syphilis. The prognosis of patients with a positive CSF-FTA test without other cerebrospinal fluid abnormalities is not known, but very likely this finding merely represents passive transfer of serum antibody into the CSF, not asymptomatic neurosyphilis. Similarly, the finding of a positive CSF-FTA test without other cerebrospinal fluid abnormalities in patients with a positive serum FTA-ABS (fluorescent treponemal antibody-absorption) associated with nonspecific neurologic findings does not necessarily prove a diagnosis of "atypical" neurosyphilis. However, a therapeutic trial of penicillin in doses adequate for neurosyphilis is warranted in any patient with a positive serum treponemal antibody test who also has unexplained neurologic findings.

SYMPTOMATIC NEUROSYPHILIS The risk of neurosyphilis is two or three times greater in Caucasians than in Negroes, and is twice as common in men as in women. Although mixed features are common, the major clinical categories of symptomatic neurosyphilis include meningovascular and parenchymatous syphilis. The latter category includes general paresis and tabes dorsalis. The average interval from infection to onset of symptoms is 5 to 10 years for meningovascular syphilis, 20 years for general paresis, and 25 to 30 years for tabes dorsalis. However, many patients with symptomatic neurosyphilis do not present a classic picture, but have mixed or incomplete syndromes. *Meningovascular syphilis* is associated with inflammation of the pia and arachnoid, together with evidence of focal or widespread cerebrovascular disease or often only with pupillary or reflex changes. The manifestations of *general paresis* reflect widespread parenchymal damage and include abnormalities corresponding to the mnemonic "paresis": *p*ersonality, *a*ffect, *r*eflexes (hyperactive), *e*ye (e.g., Argyll Robertson pupils), *s*ensorium (illusions, delusions, hallucinations), *i*ntellect (decreased recent memory orientation, calculations, judgment, insight), and *s*peech. *Tabes dorsalis* presents symptoms and signs of demyelinization of the posterior columns, dorsal roots, and dorsal root ganglia. Symptoms include ataxic, wide-based gait and footslap, paresthesias, bladder disturbances, impotence, and signs including areflexia, loss of position, deep pain, and temperature sensation. Trophic joint degeneration (Charcot's joints) and perforating ulceration of the feet may result from loss of pain sensation. The Argyll Robertson pupil, seen in both tabes dorsalis and paresis, is a small, irregular pupil which reacts to accommodation but not to light. *Optic atrophy* also occurs frequently in association with tabes.

CARDIOVASCULAR SYPHILIS Cardiovascular manifestations are limited to the large vessels in which the blood supply is provided by vasa vasorum. Endarteritis obliterans of the vasa vasorum produces medial necrosis with destruction of elastic tissue, particularly in the ascending and transverse segments of the aortic arch, resulting in uncomplicated aortitis, aortic regurgitation, saccular aneurysm, or coronary ostial stenosis. These complications do not occur following congenital syphilis or syphilis acquired before age fourteen, indicating some unexplained resistance of the large blood vessels in youth to invasion by *T. pallidum.* The onset of symptoms occurs from 10 to 40 years after infection. Cardiovascular complications are commoner and occur at an earlier age in men than in women, and in Negroes than in Caucasians. The incidence of symptomatic cardiovascular complications in late untreated syphilis is approximately 10 percent, with aortic regurgitation being two to four times as common as aneurysm. However, syphilitic aortitis can be demonstrated at autopsy in about one-half of Negro males with untreated syphilis.

Asymptomatic syphilitic aortitis may be suspected in life if linear calcification of the ascending aorta is demonstrated on chest x-ray films, since arteriosclerotic disease seldom produces this sign. Aortic dilatation and a tambour quality of the sound of aortic closure are unreliable signs of aortitis. Syphilitic aneurysms are usually saccular, occasionally fusiform, and do not lead to dissection. Approximately 1 in 10 aortic aneurysms of syphilitic origin may involve the abdominal aorta, but tend to occur above the renal arteries, whereas arteriosclerotic abdominal aneurysms usually are found below the renal arteries. The nervous system is also affected in 40 percent of patients with cardiovascular syphilis.

LATE LESIONS OF THE EYES Iritis associated with pain, photophobia, and dimness of vision or chorioretinitis occurs not only during secondary syphilis, but also as a relatively common manifestation of late syphilis. Adhesions of the iris to the anterior lens may produce a fixed pupil, not to be confused with Argyll Robertson pupil.

LATE BENIGN SYPHILIS (GUMMA) Gummas may be multiple or diffuse, but are usually solitary lesions which range from microscopic size to several centimeters in diameter, and histologically consist of nonspecific granulomatous inflammation with central necrosis surrounded by mononuclear, epithelioid, and fibroblastic cells, occasional giant cells, and perivasculitis. Although *T. pallidum* cannot be demonstrated microscopically, it can be recovered from the lesions by rabbit inoculation. The most commonly involved sites are the skin and skeletal systems, mouth and upper respiratory tract, larynx, liver, and stomach. Virtually any organ may be involved. Gummas of skin produce painless nodular, papulosquamous, or ulcerative lesions, which are indurated, and form characteristic circles or arcs, with peripheral hyperpigmentation. The lesions are usually indolent, and may heal spontaneously with scarring, but may also be explosive in onset and are often destructive. These lesions may resemble many other chronic granulomatous conditions, including *tuberculosis* and *sarcoidosis* of skin, leprosy, and *deep fungal infections.* Skeletal gummas involve long bones of the legs with greatest frequency, although any bone may be affected. Trauma may predispose to involvement of a specific site. Presenting symptoms usually include focal pain and tenderness. When sufficiently advanced to produce radiographic abnormalities, the findings may include periostitis or destructive or sclerosing osteitis. Gummas of the upper respiratory tract can lead to perforation of the nasal septum or palate. Gummatous hepatitis may produce epigastric pain and tenderness and low-grade fever, and may be associated with splenomegaly and anemia.

The histopathology and extensive tissue necrosis associated with gummas suggest that cellular hypersensitivity to relatively few treponemes produces these lesions. This response might result from transient treponemia with seeding of sensitized tissues or from reinfection of a previously sensitized individual. This has been reported in areas where syphilis is endemic in childhood; when one member of a household acquires a fresh infection, other members of the household who then become reinfected develop gummas. Experimental inoculation of *T. pallidum* into individuals with latent or late syphilis also sometimes results in gumma formation at the site of inoculation.

Since the histologic changes may be suggestive but are nonspecific, the diagnosis of late benign syphilis is confirmed by serologic testing and by therapeutic trial. Treatment with penicillin results in rapid healing of active gummatous lesions.

Congenital syphilis The fetus becomes susceptible to congenital syphilis only after the fourth month of gestation or later, when atrophy of the Langhans' cell layer of the placenta is completed, and also when immunologic competence begins to develop. This suggests that the pathogenesis of congenital syphilis may depend upon the immune response of the host rather than upon a direct toxic effect of *T. pallidum.* The risk of infection of the fetus during untreated early maternal syphilis is estimated to be 80 to 95 percent, decreases to about 70 percent at four years, and is still lower during late latent maternal syphilis. Adequate treatment of the mother before the sixteenth week of pregnancy prevents infection of the fetus. During the past decade, the number of reported cases of congenital syphilis in the United States has remained steady at about 6 cases per 100 reported cases of primary and secondary syphilis in women. A study of cases reported in 1972 showed that 37 percent of the mothers of infected children had not sought prenatal examination, while 44 percent had had a nonreactive serologic test during the first trimester, presumably due either to false negative first trimester tests or to acquisition of syphilis during pregnancy. Syphilis acquired during pregnancy is likely to remain subclinical in the mother while nearly always causing serious fetal infection. Untreated early maternal infection may result in up to 40 percent fetal loss (stillbirth is more common than abortion, because of the late onset of fetal infection), prematurity, neonatal death, or nonfatal congenital syphilis. Therefore, routine serologic testing in early pregnancy as well as at delivery and repeat serologic testing of "high risk" pregnant women in the third trimester are fully justified.

Only fulminant cases of congenital syphilis are clinically apparent in live infants at birth, and these babies have a very poor prognosis. The most common clinical problem is the healthy appearing baby born to a mother who has a positive serologic test.

The manifestations of congenital syphilis can be divided into (1) early manifestations, which appear within the first two years of life often between two and ten weeks of age, are infectious, and resemble severe secondary syphilis in the adult; (2) late manifestations, which appear after 2 years, and are noninfectious; and (3) the residual stigmata of congenital syphilis. Only about 25 percent of cases of congenital syphilis are diagnosed during the first year of life.

The earliest sign of congenital syphilis is usually rhinitis ("sniffles"), soon followed by other mucocutaneous lesions. These may include bullae (syphylitic pemphigus), vesicles, superficial desquamation, petechial, and later, papulosquamous lesions, mucous patches, and condyloma latum. The most common early manifestations are osteochondritis and osteitis, particularly involving the metaphyses of long bones, progressing in severity during the first six months of life, then spontaneously subsiding; and periostitis, which continues to progress after the first six months. Hepatosplenomegaly, lymphadenopathy, hemolytic anemia, jaundice, thrombocytopenia, and leukocytosis are common. The nephrotic syndrome in early congenital syphilis, as in adult secondary syphilis, represents an immune complex–induced glomerulonephritis.

Neonatal congenital syphilis must be differentiated from other generalized congenital infections, including rubella, cytomegalovirus infection, and toxoplasmosis, and also from erythroblastosis fetalis. Neonatal death is usually due to pulmonary hemorrhage, secondary bacterial infection, or severe hepatitis. Pathologic findings include interstitial and perivascular inflammation followed by variable fibroblastic proliferation, involving skin, bones, liver, kidneys, pancreas, spleen, lungs, and intestines, and extramedullary hematopoiesis.

Late congenital syphilis is defined as congenital syphilis which remains untreated after two years of age. In perhaps 60 percent of cases, the infection remains latent, while the clinical spectrum in the remainder differs in certain respects from that of acquired late syphilis in the adult. For example, cardiovascular syphilis rarely develops in late congenital syphilis, whereas interstitial keratitis is much more common and occurs between ages five and twenty-five. The onset is acute with photophobia, pain, and circumcorneal injection, followed by superficial and deep vascularization of the cornea, which progresses despite antibiotic therapy, and eventually becomes bilateral. The symptoms and signs may be suppressed with corticosteroid therapy. Although treponemes have occasionally been demonstrated in aqueous humor in interstitial keratitis, the pathogenesis is obscure and is ascribed to "hypersensitivity." Other manifestations associated with interstitial keratitis are eighth-nerve deafness and recurrent arthropathy. Bilateral knee effusions are known as *Clutton's joints.* Examination of CSF discloses asymptomatic neurosyphilis in about one-third of untreated patients without other late clinical manifestations, and clinical neurosyphilis occurs in a quarter of individuals with congenital syphilis over six years of age. The clinical manifestations of congenital neurosyphilis correspond to those seen in adult neurosyphilis. Gummatous periostitis occurs between ages five and twenty and, as in endemic nonvenereal childhood syphilis, tends to cause destructive lesions of the palate and nasal septum.

Characteristic stigmata include Hutchinson's teeth, the centrally notched, widely spaced, peg-shaped upper central incisors, and "mulberry" molars, sixth-year molars which have multiple, poorly developed cusps, rather than the usual four. The abnormal facies, which includes frontal bossing, saddlenose, and poorly developed maxilla, may also be seen in congenital ectodermal dysplasia. Saber shins, or anterior tibial bowing, are rare but were probably more common in the past when syphilitic periostitis of the anterior tibia was associated with vitamin D deficiency. *Rhagades* are linear scars at the angles of the mouth and nose caused by secondary bacterial infection of the early facial eruption. Other stigmata include unexplained nerve deafness, old chorioretinitis, optic atrophy, and corneal opacities due to past interstitial keratitis.

LABORATORY EXAMINATIONS **Dark-field examination technique** Dark-field examination is essential in evaluating moist lesions, such as the chancre of primary syphilis, or condyloma lata of secondary syphilis. Although it is difficult to demonstrate *T. pallidum* in dry maculopapular lesions in secondary syphilis by dark-field examination, the organism may be demonstrated by saline aspiration of lymph nodes during this stage. The surface of the suspected ulcerated lesion should be cleaned with saline and gauze, then gently abraded further with dry gauze, without production of bleeding. The lesion is then squeezed to express a serous transudate, and a drop of the transudate is picked up on the surface of a glass slide. A drop of saline (without bacteriostatic additives) may be mixed with the transudate if necessary, and this is then covered with a cover slip and examined for *T. pallidum* with a dark-field or phase contrast microscope by an experienced individual. A single negative examination does not exclude syphilis, since at least 10^4 treponemes per milliliter transudate must be present to be detected, and prior use of topical antiseptic or cleansing by the patient may obfuscate the examination. Cleansing or use of topical medication should, therefore, be avoided, and the dark-field examination should be repeated on three successive days before being considered negative.

Serologic tests for syphilis The profusion of serologic tests for syphilis causes much unnecessary confusion. Syphilitic infection produces two types of antibodies, the *nonspecific reaginic antibody* and *specific antitreponemal* antibody.

The term *reagin* is unfortunate, since the unrelated gamma-E globulin (IgE) antibody involved in certain allergic phenomena is also known as *reagin.* The nontreponemal reaginic antibodies produced in syphilis contain both IgG and IgM immunoglobulins directed against a lipoidal antigen that results from the interaction of *T. pallidum* with host tissues, and possibly against a lipoidal antigen of *T. pallidum* itself. The cardiolipin antigens initially used in the detection of reaginic antibody were relatively crude extracts of beef heart, and it is not surprising that false positive reactions were extremely common in many conditions other than syphilis. The cardiolipin-cholesterol-lecithin antigen now in use in a variety of tests for reaginic antibody (Table 164-1) is more purified and gives fewer false positive reactions than did earlier antigens. The tests for treponemal antibody employ antigens derived from *T. pallidum,*

TABLE 164-1
Common serologic tests for syphilis

Nonspecific (reagin) antibody tests
Flocculation: VDRL
Complement fixation: Kolmer
Agglutination: rapid plasma reagin (RPR)
Specific treponemal antibody tests
Immunofluorescence: fluorescent treponemal antibody-absorption (FTA-ABS)
Immobilization: *Treponema pallidum* immobilization (TPI)
Hemagglutination: *T. pallidum* hemagglutination assay (TPHA)

rather than from tissues, and detect antibody related only to past or present treponemal infections.

The most widely used reagin antibody tests are the sensitive rapid plasma reagin (RPR) tests, which can be automated and are used to screen large numbers of serums, and the VDRL slide flocculation test, which is used to determine quantitatively the exact titer of serum reagin antibody. The reagin titer reflects the activity of the disease: false positive VDRL titers usually do not exceed 1:8; a fourfold or greater rise in titer may be seen during the evolution of primary syphilis; VDRL titers usually reach 1:32 or higher in secondary syphilis; a persistent fall in titer following treatment of early syphilis provides essential evidence of an adequate response to therapy.

The standard antitreponemal antibody test is the FTA-ABS test. The patient's serum is first absorbed with a nonpathogenic treponemal antigen (sorbent) to remove group-specific antibody which may be produced against saprophytic oral and genital treponemes. The patient's absorbed serum is then placed on a slide which contains dried *T. pallidum.* If specific antibody to *T. pallidum* remains in the patient's serum after the absorption step, it is fixed to the dried treponemes, and then is detected by the addition of fluorescein-labeled antihuman gamma-globulin and subsequent examination of the slide by fluorescence microscopy. The *T. pallidum* immobilization (TPI) test, in which immobilization of live *T. pallidum* is produced by immune serum plus complement, is more laborious and is no longer in use in most laboratories. The *T. pallidum* hemagglutination assay (TPHA) is a convenient test for treponemal antibody but is less sensitive than the FTA-ABS test for detection of early primary syphilis. Both the TPHA and FTA-ABS test are very specific when used for confirmation of positive reaginic antibody tests but give false positive rates as high as 1 percent when used for screening normal populations which have a low prevalence of syphilis. The relative sensitivities of the VDRL, FTA-ABS, and TPI tests in the various stages of syphilis are shown in Table 164-2.

The VDRL is negative in nearly one-third of patients with primary or late syphilis. Obtaining a reagin antibody test alone is not sufficient in evaluating late syphilis; the more sensitive FTA-ABS test should be routinely obtained in suspected late syphilis. In early primary syphilis, the detection of antibody can be maximized either by performing an FTA-ABS test or simply by repeating a VDRL test after 1 to 2 weeks if the initial VDRL was negative. However, both tests are always positive during secondary syphilis, and a negative VDRL or FTA-ABS virtually excludes syphilis in a patient with otherwise compatible mucocutaneous lesions. (An estimated 1 percent of patients with secondary syphilis have a negative VDRL test with undiluted serum which becomes positive in higher dilutions—the *prozone* phenomenon.)

TABLE 164-2
Frequency of positive tests in untreated syphilis

	VDRL, %	*TPI, %*	*FTA-ABS, %*
Primary syphilis	70	50	85
Secondary syphilis	100	95	100
Latent or late syphilis	70	95	98

False positive serologic tests for syphilis An estimated 20 to 40 percent of all positive reagin tests are false positive tests, but the percentages vary widely depending upon the population being examined. False positive reagin tests are classified as acute if they become negative within 6 months. Acute false positive reagin tests occur during mycoplasma pneumonia, malaria, and various acute bacterial or viral infections, and following smallpox vaccinations. Chronic reactions, which persist 6 months or longer, occur in addiction, autoimmune diseases, and aging. False positive reagin tests occur in 25 percent of narcotics addicts, and in 10 to 20 percent of patients with active systemic lupus erythematosus. Other antibodies which have been found with great frequency in serums from chronic false positive reactors include antinuclear, antithyroid, and antimitochondrial antibodies, as well as rheumatoid factor and cryoglobulins. The Donath-Landsteiner antibody responsible for paroxysmal cold hemoglobinuria is a hemolysin which appears in syphilis. The autoimmune nature of the false positive reagin test is further suggested by the occurrence of systemic lupus erythematosus or other connective tissue diseases in 15 to 45 percent of chronic false positive reactors. The prevalence of false positive reagin tests increases with advancing age, and 10 percent of people over seventy years of age have false positive reactions. Other diseases associated with hyperglobulinemia, such as leprosy, may also produce chronic false positive reactions.

In the patient with a false positive reagin test, syphilis is excluded by obtaining a negative FTA-ABS or TPHA test. The results of the FTA-ABS test are reported as negative, borderline, or positive. *Borderline* results are more common in patients who are pregnant or have diseases associated with abnormal or increased globulins, and are frequently not associated with either clinical, historical, or other serologic evidence of syphilis. Borderline results should, therefore, always be repeated in questionable cases and interpreted with caution. A typical "positive" FTA-ABS occurs infrequently in conditions other than syphilis. Although false positive FTA-ABS tests have been reported in 15 percent of patients with active systemic lupus erythematosus, the fluorescent staining is "borderline" or has an atypical "beaded" appearance in most cases (thought to be due to attachment of antinuclear antibody to treponemal DNA or nucleoprotein leaked through breaks in the outer treponemal membranes). However, because of the occasional occurrence of false positive FTA-ABS tests, only a positive TPI provides conclusive proof of past or present treponemal infection. Both the FTA-ABS and TPI tests are positive in patients who have had yaws or pinta.

For practical purposes, most clinicians need to be familiar with the three serologic tests: (1) For screening large numbers of serums for reaginic antibody (e.g., RPR); (2) for quantitative measurement of reaginic antibody titer in order to assess the clinical activity of syphilis, and to follow the reagin titer in response to therapy (e.g., VDRL); and (3) to confirm the diagnosis of syphilis in a patient with a positive reagin antibody test or with a suspected clinical diagnosis of syphilis (e.g., FTA-ABS).

IgM-FTA-ABS test for active congenital syphilis in the newborn All newborn infants of mothers with reactive VDRL or FTA-ABS tests will themselves have reactive tests whether or not they have become infected, because of passive transplacental transfer of maternal IgG immunoglobulins which are reactive in these tests. However, if IgM antitreponemal antibody is present in the infant's serum, it reflects fetal antibody production in response to intrauterine infection, particularly if there is a rise in titer, since maternal IgM antibody does not cross the intact placental barrier. Neonatal IgM antibody is detected in cord or neonatal serums in a modified FTA-ABS test, employing fluorescein-labeled antihuman IgM to detect antitreponemal IgM antibody. Similar tests have been developed for detection of congenital toxoplasmosis, rubella, and cytomegalovirus infections. The IgM-FTA-ABS test is sensitive and is positive in most infants with active congenital syphilis, except when the mother and fetus become infected very late during pregnancy. However, the specificity of this test is in doubt because of evidence that infants with a variety of congenital infections may produce IgM antibody to maternal allotypes of IgG. Thus, IgM antibody detected in the IgM-FTA-ABS test may be directed against maternal IgG antibody bound specifically to *T. pallidum*, rather than against *T. pallidum* itself.

TREATMENT AND FOLLOW-UP MANAGEMENT Penicillin G is the drug of choice for most forms of syphilis. *Treponema pallidum* is killed by very low concentrations of penicillin G, although a long period of exposure to penicillin is required for treatment because of the unusually slow rate of multiplication of the organism. The efficacy of penicillin for syphilis remains undiminished after 30 years of use. Other antibiotics which are effective in syphilis include the tetracyclines, erythromycin, chloramphenicol, and the cephalosporins. Streptomycin inhibits *T. pallidum* only in very large doses, and the sulfonamides are inactive. The optimal dose and duration of therapy have not been established for any antimicrobial for any stage of syphilis. The United States Public Health Service recommendations are based on limited therapeutic trials and should be interpreted in light of the considerations noted below.

Recurrence rates for a given regimen increase as infection progresses from incubating syphilis to seronegative primary to seropositive primary to secondary to late syphilis. Therefore it is probable, but unproved, that a longer duration of therapy is required to effect cure as the lesion progresses. For these reasons some authorities use more prolonged penicillin therapy than that recommended by the United States Public Health Service when treating secondary, latent, or late syphilis.

The optimal dose and duration of therapy have not been carefully evaluated in well-controlled studies. A variety of data suggest that it is necessary to achieve serum levels of penicillin G ≥ 0.03 μg per ml for at least 7 days to effect cure of early syphilis. Other tentative conclusions which can be gleaned from published studies include the following: (1) Extending therapy with aqueous procaine penicillin G beyond 2 weeks does not improve cure rates for primary or secondary syphilis; (2) studies of experimental syphilis show that *T. pallidum* begins to regenerate if penicillinemia is allowed to fall to subinhibitory levels for periods of 18 to 24 h; (3) in humans, increases in the dosage of crystalline penicillin G administered over 9 h from 0.03 to 0.6 mg per kg progressively increased the rate of disappearance of *T. pallidum* from chancres, but further increases in dosage did not further speed the disappearance of treponemes; and (4) the serum concentration of penicillin G achieved after one injection of 2.4 million units of benzathine penicillin G probably does not kill *T. pallidum* at the maximum rate.

The treatment regimens currently recommended for syphilis by the Center for Disease Control are summarized in Table 164-3 and described below.

Early syphilis In very early incubating syphilis, treatment of concurrently acquired gonorrhea with 4.8 million units of procaine penicillin G (plus 1.0 g probenecid) aborts the syphilis. For this reason follow-up serologic testing for syphilis is unnecessary in patients treated for gonorrhea with the recommended dose of procaine penicillin G. Preventive (abortive, "epidemiologic") treatment is recommended for seronegative individuals without signs of syphilis who were exposed to syphilis when the contact was infectious and the exposure occurred within the previous 3 months. Before treatment is given, every effort should be made to establish a diagnosis by examination and serologic testing. The regimens recommended for preventive treatment are the same as those recommended for early syphilis.

Benzathine penicillin G is the most widely used form of treatment for early syphilis, although it is more painful on injection than procaine penicillin G. A single dose of 2.4 million units cures over 95 percent of cases of primary syphilis. Because efficacy for secondary syphilis may be slightly lower, some physicians administer a second dose of 2.4 million units 1 week after the initial dose for secondary syphilis.

Pregnant patients with early syphilis should receive penicillin in the same doses used for nonpregnant patients. If they have well-documented penicillin allergy, alternative treatment should include erythromycin base, stearate, ethyl succinate (of uncertain efficacy in preventing congenital syphilis), or possibly a cephalosporin (potentially cross allergenic with penicillin). Erythromycin estolate and tetracycline are toxic in pregnancy and should not be used. After treatment, a quantitative reagin test should be repeated monthly throughout pregnancy, and if a fourfold use in titer occurs, treatment should be repeated.

If adequate treatment of the mother is accomplished during pregnancy, the risk of congenital syphilis in the newborn is minimal; the child should then be examined monthly after delivery until his reaginic antibody test becomes negative. However, if the seropositive mother received inadequate penicillin treatment or treatment other than penicillin, or her treatment status is unknown, or if the infant may be difficult to follow, treatment should be given promptly. It is unwise to require proof of diagnosis before treatment in such cases. Similarly, every infant with suspected or proved congenital syphilis should be treated promptly. The CSF should be examined as a base line before treatment of such infants. The calculation of penicillin dosage for treatment of late congenital syphilis is the same as for that used in the infant, until dosage based upon body weight reaches that used for adult neurosyphilis.

The response of early syphilis to treatment should be determined by following the quantitative VDRL titer 1, 3, 6, and 12 months after treatment. Because the FTA-ABS and TPHA tests remain positive after 2 years in nearly all patients treated for seropositive early syphilis, this test is not useful in following the response to therapy. However, IgM antibody detected in the FTA-ABS test is uniformly present in untreated syphilis in all stages, but disappears over a period of several months after successful treatment. After successful treatment of seropositive primary or secondary syphilis, the VDRL titer progressively declines, becoming negative within 3 to 12 months in about 75 percent of seropositive primary cases and 40 percent of secondary cases. After 2 years, nearly all patients with primary syphilis have a negative VDRL, although 25 percent of secondary cases and a higher proportion of those treated for early latent syphilis still maintain low titers of reagin. If the VDRL becomes negative or reaches a fixed low titer within 1 or 2 years, performing a lumbar puncture is unnecessary at that time, since the spinal fluid examination is invariably normal and there is no risk of subsequent neurosyphilis. However, if a VDRL titer ≥1:8 fails to fall at least fourfold within 12 months, the VDRL titer rises fourfold, or clinical symptoms persist or recur, retreatment is indicated. Every effort should be made to differentiate treatment failure from reinfection. If signs of secondary syphilis recur, the CSF should be examined. Suspected treatment failures, especially those with abnormal CSF, should be treated as described for neurosyphilis. If the patient remains seropositive but asymptomatic after such retreatment, no further therapy is necessary.

Asymptomatic neurosyphilis The activity of asymptomatic neurosyphilis correlates best with the degree of cerebrospinal fluid pleocytosis. Changes in the cerebrospinal fluid cell count, and to a lesser extent, in cerebrospinal fluid protein concentration, provide the most sensitive index of response to treatment. Spinal fluid examination should be performed every 3 to 6 months for 3 years after treatment of asymptomatic neurosyphilis. An elevated cerebrospinal fluid cell count falls to 10 or less per mm³ within 3 to 12 months in 95 percent of adequately treated cases, and becomes normal in all cases within 2 to 4 years. Elevated levels of cerebrospinal fluid protein fall more slowly, and the cerebrospinal fluid reagin titer declines slowly over a period of several years. Since benzathine penicillin G given in single doses of 2.4 million units to adults or 50,000 units per kg to infants does not produce detectable concentrations of penicillin G in cerebrospinal fluid, this form of penicillin is unreliable for the treatment of neurosyphilis in the adult, or for congenital syphilis, and asymptomatic neurosyphilis has been found to relapse in nearly one-quarter of patients treated with 2.4 million units benzathine penicillin. Symptomatic neurosyphilis has rarely, if ever, occurred in patients who received a total dose of 6,000,000 units or more of other forms of penicillin G for

TABLE 164-3
Recommended therapy for syphilis

Stage of syphilis	*Patients without penicillin allergy*	*Patients with penicillin allergy*
Primary, secondary, or early latent	Benzathine penicillin G 2.4 million units single dose (1.2 million units in each hip) or Aqueous procaine penicillin G, 600,000 units daily for 8 days	Erythromycin base, stearate, or ethyl succinate, 2 g daily for 15 days or Tetracycline hydrochloride 2 g daily for 15 days
Late latent or latent of uncertain duration	CSF normal: Treat as primary CSF abnormal: Treat as neurosyphilis	Lumbar puncture CSF normal: Treat as primary CSF abnormal: Treat as neurosyphilis
Late neurosyphilis* (asymptomatic or symptomatic)	Aqueous procaine penicillin G, 600,000 units daily for 14 days or Aqueous penicillin G 12 to 24 million units per day intravenously for at least 10 days	Erythromycin base, stearate, or ethyl succinate 2 g daily for 30 days or Tetracycline hydrochloride 2 g daily for 30 days
Late cardiovascular or benign tertiary	Benzathine penicillin G 2.4 million units weekly for 3 weeks or Aqueous procaine penicillin G, 600,000 units weekly for 10 days	Treat as for neurosyphilis
Congenital (treat *all* neonates with either proved *or* suspected congenital syphilis)	Aqueous procaine penicillin G, 50,000 units/kg/day for at least 10 days or Aqueous penicillin G, 50,000 units/kg/day in two divided daily doses for at least 10 days or *Only if CSF normal:* Benzathine penicillin G, 50,000 units per kg in a single dose	Antibiotics other than penicillin should not be used

* *Benzathine penicillin G has given inferior results for treatment of symptomatic neurosyphilis. Although only erythromycin or tetracycline was recommended by the CDC Syphilis Therapy Advisory Committee for CNS Syphilis, chloramphenicol may be theoretically preferable, since it reaches higher concentrations in the CSF.*

SOURCE: *From CDC recommendations, revised 1976.*

asymptomatic neurosyphilis. Chloramphenicol would be a logical choice for the treatment of neurosyphilis in the penicillin-allergic patient but has not been evaluated definitively.

Late syphilis Lumbar puncture should be performed even in the evaluation of late complications other than symptomatic neurosyphilis, since asymptomatic neurosyphilis may coexist with other late complications, and abnormal cerebrospinal fluid findings can then be followed serially as a guide to therapy. No studies of benzathine penicillin G for cardiovascular syphilis have ever been reported, and the efficacy of penicillin therapy in any form for cardiovascular syphilis has not been proved. The response of cardiovascular syphilis to penicillin is seldom dramatic because aortic aneurysm and aortic regurgitation cannot be reversed by antibiotic treatment, although further progression of these lesions may be arrested by treatment.

In contrast, the response of benign tertiary syphilis and of meningovascular syphilis to penicillin G is usually impressive. The response of parenchymal neurosyphilis has been variable. In a cooperative study of the treatment of 1,086 general paretics with penicillin, the frequency of clinical improvement or termination of progression ranged from 38 percent of those with severe involvement to 81 percent of those with mild involvement. All patients who relapsed following initial improvement in cerebrospinal fluid pleocytosis had received less than 6,000,000 units penicillin, and all improved with subsequent therapy. Tabes dorsalis or optic atrophy respond less often. In general, treatment of inactive neurosyphilis in which permanent neurologic damage has already occurred may not produce any clinical change, and retreatment of such cases is not warranted. However, persistence of cerebrospinal fluid pleocytosis, or recurrence following initial response to treatment, indicates continuing active infection, which should respond to additional treatment. The optimal dose and duration of penicillin for neurosyphilis has not been determined, but administration of 600,000 to 900,000 units procaine penicillin G daily for 10 days has been about 90 percent effective. Some physicians advocate administration of intravenous penicillin G in doses ≥ 12 million units per day for 10 days or longer, to ensure maximally treponemacidal concentrations of penicillin G in cerobrospinal fluid. Such therapy has occasionally cured patients who failed to respond to conventional therapy. There are no data to support the use of antibiotics other than penicillin G for the treatment of neurosyphilis. Therefore follow-up for at least 3 years, with reexamination of spinal fluid every 3 to 6 months, is especially important if antibiotics other than penicillin were used.

Jarisch-Herxheimer reaction A dramatic reaction consisting of fever (average temperature elevation 1.5°C), chills, myalgias, headache, tachycardia, increased respiratory rate, increased circulating neutrophil count (average 12,500 total white blood cell count per mm^3), and vasodilatation with mild hypotension, may occur following initiation of treatment of syphilis. This reaction occurs in approximately 50 percent of patients with primary syphilis, 90 percent with secondary, and 25 percent with early latent syphilis. The onset occurs within 2 h of treatment, the peak temperature occurs at about 7 h, and defervescence takes place within 12 to 24 h. In patients with secondary syphilis, an increase in erythema and edema of the mucocutaneous lesions occurs; occasionally subclinical or early mucocutaneous lesions may first become apparent during the reaction. The pathogenesis of this reaction may involve release of endotoxin in tissues. Patients should be warned to expect such symptoms, which can be managed by bedrest and aspirin. The Jarisch-Herxheimer reaction in neurosyphilis or cardiovascular syphilis has, on very rare occasions, been associated with acute progression of irreversible organ damage.

Persistence of treponemal forms The persistence of *T. pallidum* in the aqueous humor, cerebrospinal fluid, lymph nodes, brain, inflamed temporal arteries, and other tissues following "adequate" penicillin treatment of latent or late syphilis has been suggested by dark-field microscopy and by immunofluorescent antibody and silver staining techniques. Treponemal forms have also been demonstrated in patients with various clinical findings suggestive of syphilis, but in whom serologic tests, including the FTA-ABS test, were negative. Although many of these findings could be explained by artifact or by the coincidental presence of nonpathogenic treponemes, in a few cases the persistence of pathogenic *T. pallidum* after antibiotic treatment was proved by rabbit inoculation experiments. The question has been raised as to whether the life-long persistence of antitreponemal antibody measured in the TPI and FTA-ABS tests following treatment of latent or late syphilis represents prolonged immunologic memory or continued antigenic stimulation by persisting treponemes in lymph nodes and other tissues.

It is not surprising that *T. pallidum* might persist in the aqueous humor or cerebrospinal fluid despite penicillin treatment, because of poor penetration of the antibiotic, but persistance in lymph nodes and other sites remains unexplained. Limited evidence indicates no increase in resistence to penicillin of such persistent treponemes. Since the data on persisting treponemes are scanty, no modification of the treatment recommendations for latent or late syphilis seems warranted.

IMMUNITY AND PREVENTION OF SYPHILIS Only about 50 percent of the named contacts of primary and secondary syphilis become infected. The actual risk of infection from a single exposure is probably much lower. The relative importance of variations in sexual and hygienic practices, inoculum size, body and environmental temperature, and other local and systemic factors affecting transmissibility of syphilis remains undefined. There is some interest in the possible efficacy of intravaginal contraceptive gels as prophylactics against venereal diseases including syphilis, since many available preparations have bacteriostatic as well as spermicidal properties.

Man has no natural resistance to infection by pathogenic treponemes. The rate of development of acquired resistance to *T. pallidum* following natural or experimental infection is quantitatively related to the amount of the antigenic stimulus, which depends upon both the size of the infecting inoculum and the duration of infection prior to treatment.

Resistance to reinfection or superinfection by challenge inoculation develops about three months after the primary (immunizing) infection in animals with experimental syphilis. Resistance of human beings to reinfection by intradermal inoculation of *T. pallidum* was studied in volunteers. Those who had previously been treated for *early* syphilis developed a primary lesion and a serologic response, while the majority of those who had previously been treated for *late latent* syphilis and all those with *untreated latent* syphilis developed neither primary lesions nor serologic response following inoculation. Two patients treated for late latent or late congenital syphilis developed gummas at the site of inoculation.

The role of serum antibody in conferring immunity to syphilis remains controversial. Reagin antibody is not protective, and the evidence is equivocal that antibody directed against specific treponemal antigens confers immunity. Nonetheless, passive transfer of serum antibody from rabbits recovering from experimental syphilis partially protects antibody-recipient rabbits from experimental infection with *T. pallidum.* Delayed hypersensitivity to *T. pallidum* has been demonstrated by skin test in late syphilis, and lymphocytes from patients with syphilis have been demonstrated to undergo blast transformation when exposed to treponemal or cardiolipin antigen. The histopathology of gummas suggests that the cellular immune response is somehow involved in the pathogenesis of these lesions.

Inability to cultivate pathogenic treponemes in vitro has hindered analysis, purification, and concentration of treponemal antigens, and attempts to induce immunity to syphilis by vaccination have shown limited promise. Injection of rabbits with motile strains irradiated with x-rays or with strains of *T. pallidum* inactivated during cold storage has conferred limited immunity, but many injections over long periods of time were required. Attempts to provide cross-resistance by immunization of rabbits with cultivated nonpathogenic treponemes have been unsuccessful. Experiments in man have shown that varying degrees of cross-immunity exist in patients infected with *T. pallidum, T. pertenue,* and *T. carateum,* but chimpanzees with experimental pinta have not developed cross-resistance to syphilis. These findings indicate that the prospects for a syphilis vaccine remain remote, and that the prevention of syphilis depends upon use of mechanical or antiseptic prophylactic agents, and upon detection and treatment of infectious cases.

REFERENCES

BHORADE MS et al: Nephropathy of secondary syphilis: A clinical and pathological spectrum. JAMA 216:1159, 1971

BROWN WJ: Status and control of syphilis in the United States. J Infect Dis 124:428, 1971

CLARK EG, DANBOLT N: The Oslo study of the natural course of untreated syphilis. Med Clin North Am 48:613, 1964

IDSOE O et al: Penicillin in the treatment of syphilis. Bull WHO 47 (Suppl):1, 1972

MAGNUSON HJ et al: Inoculation syphilis in human volunteers. Medicine 35:33, 1956

MERRITT HH et al (eds): *Neurosyphilis,* New York: Oxford, 1946

O'NEILL P, NICOL CS: IgM class antitreponemal antibody in treated and untreated syphilis. Br J Vener Dis 48:460, 1972

PREWITT T: Cardiovascular syphilis. Med Aspects Hum Sexuality 12:68, 1972

REIMER CB et al: The specificity of fetal IgM: Antibody or anti-antibody? NY Acad Sci 254:77, 1975

SCHROETER AL et al: Treatment for early syphilis and reactivity of serologic tests. JAMA 221:471, 1972

SHERLOCK S: The liver in secondary (early) syphilis. N Engl J Med 284:1437, 1971

SHORT DH et al: Neurosyphilis, the search for adequate treatment: A review and report of a study using benzathine penicillin G. Arch Dermatol 93:87, 1966

SMITH JL: *Spirochetes in Late Seronegative Syphilis, Penicillin Notwithstanding,* Springfield, Ill.: Charles C Thomas, 1969

SPARLING PF: Diagnosis and treatment of syphilis. N Engl J Med 284:642, 1971

TURNER TB: *Syphilis and the Treponematoses, Infectious Agents and Host Reaction,* ed S Mudd, Philadelphia: Saunders, 1970, p. 346

WORLD HEALTH ORGANIZATION: Treponematosis research: Report of a WHO scientific group. WHO Tech Rept Ser 455, 1970

165 NONVENEREAL TREPONEMATOSES: YAWS, PINTA, AND ENDEMIC SYPHILIS

KING K. HOLMES
JAMES P. HARNISCH

GENERAL CONSIDERATIONS Nonvenereal treponematoses occur in remote, impoverished areas of the world. Yaws, pinta, and endemic syphilis are distinguished from venereal syphilis solely by clinical and epidemiologic features. Yaws and pinta are caused by treponemes which are conventionally designated as unique species (*Treponema pertenue* causes yaws, and *T. carateum* causes pinta), but no convincing morphologic or antigenic differences have yet been demonstrated among *T. pertenue, T. carateum,* and *T. pallidum.* The etiologic agent of endemic syphilis is generally held to be identical with *T. pallidum* and is sometimes designated as *T. pallidum endemicum.* Pinta involves the skin alone; yaws affects skin and bones; and endemic syphilis involves the skin, bone, and mucous membranes. Congenital infections and cardiovascular and central nervous system involvement occur rarely if ever in the nonvenereal treponematoses but are common in syphilis. It remains unclear whether the clinical and epidemiologic differences among yaws, pinta, endemic syphilis, and venereal syphilis are solely determined by environmental and host factors or are attributable to undefined biological differences among the causal treponemes. The relationship of the treponematoses is summarized in Table 165-1.

EPIDEMIOLOGY Treponemal antibodies are demonstrable in a high proportion of nonhuman primates in regions of Africa where human yaws and endemic syphilis are common, and pathogenic treponemes have been found in skin lesions and lymph nodes of seropositive animals. These treponemes have produced yaws-like lesions in susceptible monkeys and hamsters. Treponemes related to or identical with *T. pertenue* thus may antedate *Homo sapiens.*

Yaws and endemic syphilis are diseases of young children. Yaws occurs throughout the world between the Tropics of Cancer and Capricorn, in humid, warm environments. Transmission of yaws among children is favored by scanty clothing, poor hygiene, and frequent skin trauma. Spread occurs by direct contact with infected lesions and perhaps by passive transfer of treponemes by insects. Endemic syphilis occurs in arid subtropical or temperate climates in Africa, the eastern Mediterranean, the Arabian Peninsula, Central Asia, and Australia. It is not observed in the Western Hemisphere. Skin-to-skin transmission is less important than in yaws; instead, infection of mucous membranes results from direct mouth-to-mouth contact or from contaminated fomites, such as shared drinking or eating utensils. Household outbreaks of endemic childhood syphilis still occur in modern cities when crowding and poverty favor childhood transmission of *T. pallidum.*

Although cutaneous pigmentary changes resembling pinta occur in yaws or endemic syphilis, most authorities believe pinta is a separate, more benign disease which occurs only in the Western Hemisphere. The onset is typically later than in yaws or endemic syphilis, usually when the person is between ten and twenty years of age. The method of transmission is not well defined.

The WHO/UNICEF-assisted mass campaign for eradication of endemic nonvenereal treponematosis from 1948 to 1965 was an unusually successful public health campaign. Over 160 million people were examined in 46 countries, and approximately 50 million cases, contacts, and latent infections were treated. The impact of this program was remarkable. The prevalence of active yaws lesions was reduced from over 20 percent to less than 1 percent in many rural areas. In Bosnia, Yugoslavia, endemic syphilis was eradicated—the only example of eradication of endemic treponematosis.

Unfortunately, relaxation of active surveillance activities after the mass campaigns has led to a resurgence of yaws. For example, in Ghana, reported cases of yaws increased fivefold from 1970 to 1974. Yaws has not been eradicated in any large area.

Antitreponemal and reaginic seroreactivity has been detected recently in a small percentage of children without clinical disease born after the mass campaigns in some areas (e.g., Nigeria, New Guinea, and Bosnia). This may represent asymptomatic infection or may simply reflect the decreased predictive value of serologic tests (probability that disease is present if the test is positive) when the prevalence of disease is sharply reduced.

In the Americas, the major residual foci of yaws are Haiti; Trinidad-Tobago, Dominica, St. Lucia, and St. Vincent; Colombia and Ecuador; and probably Brazil. Pinta is confined to Central America and Northern South America, where it appears to have regressed to remote Indian villages.

BIOLOGIC RELATIONSHIPS Specific humoral antibodies to *T. pallidum* are produced in individuals with yaws, pinta, or endemic syphilis, but the time of appearance of antibodies after onset of infection is variable. The fluorescent treponemal antibody absorption (FTA-ABS) test, the *T. pallidum* hemagglutination test (TPHA), and the *T. pallidum* immobilization (TPI) test cannot differentiate among the treponematoses.

In addition to the clinical and epidemiologic differences among the treponematoses in humans, the range of susceptible animal hosts and some manifestations of experimental infection are also different. In particular, *T. carateum* has produced an infection in chimpanzees which resembles pinta, but attempts to infect other experimental animals have usually been unsuccessful. Turner and Hollander reported differences between *T. pallidum* and *T. pertenue* in infections produced in the rabbit and golden hamster, and also found that experimental rabbit infection with one species conferred greater immunity to reinfection with the homologous species than with the heterologous species. However, these interspecies differences in superinfection immunity are no greater than intraspecies differences which exist among different strains of *T. pallidum.* Individuals who have had yaws or pinta are considered relatively immune to syphilis, and the extensive studies of Medina in Caracas show that persons with active pinta or syphilis cannot be superinfected with *T. pertenue* by experimental inoculation.

TABLE 165-1
Etiology, epidemiology, and clinical manifestations of the treponematoses

	Venereal syphilis	*Endemic syphilis*	*Yaws*	*Pinta*
Organism	*T. pallidum*	*T. pallidum endemicum*	*T. pertenue*	*T. carateum*
Transmission	Sexual, transplacental*	Household contacts: Mouth-to-mouth or via drinking, eating utensils	Skin-to-skin ? Insect vector	Skin-to-skin ? Insect vector
Usual age	Adult	Early childhood	Early childhood	Adolescent
Primary lesion	Cutaneous ulcer (chancre)	Rarely seen	Framboise (raspberry), or "mother yaw"	Nonulcerating papule with satellites
Secondary lesion	Mucocutaneous; occasional periostitis	Florid mucocutaneous lesions (mucous patch, split papule, condyloma latum); osteoperiostitis	Cutaneous papulosquamous lesions	Pintides
Tertiary	Gumma, cardiovascular, and CNS lues	Destructive cutaneous osteoarticular gummas	Destructive cutaneous osteoarticular gummas	Dyschromic, achromic macules

* *Since the nonvenereal treponematoses are usually acquired in childhood and treponemal bacteremia ceases with time, only in adult-onset venereal syphilis is there any likelihood of a mother giving birth to an infected child.*

CLINICAL MANIFESTATIONS **Yaws** Also known as pian, framboesia, buba, or bouba, yaws is a chronic infectious disease of childhood caused by *T. pertenue.* The disease is characterized by an initial skin lesion followed by relapsing, nondestructive, secondary lesions of skin and bone. In the late stages, destructive lesions of skin, bone, and joints occur.

The incubation period following experimental inoculation of susceptible human beings is 3 to 4 weeks. Disruption of the skin by insect bites, abrasions, or injuries promotes acquisition of natural infection from infected contacts. The initial early lesion is a single papule which is usually located on a leg. The lesion enlarges and becomes papillomatous. This lesion is known as a framboise (raspberry) or "mother yaw." It becomes superficially eroded and covered by a thin yellow crust of serous exudate containing *T. pertenue.* Erythema and induration are not common. The lesion is pruritic, and regional lymphadenopathy occurs. The initial lesion usually heals in 6 months. As a result of treponemal bacteremia, a generalized secondary eruption of similar lesions appears either before or after the initial lesion has healed and is most extensive on the exposed surfaces of the body. These early cutaneous lesions of yaws have a variety of forms including desquamative macular and papular as well as papillomatous types. Painful papules on the soles of the feet result in a crablike gait referred to as *crab yaws.* Early lesions are infectious and heal slowly; they may result in scarring, hyperpigmentation, or depigmentation, resembling the pigmentary changes seen in pinta. Histologic findings are mononuclear-cell infiltration, acanthosis, hyperkeratosis, and the presence of many treponemes. Other manifestations of early yaws include lymphadenopathy, and nocturnal bone pain and polydactylitis due to periostitis. Fever and other constitutional symptoms may occur. Infectious cutaneous relapses may occur any time during the first 5 years after infection. Late yaws lesions occur 5 years or more after infection and differ histologically from early lesions in showing endarteritis. Late lesions include gummas of the skin and long bones, particularly of the legs, hyperkeratoses of the soles and palms, osteitis, periostitis, juxtaarticular fibromatous nodes, and hydrarthrosis.

Late lesions of yaws are characteristically extensive and usually destructive. Destruction of the nose, maxilla, palate, and pharynx, termed *gangosa,* or *rhinopharyngitis mutilans,* occurs in late yaws, as well as in leprosy and leishmaniasis. Hypertrophic paranasal maxillary osteitis produces distinctive facies known as *goundou.*

The clinical features of yaws have become less reliable for diagnosis as the prevalence of yaws has decreased, necessitating the use of easily performed serologic tests, such as the rapid plasma reagin (RPR) card test, by paramedical field workers engaged in the consolidation phase of yaws surveillance.

Treponema pertenue can be demonstrated by dark-field examination in early cutaneous lesions but should not be confused with other spirochetes found in tropical ulcers. The serum reagin antibody tests become positive after 1 month, and the FTA-ABS test is also positive.

Endemic syphilis Synonyms for endemic syphilis are Bejel, Siti, Dichuchwa, Njovera, Belesh, and Skerljevo. It is a chronic, nonvenereal, treponemal infection of childhood characterized by early mucous membrane or mucocutaneous lesions, a latent period of indeterminate duration, and late complications including gummas of bone and skin. The causative organism is indistinguishable from *T. pallidum.* Endemic syphilis differs from congenital syphilis in that dental changes, interstitial keratitis, and neurosyphilis rarely occur. Cardiovascular complications are considered rare in both endemic and congenital syphilis.

Primary cutaneous lesions are infrequent and when present are extragenital. The earliest manifestation of endemic syphilis is usually an intraoral mucous patch or mucocutaneous lesion resembling the split papules or condylomata of secondary syphilis. Periostitis is common. Regional lymphadenopathy occurs, but generalized lymphadenopathy is unusual. Treponemes are abundant in the moist early lesions and in aspirates from regional lymph nodes. After a variable latent period, late lesions may develop and are the most frequent clinical manifestations. These resemble the lesions of late benign syphilis and include osseous or cutaneous gummas. Destructive gummas, osteitis, and periostitis of nasopharyngeal structures are more common than in late yaws. Gummas occur on the nipples of mothers who have themselves previously had endemic syphilis who breastfeed infants with oral lesions. Both early and late forms of endemic syphilis thus may coexist in the same family. The tertiary lesions of endemic syphilis sometimes may be a consequence of repeated reexposure of a previously sensitized host to reinfection.

Pinta Also known as mal del pinto, carate, azul, or purupuru, pinta is an infectious disease of the skin caused by *T. carateum.* This disease has three cutaneous stages characterized by marked changes in the skin color, does not involve the viscera, and causes no disability other than that associated with cosmetic disfigurement.

The initial lesion is a small papule which appears 7 to 30 days after exposure and is located most often on the extremities, face, neck, or buttocks. It increases in size slowly by peripheral extension and by coalescing with smaller satellite papules. Regional lymphadenopathy occurs. A secondary eruption not associated with generalized lymphadenopathy appears 1 month to 1 year after the appearance of the initial lesion. The secondary lesions are termed *pintides,* may be numerous, and evolve into a psoriatic or circinate configuration. Pintides are initially red but become deeply pigmented, reaching a slate-blue color after a period of time which is related to exposure to sun. Pigmentation occurs most rapidly on the exposed parts of the body. These pigmented lesions are known as dyschromic macules and contain treponemes which are located principally in the epidermis in older lesions. Histologically there is deposition of pigment in the dermis with decreased melanin pigment in the basal-cell layer. Within 3 months to a year, most of the pintides show varying degrees of depigmentation, becoming brown and finally white and giving the skin a mottled appearance. The porcelain-white achromic lesions represent the "late" stage of the disease in which the epidermis is atrophic and melanocytes and melanin are absent. *Treponema carateum* can be demonstrated in transudates from initial, early secondary, or dyschromic lesions. Serologic reaginic and antitreponemal antibody tests are positive, but may take four times longer to become positive in pinta than in venereal syphilis.

TREATMENT Treatment is similar for all the treponematoses. Intramuscular injection of 2.4 million units benzathine penicillin G in adults and half this dose in children results in rapid resolution of lesions and prevents recurrence. Procaine penicillin G in oil and 2 percent aluminum monostearate (PAM) has been used extensively. In persons who are allergic to penicillin, tetracycline hydrochloride in a dose similar to that used for infectious syphilis (Chap. 164) is effective. In areas where less than 5 percent of the population has active disease, cases are managed on an individual basis, and all contacts of infected persons are treated with antibiotics.

REFERENCES

Bibliography on Yaws 1905–1962, Geneva: WHO, 1963

FURTADO T: Some problems of late yaws. Int J Dermatol 12:123, 1973

GRIN EI, GUTHE T: Evaluation of a previous mass campaign against endemic syphilis in Bosnia and Herzogovina. Br J Vener Dis 49:1, 1973

GUTHE T: Clinical, serological and epidemiological features of framboesia tropica (yaws) and its control in rural communities. Acta Derm Venereol 49:343, 1969

HACKETT CJ: An international nomenclature of yaws lesions. Geneva: WHO, 1957

HUDSON EH: *Nonvenereal Syphilis,* Edinburgh: E. and S. Livingstone, 1958

MARQUEZ F et al: Mal del pinto in Mexico. Bull WHO 13:299, 1955

TANEJA BL: Yaws: Clinical manifestations and criteria for diagnosis. Indian J Med Res 56:100, 1968

Treponematoses research: Report of a WHO scientific group. WHO Tech. Rept. Ser. 455:1, 1970

TURNER TB, HOLLANDER DH: Biology of the treponematoses. Geneva: WHO Monograph Ser. 35, 1957

WILLCOX RR: Changing patterns of treponemal disease. Br J Vener Dis 50:169, 1974

166 LEPTOSPIROSIS

JAY P. SANFORD

DEFINITION Leptospirosis is a term applied to disease caused by all leptospiras regardless of specific serotype. Correlation of clinical syndromes with infection by differing serotypes leads to the conclusion that a single serotype of *Leptospira* may be responsible for a variety of clinical features; conversely, a single syndrome, e.g., aseptic meningitis, may be caused by multiple serotypes. Hence there is a preference for the general term leptospirosis rather than the synonyms such as Weil's disease and canicola fever.

ETIOLOGY The genus *Leptospira* contains only one species, *L. interrogans*, which may be subdivided into two complexes, interrogans and biflexa. The interrogans complex includes the pathogenic strains, while the biflexa complex includes saprophytic strains. Within each complex the organisms show antigenic variations that are stable and allow them to be classed as serotypes (serovars). Serotypes with common antigens are arranged in serogroups. Despite contrary common usage, an example of the correct designation of *Leptospira* is as follows: pomona serogroup of *L. interrogans* or *L. interrogans* serovar pomona, not *L. pomona*. The interrogans complex now contains about 130 serotypes arranged in 16 serogroups (the number in parentheses refers to number of serotypes within the serogroup): icterohemorrhagiae (13), hebdomadis (28), autumnalis (13), canicola (11), australis (10), tarassovi or hyos (10), pyrogenes (9), bataviae (8), javanica (6), pomona (6), ballum (3), cynopteri (3), celledoni (2), grippotyphosa (2), panama (2), and shermani (1). At least 22 serotypes of *Leptospira* occur naturally in the United States.

EPIDEMIOLOGY Although leptospirosis is not a common disease, it has been reported from all regions of the United States. Between 1964 and 1974, approximately 50 to 150 cases were reported annually. Occasional upswings in number of cases have been the result of common-source outbreaks. Infection in human beings is an incidental occurrence and is not essential to the maintenance of leptospirosis. The disease occurs in a wide range of domestic and wild animal hosts. In many species, such as opossums, skunks, raccoons, and foxes, infectivity ratios in the range of 10 to 50 percent are not unusual. Interspecies spread of specific serotypes of leptospiras between animal hosts is frequent, e.g., pomona, a serotype principally associated with livestock, has been demonstrated in dogs. Infection in animals may vary from inapparent illness to severe fatal disease. The carrier state, in which the host may shed leptospiras in its urine for months to years, may develop in many animals. Immunization of dogs may not prevent the carrier, or shedder, state.

Survival of pathogenic leptospiras in nature is governed by factors including pH of the urine of the host, pH of soil or water into which they are shed, and ambient temperature. Acid urine permits only limited survival; however, if the urine is neutral or alkaline and is shed into a similar moist environment which has low salinity, is not badly polluted with microorganisms or detergents, and has a temperature above 22°C, leptospiras may survive for several weeks. Human infections can occur either by direct contact with urine or tissue of an infected animal or indirectly through contaminated water, soil, or vegetation. The usual portals of entry in humans are abraded skin, particularly about the feet, and exposed conjunctival, nasal, and oral mucous membranes. The previously held concept that organisms could penetrate intact skin has been questioned. While leptospiras have been isolated from ticks, these arthropods appear to be unimportant in transmission.

With the ubiquitous infection of animals, leptospirosis in human beings can occur in all age groups, at all seasons, and in both sexes. However, it is primarily a disease of teen-age children and young adults (about one-half of patients are between ages ten and thirty-nine years), occurs predominantly in males (80 percent), and develops most frequently in hot weather (in the United States two-thirds of infections occur from June to October). The wide spectrum of animal hosts results in both urban and rural human disease. Leptospirosis has been considered an occupational disease; however, improved methods of rat control and better standards of hygiene have reduced the incidence among occupational groups such as coal miners and people who work in sewers. Currently less than 20 percent of patients have direct contact with animals; they are mostly farmers, abattoir workers, or veterinarians. In the majority of patients exposure is incidental; two-thirds of cases occur in children, students, or housewives. Swimming or partial immersion in contaminated water, e.g., riding motorcycles through contaminated pools of water, has been implicated in one-fifth of patients and has accounted for most of the recognized common-source outbreaks.

PATHOLOGY In patients who have died with either hepatic involvement (Weil's syndrome), renal involvement, or both, the significant gross changes include hemorrhages and bile staining of tissues. The hemorrhages, which vary from petechial to ecchymotic, are widespread and are most prominent in skeletal muscle, kidneys, adrenals, liver, stomach, spleen, and lungs.

In skeletal muscle, focal, necrotic, and necrobiotic changes thought to be rather typical of leptospirosis occur. Biopsies early in the illness demonstrate swelling, vacuolation, and subsequently hyalinization. Leptospiral antigen has been demonstrated in these lesions by the fluorescent antibody technique. Healing ensues by the formation of new myofibrils with minimal fibrosis. The renal lesions in the acute phase involve predominantly the tubules and vary from simple dilatation of distal convoluted tubules to degeneration, necrosis, and basement membrane rupture. Interstitial edema and cellular infiltrates consisting of lymphocytes, neutrophilic leukocytes, histiocytes, and plasma cells are uniformly present. Glomerular lesions either are absent or consist of mesangial hyperplasia and focal foot process fusion which are interpreted as representing nonspecific changes associated with acute inflammation and protein filtration. Microscopic alterations in the liver are not diagnostic and correlate poorly with the degree of functional impairment. The changes include cloudy swelling of parenchymal cells, disruption of liver cords, enlargement of Kupffer cells, and bile stasis in biliary canaliculi. The changes in the brain and meninges are also minimal and are not diagnostic. Thickening of the meninges with a polymorphonuclear leukocytic infiltration has been observed. Microscopic evidence of myocarditis, including focal hemorrhages, interstitial edema, and focal infiltration with lymphocytes and plasma cells, has been recorded. Pulmonary findings consist of a patchy, localized hemorrhagic pneumonitis. Special staining techniques utilizing silver impregnation methods have demonstrated organisms in the lumina of renal tubules but rarely in other organs.

CLINICAL MANIFESTATIONS **General features** The incubation period following immersion or accidental laboratory exposure has shown extremes of 2 to 26 days, the usual range being 7 to 13 days and the average 10 days.

Leptospirosis is a typically biphasic illness. *During the leptospiremic* or *first phase*, leptospiras are present in the blood and cerebrospinal fluid. The onset is typically abrupt, and initial symptoms include headache, which is usually frontal, less often retroorbital, but occasionally may be bitemporal or occipital. Severe muscle aching occurs in most patients, the muscles of the thighs and lumbar areas being most prominently involved, and often is accompanied by severe pain on palpation. The myalgia may be accompanied by extreme cutaneous hyperesthesia. Chills followed by a rapidly rising temperature are prominent. Following the abrupt onset, the leptospiremic phase typically lasts 4 to 9 days. Features during this interval include recurrent chills, high spiking temperatures (usually 102°F or greater), headache, and continued severe myalgia. Anorexia, nausea, and vomiting are encountered in one-half or more of the patients. Occasional patients have diarrhea. Pulmonary manifestations, usually either cough or chest pain, have varied in frequency of occurrence from less than 25 percent to 86 percent. Hemoptysis occurs but is rare. Examination during this phase reveals an acutely ill, febrile patient, with a relative bradycardia and normal blood pressure, although European authors comment on early hypotension. Disturbances in sensorium may be encountered in up to 25 percent of patients. The most characteristic physical sign is conjunctival suffusion, which usually first appears on the third or fourth day. It may be lacking in some patients but more often is overlooked. This may be associated with photophobia, but serous or purulent secretion is unusual. Less common findings may include pharyngeal injection, cutaneous hemorrhages, and skin rashes that are usually macular, maculopapular, or urticarial and usually occur on the trunk. Uncommon findings are splenomegaly, hepatomegaly, lymphadenopathy, or jaundice. A palpably enlarged gallbladder, reflecting acalculous cholecystitis, has been observed in children with leptospirosis. The first phase terminates after 4 to 9 days, usually with defervescence and improvement in symptoms. This coincides with the disappearance of leptospiras from the blood and cerebrospinal fluid.

The second phase has been characterized as the "immune" phase and correlates with the appearance of circulating IgM antibodies. The concentration of C-3 in serum has remained within normal range during this phase. The clinical manifestations of this phase show greater variability than those during the first phase. After a relatively asymptomatic period of 1 to 3 days, the fever and earlier symptoms recur and meningismus may develop. The fever rarely exceeds 102°F and is usually of 1 to 3 days' duration. It is not uncommon for fever to be absent or quite transient. Even when symptoms or signs of meningeal irritation are absent, routine examination of cerebrospinal fluid after the seventh day has revealed pleocytosis in 50 to 90 percent of patients. Less common features include iridocyclitis, optic neuritis, and other nervous system manifestations, including encephalitis, myelitis, and peripheral neuropathy.

Some clinicians recognize a third or convalescent phase, usually between the second and fourth weeks, when both fever and aching may recur. The pathogenesis of this stage is not understood.

Leptospirosis during pregnancy may be associated with an increased risk of fetal loss.

Specific features WEIL'S SYNDROME Weil's syndrome, which may be due to serotypes other than icterohemorrhagiae, is defined as severe leptospirosis with jaundice, usually accompanied by azotemia, hemorrhages, anemia, disturbances in consciousness, and continued fever. There is uncertainty as to the pathogenesis of the syndrome, i.e., whether it represents direct toxic damage due to leptospiras or whether it is the consequence of immune response to leptospiral antigens. The consensus favors toxic damage.

The onset and first stage are identical with the less severe forms of leptospirosis. The distinctive features of Weil's syndrome appear from the third to the sixth days but do not reach their peak until well into the second stage. As in milder forms of leptospirosis, there is a tendency for defervescence about the seventh day; however, with recurrence, fever is marked and may persist for several weeks. Either renal or hepatic manifestations may predominate. Hepatic disturbances include tenderness in the right upper quadrant and hepatic enlargement, both of which are common when jaundice is present. Serum glutamic oxaloacetic transaminase (SGOT) values are rarely increased more than two- to threefold regardless of the degree of hyperbilirubinemia, which is predominantly conjugated (direct); e.g., serum bilirubin 40 mg per 100 ml, SGOT 170 IU. The predominant mechanism appears to be an intracellular block to bilirubin excretion.

Renal manifestations consist primarily of proteinuria, pyuria, hematuria, and azotemia. Dysuria is rare. Serious renal damage usually occurs in the form of acute tubular necrosis associated with oliguria. The peak elevation of blood urea nitrogen usually is seen on the fifth to seventh day. Hemorrhagic manifestations are most prevalent in this group of patients and include epistaxis, hemoptysis, gastrointestinal bleeding, hemorrhage into the adrenal glands, hemorrhagic pneumonitis, and subarachnoid hemorrhage. These have been explained on the basis of diffuse vasculitis with capillary injury. In addition, in some patients hypoprothrombinemia and thrombocytopenia have been observed.

ASEPTIC MENINGITIS A leptospiral etiology has been incriminated in 5 to 13 percent of sporadic cases of aseptic meningitis. The pleocytosis is not present before the immune phase, when it develops rapidly. There are usually tens to hundreds of leukocytes, occasionally 1,000, per cubic milliliter, among which neutrophils or mononuclear cells may predominate. The cerebrospinal fluid glucose concentration is almost always normal, but occasional instances of lowered glucose levels (hypoglycorrhachia) have been recorded. In contrast to the observations with many viral causes of aseptic meningitis, with leptospirosis the cerebrospinal fluid protein may exceed 100 mg per 100 ml early in the course. Xanthochromic cerebrospinal fluid has been observed in the presence of jaundice. Each of the serotypes of leptospiras that are pathogenic for human beings is probably capable of causing aseptic meningitis. The most prevalent serotypes have been canicola, icterohemorrhagiae, and pomona.

PRETIBIAL (FORT BRAGG) FEVER An illness was observed in the summer of 1942 that had an onset identical with that of the first phase of leptospirosis. The most distinctive feature was the development on about the fourth day of a rash, characterized by 2- to 5-cm, slightly raised, erythematous lesions that were usually symmetrically distributed over the pretibial areas. In contrast to other leptospiral syndromes, splenomegaly occurred in 95 percent of these patients. This outbreak was shown to be due to the autumnalis serogroup. Subsequently, pomona has been observed in association with rashes, which are usually truncal but which have also been pretibial.

MYOCARDITIS Cardiac arrhythmias including paroxysmal atrial fibrillation, atrial flutter, ventricular tachycardia, and premature ventricular contractions have been described but are usually of little clinical significance. However, on rare occasions definite cardiac dilatation with acute left ventricular failure has been observed. Associated manifestations have included jaundice, pulmonary infiltrates, arthritis, and skin rashes. The serogroups thus far incriminated have included icterohemorrhagiae, pomona, and grippotyphosa.

LABORATORY FEATURES Leukocyte counts vary from leukopenic levels to mild elevations in the anicteric patients. In patients with jaundice, leukocytosis as high as 70,000 cells per mm^3 may be present. However, regardless of the total leukocyte count, neutrophilia of greater than 70 percent is very frequently encountered during the first stage.

Hemolytic substances have been demonstrated in cultures of pathogenic leptospiras. In contrast to many hemolysins of bacterial origin which are not hemolytic in vivo, the leptospiral hemolysins appear to be active in vivo. In patients with jaundice, anemia may be severe and is most characteristically due to intravascular hemolysis. Other mechanisms of anemia include azotemia and blood loss secondary to hemorrhage. Anemia due to leptospirosis is unusual in anicteric patients.

Rarely thrombocytopenia sufficient to be associated with bleeding is encountered. Additional hematologic abnormalities include elevation of the erythrocyte sedimentation rate in over one-half of patients, but it is usually less than 50 mm per h.

Urinalysis during the leptospiremic phase reveals mild proteinuria, casts, and an increase in cellular elements. In anicteric infections, these abnormalities rapidly disappear after the first week. Proteinuria and abnormalities in the urine sediment usually are not associated with elevations in blood urea nitrogen. Since the anicteric form of the disease often has gone undiagnosed, estimates of the frequency of azotemia and jaundice are probably high. Azotemia has been reported in approximately one-fourth of patients. In three-fourths of these patients, the blood urea nitrogen is less than 100 mg per 100 ml. Azotemia is usually associated with jaundice. The serum bilirubin levels may reach 65 mg per 100 ml; however, in two-thirds of patients the levels are less than 20 mg per 100 ml. Of the total serum bilirubin, most is conjugated (direct reacting).

DIAGNOSIS Diagnosis is based upon culture of the organism or serologic proof of its existence. The most common initial diagnostic impressions in patients with leptospirosis are meningitis, hepatitis, nephritis, fever of undetermined origin (F.U.O.), and influenza. Leptospiras may be isolated quite readily during the first phase from blood and cerebrospinal fluid or during the second phase from the urine. Leptospiras may be excreted in the urine for up to 11 months after the onset of illness and may persist despite antimicrobial therapy. Whole blood should be inoculated immediately into tubes containing semisolid medium, such as Fletcher's medium. If culture medium is not available, leptospiras reportedly will remain viable up to 11 days in blood to which anticoagulants, preferably sodium oxalate, have been added. Animal inoculation (preferably either suckling hamsters or guinea pigs) may be used and is of particular value if specimens are contaminated. Direct examination of blood or urine by dark-field methods has been employed; *however, this method so frequently results in failure or misdiagnosis that it should not be employed as the only diagnostic test.* Serologic methods are applicable during the second phase; antibodies appear from the sixth to the twelfth days of illness. Four serologic tests are available: macroscopic plate agglutination test (easy to perform but not very sensitive), hemolytic test (complex but requires only a single antigen), microscopic agglutination test (complex but most specific), and complement fixation tests. Serologic criteria for diagnosis include a fourfold or greater rise in titer during the course of illness. Cross-agglutination reactions between various serotypes commonly occur so that the infection serotype often cannot be determined with certainty without isolation of leptospiras.

PROGNOSIS The prognosis is dependent upon both the virulence of the organism and the general condition of the patient. Between 1965 and 1968, there were 10 deaths (4 percent) in the 277 patients reported in the United States. Age is the most significant host factor related to increased mortality. In a representative series, the mortality rose from 10 percent in men less than fifty years of age to 56 percent in those over fifty-one years of age. The virulence of the infecting leptospiras correlates best with the development of jaundice. In anicteric patients, mortality does not occur, but with the development of jaundice, mortality in various series has ranged from 15 to 40 percent. The long-term prognosis following the acute renal lesion of leptospirosis is good. Glomerular filtration rates have returned to normal; however, a few patients exhibit residual tubular dysfunction, e.g., a defect in renal concentrating capacity.

TREATMENT A variety of antimicrobial drugs, including penicillin, streptomycin, the tetracycline congeners, and chloramphenicol, and erythromycin, have been effective in vitro and in experimental leptospiral infections. Data concerning the efficacy of antibiotics in human beings are conflicting. If antimicrobial drugs are to have any beneficial effect, they must be administered within 4 days, and preferably within 2 days, of the onset of illness. Turner states that large doses of penicillin G (usually 600,000 units intramuscularly every 4 h) is the preferred treatment, although others have considered the tetracyclines to be effective. Within 4 to 6 h after initiation of penicillin G therapy, a Jarisch-Herxheimer type of reaction, which suggests antileptospiral activity, may occur. There is general agreement that antimicrobials administered after the fifth day of illness have no beneficial effect. There exists the clinical impression that early bedrest may minimize subsequent morbidity. Azotemia and jaundice require meticulous attention to fluid and electrolyte therapy. Since the renal damage is reversible, patients with azotemia should be considered for peritoneal dialysis or hemodialysis. From case reports exchange transfusion has been suggested to be beneficial in the management of patients with extreme hyperbilirubinemia.

REFERENCES

ALSTON JM, BROOM JC: *Leptospirosis in Man and Animals*, Edinburgh: E & S Livingstone, 1958

BARTON LL et al: Leptospirosis with acalculous cholecystitis. Am J Dis Child 126:350, 1973

BERMAN SJ et al: Sporadic anicteric leptospirosis in South Vietnam. Ann Intern Med 79:167, 1973

EDWARDS GA, DOMM M: Human leptospirosis. Medicine 39:117, 1960

FEIGIN RD et al: Human leptospirosis from immunized dogs. Ann Intern Med 79:777, 1973

HEATH CW JR, ALEXANDER AD: Leptospirosis in the United States: Analysis of 483 cases in man, 1949–1961. N Engl J Med 273:857, 915, 1965

KOCEN RS: Leptospirosis: A comparison of symptomatic and penicillin therapy. Br Med J 1:1181, 1962

OOI BS et al: Human renal leptospirosis. Am J Trop Med Hyg 21:336, 1972

TONG MJ et al: Immunological response in leptospirosis. Am J Trop Med Hyg 20:625, 1971

TURNER LH: Leptospirosis. Br Med J 1:537, 1973

167
RELAPSING FEVER

JAMES J. PLORDE

DEFINITION Relapsing fever refers to a group of acute infectious diseases that are characterized clinically by cyclic periods of fever and apyrexia. They are caused by spirochetes of the genus *Borrelia* and occur in two epidemiologic varieties, louse-borne and tick-borne.

ETIOLOGY Borreliae are slender helical organisms which measure 10 to 20 μm in length. They have 3 to 10 irregular coils, move in a corkscrew fashion, and divide by transverse fission. Unlike other spirochetes, they readily stain with aniline dyes. *Borrelia recurrentis* is the causative agent of louse-borne relapsing fever. Many strains of *Borrelia* have been found in tick-borne disease; *B. turicatae, B. parkeri*, and *B. hermsii* are responsible for the disease seen in this country. The organisms grow poorly on artificial media and readily in developing chick embryos.

EPIDEMIOLOGY Louse-borne relapsing fever is transmitted from person to person by the human body louse. Spirochetes that are ingested by the vector during feeding penetrate the wall of the intestine and multiply in the body cavity. Human infection occurs when the louse is crushed against an abrasion or wound. There is no known animal reservoir. The disease persists in endemic focuses in Ethiopia, South America, and the Far East. Like typhus, it occurs in epidemic form during war and famine. Major epidemics involving millions of people occurred in Europe and Africa after both the First and Second World Wars. A third, much smaller outbreak, was seen at the time of the Korean conflict.

The tick vectors of relapsing fever belong to several species of the genus *Ornithodoros*. Like lice, they ingest the borreliae during feeding. The organisms may remain viable in the ticks for several years and can be passed transovarily to the next generation, making the tick a major reservoir of the disease. It is likely that rodents and other small animals act as vertebrate reservoirs in some locales. Human beings are involved when they come into contact with an infected tick in its natural habitat. Transmission occurs if the tick's saliva or coxal fluid contaminates the feeding site. The tick-borne disease is found in localized areas throughout the world, and occurs sporadically in the United States. Recent outbreaks have occurred among Boy Scouts camping in northeastern Washington and tourists visiting the north rim of the Grand Canyon.

PATHOGENESIS AND PATHOLOGY After inoculation into a human being, the borreliae reach the bloodstream, producing spirochetemia and a febrile illness. After several days, immobilizing and borrelicidal antibodies appear, the organisms are cleared from the peripheral blood, and the fever resolves. Following a latent period of approximately 1 week, during which the spirochetes are sequestered in the body, a new antigenic variant of the organism arises. There is reinvasion of the bloodstream, causing a second paroxysm of fever and eventually, with the formation of specific antibodies, a second defervescence by crisis. The continued sequential production of new antigenic variants and specific antibodies results in the characteristic relapsing febrile course.

At autopsy follicular splenic abscesses, histiocytic interstitial myocarditis, intracranial hemorrhage, and hepatitis with focal necrosis may be seen. Spontaneous splenic rupture and hemorrhagic gastrointestinal lesions have been noted occasionally. Borreliae have been recovered from the brain, heart, spleen, liver, and skin.

MANIFESTATIONS Clinical manifestations vary from outbreak to outbreak and between the tick- and louse-borne varieties of the disease. Generally, patients with louse-borne relapsing fever are more seriously ill but have fewer relapses than those with tick-borne illnesses. After an incubation period of 4 to 18 days, the disease begins abruptly with rigors, headache, anorexia, nausea, vomiting, photophobia, and pain in the muscles and joints. The temperature rises rapidly, reaching 39 to 40°C, where it remains until the time of the crisis. The patient appears dull, apathetic, and is uncomplaining. He may have conjunctival suffusion and a macular or petechial rash. Cough, tachypnea, and rhonchi are common. A gallop rhythm and premature ventricular beats may occur in the louse-borne variety. Cardiac enlargement and heart failure are more uncommon. Upper abdominal tenderness is frequent. The liver and spleen are palpable and tender in 20 to 80 percent of cases, and may enlarge 6 to 10 cm during the course of fever. Jaundice secondary to hepatocellular destruction is present in 7 to 36 percent of patients. It is usually seen in louse-borne disease, occurs relatively late in the illness, and if severe, is often associated with purpura.

Bleeding is common in louse-borne relapsing fever. Petechiae develop in the skin and serous membranes, apparently as a result of damage to the capillary endothelium by clumps of spirochetes. Mild epistaxes and microscopic hematuria are present in many patients early in the disease. Later, with the development of liver disease, severe prolonged epistaxes and widespread ecchymoses occur. Infrequently, there may be massive gastrointestinal, urinary, or intracranial hemorrhage. Disseminated intravascular coagulation has been described. Neck stiffness, confusion, and transient focal neurologic signs may be seen even without intracranial bleeding. Patients with tick-borne disease with repeated relapses may develop iritis or iridocyclitis with permanent visual impairment. Pregnant women with relapsing fever often abort.

Three to six days after the onset of illness, the attack ends in a crisis. Clinically this is characterized by a chill and an abrupt but transient rise in temperature, heart rate, respiratory rate, and arterial blood pressure. As the spirochetes disappear, the patient becomes flushed, diaphoretic, and hypotensive. Occasionally, cardiovascular collapse and death may occur at this point. More frequently the blood pressure and temperature return to normal over several hours, leaving the patient comfortable but exhausted. After 7 to 10 afebrile days, a relapse occurs which mimics the original illness. In the louse-borne disease there is usually only a single relapse, but in tick-borne relapsing fever there may be several, each somewhat briefer and milder than the preceding one.

LABORATORY FINDINGS A moderate anemia is common. The leukocyte count is usually normal or slightly elevated. During the crisis, a marked leukopenia occurs which may be followed by a transient rebound leukocytosis. A consumptive thrombocytopenia is seen in most cases, and the prothrombin and partial thromboplastin times may be prolonged. Fibrinogen levels are increased. Liver function tests reveal disturbed hepatocellular function. In severe cases, the total serum bilirubin level may reach 16 mg per 100 ml. Azotemia unrelated to extracellular fluid depletion is common among jaundiced patients. Electrocardiogram abnormalities, including a prolonged Q-Tc interval and ST-T wave changes, may occur. Reagin tests for syphilis are positive in 5 to 10 percent of cases, and experimental data suggest that false positive FTA-ABS tests may also occur. Patients with louse-borne relapsing fever frequently develop agglutinins to *Proteus* OXK antigens.

The definitive diagnosis is made by demonstrating borreliae in the peripheral blood during a febrile episode. This is most easily accomplished by examining thick and thin films stained with Giemsa's and Wright's stains. Repeated examinations may be required, especially in tick-borne disease. Blood spun in a microhematocrit tube and examined microscopically may reveal organisms when thin and thick smears are negative. Spirochetes may also be seen in wet mounts with phase-contrast microscopy. When the direct methods are negative, blood may be injected into mice or rats and their blood examined frequently for the presence of borreliae.

DIFFERENTIAL DIAGNOSIS Many acute febrile illnesses, including malaria, salmonellosis, typhus, dengue, rat-bite fever, and Weil's disease, must be considered. Practically, there is seldom confusion if blood films are examined carefully.

TREATMENT The peripheral blood is quickly cleared of spirochetes by a variety of drugs, including penicillin, tetracycline, and chloramphenicol. Treatment with these antimicrobial agents, however, is accompanied by a Jarisch-Herxheimer–like reaction which contributes to the morbidity, and perhaps mortality, of the disease. The reaction appears both clinically and pathophysiologically to be an exaggeration of the spontaneously occurring crisis. Its mechanism is unknown, but it may be related to release of endotoxin liberated during destruction of spirochetes. It is certainly related temporally to disappearance of spirochetes from the blood, and its severity appears to depend upon the speed with which they are removed.

In louse-borne relapsing fever, where the spirochetemia is often intense and the Jarisch-Herxheimer reaction severe, the drug of choice is a repository penicillin such as penicillin aluminum monostearate (PAM). Unlike tetracycline, this drug achieves a very gradual clearing of the spirochetes and a correspondingly mild reaction. The drug is given intramuscularly in a dose of 600,000 units. If the shorter-acting procaine penicillin is used, the dose should be repeated in 12 to 24 h to prevent relapse. In epidemics, a single 0.5- to 1-g oral dose of chloramphenicol can be used with good results.

In tick-borne disease where penicillin is not effective in terminating relapses, tetracycline is most rapidly borrelicidal. This drug should be given in a dose of 0.5 g four times a day for 5 to 10 days. The Jarisch-Herxheimer reaction tends to be less severe in this form of the disease.

PROGNOSIS When epidemics strike a nonimmune population, the high mortality rate due to the louse-borne disease shows the potential menace of this disease. Most patients, however, recover quickly and completely; relapses do not occur if antibiotic therapy is adequate. Adverse signs are deep jaundice, uncontrolled bleeding, and a grossly prolonged Q-Tc interval.

Typhus and enteric fever may occur simultaneously with louse-borne relapsing fever, and they probably contribute to the mortality rate, particularly during epidemics.

REFERENCES

BRYCESON ADM et al: Louse-borne relapsing fever: A clinical and laboratory study of 62 cases in Ethiopia and a reconsideration of the literature. Q J Med 39:139, 1970

FELSENFELD O: *Borrelia: Strains, Vectors, Human and Animal Borreliasis*, St. Louis: Warren H. Green, 1971

JUDGE DM et al: Louse-borne relapsing fever in man. Arch Pathol 97:136, 1974

KELLY R: Cultivation of *Borrelia hermsi*. Science 30:443, 1971

SOUTHERN PM JR, SANFORD JP: Relapsing fever. Medicine 48:129, 1969

168
RAT-BITE FEVER (SPIRILLUM MINUS INFECTION)

ROGER BULGER

DEFINITION The term *rat-bite fever* refers to infection with either *Spirillum minus* or *Streptobacillus moniliformis* (Chap. 149). The acute infection caused by *S. minus* follows the bite of a rodent, usually a rat, and is characterized by a prolonged incubation period, followed by relapsing fever and recurrence of local inflammation at the puncture wound site, with lymphangitis and skin lesions.

ETIOLOGY AND EPIDEMIOLOGY *Spirillum minus* is a rigid spiral organism 2 to 5 μm in length, with polar flagella and from two to five spirals. It has never been cultivated on artificial media; animal inoculation is required for its isolation from patients. These organisms are readily recognized with dark-field microscopy by their quick, darting motility; they may be seen also in Wright-stained smears of blood from infected animals and patients.

Infection with *S. minus* in humans almost always follows a rat bite, although examples of infection from the bite of a mouse are known. The disease is most common in people who live or work in rat-infested areas and in laboratory workers who handle rats. It is useful to remember that rats can bite babies or sleeping or inebriated people without their realizing it. Carrier rates among wild rats have been observed to vary from 0 to 25 percent in different locales.

CLINICAL MANIFESTATIONS The incubation period is usually from 1 to 4 weeks and occasionally longer. If the original bite has healed completely, the patient may neglect to associate the bite with the illness. Usually, however, after initial healing, the wound site becomes swollen, and pain returns before or at the time of the onset of systemic symptoms of infection. Lymphangitis and swollen, tender regional lymph nodes are also usually found when chills and fever commence. During febrile periods, which usually last from 2 to 4 days, there may also be malaise, headache, photophobia, nausea, and vomiting. In more than half the cases, an asymmetric rash occurs, usually on the extremities; the rash is usually macular, and the lesions may become confluent. Arthritis is uncommon. Afebrile periods are from 2 to 4 days in length, alternating with periods of fever, and the course is protracted, usually lasting from 4 to 8 weeks. Cases have been reported in which signs and symptoms persisted for more than a year; rarely, subacute bacterial endocarditis due to this organism has been reported.

LABORATORY FINDINGS The blood leukocyte count may be normal or may be as high as 20,000 per mm^3. The organism cannot be cultured on artificial media, but can be seen in the blood of patients by dark-field microscopy or on Wright-stained smears. When this disease is suspected, the patient's blood must be inoculated intraperitoneally in mice or guinea pigs; 5 to 15 days later, *S. minus* will be found in the animal's blood or peritoneal fluid. In about half the patients, there are biologic false positive serologic tests for syphilis.

DIFFERENTIAL DIAGNOSIS It is important to inquire about rat bite in all patients with a relapsing type of fever. In patients with a history of rat bite, the principal problem is in differentiating between *S. minus* and *Strep. moniliformis* infections. This cannot be done with certainty on clinical grounds (Chap. 149), but a prolonged incubation period, relapsing instead of sustained fever, and few or no manifestations of arthritis suggest a diagnosis of *S. minus* infection. Laboratory tests should be made for both organisms. The significance of a previous rat bite may not be appreciated in cases with a long incubation period, and the disease may be confused with other infections characterized by relapsing fever, such as malaria, meningococcemia, and *Borrelia recurrentis* infection.

TREATMENT AND PROGNOSIS Penicillin, in dosage of 600,000 units twice a day intramuscularly, is the drug of choice. In patients allergic to penicillin, tetracycline in divided dosage of 2 g per day for 7 days may be used.

Patients treated with penicillin become afebrile within 24 to 72 h, and complete recovery is the rule. Prior to the availability of effective antibiotics, fatality was estimated to occur in 2 to 10 percent of those with clinical infection.

REFERENCES

(See also Chap. 149)

COLE JS et al: Rat-bite fever. Ann Intern Med 71:979, 1969

HUBBERT WT et al: *Diseases Transmitted from Animals to Man*, Springfield, Ill.: Charles C Thomas, 1975, p. 186

section 11 | Diseases caused by fungi

INTRODUCTION

ABRAHAM I. BRAUDE

Except for their etiology, fungous infections differ little from bacterial infections. The close relationship between bacteria and fungi is apparent from transitional forms connecting the two classes, and from the similarity of the pathologic changes and clinical manifestations induced by them.

The intermediate, or transitional, forms are represented by the actinomycetes. These branch as fungi do, but divide into gram-positive bacillary or coccoid forms. The acid-fast property of one species, *Nocardia asteroides*, indicates a relationship to the tubercle bacillus. The actinomycetes also differ from fungi in their susceptibility to phages, their unorganized nuclei, and their sensitivity to antibiotics, which attack bacteria, but not to the antifungal polyene antibiotic amphotericin B. The actinomycetes do not possess the sterols which complex with polyene antibiotics and injure the cell membranes of the fungi. Finally, actinomycetes, like bacteria but unlike fungi, contain neither chitin nor cellulose in their cell walls. *Although actinomycosis and nocardiosis are placed among the fungous diseases in this book, the causative agents are bacteria.*

An important characteristic of pathogenic fungi is dimorphism, i.e., growth in two distinct forms under different environmental conditions. The fungi responsible for blastomycosis, sporotrichosis, and histoplasmosis assume unicellular "yeast" forms in infected tissues but grow as mycelia and produce asexual spores on Sabouraud's agar. The reverse is true for the fungus causing moniliasis. Another type of dimorphism is found in coccidioidomycosis. The organism responsible for this infection is multicellular in vivo and in vitro, but its form differs under the two conditions. In tissues it is a sac filled with spores, but on agar it grows as a segmented mycelium. *Cryptococcus neoformans* is one pathogenic fungus that fails to change form when the environment varies.

Mycotic diseases are not transmitted from one person to another. Many fungous infections are acquired by inhalation of spores growing freely in nature. These spores may be rectangular unicellular mycelial fragments known as *chlamydospores*, or spherical bodies borne on thin mycelial stalks and called *conidia*. Some infections, such as sporotrichosis, result from inoculation of spores directly into the skin.

A few fungous diseases are endogenous in origin. *Actinomyces israelii* and *Candida albicans* are normal residents of the intestine and mouth. When resistance is lowered, endogenous infection with either agent may develop. Actinomycosis often follows tooth extraction, and overgrowth of normal saprophytic bacteria by *C. albicans* in the course of antibiotic therapy can lead to moniliasis.

The mechanisms whereby fungi produce disease are obscure. *Cryptococcus neoformans* has a polysaccharide capsule similar to that of the pneumococcus which seems to protect the yeast from phagocytosis. This capsular material also produces mechanical injury in the nervous system. It is possible that the thick walls of other fungi such as *Blastomyces dermatitidis* and *Coccidioides immitis* also protect against leukocytes. Some fungi are ingested by phagocytes but seem to flourish within them. In histoplasmosis, for example, the parasites are found in enormous numbers within reticuloendothelial cells. The endothelium of small vessels can become so packed with histoplasma organisms that blood flow is compromised.

Another possible factor in the pathogenesis of these infections is hypersensitivity. In most fungous diseases there is marked local or even systemic reactivity to intradermal injection of the causative organism. In coccidioidomycosis this type of reaction is closely associated with the development of erythema nodosum and pleural effusions. In allergic pulmonary aspergillosis, the disease results from both reaginic and precipitating antibodies against aspergillus antigens. The occurrence of necrosis at the site of injection of fungous antigens suggests that hypersensitivity may be responsible for necrosis of infected tissues. In other patients, however, widespread destruction of tissue may occur despite absence of dermal sensitivity.

Despite the differences in structure and life cycle of fungi and bacteria, both elicit similar pathologic changes and clinical manifestations. For this reason, specific diagnosis can seldom be made without demonstration of the causative organism. Fortunately, most pathogenic fungi are easily seen in infected tissues or exudates. In a few circumstances, however, it is necessary to rely upon epidemiologic and immunologic methods for diagnosis.

The following chapters deal only with those infections in which fungi penetrate beneath the skin and mucous membranes to involve the underlying tissues and viscera.

169 ACTINOMYCOSIS

ABRAHAM I. BRAUDE

DEFINITION Actinomycosis is a noncontagious infection produced by an anaerobic organism normally resident in the mouth. The disease is characterized by chronic inflammatory induration and sinus formation.

ETIOLOGY The causative agent is a branching gram-positive filamentous organism. Two separate pathogenic anaerobic species of the genus *Actinomyces* have been recognized: *A. bovis* is responsible for actinomycosis in cattle, and *A. israelii* for human actinomycosis. Another actinomycete, *Arachnia propionica*, may produce chronic abscesses and draining sinuses.

Intolerance of free oxygen and failure to grow on Sabouraud's medium on the part of *A. israelii* and *A. bovis* distinguish them from *Nocardia* and other actinomycetes. On blood agar, colonies require 4 to 6 days of anaerobic incubation at 37°C to reach a size of 1 to 2 mm. Although most strains require anaerobic conditions for isolation, some can be subcultured aerobically in 10 to 20 percent carbon dioxide. *Actinomyces israelii* has never been found outside humans or animals, and case-to-case transmission is unknown. *Ar. propionica* resembles *A. israelii* in oxygen requirements, colonial morphology, and microscopic disappearance. Distinction is based on the ability of *Ar. propionica* to produce large amounts of propionic acid and the presence of diaminopimelic acid in its cell wall.

PATHOGENESIS The oxidation-reduction potential of normal tissues is probably too high for multiplication of *A. israelii* but dead tissues allow it to reproduce and spread. The frequency of actinomycosis of the face and neck may be explained by the greater population of *A. israelii* on teeth, in carious teeth, and in tonsillar crypts and by trauma from eating, dental procedures, or infection with oral bacteria. Anaerobic conditions also prevail in atelectatic areas of the lung after aspiration of *A. israelii* so that pulmonary actinomycosis can develop. It is also possible that pulmonary actinomycosis may arise hematogenously from an infected focus in the mouth. Mediastinal actinomycosis probably spreads from the esophagus into the superior or posterior mediastinum, quickly involving the pleura to produce early pleural effusion or empyema, and then tends to attack the adjacent ribs and vertebral bodies. Eventually mediastinal actinomycosis produces abscesses which point in the paravertebral region. Ileocecal actinomycosis is the most common intestinal form, occurring after appendiceal rupture and the escape of actinomycetes to form an inflammatory mass in the right iliac fossa. The liver is the solid abdominal viscus most frequently attacked by actinomycosis.

From foci in the jaw, lung, or intestine, actinomycosis may spread by contiguity or through the bloodstream to the liver, spine, brain, kidneys, genitalia, spleen, and subcutaneous tissues. Lymphatic spread is rare.

The inflammatory reaction to *A. israelii* is characterized by three features: (1) chronic suppuration, (2) extensive necrosis, and (3) intense fibrosis. The so-called "sulfur granules" in the inflammatory lesion are composed of intertwined mycelial filaments.

CLINICAL MANIFESTATIONS The essential feature of actinomycosis is a painful, indurated swelling. This lesion may appear over the jaw a week or more after such trauma as tooth extraction or compound fracture of the mandible. As it increases in size, points of suppuration, the openings of fistulas, appear on the bluish-red surface of the edematous skin. Trismus is prominent early. Cervical lymphadenopathy is rare.

The lower lobes of the lung are frequently affected; then the disease suddenly becomes evident when the pleura and chest wall are involved by direct extension from the lung. Until then the patient may notice only fever, cough, and expectoration. Physical examination at this time reveals a diffuse, tender, indurated swelling of the chest wall with pulmonary consolidation and empyema.

Abdominal actinomycosis is often mistaken for appendicitis, carcinoma of the cecum, tuberculosis, or amebiasis. Patients with abdominal actinomycosis are subjected to surgery for drainage of a supposed appendiceal abscess, and the true nature of the disease is recognized only when an indurated draining sinus stubbornly refuses to heal. Actinomycosis may also be mistaken for tumor of the reproductive organs in women or for tuberculous psoas abscess. Rarely, peritonitis develops. Actinomycosis involving the perianal region can cause recurrent multiple draining sinuses and fistulas *in ano*.

In the rare case of hematogenous disseminated actinomycosis, lesions appear in all parts of the body. Painful indurated nodules under the skin of the legs, arms, back, and scalp are prominent, and nonsuppurative effusions of the pleura or pericardium develop.

DIAGNOSIS The disease is easily recognized by detecting *A. israelii* in pus obtained from sinuses, empyema fluid, or abscess cavities. Interpreting actinomycetes in sputum is difficult because the organisms are normal inhabitants of the mouth. Sulfur granules vary in size from several microns to 3 mm in diameter. Large granules are found if a thorough search is made by diluting the pus with saline solution and filtering through gauze. They are white, yellow, or brown and stand out sharply against the background of blood-tinged pus. Gram-positive branching filaments or bacilli which fail to grow aerobically are key findings. Granules of other organisms (staphylococci, nocardias, monosporia), fragments of caseous material, and clumps of pus cells or fibrin may be confused with actinomycotic granules. Sabouraud's medium will not support its growth. Cultural isolation of *A. israelii* is not difficult if anaerobic methods are used. A small microaerophilic gram-negative bacillus, *Actinobacillus actinomycetemcomitans*, is often associated with *A. israelii* in actinomycosis. Anaerobic streptococci, *Bacteroides*, and other anaerobes are also present frequently. Hence *actinomycosis is characteristically a mixed anaerobic infection.*

Biopsy may establish the diagnosis if the actinomycotic colony ("ray fungus") is observed microscopically. Demonstration of the organism may be difficult, requiring careful search of many sections.

Intradermal or serologic tests with *A. israelii* or its fractions are of no diagnostic aid. Radiologic examination may suggest actinomycosis if consolidation of the lungs and periosteal proliferation of the ribs are found, because this combination rarely occurs in other conditions. The appearance of the spine in lateral views may be almost pathognomonic, because the areas of absorption and newly formed bone give a picture of a coarse sieve not seen in any other vertebral disease.

TREATMENT Penicillin and the tetracycline antibiotics are so effective that the disease is disappearing through the wide use of these drugs prophylactically after dental extraction and in other conditions that might evolve into actinomycosis. When either is administered in large doses over long periods of time, remarkable improvement may be expected even when the purulent foci are inaccessible to surgical drainage. Many reports indicate that the tetracycline drugs (chlortetracycline, oxytetracycline, tetracycline) are superior to penicillin. When the tetracyclines are given in doses of 500 mg every 6 h, there is a reduction in pain and swelling within a few days as well as gain in strength, increase in weight, and prompt defervescence. Treatment should be continued for several weeks after the patient appears cured. Because penicillin is no more effective than the tetracyclines and because it requires repeated intramuscular or intravenous injection of large doses for long periods of time, it should be reserved for patients who cannot tolerate tetracycline drugs. The optimum dose of penicillin is not known, but at least 4 million units daily should be given intramuscularly.

Surgical drainage is a valuable adjunct to chemotherapy and may occasionally lead to spontaneous cure. Older

treatments such as iodides, irradiation, or the sulfonamides have no place in the treatment of actinomycosis, and amphotericin B is of no value.

REFERENCES

Brewer N, Spencer R, Nichols D: Primary anorectal actinomycosis. JAMA 228:1397, 1974

Brock DW et al: Actinomycosis caused by *Arachnia propionica.* Am J Clin Pathol 59:66, 1973

Cope VZ: *Actinomycosis*, London: Oxford, 1938

Flynn MW, Felson B: The roentgen manifestations of thoracic actinomycosis. Am J Roentgenol 110:707, 1970

Garrod LP: Actinomycosis of the lung: Etiology, diagnosis, and chemotherapy. Tubercle 33:258, 1952

McVay LV Jr, Sprunt DH: A long-term evaluation of aureomycin in the treatment of actinomycosis. Ann Intern Med 38:995, 1953

Nichols DR, Herrell WE: Penicillin in the treatment of actinomycosis. J Lab Clin Med 33:521, 1948

170 CRYPTOCOCCOSIS

ABRAHAM I. BRAUDE

DEFINITION Cryptococcosis is a pulmonary infection caused by *Cryptococcus neoformans*, an encapsulated yeast with a special predilection for the central nervous system. It occurs with increased frequency in patients with leukemia or lymphoma.

ETIOLOGY Members of the genus *Cryptococcus*, to which *C. neoformans* belongs, form neither mycelia nor spores and reproduce entirely by budding. The cells of *C. neoformans* are spherical, measure 5 to 15 μm in diameter, retain the Gram stain, and are surrounded by a capsule which may have a diameter three times that of the cell. The capsular material contains a polysaccharide which is responsible for the slimy appearance of the yeast in culture, for the myxomatous character of cryptococcal lesions, and for the serologic type. Of the four serotypes, type A is by far the commonest recovered from human infections.

The organisms grow readily on various media at room temperature and at 37°C. On Sabouraud's glucose agar, visible growth appears within a few days at 37°C and gradually becomes brownish and slimy. Unlike other pathogenic yeastlike fungi, cryptococci never form mycelia. Most cells of *C. neoformans* are killed in 24 h at temperatures of 40.6°C or higher.

PATHOGENESIS AND PATHOLOGY Cryptococci resembling *C. neoformans* have been isolated from soil, the surface of fruit, and the skin and intestinal tract of normal human beings. The most constant sources of virulent strains, however, are pigeon droppings, which provide an alkaline medium rich in nitrogen and salts that promotes survival of *C. neoformans*. In dust composed of these materials, desiccated cryptococcal cells only 1 μm in diameter can pass through the smallest airways to alveoli. These cryptococci are unencapsulated but can rapidly develop capsules upon contact with human beings. Hence it is possible for infections to be of either endogenous or exogenous origin. Although neurologic disturbances overshadow others, there is good evidence that infection is usually established in the lung and other viscera before dissemination to the brain and the meninges occurs. Often the pulmonary foci give rise to no clinical findings, although they can be detected if a careful search is made post mortem.

The cryptococcus does not evoke the active inflammatory response observed with other fungi or bacteria. The cellular reaction is very slow to develop and is seldom intense. The cryptococcus seems to meet little resistance and frequently proliferates so freely that macroscopic masses of gelatinous yeasts fill the lesions. Older lesions occasionally show granulomatous reactions. The small number of cryptococci observed within granulomas suggests that mononuclear cells can destroy the organism. This may account in part for the fact that lymphomatous diseases involving the mononuclear cells lower resistance to cryptococcal infection. At other times, however, many cryptococci are present within mononuclear and giant cells. It is unusual to see necrosis in cryptococcosis.

Granulomas or gelatinous cryptococcal masses may appear in the nervous system, lungs, bones, or skin. In the nervous system, lesions usually develop in the meninges at the base of the brain, with involvement of the brainstem, cranial nerves, and cerebellum. Large masses of yeast in the subarachnoid space may extend diffusely along perivascular spaces into the brain to produce cystic nodules. Because the fungal masses shrink after fixation of the brain in formalin, cystlike spaces remain. In the lung, scattered miliary nodules, diffuse pneumonic infiltrations, or solitary masses easily mistaken for pulmonary neoplasms may occur. Calcification or hilar lymphadenopathy is extremely rare. These characteristics of the cryptococcal pulmonary lesions are helpful in distinguishing the disease from tuberculosis, sarcoidosis, and other mycoses. In contrast to cryptococcal meningoencephalitis, serious predisposing diseases accompany pulmonary cryptococcosis in only 10 percent of patients.

CLINICAL MANIFESTATIONS Most patients with cryptococcal infection consult a physician only after the onset of neurologic manifestations. Complaints of severe headache, diplopia, dizziness, ataxia, vomiting, tinnitus, memory disturbances, or Jacksonian convulsions are common. Fever is usually absent. Many patients die within a few months, but some have lived for many years as the disease undergoes remissions and relapses.

When pulmonary infection is present in the absence of meningoencephalitis, the patient is generally free of constitutional symptoms. The disease is detected when roentgenographic examination of the chest shows a dense, usually solitary infiltration of the lower portions of the lung. Cough may be a prominent feature of diffuse cryptococcal pneumonia. Pleural effusions are unusual, but cavities are not rare.

Involvement of bones in the absence of disseminated disease is rare, and cryptococcosis of joints is almost always secondary to adjacent osseous lesions.

Disseminated infection may also produce multiple nodules or papules in the skin. These range from a few millimeters in diameter to masses resembling strawberries in size and color.

The possibility of underlying Hodgkin's disease, lymphosarcoma, leukemia, or diabetes should be considered in every patient with cryptococcosis.

DIAGNOSIS Cryptococcal meningitis must be distinguished from other diseases which present as aseptic meningitis, including brain abscess, tuberculous meningitis, coccidioidal meningitis, and carcinomatous meningitis. In each of these, the spinal fluid is sterile by ordinary cultural methods and may contain from a few to several hundred mononuclear cells, increased protein, and reduced glucose. Because *C. neoformans* is recovered with much greater ease than the etiologic agents of the other diseases, culture of the spinal fluid is the decisive procedure in differential diagnosis. The cryptococcus is isolated on Sabouraud's agar at room temperature and usually grows after 1 to 2 weeks. In tuberculous and coccidioidal meningitis positive cultures are much less common, and in uncomplicated brain abscess the spinal fluid is sterile. Cryptococcal cells may also be found by direct microscopic examination of sediment from centrifuged spinal fluid. Mixing a drop of sediment with India ink facilitates the recognition of the mucinous capsule, but artifacts resembling cryptococci develop in India ink from inflammatory cells and mislead even the experienced observer. The organism can be cultured from the blood and urine in 25 to 35 percent of patients with cryptococcal meningitis. Specimens obtained via bronchoscopy or transbronchial brush biopsy may contain cryptococci in pulmonary cryptococcosis when sputum cultures are negative. Biopsy is essential for diagnosis in most cases of pulmonary infection. In tissue, intracellular forms with small capsules may resemble *Histoplasma capsulatum* but can be differentiated by mucicarmine, which stains the capsular mucopolysaccharide peculiar to *C. neoformans*. Biopsied material should also be inoculated onto Sabouraud's glucose agar. In many cases, the patients' serums give positive tests for either cryptococcal antigen or antibody. Circulating antigens appear to indicate continuing disease, while antibodies are found only after treatment, when the cryptococcus and its antigens are disappearing from the body fluids. The finding of cryptococcal antigen in the cerebrospinal fluid may be particularly important in diagnosing meningitis, when organisms are not seen or cultured.

TREATMENT All forms of cryptococcosis usually improve after intravenous infusions of 0.75 to 1 mg per kg amphotericin B daily, and 60 percent of those with cryptococcal meningitis are cured. These maximum daily doses are reached only after gradual increments of the initial dose of 1 mg. When maintenance levels are reached, the drug should be given every other day. Patients without meningoencephalitis can be cured with total doses of less than 1.5 g, but 3 g is probably required for infections of the nervous system. If relapse occurs after intravenous treatment, amphotericin B may be dissolved in the spinal fluid and 0.5 mg injected intrathecally on alternate days in conjunction with intravenous administration. Strict precautions must be taken during intrathecal injection to avoid bacterial contamination and drug overdosage. One milligram amphotericin B intrathecally may cause fever, temporary paralysis of the bladder and legs, and arachnoiditis. Arachnoiditis can be minimized by using 10% dextrose in water as a hyperbaric solution for carrying 0.5 mg amphotericin B away from the lumbar injection site to the basilar cistern after the patient is placed in the Trendelenburg position. The chief dangers of intravenous amphotericin B are anemia, hypokalemia, and renal damage characterized by renal tubular acidosis. The anemia frequently occurs after prolonged treatment and is normocytic, normochromic, and reversible. The hypokalemia develops with or without impaired renal function and requires prophylactic potassium supplements. Disturbances in renal function should be expected. Azotemia, impaired urine concentration, and microscopic hematuria with granular casts are the main findings but are reversible if detected in time. Treatment should be discontinued if the blood urea nitrogen exceeds 40 mg per 100 ml and resumed when it approaches normal levels. Serious and permanent renal damage with nephrocalcinosis has occurred in patients given a total dosage greater than 5 g. In cryptococcal meningitis, sterility of the spinal fluid is probably the best end point of successful treatment. Dead cryptococci may be visible for years after the disease is cured and do not require more treatment. Prognosis is poorest in patients with the following manifestations: (1) lymphoreticular malignancy; (2) cerebrospinal fluids with high opening pressure, low glucose levels, fewer than 20 leukocytes per mm^3, and cryptococci seen in smear; (3) cryptococci outside the nervous system; and (4) high posttreatment titers of cryptococcal antigen in serum or cerebrospinal fluid.

Flucytosine (5-fluorocytosine) is also successful in some patients with cryptococcal infections. It is given orally in doses of 150 mg per kg per day, with little toxicity and a success rate of about 50 percent in cryptococcal meningitis. Treatment failures result from the development of drug resistance during treatment, a phenomenon not seen with amphotericin B. Since Flucytosine can be given in full doses at the start of treatment, it should be used in fulminating cryptococcal infections to produce immediate therapeutic levels in the blood and cerebrospinal fluid during the period when subtherapeutic amphotericin doses are being gradually increased.

Diamox in doses of 500 mg twice daily is valuable for lowering the cerebrospinal fluid pressure during and after antifungal therapy.

REFERENCES

Diamond R, Bennett J: Prognostic factors in cryptococcal meningitis. Ann Intern Med 80:176, 1974

Littman ML, Walter JE: Cryptococcosis: Current status. Am J Med 45:922, 1968

Powell K, Christianson C: Pulmonary cryptococcosis: Clinical forms and treatment: A Center for Disease Control cooperative mycoses study. Am Rev Resp Dis 108:1116, 1973

Utz JP: Flucytosine. N Engl J Med 286:777, 1972

Walter JE, Jones RD: Serodiagnosis of clinical cryptococcosis. Am Rev Resp Dis 97:275, 1968

171 BLASTOMYCOSIS

ABRAHAM I. BRAUDE

DEFINITION Blastomycosis is a fungous infection of the skin and viscera, caused by *Blastomyces dermatitidis* in North America and by *Paracoccidioides brasiliensis* in South America. South American blastomycosis is also termed paracoccidioidomycosis.

ETIOLOGY In infected tissues *B. dermatitidis* has the appearance of a yeast, forming single buds from 3 to 24 μm in diameter. Two features aid in recognition: (1) its thick wall, spoken of as "double-contoured," because the inner and outer margins can be seen, and (2) the wide opening between parent cell and bud at the base of attachment.

In culture, *B. dermatitidis* is dimorphic and appears as the wrinkled, waxy yeast form on blood agar incubated at 37°C, or as a mold with branching hyphae on Sabouraud's agar at room temperature. On microscopic examination the cultured yeast may be found to be identical with that in the infected lesions or may have abortive mycelia. The mycelia give rise to oval or pear-shaped exogenous spores.

Multiple buds on the yeastlike cell of *P. brasiliensis* distinguish it morphologically from *B. dermatitidis*. The tiny multiple buds have the appearance of a crown of small beads attached to the cell wall. The fungus reproduces by budding both in tissues and when cultured at 37°C. At room temperature it produces mycelia but not true spores.

PATHOGENESIS AND PATHOLOGY Although *B. dermatitidis* has seldom been cultured from the soil and soon disappears after inoculation into natural soil, this remains the most likely source of the fungus. Most infections occur in people who are in close contact with soil, especially in the Mississippi and Ohio River Valleys. A better case for such an origin can be made for *P. brasiliensis*, which is probably harbored in the soil of the warm wet forests of Colombia, Venezuela, and Brazil.

The lung appears to be the major portal of entry for both North and South American blastomycosis. Because of strong natural resistance to both *B. dermatitidis* and *P. brasiliensis*, most persons develop subclinical pulmonary infections recognizable only by skin tests. In North American blastomycosis, heavy infection in healthy persons can cause multiple benign pulmonary lesions that heal spontaneously. Benign pulmonary lesions also occur in paracoccidioidomycosis. But in both infections primary lesions may give rise to progressive disease, with or without a variable latent interval. In North American blastomycosis the pulmonary lesion may enlarge and spread to other parts of the lung before dissemination to skin and bones; or systemic dissemination may occur from a small stationary pulmonary focus. In paracoccidioidomycosis, the face, nasal mucosa, oropharynx, and gingiva are affected most commonly, presumably as a result of spread from the previous pulmonary focus. The mucosal lesions, in turn, invariably spread to the regional lymphatics to produce massive lymph node enlargement with necrosis and sinuses draining through the skin. Hematogenous spread can cause massive enlargement of the abdominal or mediastinal lymph nodes. The spleen, liver, adrenal gland, urogenital tract, and brain can also be infected. Intestinal ulcerations develop after rupture of infected submucosal lymphoid tissue.

The basic lesion in both North and South American blastomycosis is the suppurative granuloma with Langhans and foreign-body giant cells. In the skin and mucous membranes this combination of abscesses and epithelioid cell granulomas occurs in the midst of pseudoepitheliomatous hyperplasia. Characteristic cells of *P. brasiliensis* with its multiple buds, or of *B. dermatitidis* with its single broad-based bud, can be seen in these lesions.

CLINICAL MANIFESTATIONS The rare acute pulmonary form of North American blastomycosis varies from asymptomatic infection to a severe illness resembling acute histoplasmosis. Two clinical types have been recognized. The first consists of fever, productive cough, joint and muscle pains, with multiple nodular pulmonary densities in roentgenograms and budding yeast in the sputum. In the second type, pleuritic chest pain of variable severity and lasting only a few hours is the distinctive feature, but chest x-rays reveal no pleural effusions despite multiple pulmonary nodules. Both forms are benign, and the patient recovers without specific treatment. In the typical case of progressive North American blastomycosis the onset is insidious. The patient may seek medical attention because of a persistent "chest cold," low-grade fever, weight loss, or progressive disability. Physical examination and a roentgenogram of the chest disclose evidence of pneumonia, which may involve any segment or lobe of the lung. Cavitation is frequent, and mediastinal lymph nodes may be prominent. Hemoptysis, purulent sputum, chest pain, and dyspnea appear as the disease progresses. Although the pulmonary infection may subside spontaneously, extrapulmonary lesions of the skin, bones, joints, and viscera eventually call attention to dissemination. These metastatic suppurative lesions are accompanied by an increase in fever, sweats, chills, and weakness. Death in the untreated infection sometimes occurs in less than 6 months, but most patients live for a year or two. The overall mortality rate in systemic blastomycosis is said to be 92 percent in patients whose cases have been followed for 2 years or longer without specific therapy.

Infection of the skin by *B. dermatitidis* (Gilchrist's disease) first appears on unclothed areas such as the hands, face, or forearm but not the scalp, palms, or soles. The infection begins as a firm nodule surrounded by similar lesions which tend to coalesce. Suppuration in the center of the nodule is followed by partial healing and fibrosis as extension occurs peripherally. The hyperplastic epithelium gives these lesions a hard, raised, wartlike margin. When fully developed, blastomycosis of the skin presents the appearance of one or more ragged ulcers with partially healed centers and thick raised margins. The primary cutaneous infection may be confined to the skin for months or years.

South American blastomycosis may be present in a *pulmonary* or *disseminated* form. Symptoms of the pulmonary form include productive cough, hemoptysis, dyspnea, fever, fatigue, malaise, and weight loss. Dissemination is characterized by painful ulcers of the mouth and nose, hoarseness, dysphagia, cervical lymphadenopathy which may be massive and which is occasionally accompanied by sinus formation, inability to eat, abdominal pain, and cachexia. The disease may spread to viscera, bones, and central nervous system, and, if left untreated, is fatal after a few months or several years.

DIAGNOSIS Pulmonary blastomycosis closely resembles tuberculosis, carcinoma of the lung, aspiration pneumonitis, and other fungous infections, including coccidioidomycosis, actinomycosis, nocardiosis, and histoplasmosis. Differentiation must be based on the recovery of the etiologic agent, because neither clinical nor epidemiologic features are specific. Most cases of North American blastomycosis are found in the Southeastern United States and in the Mississippi River Valley, but the disease occurs throughout the United States and Canada.

It is usually possible to find either *B. dermatitidis* or *P. brasiliensis* by microscopic examination of biopsied material, sputum, or pus. The yeastlike forms can be observed if a drop of purulent material is first mixed on a slide with a drop of 10% potassium hydroxide and kept at room temperature for 30 min. The multiple buds covering the entire surface of *P. brasiliensis* are connected by a narrow neck to the parent cell, while buds of *B. dermatitidis* are connected by a wide communication. *Blastomyces dermatitidis* is isolated by culturing pus on Sabouraud's agar at room temperature and on blood agar at 37°C. *Paracoccidioides brasiliensis* can also be isolated on blood agar at 37°C but grows so slowly that more than a month may elapse before colonies appear.

The diagnostic value of the skin test for blastomycosis is limited. The complement fixation test in both North and South American blastomycosis is positive in high titer with serums of patients who have systemic infections. The results of intradermal and serologic tests may be of prognostic value. Patients with marked dermal hypersensitivity and low serum titers of complement-fixing antibody are said to have a better prognosis in North American blastomycosis than those with negative skin tests and high complement fixation titers. Patients with severe paracoccidioidomycosis are anergic to paracoccidioidin and other antigens used for measuring delayed hypersensitivity. Their lymphocytes respond subnormally to stimulation of blast transformation and they tolerate heterologous skin grafts better than normal, both evidence of acquired deficiency of cell-mediated immunity.

TREATMENT Amphotericin B is curative in both North and South American blastomycosis. North American blastomycosis also responds, but less favorably, to 2-hydroxystilbamidine, while South American blastomycosis is resistant to it. Either drug is given daily or every other day by slow intravenous drip in increasing doses. The maximum adult daily dose of amphotericin B is 40 mg, and that of 2-hydroxystilbamidine is 250 mg. North American blastomycosis should be treated with a total of 1.5 g amphotericin B; 7 to 8 g of 2-hydroxystilbamidine may be required. Anesthesia over the distribution of the trigeminal nerve is the main untoward reaction from 2-hydroxystilbamidine; it persists after treatment. Surgical excision of pulmonary cavities or destroyed tissues is sometimes necessary in addition to chemotherapy.

In South American blastomycosis the sulfonamide drugs

produce dramatic clinical remissions of most forms of the disease, but relapses invariably occur unless the patient is maintained on continuous therapy. Sulfadiazine in doses of 4 to 6 g daily or sulfisoxazole in dosage of 6 to 8 g per day has been successful in arresting the disease. In severe cases both amphotericin and sulfonamides should be used.

REFERENCES

ABERNATHY R: Treatment of systemic mycoses. Medicine 52:385, 1973

CHICK EW: Blastomycosis—the enigma of systemic mycoses. Chest 60:2, 1971

LONTERO AT, RAMOS CD: Paracoccidioidomycosis. Am J Med 52:771, 1972

MENDES NF: Lymphocyte cultures and skin allograft survival in patients with SA blastomycosis. J Allergy Clin Immunol 48:40, 1971

RESTREPO A et al: Paracoccidioidomycosis (South American blastomycosis). Am J Trop Med Hyg 19:68, 1970

SAROSI G, HAMMERMANS R et al: Clinical features of acute pulmonary blastomycosis. N Engl J Med 290:540, 1974

WITORSCH P, UTZ JP: North American blastomycosis: A study of 40 patients. Medicine 47:169, 1968

172
COCCIDIOIDOMYCOSIS

ABRAHAM I. BRAUDE

DEFINITION Coccidioidomycosis is an infection acquired by inhalation of *Coccidioides immitis,* a fungus existing only in the mycelial phase in nature and converted to a spherule in tissues. Although most infections are mild or inapparent, *C. immitis* may produce a fatal disseminated disease with destructive lesions in the lungs, lymph nodes, spleen, liver, bones, kidneys, and brain.

ETIOLOGY *Coccidioides immitis* grows readily at room temperature or at 35°C and produces white, cottony mycelia. As the culture ages, the segmented mycelium breaks up into thick-coated rectangular *arthrospores,* 2×4 μm in size. These arthrospores can survive in stored cultures and are highly infectious for laboratory personnel. The mycelium and its spores are pathogenic for various laboratory animals. The mycelial form is converted to a thick-walled spherule filled with endospores in animal tissues and under special cultural conditions.

PATHOGENESIS AND PATHOLOGY Coccidioidomycosis is acquired by inhalation of *chlamydospores* in endemic areas in the semiarid regions of the Southwestern United States and the Chaco district of Argentina. Most infections occur during the dry seasons, particularly after exposure to dust storms. The fungus grows in the soil in rainy weather and becomes disseminated in dust during dry weather. *Coccidioides immitis* is isolated from soil and from desert rodents.

The inhaled spores are carried to the terminal bronchioles and alveoli, where the first reaction is an outpouring of polymorphonuclear leukocytes, fluid, and a few mononuclear cells. In most cases, the organism is probably killed or arrested. In others, the organisms proliferate and

elicit an inflammatory response which appears to depend on their multiplication. Rapid multiplication is manifested by frequent discharge of endospores from spherules and an exudate rich in polymorphonuclear leukocytes. The phase of slow multiplication, with infrequent rupture of spherules, produces a granulomatous reaction in which epithelioid cells and giant cells predominate. Although polymorphonuclear leukocytes congregate about the point of rupture of a spherule and invade the broken capsule, phagocytosis by these cells is unsuccessful. As the released endospores develop into spherules, the neutrophilic reaction gives way to proliferating mononuclear cells which ingest the fungus.

Either phase of this inflammatory cycle may predominate, or a mixture of the two may be found. Rapidly progressive infections produce large areas of confluent suppurative pneumonia and necrosis. In contrast, granulomatous lesions contain exudates composed almost exclusively of mononuclear cells and giant cells which fill alveoli but leave their walls intact. Both reactions involve the overlying pleura and spread to the hilar and mediastinal lymph nodes. Ultimately the bronchopneumonia in most patients resolves or heals by fibrosis; in others, the lesions persist as cavities or solid nodules.

Recovery is accompanied by the development of hypersensitivity to the fungus. This hypersensitivity is apparently responsible for at least two special manifestations: (1) *erythema nodosum,* a sterile, focal nodular granulomatous reaction usually limited to the skin of the lower extremities and characterized by extravasation of red blood cells into the lesion; (2) *pleural effusion.* It is believed that rupture of a pleural granuloma discharges antigenic material onto the sensitized pleural membranes.

In patients who do not develop dermal hypersensitivity, the infection spreads to lymph nodes, spleen, bones, liver, kidney, meninges, skin, adrenals, and pericardium. In the meninges, the reaction may take two forms: (1) the granulomatous reaction is commoner and produces a firm plastic lesion which encloses the brainstem and other structures in a rigid mass of tissue; (2) the suppurative reaction results in outpouring of polymorphonuclear leukocytes with little granulomatous change. In either type, but especially in the granulomatous, involvement of the brainstem may lead to severe hydrocephalus.

CLINICAL MANIFESTATIONS The infection may be either benign or disseminated. The benign infection, so-called "desert fever," is self-limited, and as many as 50 percent of benign infections are asymptomatic. The remainder have influenza-like symptoms. After an incubation period of 1 to 3 weeks, the patient has fever, chills, fatigue, headache, severe arthralgia, a maculopapular pruritic eruption, erythema nodosum, and symptoms of respiratory infection. The most frequent complaint is poorly localized chest pain, aggravated by breathing or coughing. A nonproductive cough is common, but hemoptysis is infrequent. Although hydrothorax may be massive and require repeated thoracenteses, it eventually resorbs without further difficulty.

Despite the paucity of signs in the chest, prominent abnormalities are found in roentgenograms. These include focal areas of infiltration, hilar and mediastinal lymphadenopathy, nodules or cavities, and pleural effusion. The commonest are single or multiple infiltrates in any segment that simulate tuberculosis if the upper lobe is involved. They usually resolve after several weeks.

In about 2 percent of benign infections a solid or cavitary pulmonary lesion remains. The typical cavity of coccidioidomycosis is peripheral, has a thin wall, and gives a cystlike appearance in roentgenograms. The cavitary disease may also be indistinguishable from chronic pulmonary tuberculosis and produce chronic cough, weight loss, fever, hemoptysis, chest pain, and dyspnea. Residual solid lesions may be as large as 3 cm in diameter. Both solid and cavitary lesions are commoner in the upper lobes.

In a few individuals (0.05 to 0.2 percent), the primary infection progresses to the disseminated form of the disease, usually within a few months of infection. Dark-skinned persons and pregnant women are more vulnerable. Among blacks and Filipinos, 85 to 90 percent with dissemination die, as compared to 50 percent of Caucasians. Patients who develop progressive coccidioidomycosis do not give a history of erythema nodosum.

The course of disseminated infections is marked by fungating or ulcerating skin lesions, multiple pulmonary nodules or cavities, widespread destructive lymphadenopathy, osteomyelitis, and meningitis. Weight loss, fever, and weakness are the outstanding systemic manifestations, and the course is often rapid, with death occurring in less than a year. If vital organs are spared, however, patients with disseminated coccidioidomycosis may feel surprisingly well, continue to work, and even gain weight despite the presence of large numbers of *C. immitis* in the sputum or subcutaneous abscesses. The meningeal form is invariably fatal, but even it is compatible with survival for several years. In the presence of meningitis with progressive hydrocephalus, patients experience severe headaches, cranial nerve palsies, memory disturbances, and disorientation. The spinal fluid shows 100 to 200 cells, mostly mononuclear, elevated protein levels, and frequently a reduction in glucose concentration.

DIAGNOSIS Except in meningitis, *C. immitis* is easily recovered from the lesions of disseminated coccidioidomycosis by direct examination and cultures of exudates or biopsied tissues. The characteristic spherule is seen best in purulent material treated with 20% potassium hydroxide. Occasionally, in biopsied tissue, spherules may all be immature and contain no endospores, making them indistinguishable from *B. dermatitidis.* Cultural identification becomes essential for diagnosis. On Sabouraud's agar, mycelial growth appears in 4 to 8 days, and diagnostic spherules develop when the mycelia are incubated in Converse medium at 40°C in 20% CO_2. In meningitis, only a few spherules appear in the spinal fluid, despite the presence of large numbers in the granulomatous exudate around the brainstem. Occasionally, the culture of 20 to 30 ml of spinal fluid yields positive results, but usually the diagnosis can be based only on a positive coccidioidin complement fixation test with spinal fluid.

Serologic tests are performed with coccidioidin, a filtrate from cultures of *C. immitis.* By the third week of primary infection, precipitins are found in the serum of 91 percent of patients with symptomatic infection but in only 7 percent of asymptomatic individuals. Complement-fixing antibodies appear later and persist longer than precipitins in nondisseminated coccidioidomycosis; they are almost always present in the disseminated disease and in the spinal fluid in meningitis. The simpler serum immunodiffusion test gives nearly identical results to the complement fixation test. Intradermal tests with coccidioidin are of value in the recognition of primary benign infections because they become positive before precipitins appear, but in disseminated infection the skin test is frequently negative.

The x-ray suggests pulmonary coccidioidomycosis if hilar lymphadenopathy progresses while the parenchymal infiltrate is subsiding or if the adenopathy is associated with multiple areas of pneumonitis. A smooth, thin-walled cavity without surrounding infiltration is also characteristic of residual primary disease. Other residual lesions include calcified or noncalcified nodular foci and localized bronchiectasis. In disseminated pulmonary infection the commonest picture is that of multiple infiltrates accompanied by pleural involvement and prominent hilar or mediastinal lymphadenopathy. Acute miliary coccidioidomycosis cannot be distinguished radiographically from acute miliary tuberculosis, while chronic pulmonary coccidioidomycosis can resemble tuberculosis, with chest x-rays showing soft confluent infiltrates and single or multiple apical cavities.

The only remarkable hematologic finding is eosinophilia, which may reach 35 percent of the total leukocyte count in the primary disease, especially if erythema nodosum is present. Eosinophils may also appear in the cerebrospinal fluid in coccidioidal meningitis.

TREATMENT Intensive intravenous treatment with amphotericin B in daily doses of 1 mg per kg body weight appears to be effective in some cases of extrameningeal coccidioidomycosis. Coccidioidal meningitis should be treated with repeated intrathecal injections of 0.5 mg amphotericin B, as well. Introduction of amphotericin in a hyperbaric solution helps prevent arachnoiditis after lumbar infection and improves delivery of the drug to the brainstem. Ten percent dextrose in water is used as a hyperbaric solution for carrying amphotericin B away from the injection site to the basilar cistern by placing the patient in the Trendelenburg position. The total dose varies from less than 1 g to more than 10 g intravenously. Severe nausea, venous thrombosis, and reversible impairment of renal and hepatic function often interrupt the treatment schedule, but persistent administration of amphotericin B in the face of troublesome side effects has occasionally produced improvement. A fall in titer of complement-fixing antibodies and a return of coccidioidin skin sensitivity are evidence of effective treatment. Drug therapy may have to be supplemented by surgical removal of peripheral granulomas and by ventricular shunts to relieve hydrocephalus.

Primary surgical excision of residual pulmonary foci is indicated for secondary infection or hemoptysis. Dissemination from these foci almost never occurs.

REFERENCES

AJELLO L: *Coccidioidomycosis,* Tucson: University of Arizona Press, 1967

ALAZRAKI NP et al: Use of a hyperbaric solution for administration of intrathecal amphotericin B. N Engl J Med 290:641, 1974

FIESE MJ: *Coccidioidomycosis,* Springfield, Ill.: Charles C Thomas, 1958

SMITH CE et al: Pattern of 39,500 serologic tests in coccidioidomycosis. JAMA 160:546, 1956

173 HISTOPLASMOSIS

ABRAHAM I. BRAUDE

DEFINITION Histoplasmosis is caused by the dimorphic fungus *Histoplasma capsulatum,* found as a tiny body within reticuloendothelial cells. The disease varies from mild or unnoticed respiratory infection to widely disseminated lethal disease. African histoplasmosis, caused by *Histoplasma capsulatum* var. *duboisii,* spares the lung and attacks the skin and bones.

ETIOLOGY Although *H. capsulatum* grows on Sabouraud's agar at room temperature as a spore-bearing mold, it is transformed after animal inoculation into nonencapsulated, oval, yeastlike cells measuring 2 × 4 μm. In histologic section the protoplasm is shrunken so that the unstained space beneath the cell wall has the appearance of a capsule. The fungus also grows in the yeastlike phase if incubated at 37°C in sealed tubes of blood agar. The most distinctive cultural feature, however, is the tuberculate *chlamydospore* found only on mycelia; it is round, 10 × 20 μm in diameter, and covered with warty projections. Another smaller spore, not distinguishable from that of *Blastomyces dermatitidis,* is also present on the mycelium. *Histoplasma duboisii* resembles *B. dermatitidis* in tissues and *H. capsulatum* in culture.

PATHOLOGY AND PATHOGENESIS Infections with *H. capsulatum* are prevalent in the great river valleys of South America, Africa, India, Burma, Thailand, Cambodia, and Indonesia, but are rare in Europe. In the United States such infections are highly prevalent in the Mississippi River Valley and its tributaries. The source of human infection is probably soil containing spores of *Histoplasma.* Several studies have emphasized the isolation of the fungus from soil in areas inhabited by chickens, birds, and bats. Contamination of caves with *H. capsulatum* by bats may lead to outbreaks of "cave fever." City dwellers are often exposed to histoplasma growing in soil under trees which shelter starlings or blackbirds. The portal of entry is the lung, where a primary complex may be formed by extension of infection from the pulmonary focus to the regional lymph nodes. Most primary infections have benign self-limited dissemination, as evidenced by hepatic and splenic calcifications.

The basic pathologic process is multiplication of *H. capsulatum* in reticuloendothelial cells of the liver, lymph nodes, lung, spleen, adrenal glands, intestine, and marrow. In addition to diffuse lesions, the reticuloendothelial tissues contain nodular accumulations of epithelioid cells and giant cells of the Langhans type. Histoplasma organisms are difficult to demonstrate in the epithelioid cells of the noncaseous granuloma.

Caseous necrosis may accompany both diffuse lesions and granulomas. The adrenals, which are involved in nearly all disseminated infections, are often massively enlarged. Caseous necrosis is usually present in the center of the pulmonary granulomas, which resemble those of cavitary pulmonary tuberculosis. Necrotizing histoplasmosis may also take the form of renal papillitis. Extracellular forms of histoplasma are readily found in the necrotic areas of all organs by special stains (periodic acid-Schiff, Gridley). These extracellular organisms may be much larger than the intracellular ones, appear distorted, and occasionally assume the mycelial form.

The portal of entry for African histoplasmosis is unknown. No pulmonary foci of infection have been found in the few fatal cases examined. The earliest lesions are single granulomas of the skin, lymph nodes, and bone. Masses of large yeast cells are found in giant cells. Dissemination produces multiple lesions in skin, bone, liver, and spleen.

CLINICAL MANIFESTATIONS The signs and symptoms of histoplasmosis range from those of a slight self-limited infection to fatal disseminated disease. The high incidence of positive intradermal reactions to histoplasmosis in healthy persons in many parts of the world indicates that most infections by *H. capsulatum* are inapparent or very mild. This variability in severity is observed among different persons in the same outbreak. Severe infections are characterized by prolonged fever, dyspnea, chest pain, weight loss, prostration, widespread pulmonary infiltrates, hepatomegaly, and splenomegaly. Other infected persons may have only a benign acute pneumonitis lasting a week or less, while still others are entirely free of symptoms. Widespread ill-defined noncalcified pulmonary infiltrates of miliary size or larger are found in symptomatic infections and may also be present, although less extensively, in the asymptomatic ones. Eventually, pulmonary lesions either disappear or calcify. In the east central part of the United States there is a high incidence of pulmonary calcification in persons who have negative tuberculin and positive histoplasmin skin tests. In some epidemics of acute histoplasmosis, erythema nodosum and erythema multiforme have been prominent in middle-aged women.

Least resistance to histoplasmosis is encountered in young infants and in adults after the fifth decade. Most cases of disseminated infection have occurred at these extremes of life. In the infant there are fever, emaciation, anemia, and leukopenia, and evidence of widespread involvement of many viscera, including the liver, spleen, lung, intestine, lymph nodes, adrenals, skin, kidney, brain, eye, and endocardium. In the adult, visceral involvement is usually less widespread. Unlike the disease in infancy, adult histoplasmosis shows a marked predilection for males. Histoplasmosis of the lips, mouth, nose, and larynx occurs almost exclusively in adults and is the initial manifestation in about one-third of the fatal cases. Among the various syndromes encountered are subacute endocarditis, massive lymphadenopathy resembling tuberculosis or lymphoma, mediastinal fibrosis, superior vena cava syndrome, various forms of pneumonia, cerebral histoplasmoma, and meningitis. The last is characterized by signs of basilar localization with spinal fluid findings and a clinical course identical with those of tuberculous meningitis.

In addition to the acute benign and disseminated infections, chronic localized histoplasmosis occurs in adults. Two main clinical types of chronic localized histoplasmosis are encountered: (1) *Pulmonary.* This may resemble pulmonary tuberculosis in all respects. The patient may be asymptomatic or may complain of chronic and occasionally productive cough. Roentgenograms will show lesions identical to those of reinfection tuberculosis, sometimes with cavitation, and accompanied by consistently positive cultures of sputum for *H. capsulatum.* (2) *Mucocutaneous.* Ulcers of the mouth, tongue, pharynx, gums, larynx, penis, or bladder are rare lesions found only in adults. Regional lymphadenopathy is common in these types.

In African histoplasmosis, the predominant lesions are in the skin. These may rupture through the epidermis or encroach on underlying bone. In the disseminated form, multiple lesions involve the lymph nodes, bone, skin, liver, and spleen, but, in contrast to what happens in *H. capsulatum* infections, the lungs are spared.

DIAGNOSIS Isolation of *H. capsulatum* is not difficult in disseminated or chronic localized infections if cultures are made of bone marrow, blood, biopsied lesions, sputum, or exudate from an ulcer. After incubation of infected material on Sabouraud's agar at room temperature there appears a white cottony colony which later turns brown and produces the diagnostic tuberculate chlamydospores. Isolation from sputum is best accomplished in mice, because contaminants are suppressed and the mouse is extremely susceptible to infection by histoplasmas. The animal does not die, but subculture of the spleen 1 month later on Sabouraud's agar yields the organism. Histoplasmas may also be seen in bone marrow, material from open or biopsied lesions, and occasionally in blood smears of terminally ill patients. Special fungus stains (periodic acid-Schiff, Gridley) should be used. Certain intracellular forms of *Cryptococcus neoformans* may be indistinguishable from histoplasma in histologic sections, unless stains for the cryptococcal mucinous capsule are employed.

In cases from which *H. capsulatum* cannot be isolated indirect clues to identification are (1) history of exposure to oil or dust in an endemic area, (2) positive complement fixation or immunodiffusion tests, (3) positive histoplasmin skin tests, and (4) development of miliary calcifications in the lung and spleen. Although these criteria are not dependable individually, they are reliable when used together. The serologic and skin tests are frequently negative in culturally proved cases of histoplasmosis, and their specificity is not fully established. Histoplasmin skin tests may confuse the serologic picture by producing complement-fixing antibodies to mycelial antigens but not to yeast-phase antigens.

Histoplasmosis must be differentiated from tuberculosis, sarcoid, leukemia, infectious mononucleosis, Hodgkin's disease, brucellosis, and kala-azar. Because cortisone is frequently of value in sarcoid but can cause dissemination in histoplasmosis, differential diagnosis between these two diseases is critical and the diagnosis of sarcoid should be withheld until tissues have been examined with special fungous stains. In kala-azar the intracellular Leishman-Donovan body bears a close resemblance to *H. capsulatum,* and cultural isolation of the fungus may be important in distinguishing between the two.

TREATMENT Amphotericin B in intravenous doses of 0.50 to 0.75 mg per kg per day is of value in all forms of histoplasmosis, including African histoplasmosis. In progressive disseminated histoplasmosis caused by *H. capsulatum,* a minimal total of 40 mg per kg amphotericin should be given. But even with this dosage a low survival rate (37 percent) is to be expected unless fatal Addison's disease can be averted by early recognition and treatment of this complication. In chronic pulmonary histoplasmosis the infection is controlled in two-thirds of patients given only 0.5 g over 3 to 5 weeks, and retreatment is uniformly successful in the other third.

REFERENCES

BRODSKY A et al: Outbreak of histoplasmosis associated with 1970 Earth Day. Am J Med 54:333, 1973

COCKSHOTT W, LUCAS A: *Histoplasmosis duboisii.* Q J Med 33:223, 1964

GOODWIN RA, et al: Mediastinal fibrosis complicating healed primary histoplasmosis and tuberculosis. Medicine 51:227, 1972

SAROSI G et al: Disseminated histoplasmosis: Results of long-term follow-up. Ann Intern Med 78:511, 1971

SUTLIFF W: Histoplasmosis Cooperative Study V. Amphotericin B dosage for chronic pulmonary histoplasmosis. Am Rev Resp Dis 105:60, 1972

174 SPOROTRICHOSIS

ABRAHAM I. BRAUDE

DEFINITION Sporotrichosis is a chronic infection due to *Sporothrix schenckii.* It is characterized by the formation of suppurating nodules along the lymphatics of the skin and subcutaneous tissues. Hematogenous dissemination is rare.

ETIOLOGY The fungus *S. schenckii* is dimorphic. On Sabouraud's agar at room temperature its growth is mycelial, but in the tissue it takes the form of tiny, cigar-shaped yeast cells. The yeast phase also develops in vitro by incubation at 37°C on blood agar containing cystine.

PATHOGENESIS AND PATHOLOGY The fungus lives as a saprophyte on vegetation and penetrates the hands when the skin is broken. Many cases have followed injury by thorns; sporotrichosis is primarily an occupational disease in people working with plants. Sphagnum moss is an important source of infection, and its increased use as mulch may lead to a greater occurrence of sporotrichosis.

From 7 to 20 weeks after penetrating the skin, the fungus produces at the inoculation site a reddish-purple necrotic nodule, the sporotrichotic chancre. Occasionally the lesion at the inoculation site remains confined to the skin or epidermis without lymphatic involvement, but in the vast majority of cases the fungus spreads from the chancre up the extremities and evokes nodular lesions along the thickened lymphatics. Microscopically the nodules are granulomas with central necrosis. In rare infections the organism may become disseminated throughout the subcutaneous tissues, the liver, testicles, bone, and kidney. Disseminated disease is not usually accompanied by primary infections of the extremities, and its portal of entry is believed to be the gastrointestinal tract.

Inhalation seems to be responsible for a growing number of upper lung cavities due to sporotrichosis.

CLINICAL MANIFESTATIONS There is a marked disproportion between symptoms and findings. A chain of hard, reddened discrete lumps extends up the arm or leg to the axilla or groin, and the intervening lymphatics are red and thickened, but there is no pain, fever, or other constitutional symptom. Older nodules may rupture to produce fistulas or ulcers. In the rare patient with disseminated sporotrichosis, constitutional symptoms may be marked and the disease is rapidly fatal. Unlike other disseminated mycoses, sporotrichosis seldom involves the central nervous system. Instead, it has a predilection for bone, joints, periosteum, and muscle.

Without treatment, sporotrichosis does not heal, and the lesions often become secondarily infected with bacteria.

DIAGNOSIS The fungus cannot be seen upon microscopic examination of biopsied material or pus in most cases. Cultural isolation is invariably successful, however, if pus is aspirated from an unbroken nodule and inoculated onto Sabouraud's agar. The growth at first has the soft, creamy character of bacterial colonies and later develops a wrinkled, dark-brown appearance without the cottonlike filament of most molds. Microscopically, typical clusters of pear-shaped spores are found at the tips of conidiophores arising from the tangled mass of delicate branched mycelia. If the mold or the pus is inoculated intraperitoneally into mice or rats, numerous yeast forms will be seen in lesions of the peritoneal cavity or testicle, where they take the form of gram-positive cigar-shaped rods within polymorphonuclear leukocytes.

Recovery of the organism by these techniques permits ready differentiation of sporotrichosis from other chronic infections of the subcutaneous tissues such as syphilis, tularemia, blastomycosis, coccidioidomycosis, and mycobacterial infections. The lymphangitic forms of *Mycobacterium marinum* and *Mycobacterium kansasii* infections cannot be distinguished from sporotrichosis clinically, but skin injuries in an aquarium or swimming pool point to *M. marinum.*

Yeast antigens of *S. schenckii* have been used for immunodiffusion, complement fixation, and agglutination with patients' serums, and for intradermal tests, but these procedures are not well enough standardized for routine diagnosis.

TREATMENT The common lymphangitic form of sporotrichosis is almost invariably dramatically cured by saturated potassium iodide. This should be given orally in starting doses of 10 drops t.i.d. after meals and gradually increased to the point of maximum tolerance. Treatment should be continued for a month after lesions disappear. Additional local therapy may be required for cutaneous ulcers, which should be painted with tincture of iodine. It may also be necessary to excise the epidermal lesions, because these may not subside with oral iodides. Systemic sporotrichosis is resistant to iodides, but it responds well to intravenous

treatment with amphotericin B, given in a total dose of 1.5 to 2 g over a period of 6 to 8 weeks.

REFERENCES

DICKEY RF: Sporotrichoid mycobacteriosis caused by *M. marinum* (balnei). Arch Dermatol 98:385, 1968

KEDES LH et al: The syndrome of the alcoholic rose gardener: Sporotrichosis of the radial tendon sheath. Ann Intern Med 61: 1139, 1964

LYNCH PJ et al: Systemic sporotrichosis. Ann Intern Med 73:23, 1970

175 MONILIASIS (CANDIDIASIS)

ABRAHAM I. BRAUDE

DEFINITION Moniliasis is a common mild mucocutaneous infection due to *Candida albicans.* This fungus also causes widespread visceral infection.

ETIOLOGY Among the many species of *Candida,* only *C. albicans* is a common pathogen for human beings. On nutrient laboratory media *C. albicans* grows as a budding yeast in creamy-white colonies, but it produces both mycelia and yeastlike cells in infected tissues. *Candida parapsilosis* is important only as a cause of endocarditis. *Candida guilliermondii* and *Candida tropicalis* have also been isolated rarely in endocarditis.

PATHOGENESIS *Candida albicans* resides normally on the mucous membranes and is frequently cultured from the mouth and feces of healthy persons. The rate of cultural isolation from feces in numerous surveys has ranged from 14 to 19 percent. In debilitated patients, the fungus may produce white patches on the buccal mucosa and initiate mild inflammatory reaction. At times chronic moniliasis of the oral mucosa induces chronic hyperplastic changes that resemble leukoplakia. In pregnancy and diabetes, *C. albicans* frequently causes a mild superficial infection of the vagina. Presumably, the high glycogen content of the vaginal mucosa in pregnancy and the glycosuria of diabetes favor its growth. Although *Candida* multiplies excessively in the intestine or mouth if the normal bacterial flora is suppressed by antibiotics, true infection seldom accompanies this overgrowth. Membranous esophagitis is probably the best-defined *Candida* infection of the alimentary canal. *Candida* is usually introduced directly into the bloodstream by intravenous catheters or injections of narcotics, but *Candida* septicemia may also develop from infected burns or wounds. The kidney and brain bear the brunt of hematogenous infection, but lesions also occur in the thyroid, myocardium, endocardium, pancreas, adrenals, and liver. The visceral lesions are granulomatous nodules or abscesses containing both mycelia and yeastlike cells. Rarely, fungal masses act as "fungus balls" in the renal pelvis and obstruct the ureter. More commonly *C. albicans* causes cystitis in patients with indwelling urethral catheters.

A striking susceptibility to moniliasis of the skin and nails is seen in children with congenital hypoparathyroidism. Extensive cutaneous moniliasis occurs in infants with the Swiss type of agammaglobulinemia (alymphocytosis), but not in those with the Bruton form (Chap. 74). Chronic mucocutaneous candidiasis is also seen in other patients with diseases or therapy that depress cellular immunity.

CLINICAL MANIFESTATIONS No systemic disturbances accompany mucocutaneous infection. Infection of the mucous membranes, known as *thrush*, gives rise only to soft white patches on the tonsils, cheeks, gums, and tongue. These patches are easily removed and leave a reddened surface. Although usually self-limited, the disease may become chronic and spread to other mucosal surfaces or intertriginous areas in the groins, the antecubital fossae, the interdigital folds, the inframammary areas, the umbilicus, and the axillae. Eczematoid lesions and vesicles are also found in vulvovaginal moniliasis of pregnancy or diabetes. Bladder thrush may cause cystitis.

Painful swallowing or chest pain is the main symptom of *Candida* esophagitis. In some patients the pain may simulate myocardial infarction. This syndrome should be kept in mind in myeloproliferative diseases and during intensive courses of immunosuppressive drugs and antibiotics. Patients with esophageal moniliasis may have no oropharyngeal thrush.

Bloodstream infections are seen in the late stages of severe debilitating disease and seem to occur most commonly in children and debilitated adults given prolonged parenteral feeding or antibiotic therapy through intravenous catheters. Clinical signs range from fever alone to azotemia, depressed sensorium, and shock. *Candida* endocarditis may also develop from intravenous catheters, especially after heart surgery, but most *Candida* endocarditis is seen in narcotic addicts and affects the aortic or mitral valve.

DIAGNOSIS In thrush, the organisms are seen upon microscopic examination of the white patches as a tangled mass of mycelia and yeastlike cells. They grow readily on Sabouraud's agar. In fungemias the fungus can be isolated repeatedly from the blood and can be seen in a direct smear of the catheter tip. *Candida* organisms can be found in biopsies or aspirates of a disseminated macronodular red rash in candidemic patients suffering from hematologic malignancies. Diagnosis of candidemia may be aided by finding retinal lesions that look like colonies of *C. albicans* and often produce visual blurring and pain. *Candida* esophagitis is recognized roentgenographically by characteristic signs of mucosal irregularities, submucosal edema, and ulcerations. Endoscopy discloses a yellow-white friable pseudomembrane from which candida are obtained.

TREATMENT Oral and vaginal thrush are best treated topically. Nystatin oral suspension is used in the mouth and nystatin or candicidin tablets in the vagina. Topical therapy with nystatin ointment, miconazole cream, amphotericin B lotion, or alcoholic solutions of gentian violet is effective in cutaneous moniliasis. Nystatin oral suspension also produces marked improvement in *Candida* esophagitis. *Candida* cystitis in patients with indwelling catheters can be eliminated by bladder irrigations with 50 mg amphotericin B per liter. Candidemia usually disappears within several days after the contaminated intravenous catheters have been removed. Otherwise the disease is best treated with oral 5-fluorocytosine in doses of 150 mg per kg body weight daily if the yeast is sensitive to the drug. The heavy urinary excretion of this drug produces remarkable reversal of severe renal moniliasis not seen with other therapy. Unfortunately many strains of *C. albicans* causing candidemia are resistant to 5-fluorocytosine, and require treatment with intravenous amphotericin B in doses of 40 mg every other day for a total dose of 800 mg. A few patients with *Candida* endocarditis have been cured with 5-fluorocytosine, but this disease is best treated by surgical replacement of the infected aortic or mitral valve.

REFERENCES

BODEY G, LUNA M: Skin lesions associated with disseminated candidiasis, JAMA 229:1464, 1974

BRAUDE AI, ROCK J: The syndrome of acute disseminated moniliasis in adults. AMA Arch Intern Med 104:91, 1959

CURRY CR, QUIE PB: Fungal septicemia in patients receiving parenteral hyperalimentation. N Engl J Med 285:1221, 1971

FISHMAN L et al: Hematogenous candida endophthalmitis—a complication of candidemia. N Engl J Med 286:675, 1972

KIRKPATRICK C et al: Chronic mucocutaneous candidiasis: Model-building in cellular immunity. Ann Intern Med 74:955, 1971

176 PHYCOMYCOSIS

ABRAHAM I. BRAUDE

DEFINITION Phycomycosis is the general name given to two entirely different infections by two orders of the class Phycomycetes: (1) Mucormycosis is a malignant infection of cerebral, pulmonary, and abdominal blood vessels due to Mucorales. (2) Tropical subcutaneous and nasal phycomycosis is a benign chronic infection due to Entomophthorales.

ETIOLOGY The etiologic agent of cerebral mucormycosis has rarely, if ever, been cultured from the brain or spinal fluid even when expert mycologic techniques were used with fresh cerebral tissues known to harbor the characteristic mycelium. The mycelium is broad, branching, and aseptate, with a diameter of 6 to 15 μm. The fungus *Rhizopus oryzae*, a species of the order Mucorales, has been recovered from the paranasal sinuses of patients with fatal mucormycosis, and the mycelia in culture were identical in appearance with those in the brain. In addition to *R. oryzae*, it has been possible to isolate *Absidia corymbifera*, *Rhizopus arrhizus*, and *Mucor pusillus* from infected foci outside the nervous system. The Entomophthorales responsible for tropical phycomycosis are curious fungi capable of shooting off their conidia. Rhinoentomophthoromycosis is caused by the genus *Entomophthora coronata*, and subcutaneous phycomycosis by *Basidiobolus ranarum*, a phycomycete with septate mycelia.

PATHOGENESIS The Mucorales abound in soil, manure,

and starchy foodstuffs, but become pathogenic for man only in rare cases of diabetic acidosis and even less commonly in patients debilitated by uremic acidosis, leukemia, irradiation, radiomimetic drugs, or severe burns. The usual portal of entry appears to be the nasal turbinates or paranasal sinuses; from there the organism is thought to extend along the invaded vessels to the retroorbital tissues and cerebrum. Thrombosis of arteries and veins leads to multiple infarcts throughout the brain, but only a minimal inflammatory response is found. Cerebral mucormycosis may be associated with hematogenous spread to pulmonary and intestinal vessels. Pulmonary, gastric, and intestinal infarction may also develop as a primary infection apparently after inhalation or ingestion of the fungus. Organisms probably penetrate the walls of bronchi, stomach, or intestine and infect the adjacent hilar or mesenteric vessels. Intestinal mucormycosis takes the form of hemorrhagic segmental infarction of the ileum or colon. Invasion of coronary arteries may produce myocardial infarction.

CLINICAL MANIFESTATIONS Cerebral mucormycosis is characterized by (1) uncontrolled diabetes with acidosis. (2) ophthalmoplegia, and (3) signs of acute diffuse cerebrovascular disease. If the portal of entry is the nose, a black nasal turbinate, malar anesthesia, a necrotic palatal ulcer, and a thick, dark, blood-tinged discharge are found. When the patient is first seen, drowsiness and semistupor are usually attributed to the metabolic disturbance, but the cerebral manifestations persist and progress after the acidosis is corrected. Headache and fever are prominent, and paranasal sinusitis is frequently present. In addition to complete internal and external ophthalmoplegia, there may be edema of the eyelids and retina, proptosis, and signs of retinal vascular occlusion. Nuchal rigidity and mild mononuclear pleocytosis in the spinal fluid have also been described.

Pulmonary mucormycosis may start gradually or suddenly with chest pain, fever, hemoptysis, and a friction rub. A few cases have been described in which the orbit or sinuses were infected without extension to the brain.

In contrast to nasal mucormycosis, the African form of nasal phycomycosis does not invade blood vessels. Instead *E. coronata* causes a submucosal granuloma near the inferior turbinate that spreads along fascial planes and through sutures and foramens to produce progressive nasal obstruction and firm irregular swellings of the face without breaking through the skin. The other African phycomycete, *B. ranae* produces a woody-hard, freely movable lump in the thighs, buttocks, and forearms, with no constitutional disturbances. Most patients are children. The Sassoon Hospital syndrome, a remarkable disorder attributed to the toxin of *Rhizopus nigricans,* is characterized by epidemic polyuria and polydipsia.

DIAGNOSIS The syndrome of cerebral mucormycosis is so characteristic that it can be recognized by its clinical features alone. The fungus can be found in sections and cultures of the infarcted nasal turbinate or paranasal sinus.

PROGNOSIS Untreated cerebral mucormycosis is almost invariably fatal. Rare cases of recovery have followed control of diabetic acidosis.

TREATMENT A few patients with cerebral mucormycosis have recovered after treatment with amphotericin B in doses of 50 to 70 mg intravenously daily. The total doses were approximately 2.2 g. Treatment should also be directed toward rapid correction of the hyperglycemia and acidosis as well as local excision of infected tissue in the nose, paranasal sinuses, or orbit. Surgical removal of infected lung has been successful. Subcutaneous and nasal types of African phycomycosis improve with oral administration of potassium iodide.

REFERENCES

AMBRAMSON E, ARKY R: Rhinocerebral phycomycosis in association with diabetic ketoacidosis. Ann Intern Med 66:735, 1967

BURKITT DP et al: Subcutaneous phycomycosis: A review of 31 cases seen in Uganda. Br Med J 1:1669, 1964

177 NOCARDIOSIS

ABRAHAM I. BRAUDE

DEFINITION Nocardiosis, an infection caused by an aerobic actinomycete, may produce lung abscesses and spread to the brain and elsewhere; or it may appear as a chronic deforming granulomatous infection limited to the foot (maduromycosis).

ETIOLOGY Pulmonary and disseminated nocardiosis usually results from infection with *Nocardia asteroides.* This organism is relatively acid-fast, and its bacillary form resembles the tubercle bacillus, but *N. asteroides,* in contrast to the tubercle bacillus, grows rapidly on Sabouraud's medium or 10% blood agar at room temperature, and appears in exudates as long-branched, gram-positive mycelial forms.

PATHOGENESIS *Nocardia asteroides* can be recovered readily from soil. Nocardiosis appears, therefore, to be an exogenous infection usually having its portal of entry in the lungs. In almost every patient with nocardiosis (other than maduromycosis) the earliest and most extensive lesions are pulmonary acute suppurative foci. A well-defined wall is absent, a fact which probably accounts for the marked tendency of nocardial abscesses to spread to the brain and to a lesser extent to the spleen, skin, peritoneum, and kidney. Occasionally noncaseating granulomas are found. Susceptibility to nocardiosis is increased in Cushing's syndrome, in pulmonary alveolar proteinosis, and in some patients with lymphomas or leukemia after antitumor chemotherapy.

CLINICAL MANIFESTATIONS The chief symptom is cough, usually productive of a thick, sometimes bloody, sputum. Chest pain and dyspnea are common, as are fever, sweats, chills, leukocytosis, weakness, anorexia, and weight loss. The illness may be prolonged and present the picture of chronic pulmonary tuberculosis, lung abscess, or unresolved suppurative pneumonia. In nearly one-third of the patients this syndrome is interrupted suddenly by the acute neurologic changes of metastatic brain abscess. At this time the patient may have severe headache and focal sensory or motor disturbances. The protein, cells, and pressure of the spinal fluid are increased, but the concentration of glucose is not reduced unless the meninges are also infected. Occasionally, brain abscess is the first clinical manifestation of nocardiosis, especially in Cushing's syndrome secondary to adrenal steroid therapy. Infection of the skin is frequent and produces numerous scattered abscesses or single draining sinuses of the hand, chest wall, or buttocks.

The disease is usually fatal, after months to years.

DIAGNOSIS Because patients with nocardiosis are suspected of having tuberculosis, their sputums are examined for tubercle bacilli. The usual methods for concentrating tubercle bacilli often kill *N. asteroides. Nocardia asteroides* may also be overlooked in smears stained by the Ziehl-Neelsen method, because it is less resistant than the tubercle bacillus to decolorizing by alcohol. The organism is not killed by concentrating with trisodium phosphate, and overdecolorizing can be avoided by using 1% sulfuric acid.

Although sulfur granules are not found in pulmonary or disseminated nocardiosis, the gram-positive filamentous organisms in nocardial exudates often resemble *Actinomyces israelii.* The two pathogens can be distinguished, however, by the ease with which *N. asteroides* is cultivated on Sabouraud's medium or blood agar aerobically, and by its acid-fast staining characteristics. In biopsy material the nongranulomatous and minimally fibrotic character of the nocardial suppurative reaction also helps to distinguish it from infections due to *A. israelii.* The absence of tubercles is valuable in differential diagnosis from tuberculosis.

TREATMENT The sulfonamides have cured many patients with pulmonary nocardiosis and are the treatment of choice. Sulfadiazine or trisulfapyrimidines should be given in a dose of 8 to 12 g daily. Penicillin and tetracycline appear ineffective, and resistance of nocardiosis to these drugs may be used in distinguishing it from actinomycosis due to *A. israelii* and from other pulmonary infections which respond to these antibiotics. Combinations of antibiotics, based on sensitivity tests, are said to be effective in nocardiosis if sulfonamides are unsuccessful. A combination of erythromycin and ampicillin is synergistic against *N. asteroides* and has produced clinical improvement in pulmonary nocardiosis.

Treatment of brain abscess is unsatisfactory. Only one of 42 patients with cerebral nocardiosis has survived treatment with sulfadiazine alone, and when sulfadiazine is used in combination with surgery the prognosis improves only slightly.

REFERENCES

ANDRIOLE VT et al: The association of nocardiosis and pulmonary alveolar proteinosis. Ann Intern Med 60:266, 1964

BACH M et al: Susceptibility of *Nocardia asteroides* to 45 antimicrobial agents in vitro. Antimicrob Agents Chemother 3:1, 1973

DANOWSKI TS et al: Cushing's syndrome in conjunction with *Nocardia asteroides* infection. Metabolism 11:2, 1962

WEED LA et al: Nocardiosis: Clinical, bacteriologic and pathologic aspects. N Engl J Med 253:1138, 1955

YOUNG LS et al: *Nocardia asteroides* infection complicating neoplastic disease. Am J Med 50:356, 1971

178
OTHER DEEP MYCOSES:
Aspergillosis, Geotrichosis, Mycetoma, Chromomycosis, Rhinosporidiosis

ABRAHAM I. BRAUDE

ASPERGILLOSIS

DEFINITION Aspergillosis is an infection produced by *Aspergillus fumigatus* and other species of *Aspergillus,* a group of fungi of low pathogenicity for human beings unless resistance is overcome by an overwhelming inoculum or debilitating illness. The disease may become disseminated or remain localized to the lung, ear, orbit, or paranasal sinuses.

ETIOLOGY Aspergilli assume the mycelial form both in culture and in infected tissues. They are hardy, widely prevalent organisms and grow rapidly on all culture media at room temperature or 35°C as colored, woolly colonies peppered with dark dots. They are composed of segmented mycelia that bear masses of small round spores on a knoblike swelling at the end of specialized mycelial stalks known as conidiophores.

PATHOGENESIS AND PATHOLOGY Aspergilli cause disease by superficial colonization or invasion of respiratory or alimentary tissues. In *Aspergillus* bronchitis, mycelia form small, compact masses mixed with mucus that cause localized bronchial irritation and obstruction, but no invasion. Pulmonary infection may be superimposed on existing cavities, or may become established after resistance is lowered by leukopenia, Hodgkin's disease, irradiation, transplantation therapy, and other debilitating processes. Excessive use of adrenal steroids or antibiotics is also thought to favor secondary invasion by *Aspergillus.* The most distinctive pulmonary lesion is the aspergilloma, a mycelial mass in a fibrous cavity lined with bronchial epithelium. Aspergillomas (fungus balls) often form in the upper-lobe cavities of tuberculosis, bronchiectasis, bronchogenic carcinoma, sarcoidosis, and in patients with ankylosing spondylitis. Chronic granulomatous lung lesions resembling tuberculosis have also been described. More destructive infections occur in leukemia or lymphoma and take the form of necrotizing bronchopneumonia and lung abscesses. Thrombosis of vessels by invading mycelia leads to local necrosis with hemorrhage and to hematogenous abscesses in the brain, liver, kidney, spleen, heart, and thyroid. Primary infections of the ear, orbit, and nasal sinuses may also be invasive and extend locally into the middle ear and brain. Aspergillosis of the alimentary tract produces multiple lesions, involving oropharynx, esophagus, stomach, and intestine. *Aspergillus* esophagitis is the commonest of these lesions and is more invasive than *Candida* esophagitis, causing ulcers and extending into the muscularis or even perforating into the mediastinum. Mediastinal infection and *Aspergillus* endocarditis may occur after cardiac surgery.

CLINICAL MANIFESTATIONS In pulmonary aspergillomas the chief symptom is hemoptysis. Necrotizing bronchopneumonia and hemorrhagic pulmonary infarction, the commonest forms of acute pulmonary aspergillosis in hematologic malignancies, usually present the picture of dyspnea, fever, and tachypnea. In fulminating disseminated infections, pulmonary manifestations are often overshadowed by coma and other signs of cerebral infection. Fever, joint pains, and skin eruptions lasting for a few weeks or months may also accompany disseminated aspergillosis.

A syndrome of *allergic aspergillosis* occurs in asthmatics who develop hypersensitivity to *Aspergillus* antigens. These patients are subject to recurrent episodes of migratory pulmonary infiltrations with blood eosinophilia, increased wheezing, cough, fever, and pleuritic pain. The allergic process may lead to bronchiectasis and aspergilloma. Both reaginic and precipitating antibodies are considered responsible for the pulmonary and systemic responses. Allergic aspergillosis is said to be the most frequent cause in Great Britain of transient lung infiltrates with eosinophilia. A form of allergic aspergillosis, known as hemp disease, produces asthma in people working in rope factories. In localized *Aspergillus* bronchitis, the symptoms are dyspnea, wheezing, cough, and mild hemoptysis.

DIAGNOSIS Cultures of aspergilli have no diagnostic value unless they are obtained directly from infected tissues. They may be present in the mouth and in sputum cultures in the absence of *Aspergillus* infection, and they may contaminate uninfected biopsy specimens unless strict sterile precautions are observed. Cultural findings should be confirmed by demonstration of mycelia in biopsy material. In chronic aspergillomas the sputum cultures may sometimes become negative after the fungus loses its ability to sporulate, but bronchial brushing under fluoroscopic visualization may give pure growths of *Aspergillus.*

Aspergillomas of the lung can usually be recognized by the unique appearance in roentgenograms of a crescentic radiolucency surrounding a circular mass. In other forms of pulmonary aspergillosis the roentgenogram is not diagnostic and may resemble that of bronchogenic carcinoma, bacterial lung abscess, and tuberculosis. In allergic aspergillosis, the sputum may contain small plugs of eosinophilic and mycelial fragments. *Aspergillus* antigens produce immediate intradermal wheals followed by Arthus phenomena, and serum precipitins against *Aspergillus* antigens are found by double diffusion in agar gel. These precipitins are also present constantly in pulmonary aspergillomas but not in invasive disseminated aspergillosis.

TREATMENT Localized lesions have been successfully excised from both the lung and the brain. Endobronchial infusion of amphotericin B is effective in properly selected patients with aspergillomas. The value of chemotherapy has not been established in systemic infections, but intravenous amphotericin B shows enough promise to warrant its use. Corticosteroids may cure allergic pulmonary aspergillosis by suppressing the bronchial edema and asthmatic secretions in which the fungus grows.

GEOTRICHOSIS

DEFINITION Geotrichosis is the name given to certain disorders of the mouth, bronchi, and intestinal tract from which *Geotrichium candidum* has been isolated. This fungus has not been established as a human pathogen, and the validity of geotrichosis as a disease entity remains questionable.

ETIOLOGY The fungus *G. candidum* may resemble *Coccidioides immitis* in culture because its septate mycelium fragments into large square-ended arthrospores. *Geotrichium candidum* does not form sporangia in vivo, however, and its soft, creamy colonies on solid medium are easily distinguished from those of *C. immitis.*

PATHOGENESIS Geotrichium is a normal inhabitant of the pharynx and intestine and may proliferate locally to produce visible white colonies on the mucous membranes. It may also appear in dead tissues and secretions of the nasopharynx, bronchopulmonary tree, and colon but probably not as a primary pathogen.

CLINICAL MANIFESTATIONS Geotrichosis is reported to cause pulmonary cavities and colitis. In bronchopulmonary geotrichosis, the patient coughs up gelatinous sputum tinged with blood, and in rare cases thin-walled cavities like those of coccidioidomycosis have been described. An allergic type of bronchopulmonary geotrichosis, similar to allergic aspergillosis, is said to produce symptoms of severe asthma, and *Geotrichium* can be visualized in the bronchial lumen.

DIAGNOSIS In secretions and exudates, *G. candidum* has the appearance of oval or barrel-shaped spores measuring up to 8 to 10 mm in diameter. They are easily recovered on Sabouraud's agar at room temperature.

TREATMENT Lesions resembling thrush respond to local application of 1:10,000 solution of gentian violet. Bronchopulmonary geotrichosis is said to respond to oral treatment with potassium iodide, and intestinal geotrichosis is treated by oral administration three times daily of capsules containing 0.32 mg gentian violet.

MYCETOMA

DEFINITION Mycetoma is a chronic destructive infection of the skin, subcutaneous tissues, fascia, and bone. The infection produces a localized swelling containing multiple fistulas which extrude mycotic granules.

ETIOLOGY The most frequent cause of mycetoma in the United States is a higher fungus known as *Monosporium apiospermum,* the "imperfect" form of the ascomycete *Allescheria boydii.* It grows rapidly on Sabouraud's agar as a cottony mycelium bearing asexual spores either singly or in small groups at the tips or sides of conidiophores. Other higher fungi isolated in mycetoma include members of such diverse genera as *Aspergillus, Penicillium, Madurella, Acremonium,* and *Phialophora.*

Actinomadura, Madurella, Streptomyces, and *Nocardia* are important causes of mycetoma outside the United States. *Actinomadura madurae* is found in southeastern Asia, *Nocardia brasiliensis* in South America and Mexico, and *Madurella mycetomii* in equatorial Africa.

PATHOGENESIS AND PATHOLOGY The fungi found in mycetoma are inhabitants of the soil and enter the tissues of the bare foot and leg, presumably after trauma. The chest wall is infected by sacks, contaminated with soil, carried over the shoulder. The buttocks, abdomen, and arm are also infected.

The infection begins in the outer tissues and burrows through to destroy bone, muscle, and connective tissue indiscriminately. The areas of destruction show chronic suppuration with fibrosis and are connected by multiple fistulas which rupture to the outside. Mycotic granules are seen in the suppurative foci. The prolonged proliferation of granulation and scar tissue leads to enlargement of the affected part.

CLINICAL MANIFESTATIONS The earliest sign is usually a small swelling on the sole or dorsum of the foot which undergoes a recurring cycle of swelling, suppuration, and healing. Later, similar lesions appear on other parts of the foot, and over a period of months destruction of deeper tissues is manifested by slight or moderate pain, generalized swelling, and redness. The course is intermittently progressive, and there may be periods of remission. Ultimately the foot becomes a swollen, deformed mass of destroyed tissue with many fistulous openings through which mycotic granules are discharged. The infection does not spread hematogenously to other parts, but in rare instances there is direct extension along lymphatics. Death may occur from secondary bacterial infection.

DIAGNOSIS The characteristic granules are 0.5 to 2 mm in diameter and may be white, yellow, black, or red. Nocardial granules are easily distinguished from those of *Aspergillus boydii* and other higher fungi by direct microscopic examination. They are masses of radiating gram-positive filaments; those of higher fungi contain large segmented hyphae and numerous chlamydospores. Either type of granule grows rapidly on Sabouraud's agar.

Roentgenograms disclose destruction of bone which is more extensive than the external appearance and pain might indicate.

TREATMENT Nocardial and streptomycotic mycetomas should be treated with oral sulfonamides, and those due to higher fungi with intravenous and local amphotericin B. Antibacterial chemotherapy is valuable in arresting secondary infection. There is no dependable cure, however, and many patients eventually require amputation.

CHROMOMYCOSIS

DEFINITION Chromomycosis is an infection of the skin or brain produced by several species characterized by several species of pigmented soil fungi belonging to the family Dematiaceae. The commonest infection is characterized by slowly progressive cauliflower-like lesions of the skin of agricultural workers in tropical or subtropical regions.

ETIOLOGY The three species *Fonseca pedrosi, Fonseca compactum,* and *Phialophora verrucosa* are the chief causes of the verrucous form, usually known as chromoblastomycosis. They cannot be distinguished upon microscopic examination of infected tissue, in which all appear as small clusters of spores with thick, dark-brown walls. On culture, however, the three differ in their methods of sporulation. On Sabouraud's agar all three grow very slowly and will produce deeply pigmented olive or black colonies. *Phialophora gougerotii* is the commonest cause of cystic skin lesions, and *Cladosporium bantianum* usually produces brain abscess.

PATHOGENESIS AND PATHOLOGY The fungi live in the soil or vegetation and enter the skin of agricultural workers. The disease occurs mostly on the lower extremity of barefoot workmen, but sometimes on the upper extremity or buttocks.

Three pathologic processes are found in the verrucous form: (1) microabscesses in the dermis containing numerous fungi, (2) extensive fibrosis, and (3) epidermal hyperplasia and hyperkeratosis. The lesions progress along the lymphatics but only rarely beyond them, and they do not penetrate deeply to involve bone. In the cystic form, subcutaneous or intramuscular cysts full of pigmented fungi develop after puncture wounds. The brain abscesses are hematogenous and tend to occur as opportunistic infections in debilitated patients.

CLINICAL MANIFESTATIONS The earliest verrucous lesion is a papule, which develops into a well-circumscribed bluish lesion with a warty, raised margin. Although it resembles the cutaneous form of North American blastomycosis at this early stage, it does not spread peripherally. Instead, adjacent new lesions appear over a period of years and, as the epithelial hyperplasia and hyperkeratosis increase, the entire area assumes a cauliflower-like appearance. Eventually the whole extremity is covered. Pain and constitutional symptoms are absent unless secondary bacterial infection occurs or elephantiasis develops as a result of lymphatic scarring. Cystic chromomycosis presents the picture of one or more abscesses of the skin or muscle. Cladosporiosis of the brain is indistinguishable from other forms of brain abscess.

DIAGNOSIS The typical dark-brown septate bodies are seen in large numbers in biopsied tissue or pus, and brown hyphae can be found in crusts or pus treated with 10% potassium hydroxide. For specific identification, however, it is necessary to culture the slowly growing fungus on Sabouraud's agar.

TREATMENT Early in the verrucous disease, the lesions may be removed by liquid nitrogen, electrocoagulation, or surgical excision. Later in the course, excision of the larger nodules leaves indolent ulcers which heal very slowly. Cystic chromomycosis can also be excised.

Saturated solution of potassium iodide, given to tolerance orally, as in sporotrichosis, is said to be effective when combined with weekly injections of calcipherol. Local injection into the lesions of 0.035 mg amphotericin B in 7 ml of 2% procaine solution at weekly intervals has been used because the organisms are resistant to the levels achieved after intravenous injection. This local treatment produced complete resolution of lesions in a limited trial and should be tried. Oral 5-fluorocytosine in doses up to 10 g daily is the latest treatment to show promise. In general, the treatment of dermal chromoblastomycosis has been disappointing. The disease is never fatal, however, and the usefulness of the limb is retained despite its unsightly appearance. Chromomycosis of the brain, on the other hand, has been invariably fatal.

RHINOSPORIDIOSIS

DEFINITION Rhinosporidiosis produces small tumor-like masses usually in the nose and nasopharynx, but sometimes in the eye. An endosporulating fungus seen in the tissues cannot be cultured on laboratory media.

ETIOLOGY The fungus *Rhinosporidium seeberi* is placed in the class Phycomycetes and family Coccidioidaceae because characteristic giant sporangia develop in the tissues. These thick-walled endospore-filled sporangia resemble the smaller spherules of *Coccidioides immitis.*

PATHOGENESIS AND PATHOLOGY The nasal disease is probably acquired by bathing or diving into infected water. In India, where rhinosporidiosis reaches endemic proportions, its rarity in women is attributed to social taboos that prohibit their bathing in open places. The characteristic lesion is a vascularized papillomatous proliferation of the nasal or pharyngeal mucous membrane containing sporangia in various stages of maturity. Red blood cells, inflammatory cells, and extruded endospores fill the interstitial tissue. As sporangia enlarge, they compress the columnar epithelium of the nose or the squamous epithelium of the pharynx and allow endospores to escape and reinoculate the adjacent tissue. Ocular infection occurs in dry, dusty regions and may be transmitted in dust storms. In Texas, half the cases of rhinosporidiosis are ocular.

CLINICAL MANIFESTATIONS Single or multiple pedunculated, fleshy, red masses appear in the nares or pharynx and produce symptoms of rhinitis, epistaxis, and nasal obstruction. In exceptional cases hoarseness may develop from laryngeal infection. The conjunctiva of the lids is most prominently affected in the ocular form, which tends to be unilateral and remarkably free of pain. Although usually confined to the nose or eye, the infection may infrequently be seen in the vagina, rectum, male urethra, and bronchi. Generalized rhinosporidiosis with visceral involvement has also been reported.

DIAGNOSIS The characteristic sporangia are easily identified in biopsied tissue section. Because the only endemic foci are in India, most patients are Asiatic.

TREATMENT The lesions can be completely removed surgically or by electrocautery. Electrocautery is preferred because surgery leaves open incisions in which spores can be implanted and produce recurrences.

REFERENCES

AL-DOORY Y: *Chromomycosis,* Missoula, Mont.: Press Publishing, 1972

GILBERT T, PATTERSON R: Pulmonary allergic aspergillosis. Ann Intern Med 72:395, 1970

GRCEVIC N, MATHEWS WF: Pathologic changes in acute disseminated aspergillosis. Am J Clin Pathol 35:536, 1959

MEYER RD et al: Aspergillosis complicating neoplastic diseases. Am J Med 54:6, 1973

OLIN RR: Pulmonary geotrichosis and candidiasis. Minn Med 54: 881, 1971

PURANDARE NM, DEORAS SM: Rhinosporidiosis in Bombay. Indian J Med Sci 7:603, 1953

RAMIREZ M: Treatment of chromomycosis with liquid nitrogen. Int J Dermatol 12:250, 1973

SAFIRSTEIN B et al: Five-year follow-up of allergic bronchopulmonary aspergillosis. Am Rev Resp Dis 108:450, 1973

YOUNG R, BENNETT J: Aspergillosis: The spectrum of the disease in 98 patients. Medicine 49:147, 1970

ZAIAS N et al: Mycetoma. Arch Dermatol 99:215, 1969

section 12 | The rickettsioses

179 GENERAL CONSIDERATIONS

THEODORE E. WOODWARD

The rickettsial diseases of humans consist of a variety of clinical entities caused by microorganisms of the family *Rickettsiaceae.* The rickettsias are obligate intracellular parasites about the size of bacteria and are usually seen microscopically as pleomorphic coccobacilli. Each of the rickettsias pathogenic for human beings is capable of multiplying in one or more species of arthropod as well as in animals and humans. Indeed, the majority of the rickettsias are maintained in nature by a cycle which involves an insect vector and an animal reservoir, and infection of humans is unimportant in the cycle. Epidemic typhus presents a number of points of dissimilarity to most of the other rickettsioses, because the natural cycle of the infection involves only humans and the louse.

A compendium of information on the rickettsial diseases is given in Table 179-1. Because each of the rickettsioses responds therapeutically to tetracyclines or chloramphenicol, the table mentions no therapy. Procedures for diagnostic isolation of the rickettsias are omitted because they generally are less useful than serologic methods, and the techniques which they require are highly specialized and hazardous. Information on isolation may be found in textbooks devoted to viral and rickettsial diseases.

HISTORY OF THE RICKETTSIAL DISEASES Of all the afflictions of the human race the rickettsial diseases, particularly epidemic typhus, rank among the foremost as a cause of suffering and death.

The record of deaths from epidemic typhus in this century in the Balkan countries and in Poland and Russia reaches astounding figures. Typhus ravaged Russia and eastern Poland from 1915 to 1922, infecting 30 million of the inhabitants and causing an estimated 3 million deaths.

The past two decades have seen the development of excellent methods for the prevention and treatment of the rickettsioses. In fact, these measures have been so successful that the rickettsioses have become of minor importance in the United States and in many other countries. Although

TABLE 179-1
Rickettsial diseases

Disease		*Natural cycle*			*Principal means of transmission to humans*	*Serologic diagnosis*	
Type	*Agent*	*Geographic distribution*	*Arthropod*	*Mammal*		*Weil-Felix reaction*	*Complement fixation*
SPOTTED FEVER GROUP							
Rocky Mountain spotted fever	*R. rickettsii*	Western Hemisphere	Ticks	Wild rodents; dogs	Tick bite	Positive OX-19 OX-2	Positive group- and type-specific
Boutonneuse fever	*R. conorii*	Africa, Europe, Middle East, India					
Queensland tick typhus	*R. australis*	Australia		Marsupials, wild rodents			
North Asian tick-borne rickettsiosis	*R. sibirica*	Siberia, Mongolia		Wild rodents			
Rickettsialpox	*R. akari*	United States, Russia, Africa(?)	Blood-sucking mite	House mouse, other rodents	Mite bite	Negative	
TYPHUS GROUP							
Endemic (murine)	*R. mooseri*	Worldwide	Flea	Small rodents	Infected flea feces into broken skin	Positive OX-19	Positive group- and type-specific
Epidemic	*R. prowazekii*	Worldwide	Body louse	Humans	Infected louse feces into broken skin	Positive OX-19	
Brill-Zinsser disease	*R. prowazekii*	Worldwide	Recurrence years after original attack of epidemic typhus			Usually negative	
Scrub	*R. tsutsugamushi*	Asia, Australia, Pacific islands	Trombiculid mites	Wild rodents	Mite bite	Positive OX-K	Positive in about 50% of patients
OTHER RICKETTSIAL DISEASES							
Q fever	*R. burnetii*	Worldwide	Ticks	Small mammals, cattle, sheep, goats	Inhalation of dried infected material	Negative	Positive
Trench fever	*R. quintana**	Europe, Africa, North America	Body louse	Humans	Infected louse feces into broken skin	Negative	None available

* *Some authorities no longer place the agent in the genus* Rickettsia *because it cannot be cultured on artificial media.*

conquered, the rickettsioses have not been eliminated, and they could again become rampant if the will to control them, the present high standards of sanitation, and the necessary industrial capacities for production of effective insecticides and therapeutic agents should be decreased through war or disaster.

Gerhard in 1836 differentiated typhoid fever from louse-borne typhus fever. In 1899, Maxcy described the clinical manifestations of Rocky Mountain spotted fever. In a series of studies from 1906 to 1909, Ricketts, for whom the rickettsial microorganisms are named, successfully transmitted this disease to guinea pigs, incriminated the wood tick as a vector, and observed rickettsias in smears prepared from tick tissues.

Nicolle in 1909 reproduced typhus fever in monkeys and demonstrated transmission by the body louse. Von Prowazek in 1914 and Da Rocha-Lima in 1916 demonstrated small microorganisms in the tissues of lice taken from typhus patients.

Brill in 1910 recognized a febrile disease in patients in New York City as an example of mild epidemic typhus unassociated with lousiness. Zinsser in 1934 postulated that this disease was a recurrent form of typhus occurring in patients during periods of stress or waning immunity. Subsequent studies have confirmed Zinsser's hypothesis. This entity is now called Brill-Zinsser disease.

Weil and Felix, working with typhus patients in Poland in 1915, recognized that agglutinins for certain *Proteus* organisms appeared in the serum of convalescent patients. The Weil-Felix reaction, although nonspecific, affords a simple and valuable screening method for several rickettsioses.

In 1926 Maxcy, on purely epidemiologic evidence, surmised that typhus in the United States had its reservoir in rodents and was transmitted to humans by ticks or fleas. Confirmation of Maxcy's hypothesis was obtained in Baltimore in 1930 by Dyer and others when they isolated rickettsias from the brains of rats and shortly thereafter incriminated the flea as a vector. This disease, caused by *Rickettsia mooseri* and now designated endemic or murine typhus, is distinct from epidemic typhus and Brill-Zinsser disease.

The development of suitable vaccines and specific diagnostic antigens was impeded until it was possible to prepare appreciable quantities of highly infectious rickettsial material in the laboratory. The most important steps were (1) the Weigl vaccine (1930), a phenolized suspension of gut tissue obtained from body lice which had been injected intrarectally with the rickettsias of epidemic typhus; (2) the killed murine typhus vaccine prepared by Casteneda (1939) from lung tissues of rats, injected intranasally; and (3) the inactivated Rocky Mountain spotted fever vaccine obtained by Cox (1941) from infected yolk sacs of embryonated hen eggs. The low cost and relative simplicity of the egg techniques have led to their general use for preparation of vaccines and diagnostic antigens.

The years of World War II saw many strides in the conquest of the rickettsioses; perhaps greatest among these were the highly successful attacks on the arthropod vectors. The lousicide DDT proved to be ideal for control when dusted on the clothes of infested persons. The epidemic at Naples during the winter of 1943 to 1944 established a milestone, because it was the first to be suppressed by the use of insecticides. Scrub typhus (mite-borne typhus) was creating a major problem in the Pacific area. Here, too, the major contributions to successful control were concerned with application of miticidal chemicals to the person and his clothes.

The advent of broad-spectrum antibiotics—first chloramphenicol, then chlortetracycline, and later oxytetracycline—provided dramatic therapeutic results in each of the rickettsioses.

PATHOGENESIS Rickettsial diseases develop following infection through the skin or the respiratory tract. Agents of the typhus and spotted fever group are introduced through the bite of the infected arthropod vector. Ticks and mites, which transmit the agents of spotted fever and scrub typhus, inoculate the rickettsias directly into the dermis during feeding. The louse and flea, which transmit epidemic and murine typhus, respectively, deposit infected feces on the skin; infection occurs when organisms are rubbed into the puncture wound made by the arthropod. The rickettsia of Q fever gain entry through the respiratory tract when infected dust is inhaled; moreover, the respiratory route is occasionally implicated in epidemic typhus when infection results from inhalation of dried infected louse feces.

Although organisms probably multiply at the original site of entry in all instances, local lesions appear with regularity only in certain diseases, namely, the initial cutaneous lesions of scrub typhus, rickettsialpox, and boutonneuse fever, and the pneumonitis which develops in about half the persons infected with Q fever.

Volunteers infected with either scrub typhus or Q fever develop rickettsemia late in the incubation period, often some hours before the onset of fever. Similar events probably occur in all the rickettsial diseases; circulating rickettsias can be detected during the early febrile period in practically all patients. Little is known about the pathogenesis of infection during the midportion of the incubation period. However, it is reasonable to assume that during this time in patients with typhus or spotted fever, a transient low-grade rickettsemia results from release of organisms multiplying at the initial site of infection and that this seeds infection in the endothelial cells of the vascular tree. Vascular lesions developing at such sites account for the pathologic changes, including the rash.

Rickettsias apparently invade and proliferate in the endothelial cells of small blood vessels. Endothelial cell destruction occurs from the proliferation of organisms and eventual disruption. Rickettsia may exert a cytotoxic effect on endothelial cells; in mice the rickettsial toxin causes remarkable increase in capillary permeability, independent of proliferation. Later manifestations in rickettsial diseases may result from immunopathologic mechanisms, since humoral antibodies are present during the second febrile week, when increases in capillary permeability and vascular thrombosis and ecchymoses are greatest. Also, a delayed type of hypersensitivity occurs during infection.

The underlying cause of the toxic-febrile state which characterizes the rickettsial diseases remains unknown. Several rickettsial species contain type-specific toxins which are lethal for mice; these may play a role.

PATHOLOGIC PHYSIOLOGY Peripheral vascular collapse results in death in fulminating cases during the first week, with capillary dilatation and pooling of blood without increased capillary permeability or loss of fluid into extravascular spaces. As proliferative and thrombotic lesions develop in small vessels, anoxia occurs in the areas supplied, resulting in necrosis and increased capillary permeability, with loss of water, electrolytes, proteins, and erythrocytes. This, in turn results in a decrease in blood volume, together with an increase in extravascular space and clinical edema. Edema and anoxia of the myocardium are reflected in electrocardiographic changes. Liver function is impaired. The azotemia which develops in seriously ill patients appears to be prerenal. Clinical manifestations resulting from the peripheral vascular collapse are oliguria and anuria, azotemia, anemia, hypoproteinemia, hyponatremia, edema, and coma. In spotted fever and typhus patients with hemorrhagic skin lesions, consumptive coagulopathy is present. All these alterations are absent or minimal in mild cases or in those who are given specific treatment early.

PATHOLOGY The basic changes in the spotted and typhus fever groups are vascular, with resultant widespread lesions in adjacent parenchymatous tissues throughout the body. They are most common in the skin, muscles, heart, lung, and brain. The most conspicuous and diverse are found in Rocky Mountain spotted fever. Here swelling, proliferation, and degeneration of the endothelial cells occur, frequently with thrombus formation which partially or completely occludes the lumen. The muscle cells of the arterioles undergo swelling and fibrinoid changes. The adventitial tissues are infiltrated with mononuclear leukocytes, lymphocytes, and plasma cells. The vascular damage is scattered along the arteries, veins, and capillaries, with normal architecture prevailing throughout most of the vascular bed. The changes in murine, epidemic, and scrub typhus fevers resemble those in Rocky Mountain spotted fever, but thrombosis is uncommon and involvement of the musculature is rare.

Interstitial myocarditis occurs in each of these diseases but is usually most extensive in Rocky Mountain spotted fever and in scrub typhus. In the brain glial nodules are found in all members of the group, but microinfarcts in the brain tissue or in the myocardium are most often observed in spotted fever.

A rickettsial pneumonitis occurs, at least to some extent, in many patients with spotted or typhus fever and is the characteristic pathologic change in patients with Q fever. The process is patchy and consists microscopically of areas of congestion and edema. Within the consolidated areas the alveoli are filled with compact fibrinocellular exudate containing lymphocytes, plasma cells, large mononuclear cells, and erythrocytes but few, if any, polymorphonuclear leukocytes.

Rickettsias can occasionally be observed microscopically in sections of tissue. Failure to demonstrate them is of no diagnostic significance.

LABORATORY DIAGNOSIS Diagnostic procedures which depend on isolation of the etiologic agent from blood or other clinical material are expensive, time-consuming, and hazardous to laboratory personnel. Except in unusual circumstances, currently available serologic tests are adequate for laboratory confirmation of the clinical diagnosis in each of the rickettsial diseases. The demonstration of a rise in titer of specific antibody during convalescence is of prime importance in establishing the laboratory confirmation. Table 179-2 summarizes the serologic results usually encountered in persons who have rickettsial diseases in the United States. The Weil-Felix test employing *Proteus* strains OX-19 and OX-2 gives positive results in patients with spotted fever and murine typhus and negative results in those with rickettsialpox and Q fever. It is useful as a screening procedure but cannot be relied upon to differentiate spotted fever from murine typhus. In patients with Brill-Zinsser disease the *Proteus* OX-19 reaction is usually negative or low in titer.

Complement fixation tests employing group-specific rickettsial antigens provide data which clearly differentiate the most common infections, i.e., murine typhus, Rocky Mountain spotted fever, and Q fever. Moreover, if type-specific rickettsial antigens are employed, it is generally possible to distinguish rickettsialpox from spotted fever and Brill-Zinsser disease from murine typhus.

Antibodies during response to a primary infection of epidemic typhus or Rocky Mountain spotted fever are usually 19S globulins. In patients with Brill-Zinsser disease, which

TABLE 179-2
Serologic diagnosis of rickettsial diseases of the United States

		Weil-Felix reaction				*Complement fixation tests with type-specific antigen*				
			Illustrative titer				*Illustrative titer*			
Group	*Disease*	*Proteus*	*10th day*	*20th day*	*Cases with diagnostic titer*	*Rickettsial antigen*	*10th day*	*20th day*	*30th day*	*Cases with diagnostic titer*
Spotted fever	Rocky Mountain spotted fever	OX-19 OX-2	40 20	320 160	Most	*R. rickettsii*	20	160	80	Most
	Rickettsialpox	OX-19 OX-2	0 0	0 0	None	*R. akari*	0	64	128	Most
Typhus	Murine typhus	OX-19 OX-2	160 10	640 40	Most	*R. mooseri*	0	160	160	Most
	Brill-Zinsser disease	OX-19 OX-2	160 0	20 0	Infrequent	*R. prowazekii*	1,280	640	320	Most
	Q fever	OX-19 OX-2	0 0	0 0	None None	*R. burnetii*	10	80	160	Most

is a recrudescence, antibodies occur more quickly (within several days after onset of illness), rise to a higher titer, and are 7S globulins.

Specific antibiotic therapy has little effect on the time of appearance of antibodies or on their ultimate titer, provided treatment is instituted some days after onset of the illness. However, if the illness is cut short by early and vigorous treatment, antibody production may be delayed for a week or so, and also the maximal titers attained may be below those illustrated in Table 179-2. Under these circumstances a sample of blood taken 4 to 6 weeks after onset of illness should also be tested.

Two additional serologic tests are useful. Rickettsial agglutination with specific antigens is a reliable and practical microagglutination test. Another test is based on the agglutination of sheep or human O erythrocytes after sensitization with a serologically active fraction of rickettsias designated ESS (erythrocyte-sensitizing substances). Erythrocytes exposed to the typhus ESS are specifically agglutinated by serums of patients as early as the eighth febrile day. The ESS test is simple and inexpensive.

The immunofluorescent antibody test is a very useful procedure for detecting rickettsia in the tissues of patients with the typhus group of rickettsioses, the spotted fevers, and Q fever. The technique also visualizes rickettsia in ticks and the tissues of animals.

Normochromic anemia occurs in patients severely ill with rickettsial diseases. The white blood cell count in Rocky Mountain spotted fever, rickettsialpox, murine and epidemic typhus, Brill-Zinsser disease, Q fever, and other rickettsial diseases is usually within the normal range; 6,000 to 10,000 cells per mm^3. Leukopenia is occasionally observed, and in the presence of complications, such as superimposed infections and extensive vascular lesions, moderate leukocytosis occurs. The differential blood cell count is usually normal.

Thrombocytopenia occurs in severely ill spotted and scrub typhus fever patients with extensive vascular lesions; hypofibrinogenemia, prolonged prothrombin and partial thromboplastin times, and other clotting abnormalities occur.

REFERENCES See end of Chap. 187.

180 ROCKY MOUNTAIN SPOTTED FEVER

THEODORE E. WOODWARD

DEFINITION Rocky Mountain spotted fever is an acute febrile illness caused by *Rickettsia rickettsii.* It is transmitted to humans by ticks. The disease is characterized by sudden onset with headache and chills and by fever which persists for 2 to 3 weeks. A characteristic exanthem appears on the extremities and trunk about the fourth day of illness. Delirium, shock, and renal failure occur in the severely ill.

ETIOLOGY AND EPIDEMIOLOGY The causative microbe *R. rickettsii* is the prototype for the rickettsial group of agents. The minute organisms are purple when stained by Giemsa's method or red by Macchiavello's technique; most of them are gram-negative. These organisms often occur in pairs and possess a cell wall similar in structure and chemical composition to that of gram-negative bacteria; one finds a cell membrane, cytoplasmic granules corresponding to ribosomes, and prokaryotic organization of nuclear material. The cell membrane is selectively permeable; the cell wall is the focus of important antigens and an endotoxin-like substance.

The rickettsias grow in the nucleus and the cytoplasm of infected cells of ticks, mammals, and embryonated eggs; the intranuclear situation of the organisms is shared by the other members of the spotted fever group, but not by rickettsias of the typhus group. *Rickettsia rickettsii* is readily distinguishable from the agents of the typhus fevers by cross-immunity tests in guinea pigs and by complement fixation tests employing antigens prepared from infected yolk sac tissues. The differentiation of *R. Rickettsii* from closely related members of the spotted fever group frequently requires elaborate procedures. Strains of the agent of Rocky Mountain spotted fever vary considerably in their virulence for humans and animals.

The first reports of spotted fever in Idaho and Montana during the final decade of the last century led to the name Rocky Mountain spotted fever. However, the disease has been reported in all states except Maine and Vermont, as well as in Canada, Mexico, Colombia, and Brazil. Although related diseases are found on other continents, this particular infection is limited to the Western Hemisphere. During the 1960s, about 300 cases occurred annually in the United States. In the years 1973 and 1974, 668 and 784 cases respectively were reported. The mortality rate was about 20 percent in the days before specific therapy but has decreased to about 5 percent. Although the attack rate per unit of population is highest in Wyoming, almost half the cases occur in the South Atlantic states, with the greatest number of these in Virginia, North Carolina, Georgia, and Maryland.

A number of species of ticks are found infected with *R. rickettsii* in nature, but only two are important in transmitting spotted fever to humans. These are *Dermacentor andersoni,* the wood tick, which is the principal vector in the West, and *D. variabilis,* the dog tick, which assumes this role in the East. Infected female ticks transmit the agent transovarially to at least some of their offspring. Ticks which become infected, either through the egg or at one of the stages during their development cycle by feeding on an infected mammal, harbor the rickettsias throughout their lifetime, which may be several years. Thus, the tick serves as a reservoir in addition to being a vector. Small wild mammals are suspected of playing an important role in spreading the rickettsias in nature by infecting ticks which feed on them during rickettsemia.

Disease in humans is generally acquired from the bite of an infected tick. Transmission is unlikely unless the tick remains attached for a number of hours. Infection may also be acquired through abrasions in the skin which become contaminated with infected tick feces or tissue juices; hence, the hazard associated with crushing ticks between the fingers when removing them from persons or animals.

There are seasonal variations in the incidence of cases of

spotted fever, as well as differences in age and sex distribution of cases. In each instance these differences are related to exposure to ticks. Most cases are seen during the period of maximal tick activity, i.e., late spring and early summer. About half the cases in the Western states occur in men over forty, whereas half those in the Eastern states are in children under fifteen. This age distribution is undoubtedly influenced by propinquity to the wood and dog ticks, respectively. Mortality increases with age of the patient.

CLINICAL MANIFESTATIONS Incubation period and prodromata A history of tick bite is elicited in approximately 80 percent of patients. The incubation period varies between 3 and 12 days, with a mean of 7. A short incubation period usually indicates a more serious infection.

Onset In nonvaccinated persons, the onset is usually abrupt, with severe headache, a sudden shaking rigor, prostration, generalized myalgia, especially in the back and leg muscles, nausea with occasional vomiting, and fever which reaches 103 to 104°F within the first 2 days. Pain in the abdominal muscles may be severe, and arthralgia is not uncommon. Deep muscle palpation often elicits tenderness. Occasionally the debut of illness in children and adults is mild, accompanied by lethargy, anorexia, headache, and low-grade fever. These symptoms are similar to those of many acute infectious diseases, making specific diagnosis difficult during the first few days.

Pyrexia Fever continues for approximately 15 to 20 days in untreated cases. The febrile course in children may be shorter. Hyperthermia of 105°F or greater is of unfavorable prognostic significance, although fatalities may occur when the patient is hypothermic, with concurrent vasomotor collapse. Fever generally terminates by lysis over a period of several days, but rarely does so by crisis. Recurrent fever is uncommon except in the presence of secondary pyogenic complications.

The *headache* is generalized and excruciating, and frequently more intense over the frontal area. It persists throughout the first and second weeks of illness in untreated cases. Malaise continues for the first week; irritability is notable, and the patient shuns distractions such as questioning and examination.

Cutaneous manifestations The rash which is present in practically all cases is the most characteristic and helpful diagnostic sign. It usually appears on the fourth febrile day; the range is 2 to 6 days. The initial lesions are on the wrists, ankles, palms, soles, and forearms. The first lesions are macular, nonfixed, pink, irregularly defined, and measure 2 to 6 mm. A warm compress applied to the extremity accentuates the rash in the early stages. The exanthem is most prominent when the temperature is elevated. After 6 to 12 hr, the rash extends centripetally to the axilla, buttocks, trunk, neck, and face. (This is in contrast to the eruption of typhus fever, which begins on the trunk and spreads centrifugally, rarely involving the face, palms, or soles.) The rash becomes maculopapular after 2 to 3 days (it may be felt by light palpation) and assumes a deeper red hue. By about the fourth day it is petechial and fails to fade on pressure. Not uncommonly, the hemorrhagic lesions coalesce to form large ecchymotic blemishes; these lesions tend to form over bony prominences and may ultimately slough to form indolent, slow-healing ulcers. Patients who have had the typical rash show brownish discolorations at the site for several weeks during convalescence. In milder cases, the rash does not become purpuric and may disappear within a few days. Antibiotic therapy may abort the early exanthem; the later fixed lesion fades less rapidly with specific therapy.

The application of tourniquets for several minutes, or the occasional taking of the blood pressure, may provoke additional petechiae (Rumpel-Leede phenomenon), further evidence of capillary abnormalities.

Cardiovascular and respiratory features During the early stages, the pulse is full and regular but accelerated in proportion to the height of the temperature, and the blood pressure is well sustained. During the peak of illness in seriously ill patients, the pulse is rapid and feeble, and hypotension of 90 mmHg is common. If circulatory failure is sustained, the resultant hypoxia and shock lead to agitation and delirium and contribute to the formation of ecchymoses and gangrene of fingers, toes, genitalia, buttocks, earlobes, and nose. Cyanosis of the peripheral parts of the body is common. Venous pressure determinations show no elevation. A reduction of the total blood volume is occasionally found, as are evidences of myocardial impairment as shown by low voltage of ventricular complexes, minor S-T segment deflections, and occasionally delay in atrioventricular conduction on the electrocardiogram. These changes are transient and nonspecific. Severely ill patients have a puffy appearance of the face, hands, ankles, feet, and lower part of the sacrum.

Respirations are either normal or slightly accelerated. Cough may be harrassing and nonproductive, and localized pneumonitis may occur, but pulmonary consolidation is extremely rare. Pulmonary edema may develop after injudicious use of intravenous fluids.

Hepatic and renal manifestations In the majority of patients, there is little alteration in renal or hepatic function. The liver may be enlarged, but jaundice is unusual. Oliguria commonly occurs in the seriously ill, and anuria may mark the critically ill patient. Azotemia is common; when marked, it is a very unfavorable sign. Abnormalities in liver function are probably responsible for the hypoproteinemia, with reduction in the albumin fraction.

Neurologic manifestations The principal neurologic manifestations are headache, restlessness, and varying degrees of insomnia. Stiffness of the back is common. The cerebrospinal fluid is clear, with normal dynamics and normal chemical constituents. Coma and muscular rigidity may occur. Athetoid movements, convulsive seizures, and hemiplegia are grave manifestations. Deafness during the active stages of the disease is not uncommon. As a rule, all neurologic signs abate without residua. Findings based upon follow-up examinations and electroencephalograms may be interpreted as indicative of minor residual brain damage for a year or more following recovery of certain patients from Rocky Mountain spotted fever.

Other physical manifestations Patients become dehydrated, with extreme dryness of lips, gums, tongue, and pharynx. The skin is hot and dry, the conjunctivas are frequently injected, and the eyes suffused. Photophobia is common in the early stages of illness. Petechial hemorrhages may be noted in the conjunctivas or in the retina. The spleen is enlarged in approximately one-half the cases and is firm and nontender. Abdominal distention is frequent, and occasionally some degree of intestinal ileus is observed. Constipation is usual.

COURSE In patients with mild and moderately severe cases who are given no specific antibiotic therapy, the disease abates within 2 weeks, and convalescence is rapid. In fatal cases death usually occurs during the latter part of the second week as a result of toxemia, vasomotor weakness, and shock or renal failure.

In vaccinated individuals who contract the disease, the illness is mild, with a short febrile course and an atypical rash.

COMPLICATIONS AND PROGNOSIS If the serious manifestations of spotted fever mentioned above are regarded as intrinsic parts of the disease, then complications are uncommon and consist mainly of secondary bacterial infections, namely, bronchopneumonia, otitis media, and parotitis. Thrombosis of major blood vessels may result in gangrene of a portion of an extremity. Hemiplegia and peripheral neuritis are rare sequelae.

The overall mortality rate for spotted fever was formerly about 20 percent. Death occurred in more than half of persons over forty years of age, but the mortality rate was much lower in children and young adults. Since the introduction of the broad-spectrum antibiotics and the development of more precise knowledge regarding correction of the physiologic abnormalities which develop during the disease, fewer deaths occur from this infection. Some of the fatalities can be attributed to failure to consider spotted fever in the differential diagnosis.

DIFFERENTIAL DIAGNOSIS During the early stages of infection before the rash has appeared, differentiation from other acute infections is difficult. History of tick bite while living or traveling in a highly endemic area is helpful. The rash of meningococcemia (Chap. 136) resembles Rocky Mountain spotted fever in certain aspects, because it is macular, maculopapular, or petechial in the chronic form, and petechial, confluent, or ecchymotic in the fulminant type. The meningococci skin lesion is tender and develops with extreme rapidity in the fulminant form, whereas the rickettsial rash occurs on about the fourth day of disease and gradually becomes petechial. *Spotted fever is often confused with measles.* The exanthem of rubeola rapidly becomes confluent, while that of rubella *usually remains discrete.*

Murine typhus is a milder disease than Rocky Mountain spotted fever; the rash is less extensive, nonpurpuric, nonconfluent; and renal and vascular complications are uncommon. Not infrequently differentiation of these two rickettsial infections must await the results of specific serologic tests. Epidemic typhus fever is capable of causing all the pronounced clinical, physiologic, and anatomic alterations seen in patients with Rocky Mountain spotted fever, i.e., hypotension, peripheral vascular collapse, cyanosis, skin necrosis and gangrene of digits, renal failure and azotemia, and neurologic manifestations. However, the rash of classical typhus is noted initially in the axillary folds and on the trunk and later extends peripherally, rarely involving the palms, soles, or face. The serologic patterns in these two diseases are distinctive when specific rickettsial antigens are employed in tests. Moreover, louse-borne typhus is not recognized in the United States except in the form of Brill-Zinsser disease (recurrent typhus fever). Rickettsialpox, although caused by a member of the spotted fever group of organisms, is usually readily differentiated from Rocky Mountain spotted fever by the initial lesion, the relative mildness of the illness, and the early vesiculation of the maculopapular rash. The Weil-Felix reaction is positive in Rocky Mountain spotted fever and in murine and epidemic typhus, but is negative in rickettsialpox. Agglutinins against *Proteus* OX-19 and OX-2 appear in the serum of patients with spotted fever, but only those against OX-19 are generally found in murine and epidemic typhus.

THERAPY Certain physiochemical changes occurring in the patient seriously ill with one of the diseases of the typhus-spotted fever group should be understood before a therapeutic regimen is outlined. These changes are circulatory collapse, coma, oliguria and anuria, azotemia, anemia, hypoproteinemia, hypochloremia and hyponatremia, and edema. These alterations are often absent in the mildly ill, and in them management is much less complicated. The therapeutic principles necessary for treatment of all rickettsioses are (1) specific chemotherapy and (2) supportive care. Attention to both is mandatory for the seriously ill patient first recognized late in the disease. During the first week in the moderately ill patient, supportive therapy may be less energetic, because specific chemotherapy usually suffices. The early mild case may be successfully treated at home; later in the course of the disease patients should receive hospital care.

Therapeutic measures advisable for the management of Rocky Mountain spotted fever will be described in detail. Variations of this regimen which apply to the other rickettsioses are described in subsections dealing with other diseases of the typhus-spotted fever group and Q fever.

Specific therapy Specific therapy is most effective when initiated during the early stages of disease coincident with the appearance of the rash. When therapy is delayed until the rash has become hemorrhagic and widespread, the response is less dramatic. The antibiotics of choice are chloramphenicol and the tetracyclines, which are effective because of their rickettsiostatic properties. They are not rickettsiocidal.

The following antibiotic regimen is considered optimal: for chloramphenicol, an initial dose of 50 mg per kg body weight, and for tetracycline, 25 mg per kg body weight. Subsequent daily doses are the same as the initial loading dose, with the requirement divided equally and given at 6- to 8-h intervals. Antibiotic treatment is continued until the patient has improved and has been afebrile approximately 24 h. In patients too ill to take oral medication, an intravenous preparation of one of the antimicrobials may be employed for the loading dose.

Adrenal cortical hormones may need to be utilized for their antitoxemic effects, in patients first observed late in the course of severe illness. Large doses for brief periods of about 3 to 5 days, in combination with specific antibiotics, are recommended in critically ill patients.

Therapy with antibiotics is continued until the toxemia has abated, the general condition has markedly improved, and the temperature has remained at normal levels for 24 h. In uncomplicated cases of spotted fever, there is symptomatic improvement within 24 h and temperature becomes normal in 60 to 72 h.

Supportive care Frequent turning of the patient relieves pressure from prominent bony parts and also militates against the development of aspiration pneumonia. Proper mouth care, with frequent swabbing of the oral cavity, may avert the development of parotitis and gingivitis. Sucking of the juice of a lemon or the oral use of glycerin or mineral oil is helpful.

A generous intake of protein should be provided by frequent feedings as soon as the disease is suspected, in order to avoid subsequent protein deficiency. Usually food is well tolerated by patients with rickettsial disease, and the daily diet should provide 3 to 5 g protein per kg normal body weight, with adequate carbohydrate and fat to make it palatable. When the patient is uncooperative, the diet may be supplemented by hourly liquid protein feedings via stomach tube, provided that there is no abdominal distention.

At the critical stage, when hypoproteinemia is present and changes in capillary permeability lead to edema and vascular embarrassment, careful attention must be given to parenteral hyperalimentation with high concentration of glucose and amino acids. When indicated by hematologic studies, whole-blood transfusions given slowly are helpful. The judicious administration of one of the plasma expanders at this stage may have a definite favorable effect upon impending circulatory collapse. If the patient is anuric and azotemia is pronounced, overloading the circulation with fluids should be governed by clinical judgment and very careful laboratory studies. Frequent determinations of hemoglobin, hematocrit, electrolytes, and protein, sometimes at intervals of a few hours during crucial periods, are necessary in order to ascertain abnormalities and to permit institution of corrective measures. Dialysis is indicated when there is clear-cut evidence of acute tubular necrosis (Chap. 272).

Complications *Pyogenic complications,* including otitis media and parotitis, are encountered in patients severely ill with Rocky Mountain spotted fever and other rickettsioses. These localized infections respond to therapy with appropriate antibiotics combined with ordinary supplemental surgical measures.

Pneumonitis usually develops as a result of specific rickettsial action. The sputum is scant but should be examined to determine whether superimposed bacterial infection is present. Specific therapy is guided by the results of these laboratory studies. The pneumonitis generally responds to the antibiotic therapy the patient is receiving, but if staphylococcal pneumonia is suspected, a penicillinase-resistant penicillin should be added to the broad-spectrum drug.

Circulatory failure of peripheral or central origin is combated by careful administration of plasma expanders and fluids. Heart failure may develop from the disease or as a result of overzealous intravenous therapy and is recognized by rapid pulse. gallop rhythm, and increase in venous pressure. When the clinical signs reveal unmistakable evidence of cardiac failure, digitalis should be employed. Oxygen therapy improves the cardiac and circulatory status and is helpful in hypoxemic patients with involvement of the central nervous system.

PREVENTION Prevention is attained primarily by avoidance of tick-infested areas. When this is impractical, prophylactic measures include (1) spraying the ground with dieldrin or chlordane for area control of ticks (though there are environmental objections to the use of residual insecticides in area control of ticks, under special conditions, such procedures may be warranted); (2) application of repellents such as diethyltoluamide or dimethylphthalate to clothing and exposed parts of the body, or in very heavily infested areas the wearing of clothing which interferes with attachment of ticks, i.e., boots and a one-piece outer garment, preferably impregnated with repellent; and (3) daily inspection of the entire body, including the hairy parts, to detect and remove attached ticks. In removing attached ticks great care should be taken to avoid crushing the arthropod with resultant contamination of the bite wound; touching the tick with gasoline or whisky encourages detachment but gentle traction with tweezers applied close to the mouth parts may be necessary; the skin area should be disinfected with soap and water or other antiseptics. Similarly, precautions should be employed in removing engorged ticks from dogs and other animals, because infection through minor abrasions on the hands is possible. Vaccines containing *R. rickettsii* are available commercially and should be used for those exposed to great risk, namely, persons frequenting highly endemic areas and laboratory workers exposed to the agent. Because the broad-spectrum antibiotics are such excellent therapeutic agents in spotted fever, there has been less impetus for vaccination of persons who run only a minor risk of infection.

REFERENCES See end of Chap. 187.

181
OTHER TICK-BORNE RICKETTSIAL DISEASES

THEODORE E. WOODWARD

DEFINITION Boutonneuse fever, North Asian tick-borne rickettsiosis, and Queensland tick typhus, three diseases occurring in the Eastern Hemisphere, are caused by rickettsias closely related to one another and to the agent of Rocky Mountain spotted fever. Each is transmitted by the bite of an ixodid tick. These mild to moderately severe illnesses are characterized by an initial lesion (called *tache noire* in boutonneuse fever), a fever of several days to 2 weeks, and a generalized maculopapular erythematous rash which appears on about the fifth day and usually involves the palms and soles. Specific complement-fixing antibodies appear in the patients' serums during convalescence, but agglutinins to *Proteus* OX-19 (Weil-Felix reaction) are frequently found only in low titer.

ETIOLOGY AND EPIDEMIOLOGY The etiologic agents of these three diseases are all members of the spotted fever group of rickettsias. Together with *Rickettsia rickettsii* and *R. akari* they possess common group antigens which are readily demonstrated by agglutination and complement fixation.

Boutonneuse fever, which may be regarded as the prototype of the three, is caused by *R. conorii.* Modern serologic methods employing specific rickettsial antigens have shown this rickettsia to be the causative agent for a single widely disseminated disease known by various local names. Information on the distribution and etiology of the various tick-borne rickettsial diseases is contained in Table 179-1.

In general, the epidemiology of these tick-borne rickettsioses resembles that of spotted fever in the Western Hemisphere. Ixodid ticks and small wild animals maintain the rickettsias in nature; if humans intrude accidentally into the cycle, they become a dead end in the transmission chain. In certain areas, the cycle of boutonneuse fever involves domiciliary environments, with the brown dog tick *Rhipicephalus sanguineus* as the dominant vector.

CLINICAL MANIFESTATIONS These three tick-borne rickettsioses, which occur in different parts of the Eastern Hemisphere, resemble one another closely. The clinical course is usually milder than that of spotted fever, with a shorter febrile period and fewer severe complications; fatalities are rare and generally limited to the aged and debilitated. The initial lesion, which is present in most cases at the onset of fever, heals slowly; the regional lymph nodes are enlarged. The rash usually remains papular and only in severe cases becomes hemorrhagic.

The clinical picture (including the primary lesion), the geographic location, and epidemiologic considerations are helpful in establishing the diagnosis. The typhus fevers, meningococcal infections, and measles must be considered in the differential diagnosis; the serologic reactions, i.e., Weil-Felix and complement fixation tests, are of value here.

TREATMENT AND PREVENTION Chloramphenicol and the tetracyclines are effective therapeutic agents for boutonneuse fever. Patients generally become afebrile after 2 to 3 days of treatment, and recovery is rapid. The therapeutic procedures are comparable to those used in spotted fever. Presumably these measures are also applicable to North Asian tick-borne rickettsiosis and Queensland tick typhus.

The major effective methods of control are concerned with avoidance of tick bites; these include application of new repellents and prompt removal of attached ticks. Effective vaccines are not available commercially.

REFERENCES See end of Chap. 187.

182 RICKETTSIALPOX

THEODORE E. WOODWARD

DEFINITION Rickettsialpox is a mild, nonfatal self-limited, febrile illness caused by *Rickettsia akari,* which is transmitted from mouse to humans by mites. It is characterized by an initial skin lesion at the site of the mite bite, a week's febrile course, and a papulovesicular rash.

ETIOLOGY AND EPIDEMIOLOGY Rickettsialpox was first recognized in New York City in 1946, and about 180 cases were reported annually for several years thereafter. It has been diagnosed in several other areas of the United States, and outbreaks have been reported in European Russia. The vector is a small, colorless mite, *Allodermanyssus sanguineus* (Hirst), which infests small mice and rodents. House mice serve as the reservoir of infection.

Rickettsia akari is morphologically and biologically similar to other rickettsias and is antigenically related to, but distinct from, *R. rickettsii,* the cause of Rocky Mountain spotted fever. Mice, guinea pigs, and fertile hen eggs are susceptible to experimental infection. Diagnostic antigens prepared from infected yolk sacs are used in complement fixation tests.

CLINICAL MANIFESTATIONS The initial skin lesion appears about 7 to 10 days after the mite bite as a firm red papule 1 to 1.5 cm in diameter. In a few days, the center vesiculates, and the papule is surrounded by an area of erythema. The regional lymph glands are moderately enlarged. The primary lesion, which is never painful, becomes covered with a black scab; it heals slowly, and a small scar is visible on separation of the crust.

The febrile phase begins 3 to 7 days following the initial lesion, and exanthem may accompany the fever or begin several days later. The onset of fever is sudden, with chilly sensations or frank chills, headache, sweats, myalgia, anorexia, and photophobia. The pyrexia ranges from 103 to 104°F and continues for about a week, occasionally with morning remissions.

The exanthem is maculopapular-vesicular, generalized in distribution, and may be abundant or scant. The lesions may involve the oral cavity but not the palms or soles. In a week, the vesicles dry and form scabs which eventually scale but leave no scar.

The constitutional symptoms are generally mild, and the course of illness is uncomplicated. No fatal cases have been reported.

The disease may be confused with chickenpox, which is different because it occurs usually in childhood and has no initial lesion and the papular cutaneous lesion is entirely transformed into a vesicle. Variola (smallpox) is accompanied by a more severe constitutional reaction, and the vesicles become pustules. The skin lesions of the other rickettsioses differ in their lack of vesiculation. The Weil-Felix reaction is usually negative in this rickettsial disease, but the specific complement fixation test is a useful laboratory diagnostic aid even though there is considerable crossing with materials from Rocky Mountain spotted fever.

TREATMENT AND PREVENTION Chloramphenicol and the tetracycline antibiotics are all effective for treating patients with rickettsialpox. The temperature reaches normal levels in about 2 days, and recovery is rapid.

Control measures should be directed toward elimination

of house mice and the vector mites responsible for transmitting the disease.

REFERENCES See end of Chap. 187.

183
MURINE (ENDEMIC) TYPHUS FEVER

THEODORE E. WOODWARD

DEFINITION Murine typhus fever is an acute febrile disease caused by *Rickettsia mooseri* and transmitted to humans by fleas. The clinical illness is characterized by fever of 9 to 14 days, headache, a maculopapular rash appearing on the third to fifth day, and myalgia.

ETIOLOGY AND EPIDEMIOLOGY *Rickettsia mooseri* resembles other rickettsias in morphologic properties, staining characteristics, and intracellular parasitism. Under the electron microscope *R. mooseri* is seen to contain dense masses of nuclear material in a less dense homogeneous protoplasmic substance, the whole of which is surrounded by a limiting membrane. It differs from *R. rickettsii* in that it always multiplies within the cytoplasm of cells, in contrast to the intranuclear and cytoplasmic positions of spotted fever rickettsias.

Invasion of the body by *R. mooseri* provokes specific and nonspecific immunologic responses. Utilizing highly purified antigens, specific antibodies may be demonstrated readily by complement fixation and agglutination reactions. The positive Weil-Felix reaction which occurs in this disease is nonspecific, because it is attributable to the presence of a common carbohydrate antigen in *Proteus* OX-19 and *R. mooseri* and because the reaction is also positive in epidemic typhus and spotted fever. Group-specific rickettsial antigens are common to both *R. mooseri* and *R. prowazekii.* Furthermore, both murine and epidemic rickettsias possess toxic factors which are lethal to mice and rats and can be neutralized by convalescent serum from humans or lower animals.

The common vector of *R. mooseri* for rats and humans is the rat flea (*Xenopsylla cheopis*). In nature, the rat louse (*Polypax spinulosis*) may transmit the agent among rodents. Customarily, rat fleas become infected on ingestion of blood from diseased rats; the rickettsias multiply within the intestinal cells of the arthropod and are excreted in the feces. Infection in humans occurs following the flea bite and contamination of the broken skin by rickettsia-laden feces. Dried flea feces may also infect via the conjunctivas or the upper part of the respiratory tract.

Rats and mice are naturally infected with murine typhus, and although the rodent disease is nonfatal, viable rickettsias persist in the brain for variable periods.

Murine typhus is one of the most benign and widespread of the rickettsioses in the United States. Prevalent in the Southeastern and Gulf Coast states, it has been identified in most of the other states and in harbor centers throughout the world wherever rats and fleas abound. Through control of rats and their fleas a sharp decline in incidence has occurred since 1951, particularly in the Southern United States. In urban areas the disease is more prevalent during the summer and fall months and occurs predominantly among persons working in proximity to granaries or food depots. There has been an extension to certain rural areas when changing agricultural practices have provided rats with ready access to adequate food supplies.

CLINICAL MANIFESTATIONS Incubation period and prodromata The incubation period ranges from 8 to 16 days, with a mean of 10. Common prodromata are headache, backache, arthralgia, and chilly sensations. Nausea, malaise, and transient temperature rises may precede the true onset of disease.

Onset and general symptoms A frank shaking chill and repeated rigors are present at the onset, associated with a severe frontal headache and fever. This triad of headache, chill, and pyrexia is usually followed within a few hours by nausea and vomiting. Prostration, malaise, and weakness are sufficient to enforce cessation of activity in adults, in contrast to children, whose illness is less severe. Occasionally, mild symptoms make it difficult to define the actual onset.

Pyrexia The usual febrile course in murine typhus lasts for about 12 days in adults; the temperature ranges from 102 to 104°F but may reach 105 to 106°F in children. The temperature may reach high levels abruptly after onset or ascend in a stepwise manner during the first few days. With the appearance of the rash, fever is usually sustained, with partial daily remissions which occasionally reach normal levels in the morning. Defervescence is generally by lysis over several days but sometimes occurs by crisis. Transient mild fever of 100°F is not uncommon during early convalescence. A few patients experience only low-grade fever throughout, but this does not necessarily connote a mild illness.

Cutaneous manifestations The early lesions, which are sparse and discrete, are hidden in the axillas and inner surface of the arm. Most patients then develop with surprising suddenness a generalized, dull red macular rash of the upper part of the abdomen, shoulders, chest, arms, and thighs. The individual lesions are discrete and pea size, with an ill-defined border, and fade on pressure during the first 24 h. They later become maculopapular, in contrast to the exanthem of epidemic typhus, which is persistently macular. The distribution over the trunk with sparse involvement of the extremities, palms, soles, and face differs from the peripheral distribution and facial involvement of Rocky Mountain spotted fever. The murine rash generally appears initially on the fifth febrile day, but rarely it is seen concurrently with the onset of fever or developing as late as the seventh day.

Eighty percent of patients develop a rash which persists for 4 to 8 days and fades before defervescence. The cutaneous manifestations vary greatly in intensity and duration and may be fleeting. They are readily overlooked in dark-skinned patients, in whom they should be sought by light palpation and indirect lighting.

Cardiovascular and respiratory features An irritating,

nonproductive cough is frequent and is occasionally associated with moderate hemoptysis. Early in the second week, rales may be detected in the basilar lung areas. These changes are generally rickettsial rather than bacterial in origin and respond to the broad-spectrum antibiotics. Pulmonary congestion occurs in extremely ill and elderly patients.

Accelerated pulse, hypotension, and general circulatory weakness occur in this disease, although less frequently than in patients with epidemic typhus or Rocky Mountain spotted fever.

Neurologic manifestations Headache is the most common neurologic manifestation of murine typhus and may dominate the clinical picture. It is frontal and continues into the second week of illness. Stupor and prostration may occur in the second week, and in severe cases, there may be muttering delirium, extreme agitation, or coma. Coma in elderly patients after 2 weeks of illness presages death. Nuchal rigidity and general spasticity often suggest meningitis, although the spinal fluid is normal except for slight increases in pressure and lymphocytes (5 to 30 per mm^3). Transient partial deafness occurs occasionally, but rarely is there localized neuritis or hemiplegia. Neurologic sequelae are unusual. Children experience minimal neurologic changes.

Other physical manifestations During the first 2 days of illness the patient may be nauseated and vomit, but vomiting later in the illness should arouse suspicion of an intercurrent complication. Abdominal pain is bothersome; when associated with diarrhea it responds to intravenous alimentation. Hepatomegaly and jaundice are unusual. There is splenomegaly in approximately 25 percent of patients.

Photophobia, retroocular pain, suffusion of the eyes, and congestion of the conjunctivas are common but are less severe than in the other typhus and spotted fevers.

Renal function is usually unaltered except in elderly patients with prolonged hypotension. Under these circumstances, azotemia may develop to the degree observed in epidemic typhus. In severe murine typhus, as in the epidemic typhus, hyponatremia and hypoalbuminemia are encountered.

COURSE After defervescence, murine typhus patients recover rapidly. Fatalities occur between the ninth and twelfth days in elderly or debilitated patients, usually as a result of circulatory and renal failure or intercurrent bacterial infection.

PROGNOSIS The mortality rate in murine typhus was low even before the introduction of modern specific therapy. Only one death occurred in 114 cases studied by Maxcy and none in the 180 reported by Stuart and Pullen.

DIFFERENTIAL DIAGNOSIS Because murine typhus and Rocky Mountain spotted fever occur in many of the same states, the problem of differential diagnosis often arises. Flea-borne murine typhus, which is predominantly an urban disease, is more likely to occur in late summer and autumn. In contrast, spotted fever is a rural and suburban disease in which exposure to ticks is important. Most cases occur in the spring and summer.

TREATMENT AND PREVENTION The therapeutic procedures are comparable to those used in spotted fever. Both chloramphenicol and the tetracycline antibiotics have controlled the disease.

Prevention of murine typhus in humans is attained by reducing the natural reservoir and vector by applying measures for eliminating rodents and employing appropriate insecticides in rat-infested areas to control fleas.

REFERENCES See end of Chap. 187.

184
EPIDEMIC TYPHUS FEVER AND BRILL-ZINSSER DISEASE

THEODORE E. WOODWARD

EPIDEMIC (LOUSE-BORNE) TYPHUS FEVER

DEFINITION The classical epidemic form of typhus is a severe, febrile disease caused by *Rickettsia prowazekii* and transmitted to humans by the body louse. Intense headache, continuous pyrexia of about 2 weeks, a macular skin eruption appearing on about the fifth febrile day, malaise, and vascular and neurologic disturbances represent the principal clinical features. Confirmation of the diagnosis is made by demonstration of *Proteus* OX-19 agglutinins and of specific complement-fixing antibodies in convalescence. The broad-spectrum antibiotics are specific therapeutic agents.

ETIOLOGY AND EPIDEMIOLOGY The causative microbe, *R. prowazekii,* is closely related to *R. mooseri,* which causes murine typhus; indeed, the two have a number of common antigens.

Human beings generally are infected when rickettsia-laden louse feces are rubbed into the broken skin; scratching the louse bite facilitates this process. *Pediculus humanus corporis,* which is peculiarly adapted to humans, is the only important vector of epidemic typhus. It dies of its infection and fails to transmit rickettsias to its offspring. There is no known animal habitat of *R. prowazekii.* Although successful isolation of *R. prowazekii* from flying squirrels has been reported, the organism is maintained by a cycle involving human-louse-human. New epidemics apparently originate from patients with Brill-Zinsser disease (recurrent epidemic typhus). Inhalation of dust containing dried louse feces may rarely cause infection.

Epidemic typhus, if uncontrolled, behaves as a cyclic disease in a susceptible population, extending over a 3-year period. During the first year there is a gradual seeding of cases throughout the group; during the second there is epidemic spread; and during the third the epidemic tapers off, because the majority of persons have become immune. Outbreaks of epidemic typhus last occurred in the United States in the nineteenth century, and its presence is now recognized only in the form of Brill-Zinsser disease.

CLINICAL MANIFESTATIONS Epidemic typhus resembles murine typhus but is more severe. After an incubation period of about 7 days an abrupt onset of headache, chill, and rapidly mounting fever ushers in the illness. Headache, malaise, and prostration continue unabated until the rash appears on the fifth febrile day. It is initially macular in the axillary folds but ultimately invades the trunk and extremities as a pink, irregular macular lesion which becomes fixed, petechial, and confluent in the later stages.

Neurologic features range from headache and general spasticity to extreme agitation, stupor, and coma. Circulatory disturbances consisting of tachycardia, hypotension, and cyanosis are more profound than those observed in murine typhus and are almost as severe as in Rocky Mountain spotted fever. Ultimately, in untreated cases azotemia often reaches high levels as a result of vascular and renal failure, and death occurs late in the second week of illness. Furthermore, thrombosis of major blood vessels and cutaneous gangrene develop in a manner similar to that seen in the virulent form of Rocky Mountain spotted fever.

The complications and sequelae of epidemic typhus are more severe than those in murine typhus, but not as severe as those in Rocky Mountain spotted fever. However, during certain outbreaks, epidemic typhus was fatal in 60 percent of those infected, and convalescence in survivors was prolonged. Broad-spectrum antibiotics have eradicated mortality in this dread disease, provided therapy is instituted before irreversible changes have been established in the tissues.

DIFFERENTIAL DIAGNOSIS Differentiation of epidemic typhus from the various rickettsioses and other diseases with which it may be confused is described in Chap. 180. The disease in epidemic form never occurs in the absence of lousiness in the general population. Under the conditions in which typhus epidemics are likely to occur, other diseases which may cause confusion include malaria, relapsing fever, pneumonia, and tuberculosis. Classic typhus contracted by a previously vaccinated person is usually mild and may be clinically indistinguishable from murine typhus except by serologic methods.

TREATMENT AND PREVENTION Both chloramphenicol and the tetracycline antibiotics have been found to be highly efficient therapeutic agents in epidemic typhus. Usually the patient becomes afebrile after 2 days of treatment. The therapeutic procedures are comparable to those used in spotted fever. Under field conditions, 100 mg of doxycycline in a single oral dose resulted in abatement of clinical manifestations and defervescence in epidemic typhus.

The most effective measures for controlling epidemic typhus are those which eliminate lousiness. DDT or lindane powder when dusted into clothing is suitable for this purpose. If resistant lice are found, malathion or carbaryl may prove effective.

A commercially available vaccine prepared from Formalin-treated suspensions of infected yolk sac tissue is an effective immunizing agent. A viable vaccine utilizing an attenuated strain of *R. prowazekii* is under development.

BRILL-ZINSSER DISEASE (RECRUDESCENT TYPHUS)

DEFINITION Brill-Zinsser disease is a recrudescent episode of epidemic typhus fever which occurs years after the initial attack, in persons who had recovered from the epidemic disease acquired while residing in countries where it was prevalent. *Rickettsia prowazekii* have been isolated from lice fed on patients during the active stages of illness.

CLINICAL MANIFESTATIONS The clinical entity, not always mild, resembles epidemic typhus in the character of the rash, circulatory disturbances, and hepatic, renal, and nervous system changes. Recovery is the rule. The Weil-Felix reaction with the various *Proteus* antigens is usually negative, or positive in very low titer. The specific complement fixation reaction is valuable in establishing the diagnosis. In Brill-Zinsser disease the specific complement-fixing antibodies appear as early as the fourth day after the onset of illness; the peak response is attained by the eighth to tenth days. Specific antibody titers in the primary attack of epidemic typhus begin later, about the eighth to twelfth day, with maximum titers on about the sixteenth day after onset. Antibodies in Brill-Zinsser disease and the primary attack are associated with 7S and 19S globulins, respectively. Therapy is like that used in spotted fever.

REFERENCES See end of Chap. 187.

185 SCRUB TYPHUS

THEODORE E. WOODWARD

DEFINITION Scrub typhus is limited to eastern and southeastern Asia, India, northern Australia, and the adjacent islands. It is caused by *Rickettsia tsutsugamushi* and characterized by a primary lesion at the site of the bite of an infected mite, a fever of about 2 weeks' duration, a cutaneous rash which develops about the fifth day, and the appearance late in the second week of agglutinins against the OX-K strain of *Proteus* bacillus. The broad-spectrum antibiotics are specific therapeutic agents.

ETIOLOGY The agent of scrub typhus resembles other rickettsias in its physical properties but differs from them in antigenic structure, vector, and reservoir. The disease is transmitted by larvae of several species of mites, especially *Leptotrobidium (Trombicula) akamushi* and *L. deliense.* These tiny chiggers attach themselves to the skin and during the process of obtaining a meal of tissue juice may acquire infection from the host or transmit rickettsias to the vertebrate. The infection is maintained in nature by a cycle involving mites and small rodents and by transovarial transmission in mites; human infection represents an accident attributable to propinquity.

CLINICAL MANIFESTATIONS About 10 to 12 days after infection, illness begins abruptly with chilliness, severe headache, fever, conjunctival injection, and moderate generalized lymphadenopathy which is most prominent in the nodes draining the area of the primary lesion. The initial lesion at the beginning of fever is evidenced by an erythematous indurated area 1 cm in diameter, surmounted by a multiloculated vesicle; within a few days the vesicle ulcerates and becomes covered with a black crust.

Fever increases progressively during the first week, generally reaching 104 to 105°F, but the pulse remains relatively slow, 70 to 100 beats per min. The red macular rash, which begins on the trunk about the fifth day and spreads to the extremities, sometimes becomes maculopapular but usually fades in a few days. The course of the disease and the complications resemble those of endemic and epidemic typhus; however, interstitial myocarditis is more prominent than in the other typhus fevers.

PROGNOSIS Prior to the introduction of the broad-spectrum antibiotics the mortality rate varied from 1 to 60 percent, depending on the geographic area and the virulence of the local strains of *R. tsutsugamushi,* and convalescence was prolonged. With modern therapeutic methods, deaths are extremely rare and convalescence is short.

DIFFERENTIAL DIAGNOSIS Scrub typhus is to be differentiated from the other members of the typhus and the spotted fever group of diseases as well as from measles, typhoid fever, and the meningococcal infections. The geographic localization of scrub typhus, the primary lesion, and the occurrence of OX-K agglutinins are especially useful in establishing the diagnosis.

TREATMENT AND PREVENTION Chloramphenicol and the tetracycline antibiotics are valuable specific therapeutic agents in scrub typhus. The therapeutic procedures are comparable to those used in spotted fever. In fact, scrub typhus is more amenable to drugs than are the other rickettsial infections, and patients with this disease regularly become afebrile and are decidedly improved within 24 to 36 h after beginning treatment, irrespective of the stage of disease.

Prevention of disease in the individual is accomplished by the application of miticidal chemicals (dibutyl phthalate, benzyl benzoate, diethyltoluamide, and others) to clothing and the skin. There is no satisfactory vaccine.

REFERENCES See end of Chap. 187.

186 Q FEVER

THEODORE E. WOODWARD

DEFINITION Q fever is an acute infectious disease caused by *Coxiella burnetii* and characterized by a sudden onset of fever, malaise, headache, weakness, anorexia, and interstitial pneumonitis. Rickettsemia occurs during the febrile period, and specific complement-fixing antibodies are present during convalescence. In contrast to the other rickettsioses, the disease is not associated with a cutaneous exanthem or agglutinins for the *Proteus* bacteria (Weil-Felix reaction).

ETIOLOGY AND EPIDEMIOLOGY *Coxiella burnetii* possesses the general properties of other rickettsias but is somewhat more resistant to inactivation in unfavorable environments and more pleomorphic than the others. Its infectivity after drying under natural conditions is of importance in the spread of infection to humans. *Coxiella burnetii* has a wide host range in nature, but guinea pigs and embryonated eggs are the common laboratory hosts employed for its propagation.

Human cases of Q fever are contracted by inhalation of infected dusts, by handling infected materials, and possibly by drinking milk contaminated with *C. burnetii.* The disease in Australia is enzootic in animals, especially bandicoots, and is transmitted in nature by ticks. Rickettsia-laden tick feces may contaminate cattle hides, and inhalation of this material has caused infection in humans. In the United States, a number of species of ticks are naturally infected, among them *Dermacentor andersoni* and *Amblyomma americanum,* and in North Africa transovarial transmission of the agent in indigenous ticks has been demonstrated. Sheep, goats, and cows have been found to be naturally infected in North America and in Europe, and *C. burnetii* has been recovered from the milk of such animals. Milk, as well as infected excretions from livestock, probably accounts for certain outbreaks of human disease following inhalation by cows of infected dust from barns and pens. The airborne route of dried contaminated material is the most likely method of spread. A number of epidemics have occurred among laboratory workers engaged in studies on *C. burnetii.* The disease is not transmitted between humans.

CLINICAL MANIFESTATIONS After incubation of approximately 19 days (the range is 14 to 26), the disease begins with headache, chilly sensations, fever, malaise, myalgia, and anorexia. For several days, the temperature ranges from 101 to 104°F; the entire course rarely exceeds 2 weeks and usually ranges from 3 to 6 days. There may be wide fluctuations in the fever. Respiratory and gastrointestinal symptoms are not conspicuous in the early stages. Headache and fever predominate. A dry cough and chest pain occur after about 5 days, when rales are usually audible. Roentgenographic findings indistinguishable from those of primary atypical pneumonia are present usually by the third to fourth day of disease, first as patchy areas of consolidation involving a portion of one lobe, giving a homogeneous ground-glass appearance. These manifestations persist beyond the febrile period and may appear in patients who are unaware of pulmonary involvement. Complications are rare, and coincident with defervescence the appetite begins to return. Convalescence progresses slowly for several weeks, during which time the principal disability is weakness. It is not uncommon for patients to lose 15 to 20 lb during the active stages of disease. The disease may be protracted in approximately 20 percent of cases, with fever persisting for longer than 4 weeks, particularly in elderly patients. Occasionally relapse occurs, especially in patients treated with antibiotics during the first several days of disease.

Hepatitis, with the development of clinically detectable icterus, occurs in approximately one-third of patients with the protracted form. This form of Q fever is characterized by fever, malaise, absence of headache or respiratory signs, and hepatomegaly with right upper quadrant pain. Liver biopsy specimens show diffuse granulomatous changes with multinucleated giant cells and scattered infiltrations of polymorphonuclear leukocytes, lymphocytes, and macrophages. *Coxiella burnetii* may be demonstrated in such specimens with the fluorescent antibody technique. Therefore, Q fever must be included in the differential diagnosis of liver granulomas such as tuberculosis, sarcoidosis, histoplasmosis, brucellosis, tularemia, syphilis, and others.

Endocarditis also has been reported, and *C. burnetii* has been identified by smear and isolation in vegetations on the heart valves obtained at operation or autopsy. The aortic valve is most commonly involved, often with large vegetations. It is important, therefore, to suspect the possibility of Q fever in cases of apparent subacute bacterial endocarditis with persistently negative blood cultures. Operative intervention with replacement of damaged valves may be necessary for recovery because the available antibiotics are not rickettsicidal.

A high complement-fixing antibody titer to phase I antigen is present in patients with endocarditis and granulomatous hepatitis.

PROGNOSIS Few fatalities have been recorded and, except for the patient with protracted illness and hepatic involvement or endocarditis, the course of disease is generally uncomplicated and benign.

TREATMENT AND CONTROL The tetracycline antibiotics and chloramphenicol are effective in the treatment of patients with Q fever. Most patients, when treated early in the course of disease, respond promptly and recover without relapses. The therapeutic procedures are comparable to those used in spotted fever.

Control of Q fever depends primarily on immunization of susceptible persons with specific vaccines. Vaccines made from phase I rickettsias are potent and afford considerable protection to slaughterhouse and dairy workers, herders, rendering-plant workers, woolsorters, tanners, laboratory workers, and others at risk. Measures should be taken to avoid exposure to infected aerosols; milk from infected domestic livestock must be pasteurized or boiled.

REFERENCES See end of Chap. 187.

187
TRENCH FEVER

THEODORE E. WOODWARD

DEFINITION Trench fever is a febrile disease transmitted between humans by the body louse, *Pediculus humanus corporis.* It is characterized by a sudden onset with headache and severe pain in the muscles, bones, and joints. In most cases, the fever and other symptoms assume a relapsing character. Fatalities are rare. The disease is also known as shin bone fever, Volhynia fever, His-Werner disease, and Quintan fever.

ETIOLOGY AND EPIDEMIOLOGY *Rickettsia quintana* (see footnote, Table 179-1), the etiologic agent, grows extracellularly in the louse gut, in contrast to other pathogenic rickettsias which can multiply only within cells. A European strain of *R. quintana* has been cultivated on blood agar, and typical trench fever has been induced in volunteers.

Humans are the only known reservoir of infection. The louse does not transmit the organism transovarially but acquires its infection by ingesting the blood of a person with rickettsemia. The organisms multiply extracellularly in the louse gut, without injury to this host, and are excreted in large numbers with the feces. Humans become infected by the inoculation of the contaminated feces into abraded skin or conjunctivas. *Rickettsia quintana* may be recovered periodically from human blood for several years after convalescence from an acute attack. Trench fever is known to exist in Mexico, Tunisia, Eritrea, Poland, the U.S.S.R., and possibly China, and there is serologic evidence for its occurrence in Bolivia, Burundi, and Ethiopia.

PATHOLOGY Since there have been no recorded fatalities, histologic examination has been confined to excised macules of the skin, which have shown nonspecific perivascular infiltrates without the involvement of the vessel walls that is seen in typhus fever.

CLINICAL MANIFESTATIONS A variety of clinical manifestations is displayed in trench fever, ranging from a mild afebrile disease to a debilitating illness with a protracted clinical course involving numerous relapses. Following an incubation period of 10 to 30 days the onset may be insidious or dramatically abrupt. The acute disease is characterized by malaise, headache, fever, and bone and body pain, especially severe in the shins. In some cases only one fever peak occurs; in others the fever continues for 5 to 7 days; and in others there is an initial febrile episode lasting 1 to 3 days followed by relapses which characteristically occur at 4- to 5-day intervals. In some cases the fever and symptoms are continuous for 2 or 3 weeks. Enlargement of the spleen and a red macular rash occur in 70 to 80 percent of the cases. Pain and soreness in the muscles usually recur with each febrile relapse.

The disease is marked by a persistent rickettsemia, which is present during the initial attack and which continues during the relapses, throughout the asymptomatic periods between relapses, and for months or even years after cessation of physical symptoms. A relapse has been reported 10 years after the original attack.

PROGNOSIS The disease causes no known deaths, but its duration is variable. About 85 percent of patients are able to return to work within 2 months of onset, but about 5 percent of all cases become chronic. Recovery is even more delayed in the aged and debilitated.

DIFFERENTIAL DIAGNOSIS During epidemics, typical cases are easily diagnosed on the basis of symptoms. The disease may be differentiated from influenza, typhoid, typhus, dengue, and relapsing fever by the specific laboratory tests available for the diagnosis of each of these diseases.

TREATMENT AND PREVENTION *Rickettsia quintana* is highly sensitive in vitro to the broad-spectrum antibiotics, but no reliable information has been obtained about the value of these drugs in treating trench fever. The treatment is symptomatic. Aspirin is used to control pain and discomfort, but codeine may be necessary. The patient should remain in bed for a week or more after complete cessation of subjective and objective evidence of infection. He should be kept under observation for several months and returned to bed at the first sign of relapse.

The methods employed to control epidemic typhus should be equally efficacious in controlling trench fever. These are based on the elimination of lousiness and the improvement of living conditions with provision for frequent bathing and washing of clothing. DDT or lindane powder should be applied by hand or power duster at appropriate intervals to clothes and persons of populations living under conditions favoring lousiness. If resistant lice are found, malathion or other effective lousicides may be substituted as a dusting powder.

REFERENCES

(Chaps. 179 to 187)

ANDREW R et al: Tick typhus in North Queensland. Med J Aust 2:253, 1946

BLAKE FG et al: Studies on tsutsugamushi disease (scrub typhus, mite-borne typhus) in New Guinea and adjacent islands: Epidemiology, clinical observations and etiology in the Dobadura area. Am J Hyg 41:243, 1945

DERRICK EH: The epidemiology of Q fever: A review. Med J Aust 1:245, 1953

FERGUSON IC et al: Clinical, virological and pathological findings in a fatal case of Q fever endocarditis. Br J Clin Pathol 15:235, 1962

GEAR J: The rickettsial diseases of Southern Africa: A review of recent studies. S Afr J Clin Sci 5:158, 1954

GREENBERG M: Rickettsialpox in New York City. Am J Med 4:866, 1948

HARRELL GT: Rocky Mountain spotted fever. Medicine 28:333, 1949

——: Rickettsial involvement of the nervous system. Med Clin North Am 37:395, 1953

HAZARD GW et al: Rocky Mountain spotted fever in the Eastern United States. N Engl J Med 280:57, 1969

LENNETTE EH: Epidemiology of Q fever. Arch Inst Pasteur (Tunis) 36:521, 1959

MARMION BP, STOKER MGP: The epidemiology of Q fever in Great Britain: An analysis of the findings and some conclusions. Br Med J 2:809, 1958

MAXCY KF: Typhus fever in the United States. Public Health Rep (Washington) 44:1735, 1929

MOHR CO, SMITH WW: Eradication of murine typhus fever in a rural area. Bull WHO 16:255, 1957

MOULTON FR (ed): *The Rickettsial Diseases of Man,* Washington: American Association for the Advancement of Science, 1948

MURRAY ES et al: Brill's disease: I. Clinical and laboratory diagnosis. JAMA 142:1059, 1950

——, SNYDER JC: Brill's disease: II. Etiology. Am J Hyg 53:22, 1951

ORMSBEE RA et al: The influence of phase on the protective potency of Q fever vaccine. J Immunol 92:404, 1964

PRATT HD: The changing picture of murine typhus in the United States. Ann NY Acad Sci 70:516, 1958

ROSE HM: The clinical manifestations and laboratory diagnosis of rickettsialpox. Ann Intern Med 31:871, 1949

SCHAFFNER W, KOENIG MG: Thrombocytopenic Rocky Mountain spotted fever. Arch Intern Med 116:857, 1965

SMADEL JE: Influence of antibiotics on immunologic responses in scrub typhus. Am J Med 17:246, 1954

——: Status of the rickettsioses in the United States. Ann Intern Med 51:421, 1959

—— (ed): *Symposium on Q Fever,* Med Sci Publ 6, Washington: Walter Reed Army Institute of Research, 1959

——, JACKSON EB: Rickettsial infections, in *Diagnostic Procedures for Viral and Rickettsial Diseases,* 3d ed, New York: American Public Health Association, 1964, p. 743

SNYDER JC: Typhus fever rickettsiae, in *Viral and Rickettsial Infections of Man,* 4th ed., eds FL Horsfall, Jr., I Tamm, Philadelphia: Lippincott, 1965, p. 1059

STRONG RP: Trench fever, in *Stitt's Diagnosis, Prevention and Treatment of Tropical Diseases,* 7th ed., New York: McGraw-Hill, 1944, p. 984

STUART BM, PULLEN RL: Endemic (murine) typhus fever: Clinical observations of one hundred and eighty cases. Ann Intern Med 23:520, 1945

VINSON JW: Etiology of trench fever in Mexico in *Industry and Tropical Health: V,* Boston: Harvard School of Public Health, 1964, p. 109

WOODWARD TE: Rickettsial diseases in the United States. Med Clin North Am 43:1507, 1959

——: A historical account of the rickettsial diseases with a discussion of unsolved problems. The First Maxwell Finland Lecture. J Infect Dis 127:583, 1973

section 13 | Mycoplasmal diseases

188
RESPIRATORY AND GENITAL TRACT INFECTION WITH MYCOPLASMAS

VERNON KNIGHT

INTRODUCTION The mycoplasmas, formerly called pleuropneumonia-like organisms (PPLO) after the organism that caused a highly contagious form of bovine pneumonia and pleurisy in Europe in the eighteenth century, are now designated class Mollicutes, family Mycoplasmataceae, genus *Mycoplasma.* There are 37 species, 8 of which have been isolated from man (Table 188-1).

They are small, 150 to 200 nm in diameter, lack a cell wall, and require cholesterol for the development of a limiting membrane. They grow as small colonies that penetrate deeply into the agar. *Mycoplasma hominis* and some other strains also show secondary growth around the center that gives a "fried egg" appearance. With most media, this does not occur with *M. pneumoniae.* Human mycoplasmas form colonies 200 to 300 μm in diameter except for those which form colonies 20 to 50 μm in diameter and consequently have been designated T-strain mycoplasmas (for tiny colonies). The usual growth medium is peptone-enriched beef heart infusion broth supplemented with horse serum (supplies cholesterol) and yeast extract. The T-strain mycoplasmas possess a urease system and require urea for growth. *Mycoplasma pneumoniae, M. hominis,* and T-strain mycoplasmas grow aerobically and anaerobically.

Mycoplasmas are resistant to penicillin and antibiotics known to interfere with polymerization of cell wall precursors and do not retain the dye-iodine complex of the gram stain. They are inhibited by tetracyclines, erythromycin, chloramphenicol, and some other antibiotics. Like bacteria, they grow outside the cell, possess ribonucleic and deoxyribonucleic acids, reproduce by fission, and generate metabolic energy. They are not to be confused with L forms of bacteria or protoplasts that are derived from bacteria and possess the cell wall precursors, muramic acid and diaminopimelic acid, or the capability of synthesizing these precursors. Of the human mycoplasmas, only *M. pneumoniae* has been unequivocally defined as a human pathogen. Both *M. hominis* and T-strain mycoplasmas are found frequently in the genital tract of men and women, and evidence for their role in disease is considered in a subsequent section of this chapter. The mycoplasmas that occur in the oropharynx are apparently commensals that do not cause disease.

TABLE 188-1
The human mycoplasmas

Species	*Usual site of occurrence*
Mycoplasma pneumoniae	Respiratory tract
M. salivarium	Oropharynx
M. orale 1	Oropharynx
M. orale 2	Oropharynx
M. orale 3	Oropharynx
M. fermentans	Oropharynx and genital tract (rarely detected)
M. hominis	Genital tract
T-strain mycoplasmas (ureaplasma urealyticum)	Genital tract

PNEUMONIA AND RESPIRATORY TRACT DISEASE CAUSED BY *MYCOPLASMA PNEUMONIAE* Synonyms are primary atypical pneumonia, Eaton's agent pneumonia, cold agglutinin-positive pneumonia, and "virus" pneumonia.

Definition Pneumonia caused by *M. pneumoniae* is characterized by fever, pharyngitis, cough, and pulmonary infiltration, often multilobular, in which roentgenographic signs are more extensive than indicated by physical examination. This organism also causes upper respiratory illness without pneumonia and asymptomatic infection.

Etiology *Mycoplasma pneumoniae* is distinguished from other mycoplasmas by rapid hemolysis of guinea pig erythrocytes and utilization of glucose and other sugars. It also hemolyzes human and rat erythrocytes. It may also be distinguished from other mycoplasmas by fluorescent antibody, complement fixation, growth inhibition, and indirect hemagglutination tests, all of which are useful for serologic diagnosis of human infection. In addition to growing on agar, the organism grows on the surface of cells of embryonated eggs and monkey kidney cell culture with little evidence of cytopathic effect. In human cell cultures, however, there is intracellular growth with cytopathic effects.

Epidemiology In the general population *M. pneumoniae* infection is characterized by intrafamily spread. In most cases the infection is introduced into the family by a schoolchild. Once it is introduced, most family members become infected. In family outbreaks, pneumonia occurs with greatest frequency among school-age children, with a predominance in males. The disease is rare above age forty. *Mycoplasma pneumoniae* pneumonia occurs throughout the year, although prolonged wintertime outbreaks may occur in college groups or communities. The total incidence of *M. pneumoniae* pneumonia in a study in Seattle was 1.3 per 1,000 per year, which constituted about 15 to 20 percent of pneumonia from all causes. At intervals of several years, epidemics of *M. pneumoniae* pneumonia may occur with about double the usual incidence of disease.

In the military, *M. pneumoniae* infections account for a small proportion of upper respiratory illness in recruits—in one study, 6.3 percent. However, it accounted for almost one-half of cases of pneumonia in the same military population. The disease appears to be endemic at military bases.

Mycoplasma pneumoniae is probably spread by means of infected respiratory secretions. The organisms can be cultured from sputum of naturally occurring cases and from volunteers inoculated artificially. Primary atypical pneumonia has been induced in volunteers both by nasopharyngeal inoculation and by inhalation of a small-particle aerosol containing the agent. In volunteers naturally acquired antibody is associated with a high degree of resistance to infection.

Clinical manifestations The incubation period is from 9 to 12 days, but the interval between cases in families is approximately three weeks. Illness usually begins with symptoms of upper respiratory infection, which, in a small percentage of cases, progresses to bronchitis and pneumonia. Cough is almost universal in pneumonia and is frequent in cases without pulmonary involvement. Blood-flecked sputum may occur in the more severe cases, but gross hemoptysis is rare. A variety of other respiratory and systemic complaints may occur. Fever, nasal congestion, and sore throat are common. In pneumonia, harsh or diminished sounds are frequent but bronchial breathing is uncommon. Fine inspiratory rales are found in most patients but are not impressive. Pleural rubs and pleural effusion are infrequent. Studies on the distribution of pneumonia in one large series showed more than one-half of cases were multilobular and slightly less than one-half were bilateral. Lower-lobe pneumonia was appreciably more frequent than upper-lobe pneumonia. Pulmonary infiltrates may occur as an isolated area in the lung periphery but more often spread from the hilum.

The disease is variable in severity, but high fever may persist for 1 to 2 weeks in untreated cases. X-ray changes last for as long as 3 weeks in untreated cases, but for 7 to 10 days in treated cases. Even in untreated cases, complications are rare and consist of occasional purulent sinusitis, persistent cough, and, rarely, pleurisy. Prolonged weakness and malaise follow the untreated illness in adults.

Ear involvement consisting of congestion of the tympanic membrane and of bullous and, rarely, hemorrhagic myringitis may occur in as many as 10 percent of cases of pneumonia, most often in children.

Rare complications include meningoencephalitis, monoarticular arthritis, Stevens-Johnson syndrome, pericarditis, myocarditis, and hemolytic anemia.

Studies with volunteers have revealed, in addition to pneumonia, the occurrence of febrile and afebrile upper respiratory illness characterized by nonexudative pharyngitis and tracheobronchitis, often associated with cough, headache, and nasal congestion. Recovery occurred without complications in about 2 weeks. Upper respiratory disease occurs more commonly than pneumonia with infection in children and adults. Ten to fifteen percent of patients with illness due to *M. pneumoniae,* predominantly pneumonia, may develop maculopapular, confluent, fiery-red rashes, sometimes becoming vesicular and lasting for 1 to 2 weeks.

Laboratory findings During acute illness leukocytosis in the range of 10,000 to 15,000 per mm^3 occurs in about 25 percent of cases. Increase in sedimentation rate above 40 mm per h occurs in at least two-thirds of cases. Urinalysis, electrocardiograms, and fluid and electrolyte and liver function studies show no characteristic changes. The complement fixation, fluorescent antibody, indirect hemagglutination, and growth inhibition tests all yield highly specific diagnostic information. The simplicity of the complement fixation test recommends it for general use. Fourfold rises in titer often occur within 2 weeks, and maximum rise is achieved in 4 weeks. In atypical pneumonia, agglutinins to *Streptococcus MG* have developed with varying frequency. Higher titers are correlated with more severe illness. Of probably greater diagnostic value than *Streptococcus MG* agglutination is the appearance 7 to 10 days after onset of illness of cold agglutinins for human, type O red blood cells. The test may be positive in as high as 90 percent of severely ill patients but is less often positive in mild illness.

Differential diagnosis Pneumonia due to *M. pneumoniae* needs to be distinguished from pneumonia of all other types. It is usually less severe, is associated with less dense pulmonary infiltration than pneumococcal and other bacterial pneumonias, and occurs throughout the year. Pulmonary infiltrate in the absence of symptoms or physical signs may initially suggest acute pulmonary tuberculosis. In military populations adenoviral pneumonia must be excluded. Pneumonic involvement as a direct result of influenza viral infection or its complication by pneumococcal, streptococcal, staphylococcal, or *H. influenzae* infection may cause difficulty in diagnosis. Q fever, psittacosis, and tularemia are less frequent causes of pneumonia that may be difficult to distinguish from *M. pneumoniae* infection. In children, especially young infants, pneumonia due to respiratory syncytial, parainfluenza, adenovirus, and influenza viruses may resemble *M. pneumoniae* infection.

Treatment Tetracycline derivatives and erythromycin are effective in treatment of pneumonia due to *M. pneumoniae.* Demethylchlortetracycline may be given to adults in daily doses of 0.9 g; tetracycline, 1.5 g; erythromycin stearate, 1.5 g per day. Response to treatment is characterized by prompt defervescence, rapid clearing of x-ray signs of pneumonia, and disappearance of malaise and weakness. Persistent cough, despite treatment, is a relatively common finding, especially in women.

Treatment temporarily reduces the frequency of positive cultures from the respiratory tract, but shedding may continue for several weeks after treatment, a finding similar to that in psittacosis pneumonia. Relapse of *M. pneumoniae* pneumonia occurs occasionally, but such cases respond to retreatment. In cases in which there is doubt between the diagnosis of *M. pneumoniae* and pneumococcal infection, erythromycin should be used in preference to a tetracycline.

Prevention Although antibody is apparently highly protective, effective vaccines are not available. Acutely ill patients should be isolated from very young children and persons in whom a complicating respiratory illness would constitute a special hazard.

GENITAL TRACT INFECTION WITH MYCOPLASMAS The genital tract of male and female infants frequently becomes colonized at birth with *M. hominis* and T-strain mycoplasmas, presumably from the birth canal; about 15 percent of infants have nasopharyngeal colonization with these organisms. At about one year of age, the rate of carriage of these organisms decreases, to increase again at puberty.

In the adult population the frequency of genital occurrence of mycoplasmas is higher in low socioeconomic groups and in women and men who are sexually active. Cultures from men are best obtained from urethral scrapings, but organisms can be isolated in the female from the full extent of genital mucosa, cervical os, vagina, vestibule, and distal urethra.

T-strain mycoplasmas have been inconsistently associated with nongonococcal urethritis (Chap. 137) and Reiter's syndrome. Evidence of a causal connection between these two syndromes and the organisms in men is scanty. In women, there have been inconstant associations between T-strain mycoplasmas and *M. hominis* and cervicitis, vaginitis, pelvic inflammatory disease, septic abortion, puerperal infections, spontaneous abortion, stillbirths, and infertility. Causal significance of mycoplasmas in these conditions is uncertain, particularly in pelvic inflammatory disease where other organisms seem more important. There is no evidence that treatment of these conditions must include antimicrobials active against mycoplasmas.

REFERENCES

CHERRY JD et al: *Mycoplasma pneumoniae* infections and exanthems. J Pediatr 87:369, 1975

COUCH RB: *Mycoplasma pneumoniae,* in *Viral and Mycoplasmal Infections of the Respiratory Tract,* ed V Knight, Philadelphia: Lea & Febiger, 1973

FOY HM et al: Viral and mycoplasmal pneumonia in a prepaid medical care group during an eight year period. Am J Epidemiol 97:93, 1973

FREUNDT EA: Principles of mycoplasma classification. Ann NY Acad Sci 225:7, 1973

HOLMES KK et al: Etiology of nongonococcal urethritis. N Engl J Med 292:1199, 1975

MCCORMACK WM et al: The genital mycoplasmas. N Engl J Med 288:76, 1973

MURRAY HW et al: The protean manifestations of *Mycoplasma pneumoniae* infection in adults. Am J Med 58:229, 1975

STENSTROM R et al: Mycoplasma pneumonias. Acta Radiol [Diagn] (Stockh) 12:833, 1972

section 14 | Chlamydial diseases

189
EYE INFECTIONS WITH TRACHOMA AND INCLUSION CONJUNCTIVITIS

J. THOMAS GRAYSTON
CHANDLER R. DAWSON

INTRODUCTION The eye and its adnexa may be infected during the course of many cutaneous and systemic viral diseases. Sometimes these ocular infections produce minor manifestations, such as the transient loss of accommodation of dengue and the milder forms of conjunctivitis in systemic adenovirus infections. Other virus infections, however, such as herpes simplex (Chap. 206), herpes zoster (Chap. 205), measles (Chap. 201), and vaccinia or smallpox (Chap. 204), occasionally produce serious and permanent visual loss. In addition, congenital viral infections are an important cause of blindness, particularly rubella, which leads to cataracts and microphthalmus, and cytomegalic inclusion disease with retinal involvement.

The diseases described in this chapter are caused by microorganisms that produce localized eye disease. Although they are mainly of concern to ophthalmologists, these diseases are important in the differential diagnosis of systemic disorders involving the eye. Knowledge of the epidemiology of the diseases will aid in their recognition.

TRACHOMA AND INCLUSION CONJUNCTIVITIS Definition Trachoma is a chronic conjunctival infection. It is still the most important cause of visual loss, having produced an estimated 20 million cases of blindness throughout the world. Inclusion conjunctivitis is an acute ocular inflammation caused by trachoma organisms in sexually active adults and in their newborn offspring. It is a clinical manifestation of initial infection with the organisms.

Etiology The genus *Chlamydia* has been divided into two species, *C. trachomatis* and *C. psittaci.* The *Chlamydia trachomatis* species includes two primary human pathogens, the trachoma organisms and the organisms causing lymphogranuloma venereum (LGV) (Chap. 190). While these two groups of organisms have important biological and pathogenic differences, they are identical morphologically and very closely related immunologically. *Chlamydia* are obligate, intracellular microorganisms; they are not viruses, being more closely related to bacteria, because they have cell walls with chemical and metabolic properties similar to bacteria and are affected by broad-spectrum antibiotics. Trachoma organisms grow primarily in the epithelium of the conjunctiva, urethra, and cervix. They can be identified by the typical cytoplasmic inclusion bodies in Giemsa stained smears of cells from these sites. The agents may be isolated and grown in yolk sacs of embryonated hens' eggs or now, more easily, in special tissue culture cells. Primates are the only laboratory animals susceptible to eye infections with trachoma organisms. Trachoma and LGV organisms have been classified into 15 immunotypes by immunofluorescent techniques.

Epidemiology Epidemiologically, there are two types of trachomatous eye disease: endemic and sporadic trachoma. In endemic areas, transmission is from eye to eye, while in nonendemic areas sporadic trachoma is transmitted from the genital tract to the eye. The worldwide incidence and severity of trachoma have decreased dramatically during the past 25 years in areas with improving hygienic and economic conditions. Endemic trachoma is still the major cause of blindness in North Africa, sub-Saharan Africa, the Middle East, and northern India. Transmission of the endemic disease occurs primarily through close personal contact, particularly among young children. Development of the chronic disease usually requires repeated infections. In the United States a mild form of endemic trachoma still occurs in American Indians and in Mexican Americans as well as in immigrants from areas where trachoma is endemic. Acute relapse of old trachoma may be seen occasionally following treatment with cortisone eye ointment.

Trachoma eye infection in nonendemic areas is a complication of what is now well recognized as one of the commonest venereal infections. Trachoma organisms are the most frequent cause of nongonococcal urethritis (Chap. 137), and they are often found in the female genital tract in the absence of disease. While genital tract infection with trachoma organisms is common throughout the world, sporadic trachoma eye infection is uncommon and is recognized infrequently.

Clinical manifestations Initially eye disease with trachoma organisms presents as a papillary or follicular conjunctivitis that is not clinically unique. Sporadic nonendemic trachoma usually presents as an acute or subacute follicular conjunctivitis with keratitis. Sometimes the inflammation is extremely acute and resembles acute adenovirus or herpesvirus eye infection. Usually onset follows several weeks after exposure to a new sexual partner. If inadequately treated with antibiotics or improperly treated with corticosteroids, the initial follicular conjunctivitis may progress with significant, although transient, visual loss and pannus formation. Untreated cases may persist for several months to 2 years. In the absence of reinfection scar formation and complications are rare; however, relapse of disease after insufficient treatment may prolong the course.

In endemic areas, reinfection is common. It usually results from eye-to-eye contamination among members of a household. The classic form of trachoma is a chronic follicular conjunctivitis with involvement of the cornea. As the disease progresses, scarring of the conjunctiva occurs, as well as corneal vascularization and leukocytic infiltration (pannus formation). If the scarring of the conjunctiva is severe enough, distortions of the lid result, with inversion of the entire lid margins (entropion) or of individual lashes (trichiasis). Destruction of the lacrimal glands may pro-

duce keratitis sicca and xerosis (abnormal dryness). Complete corneal pannus with visual impairment may occur as part of the primary disease process or as a result of secondary complications. Once the normal physiological function of eyelid and conjunctiva is impaired, complete blindness occurs as a result of bacterial corneal ulcers late in the course of the disease.

Diagnosis The diagnosis of trachoma should be considered in all cases of follicular conjunctivitis persisting for more than 3 weeks. Trachoma is usually a clinical diagnosis. However, laboratory diagnosis has been greatly improved. The presence of the typical cytoplasmic inclusion bodies in Giemsa-stained or fluorescent antibody-stained smears of the conjunctival epithelium is considered adequate proof of trachoma infection. Such inclusions are often found in acute disease but are difficult to demonstrate in milder or chronic disease. Isolation in eggs and cell cultures and the direct immunofluorescent test to detect serum antibodies or those from eye secretions provide evidence of infection, but these procedures are limited to a few research laboratories. Follicular conjunctivitis in Americans or Europeans exposed in countries where trachoma is endemic is rarely trachoma.

Treatment Sulfonamides, tetracycline, and erythromycin are effective against *C. trachomatis.* Most sporadic or mild endemic trachoma (such as that found in American Indians) responds to 3 to 6 weeks of full courses of these chemotherapeutic agents. The genital infection associated with sporadic trachoma is effectively treated with similar courses of drugs. It is necessary to treat the sexual partners simultaneously to prevent reinfection. Where trachoma is more severe and complicated by secondary bacterial conjunctivitis, particularly with *Hemophilus,* local treatment with tetracycline eye ointments has been used most extensively. In mass therapy campaigns, treatment for 60 days with tetracycline or erythromycin ointment locally has produced satisfactory clinical improvement. The World Health Organization has suggested intermittent therapy consisting of topical application twice daily for 1 week each month for 6 months. In countries where mass treatment programs have not been accompanied by a rise in the standard of living, trachoma and its blinding complications have not been effectively reduced. In such endemic areas, control programs frequently include provisions for surgical repair of entropion and trichiasis to prevent visual loss later in the course of the disease.

Prevention Efforts to develop a practical vaccine have not been successful. General hygienic measures associated with improved living standards are effective in the elimination of trachoma. Adequate water supply for personal cleanliness may be a key factor. In order to prevent spread of the disease to uninfected family members, treatment of healthy contacts with antibiotic ointment once daily is an effective procedure.

INCLUSION CONJUNCTIVITIS OF THE NEWBORN (INCLUSION BLENNORRHEA) In the newborn, inclusion conjunctivitis can be differentiated from gonococcal ophthalmia by its longer incubation period (5 to 14 days versus 1 to 3 days). Neonatal inclusion conjunctivitis has an acute onset and produces a profuse mucopurulent discharge with membrane formation and occasional scar formation on the conjunctiva. Inclusions usually can be demonstrated in conjunctival smears. Administration of systemic tetracycline, erythromycin, or sulfonamide controls the symptoms of the disease within 48 h but should be continued for at least 3 weeks. Recent evidence suggests that many birth canal infections are asymptomatic. Relapsing childhood trachomatous eye disease in nonendemic areas has been demonstrated in some of these cases. This disease is probably rare and is related to the original birth canal infection.

EPIDEMIC KERATOCONJUNCTIVITIS (EKC) EKC typically occurs in epidemics; the etiologic agent found in most outbreaks is adenovirus type 8 or 19, although minor forms of EKC occur with the other adenovirus types. Adenovirus spread occurs when medical personnel manipulate the eye, e.g., for foreign-body removal in industrial dispensaries or during eye examinations by an ophthalmologist. The virus, which is unusually resistant to inactivation, is transmitted on the fingers, by instruments, or in solutions. EKC presents as a moderate to severe follicular conjunctivitis which subsides spontaneously within 10 to 18 days. The incubation period varies from 5 to 12 days.

The disease is usually unilateral at onset. The more severe cases may be associated with conjunctival membrane formation and subsequent conjunctival scarring and with subconjunctival hemorrhages. Mild systemic manifestations such as low-grade fever, headache, and malaise may occur. A preauricular lymph node on the side of the affected eye is usually enlarged. With corneal involvement, about 7 days after onset, there is often a marked increase in pain (foreign-body sensation), lacrimation, and photophobia. The typical punctate corneal opacities appear to progress as the conjunctivitis subsides. These opacities may persist for as long as 2 years. If visual acuity is impaired, treatment with topical corticosteroids will temporarily suppress the opacities. There is no specific treatment. In epidemics, milder episodes of disease in adults are often recognized. In children, adenovirus type 8 infections may present as upper respiratory disease, often with otitis media, and may be overlooked as a source of infection for the eye disease. Explosive epidemics in industrial dispensaries and ophthalmologists' offices can be controlled by scrupulous hand washing and adequate cleansing of instruments to break the chain of infection.

NEWCASTLE DISEASE Human infection with this avian virus, which is related to influenza, occurs mainly in poultry workers, veterinarians, and virologists. In man, accidental introduction of contaminated material from naturally infected animals or from live virus (e.g., vaccines) is followed in 24 to 72 h by conjunctivitis, edema of the lids, and tearing. Systemic symptoms occur very rarely, and recovery is complete in 10 to 14 days. The diagnosis may be confirmed by virus isolation in embryonated eggs.

ACUTE HEMORRHAGIC CONJUNCTIVITIS Acute hemorrhagic conjunctivitis (AHC) was first described in 1969 in epidemics in Africa and Asia. The disease presents as an acute conjunctivitis with numerous punctate hemorrhages which become confluent on the bulbar conjunctiva within 24 h. There is also minor involvement of the cornea. The inflammation subsides in 4 to 5 days, but the hemorrhages do not resolve for 7 to 10 days. The only reported complication has been the rare occurrence of lumbar radiculomyelitis. In all but one epidemic, enterovirus 70 (a member of the picornavirus group) has been identified as the etiologic agent. Epidemics of AHC have occurred in the crowded urban populations of developing countries affecting all age groups and social classes. Occasional outbreaks in Europe have been centered around eye clinics. The disease has not yet been reported in the Western Hemisphere.

REFERENCES

DAWSON CR et al: Infections due to adenovirus type 8 in the United States. III. Epidemiological, clinical and microbiological features of epidemic keratoconjunctivitis. Am J Ophthalmol 69:473, 1970

——: Therapy of diseases caused by chlamydia organisms. Int Ophthalmol Clin 13:93, 1973

GRAYSTON JT et al: Epidemic keratoconjunctivitis on Taiwan. Am J Trop Med 13:492, 1964

——, WANG SP: New knowledge of *Chlamydiae* and the diseases they cause. J Infect Dis 132:87, 1975

NELSON CB et al: Outbreak of conjunctivitis due to Newcastle disease virus (NDV) occurring in poultry workers. Am J Public Health 42:672, 1952

NICHOLS RL (ed): *Trachoma and Allied Diseases,* Amsterdam, New York: Excerpta Medica, 1971

WHITCHE JP et al: Acute hemorrhagic conjunctivitis in Tunisia: Report of viral isolations. Arch Ophthalmol, Jan 1976

190 LYMPHOGRANULOMA VENEREUM

KING K. HOLMES
PETER L. PERINE

DEFINITION Lymphogranuloma venereum (LGV) is a sexually transmitted infection caused by *Chlamydia trachomatis.* The acute disease is characterized by a transient primary genital lesion followed by multilocular suppurative regional lymphadenopathy. Homosexual men and women may develop hemorrhagic proctocolitis with regional lymphadenitis. Acute LGV is almost always associated with nonspecific systemic symptoms, usually with fever and leukocytosis, and rarely with systemic complications such as meningoencephalitis. After a latent period of years, late complications include genital elephantiasis, strictures, and fistulas of the penis, urethra, and rectum.

ETIOLOGY The chlamydia are small bacteria with a distinctive obligately intracellular developmental cycle. The genus includes two pathogens, *C. psittaci* and *C. trachomatis,* which are isolated in the laboratory by inoculation of yolk sacs or tissue cell culture. The only natural host for *C.*

trachomatis is the human. Three separate epidemiologic groups of *C. trachomatis* have been differentiated by immunofluorescent antibody typing. Immunotypes A to C have been associated mainly with ocular trachoma and occasionally with genital infection. Types D to K are the predominant types encountered in the United States and England, and are associated with ocular infection, nongonococcal urethritis, and probably with cervicitis. Only three immunotypes, designated L1, L2, and L3, cause LGV. LGV immunotypes also have other distinguishing biological characteristics: They are more invasive than the other immunotypes of *C. trachomatis,* cause disease primarily in lymphatic tissue, grow more readily in tissue culture, and are pathogenic when inoculated intracerebrally into mice and monkeys.

EPIDEMIOLOGY Lymphogranuloma venereum usually is sexually transmitted, but occasional transmission by nonsexual personal contact, fomites, or laboratory accidents has been documented. The peak incidence corresponds to the age of greatest sexual activity, the second and third decades of life. The worldwide incidence of LGV is falling, for unexplained reasons, but the disease is still endemic in certain countries of Asia, Africa, and South America. In the United States, only 386 cases were reported during 1975.

The frequency of infection following exposure is believed to be much less than that associated with gonorrhea and syphilis. Early manifestations are recognized far more often in men than in women, who usually present with late complications. In the United States, where the reported sex ratio is 3.4 males to 1 female, most cases involve travelers, seamen, and military personnel returning from abroad; male homosexuals; or individuals of low socioeconomic status living in areas of low endemicity in the Southeast. The main reservoir of infection in the United States is presumed to be asymptomatically infected individuals, but attempts to isolate LGV strains from the urethra or cervix of sexually active persons without clinical LGV have been unsuccessful.

Prevalence studies of LGV are difficult to interpret. Most have employed the Frei skin test or LGV complement fixation (CF) serologic test. Since the antigens used in these tests cross-react with other strains of *C. trachomatis* which are much more widely prevalent in developed countries than the three LGV strains, the specificity of the Frei and LGV CF tests is open to question.

CLINICAL MANIFESTATIONS A *primary genital lesion* occurs from 3 days to 3 weeks after exposure. It is a small, painless vesicle or nonindurated ulcer or papule located on the penis in the male or on the labia, posterior vagina, or fourchette in the female. The primary lesion is noticed by only one-third of men with LGV and only rarely by women. It heals in a few days without scarring and even when noticed is not recognized as LGV except in retrospect when it is followed by lymphadenitis. LGV strains of *C. trachomatis* have occasionally been recovered from the male urethra and the endocervix of patients who present with inguinal adenopathy, suggesting that these areas may be the primary site of infection in some cases.

In women and homosexual men, *primary anorectal infection* occurs following rectal intercourse. In women, this may also occur by spread via the pelvic lymphatics, or by direct spread of infection from the genitalia along the perineum to the anal canal. Anorectal colonization also occurs in women with cervical infection due to non-LGV immunotypes of *C. trachomatis.* After an incubation period of unknown length, multiplication within intestinal epithelial cells leads to symptoms which include mucopurulent or bloody anal discharge, tenesmus, and diarrhea. Sigmoidoscopy reveals diffuse proctitis or discrete ulcerations limited to the rectosigmoid colon.

From the site of the primary infection, the organism spreads via the regional lymphatics. Penile, vulvar, and, occasionally, anal infection can lead to inguinal and femoral lymphadenitis. Anorectal infection produces hypogastric and deep iliac lymphadenitis. Upper vaginal or cervical infection results in enlargement of the obturator and iliac nodes. The most common presenting picture in heterosexual men is the *inguinal syndrome.* This also occurs in about 10 percent of men with anorectal infection. It is characterized by painful inguinal lymphadenopathy beginning 2 to 6 weeks after presumed exposure; rarely the onset occurs after a few months. The inguinal adenopathy is unilateral in two-thirds of cases, and palpable enlargement of the iliac and femoral nodes is often present on the same side as the enlarged inguinal nodes. The nodes are initially discrete, but progressive periadenitis results in a matted mass of nodes which become fluctuant and suppurative. The overlying skin becomes fixed, inflamed, and thinned and finally develops multiple draining fistulas. Extensive enlargement of chains of inguinal nodes above and below the inguinal ligament ("the sign of the groove") is characteristic but is present in only a minority of cases. Histologic involvement of nodes initially shows characteristic small stellate abscesses surrounded by histiocytes. These abscesses coalesce to cause large, necrotic, suppurative foci. Spontaneous healing usually occurs after several months, leaving inguinal scars or granulomatous masses of varying size which persist for life. Massive pelvic lymphadenopathy in women or homosexual men may lead to exploratory laparotomy.

Constitutional symptoms are common during the state of regional lymphadenopathy and include fever, chills, headache, meningismus, anorexia, myalgias, and arthralgias. These findings in the presence of lymphadenopathy are often mistaken for malignant lymphoma. Other systemic complications are infrequent but include arthritis with sterile effusion, aseptic meningitis, meningoencephalitis, conjunctivitis, hepatitis, and erythema nodosum. Chlamydiae have been recovered from the cerebrospinal fluid, and in one case from the blood in a patient with severe constitutional symptoms, indicating the occurrence of disseminated infection. Associated laboratory findings during the acute stage of infection include leukocytosis and mild elevation of the sedimentation rate. Abnormal liver function tests, hyperglobulinemia, mixed cryoglobulinemia, rheumatoid factor activity, and elevated IgG, IgA, and IgM have been reported in subacute and chronic LGV. False positive serologic tests for syphilis are rare, and syphilis should be suspected if these tests are positive, as is often the case.

Complications of anorectal infection include perirectal abscess, fistula in ano, and rectovaginal, rectovesical, and ischiorectal fistulas. Secondary bacterial infection probably contributes to these complications. Rectal stricture is a late complication of anorectal infection and usually occurs 2 to 6 cm from the anal orifice, within reach on digital rectal examination. The stricture may extend proximally for several centimeters, leading to a mistaken clinical and radiographic diagnosis of carcinoma.

Approximately 5 percent of cases of LGV in men present with chronic progressive infiltrative, ulcerative, or fistular lesions of the penis, urethra, or scrotum. Urethral stricture may occur and usually involves the posterior urethra, causing incontinence or difficulty with micturition.

An uncommon late complication of LGV is *genital elephantiasis,* a chronic induration and edema of the penis or vulva caused by lymphatic obstruction. Polypoid welling of the skin and large stellate hyperplastic keloidal scars of the genitalia may be associated with vulvar induration or lymphedema and are difficult to distinguish clinically from granuloma inguinale and genital tuberculosis. Chronic ulcerations of the vulva (esthiomene) and smooth pedunculated perianal growths (lymphorrhoids) also occur. The significance of reports of malignant changes associated with chronic anorectal or genital LGV is uncertain.

DIAGNOSIS Although LGV is uncommon, it frequently enters the differential diagnosis of common conditions such as inguinal lymphadenopathy; vesicular, papular, or ulcerative genital lesions; and perirectal abscess, fistula in ano, or proctocolitis. When methods for culture and serodiagnosis become more available, diagnostic testing for LGV in these conditions probably will increase.

The most reliable method of diagnosis is isolation of an LGV strain of *Chlamydia* from aspirated bubo pus or from the urethra, endocervix, or infected tissue. Isolation has been possible from bubo pus in about 30 percent of cases with both clinical and serologic evidence of LGV. The methods needed for isolation in tissue cell culture are widely available but seldom used. The most widely used immunodiagnostic tests have been the LGV complement fixation test and the Frei skin tests. The LGV complement fixation test becomes positive (serum titer $\geq$ 1:32) shortly after the bubo first appears and is positive in 80 to 90 percent of patients with the inguinal syndrome. The titer may not increase in paired serums since most patients have already been infected for several weeks when first seen. The Frei skin test is less sensitive than the LGV complement fixation test. It is performed by intradermal inoculation of 0.1 ml of a crude antigen prepared from infected yolk sac into the flexor surface of the forearm. The test is read at 72 h and is positive ($\geq$ 6 mm induration and erythema at the site of antigen inoculation, with no induration at the site of normal yolk sac control inoculation) in less than 50 percent of patients who present with the inguinal syndrome. The frequency of positive skin tests increases with the duration of untreated infection, and positive tests remain positive for life. *A negative Frei test does not exclude the diagnosis of LGV.* Conversely, a positive LGV complement fixation test or Frei skin test may not be specific for LGV, since the reactivity of these tests has not yet been systematically studied in patients who have been infected with non-LGV immunotypes of *C. trachomatis*—for example, patients with nongonococcal urethritis (NGU).

However, two serologic tests for LGV have been developed which appear to be both sensitive and specific. Limited experience indicates that the microimmunofluorescent antibody test developed by Wang detects antibody to *C. trachomatis* in nearly all patients with culture-proved LGV. Serum microimmunofluorescent antibody titers from patients with LGV exceed the highest titers that occur in chlamydial NGU and can usually be shown to be directed against immunotypes L1, L2, or L3. A counter-immunoelectrophoresis test has also been developed using the soluble *C. trachomatis*–specific antigen extracted from the LGV strain. This test is positive in over 95 percent of patients whose microimmunofluorescent test shows antibody to LGV strain, but is negative in patients with chlamydial NGU. The histopathology of excised nodes or of rectal biopsy specimens is seldom definitive, but suggestive findings may raise the question of LGV and lead to more specific tests.

TREATMENT LGV chlamydiae are susceptible in vitro to the tetracyclines, sulfonamides, erythromycin, rifampin, and chloramphenicol and are slightly sensitive to the penicillins. They are resistant to the aminoglycosides such as streptomycin, as well as to bacitracin, vancomycin, and the polymyxins. Rare isolates have been resistant to sulfonamides. Despite their in vitro activity, antibiotics do not have a dramatic effect on the duration and healing of inguinal buboes. However, acute constitutional symptoms are often terminated abruptly. Antibiotics are usually not helpful in improving late complications such as rectal stricture or genital elephantiasis unless secondary infection is also present. Genital elephantiasis and rectal, penile, and urethral strictures and fistulas require surgical correction, although sometimes urethral and even rectal strictures can be managed by repeated mechanical dilation.

The recommended treatment regimens are tetracycline hydrochloride, 0.5 g four times a day for 21 days, or a sulfonamide preparation, 4 g per day for 21 days. Sulfonamides and trimethoprim show synergistic activity against *C. trachomatis.* Fluctuant buboes should be aspirated with a syringe and 18-gage needle as often as necessary to prevent spontaneous rupture. It is not unusual for buboes to increase in size or to develop at another site after initiation of treatment. Although these seldom progress to fistula formation, they should be aspirated if fluctuant. A fourfold or greater fall in complement fixation titer occurs in most treated patients, and LGV *Chlamydia* cannot be isolated from lesions after the initiation of antibiotic treatment.

REFERENCES

Abrams AJ: Lymphogranuloma venereum. JAMA 205:199, 1968

Caldwell HD et al: Antigenic analysis of chlamydiae by two-dimensional immunoelectrophoresis II. A trachoma-LGV-specific antigen. J Immunol 115:969, 1975

Grayston JT, Wang S: New knowledge of chlamydiae and the diseases they cause. J Infect Dis 132:87, 1975

Greaves AB: The frequency of lymphogranuloma venereum in persons with perirectal abscesses, fistula-in-ano, or both. Bull WHO 29:797, 1963

Holder WR, Duncan WC: Lymphogranuloma venereum. Clin Obstet Gynecol 15:1004, 1972

Hopsu-Havu VK, Sonck CE: Infiltrative, ulcerative, and fistular lesions of the penis due to lymphogranuloma venereum. Br J Vener Dis 49:193, 1972

JAWETZ E: Chemotherapy of chlamydial infection. Adv Pharmacol 7:253, 1969

SCHACHTER J et al: Lymphogranuloma venereum, 1. Comparison of the Frei test, complement fixation test, and isolating the agent. J Infect Dis 120:372, 1969

191
PSITTACOSIS

VERNON KNIGHT

DEFINITION Psittacosis is an infectious disease of birds caused by an organism that has a number of properties in common with gram-negative bacteria. Transmission of infection from birds to humans results in a febrile illness characterized by pneumonitis and systemic manifestations. Inapparent infections or mild influenza-like illnesses may also occur. The term *ornithosis* is sometimes applied to infections contracted from birds other than parrots or parakeets, but *psittacosis* is the preferred generic term for all forms of the disease.

ETIOLOGY The causative agent *Chlamydia psittaci* is a gram-negative obligate intracellular parasite, formerly classified as a virus. Now chlamydias, along with the rickettsias, may be considered specialized bacteria. Both synthesize ribonucleic acid (RNA) and deoxyribonucleic acid (DNA), reproduce by binary fission, and are susceptible to antimicrobial drugs. In contrast to rickettsias, the chlamydias are dependent on their hosts for metabolic energy. Slight but definite homology of the DNA of members of the *Chlamydia* genus with the DNA of *Neisseria meningitidis* has been shown. The psittacosis agent is the prototype of a biologically and antigenically homogeneous class of microorganisms that includes the causative agents of lymphogranuloma venereum, trachoma, and 30 or more mammalian parasites which rarely produce human disease.

EPIDEMIOLOGY Psittacosis is widely distributed throughout the world, and almost any avian species can harbor the agent. Psittacine birds are most commonly infected, but human cases have been traced to contact with pigeons, ducks, turkeys, chickens, and many other birds. Psittacosis may be considered an occupational disease of pet-shop owners, poultry raisers, pigeon fanciers, taxidermists, and zoo attendants. The incidence of human infection in the United States rose steadily from 1930, owing in large measure to the increasing popularity of parrots and parakeets as pets and, as subsequently recognized, transmission of infection by barnyard fowl and pigeons. The number of reported cases reached a peak in 1956 and gradually declined thereafter. By 1963, with acceptance of control measures such as incorporation of tetracyclines in poultry feed, the disease had again become relatively uncommon. In 1973 only 35 cases from 14 states were reported to the Center for Disease Control. In contrast, the disease appears to be more common in England, where budgerigars are common household pets and where restrictions on the importation of these birds have been eased.

The agent is present in nasal secretions, excreta, tissues, and feathers of infected birds. Although the disease can be fatal, infected birds frequently show only minor evidence of illness such as ruffled feathers, lethargy, and anorexia. Asymptomatic avian carriers are common, and complete recovery may be followed by continued shedding of the organism for many months.

Psittacosis is almost always transmitted to humans by the respiratory route. On rare occasions the disease may be acquired from the bite of a pet bird. Intimate and prolonged contact is not essential for transmission of the disease; a few minutes spent in an environment previously occupied by an infected bird has resulted in human infection. The severity of the disease in humans bears no apparent relationship to closeness or duration of contact, although sick birds are more likely to transmit infection than healthy ones. Transmission of a psittacosis-like agent between humans has occurred among hospital personnel, with severe and sometimes fatal infections. There is evidence that these "human" strains are more virulent than native avian organisms. There is no record of infection acquired by eating poultry products.

PATHOGENESIS The psittacosis agent gains entrance to the body through the upper part of the respiratory tract and eventually localizes in the pulmonary alveoli and in the reticuloendothelial cells of the spleen and liver. Invasion of the lung probably takes place by way of the bloodstream rather than by direct extension from the upper air passages. A lymphocytic inflammatory response occurs on both the interstitial and respiratory surfaces of the alveoli as well as in the perivascular spaces. The alveolar walls and interstitial tissues of the lung are thickened, edematous, necrotic, and occasionally hemorrhagic. Histologically, the affected areas show alveolar spaces filled with fluid, erythrocytes, and lymphocytes. The picture is not pathognomonic of psittacosis unless macrophages containing characteristic cytoplasmic inclusion bodies (LCL bodies) can be identified. The respiratory epithelium of the bronchi and bronchioles usually remains intact.

MANIFESTATIONS The clinical manifestations and course of psittacosis are extremely variable. After an *incubation period* of 7 to 14 days, or longer, the disease may start abruptly with shaking chills and high fever, but the onset is often gradual with increasing fever and malaise over a 3- to 4-day period. Headache is almost always a prominent symptom; it is usually diffuse and excruciating and often the patient's chief complaint. Generalized myalgia is also common. Spasm and stiffness of the muscles of the back and neck may lead to an erroneous diagnosis of meningitis. A faint, macular rash (Horder's spots) simulating the rose spots of typhoid fever has been described. Lethargy, mental depression, agitation, insomnia, and disorientation have been prominent features of the illness in some epidemics, but not in others; delirium and stupor occur near the end of the first week in severe cases. Occasional patients are comatose when first seen, and the diagnosis of psittacosis may be missed. Gastrointestinal complaints such as abdominal pain, nausea, vomiting, or diarrhea are present in some cases; constipation and abdominal distention sometimes occur as late complications. Icterus, the result of severe hepatic involvement, is a rare and ominous finding.

Symptoms of upper respiratory tract infection are not prominent, although mild sore throat, pharyngeal infection, and cervical adenopathy are often present; on occasion they may be the only manifestations of illness. Epistaxis is encountered early in the course of nearly one-fourth of the cases. Photophobia is also a common complaint.

A dry, hacking cough is characteristic; it is usually nonproductive, but small amounts of mucoid or bloody sputum may be raised as the disease progresses. Cough may appear early in the course of the disease or as late as 5 days after the onset of fever. Chest pain, pleurisy with effusion, or a friction rub may all occur but are rare. Pericarditis and myocarditis have been reported. Most patients have a normal or slightly increased respiratory rate; marked dyspnea with cyanosis occurs only in severe psittacosis with extensive pulmonary involvement. In psittacosis, as in most nonbacterial pneumonias, the physical signs of pneumonitis tend to be less prominent than symptoms and x-ray findings would suggest. The initial examination may reveal fine, sibilant rales, or clinical evidence of pneumonia may be completely lacking. Rales usually become audible and more numerous as the illness progresses. Signs of frank pulmonary consolidation are usually absent.

Patients without cough or other clinical evidence of respiratory involvement come to the physician with fever of unknown origin. The pulse rate is slow in relation to the fever. When splenomegaly is present in a patient with acute pneumonitis, psittacosis should be considered; the reported incidence of splenomegaly ranges from 10 to 70 percent. Nontender hepatic enlargement also occurs, but jaundice is rare. Thrombophlebitis is not unusual during convalescence; indeed, pulmonary infarction is sometimes a late complication and may be fatal.

In untreated cases of psittacosis, sustained or mildly remittent fever persists for 10 days to 3 weeks, or occasionally as long as 3 months. Defervescence is by lysis and is accompanied by abatement of respiratory manifestations. Psittacosis contracted from parrots or parakeets is more likely to be a severe, prolonged illness than infections acquired from pigeons or barnyard fowl. Relapses occur but are rare. Secondary bacterial infections are uncommon. Immunity to reinfection is probably permanent.

LABORATORY FINDINGS The x-ray of the lungs in psittacosis mimics that in a great variety of pulmonary diseases. The pneumonic lesions are usually patchy in appearance but can be hazy, diffuse, homogeneous, lobar, atelectatic, wedge-shaped, nodular, or miliary. The white blood cell count is normal or moderately decreased in the acute phase of the disease but may rise in convalescence. The erythrocyte sedimentation rate is frequently not elevated. Transient proteinuria is common. The cerebrospinal fluid sometimes contains a few mononuclear cells but is otherwise normal. Cold agglutinins are rarely present.

The diagnosis can be confirmed only by isolation of the causative microorganism or serologic studies. The agent is present in the blood during the acute phase of the disease and in the bronchial secretions for weeks or sometimes years after infection, but it is difficult to isolate. Psittacosis is most readily diagnosed by the demonstration of a rising titer of complement-fixing antibody in the patient's blood. An acute and convalescent specimen should always be tested. Even a low titer of antibody during the acute febrile phase constitutes presumptive evidence of psittacosis. The prompt initiation of treatment with tetracycline has been shown to delay antibody rise in convalescence for several weeks or months. Interpretation of a single complement fixation test may sometimes be difficult because of the antigenic cross reaction between the agent of psittacosis and that of lymphogranuloma venereum.

DIFFERENTIAL DIAGNOSIS A history of exposure to birds may be the only clinical basis for differentiating psittacosis from a great variety of infectious and noninfectious febrile disorders. A partial list of pneumonic disease that may be confused with psittacosis includes *Mycoplasma* pneumonia, Q fever, coccidioidomycosis, tuberculosis, carcinoma of the lung with bronchial obstruction, and bacterial pneumonias. In the early stages, before pneumonitis appears, psittacosis may be mistaken for influenza, typhoid fever, miliary tuberculosis, and infectious mononucleosis.

TREATMENT The tetracyclines are consistently effective in the treatment of psittacosis. Defervescence and alleviation of symptoms usually occur in 24 to 48 h after instituting therapy with 2 g daily in six-hourly divided doses. To avoid relapse, treatment should probably be continued for at least 7 days after defervescence. In severe cases, oxygen and other supportive measures are indicated.

REFERENCE

CENTER FOR DISEASE CONTROL: Morbid Mortal Week Rep 23:434 (Dec 21), 1974

section 15 | Viral diseases

192
BASIC CONSIDERATIONS OF VIRAL INFECTIONS

A. MARTIN LERNER

A more complete view of the causes, manifestations, and responses of human beings to virus diseases is unfolding. Effective attenuated vaccines against measles, rubella, mumps, and poliomyelitis are available. In certain situations antiviral prophylaxis (e.g., influenza with amantadine) and chemotherapy (e.g., herpes simplex virus keratitis with idoxuridine) are now a reality, and investigations are under way in immunotherapy utilizing transfer factor, human interferon, or synthetic interferon inducers. Some human data and animal models suggest that a number of degenerating diseases of the central nervous system (progressive multifocal leukoencephalopathy, subacute sclerosing panencephalitis, multiple sclerosis), certain "collagen diseases," and some malignancies may be virus-induced.

During acute illnesses caused by viruses it is often possible to culture or visualize fleetingly the etiologic agent by fluorescence or electron microscopy at body orifices, or in secretions or excretions. To the physician caring for the patient, retrospective diagnoses based upon fourfold or greater rises in humoral antibodies are academic. The specific events of cellular immunity have not yet yielded practical diagnostic tests. A compelling need is for further development of rapid means of specific virologic diagnosis. Potent immunologic assays of components of viruses or of antibodies at sites of synthesis are needed. In this regard use of immunoelectrophoresis and radioimmunoassay for hepatitis B surface and core antigens, immune electron microscopy in the recognition of the viruses of epidemic diarrheal diseases, and the immune adherence test for detecting antibodies to hepatitis A virus have been recent important advances.

GENERAL PROPERTIES AND CLASSIFICATION Viruses are grouped according to their biophysical characteristics: (1) nucleic acid, (2) size, (3) sensitivity to ether, (4) presence of an envelope, and (5) symmetry (cubic or helical). They contain macromolecular cores of ribonucleic acid (RNA) or deoxyribonucleic acid (DNA), but not both. (On the other hand, chlamydiae, mycoplasma, and rickettsiae contain both RNA and DNA.) Viruses do not contain adenosine triphosphate–generating enzymes. Viruses have marked species and organ specificities, and on the whole, viruses infecting plants, insects, rickettsiae, bacteria, and other animals are distinct from their human counterparts.

Human viruses range in size from 17 nm (picornavirus) to 300 nm (poxvirus). They may be naked and contain only nucleic acid (genome) which is protected by a closed shell or tubing, the capsid. Other viruses have, in addition, a lipid envelope, acquired during maturation as virus evaginates from the nucleus (herpes simplex virus) or cytoplasm (influenza, herpes simplex virus). The lipid coat of these viruses surrounds the capsid. The capsid consists of protein and is composed of repeating subunits, capsomeres. Mature virus particles are called *virions* (Fig. 192-1). Specific antigens of the capsid may penetrate the lipid envelope.

The nucleic acid contains all the genetic material necessary to reproduce itself (transcription) and the code for structural proteins and enzymes (translation) important in synthesis and attachment to susceptible cells. The nucleic acid core plus the capsid is known as the *nucleocapsid* (Fig. 192-1). When the virion is stripped of its capsid, nucleic acid may enter a host foreign species and produce a single cycle of mature virus (e.g., poliovirus in mouse renal cells). Species and organ specificities of virus-cell union are functions first of complementary physical characteristics and then of covalent union between proteins of the virus and susceptible cell membranes. For instance, molecules of neuraminic acid act as receptors on human red blood cells, allowing hemagglutination by influenza virus. Within several hours after virus adsorption, neuraminidase, one of the proteins of the influenza capsid, digests the neuraminic acid. Elution of influenza virus from red blood cells follows.

At present there are seven known groups of RNA viruses (picornavirus, reovirus, arbovirus, myxovirus, rhabdovirus, coronavirus, arenovirus) and four groups of DNA viruses (papovavirus, adenovirus, herpesvirus, poxvirus) (Table 192-1).

FIGURE 192-1
Components of a complete virus particle (virion).

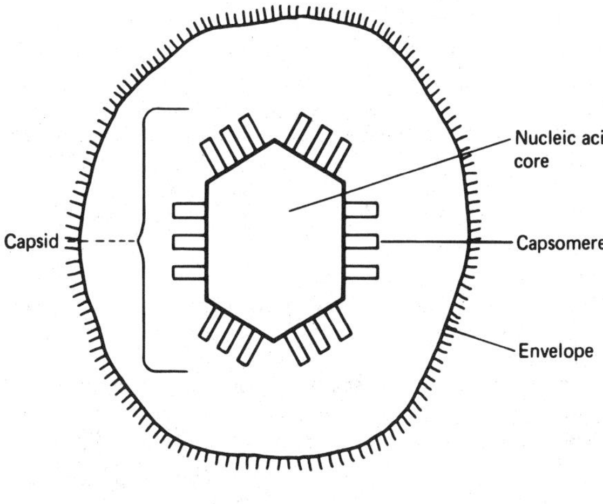

Nucleic acids of infectious and serum hepatitis viruses have not yet been identified. By electron microscopy these agents are seen to have cubic symmetry and are about 20 nm in diameter. Other viruses belonging to the parvovirus and leukovirus groups have not been shown to affect human beings.

VIRUS MULTIPLICATION Virus adsorption is a specific physical and then chemical reaction. Capsids of reoviruses and enteroviruses may contain glycoproteins. Attachment involves free carbonyl groups. Sulfhydryl groupings on enteroviruses need to be intact. After absorption, virus enters the cell by pinocytosis and is uncoated; i.e., nucleic acid is stripped from the capsid. With DNA viruses, specific virus DNA strands are transcribed into specific mRNA (messenger RNA), which is, in turn, translated to synthesize virus-specific proteins and enzymes necessary for biosynthesis of virus DNA. In the case of virus RNA, single-stranded RNA serves as its own messenger. The mRNA is translated, resulting in the formation of an RNA polymerase. Synthesis of host cell protein and nucleic acid is suppressed to variable degrees. Assembly of protein subunits around virus DNA results in formation of complete virions which may be released by cell lysis or budding from the cytoplasm. Recently, virions of RNA tumor viruses have been found to contain an enzyme which is capable of catalyzing synthesis of DNA. The product consists of small fragments of DNA, most of which are complementary in base sequence to 70S RNA of the virion. Thus, information can travel not only from DNA to RNA but also, at least in certain cases, in the reverse direction.

ROUTES OF INFECTION Viruses, like fungi, bacteria, parasites, or rickettsiae, infect humans by respiratory, enteric, or contact mechanisms. Coughs, sneezes, or ordinary speech give rise to aerosolized infectious units. From human respiratory reservoirs droplets of water over 10 μm containing virus travel short distances through the air, while droplet nuclei, minus moisture and less than 10 μm in size, waft over greater distances. Successful primary infection in a susceptible host depends upon (1) the number of virions circulating per cubic foot of air; and (2) the time of exposure, which in turn determines the total size of the inoculum. For instance, if an aerosol contains four virions per liter of air, and 30 virions are required for infection, then persons breathing this air will inspire an infectious dose within a half hour. The smaller number of respiratory infections (usually rhinoviruses) during the summer may be due in part to open windows with multiple exchanges of air.

Fecal-oral contamination is usual with enteroviruses (Coxsackie viruses A and B, polioviruses, and hepatitis A). Occasionally, they, too, are spread by droplets or their nuclei. On the other hand, rabies virus in the saliva of a rabid dog reaches the victim's brain after a bite exposes peripheral nerve endings. Contaminated urines disseminate rubella or cytomegaloviruses. Blood, plasma, or buffy coat may transmit herpesviruses and viruses of infectious or serum hepatitis. Intimate contact of mucosal surfaces is important with herpesviruses. Insect vectors (arboviruses) or life cy-

TABLE 192-1
Major groups of viruses infecting human beings

Generic name, nucleic acid, and prototype virus	*Size, nm*	*Ether sensitive*	*Envelope*	*Symmetry*
Picornavirus (RNA):	17–30	No	No	Cubic
Coxsackie viruses A and B; echo, rhino-, and polioviruses				
Reovirus (RNA)	74	No	No	Cubic
Arbovirus (RNA):	20–100	Yes	?	
Group A (equine encephalitis, Semliki Forest)				
Group B (Japanese B, Russian tick-borne, yellow fever, dengue)				
Group C (Morituba, Oriboca)				
Ungrouped (Rift Valley, Colorado tick fever, sandfly)				
Myxovirus and paramyxovirus (RNA):	80–200	Yes	Yes	Helical
Influenzas A, B, and C: parainfluenza, mumps, rubeola; respiratory syncytial				
Rhabdovirus: rabies (RNA)	65–180	Yes	Yes	
Coronavirus (RNA)		Yes	Yes	
Arenovirus (RNA):				
Togavirus: rubella (most arboviruses of groups A and B)	50	Yes	Yes	
Tacaribe-LCM: lymphocytic choriomeningitis, South American hemorrhagic fevers (Lassa, Machupo)	50–300	Yes	Yes	
Papovavirus (DNA):	45–55	No	No	Cubic
"Warts," simian virus 40				
Adenovirus (DNA)	65–85	No	No	Cubic
Herpesvirus (DNA):	120–180	Yes	Yes	Cubic
Herpes simplex, monkey B, varicella-herpes zoster, cytomegalovirus, Epstein-Barr				
Poxvirus (DNA):	150–300	Yes or no	Yes	Cubic
Variola, vaccinia, molluscum contagiosum, orf (milker's nodules)				
Human hepatitis (nucleic acid unclassified):				
Infectious hepatitis, serum hepatitis				

cles in other animal species may be important (arboviruses, lymphocytic choriomeningitis). Infection via ovum or sperm is possible but has not been demonstrated in humans.

PATHOGENESIS OF DISEASE The primary site of virus multiplication depends upon the route of acquisition and the special receptor-site complementarity of the host. Respiratory viruses (rhinovirus, myxovirus, coronavirus, rubella, adenovirus, herpesvirus) multiply in upper respiratory epithelium, injuring, denuding, and slowing ciliary movements. Respiratory viruses in the nasopharynx may involve the conjunctivas via connecting lymphatics, producing serous conjunctivitis, as in the pharyngoconjunctival fever of adenovirus, type 3. Rhinoviruses and coronaviruses usually remain within the nasopharynx. Parainfluenza viruses involve larynx and trachea. Influenza A, adenoviruses, varicella-zoster, cytomegaloviruses, and enteroviruses may produce pneumonias. Adjacent areas of atelectasis and emphysema, mixed cellular infiltrates, and thickening of alveolar septa are common. Alveoli may be free or contain edema amid red blood cells, a modest number of mononuclear cells, and a few polymorphonuclear leukocytes. Virus-specific structures (inclusion bodies) may be present within the cytoplasm (variola), nucleus (herpes simplex virus, varicella-zoster, adenovirus), or both (measles). Viremia may or may not occur. In many virus infections, in distinct contrast to bacteremias, viremia occurs during the incubation period when the patient is well. Viremia is usual with the exanthems of enteroviruses, rubeola, and varicella-zoster viruses. Herpesviruses may multiply within lymphocytes sequestered from antibodies and phagocytes.

Enteric viruses multiply in epithelium and lymphoid tissues first in the pharynx and later in the intestine. Lysis of affected cells (polioviruses) may follow. On the other hand, a slowly destructive, relatively symbiotic relationship ensues in subacute sclerosing panencephalitis (measles virus) and progressive multifocal leukoencephalopathy (papovavirus).

With enterovirus infections, viremia occurs early. Secondary sites of infection are the heart, liver, pancreas, kidneys, and brain. Echo and Coxsackie viruses multiply in the choroid plexus and seed cerebrospinal fluid; polioviruses do not grow within the choroid plexus. Therefore, echo and Coxsackie viruses are regularly isolated from cerebrospinal fluid, but polioviruses are rarely isolated from it.

Responses of the host At sites of virus multiplication extracellular virus often abounds. Macrophages and polymorphonuclear leukocytes migrate to the area producing inflammation. Interferon and B and T lymphocytes are specifically activated. Macrophages attach to antigen in the process of lymphocyte sensitization, and markedly augment the efficiency of viral inactivation by specific neutralizing antibodies or sensitized T lymphocytes.

INTERFERON Viruses, endotoxin, certain parasites, double-stranded RNA or reoviruses, synthetic polyribonucleotide complexes such as poly rI:rC (polyinosinic polycytidilic ribonucleic acid), transfer factor, and synthetic anionic polymers stimulate interferon. Within several hours after onset of virus infection, and days before humoral antibodies can be measured by ordinary methods, interferon is found in tissues where virus is synthesized, and in the blood.

A delay in the appearance of interferon in vesicular fluid has been associated with viremic dissemination in herpes zoster. Likewise, a decreased in vitro responsiveness of the patient's lymphocytes after stimulation by herpes simplex virus in the production of interferon has been found in recurrences of herpes labialis. Moreover, severe repetitive and exhausting exercise in mice infected with Coxsackie virus B-3 results in a delay in the appearance of circulating interferon and, later, in both a delay and a depression in the quantity of type-specific neutralizing antibody in serum. A marked increase in the quantity of myocardial virus and in mortality follows. Rest may be a very important factor in recovery from virus infections.

Interferons of two classes are produced. The first, a high molecular weight protein (i.e., 8.5×10^4 daltons), is preformed and released within 2 h. At 18 h, serum contains proteins with biologic activity of interferon with molecular weights of 3 to 4×10^4 daltons. Interferon is acid-stable (pH 2), trypsin-sensitive, nondialyzable, and nonsedimentable by ultracentrifuge forces sufficient to pellet viruses. Most cells tested produce interferon, but those of the reticuloendothelial system (especially the spleen) and lymphocytes are most important.

Interferon has no effect upon extracellular virus. Following entry of virus nucleic acid into a susceptible cell, the cell nucleus is stimulated to produce interferon, which is released through the cytoplasm of the infected cell to induce a second noninfected cell to release an antiviral protein distinct from interferon. This second protein is translational inhibitory protein (TIP). The TIP binds to cellular ribosomes and alters them so that virus RNA is not translated. Cellular messenger RNA (mRNA) is probably translated normally, permitting normal cell functions, but synthesis of virus-directed coat proteins and enzymes is prevented. New virus is not formed.

Interferons have activity against a wide variety of viruses and are not virus-specific. However, interferon is an effective antiviral substance only in cells of the same species in which it is produced. For instance, anti-influenza A interferon produced in hamster tissue cultures is effective against influenza in hamsters but not in humans.

Viruses vary greatly in their sensitivity to interferon. Myxoviruses are sensitive, while herpes viruses are more resistant. Likewise, the importance of interferon in recovery from virus infection varies. With Coxsackie virus B-3, interferon titers actually parallel virus. In animal models, interferon has been shown to have a prophylactic effect in a number of viral infections, but once the titers of virus are high, this natural antiviral agent is ineffective. It may be that the role of interferon in recovery from viral infections occurs very early, when the inoculum is small.

ANTIBODIES Proteins of the virus capsid stimulate B lymphocytes to synthesize humoral (IgM, IgG, IgA, IgD) and secretory antibodies (IgA). Cell-associated antibodies (IgE) are probably also produced. Immunoglobulins are synthesized in local lymph nodes, at body surfaces (saliva, respiratory secretions, colostrum) and in inflammatory exudates within organs (kidney, brain, cervix). During the first 3 to 10 days after an initial exposure to a virus, IgM antibodies predominate. Later, IgG antibodies usually prevail. Immunoglobulin M is important in clearing viremias, and remains within vascular spaces; IgG antibodies enter interstitial spaces. At surfaces, IgA antibodies contain an added secretory piece, allowing functional integrity in the presence of hydrolytic enzymes of the secretions. Many molecules of antibody combine with a single virion. Covering a critical number of essential sites on the virion renders an antigen-antibody complex noninfectious. Antigen-antibody complexes attract components of complement which are the mediators of the calling forth (chemotaxis) of polymorphonuclear leukocytes. Immune complexes may be fixed in tissues ("postinfectious" encephalitis), circulate, or precipitate at the glomerulus, in the synovia of joints, or in the skin.

Secretory IgA antibodies in respiratory secretions are vital to the bodily defenses against respiratory viruses such as influenza and rhinoviruses. During rhinovirus infections of the nasopharynx, viremia does not occur regularly. Humoral antibodies persist only for months. Immunity is transient; reinfections with the same virus at a later time are possible. On the other hand, after systemic infections, humoral antibodies and immunity persist. Likewise, after administration of killed virus vaccines immunity is briefer than with attenuated viruses.

Circulating neutralizing antibody usually affords effective protection against viremia, but a very large inoculum (or a low antibody titer) may counteract this effect. On the other hand, some viruses multiply and spread from cell to cell even in the presence of neutralizing antibodies. Herpes simplex virus, type 1, and rubeola in nervous tissues are examples. Cell-mediated immunity is the most important means of defense against herpesviruses, while antibody is vital to recovery from enteroviruses. In some cases antibodies or T lymphocytes (cytotoxic "killer" cells) may be important in continuing the pathogenic process. This appears to be the case in chronic murine Coxsackie virus B-3 myocardiopathy.

Antibodies to viruses are measured by neutralization of cytopathic effects in tissue cultures or by protection tests using embryonated eggs or animals. Complement fixation, precipitin, or radioimmunoassay techniques are also used. Certain viruses such as herpes simplex virus, type 1, and cytomegalovirus form complement-requiring neutralizing antibodies early after infection. Myxoviruses, some enteroviruses, and reoviruses hemagglutinate several species of red blood cells. In these cases antibodies can be measured by inhibition of hemagglutination. Virus capsids of nonhemagglutinating viruses may be absorbed to the surface of tanned sheep red blood cells. Antibodies are assayed by passive hemagglutination. Kinetics of rises and falls of the several antibodies suggest that different assays test separate immunoglobulin responses to distinct proteins of the capsid.

CELL-MEDIATED IMMUNITY Thymic-derived T lymphocytes confer delayed immune functions. In most virus infections, both T and B lymphocytes participate in the containment of virus replication. After a latent period, usually of 3 to 4 days, stimulated T lymphocytes transform to lymphoblasts. They release a number of nonspecific, nondialyzable effector molecules which migrate with albumin on electrophoresis. Among these effector molecules are lymphocyte-transforming factor, migration-inhibitory factor, cytotoxin factor, and interferon. Components of complement react with the surface of sensitized lymphocytes, releasing a chemotactic factor to monocytes, which are the important phagocytes of cellular immunity. After stimulation by an antigen evoking a potent T lymphocyte response, macrophages become "activated" and are able specifically to aid in the containment of viral replication before the release of effector molecules. Moreover, the increased phagocytic ability of the activated macrophage is not limited to that of the stimulating virus.

Lysates of human lymphocytes release transfer factor, a dialyzable nonantigenic macromolecule (mol wt, approximately 10,000) which endows specific and prolonged delayed hypersensitivity. Transfer factor may be a double-stranded polynucleotide or polypeptide; it has been used experimentally in treatment of several diseases where cell-mediated immunity is deficient, such as disseminated vaccinia, cytomegalovirus infections, mucocutaneous candidiasis, or in other immunodeficient patients. Inadvertently, transfer factor is "passaged" from donor to recipient during blood transfusions, relaying cellular immunity and hypersensitivity. When viruses multiply within lymphocytes, transient hypofunction probably ensues.

DIAGNOSIS Detection of virus infection depends upon isolation of the virus or recognition of virus antigen or of the immune response of the host. Etiologic associations are more secure if virus is isolated or demonstrated by electron or fluorescence microscopy in diseased tissues. For instance, a definitive diagnosis of herpes simplex virus encephalitis is possible when herpes simplex virus, type 1, is recovered from a brain biopsy. Isolations of Coxsackie virus B-5 from throat or feces in a case of acute myopericarditis are suggestive but insufficient to relate the disease in question to the recovered agent. Isolation of virus from the blood or cerebrospinal fluid offers a greater probability of an etiologic association. A fourfold rise in specific antibodies in convalescent serum is also suggestive but, likewise, insufficient for definitive diagnosis. The finding of antibodies in tissues or fluids at the site of disease is a rapid means of stronger association. Antibodies are synthesized in B lymphocytes of inflammatory exudates in the brain. Spinal fluids from patients with subacute sclerosing panencephalitis or herpes simplex virus encephalitis often contain inordinate titers of measles or herpes simplex virus antibodies, respectively, indicating that these immunoglobulins are locally produced.

When diagnosis is required, acute specimens are obtained by swabbing the nasopharynx, throat, conjunctiva, or cervix. Urine, feces, respiratory secretions, vesicular fluids, blood, buffy coat, and cerebrospinal fluid may be collected. Swabs are transferred to the laboratory in balanced salt solution containing antibiotics to inhibit bacteria. Optimally, specimens are inoculated promptly into tissue cultures for incubation at 35°C. Recognition of virus particles by electron microscopy or of antigens by fluorescence microscopy by using specific antiserums allows immediate presumptive diagnosis. Sometimes specimens may be held for 24 to 48 h prior to processing (echo viruses), but this is hazardous with many respiratory or herpesviruses. Concomitant use of human foreskin and rhesus kidney tissue cultures offers a broad spectrum for the isolation of viruses. Cell cultures must be observed for cytopathic effects daily for a minimum of 14 days. In other cases, inoculations into suckling mice (Coxsackie viruses, group A) or special techniques such as use of embryonated eggs (influenza), organ cultures (coronaviruses), or cultivation of whole infected cells (co-cultivation) are required.

In contrast to most antibodies, complement-requiring neutralizing antibodies peak early, and fall during convalescence. Current antibody responses may be noted in single acute-phase serums by finding complement-requiring or 2-mercaptoethanol-sensitive (IgM) specific immunoglobulins. Types of antibodies usually measured have been discussed above.

PROPHYLAXIS AND THERAPY Vaccine prophylaxis with live or inactivated vaccines is available for poliomyelitis, measles, smallpox, mumps, rubella, influenza, rabies, and yellow fever. Under special circumstances inactivated vaccines against adenovirus and Japanese B, equine, and Russian spring-summer encephalitis are available. Vaccinia immune globulin (VIG) is effective in reducing the risk of smallpox in exposed susceptibles: VIG is also indicated when a person at increased risk of generalized vaccinia is given smallpox vaccine. Persons at increased risk of generalized vaccinia are those with eczema, burns, neurodermatitis, pyoderma, immunologic defects, white blood cell defects, malignancy, neurologic disease, and undiagnosed febrile illness. Hyperimmune rabies antiserum is used prophylactically in bites about the face or shoulders by animals suspected of being rabid.

Chemoprophylaxis against smallpox with oral N-methylisatin β-thiosemicarbazone (Marboran) is effective. Amantadine hydrochloride (Symmetrel) taken by mouth throughout the period of exposure to influenza A is prophylactic. Amantadine is not effective against strains of influenza B. Topical idoxuridine (5-iodo-2′-deoxyuridine), cytosine arabinoside (ara-C), and adenine arabinoside (ara-A) are therapeutic in herpes simplex virus keratitis. Intravenous ara-A is useful also in the therapy of deep stromal herpetic keratitis. Ara-C is markedly immunosuppressive and is not helpful in the therapy of disseminated herpes zoster. Ara-A is now being tested in controlled trials against disseminated herpes zoster and other herpesvirus infections, particularly in immunosuppressed patients. The potential of adenine arabinoside in the treatment of herpes simplex virus, type 1, encephalitis, and disseminated infections of the newborn with herpes simplex virus, type 2, cytomegalovirus, and varicella-zoster virus is promising, but its exact role is not yet clear. Parenteral idoxuridine and ara-C are no longer used for herpesvirus infections because of their limited therapeutic potential and marked hematopoietic toxicity. Uncontrolled results with ara-A are most hopeful in cutaneous herpes simplex virus, type 1, and disseminated varicella-zoster infections. Results with ara-A are not as encouraging in herpes simplex virus, type 2, cytomegalovirus, or variola virus infections. Topical human interferon and interferon inducers have been successfully used in the treatment of rhinovirus infections, but these procedures remain experimental. Certain photodynamic dyes (proflavine, neutral red) have been tested in recurrent cutaneous herpes simplex virus disease; but an

oncogenic potential has been demonstrated, and they are not recommended. Corticosteroids suppress both T and B cells as well as chemotaxis, and should not be given during active virus multiplication.

REFERENCES

CARTER WA (ed): *Selective Inhibitors of Viral Functions,* Cleveland: CRC Press, 1973

DAVIS BD et al: *Microbiology,* 2d ed., New York: Harper & Row, 1973

HORSFALL FL JR, TAMM I: *Viral and Rickettsial Infections of Man,* 4th ed., Philadelphia: Lippincott, 1965

HOSKINS JM: *Virological Procedures,* New York: Appleton-Century-Crofts, 1967

JAWETZ E et al: *Review of Medical Microbiology,* 11th ed., Los Altos, Calif.: Lange, 1974

LAWRENCE HS: Transfer factor in cellular immunity. Harvey Lect, ser 68, pp. 239–300

LERNER AM et al: Serologic responses to herpes simplex virus in rabbits: Complement-requiring neutralizing, conventional neutralizing, and passive hemagglutinating antibodies. J Infect Dis 129(6):623, 1974

——: Enteroviruses and the heart (with special emphasis on the probable role of coxsackieviruses, group B, types 1-5). I. Epidemiological and experimental studies; II. Observations in humans. Mod Concepts Cardiovasc Dis 44(2):7, 1975; 44(3):11, 1975

RAGER-ZISMAN B, ALLISON AC: Effects of immunosuppression on coxsackievirus B-3 in mice, and passive protection by circulating antibody. J Gen Virol 19:339, 1973

STEVENS DA, MERIGAN TC: Interferon, antibody and other host factors in herpes zoster. J Clin Invest 51:1170, 1972

193 ENTERIC VIRUSES:
Coxsackie Viruses, Echo Viruses, Reoviruses

A. MARTIN LERNER

General considerations It has been over 25 years since Dalldorf and Sickles isolated the first Coxsackie viruses by inoculating suspensions of feces from two children with signs of clinical paralytic poliomyelitis into suckling mice. Subsequently, some 67 enteroviruses, including poliovirus and Coxsackie and echo viruses (Table 193-1) have been shown to multiply at various times in the gastrointestinal tracts of human beings. Enteroviruses have been recovered wherever attempts have been made; their distribution appears global. With notable exceptions such as Coxsackie virus, type A-21, and echo virus 28, which are predominantly respiratory pathogens and are only incidentally isolated from feces, enteroviruses like *Salmonella* periodically multiply within the human alimentary canal and sometimes concomitantly produce disease. Available information suggests that there is no normal enteric virus flora. In

TABLE 193-1
Classification of enteroviruses

I Picornaviruses of human origin
- *A* Enteroviruses
  - *1* Polioviruses (3 types)*
  - *2* Coxsackie virus A (24 types)
  - *3* Coxsackie virus B (6 types)
  - *4* Echoviruses (34 types)†
- *B* Rhinoviruses (see Chap. 195)
- *C* Unclassified

II Picornaviruses of lower animals

* *Typing is by neutralization of infectivity with immune serums either in suitable tissue cultures or in suckling mice.*
† *Echo virus, type 10, has been reclassified as belonging to another taxonomic group, now known as reoviruses.*

addition to enteroviruses, adenoviruses (Chap. 195) and reoviruses are commonly recovered from stools.

Coxsackie viruses are named for their site of origin, the village of Coxsackie on the banks of the Hudson River in the state of New York. Echo viruses were descriptively named: *E,* for their *enteric* residence; *C,* the filtrable agents produced *cytopathic* effects in tissue cultures of rhesus kidney; *H, human; O, orphan,* indicating that their relationship to disease remained to be established. They were viruses "in search of a disease." It is increasingly evident that a wide but definite variety of illnesses may result from enterovirus infections. As observations accumulate, these illnesses (Table 193-2) are continually being defined.

Etiologic associations are difficult to establish and usually require virologic, serologic, epidemiologic, and, when ethically possible, volunteer studies. These are especially useful if viruses are isolated from sites other than the pharynx or anus, where they often multiply without causing significant injury to tissues. More meaningful are isolations from blood, vesicular fluids of patients with rashes, urine, cerebrospinal fluid, or from tissues at biopsy or autopsy. Coxsackie or echo viruses have been recovered from lung, heart, pericardial fluid, liver, spleen, testicle, kidney, muscle, and brain. Dual virus infections and possible bacterial-virus synergisms are being defined. Until enteroviruses had been repeatedly documented in infants by isolations from pneumonic lungs, prevalent opinion was that they did not produce pneumonias. The same skepticism must remain concerning etiologic associations of enterovirus infections and chronic myocardiopathies, nonrheumatic valvular deformities, subendocardial fibroelastosis, and other congenital malformations.

Characteristics of the viruses The enterovirus group (Coxsackie viruses A and B, echo viruses, polioviruses) are icosahedral-shaped, with a particle diameter of 17 to 30 nm and a ribonucleic acid core surrounded by a capsid of pro-

TABLE 193-2
Illnesses (or syndromes) associated with Coxsackie or echo virus infections

	Coxsackie virus types		
	Group A	*Group B*	*Echo virus types*
I No illness (probably 75% of cases)	1–24	1–6	1–8,* 11–34
II Mild or moderate illness			
A Undifferentiated mild febrile illness (nonspecific)	1–24	1–6	1–8, 11–34
B Upper respiratory syndromes (rhinitis, pharyngitis, including herpangina and lymphonodular pharyngitis, conjunctivitis)	1–10, 16, 21, 22, 24†	1–5	1, 3, 6, 9, 16, 19, 20, 28
C Laryngotracheitis	9	5	11
D Exanthems (various)	5, 9, 16	3, 5	2, 4, 5, 9, 11, 16
E Lymphadenitis, with or without splenomegaly	5, 6, 9	5	4, 9, 16, 20
F Pleurodynia (sometimes with pleural effusion)	4, 6, 10	1–5	1, 6, 9
G Orchitis		1–5	9
H Gastroenteritis	9	3, 4	2, 3, 6–9, 11–14, 18, 19, 22–24
I Chronic myopathy			
III Severe or life-threatening illness			
A Hepatitis	4, 9	5	4, 9
B Hemolytic-uremic syndrome	4	4	
C Pneumonia	9	1, 4	3, 8, 9, 19, 20
D Diabetes mellitus‡		4	
E Cardiac			
1 Myocarditis/pericarditis	1, 2, 4, 5, 8, 9, 16	1–5	1, 4, 6, 8, 9, 14, 19, 22, 25, 30
2 Chronic myocardiopathy		2, 4, 5	
3 Subendocardial fibroelastosis‡		3	
4 Endocardial deformities		4	
5 Constrictive pericarditis		1, 2	
6 Congenital malformations‡	9	3, 4	
F Neurologic			
1 Aseptic meningitis/encephalitis including variants (b-f)	7, 9, 16	1–5	1–9, 11–23, 25, 30–32
2 Acute cerebellar ataxia	3, 4		
3 Benign intracranial hypertension			
4 Transverse myelitis			
5 Postencephalitic parkinsonism			
6 Guillain-Barré syndrome‡			

* *Asymptomatic infection is common with echo virus, type 9. Variation in attack rates among types (and strains of a single type) occurs.*
† *Coxsackie virus A, type 21, is also known as Coe virus.*
‡ *Suggested (and probable), but cause not established.*

tein. Enteroviruses share about 20 percent of their nucleotide sequences, while within a grouping such as Coxsackie virus B, there is 30 to 50 percent homology among types. The subunit structure of the outer protein capsid (capsomere) determines species, tissue, and age specificities for infection, as well as antigenicity. The RNA of the virus within infected cells transcribes and translates its own genetic information independent of the DNA (deoxyribonucleic acid) of the host. Enteroviruses are quite stable in acid and lipid solvents. They can be protected from thermal inactivation by certain cations.

When inoculated into suckling mice, group A Coxsackie viruses induce primarily inflammation and necrosis of skeletal muscle, whereas group B viruses cause lesions of the central nervous system and other viscera, but only focal muscular involvement. Coxsackie viruses B and echo viruses are cytopathogenic for cultures of monkey kidney cells, but this is not the case for Coxsackie viruses of group A. These distinctions are not without exception. Some strains of echo viruses, types 6 and 9, have been adapted to produce lesions in baby mice, the former in viscera and the latter in skeletal muscles. Some strains agglutinate human erythrocytes obtained from adults or umbilical cords at the time of delivery. None of the Coxsackie or echo viruses has been adapted to grow in embryonated eggs.

Epidemiology Fecal-oral contact is the usual method of transmission. Personal hygiene (particularly hand washing) inhibits the infectious cycle. Toddlers often bring enteroviruses into a household. Insects, including flies and mosquitoes, may act as passive vectors. Echo virus, type 6, may multiply in the gastrointestinal tracts of dogs. This has not been noted with other Coxsackie or echo viruses, and with echo virus 6 canine-to-human transmission has not been demonstrated. Respiratory transmission by droplets or their nuclei also occurs.

The incubation period is 2 to 5 days. Multiple concurrent infections within a family are not unusual. Clinical manifestations of infection vary within the family and community. Thus a two- to three-year-old child may have a mild fever with rash, while an older sibling may have pleurodynia, myocarditis, or one of a number of syndromes heralding involvement of the central nervous system (Table 193-2). The mechanism of the varied expression of enterovirus disease is not well understood but may relate to developmental changes in the number or availability of specific receptors on the surfaces of susceptible cells.

Enterovirus infections are most common during the summer. Prevalence is mirrored by virus isolations from samples of sewage. Serotypes present in a community vary from year to year. The level of immunity of a population as reflected by the prevalence of type-specific neutralizing antibodies in serums apparently determines the likelihood of infection by a particular enterovirus. In an individual usually one enterovirus multiplies within the intestine at any one time. Vaccination with attenuated polioviruses has virtually eliminated these interfering agents, and there may be a real increase in infections due to Coxsackie or echo viruses. Improved hygiene and urbanization have led to an "epidemiologic shift" from infants to adults. On the basis of intrahousehold spread, infectivity of Coxsackie viruses is fairly high (76 percent of exposed susceptibles and 25 percent of immunes). For echo viruses, apparent infectivity is substantially lower (43 percent of susceptibles) and immune contacts are rarely infected. At least 49 percent of Coxsackie virus and 55 percent of echo virus infections are subclinical.

An interesting correlate has been a seasonal incidence of new cases of insulin-dependent diabetes mellitus in patients under thirty years old. This autumn peak has been correlated with an annual prevalence for Coxsackie virus B-4, but does not relate to other virus infections.

Virus isolation Primary multiplication occurs in epithelial and paraepithelial lympathic cells of the pharynx. During this early period of infection the patient may be asymptomatic or have mild malaise, sore throat, or low-grade fever. Slightly later virus multiplies in the intestines. If a critical virus concentration within the pharynx results, viremia follows. During the viremic phase the patient is asymptomatic. Secondary foci of virus multiplication may occur in various tissues (skin, muscle, heart, nervous system, etc.). Major illness of moderate to serious severity sometimes results (Table 193-2). Occasionally (especially during infancy) aspiration of pharyngeal virus leads to lower respiratory infection.

Virus may be isolated from the throat during the minor illness and for as long as a week thereafter. Virus shedding persists in feces for a longer interval. Viremia can be documented during the incubation period until type-specific neutralizing antibodies appear.

Protective responses and serologic diagnosis Intracellular virus multiplication stimulates interferon production within the infected cell (Chap. 192). About 3 days after the onset of infection specific antibodies appear in saliva and serum. These immunoglobulins combine with extracellular virus to limit spead of virus. Virus-antibody complexes are eliminated by phagocytosis.

Secretory immunoglobulins in saliva and succus entericus are in the IgA class, while the earliest antibodies to appear in serum are IgM. Both species of macromolecules have complement-fixing and neutralizing qualities. Within 3 to 4 weeks complement-fixing antibodies reach their peak and decline. Neutralizing antibodies of higher avidity (IgG) replace the IgM molecule about 2 weeks after the onset of infection. IgG antibodies persist and provide permanent type-specific immunity.

This information is important in diagnosis, because IgM molecules are susceptible to reduction and resultant biologic inactivation with sulfhydryl active compounds such as 2-mercaptoethanol (2-ME). IgG immunoglobulins are resistant to 2-ME.

IgG antibodies to Coxsackie and echo viruses traverse the placenta freely. IgM immunoglobulins do not. IgA antibodies in colostrum and milk are not absorbed, but apparently provide some local protection in the intestines of nursing babies. Passively acquired antibodies in serums protect the newborn from viremia for 3 to 6 months. Since the half-life of IgG immunoglobulins is about 3 weeks, duration of firm neonatal immunity depends upon initial titers of the transferred antibodies. Passively acquired antibodies inhibit active synthesis of immunoglobulins, and also may not protect the respiratory tract. Active synthesis of secretory antibody in saliva and nasal secretions is required. The role of cellular immunity in enterovirus infections remains to be fully defined. However, in Coxsackie virus B-3 murine cardiomyopathy, antibodies inhibit virus replication. Cytotoxic T lymphocytes augment the pathologic changes.

A fourfold rise in neutralizing antibodies or a titer which is similarly diminished by 2-ME indicates recent infection. When applicable, hemagglutination inhibition tests are simpler, and the results parallel those obtained in more cumbersome neutralization tests. Complement-fixing antibodies to enteroviruses are not type-specific. Many cross reactions render these tests less useful.

The neutralizing antibody response is highly type-specific in primary or initial enterovirus infections. In subsequent infections heterotypic responses occur with increasing frequency; they presumably arise from a booster effect of the current infecting virus on the level of antibodies to other types with which the individual has previously been infected. Levels of heterotypic antibody frequently exceed the level of homotypic antibody. Neutralizing antibodies to group B Coxsackie virus, types 1 to 5, are frequently found in titers of 1/64 to 1/512 in patients without evidence of current Coxsackie virus infections.

Other laboratory findings Enterovirus infections are usually acute processes, and persistent or chronic infections are unusual [e.g., chronic myopathy (Coxsackie virus A-9) or chronic myocardiopathy (Coxsackie virus B-3)]. Hence, changes in concentrations of hemoglobin, albumin, or globulins are unusual. Occasionally hemolysis occurs (see Group A Coxsackie Virus Infections and Echo Virus Infections, further on in this chapter). White blood cell counts and the erythrocyte sedimentation rates are only mildly elevated. If there is necrosis (e.g., liver, lung), a neutrophilic leukemoid reaction may be noted. Hyperbilirubinemia, elevated transaminase and alkaline phosphatase levels, and delayed excretion of Bromsulphalein may be seen in cases of hepatitis. Albuminuria often occurs transiently, but hematuria is rare.

Treatment and prophylaxis Antiviral chemotherapy is not available. The 64 antigenic varieties of Coxsackie and echo viruses make prophylaxis by a single vaccine impractical. Pooled human gamma-globulin contains enterovirus antibodies, but during serious infections administration is not helpful. Most human enterovirus infections are mild, and gamma-globulin prophylaxis is not often warranted. As with poliomyelitis, tonsillectomy and other inoculations are probably best delayed during an outbreak of enterovirus disease. In a murine model of Coxsackie virus B-3 myocarditis, virus was isolated in higher titer from hearts of mice vigorously exercised daily by swimming, and a benign myocarditis was transformed into a lethal infection. Rest is the cornerstone of symptomatic therapy.

It has been repeatedly shown in experimental animals that during the acute phase of infection administration of steroids appreciably increases the quantity of virus in tissues and the degree of ensuing injury. Corticosteroids also depress cell-mediated immune functions, interferon and antibody synthesis, and leukocyte migration to the area of injury. Therefore, at least during the acute phase of enterovirus infections, steroids are contraindicated. Pregnancy may be associated with enhanced susceptibility to these and other infections. Alcohol, cold temperature, and chronic undernutrition are also associated with an increased virulence of Coxsackie virus and perhaps other virus infections. Alcohol depresses phagocytic function. Malnutrition suppresses T and B lymphocytes, early mononuclear cell migration, and interferon.

GROUP A COXSACKIE VIRUS INFECTIONS Group A Coxsackie viruses cause herpangina, lymphonodular pharyngitis, upper and lower respiratory disease, cutaneous eruptions, hepatitis, aseptic meningitis, paralytic disease, myopericarditis, and some sudden unexpected deaths in infancy. A chronic myopathy in an eleven-year-old girl has been associated with Coxsackie virus A-9. Picornavirus-like particles were seen at electron microscopy, and virus was isolated from the diaphragm at autopsy. Diarrheas are also probably caused by Coxsackie virus A infections. Pharyngeal multiplication may induce infection of superficial vessels or diffuse moderate erythema. Purulent exudate is not seen. More characteristic is *herpangina,* a common febrile illness characterized by small papular, vesicular, or ulcerative lesions on the anterior pillars, soft palate, tonsils, pharyngeal mucous membrane, and posterior part of the buccal mucosa. Herpangina has been seen during infections with Coxsackie viruses, group A, types 1 to 10, 16, and 22. Vesicular lesions of herpangina have also been described in patients with illnesses due to Coxsackie viruses, group B, types 1 to 5, and echo viruses, types 9 and 17. Coxsackie virus A-10 may induce *acute lymphonodular pharyngitis.* Lesions here are raised, discrete, white to yellow 3- to 6-mm papules surrounded by a zone of erythema. All the papules appear at the same time; they do not ulcerate, and they occur on the uvula, anterior pillars, and posterior pharynx.

Coxsackie virus A-21 (Coe virus) is predominantly a respiratory pathogen, being regularly isolated from the throat and occasionally from feces. It has been associated with several outbreaks of an illness resembling the common cold in military recruits.

The first enterovirus etiologically implicated in pneumonia was Coxsackie virus A-9. Subsequently, a number of other enteroviruses have been implicated (Table 193-2). Fatal cases have occurred in infants or young children. Hyperpnea, cyanosis, hyperpyrexia, leukocytosis (or leukemoid reactions), and subsequently coma have been characteristic. Interstitial diffuse polylobed bronchopneumonia with alternate areas of atelectasis and emphysema have been found. Microscopically mixed alveolar septal infiltration without necrosis or formation of giant cells is seen.

A striking cutaneous vesicular eruption, *hand-foot-and-mouth disease* (Chap. 207), has repeatedly been associated with infections due to Coxsackie virus, group A, type 16. Infants and children with Coxsackie virus, group A, type 4 (also Coxsackie virus B-4) infections have been described with respiratory or gastrointestinal symptoms, acute renal disease, thrombocytopenia, and hemolytic anemia. Reticulocytosis, albuminuria, and hematuria accompany this constellation of findings, which has been described as the *hemolytic-uremic syndrome.* Aseptic meningitis with occasional paralytic disease (especially with A-7) also occurs. Acute myopericarditis has been associated with infections with Coxsackie virus A, types 1, 2, 5, 8, and 9; there are firmer etiologic data for Coxsackie virus, types 4 and 16. One estimate suggests that 23 percent of acute virus cardiomyopathies may be caused by Coxsackie virus A. A significantly greater incidence of infection with Coxsackie virus, group A, type 9, has been reported in mothers of infants with congenital heart disease.

GROUP B COXSACKIE VIRUS INFECTIONS Infections with group B Coxsackie viruses cause a number of upper respiratory syndromes, exanthems, diarrheas, pleurodynia, orchitis (with subsequent atrophy), pneumonia, hemolytic-uremic syndrome, and cardiac and central nervous system disease. Pleurodynia and cardiac disease due to enteroviruses were first associated with this group of enteroviruses (Table 193-2). In 1965 the Public Health Service (Britain) reported 1,160 Coxsackie virus B-5 infections. Gastroenteritis (90 percent), aseptic meningitis (31 percent), myalgia and Bornholm's disease (23 percent), respiratory disorders (15 percent), and cardiomyopathies (5 percent) were included. There were 41 patients with pericarditis and 5 with myocarditis. Of 6 deaths, 2 each were due to neurologic, respiratory, or cardiac cause. During infancy, the mortality rate of patients with acute infectious myocarditis approaches 50 percent.

Pleurodynia (epidemic myalgia, Bornholm's disease, devil's grip) Prodromal symptoms of malaise, sore throat, and anorexia are interrupted by increasing debility, fever, and sudden onset of muscle, pleuritic, and abdominal pain. Pain is sharp, severe, and paroxysmal over the lower ribs or substernal area. It is accentuated by moving, breathing, coughing, sneezing, and hiccuping, and may be referred to the shoulders, neck, or scapulae. Pain and spasm of anterior abdominal muscles occur in about half the cases, often in combination with chest pain. Muscle tenderness is usually not prominent, but some patients complain of intense cutaneous hyperesthesia and paresthesia over the affected area. The illness usually lasts 3 to 7 days, but relapses may occur. Among differential diagnoses are myocardial infarction and acute surgical conditions of the abdomen. Coxsackie viruses B have been isolated from striated muscle of patients with pleurodynia during epidemics. Occasionally pleuritis is accompanied by effusion, and virus has been isolated from pleural fluid. Bornholm's disease may occur at any age, but is most common in children and young adults.

Early in the course of illness meningitis, myocarditis, or hepatitis may ensue. Liver biopsy in patients with complicating jaundice shows subacute portal triaditis and intense cloudy swelling of central-zone hepatocytes. A late complication is orchitis, occurring in 3 to 5 percent of patients with pleurodynia during relapse.

Cardiac disease Acute myocarditis may be caused by Coxsackie viruses of groups A and B as well as echo viruses. Infections with strains of Coxsackie virus, group B, have been most frequent. When congenital or neonatal infection occurs, the course is often rapidly fatal, with concomitant myocarditis, encephalitis, hepatitis, and sometimes adrenal necrosis. Later in childhood or in adult life the heart and pericardium more frequently are involved as the single site of disease. Cardiac inflammation varies in intensity and degree of muscle necrosis. Pericarditis may dominate the clinical presentation, with myalgia, fever, precordial pain, friction rub, and even cardiac tamponade. There may be prominent signs of myocarditis, with myocardial failure or arrhythmias. Illnesses may be self-limited and recovery complete. However, of 22 episodes of acute virus cardiomyopathies associated with infections due to Coxsackie viruses, group B, 12 patients developed chronic heart disease. Strict bed rest until all electrocardiographic changes have reverted to normal (or are stationary) is indicated. This may require 4 to 6 weeks. Since steroids increase virulence of Coxsackie B myocarditis in mice, they are contraindicated. Some infections may heal with significant myocardial scarring.

Coxsackie virus particles have been localized along tubules of the sarcoplasmic reticulum in infected mice with myocarditis, and Coxsackie virus B-4 has been shown to cause experimental murine valvulitis and mural endocarditis. These findings may prove to be pertinent to humans. Of 40 hearts from autopsies of patients dying before age thirty, 17 were positive by fluorescent antibody staining for Coxsackie virus antigen in the myocardium. Chronic focal interstitial myocarditis was present in each of the positive cases, and viral antigens were found in both the myocardium and mitral valve in three cases. Similarly, there is epidemiologic evidence associating Coxsackie virus B, types 3 and 4, with congenital heart disease. Most infections in pregnant mothers are subclinical and occur in the first trimester. There are other data associating group B Coxsackie viruses with congenital subendocardial fibroelastosis. These findings need confirmation, particularly because a similar study failed to demonstrate an association of echo virus, type 9, infection and congenital malformations. After experimental Coxsackie virus B infections in mice and monkeys, Aschoff bodies and Anitschkow myocytes, as well as valvular deformities, are seen. At this time strong or suggestive evidence indicates that the following conditions may be caused by infections with Coxsackie viruses belonging to group B: chronic continuing cardiomyopathies (B-2, B-4, B-5); congenital calcific pancarditis (B-3); aortic/mitral valvular incompetence (B-4); and constrictive pericarditis (B-1, B-2), with or without superior or inferior vena caval obstruction.

ECHO VIRUS INFECTIONS Echo virus infections may be asymptomatic or mild, moderate, or life-threatening (Table 193-2). Mild to moderate are undifferentiated fevers, upper respiratory infections, various rashes (Chap. 203), pleurodynia, and diarrheas. Pneumonia, myopericarditis, hemolytic-uremic syndromes, and neurologic involvement may be quite serious. They do not differ from similar illnesses caused by Coxsackie viruses.

Viral gastroenteritis Sporadic endemic cases of nonbacterial diarrheas, as well as acute outbreaks in summer or winter, occur. The latter have been termed *winter vomiting diseases* or *intestinal flu.* The majority of cases apparently do not result from enterovirus infection, but are due to a reovirus-like agent (Norwalk) in the stool. Gastrointestinal symptoms are not caused by influenza virus. Diarrhea may occur as a minor manifestation of enterovirus disease during a summer outbreak, but this is not usually the case. In individuals and in epidemiologically controlled series Coxsackie virus, types B-3 and B-4, as well as echo viruses, types 1, 3, 6 to 9, 11 to 14, 18, 19, and 22 to 24, have been implicated etiologically as a cause of gastroenteritis, as has oral attenuated poliovirus vaccine.

Attacks of vomiting and diarrhea occurring in winter outbreaks due to echo viruses are brief but debilitating illnesses. Malaise and several watery stools herald their onset. Fever is not invariably present. Typically, within 24 h repeated vomiting, retching, and chilliness ensue. Abdominal cramps and myalgia may occur. The disease is highly contagious, with multiple cases within a family at one time or following closely one upon another. Similar epidemic spread usually results in the surrounding community. Recovery from this acute but severe episode usually occurs within 48 h, but mild diarrhea and a malabsorption syndrome may persist for several weeks. During initial chilliness and cramping, echo viruses have been isolated from the blood, posterior pharyngeal wall, and rectal swabs. Shedding of virus is brief, and virus isolation is often unsuccessful by 36 h after onset. Reoviruses and adenoviruses have also been sporadically implicated in similar gastroenteritides. Leukocytes are not seen in smears of the watery feces as they are in *Shigella* or amebic infections.

Aseptic meningitis There may be a mild prodromal malaise, but major illness usually begins with fever, headache, and stiff neck. Papilledema and Kernig's and Brudzinski's signs may be present. Localizing sensory or motor deficits are unusual. Confusion and delirium are common. These acute findings may persist for 4 to 7 days. Cerebrospinal pleocytosis is usually less than 500 cells per mm^3. Early there may be as many as 90 percent polymorphonuclear leukocytes, but within 48 h the cellular response becomes completely mononuclear. Persistence of polymorphonuclear leukocytes in the cerebrospinal fluid suggests pyogenic meningitis or intracerebral, subdural, or epidural abscess. Gram stain and appropriate spinal fluid cultures must be done to exclude bacterial meningitis, tuberculosis, or mycotic meningitis. Protein concentration in the cerebrospinal fluid is moderately elevated, but glucose is normal. Early in the illness echo viruses may be isolated from spinal fluid. It usually takes several weeks before the cerebrospinal fluid reverts to normal.

For attempts at virus isolation, throat and rectal swabs, serum, and cerebrospinal fluid should be collected as early in the course as possible. Acute and convalescent serums should be studied for rises in type-specific neutralizing antibody.

It is not possible to distinguish clinically between aseptic meningitis due to various enteroviruses and mumps. Localizing findings, hemiplegia, prolonged fevers, oculogyric crises, coma, and bloody spinal fluid favor the diagnosis of herpes simplex virus encephalitis. Although echo virus aseptic meningitis most often is self-limited and recovery in persons afflicted after the first year of life complete, about 10 percent of patients have more serious involvement of the central nervous system. Minor muscle weakness with reflex changes may persist for weeks to months, but over 90 percent of patients recover completely within a year. Occasionally, choreiform movements, ataxia, nystagmus, transverse myelitis, Guillain-Barré syndrome, coma, bulbar involvement, and death result.

REOVIRUS INFECTIONS Reoviruses were discovered inadvertently in studies of the intestinal viral flora of healthy children and adults. They were initially classified as echo virus, type 10, but were later reclassified. They were named to emphasize their (1) *respiratory* or (2) *enteric* human origins, and their (3) *orphan* status.

Reoviruses are quite different from picornaviruses (Table 193-1). They are about 2½ times larger (70 nm in diameter) and show icosahedral symmetry. Their RNA is unique in that it consists of 10 discrete segments and is resistant to ribonuclease. The protein capsid consists of an inner core and 92 outer shell capsomeres. The capsid is composed of seven species of polypeptides. Unlike those of enteroviruses, reovirus cytopathic effects are nonlytic. Reoviruses multiply in primate and nonprimate tissue cultures. The particles hemagglutinate human or avian erythrocytes. On the basis of tests of hemagglutination inhibition antibodies (HIA) with type-specific serums, there are three serotypes.

Human infections with reoviruses are common, and their distribution is worldwide. Like Coxsackie and echo viruses, reoviruses spread by enteric and respiratory routes. Fifty to eighty percent of adults in the Western Hemisphere have had reovirus infections, as measured by the presence of persisting neutralizing or hemagglutinating antibodies. Infections are more frequent in winter but occur in every season. Reoviruses have been isolated from human nasal secretions, posterior pharyngeal and rectal swabs, spinal fluid, brain, and lung. They have been recovered from tissues of Burkitt's lymphoma. In addition, reovirus isolations or serologic data indicate that natural infections occur in cattle, dogs, cats, mice, horses, swine, birds, and monkeys. Although animal-to-human transmission has never been demonstrated, its possibility is likely.

Widespread evidence of infection and few associations with disease indicate that most infections with reoviruses are asymptomatic. Isolations of virus and fourfold rises in HIA in individual patients with common colds, nonspecific febrile illness, exanthem, and diarrhea suggest an etiologic role in some instances. Provocative data came from three thoroughly studied fatal cases of encephalitis, myocarditis, hepatitis, or interstitial pneumonias. In these patients reoviruses and no other bacterial or viral pathogens have been isolated.

A reovirus-like (Norwalk) particle has been visualized by electron microscopy in stool filtrates prepared from stools of persons with severe acute gastroenteritis. An antibody response in patients by the presumed agent(s) has been found by methods of immune electron microscopy and by complement fixation. The Norwalk agent is antigenically related to the epizootic diarrhea of infant mice and the Nebraska calf diarrhea virus. In volunteer studies, diarrhea was produced and biopsies of the small intestine showed an intact mucosa with blunted villi, shortening of the microvilli, and dilation of endoplasmic reticulum.

REFERENCES

General

GELFAND HM: Occurrence in nature of coxsackie and ECHO viruses. Prog Med Virol 3:193, 1961

HORSTMANN DM: Clinical virology. Am J Med 38:738, 1965
KIBRICK S: Current status of coxsackie and ECHO viruses in human disease. Prog Med Virol 6:27, 1964
KOGON A et al: The virus watch program: A continuing surveillance of viral infections in metropolitan New York families. VII. Observations on viral excretion, seroimmunity, intrafamilial spread and illness association in Coxsackie and echovirus infections. Am J Epidemiol 89:51, 1969
PHILIPSON L et al: Structural model for picornaviruses as suggested from an analysis of urea-degraded virions and procapsids of coxsackie virus B-3. Virology 54:69, 1973
WOODRUFF JF, WOODRUFF JJ: Involvement of T-lymphocytes in the pathogenesis of coxsackie virus B-3 heart disease. J Immunol 113:1726, 1974

Coxsackie A virus infection
HUEBNER RJ et al: Herpangina: Etiological studies of a specific infectious disease. JAMA 145:628, 1951
LERNER AM et al: Infections due to coxsackievirus, group A, type 9, in Boston, 1959, with special reference to exanthems and pneumonia. N Engl J Med 163:1265, 1960
TANG TT et al: Chronic myopathy associated with coxsackievirus A9. A combined electron microscopical and viral isolation study. N Engl J Med 292:608–611, 1975

Coxsackie B virus infection
BAIN HW et al: Epidemic pleurodynia (Bornholm's disease) due to coxsackie B 5 virus: The interrelationship of pleurodynia, benign pericarditis and aseptic meningitis. Pediatrics 27:889, 1961
BROWN GC, EVANS TN: Serologic evidence of coxsackievirus etiology of congenital heart disease. JAMA 199:151, 1967
BURCH GE et al: Coxsackie B viral myocarditis and valvulitis identified in routine autopsy specimens by immunofluorescent technique. Am Heart J 74:13, 1967
——, COLCOLOUGH HL: Progressive Coxsackie viral pancarditis and nephritis. Ann Intern Med 71:963, 1969
JOHNSON RT et al: Acute benign pericarditis: Virologic study of 34 patients. Arch Intern Med 108:828, 1961
KIBRICK S: Viral infections of the fetus and newborn. Perspect Virol Symp NY 2:140, 1961
LERNER AM, WILSON FM: Virus myocardiopathy. Prog Med Virol 15:63, 1973
SAINANI GS et al: Adult heart disease due to Coxsackievirus B infection. Medicine 47:133, 1968

Echo virus infection
BEHBEHANI AM, WENNER HA: Infantile diarrhea (a study of the etiologic role of viruses). Am J Dis Child 111:623, 1966
GOODWIN MH JR et al: Observations on the association of enteric viruses and bacteria with diarrhea. Am J Trop Med 16:178, 1967
HORSTMANN DM, YAMADA N: Enterovirus infections of the central nervous system. Res Publ Assoc Res Nerv Ment Dis 44:236, 1968

Reovirus infection
AGUS SG et al: Acute infectious nonbacterial gastroenteritis: intestinal histopathology. Histologic and enzymatic alterations during illness produced by the Norwalk agent in man. Ann Intern Med 79:18, 1973
EL-RAI FM, EVANS, AS: Reovirus infections in children and young adults. Arch Environ Health 7:700, 1963
JOKLIK WK: The molecular biology of reovirus. J Cell Physiol 76:289, 1970
KAPIKIAN AZ et al: Reoviruslike agent in stools: Association with infantile diarrhea and development of serologic tests. Science 185:1049, 1974
ROSEN L: Serologic grouping of reoviruses by hemagglutination-inhibition. Am J Hyg 77:29, 1963
—— et al: Reovirus infections in human volunteers. Am J Hyg 77:29, 1963
TILLOTSON JR, LERNER AM: Reovirus, type 3, associated with fatal pneumonia. N Engl J Med 276:1060, 1967

194
GENERAL CONSIDERATIONS OF VIRAL RESPIRATORY DISEASES

VERNON KNIGHT

The viral respiratory diseases as a group are responsible for one-half or more of all acute illnesses, and although influenza virus is the only agent among them which causes significant mortality in adults, several different viruses contribute to the 20 percent of childhood mortality due to respiratory disease. Respiratory disease morbidity, due primarily to virus infections, causes 30 to 50 percent of time lost from work by adults, and from 60 to 80 percent of time lost by children from school. These diseases are worldwide, and although studies in many areas are scanty, reports from Great Britain, Western Europe, U.S.S.R., Czechoslovakia, Latin America, and the Orient indicate many common denominators in cause, prevalence, and severity.

Viral respiratory diseases are associated with a spectrum of host responses ranging from asymptomatic carrier states to severe and sometimes fatal pneumonias. There is a recurring pattern of severe illness in infants and young children and of milder disease with increasing age. A few clinical and epidemiologic entities can be recognized without laboratory aids, such as acute respiratory disease (ARD) in military recruits, caused by adenovirus type 4 and rhinovirus coryza in adults. The causative agent in a large proportion of cases, however, cannot be identified with virologic study.

EPIDEMIOLOGY IN THE UNITED STATES More than 150 serotypes, representing 12 groups of viruses, have been or may be associated with the majority of acute respiratory illness in human beings. With the capacity to isolate this large group of agents and with the recognition of the role of *Mycoplasma pneumoniae* (Chap. 188) it is possible to define the cause of many respiratory illnesses. The recent identification of coronaviruses as a cause of respiratory illness increases the potential for diagnosis. Though some of the inability to identify agents is caused by lack of efficient application of known diagnostic methods, it is probable that additional viral and possibly other causes of respiratory illness remain to be discovered.

FREQUENCY AND SEVERITY Since 1957 the National Health Survey has made annual estimates from selected population samples of the incidence of acute respiratory illness in the United States. Since these estimates are designed to measure the socioeconomic impact of illness, cases are reported only if they caused restriction of daily activity or required medical care. There were 259 million cases of acute respiratory illness in the United States between July 1, 1961, and June 30, 1962, an average of 1.4

TABLE 194-1
Patterns of illness with respiratory viruses in older children and adults

Agent	*Relative frequency of occurrence*	*Rhinitis*	*Pharyngitis*	*Tracheobronchitis*	*Pneumonia*	*Constitutional*
Rhinoviruses	40	++	±	+	Rare	± (usually afebrile)
Influenza, A, B	10	+	+	++	Severe when present	++ (high fever common)
Parainfluenza viruses	8	+	++	++*	Rare	+ (low or no fever)
Respiratory syncytial virus	6	++	+	+†	?	+ (usually afebrile)
Adenoviruses	2	+	++	++	Severe, when present	++ (high fever)
Coxsackie and echo viruses	<1	±	+	+	?	++ (fever, visceral and CNS complications)
Coronaviruses	8	+	+	+	?	+
Herpesviruses	10	+	+	Rare	Rare	+
Other	13	?	?	?	?	?

Note: ++ = severe; + = moderately severe; ± = mild; ? = unknown or uncommon.
* *Laryngeal involvement common.*
† *Especially in older patients.*

TABLE 194-2
Classification of human respiratory viruses

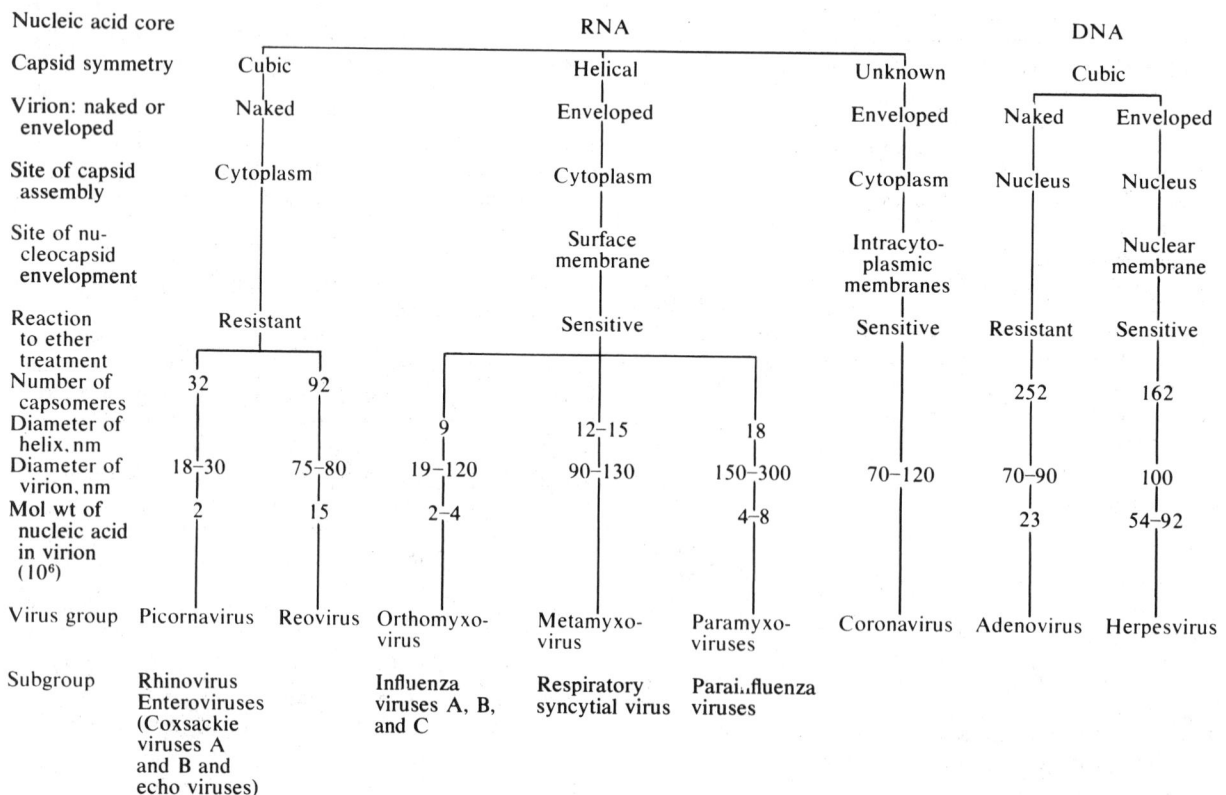

Nucleic acid core	RNA	RNA	RNA	RNA	RNA	RNA	DNA	DNA
Capsid symmetry	Cubic	Cubic	Helical	Helical	Helical	Unknown	Cubic	Cubic
Virion: naked or enveloped	Naked	Naked	Enveloped	Enveloped	Enveloped	Enveloped	Naked	Enveloped
Site of capsid assembly	Cytoplasm	Cytoplasm	Cytoplasm	Cytoplasm	Cytoplasm	Cytoplasm	Nucleus	Nucleus
Site of nucleocapsid envelopment			Surface membrane	Surface membrane	Surface membrane	Intracytoplasmic membranes		Nuclear membrane
Reaction to ether treatment	Resistant	Resistant	Sensitive	Sensitive	Sensitive	Sensitive	Resistant	Sensitive
Number of capsomeres	32	92					252	162
Diameter of helix, nm			9	12–15	18			
Diameter of virion, nm	18–30	75–80	19–120	90–130	150–300	70–120	70–90	100
Mol wt of nucleic acid in virion (10^6)	2	15	2–4		4–8		23	54–92
Virus group	Picornavirus	Reovirus	Orthomyxovirus	Metamyxovirus	Paramyxoviruses	Coronavirus	Adenovirus	Herpesvirus
Subgroup	Rhinovirus Enteroviruses (Coxsackie viruses A and B and echo viruses)		Influenza viruses A, B, and C	Respiratory syncytial virus	Parainfluenza viruses			

SOURCE: *Condensed from J. L. Melnick, Classification and nomenclature of viruses, 1972, vol. 14 in* Progress in Medical Virology, *Basel: Karger, 1972, p. 327.*

illnesses per person per year. Loss of time from work or school averaged 4.2 days for the 80 percent (207 million) of cases in which some restriction of activity was reported, and about 50 percent (or 130 million persons) sought medical attention. A similar incidence has been noted in every year of the survey. Analysis of these data indicates that two-thirds to three-fourths of the cases are caused by viruses; the remaining are divided principally among infections with *M. pneumoniae,* streptococcal sore throat, bacterial pneumonia, and sinusitis.

In other studies, milder illness has been included, with a corresponding rise in annual frequency of reported cases. The Cleveland Family Study found an annual rate of illness of 6.2 per person per year, amounting to an estimated more than 1 billion cases annually in the United States. The greatest proportion of these illnesses were so mild that they constituted no hazard to health, but they are significant in the spread of infection. In addition, it is known that wholly asymptomatic virus infections occur.

Age, sex, and seasonal variation Infants and young children have the greatest number of viral respiratory infections; children under six may have twice as many illnesses per year as the average for the entire population. Females have more illness than males. This difference is most marked in adults, where the excess is 25 percent. In children respiratory viral infections appear to affect the sexes about equally, but boys have more lower respiratory tract disease with respiratory syncytial virus infection than girls.

There are prominent seasonal differences in the frequency of acute respiratory illnesses; the rates are highest in winter, with about 30 cases per 100 persons per quarter. Illness is least frequent during the summer—about one-third of the maximum. Epidemics of influenza cause pronounced increases in wintertime frequency of respiratory illness and are the most significant cause of mortality among the respiratory viruses. In pandemic years influenza may begin in summer or fall.

Etiology The known viral causes of acute respiratory disease and their estimated relative frequency in adults and older children in relation to their common patterns of illness are shown in Table 194-1.

Viruses, as a group, cause about three-fourths of acute respiratory illness, and nearly one-half of these illnesses are due to one of the rhinoviruses. The principal nonviral causes of respiratory illness are *M. pneumoniae* and hemolytic streptococci.

Table 194-2 shows a current classification of the respiratory viruses based on size, structure, and biochemical and other properties. Adenoviruses and herpesvirus are DNA viruses, while the remainder possess RNA cores. Respiratory tract disease is not known to be associated with particular properties of the viruses except that the long incubation period of adenovirus infection may be related to its longer cycle of replication. The relatively nonspecific response of the respiratory tract to virus infection probably indicates that the target cells of the respiratory tract (i.e., the respiratory epithelium), when damaged by infection, have a limited variability of pathologic response. Classification of viruses will certainly assume greater importance, however, as new chemotherapeutic agents are developed, since many of them will act on specialized viral functions unique to single or related groups of viruses.

Clinical syndromes of viral respiratory disease including the common cold The descriptive term "common cold" was coined to describe the coryzal syndrome before its diverse causes were known. It refers to illness characterized by nasal obstruction and discharge, sneezing, moderate sore throat, and mild constitutional reaction, usually without fever. Patterns of illness shown in Table 194-1 demonstrate that most respiratory viral infections may produce this picture. However, in adults and older children, syndromes more or less restricted to these manifestations are caused by infection with rhinoviruses, respiratory syncytial virus, and coronaviruses. These three groups of viruses may account for as much as two-thirds of cases of acute respiratory viral disease. The other agents listed, while causing coryzal syndrome, also cause varying degrees of involvement of the lower part of the respiratory tract, with additional symptoms.

The following chapter (Chap. 195) considers five of the seven groups of viruses chiefly responsible for respiratory disease, i.e., rhinoviruses, adenoviruses, respiratory syncytial viruses, parainfluenza viruses, and coronaviruses. Included also is a description of the small contribution to respiratory illness of the enteroviruses, Coxsackie viruses A and B, and echo viruses, which are discussed in detail in Chap. 193. Influenza is described in Chap. 196. Respiratory diseases caused by *M. pneumoniae* and the psittacosis agent, both of which resemble viral respiratory diseases, are considered in Chaps. 188 and 191.

REFERENCE

KNIGHT V (ed): *Viral and Mycoplasmal Infections of the Respiratory Tract,* Philadelphia: Lea & Febiger, 1973

195 COMMON VIRAL RESPIRATORY ILLNESSES:

Rhinoviruses, Adenoviruses, Respiratory Syncytial Virus, Parainfluenza Viruses, Coxsackie Viruses, Echo Viruses, and Coronaviruses

VERNON KNIGHT

RHINOVIRUS INFECTIONS

ETIOLOGY More than 100 types of rhinovirus are known, and others are certain to be found. Some of the properties of rhinoviruses are shown in Table 194-2. They resemble the other picornaviruses in being small (15 to 30 nm), non-lipid-enveloped, relatively stable agents. Rhinoviruses can be distinguished from enteroviruses, the other subgroup of picornaviruses, by their loss of infectivity when exposed to an acid medium for 1 to 3 h.

EPIDEMIOLOGY Rhinovirus infection is the cause of approximately 40 percent of respiratory illness in children and adults. While it occurs throughout the year, there are peaks of high incidence in spring and fall. Infection with rhinoviruses, as with other respiratory viruses, is much more frequent in infants and children than was previously thought. Children may develop second episodes of rhinovirus infection and illness with different serotypes within a few weeks. The disease is also more severe in children, especially those under two years of age. In the young, fever, cough, croup, and occasionally pneumonia occur.

Family infections are most often initiated by children, and up to three-fourths of family outbreaks may be introduced by children of pre-school age; however, at all ages spread is much greater from ill than from well primary cases. Large families have more episodes of infection than small families. Family secondary attack rates are high at all ages, but highest in infants, of whom almost two-thirds of susceptibles may become infected. Infection occurs in about two-thirds or more of exposed persons without antibody, and about 60 percent of these develop illness. In persons with preexisting homotypic antibody, rates of infection and illness are about half that of those without antibody. However, studies in volunteers indicate that high titers of homotypic antibody are uniformly protective. Before 1970 a majority of infections were caused by lower-numbered serotypes; more recently the proportion of infections caused by higher-numbered (and also more recently identified) serotypes has increased. Virus is shed in a high percentage of patients from the day before to 6 days after onset of illness. In general, about one-half of individuals whose infection is associated with virus shedding develop a significant serologic response.

TABLE 195-1
Illness associated with rhinovirus infection

Diagnosis	*Adults (61)*	*Children (32)*	*Adult volunteers with naso-pharyngeal inoculation (31)*
	%	%	%
Common cold	58 (92)	14 (44)	26 (84)
Croup		1 (3)	
Bronchitis	1 (2)	7 (23)	2 (6)
Bronchiolitis		3 (9)	
Bronchopneumonia		3 (9)	
No disease	2 (3)	4 (12)	3 (10)

SOURCE: *Hamparian et al, Proc Soc Exp Biol Med 117:469, 1964; and Cate et al, J Clin Invest 43:56, 1964*

TABLE 195-2
Illness associated with adenovirus infection

		Order of association (serotypes)		*Respiratory tract involvement*			
Disease	*Occurrence*	*Common*	*Less common*	*Common cold*	*Pharyngitis*	*Bronchitis*	*Pneumonia*
Acute respiratory disease (ARD)	Epidemic in winter and spring in military recruits	4, 7	3, 14, 21	Often present	*Most frequent,* usually with fever, often with laryngitis	Frequent, usually with fever and laryngitis	Infrequent complication of ARD, but adenovirus pneumonia is an important type of pneumonia in recruits
Pharyngoconjunctival fever	Summer epidemics in civilians, often in school-age children, related to swimming pools. Sporadic cases of conjunctivitis may occur without pharyngitis	3, 7	4, 14	Often present	*Most frequent,* usually with fever and cervical lymphadenopathy, hoarseness	Uncommon	Rare
Febrile pharyngitis	Sporadic or epidemic, resembles ARD, often in children	3, 7	1, 2, 5	Often present	*Most frequent,* usually with fever	Frequent, especially in older children	Infrequent but severe complication
Pneumonia in children	Highly fatal illness in infants, sporadic or epidemic	3, 7		Sometimes present	Very frequent	Very frequent	Primary, with acidophilic necrosis of tracheal and bronchial mucosa resembling tissue culture cytopathogenic effect
Keratoconjunctivitis (EKC)	Epidemic disease in shipyard workers; also spread from infected eye solutions	8	11	Unusual	Uncommon	Not reported	Not reported

CLINICAL MANIFESTATIONS The incubation period for rhinovirus infections is 1 to 2 days. The first signs of disease are scratchy throat, nasal congestion and discharge, malaise, and mild headache. There is usually no fever. Nasal secretions increase sharply between days 1 and 2 and then as promptly return to pre-illness values. Recovery is rapid and complete. Virus shedding begins a few hours after inoculation and continues for a week or more.

Table 195-1 summarizes clinical experience with naturally occurring rhinovirus infections in adults and children and artificial infection in volunteers. Most adults have only a common cold syndrome, with a rare case of bronchitis the only other form of illness. In contrast, more than one-half of children develop bronchitis, bronchiolitis, or bronchopneumonia. Although these findings resemble those of respiratory syncytial (RS) virus infection, rhinovirus disease is generally milder than that due to RS virus.

LABORATORY FINDINGS In illness with rhinovirus there is usually slight neutrophilia. About one-third of volunteers develop moderate elevations in sedimentation rate.

COMPLICATIONS No serious complications have been reported with rhinovirus infections.

DIFFERENTIAL DIAGNOSIS Among the respiratory viruses, rhinovirus infection most consistently causes coryzal illness. In any one case, however, the illness cannot be distinguished from coryza due to other agents. Except for rare confusion with an atypical case of streptococcal sore throat, only respiratory viral diseases and *Mycoplasma pneumoniae* infection need be considered in differential diagnosis.

TREATMENT AND PREVENTION There is no specific treatment, and no vaccines are currently available for rhinovirus infections. Analgesics, antihistamines, and nose drops may be beneficial.

Constitutional reaction	*Other*
Headache, malaise, often high fever for several days	Usually no other involvement
Headache, malaise, high fever for several days	Acute follicular conjunctivitis, usually unilateral, occurs with varying frequency. Preauricular lymphadenopathy common with conjunctivitis
High fever, malaise, headache	Nausea, vomiting and diarrhea may occur, especially in infants
High fever, prostration	Conjunctivitis, skin rash, diarrhea, intussusception, and CNS invasion in some cases
Usually afebrile	Usually unilateral severe, acute conjunctivitis followed by corneal subepithelial keratosis; preauricular lymphadenopathy common

ADENOVIRUS INFECTIONS

ETIOLOGY The adenovirus group contains 31 human and 17 animal serotypes. Strains of types 3, 7, 11, 12, 14, 16, 18, 21, and 31 have been shown to cause sarcomas when injected into newborn hamsters.

Adenoviruses share a common antigenic determinant on a surface structure of the virus called a *hexon.* This antigen is the basis for an adenovirus group–diagnostic complement fixation test. An immunofluorescent test is also available that uses antihexon antibody to detect adenoviral group antigen present in exudates from patients or in infected cell cultures. Type specificity in neutralizing antibody tests depends primarily on antigenic determinants present on another surface structure (penton). Except for types 12 and 18, hemagglutination inhibition (HI) tests also permit type-specific identification. Adenovirus hemagglutinins, the basis for the HI test, are also associated with the penton. Human adenoviruses grow well in continuous cell lines of epithelial origin.

EPIDEMIOLOGY Adenoviruses are most prevalent in infants and children; they are found in the throat and rectum of both sick and well children. Adenovirus-associated illness occurs throughout the year and accounts for about 2 to 10 percent of all respiratory illness in infants and children, but the highest frequency is in the period from the fall through the spring. Isolations of virus from well children show a similar pattern of seasonal prevalence but a lower frequency of occurrence. Adenovirus types most commonly associated wilh illness in children are 1, 2, 3, and 5.

The second most frequent occurrence of adenovirus disease is among military recruits. In the general adult population the disease is sporadic. An appreciable prevalence of infection with many adenovirus serotypes is suggested by serologic surveys, but definite virus-associated illness is limited to about 10. These serotypes produce five major patterns of illness, all of which occur in epidemics. A summary of these is presented in Table 195-2.

Acute respiratory disease (ARD), a respiratory illness of military recruits, caused principally by adenoviruses types 4 and 7, occurs in winter and spring outbreaks. Adenoviruses account for 15 to 50 percent of ARD in military groups, but only for about 2 percent of respiratory illness in civilian adults.

Febrile pharyngitis due to adenoviruses usually occurs sporadically or in small outbreaks in children. Its manifestations are summarized in Table 195-2. *Pharyngoconjuncti-*

val fever is febrile pharyngitis associated with acute follicular conjunctivitis. This disease occurs as summer epidemics, frequently among children in relation to exposure in swimming pools. Although it is not limited to swimming pool exposure, it is believed that eye irritation from water, sun, or chlorine may be a factor in its initiation. Conjunctivitis may occur without pharyngitis.

Pneumonia due to adenovirus infection is rare in civilian adults, but occurs in military recruits, usually as an extension of ARD. In infants and children, sporadic and epidemic occurrence of highly fatal adenoviral pneumonia has been described in several parts of the world. Such outbreaks have been principally caused by types 3 and 7. The severity of disease in this young age group may reflect the lack of prior experience with these agents, but other factors such as size and route of inoculation, general health, or greater susceptibility due to immaturity may be important.

Incubation period The period of incubation for pharyngoconjunctival fever and ARD is 5 to 10 days, and is probably similar for other syndromes, since induced disease in volunteers has a similar period of incubation.

PATHOGENESIS When the conjunctival sac is swabbed with suspensions of adenovirus, conjunctivitis occurs and there is sometimes respiratory involvement. The initiation of illness appears to require a significant degree of conjunctival irritation. Administration of virus aerosol by inhalation also produces illness. Volunteers inoculated in this way have developed ARD and mild pneumonia.

These observations suggest the existence of at least two routes of inoculation for naturally occurring respiratory illness with adenoviruses: (1) ocular inoculation associated with eye irritation such as may occur in outbreaks around swimming pools, with the development of *pharyngoconjunctival fever;* (2) inoculation through inhalation of infectious aerosol generated by sneezing and coughing of ill recruits under the crowded circumstances incidental to recruit training. The route of inoculation of infants is less likely to be limited to aerosolized virus, and whatever the route of inoculation, the occurrence of pneumonia may represent primarily a lack of resistance in this young age group.

Nasopharyngeal inoculation in volunteers often produces virus infection without illness, suggesting that the high frequency of antibody to many serotypes in the population may result from asymptomatic infections. Antibody may also result from intragroup cross reactions among serotypes in the three broad immunologic groups of adenovirus.

CLINICAL MANIFESTATIONS *Acute respiratory disease* is an acute febrile illness lasting about 1 week and characterized by fever, cough, hoarseness, and sore throat. Fever has gradual onset and reaches a maximum of 103 to 104°F on the second or third day. There are associated malaise and often headache. Pharyngitis, the most prominent localized manifestation of the disease, reaches maximum severity after about 3 days. There may also be regional lymphadenopathy, pharyngeal injection, some edema, frequent lymphoid follicular hyperplasia, but little or no faucial exudate. Nasal obstruction and discharge occur in almost one-half of cases, but these abnormalities are not usually conspicuous. Cough is almost always present, and hoarseness is frequent.

Pharyngoconjunctival fever is usually a milder respiratory illness than ARD, although fever may be high for 5 or 6 days. Nontender submandibular lymphadenopathy is common even in the absence of sore throat. Lower respiratory tract involvement has not been described. Conjunctivitis is mild to moderate but may last longer than respiratory symptoms. It is an acute, nonpurulent, follicular conjunctivitis. In most cases, it is unilateral, and preauricular lymphadenopathy is rare. There is usually no involvement of the cornea or uveal tract.

Febrile pharyngitis without conjunctivitis resembles the foregoing illness, except for the absence of conjunctivitis.

Adenoviral pneumonia in children occurs as a primary illness and is associated with as much as 15 percent mortality. Pediatric texts should be consulted for further details.

DIFFERENTIAL DIAGNOSIS The differential diagnosis of ARD should include the respiratory viral diseases described in the present chapter and influenza (Chap. 196), nonpneumonic forms of *M. pneumoniae* infection (Chap. 188), streptococcal sore throat, and purulent sinusitis. Pharyngitis and upper respiratory illness may also accompany the onset of infectious hepatitis and infectious mononucleosis.

Differential diagnosis of *pharyngoconjunctival fever,* when conjunctivitis is prominent, includes leptospirosis, influenza, measles, herpangina, and the nonpurulent conjunctivitides, such as inclusion conjunctivitis and physical or chemical trauma to the eye.

TREATMENT There is no specific treatment for adenovirus infection. Treatment is limited to alleviation of general discomfort, headache, and coughing, with analgesics, cough syrup containing terpin hydrate, codeine, antihistamines, or other antitussives.

PREVENTION Communicability of adenovirus infection probably extends from a day or so before onset of illness to recovery, and conventional precautions against respiratory spread should be employed during acute illness for patients in the hospital and to the extent reasonably possible in care of patients at home. Avoidance of swimming pools during outbreaks of pharyngoconjunctival fever is recommended.

Formalin-treated vaccines against types 3, 4, and 7 afford significant protection against infection and illness, but these vaccines were withdrawn from civilian use when it was discovered that some serotypes of adenoviruses produced tumors in hamsters. A live adenovirus vaccine given orally in enteric-coated capsules is highly effective in preventing infection with adenovirus types 3, 4, and 7 in military recruits. More recently, a vaccine prepared from hexons and the fiber portion of penton demonstrated a high degree of protection against experimental infections in volunteers. No vaccine is now marketed for civilian use.

RESPIRATORY SYNCYTIAL VIRUS INFECTION

ETIOLOGY Respiratory syncytial virus (RS) is classified as a subgroup of the myxoviruses (Table 194-2). In tissue culture, it causes formation of giant cells, or syncytia, from which its name was derived. It grows well in several human primary and continuous cell lines and in primary rhesus monkey kidney culture. There is a soluble complement-fixing antigen which, with the neutralization test, permits virus identification and serologic studies. Viral antigen can also be detected by immunofluorescence of exudates from infected patients or in infected cell cultures. Respiratory syncytial virus contrasts with other myxoviruses because it does not grow in mice, guinea pigs, rabbits, or chick embryos and does not cause hemagglutination or hemadsorption.

EPIDEMIOLOGY Epidemiologic studies have delineated a very substantial role of this agent in acute respiratory disease in children. Illness in young children occurs most commonly in epidemics in the late winter and early spring. Attack rates are nearly 100 percent among susceptibles, who are mostly children under four years of age, but the peak occurrence of bronchiolitis and bronchopneumonia is observed at two to three months of age. In older children and adults, the disease appears in nonepidemic patterns. The limitation of epidemic disease to the younger age group is also evidence for unchanging antigenicity of the agent, in contrast to the situation with influenza virus, in which antigenic shifts are associated with recurrent epidemics in persons of all ages. In serologic surveys of volunteers, all were found to possess a measurable titer of neutralizing antibody to RS virus. Mild upper respiratory illness appears to be a reinfection form of the disease in adults, but the virus has been isolated from cases of acute bronchitis in older people with chronic pulmonary disease.

It is probable that RS virus is transmitted by means of infected respiratory secretions. The incubation period of naturally occurring disease in children is about 4 days, and in adult volunteers approximately 5 days. Virus was generally recovered from volunteers a day or so before the onset of illness, and throat swabs yielded a higher proportion of positive cultures than nasal swabs. Virus shedding continues for 3 to 4 days after onset of illness.

CLINICAL MANIFESTATIONS Somewhat less than one-half of infected children have symptoms defined as a common cold; the remainder have bronchiolitis or bronchopneumonia. Fever occurs in about 90 percent of ill children, with an average elevation to 102°F. Cough is almost invariably present, and severe malaise is frequent. Pharyngitis is not usually severe. Fatalities have been reported in infants.

LABORATORY FINDINGS In children, leukocytosis occurs with some frequency, but no significant hematologic changes were observed in adult volunteers. Bacterial flora of the nasopharynx and other laboratory indices show no significant alterations in either age group.

COMPLICATIONS Except for progression to overwhelming lower respiratory tract disease in a few young children, no special complications are known. There is no evidence of secondary bacterial infection or systemic invasion by the virus in children. In adults, bacterial sinusitis occasionally complicates the virus infection.

DIFFERENTIAL DIAGNOSIS The resemblance of this disease in children to influenza has been suggested. In adults, the differential diagnosis should include rhinovirus and parainfluenza infection and, less often, other respiratory viral disease and *M. pneumoniae* infection.

TREATMENT As with other respiratory viral diseases, treatment should include rest and palliative medications such as aspirin, nose drops, and medication for sleep when restlessness occurs. The possibility of bacterial sinusitis in adults should be kept in mind and antimicrobial treatment, drainage procedures, or other therapy instituted when necessary.

PREVENTION A Formalin-inactivated RS vaccine elicited a high frequency of antibody, but a few months later vaccinated children experienced more severe illness than nonvaccinated children in the same population. This paradoxical effect of vaccination is a major contraindication to further attempts to develop a vaccine. The infection spreads rapidly among children in institutions and poses a threat to debilitated or very young children.

PARAINFLUENZA VIRUS INFECTIONS

ETIOLOGY On the basis of antigenic differences, parainfluenza viruses are divided into four types, of which type 4 is divided into two subtypes. They agglutinate avian and mammalian erythroctyes and grow slowly in tissue culture; only type 2 produces readily visible cytopathic effects. Growth of these agents in tissue cultures is detected by addition of guinea pig erythrocytes, which absorb on the surface of infected cells to form rosettes, a process known as hemadsorption. Parainfluenza viruses have antigens common to Newcastle disease and mumps viruses, but influenza virus does not share these. Parainfluenza serotypes are distinguished in complement fixation, hemagglutination-inhibition, or tissue culture neutralization tests. The serotypes can also be identified and differentiated from one another by immunofluorescence.

Parainfluenza virus can be isolated in primary monkey or primary embryonic kidney cell cultures, but grows slowly or not at all in embryonated eggs.

EPIDEMIOLOGY The first three types of parainfluenza viruses have been found in many parts of the world; type 4 has so far been isolated only in the United States. Infection with parainfluenza viruses occurs early in life. By the age of eight years, a majority of children show antibody to types 1 to 3, and it appears that most adults have antibody to all four types.

In children, illness with parainfluenza viruses occurs throughout the year, with seasonal increases in the winter and spring. Type 3 virus spreads more rapidly than types 1 and 2. Heterotypic antibody rises are frequent, with antibody to type 3 developing in half the cases with type 1 infection. In both children and adults, reinfection is frequent. In one outbreak, 96 percent of children without antibody, 67 percent with low levels, and 33 percent with high levels of antibody became infected. In adults, the disease is almost invariably a reinfection and is much milder than in children.

The total contribution of parainfluenza infections to respiratory illness is variable; its frequency is increasing in institutions in which general health status is lower than average and levels of sanitation and personal hygiene are less than optimum. In studies in the United States parainfluenza infections account for 4.3 to 17 percent of respiratory illness in children. The milder illness of adults constituted less than 5 percent of respiratory illnesses.

CLINICAL MANIFESTATIONS In all age groups, the incubation period appears to be 5 to 6 days. The disease is most serious in infants and children, the characteristic syndrome being laryngotracheobronchitis, or croup. Bronchiolitis, bronchitis, and bronchopneumonia in children are also caused by parainfluenza infections. In older children the disease is less serious, usually without evidence of pulmonary involvement, and in adults, the virus produces a common cold syndrome with hoarseness and cough.

Fever is a constant feature of illness in children but is less frequent in adults. Nasal discharge is common at all ages. Cough and hoarseness are common, and stridor, indicative of croup, is present in many of the cases among infants and children.

Physical findings are not distinctive. The throat is reddened, with little or no exudate. There may be tender submandibular lymphadenopathy.

LABORATORY FINDINGS In adult volunteers given type 2 virus, leukocyte counts were not abnormal. In children there is a considerable variation in leukocyte counts early in illness, making it difficult to distinguish this disease from pneumococcal and other bacterial infections. No characteristic alterations have been reported in other laboratory indices such as liver or renal function tests, electrocardiograms, and urinalyses.

COURSE AND COMPLICATIONS In children, *otitis media* has occurred as a complication more often with parainfluenza than with the other respiratory viral infections. It may be caused by pneumococci, streptococci, or *Hemophilus influenzae.*

Parainfluenza virus infection is characterized by slow resolution of pulmonary involvement and long persistence of cough and other symptoms. In very young or debilitated children, the outcome can be fatal. In adults, bacterial sinusitis may occur, and in persons with chronic bronchitis, emphysema, or bronchiectasis, the possibility of pulmonary bacterial superinfections should be considered.

TREATMENT There is no specific treatment. Therapy is limited to symptomatic measures and efforts aimed at early detection and treatment of bacterial complications such as otitis media or pneumonia. Nursing care is important in pediatric cases, especially children with croup. In adults, analgesics, antihistamines, and small doses of codeine for cough are generally sufficient.

PREVENTION Vaccines against parainfluenza virus infections are not available. In hospitals, respiratory precautions should be carried out. At home, bed rest or room isolation during acute illness is advised, with special effort to avoid contact with very young or aged persons.

COXSACKIE AND ECHO VIRUS INFECTIONS

Diseases produced by these agents are described in Chap. 193. Table 195-3 summarizes the respiratory illnesses sometimes seen with infections caused by these viruses.

CORONAVIRUSES

ETIOLOGY The disease in humans is caused by an antigenically heterogeneous group of lipid-enveloped RNA viruses sharing morphologic and other properties with mouse hepatitis virus (MHV) and avian infectious bronchitis virus (IBV). A few serotypes of human coronaviruses recovered in tracheal organ culture share antigens with the murine agent.

EPIDEMIOLOGY The disease, characteristically a common cold syndrome, occurs in winter and spring outbreaks that vary from year to year, with maximum attack rates in the fifteen- to nineteen-year-old age group, but it may involve adults of forty years of age and older. The incubation period is 3 to 5 days.

TABLE 195-3
Respiratory illness associated with Coxsackie viruses A and B, and echo viruses

Diagnosis	*Description*	*Associated viruses*
Herpangina	Febrile pharyngitis, anorexia, and discrete vesicular eruption on anterior faucial pillars. Occurs chiefly in children in summer and early fall outbreaks. Similar illnesses without eruption caused by the same viruses probably occur. An illness with nonulcerating nodules on anterior pillars caused by Coxsackie virus A-10 has also been described	Coxsackie virus A-1 through 6, 8, 10, and 12
Febrile respiratory illness ("summer grippe")	Undifferentiated febrile illness marked by headache, sore throat, and anorexia occurring in summer or early fall. Includes epidemics in recruits with Coxsackie virus A-21 infection, in which illness patterns have been confirmed by experimental inoculation of volunteers	Coxsackie virus A-21, 24 B-2, 3, 5 (?), and echo virus 1, 3, 6, 19, 20
Upper respiratory illness associated with gastroenteritis	Cases occurring largely in infants and exposed mothers	Echo virus 1, 11, 19, 20
Acute laryngotracheobronchitis (croup)	Winter outbreaks in nurseries and institutions. Association less definite than with other syndromes	Coxsackie virus A-9, B-5, and echo virus 11
Pneumonitis and pleuritis	Largely confined to young infants and children; uncommon	Coxsackie virus A-9, B-4, 5, and echo virus 9, 19, 20

CLINICAL FEATURES The disease resembles rhinovirus common cold with profuse watery and later mucopurulent nasal discharge, sore throat, moderate cough, and mild constitutional symptoms. It is of short duration. Diagnosis is based on isolation of the agent in organ culture or human embryo kidney culture or by antibody rise. The neutralizing antibody test is more sensitive than the complement fixation test, and rises in titer persist for a longer time. Both tests, however, will provide adequate diagnostic information. There is evidence that coronaviruses causes bronchiolitis and pneumonia in the young.

TREATMENT AND PREVENTION Treatment is symptomatic; no preventive measures are available.

REFERENCES

Adenoviruses

BRANDT CD et al: Infections in 18,000 infants and children in a study of respiratory disease. II. Variation in adenovirus infections by year and seasons. Am J Epidemiol 95:218, 1972

KNIGHT V, KASEL JA: Adenoviruses, in *Viral and Mycoplasmal Infections of the Respiratory Tract,* ed V Knight, Philadelphia: Lea & Febiger, 1973

Coronaviruses

CAVALLARO JJ, MONTO AS: Community-wide outbreak of infection with 229E-like coronavirus in Tecumseh, Michigan. J Infect Dis 122:27, 1970

KNIGHT V, MAYOR HD: Coronaviruses, in *Viral and Mycoplasmal Infections of the Respiratory Tract,* ed V Knight, Philadelphia: Lea & Febiger, 1973

WENZEL RP et al: Coronavirus infections in military recruits. Am Rev Resp Dis 109:621, 1974

Coxsackie and echo viruses

SPICKARD A et al: Acute respiratory disease in normal volunteers associated with Coxsackie A-21 viral infection. III. Response to nasopharyngeal and enteric inoculation. J Clin Invest 42:840, 1963

Parainfluenza virus

CHANOCK RM et al: Newly recognized myxoviruses from children with respiratory disease. N Engl J Med 258:207, 1958

KNIGHT V: Parainfluenza viruses, in *Viral and Mycoplasmal Infections of the Respiratory Tract,* ed V Knight, Philadelphia: Lea & Febiger, 1973

MONTO AS: The Tecumseh study. V. Patterns of infection with parainfluenzaviruses. Am J Epidemiol 97:338, 1973

Respiratory syncytial virus

AHERNE W et al: Pathological changes in virus infections of the lower respiratory tract in children. J Clin Pathol 23:7, 1970

KNIGHT V: Respiratory syncytial viruses, in *Viral and Mycoplasmal Infections of the Respiratory Tract,* ed V Knight, Philadelphia: Lea & Febiger, 1973

PARROT RH et al: Epidemiology of respiratory syncytial virus infection in Washington D.C. II. Infection and disease with respect to age, immunologic status, race and sex. Am J Epidemiol 98:289, 1973

Rhinoviruses

CATE TR: Rhinoviruses, in *Viral and Mycoplasmal Infections of the Respiratory Tract,* ed V Knight, Philadelphia: Lea & Febiger, 1973

FOX JP et al: The Seattle virus watch. V. Epidemiologic observations of rhinovirus infections, 1965–1969, in families with young children. Am J Epidemiol 101:122, 1975

MINOR TF et al: Failure of naturally acquired rhinovirus infections to produce temporal immunity to heterologous serotypes. Infect Immun 10:1192, 1974

196 INFLUENZA

VERNON KNIGHT

DEFINITION Influenza is an acute respiratory infection of specific viral etiology characterized by sudden onset of headache, myalgia, fever, and prostration. The terms *influenza* and "flu" should be restricted to those cases with clear-cut epidemiologic or laboratory evidence of infection with influenza viruses.

HISTORY According to the best available records, influenza was uncommon in Europe during the nineteenth century until the pandemic of 1889. Subsequently, the frequency and severity of epidemics increased, culminating in the disastrous pandemic of 1918, which caused an estimated 20 to 40 million deaths. The isolation of the causative virus in 1933 led to the development of simple diagnostic tests, which have greatly advanced knowledge of the disease.

ETIOLOGY There are three distinct antigenic types of influenza virus, designated A, B, and C. Infection with one type confers no immunity to infection with the other two. They are approximately 100 nm in diameter, visible as spheres or filaments by electron microscopy, and are biologically related by their infectivity for chick embryos, capacity to agglutinate erythrocytes, and affinity for the respiratory epithelium of various mammals. Influenza viruses are the prototypes of the myxovirus group and are related to the larger paramyxoviruses, which include mumps, Newcastle disease, measles, and the parainfluenza viruses. Influenza viruses are composed of a helical ribonucleoprotein core with a lipid-containing envelope from which protein spikes protrude. The protein spikes, or coat proteins, are of two types, hemagglutinins and neuraminidase. The former are responsible for attachment of the virus to cell receptors; the latter enzymatically inactivate neuraminic acid, the active receptor substance. Enzyme activity frees virus from attachment sites if cell penetration is unsuccessful. Hemagglutinins and neuraminidase are antigenic and elicit protective antibody.

EPIDEMIOLOGY Influenza B usually occurs sporadically or in localized outbreaks, particularly in schools and military camps. Illness with influenza C is rarely detected, although antibody surveys indicate a wide prevalence of infection with this agent. Influenza A viruses are the cause of major epidemics that tend to recur at intervals of 2 to 4 years in the winter months. The factors responsible for this periodicity are the decline in effective immunity of a population in interepidemic periods and the emergence every few years of new strains of virus. Antigenic shifts in influenza viruses are due to changes in the coat proteins, hemagglutinins (H), and neuraminidase (N). The designation of antigenic changes, and the major occurrences of influenza for which they were responsible are described below.

Pandemic 1918	Swinelike agent
Epidemics 1933	H0N1, formerly A_0
Epidemics 1947	H1N1, formerly A_1
Pandemic 1957	H2N2, formerly A_2 (Asian)
Pandemic 1968	H3N2 (Hong Kong)

A variant of these H3N2 viruses, A/Victoria/75, was epidemic in many parts of the world, including most of the United States, in 1975–1976. In February 1976, a new strain of human influenza A virus, A/New Jersey/76 (Hsw1N1), was isolated in an outbreak of influenza among United States Army recruits at Fort Dix, New Jersey. Several hundred individuals were infected, but the outbreak did not appear to spread beyond Fort Dix, and only sporadic cases have been reported subsequent to the initial outbreak. This virus is related antigenically to the virus that is believed to have caused the severe influenza pandemic of 1918–1919, and to that which has been circulating in swine since then. The outbreak at Fort Dix represents the first documented human-to-human transmission of swine influenza since before 1930. Because this virus represents a major antigenic change from the influenza A viruses prevalent since 1968, there may be a greater hazard of its spread worldwide. However, six months after the outbreak such a spread had not occurred.

Hemagglutinins and neuraminidase of some equine, swine, and avian strains of influenza share antigenic properties with some human influenza viruses. It is not known whether the animal viruses interact in some way with human viruses, possibly by exchange of genetic material (recombination), to account for new antigenic variants. Against this possibility is the lack of evidence of natural spread of infection between human and animal hosts.

Influenza A epidemics start abruptly, reach a peak in 2 to 3 months, and subside almost as rapidly. The attack rate is variable but was noted in 1957 to exceed 50 percent of urban populations. An additional 25 percent of individuals may show serologic evidence of infection without clinical manifestations. Experiences in 1957 proved conclusively that crowding, even in summer months or in tropical countries, is the major factor predisposing to epidemics. Schoolchildren, in particular, are the primary focus and disseminators of infection in the United States. If the general immunity of a population is at low levels, communitywide epidemics may occur within a short period after the introduction of new strains of virus. If, however, immune individuals predominate, the case rate will rise slowly and may not reach epidemic proportions.

PATHOGENESIS Influenza is primarily an infection of the respiratory epithelium that is transmitted from person to person by inhalation of infective droplet nuclei. Detailed experimental studies of the pathogenesis of the disease have been made in ferrets and mice. After intranasal inoculation, the virus multiplies to maximum titers in 24 to 48 h and rapidly involves the entire tracheobronchial tree. At first, the mucosa becomes boggy and hyperemic and loses its normal ciliary activity. This may shortly be followed by necrosis of respiratory epithelium, invasion by leukocytes, pulmonary consolidation, and abnormal regeneration of metaplastic squamous epithelium in the bronchi and bronchioles. The infection is largely confined to the respiratory tract and hilar lymph nodes of adult animals; viremia is a transient and inconstant feature. However, virus has been isolated from heart, kidney, and other extrapulmonary tissues in fatal human infections, suggesting that virus products can enter the circulation and may account for systemic manifestations of the disease.

The findings at autopsy are pulmonary hemorrhages, necrosis of bronchial epithelium, bronchiolitis, squamous metaplasia of respiratory epithelium, and marked edema of alveolar septa and spaces. Fatal illness can result from influenza virus infection alone but more often results from combined viral and bacterial infection.

MANIFESTATIONS The disease assumes its typical form during major epidemics of influenza A, but clinical differentiation between influenza A and B is not possible in localized outbreaks. Sporadic infections with either influenza A or B are likely to result in relatively minor illnesses, with predominantly respiratory symptoms, similar to those of common respiratory disease. Influenza C is particularly difficult to recognize because of its mildness. Although the manifestations and severity of influenza A vary from year to year, cases in a single epidemic often follow a remarkably similar pattern. The clinical description that follows is a composite picture of epidemic influenza A of the past three decades.

The *incubation period* is usually 18 to 36 h but may be as long as 3 days. Mild prodromal symptoms of cough, malaise, and chilliness are sometimes present, but extremely sudden onset is often such a characteristic feature that many patients can recall its exact time. The most common initial symptom is severe generalized or frontal *headache*, frequently accompanied by stabbing retroorbital pain that is accentuated by lateral or upward gaze. Diffuse *myalgia*, particularly marked in the legs and over the lumbosacral area, occurs in more than half the cases. Pain and spasm of the abdominal muscles may simulate acute peritonitis, and incapacitating periarticular pains are sometimes confused with acute arthritis. *Feverishness* and *chilliness*, or occasionally true rigors, may be the first manifestations, but more often they are preceded by headache and myalgia. The temperature rises abruptly to a maximum of 100 to 103°F several hours after onset; rarely it may reach 106°F. Thereafter, the fever and pain usually subside over a 2- to 3-day period but may persist for as long as a week. A common variant in the temperature course is rapid defervescence after the initial peak, with a secondary rise to the original level on the following day. In general, severity of illness parallels the height and duration of the fever. The pulse rate is usually slow in relation to the fever, but marked tachycardia may occur in severely ill patients.

Prostration of some degree is almost invariable and is often the most prominent and alarming manifestation. The face is flushed, and the skin is hot and dry; however, profuse sweating and cold, mottled extremities are sometimes noted. Anorexia, nausea, and constipation are frequent secondary symptoms, but vomiting and diarrhea are rare. There is no evidence that influenza viruses infect the gastrointestinal tract, and the term *intestinal flu* is a misnomer. Meningoencephalitis, polyneuritis, cranial nerve palsies, transient nerve deafness, aphasia, hemiplegia, psychoses, and other neurologic disorders have been described in association with influenza but are very unusual. Hypotension, heart block, peripheral vasoconstriction, and fatal myocarditis have also been reported in a few cases. The exact relationship of these neurologic and cardiovascular disorders to influenza viral infection has not been determined.

Respiratory symptoms may be present at the onset but become most prominent when the systemic manifestations and fever begin to subside. They are frequently less pronounced than in common respiratory disease and may be entirely absent. Sneezing, watery nasal discharge, and stuffy nose occur in most cases; hoarseness and epistaxis are less frequent. Conjunctival suffusion and burning, itching, watery eyes are often noted. The throat may feel dry, and the pharynx often appears slightly injected. *Cough* develops during the course of the illness in more than three-fourths of the cases, and in about a third of these it is productive of small amounts of tenacious, mucoid sputum. *Chest pain,* usually substernal in location and accentuated by coughing but not by breathing, is present in almost half the patients. Pleurisy and pleural effusion are uncommon. Slight hyperpnea is often noted, but the most ominous, although infrequent, signs are dyspnea and cyanosis, which signal bronchiolar or pneumonic involvement. Findings on physical examination of the lungs are often negative in uncomplicated influenza but scattered rhonchi, wheezes, and showers of moist rales have been reported in 5 to 40 percent of cases in different epidemics. These changes may persist for several days after apparent recovery. Patients with uncomplicated influenza may have restrictive ventilatory defects and increased alveolar-capillary oxygen tension gradients, suggesting the regular occurrence of lower pulmonary tract involvement in the disease. Influenzal bronchiolitis should be suspected if rales persist in the absence of x-ray evidence of pneumonitis and if the patient raises mucopurulent or blood-tinged sputum.

COMPLICATIONS The chief complications of influenza are pneumonia, either primary (due to influenza virus infection alone) or secondary bacterial pneumonia superimposed on the lesions produced by the influenza virus. In addition, bacterial infections of the paranasal sinuses and middle ear may occur. The incidence of bacterial pneumonia is greatly increased during influenza epidemics; even mild or asymptomatic infections with influenza viruses predispose to pneumococcal and other types of pneumonia. The most serious complication is staphylococcal pneumonia, which tends to follow a fulminant, often fatal, course. Primary influenza virus pneumonia typically has its onset about 1 week after onset of influenza, often following a period of apparent improvement. The disease is characterized by severe dyspnea and cyanosis, scanty sputum containing gross blood, leukopenia, few physical findings in the lung, and perihilar infiltrates. The disease has a rapid course, and fatality, when it occurs, results from acute respiratory failure. Secondary bacterial pneumonia responds less well to antimicrobial treatment than pneumonia that occurs in the absence of influenza, presumably because of underlying pulmonary damage from the influenza virus infection. Superinfection with *Hemophilus influenzae,* so common in the pandemic of 1918, is rarely encountered now.

A complication of influenza B, seen increasingly in recent years, is a syndrome of encephalopathy with acute cerebral edema and fatty infiltration of the liver. This is termed *Reye's syndrome;* it occurs with several other virus infections, but is uncommon with influenza A. Reduced activity of one or two hepatic enzymes of the urea cycle is noted in these patients. The mortality is high. Treatment has consisted of dexamethasone administration under continuous monitoring to maintain intracranial pressure at tolerable levels. Peritoneal dialysis is also used to remove excess blood ammonia commonly present in these patients.

Recovery from uncomplicated influenza is often complete in 2 to 3 days or, occasionally, in a week, but convalescence may be prolonged by "postinfectious asthenia" and depression particularly in elderly persons. Minor relapses with fever may occur but are uncommon.

The *mortality* rate from all causes always increases markedly during epidemics of influenza. In the fall and winter of 1957–1958 it was estimated that 40 million persons in the United States became ill with influenza and the total number of influenza-associated deaths was reported to be in excess of 8,000. In addition, approximately 60,000 more deaths from various causes occurred during this period than would be expected under normal conditions. The greatest incidence of excessive mortality occurred among infants under one year of age and adults over sixty years of age. Data from small series of cases clearly indicate that influenza is frequently fatal in individuals with preexisting pulmonary or cardiac disease, regardless of age. Chronic rheumatic heart disease with mitral stenosis, in particular, appears to predispose to fatal influenzal pneumonia.

LABORATORY FINDINGS Virus is isolated most readily during the acute phase of the disease by inoculation of broth garglings into the amniotic cavity of chick embryos or into tissue cultures of monkey kidney or human cells. Influenza virus types A, B, and C may be identified in complement fixation tests. These tests depend on the nucleocapsid antigen found in the viral core and in soluble form in infected cells. Antiserum to whole virions readily detects the same or closely related strains by immunofluorescence in infected cell culture and, on occasion, directly in exudates from patients with infection. This methodology is useful in rapid diagnosis. Serologic diagnosis can be made most reliably by hemagglutination-inhibition or complement fixation tests, using paired serum samples obtained in both the acute and convalescent phases. Type-specific antibody against soluble complement-fixing antigens of influenza A virus also appears in the circulation of patients during the acute illness.

In uncomplicated influenza the lungs usually appear normal by x-ray but occasionally have increased vascular markings, basilar streaking, small areas of patchy infiltration, atelectasis, nodular densities, or pleural effusion. The blood leukocyte count may be low 2 to 4 days after onset of illness, but is often normal or slightly elevated. Leukocytosis with counts above 15,000 cells per mm^3 indicates secondary bacterial infection, but leukopenia may occur in severe staphylococcal pneumonia. Slight proteinuria is common during the height of the febrile illness.

DIFFERENTIAL DIAGNOSIS Many bacterial and viral infections simulate influenza at their onset, but few febrile diseases have such a self-limited course. The pattern of clinical manifestations becomes readily apparent during an epidemic. Noninfluenzal respiratory diseases are generally characterized by more gradual onset, milder systemic manifestations, and predominant symptoms of coryza, rhinorrhea, pharyngitis, and conjunctivitis.

TREATMENT Antibiotics do not affect the course of uncomplicated influenza, nor is there any evidence that they prevent complications. Specific chemotherapy should be reserved for secondary bacterial infections. Clinical trials have shown some effectiveness of amantadine, a symmetric amine that inhibits cellular penetration of influenza virus, as a chemoprophylactic and therapeutic agent, but the results are not impressive. Codeine affords relief from incapacitating cough and is more effective than salicylates for symptomatic treatment of headache and myalgia; salicylates often increase discomfort by causing drenching sweats and chills. Bed rest and gradual return to full activity are advisable.

PROPHYLAXIS Formalinized egg vaccines purified by zonal ultracentrifugation or other methods and containing a mixture of influenza A(H3N2) and B viruses are available commercially in the United States. Present purified vaccines contain larger amounts of virus than in previous years, with resulting increased potency. Current vaccines can be expected to be effective when given in suitable dosage at an interval of several weeks to several months before exposure, and when the antigens of the vaccine are still closely related to the epidemic strain.

The U.S. Public Health Service strongly recommends routine yearly immunization with polyvalent influenza vaccine for high-risk groups, including persons of all ages who suffer from chronic rheumatic heart disease, other cardiovascular diseases, chronic bronchopulmonary diseases, diabetes mellitus, or Addison's disease, and persons sixty-five years of age, or older, regardless of their previous state of health. Pregnant women should be immunized only if they fall into one of the high-risk categories. For initial immunization of adults it is advisable to administer the vaccine subcutaneously in two divided doses of 0.5 ml each, the first injection in September and the second several weeks or months later. A single subcutaneous dose of 0.5 ml given each autumn is satisfactory as a yearly booster. Intradermal injection of vaccine is far less satisfactory because a sufficient antigenic mass cannot be so administered.

Because of the possibility that the new swine influenza virus will persist and cause extensive disease, the federal government has instituted the National Influenza Immunization Program, which provides for two vaccine formulations: a bivalent vaccine containing both the A/Victoria/75 and A/New Jersey/76 strains, which is recommended for the traditional "high-risk" groups, and a monovalent vaccine, containing the A/New Jersey/76 strain, for the rest of the population. In addition to the influenza A vaccines, there will be a monovalent influenza B vaccine, which should be taken by individuals for whom annual influenza vaccination is regularly recommended.

Influenza vaccination is generally safe but not completely innocuous. Fatal anaphylactic reactions and purpura have been reported in individuals sensitive to egg proteins, and inactivated virus itself is pyrogenic and can sometimes produce an illness similar to active influenza. Infants and children have experienced severe febrile convulsions following vaccination, and vaccine should be avoided in children with a history of this syndrome. A decision to vaccinate children, especially the very young, should be made on an individual basis.

REFERENCES

Hochberg FH et al: Influenza type B–related encephalopathy, the 1971 outbreak of Reye's syndrome in Chicago. JAMA 231: 817, 1975

Kilborne ED (ed): *The Influenza Viruses and Influenza,* New York: Academic, 1975

Knight V, Kasel JA: Influenza viruses, in *Viral and Mycoplasmal Infections of the Respiratory Tract,* ed V Knight, Philadelphia: Lea & Febiger, 1973

197
LYMPHOCYTIC CHORIOMENINGITIS

HARRY N. BEATY

DEFINITION Lymphocytic choriomeningitis (LCM) is an acute systemic viral infection which is frequently accompanied by the clinical syndrome of aseptic meningitis.

ETIOLOGY The agent responsible for LCM is a small RNA virion which is the prototype for a group of viruses called arenaviruses. Included in the group are the morphologically and serologically similar Machupo and Lassa viruses. Many different strains of the virus have been identified on the basis of tissue tropism and pathogenicity, but none is antigenically distinct. The agent can be propagated readily in many mammalian cell cultures, but it produces little or no cytopathic effect.

EPIDEMIOLOGY The virus of LCM is probably worldwide in distribution, but is an uncommon cause of human disease. Although infection can be induced in a variety of animals, mice are the major natural reservoir as well as the primary host in which latent, asymptomatic infection occurs. The latency of mouse infection depends upon immunologic tolerance, and animals infected *in utero* or shortly after birth excrete the virus for life without overt disease. In humans LCM has followed direct contact with wild mice or infected rodents in experimental laboratories, and increasing numbers of cases have resulted from association with infected pet hamsters. Disease is thought to be transmitted to humans via airborne spread or contact with excrement from infected animals. LCM occurs throughout the year, but is somewhat more frequent in the colder months when human contact with wild rodents is greatest. Transmission by arthropods has been accomplished experimentally but has never been demonstrated naturally. Person-to-person transmission is extremely rare.

PATHOGENESIS In natural infection, the portal of entry of the LCM virus is probably through the respiratory tract. Virus multiplication occurs initially in the respiratory epithelium, and in some patients symptoms of an upper respiratory tract infection or influenza-like illness develop. Dissemination of virus to secondary extraneural sites of growth, possibly in reticuloendothelial cells, may be an important step in the pathogenesis of central nervous system disease. The virus multiplies in these sites, and when sustained viremia develops, crosses the blood-brain barrier and infects meningeal cells. In mice, the resulting meningitis, which is characterized by lymphocytic infiltration, is attributed to an immunologic reaction. It is postulated that this immune response is mediated by lymphocytes rather than antibody and is directed against host cells which are no longer recognized as self because of membrane alterations induced by the virus. Support for this hypothesis derives from observations that disease but not infection can be prevented in experimental animals by neonatal thymectomy, irradiation, or immunodepressant drugs. Similar pathogenetic mechanisms may operate in human beings.

CLINICAL MANIFESTATIONS Infection of humans by the LCM virus produces a variety of clinical manifestations. Serologic surveys indicate that inapparent or unrecognized infection is uncommon. It is also clear that symptomatic infection ordinarily consists of a clinically nonspecific upper respiratory tract infection which may resemble influenza. Neurologic manifestations appear only infrequently, and take the form of aseptic meningitis or encephalitis.

The exact incubation period is not known, but it is probably only a few days. Initially, symptoms consist of remittent fever, anorexia, malaise, generalized aching, headache, and respiratory manifestations ranging from pharyngitis, cough, and bronchitis to frank pneumonia. Fever and discomfort often vary in intensity, abating somewhat and then recurring over a period of 1 to 3 weeks. Many patients then recover completely. In others, however, apparent convalescence is interrupted by a recurrence of fever and the abrupt onset of headache, photophobia, and signs of meningeal irritation. This second stage of the disease ordinarily lasts 7 to 10 days, but relapses of meningeal symptoms are seen occasionally. A few patients have transient erythematous or papular rashes during the meningeal phase.

Patients with aseptic meningitis almost always recover without sequelae. With encephalitis, however, 25 to 30 percent of patients have neurologic abnormalities, and convalescence may be prolonged. Arthralgia and frank arthritis may be seen during recovery from the acute systemic illness, and in a few well-documented cases of infection with the LCM virus, orchitis has been observed.

LABORATORY FINDINGS Leukopenia with granulocytopenia and relative lymphocytosis is commonly seen in the acute systemic illness. If meningitis develops, the leukocyte count is often normal, but may be elevated with a predominance of polymorphonuclear leukocytes. Typically, cerebrospinal fluid pressure is elevated, and protein concentration increased. The glucose concentration is usually normal, but levels of 35 to 40 mg per 100 ml have been observed. Spinal fluid cell count ranges from 100 to 3,000 cells per mm^3 with 90 percent lymphocytes.

DIAGNOSIS The diagnosis of LCM can be established with certainty by recovery of the virus from blood or spinal fluid, or by serologic studies. Complement-fixing antibodies are usually detectable 1 to 2 weeks after the onset of infection, peak 5 to 8 weeks, and are gone by 6 months. Neutralizing antibodies appear after 6 to 8 weeks, increase in titer slowly, and remain high for years. Immunofluorescent studies have detected antibody to the LCM virus earlier in the course of the illness, and its appearance seems to parallel the development of the neurologic phase. The clinical manifestations of LCM cannot be differentiated from those produced by numerous other viruses. A detailed discussion of aseptic meningitis appears in Chap. 338.

TREATMENT The management of infections with the LCM virus is purely supportive and symptomatic.

REFERENCES

BAUM SG et al: Epidemic nonmeningitic lymphocytic choriomeningitis virus infection. N Engl J Med 274:937, 1966

HOTCHIN J: Virus, cell surface, and self: Lymphocytic choriomeningitis of mice. Am J Clin Pathol 56:33, 1971

LEHMANN-GRUBE F: *Lymphocytic Choriomeningitis Virus,* ed S Gard, C Hallauer, KF Meyer, New York: Springer-Verlag, 1971

198 POLIOMYELITIS

LOUIS WEINSTEIN

DEFINITION Poliomyelitis is a common acute viral infection which occurs naturally only in human beings and produces a wide variety of clinical manifestations. In its most severe form, it involves parts of the central nervous system. In most instances, the nervous system is not invaded; infection may take place without apparent illness, or it may result in the production of nonspecific syndromes or in invasion of the nervous system with or without the development of dysfunction.

ETIOLOGY The causative agent of poliomyelitis is an RNA virus of the picorna group, 8 to 30 nm in diameter, pathogenic for humans and primates. Three antigenically distinct types have been defined: type 1 (Brunhilde), type 2 (Lansing), and type 3 (Leon). Cross neutralization is demonstrable in highly immunized experimental animals, but infection in humans with one type does not protect against invasion by another. Poliomyelitis virus grows well in tissue culture.

Under proper conditions, the virus may remain viable in water or sewage for as long as 4 months. It is not killed by ether, Merthiolate, tincture of Zephiran, ethyl alcohol, low concentrations of mercury, oxidizing agents, 2% tincture of iodine, ultraviolet light, or 10-min exposure to a chlorine concentration of 0.05 ppm.

EPIDEMIOLOGY Poliomyelitis is worldwide, but epidemics have been limited to a relatively small number of areas. That infection is much more prevalent than is suggested by the number of clinically recognized cases is proved by the widespread distribution of neutralizing antibody in population groups all over the world. Poliomyelitis occurs with the highest frequency from July through September in the North Temperate Zone, although it may appear as early as April or as late as December. In tropical or subtropical regions, the "season" may be prolonged.

In areas of poor sanitation, most individuals develop

neutralizing antibodies in early childhood, whereas in other localities, the peak of immunity is not reached until fifteen years of age or older. Urban dwellers become immune earlier than those who live in rural areas. In lower-income groups, evidence of contact with poliomyelitis virus appears at a younger age than in individuals whose economic status is good.

PATHOGENESIS Human beings are the sole reservoir of poliomyelitis virus. Carriers with inapparent infection are most important in transmission of the virus. A history of contact with recognized cases is uncommon. Milk was incriminated as the source of infection in one epidemic.

Virus is recoverable from pharyngeal secretions for only a few days but is demonstrable in the feces for several weeks. The intestinal tract is the main source from which virus is disseminated. Therefore, the route of infection, fecal-oral, is the same as that in salmonellosis, shigellosis, and other enteric infections. Large quantities of virus are present in sewage drained from areas in which the infection is present. Poliomyelitis is as communicable as measles or varicella. In the 15-and-under age group, infection, with or without clinical manifestations, occurs in 100 percent of household and 87 percent of daily contacts.

The following sequence of events has been postulated for the pathogenesis of poliomyelitis: (1) The virus enters the body by way of the mouth and begins to multiply in the oropharynx and lower part of the intestinal tract. Virus is present in pharyngeal secretions and stool during the incubation period; it has been demonstrated in the feces as long as 19 days prior to onset of the disease. (2) The phase of "minor illness" (described below) develops in association with the presence of the virus in the blood, throat, and feces; the viremia persists for only a few days until antibodies make their appearance. Virus in the intestinal tract penetrates the lymphatic channels and enters the bloodstream, from which it is disseminated. (3) The final stage is invasion of the nervous system. It has been suggested that the virus enters the nervous system from the blood in the area postrema of the medulla oblongata; it has also been postulated, however, that viral invasion of the nervous system occurs at many points by direct passage of virus from capillaries to neurons. Once the infectious agent has reached the nervous system, it spreads along nerve fibers.

Strains of poliomyelitis virus vary greatly in their ability to invade nervous tissue and to destroy neurons. The early presence of detectable antibody results from multiplication of virus in nonnervous tissue and accounts for the short persistence of the agent in the pharynx and blood, sites in which antibody is demonstrable. The persistence of virus in the nervous system and intestine is probably due to the difficulty which antibody has in reaching these areas.

The most important determinant of human susceptibility to poliomyelitis is serum antibody. Previous inapparent infection and illness without invasion of the nervous system are common. Many children and most adults possess neutralizing antibody for all three types of virus; this probably accounts for the relative infrequency of the disease in older age groups. Infants under six months old rarely get poliomyelitis because immunity is passively transferred from the mother. Babies born to women in the acute phase of poliomyelitis can develop the disease shortly after birth. Among children, males are affected more often than females; the opposite is true in adults. Pregnancy increases the risk of clinically apparent poliomyelitis, and multiparous females are more susceptible than primiparas. The disease is somewhat more frequent in the second than in the first or third trimesters of pregnancy. Menstruation or ovulation appears to heighten susceptibility. Absence of the tonsils and adenoids, regardless of the time of their removal, is associated with a marked increase in incidence of bulbar poliomyelitis. Chilling or physical exertion after invasion by the virus leads to more frequent development of paralytic poliomyelitis, especially in adults.

CLINICAL MANIFESTATIONS The incubation period of poliomyelitis varies from 3 to 35 days; about 80 percent of cases occur 6 to 20 days after contact with the virus. The infection may assume one of four forms: (1) inapparent infection, (2) "minor illness," (3) nonparalytic poliomyelitis, (4) paralytic poliomyelitis.

Inapparent infection The bulk of infection with the virus of poliomyelitis (95 percent) occurs in this form. There are no symptoms, but the virus is present in the pharynx and intestine and probably also in the blood. Type-specific neutralizing antibody usually develops.

"Minor illness" The entire course of poliomyelitis may consist of a nonspecific illness without clinical or laboratory evidence of central nervous system invasion; this is "abortive" poliomyelitis. Three syndromes have been observed: (1) upper respiratory manifestations, consisting of fever of varying degree, pharyngeal discomfort, with or without coryza, and reddening and swelling of the lymphoid tissues of the throat; (2) gastrointestinal disturbances, with nausea, vomiting, diarrhea or constipation, and abdominal discomfort, accompanied by moderate fever; (3) grippelike disease with fever and symptoms resembling influenza. Virus can be demonstrated in the pharynx, feces, and blood in the early stages of these "minor" illnesses. Type-specific neutralizing and complement-fixing antibodies develop during convalescence.

Nonparalytic poliomyelitis Nonparalytic poliomyelitis consists of prodromal manifestations, signs of meningeal irritation, and abnormalities of the spinal fluid. The prodrome is similar to that of the "minor" illnesses and is usually present for several days before the onset of other signs. Stiffness of the neck and back, positive Kernig's sign, and, with severe meningeal irritation, Brudzinski's sign are present. The tripod (patient extends arms behind back with hands on bed for support when sitting up) and Hoyne's signs (head falls back when, with patient in supine position, shoulders are elevated) can be elicited in paralytic or nonparalytic poliomyelitis but are not pathognomonic. The spinal fluid usually contains between 25 and 500 cells, rarely as many as 1,000 to 2,000. Very early in the disease, there is often a preponderance of neutrophils (up to 80 percent); within a few days, however, mononuclear cells predominate. The protein is normal or slightly elevated at the beginning of the illness but may increase to between 50 and 100 mg per 100 ml. The sugar content is normal. These findings are not diagnostic of poliomyelitis. They are also present in all of the entities classified as aseptic meningitis (Chap. 338). The diagnosis of nonparalytic poliomyelitis is impossible on clinical grounds alone, because the signs, symptoms, and laboratory findings are completely nonspecific. Viral and immunologic studies suggest that fewer than 40 percent of patients in whom "nonparalytic poliomyelitis" is diagnosed actually have the disease.

The course of nonparalytic poliomyelitis is benign. Defervescence occurs in 3 to 5 days, but meningeal irritation may persist for 2 weeks. No change in muscle and nerve function is detectable. The white blood cell count may be as high as 15,000 in the early stage of the disease but is usually normal within a week.

Paralytic poliomyelitis The syndrome of paralytic poliomyelitis consists of prodromal manifestations ("minor illness"), signs of meningeal irritation, abnormal spinal fluid, and involvement of motor nerve cells in the spinal cord, brain, or cranial nerve nuclei, resulting in paresis or paralysis of various muscles. Lesions may also be present in parts of the nervous system other than anterior horn cells; the precentral gyrus, the reticular formation in the medulla, the roof nuclei and vermis of the cerebellum, Auerbach's and Meissner's plexuses, and sympathetic ganglions are usually found to be involved in fatal cases. Seldom, however, are there clinical signs pointing to disease of these parts. "Skip" areas are common in spinal paralytic disease; e.g., involvement of the cervical and lumbar cords is often present with no dysfunction of the thoracic portion.

Paralytic poliomyelitis may be subdivided into the following types:

- *I* Spinal
  - *A* Cervical
  - *B* Thoracic
  - *C* Lumbar
  - *D* Any combination of A, B, and C
- *II* Bulbar
  - *A* Upper cranial nerve involvement—III, IV, V, VI, VII, VIII
  - *B* Lower cranial nerve involvement—IX, X, XI, XII
  - *C* Involvement of cardiorespiratory centers
- *III* Bulbospinal
- *IV* Polioencephalitis, paralytic or nonparalytic
  - *A* Diffuse encephalitis
  - *B* Focal encephalitis
  - *C* Cerebellar involvement (?)
  - *D* Bulboencephalitic disease
  - *E* Spinal-encephalitic disease

Prodromal manifestations are often absent in paralytic poliomyelitis. In some cases, the illness is biphasic in character. The disease starts with fever and manifestations of one of the "minor" illnesses. After several days, all symptoms disappear; in 5 or 10 days, there is recrudescence of fever, the development of signs of meningeal irritation, and the appearance of paralysis. The commonest prodromal symptoms in adults are generalized muscle and bone discomfort. In children, upper respiratory tract syndromes are most frequent. The spinal fluid findings in paralytic poliomyelitis are the same as those in the nonparalytic disease. A completely normal spinal fluid may be present initially and, rarely, throughout the entire course of the disease.

SPINAL PARALYTIC POLIOMYELITIS In the early stages of spinal paralytic poliomyelitis, severe cramping pain in the muscles innervated by the affected neurons and hyperesthesia of the overlying skin are present. Muscle "spasm," the exact mechanism of which is not clear, is usually detectable. In some instances, progression of muscle weakness is very slow; in others, it becomes widespread within 48 h. A rapidly ascending paralysis of the Landry type may develop rarely. Age often determines the extent of involvement. In children less than five years old, paresis of one leg is most common. In patients between five and fifteen years of age, weakness of one arm, or paraplegia, is most frequent, while in adults (sixteen to sixty-five years old), quadriplegia is observed most often. Dysfunction of the urinary bladder is ten times more frequent in adults than in children. Paralysis of the muscles of respiration is most common in those over sixteen years of age. Infants under one year of age are subject to very extensive involvement. Among adults, men develop quadriplegia, respiratory paralysis, and loss of bladder function more frequently than do women. Pregnancy does not increase the severity of the disease unless parturition takes place during the acute phase. There is a definite association of inoculation of antigenic materials ("triple vaccine," for example) with involvement of the muscles around the site of injection.

When the cervical cord is involved, there is paresis or paralysis of the muscles of the shoulders, arms, neck, and diaphragm. Very early in the disease, the reflexes in the arms remain lively; they diminish rapidly, however, and are usually absent by the time paralysis has become established. Coarse twitching of the affected muscles is common. There is always danger of respiratory paralysis when the cervical cord is involved; this is related to spread of the infection to the motor nuclei of the phrenic nerves and medulla.

Weakness of the muscles of the chest, upper portion of the abdomen, and spine follows involvement of the thoracic portion of the spinal cord. Difficulty in breathing results from dysfunction of the intercostal and other thoracic muscles. The chest wall may be in "spasm" and may appear rigid despite the presence of only a minor degree of paresis.

Disease of the lumbar portion of the spinal cord produces weakness of the legs and inferior portions of the abdomen and back. Pain, tenderness, "spasm," and twitching herald the oncoming paralysis, and the reflexes are abolished with the development of flaccid paralysis. In adults, complete paraplegia is not infrequent. Paralysis of the urinary bladder, usually temporary, occurs in about one-third of patients over sixteen years of age and is rarely observed in the absence of weakness of the legs.

The abdominal and cremasteric reflexes usually disappear before muscle weakness is marked and may be absent during the entire course of the disease. An extensor plantar response is a rare finding; its persistence is incompatible with poliomyelitis. Hyperesthesia of the skin is frequent, but sensory loss does not occur. Constipation, abdominal cramps, and meteorism are common and are due to ileus resulting from involvement of the autonomic nervous system and weakness of the abdominal muscles. When the disease is severe, sympathetic nervous system disturbances are present: tachycardia, hypertension, abnormal sweating, and cyanosis and coldness of the involved extremities.

Fever in spinal paralytic poliomyelitis is usually present for the first few days of the disease and disappears by lysis. In about 90 percent of cases, there is little or no extension of paralysis after defervescence has been established for 48 h. In about 10 percent, however, noticeable progression of weakness may continue for as long as a week or more.

BULBAR POLIOMYELITIS The incidence of bulbar poliomyelitis differs from one epidemic to another and varies between 6 and 25 percent. About 85 percent of patients subjected to tonsilloadenoidectomy within 30 days of onset of the disease as well as others who have had this operation years before develop the bulbar form of infection. Pure bulbar involvement, without any signs of spinal cord involvement, is commonest in children; adults with bulbar disturbances usually have associated spinal paralysis. The syndromes which develop depend on the area of the brainstem involved, and result from damage to the medulla, pons, and midbrain. Signs and symptoms are produced by (1) dysfunction of the upper cranial nerve nuclei, (2) damage to the lower cranial nerve nuclei, and (3) disturbances of the respiratory and vasomotor regulating centers in the medulla. Combined bulbar and diffuse or focal encephalitis or spinal involvement may occur.

Upper cranial nerve nuclei—III, IV, V, VI, VII, VIII Isolated ocular nerve palsies, total external ophthalmoplegia, pupillary disorders, and Horner's syndrome occur. There may be unilateral or bilateral involvement of the fifth nerve. Paralysis of the seventh cranial nerve is common and usually unilateral; the entire face or only the upper or lower parts may be affected. Disturbances of vestibular function and deafness resulting from damage to the nucleus of the eighth nerve occur infrequently.

Lower cranial nerve nuclei—IX, X, XI, XII Life may be endangered when the muscles of deglutition are paralyzed because of involvement of the nucleus ambiguus. Hoarseness and laryngeal stridor follow weakness or paralysis of the vocal cords. Unilateral or bilateral weakness of the tongue and of the sternocleidomastoid and trapezius muscles may be present. Inability to swallow results in pooling of saliva and food in the pharynx, with obstruction of the airway. Aspiration into the larynx, reflex spasm of the glottis, and abductor paralysis of the vocal cords constitute very serious threats to life. Minor or major pareses of the soft palate and pharyngeal muscles are detectable by a nasal quality of the voice.

Disease of the medullary respiratory center This produces irregularity of the rhythm, depth, and rate of breathing. Respirations are shallow, and as the disease progresses, there are longer and longer periods of apnea until breathing stops completely. The thoracic muscles and diaphragm are not weak, unless spinal involvement is present. Hiccuping is frequent in the early phase of respiratory center dysfunction. Hypoxia, without visible cyanosis, is common and contributes to the intensity of the manifestations. In the late stages, cyanosis, not responsive to oxygen administration is common, and temperature, pulse rate, and blood pressure are elevated. The final event is usually irreversible shock.

The manifestations of involvement of the circulatory regulating center are a cherry-red color of the lips, flushed skin, rapid, irregular pulse, small pulse pressure when the blood pressure is normal, and moderate to severe hypotension. Hyperthermia, cold, mottled, clammy skin, shallow respiration, and anxiety, restlessness, and confusion appear as the circulation becomes progressively impaired.

POLIOENCEPHALITIS Encephalitic symptoms occur as isolated syndromes or together with bulbar or spinal poliomyelitis. The incidence of polioencephalitis is variable. The diffuse form is characterized by confusion, agitation, anxiety with a feeling of impending doom, or somnolence. Quivering and jerking of the facial muscles and extremities, flushing of the face, tremor of the hands, and restless movements occur. Insomnia may be severe. In fatal cases, the confusion is marked and progresses to lethargy and death.

In focal polioencephalitis, there may be clinical evidence of brain damage, or the lesions may be silent and demonstrable only at necropsy. Visual-verbal agnosia, myoclonic jerks, grand mal convulsions, which occasionally persist for a long time after recovery, spastic hemiparesis, ataxia of one arm or leg, and hydrocephalus have been described.

DIAGNOSIS The diagnosis of paralytic poliomyelitis can usually be made on clinical grounds. The outstanding manifestation is rapidly developing lower motor neuron dysfunction resulting in flaccid weakness and hypo- or areflexia. Signs of upper motor neuron disease or decreased sensation are not compatible with poliomyelitis. A number of other forms of encephalitis may present with similar manifestations. The only positive method of establishing the diagnosis of paralytic poliomyelitis is the isolation of the virus from the stool or pharyngeal secretions (spinal cord or brain at necropsy) and the demonstration of a rise in the level of neutralizing antibody to the isolated strain in acute- and convalescent-phase serums. The three type strains maintained in tissue culture may be used for serologic tests. A significant rise in titer of neutralizing antibody against a specific serotype is diagnostic.

COMPLICATIONS Complications occur most frequently when the respiratory muscles are involved. Disturbances in water and electrolyte balance are common in patients receiving continuous artificial respiration. Fever and sweating especially during the summer months, together with vomiting, diarrhea, inability to take food, and disturbances in blood gases may produce severe chemical disturbances. Edema and hyponatremia often follow overenthusiastic hydration. *Myocarditis,* probably the result of viral invasion of the heart, is not uncommon in poliomyelitis. Changes in the ECG, mainly T and ST-T and P-R abnormalities, are present in from 10 to 20 percent of cases. Interstitial infiltration of the myocardium with round cells, and mild muscle changes are not infrequent. Cardiomyopathy has been thought to be responsible for death in some cases. *Hypertension* may develop by two mechanisms: (1) transient elevation of blood pressure due to hypoxia, and (2) persistent hypertension secondary to hypothalamic involvement, which may become "malignant" and lead to retinopathy, convulsions, and mental deterioration.

Pulmonary edema and *shock,* the exact pathogenesis of which is not known, are usually the terminal events in fatal cases of poliomyelitis. Although relatively young adults are involved, phlebothrombosis of the legs with or without pulmonary embolism is not uncommon. Acute and severe dilatation of the stomach and large intestine, perforation of the cecum, acute ulceration of the duodenum, stomach, and esophagus, and multiple erosions of the entire gastrointestinal tract with considerable bleeding and paralytic ileus have been observed. Marked depression of prothrombin, with massive spontaneous hemorrhage, may result from the administration of large doses of broad-spectrum antibiotics orally. Severe bulbar (ninth and tenth cranial nerves) or bulbospinal disease with paralysis of the respiratory muscles is accompanied by the risk of atelectasis. Pneumonia is quite common in patients with paralysis of the muscles of respiration or deglutition. Its incidence is greatly increased by tracheostomy. The organisms involved most often are *Staphylococcus aureus* and gram-negative bacilli, many strains of which are not sensitive to the commonly used antimicrobial agents. Chemoprophylaxis is of no value in preventing secondary bronchopulmonary bacterial invasion.

A common site of infection in poliomyelitis is the urinary tract; this is usually related to the presence of an indwelling urethral catheter; chemoprophylaxis, even when given together with tidal drainage, is usually ineffective. Renal lithiasis, with infection, is common and is due to immobility, with mobilization of calcium. Liberal administration of fluids, decreased calcium intake, acidification of the urine, administration of salicylate, and early mobilization may reduce the incidence of stone formation.

A syndrome resembling rheumatoid arthritis, with redness, swelling, pain, and tenderness of the larger joints, may occur in the convalescent phase of paralytic poliomyelitis. Markedly paralyzed patients, especially those whose life is threatened by respiratory difficulty, frequently experience very difficult emotional problems. Disorientation, acute panic states, Korsakoff-like syndromes, and acute psychoses have been noted. Chronic anxiety and depression are almost universal in adults with severe disease, and probably reflect the sudden impact of a crippling disease, rather than brain damage due to viral invasion.

IMMUNITY One attack of poliomyelitis usually confers lifelong immunity against the same serotype. Both neutralizing and complement-fixing antibodies appear early in the disease; the latter persist for several years after infection, while the former persist throughout life. Theoretically, an individual could develop three episodes of the disease, because immunity is strictly type-specific. Most adults and many children have poliomyelitis, without nervous system invasion, two or three times, as shown by the presence in their serums of neutralizing antibody for more than one virus type. There are, however, well-documented instances of two episodes of paralyzing infection separated by a number of years in the same individual.

TREATMENT Cases of abortive poliomyelitis require no therapy. The management of nonparalytic poliomyelitis involves primarily the relief of the headache, pain in the back, and "spasm" of the legs. Rest in bed with the mattress supported by a board is helpful in reducing the back discomfort. The application of wet heat, in the form of "hot packs," to the affected muscles produces considerable relief. Analgesics such as meperidine and codeine are very useful and are preferable to morphine derivatives. Antimicrobial agents are useless, because they have no effect on the primary disease and do not decrease the risk of secondary infection. Neuromuscular examination should not be carried out more often than every 3 to 4 days. Bed rest is terminated as soon as severe discomfort is absent, in order to reduce the risk of phlebothrombosis and pulmonary embolism. Every patient thought to have nonparalytic poliomyelitis should have careful assessment of muscle function for 2 to 3 months after recovery. The purpose of this is to detect and correct minor degrees of weakness which may become apparent only when muscles which appear normal at rest are taxed by the exertion of normal physical activity.

The treatment of paralytic poliomyelitis involves (1) the use of all measures to spare the life of the patient threatened by involvement of vital areas, (2) relief of discomfort, (3) maintenance of weak muscles in as good a condition as possible, (4) immediate recognition and treatment of medical complications, (5) prophylaxis and therapy of emotional disorders, (6) surgical treatment of correctable defects, and (7) social, economic, occupational, and physical rehabilitation.

Patients with paralysis of swallowing or respiratory muscles, pulmonary edema, or shock are in great danger of death. Dysfunction of the ninth and tenth cranial nerves is most important because of the danger of fatal airway obstruction. For this reason, it has been suggested that tracheostomy be performed in all such cases. However, this procedure is followed by a much higher incidence of bronchopulmonary infections due to organisms difficult to eradicate with antibiotic agents than occurs when the procedure is not carried out. In some cases, nevertheless, tracheostomy becomes necessary, despite the risks. The indications for this operation are (1) abductor paralysis of the vocal cords; (2) pneumonia with inability to clear the lungs of exudate; (3) repeated bouts of major atelectasis requiring tracheal catheterization or bronchoscopy; (4) inability to keep the airway relatively free of secretions (this is often purely a matter of availability of experienced personnel).

Decreased function of the diaphragms or intercostal muscles necessitates frequent determination of vital capacity. When this is reduced to 50 percent of normal or less, respiratory assistance devices must be used (Chap. 268). An electrophrenic respirator is indicated when the respiratory center is involved.

Shock is easier to prevent than to treat. Assurance of adequate oxygen saturation, prevention of dehydration, and early treatment of superimposed bacterial infection are of prophylactic value. When marked hypotension and clinical evidence of shock develop, treatment is similar to that employed in other situations in which infection is responsible for the syndrome (Chap. 129). However, treatment may not be effective because of failure of the neurologic control of blood pressure and oxygen perfusion. Hypotension appearing during artificial respiration may respond to alternating positive and negative tank pressures of approximately the same magnitude.

Relief of discomfort is the same as for nonparalytic disease. Changing the position of paralyzed limbs and moving the patient about in bed are effective in reducing pain.

Weak muscles must be maintained in as good condition as possible until neural function returns; the time, degree, and extent of resumption of function are unpredictable, but treatment should be continued for at least 2 years. Daily physiotherapy is usually started 3 to 4 days after complete defervescence, and when extension of weakness has ceased.

The prevention and treatment of the emotional disorders which accompany severe paralytic poliomyelitis are often best carried out by the attending physicians and nurses. Although the help of the psychiatrist is necessary in difficult situations, the physicians, nurses, and attendants who are in constant contact with the patient and are properly oriented toward his problems should play the major role.

Maximal return of muscle function usually is established at the end of 2 years following the onset of paralysis. If there is a considerable degree of residual paralysis after this time, a program of surgical rehabilitation should be initiated.

The impact of paralytic poliomyelitis on the social and economic status of adults is often very severe. Every effort must be made to enlist the cooperation of social service agencies to minimize the disruptive effects of the disease. Many patients require occupational rehabilitation because of inability to perform the work in which they were engaged prior to being crippled. For others, the use of devices such as movable splints, hooks, etc., is very helpful in physical rehabilitation.

PROGNOSIS The overall mortality rate for poliomyelitis is about 5 percent. Patients with abortive or nonparalytic disease recover completely. About 2 to 5 percent of children and 15 to 30 percent of adults (increasing with age) with paralyzing infection die. When bulbospinal involvement, especially with medullary or phrenic and intercostal nerve dysfunction, is present, the fatality rate varies between 25 to 75 percent; in these cases, it is greatly influenced by age and the presence of shock, pulmonary edema, superimposed infection, or other medical complications.

Many persons with paralytic poliomyelitis recover completely, and in most of them muscle function returns to some degree. Only a few remain totally paralyzed. The more life-threatening the disease in the acute stage, the more frequent is complete functional recovery, if the patient survives; paralysis of the respiratory center usually disappears completely. Similarly, dysfunction of the ninth and tenth cranial nerves is followed by total recovery in most instances, although mild palatopharyngeal weakness may occasionally persist for life. Paralysis of the muscles of respiration often disappears completely, and in most cases the final vital capacity is adequate to maintain ventilation. In a very few instances chronic respirator care is necessary. Weak extremities regain about 60 percent of the total strength that they will ever recover in 3 months, and 80 percent within 6 months, but improvement may continue for as long as 2 years.

PREVENTION Because 90 to 95 percent of cases of poliomyelitis are inapparent, or "minor" infections, and are not diagnosed, the prevention of the disease by isolation is very difficult. The common practice of isolating patients with clinically evident cases is of much greater individual than public health benefit. The usual period of isolation is about 2 weeks, although virus may be present in the feces for a much longer period. Contact with persons known to have poliomyelitis should be avoided. Restriction of community activities such as swimming, gathering of people, etc., is not indicated except with large epidemics, when it is more effective in allaying panic than in reducing infection. Pregnant women should take special precaution because of the increased susceptibility to the disease during pregnancy. Tonsillectomy is contraindicated in areas where poliomyelitis is present. All individuals with "minor" illnesses during the poliomyelitis season should limit their physical activity and avoid chilling until all symptoms have disappeared.

Active immunization against paralytic poliomyelitis has been successfully produced by parenteral administration of Formalin-inactivated strains of the three viral serotypes grown in monkey kidney tissue culture. The vaccine is 60 to 70 percent effective against type 1 and 85 to 90 percent against types 2 and 3. A booster dose should be given within 2 years after the initial injection series. The effectiveness of this type of vaccine is evidenced by the fact that, in the year (1955) in which it was introduced, there were 28,985 cases of poliomyelitis in the United States. Two years later, only 2,218 cases were reported. However, this vaccine does not appear to decrease the incidence of nonparalytic poliomyelitis and has no effect on the intestinal phase of the disease. It has been practically completely replaced by "live vaccines."

Oral administration of attenuated strains of poliovirus is highly effective in stimulating antibody production and preventing infection and is the method of choice for protecting a population. The virus preparations are easily handled and are stable. They may be stored in a conventional refrigerator for up to 30 days. Once a vial has been used in part, the rest of its contents should be discarded after 7 days.

Vaccine virus multiplies in the intestinal tract and remains at this site. Viremia occurs rarely, and then only with some strains. Live vaccine virus spreads and infects contacts of vaccinated individuals. This type of immunization in the presence of epidemic poliomyelitis may lead to replacement of the "wild" paralytogenic strain by the one in the vaccine, actually aborting spread of the disease.

Significant levels of antibody develop in 90 to 100 percent of persons receiving live virus vaccine; they develop more rapidly and persist longer than those which follow the use of Formalinized vaccines. Intestinal immunity is present after feeding of the "live" preparations so that minimal or no multiplication in the intestine occurs on exposure to "wild" strains of virus.

The highest levels of poliomyelitis-neutralizing antibody appear when monovalent oral vaccines are administered. The recommended order of administration is type 1, followed after no less than 8 weeks by type 3, and at 6 or more weeks later by type 2. If the polyvalent vaccine (all three types) is given to adults, two doses are fed 8 weeks apart. If newborns are given vaccine, the viruses should be refed at a later date, because about 50 percent of neonates fail to develop significant levels of immunity if treated shortly after birth. Immunization of breast-fed infants is best delayed until they are taking regular diets. It has been suggested that a community-wide program of vaccine virus feeding followed by routine immunization of infants in the first year of life may result in eradication of poliomyelitis. Immunization with live vaccine is best carried out during the colder months of the year. The widespread prevalence of other enteroviruses in the intestinal tract, especially in children, in the summer may result in a low level of immunization because these other viruses may interfere with the implantation of the vaccine strains. Although the necessity for "booster" doses of this preparation in older children and adults has not been proved, many physicians are administering the triple vaccine 1 to 2 years after primary immunization; some are giving a second "booster" 1 to 2 years after the first.

The administration of live poliomyelitis virus vaccines to millions of persons in many areas of the world has demonstrated very convincingly the very high degree of protection (over 90 percent) against paralytic poliomyelitis conferred by this preparation and a tendency for epidemic strains to be replaced by those present in the vaccine. The vaccines are remarkably safe. Although instances of the disease are thought to have been associated with feeding of each of the three strains (0.4 cases per million doses for type 3; 0.16 per million doses for type 1; and 0.02 per million doses for type 2), it has been suggested that the greatest risk of production of active disease by the vaccine strain is related to the administration of the type 3 preparation to individuals in the age range of twenty to thirty-nine years. Some observers have pointed out that firm proof of the association of vaccine virus and the development of poliomyelitis is lacking. Type 1 vaccine strain has been incriminated in a case of paralytic poliomyelitis in a young child with marked hypogammaglobulinemia. Children known to have this defect probably should not receive this agent.

The incidence of paralytic poliomyelitis has been reduced in the United States to the point that only 22 cases, three of which were fatal, were recognized in 1972. Four of the patients were infected by strains present in the vaccine that they had received; in six others, the vaccine virus was acquired from contacts who had been immunized by the oral route. That this favorable state may not be maintained for very long is suggested by data that there are presently an appreciable number of persons, especially members of the disadvantaged groups, who have never been immunized against poliomyelitis. In addition, in some who have received oral vaccine, especially the polyvalent preparation, neutralizing antibody for any of the viral types has failed to appear or, when present, has decreased considerably in titer over a period of 2 to 5 years, especially against types 1 and 3. The exact status of immunity against poliomyelitis of the American population is unknown at present; therefore, longitudinal surveillance as well as continuation of an active program of immunization is mandatory. It is probably best, at this time, to give "booster" doses of oral vaccine to those who have received it previously, especially if the Formalin-treated or polyvalent oral preparations were given initially. It is of greater importance to find all individuals, especially children, who have never been immunized and to make sure that they receive the vaccines. Primary immunization of this type is best carried

out using the monovalent vaccines, followed 1 or 2 years later by oral administration of the polyvalent vaccine.

REFERENCES

HENDERSON DA et al: Paralytic disease associated with oral polio vaccines. JAMA 190:41, 1964

SABIN AB: Commentary on report on oral poliomyelitis vaccines, JAMA 190:52, 1964

——: Poliomyelitis. Accomplishments of live virus vaccine. First international conference on vaccines against viral and rickettsial diseases. Bull WHO 171, 1967

SPECIAL ADVISORY COMMITTEE TO THE SURGEON GENERAL: Oral poliomyelitis vaccines. JAMA 190:49, 1964

Symposium on poliomyelitis. Pediatr Clin North Am 1:1, 1953

WEINSTEIN L: Diagnosis and treatment of poliomyelitis. Med Clin North Am September: 1377, 1948

——: The influence of muscular fatigue, tonsilladenoidectomy and antigen injections on the clinical course of poliomyelitis. Boston Med Q 3:11, 1952

——: Influence of age and sex on susceptibility and clinical manifestations in poliomyelitis. N Engl J Med 254:47, 1957

——: Cardiovascular disturbances in poliomyelitis. Circulation 15:735, 1957

——: Poliomyelitis—a persistent problem. N Engl J Med 288:369, 1973

199 RABIES

ROBERT H. RUBIN

DEFINITION Rabies is an acute viral disease of the central nervous system that affects all mammals and is transmitted from one to another by infected secretions, usually saliva, or tissue. The common mode of transmission is by the bite of an infected animal, but on occasion a virus aerosol or the ingestion of infected tissues may also initiate the disease process.

ETIOLOGY The rabies virus is a bullet-shaped RNA virus belonging to the rhabdovirus group, with a diameter of 750 to 800 Å and varying lengths. Excrescences, 60 to 70 Å long, each with a knoblike structure at the distal end, cover the surface of the virion. These surface structures elicit neutralizing and hemagglutination-inhibiting antibodies, while a nucleocapsid antigen induces a complement-fixing antibody. Following immunization or active infection a third group of antibodies is elicited, which, together with complement, reacts with surface membranes of infected cells to produce lysis and cell death. Whereas the first two classes of antibody appear to correlate with protection against the disease, the third may have an important injurious effect. Only one serologic type of rabies virus has been identified, but multiple passages of the virus through animals or tissue culture can change tissue infectivity. Interferon is induced by rabies virus, particularly in those tissues with high virus concentrations, and may play some role in retarding progressive infection.

EPIDEMIOLOGY Rabies exists in two epidemiologic forms: *urban,* propagated chiefly in unimmunized domestic dogs, and *sylvatic,* propagated in skunks, foxes, raccoons, mongooses, wolves, and bats. Infection in domestic animals usually represents a "spillover" from sylvatic reservoirs of infection, and human beings can be infected by either. Hence, human infection tends to occur in locales where rabies is enzootic or epizootic, where there is a large population of unimmunized domestic animals, and where human contact with the outdoors is common. Approximately one thousand human cases are reported to the World Health Organization each year, with many times that number believed to go unreported. Southeast Asia, the Philippines, Africa, and the Indian subcontinent are areas with an especially great problem. In contrast, the United States has noted less than three cases per year for more than a decade.

In most areas of the world the dog is the important vector of rabies virus, but the wolf (Eastern Europe, Arctic regions), the mongoose (South Africa, the Caribbean), the fox (Western Europe), and the vampire bat (Latin America) have an even greater impact in some places. In the United States, in recent years, the skunk has been the most important source of human disease, with raccoons, bats, and unimmunized dogs and cats also playing a role. These species come into close proximity with human populations, are quite aggressive when ill, and tend to have quite high titers of virus in their saliva. Aerosol transmission of the disease has occurred as a laboratory accident, and, in nature, in the unique ecologic conditions of the bat caves of Texas.

PATHOGENESIS The essential first event is the introduction of live virus into intimate contact with nerve tissue. Virus may persist here for up to 96 h, with initial replication within myocytes at the site of inoculation. It then spreads centripetally up the nerve to the central nervous system, probably via peripheral nerve axoplasm. Experimentally, viremia has been shown to occur, but it is not thought to play a role in naturally acquired disease. Once the virus reaches the central nervous system, it replicates almost exclusively within the gray matter, and then passes centrifugally along autonomic nerves to reach other tissues—the salivary glands, adrenal medulla, kidney, lung, liver, skeletal muscle, skin, and heart. Passage to the salivary glands allows for further transmission of the disease via infected saliva. The amount of time this process takes is exceedingly variable, with incubation periods of 10 days to 1 year (mean, 1 to 2 months). This time period appears to depend more upon the amount of virus introduced, the type of tissue and tissue injury involved, and host defense mechanisms than the actual distance from site of inoculation to central nervous system that the virus has to travel.

The important point about the neuropathology of rabies is that it resembles that of any other viral encephalitis. These nonspecific findings include hyperemia; varying degrees of chromatolysis, nuclear pyknosis, and neuronophagia of the nerve cells; infiltration by lymphocytes and plasma cells of the Virchow-Robin spaces; and parenchymal areas of nerve cell destruction. The pathognomonic lesion of rabies is the Negri body, which is an eosinophilic mass approximately 10 mm in size, found in relatively undamaged nerve cells and distributed particularly in Ammon's horn, cerebral cortex, medulla, and the Purkinje cells of the cerebellum. The Negri body is a site of virus replication. Failure to find the Negri body on light microscopy of brain material from at least 20 percent of rabies victims has been correlated with a higher degree of cellular damage and degeneration than is present in cells that show the characteristic structures. The absence of Negri bodies does not rule out the diagnosis of rabies.

MANIFESTATIONS The clinical manifestations of rabies can be divided into three stages: a nonspecific prodrome; an encephalitis similar to other viral encephalitides; and a profound dysfunction of brainstem centers. It is this last which causes the classic features of rabies encephalitis.

The prodromal period usually persists for 1 to 4 days and is marked by fever as high as 102°F, headache, malaise, increased fatigability, anorexia, nausea and vomiting, sore throat, and a nonproductive cough. Characteristically, there are paresthesias at or about the site of inoculation of the virus in over 80 percent of patients during this period.

The encephalitic phase is usually ushered in by periods of excessive motor activity, excitation, and agitation. Quickly, confusion, hallucinations, combativeness, bizarre aberrations of thought, muscle spasms, meningismus, opisthotonic posturing, seizures, and focal paralysis appear. Characteristically, the periods of mental aberration are interspersed with completely lucid periods, but as the disease progresses, the lucid periods get shorter until the patient lapses into coma. Hyperesthesia, with sensitivity to bright light, loud noise, touch, and even gentle breezes, is very common. On physical examination the temperature may be found to be as high as 105°F. Abnormalities of the autonomic nervous system, with dilated, irregular pupils, increased lacrimation, salivation, and perspiration, and postural hypotension may be seen. Evidence of upper motor neuron paralysis with weakness, increased deep tendon reflexes, and extensor plantar responses is the rule. Paralysis of the vocal cords is common.

The manifestations of brainstem dysfunction begin shortly after the onset of the encephalitic phase. Cranial nerve involvement causes diplopia, facial palsies, optic neuritis, and the characteristic difficulty with deglutition. The combination of excessive salivation and difficulty in swallowing produces the traditional picture of "foaming at the mouth." The first manifestation of difficult swallowing is usually painful spasms of the muscles of deglutition, rapidly progressing to frank paralysis. If the patient is still lucid during this period, he avoids swallowing water and manifests classic hydrophobia. From this point the patient quickly lapses into coma, and involvement of the respiratory centers produces an apneic death. The prominence of early brainstem dysfunction distinguishes rabies from other viral encephalitides and accounts for the rapid downhill course. The median survival after the onset of symptoms is 4 days, with a maximum of 20, unless artificial supporting measures are instituted.

An atypical form of rabies, resembling the Landry-Guillain-Barré syndrome, has been described and has been especially correlated with illness occurring after the bite of the vampire bat.

LABORATORY FINDINGS The hematocrit reading and findings on urinalysis and routine blood chemistry tests are usually normal. Typically the white blood cell count is moderately elevated (12,000 to 17,000 per mm^3), but may be normal or as high as 30,000. The electrocardiogram may show evidence of a myocarditis. Cerebrospinal fluid findings include normal pressures, a few hundred cells (usually less than 100) with a predominance of lymphocytes, a normal sugar level, and a moderately increased protein level (60 to 85 mg per 100 ml). Virus has rarely been isolated from the cerebrospinal fluid, but not uncommonly from saliva.

Specific diagnosis of rabies depends on either serologic testing or examination of brain material. If the patient has not received antirabies immunization, then a greater than fourfold change in neutralizing antibody titer in serial specimens, as in any viral disease, is diagnostic of rabies. If the patient has received antirabies immunization, a clue to the diagnosis of rabies may be the absolute titer of neutralizing antibody found; immunization rarely produces titers greater than 1:5,000. Recently, fluorescent antibody staining of skin biopsies, corneal impression smears, and saliva has been done in living patients, and may be useful in diagnosing rabies during life. At this point, however, definitive diagnosis depends upon examination of brain material.

Samples of brain, obtained either on postmortem examination or from brain biopsy, are tested in three ways: special histologic staining for Negri bodies, fluorescent antibody staining for viral antigen, and mouse inoculation tests. If any one of these is positive, a definitive diagnosis can be made. Negri body tests have an incidence of 20 percent false negatives. Mouse inoculation tests and fluorescent antibody staining are quite reliable in the usual case of rabies, but if the patient's life is prolonged for a long period of time, "auto-sterilization" may occur and these tests become negative.

DIFFERENTIAL DIAGNOSIS There is little to distinguish rabies from other viral encephalitides, and the most helpful point in diagnosis is the history of exposure. Other problems to be considered include hysterical reactions to animal bites (pseudohydrophobia), Landry-Guillain-Barré syndrome, poliomyelitis, and allergic encephalomyelitis to rabies vaccine. The latter condition occurs most commonly after use of nerve tissue–derived vaccine, and usually begins 1 to 4 weeks after vaccination.

PREVENTION AND TREATMENT Approximately thirty thousand persons in the United States and approximately one million in the world are given postexposure therapy for rabies each year. The general principle in postexposure therapy is to minimize the amount of virus at the site of inoculation with local wound treatment, and then to have as high a titer of neutralizing antibody present as early and as long as possible. To this end, the following therapeutic regimen is presently employed:

1. *Local wound therapy* with generous scrubbing with soap and then flushing of the wound with water or ethyl alcohol, removing all vestiges of the soap. This is followed by a second scrubbing with a quaternary ammonium compound such as 1 to 2% benzalkonium chloride (Zephiran) or 1% cetrimonium bromide (Cetavlon). Lacerations should not be sutured primarily.
2. *Active immunization* with either nerve tissue–derived vaccine (NTV) or duck embryo–derived vaccine (DEV). When vaccine is given alone 14 daily doses is sufficient; when vaccine is given with antiserum, 21 daily injections of 1 ml vaccine subcutaneously, followed by boosters 10 and 20 days after the initial series, is required.
3. *Passive immunization* with antirabies antiserum of either equine or human origin. The latter is preferred when available, because of the absence of the adverse reactions seen with the equine product. Fifty percent of the dose (20 units per kg for the human product, 40 units per kg for the equine) is given by local infiltration of the wound, and the rest intramuscularly.

In the future the availability of more potent vaccines and the possible employment of interferon or interferon inducers may improve on this currently recommended regimen.

The critical problem with antirabies treatment is the reactions to therapy. Because of the exceedingly rare occurrence of severe neurologic reactions when DEV is used, this is the vaccine favored by the United States Public Health Service (USPHS). Less serious reactions seen with DEV include the following: rare anaphylaxis, occasional gastrointestinal upset, and very common (up to 50 percent) local skin reactions with or without adenopathy, fever, chills, and myalgias. Treatment of such reactions is symptomatic, with salicylates and antihistamines. Life-threatening neurologic reactions should be treated with steroids, but the use of steroids must be tempered by the awareness that they interfere with immunologic defenses and may activate latent rabies infection.

Although the therapy of a bona fide rabies exposure is relatively simple, the major difficulty is in deciding whether therapy is indicated. Table 199-1 presents the guidelines suggested by the USPHS. In making this decision, the following questions should be asked: What was the nature of

TABLE 199-1
Antirabies postexposure prophylaxis guide of the Advisory Committee on Immunization Practices of the United States Public Health Service*

		Treatment†	
Species	*Condition at time of attack*	*For bite*	*For nonbite exposure*
WILD			
Skunk	Regard as rabid	S,V,1	S,V,1
Fox	Regard as rabid	S,V,1	S,V,1
Raccoon	Regard as rabid	S,V,1	S,V,1
Bat	Regard as rabid	S,V,1	S,V,1
DOMESTIC			
Dog	Healthy	None,2	None,2
	Escaped (unknown)	S,V	V 3
Cat	Rabid	S,V,1	S, V, 1
Other		Consider individually	

* *The recommendations are only a guide. They should be used in conjunction with knowledge of the animal species involved, circumstances of the bite or other exposure, vaccination status of the animal, and presence of rabies in the region.*
† V *indicates rabies vaccine;* S, *antirabies serum;* 1, *discontinue vaccine if fluorescent antibody tests of animal killed at time of attack are negative;* 2, *begin serum and vaccine at first sign of rabies in biting dog or cat during holding period (10 days);* 3, *14 doses of duck embryo vaccine.*

the exposure? Was the attack provoked or unprovoked? What is the status of animal rabies in the locale where the exposure took place? What is the immunization status of the animal involved? What species inflicted the injury? Is the animal available for examination? What is the state of health of the animal? Most animals can transmit rabies virus in their saliva only a few days before becoming ill, although bats may do so for months. Bites of wild animals, especially skunks, foxes, raccoons, and bats, should always be regarded as highly suspect and should be dealt with as significant exposures, unless examination of the brain tissues of the animal in question fails to demonstrate the presence of rabies virus.

The availability of the relatively safe DEV has permitted the initiation of preexposure therapy for individuals with a high risk of contact with rabies virus: veterinarians, spelunkers, laboratory workers, animal handlers, etc. Such preexposure therapy consists of two 1-ml subcutaneous injections of DEV given 1 month apart, followed by a 1-ml booster 7 months later. At the completion of the three-shot series a neutralizing antibody titer should be checked through the state health department.

Until recently, rabies in humans had been regarded as being 100 percent fatal. However, since abortive rabies infection with full recovery was recognized in animals, and since neuropathologic changes from the virus itself are relatively minor, it was suggested that survival might be possible if prolonged intensive cardiorespiratory assistance were employed to counteract brainstem dysfunction. There has now been a human survivor of clinical rabies as a result of this mode of therapy. For the first time in history there is now hope in this dreaded disease.

REFERENCES

COREY L et al: Treatment of persons exposed to rabies. JAMA 232:272, 1975

DEBBIE JG: Rabies. Prog Med Virol 18:241, 1974

HATTWICK MA et al: Recovery from rabies: A case report. Ann Intern Med 76:931, 1972

RUBIN RH et al: Adverse reactions to duck embryo vaccine. Ann Intern Med 78:643, 1973

WHO EXPERT COMMITTEE ON RABIES: Sixth Report, WHO Tech Rep Ser 523, 1973

200
DISEASES CAUSED BY SLOW VIRUSES

DONALD H. HARTER

Slow virus diseases are characterized by a long asymptomatic period, often on the order of months or years, between the introduction of the infectious agent and the appearance of clinical illness.

The factors responsible for this protracted incubation period have not been defined. Viruses causing slow infections do not appear to have any unique or common features, and the slowness of the disease may be due in large measure to the manner in which the host reacts or accommodates to the virus.

Some slow viruses provoke a conventional inflammatory response during the time they are clinically silent; others are able to reside within cells for long periods without causing detectable cytopathic changes. The role of immunity in slow virus infection is largely unknown. Some slow virus infections occur in the presence of elevated levels of circulating antibodies; in others, there may be no detectable immune response.

In animals, slow viruses are known to produce a variety of pulmonary, hepatic, renal, and neurologic disorders. At present, there are only five definitely identified slow virus infections of human beings. These are five infrequently encountered neurologic diseases: *kuru, Creutzfeldt-Jakob disease, progressive multifocal leukoencephalopathy, subacute sclerosing panencephalitis,* and *progressive rubella encephalitis.* Kuru and Creutzfeldt-Jakob disease share common neuropathologic features and are referred to as the *subacute spongiform virus encephalopathies.* Although these diseases have been shown to be of infectious etiology by the transmission of neurologic illness to higher primates, the causative agents are still incompletely characterized. Viruses have been recovered from the nervous system of patients with subacute sclerosing panencephalitis, progressive multifocal leukoencephalopathy, and progressive rubella encephalitis, but the pathogenesis of these disorders is still largely unknown. At present, there is no consistently effective therapy for any of the five diseases.

KURU Kuru, or "trembling with fear," is a progressive and fatal neurologic disorder which occurs exclusively among natives of the New Guinea Highland.

Difficulty in walking is usually the first sign of kuru. This usually progresses from a minor disturbance in gait rhythm to marked side-to-side lurching and staggering. Eventually, ambulation becomes incoordinated, and the patient is unable to use his limbs. As the disease progresses, cerebellar involvement (intention tremor, inability to perform rapid alternating movements, slurring of speech, hypotonia), abnormal involuntary movements resembling myoclonus, athetosis, or chorea, and convergent strabismus appear. There are no blood or cerebrospinal fluid abnormalities. Dementia develops in the later phases of the disease. The illness terminates fatally in 4 to 24 months, usually from decubitus ulcers or bronchopneumonia. Approximately 80 percent of adults afflicted with the disease are women.

Pathologic changes are limited to the central nervous system and include widespread neuronal loss, intense astrocytic and microglial proliferation, loss of myelinated fibers, and the presence of plaque-like bodies. Perivascular cuffing by lymphocytes and mononuclear cells has been observed occasionally.

It was the close similarity between the neuropathologic and clinical findings found in kuru and in scrapie, a slow infectious disease to sheep, that suggested the possibility that kuru was caused by a virus or other infectious agent. The infectious origin of kuru was confirmed subsequently by the appearance of a kuru-like syndrome in chimpanzees 14 to 38 months after intracerebral inoculation of suspensions of brain from human cases. Disease has also been produced in chimpanzees by inoculation of tissues other than brain. The clinical illness in chimpanzees lasts 3 to 11 months. The disease has also been successfully transmitted to a number of New World and Old World monkeys. Although a number of known and novel viruses have been recovered from tissue explants prepared from chimpanzees with the kuru syndrome, the specific agent responsible for the disease has not been fully characterized.

Cannibalism has been considered as a possible mode of transmission of kuru. Native custom in New Guinea dictates that marrow, viscera, and brain be cooked and eaten. The marked predilection of kuru for the adult female may be explained by the observation that cannibalism appears more prevalent among women and that males who practice cannibalism seldom eat the bodies of women. The recent influx of foreign settlers into the kuru area has led to increasing rejection of cannibalistic practices, and this, in turn, may be responsible for the progressive decline in the number of cases of kuru since 1960. Oral feeding of kuru brain to chimpanzees has not yet been reported to produce disease.

CREUTZFELDT-JAKOB DISEASE Creutzfeldt-Jakob disease is a fatal degenerative disease of the central nervous system which afflicts persons between forty and sixty years of age and presents as a rapidly evolving dementia with myoclonic seizures. Unlike kuru, the disease is not geographically limited.

Although Creutzfeldt-Jakob disease may have a diverse clinical presentation, it is usually first manifested by organic mental changes similar to those seen in the presenile dementias. The earliest changes include impairment of reasoning and judgment, memory disturbances, and bizarre behavior. The patient may complain of distortions in the shape and appearance of objects. Hallucinations, delusional ideas, and confusion occur as the disease progresses, and myoclonic movements and convulsive episodes develop. Ataxia, dysarthria, muscular atrophy, and other signs of anterior horn cell damage may be noted in some cases. Spasticity and rigidity appear later. The disease progresses rapidly to death within 3 to 12 months, often from intercurrent infection. There are no abnormalities in the cerebrospinal fluid, but the electroencephalogram is usually abnormal.

The cerebrum and cerebellum are affected predominantly. Widespread status spongiosus in gray matter and intense gliosis are seen. Vacuoles are located within the neuropil, within and around neurons. There is a marked proliferation of astrocytes and disappearance of nerve cells. Inflammatory changes are absent. In the spinal cord, anterior horn cells may be damaged or lost, and there may be degeneration of the corticospinal tracts.

A neurologic disease with the clinical and pathologic features of Creutzfeldt-Jakob disease occurs in chimpanzees 10 to 14 months after inoculation with brain suspensions from patients with Creutzfeldt-Jakob disease. The duration of the chimpanzee's illness varies from 1 to 3 months. It is also possible to transmit the disease to monkeys and the domestic cat. The agent persists for many months in tissue cultures of human brain cells without loss of virulence. Neutralizing antibodies to the Creutzfeldt-Jakob agent have not yet been demonstrated in the serums of patients with the disease or of primates with the experimental disease.

PROGRESSIVE MULTIFOCAL LEUKOENCEPHALOPATHY
This rare neurologic condition, first described in 1958, usually occurs in patients who have leukemia, malignant lymphomas, carcinomatosis, or a variety of other chronic disease processes. The disease is consistently associated with disorders of cell-mediated immunity in which deficits in humoral antibody response may or may not coexist.

The disease affects adults of both sexes, and its duration from onset of symptoms to death is 1 to 4 months. The neurologic signs and symptoms show diffuse, asymmetric involvement of the cerebral hemispheres. Hemiplegia, hemianopsia, aphasia or dysarthria, and organic mental changes are frequent, and complete or incomplete transverse myelitis may develop. Headache and convulsive seizures are rare, but electroencephalographic abnormalities consisting of diffuse or focal abnormalities are often present. Cerebrospinal fluid is normal in most cases.

The pathologic changes consist of multiple areas of demyelination with little or no perivascular infiltration. The presence of distinctive intranuclear inclusions in oligodendrocytes first suggested that the disease was of a viral etiology. Electron microscopic observations show the intranuclear inclusion bodies to be composed of closely packed spheres, which have the physical dimensions and properties of the polyomavirus genus of the papovaviruses.

By employing tissue cultures derived from human fetal brain it has been possible to recover a new human polyomavirus serotype (JC virus) from the brains of patients with progressive multifocal leukoencephalopathy. Abundant numbers of virus particles are present in brain, and some patients with the disease have antibodies directed against the virus recovered from their brain. Rapid identification of the virus in brain is possible using fluorescence antibody staining or electron microscopic agglutination with monospecific hyperimmune rabbit serum. Serologic diagnosis using the patient's serum is unreliable.

The virus has not been demonstrated in tissues other than brain; the disease has not been transmitted to animals.

Progressive multifocal leukoencephalopathy may result from the activation of a polyomavirus which has been latent in brain or other tissues since childhood infection. Alternatively, there may be certain individuals who fail to acquire immunity in childhood and have their first encounter with the virus when a disease which interferes with cell-mediated immunity develops. The demyelination which occurs may be related to virus-induced damage of oligodendroglia, cells which appear to be required for the normal maintenance of myelin.

SUBACUTE SCLEROSING PANENCEPHALITIS (INCLUSION-BODY ENCEPHALITIS) This progressively fatal disease of children and adolescents has been suspected to be of viral origin since its initial description by Dawson in 1932. Measles virus or a virus very closely related to measles virus has been recovered from the brains of patients with the disease. The disorder may be considered to be a "slow" form of measles encephalitis.

Subacute sclerosing panencephalitis occurs between four and twenty years of age; 80 percent of patients are under eleven. The disease affects boys three to ten times as frequently as girls. Most patients are from rural areas or small towns. They are entirely well until the disease begins. Onset is usually insidious, and mental deterioration, often expressed by a decline in the patient's schoolwork, is the presenting symptom. Incoordination, ataxia, and myoclonic jerks develop along with abnormalities of the pyramidal and extrapryamidal motor systems. Cortical blindness, papilledema, and optic atrophy may be present, and focal chorioretinitis has been described.

The patient becomes bedridden within 6 to 9 months. Death occurs from superimposed pulmonary or urinary tract infections or from decubiti. Signs of meningeal irritation do not occur.

The cerebrospinal fluid gamma-globulin level, as determined by electrophoresis, quantitative immunochemical assay, or colloidal gold curve, is elevated, but the fluid is otherwise normal. The electroencephalogram typically shows a "burst suppression" pattern characterized by synchronous and symmetric spike and high-voltage slow wave activity. Elevated levels of measles antibody are found in serum and cerebrospinal fluid. Brain biopsy may be required to make a definitive antemortem diagnosis.

Pathologic findings include round-cell infiltration about small cerebral arteries and veins, intranuclear and intracytoplasmic inclusions in neurons and glial cells, and varying degrees of demyelination.

Measles virus is now considered to be the etiologic agent. Electron microscopic studies show that the intranuclear inclusions in brain cells are composed of hollow tubular filaments resembling paramyxovirus internal nucleocapsid component. Staining of brain tissue from patients with the disease demonstrates measles virus antigen in the inclusions. An agent serologically identical to measles virus and having measles virus properties has been recovered from brain by cocultivating cell cultures originated from brain tissue with established laboratory cell lines.

Attempts to transmit the disease to animals have met with variable results. Ferrets inoculated with suspensions of brain from patients with the disease develop a nonfatal neurologic disorder with electroencephalographic changes.

Subacute sclerosing panencephalitis appears many years after the patient's initial experience with rubeola. There is evidence that subacute sclerosing panencephalitis patients have clinical measles at an unusually early age. A few reported cases may have been related to measles vaccination. The disorder appears to represent an unusual response of the nervous system to measles infection. It is possible that the virus is present in a defective form or that a carrier state is produced wherein cells may continue to elaborate intracellular viral antigen without producing detectable amounts of mature infective virus. One can speculate that similar virus-cell interactions may be important in the development of other diseases of the central nervous system such as parkinsonism and multiple sclerosis.

PROGRESSIVE RUBELLA ENCEPHALITIS A chronic progressive encephalitis developing in the second decade of life and sharing some of the features of subacute sclerosing panencephalitis has been described in patients with congenital rubella.

Deterioration of mental and motor functions begins after a stable period of 10 or more years. The cerebrospinal fluid has an increased cell count and the protein and IgG levels are elevated. High titers of antibody to rubella virus can be detected in both serum and cerebrospinal fluid. Rubella virus has been recovered from the brain by use of the cocultivation technique.

Unlike subacute sclerosing panencephalitis, patients with rubella panencephalitis have the stigmata of congenital rubella before the onset of progressive disease. Myoclonus is less constant, and the electroencephalogram does not show the "burst suppression" observed in subacute sclerosing panencephalitis. Histologic examination of the brain shows mineralization, but not the inclusion bodies characteristically found in subacute sclerosing panencephalitis.

The progressive rubella encephalitis also resembles the rare cases of juvenile paresis which may occur in patients with congenital syphilis. The immune status of patients with this disorder has not been fully defined, and the pathogenesis of the disease remains obscure.

REFERENCES

FREEMAN JM: The clinical spectrum and early diagnosis of Dawson's encephalitis. J Pediatr 75:590, 1969

FUCILLO DA et al: Slow virus diseases. Ann Rev Microbiol 28:231, 1974

GIBBS CJ JR, GAJDUSEK DC: Experimental subacute spongiform virus encephalopathies in primates and other laboratory animals. Science 182:67, 1973

JABBOUR JT et al: Epidemiology of subacute sclerosing panencephalitis (SSPE): A report of the SSPE registry. JAMA 220:959, 1972

LAMPERT PW et al: Subacute spongiform virus encephalopathies. Scrapie, kuru and Creutzfeldt-Jakob disease: A review. Am J Pathol 68:626, 1972

MEULEN V TER et al: Subacute sclerosing panencephalitis: A review. Curr Top Microbiol Immunol 57:1, 1972

NARAYAN O et al: Etiology of progressive multifocal leukoencephalopathy: Identification of papovavirus. N Engl J Med 289:1278, 1973

RICHARDSON EP: Progressive multifocal leukoencephalopathy. N Engl J Med 265:815, 1961

ROOS P et al: The clinical characteristics of transmissible Creutzfeldt-Jakob disease. Brain 96:1, 1973

WEIL ML et al: Chronic progressive panencephalitis due to rubella virus simulating subacute sclerosing panencephalitis. N Engl J Med 292:994, 1975

ZURHEIN GM: Association of papova-virions with a human demyelinating disease (progressive multifocal leukoencephalopathy). Prog Med Virol 11:185, 1969

201 MEASLES (RUBEOLA)

C. GEORGE RAY

DEFINITION Measles, or rubeola, is an acute febrile eruption which has been one of the most common diseases of civilization. With the development of effective prophylactic measures it should become a rarity.

HISTORY Measles probably was not a significant problem before the building of large cities. Rhazes wrote about it in the tenth century, and Sydenham in the seventeenth century wrote a full account of the disease and differentiated it from other exanthems. In 1905 measles was transmitted by the blood of infected persons to human volunteers and in 1911 to monkeys by both blood and nasopharyngeal secretions that had previously been passed through bacteria-retaining filters. In 1954, Enders and Peebles obtained an agent from patients with measles that produced cytopathic changes in cell cultures. This achievement allowed the investigation of the characteristics of the measles virus and of the pathogenesis of the disease, with subsequent development of diagnostic and prophylactic measures.

ETIOLOGY The measles virion is composed of a central core of ribonucleic acid with a helically arranged protein coat surrounded by a lipoprotein envelope with small, spike-like structures. The virion is 120 to 250 nm in diameter, and is classified as a paramyxovirus.

The measles virus is isolated most easily from infected persons in the first 4 or 5 days of illness, by utilizing primary cell cultures of monkey or human kidney, although primary isolations have been accomplished by using cells from human amnion or chorion or dog kidney. After several passages, the virus can be propagated on a number of types of cell cultures, including chick embryo cells, upon which many of the vaccine strains are grown.

Measles virus infection of cells in culture results in the formation of multinucleated giant cells, many with eosinophilic intranuclear and intracytoplasmic inclusions.

EPIDEMIOLOGY Measles occurs naturally only in human beings, although infection with the virus can be demonstrated in laboratory colonies of monkeys exposed to infected individuals. Before active immunization was available, epidemics of measles occurred in 2- to 3-year cycles, and about 95 percent of town and city dwellers developed the disease before the age of fifteen years. The virus is transmitted by transfer of nasopharyngeal secretions, either directly or in airborne droplets, to the respiratory mucous membranes or conjunctivas of susceptible individuals. Persons infected with the virus may transmit the disease during a period which extends from 5 days after exposure until 5 days after skin lesions have appeared. The virus is highly contagious, with secondary attack rates among susceptible household contacts usually exceeding 90 percent; asymptomatic primary infections are rare. Measles is a disease of childhood in populous areas, but may occur at any age in remote isolated communities if the disease is introduced. Infants are uncommonly affected under the age of six to eight months, presumably because of the persistence of maternal antibody acquired by transplacental transmission.

PATHOGENESIS AND PATHOLOGY It is probable that, after infection, measles virus multiplies in the epithelium of the respiratory tract and is disseminated by way of the blood to distant sites. For a few days before the rash appears, and for 1 or 2 days after, the virus can be isolated from blood or washed white blood cells, conjunctiva, lymphoid tissue, and respiratory mucous membranes and secretions. The virus can be obtained from urine for as long as 4 days after the onset of the eruption.

The mucous membrane lesions (Koplik's spots) consist of vesicle formation and epithelial necrosis. Histology of the Koplik's spots reveals cytoplasmic and intranuclear inclusions, giant cells, and intercellular edema. Electron microscopy of the Koplik's spots and skin lesions has demonstrated microtubular aggregates which are thought to be the measles virus, and suggests that both the exanthem and enanthem are associated with local viral replication. Large multinucleated epithelial giant cells can be found during the prodrome and acute stages of illness in the buccal mucosa, pharynx, tracheobronchial mucosa, and occasionally in the urine. In addition, reticuloendothelial giant cells (Warthin-Finkeldey cells) are found in hyperplastic lymphoid tissues, including lymph nodes, tonsils, spleen, and thymus. An unusually high number of white blood cells from patients with the disease contain broken chromosomes. The epithelium of the respiratory passages may become necrotic and slough, leading to secondary bacterial infection; in addition, interstitial pneumonia with giant-cell infiltration may be observed. Changes in the brain of patients with encephalitis resemble those seen in other postviral encephalitides and consist of focal hemorrhage, congestion, and perivenous demyelination.

MANIFESTATIONS The time from exposure to the development of the first symptoms of measles infection is usually 9 to 11 days, and from exposure to the appearance of rash is about 2 weeks. The initial manifestations of the disease are malaise, irritability, fever as high as 105°F, conjunctivitis with excessive lacrimation, edema of the eyelids and photophobia, moderately severe hacking cough, and nasal discharge. The prodromal period usually lasts 3 to 4 days, with a range of 1 to 8 days before the onset of a rash. Koplik's spots—small, red, irregular lesions with blue-white centers—appear 1 or 2 days before the onset of the rash on the mucous membranes of the mouth and occasionally on the conjunctiva or intestinal mucosa. The findings of the prodromal illness subside or disappear within 1 or 2 days after the appearance of skin lesions, although the cough may persist throughout the course of the disease.

The red maculopapular rash of measles breaks out first on the forehead, spreads downward over the face, neck, and trunk, and appears on the feet on the third day. The density of lesions is greatest on the forehead, face, and shoulders, where coalescence of individual spots usually occurs. The lesions in each area persist for about 3 days and disappear in the same order in which they appeared, resulting in total duration of rash of about 6 days. As the maculopapules fade, a brown discoloration of the skin may be noticed, and finely granular desquamation may occur. In adults the duration of fever may be longer, the rash more prominent, and the incidence of complications higher.

The course of measles can be altered by the administration of gamma-globulin soon after exposure. The incubation period may be prolonged for as long as 20 days. The prodromal period of the modified disease may be shorter, the fever, respiratory symptoms, and conjunctivitis milder, and the rash less marked; Koplik's spots may not be present. An atypical, severe form of measles is seen in some persons who received inactivated measles vaccine several years before exposure. The prodromal period with prominent fever, headache, myalgias, and abdominal symptoms lasts for 2 or 3 days and is followed by an eruption of maculopapules, vesicles, and petechiae. In contrast to natural measles, the rash begins on the feet and progresses toward the head and is especially prominent on the legs and in the body creases. Peripheral edema and pneumonia have been prevalent in this form of atypical measles. The pneumonia is lobar or segmental; hilar lymphadenopathy and pleural effusion are frequent. Ill-defined nodular shadows may persist at the periphery of the lung for as long as 1 to 2 years.

COMPLICATIONS Measles, usually a benign self-limited disease, may be associated with a number of complicating illnesses. Viral involvement of the respiratory tract may lead to croup, bronchitis, bronchiolitis, or rarely to *interstitial giant-cell pneumonia,* which is seen most often in children suffering from severe systemic disease such as leukemia or congenitial immunodeficiency and which is characterized by severe respiratory symptoms, pulmonary infiltrations, and the presence in the lungs of multinucleated giant cells. It may occur in the absence of the typical measles exanthem. *Conjunctivitis,* which is seen regularly in the course of uncomplicated measles, may occasionally progress to permanent corneal ulceration, keratitis, and blindness. *Myocarditis,* characterized by transient changes in the electrocardiogram, occurs in about 20 percent of patients with measles, but clinical evidence of cardiac dysfunction is rare. Viral involvement of the mesenteric lymph nodes and appendix may result in abdominal pain and signs of peritoneal inflammation so severe that surgical exploration is considered. The situation is especially confusing if the evidence of appendiceal involvement becomes manifest during the preeruptive phase of the disease. Measles infection of pregnant women results in death of the fetus in about 20 percent of the cases; however, a teratogenic effect such as that observed in rubella has not been demonstrated.

Superimposed bacterial pneumonia caused by streptococci, pneumococci, staphylococci, or *Hemophilus influenzae* is considerably more common than giant-cell pneumonia and occasionally may progress to formation of empyema or lung abscess. Bacterial otitis media is a frequent sequel of measles infection in children. In tropical areas, stomatitis, probably of bacterial origin, progressing to cancrum oris may be encountered during the course of the disease.

In addition to conditions associated with the viral infection and the complications resulting from superimposed bacterial infection, several situations may arise after measles infection which are of uncertain pathogenesis. Clinically apparent *encephalomyelitis* occurs in 1 of 1,000 patients with measles. It usually begins 4 to 7 days after the appearance of the eruption, but may precede the rash by 10 days or follow it by 24 days. It is characterized by high fever, headache, drowsiness, and coma, and in some patients by focal brain or spinal cord involvement. Death occurs in about 10 percent of affected individuals, and persistent signs of central nervous system damage, including mental changes, epilepsy, and paralysis, are encountered. Electroencephalographic abnormalities without other signs of central nervous system dysfunction may be demonstrated in 50 percent of patients with otherwise uncomplicated measles. Though it is generally postulated that the encephalomyelitis is "postinfectious" or allergic in origin, a recent report of isolation of the virus from the brain of a patient with a fatal case suggests direct viral invasion of the central nervous system. Other, more unusual neurologic complications include transverse myelitis and ascending myelitis. An extremely rare condition, *subacute sclerosing panencephalitis* (Chap. 200), is now thought to be a late complication of measles. *Thrombocytopenia* may occur 3 to 15 days after the onset of the rash and results in purpura as well as bleeding from mouth, intestine, and genitourinary tract. Measles is also associated with transient suppression of delayed hypersensitivity to tuberculin, exacerbation of existing tuberculosis, and an increased incidence of new tuberculous infections.

LABORATORY FINDINGS Leukopenia is frequent in the prodromal phase of measles, and the appearance of leukocytosis suggests bacterial superinfection or another complication. During the prodrome and in the early eruptive phase, multinucleated giant cells can be identified in stained preparations of sputum, nasal secretions, or urine, and the measles virus can be isolated by inoculation of the same materials into appropriate cell cultures. Complement fixation, neutralization, and hemagglutination-inhibition tests are available for serologic confirmation of measles. Spinal fluid protein of patients with encephalomyelitis ranges from 48 to 240 mg per ml, and lymphocyte counts are usually in a range of 5 to 99 per mm^3, although counts as high as 1,000 per mm^3 have been reported. Bacterial infection can be identified by appropriate cultures.

DIFFERENTIAL DIAGNOSIS Measles, with its prodrome, Koplik's spots, and characteristic rash, is infrequently confused with other diseases. Rubella is a milder disease of shorter duration with mild respiratory complaints or none at all. Infectious mononucleosis and toxoplasmosis can be identified by the presence of atypical lymphocytes and by serologic tests. Secondary syphilis may display skin lesions similar to the measles rash. Other infections which can sometimes mimic measles include those caused by adenoviruses, enteroviruses, *Mycoplasma pneumoniae,* and *Streptococcus pyogenes,* e.g., scarlet fever. Drug reactions, particularly those associated with ampicillin and Dilantin, can also produce a morbilliform rash. The atypical form of measles in patients previously immunized with inactivated vaccine may suggest Rocky Mountain spotted fever.

PROPHYLAXIS Measles can be prevented by the administration of 0.25 ml per kg gamma-globulin within 5 days of exposure. Passive immunization should be considered for any susceptible person exposed to the disease, but is especially important for children under three years of age, for pregnant women, for patients with tuberculosis, and for those patients in whom immune mechanisms are impaired. A modified, less severe form of the disease which results in some degree of active immunity may be observed if 0.04 ml per kg gamma-globulin is given within 5 days of exposure (see Manifestations, above). Prophylactic administration of antibiotics does not decrease the frequency or severity of bacterial superinfections.

Active immunity can be induced by the use of live, attenuated measles virus without spread to contacts of vaccinated individuals. Further attenuated vaccine strains (Schwarz, Attenuvax) derived from additional chick cell culture passages of the original Edmonston B strains are currently recommended, are associated with few local or systemic reactions, and are administered without gamma-globulin. Vaccination with these preparations induces antibody formation in more than 95 percent of susceptible individuals. Vaccination results in protection for at least 8 years, but the total duration of immunity is not known. Live measles vaccine should not be given to pregnant women, to patients with untreated tuberculosis, to patients with leukemia or lymphoma, or to those who are receiving therapy which depresses immune response. Though adverse effects have not been observed in egg-sensitive patients, the vaccine should be used with caution in such individuals, or the use of a vaccine produced in dog kidney rather than chick cells should be considered. Except in unusual circumstances, vaccination should not be given in the first 12 months of life. However, if epidemiologic circumstances suggest a risk to infants in the six- to twelve-month age group, the vaccine may be used, and a second dose administered at fourteen to eighteen months of age to ensure adequate seroconversion. The vaccine seems equally effective when administered alone or simultaneously in combination with rubella and mumps vaccines. Measles vaccination has been very effective in decreasing the incidence of measles in the United States without producing serious side effects. Measles occurs almost exclusively among the unvaccinated, who, for the most part, are members of low socioeconomic groups. The disease rarely occurs in those who have been vaccinated, although there have been vaccine failures. These failures are related, in part, to early vaccination of infants who still have maternal neutralizing antibody or to the use of improperly stored vaccine.

There is no indication for the use of *inactivated* vaccine because of severe atypical measles which has been observed in persons immunized with it (see Manifestations, above).

TREATMENT No therapy is indicated for uncomplicated measles. Gamma-globulin, although effective in prophylaxis, is of no value once symptoms are evident. Patients should be monitored for the development of bacterial superinfections, with specific antibiotic selection based on clinical and bacteriologic findings.

REFERENCES

CHERRY JD et al: Urban measles in the vaccine era: A clinical, epidemiologic and serologic study. J Pediatr 81:217, 1972

ENDERS JF, PEEBLES T: Propagation in tissue cultures of cyto-

pathogenic agents from patients with measles. Proc Soc Exp Biol Med 86:277, 1954

KRUGMAN S: Present status of measles and rubella immunization in the United States: A medical progress report. J Pediatr 78:1, 1971

MEULEN V et al: Isolation of infectious measles virus in measles encephalitis. Lancet 2:1172, 1972

WITTE JJ: The epidemiology and control of measles. Am J Epidemiol 100:77, 1974

202
RUBELLA ("GERMAN MEASLES")

C. GEORGE RAY

DEFINITION Rubella ("German measles," "3-day measles") is usually a benign febrile exanthem, but when it occurs in pregnant women, it may lead to serious chronic fetal infection and malformations.

ETIOLOGY In the late 1930s and 1940s rubella was transmitted to humans and monkeys, and in 1962 a viral agent was recovered in cell cultures inoculated with nasopharyngeal secretions of infected persons. Human primary amnion cells infected with rubella virus display rounding, clumping of nuclear chromatin, and eosinophilic intranuclear inclusions. Rabbit kidney and some other cell lines also display cytopathic effects. Rubella virus can be detected indirectly in African green monkey kidney cells by the interference or exclusion method. In this system, cells infected with rubella appear normal but are resistant to superinfection with viruses such as echo 11 or Coxsackie A-9 that ordinarily produce a cytopathic effect in these cells. Complement-fixing antigen and a hemagglutinin have been identified.

The rubella virion, 50 to 85 nm in diameter, is a somewhat spheroidal RNA virus which has been tentatively classified in the togavirus family.

PATHOGENESIS AND PATHOLOGY Rubella can be induced in susceptible persons by the instillation of virus into the nasopharynx, and natural infection is probably induced in the same way. Virus is present in blood, throat washings, and occasionally feces for several days before the exanthem becomes apparent. It can be detected in blood for 1 or 2 days, and in throat washings for as long as 7 days before appearance of rash, to 2 weeks after onset. Lymph nodes show edema and hyperplasia.

Congenital rubella results from transplacental transmission of virus to the fetus from an infected mother, and may be associated with growth retardation, infiltration of liver and spleen by hematopoietic tissue, interstitial pneumonia, decreased number of megakaryocytes in the bone marrow, and various structural malformations of the cardiovascular and central nervous systems. The virus can persist in the fetus during intrauterine life and may be excreted for 6 to 31 months after birth.

EPIDEMIOLOGY Rubella is not as contagious as measles, and immunity to the disease is not so widespread. Estimates of susceptibility to rubella among women of childbearing age range from 10 to 25 percent. Prior to the routine introduction of vaccine in 1969, epidemics occurred at 6- to 9-year intervals; however, it is not known as yet whether this cyclical pattern will continue in the future. In 1964 more than 1.8 million cases of rubella were reported in the United States; in 1973, 27,901 cases were reported in this country. Rubella is most frequent among children five to nine years of age, but with the advent of immunization programs often directed primarily at this age group as well as at preschoolers, a greater proportion of cases is now being reported among older school children and young adults.

MANIFESTATIONS The time from exposure to the appearance of the rash of rubella is 14 to 21 days, usually about 18 days. In adults there may be a prodromal illness preceding the exanthem by 1 to 7 days and consisting of malaise, headache, fever, mild conjunctivitis, and lymphadenopathy. In children the rash may be the first manifestation of disease. It is apparent from serologic studies that rubella infection may be associated with no signs or symptoms, or may result in lymph node enlargement without skin lesions; however, rash without lymphadenopathy is uncommon. Respiratory symptoms are mild or absent. Small, red lesions (Forchheimer's spots) occasionally may be seen on the soft palate but are not pathognomonic of the disease.

The rash begins on the forehead and face and spreads downward to the trunk and extremities. The small maculopapular lesions, of lighter hue than those of measles, are usually discrete but may coalesce to form a diffuse erythema suggestive of scarlet fever. The rash may last from 1 to 5 days, but is most commonly present for 3 days. Enlarged, tender lymph nodes appear before the rash, are most impressive during the early eruptive phase, and may persist several days after the rash has disappeared. Splenomegaly or generalized lymphadenopathy may occur, but the postauricular and suboccipital nodes are most strikingly involved. Arthralgias and slight joint swellings may be a complication of rubella, especially in young women. The pain and swelling, usually in the small joints, are most marked during the period of rash and may persist for 1 to 14 days after other manifestations of rubella have disappeared. Recurring joint symptoms for a year or more have also been reported. Purpura with or without thrombocytopenia may occur and may be associated with hemorrhage. Encephalomyelitis following rubella resembles other postinfectious encephalitides and is much less common than encephalitis following measles.

Congenital rubella The syndrome of congenital rubella has conventionally been thought to consist of heart malformations—patent ductus arteriosus, interventricular septal defect, or pulmonic stenosis; eye lesions—corneal clouding, cataracts, chorioretinitis, and microphthalmia; microcephaly, mental retardation, and deafness. In the American epidemic of 1964, thrombocytopenic purpura, hepatosplenomegaly, intrauterine growth retardation, interstitial pneumonia, myocarditis or myocardial necrosis, and metaphyseal bone lesions were encountered frequently in association with the previously recognized manifestations, leading to the term *expanded rubella syndrome.* Some infants have also been found to have significant humoral and/or cellular immunodeficiency, which generally resolves as chronic viral excretion diminishes and eventually ceases. Any combination of lesions may be seen in an individual infant, and the severity is highly variable.

Later complications include an apparent higher risk of subsequent development of diabetes mellitus. In addition, there are reports of patients with congenital rubella who develop a progressive, subacute panencephalitis, with onset in the second decade of life. This is characterized by intellectual deterioration, ataxia, seizures, and spasticity.

Congenital rubella is usually the result of maternal infection during the first trimester of pregnancy, although well-documented cases have resulted from infection several days prior to conception; deafness may occur as a result of infection in the fourth month. In the 1964 epidemic, about 10 percent of women with clinically recognized rubella during the first trimester gave birth to infants with the rubella syndrome. Serologically identified, asymptomatic maternal rubella can also result in severe fetal disease. If exposure of a pregnant woman occurs in the first trimester, serum rubella antibody titers should be obtained immediately and 2 or 3 weeks later. The combination of determinations may allow the detection of seroconversion occurring in subclinical infection, aid in the diagnosis of rubella if an exanthematous disease develops, or suggest infection in the past, with immunity to the agent.

DIAGNOSIS Rubella is frequently confused with other diseases associated with maculopapular exanthems such as those described in Chap. 203, and with infectious mononucleosis (Chap. 209), as well as with drug eruptions and scarlet fever. *A certain diagnosis of rubella can be made only by virus isolation and identification, or by changes in antibody titers.* Rubella hemagglutination-inhibiting antibodies may be present by the second day of rash and increase in quantity over the next 10 to 21 days. Patients with the congenital rubella syndrome may lose hemagglutination-inhibiting antibodies at age three or four years. Therefore a negative serologic test in a child over three years does not exclude the possibility of congenital rubella. There are no other laboratory findings helpful in the diagnosis of rubella, although lymphocytosis with atypical lymphocytes may occur. Congenital rubella should be differentiated by appropriate serologic tests from congenital syphilis, toxoplasmosis, and cytomegalic inclusion virus disease.

PREVENTION In adults and children rubella is usually a mild disease with infrequent complications. However, the severity of congenital infection has prompted efforts to prevent the disease. Administration of gamma-globulin to exposed persons can abort the clinical disease, but seroconversion and transmission of the disease from mother to fetus may occur despite the administration of large amounts of gamma-globulin soon after exposure.

Active immunization with live attenuated rubella vaccines prepared in duck, dog, rabbit, or human diploid fibroblast cells has been practiced in this country since 1969, especially among young children. The aim has been to decrease the frequency of the infection in the population, thus decreasing the chance that susceptible pregnant women will be exposed. Because of concern for a possibly enlarging pool of susceptible adolescents and adults, there has been increasing enthusiasm for serologic screening of females with no history of immunization, followed by selective immunization of those who are seronegative. Such immunization must of course be done with appropriate precautions, as noted below.

The attenuated virus can be detected in the respiratory secretions of vaccinees for as long as 4 weeks after immunization, but transmission to other susceptible individuals almost never occurs. This has not been shown to be a problem, even in households where susceptible pregnant women are in contact with children who are being vaccinated. The vaccine induces antibodies in about 95 percent of recipients, but the degree and duration of protection are still being evaluated. After heavy exposure in closed populations, vaccinated individuals sometimes develop subclinical infections (diagnosed by antibody rises and virus isolation). However, viremia has not been demonstrated in immunized persons, which suggests that previously vaccinated pregnant women will not infect their fetuses even if they acquire subclinical rubella.

Side effects of fever, rash, lymphadenopathy, polyneuropathy, or joint pains occur very seldom in vaccinated children, but joint pain and swelling were seen in more than 25 percent of women who were immunized with the earlier available vaccines. The risk has been considerably reduced with the advent of vaccines prepared in rabbit or human embryonic fibroblast cell cultures. The joint symptoms may begin as long as 2 months after vaccination, and they may be confused with other forms of arthritis. *Rubella vaccine must never be given to pregnant women or to those who may become pregnant within 2 months of immunization.* This precaution is necessary because the vaccine virus may have the potential to damage the fetus of susceptible women.

REFERENCES

COOPER LZ et al: Loss of rubella hemagglutination inhibition antibody in congenital rubella. Am J Dis Child 122:397, 1971

FLEET WF et al: Gestational exposure to rubella vaccines: A population surveillance study. Am J Epidemiol 101:220, 1975

HORSTMANN D: Rubella: The challenge of its control. J Infect Dis 123:640, 1971

MODLIN JF et al: A review of five years' experience with rubella vaccine in the United States. Pediatrics 55:20, 1975

PLOTKIN SA et al: Immunologic properties of RA 27/3 rubella virus vaccine. JAMA 225:585, 1973

SEVER JL et al: Rubella epidemic, 1964: Effect on 6,000 pregnancies. Am J Dis Child 110:395, 1965

TOWNSEND JJ et al: Progressive rubella panencephalitis: Late onset after congenital rubella. N Engl J Med 292:990, 1975

WEIL ML et al: Chronic progressive panencephalitis due to rubella virus simulating SSPE. N Engl J Med 292:994, 1975

203 OTHER VIRAL EXANTHEMATOUS DISEASES

C. GEORGE RAY

In addition to the diseases such as measles, rubella, and chickenpox which historically have been associated with prominent skin lesions, there are other virus infections in which skin manifestations may occur. Table 203-1 lists the other more commonly recognized causes of maculopapular eruptions. Some of them, particularly the enteroviruses, can also occasionally cause papulovesicular or petechial rashes; others are capable of provoking erythema multiforme–like eruptions. One helpful aspect of the physical examination is the observation that viral-caused maculopapular (not vesicular) exanthems usually *relatively* spare the palms and soles. This is in contrast to eruptions associated with drug reactions, bacteria, *Mycoplasma,* and *Rickettsia,* in which a prominent palmar or plantar eruption is often noted.

EXANTHEM SUBITUM (ROSEOLA INFANTUM) Exanthem subitum is a benign disease of infants six to twenty-four months of age that is characterized by a high fever and rash. The disease can be transmitted to humans and monkeys by the transfer of blood obtained from a patient during the first few days of illness. The infectious agent is probably a virus, although it has not been isolated. The first manifestations of disease, after an estimated incubation period of 5 to 15 days, are the abrupt onset of irritability and fever, which lasts for 3 to 5 days; the temperature may be as high as 105°F. There may be mild pharyngitis and slight lymph node enlargement; convulsions may occur during the height of the fever. On the fourth to fifth day of illness, there is a sudden drop in temperature to normal or below normal; several hours before or after defervescence the rash suddenly and surprisingly appears. It is characterized by faint 2- to 3-mm macules or maculopapules over the neck and trunk and may extend to the thighs and buttocks; it may last for only a few hours or may be present for a day or two. Leukopenia is frequently noted later in the febrile period. The disease is benign and not associated with complications, although occasionally an infant may show sequelae as a result of febrile convulsions.

TABLE 203-1
Causes of maculopapular eruptions

Viral	*Other*
Measles	*Mycoplasma pneumoniae*
Rubella	Syphilis
Exanthem subitum	Typhoid fever
Erythema infectiosum	Bacterial toxins--streptococci and staphylococci
Enteroviruses—Coxsackie, echo	Rat-bite fever
Infectious mononucleosis	*Rickettsia*
Adenoviruses	Live-virus vaccines
Reoviruses	Drug eruptions
Arboviruses	

In the early, preeruptive phase, the disease may be difficult to differentiate from an acute, occult bacteremia, particularly from one associated with *Streptococcus pneumoniae.* Though a leukocytosis with an increase in band forms is often seen in occult bacteremias presenting in this fashion, blood cultures are necessary to aid in precise diagnosis.

ERYTHEMA INFECTIOSUM (FIFTH DISEASE) Erythema infectiosum is a mild febrile exanthematous disease without a prodrome. The incubation period is probably 5 to 10 days. The first manifestations are low-grade fever and the appearance of indurated, confluent erythema over the cheeks, giving a "slapped face" appearance. A day or so later, a bilaterally symmetric eruption is seen on the arms, legs, and trunk, but rarely on the palms or soles. The lesions are maculopapular and tend to be confluent, forming slightly raised blotchy areas and reticular or lacy patterns. The rash usually lasts about a week, and during this time it may disappear, only to reappear in the same areas a few hours later. The waxing and waning eruption may occasionally persist for several weeks, and can be brought on by fever, heat, exercise, sunlight exposure, or emotional stress. Mild joint pain and swelling have been observed in a large proportion of adults with the disease. Erythema infectiosum affects all ages but is most common in children of school age and may occur in epidemic form. The mode of transmission of the disease is not known, and an infectious agent has not been recovered. A clinical diagnosis of this disease must sometimes be made with caution, since rubella and some enteroviruses have also been shown occasionally to cause a nearly identical syndrome.

ENTEROVIRAL EXANTHEMS Many individual enteroviruses have been associated with rash. Of these, polioviruses are rarely implicated. More commonly, echo virus serotypes 1 through 7, 9, 11, 12, 14, 16, 18, 19, 20, 25, and 30, Coxsackie virus serotypes A-4, 5, 6, 9, 10, 16, and B-2, 3, and 5 have all been implicated. With the exception of hand-foot-and-mouth disease, usually associated with Coxsackie A-16 virus infection (Chap. 193), there is no set of clinical or epidemiologic features that aid in differentiating the specific enteroviral agent involved in a specific case. All are capable of producing maculopapular rashes which vary in intensity and duration, and can also occasionally produce petechial or papulovesicular exanthems and enanthems. In community and household outbreaks, younger children and infants are usually more likely to manifest exanthems, while other features of enteroviral infection, such as fever, myalgia, and aseptic meningitis, are more prominent among older children and young adults. Two enterovirus infections which have been frequently associated with rashes and have been studied extensively are described here as examples of epidemic enteroviral infections.

Boston exanthem (infections with echo virus 16) Echo virus 16 infection was described first and most extensively during an epidemic in Boston in 1951. Children who were infected usually had a disease characterized by exanthem and low-grade fever, while adult family contacts often developed high fever, prostration, and signs of aseptic meningitis with absent or fleeting rash. The first manifestation of the disease in children was fever of 101 to 102°F, lasting for a day or two, pharyngitis with small ulcerated lesions resembling herpangina, and slight enlargement of the cervical and postauricular lymph nodes. The rash appeared during fever or after defervescence and consisted of small pink maculopapules on the face, upper part of the chest, and occasionally on the whole body, including the palms and soles. The rash lasted for 1 to 5 days, and there were no important complications or sequelae. The disease resembled exanthem subitum but occurred in children of all ages and in adults.

Infection with echo virus 9 Infection with this virus in children and adults has been characterized by a febrile illness with a high incidence of aseptic meningitis. The incubation period is 5 to 8 days. About 30 percent of patients have a rash, which may occur with or without meningitis. It is usually maculopapular, developing at the onset of fever. The exanthem appears first on the face and neck, spreads to the trunk and extremities, may involve the palms and soles, although slightly, and persists for 3 to 5 days. Petechiae with or without maculopapules have been recognized; when they are seen in association with meningitis, there may be confusion with meningococcal meningitis. This can be a point of some concern, since concurrent outbreaks of echo virus 9 and meningococcal disease have been observed. A vesicular eruption with crusting lesions has been seen occasionally. An exanthem on the buccal mucosa and soft palate occurs in about 30 percent of patients and consists of small red areas with white centers which resemble Koplik's spots. The disease is usually benign but rarely has been associated with permanent central nervous system damage.

REFERENCES

BALFOUR HH: Erythema infectiosum: Clinical description of 91 cases seen in an epidemic. Clin Pediatr 8:721, 1969

BALFOUR HH et al: Erythema infectiosum: Recovery of rubella virus and echovirus 12. Pediatrics 50:285, 1972

LERNER AM et al: New viral exanthems. N Engl J Med 269:678, 1963

NEVA FA et al: Clinical epidemiological features of unusual epidemic exanthem. JAMA 155:544, 1954

WENNER HA: Virus diseases associated with cutaneous eruptions. Prog Med Virol 16:269, 1973

204
SMALLPOX, VACCINIA, AND COWPOX

C. GEORGE RAY

Poxviruses are a group of large (200 to 320 nm), brick-shaped, DNA-containing viruses that possess a common antigen and have a predilection for skin. Many of the poxviruses, such as myxoma and fowl pox agents, cause disease mainly in lower animals. Smallpox (variola major), alastrim (variola minor), vaccinia, and cowpox agents are closely related members of the poxvirus group that cause human disease. All these viruses grow and produce pox on the chorioallantoic membrane of chick embryos and can be cultivated in cells from various mammalian tissues with formation of intracytoplasmic inclusions, rounding fusion, and heaping up of cells, and eventual degeneration of the infected area. The poxviruses responsible for human disease may be distinguished from one another by minor antigenic differences and by the type and severity of lesions they induce in experimental animals and humans. Smallpox and alastrim viruses produce smaller pox on the chorioallantoic membrane than vaccinia, and there are differences in incubation temperatures at which poxviruses produce lesions.

SMALLPOX (VARIOLA)

DEFINITION Smallpox is a severe, contagious, febrile disease characterized by a vesicular and pustular eruption. Alastrim is a similar but milder illness, with a lower mortality rate. Though the difference in severity between these diseases is apparent, the agents of smallpox and alastrim are biologically and immunologically indistinguishable from each other in the laboratory.

PATHOGENESIS AND PATHOLOGY The virus gains access to the body by the respiratory tract and multiplies in unidentified sites, probably in lymph nodes or liver. After several days, during which there is no evidence of infection, viremia ensues, with swelling of the endothelium of blood vessels in the corium and perivascular inflammation. Loculated vesicles are the result of cellular destruction and exudation of serum. The infected epithelial cells are swollen and contain intracytoplasmic inclusions surrounded by a halo (Guarnieri bodies). The extent of skin involvement is greater in smallpox than in chickenpox and reaches into the corium. Pitting, most commonly seen on the face, is said to result from destruction of sebaceous glands, which are abundant in this area. The liver, spleen, and lymph nodes may be enlarged and may show focal accumulations of large mononuclear cells.

EPIDEMIOLOGY Smallpox is not as contagious as measles or influenza, and ordinarily face-to-face contact with an infected person is required to transmit the disease; however, airborne dissemination from contaminated fomites has also been shown to occur. A patient with smallpox is infectious from a day before the rash appears until all lesions have healed and the scabs have fallen off. During the early phase of the illness, the virus is transmitted in nasopharyngeal secretions; when the eruption is fully formed, the lesions themselves are a major source of infectious material. Variola virus may contaminate clothing, bedding, dust, or other inanimate objects and remain infectious for months, necessitating disinfection of articles in the patient's environment. The World Health Organization's program to eradicate smallpox has resulted in marked decrease in the incidence of the disease since 1966, and the prospects for ultimate eradication seem bright. Two important epidemiologic factors which would suggest that this is possible are the absence of nonhuman reservoir for the virus, and the apparent nonexistence of completely asymptomatic human carriers. Control and the ultimate eradication of the disease, therefore, rely on complete reporting of cases and identification of even very mild ones, as a prelude to specific quarantine and selective immunization. By the end of 1975, endemic smallpox was confined to Ethiopia.

MANIFESTATIONS The incubation period of smallpox, from the time of exposure to the onset of the prodrome, is about 12 days, with extremes of 7 to 17 days. The disease can be divided into a prodrome, an early eruptive phase, and a period of vesiculation and pustule formation. The prodrome is characterized by a temperature of 102 to 106°F, headache, myalgia especially in the back, abdominal pain, vomiting, and in some patients by a transient, blotchy, erythematous eruption. After 3 or 4 days the fever subsides, the symptoms decrease, and the patient seems to recover. It is at this time, when the patient is afebrile, that the focal eruption begins. Early manifestations are painful ulcers on the buccal mucosa and macules which appear first on the face and forearms, and rapidly become firm, shotty papules. The papules increase in number and spread from the face and distal extremities to involve the trunk. The individual lesions may remain discrete and scattered, or they may become confluent and involve most of the body. They are most concentrated on the face and distal extremities, including the palms and soles, and are relatively sparse in the axilla. On the third or fourth day after the appearance of the focal rash, the papules progress to vesicles containing clear fluid, which, over the next few days, becomes cloudy because of infiltration by pus cells and desquamated epithelial cells; hemorrhage into the vesicles and surrounding skin may also be seen. During the course of smallpox, the lesions at any one time, in one area, are all at the same stage of evolution. At the time the vesicles become pustular, there is recurrence of fever, which may persist until healing occurs. The pustules umbilicate and form crusts and scabs which usually fall off 3 weeks after the beginning of illness, leaving small scars or deep pits.

The above description applies to disease of moderate severity. A milder illness may occur in previously immunized persons or in some who have no history of vaccination. It is characterized by the usual incubation period and prodrome, but is followed either by focal eruption of fewer than 100 papules, or by a rash resembling chickenpox. Smallpox with prodrome but with no eruption of any kind has been recognized (variola sine eruptione). The disease may also occur in a rapidly fulminating form ("sledgehammer" smallpox). After the usual incubation period, the patient develops an initial illness characterized by severe prostration, fever, bone marrow depression, hemorrhagic skin lesions, and bleeding. The disease progresses from inception to death within 3 or 4 days without evidence of the typical focal skin lesions.

Alastrim is similar to mild and moderate forms of variola major in that it has the same incubation period and prodromal illness, but the skin eruption is less extensive, and fatalities are rare and usually related to secondary bacterial infections.

COMPLICATIONS Bacterial superinfections of the lesions, usually with *Staphylococcus aureus,* may occur in the late pustular stage. Bacterial pneumonia and sepsis may be seen in severe forms of smallpox. Mild conjunctivitis is quite common, and iritis and keratitis have been recognized. Encephalomyelitis may occur in the late stage of the disease and is similar to other postinfectious encephalitides. Osteomyelitis and joint effusions may complicate the disease, and orchitis has also been reported.

LABORATORY FINDINGS Leukopenia is present during the prodromal illness, and there is usually leukocytosis during the pustular stage. Rapid diagnosis of poxvirus infection can be made by the finding of characteristic brick-shaped particles in preparations of vesicle fluid examined by electron microscopy. Specific precipitation in agar by use of antigen prepared from lesions and antivariola or antivaccinia immune serum may also allow detection of poxvirus within a few hours. These tests do not distinguish variola from vaccinia or other poxviruses but do allow rapid differentiation from herpes simplex and varicella-zoster viruses. For definitive identification the virus must be grown in cell culture or on the chorioallantoic membrane and neutralized with specific antiserum.

DIFFERENTIAL DIAGNOSIS The major problem in differential diagnosis is in distinguishing smallpox from chickenpox. Smallpox is preceded by a longer prodrome than chickenpox, and the eruption vesiculates over a period of days instead of hours. The smallpox lesions are all characteristically in the same stage of development, whereas those of chickenpox may, in one area, display all stages of evolution. Electron microscopy and agar precipitation techniques (see above) are especially useful in distinguishing between smallpox and chickenpox. Cytologic examination of scrapings of the base of a vesicle can also be helpful in the differential diagnosis. The presence of multinucleated giant cells and/or intranuclear inclusions strongly suggests a herpes group infection (varicella-zoster or herpes simplex); such findings are not seen with poxvirus infections.

Other conditions which are sometimes confused with smallpox include eczema vaccinatum, eczema herpeticum, rickettsialpox, drug eruptions, some cases of contact dermatitis, and Stevens-Johnson syndrome. The fulminant, hemorrhagic smallpox may closely resemble meningococcemia, typhus, and hemorrhagic fevers.

PROPHYLAXIS Smallpox may be prevented among the patient's contacts by vaccination. Because this procedure is most successful if carried out during the early part of the incubation period, all exposed persons, regardless of previous immunization, should be vaccinated immediately upon recognition of exposure. Large, controlled, clinical trials have demonstrated that oral administration of N-methylisatin 3-thiosemicarbazone (methisazone), a drug which interferes with poxvirus multiplication, can prevent smallpox and alastrim in patients exposed to these diseases. The use of a drug together with prompt vaccination results in greater chance of protection than either measure alone. A drawback to the use of methisazone is its tendency to induce vomiting. The combined use of vaccination and parenteral administration of vaccinia immune globulin early in the incubation period is also effective in the prevention of smallpox in exposed individuals. It is now usual to apply these control measures selectively to the primary and secondary contacts of a patient rather than to all the inhabitants of a community.

TREATMENT There is no specific therapy for smallpox. Thiosemicarbazone, although effective in prophylaxis, has not been shown to be of value in the treatment of established cases. Fluid deficits should be replaced by the administration of appropriate solutions. During the vesicular and pustular phases of the disease, an attempt should be made to prevent bacterial infection by the use of sterile sheets and aseptic nursing procedures. Antihistamines may be helpful in decreasing pruritus. Application of lotions or ointment should be avoided. Later in the course of the illness, when desquamation has begun, showers or baths may be helpful in removing desquamating tissue. If bacterial infection develops, an antibiotic active against the infecting organism should be given by the parenteral route. Topical antibiotics should be avoided.

VACCINIA

Vaccinia is a virus disease of the skin which is induced by inoculation for the prevention of smallpox. The exact origin of the vaccinia virus is obscure. The material first used by Jenner in 1796 was derived from cowpox lesions, and the infectious agent was propagated for many years by successive passage from person to person through use of exudate from fresh skin lesions. The original agent possibly became contaminated with variola virus during the period when transfer was being carried out without strict controls. It has been suggested that vaccinia virus is a hybrid of cowpox and variola agents, a contention supported by the finding that laboratory-induced hybrids of variola and cowpox viruses have many of the characteristics associated with vaccinia.

VACCINATION Live, lyophilized vaccinia virus prepared from vesicle fluid of infected calves is commercially available and maintains potency for 18 months at 46°F. It is dissolved in a diluent solution just prior to use. The usual method for vaccination is to apply a small drop of vaccine to the skin over the deltoid muscle and to press a sterile needle through the vaccine several times in such a way that only the superficial layer of skin is entered, or by simultaneous puncture utilizing a plastic tine device. Vaccination should always induce some form of skin reaction; complete absence of any kind of lesion indicates that the vaccine was not viable or was not administered properly. The reaction which occurs in nonimmune individuals is characterized by a red papule at the site of inoculation 3 to 5 days after vaccination. The papule becomes vesicular on about the fifth or sixth day and pustular by the ninth or eleventh day after inoculation. The vesicle and pustule may be surrounded by a large area of erythema. About 2 weeks after vaccination, the pustule dries and develops a crust which falls off by the end of the third week, leaving a scar. Fever, malaise, and irritability are common in children during the vesicular and pustular phases, and axillary lymphadenopathy may develop and persist for several months. In the partially immune person, a modified reaction develops without fever or constitutional symptoms. A papule appears on the skin within 3 days, vesiculates in 5 to 7 days, and heals without much scarring. The so-called "immune" reaction described by some, where a papule and/or erythema appears in a few days, then recedes without vesiculation, is an "equivocal" reaction, and may simply represent allergy to the components of an inadvertently inactivated vaccine. A successful vaccination is defined as the presence of a Jennerian vesicle (vesicular, pustular, or crusted) 7 days after inoculation. If this criterion is not met, the patient should be revaccinated, preferably with vaccine from a different lot.

Revaccination every 3 years is required to ensure protection. Vaccination is currently recommended only for individuals traveling to areas which are infected with or endemic for smallpox, for health workers, and for primary and secondary contacts of smallpox cases. *Absolute* contraindications to vaccination include individuals with congenital or acquired immune deficiencies, lymphoma, leukemia or other blood dyscrasias, patients being treated with steroids, antimetabolites, alkylating agents, or ionizing irradiation, and individuals with a history of vaccinia encephalitis. *Relative* contraindications include patients or household contacts with eczema or a history of eczema, severe acne, or other similar dermatologic problems, pregnancy, and infants under twelve months of age. If the necessity to vaccinate any individual in this latter group is great, simultaneous administration of vaccinia immune globulin (VIG), 0.3 ml per kg, is suggested, to be given at a separate site intramuscularly at the time of immunization.

COMPLICATIONS Healing of the primary vaccinal lesion may not occur, and some patients go on to develop slowly progressive necrosis with destruction of large areas of skin, subcutaneous tissue, and underlying structures *(vaccinia gangrenosum).* In addition to the local destruction, there may be metastatic lesions on other parts of the skin surface and in bone and viscera. Vaccinia gangrenosum occurs most frequently in persons with disorders of immunity and, if untreated, is nearly always fatal. *Eczema vaccinatum* is a serious complication that is seen in persons with eczema or other types of chronic dermatosis. Widespread infection in the previously affected areas, as well as in normal skin, may result from direct vaccination of an eczematous patient or from exposure to a recently vaccinated individual. *Generalized vaccinia* in patients without preexisting skin disease is characterized by a few satellite lesions surrounding the inoculation site or by widely disseminated pox resembling the primary vaccination lesion. This condition is usually mild with generally complete recovery. Vaccinia virus may be transferred from the primary inoculation site to the eye or other sites by scratching. *Postvaccinal encephalomyelitis* appears from 2 to 25 days after vaccination. The patient becomes severely ill quite suddenly, with nuchal rigidity, drowsiness, vomiting, convulsions, coma, and signs suggesting disease of the spinal cord. The period of coma lasts for a few days, and in those who recover there are usually no permanent sequelae. Death occurs in about 30 to 40 percent of the patients with encephalomyelitis. Erythema multiforme bullosum, or diffuse blotchy erythema, may occur in vaccinated patients 7 to 10 days after vaccination, and is thought to be an allergic reaction to the virus or other components of the vaccine.

The incidence of complications was compiled for 1968 by the Center for Disease Control. The rates of adverse effects per million primarily vaccinated persons were vaccinia gangrenosum, 0.9; eczema vaccinatum, 10.4; generalized vaccinia, 23.4; vaccinal lesions resulting from accidental implantation of virus, 25.4; postvaccinal encephalitis, 2.9; other complications, 11.8; the death rate was one per million. In view of the current status of smallpox in the world, the risks of widespread routine immunization seem far greater than the risk of inadvertent introduction of disease in this country. Because of this, the sharp modification of indications for vaccination as noted above appears to be justified.

Active treatment of vaccinia complications, aside from control of bacterial superinfection and treatment of any underlying defects, is rather limited. VIG is of possible value in accidental inoculation into secondary sites such as the eye, vaccinia gangrenosum, eczema vaccinatum, and generalized vaccinia. Dosage is usually 0.6 ml per kg intramuscularly, although much larger doses are sometimes used in severe cases. VIG is of no use in erythema multiforme or postvaccinal encephalitis. Thiosemicarbazone has apparently been of benefit in some cases of progressive vaccinia necrosum. 5-Iodo-2′-deoxyuridine, while not yet proved to be effective, is suggested for topical treatment of vaccinial keratitis and conjunctivitis.

COWPOX

Cowpox is primarily a disease of the teats and udders of cows. Humans are almost always infected by milking, but occasional spread to contacts may occur from an infected person. The human disease is characterized by low-grade fever and by small papules on the fingers and hand, which go through vesicular and pustular stages resembling the course of vaccinia infection. The lesions may be ruptured by trauma and spread to immediately adjacent areas on the hand and continue to ulcerate for several weeks. Edema, lymphangitis, and axillary lymph node enlargement are common. Very rare cases of post-cowpox encephalitis and serious infections of eczematous persons have been reported. In general, the disease is benign, heals without scarring, and is usually uncomplicated.

PARAVACCINIA (MILKERS' NODULES)

Paravaccinia is a poxvirus which is antigenically unrelated to cowpox, but produces similar lesions in humans. It is primarily a disease of calves and milk cows, producing lesions on the teats of the cows and oral lesions in the suckling calf. Humans acquire infection through the skin by direct contact. The lesion is usually solitary, beginning as a macule on the finger, hand, or wrist, and progressing to a firm nodule, 1 to 2 cm in diameter, in 10 days. It then crusts and heals without scarring in 2 to 3 weeks. Occasionally, there is associated lymphadenitis. The lesion and its evolution are closely similar to ecthyma contagiosum (orf), a poxvirus of sheep, which can also infect humans by direct inoculation.

REFERENCES

BEDSON HS, DUMBELL K: Smallpox and vaccinia. Br Med Bull 23:119, 1967

BROWN GC (ed):Symposium: Is routine smallpox vaccination necessary in the United States? Am J Epidemiol 93:221, 1971

DIXON, CW: *Smallpox,* London: J. & A. Churchill Ltd., 1962

DOUGLAS RG et al: Treatment of progressive vaccinia. Arch Intern Med 129:980, 1972
GOLDSTEIN JA et al: Smallpox vaccination reactions, prophylaxis, and therapy of complications. Pediatrics 55:342, 1975
JOKLIK WK: The poxviruses. Bacteriol Rev 30:33, 1966
LANE JM et al: Smallpox and smallpox vaccination policy. Ann Rev Med 22:251, 1971
RENNIE AGR et al: Ocular vaccinia. Lancet 2:273, 1974
WENNER HA: Virus diseases associated with cutaneous eruptions. Prog Med Virol 16:269, 1973

205
CHICKENPOX (VARICELLA) AND HERPES ZOSTER

C. GEORGE RAY

DEFINITION Chickenpox is a contagious disease characterized by fever and a disseminated vesicular eruption. Herpes zoster, or shingles, is characterized by segmental inflammation of the spinal or cranial nerves and their ganglions, and by a painful localized vesicular eruption of the skin along the distribution of the involved nerve. Chickenpox and herpes zoster are different manifestations of infection with the same viral agent.

ETIOLOGY In 1953 a virus was recovered from patients with chickenpox and herpes zoster that produced intranuclear, eosinophilic inclusions and multinucleated giant cells in lines of cells derived from various monkey and human tissues. The infectivity of varicella-zoster virus in culture is closely cell-associated, and ordinarily can be passed to other tissue cultures only by transfer of infected, intact cells. The structure of the varicella-zoster virion resembles that of herpes simplex and the other viruses of the herpes group.

PATHOGENESIS AND PATHOLOGY Varicella is presumably transmitted by the respiratory route, although the virus has only rarely been isolated from nasopharyngeal secretions of infected persons. Virus multiplication occurs at some unidentified site and probably results in intermittent viremia, as suggested by the successive crops of widely spaced lesions. Focal viral infection of blood vessels in the corium, with intranuclear inclusions in endothelial cells, results in degeneration of the epidermis and formation of vesicles containing serum, polymorphonuclear leukocytes, and multinucleated giant cells. Virus can be isolated from vesicle fluid, but not usually from crusting lesions or scabs, for 3 to 4 days after eruption. In patients with varicella pneumonia, the tracheobronchial mucosa, the alveolar septa, and the interstitial areas of the lungs are edematous and contain monocytic inflammatory cells, cells with intranuclear inclusions, and giant cells. The nodular areas of pneumonia may eventually become calcified. The changes in the central nervous system in patients with postinfectious varicella encephalomyelitis resemble those seen in measles. Rarely, encephalomyelitis with inclusion bodies resembling herpes simplex infection may occur, and varicella-zoster virus can be recovered from the central nervous system. In infants and children, acute encephalopathy with fatty infiltration of the viscera (Reye's syndrome) sometimes follows the acute phase of varicella; in this condition, only cerebral edema is found on pathologic examination of the brain.

The pathogenesis of herpes zoster is not clear (see Epidemiology, below), but the tissue changes are well documented. The dorsal root ganglion of the affected nerve is swollen and hemorrhagic; the edema spreads along the peripheral nerve and may reach the spinal cord. The nerve tissue shows hemorrhagic infarction, inflammation, and necrosis of many of the ganglion cells, some of which contain intranuclear inclusions. The microscopic appearance of zoster skin lesions is almost identical to that described for chickenpox vesicles. Virus can be cultured from the lesions for as long as 8 days after onset.

EPIDEMIOLOGY Chickenpox is a highly contagious disease with attack rates of 80 percent or more among susceptible household contacts of an index case. The infectious period extends from a day or two before the rash until as long as 6 days after the appearance of new skin lesions, or until all vesicles have crusted over. Patients with herpes zoster may be the source of an outbreak of chickenpox among susceptible contacts. Children from five to eight years of age are most commonly affected, but younger children, including newborn infants, and adults may develop chickenpox; an estimated 2 to 20 percent of cases occur in persons over the age of 15 years. In the United States the disease is endemic, with superimposed epidemics every 2 to 5 years, usually in the winter or spring.

Herpes zoster is mainly a disease of adults who have previously had chickenpox. The epidemiologic evidence strongly suggests that herpes zoster results from reactivation of virus that has remained dormant in spinal ganglia since an episode of chickenpox. Exogenous acquisition of infection directly resulting in herpes zoster rarely, if ever, occurs. Most patients with zoster have had no recent exposure to patients with zoster or varicella, and the incidence of the disease does not increase during seasonal chickenpox epidemics.

Zoster occurs commonly in patients with neoplasms, most frequently in those with Hodgkin's disease, where the incidence may be as high as 25 percent. Advanced disease, cutaneous anergy, recent x-irradiation of affected nodes, and possibly splenectomy predispose patients with Hodgkin's disease to zoster. The most significant common factor responsible for the development of zoster in these patients appears to be depressed cell-mediated immunity; there is no clear correlation with humoral immune status.

Recurrent herpes zoster is distinctly rare. If such a recurrence is documented, the likelihood of an underlying malignancy or immunodeficiency is great. When episodes of so-called recurrent zoster in healthy individuals have been carefully studied, herpes simplex virus has usually been found to be the causative agent. Like varicella-zoster virus, herpes simplex can cause zoster-like disease, but can also cause recurrent lesions.

MANIFESTATIONS **Chickenpox** The incubation period from the time of exposure to the appearance of varicella rash is 10 to 21 days, most often 14 to 17 days. There may be a 1- or 2-day prodrome with fever and malaise, but these symptoms usually begin when the rash appears. The first skin manifestations are pruritic maculopapules that evolve in a few hours to thin-walled vesicles which contain clear fluid and are surrounded by a red border. During the next day the erythema diminishes and the vesicles collapse in the center, forming annular or umbilicated lesions which dry further and form scabs that fall off, after several days, without scarring. New maculopapules continue to erupt during the first 3 or 4 days of illness and go through a similar evolution. The findings at one time, in one area, of skin lesions in all stages of development—maculopapules, vesicles, umbilicated lesions, and scabs—is characteristic of chickenpox. The rash is most concentrated on the trunk, but pox are frequently seen on the face and scalp, occasionally on the mucosal surface of the mouth or conjunctiva, and rarely on the palms and soles.

Chickenpox in adults is often more severe than in children, with more profuse rash, higher fever, and a greater incidence of pneumonia.

Herpes zoster Herpes zoster is a disease of nerves of the skin and other tissues that they supply. It most commonly affects the thoracic (55 percent of cases), cervical (20 percent), lumbar and sacral nerves (15 percent), and the ophthalmic division of the trigeminal nerve.

Fever and pain that is localized to the areas served by the affected nerves may begin 4 or 5 days before or be concomitant with the appearance of the skin eruption. Rarely, characteristic pain and serologic evidence of zoster occur with no clinical involvement of the skin (zoster sine eruptione). The discomfort is mild to severe and can be sharp, burning, or dull. In addition to disorders of sensation, herpes zoster is occasionally associated with motor paralysis of arms, legs, intercostal muscles, or muscles innervated by cranial nerves. The skin lesion starts with local redness followed by red papules that progress over the next 2 weeks through vesicular, pustular, and crusting stages that resemble the evolution of individual pox of varicella. The lesions are arranged unilaterally in characteristic bandlike clusters which follow radicular lines. They may run transversely along the hemithorax or vertically over the arm or leg.

Disease of the individual cranial nerves leads to characteristic groups of symptoms. If the trigeminal (Gasserian) ganglion is affected, there will usually be pain in the distribution of the nerve, headache, weakness of the eyelid muscles, and occasionally Argyll Robertson pupil. Lesions appear on the face, in the mouth, on the tongue, and frequently on the cornea. Iridocyclitis, anesthesia of the cornea, and scarring may result. If the geniculate ganglion is involved, there may be Bell's palsy, disorders of hearing, and vertigo, with unilateral herpetic lesions of the external ear and canal and of the anterior portion of the tongue. Central nervous system inflammation is prominent when herpes zoster attacks the cranial nerves, and meningeal signs and symptoms are frequent.

COMPLICATIONS Hemorrhage into vesicles and surrounding skin may be seen in adults with severe chickenpox or in children receiving adrenal steroids. Infection of the varicella lesions by bacteria, most commonly *Staphylococcus aureus,* results in delayed healing and scarring of skin, and occasionally in bacteremia.

Of adults with chickenpox, 15 percent develop primary *varicella pneumonia,* and adult patients account for 90 percent of the patients who develop this complication. Pneumonia is invariably associated with skin lesions and appears 1 to 6 days after onset of rash. The degree of pulmonary involvement correlates to some extent with the severity of the rash; patients may be virtually asymptomatic or may develop serious, life-threatening disease. Tachypnea, dyspnea, cough, and fever, with a temperature of 102°F or more, are present in most patients with symptomatic pneumonia; cyanosis, pleuritic chest pain, and hemoptysis each occur in 20 to 40 percent of the recorded cases. The physical examination may disclose no abnormalities, or there may be intercostal retractions, a few rhonchi, wheezes, scattered rales, and, rarely, evidence of pleural effusion. In contrast to the paucity of physical signs, roentgenograms demonstrate widespread nodular infiltration of both lungs, most prominent at the hila and least evident at the apices. Vital capacity is decreased, arterial oxygen saturation is diminished, and the airways may be blocked by tenacious bronchopulmonary secretions. Most patients with varicella pneumonia show symptomatic improvement when the rash begins to wane; however, seriously ill patients may remain febrile and dyspneic for as long as 2 weeks. Roentgenographic evidence of disease diminishes at the time of clinical improvement, but may persist for several weeks, followed in some cases by persistent miliary calcifications. Persistent abnormalities of pulmonary gas diffusion have been demonstrated several months after apparent recovery.

Central nervous system complications occur most frequently in children, with estimated rates as high as 1 in 200 cases. The most common manifestation is acute cerebellar ataxia, which usually begins 3 to 21 days after onset of rash and is usually benign. Other, less common manifestations include acute encephalomyelitis, polyneuritis, ascending or transverse myelitis, optic neuritis, and Reye's syndrome.

Patients who contract *varicella while receiving steroids* may have recurrent crops of new skin lesions for as long as 3 weeks. They have a higher incidence of hemorrhagic and progressive gangrenous lesions and occasionally develop a fatal disseminated disease with viral infection in all the viscera. The fatal form of the disease has been encountered most frequently in children being treated with steroids for leukemia or other disease of the hematopoietic system, but it has also been seen in those receiving therapy for rheumatic fever and allergic disorders. Children with the rare syndrome of cartilage-hair hypoplasia may suffer from unusually severe and occasionally fatal chickenpox. *Other complications of chickenpox* such as myocarditis, corneal lesions, iritis, nephritis, nephrosis, monoarticular arthritis or polyarthritis, thrombocytopenic purpura, purpura fulminans, orchitis, and appendicitis have been recognized but are rare. Like measles, chickenpox can transiently produce anergy to tuberculin, and occasionally there may be reactivation of latent tuberculosis. Congenital infection with varicella can occur, and infants born of mothers with chickenpox may display the typical skin lesions. Congenital malformations as a result of infection in early pregnancy have been reported but are rare. The greatest mortality risk to the newborn infant appears to occur when onset of the maternal rash occurs in the 4-day period immediately prior to delivery. It has been suggested that, in this situation, high doses of pooled gamma-globulin be given to the infant immediately after birth in an effort to modify severity of the disease.

Postherpetic neuralgia may last for several months or years and become the most troublesome part of the disease. In nearly all patients with zoster, healing with loss of scab is complete within 2 to 3 weeks. In the young, pain persists for only a week or two after healing and then usually disappears, although hypo- or hyperesthesia may remain. However, in patients over sixty years of age, moderate to severe pain persists for more than 2 months in as many as 70 percent, even though the skin lesions have healed normally.

Zoster skin lesions do not always remain localized. *Generalized zoster* occurs in 5 percent of zoster patients with no underlying disease, and in as many as 70 percent of those with Hodgkin's disease, and is characterized by dissemination to all parts of the skin, producing a picture similar to that of chickenpox. The scattered lesions last 6 to 9 days in normal hosts, but they may persist for 3 to 4 weeks in those with serious underlying disease. In these patients dissemination may also involve the visceral organs (including the lungs) and frequently results in death.

LABORATORY FINDINGS Multinucleated giant cells and epithelial cells with eosinophilic intranuclear inclusions can be identified in material scraped from the base of a vesicular lesion or in sputum from patients with varicella pneumonia. For specific diagnosis, virus can be isolated from vesicular fluid, and antigens can be demonstrated in vesicular fluid and in crusts of lesions by the use of a simple gel-precipitin technique. The white blood cell count in patients with uncomplicated chickenpox or zoster is normal. Mononuclear pleocytosis is present in the cerebrospinal fluid of patients with herpes zoster, especially those with involvement of the cranial nerves. The spinal fluid in varicella-zoster encephalomyelitis often contains increased protein, and cell counts may range from zero to 3,000 lymphocytes per mm^3.

DIFFERENTIAL DIAGNOSIS Chickenpox can usually be diagnosed by the history of recent exposure and the character of the rash. In situations where smallpox is a possibility, differentiation from chickenpox can be attempted by noting the distribution and evolution of the rash and by examining the cells from vesicles, but definitive diagnosis can be made only by identification of the virus or by serologic methods. Disseminated vaccinia lesions similar to chickenpox lesions may occur in patients, especially those with disorders of immunity or eczema, who have recently been vaccinated or exposed to a vaccinated person. Herpes simplex infection in patients with chronic eczema or neurodermatitis may present as a varicelliform eruption confined to previously involved areas of skin. The diagnosis can be confirmed by virus isolation. Rickettsialpox can be differentiated from chickenpox by the presence of an eschar in the area of mite bite, prominent headache, and specific complement-fixing antibodies to *Rickettsia akari.* Rarely, Coxsackie viruses can produce a similar eruption in young children, although the lesions all tend to be in the same stage of development in one area. Stevens-Johnson syndrome has also been occasionally confused with chickenpox.

In the preeruptive stage, the diagnosis of herpes zoster is difficult, and the disease is usually confused with other causes of pain, such as pleurisy, appendicitis, pleurodynia, or collapsed intervertebral disk. After the unilateral eruption appears, the clinical features are so characteristic that the diagnosis is simple. Occasionally, localized herpes simplex along the distribution of a segmental nerve may simulate zoster, including the localized pain and tenderness. The diagnosis of herpes simplex infection can be confirmed in the laboratory by virus isolation.

PROPHYLAXIS Chickenpox can often be prevented by the administration of specific zoster immune globulin (ZIG) derived from the serum of patients recovering from herpes zoster. It should be given within 72 h of exposure to susceptible individuals who have leukemia or lymphoma, or who are receiving large doses of adrenal steroids or immunosuppressive drugs. Its use may also be justified in pregnant women and newborn infants who are exposed to chickenpox. This material should not be used for healthy children who are exposed to the disease. ZIG has not been evaluated in the treatment of chickenpox after lesions have developed, nor is its usefulness in prevention or treatment of herpes zoster known. Large doses of pooled human gamma-globulin have also been shown to modify the disease if given shortly after exposure, but the quantity required to do so is so great (0.6 to 1.2 ml per kg) that this is not generally recommended. Transfusion of plasma from donors recently convalescent from varicella or zoster has also been suggested for modification, and perhaps treatment, but there is no evidence at present to document its efficacy.

TREATMENT The patient with uncomplicated chickenpox seems to benefit most from cool, wet compresses or tepid water baths, rather than drying lotions, for the relief of itching. Secondary bacterial infections should be treated with appropriate antibacterial agents. Patients with varicella pneumonia require skillful nursing care, removal of excessive bronchial secretions, administration of oxygen, and on occasion ventilatory assistance, such as positive pressure breathing. Adrenal steroids have been considered by some to be beneficial in the treatment of varicella pneumonia, but convincing evidence of their efficacy in this condition is not available. Patients suspected of having varicella-zoster infection of the eye should be promptly treated by an ophthalmologist. The therapy consists of analgesics for severe pain and the use of atropine to prevent synechiae. Some ophthalmologists recommend the use of adrenal steroids if uveitis is present. Topical 5-iodo-2′-deoxyuridine is of possible value for corneal or conjunctival ulcerative lesions.

The use of cytosine arabinoside should *not* be considered for the treatment of patients whose lives are threatened by severe chickenpox, inasmuch as this drug may adversely affect the outcome of the disease in seriously ill individuals. It is possible that adenine arabinoside may have a beneficial effect on the course of serious disseminated herpes zoster, but conclusive data are not yet available.

It has been claimed that in older patients with herpes zoster and no underlying disease, the administration of a short course of adrenal steroids by mouth during the early eruptive phase of the disease reduces the incidence and duration of postherpetic neuralgia without inducing dissemination or other complications. Steroids should *not* be used for this purpose in patients with neoplasms or other underlying disease.

REFERENCES

BRUNELL PA, GERSHON AA: Passive immunization against varicella-zoster infections and other modes of therapy. J Infect Dis 127:415, 1973

EAGLESTEIN WH et al: The effects of early corticosteroid therapy on the skin eruption and pain of herpes zoster. JAMA 211:1681, 1970

GOFFINET DR et al: Herpes zoster-varicella infections and lymphoma. Ann Intern Med 76:235, 1972

GOLD E: Serologic and virus isolation studies of patients with varicella or herpes-zoster infection. N Engl J Med 274:181, 1966

JUDELSOHN RG et al: Efficacy of zoster immune globulin. Pediatrics 53:476, 1974

KREBS RA, BURVANT MU: Nephrotic syndrome in association with varicella. JAMA 222:325, 1972

MILLER LH, BRUNELL PA: Zoster, reinfection or activation of latent virus? Am J Med 49:480, 1970

MINKOWITZ S et al: Acute glomerulonephritis associated with varicella infection. Am J Med 44:489, 1968

MULHERN LM et al: Arthritis complicating varicella infection. Pediatrics 48:827, 1971

NORRIS FH et al: Herpes-zoster meningoencephalitis. J Infect Dis 122:335, 1970

RAIDER, L: Calcification in chickenpox pneumonia. Chest 60:504, 1971

SCHIMPFF S et al: Varicella-zoster infection in patients with cancer. Ann Intern Med 76:241, 1972

STEVENS DA et al: Adverse effect of cytosine arabinoside on disseminated zoster. N Engl J Med 289:873, 1973

TRIEBWASSER JH et al: Varicella pneumonia in adults: Report of seven cases and a review of literature. Medicine 46:409, 1967

206
INFECTIONS WITH HERPES SIMPLEX VIRUS

A. MARTIN LERNER

Herpes simplex virus, types 1 and 2, sometimes known as *Herpesvirus hominis,* establishes diverse relations with humans. Acute disseminated primary infection (gingivostomatitis), chronic infection with continual virus shedding (herpes keratitis and herpes labialis), and clinical reactivation occur. Virus multiplies in many tissues, including lymphocytes, and by its intracellular locus is able to escape antiherpesvirus antibodies. Herpesvirus antibody complexes may be infectious, and when this is the case, are called "sensitized virus." Interactions with the complement system are important in neutralizing sensitized virus. Since the decline of poliomyelitis with the development of an effective vaccine, herpes simplex virus encephalitis is the most frequent endemic encephalitis in this country. Type 2 herpes simplex virus (HSV) has been associated with carcinoma of the cervix.

ETIOLOGY The virus particle consists of DNA, protein, lipid, and carbohydrate. On an average there are 100 parts DNA, 25 parts carbohydrate, and 320 parts phospholipid to 1,000 parts protein. Virus DNA is double-stranded with densities of 1.727 (type 1) and 1.729 (type 2). The base composition (guanine plus cytosine per 100 ml) of HSV type 1 (HSV-1) is 68.3, and that for HSV type 2 (HSV-2) is 70.4. The molecular weight of the virion is about 100×10^6 daltons. On phosphotungstic acid staining by electron microscopy the virion is seen to consist of a roughly spheric central area or "core" of DNA which measures 75 nm in diameter, and a stable "capsid" which measures 100 nm in diameter; it appears to be an icosahedron with a 5:3:2 axial symmetry consisting of 162 capsomeres (9 to 10 nm by 12 to 13.5 nm) of which 150 are hexagonal and 12 pentagonal in cross section, and a surrounding envelope derived from host cell membranes, 145 to 200 nm. Particles appear with or without envelopes [enveloped and/or with or without cores ("full" or "empty")].

Although complete virions are more efficient, both "enveloped" and "naked" particles can infect cells. Phagocytosis of virions by susceptible cells, viropexis, precedes the digestion of virus envelopes and proteins. After initiation of infection, virus absorption is complete in 3 h. New virus infectivity rises sharply from the sixth to the ninth hour, when it levels off. Viral DNA enters the nucleus where new virus DNA is synthesized. Virus proteins are synthesized in the cytoplasm and migrate to the nucleus. To date, from 9 to 24 distinct proteins (or polypeptides) are identified. The complete virion has a triple-layered envelope. The inner envelope is made within the nucleus, while the second and third are formed by evagination processes at the nuclear and cytoplasmic membranes, respectively. Host materials make up major portions of the envelope. Virus envelope contains adenosine triphosphatase (ATPase), which also is present in host membranes. Antihost serum agglutinates "enveloped," but not "naked," particles. An infected cell produces about 1,000 virus particles, but only 5 to 10 percent are infectious.

BIOLOGIC CHARACTERISTICS By means of neutralization kinetics, hyperimmune unitypic serums in conventional neutralization tests or direct immunofluorescent methods, strains of herpes simplex virus can be readily typed. Type 1 strains are recovered from the nasopharynx, skin (other than thigh or buttocks), and brain in cases of postnatal encephalitis. Type 2 strains are usually related to the adult genital tract. Isolates have been recovered from the penis, cervix, endocervix, vagina, vulva, skin, and spinal fluid. In infections of the newborn, HSV-2 has been recovered from brain, liver, adrenal, and lung.

Optimal virus isolation occurs in rabbit or baby hamster kidney and human foreskin tissue cultures. Cytopathic effects are usually evident within 72 h after inoculation. However, when isolation of virus by brain biopsy is attempted, trypsinized suspensions of cells, rather than ground tissue suspensions, should be planted, both for primary growth and for cocultivation with herpesvirus-susceptible tissue cultures. Typical of in vitro and in vivo cytopathic effects is the type A inclusion of Cowdry, an eosinophilic mass surrounded by a halo in a nucleus with marginated chromatin (Fig. 206-1). After infection of rabbit kidney cells with HSV-1 a cell factor is released which, upon incubation with serum, cleaves the fifth component of complement. The product of this cleavage, C5a, is chemotactic for polymorphonuclear leukocytes which accumulate at the site of herpetic lesions.

In addition to site of recovery, a number of other properties separate type 1 from type 2 herpes simplex virus: HSV-2 produces (1) larger pocks on the chorioallantoic membrane of embryonated eggs, (2) greater virulence for female mice which have been infected by the genital route, and (3) greater tendency toward formation of giant cells in tissue cultures. These strains also exhibit (4) difference in density and base composition of DNA and (5) antigenic distinctiveness. Likewise, (6) minimal inhibitory concentrations (MIC) of idoxuridine (IDU; 5-iodo-2′-deoxyuridine) for type 1 strains are 2.5 to 10 μg per 0.4 ml, while similar values for type 2 herpesviruses are 25 to 50 μg per 0.4 ml.

IMMUNOLOGY Following primary exposure to herpes simplex virus, humoral antibodies appear. Different polypeptides of the virus capsid probably stimulate distinct antibodies which rise and fall, describing separate kinetic curves. In contrast to other antibodies (conventional neutralizing, complement-fixing, passive hemagglutinating), complement-requiring neutralizing antibodies peak during the acute phase of primary infections with HSV-1 and fall during convalescence. Complement apparently enhances the immunoaggregation of the virus. In early immune serum, complement-requiring antibody behaves like monovalent antibody, sensitizing virus to the action of complement. Immunoaggregates form when complement is added. Each virus-antibody-complement aggregate functions as a single infectious unit. Late immune serum is polyvalent, and convalescent serum alone aggregates and neutralizes virus. IgM and early IgG antibodies to HSV-1 may be complement-requiring. Several strains of HSV-2 have been tested and have not been shown to stimulate homotypic complement-requiring neutralizing antibodies.

FIGURE 206-1
Cowdry, type A (owl-eye) intranuclear inclusions are seen in this hematoxylin and eosin section (855) obtained at biopsy from the right temporal lobe of a fifty-seven-year-old woman in coma. Herpes simplex virus (4,000 fifty-percent tissue culture doses) was recovered from the specimen.

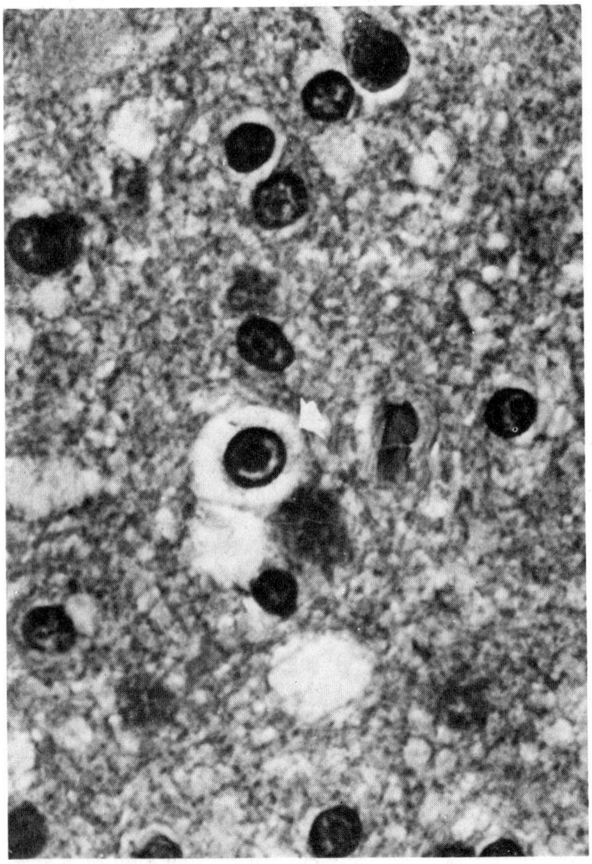

After initial exposure immunoglobulin M antibodies appear in serum within 1 week. In respiratory secretions IgA antibodies form. In cases of encephalitis, passive hemagglutinating antibodies can be measured in cerebrospinal fluid. Seven days after infection IgG antibodies appear and antiherpesvirus IgM synthesis decreases. Complement-fixing antibodies appear in 14 days.

Antiherpesvirus IgM antibodies may be measured by conventional or complement-requiring neutralization techniques, fluorescent microscopy, or passive hemagglutination.

After an initial exposure, complement-fixing antibodies fall to low levels within several months, while neutralizing antibodies persist for many years. Reactivations of infection evoke variable rises in serums of conventional neutralizing or complement-fixing IgG antibodies. Low titers of heterologous antibodies to HSV-1 and HSV-2 are also found by complement-fixing and passive hemagglutination tests. There are some low-titered cross-reactions when anti-HSV antibodies are measured against varicella-zoster or cytomegalovirus.

By means of the passive hemagglutination technique, herpesvirus protein is indiscriminately absorbed to the surface of tannic acid–treated sheep red blood cells, providing a comprehensive measure of several antibodies and increasing sensitivity. For strains of HSV, type 1 and type 2, respectively, titers of passive hemagglutinating antibodies are 2.6 to 14 times and 4 to 22 times greater than conventional neutralizing antibodies.

Herpes simplex virus IgA complexes are generally noninfectious, while HSV-1 IgC complexes (sensitized virus) are infectious. Complete covering of the virion and a resulting steric hindrance to absorption may be important in order to neutralize sensitized virus. Thus, antibody to gamma-globulin, papain-derived Fab fragments of IgG anti-HSV-1 serums, IgM rheumatoid factor, and components of complement (C1 plus C4) can neutralize sensitized virus. There is every likelihood that during herpesvirus infections of human beings, sensitized virus is present in the circulation and is fixed in tissues. It remains to be determined what role these infectious antigen-antibody complexes have in disease.

CLINICAL FINDINGS: HSV-1 Primary infection with HSV-1 causes *acute gingivostomatitis, rhinitis, keratoconjunctivitis, meningoencephalitis, eczema herpeticum* (Kaposi's varicelliform eruption), and *traumatic herpes,* including *herpetic* *whitlow* and *generalized herpes simplex* in burned patients or wrestlers. In immunosuppressed patients initial infection or clinical reactivation may induce esophageal ulceration or interstitial pneumonia.

The incubation period is 2 to 12 days, averaging 6 or 7 days. The route of infection is usually respiratory. During acute herpetic gingivostomatitis there are fever, irritability, red swollen gums, a vesicular eruption on the mucous membranes of the mouth, oral fetor, and local submaxillary adenopathy. A visit to the dentist may precede an attack. Any portion of the oral mucosa may be affected. Viremia may occur. A generalized vesicular eruption may follow and appear in crops. Lesions are generally smaller than those of varicella. In the eczematous infant (Kaposi's varicelliform eruption) large quantities of fluid, electrolytes, and protein may be lost.

Within the tense vesicles is a clear fluid. An impression smear of an opened vesicle demonstrates syncytial giant cells undergoing ballooning degeneration. Intranuclear inclusions are seen. Virus can readily be isolated from the fluid; no bacteria are seen by Gram's stain and none may be cultured. Later, vesicles collapse and ulcerate. Sometimes the nose is the site of primary infection. Tiny vesicles surrounding reddened areolae appear in the nostrils. Usually, there is fever and the anterior cervical lymph nodes enlarge.

Infected secretions from patients contaminate the fingers of hospital personnel through unnoticed abrasions, producing *herpetic whitlow*. Painful deep vesicles appear suddenly and spread locally for about a week. The nail may be separated from its matrix by a lesion at its base.

Follicular conjunctivitis (often unilateral) with chemosis, edema of the lids, and conjunctival ulcers may be seen. The cornea may be involved in primary or recurrent infections. When the cornea is affected, a diffuse epitheliolitis develops with superficial punctate erosions which extend into small dendritic ulcers. If untreated, this ulcer increases in size to form a large, anesthetic "geographic" ulcer. Erosions of the cornea recur. *Deeper interstitial keratitis* with secondary bacterial invasion, hypopyon, iridocyclitis, synechia, and opacification of the lens follows.

Others with preexisting neutralizing antibodies in serums may suffer *recurrent attacks of herpes labialis* or trigeminal neuralgia. Pneumococcal and meningococcal, but not gram-negative infections; menstruation; emotional upset; and other little-understood events seem to trigger recurrent localized episodes. Quiescence and recurrences of herpes labialis may be associated with alternating low and higher titers of virus shedding, but reactivation of latent infection also occurs. Herpes simplex virus resides in a quiescent state within paraspinal or cranial nerve ganglia for years, intermittently releasing virus along nerve fibers. After traversing the axon, HSV reaches the skin, and vesiculation occurs.

Encephalitis Occasionally, and for as yet ill-defined reasons, HSV-1 begins an ascent from the respiratory epithelium of the nose up the olfactory tract to reach the frontal and temporal areas of the brain. An often fatal or severely damaging necrotizing encephalitis results. Immediate mortality of patients with seizures who are in coma is about 38 percent, but the majority of the survivors are markedly impaired.

Patients of any age, either sex, and of any socioeconomic status may be affected. About 15 percent of patients who develop herpes simplex virus encephalitis have histories of recurrent herpes labialis. Prodromal illnesses begin 3 to 4 days before admission to the hospital. Various combinations of headache, rhinorrhea, sore throat, fever, nausea, or vomiting are noted. Less frequently photophobia, vertigo, insomnia, or anorexia occurs. One-third of the patients have concurrent fever blisters during the course of their illness. Neurologic symptoms necessitate hospitalization. In order of frequency, disorientation, personality change, hallucinations, photophobia, ataxia, facial weakness, incontinence of stool or urine, tremors, and amnesia appear. Patients with proved herpes simplex virus encephalitis have been mistaken for inebriates or psychotics. Neurologic signs include stupor, seizures (Jacksonian or generalized), coma, extensor plantar reflexes, nuchal rigidity, motor deficit, cranial nerve palsies, sensory deficit, decorticate and decerebrate posture, abnormal conjugate deviation of eyes, frontal lobe signs (glabella, snout, sucking), asymmetric deep tendon reflexes, and dysphasia. Coma (absence of response to all stimuli) indicates an ominous prognosis.

Leukocyte counts average 13,000 per mm^3 with concomitant "shifts to the left." Cerebrospinal fluid samples are completely normal or contain only a few to several hundred leukocytes which may be predominantly mononuclear or polymorphonuclear. Grossly bloody spinal fluid is an ominous sign. Cerebrospinal fluid protein is normal or elevated as high as 250 mg per 100 ml. Glucose in cerebrospinal fluid is usually normal, but may be low. In every case electroencephalograms are diffusely abnormal, or show focal lesions in the temporal or frontal regions. The abnormal electroencephalogram is an especially important finding, particularly in cases in which the cerebrospinal fluid is normal. Bilateral carotid angiograms are indicated to rule out an epidural, subdural, or intracerebral hematoma, abscess, or tumor. In a few cases of HSV-1 encephalitis, the focal hemorrhagic necrotic mass deviates carotid vessels, and craniotomy is necessary for diagnosis.

The following criteria are used to make a presumptive or definitive diagnosis of herpes simplex virus encephalitis: (1) Encephalitis is present clinically and confirmed by an abnormal electroencephalogram, often with focal changes in the frontal or temporal lobes. (2) Cerebrospinal fluid is sterile for bacteria (including *Mycobacterium tuberculosis*), fungi, and other viruses. (3) Carotid angiograms are done when focal signs persist. When cerebral vessels are found to be displaced at angiography, craniotomy is done to exclude a diagnosis of subdural, epidural, or intracerebral abscess, hematoma, or tumor. (4) A fourfold rise (or occasionally fall) in complement-fixing, conventional neutralizing, or passive hemagglutinating antibodies is demonstrated in acute and convalescent phase specimens of serum in all the survivors. In addition, a single serum with a ratio of complement-requiring to conventional neutralizing antibodies to HSV-1 of 4 or more is considered equal to information gleaned through retrospective rises in complement-fixing, conventional neutralizing, or passive hemagglutinating antibodies. In every patient with a presumptive diagnosis of HSV encephalitis, the same serums are tested for concomitant rises in complement-fixing antibodies to mumps or rubeola viruses; they must be negative. Passive hemagglutinating antibodies have been found in cerebrospinal fluids of several patients with definitive HSV encephalitis. To date, these antibodies, at a ratio in CSF to serum of greater than 1:100, have not been found in cerebrospinal fluids of controls. (5) Isolation of herpes simplex virus from the brain at biopsy or autopsy is diagnostic. Cowdry, type A (owl-eye) intranuclear inclusions may be demonstrated from the brain (Fig. 206-1). (6) Cases are excluded if the course suggests another diagnosis or if the above criteria are not met. Attempts at isolation of viruses from throat or rectal swabs, urine, and cerebrospinal fluid as well as, when possible, from brain, spinal cord, and vesicular fluid should be made.

CLINICAL FINDINGS: HSV-2 Infection with HSV, type 2, is a venereal disease. In one study seven of eight female contacts of men with penile herpetic infection showed evidence of current HSV genital infection. Similarly, 63 of 64 HSV isolates from male genitalia and 155 of 162 from the female genital tract were HSV-2. This infection is the most common cause of genital vesicles and/or ulcers found in women, and is second only to primary syphilis as the cause of such lesions in males. Teenagers make up one-fourth to one-half of patients with genital herpetic infections.

Neutralizing antibodies to HSV-2 are reported to be present in 35.7 percent of patients who subsequently develop carcinoma *in situ* of the cervix, and are found in only 7.1 percent of matched controls. However, an etiologic relation between carcinoma of the cervix and infection with HSV-2 is not established.

During primary infections fever, malaise, and inguinal adenopathy may be seen and viremia may follow. A benign aseptic meningitis has resulted. In the male there may be tiny vesicles on the glans or shaft of the penis, burning, urgency, frequency, and watery discharge. Herpesvirus is easily cultivated from vesicular fluids.

In women there are tiny vesicles on the labia minora and inner surfaces of the labia majora and cervix. They rapidly ulcerate to round and oval, discrete, and coalescent gray-white lesions. Typical cytologic changes of infection with herpes simplex virus, which may be recognized with a Papanicolaou preparation, occur. If initial infection occurs during pregnancy, transplacental infection of the fetus may ensue.

Recurrent attacks may be associated with neurologic pain and vesicles on the penis or vulva, thighs, or buttocks. If the cervix or vulva is affected at the time of delivery, perinatal infection of the infant may occur during transit through the birth canal. The newborn infant may show signs of illness by the fourth to seventh day of life. Viremia is usual. Cutaneous vesicles may occur at diverse sites. The lungs, liver, brain, and adrenals may be affected. A diffuse encephalitis, respiratory failure, severe hepatic destruction with increasing jaundice, and adrenal insufficiency may follow. If hepatic necrosis is marked, most of these infants die.

TREATMENT Neither killed nor attenuated vaccine has been shown to be effective. When there is a history of recurrent herpetic vulvovaginitis coupled with a clinical exacerbation at term, delivery by cesarean section must be considered. If primary herpetic vulvovaginitis is documented during gestation, the fetus may be infected during the mother's viremia, and the indication for cesarean section is less clear.

Idoxuridine (5-iodo-2′-deoxyuridine, IDU) and adenine arabinoside (9-β-D-arabinofuranosyladenine, vidarabine, ara-A) are effective topically in herpes simplex virus keratitis. For herpetic keratitis topical IDU is applied in a 0.1% solution every hour during the day and every 2 h during the night. A simpler means of application is a 0.5% ointment four or five times a day. Patients have used this ointment locally in recurrent herpes labialis and progenitalis. There are no controlled data, but patients state that pain and morbidity are shortened. Several patients with herpetic vulvovaginitis have been treated with idoxuridine (100 μg per ml) or adenine arabinoside (100 μg per ml) in water as a sitz bath four times a day, with rapid relief of fever and pain. In these uncontrolled observations, lesions have healed.

IDU is more toxic than ara-A, and intravenous ara-A is being evaluated in disseminated perinatal infections and encephalitis. In a carefully done placebo-controlled trial, cytosine arabinoside (ara-C) has been shown to be ineffective in herpes zoster infections. It should also not be used parenterally in herpes simplex virus infections. Interferon, interferon inducers, transfer factor, and corticosteroids have not yet been shown to be useful in herpesvirus infections.

On account of the development of resistance of strains of herpes simplex virus to photoactive heterotricyclic dyes (proflavine, neutral red) and the possible induction of malignant transformation by these agents, this treatment is not recommended.

Adenine arabinoside is the most promising antiherpesvirus agent presently being tested. Multicenter controlled clinical trials are underway. Ara-A is not yet licensed, but since 1971 it has been used extensively in several university centers. It is active in preventing cytopathic effects in tissue culture of herpes simplex virus, type 1, herpes simplex virus, type 2, varicella-zoster (V-Z) virus, cytomegalovirus, and herpes B and vaccinia viruses. It is much less depressive to the bone marrow than idoxuridine or cytosine arabinoside. To date, ara-A has not been shown to be an immunosuppressive agent. Moreover, it is immediately converted within cells by the ubiquitous enzyme adenosine deaminase to hypoxanthine arabinoside (ara-Hx), which, in turn, also has antiviral activity, albeit less than the parent compound. On the other hand, the immediate metabolic products of ara-C and IDU have no antiviral properties. Experience, to date, suggests but does not prove that ara-A is useful in disseminated cutaneous HSV-1 and V-Z infections, but is of dubious value in recurrent cutaneous HSV-2 or cytomegalovirus infections. Permission must be obtained prior to each experimental usage.

Ara-A is diluted in 5% dextrose solutions at a ratio of at least 2 ml for each milligram of antiviral compound. Adenine arabinoside is given by slow, continuous intravenous infusions at a dose of 10 mg per kg per day for 5 to 10 days. Slight depressions in hemoglobin have been noted, and megaloblasts have been seen in the bone marrow. When patients are receiving other immunosuppressive or cytotoxic treatments, toxicity of ara-A may be greater. Approximately 40 percent of the daily dose of ara-A is excreted in the urine within 24 h.

REFERENCES

CATALANO LW, JOHNSON LD: Herpesvirus antibody and carcinoma *in situ* of the cervix. JAMA 217:447, 1971

CHIEN LT et al: Effect of adenine arabinoside on severe *Herpesvirus hominis* infections in man. J Infect Dis 128:658, 1973

DOWDLE WR et al: Association of antigenic type of *Herpesvirus hominis* with site of viral recovery. J Immunol 99:974, 1967

KAPLAN AS (ed): *The Herpesviruses,* New York: Academic, 1973

LERNER AM, BAILEY EJ: Concentrations of idoxuridine in serum, urine and cerebrospinal fluid of patients with suspected diagnoses of *Herpesvirus hominis* encephalitis. J Clin Invest 51:45, 1972

—— et al: Serologic responses to herpes simplex virus in rabbits: complement-requiring neutralizing, conventional neutralizing, and passive hemagglutinating antibodies. J Infect Dis 129:623, 1974

NAHMIAS AJ et al: Genital infection with type 2 *Herpesvirus hominis*: A commonly occurring venereal disease. Br J Vener Dis 45:294, 1969

NOLAN DC et al: *Herpesvirus hominis* encephalitis in Michigan: Report of 13 cases, including 6 treated with idoxuridine. N Engl J Med 282:10, 1970

STEVENS DA et al: Adverse effect of cytosine arabinoside on disseminated zoster in a controlled trial. N Engl J Med 289:873, 1973

TERNI M et al: Aseptic meningitis in association with herpes progenitalis. N Engl J Med 285:503, 1971

WHEELER CE, HUFFINES WD: Primary disseminated herpes simplex of the newborn. JAMA 191:455, 1965

207 MINOR VIRAL DISEASES OF THE SKIN AND MUCOSAL SURFACES

ALVIN E. FRIEDMAN-KIEN

HERPANGINA Herpangina is a specific, benign, infectious disease of childhood, although it is not uncommon in young adults. It is caused by group A Coxsackie viruses types 2, 3, 4, 5, 6, 8, and 10. It occurs throughout the world in epidemic form, usually in the summer and early fall. Similar disorders have been attributed to echo types 9 and 17, and Coxsackie B viruses types 1 to 5 (Chap. 193).

The incubation period for herpangina is about 3 to 6 days. Children between the ages of one and seven years are most commonly afflicted. Immunity persists for at least 1 year; reinfection with another strain of the virus can occur.

Herpangina is characterized by sudden onset of fever, temperatures often rising to 104°F, severe sore throat, nausea, and vomiting. Anorexia, dysphagia, excessive salivation, and severe malaise are common. The throat and posterior portions of the mouth are usually quite red and injected and are covered with numerous minute vesicles (1 to 2 mm in diameter), which quickly rupture, erode, and enlarge to form 3- to 4-mm punched-out, shallow ulcers with grayish centers surrounded by deep-red areolas. The number and size of the lesions increase for 2 to 3 days and heal within 4 or 5 days. The anterior faucial pillars of the pharynx, the tonsils, and the soft palate are usually involved. Occasionally, similar vesicles are found in the vaginal mucosa.

The systemic and local symptoms begin to regress within 4 to 5 days, and total recovery occurs within 7 to 10 days.

Headache, coryza, and other respiratory tract symptoms are absent. Myalgia and arthralgia are rare. Mild cervical lymphadenopathy is sometimes noted. Parotitis and aseptic meningitis have been reported.

Recovery from the illness is always uneventful. Treatment is confined to topical symptomatic measures; frequent mouthwashes and gargles with topical anesthetics such as Benadryl elixir or butacaine are soothing. A fluid or soft diet is advisable. Demonstration of a Coxsackie virus from one of the vesicles, or isolation from pharyngeal washing and/or stool may be helpful, especially when combined with a demonstrable rise in antibody titer in the convalescent as compared with the acute serum.

Differential diagnosis should include a primary herpes simplex infection which may produce a severe oropharyngeal eruption. However, herpes does not usually occur in epidemics, and the herpetic lesions are more typically confined to the anterior portions of the mouth, such as the lips and tongue. With herpes, the gingiva are typically red and edematous. Aphthous stomatitis, bacterial pharyngitis, and the oropharyngeal lesions of viral exanthems, such as chickenpox and measles, may be confused initially with herpangina. The natural course of the disease will help clarify the diagnosis.

FOOT-AND-MOUTH DISEASE (Aphthous Fever) Foot-and-mouth disease is a fairly common epidemic viral disease of farm animals in Europe, Asia, and Africa. It is rarely known to affect humans. The causative agent is the smallest virus known to infect animals. A few cases have been reported in children and adults who had been exposed by contact with an infected stock of animals, by ingestion of meat or dairy products, or from exposure to the hides or excretions of sick animals. The incubation period seems to range between 2 and 18 days. Multiloculated vesicles appear on the skin and mucous membranes. Intranuclear inclusion bodies have been observed in the epidermal cells at the base of the vesicles and in the surrounding tissue.

The onset of the infection is characterized by fever, headache, malaise, and dryness and burning sensation of the oral mucosa. Within 2 to 3 days loculated vesicles develop on the lips, tongue, and buccal mucosa. The palms, soles, and interdigital skin may also show such lesions. Generalized pruritus may occur. The vesicles go on to develop into irregularly shaped, painful ulcers which may become edematous and bleed easily. At times either the mouth or the hands alone may be involved. Rarely, other areas of the skin may be affected. The course of the disease is usually mild; the temperature falls rapidly, and the lesions begin to heal after 6 or 7 days. Total healing is complete by 2 to 3 weeks; there are no scars.

Diagnostic confirmation depends upon a rise in specific complement-fixing antibody titers. The virus can be isolated in tissue cultures, guinea pigs, and chick embryos. In the United States, strict regulations of quarantine and meat inspection have limited the occurrence to a few outbreaks near the Mexican border. Treatment is symptomatic.

HAND-FOOT-AND-MOUTH DISEASE Hand-foot-and-mouth disease represents a syndrome characterized by a vesicular eruption of the skin and the mouth. It has been reported to occur in epidemics in the United States, England, and Australia. Laboratory studies suggest that the disease is associated with Coxsackie A viruses, types 4, 5, 9, 10, and 16. The infection occurs primarily in children. The incubation period is 3 to 5 days. The disease is mild, running its course in 4 to 8 days. A transient, low-grade fever may be present at the onset. The most troublesome symptom is stomatitis. Initially vesicles appear in random distribution on the tongue, buccal mucosa, gingiva, and palate, usually sparing the pharynx. These vesicles are few in number and are somewhat larger than those seen in herpangina. The vesicles quickly develop into shallow, whitish ulcerations with red areolas.

Lesions on the skin are not always present, but are typically vesicular, approximately 4 or 5 mm in size. They are characteristically few in number, ovoid or elongated in shape, grayish in color, surrounded by a fine, red margin. These vesicles appear on the dorsum of the fingers and especially about the periungual region and the heel margin. Occasionally vesicles may be found on the palms or soles. They usually start to disappear within a few days after onset. On rare occasions a more diffuse, vesicular eruption and exanthematous rash have been reported, with particular concentration of such lesions on the buttocks.

The differential diagnosis includes herpangina, aphthous stomatitis, and other Coxsackie and echo virus infections. The confirmation of the exact diagnosis depends upon viral and serologic studies.

VESICULAR STOMATITIS Vesicular stomatitis is a viral illness of horses, cattle, and pigs, but it occasionally affects humans. The disease occurs in the United States and South America. The mode of natural spread among livestock is unknown, but the disease is probably transmitted by direct and indirect contact. Epidemics do not occur in freezing weather, and it is therefore assumed that the virus is arthropod-borne in nature. The virus has been isolated from flies and mosquitoes. Two antigenically distinct viruses are known to cause the disease in the United States, the Indiana type and the New Jersey type. The incubation period is 2 to 6 days. In humans the disease is mild and self-limited; the symptoms are similar to those of influenza. The virus has been studied and used extensively in experimental laboratories. Consequently, several cases have been reported in laboratory personnel as well as farm workers.

The sudden onset is characterized by fever up to 104°F, lasting 24 h, chills, and profuse sweating. Myalgias, malaise, headache, and aching of the eyes are common. The symptoms are worse on the second day. One-third of the patients develop sore throats with cervical and submandibular adenopathy. The tongue and mucous membranes may become sore as well, and conjunctivitis may occur. In a few cases, small, subcorneal, intraepithelial vesicles appear on the fingers. Symptoms last only 3 to 4 days, but relapses can occur. Inapparent infections have been demonstrated by a rise of both complement-fixing and neutralizing-serum antibodies in laboratory workers. Differential diagnosis must include hand-foot-and-mouth disease, herpangina, and other mucocutaneous syndromes. Viral isolation from patients is rare, but the comparison of acute and convalescent serums in a suspected case will help to confirm the diagnosis.

WARTS (Verrucae) Warts are an infectious disease of the skin and contiguous mucous membrane. The etiologic agent is a member of the papova group of viruses that includes the animal papilloma viruses, the polyoma, and simian vacuolating viruses, such as SV40 and SV5. These viruses have been shown to induce tumors in experimental animals and to cause in vitro transformation of tissue cultures.

The human wart virus, which is a DNA virus measuring about 45 nm in diameter, has been extracted from human lesions and has been used experimentally to induce the formation of warts at inoculated sites in the skin of human volunteers. The incubation period based on experimental inoculations varies from 1 to 20 months, averaging about 4 months. The virus has been shown by electron microscopy to parasitize the nuclei of epidermal cells. The successful isolation of the human wart virus in tissue culture has recently been accomplished.

The skin lesions induced by the wart virus are due to an abnormal proliferation of epidermal cells. The lesions, which are skin-colored, may occur as single lesions or in multiples widely disseminated over the entire body. Although the same virus is thought to cause all varieties of human warts, the character of the lesion depends upon the local response of the affected skin to the virus. Immunity may also play a role. For convenience, lesions are classified according to location and morphology.

Common warts (verrucae vulgares) are usually seen on the hands or under and about the fingernails. These lesions are rough-surfaced, horny papules which can vary in size from 1 mm to 2 cm in diameter. Confluency of clustered lesions occurs frequently. The lesions are asymptomatic.

Plantar warts occur mostly beneath pressure points on the soles of the feet and are frequently quite painful. The surface lesions are flat, firm, stippled, and horny. They may occur individually or in a mosaiclike cluster. The mass of a plantar wart is beneath the skin surface. These warts are generally larger than one might expect. They have a conical shape, the pointed end projected inward. This configuration is probably due to the pressure imposed by walking. Plantar warts are most common in teen-agers; females seem slightly more susceptible than males.

The differential diagnosis of plantar warts includes calluses and corns. The normal epidermal ridges are continuous across the surface of calluses and corns, whereas the surface of warts disrupts the normal pattern. Local foreign body reactions and congenital keratotic lesions of the palms and soles also have to be ruled out.

Flat warts (verrucae planae) are skin-colored, smooth, flat or slightly elevated, round or polygonal papules that vary between 1 and 5 mm in diameter. They almost always occur in multiples, up to several hundred. The common sites are the face, neck, chest, dorsum of the hands, flexor surface of the forearms, and shins. The mucous membranes are rarely involved. The surface of these lesions shows a stippled appearance when examined under a magnifying glass. Flat warts are most frequently confused with the lesions of lichen planus. Multiple lesions on the dorsum of the hands may be mistaken for one of the inherited disorders known as acrokeratosis verruciformis, epidermodysplasia verruciformis, or Darier's disease.

Filiform warts are most frequently seen in adult males, and usually occur in the bearded area of the face. The lips and eyelids are often involved. The lesions are horny, fingerlike projections which may grow to considerable length if left unattended. They occur in multiples, but are seen occasionally as individual lesions. Differential diagnosis includes cutaneous horns.

Digitate warts are seen on the scalp of adults as clusters of fleshy fingerlike projections. They must be differentiated from epidermal nevi.

Condylomata accuminata (moist warts), also known as *venereal* or *fig warts,* are the lesions which occur at the mucocutaneous junctions of the skin in the genital and perianal areas. Rare cases have been seen about the areola of the nipple in females, the margins of the mouth, both the inguinal and axillary folds, and in the interdigital skin between the toes.

These warts are pink to red in color and moist and soft. They may be pedunculated or elongated. Clusters of these warts may resemble a cauliflower in appearance. They may occur in great numbers and can become macerated and malodorous because of their location. These warts are most often seen in young adults, but children as well as adults are affected. The eruption of moist warts is frequent and most severe in pregnancy. Although the lesions have been known to be transmitted between sexual partners, it is a misconception that these lesions are usually venereal in origin.

Condylomata accuminata, unlike other warts, are most effectively treated with the repeated topical application of a 25 percent podophyllum resin in tincture of benzoin. A single, persistent, fungating lesion on the penis, resistant to this treatment, should be biopsied to rule out a malignancy, such as squamous-cell carcinoma or a rare, abnormal growth, known as the Buschke-Löwenstein tumor. The more sessile condylomata lesions of secondary syphilis may be confused with viral-induced and genital warts.

Warts often tend to recur, even after apparently adequate treatment. The variety of methods used for removal are primarily destructive, such as electrodessication and curettage, surgical excision, x-ray, or cryosurgery by applying liquid nitrogen or dry ice. Repeated paring of warts, followed by the application of caustic agents such as mono- or trichloracetic acid, salicylic acid, cantharidin, or silver nitrate is very helpful. It is important to avoid radical means of therapy, because all warts will eventually disappear spontaneously, leaving no scar, suggesting the development of an immune response. However, warts may persist and spread within the same host for several years. Warts may recur in individuals several years after a total remission. The development of warts is frequently seen as a complication in patients with primary or secondary immunologic deficiencies as well as in those undergoing immunosuppressive therapy.

ORF (Ecthyma Infectiosum) Orf is an infectious disease which primarily affects the mouth and lips of sheep. It is caused by a specific virus which has been isolated in tissue culture. The disease is transmitted between animals and also from virus-contaminated, dried crusts of lesions found in grazing pastures. The virus may remain in an infective state for several months or years. The disease has a worldwide distribution. The mouths of young lambs are most often affected; infection occurs in shepherds, butchers, veterinarians, and children who play with sheep.

In humans, the incubation period is about 5 to 6 days. The eruption may occur as single or multiple lesions on the hands and other exposed parts of the body. Initially, a small, reddish-blue papule appears and rapidly enlarges to form a 2- to 3-cm hemorrhagic bulla. Itching is intense, and the bulla ruptures to form an umbilicated, erythematous ulcer which develops a gray-white crust. Systemic manifestations are rare, except for occasional low-grade fever and mild regional lymphangitis and lymphadenopathy. A transient macular and papular red rash may occur on the trunk during the second week of the disease. Spontaneous healing occurs within 3 to 6 weeks.

The disease should be suspected when the characteristic lesions develop in individuals exposed to sheep. The diagnosis can be confirmed by virus isolation in the laboratory as well as by a comparative rise of antibody titers in acute and convalescent serums.

Differential diagnosis must include milkers' nodule, anthrax, tularemia, primary inoculation tuberculosis, cowpox, and pyogenic granuloma.

MILKERS' NODULE (Paravaccinia, Milkers' Warts) Milkers' nodule is a benign, poxvirus disease contracted from infected cows. The disease has a worldwide distribution. Nodules and ulcers occur on the teats of infected dairy cattle. In humans, lesions appear within 5 to 7 days after milking an infected cow. They usually occur on the hands, but other exposed parts of the body, such as the face, may be inoculated. The virus has been isolated in bovine kidney tissue culture and resembles the orf virus. The early, flat, dark-red papules enlarge up to 1 to 2 cm in diameter within a week and develop into solid, elastic, shiny, brownish-purple, highly vascular nodules. No pus or fluid accumulates. The nodules may be slightly tender, and mild regional lymphadenopathy may occur. Mild temperature elevations have been reported. Gradually an opaque, gray, slightly depressed eschar develops over the surface of the nodules' red granulation tissue. The lesion is surrounded by an areola of erythema. Resolution occurs within 5 to 6 weeks without scarring. One infection provides permanent immunity. The virus can be isolated in tissue culture, but this is not a practical routine procedure. There is no cross-immunity between milkers' nodule, cowpox, and vaccinia.

Differential diagnosis between milkers' nodule and warts may not be possible on clinical grounds. Pyogenic granuloma and cowpox should also be considered.

MOLLUSCUM CONTAGIOSUM Molluscum contagiosum is an infectious disease of the skin and mucous membranes caused by one of the largest known viruses. It is limited to humans and most frequently occurs in childhood. Although the virus has not been grown in the laboratory, it has been classified morphologically on the basis of electron microscopy with the pox group of viruses. No cross-antigenicity with other pox viruses has yet been demonstrated.

The mode of transmission is unknown. The disease has a worldwide distribution and has occurred in epidemics within children's institutions, between wrestlers, and among members of the same family. Infections have been transmitted between genitalia during sexual intercourse and from the mouth of a suckling baby to its mother's breast. Successful experimental inoculation of lesion extracts to the skin of human volunteers has been reported. The incubation period varies between 2 weeks and 2 months. Recent fluorescent-antibody and gel-diffusion immunologic studies have shown demonstrable antibody in the serum of infected individuals.

The lesions may vary in number and size, ranging from 1 mm up to "giant" lesions of 1 to 2 cm in diameter, and average about 4 mm. They are elevated, waxy, pearly-white papules which show an umbilicated central pore. By squeezing such a papule, one can express from the pore a curdlike, cheesy material, which, upon electron microscopic examination, proves to be loaded with virus particles. Ordinary light microscopy smears of the curd show a specific diagnostic picture of clusters of cells containing eosinophilic, giant cytoplasmic inclusion bodies. The papules may appear alone or in groups. Autoinoculation is frequent; the lesions are usually present for 6 months to a year, but may persist and spread for 3 to 4 years. The face, especially the eyelids, the trunk, and the anogenital areas are most commonly involved. The conjunctiva, lips, and buccal mucosa may rarely be involved. Molluscum lesions are frequently traumatized and become secondarily infected, but injury seems to cause individual lesions to resolve. Spontaneous regression eventually occurs without scarring. Treatment by sharp curettage clears up the lesions with little, if any, scarring.

Diagnosis of multiple lesions is fairly simple. A single lesion may be confused with a keratoacanthoma, basal-cell epithelioma, or pyogenic granuloma. The diagnosis can be made histologically.

REFERENCES

CHERRY JD, JAHN CL: Herpangina: Etiologic spectrum. Pediatrics 36:623, 1965

EISINGER M et al: Propagation of human wart virus in tissue culture. Nature 256:432, 1975

EVANS AD, WADDINGTON E: Hand, foot and mouth disease in South Wales, 1964. Br J Dermatol 79:309, 1967

FRIEDMAN-KIEN AE et al: Milkers' nodule: Isolation of a virus from a human case. Science 140:1335, 1963

——, VILCEK J: Induction of interference and interferon synthesis by non-replicating molluscum contagiosum virus. J Immunol 99:1092, 1967

HUEBNER RJ et al: Herpangina: Etiological studies of a specific infectious disease. JAMA 145:628, 1951

KIBRICK S: Current status of Coxsackie and ECHO viruses in human disease. Prog Med Virol 6:27, 1964

LEAVELL UW et al: Orf. Report of 19 human cases. JAMA 204: 657, 1968

PATTERSON WC et al: A study of vesicular stomatitis in man. J Am Vet Med Assoc 133:57, 1958

POSTELETHWAITE R: Molluscum contagiosum: A review. Arch Environ Health 21:432, 1970

208 CAT-SCRATCH DISEASE

ROBERT G. PETERSDORF

DEFINITION Cat-scratch disease is an infection characterized by indolent, occasionally suppurative, regional lymphadenitis, secondary to a primary cutaneous lesion at the site of inoculation, usually a cat scratch. Because more than 90 percent of the reported cases have originated from cat scratches and a history of close contact with cats is often elicited, the name *cat-scratch disease* has become popular. However rarely, a similar disorder has been acquired from injury due to splinters, thorns, beef-bone fragments, and dog and monkey scratches, and in some patients no inciting trauma is recalled.

ETIOLOGY A specific etiologic agent has not been identified. Among the agents that have been incriminated are atypical acid-fast bacteria, organisms of the psittacosis-lymphogranuloma group, and herpes-like (EB) virus. The evidence for ascribing a definitive causative role to any of these is not convincing.

EPIDEMIOLOGY Cats act only as vectors for the diseases. They are not ill, and have negative skin tests. The disease occurs mostly in children (75 percent), and several cases have been described in siblings, because of contact with the same cat. The disease is most common in fall and winter. Cats may act as long-term carriers, a hypothesis supported by the familial occurrence of several infections interspersed by months or years.

PATHOLOGY The histopathologic appearance of lymph nodes is not specific. Three stages have been described: (1) Early lesions show reticulum-cell hyperplasia; (2) intermediate lesions show granuloma formation; and (3) late lesions show microabscesses. These reactions are not readily distinguished from those induced by the tubercle bacillus. However, acid-fast bacilli are invariably absent.

MANIFESTATIONS The incubation period lasts a few days to several weeks, with an average of 3 to 10 days. In a typical case the primary lesion consists of a raised, slightly tender, nonpruritic papule crowned by a small vesicle or eschar; it often resembles an indolent furuncle or insect bite. Multiple primary lesions have been described. In some patients a primary lesion cannot be found.

Regional lymphadenopathy becomes evident in a few days or as long as 6 weeks after infection. Adenopathy is unilateral and asymmetric; in most instances only one node is involved. The axillary, cervical, preauricular, submandibular, epitrochlear, femoral, or inguinal nodes (in decreasing order of frequency) on one side become visibly swollen and tender, often with redness of the overlying skin. The nodes occasionally suppurate, soften, and drain spontaneously; fistulas heal completely with only slight scarring. Usually the tenderness subsides gradually, and nontender, firm, enlarged nodes remain palpable for some weeks or even months. With rare exceptions, there is no generalized glandular enlargement, and the spleen is not palpable.

Systemic symptoms are usually mild and consist of headache, fever, and malaise, which subside within a few days.

Shaking chills and fever with temperatures as high as 104°F can occur but are unusual. Many patients are entirely symptom-free. A transient macular or vesicular rash which subsides within 48 h is rarely present during the early stages. Erythema nodosum and multiforme have been reported.

Clinical forms of this disease other than that described above may be delineated. These include (1) encephalitis characterized by fever, convulsions, alterations in consciousness, mild cerebrospinal fluid pleocytosis and elevation in protein, and complete recovery; (2) Parinaud's oculoglandular syndrome characterized by granulomatous conjunctivitis and enlargement of the homolateral preauricular node; more rarely, mesenteric lymphadenitis; osteolytic bone lesions, which subside spontaneously, and thrombocytopenic as well as nonthrombocytopenic purpura. In all these syndromes the diagnostic criteria for cat-scratch disease must be present before the illness can be ascribed to cat-scratch disease.

DIAGNOSIS The following criteria should be fulfilled before a diagnosis of cat-scratch disease is established: (1) history of contact with cats, (2) finding of a primary lesion, (3) regional lymphadenopathy, (4) positive intradermal skin test, (5) biopsy of lymph node with demonstration of histopathologic changes consistent with cat-scratch disease (this may not be necessary if the skin test is positive), and (6) failure to demonstrate other causative agents.

The specific diagnosis is made by means of a skin test. Antigen for this is prepared by mixing one part pus aspirated from infected lymph nodes with three parts saline solution, and inactivating the mixture by heating. A positive reaction is of the delayed tuberculin type, consisting of 5-mm induration and 1-cm erythema, that appears in 24 to 48 h. Although batches of antigen vary in potency, in general, patients reacting to one batch react to another. Skin test material can be preserved by freezing. The test becomes positive within 30 days after infection and may persist for many years. Each batch of antigen must be tested against patients known to have had the disease. A well-standardized batch should provide highly reliable results. Approximately 10 percent of normal individuals have false positive reactions. The chance of carrying hepatitis virus in the antigen is remote.

Other laboratory abnormalities include mild leukocytosis (up to 15,000 cells per mm^3), occasional mild eosinophilia, and an elevated sedimentation rate. The Frei test is negative.

Patients with cat-scratch disease show significantly depressed lymphocyte transformation responses to phytohemagglutinin and *Candida albicans*. These reactions revert to normal as the disease subsides.

Cat-scratch disease is a benign illness, and the prognosis is uniformly good. Its main clinical importance lies in its possible confusion with other more serious diseases of the lymphatics. Diseases to be considered are tularemia, lymphatic tuberculosis, sporotrichosis, histoplasmosis, coccidioidomycosis, toxoplasmosis, and bacterial adenitis. Because of the indolent character of the adenopathy, Hodgkin's disease or other lymphomas may be suspected. Neck masses may be confused with thyroglossal duct cysts, bronchial cleft cysts, dermoids, cystic hygromas, thyroid and parathyroid adenomas, salivary gland tumors, carotid body tumors, aneurysms, pharyngeal or esophageal diverticula, and mesodermal tumors, as well as lymphomas. Appropriate serologic and cultural tests serve to rule out other infections; biopsy may be needed to exclude tumor, but a positive skin test with cat-scratch antigen effectively rules out the necessity for biopsy. Cat-scratch disease must be differentiated from tularemia, which occasionally can be transmitted by cats.

TREATMENT In instances of node suppuration, aspiration of accumulated pus affords relief of pain (and incidentally, serves as a source of material for the preparation of skin-test antigen). Aspiration is required in only a few cases. Antibiotics and steroids are ineffective.

REFERENCES

Carithers HA et al: Cat-scratch disease: Its natural history. JAMA 207:312, 1969

Futrell JW et al: Unsuspected etiology of lateral neck masses. Arch Otolaryngol 95:277, 1972

Lyon LW: Neurologic manifestations of cat-scratch disease. Arch Neurol 25:23, 1971

Margileth AM: Cat-scratch disease: Nonbacterial regional lymphadenitis. The study of 145 patients and a review of the literature. Pediatrics 42:803, 1968

Schulkind ML, Ayoub EM: Cell-mediated immunity in cat-scratch disease. J Pediatr 85:199, 1974

Warwick WJ: The cat-scratch syndrome: Many diseases or one disease? Prog Med Virol 9:256, 1967

209 INFECTIOUS MONONUCLEOSIS

JAMES C. NIEDERMAN

DEFINITION Infectious mononucleosis (IM) is an acute and usually benign infectious disease caused by the Epstein-Barr virus (EBV). It occurs most commonly among adolescents and young adults, who have a characteristic clinical picture consisting of fever, pharyngitis, lymphadenopathy, an increase of peripheral lymphocytes with a high proportion of atypical cells, and the development of transient heterophil and persistent EBV antibody responses.

HISTORY Idiopathic lymphadenopathy in children was mentioned in the medical literature by Filatov, a Russian pediatrician, in 1885. Pfeiffer first described glandular fever (*Drüsenfieber*) as a clinical entity in 1889. It was not until 1920 that the term *infectious mononucleosis* was employed by Sprunt and Evans; shortly thereafter the condition they described was recognized to be the same disorder as glandular fever.

In 1932, a diagnostic test was introduced by Paul and Bunnell, who demonstrated the development of heterophil antibodies during the course of the disease; the characteristic absorption patterns of this antibody were described by Davidsohn and Walker several years later. Evidence of the etiologic role of EBV was first recognized by Henle et al early in 1968.

ETIOLOGY EBV, which has the structural and immunologic characteristics of a member of the herpes group, was originally discovered by electron microscopic studies of tumor cells from biopsies of Burkitt's lymphoma grown in tissue culture. EBV antibodies measured by immunofluorescence techniques, complement fixation, immunodiffusion, and virus neutralization are consistently absent prior to infectious mononucleosis, regularly develop during the course of the disease, and persist with little change for many years thereafter. In addition to IgG, EBV-specific IgM antibody has been demonstrated during acute infectious mononucleosis in serums obtained 7 to 70 days after onset, and in one instance persisted for 6 months in association with protracted clinical symptoms.

Further evidence of a causative relationship is the presence of EBV in leukocytes cultured from serums of patients with acute cases of mononucleosis as well as from subjects with a past history of the disease. The classical heterophil antibody of infectious mononucleosis has been produced experimentally in squirrel monkeys inoculated with EBV-transformed autologous leukocytes. In addition, inadvertent transmission of EBV by transfusion has been reported and in several instances was associated with the development of clinical infectious mononucleosis, including heterophil antibody.

EPIDEMIOLOGY Infectious mononucleosis has been recognized in all parts of the world. Although no yearly or seasonal trends are present in the general population, early fall and spring are periods of high frequency among college students. The most characteristic epidemiologic feature of the disease is its occurrence among young adults, especially in the fifteen- to twenty-five-year age group.

Seroepidemiologic studies have demonstrated that the absence of EBV antibody correlates with susceptibility to infectious mononucleosis and its presence indicates immunity. The age at which infection is acquired is related to socioeconomic factors and hygienic environment. Among disadvantaged groups such as children living in certain tropical countries, antibody is acquired early. In contrast, in middle and upper socioeconomic groups, only 50 to 60 percent have detectable antibody during adolescent years and at the time of entry into college. Among these individuals, infectious mononucleosis is a well-recognized disorder. Studies measuring both apparent and inapparent infections suggest a clinical/subclinical ratio of 1:2 to 1:3 in young adults.

When EBV infection develops in early childhood, a mild and nonspecific or an inapparent illness occurs, both of which are associated with the appearance and persistence of specific antibody. If primary infection is delayed until adolescence or young adulthood, the clinical response is frequently typical infectious mononucleosis with the development of both heterophil and EBV antibodies.

Epidemiologic and laboratory evidence has suggested that transmission of EBV occurs through the oropharyngeal route during close personal contact. Table 209-1 indicates that EBV is present in small amounts in throat washings from 1 week to many months after clinical illness.

This prolonged carrier state following clinical infectious mononucleosis, and perhaps also after inapparent EBV infection, may serve as a principal source of transmission. Investigations utilizing the presence of EBV antibody as an index of immunity have confirmed the low contagiousness of both the infection and the disease among susceptible college roommates; secondary attack rates for EBV infection within family units have also been low.

Pathology Generalized involvement of lymphoid tissue with lymphadenopathy, nasopharyngeal lymphoid hyperplasia, and splenomegaly is the outstanding pathologic feature. Widespread focal and perivascular aggregates of mononuclear cells, including atypical lymphocytes, are found throughout the body. Nonspecific hyperplastic changes in lymph nodes are present without infiltration of the capsule or surrounding tissues. Nonlymphoid organs and tissues, including liver, heart, kidneys, and central nervous system, are also infiltrated, and changes in these organs may be associated with functional disturbances. Bone marrow hyperplasia develops, and occasionally small granulomas are present.

MANIFESTATIONS In young adults an incubation period of 30 to 50 days has been suggested on the basis of contact infection studies. Infectious mononucleosis associated with the development of heterophil and EBV antibody has occurred in several patients 5 weeks following blood transfusion. Children appear to have shorter incubation periods, in the range of 10 to 14 days, but there is relatively little information on this point.

During a prodromal period of 3 to 5 days, mild symptoms, including headache, malaise, and fatigue, are common. Frank clinical features usually present over the next 7 to 20 days; they are variable in severity, but in over 80 percent of cases include fever, sore throat, and cervical adenopathy. In adults, temperature elevations which peak at 101 to 103°F may persist for 7 to 10 days. In severe cases, a daily rise in temperature to 105°F may continue even longer. On the other hand, children often have little or no fever accompanying the infection.

Sore throat occurs in the first week and is the most common feature of infectious mononucleosis. Hyperplasia of pharyngeal lymphoid tissue with inflammation and edema develops. A grayish-white exudative tonsillitis persisting for 7 to 10 days is present in approximately 50 percent of cases. The uvula and palatal arch frequently have a gelatinous appearance. *Palatine petechiae,* located near the border of the hard and soft palate, are observed in about one-third of patients toward the end of the first week of illness. Although highly suggestive, their presence is not pathognomonic of the disease.

TABLE 209-1
Recovery of EBV in pharyngeal excretions from 25 cases of infectious mononucleosis

Time after onset of symptoms, days	*No. specimens tested*	*No. specimens positive*	*Percent positive*
0–14	16	13	81.3
15–28	12	10	83.3
29–150	11	11	100.0
>150	3	2	66.7
Total	42	36	85.7

SOURCE: *G Miller et al.*

Lymph node enlargement is a hallmark of infectious mononucleosis. The onset is gradual, and anterior and posterior cervical chains are most commonly involved. Generalized adenopathy, including axillary, epitrochlear, and inguinal nodes, may also develop during the course of the disease. The nodes are affected singly or in groups and may be small or grape-sized; they are firm, discrete, and moderately tender on palpation.

Splenomegaly occurs in approximately one-half the patients, and enlargement is greatest during the second and third weeks of illness. Although extremely rare, splenic rupture is one of the few potentially fatal complications of the disease.

Percussion tenderness over the liver and hepatomegaly develop in only about 10 percent of patients, but the majority (90 percent) have abnormal liver function test results which persist for several weeks. Jaundice occurs in no more than 4 to 5 percent of cases and is usually mild and uncomplicated.

During early stages of the disease a transient faint erythematous maculopapular eruption on the trunk and extremities is present in about 10 percent of patients. The rash often resembles rubella, but may be urticarial, hemorrhagic, or scarlatiniform in nature. *Bilateral supraorbital edema* may also be a transient finding early in the course.

A wide variety of neurologic manifestations has been described, but they occur only rarely. Aseptic meningitis, encephalitis, blurred vision, coma, acute cerebellar syndrome, and the Guillain-Barré syndrome may appear at any time during the illness. Most patients experience complete recovery from central nervous system involvement; however, severe paralysis and/or respiratory incapacity occur in rare instances and are potentially fatal complications.

LABORATORY FINDINGS **Blood picture** Essential to the diagnosis of infectious mononucleosis is an increase in relative and absolute numbers of lymphocytes and monocytes, including 10 to 20 percent atypical forms. Early in disease this is the result of increased numbers of both B and T cells, and later of a predominance of T lymphocytes. The atypical lymphocytes are large cells with oval, horseshoe-shaped, or indented nuclei and basophilic, vacuolated foamy cytoplasm. Nuclear chromatin is usually dense and irregular, and nucleoli are rarely seen. During the first week of illness, either the total leukocyte count is normal or there may be a leukopenia due to granulocytopenia. The total count then rises to between 10,000 and 20,000 leukocytes per mm^3 by the second or third week of illness; rarely, the number of leukocytes may range as high as 50,000 per mm^3. Characteristic leukocyte changes often persist for 4 to 8 weeks or more. Anemia is rare in infectious mononucleosis, but hemolytic anemia has been reported as a complication. Slight to moderate thrombocytopenia, which is usually symptomless, has been recognized during the early weeks of disease. In a few reported cases, the clinical picture has suggested idiopathic thrombocytopenic purpura.

Serologic diagnosis The serum of IM patients characteristically contains heterophil antibodies, i.e., agglutinins against sheep red blood cells, in high titer. Heterophil antibody is associated with the IgM fraction of serum and usually declines over a period of 3 to 6 months. In general, the higher the titer developed during clinical illness, the longer the antibodies will remain detectable in convalescence. Though a nonspecific serologic response, the heterophil antibody of infectious mononucleosis differs from other antibodies in human serums that also agglutinate sheep red blood cells. The latter are found at low levels in normal human serums and in high titers in serum sickness. Differentiation is based on absorption techniques utilizing guinea pig kidney and beef erythrocytes. The sheep cell agglutinins of infectious mononucleosis are completely absorbed by beef red blood cells but not by guinea pig kidney. Serum sickness agglutinins are absorbed by both, whereas nonspecific Forssman agglutinins are absorbed only by guinea pig kidney. A high order of specificity has now been achieved with other qualitative heterophil antibody tests which utilize Formalin-treated horse red blood cells, ox red blood cells, and enzyme-treated and -untreated sheep cells.

Usually sheep cell agglutinins are present in the first week of illness, but they may be delayed in appearance. During the first 2 weeks after onset of the illness, 60 percent of young adult patients develop a positive heterophil antibody test. This percentage increases to 80 to 90 percent by the end of 1 month. The height of the titer is not related to severity of the disease or to the degree of lymphocytosis. In the presence of clinical and hematologic findings, a sheep cell agglutinin titer of 1:224 or higher before guinea pig kidney absorption and 1:28 after absorption has diagnostic significance. In the beef cell hemolysin test, a titer of 1:280 or higher may be considered significant. A rising titer in early stages of disease is the best criterion.

During acute infectious mononucleosis an increase in total serum IgM levels up to 100 percent over control values and a 50 percent increase in IgG levels has been observed. Other protein alterations associated with the IgM fraction which may be present in the disorder include cold agglutinating antibody and transiently positive serologic tests for syphilis and rheumatoid factor. In IM, the presence of EBV antibody is a regular feature. Prospective clinical studies have shown that the disease occurs only in individuals who lack antibodies to EBV; patients become seropositive in almost all cases by the time acute symptoms appear. As measured by immunofluorescence techniques, levels of 1:80 to 1:320 are often found during early illness, and in only 15 to 20 percent of cases are significant antibody rises demonstrable. Rarely, the development of both EBV and heterophil antibodies is delayed several weeks following onset of symptoms. The relationships between clinical features and antibody levels in a typical heterophil positive case are shown in Fig. 209-1. In addition to development of antibody to EB viral capsid antigen, which is the most widely used clinically, antibodies to early antigen and EBV-specific IgM occur in 75 to 85 percent of patients with acute mononucleosis. Antibodies to other EBV-associated antigen systems (membrane, nuclear, complement-fixing, neutralizing, and immunoprecipitating) are also absent before infection and appear during the course of disease.

No direct correlation has been found between the levels of EBV and heterophil antibodies, nor between the anti-

EBV titer and severity of clinical symptoms or hematologic findings. Heterophil antibody levels are highest during the first 4 to 6 weeks after onset, and then decline or disappear after several months. EBV antibodies also reach peak titers within 3 to 4 weeks but persist at lower levels for many years thereafter, if not for life. Antibody titers of 1:20 to 1:40 have been demonstrated in serum collected 45 years after laboratory documentation of heterophil-positive IM.

The appearance of EBV antibody has also been demonstrated in cases which have the clinical and hematologic characteristics of IM but do not develop heterophil antibody. These EBV-positive, heterophil-negative cases are apparently frequent in infants and children but rare in adults.

Other laboratory abnormalities These consist primarily of abnormal liver function tests and may include an elevation in alkaline phosphatase level, retention of Bromsulphalein, mild abnormalities in serum glutamic oxaloacetic transaminase and serum glutamic pyruvic transaminase, and mild icterus. With recovery, all these values return to normal.

Acute infectious mononucleosis is associated with depressed cell-mediated immunity manifested by loss of skin hypersensitivity and lymphocyte hyporesponsiveness to in vitro stimulation by a variety of mitogens and specific antigens.

DIAGNOSIS The main diagnostic features of infectious mononucleosis are (1) irregular fever, sore throat, and lymphadenopathy; (2) an absolute increase in lymphocytes and monocytes exceeding 50 percent and including more than 10 percent atypical lymphocytes in the peripheral blood; (3) the transient appearance of sheep cell agglutinins and beef cell hemolysins; (4) the development of persistent antibody against Epstein-Barr virus; and (5) abnormalities of liver function tests.

Since many of these features are also seen in other dis-

FIGURE 209-1
Relationships between clinical features, hematologic changes, and antibody levels in a typical case of infectious mononucleosis.

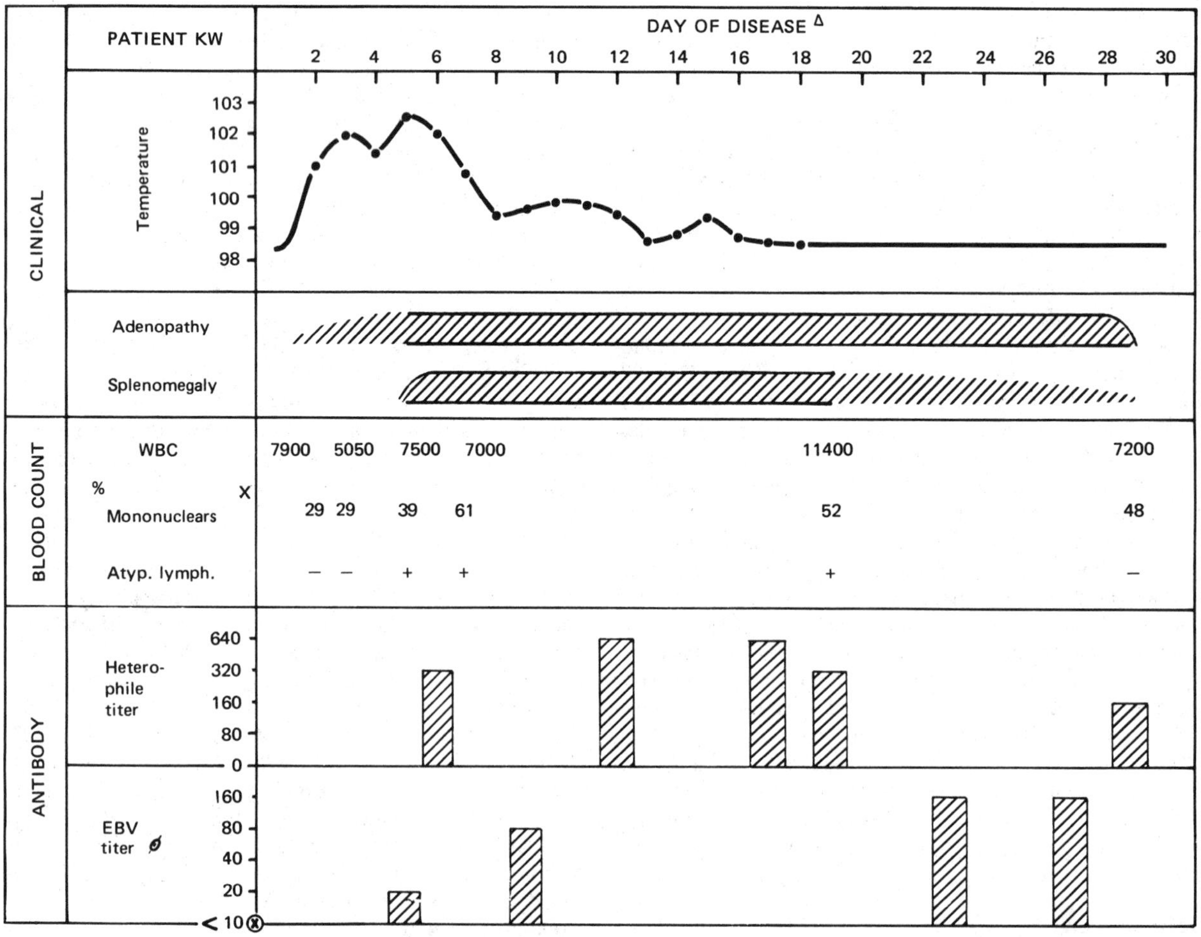

° After adsorption
X % Mononuclears = lymphocytes + monocytes
Δ Day 1 = (30/IV/64)
ø Antibody titer expressed as reciprocal of serum dilution
⊗ EBV titer of patient's pre-illness serum = < 10

ease, IM may resemble a number of febrile disorders, especially those associated with fever, sore throat, adenopathy, and leukocytosis. In early stages of the disease, it is often difficult to distinguish IM from other forms of febrile exudative pharyngotonsillitis such as *streptococcal infections, exudative tonsillitis of viral etiology, Vincent's angina,* and *diphtheria.* Differentiation depends on the results of throat cultures and the development of the hematologic and serologic features characteristic of infectious mononucleosis.

Diseases with some similarities in hematologic abnormalities such as *acute leukemia* and other lymphoproliferative disorders may be mistaken for IM. Demonstration of very immature leukocytes in blood or bone marrow and the presence of anemia, severe thrombocytopenia, and a negative heterophil antibody test distinguish these disorders from IM.

Cytomegalovirus (CMV) mononucleosis usually involves a slightly older age group, i.e., twenty to thirty years. Splenomegaly, hepatic involvement, and the presence of atypical lymphocytes in blood are common features of this disease, whereas sore throat and cervical adenopathy are usually absent. In transfusion-associated CMV infections, cytomegalovirus is excreted in the urine and a rise in complement-fixing antibody can be demonstrated.

Acute infectious lymphocytosis, a benign disorder of children, should be considered in the differential diagnosis among younger age groups. The majority of these cases are associated with signs of an upper respiratory tract infection; adenopathy is minimal, and splenomegaly is absent. The major feature is leukocytosis consisting of small mature lymphocytes; this abnormal blood picture may persist for 4 to 5 weeks, and occasionally for several months. The heterophil antibody test is negative, and no relationship to EBV antibody has been found.

The prodromal stage of *rubella,* associated with fever, malaise, postauricular and posterior cervical adenopathy, and lymphocytosis, may be indistinguishable from early infectious mononucleosis. A distinguishing feature of the rash of rubella is its invariable presence on the face, while that of IM is prominent on the trunk and usually spares the face; it is rarely as florid as in typical rubella. The appearance of large numbers of atypical lymphocytes in the blood and the development of heterophil and/or EB viral antibodies indicate infectious mononucleosis. Isolation of rubella virus from the throat and demonstration of a rising rubella antibody titer will confirm a diagnosis of rubella.

Acquired *toxoplasmosis* may be associated with fever, generalized adenopathy, splenomegaly, and lymphocytosis. A definitive diagnosis is based on direct isolation of *Toxoplasma gondii* and/or the demonstration of the development of specific serologic responses.

Infectious mononucleosis with jaundice can frequently be confused with *infectious hepatitis.* In hepatitis, fever is often lower and disappears when jaundice develops. Similarly, the presence of atypical lymphocytes is usually transitory during the preicteric phase of hepatitis, and the disease is rarely associated with splenomegaly and leukocytosis.

TREATMENT Therapy is symptomatic. Antibiotics have no effect on uncomplicated cases of infectious mononucleosis. During the febrile period rest in bed is advisable. Salicylates or other analgesics are usually sufficient to control headache and discomfort from sore throat. Gargling and irrigation with saline solutions provide symptomatic relief of pharyngitis and stomatitis. As a rule, most patients recover uneventfully on this regimen in 2 to 4 weeks, with gradual return to normal activities. Patients with splenomegaly should be cautioned against heavy lifting and strenuous athletics until splenic enlargement has disappeared.

In patients with severe toxic exudative pharyngotonsillitis associated with extensive pharyngeal edema, corticosteroids are useful to induce a prompt anti-inflammatory effect. A short course of prednisone may be administered, starting with 40 to 60 mg the first day and decreasing this total dose 5 mg daily over 7 to 10 days. Steroids are not necessary in treatment of the usual patient with IM. However, full dosages of steroids should be employed in the management of severe complications, including (1) airway obstruction, in which a tracheostomy may also be required, (2) neurologic complications, (3) hemolytic anemia and thrombocytopenic purpura, and (4) myocarditis and pericarditis.

Severe abdominal pain is rare in IM except in association with splenic rupture. This serious complication requires massive transfusions and immediate splenectomy.

REFERENCES

Carter RL, Penman HG: *Infectious Mononucleosis,* Oxford: Blackwell Scientific Publications, Ltd., 1969

Evans AS et al: Seroepidemiologic studies of infectious mononucleosis with EB virus. N Engl J Med 279:1121, 1968

Henle G et al: Relation of Burkitt's tumor associated herpes-type virus to infectious mononucleosis. Proc Natl Acad Sci USA 59:94, 1958

——: Antibodies to Epstein-Barr virus–associated nuclear antigen in infectious mononucleosis. J Infect Dis 130:231, 1974

Hoagland RJ: *Infectious Mononucleosis,* New York: Grune & Stratton, 1967

Mangi RJ et al: Depression of cell-mediated immunity during acute infectious mononucleosis. N Engl J Med 291:1149, 1974

Miller G et al: Prolonged oropharyngeal excretion of Epstein-Barr virus following infectious mononucleosis. N Engl J Med 288:299, 1973

Niederman JC et al: Prevalence, incidence and persistence of EB virus antibody in young adults. N Engl J Med 282:361, 1970

—— et al: Infectious mononucleosis: Clinical manifestations in relation to EB virus antibodies. JAMA 203:205, 1968

210 MUMPS

C. GEORGE RAY
ROBERT G. PETERSDORF

DEFINITION Mumps is an acute communicable disease of viral origin characterized by painful enlargement of the salivary glands and sometimes by involvement of the gonads, meninges, pancreas, and other organs.

ETIOLOGY The causative agent of mumps is a paramyxovirus of intermediate size (150 to 250 nm in diameter). It has a tight helical inner core (RNA) enclosed in an outer shell of lipid and protein. Serologic cross reactions have been demonstrated between viruses. The virus of mumps causes in vitro agglutination of erythrocytes of fowl, human beings, and some other species, produces hemolysis, and has two components capable of fixing complement. These are the soluble, or S, antigens derived from the nucleocapsid, and the V antigen derived from the surface hemagglutinin. It elicits a delayed allergic reaction when used as an antigen in persons who have had mumps infection.The virus can be cultivated in chick embryos and in a variety of mammalian cell cultures, including HeLa and monkey kidney cells.

EPIDEMIOLOGY Human beings are the only natural host for mumps. The disease is worldwide and is endemic in urban communities. Epidemics are relatively infrequent and are confined to closely associated groups who live in orphanages, army camps, or schools. The disease is most frequent in the spring, particularly during April and May. Although mumps is generally considered less "contagious" than measles and chickenpox, this difference may be more apparent than real because many mumps infections (at least 25 percent) tend to be inapparent clinically. In some surveys, 80 to 90 percent of an adult population had serologic evidence of previous infection with mumps.

Infections are rare before the age of two years and then increase rapidly in frequency, reaching a peak at ages six to ten. Clinical mumps may be more common in males than in females. Adults are usually infected through direct contact. In North American cities, most infections are contracted from schoolmates and infected family members. The virus is transmitted in infected salivary secretions, although its isolation from urine suggests that the virus may also spread via this route. Mumps virus is rarely isolated from stools. The saliva is infectious for approximately 6 days prior to the onset of parotitis, and virus has been recovered from this site for as long as 2 weeks after onset of parotid swelling. Viruria also persists for 2 to 3 weeks in some patients. Despite this prolonged secretion of virus, the peak of infectivity occurs a day or two before onset of parotitis and subsides rapidly after the appearance of glandular enlargement.

One attack of clinical or subclinical mumps confers lasting immunity, and second attacks are most unusual. Unilateral parotitis affords protection just as effectively as does bilateral disease.

PATHOGENESIS The virus enters via the respiratory route; during the incubation period of 15 to 21 days it presumably replicates in the upper respiratory tract and cervical lymph nodes, from which it is disseminated via the bloodstream to other organs, including the meninges, gonads, pancreas, breasts, thyroid, heart, liver, kidneys, and cranial nerves. The salivary adenitis is thought by many to be secondary to viremia, but primary spread from the respiratory tract has not been ruled out as an alternative mechanism.

MANIFESTATIONS **Salivary adenitis** The onset of typical parotitis is usually sudden, although it may be preceded by a prodromal period of malaise, anorexia, chilly sensations, feverishness, sore throat, and tenderness at the angle of the jaw. In many cases, however, parotid swelling is the first indication of illness. The glands enlarge progressively over a period of 1 to 3 days, and the swelling resolves within a week after maximal enlargement. The swollen gland extends from the ear to the lower portion of the mandibular ramus and to the inferior portion of the zygomatic arch, often displacing the ear upward and outward. The skin over the gland is usually not warm or erythematous, in contrast to what happens in bacterial parotitis. There may be reddening and pouting of the orifice of Stensen's duct. Usually, pain and tenderness are marked, although at times they are absent. The edema of mumps has been described as "gelatinous," and when the involved gland is tweaked, it rolls like jelly. Swelling may involve only the submaxillary and sublingual glands and may extend over the anterior part of the chest, producing *presternal edema.* Involvement of submaxillary glands alone can cause difficulty in distinguishing mumps from acute cervical adenitis. Swelling of the glottis occurs rarely but may require tracheostomy. Parotitis is bilateral in two-thirds of cases and remains confined to one side in the remainder. The second gland tends to swell as the first is subsiding, usually 4 to 5 days after onset. In general, parotitis is accompanied by a temperature of 100 to 103°F, malaise, headache, and anorexia, but systemic symptoms may be virtually absent, particularly in children. In most patients, the chief complaints refer to difficulty in eating, swallowing, and talking.

Epididymoorchitis Mumps is complicated by orchitis in 20 to 35 percent of postpubertal males. Testicular involvement usually appears 7 to 10 days after onset of parotitis, although it may precede it or appear simultaneously. Occasionally, orchitis occurs in the absence of parotitis. Gonadal involvement is bilateral in only 2 to 12 percent of patients. Orchitis is heralded by recrudescence of malaise and appearance of chilly sensations, headache, nausea, and vomiting. Shaking chills and high fevers, with temperatures between 103 and 106°F, are frequent. The testicle becomes greatly swollen and acutely painful. The epididymis is often palpable as a swollen tender cord. Occasionally there may be epididymitis without orchitis. Swelling, pain, and tenderness persist for 3 to 7 days and gradually subside; lysis of fever usually parallels abatement of swelling. Occasionally, the temperature falls by crisis. Mumps orchitis is followed by progressive atrophy of the testicle in one-half the cases. Even after bilateral orchitis, sterility is unusual, provided no significant atrophy has taken place. However, if bilateral testicular atrophy occurs after mumps, sterility or subnormal sperm counts are quite common. *Pulmonary infarction* has been noted to follow mumps orchitis. This may be the result of thrombosis of the veins in the prostatic and pelvic plexuses in association with the testicular inflammation. Priapism is a rare but painful complication of mumps orchitis.

Pancreatitis Pancreatic involvement is a potentially serious manifestation of mumps, which may rarely be complicated by shock or pseudocyst formation. It should be suspected in patients with abdominal pain and tenderness together with clinical or epidemiologic evidence of mumps. It is difficult to document, since hyperamylasemia, the hallmark of pancreatitis, is also often present in parotitis. Many times the symptoms resemble those of gastroenteritis, and it is conceivable that the high incidence of gastrointestinal symptoms seen in association with the mumps epidemic in Great Britain in 1961 was due to involvement of the pancreas. Although diabetes or pancreatic insufficiency rarely follows mumps pancreatitis, several children have developed "brittle" diabetes a few weeks after mumps.

Central nervous system involvement Nearly half the patients with mumps have an increased number of cells, usually lymphocytes, in the cerebrospinal fluid (CSF), although symptoms of meningitis, stiff neck, headache, and drowsiness are less common. In typical cases, the onset of overt central nervous system signs and symptoms occurs 3 to 10 days after the onset of parotitis; however, the onset has also been noted to develop prior to the parotitis or 2 to 3 weeks later. In approximately 30 to 40 percent of laboratory-proved cases, there is *no* associated salivary gland involvement at any time in the course of illness. The CSF protein is moderately elevated, and CSF glucose tends to be normal, although in as many as 10 percent of patients low CSF glucose concentrations, in the range of 20 to 50 mg per 100 ml, may be seen. True encephalitis is unusual, although it is responsible for most of the central nervous system sequelae, including behavioral disturbances, headaches, seizures, deafness (usually unilateral), and visual disturbances. At least two cases of aqueductal stenosis and hydrocephalus have been reported as possible late sequelae to mumps encephalitis, but the association remains unproved. Mumps should also be recognized as capable of presenting a picture of mild paralytic poliomyelitis; definition of the cause depends on isolation of virus or serologic confirmation of mumps in the absence of changing antibody titers to poliomyelitis viruses. Rarely, mumps may produce a transverse myelitis, cerebellar ataxia, or the Guillain-Barré syndrome. Mumps meningitis, without clinical encephalitis, is generally thought to be benign.

Other manifestations Mumps virus tends to involve glandular tissues; inflammation of the lacrimal glands, thymus, thyroid, breasts, and ovaries occurs occasionally. *Oophoritis* may be recognized by persistence of pain in the lower part of the abdomen and fever. It does not result in sterility. Mumps virus has been implicated in the causation of subacute thyroiditis; the diagnosis can be made serologically, and occasionally the virus can be isolated from the thyroid gland. A case of myxedema following mumps thyroiditis has been reported. Ocular manifestations of mumps include dacryadenitis, optic neuritis, keratitis, iritis, conjunctivitis, and episcleritis. Although these conditions may transiently interfere with vision, complete resolution is the rule. Mumps *myocarditis,* evidenced primarily by transient abnormalities in the electrocardiogram, is relatively common but does not usually produce symptomatic disease or impair cardiac function. Similarly, *hepatic* involvement may be manifested by mild abnormalities in liver function, but icterus and other clinical signs of hepatic damage are extremely rare. *Thrombocytopenic purpura* as a complication of mumps has been described, and an occasional patient has a leukemoid reaction involving predominantly lymphocytes. Tracheobronchitis and interstitial pneumonia have also been associated with mumps infection, particularly among young children.

A rare but interesting manifestation of mumps is *polyarthritis* which is often migratory. It is most common in males between the ages of twenty and thirty. Joint symptoms begin 1 to 2 weeks after subsidence of parotitis; usually the large joints are involved. The illness lasts 1 to 6 weeks, and complete recovery is the rule. It is not clear whether arthritis is due to viremia or whether it is a "hypersensitivity reaction."

Acute hemorrhagic glomerulonephritis in the absence of streptococcosis has been reported after mumps. The relationship of these two diseases is not clear.

Late complications With the exception of the rare central nervous system sequelae which follow mumps encephalitis, and the occasional patient who is sterile following bilateral testicular involvement, mumps leaves no sequelae. There is no firm evidence that stillbirths and offspring with congenital defects are more common among mothers who have mumps during pregnancy. Likewise, the causal relationship between intrauterine mumps infection and endocardial fibroelastosis has not been clearly established.

LABORATORY FINDINGS In uncomplicated parotitis, the blood leukocyte count is normal, although there may be mild leukopenia with relative lymphocytosis. Patients with mumps orchitis, however, may have a marked leukocytosis with a shift to the left. In meningoencephalitis, the white blood cell count is usually within normal limits. The erythrocyte sedimentation rate is usually normal but may rise with testicular or pancreatic involvement. The serum amylase level is elevated both in pancreatitis and in salivary adenitis. It may also be elevated in some patients in whom the sole evidence of mumps is meningoencephalitis, and probably reflects subclinical involvement of the salivary glands. In contrast to the amylase, the serum lipase level is elevated only in pancreatitis, in which hyperglycemia and glucosuria also may occur. The cerebrospinal fluid contains 0 to 2,000 cells per mm^3, almost all mononuclears, although occasionally polymorphonuclear cells will predominate in the early stages. The pleocytosis in mumps meningitis tends to be greater than in aseptic meningitides caused by the poliomyelitis, Coxsackie, and echo viruses. There is no relationship between the cell count and the severity of central nervous system involvement. Transient hematuria and mild reversible abnormalities in renal function, including inability maximally to concentrate the urine and to clear creatinine, occur in association with the viruria of mumps.

DIAGNOSIS The definitive diagnosis of mumps depends on isolation of the virus from blood, throat swabs, secretions from Stensen's duct, cerebrospinal fluid, or urine. However, even with the simplification of viral isolation by means of tissue culture techniques, culture of the virus is rarely necessary in the typical case with associated parotitis. When an etiologic diagnosis is needed, as in aseptic meningitis or in atypical cases of parotitis, the complement fixation test is most commonly employed. Antibodies to the S antigen develop rather rapidly, often reaching a peak within 1 week after the onset of symptoms, and usually disappearing in 6 to 12 months. Complement-fixing antibodies to the V antigen follow a more typical pattern, reaching a peak titer within 2 to 3 weeks after onset, remaining elevated for at least 6 weeks, then persisting at lower levels for years afterward. Paired serums obtained 2 to 3 weeks apart are recommended. A fourfold increase in titer confirms recent infection. In cases where an acute serum is not obtained until later in the course of illness, an elevation of antibodies to the S antigen which exceeds the V antibody titer also suggests recent infection. The hemagglutination inhibition reaction is demonstrable somewhat later and persists for several months. The serum neutralization test is the most sensitive indicator of previous mumps infection, although it is more complicated to perform. However, it is a much better indicator of previous mumps infection than the skin test, and individuals with detectable specific neutralizing antibody are highly unlikely to contract mumps. The *skin test* consists of intradermal injection of killed mumps virus; previous exposure will result in a delayed reaction of the tuberculin type and an anamnestic antibody titer rise to mumps. The skin test is unreliable when used alone in determining the immune status of an individual and is useless in the diagnosis of acute mumps.

The diagnosis of mumps during an epidemic is usually obvious. Sporadic cases, however, must be distinguished from other causes of parotid enlargement. Parotitis may be caused by other viruses, notably parainfluenza. *Bacterial parotitis* usually occurs in debilitated patients with severe underlying diseases such as uncontrolled diabetes mellitus, cerebrovascular accidents, or uremia. It may also follow surgical operations. The parotid glands are swollen, warm, and tender, and pus can be expressed from the orifices of Stensen's ducts. Marked polymorphonuclear leukocytosis is present. The disease is usually acquired in the hospital, and *Staphylococcus aureus* is the usual causative organism. Dehydration followed by inspissation of secretions in the salivary ducts is an important predisposing factor. *Calculus* in a salivary duct is usually detectable by palpation or by injection of radiopaque media into Stensen's duct. *Drug reactions* may produce tender swelling of the parotid and other salivary glands. "Iodine mumps" is the commonest type; it may follow such procedures as intravenous urography. Mercurialism and the antihypertensive agent guanethidine may also cause parotid enlargement and tenderness. A careful history usually serves to clarify the cause of these reactions. *Cervical adenitis* caused by streptococci, "bullneck" diphtheria, infectious mononucleosis, cat-scratch disease, sublingual cellulitis (Ludwig's angina), and cellulitis of the external auditory canal are usually easy to distinguish from mumps by careful examination. Parotid tumors and chronic infections such as actinomycosis tend to follow a more indolent course, with slowly progressive swelling. The common "mixed tumor" of the parotid is well circumscribed, nontender, and very firm, almost cartilaginous on palpation. Parotid swelling and fever, often accompanied by lacrimal adenitis and uveitis (Mikulicz's syndrome), may occur in tuberculosis, leukemia, Hodgkin's disease, and lupus erythematosus. The onset may be sudden, but the process is usually painless and of long duration. "Uveoparotid fever" of similar type may be the first manifestation of sarcoidosis; in this disease parotid swelling is frequently accompanied by single or multiple palsies of cranial nerves, particularly the facial nerve, and is referred to as Heerfordt's syndrome. Presternal edema may also be a manifestation of malignant lymphoma involving retrosternal lymph nodes. Bilateral painless parotid swelling unassociated with fever is found in patients with Laennec's cirrhosis, chronic alcoholism, malnutrition, diabetes mellitus, pregnancy and lactation, and hypertriglyceridemia.

Sjögren's syndrome (Chap. 366) is a chronic inflammation of the parotid and other salivary glands which is often associated with atrophy of the lacrimal glands and occurs most commonly in women past the menopause. With cessation of lacrimal and salivary function, there may be striking dryness of the conjunctiva and the cornea (keratoconjunctivitis sicca) and of the mouth (xerostomia). These patients may also have a variety of systemic manifestations, including arthritis of the rheumatoid type, splenomegaly, leukopenia, and hemolytic anemia. The chronicity of the process and its occurrence in elderly women make confusion with mumps unlikely. Finally, benign hypertrophy of both masseter muscles, presumably due to habitual clenching and grinding of teeth, may be confused with painless parotid swelling. The causes of aseptic meningitis are listed in Chap. 338.

Orchitis occurring in the absence of parotitis is likely to remain undiagnosed. Serologic testing may later confirm the diagnosis of mumps. Orchitis may occur in association with acute bacterial prostatitis and seminal vesiculitis. It is a rare complication of gonorrhea. Occasionally testicular inflammation accompanies pleurodynia, leptospirosis, melioidosis, relapsing fever, chickenpox, brucellosis, and lymphocytic choriomeningitis.

TREATMENT There is no specific treatment for infections with the mumps virus. Patients with parotitis should receive mouth care, analgesics, and a bland diet. Bed rest is advisable only as long as the patient is febrile; contrary to popular belief, physical activity has no influence on the development of orchitis or other complications. Patients with epididymoorchitis may be acutely ill and in great pain. Many forms of treatment, including surgical decompression of the testicle, infiltration of the spermatic cord with local anesthetics, estrogens, convalescent serum, and broad-spectrum antibiotics, have not been regularly effective. Despite failure to document their effectiveness in controlled studies, adrenal steroids have been of considerable benefit in diminishing fever, as well as testicular pain and swelling, and in restoring the sense of well-being in a number of patients. It is important to give a single large dose corresponding to 300 mg cortisone or 60 mg prednisone, initially. During the ensuing 24 h the same quantity should be given in divided doses. Subsequently, administration of the hormone can be tapered off over 7 to 10 days. Adrenal steroids have not exerted an adverse effect on concomitant pancreatitis or meningitis, although they have not benefited patients with meningeal involvement, and their withdrawal has usually been accompanied by a sharp recrudescence of symptoms. Adrenal steroids have not prevented the appearance of parotid involvement on the contralateral side. Mumps arthritis is usually mild and requires no treatment. Mumps thyroiditis may subside spontaneously, but excellent relief has been obtained with adrenal hormones.

PREVENTION A live attenuated mumps virus vaccine (Jeryl Lynn strain) has been highly effective in producing significant rises in mumps antibody in individuals who are seronegative prior to vaccination, and has afforded 95 percent protection to individuals subsequently exposed to mumps. The vaccine also has boosted antibody levels in seropositive vaccines. The vaccine produces an inapparent, noncommunicable infection which is not associated with fever or mumpslike symptoms. It has conferred excellent protection for at least 6 years and has not interfered with vaccines against measles, rubella, and poliomyelitis or with smallpox vaccination given simultaneously. Protection has been demonstrated in both children and adults.

Live mumps vaccine can be administered at any time after one year of age, and should be particularly considered for children approaching puberty, adolescents, and adult males who have not had clinical mumps or live mumps vaccine in the past. Individuals living in groups or in institutions should be vaccinated, particularly because it has been shown that physical isolation of mumps patients does not effectively prevent transmission of the infection.

Vaccination is contraindicated in babies under the age of one year because of the interfering effect of maternal antibody; in individuals with a history of hypersensitivity to egg proteins; in patients with febrile illnesses, leukemia, lymphoma, or generalized malignancies; in those receiving steroids, alkylating drugs, antimetabolites, or irradiation; and during pregnancy.

It is not known whether the vaccine will prevent infection when administered after exposure, but no contraindication to its use in this situation exists. Specific mumps-immune globulin in large quantity is of questionable efficacy in aborting orchitis when given 1 to 2 days after exposure, and does not prevent parotitis. Ordinary gamma-globulin is not at all effective.

REFERENCES

BRAY PF: Mumps—a cause of hydrocephalus? Pediatrics 49:446, 1972

BRUNNELL PA et al: Ineffectiveness of isolation of patients as a method of preventing the spread of mumps. N Engl J Med 279: 1357, 1968

CARANASOS GH, FELKER JR: Mumps arthritis. Arch Intern Med 119:394, 1967

KALTREIDER HA, TALAL N: Bilateral parotid gland enlargement and hyperlipoproteinemia. JAMA 210:2067, 1969

KARCHMER AW et al: Simultaneous administration of live virus vaccines. Am J Dis Child 121:382, 1971

KOCEN RS, CRITCHLEY E: Mumps epididymo-orchitis and its treatment with cortisone. Br Med J 2:20, 1961

LERNER AM: Guide to immunization against mumps. J Infect Dis 122:116, 1970

LEVITT LP et al: Central nervous system mumps: A review of 64 cases. Neurology 20:829, 1970

ST GEME JW JR et al: Immunologic significance of the mumps virus skin test in infants, children and adults. Am J Epidemiol 101:253, 1975

UTZ JP et al: Studies of mumps: IV. Viruria and abnormal renal function. N Engl J Med 270:1283, 1964

WILFERT CM: Mumps meningoencephalitis with low cerebrospinal fluid glucose, prolonged pleocytosis and elevation of protein. N Engl J Med 280:855, 1969

211
CYTOMEGALIC INCLUSION DISEASE (SALIVARY GLAND VIRUS DISEASE)

C. GEORGE RAY

DEFINITION Cytomegalic inclusion disease (CID) is a viral infection which can affect human beings at all ages beginning with conception. The agent was initially called *salivary gland virus* and was thought to be primarily responsible for occasional cases of disseminated, fatal illness in newborn infants, or subclinical salivary gland involvement only. Since its initial cultivation in 1956, the virus has been demonstrated to cause a broad spectrum of disease in humans. In adults the manifestations are frequently those of an illness like infectious mononucleosis, or may constitute a terminal complication of chronic debilitating disease.

ETIOLOGY Cytomegalovirus (CMV) belongs to the herpes-virus group and produces large, intranuclear (10 to 15 nm), and inconspicuous cytoplasmic (2 to 4 nm) inclusions which occur in all types of normal and neoplastic tissues. The agent is affected by temperature and other environmental factors. Low temperatures (−80°C) with added stabilizers are needed for shipment and storage. Several antigenically heterogeneous, but closely interrelated, strains have been isolated which are largely species-specific for man and grow in human fibroblast cultures. Of the various immunologic procedures available for diagnosis, the complement fixation test is most widely used, since the different human strains share a common complement-fixing antigen. Species-specific CMV occurs in many different animals and animal models. The mouse CMV systems are particularly important in the experimental study of the infection.

EPIDEMIOLOGY The infection is worldwide and, in this country, highest prevalence rates are found among young, preschool children of low socioeconomic background. CMV infection may be congenital but is more often acquired during the first year of life. At birth 0.5 to 2 percent of infants have been found to be excreting virus in the urine, and by 12 months of age, between 9 and 60 percent of infants in various population groups have acquired infection, with viruria. Among healthy adults, asymptomatic excretion rates are usually less than 1 percent; in late pregnancy, urine and/or uterine cervical virus excretion increases to between 2 to 13 percent. Complement-fixing antibody is relatively infrequent in infancy, increases during childhood, and is present in about 35 to 80 percent of adults. The virus persists in the host for a long time, perhaps indefinitely, and is excreted in saliva, urine, and semen even in the presence of antibody. Breast milk and feces may also transmit the infection. Close and prolonged contact appears necessary for efficient transmission of the infection. Venereal transmission appears to be common among young adults. Transplacental passage of the virus produces congenital infection, and perinatal infection may follow exposure to the virus in the infected cervix uteri during delivery. In adults CID may represent either activation of latent infection or may be newly acquired. It can also be transmitted by transfusion of whole blood; the risk of infection per unit of fresh blood transfused has been estimated as between 5 and 7 percent. The majority of these infections, however, are subclinical, and only detectable by serologic conversion.

PATHOGENESIS Localized or systemic CID which may be latent or active occurs in hematopoietic and lymphocytic-reticular disorders (various anemias, leukemias, lymphomas), other chronic debilitating diseases, and often during immunosuppression. It is a potential complication of any therapy which results in an impairment of humoral and/or cellular immunity. Physiologic factors related to age or late pregnancy favor viral proliferation and dissemination. CID may be associated with stillborn, premature, or low-birth-weight infants. Self-limited forms with generally mild clinical manifestations are being increasingly recognized in apparently normal persons.

PATHOLOGY Enlarged cells, 25 to 40 nm in diameter, with the distinctive nuclear inclusions, are the morphologic hallmark of the infection, and are similar in all forms and sites of infection. Infected cells elicit an inflammatory cell response only after cell death. In adults localized infection most commonly consists of interstitial pneumonitis and gastrointestinal ulcers. Less frequently affected are the nasal mucosa, salivary glands, liver, and adrenals. Hepatitis with the distinctive inclusions has been related to CID by serologic studies. In the disseminated form nearly every tissue may be affected, including the central nervous system. Involvement of the latter, however, has been noted most often in the immunosuppressed adult. In infancy the localized form is largely confined to the salivary glands, hence the original designation of salivary gland virus disease. In disseminated disease the more common sites are salivary glands, kidney, liver, lung, pancreas, gastrointestinal tract, thyroid, adrenal, and central nervous system. Multiple infections are frequently associated with CID. Bacterial, fungal, and various forms of other herpesvirus infections are common. Concomitant infection with pertussis, toxoplasmosis, and *Pneumocystis carinii* are frequent. Interesting interactions between CMV and toxoplasmosis and Newcastle disease virus have been noted experimentally.

CLINICAL MANIFESTATIONS In adults CMV infection is generally latent. It most often becomes clinically manifest in chronic disorders with impaired host resistance, but has been encountered in the absence of demonstrated underlying disease. The manifestations are nonspecific and vary according to the principal organ involved. Acute interstitial pneumonia is the most common presentation, but chronic lung disease and gastrointestinal disorders have been noted. The course of disseminated CID is often fatal.

Congenital CMV infection produces the constellation of hepatosplenomegaly with hepatitis and cirrhosis, purpura, and encephalitis with microcephaly and microgyria. Despite the common occurrence of viruria and inclusion-bearing cells in the kidney, progressive renal disease has not been noted at any age.

CMV mononucleosis is an acute febrile illness with relative or absolute lymphocytosis and many atypical lymphocytes. The patient often complains of headache, back and abdominal pain, and sore throat. Rubella-like rashes, usually lasting only 1 or 2 days, have also been noted. The appearance of extensive rash and prolongation of its duration can be aggravated by inadvertent treatment with ampicillin, an event similar to that seen in infectious mononucleosis treated with the same agent. Other findings have included hepatitis with icterus, hemolytic anemia, thrombocytopenia, purpura, acute polyneuritis, pneumonitis, myocarditis, pericarditis, and occasional splenomegaly. The heterophil test and ox cell hemolysins are negative, but liver function tests are frequently abnormal. Elevated cold agglutinin titers are found in severe cases. The disease occurs spontaneously or after perfusion with fresh whole blood (the postperfusion syndrome) and usually resolves without residua in 3 to 6 weeks. On the basis of observations of the postperfusion syndrome, the incubation period has been estimated to be 21 to 50 days.

Among debilitated or extremely immunosuppressed patients, particularly recent recipients of organ or bone marrow transplants, CMV infection may be particularly virulent, and progressive interstitial pneumonia is a major cause of death.

The differential diagnosis of acquired CMV mononucleosis most commonly includes infectious mononucleosis and toxoplasmosis. Unlike infectious mononucleosis, CMV infection does not evoke a heterophil antibody titer, and exudative pharyngitis and significant lymphadenopathy are unusual. CMV mononucleosis is more commonly seen among adults 19 to 34 years of age, while infectious mononucleosis typically affects a slightly younger, although overlapping, age group. Acquired toxoplasmosis can usually be differentiated by appropriate serologic testing.

CID in infancy is extremely variable in its presentation. Most infections are asymptomatic, or are characterized by mild hepatomegaly, occasional jaundice, and moderately abnormal liver function tests. In the congenital disease, the clinical manifestations range from these minor findings to severe, disseminated disease, which can include growth retardation, severe jaundice, hepatosplenomegaly, encephalitis, microcephaly, chorioretinitis, pneumonitis, thrombocytopenic purpura, maculopapular or hemorrhagic skin rash, and hemolytic anemia. The most common sequelae of congenital infection include sensorineural deafness and mental retardation. It has been estimated that 10 percent of newborns with virologically proved infection at the time of birth will develop significant neurologic impairment.

DIAGNOSIS Virus isolation from blood, body fluids, or tissues establishes the presence of active infection but cannot always be equated with disease, particularly in groups where high asymptomatic infection rates are known to occur. Demonstration of significantly rising antibody titers are of some help, particularly in cases of acquired disease. However, spontaneous, wide fluctuations of complement-fixing antibody titers in healthy individuals have been demonstrated in one longitudinal study, and this rather unique lability of specific antibody tests should also be kept in mind when interpreting results. In congenital infections, the finding of elevated IgM-specific CMV antibody in the newborn generally correlates well with active disease. Morphologic demonstration of CMV inclusions is a relatively insensitive method of diagnosis, as compared with cultures and serology. Roentgenographic and laboratory findings are nonspecific except for the lymphocytosis and atypical lymphocytes in CMV mononucleosis.

TREATMENT No specific therapy is available. No clearly beneficial results have been obtained with interferon or with viral antagonists such as idoxuridine or cytosine arabinoside.

REFERENCES

HANSHAW JB: Congenital cytomegalovirus infection: A fifteen year perspective. J Infect Dis 123:555, 1972

JORDAN MC et al: Spontaneous cytomegalovirus mononucleosis. Clinical and laboratory observations in nine cases. Ann Intern Med 79:153, 1973

REYNOLDS DW et al: Congenital cytomegalovirus infection: Relation to auditory and mental deficiency. N Engl J Med 290:291, 1974

STAGNO S et al: Cervical cytomegalovirus excretion in pregnant and nonpregnant women: Suppression in early gestation. J Infect Dis 131:522, 1975

WANER JL et al: Patterns of cytomegaloviral complement-fixing antibody activity: A longitudinal study of blood donors. J Infect Dis 127:538, 1973

WELLER TH: The cytomegaloviruses: Ubiquitous agents with protean clinical manifestations. N Engl J Med 285:203 and 269, 1971

212 ARBOVIRUS AND ARENAVIRUS INFECTIONS

JAY P. SANFORD

Most viral infections in humans are either asymptomatic or present as undifferentiated illnesses characterized by fever, malaise, headache, and generalized myalgia. The similarities in clinical features between infections caused by viruses as dissimilar as the myxoviruses (e.g., influenza), the enteroviruses (e.g., poliovirus, Coxsackie virus, echo virus), some of the herpesviruses (e.g., cytomegalovirus), and the arboviruses usually preclude an etiologic diagnosis based entirely on clinical manifestations without ancillary information regarding epidemiologic features and serologic findings. The purpose of this chapter is to direct attention to the ever-expanding list of viruses which produce febrile disease in humans. Because the number of agents is large, mention will be made of those which have been best documented, have demonstrated unusual features, or seem to be of greatest potential significance.

ARBOVIRUSES

Definition and classification

It has not always been easy to determine that an agent is an arbovirus; hence with further characterization some agents which were initially registered as arboviruses have been reclassified, e.g., the zoonotic agents which have unique morphology on electron microscopy have been classified as arenaviruses. Similarly, vesicular stomatitis virus and Lagos bat virus, provisionally registered as arboviruses, were found to be related to rabies virus morphologically or serologically, and both are now classified as rhabdoviruses. The currently accepted definition of an arthropod-borne virus was published in 1967 by the World Health Organization:

Arboviruses are viruses which are maintained in nature principally, or to an important extent, through biological transmission between susceptible vertebrate hosts by hematophagous arthropods; they multiply and produce viremia in the vertebrates, multiply in the tissues of arthropods, and are passed on to new vertebrates by the bites of arthropods after a period of extrinsic incubation.

From this definition it can be appreciated that the term *arbovirus* is used in the ecological sense. Transmission by vectors is not correlated with virus architecture, which forms an important basis for current classification. Thus, the broad category arbovirus is being subdivided, and structurally related non-arthropod-borne agents may be classified with agents designated as arboviruses. Casal's serologic groups A and B arboviruses have been shown to be enveloped RNA agents with a spherical nucleocapsid forming the viral core, probably of icosohedral symmetry. Agents with these characteristics are now classified as Togaviruses, with group A designated as alphaviruses and group B as Flavoviruses. Other members of the Togavirus group which are not transmitted by arthropods include rubella virus, equine arteritis virus, European swine fever/hog cholera virus, and viral disease of cattle agent.

There are more than 250 distinct arboviruses, which have been grouped into four families with some agents yet remaining unclassified. Within each family, the agents have been subdivided on the basis of antigenic differences (Table 212-1). The characteristics of individual members of this large group of viruses are not uniform; those in group A are 40 to 60 nm in diameter, and those in the Bunyamwera group are about 100 nm in diameter. The majority of agents contain single-stranded RNA, although some, such as Colorado tick fever, contain double-stranded RNA.

Arboviruses are of importance in both temperate and tropical zones. Representative viruses have been isolated in almost every geographic area outside the polar region.

Arbovirus infection of vertebrates is usually asymptomatic. The viremia stimulates an immune response which sharply limits the duration of the viremia. In arbovirus infections other than urban yellow fever, phlebotomus fever, and dengue, infection of humans represents an incidental occurrence which is tangential to the basic maintenance cycle of the virus. Hence, the isolation of virus from arthropod vectors or the detection of infection in the natural vertebrate host may provide a means for early detection and enable control of epizootic infection before significant spread to humans occurs.

As determined by serologic evidence of host responses,

at least 80 immunologically distinct arboviruses are capable of infecting humans, while somewhat fewer have been incriminated as causing clinical disease. The spectrum of clinical illness produced by the arboviruses is varied both in predominant features and in severity. Five broad, often overlapping, and somewhat arbitrary clinical syndromes may be delineated (Table 212-2).

TABLE 212-1
Classification of arboviruses

Family	*Group*	*Specific agent*	
Toga-viruses	A (alpha-viruses)	Chikungunya* Eastern equine* Mayaro (Uruma)* Mucambo O'nyong-nyong*	Ross River* Sindbis* Venezuelan equine* Western equine*
	B (Flavo-viruses)	Banzi Bat salivary gland* Bussuquara Central European encephalitis Dengue 1,2,3,4* Ilheus Japanese (B)* Kunjin Kyasanur Forest* Louping ill Murray Valley	Negishi Omsk hemorrhagic* Powassan Russian spring-summer Spondweni St. Louis* Usutu Wesselbron West Nile* Yellow fever* Zika*
Bunya-viruses	C	Apeu* Caraparu* Itaqui* Madrid* Marituba*	Murutucui* Oriboca* Ossa* Restan*
	Bunyamwera	Bunyamwera Germiston Guaroa	Ilesha Wycomyia
	Bwamba	Bwamba	
	California	Califoruis LaCrosse*	Tahyna
	Guama	Catu	Guama
	Sandfly fever (Phlebotomus)	Candiru* Chagres* Naples type*	Punta Toro* Sicilian type*
	Simbu	Shuni	Oropouche
	Ungrouped	Crimean hemorrhagic/Congo* Dugbe Ganjam	Rift Valley* Nairobi sheep disease Thogoto
Orbi-viruses	Changuinola Kemerovo Ungrouped	Changuinola Kemerovo Colorado tick fever*	 Tribec Lipovnik
Rhabdo-viruses	Vesicular stomatitis	Vesicular stomatitis (Indiana & New Jersey)* Chandipura	Piry
Not classified		Nyando	Quaranfil

* *Discussed in the text.*

Arbovirus infections presenting chiefly with fever, malaise, headache, and myalgia

PHLEBOTOMUS FEVER Phlebotomus (sandfly, pappataci, or 3-day) fever is an acute, relatively mild, self-limited infection caused by at least five immunologically distinct arboviruses (Naples, Sicilian, Punta Toro, Chagres, and Candiru). Serologic evidence of human infection has been demonstrated for four additional agents (Bujaru, Cacao, Karimabad, and Salehabad). The viruses have been adapted to white mice, but there is no evidence of an animal reservoir in nature.

Prevalence The disease occurs throughout the Mediterranean Basin, the Balkans, the Near and Middle East, the eastern part of Africa, the Soviet republics of Central Asia, West Pakistan, and possibly certain parts of southern China. Recently, sandfly fever has been recognized in Panama and Brazil. In the Middle East and Central Asia native populations acquire the disease at an early age and develop and maintain high levels of immunity. Cases in Panama and Brazil are sporadic, occurring mainly in persons entering the forest. The apparent absence of phlebotomus fever in indigenous adult populations residing in areas where sandflies are abundant may present a deceptive picture of the actual risk to susceptible persons.

Epidemiology In the Middle East and Central Asia, the disease occurs during the hot, dry season (summer or autumn months) and is transmitted to human beings by the bite of infected sandflies (*Phlebotomus papatasi*). *Phlebotomus papatasi* is a small urban fly which can penetrate ordinary house screens. Only the female bites and usually does so during the night. In persons who are not sensitive, there is neither pain nor local irritation after the bite; hence only about 1 percent of patients will remember having been bitten. In contrast, most of the man-biting sandflies of tropical America are sylvan in their habits. Approximately 7 days after feeding on an infected individual, the fly acquires the capacity to transmit infection and remains infectious for its life span. Transovarial transmission of the virus to the next generation has been demonstrated and offers the best explanation for the mechanism of overwinter survival of the virus. In humans, the incubation period may be as short as 3 days. Viremia is present for at least 24 h before the onset of fever, but is not detectable for more than 2 days after the onset of illness.

Clinical manifestations The onset of symptoms is abrupt in over 90 percent of patients, with the temperature rapidly rising to its highest point, which may vary from 100 to 105°F. Headache is nearly always present and often is accompanied by pain on moving the eyes and by retroorbital pain. Myalgia is common and may be localized to the chest, resembling pleurodynia, or to the abdomen. Other symptoms may include vomiting, photophobia, giddiness, neck stiffness, alteration or loss of taste, and arthralgia. Conjunctival injection is present in approximately one-third of patients. Small vesicles may be seen on the palate, and macular or urticarial rashes occur. The spleen is rarely palpable, and lymphadenopathy is absent. The pulse rate may be elevated in proportion to the temperature on the

TABLE 212-2
Summary of clinical and epidemiologic features of arboviruses and arenaviruses associated with disease in humans

Syndrome	*Virus*	*Vector*	*Known geographic range of infection*
Fever with malaise, *headaches,* and *myalgia*	Mayaro	Mosquito	Trinidad, Colombia, Brazil
	Mucambo	Mosquito	Brazil
	Uruma		Lowland forest, Bolivia
	Venezuelan equine encephalitis	Mosquito	Florida, Texas, Louisiana, Mexico, Central America, Ecuador, Colombia, Venezuela, Brazil, Trinidad, Surinam, Guyana, French Guiana
	Kunjin	Mosquito	Northern Australia
	Spondweni	Mosquito	South Africa, Mozambique, Nigeria
	United States bat salivary gland	?	California, Texas, Sonora in Southwest North America
	Wesselbron	Mosquito	South Africa, Bechuanaland
	Yellow fever	Mosquito	Africa, Central and South America
	Zika	Mosquito	Uganda, Nigeria
	Apeu	Mosquito	Brazil
	Anhembi	Mosquito	Brazil
	Caraparu	Mosquito	Brazil, Panama, Trinidad
	Itaqui	Mosquito	Brazil
	Madrid	?	Panama
	Marituba	Mosquito (?)	Brazil
	Murutucui	Mosquito (?)	Brazil
	Oriboca	Mosquito	Brazil
	Ossa	?	Panama
	Restan	Mosquito	Trinidad
	Calovo	Mosquito	Czechoslovakia
	Germiston	Mosquito	South Africa, Angola
	Ilesha	Mosquito (?)	Nigeria
	Guaroa	Mosquito	Colombia, Brazil
	Tahyna	Mosquito	Czechoslovakia, Yugoslavia
	Catu	Mosquito	Brazil, Trinidad
	Guama	Mosquito	Brazil, Trinidad
	Oropouche	Mosquito	Brazil, Trinidad
	Bwamba	Mosquito	Uganda
	Phlebotomus, Naples	Sandfly	Italy, Egypt, Iran, West Pakistan
	Phlebotomus, Sicilian	Sandfly	Italy, Egypt, Iran, Pakistan, Yugoslavia
	Chagres	Sandfly	Panama
	Candiru	Sandfly	Brazil
	Punta Toro	Sandfly	Panama
	Colorado tick fever	Tick	Western United States
	Nairobi sheep disease	Tick	Kenya, Congo
	Rift Valley fever	Mosquito	Africa
	Quaranfil	Tick	Egypt, South America
	Dugbe	Tick	Nigeria
Fever with malaise, headaches, myalgia, *arthralgia,* and *rash*	Chikungunya	Mosquito	South, East, West, Central Africa; India, Thailand, Vietnam, Malaya
	Mayaro	Mosquito	Brazil, Trinidad
	O'nyong-nyong	Mosquito	East Africa, Senegal
	Sindbis	Mosquito	South and East Africa; Egypt, Israel, India, Malaya, Philippines, Australia
	Bunyamwera	Mosquito	South, East, West Africa
	Changuinola	Phlebotomus	Panama
	Ross River	Mosquito	Australia
Fever with malaise, headaches, myalgia, rash, and *lymphadenopathy*	Dengue 1	Mosquito	Hawaii, Oceana, New Guinea, Japan, Malaysia, Thailand, India
	Dengue 2	Mosquito	Circumglobal
	Dengue 3	Mosquito	Caribbean, Oceana, Philippines, Thailand
	Dengue 4	Mosquito	Philippines, Thailand, India
	West Nile	Mosquito	South and West Africa, Rhone delta, Near East, Israel, India, Malaysia, Borneo
Fever with *central nervous system involvement* (meningitis to encephalitis)	Eastern equine encephalitis	Mosquito	Eastern Canada, United States, Mexico, Dominican Republic, Jamaica, Panama, Trinidad, Brazil, Colombia, Argentina
	Western equine encephalitis	Mosquito	Canada, United States, Mexico, Brazil, Argentina
	Venezuelan equine encephalitis	Mosquito	Florida, Texas, Louisiana, Mexico, Central America, Ecuador, Colombia, Venezuela, Brazil, Trinidad, Surinam, Guyana, French Guiana
	Apoi	?	Hokkaido, Japan
	Ilheus	Mosquito	Northern South America, Trinidad, Central America, Florida
	Japanese encephalitis	Mosquito	Japan, China, Malaya, Taiwan, Thailand, Vietnam, Burma, Guam, Philippines, Korea, Australia, New Zealand
	Kyasanur Forest disease	Tick	India
	Louping ill	Tick	Great Britain, Eire
	Medoc	?	United States

TABLE 212-2 *(continued)*

Syndrome	*Virus*	*Vector*	*Known geographic range of infection*
Fever with *central nervous system involvement* (meningitis to encephalitis) (continued)	Murray Valley encephalitis	Mosquito	Australia, New Guinea
	Negishi	?	Japan
	Powassan	Tick	Canada, New York
	St. Louis encephalitis	Mosquito	United States, Caribbean Islands, Panama, Brazil, Argentina
	Tick-borne encephalitis	Tick	Central and Eastern Europe, U.S.S.R.
	West Nile	Mosquito	South and West Africa, Rhone delta, Near East, Israel, India, Malaysia, Borneo
	California encephalitis	Mosquito	United States
	Phlebotomus, Naples	Sandfly	Italy, Egypt, Iran, West Pakistan
	Congo—Crimean hemorrhagic fever	Tick	Central Africa, West Pakistan, Bulgaria, U.S.S.R.
Fever with malaise, headaches, myalgia, and *hemorrhagic signs*	Chikungunya	Mosquito	Thailand, Malaysia, India, Vietnam
	Dengue 1	Mosquito	Thailand, India
	Dengue 2	Mosquito	Philippines, Vietnam, Thailand, Malaysia, India, Puerto Rico
	Dengue 3	Mosquito	Philippines, Thailand
	Dengue 4	Mosquito	Philippines, Thailand
	Kyasanur Forest disease	Tick	India
	Omsk hemorrhagic fever	Tick	Western Siberia, U.S.S.R.
	Yellow fever	Mosquito	Africa, Central and South America
	Central Asian hemorrhagic fever	Tick (?)	Central Asia, U.S.S.R.
	Congo—Crimean hemorrhagic fever	Tick	Southern U.S.S.R., Central Africa, West Pakistan, Bulgaria
	Far Eastern or Korean hemorrhagic fever	Rodent, mite (?)	U.S.S.R., Manchuria, China, Korea

first day; thereafter bradycardia is often present. The fever persists 3 days in most patients, with gradual defervescence. Giddiness, weakness, and feelings of depression are frequently encountered during convalescence. Second attacks 2 to 12 weeks after the first occur in 15 percent of cases.

In common with other arbovirus infections, phlebotomus fever may be associated with *aseptic meningitis.* In one series, 12 percent of patients had symptoms and signs sufficient to warrant a lumbar puncture. Findings in these patients included pleocytosis, with an average cell count of 90 per mm^3 and a predominance of either polymorphonuclear or mononuclear leukocytes. Spinal fluid protein concentration ranged from 20 to 130 mg per 100 ml. In another series mild papilledema was observed in a few patients with severe illness.

Laboratory findings The changes in leukocyte count constitute the only positive laboratory findings. Total leukocyte counts of less than 5,000 per mm^3 are observed in 90 percent of patients if daily counts are done during the febrile period and convalescence. The leukopenia may not appear until the last day of fever or even after defervescence. The differential leukocyte count will reveal an absolute decrease in lymphocytes on the first day, accompanied by an increase in nonsegmented neutrophils. During the second or third day, the number of lymphocytes begins to return to normal and may constitute 40 to 65 percent of the total count. Concurrently, there is a reversal in proportion of segmented and band neutrophils. The differential count usually returns to normal within 5 to 8 days after defervescence. Erythrocyte values and urinalyses are usually normal.

Diagnosis In the absence of a specific serologic test, the diagnosis must be made on clinical and epidemiologic grounds.

Treatment The disease is self-limited, and no specific therapy is available. Symptomatic care, including bed rest, adequate fluid intake, and analgesia with aspirin, is recommended. Convalescence may require a week or longer.

Prognosis No fatalities have been recorded among the tens of thousands of cases.

COLORADO TICK FEVER Colorado tick fever is one of the two tick-transmitted virus diseases of human beings recognized in the Western Hemisphere, Powassan virus being the other. Though "mountain fever" had been described ever since the advent of immigrants to the Rocky Mountain region, Becker in 1930 differentiated it from mild Rocky Mountain spotted fever, established the clinical picture of disease, and renamed it Colorado tick fever.

Etiology Colorado tick fever virus is classified as an arbovirus because it replicates in ticks, but is a reovirus (orbivirus) on the basis of both its structure and its content of double-stranded RNA.

Prevalence The disease has been contracted in Colorado, Idaho, Nevada, Wyoming, Montana, Utah, the eastern portions of Oregon, Washington, California, and the northern portions of Arizona and New Mexico. However, the virus of Colorado tick fever has been reported to have been isolated from the dog tick, *Dermacentor variabilis*, obtained from Long Island. This observation has not been confirmed, but suggests the possibility that Colorado tick fever may occur over a wider geographic area. The actual prevalence is difficult to assess, but the disease is relatively common. Mild and clinically inapparent forms of the disease occur, but its frequency has never been determined. The number of cases of Colorado tick fever reported in Colorado is twenty times greater than that of Rocky Mountain spotted fever. In fact, almost one-half of the patients diagnosed as having Rocky Mountain spotted fever in Utah were subsequently shown to have Colorado tick fever.

Epidemiology Colorado tick fever is transmitted to humans by the adult hard-shelled wood tick, *Dermacentor andersoni*. The virus has been found in as many as 14 percent of this species of ticks collected in endemic areas. Transovarial transmission of the virus in the tick has been established. Illness occurs primarily in the spring and summer months, with a predilection for April and May at lower altitudes and for June and July at higher altitudes. Virus has been obtained from both the blood and the spinal fluid of patients during the acute illness. The virus persists within erythrocytes of convalescent patients for as long as 120 days. Virus can be readily isolated from washed erythrocytes 100 days following infection. This makes transfusion-associated Colorado tick fever theoretically possible.

Clinical manifestations The incubation period is usually 3 to 6 days, and in most cases a history of tick bite can be obtained. Persons affected usually are those whose occupational or recreational activities bring them in contact with ticks. The disease may occur at any age. The clinical picture is characterized by the sudden onset of severe aching of the muscles of the back and legs, chilliness without true rigors, a rapid increase in temperature, which usually reaches 102 to 104°F, headache with pain on ocular movement, retroorbital pain, and photophobia. Occasionally nausea and vomiting occur. The physical findings are not specific. Tachycardia in proportion to the temperature, flushed facies, and variable conjunctival injection may be present. Occasionally the spleen is palpable. A rash is usually not present, but on occasion a petechial rash involving primarily the arms and legs or a maculopapular rash over the entire body may occur. Rarely, punched-out ulcers may form at the site of tick bite. The fever with the associated symptoms lasts about 2 days, then abruptly lyses to normal or subnormal, leaving the patient very weak. After an afebrile period of about 2 days, the temperature recurs, may be higher than in the first phase, and may last as long as 3 days. Over 90 percent of patients show this saddleback pattern of temperature. Rarely there may be three febrile phases. The febrile episode may be followed by a period of weakness of several weeks' duration.

Evidence of central nervous system involvement has been recorded in a few patients. The findings are those of either an aseptic meningitis with stiffness of the neck or encephalitis with clouding of the sensorium, delirium, and coma.

Laboratory findings The most important laboratory feature is moderate to marked leukopenia. On the first day of illness, the total leukocyte count may be at normal levels, but usually by the fifth or sixth day there has been a decrease to 2,000 to 3,000 per mm^3. Characteristically there is a proportionate decrease in lymphocytes and granulocytes. A moderate "left shift" in the neutrophilic series is usually apparent. Toxic changes in neutrophils are often conspicuous, and "virocyte" types of lymphocytes are frequently observed. Bone marrow examination reveals "maturation arrest" in the granulocytic series. Erythrocyte values remain normal. Thrombocytopenia has been recorded in an isolated case report. The blood picture returns to normal within a week after the fever subsides.

Diagnosis The diagnosis of Colorado tick fever is suspected on the basis of the epidemiologic history and clinical findings. The usual methods for confirming Colorado tick fever are mouse inoculation and fluorescent antibody (FA) staining of patients' erythrocytes; a combination of the two is best. Special handling of blood is not necessary for the FA test which remains positive during as well as several weeks after clinical illness.

Treatment Treatment is entirely symptomatic.

Prognosis The prognosis is excellent.

Prevention No patients have been reported as having the disease twice. Active immunity with an attenuated virus has been produced, but the immunization itself frequently produced mild disease. Colorado tick fever is best prevented by avoiding contact with the wood tick. Convalescent individuals should be excluded as blood donors for at least 6 months.

VENEZUELAN EQUINE ENCEPHALITIS Venezuelan equine encephalitis (VEE) was first noted in equines in Colombia in 1935.

Etiology Like other group A arboviruses, the causative agent of VEE is a relatively small, 40 to 45 nm, RNA virus. On the basis of serologic tests, differing serotypes have been identified, IA-E, II, III, and IV. Strains ID, IE, II, III, and IV have remained sylvatic in distribution. IA was the original epidemic strain which occurred in Venezuela, and IB, which was recognized in Ecuador in 1963, spread through Central America into Mexico and was responsible for the epidemic in Mexico in 1971 which spread into southern Texas, with the occurrence of at least 76 laboratory-confirmed human cases. In early 1973, almost 4,000 cases occurred in Peru.

Epidemiology VEE has been primarily a disease of equines and other mammals, although occasionally the agent has infected humans. Evidence of human infection (virus isolation or specific neutralizing antibodies) has been found in Colombia, Ecuador, Panama, Surinam, Guyana, French Guiana, Mexico, Brazil, Curacao, Trinidad, Argentina, Florida, and Texas. The VEE virus complex in nature has been associated with numerous mosquitoes (at least 9 genera and 37 species), including *Aëdes, Mansonia, Psorophora,* and *Culex.* In this respect it differs markedly from other mosquito-borne encephalitogenic arboviruses, which usually are associated with only one to three vector species. VEE apparently has different vectors for its endemic-epizootic and its epidemic-epizootic cycles. The virus has a wide host range in wild mammals, with at least 20 genera, including capuchin monkeys, rats, mice, oppossum, jackrabbit, fox, and bats being naturally infected. Domestic animals other than equines which have been shown to be infected include cattle and pigs in Mexico and goats and sheep in Venezuela. VEE appears to multiply well in mammals with high titers of virus in the blood; e.g., infected horses may have titers of up to $10^{7.5}$ mouse intraperitoneal lethal doses per milliliter of blood. Though 29 species of wild birds have been shown to be naturally infected with VEE (20 percent of which are colonial nestling herons and related species), whether the VEE-viremia levels in birds are high enough to infect vector mosquitoes is not yet known. During the initial 3 days of illness, viremia has been detected in approximately two-thirds of patients. The levels of viremia are sufficiently high that humans could serve as a reservoir. VEE virus also has been isolated by pharyngeal swab in a few patients, suggesting the potential for person-to-person transmission. The available observations make it reasonable to consider that the natural vector is a mosquito, with the primary reservoir being either wild or domestic terrestrial mammals. However, natural infection can probably take place without an arthropod vector. Laboratory infections have occurred and are probably due to inhalation of aerosols.

Clinical manifestations In humans, infection with VEE virus usually results in a mild acute febrile illness without neurologic complications. No age is spared, and there is no sex preponderance. The incubation period is 2 to 5 days, followed by the abrupt onset of headache, fever often associated with rigors, malaise, and myalgia. Other common symptoms may include nausea, vomiting, diarrhea, and sore throat. Uncommon features include seizures, mental confusion, coma, tremors, and diplopia. On laboratory examination the cerebrospinal fluid may reveal pleocytosis with modest increases in protein concentration and normal glucose concentration. Virus may be isolated both from blood and from cerebrospinal fluid. The symptoms usually last 3 to 5 days in mild cases and up to 8 days in more severe cases, although one patient reported from Florida was febrile for 3 weeks. A biphasic course of illness may be encountered, with recrudescence of symptoms at the sixth to the ninth day. In one case report, palatine petechiae were noted and the patient vomited "coffee-grounds" material. In an epidemic in Venezuela in 1962, almost 16,000 cases of acute disease were evaluated; 38 percent were classified as encephalitis, but only 3 to 4 percent had severe neurologic abnormalities: convulsions, nystagmus, drowsiness, delirium, or meningitis. The mortality rate was estimated to be less than 0.5 percent, and nearly all deaths occurred in young children.

RIFT VALLEY FEVER Rift Valley fever is an acute disease principally of sheep and cattle and first described in humans during an extensive epizootic of hepatitis in sheep in the Rift Valley in East Africa. During this epizootic in 1930, workers associated with the investigations contracted a severe but limited febrile disease. A similar syndrome was common among the herders of infected flocks. More than 200 cases of human disease were originally recognized. The infection is widespread throughout East and South Africa. During an epizootic in South Africa in 1950–1951, an estimated 20,000 human beings became infected.

Virus has been found in several species of mosquitoes: *Eretmapodites chrysogaster, Aëdes caballus, Aëdes circumluteolus,* and *Culex theileri.* Antibodies to Rift Valley fever have been found in wild field rats in Uganda. Humans appear to be incidentally infected during the course of an epizootic. Although humans presumably can be infected by arthropods, many infections occur as a result of handling infected animal tissues. In addition, laboratory-acquired infections have been common, which suggests a respiratory route.

The incubation period is usually 3 to 6 days. The onset is abrupt, with malaise, chilly sensation or rigors, headache, retroorbital pain, and generalized aching and backache. The temperature rises rapidly to 101 to 104°F. Later complaints include anorexia, loss of taste, epigastric pain, and photophobia. Findings on examination are usually unremarkable except for flushing of the face and conjunctival injection. The temperature curve is often saddleback in type, with an initial elevation lasting 2 to 3 days, followed by a remission and second febrile period. Convalescence is typically rapid. Complications are rare; jaundice has not been seen in man. Macular exudates, with decreased vision, have been reported. One of the most characteristic findings is the initial normal total leukocyte count followed by leukopenia with a decrease in neutrophils associated with an increase in band forms. The diagnosis is made by isolating the virus from the blood by inoculation of mice. In human beings, viremia is present during the first 3 days. Neutralizing antibodies have been demonstrated as early as 4 days after onset. There is no specific treatment. The prognosis in human infections is good. Only one fatality has been recorded, and in this instance death was not due directly to the infection.

MAYARO-SEMLIKI FOREST VIRUS DISEASE Mayaro virus was initially isolated from humans in Trinidad in 1954. Outbreaks involving a number of persons subsequently have occurred in Brazil and Bolivia. Mayaro virus has been isolated from a wild mosquito, *Mansonia venezuelensis,* and can be maintained serially in *Aëdes aegypti* and *Anopheles quadrimaculatus.* Semliki Forest virus has been isolated from *Aëdes abnormalis* mosquitoes in Uganda and from various *Eretmapodites* mosquitoes in West Africa. Serologic surveys in humans document widespread virus activity. Antigenically these two group A arboviruses are very closely related, suggesting that these two viruses may have been derived from one strain, with geographic separation having led to some antigenic variation. The mechanism of spread has not been determined, but the presence of viremia favors a biting arthropod vector. The predominance of illness and greater incidence of immunity in males suggest a forest infection.

Symptoms include fever of several days' duration, which may be marked during the first 1 to 2 days. Systemic complaints include severe frontal headache, epigastric pain, backache, nausea, photophobia, and vertigo. Signs have included conjunctival injection, mild icterus in a few patients, and arthritis in at least one patient. The leukocyte count is in the range of 5,000 to 8,000 per mm^3. The fever lasts 3 to 5 days in most patients. Recovery is usually complete, although in Bolivia the illness was more severe, and several fatalities were reported.

BAT SALIVARY GLAND VIRUS During the course of a survey of rabies infection in bats, an agent was obtained from the salivary glands of Mexican free-tailed bats in Texas. The virus is related to the St. Louis encephalitis complex of viruses (group B). It is not known how the virus is maintained in nature. Five laboratory-acquired human infections have been recorded. The illnesses were characterized by fever associated with headache, myalgia, and a mild nonproductive cough. In two patients, there was evidence of central nervous system involvement with encephalitis and aseptic meningitis. One patient had oophoritis, and two developed orchitis. By the sixth to seventh day of illness, leukopenia in the range of 2,000 to 3,000 per mm^3 was observed in two individuals.

ZIKA VIRUS Zika virus was first isolated from a captive rhesus monkey in Uganda and subsequently from wild mosquitoes. On the basis of serologic surveys, it is known to infect humans in Uganda and Nigeria. During investigation in eastern Nigeria of an outbreak of jaundice that was suspected of being yellow fever, physicians isolated Zika virus from one patient and noted that two others had a rise in neutralizing antibodies. The symptoms in these patients included fever, arthralgia, and headache with retroorbital pain. Jaundice was present in one, and bile was demonstrated in the urine of another. Albuminuria was noted in one patient. Prothrombin times were normal. The clinical syndrome appears to simulate mild yellow fever.

GROUP C ARBOVIRUSES Currently 11 viruses are classified as Bunyaviruses, group C, of which 9 have been isolated from blood obtained from humans. The geographic distribution includes Brazil (Apeu, Caraparu, Itaqui, Marituba, Murutucui, Oriboca), Trinidad (Caraparu, Restan), and Panama (Madrid, Ossa). Several of these viruses have been isolated from Culicine and Subethine mosquitoes, as well as from several species of rodents. Isolates have been obtained mostly from forest workers and laboratory technicians. Epidemics have not been recognized. The disease begins with headache, fever (with temperature up to 105°F), and myalgia. Additional symptoms include malaise, photophobia, vertigo, and nausea. Illness is generally mild, lasting 2 to 4 days, and is occasionally followed by a relapse. No fatalities have been reported. Occasionally a prolonged period of convalescence ensues. Leukopenia, with total leukocyte counts as low as 2,600 per mm^3, is a common finding. Diagnosis has been established mainly by virus isolation.

BUNYAMWERA GROUP Representative viruses of this group are found in all inhabited continents except Australia. Only five viruses of the group—Bunyamwera itself, Germiston, Ilesha, Guaroa, and Wycomyia—have been associated with clinical disease. Serologic surveys give evidence of a high prevalence of inapparent infection in some areas. The clinical patterns of infection due to Germiston, Ilesha, and Guaroa viruses seem similar, while infection

due to Bunyamwera virus is associated often with arthralgia and sometimes with a rash. The mild clinical illness is characterized by low-grade fever, headache, and myalgia which last several days, and it may be followed by weakness during convalescence.

Arbovirus infections presenting chiefly with fever, malaise, arthralgia, and rash

CHIKUNGUNYA In 1952 an epidemic of a disease similar to dengue occurred in Tanzania, an area in which dengue had never been observed. The disease was given the name *chikungunya* ("that which bends up") because of the local description of the sudden onset of distinctive joint pains. A group A arbovirus was isolated in 1956 both from serum of patients ill with the disease and from a pool of *Aëdes aegypti* mosquitoes.

Chikungunya virus is responsible for a dengue-like illness in South Africa, India, and Southeast Asia, as well as for a rather mild form of hemorrhagic fever in Asiatic children. Outbreaks have been associated with high attack rates, with as many as 80 percent of the inhabitants in some settlements becoming ill. It is not known definitely what vertebrates and arthropods are involved in the wild transmission cycle. Because the virus has been isolated from *Aëdes africanus* and because antibodies against the virus can be detected in chimpanzees, it appears that these may play a role in the natural cycle in Africa.

After an incubation period estimated at no less than 9 days, the onset is typically abrupt, with a rapid rise in temperature to 102 to 105°F, often associated with a rigor and headache. Pain in large joints occurs early, incapacitating some individuals within a few minutes of onset. The pain is frequently severe enough to prevent sleep. The arthralgia is often associated with objective arthritis. Sites of involvement include knees, ankles, shoulders, wrists, or proximal interphalangeal joints. Myalgia, especially backache, and malaise occur frequently. In 60 to 80 percent of patients a maculopapular eruption, which may appear at any time during the febrile course, is noted on the trunk or on the extensor surfaces of the extremities. Mild lymphadenopathy, predominantly in the axillary or inguinal areas, may be evident. Pharyngitis and conjunctival suffusion may be observed in a few patients. Elevated temperatures continue for 1 to 6 days, and in some patients an afebrile interval of 1 to 3 days is followed by a secondary rise in temperature. The joint pains sometimes continue after the temperature has returned to normal. In a few individuals joint pains have persisted for up to 4 months. Hematocrit values remain normal. Total leukocyte counts may be less than 5,000 per mm^3 in some patients, while in others they remain normal. Urinalyses are normal. There is no specific antiviral treatment. Anti-inflammatory agents such as aspirin or indomethacin have been utilized. No second attacks have been recognized, and in the absence of the hemorrhagic fever syndrome, no deaths have been described.

O'NYONG-NYONG FEVER O'nyong-nyong fever was first noted as an epidemic illness characterized by joint pains, rash, and lymphadenopathy in the northern province of

Uganda in 1959. The agent is a group A arbovirus which shows close antigenic relationships with chikungunya and Semliki Forest viruses. The original outbreak was associated with an explosive epidemic which spread to Tanzania and other areas in East Africa. By 1961, 2 million cases were recorded. In some areas, 91 percent of the population had either clinical disease or inapparent infection. Local outbreaks extended over the entire year. All age groups were affected. The most likely vector is *Anopheles funestus.* The clinical features are similar to those of chikungunya virus infection.

SINDBIS VIRUS Sindbis virus infection in humans rarely presents as a clinical disease. Of five cases from Uganda, one patient gave a history of joint pain. In the only well-studied clinical illness, a South African woman had arthritis as a prominent finding. Two days after a headache she noted swelling in her hands and feet. Soon thereafter she developed a confluent macular rash, followed by vesicle formation. The small joints of the hands and feet were swollen at the time of examination. Slight swelling of the fingers was present at 10 weeks, although she had otherwise recovered.

ROSS RIVER VIRUS Epidemics of polyarthritis associated with rashes have been observed in Australia since 1928. Outbreaks occur almost entirely in the period December to June. There is a predilection for women, and children are seldom involved (an obvious similarity with rubella, another Togavirus). The onset is characterized by headache, mild catarrh, and occasionally tenderness of the palms and soles. Initially fever may be absent or minimal (highest 100.4°F). In about one-half of patients, the occurrence of arthritis which involves mainly the small joints, wrists, and ankles and is sometimes associated by swelling and paresthesias precedes the rash by 1 to 15 days. In the other half, the rash precedes the arthralgia. The rash, which lasts 2 to 10 days, is usually maculopapular, appears on the cheeks and forehead, occasionally spreads to the trunk, or may be restricted to the limbs. The rash may be pruritic. Vesicles occur rarely. Tender lymphadenopathy occurs in one-fifth of the patients. Joint symptoms persist for 3 weeks to 3 months. Patients with this syndrome have shown serologic evidence of infection with Ross River virus, although virus has not been isolated from synovial fluid.

OTHER ARBOVIRUSES Mayaro and Bunyamwera viruses have been associated with the syndrome of rash and arthralgia.

Arbovirus infections presenting chiefly with fever, malaise, lymphadenopathy, and rash

DENGUE FEVER Dengue is endemic over large areas of the tropics and subtropics. Localized outbreaks of dengue have occurred annually in Puerto Rico since the 1969 epidemic. A number of travelers returned to the mainland United States in 1969 with clinical illness. In these areas a high proportion of infections are inapparent or represent undifferentiated febrile illnesses. It is now recognized that the dengue syndrome can be caused by other arboviruses; hence the exact etiology of some of the earlier epidemics is uncertain.

Etiology There are four distinct serogroups of dengue viruses, types 1, 2, 3, and 4, all of which are group B arboviruses. The existence of at least two further antigenic types has been suggested. They are transmitted solely by mosquitoes of the genus *Aëdes.*

Epidemiology So far as is known, dengue infections in nature involve only human beings and *Aëdes* mosquitoes. Attempts have been made to implicate lower vertebrates, especially monkeys, as reservoir sylvatic hosts, but the data are inconclusive. *Aëdes aegypti* is the most important worldwide vector species. This species, as well as the less common vector species, bite humans readily or even preferentially, breed in small collections of water such as cisterns and backyard litter, and are peridomestic in nature. They fly during the day. Humans appear to be uniformly susceptible, and susceptibility is not influenced by age, sex, or race. The disappearance of dengue from an area may be the result either of elimination of the vector or of exhaustion of the susceptible population. During outbreaks, attack rates may be very high; in Puerto Rico (1969) the overall rate of clinical illness was 24 per 100 persons in some areas, with infection rates as determined by serologic survey as high as 79 per 100.

Pathology Biopsy of skin lesions in volunteers demonstrated endothelial swelling, perivascular edema, and infiltration of small blood vessels with mononuclear cells. Since the disease is self-limited, other studies have not been made.

Clinical manifestations Dengue viruses frequently produce inapparent infections in humans. When symptoms develop, three broad clinical patterns may be encountered: classic dengue, hemorrhagic fever, and a mild atypical form. Classic dengue (breakbone fever) occurs primarily in nonimmune individuals, specifically nonindigenous adults and children. The usual incubation period is 5 to 8 days. Prodromal symptoms such as mild conjunctivitis or coryza may occur, followed in hours by the abrupt onset of a severe splitting headache, retroorbital pain, backache, especially in the lumbar area, and leg and joint pains. The headache is aggravated by movement. At least three-fourths of patients have ocular soreness, with pain on moving the eyes. A few have mild photophobia. Though true rigors are common during the course, they are usually not present at the onset. Additional symptoms include insomnia, anorexia with loss of taste or bitter taste, and weakness. Mild transient rhinopharyngitis occurs in as many as one-quarter of the individuals. Cough is almost never seen. Epistaxis has been observed. Examination reveals scleral injection (90 percent), tenderness upon pressure on the ocular globe, and nontender posterior cervical, epitrochlear, and inguinal lymphadenopathy. Over one-half of patients have an enanthem characterized initially by pinpoint-sized vesicles over the posterior half of the soft palate. The tongue is often coated. Skin rashes, varying from diffuse flushing to scarlatiniform and morbilliform, are frequently present over the thorax and inner aspects of the arms. These are transient and fade, only to be followed by a more apparent maculopapular rash which appears on the trunk on the third to the fifth day and spreads peripherally. The rash may be pruritic and generally terminates with desquamation. Extreme bradycardia is not observed. Within 2 to 3 days after the onset, the temperature may decrease to nearly normal and other symptoms disappear. The remission typically lasts 2 days and is followed by return of fever and the other symptoms, although they are generally less severe than during the initial phase. This "saddleback" diphasic febrile course is considered characteristic, but often is not encountered. The febrile illness usually lasts 5 to 6 days and terminates by crisis. Complaints of fatigue for several weeks after infection are common.

In addition to this "classic" syndrome, an atypically mild illness may occur. Symptoms include fever, anorexia, headache, and myalgia. On examination, evanescent rashes may be seen, but lymphadenopathy is usually absent. The course is usually less than 72 h in duration.

At the onset both in classic and in mild dengue, the leukocyte counts may be low or normal; however, by the third to the fifth day, leukopenia, usually with counts of less than 5,000 per mm^3, and neutropenia are usually seen. Occasionally albuminuria of moderate degree occurs.

Diagnosis Virus isolation in tissue culture of serum obtained during the first days of illness is definitive. Diagnosis can be made by serologic tests employing paired serums for hemagglutination inhibition tests and complement fixation tests. Specific serologic diagnosis is complicated by cross reactions with other group B arbovirus antibodies such as those following immunization with yellow fever vaccine.

Treatment The treatment is entirely symptomatic.

Prognosis Mortality is nil.

Prevention Attenuated vaccines are undergoing experimental evaluation but are not available. The hypothesis of "second infections" being responsible for the dengue hemorrhagic fever syndrome raises further questions about a program of active immunization. Control depends upon mosquito abatement.

WEST NILE FEVER West Nile virus is distributed from South Africa to southeastern India, but has been shown as a cause of significant disease only in the Near East, where it can produce a clinical picture closely resembling dengue.

Etiology West Nile virus is a group B arbovirus with pathogenicity for common laboratory animals. The virus multiplies and causes cytopathic effects in a variety of cells in tissue culture.

Prevalence In 1940 the virus was isolated from the blood of a febrile patient. Subsequent serologic surveys demonstrated neutralizing antibodies against the virus to be widely prevalent in the native populations of Uganda, Kenya, the Congo, and the Sudan. However, the clinical manifestations were unknown until the virus was isolated from the blood of a child during an epidemic of febrile disease in Israel in 1951. Outbreaks of disease involving several hundred patients occurred in Israel in 1950 to 1952. In one outbreak, over 60 percent of the population developed overt disease.

Epidemiology The disease is highly endemic in Egypt but goes largely unrecognized. Presumably the adult population is for the most part immune, and the infection in childhood is an undifferentiated mild febrile illness, whereas in Israel it mainly affects adults. The infection occurs in the summer both in Israel and in Egypt. The transmission cycle in Egypt is believed to be bird-to-mosquito-to-bird, with *Culex univittatus* as the principal vector. Although humans and a variety of other vertebrates are infected by the virus, their involvement is believed to be tangential. In Israel, the most probable vectors are *Culex molestus* and *C. univittatus.*

Clinical manifestations Most of the patients in Israel have been young adults, with neither sex predominating. The onset is usually abrupt and without prodromal symptoms. The temperature quickly rises to 101 to 104°F, with chills occurring in one-third of patients. Symptoms include drowsiness, severe frontal headache, ocular pain, and pain in the abdomen and back. A small number of patients have anorexia, nausea, and dryness of the throat. Cough is uncommon. Signs observed include flushing of the face, conjunctival injection, and coating of the tongue. The prominent finding is general enlargement of lymph nodes, which are of moderate size but are not hard and are only slightly tender. Occipital, axillary, and inguinal nodes are usually involved. The spleen and liver are slightly enlarged in a small proportion of patients. In one-half the patients a rash may appear from the second to the fifth day of illness and may persist for several hours or until defervescence. The rash occurs predominantly over the trunk and consists of pale roseolar maculopapular lesions. The illness is self-limited and lasts 3 to 5 days in 80 percent of patients.

In a few patients, transitory meningeal involvement may be encountered. Spinal fluid examinations may reveal a pleocytosis and some increase in protein concentration.

Leukopenia occurs in the majority of patients, and total leukocyte counts are lower than 4,000 per mm^3 in one-third. Differential counts vary from a moderate shift to the left to a slight lymphocytosis.

Convalescence is often prolonged, lasting 1 to 2 weeks, with prominent symptoms of fatigue. Enlargement of lymph nodes subsides over several months. Only rarely have complications, sequelae, or fatalities been seen in natural infections, although in one outbreak in a group of elderly patients a high proportion of patients developed meningoencephalitis, and four fatalities ensued.

Accurate diagnosis rests on virus isolation, which can be accomplished because viremia persists for as long as 6 days, or the demonstration of a rising specific antibody titer.

The treatment is symptomatic.

Arbovirus infections presenting chiefly with CNS involvement

Four arboviruses are presently recognized as numerically important causes of central nervous system disease in the United States: St. Louis encephalitis virus, Eastern equine encephalitis virus, Western equine encephalitis virus, and the California encephalitis group of viruses. The spectrum of infection caused by these agents includes inapparent infection, fever with headache, aseptic meningitis, and encephalitis. Of the more than 1,967 patients reported with encephalitis during 1973, 18 percent were classified as postinfectious. This is a broad category which includes measles, mumps, chickenpox, rubella, and cytomegalovirus. An enteroviral etiology (poliovirus, Coxsackie virus, and echo virus) was confirmed in 0.7 percent of cases, while 4.5 percent were due to arboviruses. In 74 percent, the etiology was unknown. For 8 of the 12 years from 1955 to 1966, St. Louis encephalitis virus was the most common cause of arboviral encephalitis in the United States. In contrast, from 1967 through 1973, the California encephalitis group of viruses accounted for 50 to 81 percent of the reported cases of human arthropod-borne encephalitis.

Etiology Despite the diversity of specific viral etiologies (Table 212-2), in individual patients the clinical manifestations of aseptic meningitis and encephalitis are very similar, and preclude an etiologic diagnosis without ancillary information regarding epidemiologic and serologic features. The clinical features of aseptic meningitis due to arboviruses are indistinguishable from those due to the more prevalent enteroviruses, which are discussed in Chap. 193. The broad clinical picture of arbovirus encephalitis will be discussed; then the specific epidemiologic and prognostic features which characterize the major types will be presented.

Clinical manifestations The clinical features of arbovirus encephalitis differ among age groups. In infants under one year of age, the only consistently noted symptoms are sudden onset of fever, which is often accompanied by convulsions. Convulsions may be either generalized or focal. Typically the fever ranges between 102 and 104°F. Other physical findings may include bulging of the fontanelle, rigidity of the extremities, and abnormalities in reflexes.

In children between five and fourteen years of age, subjective symptoms are more easily elicited. Headache, fever, and drowsiness of 2 to 3 days' duration before medical attention is sought are common. The symptoms may then subside or become more intense and may be associated with nausea, vomiting, muscular pain, photophobia, and, less frequently, convulsions (less than 10 percent except in California encephalitis). On examination, the child is found to be acutely ill, febrile, and lethargic. Nuchal rigidity and intention tremors are often present, and on occasion muscular weakness can be demonstrated.

In adults, the initial symptoms commonly include the fairly abrupt onset of fever, nausea with vomiting, and severe headache. The headache is most often frontal but may be occipital or diffuse in location. Mental aberrations, represented by confusion and disorientation, usually appear within the subsequent 24 h. Other symptoms may include diffuse myalgia and photophobia. The abnormalities found on physical examination predominantly relate to the neurologic examination, although conjunctival suffusion is frequently seen and skin rashes may occur. Disturbances in mentation are among the most outstanding clinical features. These range from coma through severe disorientation to subtle abnormalities detected only by cerebral function tests such as the subtraction of serial 7s. A small proportion of patients show only lethargy, lying quietly, apparently asleep unless stimulated. Tremor is common and is observed more frequently in individuals over forty years of age. The tremors vary in location and may be continuous or intention in type. Cranial nerve abnormalities resulting in oculomotor muscle paresis and nystagmus, facial weakness, and difficulty in deglutition may occur, and are usually present within the initial several days. Objective sensory changes are unusual. Hemiparesis or monoparesis may occur. Reflex abnormalities are also common; these include exaggerated palmomental reflexes, and suck and snout reflexes. Superficial abdominal and cremasteric reflexes are usually absent. Changes in the tendon reflexes are variable and inconstant. The plantar response may be extensor and fluctuates almost hourly. Dysdiadochokinesia often exists.

The duration of the fever and neurologic symptoms and signs varies from several days to a month but usually ranges from 4 to 14 days. Clinical improvement generally follows the subsidence of the fever within several days unless irreversible anatomic changes have occurred.

Laboratory findings Erythrocyte values are usually normal. Total leukocyte counts often reveal both a slight to moderate leukocytosis (occasionally greater than 20,000 per mm^3) and neutrophilia. Examination of the cerebrospinal fluid usually reveals several hundred cells per cubic millimeter, but on occasion cloudy cerebrospinal fluid with cells in excess of 1,000 per mm^3 may be seen. Within the first several days of illness, polymorphonuclear neutrophils may predominate. The initial cerebrospinal fluid protein is usually only slightly elevated but on occasion may exceed 100 mg per 100 ml. The level of spinal fluid sugar is normal; a significant decrease should raise serious consideration of an alternative diagnosis. As the illness progresses, mononuclear cells in the cerebrospinal fluid tend to increase so that they predominate and the protein concentration may increase. Other laboratory studies have been performed only sporadically, but abnormalities may include hyponatremia, often due to the inappropriate secretion of antidiuretic hormone, and elevations in serum creatine phosphokinase.

Diagnosis Specific diagnosis requires the isolation of the virus or detection of antibodies with a rising titer between the acute phase of disease and convalescence. Antibodies can be detected by hemagglutination inhibition, complement fixation, or virus neutralization techniques.

Treatment Treatment is entirely supportive and requires meticulous attention in the comatose patient.

EASTERN EQUINE ENCEPHALITIS Eastern equine encephalitis, a group A arbovirus, was first isolated in 1933 from the brain tissue of horses during an outbreak of equine illness in New Jersey. The first recognized human outbreak occurred in Massachusetts in 1938.

Epidemiology The virus is distributed along the eastern coast of the Americas from Northeastern United States to Argentina. Viral isolations also have been reported in the Philippines, Thailand, Czechoslovakia, Poland, and the U. S. S. R., but the question of type specificity has not been resolved. In the Northeastern United States, epidemics occur in the late summer and early fall. Epizootics in horses precede the occurrence of human cases by 1 to 2 weeks. The disease affects mainly infants, children, and adults over fifty-five years of age. There is no sex preponderance. Inapparent infection occurs in all age groups, suggesting that the decreased likelihood of developing overt infection in the fifteen- to fifty-four-year age group is not the result of decreased exposure. The ratio of inapparent infection to overt encephalitis approximates 25:1.

The natural reservoir is unknown. Isolations have been made from numerous species of wild birds and also from amphibians, reptiles, and mammals. The natural vector is the mosquito, including *Aëdes sollicitans* and *Culiseta melanura. Aëdes sollicitans,* a salt-marsh mosquito which is an avid human feeder, has been postulated as the epidemic vector, while *C. melanura* is important in bird-to-bird transmission. Equine animals and human beings are probably "dead ends" in the transmission cycle, and infection in them is accidental.

Clinical manifestations Though human infections have been thought usually to result in serious, if not fatal, central nervous system involvement, the detection of inapparent infection as well as relatively mild disease establishes the occurrence of milder forms. In many patients, the cerebrospinal fluid is cloudy and contains in excess of 1,000 cells per mm^3.

Diagnosis The hemagglutination-inhibition or neutralization tests are the serologic methods of choice. The complement fixation test may be negative in patients with confirmed infections.

Prognosis The mortality rate in clinical infection exceeds 50 percent. In the most severe cases, death occurs between the third and fifth days. Children under ten years of age have a greater likelihood of surviving the acute illness, but they also have a greater likelihood of developing severe disabling residuals: mental retardation, convulsions, emotional lability, blindness, deafness, speech disorders, and hemiplegia.

WESTERN EQUINE ENCEPHALITIS Western equine encephalitis (WEE) virus is a group A arbovirus which was isolated in 1930 in California from horses with encephalitis. In 1938 it was recovered from a fatal human infection.

Epidemiology WEE virus has been isolated in the United States, Canada, Brazil, Guyana, and Argentina. Human disease has been diagnosed only in the United States, Canada, and Brazil. In the United States, the virus is found in virtually all geographic areas. The central valley of California represents an important endemic area. The disease occurs mainly in early summer and midsummer. Wild birds, which develop viremia of sufficiently high titer to be able to infect mosquitoes that feed on them, are the basic reservoir, although nonavian vertebrate hosts may be important. *Culex tarsalis* is the principal vector in the Western United States. In areas east of the Appalachian Mountains, another vector must be operative. The virus has been repeatedly isolated from *Culiseta melanura;* however, the importance of this species has been questioned, since it is not primarily a human-biting mosquito. The ratio of inapparent infection to disease, as evidenced by serologic survey studies, varies from 58:1 in children to 1,150:1 in adults. Approximately one-fourth of patients are less than one year of age. The highest attack rates occur in persons fifty years or older. In the summer of 1975, 46 cases of WEE were reported from North Dakota and northwestern Minnesota.

Prognosis The fatality rate approximates 3 percent in laboratory-confirmed cases. The incidence and severity of sequelae are related to age. Sequelae among very young infants are frequent (appearing in 61 percent of a group of patients less than three months old) and severe; they consist of upper motor neuron impairment, involving the pyramidal tracts, extrapyramidal structures, and cerebellum, and result in behavioral problems and convulsions. Both the incidence and severity of sequelae diminish rapidly after one year of age. Adults may complain of nervousness, irritability, easy fatigability, and tremulousness for 6 months or longer after the acute illness. Probably not more than 5 percent of adults have sequelae which are sufficiently severe to be of practical significance. Postencephalitic seizures are rare.

JAPANESE ENCEPHALITIS The name Japanese B encephalitis was employed during an epidemic which occurred in 1924 to distinguish it from von Economo's disease, which was designated as type A encephalitis (Chap. 338). The designation as Japanese B no longer seems useful, and the term Japanese encephalitis will be employed.

Epidemiology Japanese encephalitis virus infection is known to occur in eastern Siberia, China, Korea, Taiwan, Japan, Malaya, Vietnam, Thailand, Singapore, Guam, and India. In temperate climates, the disease shows a late-summer early-fall seasonal incidence. In tropical climates there is no seasonal variation. The mosquito *Culex tritaeniorhynchus* is the major vector species. It is a rural mosquito which breeds in rice fields and preferentially bites large domestic animals, such as pigs, but also feeds on birds and humans. The human is an accidental host in the transmission cycle. In several outbreaks, a higher incidence of cases has been reported in children than in adults. The ratio of inapparent infection, as evidenced by a serologic survey study of Australian troops in Vietnam, was 210:1.

Clinical manifestations The occurrence of severe rigors at the onset has been noted in almost 90 percent of patients. On admission, most patients are alert, but deterioration of mental status occurs in about three-fourths of patients within 3 to 4 days. Localized paresis is found more often than with other arboviral encephalitides, e.g., in 31 percent of cases, with predominantly upper extremity involvement; however, it resolves rapidly with defervescence. Weight loss has been very striking. The failure of the temperature to lyse, appearance of diaphoresis, tachypnea, and the accumulation of bronchial secretions are grave prognostic signs.

Prognosis The immediate mortality rate has varied from

7 to 33 percent or higher. The rate of occurrence of sequelae varies inversely with the fatality rate; in those series with high fatality rates (33 percent), sequelae occurred in 3 to 14 percent. In another series with a fatality rate of 7.4 percent, the sequelae rate was 32 percent. Individuals who had neurologic abnormalities during the acute phase but survived have no more than an 80 percent chance for complete recovery. Sequelae consist of seizures, persistent paralysis, ataxia, mental retardation, and behavioral disorders.

ST. LOUIS ENCEPHALITIS St. Louis encephalitis (SLE) was first recognized as an entity during a major outbreak in St. Louis, Mo., and the surrounding area in 1933. Sporadic, unpredictable outbreaks occurred, for example, in Houston, 1974, Dallas, 1966, Memphis, 1974, Northern Mississippi and Illinois, 1975.

Epidemiology In the United States, epidemics of SLE fall into two epidemiologic patterns. One pattern is found in the West, where mixed outbreaks of Western equine encephalitis and SLE have occurred primarily in irrigated rural areas. The vector has been *Culex tarsalis.* The second pattern occurred in the original St. Louis outbreak and the numerous subsequent epidemics in the Midwest, New Jersey, and Florida. These outbreaks have been more urban in location and are characterized by a marked tendency for the development of encephalitis in older persons. In such urban-suburban epidemics, the epidemic vectors have been mosquitoes of the *Culex pipiens-quinquefasciatus* complex, with the exception of the Florida epidemic, in which *Culex nigripalpus* was incriminated. The presence of SLE virus outside the United States has been proved by isolations in Trinidad, Panama, and Jamaica. However, except in Jamaica, no case of SLE has been reported outside the United States. The basic transmission cycle is that of wild bird-mosquito-wild bird. The mechanism by which the virus overwinters has not been defined. The disease in humans usually appears in midsummer to early fall. There is no sex preponderance. The human represents an accidental host and plays no role in the basic transmission cycle. Serologic studies following most urban epidemics indicate that infection rates are similar in all age groups, and that the increasing age-specific attack rate for clinical encephalitis which is typical of urban St. Louis encephalitis is probably due to age differences in host susceptibility to overt disease rather than to a higher rate of infection.

Clinical manifestations Infection with SLE virus most commonly results in an inapparent infection. Of the patients with confirmed disease, approximately three-fourths have clinical encephalitis; the remainder present with aseptic meningitis, febrile headaches, or nonspecific illness. Virtually all patients over forty years of age have encephalitic manifestations. Urinary frequency and dysuria have been symptoms in approximately 20 percent of patients despite sterile routine aerobic urine cultures. The basis for the urinary tract symptoms is not understood.

Diagnosis The occurrence of either encephalitis or aseptic meningitis as manifested by febrile illness with cerebrospinal fluid pleocytosis in the months of June through September in an adult, especially over thirty-five years of age, should raise the suspicion of St. Louis encephalitis. Because approximately 40 percent of patients with SLE have antibodies detectable by hemagglutination inhibition at the onset of illness, acute serum for serologic studies should be submitted promptly to a competent laboratory.

Prognosis The case fatality ratio in the original St. Louis epidemic was 20 percent. In most subsequent outbreaks the mortality rate has varied from 2 to 12 percent. Subjective nervous complaints, including nervousness, headaches, and easy fatigability and excitability, appear to be the most common residuals. Late organic defects such as speech defects, difficulty in walking, and disturbances in vision were demonstrated in approximately 5 percent of patients 3 years following infection.

CALIFORNIA (LACROSSE) ENCEPHALITIS A previously undescribed virus was isolated in 1943 from mosquitoes in Kern County, California. Since 1963, a large number of agents now designated as the California group of viruses have been isolated. Almost all the isolates have been La-Crosse virus.

Since 1966 in the Midwest United States, California (La-Crosse) encephalitis has been incriminated in 5 to 6 percent of cases of acute central nervous system disease, ranking above all agents except the enteroviruses.

Epidemiology Infection has been demonstrated to occur in the Midwest, especially in Ohio, Indiana, and Wisconsin, in wooded areas of eastern Texas and Louisiana, and along the Eastern Seaboard. The principal animal reservoir is the squirrel. The mosquito vectors are primarily woodland mosquitoes belonging to *Aëdes* species except for *A. sollicitans,* which is a saltwater swamp mosquito. California encephalitis occurs during the summer months (June to October), most often involving boys (60 percent) 5 to 10 years of age (60 percent) who live in rural areas.

Clinical manifestations Two clinical patterns have been defined. One is a mild form with a 2- to 3-day prodrome of fever, headache, malaise, and gastrointestinal symptoms. About the third day the temperature increases to 104°F, and the patient becomes lethargic and develops meningeal signs. These findings abate gradually over a 7- to 8-day period without overt sequelae. The second pattern, a severe form which occurs in at least one-half of the patients, begins abruptly with fever, headache, and vomiting, followed shortly by lethargy and disorientation. During the first 2 to 4 days the course is rapidly progressive with the occurrence of seizures (50 to 60 percent), focal neurologic signs (20 percent), pathologic reflexes (10 percent), and coma (10 percent). Focal neurologic signs may include asymmetrical flaccid paralysis. Uncommon findings have included arthralgia and rash. Clinical laboratory features include peripheral leukocyte counts ranging from 7,000 to 30,000 per mm^3 (median 16,000 per mm^3) with neutrophilia. Cerebrospinal fluid examination reveals 10 to 500 cells per mm^3, usually with a predominance of mononuclear cells, protein concentrations of less than 100 mg per 100 ml, and normal sugar concentrations. Electroencephalograms are abnormal in at least 80 percent of patients, revealing slow delta-wave activity. In one-half of the patients the abnormality is asymmetrical, suggesting focal destructive lesions. Brain scans using ^{99M}Tc pertechnetate also may be abnormal, and localized asymmetrical increased uptake has been observed. Beginning about the fourth day and proceeding over the next 3 to 7 days, there is progressive improvement, with almost all patients becoming afebrile, seizure-free, and ready for discharge from the hospital within 2 weeks after onset.

Diagnosis Neutralizing and hemagglutination-inhibition antibodies usually are present a few days after the onset. Complement-fixing antibodies become detectable 10 to 12 days after onset.

Treatment Initial seizure activity is frequently prolonged and difficult to control. The most effective anticonvulsant medication has been parenteral diazepam. Patients with the severe form of disease should be discharged on anticonvulsants such as phenobarbital for 6 to 12 months.

Prognosis The case fatality ratio is low (2 percent or less); however, one-third of patients may have abnormal neurologic findings at the time of discharge. During the early convalescent period, emotional lability and irritability are common. In one series, recurrent seizures occurred in one-quarter of the patients who had seizures during the acute phase. In this same series EEGs were abnormal in one-third of patients evaluated 1 to 8 years after their acute illness. In another series, 15 percent had sequelae, predominantly personality or behavioral problems.

OTHER ARBOVIRUSES WITH CNS INVOLVEMENT A large group of additional arboviruses have been associated with encephalitis or aseptic meningitis. Some of these agents are listed in Table 212-2. Though the epidemiologic picture of each of these agents is unique, the general features are sufficiently similar to require laboratory support for their differentiation.

Arbovirus diseases presenting chiefly with hemorrhagic manifestations

For 300 years, yellow fever was the only epidemic viral disease known to be accompanied by grave hemorrhagic manifestations. Since the 1930s diverse viral etiologies of the hemorrhagic fever syndrome have been recognized and are now known to be responsible for the variety of epidemiologic situations in which this syndrome occurs (Table 212-2). One or more illnesses so named occurs on three continents. Despite the diverse viral etiology, there are many similar clinical manifestations. The onset is usually sudden, with headache, backache, generalized myalgia, conjunctivitis, and prostration. From approximately the third day, the initial stage is followed by hypotension, and hemorrhagic manifestations may occur; these are characterized by bleeding gums, epistaxis, hemoptysis, hematemesis, melena, petechiae, ecchymoses, and hemorrhages into most visceral organs. Early mild leukopenia develops, but with the appearance of hemorrhagic manifestations, leukocytosis may occur. The pathophysiology of the cardinal signs is attributable to hematopoietic and capillary damage, with variable localization of lesions. On the basis of limited confirmatory observations, variable degrees of disseminated intravascular coagulation may be responsible for a significant part of the pathophysiology of the hemorrhagic fever syndromes. Death usually occurs in the second week of disease, at which time a high titer of antibody has developed and the patient may have become afebrile. Death is usually associated with coma, which is due not to encephalitis but to an encephalopathy. The pathologic changes may be similar despite diverse viral etiologies, with midzonal hepatic necrosis and acidophilic cytoplasmic inclusions similar to the Councilman bodies of yellow fever.

YELLOW FEVER Yellow fever is an acute infectious disease of short duration and extremely variable severity; it is caused by a group B arbovirus and is followed by lifelong immunity. The classic triad of symptoms—jaundice, hemorrhages, and intense albuminuria—is present only in severe infections, which now compose only a small proportion of the total.

Prevalence Yellow fever remains the most dramatically serious arbovirus disease of the tropics. For more than 200 years, after the first identifiable outbreak occurred in Yucatan in 1648, it was one of the great plagues of the world. As late as 1905, New Orleans and other Southern United States ports experienced at least 5,000 cases and 1,000 deaths. Because of the existence of the sylvatic form of the disease, protective measures must be maintained against human disease, as demonstrated by recent outbreaks in Trinidad in 1954, Central America in 1948 to 1957, the Congo in 1958, the Sudan and Ethiopia in 1959 to 1962, Senegal in 1965, central West Africa in 1969, Panama and Colombia in 1974, and Ecuador in 1975.

Epidemiology Human infection results from two basically different cycles of virus transmission, urban and sylvatic. The urban cycle is human-mosquito-human, i.e., *Aëdes aegypti*-transmitted yellow fever. After a 2-week extrinsic incubation period, mosquitoes can transmit infection. Sylvan yellow fever differs under various ecologic circumstances. In the rain forests of South and Central America, species of treetop *Haemagogus* or *Sabethes* mosquitoes maintain transmission in wild primates. Once infected, the mosquito vector remains infectious for life; hence it may serve as a reservoir as well as a vector. When humans come into proximity with the forest-canopy mosquitoes, sporadic cases or focal outbreaks may occur. In East Africa, the mosquito-primate cycle is maintained by the forest-canopy mosquito *A. africanus,* which seldom feeds on humans. The peridomestic mosquito *A. simpsoni* feeds upon primates entering the village gardens and can then in turn transmit the virus to humans. Once yellow fever is reintroduced into urban areas, the urban cycle can be reinitiated, with the potential for epidemic disease. Why yellow fever has never invaded Asia despite widespread distribution of human-biting *A. aegypti* mosquitoes has never been satisfactorily explained.

Pathology The lesions are predominantly visceral. The diagnosis of yellow fever in the experimental animal may be suspected by the presence of acidophilic degeneration in Kupffer's cells of the liver within 24 h after inoculation. By the fourth day necrobiosis and acidophilic necrosis of the parenchymal cells of the liver with the formation of Councilman bodies may occur in a characteristically discontinuous fashion in the midzones of the liver lobules. In the kidney, the virus produces fatty changes, necrobiosis, and necrosis of the tubular epithelium. Multiple minute hemorrhages occur in the gastrointestinal tract. In the brain, the chief lesion is perivascular hemorrhage, which is most frequently found in the subthalamic and periventricular regions at the level of the mammillary bodies.

Clinical manifestations The incubation period is usually 3 to 6 days. In accidental laboratory- or hospital-acquired infections longer incubation periods (10 to 13 days) have been reported. In considering the clinical features, it is advantageous to classify the illness as to severity: inapparent, mild, moderately severe, and malignant. In mild yellow fever the only symptoms may be the abrupt onset of fever and headache. Additional symptoms may include nausea, epistaxis, relative bradycardia known as Faget's sign (e.g., with a temperature of 102°F the pulse may be only 48 to 52 beats per min), and slight albuminuria. The mild illness lasts only 1 to 3 days and resembles influenza except that coryzal symptoms are lacking.

Moderately severe and malignant attacks of yellow fever are characterized by three distinct clinical periods: the period of infection, the period of remission, and the period of intoxication. Prodromal symptoms are usually absent. The onset is characteristically sudden, with headache, dizziness, and temperature elevations to 104°F without a relative bradycardia. Young children may have febrile convulsions. The headache is followed quickly by pains in the neck, back, and legs. Often there is nausea with vomiting and retching. Examination reveals a flushed face and injection of the conjunctiva. The congestion of the eyes persists until the third day. The tongue characteristically shows bright red margins and tip and a white furred center. Faget's sign appears by the second day. Epistaxis and gingival bleeding are common. On the third day of illness, the fever may fall by crisis and the patient enters remission, or, in the malignant form, copious hemorrhages, anuria, or delirium may occur. The stage of remission lasts from several hours to several days. In the third stage, the "classic" symptoms develop; the fever returns but the pulse remains slow. Jaundice becomes detectable about the third day; however, jaundice often is not prominent even in fatal illnesses. Increased epistaxis, melena, and uterine hemorrhages are common, but gross hematuria is rare. Of the classic signs, "black vomit" is more characteristic than is jaundice. Hematemesis usually does not occur before the fourth day and is often associated with a fatal outcome. Albuminuria, which rarely develops before the third day, occurs in 90 percent of patients and may be quite marked (3 to 20 g albumin per liter). In spite of this massive albuminuria, edema or ascites has not been reported. In malignant infections, coma frequently occurs 2 to 3 days before death. Shortly before death, which usually occurs between the fourth and the sixth days, it is not uncommon for the patient to become delirious and wildly agitated. Though the duration of fever in the third stage is usually 5 to 7 days, the period of intoxication is the most variable of the stages and may last up to 2 weeks. Clinical yellow fever is relatively free from complications, suppurative parotitis being the most striking of those which do occur. Clinical relapses are not characteristic of yellow fever.

Laboratory findings Early in the disease, progressive leukopenia may occur. By the fifth day, total leukocyte counts of 1,500 to 2,500 per mm^3 often are found, the decrease being due mostly to a decrease in neutrophils. Total leukocyte counts return to normal by the tenth day, and in fatal cases there may be a marked terminal leukocytosis. Hemoglobin values remain normal except terminally, when hemoconcentration or bleeding may occur. Platelet counts are reported to be normal. Detailed coagulation studies have been performed only in rhesus monkeys experimentally infected with yellow fever. Within 72 h after viral inoculation and prior to apparent clinical illness, a coagulation defect was observed. This was characterized by a prolonged one-stage prothrombin time and a prolonged partial thromboplastin time, reflecting measured deficiencies in factors II, V, VII, VIII, IX, X, and XI. Both the euglobulin lysis time and the thrombin time were prolonged, suggesting a depression of plasminogen activation and accumulation of fibrinogen degradation products. At this time platelet counts and chemical measurements of fibrinogen were normal. During the subsequent 48 h, these coagulation defects worsened as the monkeys developed clinical illness; terminally, depression of platelet counts and fibrinogen levels occasionally was observed. The disturbances in coagulation occurred during the stage of viremia and existed before the stage of hepatic necrosis in liver biopsy specimens. These data suggest that the *hemorrhagic manifestations are primarily caused by a disseminated intravascular coagulation rather than by hepatic failure.* Also, in experimental infections in primates, modest increases in total bilirubin and alkaline phosphatase levels and marked increases in serum glutamic oxalacetic transaminase occur. Electrocardiograms may show T-wave changes. Clinical examinations of cerebrospinal fluid have not revealed abnormalities.

Diagnosis There are three established procedures for the laboratory diagnosis of yellow fever: (1) Isolation of the virus from blood. This must be done early, preferably during the first 3 days. Caution must be exercised to avoid autoinoculation. (2) Demonstration of increase in neutralizing antibody. (3) Demonstration of the typical, although not completely specific, histopathologic lesions on liver biopsy.

Treatment The management has been symptomatic and supportive and should be based upon assessment and correction of the circulatory abnormalities. If evidence of disseminated intravascular coagulation is present, the administration of heparin should be considered. Close attention to fluids and electrolytes is essential.

Prognosis The overall fatality rate in yellow fever is between 5 and 10 percent of clinical cases; it may be less now since many infections are mild or inapparent.

Prevention Effective control measures are available. Immunization has been effective in the prevention of outbreaks. With the occurrence of sylvatic outbreaks, work in the area of epizootic activity should be discontinued and intensive mosquito abatement measures should be instituted. These measures may provide the time necessary for a mass immunization program.

MOSQUITO-BORNE HEMORRHAGIC FEVERS The term *hemorrhagic fever* was first applied to illness in Southeast Asia in the Philippines in 1953. Subsequently the hemorrhagic fevers have grown steadily as a disease problem. Initially they were classified on the basis of geography as Philippine, Thai, and Southeast Asian hemorrhagic fevers. With further study it appeared more rational to classify the syndromes as hemorrhagic dengue or chikungunya, depending upon the etiology. These diseases are caused by viruses transmitted by *A. aegypti.*

Etiology At least four (dengue types 1, 2, 3, 4) and possibly six types of dengue and chikungunya virus have been isolated from arthropods and humans during outbreaks of hemorrhagic fever.

Prevalence The reasons for the apparent sudden "appearance" of the syndrome in the past 15 years are completely obscure. However, during the 1922 epidemic of dengue fever in Louisiana, hemorrhagic manifestations, including epistaxis, bleeding gums, melena, menorrhagia, and even "black vomit," were observed. Hemorrhagic disease with dengue also was seen in Durban in 1927, in Athens in 1928, and in Curacao in 1968. Yet no deaths were attributed directly to the dengue, which is at variance with the observations in Southeast Asia. Outbreaks have tended to recur at the original site and to spread to other *A. aegypti*-infested areas. Outbreaks have occurred in the Philippines, Vietnam, Cambodia, Thailand, Malaysia, Singapore, and India. Hemorrhagic fever is a disease of children, with virtually all cases occurring in children under age fourteen years. In 1962 in Bangkok and Thonburi, an estimated 10 to 20 percent of children under age fifteen had illness due either to dengue or to chikungunya virus. Approximately 5 percent of children with dengue or chikungunya had hemorrhagic fever. Dengue hemorrhagic fever occurs almost exclusively in indigenous populations; it has been observed only rarely in Caucasians of European descent despite the frequent occurrence of classic dengue in this group. Despite annual outbreaks of dengue-2 fever in Puerto Rico since 1969, hemorrhagic fever has not been reported.

Epidemiology *Aëdes aegypti* is the vector of both dengue and chikungunya viruses. It is an urban mosquito which breeds in artificial containers and receptacles. Outbreaks are confined to the rainy season, although in areas without marked seasonal rainfall cases may occur throughout the year. Human-mosquito-human transmission of dengue is responsible for urban epidemics. Recent isolates of chikungunya virus from *Culex tritaeniorhynchus* in Thailand where human population densities are low suggest a nonhuman reservoir for this virus.

Clinical manifestations The hemorrhagic dengue syndrome is almost exclusively a disease of children. There is no sex predominance. Illness begins abruptly with a minor stage characterized by fever, cough, pharyngitis, headache, anorexia, nausea, vomiting, and abdominal pain. This continues for 2 to 4 days. In contrast to what occurs in classic dengue, myalgia, arthralgia, and bone pain are unusual. Physical signs include fever varying from 101 to 105°F, injection of the tonsils and pharynx, and palpable lymph nodes and liver. The initial state is followed by abrupt deterioration, with the rapid onset of lassitude and weakness. On examination the child is found to be restless and to have cold clammy extremities with a warm trunk and flushing of the face. Petechiae, most frequently located on the forehead and distal extremities, are seen in half the cases. Occasionally there may be a macular or maculopapular rash. The extremities are frequently cyanotic. Hypotension, with narrowing of the pulse pressure, and tachycardia occur. Pathologic reflexes may be observed. Most fatalities occur in the fourth or fifth day of illness, melena, hematemesis, coma, or unresponsive shock being poor prognostic signs. Cyanosis, dyspnea, and convulsions are terminal manifestations. Following this critical period, survivors show steady and quite rapid improvement.

Laboratory findings In one study, hemoconcentration was found in one-fifth of the children. The majority had leukocyte counts between 5,000 and 10,000 per mm^3, with one-third showing a leukocytosis. Only 10 percent of children had a true leukopenia. The most characteristic findings were thrombocytopenia, rarely with blood platelets under 75,000 per mm^3, positive tourniquet test, and prolonged bleeding time. Prothrombin time and partial thromboplastin times were usually near normal values. Depression of clotting factors V, VII, IX, and X may be present. Bone marrow examination may reveal maturation arrest of megakaryocytes. Urinalyses are usually normal, as are cerebrospinal fluid examinations. Other abnormal laboratory findings may include hyponatremia, acidosis, elevated blood urea nitrogen levels, elevation in serum glutamic oxalacetic transaminase levels, mild hyperbilirubinemia, and hypoproteinemia. Electrocardiograms may reveal diffuse myocardial abnormalities. Two-thirds of patients have radiologic evidence of bronchopneumonia, with many showing pleural effusions.

Diagnosis Specific virologic diagnosis of dengue virus infection by serologic means often is difficult because broad antibody responses to group B arboviruses occur. Virus isolation may provide the only means of identifying the specific agent. Chikungunya virus diagnosis poses less difficulty, since it can be isolated from acute serum in suckling mice or hamster kidney cells. Serologic responses can also be demonstrated.

Pathophysiology The pathophysiologic processes that occur in dengue hemorrhagic fever (DHF) and that distinguish it from unmodified dengue fever are increased vascular permeability, decreased plasma volume, hypotension, thrombocytopenia, and a hemorrhagic diathesis. The association of DHF with secondary heterologous dengue virus infections has suggested that an immunopathologic process might be involved. Anamnestic antibody responses with high titers of antidengue IgG antibody early in the course of DHF support this concept. Activation of both the classic and alternate complement pathways, with depression of both C4 and C3 proactivator levels, has been shown in most patients. The level of depression of C3 has correlated with the severity of disease. Relatively stable transferring levels indicated that depletion of complement components was not primarily due to extravasation. Fibrinogen levels were depressed, and circulating fibrin split products increased. These data, combined with the observation that histologically vascular lesions are not found, strongly suggest that the DHF syndrome is immunologically mediated, through the release of mediators secondary to activation of the complement system.

Treatment The mainstay is correction of circulatory collapse while avoiding fluid overload. Administration of 5% glucose in 0.5 *N* saline at a rate of 40 ml per kg restored blood pressure within 1 to 2 h in one-half of patients. When stable, the rate of administration of intravenous fluids was slowed to 10 ml/kg/h. If improvement did not occur, plasma or a plasma expander (20 ml per kg) was administered. Transfusion of whole blood is not recommended. Glucocorticosteroids have been used, but doses of 25 mg per kg have not resulted in significant improvement. Since the evidence for severe disseminated intravascular coagulation is questionable, use of heparin is not clear-cut, although in a group of Filipino children with dengue-3 virus, administration of heparin (1 mg sodium heparin per kg) was associated with a dramatic rise in number of platelets and level of plasma fibrinogen. Antibiotics are not indicated, and sympathomimetic amines are contraindicated. Recovery from vascular collapse usually occurs within 24 to 48 h, at which time diuretics and digitalis may be necessary.

Prognosis Mortality has varied from 6 to 23 percent. Deaths have been most common in infants under one year of age.

Prevention At present, vector control is the only method available to prevent hemorrhagic fever.

TICK-BORNE HEMORRHAGIC FEVERS **Crimean hemorrhagic fever** At the close of World War II, a new disease entity was recognized in the Crimea region of the U.S.S.R. Retrospective studies demonstrated that an almost identical syndrome had been recognized in the south central Asian republics of the U.S.S.R. for many years. Soviet workers repeatedly isolated virus strains during 1967 to 1969.

ETIOLOGY The virus of Crimean hemorrhagic fever (CHF) has been shown to be antigenically identical with Congo virus, which has been isolated from patients, cattle, and ticks in Africa (Kenya, Uganda, Congo, and Nigeria). CHF-Congo isolates now have been made from an area extending from southwestern and central U.S.S.R. to Pakistan and across central Africa from Nigeria to Kenya.

EPIDEMIOLOGY Approximately 30 cases of CHF have been recorded annually in each of the known areas of occurrence in the U. S. S. R. The cases occur between April and September. The sex distribution of CHF is equal, and 80 percent of the cases occur in the twenty- to sixty-year age group, with the majority occurring in milkmaids and agricultural workers. The major arthropod vectors for transmission to humans are ticks which belong to the genus *Hyalomma.* Cattle and wild hares appear to be important reservoirs, and rooks and other birds have been implicated, although the detailed epidemiology has yet to be defined.

CLINICAL MANIFESTATIONS The onset is abrupt, with temperatures to 104°F, dizziness, headache, and diffuse myalgia. The course of fever is occasionally biphasic, with an average duration of 8 days. Physical signs include flushing of the face, conjunctival injection, vomiting, and, on occasion, epigastric pain. Hepatomegaly is found in half the patients. Splenomegaly has been reported in 2 to 25 percent of patients. Respiratory symptoms or signs are unusual. Hemorrhagic manifestations generally begin on the fourth day with petechiae on the oral mucosa and skin, epistaxis, gingival bleeding, hematemesis, and melena. Neurologic abnormalities, seen in 10 to 25 percent of patients, include nuchal rigidity, excitation, and coma. Laboratory findings show leukopenia, with the number of white blood cells falling as low as 1,000 per mm^3, and thrombocytopenia, which is often severe. Proteinuria and microscopic hematuria are common, but azotemia and oliguria are not. Convalescence may be prolonged. Death is usually attributed to shock or intercurrent infection. Sequelae include transient alopecia and mononeuritis or polyneuritis. Although the clinical disease seen in Africa due to Congo virus generally has not been associated with hemorrhagic manifestations, one fatal case with gastrointestinal bleeding has been reported from Uganda.

TREATMENT The major approach to therapy has been transfusions of blood or plasma. The clinical similarities to other hemorrhagic fever syndromes in which the phenomenon of intravascular coagulation seems to occur are sufficient to suggest that appropriate studies should be done. If evidence of disseminated intravascular coagulation is demonstrated, treatment with heparin should be considered.

PROGNOSIS The reported mortality rate has shown variation between 9 and 50 percent.

Omsk hemorrhagic fever OHF is an acute febrile disease which occurs in the Omsk and Novosibirsk oblasts in the U. S. S. R. and is caused by a group B arbovirus of the Russian spring-summer complex.

EPIDEMIOLOGY The seasonal occurrence of OHF shows a biphasic pattern with peaks in May and August. OHF is transmitted to humans either by the bite of infected ticks of the genus *Dermacentor* or by the handling of infected muskrats. The natural reservoir includes muskrats, other rodents, and ticks. Epidemics occurred from 1945 to 1948, but recently the disease has been less prevalent.

CLINICAL MANIFESTATIONS Following an incubation interval of 3 to 8 days, illness begins abruptly with fever, headache, and hemorrhagic manifestations, which include epistaxis and gastrointestinal and uterine bleeding. Rarely, neurologic abnormalities may occur. Laboratory features include leukopenia. In contrast to many of the other hemorrhagic fevers, OHF has a low case fatality rate (0.5 to 3.0 percent).

Kyasanur forest disease Kyasanur Forest disease was first recognized in south India in 1957 as a discrete clinical entity shown to be due to an arbovirus.

ETIOLOGY The virus is a group B arbovirus immunologically related to the Russian spring-summer complex.

EPIDEMIOLOGY Kyasanur Forest disease occurs following occupational exposure to *Haemaphysalis spinigera* ticks in the tropical forests of western Mysore in southern India. The silent reservoir cycle which infects the primate- and bird-feeding *Haemaphysalis* ticks is now believed to be *Ixodes* ticks transmitted among small forest mammals, especially the shrew. Laboratory-associated infections have been common.

CLINICAL MANIFESTATIONS The major symptoms include abrupt onset of fever, headache, fatigue, myalgia (especially of the lumbar area and calf muscles), and retroorbital pain. Cough and abdominal pain occur in half the patients. Additional symptoms may include photophobia and polyarthralgia. Epistaxis and hematemesis are observed in some patients. On examination, findings include relative bradycardia, conjunctival injection, and generalized lymphadenopathy. Fine and coarse rales are frequently heard. Hepatosplenomegaly has been encountered occasionally. During the initial phase, generalized hyperesthesia of the skin occurs occasionally. The fever usually lasts from 6 to 11 days. After an afebrile period of 9 to 21 days, approximately half the patients may develop a second phase, which lasts from 2 to 12 days. This is manifested by recurrence of fever, severe headache, neck stiffness, mental disturbance, coarse tremors, giddiness, and abnormalities in reflexes, as well as by recurrence of many of the initial symptoms. No sequelae have been observed, but convalescence is often prolonged.

Only limited laboratory studies have been performed. During the initial phase, leukopenia is a constant feature, with a total leukocyte count of fewer than 3,000 per mm^3 by the fourth to sixth day. The leukopenia is associated with neutropenia. During the second phase there is a mild leukocytosis. Lumbar puncture during the second phase has shown a pattern of aseptic meningitis.

DIAGNOSIS Diagnosis is based upon virus isolation from blood; this is readily accomplished, since viremia is prolonged. Serologic tests of paired serums also can be performed.

TREATMENT The management is supportive.

PROGNOSIS The mortality rate is approximately 5 percent.

ARENAVIRUSES

Definition and classification

The term *arenavirus* is the proposed designation for a set of 10 RNA viruses which have unique morphology (Table 212-3). The virions are round, oval, or pleomorphic with diameters between 60 and 350 nm, and contain an electron-dense membrane with projections and 2 to 10 inclusion-like dense particles (resembling ribosomes) that give the virion an appearance of having been sprinkled with sand (*arenaceus,* Latin "sandy"). A special property of arenaviruses that cause disease in humans, especially Machupo and those causing lymphocytic choriomeningitis (Chap. 197), is their capacity to induce persistent infection in their reservoir hosts, with no ill effects and in the absence of an immune response.

HEMORRHAGIC FEVER WITH RENAL SYNDROME Synonyms for this disease include Korean hemorrhagic fever, Far Eastern hemorrhagic fever, endemic or epidemic nephrosonephritis, Manchurian epidemic hemorrhagic fever, Songo fever, and Churilov's disease.

Epidemic hemorrhagic fever (EHF) is an acute febrile, often fatal, otherwise self-limited illness of unknown etiology characterized by severe toxemia, widespread capillary damage, hemorrhagic phenomena, and renal insufficiency. In 1932, the Russians first observed the disease in southeastern Siberia along the Amur River. In April 1951, a previously unknown illness, subsequently recognized as EHF, broke out among the United Nations forces in Korea.

Etiology The causative agent of EHF has not been definitively isolated in either culture or lower animal hosts, and immunologic or serologic diagnostic procedures have not been developed. On the basis of extensive clinical, pathologic, and epidemiologic studies, Smorondintsev, who led a Soviet research group, provisionally classified EHF as one of the zoonotic hemorrhagic fevers, which would suggest an arenavirus etiology.

TABLE 212-3
Classification of arenaviruses

Virus	*Clinical disease*	*Reservoir*	*Known geographic range*
Lymphocytic choriomeningitis	Aseptic meningitis, meningoencephalitis, influenzal syndrome	Mice, hamsters	Worldwide except Australia
Tacaribe		Bats	Trinidad
Junin	Argentinian hemorrhagic fever	*Calomys musculinus*	Argentina
Machupo	Bolivian hemorrhagic fever	*Calomys callosus*	Northeast Bolivia
Amapari			Brazil
Latino			Bolivia
Parana			Paraguay
Pichinde			Colombia
Tamiami			Florida
Lassa	Lassa fever	*Mastomys natalensis*	Nigeria, Liberia, Sierra Leone, Republic of Guinea, Central African Republic
?	Far Eastern hemorrhagic fever	?	U.S.S.R., Manchuria, China, Korea

Prevalence In Korea between April 1951 and January 1953, 2,070 cases of EHF were reported among United Nations personnel. The disease usually occurs as an isolated event; hence, overall attack rates have relatively less meaning. With this reservation, attack rates in two United States Army divisions stationed in Korea varied between 1.9 and 2.9 cases per 1,000 men per epidemic season. Sporadic cases have continued to occur in United States military personnel assigned to endemic areas of Korea. The U. S. S. R. reports 500 to 2,000 cases yearly.

Epidemiology In Korea the majority of cases occur in May to June and in October to November. These peaks coincide with the dry seasons. Geographically, EHF occurred among troops stationed in the vicinity of Seoul north of the 38th parallel, with only rare cases reported from the southern portion of the Korean peninsula. The epidemiology of EHF observed in Korea is compatible with the assumption that EHF is transmitted by some arthropod and that the reservoir of disease is a member of the local fauna. Trombiculid mites (chiggers), bloodsucking mites (laelaptids), fleas, and ticks may all be regarded as potential vectors, but chiggers, especially *Trombicula pallida,* correlate most closely with the epidemiology of EHF in Korea.

Since World War II, rather remarkable outbreaks have occurred in northeast Asia between November and January. In these outbreaks, the peak of the epidemic was preceded by a marked increase in forest rodent populations (usually the red-backed vole *Clethrionomys glariolus*), which migrated into the fields, barns, and even houses near the forest. On the basis of these data, Soviet investigators now believe that EHF is transmitted directly from asymptomatically infected rodents to man by means of virus-contaminated rodent excreta, an epidemiologic pattern analogous to that demonstrated for Bolivian hemorrhagic fever. Thus, EHF may represent either a zoonotic hemorrhagic fever, as postulated by Soviet investigators, or an arthropod-borne infection involving one or more species of mites.

Clinical manifestations The incubation period in EHF is usually 10 to 25 days, with possible extremes of 7 and 36 days. Individuals who contract the disease in an endemic area may easily not develop illness until their return to the United States. Inapparent or mild disease is less common than typical EHF.

The clinical course of EHF may be divided into phases on the basis of the underlying physiologic aberrations: febrile, hypotensive, oliguric, diuretic, and convalescent. There is considerable variation among patients in the severity of the illness. In one study two-thirds of the 264 cases studied were classified as mild, while 14 percent were termed severe. The illness in most patients was of comparable severity in each phase.

FEBRILE (INVASIVE) PHASE From 10 to 20 percent of patients describe vague prodromal symptoms resembling mild upper respiratory infections. The onset is then usually abrupt, often initiated by a chill and accompanied by fever, headache, backache, abdominal pain, and generalized myalgia. Anorexia and thirst are almost universal, while nausea and vomiting are common although not constant symptoms. The headache is most commonly frontal or retroorbital. Eye symptoms, especially mild photophobia and pain on movement of the eyes, are characteristic. Diarrhea is not a feature. Fever is present in almost all patients; the temperature ranges from 100 to 106°F, reaches a peak on the third or fourth day after onset, and falls by lysis on the fourth to seventh day. There is a relative bradycardia. Initially the blood pressure is normal. One of the most typical early findings is a diffuse reddening of the skin, most marked over the face and V area of the neck. It may resemble a severe sunburn. The erythema blanches on pressure. Dermographism can be demonstrated in over 90 percent of patients at the same time as the flush. Slight edema of the upper eyelids causes a bleary-eyed appearance. Bulbar and palpebral conjunctivas show injection. Conjunctival petechiae may develop by the third or fifth day of illness. Subconjunctival hemorrhages may be striking. Intense pharyngeal reddening without significant sore throat is typical. The first location for petechiae is usually the palate, where they occur in half the patients. Within 12 to 24 h, petechiae appear at pressure areas such as the axillary folds, lateral chest wall, belt line, hips, and thighs. Retinal hemorrhages occur rarely. Cervical, axillary, and inguinal nodes are moderately enlarged but nontender. Abdominal and costovertebral tenderness is almost a constant finding. Splenomegaly is unusual and in Korea was generally attributable to malaria with which EHF coexisted in about 1 percent of patients. The degree of flush, fever, and conjunctival injection and the number of petechiae correlate quite well with the overall severity of illness.

Laboratory studies during this phase are often not striking. Initial hemoglobin and hematocrit values are usually normal. Prior to the fourth day, leukocyte counts range from 3,600 to 6,000 per mm^3 but are associated with neutrophilia. Early in the course urine specific gravity may be high. Albuminuria, which is an almost universal finding, appears, often abruptly, between the second and fifth days of illness. The urinary sediment reveals microscopic hematuria and hyaline, granular, red blood cell casts, and/or white blood cell casts. Erythrocyte sedimentation rates are normal during the first week. Capillary fragility tests are usually positive at the time of admission and become most abnormal by the ninth day. Electrocardiographic abnormalities may be seen in 15 to 30 percent of patients; these include sinus bradycardia and low or inverted T waves. Lumbar punctures may reveal gross blood in the spinal fluid.

HYPOTENSIVE PHASE On about the fifth day of illness, during the last 24 to 48 h of the febrile phase, hypotension or shock may occur. In mild cases, only a transient fall in blood pressure occurs; among moderately and severely ill patients shock may persist for 1 to 3 days. In 828 patients, 16.5 percent had clinical shock, and another 14 percent had hypotension without shock. Headache often diminishes, but thirst persists. In the beginning of the hypotensive phase, most patients have warm, dry skin and extremities. As the hypotensive phase progresses and the systolic blood pressure decreases and pulse pressure narrows, the skin becomes cool and moist. Tachycardia replaces the relative bradycardia.

At this stage, an increase in hematocrit with no change in total serum protein level is found. This is thought to reflect a loss of plasma through damaged capillaries. On about the fifth day, all patients develop marked proteinuria. The previously normal urine specific gravity begins to fall and in 2 to 3 days is usually around 1.010. Blood urea nitrogen concentrations begin to increase. Other laboratory findings include leukocytosis with white blood cell counts of 10,000 to 56,000 per mm^3 with neutrophilia and toxic granulation. The number of platelets often decreases to less than 70,000 per mm^3. In a single patient who became ill 30 days after leaving Korea and who was studied on the fourth day of illness (i.e., in the hypotensive phase), there was marked thrombocytopenia, hypofibrinogenemia, and hypoprothrombinemia with a prolonged thrombin time. The deficiency of multiple blood coagulation factors suggests that the bleeding defect was due to disseminated intravascular coagulation.

OLIGURIC PHASE (HEMORRHAGIC OR TOXIC PHASE) About the eighth day of illness, blood pressure returns to the normal range and in some instances increases to hypertensive levels. While oliguria may have appeared during the shock phase, it now becomes a prominent feature. Oliguria develops even though hypotension was not recognized. Symptomatically patients continue to feel weak and thirsty and have more severe backache. Protracted vomiting and hiccups may ensue.

Blood urea nitrogen levels increase rapidly and are associated with hyperkalemia, hyperphosphatemia, and hypocalcemia. Metabolic acidosis is rarely severe. Although platelets begin to return to normal, hemorrhagic manifestations become more prominent and include petechiae, hematemesis (analogous to "black vomit" in yellow fever), melena, hemoptysis, gross hematuria, and hemorrhages into the central nervous system. The enlarged lymph nodes may now become tender.

With the onset of diuresis on about the seventh day in moderately ill patients and the ninth to eleventh day in severely ill patients, symptoms of fluid and electrolyte abnormalities and central nervous system or pulmonary complications may appear. Central nervous system symptoms include disorientation, extreme restlessness, lethargy, paranoid delusions, and hallucinations. Grand mal seizures, pulmonary edema, and pulmonary infection occur in some patients.

DIURETIC PHASE With the onset of diuresis, progressive improvement is the rule. Most patients begin to eat and regain their strength. In fatal cases the diuretic phase is associated with a daily urine output of less than 4 liters and often less than 2 liters, in contrast to larger volumes in surviving patients.

CONVALESCENT PHASE The convalescent phase lasts 3 to 6 weeks. Weight is regained slowly. Complaints include muscular weakness, intention tremor, and lack of stamina. Hyposthenuria and polyuria are present; however, within 2 months most patients are able to concentrate their urine to a specific gravity of 1.023 or greater after a 12-h period of water deprivation.

Diagnosis In the absence of identification of the causative agent or agents and specific serologic methods, the diagnosis of EHF is one of exclusion. The following criteria are necessary for diagnosis: the patient must have been in the endemic area within the limits of the incubation period, and there must be a characteristic history, hemorrhagic findings, and evidence of renal involvement. In addition, studies to exclude other forms of the hemorrhagic fever syndrome must be undertaken, particularly in the sporadic cases.

Pathology The most characteristic fundamental alteration is widespread capillary and endothelial damage, with all subsequent manifestations being the result of this damage. This is manifested by dilatation of all small vessels in tissues, congestion, plasma transudation, and multiple small hemorrhages. Three features are prominent and characteristic: hemorrhage, particularly in the renal medulla, right atrium, and gastrointestinal submucosa; a peculiar type of necrosis of the renal pyramids, anterior lobe of the pituitary body, and adrenal gland; and a mononuclear cellular infiltration of the myocardium, spleen, and liver. Moderate to severe retroperitoneal edema was present in three-fourths of patients who died in the hypotensive phase of EHF.

Pathophysiology The physiologic changes correlate with the clinical features. During the early febrile phase, the cardiac index is normal. Late in the febrile phase widespread capillary dysfunction becomes evident. This is manifest by loss of protein-rich plasma through damaged capillaries and results in hemoconcentration and a progressive fall in cardiac output. Measured total peripheral resistance is low, a finding compatible with the observed capillary dilatation and refractoriness to *l*-norepinephrine. During the hypotensive phase, the increases in hematocrit values and decreases in plasma volume are accentuated. These findings have the pathologic corollary of marked retroperitoneal edema. The hypotensive phase is associated with a reduction in cardiac output and an increase in peripheral vascular resistance. The reduced cardiac output is probably the result of reduction in circulating blood volume, inadequate vasoconstriction, and possibly myocardial damage. Although adrenal hemorrhages can be seen at necropsy, adrenal insufficiency does not seem to be a contributing cause of shock. The initial pathophysiologic changes may result in impairment of circulation through various organs, with the development of functional and morphologic changes secondary to inadequate perfusion with its attendant hypoxemia. The hemorrhagic manifestations appear to be the result of capillary damage, with diapedesis of erythrocytes and the development of disseminated intravascular coagulation.

The plasma loss and arteriolar dysfunction are limited in duration, and, for unknown reasons, the sequestered plasma rather abruptly returns to the vascular system at the time of oliguric phase. During this phase, examination of nailbed capillaries reveals increased vasomotor activity and vasoconstriction. When patients who became hypertensive were divided on the basis of the presence or absence of diuresis, the clinical and hemodynamic differences became more apparent. During the hypertensive phase in anuric or oliguric patients, some individuals presented with full veins, an exaggerated cardiac apical thrust, and wide pulse pressure. In this group the cardiac index was high, and the peripheral resistance and hematocrit were low. Hypertensive patients who had begun to have diuresis had normal cardiac outputs and significantly elevated values for peripheral vascular resistance.

Although diuresis is a harbinger of convalescence, a daily urine output of 3 to 8 liters contributes to further serious fluid and electrolyte imbalances. If fluid output exceeds intake, low cardiac indexes may be seen and shock may ensue. Conversely, if fluid intake exceeds output, hypertension and pulmonary edema may develop.

Treatment Clinical management primarily revolves around meticulous supportive care. Trials with a variety of agents including antibiotics, adrenocortical steroid hormones, antihistamines, and convalescent serum were without significant beneficial effect during the Korean epidemics. The treatment of shock is discussed in Chap. 129, and that of acute tubular necrosis in Chap. 272.

Prognosis The Soviet experience indicates a mortality rate of 3 to 32 percent; in other early reports the mortality has ranged from 10 to 15 percent. Between April 1951 and January 1953, the overall case fatality ratio in Korea was 5.9 percent; however, during 1967–1968, there were no fatalities among 44 patients admitted to the Hemorrhagic Fever Center.

Residua are uncommon. Of 783 surviving patients cared for at the Hemorrhagic Fever Center in Korea between April and December 1952, only 16 were unable to return to duty within a period of 4 months. Fifteen of these individuals still had hyposthenuria. Follow-up studies on former EHF patients 3 to 5 years later showed that they had many more subsequent hospital admissions for urologic problems than did a control group and that the relative frequency correlated with the severity of the acute episode of EHF. Asymptomatic residual renal tubular dysfunction may be more common than has been appreciated.

ARGENTINIAN AND BOLIVIAN HEMORRHAGIC FEVERS

The first cases of a new American hemorrhagic disease were seen near the Argentinian town of Junin near Buenos Aires in 1953. A virus was isolated from patients' blood and from local rodents and their mites. In 1959, cases of a disease thought to resemble severe epidemic typhus were noted among rural workers in northeastern Bolivia. The similarity between these syndromes was recognized. In 1963, the causal virus was isolated from patients and rodents and named the Machupo virus. Machupo virus is serologically related to but distinct from Junin virus.

Prevalence Junin virus infections have occurred in epidemic form since 1958 with between 100 and 3,500 cases reported annually. The hemorrhagic disease in Bolivia has been particularly severe. Of a total population of 4,000 to 6,000 in the endemic area, 750 persons were affected between 1959 and 1963.

Epidemiology Argentinian hemorrhagic fever occurs in sharply endemic seasonal form, (February to August), mostly among male rural workers, especially those exposed to fields at the time of the maize harvest. Virus is transmitted in the urine of rodents with chronic infection and viruria. Humans acquire the virus through contact with items or foodstuffs which have been contaminated with infected rodent urine. The main reservoir is two species of cricetidae, *Calomys laucha* and *C. musculinus.*

Bolivian hemorrhagic fever is similarly transmitted by the urine of *C. callosus* (a mouse-like rodent) chronically infected with Machupo virus. Direct human-to-human transmission is possible and may have occurred in the outbreak in Cochabamba. Disease has not occurred in medical personnel attending infected patients.

Clinical features Argentinian hemorrhagic fever presents manifestations of renal, cardiovascular, and hematologic involvement. Inapparent infections are rare. The incubation period is estimated to be 7 to 16 days, followed by a gradual onset of chills, fever, headache, malaise, myalgia, anorexia, nausea, and vomiting. The temperature reaches 102 to 104°F, facial flushing may be prominent, and there is a painless enanthem of the pharynx. Lymphadenopathy and splenomegaly are not present. From 3 to 5 days after the onset, the signs and symptoms worsen, with the appearance of signs of dehydration, hypotension to 50 to 100 mmHg, oliguria, and relative bradycardia. In the more severe cases, hemorrhagic manifestations, including bleeding from the gums, hematemesis, hematuria, and melena, occur. Progressive oliguria and tremor of the tongue and extremities may develop. Some patients develop psychic manifestations, with agitation, delirium, or stupor. Progressive shock, hypothermia, gallop rhythm, or gastrointestinal bleeding may occur from the seventh to tenth days. In fatal cases, pulmonary edema usually is the cause of death. During convalescence a temporary alopecia has been noted. Erythrocyte counts are normal or elevated. The total leukocyte count drops to 1,200 to 3,400 blood cells per mm^3. Thrombocytopenia may occur. The urine is dark and may approach the color of mahogany, with intense albuminuria. Blood urea nitrogen levels rise rapidly.

The clinical picture of Bolivian hemorrhagic fever is similar to Argentinian, although epistaxis and hematemesis at the onset is more common.

Diagnosis Complement-fixing antibodies appear in 15 to 30 days in about 75 percent of the clinically diagnosed cases.

Treatment Available reports do not provide details as to therapy. Supportive measures, including peritoneal dialysis to correct both the azotemia and the pulmonary edema, would seem to offer the most reasonable approach.

Prognosis The mortality rate among patients with Argentinian hemorrhagic fever is usually 3 to 15 percent, while that in Bolivian hemorrhagic fever is 5 to 30 percent.

Prevention In Bolivia, rodent control measures directed primarily against *C. callosus* populations in the houses resulted in a prompt and dramatic cessation of human cases.

LASSA FEVER A new virus disease, which is both highly contagious and virulent, occurred in a missionary nurse in Lassa, a town in northeast Nigeria, in 1969.

Epidemiology Since the initial outbreak at Lassa in

1969, during which one of the patients was transferred to New York City, there have been other outbreaks near Jos in Northern Nigeria in 1970 (32 suspected cases with 10 deaths), in Zorzor, Liberia, in 1972 (11 cases with 4 deaths), and in the eastern province of Sierra Leone with 63 suspected cases admitted to two hospitals between 1970 and 1972. In Jos and Zorzor, outbreaks apparently resulted from person-to-person nosocomial spread from the index case to hospital workers or other patients. In Sierra Leone, the great majority of cases were acquired outside the hospital, although hospital workers were at high risk. *Mastomys natalensis,* a multimammate rat widespread in Africa, is known to be an animal reservoir of the virus, and primary human cases probably result from contamination of foodstuffs with rodent urine. Human-to-human transmission may occur through contact with urine, feces, vomitus, or saliva through droplets and aerosols, and particularly through wounds contaminated with blood. Intrafamilial outbreaks have occurred around several cases. There are a number of cases which have been acquired through accidental autoinoculation with needles while starting intravenous fluids. At least one laboratory-acquired infection has occurred. In Sierra Leone 6 percent of the population surveyed had complement-fixing antibody against Lassa virus, while only 0.2 percent had recognized disease, suggesting mild disease or inapparent infection.

Clinical features The incubation period is 1 to 24 days, being 10 days following accidental inoculation. Patients have ranged from 5 months to 46 years of age; approximately two-thirds are women. Three of eight women in one series were 22 to 28 weeks pregnant during their illness. The apparent predilection for women may relate to exposure to contaminated food or work in hospitals rather than to differences in susceptibility. The onset of illness was described by most patients as insidious. The most frequent initial symptoms are fever (100 percent), chilliness and true rigors, headache (50 percent), malaise (100 percent), and myalgia (50 percent). Most patients did not seek medical attention for 4 to 9 days after onset. Symptoms of a systemic viral illness then developed with anorexia, nausea, vomiting, myalgia, and pain in the chest, epigastrium, and lumbar area. Headache was usually present. Early examination reveals fever and flushing of the face and V area of the neck. Pharyngitis developed early and became progressively more severe during the first week; examination may reveal raised patches of whitish exudate occurring on the palatine arches which occasionally coalesce into a pseudomembrane. Oral ulcerations have been noted in up to one-half of cases. Generalized nontender lymphadenopathy occurred in one-half of patients. During the second week severe lower abdominal pain and intractable vomiting are common, and facial and neck swelling with conjunctival edema and infection frequently develop. Occasionally patients have tinnitus, epistaxis, bleeding from the gums and venapuncture sites, maculopapular rashes, cough, and dizziness. During the acute stage, systolic blood pressures of less than 90 mmHg with pulse pressures of less than 20 mmHg occurred in 60 to 80 percent of patients. Initially, relative bradycardia was common. During the second week, the patients who recovered defervesced, while the patients who died often developed signs of shock, clouding of the sensorium, rales, signs of pleural effusion, agitation and, on occasion, grand mal seizures. The duration of illness in surviving patients ranged from 7 to 31 days (average 15 days), while that in fatal cases was 7 to 26 days (average 12 days). The mortality rates in Jos and Zorzor were 52 percent and 36 percent, respectively, while in Sierra Leone the rate was 8 percent. During convalescence occasional flurries of rapid involuntary eye movements (oculogyric crises) occurred. Late sequelae include deafness in a number of patients (two of six in one series) and alopecia in one patient.

Laboratory features The hematologic findings include relatively normal hematocrit values and early leukopenia (less than 4,000 per mm^3 in 36 percent) with a relative neutrophilia and immature forms of leukocytes. In two cases in which it was recorded, the erythrocyte sedimentation rate was normal. Urinalyses revealed proteinuria, which was often massive. Chest radiographs may suggest basilar pneumonitis and pleural effusions. Electrocardiographic abnormalities compatible with diffuse myocardial disease have been encountered. Levels of serum enzymes, serum glutamic oxaloacetic transaminase (SGOT), creatinine phosphokinase (CPK), and lactic dehydrogenase (LDH) have been elevated.

Diagnosis Confirmation of diagnosis may be made by growth of the virus in tissue culture and by a complement fixation test; however, it is rarely positive before the fourteenth day of illness.

Treatment The management has been supportive. Infusion of immune plasma from convalescent patients resulted in a dramatic effect in three of four patients. Because of the self-limited nature of the disease, these results cannot be assessed easily. In view of the hospital association and the presence of virus in pharyngeal secretions and urine, strict isolation is required. Known contacts should be kept under medical surveillance for at least 3 weeks.

REFERENCES

Arboviruses

Definition and classification

HORZINCK MC: The structure of Togaviruses. Prog Med Virol 16: 109, 1973

THE SUBCOMMITTEE ON INFORMATION EXCHANGE OF THE AMERICAN COMMITTEE ON ARTHROPOD-BORNE VIRUSES: Catalogue of arthropod-borne and selected vertebrate viruses of the world. Am J Trop Med 20:1018, 1971

WHO STUDY GROUP: *Arthropod-borne Viruses,* WHO Tech. Rept. Ser. 219, Geneva, 1961

WHO SCIENTIFIC GROUP: *Arbovirus and Human Disease,* WHO Tech. Rept. Ser. 369, Geneva, 1967

Arbovirus infections characterized by fever, malaise, headaches, and myalgia

BECKER FE: Tick-borne infections in Colorado. Colorado Med 27:36, 1930

BRICENO ROSSIE AL: Rural epidemic encephalitis in Venezuela caused by a group A arbovirus (VEE). Prog Med Virol 9:176, 1967

DAUBNEY R et al: Enzootic hepatitis or Rift Valley Fever. J Pathol Bacteriol 34:545, 1931

DIASIO JS, RICHARDSON, FM: Clinical observation on dengue fever. Milit Surg 94:365, 1944

EHRENKRANZ NJ et al: Natural occurrence of Venezuelan equine encephalitis in USA. N Engl J Med 282:298, 1970

FLEMING J et al: Sandfly fever. Review of 664 cases. Lancet 1:443, 1947

FLORIO L et al: The etiology of Colorado tick fever. J Exp Med 83:1, 1946

HUGHES LE et al: Persistence of Colorado tick fever virus in red blood cells. Am J Trop Med Hyg 23:530, 1973

LENNETTE EH, KOPROWSKI H: Human infection with Venezuelan equine encephalomyelitis virus. JAMA 123:1088, 1943

LIKOSKY WH et al: An epidemiologic study of dengue type 2 in Puerto Rico, 1969. Am J Epidemiol 97:264, 1973

LLOYD LW: Colorado tick fever. Med Clin North Am, March 1951

SABIN AB: Research on dengue during World War II. Am J Trop Med 1:30, 1952

——et al: Phlebotomus (Papataci or sandfly) fever; disease of military importance: Summary of existing knowledge and preliminary report of original observations. JAMA 125:603, 693, 1944

SCHERER WF et al: Ecologic studies of Venezuelan encephalitis virus in Southeastern Mexico. VII. Infection of man. Am J Trop Med 21:79, 1972

SIDWELL RW et al: Epidemiological aspects of Venezuelan equine encephalitis virus infections. Bacterial Rev 31:65, 1967

SMITHBURN KC et al: Rift Valley fever. J Immunol 62:213, 1949

SPRUANCE SL, BAILEY A: Colorado tick fever. A review of 115 laboratory confirmed cases. Arch Intern Med 131:288, 1973

SULKIN SE et al: Bat salivary gland virus: Infections of man and monkey. Tex Rep Biol Med 20:113, 1962

TESH RB et al: Antigenic relationships among Phlebotomus fever group arboviruses and their implications for the epidemiology of sandfly fever. Am J Trop Med Hyg 24:135, 1975

Arbovirus infections presenting chiefly with fever, malaise, arthralgia, and rash

CLARK JA et al: Annually recurrent epidemic polyarthritis and Ross River virus activity in a coastal area of New South Wales. I. Occurrence of the disease. Am J Trop Med Hyg 22:543, 1973

DELLER JJ JR., RUSSELL PK: Chikungunya disease. Am J Trop Med 17:107, 1968

DOHERTY RL et al: Studies of epidemic polyarthritis: The significance of three group A arboviruses, isolated from mosquitoes in Queensland. Aust Ann Med 13:322, 1964

MALHERBE H et al: Sindbis virus infection in man. Report of a case with recovery of virus from skin lesions. S Afr Med J 37: 547, 1963

ROBINSON MC: An epidemic of virus disease in Southern Province, Tanganyika territory in 1952–53. I. Clinical features. Trans R Soc Trop Med Hyg 49:28, 1955

SHORE H: O'nyong-nyong fever: An epidemic virus disease in East Africa. III. Some clinical and epidemiological observations in the Northern Province of Uganda. Trans R Soc Trop Med Hyg 55:361, 1961

Arbovirus infections presenting chiefly with fever, malaise, lymphadenopathy, and rash

MARBERG K et al: The natural history of West Nile fever. I. Clinical observations during an epidemic in Israel. Am J Hyg 64:259, 1956

PERELMAN A, STERN J: Acute pancreatitis in West Nile fever. Am J Trop Med Hyg 23:1150, 1974

TAYLOR RM et al: A study of the ecology of West Nile virus in Egypt. Am J Trop Med 5:579, 1956

Arbovirus infections presenting chiefly with central nervous system involvement

ALTMAN R et al: The impact of vector-borne viral diseases in the middle Atlantic States. Med Clin N Amer 51:661, 1967

BALFOUR HH JR et al: California arbovirus (LaCrosse) infections. Pediatrics 52:680, 1973

DICKERSON RB et al: Diagnosis and immediate prognosis of Japanese B encephalitis. Observations based on more than 200 patients with detailed analysis of 65 serologically confirmed cases. Am J Med 12:277, 1952

FEEMSTER RF, HAYMAKER W: Eastern equine encephalitis. Neurology 8:882, 1958

FINLEY KH et al: Western equine and St. Louis encephalitis. Preliminary report of a clinical follow-up study in California. Neurology 5:223, 1955

GRABOW JD et al: The electroencephalogram and clinical sequelae of California arbovirus encephalitis. Neurology 19:394, 1969

HILTY MD et al: California encephalitis in children. Am J Dis Child 124:530, 1972

KETEL WB, OGNIBENE AJ: Japanese B encephalitis in Vietnam. Am J Med Sci 261:271, 1971

LUBY JP et al: The epidemiology of St. Louis encephalitis (SLE): A review. Ann Rev Med 20:329, 1969

SCHNEIDER RJ et al: Clinical sequelae after Japanese encephalitis: One year followup study in Thailand. Southeast Asian J Trop Med Public Health 5:560, 1974

WEAVER OM et al: Japanese encephalitis: Sequelae. Neurology 8:887, 1958

Arbovirus diseases presenting primarily with hemorrhagic manifestations

BOKISCH VA et al: The potential pathogenic role of complement in dengue-hemorrhagic fever syndrome. N Engl J Med 289:996, 1973

CASALS J et al: A current appraisal of hemorrhagic fevers in the USSR. Am J Trop Med 15:751, 1966

DENNIS LH, CONRAD ME: Accelerated intravascular coagulation in a patient with Korean hemorrhagic fever. Arch Intern Med 121:499, 1968

——et al: The original hemorrhagic fever: Yellow fever. Blood 30:858, 1967

GREISMAN SE: Capillary observations in patients with hemorrhagic fever and other infectious illnesses. J Clin Invest 36:1688, 1957

HALSTEAD SB: Mosquito-borne haemorrhagic fevers of South and Southeast Asia. Bull WHO 35:3, 1966

KERR JA: Clinical aspects and diagnosis of yellow fever, in *Yellow Fever,* ed GK Strode, New York: McGraw-Hill, 1951, p. 389

KIRK R: An epidemic of yellow fever in the Nuba Mountains, Anglo-Egyptian Sudan. Ann Trop Med Parasitol 35:67, 1941

LOW GC, FAIRLEY NH: Laboratory and hospital infections with yellow fever in England. Br Med J 1:125, 1931

NELSON ER: Hemorrhagic fever in children in Thailand: Report of 69 cases. J. Pediatr 56:101, 1960

PONGPANICH B et al: Management of shock associated with dengue hemorrhagic fever based on pathophysiological findings. Southeast Asian J Trop Med Public Health 6:115, 1975

POWELL GM: Hemorrhagic fever: A study of 300 cases. Medicine 33:97, 1954

RUBINI ME et al: Renal residuals of acute epidemic hemorrhagic fever. Arch Intern Med 106:378, 1960

SHEEDY JA et al: The clinical course of epidemic hemorrhagic fever. Am J Med 16:619, 1954

Arenaviruses

CASALS J: Arenaviruses. Yale J Biol Med 48:115, 1975

FRAME JD et al: Lassa fever, a new virus disease of man from West Africa. I. Clinical description and pathological findings. Am J Trop Med Hyg 19:670, 1970

JOHNSON KM et al: Hemorrhagic fevers of Southeast Asia and South America. A comparative approach. Prog Med Virol 9:105, 1967

MACKENZIE RB et al: Epidemic hemorrhagic fever in Bolivia. I. A preliminary report of the epidemiologic and clinical findings in a new epidemic area in South America. Am J Trop Med Hyg 13:620, 1964

MERTENS PE et al: Clinical presentation of Lassa fever cases during the hospital epidemic at Zorzor, Liberia, March-April 1972. Am J Trop Med Hyg 22:780, 1973

MONATH TP et al: Lassa fever in the Eastern Province of Sierra Leone, 1970–1972. II. Clinical observations and virological studies on selected hospital cases. Am J Trop Med Hyg 23:1140, 1974

213 OTHER VIRAL FEVERS

JAY P. SANFORD

RHABDOVIRUS INFECTIONS OTHER THAN RABIES The rhabdoviruses consist of a group of RNA viruses which previously were ungrouped or grouped with the arboviruses but which do not meet the revised criteria established for arboviruses, and which share a characteristic morphology. On electron microscopy, these agents are bullet-shaped, one of the extremities being pointed and the other flattened. Members of the rhabdovirus group which infect vertebrates include rabies, vesicular stomatitis virus, Marburg virus, and Mokola virus, which produce disease in humans, and Lagos bat, Cocal, Chandipura, Mount Elgon bat, Flanders, Hart Park, Kern Canyon, Piry, and Kotonkan viruses, which have not been recognized as producing human disease.

VESICULAR STOMATITIS VIRUS This virus disease of animals, which chiefly affects cattle, horses, swine, and wild animals, including deer, raccoons, skunks, and bobcats, appears in humans as an acute, self-limited infection with signs and symptoms similar to those of influenza. Two distinct serotypes, New Jersey and Indiana, have been recognized. Most of the outbreaks, especially in North America, have been due to the New Jersey strain. Although most commonly acquired as a laboratory infection in humans, it is transmissible under natural conditions. In one report, three-fourths of the laboratory personnel handling experimentally infected animals or manipulating the viruses developed neutralizing antibodies. In nature, the virus has been isolated from *Phlebotomus* sandflies collected in a tropical rain forest in Panama and from a pool of *Aëdes* sp. (probably *dorsalis*) mosquitoes during an epizootic in New Mexico. In the areas of Panama which were involved, 17 to 35 percent of the population had neutralizing antibodies against vesicular stomatitis virus (VSV). Of the laboratory workers with serologic evidence of infection, approximately one-half reported clinical symptoms. In the majority of cases the incubation period has been 2 to 6 days, although symptoms have developed within 30 h of accidental inoculation. The onset usually is sudden, with chills, fever, profuse diaphoresis, and generalized myalgia including pain on ocular movement. One-third to one-half of patients have sore throats, and 20 percent have coryza. Physical signs include a temperature of 102 to 104°F in severe cases; fever is absent in mild cases. Conjunctivitis is noted in 20 percent, and in some patients (10 percent), small, raised vesicles may be present on the buccal mucosa. Submaxillary and cervical lymphadenitis is seen in approximately one-third of patients. A diphasic course is noted in approximately 10 percent of patients. Treatment is symptomatic.

MARBURG VIRUS DISEASE From the middle of August through September, 1967, 31 individuals developed a febrile illness characterized by rash and hemorrhagic manifestations. Twenty-five of the patients had direct contact with African green monkeys (*Cercopithecus aethiops*) or tissue culture cells derived from them. The cases occurred in Marburg (23 cases) and Frankfurt (6 cases), Germany, and Belgrade, Yugoslavia (2 cases). The illness was clinically dramatic. It was associated with a 23 percent mortality, and evoked immediate worldwide concern and investigation, since thousands of monkeys are used in virologic studies and vaccine production. In February, 1975, two Australians who had hitchhiked around South Africa and had been in Rhodesia 10 days before being admitted to a hospital in South Africa, and an attending nurse, were proved to have Marburg virus disease. Noteworthy was the denial of contact with any monkeys.

Etiology The agent was propagated in guinea pigs, in which electron microscopy of liver revealed spheric particles 80 to 100 nm in diameter, filamentous forms, rods, and bullet-shaped organisms. It can be propagated in several primate tissue culture systems and has the characteristics of an RNA virus. While morphologically similar to rabies and VSV, it is serologically unrelated to 200 agents including other rhabdoviruses.

Epidemiology The outbreak related to vervet monkeys from the Lake Kyoga area of Uganda, which were shipped to London and then distributed to Europe. While there were no unusual illnesses or deaths among monkeys in the Lake Kyoga area, complement-fixing antibodies were demonstrated in up to 36 percent of *C. aethiops* trapped near Lake Kyoga; they were also present in three monkey trappers. Twenty of twenty-nine persons who had contact with blood or organs of this batch of vervet monkeys became ill, while 4 of the 13 persons exposed to tissue cultures prepared from these monkeys became ill. Infection from monkey to human occurred through direct contact with blood or organs, with no evidence for airborne spread. Secondary cases occurred reflecting human-to-human transmission, again probably through direct contact with blood or possibly body secretions (semen) from primarily infected patients.

Clinical manifestations After an incubation of 5 to 9 days, patients suddenly developed prostration, headache, myalgia, especially in the lumbar area, nausea, and vomiting. Initially the temperature rose to 103 to 104°F and often was associated with relative bradycardia. Other initial signs included conjunctivitis in at least three-fourths of patients and occasionally pharyngitis. One to two days after the onset, patients developed watery diarrhea, drowsiness, and changes in mentation. At about the fourth day of illness, an enanthem was noted, and lymphadenopathy was observed in some patients. The most reliable clinical feature was an erythematous rash which began on the fifth to seventh days on the buttocks, trunk, and outer surfaces of both upper arms. During the first week the temperatures continued in the range of 104°F, falling by lysis during the second week, to increase again between the twelfth and fourteenth days. Other clinical signs which were observed in some patients in the second week included splenomegaly, hepatomegaly, facial edema, and scrotal or labial reddening. Gastrointestinal hemorrhages occurred in approximately one-third of patients. After the sixteenth day, desquamation occurred and involved especially the palms and soles. Complications included orchitis in at least three patients, two of whom developed late testicular atrophy, and myocarditis with irregular pulse and electrocardiographic abnormalities. Fatalities occurred between the eighth and sixteenth days of illness, with an overall fatality rate of 23 percent. Late sequelae included myelitis and possible psychosis.

Laboratory findings Leukopenia was detected as early as the first day, with leukocyte counts as low as 1,000 per mm^3, with a neutrophilia by the fourth day. Subsequently between the fourth and nineteenth days, atypical lymphocytes appeared. At the end of the first week, a leukocytosis supervened. Thrombocytopenia appeared early and was most marked (often less than 10,000 cells per mm^3) between the sixth and twelfth days. In fatal cases evidence of disseminated intravascular coagulation was demonstrated. Several patients had proteinuria and azotemia. At the end of the first week, elevations in serum glutamic oxaloacetic transaminase (SGOT) were usual. Lumbar punctures performed on five patients revealed minimal pleocytosis in two.

Diagnosis The diagnosis was based upon the characteristic clinical course and epidemiologic features. With the preparation of antigens, serologic diagnosis is now possible.

Treatment The patients received a multiplicity of drugs without apparent influence on the course of the illness. Convalescent serum was administered to four patients, whose subsequent disease followed a mild course. However, similarly benign courses were observed in patients who did not receive serum.

MOKOLA VIRUS Although Mokola and rabies virus are related morphologically and serologically, neither of the two reported cases of human disease (both children) showed clinical features of classic rabies. One patient had a nonfatal illness characterized by fever, pharyngitis, and convulsions. Mokola virus was recovered from her cerebrospinal fluid. The second patient initially had fever, cough, and vomiting, followed in several days by drowsiness, confusion, and generalized flaccid weakness. Her cerebrospinal fluid was normal. She progressed to deep coma and died within 10 days of onset. Mokola virus was isolated from her brain, and histopathologic sections revealed finely granular cytoplasmic inclusions in many neurons. The inclusion bodies were easily distinguishable from Negri bodies.

ENCEPHALOMYOCARDITIS VIRUSES The encephalomyocarditis (EMC) viruses, Columbia S-K, MM, Mengo, are a group of small RNA viruses which are immunologically indistinguishable from each other. Rodents, in particular certain species of wild rats, constitute the major reservoir for EMC viruses. Strains also have been isolated from primates, swine, and other rodents from many parts of the world. Strains of Mengo virus have been isolated from mosquitoes (*Taeniorhynchus fuscopennatus*) in Uganda, but the epidemiologic evidence does not suggest that EMC viruses are arboviruses. The prevalence of neutralizing antibodies in surveys of healthy individuals in the United States, Germany, Sweden, and Mexico ranges up to 7 percent.

Human infections vary from inapparent to mild febrile illness to severe encephalomyelitis. Study of an outbreak of aseptic meningitis characterized by chills, fever, headache, stiff neck, and cerebrospinal fluid pleocytosis of 50 to 500 cells per mm^3, which involved a group of 44 U. S. Army personnel in the Philippine Islands, revealed that during convalescence 39 percent of the individuals had high titers of specific neutralizing antibodies. In this outbreak fever lasted 2 to 3 days, and all patients recovered promptly without sequelae. Sporadic EMC virus isolates have been made from adults and children with illnesses diagnosed as paralytic poliomyelitis, the Guillain-Barré syndrome, and severe meningoencephalitis. Myocarditis has not been a feature of EMC virus infection in man. Nothing is known of the pathologic findings in man. The diagnosis of human EMC virus infection depends upon isolation of the virus from blood, cerebrospinal fluid, or stool or the demonstration of a rising titer of specific antibodies during convalescence. Treatment is symptomatic and supportive.

REFERENCES

Encephalomyocarditis viruses

GAJDUSEK DC: Encephalomyocarditis infection in childhood. Pediatrics 16:902, 1955

WARREN J: Encephalomyocarditis viruses, in *Viral and Rickettsial Infections of Man,* 4th ed., eds FL Horsfall Jr, I Tamm, Philadelphia: Lippincott, 1965

Marburg virus disease

MARTIN GA, SIEGERT R (eds): *Marburg Virus Disease,* New York: Springer-Verlag, 1971

Mokola virus disease

FAMILUSI JB: Fatal human infection with Mokola virus. Am J Trop Med Hyg 21:959, 1972

Vesicular stomatitis virus

FIELDS BN, HAWKINS K: Human infection with the virus of vesicular stomatitis during an epizootic. N Engl J Med 277:989, 1967

SUDIA WD et al: Isolation of vesicular stomatitis virus (Indiana strain) and other viruses from mosquitoes in New Mexico, 1965. Am J Epidemiol 86:598, 1967

section 16 | Diseases caused by protozoa

INTRODUCTION

JAMES J. PLORDE

Protozoan diseases such as *malaria, trypanosomiasis, leishmaniasis, amebiasis,* and *toxoplasmosis* remain among the major causes of human sickness and death in the world today. Over 500 million people still live in malarious areas, and it is estimated that 100 million of these are infected at any given time. Of those infected, 1 million die of the disease annually.

In Africa, from the Sahara in the North to the Kalahari Desert in the South, human strains of *Trypanosoma brucei* cause one of the most lethal of all human diseases, *sleeping sickness.* Animal strains of this species limit food supply in the same area through their impact on animal husbandry. In South America, a related organism, *T. cruzi,* infects several million people, leaving many with severe heart and gastrointestinal lesions (*Chagas' disease*).

Leishmaniasis is found in parts of Europe, Asia, Africa, and South and Central America where it may present as a chronic, highly lethal infection of the reticuloendothelial system (kala azar), a mutilating mucocutaneous infection (espundia), or a self-limiting skin ulcer (oriental sore).

Ten percent of the world population, including 2 to 5 percent in the United States, are infected with the intestinal protozoa *Entamoeba histolytica.* Invasive disease resulting in an ulcerative colitis and/or liver abscess is particularly common in Mexico, western South America, South Asia, and West and Southwest Africa.

Toxoplasmosis, giardiasis, and *trichomoniasis* are three cosmopolitan protozoan infections well known to American physicians. The first infects perhaps one-third of the world's population. Although it is usually asymptomatic, congenital toxoplasmosis may result in abortion, stillbirth, prematurity, or severe neurologic defects. Even when there are no obvious signs at birth, chorioretinitis with visual impairment may occur years later. Asymptomatic infection may also result in fatal encephalitis during periods of immunosuppression later in life.

In contrast, giardiasis and trichomoniasis seldom result in severe disability; nevertheless their morbidity can be attested to by millions of otherwise healthy individuals.

The pathogens responsible for these diseases are unicellular and possess a true, or membrane-limited, nucleus. Morphologic differences in the cytoplasmic organelles of locomotion are useful in separating the protozoa pathogenic for human beings into four major groups: *flagellates, ciliates, amebas,* and *sporozoa.* The structures concerned with the motility of the first two groups are self-evident. Amebas move by means of pseudopodia, while the sporozoa generally lack any specific locomotor structures. Nuclear morphology, particularly the distribution pattern of the chromatin and karyosome (nucleolus), is used in distinguishing the species of certain organisms in the above groups.

Characteristically, the flagellates, ciliates, and amebas reproduce by asexual binary fission, while the sporozoa have alternating cycles of asexual (*schizogony*) and sexual (*sporogony*) reproduction. In the process of asexual multiplication the nucleus of the intracellular trophozoite first divides into several portions to form a schizont. Cytoplasmic division then occurs, resulting in the formation of daughter cells, or *merozoites.* These invade new host cells in which they become trophozoites, thus completing the asexual cycle. After one or more such cycles some merozoites initiate the sexual phase of reproduction by differentiating into male and female gametocytes. These mature and effect fertilization; the fertilized zygote, upon encysting, becomes known as an *oocyst. Sporozoites* formed within the oocyst are released, penetrate tissue cells, and begin another asexual cycle as trophozoites. These alternating sexual and asexual cycles may occur within the same (*Toxoplasma* spp., *Isospora* spp.) or different hosts (*Falciparum* spp.).

The mode of transmission of these protozoa depends upon whether they are luminal or tissue parasites. Those which inhabit human gastrointestinal or genitourinary tracts are passed from human to human either directly as in the case of *Trichomonas vaginalis* or indirectly by the ingestion of contaminated food or water (fecal-oral transmission), e.g., *E. histolytica* and *Giardia lamblia.* In the former situation the infecting agent is the vegetative form, or trophozoite; in the latter it is a cyst capable of survival in the external environment for prolonged periods. Blood and tissue parasites, on the other hand, are generally transmitted via an arthropod which functions as both a vector and a second host. In the case of *Falciparum* spp. this alternation of human and arthropod host is associated with the alternation of asexual and sexual generations described above.

These differences in transmission have a profound effect on both the distribution and control of protozoan diseases. Those spread by the fecal-oral route are essentially diseases of poverty and are found throughout the world wherever there is inadequate hygiene and sanitation. Their control depends upon the improvements in these areas which invariably accompany economic development. In contrast, the geographic distribution of the blood and tissue parasites is determined by the ecologic factors, particularly climate, responsible for the persistence of the arthropod vector. Attempts at disease prevention are characteristically directed at the control or elimination of the specific vectors. However, malaria, trypanosomiasis, and leishmaniasis can also be passed from person to person via blood transfusion, and careful screening of donors from endemic areas is important.

Clinically, protozoa exert their effects in a number of ways. In diseases such as malaria, the primary pathogenic mechanism appears to be the invasion and subsequent alteration or destruction of erythrocytes by the parasite. *Entamoeba histolytica* destroys host cells via enzymes or toxins without actual cellular invasion. In still other diseases, clinical manifestations are the result of a host-mounted inflammatory reaction, and in several, immunologic mechanisms are responsible for clinical findings, e.g., nephrotic syndrome in quartan malaria. *Giardia lamblia*, on the other hand, is thought by some to produce malabsorption by simply covering a significant proportion of the microvilli in the small bowel.

By themselves, the clinical manifestations of disease are not always specific enough to ensure prompt diagnosis. Furthermore, general laboratory findings are often of little diagnostic aid. Although eosinophilia has been recognized as an important clue to the diagnosis of parasitic diseases, this phenomenon is characteristic of helminthic, not protozoan, infections. A carefully elicited travel, transfusion, and socioeconomic history often first suggests to the physician the possibility of a protozoan infection.

Reliable serologic tests have recently become available in the United States for many of the protozoan infections including malaria, amebiasis, toxoplasmosis, leishmaniasis, and South American trypanosomiasis. However, the definitive diagnosis usually rests upon the recovery and morphologic identification of the parasite from the genitourinary tract, intestinal contents, tissue, or blood.

Many of the drugs used to treat protozoan infection are either not generally available or have not yet been approved for use in the United States. Fortunately, many of these agents are available through the Parasitic Disease Drug Service of the Center for Disease Control, Atlanta, Georgia. These drugs are listed below.

Antiprotozoal agents available through the Parasitic Disease Drug Service*

Infection	*Therapeutic agent*
Amebiasis (severe forms in which metronidazole has failed)	Dehydroemetine
Chagas' disease (*Trypanosoma cruzi*)	Bayer 2502 (Lampit)
Leishmaniasis	Sodium antimony gluconate (Pentostam)
Malaria	Parenteral chloroquine hydrochloride Parenteral quinine dehydrochloride
Pneumocystosis	Pentamidine isothionate
Sleeping sickness (*Trypanosoma brucei*)	Melarsoprol (Mel B) Pentamidine isothionate Suramin (Antrypol)

* *Parasitic Disease Branch, Bureau of Epidemiology, Center for Disease Control, Atlanta, Ga. 30333. Day telephone: (404) 633-3311, ext. 3496; nights, weekends, and holidays: (404) 633-2176.*

REFERENCES

BROWN HW: *Basic Clinical Parasitology*, 4th ed., New York: Appleton Century Crofts, 1975

FAUST EC, RUSSELL PF: *Clinical Parasitology*, 8th ed., Philadelphia: Lea & Febiger, 1970

MAEGRAITH BG: *Clinical Tropical Medicine*, 5th ed., Oxford: Blackwell Scientific Publications, 1971

WILCOKS C, MANSON-BAHR PEC: *Manson's Tropical Diseases*, 17th ed., Baltimore: Williams & Wilkins, 1972

214
AMEBIASIS

JAMES J. PLORDE

DEFINITION Amebiasis is an infection of the large intestine produced by *Entamoeba histolytica*. It is an asymptomatic carrier state in most individuals, but diseases ranging from chronic, mild diarrhea to fulminant dysentery may occur. Among extraintestinal complications, the commonest is hepatic abscess, which may rupture into peritoneum, pleura, lung, or pericardium.

ETIOLOGY There are seven different species of ameba that naturally parasitize the human mouth and intestine, but of these only *E. histolytica* causes disease. *Entamoeba coli* and *E. hartmanni* are the two species with which it is most likely to be confused in examination of stools.

Entamoeba histolytica exists in two forms: the motile trophozoite and the cyst. The trophozoite is the parasitic form and dwells in the lumen and/or wall of the colon, divides by binary fission, grows best under anaerobic conditions, and requires the presence of either bacteria or tissue substrates to satisfy its nutritional requirements. When diarrhea occurs, the trophozoites are passed unchanged in the liquid stool, where they can be distinguished by their size (10 to 20 μm in diameter), directional motility, sharply demarcated clear ectoplasm with slender finger-like pseudopodia, and finely granular endoplasm. In dysentery, the trophozoites are larger (up to 50 μm in diameter), and often contain ingested erythrocytes. In the absence of diarrhea, the trophozoites usually encyst before leaving the gut. The cysts are highly resistant to environmental changes and are responsible for transmission of disease. Young cysts have a single nucleus, a glycogen vacuole, and sausage-shaped chromatoid bodies. As the cyst matures, it absorbs its cytoplasmic vacuoles and becomes quadrinucleate. The cysts of *E. histolytica* can be distinguished from those of *Entamoeba coli* by the presence of one to four nuclei with small centric karyosomes and fine peripheral chromatin and by their thick chromatoid bodies with round ends.

Entamoeba histolytica had been classified into large and small races depending upon whether they form cysts measuring more or less than 10 μm in diameter. Strains of the small race, however, are not pathogenic for human beings and are now considered as a distinct species, *Entamoeba hartmanni*.

Entamoeba histolytica–like amebas are organisms isolated from humans that are morphologically indistinguishable from true *E. histolytica*. However, unlike *E. histolytica* they are nonpathogenic, grow best at 20°C, and can multiply indefinitely in hypotonic solutions.

Entamoeba histolytica can be cultivated in artificial media, a procedure that is useful in direct diagnosis and in the preparation of purified antigens for serologic testing.

EPIDEMIOLOGY Infection with *E. histolytica* is worldwide. Stool surveys indicate that the prevalence of infection in the United States is between 1 and 5 percent. Rates as high as 50 percent may occur in areas where the level of sanitation is low. Reports of amebic liver abscess suggest that invasive amebiasis is concentrated in comparatively few parts of the world, most notably Mexico, western South America, South Asia, and West and Southwestern Africa. In this country, the incidence of amebiasis has decreased sharply in the past 20 years. Furthermore, an increasing proportion of reported cases are now acquired outside the United States. Cases of dysentery and liver abscess still occur, however, in institutions for the mentally retarded. Although the parasite can sometimes infect rats, cats, dogs, and primates, human beings are the principal host and reservoir. Because trophozoites die rapidly after leaving the intestine, patients with amebic dysentery do not play a major role in transmission of the disease. Asymptomatic cyst passers are the source of new infections. The cysts are usually spread through contaminated food or water. Direct fecal spread may occur in situations where there is massive contamination of the environment. Cases of amebic dysentery are usually sporadic, but epidemics, which are sometimes waterborne, have occurred. Outbreaks of amebiasis are never explosive, as are those produced by pathogenic intestinal bacteria. Symptomatic amebiasis is unusual below the age of ten years in temperate climates, and both intestinal and hepatic lesions predominate in adult males to an extent that is not readily explainable on the basis of different rates of exposure to infection.

PATHOGENESIS AND ANATOMIC CHANGES After ingestion, cysts undergo further nuclear division. In the small intestine, the cyst wall disintegrates, and trophozoites are released. The immature amebas are carried to the large intestine, where they live in the lumen of the gut as commensals feeding on bacteria and superficial mucosal cells. On occasion the amebas may invade the mucosa, causing ulcerations that are sufficiently extensive to produce symptoms. The factors responsible for this are not completely understood, but the state of the host and the virulence of the infecting organism both play roles. Epidemiologic evidence suggests that amebic strains indigenous to temperate climates are usually avirulent. It has also been shown, however, that invasiveness is not a stable strain characteristic. It can either be lost after continued cultivation in vitro or enhanced by rapid animal passage. The virulence of various strains of *E. histolytica* is dependent upon the association with living bacteria. This suggests that an episome-like factor provided by certain strains of bacteria may be required to maintain virulence of *E. histolytica*.

Amebic ulceration of the intestinal wall is characteristic. A small mucosal defect overlies a larger, burrowing area of necrosis in the submucosa and muscularis, producing a bottle-shaped lesion. There is little acute inflammatory response, and in contrast to the picture in bacillary dysentery, the mucosa between ulcers is normal. The sites of involvement in order of frequency are cecum and ascending colon, rectum, sigmoid, appendix, and terminal ileum. In the cecum and sigmoid, chronic infection may lead to the formation of large masses of granulation tissue or *amebomas*. Amebas can enter the portal circulation and lodge in venules; liquefaction necrosis of liver tissue leads to the formation of an abscess cavity. Rarely, embolization results in lung, brain, or splenic abscess.

CLINICAL MANIFESTATIONS **Asymptomatic cyst passer** In the majority of patients with this common form of amebiasis, *E. histolytica* probably lives as a commensal in the bowel lumen. Individuals infected in temperate climates are unlikely to develop significant tissue invasion. However, invasion does occur occasionally, so treatment of cyst passers is warranted.

Symptomatic intestinal amebiasis In some patients there is intermittent diarrhea consisting of one to four foul-smelling loose or watery stools daily. The stools sometimes contain mucus and blood. Loose stools alternate with periods of relative normality and may persist for months or years. Flatulence and abnormal cramping are frequent. The only physical findings are occasional tender hepatomegaly and slight pain when the cecum and ascending colon are palpated. Sigmoidoscopy sometimes reveals typical ulcerations with areas of normal mucosa interspersed. The diagnosis depends upon finding the organism in the feces or in ulcers.

Fulminating attacks of amebic dysentery are less common. Waterborne outbreaks may occur, but fulminating dysentery is more likely to occur spontaneously in debilitated individuals. Attacks may be precipitated by pregnancy or corticosteroids. The onset in half the cases is abrupt with high fever, between 104 and 105°F, severe abdominal cramps, and profuse, bloody diarrhea with tenesmus. There is diffuse abdominal tenderness, often so severe that peritonitis is suspected. Hepatomegaly is very frequent, and sigmoidoscopy almost always demonstrates extensive rectosigmoid ulceration. Trophozoites are numerous in stools and in material obtained directly from the ulcers.

In some cases there may be extensive destruction of the colonic mucosa and submucosa, massive hemorrhage or perforation of the bowel wall, with resultant peritonitis. Repeated severe attacks of intestinal amebiasis can lead to an ulcerative postdysenteric colitis. Amebas can usually not be demonstrated in this condition, but serologic tests are strongly positive. Invasion of the appendix may lead to a clinical picture of *appendicitis*. Penetration of trophozoites through the muscle wall of the bowel may result in the development of large masses of granulation tissue. When the entire circumference of the intestine is involved, there may then be partial obstruction, and a movable, tender, sausage-shaped mass is often palpable. This lesion or ameboma is most frequently seen in the cecum where a palpable mass and radiologic demonstration of a ragged encroachment of the lumen may lead to a mistaken diagnosis of adenocarcinoma.

Hepatic amebiasis The parasites usually reach the liver through the portal vein; rarely, they may traverse the lymphatic vessels. It has been believed for a long time that amebas which lodged in the liver could produce a diffuse hepatitis. Careful postmortem and biopsy studies indicate that the syndrome of tender hepatomegaly, right upper quadrant pain, fever, and leukocytosis in patients with amebic colitis is not a result of amebas in hepatic tissues, is accompanied by nonspecific periportal inflammation, and is rarely, if ever, a prelude to hepatic abscess. It is evident, then, that these manifestations are best regarded as an accompaniment of colitis and do not merit a separate diagnosis of "diffuse amebic hepatitis."

Hepatic abscess may develop insidiously, with fever, sweats, weight loss, and no local signs other than painless or slightly tender hepatomegaly. In other patients, there is abrupt onset, with chills, fever to 105°F, nausea, vomiting, severe upper abdominal pain, and polymorphonuclear leukocytosis. Initially, cholecystitis, perforated ulcer, or acute pancreatitis may be suspected.

Most commonly, the abscess occurs singly and is localized in the posterior portion of the right lobe of the liver, because this lobe receives most of the blood draining the right colon through the "streaming" effect in portal vein flow. This location is responsible for several features that aid in diagnosis. *Point tenderness* in the posterolateral portion of a lower right intercostal space is frequent even in the absence of diffuse liver pain. Most abscesses enlarge upward, producing a bulge in the diaphragmatic dome, obliteration of the costophrenic gutter, small hydrothorax, basilar atelectasis, and pain referred to the right shoulder. Liver function tests may be mildly to moderately disturbed but are of little diagnostic aid. Jaundice is uncommon. Radiologically, unruptured abscesses do not show a fluid level, and calcification of the liver parenchyma is very rare. Isotope liver scan utilizing two, or preferably three, projections is invaluable in confirming both the presence and location of a liver abscess. Ultrasonic scanning will confirm that the lesion is fluid-filled. It has been reported that hepatic tomograms will visualize amebic abscesses following intravenous Hypaque infusion. Serologic tests are positive in over 90 percent of patients.

Needle puncture results in the withdrawal of "pus" which consists of liquefied, necrotic liver, the classic "chocolate syrup" or "anchovy paste" exudate; the pus contains no polymorphonuclear leukocytes (barring secondary bacterial infection) and, usually, no amebas. The parasites are localized in the cyst wall and may be demonstrated at times by a Vim-Silverman needle biopsy of the cyst wall following aspiration of the abscess.

Hepatic abscess complicates asymptomatic infection of the colon more often than symptomatic intestinal disease, another factor making recognition difficult. Trophozoites or cysts are demonstrable in the feces of only about one-third of patients with abscess, and fewer than one-half can recall significant diarrheal illness.

Pleuropulmonary amebiasis The right pleural cavity and lung are involved by direct extension from the liver in 10 to 20 percent of patients with liver abscess. Rarely, amebic lung abscess has resulted from embolization rather than direct extension.

Manifestations are those of massive pleural effusion; aspiration of chocolate fluid is diagnostic, or if the lung parenchyma is involved and perforation into a bronchus occurs, patients expectorate large amounts of the typical exudate, some patients even commenting that the sputum "tastes like liver." Cough, pleural pain, fever, and leukocytosis are the rule, and secondary bacterial infection is frequent.

Other extraintestinal lesions Rupture of liver abscess into the *pericardium* with pericardial tamponade has occurred. These patients are often thought initially to have tuberculous pericarditis. *Peritonitis* is a result of perforation of colonic ulcer or rupture of liver abscess. Painful ulcers of the genitalia, perianal skin, or abdominal wall (draining sinuses), vaginitis, urethritis, and prostatitis are unusual complications resulting from extension of intestinal disease. Metastatic brain abscess is rare, and an etiologic diagnosis is seldom made clinically. Splenic abscess has been reported but is very unusual.

DIAGNOSIS The diagnosis of intestinal amebiasis depends upon *identification of the organism in the stool or tissues.* Formed stools are examined initially in saline and iodine mounts for amebic cysts; concentration methods such as the formalin-ether technique increase the yield two- to threefold. Liquid or semiformed stools should be examined immediately in saline solution for the presence of motile hematophagous trophozoites. If there is any delay in examination of the stool, a portion of the specimen may be refrigerated for a few hours at 4°C or placed in a fixative solution. Polyvinyl alcohol and 10% formalin not only preserve amebas for better identification but permit preparation of permanently stained smears. Careful examination of four to six stool specimens may be required for diagnosis. If possible, the stool should be examined before the administration of antimicrobial, antidiarrheal, or antacid preparations, because all these agents may interfere with the recovery of amebas. Likewise, enemas and radiographic procedures utilizing barium sulfate are best postponed until after a thorough search for *E. histolytica* has been made.

Sigmoidoscopy is of value in symptomatic cases. The mucosal lesions should be aspirated and the material examined for trophozoites. Biopsy material obtained from such lesions and stained with periodic acid–Schiff solution also will frequently reveal trophozoites.

The diagnosis of extraintestinal amebiasis is difficult. The parasite usually cannot be recovered from stool or tissue. Cultivation of amebas from feces or pus is possible but is not practical in most laboratories. The most important diagnostic procedure in suspected liver abscess is a *therapeutic trial of antiamebic drugs*. The response is often dramatic within 3 days. In the event that demonstrating parasites is difficult, the therapeutic trial should be instituted without hesitation.

Serologic tests employing purified antigens are positive in nearly all patients with proved amebic liver abscess and in a great majority of those with acute amebic dysentery. However, the persistence of significant anitbody titers for months to years after complete cure makes serology, particularly in endemic areas, of more value in excluding the diagnosis than in confirming it. The tests are generally negative in asymptomatic cyst passers, suggesting that tissue invasion is required for antibody production. Of the available tests, the indirect hemagglutination appears to be the most sensitive. A number of rapid tests such as latex agglutination and cellulose acetate diffusion have made serologic testing available to most laboratories. Intradermal tests have been shown to be helpful in epidemiologic surveys, but their value in the diagnosis of amebiasis remains to be determined.

TREATMENT Treatment should be aimed at relief of symptoms, replacement of fluid, electrolyte, and blood losses, and eradication of the organism. Amebas may be found in the lumen of the bowel, in the intestinal wall, or extraintestinally. Most amebicides are not effective at all sites or when used alone, and a combination of drugs is often necessary to achieve cure. The available drugs based on their site of action fall into several different categories, as described below.

Luminal amebicides These oral agents act by direct contact with trophozoites dwelling in the bowel lumen but are ineffective against amebas in tissue. Of the large number of available drugs, diloxanide furoate (0.5 g three times daily for 10 days) is one of the most effective and well tolerated but is not presently available in the United States.

Tetracycline, when given in dosage of 1 to 2 g daily for 5 days, is effective against amebas residing in the intestinal wall as well as in the lumen. It probably has a direct amebicidal action as well as acting indirectly by altering the bacterial flora of the intestine.

Tissue amebicides *Chloroquine diphosphate* (Aralen) is a systemic amebicide which is useful in hepatic disease because of its high concentration in the liver. It has little activity elsewhere. The dose is 0.6 g base initially, 0.3 g base 6 h later, and then 0.3 g base twice daily for 14 to 28 days.

Emetine is an alkaloid derivative of ipecac. When given intramuscularly (1 mg per kg with a maximum of 65 mg daily for 10 days), it is highly effective in destroying trophozoites in tissue including those in the wall of the intestine. It is ineffective against luminal amebas. Emetine is relatively toxic and may produce vomiting, diarrhea, abdominal cramping, weakness, muscle pain, tachycardia, hypotension, precordial pain, and electrocardiographic abnormalities. The common ECG changes include T-wave inversion and prolongation of the Q-Tc interval. Rarely arrhythmias and prolongation of the QRS complex are seen. A synthetic derivative, dehydroemetine, is thought to be less toxic by virtue of its more rapid excretion and lower concentration in myocardial tissue. The drug is given intramuscularly in the dose of 1.25 mg per kg (maximum 90 mg) daily for 10 days. It is not free of toxicity, however, and patients treated with either drug should be at bed rest with ECG monitoring. Neither drug should be used in patients with renal, cardiac, or muscle disease, during pregnancy, or in children unless other drugs fail.

Metronidazole (Flagyl) is unique because it is both safe and effective against trophozoites at all sites, intestinally and extraintestinally. It is the drug of choice in most forms of amebiasis. For intestinal amebiasis it is given in dosage of 750 mg three times daily for 5 to 10 days. Smaller doses are effective in hepatic amebiasis. Metronidazole has an Antabuse-like action, and alcohol should be avoided during its administration. The recent evidence that this drug is carcinogenic and possibly teratogenic in animals when given in large doses is disturbing. The potential risk in human beings must be weighed against the severity of the disease, particularly in pregnant women.

Management A course of tetracycline or diloxanide furoate should be given in asymptomatic or mildly symptomatic patients. Stools should be examined monthly for 6 months to detect relapse. If it occurs, retreatment should consist of tetracycline. Chloroquine can be added for its potentiating effect on tetracycline as well as its ability to eradicate subclinical hepatic infection. Metronidazole appears to be somewhat less effective than the above programs in asymptomatic patients.

Treatment of acute dysentery involves control of symptoms as well as eradication of the organism. A number of regimens can be used:

For both mild and moderate dysentery, metronidazole given in a dose of 750 mg three times daily for 5 to 10 days is the simplest and least toxic regimen. This drug will cure about 90 percent of patients. The addition of tetracycline will raise the cure rate close to 100 percent. Of some concern is the occurrence of amebic liver abscess in a few patients treated for dysentery with metronidazole. It is probable that this results from failure of metronidazole to eliminate luminal organisms in a small proportion of cases. For this reason, the routine addition of tetracycline seems indicated.

In severe dysentery, emetine or dehydroemetine should be added to the above regimen. These intramuscular agents rapidly control the acute attack, but because of their toxicity administration should be discontinued as soon as symptoms abate. Tetracycline should be given in the dosage of 2 g daily.

If hepatic abscess is suspected, chloroquine is the drug of choice. It is effective, nontoxic, and produces symptomatic relief in 48 to 72 h. Even larger abscesses subside, but relapse is relatively frequent. If aspiration or a dramatic response to chloroquine proves that a hepatic abscess is of amebic origin, the drug should be continued for 3 or 4 weeks. In addition, emetine or dehydroemetine should be given for 10 days to prevent relapse. Alternatively, metronidazole may be administered. In dosage of 750 mg three times daily for 5 days, it is less toxic and probably just as effective as the chloroquine-emetine combination. Although lower doses have been shown to be effective in hepatic amebiasis, they are not consistently effective in eradicating intestinal trophozoites that might lead to relapse. For this reason, the larger dose is recommended, and the drug should probably be combined with a luminal amebicide. Luminal amebicides must always be given with the chloroquine-emetine regimen. Treatment failures have been reported for both emetine-chloroquine and metronidazole. They appear to be unrelated to the organism's resistance.

A diagnostic trial of metronidazole in patients with suspected amebic liver abscess may lead to serious error, because this drug readily inhibits anaerobic bacteria, common causes of pyogenic liver abscess.

Drainage of an amebic abscess usually is not necessary and should be performed only if there is localized swelling over the liver, marked elevation of the diaphragm, severe localized liver tenderness, and failure to respond to systemic amebicides. Adequate drainage can usually be accomplished by needle alone, and surgical drainage is rarely necessary. The greatest hazard in needling an abscess is secondary bacterial infection.

Amebiasis in locations other than the intestine and liver should be treated with emetine, dehydroemetine, or metronidazole and a luminal amebicide.

PROGNOSIS Intestinal amebiasis usually responds readily and completely to appropriate drugs. Parasitologic relapses sometimes occur, and posttreatment stools should be checked monthly for 6 months. Repeated relapses, however, are usually a manifestation of reinfection, complicating illness, inadequate therapy, or incorrect diagnosis. The fatality rate is less than 5 percent.

Hepatic and pulmonary amebiasis are still accompanied by an appreciable mortality, but no reliable figures are available.

PREVENTION For the individual, avoidance of contaminated food and water, scalding of vegetables, and the use of iodine-releasing tablets in drinking water (chlorine, in the form of halazone, is ineffective) are important measures. Globaline tablets, containing tetraglycine hydroperiodide, are convenient and effective.

Improvements in general sanitation and the detection of cyst passers and their removal from food-handling duties are general measures in prophylaxis, but such segregation of carriers is rarely practiced. Community control of amebic disease by periodic mass treatment with metronidazole and diloxanide furoate has been successful in some areas. At the present time, however, personal chemoprophylaxis for travelers is not recommended.

PRIMARY AMEBIC MENINGOENCEPHALITIS

Primary amebic meningoencephalitis is caused by free-living amebas, usually of the genus *Naegleria*. It most often affects children and young adults, appears to be acquired by swimming in fresh warm water, and is almost invariably fatal.

Free-living amebas are ubiquitous in nature where they are commonly found in soil and water. Although generally considered harmless, some varieties are clearly pathogenic for the central nervous system of mammals. Early reports incriminating *Hartmanella* and *Acanthamoeba* in human meningoencephalitis were based on the morphologic appearance of the trophozoites in histologic preparations. In those instances where the responsible organism has been isolated and cultured, however, it has, with few exceptions, been identified as an amoeboflagellate and has been assigned the name *Naegleria fowleri*.

Over 60 cases have been reported from different parts of the world including Australia, Czechoslovakia, Great Britain, New Zealand, and the United States. Most of the cases recognized in this country have occurred in the Southeastern states, particularly Florida, Georgia, and Virginia. Characteristically the patients have fallen ill during the summer months approximately 1 week after swimming in fresh or brackish water. The 16 Czechoslovakian cases followed swimming in an indoor pool with chlorinated water maintained at 24°C, and 5 cases have been acquired apparently after bathing in hot mineral water. Histologic evidence suggests that the amebas reach the central nervous system directly via the nasal mucosa at the level of the cribriform plate. Clinically, the illness is rapid in onset, brief in duration, and inexorable in course. The initial symptom is a severe, persistent, frontal headache followed by nausea, vomiting, fever, and nuchal rigidity. Unusual tastes or smells may be noted. Later, drowsiness, confusion, convulsions, and coma appear. Focal neurologic findings may occur late in the course of the illness. Whether the few reports of the more benign meningoencephalitis occurring in patients with underlying disease represents *Acanthamoeba* rather than *Naegleria* infections remains uncertain.

A careful examination of the cerebrospinal fluid is the single most helpful diagnostic procedure. The fluid is usually bloody or sanguinopurulent and demonstrates an intense neutrophilic response. The protein is elevated and the glucose diminished. No organisms are demonstrated on Gram's stain or routine culture. Early examination of a wet preparation of unspun spinal fluid will usually reveal viable trophozoites. They are 10 to 20 μm in diameter, possess a granular cytoplasm, a distinct ectoplasm, and bulbous pseudopodia. If the specimen is allowed to cool, the trophozoites may become immobile and more difficult to recognize. Although the amebas may be easily grown on ordinary culture media which have been seeded with coliform bacteria, this is not helpful in clinical management, so rapidly progressive is the disease. Treatment with standard antiprotozoal agents seems completely ineffective. *Naegleria*, however, is highly sensitive to amphotericin B in vitro, and to date the only patient who has survived a *Naegleria* infection was diagnosed early and treated with this agent. Intracisternal, as well as intravenous, administration of amphotericin is probably essential to rapidly obtain effective levels in the cerebrospinal fluid. The intraventricular dose is 0.5 to 1 mg for the first few days. The intravenous dose is similar to that for cryptococcal meningitis (Chap. 170).

If the source of the infection can be determined, further cases might be prevented by closing the area to bathing.

REFERENCES

Amebiasis

BARBOUR GL, JUMPER K JR: A clinical comparison of amebic and pyogenic abscess of the liver in sixty-six patients. Am J Med 53:323, 1972

COHEN HG, REYNOLDS TB: Comparison of metronidazole and chloroquine for the treatment of amebic liver abscess. Gastroenterology 69:35, 1975

ELSDON-DEW R: The epidemiology of amebiasis. Adv Parasitol 6:1, 1968

GRIFFIN FH, JR: Failure of metronidazole to cure hepatic amebic abscess. N Engl J Med 288:1397, 1973

HEALY GR: Laboratory diagnosis of amebiasis. Bull NY Acad Med 47:478, 1971

JUMPER K JR et al: Serologic diagnosis of amebiasis. Am J Trop Med Hyg 21:157, 1972

MOST H: Drug therapy: Common parasite infections of man. N Engl J Med 287:698, 1972

NEAL RA: Pathogenesis of amebiasis. Bull NY Acad Med 47:462, 1971

POWELL SJ et al: Metronidazole combined with diloxanide furoate in amebic liver abscess. Ann Trop Med Parasitol 67:367, 1973

SODEMAN WA JR, DOWDA MC: Rapid serologic methods for the demonstration of *Entamoeba histolytica* activity. Gastroenterology 65:604, 1973
WHO EXPERT COMMITTEE: Amebiasis, WHO Tech Rep Ser 421, Geneva, 1969
WILMOT AJ: *Clinical Amebiasis*, Philadelphia: Davis, 1962

Primary amebic meningoencephalitis
CARTER RF: Primary amoebic meningoencephalitis: An appraisal of present knowledge. Trans R Soc Trop Med Hyg 67:193, 1972
DUMA RJ et al: Primary amebic meningoencephalitis caused by *Naegleria*. Ann Intern Med 74:861, 1971
GILBERTSON CG et al: Pathogenic *Naegleria* sp.: Study of a strain isolated from human cerebrospinal fluid. J Protozool 15:353, 1968
ROBERT VB, RORKE LB: Primary amebic encephalitis, probably from *Acanthamoeba*. Ann Intern Med 79:174, 1973

215
MALARIA

JAMES J. PLORDE

DEFINITION Malaria is a protozoan disease transmitted to humans by the bite of *Anopheles* mosquitoes. It remains the major infectious disease problem in the world. The increased import of malaria into the United States by travelers and military personnel in recent years has caused a resurgence of interest in this disease. Malaria is characterized by *rigors, fever, splenomegaly, anemia,* and *a chronic relapsing course.*

ETIOLOGY *The causative organisms are protozoa of the genus Plasmodium.* The four species known to infect human beings do not produce disease in lower animals, although many species affecting animals and birds are known. *Plasmodium vivax* causes tertian malaria; *P. malariae* causes quartan malaria; *P. falciparum* causes malignant tertian malaria; *P. ovale* causes ovale tertian malaria, a relatively rare and mild illness largely confined to Africa.

The human being is the intermediate and the mosquito the definitive host. In humans, after a stage of exoerythrocytic development in the liver, the parasites invade circulating erythrocytes where they reproduce asexually. They first appear in the red cells as ring-shaped trophozoites which later enlarge and assume an irregular or ameboid shape. Following mitotic division of the nucleus, the organism is known as a *schizont.* After several divisions, daughter cells (*merozoites*) fill the corpuscle, which ruptures and releases them (*sporulation*) to parasitize additional erythrocytes. With repetition of this cycle, some of the red cells become filled with *sexual forms* (*gametocytes*); these do not induce cell lysis and are unable to undergo further development unless ingested by an appropriate mosquito during a blood meal. In the stomach of the mosquito fertilization occurs, and the resulting *ookinete* encysts on the outer surface of the stomach and releases myriads of *sporozoites.* These migrate to the salivary glands and, if inoculated into a human subject, lead to repetition of asexual multiplication.

The asexual cycle in the erythrocyte requires 36 to 48 h for *P. falciparum*, 48 h for *P. vivax* and *P. ovale*, and 72 h for *P. malariae*. The periodicity of febrile paroxysms in

infections by the different species coincides with the cyclic discharge of merozoites. The incubation period between the bite of an infected mosquito and onset of symptoms is 10 to 14 days in vivax and falciparum malaria and 18 days to 6 weeks in quartan infections. The incubation period may be prolonged for weeks or months with certain strains of *P. vivax* and in persons who have taken antimalarial suppressants. Occasionally the infection may remain asymptomatic. There is good evidence of the existence of several strains of each species of human malarial *Plasmodium*, and greater virulence of some strains is suggested by the consistent severity of clinical illness which they produce.

EPIDEMIOLOGY Malaria survives only in areas of South and Central America, Africa, and Asia where the mosquito and the infected human populations remain above a *critical density* for each other (Fig. 215-1). These two critical densities are interdependent, but either may fluctuate in a given area. Control measures are directed toward reducing both populations to levels that are too low for the infection to survive. Important procedures include drainage or filling of breeding areas, use of residual insecticide sprays (this has largely replaced the use of oil or other antilarval measures), screening, use of skin repellents, effective treatment of cases, and large-scale suppressive drug programs in some human populations.

An active international cooperative program aimed at the eradication of malaria has resulted in a significant decline in the incidence of the disease since 1945. In over three-quarters of the original malarial areas of the world, the disease has been eradicated or active eradication programs have been instituted. The presence of mobile populations, outdoor biting mosquitoes, and high levels of disease transmission make successful eradication in the remaining areas less certain. Furthermore, the emergence of insecticide-resistant mosquitoes and drug-resistant parasites as well as a variety of administrative and socioeconomic problems has produced serious setbacks to several previously successful eradication programs. The demonstration of naturally occurring simian malaria in humans has raised the question of an animal reservoir of the disease. Although this may not prove to be a major problem, the global eradication of malaria remains today a distant goal. In areas of the world such as Africa where eradication is presently impractical, limited control programs utilizing residual insecticides plus chemoprophylaxis for pregnant women and small children are recommended.

Endemic malaria did not disappear from the United States until the 1950s. Imported cases and occasional outbreaks of malaria acquired by mosquito transmission from imported infections (*introduced malaria*) continued to occur, but until 1966 the total never exceeded 200 cases a year. This number rapidly increased with the return of infected military personnel from Southeast Asia, reaching a peak of over 4,000 in 1970. Associated with this wave of imported malaria was a smaller increase in the number of infections induced by blood transfusion and intravenous heroin use. Fortunately this epidemic has now waned, but the continued increase in international travel will ensure the presence of this disease in the United States until malaria is eradicated on a worldwide basis.

PATHOGENESIS AND PATHOLOGY The invasion, alteration, and destruction of red cells by malaria parasites, systemic and local circulatory changes, and immune phenomena are probably all important in the pathophysiology of malaria. Malaria species differ significantly in their ability to invade red cells. *Plasmodium vivax* and *P. ovale* attack only immature erythrocytes; *P. malariae*, only senescent ones. During infection with these species, therefore, no more than 1 or 2 percent of cells are involved at any one time. *Plasmodium falciparum* invades red cells regardless of age and may cause extremely high levels of parasitemia. Only the presence of certain abnormal hemoglobins, notably S, is capable of limiting parasitemia produced by the species. The same protective effect may be exerted in hemoglobin C, D, E thalassemia, and glucose 6-phosphate (G-6-PD) deficiency, since these abnormalities are found more commonly in malarious areas.

Once parasitized, the cells may be destroyed at the time of sporulation or in the presence of specific opsonizing antibody phagocytosed in the liver or spleen. In the spleen the parasites are also removed from some cells, and the intact erythrocytes are returned into the circulation. However, anemia usually develops and, in the case of falciparum malaria, may be severe. This species also induces physical changes in parasitized cells resulting in intravascular agglutination and sludging.

Although paroxysms of fever coincide with sporulation and the destruction of red cells, the cause of the fever remains obscure and may be related to release of an endogenous pyrogen from injured cells.

The circulatory changes in malaria are characterized by vasoconstriction during the "cold" stage followed by vasodilation during the "hot" stage. In falciparum malaria vasodilation in the skin is accompanied by hypotension, decreased central venous pressure, increased radioiodinated serum albumin space, and increased excretion of aldosterone, suggesting a decrease in effective circulating blood volume due to enhanced vascular permeability and/or capacitance. On the other hand, there may be localized vasospasm, increased capillary permeability with a resulting increase in blood viscosity, obstruction of capillaries with agglutinated red cells, and, occasionally, intravascular coagulation which may compromise perfusion to vital organs such as the kidney, brain, liver, and lung.

Normal as well as parasitized red cells are destroyed in malaria. The explanation for this phenomenon is unknown, although immunologic mechanisms including autoantibody production and adherence of antigen-antibody complexes to uninfected red cells have been suggested. The destruction is most profound in blackwater fever where there is massive intravascular hemolysis. More commonly, however, the red cells are sequestered and destroyed in the reticuloendothelial system of the liver and spleen. Thrombocytopenia is related to splenic pooling and shortened platelet life span. Both direct parasitic invasion and immune mechanisms may be operative in platelet destruction. Host γ- and β-1C-globulin deposits have been noted along

FIGURE 215-1
Areas of risk for malaria transmission as of December 1974. (WHO Weekly Epidemiologic Record No. 45, *1975)*

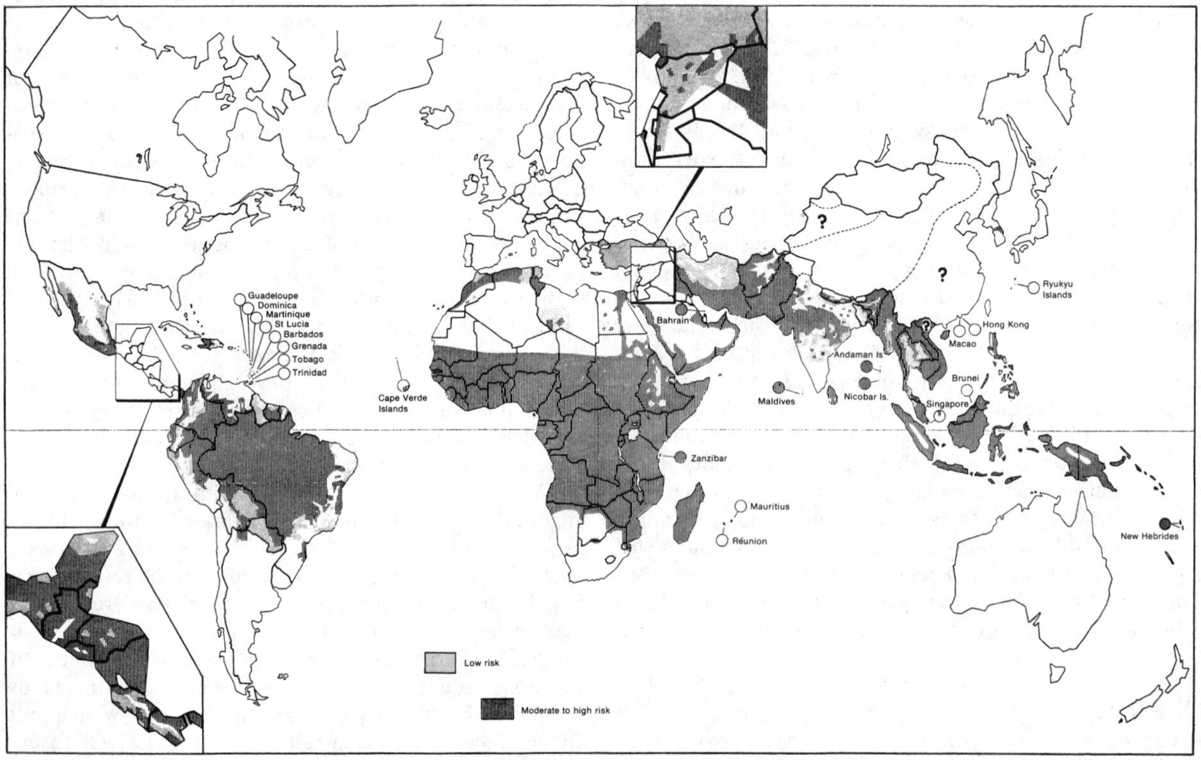

the glomerular capillary basement membrane of patients with the acute transient glomerulonephritis of falciparum malaria and the progressive nephrosis of chronic quartan malaria, establishing these as immune-complex nephropathies.

Protective immunity in malaria is mediated by species-specific IgG and IgM antibodies which appear early in malaria infection in response to the erythrocytic phase of parasitemia. These antibodies have an antiplasmodial effect, but it is uncertain whether they act simply as opsonizing antibodies or are directly lethal as well. The relative rarity of malaria in young infants has been attributed to transplacental passage of IgG antibodies. While immunity in malaria has been thought to be strain-specific, different strains appear to share common antigens. Furthermore, there appear to be antigenic changes in the parasites during chronic simian malaria which may provide an explanation for the relapsing course of malarial infection. The role of T cell–mediated immunity is unknown.

Blacks seem to be peculiarly resistant to *P. vivax* infection; the mechanism for this is unknown.

MANIFESTATIONS General There is some variation in malaria produced by the different plasmodia, but in all, chills, fever, headache, muscle pains, splenomegaly, and anemia are common. Herpes labialis is frequent and usually appears after the infection is well established. Hepatomegaly, mild icterus, and edema are often observed, especially in falciparum infections. Urticaria is common in patients with chronic malaria.

The hallmark of the disease is the malarial *paroxysm*, which recurs regularly in all but falciparum infections. The typical paroxysm begins with a rigor that lasts 20 to 60 min—the "cold stage"—followed by a "hot stage" of 3 to 8 h with temperature of 104 to 107°F. The "wet stage" consists of defervescence with profuse diaphoresis and leaves the patient exhausted.

First attacks are often severe, but repeated episodes become milder, although debilitation may be progressive. In untreated cases, the attacks may persist for weeks. The paroxysms eventually become more irregular and less frequent and finally cease, corresponding with the disappearance of parasites from the blood and marking the end of the primary attack. Relapses occur when exoerythrocytic parasites persisting in the liver reinvade the bloodstream.

Tertian malaria (*P. vivax* or *P. ovale*) This infection is rarely fatal, although relapses are common, and it is the most difficult to cure. A prodrome of myalgia, headache, chilliness, and low-grade fever for 48 to 72 h heralds the onset of the acute illness. Initially, the fever may be irregular because the maturation cycle of the parasite is not synchronized. Synchronization usually occurs toward the end of the first week, and typical paroxysms then occur on alternate days. The spleen becomes palpable at the end of the second week. Infections with *P. ovale* tend to be milder, and primary attacks shorter than those caused by *P. vivax*.

Quartan malaria (*P. malariae*) Paroxysms occur every third day and tend to be regular. The disease is usually more disabling than tertian but responds well to treatment. Edema, albuminuria, and hematuria (*not* hemoglobinuria) a clinical state similar to acute hemorrhagic nephritis, occasionally appear during the course. This complication should not be confused with *blackwater fever*. Chronic *P. malariae* infection may be associated with a clinically and histologically unique nephrosis.

Falciparum malaria (*P. falciparum*) Because of an asynchronous cycle of multiplication, onset may be insidious and fever continuous, remittent, or irregular. Typical paroxysms occur in a minority of patients. Splenomegaly occurs rapidly, and mental confusion, postural hypotension, edema, and gastrointestinal symptoms are common. If the acute attack is treated rapidly, the disease is usually mild and recovery uneventful. If left untreated, anemia becomes severe, and the decreased effective circulating blood volume results in capillary blockage that can give rise to serious complications. This feature of *P. falciparum* infections accounts for the protean manifestations of this form of malaria, and the high morbidity and mortality associated with it. Depending upon the organ system involved, several so-called *pernicious syndromes* are seen. *Cerebral malaria* can lead to hemiplegia, convulsions, delirium, hyperpyrexia, coma, and rapid death. When the *pulmonary* circulation is involved, there may be cough and blood-streaked sputum, leading to confusion with many other diseases of the lung. Severe pulmonary insufficiency closely resembling the "shock lung" syndrome frequently accompanies cerebral malaria. The splanchnic capillaries can be obstructed, with consequent vomiting, abdominal pain, diarrhea, or melena. Such patients are sometimes thought to have bacillary dysentery or cholera. Fever in these disorders may be low or absent. Indeed, in patients with predominantly gastrointestinal manifestations, there are usually cold, clammy skin, hypotension, profound weakness, and repeated syncopal attacks, so-called *algid malaria*. Tender hepatomegaly, with or without jaundice, and acute renal failure are common. The pernicious syndromes should be anticipated if more than 5 percent of red cells are parasitized.

Blackwater fever This is a disorder that occurs in association with malaria, particularly and perhaps only with *P. falciparum* infections. The usual attack begins with a rigor and fever followed by massive intravascular hemolysis, icterus, hemoglobinuria, collapse, and often acute renal failure and uremia. The pathologic findings in the kidney are necrosis of tubules and occasionally hemoglobin casts. The mortality is 20 to 30 percent, and survivors are very likely to experience hemolytic episodes with subsequent malarial infections.

Although blackwater fever is often classified as one of the "pernicious" complications of falciparum malaria, its cause is obscure. In many patients, parasitemia is absent at the time hemolysis occurs. Because blackwater fever has usually occurred in patients with chronic falciparum infections who were treated with quinine, it was suggested that the hemolysis results from an autoimmune reaction to the red cells that have been altered by the drug, parasite, or both. However, blackwater fever can occur in patients not given drugs. The institution of an appropriate regimen for acute renal failure (Chap. 272) will reduce the fatality rate considerably.

Complications In addition to the several complications already mentioned, others deserve comment. Rupture of the spleen is relatively rare, but malaria is by far the commonest cause of spontaneous rupture and predisposes to traumatic rupture of this organ.

Chronic malaria or repeated infection in an endemic area leads to anemia, debility, and cachexia. These manifestations are particularly severe in children under the age of three and in pregnant women. Secondary bacterial infection is often the immediate cause of death. Bacillary dysentery, cholera, and pyogenic pneumonia are common. Tuberculous foci often extend in malarial patients, and miliary tuberculosis is occasionally observed.

Patients living in endemic malarious areas commonly present with chronic hepatosplenomegaly of unknown cause. In some of these, liver biopsies reveal sinusoidal lymphomatosis, and serologic tests for malaria are positive. Long-term antimalarial therapy leads to a decrease in spleen size and a disappearance of hepatic sinusoidal lymphocytosis. It has been suggested that this syndrome represents an abnormal immune response to malaria. The epidemiologic evidence implicating malaria as a contributory factor in the etiology of Burkitt's lymphoma has increased. It has been suggested that continuous stimulation of the lymphoid system in chronic malaria makes it more susceptible to neoplastic transformation in the presence of EB virus.

LABORATORY FINDINGS The blood leukocyte count is low or normal. The platelet count is often reduced, especially in falciparum malaria. The erythrocyte sedimentation rate is elevated. Plasmodia are demonstrable in smears of peripheral blood from the vast majority of patients with symptomatic malaria. When the disease is suspected, appropriately stained blood films should be examined diligently. For the inexperienced examiner, a thin smear of fingertip blood on a clean glass slide should be stained with Wright's or Giemsa's stain. Parasitized erythrocytes are most frequent at the edges of a smear; extracellular parasites are not found. Thick smears should be thoroughly dried and stained with diluted Giemsa's or Field stain. This method has the advantage of concentrating the parasites, but artifacts are numerous, and correct interpretations of these preparations require much experience.

The morphology of the four species of plasmodia that infect humans is specific enough to allow identification in blood smears. The parasitized red cells in *P. vivax* infections are enlarged and pale and may contain diffuse bright red dots (Schaffner's dots), and the parasite presents in a wide variety of shapes and sizes; in *P. ovale* infections, the red cells containing parasites are oval but otherwise resemble those in *P. vivax*; in *P. malariae* the red cells are of normal size and do not contain dots. The parasites often present in "band" forms, and the merozoites are arranged in a rosette around central pigment; in *P. falciparum* infections the rings are very small, may contain two rather than one chromatin dot, and often are found lying flat against the margin of the cell. Only the ring stages of the asexual forms are found in the peripheral smear, and there may be more than one ring in a single red cell. The gametocytes are distinctively large and banana-shaped.

There is no advantage of blood over material obtained by splenic or sternal puncture. The administration of epinephrine with the idea of dislodging parasites by producing contraction of the spleen has been advocated, but results are irregular. Serologic tests are used primarily for epidemiologic rather than diagnostic purposes but are also helpful in speciation of the infecting organism and in detection of occult malaria in the bloodstream. The indirect immunofluorescent test seems to be the most sensitive and specific.

DIAGNOSIS The most important diagnostic test is the search for parasites in peripheral blood. Because the intensity of parasitemia varies greatly from hour to hour, particularly in *P. falciparum* infections, blood smears should be examined for 2 or 3 days before the diagnosis is abandoned. History of residence in an endemic area, previous attacks of malaria, typical malarial paroxysms, or some artificial exposure (blood transfusion, narcotic injections in an addict) should suggest the disease. Splenomegaly is an almost invariable finding during the second week of illness. Leukocytosis is *not* a feature of malaria.

While final cure of malaria may be difficult, particularly in *P. vivax* infections, almost all cases will respond symptomatically to quinine or one of the newer antimalarial drugs, and failure of response to a therapeutic trial argues strongly against the diagnosis.

TREATMENT The use of appropriate chemotherapy can suppress symptoms in individuals exposed in endemic areas or cure malarial infection completely. However, the emergence of drug-resistant falciparum malaria in Southeast Asia, including Burma, Indonesia, and the Philippines, in South America, and in adjacent areas of Central America necessitates the use of drug combinations in the treatment of this infection.

Treatment of acute attack Treatment of an acute attack can be accomplished with chloroquine for all types of malaria except drug-resistant falciparum infection. Administration of 0.6 g chloroquine base (four tablets) followed by 0.3 g 6 h later and then 0.3 g daily for 2 days usually produces complete subsidence of symptoms and destruction of the erythrocytic forms of the parasite. If vomiting is present, chloroquine hydrochloride should be given intramuscularly in dosage of 0.2 to 0.3 g base every 6 h (maximum 900 mg per day). Oral therapy should be resumed as soon as possible.

If patients have contracted malaria in an area known to harbor drug-resistant *P. falciparum*, they should be treated with a combination of quinine, pyrimethamine, and one of the sulfonamides or sulfones. *Quinine sulfate*, 0.6 g orally three times a day, should be given for 14 days. If nausea and vomiting preclude oral therapy, quinine dihydrochloride diluted in saline solution or glucose can be given very slowly intravenously. The dose may be repeated every 6 h, but oral therapy should be instituted as soon as possible. In the presence of renal failure, the dose of quinine should be limited to 0.6 g a day. An overdose of quinine produces cinchonism of which tinnitus is an early manifestation. The drug may also cause mild hemolysis, allergic purpura, and drug fever. Pyrimethamine should be given orally in dosage of 25 mg two times daily for 3 days. This is an antifolate agent and may cause megaloblastic anemia. Sulfisoxazole or sulfadiazine, 2.0 g initially and then 0.5 g every 6 h for 5 days, should be given concurrently with the other two drugs. A variety of other combinations of antifolate agents with sulfonamides or sulfones have also been used alone or with quinine to good effect. The combination of tetracycline (1.0 g per day for 10 days) or clindamycin (450 mg every 6 h for 3 days) plus quinine has been suggested for the treatment of drug-resistant malaria.

Patients should be followed for 1 month to detect recrudescence of the infection, and if there is evidence of recurrence, retreatment with pyrimethamine and a sulfonamide should be instituted.

Radical cure *Plasmodium vivax, P. ovale*, and *P. malariae* all persist in the liver in the exoerythrocytic stage and in this form are not affected by drugs used in the treatment of the acute attack. Unless destroyed, they will eventually reinvade the bloodstream. Primaquine base, 15 mg by mouth daily for 14 days, will effect a radical cure in most cases. If relapse occurs after primaquine therapy, a second course of the drug at twice the dosage should be given. Alternatively, 45 mg primaquine base can be given in combination with 300 mg chloroquine once weekly for 8 weeks. Primaquine may cause hemolysis in patients with G-6-PD deficiency, but in the dosage recommended this is rare and usually mild.

Treatment of complications This includes careful attention to fluid and electrolyte balance, prevention of fluid overload in patients with oliguria, and early diagnosis and treatment of renal failure. In severe hemolysis large doses of steroids may be helpful. Transfusions should be given in severe hemolysis, care being taken to match the donor's cells and plasma with those of the recipient. Intravenous low-molecular-weight dextran may be helpful in increasing capillary blood flow in cerebral malaria. Dexamethasone is used in management of cerebral edema. The value of heparin in this syndrome, even when evidence suggestive of intravascular coagulation is present, remains controversial.

Suppressive therapy Although it is not possible to prevent infection with chemotherapeutic agents, it is possible to suppress symptoms while the patient is residing in an endemic area by the administration of chloroquine base in dosage of 300 mg weekly (2 tablets Aralen). If the medication is continued for 6 weeks after the patient has left the area, sensitive strains of *P. falciparum* will be eradicated. *Plasmodium ovale, P. malariae*, and *P. vivax* will produce clinical manifestations some weeks or months after chloroquine is discontinued because of their persistence outside red cells. This can be circumvented by administration of primaquine after chloroquine is discontinued. Chloroquine is not effective in suppressing drug-resistant *P. falciparum*. In areas of the world where this is a problem pyrimethamine, 25 mg, plus sulfadoxine, 500 mg, can be taken orally once weekly. These drugs are available in combination form in most endemic areas. Leukopenia occurs in approximately 10 percent of patients using this regimen.

REFERENCES

BROWN HW: *Basic Clinical Pathology*, 4th ed., New York: Appleton Century Crofts, 1975

BRUCE-CHAWATT LJ: Transfusion malaria. Bull WHO 50:337, 1974

CAHILL KM (ed): Symposium on malaria. Bull NY Acad Med 45:997, 1969

HEINEMAN HS: The clinical syndrome of malaria in the United States. Arch Intern Med 129:607, 1972

HENDRICKSE RG et al: Quartan malarial nephrotic syndrome. Lancet 1:1143, 1972

KAGAN IG: Malaria: Seroepidemiology and serologic diagnosis. Exp Parasitol 31:126, 1972

MCGREGOR IA: Immunology of malarial infection and its possible consequences. Br Med Bull 28:22, 1972

NEVA FA: Malaria: Recent progress and problems. N Engl J Med 277:1241, 1967

PETERS W: Advances in malariology relating to control and eradication. Br Med Bull 28:28, 1972

WILSON M et al: Comparison of the complement fixation, indirect immunofluorescence and indirect hemagglutination tests for malaria. Am J Trop Med Hyg 24:755, 1975

216
LEISHMANIASIS

JAMES J. PLORDE

DEFINITION Leishmaniasis designates a human disorder produced by flagellated tissue protozoa of the genus *Leishmania*. It is transmitted from animal to human being or sometimes from human to human by the bite of sandflies (*Phlebotomus*). The infection may be either visceral or cutaneous. The former, or kala azar, is characterized by chronic recurrent fever, splenomegaly, pancytopenia, weight loss, and high mortality. Cutaneous leishmaniasis may present as single or multiple chronic skin ulcers, destructive mucocutaneous lesions, or a disseminated infection resembling leprosy.

ETIOLOGY AND PATHOGENESIS There is confusion over speciation of *Leishmania*. These organisms appear morphologically identical and must be differentiated on serologic, immunologic, nosologic, and behavioral grounds which are not entirely satisfactory. Four main groups are generally recognized: *L. donovani, L. tropica, L. mexicana*, and *L. brasiliensis*. Each group contains a variety of strains which have been accorded separate species or subspecies status by some workers.

Leishmania donovani is the cause of kala azar, the visceral form of leishmaniasis.

Leishmania tropica causes Old World cutaneous leishmaniasis, or oriental sore, also known as Delhi boil, Bagdad boil, Aleppo button, and Salek and Pendeh sore. A variety of this organism, *L. tropica aethiopica*, causes both oriental sore and diffuse cutaneous leishmaniasis in Ethiopia.

Leishmania mexicana produces a cutaneous leishmaniasis known as forest yaws, bay sore, and *chiclero ulcer* as well as the South American form of disseminated cutaneous disease. *Leishmania brasiliensis* is the cause of American mucocutaneous leishmaniasis also known as *espundia*.

Leishmania brasiliensis peruviana produces *uta*, another type of cutaneous leishmaniasis.

In the sandfly, the parasites assume the flagellated leptomonas form, but in humans the organisms lose their flagella, enter mononuclear phagocytes, and multiply as small, rounded leishmanial forms 2 to 3 μm in diameter, containing a nucleus and kinetoplast, the pathognomonic Leishman-Donovan bodies.

In humans continued intracellular multiplication of the parasite leads to rupture of the affected phagocyte and invasion of other cells, resulting in extensive histiocytic proliferation. The course of the disease from this point is apparently determined by the host's cellular immunity as well as the species of the parasite. In cutaneous leishmaniasis, there is a marked lymphocytic infiltration associated with a reduction in the number of parasites, the development of a delayed skin (leishmanin) reaction, and spontaneous cure. In the mucocutaneous form, the spontaneous disappearance of the primary lesion may be followed by metastatic mucocutaneous lesions at some later date. The destructiveness of the cutaneous lesions is attributed to the development of hypersensitivity to parasitic antigens. An interesting exception to the general pattern in cutaneous disease is disseminated cutaneous leishmaniasis (*leishmaniasis tegumentaria diffusa*) in which there is no infiltration of lymphocytes and plasma cells or reduction in the number of parasites, the leishmanin reaction is negative, and the skin lesions become chronic, progressive, and disseminated. In visceral leishmaniasis, the cellular changes are similar but the parasites spread to reticuloendothelial cells throughout the body. This spread is associated with development of marked hyperglobulinemia. As in the mucocutaneous form of the disease, circulating antibodies are detectable but do not seem to have a protective function. They may, in fact, be responsible for the pancytopenia and glomerulonephritis seen in visceral disease. A positive skin test develops in the visceral form after successful treatment.

KALA AZAR

DISTRIBUTION AND EPIDEMIOLOGY Kala azar occurs in China, Russia, India, the Middle East, Egypt, Sudan, East Africa, several Mediterranean countries, including Greece, Crete, and Malta, and a few areas of South and Central America. Although the manifestations of the disease throughout this area, which touches all continents but Australia, are basically similar, certain definite peculiarities in its behavior justify classification of visceral leishmaniasis into at least three main types. These differences are attributed to variations in the strains of *L. donovani* in a given area and, perhaps more important, to the length of time that the disease has been endemic in a population. It is believed that kala azar (and also infection by *L. tropica*) is introduced into a new area from animal reservoirs and that this "primitive" or zoonotic infection is likely to result in many cases of acute, rapidly fatal illness among the population coming into contact with the parasites for the first time. After generations, kala azar becomes endemic, the disease assumes a more chronic form, and the domestic dog becomes an important reservoir.

Mediterranean, or *infantile, kala azar* is seen primarily in the Mediterranean area, China, Russia, and Latin America. It is a disease of children under the age of four, but adults, particularly travelers to endemic areas, are not spared. Dogs, jackals, and foxes serve as reservoirs, and human-to-human transmission is thought to be rare. The strains responsible for the Eurasian and American diseases are sometimes referred to as *L. infantum* and *L. chagasi* respectively.

Indian kala azar affects older children and young adults, and males are involved more commonly than females. The human being is the only known reservoir, and transmission is carried out by anthropophilic species of sandflies. This form of disease has become uncommon as a result of antimalarial spraying.

African kala azar is found in the Eastern half of Africa from the Sahara in the North to the equator in the South. Its age and sex distribution is similar to that of Indian kala azar. It is endemic in gerbils and other rodents in many areas and is more resistant to therapy with antimony compounds than that found in the rest of the world.

MANIFESTATIONS The incubation period varies from 10 days to 1 year but is usually about 3 months. No lesion appears at the site of the infecting bite in most cases, but a primary "chancre" which heals with scarring before the onset of systemic symptoms is commonly noted in the African disease. The organisms multiply extensively in the macrophages of spleen, liver, bone marrow, lymph nodes, skin, and small intestine, accounting for many of the manifestations of the disease. Organisms may be found in the blood for several months before the onset of symptoms.

Fever, which is characterized at times by two daily spikes, may be abrupt or gradual in onset. It persists for 1 to 6 weeks and then disappears, only to reappear at irregular intervals during the course of the illness. Although prostration is absent even during periods of high fever, there is progressive weakness, pallor, weight loss, and tachycardia. Gastrointestinal disturbances are frequent in Indian cases. Physical findings include enormous splenomegaly, lymphadenopathy, hepatomegaly with signs of portal hypertension, and often edema, which tends to conceal the extent of the wasting. Hyperpigmentation is noted in light-skinned individuals, and mucocutaneous lesions similar to those seen in espundia occur in the African form of the disease. Anemia is the rule, and thrombocytopenia with gingival and other mucosal bleeding is common. The peripheral leukocyte count is low (usually less than 4,000 per mm^3); in children, agranulocytosis with cancrum oris (noma) and secondary pulmonary or intestinal infections contribute to the high mortality. The presence of a short erythrocyte life span, anti-red blood cell antibodies, positive Coombs test, and antibody against white blood cells and platelets suggests an autoimmune basis for the pancytopenia.

Hypergammaglobulinemia is universally present. Proteinuria and hematuria are frequent in the course of kala azar and are thought to be related to the glomerular deposition of poorly soluble immune complexes. Uremia due to renal amyloidosis and symptoms of heart failure can occur.

Post-kala azar dermal leishmaniasis Patients treated successfully with antimony compounds for kala azar may develop cutaneous lesions called *leishmanoids*, in which *Leishmania* organisms are demonstrable. These are rare in Mediterranean or Chinese kala azar but develop in 3 percent of African cases almost immediately after systemic symptoms subside. They occur after a latent period of 1 to 2 years in as many as 10 percent of Indian cases. The lesions range from patchy areas of depigmentation to erythematous papules and confluent nodules which may involve the ears and mucous membranes and have been mistaken for leprosy. They are short-lived in African kala azar but may persist for years in the Indian variety, creating a persistent reservoir of infection.

DIAGNOSIS The diagnosis is made by finding *Leishmania* organisms in stained preparations of blood (often possible in Indian but rarely so in other forms), bone marrow, lymph nodes, or material obtained by splenic puncture. The last is the best source of organisms, but the spleen should be needled only when it is firm and enlarged well below the left costal margin. The organisms will grow out as flagellated forms in Nicolle-Novy-MacNeal (NNN) medium containing defibrinated rabbit blood incubated at 22°C.

A complement fixation test using an antigen from *Mycobacterium phlei* gives positive results in 95 percent of patients with kala azar, but tuberculosis gives positive results also. Fluorescent antibody and indirect hemagglutination tests with leishmanial antigens are more specific but are not generally available. The leishmanin skin test is negative during active kala azar but becomes positive several months after successful treatment of the disease.

TREATMENT Rest, good diet, transfusions, and treatment of complicating infections, of which tuberculosis, bacterial pneumonia, amebiasis, and bacillary dysentery are more important, must supplement or precede specific therapy. Pentavalent antimony compounds are highly effective against the parasites. Owing to its lack of toxicity, Pentostam (sodium antimony gluconate) given intravenously or intramuscularly is the drug of choice. The adult dose is 0.6 g (6 ml) daily for 6 days in Indian kala azar and for 30 days in other forms. Neostibosan (ethylstibamine) can also be used. Urea stibamine is popular in India.

More than 90 percent of cases respond promptly to antimony, except in Africa, where the cure rate is as low as 70 percent. Resistant cases can be treated with either one of the more toxic diamidines or with amphotericin B. Pentamidine is given intramuscularly in the dose of 4 mg base per kg body weight dissolved in 3 to 4 ml water daily for 10 days. The course may be repeated twice after intervals of 10 days. Hypotension, hypoglycemia, and diabetes mellitus can complicate therapy with this drug. The more effective hydroxystilbamidine is given intravenously in 10 daily injections of a fresh solution in dosage of 0.25 g daily. The course may have to be repeated in African kala azar. Amphotericin B is given in the manner described for cryptococcosis (Chap. 170) to a total dose of 2 g.

PROGNOSIS AND CONTROL The mortality in untreated kala azar is 95 percent in adults and 80 percent in children. This has been greatly reduced by treatment with antimony and the aromatic diamidines. Relapses, occasionally several in number, occur in 5 to 15 percent of African and Mediterranean cases up to 2 years after treatment. Both relapses and post-kala azar dermal leishmaniasis should be re-treated in the same fashion as the initial illness.

The treatment of the disease in humans, the elimination of diseased dogs, and the use of DDT residual sprays against sandflies are the important preventive measures. Incidence of the disease has diminished greatly in many areas where DDT has been used to eradicate malaria—an unexpected added benefit of this program. When the vectors are exophilic, control is difficult. Attempts at vaccination with avirulent strains of *L. donovani* have been unsuccessful.

AMERICAN CUTANEOUS LEISHMANIASIS

These diseases occur in every country of Central and South America except Chile. In some areas, 10 to 20 percent of the population is infected. There are four varieties of American cutaneous leishmaniasis. All begin with a local lesion at the site of the infecting sandfly bite after an incubation period of from 10 days to 3 months.

Chiclero ulcer, which is found in Mexico, Guatemala, British Honduras, and possibly other parts of Central America, is a zoonosis caused by *L. mexicana*. The disease occurs naturally in several arboreal rodents. It is occasionally transmitted to persons entering forests to harvest chicle. In immunocompetent individuals, it is a relatively mild infection characterized by a single cutaneous lesion on the ear, face, or hand which is chronic and shows little tendency to ulceration. The leishmanin skin test is positive. Spontaneous healing usually occurs within 6 months. The parasites are never numerous in the lesions. Mucosal ulceration does not occur. Ear lesions cause extensive destruction of the pinna and should be treated with a single 350 mg intramuscular dose of cycloguanil pamoate. Immunization with live cultures of *L. mexicana* has been effective in forest workers.

Diffuse cutaneous leishmaniasis is found in Venezuela. It apparently results from a specific deficiency of cell-mediated immunity to leishmanial antigen. In South America, it is caused by members of the *L. mexicana* complex, usually *L. mexicana amazonensis*. This remarkable disease is characterized by massive dissemination of skin lesions without visceral involvement. The clinical picture often bears a striking resemblance to lepromatous leprosy. The diagnosis is not difficult, because the lesions contain a large number of organisms. In contrast to all other types of cutaneous leishmaniasis, the leishmanin skin test is negative. The disease is progressive and very refractory to treatment. Amphotericin B and pentamidine have been used to produce remissions, but cure is rare.

Uta, which occurs in cooler climates and at altitudes of more than 2,000 ft, consists of single or multiple skin ulcers of the nose and lips in which parasites are readily demonstrable. Spontaneous healing within 3 months to a year is the rule, and mucosal spread is unusual. The etiologic agent is *L. peruviana,* a member of the *L. brasiliensis* group, and the reservoir is the domestic dog. With widespread use of insecticides in Peru, the disease has almost disappeared.

In tropical Latin America, *L. brasiliensis* causes the better-known and more serious *espundia*. The organism causes a natural infection in large forest rodents and is transmitted to human beings by sandflies when new settlements are made in jungle areas. The initial skin lesion enlarges progressively, and secondary bacterial infection is frequent. The disease may spread by direct extension or by lymphatics to the mucosal surfaces of the mouth and nose, where, after the primary lesion has healed, painful, destructive, and mutilating erosions scar and distort the involved structures. Fever, anemia, and weight loss accompany these mucosal complications. Destruction of the nasal septum produces a characteristic deformity called *tapir nose* or *camel nose*. The hard palate may be destroyed, and laryngeal erosion can lead to aphonia. In blacks, the lesion is often hypertrophic, and large polypoid masses deform the lips and cheeks, perhaps representing a type of keloid reaction. This can be mistaken for South American blastomycosis (Chap. 171). Secondary bacterial infection, inanition, and respiratory obstruction lead to death.

The diagnosis is made by finding the organisms in scrapings or by culture. The leishmanin skin test is specific and highly useful. Treatment consists of antibiotics for bacterial infections and pentavalent antimonials used as in kala azar. Cases that fail to respond to antimonials should be treated with amphotericin B.

The early lesions respond well, but even with repeated courses of antimony the mucosal complications of the espundia type heal slowly. In advanced cases, the prognosis is very poor.

OLD WORLD CUTANEOUS LEISHMANIASIS: ORIENTAL SORE

This, the least serious form of human leishmaniasis, consists of localized cutaneous ulceration which heals spontaneously and is endemic in the European countries bordering the eastern Mediterranean, in Africa, in Asia Minor, in Southwest Asia, and in India. Two major strains of the causative organism, *L. tropica*, produce similar but distinctive clinical syndromes. Homologous immunity after recovery from infection by either strain is solid and lifelong. Infection with *L. tropica major* protects against *L. tropica minor*, but the opposite is not the case. The rural type, caused by *L. tropica major*, has its reservoir in gerbils and other small rodents; the ulcers usually appear on the extremities 2 to 6 weeks after the bite of the sandfly and are accompanied by regional lymphadenopathy in a majority of cases. Spontaneous healing occurs within 3 to 6 months, leaving a depigmented, pitted scar.

The incubation period in the *urban*, or *dry*, type ranges from 2 months to more than a year. The lesion is usually facial and begins as a pruritic, purplish nodule (the Aleppo button), which slowly enlarges and finally breaks down after 3 or 4 months. Lymphatic involvement is uncommon. Healing of the indolent, granulomatous ulcer may require a year or more. Occasionally, healing fails to occur, which results in lesions closely resembling lupus vulgaris. This condition, known as *leishmaniasis recidiva*, is thought to be the result of an exaggerated delayed hypersensitivity to leishmanial antigens. Humans and the domestic dog serve as the reservoirs of infection.

The typical oriental sore is a sharply punched-out, ragged ulcer about 1 in. in diameter, surrounded by an erythematous rim. Satellite lesions which fuse with the original are not rare. The center of the granulating base of the ulcer frequently contains a hard excrescence called the *Montpellier sign* or the *rake* beneath which the parasites are most likely to be found when scrapings are examined.

The rural and urban types occur together in Asia Minor; indeed, it is not rare to find simultaneous infections in the same patient. In Southeastern Europe, India, and North Africa, the urban type is prevalent, while in the remainder of Africa the disease is predominantly rural.

A form of diffuse cutaneous leishmaniasis is seen in Ethiopia. It closely resembles the disease in Venezuela and appears to have a sylvatic reservoir.

Diagnosis is usually made on clinical grounds and is confirmed by finding the parasites, which occur both intra- and extracellularly. Pyogenic infection makes direct visualization difficult, but *L. tropica* can be cultured in NNN medium at room temperature, and a skin test using *L. tropica* antigen becomes positive in the vast majority of patients with the disease.

Treatment should include vigorous measures for bacterial infection, such as hot soaks and appropriate systemic antibiotics. Infrared heat treatment has also been suggested, as the leishmanial organisms are very heat-sensitive. Systemic antimonials may be required where ulceration is extensive or multiple. Pentostam is used as in kala azar in a course of 10 daily injections totaling 6 g. It may be injected locally in dosage of 0.6 g three to four times on alternate days. In endemic areas the custom is to withhold treatment directed against the parasite until the initial nodule ulcerates, to assure the development of immunity against reinfection.

Prevention consists of use of insect repellents on exposed parts of the body, residual DDT sprays, and fine-mesh screening for dwellings. The lesions should be covered to prevent infection of vectors and, of course, contact with the lesion or its discharges should be avoided.

REFERENCES

BRAY RS: Leishmaniasis in the Old World. Br Med Bull 28:39, 1972

——: Leishmania. Ann Rev Microbiol 28:189, 1974

BRYCESON ADM: Diffuse cutaneous leishmaniasis in Ethiopia. Trans R Soc Trop Med Hyg 64:369, 1970

CONVIT J, KERDEL-VEGAS F: Disseminated cutaneous leishmaniasis. Arch Dermatol 91:439, 1965

HUNTER GW et al: *A Manual of Tropical Medicine*, 4th ed., Philadelphia: Saunders, 1966

KERN F, PEDERSEN JK: Leishmaniasis in the United States: Report of ten cases in military personnel. JAMA 226:872, 1973

LAINSON R, SHAW JJ: Leishmaniasis of the New World: Taxonomic problems. Br Med Bull 28:44, 1972

MAEGRATH BG, GILES HM: *Management and Treatment of Tropical Diseases*. Oxford: Blackwell Scientific Publications, 1971

WOODRUFF AW et al: The anemia of kala azar. Br J Haematol 22:319, 1972

217 TRYPANOSOMIASIS

JAMES J. PLORDE

SLEEPING SICKNESS

DEFINITION African trypanosomiasis, or sleeping sickness, is a disease caused by the hemoflagellate *Trypanosoma brucei*, which is transmitted to human beings by several species of tsetse fly belonging to the genus *Glossina*. Clinically, the untreated disease is characterized by an acute febrile lymphadenopathy followed, after a variable period, by a chronic lethal meningoencephalomyelitis. It occurs in two principal epidemiologic patterns: Gambian, or Mid- and West African, sleeping sickness, and Rhodesian, or East African, sleeping sickness.

ETIOLOGY Trypanosomes are fusiform protozoa recognized by an undulating membrane which extends along the length of the cell and terminates in an anterior flagellum. The morphologic characteristics of many varieties are so nearly identical that they are distinguishable only by their pathogenicity for certain animals, differences in biochemical requirements, and ability to multiply in insects. *Trypanosoma brucei* strains are polymorphic organisms varying in shape from slender to stumpy and in length from 8 to 30 μm. The slender forms have a long flagellum that in the shorter types is rudimentary or absent. The Gambian and Rhodesian forms of sleeping sickness were previously thought to be caused by two distinct species of trypanosomes, *T. gambiense* and *T. rhodesiense*. It is felt now, however, that they, along with the animal trypanosome responsible for *nagana* in cattle, are all variants of a single species. The individual varieties are referred to as *T. brucei gambiense, T. brucei rhodesiense*, and *T. brucei brucei*.

Trypanosomiasis in animals is a great economic problem in many parts of the world. It is probable that an area of approximately 4 million square miles in Africa is not populated because of the impossibility of keeping animals in sites where tsetse flies are infected with trypanosomes.

EPIDEMIOLOGY Gambian sleeping sickness occurs in tropical, West, and Central Africa extending from the Sahara to the Kalahari Deserts and east to the Rift Valley. The incidence of disease is particularly high in Zaire. Rhodesian trypanosomiasis is found in tropical East Africa from Ethiopia in the north to Botswana in the south.

Transmission of the trypanosomes of sleeping sickness occurs by what is referred to as the "anterior station." After ingestion by a feeding tsetse, the parasites first develop in the intestine of the fly and then migrate to the salivary glands, where they are discharged when the host is bitten. In some situations it is possible that the trypanosomes can be mechanically transmitted from host to host by the tsetse and other hematophagous arthropods. This may be of importance during epidemics.

The Gambian strains of *T. brucei* are transmitted mainly by *G. palpalis* and *G. tachinoides*. These species live in shaded areas near water. Less than 5 percent of the flies are infected even in the most notorious endemic foci. Although *G. palpalis* and *G. tachinoides* are not exclusively anthropophilic, human beings are thought to be the only reservoir for Gambian sleeping sickness.

Rhodesian sleeping sickness, on the other hand, is primarily a zoonosis. It is transmitted to humans from the bushbuck, a small antelope, by the bite of *G. morsitans*, a savannah tsetse. It is seen typically in individuals who travel away from their villages to hunt or fish. Domestic cattle and sheep may also serve as reservoirs, and transmission from human to fly to human can occur.

PATHOLOGY AND PATHOGENESIS The tsetse fly inoculates the organism into the subcutaneous pool of blood that forms during its feeding. Some of the parasites may reach the bloodstream directly, but most remain at the site of inoculation, where they multiply to produce a local chancre. Following the appearance of this lesion, the trypanosomes spread through tissue spaces and lymphatics, eventually spilling over into the general circulation where they continue to multiply by longitudinal fission. The parasitemia is of low intensity and typically occurs in waves; each wave disappears coincidentally with the production of antibody to an exoantigen of the protozoan and reappears as a new antigenic variant arises. These waves of parasitemia, which are accompanied by fever and mononuclear leukocytosis, tend to become more infrequent and irregular in the later stages of the disease. At some time during this stage of dissemination, trypanosomes localize in the tissues of the central nervous system. This is first manifested as a diffuse leptomeningitis and later by a perivascular cerebritis. If untreated, this parenchymal inflammation gives rise to a demyelinating panencephalitis. Leishmanial or short forms have been demonstrated in experimental *T. brucei* infections, suggesting that this organism has an intracellular tissue phase in its developmental cycle. This could be of significance in occult infections.

The mechanism by which the trypanosome elicits tissue damage is unknown. It has been suggested that antigen-antibody reactions lead to the release of kinins. The release of proteolytic enzymes by degenerating phagocytes may be important. The parasitemia stimulates the production of large quantities of IgM immunoglobulin, perhaps in response to the rapid antigenic variation of the parasite. It seems likely that these antibodies are not protective and may, in fact, contribute to the pathogenesis of the anemia and thrombocytopenia sometimes seen in this disease. Cell-mediated immunity is probably important.

CLINICAL MANIFESTATIONS The Gambian and Rhodesian forms of sleeping sickness differ somewhat in symptoms, severity, and duration. Rhodesian trypanosomiasis is the more acute and severe of the two forms, usually terminating fatally within a year. Fever is higher, emaciation more rapid, and lymphatic involvement less evident. Death from intercurrent infections or myocarditis usually occurs before the typical sleeping sickness syndrome appears. In the Gambian variety there are often successive bouts of clinical activity with intervening latent periods that persist for a number of years. The early stages may be mild, and the disease may go unrecognized until the central nervous system is involved. In both forms of the disease, however, an entry lesion, a febrile period of dissemination, and a stage of central nervous system involvement are found to some degree. The *trypanosomal chancre* appears as an erythematous nodule at the site of inoculation 2 or 3 days after the bite of an infected fly. It may occur anywhere in the body but is most commonly seen on the head or limbs and is accompanied by regional lymphadenopathy. The lesion, which subsides spontaneously, is noted more frequently in Rhodesian sleeping sickness, perhaps because of the acute nature of the disease.

The incubation period is usually about 2 weeks, but in *T. brucei gambiense* infections may be several years. Systemic manifestations generally become apparent during the hematogenous dissemination of the trypanosomes. In the usual case the patient develops a high remittent fever, severe headache, insomnia, and inability to concentrate. In Caucasians a characteristic circinate erythema resembling erythema marginatum is frequent. Transient firm areas of painful subcutaneous edema localized to the hands, feet, and periorbital tissues may appear. All these signs and symptoms may disappear and reappear intermittently over a period of months to years. Tender lymphadenopathy with gradual induration of the nodes and splenomegaly are almost invariably present in Gambian sleeping sickness. The lymph nodes of the posterior cervical triangle are frequently prominent. This is referred to as *Winterbottom's sign*. Eventually the parasites enter the central nervous system. This may occur early in the course of the disease or may be delayed for as long as 8 years. Cerebral trypanosomiasis can be explosive, causing repeated convulsions or deep coma and death within a few days. Most patients show gradual progression to the classic picture of *sleeping sickness*. The patient develops a vacant expression, the eyelids droop, the lower lip hangs loosely, and it becomes more and more difficult to gain his attention or prod him to any activity. Patients will eat when offered food, but they never ask for it or engage in spontaneous conversation, and speech gradually becomes blurred and indistinct. Tremors of the hands and tongue, choreiform movements, seizures with transient paralysis, loss of sphincter control, ophthalmoplegia, extensor plantar responses, and finally death in coma, in status epilepticus, or from hyperpyrexia follows inexorably.

Death may also occur from intercurrent infection, of which bacillary and amebic dysentery, malaria, and bacterial (often pneumococcal) pneumonia are the most important.

DIAGNOSIS AND LABORATORY FINDINGS *Anemia* and *hypermacroglobulinemia* are invariably present, and spontaneous clumping of erythrocytes in blood specimens is grossly evident in many cases. The sedimentation rate is rapid, and peripheral monocytosis is frequent. When there has been invasion of the central nervous system, the *cerebrospinal fluid* shows mononuclear pleocytosis and increased protein concentration. The protein concentration is a better index of severity of disease and therapeutic response than the number of cells. The presence of IgM in the spinal fluid is almost pathognomonic of cerebral trypanosomiasis.

The definitive diagnosis depends upon finding the trypanosomes in the blood, aspirate of lymph node, or cerebrospinal fluid. These should be examined first in wet mounts; actively motile organisms are seen easily under high power. For final identification thin and thick blood films should be stained with Wright's or Giemsa's stain. If the blood smears are negative, citrated blood should be centrifuged at 1,000 rpm for 10 min, the supernatant (including the leukocytes) recentrifuged at 2,000 rpm for 15 min, and the sediment examined. Cerebrospinal fluid should be centrifuged at 2,000 rpm for 15 min before examination. Alternatively the blood and spinal fluid may be centrifuged in a heparinized capillary tube at 12,000 rpm for 4 min and the tubes examined under a microscope using a 10-power objective. The trypanosomes are found at the junction of the plasma and buffy layer in centrifuged blood and near the sealed end of the tube in centrifuged spinal fluid. If these methods are negative, inoculation of rats or mice can be helpful in the diagnosis of Rhodesian disease. A severalfold increase in IgM globulins in the serum is of confirmatory value. Complement fixation and indirect fluorescent antibody tests utilizing stable antigens are useful in endemic areas.

TREATMENT *Suramin* (Bayer 205, Antrypol) is the most effective agent before central nervous system involvement has occurred. The initial dose should be limited to 0.2 g intravenously because of possible idiosyncrasy. If there is no evidence of sensitivity, a full course of therapy can be instituted the following day. One gram (10 ml fresh 10% solution) is given intravenously on the first, third, seventh, fourteenth, and twenty-first days for a total of 5 g. If red blood cells, casts, or significant amounts of protein occur in the urine, therapy should be discontinued. Pentamidine given in water intramuscularly each day for 10 injections is also effective in early disease. The dose is 3 to 4 mg pentamidine base per kg for each injection. When the agent is given too rapidly by the intravenous route, it may cause hypotension.

Lumbar puncture should always be performed in patients who are about to undergo therapy for trypanosomiasis. If the central nervous system is involved, agents that will penetrate the blood-brain barrier must be used; for this purpose the most effective agent is *melarsoprol* (Mel B). This drug, an arsenic derivative of British antilewisite (BAL), is effective at all stages of the disease but is more toxic than suramin. It is given intravenously in a 3.6% solution. The initial dose is 0.5 ml. Each subsequent dose is increased by 0.5 ml until the maximum single dose of 5 ml is reached. The first three doses are given at daily intervals followed by a 7-day rest. This schedule is repeated until a total of 37.5 ml has been given over a period of 1 month. If signs of arsenic toxicity occur, the drug should be discontinued. A reactive encephalopathy, probably due to the release of trypanosomal antigen, may occur early in the course of treatment. Pretreatment with suramin may help avert this complication. A hemorrhagic encephalopathy, a direct arsenic toxic reaction, may also occur and is usually fatal. BAL may be of some use in this situation.

Nitrofurazone can also be given for cerebral trypanosomiasis in an oral dose of 0.5 g three times a day for 7 days, but is more toxic than melarsoprol, and it should not be used unless the patients have failed to respond to this drug. The increasing incidence of drug-resistant parasites has limited the usefulness of *tryparsamide* in the treatment of certain *T. brucei gambiense* infections.

PROGNOSIS The disease is probably always fatal if untreated. If the infection is treated with suramin prior to central nervous system involvement, the cure rate is high and recovery is rapid and complete. When the nervous system becomes involved, the prognosis is less bright, and in far-advanced disease the survivors may suffer neurologic damage. Relapses may occur, particularly following treatment with suramin, if the central nervous system was already involved at the time therapy was instituted. Less commonly they may be the result of drug resistance. Examination of the spinal fluid 6 and 12 months after therapy, or earlier if symptoms recur, is helpful in detecting relapse. Such patients must be re-treated with a second therapeutic agent.

PREVENTION Personal protection is best achieved by the use of repellents and protective clothing. A single intramuscular injection of pentamidine in dosage of 3 to 4 mg base per kg (maximum 300 mg) will protect against the Gambian form of disease for 6 months or more; its usefulness in Rhodesian trypanosomiasis is controversial. Because of the danger of cryptic infections occurring during chemoprophylaxis, it has been generally restricted to mass prophylactic campaigns. Other methods of disease control include clearing vegetation and the use of insecticides.

CHAGAS' DISEASE

DEFINITION American trypanosomiasis is an infection caused by *T. cruzi* that is characterized by an acute, often asymptomatic illness that is followed by chronic cardiac and gastrointestinal sequelae.

ETIOLOGY *Trypanosoma cruzi* circulates in the blood as a slender, fusiform hemoflagellate measuring 20 μm in length. In stained preparations, its narrow undulating membrane, large kinetoplast, and characteristic C shape are easily recognized. Unlike the trypanosomes of sleeping sickness, it does not multiply within the bloodstream. After invading tissue cells, it loses its undulating membrane and flagellum, assumes its leishmania form, and divides by binary fission. Eventually, new flagellated forms are produced which reenter the general circulation to initiate another cycle.

Strains of *T. cruzi* vary widely in both virulence and tissue tropism.

EPIDEMIOLOGY This infection is found from Chile and Argentina to Mexico, where it affects more than 7 million people. *Trypanosoma cruzi* has been found in insect vectors and wild animals in several areas of the Southern United States and serologic studies have documented that acquisition of human infection occurs within this country. There are to date, however, only a handful of clinically apparent autochthonous cases reported from Texas.

The disease is transmitted to humans by reduviid ("assassin" or "kissing") bugs, primarily those of the genera *Triatoma, Panstrongylus,* and *Rhodnius*. These winged, hematophagous insects can be found in the burrows of animals and in the cracks and thatch of poorly constructed rural dwellings. The insect attacks human beings at night, usually biting the face at the mucocutaneous junction (most frequently the lip or outer canthus of the eye). The flagellated trypanosomes are ingested by the bug while feeding, and after multiplying and developing in the midgut of the insect for 8 to 10 days, are discharged in the feces; human infection occurs through contamination of the bite wound. This is referred to as transmission by the "posterior station." The reduviid may remain infected as long as 2 years.

Human beings, domestic animals (cats and dogs), and wild animals, especially the opossum and armadillo, may serve as reservoirs for the infection. The close association of human beings, domestic animals, and the vector within human dwellings is of prime epidemiologic importance, but the disease is occasionally transmitted by a blood transfusion and via the placenta to newborn infants.

PATHOGENESIS AND CLINICAL MANIFESTATIONS A local inflammatory reaction, manifested clinically as an erythematous nodule or *chagoma*, appears within a few days at the site of inoculation of the protozoan. If, as is commonly the case, the portal of entry has been the conjunctiva, the presenting manifestations are a unilateral, painless conjunctivitis, palpebral edema, and preauricular lymphadenopathy (Romaña's sign). This primary complex may persist for 1 to 2 months during which parasites can be demonstrated in the lesion.

Following an incubation period of 2 weeks, trypanosomal forms reach the general circulation, producing a parasitemia and initiating the acute phase of the illness. After circulating in the blood for some time, the trypanosomes invade tissue cells, and, in the leishmanial form, multiply, producing intracellular pseudocysts. In 4 to 6 days these pseudocysts rupture, releasing both leishmanial and newly formed trypanosomal organisms. The leishmanial forms disintegrate, eliciting an intense inflammatory reaction, while the trypanosomal forms regain the bloodstream to maintain the infection and invade new tissues, particularly the heart, skeletal muscle, smooth muscle, and nervous system.

Clinically, the patient experiences a continuous or recurrent fever, generalized lymphadenopathy, hepatosplenomegaly, and in some cases extensive gelatinous edema of the face and trunk. A transient morbilliform or urticarial skin eruption may occur early in the acute phase. Rarely, in newborn infants and young children, an acute meningoencephalitis may complicate the acute illness. Myocarditis characterized by tachycardia and electrocardiographic changes is very common. In severe cases, there may be conduction disturbances, cardiac dilatation, and heart failure. The duration of the acute illness is variable. In 5 to 10 percent of cases, meningoencephalitis or severe heart disease results in a fatal outcome within a few days or weeks. Most often it resolves slowly over a period of several weeks. Parasites become extremely scanty in both the tissues and blood, and the patient remains asymptomatic until the onset of the chronic phase 1 or 2 years later. Most patients presenting with late manifestations, however, deny a history of acute illness, suggesting that subclinical infections often result in chronic disease. It has been suggested that the basic pathogenetic mechanism is a hypersensitivity or autoimmune inflammatory reaction involving mesenchymal tissues. A diffuse myocarditis is usually present in chronic Chagas' disease, and recently antibodies reactive with endocardium, striated muscle, and vascular tissues have been described. It is generally felt, however, that the late manifestations of disease are primarily due to neuropathies caused by the destruction of ganglionic nerve cells during the acute phase of the disease and resulting in the dilatation and malfunction of the affected organs.

The most important late manifestation is heart disease which may affect as much as 10 percent of the rural population in endemic areas. Symptoms and signs range from arrhythmias and heart block to chronic congestive heart failure (predominantly right-sided). Thromboembolic phenomena and sudden cardiac arrest are relatively common. At autopsy the hearts of patients with Chagas' disease may show a peculiar herniation of the endocardium through the apical muscle bundles. Megacolon and megaesophagus are sequelae seen in southern South America, but they are less common in Central America and in northern South America.

DIAGNOSIS The diagnosis depends on the demonstration of *T. cruzi* in the patient or upon serologic tests. In the acute phase of the disease the parasite may be seen in the peripheral blood by means of the same direct methods described for African trypanosomiasis. If these are negative, blood may be cultured in Nicolle-Novy-MacNeal (NNN) medium or inoculated into rats, mice, or guinea pigs.

Trypanosoma cruzi is easily grown in blood broth and incubated at 28°C; a more sensitive tissue culture method has been described recently. The technique of *xenodiagnosis* is often used in endemic areas; a laboratory-reared vector, known to be parasite-free, is allowed to feed on subjects with suspected cases, and 2 weeks later, the insect's intestinal contents are examined for parasites. Confusion sometimes arises from the finding of trypanosomes in blood. Many children in Venezuela and other South American countries are infected with a harmless species *T. rangeli*, which produces no symptoms but may be present in the blood for many months. By utilization of both culture and xenodiagnosis repeatedly, organisms can be recovered from most acute cases and from up to 40 percent of chronic ones. Biopsy of an involved lymph node or calf muscle may reveal the organism during the initial illness when the parasites cannot be recovered from the blood. The Machado-Guerreiro test (a complement fixation reaction) is most helpful in the diagnosis of chronic cases and in survey work. Fluorescent antibody and hemagglutination inhibition tests appear useful.

TREATMENT AND PREVENTION There is still no satisfactory treatment for Chagas' disease, although several drugs, including primaquine given in dosage suggested for malaria, will clear the blood of trypanosomes, but they do not affect the intracellular parasites. Bayer 2502 (Lampit), a nitrofurazone derivative given in dosage of 10 mg per kg per day for 3 or 4 months, shows promise as a curative agent. Chronic organ damage, however, is generally thought irreversible. Prevention consists of using residual insecticide sprays—of which benzene hexachloride (BHC) is the most effective—on the walls of houses, the main habitat of the vectors. Reinfestation, however, may occur within a year or two of spraying. Transfusion infections can be prevented by serologic screening of blood donors in endemic areas and by adding gentian violet to the blood. Immunosuppression may reactivate Chagas' disease, and patients from endemic areas should be serologically screened before such treatment is instituted.

REFERENCES

BARRETT-CONNOR E: Chemoprophylaxis of amebiasis and African trypanosomiasis. Ann Intern Med 77:797, 1972

BROWN HW: *Basic Clinical Parasitology*, 4th ed., New York: Appleton Century Crofts, 1975

GOODWIN LG: The pathology of African trypanosomiasis. Trans R Soc Trop Med Hyg 64:797, 1970

KABERLE F: Chagas' disease and Chagas' syndromes: The pathology of American trypanosomiasis. Adv Parasitol 6:63, 1968

LUMSDEN WHR: Trypanosomiasis. Br Med Bull 28:34, 1972

MAEGRATH BG, GILES HM: *Management and Treatment of Tropical Diseases*, Oxford: Blackwell Scientific Publications, 1971

MARTINI-CAMPOS JV, TAFURI WL: Chagas' enteropathy. Gut 14: 910, 1973

MULLIGAN HW (ed): *The African Trypanosomiasis*, London: Allen & Irwin, 1970

SPENCER HC JR et al: Imported African trypanosomiasis in the United States. Ann Intern Med 82:633, 1975

WHO: Comparative studies of American and African trypanosomiasis, WHO Tech Rep Ser 411, Geneva, 1969

WHO MEMORANDA: Immunology of Chagas' disease. Bull WHO 50:549, 1974

WILCOX C, MANSON-BAHR PEC (eds): *Manson's Tropical Diseases*, 17th ed., Baltimore: Williams & Wilkins, 1972

218
TOXOPLASMOSIS

HARRY A. FELDMAN

DEFINITION Toxoplasmosis is caused by *Toxoplasma gondii*, an obligate intracellular protozoan parasite which is widely distributed among mammals and birds. In humans it produces either acquired (often asymptomatic) or congenital infections.

HISTORY Toxoplasma was first demonstrated in animals in 1908, but was not proved to cause human disease until 1939, when several cases of fatal neonatal encephalomyelitis were shown to have resulted from congenital infections with this parasite. The development of the dye and complement fixation tests, and subsequently other serologic procedures, led to the demonstration that toxoplasma frequently infects humans and animals, but that disease is uncommon. Congenital toxoplasmosis, if symptomatic, represents only one form of clinical expression.

ETIOLOGY *Toxoplasma gondii*, an obligate intracellular protozoon, is a coccidian of cats, its definitive host. All strains are antigenically similar, and there is only one species. Trophozoites measuring about 2 by 5 μm and appearing crescentic, oval, or round may be found free in tissues, but usually move through the host within cells. They divide by endodyogeny and are best stained with Wright or Giemsa stains. Toxoplasma is unique in that it can infect any nucleated cell of any warm-blooded animal. Parasites can be maintained in mice, tissue cultures, or embryonated eggs, but require living cells, in whose cytoplasm they multiply. Under special conditions toxoplasma can be frozen and stored, but ordinary freezing kills them. They remain alive within cysts in tissues, especially muscle and the central nervous system. Such cysts do not calcify, have sharply demarcated tough elastic surrounding membranes, and may reach 100 μm in size, containing thousands of zoites.

Following the ingestion of toxoplasma cysts in meat or oocysts from cat feces, susceptible cats acquire infections, antibodies, and immunity. Such material is infective for other animals as well, but in the cat (and in other Felidae but no other species) schizogonic and gametogonic cycles follow in their intestinal epithelium. Subsequently, oocysts containing two sporocysts are excreted, which on maturation develop into four sporozoites resembling trophozoites. Sporocysts are shed for about 1 to 2 weeks but are not infectious until exposed to temperature, air, and moisture conditions which permit sporulation. This usually requires 1 to 5 days. With suitable humidity and temperature, oocysts can retain their infectivity for a year or more, but they are killed by drying, boiling water, and certain chemicals.

EPIDEMIOLOGY Serologic surveys indicate that toxoplasma infections are worldwide in distribution. With the dye test, the most sensitive indicator of specific antibody, it was demonstrated that approximately one-third of the inhabitants of several American cities, two-thirds of Hondurans, and 70 percent of Tahitian natives had positive tests, as compared with 1 percent of residents of several islands off the northern coast of Australia and 4 percent of Navajo Indians. American military recruits, originating in different areas of the United States, have marked differences in antibody prevalence. Among East Coast recruits, 20 percent were positive in contrast with only 3 and 8 percent, respectively, from the Mountain and Pacific Coast regions. Overall, 14 percent of Americans had antibodies, compared with 51 and 56 percent, respectively, of Colombian and Brazilian recruits.

Two longitudinal studies of seroconversion in American families were especially informative. In a Cleveland population, it was found during a 10-year observation period that only four individuals who had no indirect hemagglutinating antibodies at the start acquired them subsequently. During a 4-year period, seroconversion (as indicated by the dye test) occurred in only three persons in a group of Syracuse families, i.e., 1 in 2,392 person-months of observation. In neither study was an associated clinical illness identified in any person in whom seroconversion took place.

In animal surveys, cats, dogs, goats, guinea pigs, sheep, swine, rabbits, pigeons, and many others have been found to have different prevalences of positive tests. Many wild animals are infected. These surveys show that toxoplasma infections are frequent in humans and animals, but that their prevalence varies considerably from place to place and in different species in the same general locale.

The pathways whereby humans and animals usually acquire toxoplasma are unknown. Person-to-person transfer seems not to occur except from mother to fetus. Rarely, it has followed organ transplantation or the transfusion of fresh blood. It has long been known that animals can acquire parasites by cannibalizing others which are infected. This also applies to humans. Children without antibodies were demonstrated to acquire them following the ingestion of undercooked mutton and beef, but no clinical illnesses were noted. Unfortunately, this would not explain the route by which herbivores acquire toxoplasma. More recently, it has been demonstrated that newly infected cats excrete oocysts which under proper circumstances are infectious for other animals, including humans. Human infections are contracted in all seasons, usually with equal frequency by the two sexes. High infection rates have been noted in some areas where there are no cats, pointing again to the probable multiplicity of sources of human infections.

CLINICAL MANIFESTATIONS **Congenital toxoplasmosis** Congenitally infected infants may be born prematurely or at term and stillborn or alive with active disease, which can be expressed by fever, rash, icterus, hepatomegaly, splenomegaly, chorioretinitis, convulsions, and xanthochromic spinal fluid, in various combinations. The newborn infant may have none of these signs, but subsequently hydrocephaly or microcephaly, chorioretinitis, psychomotor retardation, cerebral calcifications, and convulsions may appear, either singly or together. The most common residuals in congenitally affected children are chorioretinitis, cerebral calcifications, psychomotor retardation, hydro- or microcephaly, and convulsions. Chorioretinitis is by far the most frequent. Any, or all, of these may follow other congenital infections, especially those due to cytomegalovirus (Chap. 211). The mothers of congenitally infected offspring ordinarily are unaware of having had any specific illness during the pregnancy. They should be advised that for all practical purposes, the risk of producing a second such baby is nil. Thus, future pregnancies can be undertaken without fear of having another affected child. This complication occurs only in a female who happens to be pregnant when she has a parasitemia with her initial, usually asymptomatic, toxoplasma infection. Congenital cases should be most rare in those areas where childhood infection rates are high. A recent prospective study of 183 pregnant women who acquired toxoplasma infections during pregnancy has shown that 60 percent of the offspring were found not to be infected at all and of those that were, more than two-thirds were normal. Most of the others had only isolated areas of chorioretinitis. It appears, therefore, that more than 80 percent of the offspring of such pregnancies are uninfected or unaffected. Elevated IgM levels have been noted in neonates with congenital toxoplasma infections, but specific IgM often is lacking at birth.

Acquired toxoplasmosis Although the clinical features show great variability, certain manifestations may be suggestive of this disease. Maculopapular rashes may appear soon after the clinical onset of illness, but tend to disappear in 3 to 4 days. Nonsuppurating lymphadenopathy, especially cervical, is common and may be present alone or in combination with other signs. Myalgias, arthralgias, myocarditis, pericarditis, pneumonitis, and encephalitis also have been noted. Splenomegaly usually is absent, but has been reported irregularly. Acquired toxoplasmosis may resemble infectious mononucleosis or cytomegalovirus disease because of lymphadenopathy, lymphocytosis, and atypical lymphocytes, but the heterophil test is negative.

Parasites have been demonstrated in lymph nodes removed from such patients, even when they were afebrile.

Toxoplasma has been isolated from several patients with posterior granulomatous uveitis, usually the result of congenital infections. The proportion of such cases which is caused by toxoplasma has not been established. In contrast to congenital chorioretinitis, which is usually bilateral, the acquired form more often is unilateral. Cerebral calcifications are not found in postnatally acquired infections. The incubation period, mortality rate, average duration of illness, and the residual defects resulting from acquired toxoplasmosis remain undefined.

Increasingly, disseminated toxoplasmosis has come to take its place alongside herpesviruses, cytomegalovirus, varicella, *Pneumocystis carinii,* and various fungi and bacteria as frequent causes of death among those with profound debilitating diseases or receiving immunosuppressive treatment. In these instances toxoplasma most often affects brain, diffusely or localized, myocardium, and lungs. If it is suspected and demonstrated (serologically or biopsy), chemotherapy may be of value, providing the patient can tolerate such treatment. Whether these cases represent primary infections or dissemination from a localized site is usually indeterminable.

LABORATORY DIAGNOSIS A specific diagnosis may be made by serologic methods, by demonstrating the organism in smears, or by its cultivation in mice. Toxoplasma can be identified in cerebrospinal fluid sediment with Wright's or Giemsa's stain or occasionally in biopsied lymph node or muscle. Laboratory-reared mice are best for isolation trials from fresh spinal fluid sediment (when acute central nervous system signs are present) or suspensions of tissue.

Serum antibodies can be detected with the dye, immunofluorescence, complement fixation, direct agglutination, and indirect hemagglutination tests. The results are most helpful when they are negative or when a rising titer is demonstrated. Dye test antibodies appear and persist for many years. This is paralleled most closely by the results of the immunofluorescent antibody test. Complement-fixing antibodies are slower to develop and disappear more rapidly. A high dye test titer (1:256 or more) and a negative complement fixation reaction in the same serum suggest either very recently acquired infection or the serologic residual of a previous one. Hemagglutinating antibodies often parallel the dye test, but on occasion the two are quite divergent.

Antibodies of the IgM class are demonstrable by immunofluorescence and can help to identify an active or recent infection. Authenticated, specific reagents are a requisite. On occasion, IgM antibodies seem to appear temporarily, even several years after infection, for reasons which are obscure. This reaction is especially useful in the differentiation of passively transferred antibodies from congenital infection in newborns.

Skin test antigens prepared from mouse peritoneal fluid or embryonated eggs yield reactions of the delayed type. Once quite popular, they are insensitive and nonstandardizable, and their use is not recommended.

TREATMENT There is evidence from the treatment of experimental infections that a combination of sulfonamide and 5-*p*-chlorophenyl-2, 4-diamino-6-ethylpyrimidine (Daraprim) is more effective than either drug by itself. Combinations of sulfadiazine or triple sulfonamides (not sulfisoxazole) and Daraprim have been reported to yield excellent results in some cases of uveitis but have not affected the course of others at all. Information on the effectiveness of this regimen in systemic toxoplasmosis is inadequate; it does appear to shorten the clinical course of acute infections, but does not eradicate encysted organisms. This combination of drugs is not specific for toxoplasmosis, so that the patient's favorable response does not prove the diagnosis. The sulfonamide should be administered in dosage of 2 to 4 g daily with 50 mg Daraprim daily in adults. Since Daraprim is an antifolic agent, leukocyte counts should be determined at least twice weekly. The dosage of Daraprim should be halved after 3 days, and 1 month of treatment certainly constitutes an adequate trial. The leukopenia and thrombocytopenia which may result from Daraprim administration may be helped by the simultaneous administration of leucovorin factor without interfering with the antitoxoplasmic effect of the drug.

Recent experimental data suggest that clindamycin may offer some therapeutic advantages, but its effectiveness in human toxoplasmosis remains to be determined.

REFERENCES

DESMONTS G, COUVREUR J: Congenital toxoplasmosis: A prospective study of 378 pregnancies. N Engl J Med 290:1110, 1974

FELDMAN HA: Toxoplasmosis: An overview. Bull NY Acad Med 50:110, 1974

GLEASON TH, HAMLIN WB: Disseminated toxoplasmosis in the compromised host. Arch Intern Med 134:1059, 1974

MAUMENEE AE, SILVERSTEIN AM: *Immunopathology of Uveitis,* Baltimore: Williams & Wilkins, 1964

REMINGTON JS: Toxoplasmosis in the adult. Bull NY Acad Med 50:211, 1974

TOWNSEND JJ, WOLINSKY JS, et al: Acquired toxoplasmosis: A neglected cause of treatable nervous system disease. Arch Neurol 32:335, 1975

219 PNEUMOCYSTIS CARINII PNEUMONIA (PNEUMOCYSTOSIS, INTERSTITIAL PLASMA CELL PNEUMONIA)

C. GEORGE RAY

DEFINITION *Pneumocystis carinii* pneumonia occurs in patients with impaired antibody and/or cellular immune responses, or severe debility with protein-calorie malnutrition. Progressive pulmonary insufficiency is the cardinal clinical manifestation.

ETIOLOGY *Pneumocystis carinii* has not been cultured, and its taxonomic position remains uncertain; most now consider it to be a protozoan. Histologically, 1 to 2 μm oval or crescentic "merozoite" forms with a single nucleus-like, chromatoid body can be seen. These are usually arranged in groups of two to eight within cysts measuring 5 to 10 μm. Cyst rupture permits release of mature trophozoites, measuring 2 to 4 μm, into alveoli. The crescentic appearance of the cysts is thought to be due to partial collapse after encystment of trophozoites. Electron microscopic studies reveal a complex structure and suggest the capacity for protein synthesis and oxidative metabolism, while structures usually associated with phagocytosis are lacking. The agent can be best visualized with special stains, particularly methenamine silver or Giemsa stains (but not with hematoxylin-eosin), with phase microscopy, and with fluorescent antibody. The organism seen in human beings is morphologically similar to that in animals but species-specific antigenic differences may exist.

EPIDEMIOLOGY Because of the lack of in vitro culture and readily applicable serologic tests, the incidence of *P. carinii* infection is uncertain, and epidemiologic data are based on indirect evidence. It appears that latent infection is not rare in humans and is frequent in many wild, domestic, and laboratory animals. In humans the disease is worldwide and occurs in all age groups either as epidemics in nurseries or as isolated cases. Clinical observations suggest that the disease can be contagious. This is based on evidence suggesting aerosol transmission in nurseries with debilitated and malnourished infants under six months of age, possible spread among patients in cancer hospitals, and isolated reports of intrafamilial spread. However, while it is possible that person-to-person or even animal-to-person spread of infection may occur, the presence of an underlying immunologic or nutritional deficiency is usually required for the development of overt disease. Intrauterine *P. carinii* pneumonia probably acquired by transplacental transmission has also been reported. The incubation period is estimated to be 1 to 2 months.

PATHOGENESIS The organism is of low virulence, proliferates slowly, and may require the presence of another microbial agent for multiplication. When affecting persons in the first year of life, the disease is usually associated with congenital immunodeficiency syndromes or severe protein-calorie malnutrition; in patients over one year of age, it is most commonly a complication of neoplasia, particularly of malignant lymphoreticular disorders, cyclic neutropenia, various anemias, collagen vascular and autoimmune diseases, renal failure, and in patients with transplants who are receiving immunosuppressive drugs and adrenal steroids. Surprisingly, among patients with acute lymphocytic leukemia, the clinical manifestations of infection are most frequently found during periods of remission. *Pneumocystis carinii* pneumonia has also been reported occasionally in the absence of demonstrated underlying disease. Progressive *P. carinii* infection has been produced in various laboratory animals by corticosteroid-induced immunosuppression or malnutrition, both of which apparently activated latent infection.

The largest group of patients with *P. carinii* pneumonia in the past were premature or debilitated newborns in whom the disease, first described as interstitial plasma-cell pneumonia, occurred at about the age of three to four months, often in nursery epidemics. These epidemics are virtually unheard of in this country, and are becoming increasingly rare in other areas, presumably as a result of improved infant nutrition and less crowding. However, cases continue to be reported, now often involving young infants from orphanages in southeast Asia.

Many infections occur together with *P. carinii* pneumonia, and these are often multiple. Acute and chronic bacterial infections are common, and a wide range of concurrent viral, fungal, and some protozoan infections has been observed. Localized and disseminated cytomegalic inclusion disease is a particularly frequent concomitant infection.

PATHOLOGIC FINDINGS In widespread disease the lungs are massively consolidated. The consolidation may be focal and confined to the central or dorsal lung areas. The alveoli are distended by a foamy material which suggests the diagnosis, and, when stained appropriately, the organisms can be seen. Hyaline membranes may be present. The sparse cellular response consists of mononuclear cells. Alveolar septal infiltration with plasma cells (interstitial plasma-cell pneumonia) is prominent in many cases and absent in others. Septal fibrosis is generally slight. The changes appear reversible. Granuloma formation, calcification, and focal and diffuse persistent fibrosis have also been noted. In latent infection the lesions are few and minute, organisms are scanty, the foamy intraalveolar material is lacking, and the cellular response is sparse. The infection is generally confined to the lung, but organisms have been seen in the regional lymph nodes. Pleuritis is characteristically absent, and systemic dissemination with focal lesions in distant sites is extremely rare.

CLINICAL MANIFESTATIONS Generally the onset is insidious. The fully developed clinical picture includes severe dyspnea and tachypnea. The patient displays all signs of extreme air hunger and is anxious and cyanotic. There may be a dry cough which, together with the cyanosis, is aggravated by any movement. Fever is absent or slight. Pulmonary physical findings are scanty in contrast with the grave clinical state and the extensive lung involvement seen roentgenologically. Roentgenograms show hazy alveolar infiltrates spreading from the hilum and eventually affecting most of the lung. Some patients may develop peripheral, somewhat nodular infiltrates, which can be confused with other infections or malignant processes and usually require biopsy for confirmation of the diagnosis. Focal emphysema may be present, but pleural effusions are rare. Blood gas studies indicate impaired diffusion, with severe hypoxemia and normal or only slightly elevated P_{CO_2} values. Other laboratory studies are generally nonrevealing, except for a frequently observed lymphopenia. In young infants with combined immunodeficiency and *P. carinii* infection, significant eosinophilia has been observed. Complications include pneumothorax from a ruptured emphysematous bleb and rib fractures from forced respiratory movements. Death occurs by progressive asphyxia or cardiac failure within 1 to 10 weeks in untreated cases.

The differential diagnosis usually includes viral infection, particularly cytomegalovirus, disseminated pulmonary aspergillosis, and occasionally other bacterial and mycotic infections. In addition, pulmonary alveolar proteinosis, desquamative interstitial pneumonia, pulmonary hemorrhage, and pulmonary fibrosis, either idiopathic or secondary to irradiation or drugs, such as bleomycin, methotrexate, busulfan, cyclophosphamide, or nitrofurantoin, must be considered. The best way to resolve this differential is to do open lung biopsy, whenever possible.

DIAGNOSIS The diagnosis depends on the morphologic demonstration of the organism. Bronchial secretions, tracheal lavage, and various biopsy techniques have been used. Examination of secretions has, in general, yielded poor results but may be improved by fluorescent antibody methods. Needle or open lung biopsy is often diagnostic but carries some risk, particularly in far-advanced cases. Endobronchial brush biopsy has been reported as a simple, frequently successful procedure. Complement fixation and indirect fluorescent antibody tests are also used by some, but have been positive in only 20 to 33 percent of confirmed cases.

PROGNOSIS Morbidity and mortality figures are uncertain. *Pneumocystis carinii* infection is not rare at any age, and it seems likely that it will be recognized more frequently. The prognosis of *P. carinii* pneumonia is grave since it is generally a complication of a severe underlying disorder. A mortality of 40 to 50 percent has been suggested. However, remissions and spontaneous cures have been reported. The outcome is heavily dependent on the course of the underlying disease.

TREATMENT Pentamidine isethionate appears to be effective in the treatment of *P. carinii* infection, and clinical recovery has been reported in a substantial number of treated patients. The drug may be obtained from the Parasitic Disease Drug Service of the National Communicable Disease Control Center in Atlanta, Georgia. The recommended daily dose is 4 mg per kg body weight given by a single intramuscular injection for 12 to 14 days. In desperately ill patients the drug has been given intravenously. The drug is toxic and may produce abscesses and ulcers at the site of injection. Approximately 40 percent of patients also develop systemic side effects including azotemia, hypoglycemia, changes in liver function, and pulmonary fibrosis. Pyrimethamine, 25 to 75 mg daily, and sulfadiazine, 2 to 6 g daily, administered orally in divided dosage, may be effective alternative therapy. In patients with malnutrition and the histopathology of interstitial plasma-cell pneumonia, response to either form of therapy is often very slow. It has been suggested that concomitant corticosteroid therapy might benefit these patients by suppressing the alveolar inflammatory response until the organisms are eradicated. Antibiotics, convalescent serum, and commercial immunoglobulin have no effect. Symptomatic treatment with oxygen and digitalis may be indicated.

REFERENCES

BURKE BA, GOOD RA: *Pneumocystis carinii* infection. Medicine, 57:23, 1973

CROSS AS, STEIGBIGEL RT: *Pneumocystis carinii* pneumonia presenting as localized nodular densities. N Engl J Med 291:831, 1974

DUTZ W: *Pneumocystis carinii* pneumonia. Pathol Annu 5:309, 1971

HUGHES WT et al: *Pneumocystis carinii* pneumonitis in children with malignancies. J Pediatr 82:404, 1973

——: Treatment of pneumocystis carinii pneumonitis with trimethoprim-sulfamethoxazile. Canad Med Assoc J 112:475, 1975

KIRBY HB et al: *Pneumocystis carinii* pneumonia treated with pyrimethamine and sulfadiazine. Ann Intern Med 75:505, 1971

RUSKIN J, REMINGTON JS: The compromised host and infection: I. *Pneumocystis carinii* pneumonia. JAMA 202:1070, 1967

WALZER PD et al: *Pneumocystis carinii* pneumonia in the United States: Epidemiologic, diagnostic and clinical features. Ann Intern Med 80:83, 1974

220
MINOR PROTOZOAN DISEASES

JAMES J. PLORDE

TRICHOMONIASIS Trichomoniasis is a venereal infection caused by the protozoan *Trichomonas vaginalis*. Of the many members of the genus *Trichomonas*, three are parasites of human beings: *T. hominis* in the intestine, *T. tenax* in the oral cavity, and *T. vaginalis*, the only one capable of producing disease, in the vagina, urethra, and prostate. All three exist only in the trophozoite stage and resemble one another morphologically. *Trichomonas vaginalis* is the largest, however, and confusion in diagnosis is rare because of the anatomic specificity of their habits.

Trichomonas vaginalis is transmitted by sexual intercourse. Although the organism may survive on moist washcloths for a few hours, transmission of fomites has not been convincingly demonstrated and is probably rare. Newborn children of infected mothers have, on occasion, acquired the infection. The parasite is cosmopolitan in its distribution, and estimates hold that up to 25 percent of the sexually active population may be infected.

In the female, trichomoniasis usually presents as a persistent vaginitis. Initial manifestations include itching, burning, and profuse, creamy yellow, frothy leukorrhea. This acute stage may persist for a week or months, often fluctuating in intensity; it may worsen following menstruation. Eventually the discharge and other symptoms subside and may actually disappear completely, even though the patient still harbors trichomonads. Examination shows inflammation ranging from mild hyperemia of the vaginal vault to extensive erosion, petechial hemorrhages, and perianal intertrigo.

The prostate and urethra are the usual sites of infection in the male. It may present as persistent or recurring nonspecific urethritis, or, more commonly, it may be completely asymptomatic. Acute purulent urethritis may occur.

The diagnosis is made by examining vaginal, prostatic, or urethral secretions for the presence of *Trichomonas*. The organism may also be found in the sedimented urine. A wet mount will usually reveal numerous motile organisms. A Giemsa-stained preparation is confirmatory. *Trichomonas vaginalis* may be grown in culture, but this technique is not generally available. A variety of serologic tests, including a complement fixation, an indirect hemagglutination, and an immunofluorescent reaction, have been described, but are not generally available or completely reliable.

Trichomonas is sometimes responsible for confusing changes in the cytologic pattern of exfoliated vaginal cells. Moreover, ordinary Papanicolaou preparations are not well suited to the diagnosis, and when trichomoniasis is suspected, fresh material should be looked at immediately.

Oral metronidazole (Flagyl), given either in dosage of 250 mg three times daily for 10 days or in a single 2-g dose, is an extremely effective therapeutic agent. In women, the supplemental use of a 500-mg vaginal insert once daily for 10 days has been recommended. Recurrent treatment of sexual partners will minimize recurrent infections.

The recent evidence that metronidazole is carcinogenic in rodents and mutagenic in bacteria has placed the role of this agent in trichomonas infections in doubt. The drug should not be used in pregnancy until further information on its teratogenicity is available. Some authorities suggest that the drug should not be used at all unless patients cannot be rendered asymptomatic by other means.

GIARDIASIS *Giardia lamblia* is a pear-shaped multiflagellar protozoan that parasitizes the human duodenum and jejunum where it multiplies by longitudinal fission. Under a microscope, its two nuclei give the organism the appearance of a face with two large eyes. It is actively motile but may attach itself to the intestinal mucosa by means of a large ventral sucker. Encystation occurs in transit through the colon. The resulting ovoid cysts are the infective form of the parasite and are transmitted by the fecal-oral route. Waterborne outbreaks of giardiasis have been reported. Two followed ingestion of water from remote mountain streams or ponds, suggesting that wild animals may serve as alternate hosts.

The response to infestation is highly variable and seems related at least in part to host factors. Children are three times more likely to be parasitized than adults and probably have more prominent clinical manifestations. Gastrectomy or decreased gastric acidity in adults may increase their susceptibility. Giardiasis also has been reported frequently in patients with immunoglobulin deficiencies, and may be a major cause of intestinal abnormalities in these patients. Similarly, *G. lamblia* infections appear to be a significant cause of travelers' diarrhea. Unlike the typical syndrome seen in travelers, however, the diarrhea usually begins late in the course of travels and may persist for several weeks.

Most often the infection is asymptomatic, but in some patients nausea, flatulence, epigastric pain, abdominal cramps, distention, and watery diarrhea occur. After a few days the stools may become semisolid, bulky, and malodorous. Symptoms and accompanying weight loss may persist for several weeks. These symptoms are more common in children and are usually self-limited. Rarely, fulminating and extensive duodenal ulceration has been described. Radiographically, asymptomatic carriers may show irritability of the duodenal bulb. Chronic giardiasis may lead to malabsorption of carbohydrate, fat, and vitamin B_{12}. Lactase intolerance and disaccharidase deficiencies have been described. The pathogenesis of these abnormalities is poorly understood. Mechanical blockage of microvilli by the parasites, competition between the organisms and host for nutrients, altered motility, and mucosal invasion have been suggested as possible mechanisms. Jejunal biopsy of patients infested with *Giardia* sometimes shows flattening of the microvilli and an inflammatory infiltrate. Both malabsorption and the jejunal lesions have been reversed with specific treatment.

The diagnosis is made by finding the trophozoite stage of the parasite in duodenal washings, jejunal biopsies, or diarrheal stools. Cyst forms are often passed in solid stool; they contain two to four nuclei and are readily identified when stained with iodine.

Treatment consists of the administration of 0.1 g Atabrine Hydrochloride three times daily for 3 days, a regimen which eliminates the organisms in 90 percent of the cases. Metronidazole 250 mg three times daily for 10 days is tolerated better but may be slightly less effective.

COCCIDIOSIS This is an infrequently recognized disease characterized by fever, diarrhea, abdominal pain, and weight loss which results from ingestion of the oocysts of coccidia belonging to the genus *Isospora*. Coccidia are widespread in the animal kingdom; each vertebrate host harbors a specific species. *Isospora hominis* and *I. belli* are the two that most commonly infect human beings. Parasitization is much more common in children and is worldwide in distribution, particularly in tropical areas.

Like the related plasmodia, there is both an asexual and sexual stage of multiplication. Unlike plasmodia, however, both occur within a single host. Following the ingestion of an oocyst, *sporozoites* are released which invade the epithelial cells of the intestine to become trophozoites. These multiply asexually producing a large number of *merozoites*, which in turn invade other epithelial cells to continue the cycle. In some cells sexual gametocytes are produced. With the fertilization of the female gametocyte, an oocyst is formed which is then passed in the stool. Transmission is by the fecal-oral route. Volunteers develop symptoms about 1 week after the ingestion of viable oocysts. The illness usually has an acute onset with fever, headache, abdominal cramps, and diarrhea. Stools are often fatty and weight loss is common. Coccidiosis may be associated with a malabsorption syndrome and abnormalities of the mucosa in the small bowel. Symptoms, which presumably continue as long as the asexual cycle of multiplication continues, usually subside spontaneously within a few weeks. In some cases, however, they may persist for months or even years, eventually resulting in death.

A peripheral eosinophilia occurs in approximately half of the infected patients. The diagnosis can be made by examination of stool for oocysts. These are often scanty, and concentration techniques such as zinc sulfate flotation or the formol-ether method must usually be employed. Incubation of the stool for 2 days at room temperature improves the recovery rate. Duodenal aspiration and jejunal biopsy are less cumbersome and more reliable.

BALANTIDIASIS *Balantidium coli*, the largest protozoon of human beings, inhabits the large intestine. In addition to producing an asymptomatic carrier state, it elicits disease ranging from mild recurrent diarrhea to fulminant ulceration with perforation and death. In many repects the disease is similar to amebiasis in its range of manifestations, exclusive of spread to the liver.

The illness has been reproduced by feeding the organism

to volunters. The diagnosis is made by finding the trophozoite or cyst in the stool, but repeated examinations may be required because shedding of *Balantidium* is intermittent. The disease is more likely to occur in tropical areas, but at least 60 cases have been reported in the United States. Swine are frequent carriers of *B. coli* and may play an important role in the spread of the disease to humans. Outbreaks have been noted in mental institutions where coprophagy implicated direct person-to-person transmission.

The tetracyclines in ordinary doses are highly effective in treatment, as is metronidazole given in dosage of 750 mg three times daily for 5 or 6 days.

REFERENCES

Balantidiasis

WALZER PD et al: Balantidiasis outbreak in Truk Islands. Am J Trop Med Hyg 22:33, 1973

Coccidiosis

BRANDBORG LL et al: Human coccidiosis: A possible cause of malabsorption. N Engl J Med 283:1306, 1970

SMITSKAMP H, OEY-MULLER E: Geographical distribution and clinical significance of human coccidiosis. Trop Geogr Med 18: 133, 1966

TRIER JS: Chronic intestinal coccidiosis in man: Intestinal morphology and response to treatment. Gastroenterology 66:923, 1974

Giardiasis

AMENT ME, RUBIN CE: Relation of giardiasis to abnormal intestinal structure and function in gastrointestinal immunodeficiency syndromes. Gastroenterology 62:216, 1972

BRADY PG, WOLFE JC: Waterborne giardiasis. Ann Intern Med 81:498, 1974

HOSKINS LC et al: Clinical giardiasis and intestinal malabsorption. Gastroenterology 53:265, 1967

JOKIPII L, JOKIPII AMM: Giardiasis in travelers: A prospective study. J Infect Dis 130:295, 1974

KAMATH KR, MURUGASU R: A comparative study of four methods for detecting *Giardia lamblia* in children with diarrheal disease and malabsorption. Gastroenterology 66:16, 1974

Trichomoniasis

JIROVEC O, PETRU M: *Trichomonas vaginalis* and trichomonas, in *Advances in Clinical Parasitology*, vol. 6, ed B Dawes, London: Academic, 1968, p. 117

KEIGHLEY EE: Trichomonas in a closed community: Efficacy of metronidazole. Br Med J 1:207, 1971

section 17 | Diseases caused by worms

INTRODUCTION

JAMES J. PLORDE

Helminths that parasitize humans can be divided into three major groups: roundworms (nematodes), tapeworms (cestodes), and flukes (trematodes). In contrast to the protozoa, helminths are large, multicellular organisms which have excretory, nervous, and reproductive systems. Of these, trematodes are the most highly differentiated, possessing fully developed male and female sexual organs capable of producing enormous numbers of offspring in the form of eggs, or larvae. With few exceptions these offspring must pass out of the *definitive host* harboring the sexually active adults before they can mature into forms capable of infecting their next host. The eggs of *Enterobius vermicularis* require only a few hours of embryonation on the perianal skin before they become infective. The eggs and larvae of most of the intestinal nematodes, however, require a prolonged period of incubation in soil under appropriate conditions of temperature and humidity, while those of the cestodes and trematodes must undergo developmental changes in one or more *intermediate hosts* before they are capable of completing their life cycle.

These differences in life cycle have a determinative influence on the epidemiology of helminthic parasites. *Enterobius vermicularis,* which can be spread directly from host to host because of its brief embryonation time in the external environment, has a cosmopolitan distribution. The remainder of the intestinal nematodes are spread via contamination of soil by eggs or larvae-containing human excrement. They are thus found in all areas of the world with poor sanitation where the appropriate conditions of temperature and humidity pertain. Finally, the distribution of trematodes such as the various species of *Schistosoma* are limited by the ecologic niches of their intermediate hosts.

Human disease can result when humans serve as either the definitive host, harboring the mature adults (e.g., *Taenia saginata*), or the intermediate host to the larval stages of the worm (e.g., echinococcosis). Occasionally a person may function as both the definitive (*T. solium*) and intermediate host (cysticercosis) for the same helminth. Since most adult helminths are incapable of multiplying within their definitive host, the manifestations of illness are related to the total number of worms acquired by the host. Most small worm load infections are, in fact, asymptomatic, and many need not even be treated. As helminths are usually long-lived, however, repeated infections can result from very high worm loads with disability typical of infections, particularly in endemic areas.

The pathogenesis of helminthic disease is variable. *Diphyllobothrium latum* competes with the host for nutrients, *Strongyloides stercoralis* and *Capillaria philippinensis* interfere with the absorption of food across the intestinal mucosa, and hookworm causes loss of iron, an essential mineral. Other parasites such as *Clonorchis sinensis* and *Schistosoma haematobium* compromise the function of important organs by obstruction and secondary bacterial infections. Long-term infections with both of these organisms can also be carcinogenic. Disease can result from simple mass effect as in the case of echinococcosis. Actual tissue invasion and destruction by larval forms occur in many infections. Immunologic mechanisms are undoubtedly responsible for tissue damage and clinical manifestations in many helminthic diseases.

Once the clinician thinks of the possibility of a helminthic infection, the diagnosis is usually straightforward. Although these infections are not common in this country, the continuous arrival of travelers and immigrants and the importation of food from endemic areas of the world make it necessary to consider them in the differential diagnosis. Patients should be carefully questioned about their travels and food intake. Many helminths can survive within the host for a decade or more after he leaves an endemic area.

Although eosinophilia has long been recognized as a clue to the presence of helminthic infections, the failure to detect it does not preclude this diagnosis. The eosinophilia presumably reflects an immunologic response to the complex foreign proteins of the worm and is most marked during the early stages of tissue migration and invasion. Once migration ceases and the worm matures to adulthood, the eosinophilia may diminish or disappear.

The definitive diagnosis ususally rests upon the recovery and morphologic identification of the parasite in stool, urine, sputum, blood, or tissues. Because these parasites are so antigenically complex, serologic and skin tests have been much less reliable than in the case of microbes or protozoa. They are very helpful, however, in the diagnosis of a few helminthic diseases such as trichinosis and echinococcosis.

The goal of treatment is the reduction of worm load. Since most helminths do not multiply within the body and because disability is usually related to the intensity of infection, total eradication of the parasite is often unnecessary. Moreover, the toxicity of many of the anthelmintics makes attempts at cure unwise. When, as in the case of strongyloidiasis, the presence of even a light worm load can be dangerous, when the chance of reinfection is slight, and/or when the anthelmintic agent in question is without serious side effects, cure should be pursued.

Many anthelmintics are not generally available in the United States or have not yet been approved for use in that country. Fortunately, many of these are available through the Parasitic Disease Drug Service of the Center for Disease Control in Atlanta, Georgia (Table 1).

TABLE 1
Anthelmintics available from the Parasitic Disease Drug Service*

Infection	*Therapeutic agent*
Dracunculosis	Niridazole (Ambilhar)
Onchocerciasis	Suramin (Antrypol)
Schistosomiasis	Sodium antimony dimercaptosuccinate (Astiban)
Tapeworms (*T. saginata, T. solium, Hymenolepis nana, H. diminuta, Diphyllobothrium latum, Dipylidium caninum*)	Niclosamide (Yomesan)

* *Center for Disease Control, Atlanta, Ga. 30333.*

NEMATODE INFECTIONS

Nematodes are elongated, cylindrical, unsegmented organisms that vary in size from the tiny *Trichinella spiralis* and *Strongyloides stercoralis,* which are a few millimeters in length, to *Dracunculus medinensis,* which may measure more than a meter. They have a simple tubular digestive tract running from the mouth in the anterior end to the anus located ventrally near the tail. The sexes are separate, and the male, which is usually smaller than the female, generally has a curved posterior end. The life span varies from 1 to 2 months in the case of *T. spiralis* and *Enterobius vermicularis* to 10 years or more for hookworms. During this time the gravid female produces enormous numbers of progeny either as fertile eggs or larvae. With the sole exception of *Trichinella,* these offspring must undergo a period of development outside the definitive host.

Among the intestinal nematodes, this period of development occurs without the benefit of intermediate hosts. The eggs of *E. vermicularis,* or pinworm, are fully embryonated when laid and become infective within hours of being deposited on the perianal skin. After being ingested, these eggs mature into adult worms within the alimentary tract of humans. The life cycle of the whipworm, *Trichuris trichiura,* is similar except that the eggs must pass in the stool and incubate several weeks in soil before becoming infective for humans on ingestion. The external devel-

TABLE 2
Life cycle of intestinal nematodes

Species	*Route of infection*	*Migration in body*	*Diagnostic form*	*Site of larval development*	*Infective form*	*Free-living stage*
Enterobius vermicularis	Mouth	Intestinal	Egg	Perineum	Egg	No
Trichuris trichiura	Mouth	Intestinal	Egg	Soil	Egg	No
Ascaris lumbricoides	Mouth	Pulmonary	Egg	Soil	Egg	No
*Necator americanus**	Skin	Pulmonary	Egg	Soil	Filariform larvae	No
Strongyloides stercoralis	Skin	Pulmonary	Rhabditiform larvae	Soil, intestine†	Filariform larvae	Yes

* *Also* Ancylostoma duodenale.
† *Intestine only in cases of autoinfection.*

opment of *Ascaris lumbricoides* eggs is identical. However, following ingestion, the embryonated eggs hatch, releasing larvae which penetrate the intestinal wall and are carried to the pulmonary capillaries via the bloodstream. Here they penetrate the alveoli, ascend the respiratory tract, and reach the glottis. Then, after completing their pulmonary migration, the larvae are swallowed, regain the intestinal lumen, and develop into mature adults.

The eggs of *Strongyloides* and of hookworm, in contrast to those of the above three, hatch shortly before (*Strongyloides*) or after (hookworm) being passed in the stool, producing rhabditiform soil larvae. Following several molts, these larvae are transformed into infective or filariform larvae, penetrate human skin, and after migrating through the lung in the manner described above for *Ascaris,* reach the intestine.

The life cycle of *Strongyloides* differs from that of hookworm in two important respects. First, rhabditiform larvae may, under certain conditions, develop into free-living adult male and female worms which reproduce in the soil. Second, rhabditiform larvae may develop into the infective filariform larvae while still within the human intestine. These may then reinfect the original host directly (autoinfection) without first going through a period of incubation in the external environment (Table 2).

The offspring of the tissue nematodes such as *Dracunculus* and the filarial worms undergo their development in a second invertebrate host before they can complete their maturation in the human.

The nematodes infecting humans are usually divided into intestinal and tissue parasites. Those which produce clinical manifestations by virtue of the presence of the adult worm within the human alimentary tract are considered intestinal nematodes; they include *Enterobius, Trichuris, Ascaris,* the hookworms, and *Strongyloides.* A number of closely related nematodes infecting animals such as *Toxacara canis* and *Ancylostoma braziliense* which may infect, but usually fail to reach maturity within, humans will also be included in this group in the following discussion. Listed among the tissue nematodes are those which produce disease by the migration of the adult and/or larval forms through tissues such as *Trichinella,* the filarial worms, and *Dracunculus.*

221 INTESTINAL NEMATODES

JAMES J. PLORDE

ENTEROBIASIS Definition Enterobiasis (pinworm, seatworm, or threadworm infection; oxyuriasis) is an intestinal infection of man caused by *Enterobius vermicularis* and characterized by perianal pruritus. It has been estimated that the worm infects 200 million people, 18 million of them in the United States and Canada.

Etiology The female averages 10 mm in length, the male 3 mm. They live with their heads attached to the mucosa of the cecum, appendix, and adjacent parts of the bowel. The gravid female migrates through the anal canal at night, deposits her 10,000 eggs on the perianal skin, and dies. In female patients the worm may enter the vagina and occasionally gain access to the peritoneal cavity through the fallopian tubes. Each egg contains an embryo which, within a few hours, develops into an infective larva. After the egg has been ingested, the larva is released in the small intestine and migrates down the bowel lumen to the cecum. In less than 1 month from the time of ingestion, newly developed gravid females are again discharging eggs. They are planoconvex and measure approximately 20 by 50 μm. The shell is clear and doubly contoured.

Epidemiology Humans are usually infected by the direct transfer of eggs from the anus to the mouth by way of contaminated fingers. Retroinfection may occur when the eggs hatch in the perianal area and the larvae migrate back into the bowel to become mature adults. The eggs, which are relatively resistant to desiccation, also contaminate nightclothes and bed linen, where they remain viable and infective for a few days. Airborne transmission is possible, and spread within family and children's groups occurs readily. Enterobiasis is found in all climates and is probably the most common helminthic infection of humans. Its low incidence in some tropical areas, however, defies explanation.

Clinical manifestations The most common symptom is pruritus ani, which is most troublesome at night, being related to the migration of the gravid female worms. Irritability, insomnia, enuresis, and other minor complaints are probably secondary to the pruritus. Scratching may lead to perianal eczema or pyogenic infection. Vaginal discharge has been reported, and rarely a chronic granulomatous salpingitis or endometritis results from the presence of ectopic adults. Other rare ectopic locations include the lung, liver, and peritoneum.

Laboratory findings Examination for ova of material obtained from the perianal skin by means of a Scotch brand cellophane tape swab is the preferable method for the detection of enterobiasis. The tape is folded sticky side out over the end of a tongue blade, pressed firmly against the perianal area, and then spread on a glass slide and examined under the lower power of a microscope. The swab should be taken at home by the patient on 3 to 5 consecutive mornings prior to bathing and brought to the laboratory for examination. Searching for ova in the feces is rarely helpful, but scrapings from under the nails may reveal ova. The diagnosis is sometimes made by finding adult worms in the perianal area or in the feces following a laxative or an enema. Eosinophilic leukocytosis is not a typical finding.

Treatment All infected individuals in a family or communal group should be treated simultaneously. The frequently recommended sanitary measures aside from hand washing before meals and after stools are of dubious benefit. It is relatively easy to eradicate the worms, but reinfection is frequent. Retreatment does not appear necessary unless symptoms recur.

Two highly satisfactory drugs are available. Pyrantel pamoate (Banminth) given in a single oral dose of 11 mg per kg (maximum 1.0 g) is probably the drug of choice. Alternatively, a single 100 mg oral dose of mebendazole (Vermox) can be used. This drug is not recommended for infants or pregnant women. Pyrvinium pamoate (Povan) and piperazine citrate are equally effective but less convenient. The former is given orally as a single dose of 5 mg per kg in tablet or liquid form. This compound turns the stool red and may stain bedclothes or undergarments. Piperazine citrate is given in dosage of 65 mg per kg (maximum 2.5 g) once daily for 8 days. When renal insufficiency is present, the dose should be reduced to avoid neurotoxicity. In heavily contaminated environments, treatment with the above drugs may be repeated after an interval of 2 weeks to eliminate any new infections.

Prevention Methods of preventing autoinfection and dissemination within a group involving children are extremely difficult to enforce. Personal environmental hygiene should be stressed, and anthelmintic and symptomatic treatment of pruritus ani should be instituted. To control infection within a group, simultaneous treatment of all cases is mandatory.

TRICHURIASIS Definition Trichuriasis (whipworm infection; trichocephaliasis) is an intestinal infection of man caused by *Trichuris trichiura* and is characterized by invasion of the colonic mucosa by the adult trichuris. Five hundred million people are thought to be infected with this parasite.

Etiology The adult whipworms are found in the large intestine with their anterior ends deeply embedded in the mucosa. They are 30 to 50 mm in length and possess a threadlike anterior two-thirds with a stouter posterior third, giving them a whiplike structure. The female produces about 5,000 eggs each day. They are characteristically barrel-shaped (20 by 50 μm), brown, thick-walled, and translucent with knoblike ends. The eggs, like those of *Ascaris,* must incubate at least 3 weeks in soil before they become infective. After ingestion, the eggs hatch in the small intestine and the larvae become embedded in the intestinal villi. After several days they migrate to the large intestine where they mature in about 3 months. The adult worms may live for 4 to 8 years.

Epidemiology Whipworm is a cosmopolitan parasite but is most commonly found in the tropics where the level of sanitation is low and environmental conditions necessary for the incubation of the eggs are optimal. In the United States, it is found throughout the rural areas of the Southeast. Its distribution is similar to that of *Ascaris* and hookworm, but the eggs are less resistant than those of *Ascaris* to sunlight and drying. Because of their general lack of sanitary habits, children have the highest incidence of infection. For example, 13 percent of patients confined to hospitals for the mentally subnormal were found to harbor *Trichuris.*

Pathogenesis and clinical manifestations Symptomatic infection generally requires the presence of large numbers of adult whipworms and may be correlated in part with the degree of mucosal involvement. Heavy infections usually occur only in children and may be accompanied by nausea, abdominal pain, diarrhea, and dysentery. It has been estimated that infected patients lose 0.005 ml blood per worm per day. Infections with more than 800 worms often results in anemia. In heavier infections, the distribution of worms throughout the colon and rectum may result in rectal prolapse while straining at stool. Some investigators also feel that *Trichuris* infections predispose to amebic dysentery and bacterial gastroenteritis.

Laboratory findings In symptomatic infection, large numbers of eggs are present in the feces, and there may be eosinophilic leukocytosis and anemia. In light infections, concentration techniques may be necessary to recover the eggs. Quantitation of egg output is helpful since only counts above 10,000 eggs per g feces are likely to be associated with symptoms. Stools should be cultured for bacterial pathogens and examined for the presence of *E. histolytica.*

Treatment Treatment is unsatisfactory. Mebendazole in the oral dose of 100 mg twice daily for 3 days is the drug of choice. Its cure rate is 60 to 70 percent, and it achieves a 90 percent reduction in egg burden. It is not recommended for children under the age of two or pregnant women. Thiabendazole, 25 mg per kg twice daily for 2 to 3 days, will cure a small percentage of cases. A single dose of 25 mg/kg/day for 11 to 30 days may be more effective. Diphetarsone, an oral pentavalent arsenical, has been found effective in trichuriasis and is undergoing further trials.

Prognosis Whipworm infection, unless characterized by severe diarrhea, blood loss, and systemic reaction, usually responds well to treatment. Serious infections may require supportive treatment as well as chemotherapy.

Prevention Measures recommended for ascariasis apply also to trichuriasis.

ASCARIASIS Definition Ascariasis is an infection of humans caused by *Ascaris lumbricoides* and characterized by an early pulmonary phase related to larval migration and a later, prolonged intestinal phase. It is estimated that 25 percent of the world's population, including 1 million Americans, are infected with this nematode.

Etiology The adult ascarids are large (15 to 40 cm in length), cylindric worms with blunt ends which maintain themselves in the lumen of the jejunum by virtue of their muscular activity. Despite a life span of only 6 to 18 months, the female releases millions of eggs, both fertile and infertile, into the fecal stream; the daily output is estimated to be 200,000 per worm. Fertilized eggs are elliptic (30 to 40 μm by 50 to 60 μm) with an irregular, dense outer shell and a regular, translucent inner shell. They require a period of soil incubation before they become infective. Under optimum conditions of warmth and moisture this occurs in 2 to 3 weeks. The eggs may then remain viable for several months. When an infective egg is ingested, the larva is liberated in the small intestine. It migrates through the wall and is carried by the bloodstream or lymphatics to the lung. After about 10 days in the pulmonary capillaries and alveoli, the larvae pass in turn up the bronchioles, bronchi, trachea, and epiglottis, are swallowed, and return to the jejunum. There they develop into mature adult worms within 2 to 3 months of ingestion. *Ascaris suum,* a roundworm of pigs, may occasionally complete a similar life cycle in humans.

Epidemiology Infection follows the ingestion of the embryonated eggs contained in contaminated food, or, more commonly, the introduction of the eggs into the mouth by the hands after contact with contaminated soil. Geophagia may produce massive infections. In endemic areas, the infection is maintained primarily by small children who defecate indiscriminately in the area of the home. In dry, windy climates, eggs may become airborne, get into the mouth, and be swallowed. Since the eggs are relatively resistant to desiccation and wide variations in temperature, the disease is worldwide. In the developing areas of the world where the lack of sanitary facilities exposes populations to the greatest risk, the prevalence of infection may be as high as 80 to 90 percent; children are almost universally infected in these areas. In temperate areas, the infection occurs in family clusters.

Pathogenesis and clinical manifestations Because of the extensive migration of which both the larvae and adults are capable, the manifestations may be diverse. Bronchopneumonia characterized by fever, cough, wheeze, eosinophilic leukocytosis, and migratory pulmonary infiltrates may occur during the passage of the larvae through the lung. The severity of symptoms is apparently related to both intensity of infection and the degree of sensitization resulting from previous exposures. Significant arterial oxygen desaturation and, rarely, death may occur. Adult worms may produce no symptoms if the infection is light and may be detected accidentally when the adult worm is vomited or passed in the stool. Heavier infections may cause abdominal pain, and occasionally a bolus of worms may result in volvulus, intussusception, or intestinal obstruction in the iliocecal area. Children are most likely to have these complications because of their anatomically smaller intestine and larger worm loads. Up to 2,000 worms have been found in children, although the usual load is less than 50. Obstruction often follows a febrile illness or drug therapy which stimulates the worms to increase motility. Rarely, an adult worm will migrate into the appendix, bile ducts, or pancreatic ducts, causing obstruction and inflammation of these organs. Biliary tract obstruction may be associated with bacterial cholangitis and liver abscess. Worms may also penetrate the intestinal wall, particularly at a site of surgical anastomosis, and patients should be dewormed prior to elective surgery. Migration of the worms into the oral pharynx and mouth may lead to acute respiratory distress.

It seems likely that large worm loads may interfere with the growth of marginally nourished children, probably by competing for nutrients.

Laboratory findings The diagnosis is usually made by finding the ova in the feces. The fertilized eggs are usually numerous, characteristic, and not easily confused with those of other helminths. The occasional unisexual infection may pose diagnostic problems. The male produces no eggs, and the unfertilized ova produced by a single female may be atypical and difficult to recognize. Occasionally the worms may be seen after a barium meal, either as negative images or after ingesting barium themselves. Ascaris pneumonia may be diagnosed by finding larvae and eosinophils in the sputum or gastric aspirate. Eggs will usually not be found until after the larvae have matured in the intestine. Eosinophilic leukocytosis is usually noted during larval migration, but diminishes and often disappears during the chronic intestinal phase of infection.

Treatment Only symptomatic treatment can be used during the period of pulmonary involvement by the migrating larvae. For removal of the adult worms from the intestines, piperazine citrate, as a flavored syrup administered in a single dose after breakfast on two successive days, will cure the majority of cases. The drug acts by paralyzing the ascarids, which are then passed in the stool. The dose of piperazine is 75 mg per kg with a maximum of 4 g. No particular dietary regulation is necessary. The drug must be administered with caution to patients with renal insufficiency, because impaired elimination may produce neurotoxic signs. In intestinal obstruction, nasogastric suction should be initiated. After vomiting is controlled, piperazine should be given through the nasogastric tube every 12 to 24 h in dosage of 65 mg per kg (maximum 1.0 g) for six doses. Surgery usually is not required.

Two newer drugs, pyrantel pamoate and mebendazole, have both been highly effective. Pyrantel is given in the dose of 11 mg per kg (maximum 1.0 g) once daily for 3 days. Mebendazole is given as described for trichuriasis, above. Thiabendazole (see Strongyloidiasis below) or biphenium hydroxynaphthoate (see Hookworm Disease below) may also be used. When both ascariasis and trichuriasis are present, treatment with mebendazole is effective. When both ascariasis and infection with *Ancylostoma duodenale* are present, treatment with pyrantel, mebendazole, or biphenium hydroxynaphthoate is recommended.

Prognosis The prognosis in intestinal infection is generally good. When acute or chronic obstruction of ducts of hollow viscera has occurred, the immediate prognosis is determined by the promptness of diagnosis and treatment.

Prevention Ascariasis is primarily a household infection of rural areas. All infections should be treated, personal hygiene stressed, and adequate toilet facilities provided.

TOXOCARIASIS (VISCERAL LARVA MIGRANS) Definition This is a human infection with *Toxocara canis* or *T. cati.* The animal ascarids are usually unable to complete their life cycle in humans, but they may be widely disseminated in the body, producing a variety of clinical manifestations, collectively referred to as *visceral larva migrans.*

Etiology and epidemiology The large adult toxocaral worms live in the intestine of cats and dogs. Their eggs must be passed in the stool and incubate in soil for 2 to 3 weeks before they become infective. If the ova are then ingested by a human, larvae are liberated in the intestine, penetrate the wall, and are carried in the blood to the liver, where most remain, and lung. At the time the larvae reach the pulmonary capillaries, they are still very small (approximately one-half the size of *A. lumbricoides*), and many pass through the lungs to reach the systemic circulation. Larvae penetrate the tissues where their gradually increasing size approaches the diameter of the vessel through which they are traveling. Rarely the organisms break into the alveoli, ascend the respiratory tract, and are swallowed to reach the small intestine where they mature into adult worms. *Toxocara* infections of cats and dogs are common and widespread; viable ova were found in 25 percent of soil samples taken from public parks in Great Britain. Although most human infections have been reported from the United States and Europe, it seems likely that the disease is present in other areas of the world as well. Children from the age of two to five years, because of their sanitary habits and intimate association with domestic pets, are most frequently involved. In Great Britain, 4 percent of children who play in public parks have positive skin tests to *Toxocara* antigens.

Pathogenesis and clinical manifestations The larvae migrate freely in tissues, causing hemorrhage, necrosis, eosinophilic inflammatory reaction, and eventually granuloma formation. The most frequently involved organs are the liver, lungs, brain, eye, heart, and skeletal muscles. Symptoms and signs are related to the number and location of the granulomas as well as sensitization to the parasite antigen. Most frequently, patients present with fever and tender hepatomegaly. Splenomegaly, skin rash, and recurrent pneumonitis with wheezing respirations may occur in more severe infections. Respiratory failure with death has been reported. There is often a history of dirt eating and contact with cats and dogs. Leukocytosis with eosinophilia to high levels (over 60 percent) and hypergammaglobulinemia are common. Anti-IgG factors have been reported in the serum of children with this syndrome. These manifestations may persist for several months. At surgery or autopsy the liver may be studded with small granulomas. A granulomatous endophthalmitis, which may be mistaken for retinoblastoma, convulsions, focal neurologic defects, and myocarditis may also be observed. Asymptomatic infection is probably common.

Diagnosis The diagnosis can usually be made on the basis of clinical findings. Infections with *A. lumbricoides*, hookworm, and *Strongyloides stercoralis*, as well as other nonhuman nematodes, may also on occasion present as visceral larva migrans, making the etiologic diagnosis difficult. Eosinophilic leukemia, trichinosis, and periarteritis nodosa must be ruled out. Isoagglutinin titers of 1:1024 or greater are often present. Antibodies to *Toxocara* and *Ascaris* antigens may be found, but, as with the isoagglutinins, these tests are neither very sensitive nor specific. A standardized skin test and indirect hemagglutination and fluorescent antibody tests have been developed but are not generally available. A definitive diagnosis depends on the identification of the larvae in sputum or tissue granuloma. Biopsy of the liver with serial sections of the specimen may reveal eosinophilic granulomas or a *Toxocara* larva.

Treatment No uniformly effective therapy is available. Diethylcarbamazine as used in bancroftian filariasis (Chap. 224) is probably the drug of choice. Thiabendazole in dosage of 25 to 50 mg per kg for 7 to 10 days may be helpful. Adrenocortical steroids may be beneficial when respiratory difficulty is pronounced. Control measures are directed toward preventing ingestion of eggs. Removal and repeated worming of infected cats and dogs must be considered. Animals less than six months of age should be wormed monthly; older ones every 2 or 3 months.

ANISAKIASIS Ascarids belonging to family Anisakidae infect seals, dolphins, porpoises, whales, and other large sea mammals. Their larval stages are found in the flesh of several marine fish including cod, salmon, and herring. Humans are infected by eating raw, pickled, or slightly salted fish delicacies such as "green herring," sashimi, sunomono, creviche, and gravlax which contain the third-stage larvae. The infection may be asymptomatic and noted only when the worm is coughed or vomited up. More characteristically, the larvae burrow into the mucosa of the stomach, small intestine, or more rarely the colon. Here they produce eosinophilic granulomatous tumors with edema, thickening, and induration of the bowel wall which may be mistaken for gastric carcinoma or regional enteritis. Occasionally, larvae may penetrate the intestinal wall to involve other abdominal organs. Perforations of the bowel with peritonitis have also been described. The pathologic changes are thought to be the result of a hypersensitivity reaction. In these invasive forms of the disease the patient may develop epigastric pain, nausea, and vomiting within a few hours of ingesting infected fish, and the clinical picture may be severe enough to simulate an acute surgical abdomen. More commonly, colicky pain, diffuse abdominal tenderness, fever, and leukocytosis develop a week or more after the ingestion of fish. Peripheral eosinophilia is not always present, and a definitive diagnosis can be made only by the identification of larvae in tissue. Serologic tests are being developed, but are neither highly reliable nor generally available. The disease usually subsides spontaneously with conservative therapy. Occasionally, a chronic illness develops which requires surgical resection of the lesion.

Hundreds of cases have been recognized in the Netherlands and Japan, and several cases have been reported from North America. The disease can be prevented by storing marine fish at $-20°C$ for a single day or by cooking it at normal cooking temperatures.

HOOKWORM DISEASE Definition Hookworm disease is a symptomatic infection caused by *Ancylostoma duodenale* or *Necator americanus*. Asymptomatic infection may be termed simply *hookworm infection*, and the individual with such infection is called a *carrier*.

Etiology *Ancylostoma duodenale*, also known as the "Old World" hookworm, possesses four prominent hooklike teeth in its adult stage. The adults are about 1 cm long and inhabit the upper part of the human small intestine, where they attach to the mucosa by means of the mouth parts and suck blood. Each adult extracts approximately 0.20 ml blood daily. The adults migrate within the small intestine, and each site of attachment persists temporarily as a bleeding point. Following fertilization, the female liberates approximately 20,000 eggs per day. They measure about 40 to

60 μm and are usually in the two-to-four-celled stage when discharged in the feces.

Necator americanus, the "New World" hookworm, has a buccal capsule containing dorsal and ventral plates rather than teeth. It is slightly smaller, deposits fewer eggs, and causes much less blood loss than *A. duodenale* (0.03 ml per worm daily). *Ancylostoma cylonicum,* a hookworm of cats found in the Far East, may occasionally reach maturity in humans.

The life cycles of both hookworms are similar. Under appropriate conditions, the eggs hatch in 24 to 48 h, releasing free-living or rhabditiform larvae. Within a few days, these develop into infective or filariform larvae which may remain viable in the soil for several weeks. These, in turn, penetrate the skin to enter vessels which carry them to the lungs. The larvae leave the alveolar capillaries, enter the alveoli, ascend the respiratory tree, enter the pharynx, and are swallowed. They reach the intestine about 1 week after penetration of the skin and mature within 5 weeks. Adults have been known to survive in the human intestine for as long as 14 years, but *A. duodenale* seldom persists beyond 6 to 8 years, and most *N. americanus* infections are eliminated within 2 to 4 years.

Epidemiology It has been estimated that hookworms infect 700 million people and cause the loss of 7 million liters of blood daily throughout the world from 45°N to 30°S latitude. *Necator americanus* is found predominantly in the tropical areas of Africa, Asia, and the Americas, while *A. duodenale* occurs in the Mediterranean Basin, the Middle East, northern India, China, and Japan. In many areas both species are found. In general, *Ancylostoma* presents a greater public health hazard than *N. americanus,* the species which is most prevalent in the southern United States, because it is most persistent in the environment, more harmful to the host, and less amenable to treatment. Conditions conducive to the development of the hookworm egg into infective filariform larvae are a mean temperature between 23 and 33°C, abundant rainfall, shade, and well-drained sandy soil. Hookworm infection occurs where there is opportunity for disease contact of the skin with soil contaminated by promiscuous defecation. The disease may also be acquired by oral ingestion of infective larvae, particularly those of *A. duodenale.* Probably because of greater exposure, males show a higher incidence of infection than females. Infections are particularly common in closed, heavily populated communities such as coffee or tea plantations.

Repeated infections of hookworm in dogs result in immunity and elimination of the parasite. It seems probable that a similar phenomenon occurs in human infections. When the possibility of reinfection is eliminated, the majority of worms is eliminated spontaneously within 1 or 2 years.

Pathogenesis and clinical manifestations During the invasion of the exposed skin by the larvae, there may be an erythematous maculopapular skin rash and edema with severe pruritus. These manifestations, which may persist for several days, are more marked in *N. americanus* infection. The lesions are most common about the feet, particularly between the toes, and have been termed "ground itch."

During migration through the lungs, cough, pneumonia, and, in severe infections, fever may occur. Usually, however, pulmonary involvement does not give rise to clinical symptoms.

Various gastrointestinal symptoms, ranging from vague epigastric distress and pica to typical ulcer pain, have been reported in association with hookworm infection. Roentgenographic studies may reveal nonspecific changes such as excessive peristalsis and "puddling," particularly in the proximal jejunum. However, gross and microscopic examination of the bowel itself reveals conspicuously little damage. Previous reports of absorptive abnormalities in hookworm infection have not been supported.

The major clinical manifestations of hookworm disease clearly are those of iron-deficiency anemia and hypoalbuminemia consequent to chronic intestinal blood loss. Whether anemia develops and how severe it becomes depends on the balance between iron lost in the gut and iron absorbed from the diet. In many endemic areas, dietary iron is largely of vegetable origin and is absorbed poorly. General dietary deficiency also may lower resistance to parasitic infections. The severity of the disease and the prognosis depend on such factors as the age of the patient, the magnitude of the worm burden, the duration of the disease, and diet. Young children often have extreme anemia, with cardiac insufficiency and anasarca. These conditions may precipitate kwashiorkor. Those who survive to puberty show retarded physical, mental, and sexual development. Milder degrees of the disease, as seen in older children and adults, are characterized by lassitude, dyspnea, palpitation, tachycardia, constipation, and pallor of the skin and mucous membranes.

Asymptomatic infections outnumber symptomatic infections, considering all age groups, 20 to 40 times in endemic areas. The worm burden is small in asymptomatic infections, and the carrier state may be indicative of some degree of acquired host resistance.

Laboratory findings In symptomatic infection, hookworm eggs are usually numerous enough to be detected by microscopic examination of a direct or concentrated fecal smear. A quantitative egg count, using the Stoll or Beaver technique, allows an estimation of the intensity of infection. If a stool specimen is allowed to stand for several hours before examination, the eggs may hatch, releasing larvae which are easily confused with those of *Strongyloides.* The eggs must be differentiated from those of *Trichostrongylus* and *Ternidens diminutus,* which are larger and in a later stage of maturation when observed in a fresh fecal specimen than are those of *Necator* or *Ancylostoma.* Abdominal and pulmonary symptoms appear before the eggs are discharged, although a presumptive diagnosis may be made on the basis of the clinical history and the eosinophilic leukocytosis. The feces seldom contain gross blood in hookworm disease, although tests for occult blood are usually positive.

Generally, the leukocyte count is normal. However, in some early cases, leukocytosis may be marked, with an eosinophilia as high as 70 or 80 percent. The anemia is characteristically hypochromic and microcytic.

The species of hookworm may be determined by the

identification of the adult worm passed in the stool following treatment or by culturing the feces and identifying the third-stage larvae. This is seldom important in clinical practice.

Differential diagnosis Since hookworm disease occurs in areas in which beriberi and malaria are also common, these diseases must be differentiated from hookworm disease, or their coexistence must be established.

Treatment Therapy specific for the infection and directed toward the improvement of nutrition and the anemia should be considered simultaneously. In the usual case, anthelmintics may be administered immediately, followed by iron and a high-protein diet. A number of satisfactory anthelmintic agents are available, but two, pyrantel pamoate (see Ascariasis above) and mebendazole (see Trichuriasis above) are currently favored. Where expense remains a major consideration, the drug of choice is tetrachloroethylene (TCE). It is highly effective, nontoxic, inexpensive, and ideal for mass treatment. (The U. S. P. tetrachloroethylene available to veterinarians may be used.) In most instances a single dose of this agent will decrease the worm load substantially. Complete cure may require several courses of treatment but is not necessary in endemic areas; the aim of therapy is reduction of the worm load to an asymptomatic level. Tetrachloroethylene is administered as a single 5-ml oral dose. Children should receive 0.12 ml per kg (to a maximum of 5 ml) by the same route. The night before treatment, the patient is permitted a light fat-free meal. The following morning, breakfast is omitted and the drug is administered. No food is permitted for 4 h and no alcohol for 24 h. Treatment can be repeated in a week if complete cure is desired and has not been accomplished. If ascariasis is also present, it should be treated first with piperazine citrate (see Ascariasis above).

Biphenium hydroxynaphthoate (Alcopar) is also a drug of low toxicity which is said to be more effective than TCE against *A. duodenale* but possibly less effective against *N. americanus.* In mixed infections with *Ascaris* it can be used alone because it is active against both types of parasite. A single dose of 5 g biphenium hydroxynaphthoate is dispersed in water and ingested in the morning on an empty stomach. No food is permitted for 2 h, and no purgation is recommended. The dose for children is the same as for adults. In *N. americanus* infections, treatment should be repeated on three consecutive days. Another drug which has been introduced for treatment of hookworm infections is thiabendazole (Mintezol). This is a broad-spectrum drug which is effective against *Ascaris, Trichuris,* and *Strongyloides* as well as hookworm. The dose is 25 mg per kg twice a day for 2 or 3 days. Twenty-five percent of patients treated with this agent develop nausea and vomiting. Bitoscanate (Jonit) in oral dosage of 100 mg every 12 h for three doses is equally effective against *N. americanus* and *A. duodenale.* It is not available in the United States.

The anemia requires iron replacement. When anemia is severe and there is malnutrition with anasarca, blood transfusions and a high-protein diet should be given before drug treatment is begun. Blood should be given in an amount sufficient to raise the hemoglobin level to 10 g per 100 ml. In advanced cases it may be necessary to delay drug treatment for 2 to 3 weeks.

Prognosis The immediate prognosis is good. When opportunity for reinfection persists and nutrition cannot be maintained, a state of chronic debility develops. Maturation of children is impaired, and intercurrent disease is a serious problem in adults.

Prevention Many of the measures required are obvious but difficult to apply on a large scale. Even if facilities for proper disposal of feces are provided, it is no simple matter to educate the population in their use. Soil pollution must be eliminated. Avoidance of direct skin contact with the soil (by wearing shoes) is often not practical in endemic areas. Periodic mass treatment of the population has been used in some hookworm control programs.

CUTANEOUS LARVA MIGRANS (CREEPING ERUPTION)

Definition Creeping eruption is an infection of human skin caused by the larvae of the dog and cat hookworm, *A brasiliense.* The other dog hookworms, *A. caninum* and *Uncinaria stenocephala,* as well as the human parasites, *Strongyloides stercoralis* and *Necator americanus,* may also produce the disease. The larvae of *Gnathostoma spinigerum,* a nematode found in the Orient, and *Gasterophilus,* the horse bat fly, may produce a similar cutaneous infection.

Etiology *Ancylostoma brasiliense* reaches adulthood regularly only in the dog and cat. The larvae emerging from eggs discharged in the feces develop to the filariform stage and then are capable of penetrating the skin. In humans, the larvae usually remain in the skin and migrate, producing an irregular erythematous tunnel visible on the skin surface.

Epidemiology and distribution Transmission to humans requires environmental temperature and humidity appropriate for development of the egg to the infective filariform larva stage. Beaches and other moist, sandy areas are hazardous, because animals choose such areas for defecation, and the *A. brasiliense* eggs develop well in such soil. In the United States infection is found in the southern Atlantic and Gulf states.

Pathogenesis and clinical manifestations The site of penetration of the skin by the larvae becomes apparent in a few hours. The migration of the larvae in the skin is accompanied by severe itching. Scratching may lead to bacterial infection. In the course of 1 week, the initial red papule develops into an irregular, erythematous, linear lesion which may attain a length of 15 to 20 cm. The larvae may persist for weeks to months without treatment.

Loeffler's syndrome has been observed in 26 of 52 cases of creeping eruption. Transient, migratory pulmonary infiltrations associated with an increased number of eosinophils in the blood and sputum were interpreted as an allergic reaction to the helminthic infection.

Laboratory findings Eosinophils occur in the lesion, but eosinophilic leukocytosis is slight, except when Loeffler's syndrome appears. The percentage of eosinophils in the blood may then rise to 50 percent and in the sputum to 90 percent. Only rarely are larvae found on skin biopsy.

Treatment Thiabendazole is the drug of choice; it should be given orally in the dosage suggested for hookworm. It may be repeated if necessary. Alternatively, it may be applied topically as a 10% aqueous suspension. Topical administration avoids systemic toxicity. Superficial bacterial infections are improved by the application of wet dressing and elevation of the extremity. For intense itching, oral antihistaminics may be of aid.

Prognosis Untreated infections last several months. Treatment, which is usually sought because of severe pruritus, is usually successful.

Prevention Dogs and cats should be prevented from contaminating recreation areas and children's sandboxes.

TRICHOSTRONGYLIASIS Definition Trichostrongyliasis is an intestinal infection of herbivorous animals throughout the world. Humans are an intermediate host.

Etiology Almost a dozen species of *Trichostrongylus* are known to have infected humans. The disease is common in Asia, the Middle East, and South America, but few human infections have been reported in the United States. In view of the high frequency of animal infections here, the low incidence of human infections is difficult to understand. The possibility exists that some such infections are mistaken for hookworm infections.

The ova resemble those of the hookworm but are larger, have more pointed ends, and, when observed in a fresh fecal specimen, show a more advanced stage of segmentation (16- to 32-celled stage).

Pathogenesis Infection is acquired by ingestion of green leafy plants contaminated with third-stage larvae. On reaching the small intestine, they attach themselves to the mucosa and develop into adult worms within 4 weeks. The adult at that time sucks blood and maintains residence in the intestine for long periods. Sandground, who infected himself, observed infection to last more than 8 years.

Manifestations Most infections are asymptomatic, but massive infections may result in anemia. The parasite owes its importance primarily to the resemblance of its ova to those of the hookworms. Moreover, because the trichostrongylidae do not respond to anthelmintics effective in hookworm infection, it may be assumed incorrectly that one is dealing with refractory hookworm infection.

Laboratory diagnosis The diagnosis depends on the finding of the ova in the feces. Since they are few, they are usually found only when a concentration method is used. In symptomatic infections, there may be leukocytosis with marked eosinophilia (for example, 80 percent).

Treatment These infections do not respond to tetrachloroethylene. Thiabendazole 25 mg per kg twice daily for 2 or 3 days, pyrantel pamoate as used in hookworm infections, and piperazine citrate as used against enterobiasis, are effective in symptomatic infections.

Prevention Leafy vegetables should be cooked before ingestion in endemic areas.

STRONGYLOIDIASIS Definition Strongyloidiasis is an intestinal infection of humans caused by *Strongyloides stercoralis.* Extraintestinal involvement may occur in severe cases.

Etiology The tiny (2 mm in length) adult female resides and lays her eggs in the mucosa of the upper part of the jejunum. In heavy infections, the biliary and pancreatic ducts, the entire small bowel, and the colon may be parasitized. The eggs quickly hatch, releasing rhabditiform larvae which enter the lumen of the bowel and are passed in the feces. On reaching the soil, the larvae develop into the infective filariform stage. There, as in the case of the filariform larvae of hookworm, they penetrate the skin and small blood vessels of humans. They are then carried to the lungs where they leave the alveolar capillaries, ascend the respiratory tree, enter the pharynx, and are swallowed. On reaching the small intestine, they mature and copulate. The fertilized female burrows into the jejunal mucosa, while the male is excreted in the stool. Oviposition begins 17 to 28 days after the initial infection. It is likely that the females also reproduce parthenogenetically. In addition to the *direct* host-soil-host cycle, *Strongyloides* has two alternative cycles. In the first, or *indirect,* cycle, the rhabditiform larvae, after passing from the host, develop into free-living adults which reside and reproduce in the soil, thus creating a reservoir of infection independent of the human host. Under certain environmental conditions, the free-living larvae are capable of transforming back into filariform larvae which initiate a new cycle in humans. In the second, or *autoinfection,* cycle, the rhabditiform larvae develop into filariform larvae before they are passed in the stool. They may then invade the intestinal mucosa or perianal skin of the same host without first going through a soil phase. This may explain the long persistence (20 to 30 years) of strongyloidiasis in patients who have left endemic areas and may also account for the extremely heavy worm loads in some individuals. The early transformation of the filariform larvae is probably also responsible for the frequency with which strongyloidiasis is seen in crowded, unsanitary institutions for the mentally retarded.

Epidemiology The usual mode of infection is the penetration of the skin by larvae. Some infections may result from ingestion of contaminated food and drink, and some are believed to be transmitted by contact. This disease is endemic in the tropics, where the warmth, moisture, and lack of sanitation favor its spread. Sporadic cases appear among Puerto Ricans and throughout the rural south of the continental United States.

Pathogenesis and clinical manifestations The initial cutaneous penetration of the filariform larvae usually produces no symptoms. However, transitory skin eruptions characterized by blotchy erythema, serpiginous lesions, and urticaria may be seen. These may recur at irregular intervals thereafter and are particularly common following recovery from an acute febrile illness. In these situations the lesions are generally found over the lower back and buttocks and are related to episodes of autoinfection. Cough, dyspnea, gross hemoptysis, and bronchospasm may accompany migration through the lungs. Chest x-rays may show pulmonary infiltration at this time. The intestinal infestation is usually asymptomatic or productive only of vague abdominal complaints. In heavier infections, epigastric pain and tenderness, nausea, flatulence, vomiting, and diarrhea alternating with constipation may be observed. Peptic ulcer may be simulated, but food often aggravates the pain. The mucosal inflammation may be severe enough to produce subacute obstruction, segmental ileus, and impaired absorption. A severe form of ulcerative colitis, accompanied by intestinal perforation and peritonitis, has been encountered. In debilitated, immunodepressed, or steroid-treated patients massive autoinfection with widespread dissemination of larvae to the extraintestinal organs including the central nervous system may occur. This hyperinfection is often associated with severe enterocolitis and gram-negative bacteremia. Unrecognized, it usually leads to death.

Laboratory findings Although clinical findings may be suggestive, the definitive diagnosis can be made only in the laboratory. Fresh fecal specimens should be examined to avoid confusion with hookworm infection; generally, fresh specimens contain *larvae* in strongyloidiasis infections, while in hookworm infection they contain *eggs.* Since the number of larvae in the stool is small and varies from day to day, several samples should be checked, using concentration and culture techniques. If pulmonary involvement is present, the sputum should be examined for larvae. Microscopic examination of the duodenal washings and jejunal biopsies may also establish the diagnosis. Alternatively, a weighted string can be passed into the duodenum, allowed to remain for a short time, and then withdrawn. The bile-stained section of the string is stripped of fluid which is then examined for the presence of larvae. The filarial complement fixation test is positive in approximately 75 percent of patients and may be helpful in the diagnosis of light infections.

Eosinophilic leukocytosis is common, except in very severe cases. When eosinophilia occurs in association with peptic ulcer symptoms, strongyloidiasis should be suspected.

Treatment All infected patients should be treated to prevent the occurrence of severe invasive disease. The drug of choice is thiabendazole, which should be given orally in dosage of 25 mg per kg twice a day for 2 or 3 days. Lightheadedness, nausea, and vomiting are common accompaniments of therapy with this agent. Hypersensitivity reactions may occur but usually respond to treatment with antihistamines. The stools should be rechecked at intervals of 3 months because the parasite is not easily eradicated and retreatment may be necessary.

Prognosis In the usual case, the prognosis is good. Since the occurrence of hyperinfection is unpredictable, every effort should be made to eradicate the infection in each case. In severe cases with hyperinfection, the prognosis is poor.

Prevention In general, the measures are those for the control of hookworm infection. In addition, it is well to remember that infection may be contracted by ingestion of contaminated food (especially uncooked vegetables) or of contaminated drinking water and by contact. Patients who have a history of residence in an endemic area should be carefully checked for the presence of the parasite prior to the initiation of steroid or immunosuppressive therapy. Because the larvae may not appear in the stool for several weeks after the initiation of such therapy, repeated examinations are indicated.

INTESTINAL CAPILLARIASIS **Definition** Intestinal capillariasis is an infection of humans caused by the roundworm *Capillaria philippinensis.* This species of *Capillaria* was first discovered in 1963 from a fatal human infection occurring in the Philippines. The infection results in intractable diarrhea with a high mortality rate. Clinical studies have shown a severe protein-losing enteropathy and malabsorption of fats and sugars.

Etiology *Capillaria* are nematodes of the family Trichuroidea and are closely related to comembers *Trichuris* and *Trichinella.* Adult *C. philippinensis* are small, measuring 2 to 4 mm in length. The peanut-shaped eggs have flattened bipolar plugs and an average size of 42 by 20 μm. The adults inhabit the mucosa of the small intestine, especially the jejunum. Adults, larval forms, and eggs are found in the stool.

Epidemiology The infection has been found almost exclusively in persons residing in the Ilocano ethnic region in Northwest Luzon, Philippines. Two cases from Thailand have also been reported. Since 1966 the disease has occurred in epidemic form, and more than 1,000 cases and 100 deaths have been reported. Males are infected more frequently than females, perhaps because of occupational exposure. Prior to the discovery of an effective chemotherapeutic agent, the mortality rate in untreated cases was about 30 percent. With chemotherapy, the case fatality rate has been reduced to 6 percent.

The mode of transmission and life cycle of the parasite are not established. The presence of many adult worms, larviparous females, embryonated eggs, and all larval stages in human intestinal contents suggests that autoinfection may be part of the life cycle. In addition, indirect evidence indicates that man-to-man transmission occurs. The mechanism by which man originally became infected remains obscure. Because the Ilocano people of the region eat many animal foods raw or semicooked, numerous species of local fauna have been examined for *Capillaria,* and developing larvae have been recovered from 3 species of fish.

Pathogenesis and manifestations Adult worms in large numbers invade the small-intestinal mucosa and cause a severe protein-losing enteropathy and malabsorption. Hypokalemia, hypocalcemia, and hypoproteinemia are the rule. Autopsy studies have failed to show extraintestinal spread of the parasite. Initial symptoms of intestinal "gurgling" (borborygmi) and recurrent vague abdominal pain are followed, usually within 2 to 3 weeks, by a voluminous watery diarrhea. Other findings, consistent with the basic pathophysiologic process, are anorexia, vomiting, weight loss, muscle wasting and weakness, hyporeflexia, and edema. Abdominal tenderness and distention may occur. The period between onset of symptoms and death is usually 2 to 3 months. Subclinical infection has not been noted.

Diagnosis The diagnosis is made by finding ova in the stool. The ova of *C. philippinensis* must be differentiated from those of *T. trichiura,* which are similar. Care must be taken that capillaria are not overlooked in patients with *Trichuris* infections because in the endemic area most patients with capillariasis have coexistent *Trichuris* infection.

Treatment Administration of thiabendazole, combined with fluid and electrolyte replacement, leads to dramatic improvement. Thiabendazole therapy must be given over a prolonged period to prevent relapse. A divided dose of 25 mg/kg body weight/day is given for 1 month, followed by a maintenance dose of 1 g every day for 6 months. On this schedule ova disappear from the stool within 2 weeks.

REFERENCES

AUR RJA et al: Thiabendazole in visceral larva migrans. Am J Dis Child 121:226, 1971

AZIZ MA, SEDDIQUI AR: Morphological and absorption studies of small intestine hookworm disease (ancyclostomiasis) in West Pakistan. Gastroenterology 55:242, 1968

BEAVER PC: The nature of the visceral larva migrans. J Parasitol 55:3, 1969

BROWN HW: *Basic Clinical Parasitology,* 4th ed., New York: Appleton-Century-Crofts, 1975

CHITWOOD MB et al: *Capillaria philippinensis* N. (Nematoda: Trichinellida) from the intestine of man in the Philippines. J Parasitol 54:368, 1968

CROSS JH et al: Studies on the experimental transmission of *Capillaria philippinensis* in monkeys. Trans R Soc Trop Med Hyg 66:819, 1972

DAVIS CM, ISRAEL RM: Treatment of creeping eruption with topical thiabendazole. Arch Dermatol 97:325, 1968

FRANZ KH et al: Clinical trials with thiabendazole against intestinal nematodes infecting humans. Am J Trop Med 14:383, 1968

HUNTLEY CG et al: Isohemagglutinins in parasitic infections. JAMA 208:1145, 1969

KAGAN IG: Current status of serologic testing for parasitic diseases. Hosp Pract, Sept., 1974, p. 157

KAMATH KR: Severe infection with *Trichuris trichuria* in Malaysian children. Am J Trop Med Hyg 22:600, 1973

KANANI SR, REESE PH: The diagnosis of strongyloidiasis with special reference to the value of the filarial complement fixation test as a screening test. Trans R Soc Trop Med Hyg 64:246, 1970

LAYRISSE M et al: Blood loss due to infection with *Trichuris trichuria.* Am J Trop Med Hyg 16:613, 1967

MAK CH: Visceral larva migrans: A discussion based on review of the literature. Clin Pediatr 7:565, 1968

MARKETT EK: Pseudohookworm infection-Trichostrongyliasis: Treatment with thiabendazole. N Engl J Med 278:831, 1968

MARSEN JM, TURNER JA: Reinfection of enterobiasis (pinworm infection): Simultaneous treatment of family members. Am J Dis Child 118:576, 1969

MILLER MJ et al: Mebendazole. An effective anthelmintic for trichuriasis and enterobiasis. JAMA 230:1412, 1974

MOST H: Drug therapy: Common parasitic infections of man. N Engl J Med 287:495, 1972

NEEFE LI: Disseminated strongyloidiasis with cerebral involvement. A complication of corticosteroid therapy. Am J Med 55: 832, 1973

NEVA FA: Parasitic diseases of the GI tract in the United States. DM, June, 1972

PHILLS JA et al: Pulmonary abnormalities and eosinophilia due to *Ascaris suum.* N Engl J Med 286:965, 1972

PIGGOTT J et al: Human ascariasis. Am J Clin Pathol 53:223, 1970

PINKUS GS et al: Intestinal anisakiasis. First case report from North America. Am J Med 59:114, 1975

ROCHE M, LAYRISSE M: The nature and causes of hookworm anemia. Am J Trop Med Hyg 15:1029, 1966

STEMMERMAN GN: Strongyloidiasis in migrants: Pathological and clinical considerations. Gastroenterology 53:59, 1967

WHALEN GE et al: Intestinal capillariasis. Lancet I:13, 1969

WOODRUFF AW: Toxocariasis. Br Med J 3:663, 1970

222
TISSUE NEMATODES

JAMES J. PLORDE

ANGIOSTRONGYLIASIS CANTONENSIS Definition *Angiostrongylus cantonensis,* the rat lungworm, is the etiologic agent of the common form of *eosinophilic meningitis* found in Southeast Asia in the tropical areas of the Pacific.

Etiology The delicate filariform adults (20 mm in length) reside and lay their eggs in the pulmonary arterioles of rats and certain other rodents. After hatching, the larvae break into the alveoli, migrate up the respiratory tract, are swallowed, and pass in the feces. They develop into infective third-stage larvae within snails and slugs, their natural intermediate host. Viable third-stage organisms may also be found in land planarians, crabs, and freshwater prawns. These carriers appear to acquire the larvae by feeding on the tissues of infected mollusks. Humans, like rodents, become parasitized when they ingest raw intermediate or carrier hosts containing the infective stage. In rodents the larvae migrate to the brain where they grow into young adults. After a period of further maturation, the worms travel to the lungs and begin to deposit eggs. The nematode does not complete its life cycle in humans and dies after reaching the central nervous system.

Epidemiology Human infections with *A. cantonensis* have been found in Thailand, Vietnam, Cambodia, Indonesia, the Philippines, Taiwan, Hawaii, and several smaller Pacific islands from Okinawa in the north to New Caledonia and Tahiti in the south. In addition, rodent infections have been found in the islands of East Africa, Sri Lanka, India, and China. The rat lungworm may have been spread from Madagascar to Asia and to the Pacific by the recent dispersal of the giant African land snail, *Achatina fulica.*

Pathology and pathogenesis The nematode can produce extensive tissue damage by moving through the brain when alive and provokes a marked inflammatory reaction when dead. The pathologic lesions are characterized by (1) marked lymphocyte and eosinophilic infiltration of the meninges, (2) hemorrhagic and nonhemorrhagic worm tracts through the brainstem and spinal cord, (3) granuloma formation around dead parasites and necrotic debris which sheathes the worm, and (4) engorgement of almost all blood vessels, particularly the veins. Necrosis of vessel walls, aneurysmal dilatation of arteries, and perivascular hemorrhages have been noted. Living worms have been removed from the eyes of patients without central nervous system involvement.

Clinical manifestations The eosinophilic meningoencephalitis is characterized by a relatively mild fever, headache, and neck stiffness. Paresthesias of the trunk and lower extremities are a common complaint, and paralysis of the sixth and seventh nerves is seen in 3 to 7 percent of cases. Paralysis of the limbs, convulsions, and loss of consciousness are rare. The disease usually ends in complete spontaneous recovery. The cerebrospinal fluid contains several hundred cells per cubicmillimeter and many eosinophils, and the cerebrospinal fluid protein is elevated. There may or may not be an eosinophilia in the peripheral blood.

The second clinically distinct form of eosinophilic meningitis has been reported from Thailand. This presents as a radiculomyeloencephalitis with limb pain and paresis and is thought to be caused by the nematode *Girathostoma spinigerum.* The cerebrospinal fluid eosinophilic leukocytosis is less marked than in *angiostrongylus* infections. The fluid is often xanthochromic. Death may occur from cerebral hemorrhage or destruction of vital centers.

Diagnosis The diagnosis is made on the basis of the clinical manifestations in an endemic area. Angiostrongyliasis must be differentiated from other ectopic worm infections of the central nervous system including paragonimiasis, hydatid disease, schistosomiasis japonicum, trichinosis, cysticercosis, toxocariasis, and gnathostomiasis.

Treatment and prevention There is no known effective treatment. Thiabendazole might conceivably be of help in the early stages of larval dissemination. Prevention depends upon avoidance or proper cooking of such foods as snails, prawns, and crabs. Raw vegetables should be carefully inspected for the presence of planarians and mollusks before they are eaten. Freezing of crustaceans and mollusks at $-15°C$ for 12 h will destroy infective larvae of *A. cantonensis.*

ANGIOSTRONGYLIASIS COSTARICENSIS *Angiostrongylus costaricensis* is a nematode that dwells in the mesenteric arteries of Central American rats. Larvae pass in the stool and develop in slugs, the intermediate hosts. Rats, and incidentally humans, are infected when they ingest slugs or vegetables contaminated with third-stage larvae. The larvae mature in the lymphatics and move to the mesenteric radicals of the cecum. Here they may cause arterial thrombosis, ischemic necrosis, ulceration, and eosinophilic granuloma formation. Infected patients present with fever, eosinophilic leukocytosis, abdominal pain, and a right lower quadrant mass. Occasionally perforation of the bowel and generalized peritonitis occur. The fever may persist for up to 2 months. Children are more frequently involved than adults. Neither larvae nor eggs are seen in the stool of the human host. No specific therapy is available.

GNATHOSTOMIASIS Definition Gnathostomiasis is a tissue infection of humans caused by *Gnathostoma spinigerum,* an intestinal nematode of carnivores. Clinically it is manifest as migratory subcutaneous swellings, creeping eruption, or a lethal eosinophilic meningitis.

Etiology and epidemiology The parasite, which is found throughout the Far East, lives encysted in the gastric mucosa of dogs, cats, and wild felines. The ova are passed to the external environment via the feces, hatch in water, and are ingested by *Cyclops,* the first intermediate hosts. These in turn are eaten by freshwater fish, frogs, snakes, and eels in whose flesh the infective third-stage larvae develop. Ducks and chickens fed on these second intermediate hosts may also come to harbor infective larvae. Human infections, which are most commonly seen in Thailand and Japan, occur when humans ingest infected uncooked fish (somfak, sashimi), duck, or chicken.

Pathogenesis and manifestations The parasite cannot complete its cycle in humans, and the immature worms migrate through the abdominal and thoracic organs producing localized areas of inflammation and hemorrhage. Clinically, this is manifest as fever, eosinophilic leukocytosis, urticaria, and pain. Typically, the systemic manifestations subside within a month as the worms make their way to the subcutaneous tissues. Here, their continued migration results in the production of transient serpiginous pruritic swellings, subcutaneous tunnels, and abscesses. If the worm invades the epidermis, the resulting lesions closely resemble those of cutanea larva migrans. Rarely the eye may be involved with orbital cellulitis, iritis, or uveitis. Migration into the central nervous system results in a lethal eosinophilic meningitis (see Angiostrongyliasis above). This presents as a radiculomyeloencephalitis with limb pain and paresis. The cerebrospinal fluid eosinophilic leukocytosis is present but less marked than in Angiostrongylus infections. The fluid is often xanthochromic. Death may occur from cerebral hemorrhage or destruction of vital centers.

Diagnosis and treatment Painless, recurrent migratory subcutaneous swellings and eosinophilic leukocytosis occurring in an endemic area make the diagnosis likely. It must be differentiated from cutanea larva migrans, however, and from angiostrongyliasis cantonensis when the central nervous system is involved. Definitive diagnosis depends upon the removal and identification of the worm. Other than excision, there is no specific therapy. The disease can be prevented by the adequate cooking of fish, chicken, and duck in endemic areas.

DRACUNCULIASIS Definition Dracunculiasis is an infection of human connective and subcutaneous tissues by the guinea worm, *Dracuncula medinensis.* The gravid female produces symptoms when she ruptures the skin to discharge her eggs.

Etiology and epidemiology Dracunculiasis affects about 50 million people in West, Central, and Northeast Africa, the Middle East, Iran, Pakistan, India, northeastern South America, and the Caribbean Islands. Humans acquire the parasite when they ingest raw drinking water containing infected copepods (*Cyclops* sp.) which serve as the intermediate host. Shallow ponds, cisterns, and wells are the usual habitat of these crustaceans. In the stomach the copepod is digested and the larvae are released. The larva penetrates the intestinal wall and matures in the connective tissue of the retroperitoneal space. The adult male is small, seldom seen, and presumably dies after mating. In contrast, the female *Dracunculus* is one of the largest nematodes known—1 to 2 mm in diameter and 300 to 800 mm in length. The female reaches gravidity in approximately one year and then migrates to the subcutaneous tissue of the lower extremities. When the anterior end of the worm approaches the skin, a blister forms. This breaks down in a few days, forming a superficial ulcer. When the protruding portion of the worm comes in contact with water, the uterus prolapses through the body and discharges large numbers of motile rhabditiform larvae. Following ingestion by one of several species of *Cyclops,* the larvae undergo further development, becoming infective in 10 to 12 days. Mammals other than humans may be infected, but their importance as a disease reservoir is uncertain.

Pathogenesis and manifestations The infection is asymptomatic until the gravid female appears in the subcutaneous tissues where it may, on occasion, be palpable. A few days before the formation of the blister, the patient frequently has fever, generalized urticaria, periorbital edema, and wheezing. Blister formation is accompanied by intense local pain and pruritus; like the systemic manifestations, this is thought to represent an allergic reaction to prematurely liberated larvae. The local lesion is usually found over the feet and ankles but may occur on the trunk or the upper extremities. Multiple infections are common. With the rupture of the blister and the release of embryos, the systemic manifestations abate, and the worm is slowly extruded over a period of 4 to 5 weeks. Secondary infection and cellulitis are common, particularly if the worm is ruptured during the process of extraction. In Nigeria, guinea worm ulcers are a common portal of entry for the spores of *Clostridium tetani.* The female worm often fails to reach the surface and discharge her larvae. In most of these cases, it dies without producing symptoms. The calcified appearance on roentgenograms is characteristic. Occasionally the worm may invade the deep tissues, causing serious symptoms, and sterile abscesses may follow the release of embryos. Invasion of joint spaces by the adult worm or larvae results in arthritis.

Diagnosis The clinical picture is characteristic. Placing a small amount of water on the worm results in discharge of larvae which can then be examined microscopically. A fluorescent antibody test may permit the diagnosis to be made prior to emergence of the gravid female.

Treatment and prevention If the outline of the worm can be clearly seen or palpated, it may sometimes be completely removed with a single incision. The gradual extraction of the worm can be accomplished by winding a few centimeters onto a stick each day. Administration of niridazole (Ambilhar) results in prompt remission of symptoms and extrusion of the adult worms. The dose is 25 mg per kg body weight given in three divided doses for 7 days. Thiabendazole in dosage of 25 mg per kg twice daily for 2 days or metronidazole 250 mg three times a day for 7 days is also effective. Dracunculiasis can be prevented by the chemical treatment of drinking water.

REFERENCES

ALICATA JE: Present status of *Angiostrongylus cantonensis* infection in man and animals in the tropics. J Trop Med Hyg 72:53, 1969

MORERA P, CESPEDES R: Abdominal angiostrongyliasis. A new human parasitic infection. Acta Med Costarric 14:159, 1971 (Spanish)

MULLER R: Dracunculus and dracunculiasis, in *Advances in Parasitology,* vol. 9, ed B Dawes, London: Academic, 1971, p. 73

NYE SW et al: Lesions of the brain in eosinophilic meningitis. Arch Pathol 89:9, 1970

PUNYAGUPTA S et al: Eosinophilic meningitis in Thailand. Am J Trop Med 19:950, 1970

223 TRICHINOSIS

JAMES J. PLORDE

DEFINITION Trichinosis is an intestinal and tissue infection of man and other mammals caused by the nematode *Trichinella spiralis.* The disease is characterized by diarrhea during the development of the adults in the intestine and by myositis, fever, prostration, periorbital edema, eosinophilic leukocytosis, and, occasionally, evidence of myocarditis or encephalitis during the stage of larval migration in tissue.

ETIOLOGY Trichinosis in humans is contracted by ingestion of meat containing the encysted larvae of *T. spiralis.* The meat has almost always been pork, but for the past several years about 10 percent of cases reported in this country have been attributed to bear meat. This has been particularly frequent in the Northern and Western states including Alaska, California, and Idaho. There are no intermediate hosts, and both the adult and larval stages develop in the same animal. Infection has been produced or observed in the bear, wild boar, wolf, coyote, fox, muskrat, horse, cow, dog, cat, rabbit, guinea pig, mouse, and marine mammals, in addition to the rat and the pig. Humans are particularly susceptible; most fowl are resistant. Among pigs, infection is contracted following feeding of the uncooked scraps, less often by eating infected rats. The incidence of infection in pigs has been reduced by laws requiring that garbage be cooked thoroughly before being fed. Rats also feed on uncooked pork scraps and, in addition, maintain a high incidence of infection by their cannibalism.

Soon after ingestion, the larvae are liberated from their cysts by gastric digestion and migrate into the intestinal mucosa, where copulation takes place. The male dies, and within a week, the viviparous female is discharging larvae (100 × 6 μm), which enter vascular channels and are distributed throughout the body. Larviposition continues for about 4 to 16 weeks, each female producing approximately 1,500 offspring. The larvae enter skeletal muscle, grow, and begin encysting within 3 weeks; calcification of cysts begins in 6 to 18 months. The life span of the encysted organism has been estimated at 5 to 10 years. The muscles of the diaphragm, tongue, and eye, and the deltoid, pectoral, gastrocnemius, and intercostal muscles are most often affected. Larvae carried to sites other than skeletal muscles do not encyst but disintegrate. The life cycle can be carried further only if a new host ingests the encysted larvae.

EPIDEMIOLOGY Trichinosis is particularly common in Europe and North America, but with the exception of Australia and Asia it is found worldwide. In the United States its prevalence as measured by finding cysts in human diaphragms at autopsy has declined from 16.1 to 4.2 percent over the past 30 years. This decline has been accompanied by a similar reduction of trichinosis in pigs. The prevalence appears highest in the New England, Mid-Atlantic, and Pacific states. Currently, it is estimated that 1.5 million Americans carry live Trichina in their musculature and that somewhere between 150,000 and 300,000 acquire new infections annually. The overwhelming majority of these infections are asymptomatic, and many of those that become clinically manifest are never correctly diagnosed. In 1973 only 129 cases with one death were officially reported in the United States. Large outbreaks are usually caused by a consumption of ready-to-eat pork sausage prepared in noninspected facilities or at home. The incidence appears highest among Americans of Italian and German descent, presumably because of their inclination to make and eat pork sausage. Recently, an epidemic among Thais living in New York City has been reported.

PATHOLOGY The most striking lesions are in the skeletal muscles, where there is a severe myositis with basophilic granular degeneration of the invaded muscle fiber. Adjacent fibers exhibit hyalin or hydropic degeneration, and the focus becomes infiltrated with neutrophilic and eosinophilic leukocytes, some lymphocytes, and mononuclear macrophages. Hyperemia, edema, and hemorrhages are constant features.

Larvae do not encyst in cardiac muscle, but an intense myocarditis has been observed in fatal cases.

In cases of central nervous system involvement, there may be granulomatous nodules, and vasculitis involving small arterioles and capillaries of the brain and meninges. Encystment of larvae in the brain is unusual.

CLINICAL MANIFESTATIONS The first symptoms usually appear within 1 to 2 days after ingestion of the uncooked or undercooked meat containing encysted larvae. At that time diarrhea, abdominal pain, nausea, and sometimes prostration and fever develop. The next stage, that of muscular invasion, begins about the end of the first week and may last as long as 6 weeks. During this period, patients have fever, edema of the eyelids, conjunctivitis and subconjunctival hemorrhages, muscle pain and tenderness, and often severe weakness. There may be a maculopapular rash which lasts for several days and subungual "splinter hemorrhages." Central nervous system involvement may be evident as polyneuritis, poliomyelitis, myasthenia, meningitis, encephalitis, focal or diffuse pareses, delirium, psychosis, and coma. Despite the severity of central nervous system involvement in some patients, the cerebrospinal fluid remains normal.

Myocarditis is characterized by persistent tachycardia or development of congestive heart failure. There are marked electrocardiographic alterations, including ST-T-wave changes and conduction abnormalities in 20 percent of patients.

LABORATORY FINDINGS The most constant finding, and one of significance early in the course of the disease, is the eosinophilic leukocytosis (over 500 eosinophilic leukocytes per mm^3) which generally appears before the end of the second week. In cases of moderate severity, the proportion of eosinophilic leukocytes ranges between 15 and 50 percent. In severe cases, particularly terminally, the eosinophilic leukocytosis may disappear entirely.

The skin test to larval antigen becomes positive early in the third week of infection, and may remain so for up to 20 years. The usual positive response is a wheal of 5 mm or more appearing within 30 min. Unfortunately, the commercially available skin test preparations are not reliable and their use is currently discouraged.

There is a variety of serologic tests for trichinosis, including the precipitin reaction, the complement fixation test, the indirect fluorescent antibody test, and the bentonite flocculation test, which is probably the best. A commercially available latex agglutination test appears to give comparable results. These serologic tests all become positive by about the third week of the disease and may remain positive for a few years. Since each may occasionally be falsely negative, two or more tests should be used. The serologic tests are most valuable if they are negative initially and then in turn positive or if there is a change in titer.

Muscle biopsy when carried out during the third or fourth week of infection remains the most useful test for demonstration of larvae or cysts. The deltoid or gastrocnemius muscles are the most useful sites for biopsy. A small portion of the excised muscle should be compressed between glass slides and examined under a low-power microscope for the presence of larvae. Calcified cysts or larvae represent an old infection. The remainder of the biopsy should be submitted for routine processing because myositis is a significant finding even in the absence of larvae or cysts.

In severe trichinosis there may be marked hypoalbuminemia, probably because of protein leakage from damaged capillaries. During the fourth, fifth, and sixth weeks of the disease, concomitant with a rise in antibody, diffuse hypergammaglobulinemia occurs. Elevated levels of circulating IgE have been reported. There may be moderate rises in SGOT, serum aldolase, and creatine-phosphokinase, probably related to myositis; the sedimentation rate is characteristically slow.

DIFFERENTIAL DIAGNOSIS Trichinosis must be differentiated from diseases which are characterized by eosinophilia (such as Hodgkin's disease, eosinophilic leukemia, and periarteritis nodosa) and from entities which are characterized by myopathy, such as dermatomyositis. When the central nervous system is involved, the diagnosis may be very difficult.

TREATMENT Thiabendazole, in dosage of 25 mg per kg b.i.d. for 5 to 7 days, has resulted in apparent improvement in a number of patients, with relief of muscle pain and tenderness and with lysis of fever. The results have not been uniform, however, and the use of this drug in trichinosis has been associated with nausea, vomiting, abdominal discomfort, dermatitis, and drug fever.

Patients with "allergic" manifestations of trichinosis, including angioedema and urticaria as well as myocardial or central nervous system involvement, should be treated with prednisone in dosage of 20 to 60 mg per day. Response to steroids usually has been prompt, particularly in central nervous system trichinosis. Not all focal lesions have resolved, however.

Other measures should be directed at relief of pain and maintenance of adequate caloric and fluid intake.

PROGNOSIS The prognosis in trichinosis has improved markedly, and even when the central nervous system is involved, the mortality rate has fallen to under 10 percent. The overall mortality rate is probably less than 2 percent.

PREVENTION The responsibility for control rests with the consumer. Adequate cooking of pork involves heating all portions of the meat to 60°C. Freezing procedures to kill the larvae require a temperature of −15°C for 20 days or −18°C for 24 h. Proper smoking and pickling will also destroy the larvae. Important in control is the cooking of garbage fed to hogs. There is no practical method of inspection which will detect trichinous pork.

REFERENCES

BARRETT-CONNER E et al: An epidemic of trichinosis after ingestion of wild pig in Hawaii. J Infect Dis 133:473, 1976

BROWN HW: *Basic Clinical Parasitology,* 4th ed., New York: Appleton-Century-Crofts, 1975

DALESSIO DJ, WOLFF HG: *Trichinella spiralis* infection of the central nervous system. Arch Neurol 4:407, 1961

GRAY DF et al: Trichinosis with neurologic and cardiac involvement. Ann Intern Med 57:230, 1962

HALL WJ III, MCCABE WR: Trichinosis: Report of a small outbreak with observations of thiabendazole therapy. Arch Intern Med 119:65, 1967

METZLER MH et al: Second-degree atrioventricular block in acute trichinosis. Am J Dis Child 124:598, 1972

RACHÓN K et al: Serum proteins in human trichinosis. Am J Med 44:937, 1968

ROSENBERG EB et al: Increased circulating IgE in trichinosis. Ann Intern Med 75:575, 1971

SULZER AJ, CHISHOLM ES: Comparison of the IFA and other tests for *Trichinella spiralis* antibodies. Pub Health Rep 81:729, 1966

WAND M, LYMAN D: Trichinosis from bear meat. JAMA 220:245, 1972

ZIMMERMAN WJ: Prevalence of *Trichinella spiralis* in commercial pork sausage. Pub Health Rep 85:717, 1970

—— et al: Trichinosis in the U. S. population 1966–70. Pub Health Rep 88:606, 1973

224 FILARIASIS

JAMES J. PLORDE

DEFINITION Filariasis is a group of disorders produced by infection with the threadlike nematodes of the superfamily Filarioidea. These worms invade the lymphatics and subcutaneous and deep tissues of humans producing reactions ranging from acute inflammation to chronic scarring. The viviparous female discharges microfilariae into the blood or subcutaneous tissues where they live for weeks or months until taken up by hematophagous arthropods. Within these vectors they are transformed into filariform larvae which then infect a new host when the arthropod takes another blood meal. The clinical pictures produced by various species in this group are more or less specific. The term *lymphatic filariasis* is commonly used to designate the disease produced by *Wuchereria bancrofti* and *Brugia malayi,* the organisms responsible for lymphatic blockade and elephantiasis. *Loa loa* causes loiasis, a disease characterized by transient subcutaneous (Calabar) swellings, and *Onchocerca volvulus* produces the blindness and pruritic skin rash typical of onchocerciasis. *Mansonella ozzardi, Dipetalonema perstans,* and *D. streptocerca* cause infections of questionable clinical significance to humans.

These parasites are identified by the location, periodicity, and morphologic characteristics of their microfilariae. Those of *W. bancrofti, B. malayi, L. loa, D. perstans,* and *M. ozzardi* are all found in the blood, and, with the exception of the last, all display nocturnal or diurnal periodicity. *Onchocerca volvulus* and *D. streptocerca* are found in the subcutaneous tissues and are nonperiodic. Morphologically, the microfilariae are distinguished by the presence or absence of a sheath and by the distribution of their deeply staining column of nuclei. The sheath, which is an elongation of the original eggshell, can be seen extending beyond the head and tail only in the microfilariae of *W. bancrofti, B. malayi,* and *L. loa.* The nuclear column extends to the very tip of the microfilariae of *B. malayi, L. loa,* and the two species of *Dipetalonema.*

Skin and serologic tests are group-specific, lack sensitivity, and may be falsely negative in other nematode infections. In the absence of microfilariae and other helminthic infections, however, they may be helpful in establishing a diagnosis in clinically suspect cases.

LYMPHATIC FILARIASIS (BANCROFTIAN AND MALAYAN)

ETIOLOGY AND EPIDEMIOLOGY The threadlike adult worms live coiled together in human lymphatics. The male *W. bancrofti* measures 35 mm and the female 80 to 100 mm. The *B. malayi* adults are about one-half as long. Gravid females release microfilariae in large numbers into the lymphatics. These embryos, which are sheathed, measure approximately 200 to 300 μm. They eventually reach the peripheral blood, where further development depends on their ingestion by a proper mosquito vector. Species of *Culex, Aëdes,* and *Anopheles* transmit Bancroftian filariasis; *Mansonia* and *Anopheles* serve as vectors in Malayan disease. After further development in the vector, larvae migrate to the mouthparts. If the mosquito feeds on a human host, they penetrate the puncture site and reach maturity in about a year. In the absence of reinfection, man harbors microfilariae for 5 to 10 years, the reproductive life of the adult worms. In most *W. bancrofti* and *B. malayi* infections, the microfilariae are found in the blood in greatest numbers between 9 P.M. and 2 A.M. During the day, apparently in response to changes in oxygen tension, they accumulate in the pulmonary vessels and disappear from the peripheral blood. However, in Polynesia and New Caledonia there is an *Aëdes*-transmitted variety of *W. bancrofti* (*W. pacifica*) that displays a diurnal periodicity in which the peak occurs in the early evenings (subperiodic form). Periodicity is of epidemiologic significance because it determines which species of mosquito serves as the vector. Furthermore, several subperiodic forms of *B. malayi* have been found in animals, suggesting the possibility that this disease has an animal reservoir. The human is the only known vertebrate host for *W. bancrofti.*

More than 250 million people throughout the world are presently infected, and both the prevalence and distribution of the disease seem to be increasing in many parts of Africa and Asia.

Wuchereria bancrofti infection is endemic between latitudes 41°N and 30°S involving primarily Africa, the Pacific Islands, and Southeastern Asia from Korea on the north to India in the West. The West Indies, Central America, and the eastern coastal plains of South America are also involved. Distribution is irregular, and there are many peculiar "skip areas" in this geographic pattern, presumably because the endemic disease can be maintained only where human infection and mosquitoes are prevalent. *Brugia malayi* infection is much more restricted in its distribution and occurs in India, Burma, Thailand, Vietnam, China, South Korea, Japan, Malaysia, Indonesia, Borneo, New Guinea, and the Philippines. The parasite has recently disappeared from Sri Lanka.

Two new types of microfilaria have been described recently. One, found in Brazil, has been named *W. lewisi,* while the taxonomic status of the strain from Portuguese Timor has not been settled.

There were approximately 15,000 *W. bancrofti* infections among American military personnel in World War II. A small endemic focus of *W. bancrofti* once existed near Charleston, South Carolina, but no new cases have been observed since 1930.

PATHOGENESIS Pathologic changes are caused primarily by the presence of the adult worm in the lymphatics and may be divided into inflammatory and obstructive. The inflammatory response, most marked around molting larvae and dead or dying adult worms, consists of infiltration with lymphocytes, plasma cells, and eosinophils. This is followed by a granulomatous reaction which may lead to lymphatic obstruction. There are hyperplasia of lymphatic endothelium, acute lymphangitis, and thrombosis. Repetition of this process over a period of years leads to permanent lymphatic obstruction. The tissues become edematous, thickened, and fibrotic. Secondary streptococcal infections are common. Dilated lymphatics may rupture into surrounding tissue. Elephantiasis is actually a relatively unusual complication of filarial infections. If repeated reinfections do not occur, the disease is self-limited.

MANIFESTATIONS The clinical manifestations vary with the geographic area, species of parasite, and intensity of infection. Light infections may be completely asymptomatic. Symptoms may occur within 3 months of infection, but ordinarily the incubation period is 8 to 12 months. The clinical findings closely reflect the pathologic changes, with inflammation early in the disease followed by obstruction later. Inflammatory filariasis consists of a series of brief febrile attacks occurring over a period of weeks. Fever is usually low grade but may reach 105°F and be accompanied by chills and sweats. Other symptoms include headache, nausea and vomiting, photophobia, and muscle pain. If the involved lymphatics lie close to the surface, the local symptoms dominate the clinical picture. Lymphangitis is very common, involving the legs more frequently than the arms. It often begins as a tender spot in the region of the malleoli or femoral area and spreads centrifugally. The involved vessels are palpably tender and painful. The overlying skin is red and swollen. When abdominal lymphatics are involved, the picture may simulate that of an acute abdomen. In Bancroftian filariasis the vessels of the spermatic cord and testes may be involved, resulting in painful orchitis, epididymitis, or funiculitis. Lymphadenitis almost always accompanies and may sometimes precede lymphangitis. The inguinal, femoral, and epitrochlear nodes are involved. Abscesses which may form about involved lymphatics and lymph nodes may discharge to the surface, resulting in persistently draining sinus tracts. The acute manifestations last only a few days and then subside spontaneously, only to recur at irregular intervals over a period of weeks or months. Recovery finally ensues. With repeated infections, slowly progressive lymphatic obstruction may develop in areas where the inflammatory reactions have occurred previously. Edema, ascites, lymph scrotum-hydrocele, pleural effusion, or joint effusion may appear as a result of interference with lymphatic drainage. Lymphadenopathy persists. The lymphatic vessels become palpably enlarged as tense elastic masses beneath the skin, especially in the femoral, inguinal, and scrotal areas. They may rupture and form draining sinuses. Internal rupture of lymphatics may give rise to chylous ascites or chyluria. In a small percentage of cases elephantiasis develops. This complication is rare below the age of twenty even in natives of heavily infested areas. The chronic obstructive phase of the disease often is punctuated by acute inflammatory episodes.

Attention has recently been focused on an aberrant type of filariasis which is characterized by the presence of hypereosinophilia, complement-fixing filarial antibodies, microfilariae in tissue but *not in the blood,* and a chronic, clinical course that can be terminated with specific antifilarial treatment. These amicrofilaremic forms were originally thought to be caused by zoontic parasites, but it is more likely that they represent an atypical host response to various filariae including *W. bancrofti* and *B. malayi.* Experience with filariasis in American servicemen during World War II suggests that this response is the rule in individuals who have their first contact with the disease. Clinically there may be marked enlargement of the lymph nodes and spleen (Meyers-Kouwenaar syndrome) and/or chronic cough, nocturnal bronchospasm, and miliary pulmonary infiltrates (tropical eosinophilia). Patients with pulmonary manifestations demonstrate both obstructive and restrictive abnormalities in pulmonary function, and irreversible pulmonary hypertension has been described in two patients with tropical eosinophilia.

DIAGNOSIS A history of exposure, the long incubation period, the occurrence of typical inflammatory episodes, and the finding of regional lymphadenopathy, thickening of the spermatic cord, or swelling of an extremity should suggest the diagnosis. There is usually eosinophilia during acute episodes. Lymphangiography may reveal dilated afferent and small efferent lymphatics. The definitive diagnosis depends on demonstration of the parasite. Although adult worms can be demonstrated in biopsied lymph nodes, biopsy is not recommended because it may interfere further with lymphatic drainage. Microfilariae are found in the blood during intermediate stages but not early or late in the disease. As they are motile, they can often be seen in a wet mount or counting chamber. Definite identification, however, requires staining with Giemsa. As in malaria, they are demonstrated best in thick smears. Concentration methods may be used if the parasite is not found in thick smears. Because the appearance of microfilariae in peripheral blood is periodic, it is essential to obtain blood at appropriate times. When this proves difficult, the oral administration of 100 mg diethylcarbamazine usually produces positive blood specimens within 30 to 60 min. Microfilariae may also be found in lymphatic fluid, hydrocele fluid, ascites, and pleural fluid. Skin tests as well as complement fixation, indirect hemagglutination, bentonite flocculation, and soluble antigen fluorescent antibody tests are available and, although not completely reliable, are helpful when microfilariae cannot be demonstrated.

TREATMENT Diethylcarbamazine (Hetrazan) rapidly eliminates microfilariae from the blood. It probably also kills or injures adult worms, impairing their ability to reproduce, and clears microfilariae permanently from the bloodstream of many patients. The drug is given in dosage of 2 mg per kg three times a day for 3 or 4 weeks. Treatment with this agent is often followed by allergic reactions to the dying parasite. These reactions may be quite severe, especially in Malayan filariasis. They can be controlled with aspirin, antihistamines, or steroid hormones. In heavy infections, it may be desirable to begin treatment with antihistamines before administration of Hetrazan.

Antimony compounds have no place in the treatment of filariasis.

Reassurance of the patient is very important in this disease. Vaccines and antiserums are valueless. Pressure bandages and surgery sometimes benefit elephantiasis. The prognosis for life is excellent, particularly if infected individuals leave endemic areas or otherwise avoid reinfections. Disease control is accomplished by combining mass treatment with mosquito control measures.

ONCHOCERCIASIS ("RIVER BLINDNESS")

DEFINITION Onchocerciasis is a cutaneous filariasis caused by *Onchocerca volvulus.* It is characterized by subcutaneous nodules, a pruritic skin rash, and ocular lesions.

ETIOLOGY AND EPIDEMIOLOGY The disease is found in focal areas within Mexico, Guatemala, Colombia, Venezuela, Surinam, and Brazil, and throughout tropical Africa. It is estimated that at least 20 million individuals are infected and that about 5 percent of these are blind as a result of the disease.

The infection is transmitted by black flies of the genus *Simulium,* which breed along fast-moving streams. An inoculated larva matures into a single male or female in approximately one year. Since larvae do not multiply within the human host, heavy parasite loads are the result of repeated infections. The adult worms are found coiled together in fibrous subcutaneous nodules. The gravid females, which may live as long as 15 years, release unsheathed microfilariae that are actively motile and migrate in the skin, subcutaneous tissue, and eye for up to 30 months or until they are ingested by a feeding *Simulium.*

PATHOGENESIS AND CLINICAL MANIFESTATIONS The subcutaneous nodules which enclose the adult worms are usually 2 to 3 cm in diameter when fully developed. They are firm, nontender, and freely movable, although occasionally they may be adherent to underlying tissue. Their location on the body is related to the biting habits of the vector. In Central America, where the fly bites on the upper part of the body, the nodules are frequently over the head; in Africa they are primarily on the trunk and thighs. They usually number less than 10, but more than 100 have been reported in a single patient.

The important pathologic changes occur as a result of a hypersensitivity reaction to the dead or dying microfilariae. The skin lesion may appear as an erysipelas-like reaction over the face or a pruritic papular rash over one extremity. In chronic cases thickening, lichenification, and depigmentation may be present. In Africa gross skin lesions are common and may be associated with large folds of skin called *hanging groins.* Some authors believe elephantiasis may occur. Children living in endemic areas may not demonstrate these changes for decades even though microfilariae are present. The most serious complications of onchocerciasis are eye lesions which are usually found in patients repeatedly infected on the upper part of the body. A punctate keratitis, iridocyclitis, or less commonly a chorioretinitis may eventually lead to blindness.

DIAGNOSIS The diagnosis is made by demonstrating microfilariae in a skin snip taken from an involved area. A thin sliver of superficial skin is removed with a razor or punch. Care must be taken to prevent bleeding and possible contamination with blood microfilariae. The skin is weighed and then is placed in saline, teased with a pair of sharp dissecting needles, and observed for emerging microfilariae over the next hour. The results should be expressed in microfilariae per milligram of tissue. Multiple skin snips may be necessary. In patients with eye lesions, microfilariae can sometimes be seen in the anterior chamber with a slit lamp. If organisms cannot be detected by the above methods, the patient may be given 50 mg diethylcarbamazine orally. The occurrence of a pruritic rash within 24 h strongly suggests the presence of cutaneous microfilariae (Mazzotti's test). One of the filarial serologic tests may also be helpful.

TREATMENT AND PREVENTION Diethylcarbamazine is effective in destroying microfilariae but has little effect on the adult worm. The drug must be used with great care as rapid destruction of the parasites may cause a severe allergic reaction. If the eye is involved, this can result in further ocular damage. The initial adult dose is 50 mg orally. It is increased to 50 mg three times daily on the second day, 100 mg three times daily on the third day, and finally 200 mg three times a day for an additional 7 days. Antihistamines, or in rare cases steroids, can be used to control allergic reactions. In ocular reactions, the pupil should be dilated and topical steroids applied.

The adult worms may be eliminated by excision of nodules on the head and neck, a procedure which is useful in preventing ocular complications, or by chemotherapy with suramin. Details of the administration and toxicity of this drug are given in Chap. 217. The dosage is 0.1 g given intravenously to detect drug idiosyncrasy, followed by 1.0 g intravenously once weekly for five to six doses.

Chemoprophylaxis is not practical, and personal protection depends upon the use of protective clothing. Insecticides, mass therapy, and nodulectomies have been used but have not been very satisfactory.

LOIASIS

This form of filariasis is produced by *Loa loa* and is prevalent in West and Central Africa. The infection is transmitted by deer flies of the genus *Chrysops.* The adult worms, which like the other filariae may live for 10 to 15 years, migrate continuously through the subcutaneous tissue. The resulting localized areas of allergic inflammation, *Calabar swellings,* are the hallmark of the disease. Occasionally the adult worms may be seen crossing the eye subconjunctivally. This usually results in intense lacrimation, pain, and anxiety, and *Loa loa* is often called the *eye worm.* Infestation may, however, be completely asymptomatic. An association between loiasis and endomyocardial fibrosis has been reported. The diagnosis can be made by finding the adult worm or by demonstrating the distinctive sheathed microfilariae in contents of the Calabar swellings or in the bloodstream during the daytime. Microfilariae are often not found. In these cases, there are usually marked eosinophilia and a positive filarial complement fixation test. Diethylcarbamazine, administered for 2 to 3 weeks in the manner described for onchocerciasis, will kill both adult worms and microfilariae. This drug taken in a dose of 200 mg twice daily for 3 days each month is also effective as a chemoprophylactic agent.

DIPETALONEMIASIS

Dipetalonema perstans (*Acanthocheilonema perstans*), is a filarial parasite of humans and other primates inhabiting the tropical areas of Africa and Latin America. The adult worm lives encysted in the subserosal tissues of the pericardium, pleura, and peritoneum, particularly the mesentery. The unsheathed microfilariae, which can be found in the peripheral blood throughout the day, have four to six nuclei in their tail. They are transmitted from host to host by blood-sucking gnats of the genus *Culicoides.* Most infections are asymptomatic, and their principal significance lies in the fact that they may be confused with other, more serious, forms of filariasis. Nevertheless, some patients complain of fever, pruritus, Calabar swellings, erysipelas-like rashes, and abdominal pain. Peripheral eosinophilia is common, but filarial complement fixation tests are generally negative. Diagnosis is made by finding the characteristic microfilariae in the peripheral blood. Treatment with diethylcarbamazine is of doubtful benefit.

Dipetalonema streptocera is found in Equatorial Africa where it inhabits the dermis and subcutaneous tissues of chimpanzees and humans. Like *D. perstans,* it is transmitted by *Culicoides.* The microfilariae inhabit the dermal collagen where they elicit a lymphocytic and eosinophilic inflammatory response, fibrosis, lymphatic dilatation, pruritus, hypopigmented macules, and a papular rash. The diagnosis is made by recovering the nonperiodic microfilariae from skin snips as described for Onchocerciasis above. They are unsheathed and possess a sharply crooked tail with nuclei. Diethylcarbamazine, as described for Bancroftian filariasis above, is effective.

MANSONELLIASIS OZZARDI

Mansonella ozzardi are found as adult worms in the mesentery and visceral fat of people living in the tropical areas of Latin America. This species is thought to be transmitted by flies of the genus *Simulium* and gnats of the genus *Culicoides.* The nonperiodic microfilariae are released into the peripheral blood where they can be identified by their lack of a sheath or caudal nuclei. This common infection is thought to be asymptomatic, but reports of patients presenting with fever, lymphadenopathy, and hydroceles have been published. Diethylcarbamazine is ineffective.

DIROFILARIASIS

Dirofilaria immitis (canine heartworm) is a large, cosmopolitan filaria of dogs which lives in their right ventricle and pulmonary arteries and releases its microfilariae into the peripheral blood. It is transmitted by several types of mosquitoes. Human infections are occasionally reported, particularly from the southern United States. The worm does not mature in humans, and hence microfilaremia is not present. Although cardiac infections have been noted at autopsy, most human infections present as well-defined pulmonary nodules. The patients may complain of cough and chest pain or, less commonly, of hemoptysis, fever, chills, and myalgia. The diagnosis is usually made by the microscopic examination of excised pulmonary nodules.

Other *Dirofilariae* may rarely invade man producing subcutaneous eosinophilic granulomas of the eyelid, trunk, or extremities. The nodules, which measure 1 to 2 cm in diameter, may be painful or completely asymptomatic. In the southern United States, the filaria most frequently involved is *D. tenuis,* a parasite of raccoons. The nodules are removed by surgical excision.

REFERENCES

AKISADA M, TANI S: Lymphangioadenopathy of filariasis. Trans R Soc Trop Med Hyg 64:885, 1970

BEAVER PC: Filariasis without microfilaremia. Am J Trop Med 19:181, 1970

BROWN HW: *Basic Clinical Parasitology,* 4th ed., New York: Appleton-Century-Crofts, 1975

CONNOR DH et al: Onchocerciasis, onchocercal dermatitis, lymphadenitis and elephantiasis in the Ubangi territory. Hum Pathol 1:553, 1970

EDESON JFB: Filariasis. Br Med Bull 28:60, 1972

HAWKING F: The 24-hour periodicity of microfilariae: Biological mechanisms responsible for its production and control. Proc R Soc Lond [Biol] 169:59, 1967

IVE FA et al: Endomyocardial fibrosis and filariasis. Q J Med 36:495, 1967

MAEGRAITH BG, GILLES HM: *Management and Treatment of Tropical Diseases,* Oxford: Blackwell, 1972

MEYERS WM et al: Human streptocerciasis. A clinico-pathological study of 40 Africans (Zaireans) including identification of the adult filaria. Am J Trop Med Hyg 21:528, 1972

NEAFIE RC, PIGGATT J: Human pulmonary dirofilariasis. Arch Pathol 92:342, 1971

ONKEL TC: Infections with *Dipetalonema perstans* and *Mansonella ozzardi* in the aboriginal Indians of Guyana. Am J Trop Med Hyg 16:628, 1967

PAK SC: The course of lung function in treated tropical pulmonary eosinophilia. Thorax 29:710, 1974

WHO EXPERT COMMITTEE ON FILARIASIS: Third Report. Tech Rept Ser 542, Geneva, 1974

225
SCHISTOSOMIASIS (BILHARZIASIS)

JAMES J. PLORDE

DEFINITION Schistosomiasis (bilharziasis) designates a group of diseases caused by three closely related species of digenetic trematodes, or blood flukes, belonging to the family Schistosomatidae—*Schistosoma mansoni, S. haematobium,* and *S. japonicum.* These blood flukes inhabit the circulatory system of humans and animals living in tropical and subtropical countries. Here they deposit large numbers of eggs, many of which are retained within the body of the host with the production of inflammatory lesions. The organs and tissues most frequently affected are the colon, urinary bladder, liver, lungs, and central nervous system.

ETIOLOGY AND LIFE CYCLE The adult worms, which grow and mature within the portal venous system of the liver, measure 1 to 2 cm in length. The male has a central trough, the gynecophoral canal, that enfolds the longer, more slender female during most of their 4- to 30-year life span. After copulation the male carries the female against the flow of portal blood to the small mesenteric vessels. *Schistosoma japonicum* ascends the superior and *S. mansoni,* the inferior mesenteric vein. Both eventually reach the submucosal vessels of the intestine; *S. japonicum* ends up in the small intestine and ascending colon and *S. mansoni,* in the descending colon and rectum. *Schistosoma haematobium* finds its way through the hemorrhoidal anastomoses to the systemic capillaries of the bladder and other pelvic organs. When they can travel no further, the female deposits her eggs in clusters (or one by one in the case of *S. mansoni*), slowly retreating down the vessel in front of them. The daily egg output of each worm pair varies from 300 for *S. mansoni* to over 3,000 in *S. japonicum* infections. The eggs, which remain viable for 3 weeks, secrete an enzymatic substance which destroys the surrounding tissue. If the eggs lie close to the mucosal surface, they rupture into the lumen of the gut (or bladder in the case of *S. haematobium*) and are carried to the outside in the urine or feces. On reaching fresh water, the embryonated eggs quickly hatch, liberating ciliated *miracidia.* These miracidia have a life span of 6 to 8 h in which to search out and penetrate the specific snail host appropriate to the species. Within the snail the miracidia are transformed by a two-generation process of asexual reproduction into thousands of infective larvae called *cercariae.* When cercariae are released 1 to 2 months after the original penetration of the snail, they swim around vigorously, and if they contact human skin within 2 days, they penetrate it and become *schistosomula.* Within 24 h the schistosomula work their way into the peripheral venules and are carried to the right side of the heart and then to the pulmonary capillaries. After some delay, they enter the systemic circulation. Those parasites that survive the passage through the mesenteric capillary bed finally reach the portal venous system, where they mature into adult flukes in 5 to 12 weeks.

EPIDEMIOLOGY AND CONTROL Schistosomiasis is possibly the most important of the helminthic diseases because of its worldwide distribution and the extensive pathologic changes produced by the parasites. It is believed that over 200 million people in 71 countries are affected by this condition, and it is likely that increasing use of land irrigation in endemic areas will increase this number substantially. Owing to the lack of appropriate snail hosts, schistosomiasis is not transmitted in the continental United States. Imported cases are seen, however, particularly among the Puerto Rican, Filipino, and Yemenite populations.

Within endemic areas, there are wide variations in both the intensity and prevalence of infection. In most patients the worm load is small, probably less than 10 worm pairs, and disease manifestations are absent. Because adult worms do not multiply within the body of their human host, heavy infections are the result of repeated reinfections occurring over a period of years. It is among this population that serious morbidity and mortality occurs.

The continuing presence of schistosomiasis depends on the disposal of infected human excrement into fresh water, the presence of suitable snail hosts, and the exposure of persons to water infested with cercarias. Promiscuous defecation, latrine drainage, and unsanitary sewage disposal are the more important sources of pollution of streams and rivers. The disease is contracted by persons washing clothes, bathing, wading, or working in contaminated water. There is a close correlation between the degree of water contact and infection rates in endemic areas. The infection rates and intensity of infection both peak in the second decade of life and then decrease with advancing age. This might be explained in part by reduced exposure to contaminated water but also may reflect slowly developing immunity. In animal models, immunity develops to reinfection with *S. mansoni* but does not seem to affect already established infections. The major stimulus to the development of this immunity seems to be the presence of live adult worms.

Of these three disease-producing blood flukes in humans, *S. mansoni* is the most widespread and the only one present in the Western Hemisphere. It was brought to the Caribbean area and South America by African slaves. It is present in Venezuela, Surinam, Brazil, Puerto Rico, Dominican Republic, St. Lucia, and several other islands in the Caribbean. In Africa, it occurs in the Nile Delta, limited areas of East and South Africa, tropical Africa, and the Middle East including Yemen, Saudi Arabia, and Israel.

Schistosoma japonicum affects the agricultural population in Japan, China, the Philippines, the Celebes, Thailand, and Laos. Men are more frequently infected than women. An important source of infection in the Orient is the use of human excreta as a fertilizer in vegetable gardens.

Schistosoma haematobium is distributed widely throughout the African continent and is found in several countries of the Middle East. In Africa, it is highly prevalent among the agricultural population of the Nile Valley.

The best attack on schistosomiasis is preventive. Public health measures, including proper disposal of human excrement, provision of pure water supplies for domestic and recreational purposes, and mass antihelmintic therapy, should be carried out in endemic areas. The effectiveness of these measures is diminished if there are significant animal reservoirs of the disease, as in *S. japonicum* and possibly in *S. mansoni* infections. Extermination of the mollusk intermediate host by chemical agents has been used in areas where infestation rates are high. Available molluscicides include *N*-tritylmorpholine, yurimin, and niclosamide (Bayluscid). This drug appears to be the most effective, but the selection of an agent is determined in large part by the nature of the habitat. Biologic snail control methods, although showing promise, have not yet been demonstrated to be effective in the field. Careful attention to the design of irrigation systems in endemic areas is important. The use of concrete-lined ditches and intermittent or fluctuant application of water can be very effective in control of the snail population. The most successful control programs have combined mass therapy with molluscicidin g and/or environmental control. Unfortunately, this approach is extremely costly and beyond the means of many countries.

SCHISTOSOMIASIS MANSONI (INTESTINAL BILHARZIASIS, SCHISTOSOMAL DYSENTERY)

ETIOLOGY *Schistosoma mansoni* is distinguished from the two other major species by the structure of its eggs and the adult flukes. The eggs are bluntly oval, have a lateral spine, and measure about 140 by about 60 μm. They are passed in feces and, rarely, in the urine. The intermediate snail hosts belong to the genera *Biomphalaria* and *Tropicorbis.* Humans are thought to be the principal host, but baboons in Kenya have been found to be infected naturally. It is not known as yet whether they constitute an important reservoir of the disease independent of humans.

PATHOGENESIS AND CLINICAL MANIFESTATIONS Schistosomiasis *mansoni* infections are usually asymptomatic. Serious disease occurs only in those who, by virtue of repeated exposures, develop and maintain heavy worm loads over prolonged periods. Clinical manifestations can be divided into three phases: (1) An early stage in which cercariae penetrate the skin and the resulting schistosomula are carried by the blood to the liver and mature into adult parasites within the intrahepatic portal veins, (2) an intermediate stage which begins with and continues through the duration of oviposition and egg extrusion, and (3) a late stage characterized by tissue proliferation and fibrosis in response to eggs that have been retained in tissue. Within a few hours of penetrating the skin, most cercariae die, producing a dermatitis characterized by round-cell infiltration, pruritus, and papular eruption. This is the result of sensitization to cercarial antigen and rarely occurs in primary infection. The rash is commonly followed by headache, myalgia, abdominal pain, and diarrhea, manifestations presumably related to the migration of the schistosomula. These may persist for 1 or 2 weeks, terminating with a modest fever.

An acute, febrile illness, resembling serum sickness and beginning 1 to 2 months after exposure, marks the onset of oviposition and the beginning of the intermediate stage of illness. This so-called *Katayama syndrome* apparently represents an allergic response to the growing antigenic mass of ova and parasites. The illness is characterized by high spiking fever, chills, cough, urticaria, abdominal pain, diarrhea, and occasionally melena. Physical examination shows lymphadenopathy, enlarged tender liver, and fine scattered rales. Sigmoidoscopy reveals an inflamed, engorged mucosa with small areas of ulceration and hemorrhage. Laboratory tests demonstrate nonspecific liver function abnormalities and a marked eosinophilic leukocytosis. Eggs may not be present in the stool initially, and the clinical manifestations, with the exception of the eosinophilia, can be mistaken for typhoid. The acute illness may last as long as 3 months and on rare occasions may result in death. The syndrome is seen in its full intensity only in previously unexposed individuals who suffer a massive cercarial exposure. In endemic areas, it is most commonly brief and mild.

The late stage of illness is caused by the reaction of local tissue to the deposited eggs. Those which are extruded into the bowel lumen elicit little damage. The 50 percent or more that are retained, however, stimulate an eosinophilic and mononuclear-cell infiltration followed by edema, granuloma formation, and vascular obstruction. This has been demonstrated to be a delayed hypersensitivity reaction to a soluble antigen secreted by the egg. Healing occurs by fibrosis, calcification, and resorption.

In the bowel, these changes produce congestion, thickening, and, in severe infections, sessile or pedunculated polyps. Clinically, abdominal pain, diarrhea with or without blood, and a mild protein-losing enteropathy may be seen. Intestinal obstruction and rectal prolapse are rare complications. These changes often regress with treatment.

Of more severe consequence is the passage of eggs back into the venous system. These are carried to portal radicles of the liver where they produce an endophlebitis, pseudotubercle formation, acute vascular obstruction, and hepatic enlargement. With time, collars of fibrosis develop around the larger portal veins resulting in shrinkage of the liver and severe presinusoidal portal hypertension. The patient presents with hepatosplenomegaly and esophageal varices. Occasionally the enlarged spleen becomes enormous, producing a visible abdominal mass and the anemia, leukopenia, and thrombocytopenia of hypersplenism. Hepatocellular function is usually well preserved, and spider nevi, gynecomastia, jaundice, and ascites are uncommon. Repeated bouts of esophageal bleeding may occur. Hepatic encephalopathy rarely results, however, and the outcome is usually favorable. When death does occur, it is the result of exsanguination.

With the development of portacaval anastomoses, some eggs are carried past the liver to the vessels of the lung where they may produce a similar histopathologic reaction in the pulmonary arterioles. Interstitial fibrosis, destruction of pulmonary capillaries, and eventually pulmonary hypertension with cor pulmonale and aneurysms of the pulmonary artery may occur. On roentgenogram the granulomas may resemble miliary tuberculosis.

Occasionally ova are carried to the spinal cord through anastomotic venous channels or are deposited there by ectopic adults resulting in a transverse myelitis.

There is impressive evidence that circulating antigen antibody complexes may produce an immune-complex nephropathy in schistosomiasis *mansoni.* This has been observed primarily in patients with the chronic hepatosplenic form of the disease and may present as asymptomatic albuminuria, the nephrotic syndrome, or progressive renal failure. There is little information on its incidence or public health significance.

DIAGNOSIS AND LABORATORY FINDINGS Diagnosis depends on finding the ova in the stools or the rectal mucosa. Stool concentration techniques such as gravity sedimentation or formol-ether centrifugation are often required for the detection of ova. Quantitation of the egg output by the Kato thick smear or similar methods is useful in estimating the severity of infection and in following response to therapy.

Rectal biopsy is probably the single most reliable method of diagnosis, and it is often positive when repeated stool examinations are negative. By means of biopsy forceps and a proctoscope, mucosal snips are obtained from the valves of Houston, compressed between two glass slides, and examined under the low-power lens of a microscope. Eggs, often numbering in the hundreds, are clearly visible. Because dead eggs may persist in tissue for a long time after the death of the adult worms, active infection is confirmed only if the eggs can be shown to be viable. This may be done by observing the eggs for movement under the high-power lens or by hatching them in water.

Eosinophilia is usually present in schistosomiasis. An intradermal test of the immediate type becomes positive within 1 to 2 months of exposure and remains so for years despite parasitologic cure. Since it is neither highly sensitive nor specific, it is of value chiefly as an epidemiologic tool. Twenty-five percent of patients with a history of swimmer's itch give a positive test.

Complement fixation, circumoval precipitin, and indirect fluorescent antibody tests can be done, but like the intradermal test, they lack sensitivity and specificity.

The complement fixation is the most reliable test available. It becomes positive early in the course of infection, often before eggs can be recovered. Positive serologic or skin tests should lead to a vigorous search for eggs by concentration methods or rectal biopsy, but are not themselves an indication for treatment.

TREATMENT No specific therapy is available for the treatment of schistosomal dermatitis or the acute illness resembling serum sickness seen in the early months of infection. Antihistamines and steroids have been used to control the manifestations of these two symptoms. Because late schistosomiasis is caused by the continued deposition of eggs by the mature worm pairs, the aim of therapy in this stage of the disease is the sterilization and destruction of these parasites. Adult schistosomicides are available for the purpose, but in light of their considerable toxicity, therapy should not be initiated unless the presence of an active infection is first proved by the recovery of *viable* eggs from the stool or rectal mucosa. Moreover, since the severity of disease is related to the intensity of infection, complete eradication of all adult worms is probably unnecessary. Appropriate therapy will usually reduce egg output by 90 percent or more, and attempts to achieve cure by repeated use of toxic agents is unwise.

Trivalent antimony compounds, including tartar emetic (antimony potassium tartrate), stibophen (Fuadin), and stibocaptate (Astiban) have been the traditional agents for this disease. Only the latter two are still widely used, and of these stibocaptate is probably the drug of choice. A new dimethylcysteine derivative of antimony sodium tartrate (NAP) which is presently undergoing trials seems to have the effectiveness of the above agents with fewer toxic side effects.

Astiban is given by intramuscular injection as a 10% solution for five doses for a total of 35 to 50 mg per kg (maximum 2.0 g). Toxic side effects are mitigated if injections are given at weekly intervals.

Temporary ECG changes are common during therapy; they consist primarily of repolarization abnormalities which disappear a few days after the drug is discontinued. However, arrhythmias, collapse, and sudden death have been reported. Antimonials also may cause hepatitis, acute nephritis, hemolytic anemia, and thrombocytopenic purpura. Any of these complications calls for immediate discontinuation of therapy. Nausea and joint pains can usually be controlled by decreasing the individual dose or increasing the intervals between doses. Heart, renal, or liver disease constitutes a contraindication to therapy with this group of agents.

Ambilhar (niridazole) can be taken orally, 25 mg per kg every day in divided doses for 7 days. Since it is less toxic than the antimonials and probably just as effective, this drug is rapidly replacing the antimonials for the treatment of *S. mansoni* infections. Although ECG changes occur with this drug also, they are less common than with antimonial therapy. However, there has been a high incidence of neurologic abnormalities, and as many as 80 percent of patients receiving the drug show electroencephalographic changes. Psychotic episodes or convulsions, which disappear when the drug is discontinued, have also been reported, particularly in adults. The incidence of neurologic reactions seems to increase if there is serious liver disease with portacaval shunting. Niridazole should not be used in patients with a prior history of seizures.

Hycanthone is a new thioxanthone preparation that can be administered in a single intramuscular injection. Its hepatotoxicity and mutagenic properties may limit its usefulness. It is not available in the United States.

Success of treatment is judged by the disappearance of eggs from the stool, reduction in eosinophils, and alleviation of symptoms. Patients should be examined monthly for 6 to 12 months to detect relapses. The decision to retreat is based on factors such as intensity of egg output, presence of potentially reversible clinical manifestations, and the likelihood of reinfection.

Treatment of the patient with severe hepatic or pulmonary disease is largely symptomatic. There is little enthusiasm for portacaval shunting in the presence of esophageal varices. These patients usually have good hepatocellular function and, if treated carefully, will probably survive longer with repeated bleeding episodes than with surgery. Additionally, splenectomy makes these patients more susceptible to the recrudescence of chronic malaria.

PROGNOSIS The prognosis is good. Many patients never develop symptoms, and early states of colonic, hepatic, pulmonary, and central nervous system disease are completely reversible with adequate therapy. In the late fibrotic stage, the prognosis is worse.

SCHISTOSOMIASIS JAPONICA (KATAYAMA DISEASE)

ETIOLOGY The oval eggs are shorter, wider, and smaller than those of the other two species, measuring about 90×70 μm. Mature eggs have a minute hook, or spine, laterally situated and smaller than that of *S. mansoni.* The ova are passed in the feces only. The life cycle is similar to that of *S. mansoni,* except that amphibious snails of the genus *Oncomelania,* which are capable of prolonged existence away from water, are utilized as intermediate hosts, and water buffalo, horses, cattle, pigs, dogs, and cats as well as humans may harbor the adult worms. Both factors add to the difficulty in disease control. *Schistosoma japonicum* lives in the superior mesenteric venules and frequently migrates to those of the colon for oviposition.

PATHOGENESIS AND CLINICAL MANIFESTATIONS The early manifestations of infection such as the pruritic dermatitis, cough, angioneurotic edema, diarrhea, and fever produced by the penetration and migration of the schistosomula are generally similar to that seen in schistosomiasis *mansoni.* However, because *S. japonicum* eggs are deposited in greater number and in closer proximity to the liver than are those of *S. mansoni,* the intermediate and late manifestations of disease are usually more severe.

The allergic manifestations accompanying oviposition are particularly frequent and severe in japonicum infections and are generally referred to as Katayama fever. Four to six weeks after exposure the patient notes the onset of a high spiking fever, chills, cough, urticaria, generalized lymphadenopathy, tender hepatosplenomegaly, and eosinophilic leukocytosis. The deposition of large numbers of eggs in the intestinal wall results in ulcerations, bloody mucoid stools, and abdominal pain. The acute illness may persist for 1 to 2 months but usually subsides leaving the patient relatively well. Death may occur in severe cases.

With continued oviposition fibrosis of the small bowel and liver develops. These changes are seen earlier than in *mansoni* infections, and as a result the entire disease may run its course in 2 to 5 years, ending in death.

In advanced cases the gross postmortem findings are emaciation and pallor; a large or contracted liver with periportal fibrosis; splenomegaly, with fibrosis of pulp; ascites; fibrotic nodules over the colonic peritoneum; fibrous thickening and rigidity of the colon, with small polyps projecting from the mucosa; and thickening and fibrosis of the omentum.

Clinically, signs of portal obstruction such as engorgement of superficial abdominal veins, ascites, etc., appear. Some individuals present marked splenomegaly, a small contracted liver, profound anemia, leukopenia, and thrombocytopenia associated with severe malnutrition and hypoproteinemia. The majority of individuals suffering from schistosomiasis japonica die of cirrhosis and cachexia, massive hemorrhage from rupture of esophageal varices, or intercurrent infections.

Central nervous system lesions occur more frequently in the brain than in the spinal cord and appear clinically as an expanding tumor.

DIAGNOSIS AND LABORATORY FINDINGS The characteristic ova must be found in the stools in order to establish the diagnosis. In established cases, ova are more difficult to demonstrate in the stools or in rectal biopsy; positive intradermal and serologic tests in suspected cases should lead to an intensive search for the egg.

TREATMENT In general, *S. japonicum* infections are more difficult to treat, and relapses are more frequent. The drug of choice is probably potassium antimony tartrate. It is administered as a freshly prepared 0.5% solution. The drug must be given slowly. Extravasation into surrounding tissue leads to painful necrosis. The initial dose is 0.04 g; subsequent doses are given on alternate days and gradually increased to a maximum of 0.12 g by the fifth dose. A total of 2.2 g should be given. The patient should be hospitalized during treatment and remain at bed rest for a few hours after each injection. Astiban, given as outlined above for *S. mansoni* infections, may also be used. Recent experience with niridazole (Ambilhar) is encouraging, and it may now be considered an acceptable alternative to the trivalent antimonials. If a lesion is present in the brain, prompt treatment may forestall the need for surgical intervention.

PROGNOSIS If the condition is not treated early, prognosis is poor in the majority of cases encountered in endemic communities.

SCHISTOSOMIASIS HAEMATOBIA (GENITOURINARY SCHISTOSOMIASIS, ENDEMIC HEMATURIA)

ETIOLOGY AND LIFE CYCLE The eggs are compact, elongated spindles, dilated in the middle and measuring about 140 by 50 μm. At one pole they present a short terminal spine. The ova are passed in the urine, and occasionally in the feces. The life cycle is similar to that of *S. mansoni.* The adult worms live in the hemorrhoidal plexus of veins, some going to the rectum for oviposition but most of them passing on to the vesical plexus. The intermediate hosts are snails of the genera *Bulinus, Physopsis,* and *Biomphalaria.*

PATHOGENESIS AND CLINICAL MANIFESTATIONS Large numbers of ova are deposited in the submucosa of the bladder where they incite an eosinophilic granulomatous reaction. The trigone is involved at first, but soon the entire mucosa is thickened and ulcerated. In chronic infections, the other coats become scarred and the muscularis hypertrophies. Pedunculated papillomas often develop at the trigone and about the urethral orifices. The bladder capacity becomes greatly reduced as the organ loses its contractility. Lesions occur in the distal third of the ureters in many cases, causing vesicoureteral reflux, obstruction, and hydronephrosis. Bacterial pyelonephritis may occur. In about 10 percent of cases, calculi develop in the bladder, renal pelvis, or ureters, and occasionally the entire calcified bladder can be visualized on roentgenograms. Fistulas between the urogenital tract and intestines may develop. The prostate and seminal vesicles in men and the cervix and vagina in women may be affected; lymphatic blockade with elephantiasis of the genitalia occurs rarely. Carcinoma of the bladder is a frequent late complication in Egypt but not in other areas. Because the ova are deposited in the vesical plexus, ectopic eggs are carried to the lungs where they produce miliary granulomas. Although in endemic areas the egg output usually decreases in adolescence, the pathologic changes continue to progress in untreated infection.

MANIFESTATIONS Painful micturition, frequency, and terminal hematuria are the leading symptoms. Secondary bacterial infection of the urinary tract is frequent, and repeated hemorrhages from the bladder produce severe anemia. Chronic *Salmonella* bacteriuria with recurrent bouts of bacteremia have been reported from Egypt. An associated nephrotic syndrome which responds to antibiotic and anthelmintic therapy also occurred. With progressive obstruction, renal failure and uremia ensue.

DIAGNOSIS AND LABORATORY FINDINGS As in the other types of schistosomiasis, diagnosis is made by finding the characteristic ova in the urinary sediment, in tissues obtained from vesical mucosa, or, less frequently, in the stools. Egg output is highest in midmorning. Cystoscopy and biopsy of the bladder are usually diagnostic. In long-standing infections, urine cultures and intravenous urograms should be obtained.

TREATMENT Chemotherapy is very effective early in the disease and often results in dramatic reversal of symptoms and obstructive phenomena. The drugs are the same as those recommended for *S. mansoni.* Niridazole (Ambilhar) is the drug of choice. Surgery may be required for abscesses, fistulas, strictures, papillomas, and various other complications involving the bladder, but it should not be undertaken until the extent to which the lesions will resolve with medical treatment is known. Chemotherapy is indicated for secondary bacterial infections of the urinary tract, especially those caused by *Salmonella.* The criteria of cure are the absence of ova in the urine and bladder wall and the disappearance of ulcerative granulomatous lesions, as revealed by cystoscopic examination.

PROGNOSIS Provided treatment is started without delay, prognosis is good in recent infection, and fair when damage to the bladder and urinary infection have already occurred. Prognosis is very poor in chronic, late infections. After age forty-five, the mortality rate increases fourfold. The frequent coexistence of infection with *S. mansoni* aggravates prognosis and the clinical picture.

SCHISTOSOME DERMATITIS

DEFINITION AND GEOGRAPHIC DISTRIBUTION Certain nonhuman schistosome cercariae are capable of penetrating human skin but are unable to develop further. This results in a schistosome dermatitis similar to that seen with the species pathogenic for humans. This condition is also known as "swimmer's itch" and is common in many parts of the world. It apparently does not develop after a single contact with cercariae, but it ensues following multiple exposures. Definitive hosts of some of the schistosomes producing dermatitis are the muskrat and migratory birds. Both fresh- and saltwater mollusks serve as intermediate hosts.

Schistosome dermatitis has been reported from the freshwater areas of North Central and Western United States, Alaska, Canada, Central and South America, Western Europe (particularly Switzerland), and the Far East.

A seawater dermatitis believed to be produced by nonhuman schistosome cercariae has been reported in clam diggers and bathers along the coasts of New York, Rhode Island, California, Hawaii, and Florida.

PATHOGENESIS AND CLINICAL MANIFESTATIONS Because the dermatitis develops only after multiple exposures it is believed to represent an allergic reaction, the nonhuman cercariae being the sensitizing agents. Exposed individuals show a positive intradermal reaction when tested with cercarial antigen. The initial symptom is usually a prickling sensation; occasionally urticaria is noted as the water evaporates from the skin. These manifestations disappear within an hour, leaving only a few macules to mark the site of cercarial penetration. Several hours later an intense itching accompanied by a papular and occasionally a vesicular rash begins. This is most intense on the second or third day and gradually subsides.

TREATMENT Local application of antipruritic lotions such as calamine with menthol or phenol is used to allay itching and thereby reduce the likelihood of secondary infection. Treatment with antihistaminic drugs will relieve the pruritus.

PREVENTION Immediate drying of the skin after swimming has been recommended as a prophylactic measure. This will not completely prevent lesions, since some penetration occurs during immersion. Dimethylphthalate cream has been reported as an effective cercarial repellent.

In some areas, control has been effected by destruction of snails. Copper sulfate and copper carbonate have been used for this purpose. Treatment of shallow waters where snails are abundant has been moderately effective.

REFERENCES

BROWN HW: *Basic Clinical Parasitology,* 4th ed., New York: Appleton-Century-Crofts, 1975

CHEEVER AW: A quantitative post-mortem study of schistosomiasis mansoni in man. Am J Trop Med 17:38, 1968

CLARK WD et al: Acute schistosomiasis mansoni in 10 boys—An outbreak in Caguas, Puerto Rico. Ann Intern Med 73:379, 1970

FALCAO HA, GOULD DB: Immune complex nephropathy in schistosomiasis. Ann Intern Med 83:148, 1975

JORDAN P: Epidemiology and control of schistosomiasis. Br Med Bull 28:55, 1972

KAGAN IG: Serologic diagnosis of schistosomiasis. Bull NY Acad Med 44:262, 1968

LEHMAN JS JR et al: Urinary schistosomiasis in Egypt: Clinical, radiological, bacteriological, and parasitological correlations. Trans R Soc Trop Med Hyg 67:384, 1973

MARCIAL-ROJAS RA, FIAL RE: Neurologic complications of schistosomiasis: Review of the literature and report of two cases of transverse myelitis due to *S. mansoni.* Ann Intern Med 59:215, 1963

ORRIS L, COMBES FC: Clam digger's dermatitis: Schistosome dermatitis from sea water. AMA Arch Dermatol Syphilol 66:367, 1952

SMITHERS SR: Recent advances in the immunology of schistosomiasis. Br Med Bull 28:49, 1972

WARREN KS: The immunopathogenesis of schistosomiasis: A multidisciplinary approach. Trans R Soc Trop Med Hyg 66:417, 1972

——: Regulation of the prevalence and intensity of schistosomiasis in man: Immunology or ecology. J Infect Dis 127:595, 1973

WHO EXPERT COMMITTEE: Schistosomiasis control. WHO Tech Rept Ser 1973

226
OTHER TREMATODES OR FLUKES

JAMES J. PLORDE

INTRODUCTION The trematodes of humans are long-lived parasites which produce progressive damage to the tissues of their hosts. With the exception of schistosomes, they are similar in morphology and life cycle. The adult flukes are flat, leaflike hermaphrodites that vary in length from a few millimeters to several centimeters. Their digestive tract, unlike that of the nematodes, ends blindly. As their name indicates, they have two "holes" in the form of oral and ventral suckers which are used as organs of attachment and locomotion. The operculated eggs, which are passed in the feces or sputum, hatch in the water to produce a ciliated, free-swimming *miracidium.* The miracidium reaches and penetrates the tissue of an intermediate snail host to undergo a period of development, eventuating in the release of thousands of swarms of free-living *cercariae* from the snail.

These thousands of tail-bearing larvae must, in turn, reach a second intermediate host, usually an aquatic animal or vegetation, where they encyst forming *metacercariae.* The definitive host is infected when he ingests the parasitized second intermediate host. The distribution of flukes is usually limited by the location of their molluscan intermediate host. With the exception of *Opisthorchis* and *Fasciola,* most hermaphroditic flukes are found only in tropical or subtropical areas.

PARAGONIMIASIS Definition Paragonimiasis (endemic hemoptysis) is a chronic infection of the lung caused by trematodes of the genus *Paragonimus.* Clinically, the disease is characterized by cough and hemoptysis. Ectopic worms may cause a variety of other manifestations. Geographically, it is probably the most widely distributed disease caused by hermaphroditic flukes.

Etiology and epidemiology Although *P. westermani,* which is widely distributed in the Far East, is the most common cause of human paragonimiasis, a number of other species, including *P. skrjabini, P. heterotremus* (China), *P. africanus* (Cameroons, Nigeria, Zaire), *P. mexicanus, P. peruvianus,* and *P. caliensis* (Central and South America), may cause the disease. The short, plump adults (7 to 12 mm in length, 4 to 6 mm in width) have a life span of 4 to 5 years which they typically spend encysted in the lung parenchyma of the host. Their golden-brown operculated eggs (50 by 90 μm) reach the bronchioles from where they are coughed up and excreted in the sputum or swallowed and passed in the feces. They must embryonate several weeks in fresh water before hatching to release the miracidium.

The infection is acquired by ingestion of cysts in the second intermediate host, a crab or crayfish. The metacercariae excyst in the duodenum, burrow through the intestinal wall into the peritoneal cavity, and then usually migrate through the diaphragm and into the lung. The worms also may be found in the liver, pancreas, kidney, mesentery, skeletal muscle, subcutaneous tissues, and central nervous system, particularly the brain. The dog, cat, pig, rat, and wild carnivores are definitive hosts for the parasite in addition to humans.

The incidence of paragonimiasis is often affected by food shortages or local customs. The metacercariae survive in vinegar, and lightly pickled or inadequately cooked food usually serves as the source of infection in the Far East. Fresh crab juice used for the treatment of measles in Korea and for infertility in the Cameroons may also transmit the parasite. Children may acquire the disease in endemic areas while handling or eating raw crabs during play.

Pathogenesis and clinical manifestations An eosinophilic granuloma forms about the adult worm, eventually leading to the formation of a fibrous cyst. The pulmonary lesions which measure up to 1 cm in diameter frequently communicate with a bronchiole, resulting in secondary bacterial infection. Small, fibrous nodules representing reaction around deposited eggs also occur. Clinically the picture is one of chronic bronchitis and bronchiectasis with production of brownish sputum and hemoptysis. A poorly resolving pulmonary infiltrate, lung abscess, or pleural effusion may be present in heavy infections. The roentgenographic findings vary with the stage of infection. Initially one or more soft infiltrates may be seen anywhere in the lungs excepting the apexes. These are then gradually replaced by round nodules which not infrequently cavitate. Eventually, fibrosis and calcification occur, presenting a picture closely resembling tuberculosis, a disease which often coexists with paragonimiasis.

An abdominal mass, pain, and dysentery characterize intestinal or peritoneal infections. Various types of paralysis and epilepsy occur in cerebral involvement. Homonymous hemianopsia, optic atrophy, and papilledema are common. The cerebrospinal fluid usually shows an eosinophilic leukocytosis and elevated protein. Cerebral calcifications are seen on x-ray in 50 percent of cases. *Paragonimus skrjabini* infections are characterized by migratory subcutaneous nodules that contain adult flukes.

Laboratory findings Eosinophilia is a constant finding. Definitive diagnosis depends upon finding the characteristic operculated ova in the sputum, stool, pleural fluid, or tissue. Eggs may be rare or totally absent from the sputum during the first 3 months of infection but are eventually found in 75 to 85 percent of infected patients. Even later, however, repeated examinations using concentration techniques may be required for their recovery. Ziehl-Neelsen staining, often carried out for suspected tuberculosis, usually will not demonstrate the eggs. In fact, the sputum concentration techniques for tuberculosis may destroy the eggs that are present. Stool examination is frequently helpful in children. A complement fixation test is available, and the results correlate well with active infection. It usually becomes negative within 6 months of successful therapy. The skin test does not distinguish present and past infections and is used primarily for epidemiologic purposes.

Treatment and prevention Bithionol is the drug of choice. From 30 to 40 mg per kg in divided doses should be given every other day for a total of 10 to 15 treatment days. The symptoms disappear rapidly, and most infiltrates resolve within 3 months. Side effects are minor and consist of nausea, vomiting, and urticaria. Concomitant bacterial infection must be treated. Prevention of superinfection by the same parasite is important, because the disease is self-limiting.

The most practical control measure is the adequate cooking of all shellfish before they are eaten.

CLONORCHIASIS Definition Clonorchiasis is an infection of the biliary passages caused by *Clonorchis sinensis,* the most important liver fluke of man. Although the infection is usually asymptomatic, heavy worm loads may produce manifestations of biliary obstruction.

Etiology and epidemiology *Clonorchis sinensis* is a small fluke (5 × 15 mm) that lives as long as 25 years in the biliary tree of its host. Here the flukes feed on mucosal secretions and pass operculated eggs into the feces. On reaching fresh water, the eggs are ingested by the intermediate snail host. After multiplication and development within the snail, the cercariae are released and penetrate freshwater fish. Infections result from ingestion of the raw, dried, slated, or pickled flesh of freshwater fish containing encysted metacercariae. The larva is released in the duodenum. It enters the common bile duct and migrates to the small bile capillaries, where it develops into the adult form in about 1 month. In addition to humans, dogs, cats, pigs, and rats serve as disease reservoirs. The main endemic areas are Korea, Japan, China, and Vietnam where clonorchiasis may be perpetuated by the practice of fertilizing fish ponds with manure and human feces. Twenty-five percent of the population of Hong Kong and a small proportion of Chinese immigrants to this country have been shown to be infected. The disease may also be acquired in the United States by the ingestion of infected, dried, frozen, or pickled fish imported from the Far East. Clinically, apparent cases are restricted to the adult population in whom the accumulated worm load eventually produces pathologic effects.

Pathogenesis and clinical manifestations During the migration of the larvae, the patient may have fever, chills, tender hepatomegaly, mild jaundice, and eosinophilia. The mature worm causes proliferation of the biliary epithelium, periductal fibrosis, chronic pericholangitis, and atrophy of the parenchyma. Light infections are usually asymptomatic, but worm loads of 500 to 1,000 flukes often result in periportal fibrosis with the clinical manifestations of portal hypertension. Recurrent attacks of suppurative cholangitis with or without intrahepatic choledocholithiasis may follow biliary obstruction with dead flukes. These occasionally present as hypoglycemic coma. Cholangiocarcinoma may occur in patients with severe, long-standing infections. The adult worms may infest the pancreatic ducts, where they can cause squamous metaplasia, periductal fibrosis, and acute pancreatitis.

Laboratory diagnosis Clinical and epidemiologic findings often suggest the diagnosis. There may be elevation of the alkaline phosphatase and hyperbilirubinemia. Eosinophilia is variable. Occasionally, a plain film of the abdomen will demonstrate intrahepatic calcification. Definitive diagnosis depends on the demonstration of the eggs in the feces or the duodenal contents. They measure 29 by 16 μm, possess a conspicuous opercular rim as well as a posterior knob, and can be distinguished from the eggs of *Metafonimus, Heterophyses,* and *Opisthorchis* only with difficulty. An antigen extracted from adult worms can be used in a complement fixation test for the detection of the host's antibody response. Skin tests are also useful.

Treatment and prevention No consistently effective treatment is known, but some success has been noted with chloroquine diphosphate. Chloroquine is prescribed in a dose of 0.25 g three times daily for 6 weeks. Infections which do not respond to this dosage should be treated for an additional 2- to 3-month period. Thorough cooking of freshwater fish will prevent infection.

OPISTHORCHIASIS Opisthorchiasis is caused by *Opisthorchis felineus* or *O. viverini* and is characterized by hepatic lesions produced by adult worms in the larger bile ducts. The life cycle resembles that of *C. sinensis.* The geographic distribution differs in that *O. felineus* is endemic in Eastern and Central Europe and in Siberia and occurs in some parts of Asia, while *O. viverini* is found in Thailand and Laos. Cats and wild carnivores act as the principal reservoir hosts, and the infection is found most commonly along rivers and lakes which harbor an abundant fish life. Up to 25 percent of inhabitants of northeastern Thailand are purported to carry the parasite. The clinical lesions are similar to those seen in clonorchiasis except that gallstones are rare. The diagnosis usually is based on the finding of the eggs in the feces or duodenal contents. Treatment as recommended for clonorchiasis may be used. Infection can be prevented by eating only well-cooked fish.

FASCIOLIASIS Fascioliasis is caused by *Fasciola hepatica,* which like *Clonorchis,* inhabits the bile ducts of the definitive host. When fully matured, the adult measures about 3 by 1 cm and discharges large operculate eggs 140 by 70 μm which must embryonate in fresh water before hatching.

Fascioliasis produces so-called "liver rot" in sheep, the principal definitive host. The disease is most common in sheep and cattle-raising countries but has been reported from many parts of the world. In North America it occurs in the Southern and Western United States, Central America, and in the Caribbean Islands.

Infection is contracted by ingestion of the encysted forms of the fluke attached to edible aquatic plants such as watercress. The larvae excyst in the duodenum, migrate through the intestinal wall, pass into the peritoneal cavity, penetrate the liver capsule, and finally reach the bile ducts, where they mature. Occasionally larvae may migrate to and mature in ectopic locations including subcutaneous tissue, chest cavity, or brain.

Early clinical manifestations are related to the migration of the larval form to and within the liver. Epigastric pain, fever, diarrhea, jaundice, urticaria, pruritus, arthralgia, and eosinophilia may be observed during this stage. Fibrosis of the liver similar to that found in clonorchiasis appears only after prolonged residence of many adult worms in the bile ducts. Obstruction of the bile duct occurs frequently and may be the presenting manifestation of disease. A pharyngeal form of the disease, called *halzoun,* can result from eating infected raw liver, the young adults attaching themselves to the pharyngeal mucosa, occasionally interfering with respiration.

The diagnosis usually is based on the finding of the eggs in the feces or in the duodenal contents. It is difficult to distinguish the eggs from those of *Fasciolopsis buski.* Complement fixation, hemagglutination, and precipitin tests have been reported to be helpful. A skin test is also available.

Treatment is unsatisfactory. Dehydroemetine dehydrochloride, 1 mg/kg/day intramuscularly for 10 days, may be helpful and at times curative. The drug should not be given to patients with chronic cardiac or renal disease or to children. Bithionol in an oral dose of 50 mg per kg every other day for 10 to 15 doses has also been effective and may be less toxic.

To prevent infection, aquatic plants such as watercress should not be eaten, vegetables grown in fields irrigated with polluted water should be boiled, and safe drinking water should be provided.

FASCIOLOPSIASIS Fasciolopsiasis is caused by the large intestinal fluke *Fasciolopsis buski,* which inhabits the upper part of the intestine of its definitive host. The principal definitive host is the pig. In parts of China, India, and other areas in the Far East, infection of humans occurs following ingestion, or peeling with the teeth, of water chestnuts and other edible aquatic plants. The large adults attach themselves to the intestinal mucosa, and these sites may later ulcerate. The infection is usually asymptomatic. In heavy infections, diarrhea and abdominal pain appear early. Later, asthenia with ascites and anasarca occurs. Diagnosis is based upon the history and the finding of eggs in the feces. The eggs resemble those of *Fasciola hepatica.* The prognosis in untreated heavy infections, especially in children, is poor. Tetrachloroethylene as given for hookworm infections is effective. Hexylresorcinol can also be expected to cure or markedly reduce the worm burden in the majority of cases.

REFERENCES

Chan PH, Teoh TB: The pathology of *Clonorchis sinensis* infestation of the pancreas. J Pathol Bacteriol 93:185, 1967

Farcey RV, Marsden PD: Fascioliasis in man: An outbreak in Hampshire. Br Med J 2:619, 1960

Koenigstein RP: Observations on the epidemiology of infections with *Clonorchis sinensis.* Trans R Soc Trop Med Hyg 42:503, 1949

Komiya V: Clonorchis and clonorchiasis, in *Advances in Parasitology,* vol. 4, ed B Dawes, London: Academic, 1966, p. 53

McFadzean AJS, Yeung RTT: Hypoglycemia in suppurative pancholangitis due to Clonorchis sinensis. Trans R Soc Trop Med Hyg 59:179, 1965

Okunda K et al: Clonorchiasis studied by percutaneous cholangiogram and a therapeutic trial of 2, 4-diisothiocyanate. Gastroenterology 65:457, 1973

Plant AG et al: A clinical study of *Fasciolopsis buski* in Thailand. Trans R Soc Trop Med Hyg 63:470, 1969

Sadun EH, Buck AA: Paragonimiasis in South Korea—Immunodiagnostic, epidemiologic, clinical, roentgenologic and therapeutic studies. Am J Trop Med 9:562, 1960

Yokogawa M: *Paragonimus* and paragonimiasis. Exp Parasitol 10:81, 139, 1960

——: *Paragonimus* and paragonimiasis, in *Advances in Parasitology,* vol. 7, ed B Dawes, London: Academic, 1969, p. 375

227 CESTODE (TAPEWORM) INFECTIONS

JAMES J. PLORDE

INTRODUCTION The tapeworms, or cestodes, are segmented ribbon-shaped hermaphroditic worms which inhabit the intestinal tract of many vertebrates. Unlike other helminths, these parasites lack a digestive tract, and they absorb food through their entire surface. Attachment to the host's intestinal mucosa is effected by means of sucking cups or grooves located on the head, or *scolex.* In some species, the head is also armed with hooklets which aid in attachment. Behind the globular scolex lies a short, narrow neck from which segments or *proglottides* develop one at a time to form the chainlike *strobila* of the worm. These proglottides progressively mature as they are displaced further and further from the neck by the formation of newer segments. As each section reaches gravidity, it releases its mass of eggs by passing them through a uterine pore, by splitting open, or by simply disintegrating. Because the eggs of many tapeworms appear identical, species identification depends on the morphologic characteristics of the scolex or gravid proglottides.

Except for *Hymenolepis nana* the tapeworm parasites of humans require one or more intermediate hosts for larval development. Among the *Taenia* group, there is a single intermediate. The eggs or *onchospheres* are passed onto the soil and ingested by the intermediate host in whose tissues they develop into cystlike structures. If the cyst contains a single scolex, it is referred to as a *cysticercus,* or *cysticercoid* in the case of *H. nana.* If several scolices develop within the cyst, it is called a *coenurus* (see Coenurosis below). However, if daughter cysts, each containing several scolices are formed, the structure is referred to as a hydatid (see Echinococcosis below).

Organisms belonging to the *Diphyllobothrium* genus require two intermediate hosts. The eggs, unlike those of the *Taenia* group, are operculated and must be deposited in fresh water. Here they hatch, releasing a free-swimming larva or *coracidium.* This is ingested by a suitable crustacean, the first intermediate host, and is transformed into a procercoid larva. If the infected crustacean is then swallowed by a freshwater fish, the larva invades the tissues of this second intermediate and develops into a plerocercoid larvae or sparganum (see Sparganosis below). In both the *Taenia* and *Diphyllobothrium* groups the definitive host is infected after ingesting the flesh of an intermediate host containing the infective larval form.

Human tapeworm infections fall into one of two major clinical groups. In the first, represented by taeniasis *saginata,* humans act as the definitive host, harboring the adult tapeworm in their intestine. In the second, humans are an intermediate host, and harbor the larval forms in their tissues. This is exemplified by sparganosis, coenurosis, and echinococcosis. Taeniasis *solium* is unique because the human may act both as the definitive and intermediate host.

TAENIASIS SAGINATA Definition Taeniasis saginata is an intestinal infection of humans caused by the beef tapeworm.

Etiology and pathogenesis In its adult stage, *Taenia saginata* inhabits the upper jejunum where it may survive for as long as 25 years. The cestode is 5 to 10 m in length and possesses a small, unarmed scolex with 4 prominent suckers and between 1,000 to 2,000 proglottides. The gravid segments are longer than they are wide (5×20 mm) and have 15 to 30 lateral uterine branches, thus distinguishing it from *T. solium,* which has 8 to 12. The eggs, which are passed within the intact proglottid, measure 30×40 μm, have a thick brown radially striated shell, and contain a fully developed embryo with three pairs of hooklets. They are indistinguishable from those of *T. solium.* After the eggs are deposited on soil or vegetation, they are ingested by cattle or other herbivores. The embryo is released in the intestine, invades the intestinal wall, and is carried by vascular channels to striated muscle in the hind limbs, diaphragm, and tongue. Here it is filtered out and is transformed over a period of 3 or 4 months into an ovoid bladder worm, or cysticercus. This form, which may remain viable for 1 to 3 years, measures about 5×10 mm and consists of a scolex held in a cystlike structure. After ingestion of the cyst in raw or undercooked beef by humans, about 2 months is required for the adult worm to develop in the intestine.

Epidemiology Taeniasis saginata occurs in all countries in which it is the custom to eat raw or undercooked beef. It is particularly prevalent in Ethiopia, Kenya, the Middle East, Yugoslavia, Mexico, and parts of South America and the U. S. S. R. Beef tapeworm transmission, although uncommon, continues to occur in the United States, particularly in the Northeastern and Western parts of the country.

Clinical manifestations In probably the majority of cases the disease is asymptomatic. Epigastric discomfort, diarrhea, hunger sensations, weight loss, irritability, nausea, and rarely an increase in appetite have been reported in association with *T. saginata* infections.

Movements of the worm are sometimes apparent, and occasionally proglottides may crawl through the anus, appearing in the bed linen or underclothing of the distraught host. Rarely, segments become impacted in the appendix or cystic or pancreatic duct producing obstruction and inflammation of these organs.

Laboratory findings The diagnosis is usually made by the finding of proglottides in the feces. Several proglottides are shed daily, making their recovery relatively easy. Eggs may be distributed on the stool or perianal area if a proglottid ruptures during defecation, and should be looked for in the absence of segments. The perianal region may be examined as for pinworm infection, using the Scotch-brand tape swab. By this method 85 to 95 percent of infections may be detected, whereas by stool examination only 50 to 75 percent can be recognized. Since the eggs cannot be distinguished from those of *T. solium,* it is necessary to examine carefully either the proglottides or the scolex to identify the tapeworm species correctly.

Treatment Niclosamide (Yomesan) is a highly effective taenicide which kills the scolex and immature segments of the worm on contact. This drug may be given without preparation or purge in a single 2-g dose. Four 0.5-g tablets are thoroughly chewed at one time and swallowed with a small amount of water. Few side effects have been reported. As the worm is digested before it is passed in the stool, no attempt should be made to recover the scolex. The stool should be checked at 3 and 6 months to be certain a cure has been obtained. Alternatively, quinacrine (Atabrine) may be used. This drug, for many years the standard medication for tapeworm, is inconvenient to administer. The evening before treatment, the patient takes 30 g sodium or magnesium sulfate in a glass of water. The following morning, while still fasting, he takes 0.8 g quinacrine as 2 tablets of 0.1 g each at 10-min intervals. Nausea, vomiting, and abdominal pain are common. This may be alleviated somewhat by taking 600 mg sodium bicarbonate with each dose of quinacrine. The entire 0.8-g dose can be mixed in water and given as a single dose through a duodenal tube. Two hours later a second dose of sodium or magnesium sulfate is taken. When successful, such treatment will remove the entire worm, which will be found to be stained yellow. If the scolex has not been removed, the tapeworm will regenerate after 2 or 3 months.

Bithional given in two oral 1-g doses 1 h apart and followed by a purge 2 to 8 h later has been found to be highly effective by Japanese workers. Paromomycin, 1.0 g orally every 4 h for four doses, has also been recommended.

Prevention The only practical means of preventing infection is the thorough cooking of beef. Temperatures as low as 56°C for as little as 5 min will destroy cysticerci. Refrigeration and salting for prolonged periods or freezing at −10°C for 5 days also destroys the cysticercus. Adequate meat inspection and proper disposal of human excreta also aid in control.

TAENIASIS SOLIUM AND CYSTICERCOSIS Definition *Taenia solium,* the pork tapeworm, inhabits the intestinal lumen of humans, its only definitive host. The usual intermediate host is the hog, but in some circumstances, the larval or intermediate stages may also develop in humans, resulting in a condition referred to as *cysticercosis.*

Epidemiology Taeniasis solium is worldwide but is most common in the U. S. S. R., Eastern Europe, Asia, Africa, Mexico, and South America. At the present time the disease is practically nonexistent in the United States.

Etiology and pathogenesis The hermaphroditic adult resides in the upper jejunum and like *T. saginata* may live for decades. It is about 3 m in length and possesses a globular scolex containing a rostellum with two rows of hooklets. There are seldom more than 1,000 proglottides. The gravid proglottid measures about 6 × 12 mm and contains a uterus with 8 to 12 lateral branchings. The eggs resemble those of *T. saginata* but are infective for both human and hog. Although humans may be autoinfected when gravid segments are returned to the stomach by reverse peristalsis, the eggs are more commonly transmitted by the fecal-oral route. When ova are ingested by the intermediate host, the embryo is released from the egg, penetrates the intestinal wall, and is carried by vascular channels to all parts of the body. Localization with development over a period of 2 to 3 months to the encysted larval stage ("bladder worm") occurs predominantly in striated muscle of the tongue, neck, and trunk. The cysticerci are ovoid, gray-white opalescent structures about 1 cm in diameter. They may survive for up to 5 years. Humans become infected with the adult stage following ingestion of undercooked pork containing cysticerci. The scolex is freed and attaches itself to the intestinal mucosa; development to the adult stage begins at this time.

Clinical manifestations Clinical manifestations of adult worm infestation resemble those associated with *T. saginata.* The clinical picture is entirely different when humans serve as the intermediate host. Cysticerci develop in the subcutaneous tissues, in muscles, in viscera, and—of most significance—in the eye and brain. Only a moderate tissue reaction occurs while the scolex is viable, but symptoms occur only in heavy infections. The dead larva, however, behaves as a foreign body and provokes a marked tissue response with muscular pains, weakness, fever, and eosinophilia. The involvement in the brain may be in the form of a meningoencephalitis when the cysticerci are widely distributed. However, epilepsy, brain tumor, encephalitis, and other types of neurologic or psychiatric disorders may be simulated. Degenerated cysticerci ultimately calcify.

Infection with the adult worm can be detected by finding eggs in perianal scrapings or in the feces. However, to differentiate *T. solium* from *T. saginata* infection, proglottides or the scolex must be examined. Cysticercosis should be suspected in an individual who has lived in a hyperendemic area and who develops neurologic findings. Biopsy of subcutaneous nodules may lead to the identification of typical encysted larvae. Roentgenograms of the soft tissues also often reveal calcified cysticerci. The cysticercosis hemagglutination or complement fixation test may be of help in the diagnosis. The prognosis is in large part determined by the stage and location of the parasite. Surgery may be necessary in cerebral and ocular cysticercosis.

Treatment For removal of the worm in the adult, quinacrine is given as for taeniasis saginata, above. It is well to administer an antiemetic before giving quinacrine, to prevent reverse peristalsis, with return of the eggs to the stomach and release of the embryos. Niclosamide and paromomycin are also effective against *T. solium.* However, because these drugs result in the maceration of worms with release of ova, cysticercosis could theoretically occur. If they are used, a saline purge should be administered 1 h after completion of therapy.

COENUROSIS This is a rare infection of humans by the larval stage, or *coenurus,* of the dog tapeworm *Multiceps multiceps.* As in cysticercosis, the subcutaneous tissue, eye, and central nervous system may be involved. Over 60 cases have been reported from around the world. In tropical areas the brain has usually been involved and the cases have ended fatally. Clinically, the presentation is one of a slowly growing tumor. Diagnosis and treatment both rely on surgical excision of the lesion.

HYMENOLEPIASIS NANA Definition Hymenolepiasis nana is an intestinal infection of humans, mice, and rats by *Hymenolepis nana,* the dwarf tapeworm. The infection is particularly common in children in whom it is usually asymptomatic.

Etiology The life cycle is unique in that both the larval and adult phases occur in the same host. The small, 2-cm adult lives only a few weeks, during which time it can be found in the proximal ileum. Its proglottides are wider than they are long and may number 100 to 200. The gravid segments break apart in the fecal stream releasing their spherical eggs. These measure 30 × 44 μm in diameter and have a double membrane enclosing the embryo with six hooklets. The inner vitelline membrane has four to eight slender filaments arising from each pole. The eggs are immediately infective and when ingested by a new host, the freed oncospheres penetrate the intestinal villi, becoming cysticercoids. Approximately 2 weeks later, the larvae migrate back to the intestinal lumen, attach themselves to the mucosa, and mature into adult worms. In some situations, the eggs hatch before passing in the stool, causing internal autoinfection.

Distribution Dwarf tapeworm infection has been reported in temperate and tropical regions around the globe. It is the most common tapeworm found in the United States, most of the infections occurring in the Southern states. The infection is spread by the direct fecal-oral route and is most common in children and institutional populations.

Clinical manifestations This tapeworm infection is characterized by the presence of many adult worms in the host's intestine. When infection is massive, diarrhea and abdominal pain occur.

Treatment Niclosamide, as prescribed for taeniasis saginata above, is given each day for five consecutive doses. Children under eight should receive one-half the adult daily dose and infants one-fourth the adult dose. Cure is obtained in 90 percent of patients. Paromomycin, 45 mg per kg daily for 5 to 7 days, may also be effective.

Prevention This is a difficult problem, similar to that encountered in enterobiasis. Only a single host is involved, and the eggs are immediately infective. Personal hygiene should be stressed. The contamination of food by rats and mice should be prevented.

HYMENOLEPIASIS DIMINUTA *Hymenolepis diminuta* is a short-lived cestode of rats and mice that occasionally infects small children. Larval development occurs in a wide variety of insect hosts including fleas and mealworms. Humans become infected with the adult tapeworm when they ingest uncooked cereal foods contaminated with these insects. Infection is usually asymptomatic, and the diagnosis is made only when the characteristic eggs are found in the stool. They resemble those of *H. nana,* but are longer (58 × 86 μm) and lack polar filaments. Niclosamide as prescribed for hymenolepiasis *nana* is the treatment of choice.

DIPYLIDIASIS *Dipylidium caninum* is the common tapeworm of cats and dogs. The orange-brown proglottid, which resembles a pumpkin seed, is often passed intact in the stool or migrates through the anal canal. This may cause animals harboring this parasite to drag their buttocks across the floor. The characteristic egg packets are then expelled by the proglottides and ingested by fleas to develop into infective larval forms. The definitive host becomes infected by swallowing involved fleas. Human infections occur primarily in small children who ingest fleas in the process of playing with their pets. The diagnosis is made by recovering the characteristic proglottid or egg packet. Treatment is the same as for *T. saginata* above. Prevention consists of periodic deworming of pets.

DIPHYLLOBOTHRIASIS LATUM Definition *Diphyllobothrium latum,* the fish tapeworm or broad tapeworm, produces a disease in its definitive host, including humans, characterized by the presence of the adult worm in the intestinal lumen.

Etiology and pathogenesis The adult *Diphyllobothrium* lies attached to the mucosa of the ileum and occasionally jejunum by a pair of sucking grooves located on the scolex. It may live up to 20 years and achieve a length of 10 to 30 ft. The 3,000 to 4,000 proglottides are wider than they are long. Unlike *Taenia,* the gravid segments are retained by the worm, and each day a million operculated ova are passed directly in the stool. On reaching water, the egg hatches, releasing a free-swimming embryo. This is eaten by small freshwater crustaceans belonging to the species *Cyclops* or *Diaptomus,* in which it develops into a *procercoid.* When the infected crustacean is swallowed by a fish, the larva migrates into the flesh and grows into a *plerocercoid,* or *sparganum,* larva. Humans are infected by ingesting raw infected fish. The tapeworm matures in the intestine and after 3 weeks is an adult capable of discharging eggs.

Epidemiology The infection is common in the Baltic and Scandinavian countries, Switzerland, Italy, Russia, Japan, Chile, and Central Africa. It also occurs in the north central United States, south central Canada, and Florida. The maintenance of infection in these areas depends upon the continued disposal of raw sewage into freshwater lakes and the ingestion of improperly prepared fish. Women who sample lutefish or gefilte fish as they prepare these dishes often become infected. Among Ontario Indians, the infection is acquired by the ingestion of salted fresh fish.

Clinical manifestations Most infections are asymptomatic or produce slight, transient abdominal discomfort. Rarely, there may be severe cramping abdominal pain, vomiting, weakness, and loss of weight. Intestinal obstruction has been reported in multiple infections.

In a small percentage of infected patients, a tapeworm anemia develops which has many features in common with Addisonian pernicious anemia, including central nervous system involvement. The location of the worm in the intestine is important, anemia occurring only when the tapeworm is in the proximal small intestine. Large amounts of vitamin B_{12} have been demonstrated in the tapeworm, presumably absorbed from the host's intestine. *Taenia saginata,* which does not produce pernicious tapeworm anemia, contains about 2 percent as much vitamin B_{12} as *D. latum.* The appearance of anemia is certainly related to vitamin B_{12} absorption and possibly also to decreased production of intrinsic factor or inadequate extrinsic factor. It is apparent that the tapeworm and the host compete for vitamin B_{12}.

Diagnosis The characteristic eggs are discharged into the stools in large numbers, making the diagnosis quite easy. They measure 55 to 76 by 41 to 56 μm and possess a single shell with an operculum at one end and a knob on the other. Eosinophilia is often present.

Treatment Treatment as prescribed for taeniasis saginata will cure most infections. In the presence of severe macrocytic anemia, parenteral vitamin B_{12} should be given.

Prevention The most practical control measure is prohibiting the disposal of untreated sewage into freshwater lakes. Personal protection consists of thorough cooking of all freshwater fish. Freezing of fish at −10°C for 24 to 48 h will also prevent transmission.

SPARGANOSIS The *sparganum,* or plerocercoid larva, of *Diphyllobothrium mansoni* will develop in humans following ingestion (usually in drinking water) of a *Cyclops* bearing the procercoid larva. Sparganosis also follows ingestion of infected frogs or application of infected fresh frog flesh as a poultice. The frog tissues contain the sparganum, which is capable of invading human tissues. The dog and cat are definitive hosts for *D. mansoni.* The infection often presents as a painful subcutaneous swelling. The periorbital tissues may be involved with marked palpebral edema and destruction of the globe. A marked eosinophilia is usually present. The location of the larvae determines the prognosis of the infection in humans. Surgery and injection of ethyl alcohol with epinephrine-free procaine to kill the worms is the preferred method of treatment. Novarsenobenzol given intravenously is also said to be effective.

ECHINOCOCCIASIS **Definition** Echinococciasis is a tissue infection of humans caused by the larval stage of *Echinococcus granulosus* or *E. multilocularis.* These species of echinococcus are distinct morphologically and biologically. In humans, *E. granulosus* produces cystic, expanding lesions, involving the liver and lungs primarily, whereas the lesions of *E. multilocularis* are destructive because of their invasive character.

Etiology The adult *E. granulosus* is found in the jejunum of dogs, wolves, and other canines, where it may live for 5 to 20 months. It is a small worm measuring 5 mm in length. In addition to the scolex and neck, it has three proglottides, one immature, one mature, and one gravid. The gravid segment splits, either before or after passage in the stool, to release eggs, which appear identical to those of *T. saginata.* When ingested by an appropriate intermediate host such as sheep, cattle, hogs, deer, or humans, the embryos escape from the eggs, penetrate the intestinal mucosa, and enter the portal circulation. Approximately 60 percent are filtered out by the liver; 25 percent lodge in the lung, and the rest are carried into the general circulation to involve the brain, kidney, bones, and other tissues. The larvae that are not phagocytosed and destroyed develop into hydatid cysts, reaching the diameter of 1 cm within 5 months. Most cysts are unilocular and consist of an external laminated cuticula and an inner germinal layer. Fluid fills and distends the cyst. Brood capsules and second- or third-generation daughter cysts develop from the germinal layer. "Hydatid sand" found in the cyst consists of scolices liberated from ruptured brood capsules. Occasionally, evagination of the cyst wall occurs, with the development of a multilocular or alveolar type of lesion. In bone, the cysts are semisolid, invade the medullary cavity and slowly erode bone, producing pathologic fractures. The cycle is completed when the hydatid cyst is ingested by a carnivore. The enormous number of scolices are released in the intestine and develop into adult worms. The life cycle of *E. multilocularis* is similar except that small rodents serve as the natural intermediate hosts, and the hydatid cyst is always of the multilocular or alveolar type. Most of the cysts develop in the liver, and progressive invasion of that organ usually occurs. The lesions may metastasize when growth extends into blood vessels.

Epidemiology The dog is the principal definitive host of *E. granulosa,* and sheep and cattle are common intermediates. Human echinococciasis, which is often acquired in childhood, has its highest incidence in countries where sheep and cattle raising is carried out with the help of dogs, particularly in East and South Africa, the Middle East, Central Europe, South America, Australia, and New Zealand. It has been reported from 15 states in this country, but most of these infections were probably contracted outside the United States. Autochthonous cases have been reported among Southwestern Indians and Basque sheep farmers in California and Utah. A "sylvatic" focus of *E. granulosa* (var. *canadensis*) exists in Alaska and western Canada, where wolves act as the definitive host and caribou and moose as the intermediate host. A second sylvatic cycle involving deer and coyotes has been reported from California. When man kills these herbivores and feeds their viscera to dogs, a domestic cycle is initiated.

In *E. multilocularis* infection, rodents and deer mice are the natural intermediate hosts, while wolves, foxes, and coyotes serve as definitive hosts. A domestic dog and cat may also harbor the adult worms, and an urban cycle involving the cat and common house mouse has been described. Human infections have been reported from Russia, Central Europe, Canada, and Alaska. An extensive sylvatic focus has been described in the north central United States.

Clinical manifestations Enlarging hydatid cysts usually produce tissue damage by mechanical means. The resulting symptoms depend upon the site, type, and rate of growth of the cystic lesions. Most patients harbor a single hydatid, but as many as 20 percent may have multiple cysts involving more than a single site. The hydatids of *E. granulosa* var. *canadensis,* which occur principally in the lung, are small, grow very slowly, and seldom cause symptoms. The unilocular hydatids produced by other strains of *E. granulosa* grow somewhat more rapidly (0.25 to 1 cm per year) and eventually may reach enormous size. Hepatic lesions may remain asymptomatic for 5 to 20 years, finally presenting as a palpable abdominal mass or abdominal pain. Obstruction of the bile duct may result in jaundice. Cough, chest pain, and hemoptysis are the most common presenting symptoms of pulmonary echinococcosis. Asymptomatic cysts are frequently discovered on routine chest x-ray. Bone lesions with pathologic fractures occur, and central nervous system involvement may be manifested by epilepsy or blindness. Cardiac cysts may produce embolic metastases. Unilocular lesions may be secondarily infected, resulting in abscess formation and sterilization of the cyst. Rupture of a hydatid into the bile duct, peritoneal cavity, lung, pleura, or bronchus may produce fever, pruritus, urticarial rash, or an anaphylactoid reaction which is occasionally fatal. Release of the numerous scolices leads to dissemination of echinococcal infection. The multilocular or alveolar cyst of *E. multilocularis* usually presents as a slowly growing hepatic tumor, with jaundice and portal hypertension.

Diagnosis and treatment The clinical picture is seldom sufficiently characteristic to suggest the diagnosis. When eosinophilia is present, it is helpful. Pulmonary lesions usually present as round, somewhat irregular, masses of uniform density. Occasionally hepatic calcifications are seen in plain x-rays of the abdomen. A liver scan with radioactive isotopes is extremely helpful in detecting the presence of hepatic lesions and should always be done in suspected cases. Ultrasonic scanning will reveal the lesion to be fluid-filled. Liver hydatids often show a characteristic rim of opacification on celiac arteriography. The skin test (Casoni's test) is usually positive, but lack of a standard antigen and testing technique limits its usefulness. Moreover, patients with other helminthic diseases, particularly schistosomiasis, may give false positive results. Of the serologic tests, the indirect hemagglutination test seems to be the most sensitive and reliable and gives positive results in up to 90 percent of patients with hepatic hydatid disease. The results are less encouraging in patients with lung disease. The latex agglutination and bentonite flocculation tests are simpler but not as reliable. Occasionally scolices may be demonstrated in the sputum with the Ziehl-Neelsen stain. Because of serious reactions to the leakage of cyst fluid into the tissues and body cavities, diagnostic aspiration should not be attempted.

There is no established medical therapy. Experimentally, prolonged administration of mebendazole has been shown to be larvicidal, but this treatment cannot be recommended until more information has become available. When the cysts become symptomatic, surgical treatment offers the only hope of cure. The size and location of the lesion will determine whether complete excision or sterilization and drainage should be performed. The contents of the cyst should be sterilized with 10 ml of 10% Formalin, 1% iodine, or 0.5% silver nitrate before an attempt to drain or excise the lesion is made.

Prevention In prevention, (1) contact with infected dogs should be avoided, particularly fecal contamination of the hands and food; (2) infected carcasses and offal should be burned or buried, in order to prevent access of dogs to material containing scolices; and (3) dogs should be treated if found to be infected. The reduction of the incidence of echinococciasis in Iceland is an example of the efficacy of control measures.

REFERENCES

BROWN HW: *Basic Clinical Parasitology,* 4th ed., New York: Appleton-Century-Crofts, 1975

CALAMAI G et al: Hydatid disease of the heart: Report of 5 cases and review of the literature. Thorax 29:451, 1974

GELFAND M, JEFFREY C: Cerebral cysticercosis in Rhodesia. J Trop Med Hyg 76:87, 1973

HERMOS JA et al: Fatal human cerebral coenurosis. JAMA 213:1461, 1970

KAGAN IG et al: Evaluation of intradermal and serologic tests for the diagnosis of hydatid disease. Am J Trop Med 15:172, 1966

KEELING JED: in *Advances in Chemotherapy,* eds A Goldin et al, vol. 3, New York: Academic, 1968, p. 109.

MOST H: Drug therapy: Common parasitic infections of man. N Engl J Med 287:495, 1972

NEWMAN CM, ARON BS: Roentgen diagnosis of tapeworm infestation. J Mt Sinai Hosp NY 28:91, 1961

PAWLOWSKI Z, SCHULTZ MG: Taeniasis and cysticercosis *Taenia (Taenia saginata).* Adv Parasitol 10:269, 1972

PERERA DR et al: Niclosamide treatment of cestodiasis: Clinical trials in the United States. Am J Trop Med 19:610, 1970

RAUSCH RL: Echinococcosis. Bull WHO 39:1, 1968

SAUDI F, NAZARIAN IJ: Surgical treatment of hydatid cysts by freezing of cyst wall and instillation of 0.5 percent silver nitrate solution. N Engl J Med 284:1346, 1971

SCHULTZ MG et al: Epidemiology of beef tapeworm infection in the United States. Public Health Rep 85:169, 1970

SWARTZWELDER JC et al: Sparganosis in southern United States. Am J Trop Med 13:43, 1964

VON BONSDORFF B et al: Vitamin B_{12} deficiency in carriers of the fish tapeworm, *Diphyllobothrium latum.* Acta Haematol 24:15, 1960

WILLIAMS JF et al: Current prevalence and distribution of hydatidosis with special reference to the Americas. Am J Trop Med 20:224, 1971

WILSON JF et al: Cystic hydatid disease in Alaska. Am Rev Resp Dis 98:1, 1968

XANTHAKIS D et al: Hydatid disease of the chest. Report of 91 cases surgically treated. Thorax 27:517, 1972

section 18 | Diseases of uncertain etiology

228 SARCOIDOSIS

CAROL J. JOHNS

INTRODUCTION At the 1975 Seventh International Conference on Sarcoidosis it was proposed that sarcoidosis be described as "a multisystem granulomatous disorder of unknown etiology most commonly affecting young adults and presenting most frequently with bilateral hilar lymphadenopathy, pulmonary infiltration, skin or eye lesions." Other organs commonly involved include peripheral lymph nodes, liver, spleen, mucous membranes, parotid glands, phalangeal bones, muscles, heart, and nervous system. The diagnosis is established most securely when there is involvement of more than one organ system with clinical and radiographic findings, supported by histologic evidence of widespread noncaseating epithelioid-cell granulomas, with the absence of known agents capable of inducing similar granulomatous lesions (beryllium, tubercle bacillus, fungi, etc.). The Kveim-Siltzbach reaction is frequently positive and lends support to the diagnosis. Impairment of cell-mediated immunity is manifest by depression of tuberculin-type delayed hypersensitivity but well-maintained or increased production of humoral antibodies (immunoglobulins). Impaired regulation of the cell functions of thymus-derived lymphocytes (T cells) and bone-marrow-derived lymphocytes (B cells) is suspected. The clinical course varies from that of a self-limited one, with spontaneous resolution, to that of progressive widespread granulomatous inflammation and fibrosis. Corticosteroids produce clinical remissions and suppress inflammation and granuloma formation. Long-term treatment for many years may be required to prevent clinical relapse.

ETIOLOGY The cause of sarcoidosis remains unknown. It is unclear whether there is a single inciting infectious or other exogenous agent. The immunologic features and abnormalities have attracted increasing attention. Defects in immunologic regulation of the cell function of B and T lymphocytes could be primary or secondary. There are other possible factors of genetic susceptibility, but no pattern of histocompatibility antigens has been identified in sarcoidosis. A possible role of the tubercle bacillus has been debated. In some cases, sarcoidosis may be related in some way to a mycobacterial infection. The disease may be a result of an interaction between an infective agent and a subject with unusual immunologic responses. It cannot be assumed that all cases of sarcoidosis are associated with the same inciting agent. Studies in mice suggest a transmissible agent from human sarcoid tissue.

EPIDEMIOLOGY Sarcoidosis has been observed in virtually every country in which it has been sought. Blacks are ten times more affected than Caucasians in the United States, and the incidence in females is usually double that in males. An increased incidence in relation to pregnancy and lactation has been noted, especially in patients with erythema nodosum. The disease is most frequent in the third and fourth decades of life, but the range begins in childhood, particularly around adolescence, and extends to the sixth and seventh decades. Familial associations are noted occasionally.

PATHOLOGY Granulomatous inflammatory changes of sarcoidosis may occur in almost any organ. Disseminated granulomas are probably often present even with clinically localized disease, i.e., hepatic granulomas with only asymptomatic hilar adenopathy. The hard tubercles are generally sharply demarcated from surrounding tissues but may coalesce. Some central fibrinoid or granular necrosis may occur, especially in association with systemic active febrile disease, but caseation is usually absent, and inflammatory reaction is minimal. Giant cells containing laminated calcific Schaumann bodies or stellate "asteroid" bodies are frequent, but neither of these inclusions is found solely in sarcoidosis.

Similar histologic changes may be seen in tuberculosis, fungous infections, leprosy, tertiary syphilis, beryllium disease, "farmer's lung," foreign-body reactions, lymphomas, and lymph nodes draining malignant tumors. The histologic picture in sarcoid is not specific for that disease alone, and the above-mentioned possibilities cannot be excluded in the absence of other data.

Adrenal corticosteroids cause a prompt reduction in the nonspecific cellular inflammatory reaction of an acute or subacute process and hasten involution and resorption of the "sarcoid" tubercles. It seems likely that these hormones prevent or lessen but do not erase progressive scarring.

Autopsy material on patients with long-standing sarcoidosis may reveal widespread tubercles in many organs, a few scattered tubercles or focal hyaline scarring, or, rarely, no residual changes.

MANIFESTATIONS Clinical manifestations of sarcoidosis generally depend on the activity, degree, and site of tissue involvement and vary from incidental radiographic findings without associated symptoms, to severe incapacity and death. Impaired function is caused both by active granulomatous disease and by secondary fibrosis.

Constitutional symptoms Fever, weight loss, and fatigue are often nonspecific presenting complaints, occasionally without other localizing symptoms. Persistent daily spiking fever to 101°F may be observed and necessitates careful exclusion of tuberculosis. This is most commonly observed in association with active granulomatous inflammation in the liver. Fever in association with erythema nodosum is another form in which sarcoidosis may become evident. This syndrome includes transient tender erythematous subcutaneous nodules over the pretibial areas, arthralgias, and pulmonary hilar adenopathy on x-ray. Hepatic tubercles and a positive Kveim reaction are frequent. This syndrome has been regarded as an early manifestation of sarcoidosis and noted frequently in young women in Scandinavia and Great Britain. It is also observed in the United States, may be overlooked easily, and has a favorable prognosis.

Lymph nodes Mediastinal and hilar nodes are most frequently involved. Vague substernal discomfort may be present. Readily palpable peripheral nodes which are discrete, firm, and nontender are often prominent. There may be generalized lymphadenopathy, or involvement may be localized to the cervical, axillary, and femoral nodes. Usually, the changes are symmetrical and the epitrochlear nodes are palpable.

Lungs Pulmonary involvement is the most common and, perhaps, the most important manifestation of sarcoidosis. Spontaneous permanent remissions are observed, but significant lung disease represents the most frequent indication for treatment. Serious parenchymal changes, with or without hilar adenopathy, are evident on x-ray in about 50 percent of all patients. Varying and impressive degrees of dyspnea and cough are noted. A discrepancy in which the radiographic changes exceed the symptoms and signs is a diagnostic clue in early sarcoidosis. In some patients, usually Caucasian, striking radiographic changes may be associated with no symptoms and ventilatory and diffusion measurements are normal. In others, often blacks, pathologic and physiologic abnormalities may be present when the x-ray shows only hilar adenopathy. Dyspnea may be severe and is present in approximately half the patients with parenchymal disease. This results from extensive interstitial changes which impair oxygenation by disturbances of ventilation and perfusion ratios and loss of effective diffusing surface. Compensatory hyperventilation is often noted. Large rounded intrapulmonary masses which may resemble metastatic tumor are probably a result of primary involvement of lymphoid tissue or localized infiltrates producing minimal physiologic disturbance and minimal symptoms despite their dramatic x-ray appearance. Pleural effusions are unusual and should lead to the suspicion that other disease is present.

Cough may be severe and incapacitating and may occur in paroxysms which can even lead to vomiting. Sputum is scanty; occasional blood streaking results from the strain of coughing or endobronchial granulomas or in association with a picture that resembles bronchiectasis. Wheezing is occasionally produced by localized bronchial lesions with stenosis. Pulmonary obstruction is noted in late fibrotic chronic sarcoidosis. Physical findings are variable and nonspecific. Respiratory excursion may be restricted, crackling rales may be heard diffusely or at the lung bases, and the P_2 may be accentuated or split if pulmonary hypertension develops.

Bronchoscopy generally reveals normal mucosa, although in a few cases it shows granulomatous inflammatory changes with endobronchial narrowing. Granuloma may be demonstrated occasionally in grossly normal-appearing mucosa.

In some patients sarcoidosis is a chronic progressive disease, and pulmonary insufficiency and cor pulmonale occur as late features. Bronchiolostenosis, resulting from peribronchial fibrosis and mucosal changes, may result in localized emphysema, giving rise to cystic changes, usually in the upper lung fields. With superimposed bacterial infection, a bronchiectasis-like picture results. Large cavitary or bullous lesions are rare but may lead to large and repeated hemoptyses, which are occasionally fatal. Such lesions may also form the locus for an aspergilloma, with which hemoptyses or disseminated *Aspergillus* infection are hazards. However, these "fungous balls" are usually saprophytic and often multiple. They may vary spontaneously in size and number over periods of 10 or more years, without invasive disease, even when steroid maintenance treatment is required. Surgical management is rarely feasible because of the diffuse and restrictive nature of the disease. Spontaneous pneumothorax is an occasional complication of lung involvement.

Eyes Acute granulomatous uveitis may be the initial manifestation of sarcoidosis. Ocular disease may progress to severe visual impairment and blindness with corneal and lenticular opacities and secondary glaucoma. A careful slit-lamp examination is worthwhile in all patients with sarcoid to detect early evidence of anterior uveitis. Lacrimal gland enlargement, conjunctival infiltrations, and keratoconjunctivitis sicca of the type seen in Sjögren's syndrome (Chap. 366) are common. Exophthalmos has been observed, as have retinal lesions with vasculitis producing papillitis and periphlebitis.

Skin Lesions occur in about 30 percent of patients, most dramatically around the nose, eyes, and mouth, and vary from extensive erythematous, infiltrated, and raised lesions to small nondescript plaques and papules. Mucosal lesions are often associated, extending into the nose, sinuses, and the hard palate. Increased or decreased pigmentation is frequently noted. Sarcoid changes often occur at sites of old scars or tattoos or recent injury. Subcutaneous nodular infiltrations occur, and in rare instances calcification of such lesions has been observed. Alopecia occurs if the scalp is affected. Skin lesions are associated with chronicity but often with otherwise mild disease. Erythema nodosum in early sarcoidosis usually presents a histologic picture of a nonspecific vasculitis.

Liver Clinical manifestations of hepatic sarcoidosis are present in only about 20 percent of cases. Nevertheless, hepatic tubercles can be found by biopsy in about 75 percent. Asymptomatic hepatomegaly is frequent. Severe jaundice is unusual, but mild increase in bilirubin and striking elevation of serum alkaline phosphatase level are observed. Intense pruritus may be the presenting manifestation. Intrahepatic cholestasis may occur with a picture resembling biliary cirrhosis. The spectrum of hepatic sarcoid includes the incidental tubercle, tubercles with surrounding nonspecific inflammatory reaction, chronic active granulomatous hepatitis, postnecrotic cirrhosis with or without portal hypertension, and portal hypertension without significant cirrhosis. Esophageal varices have been demonstrated in patients with portal hypertension, and shunt procedures occasionally have been required. Response to steroids has been disappointing in severe hepatic sarcoid, but steroids are indicated with a significant active inflammatory process. In some patients the granulomatous disease is limited to the liver, spleen, and abdominal nodes without other clinical or radiographic evidence of sarcoidosis.

Spleen Mild splenomegaly occurs in 20 to 30 percent of cases and often regresses promptly with administration of corticosteroids. Enlargement may be striking and associated with "hypersplenism," anemia, leukopenia, and thrombocytopenia. It may persist for 10 to 20 years without undue complications, although splenectomy will result in hematologic improvement.

Kidneys Impaired renal function may occur secondary to hypercalcemia and hypercalciuria, secondary to hyperuricemia, and, less commonly, because of direct granulomatous involvement. Nephrocalcinosis and renal calculi are observed.

Heart Effects are usually secondary to lung disease, with pulmonary hypertension and cor pulmonale. Primary myocardial sarcoidosis often is not recognized and is most commonly manifested by conduction disturbances, paroxysmal arrhythmias and infiltrative cardiomyopathy.

Salivary glands Asymptomatic enlargement of the parotid, sublingual, and submaxillary glands occurs in about 6 percent of cases. Spontaneous regression commonly occurs. A syndrome of fever, uveitis, and lacrimal and salivary gland enlargement is known as uveoparotid fever, or Heerfordt's syndrome. Facial nerve palsies may be associated with parotid disease.

Muscle Sarcoid granulomas occur in muscles far more frequently than is clinically indicated by pain and weakness. In a few cases symptoms may be severe and incapacitating. Muscle biopsy is likely to be positive in such patients and also in those with polyarthralgias.

Joints Arthralgias may occur independently as an early prominent feature and are common in association with erythema nodosum and fever. Sarcoid tubercles have been observed in biopsies of synovium. Transient knee effusions are occasionally noted. Chronic periarticular swelling and tenderness may be associated with bony changes in the fingers and toes and skin lesions. Monoarticular arthritis raises the suspicion of tuberculosis.

Bones Asymptomatic, punched-out lesions in the distal phalanges of the hands and feet are visible in roentgenograms in about 10 percent of cases. Associated overlying skin changes are common. Radiolucent skull lesions have been noted in a few patients. "Routine" hand x-rays are not likely to be abnormal in the absence of overlying skin changes.

Nervous system Neurologic manifestations are variable. Cranial and peripheral nerves may be affected by direct involvement of the nerve sheaths or roots. Facial nerve palsies, which may be bilateral and sequential, are the commonest neurologic finding and may undergo full remission. Swallowing disorders are observed. A granulomatous basilar meningitis can affect the cranial nerves and produce pleocytosis and elevation of the spinal fluid protein level. Pituitary involvement produces diabetes insipidus. Involvement of the choroid plexuses may obstruct the ventricles. Cortical changes may result in convulsive seizures.

Other tissues Involvement of the tonsils and laryngeal, buccal, and nasal mucosa (often with associated sinusitis) has been encountered. Bilateral nasal obstruction may be a presenting complaint. Submucous resections are contraindicated as they frequently result in septal perforations. Sarcoid lesions have been found in thyroid, parathyroid, and pancreatic tissues, and gastric granulomas have resulted in bleeding and perforation. Sarcoid involving the adrenal, cervix, uterus, epididymis, or testis is very unusual.

LABORATORY FINDINGS Mild anemia, leukopenia, eosinophilia, and elevated sedimentation rate are common in active disease. Thrombocytopenia is unusual but may be severe.

Delayed skin reactions Tuberculin anergy is noted in about two-thirds of patients, but a positive tuberculin reaction occurs if active tuberculosis supervenes. A previously known positive tuberculin reaction may become less reactive with active sarcoidosis. Associated generalized cutaneous anergy to other commonly occurring antigens such as *Candida albicans, Trichophyton,* and mumps virus has been noted. This depression of delayed skin reactivity is considered to be an important feature of sarcoidosis, but it varies with the duration and activity of the disease.

Chemical studies Hypergammaglobulinemia and reduction of serum albumin are common. Hypercalcemia and hypercalciuria are infrequent but apparently result from increased intestinal absorption of calcium, which is possibly related to increased sensitivity to vitamin D. Serum uric acid level may be elevated even in the absence of renal insufficiency. Elevation of serum alkaline phosphatase level is attributable to intrahepatic tubercles, rather than to bone lesions, and may reach very high levels.

Other studies Serum lysozyme levels are elevated in sarcoidosis (also tuberculosis) and are thought to reflect active granuloma formation. Levels seem to return to normal with corticosteroid therapy and inactivity of the disease. Elevated levels of serum angiotensin-converting enzyme (ACE) are similarly reported to correlate with the diagnosis of active sarcoidosis. The specificity and usefulness of this observation are not fully determined. Elevated levels also have been observed in Gaucher's disease.

Roentgenographic studies Approximately 90 percent of patients show intrathoracic disease on chest x-ray. Bilateral hilar adenopathy, often with associated right paratracheal adenopathy, is a common feature. Unilateral hilar adenopathy is unusual and should initiate a search for other diseases. Patients may be grouped according to the apparent extent and chronicity of the radiologic picture as follows: group I—hilar adenopathy with no parenchymal changes; group II—hilar adenopathy and diffuse parenchymal changes; group III—diffuse parenchymal changes without hilar adenopathy; group IV—chronic parenchymal changes of more than 2 years' duration with pulmonary fibrosis. The pulmonary changes are generally symmetrical, and may present a diffuse ground-glass appearance, fine reticular or miliary lesions, large nodular lesions, or multiple large confluent infiltrates resembling metastatic tumors. Fine diffuse interstitial fibrosis may be present. Pulmonary fibrosis may produce contraction and distortion, and extensive cystic and bullous lesions are common in the late stages. Bony changes in the phalanges and skull may occur.

Pulmonary function tests These tests commonly demonstrate restriction, decreased compliance, and loss of effective diffusing surface. Vital capacity is reduced. Measurements of oxygen- and carbon monoxide-diffusing capacity are frequently reduced even in the absence of demonstrable radiographic changes or clinical symptoms. Measurements of vital capacity and diffusing capacity may serve as indicators of progression of disease and response to treatment. In diffuse disease, arterial blood studies reveal with exercise a reduced P_{O_2} because of perfusion of poorly ventilated areas of the lung. The arterial P_{CO_2} is commonly below normal because of contemporary hyperventilation. Because ventilatory obstruction occurs only occasionally, and then in severe, late stages of pulmonary fibrosis, carbon dioxide retention with elevation of arterial P_{CO_2} is a late and unusual feature. Significant impairment of pulmonary function frequently remains even after radiographic clearing. Following steroid therapy or a spontaneous remission, the vital capacity tends to return toward normal, but may remain somewhat reduced. The diffusing capacity may improve significantly but usually stabilizes well below normal despite complete remission of all symptoms. Improvement in diffusing capacity is less frequent than is that of the vital capacity. Deterioration of pulmonary function may occur gradually and progressively.

DIAGNOSIS The diagnosis depends on the clinical features along with histologic evidence of epithelioid tubercles from tissue biopsy or from a positive Kveim reaction. The amount of histologic support required varies inversely with the certainty with which the pattern of clinical features is recognized. It is essential to exclude other recognized causes of granulomatous disease. To exclude local sarcoid tissue reaction, as in nodes draining a malignant tumor, evidence of involvement of more than one site is desirable. Careful search for tubercle bacilli, fungi, and foreign bodies must be made in all histologic sections. A positive Kveim reaction is a special feature and helps to exclude other granulomatous processes, but the specificity and selectivity of this reaction are uncertain. Tissue biopsy for histologic diagnosis is most readily and easily obtained from superficial or palpable lesions in skin, lymph nodes, conjunctiva, and nasal, buccal, and bronchial mucosa. Almost any palpable lymph node is likely to be positive. Liver biopsies reveal granulomas in 70 to 80 percent of cases even without clinical evidence of impaired hepatic function. Biopsy of the gastrocnemius muscle frequently reveals granulomatous changes in patients with arthralgias and erythema nodosum. In the absence of palpable peripheral lymph nodes, or dermal lesions, mediastinoscopy and node biopsy or biopsy of liver or muscle are in order. Transbronchial lung biopsy appears useful. Open lung biopsy is generally reserved for patients in whom other diagnostic maneuvers have not been successful or in whom the exclusion of other diseases is urgent. The indicated tissue biopsy is that which combines the least risk with the greatest likelihood of diagnostic yield. With typical clinical features with asymptomatic bilateral hilar adenopathy, a presumptive diagnosis may be justified, without histologic support.

Kveim reaction In 50 to 80 percent of patients with sarcoidosis, the intracutaneous injection of a heat-sterilized suspension of human sarcoid tissues (spleen or lymph nodes) produces a papulonodular lesion with epithelioid tubercles. The nodule must be biopsied in 4 to 6 weeks for routine histologic study. This reveals a spectrum from positive to negative, and includes a middle equivocal group. A positive reaction is limited to those with well-formed *epithelioid tubercles.* Test material must be assayed in patients of known reactivity, and experienced interpretation is essential. The Kveim reaction is very likely to be positive in the presence of sarcoid lymphadenopathy, in association with erythema nodosum, and when sarcoid skin lesions are present. The reaction is less likely to be positive in the absence of lymph node involvement and during steroid therapy. Tests in patients with a variety of granulomatous and collagen vascular diseases have revealed only 2 to 5 percent false positive reactions, but many false negative results are encountered in patients later shown to have sarcoidosis. The nature of the Kveim reaction is not understood, and its selectivity must be interpreted with clinical findings and demonstrated performance of the particular Kveim preparation.

COURSE Sarcoidosis is frequently no more than an incidental radiographic finding on routine chest x-ray. The course is often one of spontaneous remission over a period of 6 to 24 months, with little or no evidence of residual disease and with normal life expectancy. However, there may be persistent abnormalities with varying disability or progressive deterioration. Death related to sarcoidosis may ensue in 5 to 10 percent of cases and is most frequently related to advanced pulmonary disease. There may be impressive clearing of radiographic lesions, especially when the disease seems limited to the thorax. Following a spontaneous remission, recurrence is most unusual. Remissions are most frequent in the syndrome of erythema nodosum and hilar adenopathy. This "benign" form is more common in Caucasians than in blacks where chronic progressive diffuse systemic disease is more frequently encountered. Systemic manifestations in skin, bone, eyes, and salivary glands and hepatosplenomegaly herald a less favorable prognosis. Severe uveitis may progress to glaucoma, cataract formation, and blindness.

The influence of steroids is probably favorable when there is significant incapacitating disease and an active inflammatory process.

TREATMENT Relatively asymptomatic patients often require no treatment. *Adrenal corticosteroids* dramatically suppress the active inflammatory reaction and provide important symptomatic improvement. Indications for treatment are (1) active ocular disease; (2) persistent or progressive pulmonary involvement; (3) persistent hypercalcemia or hypercalciuria; (4) central nervous system involvement with significant functional impairment; (5) significant evidence of myocardial disease; (6) persistent systemic evidence of illness such as fever and weight loss; and (7) significant and progressive involvement of a vital organ. The disease remains in remission in some patients after administration of steroids, but it commonly recurs as the dose is reduced, even when therapy has been continued for 2 or more years. It is thought that steroids prevent the progression of disease, but healing may occur with hyaline scarring. Steroids clearly cannot reverse a fibrotic process. Early steroid therapy offers more hope than that initiated after 1 or 2 years of disease.

Steroids are most frequently required and beneficial for symptomatic lung disease. Uncertainty as to the value of steroids may stem from attempted evaluation of benefits in patients with asymptomatic minimal disease which probably required no treatment. Even relatively asymptomatic but significant lung disease should be treated if there is no evidence of spontaneous regression in 6 to 12 months, or if there is progression in 3 months. One should not wait for the appearance of symptoms when lung function is persistently and significantly reduced. Asymptomatic hilar adenopathy without evidence of pulmonary parenchymal disease does not require therapy.

Prednisone is administered in initial divided daily doses of 40 mg, with 2-week periods on daily doses of 40, 30, and 25 mg, and then in single 8 A.M. daily maintenance doses of 20 to 10 mg. Symptomatic improvement occurs in 1 to 2 weeks, and the disease regresses over a period of several months. Therapy probably should be continued for a minimum of 6 to 8 months, with periodic attempts thereafter to reduce dosage or eliminate the drug. Objective criteria such as x-rays and measurements of pulmonary function are important. Maintenance therapy for many years has proved necessary in many patients in whom relapses recur at a dose below 10 to 15 mg. Dosage must be tapered slowly, with decrements of 2.5 mg no oftener than at 2- to 4-week intervals if long-term treatment has been used. Lifelong therapy may be required. Careful documentation and observation during tapering are essential in planning treatment. Alternate-day dosage may be used for maintenance therapy. It is probably not advisable for initial management. Endocrine side effects, with weight gain of 20 to 50 lb, have been observed in some women. Diabetes has appeared in some patients, particularly in association with significant hepatic involvement. Local steroid therapy has been effective in ocular sarcoid with anterior uveitis or iritis, although there is the risk of glaucoma. Intradermal steroids have been used with some success for disfiguring cutaneous lesions. Such lesions are not usually considered justification for systemic steroids.

Chloroquine (Aralen), in doses of 250 to 500 mg daily, has been observed to induce dramatic improvement in skin and mucosal lesions over periods of several weeks, but relapse is the rule when the drug is withdrawn. With periodic ocular examinations and intermittent treatment periods of 6 months, no irreversible retinal damage has been encountered. Remission may be maintained with as little as 125 mg daily. Response to hydroxychloroquine (Plaquenil) has been slower and less satisfactory. Hypercalcemia has also appeared to respond to chloroquine.

Antituberculous therapy is ineffective in sarcoidosis. However, prophylactic isoniazid in association with corticosteroids is often recommended for black patients with extensive pulmonary disease, in areas with high risks of exposure to tuberculosis, and always for patients who are tuberculin-positive. If tuberculosis is really suspected, two drugs should be employed, e.g., isoniazid and ethambutol, especially if corticosteroids are to be administered.

COMPLICATIONS The complications are related to the effects of severe and progressive disease in various organs, the side effects of therapy, and superimposed infection. An increased incidence (2 to 5 percent) of tuberculosis in association with sarcoidosis has been recognized. Associated fungous infections seem to be increasing. Saprophytic *aspergillus* fungous balls (mycetomas) have been noted in pulmonary cysts. Candidiasis and cryptococcosis in association with sarcoidosis have also been noted. It is highly probable that long-term steroid and antimicrobial therapy predispose to these fungous infections.

REFERENCES

HEDFORS E: Immunological aspects of sarcoidosis. Scan J Resp Dis 56(1):1, 1975

JAMES DG et al: Immunology of sarcoidosis. Am J Med 59:388, 1975

JOHNS CJ et al: A ten-year study of corticosteroid treatment of pulmonary sarcoidosis. Johns Hopkins Med J 134:271, 1974

KOERNER SK et al: Transbronchial lung biopsy for the diagnosis of sarcoidosis. N Engl J Med 293:268, 1975

LIEBERMAN J: Elevation of serum angiotensin-converting-enzyme (ACE) level in sarcoidosis. Am J Med 59:365, 1975

LONGCOPE WT et al: A study of sarcoidosis: Based on a combined investigation of 160 cases including 30 autopsies from the Johns Hopkins Hospital and Massachusetts General Hospital. Medicine 31:1, 1952

MADDREY WC et al: Sarcoidosis and chronic hepatic disease: A clinical and pathologic study of 20 patients. Medicine 49:375, 1970

MAYOCK RL et al: Manifestations of sarcoidosis: Analysis of 145 patients, with a review of 9 series selected from the literature. Am J Med 35:67, 1963

MILLER A et al: Airway function in chronic pulmonary sarcoidosis with fibrosis. Am Rev Resp Dis 109:179, 1974

MITCHELL DN et al: Sarcoidosis. Am Rev Resp Dis 110:774, 1974

Proceedings of the VI International Conference on Sarcoidosis, eds K Iwai, Y Hosoda, Tokyo: University of Tokyo Press, 1974

SHARMA OP: *Sarcoidosis—A Clinical Approach,* Springfield, Ill.: Charles C Thomas, 1975

SILTZBACH LE et al: Course and prognosis of sarcoidosis around the world. Am J Med 57:847, 1974

Transactions of the N.Y. Acad. Sci. Seventh Int'l Conf. on Sarcoidosis and Other Granulomatous Disorders, 1975 (in press)

WINTERBAUER RH et al: A clinical interpretation of bilateral hilar adenopathy. Ann Intern Med 78:65, 1973

229 FAMILIAL MEDITERRANEAN FEVER (FAMILIAL PAROXYSMAL POLYSEROSITIS)

SHELDON M. WOLFF

DEFINITION Familial Mediterranean fever (FMF) is an inherited disorder of unknown etiology, characterized by recurrent episodes of fever, peritonitis, and/or pleuritis. Arthritis, skin lesions, and amyloidosis are seen in some patients.

HISTORY Although the first report of FMF was by Janeway and Mosenthal in 1908, it was not until the report of five cases by Siegal in 1945 that attention was focused on FMF as a distinct entity. Subsequently, some authors have not applied strict clinical criteria, and many patients with other diseases have been reported as having FMF. The detailed and extensive descriptions by Heller and Sohar have clarified many of the clinical aspects of FMF.

TERMINOLOGY The variety of names given to FMF has led to confusion concerning its clinical features. None of the names, including FMF, is completely satisfactory, but FMF has received the widest acceptance. Such terms as *periodic disease, periodic peritonitis, la maladie periodique* are inaccurate because the disease often is not cyclical. *Benign paroxysmal peritonitis* is inappropriate because many of the patients have involvement of serosal surfaces other than the peritoneum, and some die of amyloidosis. *Familial paroxysmal polyserositis* is an acceptable alternative for the term *familial Mediterranean fever.*

ETHNOLOGY AND GENETICS FMF occurs predominantly in patients of non-Ashkenazic (Sephardic) Jewish, Armenian, and Arabic ancestry. However, the disease is not restricted to these groups, and has been seen in patients of Italian, Ashkenazic Jewish, and Anglo-Saxon descent as well as others.

The best studies of the genetics of FMF have been done in Israel, where relatively homogeneous population groups exist. In Israel, the disease appears to be inherited as an autosomal recessive. Nevertheless, approximately 50 percent of patients give no family history of the disease. Consanguinity among the parents of FMF patients is as high as 20 percent, a figure which may be an underestimate because most patients came from very inbred ethnic groups. Approximately 60 percent of patients are male.

ETIOLOGY Although numerous pathogenetic mechanisms have been suggested, the etiology of FMF is unknown. Fever and inflammation are such prominent signs that frequent attempts have been made to implicate infectious agents and/or their products. It has been suggested that FMF is a form of brucellosis or tuberculosis. Suffice it to say that extensive studies utilizing modern microbiologic and serologic techniques have failed to implicate these or any other specific infectious agents.

It has been reported that FMF is due to an allergy or to hypersensitivity, but such hypersensitive states have not been substantiated. There is no firm evidence favoring an autoimmune etiology.

Reimann has suggested that FMF, like many other recurring illnesses (periodic disease), may be a pathologic exaggeration of normal periodic temperature rhythmicity. However, extensive studies of temperature and other circadian rhythms in FMF patients have failed to demonstrate alterations from normal.

Because many FMF patients note that certain emotional or environmental changes may have profound effects on the frequency with which episodes of their disease occur, a psychosomatic basis has been suggested for the illness. There is no question that most patients eventually have transient or even permanent psychologic alterations, which probably reflect their reaction to a chronic recurring illness that is forever threatening their social, economic, and personal well-being, but there is no evidence for a functional etiology for FMF.

The demonstration that FMF is inherited as an autosomal recessive disorder has led to the thesis that it is another inborn error of metabolism. Originally it was thought that the disorder might be one of altered lipid metabolism. Despite extensive studies, no such error has been found. Reported instances of excessive urinary excretion of porphyrins in FMF are probably examples of true porphyria and not FMF.

It has been reported that blood levels of unconjugated etiocholanolone were elevated during fever in 6 patients with FMF. Subsequent studies, however, showed no correlation between levels of etiocholanolone and fever.

PATHOLOGY Despite the striking clinical manifestations during an acute attack of FMF, no specific pathologic alterations have been found. Most FMF patients undergo at least one laparotomy, and only acute peritoneal inflammation in which the exudate contains a predominance of polymorphonuclear leukocytes is found to be present. A disproportionately large number of male patients develop gallbladder disease with and without cholelithiasis, but extensive histopathologic examination has failed to reveal any specific pathologic changes. Pleural and joint inflammation are also nonspecific.

In the amyloidosis which accompanies FMF, amyloid is deposited in the intima and media of the arterioles, the subendothelial region of venules, the glomeruli, and the spleen. Aside from their vessels, the heart and liver are uninvolved.

MANIFESTATIONS In the majority of patients, the symptoms of FMF begin between the ages of five and fifteen, although attacks sometimes commence during infancy, and onset has occurred as late as age fifty-two. The duration and frequency of attacks vary greatly in the same patient, and there is no set rhythm or periodicity to their occurrence. The usual acute episode lasts 24 to 48 h, but some may be prolonged for 7 to 10 days. The attacks range in frequency from twice weekly to once a year, but 2 to 4 weeks is the commonest interval. Spontaneous remissions lasting years have been seen. In the majority of cases, pregnancy is associated with an absence of acute episodes and many patients note less frequent attacks in the summer than in the winter. There may be a decrease in the severity and frequency of the attacks with age or with development of amyloidosis.

Fever Fever is a cardinal manifestation of FMF and is present during most but not all attacks. Rarely, fever may be present without serositis. The temperature may be preceded by a chill, and will peak in 12 to 24 h. Defervescence is often accompanied by diaphoresis. The fever ranges from 38.5 to 40°C but is quite variable.

Abdominal pain Abdominal pain occurs in more than 95 percent of patients, and may vary in severity in the same patient. Minor premonitory discomfort may precede an acute episode by 24 to 48 h. The pain usually starts in one quadrant and then spreads to involve the whole abdomen. The initial site is usually very tender. Tenderness may remain localized with referred pain in other areas, and there may be radiation to the back. There may be splinting of the chest and pain in one or both shoulders, typical of diaphragmatic irritation. Nausea and vomiting sometimes occur. The abdomen is usually distended, and may become rigid with decreased or absent bowel sounds. On x-ray, the wall of the small intestine may appear edematous, transit of barium is slowed, and fluid levels may be seen. Because the manifestations of an acute abdominal attack can simulate those of a perforated viscus so closely, patients should be advised to have an elective appendectomy between attacks so that acute appendicitis will not obfuscate the picture at a later date. An abdominal operation may precipitate an acute attack of FMF which may be confused with other postoperative complications.

Chest pain Most patients with abdominal attacks have referred chest pain at one time or another, and 75 percent also develop acute pleuritic pain with or without abdominal symptoms. In 30 percent, the attacks of pleuritis precede the onset of abdominal attacks by varying periods of time, and a small number of patients never develop abdominal attacks. Chest pain is usually unilateral and is associated with diminished breath sounds, a friction rub, or a transient pleural effusion.

Joint pain In Israel, 75 percent of patients report at least one episode of acute arthritis. Arthritis can be distinct from abdominal or pleural attacks, can be acute or, rarely, chronic, and may involve one or several joints. Effusions are common and the large joints are involved most frequently. Radiologic findings are nonspecific. Despite careful search, frank arthritis rarely has been seen in the United States. Some patients have a history of rheumatic fever-like illness in childhood, but in a large series of patients, including 30 from the Middle East, acute arthritis was not observed. Mild arthralgia is common during acute attacks but is nonspecific and can be seen in many febrile illnesses, including experimentally induced hyperthermia.

Skin manifestations Skin involvement is reported by 25 to 35 percent of patients. These lesions consist of painful, erythematous areas of swelling from 5 to 20 cm in diameter, usually located on the lower legs, the medial malleolus, or the dorsum of the foot. They may occur without abdominal or pleural pain and subside within 24 to 48 h.

Other signs and symptoms Involvement of other serosal membranes has been reported, but pericarditis is rare, and it is probable that descriptions of recurrent meningitis have been diseases other than FMF. Hematuria, splenomegaly, and small white dots called "colloid bodies" in the ocular fundus are among the findings of questionable significance. Rarely migraine-like headaches accompany acute abdominal attacks, and some patients have become somewhat irrational or show extreme emotional lability during attacks. Whether these are primary manifestations of FMF or secondary effects of pain and fever is not known.

Complications The most serious complication of FMF in the United States is drug addiction or habituation, and obviously efforts should be made to avoid use of narcotics. Depression and lack of motivation are common, and patients with FMF require considerable encouragement and support. A striking number of patients in one American series have developed gallbladder disease.

Another major complication of FMF is *amyloidosis.* Some investigators believe that few patients in Israel escape this complication and that it is an expression of the same gene that is responsible for the other manifestations of FMF. If the attacks occur first, as they do in over 90 percent of the patients, the patients are classified as being of phenotype I. Amyloidosis also occurs in siblings of FMF patients or precedes the abdominal attacks (phenotype II). The infiltration by amyloid involves the kidneys, and death is often attributable to renal failure.

Amyloidosis has been reported in Israel and North Africa, but there have been only two reported instances of amyloidosis complicating FMF in the United States. These findings are even more striking because there are probably as many known FMF patients in the United States as in Israel. These differences are unexplained and suggest that environmental or nutritional, as well as genetic, factors may play a role in the development of amyloidosis in FMF.

LABORATORY FINDINGS There is no specific diagnostic test. Polymorphonuclear leukocytosis ranging from 15,000 to 30,000 per mm^3 is almost invariable during acute attacks. The erythrocyte sedimentation rate is elevated during attacks but returns to normal between attacks. Plasma fibrinogen, serum haptoglobin, ceruloplasmin, and C-reactive protein increase during the episodes. Plasma lipids are normal, and there are no consistent abnormalities of hepatic or renal function. When amyloidosis is present, laboratory findings are typical of a nephrotic syndrome followed by renal insufficiency. Electrocardiographic and electroencephalographic changes are inconstant and nonspecific.

DIAGNOSIS When the typical acute attacks of FMF occur

in an individual of appropriate ethnic background who has a family history of FMF, the diagnosis is easy. On the other hand, if the disease has not been present in the family and the patient resides in a community where FMF is rare, the diagnosis can be very difficult.

Most patients with undiagnosed FMF have had one or more abdominal operations with no relief of symptoms. When a patient is seen for the first time, a variety of other febrile illnesses must be excluded by appropriate study or observation. These include acute appendicitis, acute pancreatitis, porphyria, cholecystitis, intestinal obstruction, and other major abdominal catastrophes.

Some of the inherited forms of the hyperlipidemias (Chap. 113) may mimic the clinical picture of FMF, but measurement of serum cholesterol and triglycerides will eliminate them from consideration. The patient with FMF is not immune to the other diseases, and when an attack differs from the usual pattern or is more prolonged, consideration should be given to other diagnostic possibilities. The pleural form of the disease is sometimes difficult to differentiate from acute pulmonary infection or infarction, but the rapid disappearance of signs and symptoms resolves the problem. The joint manifestations may be more prolonged than other forms of FMF, and differentiation from septic arthritis, gout, and acute rheumatoid disease may be necessary. The erythema is sometimes difficult to differentiate from superficial thrombophlebitis or cellulitis.

Whether or not the patient is of the appropriate ethnic group, the most difficult diagnostic problem in FMF is the patient who presents with fever alone. In this situation, an extensive diagnostic work-up for fever of unknown origin may be required. Fortunately, such patients are rare, and all eventually develop serosal involvement. Until specific diagnostic tests for FMF are available, patients with recurrent fever but without signs of inflammation of one of the serosal membranes should not be categorized as having FMF.

PROGNOSIS The prognosis of the patient with FMF varies greatly according to the country in which he lives. In the United States, the prognosis for long life is excellent. Despite the severity of the symptoms during some acute attacks, most patients are remarkably free of any debilitation during the intervals between attacks. With encouragement and an understanding of their disease, most FMF patients lead fairly normal lives. The greatest hazard to patients is prolonged periods of hospitalization due to erroneous diagnoses or failure to understand the disease. The liberal and injudicious use of narcotics for analgesia in these patients can lead to major psychologic and health problems. Establishment of a reasonable doctor-patient relation and education of the patient will avoid this hazard. In the United States, the prognosis of patients with FMF does not seem to be different from that of patients with other chronic nonfatal illnesses. Death usually results from causes unrelated to the underlying disease.

The complication of amyloidosis in Israel, parts of North Africa, Turkey, and other parts of the Middle East makes the prognosis quite different from that in America. Approximately 25 percent of FMF patients in Israel are known to have amyloidosis, and this complication usually leads to death. Because a majority of patients under observation in Israel are under forty years of age, it has been suggested that fatal amyloidosis may eventually occur in nearly all patients. This would explain the rarity of older patients in that area.

TREATMENT Many forms of therapy had been tried in FMF, but until recently, nothing was effective. Among the therapies tried have been antibiotics, hormones (including estrogens and adrenal corticosteroids), antipyretic drugs, immunotherapy, psychotherapy, elimination and low-fat diets, chloroquine, and phenylbutazone. When carefully studied and followed up, none of these therapies proved effective.

Recently a major advance was made. Goldfinger reported in 1972 that the prophylactic use of colchicine in five patients dramatically reduced the number of attacks. Subsequently, controlled trials in the United States and Israel have shown that chronic administration of colchicine will greatly reduce the number of acute attacks of FMF. It is recommended that 0.6 mg colchicine be taken by mouth three times a day. Patients often develop gastrointestinal side effects on this dose, however, in which case the dose should be reduced to 0.6 mg taken twice a day. Although an occasional patient will respond to 0.6 mg taken only once a day, this amount is less likely to be beneficial. Most but not all FMF patients will respond favorably to colchicine prophylaxis.

Since colchicine is known to result in nondisjunction of chromosomes and in azospermia in some patients, it should not be given to any patient, especially a young one, unless the disease is severe enough to warrant taking the risk. In addition, everyone who requires therapy should first be tried on a course of intermittent colchicine. The patient should take 0.6 mg colchicine by mouth every hour for 4 h, then every 2 h for 4 h, and every 12 h thereafter for 48 h. The colchicine should be given at the first premonitory sign of an attack. When colchicine is taken on such a schedule, many patients will experience aborted attacks or no symptoms at all. If both acute and prophylactic colchicine therapy fail, supportive therapy is all that can be offered. Except for unusual circumstances, narcotics should not be given to FMF patients.

The mechanism of colchicine's action against acute attacks of FMF is unknown. It is postulated that it may work by preventing the normal cellular response to inflammation.

REFERENCES

DINARELLO CA et al: Colchicine therapy for familial Mediterranean fever. A double-blind trial. N Engl J Med 291:934, 1974

EHRENFELD EN et al: Recurrent polyserositis (familial Mediterranean fever: periodic disease): A report of fifty-five cases. Am J Med 31:107, 1961

REIMANN HA: *Periodic Diseases,* Philadelphia: Davis, 1963

SCHWABE AD, PETERS RS: Familial Mediterranean fever in Armenians. Analysis of 100 cases. Medicine 53:453, 1974

SOHAR E et al: Familial Mediterranean fever. Am J Med 43:227, 1967

230 MIDLINE GRANULOMA

SHELDON M. WOLFF

DEFINITION Midline granuloma is an uncommon disease characterized by localized inflammation, destruction, and often mutilation of the tissues of the upper respiratory tract and face. This condition has also been referred to as *lethal midline granuloma, malignant granuloma,* and *granuloma gangrenescens,* none of which is an appropriate term. The disease was first described by McBride in 1897.

ETIOLOGY The etiology of midline granuloma is unknown. In view of the intense granulomatous inflammation, the disease is thought to represent a localized hypersensitivity reaction which leads to tissue destruction and mutilation. However, the responsible antigen(s) is unknown, and there is no immunologic evidence supporting this hypothesis. A variety of microorganisms have been considered as possible causative agents, but detailed microbiologic investigations have failed to detect the consistent presence of pathogenic organisms. In view of the clinical and pathologic features of the illness as well as the fact that some upper airway tumors can elicit a similar intense inflammatory response, some authors have suggested a neoplastic basis for midline granuloma. However, when malignant tissue (usually of a lymphomatous nature) is found in the lesions, the diagnosis of midline granuloma is no longer tenable.

PATHOLOGY The most characteristic pathologic findings are acute and chronic inflammation with necrosis. Superimposed pyogenic infection of the involved tissues, including the sinuses, may contribute to nonspecific histologic findings. The pathologic hallmark, noncaseating granulomas, with or without giant cells, may be obscured by the inflammatory reaction, but when present is strong evidence in favor of the diagnosis. Primary vasculitis is seen rarely, and when it occurs, a search for other causes, most notably Wegener's granulomatosis, should be made. The presence of malignant cells makes the diagnosis of midline granuloma unacceptable. Until an etiology is established, the diagnosis of midline granuloma will rest on the characteristic clinical features outlined below.

CLINICAL FEATURES The disease may occur at any age, but the majority of patients are in the fifth and sixth decades. It is more common in women than men and has been reported in all races. Many patients report recurrent "sinus" problems, and some have histories of allergic rhinitis, although the significance of these features is unknown.

The major symptoms are usually related to the nose. Patients frequently complain of nasal stuffiness and occasionally of discharge. The first symptom in a smaller percentage of patients relates to ulceration of the mucosa of the nose, the buccal mucosa, or the gums. This has led to loosening of the teeth, and dentists are often first consulted by these patients. Rarely, patients will present first with eye findings related to conjunctival inflammation or even ulceration. Although the progression of symptoms in some patients may be slow, all too often the disease steadily, and sometimes rapidly, progresses. The characteristic symptoms of nasal discharge, difficulty in breathing through the nose, and pain over the sinuses, nose, or eye become more prominent with time. Once ulceration begins, the disease often progresses rapidly. The ulcers frequently involve the nasal septum and will lead to the characteristic septal perforation and a "saddlenose" deformity. The majority of patients develop ulceration and eventually perforations of the soft and hard palates. Untreated, the disease can lead to massive destruction and mutilation of the tissues involved, including the skin of the face and the eyes. Frequently, the necrotic tissue becomes infected, and systemic symptoms such as fever and anorexia appear. The destructive lesions can become very malodorous. The disease extends to involve local tissues and does not progress below the neck; if this happens, other diseases should be considered. As the necrotic process progresses and involves vital organs, patients may lose sight in the affected eye, experience dysphagia, and have difficulty in speech. Although spontaneous temporary remissions have been reported, untreated midline granuloma is fatal. The progression of the disease can be rapidly accelerated by surgical procedures in the affected areas. The patient usually dies from secondary infection, although erosion by the process into a major blood vessel or penetration into the central nervous system with superimposed meningitis can also cause death.

Aside from the granulomatous inflammation, necrosis, and destruction, no other specific clinical or pathologic findings are associated with midline granuloma. Occasionally, with superimposed infection, local lymphadenopathy may be noted, but it is not characteristic of the disease per se.

LABORATORY FINDINGS With progression of the disease, a variety of nonspecific abnormalities may be noted. These changes are characteristic of inflammatory processes in general or of secondary infections. For example, mild anemia, leukocytosis, elevated sedimentation rate, and hyperglobulinemia are common in these patients. Radiographic examination reveals pansinusitis, and as the disease advances, destruction of bone in the involved areas is characteristic.

DIFFERENTIAL DIAGNOSIS The diagnosis of midline granuloma is made by finding the characteristic histologic lesions in biopsies of the affected tissues. When the specimens show only inflammatory tissue, a presumptive diagnosis of midline granuloma can be made only when the characteristic clinical picture is present and other diseases with similar presentation have been excluded. The diagnosis of Wegener's granulomatosis is ruled out by the absence of vasculitis in the biopsy specimens and the localized nature of midline granuloma (i.e., no pulmonary or renal involvement). In addition, Wegener's granulomatosis rarely, if ever, causes erosion through facial tissues. It is often difficult to differentiate true midline granuloma from neoplasms of the upper airways such as malignant reticulosis and certain lymphomas. These may be clinically similar to midline granuloma and are often associated with granulomatous inflammation. Careful examination of generous biopsy material as well as concomitant work-up for disseminated neoplasm often provides the clinicopathologic distinction. Other diseases to be excluded by appropriate laboratory techniques are histoplasmosis, blastomycosis, coccidioidomycosis, leprosy, tuberculosis, syphilis, mucocutaneous leishmaniasis, rhinoscleroma, and pseudotumor of the orbit.

TREATMENT The complications of midline granuloma such as superimposed infections can be treated specifically. Although adrenal corticosteroids are often used in the therapy of midline granuloma, they are of no value and probably are contraindicated if infection is present. Sporadic reports of therapy with cytotoxic agents are difficult to interpret, since some of the patients reported clearly had lymphoma or Wegener's granulomatosis, diseases where such agents are of definite value. Surgical removal of the involved tissue has been attempted but is useless and may, in fact, cause rapid progression of the disease.

The treatment of choice is radiotherapy to the local lesion. Although low dosages (1,000 rd and below) have been reported to be effective, many patients relapse after such therapy. Radiotherapy should be given in a dose of 5,000 rd to the involved areas. Where such a regimen is employed, long-lasting (more than 10 years) remissions and possible cures have been achieved. Following irradiation and after an appropriate period to allow for tissue healing (usually 1 year), reconstructive and plastic surgery, which may be of enormous cosmetic and functional value, can be undertaken.

REFERENCES

Blatt IM et al: Fatal granulomatosis of the respiratory tract (lethal midline granuloma—Wegener's granulomatosis). AMA Arch Otolaryngol 70:707, 1959

Fauci AS et al: Wegener's granulomatosis: Studies in eight patients and a review of the literature. Medicine 52:535, 1973

——et al: Radiation therapy of midline granuloma. Ann Intern Med (in press)

Fechner RE, Lamppin DW: Midline malignant reticulosis. Arch Otolaryngol 95:467, 1972

Walton EW: Reticuloendothelial sarcoma arising in the nose and palate (granuloma gangrenescens). J Clin Pathol 13:279, 1960

PART SEVEN DISEASES OF THE ORGAN SYSTEMS

section 1 Disorders of the heart

231
APPROACH TO THE PATIENT WITH HEART DISEASE

EUGENE BRAUNWALD

The initial symptoms of the patient with heart disease result most commonly from myocardial ischemia, from disturbance of the contractile activity of the myocardium, or from an abnormal cardiac rhythm or rate. Ischemia is manifest most frequently as chest pain, while reduction of the pumping ability of the heart commonly leads to weakness and fatigability or, when severe, produces cyanosis, hypotension, syncope, and elevated intravascular pressure upstream to a failing ventricle; the latter results in abnormal fluid accumulation, which in turn leads to dyspnea, orthopnea, and edema. Cardiac arrhythmias often develop suddenly, and the resulting signs and symptoms—palpitation, dyspnea, angina, hypotension, and syncope—generally occur abruptly and may disappear as rapidly as they develop.

A cardinal principle useful in the evaluation of the patient with suspected heart disease is that myocardial or coronary function which may be quite adequate at rest may be totally inadequate during exertion. Thus, a history of chest pain and/or dyspnea which appears only during activity is characteristic of heart disease, while the opposite pattern, i.e., the appearance of these symptoms at rest and their remission during exertion, is rarely observed in patients with organic heart disease.

Patients with cardiocirculatory disease may also be entirely asymptomatic, both at rest and during exertion, but may present an abnormal physical finding, such as a heart murmur, elevated systemic arterial pressure, or an abnormality of the electrocardiogram or of the cardiac silhouette on the chest roentgenogram.

Diseases of the heart and circulation are so common and the laity is so well acquainted with the major symptoms resulting from these disorders that patients, and occasionally physicians, erroneously attribute many complaints to organic cardiovascular disease. Furthermore, the combination of the widespread fear of heart disease in the Western world with the deep-seated emotional connotations concerning this organ's function results in the frequent development in persons with normal cardiovascular systems of symptoms which mimic those of organic disease. The correct interpretation of symptoms in patients with recognized organic cardiovascular disturbances is occasionally quite difficult. Such persons, in addition to having symptoms resulting from their disease, may also develop functional complaints referable to the cardiovascular system. The unraveling of symptoms and signs due to organic heart disease from those which are not directly related is an important and challenging task in these patients.

It must be recognized that dyspnea, one of the cardinal manifestations of diminished cardiac reserve, is not limited to disease of the heart, but is also characteristic of conditions as diverse as pulmonary disease, marked obesity, and anxiety (Chap. 30). Similarly, chest pain (Chap. 7) may result from a variety of causes other than myocardial ischemia. Whether heart disease is responsible for these symptoms can frequently be determined by carrying out a detailed clinical examination. The electrocardiogram and roentgenogram provide additional helpful information; more specialized examinations are often helpful but only occasionally essential.

In every branch of medicine the establishment of the prognosis and development of a rational plan of management are based on a correct diagnostic appraisal. However, in the case of patients with disorders of the cardiocirculatory system, particular care must be taken to establish not only a correct but also a *complete* diagnosis. As outlined by the New York Heart Association, the elements of a complete cardiac diagnosis include consideration of:

1 The underlying etiology. Is the disease congenital, rheumatic, hypertensive, or arteriosclerotic in origin?
2 The anatomic abnormalities. Which chambers are enlarged? Which valves are affected? Is there pericardial involvement? Has there been a myocardial infarct?
3 The physiologic disturbances. Is an arrhythmia present? Is there evidence of congestive heart failure or of myocardial ischemia?
4 The extent of functional disability. How strenuous is the physical activity required to elicit symptoms?

Two simple examples may serve to illustrate the importance of establishing a complete diagnosis. The identification of exertional chest pain caused by myocardial ischemia is of crucial significance. However, this diagnosis is insufficient to develop either a strategy of specific treatment or prognosis until the underlying disease process, e.g., coronary atherosclerosis, aortic stenosis, severe anemia, thyrotoxicosis, or atrial tachycardia, which is responsible for the myocardial ischemia, is identified. Similarly, determining that heart disease is congenital provides an important starting point, but the decision as to whether surgical treatment is advisable generally depends upon the specific anatomic defect present and often upon the nature of the physiologic disturbance and the functional impairment.

The establishment of a correct and complete cardiac diagnosis often requires the use of six different methods of examination: (1) history, (2) physical examination (Chap. 232), (3) chest roentgenogram (Chap. 234), (4) electrocardiogram (Chap. 233), (5) noninvasive graphic examinations (echocardiogram, phonocardiogram, arterial and venous pulse tracings, Chap. 234), and occasionally (6) specialized examinations, such as cardiac catheterization or angiocardiography (Chap. 235). In order to be most effective, each of these six approaches should be employed independently of one another as well as with the information derived from the other methods clearly in mind. Only in this way can one avoid overlooking a subtle, though extremely significant, finding. For example, an electrocardiogram should be obtained in every patient suspected of having heart disease. It may provide the critical clue in establishing the correct diagnosis, e.g., the finding of an atrioventricular conduction disturbance in a patient with unexplained syncope, even when all other methods of examination reveal no abnormal findings. On the other hand, when combined intelligently with the results of other methods of examination, the electrocardiogram may provide essential confirmatory data. Thus, the knowledge that a patient has an apical diastolic rumbling murmur may direct particular attention to the P waves, and the recognition of left atrial enlargement electrocardiographically would support the suggestion that the murmur is caused by mitral stenosis. Under these circumstances the additional finding of right ventricular hypertrophy suggests that pulmonary hypertension is present. Although the electrocardiogram is an invaluable aspect of every cardiovascular examination, with the exception of the identification of arrhythmias it rarely permits establishment of a specific diagnosis. In the absence of any other abnormal findings, electrocardiographic changes must not ever be interpreted. The range of normal electrocardiographic findings is wide, and the tracing can be affected significantly by many noncardiac factors, such as age, body habitus, and serum electrolyte concentrations.

In obtaining the history of the patient with known or suspected cardiovascular disease, particular attention should be directed to the family history. Familial clustering is common in many forms of heart disease. Genetic transmission may occur, as in hypertrophic subaortic stenosis (Chap. 247) or Marfan's syndrome (Chap. 367). In patients with essential hypertension or coronary atherosclerosis the genetic component may be less obvious but is also of considerable importance. The nature of the response of the myocardium to an increased hemodynamic load, such as hypertension, or a valvular lesion may also be conditioned by hereditary factors. Familial clustering of cardiovascular diseases may not only occur on a genetic basis but may also be related to familial, dietary, or behavior patterns.

When an attempt is made to ascertain the severity of functional impairment in a patient with heart disease, it is essential to determine the precise extent of activity and the rate at which it is performed before symptoms develop. Thus, breathlessness which occurs after running up two long flights of stairs denotes far less functional impairment than similar symptoms occurring after taking a few steps on the level. Also, the degree of customary physical activity at work and during recreation should be considered. Similarly, the history must include a detailed consideration of the patient's therapeutic regimen. For example, the persistence or development of edema in a patient whose diet is rigidly restricted in sodium content and who is receiving optimum doses of digitalis and diuretics must be interpreted quite differently from the finding of edema in the absence of these measures.

The phonocardiogram and the graphic indirect recording of pulse tracings, such as the jugular venous pulse, the carotid arterial pulse, and the apex cardiogram (Chap. 234), may in some instances provide information of considerable diagnostic value by amplifying the physical findings. It must be appreciated, however, that these techniques are primarily of aid in the precise timing of specific events, such as heart sounds, murmurs, and pulsations, which are easily elicited on physical examination.

PITFALLS IN CARDIOVASCULAR MEDICINE Increasing subspecialization in internal medicine and the perfection of advanced diagnostic techniques in cardiology may sometimes be accompanied by several undesirable consequences, which can be summarized as follows:

1 Failure by the noncardiologist to recognize cardiac manifestations of systemic illnesses. The latter include: (a) mongolism (often associated with endocardial cushion defect); (b) gonadal dysgenesis, i.e., Turner's syndrome (associated with a variety of congenital defects, particularly coarctation of the aorta); (c) bony abnormalities of the upper extremities (associated with atrial septal defect); (d) muscular dystrophies (associated with cardiomyopathy); (e) hemochromatosis and glycogen storage disease (associated with myocardial infiltration); (f) congenital deafness (associated with serious cardiac arrhythmias); (g) Raynaud's disease (associated with primary pulmonary hypertension); (h) connective tissue disorders, i.e., Marfan's syndrome, Ehlers-Danlos syndrome, Hurler's syndrome, and related disorders of mucopolysaccharide metabolism (aortic dilatation, billowing mitral valve, a variety of arterial abnormalities); (i) chronic hemolytic anemia (cardiac dilatation); (j) Refsum's disease (myocardial failure and conduction defects), (k) acromegaly (accelerated coronary atherosclerosis, conduction defects, myocardial fibrosis); (l) hyperthyroidism (heart failure, atrial fibrillation); (m) rheumatoid arthritis (pericarditis, aortic valve disease); (n) Whipple's disease (pericarditis and endocarditis); (o) scleroderma (cor pulmonale, myocardial fibrosis, pericarditis); (p) lupus erythematosus (valvulitis, myocarditis); (q) polymyositis (pericarditis, myocarditis); (r) sarcoidosis (arrhythmias, heart failure); (s) Fabry's disease (myocardial ischemia, heart failure); (t) exfoliative dermatitis (high-output heart failure). In patients in whom these and related systemic disorders with cardiovascular involvement are present or suspected, detailed cardiovascular examination should be carried out.

2 Failure by the cardiac specialist to recognize systemic illnesses in patients with cardiac disorders. Patients known or suspected of having heart disease require a detailed general assessment and a search for the frequent noncardiac manifestations of cardiac disorders. Indeed, the cardiovascular abnormality may provide the clue critical to the recognition of these disorders. Closely related is the failure to appreciate the profound effects of stress, such as that resulting from an intercurrent infection, of pregnancy, or from emotional disturbances, on cardiovascular performance and symptoms.

3 Overreliance on and overutilization of laboratory tests, particularly specialized invasive techniques.

The examinations noted above, such as catheterization of the right and left sides of the heart, selective angiography, and coronary arteriography (Chap. 235), provide precise diagnostic information under many circumstances. For example, they aid in establishing a specific anatomic diagnosis in patients with congenital heart disease, in patients with chest pain of uncertain etiology in whom coronary artery disease is suspected, and in determining the functional significance of valvular abnormalities in patients with rheumatic heart disease being considered for surgical treatment. Although a great deal of attention has been lavished on the newer specialized laboratory examinations, it should be recognized that they serve to *supplement,* not *supplant,* a careful clinical examination. There is an unfortunate tendency to carry out procedures such as coronary arteriography instead of taking a detailed and thoughtful history; the results often do not provide a definite answer to the question of whether a patient's complaint of chest pain is clearly attributable to coronary arteriosclerosis. Similarly, catheterization of the left side of the heart is all too frequently employed to determine whether operative treatment of valvular disease is indicated, even before the patient has had a trial of medical therapy. Despite their enormous value, it must not be overlooked that these specialized examinations entail some risk to the patient, involve discomfort and cost, and place a strain on existing medical facilities. Therefore, *they should be carried out only if there is a specific indication and if the results can be expected to modify or aid in the patient's management.*

REFERENCES

DRESSLER W: *Clinical Aids in Cardiac Diagnosis,* New York: Grune & Stratton, 1970

FOWLER NO : *Cardiac Diagnosis and Treatment,* 2d ed, Hagerstown: Harper & Row, 1976, 1133 pp

FORMEL PF: Neurologic manifestations of cardiac disease. NY State J Med (April) 968–971, 1973

GAZES PC: *Clinical Cardiology: A Bedside Approach,* Chicago: Year Book Medical Publishers, 1975, 384 pp

HURST JW (ed): *The Heart,* 3d ed., New York: McGraw-Hill, 1974

NEW YORK HEART ASSOCIATION, INC., CRITERIA COMMITTEE: *Nomenclature and Criteria for Diagnosis of Diseases of the Heart and Great Vessels,* 7th ed., Boston: Little, Brown, 1973

SELZER, A: *Principles of Clinical Cardiology: An Analytical Approach,* Philadelphia: Saunders, 1975

232
PHYSICAL EXAMINATION OF THE HEART

ROBERT A. O'ROURKE
EUGENE BRAUNWALD

The physical examination of the patient with cardiac disease includes careful evaluation of both the arterial pressure pulse and the jugular venous pulse, as well as deliberate precordial palpation and attentive cardiac auscultation.

ARTERIAL PRESSURE PULSE The normal central aortic pulse wave is characterized by a fairly rapid rise to a somewhat rounded peak (Fig. 232-1). The anacrotic shoulder, present on the ascending limb, occurs at the time of peak rate of aortic flow just before maximum pressure is reached. The less steep descending limb is interrupted by a sharp downward deflection, synchronous with aortic valve closure, called the *incisura.* As the pulse wave is transmitted peripherally, the initial upstroke becomes steeper, the anacrotic shoulder becomes less apparent, and the incisura is replaced by the smoother dicrotic notch. Accordingly, palpation of a peripheral pulse (e.g., the brachial arterial) frequently gives less information than examination of a more central pulse (e.g., the carotid arterial) regarding alterations in left ventricular ejection or aortic valve function. However, certain findings such as the bounding pulses of aortic regurgitation or pulsus alternans are more readily evident in peripheral than in central arteries. In order to examine the carotid arteries, the sternocleidomastoid muscle should be relaxed and the head rotated slightly

FIGURE 232-1

A *Simultaneous recordings of electrocardiogram, aortic pressure pulse (AOP), phonocardiogram recorded at the apex, and apex cardiogram (ACG). On the phonocardiogram, S_1, S_2, S_3, and S_4 represent the first through fourth heart sounds; OS represents the opening snap of the mitral valve, which occurs coincident with the O point of the apex cardiogram. S_3 occurs coincident with the termination of the rapid-filling wave (RFW) of the ACG, while S_4 occurs coincident with the A wave of the ACG.* B *Simultaneous recording of electrocardiogram, indirect carotid pulse (CP), phonocardiogram along the left sternal border (LSB), and indirect jugular venous pulse (JVP). ES, ejection sound; SC, systolic click.*

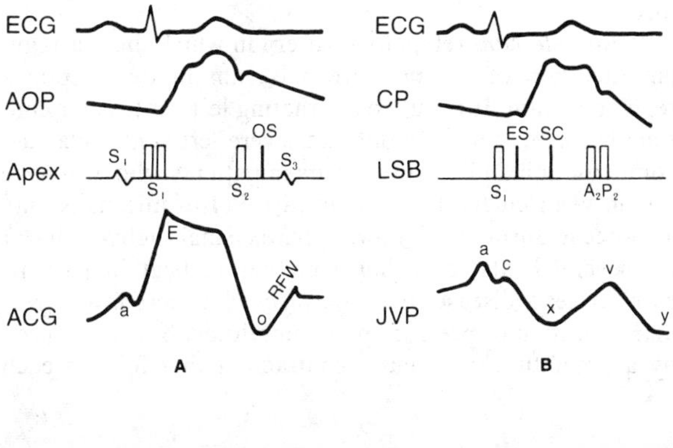

toward the examiner. The application of varying amounts of pressure with either the forefinger or the thumb may permit appreciation of the ascending limb, the systolic peak, and the descending limb of the pressure pulse. In most normal persons a dicrotic wave is not palpable.

A small weak pulse, *pulsus parvus,* is frequently present in conditions with a diminished left ventricular stroke volume, a narrow pulse pressure, and increased peripheral vascular resistance. This may be due to hypovolemia, to left ventricular failure secondary to myocardial disease or myocardial infarction, to restrictive pericardial disease, or to mitral valve stenosis. In aortic valve stenosis the delayed systolic peak, *pulsus tardus,* is the result of mechanical obstruction to left ventricular ejection and is often accompanied by the transmission of a coarse systolic thrill. In contrast, a large bounding pulse is usually associated with an increased left ventricular stroke volume, a wide pulse pressure, and a decrease in peripheral vascular resistance. This occurs characteristically in patients with abnormally elevated stroke volumes as in complete heart block, hyperkinetic circulation due to anxiety, anemia, exercise, or fever, or in patients with an abnormally rapid run-off of blood from the arterial system (patent ductus arteriosus, peripheral arteriovenous fistula). Patients with mitral regurgitation or a ventricular septal defect may also have a bounding pulse, since vigorous left ventricular ejection produces a rapid upstroke in the arterial pulse even though the duration of systole and the forward stroke volume may be diminished. In aortic regurgitation the rapidly rising, bounding arterial pulse results from increased left ventricular stroke volume and the associated increased rate of ventricular ejection.

The *bisferiens pulse,* which consists of two systolic peaks, is characteristic of aortic regurgitation (with or without accompanying stenosis) and of idiopathic hypertrophic subaortic stenosis (Chap. 247). In the latter the pulse wave upstroke rises rapidly and forcefully, producing the first systolic peak ("percussion wave"). A brief decline in pressure follows, because of the sudden decrease in the rate of left ventricular ejection as severe obstruction develops during midsystole. This pressure trough is followed by a smaller and more slowly rising positive pulse wave ("tidal wave") produced by continued ventricular ejection and by reflected waves from the periphery. When the second positive wave is produced by an accentuated and palpable diastolic wave, the pulse is called *dicrotic.* It has been recorded in patients who have a low diastolic pressure and systemic vascular resistance such as those with fever or mild aortic regurgitation and in patients with a very low stroke volume, particularly those with diffuse myocardial disease.

Pulsus alternans refers to a pattern in which there is regular alteration of the pressure pulse amplitude, despite a regular rhythm. It is due to alternating left ventricular contractile force; it usually denotes severe left ventricular decompensation and usually occurs in patients who also have a loud ventricular filling sound (S_3). Pulsus alternans may also occur during or following paroxysmal tachycardia or for several beats following a premature beat in patients without heart disease. In *pulsus bigeminus* there is also regular alteration of pressure pulse amplitude, but it is caused by a premature ventricular contraction that follows each regular beat; auscultation can reveal the cardiac irregularity. *Pulsus paradoxus* is an accentuation of the decrease in systolic arterial pressure accompanying the reduced amplitude of the arterial pulse which normally occurs during inspiration. In patients with pericardial tamponade, airway obstruction, or superior vena cava obstruction, the decrease in systolic arterial pressure frequently exceeds the normal of 10 mmHg and the peripheral pulse may disappear completely during inspiration.

Simultaneous palpation of the radial and femoral arterial pulses, which normally are virtually coincident, is important to rule out aortic coarctation, in which the latter is weaker and delayed (Chap. 241).

JUGULAR VENOUS PULSE (JVP) The two main objectives of the bedside examination of the neck veins are inspection of their wave form and estimation of the central venous pressure (CVP). In most patients, the right internal jugular vein is superior for both purposes, but occasionally examination of the left internal jugular vein, the external jugular veins, or the venous pulsations in the supraclavicular fossae may yield more information. In most normal subjects, maximum pulsation of the internal jugular vein is observed when the trunk is inclined by less than 30°. In patients with elevated venous pressure it may be necessary to elevate the trunk further, sometimes to as much as 90°. When the neck muscles are relaxed, shining a beam of light tangentially across the skin overlying the vein exposes the pulsations of the internal jugular vein. Simultaneous palpation of the left carotid artery aids the examiner in deciding which pulsations are venous and in relating the venous pulsations to their timing in the cardiac cycle.

The normal JVP reflects phasic pressure changes in the right atrium and consists of three positive waves and two negative troughs (Fig. 232-1). In considering this pulse, it is useful to refer to the events of the cardiac cycle (Fig. 234-2). The positive presystolic A wave is produced by venous distention consequent to right atrial contraction and is the dominant wave in the JVP, particularly during inspiration. Large A waves indicate that the right atrium is contracting against an increased resistance, such as occurs with obstruction at the tricuspid valve (tricuspid stenosis or right atrial myxoma) or more commonly with increased resistance to right ventricular filling (pulmonary hypertension or pulmonic stenosis). Large A waves also occur during arrhythmias whenever the right atrium contracts while the tricuspid valve is closed by right ventricular systole. Such "cannon" A waves may occur regularly (as during junctional rhythm) or irregularly (as in atrioventricular dissociation with ventricular tachycardia or complete heart block). The A wave is absent in patients with atrial fibrillation, and there is an increased temporal delay between the A wave and the carotid arterial pulse in patients with first degree AV block.

The C wave, often observed in the JVP, is a positive wave produced by the bulging of the tricuspid valve into the right atrium during right ventricular isovolumetric systole and by the impact of the carotid artery adjacent to the jugular vein. The X descent is due to a combination of atrial relaxation and the downward displacement of the tricuspid valve during ventricular systole. In patients with constrictive pericarditis, there is often increased prominence of the X descent wave during systole, but this wave is reduced in dilatation of the right side of the heart and may even be reversed in tricuspid regurgitation. The positive, late systolic V wave results from the increasing volume of blood in the venae cavae and right atrium during ventricular systole when the tricuspid valve is closed. After the peak of the V wave is reached, the right atrial pressure diminishes because of the decreased bulging of the tricuspid valve into the right atrium as right ventricular pressure declines followed by tricuspid valve opening. With mild tricuspid regurgitation the V wave becomes more prominent, and when tricuspid regurgitation becomes severe, the prominent V wave and the obliteration of the X descent result in a single large positive systolic wave ("ventricularization").

Following the summit of the V wave there is a negative descending limb, referred to as the Y descent or "diastolic collapse," which is produced mainly by tricuspid valve opening and the rapid inflow of blood into the right ventricle. A rapid, deep Y descent in early diastole occurs with severe tricuspid regurgitation. A venous pulse characterized by a sharp Y descent, a deep Y trough, and a rapid ascent to the base line is seen in patients with constrictive pericarditis or with severe failure of the right side of the heart and a high venous pressure. A slow Y descent in the JVP suggests an obstruction to right ventricular filling, as occurs with tricuspid stenosis or right atrial myxoma.

For accurate estimation of the CVP, the right internal jugular vein is best utilized, with the sternal angle as the reference point, since in the average patient the center of the right atrium lies approximately 5 cm below the sternal angle, regardless of body position. The patient is examined at the optimum degree of trunk elevation for visualization of venous pulsations. The vertical distance between the top of the oscillating venous column and the level of the sternal angle is determined and generally found to be less than 3 cm (3 cm + 5 cm = 8 cm blood). The most common cause of an elevated venous pressure is an elevated right ventricular diastolic pressure. In patients suspected of having right ventricular failure who have a normal CVP at rest, the hepatojugular reflux test may be helpful. The palm of the hand is placed over the right upper quadrant of the abdomen, and firm pressure is applied for 30 to 60 s. Normally, the jugular venous pressure is not significantly altered, but with impaired function of the right side of the heart the upper level of venous pulsation usually increases. The increased abdominal pressure most likely enhances systemic venous return, and the abnormal right ventricle is unable to accept this additional blood volume, causing pressure in the great veins to rise. Also, abdominal compression may elicit the typical JVP of tricuspid regurgitation when the resting pulse wave is normal.

PRECORDIAL PALPATION This is best accomplished while auscultating the heart in order to time the cardiac movements. The location, amplitude, duration, and direction of

FIGURE 232-2
Simultaneous recordings of ECG, aortic pressure (AOP), left ventricular pressure (LVP), and left atrial pressure (LAP). HSM is a holosystolic murmur; PSM, a presystolic murmur; MDM, a middiastolic murmur; SEM, a systolic ejection murmur; and EDM, an early diastolic murmur.

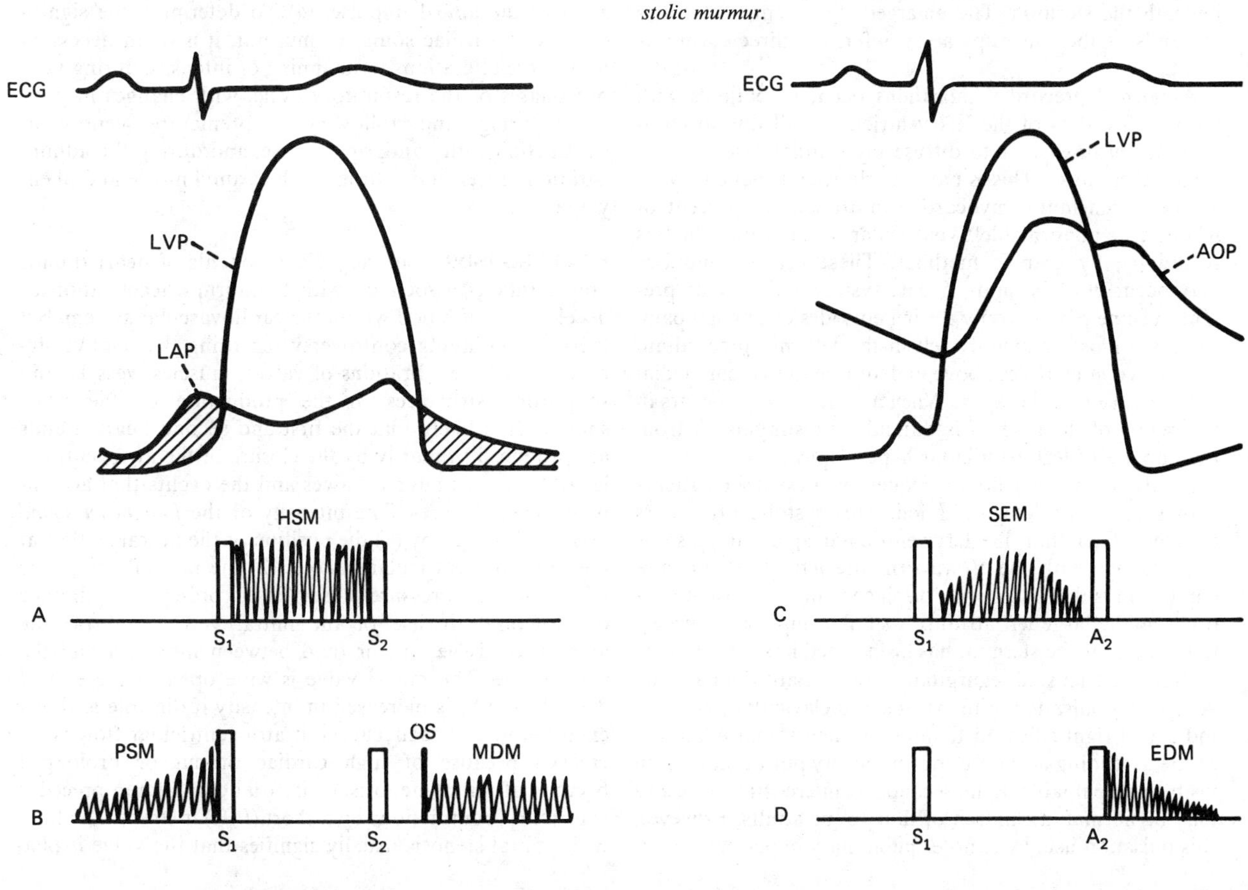

the impulse can usually be best appreciated by using the fingertips. The normal left ventricular apex impulse is located at or medial to the left midclavicular line in the fourth or fifth intercostal space and is a tapping, early systolic outward thrust localized to a point not more than 2 to 3 cm in diameter. It is due primarily to recoil of the heart as blood is ejected, and it is best evaluated with the patient lying supine. Left ventricular hypertrophy results in an exaggerated amplitude and duration of the normal left ventricular thrust. The impulse may be displaced laterally and downward into the sixth or seventh interspace, particularly in patients with a left ventricular volume load such as occurs in aortic regurgitation.

Additional abnormal features of the left ventricular apex impulse may become more obvious when the patient is turned on his left side. These include marked presystolic distention of the left ventricle, often accompanying a fourth heart sound in patients with an excessive left ventricular pressure load, and a prominent early diastolic rapid-filling wave, often accompanying a third heart sound in patients with left ventricular failure or mitral valve regurgitation (Fig. 232-1). A double systolic impulse is frequently palpable in patients with idiopathic hypertrophic subaortic stenosis.

Right ventricular hypertrophy results in a sustained systolic lift at the lower left parasternal area which starts in early systole and is synchronous with the left ventricular apical impulse. In patients with chronic obstructive pulmonary disease a right ventricular impulse may often be detected by sliding the fingers up under the rib cage just beneath the sternum. The enlarged right ventricle strikes the ends of the fingertips as an inferiorly directed movement.

Abnormal precordial pulsations occur in patients with motion disorders of the left ventricular wall due to coronary artery disease or to diffuse myocardial disease from some other cause. This is particularly true in patients with a recent transmural myocardial infarction, 70 percent of whom have abnormal left ventricular wall motion which is recordable by graphic methods. These ectopic impulses may occur in early, mid-, or late systole and may be present in some patients only during episodes of anginal pain. They are most commonly felt in the left mid-precordium one or two interspaces above and/or one to two cm medial to the left ventricular apex. When a systolic bulge occurs in the region of the apex, it is difficult to distinguish it from the impulse of left ventricular hypertrophy.

A left parasternal lift is frequently present in patients with severe mitral regurgitation. This systolic lift occurs distinctly later than the left ventricular apical impulse, is synchronous with the V wave in the left atrial pressure curve, and is due to anterior displacement of the right ventricle by the large left atrium. A similar impulse occurring to the right of the sternum has been noted in some patients with severe tricuspid regurgitation and a giant right atrium. A vigorous pulsation of the right sternoclavicular joint may indicate a right-sided aortic arch or aneurysmal dilatation of the ascending aorta. Pulmonary artery pulsation is often visible and palpable in the second left intercostal space and may be normal in children or thin young adults. However, this pulsation usually denotes pulmonary hypertension, increased pulmonary blood flow, or poststenotic pulmonary artery dilatation.

Thrills are palpable low-frequency vibrations associated with heart murmurs. The diastolic rumble of mitral stenosis and the systolic murmur of mitral regurgitation may be palpated at the cardiac apex. When the palm of the hand is placed over the precordium, the thrill of aortic stenosis crosses the palm of the hand toward the right side of the neck, while the thrill of pulmonic stenosis tends to radiate more often to the left side of the neck. The thrill due to a ventricular septal defect is usually located in the third and fourth intercostal spaces near the left sternal border.

Percussion adds little to careful inspection and palpation in the recognition of cardiac enlargement. Occasionally, however, it is useful in detecting an abnormal rightward position of the heart, such as occurs in dextrocardia, dextroversion, right lung atelectasis, and left pneumothorax, as well as in demonstrating an increased area of dullness or flatness to the right of the sternum and at the upper left sternal border in patients with a large pericardial effusion.

CARDIAC AUSCULTATION To obtain maximal information from cardiac auscultation, the observer should keep in mind several principles: (1) This portion of the examination should be carried out in a quiet room to avoid the distractions caused by the noises of normal activity. (2) In order to hear a faint heart sound or murmur, it is necessary to focus attention on that phase of the cardiac cycle during which the auscultatory event may be expected to occur. (3) The accurate timing of a heart sound or murmur necessarily involves ascertaining its relation to other observable events in the cardiac cycle—the carotid arterial pulse, the JVP, or the apical impulse. (4) To determine the significance of a cardiac sound or murmur, it is often necessary to observe alterations in its timing or intensity during various phases of the respiratory cycle, with changes in position, during and following a premature ventricular contraction with handgrip exercise, and during the administration of vasoactive drugs such as amyl nitrite and phenylephrine.

HEART SOUNDS The major components of heart sounds are vibrations associated with the abrupt acceleration or deceleration of blood within the cardiovascular system, but there is continuing controversy regarding the relative significance of the vibrations of valves, muscles, vessels, and supporting structures in the production of the heart sounds. It is likely that the first and second heart sounds are produced primarily by the closure of the atrioventricular (AV) and semilunar valves and the events that accompany these closures. The intensity of the *first heart sound* (S_1) is influenced by (1) the position of the mitral leaflets at the onset of ventricular systole; (2) the rate of rise of the left ventricular pressure pulse; (3) the presence or absence of structural disease of the mitral valve; and (4) the amount of tissue, air, or fluid between the heart and the stethoscope. The mitral valve is wide open at the end of diastole and S_1 is increased in intensity if diastole is shortened because of tachycardia, if atrioventricular flow is increased because of high cardiac output or prolonged because of mitral stenosis, or if atrial contraction precedes ventricular contractions by a short (P-R) interval. The loud S_1 in mitral stenosis usually signifies that the valve is pliable and that the valve remains wide open at the onset of isovolumetric contraction due to the elevated left atrial pressure. A reduction in the intensity of S_1 may be due to poor conduction of sound through the chest wall, a slow rise of the left ventricular pressure pulse, a long P-R interval, or imperfect closure due to reduced valve substance, as in mitral regurgitation. S_1 is also soft when the anterior mitral leaflet is immobile because of rigidity and calcification even in the presence of predominant mitral stenosis.

Splitting of the two high-pitched components of S_1 by 10 to 30 ms is a normal phenomenon (Fig. 232-1). The first component of S_1 normally is attributed to mitral valve closure and the second to tricuspid valve closure. A widened split of S_1 is most often due to complete right bundle branch block and the resulting delay in onset of the right ventricular pressure pulse. Reversed splitting of the S_1 with the mitral component following the tricuspid component has occasionally been noted in complete left bundle branch block and is frequently present in patients with severe mitral stenosis or a left atrial myxoma.

Splitting of S_2 into audibly distinct aortic (A_2) and pulmonic (P_2) components occurs normally during inspiration when augmented inflow into the right ventricle increases its stroke volume and ejection period and delays closure of the pulmonary valve. Audible expiratory splitting, heard best at the pulmonic area or left sternal border, is usually abnormal when the patient is in the upright position. Such splitting may be due to delayed activation of the right ventricle (right bundle branch block), to prolongation of right ventricular contraction with an increased right ventricular pressure load (pulmonary embolism or pulmonic stenosis), or to delayed pulmonic valve closure because of an increased right ventricular flow load (atrial septal defect). In pulmonary hypertension, P_2 is increased in intensity and splitting of the second heart sound may be diminished, normal, or accentuated, depending on the cause of the pulmonary hypertension and the presence or absence of right ventricular decompensation. Early aortic valve closure, occurring with mitral regurgitation or a ventricular septal defect, may also produce audible expiratory splitting. In patients with large atrial septal defects the proportion of right atrial filling contributed by the left atrium and the venae cavae varies reciprocally during the respiratory cycle so that right atrial inflow remains relatively constant. Therefore, the volume and duration of the right ventricular ejection are not significantly increased by inspiration, and there is little inspiratory exaggeration of the splitting of S_2. This phenomenon, termed "fixed splitting" of the second heart sound, is of considerable diagnostic value. Fixed splitting of the second heart sound may also occur with impaired right ventricular function, when right ventricular stroke volume cannot rise even with augmented inspiratory inflow.

A delay in aortic valve closure causing P_2 to precede A_2 results in so-called reversed (paradoxic) splitting of S_2. Splitting is then maximal in expiration, and decreases during inspiration with the normal delay of pulmonic valve closure. The commonest causes of reversed (paradoxic) splitting of S_2 are left bundle branch block and delayed excitation of the left ventricle from a right ventricular ectopic beat. Mechanical prolongation of left ventricular systole, resulting in reversed splitting of S_2, may be caused by severe aortic outflow obstruction, a large aorta-to-pulmonary artery shunt, systolic hypertension and ischemic heart disease, or cardiomyopathy with left ventricular failure. P_2 is normally softer than A_2 in the second left intercostal space; when P_2 is greater than A_2 in this area, it suggests pulmonary hypertension, except in patients with atrial septal defect.

The *third heart sound* (ventricular protodiastolic gallop) is a low-pitched sound produced in the ventricle 0.14 to 0.15 s after A_2, at the termination of rapid filling. This protodiastolic sound is frequent in normal children and in patients with high cardiac output. However, in patients over forty, an S_3 usually indicates ventricular decompensation, AV valve regurgitation, or other conditions which increase the rate or volume of ventricular filling. The left-sided S_3 is best heard with the bell piece of the stethoscope at the left ventricular apex during expiration and with the patient in the left lateral position. The right-sided S_3 is best heard at the left sternal border or just beneath the xiphoid and is increased with inspiration. Often there are physical findings of functional tricuspid regurgitation. Ventricular protodiastolic gallops often disappear with treatment of heart failure.

An earlier (0.10 to 0.12 s after A_2), higher-pitched third heart sound (pericardial knock) often occurs in patients with constrictive pericarditis; its presence is dependent upon the restrictive effect of the adherent pericardium, which halts diastolic filling abruptly.

The opening snap (OS) is a brief, high-pitched, early diastolic sound which is usually due to stenosis of an AV valve, more commonly the mitral valve. It is usually heard best at the lower left sternal border and radiates well to the base of the heart. The A_2-OS interval during exercise is inversely related to the height of the mean left atrial pressure, and ranges from 0.04 to 0.12 s. At the base an OS is often confused with P_2. However, careful auscultation at the upper left sternal border will reveal both components of the second heart sound, followed by the opening snap. The OS of tricuspid stenosis occurs later in diastole than the mitral OS. Since most patients with tricuspid stenosis also have severe mitral valve disease, the tricuspid OS is often overshadowed by the diastolic rumble and OS originating in the stenotic mitral valve. An OS also may occur when there is increased flow across an AV valve, such as exists with left-to-right intracardiac shunts and mitral or tricuspid regurgitation.

The *fourth heart sound* (atrial or presystolic gallop) is a low-pitched, presystolic sound produced in the ventricle during ventricular filling, associated with an effective atrial contraction, and is heard best with the bell piece of the stethoscope. The sound is absent in patients with atrial fibrillation. The atrial sound occurs when there is diminished ventricular compliance, which increases the resistance to ventricular filling, and it is frequently present in patients with systemic or pulmonary hypertension, aortic stenosis, hypertrophic cardiomyopathies, coronary artery disease, and acute mitral regurgitation. Most patients with an acute myocardial infarction and sinus rhythm have an audible S_4. The atrial sound is frequently accompanied by visible and palpable presystolic distention of the left ventricle. It is maximal in intensity at the left ventricular apex with the patient in the left lateral position, and is accentuated by mild supine exercise. The right-sided S_4 is present in patients with right ventricular hypertrophy, secondary to either pulmonary stenosis or pulmonary hypertension, and frequently accompanies a prominent presystolic A wave in the JVP.

Audible atrial sounds may be present during increased ventricular filling and normal ventricular compliance such as occurs in patients with severe anemia, thyrotoxicosis, or a peripheral arteriovenous fistula. An S_4 frequently accompanies delayed AV conduction even in the absence of clinically detectable heart disease. The incidence of an audible atrial sound increases with increasing age. Whether an audible S_4 in adults without other evidence of cardiac disease is abnormal remains controversial.

The *systolic ejection sound* is a sharp, high-pitched event occurring in early systole closely following the first heart sound. Ejection sounds occur in the presence of semilunar valve stenosis, i.e., opening snaps of the aortic or pulmonic valves, and in conditions associated with dilatation of the aorta or pulmonary artery. The aortic ejection sound is usually heard best at the left ventricular apex and the second right interspace; the pulmonary ejection sound is of maximal intensity at the upper left sternal border. The latter, unlike most other right-sided acoustical events, is heard better during expiration.

Nonejection systolic clicks, occurring with or without a late systolic murmur, often denote mitral valve regurgitation due to prolapse of the posterior leaflet (Chap. 243). They probably result from functional unequal length of the chordae tendineae of the mitral valve and are heard best along the lower left sternal border and at the left ventricular apex. Systolic clicks may be single or multiple, and they may occur at any time in systole but usually later than the systolic ejection sound. Frequently the midsystolic click is misinterpreted as S_2, and the actual second heart sound is called an OS or S_3.

Heart murmurs Cardiac murmurs result from vibrations set up in the bloodstream and the surrounding heart and great vessels as a result of turbulent blood flow, the formation of eddies, and cavitation (bubble formation as a result of sudden decrease in pressure).

The intensity or loudness of murmurs may be graded from I to VI. A grade I murmur is so faint that it can be heard only with special effort, and a grade VI murmur is audible with the stethoscope removed from contact with the chest. The configuration of a murmur may be crescendo, decrescendo, crescendo-decrescendo (diamond-shaped), or plateau. The precise time of onset and time of cessation of a murmur depend on the instant in the cardiac cycle at which an adequate pressure difference between two chambers appears and disappears (Fig. 232-2).

Accentuation of a murmur during inspiration with the augmentation of systemic venous return implies that it originates on the right side of the circulation; expiratory exaggeration has less significance. Prolonged expiratory pressure against a closed glottis, the Valsalva maneuver, reduces intensity of most murmurs by diminishing both right and left ventricular filling. The systolic murmur associated with *idiopathic hypertrophic subaortic stenosis* and the late systolic murmur due to a *prolapse of the mitral valve* are exceptions and may be accentuated during the Valsalva maneuver. Murmurs due to flow across a normal or obstructed semilunar valve increase in intensity in the beat following a premature ventricular contraction or a long R-R interval in atrial fibrillation. In contrast, murmurs due to AV valve regurgitation or a ventricular septal defect do not change appreciably during the beat following a prolonged diastole. Standing, which decreases heart size, accentuates the murmur of hypertrophic subaortic stenosis and occasionally the murmur due to a prolapse of the mitral valve. Squatting, which increases both venous return and systemic arterial resistance, increases most murmurs, except those due to idiopathic subaortic stenosis and mitral regurgitation due to a prolapsed mitral valve, which often decrease. Sustained handgrip exercise, which increases the systemic arterial pressure and heart rate, often accentuates the murmurs of mitral regurgitation, aortic regurgitation, and mitral stenosis but usually diminishes those due to aortic or subaortic stenosis.

Pansystolic (holosystolic) murmurs are generated when there is a flow between two chambers which have widely different pressures throughout systole, such as the left ventricle and either the left atrium or the right ventricle. The pressure gradient is established early in contraction and lasts until relaxation is almost complete. Therefore, holosystolic murmurs begin before aortic ejection, and at the area of maximal intensity they begin with S_1 and end after S_2. Pansystolic murmurs accompany mitral or tricuspid regurgitation, ventricular septal defect, and, under certain circumstances, aorta-pulmonary shunts. Although the typical high pitch of murmur or mitral regurgitation usually continues throughout systole, the shape of the murmur may vary considerably. The pansystolic murmurs of mitral regurgitation and ventricular septal defect are augmented by raising the arterial pressure with intravenous phenylephrine and are diminished by lowering the left ventricular systolic pressure by inhalation of amyl nitrite. The murmur of tricuspid regurgitation associated with pulmonary hypertension is holosystolic and frequently increases during inspiration, a feature of diagnostic importance. Not all patients with mitral or tricuspid regurgitation or ventricular septal defect have pansystolic murmurs (Chap. 243).

Midsystolic murmurs occur when blood is ejected across the aortic or pulmonic outflow tracts. The murmur starts shortly after S_1 when the ventricular pressure rises sufficiently to open the semilunar valve. Ejection then begins and with it the onset of the murmur; as ejection increases, the murmur is augmented, and as ejection declines, it diminishes. The murmur ends before the ventricular pressure falls enough to permit closure of the aortic or pulmonic leaflets. In the presence of normal semilunar valves and increased flow rate, as may occur in states of elevated cardiac output, ejection into a dilated vessel beyond the valve, or increased transmission of sound through a thin chest wall, may be responsible for the production of this murmur. Most benign, functional murmurs are midsystolic and originate from the pulmonary outflow tract. Valvular or subvalvular obstruction to either ventricle may also cause such a midsystolic murmur, the intensity being related to the flow. Thus, the murmur of aortic stenosis may become faint or disappear during heart failure and return when compensation has been restored.

The murmur of aortic stenosis is the prototype of the left-sided midsystolic murmur. The location and radiation of this murmur appear to be influenced by the direction of the high-velocity jet within the aortic root. In *valvular aortic stenosis* the murmur is usually maximal in the second right intercostal space, with radiation into the neck. In *supravalvular aortic stenosis* the murmur is occasionally loudest even higher, with disproportionate radiation into the right carotid artery. In idiopathic hypertrophic subaortic stenosis, the murmur originates within the left ventricular cavity, and is usually maximal at the lower left sternal edge and apex, with relatively little radiation to the carotids. When the aortic valve is immobile (calcified), the aortic closure sound (S_2) may be soft and inaudible so that the length and configuration of the murmur are difficult to determine.

The patient's age and the area of maximal intensity aid in determining the significance of midsystolic murmurs. Thus, in a young adult with a thin chest and high velocity of blood flow, a faint or moderate ejection murmur heard only in the pulmonary area is usually without clinical significance, while a somewhat louder murmur in the aortic area may indicate congenital aortic stenosis. In elderly patients pulmonary flow murmurs are rare, while aortic systolic murmurs are frequent and may be due to aortic dilatation, to a significant degree of valvular aortic stenosis, or to nonstenotic deformity of the aortic valve. Systolic ejection murmurs are intensified by amyl nitrite inhalation and during the cardiac cycle following a premature ventricular contraction. Aortic systolic murmurs are diminished by interventions which increase systemic arterial resistance such as intravenous phenylephrine. Cardiac catheterization may be necessary to separate a prominent and exaggerated functional murmur from one due to congenital semilunar valve stenosis.

Early systolic murmurs begin with the first heart sound and end in midsystole. They may be due to a very small *ventricular septal defect, a large defect with pulmonary hypertension,* or *severe acute mitral* or *tricuspid regurgitation.* In large ventricular septal defects with pulmonary hypertension the shunting at the end of systole may be small or absent, resulting in an early systolic murmur. A similar murmur may occur with very small muscular ventricular septal defects, the shunt being interrupted in late systole. An early systolic murmur is a feature of tricuspid regurgitation occurring in the absence of pulmonary hypertension. This lesion is common in drug addicts with bacterial endocarditis, in whom a tall regurgitant right atrial V wave reaches the level of the normal right ventricular pressure in late systole, confining the murmur to early systole. In patients with acute mitral regurgitation and a large V wave in a noncompliant left atrium, a loud early systolic murmur is frequently heard which diminishes as the pressure gradient between left ventricle and left atrium decreases in late systole (Chap. 243).

Late systolic murmurs are faint or moderately loud high-pitched apical murmurs, which start well after ejection and do not mask either heart sound. They are probably related to papillary muscle dysfunction caused by infarction or ischemia of these muscles or to their distortion by left ventricular dilatation. They may appear only during angina but are common in patients with myocardial infarction or diffuse myocardial disease. Late systolic murmurs following midsystolic clicks are associated with late systolic mitral regurgitation caused by prolapse of the mitral valve into the left atrium (Chap. 243).

Early diastolic murmurs begin with or shortly after the second heart sound as soon as the corresponding ventricular pressure falls sufficiently below that in the aorta or pulmonary artery. The high-pitched murmurs of aortic regurgitation or pulmonic regurgitation due to pulmonary hypertension are generally decrescendo, since there is a progressive decline in the volume or rate of regurgitation during diastole. They may be musical when the regurgitation is associated with a flail, everted semilunar valve cusp. Faint, high-pitched murmurs of aortic regurgitation are difficult to hear unless they are specifically sought by applying firm pressure with the diaphragm over the mid-left-sternal border while the patient sits, leans forward, and holds his breath in full expiration. The diastolic murmur of aortic regurgitation is enhanced by an acute elevation of the arterial pressure such as occurs with handgrip exercise; it diminishes with a decrease in arterial pressure such as occurs during amyl nitrite inhalation. The diastolic murmur of congenital pulmonic regurgitation in the absence of pulmonary hypertension is low to medium pitched. The onset of this murmur is delayed because at the time of pulmonic valve closure the regurgitant flow is minimal, since the reverse pressure gradient responsible for the regurgitation is negligible at this time.

Middiastolic murmurs usually arise from the AV valves, occur during early ventricular filling, and, like ejection murmurs, are due to disproportion between valve orifice size and flow rate. Such murmurs may be loud despite only slight AV valve stenosis when there is normal or increased blood flow. Conversely, the murmur may be soft or even absent despite severe obstruction if the cardiac output is significantly reduced. When stenosis is marked, the diastolic murmur is prolonged and the duration of the murmur is more reliable than its intensity as an index of the degree of valve obstruction.

The low-pitched middiastolic murmur of mitral stenosis characteristically follows the opening snap. It should be specifically sought by placing the bell of the stethoscope at the site of the left ventricular impulse, which is best localized with the patient on his left side. Frequently the murmur of mitral stenosis is present only at the left ventricular apex, and it may be increased in intensity by mild supine exercise or by inhalation of amyl nitrite. In tricuspid stenosis the middiastolic murmur is localized to a relatively limited area along the left sternal edge and may increase in loudness during inspiration.

Middiastolic murmurs may be generated across the mitral valve in ventricular septal defect, patent ductus arteriosus, or mitral regurgitation, and across the tricuspid valve in atrial septal defect or tricuspid regurgitation. These murmurs are related to the torrential flow across an AV valve, usually follow a third heart sound, and tend to occur with large left-to-right shunts, or severe AV valve regurgitation. A soft middiastolic murmur may sometimes be heard in patients with acute rheumatic fever (Carey-Coombs murmur). It has been attributed to inflammation of the mitral valve cusps or excessive left atrial blood flow as a consequence of mitral regurgitation.

In acute aortic regurgitation, the left ventricular diastolic pressure may exceed the left atrial pressure, resulting in a middiastolic murmur due to "diastolic mitral regurgitation." In severe chronic aortic regurgitation a murmur is frequently present which may be either middiastolic or presystolic (Austin Flint murmur). This murmur appears to originate at the anterior mitral valve leaflet when blood simultaneously enters the left ventricle from both the aortic root and the left atrium.

Presystolic murmurs begin during the period of ventricular filling that follows atrial contraction and therefore occur in sinus rhythm. They are usually due to AV valve stenosis and have the same quality as the middiastolic filling rumble but are usually crescendo, reaching peak intensity at the time of a loud S_1. The presystolic murmur corresponds to the AV valve gradient, which may be minimal until the moment of right or left atrial contraction. It is the presystolic rather than the middiastolic murmur which is most characteristic of tricuspid stenosis and sinus rhythm. A right or left *atrial myxoma* may occasionally cause either middiastolic or presystolic murmurs that resemble the murmurs of mitral or tricuspid stenosis.

Continuous murmurs begin in systole and persist through S_2 into all or part of diastole. These murmurs signify continuous flow due to communication between high- and low-pressure areas which persists through the end of systole and the beginning of diastole. A *patent ductus arteriosus* causes a continuous murmur as long as the pressure in the pulmonary artery is much below that in the aorta. The murmur is intensified by elevation of the systemic arterial pressure and is reduced by amyl nitrite inhalation. When pulmonary hypertension is present, the diastolic portion may disappear, leaving the murmur confined to systole. A continuous murmur is uncommon in aortopulmonary septal defects, since this malformation is generally associated with severe pulmonary hypertension. Surgically produced aortopulmonary connections, such as subclavian-pulmonary artery anastomosis, result in murmurs similar to that of a patent ductus.

Continuous murmurs may result from congenital or acquired *systemic arteriovenous fistula, coronary arterial fistula,* anomalous origin of the left coronary artery from the pulmonary artery, and communications between the *sinus of Valsalva and the right side of the heart.* Continuous murmurs may also occur when high left atrial pressure results in continuous flow across a small defect in the atrial septum. Murmurs associated with *pulmonary arteriovenous fistulas* may be continuous but are usually only systolic. Continuous murmurs may also be due to disturbances of flow pattern in constricted systemic (e.g., renal) or pulmonary arteries when marked pressure differences between the two sides of the narrow segment persist; a continuous murmur in the back may be present in *coarctation of the aorta; pulmonary embolism* may cause continuous murmurs in partially occluded vessels.

In nonconstricted arteries continuous murmurs may be due to rapid flow through a tortuous bed. Such murmurs typically occur within the bronchial arterial collateral circulation in cyanotic patients with severe pulmonary outflow obstruction. The "mammary souffle," an innocent murmur heard during late pregnancy and early post partum, may be systolic or continuous. The innocent cervical venous hum is a continuous murmur usually heard over the medial aspect of the right supraclavicular fossa with the patient upright. The hum is usually louder during diastole and can be instantaneously abolished by digital compression of the ipsilateral internal jugular vein. Transmission of a loud venous hum to the area below the clavicles may result in a mistaken diagnosis of patent ductus arteriosus.

The *pericardial friction rub,* which may have presystolic, systolic, and early diastolic scratchy components, may be confused with a murmur or extra cardiac sound when heard only in systole, It is best appreciated with the patient upright and leaning forward and may be accentuated during inspiration.

REFERENCES

FOWLER NO (ed): Diagnostic methods in cardiology. Cardiovascular Clinics, Philadelphia: Davis, 1975

—— (ed): Cardiac auscultation, chap 6 in *Cardiac Diagnosis and Treatment,* 2d ed, Hagerstown: Harper & Row, 1976, p 158

HURST JW (ed): *The Heart,* 3d ed., part IV: Methods Used to Obtain a Cardiovascular Data Base, sections A & B (chaps. 11–19), New York: McGraw-Hill, 1974, p. 138

LEATHAM A: *Auscultation of the Heart and Phonocardiography,* 2d ed., New York: Churchill-Livingston, 1976

LEON DF, SHAVER JA: Physiologic principles of heart sounds and murmurs. AHA Monograph 46:220, 1975

REDDY PS et al: Cardiac systolic murmurs: Pathophysiology and differential diagnosis. Prog Cardiovasc Dis 14:1, 1971

233 ELECTROCARDIOGRAPHY

ROBERT J. MYERBURG

CARDIAC ELECTROPHYSIOLOGY The electrocardiogram (ECG) is a graphic recording of the electrical activity of the heart as detected on the body surface by a group of electrodes positioned to reflect activity in various areas of the heart. The source of cardiac electrical activity resides at a cellular level. Most cardiac cells maintain a *resting* membrane *polarization* of 90 mV, the inside of the cell negative with respect to the outside (that is, −90 mV); but the cells are electrically active, and a sufficient stimulus is able to initiate a *depolarization.* Cardiac tissue is unique among other electrically active tissues in its significant time delay between depolarization and the completion of recovery of excitability or *repolarization.* This results in refractory periods—the minimum intervals required for two successive responses to occur—which are relatively long. After repolarization and before the next depolarization, most cells maintain the state of resting polarization; but certain cardiac tissues undergo slow, *spontaneous depolarization.* If this continues to threshold potential, an impulse is initiated. It is this mechanism which permits the sinoatrial (SA) node to function as the pacemaker of the heart and other regions to provide normal backup pacemakers, or to usurp this function abnormally.

Under resting, steady-state conditions, ionic gradients are maintained across cardiac cell membranes. The extracellular concentration of Na^+ is about ten to fifteen times the intracellular concentration, and the intracellular concentration of K^+ is thirty to thirty-five times its extracellular concentration. The K^+ gradient is responsible for the resting transmembrane potential. During depolarization of most normal cardiac tissue, on the other hand, specific

Na^+ channels in cell membranes open, permitting the rapid influx of Na^+ down its electrochemical gradient and very rapid depolarization, which is paralleled by rapid impulse conduction. Stimulation of partially depolarized tissue causes a slower rate of depolarization and a more slowly conducted impulse. The Na^+ channel is inactivated at membrane potentials less negative than −55 mV. Depolarization initiated at resting potentials less than −55 mV appears to result from ionic currents across a different channel—the so-called "slow channel"—carried by Ca^{2+} ions. Such impulses are conducted more slowly. At levels of partial depolarization between −90 and −55 mV, slow depolarizations could probably result from either the partially inactivated fast (Na^+) channel or slow channel impulses.

In addition to the uniquely long delay between depolarization and repolarization in cardiac tissue, there is considerable variability in the electrical properties among the various cardiac tissues, including important variations in refractory periods. The electrically active tissues may be conveniently divided into two general types: (1) the ordinary muscle, and (2) the specialized conducting tissue (SCT). The ordinary muscle of the atria and ventricles accounts for most of the cardiac mass. These tissues conduct impulses at a velocity much lower than the intraventricular SCT (the His-Purkinje system), but considerably faster than the atrioventricular (AV) node. The refractory periods of muscle are shorter in duration than SCT, and the SCT of the heart has a broader range of functional properties than does muscle. The primary function of the SA node is initiation of the cardiac impulse, and the cells are highly specialized for the purpose of impulse formation (automaticity). Spontaneous depolarization is the most prominent feature.

The AV node is a complex structure, in which the electrical activity may be predominantly or entirely dependent upon "slow channel," Ca^{2+}-dependent currents. Impulses propagating from the atria into the AV node undergo abrupt slowing in conduction, a phenomenon termed *decremental conduction;* i.e., the amplitude and velocity of the impulse diminish as it is conducted into an area which is less responsive, causing a still weaker response, which acts as a yet weaker stimulus for continued propagation. Should this sequence continue, the impulse would eventually be extinguished.

However, at some point within the AV node the process reverses, responses to the weakly conducted impulse becoming stronger and propagating into more responsive tissue. After approximately 90 to 100 ms, propagation across the AV node is complete, and the impulse enters the next area of specialized conducting tissue, the bundle of His. Propagation through the bundle of His is very rapid as this structure moves through the lower portion of the interatrial septum, giving off fibers which become the left bundle branch (LBB) as they pierce the membranous ventricular septum below the aortic ring. The rest of the bundle of His continues across the crest of the interventricular septum and courses down the right side of the septum as the right bundle branch (RBB). When the RBB reaches the apex of the right ventricle, it fans out onto the free wall as the Purkinje network.

The main LBB is a relatively short structure on the upper portion of the interventricular septum which bifurcates into two general collections of fibers, forming structures which have been referred to as the anterior (superior) and

posterior (inferior) divisions of the LBB. The two divisions are not isolated end structures, there being numerous interconnections between them on the surface of the left ventricular septum. The cells of the RBB and LBB systems are highly specialized and conduct more rapidly than any other within the heart. Specialization for rapid conduction achieves an orderly and appropriately synchronous sequence of activation of the ventricles.

The magnitude and direction of the electrical activity on the body surface may be viewed conveniently as an average of the numerous cell depolarizations or repolarizations occurring at a given instant. Although much of the electrical activity from individual cells is canceled out at the body surface by opposing forces from other cells, the resultant recording is a reasonably reproducible and accurate approximation of net cardiac electrical activity.

Early in the development of the ECG, Einthoven popularized the concept that the human body represents a large volume conductor having the source of cardiac electrical activity at its center. While this theory is not strictly true, it still provides the clinician with a practical point from which to work. As an extension of this concept, the *net* electrical activity at any instant in the cardiac cycle may be viewed as originating from a polarized point source at a theoretical "electrical center" of the heart. Since this "equivalent dipole" would have direction and magnitude, one might then extend the pattern into a sequence of instantaneous vectors recordable from the body surface. The application of this concept to ECG analysis is discussed below.

LEAD SYSTEMS The ECG lead system is composed of five electrodes, one on each of the four limbs and one placed at various sites on the precordium. Each lead is a continuous recording of the change in electrical potential during the cardiac cycle between two of the electrodes, or between one electrode and a combination of the others. The right-leg electrode is an inactive ground electrode in all leads.

The original lead system developed by Einthoven is based on assumptions of (1) the homogeneity of the body volume conductor, (2) the symmetry of the leads, and (3) a single equivalent dipole at the center of the volume conductor. The *standard limb leads* (I, II, and III) are composed of three permutations of the right arm (RA), left arm (LA), and left leg (LL) electrodes [Fig. 233-1*A* (1)]. Lead I records the potential difference between the LA and the RA, the positive electrode on the LA, and the negative electrode on the RA [Fig. 233-1*A* (2)]. Lead II records the potential difference between the electrodes on the RA and the LL, the positive electrode on the LL. Lead III records the potential difference between the LA and the LL, with the positive electrode placed on the LL. It is likely that Einthoven arbitrarily selected the relationships between positive and negative electrodes in the three leads in order to have the major deflection of the QRS complex (see below) moving in an upward (positive) direction in most individuals.

The central terminal of Wilson (CTW) is constructed by connecting the RA, LA, and LL electrodes through 5,000 Ω

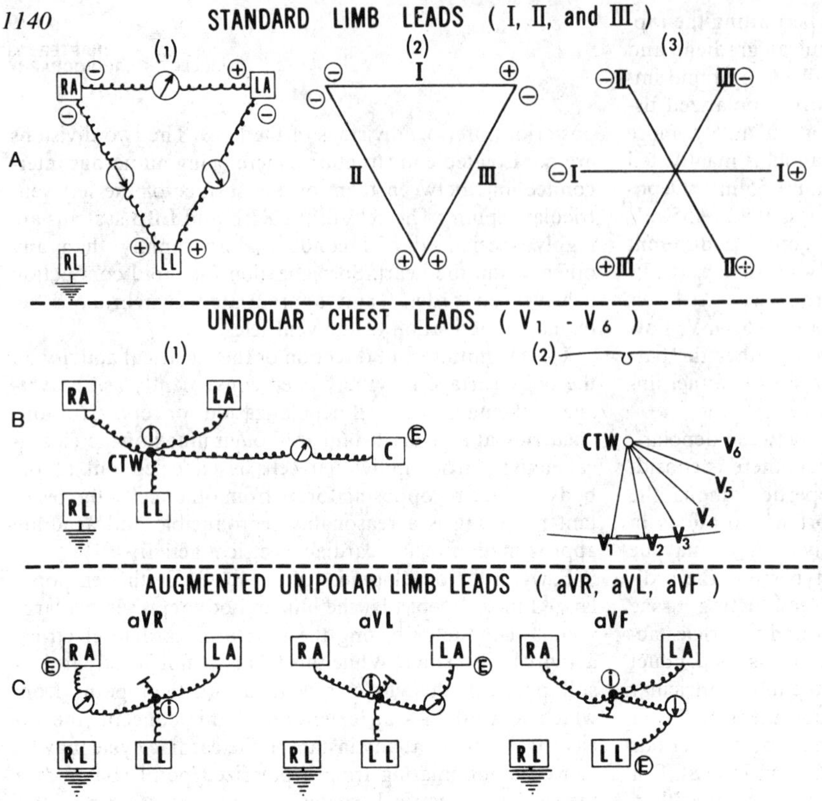

FIGURE 233-1

Lead systems. A *Standard limb leads, showing (1) electrode positions, (2) the equilateral triangle of Einthoven, and (3) the conversion of the triangle to a triaxial reference system with positive (+) and negative (−) polarity.* B *The unipolar chest leads, showing (1) the central terminal of Wilson (CTW) (or the indifferent electrode −i) and the chest electrode (C) (or the exploring electrode −E). The 5,000 Ω between CTW and each limb electrode is not shown. The relationship between CTW and V_1–V_6 in the horizontal plane is shown in* B*(2).* C *The augmented unipolar limb leads, using the modified CTW.*

resistance, in order to cancel out the potentials from these three points. With the forces canceled out, the CTW theoretically remains inactive during the entire cardiac cycle, and an exploring electrode will function as a unipolar lead [Fig. 233-1*B* (1)]. The selection of the positions for the six *unipolar chest leads* [Figs. 233-1*B* (2) and 233-2] was based on the concept that the proximity of the heart to the anterior chest wall resulted in the unipolar chest leads functioning as semidirect leads, being influenced primarily by the tissue immediately beneath the electrode. While this concept does not have the quantitative significance originally assigned to it, and the recordings from such leads do reflect the activity of the total heart, there is considerable weighting of these recordings by the tissue closest to the exploring electrode. The six standard chest leads (V_1 to V_6) are recorded by positioning the exploring chest electrode as follows: V_1 in the fourth intercostal space (4-ICS) at the right sternal border; V_2 in the 4-ICS at the left sternal border; V_4 in the 5-ICS at the midclavicular line; V_3 midway between V_2 and V_4; V_5 at the left anterior axillary line at the level of V_4 horizontally; and V_6 at the left midaxillary line at the level of V_4 horizontally (Fig. 233-2). The CTW is the indifferent electrode, and the exploring chest electrode is the active electrode.

FIGURE 233-2

The unipolar chest leads. A *The position of the chest electrode for V_1–V_6.* B *The relationship between the CTW and the chest electrode (C) in the horizontal plane.*

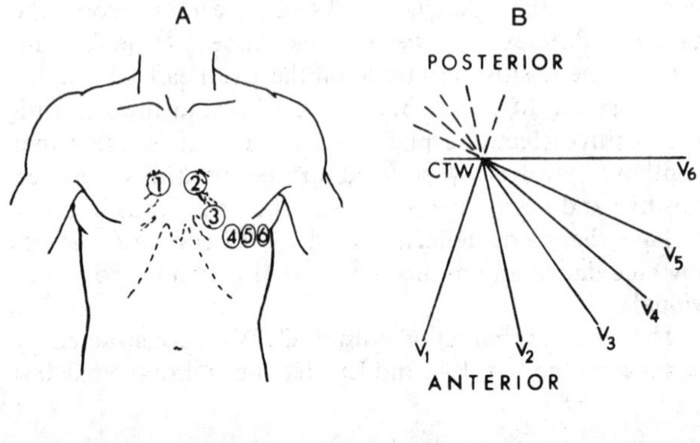

Unipolar limb leads may be recorded by a system in which the CTW constitutes the indifferent electrode and the exploring is one of the three active limb electrodes. These leads are referred to as VR, VL, and VF. By disconnecting the input to the CTW from the extremity being explored, an augmentation of the voltage of the unipolar limb leads by as much as 50 percent occurs. This modification is universally used for clinical ECGs, and the leads are labeled aVR, aVL, and aVF (Fig. 233-1*C*).

ELECTROCARDIOGRAPHIC WAVEFORMS, DURATIONS, AND INTERVALS Clinical ECGs are recorded on paper having a graphic background (Fig. 233-3) to permit rapid measurement of standardized time intervals and voltages. Time lines are 1 mm apart, with every fifth line emphasized. Standard paper speed is 25 mm per s. Thus, 1 mm = 0.04 s (lighter lines), and 5 mm = 0.20 s (darker lines). The horizontal lines, 1 mm apart, permit calibration of the voltage deflections of the ECG. Normal standardization is ↑ 10 mm = +1 mV (Fig. 233-3).

The P wave of atrial depolarization is normally the initial wave of activity during the cardiac cycle (Fig. 233-4). Ventricular muscle depolarization is represented by the *QRS complex.* A Q wave is an initial negative wave; an R

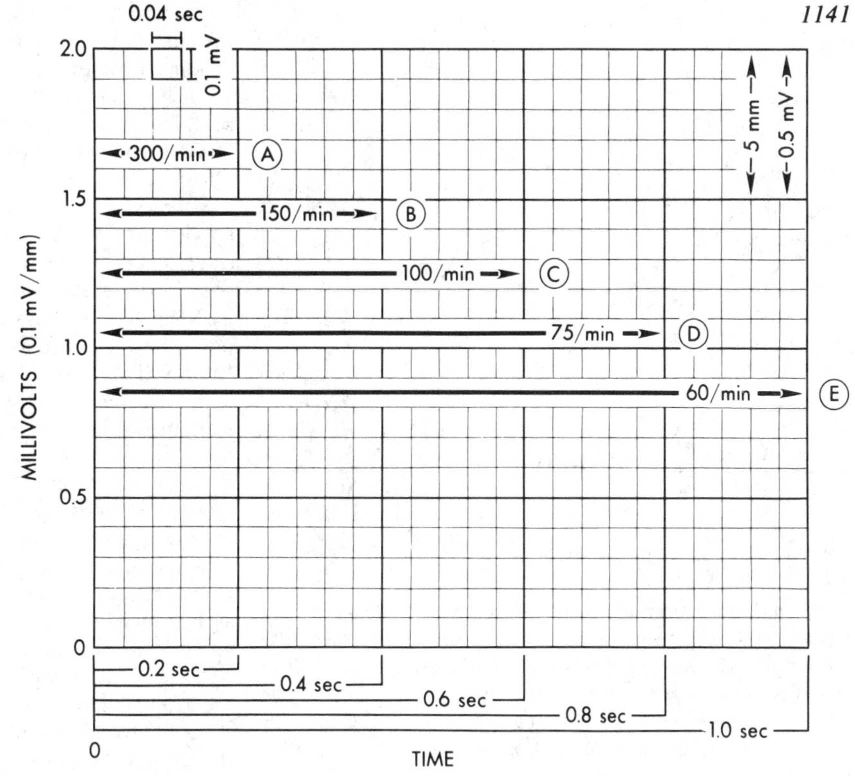

FIGURE 233-3

Standardization of the ECG. Standard time calibration is 1 mm = 0.04 s or 5 mm = 0.20 s. Standard voltage is 0.1 mV per mm. A repetitive event occurring every 5 mm (A) on time axis (0.20 s) is occurring at 300 per min. A repetitive event occurring every 10 mm (B) (0.40 s) is occurring at 150 per min. C, D, and E indicate that repetitive events at 0.60, 0.80, and 1.00 s are occurring at rates of 100, 75, and 60 per min, respectively.

wave is an initial positive wave or a positive wave following a Q wave; and an S wave is a negative deflection following an R wave (Fig. 233-4). A QRS complex having a Q wave which returns to the base line but does not produce a positive wave is labeled a QS complex, and a second R wave in a QRS complex composed of more than one R wave is labeled R′. The T wave represents ventricular muscle repolarization, and is sometimes followed by a small wave, the U wave, the mechanism of which remains uncertain. Repolarization of atrial muscle is represented by the T_a (or T_p) wave, which occurs during the P-R interval and QRS complex, and is often difficult to identify. The interval between the end of the QRS complex and the onset of the T wave is the S-T segment, representing the period of time between depolarization of the ventricles and the period of rapid repolarization.

The interval between the P wave and the QRS complex is the P-R (or P-Q) interval, measured from the *onset* of atrial depolarization (P) to the *onset* of ventricular depolarization (Q) (Fig. 233-4). The duration is 0.12 to 0.20 s in the adult. Since AV nodal activation begins before the end of depolarization of atrial muscle, the P-R interval may be used as a rough approximation of AV conduction time.

The duration of the QRS complex (0.04 to 0.10 s) reflects the time required for depolarization of ventricular muscle. It may be slightly prolonged by regional block in a portion of the intraventricular SCT or by delayed conduction in a region of ventricular muscle. Block in a bundle branch prolongs it to a greater extent. An approximation of the refractory period of the ventricles may be obtained by measuring the Q-T interval (from the onset of the QRS to the end of the T wave) (Fig. 233-4). The Q-T interval is rate dependent, and may be affected by numerous pathophysiologic influences.

THE VECTOR CONCEPT AND ELECTRICAL AXIS The representation of a force by a graphic description of its direction and magnitude is referred to as a *vector*. In specific reference to cardiac electrical activity, a vector may be projected onto a two-dimensional plane as a scalar vector (Fig. 233-5), or considered in three dimensions as a spatial vector (Fig. 233-6). It may be used to represent instantaneous forces in the sequence of the cardiac electrical cycle (Figs. 233-5*A* and 233-6*A*), or it may represent either the mean or maximum axis during the cardiac cycle (Fig. 233-6*D*).

FIGURE 233-4

The waves of the electrocardiogram—P, QRS, T, and U—are indicated. The measurements of the P-R interval, QRS complex, S-T segment, and QT interval are identified on the right.

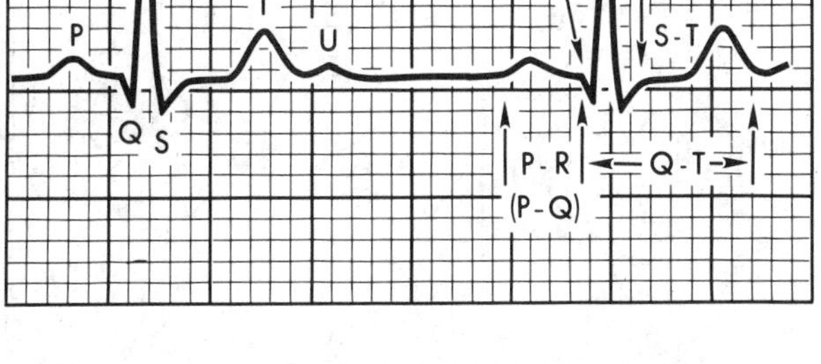

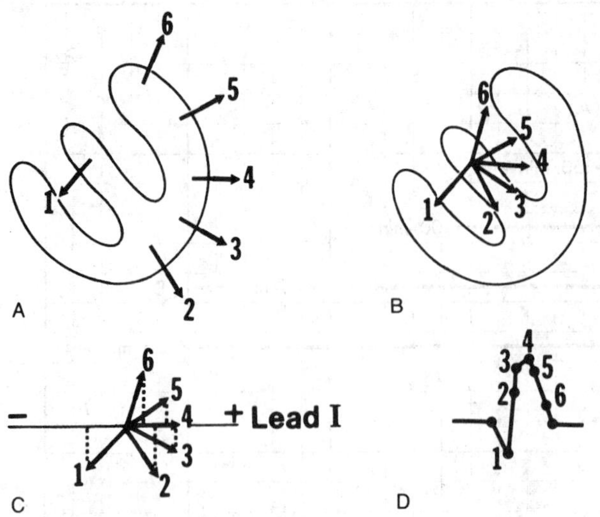

FIGURE 233-5

A *Frontal plane scaler projection of six instantaneous QRS vectors.* B *Vectors originating from a point source at the electrical center of the heart.* C *Projection of the vectors on the lead I axis.* D *Lead I QRS produced by the instantaneous vectors in panel C (see text). (From JW Hurst, RJ Myerburg, Introduction to Electrocardiography, 2d ed., New York: McGraw-Hill, 1973; reproduced with permission of the publisher)*

Mean, maximum, and instantaneous vectors are most commonly applied to the analysis of the QRS complex, but the same principles may be applied to the P wave, S-T segment, or T wave.

When an instantaneous electrical force recorded from the body surface is oriented in a direction perpendicular (or nearly so) to one of the leads (Fig. 233-5*C*, vector 6), the potential recorded by that lead at that instant will be minimum or isoelectric (Fig. 233-5*D*, point 6). Conversely, if the lead system is oriented parallel to the direction of an instantaneous electrical force (Fig. 233-5*C*, vector 4), the potential recorded by that lead will be maximum (Fig. 233-5*D*, point 4). An intermediate direction will record an intermediate voltage (for example, Fig. 233-5*C* and *D*, vector 2). If the instantaneous electrical force is oriented to the positive side of the lead, the deflection will be positive (4 in Fig. 233-5*C* and *D*); if the direction is oriented to the negative side, the deflection will be negative (1 in Fig. 233-5*C* and *D*). These general considerations may be applied to either instantaneous vectors occurring at any point during the inscription of the QRS complex, or the mean vector produced by total depolarization (see below).

In Fig. 233-6, seven instantaneous vectors are represented in three dimensions, indicating the spatial sequence of ventricular depolarization. In panel D, the mean spatial QRS vector, representing the net vector of all instantaneous forces, is shown. If the principles described above were applied, the QRS voltage would be large in lead I and small in aVF in the frontal plane (limb leads), and oriented posteriorly in the horizontal plane (chest leads).

When a triaxial system representing the augmented unipolar limb leads is superimposed on the triaxial system of Einthoven, a hexaxial system is obtained which is convenient for estimating the mean QRS axis, or any of the instantaneous vectors, in the frontal plane (Fig. 233-7). When the appropriate positive and negative voltage orientations are assigned to each of the leads, the hexaxial reference system becomes a simple means of scalar vector analysis, requiring a minimum of two leads for estimation of the mean axis. An ECG which reveals a maximum positive QRS deflection in lead I and an isoelectric deflection in aVF would be oriented at 0°. Conversely, if the QRS voltage is positive and maximum in lead II and isoelectric in aVL, it would be oriented at +60°. The mean QRS axis in the frontal plane in normal adults ranges from −30 to +110°. Overlap between normal and abnormal occurs in the range of +90 to +110°. Generally, an axis > +90° is referred to as *right axis deviation,* and more negative than −30° as *abnormal left axis deviation.* The determination of the mean QRS axis in the horizontal plane (Fig. 233-2*B*) is similarly derived, normal orientation being to the left and posteriorly.

Three normal ECGs are shown in Fig. 233-8. Analysis of the mean QRS axis in the *frontal plane* (I, II, III, aVR, aVL, aVF) reveals the axis of *A* to be oriented horizontally, of *C* to be oriented vertically, and of *B* to be oriented in an intermediate range. In *A* the net voltage of the QRS complex is largest in lead I, almost isoelectric in lead III, and low in aVF, placing the mean axis in a direction almost perpendicular to lead III. In *B,* the voltages in lead I and aVF are almost identical, and maximum in lead II and aVR. The mean QRS axis is between lead II (+) and aVR (−). In *C,* net voltage is largest in leads II and aVF and almost isoelectric in lead I, placing the mean QRS axis almost perpendicular to lead I. A similar approach is ap-

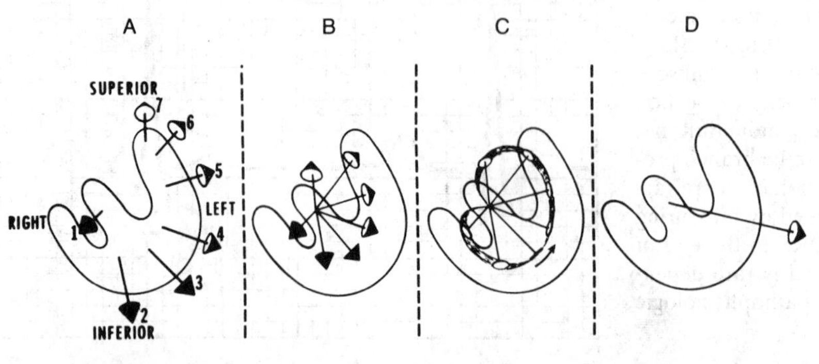

FIGURE 233-6

Spatial representation of ventricular depolarization. A *Seven instantaneous vectors in the sequence of depolarization indicated in spatial orientations.* B *Vectors originating from the electrical center of the heart.* C *A line drawn through the terminations of the spatial vectors produces a spatial QRS loop (vector loop).* D *The mean spatial QRS vector, average of all the instantaneous vectors—to the left, slightly inferiorly, and posteriorly. (See text.) (From JW Hurst, RJ Myerburg, Introduction to Electrocardiography, 2d ed., New York: McGraw-Hill, 1973; modified and reproduced by permission of the publisher)*

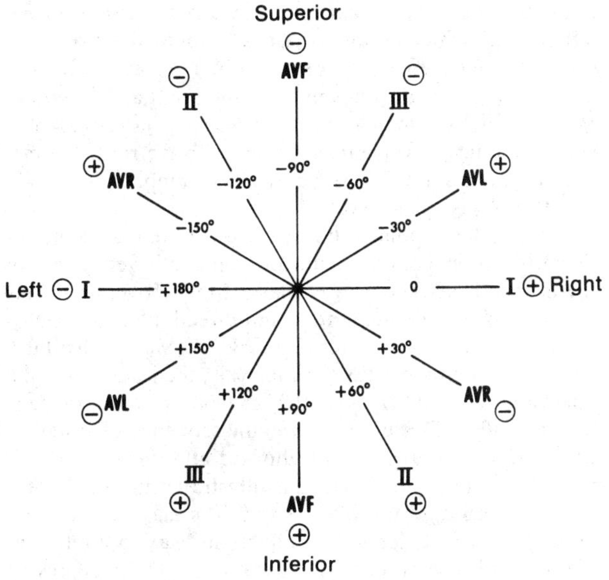

FIGURE 233-7

The hexaxial frontal plane reference system. Normal ranges are described in the text, and applications are derived in Figs. 233-5, 233-6, and 233-8.

plied to QRS-axis determination in the *horizontal plane.* In *C,* the lead in which the net forces are isoelectric is V_3. Therefore, as shown in the axial representation of the horizontal plane of tracing *C,* the QRS is oriented to the left and posteriorly. If this information is added to that obtained from the frontal plane axis, it is apparent that the mean QRS vector of electrocardiogram *C* is oriented inferiorly, to the left, and posteriorly. Similar principles may be applied to the analysis of the mean T-wave axis, which is normally oriented in the same general direction as the QRS axis. An angle between the QRS and T axis of $>45°$ in the frontal plane, or $>60°$ in the horizontal plane, is abnormal.

ELECTRICAL ACTIVITY OF THE ATRIA The mean P-wave vector is normally directed to the left, inferiorly, and slight-

FIGURE 233-8

Three normal ECGs demonstrating: (A) *horizontal,* (B) *intermediate, and* (C) *vertical mean QRS axes constructed on the frontal plane hexaxial system. The horizontal plane vector in* C *is constructed on an axial system and is posteriorly oriented. T-wave vectors are similarly constructed.*

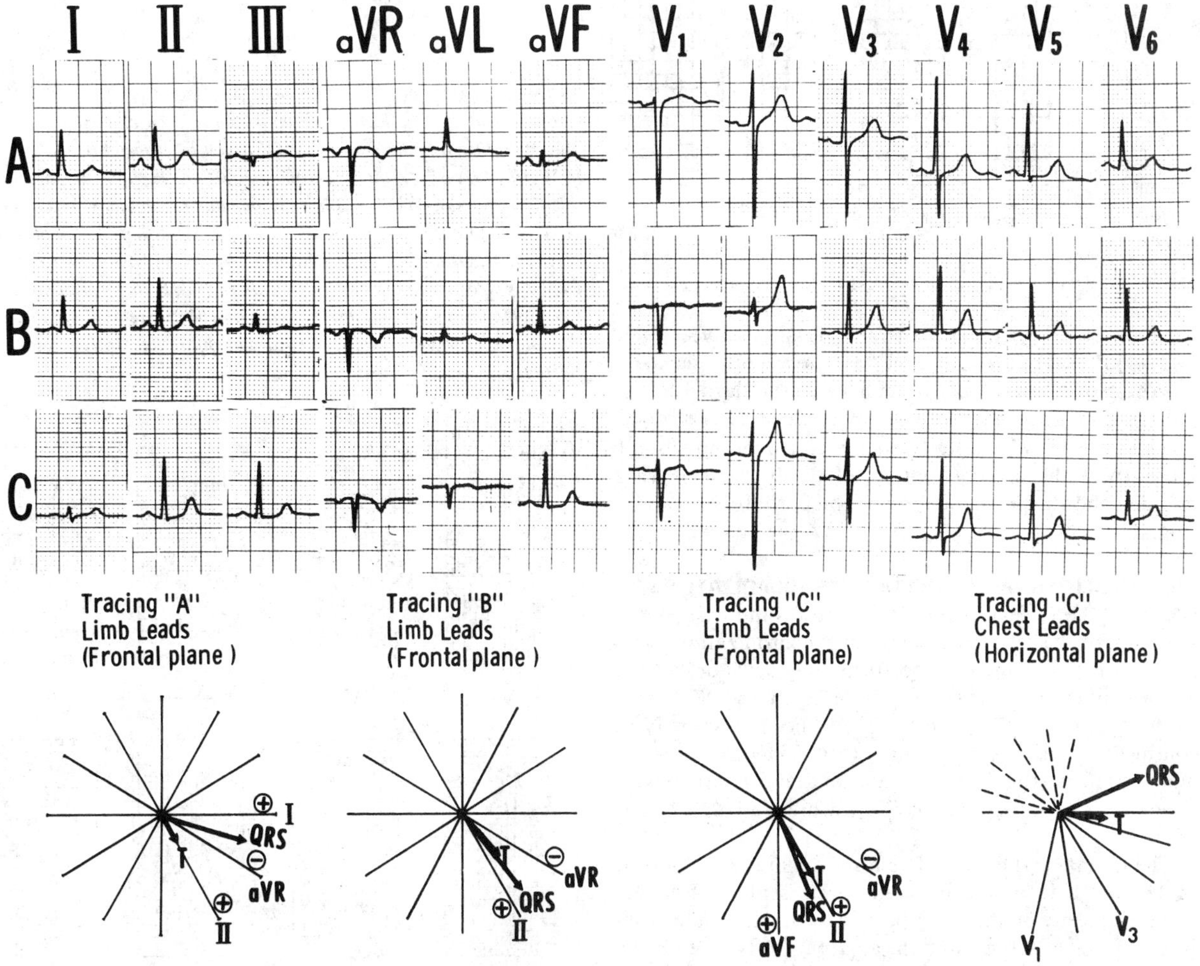

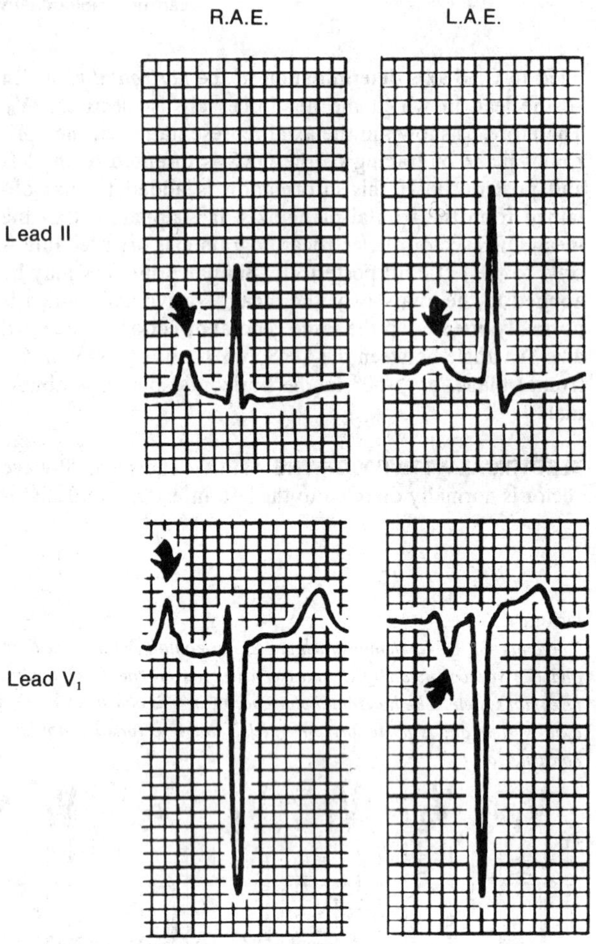

FIGURE 233-9
P waves of right atrial enlargement (RAE) and left atrial enlargement (LAE).

ly anteriorly, the frontal plane axis usually between +30 and +60°. Right atrial enlargement causes tall, peaked P waves (≥0.25 mV), most prominent in standard leads II and V_1 (Fig. 233-9). Left atrial enlargement causes broad, notched P waves in lead II, and inverted or biphasic P waves (with the inverted portion of the biphasic P wave broader and deeper than the upright portion) in lead V_1 (Fig. 233-9).

ABNORMALITIES OF VENTRICULAR DEPOLARIZATION: QRS COMPLEX Since the QRS complex is the ECG representation of the sequence, time, and synchronization of total ventricular muscle depolarization, focal or diffuse abnormalities in ventricular muscle or in the SCT may cause changes in QRS morphology. Abnormalities may be confined to initial depolarization (Fig. 233-10*B*), terminal depolarization (Fig. 233-10*C*), and mid and late depolarization (Fig. 233-10*D*), or may be diffuse (Fig. 233-10*E* to *G*).

The normal earliest site of activation is in the midportion of the left side of the interventricular septum, followed closely by a site on the lower portion of the right side of the interventricular septum and the adjacent free wall endocardium. The dominant wavefront is that one arising on the left septum, which results in a small initial R wave in V_1 (anterior movement), and a small initial Q wave in I, aVL, and/or V_6 (rightward movement). Small initial Q waves in II, III, and aVF may be observed as an indication of a small superior movement of the initial wavefront. Normal septal Q waves are ≤0.02 s and of low amplitude. A normal R in V_1 is ≤0.4 mV.

After septal depolarization has been initiated, rapid endocardial propagation occurs through both ventricles. In the normal heart, the greater mass of the left ventricle predominates, and the magnitude and direction of the electrical vectors reflect this fact (Fig. 233-8). Most individuals will have maximum QRS duration (i.e., the lead having the longest measurable QRS) of 0.05 to 0.08 s (normal range is 0.04 to 0.10 s). During this time, the sequence of instantaneous vectors rotates from rightward and anterior to leftward, posterior, and superior, as illustrated in Fig. 233-6*A* to *C*. A QRS duration of 0.09 or 0.10 s may be a normal variant or may represent a conduction delay to limited regions of either ventricle. QRS durations ≥0.12 s represent left or right bundle branch block or severe degrees of diffuse intraventricular conduction delay (see below).

Abnormal initial Q waves or an abnormal initial R in V_1 usually represents either: (1) a loss of muscle mass; (2) abnormal sequence of depolarization; or (3) a change in the relative muscle mass in the two ventricles.

The *intrinsicoid deflection* of the QRS complex is the major deflection *returning* to the base line in a left (for exam-

FIGURE 233-10
QRS complexes. The lead is indicated above each example. A *Normal.* B *Prolongation due to* initial *QRS delay between arrows (1→2) in Wolff-Parkinson-White syndrome (see Chap. 238).* C *Prolongation due to* terminal *delay (1→2) in right bundle branch block.* D *Prolongation due to mid (1→2) and late (2→3) delay in left bundle branch block.* E *Minor uniform prolongation (1→2) in left ventricular hypertrophy.* F *Distortion of total QRS pattern (1→2) in a cardiomyopathy.* G *Uniform prolongation (1→2) in an electrolyte abnormality.* H *Pathologic Q wave (1→2) in myocardial infarction. Intrinsicoid deflection = 2→3 in* D *and S→2 in* E.

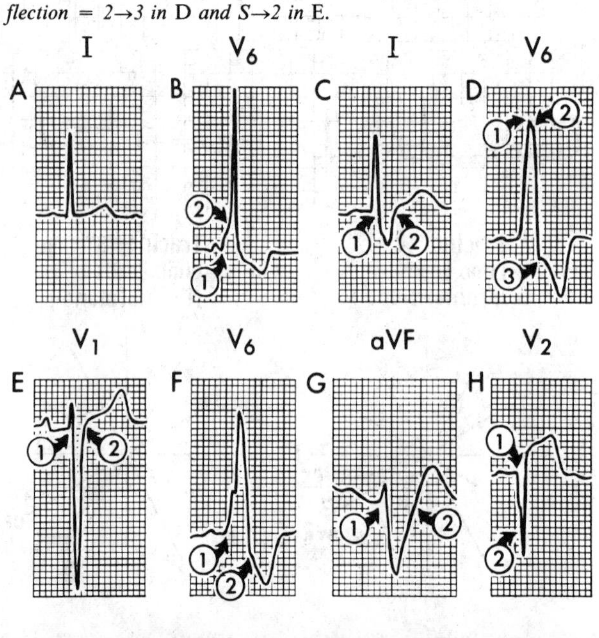

ple, 2→3 in Fig. 233-10*D*) or a right (S-wave→2, Fig. 233-10*E*) precordial lead. Its *onset* does not exceed 0.035 s from the *onset* of the QRS complex in V_1, or 0.055 s from the *onset* of the QRS in V_5 or V_6. Delayed onset of the intrinsicoid deflection may indicate hypertrophy or conduction abnormalities (see below and Fig. 233-10).

ABNORMALITIES OF VENTRICULAR REPOLARIZATION: S-T SEGMENT, T WAVE, AND U WAVE In the normal ECG, the S-T segment is "isoelectric," resting at the same potential as the interval between the T wave and the next P wave. Deviations of the S-T segment from the base line may occur as a result of injury to cardiac muscle, changes in the synchronization of ventricular muscle depolarization, or drug or electrolyte influences. Elevations of the S-T segment, in association with an elevation of the takeoff point of the S-T segment from the QRS complex (the J point), may occur as a normal variant, especially in young individuals (Fig. 233-11*A*). The most common pathologic causes for S-T segment elevation are acute myocardial infarction and pericarditis (Fig. 233-11*B* to *F*), and the normal variant must be differentiated from these. Horizontal depression or downsloping of the S-T segment with merger into the T wave occurs as a result of ischemia, ventricular strain, changes in the pattern of ventricular depolarization, or drug effects (Fig. 233-11*H, I, M, N, Q,* and *R*).

Since the sequence of ventricular muscle *de*polarization is from endocardium to epicardium, and *re*polarization represents an electrical current opposite in direction to depolarization, the T wave would be in the opposite direction to the QRS complex if the sequence of repolarization were in the same direction as depolarization. However, T waves generally assume the same direction as the major deflection of the QRS complex (see Fig. 233-8). It is assumed, therefore, that the direction of repolarization is opposite to the wave of depolarization—from epicardium to endocardium. T waves are generally considered abnormal when they are of low voltage, flat, or inverted in leads in which they are normally upright, or when they are abnormally tall and peaked. T-wave inversions are reflected vectorially by a widening of the angle between the QRS vector and the T vector (Fig. 233-8). Common causes for abnormalities of the T waves include ischemic heart disease, ventricular hypertrophy and strain, abnormal sequences of depolarization, electrolyte abnormalities, and drug influences (see Fig. 233-11*C, D, F, I, K, L, N, O, P, Q,* and *R*). However, T-wave changes are often not specific.

The U wave is usually positive in leads in which the QRS complex is positive. The abnormal U wave is manifested as either an exaggeration of the U-wave voltage, the appear-

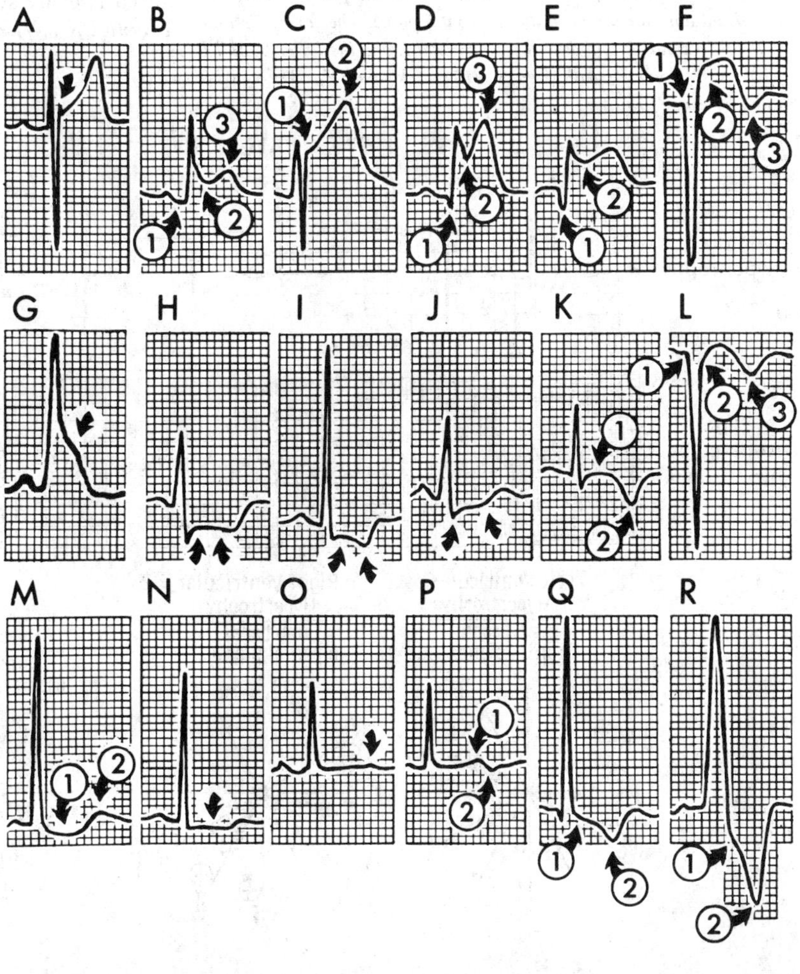

FIGURE 233-11
ST-T wave changes. Arrows in each panel indicate the major features of each complex. A *Early repolarization (J-point elevation), normal variant.* B *Acute pericarditis: (1) depressed* T_a*; (2) elevated ST; (3) normal T.* C *Early acute myocardial infarction (A.M.I.): (1) elevated ST; (2) tall, peaked T wave; steep angle between 1 and 2.* D *A.M.I.: (1) small Q wave; (2) elevated S-T segment; (3) tall, peaked T wave with steep 2→3 angle.* E *A.M.I.: (1) pathologic Q wave; (2) elevated S-T segment.* F *A.M.I.: (1) Q wave; (2) elevated S-T segment; (3) terminal T-wave inversion.* G *Angina pectoris (Prinzmetal variant) with S-T elevation during pain.* H *and* I *Angina pectoris (usual form) with horizontal or downward sloping S-T segment during pain or exercise.* J *J-point depression with upsloping S-T segment during exercise, normal response.* K *Primary T-wave inversion (2) in ischemia or primary muscle disease.* L *Myocardial infarction (healed): (1) pathologic Q; (2) S-T returning to base line; (3) symmetrically inverted T wave.* M. *Digitalis effect: (1) downward coving of S-T segment, merging into (2) an upright T wave.* N *to* P *Nonspecific ST-T-wave changes often seen in chronic ischemic heart disease.* Q *Left ventricular strain pattern with (1) downsloping S-T segment and (2) asymmetrically inverted (secondary) T wave.* R *Downsloping S-T segment merging into a deeply inverted T wave in ventricular conduction abnormality.*

ance of a U wave in leads in which it is not normally seen, or inversion of a U wave. U wave abnormalities occur in ischemic heart disease, left ventricular strain, and electrolyte disturbances.

ECG MANIFESTATIONS OF VENTRICULAR HYPERTROPHY The normal dominance of the left ventricle on the features of the QRS complex is decreased or reversed in right ventricular hypertrophy (RVH) and exaggerated in left ventricular hypertrophy (LVH) (Fig. 233-12). RVH causes a shift of the net forces of depolarization from left and posterior toward the right and anteriorly. On the ECG, this produces tall R waves in V_1 ($\geq$0.5 mV), with an abnormal S wave in V_5 or V_6 ($\geq$0.7 mV). In the frontal plane, the mean QRS axis shifts to the right of vertical (usually >110°). Less extreme degrees of RVH may result in preservation of a moderately deep S wave in V_1, with an R-wave voltage exceeding the S-wave voltage, or a normal R wave with a shallow S wave and prominent terminal S waves in V_5 and V_6. The primary QRS manifestation of LVH is an increase in voltage in those leads which represent the electrical activity of the left ventricle. R waves in the standard limb leads may increase beyond the normal limit of 2.0 mV. Concomitantly, there is a tendency for a shift of the frontal plane QRS axis to the left. It is not likely that LVH alone will cause a shift in the QRS axis beyond −30°, but it commonly causes a shift in the range of 0 to −30° (Fig. 233-12). LVH causes a deep S wave in lead V_1 or V_2 (>2.5 mV), or an abnormal R wave in lead V_5 or V_6 (>2.5 mV). When T waves are normal, the presence of voltage criteria for LVH must be interpreted in terms of body habitus of an individual. Young, healthy, thin-chested individuals will frequently exceed the voltage criteria for LVH in its absence. However, when the ST-T changes associated with "strain" are present (Figs. 233-11*Q* and 233-12), the voltage criteria must be accepted. Similarly, borderline voltage criteria carry more significance when associated with the ST-T wave changes of left ventricular strain.

ACUTE MYOCARDIAL INFARCTION Three pathophysiologic events occur, either in sequence or simultaneously, in an acute myocardial infarction—ischemia, injury, and infarction. The ECG manifestations of these processes involve changes in the T waves (ischemia), S-T segments (injury), and QRS complexes (infarction). The earliest T-wave changes of acute myocardial ischemia are tall, peaked T waves ("hyperacute") (Fig. 233-11*C* and *D*), followed later by symmetrically inverted T waves (Fig. 233-11*F* and *K*). When the electrical integrity of the cell mem-

FIGURE 233-12

Ventricular hypertrophy. Left ventricular hypertrophy and strain with R wave >2.0 mV in limb leads; R >2.5 mV in V_5 and V_6, and S in V_1 >2.5 mV. The sum of S-V_1 or S-V_2 and R-V_5 or R-V_6 exceeds 3.5 mV. Strain is indicated by the downsloping S-T segments and asymmetrically inverted T waves, especially in the lateral chest leads. The QRS-T vector angle is abnormally wide. Right ventricular hypertrophy is indicated by right axis deviation in the frontal plane and abnormal anterior forces in the horizontal plane. The former is indicated by a small R and deep S wave in lead I, and the latter by tall R waves in V_1 and V_2 with deep S waves in V_5 and V_6. The QRS-T angle is wide (strain).

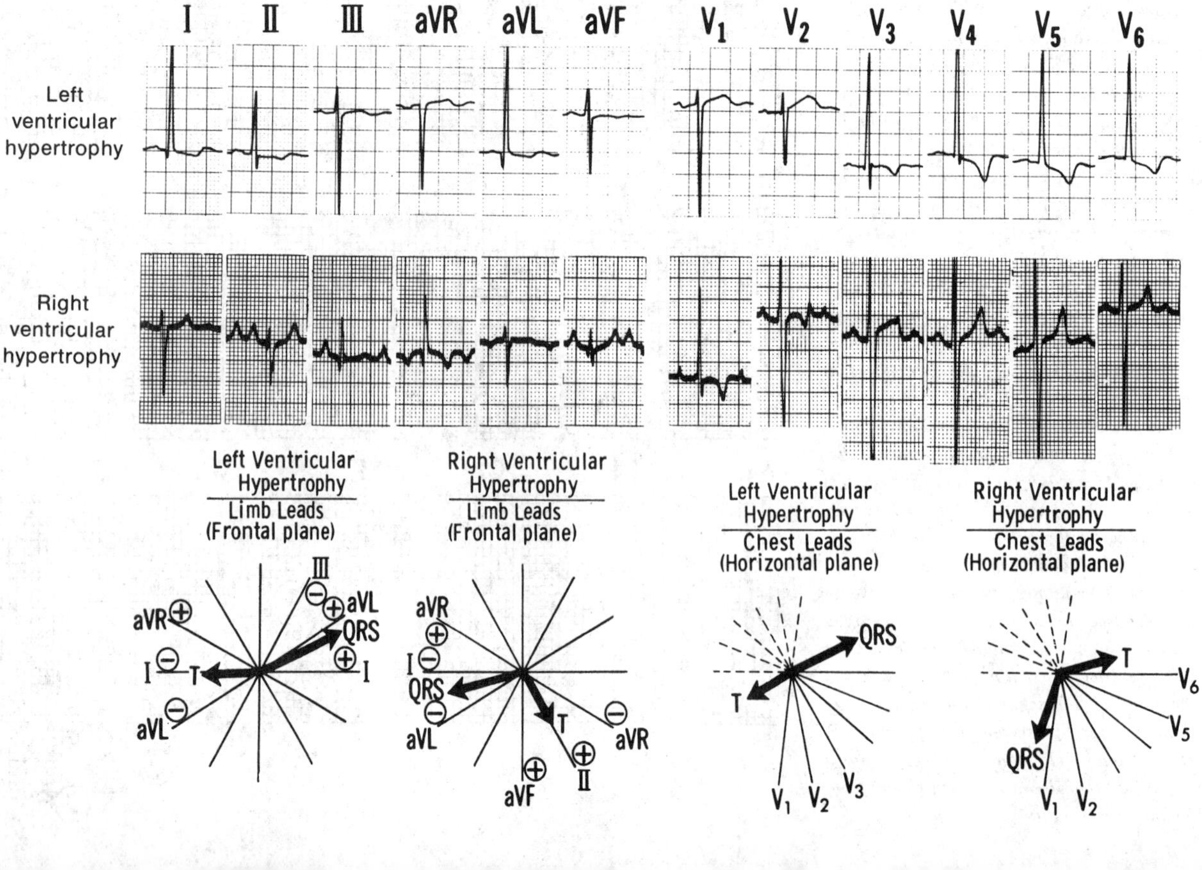

branes is affected, currents of injury develop. The injury pattern during evolution of a transmural infarction is an elevation of the S-T segments in the leads facing the infarcting area (Fig. 233-11*C* and *F*). The combination of ischemia and injury causes elevated S-T segments, followed by either tall, peaked T waves (in the very early stages) or inverted T waves (Fig. 233-13). In leads opposite the region of the acute infarction, reciprocal changes occur: depressed S-T segments and upright T waves (Figs. 233-13 and 233-14). As the period of active injury resolves, the S-T segments return to the base line, but the inverted T waves may persist for months or years (Fig. 233-11*L*). Pathologic Q waves are the QRS manifestation of a transmural myocardial infarction. Q waves are pathologic when they appear in a lead in which Q waves were previously not present, or when the Q waves of normal septal depolarization become exaggerated.

The ECG in an acute inferior wall myocardial infarction is shown in Fig. 233-13. Leads II, III, and aVF, which face the inferior surface (see Fig. 233-7), demonstrate the direct patterns of infarction (pathologic Q waves), injury (elevated S-T segments), and ischemia (inversion of the T waves). Reciprocal changes (depressed S-T, tall T) are demonstrated in aVL. The evolution of an acute anterior myocardial infarction is demonstrated in Fig. 233-14. The most obvious direct changes occur in aVL, V_2, and V_3, and reciprocal changes in II, III, and aVF. In the tracing of 4/11, S-T elevations (most prominent in aVL, V_2, and V_3) are accompanied by "hyperacute" peaked T waves in V_2 and V_3. On 4/12, deeper Q waves are present in aVL and V_{1-3}, and T waves have inverted in aVL and V_{2-5}. S-T elevations persist but less prominently. On 4/25, the pattern of a healing infarction—pathologic Q waves and ischemic T waves—is present. Eventually, the T waves might become partially or completely normal, with persistence of the Q waves. A nontransmural (subendocardial or subepicardial) myocardial infarction may cause S-T segment and T-wave evolutionary changes similar to those seen in transmural infarctions. However, pathologic Q waves do not appear on the QRS complex, although R-wave and/or S-wave voltages may change. The S-T and T-wave changes are common in leads I, II, III, aVL, aVF, and/or V_{4-6}. Similar, but transient, changes may occur during the pain of angina pectoris, in shock, after pulmonary embolism, and secondary to acute central nervous system lesions.

CHRONIC MYOCARDIAL ISCHEMIA The ECG in chronic myocardial ischemia is often nonspecific. The patterns of chronic myocardial ischemia are intrinsically variable, and this is compounded by the problem of coexistent ECG changes related to pharmacologic interventions and/or LVH. Chronic myocardial ischemia causes a broad range of ST-T changes (Fig. 233-11*G* to *I, K, L, N* to *P*). There may be moderate degrees of horizontal S-T segment depression or a downward sloping S-T segment, flattening of inversion of T waves, and prominent U waves. It is difficult to define an abnormal S-T segment depression in precise quantitative terms. However, if the J point is more than 0.5 mm below the isoelectric line, the S-T segment is horizontal or downsloping, and there is an associated T-wave abnormality, myocardial ischemia should be considered. The common clinical expression of chronic ischemic heart dis-

FIGURE 233-13
Acute inferior wall myocardial infarction. The tracing of 11/29 shows minor nonspecific ST-T wave changes. On 12/5 an acute myocardial infarction occurred. There are pathologic Q waves (1), S-T segment elevation (2), and terminal T-wave inversion (3) in leads II, III, and aVF indicating the location of the infarct on the inferior wall (see text). Reciprocal changes in aVL (arrow). Increasing R-wave voltage with S-T depression and increased voltage of the T wave in V_2 is characteristic of true posterior wall extension of the inferior infarction.

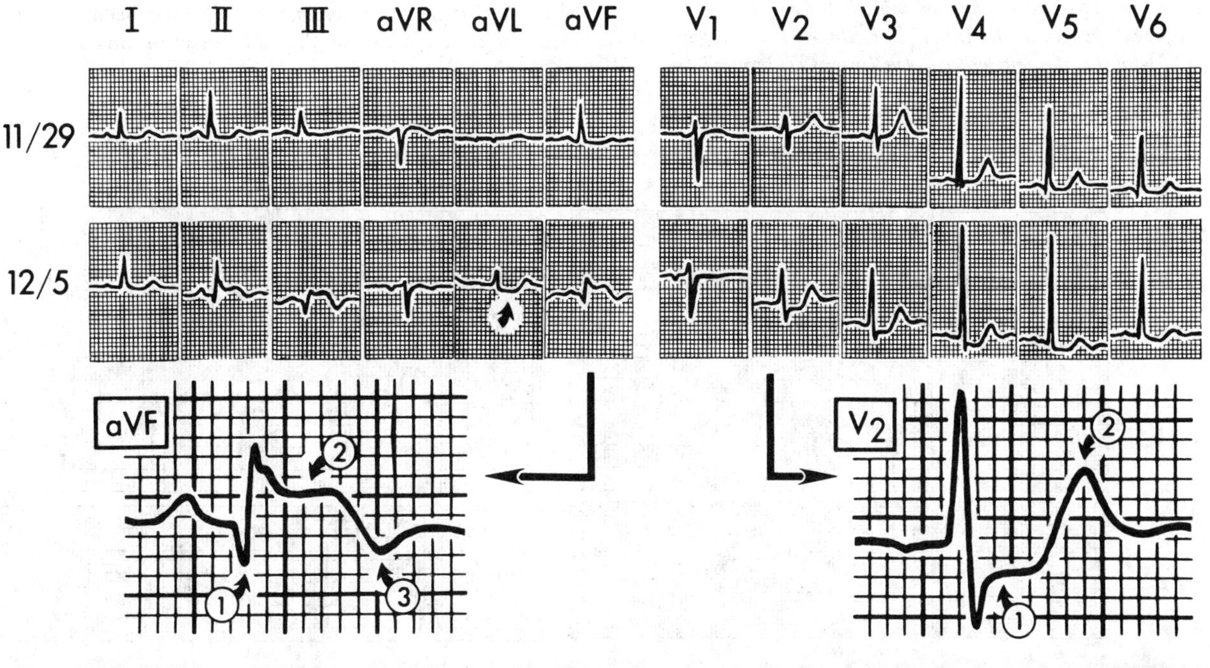

ease, angina pectoris, may be accompanied by a normal resting ECG or nonspecific ST-T-wave changes. However, during spontaneous or exercise-induced pain, the ECG may demonstrate the horizontal or downward sloping S-T depressions shown in Fig. 233-11*H* and *I*, or rarely the variant pattern of spontaneous transient S-T elevations (Prinzmetal variant) (Fig. 233-11*G*).

INTRAVENTRICULAR CONDUCTION DISTURBANCES The complex anatomy of the specialized conducting system of the ventricles, in conjunction with the focal nature of most cardiac diseases, is reflected in the multiplicity of ECG patterns which result from disorders of the sequence of activation of the ventricles. Disease of both the SCT and ventricular myocardium plays a role in the various patterns. The universal feature of ventricular conduction disturbances is a prolongation of the time required for depolarization of a portion of a ventricle, an entire ventricle, or both ventricles. Delayed or slow conduction may be diffuse or may be confined to a portion of the QRS complex (Fig. 233-10). Prolongation of the QRS may be modest as in left ventricular hypertrophy or extremely prolonged as in cardiomyopathies or metabolic abnormalities (Fig. 233-10).

The classic bundle branch block patterns are associated with specific lesions in the left or right bundle branch in the majority of cases. Complete right bundle branch block (RBBB) (Fig. 233-15) is characterized by prolongation of the QRS complex ($\geq$0.12 s) with the delayed activation of the right ventricle accounting for a terminal delay on the ECG. Since septal activation from the left bundle branch normally precedes right ventricular activation, the initial forces of ventricular depolarization are not disturbed in RBBB, and the ability to identify coexistent pathologic Q waves is not hindered. The delayed activation of the right ventricle is reflected by the presence of terminal forces directed anteriorly and to the right.

The rightward direction of the slow terminal forces are indicated by the broad S wave in leads I, aVL, and V_6 (Fig. 233-15). The anterior orientation of these forces is indicated by a large terminal R wave (R′) in V_1. Since initial forces are not disturbed, the normal initial R wave in V_1, followed by an S wave, persists. Incomplete RBBB is present when morphologic criteria for RBBB are present, but the QRS duration is $<$0.12 s.

Left bundle branch block (LBBB) is also characterized by a QRS duration $\geq$0.12 s. However, since normal initial ventricular depolarization is dependent upon the LBB to deliver the impulses of initial depolarization to the left septum, the patterns produced by LBBB are more complex. Normal septal depolarization is disturbed, and delay of the normally dominant left ventricular forces produces a more generalized disturbance of QRS morphology. The septal Q wave in standard leads I, aVL, and V_6 is typically lost. In addition, the initial anterior force reflected by the small R wave in lead V_1 may be lost because of a less anterior orientation of the initial forces. The delay in left ventricular activation produces the greatest degree of slowing in the mid and late portion of the QRS complex. This often results in notching at the peak of the upstroke in leads I and V_6 (see Figs. 233-10*D* and 233-16), with a late intrinsicoid deflection ($>$0.055 s) in V_5 and V_6. Most cases of LBBB produce secondary T-wave abnormalities as demonstrated in Fig. 233-16. Because of the changes in the initial forces, and the secondary ST-T-wave changes, it is difficult to evaluate the QRS, S-T, and T-wave changes of coexistent ischemic heart disease. When the intrinsicoid deflection is delayed in leads V_5 or V_6, but the QRS duration is $<$0.12 s, incomplete LBBB may be present. LBBB may be associated with either a normal QRS axis (Fig. 233-15) or left axis deviation.

In recent years a great deal of attention has been given to the ECG patterns referred to as the *left* hemiblocks. As the name implies, *left anterior hemiblock* (LAH) has been proposed to result from disease in the anterior division of the LBB. *Left posterior hemiblock* (LPH) has been assumed to result from disease in the left posterior division. The

FIGURE 233-14
Acute anterior wall myocardial infarction. On 2/11, changes of a very early acute myocardial infarction in leads I, aVL, V_2, and V_3, with reciprocal changes in II, III, and aVF. On 4/12, S-T segments are still elevated in the anterior leads, but T waves are inverted. On 4/25, a completed large anterior myocardial infarction is recorded—Q in I, aVL, V_{1-4}.

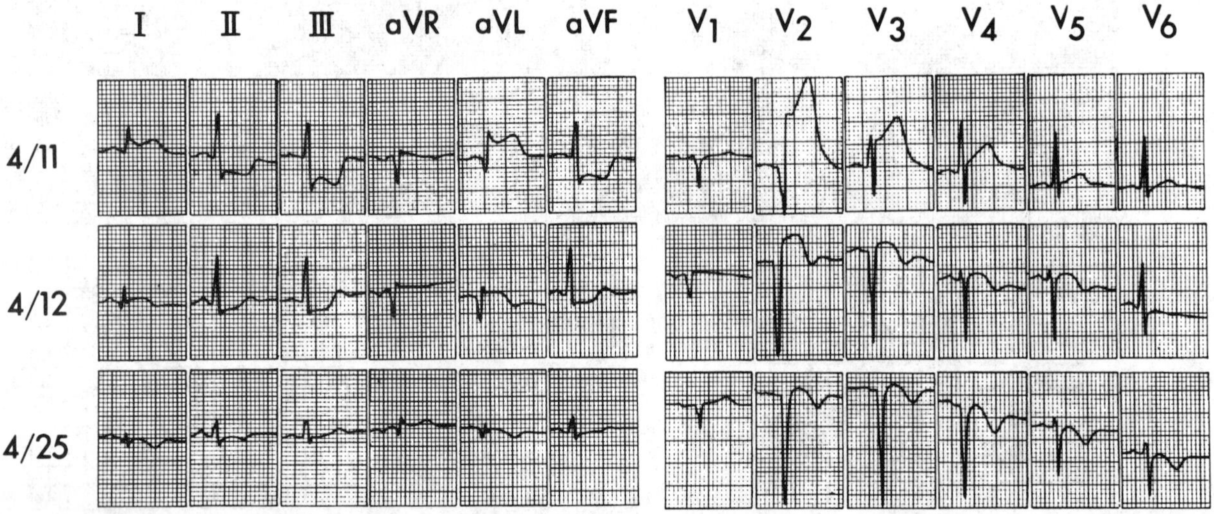

complex nature of the LBB system has thus far defied a determination of whether focal proximal disease or diffuse distal disease in the distribution of these portions of the LBB is the mechanism responsible for the hemiblock patterns.

LAH results in a moderate delay of activation of the superior portion of the left ventricular free wall, causing a modest prolongation of the QRS complex and shift of the front plane axis to the left. Initial septal depolarization is undisturbed (Fig. 233-15), and the QRS complex rarely exceeds 0.09 to 0.10 s. The differentiation between LAH and LPH may occasionally be difficult. In general, LPH alone will not produce a left axis shift beyond $-30°$, and LAH will often produce left axis deviation $\geq -60°$. The key QRS features in left anterior hemiblock include a small Q wave in leads I and aVL, with small initial R waves and deep S waves in leads II, III, and aVF.

LPH results in a moderate delay of activation of the posterior inferior portion of the left ventricular free wall. Again, there is a modest prolongation of the QRS complex, but a shift of the frontal plane QRS axis to the *right*. Thus, the initial septal forces, though generally undisturbed, may be oriented more superiorly, producing small initial Q waves in leads II, III, and aVF. Since the specificity of the ECG manifestations of LPH is not very reliable, many clinicians will not make a diagnosis of isolated LPH without demonstrating a right axis shift on serial ECGs, plus positive exclusion of other causes of right axis shift. Of all the intraventricular conduction disturbances, isolated LPH is the most difficult to diagnose.

The hemiblocks frequently coexist with disease in the RBB system. The combination of RBBB, plus LAH or LPH, is referred to as *bifascicular block*—the implication being that two fascicles of the trifascicular model of the intraventricular SCT are diseased. As stated earlier, this probably represents a pathophysiologic oversimplification, but is useful for clinical purposes. Since RBBB alone does not produce abnormal axis deviation either to the left or to the right, the coexistence of RBBB with abnormal left axis deviation (Fig. 233-16) is usually interpreted as LAH plus RBBB. Similarly, abnormal right axis deviation in association with RBBB is usually interpreted as the coexistence of LPH with RBBB, when the QRS criteria for LPH are met (Fig. 233-15). As is the case in isolated LPH, the diagnosis of LPH plus RBBB is difficult because a number of clinical

FIGURE 233-15
Intraventricular conduction abnormalities. Illustrated are right bundle branch block (RBBB); left bundle branch block (LBBB); left anterior hemiblock (LAH); right bundle branch block with left anterior hemiblock (RBBB + LAH); and right bundle branch block with left posterior hemiblock (RBBB + LPH).

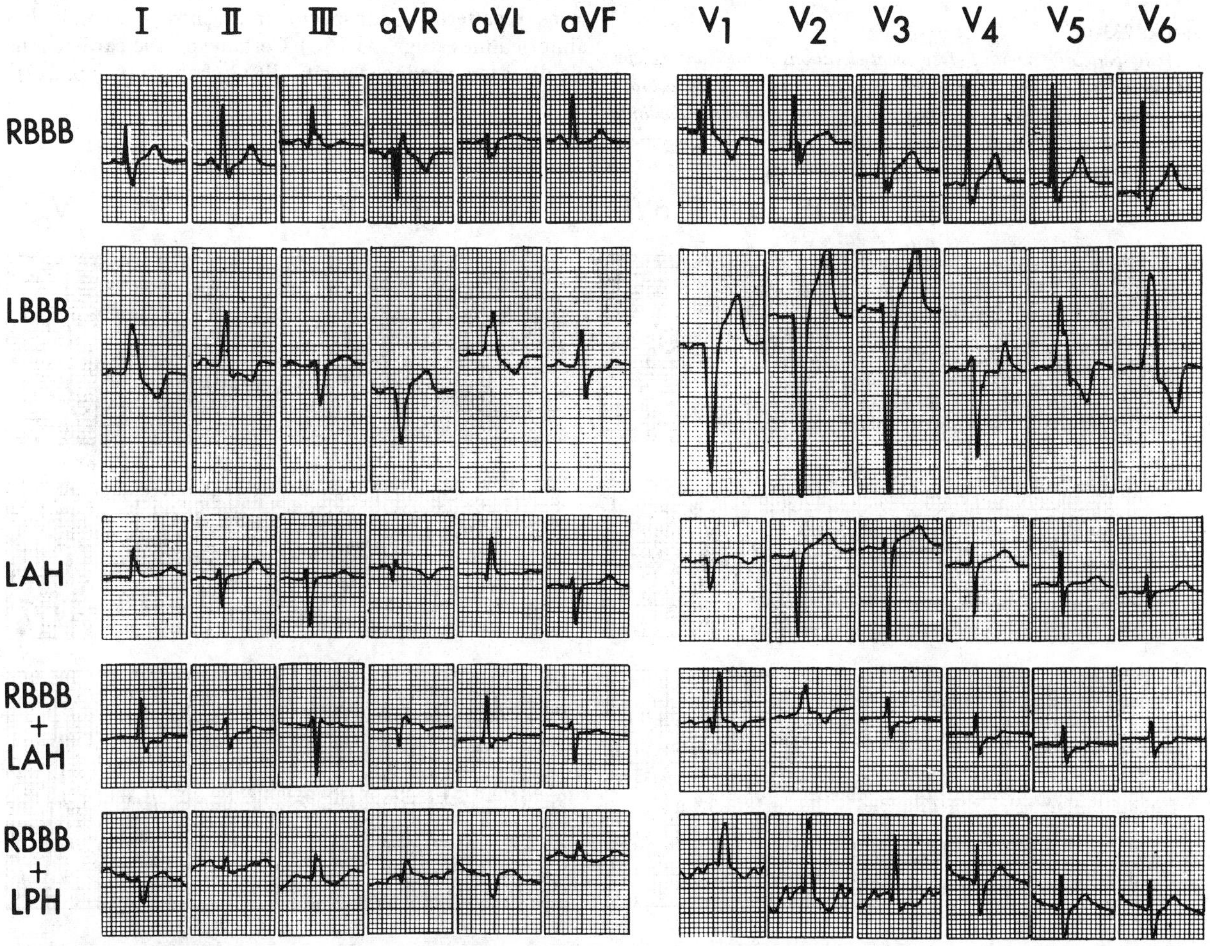

settings may cause abnormal right axis deviation in conjunction with RBBB.

Trifascicular block describes abnormal conduction in all three divisions of the intraventricular SCT. The ECG diagnosis can be made only by inference, when a patient has bifascicular block and a prolonged P-R interval. Confirmation can be achieved only with His bundle electrocardiography (Chap. 238).

PERICARDITIS, MYOCARDITIS, AND THE CARDIOMYOPATHIES Acute pericarditis causes elevation of the S-T segments in many leads without the reciprocal changes seen in acute myocardial infarction (Fig. 233-16*A*). S-T elevation may occur in all leads except aVR, and rarely involves V_1. After a period of days to weeks, the diffuse S-T elevations return to the base line, and T-wave inversions may occur. Coexistent S-T elevations and T-wave inversions rarely occur as they do in myocardial infarction (compare Figs. 233-13 and 233-16*A*). T-wave abnormalities may persist for weeks or months after the acute episode of pericarditis. If the pericarditis is accompanied by significant degrees of pericardial effusion, electrical alternans may occur. On alternate beats, ECG voltage shifts in magnitude. There also may be low voltage of the QRS complexes and T waves in all leads. Finally, the T_a waves may be transiently depressed because of atrial involvement by the inflammatory process [see Fig. 233-11*B* (1)].

The ECG changes of myocarditis and the cardiomyopathies may be either vague or dramatic, but are usually nonspecific (Chap. 247). It is often difficult to differentiate myocarditis (Fig. 233-16*B*) from the late phase of pericarditis in which symmetrical T-wave inversions are present. However, myocarditis may occur in many other settings, and an appreciation of the range of the ECG changes is important. Almost all systemic infections may produce minor myocardial involvement. Measles, mumps, influenza, hepatitis, infectious mononucleosis, and scarlet fever, just to name a few diseases, may be associated with ECG abnormalities and with histopathologic evidence of myocardial inflammation. When the myocardial involvement is subclinical, the ECG changes are usually very subtle and nonspecific. There are minor T-wave changes, manifested as flattening or perhaps shallow inversion of the T waves in multiple leads (Fig. 233-11*O* and *P*). The conducting system may be involved, and prolongation of the P-R interval may be noted.

In more obvious myocarditis, the ECG demonstrates symmetrically inverted T waves in most of the standard limb leads and in the lateral precordial leads (Fig. 233-16*B*). When the specialized conducting system is involved, bundle branch block may occur, and patterns of diffuse nonspecific intraventricular conduction defects may occur.

The cardiomyopathies may be accompanied by striking ECG changes. The patterns observed may mimic the diffuse T-wave abnormalities which accompany myocarditis, there may be pathologic Q waves which are difficult to differentiate from the Q waves of healed myocardial infarctions, or there may be either bundle branch block patterns or patterns of nonspecific intraventricular conduction abnormalities (Fig. 233-16*C*). Certain specific cardiac muscle disorders produce specific ECG changes (Chap. 247).

FIGURE 233-16

A *Acute pericarditis with S-T segment elevations in all leads except III, aVR, and V_1, and T_a depression in I, II, and aVF.* B *Myocarditis: diffuse ST-T-wave changes, with low-voltage T waves in the limb leads and primary T-wave changes in the chest leads.* C *Concentric cardiomyopathy: gross distortion of the QRS complex.*

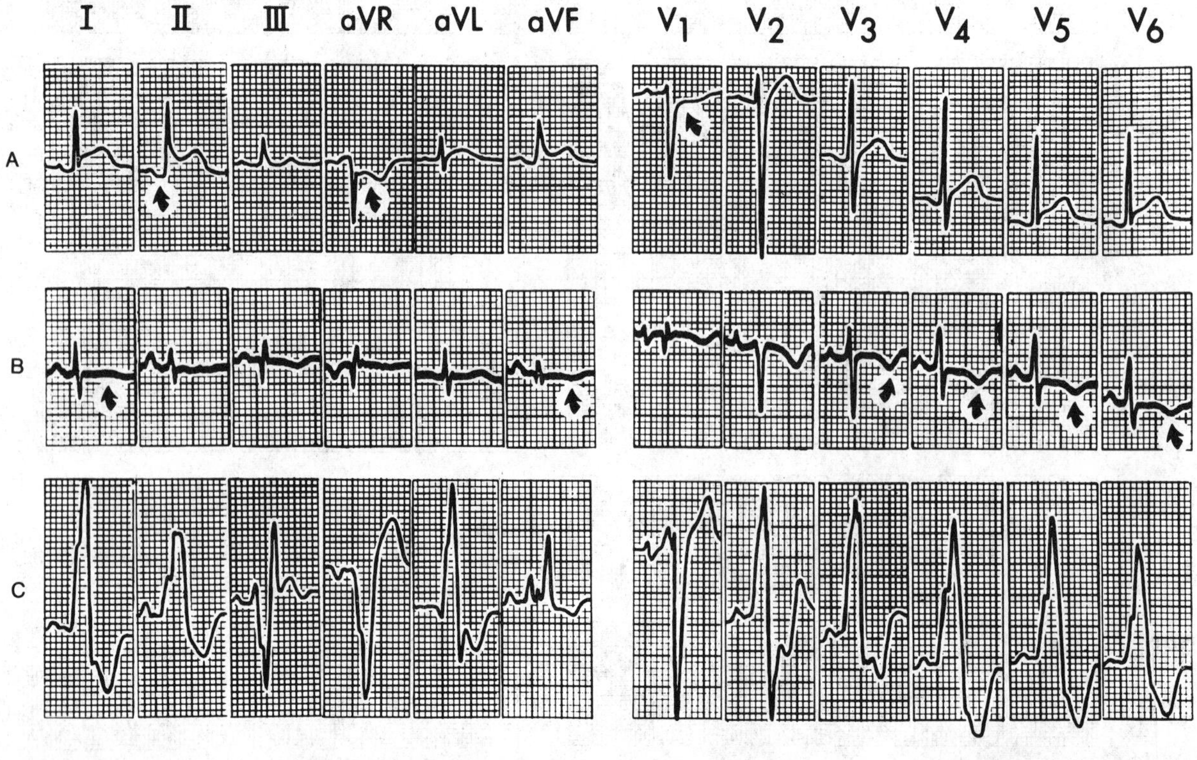

ECG ABNORMALITIES IN METABOLIC AND ELECTROLYTE DISTURBANCES The electrically active tissues of the heart are particularly sensitive to changes in the extracellular concentration of K^+, and dramatic ECG changes may accompany abrupt changes in K^+. The initial effect of acute *hyper*kalemia is the appearance of tall, peaked T waves (Fig. 233-17). As the severity of hyperkalemia increases, the QRS complex blends into the tall, peaked T waves, P-wave voltage decreases and may disappear entirely, and the P-R interval prolongs. As these changes evolve, there is marked prolongation of the QRS complex (Fig. 233-17) with the evolution of continuity between the S wave and T wave, giving a sine wave configuration. This pattern is a very late and ominous manifestation of hyperkalemia. Equally dangerous is the occurrence of severe *hypo*kalemia, which also produces characteristic ECG changes. Instead of the tall, peaked T waves of hyperkalemia, hypokalemia produces a flattening or inversion of the T wave, but at the same time a prominence of the U wave. In its fully developed state, the ECG gives the appearance of a very long Q-T interval. Careful analysis reveals that the Q-T interval is not so prolonged, and the U wave has assumed the appearance of the T wave (Fig. 233-17). Thus, the major prolongation is a "Q-U" prolongation. This ECG manifestation of hypokalemia may forewarn of the occurrence of serious ventricular arrhythmias, especially in the presence of digitalis. One must be careful to differentiate the ECG effects of hypo*calcemia* from hypo*kalemia*. Whereas hypokalemia may produce the appearance of a long S-T segment and late T wave because of flattening of the T wave and prominence of the U wave, hypocalcemia does, in fact, produce prolongation of the S-T segment with a late T wave (Fig. 233-17). Most of the other electrolyte imbalances produce ECG changes too nonspecific to be clinically useful.

FIGURE 233-17
Electrolyte disturbances. Hyper*kalemia (K^+ = 6.8) with tall, peaked T waves. Severe hyperkalemia (K^+ = 9.1) with (1) flattening of the P wave, and ↑P-R interval (1→2), (2) marked widening of the QRS complex (2→3), and (3) merging of the S wave into the T wave.* Hypo*kalemia produces flat or inverted T waves with prominent U waves, causing prolonged "Q-U" interval, while hypocalcemia produces true prolongation of the S-T segment with marked Q-T prolongation.*

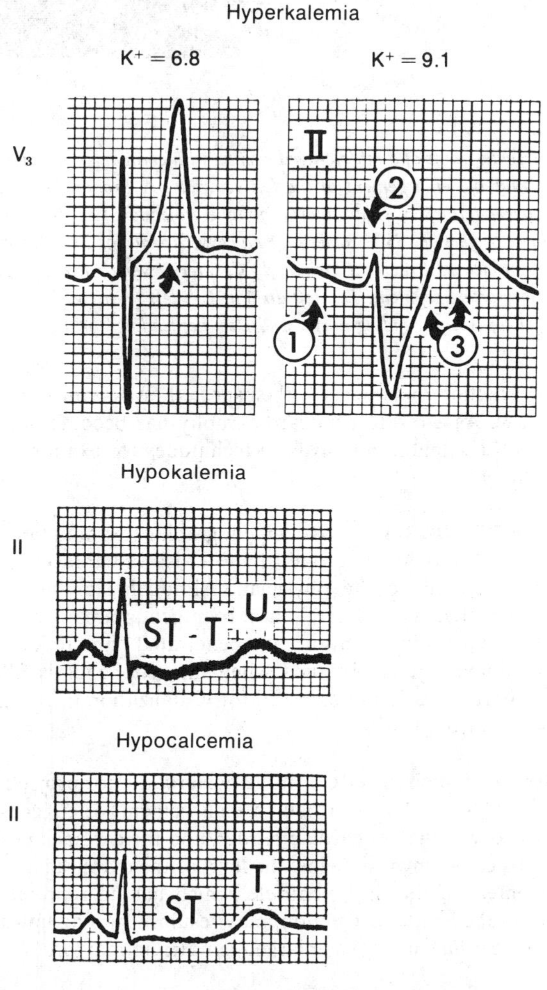

Abnormalities of metabolism, such as hyper- or hypothyroidism, Addison's disease, diabetic ketoacidosis, and the infiltrative diseases such as amyloidosis and hemachromatosis, all may produce ECG abnormalities which may be helpful in the recognition of the disease process, but are often nonspecific.

REFERENCES

CRANEFIELD PF: *The Conduction of the Cardiac Impulse,* Mt. Kisco, N. Y.: Futura, 1975

FISCH C (ed): Complex electrocardiography (I & II). Cardiovasc Clin 5 (3) and 6 (1), Philadelphia: Davis, 1973 and 1974

HOFFMAN BF, CRANEFIELD PF: *Electrophysiology of the Heart,* New York: McGraw-Hill, 1960

HURST JW, MYERBURG RJ: *Introduction to Electrocardiography,* 2d ed., New York: McGraw-Hill, 1973

LIPMAN BS et al: *Clinical Scalar Electrocardiography,* 6th ed., Chicago: Year Book, 1972

MARRIOTT HJL: *Practical Electrocardiography,* 4th ed., Baltimore: Williams & Wilkins, 1968

SCHLANT RC, HURST JW (eds): *Advances in Electrocardiography,* 2d ed., New York: Grune & Stratton, 1976

234
ECHOCARDIOGRAPHY AND OTHER NONINVASIVE METHODS OF CARDIAC EXAMINATION

ROBERT A. O'ROURKE
JOHN ROSS, JR.

The indirect methods for examination of the heart, which encompass special diagnostic approaches other than cardiac catheterization or injection of radiographic contrast medium into the circulation, include electrocardiography (Chap. 233), roentgenography, phonocardiography, external recordings of pulse wave forms, and the use of radioisotopes. Recently, there have been important advances in the use of reflected ultrasound to define cardiac anatomy

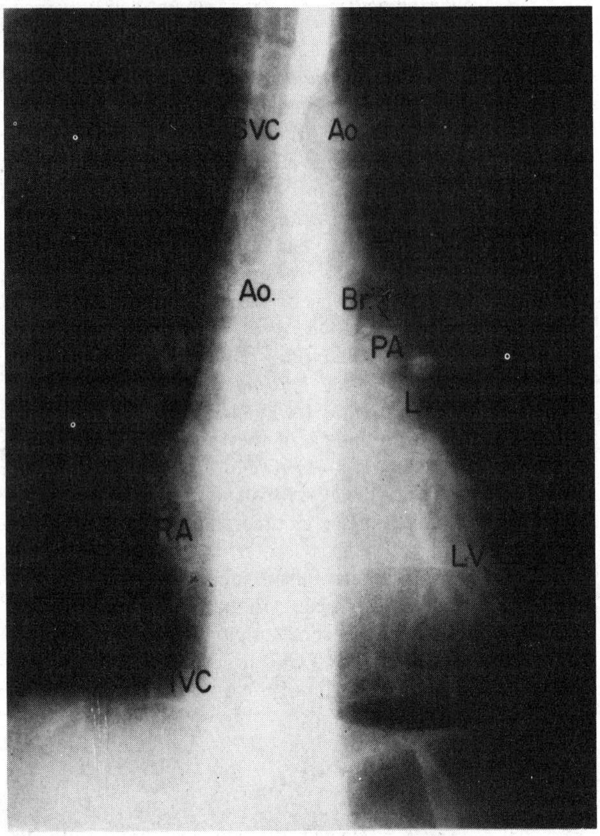

A

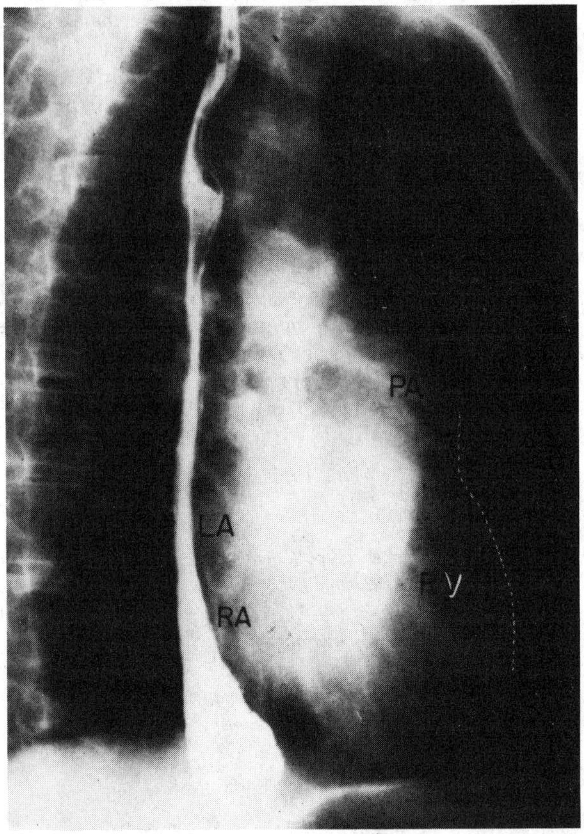

B

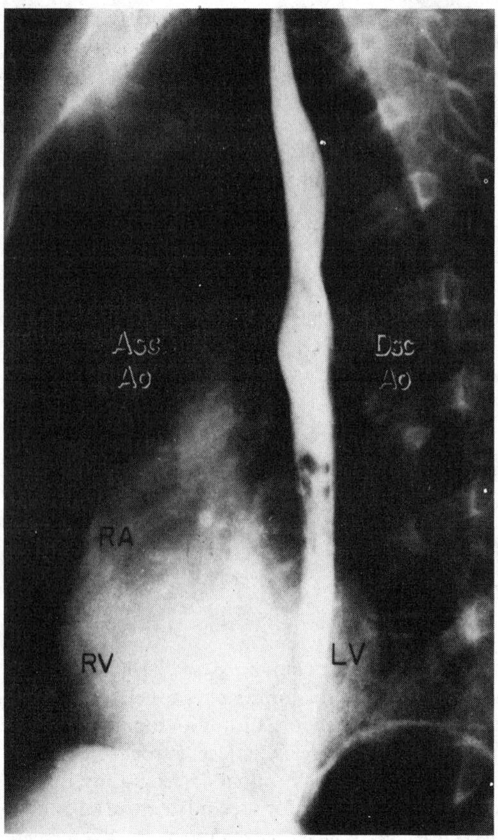

C

FIGURE 234-1
Roentgenograms of a middle-aged woman with coronary heart disease and minimal enlargement of the left ventricle. A *Frontal projection (posteroanterior).* B *Right anterior oblique projection.* C *Left anterior oblique projection. SVC, superior vena cava; Ao, aorta; Br, left main-stem bronchus; RA, right atrium; IVC, inferior vena cava; PA, pulmonary artery segment; LA, left atrium; LV, left ventricle; RV, right ventricle; Asc, ascending aorta; and Dsc, descending aorta.*

and function in subjects with suspected or definite cardiac disease. As a result, echocardiography has become one of the most valuable noninvasive techniques for examination of the heart.

ROENTGENOGRAPHY Roentgenographic examination of the heart and lungs is one of the most valuable indirect tools available to the physician. Although standard 6-ft posteroanterior and lateral chest roentgenograms may provide adequate information, overpenetrated frontal, lateral, and oblique views obtained when the esophagus is filled with barium paste are essential for visualization of specific regions of the heart.

The cardiac silhouette In the posteroanterior projection (Fig. 234-1*A*), left ventricular enlargement often causes convexity of the left cardiac border, and the cardiac apex is displaced downward, below the level of the diaphragm. Enlargement of the right ventricle, which has no representation in the frontal projection, may result in tipping upward of the cardiac apex. An enlarged left atrium may produce a round "double density" in the center of the cardiac silhouette and upward displacement of the left main stem bronchus.

In the right anterior oblique (RAO) projection (Fig. 234-1*B*), the barium filled esophagus courses directly adjacent to the left atrium. This projection is helpful for detecting right ventricular enlargement and is of particular value for recognizing compression or posterior displacement of the esophagus by an enlarged left atrium.

In the left anterior oblique (LAO) projection (Fig. 234-1*C*), the posterior aspect of the left ventricle normally clears the spine with the patient rotated to an angle of 60° or less relative to the plane of the film. When the left ventricle is enlarged, it overlaps the spine when the patient is rotated 60° or more from the posteroanterior position, but it should be appreciated that marked right ventricular enlargement alone can cause posterior displacement of the left ventricle.

The dimensions of the cardiac silhouette relative to the bony thorax can be measured directly from the standard 6-ft chest roentgenogram. The measurement most commonly made is the cardiothoracic ratio, which is obtained by dividing the transverse diameter of the heart (defined as the distance from the outermost point of the right cardiac border to the midsternal line, plus the distance from the outermost point of the left cardiac border to the midsternal line) by the internal diameter of the thorax at its widest point above the diaphragm. Although the cardiothoracic ratio is dependent on the configuration of the chest, generally it is less than 0.5 in normal subjects.

Image-intensification fluoroscopy may be employed to define further the size and the pulsations of the cardiac chambers and great vessels. It also is useful for detecting areas of calcification within the cardiac valves, coronary arteries, or pericardium. The characteristic motion of the cardiac valves observed on fluoroscopy aids considerably in identifying the site of a calcification.

The pulmonary vasculature The size of the central and peripheral pulmonary blood vessels can be evaluated from the standard chest roentgenogram. Estimation of the degree of pulmonary vascularity may be of great diagnostic importance, particularly in patients suspected of having congenital heart disease, and a disproportion between the size of the central and peripheral pulmonary arteries (enlarged main vessels that taper sharply) may suggest an elevated pulmonary vascular resistance.

An unusually prominent pulmonary vascular pattern is observed in lesions associated with left-to-right shunting of blood, and the main pulmonary artery segment often is enlarged. Examination of the heart for specific chamber enlargement often aids in determining the location of the shunt. For example, in patients with atrial septal defect there is right ventricular enlargement, but the left atrium and left ventricle are small because the defect allows decompression of those chambers. In contrast, in patients with ventricular septal defect both the left atrium and left ventricle are enlarged.

A selective increase in the caliber of the upper lobe pulmonary veins can be observed with lesions such as mitral stenosis that produce left atrial hypertension. In addition, the normal pattern in the upright subject, a more prominent vascular pattern at the lung bases than at the apexes, may be reversed in patients with an elevated left atrial pressure. Higher levels of pulmonary venous pressure (exceeding 15 to 20 mmHg) may also be associated with interstitial edema or fibrosis in the interlobular septa, resulting in the Kerley B lines, horizontal markings about 1 cm in length appearing above the diaphragm near the rib cage. Pulmonary edema (fluid within the alveoli) may be secondary to acute left atrial hypertension or left ventricular failure and is characterized by bilateral, confluent "butterfly" densities in the central lung fields.

Decreased pulmonary vascularity is observed most commonly with lesions that cause both obstruction to right ventricular outflow and right-to-left shunting of blood. The reduction in pulmonary blood flow results in diminished caliber of the pulmonary arteries and veins, and the left atrium also may be small; such findings are present in patients with tetralogy of Fallot. In patients with pure valvular pulmonic stenosis, the pulmonary vascularity often is not diminished, since the pulmonary blood flow may be normal.

Radioisotopes The intravenous injection of macroaggregated ^{131}I-labeled albumin, with subsequent scanning of the lung fields for underperfused areas, is valuable in the detection of pulmonary emboli (Chap. 266). Another application of this approach is to scan the cardiac silhouette after intravenous injection of the radioisotope; the area of the cardiac silhouette occupied by the labeled intracardiac blood pool is then compared with the cardiac silhouette on the chest roentgenogram for the detection of pericardial effusion. The intravenous injection of a small bolus of a gamma emitter such as ^{99m}Tc pertechnetate permits rapid, sequential visualization of the heart, great vessels, and pulmonary vasculature by use of an Anger scintillation camera. The image usually is recorded, stored on tape, replayed, and photographed. This technique is used in the diagnosis of a variety of congenital and acquired cardiac lesions, as well as for detecting pulmonary emboli and pericardial effusion. Radionuclide angiography is useful for detecting abnormalities in left ventricular wall motion and mitral regurgitation in patients with coronary artery disease, as well as for the noninvasive estimation of left ventricular volumes and ejection fraction. In addition, radioisotopes are being used for "myocardial imaging." Since radioactive substances such as ^{43}K (potassium), ^{81}Rb (rubidium), or ^{201}Tl (thallium) concentrate in normal myocardium but not in regions of the myocardium that are unperfused, "cold" defects may be found during isotope scanning after the intravenous injection of such radionuclides in patients with a recent or previous myocardial infarction. Other isotopes, such as ^{99m}Tc pyrophosphate, appear to be taken up in increased concentrations in regions of recent myocardial necrosis (observed as "hot" areas), and these substances have been advocated for the diagnosis of acute myocardial damage.

PHONOCARDIOGRAPHY The phonocardiogram provides a graphic display of heart sounds and murmurs, and enhances considerably the assessment of auscultatory events. The modern phonocardiograph is capable of recording sounds in a manner that resembles their detection by the ear. In order to simulate the relative insensitivity of the human ear to low-frequency vibrations and its great sensitivity to high-frequency signals, so-called logarithmic or high-frequency recordings are used to provide relatively greater amplification of high-frequency components. Filters also are employed to allow selective passage of low- and high-freqency sounds, perhaps the most satisfactory system consisting of a series of bandpass filters which encompass the frequency fields from 15 to 1,000 Hz. The transducer of the phonocardiograph consists of a crystal (piezoelectric) microphone applied directly to the skin, or attached indirectly through an air-coupled diaphragm or bell. The crystals within the microphone alter their electrical properties when stressed by sound pressure waves, and the resulting electrical signal is amplified and recorded on a high-frequency oscillograph.

Although the phonocardiogram is useful for determining the configuration and frequency composition of individual cardiac mumurs, its most important application is in the precise timing of cardiac sounds and murmurs (see Chap. 232). Thus, it allows clear definition of a sequence of events, such as the variation in the splitting of the second heart sound which occurs during respiration, or the differentiation of separate systolic and diastolic murmurs from a continuous murmur which continues throughout late systole and early diastole. The phonocardiogram also may provide quantitative information of significance, such as the precise duration of the interval between the aortic closure sound and the mitral valve opening snap in patients with mitral stenosis, an interval that correlates inversely with the atrioventricular pressure gradient (Chap. 243).

The electrocardiogram is recorded simultaneously with the phonocardiogram to provide a reference signal. Other externally recorded variables that are extremely helpful in timing auscultatory events are the venous pulse tracing (jugular phlebogram), the carotid pulse wave, and the apex cardiogram, each of which is discussed below.

In order to appreciate the significance of alterations in the timing of heart sounds which occur in various disease states and the relation that these sounds bear to external pulse tracings, it is essential to understand the normal temporal relations between the electrical and mechanical events of the cardiac cycle (Fig. 234-2). The normal cycle begins with the P wave of the electrocardiogram, which is followed by right atrial contraction, the initial mechanical event. Left atrial contraction occurs shortly thereafter. The QRS complex ensues, initiating the onset of isovolumetric left ventricular contraction 0.04 to 0.06 s after the the onset of the QRS complex. Right ventricular contraction then starts, and the brief period of isovolumetric right ventricular contraction is followed by the onset of right ventricular ejection. The onset of left ventricular ejection is the next event, and since the duration of ejection is shorter on the left side than on the right, closure of the aortic valve precedes pulmonic valve closure. Isovolumetric relaxation of the ventricles terminates earlier on the right side than on the left (at the peak of the atrial V wave). A convenient way to remember this normal sequence of mechanical events in the two ventricles (onset of isovolumetric contraction, onset of ejection, end of ejection, end of isovolumetric relaxation) is to recall that isovolumetric phases of left ventricular contraction and relaxation completely encompass those of the right ventricle (Fig. 234-2).

The jugular venous pulse tracing is obtained by applying a cup transducer over the jugular bulb with slight suction; an inner chamber transmits the pressure changes induced by the venous pulsations to a crystal microphone. The nomenclature of the venous waves is the same as that employed in describing intraatrial pressure pulse contours recorded directly (Figs. 232-1 and 235-3). Although some difficulty may be introduced by a variable delay in transmission of the venous waves to the neck (this delay generally averages 0.02 s), the venous tracing may be extremely helpful in studying the dynamics of the right side of the heart (see Chap. 232).

The indirect carotid arterial pulse wave is recorded with a transducer similar to that employed for obtaining the jugular venous tracing. This signal provides an important means of analyzing the carotid pulse contours and for timing the sounds of aortic and pulmonic valve closure (Fig. 232-1). Alterations in the contour of the carotid arterial pulse are often helpful in the diagnosis of aortic valve disease, idiopathic hypertrophic subaortic stenosis, and left ventricular failure (see Chap. 232). Normally, the ascending limb of the systolic carotid wave is steeper than the descending limb; the upstroke time from onset to peak averages 100 ms (range, 60 to 140 ms),[1] and the normal duration of ejection averages 300 ms (range, 260 to 310 ms).[1]

The aortic component of the second heart sound (A_2), generated at the closure of the aortic valve, can be identified by using the incisura of the carotid pulse wave as a reference point (Fig. 232-1). Since there is a slight delay in the transmission of the pulse wave to the neck, the recording of this sound precedes the incisura by approximately 0.02 s. In the normal person, closure of the pulmonic valve (P_2) always follows A_2 (Chap. 232). Although this interval is narrow during expiration (0.02 s) and the splitting may be inaudible, it may be recorded on the phonocardiogram.

Lesions that result in prolongation of left ventricular ejection may cause reversal of the normal sequence of aortic and pulmonic valve closure, termed *reversed splitting* of the second heart sound (Chap. 232). That A_2 follows P_2 may be verified on the phonocardiogram using the carotid pulse tracing for timing.

Systolic time intervals are calculated from the simultaneous recording at rapid paper speed of a high-frequency phonocardiogram, the indirect carotid arterial pulse wave, and the electrocardiogram. These measurements may be employed in the noninvasive evaluation of left ventricular performance. The intervals measured include electromechanical systole ($Q\text{-}S_2$), the period from the onset of the QRS complex to the first high-frequency deflection of S_2; the left ventricular ejection time (LVET), which begins with the upstroke of the carotid arterial pulse and ends with the incisura; and the preejection period (PEP), the difference between the duration of left ventricular electromechanical systole and LVET [$PEP = (Q\text{-}S_2) - LVET$] (Fig. 234-2). Factors which influence the LVET include the heart rate, stroke volume, left ventricular afterload, the inotropic state of the myocardium, and the sex of the patient. Factors which influence the PEP include heart rate, aortic

[1] *Corrected for heart rate by dividing the measured interval by the square root of the cycle length in seconds.*

diastolic pressure, intraventricular conduction, and myocardial inotropic state. Systolic time intervals can be corrected both for heart rate and the patient's sex by using regression equations derived from data obtained in a large number of resting subjects without evidence of heart disease. However, the ratio of the PEP to the LVET (PEP/LVET) need not be corrected for heart rate or sex (normal = 0.345 ± 0.036 SD). In the presence of left ventricular failure, the PEP lengthens (reflecting primarily a decreased rate of ventricular pressure development) and the LVET diminishes (reflecting a decreased stroke volume), while the duration of electromechanical systole remains unchanged. These altered relationships during left ventricular failure may be expressed as an increase in the PEP/LVET ratio. An inverse linear correlation has been demonstrated between the PEP/LVET ratio and the ejection fraction (stroke volume/end-diastolic volume), the latter being obtained by left ventricular cineangiography in patients with a variety of cardiac diseases.

The apex cardiogram, a graphic recording of the precordial movements, provide a reference signal that is of particular value in the analysis of diastolic events and heart sounds. The apex cardiogram is recorded using a bell-type, linear crystal microphone and a filter designed to pass only low frequencies (between 0.1 and 20 Hz). The O point on the apex cardiogram occurs at the end of isovolumetric left ventricular relaxation and at the onset of ventricular filling (Fig. 232-1). Thus, it corresponds closely in time to the opening of the mitral valve and is useful as a reference point for identifying the opening snap in patients with mitral stenosis. Normally, a rapid-filling wave of about 0.08 s follows the O point. In the presence of mitral stenosis this event is replaced by a slow-filling wave. On the other hand, in patients with myocardial failure, mitral regurgitation, or

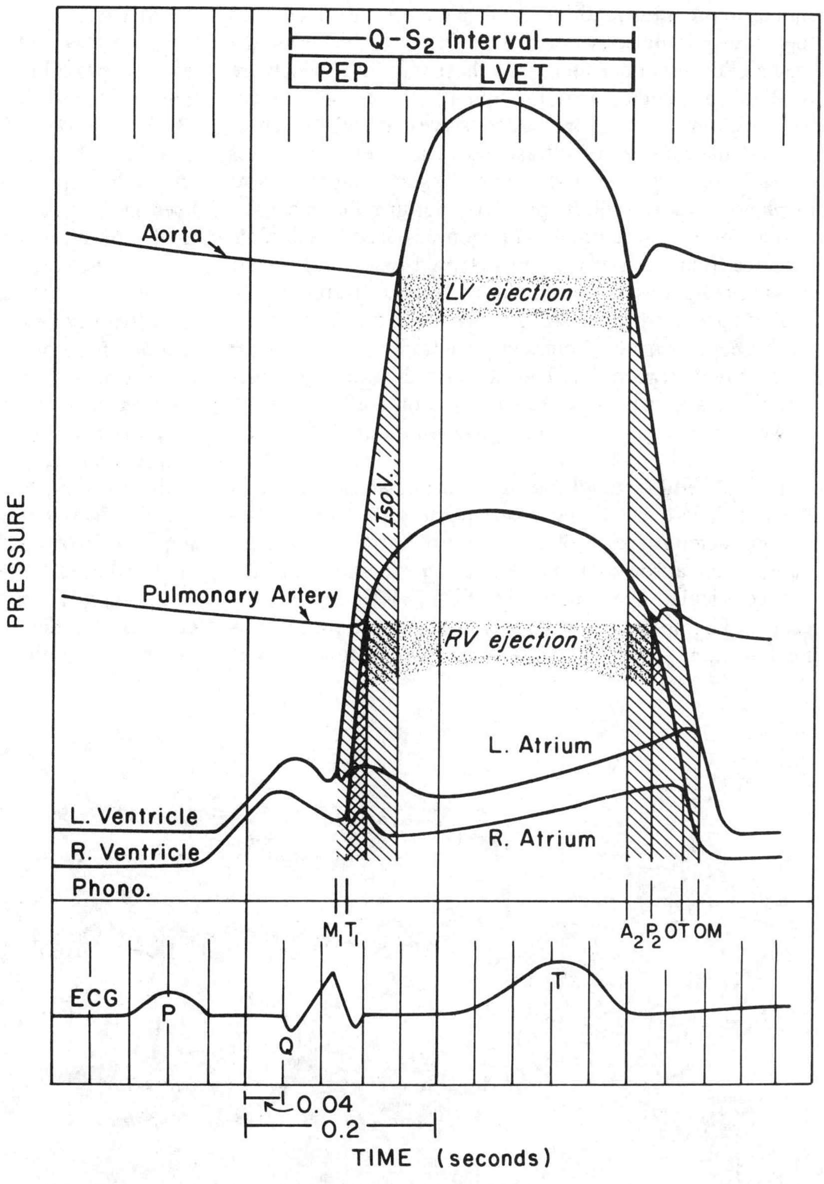

FIGURE 234-2
Diagrammatic representation of pressure tracings recorded within the left and right ventricles correlated with the ECG and the phonocardiogram (Phono). The striped areas labeled IsoV. represent the isovolumetric phases of left ventricular contraction and relaxation; isovolumetric right ventricular contraction and relaxation are shown as cross-hatched areas. M_1 and T_1, sounds produced by closure of the mitral and tricuspid valves, respectively; A_2 and P_2, sounds produced by the closure of the aortic and pulmonic valves, respectively; OT and OM, sounds produced by opening of the tricuspid and mitral valves, respectively. The Q-S_2 interval includes the preejection period (PEP) and the left ventricular ejection time (LVET), the latter being measured noninvasively from the delayed indirect carotid pulse tracing (see text).

constrictive pericarditis, an exaggerated rapid-filling wave may terminate in a ventricular diastolic gallop or third heart sound (Chap. 232).

The A wave of the apex cardiogram is absent in patients with atrial fibrillation or mitral stenosis. This wave may be augmented and accompanied by a fourth heart sound in the presence of lesions, such as aortic stenosis, that produce left ventricular hypertrophy. In patients with hypertrophic subaortic stenosis, the apex cardiogram often exhibits a double systolic wave, or even a triple contour if the A wave is prominent as well.

ECHOCARDIOGRAPHY Single-probe unidirectional ultrasound is widely used in the noninvasive diagnosis of a variety of cardiac diseases such as pericardial effusion, mitral valve disease, idiopathic hypertrophic subaortic stenosis, left atrial myxoma, congestive cardiomyopathy, and a wide spectrum of congenital cardiac disorders. With this technique, a ceramic compound such as barium titanate is excited by short, high-frequency (1.6 to 2.5 mHz) electrical signals to provide inaudible ultrasonic pulses. Reflection of the ultrasonic pulses occurs at an interface between two media of different densities, only those interfaces which are relatively perpendicular to the sound beam being sampled. The electromechanical transducer serves as both the emitter and the receiver of ultrasound at a repetition rate of 1,000 impulses per second. The echoes are amplified and displayed on an oscilloscope. For recording the echoes, a "time-motion" presentation commonly is used which plots distance from chest wall against elapsed time and displays moving structures as undulating lines. Photographs of the echo display can be taken directly from the face of the oscilloscope, but more commonly the tracings are recorded on a strip chart recorder. The electrocardiogram and time-distance markers usually are displayed on the oscilloscope as well and used as reference signals on the recorded tracing.

Tilting the ultrasound transducer cephalad or caudad in the fourth left intercostal space permits the echocardiographic demonstration of a number of cardiac structures between the aortic root and left atrium superiorly and the left ventricular apex inferiorly (Fig. 234-3). During the echocardiographic "sweep" the anterior aortic root is normally continuous with the interventricular septum inferiorly and the posterior aortic root with the anterior leaflet of the mitral valve. In position 1 (Fig. 234-3) the ultrasound beam traverses from anterior to posterior the right ventricular outflow tract, aortic root, and left atrium. Echoes from the right and noncoronary aortic cusps are often included in the ultrasound tracing; measurement of the width of the aortic root, the dimensions of the left atrium, and the excursion of aortic leaflets can be made from the echocardiographic recording. Marked dilatation of the aortic root can be demonstrated in Marfan's syndrome or aortic aneurysm; decreased excursion of aortic leaflets is evident when the stroke volume is low; thickening of the aortic leaflets can be seen in calcific aortic stenosis; and a large left atrium may accompany mitral stenosis and/or regurgitation. Furthermore, eccentric motion of aortic leaflets may be recorded in patients with bicuspid aortic valves, and thickened irregular systolic or diastolic echoes from aortic leaflets may occur in patients with aortic regurgitation due to endocarditis. Dense echoes within the left atrial cavity may be due to thrombus, tumor, vegetation, or ruptured mitral chordae.

In position 2 (Fig. 234-3) the echo beam passes through the right ventricle, interventricular septum, and left ventricle at the level of the anterior and posterior mitral valve leaflets, providing important information regarding the motion of both leaflets during systole and diastole (Figs. 234-3 and 234-4). The ultrasound tracing from the normal anterior mitral leaflet is easily recorded and has a characteristic M shape. Various points on the echogram have been labeled A through F by convention and correspond to the positions of the anterior mitral leaflet at specific times in the cardiac cycle (Figs. 234-3 and 234-4). Following the onset of left ventricular diastole at point D, the mitral valve opens and the anterior leaflet reaches its most anterior position (toward the chest wall) at point E. The initial opening of the mitral valve in diastole is normally followed by a partial closure of the valve which is recorded as a downward (posterior) deflection of the anterior leaflet on the ultrasound tracing. The end point of partial closure is the F point, and the speed of this semiclosure of the anterior leaflet during diastole can be measured by the slope (ratio of distance to time) of the E-F segment (normally 80 to 150 mm per s). Subsequently, during left atrial contraction the mitral valve again opens farther, and this event is recorded as another anterior movement terminating in the A point on the echocardiogram. The valve leaf-

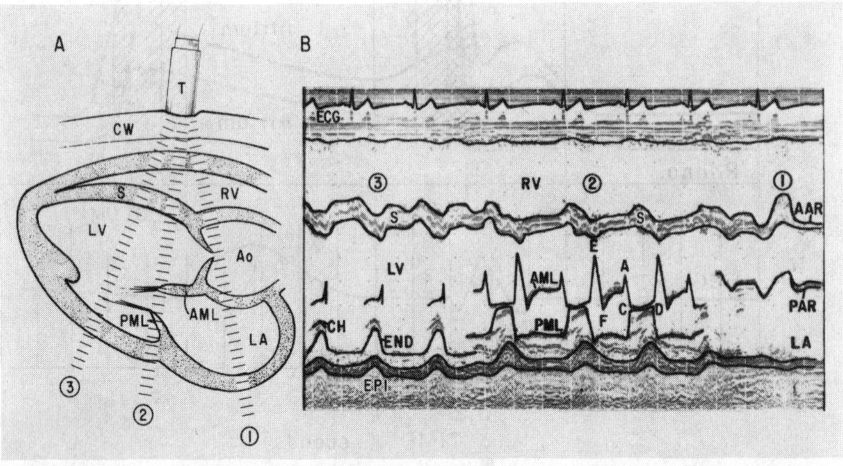

FIGURE 234-3
A schematic presentation of the cardiac structures traversed by three echo beams (A) is shown with a continuous echo "sweep" from a normal subject (B). T, transducer; CW, chest wall; RV, right ventricle; S, interventricular septum; Ao, aorta; LA, left atrium; and LV, left ventricle. AML, anterior mitral leaflet; PML, posterior mitral leaflet; AAR, anterior aortic root; PAR, posterior aortic root; CH, chordae tendineae; END, endocardium; and EPI, epicardium.

lets then return to their intermediate position, and shortly after the onset of ventricular systole at B the anterior mitral leaflet reaches its most posterior (closed) position at point C. Depending upon the exact transducer position, various portions of the posterior mitral valve leaflet are also commonly detected. The normal movements of this leaflet are approximately opposite in direction to those of the anterior mitral valve leaflet during diastole. Shortly after the onset of systole (point C) both leaflets come together and stay in apposition until point D is reached, at which time valve opening begins. This anterior motion of the closed mitral leaflets from C to D is probably related to emptying of the left ventricle during ejection.

Echocardiographic recordings of the motion of the anterior leaflet of the mitral valve have been particularly valuable in evaluating the status of patients with mitral stenosis, idiopathic hypertrophic subaortic stenosis (Chap. 247), left atrial myxoma, or mitral regurgitation due to a prolapsing mitral leaflet; characteristic movements of the mitral valve leaflet can be observed with each of these lesions (Fig. 234-4). *Mitral stenosis* frequently causes a decrease in the amplitude of anterior leaflet movement (normal = over 20 mm), a reduction of the EF slope (less than 40 mm per s), and a sustained anterior position during diastole (Fig. 234-4*A*). In addition, the posterior mitral valve leaflet usually maintains an anterior position during diastole instead of moving away from the transducer as it does normally. These phenomena result from the continued pressure gradient and sustained slow forward flow across the stenotic, domed valve, as well as from reduced mitral valve mobility consequent to thickening of the cusps and fusion of the commissures. Ultrasonic evaluation of mitral valve motion is particularly valuable in diagnosing patients with mitral stenosis in whom there is no audible diastolic murmur, despite evidence of severe pulmonary hypertension and a low cardiac output. It also is useful in distinguishing an Austin Flint murmur due to severe aortic regurgitation from the murmur of mitral stenosis. Fine high-frequency oscillations of the anterior mitral leaflet occur with aortic regurgitation, and premature closure of the mitral valve can be demonstrated by ultrasound in patients with acute severe aortic regurgitation and a very high left ventricular diastolic pressure.

Abnormal anterior movement of the mitral valve leaflet during systole occurs in patients with *idiopathic hypertrophic subaortic stenosis* (IHSS) (Fig. 234-4*B*). The abnormal systolic movement begins with the onset of ventricular ejection and reaches a peak with the initial peak in the arterial pulse. The characteristic abnormality often can be provoked by maneuvers which increase ventricular contractility or decrease left ventricular volume (e.g., amyl nitrite, Valsalva maneuver). The systolic anterior movement of the mitral valve is probably related to abnormal papillary muscle position and pulling forward of the anterior leaflet into the left ventricular outflow tract as the obstruction to ejection develops. There is also a moderately reduced EF slope, reflecting a reduced rate of left ventricular filling due to diminished ventricular compliance. This phenomenon may be seen in other forms of left ventricular hypertrophy as well. An additional echocardiographic finding usually present in patients with IHSS is marked thickening of the interventricular septum which exceeds 12 mm in diastole and results in an increased septum to left

FIGURE 234-4
A schematic presentation of the normal echocardiographic (ECHO) recording of anterior (AML) and posterior mitral leaflet (PML) motion is shown in the center with the simultaneous ECG. Abnormal mitral echocardiograms which occur in (A) *mitral stenosis,* (B) *idiopathic hypertrophic subaortic stenosis,* (C) *left atrial myxoma, and* (D) *mitral valve prolapse are also depicted. In the ECHO, the A point represents the end of anterior movement resulting from left atrial contraction, the C-D segment represents the closed position of both mitral leaflets during ventricular systole, and point E ends the anterior movement as the leaflet opens. The slope EF results from posterior motion of the AML during rapid ventricular filling. In idiopathic hypertrophic subaortic stenosis, SAM represents systolic anterior movement.*

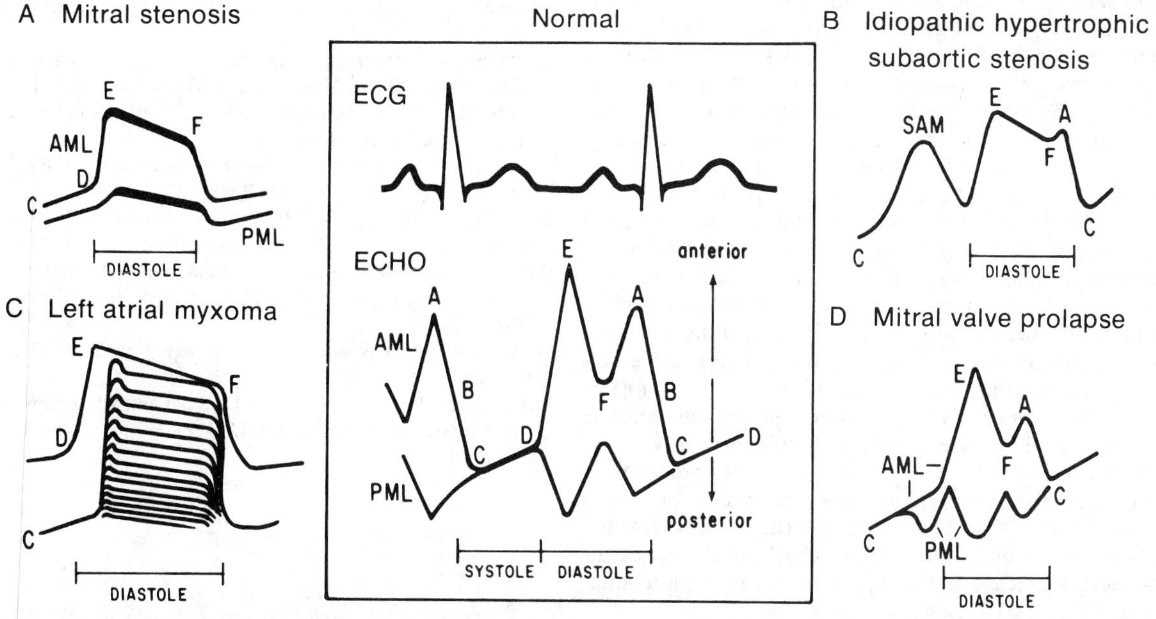

ventricular posterior wall thickness ratio of >1.3:1 (see below). This finding of asymmetrical hypertrophy has been reported as the only abnormal finding in relatives of patients with idiopathic hypertrophic subaortic stenosis, supporting the familial incidence of this syndrome. However, its specificity remains to be determined.

Ultrasound is a useful technique in detecting left atrial tumors, particularly if the tumor advances partially into the mitral valve orifice at some time during the cardiac cycle. Either mitral valve obstruction or regurgitation may result. A *left atrial myxoma* may be recognized as an aggregation of multiple echoes behind the anterior leaflet (Fig. 234-4*C*), and there may be a diminished EF slope because of mitral valve obstruction.

Patients with a *prolapsing mitral valve,* in many of whom a midsystolic click and/or late systolic murmur is heard on auscultation, often have a characteristic echocardiogram. Normally, during diastole the posterior mitral valve leaflet echo moves in a direction exactly opposite to that of the anterior leaflet echo (away from the ultrasonic transducer), while during systole the two leaflets come together. In patients with billowing or prolapsing mitral valve leaflets, the echocardiogram may show displacement of the posterior mitral leaflet (Fig. 234-4*D*) or both leaflets during late systole, or there may be separation of the two leaflets during both early and late systole resulting in pansystolic bowing.

In ultrasound position 3 (Fig. 234-3) the beam traverses the right ventricle, interventricular septum, and left ventricle at the level of mitral valve chordae tendineae. With proper technique both sides of the septum can be recorded as well as the endocardial and epicardial surfaces of the posterior left ventricular wall. Measurements of right ventricular size, left ventricular end-diastolic and end-systolic dimensions, and septal and posterior wall thickness can be made from the echocardiographic tracing. The interventricular septum normally moves posteriorly, and the posterior wall moves anteriorly during systole as the left ventricle shortens in its transverse diameter. Paradoxical systolic septal motion (toward the transducer) occurs together with an enlarged right ventricle in disorders associated with right ventricular volume overload, such as atrial septal defect or tricuspid regurgitation. Diminished or paradoxical septal motion is often recorded by ultrasound in patients with anteroseptal myocardial infarction, congestive cardiomyopathy, or left bundle branch block. Increased thickness of the septum and posterior wall is frequently demonstrated in patients with a chronic left ventricular pressure overload (e.g., aortic stenosis, systemic hypertension), and enlarged left ventricular end-diastolic and end-systolic diameters may be recorded in patients with left ventricular volume overload (e.g., aortic or mitral regurgitation) or diffuse myocardial disease. From echocardiographic measurements of left ventricular end-diastolic and end-systolic dimensions left ventricular performance can be estimated with a high degree of accuracy in subjects with normal ventricular wall motion, but this estimation is of lesser value in patients with ventricular asynergy.

Echocardiography also provides a simple, noninvasive method of reliably distinguishing *pericardial effusion* from a dilated heart (Chap. 246). In the presence of a pericardial effusion, the prominent posterior echo from the pericardial-pleural surface is stationary, while a second, more anterior echo of lower amplitude originating from the posterior left ventricular wall moves with the heartbeat. The echo-free space between the two posterior echoes is roughly proportional to the amount of pericardial fluid present.

An echocardiographic tracing of the tricuspid valve can be recorded by angulating the ultrasound transducer medially. A reduced EF slope of the tricuspid leaflets occurs in tricuspid stenosis, an increased leaflet excursion and delayed valve closure in Ebstein's malformation, and systolic posterior displacement of the leaflet in tricuspid valve prolapse.

Movement of the posterior pulmonic valve leaflet away from the chest wall can often be recorded with the transducer positioned in the second or third left intercostal space. A reduced diastolic or reversed EF slope, a diminished presystolic A dip, and midsystolic notching during the posterior excursion of the pulmonic leaflet occur in pulmonary hypertension. A marked increase in the A-dip amplitude is an echocardiographic feature of moderate to severe valvular pulmonic stenosis.

Recent advances in echocardiography have been particularly helpful in defining the anatomic defects in infants with cyanotic heart disease (e.g., positions of the aorta and pulmonary artery), and the continued development of cross-sectional or two-dimensional echocardiography should further enhance the value of reflected ultrasound in the diagnosis of various forms of congenital and acquired cardiac disease.

REFERENCES

CHANG S: *M-Mode Echocardiography Techniques and Pattern Recognition,* Philadelphia: Lea & Febiger, 1976

CHUNG EK: *Non-invasive Cardiac Diagnosis,* Philadelphia: Lea & Febiger, 1976

FOWLER NO (ed): Diagnostic methods in cardiology. Cardiovascular Clinics, Philadelphia: Davis, 1975

—— (ed): Non-invasive methods of cardiac diagnosis, chap. 11 in *Cardiac Diagnosis and Treatment,* 2d ed, Hagerstown: Harper & Row, 1976, p. 214

GRAMIAK R, WAAG RC: *Cardiac Ultrasound,* St. Louis: Mosby, 1975

MURPHY KF, KOTLER MN, REICHEK N, PERLOFF JK: Ultrasound in the diagnosis of congenital heart disease. Am Heart J 89:638–656, 1975

SIEGEL W: Non-invasive graphic methods, chap. 25 in *The Heart,* 3d ed., ed JW Hurst, New York: McGraw-Hill, 1974, p. 386

STRAUSS HW, PITT B, JAMES AE JR (eds): Cardiovascular nuclear medicine, St. Louis: Mosby, 1974

TAVEL ME: *Clinical Phonocardiography and External Pulse Recording,* 2d ed., Chicago: Year Book, 1972

WAGNER HN, RHODES BA: Radioactive tracers in diagnosis of cardiovascular disease. Prog Cardiovasc Dis 15:1, 1972

WEENS HS, GAY BB: Radiologic examination of the heart, chap. 22 in *The Heart,* 3d ed., ed JW Hurst, New York: McGraw-Hill, 1974, p. 323

WEISSLER AM (ed): *Non-invasive Cardiology,* New York: Grune & Stratton, 1974

ZARET BL et al: Radionuclides and the patient with coronary artery disease. Am J Cardiol 35:112, 1975

235 CARDIAC CATHETERIZATION AND ANGIOGRAPHY

JOHN ROSS, JR.
KIRK L. PETERSON

In 1929, Werner Forssman described the insertion of a catheter through his own arm vein into the right atrium and proposed that the procedure might prove useful for physiologic studies. A little more than a decade later, Andre Cournand and his associates introduced the modern era of cardiac catheterization in man by showing that it was possible to advance the catheter with safety further into the right ventricle and pulmonary artery and to perform hemodynamic studies by measuring intracardiac pressures and cardiac output. The technique of angiography also was developed rapidly in the period between 1930 and 1940, as relatively nontoxic opaque organic iodide media were discovered, and their intravascular injection provided definition of a number of congenital and acquired cardiovascular malformations. Since then, the development of techniques for catheterizing the left side of the heart and the coronary arteries, and for selective injection of contrast media into the cardiac chambers combined with exposure of high-speed x-ray motion pictures (cineangiography), has provided understanding of the dynamic anatomy of the heart, cardiac valves, and coronary arteries in the normal state and a variety of cardiac disorders. By permitting accurate anatomic and functional diagnoses of complex cardiac lesions, these procedures now have placed the selection of patients for surgical treatment on a firm, objective basis.

INDICATIONS

There are several types of problems for which hemodynamic or angiographic investigations commonly are performed, although other specific indications and contraindications may exist in the individual patient. These broad areas may be summarized as follows:

1 In patients with acquired valvular heart disease, hemodynamic assessment and angiographic studies often are required to determine whether the nature and severity of a mechanical valvular defect render it amenable to surgical treatment. In particular, cardiac catheterization studies may be indicated when both the mitral and aortic valves are involved, or when associated tricuspid valve disease is suspected to be of significance.
2 In patients with congenital heart disease, hemodynamic studies and angiography usually are necessary to characterize the primary defect and to determine whether associated lesions are present.
3 In patients with chest pain of undetermined cause, angiographic visualization of the coronary arteries may be indicated, and in patients with known coronary heart disease such studies may provide information that is useful prognostically and helpful in determining whether operative treatment is feasible.
4 In patients who have undergone cardiac operations, cardiac catheterization studies may be indicated to evaluate the success of the operation, particularly when residual symptoms are present. Such studies may reveal malfunction of a prosthetic valve, loss of patency of a coronary artery bypass graft, inadequate correction of a congenital defect, or residual disease of the ventricular myocardium.
5 In patients with suspected myocardial or pericardial disease, cardiac catheterization may be undertaken in an effort to exclude lesions potentially amenable to surgical treatment such as mitral regurgitation, coronary heart disease, constrictive pericarditis, and hypertrophic subaortic stenosis.
6 In patients with evidence of pulmonary hypertension, cardiac catheterization should be performed to search for such lesions as mitral stenosis, left-to-right shunts, multiple pulmonary emboli, or peripheral pulmonic stenosis.

GENERAL METHODS OF USE

CATHETERIZATION OF THE RIGHT SIDE OF THE HEART

Catheterization of the right side of the heart is now a well-standardized procedure. Using local anesthesia, an antecubital or saphenous vein is isolated and a long, flexible radiopaque catheter is introduced. Alternatively, the percutaneous approach is employed, in which a needle is positioned in the vessel, a flexible wire passed through the needle, the needle removed, and a tapered-tip catheter advanced over the guide wire. Using fluoroscopic control, the cardiac catheter is guided into the right ventricle, the pulmonary artery, and the pulmonary arterial wedge position. Blood samples may then be obtained and intracardiac pressures and indicator-dilution curves determined sequentially within the chambers of the right side of the heart in the diagnosis of congenital and acquired lesions, as discussed subsequently in this chapter. The course of the cardiac catheter alone may provide a clue to the diagnosis of certain congenital malformations. The catheter may enter an anomalous pulmonary vein or left superior vena cava; it may directly traverse a patent ductus arteriosus or an atrial septal defect; and inability to cross the tricuspid valve may indicate tricuspid atresia.

CATHETERIZATION OF THE LEFT SIDE OF THE HEART

Various methods for catheterization of the left side of the heart have been devised, and each has found application under certain circumstances. Currently, the retrograde arterial approach is used most widely for catheterization of the aorta and left ventricle. The catheter usually is inserted via the femoral artery using the percutaneous method, or through a small incision directly into the exposed brachial artery. The transseptal approach often is employed to gain access to the left atrium and left ventricle, particularly when disease of the mitral valve is suspected. With this method, a catheter is inserted via the right saphenous or femoral vein, and its tip is positioned in the right atrium. A long, curved needle is introduced through the catheter and employed to puncture the intact interatrial septum in the region of the fossa ovalis. Commonly, the catheter then is advanced over the needle into the left atrium and ventricle. Other methods of catheterization of the left side of the heart are used less commonly; e.g., with the anterior percutaneous approach a needle is introduced directly into the left ventricle in the region of the cardiac apex. This procedure sometimes is useful for measuring the left ventricular pressure in patients with valvular aortic stenosis or in postoperative patients with prosthetic valves in both the aortic and mitral positions.

CARDIAC ANGIOGRAPHY **Right side of heart** Selective injection of radiopaque contrast media (solutions of organic iodides of high sodium content) at various sites within the right side of the heart also may be performed during cardiac catheterization. Injections into the superior or inferior vena cava are useful for detecting the thickened right atrial wall of constrictive pericarditis and for defining certain congenital lesions such as Ebstein's malformation of the tricuspid valve and tricuspid atresia. Selective right ventriculography is used commonly in the delineation of congenital cardiac lesions such as pulmonic stenosis and tetralogy of Fallot. Injection into the main pulmonary artery permits visualization of pulmonary thromboemboli, congenital pulmonary arterial branch stenosis, and anomalous pulmonary venous connections, and may be useful in the detection of tumor or thrombus within the left atrium.

Left side of heart Selective left ventriculography is employed generally to define congenital and acquired lesions affecting the mitral valve and the left ventricular outflow tract and to assess the adequacy of left ventricular function. Mitral stenosis may be detected by left ventriculography as thickening and/or calcification of the valve leaflets, shortening of the chordal subvalvular apparatus, and reduced excursion and delayed closure of the leaflets. Mitral regurgitation may be detected and quantified subjectively by noting the amount and density of contrast agent which enters the left atrium (Fig. 235-1). In addition, systolic prolapse into the left atrium of one or both of the mitral valve leaflets, secondary to either chordal malfunction or primary myxomatous degeneration and redundancy of the leaflets themselves, may be identified. The site of discrete subvalvular, valvular, or supravalvular aortic stenosis may be visualized, and the abnormal apposition of the ventricular septum and the anterior mitral valve leaflet in hypertrophic subaortic stenosis can be defined. Congenital lesions such as the anomalous origin of the pulmonary artery from the left ventricle in d-transposition of the great vessels are also confirmed by left ventriculography.

Both regional as well as global left ventricular function can be determined from analysis of the left ventricular cavity silhouette on the left ventriculogram. Regions of absent contraction (akinesia), reduced contraction (hypokinesia), or paradoxical systolic expansion (dyskinesia), as well as frank aneurysm formation, can thereby be detected and assessed as to severity (Fig. 235-2). Mural thrombi also may be visualized within such areas of wall motion disorder. In addition, by determination of a magnification factor, the area of the left ventricular cavity can be measured accurately, and by assumption of a geometric model of an ellipse, the volume of the chamber at end-diastole and end-systole can be determined (Fig. 235-1), and the total stroke volume can be calculated. The total stroke volume minus the forward stroke volume (calculated by an independent method for determining cardiac output, as discussed below), can then be used to derive the amount of aortic or mitral regurgitation per beat.

Values for end-diastolic volume greater than 90 ml per m^2 body surface area (average normal, plus one standard deviation) generally indicate left ventricular dilatation due to heart failure, or to a volume overload such as occurs in aortic regurgitation. The ejection fraction, the ratio of stroke volume to end-diastolic volume, reflects the percent shortening of the left ventricular myocardium (normal range 0.56 to 0.78). When the ejection fraction is reduced, the presence of depressed left ventricular contractile function is suggested. A further useful index of myocardial function is the mean velocity of circumferential fiber shortening (mean Vcf) or the fractional shortening per unit time of the minor axis of the left ventricular chamber (Fig.

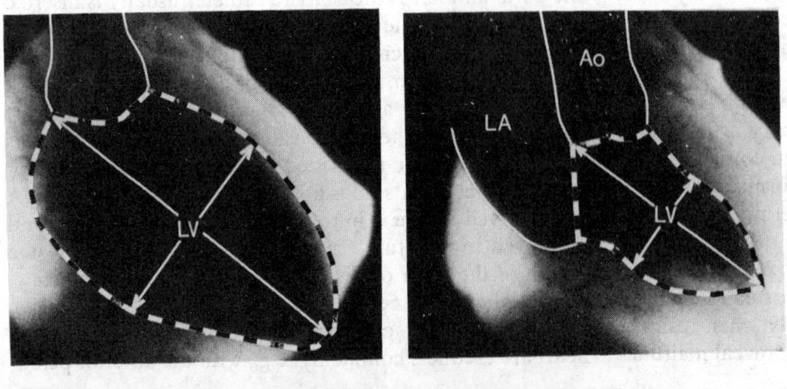

FIGURE 235-1
Cineangiogram with injection of contrast medium into the left ventricle (LV). End-diastole is on the left and end-systole on the right. Study is performed in the right anterior oblique projection in a patient with severe mitral regurgitation in whom the left atrium (LA) is densely opacified simultaneously with the aorta (Ao) during ventricular systole.

Volume of LV is determined by planimetry of chamber area (enclosed by dashed line) and measurement of longest length (solid line between base and apex), using a geometric model of an ellipsoid. Thus, $D = 4A/\Pi L$ *and* $V = \Pi(D^2 L/6)$ *where D = calculated diameter, L = longest measured length, A = area, and V = LV volume.*

Mean velocity of circumferential fiber shortening (mean Vcf, normalized to per unit circumference) can also be calculated by direct measurement of the minor axis (indicated by line with arrows) perpendicular to the midpoint of the long axis, and determination of the ejection time from cine frame rate and number of frames exposed from the beginning to the end of ejection.

$$\text{Mean } Vcf = \frac{\text{end-diastolic } D - \text{end-systolic } D}{\text{end-diastolic } D \times \text{ejection time}}$$

where D = minor axis diameter

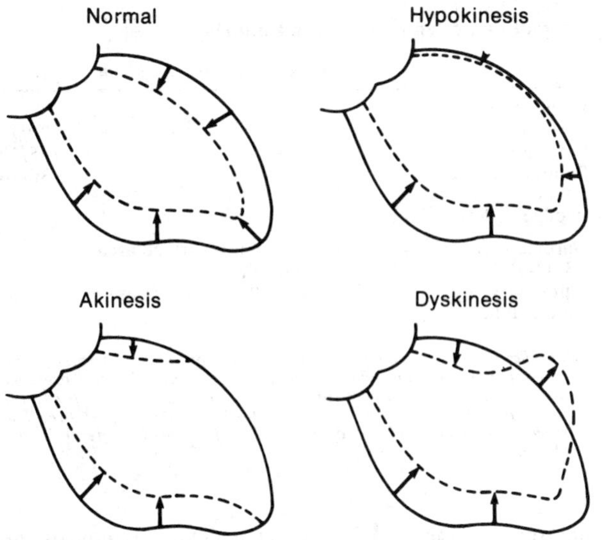

FIGURE 235-2
Diagrammatic representation of end-diastolic (solid line) and end-systolic (dashed line) silhouettes of left ventricular cineangiograms in various forms of localized wall motion disorders. Normal patient exhibits relatively symmetrical contraction; patient with hypokinesis exhibits reduced contraction over anterior and apical surfaces; patient with dyskinesis exhibits paradoxic, outward movement over anterior surface during systole.

235-1). Mean Vcf values below 1.2 end-diastolic circumferences per second are considered indicative of depressed myocardial contractility. (Other measures of depressed contractility are discussed below under intravascular pressures.)

Selective ascending aortography is used for assessing the severity of aortic regurgitation, for determining the size and location of aortic aneurysms, and for the visualization of less-common malformations such as sinus of Valsalva aneurysm. Direct injection into the left atrium has been used to study the movement of the mitral valve as well as to detect thrombi and tumors (myxoma) within that chamber.

Coronary arteriography Selective angiographic visualization of the coronary arterial tree was proved to be feasible and acceptably safe in the early 1960s, and it has since become one of the most commonly applied diagnostic procedures in the cardiac catheterization laboratory. Accurate visualization of coronary artery atherosclerotic lesions has significantly increased understanding of the pathogenesis and natural history of coronary heart disease. Moreover, this procedure has contributed in large measure to the advent of surgical procedures for bypassing obstructive lesions within the coronary arteries. Visualization of coronary artery anatomy is useful, likewise, for defining congenital abnormalities such as anomalous origin of the coronary arteries, or a coronary arteriovenous fistula.

Coronary arteriography is performed by the selective injection of 5 to 10 ml contrast medium directly into each coronary artery orifice with cinefilming at 30 to 60 frames per s and/or large film or photospot exposures at 4 to 6 per s, thereby obtaining dynamic as well as high-resolution images of the coronary arterial tree. Specially designed catheters are used: one type, which has an open, tapered tip and multiple side holes, is inserted via a brachial arteriotomy (Sones technique); another type is advanced over a guide wire inserted percutaneously via the femoral artery and is preshaped to allow ready access to the right or left coronary artery orifices (Judkins technique). Both techniques allow injections to be made with the patient in multiple oblique views and provide visualization of obstructive lesions within the main branches of the coronary vessels (Figs. 235-3*A* and *B*). In addition, collateral vessels, or new vascular pathways which serve to carry blood around a significant obstruction, can often be seen, and the vessel beyond a complete obstruction thereby visualized (Fig. 235-3*C*). The latter finding has obvious importance in determining the site for implantation of the distal end of a bypass graft.

COMPLICATIONS It is generally recognized that cardiac catheterization and angiography are invasive procedures which are associated unavoidably, although uncommonly, with serious complications. Nevertheless, diagnostic cardiac catheterization procedures have been increasingly applied in recent years, primarily in response to the need for precise functional and anatomic information prior to carrying out cardiac operations. A comprehensive analysis of the incidence and types of complications of cardiac catheterization and angiography, a cooperative prospective 5-year study, was reported in 1968, and the incidence of important complications in patients of all ages (including cardiac perforation, major arrhythmias, hemorrhage, serious hypotension, vascular thrombosis, cerebral embolism, myocardial infarction, as well as death) was 3.6 percent. The mortality rate was 0.3 percent in patients over sixty years of age but was 0.05 percent in patients between the ages of five and fourteen years. Nearly 24 percent of all reported complications occurred in infants under one year of age, although they constituted only 9 percent of the total population, and mortality under age 60 days was 6 percent. In recent years, however, in the pediatric age group greater attention has been paid to preventing metabolic disorders (hypoxia and acidemia) and pulmonary difficulties, utilization of smaller amounts of contrast agents, and use of more flexible catheters; such precautions have significantly reduced the incidence of major complications and decreased the overall mortality rate in infants markedly. In adults, the advent of coronary artery bypass graft surgery has brought about a marked predominance in the application of coronary arteriography and left ventriculography by retrograde aortic catheterization, compared with other catheterization procedures. A nationwide survey of complications due to coronary arteriography reported in 1973 showed an overall mortality rate of 0.45 percent and a morbidity rate of 4.1 percent. However, both mortality and morbidity figures were significantly less in cardiac laboratories where a large number of examinations were performed, and also varied with the approach employed, mortality with the percutaneous femoral artery approach being considerably higher than with brachial arteriotomy. For example, in institutions performing over 200 studies per year, mortality with the brachial approach averaged

0.13 percent, and with the femoral approach it averaged 0.47 percent. It seems clear that specialized invasive cardiac procedures in any age group should be performed only in well-equipped laboratories by highly experienced personnel, and the risks of cardiac catheterization and angiography should be weighed carefully in relation to the potential therapeutic benefits to be derived from an accurate anatomic and functional diagnosis.

MEASUREMENT OF INTRAVASCULAR PRESSURES

The pressures within the great vessels and chambers of the heart ordinarily are measured by means of a catheter-transducer system. The tip of the cardiac catheter is in communication with the transducer by means of the fluid column contained within the catheter lumen. A number of factors, such as movement of the catheter and the presence of air bubbles, can influence the dynamic accuracy of these catheter-transducer systems, and miniature pressure gages attached directly to the tip of the cardiac catheter are finding increasing application. These microtransducers have frequency-response characteristics greatly superior to those of conventional catheter-transducer systems.

INTRACARDIAC PRESSURE PULSES The upper limits of normal for intracardiac pressures and certain other hemodynamic variables are shown in Table 235-1. In understanding the contours of the intracardiac pressure pulses, thorough knowledge of the temporal relations between the electrical and mechanical events of the cardiac cycle is important (see Fig. 234-2). Although detailed study of the contours of the atrial pressure pulses has proved less reliable in predicting relative degrees of mitral valve stenosis and regurgitation than once was anticipated, a general understanding of the atrial pressure pulses is useful in the hemodynamic evaluation of a number of cardiac lesions.

The A wave in the right atrium normally is larger than the V wave, whereas in the left atrium the V wave is dominant (Table 235-1). Therefore, when the V wave in the right atrial pressure pulse exceeds the A wave, abnormal filling of the right atrium during ventricular systole, as occurs in tricuspid regurgitation or atrial septal defect, should be suspected. A characteristic right atrial pressure pulse also may be seen in the presence of tricuspid stenosis, the contour resembling that of mitral stenosis (see below), as well as in constrictive pericarditis, when an early diastolic "dip" and "plateau" elevation of pressure in mid- and late diastole occur. In many patients, the *mean* level of pressure in the left atrium is reflected with reasonable accuracy by the pulmonary artery wedge pressure (also sometimes termed the pulmonary "capillary" pressure), although the excursions of the wedge tracing often do not coincide with those measured directly within the left atrium. The characteristic contours of the left atrial pressure pulse in a normal subject and in patients with several forms of mitral valve disease

TABLE 235-1
Normal hemodynamic values,* mmHg

	A wave	*V wave*	*Mean*	*S/D*
Right atrium	8	7	6	
Right ventricle				30/7
Left ventricle				145/12
Pulmonary artery			17	30/14
Pulmonary artery wedge or left atrium	10	15	12	

Cardiac index = 2.4–3.8 L/min/m² body surface area.
AV O_2 difference: 3.5–5.0 ml/100 ml.
Pulmonary vascular resistance: 250 dynes/s/cm^{-5} (3 resistance units).

* *The figures shown indicate the upper limits of pressure (mmHg) and resistance in normal adult subjects. The values for the pressure waves, the mean pressures, and the systolic and diastolic pressures (S/D) are shown; in the ventricles, D = end-diastolic pressure. The ranges for cardiac index and arterial-mixed venous O_2 differences are shown.*

FIGURE 235-3
Selective coronary arteriograms obtained in the right anterior oblique projection. A *and* B *show a normal subject and* C *a patient with severe stenosis of the right coronary artery. LMCA, left main coronary artery; CCA, circumflex coronary artery; LADCA, left anterior descending coronary artery; RCA, right coronary artery. In* C, *arrow 1 indicates the area of narrowing in the right coronary artery, and arrow 2 shows retrograde filling of the anterior descending coronary artery via collateral vessels, indicating that a severe obstruction is present in that vessel as well. (Courtesy of Melvin P. Judkins, Loma Linda University, Loma Linda, Calif.)*

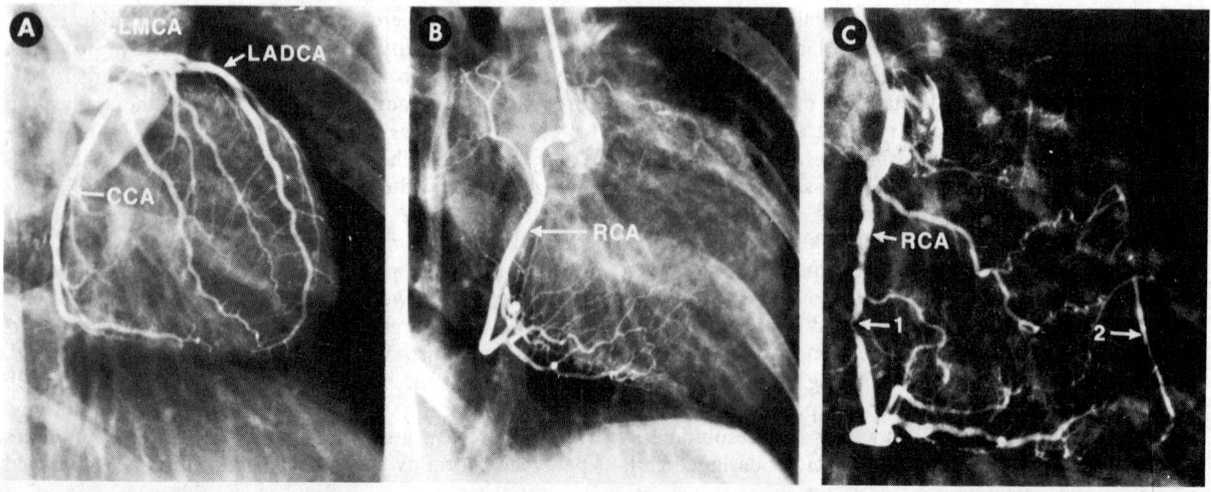

are shown in Fig. 235-4. In the normal pressure pulse, or in the presence of mitral regurgitation without stenosis, there is a rapid fall in pressure during early diastole (the Y descent), and a slow rise in pressure occurs during late diastole (diastasis), reflecting equilibration between the atrial and ventricular pressures during this slow phase of ventricular filling (Fig. 235-4*A*). In contrast, in patients with mitral stenosis the Y descent is slow and prolonged; pressure in the left atrium continues to fall throughout diastole, and evidence of diastasis on the left atrial pressure pulse is absent because of the persistent atrioventricular pressure gradient (Fig. 235-4*B*). When mitral stenosis is present with normal sinus rhythm (Fig. 235-4*C*), the A wave is present, and a large pressure gradient accompanies atrial contraction (often associated with a loud presystolic murmur in such patients). In patients with pure mitral regurgitation, the V wave is prominent and the descending limb of this wave (the Y descent) is rapid (Fig. 235-4*D*).

The left ventricular end-diastolic pressure immediately precedes the onset of isometric contraction in the left ventricular pressure pulse. This pressure point therefore follows the A wave and precedes the C wave, and the coincident pressure point in time in the left atrial tracing is termed the Z point (Fig. 235-4*A*). The left ventricular end-diastolic pressure may be elevated in several situations: (1) in the presence of myocardial failure, (2) when the ventricle bears a high flow load (as in aortic regurgitation), (3) when the ventricle is hypertrophied and relatively noncompliant (restrictive myocardial disease), and (4) in the presence of constrictive pericarditis.

The systolic pressure in the left ventricle is elevated over that in the aorta when any of the various forms of aortic stenosis obstruct outflow. In patients with valvular aortic stenosis, the left ventricular pressure pulse resembles that of an isometric contraction, the contour being more sym-

FIGURE 235-4
Simultaneously recorded left ventricular (LV) *and left atrial* (LA) *pressure tracings in a normal subject* (A) *and in patients with various forms of mitral valve disease* (B *to* D). *The tracings are recorded at high sensitivity (0 to 40 mmHg), and therefore the top portion of the left ventricular pressure tracing is cut off. The electrocardiogram is recorded in the upper portion of each panel.*

A *In the normal heart, diastole is initiated by a rapid-filling wave, which is followed by a period of slow ventricular filling or diastasis (bracket D), in which atrial and ventricular pressure rise together slowly. This period of diastasis is followed by the atrial contraction wave (A), which precedes the onset of isometric contraction in the ventricle, the end-diastolic pressure. The C wave occurs during the phase of isometric ventricular contraction and is followed by the X descent. The V wave occurs during late systole and the downslope of the V wave, constituting the Y descent, occurs immediately after opening of the mitral valve.*

B *Tracings obtained in a patient with mitral stenosis and atrial fibrillation. The pressure gradient from left atrium to left ventricle during diastole is indicated by the diagonally shaded area. The A wave is absent, and the CV wave is prominent.*

C *Tracings from a patient with mitral stenosis and normal sinus rhythm. The pressure gradient is indicated by the diagonally shaded area. A large pressure gradient occurs at the time of atrial contraction. No pressure rise during the period of diastasis is evident in the left atrial pressure tracings of panels* B *and* C.

D *Tracings from a patient with isolated, severe mitral regurgitation and atrial fibrillation. The C wave is not evident, and the giant V wave in the left atrial pressure pulse is nearly 70 mmHg. There is small pressure gradient during the phase of rapid ventricular filling, because of the large volume of antegrade flow across the mitral valve.*

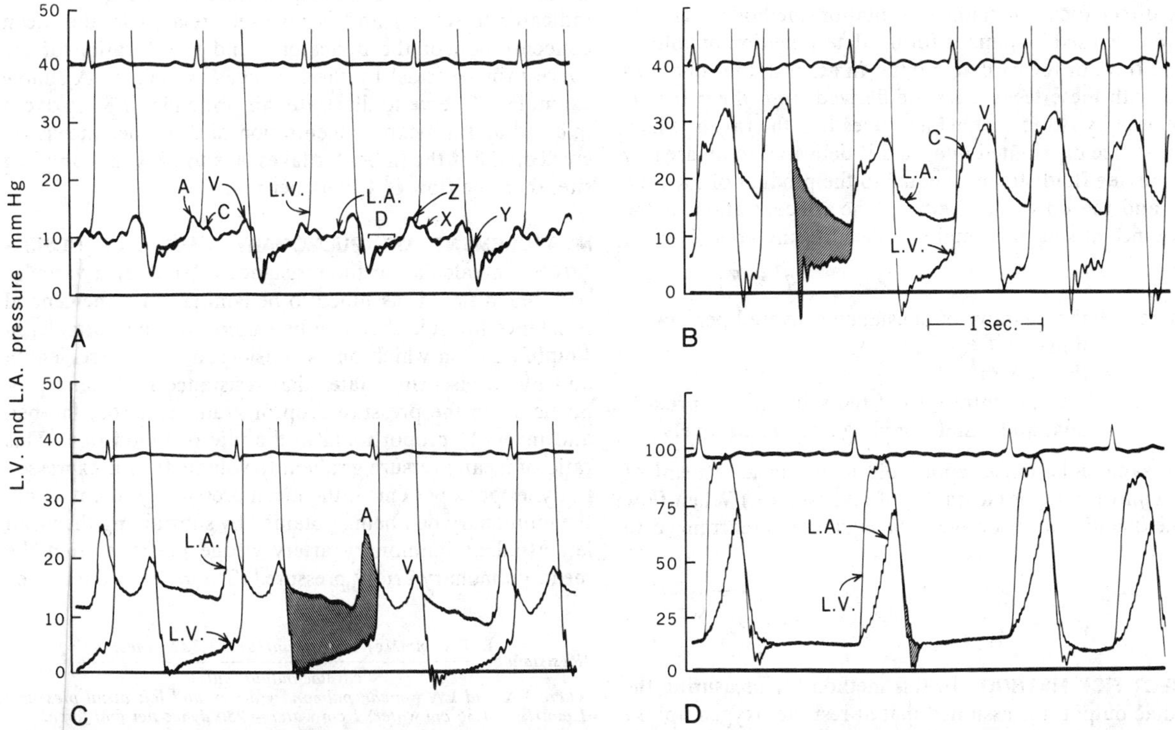

metric and the pressure peak more delayed than normal (a similar phenomenon is observed in the right ventricle in patients with pulmonic stenosis). The characteristics of the peripheral arterial pressure tracing also may be distinctive in patients with different types of aortic stenosis. Thus, when valvular stenosis is present, a slow and delayed rise of the peripheral arterial pulse wave is seen, while in hypertrophic subaortic stenosis an initially sharp upstroke is followed first by a rapid decline in pressure and then by a secondary positive wave, which reflects the development of the obstruction during systole.

Derivatives of pressure pulses The rate of change, or slope, of the isovolumetric phase of the right or left ventricular pressure pulse, often called the first derivative or *dp/dt*, frequently is used in addition to ejection phase measures mentioned above (ejection fraction, mean Vcf) to characterize the contractile behavior of the ventricular myocardium. The *dp/dt* may be measured manually by determining the slope of the pressure rise, but it is recorded more accurately by means of an electronic circuit or by computer processing. The peak of this derivative tracing (maximum *dp/dt*) as well as the maximum value of the ratio of *dp/dt* to the corresponding instantaneous ventricular pressure [peak $(dp/dt)/p$] provide indexes of the speed of contraction of the ventricle and therefore can help to define the level of the inotropic or contractile state of the heart. These measures tend to be below 1,200 mmHg per s and 32 s^{-1}, respectively, in the left ventricles of patients with disease of the left ventricular myocardium, and they may be augmented strikingly by agents which improve the contractility of the heart, such as digitalis or catecholamines.

MEASUREMENT OF CARDIAC OUTPUT

The direct Fick and indicator-dilution methods presently are widely used in humans for the determination of volume blood flow, or the cardiac output. In general, the equations used with these techniques are derived from the principle proposed by Adolf Fick which states that the rate at which a substance distributed in a fluid is delivered to an area by the moving fluid stream is equal to the product of the flow rate and the difference between the concentration of the substance at sites proximal and distal to the area. Thus,

$$q = F(C_a - C_v)$$

where q = the quantity of substance delivered per unit time
F = the flow rate
$C_a - C_v$ = the concentrations of the substance at proximal and distal sampling sites, respectively

(The same equation is applicable to the measurement of the removal rate, or clearance, of a substance.) When flow is the quantity to be derived, the equation is rearranged to

$$F = \frac{q}{C_a - C_v}$$

DIRECT FICK METHOD In this method for measuring the cardiac output it is assumed that at rest the oxygen uptake in the lungs is equal to that used by the tissues, and systemic flow, i.e., left ventricular output, therefore is equated with blood flow through the lungs. It is essential to this method that a sample of mixed venous blood be obtained, because blood samples in the venae cavae and the coronary sinus have widely differing oxygen concentrations, and therefore the venous blood sample generally is withdrawn from the right ventricular outflow tract or the pulmonary artery. In practice, arterial and venous blood samples ($C_a - C_v$) are obtained during the measurement of oxygen consumption, q, over a 3-min period by spirometry and subsequent chemical analysis of the expired gas. Flow F or cardiac output is then calculated. The subject must be in a steady state throughout the period of measurement to avoid transient changes in systemic blood flow or in the rate of ventilation that can negate the assumption that oxygen uptake in the lungs equals that taken up in the tissues.

INDICATOR-DILUTION METHOD This is a special application of Fick's principle. A variety of relatively nondiffusible indicators have been employed, the indicator substance being injected into the circulation and its concentration measured at a downstream sampling site by a suitable detector. For example, the dye indocyanine green is injected intravenously and blood is withdrawn from an artery at a constant rate through a calibrated densitometer, which provides direct measurement of the dye concentration. Generally, a single bolus of the indicator is injected rapidly and is thoroughly mixed in one of the vascular spaces such as a ventricular chamber; the concentration versus time curve then provides a measure of the rate at which indicator was washed out of the mixing site. Prior to recirculation of the indicator, the downslope of this curve is exponential, and therefore extrapolation of the curve using semilog paper permits the elimination of recirculated indicator. The mean concentration $\bar{c}$ of the dye is determined from the area of this corrected curve and its duration. The rate of blood flow F then is directly related to the quantity of indicator injected i and is inversely related to the mean concentration of the indicator $\bar{c}$ and the duration of the curve t (in seconds) by the formula $F = 60i/\bar{c}t$. A simple example will serve to illustrate this principle: if 8 mg dye is injected and a mean concentration of 2 mg per liter is recorded, and if the indicator takes 60 s to pass the sampling site, then the flow is 4 liters per min.

MEASUREMENT OF PULMONARY VASCULAR RESISTANCE In calculating the resistance offered by a vascular bed, blood flow is assumed to be laminar, and the general resistance formula then can be employed. This formula, in simplified form which omits consideration of vessel length and blood viscosity, states that resistance is directly proportional to the pressure drop or gradient across the bed and inversely proportional to the rate of blood flow. This ratio of mean pressure gradient to volume flow is expressed in dynes per s per cm^{-5}, the mean pressure gradient across the pulmonary bed being obtained by subtracting the mean left atrial or pulmonary artery wedge pressure from the mean pulmonary artery pressure.[1] The *resistance unit* (i.e.,

[1] $\text{Resistance} = \dfrac{\text{PA (mmHg)} - \text{LA (mmHg)} \times 1{,}332 \text{ dynes/cm}^2}{\text{cardiac output (ml/s)}}$

where PA *and* LA *= mean pulmonary artery and left atrial pressures. 1 mmHg = 1.36 cm water; 1 cm water = 980 dynes per cm² force.*

the pressure gradient in millimeters of mercury divided by the cardiac output in liters per minute and expressed in arbitrary units) also is commonly employed as an index of arteriolar resistance (Table 235-1). Estimation of the pulmonary vascular resistance, which normally is about 15 percent of that in the systemic vascular bed, is of importance in patients with congenital heart disease and circulatory shunts, as well as in certain forms of acquired cardiac and pulmonary diseases. Its calculation provides a useful means of interpreting the level of pulmonary arterial pressure relative to pulmonary blood flow, high pressure and high flow obviously bearing a different connotation than high pressure and low flow.

VALVE ORIFICE SIZE AND VALVULAR REGURGITATION

When the cardiac output is normal, the severity of a stenotic valve lesion may be estimated from the magnitude of the pressure gradient across the valve. When the cardiac output is elevated or reduced, however, reliance on the pressure gradient alone may lead to an erroneous estimate of the degree of mechanical obstruction. In addition, it is of importance to consider the heart rate in assessing the significance of a pressure gradient. When the heart rate is rapid, systole occupies a disproportionate amount of time in each cardiac cycle, diastole filling time is limited, and a large pressure gradient across the atrioventricular valve may exist in the face of relatively mild stenosis. The application of the hydraulic formula devised by Gorlin and Gorlin to the calculation of valve orifice size has proved helpful in analyzing the degree of valve stenosis in these situations. In simplest terms, this formula states that the area of a short-bore orifice is directly proportional to the rate of blood flow across the orifice and inversely proportional to the square root of the pressure gradient. For example, if the flow rate across a narrowed valve orifice of fixed size doubles, as may occur when the cardiac output increases during exertion, the pressure gradient will quadruple. Conversely, when the flow rate is reduced, as in patients with heart failure, a small pressure gradient may exist in the presence of a severe degree of valve stenosis. This relationship differs from the general resistance equation discussed above and reflects the fact that the kinetic energy losses across a stenotic valve are high, a large pressure head being expended in developing a rapid flow velocity across the narrowed orifice.

It should be pointed out that use of the orifice formula is not valid when significant valvular regurgitation is present and forward cardiac output alone is measured, since an unknown volume of blood is regurgitated and recrosses the valve during the subsequent cardiac cycle. Application of the formula under these circumstances leads to an underestimation of the valve orifice area, since forward flow across the valve is underestimated.

DIAGNOSIS OF CIRCULATORY SHUNTS

When a communication exists between the left and the right sides of the heart, and when pulmonary vascular resistance is lower than that in the systemic vascular bed, a left-to-right shunt of oxygenated blood will occur. Conversely, when the resistance in the pulmonary bed is higher than that in the systemic circulation, or an obstruction such as pulmonic stenosis exists distal to an intracardiac communication, a right-to-left shunt of venous blood may occur. These shunts can be readily visualized and localized by exposure of cineangiograms during selective injections of contrast medium.

Many types of indicators have been employed in the quantification and detection of circulatory shunts. The indicator may be the oxygen in room air, blood samples being withdrawn and analyzed for oxygen manometrically or by an oximeter. Foreign, inert gases such as hydrogen or krypton-85 may be employed; these, like oxygen, are "injected" into the pulmonary circulation by inhalation and sampled from the right side of the heart. They may be measured by a catheter-tip sensor (hydrogen) or by withdrawal of blood samples for analysis. In obtaining indicator-dilution curves, the substance most commonly injected is indocyanine green dye, detected by withdrawing blood through a densitometer.

The techniques used for localizing and quantifying shunts at cardiac catheterization may be divided into two basic categories: (1) Those methods in which an indicator is delivered distal to the site at which blood is sampled (the so-called upstream sampling method), e.g., indicator is injected into the pulmonary artery or is inhaled to enter the pulmonary veins and left side of the heart. Blood samples are then obtained upstream in the right side of the heart and analyzed for concentration of the indicator. (2) Those methods in which an indicator is delivered proximal to the sampling site (the so-called downstream sampling method), in which most frequently an indicator-dilution curve is obtained by intracardiac dye injection with sampling from a peripheral artery. This approach permits detection of right-to-left as well as left-to-right shunts.

UPSTREAM SAMPLING METHOD Blood samples are withdrawn in serial fashion from the pulmonary artery, right ventricle, right atrium, and venae cavae, the indicator being introduced downstream (in the case of oxygen into the lungs). This approach permits localization of the site of a left-to-right shunt. With the oxygen sampling method, a step-up of 2.0 ml per 100 ml from the venae cavae to the right atrium, of 1.0 ml per 100 ml from the right atrium to the right ventricle, or of 0.5 ml per 100 ml from the right ventricle to the pulmonary artery, is considered to be evidence of a left-to-right shunt. The use of a foreign gas improves the sensitivity of this approach, even a small left-to-right shunt being readily detected by appropriate sampling within the right side of the heart using a catheter-tip hydrogen electrode, for example.

For determination of the size of a left-to-right shunt, samples of venous blood proximal to the shunt and samples from the pulmonary artery and a systemic artery are obtained in close time sequence. The oxygen uptake at the lungs is measured simultaneously, or estimated, and the pulmonary and systemic blood flow rates (and hence the magnitude of the left-to-right shunt relative to systemic flow) can be calculated using Fick's equations. Generally a pulmonary to systemic flow ratio of 1.5:1 or greater is considered to indicate a left-to-right shunt of substantial magnitude.

DOWNSTREAM SAMPLING METHOD A needle is placed

into a systemic artery and a time-concentration curve is recorded following upstream injection of the indicator. This technique is particularly useful for localizing the site of a right-to-left shunt. For example, when a right-to-left shunt exists at the ventricular level, an injection into the right ventricle and at all sites proximal to the right ventricle will result in an early appearance time of dye that has immediately traversed the defect (Fig. 235-5). However, an injection into the pulmonary artery, distal to the right-to-left shunt, shows a normal appearance time. A left-to-right shunt also may be detected, but not localized, by injection of indicator into the right side of the heart using peripheral arterial sampling. The indicator-dilution curve will show a reduced peak concentration of dye and a break on the downslope when compared with a normal indicator-dilution curve (Fig. 235-5). This contour occurs because a portion of the indicator traverses the left-to-right shunt during its initial passage to the left side of the heart, recirculates rapidly through the right side of the heart and lungs, and reappears at the peripheral artery before the downslope of the primary curve has been completely inscribed.

OTHER SPECIAL MEASUREMENT TECHNIQUES Miniaturization of electronics has permitted the construction and application of cardiac catheters with special measuring devices mounted on, or close to, the tip. For example, a catheter-tip micromanometer permits the measurement of intracardiac pressure free of the artifacts produced by fluid filled manometer systems and catheter motion. Accurate high-fidelity pressure measurements are of particular utility in the assessment of the contractile and distensibility properties of the left ventricle. Micromanometer-tipped catheters also can be used for highly sensitive recordings of intracardiac sounds, murmurs, and clicks. In fact, an intracardiac phonocardiogram in the right ventricle is perhaps the most reliable method for documenting pulmonic insufficiency as the source of a diastolic, decrescendo murmur along the left sternal border. Other special catheters have been designed to record the intracardiac electrocardiogram and have made it possible to record selective potentials from the right atrium, right ventricle, and along the bundle of His. Recordings from the latter area are useful, for example, in determining whether a conduction delay or block on the surface electrocardiogram is located at or below the atrioventricular junction. His bundle recordings also have improved understanding of the mechanisms underlying paroxysmal atrial tachycardia and the preexcitation syndromes. Electromagnetic or ultrasonic catheter-tip velocity probes also are available and have proved useful for study of phasic blood flow patterns in the venae cavae and pulmonary artery in patients with constrictive pericarditis and cardiac tamponade, and for analysis of the pattern and velocity of left ventricular ejection into the ascending aorta in patients with disorders of left ventricular function.

FIGURE 235-5
Diagrammatic representation of indicator-dilution curves using the downstream sampling method. The time of injection (Inj.) of an indicator, such as cardiogreen dye, is indicated by the arrow and by the square wave response on the recorded tracing. With right atrial (RA) injection and sampling at a peripheral artery, the normal appearance time is about 8 s, and the normal contour of the indicator-dilution curve is represented by the solid line. In a patient with a right-to-left (R-L) shunt at the atrial, ventricular, or pulmonary arterial levels, early appearance time of the dye is indicated by the dashed line. In a patient with a left-to-right (L-R) shunt, the appearance time need not be altered, but there is a reduced peak concentration of dye, and a break on the downslope, indicating early recirculation of the indicator.

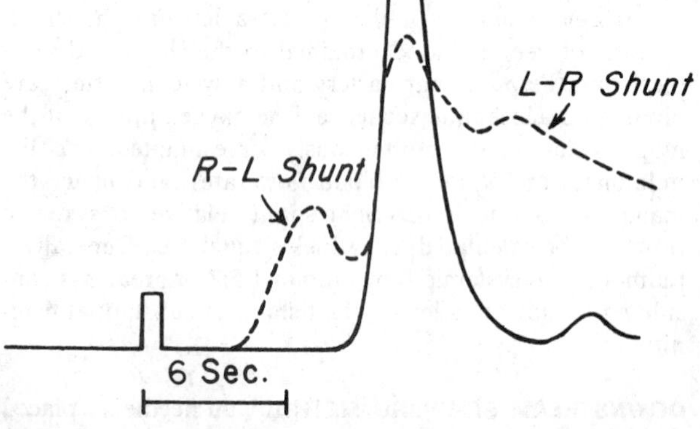

STRESS TESTING Exercise in the supine position using a bicycle ergometer may be performed during cardiac catheterization and can provide important information concerning the ability of the heart to respond to this mode of stress. For example, certain patients with heart disease may have normal intracardiac pressures at rest but exhibit an abnormal elevation of ventricular diastolic or atrial mean pressures during exercise. Similarly, the cardiac output at rest may be normal, but the exercise factor (the increase in cardiac output per 100 ml increase in total body oxygen consumption) may be reduced (normal equals 600 ml or greater), indicating a compromised cardiac reserve. Infusion of a pressor agent also has been employed to test the cardiac response to increased afterload. Electrical pacing of the heart to induce mild tachycardia may be used to induce ischemic changes in the electrocardiogram in patients with coronary heart disease.

REFERENCES

ABRAMS HL: *Angiography,* 2d ed., Boston: Little, Brown, 1971

ADAMS F et al: The complications of coronary arteriography. Circulation 48:609, 1973

BRAUNWALD E, SWAN HJC: *Cooperative Study on Cardiac Catheterization* (monograph), New York: The American Heart Association, 1968

DODGE HT, BAXLEY WA: Left ventricular volume and mass and their significance in heart disease. Am J Cardiol 23:528, 1969

GROSSMAN W (ed): *Cardiac Catheterization and Angiography,* Philadelphia: Lea & Febiger, 1974

SHABETAI R, ADOLPH RJ: Principles of cardiac catheterization, chap. 5 in *Cardiac Diagnosis and Treatment,* 2d ed, ed NO Fowler, Hagerstown: Harper & Row, 1976, p. 84

SONES FM JR.: Cine coronary arteriography, chap. 24 in *The Heart*, 3d ed., ed JW Hurst, New York: McGraw-Hill, 1974, p. 377

TAKARO T et al: An analysis of deaths occurring in association with coronary arteriography. Am Heart J 86:587, 1973

236 DISORDERS OF MYOCARDIAL FUNCTION

EUGENE BRAUNWALD
JOHN ROSS, JR.
EDMUND H. SONNENBLICK

CELLULAR BASIS OF CARDIAC CONTRACTION

The myocardium is composed of individual striated muscle cells (fibers), normally 10 to 15 μm in diameter and 30 to 60 μm in length. Under the light microscope, each fiber is seen to contain multiple cross-banded strands (myofibrils), which run the length of the fiber and are composed of a serially repeating structure, the sarcomere. The remainder of the cytoplasm, lying between the myofibrils, contains other cell constituents, such as the single centrally located nucleus, numerous mitochondria, and intracellular membrane systems.

The sarcomere, the fundamental structural and functional unit of contraction, is delimited by two adjacent dark lines, the Z lines (Fig. 236-1). The distance between Z lines varies with the degree of contraction or stretch of the muscle and ranges between 1.5 and 2.2 μm. Within the confines of the sarcomere, alternating light and dark bands are seen, giving the myocardial fibers their striated appearance under the light microscope. At the center of the sarcomere is a broad dark band of constant width (1.5 μm), the A band, which is flanked by two lighter bands, the I bands, which are of variable width. The sarcomere of heart muscle, like that of skeletal muscle, is made up of two sets of myofilaments. Thicker filaments, composed principally of the protein myosin, traverse and are limited to the A band. They are about 100 Å in diameter, with tapered ends, and measure 1.5 to 1.6 μm in length. Thinner filaments, composed primarily of actin, course from the Z line through the I band into the A band. They are approximately 50 Å in diameter and 1.0 μm in length. Thus, there is overlapping of thick and thin filaments only within the A band, while the I band contains only thin filaments (Fig. 236-1). On electromicroscopy, bridges may be seen to extend between the thick and thin filaments within the confines of the A band.

The "sliding" model for muscle rests on the fundamental observation that both the thick and thin filaments are constant in overall length, both at rest and during contraction. With activation of the sarcomere, repetitive interactions take place at the bridges between the actin and myosin filaments, and the actin filaments are propelled further into the A band. In the process, the A band remains constant in width, whereas the I bands become more narrow and the Z lines move toward one another.

The myosin molecule is a complex, asymmetric fibrous protein with a molecular weight of about 500,000; it has a rodlike portion that is about 1500 Å in length with a globular portion at its end. This globular portion contains the ATPase activity and forms the bridges. In forming the thick myofilament, the rodlike portions of the myosin molecules are laid down in an orderly, polarized manner, leaving the globular portions projecting outward so that they can interact with actin to generate force and shortening. Actin has a molecular weight of 47,000. The thin filament is composed of a double helix of two chains of actin molecules wound about each other, intimately associated with the protein tropomyosin, which appears to form the central core of this filament. Another protein complex, troponin, which can be separated into three components, is located periodically along the actin filament. In contrast to myosin, actin has no intrinsic enzymatic activity, but it has the ability to combine reversibly with myosin in the presence of ATP and Mg^{2+}, which activates the myosin ATPase. In relaxed muscle this interaction is inhibited by one of the components of troponin. During activation, Ca^{2+} becomes attached to another of the components and removes this inhibition. As a result, ATP is split, and linkages between actin and myosin filaments are made and broken cyclically. Mechanical forces are generated by these reactions, with resultant shortening of the sarcomere.

The sarcoplasmic reticulum, a complex network of anastomosing, membrane-lined intracellular channels, which invests the myofibrils, and which is less profuse in cardiac than in skeletal muscle, consists of a series of interconnecting longitudinally disposed membrane tubules closely applied to the surfaces of the individual sarcomeres; it has no direct continuity with the outside of the cell. Closely related, both functionally and structurally, are the transverse tubules or T system, formed by tubelike invaginations of the sarcolemma, which extend into the myocardial fiber, along the Z lines, i.e., the ends of the sarcomeres.

At rest, the cardiac cell is polarized; i.e., the interior has a negative charge relative to the outside of the cell, with a transmembrane potential of −80 to −100 mV (Chap. 233). The sarcolemma, which in the resting state is largely impermeable to Na^+ and has a Na^+-K^+-stimulated pump requiring ATP which extrudes Na^+ from the cell, plays a critical role in establishing this resting potential. Thus, the inside of the cell contains mainly K^+ with little Na^+, while the extracellular milieu is high in $[Na^+]$ and low in $[K^+]$. At the same time, in the resting state, the extracellular $[Ca^{2+}]$ greatly exceeds the free intracellular $[Ca^{2+}]$.

During the plateau of the action potential (phase 2) there is a slow inward current which reflects a movement of Ca^{2+} into the myoplasm. However, the absolute quantity of Ca^{2+} that crosses the surface membrane is relatively small and in and of itself appears to be incapable of bringing about full activation of the contractile apparatus. However, the depolarizing current not only extends across the surface of the cell but penetrates deeply into the cell by way of the ramifying T system. A flux of Ca^{2+} as well as Na^+ into the cell takes place, which may then lead to depolarization of the sarcoplasmic reticulum; this in turn leads to the release of much larger quantities of Ca^{2+} from the sarcoplasmic reticulum.

The Ca^{2+} then diffuses toward the sarcomere, combines with troponin, and, by repressing the inhibitor of contraction, activates the myofilaments to produce contraction, the strength of which is dependent on the quantity of Ca^{2+} which reaches the contractile sites. The sarcoplasmic reticulum then appears to reaccumulate Ca^{2+}, thereby lowering its concentration in the myofibril to a level that inhibits the actin-myosin interaction which is responsible for contraction, and in this manner leads to relaxation. Thus, the cell membrane, transverse tubules, and the sarcoplasmic reticulum, with their ability to transmit an action potential, to release and then reaccumulate Ca^{2+}, appear to play a fundamental role in the rhythmic contraction and relaxation of heart muscle.

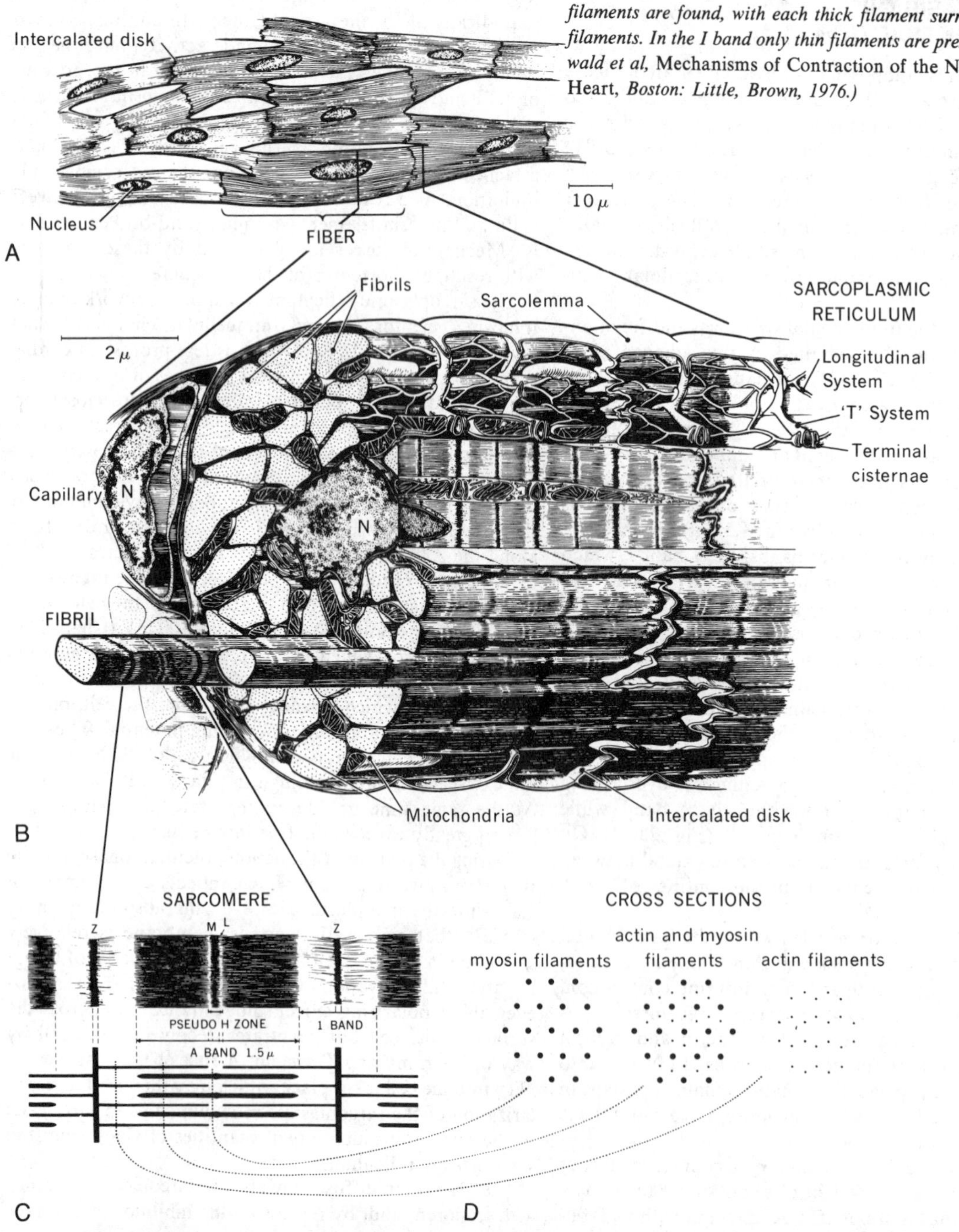

FIGURE 236-1

Microscopic structure of heart muscle. A *Myocardium as seen under the light microscope. Branching of fibers is evident. Each fiber, or cell, contains a centrally located nucleus.*

B *Myocardial cell, reconstructed from electron micrographs. Each cell is composed of multiple parallel fibrils. Each fibril is composed of serially connected sarcomeres (N, nucleus).*

C *Sarcomere from a myofibril, with diagrammatic representation of myofilaments. Thick filaments (1.5 μm long, composed of myosin) form the A band, and thin filaments (1 μm long, composed primarily of actin) extend from the Z line through the I band into the A band. The overlapping of thick and thin filaments is seen only in the A band.*

D *Cross sections of the sarcomere indicate the specific lattice arrangements of the myofilaments. In the center of the sarcomere only the thick, or myosin, filaments arranged in a hexagonal array are seen. In the distal portions of the A band, both thick and thin, or actin, filaments are found, with each thick filament surrounded by six thin filaments. In the I band only thin filaments are present. (From Braunwald et al,* Mechanisms of Contraction of the Normal and Failing Heart, *Boston: Little, Brown, 1976.)*

The ATP formed from substrate oxidation is the principal source of energy for almost all the work performed by the myocardial cell. In the normally functioning heart the major fraction of energy is expended in the mechanical work of contraction. The high-energy phosphate stores in ATP are in equilibrium with those in the form of creatine phosphate.

In all forms of striated muscle, including cardiac muscle, the force of contraction depends on initial muscle length. The sarcomere length associated with the most forceful contraction is 2.2 μm. It is at this length that the two sets of myofilaments of the sarcomere are most ideally situated to provide the greatest area for their interaction. In support of the sliding-filament hypothesis, force development diminishes in direct proportion to the decrease in the overlap between thick and thin filaments, and the resultant decrease in the number of reactive sites. At a sarcomere length of 3.65 μm, developed tension falls to zero, and it is at this point that the thin filaments are entirely withdrawn from the A band. Similarly, when the sarcomeres are shorter than 2.0 μm, the thin filaments bypass one another, producing a double overlap of the thin filaments (Fig. 236-2), and force also falls.

The relation between the initial length of the muscle fibers and the developed force is of prime importance for the function of heart muscle. This forms the basis of the Frank-Starling relation (Starling's law of the heart), which states that, within limits, an augmentation of initial volume of the ventricle, which is a function of the initial length of the muscle, results in an increase in the force of ventricular contraction. It has been shown for heart muscle that sarcomere length is directly proportional to muscle length along the ascending limb of the length–active tension curve. As muscle length decreases to the point at which developed tension approaches zero and at which sarcomere length approaches 1.5 μm, the I bands at first narrow, then disappear while the A band remains constant in length. At this latter point, the Z line abuts on the edges of the A band. Thus, the sarcomere length–active tension curve forms the ultrastructural basis of Starling's law of the heart.

FIGURE 236-2
Relation between sarcomere length and band patterns in skeletal muscle (frog sartorius). A *Band patterns as seen electromicroscopically.* B *Disposition of the thick and thin filaments that create band patterns. The vertical arrows in both panels denote the ends of the thin filaments that insert at the Z line at the left. Line 3 represents the sarcomere at the apex of the length-tension curve, i.e., at L_{max}. In lines 1 and 2, sarcomere length has been progressively decreased, whereas in 4 and 5 it has been progressively elongated. Throughout, the A band remains constant in width. The placement of filaments to provide for maximum overlap is shown in* B *(3). Line 1 shows the sarcomere pattern in the contracted muscle; the I band has disappeared, and a secondary dark band has been formed at the center of the sarcomere, termed the C contraction band, which is due to the passage of thin filaments through this area as in* B *(1). In* A *(4 and 5), an expanding H zone has appeared, owing to the withdrawal of the thin filaments from the A band, as shown diagrammatically in* B *(4 and 5). (From Braunwald et al,* Mechanisms of Contraction of the Normal and Failing Heart, *Boston: Little, Brown, 1976)*

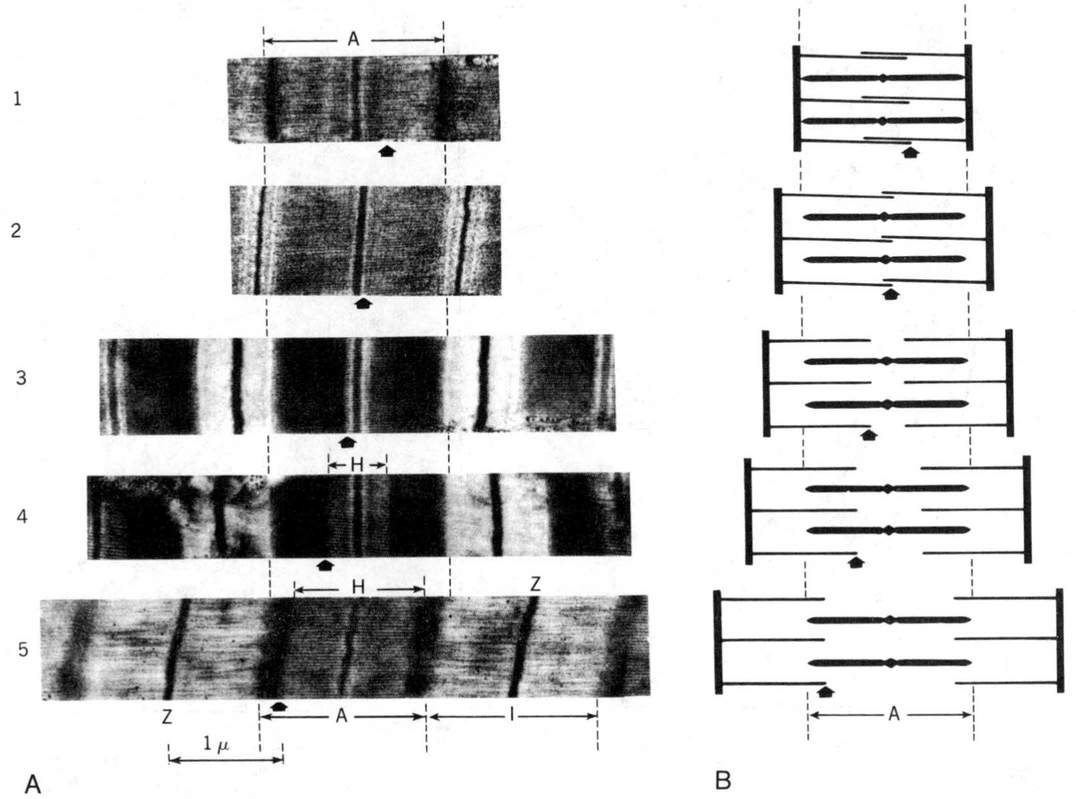

MYOCARDIAL MECHANICS

Extremely helpful methods for examining the behavior of muscle were provided by the skeletal muscle physiologists early in this century. The mechanical activity of all muscle may be expressed externally in only two ways: shortening and the development of tension. A. V. Hill showed in skeletal muscle that the velocity of shortening is inversely related to the magnitude of tension development, an expression of the so-called force-velocity relation, now acknowledged to be a fundamental property of muscle. Expressed simply, the greater the load the muscle is called upon to lift, the lower the velocity of shortening and vice versa. More recently, the concept of the force-velocity relation has been extended from skeletal to cardiac muscle. However, in this respect there is a basic difference between skeletal and cardiac muscle. Skeletal muscle has a single, essentially fixed, force-velocity curve; i.e., at any given muscle length, force and velocity are always related to each other in the same manner. The contractile activity of skeletal muscle is increased by the recruitment of additional muscle fibers, i.e., motor units, and by increasing the frequency of nerve impulses, while the contractility of each individual fiber remains constant. Although resting length also influences the characteristics of contraction, this variable remains essentially fixed in vivo. In contrast, the number of cardiac cells activated remains constant during each contraction. However, the contractile activity of the myocardium may be readily altered under physiologic conditions by changes in resting fiber length and by changes in the inotropic state, i.e., the contractility, both of which shift the myocardial force-velocity curve.

Variations in myocardial contractile activity may be expressed as displacements of the force-velocity curve. However, there are two fundamental ways in which the force-velocity curve can be shifted. Figure 236-3*A* shows a family of force-velocity curves obtained from an isolated cardiac muscle; each curve was obtained at a different preload, i.e., with a different degree of stretch on the muscle. Note that changing the preload alters the intercept of the force-velocity curve on the horizontal axis; i.e., it increases the isometric force developed by the muscle. However, within limits, these alterations in preload do not appear to alter the intrinsic velocity of shortening, since all the curves extrapolate to the same intercept on the vertical axis. Thus, a change in initial length of heart muscle shifts the force-velocity curve primarily by altering the total force which can be developed by the muscle, as illustrated by the isometric length-tension curve, shown in the insert of Fig. 236-3*A*.

This type of shift in the force-velocity curve may be contrasted with that obtained when a positive inotropic agent,

FIGURE 236-3

A *Effects of increasing initial muscle length on the force-velocity relation of the cat papillary muscle. Initial velocity of shortening has been plotted as a function of load for five different muscle lengths. The maximum velocity of shortening* (V_{max}) *is essentially unchanged, whereas the maximum force of contraction* (P_o) *is augmented. The insert shows the places along the length-tension curves at which these force-velocity curves were determined.* B *Effects of norepinephrine on the force-velocity relation of the cat papillary muscle. Both* V_{max} *and* Po_2 *have been increased. (From Braunwald et al,* Mechanisms of Contraction of Normal and Failing Heart, *Boston: Little, Brown, 1976)*

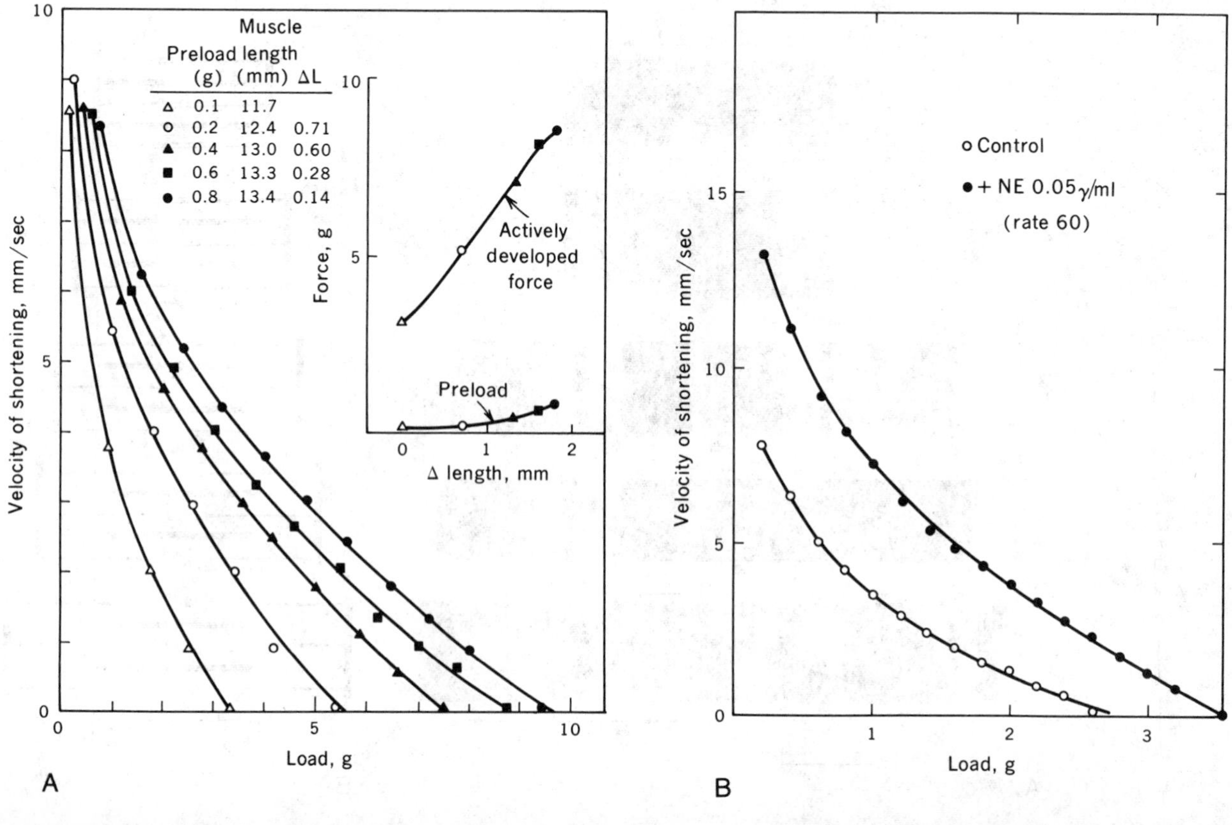

such as Ca^{2+}, digitalis, or norepinephrine, is added to the muscle while the initial length is held constant (Fig. 236-3*B*). These agents not only increase the force which the muscle is capable of lifting, i.e., the intercept of the force-velocity curve on the horizontal axis, therefore shifting the isometric length-tension curve upward, but also increase the velocity of shortening of the unloaded muscle, i.e., the extrapolated intercept on the vertical axis.

It has been postulated that an increase in initial muscle length brings about an increase in the number of effective force-generating sites without any alteration in the qualitative character of the cyclic process at these contractile sites. Such a change would be anticipated from a more advantageous overlap of interdigitating contractile filaments within the sarcomere. On the other hand, a change in the inotropic state, characterized by an increase in the velocity of shortening of the unloaded muscle, could result from an increase in the rate of cyclic force-generating processes at the contractile sites, without a change in the number of these sites, or alternatively from a greater number of sites that are activated. Increased contractility appears to be related to an increased availability of Ca^{2+} within the cell.

CONTRACTION OF THE INTACT VENTRICLE

Analysis of the heart as a pump has classically centered upon the relation between the filling pressure, or diastolic volume, of the ventricle (length of the muscle fibers) and its stroke volume (the Frank-Starling relation). It was shown clearly in the heart-lung preparation that the stroke volume is a function of diastolic fiber length, and that the failing heart delivers a smaller-than-normal stroke volume from a normal or elevated end-diastolic volume. Later, the concept of measuring stroke work (the product of stroke volume and mean aortic pressure) over a range of mean atrial or ventricular end-diastolic pressures, using one of these pressures as an index of diastolic volume, was expanded by Sarnoff and his collaborators. They concluded that this relation between the mean atrial or the ventricular end-diastolic pressure and the stroke work of the corresponding ventricle (the ventricular function curve) provided a definition of the level of the contractile, or inotropic, state of the ventricle. Significant increases in the level of ventricular contractility were accompanied by shifts of the ventricular function curve upward and to the left, while depression of contractility was identified by downward and rightward displacement of this relation.

Considerable effort also has been directed toward a study of the responses of the intact, unanesthetized animal, and it has been observed that during the adrenergic stimulation of the myocardium accompanying a stress such as exercise, relatively little change in ventricular end-diastolic size occurs, while minute cardiac output, aortic flow velocity, and the rate of ventricular pressure development are augmented. Thus, reflex and humorally mediated changes in myocardial contractility, heart rate, venous return, and peripheral vascular resistance may be more important in circulatory adaptation than changes in ventricular end-diastolic volume and the operation of the Frank-Starling mechanism.

The important influence of the neurotransmitter substance norepinephrine on the mechanical properties of the myocardium has long been recognized. Direct stimulation of the stellate ganglia has been shown to elevate the ventricular function curve, as a consequence of the release of norepinephrine from sympathetic nerve endings in the heart. In the intact animal, these adrenergic effects are evidenced by tachycardia, a reduction in cardiac dimensions, increased velocity of ejection, and an enhanced rate of tension development.

Surgically denervated hearts *in situ,* or isolated papillary muscles taken from such hearts, do not exhibit depression of their intrinsic inotropic state despite depletion of the norepinephrine stores within the sympathetic nerve endings of the muscle. The surgically or pharmacologically denervated heart of the intact organism, if otherwise normal, also appears capable of meeting many of the demands of muscular exercise. However, since it cannot be stimulated by neuronally released norepinephrine in the heart, the mechanisms by which the denervated heart increases its output differ from those of the intact animal. Thus, tachycardia is less marked, and the stroke volume and cardiac output rise more gradually than normal, and as a consequence of elevation of ventricular end-diastolic volume. In all these respects the activity of the heart muscle fiber differs from the activity of skeletal muscle fiber, the latter being totally dependent on its nerve supply and unable to contract effectively when denervated.

CONTROL OF CARDIAC PERFORMANCE AND OUTPUT

The extent of shortening of mammalian heart muscle and, therefore, the stroke volume of the intact ventricle are, in the final analysis, determined by four influences: (1) the length of the muscle at the start of contraction, i.e., the preload; (2) the inotropic state of the muscle, i.e., the position of its force-velocity-length relation or function curve; (3) the tension which the muscle is called upon to develop during contraction, i.e., the afterload; and (4) the heart rate, which determines the cardiac output at any stroke volume as long as ventricular filling is maintained.

VENTRICULAR END-DIASTOLIC VOLUME (PRELOAD) At any level of its inotropic state, the performance of the myocardium is influenced profoundly by ventricular end-diastolic fiber length and therefore by diastolic ventricular volume. The following are the major determinants of ventricular end-diastolic volume in the intact organism (see also Fig. 236-4).

1 *Total blood volume.* When depleted, as in hemorrhage, venous return to the heart declines and ventricular end-diastolic volume falls, as does ventricular performance, as reflected in ventricular work.
2 *Distribution of blood volume.* At any given total blood volume, the ventricular end-diastolic volume is influenced by the distribution of blood between the intra- and extrathoracic compartments. This distribution in turn is influenced by:
   a *Body position.* Gravitational forces tend to pool blood in dependent portions. The upright posture augments extrathoracic at the expense of intrathoracic blood volume, and reduces ventricular work.

b Intrathoracic pressure. Normally, mean intrathoracic pressure is negative, a factor which acts to increase thoracic blood volume and ventricular end-diastolic volume, particularly during inspiration. Elevation of intrathoracic pressure, as occurs in a tension pneumothorax, during the Valsalva maneuver, or in prolonged bouts of coughing, tends to impede venous return to the heart, diminish intrathoracic blood volume, and ultimately reduce ventricular work.

c Intrapericardial pressure. When elevated, as in pericardial tamponade, there is interference with cardiac filling, and the resultant reduction in ventricular diastolic volume lowers ventricular work.

d Venous tone. The veins are not a simple system of passive conduits between the systemic capillary bed and the right atrium. Instead, the smooth muscle in venous walls responds to a variety of neural and humoral stimuli. Venoconstriction occurs during muscular exercise, deep respiration, fright, or marked hypotension, tending to diminish extrathoracic and to augment intrathoracic blood volume, venous return to the heart, and ventricular performance.

e The pumping action of skeletal muscle. During exercise the contracting skeletal muscles tend to squeeze blood out of the veins and, with the aid of the venous valves, to displace it centrally, thereby increasing intrathoracic blood volume, ventricular end-diastolic volume, and ventricular work.

3 Atrial contraction. Vigorous, appropriately timed atrial contraction augments ventricular filling and end-diastolic volume. The atrial contribution to ventricular filling is of particular importance in patients with ventricular hypertrophy, in whom the loss of atrial systole (as in atrial fibrillation) tends to reduce ventricular end-diastolic pressure and volume, ultimately lowering myocardial performance.

INOTROPIC STATE (MYOCARDIAL CONTRACTILITY) A number of factors determine the level of ventricular performance at any given ventricular end-diastolic volume, i.e., the position of the ventricular function curve (Fig. 236-5). These influences may be considered to operate by modifying myocardial force-velocity-length relations.

Sympathetic nerve activity The quantity of norepinephrine released by sympathetic nerve endings in the heart is, under ordinary circumstances, dependent on the sympathetic nerve impulse traffic, and variations in the frequency of nerve impulses modify the quantity of norepinephrine released and acting upon the beta-adrenergic receptors in the myocardium. This mechanism is the most important one which acutely modifies the position of the force-velocity and ventricular function curves under physiologic conditions.

Circulating catecholamines The adrenal medulla and other sympathetic ganglia outside the heart, when properly stimulated by sympathetic nerve impulses, release catecholamines, which augment the inotropic state of the myocardium.

The force-frequency relation The position of the myocardial force-velocity curve is influenced by the rate and rhythm of cardiac contraction; e.g., ventricular extrasystoles result in post-extrasystolic potentiation.

Exogenously administered inotropic agents The cardiac glycosides, isoproterenol and other sympathomimetic agents, calcium, caffeine, theophylline, and their derivatives, all improve the myocardial force-velocity relation (Chap. 239) and therefore may be used therapeutically to augment ventricular performance at any given ventricular end-diastolic volume.

Physiologic depressants Included among these are severe myocardial hypoxia, hypercapnea, and acidosis. Acting either singly or in combination, these influences exert a depressant effect on the myocardial force-velocity curve

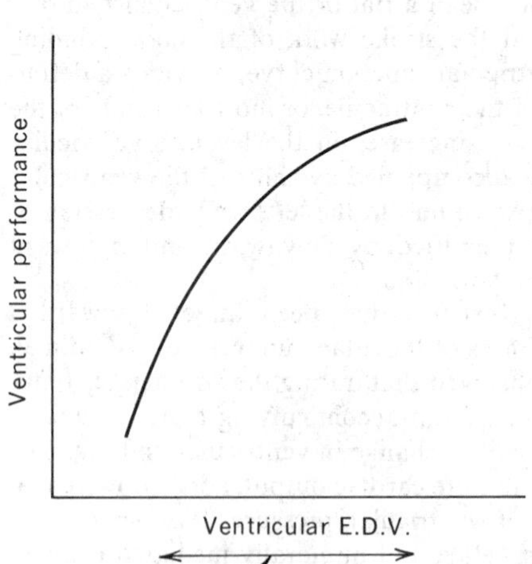

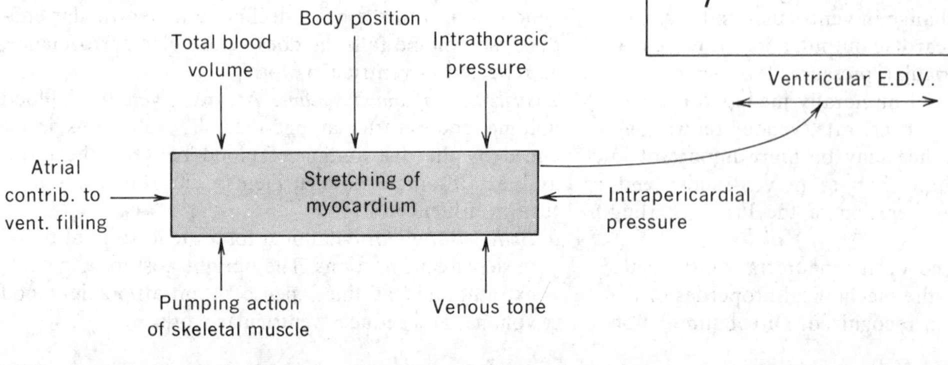

FIGURE 236-4
Diagram of a Frank-Starling curve, relating ventricular end-diastolic volume (E.D.V.) to ventricular performance (top right) and the major influences that determine the degree of stretching of the myocardium, i.e., the magnitude of the E.D.V. (bottom left). (From Braunwald et al, Mechanisms of Contraction of the Normal and Failing Heart, *Boston: Little, Brown, 1976)*

and lower the level of the left ventricular work at any given ventricular end-diastolic volume.

Pharmacologic depressants These include quinidine, procainamide, barbiturates, and other local and general anesthetics (Chap. 239), as well as many other drugs.

Loss of ventricular substance When a portion of ventricular myocardium becomes nonfunctional or necrotic, as occurs temporarily in bouts of ischemia, and permanently in myocardial infarction, total ventricular performance at any given level of end-diastolic volume is depressed, even if the remaining myocardium functions normally.

Intrinsic myocardial depression Although the fundamental mechanisms responsible for depression of myocardial contractility in heart failure still remain to be elucidated, it is now apparent that in this condition the inotropic state of each unit of myocardium is depressed and that the level of ventricular performance at any ventricular end-diastolic volume is thereby lowered.

VENTRICULAR AFTERLOAD The stroke volume is ultimately a function of the extent of ventricular fiber shortening. As in isolated cardiac muscle, the velocity and extent of shortening at any given level of diastolic fiber length and myocardial inotropic state is inversely related to the afterload imposed on the muscle. The afterload on the intact heart is dependent on the level of aortic pressure but it may be defined as the tension or stress developed in the wall of the ventricle during ejection. Therefore, the afterload on the ventricular muscle fibers also is dependent on the size of the heart, according to the Laplace principle, which indicates that the tension of the myocardial fiber is a function of the product of intracavitary ventricular pressure and the ventricular radius. Thus, at the same level of aortic pressure, the afterload faced by an enlarged left ventricle is higher than that encountered by a ventricle of normal size. The aortic pressure, in turn, is influenced largely by the peripheral vascular resistance, the physical characteristics of the arterial tree, and the volume of blood it contains at the onset of ejection. At any given ventricular end-diastolic volume and level of the myocardial state, the left ventricular stroke volume is a function of the afterload.

The critical role played by the ventricular afterload in cardiovascular regulation is summarized in Fig. 236-6. As already noted, increases in both preload and contractility increase myocardial fiber shortening, while increases in afterload reduce it. The extent of myocardial fiber shortening and left ventricular size are the determinants of stroke volume. Arterial pressure, in turn, is related to the product of cardiac output and systemic vascular resistance, while afterload is a function of left ventricular size and arterial pressure. An increase in arterial pressure induced by vasoconstriction, for example, augments afterload, which through a negative feedback depresses myocardial fiber shortening, stroke volume, and cardiac output; this in turn tends to restore arterial pressure to its previous level.

When left ventricular function becomes impaired, impedance to left ventricular ejection becomes increasingly important in determining cardiac performance. Increases in impedance may result from the influence on the arterial bed of neural, humoral, or structural changes which can occur in response to a fall in cardiac output. This increased impedance may further reduce cardiac output while myocardial oxygen requirements are increased. In this way, alterations in the peripheral vascular bed probably play an important role in the hemodynamic and metabolic events which usually are attributed to progressive impairment of the myocardium.

All the influences acting on cardiac performance enumerated above interact in a complex fashion to maintain

FIGURE 236-5
Diagram showing the major influences that elevate or depress the inotropic state of the myocardium (top right), and the manner in which alterations in the inotropic state of the myocardium affect the level of ventricular performance at any given level of ventricular end-diastolic volume (bottom left). (From Braunwald et al, Mechanisms of Contraction of Normal and Failing Heart, *Boston: Little, Brown, 1976)*

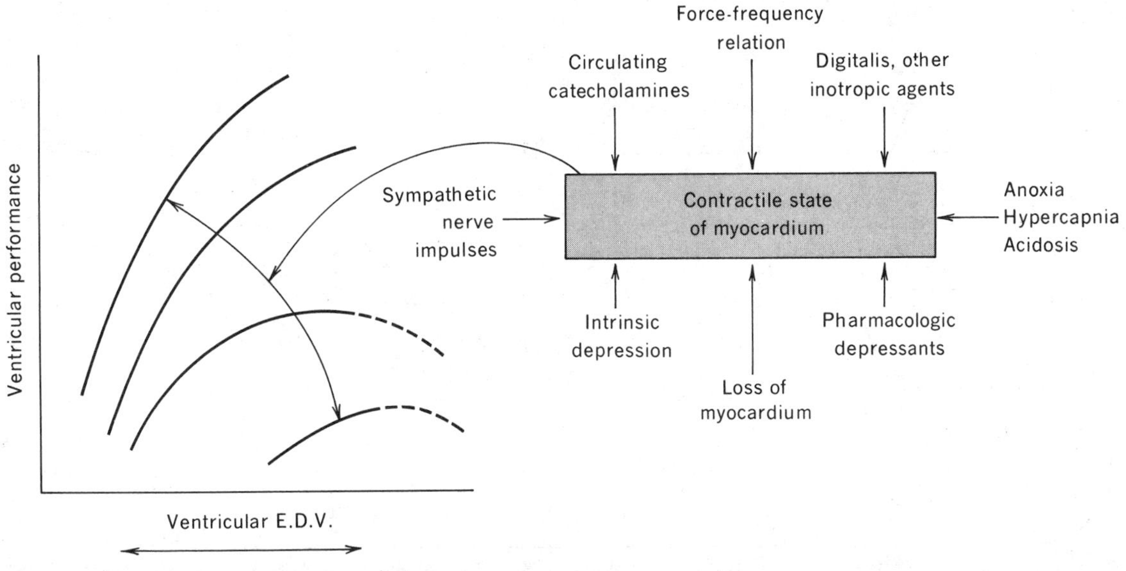

cardiac output at a level appropriate to the requirements of the metabolizing tissues, and in a normal person interference with one of these mechanisms may not influence the cardiac output. For example, a moderate reduction of blood volume or the loss of the atrial contribution to ventricular contraction can ordinarily be sustained without a reduction in the resting cardiac output. Presumably other factors, such as an increase in the frequency of sympathetic nerve impulses reaching the heart and an increase in heart rate, will, in the normal person, augment contractility and sustain output under these circumstances. Mechanisms are also available which prevent elevation of the cardiac output when there is no physiologic demand for augmented flow. For example, expansion of blood volume or augmentation of myocardial contractility by means of cardiac glycosides does not increase the cardiac output in normal man. Thus, in analyzing the effect of an intervention on cardiac output, it is important to recognize that it is the venous return, rather than the inotropic state, of the myocardium which limits cardiac output in the normal individual and that an improvement of myocardial contractility by a drug such as digitalis should not be expected to elevate the output in a normal subject. On the other hand, in the presence of congestive heart failure, the cardiac output usually is limited by the depressed contractile state of the myocardium, and a positive inotropic influence would be expected to raise cardiac output, and, indeed, does so.

EXERCISE The hemodynamic changes which normally occur during muscular exercise are complex (Fig. 236-7). The hyperventilation of exercise, the pumping action of the exercising muscles, and the venoconstriction which occur, all tend to augment venous return and hence ventricular filling. Simultaneously, the increase in the sympathetic nerve impulses to the myocardium, the increased concentration of circulating catecholamines, and the tachycardia which occur during exercise, all result in an augmentation of the contractile state of the myocardium (Fig. 236-7, curves 1 to 2) and an elevation of stroke volume, with no change or even a decrease of end-diastolic pressure and volume (Fig. 236-7, points *A* to *B*). Vasodilatation occurs in the exercising muscles, thus reducing the afterload. This ultimately allows the achievement of a greatly elevated cardiac output during exercise, at an arterial pressure greatly different from that in the resting state.

In heart failure, the fundamental abnormality resides in depressions of the myocardial force-velocity relationship and of the length–active tension curve, reflecting reductions in the contractile state of the myocardium (Fig. 236-7, curves 1 to 3). In many instances, cardiac output and external ventricular performance at rest are within normal limits but are maintained at these levels only by an increased end-diastolic fiber length and an elevated ventricular end-diastolic volume, i.e., through the operation of the Frank-Starling mechanism (Fig. 236-7, points *A* to *D*). The elevations of left ventricular end-diastolic volume and pressure are associated with similar changes in the pulmonary capillary pressure, contributing to the dyspnea experienced by patients with heart failure. The normal improvement of contractility due to augmented sympathetic activity during exercise is attenuated or even prevented by norepinephrine depletion which occurs in heart failure (Fig. 236-7, curves 3 and 3′). The factors which tend to augment ventricular filling during exercise in the normal subject push the failing myocardium even farther along its flattened length–active tension curve, and although the left ventricle may perform somewhat better, this occurs only as a consequence of an inordinate elevation of ventricular end-diastolic volume and pressure and therefore of the pulmonary capillary pressure. The elevation of the latter intensifies dyspnea and therefore plays an important role in limiting the intensity of exercise which the patient can perform. Left ventricular failure becomes fatal when the myocardial length–active tension curve is depressed (Fig. 236-7, curve 4) to the point at which cardiac performance fails to satisfy the requirements of the peripheral tissues even at rest, and/or the left ventricular end-diastolic and pulmonary capillary pres-

FIGURE 236-6
Scheme of interactions between various components that regulate cardiac activity. Solid lines indicate an augmenting effect; broken line represents an inhibiting effect. (From E Braunwald, Regulation of the circulation. *N Engl J Med 290:1124, 1420, 1974)*

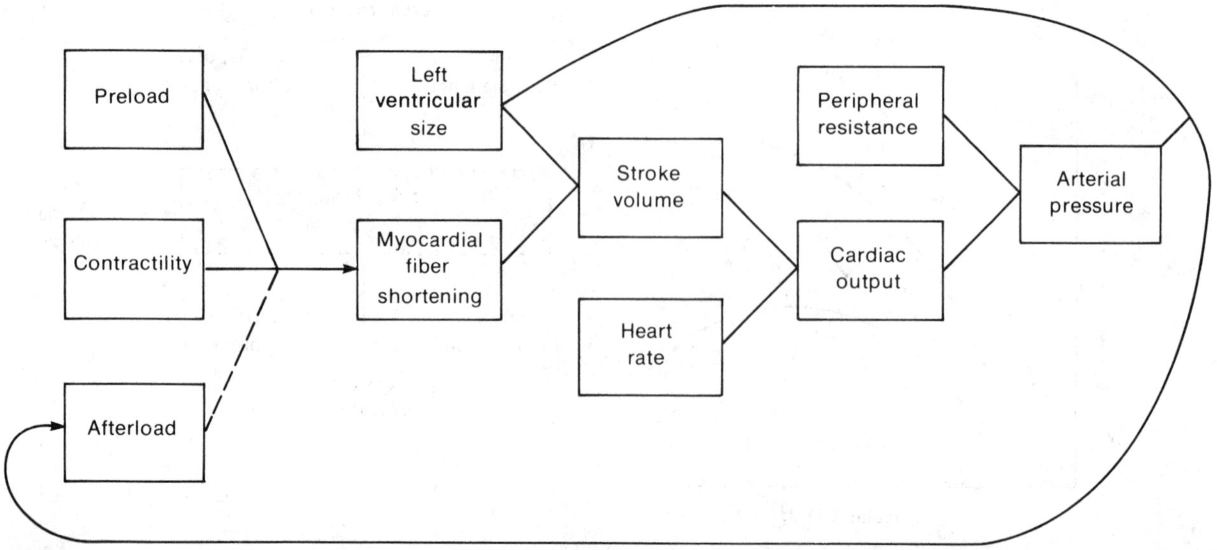

sures are elevated to levels which result in pulmonary edema (Fig. 236-7, point *E*).

THE FAILING HEART

Though heart failure may be readily described as a clinical syndrome, characterized by well-known symptoms and physical signs, a precise physiologic or biochemical definition is far more difficult. However, from the clinical point of view, heart failure may be considered to be the disease state in which an abnormality of cardiac function is responsible for the inability of the heart to pump blood at a rate commensurate with the requirements of the metabolizing tissues. Though a defect in myocardial contraction is characteristic of heart failure, this defect may result from a primary abnormality in the heart muscle, or it may be secondary to a chronic excessive work load. It is important to distinguish heart failure from (1) states of circulatory insufficiency in which myocardial function is not primarily impaired, such as cardiac tamponade, hemorrhagic shock, or tricuspid stenosis, (2) conditions in which there is circulatory congestion because of abnormal salt and water retention but in which there is no serious disturbance of myocardial function, and (3) conditions in which the normal heart is suddenly presented with a load which exceeds its capacity, e.g., accelerated hypertension, before the intrinsic state of the myocardium is altered.

Acute heart failure in the intact canine heart, studied *in situ* or in the heart-lung preparation, is characterized by a depression of ventricular stroke volume or stroke work at any given level of left ventricular end-diastolic volume or filling pressure. Further, as diastolic volume is augmented in the failing heart, an abnormally small increase or no change in stroke volume occurs. Thus, in order to maintain stroke volume at a normal level, the heart dilates and the Frank-Starling mechanism therefore might be considered one of the first lines of defense called upon to maintain cardiac output when myocardial contractility declines. An increase in the end-diastolic volume of the ventricle permits the ejection of a larger stroke volume, even when the extent of shortening of individual muscle fibers remains constant. The fact that when end-diastolic volume is augmented in the failing heart, stroke volume shows little change or is actually diminished clearly indicates that the relative degree of muscle fiber shortening must have decreased. Thus, an important mechanical defect which can be delineated in acute heart failure is a decrease in the extent of shortening of cardiac muscle fibers.

The intrinsic contractile state of myocardium removed from normal, hypertrophied, and failing animal hearts has been evaluated, and both ventricular hypertrophy and heart failure were shown to reduce the maximum isometric tension and velocity of shortening to subnormal levels; the changes were more marked in the myocardium of animals in which heart failure had been present than in those with hypertrophy alone. However, ventricular hypertrophy, in the absence of heart failure, also appears to be associated with a depression of the inotropic state per unit of myocardium, although the absolute increase of total muscle mass

FIGURE 236-7
Diagram showing the interrelations between influences on ventricular end-diastolic volume (E.D.V.) through stretching of the myocardium and the contractile state of the myocardium. Levels of ventricular E.D.V. associated with filling pressures that result in dyspnea and pulmonary edema are shown on the abscissa. Levels of ventricular performance required when the subject is at rest, while walking, and during maximal activity are designated on the ordinate. The dotted lines are the descending limbs of the ventricular-performance curves, which are rarely seen during life but which show the level of ventricular performance if end-diastolic volume could be elevated to very high levels. (From Braunwald et al, Mechanisms of Contraction of Normal and Failing Heart, *Boston: Little, Brown, 1976)*

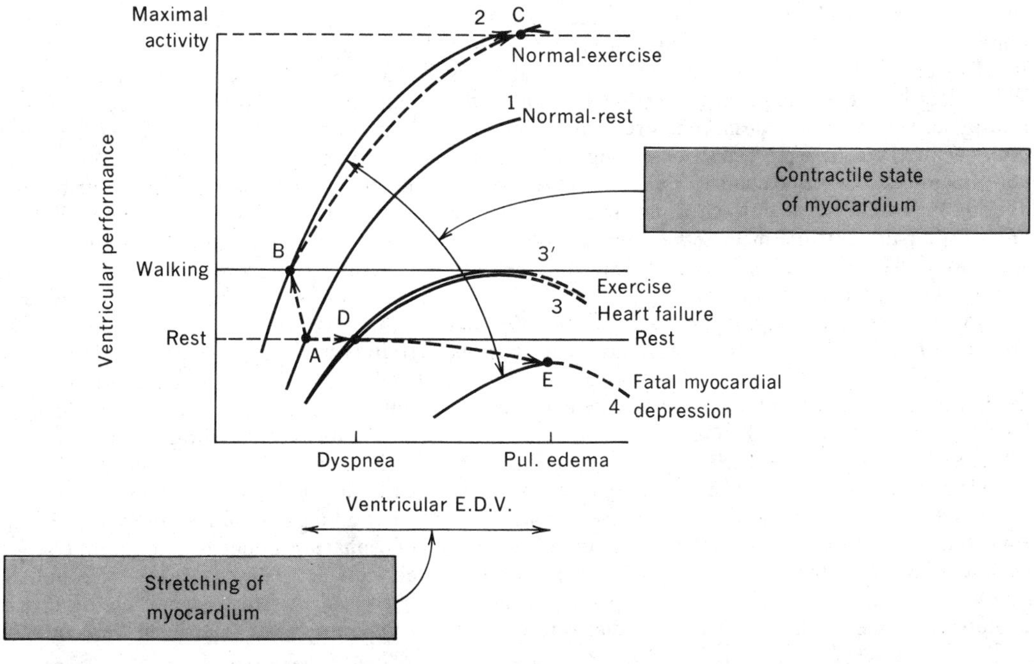

maintains cardiac compensation. Papillary muscles removed from the left ventricles of patients with heart failure have also shown a depression of the maximum degree of active tension which they can develop. Electromicroscopic analysis of failing cat papillary muscles fixed at the apexes of the length–active tension curves revealed sarcomere lengths averaging 2.2 μm. Thus, the abnormalities of contractility do *not* appear to be produced by an alteration in the overlap of filaments within the sarcomere.

The failing ventricle may still eject a normal or nearly normal stroke volume despite considerable depression of function, when its end-diastolic volume increases, i.e., through the operation of the Frank-Starling mechanism. As outlined above, an increase in the initial volume of the ventricle is associated with stretching of the sarcomere, a process which augments the number of sites at which the actin and myosin filaments can interact. Furthermore, the development of ventricular hypertrophy may be considered to provide additional contractile units, and thereby constitutes an important compensatory mechanism when the intrinsic myocardial inotropic state is depressed.

Several techniques are available for defining impaired ventricular contractility in intact man. With the patient at rest, the cardiac output and stroke volume may be depressed, but not uncommonly these variables are within normal limits. A more sensitive index is the ejection fraction, i.e., the ratio of stroke volume to end-diastolic volume, which may be estimated by biplane angiography (Chap. 235), and which is frequently depressed in heart failure even when the stroke volume itself is normal. An even more sensitive method for detecting impaired ventricular performance is based on the measurement of the circulatory changes occurring during stresses such as exercise or increased afterload. Thus, left ventricular performance may be estimated accurately by measuring the left ventricular end-diastolic pressure, cardiac output, and total body O_2 consumption at rest and during exercise. In normal persons, the cardiac output rises by more than 500 ml per min for each 100 ml increase in minute O_2 consumption. The left ventricular end-diastolic pressure at rest is less than 12 mmHg and rises slightly, remains unchanged, or decreases slightly during exercise, while stroke volume usually rises. The failing left ventricle, on the other hand, is characterized by an elevation of end-diastolic pressure during exercise, which reaches a value exceeding 12 mmHg, accompanied by either no change or a fall in stroke volume and a subnormal increase in cardiac output. Various degrees of impairment intermediate between the normal response and that of the failing left ventricle during the stress of exercise also have been described.

Another method consists of the measurement of stroke volume, arterial pressure, and ventricular end-diastolic pressure before and after ventricular afterload is increased by means of an infusion of a pressor agent such as angiotensin or by a sustained handgrip (isometric exercise). Though the normal left ventricle responds to this stress by increasing its stroke work and end-diastolic pressure, in the failing left ventricle the end-diastolic pressure rises markedly, but stroke work either remains constant or actually declines. Thus, as in the acutely failing experimental preparation, the failing human left ventricle appears to exhibit a depression of the relation between end-diastolic pressure and the stroke volume and stroke work which can be achieved. The potential value of stressing the left ventricle in some manner is emphasized by the fact that the basal values for left ventricular end-diastolic pressure, cardiac index, and ventricular stroke work may be in the same range in patients with depressed ventricular function as in normal persons. The response to these stresses may prove useful not only in the detection of the impairment of myocardial function, but also in expressing the severity of this impairment quantitatively.

The performance of the left ventricle in man may also be characterized by examining the instantaneous myocardial force-velocity relations and the extent of shortening during individual cardiac cycles. Angiocardiographic studies and analyses of the rate of change of intraventricular pressure (dp/dt) as a function of the simultaneously recorded pressure during isovolumetric contraction have shown that depressions in the velocity of myocardial fiber shortening and of tension development exist in human heart failure. Further evidence for the decreases in the velocity of myocardial fiber shortening is provided by the finding of a reduced mean systolic ejection rate in patients with heart failure and a failure of the mean systolic ejection rate to rise normally during muscular exercise. Noninvasive, graphic techniques, particularly echocardiography and the determination of systolic time intervals, are of great value in the clinical assessment of myocardial function (Chap. 234).

CARDIAC METABOLISM IN HEART FAILURE

The common forms of low-output heart failure, secondary to arteriosclerosis, hypertension, and certain valvular and congenital lesions, are characterized by an absolute or a relative decrease in the useful external work delivered by the heart. Considerable effort has been directed to the question of whether cardiac failure is due to a defect in the production of energy, its conservation, or its utilization. Only in isolated instances of heart failure, such as those associated with beriberi, are there clear-cut disturbances of myocardial energy production. The major pathway by which pyruvate enters the citric acid cycle and some reactions within the cycle itself are dependent on the presence of adequate concentrations of thiamine (Chap. 84). Thiamine deficiency results in diminished pyruvic acid utilization by heart slices, and in abnormally low pyruvate extraction coefficients in intact dogs and in man.

The principal defect in the common forms of low-output heart failure does not appear to be in an impairment of energy production by the myocardium through the oxidation of substrate. In the second phase of cardiac metabolism, energy conservation, the energy of substrate oxidation is then converted into the terminal-bond energy of creatine phosphate (CP) and of ATP, the immediate source of chemical energy utilized by heart muscle. This process, known as oxidative phosphorylation, occurs in the mitochondria. The effectiveness of the combined energy production-conservation mechanisms may be studied by measuring the stores of ATP and CP existing in the myocardium, while energy conservation may be evaluated by determining (1) the P:O ratio, i.e., the ratio of high-energy phosphate produced to oxygen consumed in the mitochondria, and (2) the degree of coupling between electron transport and the generation of high-energy phosphate compounds. Although lively controversy exists concerning the status of this phase of metabolism in heart failure, it now appears that severe impairment of myocardial performance may occur without disturbances of mitochondrial function or reduction of high-energy phosphate stores, although abnormalities in these processes do occur in some forms of experimental heart failure.

In the absence of a definitive abnormality of energy liberation or conservation in the failing myocardium, attention has naturally been directed to the possibility that energy utilization is abnormal. An abnormality of energy liberation could certainly occur if the contractile proteins themselves were altered, and indeed this was once believed to be the basic biochemical abnormality occurring in congestive heart failure, a theory no longer supported. However, it has been shown that myofibrillar, actomyosin, and myosin ATPase activity are depressed in some forms of experimentally produced heart failure, and it is possible that this depression may be responsible for a defect in energy utilization, i.e., in the breakdown of ATP, the process which leads to the shortening and tension development by the contractile filaments. In addition, substantial evidence has been obtained that in heart failure there is an abnormality of excitation-contraction coupling, which alters the delivery of Ca^{2+} to the contractile sites, thereby impairing cardiac performance.

THE ADRENERGIC NERVOUS SYSTEM IN HEART FAILURE

In view of the importance of the adrenergic nervous system in stimulating the contractility of the normal myocardium, the activity of this system has also been studied intensively in patients with congestive heart failure. An index of the activity of this system, at rest and during exercise, is provided by measurements of the concentration of norepinephrine (NE) in arterial blood. No change or very little increase in the NE concentrations occurs during exercise in normal subjects; much greater increases are seen in patients with congestive heart failure, presumably because of an increased activity of the adrenergic nervous system during exercise in these patients. Marked elevations of a 24-h urinary NE excretion occur in patients with heart failure, indicating that the activity of their adrenergic nervous systems is also augmented at rest.

The importance of the increased activity of the adrenergic nervous system in maintaining ventricular contractility when the function of the myocardium is depressed in congestive heart failure also is shown by the effects of adrenergic blockade in patients with heart failure. Antiadrenergic drugs such as propranolol or guanethidine may cause sodium and water retention, as well as intensify heart failure. The adrenergic nervous system thus plays an important compensatory role in the circulatory adjustments of patients to congestive heart failure, and caution must be exercised in the use of antiadrenergic drugs in the treatment of patients with limited cardiac reserve (Chap. 237).

Both the concentration and content of the NE in atrial and ventricular tissue in patients with heart failure are less than one-third of normal. This is a reduction in NE content in the heart and is not the result of a simple dilution of sympathetic nerve endings in a hypertrophied muscle mass.

The biosynthesis of NE proceeds through a series of steps from tyrosine to dopa to dopamine, the immediate precursor of the neurotransmitter. It is now known that tyrosine hydroxylase, which catalyzes the first reaction (tyrosine to dopa), is the rate-limiting enzyme in the synthesis of NE. Marked reductions in the activity of this enzyme recently have been shown to accompany the NE depletion in failing hearts, and it appears likely that this is responsible for the cardiac NE depletion in heart failure.

Although the mechanism ultimately responsible for this reduction of tyrosine hydroxylase in the heart in congestive heart failure remains to be elucidated, some of the consequences of cardiac NE depletion in heart failure are evident. In view of the strongly positive inotropic effect exerted by the NE released from these nerves, the adrenergic nervous system may be considered to provide an important potential source of support to the failing myocardium. However, the increments of heart rate and contractile force which occur in animals with experimental heart failure and cardiac NE depletion are abolished or markedly reduced with stimulation of the cardiac sympathetic nerves. Thus, it is likely that when congestive heart failure is accompanied by depletion of cardiac NE stores, the quantity of NE released by the sympathetic nerve endings in the heart is deficient relative to the impulse traffic along these nerves.

Cardiac stores of NE are not fundamentally necessary for maintaining the intrinsic contractile state of the myocardium. However, since the reduction of NE stores in heart failure is associated with a diminished release of neurotransmitter, this depletion of NE may be responsible for loss of the much-needed adrenergic support in the failing heart.

REFERENCES

BRAUNWALD E: Regulation of the circulation. N Engl J Med 290:1124, 1420, 1974

——: *The Myocardium: Failure and Infarction,* New York: HP Publishing Co., 1974

—— et al: *Mechanisms of Contraction of the Normal and Failing Heart,* 2d ed., Boston: Little, Brown, 1976, 417 pp

GUYTON AC et al: *Circulatory Physiology: Cardiac Output and Its Regulation,* 2d ed., Philadelphia: Saunders, 1973

JAMES TN, SHERF L: Ultrastructure of the myocardium, chap. 6 in *The Heart,* 3d ed., ed JW Hurst, New York: McGraw-Hill, 1974, pp. 63–79

LANGER GA, BRADY AJ: *The Mammalian Myocardium,* New York: Wiley, 1973

MIRSKY I et al: *Cardiac Mechanics: Physiological, Clinical and Mathematical Considerations,* New York: Wiley, 1973

Symposium: Neural regulation of the cardiovascular system. Fed Proc 31:1197, 1972

VASSALLE M (ed): *Cardiac Physiology for the Clinician,* New York: Academic, 1976

237
HEART FAILURE

EUGENE BRAUNWALD

INTRODUCTION

Heart failure can be readily described as a clinical symptom, characterized by well-known symptoms and physical signs, but a precise physiologic definition is more difficult to provide. However, for the purposes of this discussion, heart failure is considered to be the pathophysiologic state in which an abnormality of *cardiac* function is responsible for the failure of the heart to pump blood at a rate commensurate with the requirements of the metabolizing tissues. Heart failure is frequently, but not always, caused by a defect in myocardial contraction, and then the term *myocardial failure* is appropriate. The latter may result from a primary abnormality in the heart muscle, or it may be secondary to ischemia. Myocardial failure may also result from an extramyocardial abnormality, such as anatomic lesions of the heart valves or pericardium, which interferes with cardiac filling or emptying. For example, in many patients with rheumatic valvular disease and heart failure, the heart muscle has been damaged by the long-standing excessive hemodynamic burden imposed by the valvular abnormality, and/or by the rheumatic process (Chap. 243). In patients with chronic constrictive pericarditis, myocardial damage resulting from infiltration of the heart muscle by pericardial inflammation and calcification is common (Chap. 246).

In other patients with heart failure, however, a similar clinical syndrome is present, but without any detectable abnormality of *myocardial* function. These patients exhibit conditions in which the normal heart is suddenly presented with a load that exceeds its capacity, such as an acute hypertensive crisis, rupture of an aortic valve cusp, or massive pulmonary embolism, as well as chronic conditions in which there is impairment of filling of the ventricles due to tricuspid and/or mitral stenosis, constrictive pericarditis without myocardial involvement, and endocardial fibrosis. These are instances of *heart* failure, as opposed to *myocardial* failure.

Heart failure should be distinguished from conditions in which there is circulatory congestion consequent to abnormal salt and water retention but in which there is no disturbance of cardiac function per se. The latter syndrome, termed the *congested state,* may result from the abnormal salt and water retention of renal failure, or from excess parenteral administration of fluids and electrolytes.

CAUSES OF HEART FAILURE

It is important to identify not only the *underlying cause* of the heart disease but the *precipitating cause* of heart failure as well. The cardiac abnormality produced by a congenital or acquired lesion may exist for many years and produce no or only trivial disability. Frequently, however, serious manifestations of clinical heart failure appear for the first time in the course of some acute disturbance which places an additional load on a myocardium that chronically is excessively burdened, resulting in further deterioration of cardiac function. Identification of such precipitating causes is of critical importance because their prompt alleviation may be lifesaving. However, in the absence of underlying heart disease these acute disturbances do not usually, by themselves, lead to heart failure.

PRECIPITATING CAUSES

1. *Pulmonary embolism.* Patients with low cardiac output, circulatory stasis, and physical inactivity are likely to develop thrombi in the veins of the lower extremities or the pelvis. Pulmonary embolization may result in further acute elevation of pulmonary arterial pressure, which in turn may produce or intensify distention and failure of the right ventricle and may lower the cardiac output further. In the presence of pulmonary vascular congestion, such emboli may lead to infarction of the lung (Chap. 266).
2. *Infection.* Patients with pulmonary vascular congestion are particularly susceptible to pulmonary infections, but an infection anywhere in the body may precipitate heart failure. The resulting fever, tachycardia, hypoxemia, and the increased metabolic demands may place a further burden on the overloaded, but compensated, myocardium of a patient with chronic heart disease.
3. *Anemia.* The development of a significant reduction in the oxygen-carrying capacity of the blood may precipitate heart failure because in the presence of anemia the oxygen needs of the metabolizing tissues can be satisfied only by an increase in the cardiac output (Chap. 60). Though such an increase in the cardiac output might be sustained by a normal heart, a diseased, overloaded, but otherwise compensated heart may be unable to augment the volume of blood which it delivers to the periphery.
4. *Thyrotoxicosis and pregnancy.* As in anemia and fever, in these conditions adequate tissue perfusion requires an increased cardiac output. The development or intensification of heart failure may actually be one of the first clinical manifestations of hyperthyroidism in a patient with underlying heart disease (Chap. 92). Similarly, heart failure not infrequently occurs for the first time during pregnancy in women with rheumatic valvular disease; in such women cardiac compensation may return following delivery, after the excessive burden has been eliminated (Chap. 243).
5. *Arrhythmias.* Cardiac arrhythmias are among the most frequent precipitating causes of heart failure in patients with underlying but compensated heart disease for a variety of reasons: *(a)* tachyarrhythmias reduce the time period available for ventricular filling; *(b)* the dissociation between atrial and ventricular contractions characteristic of many supraventricular and ventricular arrhythmias result in the loss of the atrial booster pump mechanism, thereby tending to raise atrial pressures; *(c)* in ventricular tachycardia or any arrhythmia associated with abnormal intraventricular conduction, myocardial performance may become further impaired because of the loss of normal synchronicity of ventricular contraction; *(d)* the marked bradycardia associated with complete atrioventricular block requires a greatly elevated stroke volume if a

marked reduction in cardiac output is to be prevented (Chap. 238).

6 *Rheumatic and other forms of myocarditis.* The development of acute rheumatic fever and a variety of allergic or infectious processes affecting the myocardium may further impair myocardial function in patients with preexisting heart disease (Chap. 242).

7 *Bacterial endocarditis.* The anemia, fever, additional valvular damage, and myocarditis which often occur as a consequence of bacterial endocarditis may, singly or in concert, precipitate heart failure (Chap. 132).

8 *Physical dietary, environmental, and emotional excesses.* The augmentation of sodium intake, the discontinuation of diuretics or digitalis glycosides, physical overexertion, excessive environmental heat or humidity, and emotional crises may all precipitate cardiac decompensation.

9 *Systemic hypertension.* Rapid elevation of arterial pressure, as may occur in some instances of hypertension of renal origin or upon discontinuation of antihypertensive medication, may result in cardiac decompensation (Chaps. 35, 250).

10 *Myocardial infarction.* In patients with chronic but compensated ischemic heart disease, a fresh infarct, often silent clinically, may further impair ventricular function and precipitate heart failure (Chap. 245).

A careful and systematic search for one or more of these precipitating causes should be made in every patient with heart failure, particularly if it is refractory to the usual methods of therapy. If properly recognized, the precipitating cause of heart failure can usually be treated more effectively than the underlying cause. Furthermore, the prognosis in patients with heart failure in whom a precipitating cause can be identified and treated is far more favorable than in patients in whom the underlying disease process has advanced to the point of producing heart failure.

FORMS OF HEART FAILURE

Heart failure may be described as *high-output* or *low-output, acute* or *chronic, right-sided* or *left-sided,* and *forward* or *backward.* Although these terms may be useful in a clinical setting, they are entirely descriptive and do not signify fundamentally different disease states.

HIGH-OUTPUT VERSUS LOW-OUTPUT HEART FAILURE

With the development of methods for the measurement of cardiac output, it became useful to classify patients with heart failure into those with a low cardiac output, i.e., *low-output heart failure,* and those with an elevated cardiac output, i.e., *high-output heart failure.* The cardiac output is often depressed in patients with heart failure secondary to coronary artery disease, hypertension, primary myocardial disease, valvular disease, and pericardial disease, but it tends to be elevated in patients with heart failure and hyperthyroidism, anemia, arteriovenous fistulas, beriberi, Paget's disease, and pulmonary emphysema. In clinical practice, however, it may be difficult to distinguish between low-output and high-output heart failure. The normal range of cardiac output is wide (2.6 to 3.6 liters per min per m^2), and in many patients with so-called low-output heart failure the cardiac output may actually be within normal limits at rest, although it may fail to rise normally during exertion. On the other hand, in patients with so-called high-output heart failure the output may not be excessive but rather may be close to the upper limit of normal, particularly when heart failure is severe. Regardless of the absolute level of the cardiac output, however, cardiac failure may be said to be present when the characteristic clinical manifestations described below are accompanied by a depression of the curve relating ventricular end-diastolic volume to cardiac performance (Fig. 236-5).

An integral part of the heart failure syndrome is evidence that the heart does not deliver the quantity of oxygen required by the metabolizing tissues. In the absence of peripheral shunting of blood, such inadequate delivery of oxygen to the metabolizing tissues is reflected in an abnormal widening of the normal arterial-mixed venous oxygen difference (3.5 to 5.0 ml per 100 ml in the basal state), relative to the total body oxygen consumption. In mild cases, this abnormality may not be present at rest and may become evident only during exertion. In patients with the high-output cardiac states associated with conditions such as arteriovenous fistula, beriberi, thyrotoxicosis, and Paget's disease, the arterial-mixed venous oxygen difference is often abnormally low, because the mixed venous oxygen saturation is raised by the admixture of blood which has been shunted away from some of the metabolizing tissues, and it may be presumed that even in these patients the delivery of oxygen to the metabolizing tissues is reduced. When heart failure occurs in such patients, the arterial-mixed venous oxygen difference may be normal or even reduced, but it still exceeds the level which existed prior to the development of heart failure, and therefore the cardiac output, though normal or elevated, is lower than before heart failure occurred.

The mechanisms responsible for the development of heart failure in patients whose cardiac outputs are initially high are complex and depend on the underlying disease process. In most of these conditions the heart is called upon to pump abnormally large quantities of blood in order to deliver the normal quota of oxygen to the metabolizing tissues. The burden placed on the myocardium by the increased flow load resembles that produced by regurgitant valvular lesions. In addition, thyrotoxicosis and beriberi may impair myocardial metabolism directly, and severe anemia and chronic pulmonary emphysema may interfere with myocardial function by producing myocardial anoxia.

ACUTE VERSUS CHRONIC HEART FAILURE The prototype of acute heart failure develops in patients with large myocardial infarctions or valve rupture, while chronic heart failure is typically observed in patients with multivalvular heart disease. Frequently, however, there is no fundamental distinction between these two conditions. For example, intensive efforts to prevent expansion of blood volume by means of dietary sodium restriction and the administration of diuretics will frequently delay the development of exertional dyspnea and ankle edema in patients with severe hypertension until an acute episode, such as a small myocardial infarction, an arrhythmia, or further elevation of arterial pressure, results in acute heart failure. Without intensive efforts to restrict blood volume the same patients would have been considered to have been suffering from chronic heart failure, even though their underlying myocardial disease were no further advanced.

RIGHT-SIDED VERSUS LEFT-SIDED HEART FAILURE Many of the clinical manifestations of heart failure result from the accumulation of excess fluid behind one or both ventricles. This fluid usually localizes upstream to the specific cardiac chamber which is initially affected. For example, patients in whom the abnormal load is placed on the left ventricle develop dyspnea and orthopnea as a result of pulmonary congestion, a condition referred to as *left-sided heart failure.* When heart failure has existed for months or years, such localization behind the failing ventricle may no longer exist. For example, patients with long-standing aortic valve disease or systemic hypertension may have ankle edema, congestive hepatomegaly, and systemic venous distention late in the course of their disease, even though the abnormal hemodynamic burden initially was placed on the left ventricle. In contrast, when the underlying abnormality affects the right ventricle primarily, e.g., valvular pulmonic stenosis or pulmonary hypertension secondary to pulmonary thromboembolism, symptoms resulting from pulmonary congestion such as orthopnea or paroxysmal nocturnal dyspnea are less common. However, severe exertional dyspnea may be observed in such patients.

Thus, although specific lesions may place an abnormal load on one or the other ventricle, when this load is excessive and applied for prolonged periods, failure of the heart as a whole occurs. Perhaps this is because the muscle bundles composing both ventricles are continuous and both ventricles share a common wall, the interventricular septum. Also, biochemical changes which occur in heart failure and which may be involved in the impairment of myocardial function, such as norepinephrine depletion and alterations in the activity of myofibrillar ATPase, occur in the myocardium of both ventricles, regardless of the specific chamber on which the abnormal hemodynamic burden is placed.

BACKWARD VERSUS FORWARD HEART FAILURE For many years a controversy has revolved around the question of the mechanism of the clinical manifestations resulting from heart failure. The concept of *backward heart failure,* originated by James Hope in 1832, contends that when heart failure occurs, one or the other ventricle fails to discharge its contents normally, the end-diastolic volume of the ventricle rises, and the pressures and volumes in the atrium and venous system behind the failing ventricle become elevated. According to this concept, retention of sodium and water occurs as a consequence of the elevation of systemic venous and capillary pressures and the resultant transudation of fluid into the interstitial space, as well as from increased renal tubular reabsorption of sodium associated with an elevation of renal venous pressure.

In contrast, the proponents of the *forward heart failure* hypothesis, expounded by MacKenzie in 1913, maintain that the clinical manifestations of heart failure result directly from an inadequate discharge of blood into the arterial system. Salt and water retention, according to this concept, is a consequence of diminished renal perfusion and/or excessive tubular sodium reabsorption through activation of the renin-angiotensin-aldosterone system.

A rigid distinction between *backward heart failure* and *forward heart failure* is artificial, since both mechanisms appear to operate to varying extents in most patients with chronic heart failure. However, the rate of onset of heart failure often influences the clinical manifestations. For example, when a large portion of the left ventricle is suddenly destroyed, as in myocardial infarction, acute pulmonary edema may develop rapidly, and although stroke volume is reduced, the patient may die of acute pulmonary edema before the reduced cardiac output can be responsible for the renal retention of salt and water. However, if this patient survived the acute insult, clinical manifestations resulting from the abnormal retention of fluid within the systemic vascular bed might develop. Similarly, the right ventricle may dilate and the systemic venous pressure may rise to high levels immediately following acute massive pulmonary embolism, but this state may have to be maintained for some days before sodium and water retention sufficient to produce edema occurs.

REDISTRIBUTION OF CARDIAC OUTPUT The redistribution of left ventricular output also serves as an important compensatory mechanism in the presence of severe impairment of cardiac function. This redistribution is most marked when, in a patient with heart failure, an additional burden is imposed, such as exercise, fever, or anemia, but as heart failure advances, redistribution occurs even in the basal state. Blood flow is redistributed so that the delivery of oxygen to vital organs, such as the brain and myocardium, is maintained at normal or near-normal levels, while blood flow to less critical areas, such as the cutaneous and muscular beds, is reduced. Vasoconstriction mediated by the sympathetic nervous system is largely responsible for this redistribution of peripheral blood flow.

SALT AND WATER RETENTION IN CHRONIC HEART FAILURE

When the volume of blood pumped by the left ventricle into the systemic vascular bed is chronically reduced, and when one or both of the ventricles fail to expel the normal fraction of their end-diastolic volume, a complex sequence of adjustments occurs which ultimately results in the abnormal accumulation of fluid. Though, on the one hand, many of the clinical manifestations of heart failure are secondary to this excessive retention of fluid, on the other hand, this abnormal fluid accumulation constitutes an important compensatory mechanism which tends to maintain cardiac output and therefore perfusion of the vital organs. Except in the terminal stages of heart failure, the ventricle operates on an ascending, albeit depressed and fattened function curve (Fig. 236-7), and the augmented ventricular end-diastolic volume and pressure characteristic of heart failure must be regarded as aiding the maintenance of cardiac output. The expansion of the intravascular blood volume, regardless of the mechanism responsible, tends to elevate ventricular end-diastolic volume, and, in accordance with the Frank-Starling principle, tends to augment ventricular performance. On the other hand, the maintenance of right ventricular end-diastolic volume and pressure at elevated levels raises systemic venous and capillary pressures, resulting ultimately in transudation of fluid from the vascular bed and edema formation (Chap. 32). Similarly, the elevation of left ventricular end-diastolic volume and pressure will augment blood volume and, if the latter condition is severe, result in pulmonary edema.

In the presence of heart failure, effective filling of the systemic arterial tree is reduced, a condition which initiates the complex hemodynamic and hormonal adjustments that interact to promote reduced renal sodium and water excretion. These are described in Chap. 32). Patients with very severe heart failure often exhibit a reduced capacity to excrete a water load, which may result in dilutional hyponatremia. These abnormalities may be caused, in part, by excess antidiuretic hormone activity and/or factors that prevent sodium reabsorption in the distal tubule, such as avid proximal tubular reabsorption of sodium or the action of a diuretic acting on the distal tubule.

The importance of elevated systemic venous pressure and of the alterations of renal and adrenal function characteristic of heart failure vary in their relative importance in the production of edema in different patients with heart failure. In patients with tricuspid valve disease or constrictive pericarditis the elevated venous pressure appears to play the dominant role. On the other hand, severe edema may be present in patients with ischemic or hypertensive heart disease, in whom systemic venous pressure is within normal limits or is only minimally elevated. In such patients, the fluid retention is probably due primarily to a redistribution of cardiac output and a concomitant reduction in renal perfusion. Regardless of the mechanisms involved in fluid retention, untreated patients with congestive heart failure have elevations of total blood volume, interstitial fluid volume, and body sodium. These abnormalities diminish, but may not disappear even after clinical compensation has been achieved by treatment.

CLINICAL MANIFESTATIONS OF HEART FAILURE

DYSPNEA *Dyspnea,* or respiratory distress which occurs as the result of increased effort in breathing, is the most common symptom of heart failure (Chap. 30). It is at first observed only during activity, when it may simply represent an aggravation of the breathlessness which normally occurs under these circumstances. As heart failure advances, however, dyspnea appears with progressively less strenuous activity. Ultimately, breathlessness is present even when the patient is at rest. Thus, the chief difference between exertional dyspnea in normal persons and in cardiac patients is the degree of activity necessary to induce the symptom. Cardiac dyspnea is observed most frequently in patients with elevations of left atrial, pulmonary venous, and pulmonary capillary pressures. Such patients have engorged pulmonary vessels and interstitial pulmonary edema, which reduces the compliance of the lungs and thereby increases the work of the respiratory muscles required to inflate the lungs. The Hering-Breuer reflex, which inhibits inspiration, is enhanced, resulting in the rapid, shallow breathing of cardiac dyspnea. The oxygen cost of breathing is increased because of the excessive work of the respiratory muscles. This is coupled with the diminished delivery of oxygen to these muscles, which occurs as a consequence of the reduced cardiac output and which may contribute to the sensation of shortness of breath.

ORTHOPNEA The patient with orthopnea, i.e., dyspnea in the recumbent position, generally elevates his head on several pillows at night and frequently awakens short of breath if his head has slipped off the pillows. The sensation of breathlessness usually is relieved by sitting bolt upright, and many patients report that they find relief from sitting in front of an open window. As heart failure advances, orthopnea may be so severe that patients cannot lie down at all and must spend the entire night in a sitting position. On the other hand, in other patients with long-standing, severe heart failure, symptoms of pulmonary congestion may actually diminish with time as the function of the right ventricle becomes impaired.

PAROXYSMAL (NOCTURNAL) DYSPNEA This term refers to attacks of severe shortness of breath which generally occur at night and usually awaken the patient from sleep. Though simple orthopnea may be relieved by sitting upright at the side of the bed with legs dependent, in the patient with paroxysmal nocturnal dyspnea coughing and wheezing often persist in this position. The depression of the respiratory center during sleep may reduce ventilation sufficiently to lower arterial oxygen tension, particularly in patients with interstitial lung edema and reduced pulmonary compliance. Also, ventricular function may be further impaired at night because of reduced adrenergic stimulation of myocardial function. Acute pulmonary edema is a severe form of cardiac asthma due to further elevation of pulmonary capillary pressure and associated with extreme shortness of breath, rales over both lung fields, and the transudation and expectoration of blood-tinged fluid. If not treated promptly (page 1187) acute pulmonary edema may be fatal.

CHEYNE-STOKES RESPIRATION Also known as *periodic* or *cyclic respiration,* Cheyne-Stokes respiration is characterized by diminished sensitivity of the respiratory center. In this form of respiration there is an apneic phase, during which the arterial P_{O_2} falls and the arterial P_{CO_2} rises. This combination of changes in the arterial blood stimulates the depressed respiratory center, resulting in hyperventilation and hypocapnia, followed in turn by apnea. Cheyne-Stokes respiration occurs most often in patients with cerebral atherosclerosis and other cerebral lesions, but the prolongation of the circulation time from the lung to the brain which occurs in heart failure, particularly in patients with hypertension and coronary artery disease and associated cerebral vascular disease, also appears to precipitate this form of breathing.

FATIGUE AND WEAKNESS These are nonspecific but common symptoms of heart failure and are related to the reduction of cardiac output. Anorexia and nausea associated with abdominal pain and fullness are frequent complaints in patients with severe heart failure; they may be related to the enlarged congested liver.

CEREBRAL SYMPTOMS In severe heart failure, particularly in elderly patients with accompanying cerebral arteriosclerosis and arterial hypoxemia, there may be alterations in the mental state characterized by confusion, difficulty in concentration, and impairment of memory, headache, insomnia, and anxiety.

PHYSICAL FINDINGS IN HEART FAILURE

In moderate heart failure the patient appears to be in no distress at rest except that he may become uncomfortable if asked to lie flat for more than a few minutes. In more severe heart failure the pulse pressure may be diminished, reflecting a reduction in stroke volume, and occasionally the diastolic arterial pressure may be elevated as a consequence of generalized vasoconstriction. There may be cyanosis of the lips and nail beds. Sinus tachycardia is common, as well as evidence of congested neck veins, which fill from below and which become distended with sustained pressure on the liver (positive hepatojugular reflux). *Systemic venous pressure* is often abnormally elevated in heart failure and may be recognized most readily by observing the extent of distention of the jugular veins. In the early stages of heart failure the venous pressure may be normal at rest but may become abnormally elevated during and immediately after exertion.

Early diastolic and presystolic gallop sounds (Chap. 232) are often audible but are not specific for heart failure, and *pulsus alternans,* i.e., a regular rhythm in which there is alternation of strong and weak cardiac contractions and therefore alternation in the strength of the peripheral pulses, may be present. Pulsus alternans may be detected by sphygmomanometry and in more severe instances by palpation; it frequently follows an extrasystole and is observed most commonly in patients with cardiomyopathy or with hypertensive or ischemic heart disease. It is caused by a reduction in the number of contractile units during weak contractions and/or by alternation in the ventricular end-diastolic volume.

BASAL PULMONARY RALES Moist, inspiratory, crepitant rales and dullness to percussion over the posterior lung bases are common in patients with heart failure and elevated pulmonary venous and capillary pressures. In patients with pulmonary edema, rales may be heard widely over both lung fields; they are frequently coarse and sibilant and may be accompanied by expiratory wheezing. Rales may, however, be caused by many other conditions.

CARDIAC EDEMA Cardiac edema is usually dependent, occurring in the legs symmetrically, particularly in the pretibial region and ankles in ambulatory patients, and in the sacral region of individuals at bed rest. Pitting edema of the arms and face occurs rarely and only late in the course of heart failure.

HYDROTHORAX Pleural effusion in congestive heart failure results from the elevation of pleural capillary pressure and transudation of fluid into the pleural cavities. Since the pleural veins drain into both the systemic and pulmonary veins, hydrothorax is observed most commonly in patients with marked elevation of pressure in both venous systems, but may also occur with marked elevation of pressure in either venous bed. It is noted more frequently in the right pleural cavity than the left.

ASCITES This also occurs as a consequence of transudation and results from increased pressure in the hepatic veins and the veins draining the peritoneum (Chap. 44). Ascites occurs most frequently in patients with tricuspid valve disease and with constrictive pericarditis.

CONGESTIVE HEPATOMEGALY An enlarged, tender, pulsating liver also accompanies systemic venous hypertension and is observed not only in the same conditions in which ascites occurs, but also in milder forms of heart failure from any cause. When systemic venous hypertension and hepatomegaly are prolonged and severe, enlargement of the spleen may also occur.

JAUNDICE This is a late finding in congestive heart failure and is associated with elevations of both the direct- and indirect-reacting bilirubin levels; it results from impairment of hepatic function secondary to hepatic congestion and the hepatocellular hypoxia associated with central lobular atrophy. Serum enzyme concentrations, particularly SGOT and SGPT, are frequently elevated.

CARDIAC CACHEXIA With severe chronic heart failure there may be serious weight loss and cachexia because of (1) elevation of the metabolic rate, which results in part from the extra work performed by the respiratory muscles, the increased oxygen needs of the hypertrophied heart, and the discomfort associated with severe heart failure; (2) anorexia, nausea, and vomiting due to central causes or to congestive hepatomegaly and abdominal fullness; (3) some impairment of intestinal absorption due to congestion of the intestinal veins; and (4) rarely, in patients with particularly severe failure of the right side of the heart, a protein-losing enteropathy.

OTHER MANIFESTATIONS With reduction of blood flow the extremities may be cold, pale, and diaphoretic. Urine flow is depressed, and the urine contains protein and has a high specific gravity and a low concentration of sodium. In addition, there is prerenal azotemia.

ROENTGENOGRAPHIC FINDINGS IN HEART FAILURE

In addition to the enlargement of the particular chambers characteristic of the lesion responsible for heart failure, vascular changes in the lung fields are common in patients with heart failure and elevated pulmonary vascular pressures. These are described in Chap. 234. Also, pleural effusions may be present and associated with interlobar effusions.

CLINICAL MANIFESTATIONS OF HIGH CARDIAC OUTPUT STATES ASSOCIATED WITH HEART FAILURE

THYROTOXICOSIS The characteristic clinical features of hyperthyroidism may be so conspicuous even after the development of heart failure that the diagnosis is simple on clinical grounds (Chap. 92). In other cases, when eye phenomena and thyroid enlargement are not striking, the overactivity of the thyroid is hardly discernible. Thyrotoxicosis should be suspected as a contributing factor in patients with cardiac disease under the following circumstances:

tachycardia that persists after prolonged rest and during sleep; any suggestion of heart failure with a high cardiac output in the absence of other recognizable causes; failure of the usual treatment measures to bring about a satisfactory response; attacks of paroxysmal atrial fibrillation or chronic atrial fibrillation in a person without obvious cause such as mitral valve disease and/or left atrial enlargement, particularly when the ventricular rate is resistant to the slowing effect of full doses of digitalis. The diagnosis is discussed fully in Chap. 92.

After treatment has restored the euthyroid state, remarkable improvement in a previously intractable form of heart disease usually follows. In about one-third of patients with atrial fibrillation the rhythm reverts spontaneously to a normal sinus mechanism; angina and congestive failure disappear or become easily controllable.

HEART FAILURE SECONDARY TO ANEMIA The clinical picture is that of high-output failure with anemia. One may find cardiac enlargement, occasionally with hypertrophy; systolic murmurs resulting from the combined effects of decreased viscosity, increased flow, or an aortic diastolic blowing murmur, presumably due to dilatation of the aortic ring. The latter may present a confusing problem of diagnosis. Furthermore, when slight fever is also present, subacute bacterial endocarditis may be mimicked. In patients with sickle-cell anemia with fever and joint pains, acute rheumatic fever may be suspected.

When there is an organic obstruction in a coronary artery, the compensatory increase in coronary flow that would otherwise take place in anemia is prevented and angina may appear; alternatively, anemia may aggravate already existing angina.

HEART FAILURE SECONDARY TO THIAMINE DEFICIENCY (BERIBERI) Thiamine deficiency (Chap. 84) leads to a deficiency of cocarboxylase, resulting in impaired myocardial energy production. The defect in the peripheral tissues causes peripheral vasodilatation, increased venous return and cardiac output, and, consequently, an increased load on a heart already handicapped by the metabolic defect. Cardiac failure is more likely to occur in persons who have the least involvement of the nervous system and a greater capacity for work, i.e., who have a greater opportunity to develop an increased load on the heart.

The usual clinical picture of beriberi heart disease, as seen in the Orient, is characterized by enlargement of the heart, absence of arrhythmia, systemic venous hypertension, bounding arterial pulsations, and the classic phenomena of heart failure with a high cardiac output.

This picture is rarely encountered in the occidental countries; in these areas the more common description is that of a person who has been on a clearly deficient diet over a long period of time, who has had an excessive consumption of alcohol, who has heart disease of uncertain origin, heart failure that does not respond to the usual methods of treatment, signs of mild peripheral neuritis or other manifestations of dietary deficiency, and whose heart failure and cardiac enlargement disappear with the administration of thiamine.

The diagnosis depends mostly on securing a good dietary history and on observing the response to treatment. Beriberi heart disease should be suspected when heart failure with a normal or elevated cardiac output is observed in the absence of thyrotoxicosis or anemia. Furthermore, thiamine deficiency may contribute to the development of heart failure in all alcoholics.

Differential diagnosis

The diagnosis of congestive heart failure may be established by observing some combination of the clinical manifestations of heart failure, enumerated above, together with the findings characteristic of one of the etiologic forms of heart disease. Since heart failure is usually associated with an enlarged heart on physical examination and/or roentgenography, the diagnosis should be questioned, but is by no means excluded, when all chambers are normal in size. Heart failure may be difficult to distinguish from pulmonary disease, and the differential diagnosis is discussed in Chap. 30. Pulmonary embolism also presents many of the manifestations of heart failure, but fixed splitting of the second heart sound, a right ventricular lift, hemoptysis, pleuritic chest pain, and the characteristic mismatch between ventilation and perfusion on lung scan should point to this diagnosis (Chap. 266).

Ankle edema may be due to varicose veins, cyclic edema, or gravitational effects (Chap. 32), but in these patients there is no generalized systemic venous hypertension at rest, following exertion, or with pressure over the liver. Edema secondary to renal disease can usually be recognized by appropriate renal function tests and urinalysis and is rarely associated with elevation of the venous pressure. Enlargement of the liver and ascites occur in patients with hepatic cirrhosis, but may also be distinguished from heart failure by normal jugular antecubital venous pressures and absence of a positive hepatojugular reflux.

TREATMENT OF HEART FAILURE

The treatment of heart failure may be divided into three components: (1) removal of the precipitating cause; (2) correction of the underlying cause; (3) control of the congestive heart failure state. The first two are discussed elsewhere, together with each specific disease entity or complication. The third component of the treatment of heart failure may, in turn, be divided into three categories: *(a)* reduction of the cardiac work load; *(b)* enhancement of myocardial contractility; and *(c)* control of excessive fluid retention. The first two of these forms of therapy should be utilized simultaneously, and if abnormal fluid accumulation persists, the third should be applied. The vigor with which each of these measures is pursued in any individual patient should depend upon the severity of the heart failure state. Following effective treatment, recurrence of the clinical manifestations of heart failure may be prevented by continuing those measures that were originally effective.

Reduction of the cardiac work load

A reduction in physical activity in mild cases and rest in bed or in a chair in severe failure remain cornerstones in the treatment of heart failure. Meals should be small in quantity, and every effort should be made to diminish the patient's anxiety. Physical and emotional rest tend to lower arterial pressure, and reduce the load on the myocardium by diminishing the requirements for cardiac output. These influences act in concert to diminish the need for redistribution of the cardiac output, and in many patients, particularly those with mild heart failure, simple bed rest and mild sedation often result in an effective diuresis.

Rest at home or in the hospital should be maintained for 1 to 2 weeks in patients with overt congestive failure and should be continued for several days after the patient's condition has stabilized. The hazards of phlebothrombosis and pulmonary embolism which occur with bed rest may be reduced with anticoagulants, leg exercises, and elastic stockings. Heavy sedation should be avoided, but small doses of barbiturates or tranquilizers may be helpful in calming the emotionally disturbed patient with heart failure through the first few days of therapy and in permitting much-needed sleep. In patients with chronic, mild heart failure, bed rest on weekends will frequently allow continuation of gainful employment. Following recovery from heart failure, the patient's activities must be carefully assessed, and in many instances his work load and responsibilities must be reduced. Intermittent rest during the day and the avoidance of strenuous exertion are helpful. Weight reduction by restriction of caloric intake in the obese patient with heart failure also diminishes cardiac work load and is an essential component of the therapeutic program.

Enhancement of myocardial contractility

The improvement of myocardial contractility by means of cardiac glycosides is the second of the three cornerstones in the control of the heart failure state. The pharmacology, indications, contraindications, and methods of administration of glycosides are considered in detail in Chap. 239. Digitalis is most effective in the common forms of heart failure associated with an excessive hemodynamic burden, such as hypertension and valvular heart disease, as well as in ischemic heart disease. It is particularly effective in the treatment of euthyroid patients with atrial fibrillation or atrial flutter and rapid ventricular rates associated with heart failure. In such patients the slowing of the ventricular rate, resulting from prolongation of the refractory period of the atrioventricular node combined with the improved inotropic state of the myocardium, results in striking and rapid clinical improvement. However, even in patients without these arrhythmias digitalis produces considerable clinical improvement as a consequence of its positive inotropic action.

Cardiac glycosides are less effective in diseases primarily affecting the myocardial cell, such as the toxic and infectious myocarditides, the various forms of cardiomyopathy and fibroelastosis, and in those forms of heart failure which are precipitated by infection, fever, anemia, thyrotoxicosis, beriberi, acute rheumatic fever, complete atrioventricular block, and cor pulmonale. Digitalis is contraindicated in patients with second degree or unstable atrioventricular block, unless a pacemaker has been inserted, and in patients with idiopathic hypertrophic subaortic stenosis (Chap. 247).

Three sympathomimetic amines which act largely on beta-adrenergic receptors—epinephrine, isoproterenol, and dopamine—improve myocardial contractility in various forms of heart failure. Dopamine, the immediate precursor in the biosynthesis of norepinephrine, appears to be most effective, since it also produces renal vasodilatation by a nonadrenergic mechanism and thereby augments sodium excretion. It increases cardiac output substantially but lowers peripheral resistance slightly. It is administered by constant intravenous infusion, in doses ranging from 100 to 1,000 μg per min, and has been found useful in intractable heart failure, particularly in patients with myocardial infarction and shock or pulmonary edema (Chap. 245).

Control of excessive fluid retention

Many of the clinical manifestations of heart failure are secondary to hypervolemia and expansion of the interstitial fluid volume. When fluid retention due to heart failure first becomes clinically evident, considerable expansion of the extracellular space has already occurred, and heart failure is already advanced. The quantity of extracellular fluid volume is largely dependent on the extracellular sodium content, and treatment aimed at reducing extracellular fluid volume is dependent primarily on lowering total body sodium stores, while fluid restriction, per se, is of less importance. A negative sodium balance can be achieved by reducing the dietary intake and increasing the urinary excretion of this ion with the aid of diuretics. In severe heart failure mechanical removal of extracellular fluid by means of thoracentesis, paracentesis, hemodialysis, or peritoneal dialysis may also be employed.

DIET In patients with mild heart failure, considerable improvement in symptoms may result from the simple reduction of sodium intake, particularly if this measure is accompanied by bed rest. In patients with more severe failure the sodium intake must be controlled more rigidly, even when other measures such as cardiac glycosides and diuretics are used, and following recovery from a bout of heart failure, at least moderate sodium restriction should be maintained. The normal diet contains approximately 6 to 10 g sodium chloride; this intake can be reduced by half simply by excluding salt-rich foods and salt which is added at the table. Reduction of the ordinary dietary intake to approximately one-fourth of normal may be achieved if, in addition, all salt is omitted from cooking. In patients with severe heart failure, in whom the daily sodium chloride intake is reduced to between 500 and 1,000 mg, milk, cheese, bread, cereals, canned vegetables and soups, some salted cuts of meat, and fresh vegetables, including spinach, celery, and beets, must be eliminated. A variety of fresh fruit, green vegetables, specially processed breads and milk, and salt substitutes are permissible, but such diets are difficult to keep palatable outside the hospital. Water intake may be *ad libitum* in all but the most severe forms of congestive heart failure. However, late in the course of heart failure, dilutional hyponatremia may develop in patients who are unable to excrete a water load, sometimes because of excessive secretion of antidiuretic hormone. In such cases water intake as well as sodium intake must be restricted.

Attention must also be directed to the caloric content of the diet. Substantial improvement can result from caloric restriction in obese patients with heart failure, in whom weight loss will reduce the load placed on the myocardium. On the other hand, in individuals with severe heart failure and cardiac cachexia, an attempt must be made to maintain nutritional intake and to avoid caloric and vitamin deficiencies.

DIURETICS A variety of diuretic agents is available, and in the patient with mild heart failure almost all are effective. The choice of the particular diuretic to be employed depends to some extent on convenience. However, in the more severe forms of heart failure, the selection of diuretics is more difficult, and any existing abnormalities in the serum electrolytes must be taken into account. Overtreatment and resultant hypovolemia must be avoided, since excessive reduction of blood volume may reduce cardiac output, interfere with renal function, and produce profound weakness and lethargy.

Thiazide diuretics These agents are widely used in clinical practice because of their effectiveness when administered orally. In patients with chronic heart failure of mild or moderate severity the continued administration of chlorothiazide or one of its many analogues abolishes or diminishes the need for rigid dietary sodium restriction. Thiazides are well absorbed following oral administration; chlorothiazide and hydrochlorothiazide reach their peak action in 4 h, and diuresis persists for approximately 12 h. Thiazide agents reduce the tubular reabsorption of sodium, and chloride and water follow the unreabsorbed sodium into the more distal tubule. Here, potassium-sodium exchange is enhanced, with augmented kaliuresis the result. Thiazides fail to increase free water clearance, and in some instances reduce it, supporting the hypothesis that these drugs inhibit selective sodium chloride reabsorption in the cortical diluting segment, at a site where the urine is normally diluted. This results in the excretion of a hypertonic urine and may contribute to dilutional hyponatremia. As a consequence of the increased delivery of sodium to the distal nephron, sodium-potassium ion exchange is accelerated and kaliuresis results. The carbonic anhydrase-inhibiting properties of the thiazides are of limited importance and need not be invoked to account for most of the diuretic action. Chlorothiazide is administered in doses of up to 500 mg every 6 h. Many derivatives of this compound are available but differ principally in dosage and duration of action and therefore offer few, if any, significant advances over the parent compound. Potassium depletion is the chief adverse effect following prolonged administration of chlorothiazide, and may seriously enhance the dangers of digitalis intoxication. Hypokalemia may be prevented by the oral supplementation of potassium chloride solution. However, this is not palatable and may be hazardous in patients with renal failure. Therefore, to control potassium depletion produced by thiazides (as well as by ethacrynic acid and furosemide), intermittent dosage schedules, e.g., omitting the diuretic every third day, and the addition of a potassium-retaining diuretic, such as a spironolactone or triameterene, may be preferable. Other side effects of thiazides include reduction of the excretion of uric acid, which may lead to hyperuricemia, and a hyperglycemic effect, which is particularly troublesome in patients with overt or latent diabetes mellitus. Skin rashes, thrombocytopenia, and granulocytopenia have also been reported.

Ethacrynic acid and furosemide These two diuretics are similar physiologically but differ chemically. Ethacrynic acid is an unsaturated ketone derivative of aryloxyacetic acid, while furosemide differs from the thiazides in that the thiadiasine ring has been replaced by a furfuryl group on the amino nitrogen of the anthranilic acid.

These are extremely powerful diuretics which reversibly inhibit the reabsorption throughout the nephron, but especially inhibit active chloride reabsorption in the thick ascending limb of the loop of Henle. These agents produce rates of urine formation which may be as high as one-third of the glomerular filtration rate. They may induce renal cortical vasodilatation. While other diuretics lose their effectiveness as blood volume is restored to normal levels, ethacrynic acid and furosemide remain effective despite the elimination of excessive extracellular fluid volume. The major side effects of these agents are due to this marked diuretic potency, which may result in circulatory collapse and in reductions in the renal blood flow and glomerular filtration rate. There is an inability to generate a dilute urine; alkalosis is produced by a large increase in the urinary excretion of chloride, hydrogen, and potassium ions. Hypokalemia and hyponatremia may occur, and hyperuricemia and hypoglycemia are observed occasionally, as with thiazide diuretics.

Both drugs are readily absorbed orally and are excreted in the bile and urine. They are usually effective by mouth, in doses of 25 to 100 mg two or four times daily, and intravenously in doses ranging from 10 to 100 mg. Both drugs can be given intravenously, and furosemide intramuscularly as well. Weakness, nausea, and dizziness may accompany both diuretics; ethacrynic acid has been associated with skin rash and granulocytopenia, as well as with transient or permanent deafness.

These extremely effective diuretics are useful in all forms of heart failure, particularly in otherwise refractory heart failure and pulmonary edema. Both agents have been shown to be effective in patients with hypoalbuminemia, hyponatremia, hypochloremia, hypokalemia, and reductions in the glomerular filtration rate, and to produce a diuresis in patients in whom mercurial and thiazide diuretics are ineffective.

The effectiveness of ethacrynic acid or furosemide may be potentiated by spironolactone, triameterene, a thiazide diuretic, a carbonic anhydrase inhibitor, or an osmotic diuretic, such as mannitol. In turn, when used in combination with mercurials or thiazides, ethacrynic acid or furosemide increases the effectiveness of these agents.

Organomercurials Presumably these diuretics act by releasing inorganic mercury within the tubule cell, which then combines with sulfhydryl enzymes essential for active sodium transport in the ascending limb of Henle's loop. Mercurial diuretics reduce sodium reabsorption and make a greater quantity of sodium available for exchange with potassium in the distal tubule, thus tending to increase the excretion of potassium. Since these compounds produce a hypotonic diuresis, they may be useful in the treatment of patients with heart failure and dilutional hyponatremia. Mercurial diuretics result in a metabolic alkalosis which limits the effectiveness of further administration. Effectiveness may be restored, however, in a patient whose condition is refractory to further mercurial administration, by raising the serum chloride concentration with oral ammonium chloride, 6 to 12 g orally, in divided doses for 3 to 4 days prior to the administration of the mercurial. The most commonly used mercurial diuretic, Mercuhydrin, also contains theophylline.

A serious disadvantage of mercurial diuretics is that they are not particularly effective when given by mouth and require parenteral administration. They are usually administered intramuscularly in doses of 0.5 or 1.0 ml, but may be given intravenously in patients with severe and refractory heart failure. One commonly available mercurial diuretic, Thiomerin, may be administered subcutaneously. Rare fatal reactions following intravenous injection have been reported and presumably are due to cardiac arrhythmias. Mercurial diuretics should be administered with caution to patients with renal insufficiency in whom clinical manifestations of mercurialism, i.e., stomatitis, colitis, further renal damage, and salivation, have been reported. Skin rash and fever occur rarely.

Aldosterone antagonists The 17-spironolactones resemble aldosterone structurally and act on the distal renal tubule by competitive inhibition of aldosterone, thereby blocking the exchange between sodium and both potassium and hydrogen in the distal tubules and collecting ducts. These agents produce a sodium diuresis, and, in contrast to the thiazides, ethacrynic acid, and furosemide, they tend to result in potassium retention. Although secondary hyperaldosteronism exists in some patients with congestive heart failure, the spironolactones are effective even in patients in whom the serum aldosterone concentration is within normal limits. Aldactone A may be administered in doses of 25 to 100 mg three to four times daily by mouth. The maximal effect of this regimen is not observed for approximately 4 days. Spironolactones are most effective when administered in combination with thiazide diuretics, ethacrynic acid, or furosemide. The opposing action of these drugs on urine and serum potassium makes possible a sodium diuresis without either hyper- or hypokalemia when spironolactone and one of these other agents are administered in combination. Also, since spironolactone (and triamterene) act on the distal tubule, they are particularly effective when used in combination with one of these other diuretics which acts more proximally.

Spironolactone should not be administered alone to patients with hyperkalemia, renal failure, or hyponatremia. Reported complications include nausea, epigastric distress, mental confusion, drowsiness, gynecomastia, and erythematous eruptions.

Triamterene A pteridine derivative, triamterene exerts a renal effect similar to that of the spironolactones; i.e., it prevents sodium reabsorption and interferes with sodium-potassium exchange in the distal tubules. However, its fundamental mechanism of action differs from that of the spironolactones, since it is active in adrenalectomized animals. The effective dose is 100 mg once or twice daily. Side effects include nausea, vomiting, diarrhea, headache, granulocytopenia, eosinophilia, and skin rash. Although it resembles Aldactone A in that its diuretic potency is not great, it is extremely effective in preventing the hypokalemia characteristic of thiazide administration.

Choice of a diuretic The thiazides, administered orally, are the agents of choice in the treatment of chronic cardiac edema of mild to moderate degree in patients without hyperglycemia or hyperuricemia. Spironolactones and triamterene are not potent diuretics when used alone, but they are particularly effective when administered along with other diuretics, particularly the thiazides, ethacrynic acid, and furosemide, which by themselves may produce marked potassium loss. However, in patients with heart failure and severe secondary aldosteronism, spironolactone may be extremely effective. Ethacrynic acid or furosemide, given alone or with spironolactone or triamterene, is the agent of choice in patients with severe heart failure refractory to other diuretics. Mercurial diuretics are useful when a rapid diuresis is desired in patients with hyperglycemia or hyperuricemia.

Refractory heart failure

When the response to treatment is inadequate, heart failure is considered to be refractory. Before assuming that this state simply reflects advanced, perhaps preterminal, myocardial depression, careful consideration must be given to several possibilities: (1) an underlying and overlooked cause of the heart disease that may be amenable to specific surgical or medical therapy, such as silent aortic or mitral stenosis, constrictive pericarditis, bacterial endocarditis, hypertension, or thyrotoxicosis; (2) one or a combination of the precipitating causes of heart failure, such as pulmonary or urinary tract infection, recurrent pulmonary emboli, arterial hypoxemia, anemia, or arrhythmia; (3) complications of overly vigorous therapy, such as digitalis intoxication, hypovolemia, or electrolyte imbalance.

As pointed out in Chap. 232 (Fig. 232-6), afterload is a major determinant of cardiac function. A modest elevation in afterload will not necessarily alter stroke volume when cardiac function is normal, because the resultant small increase in preload can be tolerated easily. However, when myocardial function is impaired, such an increase in preload evoked by an elevation of afterload may raise ventricular end-diastolic and pulmonary capillary pressures to levels that may produce pulmonary congestion and pulmonary edema. In many patients with heart failure, the ventricle already is operating at the peak, flat portion of its Frank-Starling curve (Fig. 236-7), and any additional increase in afterload will reduce stroke volume (page 1173). Conversely, a reduction of afterload will elevate stroke volume.

In heart failure, left ventricular afterload is increased as a consequence of the many neural, humoral, and/or structural changes which constrict the peripheral vascular bed, and as the elevation of ventricular end-diastolic volume compensates for impaired cardiac function as a consequence of the operation of Laplace's law. The maintenance or even the elevation of arterial pressure is generally considered to be a useful compensatory mechanism which allows blood flow to vital organs to be maintained despite the marked inadequacy of total cardiac output, which occurs particularly during exertion. However, in the presence of severely impaired cardiac function, the increase in afterload may reduce cardiac output and elevate myocardial oxygen consumption further. The pharmacologic reduction of impedance to left ventricular ejection, i.e., of afterload, with vasodilator drugs may be an important adjunct in the management of heart failure of diverse etiologies; this approach may be particularly helpful in patients shortly after the onset of an acute myocardial infarction (Chap. 245) and in patients with mitral regurgitation. The reduction of afterload by means of a variety of vasodilators, including intravenous nitroprusside, sublingual nitroglycerin, or isosorbide dinitrate and oral phenoxybenzamine, or mechanically by intraaortic balloon counterpulsation, reduces left ventricular end-diastolic pressure and oxygen consumption, while raising stroke volume and cardiac output and causing only modest reductions in aortic pressure.

In patients with chronic intractable heart failure secondary to coronary artery disease or cardiomyopathy who are treated with intravenous sodium nitroprusside, cardiac output increases substantially, the pulmonary wedge pressure falls, the signs and symptoms of heart failure are relieved, and a new steady state is generated in which cardiac output is higher and afterload lower with only mild reduction of arterial pressure. Furthermore, it has been proposed that the reduction of elevated left end-diastolic pressure might improve subendocardial perfusion. Afterload reduction should therefore be considered in the management of patients with intractable heart failure, but it requires careful hemodynamic monitoring.

Treatment of acute pulmonary edema

Pulmonary edema secondary to left ventricular failure or mitral stenosis is described in Chap. 30. It is life-threatening and must be considered a medical emergency. As is the case for the more chronic forms of heart failure, in the treatment of pulmonary edema, attention must be directed to identifying and removing any precipitating causes of decompensation, such as an arrhythmia or infection. However, because of the acute nature of the problem, a number of additional measures are necessary: (1) Morphine is administered by the subcutaneous, intramuscular, or intravenous routes in doses from 5 to 20 mg, depending upon the severity of the problem. This drug reduces anxiety, which tends to perpetuate pulmonary edema, and thereby breaks a vicious cycle. Also, morphine exerts a positive inotropic effect and tends to reduce venous return. Naline should be available in case respiratory depression occurs. (2) High concentration of oxygen must be inhaled because the alveolar fluid interferes with oxygen diffusion, resulting in arterial hypoxemia. Therefore, 100 percent oxygen should be administered, preferably under positive pressure. The latter increases intraalveolar pressure and therefore reduces transudation of fluid from the alveolar capillaries and impedes venous return to the thorax, reducing pulmonary capillary pressure. (3) The patient should be maintained in the sitting position, which also tends to reduce venous return to the heart. (4) Rotating tourniquets should be applied to the extremities and may be followed by a phlebotomy of 500 ml. (5) Aminophylline (theophylline ethylenediamine), 240 to 480 mg intravenously, is effective in diminishing bronchoconstriction, increasing renal blood flow and sodium excretion, and augmenting myocardial contractility. (6) If digitalis has not been administered previously, three-fourths of a full dose of a rapidly acting glycoside, such as ouabain, digoxin, or lanatoside C, should be administered intravenously (Chap. 239). (7) Intravenous diuretics, such as furosemide or ethacrynic acid (25 to 50 mg), will, by rapidly establishing a diuresis, reduce circulating blood volume and thereby hasten the relief of pulmonary edema.

Prognosis

The prognosis in heart failure depends primarily on the nature of the underlying heart disease and on the presence or absence of a precipitating factor which can be treated. When one of the latter can be identified and removed, the outlook for immediate survival is far better than if heart failure occurs without any obvious precipitating cause. The prognosis can also be estimated by observing the response to treatment. When clinical improvement occurs with only modest dietary sodium restriction and/or digitalis without the administration of diuretics, then the outlook is far better than if, in addition to these measures, intensive diuretic therapy is necessary. The long-term prognosis for heart failure is most favorable when the underlying forms of heart disease can be treated.

REFERENCES

BRAUNWALD E et al: *Mechanisms of Contraction of the Normal and Failing Heart,* 2d ed., Boston: Little, Brown, 1976

BURG MB: Mechanisms of action of diuretic drugs, chap. 19 in *The Kidney,* eds BM Brenner, FC Rector, Philadelphia: Saunders, 1976, p. 737

CHERNIACK NS, LONGOBARDO GS: Cheyne-Stokes breathing: An instability in physiologic control. N Engl J Med 288:952, 1973

FOWLER NO (ed): Treatment of congestive heart failure, chap. 13 in *Cardiac Diagnosis and Treatment,* 2d ed, Hagerstown: Harper & Row, 1976, p. 248

FRIEDBERG CK (ed): Symposium on congestive heart failure. Prog Cardiovasc Dis 12:313, 1970

HURST JW (ed): *The Heart,* 3d ed., part V, section A: Heart Failure (chaps. 27–31), New York: McGraw-Hill, 1974, p. 416

KATZ AM: Congestive heart failure: Role of altered myocardial cellular control. N Engl J Med 293:1184, 1975

MUDGE GH: Diuretics and other agents employed in the mobilization of edema fluid, chap. 39 in *The Pharmacological Basis of Therapeutics,* 5th ed, eds LS Goodman, A Gilman, New York: Macmillan, 1975

NAYLER WG: The ionic basis of contractility, relaxation and cardiac failure, chap. 6 in *Modern Trends in Cardiology—3,* ed MF Oliver, London: Butterworth, 1975

238
CARDIAC DYSRHYTHMIAS

BURTON E. SOBEL
EUGENE BRAUNWALD

The term *dysrhythmia* is not limited to irregularities of the heartbeat but is applied also to disturbances of rate and of conduction. We shall first present certain broad considerations and then deal with specific disorders. The mechanism of action of the most important drugs utilized in the treatment of dysrhythmias is considered in Chap. 239; treatment by electrical methods is the topic of Chap. 240.

GENERAL CONSIDERATIONS

Etiologic factors

Certain dysrhythmias are especially likely to occur in the absence of detectable structural disease of the heart. These include sinus arrhythmias, sinus bradycardia, and sinus tachycardia; atrial and ventricular premature beats; milder forms of first degree atrioventricular (AV) block (that is, P-R intervals of 0.21 to 0.25 s), and paroxysmal atrial tachycardia. Only rarely can a specific agent such as tobacco, coffee, or ethanol be identified as an inciting cause of sinus or atrial tachycardia.

Other dysrhythmias are particularly likely to occur in persons with organ disease of the heart. These include ventricular tachycardia and fibrillation, atrial flutter and fibrillation, and second and third degrees of AV block. Although any type of structural cardiac disease may underlie any dysrhythmia, certain disturbances of rhythm are commonly associated with specific underlying processes, for example, atrial fibrillation in patients with hypertension, thyrotoxicosis, mitral valve disease, and left atrial enlargement; and ventricular tachycardia in those with ischemic heart disease. Still other disturbances of rhythm should immediately arouse the suspicion that a drug is responsible. Ventricular bigeminy—a disorder in which a ventricular premature beat follows every supraventricular beat—and atrial tachycardia with atrioventricular block are often due to digitalis excess, especially when there is coexistent potassium deficiency induced by diuretics (Chap. 239). Bradycardia associated with suppression of sinus node and atrial activity and prolongation of AV and intraventricular conduction may reflect procainamide or quinidine toxicity.

A cardiac dysrhythmia may be a manifestation of a serious circulatory or metabolic disturbance and should result in a careful, deliberate search for the underlying abnormality, which may be (1) a pathologic process in the myocardium, e.g., a myocardial infarction or myocarditis; (2) a vascular event such as leakage from an aortic aneurysm, or pulmonary embolization; (3) a sudden drop in blood volume due to hemorrhage such as gastrointestinal bleeding; (4) an endocrine disturbance such as thyrotoxicosis or pheochromocytoma; (5) drug toxicity, especially evoked by cardioactive agents, including digitalis, glycosides, catecholamines, methyl xanthines, and antiarrhythmics (Chap. 239); (6) systemic infections; (7) a neoplasm with cardiac metastases such as carcinoma of the lung, lymphoma, or melanoma; and (8) the rapid development of sudden severe hypoxemia or hypercapnia.

Electrolyte disturbances are of particular importance in the genesis of cardiac dysrhythmias and deserve special consideration. They occur frequently in combination. Therefore, in practice it may be difficult to determine the specific ion abnormality responsible. *Hyperkalemia* leads to AV block, impairment of intraatrial and intraventricular conduction with prolonged P waves and QRS complexes, and rarely sinoventricular conduction. Death may occur from ventricular fibrillation or, less commonly, from ventricular asystole. *Hypokalemia* may produce atrial and ventricular extrasystoles, couplets, and tachycardias, as well as mild atrioventricular and intraventricular conduction defects; severe hypokalemia may lead to multifocal premature ventricular contractions deteriorating into ventricular fibrillation. *Hypercalcemia* diminishes conduction velocity and shortens the refractory period, thereby facilitating reentry and the development of coupled ventricular beats, ventricular tachycardia, and ventricular fibrillation.

The treatment of dysrhythmias per se, without identification and management of the underlying abnormality, is often unrewarding. Also, often relatively little may be gained when treatment is directed toward a cardiac dysrhythmia which results from a structural abnormality, e.g., a greatly enlarged left atrium in a patient with mitral valvular disease. Effective control of atrial fibrillation under these circumstances might require surgical relief of the valvular abnormality.

Mechanism of dysrhythmias

Many cardiac dysrhythmias result from abnormalities in the automaticity of cardiac tissue. Increases in automaticity may result from (1) a more rapid rate of diastolic depolarization (Chap. 233); (2) a more negative threshold potential diminishing the change in potential required for excitation; (3) a less negative resting potential, which is therefore closer to the threshold potential; or (4) some combination of these abnormalities. Reductions in automaticity are produced by the opposite changes. Diminution of the resting potential and altered ionic composition of interstitial fluid may unmask automaticity due to slow, calcium-dependent current, which may be associated with afterpotentials giving rise to repetitive depolarizations. Certain dysrhythmias, e.g., sinus tachycardia and some ectopic tachycardias, appear to result from increases in automaticity of the sinoatrial node or of pacemaker tissue elsewhere in the heart. Other disturbances, such as atrioventricular junctional rhythm or idioventricular rhythm, usually result from reduction in the automaticity of the sinoatrial node, with control of the cardiac rhythm assumed by a pacemaker which ordinarily exhibits a lower degree of automaticity.

Disturbances in the conduction of the action potential provide another important physiologic basis for cardiac dysrhythmias. Pathologic slowing or failure of propagation of the impulse from the atrium and AV junctional tissue to the ventricles results in various degrees of AV block. Cells with low resting potentials, low amplitude and slowly rising action potentials, delayed recovery of excitability, and summation in response to spatially separated stimuli are found in the sinus and AV nodes, and have properties associated with slow-current, calcium-mediated responses. The decremental nature of conduction in the AV-nodal cells may lead to unidirectional AV block. The same phenomenon may occur when exposure of other cells to abnormal local metabolic conditions leads to slow-current depolarization. Slowed conduction may also set the stage for the development of tachyarrhythmias. Local ischemia or mechanical stresses may diminish conduction through segments of the myocardium so that when an impulse leaves the area of reduced conduction velocity, it finds the adjacent myocardium no longer refractory and restimulates it. This phenomenon is termed *reentry,* and it can result from either focal reexcitation due to the flow of current between adjacent portions of myocardium which are repolarized at different times (asynchronous recovery) or from circus current movement due to local impairment of conductivity. Reentry may occur within the AV or rarely sinus nodes giving rise to supraventricular tachycardia. Reentry within accessory pathways occurs in some patients with preexcitation syndromes. In the arborizing fibers of the distal Purkinje system, reentry may be related to the "false-tendon" insertions of Purkinje fibers on ventricular myocardium. The action potential and effective refractory period are prolonged in these regions, which function as "gates" in prohibiting propagation of premature impulses. However, impulses blocked at a gate in one region may be conducted slowly through another gate into ventricular myocardium, and return in retrograde fashion through the first fiber, initiating a reentry rhythm. Reentry is frequently responsible for coupled beats, and hence some instances of bigeminal rhythm. Sometimes, conduction is slowed in a diseased area so that unidirectional block is present. When this occurs, reexcitation of normal tissue may be followed by retrograde repetitive excitation of the diseased area and a self-sustaining tachycardia may result. Electrocardiographically, such rhythms appear to be initiated by a rapid ectopic pacemaker. In fact, however, although the dysrhythmia may be initiated by an ectopic impulse, it may be sustained by reentrant mechanisms. With recently available electrophysiologic techniques utilizing programmed electrical stimulation, several criteria of reentry rhythm have been established, including initiation and termination of tachyarrhythmia by appropriately timed premature beats and the appearance of a less than compensatory pause when interpolated beats are initiated during the tachycardia. Bigeminy due to digitalis, however, is probably due *not* to reentry but rather to increased automaticity associated with instability of Purkinje cells during repolarization, possibly due to slow-current, calcium-mediated depolarizations induced by the drug.

For a number of years considerable evidence supported the prevailing view that a *circus movement* is responsible for atrial flutter and fibrillation. However, some instances of these rhythms now appear to result from very rapid and irregular stimuli being discharged from a single focus. At the present time conflicting evidence favors and refutes both concepts; it is likely that each applies in different instances.

Concealed conduction is an additional important mechanism involved in complex dysrhythmias. This phenomenon usually affects the AV junction and occurs when an impulse penetrates the junction without traversing it. Thus, it may lead to apparent AV block or augmentation of the severity of block but in reality is due to concealed conduction of ectopic impulses and "resetting" of the refractory period of the junction. Concealed conduction is probably responsible for the nature of the irregularity of the ventricular response in the presence of atrial fibrillation.

Other important physiologic mechanisms which underlie complex dysrhythmias are the *Wedensky effect* (protracted enhancement of excitability after a stimulus of abnormally large amplitude); *Wedensky facilitation* (enhancement of excitability distal to the site of block of propagation of a preceding impulse); and *supernormal conduction* (enhancement of conduction occurring near the end of the relative refractory period of the preceding depolarization); temporal dispersion of depolarization, refractoriness, and recovery; and "gating," or the normally prolonged refractory period at the insertions of Purkinje fibers on ventricular myocardium. The Wedensky effect probably accounts for appearance of ventricular dysrhythmias after electrical cardioversion (Chap. 240) in the presence of occult digitalis toxicity. Wedensky facilitation probably accounts for the occurrence of enhanced AV conduction immediately after the dropped beat in a Wenckebach period (page 1203). *Supernormal conduction* is recognizable in patients with artificial pacemakers when a subthreshold impulse arising endogenously or initiated by another artificial pacemaker is conducted only when it occurs during the supernormal period of the preceding beat.

Temporal dispersion may lead to local reexcitation, reentry due to disparities in refractory periods with fragmentation of impulse transmission, slow current, calcium-mediated responses due to stimulation of partially repolarized cells, and increased vulnerability of ventricular myocardium to fibrillation. Prolonged action potentials and refractory periods in the "false tendons" may serve to preclude conduction of premature impulses by serving as gates under physiologic conditions. Type I antiarrhythmic drugs, such as quinidine and procainamide (Chap. 239), prolong the refractory period at the gate and may thereby inhibit premature stimulation. However, the increased temporal dispersion may set the stage for reentry rhythms. Type II antiarrhythmics, such as lidocaine and diphenylhydantoin, reduce action potential duration at the gate and may diminish the likelihood of reentry rhythms by decreasing temporal dispersion. However, they may set the stage for premature stimulation of ventricular myocardium by impulses initiated in ectopic foci.

Circulatory derangements associated with dysrhythmias

Dysrhythmias alter cardiac function by a variety of mechanisms.

EFFECTS OF CHANGES IN HEART RATE In a resting person with a normal heart, because of compensatory changes in stroke volume, cardiac output remains constant, or almost so, despite variations in heart rate from approximately 40 to 160 contractions per min; output decreases progressively at extremes beyond this range. However, in patients with significant myocardial, valvular, coronary arterial, or pericardial disease, such changes may seriously depress cardiac output because ventricular functional reserve mechanisms cannot compensate for altered stroke volume. The effect of bradycardia on cardiac output depends in part on its duration. Thus, in chronic long-standing AV block, cardiac output may be sustained even at rates as low as 35 beats per min. When increased demands are placed on the normal heart, as during exertion, infection, or anemia, the acceleration of heart rate contributes substantially to the circulatory adjustment to the stress. However, when third degree AV block is present with a fixed, slow ventricular rate, the cardiac output fails to rise normally, and the patient becomes especially symptomatic during the period of stress.

LOSS OF APPROPRIATELY TIMED, VIGOROUS ATRIAL CONTRACTION The atria are not merely passive conduits for returning blood from the systemic and pulmonary venous beds to the ventricles. Rather, they should be considered as booster pumps which augment ventricular filling. In many dysrhythmias the normal temporal sequence between atrial and ventricular systole is lost. These include all degrees of AV block, AV junctional rhythms, ventricular tachycardia, and many instances of atrial tachycardia and flutter. In atrial fibrillation, effective atrial contraction does not occur.

Loss of atrial booster pump function will not usually lower the cardiac output in persons with otherwise normal cardiac function, since compensatory mechanisms such as augmented sympathetic stimulation of the myocardium help to maintain the output. However, loss of atrial function reduces the maximal cardiac output which can be achieved during marked exertion. On the other hand, in patients with impaired myocardial function (particularly those with overt or incipient chronic heart failure) or with acute myocardial infarction, atrial function is more critical, and loss of the atrial booster pump results in a lowering of cardiac output by as much as 40 percent, elevation of atrial pressures, or both. In patients with marked ventricular hypertrophy, such as occurs in hypertension, aortic stenosis, idiopathic hypertrophic subaortic stenosis, and the related cardiomyopathies, characterized by ventricular hypertrophy, the atrial contribution to ventricular filling is particularly important, since the thickened ventricular wall impedes the inflow of blood. In patients with these lesions the sudden development of one of the aforementioned dysrhythmias may seriously impair cardiac performance and depress cardiac output and arterial pressure.

EFFECTS ON MYOCARDIAL OXYGEN CONSUMPTION AND CORONARY BLOOD FLOW The frequency of cardiac contraction is one of the major determinants of myocardial oxygen consumption (Chap. 7). Hence, when all other factors are constant, tachycardia increases and bradycardia reduces the need of the heart for oxygen. Coronary blood flow occurs predominantly during diastole, and since the total number of seconds of diastole per minute is reduced during tachycardia, a rapid heart rate may precipitate myocardial ischemia in the presence of coronary arterial narrowing. In turn, the ischemia may result in angina and in impairment of myocardial function. Thus, the development of AV block and a slow ventricular rate may diminish the severity of angina in patients with ischemic heart disease. On the other hand, excessive slowing of the heart rate associated with decreased cardiac output and impaired coronary perfusion may occasionally increase the severity of angina.

EFFECTS ON THE VENTRICULAR CONTRACTION SEQUENCE Ventricular function depends on a synchronous, nearly simultaneous ventricular contraction. Though the ventricular myocardium contracts in ventricular fibrillation, the chaotic nature of the contraction prevents the development of sufficient intraventricular pressure to propel blood forward. Lesser degrees of asynchrony occur in dysrhythmias associated with intraventricular conduction abnormalities, such as ventricular tachycardia, ventricular extrasystoles, and supraventricular tachycardias with bundle branch block. Such asynchrony of contraction will not impair the cardiac output in an individual with an otherwise normal heart but may exert a significant depressant effect in patients with serious cardiac disease.

EFFECTS ON MYOCARDIAL FUNCTION Although the responsible mechanism has not been identified, prolonged severe tachycardia can depress myocardial function directly, and this depression may persist even after sinus rhythm has been restored.

Methods of examination

The most precise methods of diagnosis of the various dysrhythmias include electrocardiographic examination and recordings of His bundle electrograms. However, physicians who have regularly correlated their observations by simple physical examination with electrocardiographic tracings can usually recognize many dysrhythmias at the bedside.

The exact ventricular rate should be measured by auscultation for a full minute. Pulse rate may be misleading because of a pulse deficit. The presence or absence of irregularity should be noted. The intensity of the first heart sound and the amplitude of the peripheral pulse should be observed, and it should be especially noted whether they are constant, as in dysrhythmias in which the normal temporal relation between atrial and ventricular contraction is maintained (as in sinus, paroxysmal atrial, or junctional tachycardias), or variable, as in dysrhythmias in which the normal temporal relation between atrial and ventricular contraction is lost (e.g., in complete AV heart block, ventricular tachycardia, or atrial flutter). Atrial sounds independent of the first and second heart sound are frequently audible in patients with third degree AV block. If the rhythm is irregular, one should distinguish between a basic cadence that is predictable (regular irregularity, e.g., premature beats) and one that is entirely unpredictable (irregular irregularity, e.g., atrial fibrillation). In some instances the effect of mild exercise on the ventricular rate, and likewise on the degree of irregularity, should be observed; whether the deceleration immediately after exercise occurs in the normal gradual fashion (sinus tachycardia) or in one or more abrupt steps (atrial flutter) should also be noted.

Inspection of the jugular venous pulse is helpful, especially when, in a patient with a very slow or rapid rate, an occasional abrupt large venous excursion—"cannon wave"—is seen. This giant A wave occurs when the atria contract simultaneously with or after the ventricles and results from atrial contraction when the tricuspid valve is closed. Occasionally the jugular venous pulse will be of aid in the recognition of atrial flutter, with A waves perceptible at a frequency of 250 to 350 beats per min. Observation of the effect of *carotid sinus massage* on the electrocardiogram may also be valuable. This maneuver elicits vagal efferent impulses which influence automaticity and conduction. After excluding occlusive carotid disease by examination, one may massage for a few seconds on one side. This may cause (1) no change in rate (ventricular tachycardia); (2) an abrupt slowing which persists after discontinuation of massage (atrial tachycardia); (3) a temporary slowing which lasts only during the massage (atrial flutter or sinus tachycardia), the rate then returning to the previous level either gradually (sinus tachycardia), or at once or following a brief period of irregular acceleration (atrial flutter). Carotid massage acts on the atrial mechanism (1) by gradually and temporarily slowing sinus rhythm or by abruptly interrupting a paroxysmal supraventricular tachycardia and/or (2) by increasing AV block.

The *electrocardiogram* should be studied systematically. The first and most important problem is to determine whether the dysrhythmia is ventricular or supraventricular in origin, a decision often made difficult by the presence of intraventricular conduction disturbances. The presence of P waves or flutter waves and their relation to the QRS complex in the tracing is especially important. P waves most often can be seen best in leads II, III, aVF, and/or those leads taken over the right precordium. Occasionally, other types of tracings may be necessary. For example, paroxysmal atrial tachycardia in the presence of a bundle branch block is exceedingly difficult to distinguish from ventricular tachycardia. Similarly, flutter impulses may be superimposed on the QRS complex or upon the T wave and make diagnosis difficult. In these instances, it may be necessary to employ esophageal electrodes or a bipolar anteroposterior lead. The right arm lead is placed over the right ventricle, the left arm lead on the back, and the electrocardiograph is set on lead I. Another bipolar chest lead may be used by placing the left arm lead at the cardiac apex and the right arm lead over the right ventricle. Intra-atrial electrograms, esophageal, or surface electrocardiograms recorded during carotid sinus massage are often helpful in unraveling complex dysrhythmias.

Difficult diagnostic problems may necessitate evaluation with *His bundle electrograms,* recorded with the use of a transvenous electrode catheter positioned with its tip in the right ventricle adjacent to the tricuspid valve. Ordinarily, atrial depolarization (A), His bundle depolarization (H), ventricular depolarization (V), and ventricular repolarization produce well-defined characteristic wave forms on the electrogram (Fig. 238-1). Recognition of each is facilitated by reference to a simultaneously recorded standard surface electrocardiogram and by knowledge of the usual temporal relationships between components of the electrogram. Junctional beats with aberrant ventricular conduction are preceded by an H spike, and the H-V interval is the same as in sinus beats. Ventricular premature beats are not preceded by an H spike, and in fact may be followed by an H depolarization and an A spike indicative of retrograde atrial depolarization. His bundle electrograms are useful in characterizing the nature of AV block. Prolonged A to H intervals are typical of AV junctional disease; prolonged H-V intervals are typical of delayed conduction in more distal portions of the conduction system and hence of trifascicular block. The latter is far more common than the former, and since it is more likely to evolve into sudden third degree block associated with syncope or sudden death, its recognition is of considerable importance.

Atrial or His bundle electrograms may reveal concealed conduction of ectopic impulses originating in the His-Purkinje system which mimic AV block by depolarizing the AV node without spreading into ventricular myocardium. The differentiation is important because treatment requires suppression of ectopic foci rather than facilitation of conduction. Intracardiac electrograms and characterization of the length of the refractory period in the AV node and in accessory pathways in patients with preexcitation syndromes are useful in selection of pharmacologic agents to prevent or treat tachycardia. Diagnosis may be facilitated

FIGURE 238-1
The relationship between deflections on the conventional electrocardiogram (II) and potentials evident on a simultaneously obtained His bundle recording (H). Three components are readily recognizable on the His bundle recording. The A spike follows the onset of the P wave and represents the atrial electrogram. The H spike represents depolarization of the His bundle. The V potential represents the recording of ventricular depolarization from the catheter electrode. The P-R interval on the simultaneously recorded electrocardiogram is divided conveniently into two components on the basis of the time of occurrence of the H spike. Thus the P-H component represents the time from the onset of atrial depolarization to His bundle depolarization and reflects the duration of conduction through atrial myocardium and the AV junction. The subsequent component of the P-R interval, namely, the H-V component, represents the time required for conduction of the impulse from the common His bundle to the ventricular myocardium. Normally, the P-H interval is between 80 and 140 ms and the H-V interval is between 35 and 55 ms. Prolongation of the PH interval is usually indicative of delay of conduction in the proximal AV junction and is often associated with Möbitz type I AV block. Prolongation of the H-V interval is usually indicative of conduction delay in the His bundle, or in both bundle branches or all three fascicles of the distal conduction system, and is frequently associated with Möbitz type II AV block. Premature supraventricular beats with aberrant conduction are preceded by an H spike at the usual interval prior to the onset of QRS complex on the conventional electrocardiogram. On the other hand, premature ventricular beats are recognized by appearance of a V spike occurring prematurely after an H spike, prior to an H spike, or without any association with an H spike.

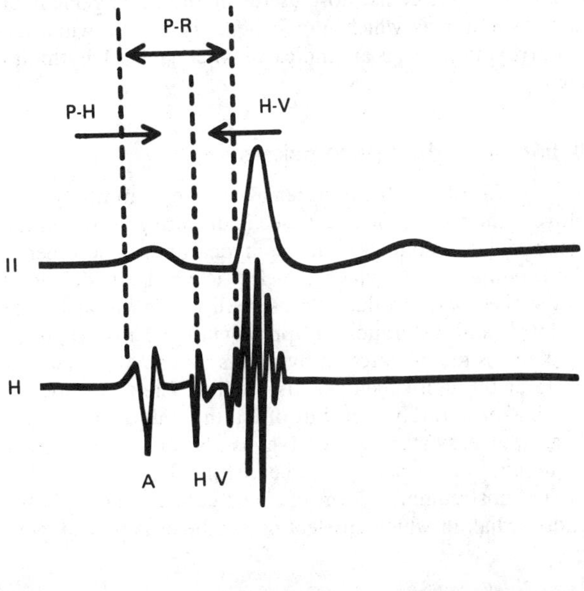

by unmasking delta waves indicative of preexcitation when atrial pacing or programmed electrical stimulation increases the A to H intervals, permitting expression of conduction through accessory pathways. Intraatrial electrical stimulation is also useful for detection and evaluation of impaired sinus node function reflected by prolonged sinus node recovery time after atrial paced rhythm.

Detection of dysrhythmias and assessment of their significance has been improved with the use of continuous, tape-recorded electrocardiographic monitoring of ambulatory patients. This approach also provides a tool for individualized evaluation of precipitating factors and antiarrhythmic therapy.

Treatment

GENERAL MEASURES The success or failure of specific treatment by drugs or by electric shock may be conditioned by appropriate systemic management. A precipitating cause of the dysrhythmia should be sought and treated. Obstruction of the air passages, hypoxia, and disturbances of pH and of electrolyte balance should be corrected. The coexistence of circulatory shock, whether of cardiac or peripheral origin, may render the patient's heartbeat refractory to the usual antiarrhythmic drugs. Thus, it may be necessary first to improve hemodynamics by blood or fluid replacement, or to administer agents with positive inotropic effects when depressed contractility is a contributing factor. Since pressor amines tend to induce ectopic rhythms at elevated blood pressure levels, the arterial pressure as well as the electrocardiogram should be observed frequently.

Rapidly acting cardiac glycosides such as digoxin, ouabain, or lanatoside C are useful for the treatment of any of the supraventricular tachycardias except, of course, paroxysmal atrial tachycardia with block, which is frequently caused by digitalis intoxication (Chap. 239). The roles of antiarrhythmic drugs and of electrical reversion in the treatment of arrhythmias are discussed in Chaps. 239 and 240 and in this chapter in relation to individual arrhythmias. The management of arrhythmias occurring with acute myocardial infarction is discussed in Chap. 244. In general, electrical reversion is most useful in the management of tachyarrhythmias which impair hemodynamics, while the antiarrhythmic drugs are indicated when tachyarrhythmias recur.

Artificial cardiac pacemakers

Two types of electrical pacemakers are commonly employed: the most commonly used is the *direct,* in which the electrode is in contact with the myocardium; the other is the *transthoracic,* in which the electrical pulse is delivered to the chest wall. In the latter, stimuli with a voltage of 25 to 150 V and a duration of approximately 2 ms are delivered across the precordium by means of a small plate electrode or through subcutaneous needles. The transthoracic pacemaker is rarely used but offers the unique advantage of a rapid, easy start-up; it serves as a useful standby technique until direct pacing can be instituted.

The most common form of *direct* cardiac pacing is the endocardial, in which an electrode catheter is placed, generally in the right ventricle, through the venous route; it is employed with an external power supply for temporary pacing or one that is implanted subcutaneously for permanent pacing. Endocardial pacing of the atrium is more difficult to achieve on a long-term basis, because of electrode instability. Epicardial pacing may be carried out by suturing wire leads to the atrial or ventricular myocardium at the time of thoracotomy, or by application of sutureless electrodes which screw into the myocardium. For permanent direct pacing the power supply is totally implanted.

Transvenous insertion of a permanent endocardial pacemaker entails minimal postoperative mortality (1 to 3 percent), but a high incidence of displacement (5 to 20 percent), maximum in the first month and especially in patients with a large right ventricle. Insertion at thoracotomy of an epicardial pacemaker entails a higher perioperative mortality (2 to 5 percent), virtually no incidence of displacement, but a high incidence of electrode breakage (approximately 20 percent) which may be diminished with newer sutureless electrodes. Increases in threshold with exit block occur more often with epicardial pacemakers and perforation of the heart (approximately 5 percent) more often with endocardial pacemakers. Infection (5 to 10 percent) is probably more common with epicardial devices. Transvenous endocardial pacing is still generally preferred except when atrial or sequential atrial and ventricular pacing are required.

Two principal modes of direct myocardial pacing may be employed. In *fixed-rate* pacing, cardiac stimulation is carried out continuously at a preset rate and is independent of the intrinsic electric activity of the heart. Consequently, if AV conduction is reestablished in patients with AV block, competition between the paced beats and the patient's intrinsic rhythm may occur. This competition may result in chaotic rhythms with an attendant, if small, hazard of the development of ventricular fibrillation.

Noncompetitive (demand) pacemakers fire only when the patient's ventricular rate falls below the preset rate of the pacemaker. In the ventricular-inhibited type the output of the pacemaker is inhibited when the frequency of spontaneous ventricular depolarizations is above this level. In the ventricular-activated type the pacemaker discharge is triggered by each spontaneous ventricular depolarization. In the absence of spontaneous depolarization the pacemaker discharges after a preset delay interval. These devices are designed with a refractory period in the range of 400 ms to preclude rapid repetitive pacemaker discharge triggered by the T wave. With triggered pacemakers evaluation of the sensing function is simplified because the stimulus artifact is present with each spontaneous ventricular depolarization.

The advantage of noncompetitive pacing is that if AV conduction returns, the hazards of competitive, fixed-rate pacing are eliminated. It is also useful in patients with paroxysms of symptomatic bradyarrhythmias other than AV block (including sinus bradycardia, SA block, the so-called sick sinus syndrome) and in patients in whom bradycardia alternates with tachycardia. In patients with bradyarrhythmias the implantation of a demand pacemaker permits the administration of antiarrhythmic drugs to suppress the development of ventricular tachyarrhythmias. Since the functional longevity and electronic reliability of current noncompetitive pacemakers are essentially equivalent to fixed-rate devices, the former are generally utilized.

SPECIFIC DISORDERS OF RATE AND RHYTHM

Derangements arising in the sinus node

SINUS BRADYCARDIA This is characterized by a slow heart rate (below 60 beats per min) with a normal spread of atrial excitation. It is frequent in athletes and is usually a sign of excellent physical fitness. However, in elderly subjects with symptoms attributable to failure of impulse formation or propagation, it may be one manifestation of sinus node dysfunction and may be associated with latent or overt AV conduction abnormalities as well. It occurs also in patients with increased intracerebral pressure, myxedema, or hypothermia.

SINOATRIAL ARREST This is due to a sporadic failure of the sinus impulse, and, therefore, there is no sinus node–initiated ventricular excitation. The electrocardiogram shows a prolonged pause between two P waves. Sinoatrial arrest is most frequently due to digitalis or to some other cause of vagal stimulation but may result from myocardial disease. Aside from withholding digitalis and the occasional use of atropine, treatment is usually unnecessary.

SINOATRIAL BLOCK In this dysrhythmia regular sinus impulse formation occurs but there are no atrial or ventricular depolarizations because the impulse is blocked from reaching these structures. The P-P interval is prolonged, usually to some multiple of the regular intervals, but may progressively and periodically shorten, prior to a dropped P wave, when sinoatrial Wenckebach exit block is present. Sinoatrial block is infrequently accompanied by AV block; it may be precipitated by digitalis, quinidine, hyperkalemia, or acute myocardial infarction.

SINUS ARRHYTHMIA This dysrhythmia is present in most healthy young persons at rest; it consists of a quickening of the heart rate during inspiration and a slowing during expiration, tends to be intensified by deep breathing, and tends to disappear when the breath is held or when the heart rate is increased by exercise or fever. It has no pathologic significance.

SINUS TACHYCARDIA (Fig. 238-2*B*) Defined as a sinus-initiated heart rate faster than 100 beats per min, this dysrhythmia must be distinguished from the various ectopic tachycardias. The latter group will usually respond to therapy aimed directly at the heart; in sinus tachycardia, the treatment of the rapid rate depends on the management of the underlying condition. A reliable history of abrupt onset and cessation suggests that the attack represents an ectopic tachycardia, rather than sinus tachycardia. However, the patient is often unable to make this differentiation with certainty. When the rate is less than 140 beats per min, the odds favor sinus tachycardia, but a ventricular rate below 140 is also frequent in patients with digitalis-induced atrial tachycardia with AV block and is seen in some persons with atrial flutter or ventricular tachycardia. Rates of 170 or more per minute are almost invariably the result of ectopic rhythms. Difficulty in distinguishing ectopic rhythms from sinus tachycardias occurs chiefly with heart rates between 140 and 170 beats per min. In sinus tachycardia the rate is less constant than in ectopic tachycardia and is altered somewhat by changes in posture and activity. Anxiety, fever, blood loss, thyrotoxicosis, pregnancy, pheochromocytoma, or some other cause of the tachycardia is usually evident. The response to manual carotid sinus stimulation may help in the differentiation. As described above under Methods of Examination, sinus tachycardia is usually slowed slightly but gradually by such massage.

Extremely rapid sinus tachycardia with heart rates exceeding 130 beats per min is usually due to marked elevation of body temperature, severe thyrotoxicosis, profound circulatory collapse, or electrolyte imbalance. Frequently, patients with severe advanced chronic airway disease have a sustained tachycardia, usually not over 120 beats per min; however, during episodes of respiratory decompensation initiated by intercurrent pulmonary infections, heart failure, or obstruction of the airways, the tachycardia may reach 160 beats per min. Consequently, correcting the underlying systemic abnormality is paramount. A similar problem is often present in patients with chronic lung disease following a pneumonectomy or lobectomy. Maintaining airway patency, ventilation, and oxygenation is of great importance. Digitalis or other cardiac therapy is of no therapeutic value in patients with sinus tachycardia unless there are manifestations of congestive heart failure. Since the response of the sinus node to pharmacologic agents may reflect the dependence of its automaticity on slow current, calcium-mediated depolarization, preferential sinus slowing may be possible with agents such as verapamil which may block calcium transport. On the other hand, the calcium dependence and sodium current independence of sinus node automaticity may account for its remarkable resistance to conventional antiarrhythmic agents such as lidocaine. However, effective management of sinus tachycardia generally requires discovering its basic cause and correcting it.

Derangements arising in the atrium

ECTOPIC ATRIAL BEATS (Fig. 238-2*A*) Also known as premature atrial beats, these originate from an abnormal focus in the atrium rather than the sinus node. Ectopic atrial beats have little clinical significance, but they may precede the onset of sustained atrial dysrhythmias, such as atrial tachycardia, flutter, or fibrillation. Also, their suppression may prevent the onset of these sustained tachyarrhythmias. Recognition of atrial ectopic beats is important, since they may be confused at the bedside with the often more serious ectopic ventricular beats; an electrocardiogram is usually necessary to distinguish between these two disorders. Ectopic atrial beats are best recognized on the electrocardiogram when a P wave can be detected preceding a QRS complex of normal duration and configuration. They usually occur prematurely after a normal beat and are followed by an incomplete compensatory pause; however, they are not always premature, and therefore the term *ectopic atrial beat* is preferred. Aberrant intraventricular conduction may alter the QRS complex in amplitude or configuration. Patterns resembling the QRS complex of right bundle branch block occur often. Aberrant conduction increases with prematurity. Definitive differentiation of supraventricular beats with aberrant conduction from ventricular ectopic beats may require His bundle electrograms.

PAROXYSMAL SUPRAVENTRICULAR TACHYCARDIA (Fig. 238-2*C*) This dysrhythmia has often been attributed to rapid discharges from an abnormal atrial pacemaker and is therefore classically called *paroxysmal atrial tachycardia.* However, recent evidence suggests that many, if not all, instances of paroxysmal supraventricular tachycardia are the consequence of sustained reentry and are really manifestations of reciprocating rhythms. Initiation and termination of appropriately timed atrial extrastimuli induced by programmed electrical stimulation, the pattern of low to high atrial activation during tachycardia, and delineation of echo zones corresponding to intervals or "windows" between refractory periods of components of the reentry

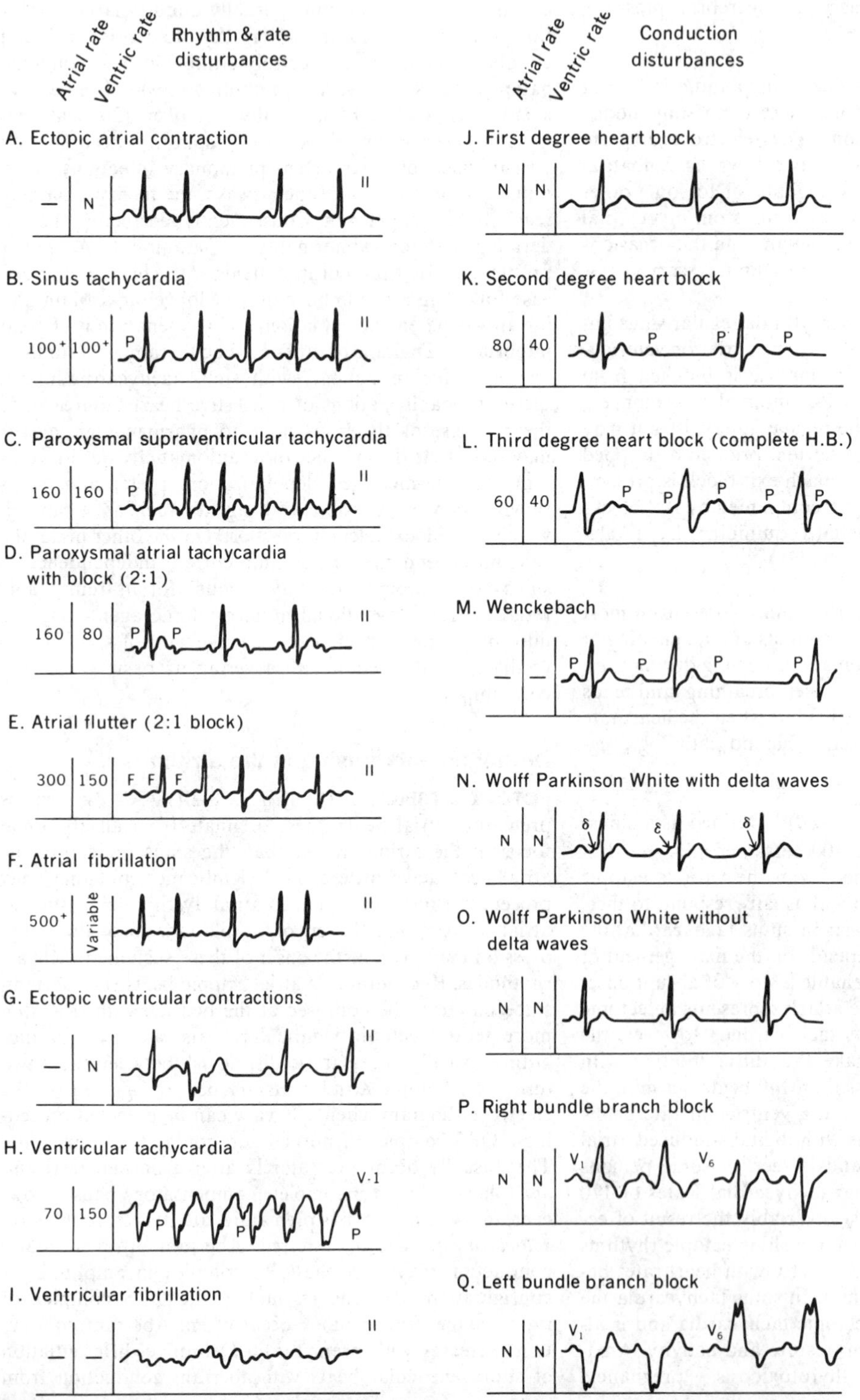

FIGURE 238-2

pathways support this interpretation. This concept is discussed in connection with the Wolff-Parkinson-White syndrome later in this chapter. When reentry occurs as the mechanism of sustained supraventricular tachycardia, it usually involves functional longitudinal stratification in the AV junction, with the reentry pathway encompassing the AV node (Fig. 238-3). In other cases reentry occurs in the sinus node or atrium. Sustained reciprocation may be initiated or terminated by an ectopic beat which precipitates or interrupts the circus current propagating the reentrant pathway. Tachycardia usually appears first in youth, and attacks may recur throughout life. Many patients with this disorder display no evidence of any other cardiac abnormality, and in the absence of structural disease, supraventricular tachycardia should be considered benign unless the rate is extremely rapid or the episodes unusually prolonged. Occasionally, the patient presents a history of precipitating events, such as emotional upset, nervousness, fatigue, indigestion, or alcohol ingestion; polyuria may occur after several hours of tachycardia. This arrhythmia may produce great anxiety on the part of the patient and his family. When a patient is seen during an attack, the

FIGURE 238-3

Diagrammatic representation of possible conduction pathways in a heart exhibiting functional bypass pathways under two conditions: sinus rhythm and reentrant tachycardia. Examples of the electrocardiogram that might be seen in each condition are included below the diagrams. AV, LBB, and RBB represent the AV junction, left bundle branch, and right bundle branch, respectively. During sinus rhythm, impulses are initiated at the SA node and propagated simultaneously through the functional bypass pathway and the AV junction. Because of the absence of delay in the bypass tract, the impulse reaches the His bundle first by spread through the ventricular myocardium, accounting for the slurred upstroke in the conventional electrocardiogram as seen in V_6 and leading to both antegrade and retrograde conduction of the impulse in the His bundle. The subsequent portion of the ventricular depolarization occurs conventionally, since impulse transmission through the main branches of the conduction system is more rapid than that resulting from spread of the impulse from the bypass pathway. During reentry tachycardia, perhaps initiated by an appropriately timed supraventricular beat which might find the accessory pathway refractory but the proximal AV junction capable of transmitting the impulse, impulse transmission to the ventricle occurs via the main branches of the conduction system. However, each impulse fragments, with propagation occurring retrograde through the bypass pathway, reentering the atrium, and returning once again to the ventricle through the AV junction, His bundle, and bundle branches. Accordingly, a repetitive reentrant tachycardia results from each QRS complex showing normal morphology and failing to demonstrate the slurred upstroke which was present with sinus rhythm. The horizontal arrows in the conventional electrocardiographic representations indicate that in both sinus rhythm and reentrant tachycardia the "P-J" intervals (from the onset of atrial depolarization to the termination of ventricular depolarization) are identical because in each case the terminal portion of ventricular depolarization results from spread of the impulse through the main branches of the conducting system.

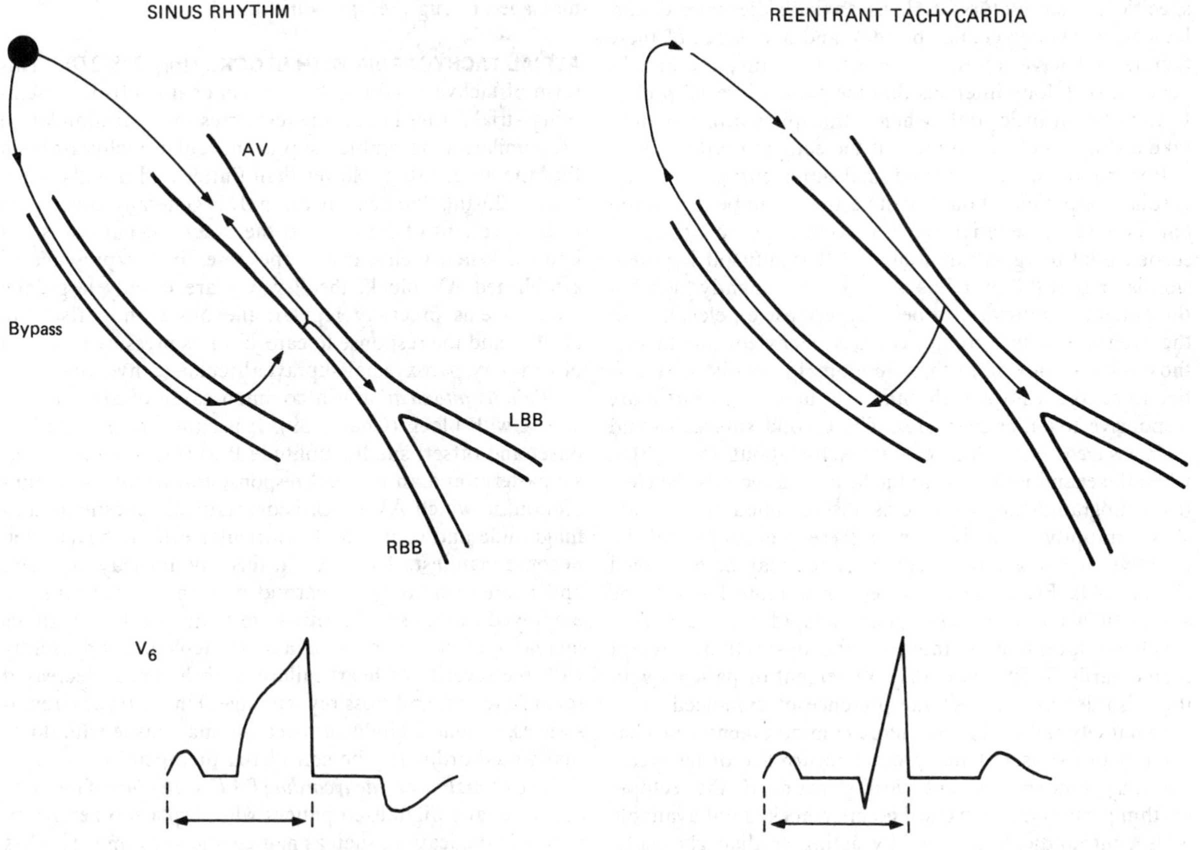

heart is found to be perfectly regular and the rate ranges from 140 to 250 beats per min. Carotid sinus pressure or other types of vagal stimulation either have no effect or will terminate the attack abruptly. Supraventricular tachycardia in the presence of intraventricular conduction disturbances may resemble ventricular tachycardia electrocardiographically, and the differentiation may be difficult. In these instances physical signs may be helpful. For example, varying intensity of the first heart sound and irregularly occurring cannon waves in the jugular venous pulse may be sufficient to establish the diagnosis of ventricular rather than atrial tachycardia. Esophageal, intra-atrial leads or His bundle recordings may be required to demonstrate the sequence between atrial and ventricular depolarization and thereby differentiate between these two entities.

The causes of supraventricular tachycardia are not known, since most patients have no signs of organic disease. However, the possibility of underlying causes, such as atrial septal defect, mitral valve disease, and the Wolff-Parkinson-White syndrome, should be considered. Prognosis is excellent unless the attack brings on congestive failure or myocardial ischemia. The keystone of therapy is reassurance, coupled with attempts to prevent recurrences and to terminate the disorder when it occurs. For many patients digitalis is the most effective drug for the prevention of the attacks; in others, quinidine or propranolol alone or in combination with digitalis is more useful. Certain patients notice that the attacks are regularly precipitated by specific trigger factors, such as anxiety, digestive disturbances, or hypoglycemic episodes, and avoidance of these factors will have a salutary effect. In many, the attacks occur at such long intervals that the patient himself prefers to treat the disorder only when it transpires rather than to take a drug regularly to prevent the ectopic rhythm.

For the treatment of paroxysmal supraventricular tachycardia, the patient should assume the recumbent position and be given a sedative, such as sodium pentobarbital or secobarbital 0.2 g intramuscularly. If significant hypotension is present (90 mmHg systolic or less, slightly higher if the patient has previously been hypertensive), elevation of the arterial pressure by intravenous phenylephrine or methoxamine to not more than 160 mmHg systolic may suffice to restore a normal rhythm or to make the heart more responsive to other measures. The carotid sinuses should be massaged, each one separately, for about 15 to 20 s, while the examiner listens to the heart and records the electrocardiogram; the massage is discontinued if the rate slows abruptly. Usually, one of these procedures will be effective; if not, electrical countershock may be employed (Chap. 240). Electrical cardioversion is more likely to be successful when the atrial response is rapid. Failure of electrical cardioversion to interrupt the dysrhythmia except momentarily in approximately 30 percent of patients with this disorder may reflect the presence of enhanced atrial automaticity rather than the more common reentry mechanism in this subset. Thus, prompt recurrence of tachycardia may follow transient cardioversion. If the ectopic rhythm persists and electrical countershock is not available or is contraindicated, a rapidly acting cardiac glycoside, such as lanatoside C, 0.8 to 1.2 mg, may be given slowly intravenously, provided, of course, that the patient has not received digitalis during the preceding 2 weeks. The digitalis acts as a vagal stimulant. If after 1 h the tachycardia continues, carotid sinus pressure should again be attempted, and if this fails, cholinesterase inhibitors—neostigmine (Prostigmine), 0.5 to 1.0 mg intramuscularly, or Tensilon (edrophonium sulfate), 10 mg intravenously—may be administered, followed again by carotid sinus massage. Among the cholinesterase inhibitors, Tensilon is generally preferred because of its rapid onset and short duration of action. In patients with asthma, these agents must be used cautiously because they may exacerbate bronchoconstriction or increase bronchial secretions. Some physicians prefer to employ cholinesterase inhibitors or propranolol before electrical cardioversion or digitalis. If all these measures fail, morphine sulfate, 10 to 15 mg subcutaneously, may be given; during the ensuing sleep, the attack will often cease.

Quinidine, propranolol, or procainamide may be given by mouth to prevent recurrences. In patients with recurrent supraventricular tachycardia resistant to drugs, the insertion of a temporary or permanent pacemaker, which is activated when tachycardia occurs and which stimulates the right atrium or ventricle and thereby interrupts the reentrant pathway, has been found to be effective.

The treatment outlined above refers to the measures taken by the physician. Often, however, the patient has previously learned how to terminate the attack by utilizing carotid sinus pressure, or by inducing gagging and vomiting, or by the Valsalva maneuver (attempting to expire against a closed glottis). Naturally, these simple methods can also be employed by the physician before carotid sinus massage or drug therapy is instituted.

ATRIAL TACHYCARDIA WITH BLOCK (Fig. 238-2*D*) This form of tachyarrhythmia has certain characteristics resembling atrial flutter in that the responses to vagal stimulation are similar; it resembles supraventricular tachycardia in that the atrial rate is slower than flutter and usually is between 120 and 250 beats per min. It is generally considered to be a variant of flutter, and the exact mechanism is not known. When tachycardia supervenes in the presence of established AV block, the P waves are usually large, the atrial rate is precisely regular, the onset and offset are abrupt, and the response to carotid sinus pressure is typical of ordinary paroxysmal supraventricular tachycardia.

Digitalis intoxication is a common cause of atrial tachycardia with block (Chap. 239). It usually exhibits gradual onset and offset; small-amplitude P waves, often in a phasic pattern; and an unusual response to carotid sinus stimulation, in which AV block is dramatically accentuated in magnitude and degree and ventricular ectopic beats often become manifest. AV block in this rhythm may be latent and made overt only by carotid massage, which must be employed cautiously. Sensitivity to toxic effects of digitalis increases markedly with potassium depletion, apparently with the severity of heart failure, with hypoxia, decreased renal function, and possibly with age. Under these circumstances, serious digitalis intoxication may ensue with doses that would ordinarily be considered therapeutic.

Paroxysmal atrial tachycardia (PAT) with block should be sought in any digitalized patient who displays other symptoms of intoxication, such as nausea and vomiting, who has received vigorous diuretic treatment, who may otherwise have lost potassium as a result of vomiting or diarrhea, or whose heart rate increases after he has received full doses of digitalis. The electrocardiogram displays an atrial rate of 120 to 250 beats per min, an isoelectric line between P waves of unusual configuration, and some degree of AV block.

The earliest stage is an alteration in the form of the P wave and an increase in the atrial rate, usually with a 1:1 ventricular response. Thus, the ventricular rate may increase to 120 to 140 beats per min and still resemble normal sinus rhythm. At higher atrial rates, 2:1 block usually appears. However, the impaired AV conduction remains inapparent, except when carotid sinus pressure is applied, because every other P wave may be masked by the T deflections of the previous beat. The danger of this abnormal rhythm comes from the fact that although it may be a manifestation of serious digitalis intoxication, it is likely to be confused with sinus tachycardia or atrial flutter and, because of the frequent presence of congestive failure, may be treated with even larger doses of digitalis, or with electrical shock. The proper treatment is prompt cessation of digitalis and of potassium-wasting diuretic drugs and the administration of potassium by mouth or parenterally, depending on the urgency. The serum potassium level must not be relied on as an absolute criterion of diagnosis; most patients with this form of disturbed heart action have little or no diminution in the level of serum potassium. Dilantin or procainamide (Chap. 239) may also be effective.

About one-fourth of patients with atrial tachycardia and block do not suffer from digitalis intoxication and/or potassium depletion. Typically digitalis-induced PAT with block responds to administration of potassium (not to be used if hyperkalemia is present) or Dilantin with slowing of the atrial rate and a decrease in AV block. If intravenous administration of 250 mg Dilantin over 5 min or 40 meq of potassium over 2 to 4 h fails to elicit this response, the dysrhythmia is not likely to be digitalis-induced and can be treated similarly to atrial flutter.

ATRIAL FLUTTER (Fig. 238-2E) This dysrhythmia is less common than atrial fibrillation. There is considerable controversy regarding its mechanism. A reciprocating rhythm or circus current movement is most likely. The atria contract at a rate of 250 to 350 beats per min. AV block is almost always present, and its ratio is usually even-numbered (e.g., 2:1 or 4:1), with corresponding ventricular rates in the neighborhood of 150 or 75. In a common variation of flutter the ventricular rate is not a constant multiple of atrial rate. This occurs with two sites of block in the AV junction; high junctional 2:1 and low junctional 3:2 Wenckebach block. When the AV block is constant but the ratio is odd (3:1, 5:1, etc.), concealed retrograde conduction of ectopic ventricular beats with antegrade block should be suspected. When the block is constant and of high degree, atrial flutter is usually not suspected without an electrocardiogram. If it is suspected, its presence may be confirmed by the fact that exercise increases the rate suddenly and stepwise rather than gradually, and in the post-exercise period slowing occurs suddenly, not gradually. This occurs because exercise has no influence on the rate of the fluttering atrium, but the decrease in vagal tone during exercise reduces the degree of AV block, 4:1 giving way to 2:1 block, for example. Thus, the acceleration of ventricular rate occurs promptly, within one beat; the reverse takes place as vagal tone is restored in the postexercise period. Usually, 2:1 block is present when the ventricular rate is between 120 and 160 beats per min. This fact alone would lead to the suspicion of flutter, because other types of tachycardias are likely to be associated with faster ventricular rates. Carotid sinus pressure slows the ventricular rate in flutter by increasing vagal tone and hence increasing the degree of AV block. The slowing is maintained only for the brief period of pressure, and both the slowing and quickening tend to occur in stepwise fashion rather than gradually, as would be the case with sinus tachycardia if there were any response at all. Occasionally, the block is so variable that the ventricular irregularity is virtually identical to that observed in atrial fibrillation. However, after exercise, the irregularity of flutter tends to disappear, whereas that seen with fibrillation is enhanced.

Careful auscultation frequently reveals an appreciable difference in the intensity of the first heart sound in atrial flutter, because of slight variations in timing of the ventricular contraction in relation to the preceding atrial contraction. The variation in the intensity of the first sound is never present in sinus tachycardia or paroxysmal atrial tachycardia (paroxysmal atrial tachycardia with variable block excepted), but it occurs frequently in ventricular tachycardia and thus serves to help limit the diagnostic possibilities. Atrial flutter is unlike paroxysmal atrial tachycardia without block, but resembles atrial fibrillation and atrial tachycardia with block because it usually occurs in patients with organic heart disease. It occurs most commonly with rheumatic mitral stenosis, but may also be seen with thyrotoxicosis, coronary disease, atrial septal defect, and chronic obstructive pulmonary disease.

The *usual treatment of atrial flutter is the administration of digitalis,* which slows the ventricular rate, by increasing the degree of AV block, and commonly converts flutter to fibrillation. When the drug is withdrawn, atrial flutter will frequently revert spontaneously to normal sinus rhythm; if this does not occur, quinidine may be employed to restore sinus rhythm; if this is unsuccessful, the patient may be maintained in chronic atrial fibrillation and treated appropriately (see below). Atrial flutter may be a difficult dysrhythmia to revert with drugs, but acute episodes frequently respond to intravenous propranolol (1 mg every 1 to 2 min with total dose generally not exceeding 0.15 mg per kg), with slowing of the ventricular response due to increased AV block often followed by reversion to sinus rhythm. Congestive heart failure or asthma are relative contraindications because of the possible cardiodepressant or bronchoconstrictive effects of the drug. Electrical reversion is often effective (Chap. 240). When flutter persists or recurs, increasing the AV block with digitalis (and when this is ineffective, with propranolol as well) may be necessary for long-term therapy similar to that used to manage atrial fibrillation. Atrial flutter in patients with suspected or latent digitalis toxicity can often be converted to sinus rhythm by rapid atrial pacing, usually requiring stimulation at a rate exceeding 125 percent of the spontaneous atrial rate for at least 30 s after atrial capture has been accomplished. Abrupt cessation of pacing usually results in restoration of sinus rhythm, presumably because the reentrant flutter pathway has been interrupted. Occasionally, atrial fibrillation ensues, but generally the ventricular response can be managed more easily in this dysrhythmia than with flutter. Atrial fibrillation in this setting often reverts spontaneously to sinus rhythm.

In the presence of atrial flutter, quinidine may slow the atrial rate from about 300 to 200 beats per min. Under these circumstances, the ventricular rate may suddenly increase paradoxically, as the previous 2:1 ratio is replaced by a 1:1 response. Furthermore, vagolytic effects of quinidine may lead to increased ventricular rates, because of enhanced AV conduction, even when the flutter rate remains constant. Accordingly, *quinidine should not be used in patients with flutter without prior or concomitant administration of digitalis or propranolol.*

ATRIAL FIBRILLATION (Fig. 238-2*F*) This is a dysrhythmia in which the effective contraction of the atria is abolished and the AV node and the ventricles are bombarded with a very rapid and irregular series of stimuli. Many of these impulses are blocked at the AV node, but many are passed through, so that the ventricular contractions in the untreated patient are usually rapid and irregularly irregular.

The untoward effects of atrial fibrillation depend on the rapidity of the ventricular rate and the extent of the pulse deficit (i.e., on the proportion of the ineffective and wasted ventricular beats), on the prior state of the affected heart, on the duration of the dysrhythmia, and on the absence of effective atrial contraction. Cardiac output may be diminished, and heart failure may occur. Stagnation of blood in the atria tends to predispose to the development of thrombi and hence to embolism in both the pulmonary and systemic circulations. Finally, the cardiac irregularity may give an unpleasant consciousness of palpitation (Chap. 33).

When the ventricular rate is rapid, 120 beats or more per minute, the diagnosis is readily made by clinical examination, because atrial fibrillation is the only common condition in which one observes the combination of a marked tachycardia with a gross irregularity. When the rate is normal or only slightly increased, as in digitalized patients, the diagnosis is less apparent on clinical examination alone. The distinction from numerous extrasystoles can be made by noting that it is only in atrial fibrillation that abnormally long pauses occur, in groups of two or more. Moreover, exercise may abolish extrasystoles, whereas it exaggerates the irregularity of atrial fibrillation. More difficult, and frequently impossible, is the differentiation by physical examination of fibrillation from atrial flutter with varying block, and from a shifting pacemaker associated with multifocal atrial ectopic beats. Paroxysmal atrial tachycardia with block is also sometimes confused with atrial fibrillation.

Atrial fibrillation may be paroxysmal or persistent. Occasionally, the paroxysmal form occurs in healthy persons in whom no evidence of structural cardiac disease can be found. These patients (lone fibrillators) may have a variant of the preexcitation syndrome (page 1202), and their dysrhythmia may be due to functional AV junctional reentry pathways. Atrial fibrillation is also encountered in persons who, otherwise normal, develop acute infections such as pneumonia, or in patients with rheumatic heart disease or acute myocardial infarction. Rarely, paroxysmal atrial fibrillation may be the consequence of administration of anesthesia, surgical manipulation within the chest, potassium deficiency, digitalis intoxication, or other forms of poisoning. Most frequently, however, paroxysmal atrial fibrillation is seen in thyrotoxicosis, mitral stenosis, or in elderly persons, many but not all of whom have ischemic heart disease. The paroxysmal attacks frequently occur before the dysrhythmia is permanently established. The bouts may last for a few seconds to a few days, and, as in most types of paroxysmal rapid heart action, the onset and offset are sudden. Unless the patient happens to be observed during an attack, the physician must rely on the patient's observation that the onset was abrupt and that the heart action was highly irregular during the episode.

Permanent atrial fibrillation is confined almost exclusively to patients with myocardial disease, mitral stenosis, constrictive pericarditis, ischemic heart disease, hypertension, and thyrotoxicosis. In patients with thyrotoxicosis the clinical signs may be absent and the arrhythmia may be the only feature suggesting the possibility of thyroid disease. Rarely, chronic atrial fibrillation may be the sole cause of congestive failure that persists despite full digitalization, and in such instances reversion to normal rhythm improves ventricular performance markedly because of the reestablishment of the atrial transport function. When the ventricular rate fails to slow in the usual fashion after full doses of digitalis, fever may be present, or thyrotoxicosis, a recent silent coronary occlusion, multiple pulmonary infarcts, or acute rheumatic carditis. The onset of this dysrhythmia in a patient who has received therapeutic doses of digitalis and of diuretic drugs may be a manifestation of potassium deficiency and an indication for potassium therapy. Rarely, persistent atrial fibrillation occurs in individuals without other evidence of heart disease.

Treatment In a patient with atrial fibrillation, several choices of therapy are available: (1) allowing the rhythm to remain irregular but attempting to control the ventricular rate with digitalis; (2) abolishing the arrhythmia by quinidine or other antiarrhythmic drugs (Chap. 239); and (3) reverting the arrhythmia by electrical means (Chap. 240). In patients with mitral stenosis, or with marked cardiac enlargement with heart failure, it is rarely possible to restore normal sinus rhythm more than transiently. In other patients with chronic atrial fibrillation, normal sinus rhythm can be restored with large, nearly toxic doses of quinidine. Moreover, it can usually be maintained only with persistent large maintenance doses of quinidine, and even then, for only variable intervals before the dysrhythmia recurs. Quinidine frequently transforms atrial fibrillation into atrial flutter, with the risk of increased ventricular rate. Electrical reversion is usually the treatment of choice for atrial fibrillation (Chap. 240). However, the problem of maintaining sinus rhythm subsequently still remains. In some patients with chronic atrial fibrillation ventricular rate must be controlled with digitalis. Hence, reversion to sinus rhythm with electrical countershock or quinidine is likely to be of value in patients with fibrillation of recent development who are known to have had no evidence of congestive failure prior to the onset of the arrhythmia. Reversion to sinus rhythm should also be considered when the ventricular rate is not well controlled by digitalis, and it may be attempted in patients with intractable heart failure. In patients who cannot be maintained in sinus rhythm and in whom the ventricular rate cannot be slowed sufficiently with digitalis, small doses (5 to 10 mg q.i.d.) of propranolol will often control the ventricular rate. In all cases of atrial fibrillation, therapeutic doses of digitalis should be administered before quinidine is given, but reversion should not be attempted if occult or overt digitalis intoxication is suspected. When atrial fibrillation follows acute myocardial infarction, the first and most important objective is to slow the ventricular rate with digitalis. For the treatment of paroxysmal atrial fibrillation, a rapidly acting digitalis glycoside is preferable; for the control of established atrial fibrillation, one of the slower-acting digitalis preparations should be used.

In many instances of transient atrial fibrillation the administration of digitalis is followed by the disappearance of the dysrhythmia. This probably results from overall hemodynamic improvement, diminished sympathoadrenal myocardial stimulation, and diminution of atrial size, rather than from a direct pharmacologic effect of digitalis on the atria. When atrial fibrillation is of long duration, digitalis rarely abolishes it. Under these circumstances, the ventricular rate slows and becomes less obviously irregular unless complete AV block and a regular idioventricular or AV junctional rhythm develop; but electrocardiographic tracings reveal that the atria continue to fibrillate.

Thromboembolism is one of the dreaded complications in patients with atrial fibrillation (or less commonly with atrial flutter), particularly when the dysrhythmia is chronic and when mitral stenosis is present. Thromboembolism is responsible for about 20 percent of the deaths in patients with mitral stenosis. To prevent such catastrophes, long-term anticoagulant therapy is advocated in patients with atrial fibrillation, and is especially important in patients who have already experienced one or more episodes of embolism. When possible, anticoagulants should be administered for at least 2 weeks prior to attempts to reestablish sinus rhythm in order to minimize thromboembolic episodes associated with pharmacologic or electrical cardioversion.

COMPLEX ATRIAL DYSRHYTHMIAS Multifocal atrial tachycardia (MAT) This is a rapid, grossly irregular atrial dysrhythmia with a rapid ventricular response (from 120 to 200 beats per min). Electrocardiographically it can be differentiated from atrial fibrillation by the presence of three or more types of morphologically distinct P waves. Numerous atrial premature complexes, AV block, and aberrant intraventricular conduction are generally present. Atrial flutter or fibrillation may supervene. MAT is generally a manifestation of advanced cardic and/or pulmonary disease and hypoxemia. Specific antiarrhythmic therapy is generally ineffective, and digitalis may aggravate dysrhythmia further; treatment should focus on the underlying disorder.

Sick sinus syndrome The sick sinus syndrome, or sinoatrial dysfunction, generally results from arteriosclerotic, hypertensive, or rheumatic heart disease, although it may be idiopathic. Its manifestations include intermittent sinus arrest; sinus bradycardia which persists despite exercise, atropine, or isoproterenol; sinoatrial block; AV junctional escape rhythm; and ectopic atrial complexes. Marked carotid sinus sensitivity may trigger bradycardia. Paroxysmal supraventricular tachycardia, atrial fibrillation, atrial flutter, and episodes of alternating bradycardia and tachycardia (the bradycardia-tachycardia syndrome) are common concomitants. Asynchronous atrial repolarization favoring reentry may predispose to the episodes of paroxysmal tachycardia. On the other hand, tachycardia may precipitate asystole or severe bradycardia because of impaired sinus node recovery and the commonly associated atrioventricular and intraventricular conduction defects. Syncope and chest pain often accompany episodes of bradycardia and tachycardia. Long-term electrocardiographic monitoring, analysis of the response of heart rate to carotid sinus massage, stress testing, or drugs, and detection of abnormal sinus node suppression by atrial pacing are most helpful diagnostically. Permanent pacing is often required to treat bradycardia and permits safe suppression of tachycardia with agents such as digitalis and propranolol. Because of the high incidence of thromboembolic phenomena, long-term anticoagulation may be indicated.

Repetitive paroxysmal tachycardia This dysrhythmia (the Parkinson, Papp syndrome) comprises innumerable brief bursts of tachycardia, most frequently paroxysmal supraventricular tachycardia, atrial fibrillation, or atrial flutter, interspersed with brief episodes of sinus rhythm punctuated with multiple atrial premature complexes. Its etiology is often obscure. Hundreds and even thousands of episodes may occur daily with disabling symptoms including chest discomfort and syncope. Overdrive suppression with pacing has not been helpful. Digitalis and conventional antiarrhythmic agents are often ineffective, but propranolol alone or in combination with digitalis or quinidine may be beneficial.

Chaotic atrial mechanism This is a general term that has been used to refer to several complex atrial dysrhythmias including MAT, sick sinus syndrome, and repetitive paroxysmal tachycardia.

SINOVENTRICULAR CONDUCTION This unusual dysrhythmia, sometimes a manifestation of severe hyperkalemia, arises in the atria. It is characterized by impulse initiation in the sinoatrial node in a normal fashion and propagation via internodal pathways to the AV junction. However, spread of the impulse through atrial myocardium fails to occur, and hence no P wave is seen on the electrocardiogram, and atrial contraction is absent. Although the ventricular electrocardiographic complexes may be distorted because of aberrant conduction, ventricular rate varies, as it does in normal sinus rhythm when maneuvers such as carotid sinus stimulation are performed, with exercise, and following drug administration. The major significance of the dysrhythmia is loss of atrial transport function; also, when bizarre QRS complexes are present, there is the possibility of misdiagnosis as ventricular tachycardia.

Derangements arising in the AV junction

ECTOPIC JUNCTIONAL BEATS The AV junction refers to fibers adjacent to the node in the low right atrium, the AV node itself, and the His bundle. Cells in the N region, i.e., in the AV node itself, do not appear to initiate impulse formation spontaneously. Decremental conduction and the physiologic delay in AV impulse transmission occur in this region. The cephalad (AN) and caudad (NH) regions of the node appear to contain cells capable of spontaneous impulse formation, presumably dependent on slow-current, calcium-mediated depolarizations giving rise to ectopic beats. Other ectopic beats may originate in atrial and His bundle components of the AV junction. Ectopic beats originating in the low atrium or AN region exhibit a short P-R interval and P waves of unusual configuration which precede a ventricular complex normal in configuration, unless there is aberrant ventricular conduction. When the impulse arises in the His bundle, retrograde atrial conduction causes impulse propagation into the atrium at about the same time that the impulse is propagated antegrade into the ventricular conduction system. Consequently, there is no visible electrocardiographic wave of atrial depolarization; again, the QRS complex is usually normal in configuration and duration, resembling a normal supraventricular beat but without a preceding visible P wave. Beats originating at a more distal site in the His-Purkinje system or those associated with delayed retrograde conduction into the atrium exhibit an abnormal P wave that regularly follows the QRS complex.

AV JUNCTIONAL TACHYCARDIAS These are of two types: *idiojunctional tachycardia,* with a ventricular rate usually between 100 and 140 beats per min; and *extrasystolic* (or paroxysmal) *AV junctional tachycardia,* with a ventricular rate generally between 140 and 200 beats per min. In the former there is acceleration of the inherent idiojunctional rhythm, which becomes evident when its rate exceeds that of the SA pacemaker. It may be a manifestation of digitalis toxicity, and has also been noted in patients with acute myocardial infarction and acute rheumatic fever. When idiojunctional tachycardia is due to digitalis toxicity, it may be particularly grave, because it may degenerate into ventricular tachycardia and ventricular fibrillation. Reversion may occur after discontinuation of digitalis or administration of intravenous potassium. However, occasionally in critical situations, more vigorous therapy is required; in these instances lidocaine, procainamide, diphenylhydantoin, or propranolol may be effective. Paroxysmal AV junctional tachycardia resembles paroxysmal atrial tachycardia in its clinical significance and management, but is much less common.

AV JUNCTIONAL RHYTHM This is an escape rhythm which occurs when the sinus impulse fails to arrive at the AV junction because of sinoatrial depression, standstill, or block of the sinus impulse proximal to the AV junctional pacemaker. The ventricular rate is 40 to 60 beats per min, and the rhythm is regular. The QRS complex is generally identical to that of the conducted sinus impulses. No treatment is necessary, as the circulation is usually adequate, but atropine or isoproterenol may be helpful to speed the sinus rate if the circulation is compromised by a ventricular rate below 50 beats per min. The presence of AV junctional rhythm is generally a manifestation of a safety mechanism, rather than a primary derangement affecting the junctional pacemaker. However, it may be a manifestation of digitalis toxicity.

Derangements arising in the ventricles

ECTOPIC VENTRICULAR BEATS (Fig. 238-2*G*) These are relatively more frequent in patients with structural cardiac disease than ectopic atrial beats, but they are so common in healthy individuals that their presence has no diagnostic significance unless they are unusually frequent, related to exercise, originate from the left ventricle, occur during the vulnerable period, or occur in pairs or salvos (Chap. 36). Their prevalence increases markedly with age. They are frequent concomitants of conditions with abnormal ventricular repolarization such as hereditary Q-T prolongation (syncope, sudden death, with or without congenital deafness), mitral valve prolapse, and cerebrovascular accidents. In the absence of organic heart disease, premature beats may be due to excessive use of tobacco, coffee, tea, and occasionally alcohol or to reflexes from the gastrointestinal tract; often they are caused by emotional stress, but in many patients the cause cannot be ascertained.

Ventricular ectopic beats are often easily recognized, as the ventricular depolarization and contraction occur before the next beat would ordinarily occur and are commonly followed by a compensatory pause. The patient may or may not be conscious of the premature beat. When extrasystoles are frequent, they may be confused with atrial fibrillation on clinical examination, an error that may sometimes be avoided by noting that the rhythm becomes regular when the heart rate is accelerated by exercise. There is still uncertainty whether ectopic ventricular beats are produced by an abnormal pacemaker or by reentry; probably each mechanism accounts for some instances of this disorder. In some patients ectopic ventricular beats and even ventricular tachycardia occur during episodes of severe bradycardia. When ectopic ventricular beats arise in an abnormal pacemaker, the latter is probably located in Purkinje cells rather than in myocardial cells per se. Ectopic beats may originate in a *parasystolic focus,* i.e., one "protected" from depolarization initiated elsewhere in the heart. The manifest rate of the parasystolic focus will depend on the degree of exit block from it, the refractoriness of surrounding myocardium, and the interplay between the rate of the focus and other pacemakers which are initiating impulses. Other ectopic beats originate in extrasystolic ventricular pacemakers which are not completely protected from depolarization by impulses arising in other pacemaker cells.

BIGEMINAL RHYTHM This is a state in which every alternate beat is premature; it may be caused by digitalis overdosage and disappears within a few days after the drug has been withheld. It should not be confused with *pulsus alternans* or with *paradoxic pulse,* conditions in which the rhythm remains regular. Bigeminy not due to digitalis is usually, though not always, associated with structural heart disease. Bigeminy probably results from several mechanisms, including electrical instability of the ectopic pacemaker during repolarization, reentry, and enhancement of spontaneous depolarization of the ectopic pacemaker by the preceding beat.

The *treatment of ectopic ventricular beats* depends on the clinical circumstances. When these beats occur occasionally, and evidence of cardiac disease is lacking, no treatment is necessary. If there is reason to believe that tobacco or coffee is a precipitating factor, its use should be discontinued or curtailed. In excitable patients, extrasystoles may disappear following the administration of a mild sedative, barbiturates, reserpine, or other tranquilizers. Ectopic ventricular beats, if caused by digitalis, will disappear if the drug is withdrawn; or if the irregularity occurs after the ingestion of a high-carbohydrate meal, it will be abolished by the administration of potassium. The occurrence of extrasystoles in undigitalized patients does not constitute a contraindication to the use of digitalis if the patient has congestive heart failure. Indeed, with the restoration of myocardial function, the irregularity will often disappear. Lidocaine, procainamide, diphenylhydantoin, and quinidine are all effective in the treatment, and the relative efficacy of each drug varies in different patients. In patients in whom the development of ventricular ectopic beats or ventricular tachycardia is precipitated by bradycardia, increasing the atrial rate with atropine or by pacing may be helpful.

Although ectopic ventricular beats may ordinarily be considered a benign form of irregularity, the occurrence of numerous such beats may diminish the efficiency of the heart with an impaired cardiac reserve. Moreover, the appearance of ventricular extrasystoles following an acute myocardial infarction should not be viewed with complacency, since they may herald the onset of ventricular tachycardia. An isolated ventricular beat may occur in the "vulnerable" period at the end of the previous systole (the time during ventricular repolarization when recovery is asynchronous, opportunity for reentry is maximized, and hence the ventricles are especially likely to develop ventricular fibrillation). Such beats are likely to initiate ventricular fibrillation and sudden death. It is for this reason that premature ventricular contractions occurring in patients with acute myocardial infarction should be treated vigorously, with intravenous lidocaine, procainamide, or diphenylhydantoin (Chaps. 239 and 244). Pharmacologic suppression of ventricular ectopic beats is less effective when the prevailing heart rate is high (greater than 120 beats per min). Thus, concomitant therapy should be directed toward correction of factors responsible for the tachycardia or toward decreasing the sinus rate with beta-adrenergic blocking agents. The treatment of premature ventricular contractions in other patients is discussed in Chap. 36.

VENTRICULAR TACHYCARDIA (Fig. 238-2*H*) This dysrhythmia is much less frequent and far more serious than paroxysmal atrial tachycardia. The commonest cause is ischemic heart disease, and ventricular tachycardia frequently occurs within a few days following the development of an acute myocardial infarction (Chap. 244). Less commonly, it is induced by digitalis or quinidine intoxication, and very rarely the arrhythmia appears spontaneously in otherwise healthy persons without any evidence of cardiac disease. The diagnosis should be suspected when the following clinical features are observed: (1) The patient has evidence of coronary disease or has been receiving digitalis or quinidine in large doses. (2) As a rule, there is no history of numerous previous attacks. (3) During the attack, the ventricular rate is usually between 150 and 210 beats per min, and although the rhythm is essentially regular, there are often slight variations in it. (4) Carotid sinus stimulation has no effect on the rate. (5) An intermittent jugular cannon A wave is present. (6) The first heart sound varies in intensity, because the relationship between atrial and ventricular contractions is inconstant. (7) Systolic blood pressure varies because of inconsistent contributions to ventricular filling by fortuitously timed atrial contractions.

Although these clues are useful, the clinical impression should be confirmed by an electrocardiogram, but the interpretation even of the ECG may be rendered difficult because atrial tachycardia may be associated with intraventricular conduction defects (aberrant QRS complexes) which cause the tracing to resemble that of ventricular tachycardia. The diagnosis is supported by evidence that the P-wave rate is independent of the ventricular rate, by evidence that in the intervals between attacks ventricular premature beats occur which are identical in form with the complexes seen during the paroxysm, and by the presence of fusion beats composing components of depolarization initiated by impulses arising in a supraventricular pacemaker and in the ectopic ventricular site. Nevertheless, the electrocardiographic diagnosis frequently cannot be made with certainty. Esophageal, atrial, or His bundle electrograms may be helpful. In ventricular tachycardia H spikes (originating from the bundle of His) may be shown to follow rather than precede the QRS complex. In as many as one-third of cases AV dissociation does not occur. Thus, atrial depolarization follows each ventricular depolarization. The dysrhythmia can be readily differentiated from junctional tachycardia, however, since the R-P interval is consistently greater than 0.11 s.

Bidirectional ventricular tachycardia is a rare dysrhythmia with a grave prognosis associated with severe digitalis intoxication and advanced cardiac disease. The rapid, regular ventricular response at a rate of 120 to 220 beats per min exhibits alternating electrocardiographic complexes with marked left and right axis deviation. Since all complexes generally exhibit a right bundle branch block pattern, the disturbance may reflect ectopic impulse formation in a left ventricular focus with alternating transmission along the posterior and anterior divisions of the left bundle. Treatment entails the discontinuation of digitalis and administration of Dilantin or lidocaine. Electrical cardioversion should not be attempted because of the risk that ventricular fibrillation will result.

Since it is but one step removed from the frequently fatal *ventricular fibrillation*, ventricular tachycardia is the most serious of the ectopic tachycardias. If the attack occurs during a bout of acute myocardial infarction, immediate electric countershock is utilized (Chap. 240), but there is a strong possibility that another episode will occur soon after the first. Hence, a maintenance dose of an antiarrhythmic drug (e.g., intravenous lidocaine, procainamide, or diphenylhydantoin, parenteral or oral) should be continued until cardiac electrical activity has become demonstrably stable. When heart failure occurs in an undigitalized patient with ventricular tachycardia, digitalis should be administered despite the dysrhythmia, since the drug is not necessarily more hazardous in such patients than in those without the disturbance.

The cardiac rhythm of patients with ventricular tachycardia who are receiving large doses of quinidine or of procainamide may fail to revert to the normal sinus mechanism, but the ventricular rate may still show marked slowing, to 120 beats per min or less. Under these circumstances the administration of large doses of atropine (up to 2 mg intravenously) may increase the atrial rate to a level above that of the ectopic rhythm, which may permit the sinoatrial node to resume its normal role as pacemaker and restore the normal sinus mechanism; alternatively, atrial overdrive, i.e., electrical stimulation of the atria with an electrode catheter at a rate exceeding that of ventricular tachycardia, may exert a similar effect. The extracardiac toxicities of procainamide and quinidine are not necessarily additive, and therefore it may be desirable to use the drugs simultaneously in patients who are especially liable to such side effects as diarrhea and tinnitus (quinidine) or hypotension, nausea, or a lupus-like syndrome (procainamide). Monitoring of serum levels of these agents to ensure adequate dosage and avoid toxicity is particularly important when vigorous treatment is required for refractory dysrhythmias.

Refractory, recurrent ventricular tachycardia has been successfully treated by surgical interruption of a reentry pathway documented by epicardial mapping studies at operation and identified preoperatively by electrophysiologic investigation utilizing programmed electrical cardiac stimulation and intracardiac electrograms. Occasionally, aneurysmectomy has led to cessation of recurrent ventricular tachycardia presumably by the same mechanism, although excision of an ectopic focus cannot be excluded.

VENTRICULAR FIBRILLATION (Fig. 238-2*I*) This chaotic rhythm may occur in very brief bursts, last for a few seconds, and then subside spontaneously, following which the rhythm previously present is resumed. These episodes are responsible for some of the Stokes-Adams attacks that occur in patients with prevailing slow rates due to high-grade AV block. Usually, however, unless it is recognized and treated immediately, ventricular fibrillation is synonymous with practically instantaneous death, since effective ventricular contraction and circulation cease (Chap. 36). Aside from AV block, ischemic heart disease is the most common cause of the dysrhythmia, particularly during attacks of acute myocardial infarction. It may also occur in patients with abnormal ventricular repolarization with Q-T prolongation associated with the hereditary Q-T prolongation syndrome, hypothermia, phenothiazine toxicity, mitral valve prolapse, or "quinidine syncope." Sympathetic nerve stimulation may provoke fibrillation, and stellate ganglion ablation or postganglionic sympathetic blockade with bretylium has been occasionally useful for prevention. Type I antiarrhythmic drugs (i.e., quinidine and procainamide) are contraindicated when ventricular fibrillation occurs as a manifestation of these unusual disorders because they slow repolarization further and probably increase temporal dispersion of recovery. There was no treatment for this calamitous disorder until introduction of externally applied electric shock (Chap. 240). Needless to say, this form of therapy must be applied promptly, because cessation of the circulation beyond 2 to 4 min leads to irreversible damage in the brain and heart. Thus, in individuals particularly susceptible to ventricular fibrillation, such as those with acute myocardial infarction or those with a history of Stokes-Adams attacks, the rhythm must be monitored constantly, and immediate availability and preparedness to apply external electric shock must be assured. Such precautions may be required for weeks, until cardiac electrical stability has been reestablished. In the absence of special equipment for delivering the countershock, closed-chest massage should be employed. This involves manual rhythmic compression of the sternum once per second, plus mouth-to-mouth respiration. Such maneuvers, described in Chap. 36, may be effective in sustaining life during the crucial time required to secure and apply the apparatus needed for countershock.

AV dissociation

As its name implies, in this dysrhythmia the atria and ventricles are controlled by two independent pacemakers. Fundamentally, it may occur in two forms, with antegrade AV block and without it. In the first type, the ventricles are excited by a pacemaker in the AV junction, or the Purkinje system, because impulses arising in the sinoatrial node or atria are blocked in the AV conduction system. In AV dissociation *without* antegrade block the automaticity of the AV junction or ventricle exceeds that of the supraventricular pacemaker, and the impulses from the atrium, while normally conducted to the ventricles, usually find these tissues refractory. Occasionally, the regular ventricular rhythm may be interrupted by a normally conducted impulse which arrives fortuitously, at an instant when the ventricle is not refractory. More precisely, this rhythm should be termed *AV dissociation without antegrade block with capture.* This dysrhythmia must be associated with some degree of retrograde block, or else the atria would be depolarized by the more rapidly firing AV junctional or ventricular pacemaker.

Abnormalities of conduction

Sinoatrial block, which represents a disorder of excitation, has been considered above (page 1193). The term *heart block* as herein employed refers to a condition in which the wave of excitation from the atria is delayed pathologically (or blocked) at the junctional tissues (AV node and His bundle). The P-R interval represents the time required for the impulse to traverse the atrium, the AV node, His bundle, and the bundle branches. The generally accepted upper limit of normal in adults is 0.20 s; it is somewhat shorter in children. When the P-R interval exceeds the normal duration and all the atrial beats are followed by ventricular beats, *first degree AV block* exists. A more advanced disturbance in the conduction system, *second degree block,* is present when from time to time the atrial impulses are incapable of penetrating the conduction system sufficiently to excite the ventricles. *Third degree* or *complete AV block* describes the condition in which the conduction system is so altered that no atrial impulses reach the ventricles, and the atria and ventricles maintain separate and independent rhythms (atrioventricular dissociation due to third degree antegrade AV block).

AV block is a general term referring to impaired conduction. The actual site(s) of impairment is not necessarily in the AV node itself. Block may exist because of impaired conduction in the atrial myocardium adjacent to the node (AN region); the node itself (N region); or the bundle of His adjacent to the node (NH region). Furthermore, block may exist only in more distal portions of the conduction system, i.e., the His bundle, the right or left bundle branches, or the anterior or posterior fascicles of the latter (Chap. 233). Proximal block is generally benign, and distal block more malignant. At each site block may be partial (first or second degree) or complete (third degree), and various sites of block may occur singly or in combination. As discussed below, bundle branch or fascicular block is generally associated with pathologic conditions other than those associated with AV junctional block proper, and it generally indicates a different prognosis. Congenital AV block generally exhibits impaired conduction high in the AV junction and narrow electrocardiographic QRS complexes. However, familial AV block may occur with trifascicular block with widened QRS complexes as well as proximal (high AV) block among individuals in the same family. Definitive differentiation between fascicular block and AV junctional block is possible with the aid of His bundle recordings (Fig. 238-1). In third degree trifascicular block (involving the right bundle and both fascicles of the left bundle branch) ventricular depolarizations occur independently of His bundle depolarizations. However, when block occurs in the AV junction proximal to the His bundle, each ventricular depolarization is preceded by a His bundle depolarization separated from it by the normal interval of approximately 50 ms.

FIRST DEGREE AV BLOCK (Fig. 238-2*J*) This is usually due to impaired conduction in the AV junction, i.e., proximal to the His bundle, but, rarely, it may be a reflection of trifascicular block. It may be caused by digitalis or by any of the inflammatory, toxic, degenerative, or vascular processes that may affect the heart. Prolongation of the P-R interval, for example as seen in patients with acute rheumatic fever, may be suspected when the intensity of the first heart sound suddenly declines without any other change in the clinical picture and without evidence of fluid in the pericardium, or in patients with mitral stenosis when a presystolic murmur becomes middiastolic in the absence of atrial fibrillation. P-R prolongation may be due to increased vagal tone in a healthy, normal, person. In the absence of any other evidence of disease, this one electrocardiographic deviation from an arbitrary norm should not be construed as evidence of organic heart disease, and it requires no treatment.

SECOND DEGREE, OR PARTIAL, AV BLOCK (Fig. 238-2*K*) This form may be divided into two groups. In the *Möbitz type I block* (also called Wenckebach block) the P-R interval increases progressively until finally a propagation of an impulse originating in the atrium is completely blocked, the corresponding ventricular beat dropping out (Wenckebach block, Fig. 238-2*M*). His bundle electrograms generally, but not always, reveal impaired conduction proximal to the His bundle. The ventricular rate generally increases prior to the dropped beat because the prolongation of AV conduction exhibits progressively smaller increments. The P-R interval after the pause shortens to within the normal range. Accordingly, the pause resulting from the dropped beat is less than the duration of any two preceding cycles. After the resumption of conduction each successive P-R interval lengthens, and the cycle is repeated periodically. The dropped beat may occur after six to eight conducted beats, or after every second atrial impulse, thus giving rise to 2:1 AV block and simulating the other type of 2:1 block (Möbitz type II), to be described below. With type I block the QRS duration is usually normal. Inhibition of vagal tone, as by intravenous injection of atropine (1 to 2 mg) or exercise, may help to differentiate these two types of block. In type I, the block often diminishes or disappears with such a procedure, whereas with Möbitz type II block it increases or it may temporarily change into a complete AV block. Möbitz type I second degree block is often due to abnormal conduction in the AV junction proximal to the His bundle; it is frequently accentuated or precipitated by heightened vagal tone, occurring spontaneously or after carotid sinus pressure or following digitalis therapy. It is usually a transitory phenomenon and requires no treatment unless hemodynamic disturbances result or the extent of block increases. It is a frequent complication of inferior myocardial infarction, presumably with ischemia of the junction.

Möbitz type II block is usually a more serious disorder. The P-R interval is either normal or increased but fixed except when beats are dropped; QRS duration is often prolonged. The dysrhythmia exhibits dropped beats, that is, 2:1, 3:1, or 4:1 block or irregular ratios. This form of block usually results from block in the His bundle or trifascicular block and may be caused acutely by anterior myocardial infarction or myocarditis. Although it may be transient, it may progress suddenly to complete block. Idiopathic sclerosis producing damage of the conduction system (Lenegre's disease) and fibrocalcific degeneration of the myocardium involving the conduction system as well (Lev's disease) are perhaps the most common causes of chronic Möbitz type II block. It may also result from coronary narrowing in the absence of an acute episode of infarction; calcification of the mitral annulus; extension of the lesion of calcific aortic stenosis into the septum; any of the diffuse disorders of the myocardium such as cardiac amyloidosis; or congenital heart disease, usually an interventricular septal defect. This type of second degree block is sometimes characterized by a unique phenomenon, a slowing of the ventricular rate during exercise as 2:1 block suddenly appears when the atrial rate increases.

Syncopal attacks (Stokes-Adams attacks) are common in type II block, and they have the characteristics of all such syncopal attacks that are due to a sudden cessation of the circulation (Chap. 16). The attacks occur suddenly and without warning, with the patient in either the upright or recumbent posture. In contrast, premonitory light-headedness, faintness, and "blacking out" usually precede simple emotional vasovagal syncope, which develops with the patient in the upright position and is relieved by the recumbent posture. If the heart of a patient with Möbitz type II 2:1 block is monitored during or shortly after the lapse of consciousness, ventricular standstill (or less commonly fibrillation) will be recorded during the syncopal period, often followed by complete block in the early recovery state, 2:1 block being restored after a variable interval. When a person with a slow heart rate or with an electrocardiogram showing second degree block develops a characteristic syncopal attack, the diagnosis should be simple. However, in a number of patients, syncopal attacks may appear at relatively long intervals over a number of years, during which time the electrocardiogram between episodes remains normal and the P-R interval stays well within the normal range. Ambulatory electrocardiographic monitoring or demonstration of latent conduction abnormalities with atrial pacing and His bundle recordings may be particularly useful in unmasking the diagnosis. Intravenous administration of atropine in such persons may reveal concealed block, since the AV conduction system may be unable to follow the accelerated sinus rate. Eventually, most people with type II block, whether overt or concealed, will develop complete block if they do not first succumb in a Stokes-Adams attack.

COMPLETE OR THIRD DEGREE AV BLOCK (Fig. 238-2*L*) This advanced form of block is caused by any of the disorders responsible for type II second degree block, as well as by accidental surgical trauma to the AV node or His bundle. Occasionally, one encounters an otherwise normal person with congenital AV block, and rarely a patient with persistent complete block will be found at autopsy to display no demonstrable microscopic lesion in the conduction system. A transitory form, lasting a few seconds, may follow carotid sinus pressure, and it may also be a consequence of digitalis intoxication, disappearing a week or two after the drug is withdrawn. Most cases of chronic and persistent complete heart block are infra-AV nodal, i.e., due to block in the bundle of His or bilateral bundle branch block. When block occurs within the bundle of His, two depolarizations of the His bundle may be recognized on His bundle electrograms—one proximal to the block and following each nonconducted P wave, and the other distal to the block and temporally associated with each QRS complex. In the presence of complete heart block the ventricular rate is usually 45 beats per min or less, although in congenital heart block, which is usually due to AV junctional block proximal to the His bundle, the rate may be as rapid as 60 beats per min. In either case the rhythm is regular, and the rate increases only slightly or not at all after exercise. The lesion tends to occur proximal to the bifurcation of the bundle of His in patients with congenital heart block, while acquired third degree AV block and Möbitz type II second degree block are usually bilateral bundle branch or trifascicular blocks. When the subsidiary pacemaker is in the AV node or the bundle of His, as is usual in congenital heart block, the QRS complex is usually normal; when it is below the bifurcation of the bundle of His, i.e., within the Purkinje system, as is usual in acquired heart block, the QRS complex is prolonged, notched, and slurred. The intensity of the first heart sound varies from beat to beat, being sometimes almost inaudible and at other times so loud as to merit the term *bruit de canon;* faint atrial contractions can also often be heard, possibly because of diastolic mitral regurgitation caused by atrial relaxation with a momentary reduction of atrial pressure below the ventricular level.

Acute myocardial infarction often precipitates AV block (Chap. 244). Infarcts associated with ischemia in the distribution of the right coronary artery (e.g., inferior or posterior infarctions) commonly cause AV junctional block which is due to impaired conduction proximal to the His bundle bifurcation, is transient, and is usually first or second degree (Möbitz type I block). Even when third degree block occurs in this setting, recovery of conduction may generally be anticipated. On the other hand, heart block associated with infarcts due to ischemia in the distribution of the left coronary artery is less common and more grave. It usually results from extensive damage of the His bundle and/or all three fascicles of the conduction system, is persistent, and presents as second degree Möbitz type II or third degree trifascicular block. The mortality rate associated with infarcts producing this type of block is high, even despite the indicated pacemaker therapy, because of the massive nature of the infarct responsible.

Because myocardial infarction is so common, it is by far the commonest cause of acute AV block. However, coronary artery disease is responsible for only a minority of cases of chronic and persistent complete heart block, which is usually due to primary or secondary degeneration or inflammation of the conduction system.

The prognosis of first and second degree, Möbitz type I, AV block is favorable. The outlook for high grades of block (second degree Möbitz type II or complete AV block) is always uncertain, since the patient is constantly subject to the risk of Stokes-Adams attacks, any of which may be fatal. When such attacks occur frequently in patients with complete block and are uncontrolled, death usually occurs within a year. AV block occurring in the course of acute myocardial infarction is often transient (Chap. 245). Temporary transvenous pacemakers are useful when the block is progressive, when it leads to impaired cardiac performance with hemodynamic sequelae, or when it sets the stage for demonstrable increases in ectopic ventricular dysrhythmias. Patients who survive acute infarction with or without the aid of a transvenous pacemaker generally exhibit eventual restoration of sinus rhythm within several days. Since bifascicular block may progress to complete block, prophylactic insertion of a temporary transvenous pacemaker is often performed when the condition develops in association with acute myocardial infarction pending evolution or regression of block or the results of thorough subsequent electrophysiologic evaluation. Trifascicular block may require implantation of a permanent pacemaker, but most patients with infarction who develop this condition have sustained extensive infarction associated with profound hemodynamic impairment and high early mortality.

TREATMENT OF HEART BLOCK The important problem is the prevention of the Stokes-Adams attacks. Accordingly, in all patients with symptomatic or high-grade block, definitive therapy and the treatment of choice consist of implantation of a permanent pacemaker. Despite the occurrence of complications with this mode of therapy including infection, failure to pace due to electrode displacement or fracture, or perforation of the heart, therapy with permanent pacemakers has dramatically improved the outlook for patients with symptomatic AV block. Mortality in treated cohorts is in the range of 5 percent per year. It approximates mortality in age- and sex-matched normal subjects except for death due to the higher prevalence of other disorders and not resulting from conduction system disease in the patient group.

In emergency situations, every effort should be made for prompt institution of pacemaker therapy without undue reliance on drugs. Atropine and isoproterenol or epinephrine are useful adjuncts to accelerate ventricular rate acutely and temporarily. However, since the latter two agents increase myocardial oxygen demand, they may increase ischemic injury or lead to prolonged anginal attacks, if used chronically. Other adjuncts employed in the past include corticotropin and corticosteroids, although the mechanism of their beneficial effect is uncertain. Because potassium depletion accelerates conduction, chlorothiazide, 500 to 1,000 mg, combined with sodium bicarbonate, 10 g, given t.i.d., has been found to exert a favorable effect in some patients with incomplete heart block. In life-threatening situations, external countershock may be applied for ventricular fibrillation, and life may be sustained by these measures and by closed-chest cardiac massage until intracardiac pacing by means of a catheter electrode has been achieved.

When AV block is not complete, digitalis therapy may either improve or worsen its degree. Hence the drug should be withheld unless congestive failure fails to respond to other measures and until a pacemaker has been implanted. Under no circumstances should quinidine, procainamide, or beta-adrenergic blockers be used in the presence of high-grade block unless the ventricular rhythm is first controlled by an artificial electrical pacemaker. However, these agents are useful in patients with complete heart block who manifest frequent ventricular premature contractions despite continued ventricular pacing.

BUNDLE BRANCH BLOCK DISORDERS (Fig. 238-2*P* and *Q*) These are examples of impaired conduction in a specific portion of the conducting system (Chap. 233). When the duration of the QRS complex exceeds 0.12 s and when the main deflection is positive in leads I and V_6 and negative in leads III and V_1, left bundle branch block is said to be present. Similar prolongation but with opposite directional deflections in the leads mentioned is characteristic of right bundle branch block. Lesser degrees of QRS lengthening are often designated as incomplete left or right bundle branch block. In some instances the ventricular complex may be markedly prolonged without these typical changes; such disturbances are usually considered to be *intraventricular blocks.*

THE WOLFF-PARKINSON-WHITE (WPW) SYNDROME (ANOMALOUS ATRIOVENTRICULAR EXCITATION) (Fig. 238-2*N*) This example of a group of *preexcitation syndromes* is a congenital or acquired disorder characterized by the presence of normal P waves, a P-R interval of 0.11 s or less, increased QRS duration, a slur on the initial phase of the QRS complex (delta wave), and a pronounced tendency for the occurrence of atrial tachyarrhythmias, especially paroxysmal tachycardia, atrial flutter, and atrial fibrillation. The pathophysiologic common denominator of these disorders is premature activation of a portion of ventricular muscle in relation to atrial depolarization. Variations include the presence of some of but not all these electrocardiographic features, such as the *Lown-Ganong-Levine syndrome* (LGL syndrome), which is manifested by a short P-R interval but no delta wave or QRS widening. Recent anatomic and electrophysiologic studies have led to a general concept embracing these disorders. The common denominator appears to be the presence of an anatomic and/or functional anomalous conduction pathway which bypasses the AV node (Fig. 238-3), often apparently because of persistent muscular bridges reflecting defects in embryologic partitioning of atria from ventricles. Conduction through the anomalous pathway may be manifest or occult. In the classic Wolff-Parkinson-White syndrome the sinus impulse is conducted concomitantly down the anomalous pathway and the normal pathway. Accordingly, the impulse fragments longitudinally. Ventricular excitation is a composite of early excitation (preexcitation) by the impulse traversing the anomalous pathway and hence not delayed in the AV node, and normal excitation by the impulse conducted normally through the AV node. Thus, "normal" beats are fusion beats containing a delta (preexcitation) wave, accounting for QRS prolongation. The activation from the preexcitation impulse travels more slowly through ventricular myocardium than does the normal impulse through the specialized His-Purkinje system once it has traversed the AV node. Accordingly, a large portion of ventricular depolarization is due to normal conduction, and the preexcitation wave is extinguished by the activation front of the normally conducted impulse.

Accessory pathways of anomalous conduction (classically the bundle of Kent, bypass tracts of James, and fibers of Mahaim) underlie the genesis of the supraventricular tachyarrhythmias so common in patients with these disorders. An important feature is the disparity between the duration of the refractory period of the AV node and accessory pathway. Although conduction through the accessory pathway occurs more rapidly, generally its refractory period is longer than that in the AV node. The tachycardia, usually paroxysmal supraventricular tachycardia, is initiated by a premature supraventricular beat which finds the anomalous pathway refractory and the normal pathway excitable. Accordingly, impulse transmission proceeds antegrade through the normal pathway; the impulse fragments in the AV node; *antegrade* conduction proceeds within one fragment, leading to ventricular excitation; *retrograde* conduction of the other fragment proceeds through the anomalous pathway, which has become excitable by this time; and the tachyarrhythmia persists because when the impulse reaches the normal pathway again it can be retransmitted antegrade in a persistently reciprocating manner. Thus, during the tachycardia QRS complexes are normal and do not exhibit a delta wave. A fortuitously timed or induced premature beat will terminate the tachycardia by resetting the refractory period of one or both pathways so that the circus movement is interrupted. Termination may occur also by block in one or the other of the pathways, or in both of them, sufficient to interrupt the reciprocating impulse and allow reemergence of sinus pacemaker activity. When the refractory period of the accessory pathway is less than that of the AV node, premature atrial depolarizations may not initiate supraventricular tachycardia probably because of concealed conduction in the AV node, although premature ventricular depolarizations do initiate supraventricular tachycardia. Preexcitation manifested by atrial fibrillation with unusually rapid ventricular response is associated with accessory pathways with short refractory periods. Marked variation of QRS morphology occurs, reflecting changing contributions from accessory pathway and AV nodal conduction. The rate of the ventricular response is inversely related to the duration of the accessory pathway refractory period.

A similar mechanism probably underlies many so-called ectopic supraventricular tachyarrhythmias in patients without electrocardiographic evidence of preexcitation. In such cases the anomalous pathway may simply represent longitudinal functional stratification within the AV junction, allowing for fragmentation of impulse propagation because of disparity between recovery times of two or more longitudinal pathways. In many patients with preexcitation syndromes the electrocardiogram shifts between the abnormal preexcitation and the normal intraventricular conduction pattern. The normal pattern may reveal abnormalities masked by the preexcitation form.

Two classic Wolff-Parkinson-White patterns have been recognized. In group A the delta wave is directed anteriorly and QRS complexes are dominantly positive in the right precordial leads. In some instances deep Q waves are present in lead aVF. In group B the delta wave is directed to the left and posteriorly, resulting in dominantly negative right precordial QRS complexes. Therefore, in both types, the tracing may be mistaken for QRS abnormalities indicative of myocardial infarction. The shift to anomalous conduction can sometimes be induced by vagal stimulation, such as that produced by carotid sinus pressure or by digitalis given intravenously. The normal type of conduction may be elicited by vagal inhibition with atropine or exercise, and also by quinidine and procainamide. As noted earlier, during paroxysms of tachycardia, the widened ventricular complexes usually assume a normal configuration.

Intracardiac electrograms, programmed electrical stimulation of the heart, and epicardial mapping in those patients requiring surgery are essential for localization of the anatomic sites of accessory pathways. Recurrent paroxysmal supraventricular tachycardia, or atrial fibrillation refractory to medical management, may require surgical section of the accessory pathway, which also often normalizes the P-R interval and QRS duration. Adequate electrophysiologic diagnostic studies are needed since (1) multiple accessory pathways may be present and identification of the one(s) responsible for the tachycardia is necessary, (2) tachycardia may be due to reentry through the AV node rather than through a demonstrable but clinically insignificant accessory pathway, and (3) the responsible accessory pathway may not correspond to the locus suggested by a delta wave on the electrocardiogram.

The preexcitation syndrome should be suspected in any person subject to paroxysms of tachycardia, particularly when they have occurred from youth. Although preexcitation has been associated with Ebstein's and other congenital cardiac abnormalities, mitral valve prolapse, hypertrophic cardiomyopathy, and hyperthyroidism, it is generally an isolated disorder. Any patient with a supraventricular tachyarrhythmia in which the ventricular rate exceeds 200 beats per min is a likely candidate, because normal AV nodal delay of conduction usually precludes rates this rapid. Pharmacologic therapy is designed to reduce the incidence of premature depolarizations potentially capable of initiating reentrant tachycardia, to diminish the disparity in length between effective refractory periods in the AV node and accessory pathways, or to prolong refractoriness in a portion of the tachycardia circuit so that propagation of the reentrant impulse is blocked. Digitalis may terminate a paroxysm of rapid heart action by increasing the AV nodal refractory period. However, with atrial fibrillation it may paradoxically increase the ventricular rate by facilitating conduction through the AV node–bypass pathway, and procainamide or propranolol is more effective. Procainamide and quinidine control attacks in some patients, perhaps by diminishing the incidence of the precipitating premature beats. Repetitive attacks may be disabling, and rarely sudden death occurs during an attack. If maintenance propranolol or other pharmacologic prophylaxis is ineffective, two procedures merit consideration: implantation of a transvenous atrial, coronary sinus, or ventricular pacemaker which can be activated to interrupt the tachycardia by initiating an appropriately timed beat; and surgical interruption of the anomalous pathway, based on results of definitive electrophysiologic studies.

REFERENCES

CHARDACK WM: Cardiac pacemakers and heart block, chap. 50 in *Gibbon's Surgery of the Chest,* 3d ed, eds DC Sabiston, FC Spencer, Philadelphia: Saunders, 1976, p. 1252

DURRER D, WELLENS HJJ: Medical and surgical treatment of the Wolff-Parkinson-White syndrome. Annu Rev Med 27, 1976

FOWLER NO (ed): Cardiac arrhythmias: Premature beats and the paroxysmal tachycardias, chap. 45 in *Cardiac Diagnosis and Treatment,* 2d ed, Hagerstown: Harper & Row, 1976, p. 889

GETTES LS: Electrophysiologic basis of arrhythmias in acute myocardial ischemia, in *Modern Trends in Cardiology*—3, ed MF Oliver, London: Butterworth, 1975, p. 219

KRIKLER DM, GOODWIN JF: *Cardiac Arrhythmias: The Modern Electrophysiological Approach,* Philadelphia: Saunders, 1975

LINDSAY AE: *The Cardiac Arrhythmias: An Approach to Their Electrocardiographic Recognition,* 2d ed., Chicago: Year Book, 1975

LOWN et al: Paroxysmal atrial tachycardia with block. Circulation 21:129, 1960

MUNDTH ED et al: Surgical treatment of ventricular irritability. J Thorac Cardiovasc Surg 66:943, 1973

NARULA OS: *His Bundle Electrocardiography and Clinical Electrophysiology,* Philadelphia: Davis, 1975

ROSEN KM: Cardiac electrophysiology symposium. Arch Intern Med 135:387, 1975

SOWTON E et al: Ten-year survey of treatment with implanted cardiac pacemaker. Br Med J 20:155, 1974

WELLENS HJJ, LIE HI: *The Conduction System of the Heart,* Philadelphia: Lea & Febiger, 1976

ZIPES DP et al: Role of the slow current in cardiac electrophysiology. Circulation 51:761, 1975

239
PHARMACOLOGIC TREATMENT OF CARDIOVASCULAR DISORDERS

EUGENE BRAUNWALD
PETER E. POOL

The clinical pharmacology of positive inotropic agents (digitalis glycosides and sympathomimetic agents), antiarrhythmic drugs, and antianginal agents is presented in this chapter. Diuretics are discussed in Chap. 237 and antihypertensive agents in Chap. 250.

The *direct* cardiac action of drugs may be divided into four major areas: (1) An effect on contractility (inotropic effect), reflecting alterations in the myocardial force-velocity relation at any given initial muscle length (Chap. 236); (2) an effect on heart rate, expressed as an alteration in the rhythmicity, i.e., the frequency of discharge of normal pacemaker tissue, generally that in the sinoatrial node; (3) an effect on conductivity, i.e., on the velocity with which the depolarization wave travels through the myocardium and the atrioventricular conduction system; (4) an effect on irritability, i.e., the tendency to develop ectopic pacemaker activity, which is dependent on the rate of diastolic depolarization and the threshold potential (Chap. 238). In addition to these direct effects, drugs may also affect any of or all these four properties *indirectly* by altering (1) autonomic influences acting on the heart directly or reflexly, or (2) the relationship between myocardial oxygen supply (determined largely by coronary blood flow) and oxygen needs (Chaps. 7 and 244).

DIGITALIS GLYCOSIDES

The basic molecular structure of the digitalis glycosides is a steroid nucleus to which an unsaturated lactone ring is attached at C_{17} (Fig. 239-1*A*). These two elements together are called *aglycone* or *genin,* and it is this portion of the molecule which is responsible for the cardiotonic activity. The addition of a sugar to this basic structure enhances both the potency and duration of action of the glycoside, probably as a result of increasing solubility. The sugar residue may prevent alterations in the steric structure of the molecule, which would result in a loss of cardiotonic activity.

PHARMACOKINETICS Although, in the absence of severe malabsorption, digitalis is adequately absorbed from the

FIGURE 239-1
Chemical structure of various cardioactive drugs.

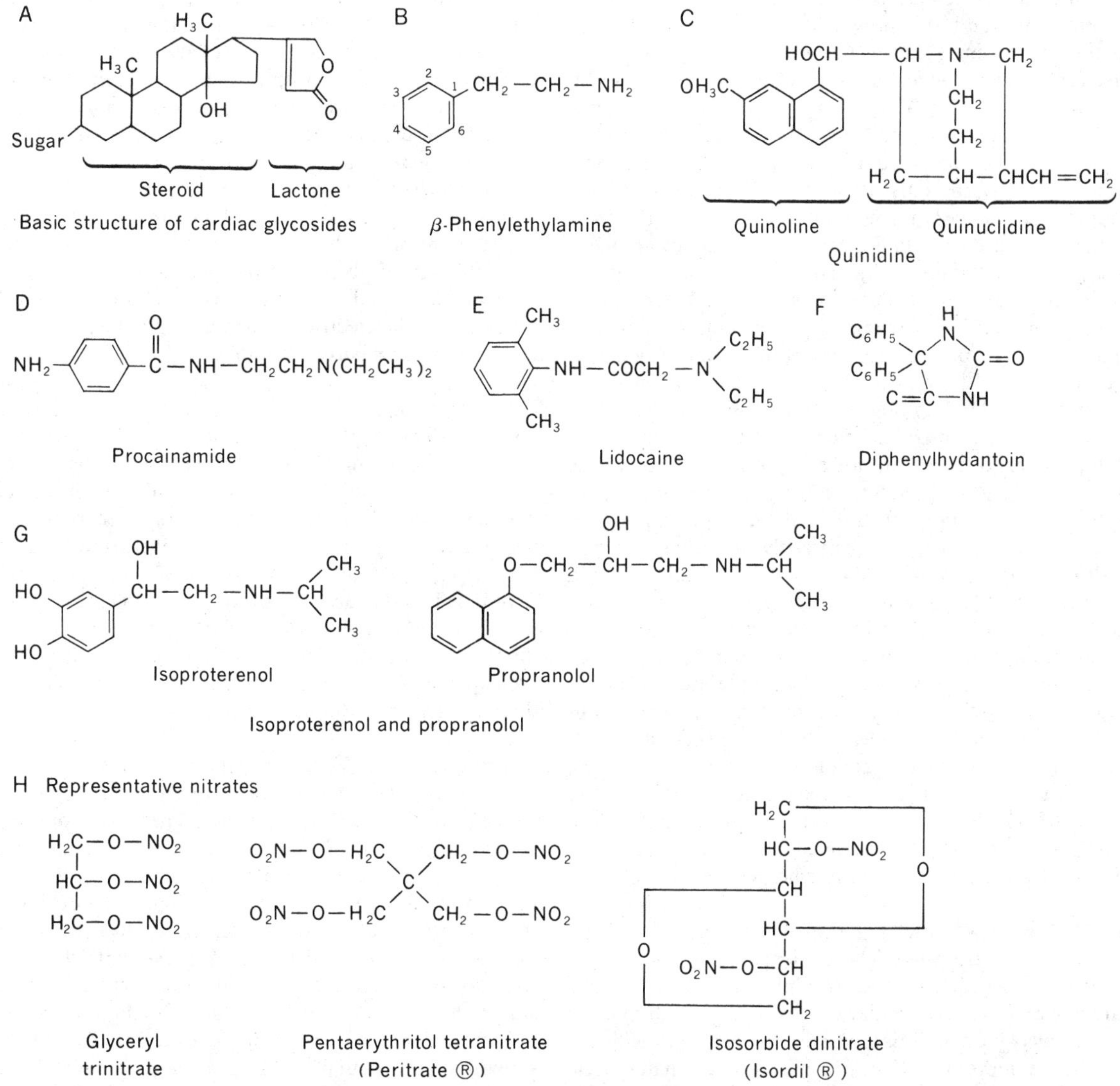

intestinal tract even in the presence of vascular congestion secondary to heart failure, some glycosides, including ouabain, are poorly absorbed and therefore are effective only when administered parenterally; the intravenous route is preferable to the intramuscular, since absorption is erratic with the latter. When they are administered orally, absorption is close to complete within 2 h. The fraction of orally administered glycoside which is absorbed varies. Approximately 40 percent of digitalis powder is absorbed, almost 100 percent of digitoxin, and up to 85 percent of digoxin. Considerable variability of bioavailability has been found in different commercial preparations of digoxin. Cholesterol-lowering resins, antidiarrheal agents containing pectin and kaolin, nonabsorbable antacids, and neomycin can reduce the absorption of digoxin and digitoxin. Varying degrees of protein-binding of glycosides occur in the bloodstream (for example, 97 percent for digitoxin and 23 percent for digoxin), and though these differences may account in part for the varying durations of the effect of different glycosides, they are not related to the speed of action of these drugs. The plasma contains only approximately one percent of the body stores of digoxin; the major fraction of the glycosides is directly bound by various tissues including the heart, in which the concentration is approximately 30 times that in the plasma for digoxin and 7 times for digitoxin, which is less polar and more lipid-soluble than digoxin.

Digoxin, which has a half-life of 1.6 days, is filtered in the glomeruli, and 85 percent is excreted in the urine, most in unchanged form; only 10 to 15 percent of digoxin is eliminated in the stool through biliary excretion. The ratio of digoxin clearance to endogenous creatinine clearance is 0.8, and the percentage of the body's total stores of digoxin lost per day can be calculated as $14 \pm 0.2 \times$ creatinine clearance in milliliters per minute. In patients with normal renal function a plateau concentration in the blood and tissue is reached after 6 days of daily maintenance treatment without a loading dose. Therefore, significant reductions of the glomerular filtration rate reduce the elimination of digoxin (but not of digitoxin) and therefore may prolong digoxin's effect, allowing it to accumulate to toxic levels. The administration of diuretics does not alter the excretion of digoxin significantly. *Digitoxin,* with a half-life of approximately 5 days, is metabolized chiefly in the liver; only 15 percent is excreted in the urine unchanged and an equal fraction in the stool. Drugs such as phenobarbital and phenylbutazone that increase activity of hepatic microsomal enzymes accelerate the metabolism of digitoxin. To reach a steady state, digitoxin requires maintenance doses for 3 to 4 weeks. *Ouabain* is very rapid acting, exhibiting an onset of action 5 to 10 min and a peak effect 60 min following intravenous injection. It is poorly absorbed from the gastrointestinal tract and therefore not suitable for oral use; it is excreted by the kidneys, has a half-life of 21 h, and is useful in emergencies.

MECHANISM OF ACTION The cardiac actions of all digitalis glycosides are alike. The clinical effects result from augmenting contractility and irritability and from slowing heart rate and atrioventricular conduction. In addition, the cardiac glycosides potentiate vagal influences on the heart.

The most important effect of digitalis on cardiac muscle is to shift its force-velocity relation upward (Chap. 236). This positive inotropic effect is exhibited in normal, nonfailing hypertrophied as well as in failing hearts. In the absence of heart failure, however, when cardiac output is not limited by cardiac contractility, the drug does not elevate the output. The finding that digitalis increases the contractility of the nonfailing heart has led to its use (1) in patients with heart disease but without heart failure prior to operation or other stressful situations such as serious infections, and (2) in the presence of a chronically increased load, such as hypertension without heart failure. However, definitive evidence of its efficacy in these circumstances has not been provided.

Excitation-contraction coupling is the membrane and intracellular process most likely involved in producing the positive inotropic effect of digitalis glycosides. These drugs inhibit transmembrane sodium and potassium movement by inhibition of the magnesium and ATP-dependent sodium- and potassium-activated transport enzyme complex. The latter, localized to the sarcolemma, and termed Na^+- and K^+- stimulated ATPase, appears to be the receptor for cardioactive glycosides. The resulting altered transmembrane distribution of sodium, i.e., the elevation of the intracellular concentration of this ion, according to one theory, then competes with calcium for efflux at internal membranes, so that less calcium is transported out of the cell and more is available to activate contractile sites. According to another concept, the increased intracellular sodium concentration enhances transmembrane exchange of sodium and calcium. Regardless of the precise mechanism involved, there is an increased myocardial uptake of calcium, which augments calcium released to the myofilaments during excitation and therefore invokes a positive inotropic response.

The action of glycosides on the inhibition of the sarcolemmal Na^+- and K^+-stimulated ATPase also produces alteration in the electrical properties of both the contractile cells and the specialized automatic cells. While low concentrations of glycosides produce little effect on the action potential, high concentrations result in a reduction in the resting potential (phase 4) with an augmented rate of diastolic depolarization (Chap. 238). The reduction in the resting potential brings the cell closer to the threshold for depolarization. These two effects lead to increased *rhythmicity* and ectopic impulse activity. With the lowering of the resting potential, the rate of rise of the action potential is reduced, resulting in a slowing of conduction velocity, which is conducive to the development of reentry. Thus, the known electrophysiologic effects of digitalis glycosides are capable of explaining both reentry and ectopic foci and the resultant arrhythmias associated with digitalis intoxication.

The glycosides also prolong the *functional refractory period* of the atrioventricular node, through a direct action, as well as an enhanced vagal effect. Digitalis also shortens the refractory period of the atrial and ventricular muscle. Small action potentials are propagated in a decremental fashion in the atrioventricular junction. Most do not reach the ventricles, but leave some of the atrioventricular junctional cells in a refractory state. Together with the action of digitalis to augment vagal activity, this helps to explain the slowing of ventricular rate produced by digitalis glycosides in supraventricular tachycardias. In atrial fibrillation, the slowing of ventricular rate is explained by several factors, in addition to prolongation of the functional refractory period of the atrioventricular node, including increased fibrillation rate (shortened atrial refractory period) and increased concealed conduction with fewer impulses penetrating the atrioventricular junction due both to direct and vagal effects of glycosides on junctional tissue.

Digitalis exerts a negative chronotropic action, which in part is a vagal effect and in part is due to a direct action on the sinus pacemaker. In heart failure, slowing of the sinus rate following the administration of digitalis results also from withdrawal of sympathetic activity secondary to general improvement in circulatory status due to the positive inotropic effect of the glycoside. In the nonfailing heart the slowing effect is negligible, and digitalis should not be used for the treatment of sinus tachycardia unless heart failure is present. The apparent suppression of pacemaker activity which may take place following high doses of digitalis is probably due not to arrest of the pacemaker but rather to a sinoatrial block related to a depression of conduction.

In addition, the digitalis glycosides also exert an action on the peripheral vasculature, causing venous and arterial constriction in normal individuals and reflex dilatation in patients with congestive heart failure.

INDICATIONS The most important indication for the administration of digitalis is congestive heart failure (Chap. 237). By stimulating the contractile function of the heart, digitalis improves ventricular emptying; i.e., it augments the ejection fraction, increases cardiac output, promotes diuresis, and reduces the elevated diastolic pressure and volume of the failing ventricle with consequent reduction of symptoms resulting from pulmonary vascular congestion and central venous pressure. Digitalis is also indicated in both the prevention and the abolition of recurrent episodes of paroxysmal supraventricular tachycardia. It is helpful in slowing the rapid ventricular rate of patients with atrial flutter and fibrillation (Chap. 238). It is of relatively little value in most forms of cardiomyopathy, myocarditis, beriberi with heart failure, mitral stenosis, thyrotoxicosis and sinus rhythm, cor pulmonale when the lung disease is not being treated concurrently (Chap. 267), and chronic constrictive pericarditis (Chap. 246). Nonetheless, it is not contraindicated in these disorders and is frequently used since it often does exert a beneficial effect, albeit not a striking one.

Digitalis is of little hemodynamic or clinical benefit in cardiogenic shock but is usually moderately effective in pulmonary edema and milder forms of heart failure secondary to myocardial infarction (Chap. 245). Digitalis has variable effects on angina pectoris, reducing this symptom in the presence of cardiomegaly and heart failure but tending to increase it in their absence. In patients with second degree atrioventricular block, digitalis may be harmful by inducing complete (third degree) block, and in those with idiopathic hypertrophic subaortic stenosis (Chap. 247) by increasing obstruction to left ventricular outflow.

DIGITALIS INTOXICATION Although digitalis is one of the cornerstones of the treatment for heart failure, it is a two-edged sword, because intoxication due to digitalis excess is a common, serious, and potentially fatal complication of its use. The therapeutic-to-toxic ratios are identical for all cardiac glycosides. In most patients with heart failure the lethal dose of most glycosides is probably 5 to 10 times the minimal effective dose and only about twice the dose which leads to minor toxic manifestations. In addition, old age, acute myocardial infarction, acute myocardial ischemia, hypoxemia, magnesium depletion, renal insufficiency, hypercalcemia, carotid sinus massage, electrical cardioversion (Chap. 240), and hypothyroidism all may reduce the tolerance of the patient to the digitalis glycosides or provoke latent digitalis intoxication. The most common precipitating cause of digitalis intoxication, however, is depletion of potassium stores, which often occurs as a result of diuretic therapy and secondary hyperaldosteronism. Since it is not necessary for a patient to receive a maximally tolerated dose of digitalis to derive a beneficial effect, even small doses provide some therapeutic action; this point should be considered if these drugs are to be used in patients prone to toxicity.

Anorexia, nausea, and vomiting, which are among the earliest signs of digitalis intoxication, are caused by direct stimulation of centers in the medulla and are not of gastrointestinal origin. The most frequent disturbance of cardiac rhythm caused by digitalis is premature ventricular beats, which may take the form of bigeminy because of increased myocardial irritability or facilitation of reentry. Atrioventricular block of varying degrees of severity may occur. Nonparoxysmal atrial tachycardia with variable atrioventricular block is quite characteristic of digitalis intoxication. Finally, sinus arrhythmia, sinoatrial block, sinus arrest, and atrioventricular junctional and multifocal ventricular tachycardia may also occur. Chronic digitalis intoxication may be insidious in onset and characterized by exacerbations of heart failure, weight loss, cachexia, neuralgias, gynecomastia, yellow vision, and delirium. Digitalis-toxic cardiac arrhythmias precede extracardiac (gastrointestinal or central nervous system) toxicity in about one-half of cases.

Digitalis intoxication has been reported to occur in more than 20 percent of hospitalized patients receiving a cardiac glycoside, which emphasizes the importance of the ability to diagnose this condition. The radioimmunoassays for digoxin and digitoxin make possible the correlation of serum glycoside levels with the presence of toxicity. In patients receiving standard maintenance doses of digoxin and digitoxin and in whom no sign of intoxication is present, serum concentrations approximate 1 to 1.5 and 20 to 25 ng per ml, respectively. When signs of intoxication are present, serum levels of more than 2 and 30 ng per ml, respectively, of these glycosides are often found. Since many factors other than the serum concentration determine digitalis intoxication, and since there is overlap in serum glycoside concentrations in patients with and without toxicity, it is clear that these levels cannot be used as a sole guide to digitalis dosage. However, when taken together with findings on the clinical examination and electrocardiogram, they add useful information to the clinical evaluations of digitalis intoxication.

Treatment of digitalis intoxication When tachyarrhythmias result from digitalis intoxication, withdrawal of the drug and treatment with potassium, diphenylhydantoin, propranolol, or lidocaine are indicated. Potassium should be administered if hypokalemia is present, but small doses may also be helpful when serum potassium levels are normal; *potassium must not be employed in the presence of atrioventricular block or hyperkalemia,* when diphenylhydantoin is more appropriate. Propranolol should not be used to treat digitalis toxicity in the presence of severe heart failure or atrioventricular block. A cardiac pacemaker may be required in digitalis-induced atrioventricular block. Electrical conversion may not only be ineffective in treating these arrhythmias but may induce more serious arrhythmias (Chap. 240). Quinidine and procainamide are not useful in the treatment of digitalis intoxication. Fab fragments of purified, intact digitalis antibodies represent a potentially lifesaving approach to the treatment of severe intoxication.

CATECHOLAMINES AND SYMPATHOMIMETIC DRUGS

Catecholamines are normally found in sympathetic nerve endings in the heart as well as in arterioles and venules. A large fraction of the endogenous stores of catecholamines in the heart is synthesized within the cardiac sympathetic postganglionic nerve endings; the remainder is taken up from the circulation. The principal catecholamine in the heart is norepinephrine, which is protected from enzymatic degradation because it is stored in granules found in the postganglionic nerve endings. The heart is capable of functioning normally in the absence of endogenous catecholamines, and in the presence of congestive heart failure, these stores are depleted (Chap. 237). However, sympathetic nerve stimulation is an important supporting mechanism for the heart in the presence of stress.

Catecholamines and other sympathomimetic drugs act upon the circulation by stimulating adrenergic receptors in the effector organs. Activation of α-adrenergic receptors results in vasoconstriction, leading to a pressor response. Stimulation of β_1-adrenergic receptors results in stimulation of cardiac contractility, automaticity, conduction velocity, and irritability, while stimulation of β_2-receptors results in relaxation of smooth muscle in the vascular bed and the tracheobronchial tree (Table 239-1).

An intimate relation between changes in cyclic AMP (cyclic 3′,5′-adenosine monophosphate) and contractility has been suggested but remains to be defined. It is clear that adenylate cyclase, a membrane-bound enzyme which catalyzes the production of cyclic AMP from ATP in the presence of Ca^{2+}, is activated by sympathomimetic amines which attach to β-receptors on the cell membrane. Cyclic AMP, in turn, activates a class of enzymes in the cell known as *protein kinases* which phosphorylate a number of proteins in the cell and stimulate the transport of Ca^{2+} into the cell. Blockade of β-receptors interferes with both the inotropic response to the drug and the augmentation of cyclic AMP concentration in the heart.

The catecholamines are based on the β-phenylethylamine molecule, an aromatic nucleus consisting of a benzene ring and an aliphatic portion, ethylamine (Fig. 239-1*B*). In general, these compounds have a brief duration of action. When administered orally, they are rapidly inactivated in the intestinal wall and liver and are therefore ineffective. Epinephrine is rapidly absorbed after intramuscular injection. However, norepinephrine should be administered only intravenously, because it produces necrosis of tissue consequent to intense vasoconstriction when given intramuscularly or subcutaneously. Isoproterenol may be administered parenterally, as an aerosol, or sublingually.

Catecholamines may be inactivated by orthomethylation by the enzyme catechol ortho-methyl transferase (COMT), or they may be deaminated by monoamine oxidase (MAO). The combined actions of MAO and COMT on epinephrine or norepinephrine lead to the production of vanillylmandelic acid (VMA), elevated urinary levels of which are useful in the diagnosis of pheochromocytoma (Chap. 94).

The specific effects of a catecholamine or a sympathomimetic amine depend on whether the drug is of the α- or β-adrenergic or mixed type, and whether its action is direct or due to release of stored catecholamines. Certain sympathomimetic drugs, similar in structure to the catecholamines but lacking the catechol nucleus, act by varying combinations of a direct action on the sympathetic receptor as well as by causing the release of stored catecholamines. Examples of this type are *metaraminol* (Aramine) and *mephentermine* (Wyamine), which have both direct and catecholamine-releasing action. Tyramine, on the other

TABLE 239-1
Electrophysiologic and electrocardiographic effects and pharmacokinetics of antiarrhythmic drugs*

Drug	*Automaticity*	*Conduction velocity*	*Effective refractory period*	*Action-potential duration*	*Interval* PR	QRS	QT	*GI absorption, %*	*Half-life, h*	*Therapeutic plasma levels, μg/ml*
Quinidine	↓	↓	↑	↑	= ↑	↑	↑	> 95	6.5	2.5–8.0
Procainamide	↓	↓	↑	↑	= ↑	↑	↑	85	3.5	3–10
Lidocaine	↓	= ↑	↓	↓	= ↓	=	= ↓	< 30	0.5–2	1–5
Diphenylhydantoin	↓	= ↑	↓	↓	= ↓	=	↓	Slow	24–36	5–20
Propranolol	↓	↓	↑	↑	= ↑	=	↓	> 95	3–6	30–100

* *Explanation of symbols:* ↑, *increased or prolonged;* ↓, *reduced or shortened;* =, *unchanged;* = ↑, *unchanged or prolonged;* = ↓, *unchanged or shortened.*

hand, acts solely by releasing stored catecholamines. In addition, sympathomimetic agents may be used for the reflex effects which they frequently induce. *Methoxamine* (Vasoxyl) and *phenylephrine* (Neo-Synephrine), for instance, are essentially pure α-adrenergic stimulators and produce arteriolar constriction, thereby augmenting systemic vascular resistance. *Norepinephrine* (Levophed), on the other hand, exerts a predominant α-adrenergic action on the peripheral vascular bed but also stimulates cardiac β-receptors. Its effects include an increase in systolic and diastolic blood pressures, as well as an increase in total peripheral resistance with compensatory reflex slowing of the heart similar to that produced by methoxamine. Stroke volume is increased and cardiac output is essentially unchanged. Coronary blood flow is increased, but blood flow through kidney, brain, liver, and skeletal muscle is usually reduced. *Isoproterenol* (Isuprel) has pure β-adrenergic activity. Its administration therefore leads to a reduction in peripheral vascular resistance with an increase in heart rate and contractility and, thus, an increase in cardiac output. Tachycardia and ventricular ectopic rhythms may also occur.

INDICATIONS Sympathomimetic amines are useful in the management of a variety of cardiovascular disorders. Isoproterenol is indicated in the treatment of a number of arrhythmias characterized by reduced automaticity and conductivity. It may be administered as a continuous intravenous infusion (1 to 6 μg per min) or sublingually (10 to 20 mg q. 2 to 4 h) in patients with sinus arrest, sinoatrial block, sinus bradycardia, various forms of atrioventricular conduction defects, and Stokes-Adams attacks (Chap. 238). This amine is also indicated in a variety of low cardiac output states, including those following cardiac operations and those associated with septic and hemorrhagic shock, unless the peripheral vascular bed is already dilated; during isoproterenol infusion expansion of circulating volume is often necessary because the vasodilatation produced by the drug may greatly reduce central venous pressure and ventricular preload. Adverse effects include the development of arrhythmias and increases in myocardial oxygen consumption due to enhanced myocardial contractility and heart rate; this may intensify myocardial ischemia if it is present.

Methoxamine and phenylephrine, which act almost exclusively by stimulating α-receptors, are indicated in hypotensive states such as occur during spinal anesthesia secondary to loss of vasoconstrictor tone, when it is desired to augment peripheral resistance without increasing cardiac contractility or automaticity. These agents are not beneficial in shock due to myocardial infarction and other conditions in which depression of cardiac contractility plays an important role in the genesis of the hypotension, except when it is desired to induce hypertension and augment vagal tone while reducing adrenergic tone reflexly in patients with supraventricular tachycardia.

Agents which stimulate both α- and β-receptors, such as *norepinephrine, epinephrine,* and *metaraminol,* may be used to elevate arterial pressure when hypotension is secondary to both a depression of myocardial contractility and an inadequate vasoconstrictor response. However, in most hypotensive states peripheral vascular resistance is already increased, and the α-receptor stimulation provided by norepinephrine may actually be deleterious. In low doses (norepinephrine <0.03 mg/kg/min; epinephrine <0.01 mg/kg/min), however, these agents stimulate β-receptors almost exclusively. In higher doses, both α- and β-receptors are activated although norepinephrine is a predominant α-adrenergic agent while epinephrine is a dominant β-stimulant. *Dopamine,* the naturally occurring immediate precursor of norepinephrine, has a combination of actions which make it particularly useful in the treatment of a variety of hypotensive states and congestive heart failure. At very low doses, that is, 1 to 2 μg/kg/min, it dilates mesenteric and renal blood vessels through stimulation of specific dopaminergic receptors, thereby augmenting renal blood flow and sodium excretion. In the range of 2 to 10 μg/kg/min dopamine stimulates myocardial β-receptors but induces little tachycardia, while at higher doses it also stimulates adrenergic receptors and elevates arterial pressure.

Undesirable reactions to the catecholamines include headache, anxiety, severe hypertension, and cardiac arrhythmias. When norepinephrine extravasates from its site of intravenous administration, tissue necrosis and sloughing may occur. Infiltration of the area with an α-adrenergic blocking agent such as phentolamine (Regitine) may prevent necrosis by blocking vasoconstriction. Following prolonged administration of sympathomimetics for the support of arterial pressure, the dose may have to be tapered slowly and the blood volume expanded to prevent vascular collapse. The replacement of endogenous catecholamine stores with nonreleasable congeners such as metaraminol may explain in part the difficulties of weaning patients from these drugs.

Protein binding, %	*Percentage excreted unchanged*	*Adverse effects*
80	20–50	GI symptoms, cinchonism, rashes, thrombocytopenia, hypotension, heart block, ventricular fibrillation
15	50–60	Lupus-like syndrome, GI symptoms, hypotension, heart block
30	< 10	Drowsiness, disorientation, agitation, convulsions, coma, paresthesias, myocardial depression
> 50	< 5	Ataxia, nystagmus, hypotension, bradycardia, skin rash
90	< 2	Asthma, heart block, asystole, hypotension, heart failure, weakness, insomnia, lethargy

ANTIARRHYTHMIC AGENTS

QUINIDINE This drug, the D-isomer of quinine (Fig. 239-1*C*), is one of some twenty alkaloids derived from the bark of the cinchona tree, found in certain regions of South America and the Far East.

The *electrophysiologic effects* of quinidine on ventricular and Purkinje fibers are shared by *procainamide* (Pronestyl), and the following summary applies equally to both drugs (Table 239-1). The durations both of the effective refractory period and of the action potential are prolonged, the former more than the latter. Quinidine also reduces the slope of phase 4 of the action potential, and it is this effect which is responsible for reducing the spontaneous frequency of discharge of ectopic pacemakers. The drug also has negative chronotropic effects, depressing the activity of both the sinoatrial node and ectopic pacemakers. However, this direct negative chronotropic effect of quinidine is often counteracted by its vagal blocking action, which may lead to no change, or an actual increase in heart rate, and reduce the refractory period of the atrioventricular junction. Quinidine slows conductivity in the atrioventricular junction; therefore, in the presence of depressed atrioventricular conduction, it must be used with great caution. However, in the absence of depressed conduction, its potent vagal blocking action may actually facilitate conduction through this system. Quinidine prolongs conduction in depressed portions of a reentrant pathway so that conduction is further delayed and block occurs, thereby terminating reentrant ventricular arrhythmias. Quinidine also increases the threshold of excitability, thereby making atrial, ventricular, and Purkinje tissue less irritable. Quinidine exerts a negative inotropic effect. In addition, large doses, especially when given parenterally, produce peripheral vasodilatation, which together with a decreased cardiac output may lead to hypotension.

There are various interpretations of the means by which quinidine is effective in converting atrial fibrillation to normal sinus rhythm. If atrial fibrillation results from the formation of rapid waves of depolarization in the atrium (Chap. 238), then by diminishing the rate of impulse of an ectopic pacemaker, quinidine may slow this rate below the frequency at which atrial fibrillation occurs. If, on the other hand, atrial fibrillation results from a circus movement of impulses around the atrium, the prolongation of the atrial refractory period by quinidine would interrupt the circus movement, even though the velocity of impulse transmission is also decreased.

Diminished intraventricular conduction velocity is reflected in an increase in the duration of the QRS complex, while the delayed repolarization is reflected in the prolongation of the Q-T interval of the electrocardiogram. The anticholinergic action of quinidine may produce sinus tachycardia. The drug may also lead to an increase in ventricular rate when it alone is used for the treatment of atrial flutter or fibrillation; the slowing of atrial rate produced by quinidine may reduce the repetitive concealed conduction of atrial impulses in the atrioventricular junction. As a consequence, a greater fraction of the impulses entering the AV junction may propagate to the ventricle. Therefore, digitalis should be administered in doses sufficient to increase the effective refractory period of the atrioventricular junction before treating either atrial flutter or fibrillation with quinidine.

Indications Although quinidine had been used for years to convert atrial fibrillation to sinus rhythm, electrical countershock is now employed more frequently because of its safety and effectiveness (Chap. 240). Quinidine is used most frequently for prevention of recurrent atrial fibrillation after sinus rhythm has been restored. It may also be used in atrial flutter after a trial of digitalis therapy has failed to convert this rhythm to normal sinus rhythm. In the treatment of atrial flutter, however, quinidine frequently leads to a progressive reduction in the degree of block from 4:1 or 2:1 to 1:1, and when this occurs the rapid ventricular response may be hazardous. Quinidine or procainamide is frequently used to prevent supraventricular and ventricular tachycardia and fibrillation in patients who have had episodes of these arrhythmias. However, if atrioventricular block is associated with ventricular tachycardia, quinidine is contraindicated, because suppression of the ventricular focus in the presence of complete heart block may lead to ventricular standstill or fibrillation. Quinidine and procainamide are also used in the treatment of ectopic premature supraventricular and ventricular beats, but are not indicated unless the frequency of these ectopic impulses seriously disturbs the patient or unless the onset of a more serious arrhythmia is feared, as in acute myocardial infarction (Chap. 245). When given orally these drugs are useful in maintaining control of ventricular extrasystoles in patients with an acute myocardial infarction when a lidocaine infusion is to be terminated.

Pharmacokinetics These differ for quinidine and procainamide. Quinidine may be administered orally or intramuscularly; absorption of the drug is essentially complete following oral administration which produces maximum effects in 1 to 2 h. If the drug is given at intervals of 2 to 4 h, effects will be cumulative. Effects are negligible 8 h following administration. This point may be especially important in the prophylaxis of recurrent supraventricular arrhythmias. If doses are spaced more than 6 h apart, less than therapeutic serum levels may occur between doses and prophylaxis may fail. More frequent rather than increased doses may avert this problem. Sustained-release preparations may also be used. Peak effects occur 30 to 90 min following intramuscular administration. Intravenous administration, however, does not produce instantaneous effects; therefore, when it is given by this route, the drug should be administered slowly and the dose should not be repeated before peak effect has been achieved.

In therapeutic concentrations approximately 80 percent of quinidine is bound by plasma albumin. Blood concentrations may be measured easily; concentrations of the order of 2.5 μg per ml are necessary for therapeutic effects; approximately 10 μg per ml usually produces toxicity. Although metabolic degradation of quinidine, mostly to hydroxy derivatives, occurs in most tissues, particularly in the liver, hepatic injury does not appear to influence the rate at which quinidine leaves the plasma. Both the metabolic end product (2-hydroxyquinidine) and the unchanged drug normally are rapidly excreted by the kidneys.

Adverse reactions to quinidine include cinchonism, consisting of tinnitus, headache, nausea, and distorted vision. Diarrhea, anorexia, nausea, and vomiting are common side effects but may be controlled with the phenothiazines. Frequently, in order to convert atrial fibrillation to normal sinus rhythm, it may be necessary to accept moderate levels of toxicity, entailing nausea, vomiting, tinnitus, and minor widening of the QRS complex. Idiosyncratic reactions, thrombocytopenic purpura, and severe hypotension may occur. The myocardial depressant action of quinidine limits its usefulness in the presence of congestive heart failure and hypotensive states. Its use is also contraindicated in patients with a history of thrombocytopenic purpura or in individuals with digitalis intoxication who have an atrioventricular conduction disorder. Widening of the QRS complex by 50 percent or greater of control values and reduction of arterial pressure by more than 20 mmHg are serious warning signs and necessitate discontinuation of the drug. The greatest hazard of quinidine is sudden death due to ventricular fibrillation. This may occur even in patients treated with moderate therapeutic doses.

PROCAINAMIDE In 1936 the discovery was made that procaine, applied directly to the heart, elevates the threshold of ventricular muscle to electrical stimulation. Its prominent central nervous system–stimulating effect and rapid enzymatic hydrolysis make it undesirable clinically. Procainamide (Pronestyl), which differs from procaine in that an amide structure (—CONH—) is present instead of an ester linkage (—COO—) (Fig. 239-1*D*), has negligible central nervous system effects and is protected from enzymatic hydrolysis by plasma esterases.

The electrophysiologic effects of procainamide on the heart are similar to those of quinidine (Table 239-1). Clinically, procainamide is generally used in the treatment or prevention of ventricular tachyarrhythmias, in which it appears to be slightly more effective than quinidine. Procainamide, especially when given by the intravenous route, may cause hypotension, and α-adrenergic stimulators should be available to counteract this effect.

Pharmacokinetics Procainamide may be administered by the oral, intramuscular, or intravenous routes. It is rapidly and almost completely absorbed from the gastrointestinal tract and has a peak effect in approximately 1 h. If given intravenously for rapid control of arrhythmia, it can be administered in doses of 100 mg at intervals of 5 min while blood pressure and ECG are continuously monitored. An intravenous infusion of 0.3 to 1.0 mg/kg/min is begun simultaneously. It is concentrated in most tissues to levels greater than in the plasma. Approximately 15 percent of procainamide is bound to plasma proteins. It is eliminated by both hepatic metabolism and renal excretion. Approximately 50 percent is acetylated to *N*-acetylprocainamide. The rates of acetylation vary widely among different individuals and appear to be genetically determined.

An initial loading dose of 1 g given intramuscularly will rapidly produce effective blood concentrations (3 to 10 μg per ml) which may be maintained with an average dose of 250 mg orally or intramuscularly every 3 h. Since the half-life is only 3 to 4 h, longer intervals between doses may cause undesirably great fluctuations in concentration. Renal excretion of procainamide is important, and renal insufficiency may predispose to toxicity.

Adverse effects These include nausea, vomiting, and diarrhea. During the chronic administration of procainamide periodic blood counts should be obtained, because this drug has caused fatal agranulocytosis. It is also frequently a cause of drug fever and drug eruptions. The commonest problem encountered during chronic administration of procainamide is a lupus erythematosus-like syndrome. After several months of administration, arthralgias sometimes accompanied by fever and hepatomegaly are present in about one-third of patients; an even higher proportion have positive antinuclear antibody tests. Cross-sensitivity to procaine and other related drugs should also be anticipated. Procainamide is contraindicated in the presence of atrioventricular block and when there is a history of hypersensitivity to local anesthetics.

LIDOCAINE Although lidocaine has some similarities to procainamide in its antiarrhythmic action, it is not similar to procaine and to the other local anesthetics in the aromatic portion of its stucture (Fig. 239-1*E*). In addition, lidocaine lacks an ester linkage and may be given to persons sensitive to procaine. Unlike quinidine and procainamide, lidocaine does not prolong the effective refractory period of ventricular myocardium. It diminishes automaticity in the His-Purkinje system and raises the threshold of ventricular fibrillation. Lidocaine enhances conduction at the Purkinje fiber–myocardial junctions, an action that may diminish reentrant arrhythmias by causing their extinction (Chap. 238). Lidocaine is the drug of choice for ventricular arrhythmias complicating myocardial infarction (Chap. 245). Its use is indicated (1) if the number of unifocal premature contractions exceeds five per min and in the presence of (2) multifocal premature contractions or early (R on T wave) premature contractions; (3) couplets; and (4) runs of ventricular tachycardia. Since the incidence of ventricular tachycardia and fibrillation is diminished when lidocaine is administered prophylactically to patients with acute myocardial infarction, some physicians use it in all patients with this condition (Chap. 245).

Pharmacokinetics The absorption, metabolism, and effectiveness of oral lidocaine are unpredictable. When administered intravenously, it acts almost instantaneously, but its action is quite transient. Because of these properties, it is particularly useful when there is expectation that the inciting cause of the arrhythmia will disappear. Lidocaine, therefore, is widely used during cardiac catheterization and during cardiac operations when the stimuli which produce arrhythmias are short-lived. However, arrhythmias abolished by single injections of lidocaine may reappear in 10 to 20 min.

In order to achieve adequate blood levels, which generally range from 1 to 5 μg per ml, administration should be initiated with a bolus intravenous injection of 1 mg per kg body weight, with additional doses every 5 min until the arrhythmia is abolished or 5 mg per kg has been administered, followed by a continuous intravenous infusion of 20 to 40 μg/kg/min. It is also effective when injected intramuscularly (5 mg per kg of 10% lidocaine) into the deltoid muscle. This route is frequently used in patients with myocardial infarction while they are being transported to the hospital. The half-life of lidocaine is about one hour, and its deactivation is dependent on hepatic metabolism. In the presence of congestive heart failure, liver disease, or shock, dosage should be reduced by as much as 50 percent to avoid toxic effects, which include myocardial depression, hypotension, and neurologic abnormalities such as drowsiness, numbness, paresthesias, euphoria, disorientation, and convulsions. It is contraindicated in patients with sinoatrial block.

DIPHENYLHYDANTOIN (Dilantin, Fig. 239-1*F*) In 1938, this agent was introduced in the treatment of epilepsy. During the following 20 years a number of studies in animals reported its effectiveness in experimentally produced cardiac arrhythmias, especially those induced by digitalis. Unlike quinidine, diphenylhydantoin does not reduce atrioventricular or intraventricular conduction velocity and does not prolong the ventricular refractory period. However, like quinidine, it reduces automaticity in Purkinje fibers and raises the atrial and ventricular fibrillation thresholds. Possibly a depressant action of diphenylhydantoin on sympathetic centers in the central nervous system may play a role in its antiarrhythmic properties.

Indications Diphenylhydantoin is particularly effective in supraventricular and ventricular arrhythmias, particularly those resulting from digitalis excess, because it does not interfere with atrioventricular conduction, as do several other antiarrhythmic agents. It may also be useful in the treatment and prevention of ventricular extrasystoles and tachycardia not caused by digitalis excess, as well as acute ventricular arrhythmias associated with anesthesia, cardioversion, cardiac catheterization, and cardiac surgery if the more standard agents such as quinidine, procainamide, and lidocaine are ineffective. Less success has been reported with diphenylhydantoin in the treatment of supraventricular tachyarrhythmias not secondary to digitalis excess or when administered prophylactically in attempts to reduce ventricular arrhythmias in patients with ischemic heart disease.

Pharmacokinetics Soon after intravenous administration, the drug is concentrated in liver, kidney, and salivary glands and to a lesser extent in brain, fat, and muscle. Plasma concentrations decrease rapidly. The liver is the chief site of inactivation, and there is a substantial enterohepatic circulation of metabolites of the drug; urinary excretion of metabolites is also significant.

Diphenylhydantoin may be administered orally or intravenously. The drug is well absorbed, although slowly, when given orally. To reach antiarrhythmic plasma levels (5 to 20 μg per ml), an oral loading dose of 1,000 mg is given the first day, 500 mg on each of the next 2 days, and 400 mg per day thereafter. Intravenous doses consist of 100 mg every 5 min until the arrhythmia is abolished or until adverse effects appear; the total dosage should not exceed 1,000 mg. For emergency use, 50 to 100 mg is administered intravenously every 5 min until the arrhythmia is controlled, until 500 mg has been given, or until untoward effects appear. Lower maintenance doses are then required.

Adverse effects These include transient hypotension and bradycardia; with long-term administration, ataxia, slurring of speech, nystagmus, mild gastric upsets, and skin rashes occur in 2 to 5 percent of patients. During chronic administration, hyperplasia of the gums develops in about 20 percent of patients. Hepatocellular injury and pseudolymphoma are rare complications.

BETA-ADRENERGIC RECEPTOR BLOCKING AGENTS

Propranolol (Inderal) is similar in configuration to the pure β-adrenergic stimulant, isoproterenol, except for the addition of a benzene ring (Fig. 239-1*G*). Beta-adrenergic blockage with propranolol is basically of the competitive type and is reversible. It is capable of blocking the effects of catecholamines and sympathetic-nerve stimulation on heart rate, cardiac output, and contractility. Therefore, it tends to reduce resting heart rate, cardiac index, and arterial blood pressure in normal subjects, but impairment of cardiac performance is even more pronounced during muscular exercise because of the blockade of the augmented sympathetic activity which occurs during exercise. In addition, propranolol reduces oxygen uptake by the myocardium, and in large doses it may cause sodium retention.

INDICATIONS Propranolol, alone or in combination with nitroglycerin or long-acting nitrates, is often effective in patients with angina pectoris in whom nitrates alone have failed to provide relief (Chap. 244). Propranolol with isosorbide dinitrate is one such combination which is felt to be effective. The beneficial effects of propranolol in angina pectoris probably are achieved by preventing the increased myocardial oxygen requirements induced by sympathetic nervous discharge during physical activity, cold, or emotion. Because propranolol depresses myocardial contractility, it may intensify heart failure and should be used only with extreme caution in patients with seriously diminished cardiac reserve. Oral dosage schedules are usually begun with 40 mg per day in divided doses; 240 mg per day is often required for efficacy, and the dosage needed has reached 800 mg per day.

A second major use of propranolol is in the treatment of cardiac arrhythmias, particularly in the abolition and prevention of paroxysmal supraventricular and ventricular tachycardias, although it is usually used only if the other antiarrhythmic drugs have failed. Propranolol is effective in the treatment of tachyarrhythmias resulting from digitalis intoxication, when electric countershock is contraindicated (Chap. 240). It is particularly useful in reducing excessive ventricular rate in patients with atrial fibrillation. Its beneficial effects in this regard result from prolongation of the refractory period of the atrioventricular junction by blocking adrenergic influences on this system. In this regard the effects of propranolol are additive to those of digitalis. Although only the L-isomer of propranolol has β-adrenergic blocking activity, D-propranolol is also effective against digitalis-induced arrhythmias. Therefore, the antiarrhythmic effects of propranolol in digitalis intoxication may derive from both its β-adrenergic blocking action and its direct antiarrhythmic activity, i.e., from a "quinidine-like" effect. However, only its β-blocking effect appears to be significant in the other actions of the drug. Propranolol is useful in treating the sinus tachycardia and palpitation of anxiety neurosis (Chap. 33), the hyperkinetic heart syndrome, and thyrotoxicosis.

Propranolol is also effective in relieving many of the symptoms of idiopathic hypertrophic subaortic stenosis (Chap. 247). Its effects are related to a depression of the contractile state of the heart, leading to lessening of the severity of obstruction. Finally, propranolol is useful in the treatment of hypertension (Chap. 250), particularly in patients with labile hypertension, those with high-output states, and those with high levels of circulating renin. In very high doses (2,000 mg per day) it reduces arterial pressure even in hypertensive patients without these characteristics. In clinical practice, propranolol is a very effective antihypertensive agent in lower doses (240 mg per day), when used in combination with a diuretic and vasodilator.

PHARMACOKINETICS Propranolol is cleared by the liver, and its inactivation is dependent on hepatic blood flow. It may be administered both orally and parenterally. Even though it is completely absorbed, much larger oral than intravenous doses are necessary because the drug traverses the portal bed and is metabolized by the liver. Plasma levels and clinical effectiveness vary widely following oral administration as a consequence of variable plasma drug binding, the presence of active metabolites, and differences in bioavailability consequent to variations in hepatic blood flow and hepatic extraction. The half-life following oral administration is 3 to 6 h, and the drug should be given four times daily in order to maintain a beta-blocking effect. Half-life may be prolonged in patients with liver disease. There is considerable variation among patients in the dosage and the plasma level required to produce a given clinical effect of propranolol. Since propranolol is a competitive antagonist, its effects can be counteracted by increased activity of the adrenergic nervous system or by injected isoproterenol. The magnitude of its effect depends on the degree of sympathetic tone present at the time of administration. A blood level of 30 to 100 μg per ml is considered to be the usual therapeutic range.

ADVERSE EFFECTS These occur in less than 2 percent of patients and include nausea, visual disturbances, diarrhea, cutaneous eruptions, and insomnia. Weakness, lethargy, and easy fatigability are troublesome side effects, which are dose-dependent and commonly observed in patients receiving more than 240 mg per day. Clinically important hypoglycemia may occur in insulin-dependent diabetics in whom the sympathetic defense of hypoglycemia has been blunted. The undesirable effects of effective beta-adrenergic blockade include the production of shock and intensification of heart failure. Propranolol is specifically contraindicated in patients with second or third degree atrioventricular block, in whom it may produce serious bradycardia or even asystole. The drug is also contraindicated in patients with asthma or bronchial constriction.

VASODILATORS

Glyceryl trinitrate (nitroglycerin) and amyl nitrite have been used for more than a century for their vasodilating properties. In recent years, however, numerous other nitrate compounds have been introduced which have a longer duration of action than nitroglycerin (Fig. 239-1*H*).

MECHANISM OF ACTION The vasodilators have only one specific therapeutic effect—to relax smooth muscle. The mechanism of this action is not known, and it cannot be blocked by any known inhibitors. For example, nitrite ion can relax smooth muscle even in the presence of the alpha-adrenergic-stimulating effects of norepinephrine. Administration of organic nitrates leads to generalized arterial and venous dilation, resulting in a fall in mean systemic arterial pressure and in peripheral pooling of blood. Pulse pressure, stroke volume, and central venous pressure decline, particularly when the patient is in the erect position. The hypotension evokes a compensatory tachycardia. Dilatation of blood vessels in the skin causes marked flushing of the head, neck, and chest, and severe pounding headache may occur because of dilatation of the meningeal vessels.

Though nitroglycerin increases coronary blood flow in normal individuals, there is considerable evidence that it does not always evoke this effect in the presence of diffuse, severe coronary artery disease. Therefore, it is difficult to relate the beneficial effects of this drug in angina pectoris to a direct increase in total coronary blood flow. Myocardial ischemia, however, relates not only to the amount of blood which reaches the coronary capillaries but also to the demands for oxygen (Chaps. 7 and 244). Since nitroglycerin regularly reduces arterial blood pressure, the work performance and the oxygen requirements of the heart are diminished. The venous dilatation produced by this drug leads to a reduction in heart size, which also tends to reduce myocardial oxygen consumption. Coronary blood flow, however, is not diminished, and therefore the major effect of nitroglycerin may be to improve the relationship between myocardial oxygen delivery and myocardial oxygen requirements. There is some evidence that nitroglycerin dilates coronary collateral vessels, increasing perfusion of ischemic areas. Finally, the reduction in left ventricular end-diastolic tension consequent to the venous dilatation induced by nitroglycerin reduces the compression of subendocardial coronary vessels and may thereby induce a more favorable distribution of myocardial perfusion to the subendocardium, which is the portion of the heart wall most subject to ischemia.

INDICATIONS The nitrates are primarily used for the treatment of angina pectoris; the chest pain is relieved within 2 to 4 min by sublingual nitroglycerin. Because the effects of this drug may persist for 30 min, it may also be used prophylactically to prevent angina pectoris when the patient predicts that it will occur. However, long-term prophylaxis with the longer-acting nitrates has been relatively unsuccessful except when used in conjunction with beta-adrenergic blocking agents.

PHARMACOKINETICS The *nitrite* ion is an active vasodilator in both inorganic and organic forms, but the *nitrate* ion is active only in organic form. The organic nitrates are absorbed most effectively from the sublingual or buccal mucosa. Many of the longer-acting nitrates, however, are also absorbed from the gastrointestinal tract and may be administered orally. Despite this, oral administration is of little value because of almost complete degradation by the liver. Portions of absorbed nitrite ion may be converted to ammonia, and portions are excreted in the urine, but their metabolic fate is largely unknown.

The most useful of the longer-acting nitrates appears to be sublingual isosorbide dinitrate in doses of 2.5 to 10 mg.

When given sublingually or transcutaneously by ointment (2 percent nitroglycerin) in adequate doses, nitrates regularly produce cutaneous flushing and headache; if the patient fails to be relieved of angina but also fails to show any side effects, it is possible that the dose of the drug is not adequate or that tolerance has developed.

ADVERSE EFFECTS These include headache, hypotension, dizziness, and syncope, as well as occasional drug eruptions. In addition, the nitrate ion readily oxidizes hemoglobin to methemoglobin, which may cause severe hypoxia if large enough doses are ingested.

DOSAGE SCHEDULES The approximate dosage schedules for cardioactive drugs are summarized in Table 239-2.

REFERENCES

BRADLEY SE, CAMPBELL CL (eds): Symposium on pharmacologic and clinical control of cardiovascular drugs. Am J Med 58:449, 1975

BRAUNWALD E, POOL PE: Mechanism of action of digitalis glycosides. Mod Concepts Cardiovasc Dis 37:129, 1968

DONOSO E (ed): *Drugs in Cardiology,* parts I and II, New York: Stratton Intercontinental Medical Book Corp., 1975

EPSTEIN SE, BRAUNWALD E: Beta-adrenergic receptor blocking drugs: Mechanisms of action and clinical applications. N Engl J Med 275:1106, 1175, 1966

FOWLER NO (ed): Digitalis intoxication and electrolyte imbalance, chap. 49 in *Cardiac Diagnosis and Treatment,* 2d ed, Hagerstown: Harper & Row, 1976, p. 1009

GOLDBERG LI: Dopamine—Clinical uses of an endogenous catecholamine. N Engl J Med 291:707, 1974

GOODMAN LS, GILMAN A (eds): *The Pharmacological Basis of Therapeutics,* 5th ed., pp. 477, 653, New York: Macmillan, 1975

JEWITT DE: Antiarrhythmic drugs and their mechanisms of actions, in *Modern Trends in Cardiology,* vol. 3, ed MF Oliver, London: Butterworth, 1975, p. 333

SHAND DG: Propranolol. N Engl J Med 299:280, 1975

SMITH TW, HABER E: *Digitalis,* Boston: Little, Brown, 1974, p. 110

TARAZI RC: Sympathomimetic agents in the treatment of shock. Ann Intern Med 81:364, 1974

WIT AL et al: Electrophysiology and pharmacology of cardiac arrhythmias. Am Heart J 88:380, 515, 664, 798, 1974; ibid 89: 115, 253, 391, 526, 665, 804, 1975; ibid 90:117, 265, 397, 521, 665, 795, 1975

240
ELECTRICAL REVERSION OF CARDIAC ARRHYTHMIAS

BERNARD LOWN

Ectopic arrhythmias of the heart have generally been controlled by means of drugs. The use of antiarrhythmic drugs presents a number of problems. To reach an effective dose requires a time-consuming biologic titration involving frequent monitoring of the patient's condition. There is a high incidence of mild as well as serious toxic reactions. Furthermore, a number of rhythm disorders are refractory to drugs. A method is needed that is simple in application, restores sinus rhythm consistently, and is free from untoward side effects. These requirements are satisfied by the use of a specific type of electrical discharge across the intact chest.

TABLE 239-2
Approximate dosage schedules for cardioactive drugs*

	Initial or loading dose			
Drug	*Oral*	*Intramuscular*	*Intravenous*	*Usual maintenance dosage*
Ouabain			0.5–1.0 mg in divided doses	
Digoxin	1.0–2.0 mg		0.8–1.6 mg in divided doses	0.25–0.50 mg p.o. daily
Digitoxin	1.0–1.5 mg			0.05–0.15 mg p.o. daily
Digitalis leaf	1.0–2.0 g			0.05–0.15 g p.o. daily
Quinidine	0.2 g q.6 h; increase dose by 0.2 g until arrhythmia is controlled or dose of 0.8 g q.4 h is reached			0.2–0.4 g p.o., q.4 h
Procainamide	0.5–1.0 g	0.5–1.0 g	100 mg q.5 min up to × 10	500 mg p.o. q.6 h
Lidocaine			75 mg (1 mg/kg)	20–40 μg/kg/min
Diphenylhydantoin	250 mg q.i.d.		100 mg q.5 min up to × 5	100 mg p.o. q.6 h
Propranolol	10–80 mg p.o., q.i.d., or greater for angina 10–40 mg p.o., q.i.d., for arrhythmias		1.0 mg for arrhythmias	Same as initial dose for angina
Glyceryl trinitrate	0.3–0.6 mg sublingually			As needed
Isosorbide dinitrate				10–20 mg p.o., q.i.d. (sublingual)

* *Dosage schedules represent broad ranges and must be modified for individual patients. Initial digitalis doses are total loading doses and should be given in fractional amounts.*

THEORETIC BASIS FOR THE USE OF ELECTRICAL DISCHARGE The use of electrical energy for terminating ectopic arrhythmias is based on three propositions:

1 Chronic ventricular and atrial arrhythmias are initiated by a multiplicity of interacting factors, some of which are transient. Once initiated, the abnormal mechanisms are self-sustaining, perhaps because of a continuing passage of recirculating wave fronts of excitation over fixed or variable pathways (circus movement).
2 When an ectopic disorder is momentarily extinguished, the sinus node, which has the highest rhythmicity in the heart, resumes as dominant pacemaker.
3 The heart can be depolarized across the intact chest by electrical discharge. When effective, such depolarization abolishes the ectopic mechanism and permits restoration of sinus rhythm.

If electrical discharge were safe, it would constitute an ideal form of antiarrhythmic therapy. Ventricular fibrillation has been terminated across the intact chest by 60-Hz alternating current (ac) shocks. When this type of electrical discharge is administered to normal animals, it may induce cardiac arrest or ventricular fibrillation. The danger of provoking such serious disruptions in cardiac mechanism has deterred adoption of alternating current for the treatment of arrhythmias.

CARDIOVERSION Capacitor discharge, or direct current (dc) shock, may also be employed to defibrillate the heart. A capacitor can be made to yield a great variety of wave forms, depending on the parameters of the discharge circuit. Incorporating an inductance in the circuit reduces the peak voltage released by a capacitor and lengthens the duration of discharge. A single monophasic pulse resulting from the use of an appropriate capacitor and inductor is more effective in depolarizing the heart, induces fewer arrhythmias and less tissue damage than alternating current, and, furthermore, does not provoke cardiac standstill. The one hazard remaining is the sporadic occurrence of ventricular fibrillation.

When the dc pulse is delivered systematically through the cardiac cycle, ventricular fibrillation occurs only when the discharge is triggered during the final one-third of systole. This vulnerable period appears to be an essential physiologic property of the mammalian heart. It generally has a duration of 30 ms and just precedes the apex of the T wave of the surface electrocardiogram. When a dc discharge is triggered outside this vulnerable period, ventricular fibrillation does not occur.

Thus by employing a capacitor discharge with a specific underdamped pulse and synchronizing the release of this pulse within a safe part of the cardiac cycle, that is, 30 ms after the beginning of the QRS complex, the twin dangers of electricity, namely, ventricular standstill and fibrillation, can be avoided. The use of synchronized capacitor shock has been designated *cardioversion* and is employed for terminating a diversity of ectopic arrhythmias.

TECHNIQUE OF CARDIOVERSION The technique employed is essentially the same irrespective of the type of arrhythmia. Cardioversion can be carried out as an outpatient procedure, although brief hospitalization is preferred. No special area is required. In the treatment of atrial fibrillation or atrial flutter, quinidine in a dose of 0.3 g every 6 h is initiated 24 to 48 h prior to the procedure. The objective is fourfold:

1 To build up an adequate level of drug in the body so that the arrhythmia will not recur soon after reversion
2 To determine whether quinidine is tolerated
3 To obtain a small dividend of reversion which occurs in about 10 percent of patients with chronic atrial fibrillation who are given this dose of quinidine
4 To decrease the occurrence of postcardioversion arrhythmias

Premedication is limited to a sedative drug given about an hour before the procedure. Amnesia is induced by means of small (10 to 15 mg) intravenous doses of diazepam.

The electrical discharge is applied by means of two insulated electrode paddles. These are covered with thick layers of conductive paste. One electrode is placed below the angle of the left scapula, the other is applied over the right parasternal area of the third intercostal space. The instrument is automatically synchronized to deliver the discharge during inscription of the QRS complex. The initial energy setting is 5 to 10 W-s, depending upon the severity of heart disease and uncertainty as to the presence of overdigitalization. If reversion is not accomplished with these low-energy discharges, successive shocks are delivered without delay at increasing energies, proceeding to 25, 50, 100, 200, 300, up to 400 W-s. The patient's response consists of a single twitch of thoracic muscle, a slight jerk of the arms, and at times an audible sigh. Normal rhythm is restored instantly; at times a brief episode of nodal rhythm precedes establishment of sinus node dominance.

CLINICAL RESULTS Many thousands of patients have been treated with this method. The good results that have almost always occurred have confirmed theoretic expectations. Cardioversion has been found effective in many ectopic rhythm disorders, whether of ventricular, nodal, or atrial origin.

Ventricular tachycardia In the majority of instances, ventricular tachycardia arises in patients with serious organic heart disease; usually, it occurs in the wake of a myocardial infarction. The rapid heart action and aberrant activation of the myocardium seriously compromise cardiac function. This arrhythmia frequently constitutes a dire emergency. Antiarrhythmic drugs may reduce ventricular contractility and peripheral resistance, and thus further impair cardiac function. Cardioversion is devoid of these adverse actions. Restoration of sinus rhythm is immediate (Fig. 240-1). This method is nearly 100 percent effective and constitutes a treatment of choice for ventricular tachycardia when the disorder does not respond to a 50-mg bolus of lidocaine. In the case of the oft-recurring episodes of ventricular tachycardia which accompany acute myocardial infarction, the use of continuous intravenous infusion of lidocaine is the treatment of choice.

Atrial fibrillation This arrhythmia is the most common chronic disorder of the heartbeat. Until recently treatment has been based on the use of quinidine. Even when it is given to the point of toxicity, the heartbeat of only 50 percent of patients can be restored to sinus rhythm. With cardioversion, atrial fibrillation can be terminated in more than 90 percent of patients. Failures are encountered mainly in patients with mitral valvular disease, with giant left atria, and with continuous arrhythmia for 5 years or longer. A typical example of cardioversion is illustrated in Fig. 240-2. At times, transitional mechanisms are encountered, consisting of nodal rhythm and ectopic atrial beats which generally last for 30 to 60 s, until the SA node "warms up." Slowing the ventricular rate is one immediate effect of restoration of sinus rhythm. The P-R interval is full, and not infrequently first degree AV block is present. In patients with congestive heart failure, restoration of sinus rhythm results in an increase in the cardiac output. The patient generally feels improved and comments on the newly sensed "calm" in the chest. Compared with the use of quinidine, cardioversion is a more efficient and safer method. Nevertheless, quinidine continues as an invaluable antiarrhythmic drug for maintenance therapy. Without its use a majority of patients would experience recurrence of atrial fibrillation.

Atrial flutter and other arrhythmias Cardioversion has proved nearly 100 percent effective in chronic atrial flutter. Usually, a single low-energy discharge proves adequate. This method is also applicable to other atrial and AV nodal ectopic arrhythmias which have not responded to drug therapy.

Complications Immediate complications have been limited to the development of ventricular ectopic beats, ventricular tachycardia, and, rarely, even ventricular fibrillation. Such disorders can nearly always be avoided if the lowest effective amount of energy for reversion is employed, electrolyte deficits are corrected prior to the cardioversion, and treatment of overdigitalized patients is avoided. Furthermore, the electrical discharge should not be released in the presence of artifacts in the electrocardiogram. Such artifacts may trigger the discharge to occur during the vulnerable period, thereby precipitating ventricular fibrillation. It is probable that most, if not all, of the very rare fatalities which have been reported have been due either to neglect of these precautions or to the excessive and, at times, improper use of such drugs as digitalis and quinidine.

In many patients electrical reversion is only temporarily successful and the arrhythmia soon recurs. It is, therefore, often necessary to continue the use of the drugs mentioned in the previous chapter. Moderate to large doses of quinidine, procainamide, or both, may be needed. Agents such as reserpine or guanethidine, that deplete or antagonize catechols, may be beneficial. In refractory patients antithyroid substances such as propylthiouracil or radioiodine may be necessary as a supplement to the several antiarrhythmic drugs.

Summary Cardioversion is a simple and direct method for terminating various ectopic cardiac arrhythmias by depolarizing the heart transthoracically by means of a synchronized dc discharge. It is based on physiologic principles and is the most effective and safest means yet devised for restoring a sinus mechanism.

FIGURE 240-1
Ventricular tachycardia in a forty-two-year-old man with acute myocardial infarction. A single cardioversion discharge restores sinus rhythm.

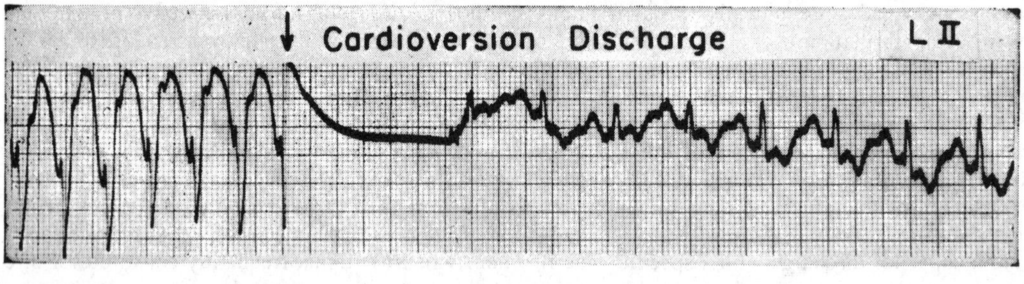

FIGURE 240-2
Restoration of sinus rhythm in a patient with long-standing atrial fibrillation. The isoelectric interval of 1.56 s represents an artifact due to the massive electrical field across the chest. Note the marked slowing in ventricular rate.

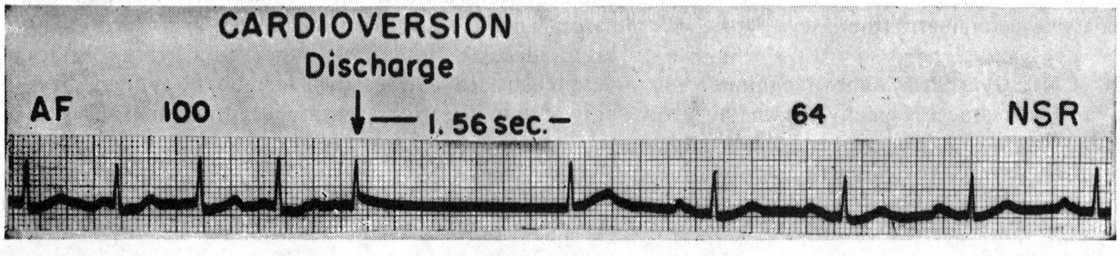

REFERENCES

HORN RH, LOWN B: Cardioversion 1975: Foremost therapy for tachyarrhythmias. Geriatrics 30:75, 1975

RESNEKOV L: Present status of electroversion in management of cardiac dysrhythmias. Circulation 47:1356, 1973

——, McDONALD L: Electroconversion of lone atrial fibrillation and flutter including haemodynamic studies at rest and on exercise. Br Heart J 33:339, 1971

241 CONGENITAL HEART DISEASE

WILLIAM F. FRIEDMAN
EUGENE BRAUNWALD

GENERAL CONSIDERATIONS

INCIDENCE Approximately 9 births in 1,000 are complicated by a cardiovascular malformation. If the problem is recognized early, these anomalies can now be diagnosed accurately, and most of these babies may be salvaged by aggressive medical and surgical management.

Children with congenital heart disease usually show an overall male preponderance. Moreover, specific defects may show a definite sex preponderance; patent ductus arteriosus and atrial septal defect are more common in females, whereas valvular aortic stenosis, coarctation of the aorta, tetralogy of Fallot, and transposition of the great arteries are more common in males. Table 241-1 demonstrates the frequency of occurrence of specific cardiovascular malformations in clinical and pathologic studies.

ETIOLOGY Congenital cardiovascular malformations are generally the result of aberrant embryonic development of a normal structure or a failure of such a structure to progress beyond an early stage of embryonic development. Malformations appear to result from a complex interaction between multifactorial genetic and environmental systems that does not allow a single specification of etiology; only rarely may a causal factor be identified. Maternal rubella and the ingestion of thalidomide early during gestation are two environmental insults that are known to interfere with normal cardiogenesis in man. The *rubella syndrome* consists of cataracts, deafness, microcephaly, and, either singly or in combination, patent ductus arteriosus, pulmonary valvular and/or arterial stenosis, and ventricular septal defect (see Chap. 202). *Thalidomide* is associated with major limb deformities and occasionally with cardiac malformations without a predilection for a specific lesion. Hypoxia, deficiency or excess of several vitamins, intake of several categories of drugs, and ionizing irradiation are teratogens that are capable of causing cardiac defects in experimental animals, but their precise relation to human malformations requires further definition.

A single gene mutation may be incriminated in the familial forms of atrial septal defect, mitral valve prolapse, ventricular septal defect, congenital heart block, situs inversus, the combination of supravalvular aortic stenosis and peripheral pulmonary arterial stenosis, and idiopathic hypertrophic subaortic stenosis (Chap. 247); Table 241-2 provides a partial list of syndromes in which cardiovascular anomalies may be manifestations of the pleiotropic effects of single genes or examples of gross chromosomal defects. Despite the long list presented in Table 241-2, it must be appreciated that recognized chromosomal aberrations and mutations of single genes account for less than 10 percent of all cardiac malformations.

The finding that, with some exceptions, only one of a pair of monozygotic twins is affected by congenital heart disease indicates that the vast majority of cardiovascular malformations are not inherited in a simple manner. Family studies indicate a two- to fivefold increase in the incidence of congenital heart disease in the siblings of affected patients. The malformations are concordant or partially concordant in at least half of such cases. Nonetheless, the incidence of congenital heart disease in the siblings of an index patient is only 2 to 5 percent. With few exceptions, therefore, patients with isolated heart defects have a negative family history for malformations and a normal chromosome pattern, and it is rarely wise to discourage the parents of one affected child from having additional children. The low recurrence rate and the increasing possibilities for effective therapy for nearly all cardiac lesions usually justify a positive approach to family counseling. If, however, two or more members of a family are affected, the recurrence risk may be quite high, and a pedigree should be obtained prior to further counseling. If a dominant or recessive mendelian pattern is established, the mendelian laws apply, and the risk of recurrence in each pregnancy is equal.

PREVENTION The feasibility of preventive programs will depend upon what is learned in the future about the cause of the 90 percent or more of cardiovascular anomalies for which no cause is now known.

A rubella vaccine has been developed that appears to be effective, and immunization of children with this vaccine may be anticipated to eradicate maternal rubella and its cardiac consequences. Strict testing in animals of new drugs that may be teratogenic when taken early in pregnancy may be expected to reduce the chances of another thalidomide tragedy. In this regard, no medications should be taken during pregnancy without prior consultation with a physician. Physicians dealing with pregnant women should be aware of known teratogens, as well as of drugs

TABLE 241-1
Frequency of occurrence of cardiac malformations at birth*

Disease	*Percent*
Ventricular septal defect	30.5
Atrial septal defect	9.8
Patent ductus arteriosus	9.7
Pulmonary stenosis	6.9
Coarctation of the aorta	6.8
Aortic stenosis	6.1
Tetralogy of Fallot	5.8
Complete transposition of the great arteries	4.2
Persistent truncus arteriosus	2.2
Tricuspid atresia	1.3
All others	16.5

**2,310 cases = 100 percent.*

TABLE 241-2
Syndromes with associated cardiovascular involvement

Syndrome	*Major cardiovascular manifestations*	*Major noncardiac abnormalities*
HERITABLE AND POSSIBLY HERITABLE		
Ellis–van Creveld	Single atrium or atrial septal defect	Chondrodystrophic dwarfism, nail dysplasia, polydactyly
TAR (thrombocytopenia-absent radius)	Atrial septal defect, tetralogy of Fallot	Radial aplasia or hypoplasia, thrombocytopenia
Holt-Oram	Atrial septal defect (other defects common)	Skeletal upper limb defect, hypoplasia of clavicles
Kartagener	Dextrocardia	Situs inversus, sinusitis, bronchiectasis
Laurence-Moon-Biedl-Bardot	Variable defects	Retinal pigmentation, obesity, polydactyly
Noonan	Pulmonary valve dysplasia	Webbed neck, pectus excavatum, cryptorchidism
Tuberous sclerosis	Rhabdomyoma, cardiomyopathy	Phacomatosis, bone lesions, hamartomatous skin lesions
Multiple lentigenes syndrome	Pulmonic stenosis	Basal cell nevi, broad facies, rib anomalies
Rubenstein-Taybi	Patent ductus arteriosus (others)	Broad thumbs and toes, hypoplastic maxilla, slanted palpebral fissures
Familial deafness	Arrhythmias, sudden death	Sensorineural deafness
Friedreich's ataxia	Cardiomyopathy	Ataxia, speech defect, degeneration of spinal cord dorsal columns
Muscular dystrophy	Cardiomyopathy	Pseudohypertrophy of calf muscles, weakness of trunk and proximal limb muscles
Osler-Rendu-Weber	Arteriovenous fistulas (lung, liver, mucous membranes)	Multiple telangiectasia
CONNECTIVE TISSUE DISORDERS		
Cutis laxa	Peripheral pulmonic stenosis	Generalized disruption of elastic fibers, diminished skin resilience, hernias
Ehlers-Danlos	Arterial dilatation and rupture, mitral regurgitation	Hyperextensible joints, hyperelastic and friable skin
Marfan	Aortic dilatation, aortic and mitral incompetence	Gracile habitus, arachnodactyly with hyperextensibility, lens subluxation
Osteogenesis imperfecta	Aortic incompetence	Fragile bones, blue sclera
Pseudoxanthoma elasticum	Peripheral arterial disease	Degeneration of elastic fibers in skin, retinal angioid streaks
INBORN ERRORS OF METABOLISM		
Pompe's disease	Glycogen storage disease of heart	Acid maltase deficiency, muscular weakness
Homocystinuria	Aortic and pulmonary arterial dilatation, intravascular thrombosis	Cystathionine synthetase deficiency, lens subluxation, osteoporosis
Mucopolysaccharidosis:		
Hurler; Hunter	Multivalvular and coronary and great artery disease, cardiomyopathy	Hurler: Deficiency of α-L-iduronidase, corneal clouding, coarse features, growth and mental retardation Hunter: Deficiency of L-idurano-sulfate sulfatase, coarse facies, clear cornea, growth and mental retardation
Morquio, Scheie, Morateaux-Lamy	Aortic incompetence	Morquio: Deficiency of N-acetylhexosamine sulfate sulfatase, cloudy cornea, normal intelligence, severe bony changes involving vertebrae and epiphyses Scheie: Deficiency of α-L-iduronidase, cloudy cornea, normal intelligence, peculiar facies Morateaux-Lamy: Deficiency of arylsulfatase B, cloudy cornea, osseous changes, normal intelligence
CHROMOSOMAL ABNORMALITIES		
Trisomy 21 (Down's syndrome)	Endocardial cushion defect, atrial or ventricular septal defect, tetralogy of Fallot	Hypotonia, hyperextensible joints, mongoloid facies, mental retardation
Trisomy 13 (D)	Ventricular septal defect, double-outlet right ventricle	Single midline intracerebral ventricle with midfacial defects, polydactyly, nail changes, mental retardation
Trisomy 18 (E)	Ventricular septal defect, patent ductus arteriosus, pulmonic stenosis	Clenched hand, short sternum, low-arch dermal-ridge pattern on fingertips, mental retardation
Cri-du-chat (short-arm deletion-5)	Ventricular septal defect	Cat cry, microcephaly, antimongoloid slant of palpebral fissures, mental retardation
XO (Turner)	Coarctation of aorta	Short female, broad chest, lymphedema, webbed neck
XXXY and XXXXX	Patent ductus arteriosus	XXXXY: hypogenitalism, mental retardation, radial-ulnar synostosis XXXXX: small hands, incurving of fifth fingers, mental retardation

for which inadequate information exists relative to their teratogenic potential. Similarly, appropriate use of radiologic equipment and techniques for reducing gonadal and fetal radiation exposure may be expected to reduce the potential hazards of this likely cause of birth defects.

The presence of a cardiac malformation as one component of a multiple system involvement that may exist in the Down's, Turner's, and trisomy 13–15 (D_1) and 17–18 (E) syndromes may be anticipated in occasional pregnancies by the detection of abnormal chromosomes in fetal cells obtained from amniotic fluid. Similarly, identification in such cells of the enzyme disorders observed in Hurler's syndrome or type II glycogen storage disease may allow one to predict the ultimate presence of cardiac disease.

THE FETAL AND TRANSITIONAL CIRCULATIONS

An understanding of the fetal and neonatal circulations is important to systematic comprehension of congenital heart disease (Fig. 241-1). The fetal circulation is a single circulation in which the pulmonary vasculature exists in parallel with the systemic circulation, not in series with it. Prenatal survival is not endangered by extremely severe cardiac anomalies as long as one side of the heart can drive blood from the great veins to the aorta. Blood can bypass the nonfunctioning lungs both proximally and distal to the heart. Inferior vena caval blood is deflected across the foramen ovale into the left atrium. Most of the blood that reaches the right ventricle bypasses the high-resistance, unexpanded lungs and passes through the ductus arteriosus into the descending aorta. In fetal life, pulmonary arteries and arterioles are surrounded by a fluid medium, have relatively thick walls and small lumens, and resemble comparable arteries in the systemic circulation.

Although fetal somatic growth may be unimpaired, the hemodynamic effects in utero of some cardiac malformations may alter the development and structure of the fetal heart and circulation. Thus, premature closure in utero of the foramen ovale may result in hypoplasia of the left ventricle. Moreover, postnatally the caliber of the aortic isthmus may be reduced in the presence of lesions in utero that divert a proportion of left ventricular output away from the ascending aorta while increasing right ventricular output and ductus arteriosus flow (e.g., aortic or subaortic stenosis with ventricular septal defect). Similarly, obstruction in utero to right ventricular outflow is associated with an increase in proximal aortic flow and diameter and almost never with aortic coarctation. In these and other examples it is important to recognize that malformations compatible with fetal survival may nonetheless result in abnormal development of the circulation in utero and also affect circulatory adjustments after birth.

Normally the fundamental change which occurs at birth is the division of this single circulation into two separate, independent circulations. Inflation of the lungs at the first inspiration produces a marked reduction in pulmonary vascular resistance. Fetal pulmonary vessels, heretofore supported by fluid media, are suddenly suspended in air, reducing extravascular pressure. New vessels are opened, and already patent vessels enlarge. Pulmonary arterial pressure falls, and pulmonary blood flow increases greatly. The systemic vascular resistance rises when clamping the umbilical cord removes the low-resistance placental circulation. Increased pulmonary blood flow increases the return of blood to the left atrium and raises left atrial pressure, which in turn closes the foramen ovale. The shift in oxygen dependence from the placenta to the lungs produces a sudden increase in arterial blood oxygen tension, which is one of the factors that initiates constriction of the ductus arteriosus, and total anatomic closure follows within a few days. As yet unclearly defined autonomic and chemical mediators may participate in these events.

Pulmonary hypertension

Pulmonary hypertension frequently complicates congenital heart disease, and the status of the pulmonary vascular bed may be the principal determinant of the clinical picture, its

FIGURE 241-1

Diagrams of the fetal, transitional (neonatal), and adult types of circulation. F.O. = foramen ovale; D.A. = ductus arteriosus. (From GS Dawes, Foetal and Neonatal Physiology, *Chicago: Year Book, 1968)*

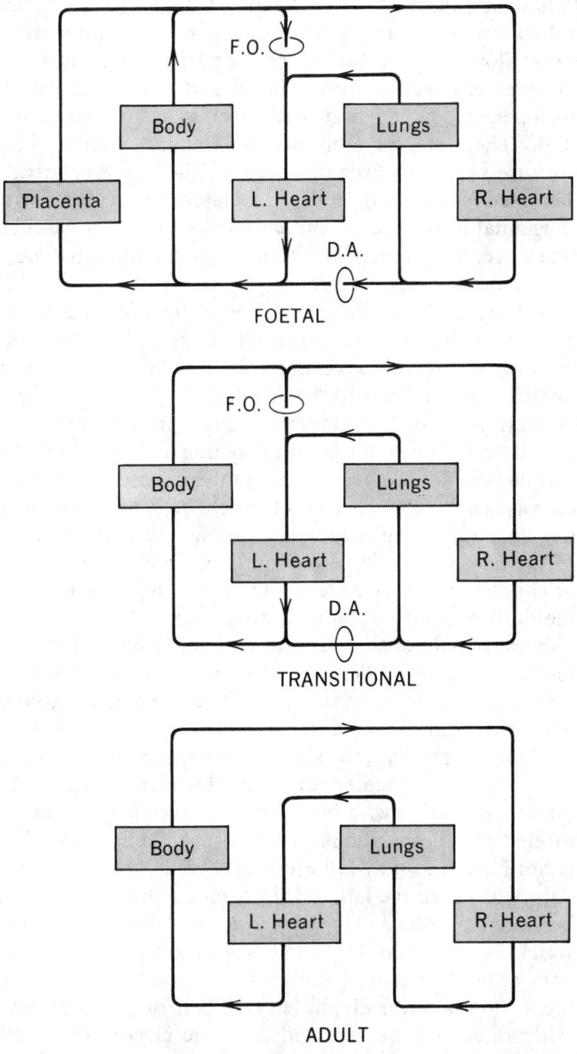

rate of progression, and whether corrective surgical treatment is feasible. Elevation of pulmonary arterial pressure results from elevation of pulmonary blood flow and/or resistance, the latter often reflecting structural alterations in the pulmonary vascular bed. Normally, following the fall in the pulmonary arterial pressure, resistance, and vasomotor tone which occurs shortly after birth, there is a gradual postnatal reduction in the thickness of the pulmonary arterial wall relative to lumen size. These changes are most prominent in the smaller pulmonary arteries and arterioles where the muscular media of the pulmonary arterioles become thin, and their lumens widen. Hence, the pulmonary circulation of the normal adult has evolved from a high-pressure, high-resistance, highly reactive vascular bed with relatively small cross-sectional area, to a low-pressure, low-resistance, less-reactive bed with a large cross-sectional area.

As in the other vascular beds, the pressure in the pulmonary artery is determined by the product of the volume of blood flow, per unit of time, and the resistance to that flow. Equalization of pressures in the systemic and pulmonary circulations may be expected if a large communication exists between the two great arteries or between the two ventricles in the absence of semilunar valve obstruction. Pulmonary vascular resistance is calculated as the transpulmonary pressure difference per unit of pulmonary blood flow (page 1164). When blood flow increases, existing patent vessels are distended and additional vessels are opened, so that calculated vascular resistance diminishes. Therefore, in a normal pulmonary vascular bed, pressure will rise substantially only if flow is very greatly increased (page 1165). In the vast majority of patients with congenital heart disease and elevated pulmonary vascular resistance, the pulmonary arterioles are the principal locus of this abnormal resistance.

A delay in the normal involution of the pulmonary vascular bed often occurs postnatally in the presence of an intra- or extracardiac communication with a large left-to-right shunt. In patients having high pulmonary arterial pressure from birth, anatomic changes in the pulmonary vessels, in the form of medial thickening and intimal proliferation, usually progress so that in the older child or adult the vascular resistance may ultimately be fixed by obliterative changes in the pulmonary vascular bed. However, if pulmonary arterial hypertension is not present in infancy or childhood, it may never occur or may not develop until the third or fourth decade, or even later.

Because pulmonary vascular obstructive disease may be the factor limiting a decision concerning the advisability of operation, it is important to quantify and compare pulmonary to systemic flows and resistances in patients with severe pulmonary hypertension. Furthermore, the lability of the pulmonary vascular resistance should be evaluated; a marked reduction with the infusion of acetylcholine or tolazoline or the inhalation of oxygen suggests that resistance is not fixed and may fall after successful operation. Some defects between the left and right sides of the heart should be closed in order to eliminate a sizable left-to-right shunt, which, in turn, may result in a significant drop in pulmonary arterial pressure because of reduction of pulmonary blood flow. Conversely, little or no benefit and high mortality rates may be expected from the closure of defects that are associated with bidirectional or predominant right-to-left shunts in patients with high-resistance and obstructive pulmonary hypertension. The designation *Eisenmenger's reaction* is applied to this condition in patients who may have a large communication between the two circulations at the aortopulmonary, ventricular, or atrial levels. The actual mechanism for the persistence, delayed reduction, or late onset of elevated pulmonary vascular resistance is not known.

The clinical manifestations of the hyperkinetic form of pulmonary hypertension, i.e., that associated with a large left-to-right shunt, reflect the specific malformation responsible. When a significant right-to-left shunt exists, the patient is cyanotic, and polycythemia and clubbing of the digits may be noted (Chap. 31). A dominant A wave in the jugular venous pulse may be seen, reflecting vigorous right atrial contraction due to diminished compliance of the right ventricle; in some instances there are large systolic C-V waves, which suggest tricuspid regurgitation. A prominent right ventricular parasternal lift and palpable systolic expansion of the pulmonary artery are present. On auscultation, one often hears a soft pulmonary systolic ejection murmur following a loud ejection sound, marked accentuation of the pulmonic component of the second heart sound, and, often, a fourth heart sound produced by right atrial contraction. The decrescendo diastolic murmur of pulmonary valvular regurgitation may be heard. The electrocardiogram shows right ventricular hypertrophy (page 1146). Roentgenologic examination reveals enlargement of the right ventricle, a conspicuously enlarged pulmonary artery, prominent hilar pulmonary vascular markings, and attenuated peripheral vessels. The site of the underlying defect may be localized by means of cardiac catheterization and angiocardiography (Chap. 235). Pressures in the right side of the heart are essentially identical to systemic pressures in cyanotic patients if the shunt is at the ventricular or aortopulmonary levels, but they are usually lower than systemic pressure in patients with an interatrial shunt. No specific treatment has proved beneficial for obstructive pulmonary vascular disease.

CIRCULATORY SHUNTS

Although equal quantities of blood flow through the pulmonary and systemic circulations in normal subjects postnatally, the systemic circulation has a flow resistance approximately six times that of the pulmonary circuit, which is reflected in the markedly higher arterial and ventricular systolic pressures in the systemic circulation; the lower compliance of the thicker left ventricle is reflected in higher ventricular end-diastolic and mean atrial pressures on the left side of the heart. Therefore, if an abnormal communication is present, blood will flow from the left to the right side of the heart. The size of the opening and the pressures on either side of it generally determine the direction and magnitude of the shunt flow. A right-to-left shunt usually requires either an obstructive lesion at some point in the right-sided circulation (i.e., tricuspid stenosis or atresia, pulmonary valvular or infundibular stenosis, elevated pulmonary vascular resistance), a mixing of systemic venous and arterialized blood (i.e., total anomalous pulmonary venous drainage, a single atrium or ventricle, or a persistent truncus arteriosus), or some form of obligatory recirculation of systemic venous blood (e.g., transposition of the great arteries). The location, direction, and magnitude of the right-to-left shunt may be determined during hemodynamic study by measuring the admixture of venous and arterial blood at various sites in the central circulation, by indicator-dilution curves, and by angiocardiography, as outlined in Chap. 235.

Clinical manifestations of right-to-left shunts

CYANOSIS AND POLYCYTHEMIA These signs are discussed in Chap. 31.

CLUBBING A prominent accompaniment of arterial hypoxemia consists of a widening and thickening of the terminal phalanges of the fingers and toes, accompanied by convex nails. These digits have an increased number of capillaries with increased blood flow through extensive arteriovenous aneurysms, and an increase of connective tissue.

SQUATTING Patients with cyanotic heart disease, especially tetralogy of Fallot, typically assume a squatting posture after exertion to obtain relief from breathlessness. Squatting appears to hasten an increase in the arterial oxygen saturation by increasing systemic vascular resistance and thereby diminishing the right-to-left shunt and by pooling markedly unsaturated blood in the legs. Also, systemic venous return and therefore pulmonary blood flow may rise.

ANOXIC SPELLS A sudden marked increase in cyanosis due to an abrupt reduction in pulmonary blood flow occurs in younger children with certain types of cyanotic heart disease, particularly tetralogy of Fallot. The spells may lead to convulsions and may even be fatal; they may be precipitated by fluctuations in intravascular volume or in arterial P_{CO_2} and pH, a sudden fall in systemic or increase in pulmonary vascular resistance, or augmented contraction of the hypertrophied muscle in the right ventricular outflow tract. Treatment consists of oxygen administration, placing the child in the knee-chest position, and intravenous administration of fluids and of sodium bicarbonate to correct the accompanying acidosis. Additional medications that may prove of value include morphine, α-adrenergic receptor stimulants such as phenylephrine or Neo-Synephrine to raise peripheral resistance and to diminish right-to-left shunting, and β-adrenergic blocking agents, which may increase ventricular volume by reducing heart rate and relieve infundibular spasm by reducing contractility.

"PARADOXIC" EMBOLUS AND BRAIN ABSCESS In patients with cyanotic heart disease, venous blood bypasses the normal filtering action of the lungs, and emboli arising in systemic veins may pass directly to the systemic circulation. Patients with severe cyanosis or polycythemia have often had previous occlusive microcirculatory damage to the central nervous system. These predisposing factors are primarily responsible for the relatively high incidence (2 to 4 percent) of brain abscess in patients with cyanotic forms of congenital heart disease, an incidence which roughly parallels the severity of cyanosis.

IMPAIRED GROWTH Physical underdevelopment and a delayed onset of adolescence are common features of many types of cyanotic and, to a lesser extent, acyanotic forms of congenital heart disease. Mental development is rarely affected. Various explanations for the mechanisms of growth interference have implicated malnutrition, tissue anoxia, diminished peripheral blood flow, hypermetabolic state, chronic cardiac decompensation, genetic and endocrine factors, and frequency of upper and lower respiratory infections. In many instances, the underdevelopment is influenced little by operative correction of the underlying cardiac anomaly. Thus, it is unwise preoperatively to guarantee to the parents of a child with heart disease that operation will result in accelerated growth and development.

SPECIFIC CARDIAC DEFECTS

Various classifications of congenital cardiovascular lesions have been proposed, depending on hemodynamic, anatomic and radiographic factors. Although there is overlapping between groups, the following arrangement of the more common anomalies is used in this chapter.

1 Communications between the systemic and pulmonary circulation without cyanosis (left-to-right shunts)
2 Obstructing valvular and vascular lesions with or without associated right-to-left shunts
3 Abnormalities in the origins of the great arteries and veins; the transpositions
4 Malpositions of the heart

Communications between systemic and pulmonary circulation without cyanosis (left-to-right shunts)

ATRIAL SEPTAL DEFECT Atrial septal defect, the most commonly recognized congenital cardiac anomaly in adults, occurs more frequently in females than in males. Defects of the sinus venosus type occur high in the atrial septum, near the entry of the superior vena cava, and are associated frequently with anomalous connection of pulmonary veins from the right lung to the junction of the superior vena cava and right atrium. Most often, an atrial defect involves the fossa ovalis, is midseptal in location, and is of the *ostium secundum* type. This type of defect should not be confused with a patent foramen ovale. Anatomic obliteration of the foramen ovale ordinarily follows its functional closure soon after birth, but residual "probe patency" is a common normal variation; atrial septal defect denotes a true deficiency of the atrial septum and implies functional as well as anatomic patency. *Ostium primum* anomalies are a form of endocardial cushion defect that lie immediately adjacent to the atrioventricular valves, either of which may be deformed and incompetent, or which may form together a common atrioventricular valve; this defect may also involve the basal portion of the interventricular septum. Ostium primum defects occur commonly in patients with *Down's syndrome* (mongolism), although the more complex endocardial cushion anomalies are more characteristic. *Lutembacher's syndrome* is the designation applied to the rare combination of atrial septal defect and mitral stenosis; this component of the malformation almost invariably is the result of acquired rheumatic valvulitis.

The magnitude of the left-to-right shunt through an atrial septal defect depends on the size of the defect, the relative compliance of the ventricles, and the relative resistances in the pulmonary and systemic circulations. In patients with a patent foramen ovale or a small atrial septal defect, the left atrial pressure may exceed the right by several millimeters of mercury, whereas the mean pressures in both atria are nearly identical when the defect is large. The left-to-right shunt causes diastolic overloading of the right ventricle and increased pulmonary blood flow. The pulmonary vascular resistance is usually normal or low in the child and young adult with atrial septal defect, and the volume load is usually well tolerated even though pulmonary blood flow may be three to six times greater than systemic. Streaming of unsaturated inferior vena caval blood from right to left is not uncommon in patients with ostium secundum defect, even in the absence of pulmonary hypertension.

Patients with atrial septal defect are usually asymptomatic in early life although there may be some physical underdevelopment (gracile habitus) and respiratory infections; cardiorespiratory symptoms occur in many of the older patients. Beyond the fourth decade, a significant number of patients develop atrial arrhythmias, pulmonary arterial hypertension, bidirectional and then right-to-left shunting of blood, and cardiac failure. Patients exposed to the chronic environmental hypoxia of high altitude tend to develop pulmonary hypertension at younger ages. Historical features suggesting that the defect is of the endocardial cushion variety include the onset of disability, pulmonary hypertension, and heart failure in infancy or childhood.

Physical examination usually reveals a prominent right ventricular cardiac impulse and palpable pulmonary artery pulsation. The first heart sound is normal or split, with accentuation of the tricuspid valve closure sound. Increased flow across the pulmonic valve is responsible for a midsystolic pulmonary ejection murmur. The second sound is widely split and is relatively fixed in relation to respiration, because of reciprocal changes in the magnitude of the left-to-right shunt and of the systemic venous inflow into the right ventricle during respiration, so that filling of the right ventricle remains constant throughout the respiratory cycle. A middiastolic rumbling murmur at the fourth intercostal space and along the left sternal border reflects increased flow across the tricuspid valve. In patients with ostium primum defects, an apical thrill and holosystolic murmur indicate associated mitral or tricuspid incompetence or a ventricular septal defect.

The *physical findings* are altered when an increase in the pulmonary vascular resistance results in diminution of the left-to-right shunt. Both the pulmonary and tricuspid murmurs decrease in intensity, the pulmonic component of the second heart sound and a systolic ejection sound are accentuated, the two components of the second heart sound may fuse, and a diastolic murmur of pulmonic incompetence appears. Cyanosis and clubbing accompany the development of a right-to-left shunt.

The *electrocardiogram* in patients with an ostium secundum defect usually shows right axis deviation, right ventricular hypertrophy, and a right intraventricular conduction defect. A coronary sinus pacemaker or first degree heart block is occasionally noted in patients with defects of the sinus venosus type; approximately 5 percent have left axis deviation. In patients with an ostium primum defect, the right ventricular conduction defect is characteristically accompanied by left axis deviation and by superior orientation and counterclockwise rotation of the QRS loop in the frontal plane. Varying degrees of right ventricular and right atrial hypertrophy may be seen with each type of defect, depending on the height of the pulmonary artery pressure; prolongation of the P-R interval is most common with defects of the ostium primum variety. Chest roentgenograms reveal enlargement of the right atrium and ventricle, dilatation of the pulmonary artery and its branches, and increased pulmonary vascular markings. Left atrial enlargement is extremely uncommon. Echocardiographic features include pulmonary arterial and right ventricular dilatation and anterior systolic (paradoxical) or "flat" interventricular septal motion if significant right ventricular volume overload is present. Prolapse of the posterior mitral leaflet has been recognized with increasing frequency in association with secundum defects. Abnormal "mitral" motion and septal-atrioventricular valve relationships are typically observed in endocardial cushion anomalies.

The diagnosis may be confirmed readily at cardiac catheterization by passage of the catheter across the atrial defect. The site at which the catheter crosses, if high in the cardiac silhouette, may suggest a sinus venosus defect, or, if low, a primum defect. Serial determinations of the oxygen saturation, or indicator-dilution curve techniques, may be used to estimate the magnitude of the shunt. In young patients, pressures in the right side of the heart are often normal despite a large shunt; pulmonary arterial hypertension occurs with greater frequency in the older patients. If an endocardial cushion defect is present, a left ventricular angiogram will frequently demonstrate a "gooseneck" deformity of the left ventricular outflow tract caused by an abnormal anterior mitral valve leaflet; it may also show mitral regurgitation. When a high oxygen saturation is found in the superior vena cava, or when the catheter enters pulmonary veins directly from the right atrium, a sinus venosus defect is likely, and indicator-dilution curves and selective angiography will aid in identifying the number and location of the anomalous veins. Partial anomalous pulmonary venous connection, although generally associated with a sinus venosus defect, may occasionally accompany primum and secundum defects.

Endocardial cushion anomalies more complex than the ostium primum defect are associated with high morbidity and mortality in infancy and childhood. Patients with atrial septal defect of the sinus venosus or secundum types rarely die before the fifth decade. During the fifth and sixth decades, the incidence of progressive symptoms, often leading to severe disability, increases substantially. Medical management should include prompt treatment of respiratory tract infections, antiarrhythmic medications for atrial fibrillation or supraventricular tachycardia, and the usual measures for heart failure (Chap. 237) if these complications occur. Although the risk of subacute bacterial endocarditis is low, antibiotics should be administered prophylactically prior to dental procedures (see Chap. 132).

Operative repair, ideally in patients between five and ten years of age, should be advised for all patients with uncomplicated atrial septal defects in whom there is evidence of significant left-to-right shunting, i.e., with pulmonary-to-systemic flow ratios exceeding approximately 1.5:1.0. Excellent results may be anticipated, at low risk, even in patients beyond forty years of age in the absence of pulmonary hypertension. The defect is closed by suture or with a patch of prosthetic material with the patient on cardiopulmonary bypass. Special attention must be given to the atrioventricular valves in patients with endocardial cushion defects; cleft, deformed, and incompetent valves may require repair or even replacement to prevent significant regurgitation and failure in the postoperative period. The operative risk and the incidence of such complications as complete heart block and the persistence of significant mitral regurgitation are significantly higher in patients with endocardial cushion defects. Electrophysiologic mapping of the course of the conduction system during operation may substantially reduce the risk of postsurgical heart block. Operation should not be carried out in patients with small defects and trivial left-to-right shunts, or in those with severe pulmonary vascular disease without a significant left-to-right shunt.

VENTRICULAR SEPTAL DEFECT Isolated defects of the ventricular septum are among the commonest cardiac malformations, and they are encountered as one component of a combination of anomalies more often than any other. Most frequently, the opening is single and situated in the membranous portion of the septum. The functional disturbance caused by a ventricular septal defect is dependent primarily on its size and the status of the pulmonary vascular bed, rather than on the location of the defect. A substantial left-to-right ventricular pressure gradient occurs in the presence of a small defect *(maladie de Roger)*, and a small shunt, limited by the size of the defect, occurs throughout systole. As the defect becomes larger, it offers less resistance to flow, until with very large defects both ventricles will function hemodynamically as a single pumping chamber with two outlets, equalizing the pressures in the systemic and pulmonary circulations. In such patients, the magnitude of the left-to-right shunt varies inversely with the pulmonary vascular resistance. In patients with large defects and large left-to-right shunts, the left ventricle is overloaded and may fail. Survival through infancy in many of these patients is predicated on delayed regression of the fetal pulmonary vascular pattern, the development of an elevated pulmonary vascular resistance, or the secondary development of infundibular hypertrophy and obstruction to right ventricular outflow. Irreversible obliterative changes in the pulmonary vessels with dominant right-to-left shunts and cyanosis become manifest in many patients with large defects after the second decade of life. Spontaneous closure of small and even large ventricular defects occurs in a significant number of patients, especially before the age of three years. In some others, the relative size of the interventricular communication may diminish as normal growth of the heart occurs with advancing age. Rarely, incompetence of the aortic valve resulting from insufficient cusp tissue or prolapse of a cusp through the interventricular defect complicates and dominates the clinical course of patients with ventricular septal defect.

The clinical picture varies greatly, depending on the patient's age, the size of the defect, and the level of the pulmonary vascular resistance. Patients with small defects are asymptomatic; moderate left-to-right shunts may be associated with effort intolerance and fatigue. Large defects are commonly accompanied by frequent pulmonary infections, growth retardation, and cardiac failure in infancy, but survival past this period is often associated with an amelioration of symptoms until adulthood. In patients with severe pulmonary vascular obstruction, symptoms develop most often in adult life and consist of exertional dyspnea, chest pain, syncope, and hemoptysis. The right-to-left shunt leads to cyanosis, clubbing, and polycythemia.

Patients with moderate-sized defects exhibit cardiomegaly with a forceful left ventricular impulse and a prominent systolic thrill along the lower left sternal border. The second heart sound is normally or closely split, with moderate accentuation of the pulmonic component; a third heart sound and diastolic rumbling murmur, reflecting increased flow across the mitral valve during rapid ventricular filling, are often audible at the cardiac apex. The characteristic holosystolic murmur results from flow across the defect; it is best heard along the third and fourth interspaces to the left of the sternum, and is widely transmitted over the precordium. A basal midsystolic ejection murmur may also be heard, because of increased flow across the pulmonic valve. In patients with pulmonary vascular obstruction and small left-to-right shunts, both the systolic thrill and murmur decrease in intensity and duration and may disappear entirely, to be replaced by a marked right ventricular precordial lift, pulmonary ejection sound and soft systolic ejection murmur, a closely split second heart sound with accentuation of the pulmonic component, and the diastolic murmur of pulmonic incompetence.

The electrocardiographic pattern, the relative size and contour of the two ventricles roentgenographically, and the appearance of the lung fields serve as indicators of the underlying pathophysiologic condition. The electrocardiogram is generally normal in patients with small defects. Left or combined ventricular hypertrophy is seen with large left-to-right shunts; right ventricular hypertrophy occurs with pulmonary vascular obstruction. The roentgenograms may be normal in patients with small defects; large defects are characterized by an enlarged left atrium, biventricular hypertrophy, a prominent pulmonary artery segment, and increased pulmonary vascular markings. Relative diminution and attenuation of the peripheral pulmonary vasculature occur in patients with obstructive pulmonary vascular disease.

In approximately 90 percent of patients with this malformation, the defect occurs in the membranous septum. A shunt from the left ventricle to the right atrium may occur with a defect in the most superior portion of the ventricular septum, since the tricuspid valve is lower than the mitral valve. The clinical, electrocardiographic, and radiologic findings in these patients often do not differ appreciably from those with a simple ventricular septal defect, although right atrial enlargement and evidence of right ventricular volume overload may be present; the diagnosis can be established by left ventriculography. Prolapse of an aortic valve leaflet through a subpulmonary ventricular defect or the combination of subcristal ventricular septal defect and underdevelopment of an aortic valve commissure may produce aortic regurgitation that is frequently progressive and is the most significant hemodynamic lesion. In these patients complete operative repair may necessitate insertion of a prosthetic aortic valve. The pathophysiology of a single or common ventricle resembles that of a large ventricular septal defect, although the two lesions are dissimilar embryologically. Single ventricle is also frequently complicated by anomalies of the atrioventricular and/or semilunar valves. There is an obligatory admixture of systemic and pulmonary venous return in patients with a single ventricle, but there is occasionally little or no cyanosis if selective streaming and increased pulmonary blood flow occur. Severe pulmonary hypertension is invariably present unless pulmonic stenosis coexists. It is imperative to differentiate a large ventricular septal defect from a single ventricle by echocardiography and angiography, because attempts at corrective operation for single ventricles have met with little success.

The risk of bacterial endocarditis is higher in patients with small or moderate-sized defects than in those with large ones, but appropriate prophylaxis is essential in all. In the small infant with a large left-to-right shunt, congestive failure may be severe and intractable despite intensive medical management; this problem is managed best beyond age six months by primary closure of the defect. Younger infants often undergo surgical constriction of the pulmonary artery, followed, when the patient is older, by a corrective operation. Closure of the defect of the ventricular septum is indicated in children and adults when there is a moderate or large left-to-right shunt with a pulmonary to systemic flow ratio which exceeds 1.5:1.0 or 2.0:1.0 regardless of the level of pulmonary artery pressure. Operation is contraindicated when the pulmonary vascular resistance is elevated to a level which eliminates the net left-to-right shunt and carries an increased risk whenever pulmonary resistance is significantly elevated. The recognition of associated cardiac anomalies is imperative if surgical treatment is contemplated. The most common of these are patent ductus arteriosus, ostium secundum atrial defects, pulmonic stenosis, coarctation of the aorta, and corrected transposition of the great arteries.

PATENT DUCTUS ARTERIOSUS The ductus arteriosus is a vessel leading from the bifurcation of the pulmonary artery to the aorta just distad to the left subclavian artery. Normal closure of the ductus immediately after birth may be due to the sudden increase in arterial oxygen tension that accompanies ventilation and/or the release of vasoactive substances. Intimal proliferation and fibrosis proceed more gradually, so that total anatomic obliteration may not occur for several months after birth. Persistent patency of the ductus after birth is a relatively common anomaly, occurring more frequently in females, in the offspring of women whose pregnancies were complicated by first-trimester rubella, in premature infants, and in children born at high altitudes. Although this anomaly occurs most frequently in the isolated form, it may coexist with other malformations, particularly coarctation of the aorta, ventricular septal defect, pulmonic stenosis, and aortic stenosis. Patency of the ductus may provide the only route for maintaining pulmonary or systemic blood flow in the presence of such lesions as pulmonary atresia or aortic arch interruption.

The flow across the ductus is determined by the pressure and resistance relationships between the systemic and the pulmonary circulations, and by the cross-sectional area and length of the ductus itself. Most commonly, pulmonary pressures are normal, and a gradient and shunt from aorta to pulmonary artery persists throughout the cardiac cycle. Physical examination reveals a characteristic thrill and a continuous "machinery" murmur, with a late systolic accentuation at the upper left sternal border. The left atrium and ventricle enlarge to accommodate the increased pulmonary venous return, and flow murmurs across the mitral and aortic valves may be detected. With large or moderate-sized left-to-right shunts, the runoff of blood through the ductus causes a widened systemic pulse pressure and bounding peripheral pulses. The hemodynamic abnormality is reflected by left ventricular and, occasionally, left atrial hypertrophy on the electrocardiogram and by left atrial and ventricular enlargement, a prominent ascending aorta and pulmonary artery, and pulmonary vascular engorgement on the chest roentgenogram. Left atrial and ventricular size determined echocardiographically provide an estimate of the magnitude of left-to-right shunting.

The clinical recognition of patent ductus arteriosus may be difficult in infancy and in patients with pulmonary hypertension or heart failure. In these circumstances, the pressure gradient between the aorta and pulmonary artery is reduced or absent, as is the typical continuous murmur, and there may be only a systolic ejection murmur at the base, a diastolic blowing murmur of pulmonary regurgitation (Graham Steell), or no murmur audible at all. When severe pulmonary vascular disease results in reversal of flow through the ductus, unoxygenated blood is shunted to the descending aorta, and the toes, but not the fingers, become cyanotic and clubbed, a finding termed *differential cyanosis.*

Delayed spontaneous closure of the ductus arteriosus has been known to occur in premature babies, even if heart failure was a problem in the neonatal period. Although a large ductus often results in cardiac failure and pulmonary edema in the premature infant, its occurrence in the full-term baby is often compatible with survival until adult life. The leading causes of death in adults with patent ductus are cardiac failure and bacterial endocarditis. In older patients, severe pulmonary vascular obstruction may cause aneurysmal dilatation, calcification, and rupture of the ductus.

In the absence of severe pulmonary vascular disease with predominant right-to-left shunting of blood, the simple presence of a patent ductus is generally considered a sufficient indication for operation, at least in patients over three years of age. Ligation or division of the ductus is associated with a low risk (under 2 percent) when it is performed electively in an otherwise healthy person. The operative risk is reduced if cardiac failure can be treated successfully before operation. Operation should be deferred for several months in patients treated successfully for bacterial endarteritis, because the ductus may remain somewhat edematous and friable.

AORTOPULMONARY SEPTAL DEFECT Aortopulmonary window, partial truncus arteriosis, and aortic septal defect are other designations applied to this relatively uncommon anomaly, which consists of a communication between the aorta and the pulmonary artery just above the semilunar valves. Such defects are usually large and are accompanied by varying degrees of obstructive pulmonary vascular disease and severe pulmonary arterial hypertension. The anomaly may be difficult to distinguish from patent ductus arteriosus with which it is often associated. However, the murmur of aortopulmonary septal defect is rarely continuous, and a basal systolic murmur is most common. Cardiomegaly is present, and pulmonary hypertension is reflected in a loud and palpable sound of pulmonary valve closure. The diagnosis of aortopulmonary septal defect should be suspected whenever a large shunt into the pulmonary artery is demonstrated at catheterization. Distinction from patent ductus and persistent truncus arteriosus is facilitated by catheter passage across the defect and selective angiocardiography, with the injection of contrast material into the left ventricle and/or the root of the aorta. Operative correction is usually indicated in children and adults with large left-to-right shunts; total cardiopulmonary bypass is required, and the defect is closed, generally with a prosthetic patch.

AORTIC SINUS ANEURYSM AND FISTULA Congenital aneurysm of an aortic sinus of Valsalva, particularly the right coronary sinus, is an uncommon anomaly with a predilection for males; it consists of a separation, or lack of fusion, between the media of the aorta and the annulus fibrosus of the aortic valve. Progressive aneurysmal dilatation of the weakened area develops but may not be recognized until the third or fourth decade of life, when rupture into a cardiac chamber occurs. The receiving chamber of the aorticocardiac fistula is usually the right ventricle, but occasionally the fistula drains into the right atrium.

The unruptured aneurysm generally does not produce symptoms or a hemodynamic abnormality, although pressure on the intracardiac conduction system by an unruptured aneurysm occasionally causes atrioventricular block, and myocardial ischemia may be caused by coronary arterial compression. Rupture is often of abrupt onset, causes chest pain, and creates continuous arteriovenous shunting and volume overloading of both right and left heart chambers, with resultant heart failure. Bacterial endocarditis may originate either on the edges of the aneurysm or on those areas in the right side of the heart which are traumatized by the jetlike stream of blood flowing through the fistula. This anomaly should be suspected in a patient with a history of recent onset of chest pain, symptoms of diminished cardiac reserve, bounding pulses, and a loud, superficial, continuous murmur accentuated in diastole when the fistula opens into the right ventricle, as well as a thrill along the right or left lower parasternal area. The electrocardiogram shows biventricular hypertrophy, and the chest roentgenogram demonstrates generalized cardiomegaly, pulmonary plethora, and sometimes evidence of heart failure. The diagnosis may be established definitively by retrograde thoracic aortography. Operation is indicated in patients with large left-to-right shunts; the aneurysm is closed and amputated, and the aortic wall is reunited with the heart, either by direct suture or with a prosthesis.

CORONARY ARTERIOVENOUS FISTULA Coronary arteriovenous fistula is an unusual anomaly that most often consists of a communication between the right coronary artery and the right atrium or ventricle. The shunt is usually of small magnitude, and myocardial blood flow is not usually compromised. Potential complications include bacterial endocarditis, thrombus formation with occlusion or distal embolization, rupture of an aneurysmal fistula, and, rarely, pulmonary hypertension and congestive failure when the left-to-right shunt is large. The finding of a loud, superficial, continuous murmur at the lower or midsternal border usually prompts a further evaluation of asymptomatic patients. Retrograde thoracic aortography or coronary arteriography permits identification of the size and anatomic features of the fistulous tract, which may be closed by suture obliteration.

ANOMALOUS PULMONARY ORIGIN OF CORONARY ARTERY In this rare malformation, the left coronary artery originates from the pulmonary artery. Myocardial infarction and fibrosis commonly develop during the first 6 months of life, leading to death within the first year. From 10 to 20 percent of patients survive to childhood or adolescence without surgical correction. As the elevated pulmonary vascular resistance declines immediately after birth, perfusion of the left coronary artery from the pulmonary artery ceases and the direction of flow in the anomalous vessel reverses. Thus, blood flows from the aorta to the right coronary artery, then through collateral channels to the left coronary artery, and finally to the pulmonary artery. Total myocardial perfusion must pass through the right coronary artery and may be sufficient for normal activity if adequate collateral channels develop between the two coronary circulations. Occasionally, in older children or adults one may find an example of mitral regurgitation which results from dysfunction of ischemic or infarcted papillary muscles. In some instances the coronary anomaly is unsuspected until a previously well adolescent or adult experiences angina, heart failure, or sudden death.

The diagnosis of anomalous origin of the coronary artery is supported by the electrocardiographic findings of an anterolateral myocardial infarction (Chap. 233). Chest roentgenograms show moderate to severe enlargement of the left atrium and ventricle. Aortic root or coronary angiography demonstrates the retrograde drainage of the coronary vessel into the pulmonary artery and the presence of a single right coronary artery arising from the aorta.

Ideal operative management of these patients consists of anastomosis of the left coronary artery to the aorta via a graft. However, if a left-to-right shunt exists and the small size of the patient precludes this approach, the disorder may be managed by simple ligation of the left coronary artery at its origin, preventing retrograde flow and allowing perfusion of the left ventricle by blood supplied through anastomoses from the right coronary artery. The outcome of operation and ultimate prognosis are influenced significantly by the degree of myocardial damage suffered preoperatively.

PERSISTENT TRUNCUS ARTERIOSUS Persistent truncus arteriosus is a rare but serious anomaly in which a single vessel forms the outlet of both ventricles and gives rise to the systemic, pulmonary, and coronary arteries. It is always accompanied by a ventricular septal defect and frequently by a right-sided aortic arch. The designation "pseudo-truncus arteriosus" refers to the condition in which a single vessel arises from the heart but is accompanied by a remnant of atretic pulmonary artery; this malformation does not differ from tetralogy of Fallot with pulmonary atresia (see below). Truncus malformations may be classified embryologically and anatomically according to the mode of origin of the pulmonary vessels from the common trunk, or, from a functional point of view, by the magnitude of flow to the lungs. Pulmonary flow is governed by the size of the pulmonary arteries and the pulmonary vascular resistance. Most often, mild cyanosis coexists with the cardiac findings of a large left-to-right shunt. The most frequent physical findings include cardiomegaly, a systolic ejection sound, a loud, single second heart sound, a harsh systolic murmur accompanied by a thrill, an early diastolic blowing murmur of truncal valve regurgitation, and a low-pitched middiastolic rumbling murmur. Biventricular (predominantly left ventricular) hypertrophy is usually present electrocardiographically, except in patients with markedly elevated pulmonary vascular resistance in whom right ventricular hypertrophy may predominate. Gross cardiomegaly with left or combined ventricular enlargement, left atrial enlargement, and a large aorta with small or absent main pulmonary artery segment with pulmonary vascular engorgement are the usual radiographic findings. The diagnosis should be suspected at catheterization if the catheter fails to enter the central pulmonary arteries from the right ventricle despite evidence of increased pulmonary blood flow; aortography is the diagnostic procedure of choice.

The early fatal course and, in patients surviving infancy, the development of pulmonary vascular obstructive disease are responsible for the poor prognosis associated with persistent truncus arteriosus. The long-term results of corrective operations employing a prosthetic tubular conduit incorporating a heterograft aortic valve to construct a pulmonary trunk have yet to be evaluated. In infants and young children, palliative banding of one or both of the pulmonary arteries may be indicated when pulmonary flow is markedly excessive. In patients with inadequate pulmonary blood flow it is occasionally possible to enhance pulmonary blood flow with a shunting operation.

Valvular and vascular lesions with or without right-to-left shunt

PULMONARY STENOSIS WITH INTACT VENTRICULAR SEPTUM Obstruction to right ventricular outflow is relatively common; it may be localized to the supravalvular, valvular, or subvalvular levels or occur at a combination of these sites. Multiple sites of narrowing of the peripheral pulmonary arteries are often a feature of rubella embryopathy and may be associated with both the familial and sporadic forms of supravalvular aortic stenosis. Valvular pulmonic stenosis is the most common form of isolated right ventricular obstruction.

The severity of the obstructing lesion, rather than the site of narrowing, is the most important determinant of the clinical course. In the presence of a normal cardiac output, a peak systolic transvalvular pressure gradient between 50 and 80 mmHg is considered to be moderate stenosis; levels below and above that range are classified as mild and severe, respectively. Patients with mild pulmonic stenosis are generally asymptomatic and demonstrate little or no progression in the severity of obstruction as they grow older. In patients with more significant stenosis, the severity of the obstruction may increase with time. Progression may be relative and may reflect disproportionate physical growth of the patient, infundibular narrowing due to progressive hypertrophy of the right ventricular outflow tract, or fibrosis of the valve cusps. Atresia of the pulmonary valve is commonly associated with a hypoplastic right ventricle and interatrial communication. Symptoms vary according to the degree of obstruction. Infants with pulmonary atresia often die from hypoxia. Fatigue, dyspnea, and syncope may limit the activity of older patients, in whom moderate or severe obstruction may prevent an augmentation of pulmonary blood flow with exercise.

In patients with severe obstruction, the systolic pressure in the right ventricle may exceed that in the left ventricle, since the ventricular septum is intact. Right ventricular ejection is prolonged in patients with moderate or severe stenosis, and the sound of pulmonary valve closure is delayed and soft. Right ventricular hypertrophy reduces the compliance of that chamber, and a forceful right atrial contraction is necessary to augment right ventricular filling. A fourth heart sound, prominent A waves in the jugular venous pulse, and, occasionally, presystolic pulsations of the liver reflect the vigorous atrial contraction. The clinical diagnosis is further supported by the presence of a right parasternal lift and harsh systolic ejection murmur and thrill at the upper left sternal border, typically preceded by a systolic ejection sound if the obstruction is valvular. The systolic murmur becomes louder, and its crescendo occurs later in systole, with more severe degrees of valvular obstruction resulting in a greater prolongation of right ventricular systole. The holosystolic decrescendo murmur of tricuspid regurgitation may accompany severe pulmonic stenosis, especially in the presence of congestive heart failure. Cyanosis usually reflects venoarterial shunting through a patent foramen ovale or atrial septal defect. In patients with supravalvular or peripheral pulmonary arterial stenosis, the murmur is systolic or continuous and is best heard over the area of narrowing, with radiation to the peripheral lung fields.

The electrocardiogram may be helpful in assessing the degree of obstruction to right ventricular output. In mild cases, the electrocardiogram is often normal, whereas moderate and severe stenoses are associated with right axis deviation and right ventricular hypertrophy. A ventricular strain pattern, as well as high-amplitude P waves in leads II and V_1, indicating right atrial enlargement, is associated with severe stenosis. The chest roentgenogram in patients with mild or moderate pulmonic stenosis often shows a heart of normal size and normal vascularity of the lungs. In the presence of valvular stenosis, post-stenotic dilatation of the main and left pulmonary arteries may be evident. In patients with severe obstruction and resultant right ventricular failure, right atrial and right ventricular enlargement are generally evident. The pulmonary vascularity may be reduced in patients with severe stenosis, right ventricular failure, and/or a venoarterial shunt at the atrial level.

Cardiac catheterization and angiocardiography with right ventricular injection are necessary to localize the site of obstruction and evaluate its severity, and to document the coexistence of additional cardiac malformations. The treatment of moderate and severe degrees of pulmonary